PROCEDURES

UNIT SIX

Assisting with Medications

UNIT SEVEN

Assisting with Medical Specialties

UNIT EIGHT

Assisting with Clinical Laboratory Procedures

UNIT NINE

Advanced Clinical Skills

UNIT TEN

Job Seeking

KINN'S

THE MEDICAL ASSISTANT

AN APPLIED LEARNING APPROACH

15th EDITION

Brigitte Niedzwiecki, MSN, RN, RMA
Medical Assistant Program Director and Instructor
Chippewa Valley Technical College
Eau Claire, Wisconsin

Julie Pepper, BS, CMA (AAMA)
Medical Assistant Instructor
Health Navigator Program Director
Chippewa Valley Technical College
Eau Claire, Wisconsin

Associate Editors

Kelli Welch Haynes, EdD, RT (R), FASRT, FAEIRS
Professor and Director of the School of Allied Health
Northwestern State University
Shreveport, Louisiana

Melanie Shearer, MS, MT (ASCP) PBTcm, CMA (AAMA)
Associate Professor, Medical Assisting
Cuyahoga Community College
Cleveland, Ohio

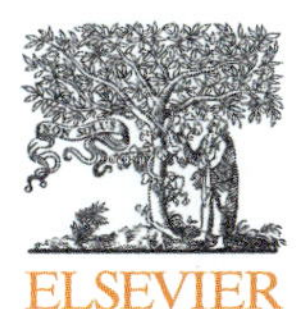

ELSEVIER

Elsevier
3251 Riverport Lane
St. Louis, Missouri 63043

KINN'S THE MEDICAL ASSISTANT: AN APPLIED LEARNING APPROACH, FIFTEENTH EDITION

ISBN: 978-0-323-87116-7

Notice

Practitioners and researchers must always rely on their own experience and knowledge in evaluating and using any information, methods, compounds or experiments described herein. Because of rapid advances in the medical sciences, in particular, independent verification of diagnoses and drug dosages should be made. To the fullest extent of the law, no responsibility is assumed by Elsevier, authors, editors or contributors for any injury and/or damage to persons or property as a matter of products liability, negligence or otherwise, or from any use or operation of any methods, products, instructions, or ideas contained in the material herein.

Previous editions copyrighted 2020, 2017, 2011, 2007, 2003, 1999, 1993, 1988, 1981, 1974, 1967, 1960, and 1956.

Content Strategist: Laura Klein
Content Development Manager: Luke Held/Danielle Frazier
Senior Content Development Specialist: Sarah Vora
Publishing Services Manager: Julie Eddy
Senior Project Manager: Abigail Bradberry
Design Direction: Ryan Cook

Printed in Canada

Last digit is the print number: 9 8 7 6 5 4 3 2 1

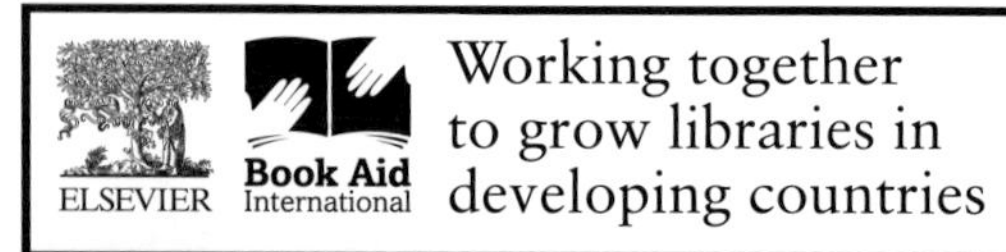

PREFACE

Medical assisting as a profession has changed dramatically since *The Office Assistant in Medical and Dental Practice,* by Portia Frederick and Carol Towner, was first published in 1956. Each subsequent edition of this textbook has reflected the age in which it was published. Now, *Kinn's The Medical Assistant: An Applied Learning Approach,* fifteenth edition, continues to represent a long-standing commitment to high-quality medical assisting education with its engaging, straightforward writing style and demonstrated positive outcomes. Hundreds of instructors in classrooms across the country have used this text to teach thousands of students over the years. Many of those students have gone on to teach students of their own with this very same trusted resource. To continue the use and growth of this text and its features, the fifteenth edition continues to offer the most comprehensive, up-to-date, and innovative approach to teaching this subject today.

This textbook has endured throughout the years because it has been able to keep pace with an ever-changing profession while producing students who are well trained and qualified to enter medical practices across the country. This dependability is the reason the market continues to rely on this text, edition after edition. Underlying this dependability is a foundation of pedagogic features that has stood the test of time and that has been expanded and improved upon yet again in this latest edition. Such features include the following:

An easy-to-read, highly interactive writing style that engages students through practical applications of medical assistant competencies

An emphasis on skill development, with procedural steps outlining each skill, supported by rationales that provide meaning to each step

A pedagogic framework based on the use of learning objectives, vocabulary terms, and supportive student supplements

A package of supportive materials to accommodate a wide variety of student learning types and instructor teaching styles

NEW TO THIS EDITION

- **New chapter** on physical medicine and rehabilitation.
- **New chapters and content** on urinary catheter insertion, intravenous therapy, and radiology for programs in states where these skills are within the medical assistant's scope of practice.
- **New content** on COVID-19, including information on the disease, vaccines, and communication concerns when wearing a mask. The medical assistant's role in telehealth and considerations when communicating virtually are addressed. Expanded information on Explanation of Benefits (EOB) and accounting terminology are included.
- **New artwork** focused on the workings of a modern medical office, with updated illustrations and photographs of office procedures and medical records.
- **Streamlined presentation** with combined chapters and an easier-to-read format.
- **More certification practice information,** with expanded and updated sample exams.

EVOLVE

The Evolve site features a variety of student resources, including Chapter Review Quizzes, new Procedure Videos, a Medical Terminology Audio Glossary, practice certification exams, and much more! The instructors' Evolve Resources site consists of TEACH Instructor Resources, including Lesson Plans, PowerPoint Presentations, Answer Keys for Chapter Review Quizzes, and a robust Test Bank.

STUDY GUIDE AND PROCEDURE CHECKLIST MANUAL

The Study Guide provides students with the opportunity to review and build on information they have learned in the text through vocabulary reviews, case studies, workplace applications, and more. The updated Procedure Checklists include Commission on Accreditation of Allied Health Education Programs (CAAHEP) and Accrediting Bureau of Health Education Schools (ABHES) competencies that can be traced to the online correlation grid.

FEATURES

A Scenario is presented at the beginning of each chapter so the student can envision a real-world situation when reading the chapter content.

Scenario questions provide a way for students to apply the concepts they are learning and think about decisions they would make in real situations.

Learning Objectives emphasize the cognitive and performance objectives presented in the chapter.

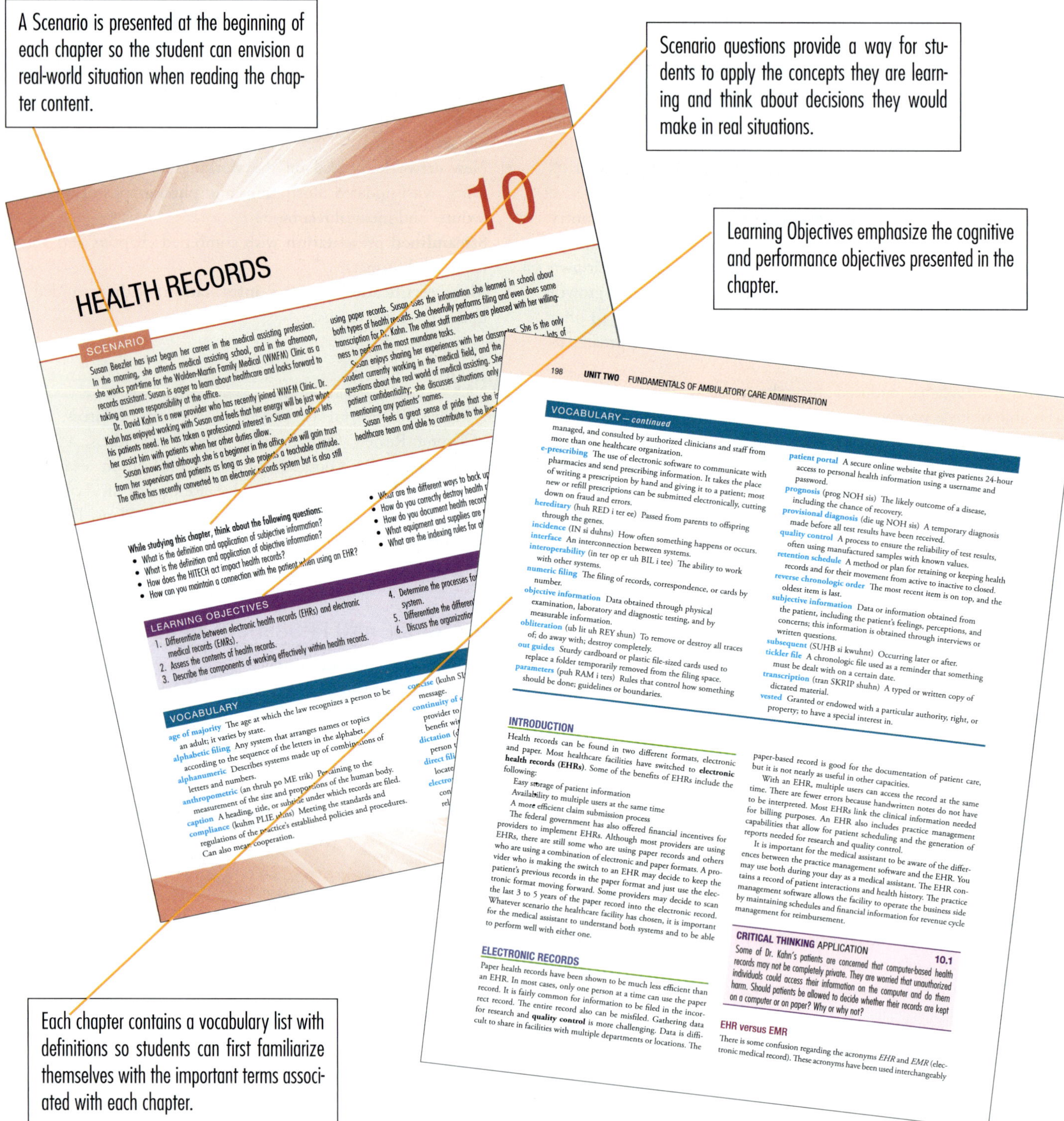

10

HEALTH RECORDS

SCENARIO

Susan Beezler has just begun her career in the medical assisting profession. In the morning, she attends medical assisting school, and in the afternoon, she works part-time for the Walden-Martin Family Medical (WMFM) Clinic as a records assistant. Susan is eager to learn about healthcare and looks forward to taking on more responsibility at the office.

Dr. David Kahn is a new provider who has recently joined WMFM Clinic. Dr. Kahn has enjoyed working with Susan and feels that her energy will be just what his patients need. He has taken a professional interest in Susan and often lets her assist him with patients when her other duties allow.

Susan knows that although she is a beginner in the office, she will gain trust from her supervisors and patients as long as she projects a teachable attitude. The office has recently converted to an electronic records system but is also still using paper records. Susan uses the information she learned in school about both types of health records. She cheerfully performs filing and even does some transcription for Dr. Kahn. The other staff members are pleased with her willingness to perform the most mundane tasks.

Susan enjoys sharing her experiences with her classmates. She is the only student currently working in the medical field, and the ... questions about the real world of medical assisting. She ... patient confidentiality; she discusses situations only ... mentioning any patients' names.

Susan feels a great sense of pride that she is ... healthcare team and able to contribute to the ...

While studying this chapter, think about the following questions:

- What is the definition and application of subjective information?
- What is the definition and application of objective information?
- How does the HITECH act impact health records?
- How can you maintain a connection with the patient when using an EHR?
- What are the different ways to back up ...
- How do you correctly destroy health ...
- How do you document health record ...
- What equipment and supplies are ...
- What are the indexing rules for ...

LEARNING OBJECTIVES

1. Differentiate between electronic health records (EHRs) and electronic medical records (EMRs).
2. Assess the contents of health records.
3. Describe the components of working effectively within health records.
4. Determine the processes for ... system.
5. Differentiate the different ...
6. Discuss the organization ...

VOCABULARY

age of majority The age at which the law recognizes a person to be an adult; it varies by state.
alphabetic filing Any system that arranges names or topics according to the sequence of the letters in the alphabet.
alphanumeric Describes systems made up of combinations of letters and numbers.
anthropometric (an thruh po ME trik) Pertaining to the measurement of the size and proportions of the human body.
caption A heading, title, or subtitle under which records are filed.
compliance (kuhm PLIE uhns) Meeting the standards and regulations of the practice's established policies and procedures. Can also mean cooperation.

198 UNIT TWO FUNDAMENTALS OF AMBULATORY CARE ADMINISTRATION

VOCABULARY—*continued*

managed, and consulted by authorized clinicians and staff from more than one healthcare organization.
e-prescribing The use of electronic software to communicate with pharmacies and send prescribing information. It takes the place of writing a prescription by hand and giving it to a patient; most new or refill prescriptions can be submitted electronically, cutting down on fraud and errors.
hereditary (huh RED i ter ee) Passed from parents to offspring through the genes.
incidence (IN si duhns) How often something happens or occurs.
interface An interconnection between systems.
interoperability (in ter op er uh BIL i tee) The ability to work with other systems.
numeric filing The filing of records, correspondence, or cards by number.
objective information Data obtained through physical examination, laboratory and diagnostic testing, and by measurable information.
obliteration (ub lit uh REY shun) To remove or destroy all traces of; do away with; destroy completely.
out guides Sturdy cardboard or plastic file-sized cards used to replace a folder temporarily removed from the filing space.
parameters (puh RAM i ters) Rules that control how something should be done; guidelines or boundaries.
patient portal A secure online website that gives patients 24-hour access to personal health information using a username and password.
prognosis (prog NOH sis) The likely outcome of a disease, including the chance of recovery.
provisional diagnosis (die ug NOH sis) A temporary diagnosis made before all test results have been received.
quality control A process to ensure the reliability of test results, often using manufactured samples with known values.
retention schedule A method or plan for retaining or keeping health records and for their movement from active to inactive to closed.
reverse chronologic order The most recent item is on top, and the oldest item is last.
subjective information Data or information obtained from the patient, including the patient's feelings, perceptions, and concerns; this information is obtained through interviews or written questions.
subsequent (SUHB si kwuhnt) Occurring later or after.
tickler file A chronologic file used as a reminder that something must be dealt with on a certain date.
transcription (tran SKRIP shuhn) A typed or written copy of dictated material.
vested Granted or endowed with a particular authority, right, or property; to have a special interest in.

INTRODUCTION

Health records can be found in two different formats, electronic and paper. Most healthcare facilities have switched to **electronic health records (EHRs)**. Some of the benefits of EHRs include the following:

Easy storage of patient information
Availability to multiple users at the same time
A more efficient claim submission process

The federal government has also offered financial incentives for providers to implement EHRs. Although most providers are using EHRs, there are still some who are using paper records and others who are using a combination of electronic and paper formats. A provider who is making the switch to an EHR may decide to keep the patient's previous records in the paper format and just use the electronic format moving forward. Some providers may decide to scan the last 3 to 5 years of the paper record into the electronic record. Whatever scenario the healthcare facility has chosen, it is important for the medical assistant to understand both systems and to be able to perform well with either one.

ELECTRONIC RECORDS

Paper health records have been shown to be much less efficient than an EHR. In most cases, only one person at a time can use the paper record. It is fairly common for information to be filed in the incorrect record. The entire record also can be misfiled. Gathering data for research and **quality control** is more challenging. Data is difficult to share in facilities with multiple departments or locations. The paper-based record is good for the documentation of patient care, but it is not nearly as useful in other capacities.

With an EHR, multiple users can access the record at the same time. There are fewer errors because handwritten notes do not have to be interpreted. Most EHRs link the clinical information needed for billing purposes. An EHR also includes practice management capabilities that allow for patient scheduling and the generation of reports needed for research and quality control.

It is important for the medical assistant to be aware of the differences between the practice management software and the EHR. You may use both during your day as a medical assistant. The EHR contains a record of patient interactions and health history. The practice management software allows the facility to operate the business side by maintaining schedules and financial information for revenue cycle management for reimbursement.

CRITICAL THINKING APPLICATION 10.1

Some of Dr. Kahn's patients are concerned that computer-based health records may not be completely private. They are worried that unauthorized individuals could access their information on the computer and do them harm. Should patients be allowed to decide whether their records are kept on a computer or on paper? Why or why not?

EHR versus EMR

There is some confusion regarding the acronyms *EHR* and *EMR* (electronic medical record). These acronyms have been used interchangeably

Each chapter contains a vocabulary list with definitions so students can first familiarize themselves with the important terms associated with each chapter.

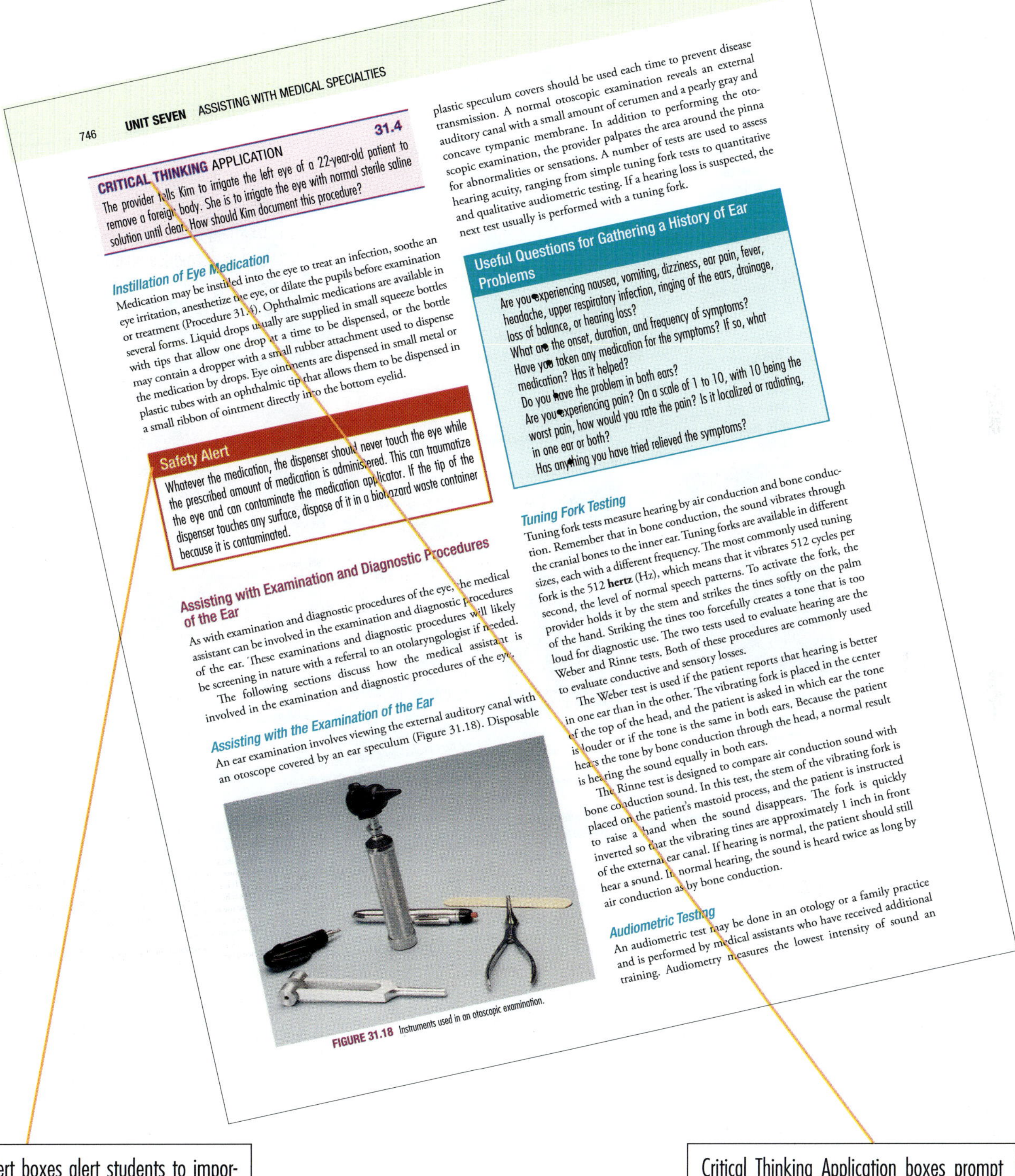

746 UNIT SEVEN ASSISTING WITH MEDICAL SPECIALTIES

CRITICAL THINKING APPLICATION 31.4

The provider tells Kim to irrigate the left eye of a 22-year-old patient to remove a foreign body. She is to irrigate the eye with normal sterile saline solution until clear. How should Kim document this procedure?

Instillation of Eye Medication

Medication may be instilled into the eye to treat an infection, soothe an eye irritation, anesthetize the eye, or dilate the pupils before examination or treatment (Procedure 31.4). Ophthalmic medications are available in several forms. Liquid drops usually are supplied in small squeeze bottles with tips that allow one drop at a time to be dispensed, or the bottle may contain a dropper with a small rubber attachment used to dispense the medication by drops. Eye ointments are dispensed in small metal or plastic tubes with an ophthalmic tip that allows them to be dispensed in a small ribbon of ointment directly into the bottom eyelid.

Safety Alert

Whatever the medication, the dispenser should never touch the eye while the prescribed amount of medication is administered. This can traumatize the eye and can contaminate the medication applicator. If the tip of the dispenser touches any surface, dispose of it in a biohazard waste container because it is contaminated.

Assisting with Examination and Diagnostic Procedures of the Ear

As with examination and diagnostic procedures of the eye, the medical assistant can be involved in the examination and diagnostic procedures of the ear. These examinations and diagnostic procedures will likely be screening in nature with a referral to an otolaryngologist if needed.

The following sections discuss how the medical assistant is involved in the examination and diagnostic procedures of the eye.

Assisting with the Examination of the Ear

An ear examination involves viewing the external auditory canal with an otoscope covered by an ear speculum (Figure 31.18). Disposable plastic speculum covers should be used each time to prevent disease transmission. A normal otoscopic examination reveals an external auditory canal with a small amount of cerumen and a pearly gray and concave tympanic membrane. In addition to performing the otoscopic examination, the provider palpates the area around the pinna for abnormalities or sensations. A number of tests are used to assess hearing acuity, ranging from simple tuning fork tests to quantitative and qualitative audiometric testing. If a hearing loss is suspected, the next test usually is performed with a tuning fork.

FIGURE 31.18 Instruments used in an otoscopic examination.

Useful Questions for Gathering a History of Ear Problems

- Are you experiencing nausea, vomiting, dizziness, ear pain, fever, headache, upper respiratory infection, ringing of the ears, drainage, loss of balance, or hearing loss?
- What are the onset, duration, and frequency of symptoms?
- Have you taken any medication for the symptoms? If so, what medication? Has it helped?
- Do you have the problem in both ears?
- Are you experiencing pain? On a scale of 1 to 10, with 10 being the worst pain, how would you rate the pain? Is it localized or radiating, in one ear or both?
- Has anything you have tried relieved the symptoms?

Tuning Fork Testing

Tuning fork tests measure hearing by air conduction and bone conduction. Remember that in bone conduction, the sound vibrates through the cranial bones to the inner ear. Tuning forks are available in different sizes, each with a different frequency. The most commonly used tuning fork is the 512 **hertz** (Hz), which means that it vibrates 512 cycles per second, the level of normal speech patterns. To activate the fork, the provider holds it by the stem and strikes the tines softly on the palm of the hand. Striking the tines too forcefully creates a tone that is too loud for diagnostic use. The two tests used to evaluate hearing are the Weber and Rinne tests. Both of these procedures are commonly used to evaluate conductive and sensory losses.

The Weber test is used if the patient reports that hearing is better in one ear than in the other. The vibrating fork is placed in the center of the top of the head, and the patient is asked in which ear the tone is louder or if the tone is the same in both ears. Because the patient hears the tone by bone conduction through the head, a normal result is hearing the sound equally in both ears.

The Rinne test is designed to compare air conduction sound with bone conduction sound. In this test, the stem of the vibrating fork is placed on the patient's mastoid process, and the patient is instructed to raise a hand when the sound disappears. The fork is quickly inverted so that the vibrating tines are approximately 1 inch in front of the external ear canal. If hearing is normal, the patient should still hear a sound. In normal hearing, the sound is heard twice as long by air conduction as by bone conduction.

Audiometric Testing

An audiometric test may be done in an otology or a family practice and is performed by medical assistants who have received additional training. Audiometry measures the lowest intensity of sound an

Safety Alert boxes alert students to important safety information and reinforce the importance of safety in the profession.

Critical Thinking Application boxes prompt students to apply what they have learned as they read and study the chapter.

454 **UNIT FIVE** FUNDAMENTALS OF CLINICAL MEDICAL ASSISTING

PROCEDURE 20.2 **Accurately Measure and Record a Temperature Using a Tympanic Thermometer**

TASK: Accurately measure and record a patient's temperature using a tympanic thermometer.

EQUIPMENT and SUPPLIES

- Patient's record
- Tympanic thermometer
- Disposable probe covers
- Alcohol wipes
- Waste container

PROCEDURAL STEPS

1. Wash hands or use hand sanitizer.
   PURPOSE: To ensure infection control.
2. Gather the necessary equipment and supplies.
3. Greet the patient. Identify yourself. Verify the patient's identity with full name and date of birth. Explain the procedure to be performed in a manner that the patient understands. Answer any questions the patient may have about the procedure.
   PURPOSE: Identification of the patient prevents errors, and explanations are a means of gaining implied consent and patient cooperation.
4. Clean the probe with an alcohol wipe if indicated. Place a disposable cover on the probe (see the following figure).
   PURPOSE: To ensure a clean surface and prevent cross-contamination.

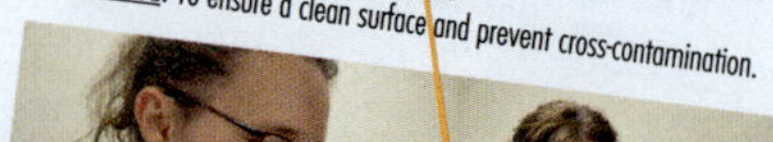

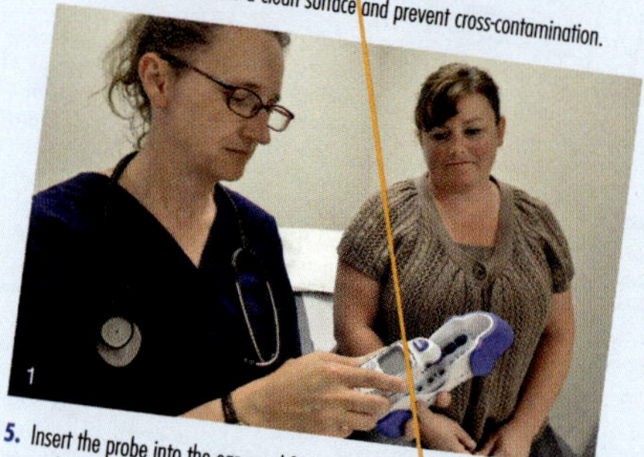

5. Insert the probe into the ear canal far enough to seal the opening. Do not apply pressure. For children younger than age 3, gently pull the earlobe down and back (see the first of the following figures); for patients older than age 3, gently pull the top of the ear (pinna) up and back (see the second of the following figures).
   PURPOSE: The external ear must be pulled gently to open the external auditory canal and expose the tympanic membrane for an accurate reading.

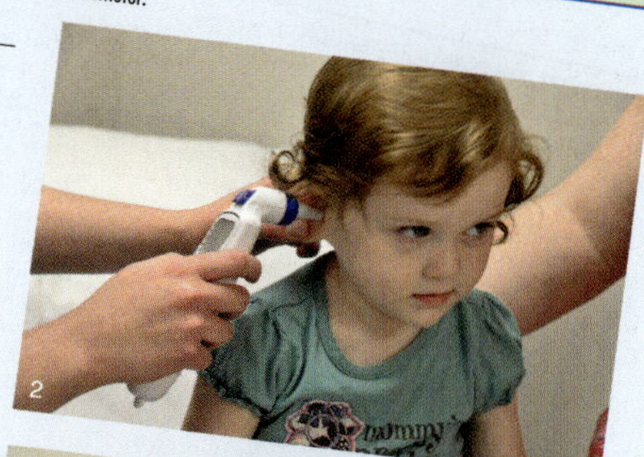

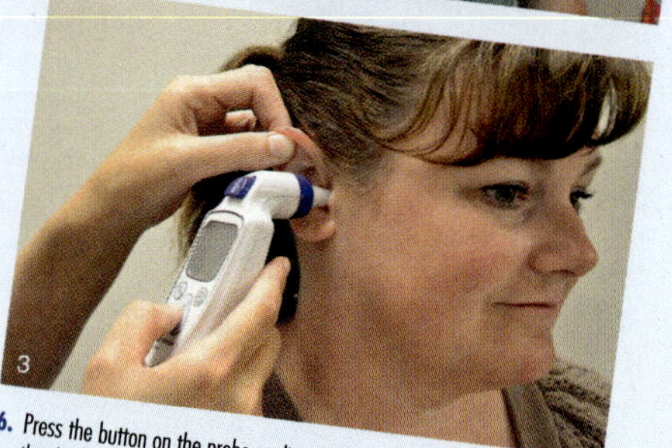

6. Press the button on the probe as directed. The temperature will appear on the display screen in 1 to 2 seconds.
7. Remove the probe, note the reading, and discard the probe cover into a waste container without touching it.
   PURPOSE: The probe cover is contaminated and must be discarded in a waste container.
8. Wash hands or use hand sanitizer and disinfect the equipment if indicated. See the manufacturer's manual for cleaning the probe tip. Many recommend cleaning the probe lens with alcohol wipes.
   PURPOSE: To ensure infection control.
9. Document the reading in the patient's medical record (e.g., T: 98.6°F [T]).
   PURPOSE: Procedures that are not recorded are considered not done.

Documentation Example

7/11/20xx 2:20 p.m. T: 101.2°F (T) ———— C. Ricci, CMA (AAMA)

Step-by-step Procedure boxes demonstrate how to perform and document procedures encountered in the healthcare setting.

188 **UNIT TWO** FUNDAMENTALS OF AMBULATORY CARE ADMINISTRATION

Angry Patients in the Reception Area

Every medical assistant eventually is confronted with an angry patient. The anger may simply reflect the patient's pain or fear of what the provider may discover during the exam. If possible, invite the patient into a room out of the reception area. Usually, the best course is to let the patient talk out the anger. Present a calm attitude and speak in a low tone of voice. Under no circumstances should the medical assistant return the anger or become argumentative. Medical assistants must use good listening skills with angry people and must be empathetic. Notify the facility's administrator of all difficult patients or ask for help from co-workers.

There should be a policy in place for dealing with potentially dangerous individuals. Policies can include the following:

Making sure that you can reach the exit if you take the patient to another room

Having another employee close by

Knowing under what circumstances you should contact the police or building security for assistance

Patient Checkout

When patients return to the front office for checkout, greet them with a friendly smile and call the individual by name. Form the habit of asking patients if they have any questions. Check the health record to determine when the provider wants the patient to return. Most providers note this information on the encounter form. Make the return appointment. Remember to give the patient choices on the time and day. Give the patient an appointment reminder card. If the copayment was not collected prior to the visit, it may be collected during checkout.

The medical assistant can convey a sense of caring by terminating the visit cordially. Thank the patient for coming. If the patient will return for another visit, the assistant can say something such as "We'll see you next week." If the patient will not be returning soon, a pleasant "I hope you'll be feeling better soon" is appropriate. In addition, tell patients to call the facility if they have any questions or if they need additional care. Whatever words of goodbye are chosen, all patients should leave the facility feeling that they have received top-quality care and were treated with friendliness, respect, and courtesy.

CLOSING COMMENTS

Patient Coaching

Providing patients with an information booklet about the healthcare facility can familiarize them with policies and procedures. Many providers compile an extensive booklet that even provides tips as to when the provider should be called immediately, listing symptoms and signs of emergencies.

Educating the patient about the healthcare facility's policies helps the facility run smoothly from day to day. All patients should be familiar with the policies about appointments. This leads to fewer misunderstandings and conflicts over bills that might include a charge for a missed appointment.

If the facility offers internet-based appointment scheduling or forms completion, patients must be taught how to use the system. A printed pamphlet or information sheet is helpful for providing instructions to the patient. A wise option is to have a special phone number that patients can call if they have problems with the system. For best results, choose a program that is simple to use, easy to understand, and does not breach patient confidentiality.

Legal and Ethical Issues

As mentioned earlier, the appointment schedule may be used as a legal record and could be brought by subpoena into a court of law. Make sure all handwriting in the book is completely legible and that information is routinely collected in a consistent manner for each entry. Do not fail to note a no-show both in the patient's health record and the appointment schedule. This often is helpful when a provider must prove that the patient did not follow medical advice or that the patient contributed to his or her poor condition by missing appointments. Old appointment schedules should be kept for a time equal to that of the statute of limitations in the state where the practice is located.

A medical assistant must never offer medical advice to a patient. The patient sees the medical assistant as an extension of the provider and tends to weigh advice and comments by the medical assistant with the same validity as if they came from the provider. Provide only information the provider has approved or that is included in the healthcare facility's policies and procedures manual.

When a patient complains, listen carefully, and try to resolve the problem or assure the patient that the issue will be discussed with the appropriate staff member to find a solution. If someone other than the patient asks for information about the patient, refrain from discussion unless the patient or provider has authorized the release of information.

Patient-Centered Care

Going to a healthcare facility can be intimidating and uncomfortable for many patients. It is important that the medical assistant try to put everyone at ease. Cultivate the habit of greeting each patient immediately in a friendly, self-assured manner. Establish eye contact and smile while introducing yourself to the patient.

Small talk can help put a patient at ease. Talking about the weather or an uncontroversial topic may make the patient more comfortable.

Asking personalized questions can also help. Providers and staff members sometimes make brief notes in the health record about the current events in the patient's life. On the next visit, the staff or provider can use this information to start a conversation with the patient. For instance, the patient may state she is going to Florida for a vacation. During the next visit, the provider may start off the visit by asking how her Florida trip was. Asking personalized questions will solidify the personal connection with patients. They may feel important, less intimidated, and more comfortable. It is a great way to provide excellent customer service.

Professional Behaviors

When working in scheduling and helping patients move through the healthcare facility, medical assistants have many opportunities to demonstrate professionalism. It is important to remember that we are often seeing patients when they are not at their best, so we must learn not to take all of the responses personally. When an angry patient approaches the reception desk, you should smile politely, ask how you can help the person, and respond in a soothing tone of voice. When a patient calls for an appointment and demands a day and time when the provider is not available, you should remain calm and explain why that day and time are not an option. As a medical assistant in the front office, you have the opportunity to make an amazing first impression on patients. Remember to always behave professionally.

Patient Coaching sections address how the MA can provide information to patients in a supportive environment that allows them to grow, change, or improve their situation.

Professional Behaviors boxes provide tips on professional behavior that are specific to each chapter's content.

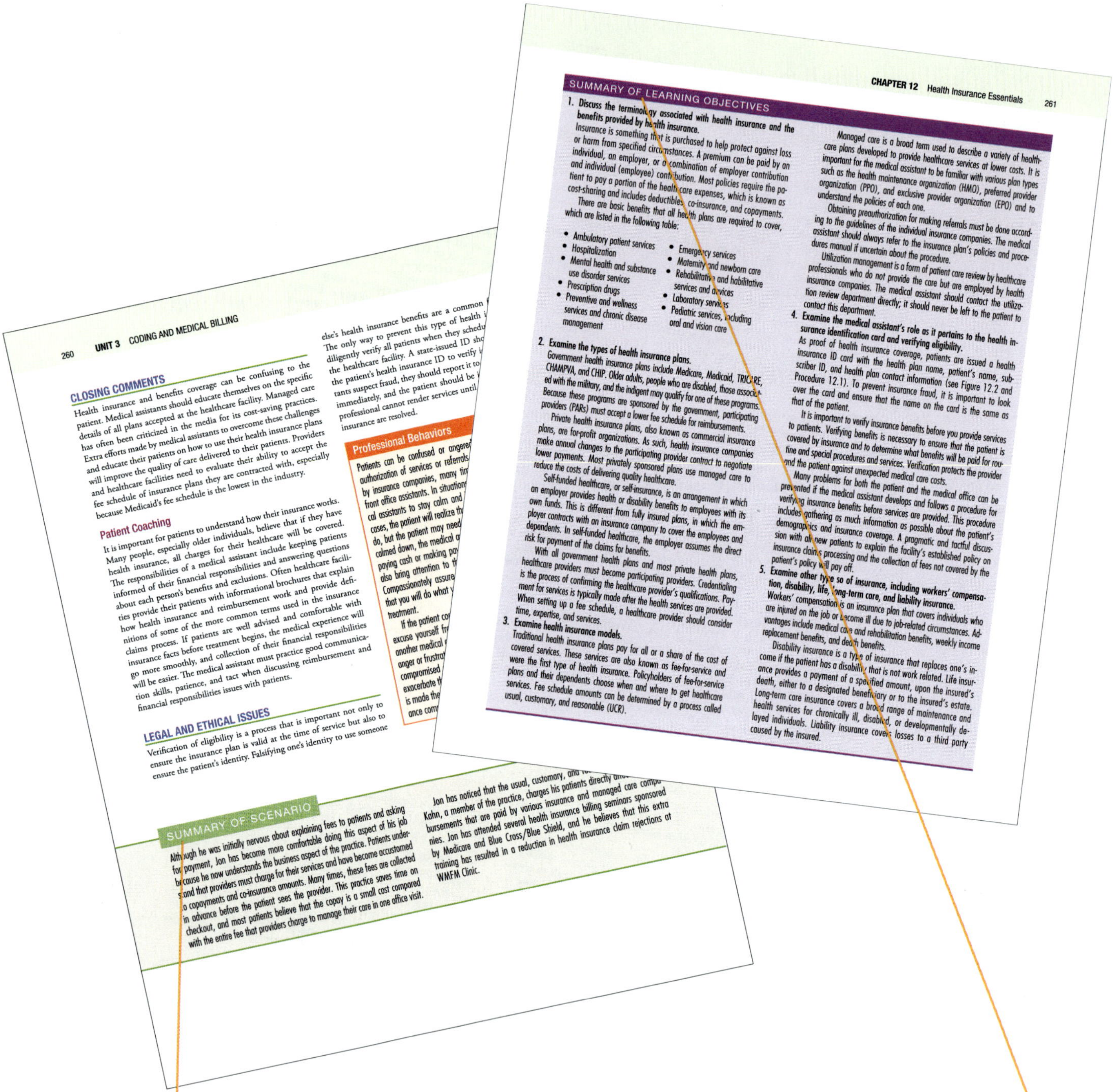

At the end of each chapter, the Summary of Scenario brings together the content of the chapter and the opening scenario in a real-world context.

The Summary of Learning Objectives reviews and reinforces the important points of the chapter's focus to help the student with content mastery.

REVIEWERS

Jamie Young Atwell, BS, MS
Adjunct Biology Instructor
Owensboro Community and Technical College
Owensboro, Kentucky

Angela Belnap, DHPE, MS, CMA (AAMA)
Associate Professor
Salt Lake Community College
West Jordan, Utah

Beverly L. Brady, CMA (AAMA), RMA (AMT), AS, BS
MDA Program Coordinator
Community College of Allegheny County
West Mifflin, Pennsylvania

Tiffany Brown, CMA (AAMA), AAS–MA, BS Ed.
Teacher
Central Arizona Valley Institute of Technology (CAVIT)
Coolidge, Arizona

Michelle Buchman, BSN, MA
Medical Assisting Program Chair and Assistant Professor
Cox College
Springfield, Missouri

Rachel Chesney, RMA
Medical Assistant and CTE Teacher
Technology and Exploration Career Center–West
Lewisville, Texas

Bryan Quincy Edmonds Sr., MBA–H, RMA, EMT
Medical Assisting Program Chair, Instructor
Milwaukee Area Technical College
Milwaukee, Wisconsin

Deborah S. Gilbert, MBA, Ed.S, RHIA
Assistant Professor, Retired
Dalton State College
Dalton, Georgia

Dustin Goldsberry, CMA (AAMA)
Certified Medical Assistant
JIS Orthopedics
Athens, Ohio

Starra Herring, MBA, MHA, BSAH, CMA (AAMA)–MA, AHI
Program Director of Medical Assisting Programs at Stanly Community College
Stanly Community College
Locust, North Carolina

Terrie Hopkins, CMA (AAMA), BS
Program Director, Medical Assisting/Phlebotomy
Practicum Coordinator
Medical Assisting Instructor
Terra State Community College
Fremont, Ohio

Catherine Howell, CCMA, CPCT, CET, CPT, CEHRS
Assistant Director
Merit Training Institute
Mount Laurel, New Jersey

Brandi Lippincott, MOS, CEHRS, BS
Director
Merit Training Institute (graduated from Rutgers School of Business)
Mount Laurel, New Jersey

Melody Miller, LPN
Medical Assistant Instructor
Lancaster County Career & Technology Center
Willow Street, Pennsylvania

Sandra Patocka, CCMA, LPN, BS
Medical Assisting Instructor
Autry Technology Center
Enid, Oklahoma

Kristen Schoville, RN/BSN
Medical Assistant Instructor
Southwest Wisconsin Technical College
Fennimore, Wisconsin

Audrey Theisen, BS, RHIA, MSCIS, PhD
Professor
Former Program Chair for Health Information Management
Front Range Community College
Westwood College
Kaplan College
ITT Technical Institute
Heritage College
Arapahoe Community College
Denver, Colorado

Miasha Torain, BS, CMA (AAMA)
Medical Assisting Department Head
Alamance Community College
Graham, North Carolina

CONTENTS

UNIT THREE

Coding And Medical Billing

UNIT FOUR

Advanced Ambulatory Care Administration

UNIT SEVEN

Assisting with Medical Specialties

THE PROFESSIONAL MEDICAL ASSISTANT AND THE HEALTHCARE TEAM

1

SCENARIO

Carmen Angelos is a new student in a medical assisting program accredited by the Commission on Accreditation of Allied Health Education Programs (CAAHEP) at Butler County Community College. Carmen is returning to school after working at a local pharmacy for 5 years, where she became interested in pursuing a career in medical assisting. She has been out of high school for a few years but is excited about her new career choice.

While studying this chapter, think about the following questions:

- Why is professionalism an important attribute in the field of medical assisting?
- What is a typical job description for an entry-level medical assistant?
- How will scope of practice and standards of care determine your role as a medical assistant?
- Why is it important to learn about professional medical assisting organizations?
- Studying may be a challenge for Carmen. What skills can she use to help her learn new material and prepare for examinations?
- Why is it important for medical assisting students to learn about the various healthcare facilities and medical specialties?
- How can Carmen show professional behavior toward all patients in the healthcare setting?
- How can time management strategies help Carmen prioritize her responsibilities as a member of the healthcare team?

LEARNING OBJECTIVES

1. Examine the typical responsibilities of a medical assistant.
2. Analyze the attributes of a professional medical assistant.
3. Differentiate between scope of practice and standards of care for medical assistants.
4. Discuss professional medical assisting organizations.
5. Examine your learning preferences and learning style.
6. Examine the history of medicine and its significance to the medical assisting profession.
7. Differentiate between various types of medical professionals.
8. Summarize the various types of allied health professionals.
9. Summarize the various types of healthcare facilities.
10. Examine the healthcare team models.
11. Explain the reasons professionalism is important in the medical field.

VOCABULARY

allopathic (al uh PATH ik) A system of medical practice that treats disease by the use of remedies, such as medications and surgery, to produce effects different from those caused by the disease under treatment; medical doctors (MDs) and osteopaths (DOs) practice allopathic medicine; also called conventional medicine.

complementary and alternative medicine (CAM) A group of diverse medical and healthcare systems, practices, and products that are not generally considered part of conventional medicine. Complementary medicine is used in combination with conventional medicine (allopathic or osteopathic); alternative medicine is used instead of conventional medicine.

conscientious (kon shee EN shuhs) Meticulous, careful.

contamination (kun tam i NAY shun) The process by which something becomes harmful or unusable through contact with something unclean.

critical thinking The constant practice of considering all aspects of a situation when deciding what to believe or what to do.

demeanor (dih MEE ner) Behavior toward others; outward manner.

detrimental (de truh MEN tl) Harmful.

holistic (hoh LIS tik) A form of healing that considers the whole person (i.e., body, mind, spirit, and emotions) in individual treatment plans.

VOCABULARY—*continued*

hospice (HOS pis) A concept of care that involves health professionals and volunteers who provide medical, psychological, and spiritual support to terminally ill patients and their loved ones.

indicator (IN di kay ter) An important point or group of statistical values that, when evaluated, indicates the quality of care provided in a healthcare facility.

initiative (i NISH eh tive) The ability to determine what needs to be done and to take action on your own.

integrity (in TEG ri tee) Adhering to ethical standards or right conduct standards.

learning style The way an individual perceives and processes information to learn new material.

mnemonic (ni MON ik) A learning device (e.g., an image, a rhyme, or a figure of speech) that a person uses to help him or her remember information.

morale (muh RAL) Emotional or mental condition with respect to cheerfulness or confidence.

negligence (NEG li jens) Failure to act as a reasonably prudent person would under similar circumstances; such conduct falls below the standards of behavior established by law for the protection of others against unreasonable risk of harm.

overlearn To learn or memorize beyond the point of proficiency or immediate recall.

patient navigator A person who identifies patients' needs and barriers, then assists by coordinating care and identifying community and healthcare resources to meet the needs. May also be called a care coordinator.

perceiving (per SEEV ing) How an individual looks at information and sees it as real.

processing (prah CES ing) How an individual internalizes new information and makes it his or her own.

reflection (ree FLEK shun) The process of thinking about new information to create new ways of learning.

reliable (ree LIE ah bul) Dependable; able to be trusted.

triage (tree AHZH) The process of sorting patients to determine medical needs and the priority of care.

What an exciting and challenging career you have chosen! Medical assistants are multiskilled healthcare workers who function under the direction of a licensed provider and are primarily employed in outpatient or ambulatory care facilities, such as medical offices and clinics. According to the US Bureau of Labor Statistics, medical assisting is one of the nation's fastest-growing careers, and employment opportunities are projected to grow 19% through 2029.

This growth in job opportunities for medical assistants is due to multiple factors, including a steady increase in the aging population as baby boomers spur demand for preventive health services from physician offices and ambulatory care centers. Because medical assistants are trained in both administrative and clinical skills, they are the perfect employee to meet the needs of this increasing population. In addition, the switch to electronic health records (EHRs) in ambulatory care centers has also opened up employment opportunities for medical assistants who are trained in EHR software.

RESPONSIBILITIES OF THE MEDICAL ASSISTANT

Medical assistants are the only allied health professionals specifically trained to work in ambulatory care settings, such as providers' offices, clinics, and group practices. That training includes both clinical and administrative skills, covering a multitude of medical practice needs. The skills performed by an entry-level medical assistant depend on his or her place of employment, but all graduates of accredited programs are taught a similar skill set.

Clinical Skills and Responsibilities

Clinical skills include the following:

- Assisting during physical examinations
- Performing patient screening procedures
- Assisting with minor surgical procedures, including sterilization procedures
- Performing electrocardiograms (ECGs)
- Obtaining and recording vital signs and medical histories
- Performing phlebotomy
- Performing tests permitted by the Clinical Laboratory Improvement Amendments (i.e., CLIA-waived tests)
- Collecting and managing laboratory specimens
- Following Occupational Safety and Health Administration (OSHA) regulations on infection control
- Administering vaccinations and medications as ordered by the provider
- Performing patient education and coaching initiatives within the scope of practice
- Documenting accurately in a paper record or an EHR
- Performing first aid procedures as needed
- Performing infection control procedures
- Applying therapeutic communication techniques
- Adapting to the special needs of a patient based on his or her developmental life stage, cultural diversity, and individual communication barriers
- Acting as a patient advocate or navigator, including referring patients to community resources
- Acting within legal and ethical boundaries

When working as a clinical medical assistant, your role is to aid both the provider and patient. By being proficient in the skills listed, you can help ensure that the patient is getting the best possible care.

Administrative Skills and Responsibilities

Administrative skills include the following:

- Answering telephones
- Managing patient scheduling
- Creating and maintaining patient health records
- Documenting accurately in a paper record and an EHR
- Performing routine maintenance of facility equipment

- Performing basic practice finance procedures
- Coordinating third-party reimbursement
- Performing procedural and diagnostic coding
- Communicating professionally with patients, family members, practitioners, peers, and the public
- Managing facility correspondence
- Performing patient education and coaching initiatives within the scope of practice
- Following legal and ethical principles
- Complying with facility safety practices

When working as an administrative medical assistant, you also support both the provider and the patient. The skills listed help to ensure that patient gets an appointment when needed and that the provider is paid appropriately for the services provided. Both the clinical and administrative skills are needed to keep patients happy and the healthcare facility running smoothly.

Another role that a medical assistant can fill is that of a scribe. With the training that a medical assistant receives, you will have the skills necessary to fulfill the role. A medical scribe works with a provider to document the patient care in the patient record. This allows the provider to focus more closely on the patient rather than the computer.

Patient Navigator Skills and Responsibilities

These lengthy lists of capabilities that make up the basic skill set are not all that is expected of entry-level medical assistants; they also play a significant role as the patient's advocate. Current research describes this role as being a **patient navigator** (Figure 1.1). If you have ever had a loved one who was very ill and required medical attention from several different practitioners and allied health specialty groups, you understand what a complex and overwhelming task it can be to make decisions and coordinate a loved one's care.

Care coordination originated from the patient navigator program. This program was established at the Harlem Hospital Center in 1990. The goal was to assist cancer patients in accessing quality healthcare. Many patient navigator positions were funded with the assistance of the Patient Navigator, Outreach, and Chronic Disease Prevention Act of 2005. Today, patient navigator positions are commonly called *care coordinators.* These positions can be found in ambulatory care settings and hospitals. In hospitals, the care coordinators help manage the acute care services and help patients transition home or to other healthcare settings.

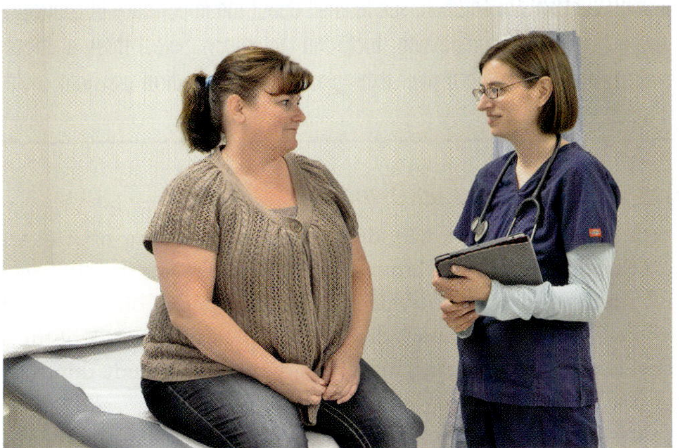

FIGURE 1.1 The medical assistant as a patient navigator.

For a medical assistant, often, the patient navigator role is embedded in the clinical and administrative responsibilities. By having an understanding of health insurance, you can help your patients understand their policy requirements. By developing trusting relationships, you allow your patients to confide in you about their concerns, even nonmedical concerns, and you can direct them to resources. Being a patient advocate is a large part of being a successful medical assistant.

CRITICAL THINKING APPLICATION **1.1**

Medical assistants have long been encouraged to act as patient advocates in the ambulatory care setting. Given their multilevel training, medical assistants can help patients navigate through a wide variety of confusing issues. Let's think about how you could help a patient and family navigate the following scenario:

Mrs. Jana Green is an 82-year-old patient at Walden-Martin Family Medical Clinic. Mrs. Green recently suffered a mild cerebrovascular accident (CVA), and her son is trying to help coordinate her care. Mrs. Green does not understand when or how to take her new medications; she is concerned about whether her health insurance will cover the cost of frequent clinic appointments and assistive devices; she doesn't understand how to prepare for the magnetic resonance imaging (MRI) the provider ordered; and, she dislikes having to have blood drawn every week.

Based on what you have learned about the job description of a medical assistant, how can you help Mrs. Green and her family navigate through this complex and challenging medical regimen? What specific actions could help Mrs. Green and her son manage her care?

Customer Service

Another aspect of being a medical assistant is providing excellent customer service. Customer service closely relates to professional behaviors. One must be professional to provide exceptional customer service. In healthcare today, many of our patients can choose where they go to seek care. The ambulatory care facility needs to attract and retain patients to remain open and for you to have a job. Two of the quickest ways to lose patients are to treat them poorly and to act in an unprofessional manner. Happy patients tend to tell others about their experiences. Great customer service leads to a successful healthcare facility and allows growth.

To understand customer service, we first need to know who our customers are. A *customer* is one who purchases goods or services. A customer can also be a person you deal with in the work environment. By that definition, we can see that patients are our customers. They choose our ambulatory care facility to seek healthcare services. They (or their insurance company) pay for the services provided. Patients are considered *external customers,* or people we do business with who are "outside" (i.e., not employed by) the healthcare facility. Other external customers include medical equipment and supply vendors and pharmaceutical representatives.

The second part of the customer definition relates to *internal customers*, or people you deal with in the work environment. These are individuals we interact with inside the facility. They include our co-workers, employees in other departments, and the administrative staff. Both internal and external customers are important for the success of the healthcare facility.

Customer service is whatever we do for our customers to improve their experience at our healthcare facility. People may have different ideas about how they should be treated during their interactions. Our goal is to provide *customer satisfaction,* or a sense of contentment with the interaction. Typically, the more we get to know the customer, the better we can provide customer service. This might not always be possible. For instance, a new patient comes for an appointment. If you are at the reception desk, you do not have a lot of time to get to know the patient. The most important things for you to do are the following:

- Be considerate and treat the patient as you would want to be treated.
- Look and act professionally.

CRITICAL THINKING APPLICATION **1.2**

During Carmen's orientation, she learned about customer service and customer satisfaction. In your own words, how would you define both of these phrases?

CHARACTERISTICS OF PROFESSIONAL MEDICAL ASSISTANTS

Medical assistants must have professional *characteristics* or distinguishing traits. You will start developing these traits while in school. You will put them into practice during practicum. They will follow you into your first job. A student who is unprofessional during practicum will find it difficult to get a job. That behavior may be **detrimental** to the medical assistant's professional career.

Professionalism

As healthcare professionals, medical assistants represent the healthcare facility. They are viewed as an extension of the provider and the facility. A healthcare professional:

- has high ethical standards
- displays **integrity**
- completes work accurately and in a timely fashion

It is important for successful professionals to show *professionalism*—that is, having courteous, **conscientious**, and respectful behaviors. This approach is used during all interactions and situations in the workplace. Our patients and co-workers expect professional behavior. Patients base much of their trust and confidence in those who show professionalism. How health professionals act is a direct reflection on the facility and provider. If a medical assistant is rude to a patient, the patient may think that the provider is rude. The perceived quality of care will be negative. Medical assistants must always display professionalism. This includes their attitude, appearance, and behavior. Regardless of the situation, they must always act professionally.

Courtesy and Respect

Courtesy, respect, and dignity often come together when discussing professionalism. *Courtesy* is having good manners or being polite. Courteous behavior is polite, open, and welcoming. *Respect* means to show consideration or appreciation for another person. *Dignity* is the state or quality of being worthy of respect.

We show our patients dignity by treating all patients the way we would want to be treated. It does not matter if the patient has bad body odor or is dressed in tattered clothes. The patient is a person worthy of respect. Patients expect to be treated as individuals who matter. They want to be respected and not treated as an annoyance or a medical condition. How can the medical assistant treat others with courtesy and respect?

- Make patients feel welcome and respected. A pleasant greeting and eye contact should be the first things patients experience. Thanking patients at the end of the visit is also important.
- Display positive nonverbal behaviors. Use a calm tone of voice, make eye contact when appropriate, and provide privacy for patients. Maintain patient confidentiality.
- Learn about other cultures in your area. When working with patients from those cultures, make sure to avoid gestures, words, and behaviors that could be perceived as disrespectful.
- Always use proper grammar, without slang words. Explain medical treatments and conditions in simple lay language. If you need to use a medical term, explain it to the patient.

Empathy and Compassion

It is important that professional medical assistants demonstrate empathy and compassion to their patients. Empathy, sympathy, and compassion can easily be confused. *Empathy* is the ability to understand another's perspective, experiences, or motivations. We can share another's emotional state. Empathy differs from sympathy. *Sympathy* is feeling sorrow, concern, or pity for what the other person has gone through. *Compassion* means we have a deep awareness of the suffering of another and wish to ease it. These characteristics will help to build positive relationships with our patients.

Tact and Diplomacy

Tact and diplomacy are extremely valuable traits in healthcare professionals. Being *tactful* means being acutely sensitive to what is proper and appropriate when interacting with others. A tactful person has the ability to speak or act without offending others. Being *diplomatic* means using tact and sensitivity when interacting with others. The medical assistant must be sensitive to the needs of others. How can a medical assistant use these traits when communicating with other people?

- Consistently be polite and honest during your communication. Show sensitivity to others through your communication and behaviors.
- Recognize the needs and rights of others. Attempt to reach a mutually beneficial resolution to the problem.
- Assess your personal response to the situation. Your personal beliefs and biases should not prevent you from interacting diplomatically and tactfully with others.

CRITICAL THINKING APPLICATION **1.3**

During Carmen's orientation, she learned about the importance of courtesy, respect, empathy, compassion, tact, and diplomacy. Select three of these words, and share with a peer examples of how a medical assistant could display these traits.

Respect for Individual Diversity

Medical assistants work with diverse populations. Your patients will come from different backgrounds. *Diversity* describes the differences and similarities in identity, perspective, and points of view among people. When talking about diversity, people usually think of things such as nationality or race, but diversity can also include things like age and economic status.

It is important to be open and nonjudgmental when working with patients and workers who are different from ourselves. Be aware and accepting of cultural differences. Be aware of your own cultural values. What preconceived ideas do you have of other diverse groups? How might your biases affect the care you provide to those in different groups?

It is important to educate yourself about other groups. Get to know their customs and practices. Culture can affect healthcare. It can influence how people describe their symptoms when healthcare is sought and how treatment plans are followed. For instance, people in some cultures eat traditional foods high in sodium. This could be an issue if a person has high blood pressure or kidney disease. Understanding and accepting the differences represented by your patients will help you provide the best care possible for them.

Honesty, Dependability, and Responsibility

Honest means to be sincere and upright. *Dependable* is the same as trustworthy and reliable. *Responsible* is defined as being trusted or depended on. These are three traits that employers value in their employees. Professional medical assistants should be honest, dependable, and responsible. When given a task, they should complete it accurately, on time, and to the best of their ability. If they make an error, they should be upfront about it. Patient safety is the number one priority. Any mistake in patient care needs to be reported immediately to the provider and the supervisor. Dependability and honesty are critical components in earning the trust and respect of others. How can medical assistants perform their duties using these three characteristics?

- Be honest and straightforward when interacting with others.
- Accept responsibility for your mistakes. Determine how to prevent them in the future.
- Follow through on your promises.
- Complete your work to the best of your abilities. Complete it on time.
- Be self-motivated. Do not wait to be asked to complete a task.
- Embrace change.

Professional Appearance

Most ambulatory healthcare facilities have dress codes for employees. Medical assistants are usually required to wear scrubs along with the facility's nametag (and a photo) clearly visible (Figure 1.2A). Table 1.1 provides a typical dress code. Dress codes will vary by facility. Some communities are more conservative, and thus the dress codes reflect this.

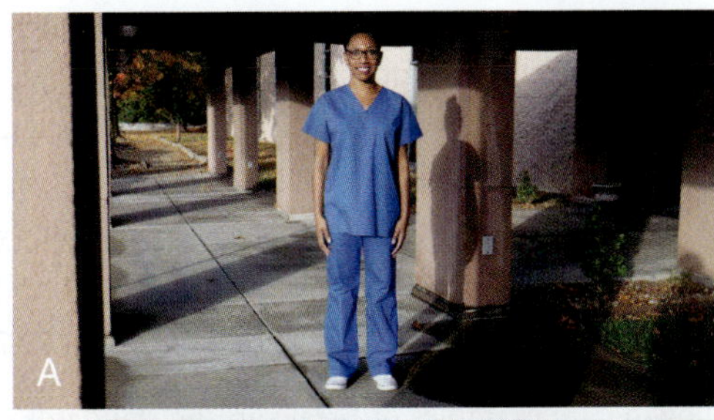
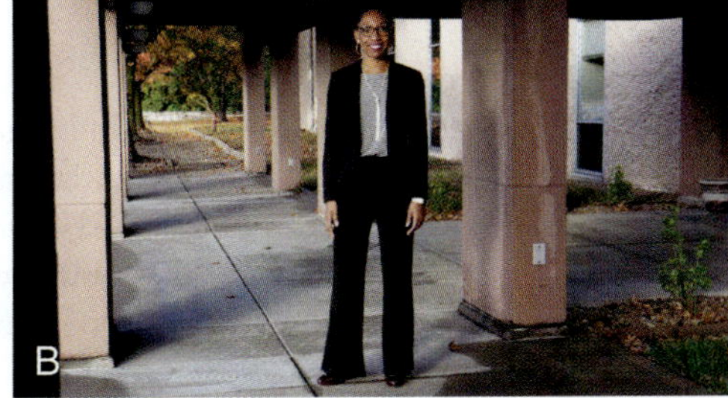

FIGURE 1.2 A professional appearance is important for a medical assistant. **(A)** Scrubs. **(B)** Business attire.

Typically, healthcare facilities include terms such as *modest* and *business attire* in describing their dress codes (Figure 1.2B). The rule of thumb is to make sure the employee does not expose too much at the neckline, the abdomen, and below the waist when bending and raising the arms. Business attire is not casual clothing. Casual clothes include jeans, T-shirts, shorts, exercise/sports clothing, and so on. Business attire is considered dressier and more professional than casual clothes. Dress pants and a dress shirt would be considered business attire for men. Dress pants, a dress shirt, modest dresses, and modest skirts and blouses would be considered business attire for women.

CRITICAL THINKING APPLICATION 1.4

Rosie, a business office employee at Walden-Martin Family Medical Clinic, is allowed to dress in business attire. She interacts with patients who have questions about their bills. Describe how Rosie should dress.

SCOPE OF PRACTICE AND STANDARDS OF CARE FOR MEDICAL ASSISTANTS

Two principles are in place to guide the actions of medical assistants. One is the scope of practice, and the other is standards of care. It is important to be familiar with both when working as a professional medical assistant.

Scope of Practice

Scope of practice is defined as the range of responsibilities and practice guidelines that determine the boundaries within which a healthcare worker practices. What is the scope of practice of a medical assistant? There is no single definition of the scope of practice for medical assistants throughout the United States, but some states have enacted scope of practice laws covering medical assistant practice. These states include Alaska, Arizona, California, Florida, Georgia, Illinois, Maine, Maryland, Montana, Nevada, New Jersey, New York, Ohio, South Dakota, Virginia, Washington, and West Virginia. Medical assistants working in those states must refer to the identified roles specified in the law. However, for those employed in states without scope of practice laws, medical assistant practice is guided by the norms of that particular location, facility policies and procedures, and individual provider-employers. In some states, medical assistants are overseen by the board of nursing, whereas in others, the board of medicine oversees medical assistants. Make sure you are aware of your state's rules governing medical assistants' scope of practice.

One fact is absolutely true about all practicing medical assistants—they are not independent practitioners. Whether certified or not, regardless of length of training or experience, every medical assistant must practice under the direct supervision of a physician or other licensed provider (e.g., nurse practitioner or physician assistant).

Earlier in this chapter, we discussed the typical tasks performed by a medical assistant, so you already know generally what duties medical assistants perform in ambulatory care centers. However, some specific tasks are beyond the scope of practice of medical assistants, including the following:

- Performing telephone or in-person **triage**; medical assistants are not legally authorized to assess or diagnose symptoms

TABLE 1.1 Typical Dress Code for Medical Assistants

DRESS CODE	PROFESSIONAL	UNPROFESSIONAL	COMMENTS
Uniform: scrubs and white shoes	• Scrubs must be clean, pressed (ironed), and fit properly. • Scrub pants must be hemmed to the appropriate length. • Closed-toed shoes must be white and clean.	• Dirty, wrinkled, ripped scrubs • Scrub pants dragging on the floor • Scruffy, dirty shoes • Open shoes (sandals), fabric shoes	• Shoes need to protect your feet. Cloth and open-toed shoes provide very little protection. • Pants dragging on floors pick up and transfer bacteria.
Hair	• Natural colors; clean and styled • Long hair must be tied back	• Unnatural colors; dirty, messy hair • Hair in face or hanging down	• Hair hanging in front can interfere with patient care, spread bacteria, and get caught in equipment.
Fingernails	• Cut short, unpolished	• Long, polished, artificial nails	• Bacteria can multiply and grow under long, artificial, or polished nails.
Cosmetics and body odors	• Professional makeup • No odors on the body	• Overuse of makeup • Wearing perfume, cologne, etc. • Using scented lotions • Smelling like a cigarette • Body odor (from not bathing)	• Too much makeup can look unprofessional. • Smells like perfumes, colognes, or cigarettes can trigger allergies in others. • Offensive body odor is unprofessional because we are in patients' intimate/personal space.
Jewelry	• Wedding band (no stones) • One pair of earrings (studs) • Watch	• Rings with stones • Multiple earrings on each ear • Necklaces, bracelets • Lanyards	• Bacteria can accumulate in rings and bracelets. • Necklaces and lanyards can be choking hazards if grabbed by a patient.
Tattoos and body piercings	• Tattoos and body piercings must follow the healthcare facility's policy	• Not following the healthcare facility's policy	• In conservative communities, body piercings and tattoos may be perceived as unprofessional.
Professional dress (street clothes) for special events	• Blouse, top, or sweater • Dress pants • Dress or skirt (to the top of the knee) • Dress shoes	• Low-cut tops; sheer tops • Jeans, ripped pants, exercise clothes • Flip-flops, tennis shoes • Miniskirts	• Clothes should look professional; should not be ripped or casual in appearance.

- Prescribing medications or making recommendations about over-the-counter drugs and remedies
- Giving out drug samples without provider permission
- Automatically submitting refill prescription requests without provider orders
- Analyzing or interpreting test results
- Operating laser equipment
- Performing laboratory tests that are not CLIA-waived
- Scheduling diagnostic or radiographic tests/procedures without provider's orders

Standards of Care

What is the difference between scope of practice and standards of care? The scope of practice for a medical assistant is what has been established by law in some states or by practice norms, institutions, or physician-employers in states without scope of practice laws. *Standards of care,* however, is a legal term that refers to whether the level and quality of patient service provided are the same as what another healthcare worker with similar training and experience in a similar situation would provide. Standards of care set minimum guidelines for job performance. They define what the expected quality of care is and provide specific guidelines on whether the care standard has been met. Medical assistants who do not meet the expected standard of care may be charged with professional **negligence** (discussed in greater detail in Chapter 3).

The following are examples of breaks in the standards of care in medical assisting:

- A patient calls reporting a persistent headache for 3 days. You tell the patient to get some rest and take ibuprofen without referring the call to a provider. What standard of care has been broken?
- A patient asks you to explain his lab report. You do your best to explain what his blood count levels mean. What is the problem here?
- An older patient tells you she cannot afford to get her prescriptions filled. The provider is busy, but you know there are samples of the prescribed drug in the medication cupboard, so you give her several packets. Does this follow standard of care?

- A patient tells you her son fell on the playground yesterday, and he is complaining that his arm hurts. You tell the mother it is probably just a strain and suggest she wrap the arm with an elastic bandage. Why is this a problem?
- You overhear a patient calling one of the other medical assistants "nurse." Should your co-worker correct the patient? Why?

Hopefully, you are beginning to see that the practice of medical assisting is limited not only by individual state laws or norms but also by the standards and scope of practice established by the supervising providers where the medical assistant is employed. Remember, the scope of practice and expected standards of care for licensed medical professionals are quite different from those for medical assisting practice. The medical assistant must refer to the provider for orders and guidance on what behaviors are expected of medical assistants in that facility. The medical assistant can *never* independently diagnose, prescribe, or treat patients. She or he must *always* have the written order of a provider or follow established policies and procedures when performing clinical skills.

PROFESSIONAL MEDICAL ASSISTING ORGANIZATIONS, CREDENTIALS, AND CONTINUING EDUCATION

Becoming a member of a professional organization, obtaining credentials, and participating in continuing education are all part of being a professional medical assistant. In this next section, you will find information about professional organizations, how to obtain a medical assistant credential, and continuing education.

Professional Organizations for Medical Assistants

Most healthcare occupations have a professional organization that sets high standards for quality and performance. A code of ethics is also developed by the organization to help guide the actions of those in that particular profession. Professional organizations provide many benefits to their members, including opportunities for continuing education, national and regional conventions, and networking opportunities. Medical assisting is no different. Becoming a member of a professional organization will also show your employer that you are committed to being the best possible medical assistant. The following sections describe three of the professional medical assisting organizations available.

American Association of Medical Assistants

The American Association of Medical Assistants (AAMA) was created in 1956 and remains the only association devoted exclusively to the medical assisting profession. According to the AAMA's website (*www.aama-ntl.org*), becoming a member includes the following benefits:

- AAMA legal counsel represents medical assistants across the United States to fight for the rights of medical assistant practice; in addition, the counsel stays abreast of federal and state laws regarding medical assisting.
- Members receive a complimentary subscription to *CMA Today*, an informative magazine devoted entirely to the medical assistant profession; each issue (six per year) offers continuing education unit (CEU) articles, medical assisting news, and healthcare information.

More information about the AAMA is available on the organization's website: *www.aama-ntl.org*.

American Medical Technologists (AMT)

The American Medical Technologists (AMT) was founded in 1939 as a nationally recognized certification agency for multiple allied health professionals, including medical assistants (RMA), medical laboratory technicians (MLT), phlebotomy technicians (RPT), medical administrative specialists (CMAS), and dental assistants (RDA).

According to the AMT's website (*www.americanmedtech.org*), becoming a member includes the following benefits:

- Professional publications
- Annual convention
- State society meetings and seminars
- Continuing education
- Career services
- Awards and scholarships

Additional information on the AMT is available on the organization's website: *www.americanmedtech.org*.

The National Healthcareer Association (NHA)

The National Healthcareer Association (NHA) was established in 1990 to offer certification examinations in a number of allied health programs; for example, certification is granted for pharmacy, phlebotomy, and electrocardiography (ECG) technicians. The NHA also offers two different medical assisting certifications: certified clinical medical assistant (CCMA) and certified medical administrative assistant (CMAA). The NHA is not involved in program curriculum standards or program accreditation. It simply offers certification if the applicant can successfully pass the NHA examination developed for each particular medical discipline. You can find out more about the certifications offered through the NHA at the association's website: *www.nhanow.com*.

Achieving a Credential

Medical assistants have several options if they choose to become credentialed. Being a credentialed medical assistant has certain benefits:

- Credentialed medical assistants have had to pass a national standardized exam. Passing the exam indicates that they have the knowledge to perform the medical assistant's duties.
- Some employers require the credential prior to hiring or within a few months after hiring.
- Some employers will pay more if a person has achieved a medical assistant credential.

There are several national agencies that will provide credentials to medical assistants upon successful completion of their exam. Table 1.2 presents some of the more common medical assistant credentials. It is important for graduating medical assistants to research whether credentials are preferred or required by local employers. It is also important to identify which credential is most wanted by local employers. Your instructors are also excellent resources if you have additional questions on credentials for medical assistants.

Continuing Education

For a professional medical assistant, it is important to stay current (up to date) with the newest medications, treatments, and diagnostic tests. Education beyond your medical assistant degree is considered continuing education. Most healthcare professionals need to do continuing education to renew their certification or license. There are many opportunities for continuing education:

TABLE 1.2 Credentialing Agencies for Medical Assistants

AGENCY/WEBSITE	CREDENTIAL	RECERTIFICATION METHODS
American Association of Medical Assistants (AAMA) http://www.aama-ntl.org	Certified medical assistant (CMA [AAMA])	Recertify every 5 years either by exam or by earning 60 continuing education points. Specific points must be achieved in the three content areas. At least 30 points must be from AAMA-approved continuing education units (CEUs).
American Medical Technologists (AMT) https://www.americanmedtech.org	Registered medical assistant (RMA)	Recertify every 3 years either by exam or by completing specific activities.
National Healthcareer Association (NHA) https://www.nhanow.com	Clinical medical assistant (CCMA) Medical administrative assistant (CMAA)	Recertify every 2 years either by exam or by earning 10 continuing education credits.
National Center for Competency Testing (NCCT) https://www.ncctinc.com	Medical assistant (NCMA)	Recertify every year either by exam or by completing 14 contact hours of continuing education.
American Medical Certification Association (AMCA) https://www.amcaexams.com	CMAC	Recertify every two years by completing 10 continuing education credits

- Reading professional journals and reputable health websites
- On-the-job educational conferences
- Local, state, and national medical assistant conferences

Typically, additional continuing education opportunities exist if a medical assistant is a member of an organization.

HOW TO SUCCEED AS A MEDICAL ASSISTANT STUDENT

You have taken the first step toward becoming a successful student by choosing your profession and field of study. Becoming a medical assistant opens the doors to a wide variety of opportunities in both administrative and clinical practice at ambulatory or institutional healthcare facilities. To become a successful medical assistant, you first must become a successful student. This section will help you discover the way you learn best, and it provides multiple strategies to assist you in your journey toward success.

Who You Are as a Learner: How Do You Learn Best?

Think about what you do when you are faced with something new to learn. How do you go about understanding and learning the new material? Over time you have developed a method for **perceiving** and **processing** information. This pattern of behavior is called your **learning style**. Learning styles can be examined in many different ways, but most professionals agree that a student's success depends more on whether the person can "make sense" of the information than on whether the individual is "smart." Determining your individual learning style and understanding how it applies to your ability to learn new material are the first steps toward becoming a successful student.

Learning Style Inventory

For you to learn new material, two things must happen. First, you must perceive the information. This is the method you have developed over time that helps you examine new information and recognize it as real. Once you have developed a method for learning about the new material, you must process the information. Processing the information is how you internalize it and make it your own. Researchers believe that each of us has a preferred method for learning new material. By investigating your learning style, you can figure out how to combine different approaches to perceiving and processing information that will lead to greater success as a student.

The first step in learning new material is determining how you perceive it, or as some experts explain, what methods you use to learn the new material. Some learners opt to watch, observe, and use **reflection** to think about and learn the new material. These students are *abstract perceivers* who learn by analyzing new material, building theories about it, and using a step-by-step approach to learning. Other students need to perform some activities, such as rewriting notes from class, making flash cards, and outlining chapters to learn new information. Students who learn by "doing" are called *concrete perceivers.* Concrete learners prefer to learn things that have a personal meaning or that they believe are relevant to their lives. So, which type of perceiver do you think you are? Before you actually learn new material, do you need time to think about it, or do you prefer to "do" something to help you learn the material?

The second step in learning new material is information processing, which is the way learners internalize the new information and make it their own. New material can be processed by two methods. *Active processors* prefer to jump in and start doing things immediately. They make sense of the new material by using it *now.* They look for practical ways to apply the new material and learn best with practice and hands-on activities. *Reflective processors* have to think about the information before they can internalize it. They prefer to observe and consider what is going on. The only way they can make sense of new material is to spend time thinking and learning a great deal about it before acting. Which type of information processor do you think you are? Do you prefer to jump in and start doing things to help you learn, or do you need to analyze and consider the material before you can actually learn it?

Using Your Learning Profile to Be a Successful Student: Where Do I Go from Here?

No one falls completely into one or the other of the categories just discussed. However, by being aware of how we generally prefer first to perceive information and then to process it, we can be more sensitive to our learning style and can approach new learning situations with a plan for learning the material in a way that best suits our learning preferences.

Your preferred perceiving and processing learning profile will fall into one of the following four stages of the Learning Style Inventory, which was created by David Kolb of Case Western Reserve University:

- *Stage 1* learners have a *concrete reflective* style. These students want to know the purpose of the information and have a personal connection to the content. They like to consider a situation from many points of view, observe others, and plan before taking action. They feel most comfortable watching rather than doing, and their strengths include sensitivity toward others, brainstorming, and recognizing and creatively solving problems. If you fall into this stage, you enjoy small-group activities and learn well in study groups.
- *Stage 2* learners have an *abstract reflective* style. These students are eager to learn just for the sheer pleasure of learning rather than because the material relates to their personal lives. They like to learn lots of facts and arrange new material in a clear, logical manner. Stage 2 learners plan to study and like to create ways of thinking about the material, but they do not always make the connection with its practical application. If you are a stage 2 learner, you prefer organized, logical presentations of material and, therefore, enjoy lectures and readings and generally dislike group work. You also need time to process and think about new material before applying it.
- *Stage 3* learners have an *abstract active* style. Learners with this combination learning style want to experiment and test the information they are learning. If you are a stage 3 learner, you want to know how techniques or ideas work, and you also want to practice what you are learning. Your strengths are in problem solving and decision making, but you may lack focus and may be hasty in making decisions. You learn best with hands-on practice by doing experiments, projects, and laboratory activities. You enjoy working alone or in small groups.

CRITICAL THINKING APPLICATION **1.5**

- Consider the two ways to perceive new material. Are you a concrete perceiver who ties the information to a personal experience, or are you an abstract perceiver, who likes to analyze or reflect on the meaning of the material? Choose the type you think most accurately describes your method of learning.
- Now, think about the way you process learning. Are you an active processor who always looks for the practical applications of what you learn, or are you a reflective processor who has to think about new material before internalizing it?
- After completing this activity, write down the combination of your perceiving and processing learning styles and share it with your instructor.

- *Stage 4* learners are *concrete active* learners. These students are concerned about how they can use what they learn to make a difference in their lives. If you fall into this stage, you like to relate new material to other areas of your life. You have leadership capabilities, can create on your feet, and usually are vocal in a group, but you may have difficulty completing your work on time. Stage 4 learners enjoy teaching others and working in groups and learn best when they can apply new information to real-world problems.

To get the most out of knowing your learning profile, you need to apply this knowledge to how you approach learning. Each of the learning stages has pluses and minuses. When faced with a learning situation that does not match your learning preference, see how you can adapt your individual learning profile to make the best of the information. For example, if you are bored by lectures, look for an opportunity to apply the information being presented to a real problem you are facing in the classroom or at home. If you are an abstract perceiver, take time outside of class to think about new information so that you are ready to process it into your learning system. If you benefit from learning in a group, make the effort to organize review sessions and study groups. If you learn best by teaching others, offer to assist your peers with their learning. By taking the time now to investigate your preferred method of learning, you will perceive and process information more effectively throughout your school career.

CRITICAL THINKING APPLICATION **1.6**

Take a few minutes to reflect on a time when you really enjoyed learning about something new. How was the material presented, and what did you do to "make it your own"? What do you need to do to become a more effective learner?

Study Skills: Tricks for Becoming a Successful Student

Let's investigate some ideas that are useful for learning new material. These study skills include memory techniques, active learning, brain tricks, reading methods, and note-taking strategies.

Organizing Content

Several techniques can help you store and remember information. The first of these involves organizing information into recognizable groups so that the brain can find it easily. You can organize information by getting the big picture first before trying to learn the details. One way to implement this strategy is to skim a reading assignment before actually reading and taking notes on the material, thus getting a general impression of what you need to learn before tackling the details. Depending on your learning style, it may also help to find a way of making the new information meaningful. Think about your educational goals and how the new material will help you achieve those goals.

Another way of remembering material is to create an association with something you already know. If new material is grouped with already stored material, the brain remembers it much more easily. For example, maybe you took a biology class in high school and learned the basics about human anatomy and physiology. Try to create a link between what you previously learned and the details of the new information you are expected to learn now. Or, maybe you have a family member who suffers from a particular disease. Think about that individual's signs and symptoms while learning more details about the disease so that you can apply your learning to his or her situation.

Being Physically Active

A useful study skill for some learners is to be physically active while learning. Some students learn best if they walk or talk out loud while studying. Besides encouraging learning, moving and talking while studying relieves boredom and keeps you awake. Another way to be actively involved in learning is to use pictures or diagrams to represent the material you are studying. Some people are visual learners, and creating pictures of the material is the easiest method for them to retain the information. Other students find that rewriting notes, making lists of information, creating flash cards, color-coding notes, or highlighting important material in a textbook helps them retain the material. Writing also helps students who need to "do" something to learn.

Studying goes much more smoothly if you work with your brain rather than against it. If you tend to get anxious and worried while studying, you may be acting as your own worst enemy. One way of dealing with a topic you are anxious about is to **overlearn** it. If material is overlearned, you are much less likely to experience test anxiety. Another method for remembering material is to review it quickly after class. This mini-review helps the new information become part of your long-term memory system.

Many students find creating songs, dances, or word associations an effective way to learn and remember new material. Putting details into a familiar song and moving to it can help trick the brain into remembering the information. This is especially helpful when trying to learn anatomy and physiology. For example, think about one of your favorite songs and "dance" your way through the blood flow through the heart. Or, if you are finding the organization of the body especially tricky to remember, such as the movement of food through the gastrointestinal (GI) system, create a **mnemonic** that helps you remember the information. The most common one suggested for the parts of the intestines is **D**ow **J**ones **I**ndustrial **C**limbing **A**verage **C**losing **S**tock **R**eport. The first letter of each word stands for an anatomic part of the intestines: *d*uodenum, *j*ejunum, *i*leum, *c*ecum, *a*ppendix, *c*olon, *s*igmoid, and *r*ectum. You can make up your own mnemonics or memory tricks to help you learn complicated material.

Teaching Back

Another excellent way of learning information is to teach it to someone else. Teaching requires you to have a good understanding of the material and the ability to describe it to others. It can be an effective reinforcement of complicated material.

A great deal of the learning process is expected to take place from assigned readings. You can use several methods to make reading assignments more meaningful. If you find a reading assignment challenging or difficult to understand, the first step is to take the time to read it again. Sometimes the first time through the material is not enough to gain an understanding. As you read, highlight important words or thoughts and stop periodically to summarize the material. Some students find outlining new material helpful. This is another way to use active learning to help you make the information your own.

If you get bored while reading, use your body; walk or talk your way through the assignment. Take the time to look up words or terms you do not understand, or ask your instructor or tutor for help. The best way to determine whether you have learned anything from your reading is to try to explain the material to someone else. For example, you can meet with other students and explain to them what you learned. If you can do that effectively, you know you have acquired the knowledge needed from the reading assignment.

Effective Note Taking

Many students find effective note taking a challenge. The big question is, "How much of what the instructor says do I actually need to write down?" The first step in effective note taking is to come to class prepared. The more familiar you are with the material, the easier it will be to determine the important parts of the instructor's lecture. Pay attention to the instructor and look for clues to what he or she thinks is important. Ask questions about the material if you do not understand it, rather than writing down information that makes no sense to you. Think critically about what you hear before you write it down so you can start to build relationships among the things you want or need to know.

If your instructor uses PowerPoint presentations to teach a lesson, request copies of the slides before the lecture, so you have an opportunity to review them as you are doing your reading. Many courses have an online website where PowerPoints or other lecture materials are available for review. Take advantage of these added materials to be prepared for each class so that you can ask questions about anything you do not understand. In addition, this textbook has an extensive online site that you can access for learning resources. Investigate the site and see whether something there can help you reach your learning goals.

When it comes to actual note taking, some strategies can make the process of recording notes an active learning tool. Organize the information as much as possible while you are writing or typing, either in an outline or a paragraph format. If you take notes on a laptop or tablet, make sure your keyboarding skills are good enough for you to keep up with the flow of information and that you review your notes shortly after class to fill in any missing details. If you take notes on paper, use only one side of the page (for easier reading) and leave blank spaces where needed to fill in details later. Use key words to help you remember the material, and create pictures or diagrams to help visualize it. If permitted, record the lecture and make sure you have copies of any handouts or notes distributed by your instructor that cover material written on the board or provided in a PowerPoint presentation. If your instructor refers the class to a YouTube video or other website, transcribe the site address correctly to refer to it at a later time. Another helpful tool is to develop your own system of abbreviations to simplify the note-taking process.

The most effective way to use your notes is to review them shortly after class and then find a time to review them every day. This is the time to add details, clarify information, or make notes about asking the instructor for explanations during the next class. You could even exchange notes with students you trust to compare information. Some students find it beneficial to create an electronic copy of their notes (if they wrote them out on paper) or to rewrite them. This gives you an opportunity to learn the material as you transcribe it. As you review your notes, you also can draw mind maps of the information or diagram outlines to help you better understand and remember the material.

Mind Maps

Creating mind maps is a way of representing the main idea of a topic and supporting important details with a figure or picture. Healthcare textbooks present complicated concepts with multiple main ideas, each with its own important details. Mind maps are a way of combining complex details and organizing them into a format that is easier to remember. The *spider map* (Figure 1.3) presents a method for including several main ideas with details in one study guide. The

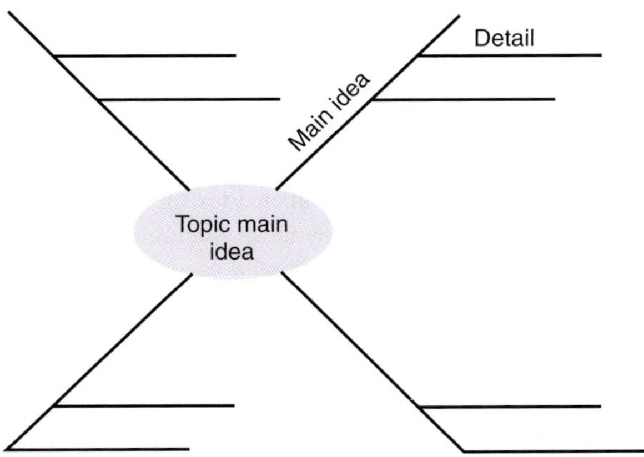

FIGURE 1.3 Spider map showing multiple main ideas with supporting details.

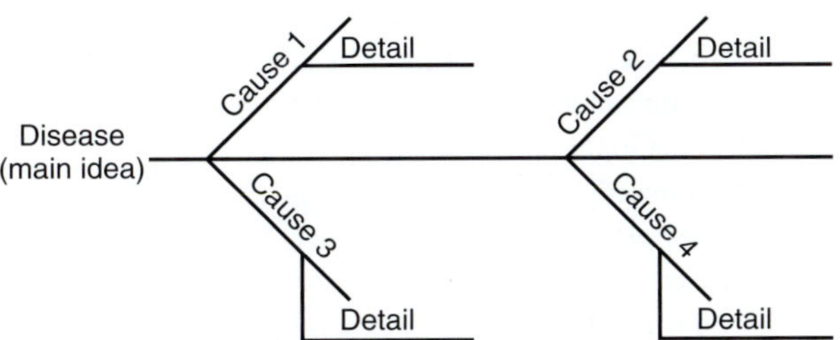

FIGURE 1.4 Fishbone map used to describe cause of disease.

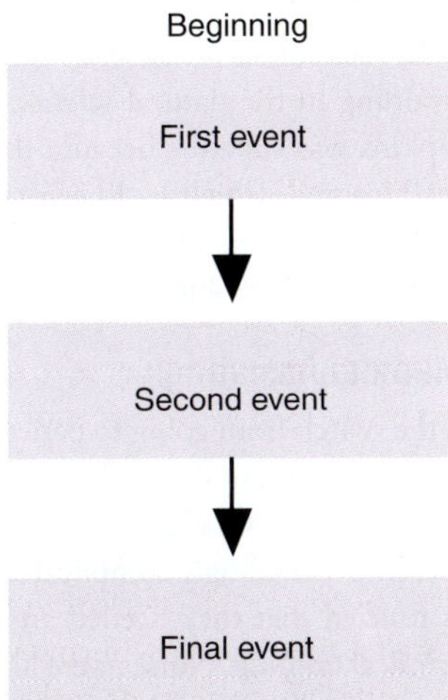

FIGURE 1.5 Chain-of-events map showing the cause and effect of events.

fishbone map (Figure 1.4) can be used to learn complicated causes of disease. The *chain-of-events map* (Figure 1.5) displays the cause and effect of events, such as infection control or the history of medicine. The *cycle map* (Figure 1.6) shows the connection between factors, such as in the chain of infection. Creating your own mind maps is a way of making the information more meaningful and easier for you to understand and remember.

Although many techniques can help you study, perhaps the most important one is your attitude toward learning. Some students fall into the "I can't possibly learn this material" trap. That type of attitude only leads to self-defeat. The way to overcome barriers is first to recognize that they exist. Once you know your weak spots, use the suggested study skills to improve in those areas. Do not be afraid to ask questions or ask for help if you do not understand the material. Use as many different strategies as necessary to become a successful student.

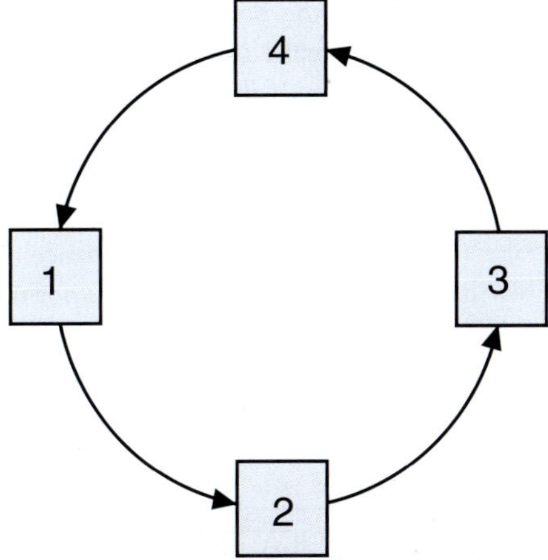

FIGURE 1.6 Cycle map illustrating the way one action leads to another.

CRITICAL THINKING APPLICATION 1.7

Write down at least two barriers to learning that you face. Review the study skills suggestions and choose four to try out. Use them over the next week to help you learn new material. Reflect on whether the chosen study skills helped you learn the material better.

Test-Taking Strategies: Taking Charge of Your Success

What happens when you do not know the answer to the first question on a test? What if you do not know the next one? Are you able to go on without panicking? Many people find taking tests the most challenging part of being a successful student. Multiple approaches are available that you can use to take charge of your success and improve your ability to take tests. These include such strategies as adequate preparation, controlling negative thoughts during test time, and understanding ways to manage various types of questions.

The first step is to go into a test adequately prepared. Use the time management skills discussed later in this chapter to prepare for the big day. Recognize and use your preferred learning style to overlearn the material and increase your confidence. Use memory tools (e.g., flash cards, checklists, and mind maps) to help you visualize the material. Form a study group if you are the type of learner who benefits from studying in groups. Schedule and plan study time, and reward yourself for your hard work. It is also important to go into the test rested and relaxed; therefore, you should eat, exercise to relieve stress, and sleep before the test so that you are as alert as possible.

Before you start the test, make sure you read the directions carefully. If possible, begin with the easiest or shortest questions to build your confidence. Be aware of the amount of time allotted for the examination, and pace yourself accordingly. As you go through the test, look for clues to answers to other questions. During test time, remember to use positive self-talk at the first indication of panic. Repeatedly remind yourself that you are well prepared; relax and think about the material before you get worried. You need to stop negative thoughts as soon as they arise and instead visualize yourself being successful. Use slow, deep breathing to relax and, if helpful, close your eyes for a minute and visualize a relaxing place before you go on with the test.

Certain strategies are useful for answering different types of questions. With multiple-choice questions, try to identify key words or clues in each question. Read the question carefully, and answer it in your head before you review the provided answers. If you are not absolutely sure of the answer, make an educated guess or follow your instincts in choosing an answer. If there are answers that you know are not correct, this knowledge can eliminate the "all of the above" answer choice. By eliminating the answers that you know are incorrect, you can focus on the other answer choices.

"True or false" questions give you a 50/50 chance of being correct. Remember that if any part of the question is not true, then the statement is false. Again, check the statements for key words that help indicate the direction of the answer. Look for qualifying terms (e.g., *always, never, sometimes*) that are the key to understanding the meaning of the true or false statement.

CRITICAL THINKING APPLICATION **1.8**

Think about a time you experienced test anxiety. Write down the details of the situation and how you felt. Choose four test-taking strategies you think would be beneficial for handling similar situations in the future.

Becoming a Critical Thinker: Making Mental Connections

The ability to process information and arrive at reasonable conclusions is crucial to all healthcare workers. The process of **critical thinking** involves (1) sorting out conflicting information, (2) weighing your knowledge about that information, (3) ignoring or letting go of personal biases, and (4) deciding on a reasonable belief or action. Critical thinking is an active search for the truth.

Critical thinking could be described as thorough thinking because it requires learners to keep an open mind to all possibilities. Successful students are thorough thinkers because they must determine the facts about a topic and come to logical conclusions about the material. Critical thinkers are also inquisitive learners; they constantly analyze and sort out conflicting information to reach conclusions.

A crucial step in critical thinking is evaluating the results of your learning. Reflection is the key to critical thinking. "How did I learn what I learned?" and "What does it mean in my life?" are questions that must be asked consistently to continue to learn. Becoming a successful student and, ultimately, a successful member of the allied health team requires critical thinking skills.

Using these tools to become the best possible medical assistant student will also help you become the best possible professional medical assistant.

THE HISTORY OF MEDICINE

Understanding the history of medicine is helpful in recognizing just how far we have come and why some things are done in the way that they are. Many historical factors have influenced how healthcare is provided today and the medical assisting profession.

History of Medicine

Although religious and mythologic beliefs were the basis of care for the sick in ancient times, evidence suggests that drugs, surgery, and other treatments based on theories about the body were used as early as 5000 BC. Moses presented rules of health to the Hebrews in approximately 1205 BC. He was the first advocate of preventive medicine and is considered the first public health officer. Moses knew that some animal diseases could be passed to humans and that **contamination** existed; therefore, a religious law was developed forbidding humans to eat or drink from dirty dishes. The people of that era believed that doing so would defile their bodies and they would lose their souls.

Hippocrates, known as the father of medicine, is the most famous of the ancient Greek physicians. He was born in 450 BC on the island of Cos in Greece. He is best remembered for the Hippocratic oath, which has been administered to physicians for more than 2000 years. To this day, most graduating medical school students swear to some form of the oath (Figure 1.7).

Hippocrates is credited with taking mysticism out of medicine and giving it a scientific basis. During this period of history, most believed that illness was caused by demonic possession; the demon had to be removed from the body to cure the illness. Hippocrates' clinical descriptions of diseases and his volumes on epidemics, fevers, epilepsy, fractures, and instruments were studied for centuries. He believed that the body had the capacity to heal itself and that the physician's role was to help nature. It is also interesting to see that Hippocrates addressed confidentiality and understood that it was important to maintain patient privacy.

Medical knowledge developed slowly, and the distribution of such knowledge was poor. In the 17th century, European academies or societies were established, consisting of small groups of men who met to discuss subjects of mutual interest. One of the earliest academies was the Royal Society of London, formed in 1662. In the United States, medical education was greatly influenced by Johns Hopkins University School of Medicine in Baltimore, Maryland, established in the early 1890s. The school admitted only college graduates with at least one year's training in the natural sciences. The clinical education at Johns Hopkins was superior because the school partnered with Johns Hopkins Hospital, which had been created expressly for teaching and research by members of the medical faculty. Table 1.3 presents selected medical pioneers and their achievements.

The History of Medical Assisting

As physicians made the switch from going to patients' homes for treatment to having the patient come to their office, some physicians hired nurses to help in their practices. Gradually, the administrative part of running a practice became increasingly complicated and time consuming, and physicians realized that they needed an assistant with both administrative and clinical training. Nurses were likely to have training only in clinical skills; therefore, many physicians began training individuals—medical assistants—to assist with all the office duties.

The first medical assistants started working in individual physicians' offices with on-the-job training to help out when an extra pair of hands was needed. Today, medical assisting is one of the most respected allied health fields in the industry, and training is readily available through community colleges, junior colleges, and private educational institutions throughout the United States.

CRITICAL THINKING APPLICATION **1.9**

- In Table 1.3, review the list of individuals who have made significant contributions to medicine. Which one do you believe had the greatest impact on modern healthcare?
- Consider how the medical assisting profession began. How do you think advances in medicine throughout history have affected the current practice of medical assistance?

I swear to fulfill, to the best of my ability and judgment, this covenant:

I will respect the hard-won scientific gains of those physicians in whose steps I walk and gladly share such knowledge as is mine with those who are to follow.

I will apply, for the benefit of the sick, all measures [that] are required, avoiding those twin traps of overtreatment and therapeutic nihilism.

I will remember that there is art to medicine as well as science and that warmth, sympathy, and understanding may outweigh the surgeon's knife or the chemist's drug.

I will not be ashamed to say "I know not," nor will I fail to call in my colleagues when the skills of another are needed for a patient's recovery.

I will respect the privacy of my patients, for their problems are not disclosed to me that the world may know. Most especially must I tread with care in matters of life and death. If it is given me to save a life, all thanks. But it may also be within my power to take a life; this awesome responsibility must be faced with great humbleness and awareness of my own frailty. Above all, I must not play at God.

I will remember that I do not treat a fever chart, a cancerous growth, but a sick human being whose illness may affect the person's family and economic stability. My responsibility includes these related problems, if I am to care adequately for the sick.

I will prevent disease whenever I can, for prevention is preferable to cure.

I will remember that I remain a member of society, with special obligations to all my fellow human beings, those sound of mind and body as well as the infirm.

If I do not violate this oath, may I enjoy life and art, respected while I live and remembered with affection thereafter. May I always act so as to preserve the finest traditions of my calling and may I long experience the joy of healing those who seek my help.

Written in 1964 by Louis Lasagna, Academic Dean of the School of Medicine at Tufts University, and used in many medical schools today.

FIGURE 1.7 Modern version of the Hippocratic oath.

MEDICAL PROFESSIONALS

Now that you have an understanding of the medical assistant profession, let's take a look at other areas in healthcare. Physicians and providers (e.g., nurse practitioners and physician assistants) are portals of entry or first contacts for patients seeking medical care. *Primary care providers* (PCPs) are healthcare practitioners who monitor a patient's overall health. Family medicine, internal medicine, and pediatrics are generally considered primary care specialties. After the initial assessment or with the diagnosis of a more complex health issue, patients may be referred to a medical specialist for further examination and treatment.

Doctors of Medicine

A medical doctor (doctor of medicine [MD]) is considered an **allopathic** physician. These individuals are the most widely recognized type of physician. They diagnose illness and disease and prescribe treatment for their patients. MDs have a wide variety of rights, including writing prescriptions, performing surgery, offering wellness advice, and performing preventive medicine procedures. Becoming an MD requires 4 years of undergraduate university training (premed) and 4 years of medical school. Regardless of where premed students attend college, a national standard of coursework is required to apply to medical school. They must take entry and advanced levels of biology, physics, organic and inorganic chemistry, mathematics, English, humanities, and social sciences. The United States has approximately 154 allopathic medical schools. After medical school, the student faces 3 to 8 years of residency programs, depending on the medical specialty he or she pursues. After completion of a residency program, a physician can obtain board certification in one or more of 37 different specialty areas recognized by the American Board of Medical Specialties (Table 1.4). An MD must have a state license to practice, and continuing education is required to maintain the license. Graduates of foreign medical schools can usually obtain a license in the United States after passing an examination and completing a residency program in this country.

Doctors of Osteopathy

An osteopathic physician (doctor of osteopathy [DO]) completes requirements similar to those of an MD to graduate and practice medicine. Osteopaths use medicine and surgery, in addition to osteopathic manipulative therapy (OMT), in treating their patients. Andrew Taylor Still is considered the father of osteopathic medicine, which he established in 1874. He believed in a more **holistic** approach to medicine, and although he was an MD, he founded the American School of Osteopathy in Kirksville, Missouri. The school originally was chartered to offer an MD degree but later focused more on the osteopathic approach. DOs stress preventive medicine and holistic patient care, in addition to a special focus on the musculoskeletal system and OMT. Premed students moving toward osteopathic medicine complete the same undergraduate coursework as allopathic candidates and 4 years of medical studies at a school for osteopathic medicine. Over the years, there have become fewer differences between allopathic and osteopathic programs, with many DO physicians earning residency programs in the same institutions as MDs.

Doctors of Chiropractic

A chiropractor (doctor of chiropractic [DC]) focuses on the relationship between the spine and the function of the body. The goal is

TABLE 1.3 Medical Pioneers and Their Achievements

NAME	ACHIEVEMENT
Andreas Vesalius (1514–1564)	Father of modern anatomy; wrote first anatomy book
William Harvey (1578–1657)	Discovered the circulatory system
Anton van Leeuwenhoek (1632–1723)	First to observe microbes through a lens; developed the first microscope
John Hunter (1728–1793)	Founder of scientific surgery
Edward Jenner (1749–1823)	Developed smallpox vaccine
Ignaz Semmelweis (1818–1865)	First physician to recommend hand washing to prevent puerperal fever; believed there was a connection between performing autopsies and then delivering babies that caused puerperal fever in new mothers
Florence Nightingale (1820–1910)	Founder of nursing
Clara Barton (1821–1912)	Established the American Red Cross
Elizabeth Blackwell (1821–1910)	First woman in the United States to earn a of medicine degree
Louis Pasteur (1822–1895)	Father of bacteriology and preventive medicine; developed pasteurization and established the connection between germs and disease
Joseph Lister (1827–1912)	Father of sterile surgery; developed antiseptic methods for surgery
Robert Koch (1843–1910)	Developed Koch's postulates, a theory of causative agents for disease; discovered the cause of cholera
William Roentgen (1845–1923)	Discovered the x-ray
Walter Reed (1851–1902)	Proved that yellow fever was transmitted by mosquito bites while in the US Army serving in Cuba
Paul Ehrlich (1854–1915)	Injected chemicals for the first time to treat disease (syphilis)
Marie Curie (1867–1934)	Discovered radium and polonium
Alexander Fleming (1881–1955)	Discovered penicillin
Albert Sabin (1906–1993)	Developed the oral live-virus vaccine for polio 10 years after Salk developed the first injected vaccine
Virginia Apgar (1909–1974)	Founded neonatology; developed the Apgar score, which assesses the status of newborns
Jonas Salk (1914–1955)	Developed the first safe and effective injectable vaccine for polio
Christiaan Barnard (1922–2001)	Performed the first human heart transplant
Edwin Carl Wood (1929–2011)	Pioneered the technique of in vitro fertilization (IVF)
David Ho (1952–)	Research pioneer in acquired immunodeficiency syndrome (AIDS)

TABLE 1.4 Examples of Medical Specialties

SPECIALTY	PRACTITIONER'S TITLE	DESCRIPTION
Allergy and immunology	Allergist/immunologist	Allergists/immunologists are trained to evaluate disorders and diseases of the immune system. This includes conditions such as adverse reactions to drugs and food, anaphylaxis, and problems related to autoimmune diseases, asthma, and insect stings.
Anesthesiology	Anesthesiologist	Anesthesiologists provide pain relief and pain management during surgical procedures and also for patients with long-standing conditions accompanied by pain.
Colon and rectal surgery	Colorectal surgeon	Colorectal surgeons diagnose and treat conditions affecting the intestines, rectum, and anal area, in addition to organs affected by intestinal disease.
Dermatology	Dermatologist	Dermatologists work with adult and pediatric patients in treating disorders and diseases of the skin, hair, nails, and related tissues. Dermatologists are specially trained to manage conditions such as skin cancers, cosmetic disorders of the skin, scars, allergies, and other disorders, both malignant and benign.

TABLE 1.4 Examples of Medical Specialties—*continued*

SPECIALTY	PRACTITIONER'S TITLE	DESCRIPTION
Emergency medicine	Emergency physician	Emergency physicians are experts in assessing and treating a patient to prevent death or serious disability. They provide immediate care to stabilize the patient's condition and then refer the patient to the appropriate professional for further care.
Family medicine	Primary care provider (PCP)	PCPs offer care to the whole family, from newborns to older adults. They are familiar with a wide range of disorders and diseases, and preventive care is their primary concern.
General surgery	Surgeon	General surgeons correct deformities and defects and treat diseases or injured parts of the body by means of operative treatment.
Genetics	Medical geneticist	Geneticists are physicians trained to diagnose and treat patients with conditions related to genetically linked diseases. They provide genetic counseling when indicated.
Internal medicine	Internist	Internists are concerned with comprehensive care, often diagnosing and treating those with chronic, long-term conditions. They must have a broad understanding of the body and its ailments.
Neurologic surgery	Neurosurgeon	Neurosurgeons provide surgical care for patients with conditions of the central, autonomic, and peripheral nervous systems.
Neurology/ psychiatry	Neurologist/psychiatrist	Neurologists diagnose and treat disorders of the nervous system. Psychiatrists are physicians who specialize in the diagnosis and treatment of people with mental, emotional, or behavioral disorders. A psychiatrist is qualified to conduct psychotherapy and to prescribe medications.
Nuclear medicine	Nuclear medicine specialist	These specialists use radioactive substances to diagnose, treat, and detect disease.
Obstetrics and gynecology	Obstetrician/gynecologist	Obstetricians provide care to women of childbearing age and monitor the progress of the developing child. Gynecologists are concerned with the diagnosis and treatment of the female reproductive system.
Ophthalmology	Ophthalmologist	Ophthalmologists diagnose, treat, and provide comprehensive care for the eye and its supporting structures. These physicians also offer vision services, including corrective lenses.
Otolaryngology	Otolaryngologist	Otolaryngologists treat diseases and conditions that affect the ear, nose, and throat and structures related to the head and neck. Problems that affect the voice and hearing are also referred to this specialist.
Pathology	Pathologist	Pathologists study the causes of diseases. They study tissues and cells, body fluids, and organs themselves to aid in the process of diagnosis.
Pediatrics	Pediatrician	Pediatricians promote preventive medicine and treat diseases that affect children and adolescents. They monitor the child's growth and development and provide a wide range of health services.
Physical medicine and rehabilitation	Physiatrist	Physiatrists assist patients who have physical disabilities. This may include rehabilitation, patients with musculoskeletal disorders, and patients suffering from pain as a result of injury or trauma.
Plastic surgery	Plastic surgeon	Plastic surgeons work with patients who have a physical defect as a result of some type of injury or condition. They perform reconstructive cosmetic enhancements and elective procedures.
Preventive medicine	Preventive medicine specialist	Preventive medicine specialists are concerned with preventing mental and physical illness and disability. They also analyze current health services and plan for future medical needs.
Radiology	Radiologist	Radiology is a specialty in which x-rays are used to diagnose and treat disease. A diagnostic radiologist specializes in using x-rays, ultrasound, nuclear medicine, computed tomography, and magnetic resonance imaging to detect abnormalities throughout the body.
Thoracic surgery	Thoracic surgeon	Thoracic surgeons are concerned with the operative treatment of the chest and chest wall, lungs, heart, heart valves, and respiratory passages.
Urology	Urologist	Urologists are concerned with the treatment of diseases and disorders of the urinary tract. They diagnose and manage problems with the genitourinary system and practice endoscopic procedures related to these structures.

to correct alignment problems and thereby alleviate pain, improve function, and support the body's natural ability to heal itself. Spinal manipulation has been shown to be beneficial for low back pain, headaches, neck pain, whiplash-associated disorders, and upper and lower extremity joint conditions. Chiropractic care is one of the most common fields of **complementary and alternative medicine (CAM)**. Examples of complementary and alternative medicine can be found in the following box.

Complementary and Alternative Medicine Therapies

- Chiropractic
- Massage therapy
- Acupuncture
- Biofeedback
- Meditation
- Guided imagery
- Healing touch
- Natural products
- Yoga, Tai Chi, or Qi Gong
- Homeopathy
- Naturopathy
- Progressive relaxation
- Hypnotherapy
- Ayurvedic medicine

Chiropractic doctors have at least 4 years of additional training beyond a bachelor's degree. The training includes both classroom and direct patient care. The doctors must pass the national licensing exam. State law regulates their practice, and many state boards require continuing education to maintain the license.

Hospitalists

Hospitalists are physicians whose primary professional focus is the general medical care of hospitalized patients. Most hospitalists are employed by the healthcare facility instead of having individual freestanding offices in which patients are seen and treated. Perhaps the most attractive benefit of becoming a hospitalist is the quality of life for the physician and his or her family. Hospitalists work a specific, set number of hours each week and receive a set salary from their employers. In addition, most institutions that employ hospitalists cover these physicians with blanket malpractice insurance, saving the practitioner the expense of costly premiums. Although the hospitalist is in charge of the patient while the person is in the hospital, if the patient has a PCP, he or she may still visit the patient. The hospitalist would still refer the patient to medical specialists as needed for more advanced care.

Nurse Practitioners

Nurse practitioners (NPs) provide basic patient care services, including diagnosing and prescribing medications for common illnesses, or they may have additional training and expertise in a specialty area of medicine. These professionals must have advanced academic training beyond the registered nurse (RN) degree and also vast clinical experience. An NP is licensed by individual states and can practice independently or as part of a team of healthcare professionals.

Physician Assistants

A physician assistant (PA) is a certified healthcare professional who provides diagnostic, therapeutic, and preventive healthcare services under the supervision of a medical doctor. Physician assistants must be licensed, which requires completion of a physician assistant program that is typically at the master's degree level. Physician assistants must pass the Physician Assistant National Certifying Examination to practice in any state. They may also complete advanced training to focus on a particular specialty practice.

ALLIED HEALTH PROFESSIONALS

In addition to doctors, nurse practitioners, and physician assistants, the healthcare team includes allied health professionals. The definition of an allied health professional can vary, but it loosely refers to those who can act only under the authority of a licensed medical practitioner (e.g., MD, DO, optometrist, dentist, pharmacist, podiatrist, or chiropractor).

Who Are Allied Health Professionals?

Allied health professionals include respiratory therapists, radiation therapists, occupational therapists, physical therapists, technologists of various types, dental hygienists, medical assistants, phlebotomists, pharmacy technicians, and other professionals who do not independently diagnose and prescribe treatment but perform diagnostic procedures, therapeutic services, and provide care.

The allied health professions fall into two broad categories, technicians (assistants) and therapists. Technicians are trained to perform procedures, and their education lasts 2 years or less. They are required to work under the supervision of medical providers or licensed therapists. This part of the allied health field includes, among others, physical therapy assistants, medical laboratory technicians, radiology technicians, occupational therapy assistants, recreational therapy assistants, respiratory therapy technicians, and medical assistants (Table 1.5).

The educational process for nurses and therapists is more intensive. These professions require a state-issued license and an advanced degree, showing that the individual is trained to evaluate patients, diagnose conditions, develop treatment plans, and understand the rationale behind various treatments (Table 1.6).

Allied Health Professionals as Part of the Healthcare Team

Allied health professionals typically work as part of a healthcare team, which is what you will do as a professional medical assistant.

As a new medical assistant, you will enter the ranks of an ever-growing group of allied health professionals who provide services for patients in a variety of settings in today's healthcare system. Allied health professionals comprise nearly 60% of the healthcare workforce. The term *allied health* is used to identify a cluster of health professions encompassing as many as 200 careers. In the United States, about 5 million allied health professionals work in more than 80 different professions; they represent approximately 60% of all healthcare providers.

TYPES OF HEALTHCARE FACILITIES

When thinking about how healthcare is provided, we have to consider the different professions involved in providing that care, and we also have to consider where that healthcare is provided. In the next section, we will be looking at the various healthcare facilities.

TABLE 1.5 Allied Health Occupations Recognized by the American Medical Association

TITLE	CREDENTIAL	JOB DESCRIPTION
Anesthesiology assistant	AA	Functions as a specialty physician assistant under the direction of a licensed and qualified anesthesiologist; assists in developing and implementing the anesthesia care plan.
Art therapist	ATR	Uses drawings and other art and media forms to assess, treat, and rehabilitate patients with mental, emotional, physical, or developmental disorders.
Athletic trainer	ATC	Provides a variety of services, including injury prevention, assessment, immediate care, treatment, and rehabilitation after physical injury or trauma.
Audiologist	CCC-A	Identifies individuals with symptoms of hearing loss and other auditory, balance, and related neural problems; assesses the nature of those problems and helps individuals manage them.
Blood bank technology specialist	SBB	Performs routine and specialized tests in blood center and transfusion services using methods that conform to the accepted standards in the blood bank industry.
Diagnostic cardiovascular sonographer/technologist	RDCS, RVT	Using invasive or noninvasive techniques (or both), performs diagnostic examinations and therapeutic interventions for the heart and blood vessels at the request of a physician.
Clinical laboratory science/medical technologist	MT, MLT	In conjunction with pathologists, performs tests to diagnose the causes and nature of disease; also develops data on blood, tissues, and fluids of the human body using a variety of methodologies.
Counseling-related professional	LPC, LMHC	Deals with human development through support, therapeutic approaches, consultation, evaluation, teaching, and research; practices the art of helping people to grow.
Cytotechnologist	CT	Works with pathologists to evaluate cellular material from all body sites, primarily through use of the microscope; examines specimens for normal and abnormal cytologic changes, including malignancies.
Dance therapist	DTR, ADTR	Uses the psychotherapeutic properties of movement as a process that furthers the emotional, cognitive, social, and physical integration of the patient as a tool for healing.
Dental assistant, dental hygienist, dental laboratory technician	CDA, RDH, CDT	Performs a wide range of tasks, from assisting the dentist to teaching patients how to prevent oral disease and maintain oral health.
Diagnostic medical sonographer	RDMS	Uses medical ultrasound to gather sonographic data, which can aid the diagnosis of a variety of conditions and diseases; also monitors fetal development.
Dietitian, dietetic technician	DTR	Integrates and applies the principles of food science, nutrition, biochemistry, physiology, food management, and behavior to achieve and maintain good health.
Electroneurodiagnostic technologist	REEG-T	Records and studies the electrical activity of the brain and nervous system; obtains interpretable recordings of patients' nervous system function.
Genetics counselor	IGC	Provides genetic services to individuals and families seeking information about the occurrence or risk of a genetic condition or birth defect.
Health information management professional	RHIA, RHIT	Provides expert assistance in the systems and processes for health information management, including planning, engineering, administration, application, and policy making.
Kinesiotherapist	RKT	Provides rehabilitation exercise and education designed to reverse or minimize debilitation and enhance the functional capacity of medically stable patients.
Massage therapist	MT	Applies manual techniques, and may apply adjunctive techniques, with the intention of positively affecting the health and well-being of a patient or client.

Continued

TABLE 1.5 Allied Health Occupations Recognized by the American Medical Association—continued

TITLE	CREDENTIAL	JOB DESCRIPTION
Medical assistant	CMA, RMA, CCMA, CMAA	Functions as a member of the healthcare delivery team and performs both administrative and clinical procedures and duties; a multiskilled health professional.
Medical illustrator	MI	Specializes in the visual display and communication of scientific information; creates visuals and designs communication tools for teaching both medical professionals and the public.
Music therapist	MT-BC	Uses music in a therapeutic relationship to address the physical, emotional, cognitive, and social needs of individuals of all ages; assesses the strengths and needs of clients and patients.
Nuclear medicine technologist	RT	Uses the nuclear properties of radioactive and stable nuclides to make diagnostic evaluations of anatomic or physiologic conditions of the body; also provides therapy with unsealed radioactive sources.
Ophthalmic laboratory technician, medical technician/technologist	COT, COMT	Collects data and performs clinical evaluations; performs tests and protocols required by ophthalmologists; assists in the treatment of patients.
Orthoptist	CO	Performs a series of diagnostic tests and measurements on patients with visual disorders; helps design a treatment plan to correct disorders of vision, eye movements, and alignment.
Orthotist/prosthetist	RTO, RTP, RTPO	Designs and fits devices (orthoses) to patients who have disabling conditions of the limbs and spine or partial or total absence of a limb.
Perfusionist	CCP	Operates extracorporeal circulation and autotransfusion equipment during any medical situation in which the patient's respiratory or circulatory function must be supported or temporarily replaced.
Pharmacy technician	CPhT	Assists pharmacists with duties that do not require the expertise or judgment of a licensed pharmacist.
Radiation therapist, radiographer	RRTD	Delivers prescribed dosages of radiation to patients for therapeutic purposes; provides appropriate patient care and maintains accurate records of the treatment provided.
Rehabilitation counselor	CRC	Determines and coordinates services to assist people with disabilities in moving from psychological and economic dependence to independence.
Respiratory therapist, respiratory therapy technician	RRT, CRT, RPFT, CPFT	Evaluates, treats, and manages patients of all ages with respiratory illnesses and other cardiopulmonary disorders. Advanced respiratory therapists exercise considerable independent judgment.
Surgical assistant	CSA	Assists in exposure, hemostasis, closure, and other intraoperative technical functions that help surgeons carry out a safe operation with optimal results for the patient.
Surgical technologist	ST, CST	Helps prepare patients for surgery and maintain the sterile field in the surgical suite, making sure all members of the surgical team follow sterile technique.
Therapeutic recreation specialist	CTRS	Uses treatment, education, and recreation services to help people with illnesses, disabilities, and other conditions develop and use their leisure in ways that enhance their health.

Hospitals

Hospitals are classified according to the type of care and services they provide to patients and by the type of ownership. There are three different levels of hospitalized care, which are interconnected.

- Primary level of care
  - smaller city or community hospitals
  - usually serve as the first level of contact between the community members and the hospital setting
- Secondary level of care
  - both PCPs and specialists provide care
  - larger municipal or district hospitals that provide a wider variety of specialty care and departments
- Tertiary level of care
  - referral system for primary or secondary care facilities
  - provide care for complicated cases and trauma
  - medical centers, regional and specialty hospitals

Private hospitals are run by a corporation or other organization and usually are designed to produce a profit for the owners or stockholders. *Nonprofit* hospitals exist to serve the community in which they are located and are normally run by a board of directors. The term

TABLE 1.6 Licensed Healthcare Professions

TITLE	CREDENTIAL	JOB DESCRIPTION
Certified nurse midwife	CNM	Registered nurse (RN) with additional training and certification; performs physical exams; prescribes medications, including contraceptive methods; orders laboratory tests as needed; provides prenatal care, gynecologic care, labor and birth care, and health education and counseling to women of all ages.
Diagnostic cardiac sonographer or vascular technologist	DCS or DVT	Assists in the diagnosis and treatment of cardiac and vascular diseases and disorders; performs noninvasive tests, including echocardiographs and electrocardiographs.
Emergency medical technician	EMT	Progresses through several levels of training, each providing more advanced skills. EMTs' medical education encompasses managing respiratory, cardiac, and trauma cases and often emergency childbirth. Some states also recognize specialties in the EMT field, such as EMT-Cardiac, which includes training in cardiac arrhythmias, and EMT-Shock Trauma, which includes starting intravenous fluids and administering specific medications.
Licensed practical or vocational nurse	LPN or LVN	Provides bedside care, assisting with the day-to-day personal care of inpatients; assesses patients, documents their progress, and administers medications and intravenous fluids when allowed by law; often works in hospitals or skilled nursing facilities and in physicians' offices.
Medical technologist	MT	Performs diagnostic testing on blood, body fluids, and other types of specimens to assist the provider in arriving at a diagnosis.
Nurse anesthetist	NA	RN who administers anesthetics to patients during care provided by surgeons, physicians, dentists, or other qualified health professionals.
Nurse practitioner	NP	Provides basic patient care services, including diagnosing and prescribing medications for common illnesses; must have advanced academic training, beyond the registered nurse (RN) degree, and also must have extensive clinical experience.
Occupational therapist	OT	Assists in helping patients compensate for loss of function.
Paramedic	Paramedic	Specially trained in advanced emergency skills to aid patients in life-threatening situations.
Physical therapist	PT	Assists patients in regaining their mobility and improving their strength and range of motion. Devises treatment plans in conjunction with the patient's physician.
Physician assistant	PA	Provides direct patient care services under the supervision of a licensed physician; trained to diagnose and treat patients as directed by the physician. In most states is allowed to write prescriptions, take patient histories, order and interpret tests, perform physical examinations, and make diagnostic decisions.
Radiology technician	RT	Uses various machines to help the provider diagnose and treat certain diseases; machines may include x-ray equipment, ultrasonographic machines, and magnetic resonance imaging (MRI) scanners.
Registered dietitian	RD	Thoroughly trained in nutrition and the different types of diets patients require to improve or maintain their condition. Designs healthy diets for patients during hospital stays and can help plan menus for home use. Also teaches patients about their recommended diet.
Registered nurse	RN	Provides direct patient care, assesses patients, and determines care plans; has many career options.
Respiratory therapist	RT	Commonly uses oxygen therapy to assist with breathing; also performs diagnostic tests that measure lung capacity. Most work in hospitals. All types of patients receive respiratory care, including newborns and geriatric patients.

nonprofit sometimes is misleading because "profit" is different from "making money." A nonprofit hospital or organization may make money in a campaign or fundraiser, but all of the money is returned to the organization. Nonprofit hospitals and organizations must follow strict guidelines in the area of finance and must account to the government for the money brought in and the purposes for which it is used.

A *hospital system* is a group of facilities that are affiliated and work toward a common goal. Hospital systems may include a hospital and a cancer center in a small community or may consist of a group of separate hospitals in a specific geographic region. Many hospital systems are designed as integrated delivery systems. An integrated delivery system (IDS) is a network of healthcare providers and organizations that provides or arranges to provide a coordinated continuum of services to a defined population and is willing to be held clinically and fiscally accountable for the clinical outcomes and health status of the population served. An IDS may own or could be closely aligned with an insurance product, such as a type of insurance policy. Services provided by an IDS can include a fully equipped community or tertiary hospital, home healthcare and **hospice** services, primary and specialty outpatient care and surgery, social services, rehabilitation, preventive care, health education and financing, and community provider offices. An IDS can also be a training location for health professional students, including physicians, nurses, and allied health professionals.

Accreditation is considered the highest form of recognition for the quality of care a facility or an organization provides. Not only does it indicate to the public that the facility is concerned with providing high-quality care, it also provides professional liability insurance benefits and plays a role in regulatory agency relicensure and certification efforts. Hospitals and other healthcare facilities are accredited by The Joint Commission, an organization that promotes and evaluates the quality of care in healthcare facilities. Standards or **indicators** have been developed to help determine when patients are receiving high-quality care. The term *quality* refers to much more than whether the patient liked the food served or had to wait to have a procedure or test performed. Categories of compliance include the following:

- Assessment and care of patients
- Use of medication
- Plant, technology, and safety management
- Orientation, education, and training of staff
- Medical staff qualifications
- Patients' rights

Accreditation by The Joint Commission is required to obtain reimbursement from Medicare, managed care organizations, and insurance companies. Besides accrediting healthcare facilities, The Joint Commission carefully evaluates patient safety. It has established the National Patient Safety Goals, which must be addressed by member facilities. The 2021 safety goals for ambulatory organizations took effect January 1, 2021, and include the following:

- Identifying patients correctly
- Using medicines safely
- Preventing infection
- Prevent mistakes in surgery

All of these safety factors are addressed in future chapters.

Ambulatory Care

Ambulatory care centers include a wide range of facilities that offer healthcare services to patients who seek outpatient health services. Physicians' offices, group practices, and multispecialty group practices are common types of ambulatory care facilities, and medical assistants can be employed in all of these practices. Group practices may involve a single specialty, such as pediatrics or may be multispecialty. A multispecialty practice might consist of an internal medicine physician, an oncologist, a cardiologist, and an endocrinologist.

Usually, the providers of the practice refer patients to each other when indicated. This is not only more convenient for the patients but also more profitable for the members of the practice. A patient seeing a provider for the first time is considered a *new* patient, whereas a patient who has seen the provider on previous occasions is called an *established* patient. Most providers charge new patients more than established patients because the levels of decision making, the extent of the physical examination, and the complexity of the medical history require that more time be directed toward the new patient.

Occupational health centers are concerned with helping patients return to work and productive activity. Often, physical therapy is used in conjunction with rehabilitation services to assist the patient in regaining as much of his or her previous level of ability as possible. Also, freestanding rehabilitation centers can assist patients with a wide range of services. Pain management centers help patients deal with discomfort associated with their condition. Sleep centers diagnose and treat people with sleep problems. Freestanding urgent or emergency care centers provide patients with an alternative to hospital emergency departments (EDs) and are typically open when traditional provider offices are closed.

Surgery has become more convenient because of the number of ambulatory surgical centers that exist today. Many insurance companies now prefer day surgery because it is more cost effective. A wide variety of outpatient surgical facilities are available, offering procedures in ophthalmology, plastic surgery, and gastrointestinal concerns, including colonoscopies.

Dialysis centers offer services to patients with severe kidney disorders, and many of the larger cities across the country have cancer centers for patients who need treatment by oncologists. Among the many other types of ambulatory care facilities are centers that provide magnetic resonance imaging (MRI), student health clinics, dental clinics, community health centers, and women's health centers.

Other Healthcare Facilities

Several other types of healthcare facilities deserve attention in the broad overview of the healthcare industry. Diagnostic laboratories offer testing services for patients referred by their providers. The enactment of CLIA in 1967 and its amendment in 1988 established that the only laboratory tests that can be performed in a physician's office lab are those designated as *CLIA waived.* You will learn how to perform many CLIA-waived tests in your medical assistant program. Larger ambulatory care centers may contain an onsite advanced diagnostic laboratory where all studies can be completed. Smaller or independent practices typically have to send non-CLIA-waived tests to an outside diagnostic facility.

Home health agencies or hospital-affiliated home healthcare organizations provide crucial services to patients who require medical follow-up but are not in a hospital setting. Home healthcare includes therapy services, administration of and assistance with medications, wound care, and other services so that the patient can remain at

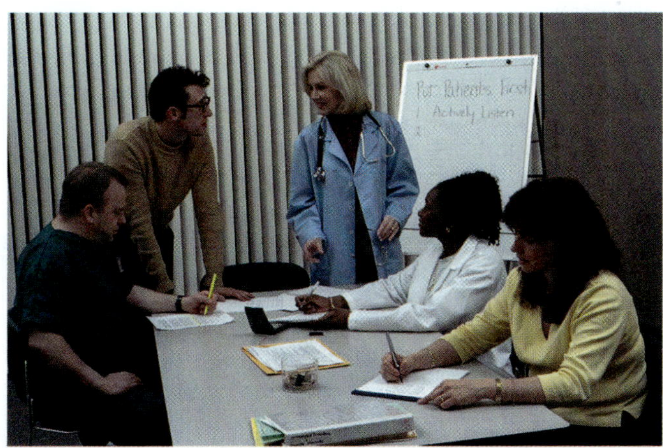

FIGURE 1.8 Teamwork is a vital part of the medical profession. All staff members must work together to care for the patient and perform required duties in the healthcare facility.

home, yet still obtain consistent medical attention. Hospice care is a type of home health service that provides medical care and support for patients facing end-of-life issues and their families. The goal of hospice is to provide peace, comfort, and dignity while controlling pain and promoting the best possible quality of life for the patient. Some communities have inpatient hospice services available either in a special unit in a hospital or in an independent hospice center.

THE HEALTHCARE TEAM

To deliver comprehensive quality care, everyone who interacts with patients, from the time they enter the facility to the time they leave, must work as a cooperative member of the healthcare team. If managers were asked to name the most important attributes for medical professionals, teamwork would be high on the list (Figure 1.8).

Teamwork

Staff members must work together for the good of the patients. They must be willing to perform duties outside a formal job description if they are needed in other areas of the office. Many supervisors frown on employees who state, "That's not in my job description." A professional medical assistant should perform the duty and later discuss with the supervisor any valid reasons that the task should have been assigned to someone else. However, if the task is illegal, unethical, or places the patient or anyone else in danger, it should not be done. If you are ever concerned about patient safety, you should discuss the situation with your supervisor before performing the task.

Although we all would enjoy working in an office where everyone gets along and likes every other employee, this does not always happen. Personal feelings must be set aside at work, and all employees must cooperate with others to get the job done efficiently. If a medical assistant has an issue with another employee, the first move would be to discuss it privately with the other person. If the situation does not improve, perhaps a supervisor (office or practice manager) should be involved for further discussions. Do not bring the provider into the discussion unless there is no choice because the facility manager is expected to deal with personnel issues (Figure 1.9).

Patient-Centered Medical Home

The concept of population health has become a valuable piece of providing healthcare. The Centers for Disease Control and Prevention

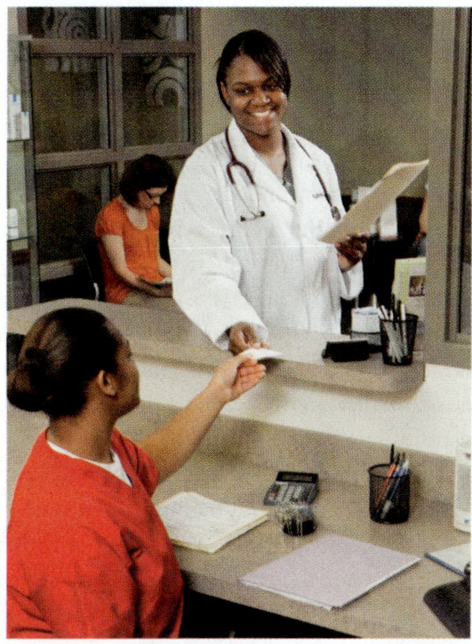

FIGURE 1.9 Knowing which employee to call when help is needed promotes goodwill among employees and often gets a task done more efficiently.

(CDC) describes population health as "an interdisciplinary customizable approach that allows health departments to connect practice to policy for change to happen locally." Many healthcare organizations look at population's health as focused on their own patient population and what can be done to provide the best possible care. The Patient Centered Medical Home (PCMH) is a model of patient care that can help facilitate the population health process. In this model, patient care is looked at from a holistic approach. The healthcare team wants to be able to assist that patient with any issues that come up about his or her care. This means having multiple team members available. The provider and the medical assistant would provide the primary care. There would also be a nurse who coordinates all of the care for the patient, including issues about home healthcare, financial issues, transportation issues, and so on. Many models include a clinical pharmacist who is available to discuss medication questions and concerns with the patient.

The healthcare team will meet with the patient and their family to determine what their needs are. This meeting could be face-to-face or in a virtual format utilizing the patient portal (discussed in Chapter 6) or another virtual meeting platform like Zoom. There may also be a home visit to better assess the needs of the patient.

Research indicates that PCMHs are saving money by reducing hospital and ED visits while at the same time improving patient outcomes. The Agency for Healthcare Research and Quality (AHRQ), which is part of the Department of Health and Human Services (HHS), believes that improving our primary care system is the key to achieving high-quality, accessible, efficient healthcare for all Americans. The agency recognizes that health information technology (IT) plays a central role in the successful implementation of the key features of the primary care medical home. According to the AHRQ, the PCMH has five core functions and attributes:

1. *Comprehensive care.* The primary care practice has the potential to provide physical and mental healthcare, prevention and wellness, acute care, and chronic care to all patients of the practice. However, comprehensive care cannot be provided by only the practicing physician. It requires a team of care providers. The

healthcare team for a PCMH includes physicians, nurse practitioners, physician assistants, nurses, pharmacists, nutritionists, social workers, educators, and medical assistants. If these specialty individuals are not readily available to smaller physician practices, virtual teams can be created online to link providers and patients to services in their communities.

2. *Patient-centered care.* The PCMH provides primary healthcare that is holistic and relationship based, always considering the individual patient and all facets of his or her life. However, establishing a partnership with patients and their families requires understanding and respect for each patient's unique needs, culture, values, and preferences. Medical assistants are trained to provide respectful patient care regardless of individual patient factors. The goal of the PCMH is to encourage and support patients in learning how to manage and organize their own care. Patients and families are recognized as core members of the care team.
3. *Coordinated care.* The PCMH coordinates care across all parts of the healthcare system, including specialty care, hospitals, home healthcare, and community services. Coordination is especially important when patients are transitioning from one site of care to another, such as from hospital to home. The PCMH works at creating and maintaining open communication among patients and families, the medical home, and members of the broader healthcare team.
4. *Accessible services.* The PCMH is designed to deliver accessible care. This is achieved by establishing policies that create shorter wait times for urgent needs, expanded office hours, around-the-clock telephone or electronic access to a member of the care team, and alternative methods of communication, such as email and telephone care.
5. *Quality and safety.* The PCMH is committed to delivering quality healthcare by providing evidence-based medicine and shared decision-making with patients and families, assessing practice performance and working on improvements, collecting safety data, and measuring and responding to patients' experiences and satisfaction. All of this information is made public to allow an open assessment of the practice and suggestions for possible methods of improvement.

The goal of the PCMH is to improve patient outcomes and reduce costs. There are accreditation processes that must be completed for a healthcare facility to be recognized as a PCMH. For further information about the PCMH model, refer to the Patient Centered Medical Home Resource Center, Department of Health and Human Services: http://pcmh.ahrq.gov.

PRACTICING PROFESSIONALISM AS A TEAM MEMBER

A *team* is a group of people organized for work or a specific purpose. In the healthcare setting, usually, the team consists of the employees working in the same department. A broader definition could include all the employees at the facility. A *team member* is loyal to the group and works well with the other people in the group. As a member, the medical assistant must help the team function. It is important to know the roles of the different team members to do this. Tables 1.5 and 1.6 describe various healthcare professionals found in ambulatory care facilities.

It is important to have several qualities to be a valuable team member. Work ethic, punctuality, cooperation, and the willingness to help are important traits in a team member. It takes all members working together to make an effective and productive team. When a member drops the ball, others must step in and do extra work.

Exceptional Customer Service

To provide exceptional customer service, medical assistants need to keep certain considerations in mind:

- Remember that patients, family members, and co-workers are all customers.
- Be professional in behavior and appearance.
- Consider cultural differences when using nonverbal communication.
- Prepare clear, concise verbal communication (written and oral).
- Use therapeutic communication, including active listening.

To help promote professionalism when you first meet a patient, it is important to GIVE:

- *G*reet the patient.
- *I*dentify yourself.
- *V*erify the patient's identity by asking for the person's full name and date of birth.
- *E*xplain the procedure to be performed in a manner that the patient understands.

The Meaning of Professionalism

Professionalism is defined as having a courteous, conscientious, and respectful approach to all interactions and situations in the workplace. It is characterized by or conforms to the recognized standard of care for the profession. Conducting themselves in a professional manner is essential for successful medical assistants. The attitude of those in the medical profession generally is more conservative than that seen in other career fields. Patients expect professional behavior and base much of their trust and confidence in those who show this type of **demeanor** in the healthcare facility (Figure 1.10).

Work Ethic and Punctuality

A *work ethic* is composed of sets of values based on hard work and diligence. The medical assistant should always display **initiative** and be

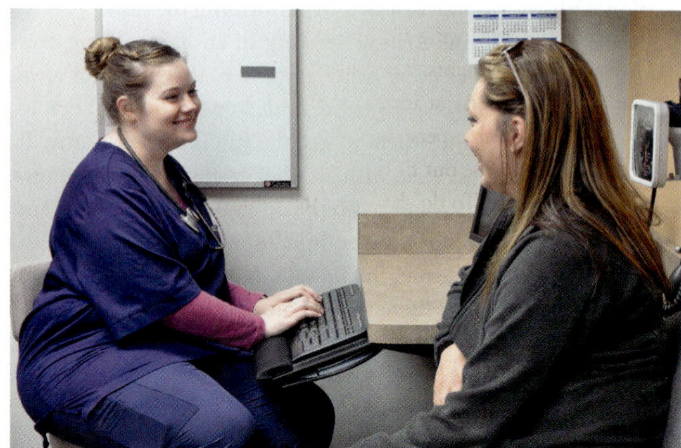

FIGURE 1.10 The professional medical assistant is an asset to the healthcare facility.

reliable. People with a good work ethic arrive on time, are rarely absent, and always perform to the best of their ability. Co-workers become frustrated if another employee consistently arrives late or is absent. This forces others to take on additional duties, and it may prevent them from completing their own work. One missing employee can disrupt the entire day. Phones may not be answered promptly. Patients may have to wait longer for appointments. Lunch breaks may be shortened to allow all the work to be done. All employees should know and follow the attendance policies of the facility as outlined in the policies and procedures manual.

Most new hires have a probationary period that may last 30 to 90 days. Excessive absences or *tardiness* (being late) will negatively affect the employee. It may be grounds for *termination* (job loss). If the medical assistant must be absent or tardy, the supervisor must be notified prior to the start time. Make sure to follow the office policy. All employees must be *punctual* (on time) every day. Providers and patients alike expect this reliability.

CRITICAL THINKING APPLICATION **1.10**

Carmen tends to arrive at the clinic with about 1 minute to spare. She realizes that she needs to change her habits and arrive about 10 minutes before her start time. This would give her a little cushion if traffic is slow. If you were Carmen, what strategies could you use to make sure to get to the healthcare facility 10 minutes before the start time?

Cooperation and Willingness to Help

Each team member must be willing to cooperate and help others on the team. It is not uncommon that one team member might be busy or handling an emergency. Other team members must be willing to step up and lend a helping hand. For instance, a medical assistant may be tied up caring for a very sick patient. Other patients who have appointments are waiting to be seen. One of the other team members needs to help room the patients (e.g., take their vital signs and histories for the provider). This is how the department can provide exceptional customer service. Team members watch out for each other. If someone is getting behind, others help out.

Through cooperation, the team is more productive. Team members have greater job satisfaction. When members cooperate and work together, there is a great sense of communication and understanding in a team. Most important, the patients are cared for, and great customer service is provided.

Prioritizing and Time Management Skills

Prioritizing duties and using time management skills are critical for the success of medical assistants. *Prioritizing* means to arrange and complete duties in the order of most importance. *Time management strategies* are methods that maximize personal efficiencies and prioritize tasks. This means that we are to use our time efficiently and concentrate on the most important duties first. To do this, we must first prioritize our duties. We must arrange our schedules to ensure that these duties can be performed. The first way to improve time management is to plan the tasks that need to be done that day. Take 10 minutes to write down the tasks for the day. This helps ensure the tasks get done. Make sure to reference the list throughout the day to keep on track. Do not schedule too much to do each day so that it is impossible to get everything done. Keep the list manageable. You need to build in some extra time in case of emergencies or urgent issues that come up. The key to managing time is prioritizing.

Time Management Strategies

- Organize and review your daily to-do list. If you honestly believe you cannot possibly get everything that is a priority done, ask for help. It is better to admit you can't do it all than to ignore a task that is important.
- Brainstorm with your peers about ways to achieve all the tasks facing everyone each day. Maybe someone can come up with a unique way to solve a problem, but if not, at least all of you will be on the same page.
- Make a master list of important tasks, so nothing is forgotten.
- Try to accomplish like tasks in the same block of time. If you have phone calls to return or insurance referrals to complete, do both at the same time to be more efficient.
- At the end of each day, create a new to-do list for the next day so that nothing important is forgotten.

When prioritizing your tasks, use a code system to indicate when they need to be done. For instance, try the following:

- Use an "M" for tasks that *must* be done that day.
- Use an "S" for tasks that *should* be done that day.
- Use a "C" for tasks that *could* be done if time permits.

Once the tasks have been divided into these categories, they can be further classified in each section. For instance, if category *M* has six tasks, they can be numbered in the order they should be performed. The same process is completed with the tasks in categories *S* and *C*. As the tasks are completed, they are checked off. At the end of each day, create a new to-do list for the next day so that nothing important is forgotten.

CRITICAL THINKING APPLICATION **1.11**

Carmen needs to practice her time management skills. Using the system described, make your to-do list. Use *M*, *S*, and *C* to categorize your activities.

Responding to Criticism

As we work, others will evaluate us. It may be informal or formal for a job evaluation. We learn from others' feedback on our performance. This criticism can be hard to take. It threatens our confidence and self-esteem. We need to realize the value of the feedback. It will help us improve our skills and refine our professional skills. When a person gives us feedback or criticism, it is important to take it as a professional. Becoming defensive or blaming others is not professional. This type of behavior will be a negative reflection on you.

Problem Solving and Chain of Command

When you are working as part of a team, it is important to understand how to solve differences with other members. Typically, it is best to talk with the person with whom you are having an issue. Try not to use statements that accuse the other person. Refrain from using sentences that start with "You are..." Try to remove the emotion from the situation if you can. Use more "I feel..." statements. If your attempt to resolve the situation is unsuccessful, then it is usually recommended that you talk with the supervisor.

If the issue is related to theft, confidentiality, or harassment, you may need to follow the chain of command in the healthcare facility. Usually, you need to start with your supervisor or the person you report to. Then, the next step is the supervisor of your supervisor, and so on. Most employee handbooks discuss the facility's chain of command.

Barriers to Professionalism

At times it is not easy to be a professional. Sometimes patients and co-workers try our patience. It can be difficult to maintain a professional attitude in these cases. Some of the obstructions to professional behavior are discussed in this section.

Attitude

A negative attitude can bring down the **morale** of the whole team. Patients can sense when the staff is unhappy, and this makes them wonder why. It is not the patient's responsibility to cheer up the medical assistants. The patients will also be less likely to share personal information with someone who has a negative attitude. Try to find the positive in any given situation.

Complaining can be considered having a negative attitude. If you have a problem, you should discuss it constructively with someone who can help resolve the situation. Sitting in the break room and complaining to another medical assistant about your schedule will not help to resolve the situation. Talking with your supervisor would be a better solution.

Procrastination

Delaying or putting off tasks can be detrimental to patient care and your relationship with your co-workers. If there is a task that you dread doing, do it quickly and efficiently, and you will not have to think about it until the next time. When you are working in healthcare, waiting to do something can put a patient at risk or require that your co-workers do it for you. Either situation can put your job at risk.

Personal Problems and "Baggage"

We all have a personal life. Sometimes things happen in our lives before we go to work. It is important that we push these issues aside and focus on our job. If we carry this "baggage" to work, it can interfere with our ability to do our job. We may be tempted to make personal calls, check emails, and so on. This takes time away from our job, and our focus is not on our job. If the baggage is so important and concerning, the medical assistant needs to speak with the supervisor. It might not be appropriate to be working if one cannot concentrate on the job at hand. The patient must be the prime concern of all the employees in the healthcare facility.

Gossip

Gossip is casual or idle chat (rumors) about other people and their business. Many times, the discussion is based on someone's opinion and not fact. Most people enjoy working in an environment in which employees cooperate and get along with each other. Rumors and gossip can cause problems with employee morale. They can affect how a team functions. A medical assistant should refuse to participate in the rumor mill (Figure 1.11). Attempting to be cordial and friendly to everyone at work is important. Supervisors regard those who gossip or spread rumors as unprofessional and untrustworthy. You should always avoid passing along work-related rumors to patients and family members.

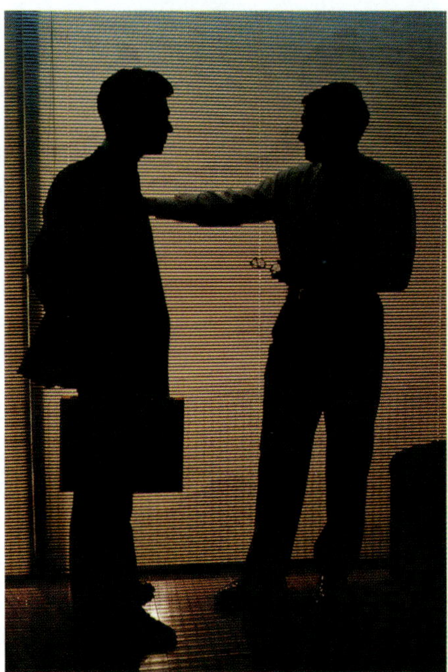

FIGURE 1.11 Gossip and rumors have no place in the medical profession. Avoid employees who participate in this type of activity.

Personal Communication

The medical assistant should not take unnecessary phone calls from friends and family at the office. The office phone is a business line and must be used as such, except in emergencies. Using personal cell phones during working hours is not acceptable. Use breaks and lunch hours to take care of business on the phone. Never take a personal call or respond to text messages on a cell phone while working with a patient. Many healthcare facilities require cell phones to be silenced and out of sight during the workday. Because most phones have cameras, facility administrators are concerned about unlawful pictures being taken. Many healthcare computer networks block certain nonhealthcare websites (e.g., social media sites). Table 1.7 describes acceptable and unacceptable activities for digital communication devices and online activities.

CRITICAL THINKING APPLICATION **1.12**

Carmen loves her phone. But, she learned quickly that her phone was to be turned off and put away during work hours. Explain why having cell phones out and turned on can create issues in the healthcare facility.

Visitors should not frequent the office, especially the area where the medical assistant is working. If someone must come to the office, always offer the reception area as a waiting room. Visitors should never be allowed to enter patient areas.

Checking personal email also should be avoided in the workplace. Any type of personal business, such as studying, looking up information on the internet for personal use, internet shopping, or using social media, should be done at home and not in the office. All of these actions distract the medical assistant from the job at hand; the

TABLE 1.7 Using Digital Communication Devices and Online Activities in Healthcare Facilities

DEVICE/ACTIVITY	ACCEPTABLE, PROFESSIONAL	UNACCEPTABLE, UNPROFESSIONAL
Phone calls/text messages	• Emergency calls only • Turn off or silence ringer • Make personal calls only on break time	• Frequent checking for calls received • Making personal calls • Have phone out and visible when working with patients • Taking pictures
Personal emails and social media	• Do not open, read, or post	• Sending and reading personal emails • Viewing social media postings
Online activities	• Work-related web-related activity	• Shopping, gaming, nonwork websites

focus should be on serving the patients in the office at all times. Many employees are fired each year for surfing or shopping on the internet for personal reasons or checking personal email. Make sure all personal business is handled outside of business hours.

Dating Co-Workers

Given the amount of time that we spend with our co-workers, it is not surprising that personal relationships can develop. Dating someone you work with can present professionalism issues. Maintaining a professional demeanor while at work becomes that much harder, especially if you are both on the same team. Other co-workers might think that there is favoritism, especially if one person is the supervisor of another. There can also be issues if the relationship ends badly, and both must continue to work together.

Self-Boundaries

When you are working in healthcare, it is important to develop a solid professional relationship with your patients. By establishing realistic self-boundaries, you can protect that relationship. It is important to keep the focus on the patient. When working with patients who are seen frequently, it is easy to start to think of them as friends. With a friend, you are likely to share personal information that is not appropriate with a patient. Patients may feel that they cannot share important health-related information because you are their friend, and it would be embarrassing to share that information.

Self-boundaries can also be thought of as professional boundaries. You need to treat patients with respect and keep the relationship professional. Be friendly to patients and always keep the focus on the patient.

CLOSING COMMENTS

Medical assisting has developed over the years into a profession that makes considerable contributions to quality patient care in ambulatory care centers. Medical assistants are uniquely trained to manage both the administrative and clinical needs of patients in physicians' offices, clinics, and outpatient facilities. One of the crucial roles of medical assistants is to act as the patient's navigator—that is, to help patients understand and comply with complex care issues. The medical assistant joins a wide range of allied health professionals as part of a healthcare team in which all members work together to best meet the needs of patients. Medical assistants can work in a variety of healthcare facilities and alongside medical specialists to care for patients. They also can act as core members of the PCMH and, along with a variety of community resources, can help provide holistic care to patients in the healthcare system. However, the medical assisting practice must align with the state and regional scope of practice laws and must meet expected standards of care. Medical assistants must always act under the direction of a physician or provider; they cannot diagnose, prescribe, or treat patients independently.

Patients expect and deserve professional behavior from those who work in medical facilities—display courtesy and respect toward patients, families, and peers. A diplomatic and tactful person always attempts to interact honestly without giving offense. By displaying these attributes, the medical assistant earns the respect of co-workers and becomes indispensable to his or her employer. Behaving in a professional manner in the medical office helps the medical assistant gain the patient's trust. Trust is one of the most important factors in preventing cases of medical liability. Treating patients with care and not subjecting them to negative behaviors keeps the patient-provider relationship strong and conducive to the health and recovery of the patient. Performing as a cooperative team member goes a long way in promoting a positive healthcare environment for the patient. Incorporating time management strategies into each day not only helps you perform tasks more efficiently but also ensures that no important tasks are left uncompleted. The entry-level medical assistant can promote professional behavior by joining one of the professional medical assistant organizations and seeking national credentialing.

Patient Coaching

Some patients have little knowledge about the healthcare industry and may need instruction and explanations about details important to their healthcare. They often call the healthcare facility with questions; therefore, medical assistants must understand the wide variety of healthcare facilities and medical resources available in the community. Become familiar with community resources to make provider-approved referrals for patients who need help from various sources. If a patient seems to have a need, speak with him or her privately and determine whether any agency or organization might help with the issues at hand. The PCMH model relies on all healthcare workers to participate in the care of patients.

Legal and Ethical Issues

Medical assistants are responsible for understanding and following the scope of practice in their communities and always meeting the expected standards of care. Not meeting these responsibilities can result in serious liability for themselves and their employers.

Remember, the medical assistant must act under the direct supervision of a physician or licensed provider. You must know the limitations placed on your practice by the state in which you live or by the facility or provider who employs you. There is nothing more important than patient safety, so always act within the guidelines of the law and according to the policies and procedures of the facility where you work. Medical assistants are multiskilled healthcare workers who can have a lasting positive effect on patient outcomes. However, never forget that you do not have the authority or education to diagnose, prescribe, or treat patients' clinical problems. Professional credentialing is becoming more important each year.

The workday should be centered around patient care, so never allow personal business to intrude on time that should be spent assisting patients and the provider. Otherwise, the patient may be left with the impression that the medical assistant or the entire staff is unprofessional, which often leads to trust issues with the individuals employed at the facility.

Patient-Centered Care

Patient-centered care involves taking care of the whole patient, not just the physical problems. As a professional medical assistant, you can be instrumental in helping the patient with coordination and integration of care, providing information and education as directed by the provider, involving the family in the patient's care, and, above all, respecting the patient's preferences.

Professional Behaviors

Much of this chapter has focused on an introduction to what it means to be a medical assistant and what you will need to learn so you can perform all the skills expected of an entry-level medical assistant. However, working with patients and providing quality care go beyond being able to perform administrative and clinical skills. Each patient must be viewed holistically. This means considering the following patient factors:

- What is the patient's physical condition, and how is it affecting his or her life?
- What is the patient's psychological state? Is it preventing the person from following treatment regimens?
- Are any communication barriers preventing the patient from understanding the diagnosis or suggested treatment?
- Is the patient's culture, age, or lifestyle preventing him or her from following the provider's orders?
- Are insurance issues or financial problems preventing the patient from following through with treatment plans?

These are just a few of the factors that can affect patient outcomes. Again, because you will be trained in both administrative and clinical duties, you will be in a unique position to understand all the factors that might affect patient care. It is your responsibility to treat all patients with respect and empathy and do whatever you can to support them throughout the healthcare experience.

SUMMARY OF SCENARIO

Carmen is a bit overwhelmed but very excited about what she has learned about the role of medical assistants in ambulatory care. She finds it hard to believe that she will become competent in all aspects of the typical medical assistant's job description, but she anticipates learning both administrative and clinical skills. She is looking forward to joining the local AAMA chapter so that she can take advantage of professional development opportunities and networking with other medical assistant professionals and students in her community. Carmen now appreciates the significance of scope of practice and meeting standards of care, and she is researching the laws affecting medical assistant practice in her state. She cannot wait until she is actually able to work with the healthcare team to meet the holistic needs of patients in the practice where she will be employed.

SUMMARY OF LEARNING OBJECTIVES

1. **Examine the typical responsibilities of a medical assistant.**
   Medical assistants are trained in both clinical and administrative skills that are applicable to ambulatory care settings, such as providers' offices, clinics, and group practices. Graduates of accredited programs are all taught a similar skill set that prepares students for an entry-level position. The actual duties will depend on the place of employment.

   Medical assistants have long been encouraged to act as patient advocates in the ambulatory care setting. That role is now described as acting as a patient navigator or care coordinator to help patients manage the complexities of their care. Given their multilevel training, medical assistants can help patients navigate through a wide variety of confusing issues.

2. **Analyze the attributes of a professional medical assistant.**
   Professional medical assistants display courteous, respectful behaviors and communicate with tact and diplomacy. They demonstrate responsible and honest behaviors and always act with integrity. Professional medical assistants view constructive criticism as a way of improving their skill level. Important assumptions are made within seconds of meeting someone based only on how the person looks. Most medical facilities require that medical assistants wear a uniform or scrubs or professional clothing that is not too tight and projects a professional, businesslike appearance. In addition, name badges should be visible, hair should be clean, longer hair should be tied back, shoes should be clean, nails should be short and without nail polish (no artificial nails), and no jewelry should be worn.

SUMMARY OF LEARNING OBJECTIVES—*continued*

It is important to recognize that diversity is more than just nationality or race. It can include age, economic status, disabilities, and so on. As professional medical assistants, we should learn as much as possible about the customs and practices of our patient population. Being informed will help us to better serve our patients.

3. **Differentiate between scope of practice and standards of care for medical assistants.**
   Scope of practice determines the range of responsibilities and practice guidelines for healthcare workers. The scope of practice for a medical assistant is what has been established by law in some states or by practice norms, institutions, or physician-employers in states without scope of practice laws. The standard of care (a legal term) sets the minimum guidelines for job performance. It defines the level and quality of patient service that healthcare workers with similar training and experience should provide in similar situations.

   Licensed healthcare professionals have a different scope of practice and expected standard of care than those expected of medical assistants. Medical assistants can never diagnose, prescribe, or treat patients. The medical assistant's actions are always done under the supervision of a provider such as a physician, nurse practitioner, or physician assistant. The medical assistant should follow the written order or established policies and procedures.
4. **Discuss professional medical assisting organizations.**
   Three professional medical assisting organizations were discussed in this chapter: the American Association of Medical Assistants (AAMA), American Medical Technologists (AMT), and the National Healthcareer Association (NHA). All three organizations offer certification and continuing education.
5. **Examine your learning preferences and learning style.**
   Learning preferences are the ways you like to learn and have proven successful in the past. Your learning style is determined by your individual method of perceiving or examining new material and the way you process it or make it your own. People are either concrete or abstract perceivers and either active or reflective processors.

   Study skills, such as memory techniques, active learning, brain tricks, effective reading methods, note-taking strategies, and mind maps, all help students to be more successful.

   Test-taking strategies include preparing adequately for the examination, controlling negative thoughts during the examination, and understanding how to deal with different types of questions.

   Critical thinking can be defined as thorough thinking because it considers all sides of the information without bias.

   Reflection is the process of thinking about or reviewing information before acting.
6. **Examine the history of medicine and its significance to the medical assisting profession.**
   The history of medicine can be traced to ancient practices as far back as 5000 BC. In 1205 BC, Moses presented rules of health to the Hebrews, thus becoming the first advocate of preventive medicine. Hippocrates, known as the father of medicine, is the most famous of the ancient Greek physicians and is best remembered for the Hippocratic oath, which has been administered to physicians for more than 2000 years. The medical assisting profession relies on previous medical discoveries to provide patients with safe care in today's healthcare environment. Table 1.3 summarizes medical pioneers and their achievements.
7. **Differentiate between various types of medical professionals.**
   Physicians and other providers (e.g., nurse practitioners and physician assistants) are portals of entry or first contacts for patients seeking medical care. Medical professionals include physicians (MDs, DOs), dentists, chiropractors, optometrists, podiatrists, pharmacists, nurse practitioners, and physician assistants. Table 1.4 presents a list of medical specialties.
8. **Summarize the various types of allied health professionals.**
   The definition of an allied health professional can vary, but it loosely refers to those who can act only under the authority of a licensed medical practitioner. Allied health professions fall into two broad categories: technicians (assistants) and therapists. Allied health professionals, including professional medical assistants, typically work as part of a healthcare team. Table 1.5 presents a list of allied health occupations, and Table 1.6 shows a list of licensed healthcare professions.
9. **Summarize the various types of healthcare facilities.**
   Healthcare facilities include different levels of hospitals, ambulatory care facilities, and a variety of other institutions that provide specialty care for patients.
10. **Examine the healthcare team models.**
    The PCMH is a concept that is transforming the organization and delivery of primary care. The healthcare team looks at patient care from a holistic approach. Improving our primary care system is the key to achieving high-quality, accessible, efficient healthcare for all Americans. The PCMH has five core functions and attributes: (1) comprehensive care, (2) patient-centered care, (3) coordinated care, (4) accessible services, and (5) evidence-based, high-quality, safe care.
11. **Explain the reasons professionalism is important in the medical field.**
    Professionalism is the characteristic of conforming to the technical or ethical standards of a profession. Professionalism is vital in the medical profession because patients expect and deserve to be treated in a professional way. When the medical assistant acts in a professional way, he or she establishes trust with the patient. Patients notice professional behavior, even when it is not directed at them specifically. They notice how others are treated in the reception room and other areas of the office. Always act in a professional manner while at work.

    Work ethics are sets of values based on the moral virtues of hard work and diligence, and they involve a whole range of activities, from individual acts to the philosophy of the entire facility.

    Each team member must be willing to cooperate and help others on the team. Through cooperation, the team is more productive.

    Medical assistants need to use time efficiently, prioritize duties, and arrange schedules to ensure that duties can be performed in a timely manner. This can be done by planning tasks that need to be done that day. Most tasks can be prioritized into three general categories: those

Continued

SUMMARY OF LEARNING OBJECTIVES—*continued*

that must be done that day, those that should be done that day, and those that could be done if time permits.

Criticism can be hard to take, but we need to realize the value of feedback. When you are working as a part of a team, it is important to understand how to resolve differences with other members. If there is an issue related to theft, confidentiality, or harassment, you may need to follow the chain of command in the healthcare facility. Everyone has a life outside the workplace, and sometimes we face challenges and difficult times that are hard to put aside. The professional medical assistant never transfers personal problems or baggage to anyone at the medical facility. The medical assistant should refuse to participate in the office rumor mill and should be cordial and friendly to everyone at work. Avoid personal phone calls and visits unless it is an absolute emergency.

Awareness of personal boundaries helps us determine the actions and behaviors we find unacceptable. Healthy self-boundaries make it possible to respect our strengths, abilities, and individuality and those of others.

THERAPEUTIC COMMUNICATION 2

SCENARIO

Christi Michelson is a newly hired medical assistant at Walden-Martin Family Medical (WMFM) Clinic. She graduated from the local community college last month. She is currently in her probationary period at WMFM Clinic. Christi has orientation for 1 month, and her probationary period will last for 3 months. Over the next 3 months, she must pass a national certification exam. At the end of 3 months, Christi will have an evaluation by her supervisor. If the evaluation is positive, she will continue in her position.

Christi is excited about her first healthcare job. In the past, she has worked as a waitress and a salesclerk. These jobs have helped her learn customer service skills, which she is now using in her current position. Christi is finding that the professionalism at WMFM Clinic is much different from her previous jobs. Christi is learning the clinic's customer service policies and procedures. She was surprised to learn that her customers include not only the patients but also her co-workers. Christi is learning new communication skills and is excited to continue learning more skills to help her provide the best patient care possible.

While studying this chapter, think about the following questions:

- What are types of nonverbal communication?
- What are styles and types of verbal communication?
- What are communication barriers, and what techniques can help overcome these barriers?
- Why do people behave the way they do?

LEARNING OBJECTIVES

1. Explain the importance of first impressions to the delivery of high-quality patient care.
2. Explain how healthcare professionals demonstrate respect when interacting with diverse populations.
3. Demonstrate appropriate responses to patients' nonverbal communication.
4. Determine how a medical assistant can communicate professionally in both written and oral forms while considering the receiver of the message.
5. Demonstrate therapeutic communication techniques when working with patients.
6. Determine strategies to overcome barriers to effective communication in healthcare.
7. Explain communication strategies to use with peers, supervisors, and providers.
8. Explain personal and professional boundaries with communication in healthcare.
9. Determine factors that impact peoples' behaviors, including needs, defense mechanisms, and coping mechanisms.

VOCABULARY

adherence The act of sticking to something.

compassion Having a deep awareness of the suffering of another and the wish to ease it.

coping mechanisms Behavioral and psychological strategies used to deal with or minimize stressful events.

defense mechanisms Unconscious mental processes that protect people from anxiety, loss, conflict, or shame.

dignity (DIG ni tee) The inherent worth or state of being worthy of respect.

diversity The differences and similarities in identity, perspective, and points of view among people.

empathy (EM pah thee) The ability to understand another's perspective, experiences, or motivations.

hierarchy (HIE er ar kee) Things arranged in order and rank.

nonverbal communication A type of communication that occurs through body language and expressive behaviors rather than with verbal or written words.

patient portal A secure online website that gives patients 24-hour access to personal health information using a username and password.

poised (poizd) Having a composed and self-assured manner; feeling confident, being patient, and maintaining good posture (standing and sitting up straight).

rapport (ra PORE) A relationship of harmony and accord between the patient and the healthcare professional.

respect To show consideration or appreciation for another person; to feel or show deferential regard for.

INTRODUCTION

Communication is the exchange of information, feelings, and thoughts between two or more people using spoken words or other methods. What we say and how we say something directly affects how the other person perceives the message. We need to communicate effectively or in a manner that is clear, concise, and easy to understand. This helps the other person to understand the message.

Therapeutic communication is a process of communicating with patients and family members in healthcare. Therapeutic communication requires healthcare professionals to have strong communication skills. It also requires an understanding of how people communicate, the importance of the first impressions, the role of diversity in communication, and what impacts behavior. This chapter provides the foundation for therapeutic communication, which will help as you develop and refine your communication skills.

FIRST IMPRESSIONS AND HIGH-QUALITY PATIENT CARE

Delivering quality patient care is the primary objective of the professional medical assistant. A patient's first impressions set the tone for the person's perceptions of the healthcare experience. The first step of delivering high-quality patient care starts with ensuring the patient's first impressions are positive.

First Impressions

The opinions formed in the early moments of meeting someone remain in our thoughts long after the first words that were spoken. The first impression involves much more than just physical appearance or dress. It includes attitude, **compassion**, and therapeutic communication skills that clearly help the patient and family members realize that the medical assistant is interested in who they are and what they need (Figure 2.1).

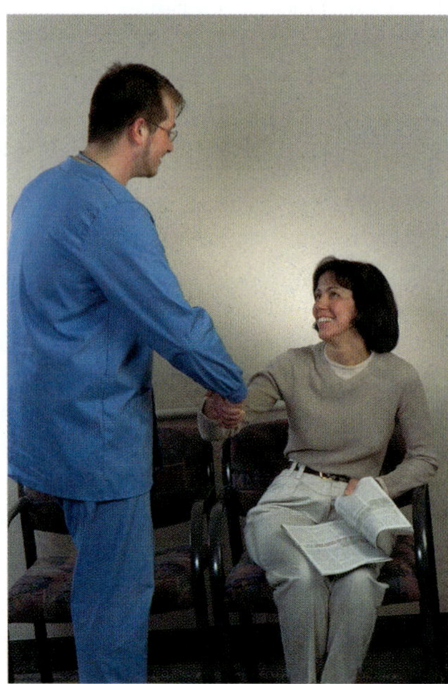

FIGURE 2.1 First impressions are critical in gaining the patient's trust.

Creating Positive Interactions with Patients

Delivering quality patient care is the primary objective of the professional medical assistant. Patients are the reason the facility exists. Each patient should be welcomed warmly by name and with a polite greeting. The medical assistant should smile and introduce himself or herself to the patient. A smile should show not only on the face but in the voice and the eyes. This small effort helps put the patient at ease in the healthcare environment.

To provide high-quality patient care, we must communicate effectively with the patient and provide a warm, caring environment. Positive reactions and interactions with the patient are vital. Because medical care by nature is extremely personal, a medical assistant must always remember that each patient is an individual with certain anxieties. Their anxieties often cause people to act and react in different ways; therefore, effective verbal and **nonverbal communication** with each patient are absolutely essential.

Healthcare professionals accept the responsibility of developing helping relationships with their patients. The interpersonal nature of the patient–medical assistant relationship carries with it a certain amount of responsibility to forget one's self-interest and focus on the patient's needs. Medical assistants can elicit either a positive or a negative response to patient care simply by the way they interact with patients. A medical assistant is usually the first person with whom the patient communicates; therefore, the medical assistant plays a vital role in initiating therapeutic patient interactions.

CRITICAL THINKING APPLICATION **2.1**

Think about an experience during which you had a favorable or unfavorable first impression of an agency. How did the first impression affect your view of that agency? Did your impression change over time? If so, how and why?

RESPECTING DIVERSE POPULATIONS

Chapter 1 discussed the importance of professionalism and respecting **diversity**. Not only does a medical assistant need to **respect** diversity, but it is also important to understand how it impacts the communication process. Your patients and co-workers will come from backgrounds that are different from your own. Their traditions, customs, beliefs, and values impact how they communicate with others. Knowing more about the diversity around you will help you become a better healthcare professional.

Types of Diversity and Influences on Patient Care

There are five types of diversity that a medical assistant should be aware of:

- *Nationality* pertains to the country where the person was born and holds citizenship. For example: John was born in Mexico, moved to the United States, and became a US citizen. Nationality can impact patient care. Some non-US citizens cannot purchase health insurance in the United States. The cost of healthcare may limit their ability to seek healthcare.
- *Race* relates to a group of people who have the same physical characteristics, such as skin color. For example, even though John was born in Mexico, his mother is Mongolian, and his father is Caucasian. John's race would be Mongolian and Caucasian.

Racism has been found to impact mental and physical health. It can make it more difficult for people to access healthcare and to receive quality healthcare.

- *Culture* includes the general customs, norms, values, and beliefs held by a group of people. For example, John has adapted to the US culture. Though he grew up in a large family (six children), he is comfortable with having two or three children. John values honesty, timeliness, punctuality, and motivation. Culture influences health beliefs, including what causes illness and how conditions are managed and treated. Patient care can be impacted if healthcare professionals assume patients will conform to the mainstream values and the patient's health beliefs are not considered.
- *Ethnicity* relates to a common ancestry, culture, religion, traditions, nationality, and language shared by a group of people. For example, John states he is Mexican. Growing up, he learned his family's Mexican traditions, which he plans to share with his children someday. He values his family and respects his grandparents and parents. The impact of ethnicity on patient care is similar to culture. Health beliefs of the patient can differ from the assumptions of the healthcare professional. This can lead to issues with patient care, including a lack of **adherence** with the treatment recommended by the provider.
- *Social factors* are all the ways a person is different from others (e.g., lifestyle, religion, tastes, and preferences). For example, John does not drink alcohol or smoke. He exercises in the gym each day. He likes to visit art museums and learn about history. Lifestyle choices, such as a lack of exercise, smoking, drinking alcohol, and doing drugs can impact a person's health. A person's lifestyle choices might influence clinical decisions and treatments for conditions. For instance, some obese patients have been denied knee replacement surgery until they lost weight.

CRITICAL THINKING APPLICATION 2.2

What types of diversity do you have in your circle of family, friends, and acquaintances?

Individual Diversity

Besides these five types, we also have individual diversity. Factors that relate to individual diversity include language, age, religion, economic status, gender, and appearance. Many times, certain stereotypes, biases, and beliefs are attached to these factors (Table 2.1). Healthcare professionals need to identify personal biases, stereotypes, and beliefs that will prevent effective communication with patients, family, and co-workers. Taking steps to overcome these negative beliefs will help healthcare professionals show respect for and honor the **dignity** of others.

Demonstrating Respect

Healthcare professionals need to show respect to others. This can be achieved with a smile, a pleasant greeting, and eye contact if appropriate when first meeting the person. During the interaction, it is important to be courteous, sincere, polite, welcoming, and professional. Using a calm tone of voice, appropriate eye contact, and proper grammar without slang or generational terms also shows respect.

Being respectful also means maintaining the person's dignity or, in other words, treating others as we would want to be treated. People expect to be treated as individuals who matter. By treating others as though they matter, you are showing them the respect they deserve.

NONVERBAL COMMUNICATION

As mentioned in the opening section, communication occurs by what we say and how we say it. These two forms of communication—verbal and nonverbal—affect how the other person perceives the message.

TABLE 2.1 Individual Diversity Factors

FACTOR	DISCUSSION
Language	Some people are fluent in more than one language. For others, English is not their primary language. It is important to be sensitive to and respectful of language differences. Using resources (e.g., translated materials, an interpreter) can also show respect to patients.
Age	There are many stereotypes about age. For instance, the older generation may not be college educated but may have "street smarts." The younger generation may be more comfortable with computers and digital devices. It is important not to stereotype a person because of age. Ask, never assume anything.
Religion	A wide range of belief systems can be observed in the United States. There are also different degrees of religious observations in the workplace. Some patients may refuse certain medical treatments based on their religion. Be sensitive to patients who refuse medical care or want to involve their shaman or healer in their care.
Economic status	Our patients may be from a variety of economic backgrounds. Some patients may be very wealthy and can afford to pay for healthcare without insurance. Other patients may rely on food banks and charities to get by. Be sensitive and respectful if your patient does not have the financial means to pay for healthcare services. Help the patient seek resources for medications, transportation, and food.
Gender	There are many stereotypes attributed to gender. We need to make sure we do not stereotype our patients and peers. Some of our patients may identify as a gender other than their birth sex. We need to respect their choices and be sensitive to any issues that arise.
Appearance	Our patients' appearances can greatly vary. If you work in a farming community, patients may come to appointments in their work clothes and smell of the barn. With the popularity of piercings, tattoos, and hair dye, we can see a variety of differences in our patients. We need to move beyond the patient's appearance and provide exceptional patient care.

TABLE 2.2 Positive and Negative Nonverbal Behaviors

NONVERBAL BEHAVIORS	POSITIVE AND OPEN	NEGATIVE AND CLOSED (COMMON INTERPRETATIONS)
Position	Be at the level of the other person, angled toward the other person	Being at a higher level (looking down on the person); leaning backward (disinterest); direct face to face (confrontational, intimate)
Arms, shoulders, and hands	Arms at the sides, shoulders relaxed	Arms are crossed in front of the body (discomfort, defensive, disagree); hands behind back (secretive, mistrustful); clenched fists (anger, aggressive); pointing at a person (accusatory); hands on hips (ready for aggressive activity); hands in the pockets (insecurity and lack of confidence)
Posture	**Poised**	Poor or slumped posture (poor self-worth, lack of confidence, unwillingness, lack of interest, less knowledgeable, unreliable); stiff, immobile (uncomfortable)
Facial expression	Smile	Rolling eyes, yawning (boredom); frowning (sadness, disagree, anger)
Gestures	Small gestures	Overuse of hands (nervousness, excitement)
Touch	Light touch on hand, appropriate touch	Inappropriate touching or hugging (makes the person feel uncomfortable or violated)
Eye contact	Movement of eyes, blinking	Staring at the person (makes it awkward); avoiding eye contact (low self-esteem, low confidence, and dishonesty)
Eyebrows	Raised eyebrows indicate surprise and openness	Lowered eyebrows (displeasure), one raised eyebrow (cynicism or doubtful)
Mannerisms	Focus on the person, nod when appropriate to acknowledge the patient	Fidgeting (nervous, impatient); looking at a watch, phone, or clock (bored, anxious, impatient)
Appearance choices	Professional appearance, well groomed, neat, and clean appearance	Unprofessional appearance; messy hair; dirty, ripped, wrinkled uniform

Experts agree that nonverbal communication greatly exceeds verbal communication. In other words, we communicate more by our body language and expressive behaviors than through our words.

Think of a time when you were talking with a person, and that person did something that left a greater impression on you than the verbal message did. Nonverbal communication is powerful. It is important that the verbal message matches the perceived nonverbal message.

With therapeutic communication, we use nonverbal communication to show respect, acceptance, and understanding. We want to appear positive and open with others. We can do this through our nonverbal communication, which involves nonverbal behaviors, nonverbal communication delivery factors, cultural differences, and spatial distance. The following sections discuss these factors along with reading others' nonverbal communication.

Nonverbal Behavior

Our nonverbal behaviors can be judged by others as positive and open or negative and closed. The professional expectation is that we appear positive and open to others. When our behaviors are judged as negative and closed, others can interpret them in ways we may not intend. Table 2.2 discusses positive and open behaviors that the medical assistant should use. It also describes common interpretations of negative and closed behavior. The next section discusses the importance of nonverbal communication while wearing a mask.

Nonverbal Communication When Wearing a Mask

A genuine smile can make others smile. Research has shown that when people are shown a smile and told to frown, they smile instead. Many times, our first message to a person is a smile. A smile is a greeting and a way to acknowledge another person. We smile to be polite and to appear approachable.

When we need to wear a mask, our smiles are covered. With our facial expressions limited, our eyes and body language must deliver the message that our smile would give. We should still smile as we also ensure that our nonverbal behaviors are positive and open.

CRITICAL THINKING APPLICATION 2.3

While working at the reception desk, Christi needs to demonstrate positive and open nonverbal behaviors. Describe the positive and open nonverbal behaviors she should be demonstrating.

Nonverbal Communication Delivery Factors

Communication delivery factors relate to how we deliver our verbal message. For instance, do we speak fast, using a high-pitched, loud voice as we deliver our verbal message? The communication delivery factors used help create the context of the message. Table 2.3 provides a list of delivery factors and the professional expectations for which medical assistants should strive.

TABLE 2.3 Nonverbal Communication Delivery Factors

NONVERBAL DELIVERY FACTORS	DEFINITION	PROFESSIONAL EXPECTATIONS
Rate	Refers to the speed at which the speaker talks	Use a moderate rate. If the rate is too fast, the message may be missed. If the rate is too slow, it may be perceived as more negative by the receiver.
Clarity	Refers to the quality of the voice	Use a clear voice when talking with others. Muffled, mumbling, or unclear speech can create inaccuracies with the message.
Volume	Refers to the loudness of the speaker's voice	Use a moderate volume. If too loud, it may be perceived as yelling, and if too soft, the message may be missed. In healthcare, we need to keep information confidential. So, using a loud voice can violate the patient's privacy.
Pitch	Refers to the highness and lowness of the voice	Using a varying pitch, or inflections, helps a person to emphasize important points. It is important to have a rhythm in your voice to help the receiver understand what is important.
Tone	Refers to the emotion in the voice	Use an accepting or a neutral tone in healthcare. An angry tone can cause the receiver to misinterpret the message or to become angry.
Pauses	Refers to a period of not talking	Using pauses helps the receiver absorb the message. Limit verbalized pauses (e.g., "ah," "um," and "er").
Intonation	Refers to the melodic pattern or the pitch variation	With statements, we usually use a medium intonation and finish the sentence on a lower pitch. Finishing the statement on a higher pitch usually indicates a question. Using correct intonation will help the correct message to be received.
Vocabulary	Refers to the word choice used	Using precise words helps the message to be correctly received. Incorrect use of words may create a negative impression of the speaker. It is important to use words that the receiver understands. If medical terminology, slang, or generational terms are used, the message may not be understood.
Grammatical structure	Refers to the sentence structure	Using incorrect grammatical sentence structure can create a negative impression of the speaker.
Pronunciation	Refers to how the word is said	Using the correct pronunciation will help ensure the correct message will be received. Incorrect pronunciation of a word (e.g., medication name) may lead to inaccuracies with the message.

Procedures 2.1 through 2.4, at the end of the chapter, provide examples of role-playing to practice responding to nonverbal communication with patients.

Cultural Differences

The meaning of nonverbal behaviors can greatly vary among cultural groups. What is acceptable to one group may be considered offensive to others. As you work with patients from diverse groups, make sure to learn about cultural differences in communication. It will reduce the likelihood of offending the other person. It also will help make the patient's experience a positive one. Here are some examples of cultural differences in nonverbal behaviors:

- Eye Contact
  - *Hispanics, Asians, Native Americans, and Middle Easterners:* Eye contact is considered rude and offensive.
  - *Females in many cultures*: May avoid eye contact with males, so it is not perceived as a sign of sexual interest.
- Touch
  - *Asians and Middle Easterners:* The head is a sacred part of the body; it is considered offensive to pat the head.
  - *Middle Easterners:* The left hand is reserved for bodily hygiene; it is inappropriate to use that hand to touch others or transfer objects.
  - *Muslims:* Consider it inappropriate to touch a person of the opposite sex.
  - *Latin Americans and Eastern Europeans:* Very comfortable with touching others, even new acquaintances.
- Gestures
  - *Many cultures*: Using the "come here" finger/hand gesture is used with dogs and considered offensive. Pointing with one finger is considered very rude.
  - *Asians and Indians*: Use the whole hand to point at something or someone.
  - *Venezuelans*: Use their lips to point; finger-pointing is impolite.
- Winking
  - *Latin Americans:* Consider winking a romantic or a sexual invitation.
  - *Nigerians:* Wink at children to indicate they should leave the room.
  - *Chinese:* Consider winking rude.

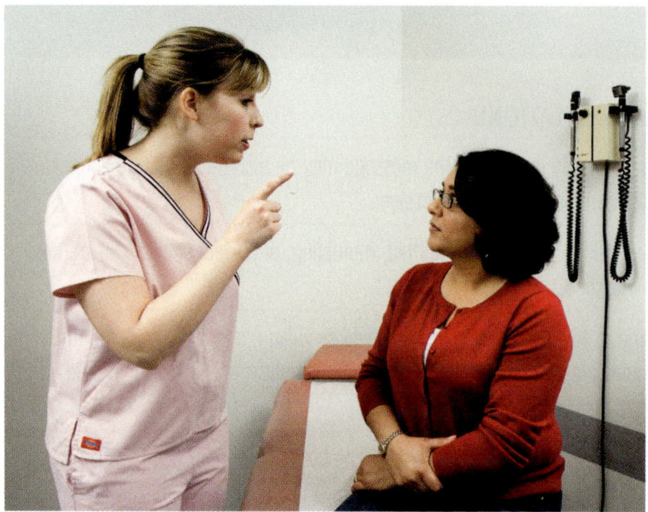

FIGURE 2.2 Pointing often is an accusatory gesture and causes discomfort.

- Posture
  - *Many cultures:* Consider poor posture disrespectful.
- Personal space
  - *Latin Americans and Middle Easterners:* Stand quite close to those they do not know.
  - *Muslim males (even providers):* Will not position themselves too close to females.

CRITICAL THINKING APPLICATION 2.4

What cultural differences have you noticed in your family, friends, and acquaintances?

Respecting Cultural Differences

If you are interacting with a person from another cultural group and you are unfamiliar with it, try following these tips:

- Follow the other person's lead in terms of nonverbal behaviors and personal space.
- Use gestures cautiously. Do not point with one finger (Figure 2.2).
- Refrain from touching a child's head.
- Remember that facial expressions can be misinterpreted (e.g., grimacing with pain may not be acceptable in some cultures, whereas other cultures encourage it).
- Lack of eye contact may be related to nervousness or the culture. It is not due to fear or dishonesty.

CRITICAL THINKING APPLICATION 2.5

Christi had heard that people from the Hmong and Vietnamese cultures do not like others commenting on their children. They fear the words might be overheard by a spirit who might try to harm the children. Christi mentions this to a co-worker. The co-worker does not believe in this. Do they need to worry about this belief when working with patients from the Hmong and Vietnamese cultures? Explain your answer.

Spatial Distance in Healthcare

Spatial distance, or the space between one person and another, is also considered to be part of nonverbal communication. The distance between ourselves and another person can vary based on our familiarity with that person. There are different types of spaces:

- *Intimate space* or *personal space* (distance of 0 to 1.5 feet): In our personal lives, we allow close family and friends into this space. In healthcare, medical assistants are in the patients' personal space for procedures such as electrocardiograms, wound care, and obtaining vital signs.
- *Casual personal space* (distance of 1.5 feet to 4 feet): In our personal lives, this space is used for conversations with friends. In healthcare, the medical assistant uses this space when talking with the patient. This may include taking a medical history or coaching a patient on home care.
- *Social-business space* (distance of 4 to 12 feet): In our personal lives, this is the acceptable space for business transactions and socializing with acquaintances. In healthcare, the medical assistant uses this space when completing business tasks, such as answering billing questions and checking in a patient at the reception desk.
- *Public space* (a distance greater than 12 feet): In our personal lives, this space is used for activities in public. In healthcare, this is the acceptable space for group events (Figure 2.3).

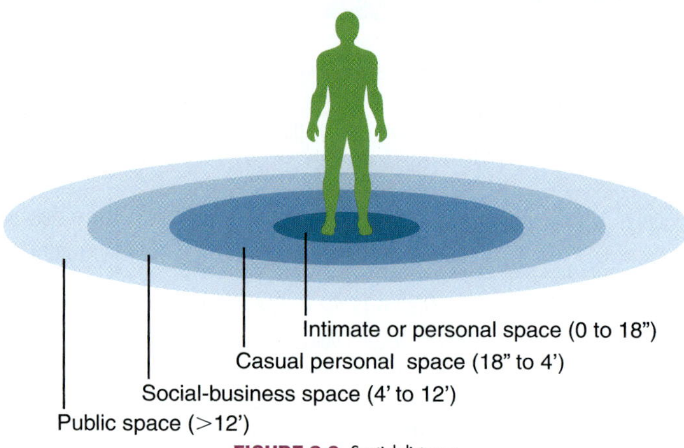

FIGURE 2.3 Spatial distance.

Respecting Spatial Distance

Research has shown that some cultural groups have different acceptable casual personal space distances. For instance, Middle Eastern cultures have about 1 foot, whereas North American and Western European cultures have about 1.5 feet. The Japanese culture has about 3 feet. You may have already experienced this when you were talking with friends. Some friends get closer to you than others. When a person is closer to us than we feel is acceptable for our culture, we may become uncomfortable.

We all have a personal space, or "bubble," around us. We may be uncomfortable and on guard, if someone we do not know well gets into our personal space. We may take a step back or move back in a chair to increase the space between the other person and us. If someone is communicating from too far away, we may also feel uncomfortable.

It is important to realize that as healthcare professionals, we move into the personal or intimate space of patients many times while providing care. We need to respect this space. We need to be aware of our grooming, appearance, and habits. When working with others, we need to watch for clues regarding the person's comfort level with distance. A person who needs more space may move backward. Leaning, shifting, or moving forward shows the person wants to reduce the distance. It is important to recognize this nonverbal communication.

CRITICAL THINKING APPLICATION **2.6**

Think about the diverse cultures in your area. What differences have you observed in the nonverbal communication among these groups?

Reading Others' Nonverbal Communication

Besides using nonverbal communication to convey acceptance and respect, we also read others' nonverbal communication. This provides us feedback on what is being said and how the person feels. The following are examples of how nonverbal behaviors are interpreted:

- *Self-confident*: The person appears confident and self-assured, has good posture, and makes appropriate eye contact.
- *Insecure*: The person is quiet, courteous, and has good listening skills but tends to focus more on others than on oneself.
- *Arrogant*: The person has increased personal space, appears to bore easily, and is a poor listener.
- *Embarrassed*: The person has a nervous giggle and tends to avoid eye contact with others.
- *Fearful*: The person has wide-open eyes, looks around, grasps their hands, and has a rigid posture.
- *Resentful*: The person hunches the shoulders, crosses the arms, and mutters or whispers.

VERBAL COMMUNICATION

Verbal communication can be defined as words used either orally or in written form. Medical assistants use verbal communication in person, on the telephone, and with virtual visit software. When we communicate with another person, we have a message to share. We hope the other person interprets the message as we intend.

The *communication cycle* is a way to describe the sender-receiver process. A breakdown of any part of the cycle can lead to a message being misunderstood. The communication cycle proceeds as follows:

1. *Sender creates the MESSAGE:* The person with a message is called the sender. The sender must organize their thoughts and communicate a clear, concise, easy-to-understand message.
2. *Receiver DECODES the message:* The person getting the message is the receiver. This person must decode or translate the message based on personal factors and subjective perceptions. If the message was correctly translated within the context of the message sent, then it matches the message the sender sent. If the message was incorrectly translated, then the receiver develops a different perception of the message than what the sender intended.
3. *Receiver creates FEEDBACK*: The receiver then provides feedback based on the perceived message.
4. *Sender DECODES feedback:* The sender gets the feedback message. Again, the feedback must be decoded correctly for the communication to be accurate (Figure 2.4).

As indicated in Figure 2.4, the verbal communication cycle exists with written and oral messages. We will examine both types of verbal communication.

Written Communication

Written communication is a type of verbal communication in which we create written messages for the receiver. Written communication includes the following types:

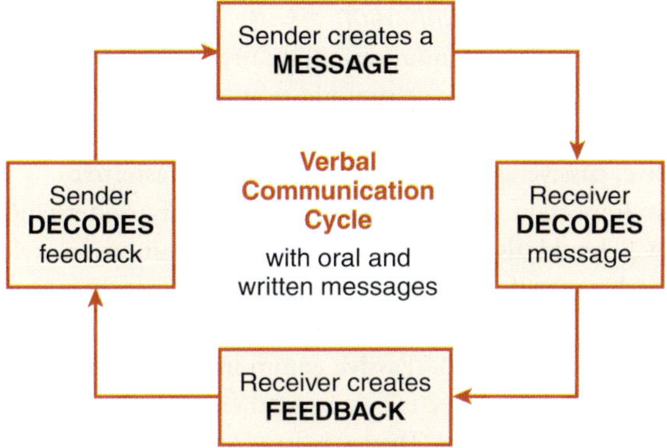

FIGURE 2.4 Verbal communication cycle.

- Written messages (e.g., written phone messages and texts)
- Letters and emails
- Online information and media (e.g., informational flyers)

It is important that we consider how we state our written message. We want the receiver to get the message we intended to send. Chapter 7 provides additional information on composing professional letters and emails.

CRITICAL THINKING APPLICATION **2.7**

Think of an email you received that had a favorable or less than favorable tone to it. Describe features of the email that gave you that impression.

Composing Written Communication

When composing all forms of written communication, the medical assistant should follow these strategies:

- Draft the message, and then read what you have written. Make sure the message is clear, concise, easy to understand, and provides the message you intended.
- Check the grammar, spelling, capitalization, punctuation, and sentence structure.
- Make sure to address the message to the correct receiver.

The use of emails has increased greatly over the years with the use of the **patient portal**. Most patient portals allow patients to send emails to the medical assistant and provider. Usually, ambulatory care facilities will have the medical assistant review the emails. After communicating with the provider regarding the patient's concerns, the medical assistant sends a return email to the patient. It is important for medical assistants to compose professional emails that can communicate their messages to the patients. Use the following strategies when composing professional emails:

- Add a few meaningful words in the subject line.
- Start with a courteous greeting.
- Write out all words. Do not use slang and use acronyms only when necessary.
- Write in complete sentences. Capitalize the first letter of the first word and end the statement with the correct punctuation.
- Do not use all capital letters. It is viewed as shouting at the receiver.

Oral Communication

Oral communication is a type of verbal communication in which we talk with others and listen to others. In the ambulatory care environment, oral communication occurs in person, over the phone, and using remote devices (e.g., webcams).

Styles of Oral Communication

Besides the types of communication, we need to discuss the styles of communication. How we communicate affects our interactions with other people. There are five main styles of communication: passive, aggressive, passive-aggressive, manipulative, and assertive.

It is important that healthcare professionals understand each type. We should also evaluate our own communication style. You should ask yourself, what style do I use? Identifying how you communicate is an important part of your professional journey.

Passive Communication. Passive communicators avoid expressing feelings or opinions. They fail to assert themselves and allow others to infringe on their rights. They may have a "victim mentality." They may feel depressed, resentful, or anxious because life seems out of their control.

Passive communicators may use these nonverbal communication behaviors:

- Speaking in a soft voice with their head down and no eye contact
- Fidgeting and hesitating
- Being self-conscious and belittling their contribution

Others may feel exasperated and frustrated with passive communicators. They may also feel that they can take advantage of the person.

When dealing with passive communicators, be assertive. Use a firm approach. Medical assistants must also ensure they take the time to reassure the person and welcome that person's suggestions and contributions.

Aggressive Communication. Aggressive communicators try to dominate others. They have low frustration tolerance, and they criticize and attack others. Aggressive communicators have poor listening skills and use "you" statements. This can cause them to be alienated from or feared by others.

Aggressive communicators may use these nonverbal communication behaviors:

- Speaking in a low voice
- Using big, sharp, and fast gestures
- Glaring and frowning
- Invading others' personal space intentionally

Others may feel hurt, fearful, afraid, humiliated, and resentful of aggressive communicators. They may lose respect for the person.

When dealing with aggressive communicators, never become aggressive and always remain calm. Do not take the person's aggression personally. Attempt to see the other's point of view, which will help you communicate yours.

Passive-Aggressive Communication. Passive-aggressive communicators deny problems. They do not confront problems or people. Passive-aggressive communicators appear to be cooperative but plan subtle sabotage or disruptions. They may become alienated from others and feel powerless.

Passive-aggressive communicators may use these nonverbal communication behaviors:

- Speaking in a sugary sweet voice
- Looking sweet and innocent
- Moving into others' personal space and touching others to pretend to be warm and friendly

Others may feel confused, angry, and hurt by the "two-faced" personality of the person.

When dealing with passive-aggressive communicators, try to refrain from drawing negative conclusions immediately. Medical assistants can use various ways to handle this approach based on the situation. Some approaches include using humor and trying to have a positive discussion.

Manipulative Communication. Manipulative communicators are cunning and try to control others. They use others to get what they want. Manipulative communicators create situations in which others feel sorry for them or guilty.

Manipulative communicators may use these nonverbal communication behaviors:

- Speaking in a high-pitched voice
- Being demeaning or condescending when talking with others

Others may feel angry, resentful, guilty, and frustrated with being manipulated.

When dealing with manipulative communicators, avoid being manipulated. Respectfully maintain your position.

Assertive Communication. Assertive communicators clearly state their needs and wants. They use "I" statements and listen without interrupting. They are relaxed, use appropriate eye contact, feel connected with others, and stand up for their rights. Assertive communicators feel in control of their lives and are mature enough to address issues.

Assertive communicators may use these nonverbal communication behaviors:

- Speaking using a medium pitch, speed, and volume of voice
- Having good eye contact (when appropriate)
- Using positive and open nonverbal behaviors
- Being respectful of others

Others feel that they can trust the individual.

When dealing with assertive communicators, know the person can handle criticism and accept compliments. A healthcare professional needs to communicate in an assertive manner. This is a healthy form of communication. It leads to better team dynamics.

CRITICAL THINKING APPLICATION **2.8**

Of the five communication styles, which one should Christi use at work? Explain your answer.

THERAPEUTIC COMMUNICATION

As mentioned before, therapeutic communication is a process of communicating with patients and family members in healthcare. It is an interactive relationship that conveys acceptance and respect without judgment or blame. It encourages healthcare professionals to build **rapport** with patients. When that bond develops and grows, patients are more comfortable with expressing their feelings, ideas, and concerns. Thus, therapeutic communication techniques are helpful in building a relationship with the patient. Active listening and other therapeutic communication techniques will be described in the following sections.

Active Listening

Active listening is the most important therapeutic communication technique. This skill takes time to master. Active listening means we fully concentrate on what is being said and how it is said. This is different from passively hearing what the speaker is saying and being distracted by our own thoughts.

When a person is actively listening, the speaker can easily see it. The listener shows interest through verbal messages, such as "yes." The listener also shows interest through nonverbal messages. As discussed earlier, nonverbal messages include eye contact, nodding your head, body position, touch, and facial expressions. Characteristics of a good listener include the following:

- Remaining nonjudgmental and neutral
- Refraining from interrupting with a comment or question
- Allowing for periods of silence
- Smiling and nodding your head to show you are listening to the message
- Using appropriate eye contact, so the speaker is not intimidated
- Leaning slightly forward or sideways toward the speaker
- Avoiding distractions (e.g., fidgeting, looking at the clock, doodling)

Showing interest at this level will encourage the speaker to be more at ease. Communication between the two people will be more open, honest, and clear.

Nontherapeutic Techniques

The following are examples of nontherapeutic techniques that must be avoided when communicating with patients:

- Overloading the patient with questions. Allow patients to answer a question before asking another question.
- Judging the patient's words or actions.
- Being unresponsive to the patient's cues or failing to give feedback. Make sure to respond to a patient who is speaking with you. Never turn your back and walk away when a patient is talking to you.
- Making false reassurance and promises, such as "The provider will make you better" or "It's going to be okay." Such statements can give the patient false hope and, in some cases, it could cause legal issues.
- Not focusing on the patient.
- Giving advice, such as "If I were you…" or "I would do…" Giving advice regarding treatments can also cause legal issues in some cases.
- Laughing nervously or at inappropriate times.
- Arguing with the patient or family members.

Closed and Open-Ended Questions

When you gather information from a patient, it is helpful to use a combination of closed and open-ended questions or statements. Closed (also called *direct*) questions ask for specific information. In many cases, this form of questioning limits the patient's answer to one or two words, including yes and no. Use this form of question when you need confirmation of specific facts, such as when asking about demographic information. Closed questions include the following examples:

- "What is the name of your insurance carrier?"
- "What is your birth date?"
- "Do you want your prescription sent to the clinic pharmacy?"

An open-ended question or statement asks for general information or states the topic to be discussed, but only in general terms. Use this communication tool to begin a conversation with a patient, to introduce a new section of questions, or whenever the person introduces a new topic. It is a very effective method of gathering more details from the patient about her or his problem. Open-ended questions include the following examples:

- "What is the reason for your appointment with Dr. Walden?"
- "How have you been getting along?"
- "You mentioned having problems with your insurance. Can you tell me more about that?"

This type of question or statement encourages patients to respond in a manner they find comfortable. It allows patients to express themselves fully and provide comprehensive information about their chief complaints.

CRITICAL THINKING APPLICATION 2.9

Christi is rooming Sam Jones, who has had a cough. List three open-ended and three closed questions she can ask Sam to gather more information about the cough and the current illness.

Other Therapeutic Communication Techniques

When you are working with patients and family members, several therapeutic communication techniques can be used. We need to make sure patients know we are listening. We also need to check that we understand the message correctly. Assuming what someone means or feels can lead to misunderstanding. Therapeutic communication techniques are detailed in Table 2.4.

Procedures 2.1 through 2.4, at the end of the chapter, provide examples of role-playing to practice communicating with patients.

BARRIERS TO EFFECTIVE COMMUNICATION

Effective communication is critical for compassionate, quality patient care. Medical assistants must understand barriers that prevent patients from understanding communication or communicating clearly with others. Taking steps to overcome these barriers will promote effective communication. Table 2.5 discusses common barriers and ways to overcome barriers. The following sections will provide additional information on communication barriers related to speech disorders, anger, age, and disease status.

Wearing a Mask

Wearing masks can make communication more challenging for people with speech or hearing impairments. Masks can muffle sounds, prevent lipreading, and cover many facial expressions. When wearing a mask in the healthcare setting, it is important to do the following:

- Make sure to face the person with whom you are speaking. Make sure nothing is blocking your view.
- Speak a little louder and a little more slowly.
- Make sure your verbal message matches your body language.
- Ask if the person understood you. If the person is struggling to understand you, write down the information or say the information in a different way.
- Know what the facility's policy is for working with people who lip-read. Are you able to remove your mask when you communicate with the person?

TABLE 2.4 Therapeutic Communication Techniques

TECHNIQUES	DEFINITION	FEEDBACK TO SPEAKER
Clarification	Allows the listener to get additional information by explaining a specific statement or topic.	Use statements such as "Can you clarify..." and "Do you mean..."
Exploring	Allows the listener to get additional information about a certain topic.	Use a phrase such as "Tell me more about..."
General leads	Allows the listener to get additional information and prompts the speaker.	Use a phrase such as "You were saying..."
Neutral	Encourages the speaker to continue and conveys you are interested and listening to the message.	Use phrases such as "Uh huh," "I see," and "That is very interesting."
Reflection	Putting words to the person's emotional reaction, which acknowledges the person's feelings. Also helps to check what the person is feeling instead of just assuming. Shows **empathy** and helps build **rapport.**	Reflect what you think was said. For example, "It sounds like you are feeling scared..." or "I understand you are having trouble with..." or "You feel that..."
Restating or paraphrasing	Rewording or rephrasing a statement to check the meaning and interpretation. Also shows you are listening and understanding the speaker.	Do not repeat the person's exact words. Use phrases such as "What I'm hearing is..." or "It sounds like you are saying..." Refrain from using "I know what you mean."
Silence	Allows time to gather thoughts and answer questions.	Can be uncomfortable to some people. Allows time to think about what was said.
Summarizing	Allows the listener to recap and review what was said.	Using a statement such as "If I understand how you feel about this situation..."

TABLE 2.5 Barriers to Communication and Ways to Overcome Barriers

TYPE OF BARRIER	PATIENT BARRIERS	WAYS TO OVERCOME BARRIERS
Environmental distractions	Noise, lack of privacy, temperature	Provide privacy for patients. Talk with patients in a quiet room with the door closed. Make sure the room temperature is comfortable.
Internal distractions	Hunger, pain, anger, tiredness	Help make the patient comfortable. Provide food and drink if available. Administer pain medications as ordered.
Visually impairment	Unable to see written communication	Use audio recordings, screen magnifiers, large-print materials, and screen reader software.
Hearing impairment	Unable to hear verbal communication	Use print materials and written instructions. Use videos with captions. Have text telephones (TTYs) available. Use a sign language interpreter.
Intellectual disability	Unable to understand what is being said; may be functioning at a lower age level	Use "functioning age"—appropriate language and materials. Provide information also to the guardian/caregiver.
Illiterate	Unable to read or write	Use pictures and models. Draw pictures and use simple language.
Non-English speaking	English is not the patient's primary language; lack of understanding of medical terminology	Use interpreters and translated materials. Limit medical terminology and define medical terms that must be used. Use culturally appropriate materials and visuals (pictures, graphs, and models).
Emotional distractions (angry, distraught, anxious)	Fear and anxiety related to being judged by the healthcare professional; inability to explain personal feelings; angry or distraught patients may not hear what is said or may not be able to communicate effectively	Provide a warm, caring environment. Make sure your body language (nonverbal behaviors) is consistent with having an open, caring manner. Gain the person's trust. Keep your voice at a normal level; raising your voice can increase the person's anger.

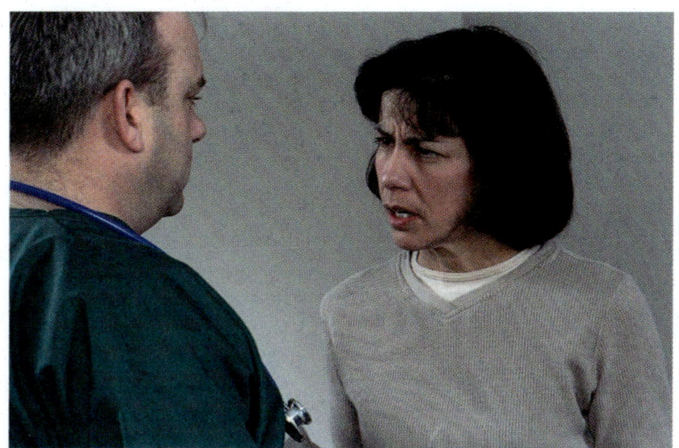

FIGURE 2.5 Remain calm, even if a patient becomes verbally aggressive. Attempt to calm the person by listening and expressing empathy whenever possible.

Speech Disorders

Speech disorders can be caused by damage to the vocal cords, brain, tongue, and mouth. Conditions that can cause speech disorders include cancer (oral, laryngeal), amyotrophic lateral sclerosis (ALS), stroke, dementia, Huntington disease, attention deficit hyperactivity disorder (ADHD), autism, and traumatic brain injury.

Common speech disorders include the following:

- *Aphasia:* Being unable to understand what is being said or to use the right words to express thoughts
- *Apraxia of speech*: Difficulty coordinating mouth movements for speech
- *Dysarthria*: Slurred speech
- *Cognitive-communication disorder*: Includes issues such as memory, attention, organization, processing speed, and problem-solving

Depending on the speech disorder, the medical assistant may need to speak more slowly. In all cases, it is important to give the patient extra time to answer. Do not pressure the patient or overload the patient with questions.

Anger

As discussed in Table 2.5, anger is a barrier to communication. Medical assistants can encounter angry patients, family members, or co-workers (Figure 2.5). It is critical to know how to handle and defuse the situation. It is important for the person to feel heard and for the medical assistant to remain safe and follow through on any promises made.

If the angry person is in a public area and the medical assistant feels safe, the person should be invited to a more private location. It is important to allow the person to talk out their anger. The medical assistant should present a calm attitude, speak in a low tone of voice, and take notes if needed. The medical assistant should demonstrate **empathy** by using active listening skills and therapeutic communication techniques. If the medical assistant responds in anger or becomes argumentative, the situation will intensify, and the person's anger may increase.

During the interaction with the angry person, the medical assistant must remain safe. There should be a policy in place for dealing with angry individuals. Policies should include the following guidelines:

- Notify the facility's administrator of all difficult patients or ask for help from co-workers.
- Keep yourself at a distance from the person (e.g., try to separate yourself from the person by a desk or another piece of furniture).

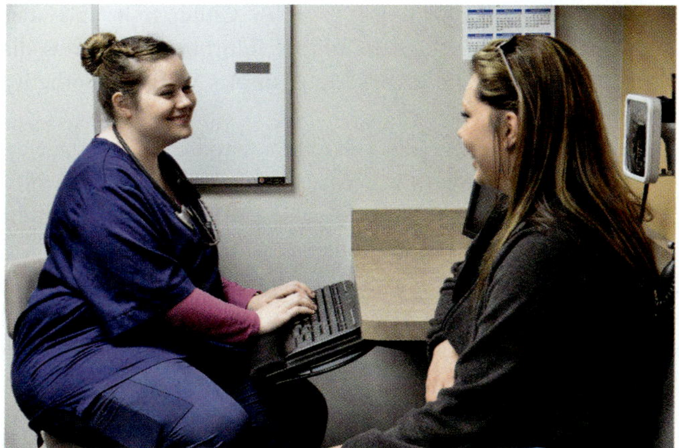

FIGURE 2.6 The medical assistant's position should be at the level of the patient.

- If you are in a room with an angry person, position yourself, so you are the closest person to the door.
- Have another employee remain close by.
- Know under what circumstances you should contact the police or building security for assistance.

Empathy

Healthcare professionals who are empathetic provide better patient care. Showing patients respect and dignity through empathetic care builds trust with patients, which increases their satisfaction and adherence to the treatment plan. It is critical when providing patient-centered care. When providers are not expressing empathy, the patients may remain anxious, feel disconnected from their care, lose trust in their healthcare team, and may have less positive health outcomes. Apply the following strategies to provide empathetic care:

- Make sure to listen to your patients and understand their experiences, perspective, and concerns.
- Use positive nonverbal behaviors. For instance, position yourself at the same level as the patient (Figure 2.6). Make appropriate eye contact. Nod your head and lean in as you communicate with the patient.
- Use therapeutic communication techniques (e.g., reflection, paraphrasing, and clarification) as you interact with the patient. Show your support.
- Interpret the patient's nonverbal behaviors and clarify any messages that differ from the verbal message received.
- Be welcoming and show your patients dignity and respect.

Developmental Stages

A person's developmental stage may be a barrier to communication. Communicating with a 3-year-old child is different from communicating with an 80-year-old adult. A medical assistant must understand developmental stages to know how to interact with people of different ages. Piaget's cognitive development stages provide information on a child's developmental stage. If a medical assistant does not consider a person's developmental stage when communicating, a barrier can occur. Piaget listed the following developmental stages:

- *Sensory motor* (age 0–2 years): Unable to process medical information.
- *Preoperational* (age 2–7 years): Does not comprehend cause and effect or the impact in the future. Children in this stage do not understand how their actions affect their health.

- *Concrete operations* (age 7–11 years): Children in this stage can begin to understand healthcare information, such as disease. They understand concrete examples versus hypothetical situations.
- *Formal operations* (12 years and older): Children in this stage can understand illness, how it occurs, and how they can control it. Typically, they understand messages at the same level as adults. Children in this stage are capable of logical reasoning.

Besides Piaget's stages, Erikson's stages also can impact communication. Erik Erikson, a psychoanalyst, described the emotional, physical, and psychological stages of human development. He stated that a person in each stage had a specific developmental task to complete. Understanding the task or goal of each stage helps healthcare professionals communicate more effectively with patients. Table 2.6 presents the developmental stages, goals of each stage, and communication tips for healthcare professionals.

Strategies When Working with Aging Patients

When medical assistants work with aging patients, it is important to keep the following suggestions in mind for effective communication:

- Address the patient by Mr., Mrs., Ms., or Miss unless permission has been given to use the patient's first name.
- Introduce yourself and explain the purpose of a procedure before performing it.
- Face and softly touch the aging person to get the individual's attention before beginning to speak.
- Use expanded speech by lowering the pitch or tone of your voice and speaking firmly, making sure to enunciate each word clearly.
- Use gestures and demonstrations to clarify communication.
- Print out instructions in block print using a larger font size to ensure aging individuals can read the information.
- If the message must be repeated, paraphrase or find other words to say the same thing.
- Observe the patient's nonverbal behavior for cues indicating whether the person understands.
- Provide adequate lighting without glare.
- Allow patients time to process information and take care of themselves unless they ask for assistance.
- Conduct communication in a quiet room without distractions.
- Involve family members as needed for continuity of care.
- When leaving a telephone message, remember to speak slowly and clearly and repeat the message in the same manner. It is difficult to interpret a message and even more difficult to write it down if the message is delivered in a hurried manner.
- Use referrals and community resources for support.

TABLE 2.6 Erikson's Stages of Psychosocial Development

DEVELOPMENTAL STAGE	GOALS OF STAGE	COMMUNICATION TIPS
Trust versus Mistrust (age range: 0–1.5 years [infancy])	Must develop trust, with the ability to mistrust should the need arise.	Use calm, soothing voice; hold child securely. Loud voices and noises can startle the child.
Autonomy versus Shame and Doubt (age range: 1.5–3 years [toddler])	Must explore and manipulate things in their "world" to develop autonomy and self-esteem.	Use simple language. Allow the child to touch and explore objects. Allow the child to play and make choices.
Initiative versus Guilt (age range: 3–6 years [preschool])	Encouraged to try new activities. Must assume responsibilities and learn new skills. Will make the child feel purposeful and increase self-esteem.	Use short, simple sentences. Encourage questions. Use imitation, play, and role-playing.
Industry versus Inferiority (age range: 6–12 years [school age])	Must seek to finish tasks. Recognition for accomplishments is important.	Use engaging simple tools to communicate information (videos, gaming software, pamphlets). Encourage discussion and questions.
Identity versus Role Confusion (age range: 12–18 years [adolescence])	To know who you are as a person and how you fit into the world around you. Creates a meaningful self-image.	Provide privacy and independence. Encourage responsible decision making. Encourage discussion and questions.
Intimacy versus Isolation (age range: 18–25 years [young adult])	Can vary. To develop friendships and take on commitments.	Identify motivating factors and use them as needed during communication. Realize person may be juggling a lot of obligations.
Generativity versus Stagnation (age range: about 25–60 years [middle adulthood])	Achieve a balance between the concern for the next generation (having a family) and being self-absorbed.	
Ego Integrity versus Despair (age range: 60 and older [late adulthood])	Reflect on one's life and come to terms with it, instead of regretting the past.	Communicate with dignity and respect. Limit slang and "generational" terms. Use simpler language. Speak clearly. Allow the patient time to respond.

CRITICAL THINKING APPLICATION 2.10

What communication tips should Christi use when communicating with the following patients?

- A 2-year-old child
- A 13-year-old teen
- A 30-year-old adult
- An 80-year-old adult

Disease Status

A person's disease status also can affect communication. For instance, think about these scenarios:

- Jim has just been notified by his provider that he may only have 3 months to live. Jim had been healthy until the past few weeks when he started to feel very ill.
- Rose has just been informed that she has type 2 diabetes mellitus. She needs to take medication, change her diet, and exercise.

If you were Jim or Rose, how would you feel? Could you understand and remember a lot of new information after hearing the diagnosis? Could you even converse normally with others, or would you be "blown away"? Would you deny the diagnosis?

Stages of Grief and Dying

Elisabeth Kübler-Ross studied people's reactions to dying. She found that people experienced similar stages as they came to terms with the situation. Over the years, these stages have been applied to grief. They can relate to patients who are informed of a chronic or terminal illness. Family and friends of the ill person can also experience these stages. Not everyone progresses through the stages at the same time, nor does everyone get to the final stage. The stages of grief and dying are as follows:

- *Denial.* The person refuses to accept the fact (e.g., diagnosis or prognosis). This is a defense mechanism that allows the person to ignore what is happening.
- *Anger.* This can be directed at oneself or others.
- *Bargaining.* The person attempts to bargain with the higher power the person believes in (e.g., God).
- *Depression.* The person feels sad, fearful, and uncertain. The person may not participate in normal activities and may distance themselves from others.
- *Acceptance.* The person comes to terms with the situation.

When you are communicating with those with a terminal or chronic illness, it is important to understand that they are working through these stages. Remember, the emotions they display may not be related to you. The emotions may be related to the grief with which they are dealing. For instance, a terminally ill patient yells at the receptionist. He is upset about his wait time, although it was under 5 minutes. His emotions may relate more to his stage of grieving than to his wait time. It is important that we provide a supportive, accepting environment. We should be empathetic to these patients.

COMMUNICATING IN THE WORKPLACE

Positive communication in the workplace is important. Keeping workplace relationships strong and healthy is an essential element of well-functioning teams.

Communication Strategies

When working with other staff members and the manager, the medical assistant should practice these guidelines:

- Be a good listener.
- Remember to use open and positive nonverbal communication. Watch the nonverbal communication of others. Many times, you will be able to determine how they are feeling by their nonverbal communication.
- Be polite, respectful, and friendly. Have a flexible, open mind.
- Make sure your message is clear and concise.
- Be confident.
- Appropriately accept positive and negative feedback. Be able to give constructive feedback to others.

Speaking with Providers

Speaking with providers can be intimidating, especially for a new medical assistant graduate. If you need to talk with the provider about a patient issue, start by writing down the information. Read back the information, and ensure you have all of the facts. Follow these guidelines:

- Make sure you are in an area where patients cannot overhear your conversation.
- Speak confidently, clearly, and concisely.
- Start with the patient's name and age if appropriate.
- Discuss the situation in an organized manner.
- If the situation is related to a series of events, start with what occurred first, then second, and so on.
- If the provider gives you information or an order, write it down. Then read it back to the provider to ensure it is correct.

PERSONAL AND PROFESSIONAL BOUNDARIES WITH COMMUNICATION

Personal boundaries (also called *self-boundaries*) are the limits people use to protect themselves. These limits include mental, emotional, physical, and social factors. In healthcare, having personal boundaries protects the healthcare professional from getting too involved with a patient's life. Getting too close to patients and their families can blur the objectivity the healthcare professional needs to have to provide the best patient care. Thus, personal boundaries also protect patients and their families (Procedure 2.5).

Professional boundaries are usually part of the facility's policies and professional association's code of ethics. Professional boundaries include legal, ethical, and facility guidelines that protect patients and healthcare professionals. Using professional communication and only having a professional relationship will help establish and maintain professional boundaries.

Professional Communication

Have you ever talked to a person who shared too much personal information? How did you feel? How did that affect your relationship with the other person? As a healthcare professional, it is important to remember our personal boundaries with professional communication. When we are talking with family and friends, the topics of our conversations can vary greatly. We can discuss many different things. When we are in the healthcare environment, we need to remember that certain topics are inappropriate. Discussions regarding relationships, politics, religion, and other such topics are not appropriate for the workplace.

Besides what we talk about, we also need to consider the phrases or words we use. Many people swear or use words that are insulting or degrading to others. Some people routinely use religious names (e.g., God) when they are surprised or upset. For some people, religious names have sacred meanings. When you say these names in their presence, it can be offensive. We need to ensure our language is professional.

Professional Relationship

The relationship between the medical assistant and the patient needs to be professional. It cannot be a dual relationship where the medical assistant also becomes a friend to the patient. When working with patients, we need to keep our lives private. It is not appropriate for the medical assistant to do the following:

- Share personal issues, struggles, life stories, or other personal, intimate information
- Contact the patient outside of the work environment
- Befriend the patient on social media
- Engage in a flirty or romantic conversation or relationship with the patient
- Gossip and share what happened in the workplace with patients and others

These behaviors cross the line between a professional relationship and a personal relationship. It is important for medical assistants to keep a professional relationship with patients and their families.

Lastly, the medical assistant should remember spatial distancing. If a patient starts to back away, the medical assistant should clue into the action. The medical assistant may be too close to the person, and the person may feel uncomfortable.

UNDERSTANDING BEHAVIOR

Throughout this chapter, we have discussed verbal and nonverbal communication. As healthcare professionals, it is important we understand why our patients and peers behave the way they do. Why do they make the choices they make? What is important to them? Many times their behaviors relate to their needs, **defense mechanisms,** and **coping mechanisms.** By understanding these factors, we can interact more effectively with others.

Maslow's Hierarchy of Needs

In 1943 psychologist Abraham Maslow proposed a **hierarchy** of needs. This is a motivational theory that depicts five levels of needs. Years later, he expanded the theory to include eight levels of needs. Maslow believed that our human needs could be categorized into these eight levels. Each level must be satisfied before we can move up to the next level. These levels are often depicted as a triangle (Figure 2.7).

Deficiency and Growth Needs

The *deficiency* needs consist of the four bottom levels. They are considered the coping behaviors. We must fulfill these needs to cope with life and survival. We all have similar needs, but when they are not met, it motivates us to get them met. Fulfillment of these needs leads to instant short-term gratification. For example, when we are thirsty, we find water to drink. We are satisfied for the moment but will be thirsty again a short time later.

The top four levels are *growth* needs. These levels relate to making ourselves a better person or being all that we can be. Achieving these levels brings long-lasting happiness. The happiness is more meaningful than the gratification achieved from meeting the lower-level needs.

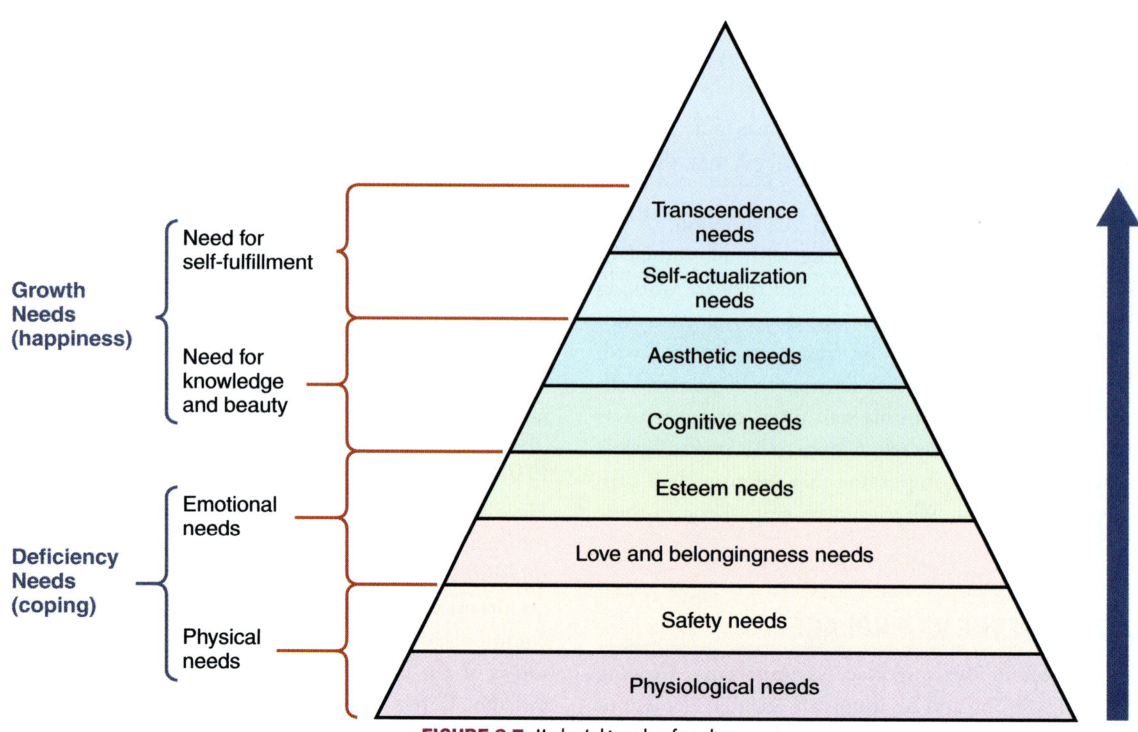

FIGURE 2.7 Maslow's hierarchy of needs.

Maslow's Eight Needs

The following are Maslow's eight needs, starting at the bottom and working upward:

1. *Physiological needs*: These include air, food, drink, shelter, warmth, oxygen, sleep, and so on. We need these things to survive. For instance, when we are hungry, we look for food.
2. *Safety needs*: These include protection from the elements, security, law, order, stability, and so forth. These needs relate to keeping us safe and secure. Unmet safety needs can lead to fear, stress, and anxiety. Some examples of meeting safety needs are as follows:
   - Staying in a job that one really dislikes for the security of the paycheck
   - Staying in an abusive relationship because it is familiar
   - Getting the brakes on your car fixed
3. *Love and belongingness needs*: These include friendship, intimacy, acceptance in a group, and receiving and giving affection and love. We need to be accepted by others. Unmet needs at this level can lead to feelings of isolation, loneliness, and depression. A person may feel anxious about going out in social situations if this need is not met.
4. *Esteem needs*: These include our self-esteem, achievement, mastery of skills, independence, status, prestige, and so on. Our needs relate to our reputation and what we think of ourselves. It is important to remember the saying, "People who matter do not judge, people who judge do not matter." The only thing we have total control over is what we think of ourselves. Some examples of how people attempt to meet this level include the following:
   - Buying the latest electronic devices to show off to others
   - Fishing for compliments
   - Cutting down others to make oneself feel better
   - Focusing on the positives about oneself
   - Setting a challenge for oneself and meeting it
5. *Cognitive needs*: These include knowledge, curiosity, understanding, and exploration. We are driven to learn more about something.
6. *Aesthetic needs*: We appreciate and search for beauty, balance, symmetry, form, and so on. Some people find true happiness when they create music, paint a picture, take a picture, or explore nature. Think of how relaxing it is to be at a beach, enjoying the sound of the water and the feeling of nature.
7. *Self-actualization needs*: We need to realize our potential, seek self-fulfillment, and experience personal growth.
8. *Transcendence needs*: We meet these needs by helping others achieve their very best, or self-actualization. This requires that we give our time and talent to help others meet their needs.

Meeting Deficiency Needs

Maslow believed that only a few people ever achieve the top levels of the hierarchy. He believed that when people did something bad (e.g., steal, put others down), they were motivated to meet their own needs. The method used to meet needs could be unhealthy or dysfunctional. It is important for medical assistants to realize that people meet their own needs in different ways. Their ways may be different and wrong by our standards. We still need to respect our patients and provide the best possible care.

A medical assistant can help patients meet their deficiency needs in the following ways:

- *Physiological needs*: Provide community resources for basic needs.
- *Safety needs*: Provide domestic abuse hotline numbers and other community resources.
- *Love and belongingness needs*: Be positive and respectful. Have a caring manner when working with patients. Acknowledge the patient's importance.
- *Esteem needs*: Encourage independence and provide sincere compliments.

Defense Mechanisms

Defense mechanisms are unconscious mental processes that protect people from anxiety, loss, conflict, or shame. We use defense mechanisms and so do our patients and peers. People use defense mechanisms to protect themselves from situations or information they cannot manage psychologically.

Defense mechanisms may hide a variety of thoughts or feelings, including anger, fear, sadness, despair, and helplessness. Dealing with a patient who uses defense mechanisms can be difficult. If medical assistants are aware of a patient's needs for psychological protection, they may be able to find a way to provide excellent care for the patient. There are many types of defense mechanisms. Table 2.7 describes several of the more common behaviors using patient and peer situations.

Coping Mechanisms

Stress is a condition that causes physical or emotional tension. Stress can be positive (e.g., learning a new job) or negative (e.g., dealing with a loved one's terminal illness). We use coping mechanisms when we are stressed. Coping mechanisms are behavioral and psychological strategies used to deal with or minimize stressful events. Two types are adaptive and maladaptive coping mechanisms.

Adaptive Coping Mechanisms

Adaptive or *healthy coping mechanisms* improve our functioning levels and reduce our stress levels. Here are some examples of adaptive coping mechanisms:

- Eating healthy, well-balanced meals
- Exercising
- Drinking water
- Getting plenty of sleep
- Taking breaks when you feel stressed
- Talking and sharing with others
- Getting help when you need it

Maladaptive Coping Mechanisms

Maladaptive coping mechanisms are also called *nonadaptive* or *unhealthy coping mechanisms.* They reduce the feelings associated with stress for a short time. Maladaptive coping mechanisms do not decrease the actual stressor and can lead to future problems. Here are some examples of maladaptive coping mechanisms:

- Hostility, aggression, manipulation
- Recognition seeking
- Passive-aggressive behavior
- Compliance, dependence
- Social withdrawal, isolation
- Denial, fantasy

TABLE 2.7 Common Defense Mechanisms

DEFENSE MECHANISM	DESCRIPTION	EXAMPLE
Denial	The person completely rejects the information.	"I couldn't possibly have kidney cancer. You must be mistaken."
Repression	The person simply forgets something that is bad or hurtful.	"I wasn't driving the car that killed my best friend."
Regression	The person reverts to an old, usually immature behavior to express feelings.	Perhaps instead of discussing the diagnosis and the need for treatment, the person just storms out of the room and slams the door.
Displacement	The person transfers the emotion toward one person to another person or thing.	After being reprimanded by a supervisor, the person goes home and screams at the children.
Projection	The person accuses someone else of having the feelings that the person has.	A patient is angry about the diagnosis and may say, "You do not have to lose your temper about this," even though the medical assistant's demeanor is completely professional.
Suppression	The person is consciously aware of the information or feeling but refuses to admit it.	"I do not think the test is accurate. My ECGs are always normal."
Splitting	The person views another person as all bad or all good and not a mixture of good and bad traits.	An abused patient may say, "She is a good wife and mother."
Reaction formation	The person expresses feelings as the opposite of what the individual really feels.	A patient is angry at the medical assistant for insisting that a biopsy be scheduled. The person expresses the opposite emotion: "I appreciate your trying to help me, but I just can't come to the clinic that day."
Rationalization	The person comes up with various explanations to justify a response.	"I think the results are wrong. I didn't follow the directions for the tests like I should have, and besides, there's no history of leukemia in my family."

- Drugs and alcohol use
- Gambling, shopping, risk-taking behaviors

Understanding the different types of coping mechanisms is important in our own lives and our role as healthcare professionals. We may have times when we are stressed and tend to use more maladaptive coping mechanisms. It is important for our health and well-being to use more adaptive strategies. Patients, family members, and co-workers are not immune to stress. They will also be using different coping mechanisms. Our role is to encourage the use of healthy coping mechanisms and provide resources for these strategies.

CRITICAL THINKING APPLICATION 2.11

Christi is starting to exercise after work each night. She has found that it helps her deal with the stress of the day. What coping mechanisms do you use when you are stressed? Are they adaptive or maladaptive coping mechanisms?

CLOSING COMMENTS

Patient Coaching

When coaching patients in the ambulatory care facility, the medical assistant must remember to adapt the teaching for the patient. This means if the patient has special needs, the medical assistant must attempt to meet those needs. For instance, a patient with a hearing impairment may struggle to hear the coaching. Writing down the information, speaking slower, and facing the patient may be helpful. When instructing patients from different age groups, the medical assistant will use different techniques. For instance, when coaching young children, the medical assistant would use play techniques and simple words to explain information. Adapting one's coaching, so it works best for the patient is an important role of the medical assistant.

Legal and Ethical Issues

Overcoming communication barriers is more than just providing great patient care. Healthcare providers are legally required to provide ways to overcome communication barriers. This legal requirement comes from the following:

- *Civil Rights Act*: Provides that all providers who accept federal funds for the healthcare provided must ensure equal access to services.
- *Americans with Disabilities Act (ADA)*: Provides that all healthcare providers must provide free effective communication to patients (and companions) with disabilities.
- *Americans with Disabilities Act Amendments Act (ADAAA)*: Expands the definition of disabilities established in the ADA.

Here are some ways that providers can meet their federal obligations for accommodating patients with communication disabilities:

- Provide informational and educational materials that have been translated into the primary languages of the patients seen in the ambulatory care facility.
- Provide large-print materials.
- Write out instructions.
- Provide a qualified medical interpreter free of charge to the patient. This can be done by having an interpreter available to the patient or by using online interpretation services during the visit. The interpreter may be present for the visit, available over the phone, or via videoconferencing. Types of interpreters used in healthcare include the following:
  - Sign language interpreter who uses American Sign Language or Signed English.
  - Oral interpreter who silently mouths speech to the hearing-impaired patient and uses gestures.
  - Cued-speech interpreter who does the same as an oral interpreter but also uses a hand code to stand for each speech sound.
  - Qualified medical interpreter who interprets between the healthcare provider and the non-English-speaking or limited-English-speaking patient. (Using a family member to interpret can be risky because the message may be changed. There is no guarantee the family member is translating exactly what the provider states.)

Patient-Centered Care

Patient-centered care focuses on creating a relationship with the patient and making the patient feel respected, involved, and knowledgeable about the plan of care. The patient has a role in decision-making, and ultimately the goal is for better health outcomes for the person seeking care.

To create this relationship, the healthcare team, which includes the medical assistant, must use therapeutic communication. This process of communication helps build a respectful, empathetic, comfortable, and accepting relationship with patients. It also gives patients the self-confidence to express their feelings, ideas, questions, and concerns. In turn, the healthcare team members can gather the information, answer questions, and share each patient's concerns and feelings with other members of the team.

Professional Behaviors

Medical assistants need to be assertive in the healthcare setting. Not every person going into the medical assisting profession is assertive. It is important to learn how to be assertive in school and your practicum (externship). Practicing assertive skills will help a medical assistant to become more confident and comfortable with that style of communication. Here are some tips for being assertive:

- Be assertive when you need to; not every situation requires it.
- Use appropriate eye contact.
- Use a medium pitch, speed, and volume of voice.
- Be respectful of others.
- Clearly state your needs; use "I" statements.
- Listen to others.
- Accept compliments graciously, and learn to handle criticism professionally.

SUMMARY OF SCENARIO

Christi is enjoying her new job. Learning how to interact with patients, peers, and providers is an essential part of her job. She is already starting to read up on the Hmong and Mexican cultures because a high percentage of her patients come from those two backgrounds. She has learned important facts about the cultures that help her understand characteristics she has seen in some of her patients. Christi enjoys learning about new cultures.

Christi realizes she has met people who communicate in different ways, and she is learning how to respond to them in a professional environment. Some days are stressful, but she is trying to eat healthy meals, get enough sleep, and use healthy coping skills.

SUMMARY OF LEARNING OBJECTIVES

1. **Explain the importance of first impressions to the delivery of high-quality patient care.**
   First impressions are very important, and they include more than just the first words that are exchanged. We must communicate effectively, both verbally and nonverbally, with the patient and provide a warm, caring environment. The medical assistant plays a vital role in initiating therapeutic patient interactions.
2. **Explain how healthcare professionals demonstrate respect when interacting with diverse populations.**
   Cultural diversity includes general customs, norms, values, and beliefs held by a group of people. Examples of cultural diversity may include values like timeliness, punctuality, honesty, and the importance of hard work. Social diversity relates to all the ways a person is different from others. Examples of social diversity include a person's lifestyle, religion, tastes, and preferences. Ethnic diversity relates to a group of people who share a common ancestry, culture, religion, traditions, nationality, and language. Examples of ethnic diversity include family traditions and values.

Continued

SUMMARY OF LEARNING OBJECTIVES—*continued*

Showing respect for individual diversity is important for healthcare professionals. Respect is shown by being courteous, sincere, polite, welcoming, and professional in both verbal and nonverbal communication.

3. **Demonstrate appropriate responses to patients' nonverbal communication.**
   Communication is the exchange of information, feelings, and thoughts between two or more people using spoken words or other methods. Nonverbal communication includes body language and expressive behaviors. More communication occurs nonverbally than verbally. Nonverbal communication occurs through our position, posture, facial expressions, gestures, touch, eye contact, and mannerisms. Nonverbal communication also occurs through the quality of our vocal expression. For instance, nonverbal communication includes the rate, clarity, volume, pitch, tone, intonation, and vocabulary we use when speaking.
4. **Determine how a medical assistant can communicate professionally in both written and oral forms while considering the receiver of the message.**
   The communication cycle is a way to describe the communication process. It involves both a sender and a receiver in addition to the message and feedback. Oral and written communications are forms of verbal communication. Oral communication means we talk with others, and we listen to others. Examples of written communication include written messages, letters, emails, and online information. It is important how we state our written message because we want the receiver to get the message that we intend to send. Always be courteous, write in complete sentences, and check grammar, spelling, and punctuation.
   Styles of verbal communication include the following communicators: passive, aggressive, passive-aggressive, manipulative, and assertive. The behaviors seen with these styles include the following:
   - *Passive communicators*: Avoid expressing feelings or opinions, fail to exert themselves, allow others to infringe on their rights and tend to speak softly.
   - *Aggressive communicators*: Try to dominate others, have low frustration tolerance, criticize and attack others, have poor listening skills, and use "you" statements.
   - *Passive-aggressive communicators*: Deny problems, do not confront problems or people, appear to be cooperative but plan subtle sabotage or disruptions.
   - *Manipulative communicators*: Are cunning and controlling of others; use others to get what they want.
   - *Assertive communicators*: Clearly state their needs and wants; use "I" statements and listen without interrupting; are relaxed, use appropriate eye contact, feel connected with others, and stand up for their rights. Healthcare professionals should use the assertive communication style.
5. **Demonstrate therapeutic communication techniques when working with patients.**
   Therapeutic communication is a process of communicating with patients and family members in healthcare. It is an interactive relationship that conveys acceptance and respect without judging or blaming. Active listening is the most important therapeutic communication technique. Active listening means we fully concentrate on what is being said and how it is said.
   When you gather information from a patient, it is helpful to use a combination of open-ended and closed questions or statements. An open-ended question or statement asks for general information or states the topic to be discussed, but only in general terms. It is a very effective method of gathering more details about the problem from the patient.
   Closed questions ask for specific information. In many cases, this form of questioning limits the patient's answer to one or two words, including yes and no. Use this form of question when you need confirmation of specific facts, such as when asking about demographic information.
6. **Determine strategies to overcome barriers to effective communication in healthcare.**
   Barriers to communication and ways to overcome the barriers include the following:
   - Environmental distractions: Provide patients with privacy.
   - Internal distractions: Help make patients comfortable.
   - Visual impairment: Use audio recordings, large-print materials, and screen reader software.
   - Hearing impairment: Use print materials, videos with captions, and sign language interpreters.
   - Non-English speaking considerations: Use interpreters and translated materials.
   - Emotional distractions: Provide a warm, caring environment.

   Erik Erikson described the emotional, physical, and psychological stages of human development. He stated that a person in each stage had a specific developmental task to complete. Understanding the task or goal of each stage helps healthcare professionals communicate more effectively with patients.
   Elisabeth Kübler-Ross studied people's reactions to dying. She found that people went through similar stages: denial, anger, bargaining, depression, and acceptance. These stages have been applied to grief and relate to patients who have chronic or terminal illnesses. Not everyone progresses through the stages at the same time, nor does everyone get to the final stage.
7. **Explain communication strategies to use with peers, supervisors, and providers.**
   When the medical assistant is working with others in healthcare, the medical assistant needs to be polite, respectful, friendly, confident, and a good listener. Speaking to providers can be intimidating. The medical assistant should confidently, clearly, and concisely deliver a message in an organized method, giving the provider the details.
8. **Explain personal and professional boundaries with communication in healthcare.**
   As a healthcare professional, it is important to remember our personal boundaries with verbal communication. When we are in the healthcare environment, we need to remember that certain topics are inappropriate. Discussions regarding relationships, politics, religion, and other such topics are not appropriate for the workplace. We also need to consider the

SUMMARY OF LEARNING OBJECTIVES—*continued*

phrases or words we use. Many people swear or use words that are insulting or degrading to others. Some people routinely use religious names when they are surprised or upset. Use of these words is not professional. The relationship between the medical assistant and the patient needs to be professional. It cannot be a dual relationship where the medical assistant also becomes a friend to the patient. When working with patients, we need to keep our personal lives private.

9. **Determine factors that impact peoples' behaviors, including needs, defense mechanisms, and coping mechanisms.**
   Maslow described what motivates people. His theory helps describe the behaviors of individuals as they cope with the world or strive for happiness. Maslow believed that our human needs could be categorized into eight levels. Each level must be satisfied before we can move up to the next level. The *deficiency* needs consist of the four bottom levels, and they are considered the coping behaviors. We must fulfill these needs to cope with life and survival, but fulfillment only leads to instant short-term gratification. The top four levels are *growth* needs, which relate to making ourselves a better person. Achieving these levels brings long-lasting happiness.
   Defense mechanisms are unconscious mental processes that patients and peers use to protect themselves from situations or information they cannot manage psychologically. Coping mechanisms are behavioral and psychological strategies used to deal with or minimize stressful events. Adaptive (healthy) coping mechanisms improve our functioning levels and reduce our stress levels. Maladaptive (nonadaptive or unhealthy) coping mechanisms reduce the feelings associated with stress for a short time, but they do not decrease the actual stressor and can lead to future problems.

PROCEDURE 2.1 Use Feedback Techniques and Demonstrate Respect for Individual Diversity: Gender and Appearance

TASKS: Use feedback techniques (e.g., reflection, restatement, and clarification) to obtain patient information. Respond to nonverbal communication. Communicate respectfully with patients who have an individual diversity related to gender and appearance. Demonstrate empathy, active listening, and nonverbal communication.

BACKGROUND: When working with a transgender patient, ask the patient privately which pronouns the person prefers. Make sure to add this information to the patient's health record for future reference.

SCENARIO: You are rooming Crystal Green. You can see that she has expertly applied her makeup, has long red fingernails, long blond hair, and is wearing at least 3-inch heels. You are surprised to see that her birth sex is male. This is the first time you have roomed a transgender patient. You are uncomfortable in this situation because you have strong personal beliefs that birth sex should be maintained throughout a person's life.

DIRECTIONS: Using the scenario, role-play with a peer the rooming process (obtain the patient's chief complaint [main reason for the visit], her allergies, her pregnancy history, and her current medications). The partner (patient) should make up any information required.

EQUIPMENT and SUPPLIES

- Patient health record
- Rooming form (optional)
- Pen

PROCEDURAL STEPS

1. Greet the patient. Identify yourself. Verify the patient's identity with full name and date of birth. Explain the procedure in a manner that the patient understands. Answer any questions the patient may have about the procedure.
   PURPOSE: It is important to identify the patient in two different ways to ensure that you have the correct patient. Explaining the procedure can make the patient feel more comfortable and reduces anxiety.
2. Demonstrate respect for the patient. Be sincere, courteous, polite, and welcoming. Maintain the patient's dignity. Demonstrate professional, nonjudgmental verbal and nonverbal communication. Ask appropriate questions as you obtain information.
   PURPOSE: It is important to provide a respectful and welcoming environment to all patients regardless of individual diversity.
3. Using appropriate closed and open-ended questions and statements, obtain the patient's chief complaint (main reason for the visit) and history of present illness, allergies, pregnancy history, medical history, and current medications. Document the information in the health record or on the history form.
   PURPOSE: Medical assistants need to gather the patient's information before the provider sees the patient.
4. Use feedback techniques, including reflection, restatements, and clarification, as information is obtained.
   PURPOSE: Feedback techniques help to ensure the information is correct.
5. Respond to the patient's nonverbal communication by using feedback techniques (e.g., reflection). If the patient's nonverbal communication is interpreted differently than the patient's oral statements, clarify the information with the patient.
   PURPOSE: Feedback techniques help to ensure the receiver's interpretation of the nonverbal and verbal communication is correct.
6. Use active listening skills. Remain neutral and refrain from interrupting. Allow for periods of silence. Smile and nod your head to show interest. Use appropriate eye contact. Focus on the patient and avoid distractions (e.g., looking at the clock, fidgeting).

PROCEDURE 2.1 Use Feedback Techniques and Demonstrate Respect for Individual Diversity: Gender and Appearance—*continued*

PURPOSE: Demonstrating active listening skills creates a trusting, welcoming environment for the patient. It helps build a trusting, caring relationship.

7. Use professional, positive nonverbal communication behaviors. Use a clear voice with a moderate rate and volume. Use a varying pitch and an accepting or neutral tone. Use words the patient can understand. Correctly pronounce the words. Be at the same eye level as the patient. Smile and have a poised posture. Use a light touch on the hand if appropriate. Maintain proper eye contact if culturally appropriate.
   PURPOSE: Demonstrating active listening skills and positive nonverbal communication behaviors creates a trusting, welcoming environment for the patient. It helps build a trusting, caring relationship.
8. Demonstrate empathy by listening to the patients and learning about their experiences and concerns. Use therapeutic communication techniques and positive nonverbal behaviors. Show your support and respect.
   PURPOSE: Being empathetic will help build a trusting relationship with the patient.

PROCEDURE 2.2 Use Feedback Techniques and Demonstrate Respect for Individual Diversity: Race

TASKS: Use feedback techniques (e.g., reflection, restatement, and clarification) to obtain patient information. Respond to nonverbal communication. Communicate respectfully with patients who have an individual diversity related to race. Demonstrate empathy, active listening, and nonverbal communication.

BACKGROUND: When working with an interpreter, allow time for the person to translate the information to the patient. Also, focus on the patient and do not look at the interpreter when speaking to the patient.

SCENARIO: You are rooming Maria Hernandez. She is always late for her appointments, and today she was 20 minutes late. She also does not speak English, and you need to use a Spanish interpreter for the visit. You are uncomfortable in this situation because you have not worked with an interpreter before. You are also feeling rushed because she was late for her appointment.

DIRECTIONS: Role-play the scenario with two peers. One peer is the patient, and the other peer is the translator. The peer who is acting as the translator can repeat the information in English. You need to obtain a brief medical history of this patient (e.g., chief complaint, allergies, and current medications). The peer who is acting as the patient should make up any information required.

EQUIPMENT and SUPPLIES

- Patient health record
- Rooming form (optional)
- Pen

PROCEDURAL STEPS

1. Greet the patient. Identify yourself. Verify the patient's identity with full name and date of birth. Explain the procedure in a manner that the patient understands. Answer any questions the patient may have about the procedure.
   PURPOSE: It is important to identify the patient in two different ways to ensure that you have the correct patient. Explaining the procedure can make the patient feel more comfortable and reduces anxiety.
2. Demonstrate respect for the patient. Focus on the patient, not on the interpreter. Pause to give the interpreter and patient time to answer. Be sincere, courteous, polite, and welcoming. Maintain the patient's dignity. Demonstrate professional, nonjudgmental verbal and nonverbal communication. Ask appropriate questions as you obtain information.
   PURPOSE: It is important to provide a respectful and welcoming environment to all patients regardless of individual diversity.
3. Using appropriate closed and open-ended questions and statements, obtain the patient's chief complaint (main reason for the visit) and history of present illness, allergies, pregnancy history, medical history, and current medications. Document the information in the health record or on the history form.
   PURPOSE: Medical assistants need to gather the patient's information before the provider sees the patient.
4. Use feedback techniques, including reflection, restatements, and clarification as information is obtained.
   PURPOSE: Feedback techniques help to ensure the information is correct.
5. Respond to the patient's nonverbal communication by using feedback techniques (e.g., reflection). If the patient's nonverbal communication is interpreted differently than the patient's oral statements, clarify the information with the patient.
   PURPOSE: Feedback techniques help to ensure the receiver's interpretation of the nonverbal and verbal communication is correct.
6. Use active listening skills. Remain neutral and refrain from interrupting. Allow for periods of silence. Smile and nod your head to show interest. Use appropriate eye contact. Focus on the patient and avoid distractions (e.g., looking at the clock, fidgeting).
   PURPOSE: Demonstrating active listening skills creates a trusting, welcoming environment for the patient. It helps build a trusting, caring relationship with the patient.

PROCEDURE 2.2 Use Feedback Techniques and Demonstrate Respect for Individual Diversity: Race—*continued*

7. Use professional, positive nonverbal communication behaviors. Use a clear voice with a moderate rate and volume. Use a varying pitch and an accepting or neutral tone. Use words the patient can understand. Correctly pronounce the words. Be in the same position as the patient. Smile and have a poised posture. Use a light touch on the hand if appropriate. Maintain proper eye contact if culturally appropriate.
   PURPOSE: Demonstrating active listening skills and positive nonverbal communication behaviors creates a trusting, welcoming environment for the patient. It helps build a trusting, caring relationship.
8. Demonstrate empathy by listening to the patient's experiences and concerns. Use therapeutic communication techniques and positive nonverbal behaviors. Show your support and respect.
   PURPOSE: Being empathetic will help build a trusting relationship with the patient.

PROCEDURE 2.3 Demonstrate Respect for Individual Diversity: Religion and Appearance

TASKS: Respond to nonverbal communication. Communicate respectfully with patients who have an individual diversity related to religion and appearance. Demonstrate empathy, active listening, and nonverbal communication.

BACKGROUND: The Sikh (sickh) religion was founded in northern India. Sikhs believe in one god, the equality of males and females, justice, and community service. Turbans and kachera are worn at all times for religious reasons. Turbans or scarves cover the uncut hair. If the turban or scarf needs to be removed, an alternative head covering should be provided. A turban or scarf should be treated with respect. Placing it on the floor or near shoes would be a sign of disrespect. Kachera are undershorts/undergarments, and at least one leg is to remain in the kachera at all times.

SCENARIO: You are preparing a patient for an examination. The patient is Sikh. The provider always wants the patient to completely undress, wear a gown, and be seated on the exam table before she comes into the room. You are uncomfortable in this situation because you have never worked with a patient who is Sikh.

DIRECTIONS Role-play the scenario with a peer. Instruct the peer (patient) on how to prepare for the examination.

EQUIPMENT and SUPPLIES

- Gown and drape sheet (optional)
- Exam table (optional)

PROCEDURAL STEPS

1. Greet the patient. Identify yourself. Verify the patient's identity with full name and date of birth. Explain the procedure (undressing) in a manner that the patient understands. Answer any questions the patient may have about the procedure.
   PURPOSE: It is important to identify the patient in two different ways to ensure that you have the correct patient. Explaining the procedure can make the patient feel more comfortable and reduces anxiety.
2. Demonstrate respect for the patient. Be sincere, courteous, polite, and welcoming. Maintain the patient's dignity. Demonstrate professional, nonjudgmental verbal and nonverbal communication.
   PURPOSE: It is important to provide a respectful and welcoming environment to all patients regardless of individual diversity.
3. Respond to the patient's nonverbal communication by using feedback techniques (e.g., reflection). If the patient's nonverbal communication is interpreted differently than the patient's oral statements, clarify the information with the patient.
   PURPOSE: Feedback techniques help to ensure the receiver's interpretation of the nonverbal and verbal communication is correct.
4. Use active listening skills. Remain neutral and refrain from interrupting. Smile and nod your head to show interest. Use appropriate eye contact. Focus on the patient and avoid distractions (e.g., looking at the clock, fidgeting).
   PURPOSE: Demonstrating active listening skills creates a trusting, welcoming environment for the patient. It helps build a trusting, caring relationship.
5. Use professional, positive nonverbal communication behaviors. Use a clear voice with a moderate rate and volume. Use a varying pitch and an accepting or neutral tone. Use words the patient can understand. Correctly pronounce the words. Be at the same eye level as the patient. Smile and have a poised posture. Use a light touch on the hand if appropriate. Maintain proper eye contact if culturally appropriate.
   PURPOSE: Demonstrating active listening skills and positive nonverbal communication behaviors creates a trusting, welcoming environment for the patient. It helps build a trusting, caring relationship.
6. Demonstrate empathy by listening to the patient's experiences and concerns. Use therapeutic communication techniques and positive nonverbal behaviors. Show your support and respect.
   PURPOSE: Being empathetic will help build a trusting relationship with the patient.

PROCEDURE 2.4 Use Feedback Techniques and Demonstrate Respect for Individual Diversity: Age, Economic Status, and Appearance

TASKS: Use feedback techniques (e.g., reflection, restatement, and clarification) to obtain patient information. Respond to nonverbal communication. Communicate respectfully with patients who have an individual diversity related to age, economic status, or appearance. Demonstrate empathy, active listening, and nonverbal communication.

SCENARIO: You are rooming Mr. Abraham Black (79 years old), who has recently been diagnosed with dementia. He likes to talk about things that happened long before you were born, and you are not interested in those events. He also has a hard time hearing your questions, and you frequently repeat questions. Mr. Black has poor personal hygiene. His clothes are dirty and torn. He has an unpleasant body odor. Mr. Black tells you he cannot afford to eat if he buys his medications. He does not believe in government programs and refuses to take "handouts." You have worked with Mr. Black in the past and have heard this numerous times. You would prefer to work with the younger generation and patients who have better hygiene.

DIRECTIONS: Using the scenario, role-play the rooming process with a peer (patient). Obtain the patient's chief complaint, allergies, and current medications. The patient should make up any information required.

EQUIPMENT and SUPPLIES

- Patient health record
- Rooming form (optional)
- Pen

PROCEDURAL STEPS

1. Greet the patient. Identify yourself. Verify the patient's identity with full name and date of birth. Explain the procedure in a manner that the patient understands. Answer any questions the patient may have about the procedure.
   PURPOSE: It is important to identify the patient in two different ways to ensure that you have the correct patient. Explaining the procedure can make the patient feel more comfortable and reduces anxiety.
2. Demonstrate respect for the patient. Be sincere, courteous, polite, and welcoming. Maintain the patient's dignity. Demonstrate professional, nonjudgmental verbal and nonverbal communication. Ask appropriate questions as you obtain information.
   PURPOSE: It is important to provide a respectful and welcoming environment to all patients regardless of individual diversity.
3. Using appropriate closed and open-ended questions and statements, obtain the patient's chief complaint (main reason for the visit), history of present illness, allergies, medical history, and current medications. Document the information in the health record or on the history form.
   PURPOSE: Medical assistants need to gather the patient's information before the provider sees the patient.
4. Use feedback techniques, including reflection, restatement, and clarification, as information is obtained.
   PURPOSE: Feedback techniques help to ensure the information is correct.
5. Respond to the patient's nonverbal communication by using feedback techniques (e.g., reflection). If the patient's nonverbal communication is interpreted differently than the patient's oral statements, clarify the information with the patient.
   PURPOSE: Feedback techniques help to ensure the receiver's interpretation of the nonverbal and verbal communication is correct.
6. Use active listening skills. Remain neutral and refrain from interrupting. Allow for periods of silence. Smile and nod your head to show interest. Use appropriate eye contact. Focus on the patient and avoid distractions (e.g., looking at the clock, fidgeting).
   PURPOSE: Demonstrating active listening skills creates a trusting, welcoming environment for the patient. It helps build a trusting, caring relationship.
7. Use professional, positive nonverbal communication behaviors. Use a clear voice with a moderate rate and volume. Use a varying pitch and an accepting or neutral tone. Use words the patient can understand. Correctly pronounce the words. Be at the same eye level as the patient. Smile and have a poised posture. Use a light touch on the hand if appropriate. Maintain proper eye contact if culturally appropriate.
   PURPOSE: Demonstrating active listening skills and positive nonverbal communication behaviors creates a trusting, welcoming environment for the patient. It helps build a trusting, caring relationship.
8. Demonstrate empathy by listening to the patient's experiences and concerns. Use therapeutic communication techniques and positive nonverbal behaviors. Show your support and respect.
   PURPOSE: Being empathetic will help build a trusting relationship with the patient.

PROCEDURE 2.5 Demonstrate Appropriate Self-Boundaries

TASKS: Use respectful and tactful communication while demonstrating the principles of self-boundaries.

BACKGROUND: For the medical assistant to have a professional therapeutic relationship with a patient, the medical assistant must guard against crossing self-boundaries, which are also called professional boundaries. The relationship between the medical assistant and the patient needs to be professional. It cannot be a dual relationship where the medical assistant also becomes a friend to the patient. This means the medical assistant cannot share intimate, personal information, contact the patient outside of the work environment, befriend the patient on social media, or engage in a flirty or romantic relationship with the patient.

SCENARIO 1: You are rooming Morgan, who frequently sees the provider you work for. You have gotten to know Morgan over the time you have worked for the provider. Today, Morgan asks you for your personal phone number and social media information.

SCENARIO 2: You are rooming Sam, who you have gotten to know well over the time you have worked for your provider. Sam is outgoing, enjoys talking, and has many of the same interests as you do. You have just split up with your significant other and have been feeling a bit down. Sam asks you if you would be available for coffee sometime.

DIRECTIONS: Role-play the scenarios with a peer. Your peer will play the patient in the scenario, and you are the medical assistant.

LEGAL PRINCIPLES

3

SCENARIO

Daniela Garcia was just hired as a part-time float receptionist at Walden-Martin Family Medical (WMFM) Clinic. As a float receptionist, she will be working with many different co-workers and providers. Besides working, Daniela is enrolled in a medical assistant program at the local community college. She is just starting a law and ethics course. The first part of the course explains legal concepts.

Daniela learned about the government in high school, but she has never been in a courtroom nor witnessed court proceedings. Learning about legal concepts is very different from what she is focusing on in her other courses. Many of her classmates did not realize that medical assistants need to learn about legal concepts and laws. Daniela hopes that she can relate what she does in the clinic to what she is learning in her course. She finds concepts are easier to remember if she can apply them to real-life situations.

Bella, a newly certified medical assistant (CMA), has offered to help Daniela study for her law course. Bella stated that she enjoyed learning about law and its importance in healthcare. Daniela is considering asking her for help on their breaks. Studying with another person also helps her retain and understand the concepts.

While studying this chapter, think about the following questions:

- What are the different sources of law?
- How do criminal and civil law differ?
- What is the difference between intentional torts and negligent torts?
- What are the requirements for a legal contract?
- How do expressed, implied, and informed consent occur in healthcare?
- What is the difference between the provider's and the medical assistant's scope of practice and practice requirements?

LEARNING OBJECTIVES

1. Examine the legal system in the United States at the federal and state level, including the balance of power and the types of laws.
2. Differentiate between criminal and civil law.
3. Differentiate between intentional torts and negligent (unintentional) torts.
4. Differentiate among the three main types of defenses used for lawsuits.
5. Examine how a civil lawsuit is resolved, including proving negligence, the stages of a lawsuit, and types of damages awarded.
6. Differentiate between types of liability insurance and types of policies.
7. Examine contracts, including the elements required for a legally binding contract, the types of contracts, and breach of contract.
8. Examine the provider-patient relationship, including termination procedures and the medical assistant's role with the relationship.
9. Examine consents, including types of consents in healthcare, elements required for informed consents, and the medical assistant's role.
10. Examine the medical assistant's role with the Patient Care Partnership (e.g., Patient's Bill of Rights).
11. Examine practice requirements for healthcare professionals and organizations.
12. Examine accreditation, including the purpose and common accreditation organizations.

VOCABULARY

arbitration (ahr bi TRAE shuhn) The process in which conflicting parties in a dispute submit their differences to a court-appointed person (arbitrator), who submits a legally binding decision.

common law Unwritten laws that come from judicial decisions based on societal traditions and customs.

damages A monetary settlement the defendant pays the plaintiff in a civil case for loss or injury. Also, one of the 4 Ds of negligence, meaning the patient suffers a legally recognized injury.

declaratory judgment A court judgment that defines the legal rights of the parties involved.

defendant (dih FEN dant) An individual or a business against whom a lawsuit is filed.

defense (di FENS) A strategy used by the defendant to avoid liability in a lawsuit.

deposition (dep ah ZISH uhn) A sworn testimony made before a court-appointed officer; it is used in the discovery process and may be used in the trial.

emancipated minor (i MANS i pa ted MIE nohr) A minor who has been granted emancipation by the court; the minor can assume the rights and responsibilities of adulthood.

expert witnesses People who are educated and knowledgeable in the area of concern; they testify in court and provide an expert opinion on the topic of concern.

fact witnesses People who observed the situation and testified in court about the facts of the case.

VOCABULARY—*continued*

incompetence (in KOM pi tahns) The state of being incompetent or lacking the ability to manage personal affairs due to mental deficiency; an appointed guardian or conservator manages the person's affairs.

injunction (in JUNGK shuhn) A court order by which an individual or institution is required to perform or refrain from performing a certain act.

interrogatory (IN tah rog ah TOOR ee) Written or oral questions that must be answered under oath.

liability (LIE ah bil i tee) The state of being liable or responsible for something.

liable Legally responsible or obligated.

licensure (LIE sen shur) A mandatory process established by state law that ensures a person has met the legal standards for practicing an occupation in that state.

litigious (LI ti jehs) Prone to lawsuits.

locum tenens (LOE kuhm TEE nenz) Latin for "to substitute for"; the term refers to physicians or advanced practice professionals who temporarily contract to provide healthcare services when a facility has a vacancy, vacation, or a leave of absence.

malpractice (mal PRAK tis) A type of negligence in which a licensed professional fails to provide the standard of care, causing harm to a person.

mature minor A person under the age of adulthood who demonstrates the maturity to make a personal healthcare decision and can give informed consent for treatment.

mediation (MEE dee ae shuhn) The process of facilitating conflicting parties to make an agreement, settlement, or compromise.

minor One who has not reached adulthood; usually age 18 or 21, depending on the jurisdiction.

negligence (NEG li juhns) Failure to act as a reasonably prudent person would under similar circumstances; such conduct falls below the standards of behavior established by law for the protection of others against unreasonable risk of harm.

patient abandonment A form of medical malpractice, also called negligent termination; the provider ends the provider-patient relationship without reasonable or adequate notification.

plaintiff (PLAIN tif) An individual or a party who brings a lawsuit to court.

precedent (PRES I dent) A prior court decision that serves as a model for similar legal cases in the future.

res ipsa loquitur (RASE ipsah low kwah tuhr) A Latin term meaning "the thing speaks for itself." A legal concept under which the plaintiff's burden to prove malpractice is minimal since the jury can clearly understand the details of the injury. For example, a surgical instrument was left in the body during surgery.

res judicata (RASE JOO di kah tah) Latin for "a thing decided." Once a case has been decided by the court, it cannot be litigated again.

respondeat superior (re SPON dee at soo PIR ee ahr) Latin for "let the master answer"; a legal doctrine by which the employer/provider is legally responsible for the wrongful actions or lack of actions of employees if done within the scope of employment.

scope of practice Range of responsibilities and practice guidelines that determine the boundaries within which a healthcare worker practices.

sentence A penalty imposed by a court of law or other authority when a person is found guilty of a crime or other offense.

subpoena (suh PEE nuh) A court order requiring a person to appear in court at a specific time to testify in a legal case.

subpoena duces tecum (suh PEE nuh DOO seez TEE kuhm) A legal document commanding a person to bring a piece of evidence (e.g., the plaintif"s health record) to court.

telemedicine (TEL i med i sin) The use of telecommunication technology to provide healthcare services to patients at a distance; it is usually used in rural communities.

tort A civil wrongdoing that causes harm to a person or property, excludes breach of contract.

tortfeasor (TORTE fee zahr) The individual or entity who committed the tort, either intentionally or as a result of negligence.

INTRODUCTION

In the United States, the number of lawsuits has increased over the years. Working in a **litigious** society requires that we know how to protect ourselves against lawsuits. This is the reason that medical assistants need to learn about the law. To avoid the risk of lawsuits, medical assistants need to practice within the guidelines of the law.

SOURCES OF LAW

Law is a custom or practice of a community. It is a rule of conduct or action prescribed or formally recognized as enforceable by a controlling authority. Law is the system by which society gives order to our lives.

The United States has both federal and state laws. The US Constitution is the supreme law of the United States. Each state has a constitution that is the supreme law of that state. State laws cannot conflict with the US Constitution. In the following sections, we will examine the makeup of the federal and state governments and the sources of law.

Balance of Power

The federal government was designed to allow for a balance of power. The three branches of government share power so that no one branch is more powerful than any other. Table 3.1 describes the three branches of the federal government. The states also have three branches of government.

When members of Congress or the state houses want new legislation, a bill is brought forward. After much debate, the bill will either die or be passed and become an act or statute. The act or statute is now part of the laws for the state or country. (The terms *act* and *statute* are used interchangeably. Most of the time, you will hear the word *act* in the name of a specific law; *statute* is used more to refer

TABLE 3.1 Branches of the Federal and State Governments

BRANCH	FEDERAL GOVERNMENT	STATE GOVERNMENT
Legislative	Made up of • Known as Congress; made up of the Senate and the House of Representatives; members of the houses are elected by eligible voters from the state they represent Roles: • Introduces legislation to become new federal laws • Declares war • Regulates interstate and foreign commerce • Can impeach the president or remove judges from office for misconduct • Must approve all appointments for judges, taxes, budget spending, and treaties • Can override the president's veto of a bill by a two-thirds vote	Made up of • Most states have two houses, although the names can differ; officials are elected Roles: • Introduces legislation to become new state laws • Can impeach state officials for misconduct • Must approve the state budget • Can override the governor's veto and amend the state constitution
Executive	Made up of • President of the United States administers this branch Roles: • Can issue *executive orders* that become law without the approval of Congress • Creates a budget • Appoints judges • Approves and passes bills from Congress (thereby making new laws) or *vetoes* (rejects) new laws • Makes treaties with other nations	Made up of • Headed by the elected governor; each state has a different executive organizational structure Roles: • Issues executive orders • Creates a budget • Appoints state court judges (in most states) • Approves and passes bills from state houses (thereby making new laws) or vetoes new laws
Judicial	Made up of • Supreme Court, which has nine justices Roles: • Interprets laws according to the US Constitution • Determines if laws from Congress and executive actions are constitutional	Made up of • State supreme court Roles: • Interprets laws according to the state constitution • Hears cases from lower courts • Determines if state laws are constitutional

to the contents of the actual law.) On the local level, an *ordinance* is a piece of legislation passed by a municipality or local government. A city ordinance to ban smoking from restaurants is an example of local legislation.

Types of Laws

There are four types of laws:

- *Constitutional law*: Derived from the federal and state constitutions, which give power to federal and state governments. Examples of constitutional law include the prohibition against slavery (based on an 1865 constitutional amendment) and the power to tax.
- *Case law*: Derived from legal **precedents** and **common law.** Common law originated in England and was used by the colonists. An example would include the right of criminal defendants to have an attorney even if they cannot afford one, which was a ruling from the Supreme Court (*Gideon v. Wainwright,* 372 U.S. 335 [1963]).
- *Regulatory* and *administrative law*: Concerns the procedures, regulations, and rules of federal, state, and local governmental administrative agencies. Examples include zoning boards, licensing agencies, the Social Security Administration, and unemployment commissions.
- *Statutory law*: Refers to the laws enacted by the state and federal legislatures. An example is the speed limits set by the state legislature.

CRIMINAL AND CIVIL LAW

Laws can be divided into two main categories:

- *Substantive law*: Laws that determine the rights and obligations of people derived from common law and statutes. Substantive laws include criminal, civil, military, and international law.
- *Procedural law*: Laws that all parties (courts, officers, and lawyers) must follow when investigating and prosecuting unlawful acts. With criminal law, procedural law ensures that a person receives due process under the US Constitution.

The following sections will explain criminal and civil law in depth as they relate to healthcare.

Criminal Law

Criminal laws are statutes that define actions or *omissions* (lack of actions) that threaten or harm public safety and welfare. These actions or omissions are prohibited by the government and are called *crimes*. Criminal law can be summarized as crimes against the state (or government). When criminal cases are brought to court, the

plaintiff is the government. The **defendant** is the person or party charged with the offense.

Criminal offenses can vary in severity, from traffic violations to murders. When a person is found guilty of a crime, the judge will determine a **sentence** for the crime. In most states, criminal offenses are classified as misdemeanors and felonies, which both appear on a person's criminal record.

Misdemeanor and Felony

A *misdemeanor* is a lesser criminal offense. Misdemeanors include the following:

- Assault, battery, and false imprisonment
- Perjury and shoplifting
- Most cases of operating while intoxicated (OWI) and operating under the influence (OUI)

A misdemeanor is punishable by a substantial fine and possible jail time under 1 year. (*Jails* are usually operated by local law enforcement and are used for short-term stays.)

A *felony* is a serious criminal offense and is classified by degree, with first degree being the most serious. Examples of felonies include the following:

- Murder, manslaughter, kidnapping, rape, and sodomy
- Robbery, larceny, burglary, and embezzlement
- Arson and mayhem
- Treason

Felonies are punishable by substantial fines and prison time of more than 1 year. (Prisons are usually operated by the state or federal government and are for long-term stays.) A felony conviction may prevent a person from voting and owning firearms (guns). A felon may have difficulty taking a certification or licensing exam and obtaining specific types of jobs, especially in healthcare.

In some cases, a criminal record can be sealed or expunged. Sealed records continue to exist but are inaccessible to the public. *Expungement* allows a way for charges, arrests, and minor convictions to be legally erased from a person's criminal record. Expungement laws vary by state, and, in some cases, the Federal Bureau of Investigation (FBI) will also expunge the information from the individual's records.

CRITICAL THINKING APPLICATION **3.1**

Bella and Daniela are reviewing criminal law concepts during their lunch break. Bella asks Daniela how criminal law would apply to medical assistants. How might Daniela respond? Discuss your response with a peer.

Civil Law

Civil laws protect and define private rights. An individual or institution can sue another person, institution (business), or the government in a civil matter (Table 3.2). Civil laws govern disputes related to contracts, property, family law, and personal injury. Common civil disputes involve contract issues, divorce, child custody, product **liability**, and accidents. There are many branches of civil law:

- *Tort law*: Applies when one person, business, or the government does a wrongdoing to an individual that causes injury or property damage. Includes intentional **tort**, **negligence**, and *strict liability* (strict duty to ensure safety of manufactured products).
- *Contract law*: Applies to agreements between two or more individuals or parties.
- *Property law*: Applies to personal property (e.g., copyrights, stocks, animals, physical goods) and real property (e.g., land, mineral rights).
- *Family law*: Applies to marriage, divorce, annulment, child custody and support, birth, and adoption.

The following sections will address tort law and contract law.

TABLE 3.2 Criminal Law Compared to Civil Law

	CRIMINAL LAW	CIVIL LAW
Plaintiff	State or federal government	Victim (individual or institution) of the wrongdoing
Defendant	Person or party accused of the criminal complaint or charge	Wrongdoer (also called **tortfeasor** [TORTE fee zahr] with tort law); could be a business, individual, or the government
Wrong Act Against	Wrongful act against the government (state or federal)	Wrongful acts against an individual or an institution (business)
Offense/Wrong Called	Crime	Tort, breach of contract (depends on the type of civil law)
Attorney	Defendant entitled to an attorney; the state must provide an attorney if the defendant cannot afford one	Defendant must pay for the attorney or defend oneself.
Court	Tried in criminal court system; almost always involves a trial by jury	Tried in a civil court system; may not involve a jury; cases are typically decided by the judge
Standard of Proof	Must prove beyond a reasonable doubt	The preponderance of evidence (more than likely it occurred)
Consequence	Substantial fine and prison time	**Damages, injunction, declaratory judgment**
Healthcare Example	A medical assistant determines a patient should have a specific medication and gives the patient the medication without a provider's order, thus practicing medicine	A medical assistant changes a sterile dressing per a provider's order but does the procedure incorrectly; the wound develops an infection, and the patient subsequently dies

TORT LAW

Tort law enforces rules that we have in our society. If these rules are violated, then an individual can sue another individual, institution (business), or government. Two types of torts will be discussed: intentional torts and negligent torts (unintentional torts).

Intentional Torts

With an *intentional tort*, the plaintiff must prove the defendant had specific intent to perform the action that caused the injury. The focus is not on whether the harm was intended, but if the action was intended. Many intentional torts are also criminal in nature. The defendant may be prosecuted in both a civil court and a criminal court for the action. Common intentional torts include the following:

- *Assault*: Intentional threat to do harm or acting in a manner that causes another to fear bodily harm. Example: A medical assistant threatens a child to behave by stating, "I will give you a 'shot' if you do not behave."
- *Battery*: Intentional, harmful, or offensive contact with another that was unconsented. This includes unauthorized administration of medical care in a nonemergent situation. Only proof of unconsented contact is required; proof of harm is not required. Example: A medical assistant gives a child a vaccination without consent from the parent or guardian.
- *False imprisonment*: Intentional restraint of another individual without consent or reason. Example: A medical assistant uses restraints to keep a patient in a wheelchair without significant reason.
- *Fraud*: Deceiving (lying to) a person or party for monetary gain. Example: A medical assistant bills an insurance company for services not provided to the patient.
- *Defamation*: Intentionally saying something false about another person, which causes harm. Written defamation is *libel*. Spoken defamation is *slander*. Example: A medical assistant posts lies about a coworker on a social media site that could cause harm to that person.
- *Invasion of privacy*: Disclosing private facts without the consent of the individual or intrusion into a person's personal life. Example: A medical assistant tells a family member or friend about a patient who was seen in the department, which is breaching confidentiality.

Legal Example: Defamation Suit

According to the complaint: In 2013, in Fairfax, Virginia, the plaintiff was to have a colonoscopy. He was told he could be groggy afterward and was concerned about recalling postprocedure instructions. Prior to the procedure, he set his mobile phone to record the postprocedure instructions. His clothing and phone ended up in the operating suite with him during the procedure. His phone recorded the entire procedure. While the plaintiff was unconscious, the doctors and medical assistant joked that he had syphilis and tuberculosis that caused a penile rash. The defendants mocked the patient for a variety of reasons and then discussed how to avoid the patient when he woke up. The medical assistant attempted to mislead the plaintiff. She indicated falsely that the physician spoke to him after surgery, but the patient must not have remembered. The plaintiff and his wife discovered the recording on their way home.

The jury awarded the plaintiff $50,000 in compensatory damages for defamation for the provider's remarks about each disease. He was also awarded $200,000 for overall medical malpractice and $200,000 in punitive damages.

From *D.B. v Ingham et al.*, 2013-16811 (2015, Fairfax Circuit Court).

CRITICAL THINKING APPLICATION 3.2

Bella and Daniela are reviewing civil law concepts after work. Bella asks Daniela, "How would civil law apply to medical assistants?" How might Daniela respond? Discuss your response with a peer.

Negligent Torts

Negligent torts, or *unintentional torts*, are more common in healthcare because they are unintentional. The harm that is caused by negligence is the result of a person's carelessness. *Negligence* results when a person's conduct falls below the standard of behavior expected of a reasonable person in the same situation.

Reasonable Person Standard and Negligent Acts

The *reasonable person standard* applies reasonable behavior as an objective test to measure another's actions or lack of actions. The accused person's actions or lack of actions are measured against what a reasonable person would or would not do in the same situation. The accused person is negligent if his or her actions or lack of actions do not measure up to the reasonable person standard.

Negligent acts can be classified as follows:

- *Malfeasance*: Performance of an unlawful, wrongful act. For instance, a medical assistant determines that a patient needs pain medication and gives a large dose without a provider's order. The patient dies from the overdose. (It is illegal for the medical assistant to practice medicine [prescribe the medication], and the dose was incorrect.)
- *Misfeasance*: Improper performance of a lawful act that causes damage or injury. For instance, a medical assistant gives an injection ordered by the provider. The injection is given in the wrong location, and the patient has lifelong pain.
- *Nonfeasance*: Failure to act when one has a legal duty to act. For instance, after a patient is given an injection, the patient starts to have an adverse reaction. The medical assistant fails to act and notify the provider. The medical assistant sends the patient home, and the patient later dies.

CRITICAL THINKING APPLICATION 3.3

Bella asks Daniela to describe negligence and the three types of negligent acts in her own words. How might Daniela respond?

Malpractice and Standard of Care

Malpractice is a type of negligence that applies to professionals. Medical malpractice occurs when a healthcare professional's performance falls below the professional minimum standard of care and thus causes harm to the plaintiff. *Standard of care* refers to the level and type of care an ordinary, prudent healthcare professional, having the same training and experience in a similar practice, would have provided under a similar situation.

The standard of care takes into account the accused person's skills and knowledge. It also considers the environment. For instance, the care provided by Dr. Walden, a family practice doctor practicing in a midsize Midwestern city, would be compared to a family practice doctor who practiced in a similar-sized city in the same geographic location. It would be unfair to compare Dr. Walden's family practice to a large family practice located on the East Coast. The resources available to the providers could be different.

Medical assistants need to be aware of the standard of care. If medical assistants identify themselves as nurses to patients, they may be held to the standard of care (including the educational level) of a nurse. If medical assistants practice beyond their **scope of practice,** they may be held to a higher standard of care. Also, medical assistants who are nationally certified may be held to a higher level than those who are not certified. It is important for credentialed medical assistants to pursue continuing education to keep updated and current in their practice. Scope of practice will be discussed later in the chapter.

Legal Example: Malpractice Case

In October 2007, in Syracuse, New York, Tina Holstein (31 years old) delivered her third child at Community General Hospital. After the delivery, she began vomiting, and the nurse administered an intramuscular (IM) injection. Ms. Holstein sued the hospital and the nurse who administered the injection, alleging malpractice. She claimed she had permanent injury of her sciatic nerve because the nurse failed to properly administer the IM injection. The case against the nurse was dropped, but the jury found the hospital **liable** for the injury. Ms. Holstein was awarded $1.69 million.

From *Holstein v. Community General Hospital Greater Syracuse,* 17 N.Y.3d 948 (2011), www.leagle.com/decision/innyco20111122672.

CRITICAL THINKING APPLICATION 3.4

Daniela asks Bella why medical assistants cannot call themselves nurses. How might Bella address this question? How might scope of practice relate to the question?

DEFENSES TO LIABILITY

When the defendant's attorney accepts a case, a **defense** is planned for the lawsuit. There are three main defenses used for lawsuits: denial, technical, and affirmative.

Denial defense is used when none of the facts are true. If even just one fact is true, then the denial defense cannot be used.

The following sections will describe technical and affirmative defenses.

Technical Defenses

When attorneys review cases, they look for ways to have the cases dismissed based on a legal technicality. Four technical defenses will be discussed: statute of limitations, Good Samaritan law, release of tortfeasor, and *res judicata*.

Statute of Limitations

The *statute of limitations* is the length of time legal action can be taken after an event has occurred. When the time has expired, the court will reject the claim or lawsuit. The statute of limitations for medical malpractice is usually 2 to 5 years, but it varies from state to state. In most states, the clock starts when the patient "reasonably should have known" the malpractice occurred. For instance, if a patient awoke after surgery to find that the operation had been performed on the wrong leg, the clock would start then. In some cases, patients do not realize the malpractice occurred for months or years after the event. For instance, something was left in the patient's body during surgery, and it was discovered on an x-ray 3 years later. According to the discovery rule, the malpractice needs to be discovered (the patient "reasonably should have known") before the clock starts on the statute of limitations. The statute of limitations for children greatly varies; some states use age 8, whereas others use age 18.

Good Samaritan Laws

The *Good Samaritan laws* vary in each state, with some states providing protection if the provider acts "in good faith." For Good Samaritan protection, a person must provide care in a true emergency. The care must be provided outside of a place with necessary medical equipment (e.g., outside of a hospital or ambulatory care facility). The person providing the care cannot bill the patient for the emergency care provided.

Release of Tortfeasor

The *release of tortfeasor* defense is used when the plaintiff has signed a release and received monetary compensation. The release indicated that the plaintiff would give up all rights to sue the defendant *(tortfeasor)* in the future in exchange for a monetary compensation. If this signed release existed and the plaintiff decided to sue the defendant at a later time, the defendant's attorney could use the release of tortfeasor defense.

Res Judicata

The final technical defense is **res judicata**, which is Latin for "a thing decided." If a case has already been decided by the court, the plaintiff cannot bring a similar suit against the defendant in the future. The defendant's attorney would use the *res judicata* defense.

Affirmative Defenses

When attorneys review cases, if the denial defense and the technical defense cannot be used, then they attempt to use the affirmative defense. An *affirmative defense* means the defendant admits to wrongdoing, but their attorney introduces facts that support the defendant's conduct. If the defense is successful, it will reduce the defendant's legal liability. The following are common affirmative defenses:

- *Contributory negligence*: The plaintiff's actions or lack of actions caused the injury. In other words, had the plaintiff used ordinary care, the injury would not have occurred. The plaintiff's carelessness (e.g., ignoring warnings or safety rules, inattention) caused the injury. (In many states, contributory negligence has been replaced by comparative negligence.)
- *Comparative negligence*: The plaintiff's action or lack of action caused the injury to a certain percentage. The damages to the plaintiff are calculated based on the percentage to which the defendant was responsible.
- *Assumption of risk*: The defendant can show evidence that the plaintiff had actual, subjective knowledge of the risks involved, and the plaintiff consented to proceed with the activity. Informed consent is critical for this defense. (Informed consent will be discussed later in the chapter.)
- *Limited or no harm*: The defendant claims the plaintiff suffered no or little harm, much less than what the plaintiff claims.
- *Intervening cause*: The defendant acknowledges the plaintiff suffered injuries due to defendant's negligence, but the injury was made worse by the plaintiff's actions following the situation.

Legal Example: Assumption of Risk

The plaintiff was being treated for bronchitis. Following his clinic visit, a coughing episode caused him to black out and hit his head at home. Upon his return to the clinic a few weeks later for a follow-up visit on the bronchitis, a medical assistant took the plaintiff into the examination room. The medical assistant instructed the plaintiff to sit on the exam table while his vital signs were obtained. The plaintiff mentioned to the medical assistant that he had fainted twice as a result of coughing episodes. After the medical assistant left to get the physician, the plaintiff had a coughing episode, fainted, and fell to the floor. He sustained injuries because of the fall.

The plaintiff sued the clinic and the medical assistant, alleging that the medical assistant was negligent for failing to move him to another location upon learning about his fainting episodes. The defendants moved for a summary judgment. They stated that an assumption of risk defense applied. The plaintiff could have chosen to sit on one of the two chairs present in the room, but he did not. The court agreed. The plaintiff appealed, and the Georgia Court of Appeals unanimously sided with the trial court's ruling. The defendants proved the plaintiff had knowledge of the danger, understood the risks associated with the danger, and exposed himself to the danger. The plaintiff lost the case.

From *Watson v. Regional First Care, Inc.*, No. A15A1708, Ga. App. (February 19, 2016), www.leagle.com/decision/ingaco20160219174.

CRITICAL THINKING APPLICATION **3.5**

Daniela is studying affirmative defenses. She asks Bella if she has any study tips for remembering the different affirmative defenses. How might Bella answer? Share your answer with a peer.

RESOLVING A CIVIL LAWSUIT

When a medical negligence suit is brought to court, four elements must be proven for malpractice to be found. A specific process must also be followed when a suit is brought to court. The suit can be resolved in different ways. Several types of damages can be awarded.

Four Ds of Negligence

The four elements (also called the *4 Ds*) of negligence include the following:

- *Duty of care*: The healthcare professional has a legal obligation to the patient. Many times, the duty of care comes from the provider-patient relationship. This will be examined in more depth later in the chapter.
- *Dereliction*: The healthcare professional *breaches* (violates) the duty of care to the patient. In other words, the professional did not follow through with the duty to the patient.
- *Damages*: The patient suffers a legally recognized injury. Examples of such an injury include physical pain, mental anguish, additional medical bills, and loss of work/earning capacity.
- *Direct cause*: The breach of duty of care (the negligent act or lack of action) directly causes the patient's injury.

The plaintiff's attorney is responsible for proving each of these four elements. In many cases, medical experts are hired by attorneys to be expert witnesses. These **expert witnesses** help establish the standard of care and some of the 4 Ds. If one of the elements is not proven, malpractice will not be found. For instance, if the provider performed below the standard of care, but the patient did not suffer any harm, malpractice cannot be found.

In a case in which there was obvious negligence, the doctrine of *res ipsa loquitur* may apply. **Res ipsa loquitur** is Latin for "the thing speaks for itself." The *res ipsa loquitur* doctrine may be used for the following:

- Cases that involve an object being left in the patient's body during surgery
- Cases that involve an operation on the wrong extremity

In these instances, the evidence shows that the plaintiff did not cause the injury. The defendant caused the injury as a result of negligence. The defendant breached the duty to the plaintiff.

CRITICAL THINKING APPLICATION **3.6**

Daniela struggles with remembering the 4 Ds of negligence. Be creative and work with a peer. How might a person remember the 4 Ds of negligence?

Stages of a Civil Lawsuit

When a situation occurs, a person may decide to sue another party. The following are stages of a civil lawsuit:

1. *Prefiling phase*: The situation occurs, and the patient seeks the advice of a civil attorney. After reviewing the person's story, medical record, and other documents, the attorney accepts the case. (Not all cases brought to attorneys are accepted. A person who wants to sue another party may have to talk with several lawyers before finding one willing to take the case.)
2. *Initial pleading phase*:
   - The plaintiff's attorney files a complaint with the clerk of the court. The complaint includes the patient's version of the situation and the *damages* (amount of money) sought from the defendant.
   - The clerk of the court issues a summons to the defendant. The summons outlines the complaint and damages and states a deadline for a response.
   - The defense attorney files an answer or motion with the court. The answer provides the courts with the defendant's version of the situation. (If the deadline is missed, the defendant may be responsible for the damages.)
3. Discovery phase:
   - Both sides exchange information and gather evidence to support their side in court.
   - A **subpoena** is issued for the healthcare professionals involved in the case. They may be required to go to court or to attend a **deposition**. They may also be required to complete an **interrogatory**. Failure to comply with a deposition or subpoena will result in a *contempt of court* charge. The person may be fined or imprisoned.
   - A **subpoena duces tecum** may also be issued.
4. *Postdiscovery phase*: At this point in the case, the judge may meet with the attorneys. Four options may occur:
   - The plaintiff may drop the case if not enough evidence is available to make the case.
   - A summary judgment may be given.
   - The judge or defendant may encourage alternative dispute resolution (ADR).
   - The case may go to trial.

The following sections describe how a case may be resolved, either by a summary judgment, by ADR, or by going to trial.

Summary Judgment

With civil litigation, either party or the judge can move for a summary judgment. A *summary judgment* is a process that can be used if there are no disputes about the facts in the case. This process speeds up cases. It allows a judgment to be made based on the facts. With a summary judgment, there is no trial.

Alternative Dispute Resolution

When a plaintiff sues the defendant, the defendant can attempt to settle outside of court or go to trial. *Alternative dispute resolution* (ADR) is the process of settling disputes outside of litigation. This process is usually cheaper and quicker than going to trial. Two types of alternative dispute resolution are **arbitration** and **mediation**. Both ADR procedures involve a neutral third party who hears both sides. With mediation, the mediator facilitates an agreement that is acceptable to both parties. With arbitration, the arbitrator listens to both sides and makes the final decision, which is *legally binding* (or a legal obligation).

Going to Trial

If the case is to be heard by a jury, the jury is selected. Expert witnesses and **fact witnesses** are questioned and cross-examined by the opposing attorney (Figure 3.1). Closing arguments are made, and the jury retires to make a decision. The verdict is read to the court, and the judge enters the judgment.

The losing party may be interested in appealing the case. During the appeal phase, the posttrial motions are filed. An appeal to a higher court may be made.

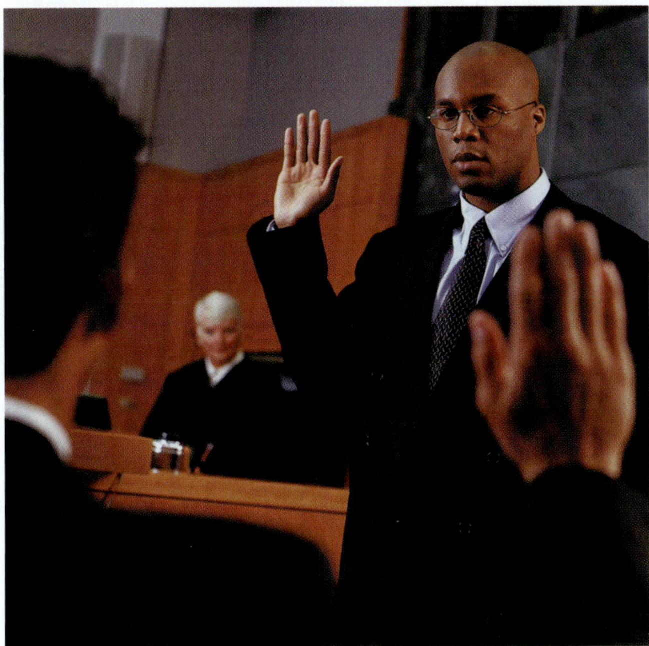

FIGURE 3.1 Witnesses must be credible and must tell the truth on the stand in court to avoid charges of perjury.

CRITICAL THINKING APPLICATION 3.7

Bella is helping Daniela study for a law exam. She asks Daniela to describe the differences between the following sets of terms. How might Daniela respond?

- Subpoena and *subpoena duces tecum*
- Fact witness and expert witness

Damages

The defendant may need to pay damages when the plaintiff wins a civil suit. *Damages* are a monetary settlement. There are several types of damages:

- *Punitive damages*: A very large payment meant to punish the defendant.
- *Nominal damages*: A very small settlement because the plaintiff's injury was slight.
- *Compensatory damages*: A settlement for losses suffered. Losses can be related to loss of income, property damage, and medical care.
- *General damages*: A settlement for emotional pain and anguish, loss of future earning power, and so on. Often sought with compensatory damages.
- *Special damages*: A settlement for a specific dollar amount that directly relates to medical bills.

PROFESSIONAL LIABILITY INSURANCE

Many people are familiar with car insurance and homeowner's insurance. When a person becomes a professional, the risk of being sued increases. Having insurance (to protect oneself in case of civil damages) is important. Providers, nurses, and, in some cases, medical assistants purchase annual insurance policies. Ambulatory healthcare facilities also must carry insurance. It is important for medical assistants to understand the types of insurance available.

The person or company purchasing the insurance policy is called the *insured* (first party). The insured pays a specific amount of money to the insurance company (second party). This payment is called a *premium*. The insurance company is the *insurer*. The insurer agrees to compensate the insured for specific losses covered in the insurance contract or policy. When the *insurer* (insurance company) pays the plaintiff, the plaintiff is known as the *third party*.

Types of Liability Insurance

Liability insurance provides protection from claims of injuries or damage to people or property. It can be referred to as third-party coverage because it covers claims from a party other than the insured. There are different types of liability insurance:

- *Professional liability insurance*: A type of liability coverage used by professionals to protect themselves against liability suits incurred because of errors and omissions while performing their professional services.
  - *Medical malpractice insurance*: A type of professional liability insurance. Protects healthcare professionals, including medical assistants, from liability related to wrongful practices resulting in injury, expense, and property damages. It also covers the cost of defending lawsuits.

- *General liability* or *commercial liability insurance*: A type of liability coverage purchased by companies. It protects businesses from lawsuits for property loss and bodily injury from nonemployees.
- *Personal injury insurance*: A type of liability coverage that protects against claims related to harm other than bodily injury. Coverage can be for invasion of privacy, slander, imprisonment, and so on.

Types of Policies

When a professional purchases a policy, it is important to understand the types of policies.

- *Claims-made policy*: An insurance policy that covers claims made during the policy year. For example, if a provider has a claims-made policy for the current year, any claims that come in this year will be covered.
- *Occurrence policy*: An insurance policy that covers claims for wrongful acts that occurred during the policy year. For example, if a provider has an occurrence policy for the current year, any wrongful acts that occur this year will be covered when the claims are filed in future years.
- *Nose coverage*: A limited-term policy purchased from the new carrier the provider is joining. The policy covers the provider between the end of the prior policy and the start of the next policy. Nose coverage can also be referred to as *retroactive* or *prior acts coverage.*
- *Tail coverage*: A limited-term policy purchased from the insurance carrier that the provider is leaving. The policy covers the provider until the new policy starts. A person would need only nose or tail coverage, not both.

CONTRACTS

Most people are aware of contracts. We sign contracts for cell phone plans, rental properties, and payment plans. We also have contracts in healthcare. The healthcare facility's business manager signs contracts for equipment and building rental, service agreements, and so on. The most common contract is the provider-patient contract.

Elements of a Legally Binding Contract

A *contract* is an agreement between two parties. For a contract to be legally binding, five elements must be present:

- *Offer*: Made by one party. Example: A family practice physician advertises complete physicals for $150.
- *Acceptance*: A second party agrees to the offer. Example: After seeing the advertisement, a patient calls to make an appointment.
- *Consideration*: Each party exchanges something of value. Example: The physician gives a physical exam, and the patient pays $150.
- *Legal subject matter*: The consideration must be legal. Example: The board-certified physician can legally perform physical exams. The payment is legal tender (money).
- *Competency* and *capacity*: A person entering a contract must have the legal capacity to be held liable for the contract obligation. If one or both parties is underage (a **minor**) or shows signs of **incompetence**, intoxication, or acting under the influence of drugs, this would invalidate a contract. An **emancipated minor** can enter into contracts. Example: Both the physician and the patient are adults with the capacity to understand the contract.

Emancipated Minors

If a minor wants to become emancipated, certain conditions must be met for the courts to declare the minor emancipated. The minors must be at least 16 years of age in most states and usually must meet one of the following conditions:

- Married
- In the US military
- Living on their own and managing their own money

When a minor is emancipated, the minor can be a part of a contract (e.g., renting housing and purchase agreements). An emancipated minor can sue. The minor can keep earned income and apply for public benefits. Lastly, an emancipated minor may make all healthcare decisions regarding oneself.

Implied and Expressed Contracts

A contract can be either an implied contract or an expressed contract.

- *Implied contract*: The parties have agreed to the terms of the contract through their actions and behaviors. The provider-patient relationship is an implied contract (Figure 3.2).
- *Expressed contract*: The parties have specifically stated the terms of the contract in writing, orally, or both. A service contract for office equipment maintenance is an expressed contract.

The *statute of frauds* is a common law concept. The statute of frauds requires that specific types of contracts must be in writing to avoid fraud and to be binding. These types of contracts are outlined in each state's statute of frauds. *Statutes of fraud* vary slightly between the states, but all indicate that contracts need to be in writing and signed by both parties. The following contracts need to be in writing:

- Contracts that are property related, such as real estate sales, real estate leases for longer than 1 year, and transfer of property upon the owner's death
- Agreements to pay another's debt
- Contracts that last longer than 1 year or last longer than the life of an individual
- Contracts over a certain amount of money (varies by state)

Breach of Contract

A *breach of contract* occurs when the terms of the contract are not fulfilled by one party without a legitimate legal reason. The breach can

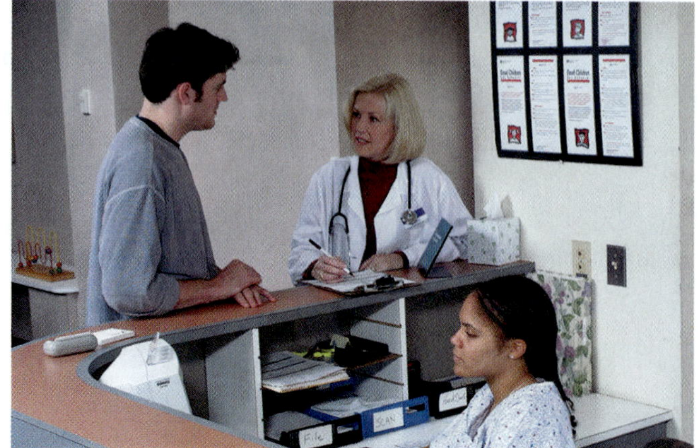

FIGURE 3.2 The provider-patient relationship is built on a strong foundation of trust, but it also is a contractual relationship.

occur when the terms are not met by the stated deadline. It can also happen when the terms are not met or performed. An allegation of a breach of contract can lead to a lawsuit. The injured party attempts to force the contract terms to be met or to receive compensation for financial loss caused by the breach.

In the healthcare field, a breach of contract can occur with the provider-patient relationship. Breach of contract may occur with improper termination and abandonment situations. Breach of contract may also occur with the business side of the facility, including the following:

- Business contracts (e.g., leases for equipment)
- Payment contracts with patients

PROVIDER-PATIENT RELATIONSHIP

The contract that is established between the provider and the patient is legally binding. The patient accepts the provider's offer when the patient makes an appointment to see the provider. This means the provider has a duty to see, diagnose, and treat the patient. The patient has the responsibility to follow the provider's recommendations and pay the bill.

As indicated earlier, duty to the patient is one of the 4 Ds in proving malpractice. The duty to the patient is established during the patient's initial visit. From that time onward, the provider has a duty to the patient. Both parties can terminate the contract or relationship. A patient can terminate the contract at any time. The patient may no longer need the provider's services. The patient may decide to use another provider.

Terminating the Provider-Patient Relationship

Providers can choose to terminate the patient relationship for a variety of reasons:

- Provider is retiring or moving
- Patient is not paying for the services provided
- Patient is not following or is noncompliant with the provider's treatment plan
- Patient's behavior has become an issue (e.g., rude, abusive, drug seeking, and not showing up for appointments)

The provider must follow the legal process to terminate the contract. Providers can be charged with **patient abandonment** if they simply stop providing care to the patient. To prevent abandonment allegations, the provider must follow the correct legal steps to terminate the provider-patient relationship:

- Provider must notify the patient in writing of the withdrawal of care.
- A date must be indicated for the termination. There must be an adequate period of coverage to allow the patient to find another provider. Fifteen to 30 days is usually recommended.
- The termination letter should be sent as a certified letter with a return receipt requested.
- A copy of the letter and the return receipt need to be placed or scanned into the patient's health record.
- Scheduling staff should be notified of the termination date so that no appointments are made after that date.

Preventing Patient Abandonment

There are many situations in which allegations of patient abandonment may occur:

- Failing to follow up with the patient. If a patient calls or emails the provider or facility, follow-up with the patient must be made in a reasonable period of time.
- Failing to have another provider cover the practice during vacations or when the facility is closed.
- Discharging a patient without proper instructions.

The medical assistant has an important role in ensuring that the patient is not abandoned. Typically, the medical assistant is responsible for answering patient calls and emails in a timely manner. Documentation in the patient health record must reflect all communication with the patient.

If the medical assistant does not follow up with the patient, allegations of abandonment can be brought against the medical assistant and the provider. **Respondeat superior** is a common law doctrine that means "let the master answer." The doctrine means that the employer/provider is liable for actions that the employee did or did not do within the scope of employment. This means that the medical assistant's actions affect the employer and the provider. The medical assistant's actions or lack of actions can lead to malpractice allegations for the provider.

CONSENTS

Consent means one party voluntarily agrees with another party's proposition or plan. This section examines the types of consents used in healthcare. Informed consents are essential in healthcare, and medical assistants must be aware of their role with informed consents.

Types of Consents in Healthcare

In healthcare, several types of consent are used.

- *Implied consent*: Consent that is inferred based on signs, actions, or conduct of the patient rather than oral communication (using words). For instance, the medical assistant asks a patient if he can obtain a blood pressure reading. The patient removes her arm from her jacket sleeve and extends it toward the medical assistant.
- *Expressed consent*: Consent that is given either by the spoken or written word. For example, the medical assistant asks the patient's preference for which arm should be used for an injection. The patient states she wants the injection in her upper right arm. The medical assistant gave the patient a choice, and the patient expressed her consent by stating her choice.
- *Informed consent*: A legal process that ensures the patient or guardian understands the treatment and gives consent for the treatment. With informed consent, the provider must educate the patient on the treatment before the patient signs the consent form. More information on the informed consent doctrine is given in the following section.

CRITICAL THINKING APPLICATION **3.8**

Daniela is studying consents. How might you define implied, expressed, and informed consents in your own words?

Doctrine of Informed Consent

With many medical procedures and treatments, informed consent is required:

- Surgical procedures; may include minor surgery done in ambulatory care facilities
- Complex procedures and tests (e.g., endoscopy, biopsy, exercise or nuclear stress test)

- Administration of high-risk medications and most vaccines
- Participation in a research study
- Cancer treatment (e.g., radiation, chemotherapy)
- Some medical laboratory testing

The provider, not the medical assistant, has a duty to provide information to the patient or guardian. The provider must educate the patient on the treatment options. Once the information has been given, the patient or guardian makes an informed decision regarding treatment.

Healthcare facilities are required to have written policies that state procedures and treatments that require informed consent. The policy should state the process of obtaining informed consents and documentation requirements. Exceptions to the policy should also be clearly described in the policy.

Elements Required for Informed Consent

Informed consent requirements may vary slightly from state to state. The requirements are usually described in the state's medical practice act. For an informed consent to occur, seven elements must be present:

1. The patient or guardian is competent to understand and decide.
2. The patient or guardian voluntarily decides to agree to or refuse the treatment.
3. The patient or guardian understands the diagnosis and reason for treatment.
4. The patient or guardian understands the proposed treatment and the risks of the treatment.
5. The patient or guardian understands the alternative treatments available and the risks of the treatments.
6. The patient or guardian understands the risks if treatment is delayed or not done.
7. The patient or guardian signs a treatment consent form.

Who Can Give Informed Consent?. Adults of sound mind can give informed consent. Married minors, minor parents, emancipated minors, and **mature minors** can also give informed consent.

Patients who cannot legally give informed consent include the following:

- Patients under the influence of alcohol or drugs
- Patients who are being treated with a preoperative medication that may affect their understanding (e.g., a sedative)
- Minors
- Patients who are mentally incompetent
- Patients who speak little or no English (an interpreter must be used for the patient to give informed consent; the interpreter will translate the information from the provider, questions from the patient, and the information on the consent form; it is important to document in the health record that an interpreter was used)

Mature Minor

Many states address the mature minor doctrine in their statutes. The definition of a mature minor and restrictions vary from state to state. Differences can be based on a variety of factors:

- A specific age, such as 14 or 16 (or no age may be specified), when one can be considered a mature minor
- The availability of the parent
- The medical concern or treatment

CRITICAL THINKING APPLICATION 3.9

Daniela is trying to distinguish between a mature minor and an emancipated minor. How would you describe each? What rights would each have in terms of healthcare?

Special Situations for Informed Consent

In special situations, such as abortion, sterilization procedures, and human immunodeficiency virus (HIV) testing, each state has specific restrictions.

Currently, with abortions, the father of the fetus has no rights. No state requires the father to give consent or be told about the abortion. State restrictions vary greatly for abortions and can include a host of factors:

- Must be performed by a licensed physician
- Mandated counseling on the possible link between abortion and breast cancer, the fetal development, or long-term mental health consequences
- Required waiting period (often 24 hours) between the counseling and performing an abortion
- Parental involvement for a pregnant minor
- Must be performed in a hospital after a certain gestational age
- Gestational limits (abortion is prohibited after a certain point in the pregnancy)

For sterilization procedures, states may have waiting periods between signing the consent form and the procedure. The patient may have to be an adult (as defined by the state).

For HIV testing, the Centers for Disease Control and Prevention (CDC) recommends that a general consent for medical care form be completed prior to HIV testing. Most states have specific language in the statutes regarding consent and counseling for HIV testing.

Informed Consent for Recording or Photographing

In many states, the patient's written consent is required to take a video or picture of the patient. Pictures are taken to show before and after images. These pictures are added to the patient's electronic health record.

According to the Joint Commission, an informed consent is required by the patient or parent/guardian if recording, filming, or photographing of patient care is used for purposes other than patient care.

The Medical Assistant's Role with Informed Consent

The medical assistant may need to prepare the informed consent form. Most informed consent forms require the following information:

- Patient's name, date of birth, and health record number
- Name of hospital or facility
- Name of provider(s) performing treatment(s)
- Risks and benefits of the treatment(s)
- Alternative treatment(s) and risks
- Risk if treatment(s) is delayed or not done
- Statement indicating the treatment was explained to the patient or guardian
- Signature of patient or guardian
- Signature and name of person who explained the treatment options
- Signature of the witness
- Date and time the consent form was completed

The medical assistant may also need to sign the form as a witness to the signature of the patient. It is important to ask patients before they sign the form if the provider discussed the treatment and if they have any questions. If patients have questions, the medical assistant should let the provider know. After all the questions have been answered, then the informed consent form can be signed. Patients should not sign in the following circumstances:

- They do not understand the treatment
- They cannot legally give consent
- They have questions

PATIENT'S RIGHTS AND RESPONSIBILITIES

Congress has attempted to create laws related to a patient's "bill of rights" for healthcare, but none of the proposed bills has passed. The Affordable Care Act's Patient's Bill of Rights focuses on rights related to insurance. With no federal laws to follow, the American Hospital Association created a patient's bill of rights for its members. In 2003 the American Hospital Association created the Patient Care Partnership. This document helps patients understand the expectations for patients and the patients' rights and responsibilities (Figure 3.3). Ambulatory care facilities may use this document or have a similarly titled document (e.g., Patient Bill of Rights) that explains these topics to patients.

CRITICAL THINKING APPLICATION 3.10

Bella is working with Daniela on the Patient's Bill of Rights. Bella asks Daniela to summarize these rights. What might Daniela say?

Choice of Treatments

A medical assistant is likely to encounter a situation in which a choice of treatments is given to a patient (Procedure 3.1). It is important that the provider discusses the treatment choices with the patient. If the medical assistant is involved, it is important to find out if the patient has any questions. Questions need to be answered before a decision is made. It is important to be respectful and professional during the discussion. Do not attempt to sway the patient in one

WALDEN-MARTIN
FAMILY MEDICAL CLINIC
1234 ANYSTREET | ANYTOWN, ANYSTATE 12345
PHONE 123-123-1234 | FAX 123-123-5678

Patient Bill of Rights

RIGHTS

1. **Medical Care and Dental Care.** The right to quality care consistent with available resources and accepted standards. The right to refuse treatment to the extent permitted by law and government regulations, and to be informed of refusal consequences. When concerned about care received, the right to request review of care adequacy.
2. **Respectful Treatment.** The right to considerate and respectful care, with recognition of personal dignity.
3. **Privacy and Confidentiality.** The right, within law and military regulations, to privacy and confidentiality concerning medical care.
4. **Identity.** The right to know, at all times, the identity, professional status, and professional credentials of health care personnel, as well as the name of the health care provider primarily responsible for his or her care.
5. **Explanation of Care.** The right to an explanation concerning diagnosis, treatment, procedures, and prognosis of illness in terms the patient can understand. When it is not medically advisable to give such information to the patient, information should be provided to appropriate family members or, in their absence, another appropriate person.
6. **Informed Consent.** The right to be advised in nonclinical terms of information (significant complications, risks, benefits, and alternative treatments) needed to make knowledgeable decisions on treatment consent or refusal.
7. **Research Projects.** The right to be advised if the facility proposes to perform research associated with care. The right to refuse to participate in any research projects.
8. **Safe Environment.** The right to care and treatment in a safe environment.
9. **Medical Treatment Facility (MTF) or Dental Treatment Facility (DTF) Rules and Regulations.** The right to be informed of facility conduct rules and regulations. The patient should be informed about smoking rules and should expect compliance with those rules from other individuals. Patients are entitled to information about the MTF or DTF mechanism for the initiation, review, and resolution of patient complaints.

RESPONSIBILITIES

1. **Providing Information.** The responsibility to provide, to the best of his or her knowledge, accurate and complete information about complaints, past illness, hospitalizations, medications, and other matters relating to his or her health. A patient has the responsibility to let his or her primary health care provider know whether he or she understands the treatment and what is expected of him or her.
2. **Respect and Consideration.** The responsibility for being considerate of the rights of other patients and MTF and DTF health care personnel and for assistance in the control of noise, smoking, and the number of visitors. The patient is responsible for being respectful of the property of other persons and of the facility.
3. **Compliance with Medical Care.** The responsibility for complying with medical and nursing treatment plans, including follow-up care, recommended by health care providers. This includes keeping appointments on time and notifying the MTF or DTF when appointments cannot be kept.
4. **Medical Records.** The responsibility for ensuring that medical records are promptly returned to the medical facility for appropriate filing and maintenance when records are transported by the patients for the purpose of medical appointment or consultation, etc. All medical records documenting care provided by any MTF or DTF are the property of the US government
5. **MTF and DTF Rules and Regulations.** The responsibility for following the MTF and DTF rules and regulations affecting patient care conduct. Regulations regarding smoking should be followed by all patients.
6. **Reporting of Patient Complaints.** The responsibility for helping the MTF or DTF commander provide the best possible care to all beneficiaries. Patients' recommendations, questions, or complaints should be reported to the patient contact representative.

FIGURE 3.3 Patient's Bill of Rights.

WALDEN-MARTIN
FAMILY MEDICAL CLINIC
1234 ANYSTREET | ANYTOWN, ANYSTATE 12345
PHONE 123-123-1234 | FAX 123-123-5678

General Procedure Consent

Patient Name: ____________________ **Date:** ________________

The doctor has discussed with you your condition and the recommended surgical or medical procedures to be performed. This discussion was intended to ensure that you had the opportunity to receive the information necessary to make a reasoned and informed decision whether or not to consent to the procedure. This document is written confirmation of the discussion and contains some of the more significant medical information discussed.

1. Based on this discussion, I understand the following condition may exist in my case:

2. I understand the procedure proposed for treating or diagnosing my condition is:

3. I have been informed of the purpose and reasonably expected benefits of the proposed procedure, the possibility of success or failure, major problems of recuperation, the reasonably anticipated consequences if the procedure is not performed, and the available alternatives.

4. I understand that all surgical and therapeutic procedures involve some risks, including pain, scarring, bleeding, and infection.

5. I am aware that in the practice of medicine, other unexpected risks or complications not discussed may or may not further acknowledge that no guarantees or promises have been made to me concerning the results of any procedures. Although the benefits are judged to outweigh the risks, should any complications occur, any one of them could be permanent. I hereby voluntarily give my authority and consent to the doctor to perform the proposed procedure described above.

6. I have been given the opportunity to ask questions about my condition, alternative forms or treatment, risk treatment, the procedure to be used, and the risks and hazards involved. I believe I have sufficient information to give this informed consent.

I have read and fully understand the contents of this form, and I understand that the disclosures referred to above were made to me and that all blanks and statements requiring insertion or completion were filled in before I signed my name below.

Patient Signature: ____________________ **Date:** ________________

If a patient is a minor or unable to give consent, signature of person authorized to consent for patient: ____________________

Relationship to Patient: ____________________

FIGURE 3.4 General Procedure Consent Form.

direction. If the patient selects a treatment that was not the provider's top choice, it is important to respect the patient's decision. The medical assistant should relay the information to the provider.

Refusal of Procedure or Treatment

A medical assistant should know how to handle the situation if a patient refuses a procedure or treatment (Procedure 3.1). It is important to follow the facility's policy and procedure in such a situation. Most times, the following applies when a patient refuses treatment or procedures:

- Show sensitivity to the patient's rights by being respectful and professional. Remember, it is the right of the patient to refuse.
- Ask if the patient has questions regarding the procedure. If so, let the provider know.
- Notify the provider of the refusal.
- Document the refusal in the health record. Make sure to include which provider was notified.

CRITICAL THINKING APPLICATION **3.11**

Daniela asks Bella how much a medical assistant really uses the Patient Care Partnership or the Patient's Bill of Rights. Bella provides this scenario for Daniela: Mrs. Ella Jones, a new patient to the practice, comes in for her 28-week pregnancy check. After the provider examines her, he comes out and gives you an order for the patient. You are to give the patient RhoGAM because she has Rh-negative blood. This is a standard practice with mothers who have Rh-negative blood. You prepare the medication and go to the exam room. You explain to Mrs. Jones what the provider ordered. She asks, "Is RhoGAM a blood product?" and you reply that it is. She refuses it, explaining that she is a Jehovah's Witness and cannot accept blood products. Bella asks Daniela, "Keeping in mind the Patient's Bill of Rights, how might a medical assistant demonstrate sensitivity to Mrs. Jones' rights in this situation?" How might Daniela answer?

WALDEN-MARTIN
FAMILY MEDICAL CLINIC
1234 ANYSTREET | ANYTOWN, ANYSTATE 12345
PHONE 123-123-1234 | FAX 123-123-5678

Vaccine Authorization

Last Name: ______________ **First Name:** ______________

Date of Birth: ______________ **Sex:** ☐ Male ☐ Female

Please answer the following questions:

1. **Are you sick, or do you have a high fever today? (If yes, you should not receive vaccine.)** ☐ Yes ☐ No ☐ Unknown
2. **Are you allergic to chicken, eggs, or egg products?** ☐ Yes ☐ No ☐ Unknown
3. **Have you ever had an allergic reaction to an injection?** ☐ Yes ☐ No ☐ Unknown
4. **Are you pregnant, or think you may be?** ☐ Yes ☐ No ☐ Unknown
5. **Do you have a blood clotting disorder, or are you taking blood thinning medication?** ☐ Yes ☐ No ☐ Unknown

CONSENT AND RELEASE STATEMENT

I, THE UNDERSIGNED, WISH TO RECEIVE A -------------------- VACCINE. I CONSENT TO THE VACCINATION BEING GIVEN TO ME. I HAVE READ THE PROVIDED INFORMATION OR HAVE HAD SUCH EXPLAINED TO ME. I UNDERSTAND THE RISKS AND BENEFITS OF THIS VACCINE. I HAVE HAD AN OPPORTUNITY TO ASK QUESTIONS, WHICH HAVE BEEN ANSWERED TO MY SATISFACTION. I HEREBY REQUEST THAT THE VACCINE BE GIVEN TO ME OR TO THE PERSON NAMED ABOVE FOR WHOM I AM AUTHORIZED TO MAKE THIS REQUEST.

Signature: ______________ **Date:** ______________

FIGURE 3.5 Vaccine Authorization Form.

PRACTICE REQUIREMENTS

Many healthcare professionals are required to complete an educational program before they can work in healthcare. Upon completion, they usually must pass an exam before practicing. This section discusses the practice requirements and scope of practice of physicians, advanced practice professionals, and other healthcare professionals (Table 3.3).

Practice Acts and State Boards

The Tenth Amendment of the US Constitution empowers each state to establish laws that protect the health and safety of that state's citizens. Each state has passed laws and regulations that govern the practice of medicine. These laws and regulations are in a state statute called the Medical Practice Act. The Medical Practice Act also outlines the responsibility of the state medical board.

Each state's medical board issues licenses to practice medicine. The board also investigates complaints and disciplines members who violate the law. The state medical board creates policies related to the practice of medicine. Other healthcare professionals (i.e., nurses) have Practice Acts and state boards with similar roles.

Licensure

Many healthcare professionals must have a state license before they begin their practice. The **licensure** process allows the state board to ensure that the healthcare professional meets the educational and training requirements. Passing the state licensing exam is a requirement for the license. Once a person gets a license, it needs to be renewed about every 1 to 2 years. Besides the renewal fee, many state boards require evidence of continuing education.

If a healthcare professional is already licensed in one state, there are different methods of obtaining a license in additional states:

- *Licensing exam*: Passing the state's licensing exam and meeting the requirements.

TABLE 3.3 Physicians, Advanced Practice Professionals, and Other Healthcare Professionals

TITLE	SCOPE OF PRACTICE	EDUCATION	CREDENTIAL AND LICENSE
Physicians			
Doctor of medicine (MD)	Trained in all areas of medicine to diagnose, treat, and prescribe medications; more focused on symptoms experienced by patient.	Beyond a bachelor's degree, must complete 4 years of medical school and 2–4 years of residency. Additional years of training may be required for specialties.	Must pass all three parts of the United States Medical Licensing Examination (USMLE). Must obtain state license to practice.
Doctor of osteopathy (DO)	Trained in all areas of medicine, like MD. Specially trained in the nervous and musculoskeletal systems and their influence on health and disease.		
Advanced Practice Professionals			
Physician assistant (PA)	Diagnoses and treats illnesses and prescribes medication; may specialize. Supervised by physician.	Must complete a 3-year PA program beyond a bachelor's degree.	Physician Assistant– Certified (PA-C) after passing the national exam. Must obtain state license to practice.
Clinical nurse specialist (CNS)	Diagnoses and treats patients. Many work in hospital and community settings.	Must complete a master's degree beyond registered nurse (RN) training; an advanced practiced registered nurse (APRN).	Must pass the national certification exam. Must obtain state license to practice.
Nurse practitioner (NP)	Diagnoses and treats patients and prescribes medication; may specialize. Depending on state law, can be more independent than a PA.		
Certified nurse midwife (CNM)	Provides prenatal and postpartum care; delivers babies.		
Certified registered nurse anesthetist (CRNA)	Gives anesthesia and related care to patients in surgery and for outpatient procedures.		
Other Healthcare Professionals			
Registered nurse (RN)	Works in a wide range of positions, including clinical and administrative; performs more advanced assessments, patient care, and treatments than LPNs.	Must have 2–4 years of education.	Must pass a licensure exam to practice.
Licensed practical nurse (LPN)	Works in long-term care, ambulatory care, and hospital settings; performs basic patient assessments, patient care, and treatments.	Must have 1 year of education.	Must pass a licensure exam to practice.
Medical assistant (MA)	Primarily works in ambulatory care settings. Performs administrative, clinical, and CLIA-waived laboratory testing under the supervision of a provider.	Varies from about 8 to 24 months; may get a diploma or an associate degree.	National certification exam is optional.

CLIA, Clinical Laboratory Improvement Amendments.

- *Endorsement*: A state board grants a license to a person who is currently licensed in another state that has the same or stricter standards.
- *Reciprocity*: A state has a written agreement with another state to recognize licenses issued by that state without additional review of the person's credentials.

In 2015 the Interstate Medical Licensure Compact was created. This compact helped create a streamlined pathway for physicians to get licensure in multiple states. With the changes in healthcare, more rural care is provided by **telemedicine**, and more physicians are becoming **locum tenens**. With these changes, the need for licensure from multiple states has increased. To be eligible for licensure through the compact's process, physicians need to meet several requirements. Eligible physicians can select the compact member states where they would like to practice. Once the verification process has been completed, the physician will get a full, unrestricted license to practice medicine in those states.

Scope of Practice

The *scope of practice* for an occupation defines the procedures, actions, and processes that individuals are permitted to perform. A state board determines the scope of practice for that state's specific occupations. In some cases, the medical state board oversees the scope of practice of other healthcare occupations. If healthcare professionals practice beyond their scope of practice, they risk being sued for malpractice.

Scope of Practice for Physicians. The scope of practice for physicians is similar across the states. Physicians diagnose, treat, prevent, or monitor disease conditions. The scope of practice differs between specialties. For instance, a family practice physician cannot perform heart surgery.

Scope of Practice for Medical Assistants. For medical assistants, the scope of practice laws varies by state. Typical duties of a medical assistant include the following:

- Obtaining and recording the patient's history and personal information
- Obtaining and recording vital signs (blood pressure, pulse, respiration rate), height, and weight
- Assisting the provider during physical exams
- Administering oral, injectable, and inhaled medications as directed by provider and as permitted by state law
- Obtaining blood samples for laboratory tests
- Performing laboratory tests that have been waived by the Clinical Laboratory Improvement Amendments (CLIA)
- Scheduling patients for appointments
- Performing receptionist duties
- Billing insurance companies and patients for services

Some states allow medical assistants to perform injections. Some states do not allow medical assistants to give certain types of injectable medications or calculate the medication amount. It is important for you to know the legal scope of practice in your state (Procedure 3.2).

Legal Example: Scope of Practice

An obstetrician-gynecologist performed a procedure on a patient in her office. A few days after the procedure, the patient had increased pain that radiated along her side to her back. The patient called the office and spoke to a medical assistant. She mentioned the increase in pain, bleeding, and changes in her bowel movements. The medical assistant thought she had a urinary tract infection, so she asked the patient if she had any of the typical symptoms. The medical assistant did not talk to the provider about the patient's pain or bleeding because she did not think the complaints were serious enough. The medical assistant did not ask more questions about the pain or bleeding. The medical assistant told the patient her symptoms could be normal and advised her to take 800 mg of ibuprofen. (The medical assistant had been instructed by the providers to advise patients to take ibuprofen, 800 mg, every 8 hours as needed, for any sort of abdominal or back pain.) Later the patient was admitted to the intensive care unit, had to undergo a hysterectomy, and later died. Two months after the procedure, the patient's antibiotic prescription was found at the front desk. (The front desk staff had failed to give the patient the prescription after the procedure.)

The plaintiff sued for damages for the doctor's professional negligence (malpractice) and sued the clinic for the medical assistant's and front desk staff's negligence. After a 16-day trial, the jury returned a verdict for the defense. The plaintiff appealed. The appeals court ruled that the complaint was ordinary negligence and not medical malpractice. The appeals court also stated that the plaintiff could sue the clinic and medical assistant. The jury would have to decide if the medical assistant had practiced medicine without a license.

From *Wong v. Chappell*, No. 333 Ga. App. 422, (2015), www.leagle.com/decision/ingaco20150713164.

Disciplinary Action

The state boards have an obligation to the public to protect consumers. To do this, state boards take disciplinary action against licensed professionals for felony convictions and unprofessional, improper, or incompetent practice. Many types of unprofessional conduct by physicians can lead to such discipline:

- Substance and alcohol abuse
- Neglect of a patient
- Sexual misconduct
- Not meeting the accepted standard of care
- Dishonesty when obtaining a license or failing to meet the continuing education requirement
- Conviction of a felony or fraud
- Inadequate record-keeping
- Delegating others to practice medicine

The following are some of the disciplinary actions state boards can take against healthcare professionals:

- *License revoked*: License is terminated, and the person can no longer practice in that occupation in the state.
- *License suspended*: Person cannot practice in that occupation for a specific period of time.
- *License surrendered*: Person voluntarily gives up license.
- *Probation*: Person's license is monitored for a specific period of time.
- *Reprimand*: Person is sent a warning or letter of concern.

Certification and Registration

For some healthcare professional occupations, certification or registry is available. *Certification* is a voluntary process indicating that a person has met predetermined criteria. The certification is granted by a nongovernmental agency, such as a national association. Most certifications require educational preparation and passing the certification exam. Medical assistants can obtain a certification. For advanced practice professionals, many state boards require certification before the professional can apply for a license. Ongoing certification requirements vary by state. In many states, the ongoing certification is voluntary.

Some healthcare occupations have registration. People working in a specific occupation have their names entered into an official registry. To become registered, a person must meet requirements. These may include educational training, passing a registry exam, participating in continuing education, and conditions of that registry.

ACCREDITATION

Accreditation differs from licensure and certification. *Accreditation* is a recognition granted by a specific organization to educational, healthcare, or managed care organizations that have demonstrated compliance with standards.

Common Accreditation Organizations

Common accreditation organizations include the following:

- *The Joint Commission*: Accredits ambulatory care facilities, hospitals, behavioral healthcare facilities, home healthcare agencies, and laboratory services
- *National Committee for Quality Assurance* (NCQA): Accredits health plans (i.e., managed care plans)

- *College of American Pathologists* (CAP) *Laboratory Accreditation Program*: Accredits medical laboratories
- *Commission on Accreditation of Allied Health Education Programs* (CAAHEP): Accredits specific allied health programs, including medical assisting
- *Accrediting Bureau of Health Education Schools* (ABHES): Accredits both schools and specific allied health programs, including medical assisting

Advantages of Accreditation

There are advantages to being accredited. Students from accredited medical assisting programs can take specific certification examinations. Agencies that have Joint Commission accreditation gain the community's confidence in the quality and safety of the care provided. Insurance companies recognize the accreditation and may reduce liability insurance costs.

CLOSING COMMENTS

Patient Coaching

As stated in Chapter 1 with GIVE (*g*reet, *i*dentify, *v*erify, and *e*xplain), it is important for the medical assistant to explain the procedure or treatment to the patient before it begins. As part of the Patient Care Partnership, patients need to be coached on what is going to occur. The medical assistant must use words that the patient understands and answer any questions the patient may have. If the medical assistant does not know the answer, it is important to talk with the provider and then make sure the patient's question is answered.

Legal and Ethical Issues

Learning about concepts of law is important for all healthcare professionals. The medical assistant is trained to perform administrative, patient care, and laboratory skills that are CLIA waived (i.e., permitted for medical assistants by the Clinical Laboratory Improvement Amendments). With this wide range of duties, it is critical that medical assistants always remember to work within the boundaries of the law and their scope of practice.

Some areas can be problematic for medical assistants and may lead to lawsuits:

- Not following up with patients who call the ambulatory care facility
- Not getting consent before giving a child a vaccination
- Not documenting phone calls, procedures, and treatments
- Identifying oneself as another type of healthcare professional (e.g., a nurse)
- Giving advice to patients without the permission of healthcare providers

With the increase in lawsuits through the years, healthcare professionals must practice within their scope of practice and ensure that patients have no grounds for lawsuits.

Patient-Centered Care

One of the elements of patient-centered care is respect for patients' preferences. The medical assistant may not understand why a patient refuses a test, procedure, or treatment. Some patients do not share their thoughts on such matters. Other patients may cite a personal belief or a religious belief. As a medical assistant, you might not agree with the patient's ideas or beliefs. To provide exceptional customer service, a medical assistant must be sensitive to the patient's rights. This means the medical assistant must be respectful of the patient's right to refuse and must notify the provider. It is not appropriate for the medical assistant to do any of the following:

- Pressure the patient into changing the refusal
- Gossip with peers about the patient's refusal
- Make fun of the patient
- Providing patient-centered care means the medical assistant respects patients and their right to refuse.

Professional Behaviors

Part of being professional is protecting the healthcare facility and the providers from lawsuits that might stem from one's own actions. The medical assistant is not exempt from being named in lawsuits. Here are some strategies that may reduce the risk of lawsuits:

- Respecting and communicating professionally with patients
- Working within one's scope of practice
- Accurately and concisely documenting all patient encounters
- Following the facility's policies and procedures

SUMMARY OF SCENARIO

Daniela enjoyed working with Bella as she studied for her midterm exam in her law class. She found that Bella had unique ways of remembering and explaining concepts. These methods helped Daniela. Daniela knew it was important for her to understand the concepts because they might appear on her national certification test.

Daniela now understands the legal importance of answering patients' calls and returning them. She knows this is important to prevent abandonment suits from patients. Daniela encourages her peers to return calls in a timely manner and has talked with her supervisor about strategies to make the reception desk more efficient.

Thanks to Bella's help, Daniela also realizes the importance of the Patient's Bill of Rights to patients and every healthcare professional. These rights must be upheld and respected. Medical assistants and other healthcare professionals must be sensitive when patients refuse tests, treatments, and procedures. Daniela is looking forward to studying more about the healthcare laws and learning how they affect her job.

SUMMARY OF LEARNING OBJECTIVES

1. **Examine the legal system in the United States at the federal and state level, including the balance of power and the types of laws.**
The legal system of the United States is made up of both federal and state laws and is designed to allow for a balance of power. The three branches of government are the legislative, executive, and judicial branches. The four types of law are constitutional, case, regulatory and administrative, and statutory law.
2. **Differentiate between criminal and civil law.**
In criminal law, the state or federal government is the plaintiff, and the defendant is the party accused. The offense is a crime, and the standard of proof is that the charge must be proved beyond a reasonable doubt. A medical assistant who gives a patient medication without a provider's order is prescribing medication, which is a criminal offense.
In civil law, the victim is the plaintiff and the person accused is the wrongdoer. The offense can be called a tort or a breach of contract. The standard of proof requires the preponderance of evidence. A medical assistant who does a task within his or her scope of practice based on a provider's order, but does it incorrectly, may be sued.
3. **Differentiate between intentional torts and negligent (unintentional) torts.**
In an intentional tort, the plaintiff must prove the defendant had specific intent to perform the action that caused the injury. Examples include assault, battery, and false imprisonment. Refer back to the Intentional Torts section to read more about the different types of intentional torts.
Negligent torts are more common in healthcare because they are unintentional. The harm that is caused by negligence is the result of a person's carelessness. Negligence results when a person's conduct falls below the standard of behavior expected of a reasonable person in the same situation.
4. **Differentiate among the three main types of defenses used for lawsuits.**
There are three main defenses used for lawsuits:
    - Denial defense: Used when none of the facts are true.
    - Technical defenses: Used to have the case dismissed based on a legal technicality. Include statute of limitations, Good Samaritan law, release of tortfeasor, and res judicata.
    - Affirmative defense: The defendant admits to wrongdoing, but the defense attorney introduces facts that support the defendant's conduct. The following are common affirmative defenses: contributory negligence, comparative negligence, assumption of risk, limited or no harm, and intervening cause.
5. **Examine how a civil lawsuit is resolved, including proving negligence, the stages of a lawsuit, and types of damages awarded.**
Negligence is the failure to act as a reasonably prudent person would under similar circumstances; such conduct falls below the standards of behavior established by law for the protection of others against unreasonable risk of harm. The 4 *D*s of negligence include the duty of care, dereliction, damages, and direct cause.
Stages of a civil lawsuit include the prefiling phase, initial pleading phase, discovery phase, and postdiscovery phase. After the postdiscovery phase, the suit may be dropped, a summary judgment may be given, the parties may use alternative dispute resolution, or the case may go to trial.
Damages are a monetary settlement. There are several types of damages including punitive, nominal, compensatory, general, and special.
6. **Differentiate between types of liability insurance and types of policies.**
Liability insurance provides protection from claims of injuries or damage to people or property. Different types of liability insurance include professional liability (which includes medical malpractice insurance), general liability or commercial liability insurance, and personal injury insurance.
When a professional purchases a policy, it is important to understand the types of policies, including claims-made, occurrence, nose coverage, and tail coverage.
7. **Examine contracts, including the elements required for a legally binding contract, the types of contracts, and breach of contract.**
A contract is an agreement between two parties. For a contract to be legally binding, these elements must be present: offer, acceptance, consideration, legal subject matter, competency, and capacity.
A contract can be either an implied contract or an expressed contract. Specific types of contracts must be in writing to avoid fraud. These types of contracts are outlined in each state's statute of frauds. A breach of contract occurs when the terms of the contract are not fulfilled by one party without a legitimate legal reason.
8. **Examine the provider-patient relationship, including termination procedures and the medical assistant's role with the relationship.**
The provider-patient relationship can be terminated if the provider is retiring or moving. It can also be terminated if the patient is not paying for the services provided, is not following or is noncompliant with the provider's treatment plan, or based on the patient's behavior.
To terminate the provider-patient relationship, the provider must notify the patient in writing of the withdrawal of care. A date must be indicated for the termination. The termination letter should be sent as a certified letter with return receipt requested. A copy of the letter and the return receipt must be placed in the health record. Scheduling staff should be notified of the termination date, so no appointments are made after that date.
The medical assistant must prevent patient abandonment by following up with patients in a reasonable period of time.
9. **Examine consents, including types of consents in healthcare, elements required for informed consents, and the medical assistant's role.**
In healthcare, implied, expressed, and informed consents are used. Informed consent is used for many medical procedures and treatments. For an informed consent to occur, the patient or guardian must meet the following conditions:
    - Is competent to understand and decide
    - Voluntarily decides to agree to or refuse the treatment
    - Understands the diagnosis and reason for treatment, the proposed treatment and the risks of the treatment, the alternative treatments available and the risks of the treatments, and the risks if treatment is delayed or not done
    - Signs a treatment consent form

    Adults of sound mind can give informed consent. Married minors, minor parents, emancipated minors, and mature minors can also give informed consent.

Continued

SUMMARY OF LEARNING OBJECTIVES—cont'd

The medical assistant prepares the informed consent form and may also be asked to sign the form as a witness to the signature of the patient. All patient questions should be answered before the form is completed.

10. **Examine the medical assistant's role with the Patient Care Partnership (e.g., Patient's Bill of Rights).**
    The Patient's Bill of Rights provides patients with information on their rights under federal and state laws. Medical assistants must ensure they uphold and respect patients' rights. See Figure 3.3 for the typical parts of the Patient's Bill of Rights.
11. **Examine practice requirements for healthcare professionals and organizations.**
    Each state's medical board issues licenses to practice medicine. The board also investigates complaints and disciplines members who violate the law. Other healthcare professionals (i.e., nurses) have practice acts and state boards with similar roles.
    Licensure is a mandatory process established by state law that ensures a person has met the legal standards for practicing an occupation in that state. If a person is already licensed in one state, different methods of obtaining a license in other states exist, including taking the licensing exam, endorsement, and reciprocity.
    The scope of practice for an occupation defines the procedures, actions, and processes that individuals are permitted to perform. The state boards define the scope of practice and also take disciplinary action against licensed professionals for felony convictions and unprofessional, improper, or incompetent practice.
    Certification is a voluntary process indicating that a person has met predetermined criteria. The certification is granted by a nongovernmental agency. To become registered, a person must meet requirements. These may include educational training, passing a registry exam, participating in continuing education, and conditions of that registry.
12. **Examine accreditation, including the purpose and common accreditation organizations.**
    Accreditation is a recognition granted by a specific organization to educational, healthcare, or managed care organizations that have demonstrated compliance with standards. Many types of healthcare programs, healthcare facilities, laboratory services, and health plans are accredited.

PROCEDURE 3.1 Apply the Patient's Bill of Rights

TASKS: Apply the Patient's Bill of Rights in scenarios related to the choice of treatment, consent for treatment, and refusal of treatment. Demonstrate sensitivity to the patients' rights.

SCENARIO 1 (CHOICE OF TREATMENT): Julia Berkley (DOB 07/05/19XX) saw Dr. Angela Perez during her entire pregnancy. Julia is experiencing some complications. Dr. Perez explained the choices Julia had for delivery. She stated that, with the complications, a cesarean delivery (C-section) might be the best option. Because you are working with Dr. Perez, you prepare the consent form for the C-section. You go into the exam room to have Julia sign the consent form. As you discuss the form, Julia tells you that she is fearful of a C-section and wants a vaginal delivery.

SCENARIO 2 (CONSENT FOR TREATMENT): Ken Thomas (DOB 10/25/19XX) sees Jean Burke, NP, before leaving for a week-long trip out of the country. He is leaving in 3 days and wants a hepatitis A vaccine injection. The area he is traveling to has a high risk for hepatitis A. Jean Burke orders immunoglobulin for Ken, which will provide immediate protection against hepatitis A. You prepare the injection and enter the exam room. As you are telling Ken about the side effects of the medication, he asks, "What is immunoglobulin?" You reply that it is a sterile medication made of antibodies from blood. Ken states that he is a Jehovah's Witness and cannot receive blood products.

SCENARIO 3 (REFUSAL OF TREATMENT): Aaron Jackson (DOB 10/17/20XX) is brought in by his mother for his well-child checkup. His records indicate that he is due for his first varicella vaccine injection. You bring the Varicella (Chickenpox) Vaccine VIS (vaccine information statement) and the Vaccine Authorization form to the exam room. As you start to discuss the vaccine, Aaron's mother, Patricia, interrupts you and tells you she is not interested in having Aaron get his chickenpox vaccination.

EQUIPMENT and SUPPLIES

- Patient's health records
- Patient's Bill of Rights (see Figure 3.3)
- General Procedure Consent form (Figure 3.4)
- Varicella (Chickenpox) VIS (available at www.cdc.gov)
- Vaccine Authorization form (Figure 3.5)

PROCEDURAL STEPS

1. Review the Patient's Bill of Rights. Apply the Patient's Bill of Rights as you role-play each of the three scenarios.
   PURPOSE: A medical assistant needs to be knowledgeable about the facility's Patient's Bill of Rights.
2. Using scenario 1, role-play the situation with a peer. You are the medical assistant. Demonstrate how a medical assistant should handle the situation. Apply the Patient's Bill of Rights to the situation by remembering the rights of the patient.
   a. Show sensitivity to the patient by being respectful and professional. Be open and accepting in your verbal and nonverbal body language.
   PURPOSE: Being open and accepting shows the patient sensitivity and respect. The medical assistant should never show any mannerisms that

PROCEDURE 3.1 Apply the Patient's Bill of Rights—cont'd

would pressure the patient into making a choice that is not what the person wants.

b. Ask the patient if she has any questions about the procedure. Let the provider know if the patient has questions.

PURPOSE: All patient questions need to be addressed before the patient can make an informed decision on the treatment.

c. Ask the patient what she would like to do. Based on her answer, follow up as necessary.

PURPOSE: If the patient wants a C-section, then the consent form should be completed. If the patient wants a vaginal delivery, then no consent form will be needed unless indicated by state laws.

d. Using the patient's health record, document the patient's decision and the name of the provider notified.

PURPOSE: Documenting the patient's refusal of treatment is important legally. It is also important that the medical assistant document that the provider was informed of the decision.

3. Using scenario 2, role-play the situation with a peer. You are the medical assistant. Demonstrate how a medical assistant should handle the situation. Apply the Patient's Bill of Rights to the situation by remembering the rights of the patient.

a. Show sensitivity to the patient regarding his right to refuse. Be respectful and professional. Be open and accepting in your verbal and nonverbal body language. Be accepting of his beliefs and his refusal.

PURPOSE: Being open and accepting shows the patient sensitivity and respect. The medical assistant should never show any mannerisms that would pressure the patient into making a choice that is not what the person wants. The patient has a right to make decisions that follow his religious beliefs.

b. When the patient refuses the medication, be respectful in your body language and words. Notify the provider.

PURPOSE: It is important to be respectful of the patient's decision and notify the provider of the refusal.

c. Using the patient's health record, document the patient's decision and the name of the provider notified.

PURPOSE: Documenting the patient's refusal of treatment is important legally. It is also important that the medical assistant document that the provider was informed of the decision.

4. Using scenario 3, role-play the situation with a peer. You are the medical assistant. Demonstrate how a medical assistant should handle the situation. Apply the Patient's Bill of Rights to the situation by remembering the rights of the patient.

a. Show sensitivity to the mother of the patient by being respectful and professional. Be open and accepting in your verbal and nonverbal body language.

PURPOSE: Being open and accepting shows the family member and the patient sensitivity and respect. The medical assistant should never show any mannerisms that would pressure the patient or guardian into making a choice that is not what the person wants.

b. Ask the mother if she has any questions about the vaccine. Let the provider know if the mother has questions.

PURPOSE: All patient and parent/guardian questions need to be addressed before an informed decision can be made on the treatment.

c. Ask the mother what she would like to do. Based on her answer, follow up as necessary.

PURPOSE: If the parent/guardian consents to the vaccination, the Vaccine Authorization form must be completed. If the parent/guardian refuses, the provider needs to be notified.

d. Using the health record, document the patient's decision and the name of the provider notified.

PURPOSE: Documenting the patient's refusal of treatment is important legally. It is also important that the medical assistant document that the provider was informed of the decision.

PROCEDURE 3.2 Locate the Medical Assistant's Legal Scope of Practice

TASKS: Search online to locate the legal scope of practice for a medical assistant practicing in your state. Summarize the scope of practice.

EQUIPMENT and SUPPLIES

- Computer
- Printer with word processing software
- Internet access

PROCEDURAL STEPS

1. Using the internet, search for the medical assistant's scope of practice in your state. Read the scope of practice for your state.

PURPOSE: Scope of practice information is available online.

2. Using the word processing software, create a short paper summarizing the medical assistant's scope of practice. Address the following points:

a. Can medical assistants give injections? If so, what type of injections?

b. Can medical assistants give oral, topical, or inhaled medications?

c. Can medical assistants calculate drug dosages?

d. What is the medical assistant's role with prescriptions?

e. Describe additional duties that a medical assistant can legally perform in your state.

f. Include the website address(es) you used for this paper.

Note: If your instructor does not provide you with different guidelines for the paper, follow these. Create at least a one-page paper, using double line spacing, a 10- or 12-point font, and 1-inch margins.

PURPOSE: Summarizing the scope of practice will help identify the duties a medical assistant can legally perform in your state.

3. After completing the paper, proofread it. Use correct spelling, punctuation, sentence structure, and capitalization. Make any changes required. Based on your instructor's directions, submit the paper to the instructor.

PURPOSE: Proofreading helps to identify mistakes.

HEALTHCARE LAWS

4

SCENARIO

Daniela Garcia was recently hired as a part-time float receptionist at Walden-Martin Family Medical (WMFM) Clinic. She works with many co-workers and providers. Daniela is attending the medical assistant program at the local community college. She is currently taking a law and ethics course. She has learned about basic law concepts. She is now learning about healthcare laws. Bella, a newly certified medical assistant (CMA), has offered to help Daniela study for her law course. Bella stated that she enjoyed learning about law and its importance in healthcare.

Many of Daniela's friends find law and ethics to be less exciting than other courses. Daniela disagrees with them. She sees the value in learning about laws that affect healthcare. She realizes it will make her a better medical assistant.

The WMFM Clinic administration created policies and procedures to follow federal and state laws. Daniela has already started to see how compliance with laws affects what she does as a receptionist. She understands the importance of following the clinic's policies and procedures. Daniela realizes that by not complying with laws, she would put her job in jeopardy. It could also raise many issues for the facility, including fines from government agencies. Daniela is excited to continue learning about healthcare laws.

While studying this chapter, think about the following questions:

- What is the importance of the Health Insurance Portability and Accountability Act (HIPAA)? Why should a medical assistant know about the Privacy Rule and the Security Rule?
- What is the impact of the Health Information Technology for Economic and Clinical Health (HITECH) Act on ambulatory care facilities?
- What important healthcare laws and regulations must be followed in the ambulatory care environment?
- What is the provider's role in compliance with public health statutes?
- What compliance programs address financial, employment, and environmental safety concerns?

LEARNING OBJECTIVES

1. Differentiate between privacy and confidentiality.
2. Examine the goals, standards, and terminology of the Health Insurance Portability and Accountability Act.
3. Analyze how to comply with the Privacy Rule when releasing patient information.
4. Examine how healthcare facilities comply with the Security Rule.
5. Examine how the Health Information Technology for Economic and Clinical Health (HITECH) Act and the Genetic Information Nondiscrimination Act (GINA) modified the Health Insurance Portability and Accountability Act (HIPAA).
6. Differentiate between the Food, Drug, and Cosmetic Act and the Controlled Substances Act.
7. Differentiate between the Occupational Safety and Health Act and the Needlestick Safety and Prevention Act.
8. Examine healthcare laws related to insurance, laboratory quality standards, emergency care, and end-of-life care.
9. Differentiate types of situations that providers must report to comply with federal and state laws.
10. Examine compliance programs, including the purpose and reporting procedures.
11. Examine illegal financial activities in healthcare, including identity theft, conflict of interest, and fraud.
12. Examine employment laws related to hiring, firing, discrimination, wage, and safety.
13. Differentiate between the laws that protect patients from discrimination.
14. Examine how incident reports and risk management protect patients and healthcare facilities.

VOCABULARY

abuse An action that purposely harms another person.

advance directives Written instructions about healthcare decisions in case a person is unable to make them.

breach Disclosure of protected health information without a reason or permission, which compromises the security or privacy of the information.

claims clearinghouse An organization that accepts the claim data from the provider, reformats the data to meet the specifications outlined by the insurance plan, and submits the claim.

coding system A system designed to use characters (i.e., numbers and letters) to represent something, such as a medical procedure or a disease.

VOCABULARY—*continued*

communicable diseases Diseases spread from person to person by either direct contact or indirect contact (e.g., insects).

dependent adults People between the ages of 18 and 64 who have a mental or physical impairment that prevents them from doing normal activities or from protecting themselves.

discrimination (dis krim eh NAE shuhn) Unfair treatment of another person based on the person's age, gender, ethnicity, sexual orientation, disability, marital status, or other selective factors.

egress (EE gress) Leaving a place; exit route.

electronic health record (EHR) An electronic record that conforms to nationally recognized standards and contains health-related information about a specific patient. It can be created, managed, and consulted by authorized clinicians and staff from more than one healthcare organization.

electronic transaction The electronic exchange of information between two agencies to accomplish financial or administrative healthcare activities.

exploitation (eks ploi TAY shuhn) The act of using another person for one's own advantage.

harassment (hah RAS ment) Continued, unwanted, and annoying actions done to another person.

neglect Failure to provide proper attention or care to another person.

precedence (PRES i dehns) The top priority.

privileged communication Communication that cannot be disclosed without authorization of the person involved; includes provider-patient and lawyer-client communications.

retaliation (ree tal ee A shuhn) Getting back at others for something they did to you.

retribution (reh trih BYOU shuhn) Punishment inflicted on someone as vengeance for a wrong or criminal act; the act of taking revenge.

whistleblower A person (usually an employee) who reports a violation of the law within an organization. The person reports the information to the public or a person in authority.

INTRODUCTION

In this chapter, we discuss federal and state laws that impact healthcare. Typically, a few people are considered to be the experts on healthcare laws in an ambulatory care setting. They work with management to create policies and procedures that follow the laws.

- *Policies* are written principles that provide goals for the employees and the facility. For instance, a policy statement may indicate that patient confidentiality is protected at all times.
- *Procedures* are step-by-step directions. They provide a consistent and repetitive approach to accomplishing a goal. For instance, there might be a procedure on how to update patient information while protecting the patient's privacy.

Following the laws is important. Not only does it safeguard patients, but it also protects employees and the facility. Facilities that do not comply with laws can be fined and have additional penalties imposed by government agencies. Therefore, medical assistants need to be knowledgeable about healthcare laws.

PRIVACY AND CONFIDENTIALITY

All states have laws related to privacy and confidentiality. If the state law is stricter than the federal law, then the state law takes **precedence**. This concept is known as *state preemption*.

Medical assistants must follow federal laws related to privacy and confidentiality, starting with their medical assistant clinical experiences. Before the federal laws are examined, it is important to have an understanding of the concepts of privacy and confidentiality.

Privacy

Privacy means being free from unwanted intrusion. Privacy was one of the principles on which our country was built. The word *privacy* does not appear in the Constitution, but privacy elements appear in the amendments. An *invasion of privacy* is the disclosing of private facts without the consent of the individual. An invasion of privacy is an intentional tort.

Confidentiality

Confidentiality is a legally protected right of patients. Healthcare professionals have the duty not to disclose medical, financial, and insurance information unless authorized by the patient. Information is shared during the provider-patient relationship, so creating a trusting relationship is critical (Figure 4.1). The patient shares sensitive, personal information with the provider, which needs to remain confidential. It cannot be discussed outside of the provider-patient relationship.

HEALTH INSURANCE PORTABILITY AND ACCOUNTABILITY ACT

The Health Insurance Portability and Accountability Act of 1996 (HIPAA) is a federal law that protects the privacy and confidentiality of patients. The following sections will examine the history, terminology, and standards of HIPAA.

Goals of HIPAA

With the anticipated changes in healthcare technology (e.g., the **electronic health record [EHR]**), Congress passed the Health

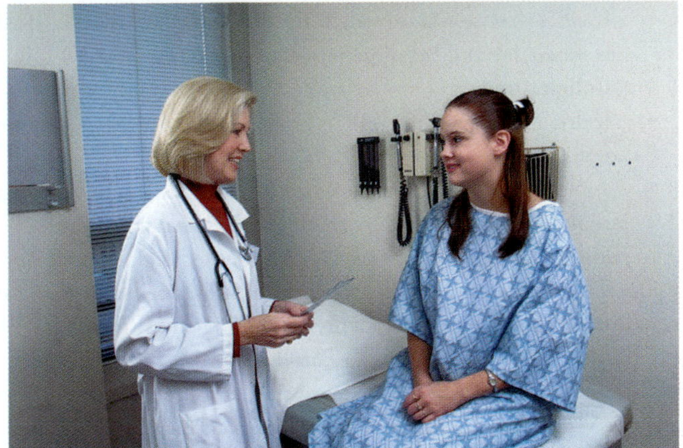

FIGURE 4.1 Patient confidentiality is the most important trust that exists between the patient and the provider.

Insurance Portability and Accountability Act of 1996 (HIPAA). The US Department of Health and Human Services (HHS) is the agency responsible for developing the specific requirements of the law. The HHS Office for Civil Rights (OCR) enforces HIPAA.

Before HIPAA, the billing and payment processes were slow. Nationwide, insurance companies used many different **coding systems.** The coding systems were used to provide information on disease and treatments for payment purposes. It took months for facilities to receive insurance payments for services provided to patients. Paper transactions and paper checks were commonly used.

One of the goals of HIPAA was to simplify the electronic exchange of information. All health plans, **claims clearinghouses,** and healthcare facilities needed to be consistent with their electronic exchange of information. This meant they all needed to use the same coding systems. They also needed to follow the same requirements for the electronic exchange of information. Today, this is called *administrative simplification.* The goal is to reduce the clerical burden and increase **electronic transaction** adoption.

Four Standards of HIPAA

With the increased electronic transactions, HIPAA also contained provisions for the privacy and security of the patients' information. Primary provisions of the law were stated in four standards:

- *Standard 1 related to transactions and code sets*: HHS adopted standard transactions for the electronic exchange of administrative healthcare information. This included insurance claims, payment, and insurance eligibility information. The goal was to speed up the process of identifying insurance benefits, submitting insurance claims, and receiving payment. Standard 1 also included mandating universal coding systems. Processes become more efficient with everyone using the same coding systems:
  - The Current Procedural Terminology (CPT) is used to code procedures and services.
  - The International Classification of Diseases (ICD) is used to code diseases and disorders.
- *Standard 2 related to the Privacy Rule*: Healthcare facilities, insurance companies, and others need to protect written, electronic, and oral patient health information.
- *Standard 3 related to the Security Rule*: Healthcare facilities, insurance companies, and others need to protect patient information that is electronically stored and transmitted.
- *Standard 4 related to unique identifiers:*
  - National Provider Identifier (NPI): Each covered healthcare provider has a unique identification number that is used for financial and administrative transactions. The NPI is a 10-digit number.
  - Health Plan Identifier (HPI): Each health plan has a unique identifier.
  - Employer Identification Number (EIN): Each employer has a unique identifier issued by the Internal Revenue Service.

In addition to these provisions, HIPAA focused on insurance portability. HIPAA states that employer health insurance plans may not exclude coverage for employees with preexisting conditions. HIPAA also allows extra opportunities to enroll in health insurance plans. For instance, a person can request special enrollment if there is a loss in coverage from another policy. HIPAA prohibited enrollment discrimination based on a person's health history or genetics.

HIPAA-Related Terminology

HIPAA has many unique terms:

- *Covered entities*: Healthcare providers, health (insurance) plans, and claims clearinghouses that transmit protected health information electronically. Examples of covered entities include these:
  - Providers (e.g., medical doctors, doctors of osteopathic medicine, nurse practitioners, physician assistants)
  - Dentists, chiropractors, and psychologists
  - Nursing homes, pharmacies, and ambulatory care facilities (e.g., clinics)
  - Health insurance companies, government insurance programs (Medicare, Medicaid), and health maintenance organizations (HMOs)
  - Claims clearinghouses and billing services
- *Protected health information* (PHI): Individually identifiable health information stored or transmitted by covered entities or business associates. Includes verbal, paper, or electronic information.
- *Business associate*: A person or business that provides a service to a covered entity that involves access to PHI. Examples include legal, billing, and management services; accreditation agencies; consulting firms; and claims processing organizations.
- *Permission*: A reason for releasing or disclosing patient information under HIPAA.
- *De-identify*: To remove all direct patient identifiers from the PHI. In other words, this is the process of removing anything that can link the information back to a specific person. Examples of direct patient identifiers include these:
  - Personal demographic information (name, date of birth, address, phone number, Social Security number)
  - Payment and insurance information
- *Limited data set*: PHI that has had all of the direct patient identifiers removed. This would include the name, contact information, Social Security number, and so on. The only information left would be health information. Examples of limited data set information include physical or mental health conditions, test results, medications currently taken, and allergies.

CRITICAL THINKING APPLICATION **4.1**

Daniela is working with Bella, a medical assistant who has been helping her with the law course. They are reviewing HIPAA. Bella asks Daniela to describe the four HIPAA standards. How might Daniela respond?

PRIVACY RULE

The HIPAA Privacy Rule has created national standards that protect health records and other patient information. The Privacy Rule's main purpose is to define and limit the situations in which a patient's information can be used or disclosed. The rule also describes patients' rights over their information. Patients have the right to do the following:

- Examine their health information
- Obtain a copy of their health records
- Request corrections to be made if the information is incorrect

Covered entities must comply with the Privacy Rule. They must safeguard all patient information. Covered entities must ensure that business associates also keep PHI private. A written agreement detailing how the business associate will safeguard the PHI must be signed. Covered entities cannot give PHI to business associates until the agreement has been signed. Only PHI required for the job of the business associates can be given.

Legal Example: HIPAA Settlement for Lack of Business Associate Agreement

In 2015 the Office for Civil Rights (OCR) of the federal Department of Health and Human Services (HHS) investigated the Center for Children's Digestive Health (CCDH). The CCDH failed to obtain a written, signed business associate agreement with Filefax. The CCDH disclosed the protected health information (PHI) of at least 10,728 patients to Filefax. In 2017 the CCDH paid the HHS $31,000 to settle the potential violations and agreed to implement a corrective action plan.

Resolution Agreement. Retrieved from www.hhs.gov/sites/default/files/ra_cap_ccdh.pdf.

Permissions Not Requiring Written Authorization

The Privacy Rule lists *permissions* or reasons that the health information can be released. The following permissions do not require written authorization from the patient to release PHI:

- *Treatment, payment, and healthcare operations* (TPO): Treatment relates to when the covered entity discloses PHI when coordinating or managing healthcare. For instance, you do not need to sign a written authorization for your provider to send a prescription to a pharmacy. Payment relates to activities related to payment or reimbursement for services. For instance, if you were not paying your bill, the healthcare facility might turn your account over to a collection agency. The facility would not need written authorization from you to disclose your information. Healthcare operations relate to the financial, legal, quality improvement, and administrative activities that healthcare facilities need to complete to run and support their business, such as patient case management.
- *Uses and disclosures with an opportunity to agree or object*: The patient can give informal permission when asked outright or can be given an opportunity to agree or object. For example, a patient comes into the exam room with a friend. You ask the patient if they want the friend to remain. The patient can say yes or no.
- *Incidental use and disclosure*: We need to take reasonable precautions, so patient information is not overheard or seen by others. The Privacy Rule does not require that we get written authorization for incidental disclosures. For instance, you take precautions, but you are overheard discussing patient PHI on the phone. There is no need for you to get a written authorization from the patient on the phone for the incidental disclosure.
- *Public interest and benefit activities*: PHI can be released when required by law, law enforcement, and public health activities. PHI can also be released for research, organ and tissue donation, and workers' compensation. Funeral directors, coroners, and medical examiners can also obtain PHI.
- *Limited data set*: The direct patient identifiers are removed from the PHI. The remaining information can be used for research, public health purposes, and healthcare operations.
- *To the individual*: A covered entity can disclose PHI to the patient. If you want a copy of your health record, you can get it without completing a written authorization (record release form).

Patients and Their Health Information

The physical part of the record belongs to the facility or provider. Under HIPAA, patients own the information in their health records. They also control when the information in their record is released to another party. There are state laws that regulate the release. In most cases, patients have a right to receive a copy of their information. The following examples illustrate cases in which patients cannot get their information immediately:

- When a provider is treating a patient for emotional or mental conditions, the provider can exercise professional judgment to determine if the records should be released to the patient. This is known as the *doctrine of professional discretion.* The provider may feel that if the patient saw the records, more harm than good would result. For instance, you are obtaining a weight on a patient with an eating disorder. The provider's policy is that you do not share the weight with the patient. The provider decides if the weight is shared. For some patients, a weight gain may harm their current success.
- Another situation in which patients cannot get health information immediately when requested relates to diagnostic tests. In the ambulatory care setting, patients have diagnostic tests done all the time. The provider must review the results before they are given to the patient. After reviewing the results, the provider instructs the medical assistant on what to tell the patient. The medical assistant contacts the patient and discusses what the provider stated. After the call, the medical assistant documents the call in the patient's health record.

Permission Requiring Written Authorization

The only permission that requires written authorization from patients is disclosing the PHI to a third party. Examples of this type of disclosure may include when the patient wants another person to be told information or when the patient wants the records transferred to another facility. This may include a life insurance company, an employer for a pre-employment health requirement, another healthcare facility, or the patient's lawyer. In both situations, the patient must sign a form allowing the information to be released. In some agencies, a *disclosure authorization form* (also called an *authorization to disclose form*) must be completed before information can be shared with another person. The patient must complete a *record release form* before the records can be transferred. The form names can differ from facility to facility. To make things more interesting, some facilities combine the forms into one document and may call it a release of information authorization or something similar.

The forms typically require the patient to indicate the information to be released/disclosed. The form must include the patient's name and the date of the request. The person or facility disclosing the information and receiving the information must be indicated. The form must include an expiration date. These forms also include a statement to notify patients of their right to revoke the release.

Disclosure Authorization Process

When patients request their information to be given to another person (e.g., family member or friend), the medical assistants can help.

They can assist patients in completing the disclosure authorization form (Figure 4.2). Once completed, this form must be added to the patient's health record.

When a person calls requesting information on a current patient, the medical assistant should first ask the caller's name. The medical assistant must check and see if the caller is listed on the patient's disclosure authorization form (Procedure 4.1). If that caller's name appears, then, per the facility's policy, the medical assistant can release information about the patient. If the caller's name is not on the form, the medical assistant has the following limitations:

- Cannot release the patient's information
- Cannot even acknowledge that that person is a patient of the facility

Applying HIPAA rules is important when protecting a patient's privacy.

In some facilities, the patient supplies a code word or number. This is documented in the patient's health record. The patient gives this code to family members. When they call the staff and give the code, the staff member can provide an update on the patient. It is understood that the patient gives consent to anyone who received the code. This helps to settle the issue of who is really calling requesting information. The code system may be seen more in the ambulatory surgical departments.

Records Release Process

Patients must complete, date, and sign a (medical) records release form for their records to be transferred to another facility (Figure 4.3; also see Procedure 4.2). No records, including images and videos, can be released without the completed form. Release forms may specifically address the release of videos and images. With these forms, patients must indicate they want these to be released. If that is not done, then the videos and images are not released.

Parts of the patient record are held at a higher level of confidentiality. Many release forms require the patient to indicate if psychotherapy notes, substance abuse information, and human immunodeficiency virus (HIV) information should be released. Such information may not be automatically released with the other records due to federal and state legislation.

WALDEN-MARTIN
FAMILY MEDICAL CLINIC
1234 ANYSTREET | ANYTOWN, ANYSTATE 12345
PHONE 123-123-1234 | FAX 123-123-5678

Disclosure Authorization

Full Name: ____________ **Date of Birth:** ____________

I hereby authorize ____________ **to use or disclose my protected health information related to** ____________

to ____________

Representative's Address:

Purpose:

- **I understand that I may inspect or copy the protected health information described by this authorization.**
- **I understand that, at any time, this authorization may be revoked, when the office that receives this authorization receives a written revocation, although that revocation will not be effective as to the disclosure of records whose release I have previously authorized, or where other action has been taken in reliance on an authorization I have signed. I understand that my healthcare and the payment for my healthcare will not be affected if I refuse to sign this form.**
- **I understand that information used or disclosed, pursuant to this authorization, could be subject to re-disclosure by the recipient and, if so, may not be subject to federal or state law protecting its confidentiality.**

Signature of Individual or Representative: ____________

Date: ____________

Authority or Relationship to Individual, if Representative: ____________

This authorization will expire on: ____________ **If no date or event is stated, the expiration date will be 6 years from the date of this authorization.**

The subject of this authorization shall receive a copy of this authorization, when signed.

FIGURE 4.2 Disclosure authorization form.

WALDEN-MARTIN
FAMILY MEDICAL CLINIC
1234 ANYSTREET | ANYTOWN, ANYSTATE 12345
PHONE 123-123-1234 | FAX 123-123-5678

Medical Records Release

Patient Name: ____________ **Date of Birth:** ____________
SSN: ____________ **Phone:** ____________
Address:

I, ____________ **authorize** ____________
to disclose/release the following information (check all applicable):

- ☐ All records
- ☐ Abstract/summary
- ☐ Laboratory/pathology records
- ☐ Pharmacy/prescription records
- ☐ X-ray/radiology records
- ☐ Other
- ☐ Billing records

****Note:*** *If these records contain any information from previous providers or information about HIV/AIDS status, cancer diagnosis, drug alcohol abuse, or sexually transmitted disease, you are hereby authorizing disclosure of this information. A copy of this signed authorization must be given to the individual.*

These records are for services provided on the following date(s): ____________

Please send the records listed above to (use additional sheets if necessary):

Name: ____________ **Phone:** ____________
Address: **Fax:** ____________

The information may be used/disclosed for each of the following purposes:

- ☐ At patient's request
- ☐ For employment purposes
- ☐ For patient's health care
- ☐ Other
- ☐ For payment/insurance

This authorization shall expire no later than: ______ **or upon the following event** ______ **, and may not be valid for greater than 1 year from the date of signature for medical records.**

I understand that after the custodian of records discloses my health information, it may no longer be protected by federal privacy laws. I understand that this authorization is voluntary and I may refuse to sign this authorization, which will not affect my ability to obtain treatment; receive payment; or eligibility for benefits unless allowed by law. By signing below I represent and warrant that I have authority to sign this document and authorize the use or disclosure of protected health information and that there are no claims or orders that would prohibit, limit, or otherwise restrict my ability to authorize the use or disclosure of this protected health information.

Patient signature
(or patient's personal representative) **Date**

Printed name of patient representative **Representative's authority to sign for patient**
(i.e. parent, guardian, power of attorney, executor)

FIGURE 4.3 Medical records release form.

Under HIPAA, psychotherapy notes are treated with higher levels of confidentiality. *Psychotherapy notes* include the patient-provider details from mental health treatment, either from a private, group, or family therapy. Psychotherapy notes include what the patient stated during the session and the provider's analysis of the patient's statements and the situation. Psychotherapy notes need to be stored separately from the patient paper health record. If the health record is electronic, the access to the psychotherapy notes is limited to those healthcare professionals who work in the mental health area. Additional information from the visit is not held at a higher level of confidentiality and includes prescriptions, session times, types and frequency of treatments, and results of clinical tests.

Drug and alcohol substance abuse and HIV content in patient records also are held at a higher level of confidentiality. There are many federal and state laws that relate to the privacy of these records. The federal statute called Confidentiality of Alcohol and Drug Abuse Patient Records, enforced by a division of HHS, is one example. This law restricts the release and use of patient records that include substance use diagnoses and services. State preemption applies to these privacy laws.

Legal Example: Disclosure of Protected Health Information

"John Doe," a man in his early 30s, was diagnosed and treated for the human immunodeficiency virus (HIV) at Spencer Cox Clinic of Mount Sinai St. Luke's Hospital in 2014. The patient had requested that his health records be sent to a post office box or his home address via regular mail. On September 11, 2014, John was handed his entire health record by his employer, who stated it was faxed to the mailroom. The health record contained HIV and mental health information, prescription drug information, and his Social Security number.

On September 12, 2014, a complaint was filed with the Department of Health and Human Services (HHS) Office for Civil Rights (OCR), alleging that John's protected health information (PHI) was faxed to his employer by an employee at St Luke's Spencer Cox Clinic. After investigating, the OCR found two instances of disclosure of PHI (that included HIV information) without patient authorization. St. Luke's agreed to pay HHS $387,200 and comply with the corrective action plan.

Resolution agreement retrieved from www.hhs.gov/sites/default/files/st-lukes-signed-ra-cap.pdf.

CRITICAL THINKING APPLICATION **4.2**

Daniela and Bella are reviewing HIPAA concepts. They start to discuss local news and a case in which a medical assistant snapped a picture of a patient record and posted it to a popular social media site. Bella asks Daniela what this action violated. How would you answer this question? Why are employee cell phones a risk in the healthcare setting?

SECURITY RULE

HIPAA's Security Rule addresses the national standards used to protect electronic protected health information (ePHI). This rule covers the records that are created, used, received, and maintained by the covered entities.

Safeguards of the Security Rule

Safeguards important to ensure the security of the ePHI include the following:

- *Administrative safeguards*: The security officer is responsible for creating and carrying out security policies and procedures. Potential risks to the ePHI must be identified. Steps must be taken to prevent any issues. Cyber attackers pose a huge risk to network security.
- *Physical safeguards*: Facility, workstation, and device security must be implemented. A security officer must create procedures for the proper use of workstations and ePHI.
- *Technical safeguards*: Only authorized employees should have access to ePHI. Safeguards include audits to track the activities of users with the ePHI and encryption of data on mobile devices. They also include safeguards to prevent improper alteration, destruction, or transmission of ePHI.

Chapter 6 provides additional information on network security procedures.

Legal Example: HIPAA Settlement for Unsecure Electronic Protected Health Information

In 2014 Touchstone Medical Imaging notified the Office for Civil Rights (OCR) that one of its servers allowed uncontrolled access to electronically protected health information (ePHI). During the OCR's investigation, it was found that over 300,000 patients' names, birth dates, Social Security numbers, and addresses were exposed on the internet. OCR also found that Touchstone failed to have business associate agreements in place for its internet technology (IT) support vendor and third-party data center provider. As a result, Touchstone paid $3 million in a monetary settlement, along with undertaking a corrective action plan.

Resolution agreement at
www.hhs.gov/sites/default/files/tennessee-diagnostic-medical-imaging-services-ra-cap.pdf.

Medical Assistant's Role

It is important for the medical assistant to follow the healthcare facility's electronic security procedures. Many facilities have policies to keep passwords confidential. Downloading personal documents puts the computer network at risk and thus is not allowed. *Audit trails* monitor who is looking at which patient's chart. If the medical assistant is not working with a specific patient, then the patient record should not be accessed. Violating this rule will cause the medical assistant to breach the patient's confidentiality and security. Many healthcare professionals, from providers to medical assistants, have breached confidentiality. They have lost their jobs and licenses or certifications. Many have also been fined. Healthcare employees cannot access their own health record or that of their family members. Most agencies require the employee to follow the patient's review of health record policy. Violating this policy can also lead to termination.

Legal Example: HIPAA Settlement for Unsecure Electronic Protected Health Information

The University of Rochester Medical Center (URMC) filed **breach** reports with the Office for Civil Rights (OCR) in 2013 and 2017 due to a loss of an unencrypted flash drive and theft of an unencrypted laptop. OCR's investigation found URMC failed to implement multiple security measures to protect electronic protected health information (ePHI). URMC had a prior OCR investigation regarding a lost unencrypted flash drive in 2010. As a result, URMC paid $3 million in a monetary settlement, along with undertaking a corrective action plan.

Resolution agreement at www.hhs.gov/sites/default/files/urmc-ra-cap-508.pdf.

Legal Example: HIPAA Settlement for Inappropriate Protected Health Information Access

In 2012 Memorial Healthcare System (MHS) submitted a breach report to the Department of Health and Human Services (HHS) indicating that two of its employees inappropriately accessed protected health information (PHI), potentially affecting 80,000 patients. Several months later, MHS notified HHS of another 12 users that inappropriately accessed PHI, which potentially affected another 105,646 individuals. As a result, some of the PHI was sold, and fraudulent tax returns were filed. In 2017 MHS paid the HHS $5.5 million to settle the potential violations and agreed to implement a corrective action plan.

Resolution agreement retrieved from www.hhs.gov/sites/default/files/memorial-ra-cap.pdf.

OTHER PRIVACY LAWS

Besides HIPAA, other federal laws protect the privacy of patients. Health Information Technology for Economic and Clinical Health (HITECH) Act and Genetic Information Nondiscrimination Act (GINA) modified HIPAA. The following sections discuss HITECH Act and GINA.

HITECH Act

One of the issues with HIPAA was the limited enforcement and penalties. In 2009, as part of the American Recovery and Reinvestment Act, the Health Information Technology for Economic and Clinical Health (HITECH) Act was passed. HITECH Act is enforced by the OCR.

The HITECH Act contains provisions that increase the enforcement of the privacy and security of electronic transmission and health information. HITECH Act modified HIPAA in the following ways:

- Made business associates directly liable for compliance with HIPAA.

- Prohibited the sale of PHI without the patient's authorization.
- Created a tiered violation category that included unknowing, reasonable cause, willful neglect–corrected, and willful neglect–uncorrected. Violation penalties range from $100 for each "unknowing" violation to $1.5 million per calendar year. The greater the violation, the greater the penalty amount. Individuals, healthcare agencies, and business associations could be penalized and fined.
- **Breach** notification requirements were increased. Individuals must be notified of the breach via mail or email. If the facility does not have up-to-date contact information for 10 or more patients, then a notice must be posted on the company's website for at least 90 days. If more than 500 individuals were affected, the media and the OCR secretary must be notified. A list of breaches reported is published on the OCR website (https://ocrportal.hhs.gov/ocr/breach/breach_report.jsf).

It is important for the medical assistant to be aware of the importance of keeping the PHI secure. Any breaches or loss/theft of computer equipment must be reported immediately to the facility's security officer.

CRITICAL THINKING APPLICATION 4.3

Daniela and Bella are reviewing HITECH Act. Daniela asks Bella why it is important for large breaches to be posted on the OCR website. How would you answer this question as an employee? How would you answer as a patient of a facility that had a posting on the OCR website?

Genetic Information Nondiscrimination Act

The Genetic Information Nondiscrimination Act (GINA) became law in 2008. GINA modified HIPAA by clarifying that genetic information is health information and prohibited the use and disclosure of genetic information by covered health plans. GINA consists of two sections or Titles:

- Title 1 of GINA: Prohibits discrimination based on genetic information in health coverage.
- Title II of GINA: Prohibits discrimination based on genetic information in employment.

DRUG LAWS

The Food, Drug, and Cosmetic Act and the Controlled Substance Act regulate medications in the United States. The following sections describe each law and how it impacts healthcare.

Food, Drug, and Cosmetic Act

In 1906, the Food and Drug Act became law. It prohibited the misbranding of food and drugs. It was replaced in 1938 by the Food, Drug, and Cosmetic Act, which is still enforced today. The US Food and Drug Administration (FDA) enforces the act. The FDA is responsible for the safety, effectiveness, security, and quality of drugs, cosmetics, and food. Some of the areas overseen by the FDA include human and veterinary drugs, vaccines, biological products (e.g., blood components), medical devices, food, cosmetics, dietary supplies, and products that give off radiation. When you see recalls of food, cosmetics, or medications, the FDA is involved with the process.

The FDA website (www.fda.gov) provides useful information for the healthcare facility. The website is the resource for information and recalls on the areas overseen by the FDA. Many times, the medical assistant is responsible for maintaining the stock medications and equipment in the department. Any medications or medical devices recalled need to be removed immediately and not used. The providers should be notified of recalls.

Controlled Substances Act

The Controlled Substances Act (part of the Comprehensive Drug Abuse Prevention and Control Act of 1970) is a federal law. The US Drug Enforcement Agency (DEA) enforces the law. The DEA oversees the manufacturing, importation, possession, use, and distribution of certain drugs and chemicals. The DEA handles both illegal and legal controlled substances. The Controlled Substances Act has five schedules of medications. These schedules are arranged from greatest to least abuse potential (Table 4.1). State statutes also address procedures related to scheduled medications. Some scheduled medication prescriptions are handled differently, which will be discussed in Chapter 28. It is important for the medical assistant to be aware of the schedule of medications.

Each provider prescribing scheduled medications needs to have a unique DEA number. The DEA number needs to be renewed every 3 years. The medical assistant may need to assist the provider in renewing or obtaining a DEA number. This can be done at the DEA website (www.deadiversion.usdoj.gov).

WORKPLACE SAFETY LAWS

The Occupational Safety and Health Act and the Needlestick Safety and Prevention Act mandate standards that help protect employees. The following sections describe each law and how it impacts the healthcare setting, making the environment safe for employees.

Occupational Safety and Health Act

The Occupational Safety and Health Act of 1970 (OSH Act) is enforced by the Occupational Safety and Health Administration (OSHA). Based on this act, OSHA sets workplace standards and conducts inspections to ensure employee safety. Employers must comply with all of OSHA's regulations. Table 4.2 addresses the OSHA standards in healthcare.

CRITICAL THINKING APPLICATION 4.4

Daniela is reading about OSHA. She thinks back to what she has heard about OSHA in other businesses. What have you heard about OSHA in other businesses? Is OSHA's role in that company similar to its role in healthcare? Explain.

Needlestick Safety and Prevention Act

The Needlestick Safety and Prevention Act was signed into law in 2000. The goal of the act was to reduce the risk of healthcare workers' exposure to bloodborne diseases. The act required OSHA to update its Bloodborne Pathogens Standard. The revised standards apply to all employees with anticipated occupational exposure to blood or other potentially infectious materials (OPIM). The impact of this act includes the following:

TABLE 4.1 Schedules of Drugs, Substances, and Chemicals

SCHEDULE	PSYCHOLOGICAL AND PHYSICAL DEPENDENCE	EXAMPLES
I	Highest potential for abuse; drugs with no currently accepted medical use	Heroin, lysergic acid diethylamide (LSD), ecstasy
II/IIN (C–II)	High level of abuse and can lead to severe psychological or physical dependence	*Schedule II narcotics:* Oxycodone (OxyContin, Percocet), fentanyl (Duragesic), codeine, morphine *Schedule IIN stimulants:* Amphetamine (Adderall), methamphetamine (Desoxyn), methylphenidate (Concerta, Ritalin LA)
III/III N (C–III)	Moderate to low physical dependence or high psychological dependence	*Schedule III narcotics:* Acetaminophen with codeine (Tylenol #3 or #4), buprenorphine *Schedule III N non-narcotics:* Ketamine, anabolic steroids (e.g., Depo-Testosterone)
IV (C–IV)	Low potential for abuse relative to substances in schedule III	*Schedule IV:* Alprazolam (Xanax), clonazepam (Klonopin), diazepam (Valium), lorazepam (Ativan)
V (C–V)	Lowest potential for abuse relative to substances listed in schedule IV; contains limited quantities of certain narcotics	*Schedule V substances:* Robitussin AC, ezogabine (Potiga)

TABLE 4.2 OSHA Standards Related to Healthcare

STANDARD	SUMMARY	EXAMPLES OF WORKPLACE APPLICATION
Bloodborne pathogens	Protects healthcare workers against the hazards caused by bloodborne pathogens.	Exposure control plans, Universal Precautions, safety needles, personal protective equipment, hepatitis B vaccination, and record keeping.
Hazard communication	Requires employers to provide information about the chemical hazards in the workplace. The General Duty Clause states that any equipment that can pose a health danger must be considered a hazard.	All chemicals are labeled. A Safety Data Sheet (SDS) must be available for each chemical in the workplace. Employees must be trained in how to handle the chemical hazards in the workplace.
Occupational exposure to hazardous chemicals in laboratories	Also called the "laboratory standard." Specifies the requirements of a Chemical Hygiene Plan (CHP).	The CHP is a written program that includes the policies, procedures, and responsibilities that protect employees from hazardous chemicals. The CHP describes the appropriate handling of chemicals in the laboratory.
Ionizing radiation	Addresses the protections needed when working with ionizing radiation (i.e., x-rays).	Signs posted where x-rays are taken. Employees wear personal radiation monitors to detect radiation amounts. X-ray rooms are built with protected areas for the employee. X-ray exposure is limited if the employee is pregnant.
Nonionizing radiation	Addresses the protections needed in place when working with nonionizing radiation (i.e., lasers).	Signs need to be posted on the door of a room where lasers are being used. Appropriate eye protection must be worn at all times by both the patient and the employees. Goal is to prevent blindness, retinal burns, and eye damage due to the radiation.
Means of **egress**	Addresses the exit routes in a building.	Employers are responsible for having appropriate building exit routes. Routes are posted. Exits are unlocked and clear in case of emergency.

OSHA, Occupational Safety and Health Administration.

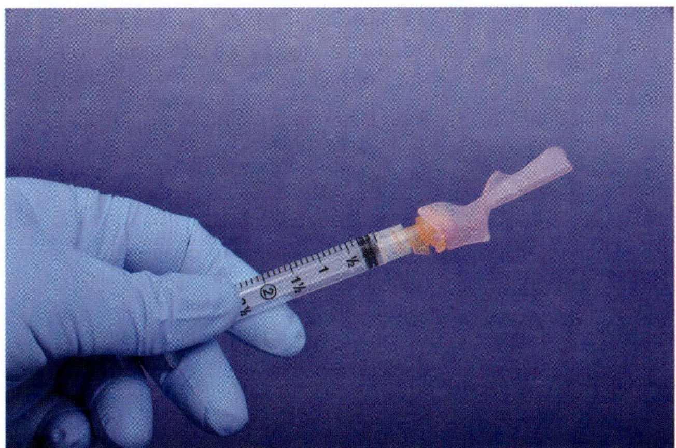

FIGURE 4.4 A safety needle device.

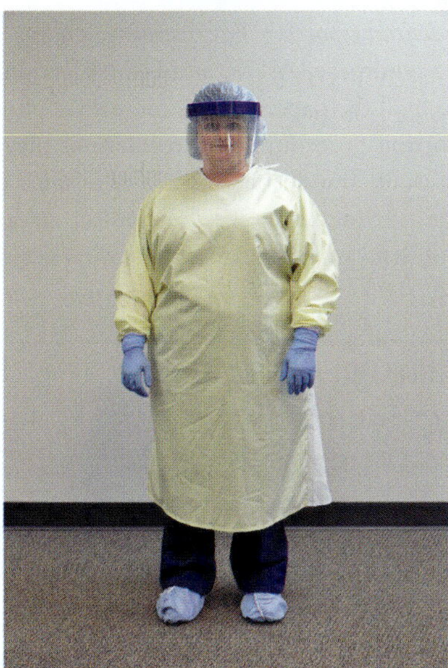

FIGURE 4.5 Personal protective equipment.

- Healthcare workers must use safer medical devices. For example, many needles can be capped with a special safety device after use (Figure 4.4).
- The facility's Exposure Control Plan must include a sharps injury log documenting all instances of injuries from sharps (e.g., used needles, blades).
- Used needles, blades, and other sharps must be put in sharps disposal containers.
- Personal protective equipment (PPE) (i.e., gloves, mask, and gown) must be worn if there is a risk of blood or body fluid exposure (Figure 4.5).

ADDITIONAL HEALTHCARE LAWS AND REGULATIONS

This section presents additional laws that affect healthcare. Throughout the textbook, these laws and others will be discussed in more depth. This chapter introduces the more common laws that impact ambulatory healthcare.

Patient Protection and Affordable Care Act

The Patient Protection and Affordable Care Act is commonly known as the Affordable Care Act. This federal statute was signed into law in 2010. The goal of the law was to provide Americans with affordable health insurance. It also attempted to reform the healthcare system and reduce healthcare spending. Some of the reforms were as follows:

- Insurance coverage of preventive services and immunizations.
- People with preexisting health conditions cannot be dropped or charged more for insurance.
- Dependents can stay on their parent's insurance plan until age 26.
- Large businesses have to provide insurance to full-time workers. Small businesses are eligible for tax credits to help offer insurance coverage to their employees.
- The Physician Payments Sunshine Act (PPSA), part of the law, increases the transparency between providers, teaching hospitals, and manufacturers of medical products (e.g., drugs and medical devices). The manufacturers must report any payments and transfers of value (e.g., gifts, meals) to the Open Payments Program of the Centers for Medicare and Medicaid Services (CMS).

Clinical Laboratory Improvement Amendments

Congress passed the Clinical Laboratory Improvement Amendments (CLIA) in 1988. CLIA establishes quality standards and regulates laboratory testing. The quality standards focus on the accuracy, reliability, and timeliness of test results. The following federal agencies are involved in administering CLIA:

- *Food and Drug Administration:* Oversees the medical laboratory tests. Categorizes the tests based on their complexity: waived, moderate, or high complexity. High-complexity laboratories can perform more tests than waived-complexity laboratories.
- *Centers for Medicare and Medicaid Services:* Inspects laboratories and issues certificates. Enforces compliance with regulations.
- *Centers for Disease Control and Prevention* (CDC): Develops standards and laboratory practice guidelines. Develops professional information and resources mostly related to health and disease topics (www.cdc.gov). (The CDC, a division of HHS, focuses on disease control and prevention, environmental health, and health promotion; thus, its overall mission is to improve the health of the people.)

All agencies providing clinical laboratory services, including ambulatory care laboratories, must meet the CLIA requirements. The laboratories must have a CLIA certificate to operate and must be certified by the state. Smaller ambulatory care laboratories have one of the following certificates:

- *Certificate of Waiver*: Allows the facility to perform CLIA-waived tests, which are simple and accurate with little risk for error if done correctly. A urine pregnancy test is a waived test.
- *Certificate for Provider-Performed Microscopy Procedures* (PPMP): Allows the provider to perform only specific microscopy procedures and waived tests.

Additional certificates are obtained by larger laboratories. These laboratories perform more complex tests.

Good Samaritan Laws

Good Samaritan laws are state laws that provide legal protection for those assisting an injured person during an emergency. If possible, the injured person needs to agree to the help. The person responding must meet the following criteria:

- Not be paid for the care given
- Act reasonably, exercising the same standard of care (for their profession) within the limitations of the emergency

- Not act negligently or recklessly; such action makes the responder liable for damages

The Good Samaritan law does not mean you cannot be sued. In some states, healthcare professionals who do not assist another person in an emergency can be held liable. It is important to be aware of your state's Good Samaritan law and find out if medical assistants have an obligation to stop and provide first aid.

CRITICAL THINKING APPLICATION **4.5**

Daniela is reviewing Good Samaritan laws. How might she describe these laws in terms of their importance during an emergency situation?

Laws for End-of-Life Issues

A medical assistant should be aware of laws that relate to end-of-life issues. The following is a brief summary of acts that relate to **advance directives,** organ donation, and determining death:

- *Patient Self-Determination Act (PSDA):* Requires most healthcare institutions to inform patients of their right to make decisions and the facility's policies respecting advance directives.
- *Uniform Determination of Death Act* (UDDA): Served as a guide for state lawmakers to create their own laws that define death.
- *Uniform Anatomical Gift Act* (UAGA): Purpose of the act was to make organ donation easier for people.
- *National Organ Transplant Act* (NOTA): Established the Organ Procurement and Transplant Network (OPTN) and also established a national registry for organ matching.

These acts are discussed in depth in Chapter 5.

COMPLIANCE REPORTING

Healthcare agencies and employees are required to comply with all federal and state laws and regulations. There are several areas of compliance on which the healthcare facility must focus. Healthcare providers need to report specific diseases, injuries, and issues with vaccines.

Compliance with Public Health Statutes

Public health statutes exist in each state to help promote the health of the residents. According to these statutes, healthcare providers have a responsibility to report specific information to various authorities:

- Births and deaths
- Specific diseases, including sexually transmitted infections (STIs)
- Specific injuries related to violence
- **Abuse, neglect,** and **exploitation**

These topics will be examined more closely in the following sections.

Per the HIPAA permission, "public interest and benefit activities," PHI can be released when required by law, law enforcement, and for public health activities. For the mandatory reporting situations based on state statutes, the provider can release PHI without the patient's authorization.

Reportable Diseases

Reportable diseases are **communicable diseases** that have a significant public health impact. When a provider diagnoses a reportable disease, the state's public health department must be notified. This notification process is called *disease reporting.* Each state has statutes that address disease reporting. Lists of reportable diseases and reporting requirements are typically available on the state's public health department website. The following are examples of reporting levels and reporting procedures, though each state may be slightly different:

- *Urgent reporting*: For diseases such as hepatitis A, food or water disease outbreaks, pertussis (whooping cough), measles, plague, and tuberculosis. Reporting must be done immediately, usually by phone or fax.
- *Less urgent reporting*: For diseases such as sexually transmitted infections; hepatitis B, C, D, and E; legionellosis, Lyme disease, mumps, bacterial meningitis, malaria, tetanus, varicella (chickenpox), and toxic shock syndrome. Reporting may be done electronically, by mail or fax. The provider usually has up to 3 days to file the report.
- *Highly confidential reporting*: For diseases such as acquired immunodeficiency syndrome (AIDS) and HIV infection. The provider may need to mail the paperwork to increase confidentiality.

Disease reporting procedures and regulations may vary by state. The medical assistant should be aware of the state's disease reporting process. The provider may ask the medical assistant to contact the public health department regarding a new reportable disease case (Procedure 4.3).

CRITICAL THINKING APPLICATION **4.6**

Daniela is learning about public health statutes and reporting obligations of providers. Why is it important for the public health services to be notified about specific diseases?

Wounds of Violence

Most state statutes require healthcare providers to report cases of violence. Statutes vary from state to state. Typically, reportable cases include wounds caused by gunshots and stabbings, specific types of burns, and nonaccidental wounds caused by a knife, an axe, or a sharp-pointed instrument. The medical assistant should be aware of the state's statutes for reporting wounds of violence. In some cases, the medical assistant may need to assist the provider in preparing documents for law enforcement for such cases.

CRITICAL THINKING APPLICATION **4.7**

Daniela is learning about public health statutes and the reporting obligations of providers. Why is it important for law enforcement to be notified about cases of violence?

Child Abuse, Neglect, and Exploitation

The Federal Child Abuse Prevention and Treatment Act (CAPTA) aided the states as state statutes were drafted. The act was updated by the CAPTA Reauthorization Act of 2010. This updated act defined child abuse and neglect as follows:

- Any recent act or failure to act on the part of a parent or caretaker that results in death, serious physical or emotional harm, sexual abuse, or exploitation; or

TABLE 4.3 Types of Child Neglect and Abuse

CHILD MALTREATMENT		DESCRIPTION
Neglect	Physical	Failure to provide adequate nutrition, clothing, shelter, and hygiene. Child has poor growth and hygiene and may hide food for later.
	Educational	Failure to enroll child in school or to home-school child. Child may have a poor school attendance record.
	Medical	Failure to provide needed care for injury, impairment, or illness. Child may have untreated injuries. May see developmental delays from lack of therapy to help with impairment.
Abuse	Physical	Bruises, fractures, or burns that are unexplained or do not match the explanation given; untreated dental or medical problems.
	Sexual	Sexual behaviors inappropriate for child's age; sexually transmitted infections, genital pain and bruising, bleeding.
	Emotional	Delayed emotional development, loss of self-confidence, social withdrawal, headaches, depression, poor school performance.

- An act or failure to act that presents an imminent risk of serious harm

These definitions set the minimum standard for describing child abuse and neglect. States typically address child maltreatment in both civil and criminal statutes.

Reporting and Reporters. All states and territories require child maltreatment to be reported. Most states mandate specific professionals to report any child maltreatment, including school personnel, social workers, healthcare providers, nurses, mental health professionals, childcare providers, medical examiners or coroners, and law enforcement officers. Some states require anyone who suspects child abuse or neglect to report the situation (Table 4.3). Mandatory reporters need to provide the facts. They do not have to prove that abuse or neglect occurred. Most state statutes do not consider abuse and neglect information as **privileged communication** between the patient and the provider. This allows the provider to report the information (and thus protect the maltreated child). The medical assistant should be aware of the state statutes regarding child maltreatment. The Child Welfare Information Gateway website (www.childwelfare.gov) can be used as a resource for state reporting information.

CRITICAL THINKING APPLICATION 4.8

Daniela is learning about child abuse and neglect. How might she describe the difference between abuse and neglect? Why is this information important for medical assistants to know?

The Unborn Victims of Violence Act. The Unborn Victims of Violence Act was signed into law by Congress in 2004. Prior to this act, babies in utero (also called *fetuses*) harmed or killed due to violence were not considered victims. This act considers babies in utero who are harmed or killed during certain acts of violence to be victims, and charges could be brought forth.

Adult Abuse, Neglect, and Exploitation

In 1965 the Older Americans Act was signed into law. The purpose of the act was to maintain the rights and dignity of the older person. It also created the Administration on Aging. Since then, several federal laws have been passed to help fund federal programs.

Abuse, neglect, and exploitation of older adults and **dependent adults** are dealt with in state statutes. All states have the following:

- Adult or elder protective services statutes that provide reporting and investigating procedures for elder abuse in the state
- Statutes that establish a Long-Term Care Ombudsman Program that advocates for the safety and rights of long-term care facility residents
- General criminal statutes on fraud, sexual assault, battery, and other abuses that can relate to elder abuse

Some states require financial institutions (banks) to report suspected financial abuse or exploitation of older adults.

Reporting and Reporters. The state statute will dictate who are mandated reporters, when to report, and how to report the situation. Many ambulatory healthcare facilities are screening older adults to identify those who do not feel safe in their living conditions. If the medical assistant suspects abuse, neglect, or exploitation of an older person, it is important to bring it to the provider's attention. Typically, the provider is a mandated reporter under state law. If the provider suspects neglect, abuse, or exploitation, then a report needs to be filed.

State statutes on domestic violence and abuse vary. In some cases, reporting injuries caused by violence covers some domestic abuse situations. Some states have mandatory reporting for domestic violence. It is recommended that providers talk to the victim of domestic violence. They should inform the person when it must be reported. In states where domestic violence is not a mandatory reporting situation, providers can encourage the victim to report the situation. Safe houses are also available in many areas for victims. Having information on local resources for domestic abuse is important in the ambulatory care setting. Providing the information in restrooms is very common. Typically, that might be the only location where the abuser does not follow the victim. It is important to remember that both males and females can be victims of domestic abuse.

Reporting Vaccination Adverse Side Effects

When a healthcare provider orders a vaccine to be given to a child, the medical assistant must provide the parent or guardian with a Vaccine Information Statement (VIS). This document reviews the reasons for and the risks of the vaccine. Prior to giving the vaccine, the medical assistant must have the parent or guardian sign a consent form allowing the administration of the immunization.

If a patient experiences an unusual side effect from a vaccine, the provider might need to file a report with the Vaccine Adverse Event Reporting System (VAERS). Patients and families can also file a report. VAERS is a national surveillance program that monitors vaccine safety. It collects information on unusual vaccine side effects. VAERS is co-sponsored by the CDC and FDA.

In 1986 the National Childhood Vaccine Injury Act was passed. It created the National Vaccine Injury Compensation Program (VICP). This program provides compensation for children injured by childhood vaccines. The VICP lifts the burden of lawsuits from vaccine manufacturers and healthcare providers. The VIS contains information about VICP for patients' families.

COMPLIANCE PROGRAMS

Administrators must have policies and procedures in place for employees to report issues. Reports need to be followed up. Documentation may need to be done for federal or state agencies regarding compliance issues. Compliance programs were instituted to make this process work.

Purpose of Compliance Programs

A *compliance program* or *corporate compliance* is a program within a business that detects and prevents violations of state and federal laws. An effective compliance program helps protect the organization from fines and lawsuits. Most compliance programs have reporting mechanisms (i.e., a toll-free number or website) where employees can report suspected violations, suspected illegal activity, fraud, abuse, safety issues, and noncompliance issues. It is important for employees to be able to report issues without fear of **retaliation** and **retribution**. Many times, reports can be submitted anonymously.

Reporting Issues

If a medical assistant needs to report a situation, it is important to follow the healthcare facility's policies and procedures. Different reporting pathways are seen in ambulatory care settings:

- *If the facility has a compliance reporting procedure*: A report can be filed through the compliance reporting mechanisms available to the employee.
- *If the facility does not have a compliance reporting procedure*: The employee may need to report the situation using the chain of command. This means the employee must report the issue to the supervisor. If the supervisor was involved with the situation, the employee must report the issue to the supervisor's supervisor.
- *For employment or conflict-of-interest issues*: Some agencies require the employee to contact the human resources supervisor.

The rest of the chapter examines specific types of compliance programs used in healthcare.

FINANCIAL CONCERNS

Financial concerns related to financial and property theft, identity theft, conflict of interest, and fraud. Theft can be of drugs, equipment, supplies, or money.

Identity Theft

Identity theft occurs when someone sells or uses another person's personal information for financial gain. In healthcare, medical identity theft occurs. When a person poses as another person during a healthcare visit, this is considered medical identity theft because the wrong person's insurance is billed for the services. To prevent medical identity theft, many agencies are doing the following:

- Requiring photo identification during the check-in process for visits and services
- Taking the patient's picture, which is uploaded to the electronic health record for future reference

Conflict of Interest

Conflict of interest relates to any financial interest, personal or professional activity, or obligation that affects a person's objectivity when performing the job. For instance, a provider owns stock in a pharmaceutical company. This provider then prescribes medications made by that company. The provider is benefiting from patients purchasing medications from that company.

Fraud

Fraud is a deceitful action that causes another to give up something of value. Healthcare fraud is prevalent. In 2020 Medicare fraud was estimated to be about $25.74 billion. Examples of healthcare fraud include the following:

- Providers and agencies bill for services that were not provided.
- Information is falsified for payment.
- Services are overcharged.
- Medical identification theft occurs.

The list of fraud examples is long. The Office of Inspector General of the HHS oversees fighting fraud and abuse in government programs.

Federal Laws Addressing Fraud

The following are federal laws that address fraud in healthcare:

- *Anti-Kickback Statute* (AKS): Since 1972, this federal statute has prohibited intentionally receiving or giving anything of value to get referrals or generate federal healthcare program business.
- *False Claims Act* (FCA): Originally signed into law during the American Civil War in 1863 and revised in 2010. It prohibits a person from submitting false or fraudulent Medicare or Medicaid claims for payment. Under this act, a person can bring a civil suit on behalf of the government when it is found that others are sending false claims to the government for payment. The individual can receive part of the settlement.
- *Stark Law* (also called the *Physician Self-Referral Law*): Became law in 1989 and became effective in 1992. Several revisions have been made since then. It prohibits a healthcare provider from referring a Medicare patient for services to a facility with which the provider or the provider's immediate family has a financial relationship.

- *Healthcare Fraud Statute*: Originated in 1996 and revised in 2010. It prohibits intentionally defrauding any healthcare benefit program.

Legal Example: False Claim Act Violations

A lawsuit alleged that Berkeley Heart Lab, Inc. paid kickbacks to physicians and patients to use the company for blood testing. The kickbacks were disguised as "processing and handling" fees. Patients received kickbacks in the form of waived copayments, which they were legally required to pay for the services provided. The government also alleged that unnecessary cardiovascular tests were charged to Medicare and TRICARE programs. Quest acquired Berkeley in 2011 and ended the practice of kickbacks. In 2017 Quest Diagnostics., Inc. agreed to pay $6 million to resolve a lawsuit by the United States.

From *United States ex rel. Mayes v. Berkeley HeartLab Inc.*, et al., Case No. 9:11-cv-01593-RMG (D.S.C.) Consolidated with U.S. EX REL. LUTZ v. BERKELEY HEARTLAB, INC.

Medical Assistant's Role

A medical assistant should be aware of the laws related to fraud and conflict of interest. If violations or illegal activities are noticed in the workplace, the medical assistant should follow the reporting procedures outlined in the facility's compliance program (Procedure 4.4). Conflicts of interest need to be reported immediately to the human resources supervisor or your supervisor.

CRITICAL THINKING APPLICATION **4.9**

Daniela and Bella are studying compliance. They start to discuss the importance of declaring a conflict of interest. Describe why being upfront and notifying administration/human resources about a conflict of interest is important in healthcare

EMPLOYMENT CONCERNS

Employment concerns relate to **discrimination**, **harassment**, retaliation and retribution, and unfair employment practices. In many states, most medical assistant positions are considered *employment-at-will*. This means that the employer can end employment at any time for any legal reason. Many states recognize this concept. It also means the employee can quit at any time for any reason, though giving a 2-week notice is considered professional. Most jobs are considered employment-at-will.

Wrongful Termination

Employers cannot fire an employee for an illegal reason. The employer needs to have a *just cause,* or legal reason, for firing an employee. Legal reasons could include terminations due to cutbacks in staffing or an employee's behavioral issues. A terminated employee may have an opportunity to sue if wrongful termination occurred. *Wrongful termination* means that the employer did not have just cause for firing the employee. For instance, an employee reported that fraud was occurring in the billing department at the facility. The facility then is under investigation for the fraud. The supervisor fires the **whistleblower.** Federal and state laws protect the whistleblower from retaliation and retribution.

Legal Example: Wrongful Termination and Invasion of Privacy

The plaintiff was a security guard at Children's Hospital. He was involved in an accident while on the job. He was examined at the emergency department, given a painkiller, and released. There was no record of intoxication or impairment. The next day, while recovering at home, he was called to the hospital to submit to a drug test. The test was positive for hydrocodone, and the hospital terminated him based on its drug-free workplace policy. He had been an employee for 18 years and had a clean record with no work-related accidents or drug abuse issues. The plaintiff sued the hospital for wrongful termination, invasion of privacy, and defamation. The case went through mediation, and the hospital offered $40,000 to settle. With no resolution, the case was brought to trial. After deliberation, the 12-member jury returned with a 12–0 decision for the plaintiff. He was awarded $385,050 for past and future economic loss and $650,000 for past and future emotional distress. The total verdict for the plaintiff was $1,035,050.

From *Mckinley Nou v. Children's Hospital Central California,* (October 16, 2014) Fresno Superior Court, Case Number: 12-CECG-02169.

Legal Example: Whistleblower Retaliation

According to a complaint, psychologist Melody Jo Samuelson was hired by Napa State Hospital in California. For 2 years, she received good reviews, and then she testified in a case in which she alleged that a patient had been improperly assessed as competent to stand trial. In court, she indicated the hospital did not use adequate methods to analyze patients. She complained that the hospital immediately retaliated against her and was fired from her job. She appealed her firing and filed a whistleblower retaliation complaint. She was reinstated, but the retaliation continued, she stated. She claimed anxiety and depression as a result of the situation. She was awarded $1 million.

From *Samuelson v. California Department of Mental Health, et. al.*, No. 26-57631 (N.D.Cal. Feb. 20, 2014).

Federal Laws Related to Discrimination

Many federal laws regulate issues regarding employment. The following laws address discrimination in the workplace:

- *National Labor Relations Act*: Also called the Wagner Act of 1935. It gave the right to most workers to organize or join a union.
- *Title VII of the Civil Rights Act of 1964* (Title VII): Prohibits employment discrimination based on color, race, gender, religion, or national origin.
- *Age Discrimination in Employment Act* (ADEA) *of 1967:* Revised several times. It protects applicants and employees 40 years and older from discrimination and includes hiring, promotion, termination, and compensation practices.
- *Rehabilitation Act of 1973*: Prohibits discrimination in employment practices based on physical or mental disabilities. This act

applies to federal employers or employers that are federal contractors (provide services to the federal government).

- *Pregnancy Discrimination Act of 1978*: Amended Title VII of the Civil Rights Act of 1964. This act prohibits sex discrimination based on pregnancy.
- *Title I* and *Title V of the Americans with Disabilities Act* (ADA) *of 1990:* Prohibits employment discrimination against qualified persons with disabilities.
- *Genetic Information Nondiscrimination Act* (GINA) *of 2008:* Prohibits employment discrimination based on the person's genetic information.
- *Civil Rights Act of 1991*: Provides punitive damages in cases of intentional employment discrimination.

Federal Laws Related to Hours, Wages, and Leave

The following federal laws address hours, pay, and leave in the workplace:

- *Federal Insurance Contributions Act* (FICA) *of 1935:* Created a payroll tax that requires a deduction from a person's paycheck. The withheld amount and an employer contribution fund the Social Security program and a portion of Medicare.
- *Fair Labor Standards Act of 1938*: Prohibits child labor and also provides overtime pay and a minimum wage.
- *Equal Pay Act* (EPA) *of 1963:* Protects against gender-based wage discrimination; requires equal pay for both males and females who are performing the same job at the same organization.
- *Employee Retirement Income Security Act* (ERISA) *of 1974:* Sets minimum standards for pension and health plans in private industry and protects individuals in these plans.
- *Family Medical Leave Act* (FMLA) *of 1991*: Provides unpaid leave time for maternity, adoption, or caring for ill family members.

State laws also protect employees in different areas. For instance, state workers' compensation laws protect employees who are injured on the job. An employee may collect money to cover lost wages, medical expenses, and retraining.

A medical assistant should be aware of the employment laws. If violations are noticed in the workplace, the medical assistant should follow the reporting procedures outlined in the facility's compliance program. If no program exists, it is important to discuss the issues with the person responsible for the human resources duties.

Interview Concerns

To prevent legal issues related to hiring practices, healthcare facilities need to stay away from specific topics during the interview process. Asking questions related to these topics can put the facility at risk for discrimination lawsuits. Here are some examples of illegal and legal questions:

- Birthplace, ancestry, or national origin: Legal to ask, "Are you eligible to work in this state?" Illegal to ask, "When did you move to the United States?"
- Marital status, children, or pregnancy: Legal to ask, "Are you able to work an 8 a.m. to 5 p.m. schedule?" Illegal to ask, "Who will look after your child when he is born?"
- Health or medical history or physical disability: Legal to ask, "Can you perform the essential job functions of a medical assistant with or without reasonable accommodations?" Illegal to ask, "What medications are you on?"
- Religion or religious days observed: Legal to ask, "Can you work on the weekends?" Illegal to ask, "Where do you attend church services?"
- Age, race, ethnicity, gender, or color: Legal to ask, "Are you 18 or older?" Illegal to ask, "How old are you?"
- Criminal records: Legal to ask, "Have you ever been convicted of a crime?" Illegal to ask, "Have you ever been arrested?"

Environmental Safety Concerns

Compliance reporting also relates to environmental safety violations. Offenses can be violations of local, state, or federal regulations. The unsafe activities or practices may cause hazardous conditions that affect the health or safety of employees, patients, and others. Recall that OSHA is involved with creating a safe environment for employees. Any situation that risks the safety of employees or patients must be reported immediately.

The Occupational Safety and Health Act of 1970 gives employees the right to file a complaint with OSHA. Employees can request an OSHA inspection if they believe their workplace has safety hazards. The employee filing the report does not need to be knowledgeable about the OSHA regulations. OSHA will keep the reporting person's information confidential.

To report a safety and health issue, the employee can file an electronic form, fax or mail a report to the local OSHA office, or call the local OSHA office. Specific information and forms are available at the OSHA website (www.osha.gov).

LAWS PROTECTING PATIENTS AGAINST DISCRIMINATION

Federal and state laws also protect patients from discrimination and unsafe situations. The following sections discuss federal and state laws that protect patients.

Americans with Disabilities Act and the Rehabilitation Act

People with disabilities have a right to accessible healthcare. The Americans with Disabilities Act (ADA) prohibits discrimination against individuals with disabilities in everyday activities, including getting healthcare. The Rehabilitation Act of 1973 prohibits discrimination against individuals with disabilities in services that receive federal financial assistance, including healthcare services. These laws require that healthcare agencies make their services accessible to people with disabilities. The following are examples of how these laws affect ambulatory care facilities:

- Patients in wheelchairs: These patients need to be moved to exam tables when the exam requires the patient to be lying down. Lifts and low exam tables are available to help in these situations. Patients with disabilities cannot be denied care on the grounds that accessible medical equipment is not available.
- Patients with disabilities: If a patient has an interpreter or a companion, it is important that the healthcare provider focuses on the patient.
- Exam table location: Patients must have a minimum of 30 inches by 48 inches of clear space adjacent to the exam table and the accessible route out of the room. This allows individuals in

wheelchairs to approach the table and be able to transfer onto it. An adjustable-height exam table should be available.

- Accessible scales: Special wheelchair scales and in-floor scales (built into the floor) are needed for patients with limited or no mobility.

Americans with Disabilities Act Amendments Act

The Americans with Disabilities Act Amendments Act of 2008 is also known as the ADA Amendment Act and the ADAAA. The original ADA narrowly defined disability. The ADA Amendment Act expanded the meaning and interpretation of the definition of disability. People with cancer, diabetes, attention deficit hyperactivity disorder, learning disabilities, and epilepsy are now included. This should ensure that individuals with disabilities receive protection under the law.

INCIDENT REPORTS AND RISK MANAGEMENT

When a person is injured or equipment malfunctions, most ambulatory care facilities require an incident report to be completed. An *incident report* is an internal document that needs to be completed whenever an unexpected event occurs (Figure 4.6). The purposes of the incident report are to gather information about the situation in case of a future lawsuit and communicate issues for risk management procedures.

Completing Incident Reports

The medical assistant should remember these points about incident reports:

- Complete an incident report for patient complaints, medication errors, medical device malfunctions, and any injury.
- Complete the incident report clearly and accurately in pen or electronically.
- List the facts. Do not speculate or draw conclusions.
- Make sure to complete it by the end of the day the situation occurs.
- Do not mention the incident report in the patient's health record. If it is mentioned, a lawyer may request a copy of the report.

WALDEN-MARTIN
FAMILY MEDICAL CLINIC
1234 ANYSTREET | ANYTOWN, ANYSTATE 12345
PHONE 123-123-1234 | FAX 123-123-5678

Incident Report

Date: ____________ **Time:** ____________

Incident Type: ☐ Staff ☐ Patient ☐ Visitor ☐ Equipment/Property

Witness: ☐ Staff ☐ Patient ☐ Visitor

Department: ____________ **Exact Location:** ____________

Medical Team: ____________

Patient Reason for Visit: ____________ **Medication Incident:** ☐ Yes ☐ No

Incident Description: ☐ **Immediate Actions and Outcome:** ☐

Contributing Factors: ☐ **Prevention:** ☐

Next of kin / guardian notified / patient? ☐ Yes ☐ No ☐ N/A **Medical staff notified?** ☐ Yes ☐ No ☐ N/A

Reported By: ____________ **Position:** ____________

Contact Phone Number: ____________

Other Persons Involved: ____________ **Position:** ____________

Contact Phone Number: ____________

Medical Report (Document patient's assessment and list investigations and treatments):

Provider: ____________ **Designation:** ____________

Provider Signature: ____________ **Date/Time:** ____________

FIGURE 4.6 Incident report form.

Usually, the incident report is given to the supervisor to review before it is sent to the risk management team. *Risk management* involves techniques used to reduce or eliminate accidental loss to the healthcare facility. It involves identifying, assessing, and controlling risks. Risks can relate to financial issues, legal liabilities, accidents, and electronic data security threats.

Patient Mistakes and Injuries

Patient safety concerns are of utmost importance in healthcare facilities. Even with careful practices, patients can be harmed. A patient can fall. The wrong medication may be given to the patient. The wrong procedure may be done. All issues of safety can lead to potential liability for injuries that result.

If a medical assistant is involved in a situation in which a person is harmed, it is important to do the following:

- Immediately notify the provider. This is especially important if the wrong medication is given to the patient. The provider must identify what steps need to be taken.
- Arrange to have the person seen by a provider immediately. The provider can assess the extent of the injuries and provide the required treatment. Information on the injuries and treatment will then be documented in the health record should future litigation occur.
- Complete the incident report (Procedure 4.5). The employee witnessing the situation should be the person completing the report if possible. The incident report communicates what occurred and provides information if future litigation occurs.
- Notify the department supervisor. The supervisor can follow up with the patient. Many agencies do not charge the injured patient for the services provided. If the wrong medication is given, many agencies do not charge for the medication and services provided.
- Notify state or federal government agencies regarding the injury, depending on the situation. Some states have medical error reporting systems in place. OSHA requires agencies to record all work-related needlestick injuries and cuts from sharp objects contaminated with another person's blood or other potentially infectious material. The case must be reported on the OSHA 300 Log (available at www.osha.gov).

CLOSING COMMENTS

Patient Coaching

When you are working with older patients, questions on record release and disclosure authorization forms can be common. Years ago, such forms did not exist. Today patients may feel they have to complete forms for everything. Make sure to take time to explain why it is important to have the forms completed. Remember that some of the older patients may have difficulty reading the forms. Some may not be able to hear as well as they once did. Take time and communicate clearly and slowly with older patients. If appropriate, use simple phrases when answering their questions. If possible, help complete whatever information you can. Be patient and respectful during your interactions with patients.

Legal and Ethical Issues

During a busy day in an ambulatory care facility, the medical assistant performs many administrative and clinical tasks. It is important for the medical assistant to perform these tasks following the facility's policies and procedures. Remember that these policies and procedures are created so that the staff complies with state and federal laws. Should it be determined that a task may conflict with a law, the medical assistant should talk with the supervisor.

Patient-Centered Care

In a patient-centered care environment, the patient is the focus. When a medical assistant does a procedure incorrectly or makes a medication error, it is very important for that assistant to notify the provider and the supervisor immediately. The provider will evaluate the situation and make a judgment on what needs to be done for the care and safety of the patient. The supervisor will help manage the situation by talking with the patient, ensuring everything is done for the patient, and eliminating charges related to the error. Being upfront and honest about the error to the provider, supervisor, and patient (per agency policy) is most important for the patient's health and safety.

Professional Behaviors

Many ambulatory care facilities do not allow medical assistants to carry personal cell phones. Limiting cell phone use can reduce the chance of employees recording or taking a picture of a patient and posting something patient related on social media sites. These situations are breaches of confidentiality and can lead to HIPAA violations and settlements. In addition to OCR concerns, the patient may choose to sue the facility. It is important to remember to maintain patient confidentiality. What you see and hear in the clinic remains there.

SUMMARY OF SCENARIO

Daniela has learned a lot about healthcare-related laws. Not only did she learn about laws that healthcare professionals must follow, but she also learned about employment laws. One of Daniela's assignments for her course was to identify three risks of HIPAA violations. Daniela and Bella talked about the assignment and the risks in their department.

Unattended computers that were open to an electronic health record were a problem. This is especially a risk in the patient examination rooms because each room is equipped with a personal computer for documenting. Daniela also mentioned conversations about patients in the medical assistants' station. Sometimes she hears medical assistants discussing a patient who came in. She feels uncomfortable about those conversations and ensures she does not take part in them.

Cell phones in the workplace and frequent use of social media sites during work hours can be risks. Bella mentioned that she had heard several stories of employees being terminated. The employees posted patient-related photos and information on social media sites. Bella and Daniela work hard to prevent HIPAA violations. They do not ever want to be named in a lawsuit for such violations.

SUMMARY OF LEARNING OBJECTIVES

1. **Differentiate between privacy and confidentiality.**
   Privacy means being free from unwanted intrusion. An invasion of privacy is the disclosing of private facts without the consent of the individual. Confidentiality is a legally protected right of patients. Healthcare professionals have the duty not to disclose medical, financial, and insurance information unless authorized by the patient.
2. **Examine the goals, standards, and terminology of the Health Insurance Portability and Accountability Act.**
   One of the goals of HIPAA was to simplify the electronic exchange of information. The goal is to reduce the clerical burden and increase the adoption of electronic transactions.
   The four standards include the following:
   - Standard 1 is related to transactions and code sets.
   - Standard 2 is related to the Privacy Rule.
   - Standard 3 is related to the Security Rule.
   - Standard 4 is related to unique identifiers.

   HIPAA-related terminology includes covered entities, protected health information, business associates, permission, de-identification procedures, and limited data sets.
3. **Analyze how to comply with the Privacy Rule when releasing patient information.**
   The Privacy Rule lists *permissions* or reasons that the health information can be released. The following permissions do not require written authorization from the patient to release protected health information PHI:
   - Treatment, payment, and healthcare operations
   - Uses and disclosures with an opportunity to agree or object
   - Incidental use and disclosure
   - Public interest and benefit activities
   - Limited data set
   - To the individual

   The only permission that requires written authorization from patients is disclosing the PHI to a third party. In some agencies, a disclosure authorization form (also called an authorization to disclose form) must be completed before information can be shared with another person. The patient must complete a record release form before the records can be transferred.
4. **Examine how healthcare facilities comply with the Security Rule.**
   Safeguards important to ensure the security of the electronic protected health information (ePHI) include the following:
   - Administrative safeguards: The security officer is responsible for creating and carrying out security policies and procedures.
   - Physical safeguards: Facility, workstation, and device security must be implemented.
   - Technical safeguards: Only authorized employees should have access to ePHI. Safeguards include audits, encryption of data on mobile devices, and measures to prevent the improper alteration, destruction, or transmission of ePHI.
5. **Examine how the Health Information Technology for Economic and Clinical Health (HITECH) Act and the Genetic Information Nondiscrimination Act (GINA) modified the Health Insurance Portability and Accountability Act (HIPAA).**
   The HITECH Act contains provisions that increase the enforcement of the privacy and security of electronic transmission and health information. HITECH Act modified HIPAA in the following ways:
   - Made business associates directly liable for compliance with HIPAA.
   - Prohibited the sale of PHI without the patient's authorization.
   - Created a tiered violation category that included unknowing, reasonable cause, willful neglect—corrected, and willful neglect—uncorrected.
   - Breach notification requirements were increased.

   GINA modified HIPAA by clarifying that genetic information is health information and prohibiting the use and disclosure of genetic information by covered health plans.
6. **Differentiate between the Food, Drug, and Cosmetic Act and the Controlled Substances Act.**
   The Food, Drug, and Cosmetic Act is enforced by the Food and Drug Administration (FDA). The FDA is responsible for the safety, effectiveness, security, and quality of drugs, cosmetics, and food. Some of the areas overseen by the FDA include human and veterinary drugs, vaccines, biological products (e.g., blood components), medical devices, food, cosmetics, dietary supplies, and products that give off radiation.
   The Controlled Substances Act is enforced by the US Drug Enforcement Agency (DEA). The DEA oversees the manufacturing, importation, possession, use, and distribution of certain drugs and chemicals. The DEA handles both illegal and legal controlled substances. The Controlled Substances Act has five schedules of medications, arranged from those with the greatest to those with the least abuse potential.
7. **Differentiate between the Occupational Safety and Health Act and the Needlestick Safety and Prevention Act.**
   Occupational Safety and Health Act (OSH Act): Enforced by the Occupational Safety and Health Administration (OSHA). Based on this act, OSHA sets workplace standards and conducts inspections to ensure employee safety.
   Needlestick Safety and Prevention Act: The goal of this act was to reduce the risk of healthcare workers' exposure to bloodborne diseases. The act required OSHA to update its Bloodborne Pathogens Standard.
8. **Examine healthcare laws related to insurance, laboratory quality standards, emergency care, and end-of-life care.**
   - *Patient Protection and Affordable Care Act:* Also known as the Affordable Care Act; it was established to provide Americans with affordable health insurance and attempted to reform the healthcare system and reduce healthcare spending.
   - *Clinical Laboratory Improvement Amendments (CLIA)*: Establishes quality standards and regulates laboratory testing. The quality

Continued

SUMMARY OF LEARNING OBJECTIVES—*continued*

standards focus on accuracy, reliability, and the timeliness of test results.

- *Good Samaritan laws*: State laws that provide legal protection for those assisting an injured person during an emergency. The person responding must not be paid for the care given; must act reasonably, exercising the same standard of care (for that person's profession) within the limitations of the emergency; and cannot act negligently.
- *Patient Self-Determination Act:* Requires most healthcare institutions to inform patients of their right to make decisions and the facility's policies respecting advance directives.
- *Uniform Determination of Death Act (UDDA):* Served as a guide for state lawmakers to create their own laws that define death.
- *Uniform Anatomical Gift Act (UAGA)*: Purpose of the act was to make organ donation easier for people.
- *National Organ Transplant Act (NOTA)*: Established the Organ Procurement and Transplant Network (OPTN) and also established a national registry for organ matching.

9. **Differentiate types of situations that providers must report to comply with federal and state laws.**

Healthcare agencies and employees are required to comply with all federal and state laws and regulations. Healthcare providers need to report births and deaths, specific diseases including sexually transmitted infections, specific injuries related to violence, abuse, neglect, exploitation, and vaccination adverse side effects.

Reportable diseases are communicable diseases that have a significant public health impact. When a provider diagnoses a reportable disease, the state's public health department must be notified. This notification process is called disease reporting. Each state has statutes that address disease reporting.

Most state statutes require healthcare providers to report cases of violence. Statutes vary from state to state. Typically, reportable cases include wounds caused by gunshots and stabbings, specific types of burns, and nonaccidental wounds caused by a knife, an axe, or a sharp-pointed instrument.

If a patient has an unusual side effect from a vaccine, the provider might need to file a report with the Vaccine Adverse Event Reporting System (VAERS). VAERS is a national surveillance program that monitors vaccine safety. It collects information on unusual vaccine side effects.

10. **Examine compliance programs, including the purpose and reporting procedures.**

A *compliance program* or *corporate compliance* is a program within a business that detects and prevents violations of state and federal laws. An effective compliance program helps protect the organization from fines and lawsuits.

Different reporting pathways are seen in ambulatory care settings:

- If the facility has a compliance reporting procedure: A report can be filed through the compliance reporting mechanisms available to the employee.
- If the facility does not have a compliance reporting procedure: The employee may need to report the situation using the chain of command.
- For employment or conflict-of-interest issues: Some agencies require the employee to contact the human resources supervisor.

11. **Examine illegal financial activities in healthcare, including identity theft, conflict of interest, and fraud.**

Financial concerns related to financial and property theft, identity theft, conflict of interest, and fraud.

- *Identity theft* occurs when someone sells or uses another person's personal information for financial gain. In healthcare, medical identity theft occurs.
- *Conflict of interest* relates to any financial interest, personal or professional activity, or obligation that affects a person's objectivity when performing the job.
- *Fraud* is a deceitful action that causes another to give up something of value. Several federal laws address fraud in healthcare, including the Anti-Kickback Statute, the False Claims Act, Stark Law, and the Healthcare Fraud Statute.

A medical assistant should be aware of the laws related to fraud and conflict of interest. If illegal financial issues occur in the workplace, the medical assistant should follow the reporting procedures outlined in the facility's compliance program.

12. **Examine employment laws related to hiring, firing, discrimination, wage, and safety.**

Employment laws related to hiring, firing, discrimination, wage, and safety include the following:

- Employers cannot fire an employee for an illegal reason. Wrongful termination means that the employer did not have just cause for firing the employee. Federal and state laws protect the whistleblower from retaliation and retribution.
- Federal laws that address discrimination in the workplace include the National Labor Relations Act (Wagner Act), Title VII of the Civil Rights Act, the Age Discrimination in Employment Act, the Rehabilitation Act, the Pregnancy Discrimination Act, Title I and Title V of the Americans with Disabilities Act, the Genetic Information Nondiscrimination Act, and the Civil Rights Act.
- Federal laws addressing hours, pay, and leave in the workplace include the Federal Insurance Contributions Act (FICA), the Fair Labor Standards Act the Equal Pay Act (EPA), the Employee Retirement Income Security Act (ERISA), and the Family Medical Leave Act (FMLA).
- Occupational Safety and Health Act: Gives employees the right to file a complaint with OSHA. Employees can request an OSHA inspection if they believe their workplace has safety hazards.

SUMMARY OF LEARNING OBJECTIVES—*continued*

13. **Differentiate between the laws that protect patients from discrimination.**
    Federal and state laws also protect patients from discrimination and unsafe situations. The Americans with Disabilities Act (ADA) prohibits discrimination against individuals with disabilities in everyday activities, including getting healthcare. The Rehabilitation Act prohibits discrimination against individuals with disabilities in services that receive federal financial assistance, including healthcare services. The ADA Amendment Act expanded the meaning and interpretation of the definition of disability.

14. **Examine how incident reports and risk management protect patients and healthcare facilities.**
    An *incident report* is an internal document that needs to be completed whenever an unexpected event occurs. The purposes of the incident report are gather information about the situation in case of a future lawsuit and to communicate issues for risk management procedures.

    If a patient mistake or injury occurs, the provider should be notified immediately. The patient should be seen by the provider immediately. An incident report needs to be completed. The department supervisor, as well as the state or federal government agencies, need to be notified regarding the injury, depending on the situation.

PROCEDURE 4.1 Protect a Patient's Privacy

TASKS: Apply HIPAA rules and protect a patient's privacy. Demonstrate active listening skills and empathy to a patient.

SCENARIO: Ken Thomas (date of birth [DOB] 10/25/19XX) saw Jean Burke, nurse practitioner (NP), this past week. He was diagnosed with acute leukemia after several tests. You work with Ms. Burke, and you were involved with arranging Ken's tests. Today, Ken's adult child, Alex Thomas, calls you. Alex wants to know what is going on with Ken. You look at Ken's health record and see that Alex is not on the disclosure authorization form. Per the facility's policy, for information to be given to a patient's family, a disclosure authorization form must be completed.

Later, Ken calls and asks why you did not update Alex on his condition. He sounds upset while he is talking with you.

DIRECTIONS: Role-play the scenario with a peer. You are the medical assistant in the scenario. Your peer will play Alex and then Ken.

EQUIPMENT and SUPPLIES

- Patient's health record
- Disclosure authorization form (electronic or paper) (see Figure 4.2)

PROCEDURAL STEPS

1. You realized that Alex is not on the disclosure authorization form. Inform Alex that his name is not on a disclosure authorization form. Discuss the purpose of the disclosure authorization form. Be professional and respectful as you apply HIPAA rules to the situation.
   PURPOSE: As a professional, you need to follow the law and yet, be professional and respectful. The patient must sign a disclosure authorization form and indicate who can be given information. If a person wants information but is not listed on the form, legally, the medical assistant cannot give any information.
2. Explain to Alex how you would be able to give him information. Encourage Alex to talk with his father about the situation.
   PURPOSE: The medical assistant can only give information if the person's name is on the disclosure authorization form.
   Scenario update: Your peer will now play the part of Ken, the patient.
3. When Ken calls, be professional and empathetic as you listen to his complaints. Inform Ken that you understand his frustration. Be respectful to his feelings and his rights. Explain why you could not give information to Alex.
   PURPOSE: Having the patient understand that you could not legally give the information to Alex is important. Speaking in a respectful tone may help Ken feel less frustrated with the situation.
4. Demonstrate active listening skills when interacting with Ken. Remain neutral and refrain from interrupting. Keep your voice even and do not raise the volume. Focus on the patient and avoid distractions.
5. Discuss with Ken how you could prepare the disclosure authorization form. Make plans for how Ken will sign the form.
   PURPOSE: Helping to develop a solution to achieve the patient's wishes is important to solving Ken's frustration.
6. Document the phone calls with Alex and Ken. Describe the facts and the plan to complete the disclosure authorization form.
   PURPOSE: All phone calls with patients or related to patients should be documented. This provides an ongoing log of what occurs with the patient and can be helpful in a court of law should something come up.

PROCEDURE 4.2 Complete a Release of Records Form for a Release of Information

TASKS: Apply HIPAA rules and complete a release of records form for a release of information.

SCENARIO: Aaron Jackson was seen at Walden Hospital for a high fever. You need to help Aaron's mother complete a records release form so his record from the emergency department visit can be sent to the clinic. She needs to request all records from the visit on the first of this month. The clinic information is on the form. The release will expire in 1 month.

AARON'S INFORMATION	WALDEN HOSPITAL'S INFORMATION
Date of birth: 10/17/20XX	Address:
Social Security number: 164-72-4618	Walden Hospital
Address:	123 Healing Way
555 McArthur Avenue	Anywhere, AL 12345-1234
Anytown, AL 12345-1234	Phone: (123) 814-4563
Phone: (123) 814-7844	Fax: (123) 814-6544
Mother: Patricia Jackson	

DIRECTIONS: You will complete the medical record release form. You will role-play the scenario with a peer. You will be the medical assistant, and the peer will be the mother.

EQUIPMENT and SUPPLIES

- Records release form (electronic or paper) (see Figure 4.3)
- Patient's health record

PROCEDURAL STEPS

1. Using the medical records release form, complete the patient information (see Figure 4.3). Add the patient's name, date of birth (DOB), and Social Security number (SSN). Include the current address and phone number found in the Patient's health record. If an electronic form is used, select the correct patient, and the fields will auto-populate.
   PURPOSE: The patient's information is required on the form. The patient's name, DOB, and SSN are direct identifiers, which will also help the hospital identify the correct patient.
2. Complete the parts of the form that specify who authorizes the release and who is to release the information.
   PURPOSE: Depending on state law and the facility's policy, the mother's name or the child's name may be the party authorizing the release. The hospital is the party that will release the information.
3. Check the box(es) of the information that needs to be released. If required, write in what other records need to be released.
   PURPOSE: Depending on state law and the facility's policy, the "Other" location might be where substance abuse and human immunodeficiency virus (HIV) records can be specifically requested. Other forms have a specific section for the release of substance abuse and HIV records.
4. Add the date of the visit. Add the name and contact information for the facility where the records need to be sent.
   PURPOSE: The release form needs to indicate where the records are being sent.
5. Indicate how the released information will be used.
   PURPOSE: This information tells the releasing facility how the information will be used. In this situation, the provider is requesting the information for healthcare purposes.
6. Indicate when the authorization should expire. Proofread the form for accuracy. If using an electronic form, save the form to the patient's health record. Print the form so the mother can sign.
   PURPOSE: In some situations, this may be an ongoing release. For example, the patient may get weekly blood tests at a local clinic, and the results need to be sent to the patient's specialist.
7. During a role-play with the patient's mother, explain what the provider is requesting. Ensure she can understand and read English. Have the mother read the form.
   PURPOSE: For the release to be legal, the mother must understand what she is signing. If she does not understand English, you will need a translator available to help in this situation.
8. Ask the mother if she has any questions. Answer any questions, and explain where she needs to sign if she agrees with the documentation.
   PURPOSE: By answering questions, you can help her understand the release process. It is important to make sure she is in agreement with the form before she signs. After the mother has signed, the form will be faxed to the hospital. The signed form should be filed in the patient record or scanned and uploaded into the electronic health record.

PROCEDURE 4.3 Perform Disease Reporting

TASKS: Research the state's disease reporting public health statutes and complete the disease reporting paperwork based on public health statutes. Document the activity in the patient's health record.

SCENARIO: Jean Burke, NP, received the test results for Ken Thomas. He tested positive for gonorrhea. She wants you to file the report with the public health department. Here is the information from his health record and the clinic. For any missing information, follow the instructor's directions (or, if no directions are provided for this exercise, make up the information).

PATIENT INFORMATION	PROVIDER AND LAB INFORMATION	HEALTH RECORD INFORMATION
Ken Thomas 398 Larkin Avenue Anytown, AL 12345-1234 Anycounty **Email:** k.thomas@anytown.mail **Phone:** (123) 784-1118 **DOB:** 10/25/19XX **Race:** Multiple races **Ethnicity:** Unknown **Marital status:** Single, living with Sandy Brown, who was not treated	**Provider:** Jean Burke, NP Walden-Martin Family Medical Clinic 1234 Anystreet Anytown, AL 12345-1234 **Phone:** (123) 123-1234 **Fax:** (123) 123-5678 **Lab:** Walden-Martin Family Medical Clinic Lab	**Diagnosis:** Gonorrhea **Symptoms:** Started 5 days ago, greenish discharge from penis, burning with urination **Test:** Urine specimen was collected yesterday; gonorrhea nucleic acid amplification test (NAAT) test done yesterday, results are positive **Treatment:** Patient treated today with ceftriaxone 250 mg intramuscular (IM) single dose and azithromycin 1 g orally single dose

EQUIPMENT and SUPPLIES

- Computer with internet access and printer
- Patient's health record (see preceding table)
- Black pen

PROCEDURAL STEPS

1. Using the internet, search for the disease reporting procedure in your state's public health department or similar facility. Read the procedure.
   PURPOSE: A medical assistant needs to be aware of the disease reporting procedure for the state.
2. Identify which form is required based on the patient's diagnosis. Print the form.
   PURPOSE: Some departments of health services agencies may have several forms available on their websites. It is important to use the correct form. Gonorrhea is a sexually transmitted infection.
3. Use a black pen to complete the form. Neatly complete the patient's demographic information section using the information from the health record.
   PURPOSE: All forms require the patient's name and contact information.
4. Complete the diagnosis, symptoms, testing, and treatment information.
   PURPOSE: The public health department needs information on the diagnosis, symptoms, test results, and the treatment provided.
5. Complete the rest of the form. Review the form for accuracy. Make any changes required before submitting the form to the instructor.
   PURPOSE: The form must be accurate and complete before it is sent to the public health department.
6. Document i the patient's health record that the disease reporting paperwork was completed and submitted.
   PURPOSE: All activities related to the patient must be documented in the patient's health record.

Documentation Example

07/25/20XX 11:05 a.m. The state's disease reporting paperwork for the Gonorrhea diagnosis (on 07/25/20XX) was completed and submitted as requested by Jean Burke, NP. —————— Bella Dickens, CMA (AAMA)

PROCEDURE 4.4 Report Illegal Activity

TASK: Report an illegal activity in the healthcare setting following proper protocol.

SCENARIO: You witness a co-worker, Sally Brown, taking medical samples from the supply cabinet. You see her sticking them into her purse. She sees you and states, "This was the same medication I had to pay $200 for the last time I was sick. I don't see why we need to pay for medications when we have samples that we give free to patients. We should be able to use them also." You know the facility's professional policy prohibits taking medical samples from the sample cabinet for personal reasons.

Continued

PROCEDURE 4.4 Report Illegal Activity—*continued*

FACILITY'S COMPLIANCE REPORTING PROTOCOL

Walden-Martin Family Medical Clinic's Compliance Program has a phone number and email address for employees to report suspected violations, suspected illegal activity, fraud, abuse, theft, and workplace safety concerns. Concerns can be left on the voice mail or emailed without fear of retribution or retaliation. Please include as many details as possible, including dates, names, and a description of the situation.

Any employee who seeks retribution or retaliation against another employee for reporting an offense needs to be aware of criminal penalties for such actions.

EQUIPMENT and SUPPLIES

- Computer with email and internet access or phone
- Instructor's email address or voice mail phone number
- Pen and paper
- Facility's compliance reporting protocol (see the previous section)

PROCEDURAL STEPS

1. Read the facility's corporate compliance reporting protocol.
   PURPOSE: Prior to reporting an illegal action, the medical assistant needs to identify the facility's protocol or the reporting chain of command. (Chain of command usually begins with your supervisor, then the supervisor of your supervisor, and so on. It is recommended you start with the lowest level that you feel comfortable with.)
2. Using paper and pen, write down the facts of what you witnessed.
   PURPOSE: Writing down the facts soon after the situation will help you remember the details.
3. Using paper and pen, compose the message you want to email or leave on the voice mail for the compliance office.
   PURPOSE: Composing a message will help you organize your thoughts and leave an accurate message.
4. Proofread the message and make any changes required. Make sure to include the date, names of people involved, and the details of the situation.
   PURPOSE: It is important to have an accurate, complete message for the compliance office. Proofreading helps to ensure the message is accurate.
5. Using your email or phone, send a message to the corporate compliance office. Use the email address or phone number provided by your instructor.
   PURPOSE: To complete the reporting process, the medical assistant must contact the corporate compliance office or the required supervisor if following the chain of command.

PROCEDURE 4.5 Complete Incident Report

TASK: Complete an incident report form for a medication error.

SCENARIO: Johnny Parker (DOB 06/15/20XX) sees Jean Burke, NP, for a well-child visit. Johnny is off schedule with his hepatitis B vaccine series, and today he is to get his last hepatitis B booster. You (a medical assistant) prepare the medication and give the injection in his right deltoid muscle. Later in the day, you realize that hepatitis B has been out of stock for 1 week. You must have given a hepatitis A booster to Johnny. You realize that you failed to read the label three times during the preparation of the medication. You report the mistake to Jean Burke and your supervisor. Your supervisor calls Lisa Parker, Johnny's mother. They will come back next week for the hepatitis B vaccine. You need to complete the incident report.

EQUIPMENT and SUPPLIES

- Incident report form (see Figure 4.6) and black pen or computer with internet access and SimChart for the Medical Office (SCMO)

PROCEDURAL STEPS

1. *SCMO method*: Access SCMO and enter the Simulation Playground. If a popup window appears, select "Return to previous session with saved patient information" and click Start. On the Calendar screen, click on the Form Repository icon. Click on Office Forms on the left Info Panel and select Incident Report. *For both methods:* Accurately complete the information from the date down to the reason for the patient's visit.
   PURPOSE: It is important to have accurate information regarding the date, time, location, incident type, and the reason for the visit. Giving the background information will help the reader understand what occurred.
2. *For both methods*: Specify the incident description, immediate action and outcome, contributing factors, and fill in the prevention boxes. Provide as much detail as possible. Be honest and concise with your facts.
   PURPOSE: It is important to give a clear, concise, and honest description of what occurred. It is hard to admit fault but doing so shows your professionalism in the situation.
3. *For both methods*: Complete the reported by, position, and contact phone number sections. Your information should be in these fields. (For this exercise, make up a contact phone number.)
   PURPOSE: It is important to have accurate information in these fields so that people can contact you if they have questions.
4. *For both methods*: Complete the other persons involved, position, and contact phone number sections. Jean Burke's information should be in these fields. (Make up her contact phone number.)
   PURPOSE: Having additional people listed on the form helps if questions arise about the situation. The rest of the form, from the Medical Reports field to the end, needs to be completed by the provider.
5. *For both methods*: Review the form for accuracy. Make any changes required before submitting the form to the instructor. (*For the SCMO method*: Save or print the form based on your instructor's directions.)
   PURPOSE: It is important to proofread the form to ensure it is accurate and complete.

HEALTHCARE ETHICS

5

SCENARIO

Daniela Garcia has just been hired as a part-time float receptionist at Walden-Martin Family Medical (WMFM) Clinic. As a float receptionist, she will be working with many co-workers and providers. Besides working, Daniela is also attending the local community college for medical assisting. She is currently taking a law and ethics course.

Daniela has completed the law part of the course. She is starting the ethics unit. Daniela grew up in a conservative family. They lived in a very small town in the Midwest. She has since relocated and finds that some of the beliefs she held as a teen are now changing as she encounters more life challenges. As she studies various topics, she has also found that what she believed to be true when she was younger is not actually true. Daniela is very interested in continuing to learn about ethics.

While studying this chapter, think about the following questions:

- What are personal and professional ethics?
- How can people separate their personal and professional ethics?
- What are the four principles of healthcare ethics?
- What are ethical issues that relate to genetics, reproductive, childhood, end-of-life, and organ donation issues?

LEARNING OBJECTIVES

1. Examine personal ethics.
2. Examine professional ethics for physicians and medical assistants.
3. Analyze how to separate professional ethics and personal ethics.
4. Analyze how medical assistants can incorporate the ethical principles of anatomy, nonmaleficence, beneficence, and justice into their work life.
5. Examine the ethical issues that relate to genetics.
6. Examine the ethical issues surrounding assistive reproductive technology and elective termination of pregnancies.
7. Examine the ethical issues surrounding childhood.
8. Examine the ethical issues related to research trials.
9. Examine end-of-life issues, including palliative medicine, hospice, and grieving.
10. Analyze the importance of the Patient Self-Determination Act and advance directives.
11. Examine ethical issues related to dying, including how death is determined, withholding life-sustaining treatments, and euthanasia.
12. Examine the ethical issues related to organ donation.
13. Differentiate between the Uniform Anatomical Gift Act and the National Organ Transplant Act.

VOCABULARY

bioethicists (BYE oh eth I sists) People who study the ethical effect of biomedical advances (e.g., drugs and genetic engineering).

cessation Bringing to an end.

chromosomes (KROE mah somes) Rod-shaped structures found in the cell's nucleus; they contain genetic information.

cryopreservation (KRIE oh pri zur vae shun) To preserve by freezing at low temperatures.

discipline A branch of knowledge, learning, or instruction—for instance, medicine, nursing, social work, and physical therapy.

embryo (EM bree oh) A developing organism from the moment of conception through the eighth week of development.

ethics (ETH iks) Rules of conduct that differentiate between acceptable and unacceptable behavior.

ethics committee A group composed of members from a variety of disciplines that analyze ethical issues.

evidence-based practice Healthcare practice that incorporates the most current and valid research results, thus providing the best patient care.

germline cells Sperm and egg cells.

morals (MORE ahls) Internal principles that distinguish between right and wrong.

oocyte (OO eh site) An immature ovum (egg).

personal ethics An individual's code of conduct.

resident A physician who has graduated from medical school and is finishing specialized clinical training.

somatic cells (soe MAT ik) Nonreproductive cells; they do not include sperm and egg cells.

surrogate (SUR ah git) A person who acts on behalf of another person or takes the place of another person. Examples include a surrogate mother or a healthcare agent.

INTRODUCTION

As you move into healthcare, you may be faced with situations in which you do not agree with a person's decision. As a healthcare professional, you need to respect a patient's decision whether or not you agree with it.

This chapter examines **ethics**. Ethical issues are different from legal issues. What may be legal may not be ethical. **Personal ethics** and their impact on professional performance will be discussed. Professional ethics differs from personal ethics. This topic is explored, along with how to handle the differences. Common ethical issues in healthcare are examined. End-of-life issues, including advance directives, are also discussed.

PERSONAL ETHICS

Personal ethics includes an individual's honesty, fairness, commitment, integrity, and accountability. It also includes doing what one considers to be correct.

Morals

Our **morals** tell us what is right and wrong. Our moral compass develops as we grow. Our first lessons on right and wrong come from those we live with. Our socialization and background shape our morals. For instance, if your parents instilled in you the importance of always being on time, you may grow up feeling that a person should always be on time. You may feel others are in error if they are late for an event. As we grow, our morals may change if our beliefs change. Our morals affect how we conduct ourselves or, in other words, our personal ethics.

Morals and Professional Performance

Our personal morals affect our professional performance. If people believe in being on time, this characteristic will transfer to the work environment. Employees will be on time for work. Being timely when rooming patients will be important to employees. Having patients wait for long periods of time in the reception area will be challenging to accept. Personal morals that align with professional characteristics will positively affect one's professional performance.

Our personal morals may also negatively affect our professional performance. Let's say a person grew up without grandparents or older adults in the family. That person may view older people as not being as knowledgeable as the younger generations. If a medical assistant had this belief, imagine how that might affect their professional performance. That person may not respect older adults and may view them as being useless, unimportant, or irrelevant individuals. This will affect how the medical assistant would treat an older patient. As professionals, we cannot let our personal morals negatively affect the care we provide to patients.

CRITICAL THINKING APPLICATION **5.1**

Daniela was working on her ethics assignment on break at the clinic. She thought about her personal ethics. She decided that some of her personal ethics would benefit her in a job. She realizes that some of her personal morals may negatively affect the care she provides to patients. She realizes that she needs to explore these morals and make some personal decisions. Think about your personal ethics and morals. What will positively influence your professional performance? What personal morals will negatively affect your professional performance?

PROFESSIONAL ETHICS

Professional ethics refers to codes of conduct stated by an employer or a professional association (Table 5.1). Many employers state how employees need to conduct themselves in the workplace. This information can usually be found in the employee handbook.

Many healthcare professional associations have published professional ethics for their members. These are called *codes of ethics.* A code of ethics is a set of rules about good and bad behavior. The association or agency will discipline any member or employee who violates a professional ethic. We will examine the codes for physicians and medical assistants.

Code of Ethics for Physicians

One of the most famous and oldest codes of ethics is the Hippocratic oath. The original oath has been around for longer than 2000 years. Some of its concepts include treating the patient, not the disease, and maintaining the patient's confidentiality. Hippocrates often called the father of medicine, is credited for the oath. The oath is a code of ethics for physicians. Over the years, the code has been modernized (see Chapter 1 for the Hippocratic Oath).

In 1847 the American Medical Association (AMA) adopted its Code of Medical Ethics. The code lists the values that physicians commit themselves to as they practice medicine. The AMA's current Code of Medical Ethics is available on its website (www.ama-assn.org). The code is a living document. This means that as medicine and technology change, the code is updated by the members. The following are key themes in the code:

- Physicians should provide competent care and continue learning.
- Physicians should respect human dignity and human rights.
- Physicians should follow the laws, be professional, and uphold the standards of the medical profession.
- Physicians should contribute to the welfare of the community.

The Council of Ethical and Judicial Affairs (CEJA) is one of the councils within the AMA. The CEJA analyzes ethical issues in healthcare and develops ethical policies and recommendations. Physicians use these recommendations, along with the Code of Medical Ethics, to guide their practice. The CEJA prompts AMA members to adhere to the Code of Medical Ethics.

TABLE 5.1 Differences Between Personal and Professional Ethics

	PERSONAL ETHICS	PROFESSIONAL ETHICS
Definition	Individual's code of conduct	Codes of conduct stated by an employer or a professional association
Ability to change	Individuals can change their own personal ethics	Individuals cannot change these codes and must comply; codes can only be changed by employer or professional association
Accountability	On the individual	On the members and organization

Medical Assisting Code of Ethics

Members of the AAMA dedicated to the conscientious pursuit of their profession, and thus desiring to merit the high regard of the entire medical profession and the respect of the general public which they serve, do pledge themselves to strive always to:

A. Render service with full respect for the dignity of humanity.
B. Respect confidential information obtained through employment unless legally authorized or required by responsible performance of duty to divulge such information.
C. Uphold the honor and high principles of the profession and accept its disciplines.
D. Seek to continually improve the knowledge and skills of medical assistants for the benefit of patients and professional colleagues.
E. Participate in additional service activities aimed toward improving the health and well-being of the community.

From the American Association of Medical Assistants: Medical assisting code of ethics, www.aama-ntl.org/about/overview#.WSDywmjytPY.

Code of Ethics for Medical Assistants

The American Association of Medical Assistants (AAMA) developed a code of ethics that provides the principles of ethical and moral conduct for the profession.

The AAMA has also written a Medical Assisting Creed, which can be used as a guideline for medical assistants facing complex ethical and moral issues in the course of their work. The Medical Assisting Creed supports the code of ethics by asking members to abide by ethical statements of belief:

- I believe in the principles and purposes of the profession of medical assisting.
- I endeavor to be more effective.
- I aspire to render greater service.
- I protect the confidence entrusted to me.
- I am dedicated to the care and well-being of all people.
- I am loyal to my employer.
- I am true to the ethics of my profession.
- I am strengthened by compassion, courage, and faith.

The Medical Assisting Creed supports the code of ethics. The above creed can be found on the AAMA's website (www.aama-ntl.org/about/overview#.WSDywmjytPY).

It is important for the medical assistant to follow the code and the creed. The care provided to others must reflect respect for that person. The medical assistant is legally and ethically obligated to keep patient information confidential. Continual learning is critical. The medical assistant must provide the best care possible and uphold the standards of the profession.

CRITICAL THINKING APPLICATION **5.2**

Daniela read the AMA Code of Medical Ethics and the AAMA Medical Assisting Code of Ethics. She notices some similarities between the codes. What similarities do you notice between the two codes?

SEPARATION PLAN

Sometimes an individual's personal ethics clash with professional ethics. It is important to take steps to separate one's personal ethics from professional ethics.

Influence of Personal Ethics

Let's examine a few situations that might affect a medical assistant. Imagine if a medical assistant has personal beliefs that vaccines are not needed and harm individuals. This medical assistant obtains a job in a pediatric department. She is required to give vaccines numerous times a day. In this situation, her personal ethics would clash with her professional ethics. She would be professionally obligated to give the vaccines to patients. She could not share her antivaccine beliefs with patients. Due to the clash of ethics, it might be a stressful job for her.

In another situation, a medical assistant believes that everything that can be done should be done when someone is dying. Professional ethics mandate that each person has a right to make end-of-life decisions. Legally and ethically, the medical assistant must follow what the patient decides. The medical assistant cannot put pressure on patients to change their decisions.

Creating a Plan

As you complete your medical assisting courses, it is important to evaluate whether your personal ethics conflict with the medical assistant code of ethics.

- Are there groups of people with whom you have issues? Maybe you do not believe in their behaviors, actions, or ideas based on your morals.
- Do you have preconceived ideas about people with differing ethnicities, sexual preferences, or specific diseases?

If you identified conflicts, how might you provide respectful care to these patients? Honestly, think about your biases. How would you approach a situation if it involved your bias? Remember, the professional code of ethics supersedes your personal code. You need to follow the professional ethics of your agency and profession (Procedure 5.1).

Before medical assistants start applying for positions, it is important that they evaluate whether personal ethics will clash with the professional ethics of an agency. If a person does not believe in vaccinations, then working in a department that gives vaccinations would not be a good job choice. If a person does not believe in abortions, then working in an agency that does abortions would not be a good choice.

CRITICAL THINKING APPLICATION **5.3**

Daniela decided to create a plan to separate her personal ethics from her professional ethics. Think about your personal ethics. What steps might you take to change your personal morals so that they better align with your professional ethics? What might you do to deal with the personal ethics that conflict with the professional ethics?

PRINCIPLES OF HEALTHCARE ETHICS

Healthcare professionals have an ethical duty to their patients. Four ethical principles summarize this ethical duty. These principles are autonomy, nonmaleficence, beneficence, and justice. Technically, all four of these principles should have equal weight in ethical decisions. Many times, autonomy overshadows the other three principles.

Besides healthcare professionals, **bioethicists** also use the principles of healthcare ethics. They apply these principles when they evaluate medical technology and procedures. Are the new technology advances ethical? Are these procedures ethical?

We will examine the four ethical principles. Ethical actions to meet the principles will be discussed for both the provider and the medical assistant.

Autonomy

Autonomy is the freedom to determine one's own actions and decisions. Patients have the right to make their own healthcare decisions. Providers need to tell patients about the risks and benefits of different procedures (informed consent). After being told what may be most successful, the patients can make their own decisions. The patient's decision-making process should be free from pressure or interference from others. Healthcare professionals must respect and honor the patient's decision.

The medical assistant must protect patients' privacy. It is important to respect the uniqueness, dignity, and decisions of others. This includes patients, families, and co-workers. Medical assistants must demonstrate these professional behaviors, which will also maintain their own dignity and self-respect:

- Help to make others around you look good without minimizing yourself. Do this by being supportive and helpful to your team members.
- Refrain from being negative and whining.
- Be assertive, not aggressive, when standing up for your rights (e.g., adequate work environment, hours, and pay).
- Collaborate and cooperate with co-workers. Do not be afraid to stand up for what is right and fair.
- Avoid bringing personal issues into the workplace.

CRITICAL THINKING APPLICATION 5.4

When Daniela learned about the autonomy principle and the role of the medical assistant, it reminded her of healthcare laws that she had learned about earlier. What healthcare laws address autonomy and the healthcare professional's role?

Nonmaleficence

Nonmaleficence means to do no harm. Healthcare professionals are obligated not to inflict intentional harm on patients. By providing the appropriate standard of care, we can reduce the risk of negligence. It is important to provide competent care to patients for both legal and ethical reasons.

The medical assistant must demonstrate professionalism by preventing harm to others—this means to intervene when a patient is at risk (e.g., falling). It is important to make sure the environment is both physically and psychologically safe for others, and that safety hazards are reported and corrected. For instance, malfunctioning equipment must never be used until fixed. Hazardous chemicals and sharps (needles) must be unavailable to patients. The medical assistant must also provide safe and competent care to all patients.

Beneficence

Beneficence refers to the moral obligation to act for the good or benefit of others. For healthcare professionals, this means promoting health in patients and assisting patients to recover from illness. Promoting health and disease prevention are professional behaviors for medical assistants. With the current focus on prevention of diseases, medical assistants help providers by identifying the immunizations and screening tests their patients need.

Justice

Justice means to treat patients fairly and give them the care that is due and appropriate. This means that patients in similar situations should receive the same services and treatments.

Professional behaviors of the medical assistant include providing equal respect and courtesy to all people. Regardless of the person's skin color, sexual preference, nationality, religion, and health history, every person must be treated respectfully. It is important that medical assistants think about their biases. Do you really feel everyone is equal? Is there any group of individuals whose ideas you do not agree with? Understanding one's biases are important. If we do not identify our biases, there is a tendency to treat others differently. As healthcare professionals, we are obligated to treat everyone equally and with respect (Procedure 5.2).

ETHICAL ISSUES RELATED TO GENETICS

The remainder of this chapter discusses ethical issues in healthcare. There are many ethical issues in healthcare. As technology and medicine evolve, additional ethical issues arise. We will examine common ethical issues and explain the CEJA's recommendations. We will start with ethical issues related to genetics.

Each person is made up of 46 **chromosomes**, 23 from each parent. Genes are the basic units of heredity or the instructions on how our bodies should develop and function. Genes provide the differences among us and the similarities in families. From genes, we get our physical appearance, in addition to our susceptibility to disease. During the process of conception and subsequent cell division, an extra chromosome (or a change in the chromosome structure) may occur, resulting in a genetic disease or disorder. The following are types of genetic diseases:

- *Monogenic disorders*: A defective gene is inherited from one or both parents. Huntington's disease, cystic fibrosis, and sickle cell anemia are examples of monogenic disorders.
- *Chromosomal disorders*: An abnormal number of chromosomes or a change in the chromosomal structure causes diseases, such as Klinefelter syndrome and Turner syndrome.

With advances in technology, we can now test for many genetic disorders, sometimes even on a baby in utero (e.g., fetus). There has also been a lot of research in the areas of cloning, genetic engineering, and gene therapy. Along with these advancements come ethical issues and questions. We will explore cloning and genetic engineering advancements and related ethical issues.

Cloning

Cloning is the process of creating a genetically identical biological entity. A clone is a copy that has the same genetic makeup as the original entity. Researchers have cloned genes, cells, tissues, and organisms. Dolly, a sheep, was the first mammal cloned. Since then, at least eight different mammals have been cloned, including horses, pigs, dogs, and cats. Advocates for human cloning discuss the need for organ transplants. Opponents of human cloning address the rights of the clone.

Genetic Engineering

Genetic engineering is the manipulation of genetic material in cells to change hereditary traits or produce a specific result. Genetic engineering is used in many areas, including agriculture and medicine. For instance, a lot of corn and soybeans are genetically modified to resist disease and insects. These foods may be labeled as genetically modified organisms (GMOs). In medicine, insulin, human growth hormone, and other drugs are genetically engineered. We will focus on genetic engineering in medicine.

A *genome* is the entire genetic makeup of an organism. The Human Genome Project, a 13-year international project, mapped the human genome. The entire human genome contains about 30,000 genes. The goal of the project was to gain information that will eventually lead to the prevention and treatment of many diseases. Genomic medicine resulted from the Human Genome Project. *Genomic medicine* is an emerging branch of medicine involved with using patients' genomic information as part of their clinical care. Genetic testing, pharmacogenetics, and stem cell transplants are important advances in genomic medicine. Gene therapy is currently being researched.

Genetic Testing

Genetic testing can identify issues with a person's chromosomes, genes, or proteins. More than 1000 genetic tests are available. The following are some of the types of genetic testing:

- *Newborn screening*: All states have newborn screening procedures to identify genetic disorders that can be treated early in life.
- *Diagnostic testing*: Used to diagnose a specific genetic or chromosomal condition. Testing can occur prior to birth or after. Not all genetic conditions have diagnostic tests.
- *Carrier testing*: Used to determine if a person is carrying one copy of a gene mutation. Two copies of a gene mutation (one from each parent) can result in a genetic disorder in a child.
- *Prenatal testing*: Used to detect genetic or chromosomal issues with a fetus (unborn baby).
- *Preimplantation testing*: Used to detect genetic issues in **embryos** that were created using assistive reproductive technology, which will be explained later in the chapter.
- *Predictive and presymptomatic testing*: Used to detect gene mutations associated with specific disorders that occur after birth. Usually done when a patient has a family member with a genetic disorder, and the patient wants to see if he or she also has it.
- *Forensic testing*: Used to identify crime or catastrophe victims, identify or rule out crime suspects, or establish biological relationships between people (e.g., paternity).

Per the CEJA, the impact of genetics on diseases is complex. Understanding genetic counseling and helping the patient to understand the results require special skills from the provider. Genetic testing is most important when it makes a meaningful impact on a person's health. The provider ordering genetic testing should have the appropriate knowledge and expertise to counsel the patient on the findings and implications. Providers must keep genetic testing information confidential.

CRITICAL THINKING APPLICATION 5.5

When Daniela learned about genetic testing, she remembered hearing about how people could trace their relatives. She also had heard about forensic testing while watching crime drama shows. What types of genetic testing are you familiar with?

Pharmacogenetics

Pharmacogenomics is a branch of pharmacology that studies the genetic factors that influence a person's response to a medication. Based on a person's genome, pharmacogenomics can determine if a specific therapy will be effective. Pharmacogenomics information is already available on more than 200 medications that have been approved by the US Food and Drug Administration (FDA). These medications include analgesics, antivirals, cardiovascular drugs, and anticancer drugs.

Stem Cell Transplants

Stem cells can differentiate or develop into specialized cells (e.g., muscle, blood, or brain cells). They can self-renew or make copies of themselves. The new cell can remain a stem cell or turn into a specialized cell. Depending on where the stem cells are located, they may constantly be repairing and replacing damaged tissue (e.g., intestinal tract). In other locations, such as the heart, they only divide in special situations.

There are two main categories of stem cells: adult and embryonic. Table 5.2 describes both types of stem cells. Stem cell research has been going on since the 1960s. New technology has helped advance the research. Many researchers are excited about the potential of stem cells. Cord blood stem cell transplants have been used to treat more than 75 diseases, including cancers, anemias, metabolic disorders, and immune system disorders.

Though both types of stem cell research have ethical issues, embryonic stem cell research has greater ethical issues. Harvesting stem cells from an embryo would mean destroying the embryo. For those who believe that life begins at the moment of conception, this means a life is lost.

Gene Therapy

Gene therapy is currently an experimental technique that uses genes to prevent or treat diseases. With this procedure, a gene is inserted into a patient's cell. The hopes are that the new gene might replace a mutated gene, prevent the mutated gene from functioning, or help fight the disease.

Gene editing or *genome editing* is a specific gene therapy. This technique can remove, add, or alter sections of the gene. With new technology emerging in this area, ethical issues have also arisen. Genome editing of **somatic cells** would only affect the individual. This treatment has already been used and is considered ethical. Genome editing of **germline cells** can cause issues that may affect future generations. Genome editing of germline cells raises ethical concerns and is illegal in the United States.

REPRODUCTIVE ETHICAL ISSUES

Ethical issues surround assistive reproductive technology used for infertility and elective termination of pregnancy. The following sections examine these two reproductive issues.

Assistive Reproductive Technology

Infertility is the inability to get pregnant after 1 year of unprotected intercourse (sex). Infertility can affect both males and females. There are many causes of infertility. With advances in technology, assistive reproductive technology (ART) has allowed many couples to have children. Assisted reproductive technology includes all procedures that involve the handling of the eggs, sperm, or embryos. Consider these common types of ART:

- *In vitro fertilization*: Involves removing mature eggs from the ovaries and fertilizing the eggs with sperm outside of the body. The fertilized eggs are then transferred to the uterus.
- *Intrauterine insemination* (IUI): Also called *artificial insemination.* Specially prepared sperm are placed into a woman's uterus using a long, narrow tube (e.g., a straw). The woman's partner's sperm or a donor's sperm can be used.
- *Surrogacy*: A woman carries and gives birth for another couple. A legal contract should be in place to protect all parties. *Traditional surrogacy* or *partial surrogacy* occurs when the egg is from a **surrogate**, and the sperm is from the father. *Gestational surrogacy* or *full surrogacy* occurs when the sperm and egg come from the intended parents or are donated, and the surrogate is not related to the baby.

One of the complications of ART is multiple births. An ethical issue can arise if the success of the pregnancy may be hindered by the number of babies in utero. If this situation occurs, the provider must inform the patient of the risks with multiple births.

The CEJA's opinions are that providers who offer assisted reproductive services should provide accurate advertising of their services. They need to provide all information, including success rates and costs, so patients can make an informed decision. Prospective donors need to be tested for infectious disease agents and genetic diseases. Donors need to provide informed consent.

Gamete Donation

Gamete (egg or sperm) donation allows others who are unable to have children to do so. Many ethical issues surround gamete donation:

- The privacy of the donors
- The rights of the child born from the donated gamete
- The relationship between the child and the donor
- The number of donations from a single donor (the more children born from the donor's gamete, the greater the risk of the children mating and conceiving children together)
- The health of the donors and the children born from the donations
- The regulations on gamete storage
- The compensation for gamete donation (many countries do not allow payment for gamete donation; however, the United States does allow it)

The CEJA's opinions are that providers who participate in the gamete donation process must inform the prospective donors about the risk of the donation, the testing involved, and whether or not the donor will receive the test results. Donors should be tested for infectious diseases and genetic disorders. The donor should be notified that all information will be kept indefinitely. The provider should discuss the storage of the gametes, compensation, and that the state law governs the relationship between the gamete donor and the child born from the gamete.

The CEJA's opinions are that providers should not allow people to donate if they have infectious diseases. The provider should also gather the donor's preferences on the use of the gametes, whether for research or reproduction. The provider should find out the donor's preferences regarding release of identifying information to any child resulting from the donor. Donors should also limit the number of pregnancies resulting from a single gamete donor.

Egg Freezing

Egg freezing, or *egg banking*, is the **cryopreservation** of **oocytes**, which is done to preserve the female's fertility. Egg freezing is done for a variety of reasons:

- A woman has been diagnosed with cancer and may become infertile with the cancer treatments.
- A woman wants to delay childbearing.
- A woman objects to freezing embryos.

The egg retrieval process requires the patient to undergo about 9 to 10 days of hormone injections to stimulate the ovaries and assist in the ripening of multiple eggs. Once the egg retrieval is completed, the eggs are frozen until needed. Usually, 10 to 20 eggs are retrieved.

With the freezing process, the eggs are dehydrated, and the water is replaced with a fluid that prevents ice from forming and destroying the egg. The eggs can be flash frozen or frozen using a slow process. When the patient wants to become pregnant, some of the eggs are thawed. They are fertilized and then transferred to the patient's uterus.

There are a number of ethical issues surrounding egg freezing:

- Safety of the procedure for both the patient and any future children that result from the eggs
- Marketing practices that focus on healthy women
- Pressures from companies for women to focus on their careers, freeze their eggs, and consider childbearing at a later time
- Disposition decisions, including egg-sharing options, for unused or unwanted eggs

The CEJA has not indicated a recommendation on egg freezing. The CEJA has provided a recommendation for cryopreservation of embryos, which is similar. Physicians who provide clinical services that include cryopreservation of embryos must discuss, with the parties involved, how the embryos will be used, thawed, or disposed of. A physician must not be involved with the sale of stored embryos.

Elective Abortion

Elective abortion is the deliberate termination of a pregnancy. Abortions can be done through medications and surgical procedures. Abortions raise many ethical questions and concerns. Some feel that women have the right to determine what occurs with their bodies, and fetuses (unborn babies in utero) have no rights until they are born. Others feel that from the moment of conception, babies have rights.

The advancement of technology has affected abortions. With greater technology, complex testing and treatments can occur. Surgery on babies in utero can treat health issues that, in the past, caused death or elected abortions. Advanced testing can diagnose issues sooner. For instance, imaging tests provide clearer pictures of babies in utero. In cases where diagnostic tests indicate major abnormalities, providers discuss the worst-case scenarios with the parents and include termination as part of informed consent. Per the CEJA's opinion, providers are not prohibited from performing an abortion in situations that do not violate the law.

TABLE 5.2 Types of Stem Cells

	ADULT STEM CELLS	EMBRYONIC STEM CELLS
Derived from	Found in infants through adults; found in many organs and tissues, including the brain, bone marrow, blood, skin, heart, teeth, testis, liver, blood vessel, and skeletal muscles. Umbilical cord blood also contains adult stem cells.	Taken from a 4- to 5-day-old human embryo
What types of cells can they become?	Variation thought to be limited; could become cell types similar to their tissue of origin. Scientists have found a way to "reprogram" some types of adult stem cells, so they act like embryonic cells.	Can become all cell types
Advantages	Thought to cause fewer rejection issues with transplants if a person's own stem cells are used.	Easy to grow in a laboratory setting
Ethical issue	Risks involved with adult stem cell use are still being evaluated.	For those believing life begins at the moment of conception, removing stem cells from an embryo would mean killing a person

CHILDHOOD ETHICAL ISSUES

Ethical issues related to childhood include making decisions regarding treatments, adoption, safe haven infant protection laws, and confidential healthcare for minors. The following sections discuss these childhood ethical issues.

Decisions on Treatments

In most cases, parents of minor children must authorize or decline treatment. In some cases, the state may need to provide the parental authority. *Parens patriae* is Latin for "father of the country." This doctrine gives the courts the power to make decisions for people who cannot make their own decisions. Many times, this doctrine is used for children or adults who are incompetent. It can be used when the parent or parents refuse healthcare for the child. The court may take over the parental rights and make decisions for the child.

There have been situations in which parents refuse procedures or treatments for their children based on religious or personal beliefs. One of the more common situations in ambulatory care is the refusal of vaccinations (see Procedure 5.2). It is important for the medical assistant to respect the Patient's Bill of Rights. If the patient provides a reason for the refusal, the medical assistant should let the provider know. The provider should also be told of the refusal, so other procedures or treatments can be discussed if needed.

The CEJA's opinion is that providers are encouraged to seek consultation with **ethics committees** in the following situations:

- The parent or guardian refuses treatment for a reversible life-threatening condition.
- There are disagreements about the minor's best interest.

The provider should only ask the courts to resolve the disagreement as the last option.

Adoption

Federal and state laws govern adoption. In healthcare, we run into adoption fairly often. Our patients may be adopted and do not know their family medical history. We need to be understanding of their situation. We may also work with pregnant women who are planning to give up their babies. Again, these are situations in which medical assistants need to be sensitive and understanding. The following are different types of adoption:

- *Adopting through an agency*: Private and public adoption agencies are regulated by the state and must be licensed to place children with adoptive parents. Public agencies usually place abandoned, orphaned, or abused children who are wards of the state.
- *Adopting independently*: The birth parents and the adoptive parents have an arrangement. Some states do not allow this type of adoption.
- *Adopting through identification*: Adoptive parents and birth parents work with an adoption agency to complete the adoption process.
- *Adopting internationally*: Adoptive parents work with an international adoption agency to adopt a child from another country. International adoption agencies must be certified by the US State Department.
- *Relative adoptions*: Relatives of a child adopt the child.
- *Closed adoptions*: There is no contact between the adoptive parents and the birth parents.
- *Open adoptions*: Adoptive parents meet and may stay in contact with the birth parents.

CRITICAL THINKING APPLICATION 5.6

For the adoptive child, what might be some advantages of open adoptions over closed adoptions? What might be advantages of closed adoptions for all parties involved?

Safe Haven Infant Protection Laws

Safe haven infant protection laws allow a person to give up an unwanted infant anonymously. The goal is to protect unwanted babies from abuse or death. The person is not prosecuted in the following circumstances:

- The infant is not abused.
- The infant is left at a designated location, as indicated by the state law.

- The infant is within the age limit, as indicated by the state law.

The designated locations vary by state. They may include hospitals, emergency departments, fire and police stations, and child welfare agencies. The age of the child varies. A few states allow children up to 1 year of age. Opponents of the safe haven laws voice concerns for fathers' rights and the lack of family medical history obtained. Supporters state that these laws save babies by providing a safe drop-off location and no questions asked.

Confidential Healthcare for Minors

Providers have an ethical duty to promote decision making in minor patients to the degree of the child's ability. Providers have a responsibility to protect the confidentiality of minor patients within certain limits. We see this in the ambulatory care setting when parents wait in the reception area while minor children (usually teens) have their physical exams. Many providers feel that the minor's answers to questions on safety, sex, drugs, and alcohol may be more truthful without the presence of parents.

In some states, laws permit unemancipated minors to request and receive confidential services. These services must relate to contraception, pregnancy testing, prenatal care, and delivery services. Additional services can include the prevention and treatment of sexually transmitted infections (STIs), substance use disorders, and mental illness. When the law does not grant minors decision-making authority for healthcare, the CEJA's opinion is that providers should do the following:

- Involve the parent or guardian in situations in which it is necessary to prevent harm to the patient or others.
- Involve the parent or guardian if the provider does not feel it will affect the patient's health.
- Explore reasons the minor does not want the involvement of the parent or guardian.
- Inform the minor that parents may learn of the treatment through insurance statements.
- Protect the confidentiality of the information from the minor, keeping it within ethical and legal standards.

CRITICAL THINKING APPLICATION **5.7**

On break one afternoon, Daniela talks to Jan, a medical assistant. She asks Jan how she handles parents who want to find out confidential information about their children. How might you professionally and respectfully handle a phone call from a parent who is requesting confidential information on their child?

RESEARCH TRIALS AND ETHICAL ISSUES

Many of the larger ambulatory healthcare facilities are involved with teaching nurse practitioner and physician assistant students and **residents** to become future healthcare providers. Typically, these facilities also are involved with research trials. These trials may relate to a treatment for a disease, such as a new surgical procedure or a new medication. Many healthcare **disciplines** use **evidence-based practice** that originated from research trials. Research on patient volunteers is critical to finding new ways of treating and managing diseases and caring for patients.

Ethical Guidelines for Research

Potentially, research trials place some people at risk of harm for the good of others. This could cause the exploitation of patient volunteers and is an ethical concern. Many ethical guidelines exist at local and national levels to protect patient volunteers. These guidelines were initiated based on past abuses. The following are some of the most influential guidelines and codes of ethics that guide clinical research.

- *Nuremberg Code*: Originated in 1947 after the Nuremberg trials, in which Nazi doctors were convicted of crimes committed during human experiments on concentration camp prisoners. The code outlined what was legal when conducting human experiments. Several of the points included the need for voluntary consent, that the results must be for the good of society, and that the experiments must be based on prior knowledge and should avoid all unnecessary physical and mental suffering.
- *Belmont Report*: Written in 1976 by the National Commission for the Protection of Human Subjects of Biomedical and Behavioral Research. The report identifies basic ethical principles and guidelines regarding human subject research.
- *Declaration of Helsinki*: A landmark document regarding research ethics developed by the World Medical Association in 1964 and revised many times. This document addressed the importance of human research, the obligations of the physicians involved, the importance of informed consent, and the protection of the participants.

Seven Principles for Ethical Research

According to the National Institutes of Health (NIH) Clinical Center (https://clinicalcenter.nih.gov/recruit/ethics.html), seven main principles are involved in ethical research:

- *Social and clinical value*: It should contribute to the knowledge base of either understanding health or preventing, treating, and caring for people with a specific disease.
- *Scientific validity*: The methods used should be valid and feasible, and the study must have clear scientific objectives.
- *Fair subject selection*: The subjects recruited should be based on the goals of the study.
- *Favorable risk-benefit ratio*: Everything must be done to minimize the risk to the research subjects and to maximize the benefits. The benefits should outweigh the risks.
- *Independent review*: The study should be reviewed by an independent review panel with no vested interest to ensure that the study is ethical and to minimize potential conflicts of interest.
- *Informed consent*: The participants need to be informed of the purpose, methods, risks, benefits, and alternatives to the research to be ethical. They need to understand the information and make a voluntary decision to participate.
- *Respect for potential and enrolled subjects*: Individuals have a right to change their minds at any time. Their information must be kept confidential, and they must be informed of information that may change their assessment of the risks and benefits of participating in the project.

Often medical assistants who are working at larger facilities may be involved with research projects. They may need to identify patients who match the project's criteria. Medical assistants may help with data collection. It is important for the medical assistant to know that all information must be kept confidential. All participants have a right to change their minds regarding their participation. Typically, the research guidelines or documents will include contact information that medical assistants can use if they have questions or concerns regarding the project.

END-OF-LIFE ISSUES

With the changes in healthcare and technology, more treatment options exist today to prolong a person's life. Ventilators assist the breathing process, and feeding tubes provide nutrition. Medications and defibrillators can help restart the heart. Legislation exists at the state and federal levels to help address death and dying issues. There are also many ethical questions that surround end-of-life issues.

It may sound like end-of-life issues are only addressed in the hospital. End-of-life issues also affect ambulatory care. Medical assistants may accompany providers in skilled nursing facility (nursing home) visits. Medical assistants provide ambulatory care to patients who have terminal illnesses. It is not uncommon for the medical assistant to process a referral for hospice care for a patient. The medical assistant should know the differences between palliative medicine and hospice care.

Palliative Medicine and Hospice Care

Palliative means to help relieve the symptoms of a serious illness. Palliative medicine is a subspecialty. The providers offer palliative care to patients who are seriously ill, regardless of age. The disease may be curable, chronic, or life threatening. Palliative care focuses on the entire person. It does not provide a cure; it just helps to reduce the symptoms.

Hospice is a type of palliative care for people who have about 6 months or less to live. The goal of hospice care is to allow patients who are dying to have dignity, comfort, and peace (Figure 5.1). Hospice programs work not only with the patient but also with the family. Hospice care can be provided in the hospital, skilled nursing facility, hospice center, and at home.

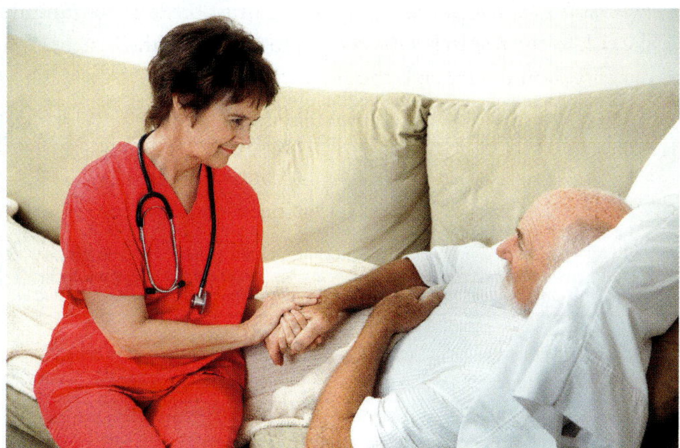

FIGURE 5.1 Hospice care is often delivered in a home environment. (From Hollen C, Stein L: Concept-based clinical nursing skills: fundamental to advanced, St. Louis, 2021, Elsevier.)

Stages of Grief and Dying

Working with patients who have a terminal illness can be emotionally challenging. It is important for the medical assistant to remember that patients and families go through the grieving process. Dr. Elisabeth Kübler-Ross defined the stages of grief and dying:

- *Denial*: Person refuses to accept the diagnosis or prognosis. Defense mechanism that protects people from being overwhelmed. Disbelief and numbness may occur.
- *Anger*: Person's anger can be directed at self or others. May blame others.
- *Bargaining*: Person attempts to bargain with the higher power the person believes in (e.g., God).
- *Depression*: Person feels sadness, fear, and uncertainty. Crying and depression may occur. Person may not participate in normal activities; distances self from others.
- *Acceptance*: Person has come to terms with the situation.

Not everyone goes through all five stages, and people may not go through the stages in the order listed. Some people may switch back and forth between the stages. Various behaviors may be seen during the grieving process:

- Sadness, loneliness, social isolation, crying, and difficulty concentrating
- Anger, guilt, denial, and confusion
- Fatigue, numbness, and appetite changes
- Sleep changes and nightmares

PATIENT SELF-DETERMINATION ACT

The Patient Self-Determination Act (PSDA) became law in 1990. This act requires most healthcare institutions at the time of admission to do the following:

- Provide patients with a written document of their rights to make decisions and the facility's policies respecting advance directives.
- Ask patients if they have advance directives and document the response in the health record.

Tuskegee Study

In 1932 the Public Health Service, working with the Tuskegee Institute, researched the natural history of syphilis. They hoped to justify treatment programs for African Americans. The study involved 399 black men with syphilis and 201 without it. The original 6-month study ended 40 years later when the Associated Press ran a story about the research study, and the public outcry led to an advisory panel investigation.

For this research study, the men had agreed freely to be examined and treated, but no informed consent was used. In compensation for the study, the men received free medical exams, free meals, and burial insurance. The men were told they were getting treated, but they did not receive proper treatment to cure syphilis, even though penicillin was available in 1947.

In 1974, a $10 million settlement was reached for the study participants and their surviving family members. The settlement also included health benefits for the participants and their family members.

Healthcare agencies must provide advance directive training to their staff. Staff members cannot discriminate against patients who have or do not have advance directives.

Per the CEJA, providers should take the following actions:

- Discuss advance care planning with all patients, regardless of health status or age.
- Explain advance directives and document in the health record information about advance care planning.
- Review advance care planning periodically with patients

If patients present advance directive paperwork, the medical assistant needs to ensure it gets into the health record. It is not uncommon for medical assistants to provide advance directive information to patients. The medical assistant must also be familiar with the different types of advance directives.

Advance Directives

Advance directives are written instructions about healthcare decisions should a person be unable to make them. Advance directives are not just for older adults to complete. It is important for everyone to consider completing advance directives. Once completed, advance directives can be modified in the future. It is important that local healthcare agencies have a copy of the person's advance directive paperwork.

Per the CEJA, providers should do the following:

- Identify if patients have advance directives, including a healthcare proxy.
- Respect the wishes of the patient's surrogate and help the surrogate understand the patient's wishes in the advance directives.
- Seek assistance from the ethics committee if a patient lacks advance directives and is unable to communicate.

Types of Advance Directives

Today most states have a multiple-page document for people to complete. The document can be found online or at healthcare agencies. The document may be called *advance directives, durable power of attorney for healthcare,* or something similar (Figure 5.2). It replaces multiple documents of the past. Generally, the advance directives document contains sections for the different types of advance directives, including the following:

- *Living will*: Provides instructions about life-sustaining medical treatment to be administered or withheld when the patient has a terminal condition.
- *Medical durable power of attorney*: May be known by other names. Similar to a living will but includes all healthcare decisions. It lasts as long as the person is not able to make decisions. This document names a healthcare proxy and can include healthcare wishes. It can be used when the situation is not terminal.
- *Healthcare proxy*: Also called *healthcare agent* or *surrogate.* Competent adults can appoint a person (called a *proxy* or

PART C: HEALTH CARE INSTRUCTIONS

NOTE: In filling out these instructions, keep the following in mind:

- The term "as my physician recommends" means that you want your physician to try life support if your physician believes it could be helpful and then discontinue it if it is not helping your health condition or symptoms.
- "Life support" and "tube feeding" are defined in PART B above.
- If you refuse tube feeding, you should understand that malnutrition, dehydration, and death probably result.
- You will get care for your comfort and cleanliness, no matter what choices you make.
- You may either give specific instructions by filling out Items 1 to 4 below, or you may use the general instruction provided by Item 5.

Here are my desires about my health care if my doctor and another knowledgeable doctor confirm that I am in a medical condition described below:

1. Close to Death. If I am close to death and life support would only postpone that moment of my death:

A. INITIAL ONE:
_______ I want to receive tube feeding.
_______ I want tube feeding only as my physician recommends.
_______ I DO NOT WANT tube feeding.

B. INITIAL ONE:
_______ I want any other life support that may apply.
_______ I want life support only as my physician recommends.
_______ I want NO life support.

2. Permanently Unconscious. If I am unconscious and it is very unlikely that I will ever become conscious again:

A. INITIAL ONE:
_______ I want to receive tube feeding.
_______ I want tube feeding only as my physician recommends.
_______ I DO NOT WANT tube feeding.

B. INITIAL ONE:
_______ I want any other life support that may apply.
_______ I want life support only as my physician recommends.
_______ I want NO life support.

PART C: HEALTH CARE INSTRUCTIONS (CONTINUED)

3. Advanced Progressive Illness. If I have a progressive illness that will be fatal and is in an advanced stage, and I am consistently and permanently unable to communicate by any means, swallow food and water safely, care for myself and recognize my family and other people, and it is very unlikely that my condition will substantially improve:

A. INITIAL ONE:
_______ I want to receive tube feeding.
_______ I want tube feeding only as my physician recommends.
_______ I DO NOT WANT tube feeding.

B. INITIAL ONE:
_______ I want any other life support that may apply.
_______ I want life support only as my physician recommends.
_______ I want NO life support.

4. Extraordinary Suffering. If life support would not help my medical condition and would make me suffer permanent and severe pain:

A. INITIAL ONE:
_______ I want to receive tube feeding.
_______ I want tube feeding only as my physician recommends.
_______ I DO NOT WANT tube feeding.

B. INITIAL ONE:
_______I want any other life support that may apply.
_______I want life support only as my physician recommends.
_______I want NO life support.

5. General Instruction.

INITIAL IF THIS APPLIES:
_______ I do not want my life to be prolonged by life support. I also do not want tube feeding as life support. I want my doctors to allow me to die naturally if my doctor and another knowledgeable doctor confirm I am in any of the medical conditions listed in Items 1 to 4 above.

6. Additional Conditions or Instructions. (Insert description of what you want done.)

FIGURE 5.2 Example of a portion of an advance directive.

agent) to make healthcare decisions in the event they are unable to do so.

- *Organ donation*: Indicates if a person wants to donate organs.
- *Do not resuscitate (DNR)*: Can be part of the living will. Indicates if the person refuses cardiopulmonary resuscitation (CPR) if they stop breathing or have no pulse.

The document can also address additional topics:

- Life-sustaining treatments (e.g., drugs, machines, medical procedures, feeding tubes)
- Desires if permanently unconscious
- Desires with terminal condition
- Mental health treatment
- Admission to a nursing home
- Desires if unconscious and pregnant
- Pain relief
- Additional desires

Remember, each state has its own advance directives form for state residents to complete.

Physician Orders for Life-Sustaining Treatment

Physician Orders for Life-Sustaining Treatment (POLST) can be known by similar names across the United States. It is promoted to work with advance directives. When a person is diagnosed with advanced illness or frailty, having a POLST may be recommended. The POLST is a one-page order sheet completed and signed by the physician. It indicates the care a person should receive. The POLST should be based on the advance directives and the person's wishes.

For some people, the POLST is concerning. The POLST can supersede a person's advance directives. Keep in mind that the POLST is a limited document, and some forms state that the healthcare staff should follow the orders listed before contacting the provider. Opponents to the POLST encourage patients to refuse it. They state that the provider should be contacted when the patient's condition changes and that the advance directives in their entirety can be followed, not the summarized version listed in the POLST.

ETHICAL ISSUES RELATED TO DYING

Death can be a difficult topic for many people. Ethical issues surrounding death include how death is legally determined, withholding or withdrawing life-sustaining treatments, and euthanasia.

Uniform Determination of Death Act

The Uniform Determination of Death Act (UDDA) was drafted in 1981. It served as a guide for state lawmakers to create their own laws. The act provided a definition of death. A person may legally be declared dead if one of the following two events occurs:

- Irreversible **cessation** of circulatory and respiratory functions
- Irreversible cessation of all functions of the entire brain, including the brainstem

This act provided an accepted definition of death. Most states have adopted the exact wording of the UDDA. Some states have added further regulations to their laws.

Withholding or Withdrawing Life-Sustaining Treatment

Withholding or withdrawing treatments that extend a person's life can be emotional for the patient and family. This situation can also be ethically challenging for healthcare providers. It is important to remember that patients have the right to decline medical intervention. They can also determine when the intervention should stop. If the patient cannot make these decisions, it is up to the patient's surrogate.

Per the CEJA's opinion, providers should identify the patient's wishes early in the treatment. Should providers have questions regarding life-sustaining treatments, they should review the patient's advance directives, support the decisions of the patient or surrogate, and seek advice from an ethics committee.

Euthanasia

Euthanasia is the act of killing a person who is suffering from an incurable disease. It can also be called "mercy killing" because it is ending the patient's suffering. There are various types of euthanasia:

- *Active euthanasia*: Killing the person using an active means (e.g., an injection).
- *Passive euthanasia*: Withholding a lifesaving treatment (e.g., feeding tube) and letting the person die.
- *Voluntary euthanasia*: The patient consents to the action.
- *Involuntary euthanasia*: The patient does not consent to the action. Patients may be unconscious or unable to communicate their wishes.
- *Self-administered euthanasia*: The patient kills himself or herself.
- *Other-administered euthanasia*: Another person kills the patient.
- *Assisted suicide/assisted euthanasia*: The patient kills himself or herself with the assistance of another person (e.g., physician-assisted suicide).

Death with dignity laws are also called *physician-assisted dying* and *aid-in-dying laws*. These laws allow providers to make available the means for a patient to end his or her life. The means can be sleeping pills in lethal doses or the administration of some other medication that affects the breathing or heartbeat. The provider is also aware that the patient wants to commit suicide. Most states make physician-assisted euthanasia illegal. Only 10 states have legalized physician-assisted suicide. Most laws indicate a minimum age of 18, a life expectancy of 6 months or less, and a required number of requests for the provider's assistance.

Proponents state that terminally ill patients have a right to end their suffering when they want to. Opponents state that providers have a moral responsibility to keep their patients alive. Per the CEJA's opinion, physician-assisted suicide is against the fundamental nature of the healer role of the provider. Providers must respond to the patient's needs at the end of life. They should respect the patient's autonomy and provide effective communication and emotional support. Providers need to make the patient comfortable and provide adequate pain medications.

ORGAN DONATION AND ETHICAL ISSUES

According to organdonor.gov, more than 106,000 people are on the national transplant list. Six people are added to the national transplant waiting list every hour. The gap between available organs and those needing organs is increasing. More people need organs than there are organs available. On average, 17 people die each day while waiting for a transplant. There continues to be a great need for organ and tissue donations.

According to Donate Life America (www.donatelife.net), one organ donor can save eight lives. A cornea donation can restore the sight of two people. Donated tissue can heal the lives of 75 people. The following organs and tissue can be donated:

- *Organs:* Kidney, liver, lung, heart, pancreas, and intestines
- *Tissue:* Hands, faces, heart valves, skin, bones, tendons, bone marrow, cord blood stem cells, blood, platelets, corneas, and eyes

Collected cord blood can be frozen and stored for years. Parents may opt to store their baby's cord blood in a private bank so it can be used in the future by the child or a close relative. Private cord banks charge fees for collection and storage. Parents could also donate the cord blood to a public bank so it can be used for a patient who needs a hematopoietic stem cell transplant.

Types of Donations

Living donations are becoming more common—people donate organs or partial organs while living. For example, they can donate a kidney, a lobe of a lung, or a partial liver, intestine, or pancreas. Living tissue donations include skin after surgeries (e.g., abdominoplasty), bone after knee and hip replacement surgeries, bone marrow, umbilical cord blood, amnion, and blood. Both blood and bone marrow can be donated more than once. There are different types of living donations:

- *Directed donation*: The donor specifically names the person to receive the donation. Usually, this is a family member or someone the donor has heard about.
- *Nondirected donation*: The donor neither knows nor is related to the recipient. The match is made based on the medical compatibility of the person and the donor. Both parties have the option to choose to meet the other person. If both agree and the transplant center's policy permits it, they can meet.
- *Paired donation*: This involves at least two pairs of living kidney donors. The transplant candidates do not match the donor they know but match the other donor; thus, the organs are swapped or traded.

A person who wishes to be a potential donor at death must first register in her or his state. Registration is available online or through local motor vehicle departments. (For more information, go to the website, www.organdonor.gov.) It is also important for potential donors to let their families know their wishes. Some advance directive forms also have areas where one can include such wishes.

Cord Blood Banking

Cord blood is found in the blood vessels of the placenta and umbilical cord. It is collected after the umbilical cord has been cut at birth. Cord blood is considered a biological product regulated by the FDA. Currently, cord blood is only used for hematopoietic stem cell transplantation procedures. Such a procedure is used for patients with leukemias and lymphomas. The cord blood has a source of stem cells that form into blood cells. If a cancer patient is given transplanted stem cells from cord blood, healthy blood cells regrow after chemotherapy has killed both cancer and healthy cells.

Xenotransplantation

With the lack of available organs and tissues, researchers are studying the use of nonhuman tissue and organs. *Xenotransplantation* is any procedure in which nonhuman cells, tissues, or organs are implanted or infused into a person.

Currently, pigs are the animals of choice for xenotransplants. Their organs are about the same size as humans, and they breed quickly. Pig heart valves are already being used to treat human heart valve issues.

Ethical Issues Related to Organ Donation

With organ donation, justice and medical utility are factors that are balanced. Justice refers to the fair consideration of the patient's situation and medical needs. Medical utility relates to trying to increase the number of transplants performed and the survival time of patients and organs.

Many factors are considered when organs are matched to patients. When an organ becomes available, patients on the waiting list are screened for blood type, height, weight, and other medical factors. The computer uses national policies to determine the order of the candidates who would be a match for the donor's organs. The right-size organ and the geographic location of the donor organ and the candidate must be considered. Children do better with pediatric donor organs. Each organ has specific factors that are also considered in the allocation. For instance, waiting time, survival benefit, and medical needs may be considered. The following sections will examine laws and ethical recommendations related to organ donation.

ORGAN DONATION LAWS

As described in the prior section, the need for organ donation is great. Two different acts influence organ donation in the United States.

Uniform Anatomical Gift Act

The Uniform Anatomical Gift Act (UAGA) was enacted in 1968. All 50 states have adopted this law. The purpose of the act was to make it easier for people to donate organs. This act has been revised several times over the years. States enacted the UAGA, but differences existed among states. In 2006 the UAGA was revised to provide uniformity in organ and tissue donations across the nation. The 2006 revisions did the following:

- Clarified who can make donation decisions for the patient
- Strengthened language on protecting the patient's decision to donate or not donate organs
- Established standards for donor registries, which will help match donors to recipients

The CEJA addressed organ donation. It is the opinion of the CEJA that providers should do the following:

- Avoid conflicts of interest and ensure that no members of the transplant team are involved in pronouncing the patient dead.
- Ensure the death is pronounced using accepted clinical and ethical standards.
- Ensure the transplantation procedures are performed by knowledgeable providers.
- Ensure the prospective recipient is fully informed about the procedure.

National Organ Transplant Act

The National Organ Transplant Act (NOTA) was passed by Congress in 1984. The act established the Organ Procurement and Transplant Network (OPTN) to be run by contract by the secretary of Health and Human Services. The act established a national registry for organ matching. NOTA also made it a criminal action for organs to be transplanted in exchange for something of value (e.g., money).

CLOSING COMMENTS

Patient Coaching

When medical assistants are working with patients who are on the organ transplant waiting list, it is important for them to coach each patient on the process and encourage the patient to get emotional support. Once the patient is on the list, the transplant center will confirm the registration. If the person is removed from the list for any reason, the transplant center sends a written letter to the patient. The length of the wait is based on how sick the person is, the availability of organs that match, and the number of donors in the local area. With the organ allocation being based on many factors, a person's wait may vary. Sadly, some people's conditions deteriorate, and they are removed from the list and never get an organ.

Waiting for an organ transplant can cause a wide range of emotions. Once on the list, the person is hopeful, but as the wait lengthens, the stress can increase. The same is true for the patient's family. It is important for the patient and family to get support during this time. Local or online support groups may be helpful.

Legal and Ethical Issues

It is important for the medical assistant to continue to learn about healthcare advances. New procedures, treatments, and medications are continually impacting patient care. As technology advances and healthcare changes, the medical assistant needs to remain updated on the ethical issues that surround the changes. Following the professional code of ethics, in addition to learning the CEJA's opinions on the new advances, will help guide the medical assistant's practice.

Patient-Centered Care

One of the key elements to providing patient-centered care is respecting the patient's decisions and preferences. When working with ethical situations, it is important for the medical assistant to remember the Patient Care Partnership (or Patient's Bill of Rights). Patients have the right to refuse treatment. They have the right to make their own decisions. Their decisions may not be our decisions in that situation, but we need to do what they want. It is important to respect patients and ensure their dignity during beginning-of-life issues through end-of-life issues.

Professional Behaviors

All healthcare professionals need to provide ethical, respectful care to all patients. Professional ethics guide healthcare employees on how to be ethical in their roles. A medical assistant should be aware of the medical assisting code of ethics and the healthcare facility's professional ethics. The medical assistant needs to practice these professional ethics in every patient situation.

SUMMARY OF SCENARIO

Daniela has completed the ethics unit in her law and ethics course. She is excited to be done with the course. What she has learned in the ethics unit has helped her consider why she believes what she believes. She is realizing that some of her values and morals were built on information that was old or inaccurate. She needs to do some research to verify the information. Daniela feels that as she continues to learn and gain experience, her moral compass may change. She hopes that this will help her to provide the best possible care to her patients.

SUMMARY OF LEARNING OBJECTIVES

1. **Examine personal ethics.**
Ethics refers to rules of conduct that differentiate between acceptable and unacceptable behavior. *Morals* are internal principles that distinguish between right and wrong. *Personal ethics* refers to individual choices and will be impacted by one's morals. *Professional ethics* refers to ethical standards that have been created by associations for members to follow. Employers also establish professional ethics for employees to follow. A medical assistant must create a plan to separate personal and professional ethics if they conflict. Our personal morals impact our professional performance in other positive or negative ways.
2. **Examine professional ethics for physicians and medical assistants.**
Professional ethics refers to codes of conduct stated by an employer or a professional association. Many healthcare professional associations have published professional ethics for their members, called *codes of ethics.* The code of ethics for physicians has been modernized over the years. The American Association of Medical Assistants (AAMA) developed a code of ethics that provides the principles of ethical and moral conduct for the profession.
3. **Analyze how to separate professional ethics and personal ethics.**
Procedure 5.1 provides an opportunity to develop a plan for separating personal and professional ethics based on the scenario provided. Procedure 5.1 also provides an opportunity to describe the impact of personal morals and ethics on the delivery of healthcare. It is important that medical assistants recognize the impact personal ethics and morals have on the delivery of healthcare.
4. **Analyze how medical assistants can incorporate the ethical principles of anatomy, nonmaleficence, beneficence, and justice into their work life.**
There are four ethical principles in healthcare:
   - *Autonomy:* The freedom to determine one's own actions and decisions
   - *Nonmaleficence:* To do no harm
   - *Beneficence:* To do good
   - *Justice:* To treat patients fairly and give them what is due to them

   These four principles need to be considered equally when evaluating ethical issues. The medical assistant has related responsibilities for each of these principles.
5. **Examine the ethical issues that relate to genetics.**
The chapter discussed the ethical issues involved with cloning, genetic engineering, genetic testing, pharmacogenetics, stem cell transplantation, and gene therapy. Many advances have occurred in genetics, and with them, many ethical issues have surfaced. Refer to each section for the ethical issues related to the topic and the CEJA's opinion for providers.
6. **Examine the ethical issues surrounding assistive reproductive technology and elective termination of pregnancies.**
Different types of assistive reproductive technology were discussed. Gamete donation and egg freezing were also addressed, along with elective abortion. Refer to the sections for the CEJA's opinion.
7. **Examine the ethical issues surrounding childhood.**
This chapter discussed many different types of adoption. With most adoptions, the child does not have information regarding the parents. This is important for the medical assistant to remember. Ethical issues surrounding adoption, safe haven infant protection laws, and confidential healthcare for minors were addressed. Refer to the chapter sections for the ethical issues surrounding these topics.
8. **Examine the ethical issues related to research trials.**
This chapter discussed the abuses and influential guidelines and codes of ethics for clinical research. Seven main principles are involved with ethical research: social and clinical value, scientific validity, fair subject selection, favorable risk-benefit ratio, independent review, informed consent, and respect for potential and enrolled subjects.
9. **Examine end-of-life issues, including palliative medicine, hospice, and grieving.**
Palliative means to help relieve the symptoms of a serious illness. The providers offer palliative care to patients who are seriously ill, regardless of age. Hospice is a type of palliative care for people who have about 6 months or less to live. The goal of hospice care is to allow patients who are dying to have dignity, comfort, and peace.
   There are stages of grief and dying, as defined by Elisabeth Kübler-Ross:
   - *Denial:* Person refuses to accept the diagnosis or prognosis.
   - *Anger:* Person's anger can be directed at self or others.
   - *Bargaining:* Person attempts to bargain with the higher power the person believes in.
   - *Depression:* Person feels sadness, fear, and uncertainty.
   - *Acceptance:* Person has come to terms with the situation.

   Not everyone goes through all five stages, and people may not go through the stages in the order listed. Some people may switch back and forth between the stages.
10. **Analyze the importance of the Patient Self-Determination Act and advance directives.**
The Patient Self-Determination Act (PSDA) requires most healthcare institutions at the time of admission to do the following:
    - Provide patients with a written document of their rights to make decisions and the facility's policies respecting advance directives.
    - Ask patients if they have advance directives and document the response in the health record.

    Advance directives are written instructions about healthcare decisions should a person be unable to make them. Types of advance directives include the following:
    - *Living will:* Provides instructions about life-sustaining medical treatment to be administered or withheld when the patient has a terminal condition.
    - *Medical durable power of attorney:* Similar to a living will but includes all healthcare decisions. Names a healthcare proxy and can include healthcare wishes.
    - *Healthcare proxy:* Also called a *healthcare agent* or *surrogate.* A competent adult can appoint a person (called a *proxy* or an *agent*) to make healthcare decisions in the event he or she is unable to do so.
11. **Examine ethical issues related to dying, including how death is determined, withholding life-sustaining treatments, and euthanasia.**
The Uniform Determination of Death Act (UDDA) served as a guide for state lawmakers to create their own laws. The act provided a definition

SUMMARY OF LEARNING OBJECTIVES—*continued*

of death. Many ethical issues surround end-of-life issues. This chapter discussed withholding or withdrawing life-sustaining treatment and euthanasia. The CEJA's opinion and the ethical issues involved with each of these topics were discussed.

12. **Examine the ethical issues related to organ donation.**
    The gap between available organs and those needing organs is increasing. More people need organs than are available. The following organs and tissue can be donated:
    - *Organs:* Kidney, liver, lung, heart, pancreas, and intestines
    - *Tissue:* Hands, faces, heart valves, skin, bones, tendons, bone marrow, cord blood stem cells, blood, platelets, corneas, and eyes

    There are different types of living donations, including direct, nondirected, and paired.

    If a person wishes to be a potential donor at death, registering in the person's state is the first step. With organ donation, justice and medical utility are factors that are balanced.
13. **Differentiate between the Uniform Anatomical Gift Act and the National Organ Transplant Act.**
    The Uniform Anatomical Gift Act (UAGA) was enacted in 1968. All 50 states have adopted this law. The purpose of the act was to make it easier for people to donate organs. The National Organ Transplant Act (NOTA) established the Organ Procurement and Transplant Network (OPTN) to be run by contract by the secretary of Health and Human Services. The act established a national registry for organ matching. NOTA also made it a criminal act to exchange organs for something of value and established the national registry for organ matching.

PROCEDURE 5.1 Develop an Ethics Separation Plan

TASK: To develop a plan for separating personal and professional ethics.

SCENARIO: You are working at WMFM Clinic. Your provider sees many children, including teens. New state laws allow confidential healthcare for minors. The agency has now adopted policies and procedures to allow providers to see teens 16 years or older without parental consent. The teens can be seen for sexually transmitted infections (STIs) and reproductive issues (including birth control). All health records related to these visits are confidential, meaning parents cannot be told about their child's visit.

Your personal belief is that parents should always be allowed to know what is occurring with their children. They are responsible for the child until age 18, and they pay the bills. You also believe that children under 18 are too young to be in an intimate relationship with others. This type of relationship should be only for adults in a committed relationship. You do not believe in birth control.

EQUIPMENT and SUPPLIES

- Paper and pen
- Medical Assisting Code of Ethics

PROCEDURAL STEPS

1. Read the code of ethics for medical assistants. Write down key themes or phrases.
   PURPOSE: Medical assistants need to follow the code of ethics for the medical assistant professional.
2. Using the scenario, write down the professional ethics involved in the situation.
   PURPOSE: Medical assistants need to follow the laws and the agency's policies and procedures. The procedures indicate how the healthcare professional needs to perform duties.
3. Using the scenario, write down the personal ethics involved in the situation.
   PURPOSE: Medical assistants need to identify their personal ethics. They need to be honest when analyzing how they think and feel about different scenarios that may occur in healthcare. Understanding one's biases is the first step in ensuring that respectful, ethical care is provided to all patients.
4. Compare the lists. Identify the personal ethics that conflict with the code of ethics and the professional ethics of the agency.
   PURPOSE: Medical assistants must identify areas where their personal ethics conflict with the code of ethics and the professional ethics of the agency. Medical assistants need to follow professional ethics. Personal ethics should not supersede professional ethics.
5. For each area of conflict, create a plan for how you will separate your personal and professional ethics. Remember, as a professional, you need to follow the professional ethics of the agency and the profession. Address how you will handle the situation and what would be your options if you were in the situation.
   PURPOSE: Medical assistants must create a plan and be aware of how they will handle situations that conflict with their personal ethics. This might mean they need to find another job. They may need to rethink their biases. Learning more about bias can help people to identify errors in their thinking.
6. Describe how personal ethics and morals in this scenario would impact patient care.
   PURPOSE: It is important that medical assistants recognize the impact personal ethics and morals have on the delivery of healthcare.

PROCEDURE 5.2 Demonstrate Professional Responses to Ethical Issues

TASKS: Identify ethical issues and demonstrate professional responses. Recognize the impact personal ethics and morals have on the delivery of healthcare.

SCENARIO 1: You are working at WMFM Clinic. You are responsible for collecting payments from patients. Mr. Smythe, who is visually impaired, paid for his visit in cash. He gives you $500 for a $402 bill. You make change and give him a receipt. At the end of the day, you notice that you have $60 more than you should have, and some of the bills were mixed up in the cashbox. You realize you gave Mr. Smythe the incorrect amount of money.

SCENARIO 2: You are setting up a laceration repair tray for Dr. Martin to use. As you are preparing the sterile equipment, one of the instruments becomes contaminated. You know Dr. Martin urgently needs the tray. You do nothing about the contamination, which you realize can cause an infection. You finish setting up the tray.

EQUIPMENT and SUPPLIES

- Paper and pen

PROCEDURAL STEPS

1. Read both scenarios. Identify and write down the ethical issues involved.
   PURPOSE: It is important to identify the issues as the first step in responding to ethical situations.
2. With a peer, role-play scenario 1. Demonstrate a professional and appropriate ethical response to this situation.
   a. Explain the situation to the supervisor.
   b. Describe how you felt the error occurred and who received the incorrect change.
   c. Explain how you would like to handle the situation and correct the error.
   PURPOSE: It is important that the medical assistant act professionally and ethically when a mistake is discovered.
3. With a peer, role-play scenario 2. During the role-play, demonstrate a professional and appropriate ethical response to this situation.
   PURPOSE: It is important that the medical assistant act ethically and notify the provider when an error is made.
4. In a written response, discuss the potential implication to the patient's health related to not reporting or correcting the error in scenario 2.
   PURPOSE: It is important that the medical assistant realize how unethical actions affect patient care.

TECHNOLOGY

6

SCENARIO

Christiana worked at Walden-Martin Family Medical (WMFM) Clinic as a clinical medical assistant for 5 years. She helped with diagnostic tests and treatment procedures. Christiana enjoyed providing patient care, but she was interested in a change and wanted to use more of her administrative skills. When a front office position opened up, Christiana moved into the administrative role. She is now the lead administrative medical assistant. Besides performing her administrative duties, Christiana is now responsible for the clinic's computer system. She is excited to continue to learn the administrative role and the computer system.

While studying this chapter, think about the following questions:

- What are the common types of hardware and software used in an ambulatory care facility?
- What is the medical assistant's role regarding maintaining computer hardware?
- How can a medical assistant apply infection control principles to a workstation?
- What are the principles of ergonomics that apply to a computer workstation?
- What are computer network security procedures?

LEARNING OBJECTIVES

1. Differentiate among various types of computers.
2. Differentiate among various input devices commonly seen in ambulatory care.
3. Differentiate among various output devices commonly seen in ambulatory care.
4. Differentiate among various internal computer components.
5. Differentiate between types of secondary storage devices.
6. Differentiate between intranet and internet access requirements.
7. Demonstrate maintaining computer hardware in ambulatory care.
8. Apply principles of ergonomics to the computer workstation.
9. Examine considerations when purchasing and installing hardware.
10. Differentiate among types of software used in ambulatory care.
11. Examine federal requirements used to maintain computer network privacy and security in healthcare.
12. Examine how to recognize and prevent phishing attacks.
13. Examine how advances in technology affect the ambulatory care environment and patient care.

VOCABULARY

anisometropia (an EYE soh mi TROE pee ah) A condition in which the refraction (focus) is different in both eyes.

astigmatism (ah STIG mah tiz um) Inability of the cornea to focus, causing blurred vision.

boot The process of starting or restarting a computer when the operating system is loaded.

business associate A person or business that provides a service to a covered entity that involves access to protected health information (PHI). Examples include legal, billing, and management services; accreditation agencies; consulting firms; and claims processing organizations.

claim An itemized statement of services and costs from a healthcare facility submitted to the health (insurance) plan for payment.

computer network A system that links personal computers and peripheral devices to share information and resources.

covered entity (KUV er ed EN ti tee) A healthcare facility, healthcare provider, pharmacy, health (insurance) plan, or claims clearinghouse that transmits protected health information electronically.

decryption (dee KRIP shun) The computer process of changing encrypted text to readable or plain text after a user enters a secret key or password.

docking station Also known as a universal port replicator, this hardware device allows a laptop to connect with other devices, turning it into a desktop computer.

dongle A small hardware device that connects to a computer device and allows access to wireless devices, such as headsets, mice, and keyboards.

downtime The interval of time during which something, such as hardware or software, is not functioning.

drive A computer device that reads data from and may write data to a storage medium.

electronic health record (EHR) An electronic record that conforms to nationally recognized standards and contains

VOCABULARY—*continued*

health-related information about a specific patient. It can be created, managed, and consulted by authorized clinicians and staff from more than one healthcare organization.

electronic medical record (EMR) An electronic record of health-related information about an individual that can be created, gathered, managed, and accessed by authorized clinicians and staff members within a single healthcare organization. An EMR is an electronic version of a paper record.

electronic transaction The electronic exchange of information between two agencies to accomplish financial or administrative healthcare activities.

e-prescribing The use of electronic software to communicate with pharmacies and send prescribing information. It takes the place of writing a prescription by hand and giving it to a patient; most new or refill prescriptions can be submitted electronically, cutting down on fraud and errors.

Ethernet (EE thuhr net) A communication system for connecting several computers so information can be shared.

file A collection of data or program records stored as a unit with a specific name.

hackers Unauthorized users who attempt to break into computer networks.

hardware Physical equipment of the computer system required for communication and data processing functions.

hyperopia (hye pur OH pee ah) Farsightedness.

interface An interconnection between systems.

intranet (IN trah net) A private computer network that can only be accessed by authorized people (e.g., employees of the facility that owns the network).

malware (MAL wair) Malicious software designed to damage or disrupt a system (e.g., a virus).

media (ME de ah) Types of communication (e.g., social media sites); with computers, the term refers to data storage devices.

modem (MOE duhm) Peripheral computer hardware that connects to the router to provide internet access to the network or computer.

myopia (mye OH pee ah) Nearsightedness.

no-show To fail to keep an appointment without giving advance notice.

operating system Software; it acts as the computer's software administrator by managing, integrating, and controlling application software and hardware. Windows is an example.

output device Computer hardware that displays the processed data from the computer (e.g., monitors and printers).

patient portal A secure online website that gives patients 24-hour access to personal health information using a username and password.

phishing A generic cyberattack toward many individuals or organizations with the intent to steal confidential data or install malware on the user's device.

point-of-care Something designed to be used at or near where the patient is seen; point-of-care tools and apps are resources for the provider to use when working directly with the patient.

practice management software A type of software that allows the user to enter demographic information, schedule appointments, maintain lists of insurance payers, perform billing tasks, and generate reports.

protected health information (PHI) Individually identifiable health information stored or transmitted by covered entities or business associates. Includes verbal, paper, or electronic information.

revenue (REV eh noo) Money collected for providing a product or service.

secondary storage devices Media (e.g., jump drive, flash drive, hard drive) capable of permanently storing data until they are replaced or deleted by the user.

server Computer hardware and software that perform data analysis, storage, and archiving; accepts and responds to requests from devices (clients) made over a network. Also called a database server or data server.

software A set of electronic instructions to operate and perform different computer tasks.

spear phishing A customized cyberattack toward an individual or organization with the intent to steal confidential data or install malware on the user's device.

spoof To assume or mimic the identity of another user to gain access to a computer system.

stylus (STI luhs) A pen-shaped device with a variety of tips that is used on touchscreens to write, draw, or input commands.

telehealth Refers to remote clinical services and nonclinical services, such as provider training, meetings, and continuing education.

INTRODUCTION

When technology was first applied in healthcare, it was used in the business departments. Computer software was used for billing and accounting procedures, registration processes, and scheduling. Data is collected once, entered, and used for many purposes. When **electronic health records** (EHRs) were introduced, agencies implemented software to increase the accuracy and efficiency of patient care. Currently, healthcare workers use "smart" devices for quick access to information to provide better patient care.

Communication has also changed over the years. Patients use emails and text messages to contact their providers. To help ensure confidentiality, administrators have created tighter network security procedures.

COMPUTERS

Many clinics are using electronic technology in both administrative and patient care areas. When you think of a computer, you likely think of laptop or desktop computers. The following section describes five types of computers and the computers typically used in the healthcare setting. Today, medical assistants must be more computer savvy than ever before to meet technological demands.

Types of Computers

Computers vary greatly in their size, function, and speed. Five types of computers are used in the healthcare setting:

- *Supercomputers*: Expensive, very large computers that have incredibly fast processing speeds. Supercomputers are used by large corporations and the government.

- *Mainframe computers*: Large tower computers that are more common and less expensive than supercomputers. Used by large organizations to store large quantities of information.
- *Minicomputers*: Large multiprocessing machines that support about 200 users at a time. Less powerful than a mainframe computer. A **server** can be a minicomputer.
- *Personal computers*: Smaller computers that have their own central processing unit (CPU).
- *Mobile computers*: Are computers that can be carried, such as laptops, netbooks, tablets, and smartphones.

Types of Personal Computers

A *personal computer* (PC) is a single-user electronic data processing device. Personal computers can also be mobile computers. They come in many types:

- *Desktop computer*: A larger unit designed for use on a desk. It is used by employees who primarily perform word processing, data entry, and business tasks (e.g., scheduling, bookkeeping, and billing).
- *Laptop computer*: A thin, lightweight, wireless, portable PC with a keyboard; it may include a touchscreen. There is currently a trend toward reducing the size and weight of laptops; those smaller, lighter laptops are often called *notebooks*. Laptops are used by providers and medical assistants in patient exam rooms and workstations.
- *Tablet PC*: A thin, lightweight, wireless, portable PC that functions with a touchscreen. The most popular **operating systems** include Android and iOS. Providers and medical assistants use tablets in patient exam rooms and at workstations. There are several types of tablet PCs:
  - *Slate-style tablet*: A thin, portable computer with no keyboard. External keyboards are available for many slate-style tablets.
  - *Convertible tablet*: Usually allows the user to use the touchscreen or the physical keyboard. The display can rotate and cover the keyboard, making it appear like a tablet, or the keyboard makes it look like a small laptop (e.g., notebook).
  - *Hybrid tablet*: May also be called a *hybrid* or *convertible notebook;* it has a removable display, making it look more like a slate tablet.

A personal computer accepts, stores, and processes data. After processing the information, it generates the data output in a specific form, such as a letter or a patient statement.

A personal computer is a *system unit*, or the primary computer equipment. All other forms of physical equipment used with the PC are called *peripheral devices*. The PC and peripheral devices are **hardware.** Computer hardware can be divided into input devices, **output devices,** internal components, **secondary storage devices,** and network and internet access devices. The following sections describe these categories.

CRITICAL THINKING APPLICATION 6.1

When Christiana transitioned into the administrative role, Dr. Kahn hired Michaela as the new clinical medical assistant. Recently the healthcare facility switched from using desktop computers to tablet computers when working with patients in the exam rooms. How might Christiana's experience using the desktop computer in the exam rooms be different from Michaela's use of the tablet computer? Think of the patient's perception; which technology might a patient prefer the medical assistant to use? Why?

INPUT DEVICES

An input device is any peripheral hardware that allows the user to provide data to the computer. Many types of input devices are available on the market. This discussion focuses on those typically used in the ambulatory care setting. Common input devices include keyboards, mice and other pointing devices, touchscreens, webcams, cameras, microphones, scanners, and signature pads.

Keyboards

Keyboards are the most common input devices. The QWERTY keyboard is the standard keyboard for computers. (Q-W-E-R-T-Y are the first six letters, from left to right, just below the number keys on the keyboard.) A wide variety of keyboards are available, including standard, internet, wireless, and ergonomic. Keyboards may have special keys that perform the same functionality as the buttons on web pages. Numeric keypads are also a feature on many keyboards. Ergonomic keyboards reduce repetitive strain injuries by minimizing muscle strain. These keyboards allow the user's hands to be in a natural position when typing. The two most common ergonomic keyboards are the split-key models and the waved or curved key layout (Figure 6.1).

Categories of Keyboard Keys

Keyboards typically have the following categories of keys:

- Typing: Include the numeric and alphabetic keys used for typing.
- Numeric: Numeric keypads are in the same position as calculators.
- Function: The 12 keys at the top of the keyboard. Each key has a specific purpose. Some software programs allow the function keys to be programmed to complete a specific function.
- Control: Allow movement of the cursor and the screen; include Home, End, Insert, Delete, Page Up, Page Down, Control, Escape, Alternate, and four arrow keys.
- Special purpose: Include Enter, Shift, Caps Lock, Num Lock, Space Bar, Print Screen, and Tab keys.

Mouse and Touchpad

The mouse is one of the most common input devices. It makes screen navigation much simpler than using the keyboard. A mouse is a palm-sized unit with a laser sensor that tracks the movement of the user's hand. It sends those messages back to the computer. The mouse is used to move the pointer (cursor) on the screen. The mouse may have left and right buttons with a wheel in between to help

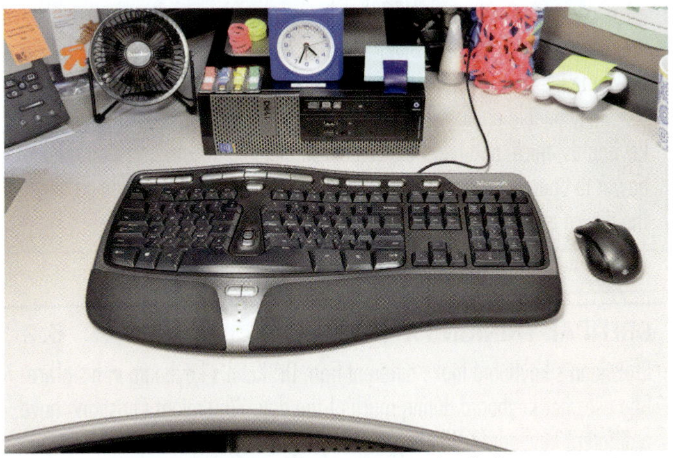

FIGURE 6.1 Ergonomic keyboards have different appearances, yet they all reduce repetitive strain injuries.

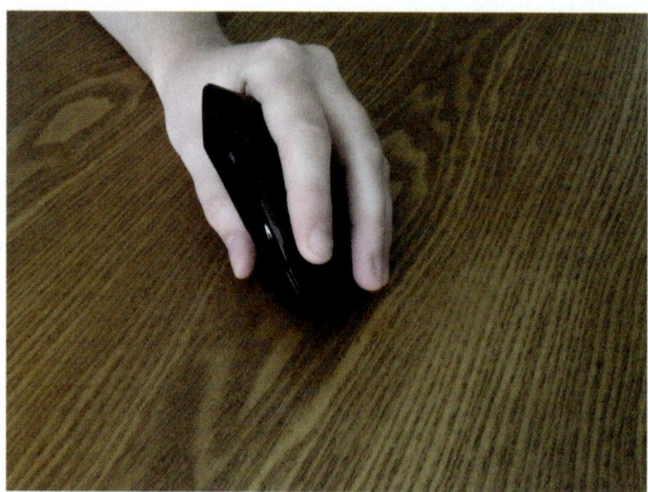

FIGURE 6.2 Left-handed, wireless vertical mouse.

with cursor/pointer navigation and functionality. A vertical mouse is ergonomically shaped, so the user's hand is in the handshake position during use (Figure 6.2). This position eliminates the wrist pressure and allows the arm to be in a neutral position. Vertical mice come wired or wireless. Left-handed and right-handed vertical mice are available.

Touchpads are touch sensitive. Touchpads move the pointer based on the user's finger movements. The functionality of touchpads can vary. Some have left- and right-click buttons like those on a mouse. Other touchpads have a finger tap or click sequence for the left- and right-click action.

Wireless Technology

The popularity of wireless technology has increased over the years. Short-range wireless communication technology allows for short-range data transfer between computer devices. Two types of technology are used for wireless keyboards, mice, and headsets:

- *2.4 GHz radiofrequency (RF) connection*: Radio frequencies transfer data between devices. For the RF connection to work, a **dongle** must be plugged into the Universal Serial Bus (USB) drive on the device (Figure 6.3). The RF connection offers a stable connection with no lag time.
- *Bluetooth*: This technology uses short-wave radio frequencies to interconnect wireless electronic devices. The computer device must support Bluetooth, or a USB dongle can also be used. Bluetooth is reliable, but if multiple Bluetooth devices are used in the same area, some lag time or momentary connection issues may occur.

Many people enjoy wireless technology until the batteries die! Wireless keyboards, mice, and headsets contain small radio transmitters that require power to operate. These devices use batteries, and if the batteries go dead, the device is not useable.

CRITICAL THINKING APPLICATION **6.2**

Christiana's keyboard looks different from Dr. Kahn's keyboard in his office. She uses her keyboard during much of the day. Why might Christiana have a different keyboard? What type of keyboard might Christiana have?

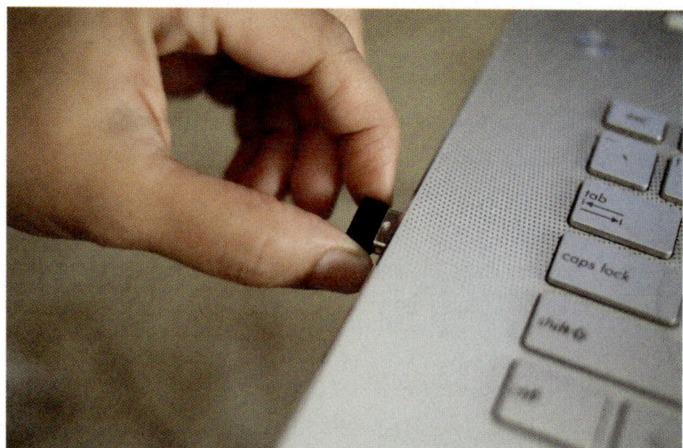

FIGURE 6.3 A dongle is plugged into the USB drive. From iStock.com/Artist's Member airdone.

Touchscreen

A touchscreen is different from a touchpad. A touchscreen allows a person to interact with the computer by touching the display screen with a finger or **stylus**. Touchscreens are found in healthcare, from mobile devices to kiosks. Touchscreens can vary, which means the compatible stylus also can vary.

- *Resistive:* Responds to the touch of almost anything that can generate pressure (e.g., finger, plastic stylus, rubber-tip stylus). Found on many handheld electronic devices.
- *Capacitive:* Responds to the electrical characteristics of a finger. Requires a specialized stylus that has more surface area at the point. Found on smartphones and other electrical devices.
- *Surface acoustic wave:* Responds to an inaudible wave of sound that is created on the screen from a finger. A stylus with a rubber or soft tip the size of a pencil eraser is required. Found on kiosks and ordering screens.

Digital Pen

A digital pen or smart pen is a battery-operated device that looks like and functions like a regular pen but can also digitally capture handwriting or a drawing. Depending on the type of pen, it can connect to a computer, smartphone, or tablet. The drawing or handwritten note appears on the mobile device or computer and can also be stored in the pen's memory. Some pens also contain a microphone that can record audio, which automatically syncs with the drawing or notes.

Camera, Webcam, and Microphone

Cameras, wireless webcams, and microphones are commonly seen in ambulatory care settings. Cameras are used to capture images of patients before and after surgery. Cameras may also be used to take a picture of a wound. These images are uploaded into the patient's health record. Regardless of if a picture is taken in the medical facility or sent by the patient to the provider using the **patient portal**, the images must remain confidential. Patients must sign a release form before the image can be given to others.

Providers can use webcams, microphones, and internet video chat software to see patients who are at a distance from the healthcare facility. The remote diagnosis and treatment of patients using technology is called *telemedicine*, a form of **telehealth**. Many times this is done using the patient portal.

Webcams and microphones are also used for meetings and continuing education opportunities. Microphones can be used for dictating notes into a patient's health record. Voice recognition software provides instant transcription into the patient's record.

CRITICAL THINKING APPLICATION 6.3

Dr. Kahn works with a home health agency. Patients and nurses can communicate with him using the internet, microphones, and webcams. How does this technology benefit the patient?

Scanner

Scanners in the healthcare setting have become more popular since the use of EHRs has increased. Documents, such are letters and laboratory results, are scanned, and the images are uploaded into the patient's EHR. Scanners convert images to digital text through a process called *optical character recognition* (OCR). Many types of scanners are available:

- *Handheld scanner*: Used in healthcare to scan identification (ID) bands prior to medication administration and procedures; may also be used for managing the inventory of supplies with the use of bar codes.
- *ID card scanner*: May have other names, including *insurance card scanner*. Used at the reception desk to scan insurance cards, driver's licenses, and so on. Usually, information is then saved in the **practice management software** for billing purposes.
- *Sheet-fed scanner*: Also called an *automatic document feeder (ADF) scanner*. Used to scan loose sheets of paper. May be used to scan test result documents to import into the patient's EHR.
- *Flatbed scanner*: Has a glass panel on which the documents are placed for scanning. May also be used to scan test result documents for importing into the EHR.

Signature Pad

In many ambulatory care settings, signature pads are used in the reception area and the exam rooms (Figure 6.4). Patients need to sign several documents, including disclosure authorization forms, consent forms, and the receipt of the Notice of Privacy Practices (NPP). Patients sign the signature pad. The signature is then imported into the EHR as part of the patient's permanent health record.

OUTPUT DEVICES

The data entered into the computer is then processed by it. The processed data is displayed using output devices. Common output devices in the healthcare setting include monitors, printers, and speakers.

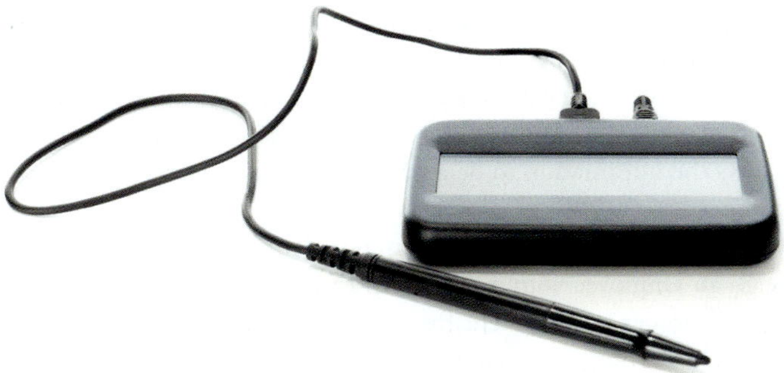

FIGURE 6.4 Signature pads allow patients' signatures to be imported into the electronic health record or practice management software.

Monitor

Monitors display the output as images. Images are created by tiny dots called *pixels*. The higher the number of pixels, the sharper the image. The most common monitor is the liquid crystal display (LCD) monitor. These monitors are easier on the eyes. They also use less electricity. LCD monitors can be built into computers, such as laptops and tablets, and are commonly called screens. LCD monitors can also be free standing and connect to desktop computers either with wires or wireless technology. They are smaller and lighter than older monitors. Some clinics use LCD monitors in the reception area. Patients can read documents on the monitor before signing the signature pad.

Printer

Printers produce the output on paper. Printers, like other computer hardware, can be wired or wireless. Inkjet and laser printers are the two most common types of printers. Inkjet printers create the images by spraying small drops of ink on the paper. Advantages of inkjet printers include their high-quality printing and that they are inexpensive to purchase. Disadvantages, when compared to laser printers, include the increased frequency of changing the ink cartridges, which gets expensive, and the slower rate of printing.

A laser printer uses a laser, electrical charges, and toner to produce images on paper. Advantages of laser printers over inkjet printers include their high-speed printing, high-quality output, and quality graphics. Laser printers can also support many fonts and font sizes. Toner cartridges are changed less often than inkjet printers. However, the initial cost of laser printers is higher than that of inkjet printers, which is a disadvantage.

CRITICAL THINKING APPLICATION 6.4

Christiana frequently prints documents, including billing statements, appointment reminders, and receipts for payment. What type of printer might be the most economical to use in the front office? Why?

Speaker

Speakers for electronic devices come in all shapes and sizes. Typically, speakers are built into the devices used (e.g., monitor, laptop, and tablet). Speakers and sound cards (which will be discussed in a later section) are needed to get sound from the computer. Speakers are used in many ways in healthcare, including listening to presentations, meetings, or patients with telemedicine.

INTERNAL COMPUTER COMPONENTS

In desktop personal computers, the internal components are found in the tower or case. Medical assistants would not need to open up the tower or case to problem-solve a computer issue. Doing so might void warranties on the computer equipment. The need to learn about internal components relates more to purchasing hardware and software.

Nonmemory Internal Components

When purchasing hardware or software, many times, the product contains the computer specifications required. If the medical assistant is responsible for the purchase, it is important to make sure the product will work with the existing computer. The following are internal components that may be of interest when purchasing new hardware or software:

- *Central processing unit* (CPU): Processor or "brain" of the computer; sits on the motherboard. It interprets and executes commands from the software (program).
- *Motherboard*: A platform that is an attachment point for all internal computer parts.
- *Sound card*: Also called an *audio card* or *audio adapter;* allows audio information to be sent to speakers or headphones.
- *Video card*: Also called a *graphic card* or *video adapter;* allows the computer to send graphic information to output devices (monitor or projectors).
- *Universal Serial Bus* (USB) *port*: A connector device that allows hardware to be plugged into the computer. There are multiple types of USB ports, including USB 2.0 standard (also called USB type A), micro-USB, and USB-C (also called USB type-C).

Memory-Related Internal Components

The primary memory consists of read-only memory, cache memory, and random-access memory. The *read-only memory* (ROM) contains hardwire instructions and is used when the computer **boots** up or starts the system diagnostic checks. The *cache memory* provides temporary use of information, and it contains data and instructions for opened programs. The cache memory allows programs to operate more quickly and efficiently. The *random-access memory* (RAM) is the main memory of the computer and is used to load and run programs. The RAM is required for the computer to operate. If the power is turned off, the memory is lost.

The *hard drive*, the C **drive** (C:) of the computer, contains the operating system and the related system fields. The C drive includes the hard disk (or disc) drive (HDD), and the hard drive as one unit. It reads and writes on the hard disk and provides the largest amount of permanent storage for the computer.

The *optical drive* reads and writes (saves) data on removable storage devices, such as compact disks (CDs), digital versatile/video disks (DVDs), and Blu-ray disks (BDs). Fewer computers have optical drives these days as the technology is changing.

SECONDARY STORAGE DEVICES AND CLOUD STORAGE

Secondary storage devices, or **media**, are capable of permanently storing data. With many types, the user can write over the existing data or delete the data. These devices can be considered removable, internal (e.g., the hard drive previously discussed), or external. The computer needs a secondary storage device to allow the user to save data. Without a storage device, the computer would be considered a *dumb terminal.* Dumb terminals provide the user access to software, the network, or the internet. They do not allow the user to save data to the hard drive of the computer.

CRITICAL THINKING APPLICATION **6.5**

Christiana would like to have a small patient education space in the reception area. She would like to have a computer there with internet access for patients so they can access health information. Christiana knows that cost is an important factor in a small healthcare facility. The computer would also have to be reasonable and reliable. What technology options might she propose to Dr. Kahn?

Types of Storage Devices

The computer storage devices are categorized as follows:

- *Magnetic storage device*: One of the oldest types of storage; uses magnetic technology to read and write data to the device. Examples of magnetic storage devices include the internal hard drive and portable hard drive.
- *Optical storage device (optical disk)*: Uses lasers and lights to read and write data onto optical storage devices. Examples of optical storage devices include the Blu-ray disk (BD), compact disk (CD), and digital versatile/video disk (DVD). Optical storage devices are not used as often today with the availability of other storage devices on the market.
  - *Recordable only* means that data can only be saved once to the disk (e.g., CD-R disk).
  - *Read/write* (RW) allows data to be saved, rewritten (resaved), and deleted many times (e.g., CD-RW).
- *Flash memory device* or *flash drive*: Portable device that has become cheaper and has gained larger storage capacity over the years; connects to the USB port in the computer. Examples of flash memory devices include the jump drive (also called the *USB flash, data stick, pen drive, keychain drive, travel drive,* or *thumb drive*), memory card, memory stick, and solid-state disk or drive [SSD]). To prevent flash drive data loss or malfunction, make sure to safely remove the drive after it is finished writing or reading data. Operating systems have different steps to do this. For instance, with Windows, a person would use the "Safely remove USB Mass Storage Device" icon.

Storage Capacity

The capacity of storage devices is also a consideration. The storage capacity is measured in *bytes.* A byte is usually considered a character, such as a number, letter, or symbol. The storage size is often estimated to simplify communication:

- 1 kilobyte (KB) equals 1024 bytes
- 1 megabyte (MB) equals 1024 KB (about 1 million bytes)
- 1 gigabyte (GB) equals 1024 MB (about 1 billion bytes)
- 1 terabyte (TB) equals 1024 GB (about 1 trillion bytes)

Over the years, the capacity of storage devices has increased, and the cost of storage has decreased. Flash drives range in size. Some now can hold more than 2 terabytes (TB), or 2 trillion bytes.

Cloud Storage

The use of cloud storage is becoming more popular. Cloud storage is also called **file** sharing or online storage. It allows computer files to be stored using the internet and a third-party service. To get started, a person signs up with a cloud storage service. Many companies allow free minimal storage. Others charge monthly fees or fees based on storage size. After signing up, individuals use the internet to send computer files to the service company's servers. The files are copied onto many servers in various locations. This is called *redundancy.* It allows the information to be accessible even if one server goes down and needs repairs.

Cloud systems are gaining in popularity. An authorized user (e.g., an employee with a password) can access the healthcare facility's computer environment from any location with web access and through a wired or wireless connection. Access can occur at any time. For instance, a patient calls the healthcare facility's after-hours number and leaves a message with the answering service. No matter the location, the provider on call can use the cloud to access the EHR when talking with the patient.

NETWORK AND INTERNET ACCESS DEVICES

Most healthcare facilities have their own private network or **intranet**. The intranet allows the employees to communicate with each other and access shared files. Local intranets are generally secure because only authorized personnel can access the network. Most healthcare facilities also have access to the internet for their employees.

Requirements for Intranet Access

The computers and output devices are usually all connected to the facility's private network. An intranet may be limited to the *local area network* (LAN). The local area network can span one building or multiple buildings. Some healthcare agencies have multiple locations over a large area. They may use *wide area network* (WAN) technology, which consists of two or more LANs. LAN and WAN technology can use telephone lines or fiberoptic cables that increase the speed of transmission.

A *router* must be used to allow multiple devices to be on the same network. Most routers used today have wireless connectivity. A router is peripheral hardware that looks like a small box. Many routers have antennas and use the **Ethernet**. The router allows multiple computers and other devices (e.g., smart devices) to use the same network to send and receive information.

Requirements for Internet Access

For the **computer network** to have internet access, the ambulatory care facility must meet the following conditions:

- Subscribe to an internet service provider (ISP)
- Have its router connected to a **modem**

Most routers have a specific port that is designed to connect to the Ethernet port of a cable or *digital subscriber line* (DSL) modem. DSL is a high-speed internet service. It uses a modem to translate the computer's digital signals into voltage that is then sent over telephone lines.

Usually, healthcare facilities have a separate network for guests that provides free internet. This protects the facility's main network, which stores confidential patient information. Nonemployees should never have access to the facility's main network.

MAINTAINING COMPUTER HARDWARE

Larger facilities usually have their own information technology (IT) department. The IT staff provides technical assistance and helps maintain the equipment. Other facilities will use external IT support companies or train an employee to handle IT issues.

The medical assistant's role involves preventing computer problems and keeping the hardware clean. The hardware should be located on a stable, even surface, away from heat sources, to prevent computer problems. The ventilation slots should be clear, allowing air to flow into the device to cool the components. The medical assistant should ensure the cables and electric cords are securely plugged in. Liquids and food should be kept away from the hardware to prevent accidental spills.

Routine Cleaning for Computer Hardware

Before cleaning the computer or peripheral components, turn off and unplug the device. Refer to the operator's manual for cleaning instructions.

- If liquids spill on the keyboard, unplug the keyboard. Tip the keyboard upside down to drain out the liquid. Let the keyboard dry overnight. Sticky liquids are more apt to damage the keyboard.
- Use a damp, lint-free cloth to wipe the hardware's casing to remove the grime and dirt.
- Wipe clean all vents and air holes.
- Spray a household glass cleaner on a lint-free cloth, and then wipe the glass monitor screen. Do not spray liquid directly on a component, as the liquid may drip into the device.
- Use a lint-free cloth dampened with water to clean nonglare or antiglare screens.
- Spray a disinfectant on a lint-free cloth or use a disinfectant cloth to disinfect the keyboard.
- Use compressed air dusters (i.e., pressurized air in a can) to blow the dirt out of the keyboard (Figure 6.5).

CRITICAL THINKING APPLICATION 6.6

Christiana works with an information technology (IT) company that provides hardware, software, and services to the healthcare facility. How might her role with her agency's computer network differ if the healthcare facility had its own IT department?

Infection Control Procedures for Computer Hardware

Many electronic devices are routinely touched by healthcare professionals and patients during the day. One study reported finding several types of harmful bacteria on keyboards. Some types could live for days or months on the keyboard surface. Another study found that keyboards in patient exam rooms were only disinfected 2% of the time, whereas the recommendation was to disinfect them on a daily basis.

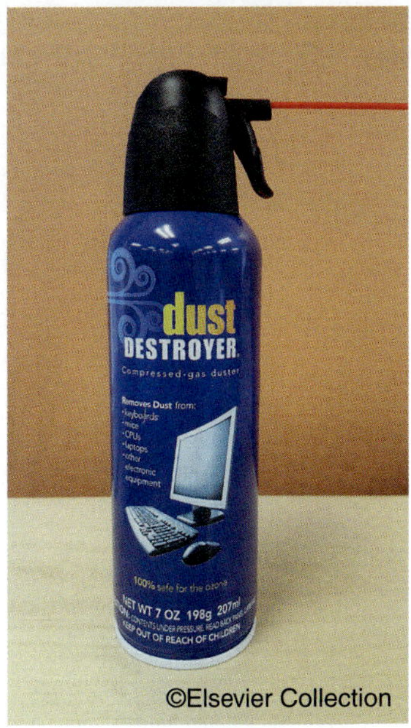

FIGURE 6.5 Compressed air dusters provide an efficient means of removing the dust and dirt from keyboards.

Kiosks are being used more often in the reception area for checking in (Figure 6.6). To help with infection control, some manufacturers are using antimicrobial coatings on kiosks and touchscreens. Some of these coatings kill 99% of all microbes. Clean Touch technology streams a UV-C light across the kiosk's touch surface for 30 seconds after the user steps away. This kills 99.9% of the bacteria and viruses on the kiosk's touch surface. Not all kiosks have infection control features.

It is important for ambulatory care facilities to have procedures for disinfecting technological devices, including kiosks, keyboards, mice, signature pads, and styluses. Procedures should follow the recommendations from the manufacturers. Usually, nonabrasive disinfectant (hospital-grade) wipes or specially made wipes (e.g., antibacterial kiosk wipes) are recommended. The following infection control practices are applied to technological devices:

- Disinfect keyboards daily. Keyboards should also be disinfected when they are contaminated with blood or visibly soiled. Using a disinfectant wipe, clean the surface using friction for 5 seconds in each area (Procedure 6.1).
- Healthcare professionals should wash their hands or use hand sanitizer before and after using the keyboard.
- Gloves should not be worn during computer use unless indicated by the facility's policy.
- Touchscreen computer monitors and signature pads should be cleaned and disinfected daily per the manufacturer's guidelines. Avoid applying excessive force to screens.
- Plastic covers can be used to enclose keyboards and other devices. These covers should be disinfected daily.

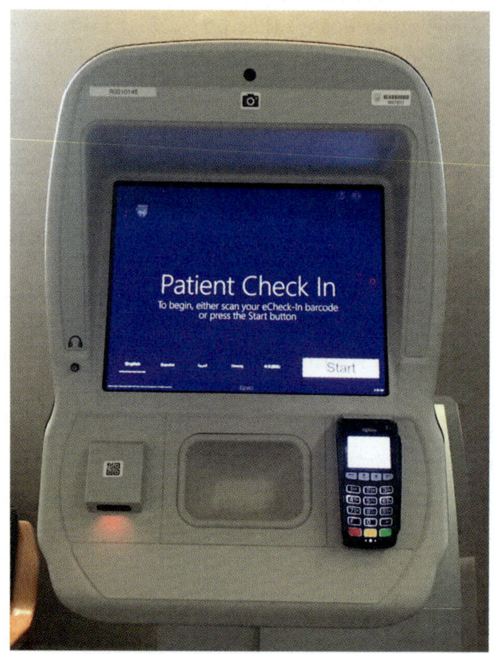

FIGURE 6.6 Many healthcare facilities use kiosks in the reception area.

COMPUTER WORKSTATION ERGONOMICS

Ergonomics is the science of designing the workplace, tools, and equipment in ways that will reduce the employee's strain and stress and will prevent work-related injuries. It is important to arrange the computer workstation correctly to avoid the risk of repetitive stress injuries. Poor posture and straining can cause physical stress and injury to the body. This results in workers' compensation **claims** for treatment and services.

An Ergonomically Friendly Workstation

For an ergonomically friendly workstation, the following factors are important:

- The torso and neck should be vertical and in line.
- The feet need to be flat on the floor or on a footrest (Figure 6.7A).
- The backrest should help support the upper body; the backrest lumbar support area should be fitted to the small of the back (Figure 6.7B; see Procedure 6.1).
- The seat should be the appropriate size and height to accommodate the person's body build so that there is no added pressure on the back of the knees or thighs.
- The armrest should support the forearms with the shoulders in a relaxed position (Figure 6.7C).
- For standing workstations, the legs, torso, head, and neck should be vertical and in line. One foot can be elevated on a step.
- The monitor should be directly in front of the person, with the top of the monitor at or just below eye level.

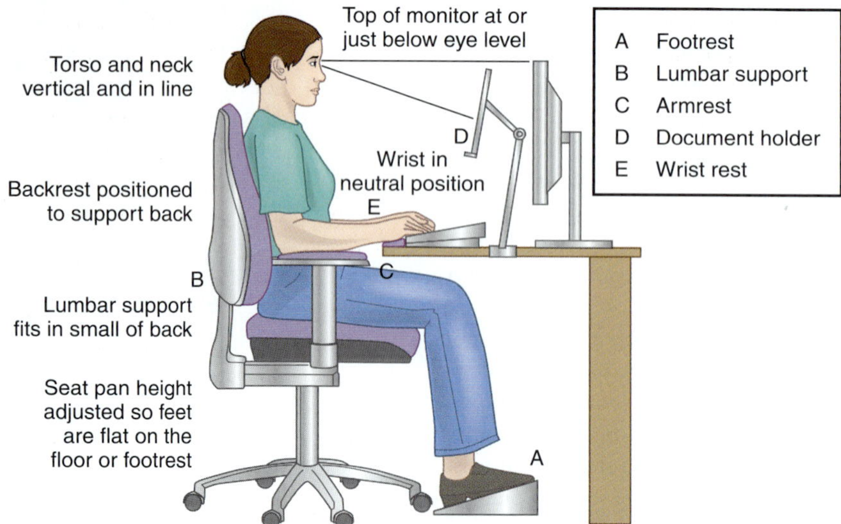

FIGURE 6.7 Medical assistants should use an ergonomically correct workstation to prevent repetitive stress injuries. Equipment that helps create this type of workstation includes a footrest **(A)**, a lumbar support **(B)**, an armrest **(C)**, a document holder **(D)**, and a wrist rest **(E)**.

- A document holder should be used so that documents are placed at the same distance and height as the monitor (Figure 6.7D).
- An ergonomic split-key or waved keyboard should be used. The keyboard should be placed at a height and an angle that allows the wrists to be in a neutral position.
- The work surface and mouse should be at elbow level for typing. The user's wrist should be supported by a foam wrist rest (Figure 6.7E).
- Headsets should be used by those answering frequent phone calls to prevent muscle strain.
- Laptop computers and tablets are not ergonomically designed for prolonged use.

Changing Positions

Whether you are standing or sitting at a workstation, it is important to change positions every 30 minutes. If you are sitting, adjustments can be made to chairs or backrests. Stretching your fingers, arms, and torso is important. Frequently look away from the computer to a distant object to prevent eyestrain. Stand up and walk around for a few minutes. Preventing repetitive stress injuries is important for all computer users.

PURCHASING AND INSTALLING COMPUTER HARDWARE

In small ambulatory care facilities, the medical assistant may help the provider with computer hardware purchases. In larger facilities, the IT department purchases and installs computer hardware.

Purchasing Hardware

If the medical assistant is helping with the purchase, identifying the equipment needed is important. This can be determined by asking the following questions when buying computers:

- Who will use it? What will be done on the computer? What operating system and other types of application software will be required? Usually, the software will indicate the amount of memory required to run it. This needs to be taken into consideration when purchasing a new computer.
- Does the computer need to be portable, or will a desktop work? If a laptop is selected, will a **docking station** be needed?
- What size processor is needed? The larger the processor, the quicker the processor will run. What type and size of hard drive are needed? Hard disk drives (HDDs) are cheaper and larger, but they are slower compared to a solid-state drive (SSD).
- What amount of RAM is needed? RAM keeps the computer working at fast speeds.
- When purchasing a printer, it is important to consider its use and how often it will be used. Ask these questions when considering keyboards:
  - Will an ergonomic version be needed?
  - Will the numeric keyboard be needed?
  - Does it need to be wireless?

Installing Hardware

If the medical assistant is installing the computer hardware, it is important to read the directions. If you are connecting cables, make sure they are properly placed and securely plugged in. Many computers will automatically detect the connected hardware and start the installation process. Other times you may be required to load the hardware using the installation directions.

SOFTWARE USED IN AMBULATORY CARE

For hardware to work, the computer must have software. The terms **software** and *program* are mostly synonymous. Programs existed before software. A *program* is a sequence of instructions. It is written in a language that the computer understands. It directs the computer to perform a specific task. *Software* contains several programs that together perform a function. Web browsers, email, games, spreadsheets, and word processors are all types of software.

The two main categories of software are system software and application software.

- *System software*: A collection of programs that operate and control the computer. The system software loads on the computer. It operates in the background while application software is used. There are two types of system software:
  - *Operating systems*: Act as the computer's software administrator by managing, integrating, and controlling application software and hardware. Windows is an example.
  - *Utility software*: Helps the computer function. Examples include file managers, screensavers, backup software, and clipboard managers.
- *Application software*: Also called an *application, app,* or *application program;* it allows the user or other applications to perform specific tasks. Application software may consist of a single program or a collection of programs. A collection can be called a *software package* or *system.* In the ambulatory care facility, several types of application software are used, including practice management software and electronic health records (Table 6.1).

PRACTICE MANAGEMENT SOFTWARE

Practice management software (PMS), sometimes called *medical practice management* (MPM) *software,* is used to run the day-to-day business side of the ambulatory care facility. This software **interfaces** with the EHR software, and each must work with the other *(interoperability).* Information is passed between the practice management software and the EHR software. For instance, a new patient calls for an appointment. During the scheduling process, the person's information is entered into the practice management software. Certain elements of the person's information then move into the EHR software, creating a new health record without requiring any additional time or action on the part of a medical assistant.

Practice management software is used for scheduling appointments, new patient registration, billing, coding, and managing finances. Some of the more useful features of many practice management software programs include the following:

- *Claim denial management and electronic claim submission*: Insurance claims from patient visits and procedures are submitted electronically using the claim submission feature. The claim denial management feature detects errors on the claim before the submission, thus preventing rejections and a loss of **revenue**.
- *Financial and management reporting*: This feature allows for customized reports to be made based on the business activities of the facility. Some of these reports may include the number of patients

TABLE 6.1 Types of Application Software Used in the Ambulatory Care Setting

TYPES OF SOFTWARE	DESCRIPTION
Virus protection software	Also called antivirus or anti-malware software. Used to protect computers against viruses (malware), which damage the computer. An example is AVG AntiVirus Free.
Database software	Allows the user to work with large amounts of data stored in the program. Examples include Microsoft Access, practice management software systems, and electronic health record (EHR) software.
Desktop publishing software	Used to create flyers and newsletters. An example is Microsoft Publisher.
Presentation software	Used to create slides and handouts for presentations. Microsoft PowerPoint and Google Slides are examples.
Spreadsheet software	Used to manage numbers, data, and expenses. Microsoft Excel and Google Sheets are examples.
Telecommunication software	Used to email patients and vendors. An example is Microsoft Outlook, which is also a personal information manager software. Besides email, it includes a calendar, contact manager, task manager, and so on.
Word processing software	Used to compose letters and documents. Examples include Microsoft Word, Google Docs, and Corel WordPerfect.

who **no-show** for appointments or the amount of revenue each provider brought into the business.

- *Scheduler*: This allows for customization of schedules, adding in providers' out-of-office times and other events. This feature is used to schedule patient appointments and procedures.
- *Medical coding or encoder*: All visits, procedures, and diagnoses need to be coded. Many practice management software programs include coding features that allow the user to easily select diagnostic and procedural codes when processing billing charges.
- *Insurance eligibility verification*: This allows the staff to verify patients' insurance benefits quickly.

Electronic Medical Records and Electronic Health Records

Many people use the terms **electronic medical record** *(EMR)* and *electronic health record (EHR)* interchangeably. However, there is a significant difference between these two types of software. When patients' records became electronic (or computerized), they were called electronic medical records. The EMR software contains limited information, usually related to medical treatment for one healthcare facility. The EMR was a digital version of the paper medical record.

The electronic health record has advantages over the EMR. The EHR allows sharing of information with other providers outside the facility, including medical laboratories, nursing homes, hospitals, and specialists. The information from all types of healthcare providers can be stored in the EHR, enhancing functionality and patient care.

Patient Portal

A patient portal is a secure online website that allows a patient 24-hour access to his or her health information. The patient needs to enter a secure username and password prior to accessing the information. The patient portal may be separate software that interfaces with the electronic health record software and the practice management software. It can also be part of the electronic health record. Patient portal features vary and may allow patients to do the following:

- View health information, such as recent visit information, medications, immunizations, allergies, laboratory results, and diagnostic imaging reports
- Securely message the provider and receive messages from the provider and staff
- Request prescription refills
- Schedule nonurgent appointments
- Make payments and check insurance benefits and coverages
- Update personal information
- Download forms and complete online forms
- View educational materials
- Attend virtual provider visits

Web-Based Video Software for Virtual Visits

Telemedicine has been done for years, but during 2020 the use of web-based video products grew quickly as patients and providers needed additional options for visits. A variety of products are available for telemedicine:

- *Online video applications*, such as FaceTime and Zoom. Security is an important aspect to consider with these online video products. Versions are available that comply with the Health Insurance Portability and Accountability Act (HIPAA).
- *Telemedicine specific software*, such as Doxy.me. Features vary with the products and may include the following:
  - No download requirements for patients. A link can be emailed or texted to a patient. The patient clicks on the link and enters his or her name before being admitted to the waiting room.
  - Virtual waiting rooms that require the provider to let the patient in for the visit.
  - Document and screen sharing, such as lab results and consent forms.
  - Payment features.
- *Video embedded patient portal*: The patient logs into the patient portal and can access the video software for the virtual visit.

The Medical Assistant's Role with Virtual Visits

A medical assistant plays an important role in helping to make virtual visits a success. This starts with scheduling the visit. The patient needs to be given directions on how to access the software used for the visit. In most cases, the patient just needs an electronic device (e.g., tablet, PC, or phone) with internet access. The medical assistant should explain the process and what will occur. At the visit, the medical assistant will initiate the visit, much like an in-person visit. The medical assistant determines the patient's reason for the visit (called the chief complaint), updates the medical history, obtains information regarding the patient's allergies, reviews the current medications, and asks if any prescriptions need to be refilled. Once this section of the visit is completed, then the provider sees the patient.

When medical assistants are working with the virtual video software, they must select a location where the patient cannot be overheard and where the patient cannot overhear others. The background the patient sees should be professional or neutral, such as a blank wall. No other patient materials should be visible. The following etiquette tips will be useful as well:

- Be punctual to the visit.
- Start by introducing yourself, and acknowledge the patient and those with the patient.
- Ask the patient if he or she can hear you and see you.
- Provide the patient with a summary of what will occur during the visit.
- If working in a nonhealthcare setting (e.g., working from home), be dressed appropriately.
- Mute your microphone when you are not talking.
- Keep lag time in mind. Allow the patient to finish talking before you start talking. Usually, wait about 2 seconds after the patient's last words before you begin to speak.
- No food should be visible.
- Stay in the patient's view and be mentally and physically present during the conversation.
- Keep your camera on and at eye level. This will help to ensure eye contact with the patient.
- Be professional, just like you would be for an in-person visit.
- Be clear when giving instructions to patients.
- Ask for feedback on the visit, either at the end of the visit or through a survey. This will help you to improve your effectiveness and provide better patient satisfaction.

COMPUTER NETWORK PRIVACY AND SECURITY

Vast quantities of confidential information are stored in computer files. Electronic security is becoming more important today. Many healthcare facilities have had their network computer systems compromised by a **hacker** and **malware**. Some hackers hold the information for ransom. Unsecured patient and employee confidential information can lead to identity theft and other criminal actions.

The Health Insurance Portability and Accountability Act (HIPAA) and the Health Information Technology for Economic and Clinical Health Act (HITECH) require privacy, security, and confidentiality of patient records. These acts mandate training and procedures to be used in healthcare facilities to keep electronic records safe. Administrators and employees must work together to keep the computer network safe.

With the anticipated changes in healthcare technology (e.g., the EHR), Congress passed the Health Insurance Portability and Accountability Act of 1996. Given the increase in **electronic transactions,** HIPAA included provisions for the privacy and security of patients' information. Primary provisions for privacy and security were stated in two standards:

- Standard 2 related to the Privacy Rule: Healthcare facilities, insurance companies, and others need to protect written, electronic, and oral **protected health information (PHI).**
- Standard 3 related to the Security Rule: Healthcare facilities, insurance companies, and others need to protect the patient information that is electronically stored and transmitted.

Of these two standards, the Security Rule will be discussed in more depth in the following sections.

HIPAA's Security Rule addresses the national standards used for electronically protected health information (ePHI). This rule covers the records that are created, used, received, and maintained by the **covered entity**. Administrative, technical, and physical safeguards are required by HIPAA and are important to ensure the security of the ePHI

Administrative Safeguards

The administrative safeguards include administrative policies, procedures, and actions to manage the security measures to protect ePHI. The facility must identify a security officer or an employee who takes on the role to develop and implement policies and procedures that address the Security Rule requirements. The security officer has the responsibility of ensuring the facility's compliance with the HIPAA Security Rule. Besides having a security officer, the facility must have additional administrative safeguards:

- *Policies and procedures for assessing and managing risk to ePHI*: The facility must develop, document, and implement policies and procedures and also have a process for periodically reviewing them. Policies and procedures must address all electronic devices and programs that contain ePHI and all users who have access to ePHI. They must also address the review of information system activity (e.g., who is looking at what information).
- *Security risk analysis*: Potential computer network breach threats are identified, the likelihood of occurrence of those threats is determined, and additional safeguards are implemented. The facility should have a plan of action in place in case a threat occurs.
- *Risk management program to prevent the impermissible use and disclosure of ePHI*: The facility must protect against unauthorized or inappropriate access to ePHI. Unauthorized access may include employees and nonemployees. Policies and procedures must include disciplinary measures for unauthorized employee access. These policies and procedures are usually given to employees during orientation and employees may be required to sign a document indicating that they were notified of them.
- *Implementation of employee training*: Employers must provide privacy and security training to new employees. Periodic refresher courses are important for current staff.
- *Execution of business associate agreements*: The healthcare facility (or covered entity) must have a signed agreement from a business associate regarding the security of confidential information before any ePHI can be given.

Physical Safeguards

The physical safeguards include the physical measures, policies, and procedures used to protect the computer network and related buildings and equipment from hazards and unauthorized access. These safeguards include the following:

- *Security policies and procedures*: The healthcare facility must implement policies and procedures that protect the agency and the equipment from unauthorized physical access, tampering, or theft. The facility should use surveillance cameras and alarms.

TABLE 6.2 Workstation Security

PHYSICAL SAFEGUARD	DESCRIPTION
Passwords	Each user should have a strong password, which has more than eight characters and uses a random combination of uppercase and lowercase letters, numbers, and symbols. Frequently change the password and use different passwords for different software. Do not share passwords.
Privacy filters	Devices attached to the monitor that allow visualization of the screen contents only if the user is directly in front of the screen, also called monitor filters or privacy screens.
Log-out procedures	Users need to log out of the network when leaving a workstation. A logged-in unsupervised workstation allows others to view confidential information. It can also allow individuals to document in an electronic health record (EHR) using your electronic signature.

Computers should have identification numbers and security cables for added protection.

- *Inventory of equipment*: The facility needs to have an inventory of all workstation equipment, portable devices, and medical devices that use, collect, or store ePHI.
- *Access restrictions*: The facility must limit what staff members can see on the computer-based on-the-job description. Not all staff members have the same access to software programs, such as EHRs and practice management software.
- *Workstation security*: These safeguards protect the workstation computer from unauthorized access (Table 6.2). Software such as the EHR allows each user to have an electronic signature, thus indicating what the person entered. When an unauthorized user gets access to a logged-in workstation, information can be looked at or added to the software (e.g., patient health record). Such activity will appear to be done by the logged-in employee, not the unauthorized user.

CRITICAL THINKING APPLICATION 6.7

As is the case in many small healthcare facilities without an IT department, Christiana must assume a leadership role with the EHRs. She has administrator rights, which means she can assign different levels of access to the various staff members. In such a small healthcare facility, what other security measures should she consider using to ensure the privacy of EHRs? What resources might she use to implement the security measures identified?

Technical Safeguards

Only authorized employees should have access to ePHI. Technical safeguards include technology and policies and procedures that protect the ePHI and access to it. Here are some examples:

- *Encryption*: Software used to encode or change the information into nonreadable or encrypted data (also called *ciphertext*), thus preventing unauthorized users from reading the information. An authorized user must enter a password for **decryption** to occur and make the text readable again.

TABLE 6.3 Additional Technical Safeguards

TECHNICAL SAFEGUARDS	DESCRIPTION
Audit trail	Record of computer activity used to monitor users' actions within software, including additions, deletions, and viewing of electronic records.
Authentication	Each employee with network access must log in using a unique password. The security officer should be able to see the employee's activity in the network and individual software.
Automatic log-off	After a period of inactivity, the workstation logs off.
Firewall	A program or hardware device that acts as a barrier or filter between the network and the internet. Data coming from the internet must pass through the firewall. Data that does not meet the firewall criteria are not allowed into the network.
Monitoring of log-in activity	Multiple incorrect log-in attempts are flagged, and often the account is then locked. Prevents hackers from cracking passwords.
Unique user identification	Each employee is assigned a unique name or number for identifying and tracking user identity. This allows the security officer to see the individual's activity on the system.
Virus protection software	Also called antivirus or anti-malware software; used to detect and remove malware. Examples include Norton and AVG AntiVirus Free.

- *Data backup*: The network may be backed up once to several times a day, depending on the size of the facility. Backing up is a process in which the network files are copied using an external hard drive, a server, or an online backup system. It is important to store the backup files offsite to protect the data from a disaster in the medical facility. When computer data is compromised, either by errors, natural causes (e.g., floods, storm damage), or human causes (e.g., fires, hackers, and malware), the data can be restored using the offsite backup copy.
- *Cloud backup services*: Many healthcare facilities contract with cloud backup services, which copy the network data on a routine basis to protect against data loss. Cloud backup services are like cloud storage services in regard to the ability to access the data anytime and anywhere. Backup companies do not typically provide file-sharing services. When computer data is compromised, the data can be restored using the backup copy.

Additional technical safeguards are listed in Table 6.3.

All facilities that are using EHRs or practice management software need to have **downtime** policies and procedures with related supplies available. When the network or a specific software is not available for use, the facility still needs to function. When the network or software becomes usable again, all the patient information collected during the downtime period must be entered into the system.

CRITICAL THINKING APPLICATION **6.8**

Some healthcare facilities store network backup copies in fireproof safes on site. Why is it important to store the backup copy offsite? What would be the advantage of using a data backup internet service that has several data storage locations around the country?

RECOGNIZING AND PREVENTING PHISHING ATTACKS

Some **phishing** attempts are easy to spot, such as those emails informing you that you won a lottery or someone you do not know left you an inheritance. With phishing, the scammer sends out a generic email to many people. Phishing attempts are usually easier to spot than **spear-phising** attempts. With spear phishing, the scammer researches someone and then addresses a personal email to that person. The goal for both phishing and spear phishing is the same—to get confidential information. Phishers may try to steal your computer passwords, bank account numbers, credit and debit card numbers, or Social Security numbers. They may try to have you download malware. If they get this information, they can access your bank accounts, charge items to your credit cards, and gain access to your computer.

Scammers are also targeting businesses, schools, and healthcare agencies. They are attempting to get personal and financial information. Some scammers lock out the legitimate users and demand *ransom* (payment) for the information. Cybercrime has increased over the years and is costly to the people and businesses impacted by it.

Recognizing Phishing Attempts

Scammers use many tricks, and it is up to you to identify phishing emails from either your personal or your business email accounts. Scammers use the following tricks when sending emails and text messages to potential victims:

- **Spoof** *an email account or website.* Scammers pretend they are from a well-known or trusted company. They may use a company's logo or make a slight variation on legitimate email or website addresses to fool people. Sometimes they will indicate a threat, such as "your account will be closed," to have you act immediately.
- *Send spear-phishing emails and text messages.* The personalized message may appear to be from someone you know, such as your boss, the human resource person, your bank, a government agency, a well-known company, or even from someone you work with. The emails are designed to trick victims into revealing confidential information. They may indicate there is a problem with your account or ask you to please confirm some personal information. They may project a sense of urgency to get you to act immediately. It might be difficult to determine if the email is legitimate.
- *Use malware.* Malicious software can infiltrate your computer system and any network (school, business) you are using. Malware can allow scammers to get access to the victim's passwords and financial account information.

Protecting against Phishing Attacks

The following actions may help to protect one against phishing attacks:

- Use virus protection software on your computer.
- Make sure security software on cell phones and computers automatically update.
- Do not respond when a text or email asks for your username or password.
- Do not click on anything in unsolicited email or text messages. Do not download any attachments from someone you do not know.
- Carefully examine the email address, website, and spelling used in any correspondence. Sometimes you can click on the sender's name or business to see the sender's email.
- Protect your accounts by using two-factor or multifactor authentication, which requires you to log onto the account using two or more credentials.
- Be careful of what information you share online and on social media. Make sure you do not share anything related to your passwords and credentials, such as pet names, schools you attended, birthdays, and family members. Make sure your security restrictions are set to limit unknown people from looking at your social media information.
- For the potential spear-phising emails, follow up with the person by using a new email or a phone call before following the directions on the questionable email.

If you accidentally respond to a phishing attack at work, report it immediately to your supervisor. If you gave your personal information to a scammer, go to IdentityTheft.gov and www.us-cert.gov/report to see specific steps to take.

CONTINUAL TECHNOLOGIC ADVANCES IN HEALTHCARE

Patients are seeing more technology in healthcare settings today. Technology is changing from the reception area to the patient care areas. Technology used at home, such as home monitoring devices, is also an important part of patient care.

Reception and Waiting Areas

Receptionists are wearing Bluetooth headsets. These headsets allow them to be more mobile when answering phone calls (Figure 6.8).

For HIPAA compliance, sign-in sheets are being replaced by sign-in kiosks. Some facilities have patients enter health information using the kiosk or a tablet computer. Some clinics use a camera to take the patient's picture for identification. The health information and the photo are then added to the EHR. Receptionists have card readers to use for collecting payments from patients using credit or debit cards. The card reader machines can be mounted on the computer monitor or are stand-alone units. Many have a printer feature that allows the receptionist to present the patient with a paper receipt.

Many healthcare facilities provide patients with wristbands that have bar code technology. This practice started in the hospital and is now moving into the ambulatory care setting. The wristband is scanned before diagnostic tests are done, or medications are administered. This scanning process creates an automatic entry in the patient's EHR. This process is another step in ensuring the patient's safety and accuracy in billing.

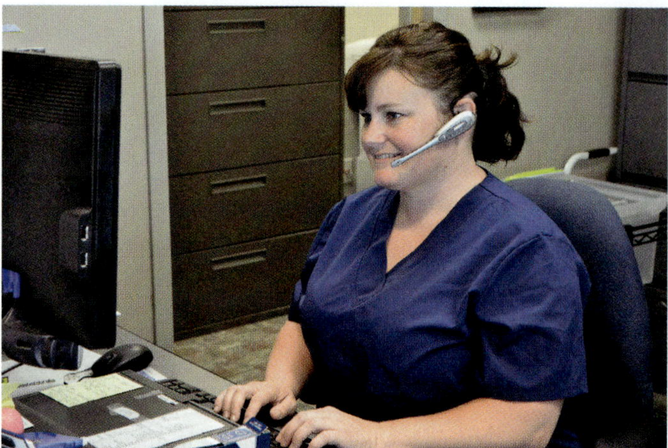

FIGURE 6.8 Bluetooth headsets are helpful for receptionists and other healthcare employees who frequently answer or make phone calls.

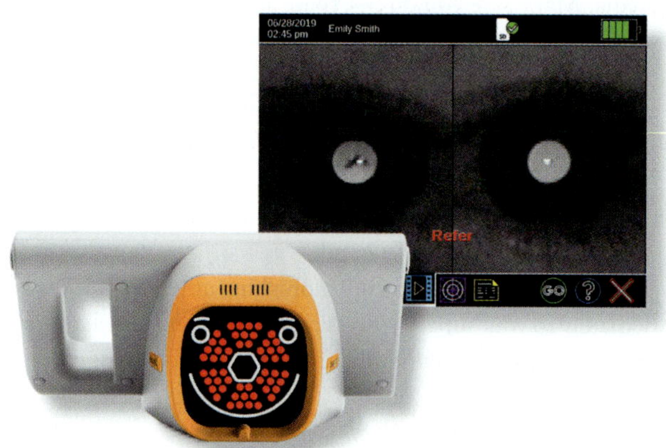

FIGURE 6.9 PlusoptiX Mobile Vision Screener. Courtesy PlusoptiX

Ambulatory surgery centers and walk-in clinics use patient tracking systems in both the reception area and the patient care area. Patients sign in or are signed into the system. Their names go into the queue. For confidentiality purposes, patients may be given a unique number. As patients move from one area of the facility to another, their progress shows on monitors in the reception area. This keeps family members informed of their progress. Patients awaiting appointments or laboratory services can see their number move up in the queue or can observe current wait times. These tracking systems provide cost-effective ways to promote patient satisfaction while improving flow and efficiency.

Patient Care Areas

Many healthcare facilities are using biometrics to log into the network. Many types of biometrics are used, including facial or voice recognition, a palm vein, or a fingerprint. Biometric data is unique and is used to provide additional security to the network.

In the exam room, healthcare workers are using more technology to provide better patient care. Some clinics use wireless mobile workstations, called *computers on wheels* (COWs) or *workstations on wheels* (WOWs). Providers and medical assistants use tablets, smart devices, and wearable computing devices to access EHRs and online resources. **Point-of-care** tools and apps are available for providers to use in the exam room with the patients. This technology gives providers the latest clinical information. Apps are available to provide patients with visuals of surgical procedures, disease processes, and anatomic structures.

Wearable computing devices allow healthcare employees to access medical records and information while moving around and providing patient care. Mobile devices and apps help providers to make quicker decisions with a lower rate of error and improved patient care outcomes. With advances in Bluetooth smart technology, more medical equipment can work with apps on smart devices.

Technology Advances and Eye Screening

During well examinations, primary care providers complete a vision screening on patients to look for potential vision problems. Typically starting about age 3, visual acuity screening is done on children during well examinations. This screening can be challenging for the medical assistant because of the child's age, behavior, and mental cognition. The provider then examines the eyes using the ophthalmoscope. The light causes the pupils to constrict, which can make the exam difficult, and patients often do not like the bright light.

With technological advances, these screening assessments can now be accurately performed in less than 1 second with the Plusoptix Vision Screener (Figure 6.9). With this device, children as young as 5 months can be screened for the most common eye disorders that also may lead to amblyopia, including **anisometropia**, **astigmatism**, **hyperopia**, **myopia**, and media opacities. Earlier screening means earlier interventions that may help prevent surgery and developmental delays depending on the child's condition.

The Plusoptix Vision Screener uses the principle of transillumination testing just like a typical ophthalmoscope. The medical assistant stands about 3.3 feet (1 meter) from the patient during the screening process. The Plusoptix Vision Screener uses infrared light, which is harmless to the patient, reduces the glare, and does not cause the pupils to constrict. The device provides immediate diagnostic feedback for the provider, along with images of the illuminated pupils for the provider to review.

Three-Dimensional Printing in Healthcare

Because it uses diagnostic imaging to provide detailed information on internal structures, three-dimensional (3D) printing has become popular in healthcare. Implants, medical devices, and prosthetics can be customized for a patient instead of using a generic model. Surgeons use 3D printing to help with virtual surgical planning. Magnetic resonance imaging (MRI) and computed tomography (CT) create detailed pictures of internal structures. An exact replica of the person's internal structures is created using 3D printing. The replica is used as the surgeons rehearse complicated surgical procedures prior to surgery.

Advancements in Software

With advancements in EHR software and practice management software, new features and programs are being used. **E-prescribing** allows providers to send prescriptions to the pharmacy electronically (Figure 6.10). With voice-recognition software, providers can dictate notes directly into the patient's EHR. Computerized provider/physician order entry (CPOE) software allows orders for medical

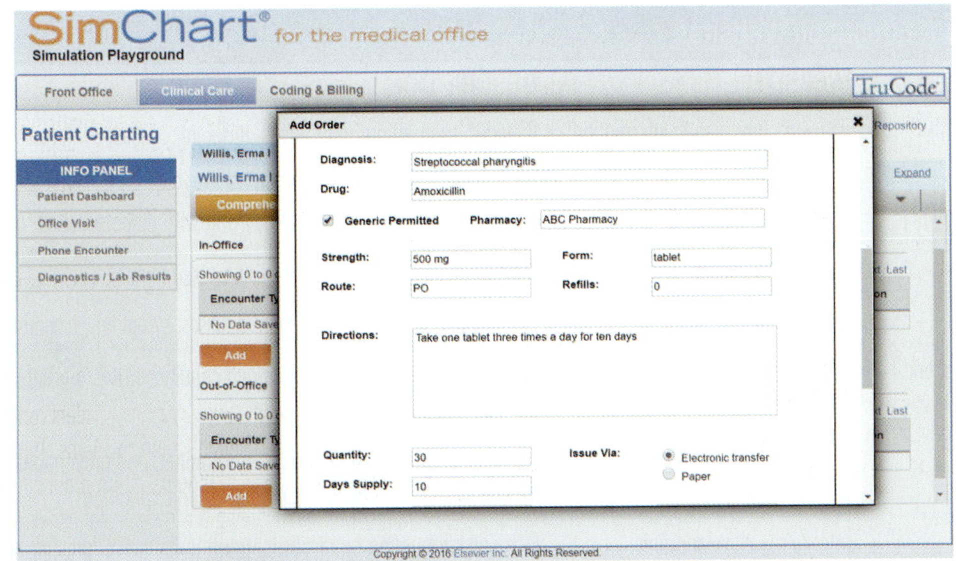

FIGURE 6.10 With e-prescribing, providers can enter the prescription information into the EHR and send it to the pharmacy. The pharmacist can easily read the information, which reduces the chance of errors.

laboratory tests, diagnostic tests, and medications to be entered into the computer. With laboratory order integration, providers can order laboratory tests, and the results are visible in the EHR. In many healthcare facilities, licensed healthcare providers and credentialed medical assistants use CPOE. This improves the efficiency of ordering tests and medications. Some healthcare agencies hire medical scribes. A medical scribe enters patient data into the EHR while the provider examines and treats the patient.

Remote Patient Monitoring

Remote patient monitoring (RPM) or *remote patient management* is a method used to gather patient data outside of the traditional healthcare environment. Technologic devices such as smartphones, smart watches, and tablets capture patient data in one location and electronically transmit it to the healthcare provider in another location. This allows healthcare professionals to monitor patients at a distance. RPM has been shown to reduce hospitalizations and readmissions. It can provide an improved quality of life for the patient and reduce costs.

Monitoring programs gather a wide range of data from point-of-care tests. These include vital signs (e.g., blood pressure and pulse), weight, blood oxygen level, blood glucose levels, and electrocardiograms.

CRITICAL THINKING APPLICATION 6.9

Christiana had considered applying for a medical scribe position at a local healthcare facility before she was promoted to lead administrative medical assistant. Why would a strong background in EHR be important for a medical scribe position?

CLOSING COMMENTS

Patient Coaching

Often, medical assistants need to research health-related topics for patients. The internet has many sites that offer information. The medical assistant must only use websites that are reliable and respected (Table 6.4). The following points should be considered when identifying reliable health websites:

- Government websites (.gov) and educational institution websites (.edu) can be trusted.
- Large, respected healthcare and educational agencies (e.g., Mayo Clinic, Cleveland Clinic, Johns Hopkins) usually have many reliable health-related resources.
- Wikipedia is not reliable.
- If you are reviewing .com or .org websites, evaluate for bias and accuracy (see Procedure 6.2). Research the site by identifying these factors:
    - What is the mission or purpose of the website? Who supports or runs the website? Is advertising present on the website pages?
    - Is the information current or less than 3 years old?
    - What is the source of the information? Who is the author of the content? Does a panel of healthcare experts (e.g., doctors, nurses) review the content?
    - Do you need to provide your personal information to view the pages? If so, what will the site do with your personal information?

When the medical assistant finds information, it is important to verify the content with the provider before using the materials to coach patients. Patients may also ask the medical assistant to recommend reputable sites for health education literature. Having a list of reputable websites for commonly seen conditions may be a timesaver for the medical assistant.

Legal and Ethical Issues

With the electronic health record, it is easy to view one's own health record and that of family and friends. Most healthcare facilities do not allow employees to view their own health records. Viewing family and friends' health records without a job-related reason is a breach of confidentiality. *Audit trails* can be done to identify what records a person views and who views a specific patient's record. Many examples can be found in which high-profile individuals were victims of

TABLE 6.4 Patient Education Websites

ORGANIZATION	WEBSITE	DESCRIPTION
National Institutes of Health (NIH)	www.nih.gov/health-information	Provides information on diseases, including causes, symptoms, and treatments. Also contains Spanish-language materials.
American Diabetes Association	www.diabetes.org	Provides information on diabetes, living with diabetes, food, and fitness.
	www.diabetesfoodhub.org	Provides recipes, a meal planner, and other resources.
Mayo Clinic	www.mayoclinic.org	Provides easy-to-read information on diseases, symptoms, diagnostic tests, and treatments.
Centers for Disease Control and Prevention (CDC)	www.cdc.gov	Provides information on diseases and conditions. It is a great resource for people who are traveling to other countries.
Johns Hopkins Medicine	www.hopkinsmedicine.org/patient-education/index.html	Provides information on diseases, treatments, and prevention. Includes additional tools for patients to learn about managing chronic conditions.
Cleveland Clinic	http://my.clevelandclinic.org/health	Provides information on diseases, treatments, procedures, drugs, supplements, diagnostic tests, videos, and tools for patients.
Drugs.com (information comes from many healthcare sources)	www.drugs.com	Provides information about medications and tools (e.g., pill identifier, symptom checker, and medication record).
MedlinePlus (hosted by NIH and US National Library of Medicine)	https://medlineplus.gov	Provides information on health topics, medications, and supplements. Also includes health and surgery videos, health check tools, and interactive games. Offers information in more than 40 languages.
Familydoctor.org (hosted by the American Academy of Family Physicians)	https://familydoctor.org	Contains information on diseases and conditions, drugs, procedures, and devices, along with prevention and wellness.
American Heart Association	www.heart.org	Includes heart disease information, management, and prevention. Includes a tracking tool for blood pressure, weight, and exercise.
American Cancer Society	www.cancer.org	Provides information on different cancers, treatment, and support.

confidentiality breaches. Regardless of their position, employees have been suspended for viewing records without job-related reasons. It is important for medical assistants to remember that others can view their activities in the EHR, and the consequences of breaches can include jail time, fines, and loss of a job.

Patient-Centered Care

One of the features of patient-centered care is coordination and integration of care. It is essential for healthcare facilities to have downtime procedures and policies when the EHR is not functioning. Most of the time, EHR system upgrades and maintenance occur outside of the normal ambulatory care hours. Unexpected downtimes that occur while patients are being seen can create chaos if policies, procedures, and supplies are unavailable. With the EHR and PMS being used for accessing lab results, prior patient information, scheduling appointments, billing, and prescriptions, everyday tasks cannot be done.

With EHR unavailability, errors can occur, including duplicate or missed testing, duplicate or missed medications, and so on. Because patient safety is critical, the Safety Assurance Factors for EHR Resilience (SAFER) guides (www.healthit.gov) recommend the following practices for facilities:

- Hardware that runs the EHR should be duplicated, and an electric generator with sufficient fuel should be available to back up the EHR during power outages.
- Paper forms need to be available during downtime to replace key EHR functions.
- Backup must be done.
- Downtime policies and procedures need to include accurate patient identification and continuity of operations with regard to patient safety and critical business operations.
- Training and testing scenarios of downtime and recovery procedures should be done.

Once the EHR system is available, all the downtime documentation and activities need to be added to the EHR. Policies and procedures must address how this should be done in a timely and accurate fashion to prevent any future issues.

Professional Behaviors

When a medical assistant is using computers while interacting with others, it is important to focus on the customer. Often, the customer feels forgotten when the employee's attention seems to be on the computer. Being attentive to our customers is important. Remember that your customers in healthcare can be co-workers, providers, patients and their family members, and vendors. It is critical that you use eye contact and body language that show your customers you are really listening:

- Turn your head and upper body toward the speaker
- Lean forward
- Tilt your head and nod
- Smile (if appropriate in the situation)

SUMMARY OF SCENARIO

Christiana has learned a great deal about the healthcare facility's computer network. She is implementing more security measures, such as training staff members to log out of their workstations before leaving the computer. She is also working with a local IT company to increase the network's protection against unauthorized users. She has contracted with an online backup service to protect the network files.

Christiana enjoys her new position and knows that she will need to stay up to date on technological advances and privacy mandates. She plans to do this by reading online articles and attending continuing education events. She understands that learning is an ongoing process that will help her to become the professional she strives to be.

SUMMARY OF LEARNING OBJECTIVES

1. **Differentiate among various types of computers.**
   Types of computers include supercomputers, mainframe computers, minicomputers, microcomputers, and mobile computers. Types of personal computers include desktop, laptop, and tablet (e.g., slate-style, convertible, and hybrid).
2. **Differentiate among various input devices commonly seen in ambulatory care.**
   An input device is any peripheral hardware that allows the user to provide data to the computer. Common input devices include keyboards, mice and other pointing devices, touchscreens, webcams, cameras, microphones, scanners, and signature pads.
3. **Differentiate among various output devices commonly seen in ambulatory care.**
   The data entered into the computer is processed by the computer. The processed data is displayed using output devices. Common output devices in the healthcare setting include monitors, printers, and speakers.
4. **Differentiate among various internal computer components.**
   Internal components found in personal computers include the central processing unit (CPU), motherboard, sound card, video card, and the Universal Serial Bus (USB) port. The primary memory consists of read-only memory (ROM), cache memory, and random-access memory (RAM).
5. **Differentiate among types of secondary storage devices.**
   Secondary storage devices are capable of permanently storing data. The computer storage devices are categorized as follows:
   - *Magnetic storage device:* Uses magnetic technology to read and write data to the device.
   - *Optical storage device (optical disk):* Uses lasers and lights to read and write data onto optical storage devices.
   - *Flash memory device:* Portable device that connects to the USB port in the computer.

   Cloud storage is also called file sharing or online storage. It allows computer files to be stored using the internet and a third-party service.
6. **Differentiate between intranet and internet access requirements.**
   The intranet allows the employees to communicate with each other and access shared files. LAN and WAN technology can use telephone lines or fiberoptic cables that increase the speed of transmission. A router allows multiple computers and other devices to use the same network to send and receive information.

   For internet access, the facility must subscribe to an internet service provider and have the router connected to the modem.
7. **Demonstrate maintaining computer hardware in ambulatory care.**
   The IT staff, whether internal or external, will provide technical assistance and help maintain the equipment. The medical assistant should help to prevent computer problems and keep the hardware clean, including routinely cleaning computer hardware.

   It is important for ambulatory care facilities to have procedures for disinfecting technology, including kiosks, keyboards, mice, and signature pad styluses. Procedures should follow the recommendations from the manufacturers. Infection control practices for technology include the following:
   - Disinfect keyboards daily. Keyboards should also be disinfected when they are contaminated with blood or visibly soiled. Using a disinfectant wipe, clean the surface using friction for 5 seconds.

Continued

SUMMARY OF LEARNING OBJECTIVES—*continued*

- Healthcare professionals should wash their hands or use hand sanitizer before and after using the keyboard.
- Gloves should not be worn during computer use.
- Touchscreen computer monitors and signature pads should be cleaned and disinfected daily per the manufacturer's guidelines. Avoid applying excessive force to screens.
- Plastic covers can be used to enclose keyboards and other devices. These covers should be disinfected daily.

8. **Apply principles of ergonomics to the computer workstation.**
To have an ergonomically friendly workstation, the following are important:
   - Torso and neck should be vertical and in line.
   - Feet need to be flat on the floor or on a footrest.
   - The backrest should help support the upper body in the upright position, and the backrest lumbar support area should be fitted to the small of the back.
   - The seat should be the appropriate size and height to accommodate the person, and the armrest should support the forearms with the shoulders in a relaxed position.
   - For standing workstations, legs, torso, head, and neck should be vertical and in line. One foot can be elevated on a step.
   - The monitor should be directly in front of the person, with the top of the monitor at or just below eye level.
   - The work surface and mouse should be at elbow level for typing. Your wrist should be supported by a foam wrist rest.
   - Use a headset, document holder, and an ergonomic split-key or waved keyboard.

9. **Examine considerations when purchasing and installing hardware.**
There are a variety of questions to ask when purchasing hardware. For example, for computers, it is necessary to know who will be using the computer, what will be done on the computer, and what operating system will be used. For printers, it is important to know what they will be used for and how often they will be used. For keyboards, you need to know if a numeric keyboard is needed, if it needs to be ergonomic, and if it needs to be wireless.

10. **Differentiate among types of software used in ambulatory care.**
The two main categories of software are system software and application software. The system software operates in the background while application software is used. Operating systems and utility software are two types of system software.
Application software allows the user or other applications to perform specific tasks. Examples of application software include anti-malware, database, desktop publishing, presentation, spreadsheet, telecommunication, and word processing. Examples of application software include the following:
    - Practice management software (PMS) (also called *medical practice management* [MPM]): Used to run the day-to-day business side of the ambulatory care facility, including scheduling appointments, new patient registration, billing, coding, and managing finances.
    - Electronic medical record (EMR): Contains limited information, usually related to medical treatment for one healthcare facility.
    - Electronic health record (EHR): Allows sharing of information with other providers outside the facility. The information from all types of healthcare providers can be stored in the EHR, enhancing functionality and patient care.
    - Patient portal: Secure online website that allows a patient 24-hour access to his or her health information.
    - Web-based video software: Used for telemedicine.

11. **Examine federal requirements used to maintain computer network privacy and security in healthcare.**
HIPAA's Security Rule addresses the national standards used to shield electronically protected health information (ePHI). This rule covers the records that are created, used, received, and maintained by the covered entities. Administrative, technical, and physical safeguards are important to ensure the security of the ePHI.
The administrative safeguards include administrative policies, procedures, and actions to manage the security measures to protect ePHI. The facility must identify a security officer who oversees compliance with the Security Rule. Physical safeguards include the physical measures, policies, and procedures used to protect the computer network and related buildings and equipment from hazards and unauthorized access. Technical safeguards include technology and policies and procedures that protect the ePHI and access to it.

12. **Examine how to recognize and prevent phishing attacks.**
Phishing and spear-phishing attacks are meant to get the victim's personal confidential information. Individuals and organizations are at risk for such attacks. Scammers spoof email accounts and websites, send spear-phishing emails, and use malware. It is important to use virus protection software on computers and have software automatically updated. Do not click on anything in unsolicited email or text messages. Examine the message if you are asked to give your personal information. Protect your accounts by using two-factor authentication.

13. **Examine how advances in technology affect the ambulatory care environment and patient care.**
This chapter addressed the use of technology in the ambulatory care facility, including in the reception and patient care areas. Technologic advances impact administrative and clinical medical assistants, along with providers.

PROCEDURE 6.1 Prepare a Workstation

TASKS: Perform infection control procedures and create an ergonomically friendly workstation.

EQUIPMENT and SUPPLIES

- Nonabrasive disinfectant (hospital grade) wipes, or specially made wipes for computer hardware, or wipes as indicated by the keyboard manufacturer
- Gloves (if required for using wipes)
- User guide for keyboard or facility's infection control procedure for computer hardware
- Desktop computer with adjustable monitor
- Office chair with an adjustable seat, armrest, and backrest
- Footrest (if needed)
- Foam wrist rest
- Document holder (optional)
- Hand sanitizer (optional)

PROCEDURAL STEPS

1. While sitting in the chair, adjust the backrest so it supports the upper body and the lumbar support area fits the small of the back. Adjust the seat pan height, so the feet are flat on the floor or footrest. Adjust the armrest to support the forearms with the shoulders in a relaxed position.
   PURPOSE: The backrest should support the back. The chair height should not add pressure on the back of the knees or thighs while allowing the feet to be flat on the floor or footrest.
2. Adjust the monitor so it is directly in front of you and the top of the monitor is at or just below eye level. If you are using a document holder, position it so it is at the same distance and height as the monitor.
   PURPOSE: Correct positioning of the monitor helps to reduce neck muscle discomfort.
3. Place the keyboard at a height and an angle to allow the wrists to be in a neutral position. Position the mouse so it is at elbow level when using it. Support the wrists with a foam wrist rest.
   PURPOSE: Supporting the wrists prevents repetitive stress injuries.
4. While sitting with your torso and neck vertical and in line, identify if everything is positioned correctly and comfortably. Make any adjustments as needed.
   PURPOSE: For ergonomics, the torso and neck need to be vertical and in line. Slouching is not considered ergonomically friendly and can lead to discomfort and potential injuries.
5. Using the keyboard user guide or the facility's infection control procedure for computer hardware, determine the product to use to disinfect the keyboard. Put on disposable gloves if needed. Using a disinfectant wipe, clean the surface using friction for 5 seconds in each area. Discard gloves if worn.
   PURPOSE: Use only the cleaning products recommended by the manufacturer or the facility when cleaning computer hardware.
6. Wash hands or use hand sanitizer before using the keyboard.
   PURPOSE: Hand sanitization is an important step for infection control.

PROCEDURE 6.2 Identify a Reliable Patient Education Website

TASKS: Research a disease or condition and evaluate a patient education website.

EQUIPMENT and SUPPLIES

- Computer with internet access, word processing software, and printer

PROCEDURAL STEPS

1. Select a disease or condition. Using the internet, find a website with information about the disease or condition. Do not use a website listed in this chapter.
2. Identify the mission or purpose of the website, who supports or runs the website, and whether there is advertising present on the page. If advertising is present, is the advertising mixed in with the content or text?
   PURPOSE: Understanding the mission or purpose of the website, along with who runs or supports it, will help determine if the website is reliable.
3. Determine if the information is current or less than 3 years old.
   PURPOSE: Healthcare content changes quickly, and it is important to have current information.
4. Identify the author(s) and the person's background. Does a panel of healthcare experts review the content?
   PURPOSE: The content is more reliable if an expert is the author or if it is reviewed by experts in the field.
5. Determine if a person needs to enter personal information to view pages of the website. If so, what does the website's host do with the personal information?
   PURPOSE: It is important to determine if the host will keep the personal information private or if the information will be sold to other companies.
6. Compose a one-page paper on your findings. Use double line spacing and a 12-point font size. Include the website you used. Discuss if the website is reliable and if the content is updated. Proofread and spell-check your document before printing it.
   PURPOSE: Professional documents need to be spell-checked and proofread.

WRITTEN COMMUNICATION 7

SCENARIO

Christiana Zwellen is a certified medical assistant (CMA) at Walden-Martin Family Medical (WMFM) Clinic. She had been working as a clinical medical assistant for 5 years. She helped with diagnostic tests and treatment procedures. Christiana enjoyed providing patient care, but she wanted to use more of the administrative skills she had learned. She is organized and enjoys challenges and technology. When a front office position opened up, Christiana moved into the administrative role. She is now the lead administrative medical assistant. Her role involves answering phones, scheduling appointments, greeting patients, and processing correspondence to patients. She is also responsible for reviewing the clinic's emails. Patients are encouraged to use email to communicate with providers through the patient portal. Christiana has seen an increase in the number of daily emails. She answers those that pertain to appointments. Other emails are forwarded to the providers or their clinical medical assistants. Christiana is excited to continue to learn the administrative role.

While studying this chapter, think about the following questions:

- What are the guidelines for using capitalization and punctuation in business communication?
- How are numbers written in business communication?
- What are the components of a business letter?
- What are the formats for business letters and memorandums?
- Why are templates used for business communication?
- What is the etiquette for professional emails?
- What postal services are used in the ambulatory care facility?

LEARNING OBJECTIVES

1. Differentiate between the parts of speech.
2. Examine common communication errors, including misused words and inconsistencies with nouns and pronouns.
3. Differentiate between the types and uses of punctuation.
4. Examine the use of capitalizations and numbers in professional communication.
5. Demonstrate how to compose a professional letter.
6. Differentiate between the various business letter formats.
7. Demonstrate how to compose a memorandum.
8. Demonstrate how to compose a professional email.
9. Examine how to fax documents while maintaining a patient's confidentiality.
10. Demonstrate how to address an envelope and fold documents to place in envelopes.
11. Examine how to handle outgoing mail, including postage and delivery services, and incoming mail to the ambulatory care facility.

VOCABULARY

authorized agent A person who has written documentation that they can accept a shipment for another individual.

bonded A term describing employees for whom an employer has obtained a fidelity bond from an insurance company, which will cover losses from any dishonest acts (e.g., embezzlement, theft) committed by those employees.

electronic health record (EHR) An electronic record that conforms to nationally recognized standards and contains health-related information about a specific patient. It can be created, managed, and consulted by authorized clinicians and staff from more than one healthcare organization.

girth The measurement around something; when referring to mail, it is the measurement around the middle of the package that is being shipped.

media (ME de ah) Types of communication (e.g., social media sites); with computers, the term refers to data storage devices.

portrait orientation The most common layout for a printed page; the height of the paper is greater than its width.

practice management software A type of software that allows the user to enter demographic information, schedule appointments, maintain lists of insurance payers, perform billing tasks, and generate reports.

template (TEM plit) A document or file that has a preset format; this is used as a starting point for composing something and eliminates the need to recreate it each time it is used.

termination letters Documents sent to patients explaining that the provider is ending the physician-patient relationship and the patient needs to see other providers.

zone A region or geographic area used for shipping.

INTRODUCTION

Communication has changed over the years. Many people have moved from writing letters to sending emails and text messages. Social media sites have gained popularity. Many of these changes have affected the ambulatory care environment. Patients use emails and text messages to contact their providers.

Written communication from an ambulatory care facility is a reflection of the provider and the facility. Medical assistants often compose emails and letters to patients and vendors. A poorly worded message or incorrect punctuation in a letter or an email gives the reader a negative impression of the sender and, thus, the clinic. A medical assistant needs to know how to properly write a letter or message to others. It is important that the sentence structure, grammar, spelling, and tone of the message are professional.

This chapter begins by covering the basics of written communication, including parts of speech, punctuation, and capitalization. Following these basics, the parts of a professional letter are discussed, along with business letter formats. The chapter closes with a discussion on outgoing and incoming mail.

PARTS OF SPEECH

When writing a letter or message to others, the medical assistant needs to properly construct the message by using the correct parts of speech.

Nouns

A *noun* is a word or phrase for a person, place, thing, or idea. A *common noun* names a general group of people, places, things, and ideas (e.g., *desk, office*). A *proper noun* names a specific person, place, or thing (e.g., *Zachary, Boston*). A proper noun should start with a capital letter. A *pronoun* is a word that takes the place of a noun (e.g., *I, he, she, it,* and *they*). A pronoun is not capitalized unless it is at the beginning of a sentence, with the exception of "I," which is always capitalized.

Subject and Verb

A *verb* is a word or a phrase that shows action or a state of being (e.g., *talks, walks, is,* and *are*). The *subject* in a sentence is a noun, pronoun, or set of words that perform the verb action.

It is important to make sure the subject and verb agree. A singular subject (e.g., provider, patient) must be matched with a singular verb (e.g., is, reads, goes). A plural subject (e.g., providers, patients) must be paired with a plural verb (e.g., are, read, go).

- Nonagreement of subject and verb examples:
  - The medical assistant talk to the patient.
  - The patients is waiting for the doctor.
- Agreement of subject and verb examples:
  - The medical assistant talks to the patient.
  - The patients are waiting for the doctor.

Sentences and Fragments

A sentence requires at least one main clause, which contains an independent subject and verb and expresses a complete thought. A *fragment* (or incomplete sentence) is a phrase without a main clause and is a major error in writing:

- Fragment: "Greeted patients before she updated their information."
- Complete sentence: "The receptionist always greeted patients before she updated their information."

Additional Sentence Elements

Many sentences also contain the following elements:

- *Independent clause*: Can stand alone as a sentence because it contains a subject and a verb. (Example: *The patient felt sick.*)
- *Dependent clause*: Often begins with words such as *although, since, when, because,* and *if.* A dependent clause needs an independent clause (e.g., subject and verb) to be a complete sentence. (Example: The receptionist immediately notified the clinical medical assistant *because the patient felt sick.*)
- *Nonessential or nonrestrictive clause*: A group of words that provides extra information and does not change the meaning of the sentence. *Which* often starts nonessential clauses. and commas are used to set off the clause. (Example: The medical assistant set out the gown, *which was made of cotton.*)
- *Essential, restrictive, or relative clause*: A group of words that includes information that is important to the meaning of the sentence. *That* is typically used with essential clauses, and commas are not used to set off the clause. (Example: The medical assistant set out a gown *that would be used during the exam.*)
- *Phrase*: A group of words without a subject or verb. (Example: A warm exam room helps keep the patient comfortable *during a physical exam.*)
- *Adjective*: A word or group of words that describe a noun or pronoun; may come before or after the noun or pronoun it describes. (Example: The *warm* room was full of patients.)
- *Adverb*: A word or group of words that answers how, where, when, or to what extent, thus further describing a verb, adjective, or other adverbs. (Example: The patient spoke *softly.*)
- *Preposition*: A word that indicates a relationship or a location between a noun or pronoun and the rest of the sentence. Commonly used prepositions include *near, besides, about, to, with, by, after,* and *in.* (Example: The student sat *beside* the receptionist.)

CRITICAL THINKING APPLICATION **7.1**

Christiana needs to compose a letter. How can she be sure she does not have any incomplete sentences in her letter? What parts of speech are required for a complete sentence?

COMMON COMMUNICATION ERRORS

When medical assistants compose professional communications, it is important to use language the reader will understand. Refrain from slang, generational terms, and abbreviations used in electronic communication. These can cause miscommunication with the reader.

To ensure that the message is clear to the reader, make the following adjustments if necessary:

- Refrain from using two negatives in the same sentence.
- Refrain from using vague expressions or overusing the same words within a paragraph.
- Avoid using run-on sentences that contain several independent clauses together without the required punctuation.

The medical assistant should review the professional communication for errors. Proper spelling, use of words, and sentence structure are important because they reflect on the writer and the healthcare facility. The following sections review common communication errors.

TABLE 7.1 Commonly Confused Words

WORDS	EXAMPLES
As: is used in comparisons *Has*: to possess, own, or experience	She is *as* fast as he is on the keyboard. The medical assistant *has* increased his keyboarding speed by using the computer every day.
Lie: to recline or rest on a surface *Lay*: to put or place	I *lie* down to sleep. I *lay* down the book.
Set: to put or place *Sit*: to be seated	She *set* the gown on the table for the patient. *Sit* on the table when you have changed into a gown.
Who: refers to people; he or she did an action *Whom*: refers to him or her	*Who* placed the order for supplies? Mike saw *whom* yesterday?
That: is used for essential clauses *Which*: starts nonessential clauses	The letters *that* are on the printer need to be signed. The letters, *which* are on the printer, need to be signed.
Like: means "similar to" *As*: means "in the same manner" and requires a verb	The child is *like* her mother. He works *as* a phlebotomist.
Farther: refers to a measurable distance *Further*: refers to an abstract length	The healthcare facility is *farther* away than I thought. *Further* research is needed before we purchase a new computer.

Homonyms and Misused Words

The medical assistant should know the proper use of commonly confused words and misused phrases (Table 7.1). *Homonyms* (i.e., words that sound alike) may not be identified by the software's spell-checker, which can lead to mistakes (Table 7.2). Here are some commonly misused words and phrases:

- Anyway (not anyways)
- Supposed to (not suppose to)
- Toward (not towards)
- Used to (not use to)

Noun and Pronoun Mismatch

A common mistake in communication is a mismatch between the noun and pronoun number. When referring to plural nouns, use plural pronouns, such as *we, us, you, they,* and *them.* For example, "When receptionists answer the phone, they need to be polite." When referring to singular nouns, use singular pronouns. Singular pronouns include *I, me, you, she, her, he, him,* and *it.*

Recently, *they* has become a singular third-person pronoun. *They* is now considered inclusive of all people, regardless of sex or gender. *They* can be used when referring to a person whose gender is unknown. When *they* is used as a subject, the verb should always be plural, even if *they* represents a single person. The pronoun *their* can be used to replace *his or her.*

TABLE 7.2 Meanings of Common Homonyms

HOMONYMS	EXAMPLES
Affect (verb): to influence or transform *Effect* (noun): a result, outcome, consequence, or appearance	The outbreak of influenza will *affect* our patients. The *effect* of influenza was devastating to the city.
Accept (verb): to receive *Except* (preposition): excluding	Will you *accept* this certified letter? She mailed all the envelopes, *except* the certified letter.
Than (conjunction): used to compare *Then* (adverb): tells when	The receptionist was busier *than* the clinical medical assistant. The receptionist finished registering the patient and *then* scheduled the appointment.
There (adverb): indicates place *Their* (pronoun): indicates possession *They're* (contraction): they are	*There* were 25 chairs in the reception area. *Their* children remained in the reception area. *They're* the only patients in the reception area.
Your (pronoun): indicates possession *You're* (contraction): you are	*Your* new job is in pediatrics. *You're* working in pediatrics today.
To (preposition): indicates direction, action, or condition *Too* (adverb): means "also" *Two* (noun): number	She went *to* answer the phone. The medical assistant's phone was ringing, *too.* Her phone has *two* lines.
Where (adverb, noun, pronoun, conjunction): to, at, or in what place *Were* (verb): past tense plural of "be" *Wear* (verb): to have something on your body	*Where* did the patient go? *Were* you finished? *Wear* the gown, please.

PUNCTUATION

Using the correct words and punctuation marks is important when you are composing written correspondence. To reduce the risk of errors, the medical assistant should perform a spelling and grammar check and proofread the document. It is important to know how to use correct punctuation because some spell-checking programs may flag incorrect issues.

This section examines the most common punctuation marks used in professional correspondence and when charting a patient's health record.

Period, Question Mark, and Exclamation Point

A sentence can end with one of three types of punctuation: a period (.), a question mark (?), or an exclamation point (also called exclamation mark) (!). Use a period for a sentence that makes a statement. Use a question mark after a direct question. Use an exclamation point for sentences that express strong emotion. An exclamation point is rarely used in professional written communication. When quotation marks are used, all punctuation goes inside the closing quotation mark (e.g., "Thank you for coming in today.").

Commas

Commas are frequently used in written communication. The following are rules regarding comma use:

- Use before a coordinating conjunction (*and, but, or, nor, yet, so,* and *for*) when joining two complete sentences. (Example: The last patient left, and the receptionist locked the door.) Do not use a comma if joining a complete sentence with an incomplete sentence.
- Use to separate items in a list of three or more things. (Example: The medical assistant escorted *the mother*, *the father*, and *the child* to the exam room.)
- Use to separate two interchangeable adjectives. (Example: The patient was a *strong, healthy* child.)
- Use after certain words at the start of a sentence (i.e., yes, no, hello). (Example: *Yes*, the bill was correct.)
- Use to set off a name or title or an expression that interrupts the flow of the sentence. (Examples: Will you, *Michaela*, want an appointment in two weeks? I am, *by the way*, very excited about the job opportunity.)
- Use after a dependent clause that starts a sentence. (Example: *If you have any questions*, let me know.)
- Use to separate the day from the year. (Example: May *24*, 20XX)
- Use to separate the city from its state. (This rule does not apply when addressing envelopes.) (Example: *Madison*, Wisconsin)
- Can be used to separate Sr. or Jr. from the person's name, but this is not mandatory. (Example: Bob Smith, *Sr.*, has arrived for his appointment.)
- Use after a degree or title and enclose the degree or title if it appears in a sentence. (Example: John Williams, *MD*, will be the speaker for the event.)
- Use to set off nonessential words or phrases. (Examples: Christiana, *the newest secretary*, has arrived. My brother, *Keith*, has an appointment to see Dr. Smith.)
- Use with direct quotations. (Example: She stated, "*I have waited too long.*")

Semicolons and Colons

A *semicolon* (;) is a common punctuation mark used in professional letters and documentation. The semicolon is used before certain words (*however* and *therefore*, for example). It is also used when separating phrases in a series or linking two complete sentences (e.g., "The provider is running late; however, our first two patients canceled this morning.").

A *colon* (:) is used to introduce a series of items either in the sentence or bulleted list. A colon is also used after the greeting or salutation in a professional letter.

Quotation Marks and Apostrophes

Quotation marks (" ") are used to set off direct quotes. They are frequently used when documenting a patient's chief complaint, the main reason for their visit. An apostrophe (') is used to show ownership. The apostrophe is placed after the "s" (e.g., patients') to show plural possession.

CAPITALIZATIONS AND NUMBERS

Besides using the correct parts of speech and punctuation, using proper capitalization is also important. Professional communication should contain correct capitalization and the right number format. As mentioned earlier, errors can reflect poorly on the writer and the facility.

Capitalization

The first letter of the first word of a sentence or question should be capitalized. The pronoun "I" is always capitalized. The first letter of proper nouns, including names of people, months, institutions, organizations, countries, and national nouns and adjectives (e.g., French, British), should be capitalized. Common nouns (e.g., girls, women, boys, men) should not be capitalized unless the word is the first word of a sentence.

Writing Numbers

A few rules apply to writing numbers. Spell out all numbers at the beginning of a sentence. Hyphenate all compound numbers from 21 to 99 (e.g., *twenty-three*) and all written-out fractions (e.g., two-thirds). For numbers with four or more digits, use commas (e.g., 1,234). It is not advised to include a decimal point or a dollar sign when writing out sums less than a dollar (e.g., 23 cents). Use noon and midnight instead of 12 p.m. and 12 a.m. The format for a.m. and p.m. can vary.

WRITTEN CORRESPONDENCE

Medical assistants are responsible for communicating with vendors or supply companies. They are also required to send a written communication to patients and other providers, as directed by their provider-employers. Knowing how to compose a professional letter is an important skill for medical assistants. To compose a letter, you must know the correct content and location for the parts of the letter.

Paper, Margins, Spacing, and Font

A professional letter uses 8.5 × 11-inch paper or letterhead paper. Letterhead paper is 20- to 24-lb. bond paper (e.g., the thicker the paper, the larger the lb. bond number). The letter typically has 1-inch margins on all four sides, though shorter letters may use larger margins. The entire letter should be written using single line spacing. Consistency in line spacing is important for a professional appearance. The font should be simple and easy to read, such as Times New Roman or Calibri in a 10- or 12-point size. Limit the use of boldface and italics in the letter.

Sender's Address

The sender's address is usually located in the letterhead (Figure 7.1). Most facilities use preprinted letterhead paper. A letterhead can also be created at the top of the document using the word processing software's header tool. The letterhead may or may not include the provider's name. It should have the clinic's name, street address or post office box, city, state, and zip code. Some letterheads have additional contact information, such as phone numbers, website addresses, and email addresses.

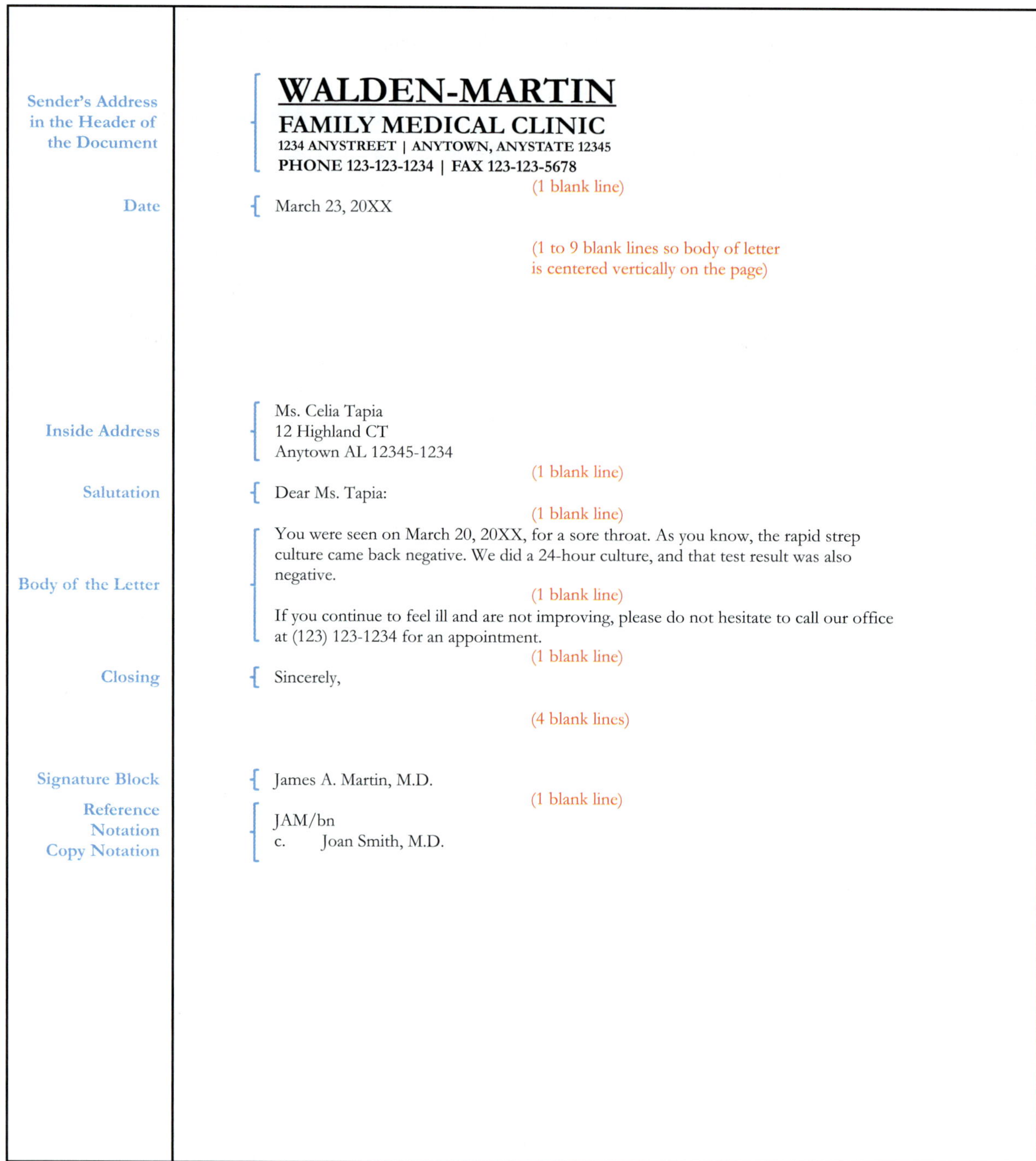

WALDEN-MARTIN
FAMILY MEDICAL CLINIC
1234 ANYSTREET | ANYTOWN, ANYSTATE 12345
PHONE 123-123-1234 | FAX 123-123-5678

March 23, 20XX

Ms. Celia Tapia
12 Highland CT
Anytown AL 12345-1234

Dear Ms. Tapia:

You were seen on March 20, 20XX, for a sore throat. As you know, the rapid strep culture came back negative. We did a 24-hour culture, and that test result was also negative.

If you continue to feel ill and are not improving, please do not hesitate to call our office at (123) 123-1234 for an appointment.

Sincerely,

James A. Martin, M.D.

JAM/bn
c. Joan Smith, M.D.

FIGURE 7.1 **Business Letter Format.** When a medical assistant types a letter for a provider, that provider must sign the letter after it has been printed.

If letterhead is not used for a professional letter, the sender's address is placed at the left margin, 1 inch from the top of the document. Use single spacing and include the facility's address. Do not include the sender's name because that is in the closing section of the letter.

Date

All professional letters must include a date. The date is located either at the left or right margin or starts at the center point of the line (see Figure 7.1). The location depends on the type of letter format used. When using letterhead, the dateline starts on the second line after the letterhead. If letterhead is not used, the dateline starts on the second line below the sender's address. In either situation, there should be one blank line between the date and the last line of the letterhead or sender's address.

When keying (typing) the date, write out the name of the month, then the number of the day, followed by a comma and the four-digit year. Make sure to have a blank space between the month and the day and after the comma (e.g., May 14, 20XX). Do not use "th" or "st" after the day (e.g., May 14th, 20XX).

Inside Address

The inside address starts between the second to the tenth line, below the dateline. The placement depends on the length of the letter (see

Figure 7.1). If the body of the letter is long, leave one blank line between the date and the inside address. If the body is short, add up to nine blank lines between the date line and the first line of the inside address. The goal is to have the body of the letter centered vertically on the page.

The inside address is always left justified. It includes the recipient's name and title on the first line. The next lines include the department and healthcare facility name. The last lines include the street address, followed by the city, state, and zip code. Always address the letter to a specific person. If the letter relates to a minor, address the letter to the patient's guardian. When writing out the person's name, include the person's personal title (e.g., Miss, Ms., Mrs., Mr., or Dr.). If you are unsure of a woman's title preference, use Ms.

If the inside address is shown through a window envelope, make sure to use the US Postal Service format and abbreviations for the address (Table 7.3). The format is explained later in the chapter.

Reference Line

The reference line may be used occasionally. It starts on the second line below the inside address at the left margin. The salutation is then placed on the second line below the reference line. The purpose of the reference line is to refer to a specific item, such as a file, case number, or product number. It provides an easy reference for the reader and sender (e.g., Reference: Invoice #44549).

Salutation

The salutation is the greeting. It starts on the second line below the inside address. It is always left justified (see Figure 7.1). For business letters, the salutation should be formal. "Dear" is followed by the person's title and name and then ends with a colon (e.g., Dear Mr. Smith:). Sometimes, the person's first name can be added (e.g., Dear Mr. Ted Smith:). If the person's gender is not known, use the first and last name without the title (e.g., Dear Sam Smith:). The phrase "To Whom It May Concern" can be used if a person's name is not known.

TABLE 7.3 US Postal Service Standard Street, Directional, and State Abbreviations

WORD	ABBREVIATION	WORD	ABBREVIATION	STATE	ABBREVIATION	STATE	ABBREVIATION
Alley	ALY	Northeast	NE	Louisiana	LA	South Carolina	SC
Avenue	AVE	Northwest	NW	Maine	ME	South Dakota	SD
Boulevard	BLVD	Southeast	SE	Maryland	MD	Tennessee	TN
Bridge	BRG	Southwest	SW	Massachusetts	MA	Texas	TX
Bypass	BYP	**State**		Michigan	MI	Utah	UT
Center	CTR	Alabama	AL	Minnesota	MN	Vermont	VT
Circle	CIR	Alaska	AK	Mississippi	MS	Virginia	VA
Court	CT	Arizona	AZ	Missouri	MO	Washington	WA
Crossing	XING	Arkansas	AR	Montana	MT	West Virginia	WV
Drive	DR	California	CA	Nebraska	NE	Wisconsin	WI
Estate	EST	Colorado	CO	Nevada	NV	Wyoming	WY
Highway	HWY	Connecticut	CT	New Hampshire	NH	**Federal District and Major Territories**	
Parkway	PKWY	Delaware	DE	New Jersey	NJ	American Samoa	AS
Road	RD	Florida	FL	New Mexico	NM	District of Columbia	DC
Route	RTE	Georgia	GA	New York	NY	Guam	GU
Street	ST	Hawaii	HI	North Carolina	NC	Northern Mariana Islands	MP
Terrace	TER	Idaho	ID	North Dakota	ND	Puerto Rico	PR
Way	WAY	Illinois	IL	Ohio	OH	U.S. Virgin Islands	VI
North	N	Indiana	IN	Oklahoma	OK		
South	S	Iowa	IA	Oregon	OR		
East	E	Kansas	KS	Pennsylvania	PA		
West	W	Kentucky	KY	Rhode Island	RI		

Subject Line

The subject line is not used very often. The purpose of the subject line is to state the main subject of the letter. It is left justified and placed on the second line below the salutation. The body of the letter starts on the second line below the subject line. The subject line should be composed using boldface, underlining, or all capital letters to draw the reader's attention (SUBJECT: ORDER NO. 45677-93).

Body of the Letter

The body of the letter starts on the second line below the salutation (see Figure 7.1). The body is single spaced and either left justified or left justified with the first word of each paragraph indented based on the letter format used. There should be one blank line between paragraphs.

The body of the letter contains the content of the letter. The first paragraph is a friendly opening and states the purpose of the letter. The remaining paragraphs support the purpose of the letter and should be concise. The final paragraph may request a specific action.

Closing

The closing is positioned vertically in the same position as the date (see Figure 7.1). There should be one blank line between the last line of the body of the letter and the closing. The first word should include a capital letter. The remaining words in the closing should be in lowercase. Typically, "Sincerely" is used; more formal closings include "Yours truly" or "Very truly yours." The word or phrase is followed by a comma.

Signature Block

The signature block includes the signature, typed name, and title of the sender. There should be four blank lines between the closing and the typed name and credentials of the sender. This space allows the person to sign the letter. The person's title is capitalized and is located on the line directly below the typed name (e.g., Director of Walden-Martin Family Medical Clinic). If the medical assistant types the letter for a provider, the provider must sign it after it has been printed (see Figure 7.1).

CRITICAL THINKING APPLICATION **7.2**

Christiana is composing several letters. Who would sign each of the following letters?

- A letter to a patient indicating her test results
- A letter to a vendor asking for specific pricing for a new computer
- A letter to a referring physician, thanking him for the patient referral

End Notations

Several items may be noted on the letter after the signature block. This may vary among healthcare facilities.

- *Reference notation*: Notes the initials of the person who composed the letter in uppercase followed by the initials of the person who keyed (typed) the letter in lowercase (see Figure 7.1). A colon (:) or a forward slash (/) divides the two sets of initials (e.g., MR:bn, MR/bn). This notation should be left justified on the second line below the last line of the signature block.
- *Enclosure/attachment notation*: Indicates the number of documents or attachments that accompany the letter. The enclosure notation is left justified. It starts on the second line below the reference notation. If the reference notation is not present, the enclosure notation is placed on the second line below the last line of the signature block. The enclosure notation can be typed in several ways. It can be indicated with either "Enclosure" or "Enc." If more than one enclosure is sent, the number of enclosures or the names of the enclosures should be indicated. Any of the following three formats can be used to indicate that an enclosure is included with the letter:
  - Enclosures: 2
  - Enclosures (2)
  - Enclosures:

  Draft of the policy statement
  Invoice #45433
- *Copy notation* (c.): Used to notify the letter's recipient who else received a copy of the letter. The "c" is left justified and goes on the line immediately following the last notation. It is then followed by a period. Use the tab tool to move a half-inch before typing the person's name (e.g., c. John Smith). Additional names should be aligned vertically on the document.
- *Blind copy* (bc.): Used if the sender does not want the recipient to know a copy was sent to another person. The format is the same as it is for "c.," but the "bc." is added only to the office copy of the letter. It is not listed on the letter going to the recipient.

CRITICAL THINKING APPLICATION **7.3**

For the letters that Christiana will sign, should she include a reference notation at the bottom of the letter? Why or why not? For the letters prepared by Christiana and signed by Dr. Walden, should she add the reference notation? Why or why not?

Subsequent Pages of a Letter

Letterhead is not used for subsequent pages of a letter. The subsequent pages should be on paper that matches in weight and color. Each sheet after the letterhead must have a heading that includes these elements on separate lines: the recipient's name, the page number, and the date. The name should be on the first line below the top margin, and all three elements should be left justified and single spaced.

Ms. Celia Tapia
Page 2
March 23, 20XX

BUSINESS LETTER FORMATS

Four main formats are used to compose a business letter. The formats vary slightly in the position of certain elements of the letter (Table 7.4). The line spacing between the elements remains the same. It is important for a medical assistant to be able to compose a professional letter.

Full Block Letter Format

The full block format is the most common type of business letter (Figure 7.2A; Procedure 7.1). All elements are left justified. This means the elements start at the left margin of the document. Typically, for business letters, closed punctuation is used. *Closed punctuation* means the document is typed using the punctuation marks described earlier in this chapter. Closed punctuation gives the letter a professional appearance.

Informal full block–formatted letters can use open punctuation. *Open punctuation* means that minimal punctuation is used in the letter. The body is the only part of the letter that contains normal grammatical punctuation. No punctuation appears in the sender's or inside addresses, date, salutation, and closing. This is a current trend with electronic technology and letters produced by word processing. Open punctuation should not be used with professional letters.

TABLE 7.4 Business Letter Formats

LETTER TYPE	FORMAT WITH VARIATIONS
Full block format	• Left justify all elements
Modified block format	• Center point (most common) or right justify (rarely used) date, closing, and signature block • Left justify all other elements
Semiblock format (or modified block with indented paragraphs)	• Center point (most common) or right justify (rarely used) date, closing, and signature block • Left justify all other elements • Indent all paragraphs five spaces
Simplified letter format	• No salutation or closing • Signature comes right after the body, followed by the sender's name in all capital letters • Left justify all elements

Modified Block Letter Format

The body and the inside address are left justified with the modified block format. If letterhead is not used, the sender's address is also left justified. The date, closing, and signature block either start at the center point of the line (most common) or are right justified (rarely used) (Procedure 7.2). If the center point is used, all three elements must start at that point (see Figure 7.2B). The text flows toward the right margin. The three elements vertically line up in the document. When you use the right-justified technique, the text for these three elements finishes in a vertical line at the right margin.

Semiblock Letter Format

The semi-block letter format can also be called the modified block with indented paragraphs (see Figure 7.2C). The semi-block format resembles the modified block format with the three elements (i.e., date, closing, and signature block) starting at the center point of the line (most common) or right justified (rarely used). The difference with the semi-block format is the indented paragraph, or paragraphs, in the body of the letter. The paragraphs should be indented five spaces (Procedure 7.3).

WALDEN-MARTIN
FAMILY MEDICAL CLINIC
1234 ANYSTREET | ANYTOWN, ANYSTATE 12345
PHONE 123-123-1234 | FAX 123-123-5678

May 23, 20XX

Ms. Celia Tapia
12 Highland CT
Anytown AL 12345-1234

Dear Ms. Tapia:

You were seen on May 22, 20XX, and had a hepatitis B titer done. Your titer showed that you are immune to hepatitis B.

If you have any questions, please do not hesitate to call our office at (123) 123-1234.

Sincerely,

James A. Martin, M.D.

JAM/cz
c. Joan Smith, M.D.

FIGURE 7.2 **(A)** Full block letter format.

WALDEN-MARTIN
FAMILY MEDICAL CLINIC
1234 ANYSTREET | ANYTOWN, ANYSTATE 12345
PHONE 123-123-1234 | FAX 123-123-5678

May 23, 20XX

Ms. Celia Tapia
12 Highland CT
Anytown AL 12345-1234

Dear Ms. Tapia:

You were seen on May 22, 20XX, and had a hepatitis B titer done. Your titer showed that you are immune to hepatitis B.

If you have any questions, please do not hesitate to call our office at (123) 123-1234.

Sincerely,

James A. Martin, M.D.

JAM/cz
c. Joan Smith, M.D.

WALDEN-MARTIN
FAMILY MEDICAL CLINIC
1234 ANYSTREET | ANYTOWN, ANYSTATE 12345
PHONE 123-123-1234 | FAX 123-123-5678

May 23, 20XX

Ms. Celia Tapia
12 Highland CT
Anytown AL 12345-1234

Dear Ms. Tapia:

You were seen on May 22, 20XX, and had a hepatitis B titer done. Your titer showed that you are immune to hepatitis B.

If you have any questions, please do not hesitate to call our office at (123) 123-1234.

Sincerely,

James A. Martin, M.D.

JAM/cz
c. Joan Smith, M.D.

FIGURE 7.2 cont'd **(B)** Modified block letter format with the three elements starting at the center point of the line. **(C)** Semiblock letter format with the three elements starting at the center point of the line.

WALDEN-MARTIN
FAMILY MEDICAL CLINIC
1234 ANYSTREET | ANYTOWN, ANYSTATE 12345
PHONE 123-123-1234 | FAX 123-123-5678

May 23, 20XX

ABC Medical Suppliers
545 Supply Ave
Anytown AL 12345-1234

Reference: PO #45938

The packing slip for this order indicated that two cases of nonsterile gauze sponges 4"x4", 10 packs (item #1583) were included in the box, but they were not. The box did contain two cases of sterile gauze sponges, though they were not ordered.

Please let me know how you would like to handle this situation. I can be reached at (123) 123-1234.

Thank you.

CHRISTIANA ZWELLEN, CMA

FIGURE 7.2 cont'd **(D)** Simplified letter with a reference line.

Simplified Letter Format

The simplified letter format is not used as often in healthcare. This format does not use a salutation and closing (see Figure 7.2D). The signature comes immediately after the body of the letter. The sender's name is keyed in capital letters. With this letter format, the elements are left justified except for the sender's information in the header. The line spacing is the same as in the other formats.

MEMORANDUMS

Memorandums, or memos, are communication documents shared within a healthcare facility. They address one topic and provide a message to the reader.

Memorandums use the **portrait orientation** for the document, single line spacing, and 1-inch margins.

Headings

Memorandums typically have four headings:

TO: Include the name of the recipient or recipients and omit the titles (e.g., Mr., Mrs.). When there are multiple recipients, each name can be followed by a comma, or each name can be on its own line.

FROM: Include the name of the sender of the memo. It is optional if the sender initials the memo before it is sent.

DATE: Spell out the month and follow it with the day and year (e.g., May 23, 20XX).

SUBJECT: Include the topic of the memo.

The headings are left justified with a blank line between each header (Figure 7.3). Boldface and capital letters are used for the headings, and a colon (:) follows the heading. The information should be in regular font, with a mix of capital and lowercase letters (Procedure 7.4). The information should be aligned vertically down the page, using the tab tool in the word processing software. The date should be written out as indicated for professional letters.

Body

The headings may be separated from the body of the memo by a centered black line. The line should extend from 2 inches to the entire width of the page. Whether or not the line is used, there should be two or three blank lines separating the headers from the body of the memo. The body of the memo should be single spaced and left justified. If it consists of multiple paragraphs, skip a single line between paragraphs. The content in the body of the letter should be clear, concise, and informative. The writer does not need to add a closing or signature. Special notations, including references, copies, and enclosures, can be added to the bottom of the memo. They should be formatted as indicated in the End Notations section.

TO:	Staff
FROM:	James Martin, M.D.
DATE:	December 15, 20XX
SUBJECT:	Holiday Office Hours

The office will be closed at noon on December 24, 20XX, through December 26. We will reopen at our normal time on December 27, 20XX. We will then close at 3 p.m. on December 31 for the holiday and will reopen at our normal time on January 2, 20XX.

FIGURE 7.3 Format for a memorandum.

PROFESSIONAL EMAILS

The use of electronic communication among ambulatory care center staff and with patients is increasing. Medical assistants need to know how to compose a professional email (Procedure 7.5). When emailing patients, copies of email communications should be uploaded to the patient's **electronic health record (EHR)** or added to the paper health record for a permanent record of the electronic communication.

Email Etiquette

Following email etiquette is important for maintaining a customer-friendly environment. Tips on writing customer-friendly emails include the following:

- When sending the email to several people, separate each email address by a semicolon (;).
- Add an email address to the cc line if another person needs to receive a courtesy copy of the email.
- If a copy of the email needs to be sent to another person without the recipient knowing, add the address to the bc line. Blind copying is used on a selected and limited basis.
- Make sure to include a subject on the subject line. Delete any messy FWD: or RE: RE: strings.
- Start with a greeting (salutation). It should include a formal greeting followed by the person's title and name (e.g., "Good morning, Mr. Jones," "Dear Mr. Jones,").
- Be courteous, polite, and respectful in your words and tone. Maintain the appropriate level of formality in the email. Be gracious by using expressions such as "please" and "thank you."
- Refrain from using all capital letters. Many people consider all capital letters to be shouting in emails.
- Write out the entire word, and refrain from using abbreviations and emoticons (emojis).
- Use proper capitalization, grammar, sentence structure, and punctuation. Check the spelling in the email before sending it. Most email software has a spell-checker.
- Be concise, accurate, and clear in your message.
- Always end your email with "Thank you," "Regards," "Kind regards," "Best," or "Sincerely," and your complete name. For business emails, include contact information after your name. The contact information should include the healthcare facility's address, phone number, and fax number.
- Leave white space (i.e., one blank line) between the salutation, paragraphs, and your complete name.
- Zip large attachments before sending the files. Zip is a computer program that compresses a file or folder, making it smaller and easier to send. The receiver uses an unzip program to extract the contents.
- Many email programs have features such as (!) urgent or a response box that sends an email back to the sender when the recipient has opened the email. Use the urgent feature only for crucial emails.
- Forward messages with caution. When forwarding messages, always read the content and ensure no confidentiality will be breached.

CRITICAL THINKING APPLICATION 7.4

Christiana receives an email from a patient that is in all capital letters. How might she perceive the situation with the patient? How could she verify her perceptions? How should she handle this situation?

Confidentiality and Emails

Some healthcare facilities may also include language in emails related about confidentiality and whom to contact if the email was sent to the wrong address. Medical assistants must adhere to the facility's confidentiality rules when communicating with or about patients.

EHR software frequently contains clinical messaging or clinical email features. This feature allows for making emails within the EHR. The clinical messaging feature provides secure communication for healthcare employees to converse about the patient. For instance, the message may be sent from the receptionist to the medical assistant regarding a patient who called requesting a refill. The medical assistant can then follow up with the provider regarding the refill.

CRITICAL THINKING APPLICATION 7.5

Christiana answers emails from patients. How might her responses differ from her personal emails to her family and friends?

Using Templates

A **template** is a sample letter or email that can be personalized for each patient. Many word processing and **practice management software** programs have prebuilt letter templates. These templates can be used, or a medical assistant can design a template. For routine communication with patients (e.g., normal laboratory results or appointment reminders), a template can be used to save time composing the entire letter or email each time.

Some templates allow the user to merge patient data to customize such things as the address, date of the visit, provider's name, and so on. Practice management software, EHR, or word processing software can be used to merge the patient's data into the letter template. This creates an individualized letter and is an efficient method of providing a customer-friendly document for a patient.

Faxed Communication

Fax (short for facsimile) machines send and receive documents using phone lines. In the healthcare facility, the fax machine may be a stand-alone unit, or it may be part of a copy machine. Many computers may have software that allows faxes to be sent and received.

Prior to the use of electronic health records, patient-related documents were faxed to and from the ambulatory care facility. As communications technology has advanced, the use of fax machines has decreased, but they are still an important piece of equipment in the ambulatory care center.

Confidentiality and Faxing Patient Documents

When sending a fax, the medical assistant must adhere to rules established by the Health Insurance Portability and Accountability Act (HIPAA) and the Health Information Technology for Economic and Clinical Health Act (HITECH). Healthcare facilities usually have a required cover sheet (the first sheet) that includes confidentiality language, which instructs the recipient, if they are not the intended party, to contact the sender (Figure 7.4). The sender usually discusses how to destroy the records to maintain confidentiality.

It is also recommended that patient records be sent to a secure, little-used fax machine. Faxes should be removed from the fax machine as soon as possible to maintain confidentiality.

Preparing a Fax Cover Sheet

Some ambulatory care facilities have their own customized cover sheets for faxing. The facility's information and the confidentiality statement are included. If a medical assistant is not using a customized cover sheet, templates of fax cover sheets are available online or with the practice management or word processing software. The

WALDEN-MARTIN
FAMILY MEDICAL CLINIC
1234 ANYSTREET | ANYTOWN, ANYSTATE 12345
PHONE 123-123-1234 | FAX 123-123-5678

Fax

To:	From:
Company:	Phone:
Fax:	Date:
Phone:	
Pages:	
Re:	

CONFIDENTIALITY NOTICE

The material enclosed with this facsimile transmission is confidential and private. The material is the property of the sender, and some or all of the information may be protected by the Health Insurance Portability & Accountability Act (HIPAA). This information is intended exclusively for the addressed person or agency indicated above. If you are not the intended individual or entity of this information, you are notified that any use, duplication, circulation, or transmission of the information is strictly prohibited under state and federal law. Please notify the sender immediately using the telephone number indicated above.

FIGURE 7.4 A HIPAA compliant fax cover sheet.

medical assistant should add the facility's information and the confidentiality statement approved by the facility to the template.

Fax cover sheets typically include the following areas for the medical assistant to complete:

- Sender's name and phone number
- Receiver's name, company, fax number, and phone number
- Number of pages, including the cover sheet
- Date and subject
- Comments

The medical assistant should proofread the fax cover sheet and verify the receiver's information (Procedure 7.6). The fax cover sheet should be the first page faxed.

PREPARING MAIL

Business letters should be enclosed in standard #10 business-sized envelopes. Standard #10 envelopes measure 4.125 × 9.5 inches. Business envelopes are available with a few variations, including the type of flap, preprinted return address, and presence or absence of a window. The window envelope and the # 6¾ envelope, which measures 3⅝ × 6½ inches, may be used for billing statements to patients. The envelopes can be white, manila, or made of recycled paper.

Addressing Envelopes

When the automated mail processing machine at the post office reads the envelope, it reads the bottom line of the recipient's address (i.e., city, state, and zip code) before moving up and reading the next line. To ensure timely delivery, use the following tips when addressing mail:

- Key (type) the envelope using a simple black font of at least 10 points in size. Use all uppercase (capital) letters and no punctuation marks (Figure 7.5).
- The address should be left justified.
- If you cannot fit the suite or apartment number on the same line as the delivery address, put it on the line above the delivery address, not below it.
- Do not write out directional and street words; instead, use the US Postal Service approved abbreviations (see Table 7.3).
- If using the # sign, have a space between # and the number (e.g., # 23).
- Put one space between the city and state and two spaces between the state and zip code.
- Use the four-code and the zip code (e.g., 55555-1111) as often as possible. This allows the piece of mail to be directed to a more precise location than when just using the zip code.
- Do not put anything (e.g., logo, slogan, attention line) below the last line of the delivery address. The machine will read it, and your letter may be misrouted or delayed. If an attention line is used, it should be at the top of the address.
- For international addresses, key (type) the name of the country in capital letters on the last line.
- Use only approved US Postal Service abbreviations.

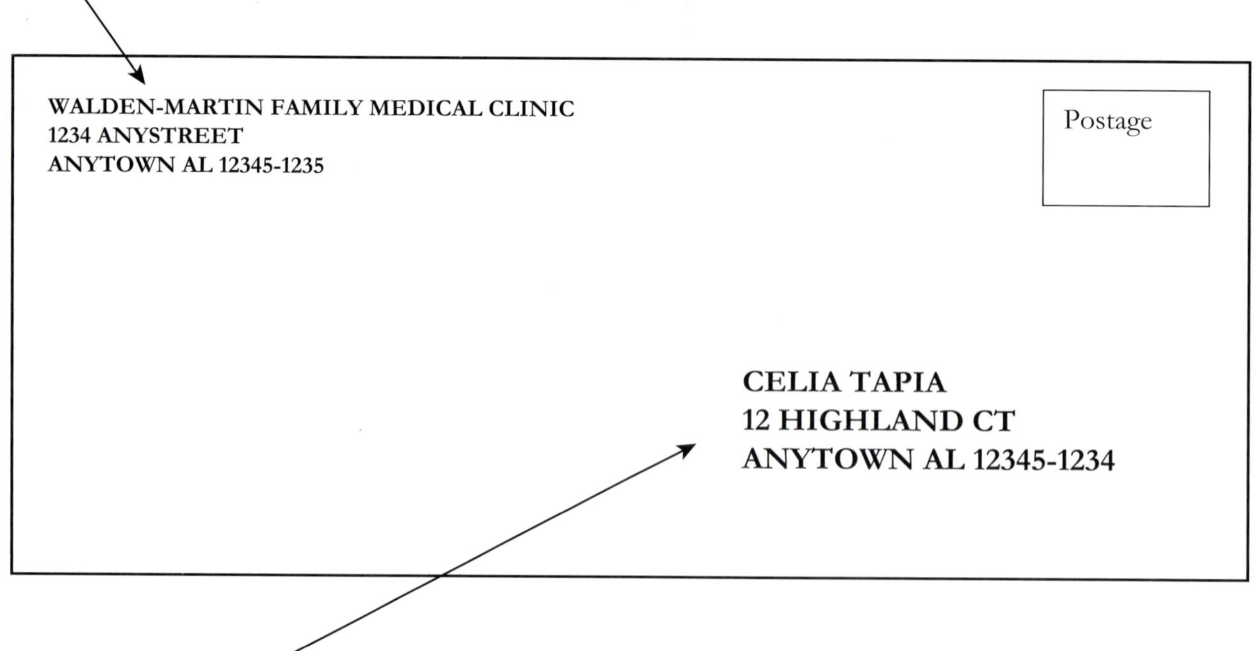

FIGURE 7.5 Address format for an envelope.

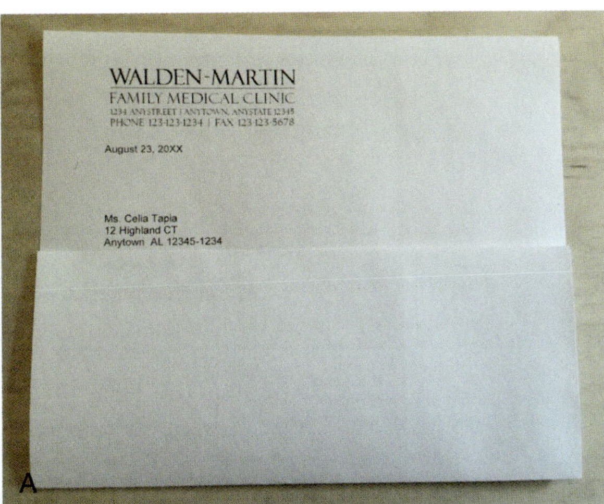

FIGURE 7.6 **(A)** For a #10 envelope, fold the bottom to just below the inside address, and crease at the fold. **(B)** Fold the top edge down to meet the bottom edge, and crease at the fold.

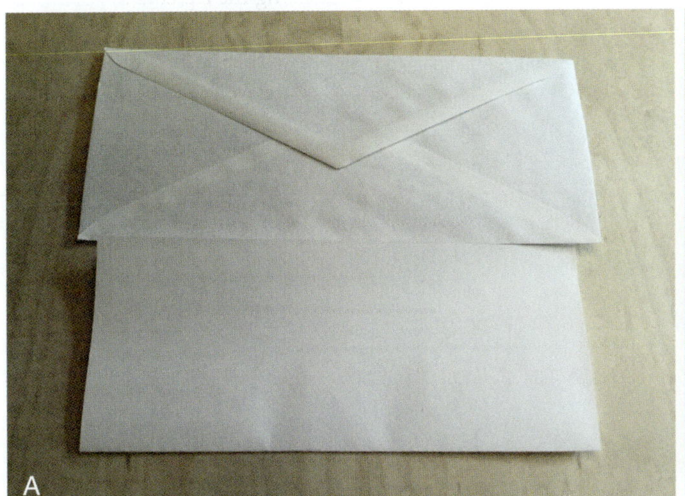

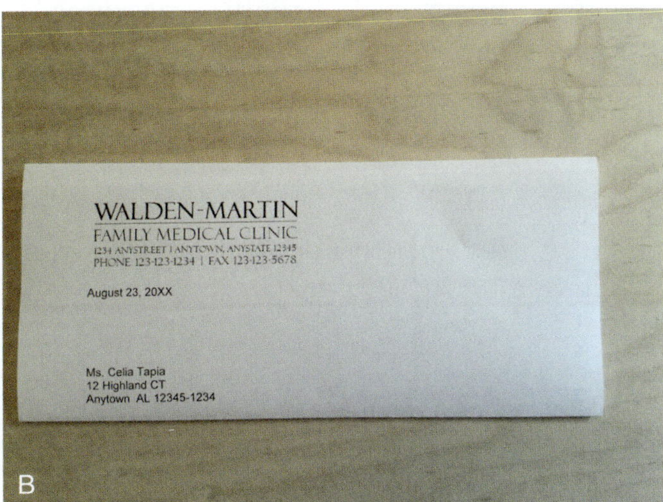

FIGURE 7.7 **(A)** For a window envelope, with the print side facing up, place the envelope over or under the top third of the letter. Fold the bottom edge up to meet the bottom edge of the envelope. Crease at the fold. **(B)** With the letter print facing down, fold the top down to the first crease line. Crease at the fold. When the letter is folded, the inside address is visible.

- If using a window envelope, the address should start and end at least one-eighth of an inch from the edge of the window.

Folding Documents

Learning Objective: Discuss how to fold documents for various types of envelopes.

Depending on the envelope size, the folding process may be different. It is important to fold the document neatly, as this is something the reader will see.

When using a #10 envelope, fold the letter by pulling up the bottom end until it reaches just below the inside address or two-thirds of the way up the letter (Figure 7.6). Crease at the fold. Then fold the top of the letter down, so it is flush with the bottom fold, and crease the paper. For window business envelopes, fold the letter in a Z pattern. With the letter's print side facing up, place the envelope over or under the top third of the letter (Figure 7.7). Fold the bottom edge of the paper up to the bottom edge of the envelope, and crease at the fold. Then remove the envelope and flip the letter over so the backside of the document is facing up. Fold the top of the letter down to the prior crease line, and crease at the fold. The letterhead and recipient's addresses should then be visible. Place the letter in the envelope so that the recipient's address shows through the window.

For a #6½ envelope, fold the letter by pulling up the bottom end until it is one-half inch from the top edge of the document (Figure 7.8). Crease at the fold. Then fold the document vertically, starting at the right edge. Bring the right edge two-thirds of the way across the width of the document and crease the paper. Then bring the left edge to the right edge, and crease at the fold. Flip the document so the left edge is on the bottom, and insert it into the envelope.

OUTGOING AND INCOMING MAIL

Medical assistants who are responsible for outgoing mail need to know the type of postage to use for mailing letters and other items. Many larger cities have delivery services that can work with healthcare facilities. When mail is delivered to the facility, the medical

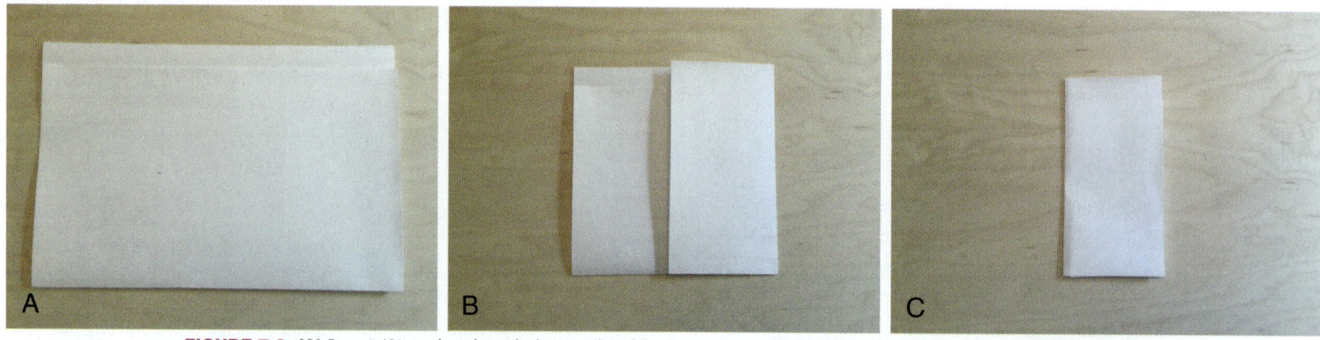

FIGURE 7.8 **(A)** For a # 6¾ envelope, bring the bottom edge of the document to one-half inch from the top edge. Crease at the fold. **(B)** Fold the document vertically. Bring the right edge two-thirds of the way across the width of the document and crease the paper. **(C)** Bring the left edge to the right edge, and crease at the fold.

TABLE 7.5 US Postal Service Domestic Shipping Sizes

DOMESTIC SHIPPING	HEIGHT (INCHES)	LENGTH (INCHES)	MAXIMUM THICKNESS (INCHES)
Postcard	3.5–4.25	5–6	0.016
Letter	3.5–6.125 (6⅛)	5–11.5	0.25
Large envelopes	6.125–12	11.5–15	0.75
Packages	Maximum length plus **girth**: 108 inches (130 inches for standard post)		

TABLE 7.6 Summary of the US Postal Service's Domestic Services

TYPE	DESCRIPTION
Priority mail express	Very expensive; 7-days-a-week delivery service with guaranteed overnight scheduled delivery. Insurance is included. For letters and packages up to 70 lb. Cost based on weight and delivery zone. Flat rate envelopes available.
Priority mail	Expensive; delivery within 3 days. Tracking and insurance are included. Cost based on weight and delivery zone. Flat rate fee for envelopes and boxes up to 70 lb.
First-class mail	Most commonly used service. Provides delivery in 3 days or fewer. For envelopes and packages weighing up to 13 oz. Cost based on size, shape, and weight. Add-on services are available for an extra fee.
USPS retail ground	Delivery in 2–8 days. Used for oversized packages weighing up to 70 lb. and measuring up to 130 inches in combined girth and length. Cost based on weight, shape, and delivery zone.
Media mail	Use for sending books, electronic **media**, and educational material, with delivery in 2–8 days. Cost based on weight.

assistant needs to know how to process the mail. These topics are explained in the following sections.

Postage

After addressing the envelope, you must add postage prior to mailing the letter. The postage depends on the weight, size, urgency for arrival, delivery **zone,** and services required (Table 7.5). For the ambulatory care facility, there are several postage options for mailings:

- *Print postage labels on the US Postal Service (USPS) website (*www.USPS.com*):* Priority Mail Express and Priority Mail shipping labels can be printed on the facility's printer.
- *Permit imprints:* Used for bulk mailing (200 or more envelopes); requires a fee and permit. Print postage information on the envelope and pay for postage when the mailing is sent.
- *Precanceled stamps:* Complete permit, place precanceled stamps on the envelopes, and mail. Cannot return unused stamps.
- *Postage meter printing:* Lease a postage meter, pay the fee, and print postage directly on the mail or on a meter tape.

The USPS website (www.usps.com) provides valuable resources for addressing and shipping mail. It allows you to buy stamps, schedule a pickup, calculate the shipping costs, look up zip codes, and track sent mail.

The medical assistant will use different types of mail services for the healthcare facility's business. It is crucial to understand the different services. For routine mail, the healthcare facility will use First-Class Mail. Table 7.6 summarizes the USPS domestic services available.

The USPS also has a host of optional services that can be added to the standard services for an additional fee. Table 7.7 summarizes additional services available. It is important to note that healthcare facilities use certified mail and return receipts. When using certified mail combined with a return receipt, the facility gets a mailing receipt showing the date when the item was mailed. It also gets additional information on when the delivery occurred and the recipient's signature. Many state laws mandate that **termination letters** be sent by certified mail with a return receipt (Figure 7.9A). The mailing receipt, return receipt, and copy of the letter are uploaded into the EHR or filed in the paper medical record (Figure 7.9B). These items provide proof that the law was followed if there is ever a question. For a complete list of services, refer to the USPS website.

TABLE 7.7 Optional Services Provided by the US Postal Service

OPTIONAL SERVICE	DESCRIPTION
Standard insurance	Protects against loss or damage. Cost is based on the item's declared value.
Registered mail	Used to protect expensive items. Mailed item can be insured up to the maximum amount. A mailing receipt is given; upon request, an electronic verification of delivery or delivery attempt can be sent.
Certified mail	Mailing receipt provides evidence the letter was mailed and, combined with the return receipt, shows delivery information and the recipient's signature.
Signature confirmation	Provides date and time of delivery or when delivery attempt was made, along with the recipient's signature. Copy of delivery record is available upon request.
Return receipt	Provides an automatic electronic or mailed delivery record showing the recipient's signature.
Adult signature restricted delivery	Addressee or **authorized agent** must verify identity and age (i.e., must be over 21); must sign for delivery.
Restricted delivery	Addressee or authorized agent must verify identity and must sign for delivery.
Certificate of mailing	Provides evidence (i.e., date and time) when an item was mailed. (Limited service because it does not provide evidence of the delivery.)
USPS tracking	Provides updates as an item is being shipped. Will include date and time of delivery or attempted delivery.
Special handling	Used to get preferential handling when shipping very unusual items or items that need extra care.
Collect on delivery (COD)	Recipient pays for merchandise and shipping when the package is received.
Hold for pickup	Option to pick up item from a specified post office within 15 days, depending on service selected.

Private Delivery Services

The USPS only handles a portion of the mail delivered in the United States. Private companies have grown by offering competitive rates and additional services compared with USPS. Some companies provide national and international services, but others are more locally based. FedEx, UPS, and DHL are very popular national options for shipping letters and packages. Some offer onsite pickups.

Larger cities have courier services that have become popular options for local deliveries. Some companies have drivers who are **bonded** and trained to handle all aspects of delivery, from medical to hazardous deliveries. These couriers provide some of the following services:

- Pickup and delivery of medical specimens (e.g., they take patient laboratory samples to a medical laboratory for testing)
- Transportation of health records and documents from one location to another, complying with HIPAA requirements
- Pickup and delivery of deposits to the bank, with a return of cash if requested

The goal for the healthcare facility is to use a mail/courier company that provides the most efficient service at the best price. The medical assistant may have to research the delivery services available in the area to identify the best fit for the facility.

CRITICAL THINKING APPLICATION 7.6

The providers at WMFM would like to use an offsite laboratory to process specimens. Christiana would like to have a local courier service pick up specimens and deliver them to the offsite laboratory. When researching potential delivery couriers for this activity, what factors should Christiana consider?

Incoming Mail

The medical assistant's responsibility with incoming mail will vary. In large facilities, designated mailroom employees handle incoming mail, and the mail is delivered to each department. The administrative medical assistant sorts the department mail. In smaller facilities, the medical assistant handles all aspects of the incoming mail.

Mail can be collected at the post office or delivered to the healthcare facility. The medical assistant must sort the mail following the facility's procedure for incoming mail. Providers may request that incoming mail be placed on their desks. In larger departments, mailboxes are used for each person in the department. The medical assistant can easily sort the mail and place it in the individual mailboxes. The mailboxes need to be safe and secure. They should not be in a patient care area.

If there is a question as to who should get a piece of mail, it is important to ask. If there is a question about opening something, it is better not to open it and ask the provider or office manager. If mail is opened accidentally, which should not have been, the medical assistant should tape the envelope shut. A note should be included with the envelope to indicate that it was accidentally opened. The note should include the name of the person who opened it and the date. The facility will have a procedure for handling the mail while the provider is on vacation.

CRITICAL THINKING APPLICATION 7.7

Christiana sorts the mail for WMFM Clinic. Because the facility is small, the staff does not use the mailbox system. Mail has gotten lost after she placed it on the providers' desks. What other options can Christiana implement to prevent mail from getting lost or misplaced on the providers' desks?

CLOSING COMMENTS

Legal and Ethical Issues

When sending letters and emails to patients, the medical assistant must ensure that a copy is added to the patient's health record. If

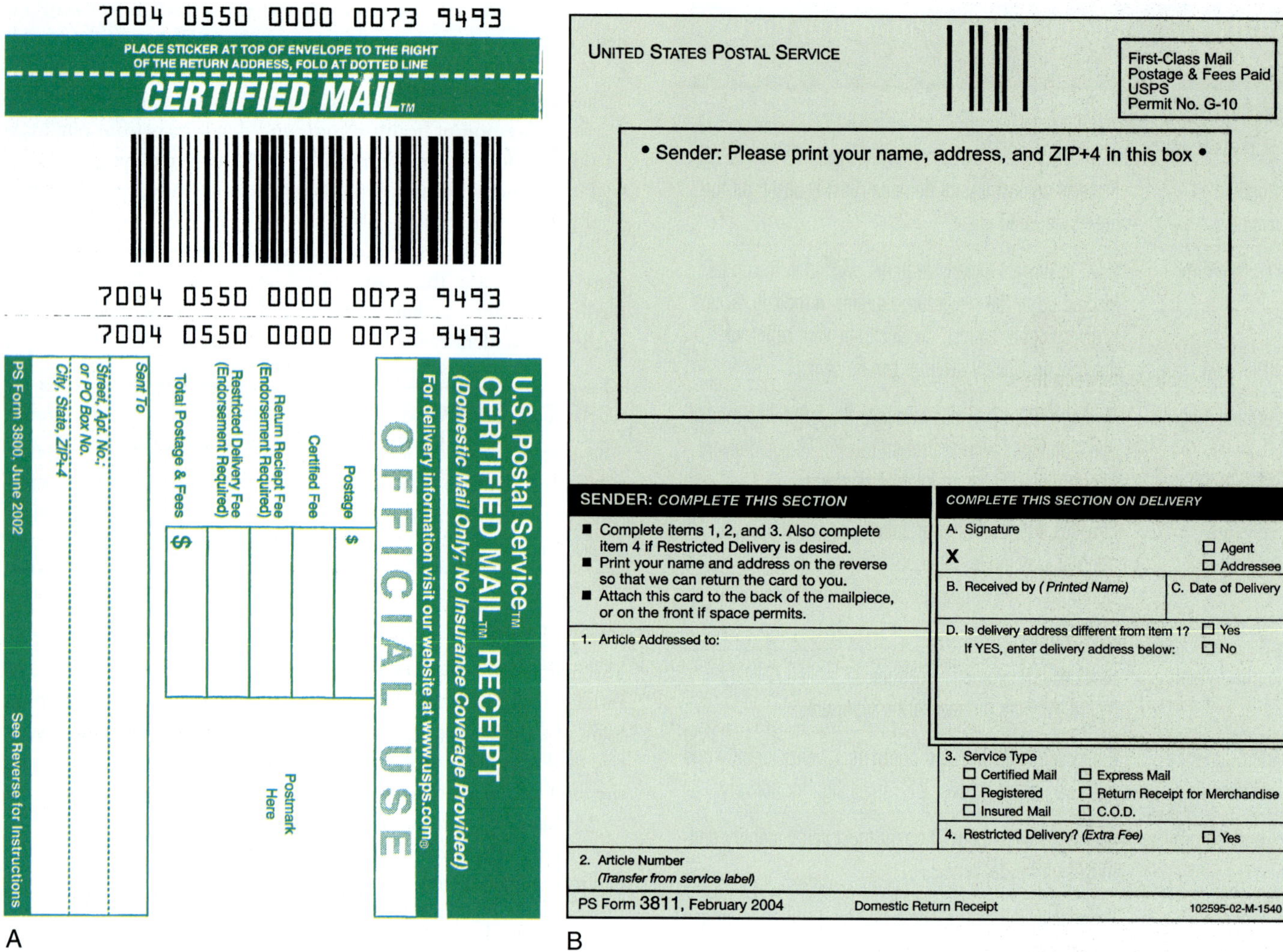
A

7004 0550 0000 0073 9493

PLACE STICKER AT TOP OF ENVELOPE TO THE RIGHT OF THE RETURN ADDRESS, FOLD AT DOTTED LINE

CERTIFIED MAIL™

7004 0550 0000 0073 9493

7004 0550 0000 0073 9493

U.S. Postal Service™
CERTIFIED MAIL™ RECEIPT
(Domestic Mail Only; No Insurance Coverage Provided)

For delivery information visit our website at www.usps.com®

OFFICIAL USE

Postage	$
Certified Fee	
Return Reciept Fee (Endorsement Required)	
Restricted Delivery Fee (Endorsement Required)	
Total Postage & Fees	$

Postmark Here

Sent To

Street, Apt. No.; or PO Box No.

City, State, ZIP+4

PS Form 3800, June 2002 See Reverse for Instructions

B

UNITED STATES POSTAL SERVICE

First-Class Mail
Postage & Fees Paid
USPS
Permit No. G-10

• Sender: Please print your name, address, and ZIP+4 in this box •

SENDER: COMPLETE THIS SECTION

- Complete items 1, 2, and 3. Also complete item 4 if Restricted Delivery is desired.
- Print your name and address on the reverse so that we can return the card to you.
- Attach this card to the back of the mailpiece, or on the front if space permits.

1. Article Addressed to:

COMPLETE THIS SECTION ON DELIVERY

A. Signature
X ☐ Agent ☐ Addressee

B. Received by (Printed Name) C. Date of Delivery

D. Is delivery address different from item 1? ☐ Yes
If YES, enter delivery address below: ☐ No

3. Service Type
☐ Certified Mail ☐ Express Mail
☐ Registered ☐ Return Receipt for Merchandise
☐ Insured Mail ☐ C.O.D.

4. Restricted Delivery? (Extra Fee) ☐ Yes

2. Article Number
(Transfer from service label)

PS Form 3811, February 2004 Domestic Return Receipt 102595-02-M-1540

FIGURE 7.9 **(A)** Receipt for certified mail. Attach the bottom portion of the receipt to the top of the package or envelope, just to the right of the return address. **(B)** Return receipt used to provide an automatic electronic or hardcopy record showing the recipient's signature.

a copy is not added to the record, then it appears that the patient was never sent the letter or email. Legally this can be a major issue for the healthcare facility. Having a paper trail of communication to the patient helps provide evidence that the staff notified the patient about test results and updates in the patient care plan.

Patient-Centered Care

When patients have a diagnostic test, it is important to let the patient know prior to the test when they will be given the results. It is also helpful to patients to let them know if the communication will be via a phone call, an email, or a letter. When a patient may receive a potentially life-changing diagnosis, waiting for the news is stressful. The medical assistant should help to ensure that test results are given to the patient as soon as possible and in the manner they were told they would be (e.g., via an email or a call).

Professional Behaviors

When communicating by email, it is important for medical assistants to watch their tone. Sharp phrases or capitalizing complete words can give the reader a sense that the sender is yelling. Keep these considerations in mind when composing an email:

- Always maintain a professional tone throughout the letter or email, even if the patient did not do so when communicating with the office originally.
- Have another staff member read an email if the medical assistant is concerned that the message may be perceived in a manner other than what is intended.
- Never send an email response when not in the office or when angry. Wait until strong emotions have calmed down before sending an email. Often it is hard to be professional when one is emotional.

SUMMARY OF SCENARIO

Since her promotion, Christiana has learned many helpful administrative procedures. She has also been implementing changes in the administrative area. Her first change was to email, rather than mail, appointment reminders. She uses the appointment reminder feature of the practice management software when emailing the notifications to patients. Not only does this save time, but it also saves postage costs.

Christiana has also learned how to create letter and memo templates. She uses templates to notify patients about laboratory and diagnostic test results. She continues to create custom letters for patients, yet she saves time by using predesigned templates. Christiana enjoys her new position, and she understands that learning is an ongoing process that will help her become the professional she strives to be.

SUMMARY OF LEARNING OBJECTIVES

1. **Differentiate between the parts of speech.**
   This chapter reviewed the parts of speech, including a noun, verb, subject, adjective, adverb, and so on. A noun is a word or phrase for a person, place, thing, or idea. A common noun names a general group of people, places, things, and ideas, and a proper noun names a specific person, place, or thing. A verb is a word or a phrase that shows action or a state of being. It is important to write using complete sentences and not fragments.
2. **Examine common communication errors, including misused words and inconsistencies with nouns and pronouns.**
   The medical assistant should know the proper use of commonly confused words and misused phrases. Homonyms may not be identified by the software's spell-checker, which can lead to mistakes. A common mistake in communication is a mismatch between the noun and pronoun number. Plural pronouns include we, us, you, they, and them. Singular pronouns include I, me, you, she, her, he, him, and it. "They" has become a singular third-person pronoun, and if used as a subject, the verb is always plural.
3. **Differentiate between the types and uses of punctuation.**
   Use a period for a sentence that makes a statement. Use a question mark after a direct question. Use an exclamation point for sentences that express strong emotion. There are many rules regarding the use of commas, including using them to separate items in a list of three or more and adding commas between the day and the year. The semicolon is used before certain words, and it is also used when separating phrases in a series or linking two complete sentences. A colon (:) is used to introduce a series of items either in the sentence or bulleted list, and it is also used after the salutation in a professional letter. Quotation marks (" ") are used to set off direct quotes. An apostrophe (') is used to show ownership.
4. **Examine the use of capitalizations and numbers in professional communication.**
   The first letter of the first word in a sentence or question should be capitalized. The pronoun "I" is always capitalized. The first letter of proper nouns should be capitalized. Spell out all numbers at the beginning of a sentence. Hyphenate all compound numbers from 21 to 99 (e.g., twenty-three) and all written-out fractions.
5. **Demonstrate how to compose a professional letter.**
   The following are components of the professional business letter:
   - *Sender's address*: Is usually in the letterhead of the document.
   - *Date*: Needs to be written out using the month, day, and year format.
   - *Inside address*: Includes the recipient's name, title, and address.
   - *Reference line*: Used occasionally to refer to a specific item (e.g., case number).
   - *Salutation*: The greeting needs to be formal for business letters.
   - *Subject line*: Used occasionally to state the main subject of the letter.
   - *Body of the letter*: Contains the message.
   - *Closing*: Usually, "sincerely" is used.
   - *Signature block*: Provides information on the sender, including the signature, typed name, and title.
   - *End notations* include the following elements:
   - *Reference notation*: The initials of the sender are followed by the initials of the person who keyed the letter. A colon or forward slash separates the initials.
   - *Enclosure/attachment notation*: Indicates the number of the documents or attachments that accompany the letter.
   - *Copy notation*: Indicates who received a copy of the letter.
   - *Blind copy*: Indicates who received a blind copy of the letter; only shows on the office copy of the letter.
6. **Differentiate between the various business letter formats.**
   - *Full block format*: Left justify all elements (Procedure 7.1).
   - *Modified block format*: Center point or right justify (rare) the date, closing, and signature block; left justify all other elements (Procedure 7.2).
   - *Semi-block format*: Center point or right justify (rare) the date, closing, and signature block; left justify all other elements; and indent all paragraphs 5 spaces (Procedure 7.3).
   - *Simplified format*: Does not use the salutation and closing. The sender's name is in all capital letters.
7. **Demonstrate how to compose a memorandum.**
   Memorandums, or memos, are communication documents shared within a healthcare facility. A memo includes the following headers: "TO," "FROM," "DATE," and "SUBJECT." The body is below the header.
8. **Demonstrate how to compose a professional email.**
   Tips on writing customer-friendly emails include the following:
   - Make sure to include a subject on the subject line.
   - Start with a greeting (salutation).
   - Be courteous, polite, and respectful in your words and tone. Maintain the appropriate level of formality in the email. Be gracious, using expressions such as "please" and "thank you."
   - Refrain from using all capital letters.
   - Write out the entire word, and refrain from using abbreviations and emoticons.

Continued

SUMMARY OF LEARNING OBJECTIVES—*continued*

- Use proper capitalization, grammar, sentence structure, and punctuation. Check the spelling in the email before sending it. Most email software has a spell-checker.
- Be concise, accurate, and clear in your message.
- Always end your email with "Thank you" or "Sincerely" and your complete name.
- Leave white space (i.e., one blank line) between the salutation, paragraphs, and your complete name.
- Zip large attachments before sending the files.
- Use the urgent feature only for crucial emails.
- Forward messages with caution.

A template is a sample letter or email that can be personalized for each patient. For routine communication with patients, a template can be used to save time composing the entire letter or email each and every time.

9. **Examine how to fax documents while maintaining a patient's confidentiality.**
When sending a fax, the medical assistant must adhere to HIPAA and HITECH rules. Healthcare facilities usually have a required cover sheet (the first sheet) that includes confidentiality language, which instructs the recipient, if he or she is not the intended party, to contact the sender. See Procedure 7.6 for details on completing a HIPAA compliant fax cover sheet.

10. **Demonstrate how to address an envelope and fold documents to place in envelopes.**
When addressing an envelope, type the address using a simple black font of at least 10 points in size. Always put one space between the city and state and two spaces between the space and zip code. Use only US Postal Service abbreviations. Procedures 7.1 through 7.3 discuss how to fold a document when using a #10 envelope. Procedure 7.2 discusses how to fold a letter when using a window envelope. Procedure 7.3 discusses how to fold a letter when using a #6{3/4 } envelope.

11. **Examine how to handle outgoing mail, including postage and delivery services and incoming mail to the ambulatory care facility.**
The medical assistant will use different types of mail services for the healthcare facility's business. For routine mail, the healthcare facility will use First-Class Mail. Table 7.7 summarizes USPS domestic services available. The medical assistant's responsibility with incoming mail will vary. In large facilities, designated mailroom employees handle incoming mail, and the mail is delivered to each department. The administrative medical assistant sorts the department mail. In smaller facilities, the medical assistant handles all aspects of the incoming mail.

PROCEDURE 7.1 Compose a Professional Business Letter Using the Full Block Letter Format

TASKS: Compose a professional letter using technology. Use the full block letter format and closed punctuation. Address the envelope and fold the letter.

SCENARIO: Jean Burke, NP (nurse practitioner), has requested that you compose a letter to the parent (Lisa Parker) of Johnny Parker (date of birth [DOB]: 06/15/20XX) to let her know that Johnny's throat culture from last Wednesday was negative. If he is not improving or if she has any questions, she should call the office. Lisa Parker's address is 91 Poplar Street, Anytown, AL 12345-1234. You are working at Walden-Martin Family Medical Clinic. The healthcare facility's address is 1234 Anystreet, Anytown, AL 12345. The phone number is 123-123-1234, and the fax number is 123-123-5678.

EQUIPMENT and SUPPLIES

- Patient's health record
- Computer with word processing software and printer
- Paper
- #10 envelope

PROCEDURAL STEPS

1. Obtain the intended recipient's contact information and determine the message you want to convey. Using the computer and word processing software, compose the letter using the full block letter format. Use 1-inch margins on all four sides, portrait orientation, and single line spacing throughout the letter. Use an easy-to-read font (e.g., Times New Roman or Calibri) in a 10- or 12-point size.
PURPOSE: Determining the message gives you a focus when composing the letter. You will need the recipient's information to create the letter.
2. Create a letterhead in the header of the document. Include the clinic's name, street address or post office box, city, state, and zip code.
PURPOSE: The information in the letterhead provides the reader with the clinic's contact information.
3. Key (type) the date, starting at the left margin. Have one blank line between the dateline and the last line of the letterhead.
PURPOSE: All letters require a date for legal purposes.
4. Key the inside address starting at the left margin and use the correct spelling and punctuation. Leave one to nine blank lines between the date and the inside address to center the body of the letter on the page.
PURPOSE: The body of the letter must be centered vertically from the top to the bottom of the document. More blank lines can be added to move the body to the correct location.

PROCEDURE 7.1 Compose a Professional Business Letter Using the Full Block Letter Format—*continued*

5. Key the salutation starting at the left margin and use the correct spelling and punctuation. Leave one blank line between the inside address and the salutation.
   PURPOSE: A proper greeting sets the tone of the letter.
6. Use your critical thinking skills to compose a concise, accurate message. Type the message in the body of the letter starting at the left margin. Leave one blank line between the salutation and the first line of the body and then between each paragraph of the body. The message should be clear, concise, and professional. Use proper grammar, punctuation, capitalization, and sentence structure.
   PURPOSE: Proper grammar helps to convey the message accurately and professionally.
7. Key a proper closing starting at the left margin and use correct spelling and punctuation. Leave one blank line between the last line of the body and the closing.
   PURPOSE: The closing helps end the message with a professional tone.
8. Key the signature block starting at the left margin and use the correct spelling and punctuation. Leave four blank lines between the closing and the signature block. If you are preparing the letter for a provider, you must include a reference notation.
   PURPOSE: The signature block provides the reader with the name of the sender of the letter. The reference notation identifies who typed the letter.
9. Spell-check and proofread the document. Check for the proper tone, grammar, punctuation, capitalization, and sentence structure. Check for proper spacing between the parts of the letter. Make any final corrections. Print the document.
   PURPOSE: The spell-checker identifies only certain errors; proofreading helps you find incorrect word use, improper tone, and errors in formatting.
10. Address the envelope using either the computer and word processing software or a pen and following the correct format.
    PURPOSE: Following the Postal Service guidelines on format helps prevent a delay in the delivery of the letter.
11. When using a #10 envelope, fold the letter by pulling up the bottom end until it reaches just below the inside address or two-thirds of the way up the letter. Crease at the fold. Then fold the top of the letter down, so it is flush with the bottom fold, and crease the paper.
    Note: If the provider needs to sign the letter, the letter is folded afterward.
    PURPOSE: The letter must be neatly folded.
12. File a copy of the letter in the paper medical record or upload an electronic copy of the letter to the electronic health record (EHR).
    PURPOSE: A copy of all correspondence should be kept in the patient's health record.

PROCEDURE 7.2 Compose a Professional Business Letter Using the Modified Block Letter Format

TASKS: Compose a professional letter using technology. Use the modified block letter format (with the center point option). Address the envelope (if needed) and fold the letter.

SCENARIO: Julie Walden, MD, has requested that you compose a letter to Carl C. Bowden (DOB: 04/05/19XX) to let him know that his hepatitis C laboratory test was negative. If he has any questions, he should call the office. His address is 19 Beale Street, Anytown, AL 12345-1234. You are working at Walden-Martin Family Medical Clinic. The healthcare facility's address is 1234 Anystreet, Anytown, AL 12345. The phone number is 123-123-1234, and the fax number is 123-123-5678.

EQUIPMENT and SUPPLIES

- Patient's health record
- Computer with word processing software and printer
- Paper
- #10 envelope or window business envelope

PROCEDURAL STEPS

1. Obtain the intended recipient's contact information and determine the message you want to convey. Using the computer and word processing software, compose the letter using the modified block letter format. Use 1-inch margins on all four sides, portrait orientation, and single line spacing throughout the letter. Use an easy-to-read font (e.g., Times New Roman or Calibri) in a 10- or 12-point size.
   PURPOSE: Determining the message gives you a focus when composing the letter. You will need the recipient's information to create the letter.
2. Create a letterhead in the header of the document. Include the clinic's name, street address or post office box, city, state, and zip code.
   PURPOSE: The information in the letterhead provides the reader with the clinic's contact information.
3. Key (type) the date starting at the center point of the line, which is usually about 3.25 inches from the margin. Have one blank line between the dateline and the last line of the letterhead.
   Note: Starting the text at the center point is not the same as the text being centered on the line. When starting the text at the center point, the text flows toward the right margin.
   PURPOSE: All letters require a date for legal purposes.
4. Key the inside address starting at the left margin and use the correct spelling and punctuation. Leave one to nine blank lines between the date and the inside address to center the body of the letter on the page. If using a window business envelope, adjust the address position to fit the window.
   PURPOSE: The body of the letter must be centered vertically from the top to the bottom of the document. More blank lines can be added to move the body to the correct location.

Continued

PROCEDURE 7.2 Compose a Professional Business Letter Using the Modified Block Letter Format—*continued*

5. Key the salutation starting at the left margin and use the correct spelling and punctuation. Leave one blank line between the inside address and the salutation.
   PURPOSE: A proper greeting sets the tone of the letter.
6. Use your critical thinking skills to compose a concise, accurate message. Type the message in the body of the letter starting at the left margin. Leave one blank line between the salutation and the first line of the body and then between each paragraph of the body. The message should be clear, concise, and professional. Use proper grammar, punctuation, capitalization, and sentence structure.
   PURPOSE: Proper grammar helps to convey the message accurately and professionally.
7. Key a proper closing. Start the closing at the center point of the line. (The first letter of the closing should align vertically with the first letter of the date.) Use correct spelling and punctuation. Leave one blank line between the last line of the body and the closing.
   PURPOSE: The closing helps end the message with a professional tone.
8. Key the signature block. Start the signature block at the center point of the line. (The first letter of the signature block should align vertically with the first letter of the date and closing.) Use the correct spelling and punctuation. Leave four blank lines between the closing and the signature block. If you are preparing the letter for a provider, you must include a reference notation.
   PURPOSE: The signature block provides the reader with the name of the sender of the letter. The reference notation identifies who typed the letter.
9. Spell-check and proofread the document. Check for the proper tone, grammar, punctuation, capitalization, and sentence structure. Check for proper spacing between the parts of the letter. Make any final corrections. Print the document. If needed, address the envelope using either the computer and word processing software or a pen and following the correct format.
   PURPOSE: The spell-checker identifies only certain errors; proofreading helps you find incorrect word use, improper tone, and errors in formatting.
10. When using a #10 envelope, fold the letter by pulling up the bottom end until it reaches just below the inside address or two-thirds of the way up the letter. Crease at the fold. Then fold the top of the letter down, so it is flush with the bottom fold, and crease the paper. For window business envelopes, have the letter's print side facing up, and place the envelope over the top third of the letter. Fold the bottom edge of the paper up to the bottom edge of the envelope, and crease at the fold. Then remove the envelope, flip the letter over, fold the top of the letter down to the prior crease line, and crease at the fold. Place the letter in the envelope so that the recipient's address shows through the window.
    Note: If the provider needs to sign the letter, the letter is folded afterward.
    PURPOSE: The letter must be neatly folded.
11. File a copy of the letter in the paper medical record or upload an electronic copy of the letter to the electronic health record (EHR).
    PURPOSE: A copy of all correspondence should be kept in the patient's health record.

PROCEDURE 7.3 Compose a Professional Business Letter Using the Semi-block Letter Format

TASKS: Compose a professional letter using technology. Use the semi-block letter format (with the center point option). Address the envelope and fold the letter.

SCENARIO: Julie Walden, MD, has requested that you compose a letter to Amma Patel (DOB: 01/14/19XX) to let her know that her thyroid test was normal, but her vitamin D level was low. Dr. Walden would like Amma to take 15 mcg of vitamin D each morning. She can purchase this over the counter. She needs to have her vitamin D rechecked in 6 months. She can call to schedule a blood test closer to that time. If she has any questions, she should call the office. Her address is 1346 Charity Lane, Anytown, AL 12345-1234. You are working at Walden-Martin Family Medical Clinic. The healthcare facility's address is 1234 Anystreet, Anytown, AL 12345. The phone number is 123-123-1234, and the fax number is 123-123-5678.

EQUIPMENT and SUPPLIES

- Patient's health record
- Computer with word processing software and printer
- Paper
- #10 envelope or # 6¾ envelope

PROCEDURAL STEPS

1. Obtain the intended recipient's contact information and determine the message you want to convey. Using the computer and word processing software, compose the letter using the semi-block letter format. Use 1-inch margins on all four sides, portrait orientation, and single line spacing throughout the letter. Use an easy-to-read font (e.g., Times New Roman or Calibri) in a 10- or 12-point size.
   PURPOSE: Determining the message gives you a focus when composing the letter. You will need the recipient's information to create the letter.
2. Create a letterhead in the header of the document. Include the clinic's name, street address or post office box, city, state, and zip code.
   PURPOSE: The information in the letterhead provides the reader with the clinic's contact information.

PROCEDURE 7.3 Compose a Professional Business Letter Using the Semi-block Letter Format—*continued*

3. Key (type) the date starting at the center point of the line, which is usually about 3.25 inches from the margin. Have one blank line between the dateline and the last line of the letterhead.
   Note: Starting the text at the center point is not the same as the text being centered on the line. When starting the text at the center point, the text flows toward the right margin.
   PURPOSE: All letters require a date for legal purposes.
4. Key the inside address starting at the left margin and use the correct spelling and punctuation. Leave one to nine blank lines between the date and the inside address to center the body of the letter on the page.
   PURPOSE: The body of the letter must be centered vertically from the top to the bottom of the document. More blank lines can be added to move the body to the correct location.
5. Key the salutation starting at the left margin and use the correct spelling and punctuation. Leave one blank line between the inside address and the salutation.
   PURPOSE: A proper greeting sets the tone of the letter.
6. Use your critical thinking skills to compose a concise, accurate message. Type the message in the body of the letter starting at the left margin. Leave one blank line between the salutation and the first line of the body and then between each paragraph of the body. Each paragraph should be indented five spaces. The message should be clear, concise, and professional. Use proper grammar, punctuation, capitalization, and sentence structure.
   PURPOSE: Proper grammar helps to convey the message accurately and professionally.
7. Key a proper closing. Start the closing at the center point of the line. (The first letter of the closing should align vertically with the first letter of the date.) Use correct spelling and punctuation. Leave one blank line between the last line of the body and the closing.
   PURPOSE: The closing helps end the message with a professional tone.
8. Key the signature block. Start the signature block at the center point of the line. (The first letter of the signature block should align vertically with the first letter of the date and closing.) Use the correct spelling and punctuation. Leave four blank lines between the closing and the signature block. If you are preparing the letter for a provider, you must include a reference notation.
   PURPOSE: The signature block provides the reader with the name of the sender of the letter. The reference notation identifies who typed the letter.
9. Spell-check and proofread the document. Check for the proper tone, grammar, punctuation, capitalization, and sentence structure. Check for proper spacing between the parts of the letter. Make any final corrections. Print the document.
   PURPOSE: The spell-checker identifies only certain errors; proofreading helps you find incorrect word use, improper tone, and errors in formatting.
10. Address the envelope using either the computer and word processing software or a pen and following the correct format.
    PURPOSE: Following the Postal Service guidelines on format helps prevent a delay in the delivery of the letter.
11. When using a #10 envelope, fold the letter by pulling up the bottom end until it reaches just below the inside address or two-thirds of the way up the letter. Crease at the fold. Then fold the top of the letter down, so it is flush with the bottom fold, and crease the paper. When using a #6¾ envelope, pull the bottom edge of the letter up until it is one-half inch from the top edge of the document and crease at the fold. Bring the right edge two-thirds of the way across the width of the document and crease the paper. Then bring the left edge to the right edge, and crease at the fold. Flip the document, so the left edge is on the bottom, and insert the letter into the envelope.
    Note: If the provider needs to sign the letter, the letter is folded afterward.
    PURPOSE: The letter must be neatly folded.
12. File a copy of the letter in the paper medical record or upload an electronic copy of the letter to the electronic health record (EHR).
    PURPOSE: A copy of all correspondence should be kept in the patient's health record.

PROCEDURE 7.4 Compose a Memorandum

TASK: Compose a professional memorandum.

SCENARIO: You are asked by the supervisor to compose a memo that can be posted in the department. You are to remind the staff about the department meeting next Tuesday, at noon, in the conference room. Staff members can bring their lunches, and beverages will be provided.

EQUIPMENT and SUPPLIES

- Computer with word processing software and printer
- Paper

PROCEDURAL STEPS

1. Determine the message you want to convey. Using the computer and word processing software, compose the memo. Use 1-inch margins on all four sides, portrait orientation, and single line spacing throughout the memo. Use an easy-to-read font (e.g., Times New Roman or Calibri) in a 10- or 12-point size.
   PURPOSE: Determining the message gives you a focus when composing the memo.
2. Left justify the headers and use boldface and capital letters, followed by a colon. Headers include TO, FROM, DATE, and SUBJECT. Leave one blank line between each header.

Continued

PROCEDURE 7.4 Compose a Memorandum—*continued*

PURPOSE: Boldface and capital letters allow the headers to stand out to the reader, making it easier to read the information.

3. Key (type) the information following the headers in regular font, using a mix of capital and lowercase letters. Using the tab tool, align the information vertically down the page. Key the date as indicated for professional letters.
   PURPOSE: Aligning the information helps the memo look professional.
4. Add a centered black line between the headers and the body (optional). Leave two to three blank lines between the headers and the body of the memo.
   PURPOSE: The line and extra blank lines help to separate the message in the body from the headers.
5. Key the message in the body of the memo. Left justify the content in the body and use single line spacing. Use proper grammar and correct spelling and punctuation. With multiple paragraphs, skip a single line between paragraphs.
   PURPOSE: For professional communication, it is important to use proper grammar and correct spelling and punctuation.
6. Write the content of the message in the body of the memo clearly, concisely, and accurately. Add special notations as needed.
   PURPOSE: Special notations may be used if the memo contains enclosures and so on.
7. Spell-check and proofread the document. Check for the proper tone, grammar, punctuation, capitalization, and sentence structure. Check for proper spacing between the parts of the memo. Make any final corrections. Print the document.
   PURPOSE: The spell-checker identifies only certain errors; proofreading helps you find incorrect word use, improper tone, and errors in formatting.

PROCEDURE 7.5 Compose a Professional Email

TASK: Compose a professional email that conveys the message to the reader clearly, concisely, and accurately.

SCENARIO: Aaron Jackson (DOB: 10/17/20XX) has an appointment at 11 a.m. next Thursday. Send his guardian an appointment reminder via email. Aaron will be seeing David Kahn, MD. The guardian should bring in any medications Aaron is currently taking. You are working at Walden-Martin Family Medical Clinic. The healthcare facility's address is: 1234 Anystreet, Anytown, AL 12345. The phone number is 123-123-1234, and the fax number is 123-123-5678. Your instructor will supply you with the guardian's name and email address.

EQUIPMENT and SUPPLIES

- Patient's health record
- Computer with email software

PROCEDURAL STEPS

1. Obtain the intended recipient's contact information and determine the message you want to convey.
   PURPOSE: Determining the message gives you a focus when composing the email. You will need the recipient's information to create the email.
2. Using the computer and email software, key (type) the recipient's email address. If the email has two recipients, use a semicolon (;) after the name of the first recipient. Double-check the email addresses for accuracy.
   PURPOSE: If the email address is incorrect, the email will not get to the recipient.
3. Key a subject, keeping it simple but focused on the contents of the email.
   PURPOSE: In many email software packages, the user can search for emails using the subject field. Keeping the subject simple and focused makes it easier for the user to find the message.
4. Key a formal greeting, using correct punctuation.
   PURPOSE: A proper greeting sets the tone of the letter.
5. Key the message in the body of the email using proper grammar, spelling, punctuation, capitalization, and sentence structure. Avoid abbreviations. The message should be clear, concise, and professional.
   PURPOSE: Using proper grammar and avoiding abbreviations will convey the message accurately and professionally.
6. Finish the email with closing remarks.
   PURPOSE: In the closing, you can thank the recipient or encourage the recipient to follow up with concerns or questions. This gives the email a professional tone.
7. Key a closing, followed by your name and title on the next line. Include the clinic's name and contact information below your name.
   PURPOSE: The email needs to clearly state who is sending it.
8. Spell-check and proofread the email. Check for proper tone, grammar, punctuation, capitalization, and sentence structure. Check for proper spacing between the parts of the email.
   PURPOSE: White space or spacing between the elements of an email helps separate the parts of the email, making it easier to read.
9. Make any final revisions, select any features to apply to the email, and then send it.
   PURPOSE: If the email is urgent (!), that feature should be selected before you send the email. If you require a confirmation email when the email is opened, this feature can also be selected.
10. Print a copy of the email to be filed in the paper medical record or upload an electronic copy of the email to the patient's electronic health record (EHR).
    PURPOSE: A copy of all correspondence should be kept in the patient's health record.

PROCEDURE 7.6 Complete a Fax Cover Sheet

TASK: Complete a fax cover sheet clearly and accurately.

SCENARIO: Lisa Parker, mother of Johnny Parker (DOB: 06/15/20XX), requested his immunization history to be sent to Anytown School, attention: Susie Payne. The school's phone number is 123-123-5784, and your instructor will supply the fax number. The release of medical records has been completed and signed by Lisa, Johnny's guardian/mother. Your phone number is the main clinic number listed on the header of the fax cover sheet.

EQUIPMENT and SUPPLIES

- Document to be faxed (optional)
- Fax machine and fax number (optional)
- Pen
- Fax cover sheet (see Figure 7.4)

PROCEDURAL STEPS

1. Using a pen and the fax cover sheet, clearly and accurately write your name, phone number, and date.
   PURPOSE: The information must be clearly written so the reader can identify who sent the fax.
2. Clearly and accurately write the name of the person receiving the fax. Also include the company, fax number, and phone number.
   PURPOSE: Being accurate with the information is important, so it gets to the correct person.
3. Write the number of pages. The cover sheet must be counted in the total.
   PURPOSE: It is important to have an accurate count of the total number of sheets faxed.
4. Complete "Re:" by indicating the subject of the fax. Be general with the subject, and refrain from including anything confidential.
   PURPOSE: It is important to be general when writing the subject. No confidential information should appear in the "Re:" line.
5. Proofread the fax cover sheet. Verify the name, agency, and contact information of the recipient. Verify that the document(s) being sent are correct. Optional: organize the documents so the coversheet is on top and fax them to the recipient.
   PURPOSE: Verifying the information and what is being sent is important for the confidentiality of the records.
   Note: Depending on the type of documents faxed and the facility's policies and procedures, the medical assistant may need to document the activity in the patient's health record.

TELEPHONE TECHNIQUES 8

SCENARIO

Ashlynn McDowell, a recent graduate of a medical assisting program, has begun her first position as a receptionist at the Walden-Martin Family Medical (WMFM) Clinic. Ashlynn is determined to perform to the best of her abilities. However, she has never held a job in a professional office. She knows that she needs to practice all of the skills that she learned in school to be an effective receptionist.

WMFM is patient-centered, care-oriented and wants its patients to feel cared for and special. Ashlynn is anxious to build trust with the patients and offer them help with the problems they encounter that fall within her realm of responsibility.

WMFM recently purchased computer software that allows Ashlynn to record telephone messages on the computer, and these messages are automatically routed both to an inbox for the provider and as an entry in the patient's health record. Although the system is new to everyone in the office, Ashlynn is determined to become proficient in its use as quickly as possible.

She knows that she must speak clearly and distinctly and be adept at following up. She plans to dress professionally each day so that she projects the right image to the patients. Ashlynn will strive to be the type of employee who has a willingness to learn, an ability to adapt, and a heart full of compassion for the patient. She is a team player who sincerely wants to cooperate with other staff members who might need her help.

All of the providers at WMFM are pleased that they have found such an eager person to add to their staff. They will assist and guide Ashlynn as she learns how to make the patients feel like part of the clinic family. Ashlynn's self-esteem has increased because she feels she is making a great contribution to healthcare.

While studying this chapter, think about the following questions:

- What are the features of a multiple-line telephone system?
- How can the principles of active listening be applied when communicating with patients?
- Why does the tone of voice play an important role in patient perception?
- What can a medical assistant do to promote a positive image of the healthcare facility when using the telephone with patients?
- How can the medical assistant reduce patients' frustration with telephone issues?

LEARNING OBJECTIVES

1. Explain the features of a multiple-line telephone system and cell phones, and describe how each can be used effectively in a healthcare facility.
2. Determine the impact of active listening and telephone personality on telephone communication.
3. Determine the importance of thinking ahead when managing telephone calls and the correct way to answer the telephone in the office.
4. Determine the various types of common incoming calls and how to deal with each type.
5. Determine various types of special incoming calls and how to deal with each type.
6. Explain how the medical assistant should handle various types of difficult calls.
7. Determine what are typical outgoing calls, and why knowledge of time zones and long-distance calling is necessary.
8. Explain the use of directory assistance.
9. Examine how answering services and automatic call routing systems are used in a healthcare facility.

VOCABULARY

answering service A commercial service that answers telephone calls for its clients.

automatic call routing A system that distributes incoming calls to a specific group or person based on customer need—for example, the customer presses 1 for appointments, 2 for billing questions, and so on.

bilingual (bie LING gwuhl) Ability to communicate effectively in two languages.

call forwarding A telephone feature that allows calls made to one number to be forwarded to another specified number.

caller ID A feature that identifies and displays the telephone numbers of incoming calls made to a particular line.

conference call A telephone call in which a caller can speak with several people at the same time.

copayment (copay) A set dollar amount that the patient must pay for each office visit. There can be one copayment amount

VOCABULARY

for a primary care provider and a different copayment amount (usually higher) to see a specialist or to be seen in the emergency department.

emergency An unexpected, life-threatening situation that requires immediate action.

enunciation (ih nuhn see EY shuhn) The use of articulate, clear sounds when speaking.

ergonomics (ur guh NOM iks) An applied science concerned with designing and arranging things needed to do a job in an efficient and safe way.

headset A set of headphones with a microphone attached, used especially in telephone communication.

intercom A two-way communication system with a microphone and loudspeaker at each station; often a feature of business telephones.

jargon (JAHR guhn) The vocabulary of a particular profession, as opposed to common, everyday terms.

monotone (MON uh tohn) A succession of syllables, words, or sentences spoken in an unvaried key or pitch.

multiple-line telephone system A business telephone system that allows for more than one telephone line.

participating provider A physician or other healthcare provider who enters into a contract with a specific insurance company or program and by doing so agrees to abide by certain rules and regulations set forth by that particular third-party payer.

pitch The depth of a tone or sound; a distinctive quality of sound.

provider An individual or company that provides medical care and services to a patient or the public.

screen A system for examining and separating into different groups; in the healthcare facility, it means determining the severity of illness that patients experience and prioritizing appointments based on that severity.

speakerphone A telephone with a loudspeaker and a microphone; it can be used without having to pick up and hold the handset.

speed dialing A telephone function in which a selected stored number can be dialed by pressing only one key.

STAT The medical abbreviation for the Latin term statum, meaning immediately; at this moment.

tactful The quality of having a sense of what to do or say to maintain good relations with others or to prevent offense.

triage (tree AHZH) The process of assigning degrees of urgency to patients' conditions.

urgent An acute situation that requires immediate attention but is not life threatening.

voice mail An electronic system that allows messages from telephone callers to be recorded and stored.

INTRODUCTION

The telephone is one of the most important pieces of equipment used in a healthcare facility. It is used to communicate with patients, other healthcare organizations, and suppliers. It would be difficult to run an office without a telephone. It is often the first point of contact with patients, and this is an opportunity to make an outstanding first impression. Developing good telephone techniques will make you a valuable asset to your employer.

TELEPHONE EQUIPMENT

Multiple-Line Telephone

Familiarity with a **multiple-line telephone system** (Figure 8.1) is a must for the medical assistant. Even the smallest healthcare facility has at least two telephone lines so that patients rarely get a busy signal when they try to contact the office. The multiple-line telephone has a button for each line, and the button flashes when a call comes in on that line. The button also flashes as a reminder for the medical assistant to check back to see whether the caller would like to remain on hold or leave a message.

The multiple-line telephone also allows you to transfer calls and possibly set up **conference calls**, which involve two or more callers. You should familiarize yourself with the multiple-line telephone system used in your healthcare practice.

Headset

Most business telephones have a handset that can be used to answer the telephone. However, the medical assistant who most frequently is responsible for answering the telephone may want to consider using a **headset** instead. Use of a headset can improve your **ergonomics** and help prevent neck strain. Also, having a headset frees your hands to use the computer or take a message.

A headset is a combination earphone and microphone that is attached to the telephone by a cord or is wireless. You can adjust the volume in the earpiece, and you may be able to adjust the volume of your voice through the microphone for callers who may have difficulty

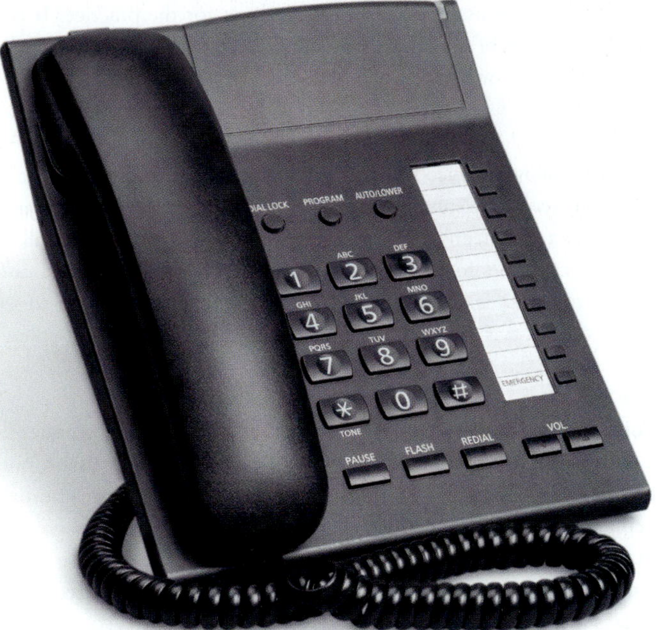

FIGURE 8.1 Multiple-line telephones allow numerous calls to come into the office at once. Each call deserves the same kind of attention and care from the medical assistant.

hearing. Bluetooth, a type of short-range wireless technology, allows you to be more mobile while on the telephone. Because this type of headset is not as visible, people may not be aware that you are on the telephone and may start a conversation with you. You should politely indicate that you are on the telephone and you will respond to the person when you can. Some healthcare facilities have a light system that indicates to a patient that you are on the phone and you will be with them when the call is complete. Also, many headsets can be muted so that you can speak with someone without the caller hearing you.

Features

Most multiple-line business telephones have many features that allow you to perform a number of different tasks in the healthcare facility.

Speakerphone

The **speakerphone** function allows you to hear and speak to the caller without using the handset or a headset. Generally, a button on the telephone is labeled "speaker" (or is indicated with an icon), and once you push it, you can hang up the handset. This can be useful if you need to have more than two people on the call using the same phone.

You should always inform callers that you will be putting them on speakerphone and let the person know who else will be listening in. You must also be conscious of protecting patient information when using a speakerphone. The speakerphone function should not be used in areas such as the patient check-in area or anywhere a conversation can be overheard. The door or reception window should be closed so that no one just walking by can overhear the conversation.

Conference Calls

As mentioned, many multiple-line telephones allow you to set up a conference call, in which you can have multiple people on the call from different locations. The person initiating the call calls one person, puts that person on hold, and continues the sequence until all parties are on the call. Conference calls can be used when the healthcare facility has more than one location, and people from all the locations must be involved in a conversation. For example, a committee may want to discuss policies and procedures for the practice. It is a much better use of time to set up a conference call than to have many people travel to one location.

Caller ID

Caller ID allows users to see who is calling before picking up the handset to answer the telephone. The caller's telephone number and name appear on a screen, and the user can decide whether to take the call. If the user subscribes to call-waiting services, another benefit, called *call-waiting caller ID,* is often available. This function allows the user to see who is calling, even when the user is already on the telephone.

Voice Mail

Voice mail affords an around-the-clock method for receiving patients' messages. Unfortunately, it can prove frustrating to those who find themselves speaking to an electronic device more often than a human being. Voice mail allows the caller to hear a recorded message that may also provide information about what to do in the case of an **emergency**. Similar to an answering machine, voice mail records a caller's message, which can later be retrieved, and allows special temporary greetings when the user is away from the office. You can keep patients happy by answering voice mail messages promptly. There is also a legal necessity for getting back to patients. It can be considered abandonment if the call is not returned. This could be cause for a potential lawsuit.

CRITICAL THINKING APPLICATION **8.1**

Ashlynn hears an employee using the speakerphone function to talk about a patient with another employee. How should she handle this situation? To whom, if anyone, should Ashlynn report this activity? What problems might be caused if this type of conversation is overheard?

Call Forwarding

Call forwarding allows the user to forward calls to another designated number, such as an **answering service**. Usually, a code is entered, then the telephone number to which the calls should be forwarded. If the medical assistant is going to be busy with a patient, the calls can be forwarded to another employee until the task is completed. This prevents the user from missing important calls when away from the main telephone.

Intercom

The business telephone in the healthcare facility may also have **intercom** capabilities. This feature allows for two-way communication within the healthcare facility, but it does not require you to pick up the handset or use a headset. This type of communication is not confidential, but it can be used to notify staff members of an emergency or ask the **provider** to come out of the exam room.

Call Hold

The multiple-line business telephone has a hold button that allows you to interrupt a call temporarily. This is often used when you have answered an incoming call, and then another line rings. You can also use this feature if you need to retrieve some information or speak to someone else to get some information. It is very important to be courteous and respectful of the caller.

Speed Dialing

Speed dialing allows you to program keys on the telephone keypad to automatically call a stored telephone number by just pressing one key. For example, if the healthcare facility uses a particular laboratory for specimen testing, the telephone number for that laboratory can be programmed for the numeral 1 on the telephone keypad; then, when you want to call that laboratory, you only need to press 1, and the call will be made. Speed dialing can be a time-saver; however, all staff members must know which telephone numbers have been programmed into particular keypad numbers.

Cell Phones

Cell (or cellular) phones, considered a luxury item in the early 2000s, have become commonplace. Many people no longer have a landline because of the expenses of having two phones, and the cell phone usually is the better buy for the money. Several of the more popular cell phone companies offer free long-distance calls in the United States and may provide users free night and weekend minutes. Most of today's smartphones even allow users to access the internet and check email on their telephone. Cell phone companies usually offer a text messaging service, which allows the user to enter a message with cell phone keys or by voice, which then is sent directly to a cell phone number.

Many people have a personal cell phone or smartphone. It is a great way to be accessible at all times, but it also can present some issues in a healthcare facility, particularly in regard to patient confidentiality. Most cell phones have a camera that can be used to take pictures of confidential information, and that information can be transmitted quickly to someone else or put on the internet. Calls can be made or taken at inopportune times and may affect the care of patients. Most healthcare facilities have a policy that prohibits employees from having their personal cell phones with them during working hours.

We have seen an increase in the number of healthcare facilities that are supplying cell phones to their providers. The communication process is improved with the provider's use of cell phones. There is ready access to the patient information needed for collaboration and care coordination. The provider's cell phone number should never be given out to patients without the provider's permission.

EFFECTIVE USE OF THE TELEPHONE

Telephones for communication are a fact of life for any business. It is important that this instrument is used effectively, especially in healthcare. The communication done on the telephone could mean life or death. This next section covers several components of effective telephone communication.

Active Listening

It may seem odd to start this section by discussing listening instead of speaking but listening well is just as important as speaking well when it comes to communicating on the telephone. When you are on the telephone, you have fewer nonverbal cues to help you determine the message. Therefore, it is important that you use good listening skills. When you use active listening skills, your patients realize that you think they are important and respect the message they are communicating to you, whether you are on the telephone or face to face.

Active Listening

- Be present in the moment.
- Focus solely on the conversation.
- Don't interrupt.
- Don't start forming your response before the person has finished speaking.
- Confirm what the speaker has said, and ask if your interpretation is correct.
- Always be respectful and professional.

Active listening involves listening to what the speaker is saying, interpreting what the message is, and restating the message to make sure that you have received the intended message. For example, you receive a telephone call from a distraught mother. Using active listening skills, you pick up on the nonverbal cues, such as her tone of voice and rate of speech, and you can tell she is upset. The mother states that her child has been very sick for the past several days, and nothing she has done has helped with the fever her child has had for 2 days. Your response should be to restate what you have heard: the child has been ill with a fever for the past 2 days, and nothing she has tried has brought the fever down. This gives the caller the opportunity to correct any misinformation or confirm that the information is correct. If it is correct, you should follow the healthcare practice's procedures for handling this situation; most likely, you will schedule an appointment for that same day.

Developing a Pleasing Telephone Personality

Each time medical assistants answer the telephone, they are representing the healthcare practice (Procedure 8.1). The manner in which the telephone is answered can influence the caller's impression of the whole office and whether the person wants to be seen there. When patients call the healthcare facility, they should hear a friendly yet professional voice. Just as active listening is an important skill to receive the message being sent, a pleasing telephone personality facilitates the sending of the message.

Although it may seem silly, you should always smile when you answer the telephone. The physical act of smiling affects how your words sound. It is as if your caller can hear you smile, and you have created a positive impression.

It is also important to be aware of nonverbal communication that occurs during a telephone conversation. Be aware of your tone of voice. Is it helping to send the message that you want to send? Your callers can tell if you are preoccupied and not focused on the current conversation. You should vary the **pitch** of your voice and avoid speaking in a **monotone**.

Enunciation is crucial when speaking on the telephone. You should speak clearly and distinctly so that the caller can understand what you are saying. Many letters of the alphabet sound similar on the telephone, such as B, P, T, F and S. You may need to clarify these letters with the caller by saying, "That is B as in bravo."

Nonvisual/Nonverbal Communication

- Tone of voice
- Speed of speech
- Pitch
- Volume
- Enunciation
- Pausing or hesitation

Phonetic Alphabet

A	Alpha	N	November
B	Bravo	O	Oscar
C	Charlie	P	Papa
D	Delta	Q	Quebec
E	Echo	R	Romeo
F	Foxtrot	S	Sierra
G	Golf	T	Tango
H	Hotel	U	Uniform
I	India	V	Victor
J	Juliet	W	Whiskey
K	Kilo	X	X-ray
L	Lima	Y	Yankee
M	Mike	Z	Zulu

It is important to always be courteous and **tactful**. Think about the words you will be using before actually speaking to them. For those working in a healthcare facility, it is easy to integrate medical terminology into our conversations. However, we must be careful not to use medical **jargon** when speaking with patients because this makes the message more difficult for them to understand. For example, if you are giving a male patient preprocedural instructions, advise him that he must not eat or drink anything for 12 hours before the procedure; do not tell him he should "stay NPO" (nothing by mouth).

To create a pleasant, friendly, and professional image of the healthcare facility, you must give the caller your full attention. Do not become distracted by other things going on around you. In addition, you should never eat, chew gum, or drink when on the telephone. Use a normal volume and tone of voice and speak directly into the mouthpiece. Be sure to speak at a moderate rate of speed because speaking too quickly makes it difficult for the caller to understand you.

CRITICAL THINKING APPLICATION **8.2**

Ashlynn has a tendency to speak a little fast in her normal conversations. How will she need to adjust as she is answering phones in the healthcare facility? She also is a friendly person and enjoys talking on the phone. What precautions should she take so that this does not become an issue on the job?

MANAGING TELEPHONE CALLS

Thinking Ahead

Whether you are answering incoming calls or placing outgoing calls, it is important to be completely prepared. Before you start answering calls, make sure you have all the supplies needed to do your job. For example, for taking messages, you should have access to a computer (if your office documents telephone messages electronically) or a paper message form, in addition to working pens and a watch or clock to record the time. You should be sure to have the healthcare facility's telephone screening guidelines available. Many offices also keep a list of commonly used telephone numbers. This list will include the number for poison control, other emergency numbers, the numbers for community resources to which patients can be referred, and so on.

For outgoing calls, have all the information you need, such as the patient's health record, the telephone number of the person you will be calling, a list of questions, and a pad and a pen to make notes during the conversation.

Confidentiality

All communication in a healthcare facility must maintain patient confidentiality. When using the telephone, you must be aware of what is going on around you and who may be able to overhear your conversation. If patient-sensitive information is discussed, place the call in an area where others cannot hear, especially other patients. Be careful when using a speakerphone because the sound can travel farther than you might think, and someone might overhear private medical information—this is a violation of the law, specifically the Health Insurance Portability and Accountability Act (HIPAA).

Answering Promptly

As mentioned earlier, telephone contact is often the first interaction with a patient. If a call is not answered promptly, this can create a negative impression before the caller even talks to someone. It is important that a call be answered within three rings. To accomplish this, you may need to do the following:

- Interrupt the call you are on by asking if you can place the person on hold for a moment.
- Answer the second call; if it is not an emergency, ask if you may place the person on hold.
- Return to the first caller.

An incoming call should never be answered with "Please hold." You should always find out the nature of the call before placing the person on hold. If it is an emergency, the second call is handled promptly before you return to the first call. If it is not an emergency, you should always ask if you can place the person on hold and wait for an answer before pushing the hold button. If the person refuses to be placed on hold, determine the reason why and assure the caller that you will return quickly.

The medical assistant who routinely answers the telephone should know how to activate emergency medical services (EMS) in the area. Generally, this means dialing 911. You may need to make this call for patients who have called the healthcare facility and are now unable to contact EMS on their own. If your phone system allows it, you can set up a conference call that includes the patient, EMS, and yourself. It is important to get a telephone number where the caller can be reached, just in case you get disconnected. It also is important to keep the patient and caregivers on the line while contacting EMS.

Identifying the Facility

When answering incoming telephone calls, medical assistants should identify the facility first, state their name, and then follow with an offer of help. For example, the medical assistant could say, "Good morning, Walden-Martin Family Medical Clinic. This is Ashlynn. How may I help you?" Medical assistants must always follow the policy of the healthcare facility when answering incoming calls. Speaking slowly and smoothly, with good enunciation, ensures that your callers understand whom they have reached.

CRITICAL THINKING APPLICATION **8.3**

Most offices dictate how the phone is to be answered. What should Ashlynn do if she is uncomfortable with the way she is asked to answer the phone? Who ultimately should decide how the phone is answered?

Identifying the Caller

If the caller does not offer a name, the medical assistant should ask, "May I ask who is calling?" It can be helpful to write down the caller's name and try to use it at least three times during the conversation if it does not compromise patient confidentiality. This helps make a strong connection and assures that the patient has been identified correctly.

Occasionally callers refuse to identify themselves to the medical assistant and insist that they speak with the provider. You must be clear, in a professional manner, that you cannot connect the caller to the provider without knowing who the caller is. Some callers may be sales representatives who know if they identify themselves, they will not get the opportunity to talk with the provider. When it becomes clear that the caller will not give a name but still insists on speaking with the provider, you can tell the person that the provider is busy with patients and has asked that messages be taken, and callers who cannot leave a name for the message may want to write a letter and mark it Personal. Most people do not want to wait for a response to a letter and will then give you their names so that a message can be taken.

Screening Incoming Calls

Most healthcare facilities expect the medical assistant answering the telephone to **screen** the calls. You must determine which calls should be routed directly to the provider, the **triage** area, and the billing office. The provider, office manager, and staff members who will be answering the telephone should work together to develop policies for screening calls.

The first step in screening calls is to determine who the caller is and the nature of the call. If the call is from a patient with a question about a recently received billing statement, the call can be transferred to the appropriate area. If the call involves determining whether a patient should be seen that day, it can be transferred to the triage area. If the caller asks to speak directly to the provider, the situation can become more complicated, and healthcare facility policies should be created to address these cases.

Healthcare facility policies often state that calls from other providers are put through immediately. If that is not possible, assure the caller that the provider will return the call as soon as possible. Some providers may also ask that calls be put through immediately for certain family members. If the provider does not want to take the calls, the medical assistant must tactfully tell the caller that the provider cannot be disturbed at this time.

Screening policies should also address how calls should be handled when the provider is out of the office. If the provider is out of the office for an extended period (e.g., for a conference or vacation), another provider is usually designated to handle calls. It should be explained that the provider the patient asked for is out of the office, but another provider is taking the calls. If the call is not an emergency, take a message, and the designated provider can return the call.

If a call is an emergency, the policies for handling emergency calls apply. Many emergency calls require judgment on the part of the person answering the telephone in the medical practice. Good judgment comes from experience and proper training by the provider. It is important to know what a real emergency is, in addition to how such calls should be handled. The person answering the telephone first should determine whether the call is truly **urgent**. If so, never hang up the telephone until an ambulance reaches the patient, or other help arrives. When necessary, ask another staff member to call 911 while remaining on the line with the patient. Emergency calls may include such conditions or symptoms as chest pain, profuse bleeding, severe allergic reactions, cessation of breathing, injuries resulting in loss of consciousness, and broken bones.

An urgent call may be an adult patient with a fever over 102°F (38.9°C), an animal bite, or an increasingly painful ear infection. Emergency calls are life threatening, whereas urgent calls require prompt attention but are not life threatening. In the case of emergencies, often, the provider instructs the patient to go straight to the closest hospital emergency department instead of the office. Policies and procedures manuals should indicate the action to take in emergency situations. When in doubt, always ask the office manager or the provider.

If the provider is in, the call may need to be transferred to the provider immediately. All offices should have a written plan of action for the times the provider is not physically present in the office. These policies should include typical questions to ask the caller to determine the validity and disposition of an emergency. Here are some examples of questions to ask:

- At what telephone number can you be reached?
- Where are you located?
- What are the chief symptoms?
- When did they start?
- Has this happened before?
- Are you alone?
- Do you have transportation?

Screening Guidelines

In a facility with multiple employees, the provider may designate one individual, such as a nurse or an experienced and trained medical assistant, as the telephone screener. Every healthcare facility would be wise to have a written telephone protocol for handling urgent situations and emergencies. The protocol should state that employees are bound by the written guidelines and that unauthorized personnel may give no advice. If advice is given, it may be grounds for dismissal.

A special sheet of instructions listing specific medical emergencies (e.g., chest pain, heavy bleeding, fainting, seizure, and poisoning) should be posted by each telephone. The telephone numbers for the nearest poison control center, hospital, and ambulance should be listed.

Emergency calls should be routed to a provider immediately. Additional instructions should include what action to take if no provider is available (e.g., sending the patient to an emergency department or calling for an ambulance). Most offices have some means of constant contact with the provider, whether by pager, cell phone, or another method.

Getting the Information the Provider Needs

Medical assistants gradually gain experience and come to know the provider better, allowing them to have a sense of the questions the provider will have for patients who call the facility. For example, the provider is interested in how long the patient has had symptoms, what makes the symptoms better or worse, what remedies have been tried, what has worked and not worked, and other specifics about the condition. If the patient complains of painful urination, the medical assistant learns to ask about pain in the back or blood in the urine. One way to learn what questions to ask is to listen to the providers carefully as they question patients about their symptoms. This can help you learn more about signs and symptoms and enable you to be a better assistant to the provider.

Remember to always be "patient with your patients." Those who call the healthcare facility for help are seldom at their best. When feeling ill, people often are short-tempered and even display poor manners. Some can be verbally abusive. Care for patients as if they were family members, and they will feel care and compassion in the medical facility.

If the provider is unavailable for only part of the day, take a message and inform the caller that the provider is currently out of the office but will return calls when they return. It is important to give the caller the time frame in which the provider will return those calls, so the patient does not waste time sitting by the phone, waiting for the call. It should be stressed that the time frame is approximate because emergencies cannot be predicted. If the caller is unavailable when the provider usually returns calls, ask what a convenient time would be and let the caller know you will try to work with that time frame.

Screening calls is an important task for medical assistants who answer the telephone. It can keep the healthcare facility running on schedule and ensure that calls that need to get to the provider are transferred immediately.

Placing Callers on Hold

When you are working with a multiple-line telephone, it is not uncommon for more than one call to come in at a time. Here is what you should to if you are on one call and another line rings:

- Ask permission to put the first call on hold.
- Answer the second call.
- Determine if it is an emergency or not.
  - If it is an emergency, follow the emergency call procedures.
  - If it is not an emergency, ask if you can place the caller on hold.
- Return to the first call.

If it has been determined through the screening process that this is a call that does not need to be put through to the provider right away, or if the call needs to be transferred to someone else in the healthcare facility and that person is not immediately available, you should ask if the caller would like to be put on hold or be called back instead. If you know that the person with whom the caller needs to speak may be busy for quite a while, inform the caller of that. The caller may still want to wait. You should check back periodically to make sure the caller still wants to remain on hold. No longer than 1 minute should pass before you check back with the caller. When you return to the call, you can use a statement such as "Thank you for waiting. Would you like to continue to hold, or should I take a message?"

Minimizing the wait for the caller shows concern, and freeing up the telephone lines is important for other people trying to contact the healthcare facility.

Transferring a Call

During the screening process, the medical assistant may determine that the call should be transferred to the provider or another person in the facility. Consider the following example: Ms. Fields calls your office because she has a billing question. You should ask Ms. Fields' permission and wait for a response before placing her on hold. It is also helpful to give Ms. Fields the name and extension of the person to whom you will be transferring her call (if it is not the provider); this way, if Ms. Fields' call happens to get disconnected, she will have that information when she calls back. Once you have Ms. Fields' permission to put her on hold, you should contact the person to whom the call is being transferred; in this case, that is Mr. Lewis in the billing department. Tell Mr. Lewis who is calling and the reason for the call; this allows Mr. Lewis to be prepared to help Ms. Fields when the connection is made. Mr. Lewis may ask for a moment to pull up information before you put Ms. Fields' call through. You should stay on the line to introduce Ms. Fields to Mr. Lewis and make sure the connection is made. If Mr. Lewis is unavailable, you should ask Ms. Fields if she would like to be connected to his voice mail. Some callers may prefer that you take a message in written form and bring it to the proper person.

Medical assistants who answer telephone calls must know who does what in the healthcare facility. An organizational chart with telephone extensions can be helpful, but it must be kept up to date so calls can be transferred successfully.

Taking a Message

Telephone messages, whether taken in a handwritten or an electronic format, are an important part of patient care (Procedure 8.2). The patient relies on the medical assistant to get the message to the appropriate person. Taking messages allows information to be delivered to a provider or an appropriate person, who can make a decision (then or later), which can be communicated back to the patient without interrupting the flow of patients through the healthcare facility. You should be sure to let the caller know when to expect a call back; for example, explain that the provider usually returns calls between 3 and 4 p.m.

Whether the message is taken in a handwritten or an electronic format, the information needed for a complete message is the same:

1. The name of the person calling
2. The name of the person to whom the call is directed
3. The caller's daytime, evening, or cell phone number
4. The reason for the call, including the telephone number of the caller's pharmacy if a medication is requested
5. The action to be taken
6. The date and time of the call
7. The initials of the person who took the call

Messages Recorded on Paper

Many types of message pads or books are available (Figure 8.2). Many are pressure sensitive, making a copy of the message and serving as a telephone call log. The original is given to the person the message is for, and the medical assistant will have a copy to use for follow-up. Having legible handwriting is a must when taking a manual, handwritten message.

Messages Recorded Electronically

Most electronic health record (EHR) systems can record telephone messages (Figure 8.3). The EHR automatically saves a copy of the message to the patient's health record and sends the message to the provider, who can either call the patient directly or give the medical assistant directions to respond to the patient. The electronic system may also be able to flag a message to indicate that it is urgent, that it requires a callback, or that a prescription refill has been requested.

Taking Action on Telephone Messages

The message process is not complete until the necessary action has been taken. If a handwritten system is used, add an identifying mark to indicate a message that requires action. If an electronic system is used, check periodically during the day to be sure you do not have to complete the response to the message, such as calling the patient back or contacting the pharmacy. For risk management purposes, the healthcare facility should have a policy on the documentation of telephone messages and the specific information that must be included. Medical assistants should become familiar with that policy.

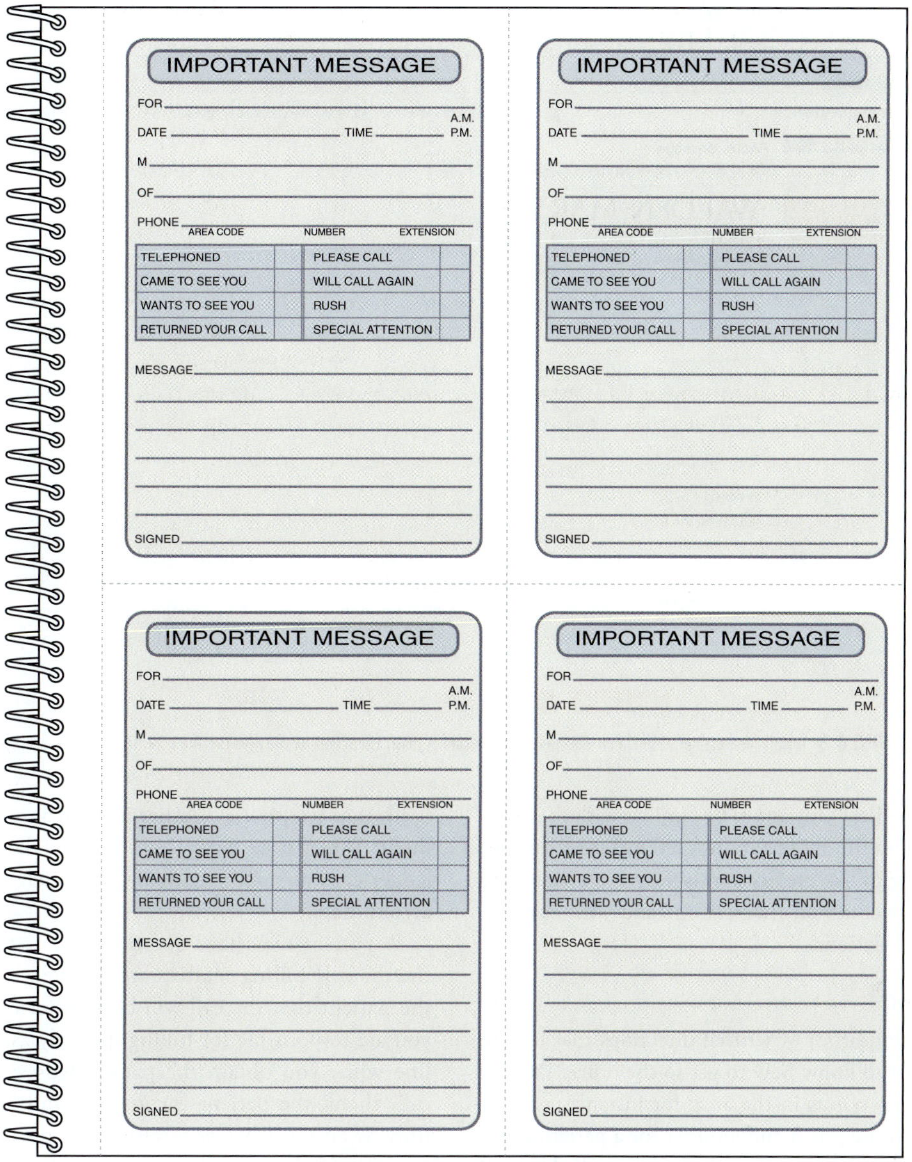

IMPORTANT MESSAGE

FOR

DATE TIME A.M. P.M.

M

OF

PHONE AREA CODE NUMBER EXTENSION

TELEPHONED		PLEASE CALL	
CAME TO SEE YOU		WILL CALL AGAIN	
WANTS TO SEE YOU		RUSH	
RETURNED YOUR CALL		SPECIAL ATTENTION	

MESSAGE

SIGNED

IMPORTANT MESSAGE

FOR

DATE TIME A.M. P.M.

M

OF

PHONE AREA CODE NUMBER EXTENSION

TELEPHONED PLEASE CALL
CAME TO SEE YOU WILL CALL AGAIN
WANTS TO SEE YOU RUSH
RETURNED YOUR CALL SPECIAL ATTENTION

MESSAGE

SIGNED

IMPORTANT MESSAGE

FOR

DATE TIME A.M. P.M.

M

OF

PHONE AREA CODE NUMBER EXTENSION

TELEPHONED PLEASE CALL
CAME TO SEE YOU WILL CALL AGAIN
WANTS TO SEE YOU RUSH
RETURNED YOUR CALL SPECIAL ATTENTION

MESSAGE

SIGNED

IMPORTANT MESSAGE

FOR

DATE TIME A.M. P.M.

M

OF

PHONE AREA CODE NUMBER EXTENSION

TELEPHONED PLEASE CALL
CAME TO SEE YOU WILL CALL AGAIN
WANTS TO SEE YOU RUSH
RETURNED YOUR CALL SPECIAL ATTENTION

MESSAGE

SIGNED

FIGURE 8.2 Telephone message forms.

Retaining Records of Telephone Messages

If a handwritten system is used for recording telephone messages, the healthcare facility must establish a policy on the retention of telephone message records. If the message relates to patient care, a copy of the message should be added to the patient's health record. If the health record is electronic, this may mean scanning in a copy of the paper message and attaching it to the EHR. The copy in the message book usually is retained for the same period that the statute of limitations runs for medical professional liability cases.

If an electronic system is used, the message is automatically saved to the patient's record, along with the response to the message. The message record can show whether the patient contacted the office, if the office responded to that contact, and what the response was. All of these are key points if a medical-professional liability case is brought against the provider. In addition, accurate telephone records can ensure quality patient care and customer service.

TYPICAL INCOMING CALLS

Handling incoming calls is often the responsibility of the medical assistant. You can handle many calls directly, but some will require the assistance of others. Knowing how to respond to the different types of calls will make you a valuable asset to the healthcare facility.

Requests for Prescription Refills

Patients will often call the healthcare facility when they need a prescription refilled. It could be that there were no refills left on the original prescription or that they have used all of the refills. Patients need to provide the following information when they request a prescription refill:

- Medication name
- Dosage
- How many pills are taken in a day
- Any issues with the medication
- Whether they want to use a pharmacy mail-order service or pick up the prescription
- Pharmacy address and phone number

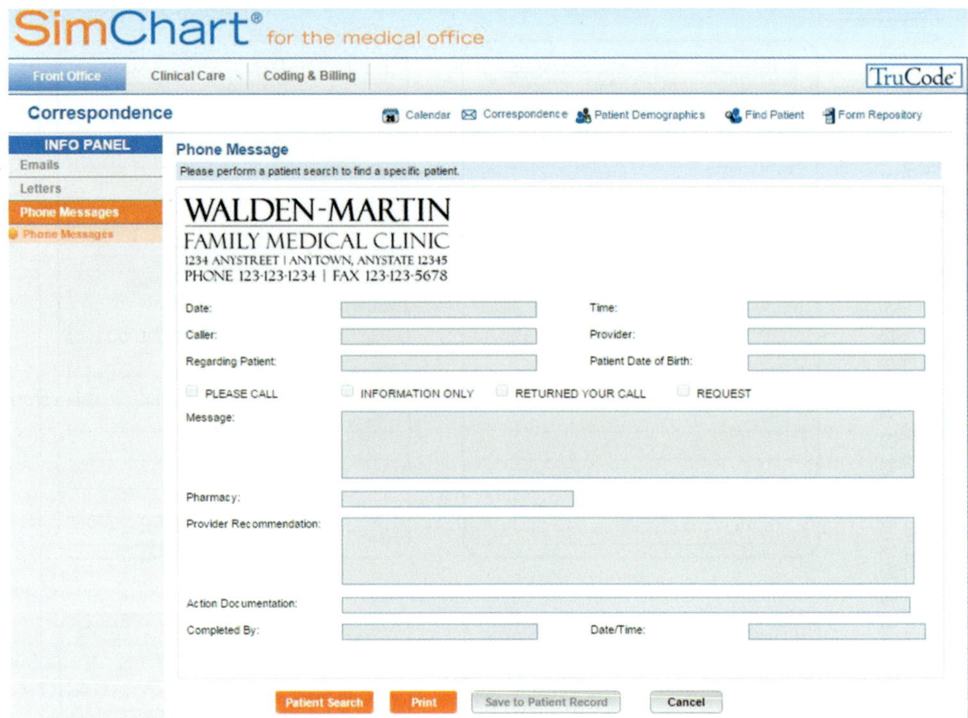

FIGURE 8.3 Telephone message screen in an electronic health record system. (*SimChart for the Medical Office,* St. Louis, 2015, Elsevier.)

It is important for a medical assistant to be familiar with the common medication names and the abbreviations used in a prescription. Using the correct spelling of the medication is very important. See Appendix A for the most common medications and their spelling and Appendix B for abbreviations.

Requests for Directions

Each office should have a clear set of written directions that can be read to a caller who wants to know how to get to the office. Prepare the directions from various points in the area; for instance, one set for a patient coming from the north and another for a patient coming from the south. Place these directions close to the telephone so that all employees can find them easily. Not all employees live close to the clinic or are familiar with the area; therefore, the written set of directions will be helpful both to staff members and to patients. Put a map on the office website and direct patients there for printable directions. Never simply suggest that callers refer to an internet map when they ask for directions.

Inquiries about Bills

A patient may ask to speak with the provider about a recent bill. Ask the caller to hold for a moment while the ledger is obtained from the computer or files. If nothing irregular is on the ledger, return to the telephone and say, "I have your account in front of me now. Perhaps I can answer your question." Most likely, the caller will have a simple inquiry (e.g., whether the insurance company has paid its portion), or the person may want to delay making a payment until the next month. Not all patients realize that the medical assistant usually makes such decisions and is the best person with whom to discuss these matters. If the healthcare facility uses an external billing service, you may need to provide the caller with that agency's telephone number. When an external billing service is used, that telephone number is often shown on the patient's statement. When necessary, post a note in the EHR or to the physical ledger card about the patient's call, such as a promise to pay on a certain date.

A patient may have questions about a statement that came in the mail. If billing matters are handled by another employee, tell the patient that the call will be transferred to the billing office. If you are responsible for billing, politely ask the patient to hold the line while you obtain the patient ledger. When returning to the call, thank the patient for waiting and explain the charges carefully. If an error has occurred, apologize, and say that a corrected statement will be sent out at once. Always remember to thank the patient for calling. If patients are properly advised about charges at the time services are rendered, the number of these calls can be reduced considerably.

Inquiries about Fees

Fees vary widely in each healthcare facility and quoting an exact fee before the provider sees the patient can be difficult. However, a good estimate should be given to patients as to what they can expect to pay, especially on the first visit. Asking a patient to just appear at the office without having an idea of the cost is unreasonable. Discuss with the provider or office manager what range should be quoted to the patient, and follow your quote with the statement that the fees vary depending on the patient's condition and the tests the provider orders.

Most healthcare facilities require patients to pay the health insurance **copayment** (or **copay**) on the day service is provided, and the caller should be informed of this. If fees are regularly discussed on the telephone, a suggested script should be included in the policies and procedures manual. Do not be evasive; have a list of fees available that you can discuss with patients.

Questions about Participating Providers

Patients may call the office to inquire whether the provider is a **participating provider** with their particular insurance plan or managed care organization. A list of the insurance plans with which the provider has a contract should be readily available to the medical assistant who answers the telephone. This is important because insurance benefits vary widely for patients based on whether they see a participating provider or a nonparticipating provider. A claim may even be denied if the provider is not a participating provider for the patient's insurance company.

Requests for Assistance with Insurance

In the ever-changing world of health insurance, patients are often confused about their coverage, how payment is determined, and what they are actually financially responsible for when it comes to their bill from the healthcare facility. A solid understanding of the basics of health insurance, including managed care, allows you to answer patients' questions about insurance. If the question is beyond your knowledge, you should know to whom to transfer the call so that the patient can get an answer.

Radiology and Laboratory Reports

Because of the increased use of EHRs, radiology and laboratory results often are available to providers as soon as the technician has completed the test. When the patient calls for those results, a message is taken, and the provider decides whether the medical assistant can relay the results or the provider needs to speak to the patient directly.

When tests are done at a facility that is not linked to the healthcare facility's EHR, the findings are usually delivered by mail to the provider's office. If the test has been marked **STAT**, reports may be telephoned, faxed, or emailed to the provider's office and an original report delivered by mail.

It is helpful to have blank laboratory results forms available that list the various tests with their normal values so that you can easily and accurately document results telephoned to the healthcare facility. This can save time, and you can be assured that the test name is spelled correctly. You should repeat the results you have been given to make sure you have written them down correctly. This report must be documented in the patient's health record and sent to the provider for review.

Satisfactory Progress Reports from Patients

Providers sometimes ask patients to telephone the office to report their condition a few days after the office visit. The medical assistant can take such calls and relay the information to the provider if the report is satisfactory. Assure the patient that you will inform the provider of the call. The report should be documented in the health record. The provider should always be immediately informed about unsatisfactory progress reports and should give instructions for the patient to follow in such situations. The provider may discuss this directly with the patient, or the medical assistant may be instructed to relay the information to the patient. All instructions given should also be documented in the health record.

Routine Reports from Hospitals and Other Sources

Routine calls may be received from hospitals and other sources reporting a patient's progress. Take the message carefully and make sure the provider sees it. The message should be placed in the patient's health record after the provider has reviewed and initialed it.

Requests for Referrals

Well-respected providers, especially primary care providers, are often asked for recommendations for referrals to other specialists. If the provider has furnished the medical assistant with a list of practitioners for this purpose, these inquiries may be handled without consulting the provider unless the patient's insurance plan requires a written referral. However, the provider should always be informed of such requests. Referrals should also be documented in the patient's health record.

Some managed care organizations require a provider referral before a patient may see a specialist; this referral should come from the provider unless the provider has authorized automatic referrals. Most providers require the patient to come in for an office visit to discuss the referral. Afterward, a staff member calls the referral provider and notifies the office staff of the referral. This process may also be done electronically. A managed care organization may offer the option of using its website to enter the referral information and then electronically forwarding the information to the new provider. Handle these calls as quickly as possible so that the patient may make an appointment to see the referral provider in a timely manner.

Non-Patient-Related Calls

Not all calls concern patients. Calls may come from the accountant or the auditor or about banking procedures, office supplies, or office maintenance, most of which the medical assistant can handle or refer to the appropriate person. For some of these calls, the medical assistant may need to gather additional information and return the call.

Pharmaceutical representatives and salespeople will often call and ask to speak to the provider. A message should be taken that includes what product they want to talk to the provider about. The provider may decide to return these calls or ask that an appointment be scheduled to talk about the new product. It is also possible that the provider will ask the office manager to talk to the salesperson.

SPECIAL INCOMING CALLS

Some incoming calls are the result of special circumstances and require special skills to handle. The following section discusses the most common special incoming calls.

Patients Refusing to Discuss Symptoms

Occasionally patients call and want to talk with the provider about symptoms they are reluctant to discuss with a medical assistant. Patients have the right to privacy, but the provider cannot be expected to take numerous calls from patients who do not want to speak to the medical assistant. Explaining that it is helpful for the provider to have the information before returning their call will sometimes convince them to give the information to the medical assistant. If the patient refuses to discuss any symptoms, follow the healthcare facility's procedures, which may include suggesting that the patient make an appointment with the provider to discuss the problem in person.

Unsatisfactory Progress Reports

Sometimes patients under treatment may report that they are still not feeling well or that the prescription the provider wrote is not helping. In such cases, do not practice medicine illegally by giving the patient medical advice. Make detailed notes about the patient's comments, and then give your notes to the provider. The provider may change the patient's medication or decide that the patient should return to the office. Follow up with the patient and convey the provider's instructions.

CRITICAL THINKING APPLICATION **8.4**

A patient calls the healthcare facility to report that she has been taking her prescribed antibiotic for 3 days and still is not feeling any better. She says she might even be feeling worse than before she started taking the pills. She asks Ashlynn if she should stop taking the pills.

- How should Ashlynn respond to this patient?
- What actions should Ashlynn take in response to this telephone call?
- What should Ashlynn document in the patient's record?

Requests for Test Results

When the provider orders special tests, the patient may be told to call the office in a couple of days for the results. It is ultimately the responsibility of the provider to notify the patient of test results, especially if they are abnormal. When a patient calls for the results, make sure the provider has seen them and has given permission before sharing the results with the patient. If specified in the office policy, the medical assistant can give test results to the patient. Patients do not always understand that the medical assistant cannot give out information without the provider's permission. If the results are unfavorable, the provider should be the one to inform the patient and give further instructions. This call must be handled tactfully; otherwise, the patient may feel as if the staff is concealing information.

Most providers prefer that medical assistants give only normal test results to patients. However, the medical assistant may give abnormal test results if authorized by the provider. For example, when a patient has an abnormal Pap test result, the medical assistant usually is the person who calls the patient with the result and further instructions from the provider. If the patient has any questions about the test result, she must be referred to the provider. The medical assistant needs good communication skills to relay information such as this without crossing the line of practicing medicine without a license.

The best policy for dealing with more serious abnormal test results is to schedule an appointment for the patient to see the provider. These results are best relayed in person instead of on the telephone.

Patients who call the office for test results must be appropriately identified before the results are given. Some offices use a special code that is documented in the patient's health record, and knowledge of this code or password gives the person access to the information. Other offices may use the patient's date of birth or other information that is known only to the patient and has been shared with the healthcare facility. You should always use at least two different methods of identifying patients.

Medical assistants must know and follow federal regulations and the laws in their state regarding the release of any information to someone other than the patient. It is important to note that this includes information about a minor. Make sure the right individual is on the line before offering results by verifying name and date of birth. It is considered a breach of confidentiality and the Privacy Rules of the Health Insurance Portability and Accountability Act if the patient is not identified correctly and information is released to the wrong individual.

Requests for Information from Third Parties

The patient must give permission before any member of the provider's staff can give information to third-party callers; this includes insurance companies, attorneys, relatives, neighbors, employers, and any other third party. HIPAA is very specific about the information that should be included in the release of information form. The patient must specify who can receive the information and exactly what information can be released. The release of information form also must include an expiration date. The medical assistant must carefully review the patient's form before releasing any information to third parties. Chapter 4 has more information regarding the release of information.

Complaints about Care or Fees

A medical assistant may be able to offer a satisfactory explanation to a patient who complains about the care they received or the charged fee. Often the patient simply does not understand a charge, and the medical assistant can provide assistance by reviewing the bill. If a patient seems angry, offer to research the problem and, if needed, discuss it with the provider. Four magic words often calm the angry patient: "Let me help you." This reassures the patient that someone is willing to talk about the problem. However, if you are unable to appease the patient easily, the provider or office manager may prefer to talk to the patient directly.

When callers complain, do not attempt to blame someone else, and never argue with the patient. Find the source of the problem, and then present options to the caller as to how the situation can be resolved. Remember to treat callers in the same manner that you would wish to be treated. A complaint may seem small and insignificant to the office staff, but it may be a serious issue to the patient. Provide good customer service to patients, and complaints will be few and far between.

Calls from Staff Members' Families or Friends

Personal calls can tie up the telephone lines. Sometimes a call is necessary in emergencies, but staff members should never monopolize the telephone for personal business and conversations. Patient emergency calls could be coming through, and the lines must be clear. Keep personal calls to an absolute minimum.

HANDLING DIFFICULT CALLS

Not all telephone calls are easy or pleasant to handle but using professional communication skills can help you in any difficult situation. The following section discusses some of the difficult situations that you might encounter.

Angry Callers

No matter how efficient the medical assistant is on the telephone or how well-liked the provider might be, sooner or later, an angry caller will be on the telephone. The anger may have a legitimate cause, or the caller's irritation may have resulted from a misunderstanding. Handling such calls is a real challenge. First, take the required actions, even if it is to say that the matter will be discussed with the provider as soon as possible and that the patient will be called back later. If answers are not readily available, a friendly assurance that the situation is important and that every attempt will be made to find the answer quickly usually calms the angry feelings.

Medical assistants may find that lowering their tone of voice and volume of speech may force the angry caller to do the same. This method does not always work, but it usually is true that when dealing with an angry person, calm promotes calm. Some patients may misread this method and become even angrier, thinking their complaint is not being taken seriously. Interpersonal skills are critical when dealing with other individuals because the more skilled the medical assistant becomes, the better able the assistant is to deal with multiple types of personalities.

Always avoid getting angry or defensive in response to an angry caller and try to get to the root of the real problem. Express interest and understanding, take careful notes and follow through with the problem to the most appropriate resolution. Never shift the responsibility by saying, "That's not my job" or "I am not the person who filed that insurance claim." No matter whose fault the problem is, it is best to deal with it and find a solution instead of placing blame. It is important to respond to the patient when you said you would, even if the call is to say that you need a bit more time to work on the problem. Keeping the patient in the loop shows that you want to come up with a solution.

CRITICAL THINKING APPLICATION **8.5**

An angry caller raises his voice at Ashlynn over an issue that happened before she began to work at the facility. She suggests that he speak with the office manager, but he refuses and continues to berate Ashlynn.

- What choices does Ashlynn have in this situation?
- Should she simply hang up on the patient?
- How can the call be handled diplomatically?

Aggressive Callers

Aggressive callers insist that they receive whatever action they feel is necessary, and they usually insist on the action immediately. Treat these callers with a calm, poised attitude but do not allow the caller's aggression to initiate inappropriate action. Reassure the caller that the concern is valid and will receive the full attention of the right person. Explain when the caller can expect a response from the office and be sure to follow up with the patient.

Unauthorized Inquiry Calls

Some individuals call the provider's office requesting information to which they are not entitled. There are circumstances under which the patient may give permission for information to be released to certain family or even friends. If patients wish to do that, they will need to complete a form that gives the healthcare facility permission to release that information. When someone calls requesting information, the medical assistant should check the record for these permissions. Callers who have not been granted permission to receive the information must be told politely but firmly that such information cannot be provided to them because of privacy laws. Insistent callers should be referred to the office manager or provider.

Sales Calls

Sales calls often are thought of as an interruption to the provider's busy day, but some salespersons may have important information on products, equipment, or services the office uses regularly. Do not disregard salespeople, but do not allow them to monopolize time or telephone lines, either. Keep these calls quick and to the point. Most professional salespeople realize that the provider's and staff's time is extremely valuable, and they respect this. It may be the healthcare facility's policy to give the salesperson an appointment, possibly over the lunch hour, to discuss the new product or service with the provider or office manager. Developing a rapport with representatives of the companies whose products the practice uses frequently may result in a discounted price and the first news of sales and promotions. In turn, these professionals rarely waste the time of office personnel.

CRITICAL THINKING APPLICATION **8.6**

Ashlynn answers the phone. The caller is a pharmaceutical representative who has been visiting the clinic for several months. She cheerfully greets him and asks if he is calling to make an appointment. He states that he wants to make an appointment with Ashlynn—for a date. How should she handle this call? What problems could arise if this was a patient and Ashlynn was to accept the date?

Callers Who Have Difficulty Communicating

Occasionally calls come into the office from patients or family members who have difficulty with the English language. In some cases, English is not the caller's primary language, so the medical assistant must use listening skills to ensure understanding. If a certain language is predominant in the area, the healthcare facility should consider hiring a medical assistant who is **bilingual**. Some patients speak English but have a heavy accent, so you should listen carefully and ask questions to be sure you have understood the person correctly. Many resources are available to assist with translation. The healthcare facility may contract with a translator who would be available to help with telephone calls and patient visits in the office. Many online services also offer translation. If the healthcare facility has a number of patients who speak a specific language other than English, it would be helpful to have a list of commonly used phrases available in that language, especially the phrase that would refer the patient to the specific translation service used by the healthcare facility.

Some providers may have patients who are deaf or hard of hearing. These patients may use a relay system to communicate with healthcare facilities over the telephone. Some relay systems have the patient use a keyboard to enter the information to an operator, who calls the office and reads the information to you; your response is then typed back to the patient. Newer technology uses an online captioned telephone service, much like closed captioning for television. Many smartphones can use a translation app to assist the caller. You should be familiar with the way this system works so that you can engage in these conversations in a professional manner.

TYPICAL OUTGOING CALLS

Most outgoing calls in the healthcare facility are responses to incoming calls. The same rules for courtesy and diction apply to calls made from the office to patients, other individuals, and businesses.

It is helpful to plan outgoing calls in advance. For instance, if the medical assistant is placing an order for office supplies, a list should be made that includes the product, the price, the quantity needed, and a catalog page number, if applicable. Questions about the various products ordered should be noted so that they can be asked while the sales representative is on the telephone.

Some medical assistants find it helpful to make all outgoing calls at once, when possible. This way, the calls can be made one after another, and if a call back is necessary, the medical assistant is likely to still be by the telephone. Organizing calls helps increase office efficiency.

Never be rude to an individual on the telephone. Remember to treat those on the other end of the telephone as you would wish to be treated. Do not forget that you are a representative of the provider and that you must behave in a professional manner at all times.

Time Zones

When making outgoing calls, it is important to keep time zones in mind, especially when calling patients. If you are trying to contact a patient who is spending the winter somewhere else, you should place that call at an appropriate time for the patient. If you are trying to get information from an insurance company, you should call when someone is available to answer your questions. The continental United States is divided into four standard time zones: Pacific, Mountain, Central, and Eastern (Figure 8.4). When it is noon Pacific time, it is 3 p.m. Eastern time. If you are calling from San Francisco to a business or professional office in New York, plan to make the call no later than 1 p.m. When it is 2 p.m. on the West Coast, it is 5 p.m. on the East Coast.

Leaving a Voice Mail for a Patient

When leaving a voice mail for a patient, it is important to protect their confidentiality. We cannot know for sure who is retrieving the voice mail. Many providers insist that messages left on voice mail do not mention the terms *doctor* or *doctor's office* for confidentiality reasons. The message should also *not* include test results or what the appointment is for. The medical assistant might say, "This Pam at Robert Welch's office confirming your appointment tomorrow at 2 p.m. Please call us if you cannot make the appointment. Our number is 555-212-0909. Thank you."

If the patient has signed the privacy policy and the policy states that messages from the provider's office may be left at certain numbers, the office certainly can leave messages at that number and mention the call is from the healthcare facility. Still, it is a good idea to have an established policy on leaving messages that do not breach the patient's confidentiality.

Long-Distance Calling

Long-distance calls are simple to place, usually inexpensive, and efficient. When information is needed in a hurry, telephoning is much more expedient than written communication. Before placing a long-distance call, have the correct number ready. If you do not have the number, you may access directory assistance by dialing 1, then the area code of the party you want to call, followed by 555-1212. In some areas, numbers are available by calling 1-411.

Some internet services, such as Skype, Jajah, or magicJack, allow the user to call long distances, and sometimes even internationally, through the computer with no long-distance charges.

USING DIRECTORY ASSISTANCE

Before placing a telephone call, have the correct number ready. If you do not have the number, you should locate it in one of the following ways.

Locate the Phone Number Using the Telephone

You may access local directory assistance by calling 411. For long-distance numbers, you can access directory assistance by doing the following:

- Dialing 1
- Entering the area code of the party you want to call
- Then entering 555-1212

Directory assistance is now an automated service in many regions. You will be asked for the name of the city and the person you

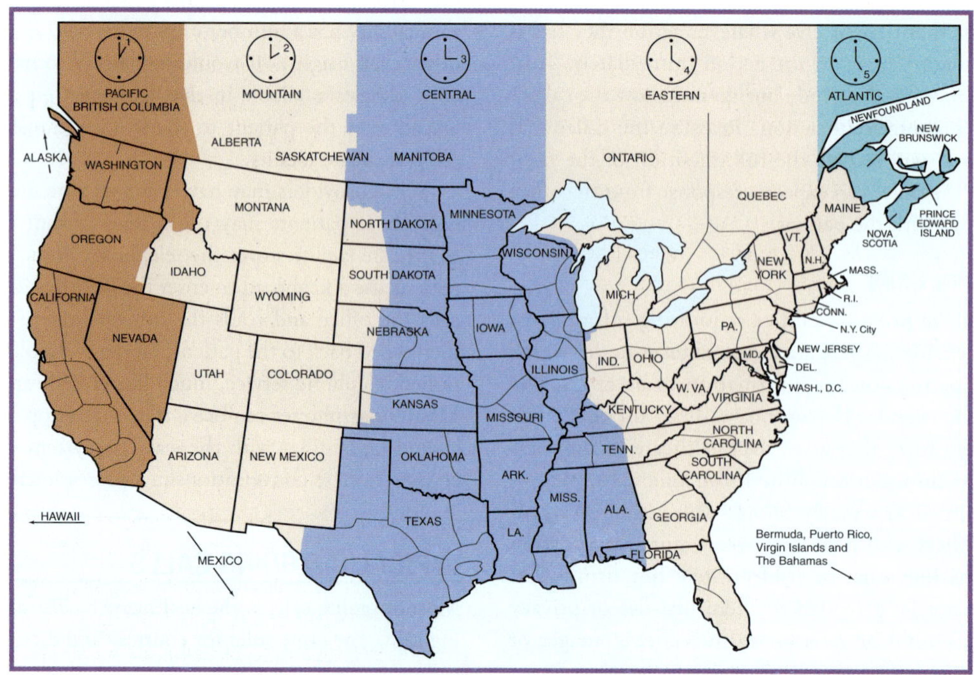

FIGURE 8.4 Time zones across the United States.

are calling. Often a fee is charged for using directory assistance, so, whenever possible, look for the telephone number using free sources.

Locate the Phone Number Using Print or Online Resources

A telephone directory would be one free source for obtaining telephone numbers. This directory is a list of those who have telephones, their telephone numbers, and, in most cases, their addresses. The Yellow Pages contain listings for businesses. Directories are found on the internet and in print format.

The internet makes searching for telephone numbers much easier. Try to find telephone numbers through websites such as www.yellowpages.com or www.whitepages.com, or use a printed telephone book to avoid directory assistance charges on the monthly phone bill. A Web search for the business or provider needed may give you the information. Companies with websites usually have a "Contact Us" page that directs users to the individual departments.

In a print telephone directory, color coding is often used to differentiate between residence listings and business listings. Governmental offices usually have their own section (commonly in blue). Some print directories include zip code maps for the local area.

TELEPHONE SERVICES

If an emergency arises, patients expect to be able to contact their provider. This means that the telephone in the healthcare facility must be answered at all times, day and night, on weekends and holidays. During normal office hours, the medical assistant is available to answer the telephone. After office hours, most healthcare facilities use an answering service or an answering machine that directs the caller to the answering service if there is an urgent issue.

Answering Services

With an answering service, a person answers the call, which can be comforting for patients. The staff at the answering service can act as a buffer for the provider after hours by screening the calls. By following the criteria given to them by the healthcare facility, they can determine whether the provider (or on-call person) should be contacted, the patient should be directed to the hospital emergency department, or whether a message can be taken and relayed to the healthcare facility in the morning.

It is common courtesy to call the answering service in the morning to let them know that you will be answering the calls and to retrieve any messages taken overnight or over the weekend. You should also call the answering service when you are leaving for the day. Answering services also can be used to cover the telephone if all staff members need to be away from the telephones at the same time during the usual working hours.

Automatic Call Routing

Many healthcare facilities have started using an **automatic call routing** system. Callers are given a menu of choices; they then press a number on the telephone keypad to direct the call to the correct department. This can be an efficient way to handle a large volume of calls, but it can also be frustrating for some patients, especially older adults who may have trouble hearing and remembering the options. Some of the frustration can be minimized by providing a number option that connects the caller with a person (e.g., "Press 0"), who can then transfer the call to the appropriate department.

CRITICAL THINKING APPLICATION 8.7

Ashlynn has had many complaints from patients about the new call routing system because it takes so long to "get to a human being." How can she help make modern call routing systems easier for her patients?

CLOSING COMMENTS

Patient Coaching

Today's telephone systems allow providers to educate patients while they are on hold; recordings may be played that offer health information on subjects from A to Z. These messages can be professionally recorded or custom designed by the provider and staff. Special events may be announced, with the option to press a certain number for more information about the event.

Legal and Ethical Issues

The guidelines for medical confidentiality apply equally to telephone conversations; therefore, take care that no one overhears sensitive information. Use discretion when mentioning the name of the caller or patient.

Do not place or receive personal phone calls during work hours. Time limitations for personal phone use should be described in the office policies and procedures manual. The telephone is a business line and should be reserved for patients and others conducting business with the office. Personal cell phones also should not be used during working hours; this takes the medical assistant's time and attention away from patient care.

Telephone message records may be brought into court as evidence; make sure all messages are complete and legible. Most offices should keep these records for at least the same period as the statute of limitations in that state.

Patient-Centered Care

When answering the telephone in a healthcare facility, the medical assistant has many opportunities to provide patient-centered care. First, you should respect the patients' preferences. This could be using the patients' cell phone numbers for returning calls or using their preferred name or nickname when talking with them. Second, telephone communication is a big part of the coordination of care. Remaining professional in all interactions will ensure that the patient's needs will be met.

Professional Behaviors

We have talked on telephones and cell phones in our own lives, and most of us have used at least some of the special features on our phones. It is important to recognize that the way we present ourselves on the phone in our professional lives is different from the style of communication we use in our personal lives. The way we speak in our personal lives may not be appropriate in the healthcare facility. We must maintain a professional tone in communications with our patients and other contacts. For example, slang should not be used; "Hello" is not a proper way to answer a business telephone; and we must take care how we use medical terminology when on the telephone (jargon should not be used when speaking with patients). The goal is always to present a positive professional image of the healthcare facility we represent.

SUMMARY OF SCENARIO

Ashlynn is quickly becoming a part of the team at WMFM and is developing into a well-liked asset to the staff. She has learned to slow down when speaking on the phone and adjust her volume and pitch, depending on the patient with whom she is speaking. Although she tends to be quite talkative, she is balancing just the right amount of friendly chatter with the business at hand. She does this by offering a friendly greeting to callers, getting to the point of the call, then being affable before ending the call. By expressing her concern and asking how she can be of help to the patients, Ashlynn shows them that she sincerely cares about their problems. She is careful about her tone of voice, realizing that patients may take her comments the wrong way if she does not treat them in a cordial manner.

Ashlynn takes care when she speaks to patients and others on the phone so that she does not breach confidentiality in any way. She has become comfortable with the way she is expected to answer the telephone. The pace of her speech and the wording are now a habit. Ashlynn is determined to maintain a professional relationship with all the people related to her work environment. She is now adept at handling calls from angry patients and can maintain control with even the most aggressive callers. She leaves callers on hold for a minimum time and reassures them frequently that she is attending to their situation. By treating callers as she would want to be treated, Ashlynn reduces frustration, and she feels that the office is more efficient at handling the large volume of calls that come in each day. She shows much promise for a long and rewarding career in the medical field and is satisfied with the current track of her career. As she continues to settle into her position, she looks forward to learning more about efficiency and time management. Her positive attitude and desire to learn will only enhance her performance at work, making her a valuable employee and one worth promoting.

SUMMARY OF LEARNING OBJECTIVES

1. **Explain the features of a multiple-line telephone system and cell phones, and describe how each can be used effectively in a healthcare facility.**

   A multiple-line telephone system has many features; most obviously, more than one telephone line comes into the office. This means that callers are less likely to get a busy signal when calling the healthcare facility. Additional features, such as speed dial, voice mail, and call forwarding, can increase efficiency.

   Medical assistants must understand how each feature of the telephone system works. For example, knowing when to use the speakerphone function and when not to use it helps protect patient confidentiality. Knowing how to use the conference call feature facilitates telephone meetings with satellite offices. Understanding how the voice mail system works is crucial to the medical assistant's work life.

   Many people have a personal cell phone or a smartphone. Although it is great to be accessible at all times, cell phones also present some issues in a healthcare facility, particularly in regard to patient confidentiality.

2. **Determine the impact of active listening and telephone personality on telephone communication.**

   A big part of communication is being able to listen. Honing your active listening skills also will increase your communication skills. Focus on the conversation by being present in the moment. Not only is interrupting rude, but it also shows that you were not listening, truly listening, because you were coming up with your response. Part of active listening is confirming what you heard to be sure that you have received the intended message.

   Medical assistants should answer the telephone promptly and professionally. A pleasing telephone personality conveys a favorable impression of the healthcare facility. Enunciate, pronouncing words clearly and distinctly. Vary the pitch of your voice and avoid a monotonous or droning manner. Courtesy to patients and other callers is vital. First impressions are important, and a medical assistant's telephone manner sets the tone for the caller's perception of the healthcare facility. Be courteous and polite to all callers. (Refer to Procedure 8.1.)

   Tone of voice can completely change the message sent. Make sure you use the correct tone of voice, so the message is not misunderstood. Enunciation also ensures that your message is not misunderstood. Communicating over the telephone has its own issues, and enunciation is crucial. Speaking clearly helps the caller to hear your message.

3. **Determine the importance of thinking ahead when managing telephone calls and the correct way to answer the telephone in the office.**

   Before you start answering calls, make sure you have all the supplies you need to do your job. Confidentiality in a healthcare facility must always be a priority.

   Medical assistants should answer the telephone promptly and professionally. The provider's image is affected by the way telephone calls are handled. Be courteous and polite to all callers. Medical assistants should identify the facility first when picking up the phone, state their name, and then offer help. If the caller does not offer a name, the medical assistant should ask who is calling.

   When working with a multiple-line telephone, it is important to know how to deal with more than one call at a time. When you are on a call and the other line rings, you need to place the first call on hold, answer the second call, determine whether or not it is an emergency (and follow proper protocol), and then return to the first call. During the screening process, the medical assistant may determine that the call should be transferred to the provider or another person in the facility. Know who does what in your healthcare facility.

   Most healthcare facilities expect the medical assistant answering the telephone to screen the calls; this is an important task. The facility's screening policies should address how calls should be handled when the

SUMMARY OF LEARNING OBJECTIVES—*continued*

provider is out of the office, and the medical assistant should always ask before placing a caller on hold or transferring a call.

If a phone call is an emergency, the policies for handling emergency calls apply. Ask for a phone number where the caller can be reached in case of a sudden disconnection. Ask about the chief symptoms and when they started. Find out whether the patient has had similar symptoms in the past and what happened in that situation. Determine whether the patient is alone, has transportation, or needs an ambulance. In severe cases, do not hang up the phone until the ambulance or police arrive. A special sheet of instructions listing specific medical emergencies (e.g., chest pain, heavy bleeding, seizure, fainting, poisoning) should be posted by each telephone.

When taking a telephone message, either in a handwritten or an electronic format, strive for accuracy. Be sure to get all the information the provider will need to act. Repeat any words or numbers that are not heard clearly. (Refer to Procedure 8.2.)

The seven elements of a correctly handled phone message are (1) the name of the person to whom the call should be directed; (2) the name of the person calling; (3) the caller's telephone number; (4) the reason for the call; (5) the medical assistant's description of the action to be taken; (6) the date and time of the call; and (7) the initials of the person taking the call, so if any question arises that person can be consulted.

If a handwritten system is used for recording telephone messages, a policy must be developed on the retention of the telephone message records. Accurate records can ensure quality patient care and customer service. (Refer to Procedure 8.2.)

4. **Determine the various types of common incoming calls and how to deal with each type.**
Knowing how to respond to the different types of calls received will make you a valuable asset to the healthcare facility. Common types of incoming calls include the following: requests for directions, inquiries about bills, inquiries about fees, inquiries about participating providers, requests for assistance with insurance, inquiries about radiology and laboratory reports, progress reports, routine report calls from hospitals or other sources, requests for a referral, and questions about office administration matters.
5. **Determine various types of special incoming calls and how to deal with each type.**
If a patient refuses to discuss symptoms with a medical assistant, the assistant should follow the healthcare facility's policies and procedures, which may suggest that the patient make an appointment with the provider to discuss the problem in person. Other types of special calls a medical assistant must know how to handle include unsatisfactory progress reports, requests for test results, requests for information from third parties, complaints about care or fees, and calls from a staff member's family or friends.
6. **Explain how the medical assistant should handle various types of difficult calls.**
If a caller becomes angry, never return the anger. Remain calm and speak in tones that are perhaps slightly quieter than those of the caller. This often prompts callers to lower their tone of voice. Offer to help the angry person, and ask questions to gain control of the conversation, moving it toward resolution. Do not argue with angry callers.

   Callers who have a complaint should be handled in a manner similar to that used for angry callers. The medical assistant should remain calm and offer to help. Take a serious interest in what the caller has to say. Let all callers know that their concerns are important to the staff and the provider. Find the source of the problem, and determine exactly what the caller wants or expects as a resolution. Always follow up on complaints and make sure they were resolved to the caller's satisfaction as much as possible.
7. **Discuss typical outgoing calls, including why knowledge of time zones and long-distance calling is necessary.**
Most outgoing calls in the healthcare facility are made in response to incoming calls. It is helpful to plan outgoing calls in advance. Organizing calls help increase office efficiency.

   The continental United States is divided into four standard time zones. Long-distance calls are simple to place, usually inexpensive, and efficient. Knowledge of both concepts is important for a medical assistant handling the telephone.
8. **Explain the use of a telephone directory.**
The primary purpose of a telephone directory is to provide lists of those who have telephones, their telephone numbers, and, in most cases, their addresses. The internet makes searching for telephone numbers much easier.
9. **Examine how answering services and automatic call routing systems are used in a healthcare facility.**
Answering services are used to answer the telephone in the healthcare facility when the staff is not available. This could be during overnight hours or regular office hours when the staff is at lunch or in a meeting. Automatic call routing systems allow the patient to select a number from a menu to reach specific departments in the healthcare facility. The system should have an option that allows patients to choose to speak to a person if they are not sure what number to press.

PROCEDURE 8.1 Demonstrate Professional Telephone Techniques

TASK: Answer the telephone in a provider's office in a professional manner and respond to a request for action.

SCENARIO: Charles Johnson, DOB 3/3/19XX, an established patient of Dr. Martin, has called to schedule an appointment to have his blood pressure checked. This will be a follow-up appointment that is 15 minutes long. He is requesting that the appointment be on a Friday during his lunchtime between 11 a.m. and noon.

EQUIPMENT and SUPPLIES

- Telephone
- Pen or pencil
- Appointment book or EHR with appointment scheduling abilities
- Computer
- Notepad

PROCEDURAL STEPS

1. Demonstrate telephone techniques by answering the telephone by the third ring.
   PURPOSE: Answering the call promptly conveys interest in the caller. This makes a positive impression on the caller.
2. Speak distinctly, with a pleasant tone and expression, at a moderate rate, and with sufficient volume for the person to understand every word.
   PURPOSE: Proper enunciation will help the patient to understand.
3. Identify the office or provider and yourself.
   PURPOSE: To assure the caller that the correct number has been reached and identify the staff member.
4. Verify the identity of the caller, and if using an electronic health record, bring the patient's health record to the active screen of the computer.
   PURPOSE: To confirm the origin of the call.
5. Screen the call if necessary.
   PURPOSE: To determine whether the caller has an emergency and needs immediate attention or referral to a hospital emergency department.
6. Apply active listening skills to assess whether the caller is distressed or agitated and determine the concern to be addressed.
   PURPOSE: To make sure the medical assistant hears and understands the message being sent by the patient and to show that the patient has the medical assistant's full attention.
7. Determine the caller's needs and provide the requested information or service, if possible. Provide the caller with excellent customer service. Be as helpful as possible. Check the appointment schedule and determine the first Friday that would have an open appointment between 11 a.m. and noon.
   PURPOSE: To allow the medical assistant to handle many calls and conserve the provider's and staff members' time and energy.
8. Obtain sufficient patient information to schedule the appointment, including the patient's full name, DOB, insurance information, and preferred contact method. Repeat the date and time of the appointment to ensure that the patient has the correct information.
   PURPOSE: By obtaining the correct patient information, the correct patient record will be pulled (if paper records are used) for the appointment. In an EHR, the appointment will be attached to the correct patient record.
9. Terminate the call in a pleasant manner and replace the receiver gently, always allowing the caller to hang up first.
   PURPOSE: To promote good public relations, provide excellent customer service, and ensure that the caller has no further questions.

PROCEDURE 8.2 Document Telephone Messages and Report Relevant Information Concisely and Accurately

TASK: Take an accurate telephone message and follow up on the caller's requests.

SCENARIO: Norma Washington, DOB 8/1/19XX, an established patient of Dr. Martin, has called to report her blood pressure (BP) readings that she has been taking at home. Dr. Martin had made a recent change to her medication and wanted her to monitor her BP at home for 3 days and call in with the results. She has taken her blood pressure in the morning and evening for the past 3 days, with the following results:

Day 1: 144/92 in the am, 156/94 in the pm
Day 2: 136/84 in the am, 142/86 in the pm
Day 3: 132/80 in the am, 138/82 in the pm

EQUIPMENT and SUPPLIES

- Telephone
- Computer
- Message pad
- Pen or pencil
- Notepad
- Health record

PROCEDURAL STEPS

1. Demonstrate telephone techniques by answering the telephone using the guidelines presented in Procedure 8.1.
   PURPOSE: Answering promptly and courteously conveys interest in the caller and promotes good customer service.
2. Using a message pad or the computer, take the phone message (either on paper or by data entry into the computer) and obtain the following information:
   - Name of the person to whom the call is directed
   - Name of the person calling
   - Caller's telephone number

PROCEDURE 8.2 Document Telephone Messages and Report Relevant Information Concisely and Accurately—*continued*

- Reason for the call
- Action to be taken
- Date and time of the call
- Initials of the person taking the call

PURPOSE: To have accurate information, which allows the staff member or provider to address the caller's issues quickly and efficiently.

3. Apply active listening skills and repeat the information back to the caller after recording the message.
   PURPOSE: To verify that all the information was recorded accurately.
4. End the call and wait for the caller to hang up first.
5. Document the telephone call with all pertinent information in the patient's health record.
   PURPOSE: To ensure that the patient's health record is kept up to date.
6. Deliver the phone message to the appropriate person.
7. Follow up on important messages.
   PURPOSE: To make sure important issues are addressed in a timely manner.
8. If using paper messaging, keep old message books for future reference. Carbonless copies allow the facility to keep a permanent record of phone messages. If using an electronic system, the message will be saved to the patient's record automatically.
   PURPOSE: To have a permanent source of messages in case the information is needed after the paper message has been discarded. This can also serve as a telephone log.
9. File pertinent phone messages in the patient's health record. Make sure the computer record is closed after the information has been documented.
   PURPOSE: To keep a permanent record of important information in the patient's chart.

SCHEDULING APPOINTMENTS AND PATIENT PROCESSING

9

SCENARIO

Ramona West is the medical assistant in charge of scheduling appointments and patient processing for Dr. Angela Perez at Walden-Martin Family Medical (WMFM) Clinic. Ramona is an extremely organized person who thinks quickly and creatively. Two of her professional goals are to ensure that the healthcare facility remains on schedule throughout the day with minimal wait time for the patients and to see to it that patient flow through the office is done in an efficient manner. She is fortunate that Dr. Perez is cooperative and time oriented, and they work well together to reach these common goals.

Ramona usually arrives at work at least 15 minutes early to begin her preparations for the day. She reviews the electronic health record for each patient to make sure test results from previous visits are available to the provider and that the medical record is complete. She pays special attention to the patients who arrive in the healthcare facility as she completes her daily tasks, remembering the importance of providing patients with good customer service. Ramona greets each patient by name and carries on a brief but cordial conversation. Patients appreciate that she goes the extra mile to remember something about them, and this promotes excellent patient relations.

Ramona leaves a little time in the morning and afternoon for emergency appointments. The healthcare facility uses an automatic call routing system to contact patients to confirm appointments in advance, which increases her show rate. She is always pleasant to the patients as they go through the check-in and checkout procedures. Her friendly, caring attitude makes her a favorite among the patients, and Dr. Perez is pleased with the relationship-building skills Ramona has developed.

While studying this chapter, think about the following questions:

- How can the medical assistant contribute to an efficient daily routine?
- How does the medical assistant contribute to keeping the daily schedule on track?
- How can the schedule be put back on track when emergencies disrupt the day?
- How does the flexibility of the medical assistant contribute to office efficiency?
- What are some ways to develop good rapport with patients?
- Why is a sign-in register a potential breach of patient confidentiality?
- What is the value of knowing some information about patients' personal lives?

LEARNING OBJECTIVES

1. Describe the guidelines for establishing an appointment schedule.
2. Explain the guidelines for establishing an appointment matrix.
3. Discuss methods of scheduling appointments.
4. Discuss the legality of the appointment scheduling system.
5. Discuss pros and cons of various types of appointment management systems.
6. Discuss the process for scheduling new and established patients.
7. Explain how the medical assistant should handle scheduling of other types of appointments.
8. Examine methods of dealing with special circumstances in scheduling.
9. Discuss methods to increase appointment show rates.
10. Explain how to handle cancellations and delays.
11. Describe how to prepare for patients' arrivals, including patient check-in procedures.

VOCABULARY

demographics Statistical data of a population. In healthcare, this includes the patient's name, address, date of birth, employment, and other details.

disruption An unexpected event that throws a plan into disorder; an interruption that prevents a system or process from continuing as usual or as expected.

established patient A patient who has been treated by the healthcare provider within the past 3 years.

expediency (ik SPEE dee uhn see) A means of achieving a particular end, as in a situation requiring urgency or caution.

follow-up (recheck) appointment An appointment type used when a patient needs to see the provider after a condition should have been resolved or to monitor an ongoing condition, such as hypertension. Also known as a recheck appointment.

integral (IN ti gruhl) Essential; being an indispensable part of a whole.

interval Space of time between events.

matrix (MEY triks) The environment in which something is created or takes shape. A base on which to build.

VOCABULARY—*continued*

no-show Failure of a patient to keep an appointment without advance notice.

Notice of Privacy Practices (NPP) A written document describing the healthcare facility's privacy practices. The patient must be provided with the NPP and sign an acknowledgment of receipt.

parameters (puh RAM it ers) Rules that control how something should be done; guidelines or boundaries.

patient portal A secure online website that gives patients 24-hour access to personal health information using a username and password.

practice management software A type of software that allows the user to enter demographic information, schedule appointments, maintain lists of insurance payers, perform billing tasks, and generate reports.

preauthorization A process required by some insurance carriers in which the provider obtains permission to perform certain procedures or services or refers a patient to a specialist.

precertification The process of determining if a procedure or service is covered by the insurance plan and what the reimbursement is for that procedure or service.

proficiency (pruh FISH uhn see) Skilled as a result of training or practice.

progress notes Documentation in the medical record to track the patient's condition and progress.

screening A system for examining and separating into different groups; in the healthcare facility, it means determining the severity of illness that patients experience and prioritizing appointments based on that severity.

triage (tree AHZH) To sort out and classify the injured; used in the military and emergency settings to determine the priority of patients to be treated.

verification of eligibility The process of confirming health insurance coverage for the patient.

INTRODUCTION

The provider's time is the most valuable asset of a medical practice. The person responsible for scheduling this time must understand the practice, be familiar with the working habits and preferences of the provider (or providers), and have clear guidelines for time management in the practice.

Appointment scheduling is the process that determines which patients the provider sees, the dates and times of appointments, and how much time is allotted to each patient based on the complaint and the provider's availability. Time management involves the realization that unforeseen interruptions and delays always occur and must be handled appropriately. In addition, the medical assistant must assign the appropriate appointment time length for the complaint, along with ensuring that the appointments are coordinated so that there are minimal gaps in the schedule. Most healthcare providers find that efficient appointment scheduling is one of the most important factors in the success of the practice. Scheduling can be done in a number of ways, and each facility must find the way that suits it best.

ESTABLISHING THE APPOINTMENT SCHEDULE

Developing a schedule that meets the needs of both the providers and the patients is the key to keeping the office running smoothly and efficiently. The scheduling team, along with the provider, should come up with scheduling **parameters**, both to meet the needs of the patients and to keep the providers' preferences and habits in mind.

Patient Needs

Consider the **demographics** of the patients when determining office hours and appointment times. The staff should answer the following questions:

- Is the office in a busy metropolitan area or a rural community?
- What type of patients are seen? Are they of a specific age or gender? Do they have common diagnoses? Is the provider a general practitioner?
- Are evening and weekend appointments needed for most of the patients served?

Knowing when the providers need to be available for patients is one of the factors involved in creating the patient schedule.

Provider Preferences and Habits

Consider the preferences and habits of the providers in the practice before establishing and implementing a scheduling plan. Ask the following questions:

- Does the provider become restless if the reception room is not packed with waiting patients?
- Does the provider worry if even one patient is kept waiting?
- Is the provider careful about being in the facility when patient appointments are scheduled to begin?
- Is the provider habitually late?
- Does the provider move easily from one patient to another?
- Does the provider require a break time after a few patients?
- Would the provider rather see fewer patients and spend more time with each one or schedule more patients each day?

All of these preferences and habits become an **integral** part of the scheduling process. Keep in mind that the provider cannot spend every moment of the day with patients. The provider also has telephone calls to make and receive, reports to examine and dictate, meetings to attend, mail to answer, and many other business responsibilities. An experienced staff can handle many but not all of these tasks.

Next, the office hours and the length of appointment time **intervals** need to be determined. Keeping in mind patients' needs and the provider's preferences and habits, decide what would be the shortest time possible for an appointment. Most healthcare facilities use 10- or 15-minute time intervals for the appointment schedule. Paper-based appointment books can be purchased with various time intervals. A computerized appointment system can also be set to the specific time interval that has been decided on. A computerized system can be customized for different providers so that one provider could have 10-minute time slots and another could have 15-minute time slots. If an appointment, such as a complete physical, needs longer than 15 minutes, multiple time slots are used to cover that appointment. Once the minimum time period has been set, then the appointment **matrix** can be established.

CREATING THE APPOINTMENT MATRIX

Setting up the appointment matrix (Procedure 9.1) involves blocking out the times during which the provider is not available to see patients (Figure 9.1), such as these:

- Lunchtime
- Hospital rounds
- Conferences
- Vacation

In a paper-based appointment book, the matrix is usually established for 6 months at a time. In a computerized system, the matrix can be set up indefinitely.

Establishing Guidelines for Appointment Scheduling

The first step in setting up the schedule matrix is to decide the length of the shortest office visit type. This visit type would usually be for a **follow-up** or **recheck appointment** for an established patient. Other specific appointment types should then be determined. General categories for appointment types are as follows:

- Follow-up or recheck
- Wellness examination
- Complete physical examination
- Urgent visit
- New patient visit
- Comprehensive visit

Each category has a specific amount of time assigned to it; for example, a follow-up or recheck appointment could be 10 to 15 minutes, and a comprehensive visit could be 30 to 40 minutes. The providers and scheduling team should work together to come up with these time periods to ensure that the office runs smoothly and efficiently. The shortest appointment time will be one line or block on the schedule. If an appointment is going to be longer than that time, multiple lines or blocks would be used. In Figure 9.1 each line on the schedule is for 15 minutes. Hospital rounds for Dr. Julie Walden are scheduled for 1 hour, or four lines. In this example, if a patient is being seen for a recheck appointment (15 minutes), only one line would be used. If the patient were being seen for a comprehensive visit (30 minutes), two lines would be used. In a paper appointment book, you may need to put arrows or a line through the additional appointment time so that another patient is not scheduled during that time (Figure 9.2).

If it is decided that a complete physical examination should be scheduled for 30 minutes, yet the provider routinely spends 45 minutes with the patient for a complete physical, then the scheduling guidelines need to be adjusted. Well-planned scheduling and sticking to that schedule allow the provider to do more than run in and out of examination rooms with little time for the patient to talk with the provider. There will be a bit of trial and error when developing the priorities for the appointment schedule.

Some providers need prompting to end the patient visit and move to the next patient. If there is a medical assistant in the examination

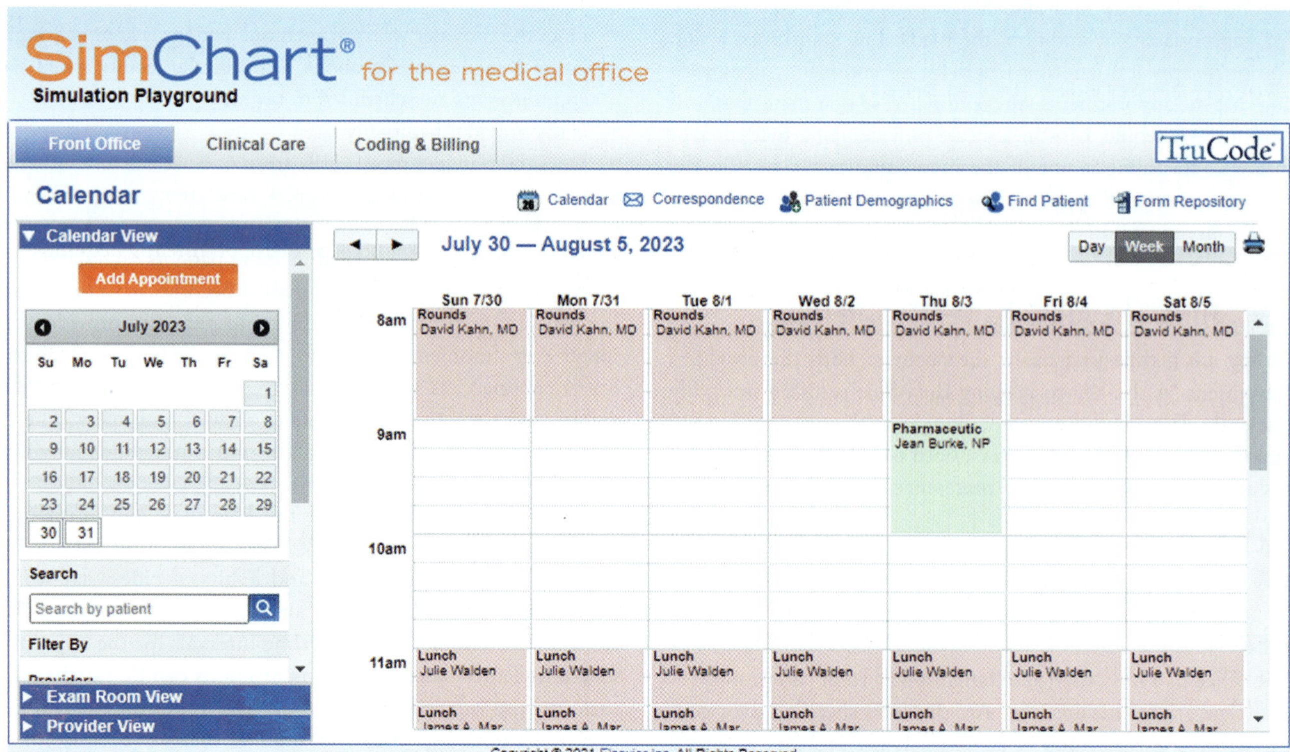

FIGURE 9.1 Schedule matrix showing provider availability.

	Monday	Tuesday	Wednesday	Thursday	Friday
8:00					
8:15					
8:30		Celia Tapia PE			
8:45		⬇			
9:00	Truong Tran Recheck				
9:15					
9:30					
9:45					
10:00					

FIGURE 9.2 Blocking off time on the appointment schedule.

room, he or she can help the provider remain on schedule by letting the provider know that the end of the appointment time is near. Some type of signal may be worked out, such as a hand gesture or phrase. A pager may be used when the medical assistant is not in room with the provider. When the provider's pager vibrates, he or she will know that it is time to wind things up with that patient. The clinical medical assistant and the administrative medical assistant must work together to keep the healthcare facility running smoothly and efficiently.

CRITICAL THINKING APPLICATION 9.1

Ramona has noticed that Dr. Perez is taking a little longer with patients than normal and that she is running consistently behind schedule by approximately 5 to 15 minutes. How can Ramona help rectify this situation?

Discuss ways of approaching the provider when he or she is the cause of the delays in the schedule. What opening remarks can the medical assistant use to start the discussion in a positive way?

Available Facilities

Another factor to keep in mind when scheduling appointments is the availability of facilities needed for a specific appointment type. Getting a patient into the office at a time when no room or equipment is available for the services needed is a waste of the patient's time. For example, suppose that a healthcare facility with two providers has only one room that can be used for minor surgery. Do not schedule two patients needing minor surgery for the same day and time, even if both doctors could be available. If the healthcare facility has only one electrocardiograph, do not book two electrocardiograms (ECGs) at the same time. As the medical assistant gains **proficiency** in scheduling, it becomes easier to match patient needs with the available facilities. Major equipment frequently used or a certain room with such equipment may need its own scheduling column in the appointment book or software system.

METHODS OF SCHEDULING APPOINTMENTS

There are two common methods of appointment scheduling:

- Computerized scheduling
- Appointment book or paper-based scheduling

Each has advantages and disadvantages. The healthcare facility should weigh the benefits and choose the method that best suits the provider and the staff.

Computerized Scheduling

The computer has replaced the appointment book in most practices. **Practice management software** ranges from relatively simple programs that merely display available and scheduled times to more sophisticated systems that perform several other functions. Information such as the following can be entered into the computer program:

- The length and type of appointment required
- The patient's day or time preferences

The computer then can select the best appointment time based on that information.

A computerized scheduling system also has the ability to search for future appointments. For example, when a patient calls and asks about a previously scheduled appointment, the system can search by the patient's name to find the time and date. Computerized scheduling allows multiple users to access the schedule at the same time, minimizing the wait time for patients.

Another advantage of computerized schedules is that reports can be generated. A hard copy of the provider's daily schedule can be created that shows the following details:

- Patients' names
- Telephone numbers
- Reasons for the visits

Some healthcare facilities print these out, and others use them on-screen. Healthcare facilities must have scheduling procedures to follow when the technology is down.

Self-Scheduling

Allowing patients to schedule their own appointments using the internet and the healthcare facility's website is becoming much more common. The patient is given limited access to the schedule, seeing only the available appointment times, not the other patients who are scheduled.

Software is available that allows the patient to self-schedule through secure links to the provider's appointment book. The software or internet site for the healthcare facility should give the patient guidelines as to the amount of time needed for certain appointments or should allow only a certain length of time to be self-scheduled, such as 15 minutes. These systems will reduce the number of calls and are available to the patient 24 hours a day. Some systems also send an automatic email reminder to the patient the day before the appointment, requesting a reply to confirm. These systems are less frustrating to patients, who do not have to wait on hold to speak to the person who does scheduling for the healthcare facility. However, lengthy or complicated appointments should be scheduled through the staff.

Although this type of system for making appointments appeals to most technologically savvy people, some patients may not be comfortable using it. It does require minimal skills and internet access. Others may object to online scheduling because they do not want their names anywhere on the internet. This is a valid concern, and the facility should allow these patients to schedule over the telephone. If this system is used, some allowance must be made for patients who choose not to use it.

Appointment Book Scheduling

Office suppliers carry a variety of appointment book styles. Some appointment books show an entire week at a glance; many are color coded, with a special color used for each day of the week (Figure 9.3). This is very helpful when the provider asks the patient to return, for instance, in 2 weeks. If Wednesdays are colored yellow, the medical assistant can flip quickly to the correct day 2 weeks later and schedule the appointment. Multiple columns may be available to correspond with the number of doctors in a group practice, and the time can be divided according to their preferences.

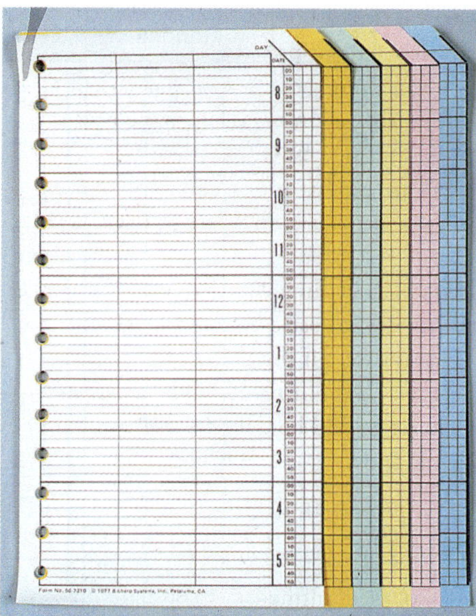

FIGURE 9.3 Color-coded appointment book pages help the medical assistant flip to the right day of the right week quickly. Appointments for multiple providers can be color coded in the book.

CRITICAL THINKING APPLICATION **9.2**

The software used at WMFM can allow patients to self-schedule. Ramona has heard about patient self-scheduling and would like to try this method in the office, but Dr. Perez is concerned that her patients will miss the personal contact and is not sold on the idea. What can Ramona say to convince Dr. Perez to try this new, time-saving method of scheduling? What challenges might the use of this system bring?

LEGALITY OF THE APPOINTMENT SCHEDULING SYSTEM

Because the paper-based appointment book can be used as a legal record, it must be accurate and maintained so that it provides correct information about the patients at the healthcare facility. Patients are expected to follow the provider's orders; this includes keeping appointments. If a patient does not show up for an appointment or cancels it and does not reschedule, this fact should be documented in the patient's health record. If a patient reschedules an appointment and subsequently keeps it, there is no need to document that it was rescheduled.

Pens are permanent, and the appointment book can become illegible if a number of patients change or cancel their appointments. To make changes to an appointment book easier, pencil should be used. The information in the book includes the patient's name and a phone number where the patient can be reached. Some healthcare facilities list the reason for the appointment, but most note only the name and phone number. Listing the reason for the visit is not necessary if the medical assistant references the time needed for the appointment and blocks off that amount of time. Because the appointment book could be evidence as a legal record, it should be kept for the number of years that constitute the statute of limitations in that individual state. If the appointment book is discarded, its contents should be shredded to protect patient privacy.

Although the appointment book can be used as a legal record, actual medical records are more likely to be used in matters of litigation. Because **progress notes** are dated, a copy of the medical record shows all pertinent information about the patient's adherence to the provider's orders, including the appointments with the provider.

Computerized scheduling systems can also be used to track patient appointments. Most computerized scheduling systems will allow the user to indicate if the patient has checked in, canceled, or missed the scheduled appointment. When a patient misses or cancels an appointment, it should be documented in the electronic patient record for legal purposes.

TYPES OF APPOINTMENT SCHEDULING

Different types of appointment scheduling are used to meet the various needs of the medical facility, the providers, and the patients. Some offices use a combination of methods to create the right mix of activity during the day and to ensure that the day runs smoothly and efficiently. The medical assistant should become proficient at managing appointments. The following section presents several methods of appointment scheduling.

No matter what appointment scheduling method is used, the medical assistant should make it a policy to leave some open time during each day's schedule. This is so that if a patient calls with a special problem that is not an immediate emergency, time will be available to book the patient for at least a brief visit. Mondays and Fridays generally are the most hectic days of the week. Keeping a time slot available in the morning and the afternoon specifically for emergencies also is a wise practice. A busy provider always fills these open slots, and having them in the schedule causes the least **disruption** during the day. If possible, set aside time in the morning and afternoon for a break. Even 15 minutes can give the provider time to return calls from patients, verify prescription calls, or answer questions.

Time-Specified (Stream) Scheduling

When each patient is given a specific time for an appointment, this is referred to as *time-specified* or *stream scheduling.* This method keeps a steady flow of patients moving through the office. This is the most common type of scheduling used in healthcare facilities. Studies have shown that providers can see more patients with less pressure when patient appointments are scheduled for a specific time slot. The medical assistant who is scheduling patients using this method should know the amount of time needed for each appointment type and keep time slots available for urgent visits.

Wave Scheduling

Wave scheduling is an attempt to create flexibility within each hour. Wave scheduling assumes that the actual time needed for all the patients seen will average out over the course of the day. Instead of scheduling patients at each 15-minute interval, wave scheduling has three patients in the office at the same time. They are then seen in the order of their arrival. This way, one person's late arrival does not disrupt the entire schedule.

Modified Wave Scheduling

The wave schedule can be modified in several ways. For example, one method is to have two patients scheduled to come in at 10 a.m. and a third at 10:30 a.m. This hourly cycle is repeated throughout the day. In another version, patients are scheduled to arrive at given intervals during the first half of the hour, and none are scheduled to arrive during the second half of the hour. This would allow time for urgent or walk-in patients to be seen.

Double-Booking

Booking of two patients to come in at the same time is sometimes used to work in a patient with an acute illness or injury when there are no open appointments. This works out best if one of the patients needs laboratory work or another procedure done before seeing the provider. The provider can see one of the patients while the other one is being prepared.

Open Office Hours

With the open office hours method, the facility is open at given hours, and the patients are told that they can come in at any time. This type of system is often used in an urgent care setting. Patients are then seen in the order in which they arrive, although a patient with an urgent condition may be seen ahead of those who arrived before him or her.

The open office hours system can have many disadvantages. The office may already be crowded when the provider arrives, resulting in an extremely long wait for some patients. Patients may arrive in waves throughout the day, which causes parts of the day to be very busy and other parts to be slow. This makes accomplishing other office duties difficult. Without planning, the facilities and staff can be overburdened.

CRITICAL THINKING APPLICATION 9.3

Dr. Perez would like to implement evening appointments one night each week and open the office every other Saturday morning. She feels this will better serve her patients with children who have difficulty making daytime appointments. If this is her primary goal, should other types of patients be seen during these time slots? Why or why not?

Grouping Procedures

Grouping, or categorizing, of procedures is another method of scheduling that appeals to many providers. For instance, an internist might reserve all morning appointments for complete physical examinations, or a pediatrician might keep that time for well-baby visits. A surgeon might devote 1 day each week to seeing only referral patients. Obstetricians often schedule pregnant patients on different days from gynecology patients. The providers and staff can experiment with different groupings until the plan that works best for the practice eventually becomes obvious. In applying a grouping system of appointments, the medical assistant may find it helpful to color-code the sections of the appointment book reserved for specific procedures.

WORKING WITH NEW AND ESTABLISHED PATIENTS TO SCHEDULE AN APPOINTMENT

A pleasant manner and a willingness to help are just as important on the telephone as when meeting patients face to face. This is especially true when making appointments. The telephone contact may be the patient's first impression of the facility. Often the way the appointment scheduling process is handled makes more of an impression than the convenience of the appointment time.

Be especially considerate if the time requested for an appointment is not available. Briefly explain why and offer a different date and time. Comply with the patient's wishes as much as possible, and do not show annoyance if the patient does not understand the scheduling process. Most people, however, understand the need for a well-managed office and are willing to cooperate.

Many offices offer the patient a choice when scheduling the appointment and let the patient decide which option suits him or her best. For example, the following dialogue might take place during the scheduling call:

Medical assistant:	"Mrs. Thomas, Dr. Perez is available to see you in the office next Tuesday or Wednesday, January 6 or 7. Which day is better for you?"
Patient:	"I will be working on Wednesday, so I would like to come in on Tuesday."
Medical assistant:	"Do you prefer a morning or afternoon appointment?"
Patient:	"The afternoon is best for me."
Medical assistant:	"Great. Would 1:30 or 3:30 be a better time?"
Patient:	"I can be there at 1:30."
Medical assistant:	"Then Dr. Perez will see you at 1:30 next Tuesday, January 6. Thank you for calling, Mrs. Thomas. We'll see you then!"

These small courtesies allow patients to have some control of their time. Always repeat the time to reinforce the appointment, and do not hesitate to ask the patient if he or she has a pen ready to jot down the time and date. While repeating the information to the patient, check the appointment book or computer screen to ensure that it was posted correctly. When you schedule appointments over the telephone, it is not possible to provide a reminder card for the appointment. Be sure to ask if the patient would like a telephone call, email, or text message reminder of the appointment.

Write legibly when using an appointment book. These records could be called into court, and the medical assistant must be able to read his or her own writing if asked to testify. The patient's daytime telephone number should be recorded for every appointment scheduled. The appointment may need to be canceled or the schedule rearranged in a hurry, and many precious minutes can be saved if the telephone number is handy. Cell phone numbers also are quite useful for quickly tracking down a patient.

Scheduling Appointments for New Patients

Arranging the first appointment for a new patient requires time and attention to detail (Procedure 9.2). This encounter provides the first impression of the healthcare facility and may set the tone for all subsequent visits. Tact, courtesy, and professionalism are extremely important. You will need to obtain information about the *chief complaint* (why the patient needs the appointment). This information will be used to determine how much time to allow for the visit. The provider may also expect the medical assistant to give general instructions to patients being seen for specific complaints. For example, the patient may be required to be fasting for certain laboratory tests. The patient's demographic information should be collected during the conversation, including the type of insurance the patient has. Some insurance carriers restrict which providers can be used.

After the necessary information has been collected, offer the patient the first available appointment. Whenever possible, offer a choice between two dates and times. Ask the patient to arrive 15 minutes before the scheduled appointment time to complete any necessary paperwork. Also ask whether he or she knows how to get to the healthcare facility or offer the physical address for those who use a GPS or an internet direction website (e.g., MapQuest). Tell the patient whether any special parking conveniences are available and whether the healthcare facility provides a token or parking validation.

The patient's options for the first payment should also be discussed. If payment is expected at the time of service, inform the patient. The staff should expect patient concerns about the amount of the first bill and should address this issue before the appointment so that there are no surprises or misunderstandings. Before ending the conversation, repeat the appointment date and time, and thank the patient for calling.

Some healthcare facilities mail an information packet/brochure to new patients, especially if the appointment is several days away. With the patient's permission and email address, this information can also be sent via the internet. An ideal tool to use to deliver this information is a new patient brochure (Procedure 9.3). This brochure can be printed with graphics and images to promote a professional impression of the healthcare facility. In addition to the brochure, the packet could include a health history form, the **Notice of Privacy Practices (NPP)**, and release of information form (to obtain records from the patient's previous provider).

If another provider has referred the patient, the medical assistant may need to call the referring provider's office to obtain additional information before the patient's appointment. This information should be printed out and given to the attending provider before the patient arrives. Remember to send a thank-you note to anyone who refers a patient to the facility.

Often, the medical assistant will need to conduct **preauthorization** or **precertification** to determine whether a patient is eligible for treatment or for certain procedures. The office manager must make certain that these procedures are being done and assigns these duties to a specific person(s). More about preauthorization and precertification is included in Chapter 12.

Scheduling Appointments for Established Patients

Scheduling appointments for established patients is a bit different than doing so for a new patient. The next sections discuss how to schedule in-person requests for appointments and also telephone requests.

In Person

Most return appointments for **established patients** are scheduled when the patient is leaving the healthcare facility. A good policy is to have all patients stop by the appointment desk to check out before leaving in case any information is needed from the patient or any outside scheduling must be done. The patient's health record can be reviewed to see whether the provider ordered any laboratory tests or procedures, and these can be scheduled and discussed with the patient. When making a return appointment, follow the same procedures as for scheduling any appointment by phone, offering the patient choices in the day and time slots (Procedure 9.4). If a certain time the patient specifically requests is not available, offer two other choices. Always give the patient an appointment card and any necessary instructions, along with a bright smile. Never forget to provide excellent customer service.

By Telephone

When scheduling an appointment over the telephone, the medical assistant usually only needs to determine when the patient must return and to find a suitable time in the schedule. Established patients do not usually need directions and parking information, unless the office has recently moved. The patient's address, telephone number, and insurance should always be verified and any changes documented in the health record. If an email address or cell phone number is not on file, obtain one so as to have a quick, easy way to notify the patient of appointments and other events.

SCHEDULING OTHER TYPES OF APPOINTMENTS

The medical assistant may also schedule services other than appointments at the healthcare facility, and these will appear on the appointment schedule:

- Surgeries the provider will perform at a hospital or other facility
- Consultations
- Outside appointments and meetings
- Skilled nursing facilities

The provider also must have time to get from one location to another, so driving time must be considered when arranging all appointments.

Some critical information is required when you schedule an admission to or treatments in other facilities. Always provide the facility with the following information:

- Patient's name, address, and phone numbers (both home and cell)
- Social Security number
- Insurance information
- Email address
- Procedures that are to be performed
- Patient's allergies
- Admitting diagnosis
- Provider's orders

Some facilities require a history form before admission. The patient will be required to bring a form of picture identification, such as a state driver's license, and his or her insurance card.

Inpatient Surgeries

- When scheduling a surgery, provide all necessary information and state any special requests the provider may have, such as the following:
- The amount of blood to have available for the patient
- A specific anesthesiologist
- An assistant surgeon
- Specific instruments

The facility may want the patient's insurance information and certainly will want a phone number so that the patient can be contacted before the surgery if necessary. Make sure all this information is available before placing the call.

Outpatient and Inpatient Procedure Appointments

A medical assistant is often asked to arrange laboratory or radiography appointments for patients. Before calling the facility to schedule the appointment, be sure all necessary information is available. Inform the patient of the time and place of the appointment, relay any special instructions, and then note these arrangements in the patient's health record. Some offices make a reminder call to the patient or send a reminder email or text message.

Outpatient testing is common because most providers do not have extensive x-ray or laboratory equipment in their offices. Magnetic resonance imaging (MRI), computed tomography (CT) scans, numerous x-ray evaluations, sonography, and simple blood tests all may need to be scheduled (Procedure 9.5). Provide the patient with the name, address, and phone number of the facility where the tests will be done.

Some patients may require a series of appointments (e.g., at weekly intervals). Try to set up these appointments on the same day each week at the same time of day. This reduces the risk of the patient forgetting an appointment.

In some cases, the medical assistant may be responsible for scheduling inpatient admissions or inpatient surgical procedures. This is similar to scheduling outpatient testing, but the medical assistant coordinates with a hospital rather than an outside facility, and this information should also be documented in the patient's health record.

It is often the medical assistant's responsibility to provide the patient with any special instructions for the procedure or test that is going to be performed. The patient also should be provided with written instructions. A patient undergoing general anesthesia will need to fast for approximately 6 to 12 hours before the procedure. If medications are to be taken the morning of the procedure, the patient may take them with a small sip of water. The provider will instruct the patient about which medications to take. The patient should also be instructed to leave valuables at home. If it is an outpatient procedure and the patient will be sedated in any way, the individual should be instructed to have someone drive him or her home.

Telemedicine Visits

In recent years there has been an increase in the use of telemedicine or telehealth visits. The Department of Health and Human Services (HHS) describes telemedicine as your doctor providing care for you without an in-person visit. These visits are done online with internet access on a computer, tablet, or smartphone.

Telemedicine can include sending and receiving messages using secure messaging, often through the patient portal; using remote monitoring where patient vital signs or other health information is sent directly to the provider; or it could be an actual visit with your provider over the phone or video chat.

If there is going to be an actual visit with the provider, this will need to be added to the appointment schedule so that provider stays on track. The time needed for a telemedicine visit will depend on what needs to be accomplished. The healthcare facility should have established guidelines so that the appropriate amount of time is allowed. Often a medical assistant will call the patient prior to the provider calling to update any changes in demographics, allergies, and medications. This can also ensure that the technology being used is working before the provider makes the call or video chat.

Outside Visits

If the provider regularly makes house calls or visits patients in skilled nursing facilities, a special block of time must be reserved in the appointment schedule. There has been an increase in the number of providers who are making house calls again, especially if they have a patient base composed of a number of older adults who are still living independently. The provider needs demographic information, such as addresses, room numbers, and the best route to each home or facility. Remember to allow for travel time.

There are a number of other situations that may have to be added to the schedule, sometimes without much advance warning. Handle these situations with care and courtesy.

Pharmaceutical Representatives

Representatives from drug companies are frequent visitors to healthcare facilities. They are well trained and bring the provider valuable information on new drugs. The medical assistant is often expected to screen these visitors and turn away those whose products would not be used in that practice. If the representative or the pharmaceutical company is unknown to the office, ask for a business card and then check with the provider. The provider will decide whether to see the representative. Many healthcare facilities are limiting and even eliminating visits from pharmaceutical representatives due to the Physician Payments Sunshine Act (part of the Affordable Care Act).

Pharmaceutical representatives will often bring samples of the medications that they are going to talk to the provider about. It is important for the medical assistant to understand the policies and procedures for the handling and dispensing of the samples. Most healthcare facilities require that these samples are stored in a locked cabinet or closet and are given to patients only with the provider's approval.

Specialists usually limit their visits with pharmaceutical representatives to their line of practice. The medical assistant, together with the provider, can prepare a list of the representatives with whom the provider is willing to spend time. The medical assistant can say whether the provider will be available that day and give an estimate of the waiting time or suggest a later time at which the representative may return. The representative then can decide whether to wait or return later. Pharmaceutical representatives are usually understanding, cooperative, and willing to wait patiently for a long time for just a brief visit with the provider. In turn, the medical assistant should treat the representative with courtesy, showing as much cooperation as possible.

Salespeople

Salespeople from medical, surgical, and office supply houses stop regularly at healthcare facilities. Sometimes they want to see the provider, but the office manager or the medical assistant in charge of ordering supplies can usually handle these visits.

Unsolicited salespeople can sometimes present a problem in the professional office. If the provider does not want to see such callers, the medical assistant must firmly but tactfully send them away. Suggest that they leave their literature and cards for the provider to study and say that the provider will contact them if further information is desired.

SPECIAL CIRCUMSTANCES

A number of special circumstances can arise when scheduling appointments for the healthcare facility. The next several sections examine how to deal with the most common special circumstances.

Late Patients

Every medical practice has a few patients who are habitually late for appointments. This seems to be a problem for which no cure has been found. Emergencies and small delays can happen to anyone, but a patient who constantly arrives late can put a strain on the practice. Such patients can be booked as the last appointment of the day. Then, if closing time arrives before the patient does, the staff has no obligation to wait, and other patients have not been inconvenienced. Some medical assistants tell the patient to come in 30 minutes before the scheduled appointment time. Try to work with patients who have occasional difficulties arriving on time, but do not allow the schedule to be constantly disrupted by late patients.

CRITICAL THINKING APPLICATION **9.4**

Seth Jones is always late for his appointments. How might Ramona approach him about this? What can Ramona do to assist Mr. Jones in arriving for appointments on time?

Rescheduling Appointments

Changes sometimes must be made to the appointment schedule. Unexpected conflicts might come up that force a patient to change the appointment time. When you reschedule an appointment, make sure the first appointment is removed from the appointment book and then set the new appointment. Otherwise, the patient will be expected in the office on 2 days, and time will be wasted with calls and follow-up, only to discover that the appointment was rescheduled. Most computerized scheduling systems will allow the medical assistant to open the appointment and change the date and time or to cut and paste the appointment into the new date and time.

Emergency Situations

Periodically, emergency or urgent calls come into the office, and an appointment needs to be scheduled. To some extent, all calls that come in go through a **screening** process to evaluate the need to see the provider, and emergencies are prioritized. Screening is an extremely important function that requires experience, knowledge of signs and symptoms, and tact.

Emergencies may involve emotional crises in addition to the more obvious physical problems. Patients with emergencies and those who are acutely ill should be seen the same day. The urgency of the call initially can be determined by having a list of questions prepared for reference. The provider should help with this list and be the one to determine what is considered an *emergency* (life threatening) and what is *urgent* (serious but not life threatening). The patient may need to be referred directly to a hospital emergency department, or the provider may want to see the patient that day in the office. If patients are unable to get themselves to the hospital, the medical assistant may need to contact the emergency medical services in the area. Remember to keep the patient on the phone until emergency medical technicians (EMTs) or other help arrives at the patient's location. Never place an emergency call on hold. Always obtain the name, phone number, and location at the start of the call so that the patient can be found if he or she loses consciousness or is disconnected.

Patients without Appointments

The provider and scheduling team should come up with a policy for patients without appointments, also referred to as *walk-in patients*. A patient who requires immediate attention most likely will be fitted into the schedule somehow. If the patient does not need immediate care, an appointment scheduled at a later time may be the answer. Be sure to follow established office policy.

Failed Appointments

Why do patients fail to keep appointments? Some are simply forgetful. Once this tendency is detected in a patient, form the habit of telephoning or emailing a reminder the day before the appointment. Automated call routing offers the patient the option of canceling an appointment and can be programmed to keep calling until the patient responds and confirms or cancels the appointment.

A patient who has been asked for payment may stay away because of an inability to pay for medical services. Do not make the mistake of classifying all such patients as "deadbeats." Many have every desire to pay, but they cannot afford to and feel embarrassed about their situation, so they avoid their appointments.

Patients may also fail to keep appointments because they are in a state of denial about their condition. For instance, if a patient recently tested positive for the human immunodeficiency virus (HIV), he or she may avoid appointments because going to see the provider forces the patient to face the reality of the disease. Take special care with such patients, and if denial is suspected, discuss this with the provider, who may want to refer the patient for counseling.

It is important to determine the reason for failed appointments and to do whatever is possible to remedy the situation. Telephone the patient to make sure no misunderstanding has occurred. If the patient's health requires ongoing care, the provider may write a letter explaining this to the patient. Send the letter by certified mail with return receipt requested. A copy of the letter needs to be added to the patient's medical record for legal protection.

For legal purposes, failed appointments need to be documented in the patient's health record and the appointment schedule. A patient may try to claim abandonment when he or she has actually been the one to miss the appointments.

No-Show Policy

Some patients may not realize the importance of keeping their appointments. The patient who does not arrive for a scheduled appointment or does not reschedule it is called a **no-show**. A busy practice must have a very specific policy on appointment no-shows and must enforce it effectively. The first time a patient fails to show, note the fact on the health record or ledger card. The second time, warn the patient, and if a third no-show occurs, consider dropping the patient by using the customary methods that provide legal protection for the provider. Another option, instead of dropping a patient, is to only allow the patient to schedule for same-day appointments.

The provider may wish to charge patients for not showing up for the appointment. Be understanding whenever possible, but do not let a patient take advantage of the provider's time. The office policy manual must state that patients may be charged for missed appointments, and this should be explained to new patients when their first appointment is made. Because the time slot was scheduled and the provider was ready and available to treat the patient, it is ethical to charge the patient for missing an appointment, especially if he or she did not call to cancel or reschedule. Many providers do not press this issue, but it is an available tool if needed.

INCREASING APPOINTMENT SHOW RATES

Everyone benefits from a full schedule of kept appointments. Appointment show rates can be increased in several ways.

Automated Call Routing

As mentioned earlier, automated call reminders can contact patients scheduled for appointments. The patient is asked to press a certain key on the phone to confirm the appointment and a different key to cancel the appointment. This same tool can be used to send messages to patients (e.g., a reminder that it is the time of year to get a flu vaccination), to introduce a new provider at the office, or to announce the availability of a new procedure. The provider can even record the call so that it sounds more personal. These systems can also be set up to send text messages to remind patients of their upcoming appointments.

Appointment Cards

Most healthcare facilities use appointment cards to remind patients of scheduled appointments and to eliminate misunderstandings about dates and times (Figure 9.4). Make a habit of reaching for an appointment card while writing an entry in the appointment book or scheduling it on the computer. After the date and time have been written on the card, double-check with the book/computer to make sure the entries agree.

Confirmation Calls

Patients who have made appointments in advance may appreciate a confirmation call to remind them that they have a time set aside to see the provider. Always note the phone number the patient prefers the office to use for such calls. Many individuals have a

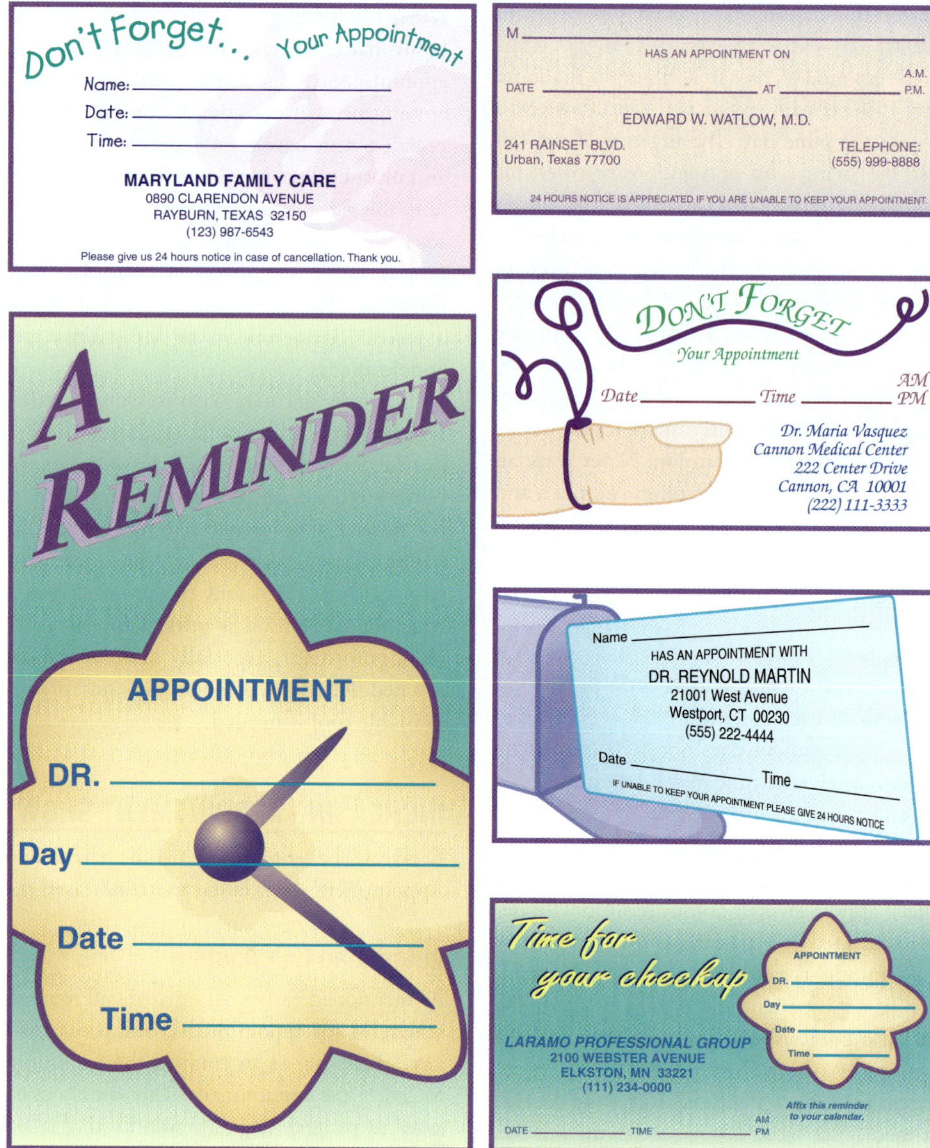

FIGURE 9.4 Examples of appointment reminder cards.

home phone, cell phone, and work phone numbers; however, they may want calls from the provider to go only to their home phone. Highlight the preferred phone number in the medical record or indicate it on the computer. The office must use caution in making calls to patients because of the significance of privacy guidelines and standards. Some offices may want to prepare a release form in which the patient grants the office staff permission to contact the patient. Many providers insist that messages left on voice mail not mention the term *doctor* or *doctor's office* for confidentiality reasons. The medical assistant might say, "This is Pam at Robert Welch's office confirming your appointment tomorrow at 2 p.m. Please call us if you cannot make the appointment. Our number is 555-212-0909. Thank you!"

If the patient has signed the privacy policy and the policy states that messages from the provider's office may be left at certain numbers, the office certainly can leave messages at that number and mention that the call is from the healthcare facility. Still, it is a good idea to have an established policy on leaving messages that does not breach the patient's confidentiality.

Email Reminders

Many computer scheduling programs can send an email to patients the day before an appointment to remind them of it. This is a great timesaver for the office staff because no time is taken to perform this duty other than the original scheduling of the appointment.

Mailed Reminders

The office staff may mail reminder letters to patients. This method is a bit time consuming with a paper-based appointment system but worth the effort if the patients show up for their appointments. Computer scheduling systems can be set up to generate the reminder letters for scheduled appointments and also to remind patients that they are due for their annual physical or influenza vaccination.

HANDLING CANCELLATIONS AND DELAYS

No matter how well planned out the scheduling procedure and matrix are, cancellations and delays will occur. The next sections explain how to handle the most common reasons for cancellations and delays.

When the Patient Cancels

Cancellations will occur in every healthcare facility. To minimize the impact of cancellations, keep a list of patients with future appointments who would like to come in sooner. The medical assistant can begin calling those patients to try to get one of them in to fill the available opening. Each cancellation should be noted in the medical record, along with a reason for the cancellation. If the patient simply reschedules an appointment, a notation does not need to be made in the health record unless a pattern develops that might be significant to the patient's medical treatment.

When the Provider Is Delayed

Some days, the provider will be delayed in reaching the office. If you are notified before patients arrive, start calling patients with early appointments and suggest that they come later. If some patients arrive before the office learns of the delay, explain that an emergency has detained the provider. Offer them the option of rescheduling, seeing another provider, or waiting for their provider.

Show concern for the patient, but do not be overly apologetic, which might imply some degree of guilt. Most patients realize that a provider has certain priorities. The patient in the office may be inconvenienced, but it is not a "life or death" matter. If this kind of situation occurs frequently, however, consider devising a different scheduling system.

When the Provider Is Called to an Emergency

Providers are conscious of their responsibilities for responding to medical emergencies, and most patients understand if the medical assistant takes time to explain what has happened. The medical assistant may say, "Dr. Wright has been called away due to an emergency. She asked me to tell you she is very sorry to keep you waiting. There will be at least a 1-hour delay." The medical assistant should then ask the patient, "Would you like to wait? If that is inconvenient, I'll be glad to give you the first available appointment on another day. Or perhaps you'd like to have some coffee or do some shopping and return in an hour." It is also possible that another provider may be able to see the patient.

As quickly as possible, call the patients scheduled for later. In many offices, especially those of obstetricians, surgeons, and general practitioners, a whole day's appointments must be canceled. For this reason, it is particularly important to have the daytime telephone number of each patient available so that the appointment can be rescheduled. If at all possible, cancel appointments before the patient arrives in the office to find that the provider is not available. The **expediency** of the office staff in contacting patients who will be affected by an emergency is appreciated.

When the Provider Is Ill or Out of Town

Providers get sick, too, and patients scheduled to be seen during the course of the provider's recovery must be informed of this and their appointments rescheduled. They do not need to be told the nature of the illness.

When the provider is called out of town for personal or professional reasons, appointments must be canceled or rescheduled. Usually, the patient is given the name of another provider, or possibly a choice of a few, who will provide care during such absences. For security reasons, only state that the doctor is unavailable. Stating over the telephone that the provider is out of town could lead to attempted burglary or other unauthorized entry on the premises.

PATIENT PROCESSING TASKS

When working at the reception desk, the medical assistant needs to screen the individuals arriving:

- *People with emergent conditions:* Individuals may be bleeding, having chest pain, or feeling very ill. It is important that the medical assistant immediately contact the **triage** nurse to see the patient. If the nurse is not available, then the medical assistant should bring the patient back to an exam room and notify the provider right away. Facilities may have procedures in place to indicate when 911 needs to be called immediately.
- *Pharmaceutical and equipment representatives:* The medical assistant should follow the facility's policies and procedures regarding when these representatives are permitted to see the providers.
- *Salespeople and visitors:* The medical assistant needs to find out the reason for the visit and then follow the facility's procedures.

The most common visitors to the facility will be patients and family members who have appointments. We will examine the tasks the medical assistant must perform when patients arrive.

Patient's Arrival

When patients arrive, two important things need to occur. First, they need to know where to go and what to do. Second, they need to be greeted as quickly as possible. Signage is helpful to indicate what patients need to do upon arrival.

Every patient has the right to expect courteous treatment in a provider's office. Regardless of the patient's economic or social status, each person who arrives should receive a cordial, friendly greeting (Figure 9.5). A personal touch, such as greeting the patient by name, is an easy way to develop patient rapport.

Using a Patient's Name

- Use the patient's last name and title (e.g., Mrs. Crawford) unless the patient insists on the use of his or her first name or nickname.
- If you do not know the person, greet the individual and then ask for his or her name.
- Learn how to pronounce each patient's name correctly. Incorrect pronunciations may offend or irritate some people.
- Make a note of the phonetic spelling in the health record for reference. Note if the patient prefers a nickname.

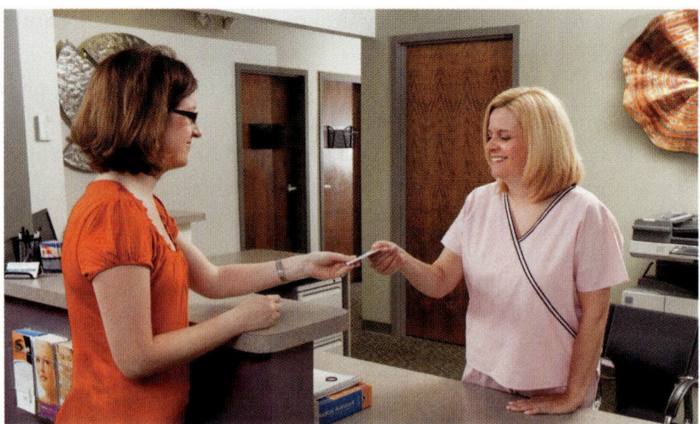

FIGURE 9.5 Greet all patients with a warm smile, and assist them with forms they need to complete for the health record.

The person sitting at the front reception desk should greet each patient as quickly as possible. Some experts say that a person should be greeted within 30 seconds of arriving. If this is not possible, a simple smile and eye contact will acknowledge the person. Make sure to greet the person verbally as soon as possible. If too much time elapses between the person's entrance and the greeting, the person may feel ignored or unimportant. This can impact a person's perception of the facility and, ultimately, the care provided. If the medical assistant must step away from the reception desk, it is important to check the reception area for new arrivals as soon as she or he returns.

In facilities where the receptionist is behind sliding glass windows, the environment can appear impersonal to patients. Although the closed glass windows increase patient privacy, they can also

Patient Sign-In

Date: ___________

Please sign-in and notify us if:

• New patient • Phone/address change • Insurance change

No.	1 Patient Name print	Appt. Time	Arrival Time	Appt. with	New patient (✓)	Phone/address change (✓)	Insurance change (✓)
1	P L E A S E						
2	2						
3	3						
4	4						
5	5						
6	6						
7	7						
8	8						
9	9						
10	10						
11	11						
12	12						
13	13						
14	14						
15	15						
16	16						
17	17						
18	18						
19	19						
20	20						
21	21						
22	22						
23	23						
24	24						
25	25						

FIGURE 9.6 Sign-in sheets contain basic information about the patient and provide information for the medical assistant about changes that need to be applied to the patient's record.

TABLE 9.1 HIPAA-Appropriate Sign-in Register

FEATURES CAUSING A HIPAA VIOLATION	FEATURES OF A HIPAA-APPROPRIATE REGISTER
• Insurance information (e.g., name, number) • Reason for visit • Demographic information (e.g., address, employer, date of birth)	• Date • Name • Arrival time • Appointment time • Appointment with • Check boxes to indicate changes (but no information can be given)

give the impression that the staff and provider are off limits to the patients. The glass window should be open as much as possible to give the appearance of openness to others. The policies and procedures manual should indicate when the glass window should be closed.

Sign-in Register

Some facilities will have the patient sign a register. A sign-in register that promotes patients' privacy should be used (Figure 9.6). Remember, other patients can read the prior patients' information. This is not considered a violation of the Health Insurance Portability and Accountability Act (HIPAA) privacy policy if the information disclosed is appropriately limited (Table 9.1). This is one type of incidental disclosure under HIPAA.

Infection Control in the Reception Area

It is vital for the medical assistant to take steps to protect the other patients in the reception area. The medical assistant may need to ask a few screening questions to identify patients who are ill with specific symptoms or at risk for specific diseases. These questions are set by the healthcare facility and usually recommended by the Centers for Disease Control and Prevention (CDC). Questions may include the following:

- "Have you traveled outside of the United States in the past 21 days?" Travel to specific countries may be included in the question. Patients who answer yes should be taken to an exam room immediately.
- "Are you coughing?" Patients who are coughing should be encouraged to use masks. This is especially important during flu season or when other respiratory infections are prevalent. Tissues, along with waste containers and hand sanitizer, should be available for patients in the reception area.

Registration for New Patients

When someone visits the provider's office for the first time, the staff must gather information from the new patient, such as demographic and the health history information. The demographic information is usually gathered using the patient information or registration form. The patient's name should appear prominently at the top of the form, followed by other pertinent facts. The patient's personal history, medical history, and family history may be obtained by using a questionnaire.

There are many ways the healthcare facility can obtain this information. Patients may be mailed the documents a few weeks prior to the appointment or directed to complete the information using the online **patient portal**. In some facilities, patients complete this information as they wait, prior to the appointment. They may complete paper forms or provide the information using an electronic device. In some cases, the medical assistant may take the patient to a private room where he or she can ask the questions and enter the information into the electronic health record (EHR).

The medical assistant must be willing to answer any questions about the form, either in person or over the phone (Figure 9.7). The medical assistant must then review the completed form and verify that the required information has been provided. The provider also reviews the health history and can then add information during the patient visit.

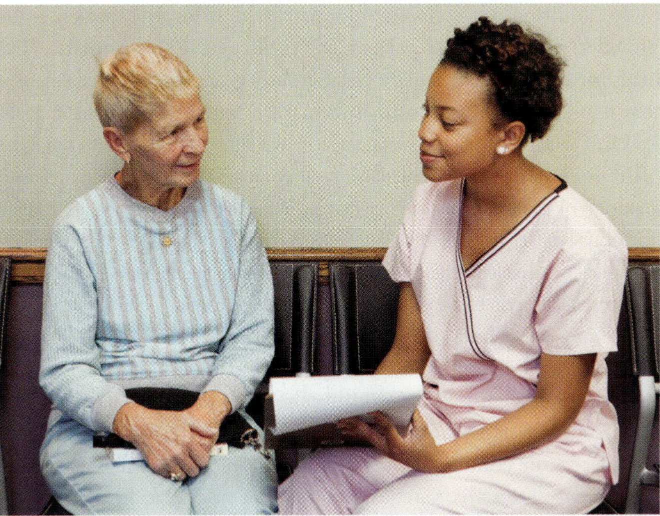

FIGURE 9.7 The medical assistant should take time to explain forms the patient does not understand and should always be willing to answer questions.

Patient Information or Registration Forms

Most patient information or registration forms contain the following:

- Patient's full name and date of birth
- Responsible person's name and relationship to the patient
- Address and telephone number
- Name, address, and telephone number of contact person
- Occupation
- Place of employment
- Social Security number
- Driver's license number
- Nearest relative not living with the patient and his or her relationship
- Source of referral, if any

CRITICAL THINKING APPLICATION 9.5

Often some time is needed to complete forms when a new patient arrives in the healthcare facility. How might Ramona keep the healthcare facility on schedule when new patients arrive who require health record construction and form completion? What are some ways to trim time from these activities?

In addition to collecting information from the patient, the provider must give the patient the facility's NPP document. The healthcare provider is legally obligated to give each patient a notice that explains how the health information may be used and shared. HIPAA requires that patients state in writing that they received the NPP document. The healthcare facility may ask the patient to sign a paper or an electronic document. This form is then kept in the patient's health record. If the patient refuses to sign, the provider can still use and disclose the health information as permitted by HIPAA. The refusal needs to be documented in the patient's health record.

Many times, new patients are given a brochure on the facility's policies and procedures. New patient brochures should be designed in a professional manner. The wording should be at a level that patients understand. When coaching a patient regarding the facility's policies, summarize the content of the brochure. Do not read the brochure to the patient. Use active listening skills. Make sure to address any questions the patient may have. Procedure 9.3 describes how to create the brochure and coach the patients regarding the policies.

New Patient Brochure Content

The following topics should be addressed in the new patient brochure:

- Description of the practice (e.g., type of practice, mission statement)
- Location or a map of the practice
- Contact information (i.e., telephone numbers, emails, and website addresses)
- Providers' names and credentials
- Services offered
- Hours of operation
- How appointments can be scheduled
- Practice policies and procedures (e.g., payment policies, appointment cancellations, medication refills, assistance after hours)

Check-in Procedures for All Patients

During the check-in process, the medical assistant must scan or copy both sides of the patient's insurance card. The medical assistant may have to perform **verification of eligibility**. (This will be described in depth in Chapter 12.) The patient's phone number and address, along with the insurance subscriber's date of birth, should also be verified. Patients must show their insurance cards and picture identification for insurance and identity verification. These verifications take place at every patient visit for eligibility and safety reasons.

Many healthcare facilities also scan or copy the patient's legal photo identification. Facilities with EHRs may require a photo of the patient to be taken. The photo is uploaded to the EHR. Between the photo identification and the EHR photo, facilities are trying to reduce the amount of healthcare identity fraud. This fraud occurs when a person obtains healthcare using another person's name and insurance.

Some healthcare facilities insist that copays be collected before the office visit. Signage in the reception area often includes a statement such as "Copayments are due at the time of the appointment." Ask the patient for payment, using phrases such as "Your copay today is $15, Mrs. Crawford. Will you be writing a check or would you like to charge this visit to your Visa?" If the facility is flexible with copayment collection, the medical assistant can give the patient an option. "Mr. Thomas, would you like to pay your copay now?"

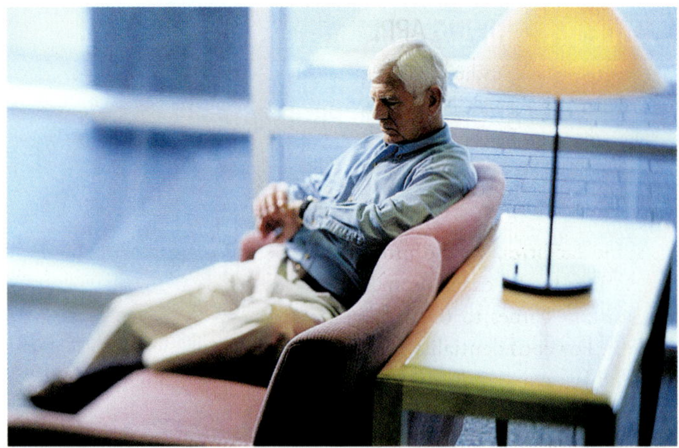

FIGURE 9.8 One of the most common patient complaints is the time spent in the reception area.

Patients with Special Needs

After a patient is checked in, the receptionist may have additional duties if the patient has special needs. Some patients arrive in wheelchairs unattended by family or friends. They may need assistance to get to the reception area. Remember to always ask patients if they need assistance before you try to assist them.

If there is a language barrier, the medical assistant may need to get translation assistance for the visit. Typical options for assistance include having a qualified translator present or using translation technology. There are many online programs that can assist with translation in many different languages. It is important for the administrative medical assistant to communicate any special needs of patients to the clinical medical assistant. In all special needs cases, it is important to remain professional and treat everyone with respect.

CRITICAL THINKING APPLICATION 9.6

A patient passes Ramona in the hallway as she is leaving for lunch and stops to greet her. The patient's face is familiar, but Ramona cannot recall the patient's name. Occasionally, Ramona sees a patient outside of the office (e.g., at the store). Everyone forgets someone's name on occasion.

- How might Ramona and her staff members remember names?
- What special tips or techniques can help you remember names?
- What can Ramona do the next time she sees a patient and does not remember the person's name?

Showing Consideration for Patients' Time

Patients expect to see the provider at the appointed time. There should be signage in the reception area stating that patients should let the receptionist know if they have been waiting for longer than 15 to 20 minutes. If the provider is delayed, the medical assistant should let the patients know (Figure 9.8). The medical assistant can also offer to reschedule the appointment. Some facilities will offer patients gift cards (e.g., coffee, gas) if an error occurred in scheduling or if the patient needs to reschedule due to a long wait time. These gestures show the patients that the staff recognizes their inconvenience. It is a great customer service practice.

CRITICAL THINKING APPLICATION 9.7

Ramona offers to reschedule patient appointments if the schedule ever falls more than 15 minutes behind. If a patient becomes belligerent about the delays, how can Ramona handle the situation in a professional manner?

Escorting Patients to the Exam Room

In some facilities, the administrative medical assistant may escort the patient to the exam room. In other facilities, the clinical medical assistant comes to the reception area and calls the name of the patient. For confidentiality, it is important to call the patient by the first and last name only. Make sure to clearly pronounce the name. If you are unsure, attempt the pronunciation and then ask the patient. Apologize for pronouncing it incorrectly. Make sure to add the pronunciation to the record for the next visit. Remember, no other information should be given in the public waiting area. When you and the patient are alone or away from the reception area, verify that the patient's date of birth matches your records. If it does not, you have the wrong patient!

Some patients may bring a family member or friend with them to an appointment. On occasion, several people may want to accompany the patient to the exam room. Based on the facility's policy, respectfully explain that the exam room has only two chairs. If the patient still insists, make every attempt to satisfy the patient's needs. Please be aware that in some cultures, it is expected that multiple people will accompany the patient to see the provider. In those situations, attempt to use a larger room if available.

Interacting with Friends and Relatives of Patients

Patients are sometimes accompanied by a relative or friend. Be cautious if they want to discuss the patient's illness. Avoid a too-casual attitude, such as "I'm sure there's nothing to worry about." A show of moderate concern and reassurance that the patient is in good hands usually takes care of the situation. Remember that health information cannot be released to anyone, including concerned friends and relatives, without the patient's consent.

It is understood that the medical assistant escorts the patient to the exam room. Ask if patients need any assistance if it appears they might. Do not assume they need assistance – ask first and ask how you can assist them. To show respect for the patient, open doors and walk at the patient's speed.

If a urine specimen is needed, direct the patient to the restroom. Always explain how to collect the specimen and where the specimen should be placed. When you get to the exam room with the patient, instruct the patient based on the provider's wishes. If the patient needs to undress, explain what clothing items need to be removed and how to put on the gown. Make sure to indicate where the patient needs to sit. If the patient has a risk of falling, have him or her sit on the chair instead of the exam table.

If you are using an EHR, make sure to log out of the software before leaving the room and then close the door. If you need to reenter the room, always knock first out of respect for the patient. Pause before opening the door. The pause allows the patient time to prepare and time to tell you to enter.

In facilities that use paper health records, often file holders are located on the door or near the door. Place the health record in the holder in such a way that the patient's name is not visible. HIPAA considers names on health records to be incidental disclosures. It is a good practice to protect the patient's privacy. Many facilities have flags on the door to indicate the status of the patient. Adjust the flagging system so the provider knows the patient is in the room and ready to be seen.

Challenging Situations

Anytime you are working with people, challenging situations can present themselves. When working in healthcare, it is especially important that these situations are handled in a professional manner. The following sections describe how to handle some of the challenging situations that can come up when working with patients.

Talkative Patients

Any professional office has problem patients. Talkative patients, for example, take up far more of the provider's time than is justified. Many times, the provider and medical assistant will devise a method to help keep everything on schedule. For instance, the medical assistant may have to page the provider after a certain time period. This alerts the provider to the time already spent with the patient. The provider can then complete the visit and move to the next patient.

CRITICAL THINKING APPLICATION 9.8

Ramona has one patient who insists on sitting close to her desk and attempting to chat the entire time she is waiting to see the provider. In addition, she comes to her appointments at least an hour early. How might Ramona subtly deal with this patient?

Children

Children frequently present special management challenges. The child may be the patient, or he or she may be accompanying the patient. Parents or guardians are responsible for their children's behavior while at the healthcare facility. If children are doing something that could be harmful, quietly speak to the parents and allow them to handle the situation. The medical assistant should not discipline the child. If the child continues to behave badly, call the parent to the exam room early. They may not be seen early, but they can wait in the exam room instead of the reception area.

In most cases (other than those that involve teens and suspected abuse situations), parents or guardians accompany the child to the exam room. Sometimes parents of older teens want to be present for the visit. Some providers find teens are more honest with their answers if parents are not present. In these situations, allowing the parent to be in the room for the interview may be helpful, but the parent can then wait in the reception area during the physical exam. This will allow the provider to ask follow-up questions, if needed, without the parent overhearing the answers. In all cases (unless indicated by state law), parental permission is required for minors to be seen.

Strategies to Use with Bad Behavior in Children

- Kneel down to the child's level and offer a book or toy.
- Lead the child away from any objects that could be broken and from other patients.
- Say to the child, "Let's come over here and play next to your dad!"

Angry Patients in the Reception Area

Every medical assistant eventually is confronted with an angry patient. The anger may simply reflect the patient's pain or fear of what the provider may discover during the exam. If possible, invite the patient into a room out of the reception area. Usually, the best course is to let the patient talk out the anger. Present a calm attitude and speak in a low tone of voice. Under no circumstances should the medical assistant return the anger or become argumentative. Medical assistants must use good listening skills with angry people and must be empathetic. Notify the facility's administrator of all difficult patients or ask for help from co-workers.

There should be a policy in place for dealing with potentially dangerous individuals. Policies can include the following:

- Making sure that you can reach the exit if you take the patient to another room
- Having another employee close by
- Knowing under what circumstances you should contact the police or building security for assistance

Patient Checkout

When patients return to the front office for checkout, greet them with a friendly smile and call the individual by name. Form the habit of asking patients if they have any questions. Check the health record to determine when the provider wants the patient to return. Most providers note this information on the encounter form. Make the return appointment. Remember to give the patient choices on the time and day. Give the patient an appointment reminder card. If the copayment was not collected prior to the visit, it may be collected during checkout.

The medical assistant can convey a sense of caring by terminating the visit cordially. Thank the patient for coming. If the patient will return for another visit, the assistant can say something such as "We'll see you next week." If the patient will not be returning soon, a pleasant "I hope you'll be feeling better soon" is appropriate. In addition, tell patients to call the facility if they have any questions or if they need additional care. Whatever words of goodbye are chosen, all patients should leave the facility feeling that they have received top-quality care and were treated with friendliness, respect, and courtesy.

CLOSING COMMENTS

Patient Coaching

Providing patients with an information booklet about the healthcare facility can familiarize them with policies and procedures. Many providers compile an extensive booklet that even provides tips as to when the provider should be called immediately, listing symptoms and signs of emergencies.

Educating the patient about the healthcare facility's policies helps the facility run smoothly from day to day. All patients should be familiar with the policies about appointments. This leads to fewer misunderstandings and conflicts over bills that might include a charge for a missed appointment.

If the facility offers internet-based appointment scheduling or forms completion, patients must be taught how to use the system. A printed pamphlet or information sheet is helpful for providing instructions to the patient. A wise option is to have a special phone number that patients can call if they have problems with the system. For best results, choose a program that is simple to use, easy to understand, and does not breach patient confidentiality.

Legal and Ethical Issues

As mentioned earlier, the appointment schedule may be used as a legal record and could be brought by subpoena into a court of law. Make sure all handwriting in the book is completely legible and that information is routinely collected in a consistent manner for each entry. Do not fail to note a no-show both in the patient's health record and the appointment schedule. This often is helpful when a provider must prove that the patient did not follow medical advice or that the patient contributed to his or her poor condition by missing appointments. Old appointment schedules should be kept for a time equal to that of the statute of limitations in the state where the practice is located.

A medical assistant must never offer medical advice to a patient. The patient sees the medical assistant as an extension of the provider and tends to weigh advice and comments by the medical assistant with the same validity as if they came from the provider. Provide only information the provider has approved or that is included in the healthcare facility's policies and procedures manual.

When a patient complains, listen carefully, and try to resolve the problem or assure the patient that the issue will be discussed with the appropriate staff member to find a solution. If someone other than the patient asks for information about the patient, refrain from discussion unless the patient or provider has authorized the release of information.

Patient-Centered Care

Going to a healthcare facility can be intimidating and uncomfortable for many patients. It is important that the medical assistant try to put everyone at ease. Cultivate the habit of greeting each patient immediately in a friendly, self-assured manner. Establish eye contact and smile while introducing yourself to the patient.

Small talk can help put a patient at ease. Talking about the weather or an uncontroversial topic may make the patient more comfortable.

Asking personalized questions can also help. Providers and staff members sometimes make brief notes in the health record about the current events in the patient's life. On the next visit, the staff or provider can use this information to start a conversation with the patient. For instance, the patient may state she is going to Florida for a vacation. During the next visit, the provider may start off the visit by asking how her Florida trip was. Asking personalized questions will solidify the personal connection with patients. They may feel important, less intimidated, and more comfortable. It is a great way to provide excellent customer service.

Professional Behaviors

When working in scheduling and helping patients move through the healthcare facility, medical assistants have many opportunities to demonstrate professionalism. It is important to remember that we are often seeing patients when they are not at their best, so we must learn not to take all of the responses personally. When an angry patient approaches the reception desk, you should smile politely, ask how you can help the person, and respond in a soothing tone of voice. When a patient calls for an appointment and demands a day and time when the provider is not available, you should remain calm and explain why that day and time are not an option. As a medical assistant in the front office, you have the opportunity to make an amazing first impression on patients. Remember to always behave professionally.

SUMMARY OF SCENARIO

Ramona is an asset to the healthcare facility because her dedication and customer service skills help her interact with patients in a positive way. She genuinely cares about the patients and makes every effort to meet their needs while following Dr. Perez's preferences. She has found that her bright smile is a valuable aid when patients have been waiting and are growing restless.

Ramona cooperates with other staff members to get the patients seen as quickly as possible and to minimize wait time. She is flexible and can change the order of the patients seen, if needed, to maximize the use of time and facilities in the office. Because she is so cheerful and friendly, patients do not seem to mind when she asks for their cooperation. She keeps current phone numbers and cell phone information so that she can notify a patient quickly if Dr. Perez is running behind schedule. Ramona's proficiency on the computer also is an asset, and she makes frequent use of email to take care of patients' problems or to reschedule requests.

Because of the cooperation she receives from staff and patients alike, Ramona successfully runs an efficient office. She contributes to that efficiency by constantly refining her knowledge about her job. She pays attention to the times during the day that do not run as smoothly as others, evaluates the problems at those times, and then corrects them. Ramona also keeps the schedule moving by communicating with the clinical medical assistants, keeping them informed about arriving patients and those who have come early or are running late. She can quickly adjust and substitute a patient who already has arrived. Ramona has learned how to manipulate the schedule to accommodate an emergency. She knows that by making minor adjustments and keeping the waiting patients informed, the staff can handle any emergency.

All medical assistants need to develop skills in flexibility. Establishing a system that works and using it correctly makes patients and staff members more content with their experience in the healthcare facility.

SUMMARY OF LEARNING OBJECTIVES

1. **Describe the guidelines for establishing an appointment schedule.**
   When appointments are scheduled, a medical assistant must consider (1) the patients' needs, (2) the provider's preferences and habits, and (3) the available facilities. Make every attempt to schedule a patient at his or her most convenient time; this helps prevent no-shows. The provider will outline his or her preferences, which should be a high priority to the medical assistant. However, most providers are flexible and make adjustments according to the needs of the office. The availability of facilities in the office is perhaps the most inflexible factor. If a certain room or piece of equipment is being used for one patient, it usually cannot be used for another.

   Refer to Procedure 9.1 to create an appointment matrix.
2. **Explain the guidelines for establishing an appointment matrix.**
   To establish the appointment matrix, certain times must be blocked out on the schedule. These times are when the provider is not available to see patients, such as during lunchtime, hospital rounds, conferences, and vacation.

   An additional step for setting up the appointment matrix is determining the length of the shortest office visit type, usually 10 to 15 minutes. This becomes one time slot on the schedule and for appointments that need more time, more than one time slot is used.
3. **Discuss methods of scheduling appointments.**
   Computerized scheduling programs are in demand because they are easy to operate and simplify both scheduling and changing of appointments. The computer can find the first available time much faster than a person scanning an appointment book. Most programs can prepare reports and even notify patients of the impending appointment automatically by email, telephone, or text message. Web-based self-scheduling programs are becoming popular; these allow a patient to see the provider's available appointments and book his or her own date and time.

   Self-scheduling can vastly reduce the number of calls to the office because a high number of everyday calls are requests to schedule appointments. With self-scheduling, patients can even make an appointment at midnight if they desire.

   Office suppliers carry a variety of appointment book styles; many are color guided.
4. **Discuss pros and cons of various types of appointment management systems.**
   Scheduling of specific appointments is the most popular method of seeing patients. Wave and modified-wave scheduling brings two or three patients to the office at the same time, and they are seen in the order of their arrival. This type of scheduling can be modified in many ways to suit the needs of the facility. Open office hours allow patients to come to the healthcare facility when it is convenient and wait their turn to see the provider. Other scheduling methods include double-booking and grouping of like procedures.
5. **Discuss the process for scheduling new and established patients.**
   Extend small courtesies to patients when on the phone with them to schedule an appointment. This contact may be the patient's first impression of the facility. Be considerate if you are not able to accommodate the date/time requested.

   Arranging the first appointment for a new patient requires time and attention to detail. Tact, courtesy, and professionalism are all extremely important. Collect the patient's demographic data, and offer the patient the first available appointment. Some healthcare facilities mail an information packet/brochure to new patients; this can also be sent via email. Often, the medical assistant will need to conduct preauthorization and precertification to determine whether a patient is eligible for treatment or for certain procedures. Refer to Procedure 9.2 to see how to schedule a new patient.

   Most return appointments for established patients are arranged when the patient is leaving the healthcare facility. Refer to Procedure 9.4. Others are reserved by telephone, and the patient's address, telephone number, and insurance should always be verified, and any changes documented in the health record.

SUMMARY OF LEARNING OBJECTIVES—cont'd

6. **Explain how the medical assistant should handle scheduling of other types of appointments.**
   The medical assistant could be responsible for setting up other appointments, such as inpatient surgeries, outpatient and inpatient procedure appointments, outside visits, and meetings with providers, pharmaceutical representatives, and salespeople. Refer to Procedure 9.5 for specific procedures on how to schedule outpatient and inpatient procedure appointments.
7. **Examine methods of dealing with special circumstances in scheduling.**
   Patients who are habitually late for appointments might be told to arrive 15 minutes before the time written in the book. Some offices book these patients as the last appointment of the day, so that if they do not arrive promptly, they do not see the provider. Usually talking with the patient and gaining an understanding of why the patient arrives late improves the situation. The office can work with the patient to choose the best times that will result in a kept appointment.

   Changes sometimes must be made in the appointment schedule. When rescheduling an appointment, make sure the first appointment is removed from the appointment book, and then set the new appointment.

   Periodically, emergency or urgent calls come into the office, and an appointment needs to be scheduled. Follow office procedures. Provider referrals and patients without appointments should also be scheduled according to office policy.

   When dealing with patients who come in without an appointment, it is important follow the facility's policy. Patients who require immediate attention will likely be seen. If not, they can be scheduled to be seen at a later date.

   It is important to determine the reason for failed appointments and to do whatever is possible to remedy the situation. Failed appointments need to be documented. A busy practice must have a specific policy on appointment no-shows and must enforce it effectively.
8. **Discuss methods to increase appointment show rates.**
   Methods to increase appointment show rates include automated call routing, appointment cards, confirmation calls, email reminders, and mailed reminders.
9. **Explain how to handle cancellations and delays.**
   Cancellations will occur for a variety of reasons (e.g., when the patient cancels, when the provider is delayed, when the provider is called to an emergency, or when the provider is ill or out of town). All situations should be handled in accordance with office policy.
10. **Describe how to prepare for patients' arrivals, including patient check-in procedures.**
    Advanced preparation helps make the day go smoothly and contributes to a more relaxed atmosphere for all. Health records should be prepared for the provider and arranged sequentially. The reception desk should be in clear view of all visitors who come to the office. Use a sign-in register that promotes patients' privacy. During the patient check-in process, it is vital for the medical assistant to take steps to protect the other patients in the reception area. Procedure 9.3 describes how to coach patients regarding office policies and how to create a new patient brochure.
    - *Show consideration for patients' time:* The medical assistant should bring the patient to the examination room for treatment or consultation as close to the appointment time as possible or explain delays.
    - *Properly treat patients with special needs:* In all special needs cases, it is important to remain professional and treat everyone with respect.
    - *Prepare for challenging situations:* For talkative patients, the patient's history could be flagged with a symbol to alert the provider. Parents are responsible for their children's behavior while at the provider's office. The medical assistant should not discipline the child. Medical assistants should use empathy and good listening skills when dealing with angry patients, and there should be a policy in place for dealing with potentially dangerous individuals. Avoid a too-casual attitude with patients' relatives and friends; show moderate concern and empathy.

PROCEDURE 9.1 Establish the Appointment Matrix

TASK: Establish the matrix of the appointment schedule.

SCENARIO: You have been asked to set up the schedule matrix for Dr. Julie Walden, Dr. James Martin, and Dr. Angela Perez. Block off the following times in the appointment schedule:

DR. JULIE WALDEN:

- Lunch: Daily from 11:30 a.m. to 12:30 p.m.
- Hospital Rounds: Mondays and Wednesdays from 8:00 a.m. to 9:00 a.m.

DR. JAMES MARTIN:

- Lunch: Daily from 12:00 p.m. to 1:00 p.m.
- Hospital Rounds: Tuesdays and Thursdays from 8:00 a.m. to 9:00 a.m.

DR. ANGELA PEREZ:

- Lunch: Daily from 12:30 p.m. to 1:30 p.m.
- Hospital Rounds: Fridays from 8:00 a.m. to 9:00 a.m.

PROCEDURE 9.1 Establish the Appointment Matrix—cont'd

EQUIPMENT and SUPPLIES

- Appointment book or computer with scheduling software
- Office procedure manual (optional)
- Black pen, pencil, and highlighters
- Calendar

PROCEDURAL STEPS

1. Using the calendar, determine when the office is not open (e.g., holidays, weekends, evenings). If using the appointment book and a black pen, draw an *X* through the times the office is not open. If using the scheduling software, block the times the office is not open.
   PURPOSE: Blocking the closed times helps prevent patients from being scheduled when the office is closed.
2. Identify the times each provider is not available. If using the appointment book, write in the providers' names on each column and then draw an *X* through their unavailable times. If using the scheduling software, select each provider and block the times the provider is unavailable indicating the reason the time is blocked.
   PURPOSE: Many providers do rounds in the hospital or long-term care facilities and cannot see patients in the clinic during those times. Providers also attend meetings and conferences during the workday. These events, along with vacations and lunchtimes, should be blocked on their schedules.
3. Using the office procedure manual or providers' preferences, determine when each provider performs certain types of examinations. In the appointment book, indicate these examinations either by writing the examination time or by highlighting the examination times. Follow the office's procedure on indicating these examination times in the appointment book. When using scheduling software, set up the times for the examinations or use the highlighting feature if available.
   PURPOSE: Some providers perform a variety of examinations. It can be more time efficient to have the same types of examinations on the same day. For instance, a provider in a women's health department may perform both gynecologic and prenatal examinations. The provider may prefer to set aside certain days to do prenatal examinations and other days to do gynecologic examinations.
4. Using the office procedure manual or the list of providers' preferences and availability, identify other times to block on the scheduling matrix. Some providers require catch-up times and these time slots are blocked. Some medical facilities save appointment times for same-day appointments. When saving time blocks for same-day appointments, make sure to use pencil so the block indicator can be erased and the patient's information entered on the day of the appointment. For the scheduling software, block those times when patients cannot be booked and indicate the times for the same-day appointments.
   PURPOSE: Allowing appointment times to be saved for same-day appointments provides the opportunity for the provider to see a patient who needs to get in immediately and prevents the patient from being turned away or double-booked.

PROCEDURE 9.2 Schedule a New Patient

TASK: Schedule a new patient for a first office visit, and identify the urgency of the visit using established priorities.

SCENARIO: Patricia Black, a new patient, calls. She just moved to the area, and her asthma has flared up over the past 24 hours, but her albuterol inhaler is empty, and she needs a new prescription for it. She states that she is doing okay, but without the albuterol she knows it will get worse within the next few days. According to your screening guidelines, she needs to be seen today, and scheduling guidelines indicate she needs a 45-minute appointment.

EQUIPMENT and SUPPLIES

- Appointment book or computer with scheduling software
- Scheduling and screening guidelines
- Pencil

PROCEDURAL STEPS

1. Obtain the patient's demographic information (e.g., full name, birth date, address, and telephone number). Write this information down or enter it into the scheduling software. Verify the information.
   PURPOSE: It is important to verify the information. If you have difficulty hearing the patient, use a system to verify the spelling (e.g., "A" as in alpha).
2. Determine whether the patient was referred by another provider.
   PURPOSE: You may need to request additional information from the referring provider, and your provider will want to send a consultation report.
3. Respectfully determine the patient's chief complaint and when the first symptoms occurred. Use the scheduling and screening guidelines as needed.
   PURPOSE: You must know the amount of time that will be required for the visit and how quickly the patient needs to be seen based on the chief complaint.
4. Search the appointment book or scheduling software for the first suitable appointment time and an alternate time. Offer the patient a choice of these dates and times. Be open to alternative times if the patient cannot make the initial options you gave. Provide additional appointment options as needed.

Continued

PROCEDURE 9.2 Schedule a New Patient—cont'd

PURPOSE: Providing the patient with a choice of dates and times and additional options as needed demonstrates sensitivity when managing appointments. It is an important customer service technique (see the following figure).

5. Enter the mutually agreeable time into the schedule. Enter the patient's name, telephone number, and add *NP* for new patient.
   PURPOSE: The *NP* in the appointment book indicates the patient is a new patient. Having the phone number available increases your efficiency if you need to contact the patient.
6. Obtain the patient's insurance information. If new patients are expected to pay at the time of the visit, explain this financial arrangement when the appointment is made.
   PURPOSE: Obtaining the patient's insurance information now ensures that the patient is seeing a provider covered by his or her insurance carrier. If you explain the payment policy before the appointment, the patient can come to the appointment prepared to pay.
7. Provide the patient with directions to the healthcare facility and parking instructions if needed.
   Note: Many facilities will email or mail new-patient paperwork to the patient, who is instructed to complete the forms before the appointment and bring them to the appointment.
8. Before ending the call, ask if the patient has any questions. Reinforce the date and time of the appointment. Politely and professionally end the call, making sure to thank the patient for calling.
   PURPOSE: It is important to restate the appointment time and date to ensure the patient knows the correct information before you end the call.
   Note: For legal and safety reasons, many healthcare practices encourage patients with urgent same-day appointments to seek emergency care immediately if the condition worsens before the appointment time.

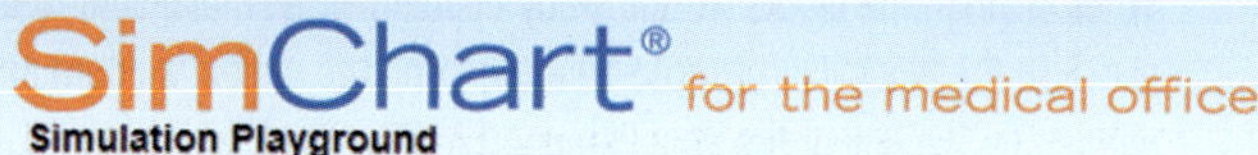

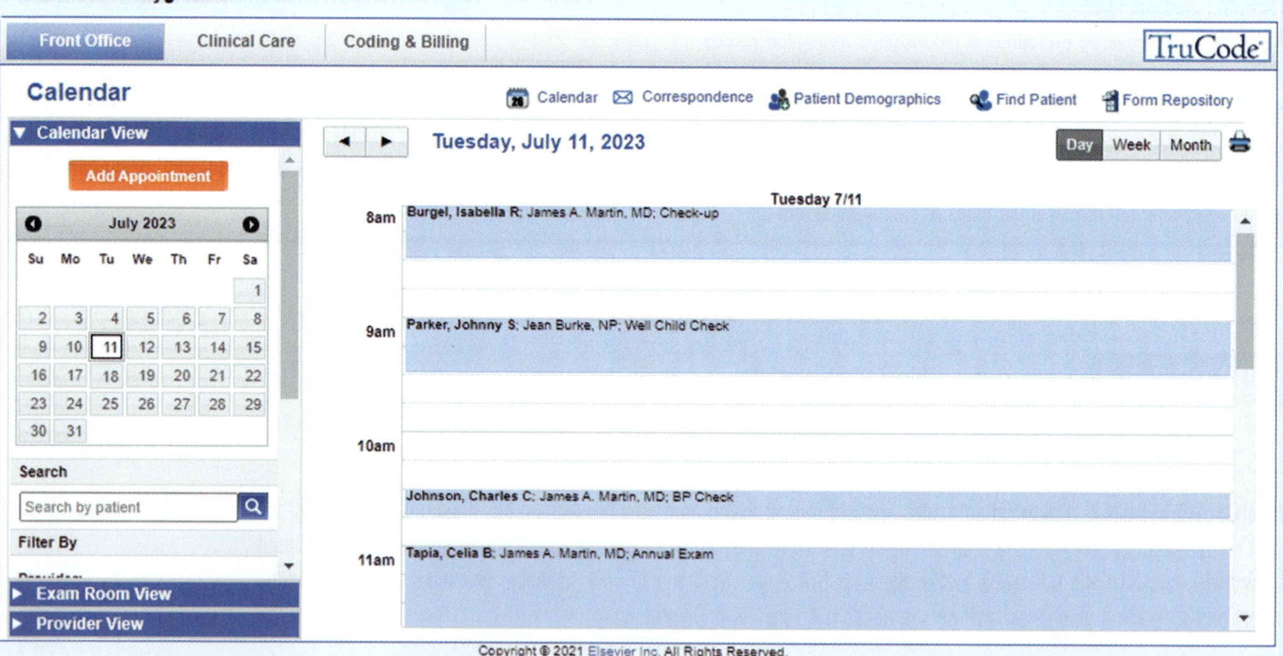

PROCEDURE 9.3 Coach Patients Regarding Office Policies

TASKS: Create a new patient brochure, and then role-play ways to coach patients regarding office policies.

SCENARIO: You work at Walden-Martin Family Medical Clinic. Your supervisor asks you to create a new patient brochure for the clinic. The clinic information is listed below. After you complete the brochure, you coach the following patients regarding office procedures:

- Mr. Charles Johnson (he has a question regarding the payment policy)
- Ms. Monique Jones (she has a question regarding the medication refill procedure)

PROCEDURE 9.3 Coach Patients Regarding Office Policies

CLINIC INFORMATION	PROVIDERS
Walden-Martin Family Medical Clinic	Julie Walden, MD
1234 Anystreet	James Martin, MD
Anytown, Anystate 12345	Angela Perez, MD
Phone: 123-123-1234	David Kahn, MD
Fax: 123-123-5678	Jean Burke, NP

EQUIPMENT and SUPPLIES

- Computer with word processing software and printer
- Office procedure manual (optional)

PROCEDURAL STEPS

1. Using word processing software, design an informational brochure for patients that provides information about the practice and describes practice procedures. At a minimum, the information should include the following:
   - Description of the practice (e.g., type of practice, mission statement)
   - Location or a map of the practice
   - Contact information (i.e., telephone numbers, emails, and website addresses)
   - Providers' names and credentials
   - Services offered
   - Hours of operation
   - How appointments can be scheduled
   - Practice policies and procedures (e.g., payment policies, appointment cancellations, medication refills, assistance after hours)

   PURPOSE: Providing patients with a written brochure listing the practice's information, policies, and procedures enables patients to use it as a reference.
2. Proofread the brochure. Make revisions as needed. Print the brochure.
   PURPOSE: It is important to proofread and revise documents as needed before they go to patients.
3. Using the scenario provided for the first patient, give a brief summary of the different parts of the brochure. Use words that the patient will understand.
   PURPOSE: By discussing each part of the brochure with the potential patient, you can help explain what is stated. Summarize the information without reading the sections to the other person.
4. Ask if the patient has any questions. Actively listen to the patient's concerns. Address the patient's concerns.
   PURPOSE: By actively listening, you will be able to identify issues or confusion the patient is experiencing. It is important that the messages during the conversation are clear for both parties.
5. Using the scenario provided for the second patient, give a brief summary of the different parts of the brochure. Use words that the patient will understand.
   PURPOSE: By reviewing the brochure, you can summarize what the policies are. If the patient has an immediate question, you can answer it.
6. Ask if the patient has any questions. Actively listen to the patient's concerns. Address the patient's concerns.
   PURPOSE: By actively listening, you will be able to identify issues or confusion the patient is experiencing. It is important that the messages during the conversation are clear for both parties.

PROCEDURE 9.4 Schedule an Established Patient

TASK: Manage the provider's schedule by scheduling appointments for an established patient and handling rescheduling and a no-show appointment.

SCENARIO: Celia Tapia has just finished seeing Dr. Martin and is checking out at your desk. You see that she needs to schedule a follow-up appointment to occur in 2 weeks. The scheduling guidelines indicate a follow-up appointment is 15 minutes long.

EQUIPMENT and SUPPLIES

- Appointment book or computer with scheduling software
- Scheduling guidelines
- Pencil, red pen
- Reminder card
- Patient's health record

PROCEDURAL STEPS

1. Obtain the patient's name and information, purpose of the visit, the provider to be seen, and any scheduling preferences. If using the scheduling software, enter the patient's name and date of birth (DOB). Verify the correct patient is selected.
   PURPOSE: To schedule an appointment, you must have the patient's information, along with the provider to be seen and the type of appointment required. Knowing any scheduling preferences or limitations will help you to efficiently find an acceptable appointment time for the patient.
2. Identify the length of the appointment by using the scheduling guidelines.
   PURPOSE: Depending on the appointment type, each provider may require a different length of time for that appointment. Ensuring you

PROCEDURE 9.4 Schedule an Established Patient—cont'd

schedule the appropriate amount of time will help facilitate the flow of patients on that day.

3. Search the appointment book or scheduling software for the first suitable appointment time and an alternate time. Offer the patient a choice of these dates and times. Be open to alternative times if the patient cannot make the initial options you gave. Provide additional appointment options as needed.
   PURPOSE: Providing the patient with a choice of dates and times and additional options as needed demonstrates sensitivity when you are managing appointments. It is an important customer service technique (see the following figure).

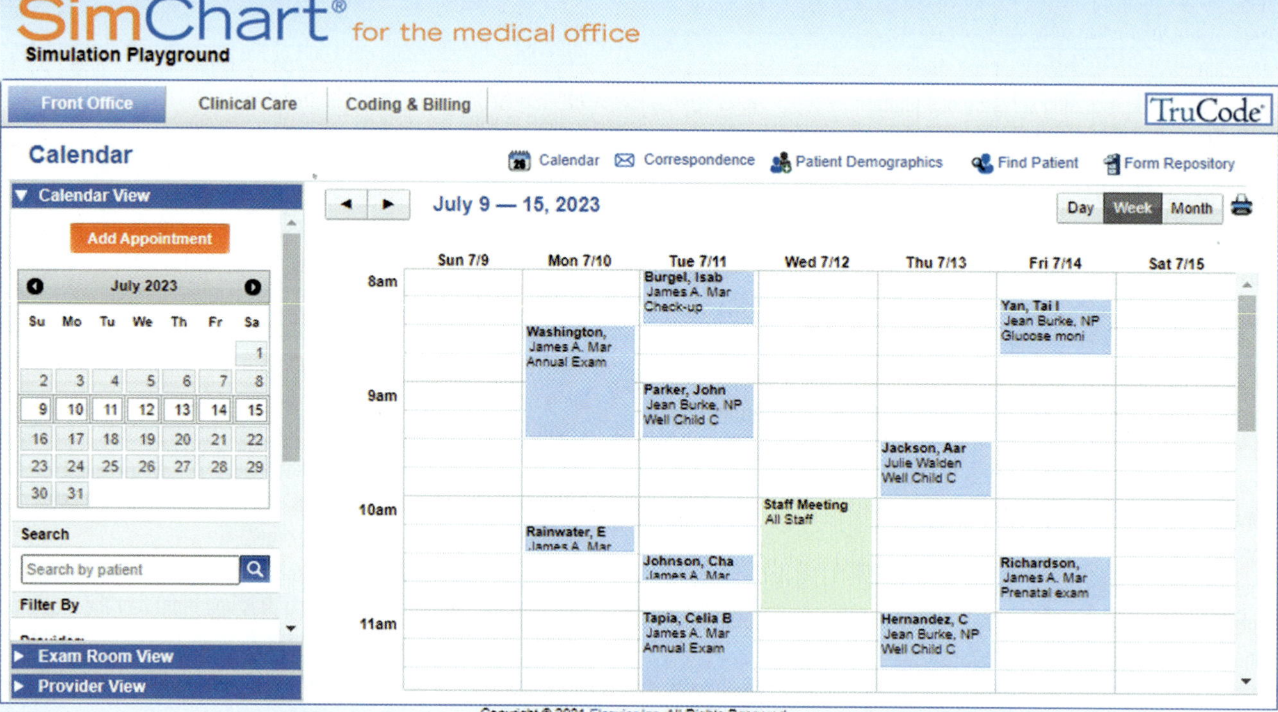

4. Using a pencil, write the patient's name and phone number in the appointment book, and block out the correct amount of time. Add in any other relevant information per the facility's procedures. If using the scheduling software, create the appointment per the facility's guidelines.
   PURPOSE: Adding the patient's phone number to the appointment book saves time if the patient needs to be contacted. Using pencil to write down the information in the book allows it to be erased if the patient cancels or reschedules for another time.
5. Complete the appointment reminder card, and ensure the date and time on the card match the appointment time. Give the card to the patient.
   PURPOSE: Using appointment reminder cards helps patients remember when their appointments are and reduces the number of no-show appointments.

CONTINUATION OF SCENARIO

Later that day, Celica Tapia calls and says she needs to reschedule her appointment for the next day at the same time.

6. When a patient calls to reschedule an appointment, follow steps 1 through 4. When the new appointment is made, make sure to erase the old appointment from the appointment log. With the scheduling software, ensure the old appointment time is removed from the schedule. Repeat the new appointment date and time to the patient.
   Note: It is important to erase the old appointment so that the patient is not expected on two different days. Erasing or deleting the old appointment opens up that time for another patient.

CONTINUATION OF SCENARIO

Celia Tapia no-shows for her follow-up appointment.

7. In the appointment book, using a red pen, indicate that the patient no-showed. Using the patient's health record, document that the patient failed to show for the follow-up examination with the provider. In an electronic system, change the appointment status to no-show and ensure that it is documented in the health record.
   PURPOSE: For legal purposes, the healthcare facility must keep a record of patients who no-show for appointments. If this is indicated in the appointment book and in the health record, the practice is covered if any issues should arise. Some medical practices have procedures that include contacting the patient regarding the no-show appointment and finding out the reason. This is then also charted in the health record.

PROCEDURE 9.5 Schedule a Patient Procedure

TASK: Schedule a patient for a procedure within the time frame needed by the provider, confirm with the patient, and issue all required instructions.

SCENARIO: Monique Jones has just seen Dr. Perez and is checking out at your desk. She gives you an order from the provider that states she needs to have a magnetic resonance image (MRI) of her left ankle within a week. The radiology department in your facility performs MRIs.

EQUIPMENT and SUPPLIES

- Provider's order detailing the procedure required
- Computer with order entry software (optional)
- Name, address, and telephone number of facility where procedure will take place
- Patient's demographic and insurance information
- Patient's health record
- Procedure preparation instructions
- Telephone
- Consent form (if required for the procedure)

PROCEDURAL STEPS

1. Obtain an oral or written order from the provider for the exact procedure to be performed.
   PURPOSE: To schedule the procedure, you will need an order from the provider for the procedure to be performed.
2. Gather the patient's demographic and insurance information. If using an electronic health record, verify you have the correct patient.
   Note: For some procedures and diagnostic tests, precertifications or preauthorizations need to be completed before the patient is scheduled. (This will be discussed in a later chapter.)

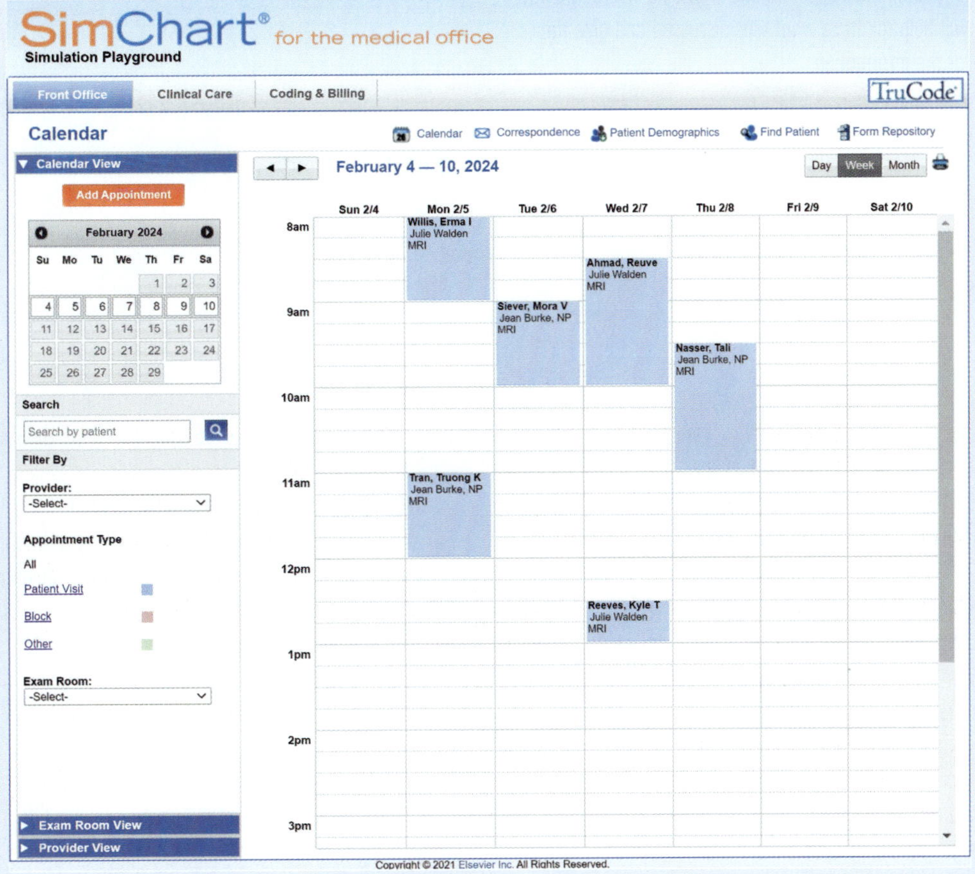

PROCEDURE 9.5 Schedule a Patient Procedure—cont'd

3. Determine the patient's availability within the time frame provided by the provider for the procedure (see the following figure).
   PURPOSE: To make sure the patient will be able to comply with the arrangements for the test, and to schedule the procedure and provide needed information.
4. Notify the patient of the arrangements, and provide the information in a written format.
   - Give the name, address, and telephone number of the diagnostic facility.
   - Specify the date and time that the patient is to report for the procedure.
   - Give instructions on preparation for the test (e.g., eating restrictions, fluids, medications, enemas).
   - If another facility is used, the patient will need to bring a form of picture identification and the insurance card.
   - If you are not using a computerized provider order entry system, explain whether the patient needs to pick up orders or whether the order will be sent to the facility in advance.
   - Ask if the patient has any questions, and answer the questions.

   PURPOSE: Make sure the patient understands the necessary preparations and the importance of keeping the appointment. Providing written instructions to the patient will help reinforce what was discussed and give the patient a reference for the information.
5. If a consent form is required for the procedure, ensure the provider has reviewed the form with the patient and the patient has signed the consent form. A copy of the consent form may be required by the diagnostic facility before the procedure. The consent form should be scanned and uploaded into the electronic health record or placed in the paper record.
   PURPOSE: The consent form is used to make sure the patient understands the risks, benefits, and alternatives to the procedure.
6. Document the details of the scheduled procedure in the patient's health record. If applicable, create a reminder to check on the procedure results after the appointment date.
   PURPOSE: Document that the procedure was scheduled. It is legally important to show that what was ordered was scheduled. Creating a reminder for yourself to check up on the results of the procedure is also important in assisting the provider.

Documentation Example

2/27/20XX Patient scheduled for colonoscopy on 3/10/20XX 8:00 a.m. at Anytown Hospital. Patient preparation instructions given, and patient verbalized understanding. —————————— Ramona West, CMA

HEALTH RECORDS 10

SCENARIO

Susan Beezler has just begun her career in the medical assisting profession. In the morning, she attends medical assisting school, and in the afternoon, she works part-time for the Walden-Martin Family Medical (WMFM) Clinic as a records assistant. Susan is eager to learn about healthcare and looks forward to taking on more responsibility at the office.

Dr. David Kahn is a new provider who has recently joined WMFM Clinic. Dr. Kahn has enjoyed working with Susan and feels that her energy will be just what his patients need. He has taken a professional interest in Susan and often lets her assist him with patients when her other duties allow.

Susan knows that although she is a beginner in the office, she will gain trust from her supervisors and patients as long as she projects a teachable attitude. The office has recently converted to an electronic records system but is also still using paper records. Susan uses the information she learned in school about both types of health records. She cheerfully performs filing and even does some transcription for Dr. Kahn. The other staff members are pleased with her willingness to perform the most mundane tasks.

Susan enjoys sharing her experiences with her classmates. She is the only student currently working in the medical field, and the others ask her lots of questions about the real world of medical assisting. She is careful not to breach patient confidentiality; she discusses situations only in general terms, never mentioning any patients' names.

Susan feels a great sense of pride that she is already a member of the healthcare team and able to contribute to the lives of her patients.

While studying this chapter, think about the following questions:

- What is the definition and application of subjective information?
- What is the definition and application of objective information?
- How does the HITECH act impact health records?
- How can you maintain a connection with the patient when using an EHR?
- What are the different ways to back up an EHR?
- How do you correctly destroy health records?
- How do you document health records?
- What equipment and supplies are needed for a paper records system?
- What are the indexing rules for alphabetic and numeric filing systems?

LEARNING OBJECTIVES

1. Differentiate between electronic health records (EHRs) and electronic medical records (EMRs).
2. Assess the contents of health records.
3. Describe the components of working effectively within health records.
4. Determine the processes for creating an efficient paper health record system.
5. Differentiate the different ways of organizing files.
6. Discuss the organization of files and health-related correspondence.

VOCABULARY

age of majority The age at which the law recognizes a person to be an adult; it varies by state.

alphabetic filing Any system that arranges names or topics according to the sequence of the letters in the alphabet.

alphanumeric Describes systems made up of combinations of letters and numbers.

anthropometric (an thruh po ME trik) Pertaining to the measurement of the size and proportions of the human body.

caption A heading, title, or subtitle under which records are filed.

compliance (kuhm PLIE uhns) Meeting the standards and regulations of the practice's established policies and procedures. Can also mean cooperation.

concise (kuhn SICE) Using as few words as possible to express a message.

continuity of care The smooth continuation of care from one provider to another. This allows the patient to receive the most benefit with no interruption or duplication of care.

dictation (dik TEY shuhn) To say something aloud for another person to write

direct filing system A filing system in which materials can be located without consulting another source of reference.

electronic health record (EHR) An electronic record that conforms to nationally recognized standards and contains health-related information about a specific patient. It can be created,

VOCABULARY—*continued*

managed, and consulted by authorized clinicians and staff from more than one healthcare organization.

e-prescribing The use of electronic software to communicate with pharmacies and send prescribing information. It takes the place of writing a prescription by hand and giving it to a patient; most new or refill prescriptions can be submitted electronically, cutting down on fraud and errors.

hereditary (huh RED i ter ee) Passed from parents to offspring through the genes.

incidence (IN si duhns) How often something happens or occurs.

interface An interconnection between systems.

interoperability (in ter op er uh BIL i tee) The ability to work with other systems.

numeric filing The filing of records, correspondence, or cards by number.

objective information Data obtained through physical examination, laboratory and diagnostic testing, and by measurable information.

obliteration (ub lit uh REY shun) To remove or destroy all traces of; do away with; destroy completely.

out guides Sturdy cardboard or plastic file-sized cards used to replace a folder temporarily removed from the filing space.

parameters (puh RAM i ters) Rules that control how something should be done; guidelines or boundaries.

patient portal A secure online website that gives patients 24-hour access to personal health information using a username and password.

prognosis (prog NOH sis) The likely outcome of a disease, including the chance of recovery.

provisional diagnosis (die ug NOH sis) A temporary diagnosis made before all test results have been received.

quality control A process to ensure the reliability of test results, often using manufactured samples with known values.

retention schedule A method or plan for retaining or keeping health records and for their movement from active to inactive to closed.

reverse chronologic order The most recent item is on top, and the oldest item is last.

subjective information Data or information obtained from the patient, including the patient's feelings, perceptions, and concerns; this information is obtained through interviews or written questions.

subsequent (SUHB si kwuhnt) Occurring later or after.

tickler file A chronologic file used as a reminder that something must be dealt with on a certain date.

transcription (tran SKRIP shuhn) A typed or written copy of dictated material.

vested Granted or endowed with a particular authority, right, or property; to have a special interest in.

INTRODUCTION

Health records can be found in two different formats, electronic and paper. Most healthcare facilities have switched to **electronic health records (EHRs)**. Some of the benefits of EHRs include the following:

- Easy storage of patient information
- Availability to multiple users at the same time
- A more efficient claim submission process

The federal government has also offered financial incentives for providers to implement EHRs. Although most providers are using EHRs, there are still some who are using paper records and others who are using a combination of electronic and paper formats. A provider who is making the switch to an EHR may decide to keep the patient's previous records in the paper format and just use the electronic format moving forward. Some providers may decide to scan the last 3 to 5 years of the paper record into the electronic record. Whatever scenario the healthcare facility has chosen, it is important for the medical assistant to understand both systems and to be able to perform well with either one.

ELECTRONIC RECORDS

Paper health records have been shown to be much less efficient than an EHR. In most cases, only one person at a time can use the paper record. It is fairly common for information to be filed in the incorrect record. The entire record also can be misfiled. Gathering data for research and **quality control** is more challenging. Data is difficult to share in facilities with multiple departments or locations. The paper-based record is good for the documentation of patient care, but it is not nearly as useful in other capacities.

With an EHR, multiple users can access the record at the same time. There are fewer errors because handwritten notes do not have to be interpreted. Most EHRs link the clinical information needed for billing purposes. An EHR also includes practice management capabilities that allow for patient scheduling and the generation of reports needed for research and quality control.

It is important for the medical assistant to be aware of the differences between the practice management software and the EHR. You may use both during your day as a medical assistant. The EHR contains a record of patient interactions and health history. The practice management software allows the facility to operate the business side by maintaining schedules and financial information for revenue cycle management for reimbursement.

CRITICAL THINKING APPLICATION 10.1

Some of Dr. Kahn's patients are concerned that computer-based health records may not be completely private. They are worried that unauthorized individuals could access their information on the computer and do them harm. Should patients be allowed to decide whether their records are kept on a computer or on paper? Why or why not?

EHR versus EMR

There is some confusion regarding the acronyms *EHR* and *EMR* (electronic medical record). These acronyms have been used interchangeably

TABLE 10.1 Electronic Health Record (EHR) versus Electronic Medical Record (EMR)

ELECTRONIC HEALTH RECORD (EHR)	ELECTRONIC MEDICAL RECORD (EMR)
• Electronic record of health-related information about a patient • Conforms to nationally recognized interoperability standards • Can be created, managed, and consulted by authorized clinicians and staff from more than one healthcare organization	• An electronic record of health-related information about an individual • An electronic version of a paper record • Can be created, gathered, managed, and consulted by authorized clinicians and staff within a single healthcare organization

for many years. The Office of the National Coordinator for Health Information Technology (ONC) has established definitions for EHR and EMR that are easy to understand. Table 10.1 shows the definitions of EHR and EMR.

EMR is being used less and less as the federal regulations regarding electronic records have been established. There is a significant push toward having all electronic records meet the definition of an EHR. There are many advantages to having an electronic record system that can be accessed by more than one healthcare organization. The continuity of patient care is much more easily established when all providers have access to the same records, regardless of what organization they are working for. There should be less running of duplicate tests and procedures, which will reduce the cost of providing healthcare.

A *personal health record* (PHR) is defined by the ONC as an electronic record of health-related information about an individual that conforms to nationally recognized **interoperability** standards and can be drawn from multiple sources, but that is managed, shared, and controlled by the individual. There are several ways that a PHR can be created. Some health insurance companies offer PHRs for those they insure, some employers offer it as a service for their employees, and some healthcare facilities offer it to their patients. It is important to remember that the patient maintains a PHR. The information from an EHR does not automatically transfer to a PHR unless it is part of the healthcare organization's EHR.

Another way for patients to access their healthcare information is through a **patient portal**. Patient portals allow patients to access their actual EHRs. At any time, a patient can view progress notes, laboratory results, medications, or immunizations. Many patient portal systems also allow the following:

- Communication between the patient and the provider
- Completion of forms online
- Requests for prescription refills
- Scheduling of appointments

By establishing effective patient portals, healthcare facilities can meet some of the meaningful use requirements.

The security of electronic records is a big part of the Health Insurance Portability and Accountability Act (HIPAA). HIPAA uses the term *protected health information* (PHI), which is any information about health status, the provision of healthcare, or payment for healthcare that can be linked to an individual patient. HIPAA requires that all PHI be safeguarded. This applies to the following:

- EHRs
- EMRs
- PHRs
- Patient portals

Capabilities of Electronic Health Record Systems

The EHR system can perform a multitude of tasks, saving time and money in the provider's office (Figure 10.1). The following are some of the features of a typical EHR system:

- *Specialty software:* Patient data is captured and processed into a system that is specialty specific. The terminology and patient care treatments are compatible with the provider's specialty. However, additional features can allow the provider to include terminology from other specialties.
- *Appointment scheduler:* The appointment scheduler (Figure 10.2) allows the staff to do the following:
  - Track and schedule appointments
  - Create the schedule matrix
  - Account for recurring time blocks

The appointments can be merged into specific types with default times so that lengthy procedures are not scheduled in short appointment blocks. The scheduler features also allow various search **parameters**; if a patient calls because they cannot remember the appointment time, a search can be initiated using the following details:

  - Date
  - Provider's name
  - Patient's name
  - Keywords
- *Appointment reminder and confirmation:* The system can be programmed to automatically remind patients with a confirmation call. The staff can record the message to be sent, and patients are prompted to choose options, such as "Press 1" to confirm or reschedule appointments.
- *Prescription writer:* The EHR system can produce electronic prescriptions, which can be printed and given to patients or automatically submitted to a pharmacy. Lists can be created with the provider's most common drug choices and dosages. An allergy function can be linked to the patient's list of allergies and alert the provider of an issue. The system can also generate a patient information sheet on new prescriptions.
- *Medical billing system:* Also known as a *practice management system.* The EHR billing system can manage all of the practice's billing and accounting systems. The system also can **interface** with clearinghouses for electronic claims submission and tracking. Reports can be generated that provide accurate details of the financial state of the practice at certain intervals or whenever requested.
- *Charge capture:* The charge capture functions can store lists of billing codes, such as the following:
  - International Classification of Diseases (ICD)
  - Current Procedural Terminology (CPT)
  - Charges for procedures, supplies, and laboratory tests

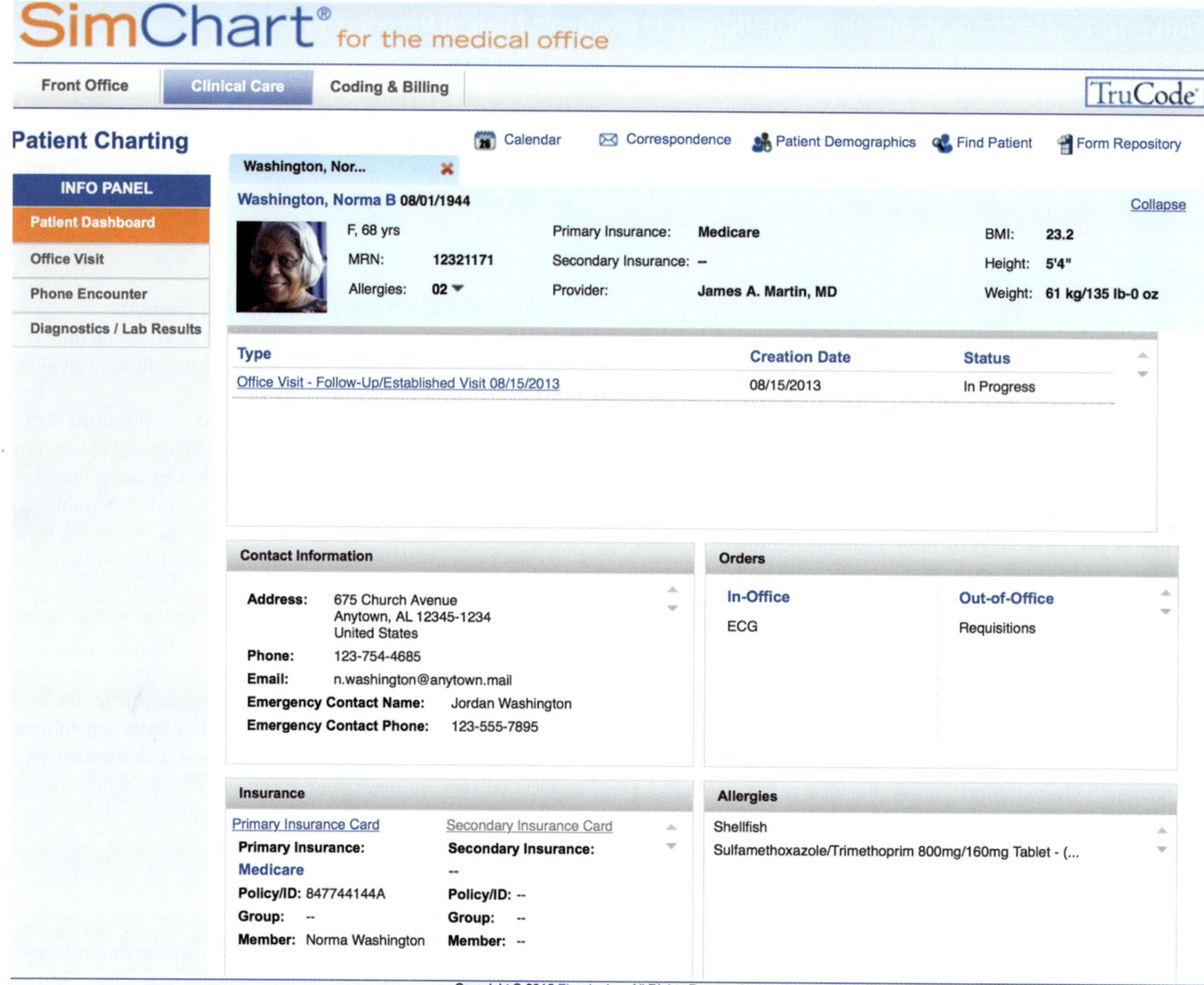

FIGURE 10.1 The electronic health record (EHR) can perform numerous tasks, in addition to displaying personal information about the patient. This allows the provider and medical assistants to interact with patients and provide better service.

Alerts can let the user know when a certain charge does not match a diagnosis code—for instance, a blood glucose test done for a sore throat. In such cases, the software alerts the user and helps prevent errors that can lead to a denial of insurance claims.

- *Eligibility verification:* EHR billing systems can perform online verification of insurance eligibility and capture demographic data.
- *Referral management:* In the case of a referral or consultation, sharing information with another provider can be done electronically. The patient does not have to obtain copies of the record and then take them to the new provider. This also eliminates the cost of making copies and is faster and more efficient than copying and mailing patients' records.
- *Laboratory order integration:* The laboratory order integration feature allows the user to interact with outside laboratories. The EHR can receive and post laboratory results to patients' records. Tests can be ordered from the provider's laptop, tablet, or smartphone. Results can be transmitted by fax, scan, or email and uploaded directly into the patient's record (Procedure 10.1).

CRITICAL THINKING APPLICATION 10.2

Jennifer, the office manager, has noticed that Susan seems overwhelmed in the training classes for the EHR system used by the clinic. During a break, Jennifer asks Susan whether she is having any specific problems with the training classes. She also asks for Susan's input on the system. Susan says that she just prefers clinical work and that her typing skills are a little rusty. She is determined to do her best to learn the system and asks if she could have extra practice time.

- How might Jennifer respond to Susan's comments?
- What can Susan do to overcome her issues with the EHR system?

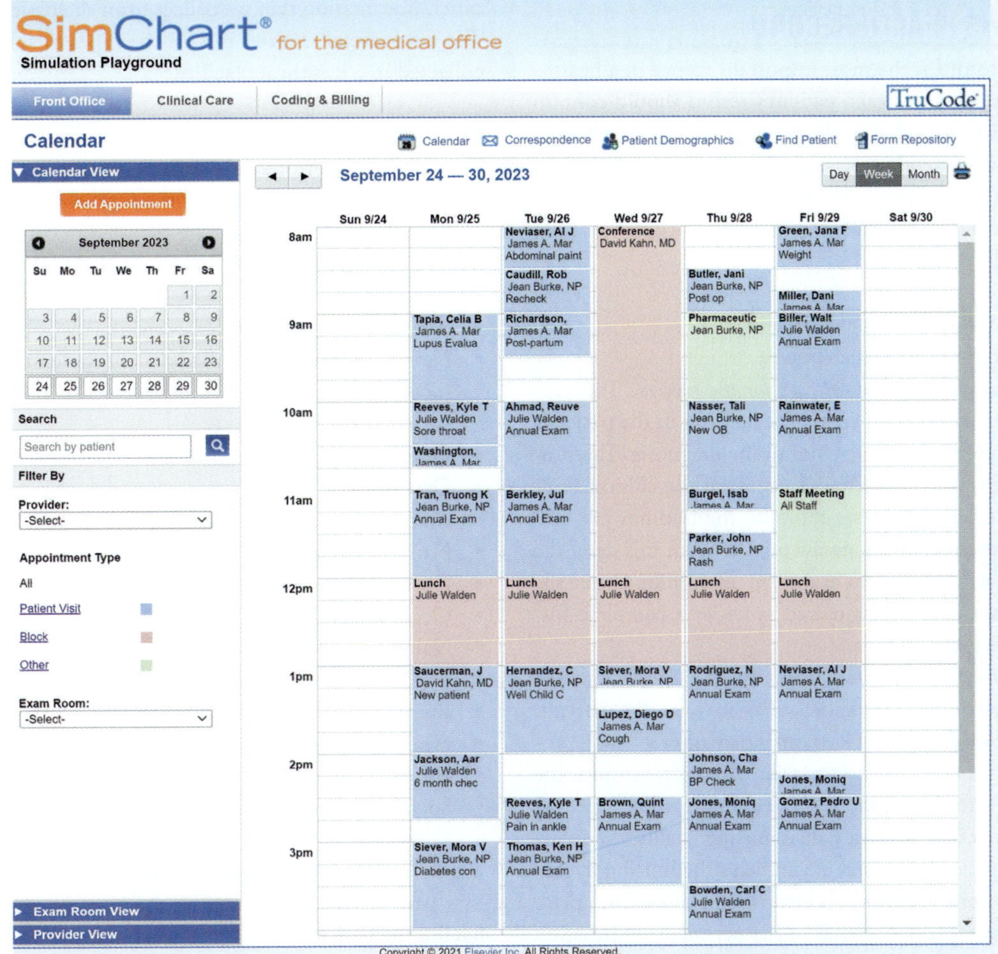

FIGURE 10.2 The EHR usually has a scheduling system that can be changed to manage the needs of the provider and office staff.

The Health Information Technology for Economic and Clinical Health Act (HITECH), Meaningful Use, and Promoting Operability

The HITECH Act provided financial incentives for the meaningful use of certified EHR technology to achieve health and efficiency goals. It was part of the American Recovery and Reinvestment Act to promote the adoption and meaningful use of health information technology. Remember, HIPAA was created in large part to simplify administrative processes using electronic devices. *Meaningful use* means that providers had to show that they were using EHR technology in ways that could be measured significantly in quality and quantity. If providers met the meaningful use requirements, they qualified for incentive payments.

In 2018, the meaningful use program was renamed "Promoting Interoperability." The focus is now on patient health data access and interoperability. There are currently four objectives:

- *Electronic prescribing:* Generate and transmit permissible discharge prescriptions electronically.
- *Health information exchange (HIE):* Encourage and leverage interoperability on a broader scale and promote health information technology (IT)–based care coordination.
- *Provider to patient exchange:* Provide patients with electronic access to their health information.
- *Public health and clinical data exchange:* Determine that an eligible hospital or critical access hospital attests yes to being in active engagement with a public health agency or clinical data registry to submit electronic public health data in a meaningful way using certified electronic health record technology.

Providers can expect reductions in the amounts they are paid from Medicare and Medicaid if they are not in **compliance**. Remember, the computer system in the medical office must be more than a tool for data recall to be considered an EHR system; the provider must use the system to meet the promoting interoperability objectives.

CRITICAL THINKING APPLICATION 10.3

Some of the patients who visit Dr. Kahn and Dr. Martin have expressed concern that electronic health records (EHRs) may not be private enough and that their health information will be "floating around on the internet." They are worried that unauthorized individuals could somehow access their information on the computer and do them harm.

- How might Susan alleviate the patients' fears about their records being available on the internet?
- What disadvantages with regard to confidentiality are associated with the EHR?

CONTENTS OF THE HEALTH RECORD

The patient's health record is the most important record in a healthcare facility. For completeness, each patient's record should contain **subjective information** provided by the patient and **objective information** obtained by the provider and staff of the healthcare facility. If all entries are complete, the health record will stand the test of time. No branch of medicine is exempt from the need to keep accurate patient health records.

Importance of Accurate Health Records

Health records are kept for five basic reasons:

- *To provide the best possible medical care for the patient:* The provider examines the patient and enters the findings in the patient's health record. These findings are clues to the diagnosis. The provider may order many types of tests to confirm the clinical findings. As the reports of these tests come in, the findings fall into place, much like the pieces of a jigsaw puzzle. With this data, the provider can prescribe treatment and form an opinion about the patient's **prognosis**. The health record provides a complete history of all the care given to the patient.
- *To provide critical information for others:* By reading through the record and discovering the methods used to treat the patient, healthcare professionals can provide **continuity of care**. Each provider knows what services have been provided and can continue the care, even from one facility to another. For example, when a patient is transferred from a hospital to a skilled nursing facility, the information from the patient's hospital record helps the nursing facility staff to better care for the patient. When patients move from place to place or caregivers change, copies of the pertinent information should move with the patient to provide this continuity of care.
- *To provide legal protection for those who provided care to the patient:* A well-documented health record is excellent proof that certain procedures were performed or that medical advice was given. An accurate record is the foundation for a legal defense in cases of medical professional liability. This is one reason why it is critical to write legibly in the paper record to document what happened to the patient and the provider's response exactly. Remember, if it is not documented, it did not happen.
- *To provide statistical information that is helpful to researchers:* The patient's record provides information about medications taken and the reactions to them. Health records may be used to evaluate the effectiveness of certain kinds of treatment or to determine the **incidence** of a given disease. Providers often take part in drug studies that track adverse reactions and side effects. The effects of various treatments and procedures can also be tracked, and statistics can be gathered from patients' records. When statistical information is tracked, the patient-specific data is removed. This information may result in a new outlook on some phases of medicine and can lead to revised techniques and treatments. The statistical data from health records are also valuable in the preparation of scientific papers, books, and lectures.
- *To provide support for claims reimbursement:* This is required by most insurance companies.

Subjective Information

Subjective information is the information gathered from the patient's point of view. We cannot see it or measure it in any way. There is much information that we collect from the patient that is subjective. The next several sections discuss the types of subjective information collected in a healthcare facility.

Personal Demographics

The patient's health record begins with routine personal data, which the patient usually supplies on the first visit when the health record is established. Most patients are required to complete a patient information form (Figure 10.3; Procedure 10.2). The following basic facts are included:

- Patient's full name, spelled correctly
- Names of parents/guardians if the patient is a child or legally incompetent
- Patient's sex
- Preferred gender pronouns
- Date of birth (DOB)
- Marital status
- Name of spouse, if married
- Home address, telephone number, and email address
- Occupation
- Name of employer
- Business address and telephone number
- Employment information for spouse
- Healthcare insurance information
- Source of referral
- Social Security number

Past Health, Family, and Social History

The past health, family, and social histories are often obtained by having the patient complete a questionnaire. Medical assistants may review the form for completeness, and they may need to clarify any questions or missing information with the patient before the patient is seen by the provider. The provider will also add information obtained during the patient interview. The responses provide information about the following issues:

- Any past illnesses (including injuries or physical defects, whether congenital or acquired)
- Hospitalizations or surgeries the patient has had (Figure 10.4)
- Patient's daily health habits

Stickers can be used on the front of paper health records to indicate allergies, advance directives, and other information (Figure 10.5). In an EHR, there will be alerts that may appear as pop-up windows when the record is accessed; these will let the provider know if the patient has allergies, if immunizations are due, or if there is no advance directive on file. The alerts are helpful for the health professional because they keep important facts about the patient in the forefront of the professional's mind while treating the individual.

Past Health History. The past health history will include information about the following:

- Previous illnesses/injuries (including childhood illnesses, such as chickenpox or measles)
- Previous hospitalizations
- Previous surgeries

The dates that these occurred will need to be documented, along with any complications that occurred. The provider needs to be aware of this information because it could affect the patient's current condition.

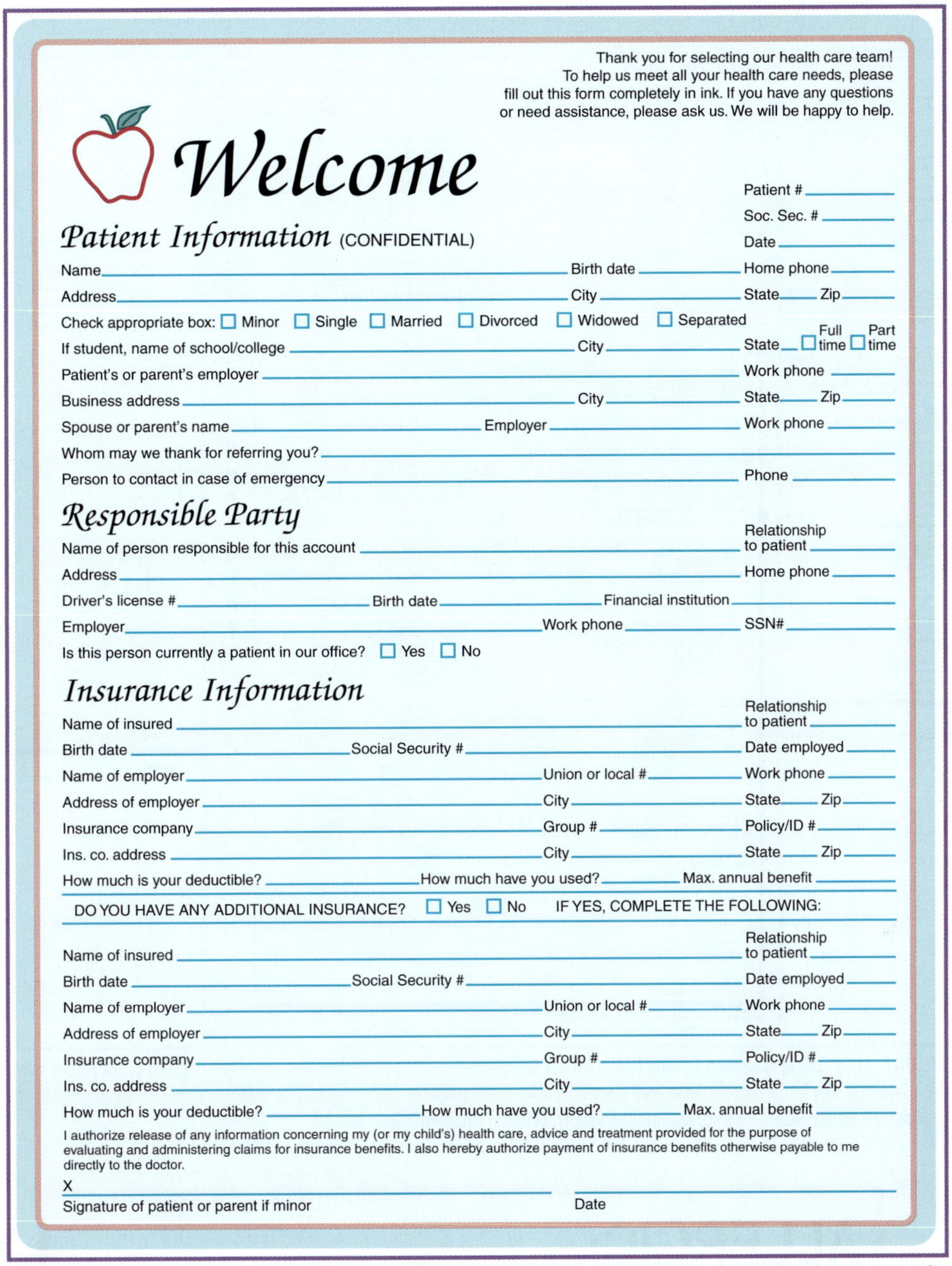

Thank you for selecting our health care team!
To help us meet all your health care needs, please fill out this form completely in ink. If you have any questions or need assistance, please ask us. We will be happy to help.

Welcome

Patient # ________
Soc. Sec. # ________
Date ________

Patient Information (CONFIDENTIAL)

Name ________ Birth date ________ Home phone ________
Address ________ City ________ State ____ Zip ____
Check appropriate box: ☐ Minor ☐ Single ☐ Married ☐ Divorced ☐ Widowed ☐ Separated
If student, name of school/college ________ City ________ State ____ ☐ Full time ☐ Part time
Patient's or parent's employer ________ Work phone ________
Business address ________ City ________ State ____ Zip ____
Spouse or parent's name ________ Employer ________ Work phone ________
Whom may we thank for referring you? ________
Person to contact in case of emergency ________ Phone ________

Responsible Party

Name of person responsible for this account ________ Relationship to patient ________
Address ________ Home phone ________
Driver's license # ________ Birth date ________ Financial institution ________
Employer ________ Work phone ________ SSN# ________
Is this person currently a patient in our office? ☐ Yes ☐ No

Insurance Information

Name of insured ________ Relationship to patient ________
Birth date ________ Social Security # ________ Date employed ________
Name of employer ________ Union or local # ________ Work phone ________
Address of employer ________ City ________ State ____ Zip ____
Insurance company ________ Group # ________ Policy/ID # ________
Ins. co. address ________ City ________ State ____ Zip ____
How much is your deductible? ________ How much have you used? ________ Max. annual benefit ________

DO YOU HAVE ANY ADDITIONAL INSURANCE? ☐ Yes ☐ No IF YES, COMPLETE THE FOLLOWING:

Name of insured ________ Relationship to patient ________
Birth date ________ Social Security # ________ Date employed ________
Name of employer ________ Union or local # ________ Work phone ________
Address of employer ________ City ________ State ____ Zip ____
Insurance company ________ Group # ________ Policy/ID # ________
Ins. co. address ________ City ________ State ____ Zip ____
How much is your deductible? ________ How much have you used? ________ Max. annual benefit ________

I authorize release of any information concerning my (or my child's) health care, advice and treatment provided for the purpose of evaluating and administering claims for insurance benefits. I also hereby authorize payment of insurance benefits otherwise payable to me directly to the doctor.

X ________ ________
Signature of patient or parent if minor Date

FIGURE 10.3 The patient information form provides all of the information that the medical assistant needs to construct the patient's record.

Family History. The family history includes the following:

- The physical condition of the various members of the patient's family
- Any illnesses or diseases individual members may have had
- Causes of death

This information is important because certain diseases may have a **hereditary** pattern. Most providers are interested in the immediate family: parents, grandparents, siblings, and children.

Social History. The social history includes information about the patient's lifestyle:

- Living situation
- Marital status
- Employment
- Tobacco use
- Alcohol and drug use
- Exercise
- Nutrition

All of these factors can have an impact on a patient's overall health; they can also help highlight risk factors.

CRITICAL THINKING APPLICATION 10.4

While taking a patient's medical history, Susan asks about the patient's social history. She asks whether the patient drinks alcohol. The patient immediately becomes defensive and accuses Susan of getting too personal.

- How might Susan explain her reasons for asking these questions? What options are available if patients refuse to discuss their social history with Susan?
- Could this opposition to questions about the social history raise suspicion in Susan's mind? What might she suspect?

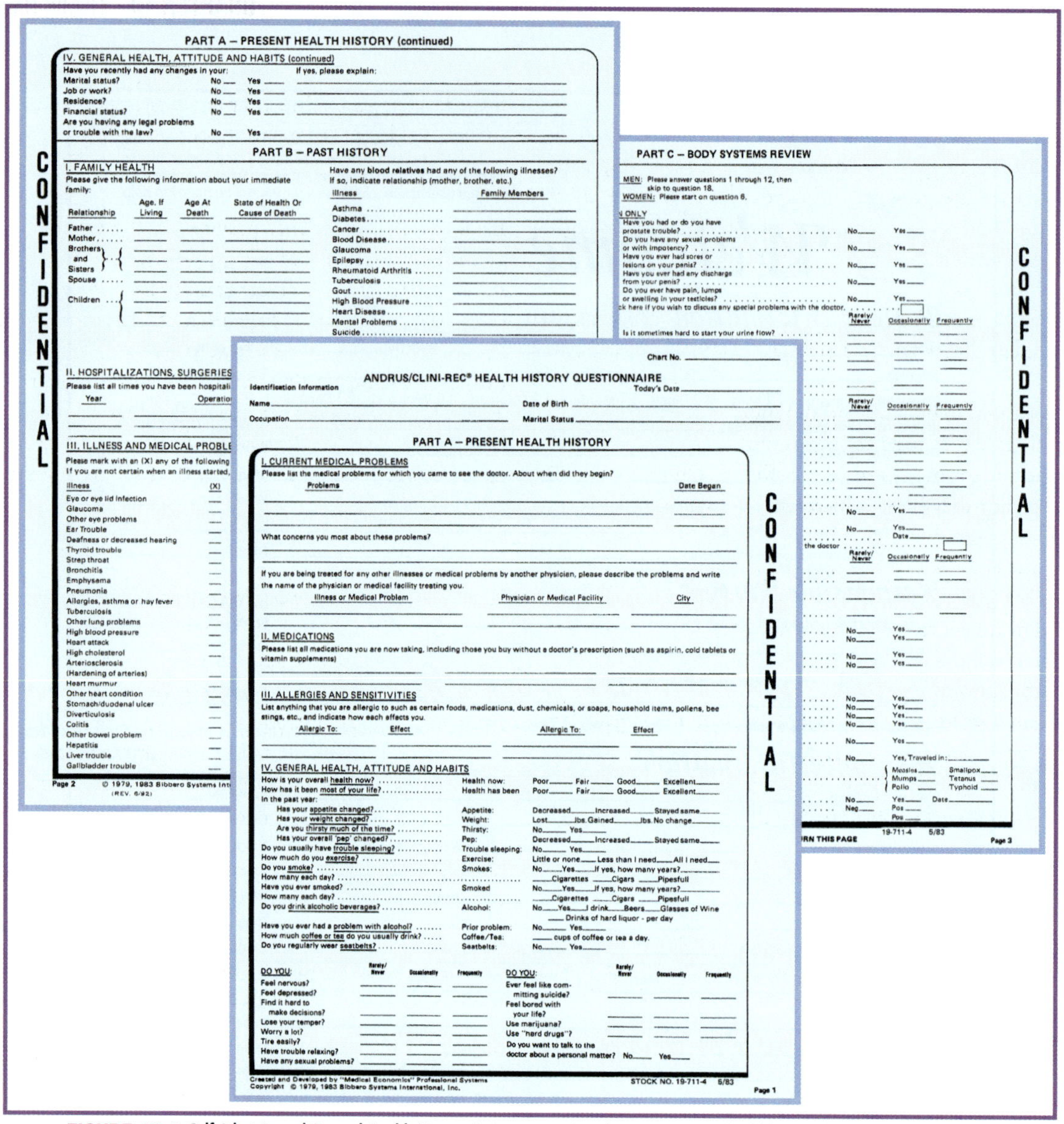

ANDRUS/CLINI-REC® HEALTH HISTORY QUESTIONNAIRE

PART A – PRESENT HEALTH HISTORY

PART B – PAST HISTORY

PART C – BODY SYSTEMS REVIEW

CONFIDENTIAL

FIGURE 10.4 Self-Administered General Health History Questionnaire. Lengthy questionnaires should be completed by the patient before the individual is seen by the provider. Either mail the questionnaire to the patient in advance or ask the patient to come in early to complete the paperwork. (Courtesy Bibbero Systems, An InHealth Company, Petaluma, CA, www.bibbero.com.)

A

ALLERGIC: ______

B

CO–PAY

C

ADVANCE DIRECTIVES

___ Durable Power of Attorney for Healthcare

___ Living Will

___ Healthcare Surrogate

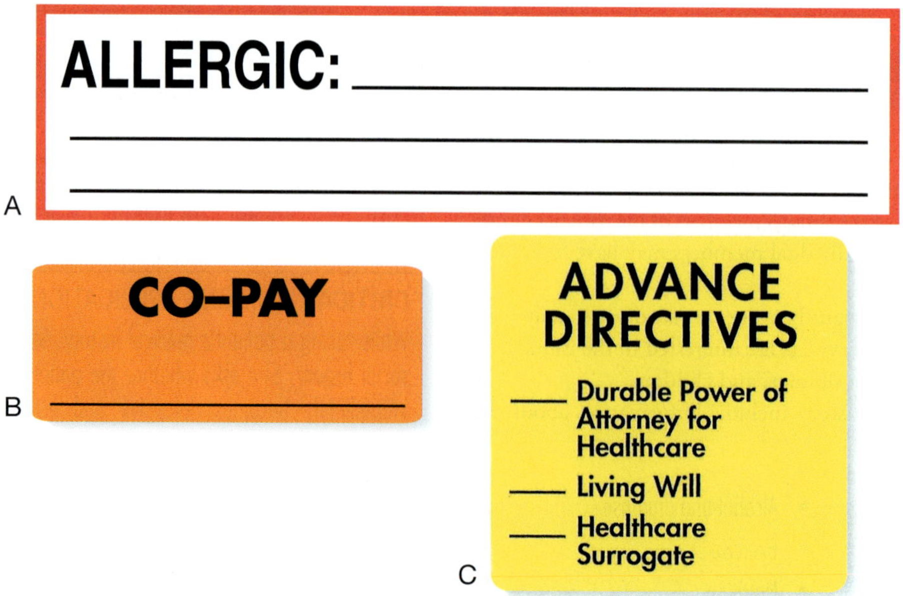

FIGURE 10.5 Record Stickers. Information on stickers on the outside of the record allows the provider and medical staff to see important information about the patient quickly. (Courtesy Bibbero Systems, An InHealth Company, Petaluma, CA, www.bibbero.com.)

Chief Complaint

The patient's chief complaint is a **concise** account of the patient's symptoms, explained in the patient's own words and describing why they have come to see the provider. When documenting the chief complaint, be sure to use quotation marks when using the patient's words to describe symptoms.

History of Present Illness

The history of present illness (HPI) describes the details of the chief complaint:

- The nature, location, frequency, and duration of pain, if any
- When the patient first noticed the symptoms
- Treatments the patient may have tried before seeing the provider and whether or not they have helped with the symptoms, when the last dose was taken
- Whether the patient has had the same or a similar condition in the past
- Other medical treatment received for the same condition in the past

Most healthcare facilities use a pain scale to determine the severity of the patient's discomfort. The medical assistant might ask, "How bad is your pain on a scale of 0 to 10, with 0 being almost no pain and 10 being the worst pain you've ever experienced?" The pain scale or wording used in individual facilities should be documented in the office policies and procedures manual and followed by the medical assistant.

Review of Systems

A review of systems is part of the history-taking procedure. This involves a list of questions arranged by the body system to help identify problems within that area. The patient may be asked to complete a questionnaire that has all of the body systems listed, and then the medical assistant or provider goes over the questionnaire with the patient to clarify any of the issues.

Objective Information

Objective findings sometimes referred to as *signs,* are findings that can be observed and measured. They can include vital signs, measurements, observations made by the medical assistant, and findings from the provider's examination of the patient.

Vital Signs and Anthropometric Measurements

The medical assistant's responsibilities include the following:

- Taking the patient's vital signs (i.e., temperature, pulse, respiration, blood pressure, and pulse oximetry reading)
- Obtaining the person's **anthropometric** measurements (i.e., height and weight)

These measurements are documented in the patient's health record and are used when the provider makes an assessment. If the medical assistant observes other signs, such as a rash, this would also be documented in the patient's health record and brought to the provider's attention.

Findings, Laboratory and Radiology Reports

After the provider has examined the patient, the physical findings are documented in the health record. The results of other tests or requests for these tests are then documented. If the tests were done elsewhere, the report is attached to the paper record. When an EHR is used, the separate sheet may be scanned so that it is in an electronic format and can be added to the patient's EHR.

Diagnosis

Based on all the evidence provided in the patient's history, the provider's examination, and any supplementary tests, the provider notes the diagnosis of the patient's condition in the health record. If some doubt remains, this may be labeled a **provisional diagnosis.** A *differential diagnosis* is a process of weighing the probability of one disease causing the patient's illness against the probability that other diseases are causative. For example, the differential diagnosis of rhinitis, or a runny nose, could indicate allergic rhinitis (i.e., hay fever), the common cold, or even abuse of drugs or nasal decongestants.

Documentation of Treatment Prescribed and Results of the Examination

The provider's suggested treatment is listed after the diagnosis. Generally, instructions for the patient to return for follow-up treatment within a specific period are also noted here. If surgery or other treatment is going to be performed during the current visit, the patient must sign a consent form.

On each **subsequent** visit, when a paper record is used, the date must be entered on the record; information about the patient's condition and the results of treatment, based on the provider's observations, must be added to the health record. Notations of all medications prescribed or instructions given, in addition to the patient's own report of how they are doing, should be documented in the health record. If the patient is hospitalized, the name of the hospital, the reason for admission, and the dates of admission and discharge are documented. Much of this information can be obtained from the hospital discharge summary.

Medication Record

An important aspect of patient care is the medications that the patient is taking. It is important to maintain a comprehensive list of the prescribed medications a patient is taking as well as any over-the-counter medications and supplements. When asking about the over-the-counter medications, you should use both the brand name (e.g., Motrin) and the generic name (e.g., ibuprofen). Vitamins, minerals, and botanicals are considered supplements and are an important part of the patient's medication list. There could be a potential interaction with over-the-counter medications or supplements and a prescribed medication. Providers who are aware of all of the medications that a patient is taking can make better decisions related to treatment plans.

Additional Content Found in the Health Record

In addition to the subjective and objective information documented in the patient's health record, forms related to patient care are included. These include consultation reports, consent for treatment forms, and release of information forms.

Consultation Reports

When a provider asks another provider for their opinion on a patient's condition is called a consultation. The consulting provider will present an opinion in the form of a consultation report. The original provider will review the consultation report, and it then becomes part of the health record. The provider will also discuss the findings with the patient.

Consent for Treatment

A patient must always consent to treatment before it is provided. In order for the consent to be valid, it must be voluntary and informed. In addition, the person giving the consent must have the capacity to consent. This means that the person understands what the treatment is, the consequences of the treatment, or of declining the treatment. This consent can be verbal, such as agreeing to a throat culture, or in writing, such as signing a consent form for a surgical procedure. Consent can even be nonverbal, as long as the patient understands the treatment, such as when a patient holds out an arm for a blood draw.

The consent should always be documented, whether it is verbal, nonverbal, or in writing. This documentation then becomes part of the patient record. More information about consent can be found in Chapter 3.

Release of Information

No information about a patient can be released to a third party without the patient's permission. A release of information form must contain specific information, including what information can be released, who it can be released to, and an expiration date. More information about the release of information can be found in Chapter 4.

The Medical Assistant's Role

It is important to ensure patient privacy when documenting the health record. If you are interviewing the patient to obtain history information, do it where the patient's answers cannot be heard by others. If privacy is not possible, the patient should be given a form to fill out. The information can be transferred to the permanent record later. When privacy is available, the medical assistant may ask the patient questions and document the answers directly into the health record. This allows you to become better acquainted with the patient while completing the necessary records. It can also ensure that the patient understands the meaning of all of the questions.

If new patients must complete a lengthy form, there are several options:

- It can be mailed to the patient. The accompanying letter can request that it be completed and returned to the provider before the appointment.
- If the record is electronic, the patient may access the record through a patient portal. The information is documented directly into the EHR system using this method. It would then be reviewed by the medical assistant and provider during the office visit.
- Another option with an EHR is for the patient to complete a paper form, and the medical assistant enters the information into the EHR while reviewing the form with the patient.

The medical assistant may document the patient's chief complaint. The provider will question the patient in more detail. Many providers write their own entries in the record in longhand if a paper record is used. Some may document the findings directly into the computer if an electronic record is used. Others may dictate the material directly into the EHR. Another option is for a medical assistant or scribe to document the provider's findings. A final option is for the provider to use a recording device. If the material is dictated and transcribed, the provider should verify each entry. The provider must initial the entry before it is entered into the patient's record. For a record to be admissible as evidence in court, the person dictating or writing the entries must be able to verify that they were true and correct at the time they were written. The best indication of this is the provider's signature or initials on the typed entry. In an EHR, the provider's electronic signature is proof of the accuracy of the entries.

Maintaining a Connection with the Patient When Using the Electronic Health Record

Many patients are required to choose a primary care provider (PCP) in order to be referred to a specialist. They also have the option of changing the PCP or specialist. Patients may decide to change providers simply because they do not feel comfortable with that particular provider.

Because the change process is relatively easy, the healthcare facility should strive to provide excellent care and service to its patients. If the care begins to seem impersonal, patients may feel a strong desire to change providers. Patients are consumers of healthcare services, and they expect quality healthcare and service.

When using the EHR, the medical assistant must make sure that his or her nonverbal communication sends the right message to the patient. Eye contact is essential (Figure 10.6). If the medical assistant constantly looks at the electronic device, the patient feels left out of the process. Make eye contact with the patient while asking questions and look at the screen only when needed to enter information. Do not shield the device from the patient's view while entering information. This can give the impression you are hiding something from the patient. Although patients may not understand anything they see on the screen, they will feel more at ease if their information is not hidden from them. Also, modify your position so that the patient feels like a part of the information process. Just as sitting in a chair across from a supervisor's desk can be intimidating, the patient may feel the same emotions sitting across from a medical assistant entering information into the EHR. Sit next to or at an angle to the patient to support the impression that those in the healthcare facility and the patient are partners in the healthcare plan.

Because patients have the right to make decisions in most aspects of their healthcare plans, offer choices wherever possible. Never expect patients to make quick decisions about their care. They may want to consult family members or give some thought to important medical decisions. The medical assistant needs to allow the patient time to think unless the patient is faced with a critical, time-sensitive decision. Providers often assume that patients will

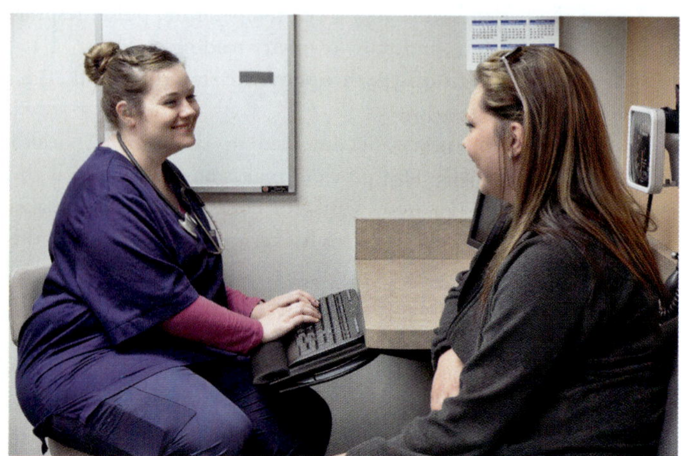

FIGURE 10.6 The medical assistant must make eye contact with the patient when using an EHR.

automatically follow their instructions or orders; however, some patients prefer some time to consider their options. Always follow up and make a note of any wait time the patient requests, notify the provider, and enter that information into the EHR. Make sure timely communication is accomplished with the patient and that any additional orders that need to be put in place are completed. The many features of the EHR allow medical assistants to be efficient and highly competent if they are willing to make an extra effort to master the EHR system.

Also, make sure patients understand all instructions given to them regarding test procedures or preparation for procedures. Most EHRs can print an instruction sheet, which the medical assistant can review with the patient. The customer service aspect of patient care is even more important when the facility uses an EHR system (Procedure 10.3).

CRITICAL THINKING APPLICATION **10.5**

Jennifer walks behind Susan's desk and notices that she is looking at the progress notes on a patient who was recently arrested and indicted for child abuse. The case has been in the newspaper and on television consistently for several weeks. Jennifer asks Susan why she has accessed that record. Susan hesitates and then says she must have entered the wrong patient ID number. Does Susan's explanation sound convincing? Why is Jennifer concerned about Susan looking at the patient's record? Just because the individual is a patient at the clinic, does that mean any employee has the right to look at the patient's EHR?

Use of a Medical Scribe

A medical scribe should have an understanding of medical terminology, excellent computer skills, and a strong attention to detail. It is important that medical scribes understand that they are not obtaining the information from the patient. Their role is to document the information obtained by the provider and enter it into the EHR, per the provider's instructions.

Healthcare facilities that have hired scribes found that both the patients and the providers are more satisfied with patient encounters. Providers are establishing a better relationship with patients because they are able to spend their time with face-to-face interaction rather than interacting with a computer.

Ownership of the Health Record

Who owns the health record? Patients often assume that because the information in the health record is about them, ownership of the record is rightfully theirs. However, the owner of the physical health record is the provider or medical facility, often called the "maker," that initiated and developed the record. The patient has the right to access the information within the record but does not own the physical record or other documents pertaining to the record. The patient has a **vested** interest and therefore has the right to demand confidentiality of all information placed in the record. The patient also has control over who has access to the health record. No information should be released to a third party without a release of information signed by the patient.

The actual paper health record should never leave the medical facility where it originated. Even the provider should refrain from taking the record from the office to the hospital or nursing facility. If information from the record is needed, copies can be made, and progress notes can be written on site and placed into the original record later. This is not an issue with an EHR because the record can be accessed by multiple users at the same time. Patients' paper records should be kept in a locked room or locked filing cabinets when the office is closed. EHRs must be protected from unauthorized access. Regulations established by the Health Insurance Portability and Accountability Act (HIPAA) state that each user must have a unique username and password; individual access is determined by the system administrator.

Written health records must be legible. Each record should be written as if the provider and staff expect it to eventually be involved in a lawsuit; therefore, every word must be legible to an average reader years after it is written. The record can help providers prove that they treated a patient in a competent manner. It can also prove that the patient was not given competent care. Every person on staff at the provider's office is responsible for writing legibly in every health record.

EHRs eliminate the issue of legibility in the record, but it is just as important to be sure that all patient care is documented in the electronic record. If care is not documented, this will leave the healthcare facility open to potential lawsuits and affect patient care. In addition, if services are not documented, they cannot be billed to the patient or the patient's insurance company.

CRITICAL THINKING APPLICATION **10.6**

On Susan's third day at work, a man comes into the office and demands to see his mother's health record. Susan accesses the record and sees that the mother has not granted permission for information to be given to her son. What should Susan do in this situation? Are there any viable reasons the son should have access to his mother's medical information?

WORKING WITH HEALTH RECORDS

Whether you are a clinical or administrative medical assistant, it is important to understand the many aspects of working within a health record. The next section of this chapter will help you gain an understanding of the organization of the health record, proper documentation in both an EHR and paper record, backup systems needed for EHRs, retention, and destruction of health records, and releasing information.

Organization of the Health Record

Whether you are working as a clinical or administrative medical assistant, it is important to understand the organization of the health record. There are two main systems used to organize information within the health record. Those systems are discussed next.

Source-Oriented Records

The traditional patient record is a source-oriented record (SOR). Observations and data are cataloged according to their source:

- Provider (progress notes)
- Laboratory

- Radiology
- Hospital
- Consultations

Forms and progress notes are filed in **reverse chronologic order** and in separate sections of the record according to the type of form or service rendered (e.g., all laboratory reports together, all x-ray reports together, and so on). Reverse chronologic order is used so that the provider and staff members do not have to search to the bottom of the record to find a recent laboratory report or a test.

Problem-Oriented Records

The problem-oriented medical record (POR) is a departure from the traditional system of keeping patient records. The POR is a method of recording data in a problem-solving system. This system is divided into four components:

- The *database* includes the chief complaint, history of present illness, patient profile, review of systems, physical examination, and laboratory reports.
- The *problem list* is a numbered, titled list of every problem the patient has that requires management or workup. This may include social and demographic troubles in addition to strictly medical or surgical ones.
- The *treatment plan* includes management, additional workups needed, and therapy. Each plan is titled and numbered with respect to the problem.
- The *progress notes* include structured notes that are numbered to correspond with each problem number.

Several companies have developed file folders for organizing patient data according to the POR. The problem list (Figure 10.7) is placed at the front of the paper record and has its own section in the EHR. Special sections are provided for current major and chronic diagnoses/health problems and for inactive major or chronic diagnoses/health problems. Progress notes usually follow the SOAP approach. SOAP is an acronym for the following:

- ***S***ubjective impressions or patient reports
- ***O***bjective clinical evidence or observations
- ***A***ssessment or diagnosis
- ***P***lans for further studies, treatment, or management

Some medical offices also use an *E* in the record to represent *evaluation* of the effectiveness of the plan; *I for intervention, medications, and education provided;* and *R* for *response* (how the patient responded). The addition of E, I, and R result in the acronym SOAPIER. The education notation shows that the patient was educated about his or her condition or given a patient information sheet. The response section is used to record an assessment of the patient's understanding of and possible compliance with the treatment plan.

The POR has the advantage of creating order and organization in the information added to a patient's health record. The records are more easily reviewed, and the likelihood of overlooking a problem is greatly reduced. The SOAP method forces a rational approach to the patient's problems and assists in forming a logical, orderly plan of patient care (Figure 10.8). The POR is especially helpful in clinics, group practices, and hospitals, where more than one person must be able to find essential information in the record.

CRITICAL THINKING APPLICATION 10.7

Susan learned about SOAP documentation in school and is eager to use it in her new job. Dr. Kahn is seeing a patient who reports to Susan that she has had nausea and vomiting for the past 3 days. Susan obtains a weight of 132.5 pounds, a temperature (T) of 101.2° F tympanically, a pulse (P) of 94 beats/min, respiration (R) of 14 breaths/min, and a blood pressure (BP) of 122/84 mm Hg in the right arm. What information would be documented in the Subjective field? What information would be documented in the Objective field? Who would document information in the Assessment field?

Documenting in an Electronic Health Record

Documentation in an EHR involves using radio buttons, drop-down menus, and free-text boxes. The radio buttons and drop-down menus allow for standardization of the content in the EHR, and the free-text boxes allow for the documentation of the unique circumstance found with each patient (Figure 10.9). Radio buttons and drop-down boxes allow for the creation of graphs using that standardized content. The information documented using the free-text boxes would not be included in those graphs. It is important to carefully review the choices made with the radio buttons and drop-down menus. Information documented using the free-text boxes should be proofread before submission.

Documenting in a Paper Health Record

When you are documenting a paper health record, the entry will always start with the date in the MM/DD/YYYY format. The date will be followed by the time. This may be written in standard or military time. If standard time is used, a colon is placed between the hour and minutes, and it must be followed by a.m. or p.m. (e.g., 2:00 p.m.). If military time is used, it is in a four-digit format without a colon (e.g., 1400). All entries must be written in black or blue ink, following the format designated by the healthcare facility. Documentation should be in the order in which the steps were completed. If a temperature, pulse, and respiration (TPR) measurement is done, it would be documented in the "O" or Objective section of the SOAP note, starting with temperature, then pulse, and, lastly, respiration.

Making Corrections and Alterations to Health Records

Sometimes corrections must be made to health records. The first step is to verify the proper procedure for making corrections in the facility's policy and procedures manual. Some providers prefer a specific method for correcting errors in the health record. Erasing, using correction fluid, or any other type of **obliteration** is never acceptable. Follow these steps to correct a handwritten entry:

1. Draw a line through the error.
2. Insert the correction above or immediately after the error in a spot where it can be read clearly.
3. If indicated by the policies and procedures manual, write "Error" or "Err." in the margin.
4. The person making the correction should write his or her initials or signature and the date below the correction. Follow the format indicated in the policy and procedures manual (Figure 10.10).

MASTER PROBLEM LIST

For use of this form, see AR 40-66; the proponent agency is the Office of The Surgeon General

MAJOR PROBLEMS

PROBLEM NUMBER	DATE ONSET	DATE ENTERED	PROBLEM	DATE RESOLVED
1.				
2.				
3.				
4.				
5.				
6.				
7.				
8.				
9.				
10.				
11.				
12.				

TEMPORARY (MINOR) PROBLEMS

PROBLEM LETTER	PROBLEM	DATES OF OCCURRENCES					
A.							
B.							
C.							
D.							
E.							
F.							
G.							
H.							

PATIENT'S IDENTIFICATION (use mechanical imprint if available; for typed or written entries give: Name, SSN, Unit, Sex, Birthdate, and Duty Phone)	SUMMARY OF PROBLEMS, ALLERGIES, MEDICATIONS, SURGERIES, AND TRAUMAS NOTE: DO NOT DISCARD FROM CHART

FIGURE 10.7 A problem list designed for a problem-oriented record (POR).

OUTLINE FORMAT PROGRESS NOTES

Patient Name

Prob. No. or Letter | DATE | S Subjective | O Objective | A Assess | P Plans | Page

Start each Progress Note (Subjective, Objective, Assessment and Plans) at the appropriate shaded column to create an outline form. Write through the intervening columns to the right margin of the page.

ANDRUS CLINI-REC ® CHART ANIZING SYSTEMS ORDER # 26-7115 • © 1976 BIBBERO TEMS, INC. • PETALUMA, CA

FIGURE 10.8 SOAP Progress Notes. The SOAP method keeps information organized and in a logical sequence. An actual progress note would include the provider's or medical assistant's signature or initials after each entry. (Courtesy Bibbero Systems, An InHealth Company, Petaluma, CA, www.bibbero.com.)

Errors made while using the computer are corrected in the usual way. However, an error discovered in an entry at a later date is corrected in the same manner as for a handwritten entry. This is sometimes called an *addendum.* Never attempt to alter health records without using this specific correction procedure because this alteration of records may indicate a fraudulent attempt to cover up a mistake made by a staff member or the provider. Do not hide errors. If the error could, in any way, affect the patient's health and well-being, it must be brought to the provider's attention immediately. An EHR system will track the changes made within the record.

Dictation and Transcription

With the increased use of EHRs and voice recognition software, there is decreased need for **transcription**. If **dictation** is still done in the healthcare facility, transcribing the dictation is a job the administrative medical assistant may sometimes perform. Transcription can be done from handwritten notes or, more likely, from machine dictation. Smooth operation of the facility may depend on the timely, accurate performance of assigned responsibilities, such as record documentation and the preparation of special reports. Accuracy and speed are the primary requirements, along with a strong grasp of medical terminology and anatomy and physiology.

Dictation may be done using a machine transcription unit or a portable transcription unit. Many healthcare facilities now use a system that is accessed by telephone; the provider calls the system, using passwords or access codes, and records the information for the health record while speaking into the telephone. Later, employees transcribe the information into the health record. The provider must acknowledge and initial all transcripts before they are placed in the health record.

Voice Recognition Software

Some healthcare facilities use voice recognition software for transcription. When first installed, the software requires the user to say several sentences into the unit so that it "learns" to recognize the user's voice. The system can be used to dictate the following:

- Progress notes
- Letters
- Emails
- Any document in the healthcare facility that needs to be created

The provider will need to approve these documents before they are permanently attached to the patient's record. Some systems have an authentication component that allows a type of electronic signature, such as those needed for hospital record dictation.

Backup Systems for the Electronic Health Record

Even the best or most expensive EHR system cannot function without power. If a natural disaster occurs and the provider's office is without electricity for several days or weeks, the provider must have

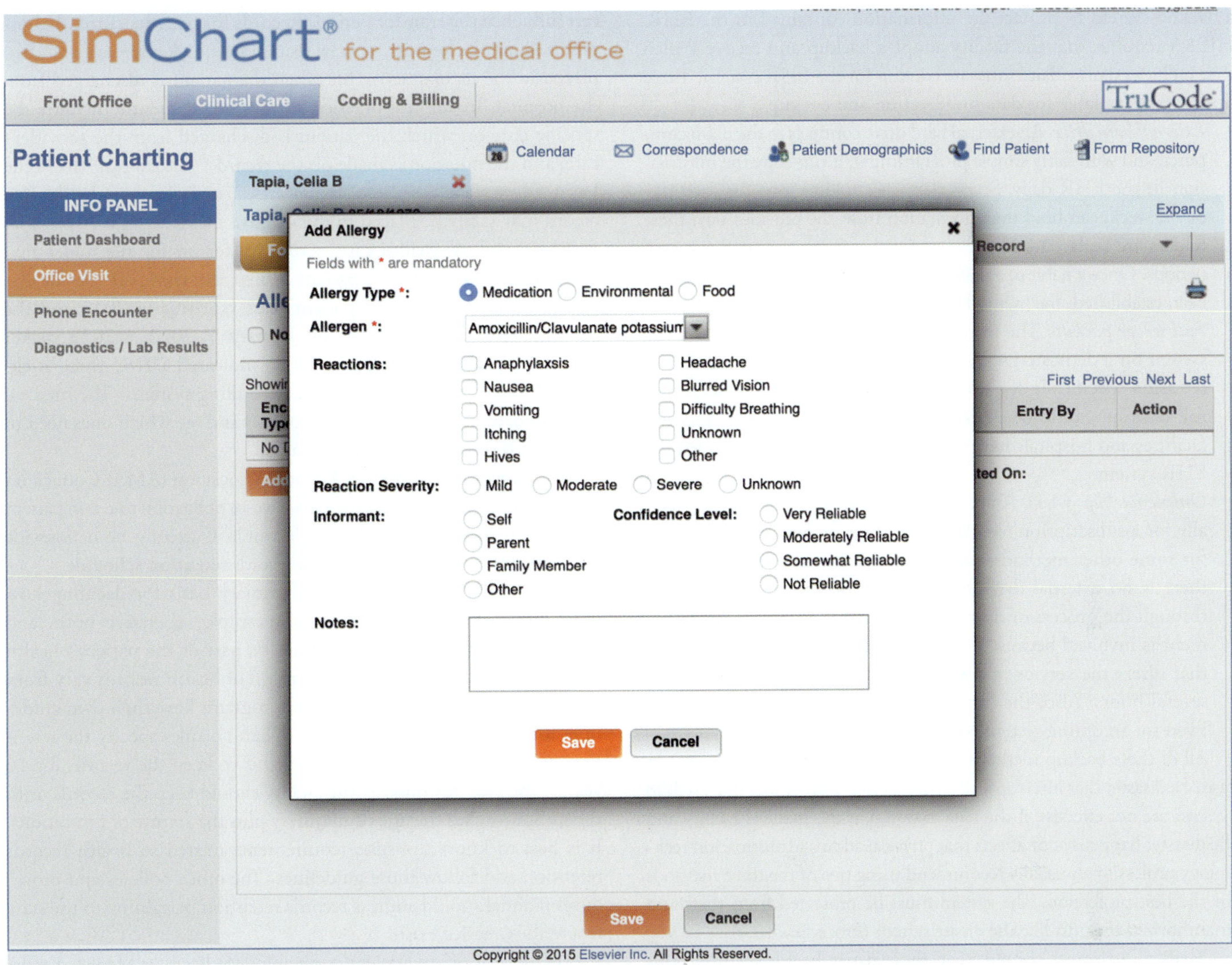

FIGURE 10.9 Documentation in an EHR is done using radio buttons, drop-down menus, and free-text boxes.

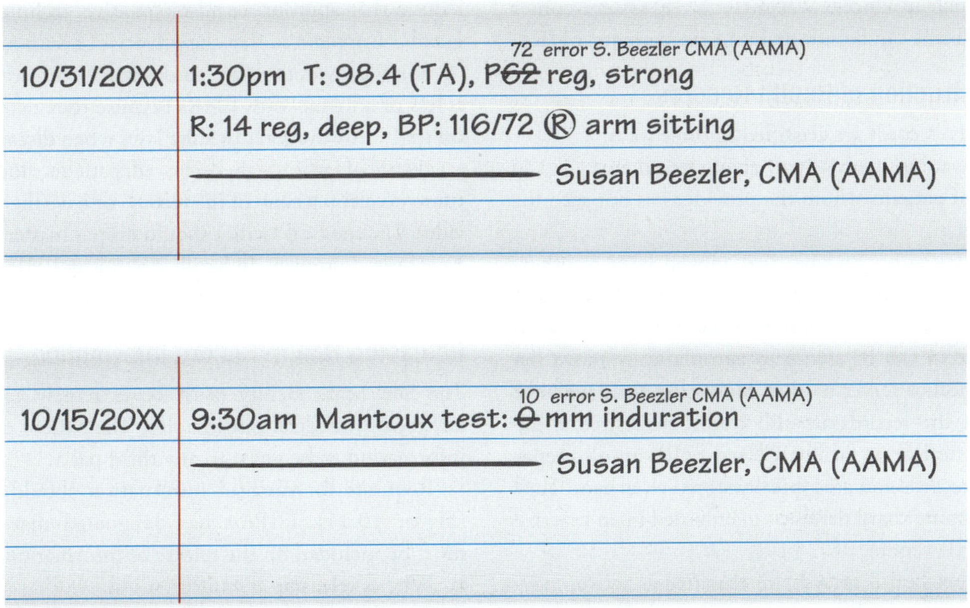

10/31/20XX 1:30pm T: 98.4 (TA), P ~~62~~ 72 error S. Beezler CMA (AAMA) reg, strong
R: 14 reg, deep, BP: 116/72 Ⓡ arm sitting
Susan Beezler, CMA (AAMA)

10/15/20XX 9:30am Mantoux test: ~~0~~ 10 error S. Beezler CMA (AAMA) mm induration
Susan Beezler, CMA (AAMA)

FIGURE 10.10 Corrections to health records must be done in a legible manner and must be clearly understood. Always initial and date corrections to health records.

a backup system to protect the information contained in the EHR. HIPAA requires that the facility adopt a backup and recovery plan that includes daily offsite software backup for the EHR system. Three options are available for data preservation and backup:

- *External hard drive:* An external hard drive connects to the main computer, and with fairly simple programming, it can copy the information in the EHR daily. Seven electronic folders, one for each day of the week, can hold the information from the previous day; these folders are replaced with new, updated information at designated periods. Once a habit of a daily backup to the external hard drive has been established, the method is relatively simple and reliable.
- *Full server backup:* The provider may want to back up the EHR system on a dedicated server, which is a large-capacity computer set aside specifically for the EHR system. With these servers, a full backup should be performed monthly. Many large medical facilities and hospitals have one or more dedicated servers for the EHR system.
- *Online backup system:* An online backup system can be used, usually for a subscription fee. Although the cost may be higher than for some other methods, online systems are easy to use because there is no external drive to carry and no thumb drive to put through the process of downloading data. However, time investment is involved because the process of contacting the company that offers the service and then downloading all the data takes several hours. Also, the initial download can take quite a while. Even so, an online system is stable and reliable.

All of these backup methods require an alternative power source in case of a disaster that interrupts electrical service. Remember that backup systems are not effective if the data is stored at the medical facility and the disaster happens at or affects that physical address. Information technology professionals usually recommend using two of the three methods for the best protection. The system must be protected from theft and unauthorized use, just like the onsite system (Procedure 10.4).

Medical assistants should keep their paper health records skills sharp in case the EHR system is down for an extended period. Always have a supply of the most commonly used forms in a paper format available for use in such instances. When the EHR system comes back up, these paper forms can be scanned into the patients' EHRs.

Retention and Destruction of Health Records

In most medical offices, records are classified in three ways:

- *Active:* Records of patients currently receiving treatment
- *Inactive:* Records of patients whom the provider has not seen for 6 months or longer
- *Closed:* Records of patients who have died, moved away, or otherwise terminated their relationship with the provider

The process of moving a file from active to inactive status is called *purging*. An EHR system can be set up to automatically move the inactive records to another server so that processing time will not be slowed down, but the records are still readily accessible if the patient returns to the healthcare facility. Closed EHRs are also separated from the active records and are typically stored elsewhere. They may be placed on computer hard drives or maintained in an inactive cloud space by the EHR vendor.

As with EHRs, paper health records are classified as active, inactive, and closed. A paper record system must have a system established for regular transfer of files from active to inactive status or possibly destruction. The expansion of records and available file space can influence the transfer period. Records for patients currently hospitalized may be kept in a special section for quick reference and then placed in the regular active file when the patient is discharged from the hospital. In surgical practice, the record frequently includes the specific date on which the patient is discharged from the provider's care, and the notation is made on the record, "Return prn" (from the Latin *pro re nata,* "as the occasion arises" or "when needed"). This record may safely be placed in the inactive file.

Most medical facilities use a year sticker on the file folder that indicates the last year the patient visited the clinic. If the file has a sticker showing that the patient's last visit was in 2018 and the patient presents to the clinic on January 5, 2022, a 2022 sticker should be placed over the one which indicated 2018. These stickers often are included with color-coded filing systems. The medical assistant can easily look at a group of files and see which ones need to be changed to inactive or closed status.

According to the American Medical Association (AMA) Council on Ethical and Judicial Affairs, providers have an obligation to retain patient records, whether they are paper or electronic. Currently, no nationwide standard rule exists for establishing a records **retention schedule**.

Medical considerations are the primary basis for deciding how long to retain health records. For example, operative notes and chemotherapy records should always be part of the patient's health record. The laws regarding the retention of health records vary from state to state, and many government programs have their own guidelines for specific records retention. When no rules specify the retention of health records, the best course is to keep the records for 10 years. However, for minors, the facility should keep the records until the minor reaches the **age of majority** plus the statute of limitations. It is best to know the state requirements related to health records retention and follow those guidelines. The office policies and procedures manual should address records retention pertaining to the state where the practice exists.

The records of any patient covered by Medicare or Medicaid must be kept for at least 10 years. The HIPAA Privacy Rule does not include requirements for the retention of health records. However, the rule does require that appropriate administrative, technical, and physical safeguards be applied so that the privacy of health records is maintained.

Some providers refuse to destroy or discard old records. Storage is less of an issue with EHRs because they take up much less physical space. Always refer to state laws when discarding health records.

Before old records are destroyed, patients should be given an opportunity to claim a copy of the records or have them sent to another provider. The medical facility should keep a master list of all records that have been destroyed. To legally destroy an EHR, the record, including the backup record, has to be overwritten using utility software.

Releasing Health Record Information

The healthcare facility must be extremely careful when releasing any type of medical information. The patient must sign a release for information to be given to any third party.

Requests for medical information should be made in writing (Figure 10.11). HIPAA has designated that specific information must be included on the release of information form:

- Who is releasing the information
- To whom the information is being released
- What specific information is to be released
- An expiration date for the release

Central Texas Dermatology Clinic • 102 Westlake Drive • Austin, Texas 78746

AUTHORIZATION TO DISCLOSE HEALTH INFORMATION

I hereby authorize the use or disclosure of information from the medical record of:
Patient Name: ______________________ Date of Birth: ______________________
Social Security# ______________________ Daytime Phone: ______________________

I authorize the following individual or organization to disclose the above-named individual's health information:
______________________ Address: ______________________

This information may be disclosed TO and used by the following individual or organization:
______________________ Address: ______________________

Please release the following:
____ Progress Notes ____ Pathology Reports ____ Lab Reports ____ Any and all Records
____ Other Diagnostic reports (specify ______________________
____ Other (specify) ______________________
Including Information (if applicable) pertaining to:
____ Mental Health ____ Drug/Alcohol ____ HIV/AIDS ____ Communicable Treatment

Purpose or Need for Disclosure:
____ Continued Patient Care ____ Personal Use
____ Attorney/Legal ____ Insurance Claim/Application
____ Disability Determination ____ Other(specify) ______________________

I understand that the information in my health record may include information relating to sexually transmitted disease, acquired immunodeficiency syndrome (AIDS), or human immunodeficiency virus (HIV). It may also include information about behavioral or mental health services, and treatment for alcohol and drug abuse.

I understand that the information released is for the specific purpose stated above. Any other use of this information without the written consent of the patient is prohibited.

I understand that I have the right to revoke this authorization at any time. I understand that if I revoke this authorization I must do so in writing and present my written revocation to the individual or organization releasing information. I understand that the revocation will not apply to information already released in response to this authorization. I understand that the revocation will not apply to my insurance company when the law provides my insurer the right to contest a claim under my policy. Unless otherwise revoked, this authorization will expire on following date, event, or condition: ______________________
____

If I fail to specify an expiration date, event or condition, this authorization will expire in six months.

I understand that authorizing the disclosure of this health information is voluntary. I can refuse to sign the authorization. I need not sign this form in order to ensure treatment. I understand that I may inspect or copy the information to be used or disclosed, as provided in CFR 164.524. I understand that any disclosure of information carries with it the potential for an unauthorized re-disclosure and the information may not be protected by federal confidentiality rules. If I have questions about disclosure of my health information, I can contact Theresa Farren at 512-327-7779.

______________________ ______________________
Signature of Patient or Legal Representative Date

______________________ ______________________
Relationship to Patient (If Legal Representative) Witness

COMPLETE ONLY IF INFORMATION IS TO BE RELEASED DIRECTLY TO PATIENT:
I understand that my medical record may contain reports, test results, and notes that only a physician can interpret. I understand and have been advised that I should contact my physician regarding the entries made in my medical record to prevent my misunderstanding of the information contained in these entries. I will not hold Central Texas Dermatology liable for any misinterpretation of the information in my medical record as a result of not contacting my physician for the correct interpretation.

______________________ ______________________
Signature of Patient or Legal Representative Date

______________________ ______________________
Relationship to Patient (If Legal Representative) Witness

Dr. review/signature/date ______________________
Date request completed ______________________ # of pages copied ______________________
Staff Signature ______________________
PHI Log completed ______________________

FIGURE 10.11 Authorization to Release Health Records. All requests for health records should be in writing, and the request should be kept in the patient's health record.

Accepting a faxed request for medical information or a faxed release of information from a patient is unwise. Even requests from the patient's attorney or insurance companies must be cleared by the patient for them to obtain information.

If a provider is involved in a liability suit, there will be a required exchange of information. As both parties to a lawsuit begin to prepare their cases, they enter the discovery process. Each side must disclose the pertinent facts of the case that may influence the final outcome of that case. On each occasion that information is needed from the provider, a separate request must be sent. Because the patient signs this request form, it serves as a release.

Most offices charge a fee to print or copy health records, whether it is a per-page charge or a per-record fee. If the records are sent electronically, no fee is charged. Follow the steps in the policies and procedures manual for the release of records. Some providers designate the office manager to handle requests for record releases.

Pay particular attention to records release requests involving a minor. In most cases, the parent or legal guardian is entitled to read through the patient's health records; however, according to the US Department of Health and Human Services (HHS), there are three situations in which the parent may not be legally entitled to review the records of his or her minor child:

- When the minor is the one who consents to care, and the parent is not required also to consent to care under state law
- When the minor obtains medical care at the direction of the court or a person authorized by the court
- When the minor, parent, and provider all agree that the doctor and minor patient can have a private, confidential relationship

If the provider believes that the minor might be in an abusive situation or that the parent or legal guardian may be harming the patient, the provider is required, both legally and ethically, to report the abuse.

Sometimes patients want to look at their own records. They certainly have a right to see this information, but some patients may not understand the terminology used in the record. A staff member should always remain with a patient who is looking at his or her health record. Remember, the original health record should never leave the medical facility. Always follow office policy when releasing health records.

When a release is presented to the office, provide only the records requested in the release. Do not provide information that is not requested. The patient must specify that substance abuse, mental health, or human immunodeficiency virus (HIV) records are to be released. Remember that the patient ultimately decides whether a record can be released. If any question arises about what is to be released, consult the office manager or the provider.

Health Information Exchanges

The demand for electronic health information exchange (HIE) between one healthcare facility and another, together with nationwide efforts to improve the efficiency and quality of healthcare, is creating a demand for HIEs. As more and more providers move to EHRs, it only makes sense to have a system in place that will facilitate the exchange of information electronically to improve the timeliness of that exchange. Patient care can be improved because all providers will have access to the information needed to treat the patient.

The ONC states that there are currently three forms of HIE:

- *Directed exchange*: The ability to send and receive secure information electronically between care providers to support coordinated care
- *Query-based exchange*: The ability of providers to find or request information on a patient from other providers, often used for unplanned care
- *Consumer-mediated exchange*: The ability of patients to aggregate and control the use of their health information among providers

The implementation of HIE varies from state to state. Some of the federal funding for the implementation of HIE is administered by the ONC.

CREATING AN EFFICIENT PAPER HEALTH-RECORDS MANAGEMENT SYSTEM

The paper health-records management system should provide an easy method of retrieving information. The files should be organized in an orderly fashion. The information must be documented accurately, and corrections should be made and documented properly. The wording in the record should be easily understood and grammatically correct. An efficient method of adding documents to the record must be established so that the provider always has the most up-to-date information. Above all, the health records management system must work for the individual facility.

Filing Equipment

For years, the traditional filing system involved a vertical, five-drawer steel filing cabinet, used with manila folders that had the patient's name on the tab. The most popular system today is color coding on open horizontal shelves. Rotary, lateral, compactable, and automated files also are available. Some records are kept in card or tray files. Several factors should be considered when selecting filing equipment:

- Office space availability
- Structural considerations
- Cost of space and equipment
- Size, type, and volume of records
- Confidentiality requirements
- Retrieval speed
- Fire protection
- Cost

Drawer Files

Drawer files should be full suspension; they should roll easily, close securely, and be equipped with a locking device. The best cabinets have a center trough at the bottom of each drawer with a rod for holding divider guides. A drawback of the vertical five-drawer files is that only one person can use a file cabinet at a time. Also, filing is slower because the drawer must be opened and closed each time a file is pulled or filed.

File cabinets are heavy and can tip over, causing serious damage or injury unless reasonable care is taken. Open only one file drawer at a time and close it when the filing has been completed. A drawer left even slightly open can injure a passerby.

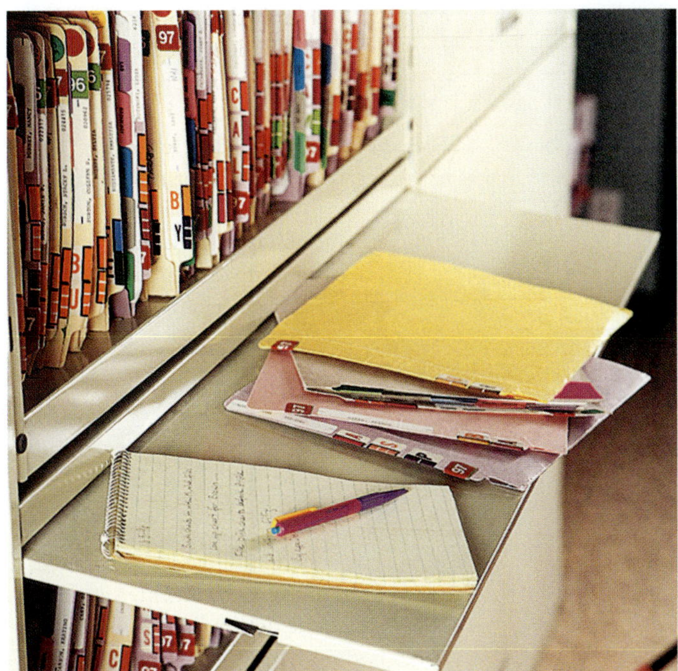

FIGURE 10.12 Open shelf filing is an efficient method, especially for color-coding filing systems. The shelf doors often can be used as a workspace.

Horizontal Shelf Files

Shelf files should have doors that lock to protect the contents. A popular shelf file has doors that slide back into the cabinet; the door from a lower shelf may be pulled out and used for workspace. Open shelf units hold files sideways and can go higher on the wall because no drawers need to be pulled out (Figure 10.12). File retrieval is faster because several individuals can work simultaneously.

Rotary Circular Files

Rotary circular files can hold a large volume of records. They save space and clerical motion. The files revolve easily; some have push-button controls. Several people can work at one rotary file and use records at the same time. One disadvantage is that they afford less privacy and protection than files that can be closed and locked.

Compactible Files

An office with little space and a large volume of records might use compactible files, which are a variation of open-shelf files. The files are mounted on tracks on the floor, and the units slide along the tracks so that access is gained to the needed records. One drawback is that not all records are available at the same time.

Automated Files

Automated files are initially very expensive, and they also require more maintenance than other types of filing equipment. They are likely to be found only in large facilities, such as clinics or hospitals. These files bring the record to the operator instead of the operator going to the record. When the operator presses a button indicating the appropriate shelf, the shelf automatically moves into position in front of the operator for record retrieval. The automated or power file is fast and can store large numbers of records in a small amount of space. However, only one person can use the unit at a time.

Card Files

Almost every office has some occasion to use a card file. This may be for patient ledgers, a patient index, a library index, an index of surgical tray setups, telephone numbers, or numerous other records. A good-quality steel box or tray is a sound investment.

Filing Supplies

Divider Guides

Each file drawer or shelf should be equipped with plenty of dividers or guides. Some authorities recommend one guide for approximately each 1 ½ inch of material or every eight to 10 folders. Guides should be of good-quality heavy cardstock or strong plastic. Less-well-constructed guides soon become bent and frayed and have to be replaced. Divider guides have a protruding tab, which may be an integral part of the card or may be made of metal or plastic. The guides reduce the area of search and serve as support for the folders. They are available in single, third, or fifth cut (i.e., one, three, or five different positions).

Out Guides

Out guides are made of heavyweight cardboard or plastic and are used to replace a folder that has been temporarily removed (Figure 10.13). They may also have a large pocket to hold any filing that may come in while the folder is out. They should be of a distinctive color for quick detection. This makes refiling simpler and alerts the file clerk that a file is missing. Several colors may be used, each color designating the temporary location of the file. The out guide may have lines for recording information, or it may have a plastic pocket for inserting an information card.

File Folders

Most records to be filed are placed in covers or tabbed folders. The most commonly used is a general -purpose, third-cut manila folder that may be expanded to three-fourths of an inch. These are available with a double-thickness, reinforced tab, which greatly extends the life of the folder. Folders kept in drawers have tabs at the top; those kept on shelves have tabs at the side. Many folder styles are available for special purposes.

Hanging or suspension folders are made of heavy stock and hang on metal rods from side to side in a drawer. They can be used only with file cabinets equipped with suspension equipment.

Binder folders have fasteners that are used to bind papers in the folder. These offer some security for the papers but filing the materials is time consuming.

The number of papers that will fit in one folder depends on the thickness of the papers and the capacity of the folder. Near the bottom edge of most folders are one or more score marks, which should be used as the contents of the folders expand. Papers should never protrude from the folder edges, and they should always be inserted with their tops to the left. When papers start to ride up in any folder, the folder is overloaded.

Labels

The label is a necessary filing and finding device. Use labels to identify each shelf, drawer, divider guide, and folder. A label on the drawer or shelf identifies the nature of its contents. It should also

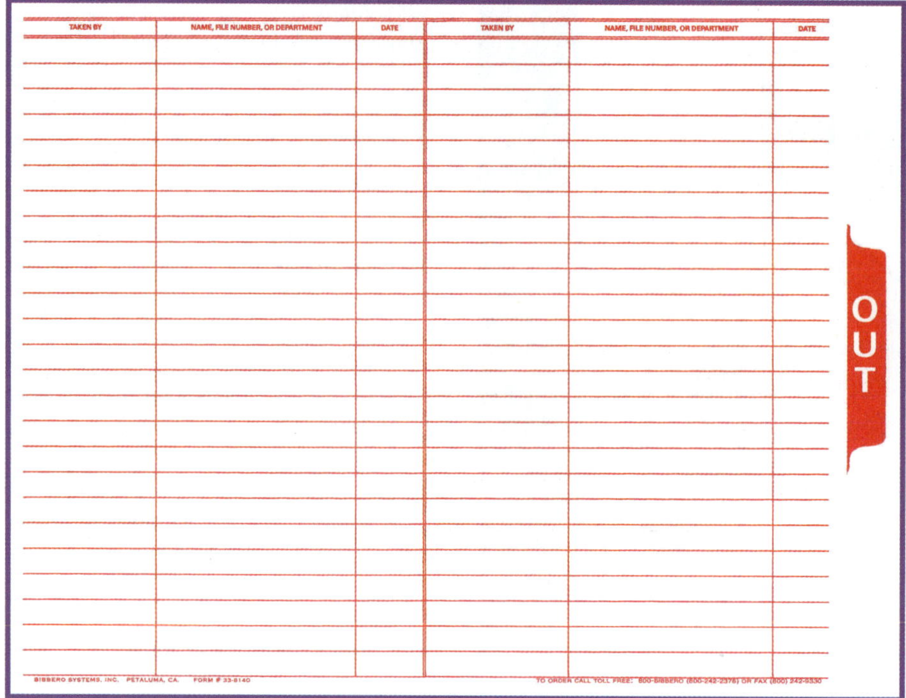

FIGURE 10.13 Out guides allow tracking of a file that is not in its proper location by providing information on the location of the file. (Courtesy Bibbero Systems, An InHealth Company, Petaluma, CA, www.bibbero.com.)

indicate the range (i.e., alphabetic, numeric, or chronologic) of the material filed in that space.

The label on the divider guide identifies the range of folder headings following that divider guide up to the next divider (e.g., Ba-Bo). The label on the folder identifies the contents of that folder only, such as the following:

- Name of the patient
- Subject matter of correspondence
- Business topic

Label a folder when a new patient is seen, existing folders are full, or materials need to be transferred within the filing system.

Labels are available in almost any size, shape, or color to meet the individual needs of any facility. Visit an office supply website and review the catalogs to find the best product to meet the needs of the facility.

A narrow label applied to the front of the folder tab is the easiest to use and is satisfactory for folders kept in a drawer file. Labels for shelf filing should be identifiable from both front and back. Always type the label before separating it from the roll or protective sheet. Type the **caption** on the label in indexing order (Procedure 10.5).

Indexing Rules

Indexing rules (Table 10.2) are standardized and based on current business practices. The Association of Records Managers and Administrators takes an active part in updating these rules. Some establishments adopt variations of these basic rules to accommodate their needs. In any case, the practices need to be consistent within the system:

1. Last names are considered first in filing; then the given name (first name), second; and the middle name or initial, third. For example, if the patient's name is Megan Grace Casper, we would start with Casper, then Megan, then Grace. Compare the names beginning with the first letter of the name. When a letter is different in the two names, that letter determines the order of filing.
2. Initials precede a name beginning with the same letter. Remember, nothing comes before something. For example, if we had two patient's, one named M.G. Casper and Megan Grace Casper. The last name is the same, so we then look at the first name. In this case, M.G. Casper will come before Megan Grace Casper.
3. With hyphenated personal names, the hyphenated elements, whether first name, middle name, or surname, are considered to be one unit. For example, if our patient's name is Adam Jones-Smith, for filing purposes we would consider the last name to be Jonessmith.
4. All punctuation is disregarded in filing.
5. When you are indexing a foreign name for which you cannot distinguish between the first and last names, index each part of the name in the order it is written. If you can make the distinction, use the surname name as the first indexing unit.
6. Names with prefixes are filed in the usual alphabetic order, with the prefix considered part of the name. Some common prefixes include Del as in Delagrosso and Mac as in MacIntyre.
7. Abbreviated parts of a name or nicknames are indexed as written if that person generally uses that form.
8. The name of a married woman who has taken her husband's last name is indexed by her legal name (her husband's surname, her given name, and her middle name or maiden surname). There should be a cross-reference, such as an out guide placed where her maiden name falls, directing you to her new name.
9. When followed by a complete name, titles may be used as the last filing unit if needed to distinguish the name from another identical name. Titles without complete names are considered the first indexing unit.

TABLE 10.2 Applying Indexing Rules

INDEXING RULE	NAME	UNIT 1	UNIT 2	UNIT 3	UNIT 4
1	Robert F. Grinch	Grinch	Robert	F.	
	R. Frank Grumman	Grumman	R.	Frank	
2	J. Orville Smith	Smith	J.	Orville	
	Jason O. Smith	Smith	Jason	O.	
3	M. L. Saint-Vickery	Saint-Vickery	M.	L.	
	Marie-Louise Taylor	Taylor	Marielouise		
4	Charles S. Anderson	Anderson	Charles	S.	
	Anderson's Surgical Supply	Andersons	Surgical	Supply	
5	Ah Hop Akee	Akee	Ah	Hop	
6	Alice Delaney	Delaney	Alice		
	Chester K. DeLong	Delong	Chester	K.	
7	Michael St. John	Stjohn	Michael		
8	Helen M. Maag	Maag	Helen	M.	
	Frederick Mabry	Mabry	Frederick		
	James E. MacDonald	Macdonald	James	E.	
9	Mrs. John L. Doe (Mary Jones)	Doe	Mary	Jones	(Mrs. John L.)
10	Prof. John J. Breck	Breck	John	J.	(Prof.)
	Madame Sylvia	Madame	Sylvia		
	Sister Mary Catherine	Sister	Mary	Catherine	
	Theodore Wilson, MD	Wilson	Theodore (MD)		
11	Lawrence W. Jones, Jr.	Jones	Lawrence	W.	(Jr.)
	Lawrence W. Jones, Sr.	Jones	Lawrence	W.	(Sr.)
12	The Moore Clinic	Moore	Clinic (The)		

10. Terms of seniority or professional or academic degrees are used only to distinguish the name from an identical name. Seniority terms include Sr., Jr., and III. If we had two people with exactly the same name except for the seniority designation, the Sr./Jr. would be considered. For example, if Jeffrey S. Saucerman, Sr., and Jeffrey S. Saucerman, Jr., were both patients, Jeffrey S. Saucerman, Jr., would come before Jeffrey S. Saucerman, Sr.

FILING METHODS

Three basic filing methods are used in healthcare facilities:
- Alphabetic by name
- Numeric
- Subject

Patients' records are filed either alphabetically by name or by one of several numeric methods. Subject filing is used for business records, correspondence, and topical materials.

Alphabetic Filing

Alphabetic filing by name is the oldest, simplest, and most commonly used system. It is the system of choice for filing patients' records in most small providers' offices.

The alphabetic system of filing is traditional and simple to set up, requiring only a file cabinet or shelf, folders, and some divider guides (Procedure 10.6). It is a **direct filing system** in that the person filing needs to know only the name to find the desired file. Alphabetic filing does have some drawbacks:
- The correct spelling of the name must be known.

- As the number of files increases, more space is needed for each section of the alphabet. This results in periodic shifting of folders to allow for expansion.
- As the files expand, more time is required for filing or retrieving each folder because of the greater number of folders involved in the search. The time can be greatly reduced by color coding.

Numeric Filing

Practically every large clinic or hospital uses some form of **numeric filing**, combined with color and shelf filing. Management consultants differ in their recommendations; some recommend numeric filing only if more than 5000 to 10,000 records are involved. Others recommend nothing but numeric filing. Numeric filing is an *indirect filing system* or one that requires the use of an alphabetic cross-reference to find a given file. Some object to this added step and overlook the advantages of numeric filing:

- It allows unlimited expansion without periodic shifting of folders, and shelves are usually evenly filled.
- It provides additional confidentiality to the record.
- It saves time in retrieving and filing records quickly. One knows immediately that the number 978 falls between 977 and 979. By contrast, an alphabetic system, even with color coding, requires a longer search to locate the exact spot.

Several types of numeric filing systems can be used:

- In a straight, or consecutive, numeric system, patients are given consecutive numbers as they first start using the practice. This is the simplest numeric system and works well for files of up to 10,000 records. It is time consuming, and the chance for error is greater when documents with five or more digits are filed. Filing activity is greatest at the end of the numeric series.
- In a terminal digit system, patients also are assigned consecutive numbers, but the digits in the number usually are separated into groups of twos or threes and are read in groups from right to left instead of from left to right. The records are filed backward in groups. For example, all files ending in 00 are grouped together first, then those ending in 01, and so on. Next, the files are grouped by their middle digits so that the 00 22s come before the 01 22s. Finally, the files are arranged by their first digits so that 01 00 22 precedes 02 00 22.
- Middle-digit filing begins with the middle digits, followed by the first digits, and finally by the terminal digits. Numeric filing requires more training, but once the system has been mastered, fewer errors occur than with alphabetic filing.

CRITICAL THINKING APPLICATION 10.8

Susan is unsure whether alphabetic or numeric filing is best in the healthcare facility. What are some advantages and disadvantages of each method?

Subject Filing

Subject filing can be either alphabetic or **alphanumeric** (e.g., A 1-3, B 1-1, B 1-2, and so on) and is used for general correspondence. The main difficulty with subject filing is indexing or classifying—that is, deciding where to file a document. Many papers require *cross-referencing*. An example would be if you had a subject folder for Laboratory Supplies and the same organization provides you with your General Medical Supplies; there should be a notation in the Laboratory Supplies folder stating, "See Also General Medical Supplies," and vice versa. All correspondence dealing with a particular subject is filed together. The papers in the folders are filed chronologically, with the most recent on top. The subject headings are placed on the tabs of the folders and filed alphabetically.

Color Coding

When a color-coding system is used, both filing and finding files is easier, and misfiling of folders is kept to a minimum. The use of color visually restricts the search area for a specific record. A misfiled record is easily spotted even from a distance of several feet. In color coding, a specific color is selected to identify each letter of the alphabet. Any selection of colors may be used, and the division of the alphabet is determined by one's own needs. However, studies have shown that the frequency with which different letters occur varies widely.

Alphabetic Color Coding

As medicine continues to consolidate into larger facilities with more patients in one system, filing patients' records become more complicated, and color coding becomes more useful. Several color-coding systems use two sets of 13 colors: one set for letters A to M and a second set of the same colors on a different background for letters N to Z.

Many ready-made systems are available for use. Self-adhesive, colored letter blocks with either two or three letters in the specific colors are supplied in rolls. The color blocks with the appropriate letter are placed on the index tab of the folder, along with the patient's full name. The letters are in pairs so that they can be seen from either side of the record. Strong, easily differentiated colors are used, creating a band of color in the files that makes spotting out-of-place folders easy (Figure 10.14).

Numeric Color Coding

Color coding is also used in numeric filing. Numbers 0 through 9 are each assigned a different color. In a terminal digit filing system, the colors for the last two numbers are affixed to the tab. If the number 1

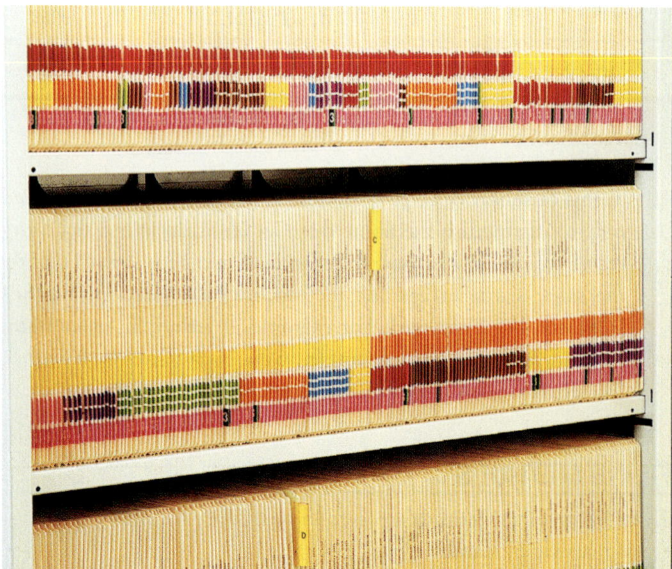

FIGURE 10.14 With color coding of patients' records, a misplaced file is easily spotted. (Courtesy Bibbero Systems, An InHealth Company, Petaluma, CA, www.bibbero.com.)

is red and 5 is yellow, all files with numbers ending in 15 have a red and yellow band. Usually, a predetermined section of the number is color coded.

Other Color-Coding Applications

Color can work in many other ways for the efficient healthcare facility. Small tabs in a variety of colors can be used to identify certain types of insured patients and other specific information. For example, a red tab over the edge of the folder may identify a patient on Medicare; a blue tab may identify a Medicaid patient; a green tab may identify a workers' compensation patient; matching tabs may be attached to the insured's ledger card; research cases may be identified by a special color tab; and brightly colored labels on the outside of a patient's record can indicate certain health conditions, such as drug allergies. In a partnership practice, a different color folder or label may identify each provider's patients. Color also can be used to differentiate dates: one color is used for each month or year.

The use of color in filing is limited only by the imagination. One word of caution: Every person in the facility who uses the files must know the key to the coding, and the key should also be written in the facility's policy and procedures manual.

ORGANIZATION OF FILES

Providers find studying a disorganized patient record very difficult. Some systematic method must be followed in placing items in the patient folder. From the filing standpoint, it should be emphasized that when a patient record is not in actual use, it should be in only one place—the filing cabinet or on the shelf. Many precious hours can be wasted searching for misplaced or lost records that were carelessly left unfiled.

The patient's full name, in indexing order, should be typed on a label and the label attached to the folder tab. A strip of transparent tape can be placed on the label to prevent smudging. The patient's full name should also be typed on each sheet in the folder. Some types of records common to the healthcare setting, other than patient records, are health-related correspondence, general correspondence, practice management files, miscellaneous files, and tickler or follow-up files.

Health-Related Correspondence

Correspondence pertaining to patients' health, such as a letter from other providers, updates on therapies, and so on, should be filed in the patient's health record. By doing this, the provider will have all the information needed to provide the best possible care to the patient. Other medical correspondence should be filed in a subject file.

General Correspondence

The provider's office operates as both a business and a professional service. Correspondence of a general nature pertaining to the operation of the office is part of the business side of the practice. Usually, a special drawer or shelf is set aside for the general correspondence. The correspondence is indexed according to subject matter or the names of the correspondents. The guides in a subject file may appear in one, two, or three positions, depending on the number of headings, subheadings, and subdivisions.

Practice Management Files

Of course, the most active financial record is the patient ledger. In facilities that still use a manual system, this is a card or vertical tray file, and the accounts are arranged alphabetically by name. At least two divisions are used: active accounts and paid accounts.

Miscellaneous Files

Papers that do not warrant an individual folder are placed in a miscellaneous folder. In that folder, all papers relating to one subject or with one correspondent are kept together in chronologic order, with the most recent on top, and then filed alphabetically with other miscellaneous material. Related materials may be stapled together. Never use paper clips for this purpose. When as many as five papers accumulate with one correspondent or subject, a separate folder should be prepared. Other business files include records of income and expenses, financial statements, income and payroll tax records, canceled checks, and insurance policies. These papers may be filed chronologically.

Tickler or Follow-Up Files

The most frequently used follow-up method is a **tickler file**, called this because it tickles the memory by reminding the health care provider that something needs to be done or followed up on a particular date. The tickler file is always in a chronologic arrangement. In its simplest form, it consists of notations on the daily calendar. If information, such as an x-ray report or a laboratory report, is expected about a patient with an appointment to come in, the medical assistant might make a note on the calendar or tickler file a day ahead to check on whether the report has arrived.

The tickler file can be a part of a computerized health record system or could be as simple as an email sent to oneself. Many people put reminders on their cell phones using an application (app) specially designed for memos and reminders. The tickler file could also be a card file: 12 guides, one for each month, are placed at the front of the cabinet, container, or other object used to hold the folders. Notations of actions to be taken are placed behind the guides for specific days of the current month. Notations for future months are placed behind the guide for that month. The tickler file must be checked first thing each day to be effective.

The tickler file can be used in many ways. It is a useful reminder of recurring events, such as payments, meetings, and so forth. On the last day of each month, all the notations from behind the next month's guide are distributed among the daily numbered guides, and the guide for the month just completed is placed at the back of the file.

CRITICAL THINKING APPLICATION **10.9**

Susan is responsible for checking the tickler file daily. What types of documents and duties might she find inside these files?

Transitory or Temporary File

Many papers are kept longer than necessary because no arrangement is made for separating those with limited usefulness. This situation can be prevented by having a transitory or temporary file. For example, if a medical assistant writes a letter requesting a reprint of the new patient brochure, the file copy is placed in the transitory folder until the reprint is received. When the reprint is received, the file copy is destroyed. The transitory file is used for materials with no permanent value. The paper may be marked with a "T" and then destroyed when the action is completed.

CLOSING COMMENTS

Just as in every aspect of the medical profession, advances in health records management are occurring rapidly, allowing providers and other caregivers to perform their duties more efficiently and accurately. A medical assistant must constantly be willing to learn and adapt to changes arising from legislation and technological advances. Computers have become generally accepted as a means of recording health information.

A primary goal of all healthcare facilities is to provide efficient, high-quality patient care. The EHR system can help the staff reach that goal. In the future, every provider's office, hospital, pharmacy, and healthcare facility may be able to access information in minutes, which will improve patient care and save lives. The medical assistant must stay abreast of news and articles related to EHR systems. The healthcare industry is one of constant growth and learning, and today's information technology provides the medical assistant with endless opportunities to make that growth rewarding and applicable to her or his current position.

Legal and Ethical Issues

The authority to release information from the health record lies solely with the patient unless such a release is required by law through a subpoena duces tecum. Ownership of the record often is a subject of controversy. The record belongs to the provider; the information belongs to the patient.

Remember that the EHR system contains information that is confidential at all times. The patient must authorize the release of health information in electronic form, just as if it were a piece of paper. EHR systems must do the following:

- Maintain the security and confidentiality of data
- Be easily retrievable
- Have safeguards against the loss of information
- Protect patients' rights to confidentiality and privacy
- Require identification and authentication for access

By supporting these requirements, the medical facility remains in compliance with applicable laws and gains the trust of patients, who are reassured that their health information is secure and safe.

Patient-Centered Care

Patients worry about the security of their information, particularly about who can access it. Lawsuits are often filed when patients discover that an unauthorized person has accessed their protected health information. The medical assistant should listen to a patient's concerns and explain the safety procedures that apply to the EHR in a language the patient can understand. Some facilities prepare a brochure to explain the conversion process to the patient and the advantages of the EHR system.

The medical assistant should expect hesitation and even reluctance from patients concerned about the privacy of their health information. Patients are concerned about the lack of control over who views their records. Be prepared to answer their questions about the safety of their records as related to the EHR. The medical assistant must know how the EHR is protected and what security measures are in place to be able to reassure the patients that their records are protected at all times.

Professional Behaviors

Once the medical assistant has been trained on the EHR system and has had the opportunity to use it for a time, daily use should become second nature. In fact, it may be difficult to imagine a workday without the system! By being open to change and willing to learn, the medical assistant can set a good example for all employees and will be more receptive to the process of change. Be encouraging to other staff members while training on the system, and if technology comes easily to you, share your knowledge with others and assist wherever possible. Do not expect to master the system in a week; instead, realize that a new system has a learning curve and be patient with and receptive to the educational process. Keep technical support phone numbers handy, and feel free to use them whenever a new or complicated issue arises. Work as a team and, if possible, help others who might find learning the system more of a struggle. Above all, while getting used to the new technology, make sure your attitude is one of enthusiasm, interest, and curiosity.

SUMMARY OF SCENARIO

Susan looks forward to attending her medical assisting classes each day and works diligently to perform to the best of her ability in the classroom. She strives to do well on each procedure check-off and each examination she completes. Her instructors provide excellent feedback and appreciate her contributions to the class.

Susan has the attitude that everything she is allowed to do in the healthcare facility is a learning tool. She regularly asks for additional responsibilities and is always ready to assist a co-worker. Dr. Kahn has recognized that she has the desire to learn, and he gives her many opportunities to glean more knowledge through the everyday activities in the office.

Although she is new to the medical profession, Susan learns quickly and thinks logically. She knows the rules and regulations on patient confidentiality and is always careful about the information she provides to those who request it. She is never hesitant about asking her office manager for guidance if she is unsure about any aspect of her duties. Susan is understanding and respectful when patients are concerned about their privacy. Her confidence and warm personality play a role in the trust she earns from the patients at the clinic.

Susan is willing to admit when she has made an error and has sought advice from Dr. Kahn and her office manager when an error needs correction. Although filing is not one of her favorite duties, she can be counted on to do her best while completing this important task. She realizes that filing is critical because the documents in the patient's health record direct the care provided to the patient. An abnormal laboratory report that is missing can make a crucial difference in

SUMMARY OF SCENARIO—cont'd

the patient's care. Susan takes pride in her work, and she is efficient and accurate where health records are concerned. When she is faced with a new task, she considers it a learning experience and asks for help if she is not completely sure about the way to handle a situation.

Susan's co-workers are supportive and always willing to help her as she learns to be the best medical assistant she can be. Her future as a professional medical assistant certainly holds opportunities and chances for advancement. Just as important, patients trust her. She has alleviated patients' concerns about EHRs by taking the time to explain privacy policies and exactly what information will be accessible to third parties. This trust also gives patients the confidence to reveal personal information and know that it will be held in the strictest confidence, not just by Susan but by each employee in the provider's office.

SUMMARY OF LEARNING OBJECTIVES

1. **Differentiate between electronic health records (EHRs) and electronic medical records (EMRs).**

   The two major types of patient records are the paper health record and the electronic health record (EHR). The EHR is much more efficient than the paper record, and most healthcare facilities have switched to EHRs for a number of reasons.

   The EHR is an electronic record of health-related information about an individual that conforms to nationally recognized interoperability standards, and that can be created, managed, and consulted by authorized clinicians and staff from more than one healthcare organization. The EMR is an electronic record of health-related information about an individual that can be created, gathered, managed, and consulted by authorized clinicians and staff within one healthcare organization.

   The HITECH act allows for financial incentives for meaningful use of certified EHR technology to improve healthcare. In 2018, promoting interoperability became the new incentive program with four objectives:

   - Electronic prescribing
   - Health information exchange (HIE)
   - Provider to patient exchange
   - Public health and clinical data exchange

   If providers are not compliant with HITECH, they can expect to have payments from Medicare and Medicaid reduced.

2. **Assess the contents of health records.**

   Health records must be accurate primarily so that patients are given the correct care. The record also helps ensure continuity of care between providers so that no lapse in treatment occurs. The record serves as indication and proof in court that certain treatments and procedures were performed on the patient; therefore, it can serve as excellent legal support if it is well maintained and accurate. Health records also aid researchers with statistical information.

   Subjective information is provided by the patient, whereas objective information is provided by the provider. Examples of subjective information include the patient's address, Social Security number, insurance information, and description of what the patient is experiencing. Objective information is obtained through the provider's questions and observations during the examination.

   Refer to Procedure 10.2 to see how to create a patient's health record and register a new patient in practice management software.

   Eye contact is critical when an EHR system is used with patients. Body language must indicate that the medical assistant is open to and listening to the patient's concerns, not just concentrating on data entry. Providers and medical assistants alike may have to relearn how to interact with patients in a natural way while using the laptop or tablet in the examination room. During the implementation period, processing and serving patients may take longer because the staff is using new technology. Most patients are understanding about this if the medical assistant explains that a new system is in place and asks for patience. Because patients are not always technologically savvy, most will be supportive and interested in the EHR system.

   The provider owns the physical health record, but the patient controls the information contained in it.

3. **Describe the components of working effectively within health records.**

   The source-oriented medical record (SOMR) categorizes the content by its sources, such as provider, laboratory, radiology, hospital, and consultation. Within each source category, the content is arranged in reverse chronologic order so that the most recent content is viewed first.

   The problem-oriented medical record (POMR) categorizes each of the patient's problems and elaborates on the findings and treatment plans for all concerns. Detailed progress notes are kept for each individual problem. This method addresses each of the patient's concerns separately, whereas a source-oriented record may address all problems and concerns at one time, usually covering one to three patient concerns per office visit. The POMR helps ensure that individual problems are all addressed.

   Documenting information in an EHR involves using radio buttons, drop-down menus, and free-text boxes. When you are documenting in a paper health record, the entry will always start with the date in the MM/DD/YYYY format. All entries must be written in black or blue ink and follow the format designated by the healthcare facility.

   A line should be drawn through the error, the correction inserted above or immediately after, and the person making the correction should write his or her initials or signature and the date below the correction to create a handwritten correction to a health record. Errors made while using an EHR are corrected in the usual way; however, an error discovered in an entry at a later date is corrected in the same manner as for a handwritten entry.

   With the increased use of EHRs and voice recognition software, there is decreased need for transcription. Transcription can be done from handwritten notes or, more likely, from machine dictation. Accuracy and speed are important. Some healthcare offices use voice recognition software for transcription.

   The provider must have a backup system for the EHR in case a medical office is without power for a significant amount of time. The EHR systems can be set to automatically back up the information at specified times during the day. This means that a minimum amount of data would be lost if the power went out. Backup options include an external hard drive, full server backup, and online backup systems. In most medical offices, records are classified in three ways: active, inactive, and closed. The process of moving a file from active to inactive is called *purging*. Providers have an obligation to retain patient records. The records of any patient covered by Medicare or Medicaid must be kept at least 10 years.

As with EHRs, paper health records are classified as active, inactive, or closed. Large healthcare facilities may find it advisable to convert their paper health records to microfilm.

The healthcare facility must be extremely careful when releasing any type of medical information; the patient must sign a release for information to be given to any third party. Requests for medical information should be made in writing. Healthcare providers must pay particular attention to records release requests involving a minor.

There are currently three kinds of health information exchange (HIE)—directed exchange, query-based exchange, and consumer-mediated exchange—and the implementation of HIE varies from state to state.

4. **Determine the processes for creating an efficient paper health record system.**
   Several types of equipment and supplies are needed to manage patients' records. Office space availability; structural considerations; cost of space and equipment; size, type, and volume of medical records; confidentiality requirements; retrieval speed; fire protection; and cost should all be considered when choosing filing equipment. Filing equipment includes drawer files, horizontal shelf files, rotary circular files, compactible files, automated files, and card files. Filing supplies include divider guides, out guides, file folders, and labels.

   Five basic steps are involved in document filing: (1) The papers are conditioned, which is the preparatory stage for filing. (2) The documents are released, which means they are ready to be filed because they have been reviewed or read and some type of mark has been placed on the document to indicate this. (3) The documents are indexed, which involves deciding where each document should be filed and coding it with some type of mark on the paper indicating that decision. (4) Sorting involves placing the files in filing sequence. (5) The actual filing and storing of the documents make up the last step. Refer to Table 10.2 for indexing rules. Refer to Procedure 10.5 for information on creating and organizing a paper health record.
5. **Differentiate various filing methods.**
   Both the alphabetic and numeric filing systems have advantages and disadvantages. Perhaps most important is the staff's preference. Some find it easier to retrieve files that are in standard alphabetic order, whereas others prefer a numeric system. The numeric system is more confidential than an alphabetic system. Some staff members prefer a combination of the two, called the alphanumeric system. Both effectively keep health records in good order and allow the medical assistant to spot a misfiled record quickly.

   Refer to Procedure 10.6 to see how to file patient health records.
6. **Discuss the organization of files and of health-related correspondence.**
   When a patient record is not in actual use, it should only be in the filing cabinet or on the shelf. Health-related correspondence, including general correspondence, should be filed appropriately. Practice management files are usually divided into active and paid accounts. Papers that do not warrant an individual folder are placed in the miscellaneous folder. Follow-up files are frequently called *tickler files*. Transitory (i.e., temporary) files can be helpful for material that has no permanent value.

PROCEDURE 10.1 Upload Documents to the Electronic Health Record

TASK: Scan paper records, and upload digital files to the EHR.

SCENARIO: A new patient brings in a laboratory report and a radiology report that he would like to have added to his EHR. You need to scan the original documents and upload them to the EHR.

EQUIPMENT and SUPPLIES

- Scanner
- Computer with SimChart for the Medical Office or EHR software
- Patient's laboratory and radiology reports

PROCEDURAL STEPS

1. Obtain the patient's name and date of birth if not on the reports.
   PURPOSE: You will need the patient's name and date of birth to find the patient's EHR.
2. Using a scanner that is connected to the computer, scan each document, creating an individual digital image for each. The uploaded file should include the patient's name (last name first), health record number, type of document, and the date.
   PURPOSE: The reports should be scanned separately and not combined to create one file. Each type of report must be uploaded separately to the correct location in the EHR.
3. Locate the file of the two scanned images in the computer drive. Open the files to ensure the images are clear.
   PURPOSE: When you are scanning and uploading documents to the EHR, it is crucial that the image of the document is clear and can be easily read by the provider. If the image is blurred, rescan the document.
4. In the EHR, search for the patient, using the patient's last and first names. Verify the patient's date of birth.
   PURPOSE: Before you begin uploading to or documenting in the EHR, it is critical to verify that the correct record has been opened.
5. Locate the window to upload diagnostic/laboratory results and add a new result. Enter the date of the test. Select the correct type of result. Browse for the image file of the laboratory file and attach it. Save the information. Select the option to add a new result and repeat the steps to upload the second report. Verify that both documents were uploaded correctly.
   PURPOSE: Errors during the upload may affect the ability to see the files. Verifying at the time of the upload will help you ensure that providers can see the results in the future.

PROCEDURE 10.2 Register a New Patient in the Practice Management Software

TASK: Register a new patient in the practice management software, prepare a Notice of Privacy Practices (NPP) form and a disclosure authorization form for the new patient, and document this in the electronic health record (EHR).

SCENARIO: The patient received both documents and signed the disclosure authorization form.

EQUIPMENT and SUPPLIES

- Computer with SimChart for the Medical Office or practice management and EHR software
- Completed patient registration form
- Scanner

PROCEDURAL STEPS

1. Obtain the new patient's completed registration form. Log into the practice management software.
   PURPOSE: The registration form will provide the information needed to create the new record in the practice management system.
2. Using the patient's last and first names and date of birth, search the database for the patient.
   PURPOSE: A search for the new patient's name must always be done before registering that person to help ensure the integrity of the practice management and EHR systems. This prevents a double record from being created if the patient had been entered into the database at an earlier time.
3. If the database does not contain the patient's name, add a new patient and enter the patient's demographics from the completed registration form.
   PURPOSE: This will create the patient's record in the practice management system. If the patient's name is in the database, you should verify the information to prevent creating two records for the same patient.
4. Verify that the information entered is correct and that all fields are completed before saving the data.
   PURPOSE: Errors during the registration process can affect the communication with the patient (e.g., if a wrong address or email is entered) or can affect billing (e.g., if the incorrect insurance information is added). Verification should also include the proper use of lowercase and uppercase letters. Accuracy is extremely important when entering the patient's information.
   Note: The software will generate a health record number for the patient.
5. Using the EHR software, prepare and print a copy of the NPP and a disclosure authorization form for the new patient. The disclosure authorization form should indicate that the disclosure will be made to the patient's insurance company.
   PURPOSE: Before the medical office can release patient information to the insurance company, the patient has to give consent in writing.
6. Using the EHR, document that the patient received a copy of the NPP and signed the disclosure authorization form. Scan the disclosure authorization form and upload it into the EHR.
   PURPOSE: Documentation in the health record provides a legal record of what was done or communicated to the patient.
7. Log out of the software upon completion of the procedure.
   PURPOSE: Logging in and out of the software helps protect the integrity of the data saved in the software and prevents unauthorized people from viewing the information.

PROCEDURE 10.3 Protect the Integrity of the Medical Record

TASK: Protect the integrity of the medical record.

SCENARIO: You are mentoring a medical assistant student who is in practicum. You notice the student routinely does not sign out of the electronic health record before leaving the desk. The facility's policy is to sign out or lock the computer before leaving it.

DIRECTIONS: Role-play the scenario with a peer who plays the student. You, the medical assistant, must explain to the "student" the facility's policy. Also, address the hazards of not protecting the medical record. If the student does not change this behavior, you will need to address the situation with the department supervisor.

PROCEDURAL STEPS

1. Professionally and respectfully discuss the situation with the student.
2. Inform the student about the facility's policy and the hazards of not protecting the electronic health record.
   PURPOSE: It is important that the student be knowledgeable about the policies and the hazards of not protecting the EHR.
3. Provide the student with strategies to protect the electronic health record.
4. Inform the student about what will occur if the electronic record is not protected.

PROCEDURE 10.4 Develop a Plan in the Event of Loss of EMR and Practice Management Software

TASK: To develop a plan to ensure information integrity and patient care when access to the EMR and practice management software (PMS) is lost for more than 24 hours.

SCENARIO: Your supervisor at WMFM Clinic has asked you to develop a plan to protect patient information in case access is lost to the EMR and PMS.

EQUIPMENT and SUPPLIES

- Paper and pen, or word processing software

PROCEDURAL STEPS

1. Using reliable internet resources, research ways to protect the information contained in the EMR and PMS.
   PURPOSE: To determine the best options to protect the integrity of the EMR and PMS.
2. Develop a list of the top four choices for protecting patient information and care.
3. Develop a pros/cons list for each of the four choices.
   PURPOSE: This will help clarify which system will work best.
4. Determine which option you would choose, and create a plan for implementing it at the WMFC clinic. Your plan should include how patients can still be seen and provided the same level of care.

PROCEDURE 10.5 Create and Organize a Patient's Paper Health Record

TASK: Create a paper health record for a new patient. Organize health record documents in a paper health record.

SCENARIO: The patient authorized his or her prior provider to send health records to your agency. You need to organize these records within the paper health record.

EQUIPMENT and SUPPLIES

- End tab file folder
- Completed patient registration form
- Divider sheets with different color labels (4)
- Progress note sheet (1)
- Name label
- Color-coding labels (first two letters of last name and first letter of first name)
- Year label
- Allergy label
- Black pen or computer with word processing software to process labels
- Health record documents (i.e., prior records, laboratory reports)
- Hole puncher

PROCEDURAL STEPS

1. Obtain the patient's first and last names.
   PURPOSE: To customize the record for the patient, the first and last names will be required.
2. Neatly write or word-process the patient's name on the name label. Left justify the last name, followed by a comma, the first name, middle initial, and a period (e.g., Smith, Mary J.).
   PURPOSE: The label should be easy to read. The last name always comes before the first name.
3. Adhere the name label to the bottom left side of the record tab. When you hold the record by the main fold in your left hand, the writing should be easy to read. (For directional purposes, assume the main record fold is on the left and the tab is at the bottom.)
   PURPOSE: Placing the labels in correct position will make it easier to find the information needed.
4. Put the color-coding labels on the bottom-right edge of the folder. Start by placing the first letter of the last name at the farthest right edge. Working left to right, place the second letter of the last name, then the first letter of the first name, and lastly, the year label. The year label should be close to the name label.
   PURPOSE: When the folders are in the file cabinet, they are sorted by the colored labels, starting with the top label (first letter of the last name), followed by the second and remaining labels.
5. Place the allergy label on the front of the record. If allergies are known, clearly write the name of the allergy on the label in red ink.
   PURPOSE: Allergies need to be clearly identified on medical records.
6. Place the divider labels on the record divider sheets if they come separately. Ensure the labels on the divider sheets are staggered, so they do not overlap. Print the name of the section on the front and back of the label. The print should be easy to read when the record is held by the main fold. (Suggested names for dividers are Progress Notes, Laboratory, Correspondence, and Miscellaneous.)
   PURPOSE: Placing divider labels on the divider sheets in a staggered pattern allows the provider to see all sections of the health record easily.
7. Using the prongs on the left-hand side of the record, secure the registration form.
   PURPOSE: The registration form should be in an easy-to-find location in the record.
8. Using the prongs on the right-hand side of the record, secure the index dividers with a progress note sheet under the progress note tab.
   PURPOSE: The provider will need the progress note sheet to document data regarding the visit.
9. Verify the name and the date of birth on the previous health record, and ensure they match the information listed on the current health record.
   PURPOSE: Before you organize and file documents in a patient's health record, it is critical to ensure the health record is for the correct patient.
10. Open the prongs on the right side of the record and carefully remove the record to the point at which the documents need to be inserted. For the documents being inserted, punch holes in the proper location. Insert the papers into the record, then reassemble the remaining part of the record. Continue to do this until all the documents are filed within the health record.
    PURPOSE: Documents need to be placed in the correct location in the record so the provider can easily find information.

PROCEDURE 10.6 File Patient Health Records

TASK: File patient health records using two different filing systems: the alphabetic system and the numeric system.

SCENARIO: The agency uses the alphabetic system. You need to file health records in the correct location.

EQUIPMENT and SUPPLIES

- Paper health records using the alphabetic filing system
- Paper health records using the numeric filing system
- File boxes or file cabinet

PROCEDURAL STEPS

1. Using alphabetic guidelines, place the records to be filed in alphabetic order.
   PURPOSE: Placing the records in alphabetic order before filing in the box or cabinet will make the filing process more efficient.
2. Using the file box or file cabinet, locate the correct spot for the first file.
   PURPOSE: It is important that you place the record in the correct spot so that others can locate the record.
3. Place the health record in the correct location. Continue these filing steps until all the health records are filed.
4. Using numeric guidelines, place the records to be filed in numeric order.
   PURPOSE: Placing the records in numeric order before filing in the box or cabinet will make the filing process more efficient.
5. Using the file box or file cabinet, locate the correct spot for the first file.
   PURPOSE: It is important that you place the record in the correct spot so that others can locate the record.
6. Place the health record in the correct location. Continue these filing steps until all the health records are filed.

DAILY OPERATIONS AND SAFETY 11

SCENARIO

Marie Van Bakel, a certified medical assistant (CMA), is a new medical assistant at Walden-Martin Family Medical (WMFM) Clinic. She was hired to work with the family medicine providers. This is Marie's first job as a new graduate from a medical assisting program. She is excited to work in family medicine. This was the same specialty she worked in during her medical assisting practicum. Because this is a small healthcare facility, Marie's responsibilities are different from what they would be in a larger facility. She and the administrative medical assistant, Catherine, are the only staff members in the office at the start of the day. The providers make hospital rounds at that time. The providers and the rest of the medical assistants come in later.

Marie and Catherine need to open the office and prepare for the patients. Marie is also responsible for the inventory of clinical supplies and administrative and clinical equipment. During Marie's interview, Dr. Walden expressed her concern about the lack of procedures for ordering and maintaining inventory. She would like Marie to develop those procedures. Having little exposure to supplies and ordering during her practicum, Marie realizes she needs to learn about these procedures.

While studying this chapter, think about the following questions:

- What are the opening and closing duties of the medical assistant?
- How is inventory performed for equipment and supplies?
- What should be considered when ordering supplies?
- How does a medical assistant use correct body mechanics when working with supplies and equipment?
- How does a medical assistant evaluate the work environment?
- How does a medical assistant respond to facility-related emergencies?

LEARNING OBJECTIVES

1. Examine the opening tasks for both the clinical and administrative medical assistants.
2. Examine the closing tasks for both the clinical and administrative medical assistants.
3. Examine equipment management, including inventory, maintenance and service calls, warranties, and purchasing.
4. Examine supply inventory management, including inventory control systems and taking inventory.
5. Examine the ordering process, including price considerations, opening an account, the purpose of the purchase order number, and payment procedures.
6. Examine how the medical assistant checks the delivered items and rotates stock.
7. Analyze the storage requirements for vaccines.
8. Demonstrate the use of proper body mechanics.
9. Analyze strategies to keep the work environment safe.
10. Demonstrate how to evaluate the work environment for potential safety issues.
11. Examine emergency response plans, including the purpose and critical elements of the plans.
12. Examine the effect of stress on the body, including the symptoms, effects, and healthy coping strategies.

VOCABULARY

accounts payable Money owed by a company to other companies for services and goods; pertains to paying the facility's bills.

answering service A commercial service that answers telephone calls for its clients.

back-ordered An order placed for an item that is temporarily out of stock and will be sent later.

billable service Assistance (i.e., service) that is provided by a healthcare provider and can be billed to the insurance company or patient.

buying cycle Refers to how often an item is purchased and depends on how frequently the item is used and the storage space available for it.

crash cart Emergency and equipment (e.g., oxygen, intravenous [IV] and airway supplies) stored in a cart and ready for an emergency.

de-escalating Reducing the level or intensity; bringing down a person's anger or elevated emotions.

depreciate To diminish in value (e.g., the value of an item) over a period of time; a concept used for tax purposes.

diluent A liquid substance that dilutes or lessens the strength of a solution or mixture; it is added to vials of powdered medications to create a solution of the drug for injection.

discrepancy A lack of similarity between what is stated and what is found; for instance, the computer inventory count is different from the physical count.

VOCABULARY—*continued*

disinfect The process of cleaning in order to destroy or prevent the growth of disease-causing microorganisms.

fire doors Doors made of fire-resistant materials; close manually or automatically during a fire to prevent it from spreading.

initiative The ability to determine what needs to be done and take action on your own.

inventory A detailed list of equipment and supplies owned and stored; the process of counting the supplies in stock.

invoices Billing statements that list the amount owed for goods or services purchased.

packing slip A document that accompanies purchased merchandise and shows what is in the box or package.

progress notes Documentation in the medical record that can be used to track the patient's condition and progress.

purchase order (PO) number A unique number assigned by the ordering facility that allows the facility to track or reference the order.

quality control A process to ensure the reliability of test results, often using manufactured samples with known values.

restock The process of replacing the supplies that were used.

sanitize The process of cleaning equipment and instruments with detergent and water in order to remove debris and reduce the number of microorganisms.

sterilize The process of removing all microorganisms.

vendors Companies that sell supplies, equipment, or services to other companies or individuals.

workplace emergencies Unforeseen situations that threaten the employees and visitors; can disrupt services provided.

INTRODUCTION

In the ambulatory healthcare facility, the medical assistant has opening tasks to accomplish to prepare the department for patients. At the end of the day, after the last patient leaves, the medical assistant has duties of closing the department for the night. Besides performing these daily duties, the medical assistant manages the equipment and supply inventories. Having adequate supplies available to use for patients is critical to the functioning of the department. These topics are addressed in this chapter.

In addition, the medical assistant must be knowledgeable about environmental safety and security. This chapter discusses workplace violence, evaluating the environment, emergency response plans, and the effects of stress. Keeping the work environment safe is an important role for every employee.

OPENING TASKS FOR THE MEDICAL ASSISTANT

Employees who are responsible for opening the ambulatory healthcare facility must arrive before the patients in the morning. These employees must prepare for the day. Preparation time will vary based on the size of the practice and the number of patients on the schedule.

The *clinical medical assistant* assists the provider with patient treatments and procedures (e.g., injections, wound care, and diagnostic tests). The *administrative medical assistant* works in the reception area and the business office. In larger facilities, both types of medical assistants have opening duties. If the healthcare facility is small, the medical assistant may be required to perform both administrative and clinical tasks. Often this is called performing "front office" and "back office" activities.

Unlocking the Facility

In smaller facilities, a few reliable employees are given keys to unlock the doors and deactivate the alarm system. In larger facilities, employees must use the locked employee entrances. Employees can unlock the doors by entering unique codes into a keypad or using unique keycards or fobs. Both systems are developed to monitor who enters the building. Usually, security, custodial, or supervisory personnel are responsible for deactivating the alarm system in larger facilities. Staff members then open the main patient doors at a set time.

Clinical Medical Assistant

It is important for the clinical medical assistant to prepare the clinical equipment and exam rooms for patient visits. An unprepared area can cause delays in patient care. Facility opening tasks for the clinical medical assistant include the following:

- Preparing the exam rooms by turning on the lights, ensuring supplies are stocked, and making sure the rooms have been cleaned appropriately and are safe for patients.
- Ensuring prescription pads (if used) are stored outside of the exam rooms, in a locked cabinet. Prescription pads should never be accessible to patients. Some patients or staff might take the pads and try to forge a prescription, which is illegal.
- Unlocking supply cabinets (with the exception of the narcotics cabinet, which remains locked).
- Ensuring restrooms have adequate supplies for patients (e.g., urine specimen containers, cleansing towelettes).
- Performing **quality control** tests on laboratory equipment and completing refrigerator and freezer temperature logs.

In addition to these tasks, the clinical medical assistant must follow up on outstanding patient issues from the prior day. The medical assistant also needs to handle new diagnostic test reports (e.g., x-ray reports). For agencies using paper health records, this would require the medical assistant to perform the following tasks:

- Obtain the patient's paper health record.
- Attach the diagnostic report to the record.
- Give the health record and report to the provider to review.

For facilities with electronic health records (EHRs), this process is completed using the electronic messaging system in the software.

Often medical assistants notify patients of normal test results and document the notification in the health record. No test result can be given to the patient unless the provider has authorized its release or the facility's procedures allow it. The medical assistant must follow the facility's procedures when notifying the patient of the results.

Administrative Medical Assistant

Opening tasks for the administrative medical assistant include the following:

- Checking the voice mail or **answering service** messages. The answering service may email or fax messages to the facility. All messages need to be addressed and documented in the patient's health record.
- Updating the voice mail message.
- Switching on the phone so that patients can reach the facility instead of the answering service.
- Turning on computers, copy machines, and other office equipment.
- Preparing the reception area for patients.
- Printing schedules of the day's appointments. A schedule is kept for the paper health record preparation. Other copies are given to the clinical medical assistants, providers, and the medical laboratory. In some facilities, the EHR allows staff to reference the schedule using the software, thus eliminating the printed schedule.

In addition to these duties, the administrative medical assistant must compile any remaining required paperwork for the day's visits. Usually, this is done the prior afternoon. A few patient visits that need to be completed may be added to the schedule. For healthcare facilities with EHRs, required patient education literature (e.g., well-child visit documents) and preprinted paper screening forms may be prepared.

For facilities with paper health records, the medical assistant must do the following:

- Pull the paper health records using a copy of the appointment schedule.
- Verify that the correct record was pulled for each patient.
- Check off the patient's name on the copy of the appointment schedule.
- Review each record.
  - Have all recently received documents (e.g., laboratory reports, radiograph readings) been placed correctly and permanently attached to the record?
  - Are documents (e.g., laboratory reports) missing that are needed for the visit?
  - Is there enough space available in the **progress notes** for the provider to write in the record? If not, additional progress note pages must be placed in the record.
- Arrange the health records in the order in which the patients will be arriving. The record for the first visit of the day should be on top. Larger facilities may alphabetize the health records.

> **CRITICAL THINKING APPLICATION 11.1**
>
> When Marie, the clinical medical assistant, opens WMFM Clinic, what jobs does she need to do? What jobs does Catherine, the administrative medical assistant, need to do to prepare for the day?

CLOSING TASKS FOR THE MEDICAL ASSISTANT

Toward the end of the workday, the staff must start the closing tasks. Some tasks must be done after all patients have left. The following sections discuss the closing tasks for both the clinical and administrative medical assistants.

Clinical Medical Assistant

At the end of the day, the medical assistant needs to help with the closing duties. The clinical medical assistant must ensure that all the patients have left by checking the exam and treatment rooms. The clinical medical assistant must complete the following duties:

- **Restock** the rooms and organize any reading materials.
- **Disinfect** the exam table, writing table, counters, computer keyboards, and chairs (i.e., those made of plastic, metal, or wood).
- Secure (put away) confidential documents.
- Turn off computers and other devices.
- **Sanitize,** disinfect, or **sterilize** equipment and instruments.
- Lock supply and medication cabinets.
- Verify and count the narcotic medication stock, following the facility's procedure.

Administrative Medical Assistant

The administrative medical assistant will complete the following closing duties:

- Prepare the patient records and documents for the next day.
- Turn off the computers, copy machine, and other office equipment.
- Switch phones to voice mail or the answering service.
- Follow office procedures for handling money at the end of the day.
- Secure (put away) any confidential documents.
- Clean up the reception area (neatly arrange the magazines, disinfect toys, and remove garbage and unsolicited advertisements) and turn off the lights, television, stereo, and other devices.

With time being short in the morning, it is important to take care of as much as possible the evening before you leave.

Depending on the facility, the medical assistant may be responsible for turning off the lights, activating the alarms, and locking the doors. In larger facilities, the custodial or security staff handles these responsibilities.

> **Daily and Monthly Duties**
>
> Custodial staff or a cleaning service is responsible for cleaning the facility. The medical assistant also is responsible for cleaning and organizing the reception area and exam rooms. During slow times, medical assistants should take the **initiative** to do extra duties, including restocking medical and office supplies, forms, and patient literature. The cabinets and drawers need to be straightened and reorganized. Medications and supplies that have expiration dates need to be checked monthly. The **crash cart** and other emergency supplies need to be inventoried monthly and after each use (Figure 11.1). Many facilities use a master list of crash cart supplies with expiration dates. This helps ensure that all supplies are in the crash cart and expiring supplies and medications can be easily identified.

> **CRITICAL THINKING APPLICATION 11.2**
>
> The office uses a local cleaning service to clean the facility's rooms. The staff members arrive after hours and are gone by the time Catherine and Marie open the office in the morning. Over the past month, Marie has noticed that the rooms do not look as clean as they should. Should she address this concern? If so, with whom should she discuss it?

EQUIPMENT MANAGEMENT

In a healthcare facility, administrative and clinical types of equipment are used. The medical assistant needs to know how to operate, maintain, and handle issues with the equipment. For financial and tax purposes, the purchase cost and age of each item need to be recorded. The process of gathering and creating a list of the equipment in the facility is called managing **inventory.**

Equipment Inventory

For all clinical and administrative equipment, records need to be maintained. These records are used to replace equipment lost in a disaster or theft. The healthcare facility's accountant also uses the information when preparing tax paperwork. For instance, records should be maintained for the following items:

- Small equipment (e.g., thermometers, glucose monitors), which is deducted as an expense for the year in which it was purchased
- Large office equipment (e.g., computer hardware, calculators, and copiers), which **depreciates** over 5 years

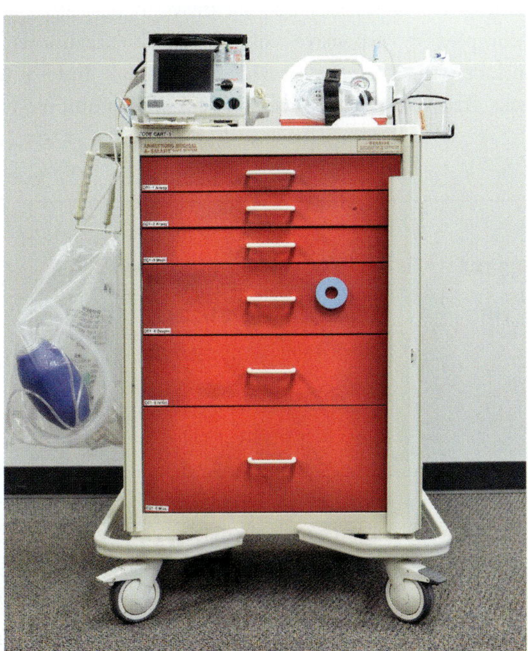

FIGURE 11.1 Crash carts must be inventoried monthly or after each use to ensure that medication and supplies have not expired and all the required supplies are available for an emergency.

- Office furniture items (e.g., desks, files, safes, exam tables), which depreciate over 7 years

The equipment inventory is also used by supervisors to identify equipment that needs to be replaced. Preplanning equipment purchases is a financial strategy for the practice. It allows the practice to be prepared and to plan for future investments.

When you are creating an equipment inventory list, it is helpful to use spreadsheet software (Figure 11.2). In some situations, you may have inventory forms that you can complete (Procedure 11.1). For all equipment, document the following information:

- Equipment name, manufacturer, and serial number
- Purchase date, cost, and supplier
- Warranty information (e.g., start and end date, warranty coverage)
- Location of the equipment (optional)
- Unique facility number is given to that piece of equipment (optional)

The owner's manual or users' guide and warranty information should be kept at a central location and available to users. Many users' guides are available online. They are used for problem-solving performance issues. They can be used to identify service schedules and routine maintenance. Many users' guides provide a list of parts or supplies needed for the operation of the machine.

CRITICAL THINKING APPLICATION 11.3

Marie needs to learn more about managing inventory. She reviews her medical assistant textbook and reads articles online. She decides to start by creating an inventory list of the equipment in the medical office. What are some advantages of having an updated list of administrative and clinical equipment?

Routine Maintenance and Safety

The medical assistant is responsible for monitoring equipment safety and proper functioning. Routine maintenance helps to ensure the best performance of the equipment. Potential issues should not be overlooked. Actions should be taken to prevent injury to staff or patients and costly damage to the equipment. The medical assistant should do the following:

- Check electrical cords on equipment for damage.
- Address any suspected overheating issues.

Equipment Name	Manufacturer / Serial Number	Location / Facility Number	Purchase Date / Supplier	Cost	Warranty Information
Laser Printer	HP / HP3598XA	Medical Assistant Desk / LP59483	08/01/20XX / Best Office Supplies	$325	Parts and labor expire 07/31/20XX
AT2 Plus ECG / Spirometry	Schiller / WA4893X	Treatment Room / ES00012	05/02/20XX / Medical Equipment Supplies	$2987	Parts and labor expire 05/01/20XX

FIGURE 11.2 An equipment inventory list can be created in a spreadsheet and provides useful information about the administrative and clinical equipment in the facility.

- Investigate any unusual noise or change in performance.
- Clean and maintain equipment routinely in accordance with the users' guide.

Routine maintenance varies with the equipment. Copiers and printers may require changing the toner or cartridges. For clinical equipment, maintenance may include changing filters or batteries.

It is important to keep track of routine maintenance. Making a schedule as a reminder for routine maintenance can be helpful. Many facilities use logs to track routine maintenance and service calls (Figure 11.3). The following information is commonly found in the routine maintenance log:

- Equipment name, serial number, location of the machine, and facility's unique equipment number (if applicable)
- Manufacturer's name
- Date of purchase
- Warranty information (e.g., start and end date, warranty coverage)
- Service provider contact information, such as telephone number
- Date and time and description of maintenance activities performed
- Signature of person performing maintenance

Procedure 11.2 explains the steps involved in creating a maintenance log, performing the maintenance, and documenting the maintenance.

CRITICAL THINKING APPLICATION 11.4

Marie realizes that the facility does not have maintenance logs for the various pieces of equipment. She decides to start making logs, but she realizes she will have to make a lot of them. How could Marie create logs in a time-efficient manner? For a small office, describe options that she could use to organize the logs, so they are easy to locate and use.

Warranties and Service Calls

When equipment is purchased, a warranty is given for a period of time. The warranty is the manufacturer's guarantee. If the piece of equipment needs to be repaired or has a defective part, the manufacturer will pay for the cost of the repair. In some cases, the item may be replaced. Warranty language includes details on what is covered. Some warranties are not honored if someone other than a recognized serviceperson attempts to fix the machine. Extended warranties lengthen the protection time and can be purchased for some equipment.

For complex or expensive equipment, the healthcare facility may contract with a service provider for repairs and routine service checks. This assistance is necessary for some equipment. It also

Maintenance Log

Equipment Name: **Laser Printer** Serial #: **HP3598XA** Location: **Medical Assistant Desk**

Facility #: **LP59483** Manufacturer: **HP** Purchased: **08/01/20XX**

Warranty Information: **Parts and labor expires 07/31/20XX**

Frequency of Inspections: **Every 6 months**

Service Provider: **Best Office Supplies**

Date	Time	Maintenance Activities	Signature
12/15/20XX	**0956**	**Replaced toner cartridge**	**Marie Van Bakel, CMA (AAMA)**
02/11/20XX	**1235**	**Service call: Office Repair Company – to fix stray ink marks on copies**	**Catherine Black, RMA**

Maintenance Log

Equipment Name: **AT2 Plus ECG/Spirometry** Serial #: **WA4893X** Location: **Treatment Room**

Facility #: **ES00012** Manufacturer: **Schiller** Purchased: **05/02/20XX**

Frequency of Inspections: **Every 12 months**

Warranty information: **Parts and labor expires 05/01/20XX**

Service Provider: **Medical Equipment Suppliers**

Date	Time	Maintenance Activities	Signature
10/23/20XX	**1123**	**Replaced battery**	**Marie Van Bakel, CMA (AAMA)**
05/02/20XX	**1445**	**No tracing, cleaned stylus with alcohol**	**Marie Van Bakel, CMA (AAMA)**

FIGURE 11.3 Equipment maintenance logs are used by the staff and outside repair agencies to track maintenance activities.

helps to extend the lifetime of those machines. For repairs on other equipment, it might be necessary to ship or bring the machine to the repair service. Usually, the cost for onsite repairs is more than if the machine is taken or shipped to the service provider for repairs. One of the main concerns when a piece of equipment breaks down is the effect on the healthcare facility. Some service providers will loan equipment to facilities while the repairs take place. This service greatly lessens the burden on the practice.

Purchasing Equipment

The process of purchasing equipment can vary depending on the size of the organization. Large agencies have purchasing departments. The purchasing staff researches the need and identifies the best equipment to purchase. The medical assistant may be involved with the process in smaller practices.

Many factors are considered when equipment is being replaced:

- Age of the equipment and availability of parts
- Frequency and cost of repairs
- Use of the machine and whether new features will lead to extra **billable services**

Leasing medical equipment is becoming a popular option for smaller facilities. The healthcare facility pays a fee to lease an item, such as monitoring equipment, diagnostic testing equipment, computer systems, and exam tables. The fee is less than what it would cost to purchase the item. The lease fees are tax deductible and allow the healthcare facility to provide extra billable services.

The medical assistant may help identify potential new equipment models to purchase or lease. Using the internet and contacting the company's salespeople are two ways to get additional information. Some salespeople will meet with the staff and demonstrate the product. In addition to research, the medical assistant may need to explain the usage of the machine and the frequency of repair checks. Usually, the supervisor or provider has the final say on whether the purchase should occur.

CRITICAL THINKING APPLICATION **11.5**

Currently, the providers are using an offsite radiology service. They are contemplating creating a small radiology room where they could take x-rays. How could Marie assist the providers with their plans for a potential purchase of x-ray equipment?

SUPPLY INVENTORY

Another medical assistant's duty is to manage the supplies in the medical office. In smaller facilities, this may involve ordering and maintaining an inventory control system. In larger facilities, purchasing department employees are hired for such roles.

Many supplies are required to run the medical office and treat patients. Supplies include administrative items (e.g., pens, paper, envelopes, and paperclips) and clinical items (e.g., bandages, vaccines, medications, slings, and splints). The medical assistant must make sure there are enough supplies to treat patients. A lack of supplies can greatly affect the services provided to patients. It can be expensive for the healthcare facility to order last-minute because of higher prices to do so. On the other hand, overstocking supplies can be a financial waste to the facility. Many supplies have expiration dates and cannot be used beyond that date. Having an adequate amount of supplies in inventory is crucial.

Inventory Management

Inventory management involves ordering, tracking inventory, and identifying the quantity of products to purchase. The goal of inventory management is to have adequate supplies on hand. It is important not to have too much stock that will expire or take a long time to use.

The medical assistant in charge of ordering and managing supplies must keep a record of each item in inventory. The record can be a manual entry written in a notebook or on index cards. It can also be computerized in a spreadsheet or inventory control system software. For each inventory item, the medical assistant must record the following:

- Item details: Item name, size, quantity, item number, supplier's name, and cost (Figure 11.4).
- *Quantity to reorder*: Number of supplies that need to be ordered. This amount reflects the product used during the **buying cycle.** For instance, the healthcare facility's buying cycle for 2 × 2 nonsterile gauze (100 per pack) is 1 month. The facility typically goes through 25 packs in 1 month. This would be the quantity used during the buying cycle. It would also be the quantity to reorder each time (see Figure 11.4).
- *Reorder point*: Point at which low inventory requires the product to be ordered. For instance, when the inventory of 2 × 2 nonsterile gauze packs gets depleted to five packs, the medical assistant must reorder (see Figure 11.4). Five is the reorder point or quantity that triggers an order to be placed to replenish the inventory. The reorder point for medical and administrative supplies can be

Item Name	Size	Quantity	Item Number	Supplier's Name	Reorder Point	Quantity to Reorder	Cost	Stock Available	Order (✓)
Nonsterile gauze sponges, 8 ply	2″x 2″	100/pkg	NG0022	Midwest Medical	5	25	$2.31/pkg		
Sterile gauze sponges, 12 ply, 2/pkg	2″x 2″	25 pkg/ box	NG0042	Midwest Medical	4	20	$3.99/box		

FIGURE 11.4 A supply inventory list shows details of items in the inventory. For efficiency, use two extra columns ("Stock Available" and "Order") as shown. This list can be duplicated and used whenever an inventory is performed.

different for each item because of the usage rate and the time it takes to receive the item after it is ordered.

Calculating the Reorder Point

The reorder point can be calculated based on the number used per day and the number of days it takes to order and receive the product.

For instance, the practice uses 0.5 packs of 2 × 2 nonsterile gauze per day. It takes 4 days to receive the order from the medical supply company. The medical practice may also want 6 extra days' worth of supplies on hand to prevent issues related to running out of the item. Here is how you would figure out the reorder point:

Stock to cover order time: 0.5 packs per day × 4 days to receive order = 2 packs

Extra stock: 6 days × 0.5 pack per day = 3 packs

Reorder point: 2 packs (stock to cover order time) + 3 packs (6-day supply) = 5 packs

Inventory Control Systems

An inventory control system helps to make inventory management work well. Large medical facilities use computerized inventory control systems. These systems monitor usage and inventory in stock. They also identify items that need to be ordered. Smaller facilities may use simple computerized or manual systems.

Barcode Inventory System

To help create an efficient computerized system, many medical facilities use barcodes to track inventory, for insurance, and for patient billing for supplies (Figure 11.5). With this system, each item has a unique barcode. The barcode is scanned with a barcode reader when items are added to or taken from inventory. Software monitors the inventory quantity. For barcodes to work successfully, the staff must be diligent in scanning the barcodes when taking a product from stock. Barcode inventory control systems work successfully in both large and small healthcare facilities.

Weight-Based Inventory System

The weight-based inventory system uses separate bins for each type of product. Each bin is connected to a scale. The weight of each type of product is entered into the software. The software monitors the weight of each bin. When an item is removed from a bin, the software reduces the inventory count.

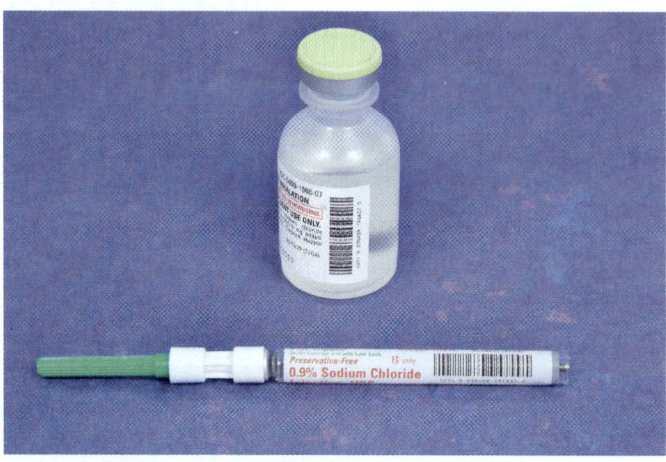

FIGURE 11.5 Using barcodes makes inventory control more efficient.

For example, the weight of a 3 mL syringe (i.e., 15 grams) is entered into the software. The bin is filled with 30 syringes and attached to the scale. The software registers 30 syringes in inventory using the weight of the bin. An employer removes two syringes, and the weight drops 30 grams. The software drops the total syringes to 28.

This type of inventory system reduces the risk of errors and also provides up-to-date inventory information without requiring employees to count supplies.

Manual Inventory Systems

Several manual systems can also be used to identify supplies that need to be ordered. The following are some of the more common methods used in medical facilities:

- When staff identifies a product that needs to be ordered, the item is written in a log. This process is like making a list of what you need at the grocery store. The person responsible for ordering supplies then prepares the order based on the information in the log.
- Another system includes using product identification slips, which contain the name of the product. The slips or cards are attached to the product or a box/package of items. When the product is used, the slip is put in a special location, such as a box or plastic pocket. The medical assistant uses the slips in the box or pocket to prepare the supply order.
- The two-bin system consists of having a main bin for each item in inventory and then a backup bin for each item. When the main bin is emptied, the backup bin is used, and the product is reordered.
- The medical assistant responsible for ordering performs a hand count of the items in stock to identify what needs to be ordered. This system is explained in the next section.

CRITICAL THINKING APPLICATION 11.6

Marie decides to implement a manual system for inventory. Of the manual systems discussed, which method might work best in the small facility? Discuss your answer.

Taking Inventory

Inventory (counting supplies) must be taken at specific times. Many businesses that use automated inventory control systems hand count their inventory at least once a year. Usually, this is done around the close of the business year. These companies compare their hand counts to the computer counts and identify **discrepancies.** The discrepancies are followed up on. The manual inventory procedure provides the company with information on the actual number of items in stock. With this information, the financial value of the inventory can be calculated and used for financial reports and taxes at the close of the business year.

Some ambulatory care facilities do not use inventory control systems. These facilities must perform inventory or count the items in stock before each buying cycle. This identifies what products need to be ordered.

One of the most frequent errors when performing inventory is to report a different quantity than what is on the supply inventory list. For instance, a medical assistant counts nonsterile sponges. Each package should be counted as 1 and not as 100 each. For example, in Figure 11.4, if there were 6 packages of nonsterile gauze sponges left in the supply cabinet, it should be noted that the stock available

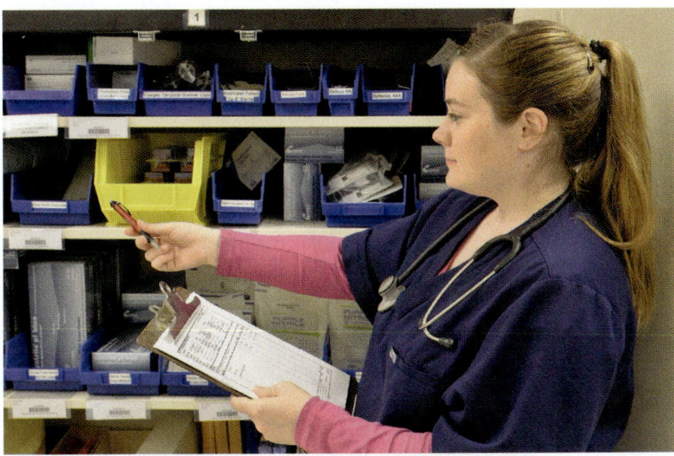

FIGURE 11.6 A medical assistant performing an inventory.

was 6 packages. It should not be indicated as 600 sponges or 600 each. Counting each item in a box or package when the product is inventoried by box or package creates conflict and confusion when looking at the reorder point.

The medical assistant should use a supply inventory list to be most efficient when counting supplies (Figure 11.6). The supply inventory list shows all the items in stock. The medical assistant can mark down the inventory counts for each item on the document (Procedure 11.3). If the supply inventory list is not available, the medical assistant needs to write down the item number, size, quantity (e.g., 100/box), manufacturer, and any other identifying information. This process takes a lot more time. Using abbreviations can be helpful:

- BTL: Bottle
- BX: Box
- CS: Case
- EA: Each
- PKG: Package
- QTY: Quantity

When you perform an inventory, work in a systematic manner. Start with one supply cabinet, working from top to bottom, before moving to another cabinet. All stock areas should be inventoried before the supply order is prepared.

ORDERING PROCESS

In larger ambulatory care facilities, employees are hired to manage the ordering and receiving duties. In smaller facilities, the medical assistant may be responsible for placing orders and reviewing orders that are received.

Price Considerations When Ordering Supplies

When you order supplies, price comparison shopping is important. The healthcare facility must balance the time it takes to get the needed supplies against the money saved when buying from various companies. Some medical offices compare prices only on more expensive items or items that are used in vast quantities. They may compare prices every 6 to 12 months. When you compare prices, consider the following factors:

- Shipping and handling charges.
- Quantity and amount (e.g., 10 per box), these must be the same among products.
- Quantity discounts or price breaks for buying a certain amount. Quantity discounts or price breaks save money. The more of an item purchased when you order, the cheaper the product becomes, as this example shows:
  - Quantity 1 to 5, $1.50 per item
  - Quantity 6 to 15, $1.25 per item

If the medical assistant purchased a quantity of 6, the price for each would be cheaper than if 4 were purchased. Before ordering extra product, consider the storage space available, how quickly the item will be used, and the shelf life or expiration date of the item. Buying too much just to get a price break may not be in the best interest of the healthcare facility.

Group Purchasing Organizations

Some medical facilities join group purchasing organizations (GPOs). These organizations combine orders from many different medical facilities. Combining orders results in volume discounts from specific **vendors.** GPOs typically purchase both supplies and medications. Physician buying groups (PBGs) offer providers potential cost-saving pricing for vaccines. The drawback is that the provider must exclusively use the vaccines from the contracted manufacturers.

CRITICAL THINKING APPLICATION 11.7

Currently, the facility orders its clinical supplies from two vendors. Marie would like to do some cost comparisons to get the best deals on supplies. She does not have a lot of time to spend on the research. How might Marie approach this situation? Where should she start? What might be a long-term goal for her?

Ordering Supplies

If the facility is not part of a buying group, the medical assistant might need to order supplies. It is important to select just a few vendors if possible. The medical assistant can use the following sources:

- The supplier's printed catalog, though it may only be printed a few times a year and may not provide accurate item availability and pricing
- The supplier's website store, which would have the most accurate prices, sale prices, and available stock

Creating an Account

Many vendors require the creation of an account before ordering. When creating an account for purchasing supplies, you should use the facility's information (address, fax number, and phone number). Be prepared to give the provider's license number when ordering medications and needles. The medical assistant may need to fax the provider's license number, if required, before ordering. If narcotics are ordered, the company will need a copy of the provider's Drug Enforcement Administration (DEA) registration. Narcotics require special tracking documentation and thus a high level of authorization when they are purchased.

Using Purchase Order Numbers

Some medical facilities use **purchase order (PO) numbers,** giving each order a unique reference number. This PO number should be included on the order sheets, added to the online information, or provided during the phone order. Vendors add the PO number to the order's documentation (i.e., **packing slip** and statement). This way, both parties can use it as a reference if questions come up. The healthcare facility uses the purchase order number to track the order.

Payment

Payment (PYMT) terms may vary among vendors. Payment methods may include credit card, check, money order, or a line of credit. Typically, the *line of credit* (preset borrowing limit) is good for 30 to 60 days. **Invoices** or billing statements are sent to the facility and should be paid after the purchases have been received. Orders can typically be placed via fax, mail, phone, or online. If the medical assistant is faxing or mailing the order, the vendor usually requires the order to be placed on the vendor's order sheet. The medical assistant should keep a copy of the phoned-in, mailed, or faxed order or a printout of the online order to verify that the order was filled correctly.

RECEIVING ORDERS

Orders can arrive via the mail, a national delivery service (e.g., FedEx, United Parcel Service [UPS]), or a local delivery service. The delivery person may require a signature from an employee. This signature is used to track who received the delivery.

Checking Deliveries

The medical assistant must check the delivery as soon as possible. Some medications, such as vaccines, are shipped in a cold environment and must remain at a cold temperature. These medications need to be placed in the refrigerator or freezer immediately upon arrival. Storage information for medications can be found in the package insert or on the manufacturer's website. If the medication warms up too much, it may be adversely affected. For instance, vaccines that get too warm can have reduced potency. This means they may not protect patients against disease.

Using the Packing Slips

When an order arrives, the medical assistant will remove the packing slip from the box, compare the items in the package to the packing slip (Figure 11.7), and check off all items received. Some vendors may indicate items that are **back-ordered** and will be arriving later. Any discrepancies or differences should be noted on the packing slip. Any items that are damaged should be noted on the packing slip. The copy of the original order should be compared against the packing slip, and any differences should be noted. Any discrepancies or damaged items should be addressed with the supply company as soon as possible.

The packing slip should be attached to the copy of the order once the supplies have been reviewed. When the complete order has been received, the copy of the order with the packing slips attached should be filed if the order was prepaid. If a line of credit was used, the copy of the order with the attached packing slips is placed in the **accounts payable** folder to wait for the invoice's arrival. The person responsible for paying the healthcare facility's bills will match the invoice with the copy of the order, ensuring everything was received before paying the bill.

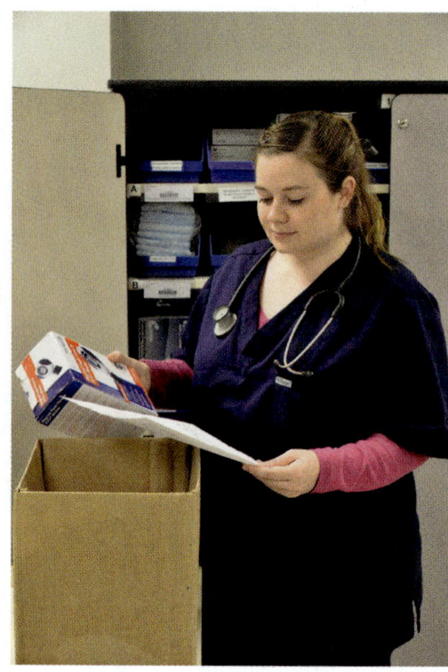

FIGURE 11.7 Comparing the packing slip to the contents in the box is an important step in receiving supplies.

Rotating Stock

The items received should be put away as soon as possible, and the boxes should be discarded. When you are putting supplies away, it is important to rotate stock. This means the new stock should go in the back, and the older stock needs to be moved forward so it can be used first. Any items with expiration dates should be placed in front with the items expiring first, so they are used first. For stock without expiration dates, consider the saying "first in, first out" (FIFO), which means when new stock comes in, it is placed behind the older stock. The older stock needs to be used first. If you are removing expired stock, remember to subtract the quantity from the inventory system.

VACCINE STORAGE REQUIREMENTS

For ambulatory care departments that administer vaccines, the Centers for Disease Control and Prevention (CDC) recommends having one person be the vaccine coordinator. The vaccine coordinator must ensure that all vaccines are stored and handled correctly. Here are some of the vaccine coordinator's duties:

- Maintaining vaccine inventory information and ordering vaccines
- Overseeing proper storage of the vaccine deliveries
- Managing and monitoring vaccine supplies, including checking expiration dates and rotating stock
- Ensuring the temperature of the refrigerator and freezer are within the normal range

Storing Vaccines

When vaccine deliveries arrive, they need to be unpacked immediately. Per the CDC:

- Each type of vaccine should be placed in its own tray; allow space between the vials to promote air circulation. Place newer vaccines behind older vaccines.
- Keep vaccine vials in their original boxes to prevent light exposure. If possible, store **diluents** with the corresponding vaccines. Never store diluents in the freezer.

- Store vaccines with similar packaging or names on different shelves to prevent mix-ups.
- Follow these practices for frozen and refrigerated vaccines:
  - Maintain refrigerator temperatures between 36°F to 46°F. The freezer should maintain temperatures between −58°F to 5°F.
  - Position vaccines and diluents 2 to 3 inches from the walls, ceiling, and floor. When using household-grade refrigerators, do not store vaccines directly under cooling vents, in drawers, or on the door shelves.
  - Do not put food or beverages in the vaccine storage refrigerator and freezer.
  - When using a household-grade refrigerator, place bottles of water on the top shelf, the floor, and the door shelves to maintain the temperature.
  - Make sure the door is closed.
  - Post a DO NOT UNPLUG warning sign on the unit and near the outlet. If possible, the unit should be connected to electrical outlets that can also be powered by backup generators.

Temperature Monitoring Equipment

The CDC recommends temperature monitoring equipment (digital data loggers [DDLs]) for all vaccine storage units. All vaccine storage units (e.g., refrigerators, freezers, transport containers) must have a temperature monitoring device (TMD). The TMD should be placed in the center of the unit, with vaccines surrounding it. Simple thermometers can show the minimum and maximum temperatures since the last reset. A DDL records a temperature at least every 30 minutes and provides the most accurate storage temperatures. The CDC recommends keeping the digital data from the DDLs for 3 years. This information may need to show compliance when the facility is involved with vaccination programs.

Temperature Monitoring Logs

The temperature of the refrigerator and freezer should be checked at the start of each workday. If a TMD is used that does not record the minimum and maximum temperature, then the CDC recommends checking the temperature at the end of the workday. Reset the thermometer if required. The temperature-monitoring log sheet needs to be completed with each temperature check (Figure 11.8). This information should be recorded:

- Date and time
- Current temperature or the maximum and minimum temperature record on the device
- Any action taken if the temperature is out of range (too high or too long)
- Name or initials of person who checked and recorded the temperature

If a temperature check was missed, leave a blank entry in the log. If the temperature is out of range, the medical assistant should notify the vaccine coordinator and the supervisor. The vaccines should be labeled DO NOT USE and placed in a separate container. The vaccine coordinator or supervisor will need to contact the immunization program or vaccine manufacturer for guidance.

CRITICAL THINKING APPLICATION 11.8

Using Figure 11.8, the temperature monitoring log, answer the following questions:

- Did all the refrigerator temperatures fall within the required range? Explain.
- Did all the freezer temperatures fall within the required range? Explain.
- If a temperature was outside the required range, what should be done?
- Were the temperatures checked twice daily?

PERSONAL SAFETY AND BODY MECHANICS

The remaining sections of this chapter focus on personal and environmental safety topics in the workplace. The provisions of the Occupational Safety and Health Act (OSH Act) of 1970 are enforced by the Occupational Safety and Health Administration (OSHA). The act requires that employers provide a workplace that is free from seriously recognized hazards. Employers must comply with OSH Act standards.

Back Injuries in Healthcare

In the healthcare environment, most injuries are sprains, strains, and tears. Back injuries are one of the most common injuries. They can result from microtrauma related to repetitive activity over time or from one traumatic experience. Back injuries have several causes:

- Improper lifting or lifting items too heavy for the back to support
- Reaching, twisting, or bending when lifting
- Bad body mechanics when lifting, pushing, pulling, or carrying items
- Poor footing or constrained posture

		Refrigerator Temperature			Freezer Temperature			
Date	Time	Max	Min	Current	Max	Min	Current	Initials
10/11/xx	0750	40°F	37°F	39°F	3°F	−13°F	−12°F	MVB
10/11/xx	1722	38°F	35°F	38°F	−8°F	−28°F	−19°F	BMN
10/12/xx	0752	42°F	36°F	39°F	−13°F	−23°F	−18°F	MVB
10/13/xx	0748	47°F	38°F	38°F	−8°F	−27°F	−22°F	MVB

FIGURE 11.8 Example of a temperature log.

Principles of Proper Body Mechanics

Proper body mechanics entails using the appropriate muscles and body movements to maintain correct posture and body alignment. Proper body mechanics will increase coordination and endurance. The risk of strain and injury to the body decreases. Medical assistants need to protect themselves from bodily harm while lifting, reaching, and carrying heavy objects. These are principles of proper body mechanics:

- To lift an object, maintain a wide, stable base with your feet. Your feet should be shoulder-width apart, and you should have good footing.
- Bend at the knees, keeping your back straight. Lift smoothly, using the major muscles in your arms and legs (Figure 11.9). Use the same technique when putting the item down. Bending over to lift or set down a heavy object increases your risk of injury.
- When lifting and carrying heavy items, keep the item directly in front of you to avoid rotating your spine. Carry the item close to your body (Figure 11.10).
- Keep your movements smooth. Jerky or uncoordinated movements increase the risk for injury.
- When you reach for an object, your feet should face the object. Twisting or turning with a heavy load can cause injury.
- Avoid reaching and straining to get an object. Clear away barriers and use a firm and level surface (e.g., a step stool) to get close to the object. Avoid standing on tiptoes.
- Get help if the item is too heavy to lift by yourself.
- Store heavy objects at waist level or below.

Using proper body mechanics is important to prevent injuries. (See Procedure 11.3, which explains how to use correct body mechanics when performing a supply inventory.)

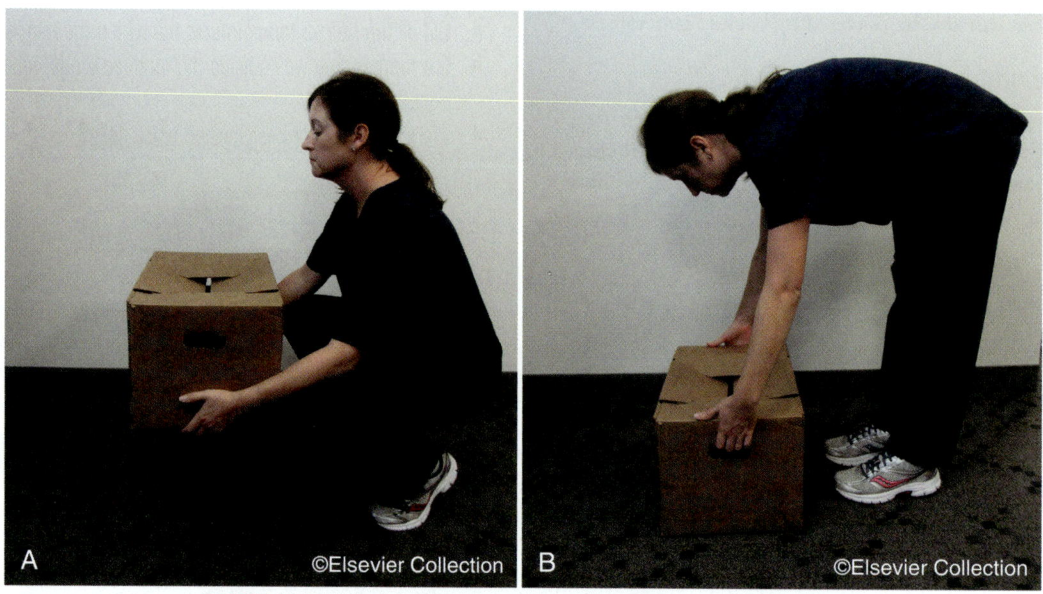

FIGURE 11.9 **(A)** Bend the knees for proper lifting technique. **(B)** Improper lifting technique.

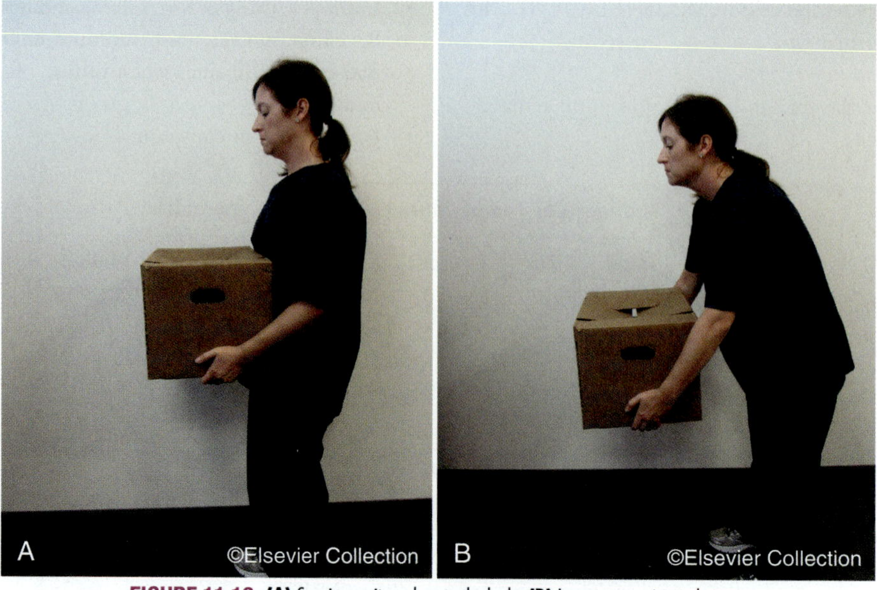

FIGURE 11.10 **(A)** Carrying an item close to the body. **(B)** Improper carrying technique.

PROVIDING A SAFE ENVIRONMENT

Security and safety are important to the well-being of the ambulatory care staff, patients, and visitors. The healthcare facility can draw unwanted attention from those seeking drugs and money. Having plans in place that can be implemented when security is in question is critical for all.

Decreasing the Risk of Theft

Ambulatory care facilities can be a target for those wanting to steal money, narcotic medications, and prescription pads. The staff should implement measures to limit the amount of money available in the building. Cash and checks from patients should be deposited daily to limit the quantities of money in the facility. Cash drawers should be stored out of the sight of patients and visitors. As mentioned earlier, prescription pads should remain out of the view and reach of patients. Narcotic medications, if present in the healthcare facility, should always be in a double-locked cabinet with the keys hidden. Depending on the type of clinic, some will post signs stating there are no narcotic medications on site.

Keeping Safe at Work

Many facilities have chosen to keep the employee entrance doors locked during business hours. The doors require either a key card or a unique code to enter the building. In high-crime areas, low-staffed clinics, or rural clinics, the doors to the patient care areas are also locked. This prevents the unauthorized entry of people to the patient care areas in the back, thereby increasing security. Follow these tips to stay safe:

- Stay alert for suspicious people.
- Listen to your instincts if a situation or person makes you feel strange or on edge.
- Try to alert another employee if a situation occurs. Many agencies have code words for those emergency situations.
- Use emergency alarms when needed. Many will notify the local police department.
- Keep yourself at a distance from the person (e.g., try to separate yourself from the person by a desk or another piece of furniture).
- Position yourself, so you are the closest to the door.
- Discuss the situation with the provider or supervisor if you are uncomfortable rooming a patient.
- Follow the facility's safety procedures.

CRITICAL THINKING APPLICATION **11.9**

Over the past 6 months, crime and break-ins have increased in the local area around the clinic. Many people believe the healthcare facility has a supply of narcotic medication in stock, which is not true. What strategies can the staff implement to increase the security of the healthcare facility?

Violence in Healthcare

Stories of workplace violence are becoming more common. Healthcare employees face an increased risk of work-related assaults, primarily from patients and visitors. In the *Guidelines for Preventing Workplace Violence for Healthcare and Social Service Workers*, published by OSHA (available at www.osha.gov/Publications/osha3148.pdf), increased risk factors for violence in healthcare include the following:

- Working with patients or family members who have a history of violence, abuse alcohol or other substances, are gang members, or carry firearms or other weapons
- Poorly designed work environments, including inadequately lit hallways, rooms, parking lots, and other areas, which can limit vision of potential situations and interfere with escape plans
- Lack of emergency communication (e.g., alarms, healthcare facility's emergency procedures) and training of employees
- Working in neighborhoods with high crime rates
- High employee turnover
- Long waits for patients in overcrowded, uncomfortable reception areas
- Unrestricted areas, allowing public access to the major areas of the building
- A perception that violence is tolerated and the police will not be called

Violence Prevention Strategies

OSHA encourages healthcare employees to take "universal precautions for violence." This means that ambulatory care facilities should be prepared for violent situations. Violence can be avoided or lessened by respecting others, protecting the dignity of others, and using teamwork to prevent violence. Medical assistants should report patient incidents or at-risk patient behaviors and situations to the manager.

Ambulatory care facilities should have violence prevention programs in place. Management and employees should work together to identify hazards and plan preventive strategies. According to OSHA, a number of strategies can be applied to secure the workplace environment:

- Physical barriers (e.g., locked doors, enclosures, bullet-proof windows, security guards)
- Bright, effective lighting and accessible exits
- Closed-circuit video (inside and outside of the building)
- **De-escalating** areas for patients and visitors
- Secure work areas for those working alone; panic buttons
- Name badges to identify employees

All employees should be trained to handle workplace violence and facility lockdown procedures. Lockdown is used when it is safer to stay where you are. This procedure is used when there is a dangerous person in the building or area:

- Lock or barricade the doors. If the person is in the area, lock windows and pull shades.
- Keep away from the windows and doors.
- If the person is in the building, silence cell phones. Contact 911 immediately and hide in a locked room.

EVALUATING THE WORK ENVIRONMENT

It is important to safeguard both the patients and the employees from injuries in the healthcare facility. The medical assistant should continually evaluate the environment for safety. From a flipped-over rug to a burned-out light in the stairway, safety risks can lead to falls and injuries. This section explains how to evaluate the work environment for unsafe working conditions. When problems are fixed or corrected, the environment becomes safer for all. Remember that for all injuries that occur to patients, visitors, and employees, an incident report form must be completed. Incident report forms are discussed in Chapter 4.

Preventing Falls and Injuries

Accidents can be expensive for the healthcare facility because costs can range from loss of employee workdays to lawsuits. Preventing accidents is therefore critical. In the healthcare facility, there are many areas that can be prone to causing slips, trips, and falls. In the winter months, depending on the facility's geographic location, slips and falls can be common because of snow and ice. The healthcare facility should have employees who oversee the sidewalks for patients and visitors.

Inside the facility, a number of high-risk situations can result in accidents:

- *Water or trash on floors*: Standing water on floors should be cleaned up. Signage should be used to indicate wet floors. Paper wrappings, covers, and other items should not be tossed on the floor during procedures due to an increased risk of injury.
- *Dim lighting*: Burned-out lightbulbs should be replaced. All stairwells should have adequate lighting.
- *Flooring and rugs*: Rugs and mats need to be smooth and flat. Flooring that is old and pulling up needs to be replaced. Carpeting with holes can catch a shoe heel, causing the person to trip and fall.
- *Cords, cables, and other objects in walkways*: Electrical cords, computer cables, boxes, and other potential tripping hazards should never be in the walkway. Hallways and **fire doors** need to be clear of debris. Unused wheelchairs and walkers should be collapsed, if possible, and moved out of the way.
- *Heavy objects placed on high shelves*: These items can fall and injure someone. Reaching for a heavy object can also cause injury. Store heavier items on lower shelves so they do not have to be lifted higher than necessary.
- *Using unsafe objects to stand on*: A chair or box could collapse or move when a person stands on it. Use a stable step stool to reach for things.

Preventing Electrical Issues and Fires

Malfunctioning equipment can also cause accidents. Any equipment that is not functioning or does not sound normal should not be used until it can be serviced and checked out. The medical assistant should follow the facility's procedure in this situation. Usually, the supervisor is notified if equipment is malfunctioning.

The medical assistant can help prevent injuries and fires in many ways:

- Checking electrical cords and plugs for cracks, fraying, or other damage
- Ensuring power strips are not overloaded
- Not using electricity near water
- Turning off equipment that appears to be overheating or malfunctioning
- Storing potentially flammable chemicals and supplies according to the manufacturers' guidelines
- Keeping combustibles (e.g., paper, cardboard, cloth, flammable chemicals) away from heat sources

Many fires are started by smoking materials. It is important to have adequate No Smoking signs at the facility's doors. Deep, non-tip ashtrays should be outside the doors so visitors have an adequate place to dispose of smoking materials.

Cautery equipment and lasers are commonly used in healthcare. Cautery equipment, by design, gets hot. Inappropriate use can cause fires. Lasers can cause health issues (e.g., burns and blindness) and fires. All staff members using or assisting with lasers should take a safety class. Signage should be on the door where the laser is being used. Water should be available if needed. Oxygen, other gases, and combustible chemicals should not be in the room when laser equipment is used.

Procedure 11.4 describes how to evaluate the environment for unsafe working conditions. Remember that when issues are found, it is important to fix them. If you cannot fix the unsafe condition, let your supervisor know immediately. Delays can increase the risk of others being injured.

EMERGENCY RESPONSE PLAN

A variety of emergency situations can occur and affect the healthcare facility. Each facility should have a plan to respond to these types of situations. An emergency response plan addresses possible **workplace emergencies.** This document guides the staff on handling emergencies and may protect the business. The occurrence of natural disasters may vary around the country. The emergency response plan should cover only potential emergencies seen at the facility and in the community (Table 11.1). Table 11.2 provides the critical elements that, at the minimum, must be included in the emergency response plan.

Having a plan is the first step. The employer also needs to train new staff on the procedures. Yearly refresher courses and mock drills help employees remain current on these procedures. The employer should document employee participation in the training sessions.

Evacuation Procedures

Evacuation procedures involve identifying exit routes and implementing procedures for moving employees, patients, and visitors to safe locations. Floor maps with evacuation exit routes and emergency equipment locations should be posted throughout the facility

TABLE 11.1 Potential Emergencies

EVENT	TYPE	EXAMPLES
Natural	Geologic hazards	Tsunami, volcano, landslide, and earthquake
	Meteorologic hazards	Flood, tornado, hurricane, and ice
	Biological hazards	Foodborne illnesses and communicable disease
Human caused	Accidental events	Hazardous spill, fire, and transportation incident (aircraft, vehicle)
	Intentional events	Robbery, lost person, bomb threat, terrorism, and weapons
	Technology-caused events	Telecommunication, electrical power, water, and cyber security issues

TABLE 11.2 Critical Elements of an Emergency Response Plan

CRITICAL ELEMENTS	INCLUDES
Methods to report a fire and other emergencies	• How to alert employees of the emergency (e.g., alarms, overhead paging system) • How to alert law enforcement and the fire department
Evacuation policy and procedure	• Evacuation conditions • Clear chain of command and designated person to order the evacuation and to account for employees (may be called an *evacuation warden*) • Patient sign-in sheets or schedules that are used to account for patients • Evacuation procedures, including routes and meeting locations; maps should be posted
Critical shutdown procedures	• Names of specific employees who must perform certain procedures before leaving • Critical shutdown procedures (describe what needs to be done); examples include turning off the water, gas, electricity, and oxygen (if piped into the exam rooms)
Emergency escape/exit routes and procedures	• Floor plan, workplace map, safe areas, and procedures
Rescue and medical duties	• Names of workers who need to perform rescue and medical duties.
Who to contact for additional information	• Names, titles, and contact information of internal and external people who can provide additional information on emergency response plans (internal people would be management and other employees; external people might be community leaders and specialists)

From How to Plan for Workplace Emergencies and Evacuations, www.osha.gov/Publications/osha3088.html.

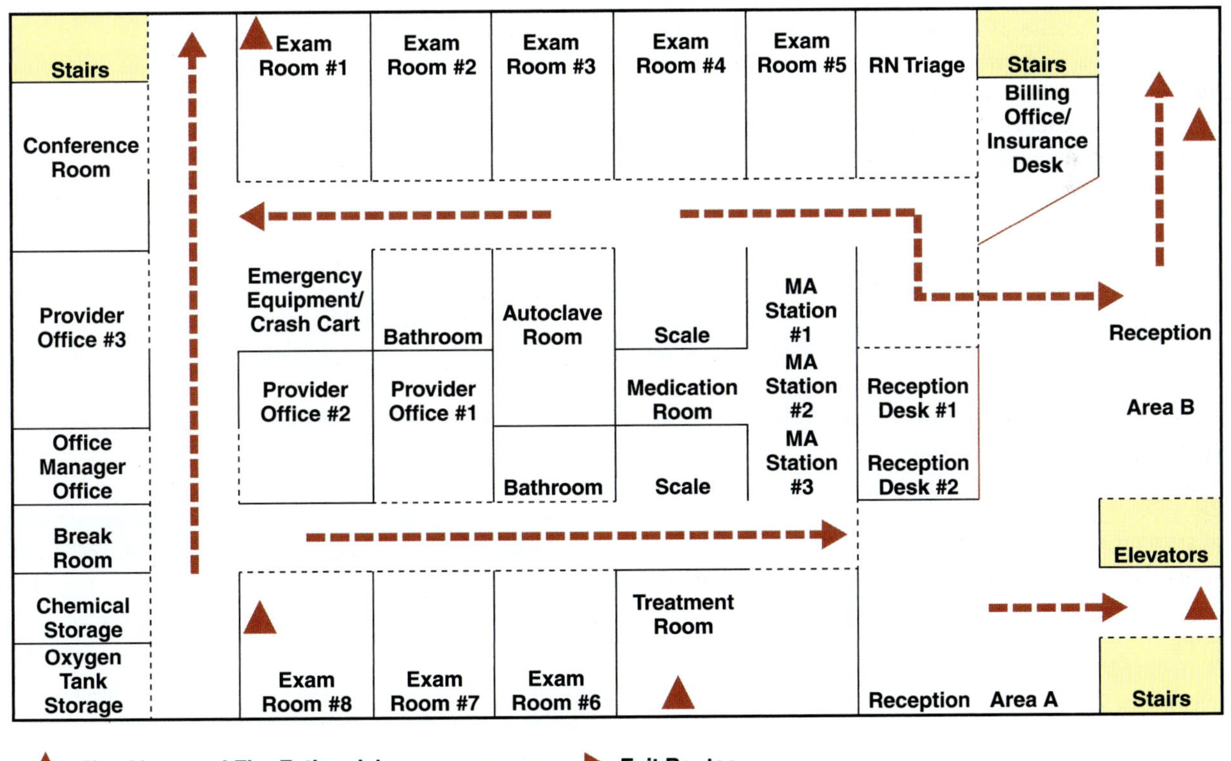

FIGURE 11.11 A floor map with exit routes and emergency equipment indicated.

(Figure 11.11). It is recommended that at least two routes should be identified, which provide a backup route if the primary route is blocked. Exit routes must follow these conventions:

- Be clearly marked and well lit
- Be wide enough to accommodate several people
- Not pass areas where flammable products (e.g., oxygen tanks, chemicals) are stored
- Be clear of debris and obstructions at all times

Evacuation Priorities

Some employees must assist those who need help evacuating. According to the Americans with Disabilities Act (ADA), safety requirements are needed for people in multistory buildings who need access to wheelchairs. Areas of rescue assistance are safe places where people in wheelchairs or those who cannot do stairs can await help in emergency situations. Typically, these areas are stairwells with alarms that communicate with emergency personnel. Evacuation chairs can be used to move people down the stairs.

Evacuation is done by priority, either by location or by people. The evacuation priority by location follows this order:

- People in immediate danger
- People located on the floor where the emergency is occurring
- People on the floors immediately above and below the floor with the situation
- People on the rest of the floors

Evacuation priority by people means the people nearest the emergency leave first, followed by the ambulatory people, and last, the nonambulatory people. As people evacuate by priority, it is important that appointed staff remain behind to verify that everyone is out. All rooms, including restrooms, need to be checked.

Types of Evacuations

Evacuation procedures vary based on the emergency (Procedure 11.5). There are five types of evacuations:

- *Shelter-in-place evacuation*: Evacuation to an interior room with no windows. In the case of tornados and other severe storms, employees, patients, and visitors should evacuate to shelter-in-place locations. Typically, these locations should be on the lowest level possible. Shelter-in-place locations are also used when a contaminant (e.g., chemical) is released into the environment.
- *Local evacuation*: Involves moving one or more people out of immediate danger (e.g., evacuating a patient from an exam room where a chemical spill occurred).
- *Horizontal evacuation*: Involves evacuating people from the same floor as the emergency situation.
- *Vertical evacuation*: Involves evacuating people located on the floors above and below the situation.
- *Building evacuation*: Involves evacuating everyone from the building to a safe location outside the building.

Fire Response

A medical assistant should be aware of the healthcare facility's fire response procedures. It is important to know how to activate the alarms, evacuate people, and use a fire extinguisher for small fires. The following are fire response actions:

- A wall-mounted fire extinguisher, manual pull station (alarm), warning alarms, smoke alarms, and automatic sprinkler systems should be located throughout the facility per state code. An employee should be assigned to routinely check this equipment and replace it as needed (Box 11.2).
- If you smell smoke or suspect a fire, think of the acronym RACE:
  - **R**escue individuals threatened by the fire.
  - **A**ctivate the alarm if you discover the fire or respond if you hear the alarm.
  - **C**onfine the fire by closing doors and fire doors to slow the spread of the fire.
  - **E**xtinguish only small fires; otherwise, evacuate individuals from the area.
- Do not use elevators if a fire is suspected. This will reduce the risk of entrapment.
- If a fire is suspected, immediately disconnect oxygen supplies or turn off oxygen tanks to prevent an explosion.
- Use the correct type of extinguisher for the fire (Table 11.3).
- For small fires, use the PASS procedure as you operate a fire extinguisher (Procedure 11.6).
  - **P**ull the pin.
  - **A**im the nozzle or hose at the base of the fire.
  - **S**queeze the handle to release the extinguishing agent.
  - **S**weep the nozzle or hose from side to side at the base of the fire until the fire is out. Evacuate if you are not successful or doubt your ability to put out the fire.

TABLE 11.3 Uses of Fire Extinguishers

LABELED CLASS	USED FOR
A	Water extinguisher: Used on *ordinary combustibles* (e.g., paper, wood, rubber, cloth, and many plastics)
B	Carbon dioxide (CO_2) extinguisher: Used on flammable liquids; fires in oils and grease
C	Dry chemical extinguisher: Used on electrical equipment; fires in wiring, fuse boxes, computers, and other electrical sources
ABC	Multipurpose dry chemical extinguisher. Used on ordinary combustibles, flammable liquids, or electrical equipment
D	Fires involving combustible metals: May be found in the medical laboratory
K	Fires involving combustible cooking oils and fats: Found in the kitchen

New Fire Extinguisher Technology

A new type of fire extinguisher, the Eliminator, has changed the way fire extinguishers are used (Figure 11.12A). This new fire extinguisher has an ergonomically designed handle and spray hose. Most fire extinguishers need to be serviced and maintained to keep them operable. This extinguisher allows facilities to maintain it more easily and cheaply than other extinguishers. When using the Eliminator, a person must follow the "TPASS" procedure (Figure 11.12B):

T: Twist the lock to break the seal.
P: Push the level down. This will pressurize the extinguisher.
A: Aim the valve nozzle at the base of the fire.
S: Squeeze the valve level.
S: Sweep the valve nozzle from side to side to put out the fire.

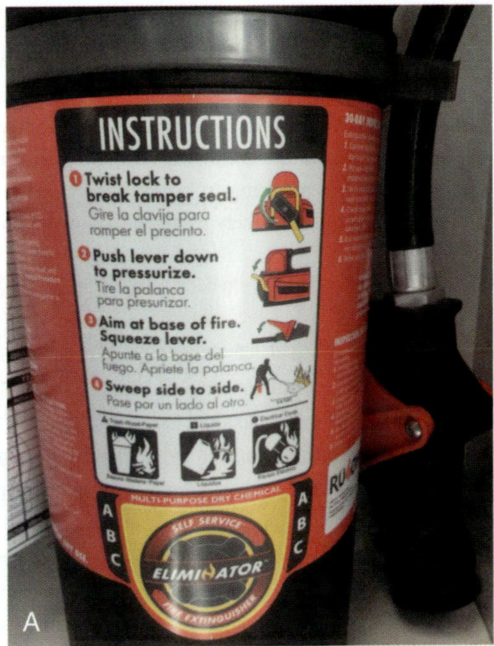

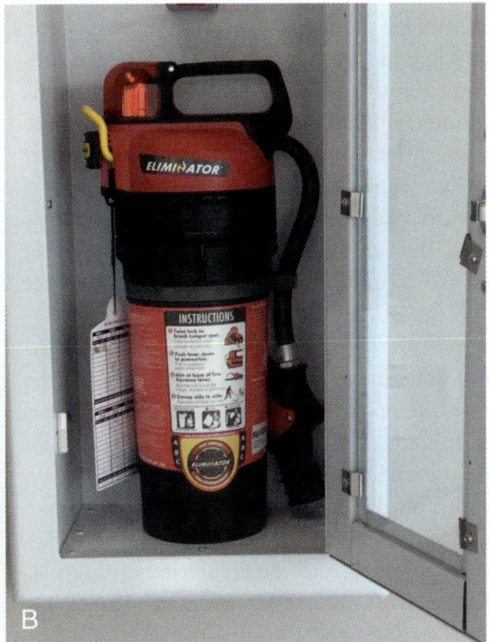

FIGURE 11.12 **(A)** The Eliminator is a new type of fire extinguisher. **(B)** Users must follow the "TPASS" procedure when using the Eliminator.

CRITICAL THINKING APPLICATION 11.10

One morning when the weather is stormy, Marie and Catherine are discussing the facility's emergency policy and procedures. How would you respond to a tornado warning and the need to evacuate to a shelter-in-place location? How would you respond if you found a wastebasket on fire in the facility?

EFFECTS OF STRESS

Stress is a person's total response to environmental demands or pressures. We have many stressors that cause stress in our lives. A *stressor* is a stimulus that provokes a stress response. It is natural to feel stressed during traumatic events or emergency situations.

Symptoms of Stress

When a person is involved in an emergency, this can cause a number of physical and emotional signs and symptoms:

- Shock, disbelief, irritability, crying, and anger
- Feelings of fear, anxiety, numbness, sadness, worry, powerlessness, or frustration
- Difficulty making decisions and trouble concentrating
- High blood pressure, high blood glucose levels
- Changes in appetite, energy, desires, and interest in normal activities
- Nightmares, sleep problems, and tension
- Headaches, body pain, stomach and intestinal problems, skin rashes
- Worsening of chronic health problems and mental health conditions
- Increase use of alcohol, tobacco, and other substances

General Adaptation Syndrome

General adaptation syndrome (GAS) is used to describe the long- and short-term effects of stress on the body. GAS was originally described by Hans Selye. He felt the syndrome affected the nervous and endocrine systems. This occurs in the following stages:

Stage 1. Alarm reaction: This is the immediate reaction to the stressor. The fight-or-flight response occurs. The body releases the hormones cortisol, adrenaline, and noradrenaline. This provides energy, preparing the body for physical activities. This stage can affect the immune system, causing the person to be more susceptible to illness.

Stage 2. Adaptation stage: If the stressor continues, the individual's body adapts to the stressor. During this stage, the body begins to repair itself, and the hormone levels gradually return to normal.

Stage 3. Exhaustion stage: At this point, the body's resistance has been diminished by the continued stress. The body is more susceptible to disease.

Healthy Coping Strategies

It is important to use healthy coping strategies to deal with stress:

- Eat healthy, well-balanced meals.
- Practice stress relievers, such as deep breathing, meditation, and stretching.
- Get adequate sleep.
- Exercise regularly.
- Avoid excessive alcohol, tobacco, and substance use.
- Talk to the support people in your life.

CLOSING COMMENTS

Patient Coaching

In the ambulatory healthcare environment, many types of supplies are available. A medical assistant may be tempted to give patients supplies to use at home for the ordered treatments, such as wound care. Many healthcare facilities do not allow this for a variety of reasons, including financial considerations. If supplies are given to patients, the low inventory may impact the care of other patients.

The medical assistant should coach the patient on what supplies are needed for the treatments prescribed. Making a list of supplies, along with specific details and where to purchase the items, is helpful for patients.

Legal and Ethical Issues

The medical assistant has important tasks when required to prepare and monitor the equipment in the healthcare facility. As mentioned in this chapter, quality control procedures are done on equipment to ensure the accuracy of test results. The medical assistant must accurately complete the quality control procedures and document the results daily or as indicated by the facility's policies and procedures. The lack of precision with quality control can lead to issues with the accuracy of test results that will impact patient care.

Besides quality control, the medical assistant is responsible for ensuring the medications that must remain cold or frozen are at the proper temperatures. This responsibility begins when the shipment of medications arrives. It is critical to open these packages very soon after delivery and place the medications in the refrigerator or freezer. The medical assistant is also responsible for monitoring to make sure the medications remain at the proper temperature. The refrigerator and freezer temperature log must be completed as directed. Any issues with the temperature must be addressed immediately. It is unethical for the medical assistant not to address the problem when medications become too warm. This can impact the quality of the medication and ultimately, the patient.

Patient-Centered Care

Safety is a concern for both patients and healthcare professionals. The medical assistant should be alert for potential situations that could turn violent. Treating patients and family members with respect, listening to their concerns, and following through with promises are especially important when working in healthcare. A person who feels respected and listened to is less likely to get angry to the point of violence.

Professional Behaviors

The medical assistant has many important duties to help the healthcare facility operate. From opening and closing the facility to managing inventory, these duties are important to the success of the facility. Paying attention to detail while performing these duties is important. Keeping the right amount of supplies in stock so providers can treat patients also requires paying attention to details.

The medical assistant also needs to be knowledgeable about the emergency policies and procedures of the healthcare facility. When an emergency occurs is not the time to read the procedure on what to do! As a medical assistant, it is important for you to be calm, cool, and composed during these times. This will help others around you to remain calm.

SUMMARY OF SCENARIO

Marie has started to implement an inventory management process that is helping her identify when to reorder and how much to reorder. Initially, she hand-counted the inventory, and then she identified how much was used in each buying cycle. It took a few months for her to identify trends. She found certain times of the year affected the quantity of products used. For instance, providers tend to use more casting products in the winter and summer months, which means Marie will need to increase her stock of those items during those times of the year. Marie knows that the more she learns, the more efficient she can become when managing inventory. She has already helped the facility save money by identifying cheaper vendors for commonly used expensive items. Marie loves her new job and the variety of responsibilities she has. She looks forward to continual learning.

SUMMARY OF LEARNING OBJECTIVES

1. **Examine the opening tasks for both the clinical and administrative medical assistants.**
   Facility opening tasks for the clinical medical assistant include preparing the exam room, ensuring the supplies are available, unlocking supplies cabinets, performing quality control tests, and completing the temperature logs for the refrigerator and freezer. Any outstanding patient issues for the prior day are completed.
   Opening tasks for the administrative medical assistant include checking the voice mail or answering service messages, updating the voice mail message, switching the phones, so patients reach ambulatory care, turning on the equipment, preparing the reception area for patients, and printing the schedule for the day.
2. **Examine the closing tasks for both the clinical and administrative medical assistants.**
   The clinical medical assistant must disinfect and restock the exam rooms, turn off the equipment, secure confidential documents, and lock cabinets. The administrative medical assistant must prepare the patient records and documents for the next day. The equipment must be turned off, and the phones must be switched to voice mail or the answering service. The reception area should be cleaned. Equipment and lights should be turned off.
3. **Examine equipment management, including inventory, maintenance and service calls, warranties, and purchasing.**
   An equipment inventory list should include the name, manufacturer, serial number, purchase date, cost, supplier, warranty information, location, and, if present, the unique facility number for that piece of equipment.
   The medical assistant is responsible for monitoring equipment safety and proper functioning. Routine maintenance helps to ensure the best performance of the equipment. Routine maintenance logs should be used to document the routine maintenance and service calls done on equipment.
   The process of purchasing equipment can vary depending on the size of the organization. Large agencies have purchasing departments, whereas the medical assistant may be involved with the process in smaller facilities.
4. **Examine supply inventory management, including inventory control systems and taking inventory.**
   Inventory management involves ordering, tracking inventory, and identifying the quantity of products to purchase. The goal of inventory manage-

SUMMARY OF LEARNING OBJECTIVES—*continued*

ment is to have adequate supplies on hand. If the medical assistant is responsible for inventory, then for each item, the name, size, quantity, item number, supplier's name, cost, quantity to reorder, and the reorder point should be documented on the supply inventory list.

An inventory control system helps to make inventory management work well. Types of inventory control systems include the barcode, weight-based, and manual systems.

When the medical assistant is completing an inventory, the supply inventory list should be used. The supplies are counted, and the count is documented on the supply inventory list. The supplies should be neatly replaced, with the older supplies in front. Procedure 11.1 discusses the steps involved with performing an equipment inventory with documentation.

5. **Examine the ordering process, including price considerations, opening an account, the purpose of the purchase order number, and payment procedures.**
When ordering supplies, price comparison is important. Group purchasing organizations can decrease the cost of supplies. To order supplies, the medical assistant can use the supplier's printed catalog or the supplier's website store. An account may need to be set up prior to ordering. Payment terms may vary among vendors.
6. **Examine how the medical assistant checks the delivered items and rotates stock.**
Orders can arrive via the mail, a national delivery service, or a local delivery service. The supplies should be checked against the packing slip to identify any discrepancies. The new stock should be placed behind the existing stock. Items expiring first should be in front of those expiring on a later date.
7. **Analyze the storage requirements for vaccines.**
When vaccine deliveries arrive, they need to be unpacked immediately. Each type of vaccine should be placed in its own tray, with space between the vials to promote air circulation. Vaccine vials are kept in their original boxes to prevent light exposure.

   For frozen and refrigerated vaccines, the refrigerators should maintain temperatures between 36°F to 46°F, and the freezer should maintain temperatures between −58°F to 5°F. Position vaccines and diluents 2 to 3 inches from the walls, ceiling, and floor. Temperature monitoring devices should be used, and the temperature should be logged daily.
8. **Demonstrate the use of proper body mechanics.**
The principles of proper body mechanics include the following:
   - To lift an object, maintain a wide, stable base with your feet. Your feet should be shoulder-width apart, and you should have good footing. Bend at the knees, keeping your back straight. Lift smoothly, using the major muscles in your arms and legs. Use the same technique when putting the item down.
   - When lifting and carrying heavy items, keep the item directly in front of you to avoid rotating your spine. Keep your movements smooth.
   - When reaching for an object, your feet should face the object. Avoid reaching and straining to get an object. Clear away barriers, and use a firm and level surface (e.g., a stepstool) to get close to the object.
   - Get help if the item is too heavy to lift by yourself.

   Procedure 11.3 discusses the steps involved when performing a supply inventory with documentation. This procedure also describes how to use proper body mechanics when performing inventory procedures.
9. **Analyze strategies to keep the work environment safe.**
Cash and checks received should be deposited daily to decrease the risk of theft. Prescription pads should remain out of view. Narcotic medications should always be in a double-locked cabinet.

   Follow these strategies to keep safe while working:
   - Stay alert for suspicious people. Listen to your instincts if a situation or person makes you feel strange or on edge.
   - Try to alert another employee if a situation occurs. Use emergency alarms when needed.
   - Keep yourself at a distance from the person. Position yourself, so you are the closest to the door.
   - Follow the facility's safety procedures.

   According to OSHA, strategies to secure the workplace environment include physical barriers, bright lighting, closed-circuit video, de-escalating areas, secure work areas, and name badges to identify employees.
10. **Demonstrate how to evaluate the work environment for potential safety issues.**
Preventing accidents is therefore critical. In the healthcare facility, there are many areas that can be prone to causing slips, trips, and falls. Inside the facility, high-risk situations for accidents include water or trash on the floor, dim lighting, flooring and rugs causing falls, and items (e.g., cords and cables) in the walkways.

    The medical assistant can help prevent injuries and fires by inspecting electrical cords, not overloading power strips, turning off malfunctioning equipment, keeping combustibles away from heat sources, and storing flammable products according to the manufacturer's guidelines.
11. **Examine emergency response plans, including the purpose and critical elements of the plans.**
An emergency response plan guides the staff in handling emergencies and may protect the business. Table 11.2 presents the critical elements that must be in an emergency response plan. These elements include the following:
    - Methods to report a fire and other emergencies
    - Evacuation policy and procedure
    - Critical shutdown procedures
    - Emergency escape/exit routes and procedures
    - Rescue and medical duties
    - Whom to contact for additional information

    Floor maps with evacuation exit routes and emergency equipment locations should be posted throughout the facility. Exit routes must be clearly marked, well lit, and free from debris. When evacuating, people in immediate danger are the highest priority, followed by people located on the same floor as the emergency. Then people above and below the floor with the emergency should be evacuated, followed by the people on the rest of the floors.

    If you smell smoke or suspect a fire, think of the acronym RACE. For small fires, use the PASS procedure as you operate a fire extinguisher (see Procedure 11.6).

Continued

SUMMARY OF LEARNING OBJECTIVES—*continued*

12. **Examine the effect of stress on the body, including the symptoms, effects, and healthy coping strategies.**
    Shock, disbelief, irritability, crying, anger, feelings of fear, anxiety, numbness, sadness, worry, powerlessness, and frustration are just some of the signs and symptoms of stress. The term *general adaptation syndrome (GAS)* is used to describe the long- and short-term effects of stress on the body. The stages include the following:
    - *Stage 1. Alarm reaction*: The body releases the hormones cortisol, adrenaline, and noradrenaline.
    - *Stage 2. Adaptation stage*: If the stressor continues, the individual's body adapts to the stressor.
    - *Stage 3. Exhaustion stage*: At this point, the body's resistance has been diminished by the continued stress.

    Healthy coping strategies are important to deal with the stress. These strategies include eating healthy, getting adequate sleep, and exercising regularly.

PROCEDURE 11.1 Perform an Equipment Inventory with Documentation

TASKS: Perform an equipment inventory. Document the inventory on the equipment inventory form.

EQUIPMENT and SUPPLIES

- Equipment inventory form
- Pens
- Administrative or clinical equipment
- Purchase information (e.g., date, cost, and supplier) and warranty information (e.g., start and end dates, warranty coverage)

PROCEDURAL STEPS

1. For the equipment to be inventoried, gather the following information for each piece of equipment:
   - Name of equipment, manufacturer, and serial number
   - Location and facility number (if applicable)
   - Purchase date, cost, supplier, and warranty information

   PURPOSE: It is important to have the essential information required when creating the spreadsheet.
2. Complete an equipment inventory form by adding the gathered information for each item inventoried (see Figure 11.2).
   PURPOSE: Creating an equipment inventory list on the computer will help you organize the information. It will also help you maintain the information easily.
3. Review the document created. Make any necessary revisions.
   PURPOSE: It is important to proofread your work to ensure it is accurate.

PROCEDURE 11.2 Perform Routine Maintenance of Equipment

TASKS: Perform routine maintenance of administrative or clinical equipment. Document the maintenance on the log.

EQUIPMENT and SUPPLIES

- Maintenance log(s)
- Pens
- Information regarding the equipment (i.e., name, serial number, location, facility number, manufacturer, purchase date, warranty information, frequency of inspections, and service provider)
- Administrative or clinical equipment (e.g., oral thermometers)
- Supplies for routine maintenance (e.g., battery)
- Users' guide or owner's manual, if needed

PROCEDURAL STEPS

1. Gather information on the piece of equipment identified for routine maintenance, including name, serial number, location, facility number, manufacturer, purchase date, warranty information, frequency of inspections, and service provider.
   PURPOSE: It is important to have the essential information required when completing the log.
2. Fill in the equipment details on the log (see Figure 11.3).
   PURPOSE: Adding the equipment details helps identify the machine. It provides a quick reference to useful information that the service provider might request. The form serves as a log for documenting the maintenance activities performed.
3. To perform the maintenance activities, gather the required supplies. If you are not familiar with the procedure or the required supplies, refer to the users' guide.
   PURPOSE: You need to be familiar with the supplies and the procedure before you start the maintenance.
4. Perform the maintenance activities as directed in the users' guide. Take any required safety precautions necessary to protect yourself and others.
   PURPOSE: Following the outlined procedure in the users' guide will help you successfully complete the maintenance without injuring yourself or others or damaging the machine.
5. Clean up the work area.
   PURPOSE: It is important to clean up after yourself.
6. Using a pen, document the date, time, and maintenance activity performed, and include your signature on the log.
   PURPOSE: The log, indicating the activities performed, will serve as a communication tool for future reference and services needed on that piece of equipment.

PROCEDURE 11.3 Perform a Supply Inventory with Documentation While Using Proper Body Mechanics

TASKS: Perform a supply inventory using correct body mechanics. Document the inventory on the supply inventory form.

EQUIPMENT and SUPPLIES

- Supply inventory form
- Pens
- Administrative or clinical supplies to be inventoried
- Purchase information (e.g., item number, cost, and supplier) for supplies in inventory
- Reorder point and quantity to reorder for each item in inventory

PROCEDURAL STEPS

1. For the supplies in inventory, gather the following information for each item:
   - Name, size, quantity (e.g., purchased individually, 100 per box)
   - Item number, supplier's name, cost
   - Reorder point and quantity to reorder

   PURPOSE: This information is required as you create the inventory form.
2. For each supply item, enter information on the inventory form. Make sure the appropriate entry is in the right location (see Figure 11.4). *Note:* The "Stock Available" column will be empty for now.
   PURPOSE: Creating a supply inventory list will help you organize the information and maintain the information easily.
3. Review the document. Make any necessary revisions.
   PURPOSE: Make sure the document is correct, so errors do not affect the inventory process.
4. Using the supply inventory list, inventory the supplies in the department. Identify how the supply should be counted (e.g., individually, by the box), and count the number of items in stock.
   PURPOSE: By identifying the correct quantity by which the item is inventoried, you will increase the accuracy of the inventory. When several individual items are included in one package, using only the word *each* can cause confusion when identifying what needs to be ordered.
5. Add the number in the appropriate row under the "Stock Available" header.
   PURPOSE: Making sure you add the number to the correct column and row will keep your inventory form accurate.
6. Compare the reorder point number to the stock available number. If the stock available number is at or below the reorder point, indicate that the item needs to be reordered by checking the appropriate column.
   PURPOSE: Identify the supplies that need to be ordered.
7. Make sure the supplies are neatly arranged. The older stock should be in front of the newer stock.
   PURPOSE: It is important to clean up your workspace. The oldest stock must be moved to the front to ensure it is used first.
8. Repeat steps 5 through 7 until all supplies are inventoried.
9. Use proper body mechanics when lifting and moving supplies by maintaining a wide, stable base with your feet. Your feet should be shoulder-width apart, and you should have good footing. Bend at the knees, keeping your back straight. Lift smoothly with the major muscles in your arms and legs. Use the same technique when putting the item down.
   PURPOSE: Correct body mechanics will reduce your risk for injury when carrying or lifting heavy objects. See Figures 11.9 and 11.10 for proper body mechanics when lifting boxes.
10. Use proper body mechanics when reaching for an object. Clear away barriers and use a step stool if needed. Your feet should face the object. Avoid twisting or turning with a heavy load.
    PURPOSE: Straining when reaching or standing on tiptoes can increase your risk for injury.

PROCEDURE 11.4 Evaluate the Work Environment

TASK: Evaluate the work environment and identify unsafe working conditions.

EQUIPMENT and SUPPLIES

- Work environment evaluation form
- Pen

PROCEDURAL STEPS

1. Observe the environment for slipping, tripping, or fall risks. Document your findings for the following questions:
   - Is the lighting appropriate? Are any lights burned out? Are any areas dim?
   - Are the flooring and carpeting ripped or pulled up? If rugs/mats are present, are they folded?
   - Is there water on the floor? Is signage present warning of the water?
   - Are items cluttering the hallway, making walking difficult?
   - Are cords, cables, and other items in the walkway?
   - Is trash on the floor?
   - Are heavy items on high shelves? Is a sturdy step stool available?

   PURPOSE: When the floor is cluttered or the flooring is damaged, the risk of falls increases.
2. Observe the environment for safety and security issues. Document your findings for the following questions:
   - Are rooms available that can be locked and used during workplace violence? Is there limited visibility from the hallway into the room?
   - Are there areas in the building with limited visibility?
   - If the building is accessible to the public, are there any safe zones or areas for staff?

PROCEDURE 11.4 Evaluate the Work Environment—*continued*

- Are the emergency call lights in the exam rooms and bathrooms functioning?
- Are the oxygen tanks (if available) checked per the facility's policy?

PURPOSE: Having a safe area in a building is important during a workplace violence situation.

3. Observe the environment for fire risks and electrical issues. Document your findings for the following questions:
   - Are electrical cords and plugs free from cracks, fraying, or other damage?
   - Are power strips overloaded?
   - Is electricity being used near a water source?
   - Are flammable chemicals and supplies stored according to manufacturers' guidelines?
   - Are combustibles (e.g., paper, cardboard, cloth, flammable chemicals) stored and kept away from heat sources?

   PURPOSE: The risk of fires increases when cords are damaged, or power strips are overloaded. Safe storage of chemicals is important to reduce the fire risk.
4. Observe the environment for fire containment and evacuation strategies. Document your findings for the following questions:
   - Are building diagrams posted on walls? Are exit routes indicated? Are two or more exit routes indicated on the map? Are fire alarms and fire extinguishers indicated?
   - Are exit routes uncluttered?
   - Are exit signs visible and lit?
   - Are fire doors unlocked and able to be closed in an emergency?
   - Are interior rooms available for severe storms?
   - Are smoke detectors located throughout the building? Are fire alarms available?
   - Are fire extinguishers available and checked routinely (per the facility's policy)?
   - Are flammable products (e.g., oxygen tanks, chemicals) stored along the exit routes?

   PURPOSE: Two or more exit routes should be available. Flammable products should not be stored in the location of the exit routes. Closed fire doors will help contain the fire.
5. Based on your observations, summarize your findings. If risks are present, create a list of issues that need to be addressed. Describe what needs to be done for each risk.

   PURPOSE: Creating a list of issues that need to be addressed is important in a professional setting.

PROCEDURE 11.5 Participate in a Mock Exposure Event

TASKS: Demonstrate self-awareness in an emergency situation. Participate in a mock exposure event and document specific steps taken. Recognize the physical and emotional effects on individuals involved in an emergency situation.

SCENARIO: You and Beth are in the autoclave room and two chemicals spill, creating toxic fumes. Beth is having trouble breathing. The following staff, patients, and visitors are present:

Rooms

1—Teen and his mother
2—Older woman in a wheelchair
3—Mother with three little children
4—Adult female
5—Empty
6—Older couple
7—Adult male
8—Empty
Procedure room—Empty

Staff and Reception Areas

Reception Area A—Four people waiting
Reception Area B—Five people waiting

Staff

Tim—In MA station 3
Rose—At the insurance desk
Dave and Patty—At the receptionist's desk
Julie Walden, MD—In provider office 1
Angela Perez, MD—In room 3
Jean Burke, NP—In room 7

DIRECTIONS: Using word processing software, write a paper and address the procedure steps. Use reliable internet resources to research the physical manifestations and emotional behaviors on persons involved in an emergency. Include your findings in the paper as indicated in the procedural steps. Use 1-inch margins, double spacing, and 12-point font. The length should be at least two pages.

EQUIPMENT and SUPPLIES:

- Paper
- Pen
- Floor map (see Figure 11.11)
- Computer with internet access

PROCEDURE 11.5 Participate in a Mock Exposure Event—*continued*

PROCEDURAL STEPS

1. Using the scenario, describe how you would handle the emergency exposure situation with Beth.
   - Identify four steps a medical assistant could take to demonstrate self-awareness while responding to this emergency situation.
   - Describe exposure control mechanisms or how you might limit the exposure to other people once you remove Beth from the room.

   PURPOSE: It is important to be self-aware of how you would respond in emergency situations. Exposure control mechanisms are ways to limit the exposure to other people. How might you contain the situation? How might you prevent others from being affected by the exposure?

   Scenario update: Dr. Walden instructs the staff to evacuate from the building. The outdoor-safe meeting location is at the back of the parking lot.
2. Document the steps to handle the exposure event and evacuation from the building.
   - Describe what each staff member and provider should do to help with the evacuation procedure and notify 911.
   - Describe the steps (evacuations) in the order they should occur.
   - Describe how the staff may ensure all individuals are out of the building.

   PURPOSE: It is important to know which individuals need to be evacuated first, second, and so on. Employees should work with individuals in their area unless they have an appointed duty. It is important to make sure all individuals are out of the building before the staff leaves the area.
3. Dr. Walden is in charge during the emergency. Describe what her responsibilities include.

   PURPOSE: The evacuation warden's name is listed in the emergency response plan. This person is in charge of the evacuation.
4. Dave took the patient registry. Describe why the patient registry is important.

   PURPOSE: The patient registry lists the patients who have checked in for appointments.

   Scenario update: Two weeks after the event, Beth confides that she is not doing well. She has recovered from the exposure, but since the event, she has had difficulty sleeping. She is anxious when she goes into the autoclave room. Beth is having trouble concentrating on her job. She mentions she has had two nightmares in which emergencies occur in the department, and she gets injured.
5. Do the following:
   - Describe what might be occurring with Beth and the symptoms that relate to it.
   - Discuss what you might encourage her to do about the situation.

   PURPOSE: It is not uncommon after an emergency that the individuals involved experience issues related to the emergency.
6. Research the physical manifestations and emotional behaviors on persons involved in an emergency. Identify four physical signs and four emotional behaviors of stress on persons involved in an emergency situation. Cite your resources.
7. Describe how the physical and emotional effects of stress would differ for Beth, you, the providers, and the other employees present.
8. Describe how a medical assistant could limit the physical and emotional effects of stress on each person/group: Beth, the providers, the other employees present in the facility, and yourself.

PROCEDURE 11.6 Use a Fire Extinguisher

TASKS: Select the correct fire extinguisher and demonstrate its use.

SCENARIOS:

a. You are working in the medical laboratory, and an electrical fire starts.
b. You are working in the clinic, and a fire starts in a wastebasket.
c. You are working in the medical laboratory, and a chemical fire starts (a combustible metal fire).

EQUIPMENT and SUPPLIES

- Fire extinguisher

PROCEDURAL STEPS

1. Using the scenario, identify the type of fire extinguisher required to put out the fire.

   PURPOSE: The correct fire extinguisher must be used to put out the fire. Using the wrong extinguisher can make the fire worse.
2. Hold the extinguisher by the handle with the hose or nozzle pointing away from you. Pull out the pin that is located below the trigger.

   PURPOSE: Pulling the pin allows the extinguisher to be used.
3. Stand about 10 feet from the fire. Aim the extinguisher hose or nozzle at the base of the fire. Keep the extinguisher in an upright position as you work.

   PURPOSE: The most efficient method of putting out fires is to work at the base of the fire.
4. Squeeze the trigger slowly and evenly.

   PURPOSE: Squeezing slowly allows the discharge to come out in a steady flow.
5. Sweep from side to side until the fire is out.

   PURPOSE: As the fire nearest to you is put out, you can move closer to the rest of the fire.

HEALTH INSURANCE ESSENTIALS 12

SCENARIO

Jon Bimmell, a registered medical assistant (RMA), has worked for Walden-Martin Family Medical (WMFM) Clinic for 3 years. Jon started with WMFM as a receptionist. Donna Potter, the office manager, recognized that Jon was very detail oriented, so 2 years ago, she asked him to take charge of the health insurance policies and procedures manual for the practice.

Jon also trains all new medical assistants on how to verify patient health insurance coverage and eligibility. Because Jon has learned quite a bit about health insurance, he can answer most of the patients' questions about their coverage, benefits, and the exclusions of their policies. He knows where to direct patients who have more complicated questions and how to follow up—one of the most important duties of a professional medical assistant. He has a great attitude about assisting patients with insurance questions and does not hesitate to call the insurance company on the patient's behalf.

He provides patients with exceptional customer service. When patients call him for assistance, he responds within 24 hours (often within 1 hour) with answers to their questions or a resource to help them. Jon is willing to help any staff member with other duties when necessary and prides himself on being a patient advocate. He is an enthusiastic team player who puts patients first.

While studying this chapter, think about the following questions:

- How important is the verification of services and benefits for reimbursement?
- How are private health insurance plans and government health insurance plans different?
- Why is it important to verify eligibility and preauthorize services before the patient appointment is scheduled?
- When and why is preauthorization necessary for patients who have a managed care health plan?
- Why is it important to educate patients on their health insurance benefits?

LEARNING OBJECTIVES

1. Discuss the terminology associated with health insurance and the benefits provided by health insurance.
2. Examine the types of health insurance plans.
3. Examine health insurance models.
4. Examine the medical assistant's role with the health insurance identification card and verify eligibility.
5. Examine other types of insurance, including workers' compensation, disability, life, long-term care, and liability insurance.

VOCABULARY

beneficiary A designated person who receives funds from an insurance policy.

capitation (ka pi TAY shun) A payment arrangement for healthcare providers in which providers receive a per person/per month payment regardless of how often the provider sees the patient.

claim A formal request for payment from an insurance company for services provided.

explanation of benefits (EOB) A document sent by the insurance company to the provider and the patient explaining the allowed charge amount, the amount reimbursed for services, and the patient's financial responsibilities.

fee schedule A list of fixed fees for services.

gatekeeper The primary care provider, who is in charge of a patient's treatment. Additional treatment, such as referrals to a specialist, must be approved by the gatekeeper.

health insurance exchange An online marketplace where people can compare and buy individual health insurance plans. State health insurance exchanges were established as part of the Affordable Care Act.

indigent (IN di jent) Poor, needy, impoverished.

online insurance web portal An online service provided by various insurance companies that allow providers to look up a patient's insurance benefits, eligibility, claims status, and explanation of benefits.

policy A written agreement between two parties in which one party (the insurance company) agrees to pay another party (the patient) if certain specified circumstances occur.

preauthorization A process required by some insurance carriers in which the provider obtains permission to perform certain procedures or services.

preexisting condition A health problem that was present before new health insurance coverage started.

VOCABULARY—*continued*

premium The amount paid or to be paid by the policyholder for coverage under the contract, usually in periodic installments.

provider network An approved list of physicians, hospitals, and other providers.

Qualified Medicare Beneficiaries (QMBs) Low-income Medicare patients who qualify for Medicaid for their secondary insurance.

referral An order from a primary care provider for the patient to see a specialist or to get certain medical services.

resource-based relative value system (RBRVS) A system used to determine how much providers should be paid for services provided by using three factors: physician work, practice expense, and malpractice expense. The geographic region is also taken into account. It is used by Medicare and many other health insurance companies.

third-party administrator (TPA) An organization that processes claims and provides administrative services for another organization. Often used by self-funded plans.

utilization management A decision-making process used by managed care organizations to control healthcare costs. It involves case-by-case assessments of the appropriateness of care.

waiting period The length of time a patient waits for disability insurance to pay after the date of injury.

INTRODUCTION

Insurance is something that is purchased to help protect against loss or harm from specified circumstances. Using automobile insurance as an example, the specified circumstances are those related to a car accident. The insurance could pay for damage done to your vehicle or other vehicles. It could also pay for medical expenses for anyone injured in the accident. With health insurance, the specified circumstances are related to the policyholder's health. This insurance would pay for hospital expenses, provider expenses, and certain supplies and equipment.

HEALTH INSURANCE BASICS

Much like the rest of the healthcare world, the health insurance industry has its own vocabulary. It is important for you, as a medical assistant, to become familiar with the terminology associated with health insurance, as patients may ask you to explain things even if you are working on the clinical side of medical assisting.

Benefits are also an area that can be very confusing for patients. Having that basic understanding of health insurance benefits will make you a better advocate for your patients.

Terminology

A health insurance **policy** is purchased with a **premium** or payment. The premium can be paid by an individual, an employer, or a combination of employer contribution and individual (employee) contribution.

The policy is considered a legal contract and will stay in force as long as the premium is being paid. The policy will specify exactly what services are covered. The more services that are covered, the higher the premium cost. The person responsible for the payment of the premium is referred to as a *subscriber*.

Regardless of who pays the premium, most policies require the patient to pay a portion of the healthcare expenses. This is referred to as *cost-sharing*, which includes the following:

- *Deductible*: A set dollar amount that the policyholder must pay before the insurance company starts to pay for services. It can be as low as $100 and as high as $5000. The higher the deductible, the lower the premium.
- *Co-insurance*: After the deductible has been met, the policyholder may need to pay a certain percentage of the bill, and the insurance company pays the rest. A typical split is 80/20—the insurance company pays 80%, and the policyholder pays 20%.
- *Copayment*: A set dollar amount that the policyholder must pay for each office visit. Copayments may differ for different types of office visits. For example, there can be one copayment amount for a primary care provider and a different copayment amount (usually higher) to see a specialist or to be seen in the emergency department.

The policy will specify the dollar amounts for the deductible, co-insurance, and copayment. The premium is not usually considered part of cost-sharing.

In order for the insurance carrier to pay for services, a **claim** must be submitted. The insurance company then reviews the claim to determine if the services provided are covered under the policy. It is important for a medical assistant to be familiar with the different types of insurance so that claims can be submitted accurately. This will result in faster payment for the healthcare facility.

Benefits

The federal government requires all health plans to cover essential health benefits. There are 10 categories of essential health benefits:

- Ambulatory patient services
- Hospitalization
- Mental health and substance use disorder services
- Prescription drugs
- Preventive and wellness services and chronic disease management
- Emergency services
- Maternity and newborn care
- Rehabilitative and habilitative services and devices
- Laboratory services
- Pediatric services, including oral and vision care

In addition to the essential health benefits, an insurance policy may cover other services. For a group policy, an employer can pick and choose the benefits it wants for employees, such as vision or dental coverage. Medical assistants should contact an insurance company to determine if certain services are covered under a patient's policy.

HEALTH INSURANCE PLANS

There are two types of health insurance plans in the United States:

- Government health insurance plans
- Private health insurance plans

Health insurance plans typically cover health services and procedures that are deemed medically necessary. *Medically necessary* services are those that are proper and needed for the diagnosis or treatment of the medical condition. Most insurance policies do not cover elective procedures. *Elective procedures* are medical procedures that are not deemed medically necessary, such as a facelift or another cosmetic procedure. The Affordable Care Act (ACA) states that health insurance plans must cover preventive care. *Preventive care* includes services provided to help prevent certain illnesses or that lead to an early diagnosis. Insurance companies must cover preventive care services and cannot impose cost-sharing for those services.

Preventive Care Services

• Alcohol misuse screening	• Hepatitis B and C screening
• Blood pressure screening	• Human immunodeficiency virus (HIV) screening
• Cholesterol screening	• Immunization vaccines
• Colorectal cancer screening	• Lung cancer screening
• Depression screening	• Obesity screening and counseling
• Diabetes (type 2) screening	• Tobacco use screening
• Diet counseling	• Sexually transmitted infection (STI) prevention counseling

Government Health Insurance Plans

Government health insurance plans provide coverage with reduced or no monthly premiums for the **indigent**, the older adult, the military, and government employees. There are a number of different plans, but patients need to qualify based on the following factors:

- Age
- Income
- Government occupation
- Health condition

A patient who is age 65 or older can qualify for *Medicare*. A low-income patient may be eligible for *Medicaid*. Dependents of military personnel are covered by *TRICARE*. Surviving spouses and dependent children of veterans who died in the line of duty are covered by the *Civilian Health and Medical Program of the Veterans Administration* (CHAMPVA).

Medicare

Medicare is a federal health insurance program that provides healthcare coverage for individuals who are age 65 or older, people who are disabled, and patients who have been diagnosed with end-stage renal disease (ESRD). Medicare refers to those covered by Medicare as *beneficiaries*. Medicare currently is the world's largest insurance program. In 2020 there were more than 62.6 million beneficiaries. The Medicare program is administered by the Centers for Medicare and Medicaid Services (CMS), a division of the Department of Health and Human Services (HHS). Laws enacted by Congress regulate the Medicare program.

The Medicare plan is divided into four parts (Table 12.1):

- Part A covers inpatient hospital charges. It is financed with special contributions deducted from employed individuals' salaries, with matching contributions from their employers. Due to these contributions and regular Social Security contributions, there is no monthly premium for Part A.
- Part B covers ambulatory care and all professional services, including primary care and specialists. Beneficiaries are required to pay a monthly premium. Beneficiaries can visit any specialist without a referral.
- Part C is a managed care option for Medicare-qualified patients to turn their Part A and Part B benefits into a private plan that can offer some additional benefits. The private plan must cover everything that would be covered under Part A and Part B.
- Part D is a prescription drug program offered to Medicare-qualified individuals that require an additional monthly premium.

Basic medical coverage for Medicare Part B is 80% of the allowed amount after the deductible. This means that patients are responsible for the remaining 20%. The allowed amount is determined using a

TABLE 12.1 Comparing Medicare Plans

	COVERED SERVICES	MONTHLY PREMIUM	DEDUCTIBLE
Part A	Inpatient hospital care, skilled nursing facilities, home health care, and hospice services	$0	$1,556 deductible for each benefit period (2022) Days 1–60: $0 co-insurance for each benefit period Days 61–90: $389 co-insurance per day of each benefit period Day 91 and beyond: $778 co-insurance per each "lifetime reserve day" after day 90 for each benefit period (up to 60 days over a lifetime) Beyond lifetime reserve days: all costs
Part B	Outpatient hospital care, durable medical equipment, provider's ser vices, and other medical services	$170.10	$233 (2022), plus 20% co-insurance for all medical services
Part C	Expanded inpatient hospital and outpatient hospital care benefits	Varies by plan	Varies by plan
Part D	Prescription drugs	Varies by income	Varies by plan

From Medicare: Medicare Costs at a Glance, www.medicare.gov/your-medicare-costs/costs-at-a-glance/costs-at-glance.html.

resource-based relative value scale (RBRVS). Some patients choose to purchase a private supplemental health insurance policy to help cover the 20%. These policies can also pay for services not covered by Medicare. These supplemental health insurance plans are known as *Medigap* policies. Federal regulations now require Medicare supplement policies to be uniform to avoid confusion for the purchaser.

CRITICAL THINKING APPLICATION **12.1**

Jana Green is a Medicare patient who has Part A and Part B coverage. Will Medicare cover her office visit with a cardiologist? What percentage of the bill will she be responsible for?

The fee schedule for Medicare Part B is determined using the RBRVS. This system consists of three parts:

- Provider work
- Charge-based professional liability expenses
- Charge-based overhead

The provider work component includes the degree of effort and time needed by a provider to perform a particular service or procedure. The professional liability and overhead components are computed by the CMS. A relative value unit (RVU) is assigned to each of the components, and the geographic practice cost index (GPCI) is used to adjust for geographic differences in market conditions and business costs.

The RBRVS fee schedule is designed to provide nationally uniform payments to healthcare providers. Payments are adjusted to reflect the differences in practice costs across geographic areas. The fee schedule includes a conversion factor, which is a single national number applied to all services paid under the fee schedule. Conversion factors are set by Congress and changed annually at the request of the CMS.

Let's use CPT code 99213 Office or Other Outpatient visit as an example. The CMS conversion factor for this code is 34.8931. You could consider this the base fee for this service. A formula is used to determine Medicare's allowed amount. The RVU for provider work, liability expenses, and charge-based overhead are each multiplied by the GPCI, and the total of those three is then multiplied by the conversion factor. The formula looks like this:

[(RVU work × GPCI work) + (RVU overhead expense × GPCI overhead expense) + (RVU liability insurance × GPCI liability insurance)] × Conversion factor = Allowed amount

For CPT code 99213, the RVU for work is 1.3, the RVU for overhead expense is 1.013, and the RVU for liability insurance is 0.10 (based on 2021 data). Let's take a look at how that impacts the allowed amount in three different cities. In Minneapolis, Minnesota, the GPCI for work is 1, the GPCI for overhead expenses is 0.55, and the GPCI for liability insurance is 0.353. Here is the calculation for the allowed amount for CPT 99213 for Minneapolis:

$(1.3 \times 1) + (1.013 \times 0.55) + (0.10 \times 0.353) = 1.3 + 0.56 + 0.04 = 1.9 \times 34.8931 = \$66.30$

In San Diego, California, the GPCI for work is 1.035, the GPCI for overhead expenses is 1.145, and the GPCI for liability insurance is 0.616. Here is the calculation for the allowed amount for CPT 99213 for San Diego:

$(1.3 \times 1.035) + (1.013 \times 1.145) + (0.10 \times 0.616) = 1.35 + 1.16 + 0.06 = 2.57 \times 34.8931 = \$89.68$

In Brooklyn, New York, GPCI for work is 1.46, the GPCI for overhead expenses is 1.223, and the GPCI for liability insurance is 2.702. Here is the calculation for the allowed amount for CPT 99213 for Brooklyn:

$(1.3 \times 1.46) + (1.013 \times 1.223) + (0.10 \times 2.702) = 1.90 + 1.24 + 0.27 = 3.41 \times 34.8931 = \$118.99$

Depending on the contract between the provider and the insurance carrier (especially Medicare, Medicaid, and other government programs), the difference between the RBRVS schedule and the provider's fee will be written off.

Contracts between the provider of service and the insurance company vary greatly, depending on the insurance. It is important for the medical assistant to know the contract terms for each insurance company. As insurance payments are received, the medical assistant should closely examine the **explanation of benefits (EOB)** to ensure that all benefits have been reimbursed correctly.

Medicaid

Medicaid is the government program that provides medical care for the indigent. This program is funded by both federal and state governments to provide medical care for people meeting specific eligibility criteria. All states and the District of Columbia have Medicaid programs, but program specifics vary by state, including the name of the program. In California, the Medicaid program is called Medi-Cal; in Colorado, it is Health First Colorado; and in Wisconsin it is ForwardHealth/Badger Care to name just a few. A person eligible for Medicaid in one state may not be eligible in another state and covered medical services may differ.

The federal government provides funding to each state for Medicaid programs. Each state is required to cover certain services to receive this funding. The individual states decide which additional services will be covered. Medicaid is always the payer of last resort. That means if the patient has any other type of insurance coverage, that insurance company will pay before Medicaid makes a payment.

An ambulatory care facility has the right to limit the number of Medicaid patients it accepts into the practice. The medical office

Mandatory Medicaid Benefits

In order to receive federal funds for Medicaid, each state Medicaid plan must cover the following services:

- Inpatient hospital services
- Outpatient hospital services
- Nursing facility services
- Early and periodic screening, diagnostic, and treatment (EPSDT) services
- Home health services
- Physician services
- Rural health clinic service
- Federally qualified health center services
- Laboratory and x-ray services
- Family planning services
- Nurse midwife services
- Certified pediatric and family nurse practitioner services
- Freestanding birth center services
- Transportation to medical care
- Tobacco cessation counseling for pregnant women

From Medicaid: List of Medicaid Benefits, www.medicaid.gov/medicaid/benefits/list-of-benefits/index.html.

personnel cannot pick and choose which Medicaid patients they are willing to see. There can be no discrimination based on age, gender, race, religious preference, or national origin. The Medicaid **fee schedule** is the lowest of all insurance companies, and it may not be in the medical office's financial interest to accept a large number of Medicaid patients. A provider who accepts Medicaid patients automatically agrees to accept Medicaid's allowed amount as payment in full for covered services. Some patients who are eligible for Medicaid are required to pay a co-payment. The provider can collect the co-payment from the patient but cannot bill for any amount over the allowed amount.

Eligibility for benefits is determined by the respective states, but members of the following groups are usually eligible for Medicaid:

- Low-income families
- Qualified pregnant women and children
- Recipients of Temporary Assistance for Needy Families (TANF)
- Individuals who receive Supplemental Security Income (SSI)
- Individuals who receive certain types of federal and state aid
- Individuals who are **Qualified Medicare Beneficiaries (QMBs)**—Medicaid pays for Medicare Part B premiums, deductibles, and co-insurance for qualified low-income elderly individuals
- Individuals in institutions or receiving long-term care in nursing facilities and intermediate-care facilities

Government Managed Care Plans

In an effort to reduce costs and increase the delivery of efficient care, Medicare and many Medicaid programs offer their members the option to join a managed care plan. These managed care plans must cover all services that would be covered under Medicare or Medicaid. The identification cards look just like those issued to people not on Medicare or Medicaid. The government-managed care plan may have a copayment for which the patient would be responsible.

Children's Health Insurance Program

The Children's Health Insurance Program (CHIP) is a state-funded program for children whose family income is above the Medicaid qualifying income limits. Although Medicaid does not typically have a premium, CHIP does. The premiums are typically 5% of the family's monthly income. State CHIP programs cover the following services:

• Routine checkups	• Dental care and vision care
• Immunizations	• Inpatient and outpatient hospital care
• Doctor visits	• Laboratory tests and x-ray services
• Prescriptions	• Emergency services

CHIP programs are similar to managed care plans in that care is covered only through the designated network of providers. There are smaller copayments for medical services for CHIP patients.

TRICARE

TRICARE is a comprehensive healthcare program for uniformed service members and retirees and their families. Members of the National Guard/Reserve and their families can also be covered under TRICARE.

The TRICARE program is managed by the military in partnership with civilian hospitals and clinics. It is designed to achieve the following goals:

- Expand access to healthcare
- Ensure high-quality care
- Promote medical readiness

All military hospitals and clinics are part of the TRICARE program and offer high-quality healthcare at a low cost. TRICARE offers two types of plans:

- TRICARE Prime
- TRICARE Select

Review Table 12.2 for a comparison of the TRICARE plans.

Civilian Health and Medical Program of the Veterans Administration

CHAMPVA, a health benefits program similar to TRICARE, provides coverage for the families of veterans who were permanently disabled or killed in the line of duty. The Department of Veterans Affairs (VA) shares the cost of certain healthcare services and supplies with eligible beneficiaries.

Private Health Insurance Plans

Health insurance plans that are available from commercial insurance companies are considered private plans. Most people are part of an employer group plan. Those who are not eligible for an employer plan can purchase insurance on their own. This is referred to as an *individual health insurance plan.* Most private plans use managed care to reduce the costs of delivering quality healthcare.

Employer Group Plans

Many businesses offer a *group policy,* a private health insurance plan purchased by an employer for a group of employees. In addition to covering the employee, these plans can cover the employee's spouse (i.e., domestic partner) and children. Typically, an employer pays a certain percentage of the premium for full-time employees. This makes the cost of the insurance plan more affordable for the employee. Employers also determine the health insurance benefits under the group policy. Health insurance monthly premiums and benefits can vary from employer to employer. For example, the health insurance plan from Aetna for Employer A covers chiropractic care, but the health insurance plan from Aetna for Employer B does not. The premium for a group policy is usually lower than that for an individual plan because of the large pool of employees. The insurance company will receive premiums from a larger number of people, and just a few of them will need a lot of services. The employees' share of the premium is often paid through payroll deductions.

Self-Funded Group Health Plans

Many large companies or organizations have enough employees that they can fund their own insurance programs. This is called a *self-funded plan.* Technically, a self-funded plan does not fit the true definition of insurance. The employer pays the employee's healthcare costs from the funds collected from the employee's monthly premiums. Usually, the costs of benefits and premiums for self-funded plans are similar to those for group plans. Self-funded plans tend to work best for companies that are large enough to offer good benefit coverage and reasonable

TABLE 12.2 Comparing TRICARE Plans

ACTIVE-DUTY FAMILY MEMBERS		
	TRICARE PRIME	**TRICARE SELECT**
Annual deductible	None	E1-E4: $52/individual or $105/family E5 and above: $158/individual or $317/family
Annual enrollment fee	None	None
Civilian outpatient visit	No cost	Primary Care • Network: $15 • Non-network: 20% Specialty • Network: $26 • Non-network: 20%
Civilian inpatient admission	No cost	Network: $63 per admission Non-network: 20%
Civilian inpatient mental health	No cost	Network: $63 per admission Non-network: 20%
Civilian inpatient skilled nursing facility care	$0 per diem charge per admission; no separate copayment/cost-share for separately billed professional charges	Network: $26/day Non-network: $52/day
RETIREES (UNDER 65), THEIR FAMILY MEMBERS, AND OTHERS		
	TRICARE PRIME	**TRICARE SELECT**
Annual deductible	None	E4 and below: $52 individual or $105 family E5 and above: $158/individual or $317 family
Annual enrollment fee	$366/individual or $732/family	$474/individual or $948 per family
Emergency services	$63	Network: $84 Non-network: 25%
Civilian inpatient	Network: $158/admission	Network: $185/admission Non-network Lesser of $317/day or 20%
Civilian inpatient skilled nursing facility care	Network: $31/day	Network: $52/day Non-network: Less or $317/day or 20%

From TRICARE: Health Plan Costs, https://tricare.mil/Costs/HealthPlanCosts.

premium rates and are able to pay large claims for expensive medical services. Often a **third-party administrator (TPA)** handles paperwork and claim payments for a self-insured group.

Self-funded healthcare is an arrangement in which an employer provides health or disability benefits to employees with its own funds. This is different from fully insured plans, in which the employer contracts with an insurance company to cover the employees and dependents. In self-funded healthcare, the employer assumes the direct risk for payment of the claims for benefits. The terms of eligibility and coverage are stated in the insurance plan document, which includes provisions similar to those found in a typical group health insurance policy.

Individual Health Insurance Plans

An individual health insurance plan is one that is not offered by an employer or another group. An individual policy can cover just one person or a family. These policies can be purchased through a **health insurance exchange** or directly from an insurance company. Premiums for an individual plan are generally higher than for a group plan.

Participating Provider Contracts

With all government health plans and most private health plans (especially managed care plans), healthcare providers must become *participating providers* (PARs). These providers are contracted with the insurance plan and have agreed to accept the contracted fee schedule as payment in full. Healthcare providers can apply to become PARs through a process called *credentialing*. Credentialing is the process of confirming the healthcare provider's qualifications, including the healthcare provider's education and professional background, license to practice medicine, and affiliated organizations.

Once the healthcare provider is credentialed, the health insurance plan issues a contract to become an in-network PAR. The contract includes a fee schedule that the health insurance company will use to reimburse the provider for health services provided. By signing the contract, the provider agrees to accept the health insurance plan's fee schedule, even if it is lower than the provider's fee schedule.

Contracted Fee Schedules

Payment for services is typically made after the health services are provided. Once the service has been provided to the patient, the healthcare provider must submit a health insurance claim, which includes the diagnosis and procedure codes, in addition to the total charges. Although healthcare providers establish their own fee schedule, health insurance plans maintain their own rates for which they reimburse. When providers become participating providers, they agree to the insurance plan's fee schedule and will not collect more than that amount.

When setting up a fee schedule, a healthcare provider considers three factors:

- Time
- Expertise
- Services

In every case, healthcare providers must place an estimate on the value of these services. Fees for medical procedures and services differ from office to office based on the type of practice. An office visit with a family practice provider may cost less than an office visit with a specialist. In the past, most providers worked on a fee-for-service basis—that is, patients were charged for the provider's service based on each individual service performed.

In recent years, health insurance plans, particularly government plans and managed healthcare organizations, have greatly influenced what healthcare providers can be reimbursed by establishing the allowable charge. The *allowable charge* is the maximum dollar amount the insurance plan will pay for a procedure or service. The patient cannot be billed for the amount above the allowable charge if the provider or the healthcare facility is a PAR.

HEALTH INSURANCE MODELS

There are basically two different models of health insurance today:

- Traditional health insurance
- Managed care organizations

You can find these options in both employer group plans and individual plans.

Traditional Health Insurance

Traditional health insurance plans pay for all or a share of the cost of covered services, regardless of which provider, hospital, or other licensed healthcare provider is used. Because providers are paid for each office visit, test, procedure, or other services they deliver, traditional insurance plans are often called *fee-for-service plans*. This was the first type of health insurance. Traditional health insurance plans provide the most flexibility for the patient but are also the costliest option.

Policyholders of fee-for-service plans and their dependents choose when and where to get healthcare services. When the policy is purchased, the subscriber is often given a fee schedule, which explains the benefit payment amounts. Benefits are usually paid to the insured unless that person has authorized payment to be made directly to the provider. This is referred to as the *assignment of benefits*.

The fee schedule amounts can be determined by a process called *usual, customary, and reasonable* (UCR). UCR is the amount paid for a medical service in a geographic area based on what providers in the area usually charge for the same or similar service.

Managed Care Organizations

Managed care organizations (MCOs) are health insurance companies whose goal is to provide quality, cost-effective care to their members. MCOs negotiate reduced rates with contracted providers and hospitals. In return, the managed care plan increases the provider's patient load. Many MCOs require the patient to choose a *primary care provider* (PCP) who coordinates the patient's care. Managed-care plans can also require **referrals** for their patients to be treated by a specialist, thus limiting patient access to more expensive care. The **preauthorization** process can further control patient care costs. Medical care, testing, or medication therapy is provided only when it is justified by the health insurance plan. It is important for medical assistants to be familiar with the various models of managed care to understand their effects on healthcare costs fully.

Models of Managed Care Organizations

Patient care is coordinated through a network of providers and hospitals. There are different types of managed care plans, such as health maintenance organizations (HMOs), preferred provider organizations (PPOs), and exclusive provider organizations (EPOs). They provide healthcare in return for scheduled payments and coordinate healthcare through a defined network of PCPs, hospitals, and other providers.

Health Maintenance Organization. HMOs are health plans that are regulated by HMO laws, which require them to include preventive care as part of their benefits package. The goal of the HMO health insurance plan is to reduce the cost of healthcare while still providing quality healthcare. HMO plans typically have the lowest monthly premiums among other health insurance plans. The patient's out-of-pocket expenses are also very low. Patients are not required to pay a deductible or co-insurance.

Patients are required to select a PCP, who acts as the **gatekeeper** to more specialized care. The insurance plan will not pay for services that are not included in its **provider network**; patients are 100% financially responsible for medical expenses incurred outside the HMO network of providers. For example, patients wanting to visit the dermatologist for eczema must visit their PCP first; they would be fully responsible financially if they made an appointment with a dermatologist directly. The PCP can either treat patients or refer them to a specialist.

PCPs receive financial incentives when they reduce the cost of patient care. In the earlier example, prescribing medicine to the patient is more cost-effective than referring the patient to a specialist. HMOs always require the following:

- Referrals from the PCP to specialists
- Precertification and preauthorization for hospital admissions, outpatient procedures, and treatments (Figure 12.1)

HMOs can be set up using several models. The payment structure can be different for each of those models (Table 12.3).

Preauthorization Request Form

TO BE COMPLETED BY PRIMARY CARE PHYSICIAN OR OUTSIDE PROVIDER

☐ Medicare ☑ Blue Cross/Blue Shield ☐ Tricare ☐ Health Net
☐ Medicaid ☐ Aetna ☐ Cigna ☐ Other
Group No.: 54098XX

Name: (First, Middle Initial, Last) Louann Campbell Date: 7-14-20XX
☐ Male ☑ Female Birthdate: 4-7-1952 Home Telephone Number: (555) 450-1666
Address: 2516 Encina Avenue, Woodland Hills, XY 12345-0439
Primary Care Physician: Gerald Practon, MD
Referring Physician: Gerald Practon, MD
Referred to: Raymond Skeleton, MD Office Telephone Number: (555) 486-9002
Address: 4567 Broad Avenue, Woodland Hills, XY 12345
Diagnosis Code: M54.5 Diagnosis: Low back pain
Diagnosis Code: M51.27 Diagnosis: Sciatica
Treatment Plan: Orthopedic consultation and evaluation of lumbar spine; R/O herniated disk L4-5
Authorization Requested for: ☐ Consult Only ☐ Treatment Only ☐ Consult/Treatment ☑ Consult/Procedure/Surgery ☐ Diagnostic Tests
Procedure Code: 99244 Description: New patient consultation
Procedure Code: Description:
Place of Service: ☑ Office ☐ Outpatient ☐ Inpatient ☐ Other Number of Visits: 1
Facility: Length of Stay:
List of Potential Future Consultants (i.e., anesthetists, surgical assistants, or medical/surgical):
Physician's Signature: Gerald Practon, MD

TO BE COMPLETED BY PRIMARY CARE PHYSICIAN

PCP Recommendations: See above PCP Initials: GP
Date Eligibility Checked: 7-14-20XX Effective Date: 1-15-20XX

TO BE COMPLETED BY UTILIZATION MANAGEMENT

Authorized: Auth. No. Not Authorized:
Deferred: Modified:
Effective Date: Expiration Date:

FIGURE 12.1 Preauthorization Request Form.

CRITICAL THINKING APPLICATION 12.2

Noemi Rodriguez, a patient, calls to make an appointment with the endocrinologist because she has trouble managing her diabetes. She tells Jon over the phone when she is making the appointment that she has the Aetna HMO. Will Jon be able to schedule Ms. Rodriguez's appointment with the endocrinologist? Why or why not? What would she need to make an appointment?

Preferred Provider Organization. A PPO is a managed care network that contract with a group of providers. The providers agree on a predetermined list of charges for all services, including those for both normal and complex procedures. The PPO model of managed healthcare uses the fee-for-service concept that many providers prefer. Typically, the patient's financial responsibilities represent, on average, 20% to 25% of the allowed charge, but this depends on the patient's health insurance policy. A provider who joins a PPO does not need to change the manner of providing care and continues to treat and bill patients on a fee-for-service basis. When a patient covered under a PPO plan comes for treatment, the provider treats the patient and bills the PPO. Patients do not need to visit their PCP to obtain a referral to a specialist for more specialized care, and they typically have more control over healthcare choices.

PPOs provide their subscribers with a list of participating providers and healthcare facilities from which they can access in-network healthcare at PPO reduced rates. Rates are quite often lower than those charged to non-PPO patients. This gives the patient more choices for providers. If the patient chooses to see a provider, not in the PPO network, the deductible, co-insurance, and copayments will be higher.

Although patients have the option to visit a specialist when they feel the need, they are still required to obtain preauthorization for more expensive services, such as diagnostic imaging.

CRITICAL THINKING APPLICATION 12.3

Diego Lupez calls Jon. He is upset because he received a patient statement with a balance owing. He tells Jon that he has full-coverage insurance through his employer and does not know why he has a balance. What information can Jon share with Mr. Lupez to explain his financial responsibility?

Exclusive Provider Organization. An EPO combines features of an HMO (e.g., an enrolled group or population, PCPs, and an authorization system) and a PPO (e.g., flexible benefit design and fee-for-service payments). Patients with EPO coverage will not be covered for services outside the designated network of providers (unless there is an emergency), but they may not need to obtain a referral for specialized care. Unlike HMO members, EPO plan members are not required to choose a PCP.

Table 12.4 compares the different types of managed care plans.

Referrals

Patients seeking specialized care must first visit their assigned PCP to obtain a referral to a specialist or for more specialized therapy or care. Patients with HMO plans can only obtain a referral to the specialist by visiting their assigned PCP. HMOs will measure how many patients are referred to specialists by individual PCPs. Approval or denial of a referral can take anywhere from a few minutes to a few days. There are three types of referrals:

- A *regular referral*, which usually takes 3 to 10 working days for review and approval. This type of referral is used when the provider believes that the patient must see a specialist to continue treatment.
- An *urgent referral*, which usually takes about 24 hours for approval. This type of referral is used when an urgent but not life-threatening situation occurs.
- A *STAT referral*, which can be approved online when it is submitted to the utilization review department through the provider's web portal. A STAT referral is used in an emergency situation as indicated by the provider.

A *regular referral* is the most common type and can be inconvenient for the patient. With most managed care plans, preauthorization needs to be obtained for a referral. Remember this cardinal rule: never tell the patient the referral has been approved unless you have a hard copy of the authorization. A referral is authorized after the approval has been received. When a referral is approved, the PCP's office and the patient should receive a copy of the authorization. Always review the authorization thoroughly and confirm details, such as approved diagnosis and procedure codes and the exact period of time the authorization lasts. The patient will receive a letter with an authorization number and details regarding the approved services. The patient must bring the authorization to the specialist's office on the appointment date.

TABLE 12.3 Health Maintenance Organization (HMO) Models

MODEL	STRUCTURE	PAYMENT STRUCTURE
Independent practice association (IPA)	General or family practice provider or provider group that practices independently and may contract with several HMOs. Can see patients outside of the HMO.	**Capitation** or fee-for-service
Staff	One or more providers hired by an HMO. Providers see only HMO patients.	Salaried
Group	Multispecialty group with or without a primary care provider (PCP; i.e., gatekeeper). May contract with several HMOs.	Capitation or fee-for-service
Network	HMOs contract with multiple provider groups. Those providers can see patients outside of the HMO. Provides wider geographic coverage for members.	Capitation or fee-for-service

Utilization Management/Utilization Review

Utilization management is a form of patient care review by healthcare professionals who do not provide the care but are employed by health insurance companies. It is a necessary component of managed care to control costs. A *utilization review committee* reviews individual cases to ensure that medical care services are medically necessary. For this committee to function properly, having the correct diagnosis code is critical. This committee also reviews all provider referrals and cases of emergency department visits and urgent care. For referrals, the committee reviews the referral and either approves or denies it, so it is important to submit accurate documentation. The medical assistant should contact the utilization review department directly; it should never be left to the patient to contact this department.

TABLE 12.4 Managed Care Plans

PLAN	PROVIDERS	ACCESS TO SPECIALIZED CARE	DEDUCTIBLE, CO-INSURANCE, COPAYMENT
Health maintenance organization (HMO)	Must see only HMO providers and choose a primary care provider (PCP).	Referral required for specialized care.	Usually no deductible or co-insurance. Copayments required for office visits and prescriptions.
Preferred provider organization (PPO)	No PCP required. There is a network of providers, but out-of-network providers can be seen.	No referral required. Preauthorization needed for expensive services.	Lower deductible and co-insurance if an in-network provider is used. Copayments required for office visits and prescriptions.
Exclusive provider organization (EPO)	Must see network providers. No PCP required.	No referral needed.	Usually no deductible or co-insurance. Copayments required for office visits and prescriptions.

THE MEDICAL ASSISTANT'S ROLE

A medical assistant can be involved in many different tasks related to health insurance. Being familiar with the technology and forms that are used will make you more efficient at your job.

Health Insurance Identification Card

A patient enrolled in a health insurance plan will be issued a health insurance identification (ID) card that supplies the following information:

- Health insurance company
- Health plan type
- Subscriber identification number
- Copay amounts
- Health plan name
- Subscriber's name and covered dependents
- Policy group number
- Health plan contact phone numbers

The medical assistant must be able to identify all of the information provided on the health insurance identification card (Procedure 12.1). To ensure that the person with the insurance card is actually the person named on the card, the medical assistant should also ask to see a photo ID. This information needs to be entered into the practice management software for accurate billing. The medical assistant will also be responsible for scanning an image of the health insurance identification card. Both sides of the card should be scanned because there is important information, usually instructions for preauthorization, on the backside of the card. Review Figure 12.2 for a sampling of different ID cards for common insurance companies.

Verifying Eligibility

Verification of eligibility is the process of confirming health insurance coverage for the patient. When you are scheduling an

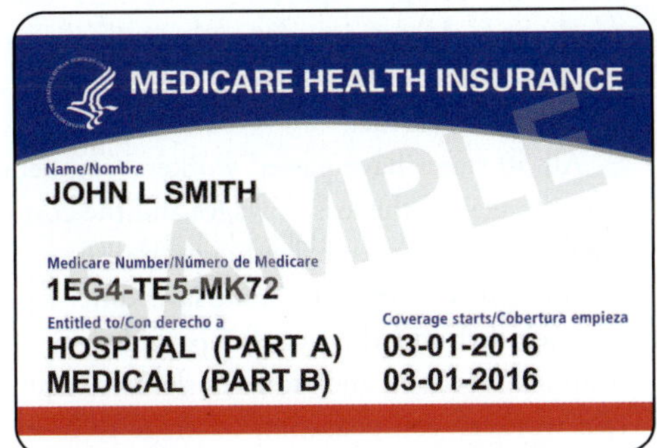

Medicare: The Medicare card uses the patient's Social Security number as the ID number. The card also details the plan coverages, in this case Part A and Part B.

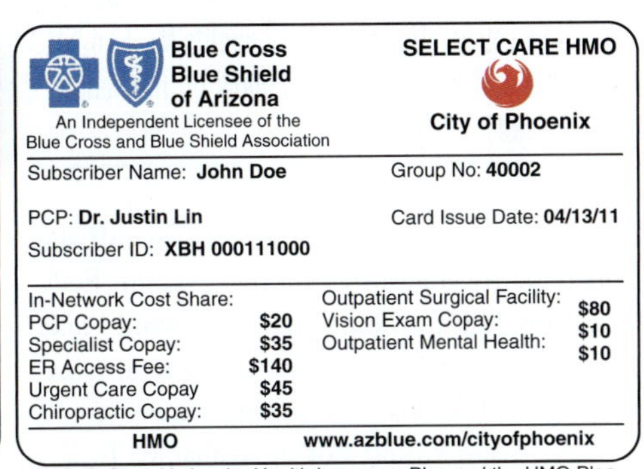

HMO ID Card: Notice the Health Insurance Plan and the HMO Plan are both listed. Common copayments are also listed. HMO members are required to choose a PCP that which is designated on their health ID card.

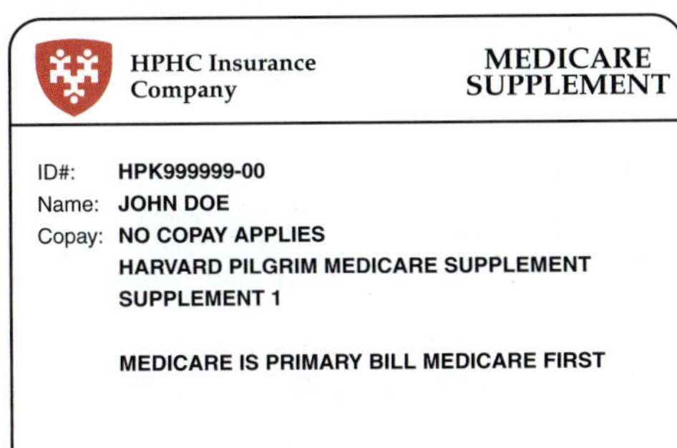

Medicare Secondary Insurance: The ID card states that it is a supplement to Medicare, thus Medicare should be billed as the primary. The ID number does not match the Medicare card.

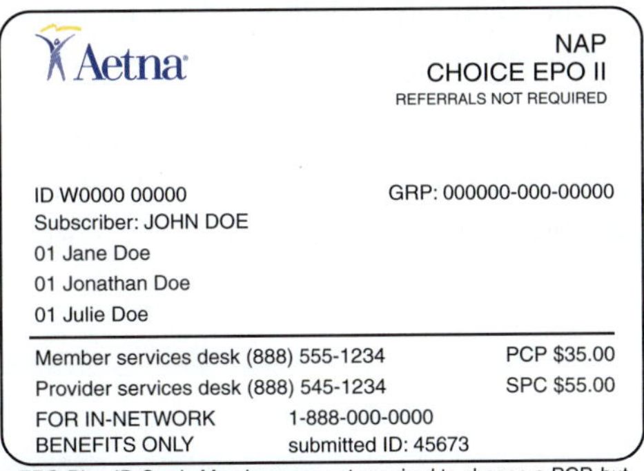

EPO Plan ID Card: Members are not required to choose a PCP, but can only use their benefits for in-network providers and facilities. Notice the ID number stays the same for the insured and all family members listed.

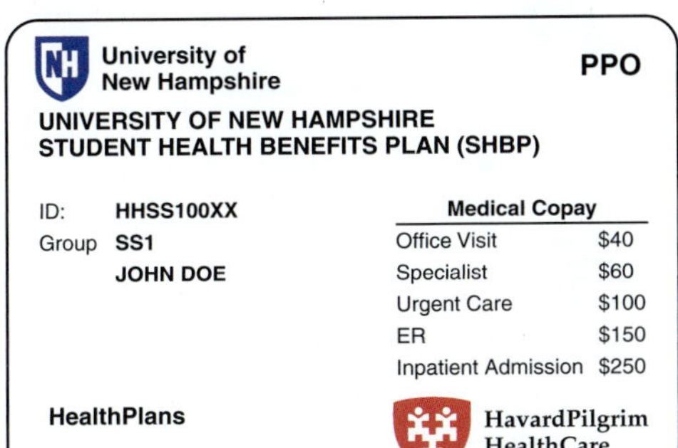

PPO plan ID card: PPO patients have the most flexibility to visit whichever provider, primary care, or specialist they choose. Notice the medical copays are slightly higher than HMO copayments.

FIGURE 12.2 A variety of different health insurance identification cards.

appointment, health insurance information should be collected (unless it is an emergency situation). If the healthcare facility is not part of the patient's network of providers, the individual should be informed of this. The patient can then decide whether to schedule an appointment. The medical assistant should also verify the *effective date,* or date the insurance coverage began, and confirm that the patient will be covered on the date the medical services are provided. The medical assistant should make it a practice to review each insurer's **online insurance web portal**, which can verify insurance eligibility, benefits, and exclusions, prior to the patient's appointment. If the online insurance web portal is not available, the medical assistant should contact the provider services desk; the phone number should be listed on the patient's health insurance ID card.

CRITICAL THINKING APPLICATION 12.4

Robert Caudill, an older adult patient, calls to make an appointment but is unsure what his benefits are. How can Jon find out what benefits Mr. Caudill qualifies for? Is it appropriate for Jon to educate Mr. Caudill on his health insurance benefits? Why or why not?

In the recent past, the medical assistant would have to call the health insurance company to verify eligibility for every patient. Each call to the health insurance company's automated system would take at least 5 minutes, and unless the medical assistant spoke to a member services agent, which would take even more time, access to all of the patient's benefit information would not be available. Today, most privately sponsored health insurance plans offer online insurance provider portals, which allow for quick and easy verification of eligibility (Figure 12.3). The healthcare facility will have to apply for access to the online web portal. Once it has been approved, a patient's benefits can be looked up in their entirety in seconds instead of minutes. Information on a patient's benefit plan can be uploaded to the electronic health record (EHR) quickly; this process reduces the use of paper in the healthcare facility.

OTHER TYPES OF INSURANCE

When you work in a healthcare facility, the most common type of insurance you will see is health insurance. However, there are other types of insurance that can require the involvement of a healthcare provider. These other types of insurance are discussed next.

Workers' Compensation

Workers' compensation is an insurance plan for individuals injured on the job or become ill due to job-related circumstances. An example of a job-related illness would be mesothelioma caused by inhaling asbestos. The insurance plan covers the following:

- Medical care and rehabilitation benefits
- Weekly income replacement benefits
- Death benefits to dependents

The provider accepts the workers' compensation reimbursements as payment in full and does not bill the patient. Time limitations are set for the prompt reporting of workers' compensation cases. The employee is obligated to promptly notify the employer. The employer must then notify the insurance company and refer the employee to a healthcare provider.

All 50 states have passed workers' compensation laws to protect workers against the loss of wages and the cost of medical care resulting from an occupational accident or disease, as long as the employee was not proven negligent. State laws differ regarding employees who are included and the benefits provided by workers' compensation insurance. Federal and state legislatures require employers to maintain workers' compensation coverage to meet minimum standards, covering most employees for work-related illnesses and injuries. The purpose of workers' compensation laws is to provide prompt medical care to an injured or ill worker so that the person may be restored to health and return to full earning capacity in as short a time as possible.

Disability Insurance

Disability insurance is a type of insurance that replaces income if the patient has a disability that is not work related. The disability

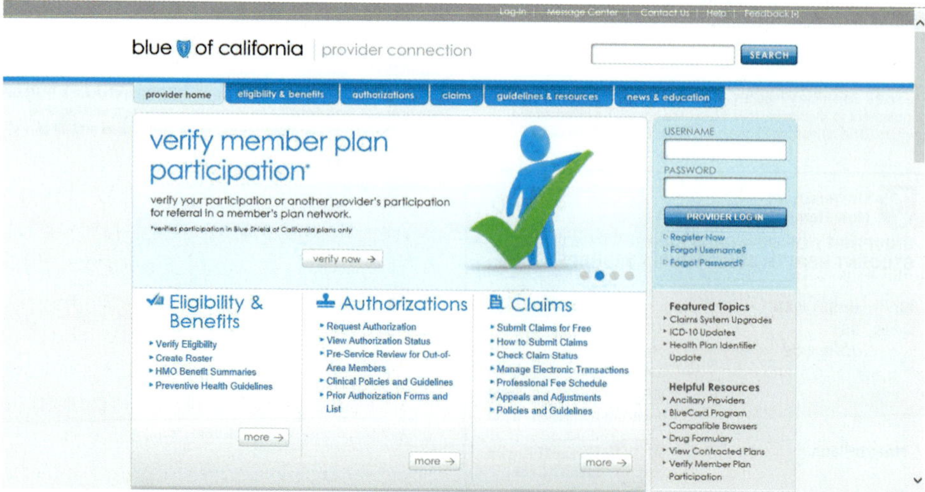

FIGURE 12.3 A provider's web portal for online health insurance. (From Fordney MT: *Insurance handbook for the medical office,* ed 14, St. Louis, 2017, Elsevier.)

means that the employee is unable to perform standard work functions or duties. It could involve either short-term or long-term disability benefits. Both provide 40% to 70% of the individual's predisability income. Many employers offer a disability policy to their employees. Generally, the employee pays the monthly premium. These policies can also be purchased by an individual.

Short-term disability means that a person is unable to work for 9 to 52 weeks. Long-term disability policies pick up when short-term benefits are exhausted. Long-term disability coverage will pay out until the patient returns to work or for the number of years specified in the policy. Some policies will pay out until the patient reaches the age of 65 and then is eligible for Social Security benefits. There may be a **waiting period** before benefits can be paid. Sick time can be used for the waiting period days.

Weekly or monthly cash benefits are provided to employed policyholders who become unable to work due to an accident or illness. The accident or illness must not be related to work because that would be covered under workers' compensation. Payments are made directly to the insured and are intended to replace lost income resulting from an illness or other disability. Disability payments are not intended for payment of specific medical bills, and a disability insurance policy should not be confused with a regular health insurance plan.

The medical office may be involved in the examination of the patient to determine the level of disability and when the disability ends. There are forms that a healthcare provider must complete and then submit to the insurance carrier. Prompt attention to the completion of these forms is important, as these patients are waiting for the benefits to pay their bills and buy groceries.

Life Insurance

Life insurance provides payment of a specified amount, upon the insured's death, either to a designated **beneficiary** or to the insured's estate. Annuity life insurance policies provide monthly cash benefits if the policyholder becomes permanently and totally disabled. Sometimes the proceeds from life insurance are used to meet the expenses of the insured person's last illness.

The healthcare facility may be required to complete physical examination forms when a patient is applying for life insurance. If there is an annuity policy, the healthcare provider may have to determine if there is a permanent disability and submit documentation.

Long-Term Care Insurance

Long-term care insurance is a relatively new type of insurance that covers a broad range of maintenance and health services for chronically ill, disabled, or developmentally delayed individuals. Medical services may be provided on an inpatient basis (e.g., at a rehabilitation facility, nursing home, or mental hospital), on an outpatient basis, or at home.

Liability Insurance

Liability insurance covers losses to a third party caused by the insured. There are many types of liability insurance, including automobile, business, and homeowners' policies. Liability policies often include benefits for the following:

- Medical expenses resulting from traumatic injuries
- Lost wages
- Sometimes pain and suffering

All liability insurance policies are payable to victims injured by the insured person's home or car, without regard to the insured person's actual legal liability for the accident.

The Affordable Care Act

In the early 2000s, it became clear that a large number of Americans lacked basic health insurance. **Preexisting conditions** made it difficult for Americans who did not work full time or were self-employed to obtain health insurance. In addition, the health insurance market was discriminating against young adults 18 years or older, who may not have been qualified to receive health benefits because they could not find full-time employment.

In 2010, the Patient Protection and Affordable Care Act, known as the *Affordable Care Act* (also Obamacare), was enacted. It increased the quality, availability, and affordability of private and public health insurance for more than 44 million uninsured Americans. The legislation included new qualifying regulations, taxes, mandates, and subsidies. The federal mandate not only has opened opportunities for more Americans to obtain affordable health insurance but also works to reduce overall healthcare spending in the long run. The following are other patient protections and provisions under the Affordable Care Act:

- Insurance companies are prohibited from dropping patient health coverage if the individual gets sick or makes an unintentional mistake on the health insurance application.
- Preexisting conditions and gender discrimination were eliminated, so patients cannot be charged more based on their health status or gender.
- Young adults can remain on their parent's or guardian's insurance policy until age 26.
- *Health insurance marketplaces* were created, where low- to middle-income Americans can compare plans and lower their costs on healthcare coverage.
- States expanded Medicaid coverage to 15.9 million Americans to include those who qualify for cost assistance through the marketplace.
- Individuals seeking health insurance can apply only during the open enrollment period, which is established by each state.

With more Americans having health insurance, the number of office visits to providers across the country is expected to increase. Thus, efficient health insurance management policies should be instituted to meet the new demand for services.

CLOSING COMMENTS

Health insurance and benefits coverage can be confusing to the patient. Medical assistants should educate themselves on the specific details of all plans accepted at the healthcare facility. Managed care has often been criticized in the media for its cost-saving practices. Extra efforts made by medical assistants to overcome these challenges and educate their patients on how to use their health insurance plans will improve the quality of care delivered to their patients. Providers and healthcare facilities need to evaluate their ability to accept the fee schedule of insurance plans they are contracted with, especially because Medicaid's fee schedule is the lowest in the industry.

Patient Coaching

It is important for patients to understand how their insurance works. Many people, especially older individuals, believe that if they have health insurance, all charges for their healthcare will be covered. The responsibilities of a medical assistant include keeping patients informed of their financial responsibilities and answering questions about each person's benefits and exclusions. Often healthcare facilities provide their patients with informational brochures that explain how health insurance and reimbursement work and provide definitions of some of the more common terms used in the insurance claims process. If patients are well advised and comfortable with insurance facts before treatment begins, the medical experience will go more smoothly, and collection of their financial responsibilities will be easier. The medical assistant must practice good communication skills, patience, and tact when discussing reimbursement and financial responsibilities issues with patients.

LEGAL AND ETHICAL ISSUES

Verification of eligibility is a process that is important not only to ensure the insurance plan is valid at the time of service but also to ensure the patient's identity. Falsifying one's identity to use someone else's health insurance benefits are a common fraudulent practice. The only way to prevent this type of health insurance fraud is to diligently verify all patients when they schedule appointments with the healthcare facility. A state-issued ID should be presented with the patient's health insurance ID to verify identity. If medical assistants suspect fraud, they should report it to the health insurance plan immediately, and the patient should be informed that the medical professional cannot render services until issues relating to the health insurance are resolved.

Professional Behaviors

Patients can be confused or angered when insurance companies deny authorization of services or referrals. Although these decisions are made by insurance companies, many times, the blame is put on the medical front office assistants. In situations such as these, it is important for medical assistants to stay calm and listen to the patient's concerns. In most cases, the patient will realize that there is nothing the medical assistant can do, but the patient may need to express frustration. Once the patient has calmed down, the medical assistant can then recommend options, such as paying cash or making payment arrangements; the medical assistant can also bring attention to the patient's insurance member services hotline. Compassionately assure patients that their health is most important and that you will do what you can, so they can receive the appropriate medical treatment.

If the patient continues to escalate the situation or becomes belligerent, excuse yourself from the discussion and ask either an office manager or another medical assistant to step in. A medical assistant should never return anger or frustration to the patient. Remember, the patient may be mentally compromised and frustrated from extensive healthcare problems, so don't exacerbate the situation by releasing your own anger. If the patient's health is made the primary concern, the healthcare facility can work with the insurance company so that the patient can receive appropriate medical care.

SUMMARY OF SCENARIO

Although he was initially nervous about explaining fees to patients and asking for payment, Jon has become more comfortable doing this aspect of his job because he now understands the business aspect of the practice. Patients understand that providers must charge for their services and have become accustomed to copayments and co-insurance amounts. Many times, these fees are collected in advance before the patient sees the provider. This practice saves time on checkout, and most patients believe that the copay is a small cost compared with the entire fee that providers charge to manage their care in one office visit.

Jon has noticed that the usual, customary, and reasonable fees that Dr. Kahn, a member of the practice, charges his patients directly affect the reimbursements that are paid by various insurance and managed care companies. Jon has attended several health insurance billing seminars sponsored by Medicare and Blue Cross/Blue Shield, and he believes that this extra training has resulted in a reduction in health insurance claim rejections at WMFM Clinic.

SUMMARY OF LEARNING OBJECTIVES

1. **Discuss the terminology associated with health insurance and the benefits provided by health insurance.**
Insurance is something that is purchased to help protect against loss or harm from specified circumstances. A premium can be paid by an individual, an employer, or a combination of employer contribution and individual (employee) contribution. Most policies require the patient to pay a portion of the healthcare expenses, which is known as *cost-sharing* and includes deductibles, co-insurance, and copayments.
There are basic benefits that all health plans are required to cover, which are listed in the following table:

• Ambulatory patient services	• Emergency services
• Hospitalization	• Maternity and newborn care
• Mental health and substance use disorder services	• Rehabilitative and habilitative services and devices
• Prescription drugs	• Laboratory services
• Preventive and wellness services and chronic disease management	• Pediatric services, including oral and vision care

2. **Examine the types of health insurance plans.**
Government health insurance plans include Medicare, Medicaid, TRICARE, CHAMPVA, and CHIP. Older adults, people who are disabled, those associated with the military, and the indigent may qualify for one of these programs. Because these programs are sponsored by the government, participating providers (PARs) must accept a lower fee schedule for reimbursements.
Private health insurance plans, also known as commercial insurance plans, are for-profit organizations. As such, health insurance companies make annual changes to the participating provider contract to negotiate lower payments. Most privately sponsored plans use managed care to reduce the costs of delivering quality healthcare.
Self-funded healthcare, or self-insurance, is an arrangement in which an employer provides health or disability benefits to employees with its own funds. This is different from fully insured plans, in which the employer contracts with an insurance company to cover the employees and dependents. In self-funded healthcare, the employer assumes the direct risk for payment of the claims for benefits.
With all government health plans and most private health plans, healthcare providers must become participating providers. Credentialing is the process of confirming the healthcare provider's qualifications. Payment for services is typically made after the health services are provided. When setting up a fee schedule, a healthcare provider should consider time, expertise, and services.

3. **Examine health insurance models.**
Traditional health insurance plans pay for all or a share of the cost of covered services. These services are also known as *fee-for-service* and were the first type of health insurance. Policyholders of fee-for-service plans and their dependents choose when and where to get healthcare services. Fee schedule amounts can be determined by a process called *usual, customary, and reasonable* (UCR).
Managed care is a broad term used to describe a variety of healthcare plans developed to provide healthcare services at lower costs. It is important for the medical assistant to be familiar with various plan types such as the health maintenance organization (HMO), preferred provider organization (PPO), and exclusive provider organization (EPO) and to understand the policies of each one.
Obtaining preauthorization for making referrals must be done according to the guidelines of the individual insurance companies. The medical assistant should always refer to the insurance plan's policies and procedures manual if uncertain about the procedure.
Utilization management is a form of patient care review by healthcare professionals who do not provide the care but are employed by health insurance companies. The medical assistant should contact the utilization review department directly; it should never be left to the patient to contact this department.

4. **Examine the medical assistant's role as it pertains to the health insurance identification card and verifying eligibility.**
As proof of health insurance coverage, patients are issued a health insurance ID card with the health plan name, patient's name, subscriber ID, and health plan contact information (see Figure 12.2 and Procedure 12.1). To prevent insurance fraud, it is important to look over the card and ensure that the name on the card is the same as that of the patient.
It is important to verify insurance benefits before you provide services to patients. Verifying benefits is necessary to ensure that the patient is covered by insurance and to determine what benefits will be paid for routine and special procedures and services. Verification protects the provider and the patient against unexpected medical care costs.
Many problems for both the patient and the medical office can be prevented if the medical assistant develops and follows a procedure for verifying insurance benefits before services are provided. This procedure includes gathering as much information as possible about the patient's demographics and insurance coverage. A pragmatic and tactful discussion with all new patients to explain the facility's established policy on insurance claims processing and the collection of fees not covered by the patient's policy will pay off.

5. **Examine other type so of insurance, including workers' compensation, disability, life, long-term care, and liability insurance.**
Workers' compensation is an insurance plan that covers individuals who are injured on the job or become ill due to job-related circumstances. Advantages include medical care and rehabilitation benefits, weekly income replacement benefits, and death benefits.
Disability insurance is a type of insurance that replaces one's income if the patient has a disability that is not work related. Life insurance provides a payment of a specified amount, upon the insured's death, either to a designated beneficiary or to the insured's estate. Long-term care insurance covers a broad range of maintenance and health services for chronically ill, disabled, or developmentally delayed individuals. Liability insurance covers losses to a third party caused by the insured.

PROCEDURE 12.1 Interpret Information on an Insurance Card

TASK: Identify essential information on the health insurance identification (ID) card to confirm copayment obligations and obtain accurate health insurance information for claims submission.

EQUIPMENT and SUPPLIES

- Patient's health insurance ID card, both sides (see the following figure)

Front

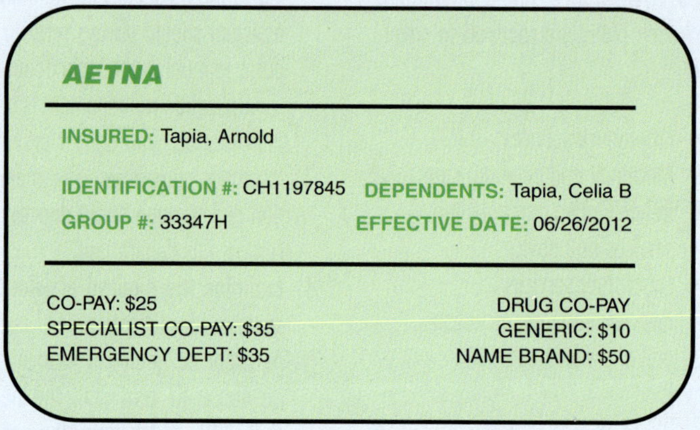

AETNA

INSURED: Tapia, Arnold

IDENTIFICATION #: CH1197845 DEPENDENTS: Tapia, Celia B

GROUP #: 33347H EFFECTIVE DATE: 06/26/2012

CO-PAY: $25
SPECIALIST CO-PAY: $35
EMERGENCY DEPT: $35

DRUG CO-PAY
GENERIC: $10
NAME BRAND: $50

Back

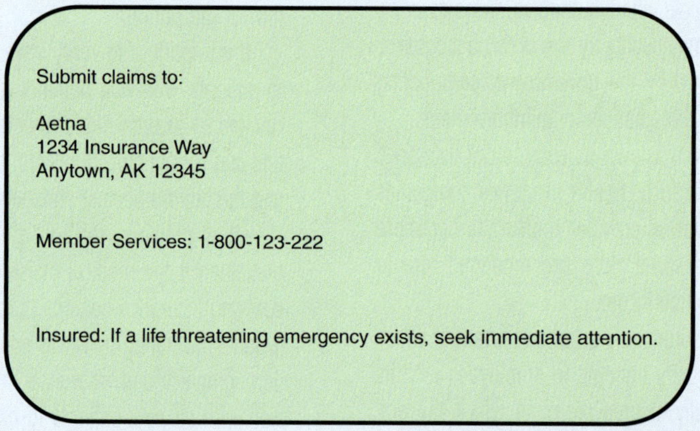

Submit claims to:

Aetna
1234 Insurance Way
Anytown, AK 12345

Member Services: 1-800-123-222

Insured: If a life threatening emergency exists, seek immediate attention.

PROCEDURAL STEPS

1. Review the patient's health insurance ID card and identify the insured on the health insurance ID card. If the patient is someone other than the insured, determine the relationship with the insured and the insured's date of birth and gender.
   PURPOSE: The insured's date of birth and gender are required to submit an accurate health insurance claim.
2. Identify the insurance plan.
   PURPOSE: To confirm that the provider is a participating provider for the insurance plan or the HMO network. If the provider is out of the network, the patient should be informed that either additional out of pocket expenses must be paid or the medical services provided will not be covered by the insurance plan.
3. Identify the insured's identification number and group number.
   PURPOSE: To accurately submit the health insurance claim under the correct insurance policy number and group number.
4. Identify the patient's copayment, which is due before the appointment. Collect the correct amount. (For example, if the provider is a specialist, collect the copayment listed for the specialist.)
   PURPOSE: To ensure that the patient pays the proper copayment.
5. On the back of the health insurance ID card, make sure that a customer service phone number and medical claims address are present.
   PURPOSE: To ensure that the provider can contact customer service and has the correct mailing address.

DIAGNOSTIC CODING ESSENTIALS 13

SCENARIO

Mike Simeone, a recent medical assistant graduate, excelled in his diagnostic coding course. He has now found an entry-level coding position at the Walden-Martin Family Medical (WMFM) Clinic.

Mike is a little nervous but also excited about starting ICD-10-CM coding. He has used encoder software in some of his classes, which helped him determine the most specific and accurate code. Mike noticed that the new software update in the medical office has the most recent ICD-10-CM codes.

Mike has had some previous experience working in health records, which gives him a strong understanding of the importance of accurate, quality documentation. He knows where to look to find diagnostic statements in providers' orders, treatment plans, progress notes, surgical reports, and other medical reports.

While studying this chapter, think about the following questions:

- How do the format, layout, and conventions of the ICD-10-CM manual help the medical assistant search for the most accurate and specific diagnostic code?
- Why is the quality of health record documentation critical to diagnostic coding?
- Why does the medical assistant need to know the steps for performing diagnostic coding?

LEARNING OBJECTIVES

1. Explain the historical use of the International Classification of Disease (ICD) in the United States.
2. Explain the structure and format of the International Classification of Diseases, 10th Revision, Clinical Modification (ICD-10-CM).
3. Explain how to abstract the diagnostic statement from a patient's health record.
4. Examine the steps involved in ICD-10-CM coding.
5. Examine the Official Coding Guidelines to assign the most accurate ICD-10-CM diagnostic code.
6. Explain the importance of maximizing third-party reimbursement.

VOCABULARY

abstract Collecting important information from the health record.

cataract (KAT ur ackt) Progressive loss of transparency of the lens of the eye.

chronic Developing slowly and lasting for a long time, generally 3 or more months.

contraindicate (kon truh IN di kayt) To specify that an agent or procedure should not be used.

dementia (di MEN shah) A mental disorder in which the individual experiences a progressive loss of memory, personality alterations, confusion, loss of touch with reality, and stupor (seeming unawareness of, and disconnection with, one's surroundings).

diagnosis (die ag NOH sis) Determining the cause of a condition, illness, disease, injury, or congenital defect.

diagnostic statement Information about a patient's diagnosis or diagnoses that have been taken from the medical documentation.

encoder Software that will apply diagnostic or procedure codes to medical conditions or procedures.

encounter form A document used to capture the services/procedures and diagnoses for a patient visit. The fees for the services/procedures are usually included on the encounter form.

epidemiology (ep i dee mee OL uh jee) The branch of medicine dealing with the incidence, distribution, and control of disease in a population. It also involves the prevalence of disease in large populations, in addition to detection of the source and cause of epidemics of infectious disease.

etiology (ee tee OL uh jee) The study of the causes or origin of diseases.

histologic Pertaining to the study of body tissues.

impending A term used in the diagnosis of a condition that can be imminently threatening. For example, a patient showing signs of prediabetes may in the near future develop diabetes; therefore, in this case, diabetes is an impending condition.

VOCABULARY—*continued*

medically necessary Accepted healthcare services that are appropriate for the evaluation and treatment of a disease, condition, illness, or injury and are consistent with the applicable standard of care.

mortality The relative frequency of deaths in a specific population.

myxedema (mick suh DEE mah) Advanced hypothyroidism in adulthood.

reimbursement (ree im BURS ment) To make repayment for an expense or a loss incurred.

sequela (si KWEL uh) (singular), sequelae (plural) An abnormal condition resulting from a previous disease.

specificity (spes uh FIS i tee) The quality or state of being specific.

INTRODUCTION

A **diagnosis** has many purposes in healthcare. Patient treatment plans are based on the diagnosis. **Reimbursement** from insurance companies is based, in part, on the diagnosis. Researchers use diagnoses for their studies. Diagnostic coding has been used to standardize the reporting of medical conditions, illnesses, and injuries. It was initially developed to study the causes of **mortality**. Over time, diagnostic coding has been expanded to include all diseases and conditions. The World Health Organization (WHO) has established the International Classification of Diseases (ICD). This classification system is in its tenth revision and is known as the *International Classification of Diseases, 10th Revision, Clinical Modification* (ICD-10-CM). These codes are used for the following:

- Mortality data
- **Epidemiologic data**
- Billing purposes

The ICD-10-CM allows providers to be much more specific when assigning diagnostic codes than was possible with previous revisions. This will, in turn, result in more accurate data collection and billing practices. Every year, the Centers for Medicare and Medicaid Services (CMS) reviews the ICD-10-CM coding manual. The update was published on October 1. Additions, revisions, and deletions are made to many of the diagnostic codes, code descriptions, and guidelines. *You must always use the current year's coding manual to ensure accurate coding and comply with regulatory guidelines.*

The Health Insurance Portability and Accountability Act (HIPAA) has mandated that specific code sets be used to help standardize the process of claims submission. The ICD-10-CM is the mandated diagnostic code set.

This chapter looks at the structure of the ICD-10-CM codes and how to accurately determine the correct code.

UNDERSTANDING DIAGNOSTIC CODING

We will start this chapter by looking at the history of medical coding. With this background, you can better understand why we do medical coding and how it has changed over time. We will also be looking at how medical coding is used in the United States.

The History of Medical Coding

Medical coding began as medical classification in 17th century England. John Graunt, a statistician, wanted to study the causes of mortality in children under age 6, so he developed a medical classification system. In the mid-1800s, William Farr, a medical statistician, established a more organized disease classification to widen the system to patients of all ages. The principles of Farr's classification method, and those of Jacques Bertillon, chief of statistics for the city of Paris, developed into the *International List of Causes of Death*, which was published in Chicago in 1893 by the International Statistics Institute. This list is revised every 10 years. After the League of Nations was established in 1920, its members saw the need for a variety of stakeholders to use the classification system, including insurers, health administrators, hospitals, and military medical providers. The name of the list was changed to the *International List of Diseases.*

In 1946 the International Commission of the World Health Organization (WHO) established codes to define specific infectious diseases, parasites, symptoms, and causes of death. This code set was called the *Manual of the International Statistical Classification of Diseases, Injuries, and Causes of Death* (ICD).

(*Note:* It is important to understand the difference between the ICD and the *Clinical Modification* versions [i.e., ICD-10-CM]. The ICD is the international version, copyrighted and published by the WHO. The WHO authorized an adaptation for use in the United States, although all modifications had to conform to WHO conventions. The adaptation currently used in the United States is the ICD-10-CM. [Other countries also may apply for adaptations.] The *Clinical Modification* version provides much more detail and sometimes has separate sections for procedures.)

In 1995 the WHO approved the development of the *International Classification of Diseases, Tenth Revision, Clinical Modification* (ICD-10-CM) code set. This code set has a different format from that of the ICD-9-CM. As of October 1, 2015, the ICD-10-CM has been used in the United States. The ICD-11 was formally adopted by the World Health Assembly on May 25, 2019 to be effective beginning January 1, 2022. The U.S. is expected to adopt ICD-11 in 2025.

Medical Coding in the United States

As history dictates, the original purpose of medical coding was to collect statistical data. The United States is the only country in the world that uses coding for health insurance reimbursement purposes. Providers are responsible for billing the insurance company for any services rendered during the *encounter* (i.e., any meeting between a patient and a healthcare provider), and the provider must use approved medical codes for these procedures and services to obtain reimbursement. This means that the provider must supply diagnostic information that demonstrates the need for the rendered procedures or services. The provider assigns a diagnosis through an assessment of the patient.

All components of the encounter (i.e., diagnostic findings, procedures, and services) are used to determine the charges and generate an insurance claim. This chapter focuses on the ways the medical assistant should gather diagnostic information and translate it into a diagnostic code. The ICD-10-CM coding manual is used for this purpose.

What Is Diagnostic Coding?

Diagnostic coding changes written descriptions of diseases, illnesses, or injuries into alphanumeric codes. The ICD-10-CM code set uses up to seven characters to identify the disease or injury. Using the ICD-10-CM can help ensure both accurate health record documentation and efficient claims processing.

The ICD-10-CM code set is available through online resources, within the electronic health record (EHR) as an **encoder** or as a print manual. The print manual is produced by several publishers and may use different layouts, symbols, color coding, and some other features. For the coding manual, however, the format, conventions, tables, appendices, content, and basic structure are the same.

When you use the ICD-10-CM, you will be choosing a standardized alphanumeric code for the **diagnostic statement** assigned by the provider. Diagnostic statements are found in the following documents:

- Operative reports
- Discharge summaries
- History and physical exam (H&P) reports
- Reports on *ancillary diagnostic services* (e.g., radiology, pathology, and laboratory reports)

All of these should provide the patient's diagnosis or diagnoses. Healthcare providers use these reports to code and report clinical information. Diagnostic coding is required for participation in Medicare and Medicaid programs and by most insurance companies. The diagnostic codes are used on insurance claims. The ICD-10-CM codes tell the insurance company why the healthcare services or procedures were done. These codes are linked to the procedures that are performed. If the diagnosis code does not match the healthcare services or procedures provided, it may not be paid for. This linking can determine if a procedure or service is paid for. The diagnostic code can show that a procedure or service was **medically necessary**. If it is not medically necessary, the insurance company will not pay for it. For example, if diabetes mellitus is the diagnosis and the procedure is a throat culture, the insurance company would not pay it as it is not medically necessary for the treatment of diabetes mellitus. The ICD-10-CM is also used to keep track of various healthcare statistics related to disease and injury. Practice management software, clearinghouses, and insurance companies recognize these codes, which simplifies the coding process and speeds reimbursement to healthcare providers.

GETTING TO KNOW THE ICD-10-CM

The ICD-10-CM is a fairly complex system for diagnostic coding. It allows for a great deal of **specificity** for the diagnosis. It is important to understand the structure and format of the ICD-10-CM codes, as well as how to use the Alphabetic Index and the Tabular List. The next sections will help you to better understand ICD-10-CM.

Structure and Format of the ICD-10-CM

The ICD-10-CM has two sections:

- Alphabetic Index (the ICD-10-CM Index to Diseases and Injuries)
- Tabular List (officially, the ICD-10-CM Tabular List of Diseases and Injuries)

Determining an ICD-10-CM code starts in the Alphabetic Index and is confirmed in the Tabular List. These codes have three to seven characters (Figure 13.1). Every ICD-10-CM code begins with an alphabetic letter that indicates the chapter in the Tabular List from which the code originates (Table 13.1). All the letters of the English alphabet are used except U, which the WHO has reserved to assign to new diseases of uncertain **etiology**. Some conditions use more than one alphabetic letter in their code ranges. For example, the codes in Chapter 1, Certain Infectious and Parasitic Diseases (A00–B99), begin with the letter A or B. The second character is always numeric. The remaining characters can be a combination of letters and numbers. A decimal is required after the third character. Only certain codes require the seventh character. The following box describes the seventh character requirements in more detail.

ICD-10-CM Seventh Character Requirements

Seventh characters are used for many ICD-10-CM codes. The following list shows the chapters that may require a seventh character and what the character identifies:

- Chapter 13: Diseases of the Musculoskeletal System—Encounter
  - A: Initial encounter for fracture
  - D: Subsequent encounter for fracture with routine healing
  - G: Subsequent encounter for fracture with delayed healing
  - K: Subsequent encounter for fracture with nonunion
  - P: Subsequent encounter for fracture with malunion
  - S: Sequela
- Chapter 15: Pregnancy, Childbirth, and the Puerperium—Fetus identification
  - 0: Not applicable or unspecified
  - 1: Fetus 1
  - 2: Fetus 2
  - 3: Fetus 3
  - 4: Fetus 4
  - 5: Fetus 5
  - 9: Other fetus
- Chapter 18: Symptoms, Signs, and Abnormal Clinical and Laboratory Findings, Not Elsewhere Classified—Coma Scale
  - 0: Unspecified time
  - 1: In the field [emergency medical technicians (EMTs) or ambulance]
  - 2: At arrival to emergency department
  - 3: At hospital admission
  - 4: 24 hours or more after hospital admission
- Chapter 19: Injury, Poisoning, and Certain Other Consequences of External Causes—Encounter
  - A: Initial encounter
  - B: Initial encounter for open fracture
  - D: Subsequent encounter
  - G: Subsequent encounter for fracture with delayed healing
  - K: Subsequent encounter for fracture with nonunion
  - P: Subsequent encounter for fracture with malunion
  - S: Sequela
- Chapter 20: External Causes of Morbidity—Encounter
  - A: Initial encounter
  - D: Subsequent encounter
  - S: Sequela
- Chapter 21: Factors Influencing Health Status and Contact with Health Services—Encounter
  - A: Initial encounter
  - D: Subsequent encounter
  - S: Sequela

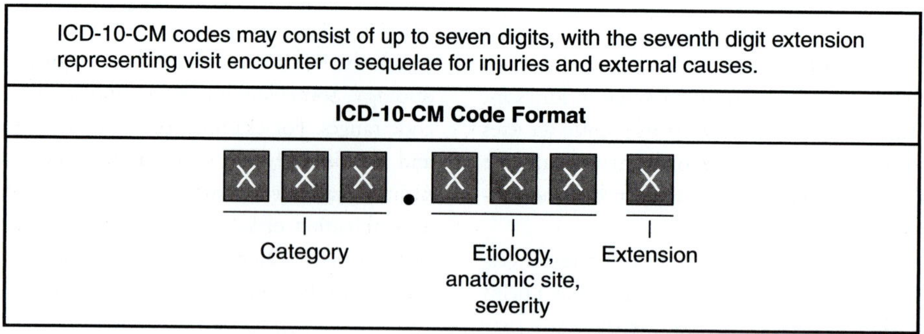

FIGURE 13.1 Code structure and format of ICD-10-CM codes.

TABLE 13.1 ICD-10-CM Tabular List of Diseases and Injuries

CHAPTER	TITLE	CODE RANGE	POSSIBLE DIAGNOSIS[a]	ICD-10-CM CODE
1	Certain Infectious and Parasitic Diseases	A00–B99	Measles	B05.9
2	Neoplasms	C00–D49	Colon cancer	C18.9
3	Diseases of the Blood and Blood-Forming Organs and Certain Disorders Involving the Immune Mechanism	D50–D89	Iron-deficiency anemia	D50.9
4	Endocrine, Nutritional, and Metabolic Diseases	E00–E89	Type I diabetes	E10
5	Mental, Behavioral, and Neurodevelopmental Disorders	F01–F99	Dementia	F03
6	Diseases of the Nervous System	G00–G99	Parkinson's disease	G20
7	Diseases of the Eye and Adnexa	H00–H59	Glaucoma	H40.9
8	Diseases of the Ear and Mastoid Process	H60–H95	Otitis media, left ear	H60.92
9	Diseases of the Circulatory System	I00–I99	Hypertensive heart disease	I11.9
10	Diseases of the Respiratory System	J00–J99	Acute sinusitis	J01.91
11	Diseases of the Digestive System	K00–K95	Inguinal hernia	K40
12	Diseases of the Skin and Subcutaneous Tissue	L00–L99	Pressure ulcer of right heel	L89.619
13	Diseases of the Musculoskeletal System and Connective Tissue	M00–M99	Rheumatoid arthritis	M05
14	Diseases of the Genitourinary System	N00–N99	Endometriosis	N80.9
15	Pregnancy, Childbirth, and the Puerperium	O00–O94	Ectopic pregnancy	O00.9
16	Certain Conditions Originating in the Perinatal Period	P00–P96	Neonatal jaundice	P59.9
17	Congenital Malformations, Deformations and Chromosomal Abnormalities	Q00–Q99	Cleft lip	Q37.9
18	Symptoms, Signs and Abnormal Clinical and Laboratory Findings, Not Elsewhere Classified	R00–R99	Abdominal pain	R10.9
19	Injury, Poisoning and Certain Other Consequences of External Causes	S00–T88	Left ankle fracture	S82.92xA
20	External Causes of Morbidity	V00–Y99	Snowboard accident	V00.318A
			Fall from cliff	W15
			Exposure to excessive natural cold	X31
21	Factors Influencing Health Status and Contact With Health Services	Z00–Z99	Pregnancy state	Z33.1

[a]All diagnoses presented are not otherwise specified (NOS).

The CMS prepares the Official Guidelines for Coding and Reporting to be used with the ICD-10-CM codes, in addition to instructions on how to report the codes on insurance claim forms. The guidelines are a set of rules that have been developed to accompany and complement the official conventions and instructions provided in the ICD-10-CM proper.

The Alphabetic Index

The Alphabetic Index consists of an alphabetic list of diagnostic terms and related codes. This index includes main terms, nonessential modifiers, essential modifiers, and subterms:

- *Main terms:* These terms appear in bold type.
- *Nonessential modifiers:* These terms follow the main term and are enclosed in parentheses. They are supplementary words or explanatory information. They do not need to be in the actual diagnostic statement.
- *Essential modifiers:* These terms are indented under the main term. They can modify the main term by describing different sites or etiology. They must be included in the diagnostic statement.

Figure 13.2 shows an example of an entry in the Alphabetic Index:

- The main term
- Nonessential modifiers
- Essential modifiers

Let's use the example of **chronic** ischemic colitis shown in Figure 13.2. You would start with the main term: Colitis. You can see that the main term is followed by the nonessential modifiers (acute, catarrhal, chronic, noninfective, hemorrhagic) that do not affect the code assignment. Follow the list to the modifying term: Ischemic. Indented under ischemic, you will find "chronic" with the code K55.1. You will look up K55.1 in the Tabular List.

You may also see the terms *see* or *see also* following the main term. *See* indicates another term should be referenced (e.g., **Bronchopleuropneumonia;** *see* Pneumonia). *See also* follows a main term and instructs that there is another main term, which may also be referenced and may provide additional Alphabetic Index entries that may be useful (e.g., **Boil**; *see also* furuncle, by site).

> **CRITICAL THINKING APPLICATION 13.1**
>
> Mike is working with the ICD-10-CM manual and is trying to refresh his memory about nonessential and essential modifiers. In your own words, define *essential modifier* and *nonessential modifier*. Compare your definitions with those of a classmate.

Supplementary Sections of the Alphabetic Index

The Alphabetic Index section includes two important tables:

- *Table of Neoplasms:* This table lists neoplasms by anatomic location. For coding purposes, neoplasms are further classified into six categories:
  - Malignant Primary
  - Malignant Secondary
  - Ca (cancer) in situ
  - Benign
  - Uncertain Behavior
  - Unspecified Behavior
- *Table of Drugs and Chemicals:* This table presents a classification of drugs and other chemical substances; it is used to identify

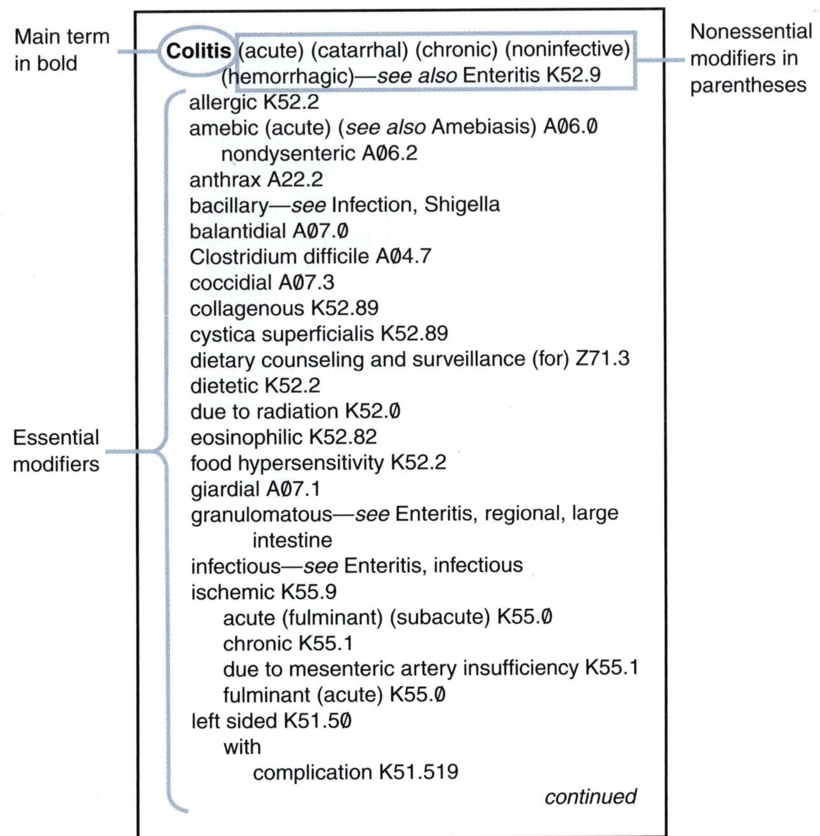

FIGURE 13.2 ICD-10-CM Alphabetic Index with main term, nonessential modifiers, and essential modifiers.

poisonings and external causes of adverse effects. There are six coding classifications:

- Poisoning, Accidental (Unintentional)
- Poisoning, Intentional Self-Harm
- Poisoning, Assault
- Poisoning, Undetermined
- Adverse Effect
- Underdosing

The Tabular List

The Tabular List is divided into 21 chapters. Most chapter titles specify a particular group of diseases and injuries, and all titles are followed by a code range in parentheses; for example, Chapter 1, Certain Infectious and Parasitic Diseases (A00–B99) (see Table 13.1). Some chapters use a body part or an organ system to group the codes:

- Chapter 7, Diseases of the Eye and Adnexa (H00–H59)
- Chapter 9, Diseases of the Circulatory System (I00–I99)

Other chapters group conditions by etiology or the nature of the disease process:

- Chapter 2, Neoplasms (C00–D49)
- Chapter 15, Pregnancy, Childbirth, and the Puerperium (O00–O9A)—groups codes related to the prenatal and postnatal periods
- Chapter 20, External Causes of Morbidity (V00–Y99)—also groups codes related to external causes of injury and poisoning
- Chapter 21, Factors Influencing Health Status and Contact with Health Services (Z00–Z99)

Each chapter is divided into subchapters or blocks, and each subchapter has a designated three-character code. These subchapter codes and code ranges form the foundation of the ICD-10-CM code set.

In each chapter, all the three-character block codes begin with the alphabetic letter assigned to that chapter. For example, in Chapter 6, Diseases of the Nervous System (G00–G99), all the block codes (and their versions) begin with G. If a chapter's code range includes two letters [e.g., Chapter 1, Certain Infectious and Parasitic Diseases (A00–B99)], each three-character block code begins with one of those two letters. The letter is followed by a two-character number. A summary of the blocks (Figure 13.3) at the beginning of each chapter provides an overview of the chapter.

As mentioned, the ICD-10-CM manual is produced by a variety of publishers, but many of the optional features are similar (remember, the important elements are always the same, regardless of the publisher). For instance, to enable the coder to better maneuver through the Alphabetic Index, each page has *guide words,* which are the first and last words on that page (this is the same arrangement used for the pages of a dictionary). Each chapter of the Tabular List has a different-colored border strip; in some manuals, this strip shows the chapter title and the range of codes found on that specific page. In the chapters in the Tabular List, the codes for each category/block are arranged alphabetically (by the initial alpha character) and then numerically. Familiarizing yourself with these tools can help you improve your proficiency as you work through the manual to find the most accurate code.

It is important to note that some codes do not need to be extended beyond the three-character code, and these are considered valid codes as is—for example, code **I10 Essential (primary) hypertension.**

If a code has only three characters, do not add a decimal after the third character. If a code has more than three characters, add a decimal point after the third character—for example, **K11.7 Disturbances of salivary secretion.** Most ICD-10-CM codes have four to seven characters.

Reporting NEC and NOS Codes

In some cases, because of limited documentation in the patient's health record, the medical assistant coder can find it difficult to assign an ICD-10-CM code with a higher **specificity**. The ICD-10-CM code set accommodates these coding circumstances by establishing "not elsewhere classified" (NEC) and "not otherwise specified" (NOS) guidelines.

- *NEC* means that the diagnostic statement contains specific wording, but no specific classification exists to match the wording. For example, an NEC code would be assigned if a patient seeks medical attention for **chronic** postoperative pain. The ICD-10-CM code would be **G89.28 Other chronic postprocedural pain.**
  - For all NEC codes, the last character is always 8.
- *NOS* means that the diagnostic statement does not contain any more specific wording. For example, sinusitis with no documentation of the specific sinus site is assigned the NOS code **J32.9 Chronic sinusitis, unspecified.**

  The coder should keep in mind that the lack of documentation does not mean that all patients' sinuses are inflamed. There must be no documentation of the exact site of the sinusitis for a non-NOS code to be assigned. As providers recognize that ICD-10-CM codes are more specific than ICD-9-CM codes, their documentation also is becoming more specific.
- For all NOS codes, the last character is always 9.

Chapter 14 *Diseases of the Genitourinary System (N00-N99)*

This chapter contains the following blocks:

NØØ-NØ8	Glomerular diseases
N1Ø-N16	Renal tubulo-interstitial diseases
N17-N19	Acute kidney failure and chronic kidney disease
N2Ø-N23	Urolithiasis
N25-N29	Other disorders of kidney and ureter
N3Ø-N39	Other disorders of the urinary system
N4Ø-N51	Diseases of male genital organs
N6Ø-N65	Disorders of male genital organs
N7Ø-N77	Inflammatory diseases of female pelvic organs
N8Ø-N98	Noninflammatory disorders of female genital tract
N99	Intraoperative and postprocedural complications and disorders of the genitourinary system, not elsewhere classified

FIGURE 13.3 Chapter blocks in the Tabular List.

CRITICAL THINKING APPLICATION 13.2

Mike is reviewing the Tabular List of the ICD-10-CM coding manual. He notices that each chapter begins with a list of diagnostic categories with a corresponding range of codes. What is this called? How can this feature be used as a tool for accurate ICD-10-CM code assignment?

Conventions Used in the Tabular List

Conventions are abbreviations, punctuation, symbols, instructional notations, and related entities that help the coder select an accurate, specific code. Conventions are found in the Tabular List but not in the Alphabetic Index. Understanding their meaning and using them as guides are crucial to accurate coding. Table 13.2 lists the most common conventions.

TABLE 13.2 Commonly Used Conventions in the Tabular List

CONVENTION	EXPLANATION	EXAMPLE
Placeholder character	ICD-10-CM uses the dummy placeholder X in two different ways. The dummy placeholder can be used as the fifth character in certain six-character codes; this allows for future expansion of the code set without interruption of the six-character structure. Specific categories have a seventh character, but may not use the fourth, fifth, or sixth characters. In these cases, the dummy placeholder X is used to fill the empty character spaces. Note that a dummy placeholder would not be needed for codes with fewer than seven characters.	T43.4X1A Poisoning by butyrophenone and thiothixene neuroleptics, accidental, initial encounter (unintentional) S50.01XA Contusion of right elbow
Punctuation	Four basic forms of punctuation are used in the Tabular List: brackets, parentheses, colons, and braces. Each form serves a different purpose to help you read and understand the code descriptions.	1. [ ] Brackets enclose synonyms, alternative wording, or explanatory phrases. 2. ( ) Parentheses are used to enclose supplementary words, which may be present or absent in the statement of a disease or procedure. 3. : Colons are used in the Tabular Index after an incomplete term that needs one or more of the modifiers or adjectives that follow to make it assignable. 4. { } Braces enclose a series of terms, each of which is modified by the statement appearing to the right of the brace.

Instructional notations	Instructional notations, which are found in both the Alphabetic Index and the Tabular List, are critical to correct coding practices. They are located directly under the main term.	• **Includes**: Further defines or gives examples of the content of the category.
		• **Excludes**: The ICD-10-CM uses two types of exclusion notes:
		  • Excludes1: This is a clear "NOT CODED HERE!" message. It means that the excluded code should never be used with the code above the Excludes1 note. For example, code **G14** **{Postpolio syndrome}** has this Excludes1 note: sequelae of poliomyelitis (B91).
		  • Excludes2: This means "not included here." The excluded condition is not part of the condition represented by the code; however, a patient may have both conditions. When an Excludes2 note is present, the coder may code both conditions if the patient presents with both. For example, code F02 **{Dementia in other diseases classified elsewhere}** has the following Excludes2 note: **vascular dementia** (F01.5). This means that vascular **dementia** is not part of the condition coded as F02; therefore, you can code both **dementia** (F02) and vascular dementia (F01.5) if the patient has both.
		• **Code first/Use additional code**: Code first notes appear under manifestation codes. Manifestation codes specify the way in which an underlying condition appears, or manifests, as a result of an underlying etiology; the main terms of most manifestation codes include the words "in diseases classified elsewhere." A Code first note indicates that the underlying condition must be coded first. For example, Code F02 **{Dementia in other diseases classified elsewhere}** states, Code first the underlying physiologic condition, such as: Alzheimer's (G30.-).

Continued

TABLE 13.2 Commonly Used Conventions in the Tabular List—continued

CONVENTION	EXPLANATION	EXAMPLE
Relational terms	These terms are used in both the Alphabetic Index and the Tabular List to clarify the context of the disease or injury.	1. *And:* In the Tabular List code titles *and* should be interpreted as meaning "and/or." 2. *With:* The term *with* should be interpreted as meaning "associated with" or "due to" when it appears in the Alphabetic Index, or in an instructional note or code title in the Tabular List. In the Alphabetic Index, the word *with* follows immediately after the main term, not in alphabetical order. 3. *Due to:* In both the Tabular List and the Alphabetic Index, the term *due to* signifies relationship between two conditions. This assumption can be made when both conditions are present or when the diagnostic statement indicates this relationship.

CRITICAL THINKING APPLICATION 13.3

Mike is looking for the ICD-10-CM code for morbid obesity. From the Alphabetic Index, Mike finds the code E66. When he goes to verify the code in the Tabular List, he finds that the main term, Overweight and obesity, has a symbol indicating that a fourth character is needed. What is Mike's next step to assign the most accurate code? Can Mike just use E66? Why or why not? Share your answer with the class.

Coding Guidelines

The coding manual begins with the ICD-10-CM Official Guidelines for Coding and Reporting. Every coding guideline for the entire ICD-10-CM code set is included in this section. The guidelines are a set of rules that have been developed to complement the official conventions and instructions provided in the ICD-10-CM proper. The guidelines are organized into four sections:

Section I. Conventions, General Coding Guidelines and Chapter Specific Guidelines: This section covers the structure and conventions of the ICD-10-CM classification system, in addition to the general guidelines that apply to the entire system. It also contains chapter-specific guidelines for each of the Tabular List's 21 chapters.

Section II. Selection of Principal Diagnosis: This section includes guidelines for the selection of a principal diagnosis for non-outpatient settings.

Section III. Reporting Additional Diagnoses: This section includes guidelines for reporting additional diagnoses in non-outpatient settings.

Section IV. Diagnostic Coding and Reporting Guidelines for Outpatient Services: As the title indicates, this section includes diagnostic coding and reporting guidelines for outpatient services.

The coding guidelines start with a table of contents for each of the four sections, including the related chapters on disease and injury. After the table of contents, the coding guidelines are presented in section order (i.e., Sections I through IV). For the purposes of outpatient medical office billing, you are most likely to need Sections I and IV.

PREPARING FOR DIAGNOSTIC CODING

Now that you have a basic understanding of the ICD-10-CM system, let's look at how you will find the information you need to determine diagnostic codes.

Abstracting Diagnostic Statements

To prepare for diagnostic coding, you must analyze the patient's health record and **abstract** the diagnostic statement documented in the various reports. Sources of diagnostic statements include the encounter form, treatment notes, discharge summary, operative report, and radiology, pathology, and laboratory reports. Let's take a look at those documents.

Encounter Form

The **encounter form** (also known as a *superbill*) can be viewed in the EHR or as a paper document. The most commonly used diagnostic and procedure codes are listed. The provider then indicates what services or procedures were done and the diagnosis code for the visit. It is important to update the encounter form annually with the new diagnostic and procedure codes. If outdated codes are used, it can delay or reduce the amount paid by the insurance company.

History and Physical Exam

The history and physical exam (H&P) are the starting point of the patient's medical evaluation. The H&P begins with a statement in the patient's own words that describes the reason for the visit. This statement, called the *chief complaint* (CC), is often abbreviated in the historical documentation of the health record. After the chief complaint, the provider documents any other pertinent history:

- Medical, current illness, and past medical history
  - History of present illness (HPI)
  - Previous illnesses
  - Previous hospitalizations
  - Previous surgeries
- Family history
  - Family members

  Current ages

  If deceased, age of death

  Any medical conditions

- Social history
  - Tobacco use
  - Alcohol use
  - Drug use

After recording the patient's history, the provider performs a physical examination. This includes both objective and subjective assessments of the patient's physical status. The final sections of an H&P include an assessment and a plan. The assessment is the provider's evaluation of the findings from the H&P, and it includes a diagnostic statement. The plan is the treatment plan for the conditions noted in the assessment; it may include x-ray studies, laboratory tests, surgery, administration of medications, or other treatments.

Progress Notes

Progress notes are the second most common medical document from which diagnostic statements are extracted. The format healthcare providers most commonly used for their notes is referred to as *SOAP notes*, a system of charting in which information is divided into ***s***ubjective findings, ***o***bjective findings, ***a***ssessment, and ***p***lan for treatment. Just as in the H&P, the diagnostic statement can most often be found in the assessment section of the SOAP notes.

Discharge Summary

The discharge summary is used primarily for abstracting diagnostic information for patients who were hospitalized rather than those seen in a provider's office. The main elements of a discharge summary are as follows:

- Admission date
- Date of discharge
- H&P findings
- Clinical course during hospitalization
- Health condition on discharge
- Discharge diagnosis
- Aftercare plan

Diagnostic statements are abstracted from the discharge diagnosis section. This diagnosis would be used to bill for the provider's visits to the patient while the person was in the hospital. The medical office can use a discharge summary as an overview of the patient's condition, especially if the discharge was recent.

Operative Report

For patients who have surgery as an outpatient or inpatient, the operative report also is used to abstract diagnostic statements. These are the elements in an operative report:

- Preliminary diagnosis
- Final diagnosis
- Detailed description of the operative procedure from start to finish

The medical assistant uses the final diagnosis when searching for and selecting a diagnostic code.

Radiology, Laboratory, and Pathology Reports

Radiology, laboratory, and pathology reports are used to support or establish the diagnostic statement. Any findings from these reports must be documented in the progress notes of the health record so they can be used for diagnostic coding, charge entry, or insurance billing purposes.

CRITICAL THINKING APPLICATION 13.4

While reviewing an encounter form, Mike noticed that the diagnostic statement indicated that the patient needed to be treated for a left inguinal hernia. However, Mike also notes that the surgical report indicates that the left inguinal hernia was obstructed. What should Mike use as the final diagnostic statement? Should he ask the provider which diagnostic statement to use?

Determining the Main Term in the Diagnostic Statement

To begin the search for the correct ICD-10-CM code, you must first find the diagnostic statement and then determine the main term in that statement. The main term is the key word or phrase that will be used in the Alphabetic Index to locate the code that will then be verified in the Tabular List. Main terms typically include the following:

- A disease (bronchitis or influenza)
- A condition (fracture, fatigue, or injury)
- An adjective (double, large, or kinked)
- A noun (a disease, disturbance, or syndrome)
- An eponym (diseases, procedures, or syndromes named after the individual who discovered or first used them, for example, Parkinson's disease)

Main terms are not anatomic sites. If the diagnostic statement was fracture of the right clavicle, the main term would be *fracture*. If the diagnostic statement was sore throat, the main term would be *sore*.

COVID-19

When the COVID-19 pandemic hit, it not only impacted the health of millions of people but also impacted diagnostic coding. This was a new disease with a wide range of complications. The World Health Organization (WHO) recognized that it could not wait until the annual update to provide codes that would cover COVID-19. Effective January 1, 2021, the following codes were implemented:

- Encounter for screening for COVID-19 (Z11.52)
- Contact with and (suspected) exposure to COVID-19 (Z20.822)
- Personal history of COVID-19 (Z86.16)
- Multisystem inflammatory syndrome (MIS) (M35.81)
- Other specified system involvement of connective tissue (M35.89)
- Pneumonia due to coronavirus disease 2019 (J12.82)

As of the writing of this textbook, these are the codes developed by the WHO. Due to the everchanging COVID-19 situation, you should review the most current coding guidelines before assigning a diagnostic code.

STEPS IN ICD-10-CM CODING

Accurate ICD-10-CM coding requires eight basic steps (Table 13.3). The first step involves abstracting the diagnostic statement from the health record and figuring out the main and modifying terms. Use the Alphabetic Index to search for the code or code ranges that best fit the diagnostic statement. The remaining steps are performed using the Tabular List to verify and confirm that the code or codes located in the Alphabetic Index fully match the diagnostic statement and that they are the most specific and accurate diagnostic codes. Procedure 13.1 details the basic coding steps using the ICD-10-CM manual and encoder software (i.e., TruCode).

TABLE 13.3 Diagnostic Coding Step-by-Step: Parkinson's Disease

Step	Action
Step 1	Determine the correct diagnosis from the diagnostic statement. • Parkinson's disease
Step 2	Use the main term to look up the diagnosis in the Alphabetic Index. • Parkinson's disease, syndrome, or tremor—see Parkinsonism
Step 3	Look up the "see" term in the Alphabetic Index. • Parkinsonism (idiopathic) (primary) G20
Step 4	Review the essential modifiers under the main term. 1. Parkinsonism (idiopathic) (primary) G20 • with neurogenic orthostatic hypotension (symptomatic) G90.3 • arteriosclerotic G21.4 • dementia G31.83 *[F02.80]* with behavioral disturbance G31.83 *[F02.81]* • due to • drugs NEC G21.19 • neuroleptic G21.11 • neuroleptic induced G21.11 • postencephalitic G21.3 • secondary G21.9 • due to • arteriosclerosis G21.4 • drugs NEC G21.19 neuroleptic G21.11 • encephalitis G21.3 • external agents NEC G21.2 • syphilis A52.19 • specified NEC G21.8 • syphilitic A52.19 • treatment-induced NEC G21.19 • vascular G21.4
Step 5	• Choose the correct essential modifier based on the diagnostic statement. • Because the diagnostic statement only indicates Parkinson's Disease, code G20 should be chosen.
Step 6	• Look up code G20 in the Tabular List. • G20 Parkinson's disease
Step 7	• Check for any coding guidelines, conventions, inclusion or exclusion notes, or an additional character symbol. Includes: Hemiparkinson's; Idiopathic Parkinsonism or Parkinson's disease; Paralysis agitans; Parkinsonism or Parkinson's disease NOS; Primary Parkinsonism or Parkinson's disease Excludes1: dementia with Parkinsonism (G31.83)
Step 8	• Assign the final ICD-10-CM code. • G20 Parkinson's disease

Using the Alphabetic Index

After the diagnostic statement has been abstracted from the health record, identify the main term and start searching for the best code, or code range, in the Alphabetic Index. It is important to note that the Alphabetic Index should be used only as a tool to locate the appropriate code or code range. The Tabular List, with its conventions, punctuation, notes, and guidelines, must always be used to confirm that the code or codes selected are accurate and specific and that there are no contraindications to the use of the code found in the Alphabetic Index. For this reason, never assign a code directly from the Alphabetic Index. Even if only one code is found in the Alphabetic Index, it may be used only if a thorough review of the conventions and instructional notations in the Tabular List does not **contraindicate** it.

Figure 13.4 shows an excerpt from the Alphabetic Index for the main term **Cyst.** The first essential modifier is *eyelid.* Note the nonessential modifier, *sebaceous,* in parentheses after eyelid. (Remember, nonessential modifiers add detail, but they do not have to be present in the diagnostic statement for the code to be acceptable for use.) Directly below the essential modifier *eyelid* are the subterms. Note that there are separate subterms for the left and right eye. In addition, the diagnostic codes for each eye are further modified by the location of the cyst (upper or lower).

Cyst—*continued*
eyelid (sebaceous) HØ2.829
infected—*see* Hordeolum
left HØ2.826
lower HØ2.825
upper HØ2.824
right HØ2.823
lower HØ2.822
upper HØ2.821

FIGURE 13.4 Excerpt from the Alphabetic Index: Cyst (main term), eyelid (essential modifier), sebaceous (nonessential modifier).

H02.82	**Cysts of eyelid**	
	Sebaceous cyst of eyelid	
	H02.821	**Cysts of right upper eyelid**
	H02.822	**Cysts of right lower eyelid**
	H02.823	**Cysts of right eye, unspecified eyelid**
	H02.824	**Cysts of left upper eyelid**
	H02.825	**Cysts of left lower eyelid**
	H02.826	**Cysts of left eye, unspecified eyelid**
	H02.829	**Cysts of unspecified eye, unspecified eyelid**

FIGURE 13.5 Excerpt from the Tabular List: H02.82 Cysts of eyelid.

Using the Tabular List

Once you have identified at least the first three characters of the code in the Alphabetic Index, turn to the Tabular List. The chapters in the Tabular List are arranged alphabetically according to the initial letter of the three-character code or codes assigned to each chapter. For example, Chapter 1 has code range A00–B99, Chapter 2 has code range C00–D49, Chapter 3 has code range D50–D89, and so on.

From the preceding example, you've determined that the code you probably need is in the H02 code range. Turn to the chapter that includes that range (Chapter 7). Figure 13.5, an excerpt from the Tabular List, shows **Cysts of eyelid** as a main term, with the code H02.82. (Note that the nonessential modifier, *sebaceous,* is not shown in parentheses; rather, it appears under the main term in the nonbold phrase "Sebaceous cyst of eyelid.")

In the coding manual, you would see the "additional character" symbol, which indicates that code H02.82 requires one more character. All possible diagnoses with six-character codes are indented below the main term. A closer look at the disorders and their codes shows that the sixth character specifies the right or left eye and the location of the cyst on the eyelid (upper or lower). For the not-specified code, 9 would be the sixth character position.

Encoder Software

Encoder software (e.g., TruCode) is a tool commonly used by coders to assist in medical coding. This software performs computer-aided coding to assign the most accurate code possible. (TruCode is especially helpful to students because it allows them to search the ICD-10-CM manual using a few key terms.) The coder types a few key words into a search box, and the software finds the most likely matches in the Alphabetic Index. The coder then clicks on a specific code, and the software searches the Tabular List. From the Tabular List, the coder can scroll up and down to determine the most accurate code. Encoder software can increase the speed and efficiency of coding for a wide variety of medical cases.

CRITICAL THINKING APPLICATION **13.5**

Mike has determined a diagnostic statement to be "Perforation of the tympanic membrane in the left ear." What key word should be used for the TruCode software search box? What main term will the encoder go to in the Alphabetic Index? What should Mike click to get to the Tabular List? At what point can Mike be sure that he has assigned the most accurate and specific code?

UNDERSTANDING CODING GUIDELINES

All ICD-10-CM coding manuals, regardless of the publisher, have comprehensive instructional notations and conventions to help the coder select the most accurate diagnostic code or codes. When there is a difference between reference sources (including this text), the current year's ICD-10-CM coding manual is the final authority—this fact cannot be emphasized enough. When coding, you must always refer to and thoroughly review the conventions, instructional notations, code definitions, and other guidelines in the Alphabetic Index and Tabular List in the current year's version of the ICD-10-CM.

The following instructions are designed to provide some additional guidance in selecting diagnostic codes from various chapters in the ICD-10-CM. But they are not to be considered a replacement for the ICD-10-CM manual, nor do they provide all the coding information, definitions, or explanations found in the manual. The steps for diagnostic coding (see Procedure 13.1) are the same for all chapters of the ICD-10-CM; however, special rules and considerations apply to some chapters that affect the code selection process.

Coding of Signs and Symptoms

Signs and symptoms are coded only if the provider has not yet determined the final diagnosis. For example, if the provider's notes state "rule out," "probable," or "suspected," the coder should use the patient's documented signs and symptoms, including subjective and objective findings. *Subjective findings* include the patient's chief complaint or statements about why the patient is seeking medical care. *Objective findings* are any measurable indicators found during the physical examination. If a provider sees a patient who comes in with a sore throat and fever occurring over the past 3 days and the provider states "suspected strep throat" as the diagnosis, you will code sore throat and fever.

In the Tabular List, ill-defined conditions, signs, and symptoms are found in Chapter 18, Symptoms, Signs, and Abnormal Clinical and Laboratory Findings, Not Elsewhere Classified (R00–R99).

Conditions, signs, and symptoms found in Chapter 18 include the following:

- Not elsewhere classified (NEC) cases, even after all the facts of the medical case has been examined
- Signs or symptoms that existed on the first encounter but were temporary and for which causes could not be determined
- Conditional diagnosis for a patient who failed to return for further care and the cause of whose condition had not yet been determined
- Medical cases referred elsewhere for treatment before a diagnosis could be made
- Not otherwise specified (NOS) cases in which a more precise diagnosis was not available for any reason
- Certain symptoms for which supplementary information is provided that represent important problems in the medical care provided

Coding the Etiology and Manifestation

Etiology refers to the underlying cause or origin of a disease. *Manifestation* describes the signs and symptoms of the disease. In the Alphabetic Index, the etiology and manifestation codes are listed together. The etiology code is always listed first, and the manifestation code is listed beside it in italics and enclosed within brackets. If the diagnosis in the health record indicated **cataract** due to **myxedema**, you would find the following listed in the Alphabetic Index:

- **cataract** (cortical) (immature) (incipient) H26.9
  myxedema E03.9 [H28]
- E03.9 is the myxedema (underlying condition/etiology)
  H28 is the cataract (condition being treated today/manifestation)

You would need to verify both codes in the Tabular List and list both codes in the documentation, and sequencing would be based on the convention "code first underlying disease."

Multiple Coding

In addition to the signs and symptoms that require two codes to fully describe a single condition affecting multiple body systems, other single conditions may require more than one code. In the Tabular List, *Use additional code* notes appear with codes that are not part of an etiology/manifestation pair but in which a secondary code is useful to fully describe a condition. The sequencing rule is the same as for the etiology/manifestation pair: *use additional code* indicates that a secondary code should be added after the condition code.

For example, consider a bacterial infection that is not included in Chapter 1, Certain Infectious and Parasitic Diseases (A00–B99). A secondary code may be required to identify the organism causing the infection. This secondary code may come from category **B95 *Streptococcus, Staphylococcus,* and *Enterococcus* as the cause of diseases classified elsewhere,** or from category **B96 Other bacterial agents as the cause of diseases classified elsewhere.**

A *use additional code* note normally is found at the infectious disease code, indicating that the organism code must be added as a secondary code.

As mentioned, *code first* notes are used for certain conditions that involve both an underlying etiology and multiple body system manifestations caused by that etiology. In such cases, the underlying condition should be sequenced first before the manifestations.

A *code, if applicable, any causal condition first* note indicates that this code may be assigned as a principal diagnosis when the causal condition is unknown or not applicable. If the causal condition is known, the code for that condition should be sequenced as the principal, or first-listed, diagnosis.

Multiple codes may be needed for sequelae, and complication codes and obstetric codes may be needed to describe a condition more fully. See the specific guidelines for these conditions.

Sequela (Late Effects) Codes

Sequelae are the lingering effects produced by a health condition after the acute phase of an illness or injury has ended. The acute phase is considered the first 30 days of a condition with no improvement. There is no time limit on when a **sequela** code can be used. The residual effect may be apparent early (e.g., another stroke) or may occur months or years later (e.g., the consequences of a previous injury). Coding of sequelae generally requires two codes sequenced in the following order: the original condition or nature of the sequela is sequenced first; the sequela code is sequenced second.

An exception to these guidelines is instances in which the code for the sequela is followed by a manifestation code identified in the Tabular List, or the sequela code has been expanded (at the fourth, fifth, or sixth character) to include the manifestation or manifestations. The code for the acute phase of an illness or injury that led to the sequela is never used with a code for the late effect. The following box presents the rules for coding **impending** or threatened conditions.

Rules for Coding Impending or Threatened Conditions

Code any condition described at the time of discharge as "impending" or "threatened."

1. If it did occur, code as a confirmed diagnosis.
2. If it did not occur, consult the Alphabetic Index to determine whether the condition has a subterm for impending or threatened; also, check main term entries for Impending and threatened.
3. If the subterms are listed, assign the given code.
4. If the subterms are not found, code the existing underlying condition or conditions, signs, or symptoms, and not the condition described as "threatened" or "impending."
   Examples: Impending myocardial infarction—I20.0; threatened labor (without delivery) O47.9

Coding Complications of Care

A complication from medical care generally requires additional procedures or services for a patient, but often the complication is not mentioned as part of the diagnostic statement; this can result in reduced reimbursement. It is important to review the medical documentation to determine whether a complication exists and to code the complication in addition to the diagnostic statement. Keep in mind, not all conditions that occur during or after medical care or surgery are classified as complications. Two criteria must be met: a cause-and-effect relationship must be established between the care provided and the condition, and the documentation must indicate that the condition is a complication, such as postprocedural hemorrhage.

Coding Infectious and Parasitic Diseases

Multiple diagnostic codes are needed to code infectious or parasitic diseases. The first code identifies the disease or condition (e.g., throat infection), and the second identifies the organism causing the disease (e.g., enterovirus). The second code can be found in the Tabular List in Chapter 1. The basic coding principles for using either combination or multiple codes apply throughout this section of the ICD-10-CM.

Coding Organism-Caused Diseases

The two-step process of coding organism-caused diseases begins with the affected anatomic site. In the case of a throat infection caused by an enterovirus, you should first assign the diagnostic code for throat infection or pharyngitis. In the Tabular List, code **J02.8 Acute pharyngitis due to other specified organisms** is accompanied by the following *Use additional code* note: "Use additional code (B95–B97) to identify infectious agent" (Figure 13.6). In the Tabular List, the B95–B97 category/block (found in Chapter 1) is titled Bacterial and Viral Infectious Agents. Starting with code B95, search for the code that specifies enterovirus; this happens to be code **B97.1 Enterovirus as the cause of diseases classified elsewhere**.

Note that code B97.1 requires a fifth character; however, no other information is provided by the medical record. Therefore, you can assign code **B97.19 Other enterovirus as the cause of diseases classified elsewhere** as the final organism code.

Coding for Specific Conditions

There are a number of conditions that require specific instructions for diagnostic coding. These conditions are described in the following sections.

Coding Human Immunodeficiency Virus (HIV) Infection and Acquired Immunodeficiency Syndrome (AIDS)

To correctly code HIV infection and AIDS, it is essential to first understand the descriptions of the codes available. The key is whether the patient has symptoms.

- HIV: This only indicates that the virus is present.
- AIDS: AIDS is a syndrome; a *syndrome* is defined as a "group of symptoms occurring together." AIDS is the manifestation of signs or symptoms that can occur as a result of HIV infection.

Never code a patient as having HIV infection unless it is clearly documented as confirmed. Probable and suspected cases are never coded; instead, the signs and symptoms present should be coded. If a patient is seen for an HIV-related condition, the principal diagnosis should be **B20 Human immunodeficiency virus [HIV] disease**, followed by additional diagnostic codes for all reported HIV-related conditions.

Remember that strict restrictions are placed on the disclosure of medical information about patients with HIV infection or AIDS. Make sure the patient has signed the appropriate release of medical information form before any disclosures are made to third parties.

Coding Neoplasms

A *neoplasm*, or new growth, is coded by the site or location of the neoplasm and its behavior. The Table of Neoplasms (Figure 13.7) is located just after the Alphabetic Index in the coding manual. This table lists the ICD-10-CM codes for neoplasms by the anatomic site in alphabetic order. Six possible code numbers exist for each anatomic site, depending on whether the neoplasm is malignant or benign, exhibits uncertain behavior, or is of an unspecified nature. In the Table of Neoplasms, malignant neoplasms are categorized into three separate subclassifications: Malignant Primary, Malignant Secondary, and Ca in situ (carcinoma in situ).

Terms Defining Malignant Neoplasm Sites

- *Malignant Primary:* Identifies the originating anatomic site of the neoplasm. A primary malignancy is defined as the original site or sites of the cancer.
- *Malignant Secondary:* Identifies sites where the primary neoplasm has metastasized (spread). A secondary malignancy is defined as a second location to which the cancer has spread from the primary location.
- *Ca in situ*: Carcinoma in situ is defined as the absence of invasion of surrounding tissues. Tumor cells are undergoing malignant changes but are still confined to the point of origin, without

• J02.8 Acute pharyngitis due to other specified organisms

Use additional code (B95-B97) to identify infectious agent
Excludes1 pharyngitis due to coxsackie virus (B08.5)
pharyngitis due to gonococcus (A54.5)
acute pharyngitis due to herpes [simplex] virus (B00.2)
acute pharyngitis due to infectious mononucleosis (B27.-)
enteroviral vesicular pharyngitis (B08.5)

FIGURE 13.6 Excerpt from the Tabular List: J02.8 Acute pharyngitis due to other specified organisms.

	Malignant Primary	Malignant Secondary	Ca in situ	Benign	Uncertain Behavior	Unspecified Nature		Malignant Primary
bladder (urinary)	C67.9	C79.11	DØ9Ø	D3Ø.3	D41.4	D49.4	marrow NEC	C96.9
dome	C67.1	C79.11	DØ9Ø	D3Ø.3	D41.4	D49.4	unspecified side	C4Ø.1Ø
neck	C67.5	C79.11	DØ9Ø	D3Ø.3	D41.4	D49.4	marrow NEC	C96.9
orifice	C67.9	C79.11	DØ9Ø	D3Ø.3	D41.4	D49.4	cartilage NEC	C41.9
ureteric	C67.6	C79.11	DØ9Ø	D3Ø.3	D41.4	D49.4	clavicle	C41.3
urethral	C67.5	C79.11	DØ9Ø	D3Ø.3	D41.4	D49.4	marrow NEC	C96.9
overlapping lesion	C67.8	—	—	—	—	—	clivus	C41.Ø
sphincter	C67.8	C79.11	DØ9Ø	D3Ø.3	D41.4	D49.4	marrow NEC	C96.9
trigone	C67.Ø	C79.11	DØ9Ø	D3Ø.3	D41.4	D49.4	coccygeal vertebra	C41.4
urachus	C67.7	—	DØ9Ø	D3Ø.3	D41.4	D49.4	marrow NEC	C96.9
wall	C67.9	C79.11	DØ9Ø	D3Ø.3	D41.4	D49.4	coccyx	C41.4
anterior	C67.3	C79.11	DØ9Ø	D3Ø.3	D41.4	D49.4	marrow NEC	C96.9
lateral	C67.2	C79.11	DØ9Ø	D3Ø.3	D41.4	D49.4	costal cartilage	C41.3
posterior	C67.4	C79.11	DØ9Ø	D3Ø.3	D41.4	D49.4	costovertebral joint	C41.3
blood vessel—*see* Neoplasm,							marrow NEC	C96.9
connective tissue							cranial	C41.Ø

FIGURE 13.7 Excerpt from the Table of Neoplasms.

invasion of surrounding normal tissue. The *Ca in situ* column is used only if the provider documents that precise terminology.

Most coding decisions on malignant neoplasms are between the primary and secondary classifications. Other terms are used in the following cases:

- *In situ* is used only when the diagnostic statement contains that exact phrase.
- *Unspecified* is used only when no pathologic study has been done, and the neoplasm is still described with a term such as *tumor* or *growth*.

Uncertain is used when the pathologic study has been done, but it cannot be determined whether the neoplasm is malignant or benign.

Definitions of Benign, Uncertain Behavior, and Unspecified Nature Neoplasms

- *Benign:* The growth is noncancerous, nonmalignant, and has not invaded adjacent structures or spread to distant sites.
- *Uncertain Behavior:* The pathologist is unable to determine whether the neoplasm is benign or malignant.
- *Unspecified Nature:* Neither the behavior nor the **histologic** type of neoplasm is specified in the diagnostic statement.

Six Steps for Coding Neoplasms. The following steps can help determine the most specific and accurate diagnostic code for a neoplasm. These steps can be used in addition to the basic diagnostic steps:

1. In the Table of Neoplasms, find the site (anatomic location) of the neoplasm.
2. Determine, from the documentation, whether the neoplasm is malignant or benign.
3. If the neoplasm is benign, select the correct column in the table by reviewing the diagnostic statement.
4. If the neoplasm is malignant, select the column in the table that best fits its behavior: Malignant Primary, Malignant Secondary, or Ca in situ.
5. Link the appropriate column to the appropriate row.
6. Check the code shown in the table with the code in the Tabular List to make sure it complies with the guidelines, conventions, and instructional notations of the latter.

The ICD-10-CM manual always provides additional information, definitions, and guidelines for coding neoplasms in the Tabular List, just as it does for all other diseases, illnesses, and injuries.

Coding for Diabetes Mellitus

Diabetes mellitus (DM) is classified as type 1 or type 2. Patients with DM type 1 develop the disease because the pancreas is unable to produce insulin. In individuals with DM type 2, the pancreas has become unable to maintain the level of insulin the body needs to function, or the person has developed target cell resistance to insulin.

The diabetes mellitus codes are combination codes. This means that they include the type of diabetes mellitus, the body system affected, and the complications affecting that body system. Use as many codes within a particular category/block as necessary to describe all the complications of the disease. These codes should be sequenced according to the reason for a particular encounter. Assign as many codes from category/block E08–E13 (Diabetes Mellitus) as needed to identify all the patient's associated conditions.

Diabetes Mellitus and the Use of Insulin. In the ICD-10-CM, the primary codes for diabetes mellitus (E08–E13) do not include whether the individual is using insulin. Therefore, if insulin use is documented in the health record, a second code is required: **Z79.4 Long term (current) use of insulin**.

Code Z79.4 should not be assigned if insulin is given temporarily during an encounter to bring the blood glucose level under control in a patient with DM type 2.

Gestational Diabetes. Gestational, or pregnancy-induced, diabetes can occur during the second and third trimesters of pregnancy in women who were not diabetic before pregnancy. Gestational diabetes can cause complications in the pregnancy similar to those of preexisting diabetes mellitus. It also puts the woman at greater risk of developing diabetes after the pregnancy. Codes for gestational diabetes are in subcategory **O24.4 Gestational diabetes mellitus** and should be used with a code from subcategory O24.4. The codes under subcategory O24.4 include diet controlled (O24.410) and insulin controlled (024.414). If a patient with gestational diabetes is treated with both diet and insulin, only the code for insulin controlled is required.

No other code from category **O24 Diabetes mellitus in pregnancy, childbirth, and the puerperium** should be assigned.

Code **Z79.4 Long-term (current) use of insulin** should also be assigned with codes from subcategory O24.4 if the patient is being treated with insulin.

An abnormal glucose tolerance level in pregnancy is assigned a code from subcategory **O99.81 Abnormal glucose complicating pregnancy, childbirth, and the puerperium**.

Coding for the Circulatory System

Providers use a wide variety of terms and phrases to identify components of the circulatory system. To code disorders of the circulatory system accurately, the coder must carefully review all inclusions, exclusions, conventions, guidelines, and instructional notations associated with each potential code selected.

Myocardial Infarction. A myocardial infarction (MI) is coded as follows:

- As *acute,* if it is documented as such in the diagnostic statement or has a stated duration of 8 weeks or less.
- As *chronic,* if it is so stated in the diagnostic statement or if symptoms persist after 8 weeks.

Other MI coding considerations include the following:

1. If an MI is specified as "old" or "healed" without any current or presenting symptoms, it should be coded using category **I21 ST elevation (STEMI) and non-ST elevation (NSTEMI) myocardial infarction.**
2. A history of an MI uses code **I25.2 Old myocardial infarction.** This code is used only if the patient has no symptoms and only if the old MI was diagnosed by means of an electrocardiogram.
3. If the patient is symptomatic, code the underlying condition or symptoms only if the underlying condition is not known: **I21.3 ST elevation (STEMI) myocardial infarction of unspecified site.**

Hypertensive Disease. A distinction is made in the ICD-10-CM between "elevated" and "high" blood pressure. High blood pressure is defined as hypertension [**I10 Essential (primary) hypertension**]. If a diagnostic statement does not contain the word *hypertension* or the phrase *high blood pressure,* the condition is coded as elevated blood pressure [**R03.0 Elevated blood-pressure reading, without diagnosis of hypertension**], not hypertension.

Hypertension frequently is the cause of various forms of heart and vascular disease; however, the mention of hypertension in the diagnostic statement does not mean that a combination code for hypertensive heart disease should be used. If a cause-and-effect relationship exists between hypertension and heart disease, it should be clearly documented in the clinical record or diagnostic statement.

The hypertension table in the ICD-9-CM was not included in the ICD-10-CM. Heart conditions classified to category **I50 Heart failure** or subcategories I51.4–I51.9 are assigned to a code from category **I11 Hypertensive heart disease** when a causal relationship is stated in the health record ("as a result of hypertension") or implied ("hypertensive"). Use an additional code from category I50 to identify the *type* of heart failure in patients with heart failure.

The same heart conditions (category I50 or subcategories I51.4–I51.9) with hypertension, but without a stated causal relationship, are coded separately. The codes should sequence according to the circumstances of the admission or encounter.

Coding for Chronic Kidney Disease

Assign codes from category **I12 Hypertensive chronic kidney disease** when both hypertension and a condition classifiable to category **N18 Chronic kidney disease (CKD)** are present. Unlike hypertension with heart disease, the ICD-10-CM presumes a cause-and-effect relationship and classifies chronic kidney disease with hypertension as hypertensive chronic kidney disease.

The appropriate code from category N18 should be used as a secondary code with a code from category I12 to identify the stage of chronic kidney disease.

If a patient has hypertensive chronic kidney disease and acute renal failure, an additional code for acute renal failure is required.

Coding for Atherosclerotic Cardiovascular Disease

The ICD-10-CM has combination codes for atherosclerotic heart disease with angina pectoris. The subcategories for these codes are **I25.11 Atherosclerotic heart disease of native coronary artery with angina pectoris** and **I25.7 Atherosclerosis of coronary artery bypass graft(s) and coronary artery of transplanted heart with angina pectoris.**

When you use one of these combination codes, you do not need to use an additional code for angina pectoris. A causal relationship can be assumed in a patient with both atherosclerosis and angina pectoris unless the documentation indicates that the angina is due to something other than atherosclerosis.

If a patient with coronary artery disease is admitted because of acute myocardial infarction (AMI), the AMI should be sequenced before the coronary artery disease.

Coding for Skin Ulcers

Codes from category **L89 Pressure ulcer** are combination codes that identify the site of the pressure ulcer and the stage of the ulcer. The ICD-10-CM classifies pressure ulcer stages based on severity, which is designated by stages 1 to 4; unspecified stage; or unstageable. Unspecified and unstageable codes are used for pressure ulcers when the stage cannot be clinically determined (e.g., the ulcer has been treated with a skin or muscle graft). These codes are also used for pressure ulcers documented as deep tissue injuries, but not documented as being due to trauma. The modifying term defines each stage, depending on the location of the ulcer (Figure 13.8).

L89.21 Pressure ulcer of right hip
- **L89.210 Pressure ulcer of right hip, unstageable**
- **L89.211 Pressure ulcer of right hip, stage I**
  - Healing pressure ulcer of right hip back, stage I
  - Pressure pre-ulcer skin changes limited to persistent focal edema, right hip
- **L89.212 Pressure ulcer of right hip, stage II**
  - Healing pressure ulcer of right hip, stage II
  - Pressure ulcer with abrasion, blister, partial thickness skin loss involving epidermis and/or dermis, right hip
- **L89.213 Pressure ulcer of right hip, stage III**
  - Healing pressure ulcer of right hip, stage III
  - Pressure ulcer with full thickness skin loss involving damage or necrosis of subcutaneous tissue, right hip
- **L89.214 Pressure ulcer of right hip, stage IV**
  - Healing pressure ulcer of right hip, stage IV
  - Pressure ulcer with necrosis of soft tissues through to underlying muscle, tendon, or bone, right hip
- **L89.219 Pressure ulcer of right hip, unspecified stage**
  - Healing pressure ulcer of right hip NOS
  - Healing pressure ulcer of right hip, unspecified stage

FIGURE 13.8 Coding Example: L89.21 Pressure ulcer of right hip.

Coding for Complications of Pregnancy, Childbirth, and the Puerperium

Coding for the obstetric patient is like using a specialty codebook within the ICD-10-CM coding manual. This is challenging for coders who do not code obstetrics often. Here are some important clinical terms regarding pregnancy:

- *antepartum*: Pregnancy (applies as soon as a pregnancy test result is positive)
- *childbirth:* Delivery
- *postpartum:* The *puerperium*, or first 6 weeks after delivery
- *peripartum:* The period from the last month of pregnancy to 5 months postpartum

Obstetrics cases use codes from Chapter 15, Pregnancy, Childbirth, and the Puerperium (O00–O9A). Additional codes from other chapters may be used in conjunction with Chapter 15 codes to further specify conditions.

If the provider documents that the pregnancy is incidental to the encounter, code **Z33.1 Pregnant state, incidental** should be used instead of any Chapter 15 codes. This would be the case if the patient were being seen for a sprained ankle. The sprained ankle is not related to the pregnancy but is an incidental diagnosis. It is the provider's responsibility to state that the condition being treated is not affecting the pregnancy. Codes from Chapter 15 are documented only in the maternal health record; they are never used in the health record of the newborn.

Most of the codes in Chapter 15 have a sixth character, which indicates the trimester of pregnancy. Assignment of the final character for the trimester should be based on the provider's documentation of the trimester (or number of weeks) for the encounter. This applies to the assignment of trimester for preexisting conditions, in addition to those that develop during or are due to the pregnancy. The provider's documentation of the number of weeks may be used to assign the appropriate code identifying the trimester. The seventh character in this chapter is used to identify the fetus when there is more than one.

Outcome of Delivery and Liveborn Infant Codes. When a delivery occurs, the principal diagnosis should correspond to the main circumstances or complications of the delivery. In cases of cesarean delivery, the selection of the principal diagnosis should be the condition assigned after the encounter that was responsible for the patient's admission. If the patient was admitted with a condition that resulted in the performance of a cesarean procedure, that condition should be selected as the principal diagnosis. If the reason for the admission was unrelated to the condition resulting in the cesarean delivery, the condition related to the reason for the admission/encounter should be selected as the principal diagnosis.

For example, a maternity patient was admitted to the hospital for pneumonia, but because of complications, a cesarean section was performed. In this case, the pneumonia would be the primary diagnosis. A code from category **Z37 Outcome of delivery** should always be included in the maternal health record when a delivery has occurred. Codes from category Z37 are not to be used in subsequent records or the newborn's health record.

Code **O80 Encounter for full-term uncomplicated delivery** should be assigned when a woman is admitted for a full-term vaginal delivery and delivers a single, healthy infant without any complications antepartum, during the delivery, or postpartum during the delivery episode. Code O80 is always a principal diagnosis.

H4: Newborn Coding. Chapter 16, Certain Conditions Originating in the Perinatal Period (P00–P96), also is used for coding and reporting purposes. The perinatal period extends from just before the birth through day 28 after the birth. When you code the birth episode in a newborn's health record, assign a code from category **Z38 Liveborn infants according to place of birth and type of delivery** as the principal diagnosis. A code from category Z38 is assigned only once to a newborn at the time of birth. If a newborn is transferred to another institution, a code from category Z38 should not be used at the receiving hospital. When a newborn is admitted to another hospital, the newborn's admitting diagnosis is the health condition that requires the hospital transfer.

Coding for Injuries

When you code injuries, assign separate codes for each injury unless a combination code is provided, in which case the combination code is assigned. Code **T07 Unspecified multiple injuries** should not be assigned in the inpatient setting unless documentation for a more specific code is not available. Traumatic injury codes (S00–T14.9) are not to be used for normal, healing surgical wounds or to identify complications of surgical wounds.

The code for the most serious injury, as determined by the provider and the focus of treatment, is sequenced first.

Superficial Injuries. Superficial injuries, such as abrasions and contusions, are not coded when they are associated with more severe injuries at the same site.

Primary Injury with Damage to Nerves or Blood Vessels. When a primary injury results in minor damage to peripheral nerves or blood vessels, the primary injury is sequenced first. Any additional code or codes for injuries to nerves and the spinal cord or injury to vessels or nerves are coded as secondary.

Coding for Traumatic Fractures

The principles of multiple coding of injuries should be followed in the coding of fractures. Fractures of specified sites are coded individually by site in accordance with the level of detail furnished by the health record. The traumatic fracture categories include the following: A02, S12, S22, S32, S42, S49, S52, S59, S62, S72, S82, S89, and S92. A fracture not indicated as open or closed should be coded as closed. A fracture not indicated as displaced or not displaced should be coded as displaced.

Coding for Burns and Corrosions

The same principles for multiple coding apply to burns. Code each burn separately unless specific combination codes are given in the Tabular List. There are many combination codes. Most burn codes are found in Chapter 19 (Injury, Poisoning, and Certain Other Consequences of External Origin); the applicable codes are T20–T32. Because burns are coded by site and degree and by the extent of body surface involvement, all burn cases should have at least two codes and a third if the wound is infected. Other types of wounds, lacerations, punctures, and so on, use a different fifth character to show that they are infected and, therefore, complicated. However, burn codes use the fifth character for other information. Therefore, these diagnoses require an additional code to indicate infection.

The ICD-10-CM makes a distinction between burns and corrosions. The burn codes are used for the following: thermal burns (except sunburns) caused by a heat source, such as a fire or hot appliance; burns resulting from electricity; and burns resulting from radiation. Corrosions, on the other hand, are burns caused by chemicals. The guidelines are the same for burns and corrosions.

Current burns (T20–T25) are classified by depth, extent, and burn agent (X code). Depth is categorized as first degree (redness), second degree (blistering), and third degree (full-thickness involvement). Burns of the eye and internal organs (T26–T28) are classified by site but not by degree.

Coding for Drug Toxicity

Chapter 19 also includes coding for the following drug toxicity classifications:

- *Poisoning* (T36–T50): A reaction to the improper use of a medication, which can be the result of an error made by the prescribing provider, intentional overdose, interaction with drugs or alcohol, or a reaction caused when a nonprescribed medication interacts with a prescribed and properly administered medication.
- *Adverse effect:* An unfavorable side effect that occurs even though medication is correctly prescribed and properly administered.
- *Underdosing:* Patient takes less of a medication than is prescribed by the provider or by the manufacturer's instructions.
- *Toxic effect:* Patient ingests or comes in contact with a toxic substance.

Codes in categories T36–T65 are combination codes that include the substance taken and the intent. No additional external cause code is required for poisonings, toxic effects, adverse effects, and underdosing codes. When you are coding, do not code directly from the Table of Drugs and Chemicals. Always refer back to the Tabular List.

Coding for External Causes of Morbidity

External cause codes are intended to provide data for research on injuries and evaluation of injury prevention strategies. These codes capture the following specifics:

- How the injury or health condition happened (cause)
- The intent (unintentional or accidental; or intentional, such as suicide or assault)
- The place where the event occurred
- The activity of the patient at the time of the event and the person's status (e.g., civilian, military)

These codes are often used for workers' compensation claims. An external cause of morbidity code can never be reported alone. It is reported in addition to the injury code and is sequenced as the last code.

Place of Occurrence Guideline

Codes from category **Y92 Place of occurrence of the external cause** are secondary codes. They are used after other external cause codes to identify the location of the patient at the time of the injury or other condition. A place of occurrence code is used only once at the initial encounter for treatment. No seventh character is used in Y92 codes. Only one code from category Y92 should be recorded on the patient's health record. Do not use place of occurrence code **Y92.9 {Unspecified place or not applicable}** if the place is not stated or if it is not applicable.

Activity Codes

Category **Y93 Activity codes** are used to define the activity the patient was involved in at the time of injury or when the health condition developed. Only one code from category Y93 should be recorded in the patient's health record. An activity code should be used in conjunction with a place of occurrence code (Y92). The activity codes are not applicable to poisonings, adverse effects, misadventures, or sequelae.

Do not assign code **Y93.9 Unspecified activity if** the activity is not stated.

A code from category Y93 can be used with external cause (Y99) and occurrence (Y92) codes if identifying the activity provides additional information about the event. For example, you are coding a closed ankle fracture that occurred while the patient was playing soccer in a public park. To begin, you must identify what should be coded first. In this case, the ankle fracture is coded first: **S92.111A Displaced fracture of neck of right talus** (remember, "A" indicates initial encounter). The second code is the activity code; the patient was playing soccer, so the code for this activity is **Y93.66 Activity, soccer.** Remember, if the report did not state an activity, do not add **Y93.9 Unspecified activity.**

Finally, when an activity code is used, a place of occurrence code should also be used. In this scenario, the patient was playing in a public park; therefore, the place of occurrence code is **Y92.830 Public park.**

Coding for Health Status and Contact with Health Services

In the ICD-10-CM, Chapter 21, Factors Influencing Health Status and Contact with Health Services (Z00–Z99), codes are used to describe circumstances or encounters with a healthcare provider when no current illness or injury exists. The 16 categories of Z codes include contact/exposure, inoculations and vaccinations, health status, history of screening, observation, aftercare, follow-up, donor counseling, encounters for obstetric and reproductive services, newborns and infants, routine and administrative examinations, and other health encounters that do not fall into any one of the mentioned categories.

MAXIMIZING THIRD-PARTY REIMBURSEMENT

The most important thing to remember in using the ICD-10-CM is to code the diagnosis to the highest level of specificity. Obtaining the correct reimbursement is important to the practice's cash flow, and it depends on proper coding and billing techniques. Here are some other crucial points to remember when submitting diagnostic codes for claims:

- Use the ICD-10-CM manual for the current year, and stay informed of all changes, revisions, and additions published for that year to both the codes and the official coding guidelines.
- Code accurately from documented information, making sure the appropriate code or codes are assigned for all parts of the diagnostic statement, with no additions or omissions.
- Be sure the diagnosis corresponds to the symptoms and treatment. Many codes are specific to age and gender.
- Review data entry to make sure no digits have been transposed.
- Know the insurance carrier's rules and requirements for completion and submission of claims.
- Remember that incomplete or inaccurate codes may result in delay or denial of reimbursement. An inaccurate diagnosis may have a lifelong negative effect on the patient.

Providers and Accurate Coding

Detailed documentation in the patient's health record can help coders code to the highest specificity. Therefore, providers should be trained in how to document patient health records appropriately. Respectfully discuss with providers that diagnostic codes cannot be assigned unless clear documentation is found in the patient's health record. Some providers may feel that because they care for the same type of cases, specialized diagnostic statements should be implied. However, the medical assistant should stress to providers the importance of detailed documentation and how developing this practice not only improves ICD-10-CM code assignment but may also result in higher health insurance reimbursements.

Staff meetings to review third-party requirements should be held regularly by the medical billing supervisor. Medical assistants should be respectful to the healthcare provider when discussing third-party requirements for more detailed documentation. An understanding and patient attitude toward the healthcare provider goes a long way in building a trusting relationship.

Ethical Standards of Medical Coding

At times coders can feel pressured by decreasing insurance reimbursements and their employers to use fraudulent coding practices. However, if a medical practice is convicted of fraudulent billing, the coders may lose their coding license and face federal fines. A number of ethical standards have been established for medical coding, and most of these can help coders identify unethical coding behaviors.

The following tips explain how to proceed in scenarios that may pose ethical dilemmas:

1. *Understand what ethical coding standards mean.* Coders face stress from all sides: financial issues, providers, and other coders. However, stress cannot be a compelling reason for coders to intentionally report diagnoses or higher specificity codes without sufficient documentation.
2. *Stand your ground.* When coding, be true to yourself, even though it can be hard in a stressful environment. When you know a record needs additional documentation to justify reporting certain codes, don't be afraid to speak up to the provider. Conduct research ahead of time to strengthen your case. For example, search through and print out applicable issues of *Coding Clinic* from the American Hospital Association website, www.ahacentraloffice.org. The more backup documentation you have, the more likely management will support your ethical coding decision.
3. *Say something.* Other coders may not follow the same ethical coding standards as you. If you observe unethical coding practices, bring it to the attention of the coder and allow them to make the needed adjustments. Broaching this issue with a colleague can be challenging but encourage the other coder to reflect on the ethics of their actions. If the unethical coding practices continue, be sure to inform the next person in command.
4. *Keep in communication with the office manager.* Some coding situations require more management involvement than others. For example, if your conversation with a colleague does nothing to dissuade unethical behavior, bring your manager into the loop. Or, if you know you need to query a provider about a health record that might yield a higher reimbursement, but that provider is on vacation for 7 days, enlist your office manager's help in flagging the health record until the provider returns to clarify it.
5. *Review notes from other health providers.* In most scenarios, coders are not allowed to code from documentation by anyone other than a provider; however, notes from ancillary staff members may encourage a coder to ask the provider whether the diagnosis does exist. For example, if a consultation with a dietitian suggests that a patient is malnourished, but the provider does not document this anywhere, you may be able to use the dietitian's clinical information as the basis for querying the provider. The diagnosis cannot be coded based solely on the dietitian's clinical information; the code can only be assigned after the provider confirms the diagnosis.

CLOSING COMMENTS

Diagnostic coding using the ICD-10-CM, with its almost 70,000 codes, can seem overwhelming. Successful medical coders follow specific steps to assign the most accurate ICD-10-CM code. Encoder software (e.g., TruCode) can search ICD-10-CM electronically to aid in faster coding. Detailed documentation in the patient's health record and accurate coding work hand in hand to maximize reimbursement for services provided. When you work with providers on issues related to coding and documentation, show respect and patience. Medical assistants are expected to follow ethical standards by assigning and reporting only codes that are clearly supported by the documentation in the patient's record. When in doubt, a medical assistant should consult the provider for clarification. Coding professionals are responsible for maintaining and continually enhancing their coding skills and staying current with the changes in the codes, guidelines, and regulations.

Patient Coaching

Most patients know very little about medical coding, so they may not understand how the codes on their encounter forms relate to their diagnosis. When patients have questions, explain that the codes representing their diagnosis to the most specific and accurate level. Because the coding system is much like a foreign language to patients, be patient when explaining this process and answering questions so that the patient can understand the insurance billing process.

Legal and Ethical Issues

Using the medical coding system allows providers to express the simplicity or complexity of a medical treatment or procedure. This specificity leads to the maximum reimbursement to the provider. The medical assistant must perform coding procedures accurately, so they exactly reflect what happened during the treatment. Codes must not be exaggerated to increase reimbursement to the provider.

Professional Behaviors

Although providers may be overly concerned about the need to maximize insurance reimbursements, coders should never feel coerced into fraudulent coding practices. Successful coders rely solely on medical documentation as the source of diagnostic statements. Coders should never assume that additional complications or conditions exist if they are not documented. In these cases, strong communication between the coder and the provider is necessary to clarify the appropriate diagnoses.

SUMMARY OF SCENARIO

Mike's experience using the ICD-10-CM coding manual and encoder software on actual medical office cases has made him even more enthusiastic about his new responsibilities, and he enjoys the coding process more. He knows that as he gains experience in ICD-10-CM coding, he will be able to set a positive example for the staff. As Mike progresses with diagnostic coding, he will also be able to help the providers and medical assistant staff be attentive to details when documenting a health record.

Although the electronic encounter form for entering billing codes is an easy tool, Mike has learned that knowing how to use the ICD-10-CM Alphabetic Index and Tabular List is a necessary skill to ensure accurate coding. He also knows that it is important when coding a diagnosis to make sure the medical documentation matches the encounter form and that all elements of the diagnostic statement are included. Furthermore, he must ensure that the diagnosis listed on the encounter form is fully documented in the patient's health record. Mike is feeling more comfortable about referring to coding guidelines to ensure the most accurate code and to make certain that every character for the ICD-10-CM code is present. Every feature of the manual provides guidance when choosing and confirming a diagnostic code that matches the diagnostic statement on the encounter form and in the health record. Searching for codes in the encoder also has helped Mike develop his coding skills more quickly.

SUMMARY OF LEARNING OBJECTIVES

1. **Explain the historical use of the International Classification of Disease (ICD) in the United States.**

   In 1946, the International Commission of the World Health Organization (WHO) established a code set called the *Manual of the International Statistical Classification of Diseases, Injuries, and Causes of Death* (ICD). Eventually, the WHO approved an adaptation of this code set for use in the United States; the ninth edition, the *International Classification of Diseases, Ninth Revision, Clinical Modification* (ICD-9-CM), was approved and put into use in 1975. The United States adopted ICD-10-CM diagnostic coding on October 1, 2015.

   The diagnostic code tells the insurance company why a procedure was done. If the diagnosis does not match the procedure, the insurance company can say that it was not medically necessary and not pay for the procedure.

2. **Explain the structure and format of the International Classification of Diseases, 10th Revision, Clinical Modification (ICD-10-CM).**

   Every ICD-10-CM code begins with an alphabetic letter that indicates the chapter of disease and injury for which the code is listed. (All the letters in the English alphabet are used except U, which the WHO has reserved to assign to new diseases with uncertain etiologies.) Codes contain up to seven alphanumeric characters; the first three characters are followed by a period. Codes that require a seventh character may use an X as a placeholder for the fourth, fifth, and sixth characters if no other code can be used for those characters.

   The ICD-10-CM Index to Diseases and Injuries (commonly called the *Alphabetic Index*) consists of an alphabetic list of diagnostic terms and related codes. This index includes main terms, nonessential modifiers, essential modifiers, and subterms. The *main term* is boldface, the *nonessential modifiers* that follow it are enclosed in parentheses, the *essential modifier* is indented one space under the main term, and the *subterm* is indented one space under the essential modifier (two spaces under the main term). The nonessential modifiers do not affect the code assignment. The hyphen (-) at the end of the code indicates that additional characters are required to complete the code.

   The ICD-10-CM Tabular List of Diseases and Injuries (commonly called simply the *Tabular List*) is divided into 21 chapters. Each chapter is divided into categories, or *blocks,* that have been assigned three-character codes. These codes form the foundation of the ICD-10-CM code set.

   In most of the chapters, the title is composed of a group of diseases and injuries, followed by a code range in parentheses. For example, Chapter 1 is Certain Infectious and Parasitic Diseases (A00–B99). *Conventions* are abbreviations, punctuation, symbols, instructional notations, and related elements that help the coder select an accurate, specific code. Conventions are found in the Tabular List but not in the Alphabetic Index. Understanding their meaning and using them as guides are crucial to accurate coding.

3. **Explain how to abstract the diagnostic statement from a patient's health record.**

   To prepare for medical coding, the medical assistant must analyze and abstract the diagnostic statements documented in the various reports in the patient's health record. Sources of diagnostic statements include the encounter form, treatment notes, discharge summary, operative report, and radiology, pathology, and laboratory reports.

4. **Examine the steps involved in ICD-10-CM coding.**

   Eight basic steps are required for accurate ICD-10-CM coding (see Table 13.3). The first step involves abstracting the diagnostic statement from the health record and determining the main and essential modifiers from the various medical reports. The next steps are performed using the Alphabetic Index to search for the code, codes, or code ranges that best fit the diagnostic statement. The remaining steps are performed using the Tabular List to verify and confirm that the code or codes located in the Alphabetic Index fully match the diagnostic statement and are the most specific and accurate diagnostic codes. The medical assistant's knowledge of accurate diagnostic coding contributes to the legal and financial health of the practice. In most cases, ICD-10-CM codes are found on the encounter form. However, with literally thousands of current diagnostic codes, it may be necessary to code from the ICD-10-CM manual. The process for diagnostic coding is outlined in Procedure 13.1.

   Encoder software is computer-aided coding, which helps determine the most accurate code possible. The coder types a few key words into a Search box, and the software matches the entry with main terms in the Alphabetic Index. The coder then clicks on a specific code to hyperlink to the Tabular List.

5. **Examine the Official Coding Guidelines to assign the most accurate ICD-10-CM diagnostic code.**

   An important section of the coding manual is the ICD-10-CM Official Guidelines for Coding and Reporting. Every coding guideline for the entire ICD-10-CM code set is included in this Coding Guidelines section at the beginning of the manual. These guidelines are a set of rules developed to accompany and complement the official conventions and instructions provided in the ICD-10-CM proper.

6. **Explain the importance of maximizing third-party reimbursement.**

   All ICD-10-CM coding manuals, regardless of the publisher, have comprehensive instructional notes and conventions to help the coder select the most accurate diagnostic code or codes. When a discrepancy occurs between reference sources, including this text, the current year's ICD-10-CM coding manual is the final authority. When coding, the medical assistant must always refer to and thoroughly review the conventions, instructional notations, code definitions, and other guidelines in the Alphabetic Index and Tabular List.

   The most important thing to remember when using the ICD-10-CM is to code the diagnosis to the highest level of specificity in order to maximize third-party reimbursement.

   At times, medical coders can feel pressure from decreasing insurance reimbursements and their employers to justify fraudulent coding practices. If a medical practice is convicted of fraudulent billing, it will lose its coding license, and it and the coder may face federal fines. A number of standards have been established for ethical coding, and most of these can help coders recognize unethical coding behaviors.

PROCEDURE 13.1 Perform Coding Using the Current ICD-10-CM Manual or Encoder

TASK: Perform accurate diagnosis coding using the ICD-10-CM manual.

SCENARIO: The encounter form and progress notes both show that the diagnosis for this patient encounter is acute colitis. Locate the most accurate ICD-10-CM code for this diagnostic statement.

EQUIPMENT and SUPPLIES

- ICD-10-CM manual (current year), or
- Encoder software, such as TruCode

PROCEDURAL STEPS

Alphabetic Index

1. Determine and locate the main terms from the diagnostic statement in the Alphabetic Index.
   PURPOSE: To provide a starting point for searching the Alphabetic Index.
2. Locate the essential modifiers listed under the main term in the Alphabetic Index.
   PURPOSE: To ensure further specificity of the codes found in the Alphabetic Index.
3. Review the conventions, punctuation, and notes in the Alphabetic Index.
   PURPOSE: To ensure that no additional searches, exclusions, or similar terms are needed to complete the search in the Alphabetic Index.
4. Choose a tentative code, codes, or code range from the Alphabetic Index that matches the diagnostic statement as closely as possible.
   PURPOSE: To prevent backtracking and repeated searches in the Alphabetic Index.

Tabular List

1. Look up the codes chosen from the Alphabetic Index in the Tabular List.
   PURPOSE: To begin the process of determining whether the codes selected from the Alphabetic Index are appropriate and accurate.
2. Review notes, conventions, and the Official Coding Guidelines associated with the code and code description in the Tabular List.
   a. Review conventions and punctuation.
   b. Review instructional notations:
      - Includes and excludes notes
      - Code first, code also, and code additional notes
      - *and, or,* and *with* statements

PURPOSE: To ensure that the code or codes selected are appropriate for use and determine whether they require additional codes or further specificity or are excluded from use.

3. Verify the accuracy of the tentative code in the Tabular List.
   a. Make sure all elements of the diagnostic statement are included in the codes selected.
   b. Make sure the code description does not include anything not documented in the diagnostic statement.

PURPOSE: To ensure that the most accurate and specific code is selected and that no contraindication exists in the use of the code or codes selected.

4. Extend the codes to their highest level of specificity (up to the seventh character, if required). If a seventh character is required, and no codes are present for the fourth, fifth, or sixth characters, it is appropriate to use the dummy placeholder X for these positions.
5. Assign the code (or codes) selected from the Tabular List as the appropriate code for the patient's condition by documenting it in the patient's health record.
   PURPOSE: To ensure that the health record and electronic encounter form contain documentation of the code or codes assigned.

Using the TruCode Encoder Software

1. Type in the main term from the diagnostic statement in the search box, as in the following figure.

PROCEDURE 13.1 Perform Coding Using the Current ICD-10-CM Manual or Encoder—*continued*

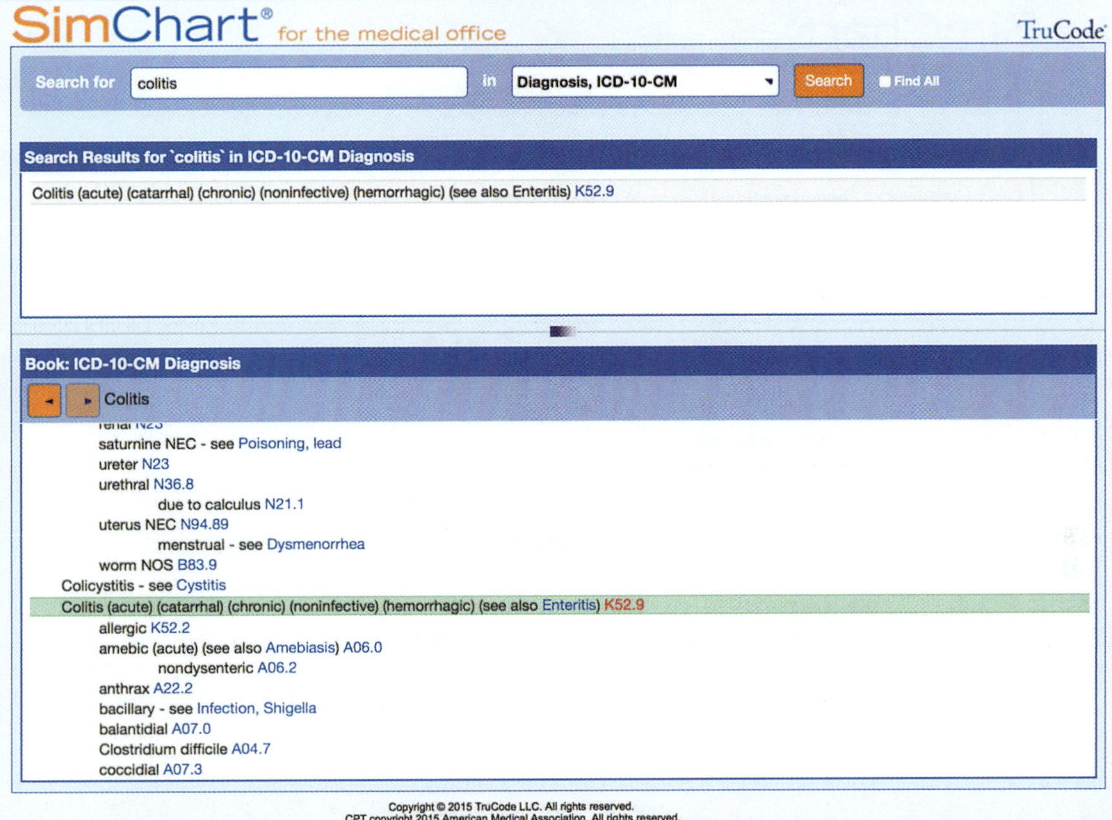

1

2. The software will provide a list of main terms that could be related to the diagnosis typed in the search box. The coder chooses the main term that best represents the diagnostic statement.
3. Based on the main term chosen, a list of essential modifiers is presented (see the following figure). The coder must review the diagnostic statement to ensure that all documented modifying terms are identified. If the provider does not document a modifying term, the coder should not assume that a modifying term was implied.

Continued

PROCEDURE 13.1 Perform Coding Using the Current ICD-10-CM Manual or Encoder—*continued*

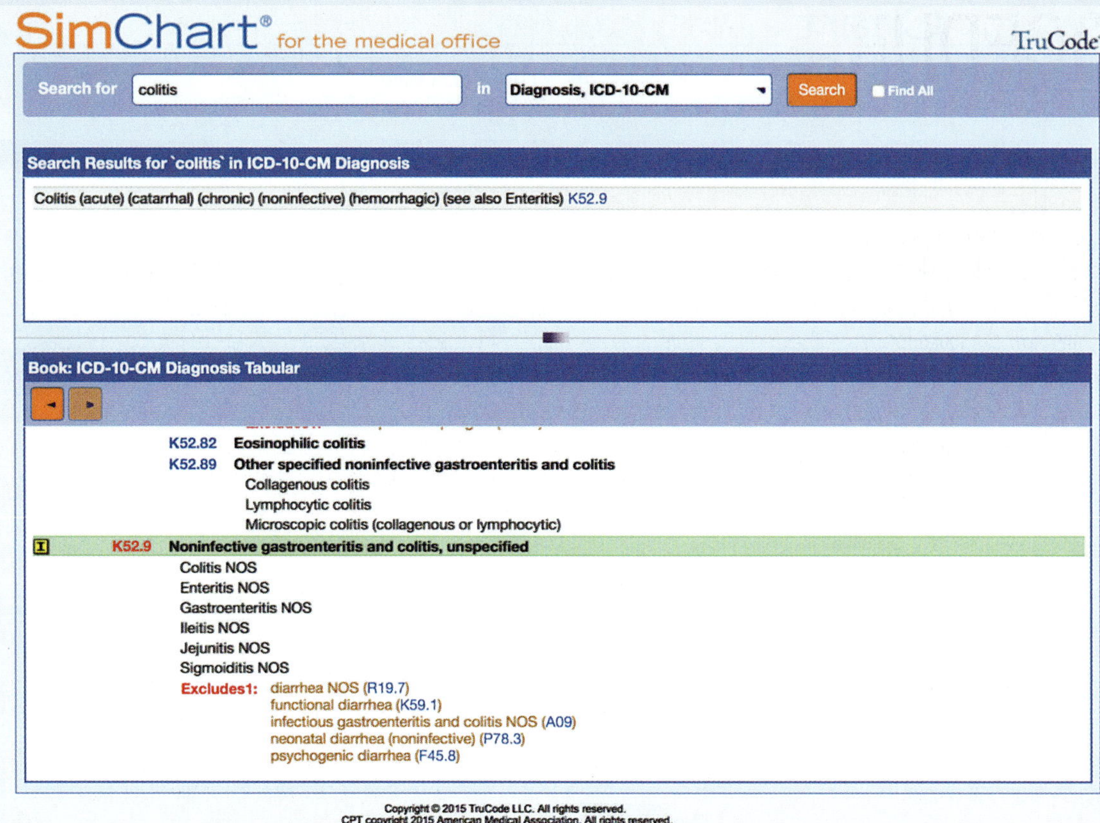

2

4. In the preceding figure, note the yellow box on the left of the chosen diagnosis. In the TruCode program, click on the yellow area, and an instructional notes textbox, which includes coding guidelines, will appear, as in the following figure. To determine the most accurate code, follow these coding guidelines.

5. Once all the menus of essential modifiers have been presented, choose the most accurate and specific code based on the diagnostic statement.

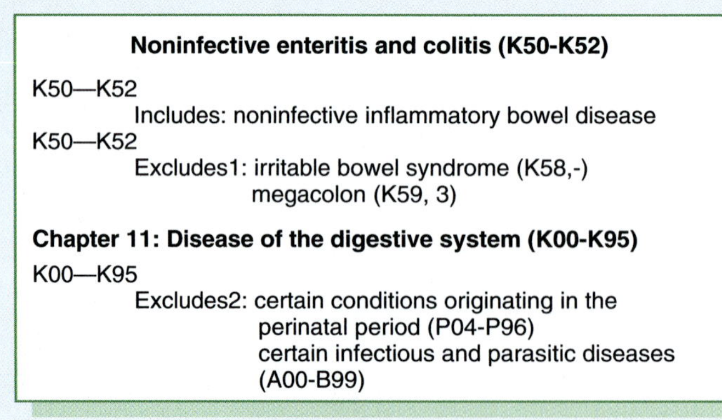

Noninfective enteritis and colitis (K50-K52)

K50—K52
Includes: noninfective inflammatory bowel disease
K50—K52
Excludes1: irritable bowel syndrome (K58,-)
megacolon (K59, 3)

Chapter 11: Disease of the digestive system (K00-K95)

K00—K95
Excludes2: certain conditions originating in the perinatal period (P04-P96)
certain infectious and parasitic diseases (A00-B99)

3

PROCEDURAL CODING ESSENTIALS 14

SCENARIO

Sherald Vogt, a medical assisting student, works at Walden-Martin Family Medical Clinic (WMFM). Sherald really enjoyed learning about diagnostic coding in the *International Classification of Diseases, 10th Revision, Clinical Modification* (ICD-10-CM), and now she looks forward to learning about procedural coding. Sherald recognizes that a strong understanding of anatomy and physiology are vital to correct diagnostic coding. She also believes that the knowledge she has gained will help her in procedural coding. Sherald will be using the *Current Procedural Terminology* (CPT) coding system for most procedures and services provided in the medical office. In addition, she will use the *Healthcare Common Procedure Coding System* (HCPCS; pronounced "hic-pix") for medical products and services not found in the CPT.

As she did with the ICD-10-CM, Sherald is learning that accurate coding begins with the proper analysis of documentation found in the health record. With that information, she will abstract the correct data to assign an accurate procedure code. As does the ICD-10-CM, the CPT has coding guidelines, symbols, and formal steps specific to procedural coding. However, unlike in ICD-10-CM diagnostic coding, in CPT and HCPCS coding Sherald must determine how and when to use modifiers. The office manager wants to give Sherald some experience, so he allows her to review some healthcare records so she can practice coding.

While studying this chapter, think about the following questions:

- What code set will be used for outpatient procedural coding?
- What will Sherald find similar to what she learned with the ICD-10-CM as she performs procedural coding?
- What will help Sherald select the most specific and accurate CPT code?
- What are the differences between CPT coding and HCPCS coding?
- How will Sherald use and apply modifiers in CPT and HCPCS coding?
- What will Sherald learn about the legal implications of inaccurate coding?

LEARNING OBJECTIVES

1. Examine the CPT manual.
2. Explain the steps for efficient CPT coding.
3. Explain the components of determining the correct evaluation and management code.
4. Explain the components determining the correct CPT codes for anesthesia.
5. Explain the components for determining the correct CPT code for surgical services
6. Explain how to determine the correct CPT codes for radiology services and pathology and laboratory services.
7. Explain what services are found in the Medicine section of the CPT manual.
8. Examine the HCPCS coding system.

VOCABULARY

bilaterally (bie LAT er uhl ee) Pertaining to, involving, or affecting two or both sides.

certified registered nurse anesthetist (CRNA) A nursing healthcare professional who is certified to administer anesthesia.

chief complaint A statement in the patient's own words that describes the reason for the visit.

CPT Assistant An online CPT coding journal, supported by the AMA, that addresses subjects such as appealing insurance denials, validating coding to auditors, training staff members, and answering day-to-day coding questions.

debridement The surgical removal of dead, damaged, or infected tissue to improve the function of healthy tissue.

eponym (EP uh nim) In medical terms, a medical diagnosis or procedure named for the person who discovered it.

global services For purposes of CPT coding, medical services and procedures performed for the patient before, during, and after a surgical procedure that are included with the assigned CPT code.

performance measurement The regular collection of data to assess whether the correct processes are being performed and the desired results are being achieved.

review of systems (ROS) A list of questions answered by the patient related to each organ system, designed to uncover potential disease processes.

special report Additional medical documentation required to confirm the need for the use of an unlisted, unusual, or newly adopted medical procedures code.

specificity (spes i FIS i tee) The quality or state of being specific.

INTRODUCTION

Procedural coding changes the written descriptions of procedures and services delivered in a healthcare facility into numeric or alphanumeric codes. These codes are used for a variety of purposes. They can be used to track the services that are being provided to patients and on claims sent for payment from insurance companies. There are three procedure code sets used for these purposes:

- International Classification of Diseases, 10th Revision, Procedural Coding System (ICD-10-PCS)
- Current Procedural Terminology (CPT)
- Healthcare Common Procedure Coding System (HCPCS)

Table 14.1 compares the three different code sets. Medical assistants most often work in an outpatient setting. This chapter focuses on the CPT and HCPCS code sets. Because ICD-10-PCS is used for inpatient coding, and medical assistants most often work in an outpatient setting, we will not review ICD-10-PCS coding in this chapter. The medical biller is responsible for maintaining accurate medical records and for processing insurance claims. This can be done efficiently by using the CPT and HCPCS codes. These codes identify procedures and services commonly used in an outpatient healthcare facility.

INTRODUCTION TO THE CPT MANUAL

The Current Procedural Terminology (CPT) system was developed and is maintained by the American Medical Association (AMA). It is updated each year and released on October 1 to become effective on January 1. The CPT coding manual consists of descriptive terms and identifying codes for reporting professional and technical services. CPT codes convert written descriptions of procedures and services into numeric codes. They establish a standard system that accurately describes medical and surgical services.

Code Categories in the CPT Manual

There are three different categories of codes in the CPT. Category I codes are used most frequently and are required for insurance claim submission. Category II and Category III codes are used for data collection.

Category I Codes

Category I codes are in the Tabular List of the CPT manual and arranged by sections. For example, codes beginning with 7 (e.g., 70100—radiologic examination of the mandible, partial, with less than four views) are in the Radiology section of the manual. Each code has a description of the service or procedure performed. These are five-digit numeric codes.

Format of the CPT Coding Manual

- Comprehensive instructions for using the manual, including the steps for coding
- Tabular List, which includes the following six sections:
  - Evaluation and Management
  - Anesthesia
  - Surgery
  - Radiology
  - Pathology and Laboratory
  - Medicine
- Coding Guidelines, Conventions, and Notes
- Appendices (16; A–P)
- The Alphabetic Index

Category II Codes

Category II codes are a set of supplemental tracking codes that healthcare facilities use for **performance measurement**. Category II codes are optional. They cannot be used as a substitute for Category I codes, and they are not used as part of the insurance billing process. When these codes are used, it can reduce the need for abstracting information from the health record. These codes describe clinical components that may be typically included in Evaluation and Management services, or clinical services. In a Category II code, the fifth digit is the letter F. If a patient was seen by the provider for asthma, a Category I code of 99213 could be used for the visit. In addition, a Category II code of 2015F Asthma impairment assessed (Asthma) could be used.

Category II codes are described and listed in their own section, which is located after the Medicine section and before the appendices. Category II codes are reviewed by the Performance Measures Advisory Group. This group is composed of members from various medical organizations and government agencies.

TABLE 14.1 Comparison of Procedural Code Sets

CODE SET	USED FOR	CODE FEATURES	EXAMPLE	DESCRIPTION	DEVELOPER	UPDATED
ICD-10-PCS	Inpatient hospital procedures	Seven-digit alphanumeric code	0TTJ0ZZ	Appendectomy	National Center for Health Statistics	Annually, October 1
CPT	Outpatient procedures; professional and technical services	Five-digit numeric code; a two-digit modifier can be added	44970	Laparoscopic appendectomy	American Medical Association (AMA)	Annually, January 1
HCPCS	Auxiliary medical treatment, including vaccines, medical transport, drugs, durable medical equipment	Five-digit alphanumeric code; a two-digit modifier can be added	A0428	Ambulance service, basic life support, nonemergency transport	Centers for Medicare and Medicaid Services (CMS)	Annually, October 1

Category III Codes

Category III codes are temporary codes used for emerging and new technology, services, and procedures that have not been officially added to the Tabular List. The fifth digit in a Category III code is the letter T. Category III codes may be used in billing and reporting under the following conditions:

- No code in the Tabular List correctly describes the technology, service, or procedure performed.
- No Category I code matches the documentation.

In most publishers' editions of the CPT manual, Category III codes are also listed in their own section, after the Medicine section and before the appendices.

Organization of the CPT Manual

The CPT coding manual is separated into the Alphabetic Index and the Tabular List. These will be discussed in the following sections.

The Alphabetic Index

CPT coding starts with the Alphabetic Index. It is found in the back of the CPT manual and is an alphabetic listing of main terms. These terms represent the type of surgery, the anatomic site, or **eponym** (Figure 14.1). Much like the Alphabetic Index in the ICD-10-CM manual, the Alphabetic Index in the CPT gives a code, codes, or a code range that must be verified in the Tabular List of the CPT manual.

CRITICAL THINKING APPLICATION **14.1**

To practice her coding skills, Sherald is reviewing a surgical report for a gallbladder removal. Will she be able to find the main term *gallbladder* in the Alphabetic Index? Why or why not? What other main term could she be looking for? Once she finds the range of codes in the Alphabetic Index, what is her next step?

Fracture

Acetabulum
  Closed Treatment 27220-27222
  Open Treatment 27226-27228
  with Manipulation 27222
  without Manipulation 27220
Alveolar Ridge
  Closed Treatment 21440
  Open Treatment 21445
Ankle
  Bimalleolar 27808, 27810, 27814
  Lateral 27786, 27788, 27792, 27808, 27810, 27814
  Medial 27760, 27762, 27766, 27808, 27810, 27814
  Posterior 27767-27769, 27808, 27810, 27814
  Trimalleolar 27816, 27818, 27822-27823
Ankle Bone
  Medial 27760-27762
Bennett's
  See Thumb, Fracture
Blow-Out Fracture
  Orbital Floor 21385-21387, 21390, 21395
Bronchi
  Reduction 31630
Calcaneus
  Closed Treatment 28400-28405
  Open Treatment 28415-28420
  Percutaneous Fixation 28406
  with Manipulation 28405-28406
  without Manipulation 28400

FIGURE 14.1 Alphabetic Index: Fractures.

The Tabular List

The Tabular List is divided into six sections, with codes listed in numeric order in each section. As in the ICD-10-CM, the codes in the Tabular List include definitions, guidelines, and notes. These enable the coder to select the most specific code based on the procedural statement and service descriptions documented in the health record. The six sections of the Tabular List and their CPT code ranges are as follows:

- Evaluation and Management (99201–99499)
- Anesthesia (00100–01999, 99100–99140)
- Surgery (10021–69990)
- Radiology, including nuclear medicine and diagnostic ultrasound (70010–79999)
- Pathology and Laboratory (80047–89398)
- Medicine (90281–99199, 99500–99607)

Sections are subdivided into *subsections*, *subsections* are subdivided into *subheadings*, and *subheadings* can be subdivided into *categories*. Each level of a section provides more **specificity** about the procedure or service performed and the anatomic site or organ system involved. Each section and subsection provides coding guidelines and, if needed, a reference to the **CPT Assistant.** In most instances, all four levels are found, although this is not a hard-and-fast rule.

Format of Tabular List

Section: Surgery (10021–69990)
Subsection: Integumentary System
Subheading: Skin Subcutaneous and Accessory Structures
Category: Debridement

In the CPT manual, the subsection is listed below the section and indented. The subsection usually describes an anatomic site or an organ system, as in the following examples:

- Anatomic site: Heart, femur, or skull
- Organ system: Digestive, integumentary, or cardiovascular

A subheading is listed below the subsection; it generally refers to a specific procedure or service, but it can also indicate a more specific anatomic site:

- Procedures: Esophagoscopy, incision and drainage, or cardiac catheterization
- Specific anatomic site: Mitral valve, distal femur, or occipital bone

Category is the lowest level of code description.

Unlisted Procedure or Service Code

Occasionally, even with the most detailed documentation, an accurate code to match the procedure or service performed cannot be found in the CPT manual. For this reason, in each section, nonspecific codes have been provided. These codes are known as Unlisted Procedures and Services. For example, code 29999 is found in the Surgery section, Musculoskeletal subsection. It describes an "unlisted procedure, arthroscopy." Unlisted codes can be used only when no other Category I or Category III code exactly matches the documentation. When an unlisted code is used, a **special report** must be sent with the insurance claim that describes the procedure or service in detail.

General CPT Coding Guidelines

At the beginning of each section and some subsections are coding guidelines. These guidelines add definitions and descriptions needed to interpret and report the procedures and services in that section or subsection. Coding guidelines enhance the coder's understanding of when and under what circumstances specific codes may be used. It is important to thoroughly read and apply the coding guidelines provided. Because coding guidelines are updated every year in October and are effective every January, it is also important to reread the guidelines after every new edition is released. Selecting a code without reading the guidelines usually leads to selection of the wrong code. Not only will this result in possibly delayed or denied reimbursement, but also, continued inappropriate code selection can be considered fraud or abuse and can result in serious civil or criminal penalties.

Terms related to inaccurate coding are upcoding and downcoding. *Upcoding* is the use of a higher-level procedure code than is supported in the documentation or medical necessity. A documentation example would be using Evaluation and Management (E/M) code 99213 (medically appropriate history and/or examination and low level of medical decision making) when the documentation supports 99212 (medically appropriate history and/or examination and straightforward level of medical decision making). As mentioned in the diagnostic coding chapter, diagnosis and procedure codes are linked on the claim. For example, a patient undergoes a rhinoplasty for cosmetic reasons, but the diagnosis code for a deviated septum is submitted. A deviated septum would be considered medically necessary and could be paid by the insurance company. It is likely that the insurance company would request the records for this procedure and see in the documentation that the patient requested a cosmetic rhinoplasty. These examples would be considered fraud.

Downcoding is the use of a lower-level procedure code than is justified. This also can be damaging to the healthcare facility because it would result in lower reimbursement.

In procedural coding, the coder must always choose the code that most accurately describes the services provided.

Modifiers

Category I code *modifiers* are two-digit, numeric codes that report or indicate specific criteria, a specific condition, or a special circumstance. Category II code modifiers are alphanumeric. Category I or Category II modifiers are used with CPT codes to indicate that a service or procedure performed was altered by specific circumstances (Table 14.2). Modifiers are included with the five-digit CPT code to supply additional information or to describe extenuating circumstances that affected the procedure or service. For instance, modifier –50 adds the detail that a procedure was performed **bilaterally**, or on both sides of the body. When assistant surgeons are needed for surgical procedures, modifier –80 should be used. This allows assistant surgeons to submit charges for their time. Modifiers can also show which side of the body a medical procedure was performed on. For example, the code 19100–RT indicates that the right breast was biopsied. A list of modifiers can be found in the CPT coding manual in Appendix A.

TABLE 14.2 Commonly Used CPT Code Modifiers

MODIFIER	DESCRIPTION
–50	Bilateral procedure. If the procedure was performed on both sides of the body (e.g., both knees, both eyes) and the code description does not indicate that the procedure or service was performed bilaterally, modifier –50 is used.
–62	Two surgeons. When two surgeons work together as primary surgeons, each performing distinct parts of a procedure, both surgeons should report the procedure they performed to the insurance carrier using modifier –62. This prevents the insurance carrier from possibly rejecting a surgical charge as a duplicate.
–26	Professional component. This modifier is used when a physician supervises the technician performing the service or provides a professional opinion.
–RT, –LT	Indicates the side of the body on which the procedure took place (e.g., 19100–LT – Breast biopsy, left side).

Symbols

▲ Revised code
● New code
▶◀ New or revised text
➲ Reference to *CPT Assistant, Clinical Examples in Radiology*, and *CPT Changes*
✚ Add-on code
⊘ Exemptions to modifier 51
⊙ Moderate sedation
✗ Product pending FDA approval
○ Reinstated or recycled code
Out-of-numerical sequence code

FIGURE 14.2 CPT conventions.

CPT Conventions

Conventions, or special symbols (Figure 14.2), are used to provide additional information about specific codes. Let's look at a skin graft procedure for a wound that is 50 sq cm:

- Code 15271, Application of skin substitute graft to trunk, arms, legs, total wound surface area up to 100 sq cm; first 25 sq cm or less wound surface area
- Code +15272, each additional 25 sq cm wound surface area, or part thereof

To accurately code for this skin graft, two codes would be used: 15271 and 15272.

In the Tabular List in most CPT manuals, the legend explaining the meanings of the convention symbols is found at the bottom of each page.

CRITICAL THINKING APPLICATION **14.2**

Sherald is trying to look up the CPT code for a left arm cyst biopsy. She has found the code, but how can she show that the procedure took place on the left side?

Sherald also came across CPT code 32440 (removal of lung, pneumonectomy), but she needs to also code for the repair of a portion of the bronchus. The code has a (+) in front of it; what does this mean?

Appendices

The CPT coding manual uses appendices to organize changes to the original code set. There are 18 appendices in 2022. A list of appendices and the codes they contain can be found in Table 14.3.

STEPS FOR EFFICIENT CPT PROCEDURAL CODING

The CPT coding process, which includes use of the Alphabetic Index and the Tabular List, applies to all sections of the CPT manual, except for the E/M and Anesthesia sections.

To start the procedural coding process, you must first determine the procedures or services that were provided. This is accomplished with two basic steps:

1. Analyze and abstract the procedural statement documented in the health record.
2. Compare it with the encounter form, operative report, or other documentation to ensure that all services and procedures have been recorded.

For practice on CPT surgery coding, refer to Procedure 14.1.

TABLE 14.3 Appendices of the CPT Manual, 2022 edition

APPENDIX	TITLE	DESCRIPTION
A	Modifiers	All modifiers applicable to CPT codes
B	Summary of Additions, Deletions, and Revisions	Shows the actual changes made to the annual CPT manual
C	Clinical Examples	Provides helpful narrative examples to aid selection of the correct and most specific level of E/M codes
D	Summary of CPT Add-on Codes	A list of CPT add-on codes
E	Summary of CPT Codes Exempt from Modifier 51	CPT codes that cannot use modifier 51, which indicates multiple procedures
F	Summary of CPT Codes Exempt from Modifier 63	CPT codes that cannot use modifier 63, which indicates procedures done on infants weighing < 4 kg
G	Summary of CPT Codes That Include Moderate (Conscious) Sedation	The summary of CPT codes that include moderate (conscious) sedation have been removed from the CPT code set
H	Alphabetic Clinical Topics Listing	The Alphabetical Clinical Topics Listing has been removed from the CPT codebook; this listing can be found on the AMA CPT website
I	Genetic Testing Modifiers	The Genetic Testing Code Modifiers has been removed from the CPT code set
J	Electrodiagnostic Medicine Listing of Sensory, Motor, and Mixed Nerves	A list in which each sensory, motor, and mixed nerve is assigned its appropriate nerve conduction study code, to enhance accurate reporting of codes 95907 to 95913
K	Product Pending FDA Approval	Vaccine products that have been assigned a CPT code in anticipation of approval from the Food and Drug Administration (FDA)
L	Vascular Families	A diagram of veins to the first, second, and third order. assuming that the starting point is catheterization of the aorta
M	Renumbered CPT Codes– Citations Crosswalk	A summary of cross-walked, deleted, and renumbered codes, in addition to descriptors with the associated *CPT Assistant* references for the deleted codes
N	Summary of Resequenced CPT Codes	A list of CPT codes that do not appear in numeric sequence, which allows existing codes to be relocated to an appropriate location
O	Multianalyte Assays with Algorithmic Analysis and Proprietary laboratory Analyses	A list of CPT codes that includes a set of administrative codes for Multianalyte Assays with Algorithmic Analyses procedures; these typically are unique to a single clinical laboratory or manufacturer

Continued

TABLE 14.3 Appendices of the CPT Manual, 2022 edition—cont'd

APPENDIX	TITLE	DESCRIPTION
P	CPT Codes That May Be Used for Synchronous Telemedicine Services	A list of CPT codes that may be used for reporting real-time telemedicine services when appended by modifier 95
Q	Severe Acute Respiratory Syndrome Coronavirus 2 (Sars-CoV-2)(coronavirus disease [COVID-19] Vaccines	A table that links the individual severe acute respiratory syndrome coronavirus 2 (SARS-CoV-2) (coronavirus disease [COVID-19] vaccine product codes to their associated immunization administration codes, manufacturer name, vaccine name(s), National Drug Code Labeler Product ID, and interval between doses
R	Digital Medicine—Services Taxonomy	A listing of digital medicine services described in the CPT code set

Documentation for CPT Coding

Medical records used for procedural coding can include any or all of the following:

- Encounter form (Figure 14.3)
- History and physical report (H&P)
- Progress notes
- Discharge summary
- Operative report
- Pathology report
- Anesthesia record
- Radiology report

When you compare the documentation to the codes, make sure all the elements of the description match substantially, with nothing added or missing. For example, review CPT codes 21315 and 21320. Both codes describe the closed treatment of a nasal bone fracture. However, 21315 indicates that there is no stabilization, and 21320 indicates that there is stabilization. The coder reviews the procedures and then assigns the CPT code with the description that most closely resembles the documentation.

Some providers have CPT and ICD-10-CM codes printed on their encounter forms; however, these codes should be treated only as a reference. Medical coders must also review the health record carefully, abstracting all the procedures and services rendered during an encounter. For example, a provider may have circled the procedure for a preventive health visit for a 4-year-old on the encounter form but forget to record the injections provided during the encounter. When the medical assistant reviews the patient's electronic health record (EHR), the provider's notes state routine injections were administered. If the medical assistant had not reviewed the EHR, the clinic would have lost reimbursement because the claim would not have included all the CPT codes for the visit. Encounter forms should be updated annually to ensure that code additions, changes, and revisions are current.

Abstracting

The term *abstract*, used as a verb in this context, is the process of collecting pertinent medical information needed to assign the correct code. Abstracting ensures that all medical procedures and services are identified, and none are omitted. The abstracted data is then broken down into main terms and modifying terms. A main term is usually the primary procedure or service performed, and a modifying term further defines or adds information to the main term. Next, the main and modifying terms are used to find the code or code ranges in the Alphabetic Index. Last, the code selected is confirmed by reviewing the guidelines, notes, and conventions in the Tabular List to verify that the most accurate code has been chosen.

Using the Alphabetic Index

Procedural coding starts with identifying the main term and then locating it in the Alphabetic Index. Although the Alphabetic Index is a comprehensive, alphabetic listing of all main terms, there are no code descriptions. It is not effective to assign a CPT code simply by finding it through the Alphabetic Index. The Alphabetic Index is not a substitute for the Tabular List. Even if an individual is only looking for one code, the Tabular List must be used to ensure the code is accurate.

The Alphabetic Index is used as a guide to search for one or more codes or code ranges. The index is similar to that found in the back of any textbook; it is an alphabetic list of main and modifying terms found in the Tabular List of the coding manual. In a typical index, the term or concept listed in the index is followed by the page numbers on which detailed information is presented in the body of the book. The Alphabetic Index in the CPT coding manual is used in the same way, except that it provides codes or code ranges rather than page numbers. As discussed earlier, the Tabular List is divided into sections, and the procedures and services are listed in numeric order by the Category I code.

The Alphabetic Index is organized by main terms and modifying terms that are indented below the main term. Modifying terms further describe and add information needed to narrow the search for an appropriate procedure or service code. A main term can be a procedure, such as an excision. Each modifying term could provide further information:

- Anatomic location
- Organ excised
- Type of instrument used
- Special technique
- Other procedures performed at the same time (e.g., obtaining biopsy tissue for examination)

Modifying terms affect the selection of appropriate codes; therefore, it is important to review the list of modifying terms when selecting a code or code range.

Searching the Alphabetic Index

Begin the search of the Alphabetic Index by using one of the four primary classifications (or types) of main and modifying terms:

- Procedure or service (e.g., examination, excision, scope, revision, repair, drainage)

Julie Walden, M.D. David Kahn, M.D.
James Marin, M.D. Jean Burke, N.P.
Angela Perez, M.D.

YOUR NAME CLINIC
Walden-Martin Family Medical Clinic,
1234 Anystreet, Anytown AK 12345
Phone: 123-123-1234 Fax: 123-123-5678

TELEPHONE:
FAX:

PATIENT'S NAME	CHART #	DATE	☐ MEDI-MEDI ☐ MEDICAL ☐ MEDICARE ☐ PRIVATE ☐ SELF PAY ☐ HMO ________

✔	CPT/Md	DESCRIPTION	FEE
	OFFICE VISIT—NEW PATIENT		
	99202	Focused Ex.	
	99203	Detailed Ex.	
	99204	Comprehensive Ex.	
	99205	Complex Ex.	
	OFFICE VISIT—ESTABLISHED PATIENT		
	99212	Focused Ex.	
	99213	Expanded Ex.	
	99214	Detailed Ex.	
	99215	Complex Ex.	
	PREVENTATIVE MEDICINE—NEW PATIENT		
	99381	< 1 year old	
	99382	1–4 year old	
	99383	5–11 year old	
	99384	12–17 year old	
	99385	18–39 year old	
	99386	40–64 year old	
	99387	65+ year old	
	PREVENTATIVE MEDICINE—ESTABLISHED PATIENT		
	99391	< 1 year old	
	99392	1–4 year old	
	99393	5–11 year old	
	99394	12–17 year old	
	99395	18–39 year old	
	99396	40–64 year old	
	99397	65+ year old	

✔	CPT/Md	DESCRIPTION	FEE
	LAB STUDIES		
	36415	Venipucture	
	81000	Urinalysis	
	81003	–w/o Micro	
	84703	HCG (Urine, Pregnancy)	
	82948	Glucose	
	82270	Hemoccult	
	85023	CBC-diff.	
	85024	CBC w/part diff	
	85018	Hemoglobin	
	88155	Pap Smear	
	87210	KOH/Saline Wet Mount	
	87430	Strep Antigen	
	87060	Throat Culture	
	80009	Chem profile	
	80061	Lipid profile	
	82465	Cholesterol	
	99000	Handling fee	
	PROCEDURES		
	92551	Audiometry	
	29705	Cast Removal	
	2900_	Casting (by location)	
	92567	Ear Check	
	69210	Ear Wax Rem. 1 2	
	93000	EKG	
	93005	EKG tracing only	
	93010	EKG. Int. and Rep	
	11750	Excision Nail	
	94375	Flow Volume	

✔	CPT/Md	DESCRIPTION	FEE
	PROCEDURES (continued)		
	93235	Holter, 24 Hour	
	10061	I & D Abscess Comp.	
	10060	I & D Abscess Simple	
	94761	Oximetry w/Exercise	
	93720	Plethysmography	
	94760	Pulse Oximetry	
	10003	Rem. Sebaceous Cyst	
	11100	Skin Bx	
	94010	Spirometry	
	92801	Visual Acuity	
	17100	Wart Removal	
	17101	Wart Removal, 2nd	
	17102	Wart Removal, 3–15	
	11042	Wound Debrid.	
	X-RAY		
	70210	Sinuses	
	70360	Neck Soft Tissue	
	71010	CXR (PA only)	
	71020	Chest 2V	
	72040	C-Spine 2V	
	72100	Lumbrosacral	
	73030	Shoulder 2V	
	73070	Elbow 2V	
	73120	Hand 2V	
	73560	Knee 2V	
	73620	Foot 2V	
	74000	KUB	

✔	CPT/Md	DESCRIPTION	FEE
	INJECTIONS		
	90724	Influenza	
	90732	Pneumococcal	
	J0295	Ampicillin, 1 gr	
	J0696	Rocephine	
	J1030	Depomedrol 40 mg	
	J2000	Lidocaine 50 cc	
	J2175	Demerol	
	J3360	Valium 5 mg	
	J1885	Toradol 30 mg IV	
	J1885	Toradol 60 mg IM	
	90720	DTP–HIB	
	90746	HEP B—HIB	
	90707	MMR	
	86580	PPD	
	86580	PPD w/control	
	90732	Pneumovax	
	90716	Varicella	
	82607	Vitamin B12 Inj.	
	90712	Polio	
	90788	TD Adult	
	95115	Allergy inj., single	
	95117	Allergy inj., multiple	

	DESCRIPTION	ICD-10-CM
___	Abdominal pain/unspec	R10.9
___	Abscess	L02._
___	Allergic reaction	T78.40_
___	Alzheimer's disease	G30
___	Anemia/unspec	D64.9
___	Angina/unspec	I20.9
___	Anorexia	R63.0
___	Anxiety/unspec	F41.9
___	Apnea, sleep	G47.30
___	Arrhythmia, cardiac	I49.9
___	Arthritis, rheumatoid	M06.9
___	Asthma/unspec	J45.909
___	Atrial fibrillation	I48.0
___	B-12 deficiency	E53.8
___	Back pain, low	M54.5
___	BPH	N40
___	Bradycardia/unspec	R00.1
___	Broncitis, acute	J20._
___	Bronchitis, chronic	J42
___	Bursitis/unspec	M71.9
___	CA, breast	C50._
___	CA, lung	C34._
___	CA, prostate	C61
___	Cellulitis	L03._
___	Chest pain/unspec	R07.9
___	Cirrhosis, liver/unspec	K74.60
___	Cold, common	J00
___	Colitis/unspec	K51.90
___	Confusion	R41.0
___	CHF	I50.9
___	Constipation	K59.00
___	COPD	J44.9
___	Cough	R05
___	Crohn's disease/unspec	K50.90
___	CVA	I63.9
___	Decubitus ulcer	L89._
___	Dehydration	E86.0
___	Dementia/unspec	F03
___	Depression, major/unsp	F32.9
___	Diab I, no complications	E10.0
___	Diab II, no complications	E11.9
___	w/kidney complic	E11.2_
___	w/ophthalmic compl	E11.3_
___	w/neurolog compl	E11.4_
___	w/circulartory compl	E11.5_
___	Insulin use	Z79.4
___	Diarrhea/unspec	R19.7
___	Diverticulitix	K57.92
___	Diverticulosis	K57.90
___	Dizziness	R42
___	Dysuria	R30.0
___	Edema/unspec	R60.9
___	Endocarditis	I38
___	Esophageal reflux	K21.0
___	Fatigue (lethargy)	R53.83
___	FUO	R50.9
___	Gastritis	K29.70
___	Gastroenteritis (colitis)	K52.9
___	G.I. bleed	K92.2
___	Gout/unspec	M10.9
___	Headache	R51
___	Health exam	200._
___	Hematuria/unspec	R31.9
___	Herpes simplex	B00.9
___	Herpes zoster	B02.9
___	Hiatal hernia	K44.9
___	HTN (HBP)	I10
___	Hyperlipidemia/unspec	E78.5
___	Hypothyroidism/unspec	E03.9
___	Impotence	N52._
___	Influenza, respiratory	J10.1
___	Insomnia	G47.0
___	IBS, diarrhea	K58.
___	Lupus, systemic erythim	M32.9
___	MI, acute	I21._
___	MI, old	I25.2
___	Migraine	G43.9
___	Myalgia	M79.1
___	Neck pain	M54.2
___	Neuropathy	G62.9
___	Nausea	R11.1
___	Nausea/vomitting	R11.0
___	Obesity/unspec	E66.9
___	Osteoarthritis (site)	M19._
___	Otitis media	H66.9_
___	Parkinson's disease	G20
___	Pharyngitis, acute	J02.9
___	Pleurisy	R09.1
___	Pneumonia	J18.9
___	Pneumonia, viral	J12.9
___	Prostatitis/unspec	N41.9
___	PVD	I73.9
___	Radiculopathyp	M54.1_
___	Rectal bleeding	K62.5
___	Renal failure	N19
___	Sciatica	M54.3_
___	Shortness of breath	R03.02
___	Sinusitis, chr./unspec	J32.9
___	Syncope	R55
___	Tachycardia/unspec	R00.0
___	Tachy., supraventric	I47.1
___	Tedinitix/unspec	M77.9
___	TIA	G45.9
___	Ulcer, duodenal/unspec	K26.9
___	Ulcer, gastric/unspec	K25.9
___	Ulcer, peptic/unspec	K27.9
___	URI/unspec	J06.9
___	UTI	N39.0
___	Vertigo	R42
___	Weight gain	R63.5
___	Weight loss	R63.4

DIAGNOSIS: (IF NOT CHECKED ABOVE)

TODAY'S FEE

AMT. REC'D.

PROCEDURES: (IF NOT CHECKED ABOVE)

RETURN APPOINTMENT INFORMATION:

(DAYS)(WKS.)(MOS.)(PRN)

REC'D BY:
☐ CASH
☐ CR. CARD
☐ CHECK
____

BALANCE

FIGURE 14.3 Encounter form.

- Organ or anatomic site (e.g., clavicle, mandible, humerus, liver, colon, uterus)
- Condition, illness, or injury (e.g., cholelithiasis, ulcer, fracture, pregnancy, fever)
- Eponym, synonym, abbreviation, or acronym (e.g., Naffziger operation, MRI [magnetic resonance imaging], TURP [transurethral resection of the prostate])

When searching the Alphabetic Index, use the following:

- The name of the performed procedure or service (anastomosis, splint, repair, stress test, therapy, vaccination)
- The organ or other anatomic site of the procedure (tibia, colon, salivary gland, aorta)
- The condition, illness, or injury (abscess, fracture, cholelithiasis, strabismus)
- The synonyms, eponyms, or abbreviations (ECG [electrocardiography], Stookey-Scarff procedure, Mohs' micrographic surgery)

Sometimes searching for a main term may not yield any results. When a main term cannot be found, search by another primary classification in the Alphabetic Index. Let's search the following procedural statement: Removal of Skin Tags on Neck. Begin by identifying the main terms that closely match the four primary classifications in the Alphabetic Index:

1. Procedure or Service: Removal
2. Organ or Anatomic Site: Neck Skin
3. Condition, Illness, or Injury: Skin Tag
4. Eponym: None in this case

Once all possible main terms have been abstracted, the coder can quickly search through the Alphabetic Index for the code or code range that matches the procedural statement.

Using See *and* See Also *in the Alphabetic Index*

The *see* statement in the Alphabetic Index points to another location in the Alphabetic Index to find the code or code range. The *see also* statement points to additional codes or code ranges in the Alphabetic Index that may be useful to the code found in the original search.

Single Codes and Code Ranges

In the Alphabetic Index, a procedure or service may list a single code or a range of possible codes that may match the documentation. Remember that the Alphabetic Index is an index; it is designed as a guide to the most suitable codes that match the documentation. At this point, the search is only for the closest match or matches to the procedural statement.

Some medical procedures and diagnostic tests can be quite complex. There may be a single code or a code range that may include one main term but has several modifying terms for the main term. For example, the code for Acromioplasty has a range of codes: 23415–23420. The same main term, Acromioplasty, with a modifying term, partial, has a single code: 23130. The code range is shown with a hyphen to indicate that all codes within that range could be appropriate.

In some cases, a single code and a range of codes are listed for the same service or procedure. For example, Craterization, femur, lists both the single code 27360 and the code range 27070–27071. Once a single code or code range has been found in the Alphabetic Index, the next step is to look up each of those in the Tabular List. Select the code or codes that most closely match the documentation.

STEPS FOR USING THE CPT ALPHABETIC INDEX

1. Abstract the procedural statement from the medical documentation, and determine the main or modifying terms.
2. Select the most appropriate main term to begin searching in the Alphabetic Index.
3. Once the main term has been located, select one or more modifying terms, if needed, to narrow the search.
4. If no main or modifying term produces an appropriate code or code range, repeat steps 2 and 3 using a different main term.
5. Find the code or code ranges that include all or most of the description of the procedure or service found in the medical record.

CRITICAL THINKING APPLICATION 14.3

Sherald is having trouble finding a procedural code in the Alphabetic Index for removal of a cataract. What are some options or alternative ways she can perform an Alphabetic Index search?

Using the Tabular List

Once the code or code ranges have been selected from the Alphabetic Index, the next stop is the Tabular List. This is where the procedural coding decision takes place. In the Tabular List, the conventions, symbols, guidelines, notes, and even the punctuation all play a part in choosing the most accurate code possible.

In the Tabular List, look up each code or code range found numerically in the Alphabetic Index. Read the description of each code thoroughly to ensure that the main terms abstracted from the procedural statement in the medical documentation are all included in the code description, with nothing substantial omitted or added. Read the section guidelines and notes to determine whether additional codes should be used, add-on codes or modifiers are required, or use of the code is contraindicated.

Use of the Semicolon

A semicolon (;) at the end of a main description indicates that modifying terms and descriptions follow. Every indented description below a stand-alone code is related to that stand-alone code. To get the full description for an indented code, you use the description of the stand-alone code up to the semicolon and then include the description of the indented code. Let's look at excision of the spleen as an example. In the CPT manual you will see the following entry:

Hemic and Lymphatic Systems
Spleen
Excision
38100 Splenectomy; total (separate procedure)
  38101 partial (separate procedure)
  38102 total, en bloc for extensive disease, in conjunction with other procedure (list in addition to code for primary procedure)

The description for code 38100 is a splenectomy, total. The description for code 38101 is splenectomy, partial. The description for code 38102 is splenectomy, total, en bloc for extensive disease, in conjunction with other procedure. If you were to use 38102, you would also have to have the code for the other procedure. You could not use just 38102.

For practice on CPT surgery coding, refer to Procedure 14.1.

Steps for Using the CPT Tabular List

Except for the special considerations required for coding from the E/M and Anesthesia sections, the following steps apply to all sections of the CPT manual:

1. Look up the code or code range from the Alphabetic Index. Search in the Tabular List numerically.
2. Compare the description of the code with the procedural statement from the documentation. Verify that all or most of the health record documentation matches the code description and that there is no additional element or information in the code description that is not found in the documentation.
3. Read the guidelines and notes for the section, subsection, and code to ensure that there are no contraindications to the use of the code.
4. Evaluate the conventions, especially add-on codes (+) and exemption from modifier −51.
5. Determine whether any special circumstances require the use of a modifier or whether a special report is required.
6. Record the CPT code selected in the health record documentation next to the procedure or service performed and in the appropriate block of the insurance claim form.

CPT CODING GUIDELINES: EVALUATION AND MANAGEMENT SECTION

Evaluation and Management codes are commonly referred to as E/M codes. These codes are used to reflect what the provider does during the time spent with the patient. To properly code for that, the medical assistant must apply different techniques from the basic steps outlined earlier. Assigning the correct E/M code includes the following:

- Identifying the following for the procedure or service:
  - Section
  - Subsection
  - Category
  - Subcategory
- Reviewing the reporting instructions and guidelines for the code chosen
- Reviewing the level of E/M service:
  - Determining the extent of the history obtained and the examination performed
  - Determining the complexity of medical decision making

The E/M section is divided into broad subsections, such as office visit, emergency room visit, hospital visit, and consultation. These subsections are further divided into subcategories, which include the place where the services were rendered, such as these:

- Provider's office
- Hospital emergency department
- Skilled nursing facility
- Patient's home
- Patient status
  - New
  - Established

Procedure 14.2, Part A, explains how to perform CPT coding for an office visit. Here are the first two steps for choosing an E/M code:

1. Identify the place of service (POS).
2. Identify the patient status (new or established).

Identifying the Place of Service

The POS is the healthcare facility where the provider delivered care to the patient. The two most common places of service are "office" and "hospital." Table 14.4 presents a list of common POS locations and their two-digit identifying numbers, or POS codes.

Identifying the Patient Status

The patient status choices are "new" or "established" patient. A new patient (NP) is one who has not received any professional services from the provider, or from another provider of the same specialty and subspecialty who belongs to the same group practice, within the past 3 years.

An established patient (EP) is one who has received professional services from the provider, or from another provider of the same

TABLE 14.4 Commonly Used Place of Service (POS) Codes

CODE	NAME
01	Pharmacy
11	Office
12	Home
13	Assisted Living Facility
14	Group Home
15	Mobile Unit
17	Walk-In Retail Health Clinic
20	Urgent Care Facility
21	Inpatient Hospital
22	Outpatient Hospital
23	Emergency Room—Hospital
24	Ambulatory Surgery Center
31	Skilled Nursing Facility
34	Hospice
51	Inpatient Psychiatric Facility
60	Mass Immunization Center
65	End-Stage Renal Disease Treatment Facility
71	Public Health Clinic
72	Rural Health Clinic
81	Independent Laboratory

specialty and subspecialty who belongs to the same group practice, within the past 3 years.

Once the POS and patient status have been established, the next step in selection of an E/M code is to determine the level of service provided.

Determining the Level of Service Provided

Key Components

The three key components for determining the level of service for E/M coding are history, examination, and medical decision making. The four contributing factors are counseling, nature of the presenting problem, coordination of care, and time; these are all secondary considerations.

History. To understand the history levels, it is important to know the definition and components of the patient's history. The history relates to the patient's clinical picture and depends on the patient for answers to specific questions.

The following are the four levels of history taking:

- *Problem-focused history:* A problem-focused history concentrates on the **chief complaint**; it looks at the symptoms, severity, and duration of the problem. It usually does not include a **review of systems (ROS)** or the family and social histories.
- *Expanded problem-focused history:* The expanded problem-focused history includes the following:
  - Symptoms, severity, and duration of the chief complaint
  - Review of systems that relate to the chief complaint

  Usually the past, family, and social histories are not included.
- *Detailed history:* The detailed history includes the following:
  - Chief complaint
  - Extended history of present illness
  - Problem-pertinent system review, including a review of a limited number of additional systems
  - Pertinent past, family, or social histories directly related to the patient's problems
- *Comprehensive history:* A comprehensive history includes the following:
  - Chief complaint
  - Extended history of present illness
  - ROS that is directly related to the problem or problems identified in the history of the present illness
  - Review of all additional body systems, in addition to complete past, family, and social histories

Examination. The examination is the objective part of the patient's visit. The provider examines the patient, obtains measurable findings, and makes notes referring to body areas or organ systems as follows:

- *Body areas:* Head, including face and neck; chest, including breasts and axillae; abdomen; genitalia, groin, and buttocks; and back, including spine and extremities
- *Organs and organ systems:* General (e.g., vital signs, general appearance); eyes; ears, nose, throat, and mouth; cardiovascular; respiratory; gastrointestinal (GI); genitourinary; musculoskeletal; skin; neurologic; psychiatric; and hematologic, lymphatic, and immunologic

The examination is divided into the following levels:

- *Problem-focused examination:* The examination is limited to the affected body area or single system mentioned in the chief complaint.
- *Expanded problem-focused examination:* In addition to the limited body area or system, related body areas or organ systems are examined.
- *Detailed examination:* An extended examination is performed on the affected body area and related body areas or organ systems.
- *Comprehensive examination:* A complete multisystem examination is performed or a complete examination of a single organ system.

Medical Decision Making. When a provider makes medical decisions, the decisions are based on many years of education and experience. Three elements constitute the medical decision-making process:

- The number of diagnoses or management options. The provider's notes during the history and examination should help identify whether the patient's problem is minor, acute, stable, or worsening. The documentation should also identify whether a new problem exists or whether the provider plans to order any diagnostic tests to further investigate the patient's illness or injury.
- The amount or complexity of data obtained, reviewed, and analyzed. The documentation should also identify what laboratory tests, x-ray diagnostic procedures, and other tests have been ordered or reviewed.
- The risk of significant complications or morbidity or mortality. Risk is often involved in medical care, either from the treatment given to the patient or from the lack of treatment and professional care. *Morbidity,* the relative incidence of disease, and *mortality,* which relates to the number of deaths from a given disease, are integral parts of the provider's assessment of risks.

After considering those three elements, the complexity of medical decision making can be determined. The complexity of medical decision making is categorized into four levels: straightforward, low complexity, moderate complexity, and high complexity. Table 14.5 presents descriptions of the different levels of complexity of medical decision making.

TABLE 14.5 Complexity of Medical Decision Making

NUMBER OF DIAGNOSES OR MANAGEMENT OPTIONS	AMOUNT OR COMPLEXITY OF DATA TO BE REVIEWED	RISK OF COMPLICATIONS, MORBIDITY, OR MORTALITY	TYPE OF MEDICAL DECISION MAKING
Minimal	Minimal or none	Minimal	Straightforward
Limited	Limited	Low	Low complexity
Multiple	Moderate	Moderate	Moderate complexity
Extensive	Extensive	High	High complexity

Other Factors That Contribute to E/M Complexity

In addition to the key components, there are some additional factors that can influence the level of service when determining the correct evaluation and management code. Those factors are discussed next.

Counseling. Counseling is a discussion with a patient or family members about diagnostic results, impressions, recommended diagnostic studies, prognosis, risks and benefits of management or treatment options, instructions for management, treatment, or follow-up.

Almost all E/M services involve a degree of counseling with the patient or family. This is factored into the E/M code.

Nature of the Presenting Problem. The presenting problem is usually explained in the chief complaint. It can range from something as simple as a cold in an otherwise healthy patient to a life-threatening problem.

Coordination of Care. Some patients need help in arranging for care beyond the visit or hospitalization. Some will need care in a skilled nursing facility or home healthcare. Others will need hospice care. The primary provider usually coordinates this care. Coordination of care is also factored into the E/M code and is a consideration for determining the level of service.

Time. Time alone can be used a determining factor for selection of the correct E/M code. It is included in the E/M code descriptions The time requirement refers to a face-to-face encounter with the provider. The times stated in the code descriptions are averages.

At first, E/M coding can be difficult to understand and put into practice. The E/M coding process provided here can serve as a guide to help medical assistants in determining place of service, patient status, and level of care provided.

You can then select the most accurate E/M code. Using the clinical examples in Appendix C of the CPT manual and comparing them to the medical documentation also can help medical assistants acquire a better understanding of E/M coding.

CPT CODING GUIDELINES: ANESTHESIA

Anesthesiologists and **certified registered nurse anesthetists (CRNAs)** use codes in the Anesthesia section. These codes always start with a zero (0) (except for Qualifying Circumstances for Anesthesia [99100–99140]) and identify the anatomic location of the surgery performed. CPT codes are used for unconscious sedation or for putting patients to sleep during the medical procedure; codes for conscious sedation are found in the Medicine section.

Anesthesia coding differs from any other form of coding in the way anesthesia services are billed. These professionals are paid a standard amount per unit compared to surgeons, who are paid by the procedure. A standard formula has been established to determine the number of units they can bill for each procedure for which they provide anesthesia.

$$\text{Basic unit value} + \text{Time units} + \text{Modifying units} \; (B + T + M)$$

Basic Unit Value (B)

The Anesthesia Society of America (ASA) publishes a Relative Value Guide (RVG) that lists the codes for anesthesia services. The RVG compares anesthesia services and assigns a numeric value to each service based on the level of complexity; this numeric value is called the *basic unit value.*

Time Units (T)

Anesthesia services are provided based on the time during which the anesthesia was administered, in hours and minutes. Typically, 15 minutes equals 1 time unit, although this can vary because insurance carriers make that determination independently. The time starts when the anesthesiology provider begins preparing the patient to receive anesthesia, continues through the procedure, and ends when the patient is no longer under the professional care of the anesthesiology provider. The hours and minutes during which anesthesia was administered are recorded in the patient's anesthesia record.

Modifying Units (M)

Modifying units reflect circumstances or conditions that change or modify the environment in which the anesthesia service was provided. The two modifying characteristics for anesthesia services are qualifying circumstances and physical status modifiers.

Qualifying Circumstances (QC)

Sometimes anesthesia is provided in situations that make administration more difficult. These types of cases include provision of anesthesia in emergency situations, to patients of extreme age, during the use of controlled hypotension, and with hypothermia. There are four qualifying circumstances (QC) codes. Each of the five-digit codes is preceded by a plus sign symbol (+), indicating that it is an add-on code; these codes are used in addition to the Category I anesthesia code. Table 14.6 presents a list of the qualifying circumstances CPT codes.

TABLE 14.6 Anesthesia Qualifying Circumstances and Physical Status Modifiers

MODIFIER	DESCRIPTION
Qualifying Circumstances CPT Codes[a]	
99100	Anesthesia for a patient of extreme age (i.e., <1 yr or >70 yr)
99116	Anesthesia complicated by utilization of total body hypothermia
99135	Anesthesia complicated by utilization of controlled hypothermia
Physical Status Modifiers[b]	
P1	A normal healthy patient
P2	A patient with mild systemic disease
P3	A patient with severe systemic disease
P4	A person with severe systemic disease that is a constant threat to life
P5	A moribund patient who is not expected to survive without the procedure
P6	A declared brain-dead patient whose organs are being removed for donor purposes

[a]Use a qualifying circumstances modifier code, if appropriate, in addition to the primary CPT Category I Anesthesia code.
[b]A physical status modifier is required for performing anesthesia calculations.

Physical Status Modifiers

Physical status modifiers are used to indicate the patient's physical condition at the time anesthesia was provided. There are five physical status modifiers, each composed of two characters: first the letter P, followed by a ranking of 1 to 6 (e.g., P1, P2, P3, and so on). P1 represents a normal, healthy patient, and P6 represents a brain-dead patient whose organs are being harvested. Table 14.6 also presents a list of physical status modifiers and their descriptions; a list also can be found in the Anesthesia section of the CPT manual.

Conversion Factors

A *conversion factor* is the dollar value of each basic unit value. Each third-party payer issues a list of conversion factors. The conversion factor for any given geographic location is multiplied by the number of basic unit values assigned to each procedure (Figure 14.4).

Calculating Anesthesia Services

Using the basic unit value (B), modifying unit (M), time unit (T), physical status (PS) modifier, if applicable, and the conversion factor (Figure 14.5), the fee for anesthesia services is calculated according to the anesthesia billing formula:

$$(B + M + T + PS) \times \text{Conversionfactor}$$

Locality Name	Anesthesia Conversion Factor
Manhattan, NY	22.65
NYC suburbs/Long I., NY	22.74
Queens, NY	22.28
Rest of New York	19.91
North Carolina	20.23
North Dakota	19.70

FIGURE 14.4 Anesthesia conversion factors.

Medical Narrative

A 25-year-old female patient in good physical condition has anesthesia services while undergoing laparoscopy (CPT-4 Code 00840). The time for the anesthesia administration was 2 hours. For the purposes of this example, the RBV basic unit value will be 4.

Basic Unit Value	= 4
+ Modifying Units: PS	= 0
+ QC	= 0
+ Time Units	= 8
= 12 Total Units	

The total units value of 12 is then multiplied by the conversion factor for the geographic location of the anesthesiologist's office. For the purposes of this exercise, the conversion factor for Manhattan, NY, will be $20.48, and for North Carolina, $15.77. For the office located in Manhattan, NY, multiply $20.48 by 12. The fee for the anesthesia services would be $245.76. For the office located in North Carolina, multiply 12 times $15.77, for a fee of $189.24.

FIGURE 14.5 Anesthesia formula and calculation.

CPT CODING GUIDELINES: SURGICAL SECTION

Specific guidelines and notes related to surgery coding must be considered when assigning a CPT code. Always review the current year's guidelines for the Surgery section for the most up-to-date information. The following sections discuss a few of the more common guidelines. When coding procedures and services, be sure to read the guidelines and notes thoroughly for accurate coding assignment.

Surgical Package Definition

The CPT code set is designed to include patient prep, surgical care, and postsurgical care in a single code. These are considered **global services** because they are already built into the surgical package cost of the assigned CPT code. Medical coders who include any of these global services as a separate CPT code are committing fraud. The CPT code descriptions of global surgical services typically include the following:

- Local infiltration, digital block, or topical anesthesia
- After the decision for surgery, one related E/M encounter on the day of, or the day before, the date of the procedure
- Immediate postoperative care, including documentation in the patient's health record and talking with family or other physicians
- Writing orders for postsurgical care
- Evaluating the patient in the post-anesthesia recovery area
- Typical postoperative follow-up care (includes care for approximately 6 to 8 weeks after surgery and is usually done at the provider's office)

NCCI Edits and Unbundled Codes

In 1996, in an effort to prevent fraudulent medical coding, the Centers for Medicare and Medicaid Services (CMS) established the National Corrective Coding Initiative (NCCI) edit list. This list contains two columns of codes, and the codes in the two columns are mutually exclusive. Submitted claims that contain mutually exclusive codes are automatically rejected.

When a CPT procedure is billed, this code includes services related to prepping the patient for the procedure, performing the procedure, and suturing to complete the procedure; the single code for the procedure is called a *bundled code* because it represents all of the stages of surgery. When each step of the procedure is listed separately, these are called *unbundled codes*. Unbundled codes are used when the components of a major procedure are separated and reported separately. When these codes are separated and used individually, a special report should be used to describe the circumstances that made the unbundling necessary; the reason for this is that unbundled CPT codes have higher reimbursements because each code is paid separately. Medical billers who regularly unbundle CPT codes may be cited for fraud or abuse.

Integumentary System: Excision of Lesions—Benign or Malignant

Excision of benign lesions includes a simple closure and local anesthesia. If a wound (incision, excision, or traumatic lesion) requires intermediate or complex closure, the repair by intermediate or complex closure is coded and reported separately from the incision or excision. For example, if the provider excised a benign lesion measuring 1 cm from the patient's arm that required intermediate repair (closure), two codes would be used:

11401 – Excision, benign lesion including margins; excised diameter 0.6 to 1 cm

12031 – Repair, intermediate, wounds of scalp, axillae, trunk and/or extremities (excluding hands and feet); 2.5 cm or less

Levels of Closure (Repair)

- *Simple repair:* Performed when the wound is superficial (epidermis, dermis, or subcutaneous) without significant involvement of deeper structures. This includes local anesthesia and chemical or electrocauterization of wounds not closed.
- *Intermediate repair:* Includes simple repair with a need for a layered closure of one or more of the deeper layers of subcutaneous tissue and superficial fascia in addition to the skin closure. Single-layer closure of heavily contaminated wounds that required extensive cleaning or removal of particulate matter also constitutes an intermediate repair.
- *Complex repair:* Includes wounds that require more than layered closure (e.g., scar revision, extensive undermining, or stents or retention sutures). Necessary preparation includes creation of a limited defect for repairs or **debridement** of complicated lacerations. Complex repair does not include excision of benign or malignant lesions, excisional preparation of a wound bed, or debridement, or the removal of damaged tissue or foreign objects from a wound, an open fracture, or an open dislocation.

Listing Services for Wound Repair

- The repaired wound or wounds should be measured and recorded in centimeters; it also should be indicated whether the wound was curved, angular, or in a starlike pattern.
- When multiple wounds are repaired, add together the lengths of those in the same classification (simple, intermediate, or complex) and from all anatomic sites that are grouped together into the same code descriptor.
- When wounds of more than one classification are repaired, list the more complicated repair as the primary procedure and the less complicated repair as the secondary procedure, using modifier –59.
- Debridement is considered a separate procedure only when gross contamination requires prolonged cleansing, when a large amount of dead or contaminated tissue must be removed, or when debridement is carried out separately without immediate primary closure.
- Wound repair that involves nerves, blood vessels, or tendons should be reported under the appropriate system for repair of those structures. The repair of these associated wounds is included in the primary procedure unless it qualifies as a complex repair, in which case modifier –59 applies.

Musculoskeletal System

When determining codes for fractures in the surgery/musculoskeletal system section of the CPT manual there a several terms that you should be aware of:

- *Closed fracture:* The fractured bone does not protrude through the dermis or epidermis.
- *Open fracture:* The fractured bone cuts through the skin layers and can be directly visualized.
- *Closed treatment:* The fracture site is not surgically opened. There are three methods of closed treatment of fractures:
  - Without manipulation
  - With manipulation
  - With or without traction
- *Manipulation:* Attempted reduction or restoration of a fracture or dislocated joint into its normal anatomic alignment by manually applied forces.
- *Open treatment:* Used when (1) the fractured bone is surgically opened or (2) an opening is made remote from the fracture site to insert an intramedullary nail across the fracture site.
- *Percutaneous skeletal fixation:* Fracture treatment that is neither open nor closed. The fracture fragments are not visualized, but a fixation device (e.g., pins) is placed across the fracture site, usually under x-ray imaging.

After determining the type of fracture and treatment, you can determine the correct code for the services provided.

Maternity Care and Delivery

The services normally provided in uncomplicated maternity cases include antepartum care, delivery, and postpartum care.

- *Antepartum* care includes the following:
  - Initial and subsequent history
  - Physical examinations
  - Recording of weight, blood pressure, and fetal heart tones
  - Routine chemical urinalysis
  - Monthly visits up to 28 weeks' gestation
  - Biweekly visits to 36 weeks' gestation
  - Weekly visits until delivery

Any other visits or services provided within this period should be coded separately, including any routine tests (e.g., sonography, routine laboratory tests).

- *Delivery* includes the following:
  - Admission to the hospital, the admission history, and the physical examination
  - Management of uncomplicated labor
  - Vaginal delivery (with or without forceps or episiotomy), or cesarean delivery

Medical problems complicating labor and delivery should be identified by using the codes in the Medicine and E/M sections in addition to codes for maternity care.

- *Postpartum* care includes the following:
  - Hospital and office visits after vaginal or cesarean section delivery

CPT CODING GUIDELINES: RADIOLOGY AND PATHOLOGY AND LABORATORY SECTIONS

Radiology services has its own section in the CPT manual, while pathology and laboratory services are combined in one section. It is important to be familiar with each section, as each has its own guidelines and those are discussed next.

Radiology Section

Assigning CPT codes for the Radiology section follows the same procedure as for the Surgery section. The Radiology section contains all diagnostic imaging codes, including x-ray studies, ultrasound, MRI, computer axial tomography (CAT) scans, and nuclear medicine procedures, in addition to radiation oncology and several other types of diagnostic imaging procedures, services, and therapies. The Radiology section is divided into subsections: head and neck; chest, spine, and pelvis; upper and lower extremities; abdomen, gastrointestinal and urinary tracts; and gynecologic, obstetric, heart, and vascular procedures. The next subdivision, categories, defines the types or functions of various procedures (e.g., diagnostic ultrasound, radiation oncology, and so on) unique to the anatomic site subsection. In addition to the radiology procedure codes, codes are included for physician supervision and interpretation of diagnostic imaging data and for clinical and radiation treatment planning and administration of contrast materials during radiologic procedures.

Pathology and Laboratory Section

Assigning CPT codes for the Pathology section also follows the same procedure as for the Surgery section. For purposes of coding from the Laboratory section, organ or disease panels are groupings of numerous tests performed to diagnose the health or disease status of specific organ systems. A panel code can be used only if all the tests listed under the code selected were performed. These are considered *bundled codes* and must be billed under the single CPT code. If they are not all present, the individual tests should be billed using a separate code for each. There are two types of drug testing, qualitative and quantitative. The codes for drug testing are *qualitative*—that is, they are based on the type of drug found. *Quantitative* assays, on the other hand, are performed to determine the amount of drug present.

CPT Tabular List Basic Metabolic Panel

80047 Basic metabolic panel (Calcium, ionized)
This panel must include the following:
- Calcium, ionized (82330)
- Carbon dioxide (bicarbonate) (82374)
- Chloride (82435)
- Creatinine (82565)
- Glucose (82947)
- Potassium (84132)

The codes in parentheses after the individual tests are CPT codes. Those CPT codes would be used if not all of these tests were ordered at the same time.
Other basic metabolic panel components:
- Sodium (84295)
- Urea nitrogen (BUN) (84520)

CRITICAL THINKING APPLICATION **14.4**

Sherald reviewed a coded medical record for a Basic Metabolic Panel with total Calcium that had listed specific CPT codes for each panel test. Is this the correct way to code for the organ panel? According to the box above, how should this organ panel be coded?

CPT CODING GUIDELINES: MEDICINE SECTION

The Medicine section of the CPT contains codes for a variety of therapeutic procedures and diagnostic testing. This section also contains codes for dialysis, ophthalmology, acupuncture, chiropractic manipulation, and conscious sedation. The steps for determining Medicine codes are similar to those for choosing Surgery codes.

Immune Globulins

When you code administration of immune globulins, identify the immune globulin product administered (CPT codes 90281–90399) and the method of administration using the codes in the hydration, therapeutic, prophylactic, and diagnostic injections and infusions subsection.

Hydration codes are intended to report a hydration intravenous (IV) infusion consisting of prepackaged fluid and electrolytes; they are not used to report the infusion of drugs or other substances. When multiple drugs are administered, report the service or services and the specific materials or drugs for each.

Immunization for Vaccines or Toxoids

The immunization for vaccines or toxoids codes (CPT codes 90460, 90461, 90471–90474) are for the administration of vaccines and toxoids only and should be reported in conjunction with the appropriate codes in the immunization administration for vaccine/toxoids subsection.

Vaccines/Toxoids Codes

These codes identify the vaccine product only (CPT codes 90476–90749). Codes in the immunization administration for vaccines/toxoids subsection must be used in addition to the vaccine or toxoid product codes. For example, if an adult patient received an influenza virus vaccine code 90471 would be used for the immunization administration and 90654 for the actual vaccine. To meet the reporting requirements of immunization registries, vaccine distribution programs, and reporting systems, the exact vaccine product administered must be reported on the insurance claim.

Home Health Procedures and Services

The home health procedures and services codes (CPT codes 99500–99602) are used by nonphysician healthcare professionals only. They are used to report services provided in a patient's residence, including assisted-living apartments, group homes, nontraditional private homes, custodial care facilities, and schools.

HCPCS CODE SYSTEM

HCPCS codes are mainly used to code drugs, supplies, and services that are not part of the CPT code system. Codes are assigned using a system similar to CPT. The next section discusses the HCPCS code set, manual, and the common coding guidelines.

HCPCS Code Set and Manual

HCPCS codes have five alphanumeric characters, beginning with one letter followed by four numbers. HCPCS uses coding conventions for special instructions relating to specific codes (Figure 14.6). The modifiers for HCPCS are codes composed of two alphanumeric characters. The HCPCS modifiers do not change the description of the code, but rather provide additional information or describe extenuating circumstances. Like the CPT manual, the HCPCS manual is divided into an Alphabetic Index and a Tabular List. As with the CPT, procedures and services are looked up in the Alphabetic Index, and the code (or codes) is then confirmed as the most accurate and appropriate using the Tabular List. The HCPCS manual has

Humidifiers/Compressors/Nebulizers for Use with Oxygen IPPB Equipment

E0550	Humidifier, durable for extensive supplemental humidification during IPPB treatments or oxygen delivery
E0555	Humidifier, durable, glass or autoclavable plastic bottle type, for use with regulator or flowmeter
E0560	Humidifier, durable for supplemental humidification during IPPB treatment or oxygen delivery
E0561	Humidifier, nonheated, used with positive airway pressure device
E0562	Humidifier, heated, used with positive airway pressure device
E0565	Compressor, air power source for equipment which is not self-contained or cylinder driven
E0570	Nebulizer, with compressor
E0572	Aerosol compressor, adjustable pressure, light duty for intermittent use
E0574	Ultrasonic/electronic aerosol generator with small volume nebulizer
E0575	Nebulizer, ultrasonic, large volume
E0580	Nebulizer, durable, glass or autoclavable plastic, bottle type, for use with regulator or flowmeter
E0585	Nebulizer, with compressor and heater

FIGURE 14.6 Healthcare Common Procedure Coding System (HCPCS) Tabular List.

no subsections, categories, or subcategories; it has only sections. An appendix contains all the HCPCS modifiers and their descriptions. The HCPCS codes are updated annually by the CMS.

The coding steps for HCPCS are almost identical to those for CPT codes. Clinical documentation is the starting point for HCPCS coding. The final code selected should add nothing to or omit anything from the description in the medical documentation. The final step is determining whether the code selected can stand alone or requires a modifier to further define or add needed information.

Sometimes HCPCS codes are used along with CPT codes, especially in the medical office setting. For example, a 67-year-old patient comes in for an annual physical examination and influenza vaccine; the visit would include the E/M code for the patient visit and also HCPCS codes for the administration of immunization. Procedure 14.2, Part B, explains how to code an office visit involving immunizations.

Common HCPCS Coding Guidelines

Ambulance transportation, medical and surgical supplies, and durable medical equipment are among the most common categories that require HCPCS codes. The guidelines for assigning those codes are discussed in the next section.

Ambulance Transport

HCPCS codes for ambulance transport range from A0021 to A0999. These codes require specific modifiers (Table 14.7) to be added to ensure code specificity. This section provides codes for various forms of medical transport, including ambulance services, nonemergency transportation, and medical supplies used during the transport. A waiting time calculation table also is available, if needed.

Medical and Surgical Supplies

HCPCS codes for medical and surgical supplies range from A4000 to A6513. The HCPCS manual provides some figures that offer guidance as to what the medical and surgical supplies look like, so that they can be billed properly. Medical assistants can code only for surgical supplies purchased by the medical office. For example, pharmaceutical and medical equipment representatives can provide the medical office with some supplies that can be used for patient care. However, it is unethical to bill the patient's insurance company for supplies that were given to the provider for free. All medical and surgical supplies used during patient care should be documented on the encounter form in the patient's health record.

TABLE 14.7 Modifiers Used for HCPCS Ambulance Transport Codes

TRANSPORTATION SERVICES MODIFIERS[a]	DESCRIPTION
D	Diagnostic or therapeutic site other than P or H when those are used as origin codes
E	Residential, domiciliary, custodial facility
G	Hospital-based dialysis facility (hospital or hospital related)
H	Hospital
I	Site of transfer (e.g., airport or helicopter pad) between modes of ambulance transport
J	Non-hospital-based dialysis facility
N	Skilled nursing facility
P	Physician's office
R	Residence
S	Scene of accident or acute event
X	Destination code only; intermediate stop at physician's office on the way to hospital

[a]Includes ambulance HCPCS origin modifiers.

Durable Medical Equipment

HCPCS codes for durable medical equipment range from E0100 to E1841. Examples of durable medical equipment include crutches, wheelchairs, walkers, and other products that assist patients with mobility. Some equipment is kept in the medical office inventory. If the practice purchases the medical equipment wholesale, it is allowed to bill patients or their insurance company for the retail value of the equipment. Just as with medical and surgical supplies, it is important for the provider to document the dispensing of durable medical equipment on the encounter form or health record (Procedure 14.3).

CLOSING COMMENTS

The CPT and HCPCS coding manuals are updated and published every year. The updated manuals should be ordered in the early fall so that they arrive in time for the medical assistant to review them. Always use the current year's manuals so that the codes are accurate. The introduction in each manual discusses and highlights changes or new coding guidelines. Annual updates should be uploaded to reflect any coding changes in the encoder to ensure that all codes are up to date for the current year.

Legal and Ethical Issues

Medical assistants are responsible for keeping up to date on CPT coding to ensure that no fraud takes place in the coding and claims submission process. Medical assistants should also ensure that proper precautions are taken to avoid incorrect coding, data entry errors, and false claims submissions, because these activities can be considered fraud.

Medical coders should be familiar with the NCCI edits, which are published every year by the CMS. Medicare can cite a healthcare facility for fraud or abuse (or both) if claims submitted by the facility regularly show unbundled codes. Not only is unbundling an unethical practice, it incurs very stiff monetary penalties. According to the Civil Monetary Penalties Law, medical practices can be cited for penalties of up to $50,000 per violation, and assessments of up to three times the amount claimed for each item or service, or up to three times the amount of remuneration offered, paid, solicited, or received.

Patient-Centered Care

It is important for anyone who does coding to be able to explain to patients what those codes mean. When statements are sent to patients, many call the healthcare facility and ask for an explanation of the charges. A common question is "Why is the charge for my office visit so high?" By looking at the CPT E/M code, you can see the level of history taking, physical examination, and medical decision making for that visit. You can help patients understand that it is not just the face-to-face time that determines the level of an office visit. If an extensive history and examination are done and a lot of tests must be reviewed, the E/M code will be at a higher level. That higher level warrants a higher charge. Most patients understand once all of the criteria have been explained to them. When you make these explanations with a pleasant attitude, patient satisfaction also improves.

Professional Behaviors

Two rules should be followed when you code any procedure or service:

1. Be as specific as possible in code selection and use all pertinent words in the description given in your documentation.
2. Never add or delete any words, modifying terms, or descriptors to the procedure or service code description that change the definition of the procedure or service or that are not documented.

SUMMARY OF SCENARIO

Sherald has learned that procedural coding using the CPT is similar in many ways to ICD-10-CM diagnostic coding. The two coding manuals have unique but similar steps, conventions, and guidelines. She has learned that proper abstraction of procedural data from the health record is equally important for ICD-10-CM and CPT coding. Sherald also has learned that HCPCS codes are used to describe procedures and services not found in the CPT, such as vaccinations, ambulance services, and durable medical equipment.

Sherald uses documentation by the provider in the encounter form to identify the procedures performed. However, she realizes that she also must know how to use the CPT manual because some procedures or services must be coded from the documentation. As with diagnostic coding, Sherald reviews the patient's health record documentation if any questions come up about a claim. She knows that coding to the highest level of specificity helps to ensure accuracy and also enables the practice to obtain the maximum reimbursement allowed. She realizes the importance of keeping up to date with the CPT and HCPCS codes, so she plans to order the updated manuals every year. As Sherald continues to learn procedural coding, she envisions herself becoming well rounded in her knowledge of the practice's administrative operations.

SUMMARY OF LEARNING OBJECTIVES

1. **Examine the CPT manual.**
   The *Current Procedural Terminology* (CPT) manual comprises three category codes: Category I, Category II, and Category III codes. Category I codes are five-digit codes that are listed in the Tabular List. Category II codes are used for performance measurement, and their use is optional. Category III codes are temporary codes for emerging medical technologies.

   The CPT has two primary divisions, the Alphabetic Index and the Tabular List. The Alphabetic Index is like any other index in a textbook; it is simply a guide for finding data in the body of the textbook. The Tabular List is divided into six sections, and codes are listed in numeric order in each section.

   The six sections of the Tabular List are Evaluation and Management, Anesthesia, Surgery, Radiology, Pathology and Laboratory, and Medicine. Sections are divided into subsections, subsections are further divided into categories, and categories can be subdivided into subcategories.

   When a bill is submitted for a service that is unlisted, unusual, or newly adopted, the third-party carrier requires a special consultation report. Modifiers are used in CPT codes to indicate that a service or procedure performed was altered by specific circumstances. Two-digit alphanumeric modifiers, included with the 5-digit CPT code, can be used to supply additional information or to describe extenuating circumstances that affected the rendered procedure or service.

   Conventions are used to provide additional information about certain codes. Examples of conventions include triangular and round symbols, which indicate that a code or description was revised, removed, or added. Medical records used for procedural coding can include any or all of the following: encounter form, history and physical report (H&P), progress notes, discharge summary, operative report, pathology report, anesthesia record, or radiology report. When the medical documentation is compared

SUMMARY OF LEARNING OBJECTIVES—cont'd

against any code description, all the elements of that code must substantially match, with nothing added or missing.

2. **Explain the steps for efficient CPT coding.**
The basic steps in procedural coding are (1) read, analyze, and abstract the procedure or service documented in the health record and (2) compare it with the encounter form, operative report, or other documentation to ensure that all services and procedures have been recorded. After searching the Alphabetic Index, the medical assistant should turn to the appropriate codes in the Tabular List to perform the final coding steps. Read the section thoroughly to determine the most accurate code to assign to the procedure or service, and then code the procedure or service. The process for procedural coding for surgery with the CPT code set is detailed in Procedure 14.1.
The Alphabetic Index is a comprehensive, alphabetic listing of all main terms used in procedural coding. However, it is not a substitute for the Tabular List. It is organized by main terms, and modifying terms are indented two spaces below that term. Begin the search of the Alphabetic Index by using one of the four primary classifications of main and modifying term entries. In the Tabular List, look up each code or code range found in the Alphabetic Index.

3. **Explain the components of determining the correct evaluation and management code.**
To properly code Evaluation and Management (E/M) services, the medical assistant must understand important differences, or variations, from the basic steps. Assigning the correct E/M code includes identifying the section, subsection, category, and subcategory of the procedure or service; reviewing the reporting instructions and guidelines for the code chosen; reviewing the level of E/M service; determining the extent of the history obtained and examination performed; and determining the complexity of medical decision making.
To code an office visit, the coder first must determine the level of all key components, which include the history, examination, and medical decision making. (See Procedure 14.2, Part A.)
Coding for HCPCS is almost identical to coding for CPT because both manuals have an Alphabetic Index and a Tabular List. After searching the Alphabetic Index, the coder turns to the appropriate codes in the Tabular List to perform the final coding steps. The coder reads the section thoroughly to determine the most accurate code to assign to the procedure or service and then codes the procedure or service. (See Procedure 14.2, Part B.)

4. **Explain the components determining the correct CPT codes for anesthesia.**
Anesthesia coding differs from any other form of coding in the way anesthesia services are billed. A standard formula has been established for payment of anesthesia services: Basic unit value (B) + Time units (T) + Modifying units (M) + Physical Status (PS): B + T + M + PS. The total number of units is then multiplied by the conversion factor.

5. **Explain the components for determining the correct CPT code for surgical services.**
Specific guidelines and notes related to surgery coding must be considered when assigning a CPT code. Always review the current year's guidelines in the Surgery section for the most up-to-date information.
Excision of benign lesions includes a simple closure and local anesthesia. Different instructions are provided for each type of wound repair. Fractures are handled according to the type. The services normally provided in uncomplicated maternity cases include antepartum care, delivery, and postpartum care.

6. **Explain how to determine the correct CPT codes for radiology services and pathology and laboratory services.**
Assigning accurate CPT codes for the Radiology section is similar to the process for the Surgery section. The Radiology section contains all diagnostic imaging codes, including x-ray studies, ultrasound, MRI, CAT scan and nuclear medicine procedures, in addition to radiation oncology and several other types of diagnostic imaging procedures, services, and therapies.
Assigning accurate CPT codes for the Pathology and Laboratory section also is similar to the process for the Surgery section. The subcategories for the Pathology section include organ panels and disease panels, drug testing, therapeutic drug assays, evocative or suppression testing, consultations, urinalysis, chemistry, molecular diagnostics, infectious agents, microbiology, anatomic pathology, cytopathology, cytogenetic studies, and surgical pathology. In the Laboratory section, organ or disease panels are groupings of numerous tests performed to diagnose the health or disease status of specific organ systems.

7. **Explain what services are found in the Medicine section of the CPT manual.**
The Medicine section contains codes for a variety of therapeutic procedures and diagnostic testing. This section also contains codes for Dialysis, Ophthalmology, Acupuncture, Chiropractic Manipulation, and Conscious Sedation. The steps for determining codes in the Medicine section are similar to those for determining codes in the Surgery section.

8. **Examine the HCPCS coding system.**
HCPCS is a collection of codes and descriptions that represent procedures, supplies, products, and services not covered by or included in the CPT coding system. HCPCS codes, like CPT codes, are updated annually by the CMS. These codes are designed to promote standardized reporting and collection of statistical data on medical supplies, products, services, and procedures.
Like the CPT manual, the HCPCS manual is divided into two parts: the Alphabetic Index and the Tabular List. As with the CPT, procedures and services are looked up in the Alphabetic Index, and the Tabular List then is used to confirm that the code is the most accurate and appropriate one. The HCPCS manual has no subsections, categories, or subcategories; it has only sections. An appendix contains all the HCPCS modifiers and their descriptions. The coding steps for HCPCS are almost identical to those for CPT Category I codes.
Ambulance Transport codes require specific modifiers to ensure code specificity. The HCPCS manual provides some figures that offer guidance as to what the medical and surgical supplies look like, so they can be billed properly. Medical assistants can only bill for surgical supplies that were purchased by the medical office. The medical office can purchase the medical equipment wholesale but still bill patients or their insurance companies for the retail value of the equipment. When the insurance company is billed, it is vital that the medical assistant fill in the "Number of Units" box on the health insurance claim form for equipment provided to the patient.

PROCEDURE 14.1 Perform Procedural Coding: Surgery

TASK: Use the steps for CPT procedural coding to find the most accurate and specific CPT surgery code.

EQUIPMENT and SUPPLIES

- CPT coding manual (current year) or
- TruCode encoder software
- Operative report (see the following figure)

Operative Report

PATIENT NAME: Sonia Sample
ROOM NUMBER: 222 West
MR NUMBER: 12-34-56

DATE OF PROCEDURE: 04/22/20XX
PREOPERATIVE DIAGNOSIS: Acute cholecystitis
POSTOPERATIVE DIAGNOSIS: Acute cholecystitis
NAME OF PROCEDURE: 1. Laparoscopic cholecystectomy
2. Intraoperative cystic duct cholangiogram
SURGEON: Claude St. John, M.D.
ASSISTANT: Mark Weiss, D.O.
ANESTHESIOLOGIST: Angela Adams, M.D.
ANESTHESIA: General

DESCRIPTION OF THE OPERATION:

The patient was placed in the supine position under general anesthesia. The oral gastric tube was placed. The Foley catheter was placed. The patient received appropriate antibiotics. The abdomen was prepped with iodine and draped in the usual fashion. Using a midline subumbilical incision, we entered the subcutaneous fat to find the aponeurosis of the rectus abdominis. Two stay sutures were placed 0.5 cm from the midline bilaterally and we left on these sutures, creating an opening in the linea alba.

Under direct vision, the catheter was placed. The Hasson cannula was placed in the abdominal cavity and all was normal except an acute necrotizing and probably gangrenous gallbladder. There were multiple omental adhesions. Three other trocars were placed in the right subcostal plane in the midline, midclavicular line, and midaxillary line using a #10, #5, and #5 mm trocar, respectively. The gallbladder was punctured and emptied of clear white bile indicating a hydrops of the gallbladder. It was grasped at its fundus and at Hartmann's pouch retracted cephalad and to the right, respectively. We found the cystic duct and the cystic artery after circumferential dissection and isolated the cystic duct completely.

When we were sure that this structure was a deep cystic duct, the clip was placed at the most distal aspect to make an opening immediately proximally and we placed a Reddick cholangiocatheter into it via #14 gauge percutaneous catheter. The cholangiogram showed normal arborization of the liver radicals. Normal bifurcation of the common hepatic duct. Normal common hepatic duct. Long large cystic duct. The common bile duct had numerous stones within it. They could not be emptied from the common bile duct. There was good flow into the duodenum.

The impression was choledocholithiasis. This was corroborated by the radiologist. The decision was made to prepare the patient most probably for endoscopic retrograde cholangiopancreatography postoperatively, and no further intervention of the common bile duct was done in this setting.

The cholangiocatheter was removed. An attempt was made to milk the bile out, but no stones came out. Three clips were placed on the proximal aspect of the cystic duct, and the duct was then cut distally. The artery was isolated and double clipped proximally and single clipped distally and cut in the intervening section. We then peeled the gallbladder off the gallbladder bed with some difficulty because of the intense edema and inflammation. It was then removed from the liver bed completely. Cautery, suctioning, and irrigation were used copiously to create a bloodless field. A last check was made, and there was no bleeding and no bile leaking. A #15 Jackson-Pratt type drain was placed into Morrison's pouch and brought out through the lateral most port. We then removed, with great difficulty, the gallbladder from the umbilicus. Because of its enormous size and a 3 cm stone within it that was very difficult to macerate, the opening of the umbilicus had to be enlarged.

As this was done, we removed the gallbladder completely and sent it for pathologic section. Two separate figure-of-eight 0 PDS were used to close the abdominal fascia. The Jackson-Pratt drain was then sutured in place with 2.0 nylon. The skin was closed throughout with subcuticular 3-0 PDS after copious irrigation of the subcutaneous plane. Mastisol and Steri-Strips were placed on the wound. The patient remained stable, although she did have bigeminy during surgery and was ona Lidocaine drip. She will be going to the intensive care unit but as she left, she was extubated in the recovery room and was fully alert. She is moving all limbs.

I will discuss with the gastroenterologist postoperative endoscopic retrograde cholangiopancreatography.

SPECIMEN: Gallbladder.

____

Claude St. John, M.D.
CSJ/ld:
D: 04/22/20XX
T: 04/22/20XX 9:21 a.m.
CC: Maria Acosta, M.D.

1

PROCEDURE 14.1 Perform Procedural Coding: Surgery—cont'd

PROCEDURAL STEPS

USING THE CPT CODING MANUAL

1. Abstract the procedures or services from the procedural statement in the surgical report.
2. Select the most appropriate main term to begin the search in the Alphabetic Index.
3. Once the main term has been located in the Alphabetic Index, review and select the modifying term or terms if required.
   PURPOSE: For additional specificity and to narrow the search for the most accurate CPT code or code range in the Alphabetic Index.
4. If the main term cannot be found in the Alphabetic Index, repeat steps 2 and 3 using a different main term, possibly based on the procedural statement.
5. Once the CPT code or code range is identified in the Alphabetic Index, disregard any code or code range containing additional descriptions or modifying terms not found in the health record.
6. Record the code or code ranges that best match the procedural statements in the surgical report.
   PURPOSE: To prevent repeated reference to the Alphabetic Index by recording all possible matches to the code or code range sought. This saves time and prevents redundant effort.
7. Turn to the Tabular List and find the first code or code range from your search of the Alphabetic Index.
   PURPOSE: To begin the process of finding the most specific and accurate code.
8. Compare the description of the code with the procedural statement in the surgical report. Verify that all or most of the health record documentation matches the code description and that there is no additional information in the code description that is not found in the documentation.
9. Review the coding guidelines and notes for the section, subsection, and code to ensure that there are no contraindications to use of the code. Review the coding conventions and add-on codes, if any.
   PURPOSE: To ensure there are no instructions that would prevent the use of the code selected.
10. Determine whether a modifier is needed.
   PURPOSE: To select any appropriate modifiers that provide additional information for the chosen code to explain certain circumstances or provide additional detail.
11. Determine whether a Special Report is required.
   PURPOSE: To clarify and add additional detail when an unusual or extenuating circumstance exists or if a Category III or unlisted procedure Category I code is used.
12. Record the CPT code selected in the health record documentation next to the procedure or service performed and in the appropriate block of the insurance claim form.
   PURPOSE: To complete the documentation and recording requirements.

USING THE TRUCODE SOFTWARE

1. Abstract the procedures or services from the procedural statement in the surgical report.
2. Type the main term into the encoder Search box, and select the CPT. Then click on Show All Results.
3. If the main term cannot be found through the search, repeat steps 2 and 3 using a different main term based on the procedural statement.
4. Choose the procedure description that is closest to the procedural statement in the surgical report (see the following figure).
   PURPOSE: To prevent upcoding or downcoding errors or other possible fraud or abuse circumstances.
5. Record the CPT code that best matches the procedural statements in the surgical report in the patient's health record.
   PURPOSE: To prevent repeated reference to the Alphabetic Index by recording all possible matches to the code or code range being sought. This saves time and prevents redundant effort.

Continued

PROCEDURE 14.1 Perform Procedural Coding: Surgery—cont'd

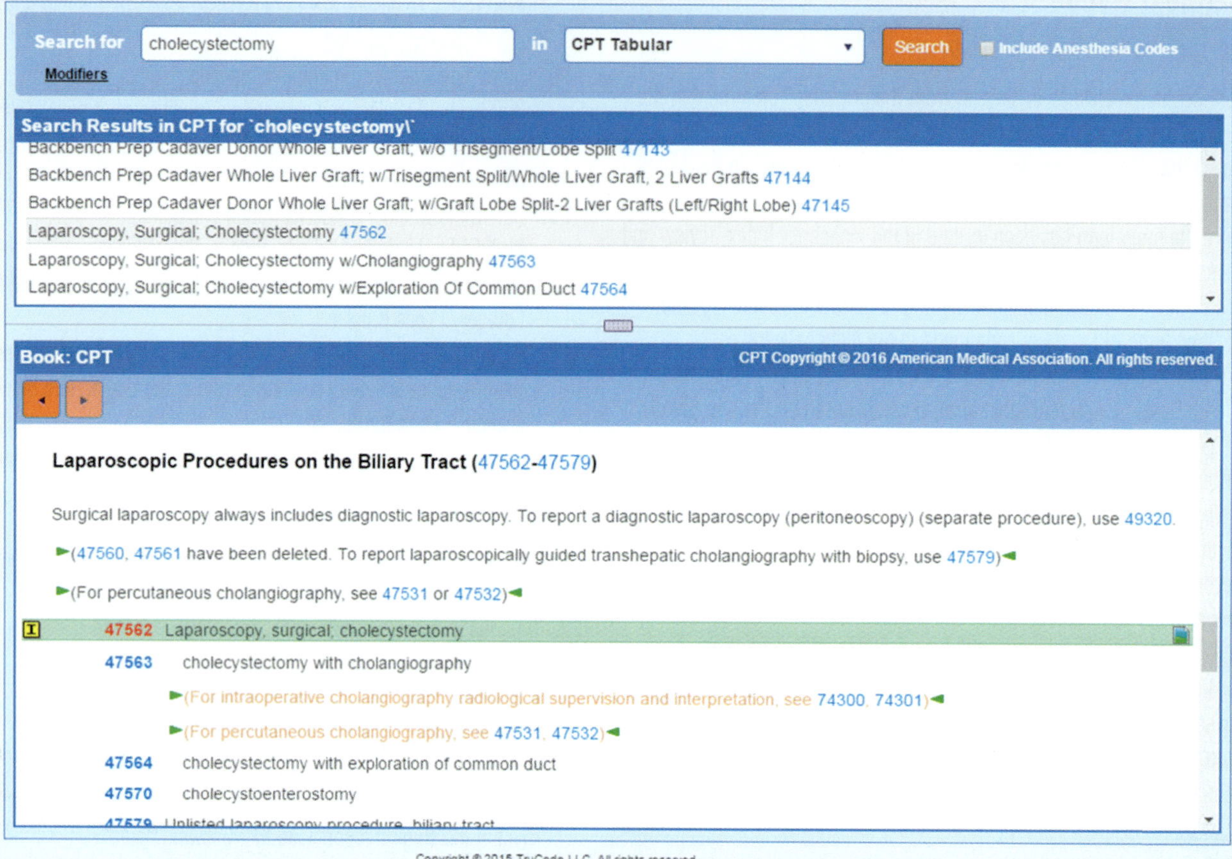

2

PROCEDURE 14.2 Perform Procedural Coding: Office Visit and Immunizations

TASK: Use the steps for CPT Evaluation and Management coding and HCPCS coding to find the most accurate and specific CPT E/M and HCPCS codes using the coding manuals or the TruCode encoder.

EQUIPMENT and SUPPLIES

- CPT coding manual (current year)
- HCPCS coding manual (current year) or
- TruCode encoder software
- Progress note

PROGRESS NOTE FOR ERMA WILLIS (DOB 12/09/19XX): 04/08/20XX Mrs. Willis was seen today for a follow-up visit for a recent case of bronchitis. The infection has completely cleared, and she would like to get the influenza vaccine. The office visit involved a medically appropriate history and examination as well as medical decision making of straightforward complexity.

PROCEDURAL STEPS

PART A: CPT E/M CODING

1. Determine the place of service from the encounter form.
   PURPOSE: To determine the most accurate CPT E/M code, the place of service needs to be identified.
2. Determine the patient's status.
   PURPOSE: To determine the most accurate CPT E/M code, the patient should be identified as new or established.
3. Identify the subsection, category, or subcategory of service in the E/M section.
   PURPOSE: To ensure that the correct place of service and patient status are used and the appropriate level of service is selected.

PROCEDURE 14.2 Perform Procedural Coding: Office Visit and Immunizations—cont'd

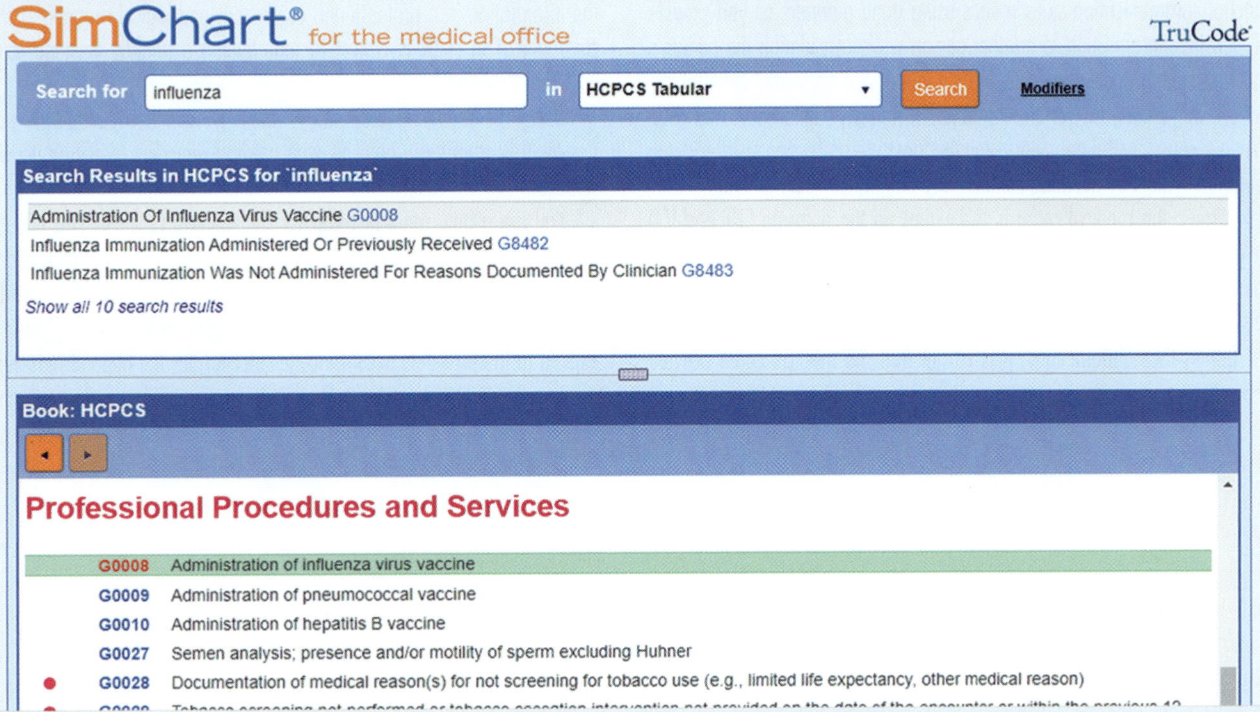

4. Determine the level of service by determining the complexity of medical decision making.
   PURPOSE: To ensure that the correct level is chosen for the level of medical decision making.
5. If necessary, compare the medical documentation against examples in Appendix C, Clinical Examples, of the CPT manual.
   PURPOSE: To help the coder select the appropriate level of service.
6. Select the appropriate level of E/M service code, and document it in the patient's health record.
   PURPOSE: To complete the documentation and reporting requirements.

PART B: HCPCS CODING WITH TRUCODE ENCODER SOFTWARE

1. Review the provider documentation.
   PURPOSE: To ensure that all procedures or services are listed on the encounter form, that all procedures and services on the encounter form match the health record, and that nothing documented in the health record is missing from the encounter form.
2. Type the main term into the Search box of the encoder, and choose the HCPCS Tabular code set for accurate coding.
3. If no modifying term produces an appropriate code or code range, repeat steps 2 and 3 using a different main term.
   PURPOSE: To help find the most appropriate code or code range by using alternative methods of searching the Alphabetic Index.
4. Compare the description of the code with the medical documentation.
   PURPOSE: To avoid upcoding and downcoding errors and to ensure there are no contraindications to use of the code selected.
5. Select the appropriate HCPCS immunization code, and document it in the patient's health record.
   PURPOSE: To complete the documentation and reporting requirements.

PROCEDURE 14.3 Work with Providers to Ensure Accurate Code Selection

Using tactful communication skills means using good manners as you provide truthful, sensitive information to another person while considering the person's feelings. Tactful communication skills include verbal and nonverbal communication that shows respect, discretion, compassion, honesty, diplomacy, and courtesy. When you use tactful behaviors, you demonstrate professionalism and you preserve relationships by avoiding conflicts and finding common ground.

Many times, the medical coder is the expert on the accurate CPT and ICD code selections. The highest level of specificity must be used when coding so that appropriate reimbursement can occur. It is not uncommon for the medical coder to interact with providers and assist them in understanding the coding process. During these interactions, it is crucial that the medical coder provide the information in a professional, organized, and logical manner. Using tactful communication skills is critical to maintaining a healthy working relationship with the providers.

Using the following case study, role-play with two peers how you would use tactful communication skills with medical providers to ensure accurate code selection.

You are a new medical coder for the medical practice. You have been on the job for 6 weeks and have been seeing a trend of downcoding charges. The required documentation is present in the health records, but the providers have been selecting less specific codes for the appointment types. Your goal is to explain to the providers accurate code selection for the appointment types.

MEDICAL BILLING AND REIMBURSEMENT ESSENTIALS 15

SCENARIO

Ann Snyder, a recent medical assisting graduate, has been hired to work in the billing office for Walden-Martin Family Medical (WMFM) Clinic. During her medical assistant program, her instructor, Grant Wilson, helped her realize that working with health insurance can be quite rewarding. Mr. Wilson worked with Ann and her classmates, answering their questions and helping them see that medical insurance is not as complicated as it may seem.

Ann is detail oriented, and she enjoys billing and coding activities. She understands that performing these duties in the provider's office is crucial because tasks related to billing have a significant effect on the healthcare facility. She also understands that the income generated is used to pay the clinic's expenses, including payroll, so the facility's staff indirectly counts on accurate and timely billing. Medical assistants who continually develop their coding skills are assets to the practice and can look forward to a long and rewarding career.

Ann gained an understanding of the insurance process while in school. Mr. Wilson showed the students several different explanations of benefits (EOB) and remittance advice (RA) forms from a variety of insurance companies so that the students could learn how the reimbursement process works for a variety of health insurance plans. Ann also learned about the importance of verifying patient billing information, in addition to the steps for obtaining precertification for medical procedures. She also learned how to discuss the patient's billing record professionally. Ann is looking forward to using all of the skills she gained in school.

While studying this chapter, think about the following questions:

- Why is it important to obtain accurate patient billing information?
- Why is it important to verify insurance eligibility and complete the precertification process before the patient receives medical services?
- What steps are needed to complete a CMS-1500 Health Insurance Claim Form?
- What information is found on an EOB/RA that is used to determine the patient's financial responsibility?
- How can you use sensitivity when informing patients of the financial responsibilities they face as a result of third-party requirements?

LEARNING OBJECTIVES

1. Explain the medical billing process, including the types of information contained in the patient's billing record and managed care policies and procedures.
2. Examine how claims are submitted to third-party payers.
3. Examine the impact of accurate coding.
4. Examine the methods for following up on claims.
5. Explain a patient's financial obligations for services rendered.

VOCABULARY

adjudicate (uh JOO di kayt) To settle or determine judicially.

Advance Beneficiary Notice (ABN) A document signed by the patient that authorizes a provider to bill the patient for services that Medicare may consider not medically necessary and may decline to cover.

allowed amount The maximum amount that an insurance company will pay for covered health services.

audit A process completed before claims submission in which claims are examined for accuracy and completeness.

capitation (ka pi TAY shun) A payment arrangement for healthcare providers. The provider is paid a set amount for each enrolled person assigned to him or her, per period of time, whether or not that person has received services.

claims clearinghouse An organization that accepts the claim data from the provider, reformats the data to meet the specifications outlined by the insurance plan, and submits the claim.

claim scrubbers Software that finds common billing errors before the claim is sent to the insurance company.

CMS-1500 Health Insurance Claim Form (CMS-1500) The standard insurance claim form used for all government and most commercial insurance companies.

copayment (copay) A set dollar amount the patient must pay for each office visit. There can be one copayment amount for a primary care provider and a different copayment amount (usually higher) to see a specialist or be seen in the emergency department.

VOCABULARY—*continued*

eligibility (el i ji BILL i tee) Meeting the stipulated requirements to participate in the healthcare plan.

endoscopy (en DOS kuh pee) A nonsurgical procedure that uses an endoscope to view inside the body.

explanation of benefits (EOB) A document sent by the insurance company to the patient explaining the allowed charge amount, the amount reimbursed for services, and the patient's financial responsibilities.

medical necessity Services or supplies (Current Procedural Terminology [CPT] and Healthcare Common Procedure Coding System [HCPCS] codes) used to treat the patient's diagnosis (*International Classification of Diseases* [ICD]codes) that meet the accepted standard of medical practice.

National Provider Identifier (NPI) An identifier assigned by the Centers for Medicare and Medicaid Services (CMS) that classifies the healthcare provider by license and medical specialties.

precertification The process of determining if a procedure or service is covered by the insurance plan and what the reimbursement is for that procedure or service.

provider web portal A secure online website that gives contracted providers a single point of access to insurance companies. This allows the provider to determine patient eligibility and deductible status, submit preauthorizations/precertifications, and check the status of claims.

release of information A form completed by the patient that authorizes the medical office to release medical records to the insurance company for health insurance reimbursement.

remittance advice (RA) A document sent by the insurance company to the provider explaining the allowed charge amount, the amount reimbursed for services, and the patient's financial responsibilities.

INTRODUCTION

Medical billing and reimbursement represent the financial lifeline of the healthcare facility. Collecting accurate patient health insurance information is essential to submitting accurate health insurance claims. Each health insurance company has its own claims submission policies and procedures for timely reimbursement. A successful medical assistant in insurance billing learns the insurance company requirements and submits accurate claims. Many health insurance companies have online **provider web portals**. This has made the process of checking the status of a claim quick and easy. The medical assistant also needs to be able to look at a patient's insurance card and interpret the information found there, including **copayment (copay)** amounts. An **explanation of benefits (EOB)/remittance advice (RA)** from the insurance carrier will indicate the patient's deductible and/or co-insurance. Clear communication with the patient about his or her financial responsibilities takes patience and sensitivity.

MEDICAL BILLING PROCESS

The *medical billing process*, also known as the *revenue cycle*, starts when a patient makes an appointment and is complete when payment for services has been received. The following steps are typically taken for medical billing:

- Collect patient information when the patient calls to schedule an appointment. This includes information about the insured, his or her employer, demographic information, and health insurance data.
- Verify the patient's **eligibility**, confirming that the patient's contract with the insurance company is valid for the date of service. Patient eligibility can be confirmed by doing the following:
  - Calling the provider services phone number on the back of the health insurance ID card
  - Using the provider web portal sponsored by the patient's health insurance company
- When the patient arrives for the appointment, you should do the following:
  - Make a copy or scan both sides of the patient's insurance card (Figure 15.1) and government-issued ID card.
  - If the patient has a copayment (copay) responsibility, collect it before services are provided
- Review patient benefits and exclusions for certain medical procedures and services.
  - If **precertification** is needed, contact the health insurance company to request it.
- After services have been provided to the patient, code the diagnosis and procedures and review the encounter form/superbill for completeness. The charges for the procedure or procedures should be provided automatically by the medical billing software.
- Complete the **CMS-1500 Health Insurance Claim Form (CMS-1500)**, or an electronic claim form. Submit the form to the insurance company. Electronic claim information may be submitted to a **claims clearinghouse**.
- Review the electronic claims submission report to ensure that the claim was submitted accurately. Correct any discrepancies through the claims clearinghouse and resubmit claims that have not been paid (denied claims).
- Meet the timely filing requirements that are outlined in the contract of each of the different health insurance carriers. These requirements can vary from carrier to carrier. Health insurance companies do not pay claims submitted after the established filing period, and this balance cannot be billed to the patient.
- Post payments in the patient's account using the EOB/RA to identify the line items that were paid, reduced, or denied. Patient account statements for the person's financial responsibility should be mailed out. Health insurance claims for patient accounts with secondary insurance should be submitted to the secondary carrier.

CRITICAL THINKING APPLICATION 15.1

The medical billing manager informs Ann that she has noticed an increase in the number of insurance claim rejections that state the patient cannot be identified. Which step of the medical billing process might be addressed to resolve this problem?

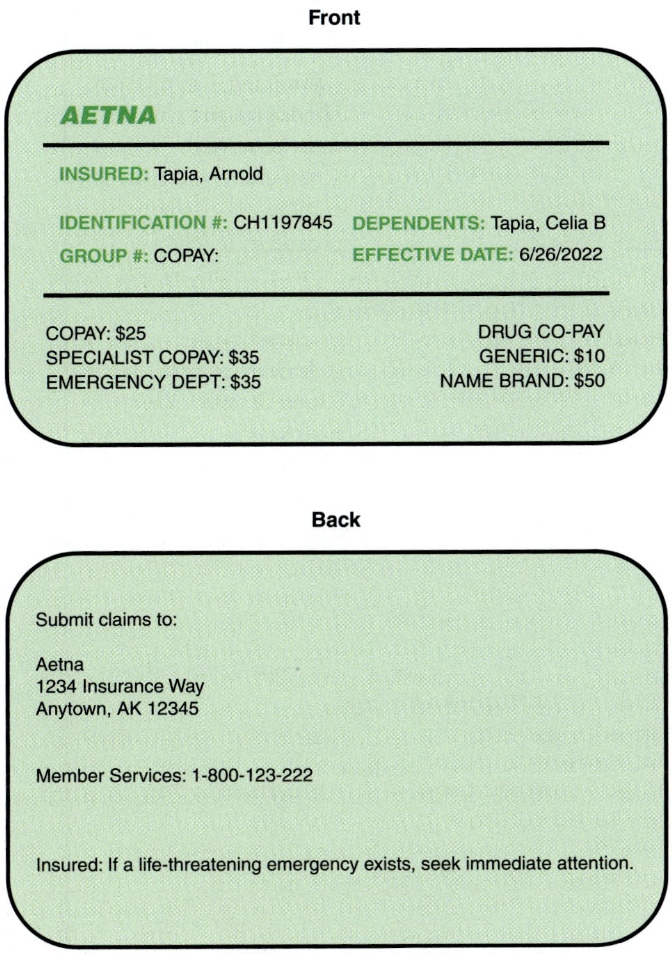

Front

AETNA

INSURED: Tapia, Arnold

IDENTIFICATION #: CH1197845 DEPENDENTS: Tapia, Celia B
GROUP #: COPAY: EFFECTIVE DATE: 6/26/2022

COPAY: $25
SPECIALIST COPAY: $35
EMERGENCY DEPT: $35

DRUG CO-PAY
GENERIC: $10
NAME BRAND: $50

Back

Submit claims to:

Aetna
1234 Insurance Way
Anytown, AK 12345

Member Services: 1-800-123-222

Insured: If a life-threatening emergency exists, seek immediate attention.

FIGURE 15.1 Insurance card.

Types of Information Found in the Patient's Billing Record

The claim submission process begins after the patient receives services from the provider. When a patient makes their first appointment, it is routine to ask the patient for insurance billing information. Much of this information is collected on the patient information form (Figure 15.2). This form can be sent to the patient ahead of time or completed when the patient comes to the medical office for the first visit. This form should always be completed for every new patient. For established patients, demographic and insurance information should be verified at every visit.

Accurate patient information for submitting a health insurance claim is important, but a medical **release of information** form, signed by the patient, should also be kept in the person's health record. The release form allows the release of medical information to the insurance company. The Health Insurance Portability and Accountability Act (HIPAA) does not require this, but some state laws do. Many healthcare facilities will have patients complete the form and keep it in their health records.

Managed Care Policies and Procedures

Medical billers should be familiar with procedures commonly used by managed care organizations (MCOs), such as precertification. If the procedures are not followed, the MCO might not pay for the services. For example, pain management services typically require a preauthorization. If a pain management facility were to provide these services to the patient without preauthorization, the MCO could deny all insurance claims. To submit accurate health insurance claims, medical assistants should follow office procedures for applying MCO policies and procedures (Procedure 15.1).

Precertification/Preauthorization

In an effort to control costs, many MCOs require precertification for certain procedures and services. The insurance company, in turn, will determine if it is a covered service and what the reimbursement will be. Precertification must be done before the procedure or service is performed.

The medical assistant will take the following steps to obtain precertification:

- Call the provider services phone number on the back of the patient's health insurance ID card or complete this process through the insurance company's web portal.
- Provide the insurance company with procedures or services requested and the diagnoses.
- Document the outcome of the call in the patient's health record, including the precertification number.

Precertification does not guarantee payment of services. The process ensures that both the healthcare provider and the patient are informed of the amount that the insurance company will pay and also the amount that the patient will have to pay.

Each insurance company has its own precertification requirements. Almost every MCO requires precertification, but medical assistants must confirm this by contacting the insurance company. Successful medical billers are diligent in obtaining precertification.

The precertification and preauthorization processes (see Procedure 15.1) are very similar. The insurance company is contacted after the primary care provider (PCP) recommends the procedure or service. In fact, many health insurance companies use the terms precertification and preauthorization interchangeably. However, precertification specifically determines whether the procedure is medically necessary, and *preauthorization* gives the provider approval to render the medical service. Precertification and preauthorization can be requested through an insurance company's online web portal (see Procedure 15.1).

Preauthorization/Precertification Examples

1. Dr. David Kahn is the primary care provider (PCP) for Janine Butler, who has heartburn that has not improved with medication.
2. Because Ms. Butler's condition is not improving, Dr. Kahn requests preauthorization for her to see Dr. Eduard Hamilton, a gastrointestinal (GI) specialist. Ms. Butler is insured by a managed care organization (MCO).
3. The MCO authorizes Ms. Butler to see Dr. Hamilton; this authorization is sent to Ms. Butler, Dr. Kahn, and Dr. Hamilton. When Ms. Butler receives the authorization, she schedules an appointment with Dr. Hamilton.
4. After evaluating Ms. Butler, Dr. Hamilton orders an esophageal **endoscopy**. However, Ms. Butler is concerned about her financial responsibility. Therefore, Dr. Hamilton's office requests precertification for the endoscopy on Ms. Butler's behalf.
5. The MCO notifies Dr. Hamilton that the plan would reimburse a total of $1500, and Ms. Butler would be financially responsible for $400. The precertification is sent to Dr. Hamilton and Ms. Butler, who agree to its financial terms and schedule the procedure.

WALDEN-MARTIN

FAMILY MEDICAL CLINIC

1234 ANYSTREET | ANYTOWN, ANYSTATE 12345

PHONE 123-123-1234 | FAX 123-123-5678

Patient Information

Patient Information (Please use full legal name.)

Last Name: Tapia
First Name: Celia
Middle Initial: B
Medical Record Number: 11012373
Date of Birth: 05/18/19XX
Age: 42
Sex: Female
SSN: 857-62-1594
Emergency Contact Name: Arnold Tapia

Address 1: 12 Highland Court
Address 2: Apt 101
City: Anytown
Country: United States State/Province: AL
Zip: 12345-1234
Email: —
Home Phone: 123-858-1545
Driver's License: —
Emergency Contact Phone: 123-200-5006

Guarantor Information (Please use full legal name.)

Relationship of Guarantor to Patient: Spouse
Guarantor/Account #: Tapia, Arnold / 12088787
Account Number: 12088787
Last Name: Tapia
First Name: Arnold
Middle Initial: —
Date of Birth: 05/18/19XX
Age: 42
Sex: Male
SSN: 812-93-1341
Employer Name: Anytown String Shop
School Name: —

Address 1: 12 Highland Court
Address 2: Apt 101
City: Anytown
Country: United States State/Province: AL
Zip: 12345-1234
Email: —
Home Phone: 123-858-1545
Cell Phone: —
Work Phone: —

Provider Information

Primary Provider: James A. Martin, MD
Referring Provider: —
Date of Last Visit: August 28, 20XX
Phone: 123-123-1234

Provider's Address 1: 1234 Anystreet
Provider's Address 2: —
City: Anytown
Country: United States State/Province: AL
Zip: 12345-1234

Insurance Information (If the patient is not the insured party, please include date of birth for claims.)

Insurance: Aetna
Name of Policy Holder: Arnold Tapia
SSN: 812-93-1341
Policy/ID Number: CT5487854
Group Number: 41554T

Claims Address 1: 1234 Insurance Way
Claims Address 2: —
City: Anytown
Country: United States State/Province: AL
Zip: 12345-1234
Claims Phone: 180-012-3222

Secondary Insurance

Insurance: —
Name of Policy Holder: —
SSN: —
Policy/ID Number: —
Group Number: —

Claims Address 1: —
Claims Address 2: —
City: —
Country: — State/Province: —
Zip: —
Claims Phone: —

"I hereby authorize direct payment of all insurance benefits otherwise payable to me for services rendered. I understand that I am financially responsible for all charges not covered by insurance for services rendered on my behalf to my dependents. I authorize the above providers to release any information required to secure payment of benefits. I authorize the use of this signature on insurance submissions."

Signature: Celia Tapia
Date: 05/06/20XX

FIGURE 15.2 Complete patient registration form.

Referrals

Patients seeking specialized care must first visit their assigned PCP to obtain a referral to a specialist or for more specialized therapy or care. Patients with HMO plans can only obtain a referral to the specialist by visiting their assigned PCP. HMOs will track how many patients are referred to specialists by individual PCPs. Approval or denial of a referral can take anywhere from a few minutes to a few days. The three types of referrals are as follows:

- A *regular referral* usually takes 3 to 10 working days for review and approval. This type of referral is used when the provider believes the patient must see a specialist to continue treatment.
- An *urgent referral* usually takes about 24 hours for approval. This type of referral is used when an urgent but not life-threatening situation occurs.
- A *STAT referral* can be approved online when it is submitted to the utilization review department through the provider's web portal. A STAT referral is used in an emergency situation as indicated by the provider.

A *regular referral* is the most common type and can be inconvenient for the patient. With most managed care plans, preauthorization needs to be obtained for a referral. Remember this cardinal rule: never tell the patient the referral has been approved unless you have a hard copy of the authorization. A referral is authorized after the approval has been received. When a referral is approved, the PCP's office and the patient should receive a copy of the authorization. Always review the authorization thoroughly and confirm details, such as approved diagnosis and procedure codes and the exact period of time the authorization lasts. The patient will receive a letter with an authorization number and details regarding the approved services. The patient must bring the authorization to the specialist's office on the date of the appointment.

SUBMITTING CLAIMS TO THIRD-PARTY PAYERS

After the registration information has been collected and coverage verified, the patient is then provided services. An encounter form is used to document the services and the diagnoses for those services, and then the encounter form is used to complete a claim to be submitted to the insurance company (third-party payers).

All health insurance companies accept the following:

- CMS-1500 as the standard claim form or the HIPAA 5010 electronic claim
- *International Classification of Diseases* (ICD)-10-CM for diagnostic codes
- **Current Procedural Terminology** (CPT) and Healthcare Common Procedure Coding System (HCPCS) procedural/supply codes

However, each health insurance company has its own policies and procedures for the submission of claims.

Guidelines for Medicare and Medicaid claims can be found on the administrator websites for each state. MCO plans associated with **capitation** agreements have specific guidelines on the types of medical services that are billable. Private health insurance plans have their own policies and procedures for submitting claims. The medical assistant should research the health plans commonly seen in the healthcare facility.

The medical assistant can successfully manage the requirements of the different insurance plans by keeping a medical billing manual. The manual should contain the billing policies and procedures for the most common third-party payers. The person in charge of the manual should make sure that every medical biller has a copy and that the policies and procedures are up to date. Whenever an update is released, the medical billing manual also should be updated.

Most providers are required to submit claims electronically for Medicare patients and are doing so for most other health insurance plans. If the majority of claims are submitted electronically, why is it important to learn the different fields of the CMS-1500 paper form? The data used to submit electronic claims is the same data used on the CMS-1500. A medical assistant who is familiar with a paper CMS-1500 will have no problem collecting the proper data for an electronic claim. Both methods are discussed in the following sections.

Generating Electronic Claims

Electronic claims are insurance claims that are transmitted over the internet from the provider to the health insurance company through *electronic data interchange*. Electronic data interchange is the electronic transfer of data between two or more entities. When submitting electronic claims, a healthcare facility transmits the data for the claim, and the health insurance company accepts it. Most medical billing software is designed to generate electronic claims.

As with paper claims, when electronic claims are submitted, accurate data is essential. When the medical assistant reviews the claim for accuracy, the claim is prepared for submission.

Electronic claims are submitted in the 5010 format established by HIPAA and can be directly transmitted to the insurance carrier or a claims clearinghouse.

Direct Billing

Direct billing is the process by which an insurance company allows a provider to electronically submit claims directly to the company. Most major insurance companies, including Medicare and Medicaid, provide software packages that are used to enter the following:

- Patient's information
- Insured's information
- Charges
- Provider details

Many carrier-direct systems are supplied free of charge to the provider, but the direct system can transmit only to specific carriers. If a majority of claims for the healthcare facility are submitted to just one insurance company, direct billing would be a good way to submit claims.

Clearinghouse Submissions

A claims clearinghouse is an organization that acts as a go-between for the healthcare facility and the insurance company. The clearinghouse takes the following actions:

- Accepts electronically submitted claims information from healthcare agencies
- **Audits** the claims for completeness
- Reformats claims to meet insurance company specifications

The claims are sorted by insurance plans and sent in batches electronically to the appropriate insurers. The insurance companies then send a report through the data clearinghouse to do the following:

- Confirm the receipt of claims

- Report the status of previously submitted claims
- Serve as a claim payment notification

A clearinghouse charges the healthcare facility a small fee to cover the following services:

- Sending and receiving claims transmissions
- Checking and preparing the claims for processing
- Consolidating claims so that one transmission can be sent to each carrier
- Submitting claims in correct data format to the appropriate insurance payer

Clearinghouses typically provide other services as well:

- Reporting the number of claims submitted, and the number of errors and their specifics
- Forwarding claims to insurance carriers that accept electronic claims (e.g., Medicare, Medicaid, Blue Cross/Blue Shield, and others) or to another clearinghouse that may hold the contracts with specific payers
- Keeping provider offices updated as new carriers are added to the database
- Generating informative statistical reports

Completing the CMS-1500 Health Insurance Claim Form

The National Uniform Claim Committee (NUCC) is a voluntary organization that is chaired by the American Medical Association (AMA) and works closely with the Centers for Medicare and Medicaid Services (CMS). The organization is tasked with maintaining national standard content related to claims submission as well as standardizing national instructions for claim form completion. NUCC is the best resource for the most up-to-date information and instructions for the completion of the CMS-1500 claim form. The CMS-1500 Health Insurance Claim Form is required by HIPAA for paper claim submission. The form has 33 blocks. These blocks are divided into three sections:

- *Section 1: Carrier.* The first section indicates the type of insurance plan to which the claim is being submitted; this section includes only Block 1.
- *Section 2: Patient and Insured Information.* The second section contains information about the patient and the insured; it includes Blocks 1a through 13.
- *Section 3: Physician or Supplier Information.* The third section contains information about the provider or supplier; it includes Blocks 14 through 33.

Section 1: Carrier—Block 1 (Figure 15.3)

Block 1 shows the type of insurance the patient has. The type of health insurance coverage for this claim is indicated by putting an X in the appropriate box, marking only one box. This information directs the claim to the correct payer.

Section 2: Patient and Insured Information—Blocks 1a through 13 (Figure 15.4)

The CMS-1500 distinguishes between the patient and the insured. The insured is the individual who is directly contracted with the insurance company. For example, if an insurance claim for Lisa Parker is submitted and Blue Cross covers her through her employer, she is both the patient and the insured. However, if the insurance claim is for Johnny Parker, her son, Lisa Parker is the insured, and Johnny Parker, her dependent, is the patient. Every CMS-1500 requires the name, gender, and birth date of both the insured and the patient, even if they are different individuals. The blocks in Figure 15.4 highlighted in yellow are for the patient's information, and the blocks highlighted in blue are for the insured's information.

Blocks 1a, 4, 7, and 11 a–d. Information required for the insured includes the following:

- Block 1a—person's health plan ID number
- Block 4—name
- Block 7—address
- Block 11—policy and group numbers
- Block 11a—birth date (MM/DD/YYYY) and gender
- Block 11b—other claim ID designated by NUCC
- Block 11c—name of the insurance plan
- Block 11d—whether the insured has another health benefit plan

Blocks 2, 3, 5, 6, and 10 a–c. Required information for the patient includes the following:

- Block 2—person's name
- Block 3—birth date (MM/DD/YYYY) and gender
- Block 5—address and telephone number
- Block 6—relationship to the insured
- Block 10 a–c—patient's status, whether the patient's condition is related to the person's job, an automobile accident, or some other accident

CRITICAL THINKING APPLICATION 15.2

Ann is preparing an insurance claim to bill to Blue Cross. She notes that the patient is the dependent of the insured, so she reviews the patient registration intake form and finds that the date of birth for the insured is not present. Can Ann accurately complete the CMS-1500?

HEALTH INSURANCE CLAIM FORM
APPROVED BY NATIONAL UNIFORM CLAIM COMMITTEE (NUCC) 02/12

PICA | PICA | CARRIER

1. MEDICARE (Medicare #) | MEDICAID (Medicaid #) | TRICARE CHAMPUS (Sponsor's SSN) | CHAMPVA (Member ID#) | GROUP HEALTH PLAN (SSN or ID) | FECA BLK LUNG (SSN) | OTHER (ID)

FIGURE 15.3 Section 1 Carrier (Block 1).

1. MEDICARE (Medicare#) MEDICAID (Medicaid#) TRICARE (ID#DoD#) CHAMPVA (Member ID#) GROUP HEALTH PLAN (ID#) FECA BLK LUNG (ID#) OTHER (ID#)
1a. INSURED'S I.D. NUMBER (For Program in Item 1)
2. PATIENT'S NAME (Last Name, First Name, Middle Initial)
3. PATIENT'S BIRTH DATE MM DD YY SEX M F
4. INSURED'S NAME (Last Name, First Name, Middle Initial)
5. PATIENT'S ADDRESS (No., Street)
6. PATIENT RELATIONSHIP TO INSURED Self Spouse Child Other
7. INSURED'S ADDRESS (No., Street)
CITY STATE
8. RESERVED FOR NUCC USE
CITY STATE
ZIP CODE TELEPHONE (Include Area Code) ( )
ZIP CODE TELEPHONE (Include Area Code) ( )
9. OTHER INSURED'S NAME (Last Name, First Name, Middle Initial)
10. IS PATIENT'S CONDITION RELATED TO:
11. INSURED'S POLICY GROUP OR FECA NUMBER
a. OTHER INSURED'S POLICY OR GROUP NUMBER
a. EMPLOYMENT? (Current or Previous) YES NO
a. INSURED'S DATE OF BIRTH MM DD YY SEX M F
b. RESERVED FOR NUCC USE
b. AUTO ACCIDENT? YES NO PLACE (State)
b. OTHER CLAIM ID (Designated by NUCC)
c. RESERVED FOR NUCC USE
c. OTHER ACCIDENT? YES NO
c. INSURANCE PLAN NAME OR PROGRAM NAME
d. INSURANCE PLAN NAME OR PROGRAM NAME
10d. CLAIM CODES (Designated by NUCC)
d. IS THERE ANOTHER HEALTH BENEFIT PLAN? YES NO *If yes*, complete items 9, 9a, and 9d.
READ BACK OF FORM BEFORE COMPLETING & SIGNING THIS FORM.
12. PATIENT'S OR AUTHORIZED PERSON'S SIGNATURE I authorize the release of any medical or other information necessary to process this claim. I also request payment of government benefits either to myself or to the party who accepts the assignment below.
SIGNED DATE
13. INSURED'S OR AUTHORIZED PERSON'S SIGNATURE I authorize payment of medical benefits to the undersigned physician or supplier for services described below.
SIGNED
PATIENT AND INSURED IN

FIGURE 15.4 Section 2: Patient and Insured Information (Blocks 1a to 13).

Block 9. Block 9 is for recording information about any secondary insurance plan that may be applicable. The data required includes the following:

- The other insured person's name
- Policy or group number
- Name of the other insurance plan

Primary and Secondary Insurance Determination

When a patient is covered by more than one insurance policy, it is important to determine which policy is considered primary. The primary insurance pays the claim first, and if there is anything left over, it is submitted to the secondary insurance company. One of the most common situations is a patient with coverage under two policies, such as a dependent whose parents each have family coverage through employer group insurance.

In the case of a child whose mother and father both carry the child as a dependent on their employer's health insurance plan, primary and secondary insurance status is determined by the *birthday rule*. Whichever parent's birth date falls first in a calendar year is considered to have the primary insurance. The year of the parent's birth is not used. If the mother's birth date is February 20 and the father's birth date is May 1, the mother's insurance is the primary insurance, and the father's insurance is the secondary. This means the claim will be submitted to the mother's insurance first, and if there is any balance left, it will be submitted to the father's insurance.

Medicare is usually the primary insurance, and there is a secondary policy to cover the patient's responsibility. In some cases, however, Medicare can be the patient's secondary insurance. This typically happens when a Medicare patient is still covered under an employer-sponsored group policy because the patient works full time.

Medicaid is always the payer of last resort. That means if there is any other type of insurance coverage for the patient, that insurance is responsible for the claim. If there is any balance left over, it will be submitted to Medicaid.

Blocks 12 and 13. Block 12 requires the signature of the *patient* or an authorized person, and Block 13 requires the signature of the *insured* or an authorized person. In Block 12, the signature authorizes the release of any medical or other information necessary to process or **adjudicate** the claim. In Block 13, the signature affirms that the healthcare organization has a signature on file authorizing payment of medical benefits directly to the provider (whose name appears in Block 31). The phrase "Signature on File" or "SOF" may be entered in these fields. The healthcare organization must actually have a signed authorization in the patient's health record.

Assignment of Benefits

In the health insurance contract between the third-party payer and the patient, the patient receives the payment when a claim is submitted. For the healthcare facility to receive the reimbursement directly from the insurance company, the patient must sign an *assignment of benefits*. The assignment of benefits transfers the patient's legal right to collect benefits for medical expenses to the provider of those services, authorizing the payment to be sent directly to the provider. In other words, the assignment of benefits authorizes the provider to not only submit the insurance claim on behalf of the patient but also to be reimbursed directly by the third-party payer. There is usually a statement about the assignment of benefits on the patient information form. When the patient has signed the assignment of benefits, the medical assistant completes Blocks 12 and 13 on the CMS-1500 form with the statement "Signature on File" or "SOF" and the claim filing date.

Section 3a: Physician or Supplier Information—Blocks 14 through 23 (Figure 15.5)

Block 14: Date of Current Illness, Injury, or Pregnancy (LMP). Block 14 requires the date of the current illness, injury, or pregnancy (LMP). The date should be the date on which the current illness

14. DATE OF CURRENT ILLNESS, INJURY, or PREGNANCY(LMP) MM DD YY QUAL.
15. OTHER DATE QUAL. MM DD YY
16. DATES PATIENT UNABLE TO WORK IN CURRENT OCCUPATION FROM MM DD YY TO MM DD YY
17. NAME OF REFERRING PROVIDER OR OTHER SOURCE
17a.
17b. NPI
18. HOSPITALIZATION DATES RELATED TO CURRENT SERVICES FROM MM DD YY TO MM DD YY
19. ADDITIONAL CLAIM INFORMATION (Designated by NUCC)
20. OUTSIDE LAB? YES NO $ CHARGES
21. DIAGNOSIS OR NATURE OF ILLNESS OR INJURY Relate A-L to service line below (24E) ICD Ind.
A. B. C. D.
E. F. G. H.
I. J. K. L.
22. RESUBMISSION CODE ORIGINAL REF. NO.
23. PRIOR AUTHORIZATION NUMBER

FIGURE 15.5 Section 3a: Physician or Supplier Information (Blocks 14 to 23).

or condition began; the date an injury occurred; or, in the case of pregnancy, the date of the last menstrual period (LMP), all in MM/DD/YYYY format.

Block 15: Other Date. This block is used for another date related to the patient's condition or treatment. Enter the applicable qualifier to identify which date is being reported.

Block 15 Qualifiers

- 454 Initial Treatment
- 304 Latest Visit or Consultation
- 455 Last X-ray
- 471 Prescription
- 090 Report Start (Assumed Care Date)
- 091 Report End (Relinquished Care Date)
- 444 First Visit or Consultation
- 439 Accident
- 453 Acute Manifestation of a Chronic Condition

Block 16: Dates Patient Unable to Work in Current Occupation. These dates help determine an employee's long- or short-term disability payments.

Blocks 17 and 17b: Name of Referring Provider or Other Source. Block 17 is for the name of the provider who referred or ordered the services or supplies. The following qualifier can be added:

- DN Referring Provider
- DK Ordering Provider
- DQ Supervising Provider

The provider's **National Provider Identifier (NPI)** is entered in Block 17b.

National Provider Identifier (NPI)

Government insurance claims require that National Provider Identifiers (NPIs) be used for the referring providers (Block 17b) and rendering providers (Block 24J). Every healthcare entity is required to have an NPI. The NPI is an identifier assigned by the CMS that classifies the healthcare provider by license and medical specialty. The Administrative Simplification provisions of the Health Insurance Portability and Accountability Act (HIPAA) required the adoption of standard unique identifiers for healthcare providers and health plans. The purpose is to improve the efficiency of electronic transmission of health information.

Some private insurance companies may require claims to be submitted with the NPI. However, each privately sponsored insurance plan in each state has its own policies and procedures. Medical assistants will find that some third-party payers require NPIs and others do not.

Block 18: Hospitalization Dates Related to Current Services. If inpatient services are provided, the admission and discharge dates are entered here.

Block 19: Additional Claim Information (Designated by the National Uniform Claim Committee [NUCC]). Some insurance plans ask for specific identifiers in Block 19. The medical assistant should check the instructions from the applicable third-party payer.

Block 20: Outside Lab Charges. This block is used for diagnostic laboratory services purchased from an independent or a separate provider (listed in Block 32). Put an X in the YES box to indicate that the diagnostic test was performed by an entity other than the provider billing for the service (i.e., the provider listed in Block 33) and that the provider in Block 33 paid the laboratory directly. Include the amount the provider was charged by the diagnostic laboratory.

Block 21: Diagnosis or Nature of Illness or Injury. The ICD-10-CM diagnosis code or codes are entered. Up to 12 diagnostic codes can be entered here. The primary diagnosis should be recorded in the first field. Do not include the decimal point in the diagnosis code. Relate lines A to L to lines of service in Block 24E by the letter of the line. This will link the diagnosis to the service provided.

Block 22: Resubmission Code and/or Original Reference Number. Both the resubmission code and the original reference number assigned by the insurance payer must be entered in this block. Here are the resubmission codes:

- 7 Replacement of prior claim
- 8 Void/cancel of prior claim

Block 23: Prior Authorization Number. The preauthorization/precertification number obtained from the insurance company is entered.

Section 3b: Physician or Supplier Information—Blocks 24 through 33 (Figure 15.6)

Procedure codes, such as the Current Procedural Terminology (CPT) or the Healthcare Common Procedure Coding System (HCPCS) codes, are listed in Block 24. Each procedure code is considered a line item; the line numbers are found to the left of Block 24. All data in one line belongs to the coordinated CPT/HCPCS code. For claims that require more than six line items, a second CMS-1500 form should be generated. Check with the insurance company to confirm how to indicate that the claim has multiple pages; some insurance companies require the statement "Continued" or "Page 1 of 2" in Block 28, Total Charges.

Block 24: Procedures and Charges

Block 24A: Date(s) of Service. Note that there is space for both "From" and "To" dates. If the service was provided on just one day, you would only enter a From date in a MM/DD/YY format. If the service was provided on multiple days, such as an inpatient hospital

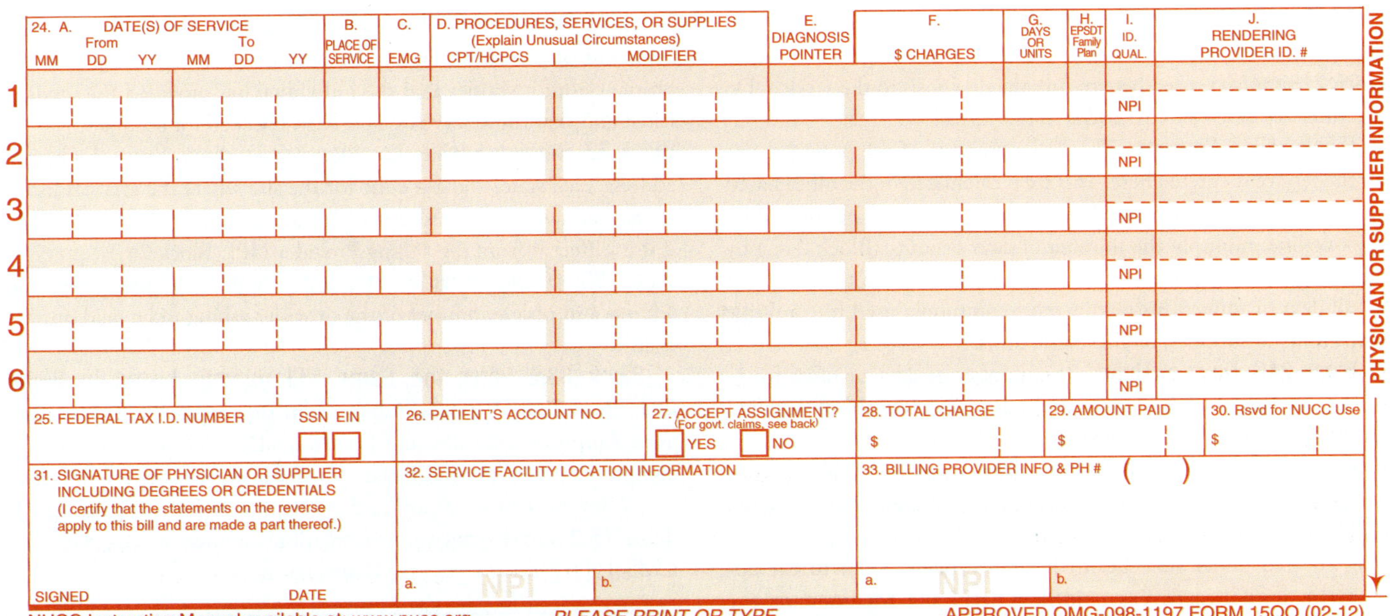

24. A. DATE(S) OF SERVICE From To MM DD YY MM DD YY | B. PLACE OF SERVICE | C. EMG | D. PROCEDURES, SERVICES, OR SUPPLIES (Explain Unusual Circumstances) CPT/HCPCS | MODIFIER | E. DIAGNOSIS POINTER | F. $ CHARGES | G. DAYS OR UNITS | H. EPSDT Family Plan | I. ID. QUAL. | J. RENDERING PROVIDER ID. #

1 NPI
2 NPI
3 NPI
4 NPI
5 NPI
6 NPI

25. FEDERAL TAX I.D. NUMBER SSN EIN | 26. PATIENT'S ACCOUNT NO. | 27. ACCEPT ASSIGNMENT? (For govt. claims, see back) YES NO | 28. TOTAL CHARGE $ | 29. AMOUNT PAID $ | 30. Rsvd for NUCC Use $

31. SIGNATURE OF PHYSICIAN OR SUPPLIER INCLUDING DEGREES OR CREDENTIALS (I certify that the statements on the reverse apply to this bill and are made a part thereof.) | 32. SERVICE FACILITY LOCATION INFORMATION | 33. BILLING PROVIDER INFO & PH # ( )

SIGNED DATE | a. NPI b. | a. NPI b.

PHYSICIAN OR SUPPLIER INFORMATION

NUCC Instruction Manual available at: www.nucc.org PLEASE PRINT OR TYPE APPROVED OMG-098-1197 FORM 1500 (02-12)

FIGURE 15.6 Section 3b: Physician or Supplier Information (Blocks 24 to 33).

TABLE 15.1 Common Place of Service Codes

CODE	DESCRIPTION	CODE	DESCRIPTION
11	Doctor's office	51	Inpatient psychiatry facility
12	Patient's home	52	Psychiatric facility—partial hospitalization
21	Inpatient hospital	53	Community mental healthcare (outpatient, 24-hour/day services, admission screening, consultation, and educational services)
22	Outpatient hospital		
23	Emergency department—hospital	54	Intermediate care facility/mentally retarded
24	Ambulatory surgical center	55	Residential substance abuse treatment facility
25	Birthing center	56	Psychiatric residential treatment center
26	Military treatment facility/uniformed service treatment facility	60	Mass immunization center
31	Skilled nursing facility (swing bed visits)	61	Comprehensive inpatient rehabilitation facility
32	Nursing facility (intermediate/long-term care facilities)	62	Comprehensive outpatient rehabilitation facility
33	Custodial care facility (domiciliary or rest home services)	65	End-stage renal disease treatment facility
34	Hospice (domiciliary or rest home services)	71	State or local public health clinic
35	Adult living care facilities (residential care facility)	72	Rural health clinic
41	Ambulance—land	81	Independent laboratory
42	Ambulance—air or water	99	Other unlisted facility
50	Federally qualified health center		

stay, the first day the service was provided would be put in the From field, and the last day the service was provided would be entered in the To field. The number of times that service was provided would be indicated in Block 24G.

Block 24B: Place of Service. The Place of Service (POS) codes indicate where the services were provided. As shown in Table 15.1, 11 would indicate that the procedure took place in a doctor's office.

Block 24C: EMG (Emergency). A Y in this field indicates that the service was an emergency.

Block 24D: Procedures, Service or Supplies. There are two sections in this block: CPT/HCPCS and Modifier. There is space for a single 5-digit code and up to four separate two-digit modifiers. No space is provided for a written description of the code; only the code is required.

Block 24E: Diagnosis Pointer. This block indicates which diagnosis is used for each line item. The letter from diagnosis listed in Block 21 should be used here to link the diagnosis to the service. Do not enter the ICD-10-CM codes in this block.

Block 24F: $ Charges. The dollar amount of the provider's fee for the service is entered here. This fee is calculated in the office based on work, expertise, and time. If a series of services was performed on any one line, multiply the number of days or units (Block 24G) by the charge for one procedure or service and enter the total amount for all days or units. This field is most commonly used for multiple visits, units of supplies, or anesthesia units.

Block 24G: Days or Units. The number of days or units is entered here. This block is used for multiple visits and units of supplies. If only one service is performed, 1 would be entered.

Block 24H: EPSDT/Family Plan. The acronym EPSDT stands for early and periodic screening, diagnosis, and treatment, the child health program under Medicaid. This block identifies specific services covered under state health insurance plans. Refer to the appropriate insurance payer's guidelines (typically Medicaid or the Medicaid intermediary) for instructions on completing this block. Leave the block blank for Medicare, TRICARE, and the Civilian Health and Medical Program of the Department of Veterans Affairs (CHAMPVA) (military insurance plans), group health plans, Federal Employees Compensation Act (FECA)/Black Lung, and most other types of insurance.

Block 24I: ID Qual. This block is used if the number in Block 24J is not an NPI. The following are the qualifiers:

- 0B State License Number
- 1G Provider UPIN Number
- G2 Provider Commercial Number
- LU Location Number
- ZZ Provider Taxonomy

Block 24J: Rendering Provider ID Number. Enter the NPI of the provider who rendered the service as identification.

Block 25: Facility Information. The federal tax ID number of the provider filing the claim can be listed as a Social Security number (SSN) or an employer identification number (EIN); mark the appropriate box with an X.

Block 26: Patient's Account Number. Enter the account number or medical record number assigned to the patient by the provider of the service. This information will be included on the EOB from the insurance company to help with posting the payment.

Block 27: Accept Assignment?. Put an X in the YES box if the provider will accept assignment; this means that the provider is a *participating provider* (PAR) and agrees to accept the terms of the agreement with the insurance company and also to accept what the plan states as an **allowed amount** for the services provided.

Block 28: Total Charge. This block shows the amount billed on the claim form for all services rendered. To arrive at this amount, add up the charges reported in Block 24F for all the lines of service on the claim form.

Block 29: Amount Paid. The amount received from the patient or other payers.

Block 30: Reserved for NUCC Use. Some secondary insurance claims use this box to claim the amount due after the primary insurance has paid.

Block 31: Signature of Physician or Supplier. This block is for the signature of the authorized or accountable person for the services on the claim; it verifies that the individual has provided the services listed and that those services have been checked for accuracy.

Block 32: Service Facility Location Information. Enter the name, address, city, state, and zip code for the site where the services listed in the claim were provided. Enter the facility's NPI in Block 32a only if it is different from the Billing Provider NPI (Block 24J).

Block 33: Billing Provider Info and Phone Number. Enter the address and phone number of the provider asking to be paid on this claim.

Block 33a: Enter the Same NPI number Listed in Block 24J. Procedure 15.2 demonstrates how to complete a health insurance claim electronically, and Procedure 15.3 demonstrates how to complete a health insurance claim form on paper using the information from an insurance card and an encounter form (Figure 15.7). Table 15.2 summarizes the information required to complete the CMS-1500 Health Insurance Claim Form.

CRITICAL THINKING APPLICATION 15.3

Ann is reviewing an encounter form that has one CPT code and two HCPCS codes with one diagnosis code for the same office visit. How many lines in Box 24 of the CMS-1500 will she need to use? Will all three CPT/HCPCS codes point to the same diagnosis? Why or why not?

IMPACT OF ACCURATE CODING

Accurate coding is an integral part of efficient claims submission. Incorrect coding can be construed as fraud or abuse. This can have a negative effect on any healthcare organization. If the wrong diagnostic or procedural codes are used, the claim can be denied and will have to be resubmitted. If coding is done incorrectly, the claim can be rejected as not medically necessary. Let's take a closer look at how to prevent fraud and abuse and the rejection of claims.

Preventing Fraud and Abuse

In any healthcare environment, accurate coding is essential to prevent fraud and abuse in reimbursement. According to HIPAA, *fraud* is defined as knowingly and willfully executing or attempting to execute a scheme to defraud any healthcare benefit program or to obtain by means of false or fraudulent pretenses, representations, or promises any of the money or property owned by any healthcare benefit program. Examples of fraud include billing for services that were not actually performed, altering the patient's diagnosis to justify tests or surgeries, and coding for a higher level of service than what was performed.

Abuse in medical billing would be actions that are contrary to ethical standards in the medical office. *Abuse* is an unintended action that directly or indirectly results in an overpayment to the healthcare provider. Abuse is similar to fraud, except that it is unclear if the unethical practice was committed on purpose. Examples of abuse include providing unnecessary clinical services and waiving copayments or coinsurance. The term *intentional* is important when determining whether fraudulent medical billing practices were done on purpose or were an accident.

HEALTH INSURANCE CLAIM FORM

APPROVED BY NATIONAL UNIFORM CLAIM COMMITTEE (NUCC) 02/12

PICA | PICA | CARRIER

1. MEDICARE ☑ (Medicare#) | MEDICAID ☐ (Medicaid#) | TRICARE ☐ (ID#/DoD#) | CHAMPVA ☐ (Member ID#) | GROUP HEALTH PLAN ☐ (ID#) | FECA BLK LUNG ☐ (ID#) | OTHER ☐ (ID#)

1a. INSURED'S I.D. NUMBER (For Program in Item 1): 123-45-6789A

2. PATIENT'S NAME (Last Name, First Name, Middle Initial): ROSE DAWSON

3. PATIENT'S BIRTH DATE MM DD YY: 02 17 XX — SEX M ☐ F ☑

4. INSURED'S NAME (Last Name, First Name, Middle Initial): ROSE DAWSON

5. PATIENT'S ADDRESS (No., Street): 123 TITANIC PLACE

6. PATIENT RELATIONSHIP TO INSURED: Self ☑ Spouse ☐ Child ☐ Other ☐

7. INSURED'S ADDRESS (No., Street): 123 TITANIC PLACE

CITY: NEW YORK — STATE: NY

8. RESERVED FOR NUCC USE

CITY: NEW YORK — STATE: NY

ZIP CODE: 10001 — TELEPHONE (Include Area Code): ( )

ZIP CODE: 10001 — TELEPHONE (Include Area Code): ( )

9. OTHER INSURED'S NAME (Last Name, First Name, Middle Initial): ROSE DAWSON

10. IS PATIENT'S CONDITION RELATED TO:

11. INSURED'S POLICY GROUP OR FECA NUMBER: 123-45-6789A

a. OTHER INSURED'S POLICY OR GROUP NUMBER: 123-45-6789

a. EMPLOYMENT? (Current or Previous) ☐ YES ☑ NO

a. INSURED'S DATE OF BIRTH MM DD YY: 02 17 XX — SEX M ☐ F ☑

b. RESERVED FOR NUCC USE

b. AUTO ACCIDENT? ☐ YES ☑ NO — PLACE (State)

b. OTHER CLAIM ID (Designated by NUCC)

c. RESERVED FOR NUCC USE

c. OTHER ACCIDENT? ☐ YES ☑ NO

c. INSURANCE PLAN NAME OR PROGRAM NAME: MEDICARE

d. INSURANCE PLAN NAME OR PROGRAM NAME: AARP SECONDARY POLICY

10d. CLAIM CODES (Designated by NUCC)

d. IS THERE ANOTHER HEALTH BENEFIT PLAN? ☑ YES ☐ NO *If yes*, complete items 9, 9a, and 9d.

READ BACK OF FORM BEFORE COMPLETING & SIGNING THIS FORM.

12. PATIENT'S OR AUTHORIZED PERSON'S SIGNATURE I authorize the release of any medical or other information necessary to process this claim. I also request payment of government benefits either to myself or to the party who accepts the assignment below.

SIGNED SIGNATURE ON FILE — DATE 01/14/20XX

13. INSURED'S OR AUTHORIZED PERSON'S SIGNATURE I authorize payment of medical benefits to the undersigned physician or supplier for services described below.

SIGNED SIGNATURE ON FILE

PATIENT AND INSURED INFORMATION

14. DATE OF CURRENT ILLNESS, INJURY, or PREGNANCY (LMP) MM DD YY — QUAL.

15. OTHER DATE QUAL. MM DD YY

16. DATES PATIENT UNABLE TO WORK IN CURRENT OCCUPATION FROM MM DD YY TO MM DD YY

17. NAME OF REFERRING PROVIDER OR OTHER SOURCE: ROBERT WILSON, MD

17a.

17b. NPI 11122233344

18. HOSPITALIZATION DATES RELATED TO CURRENT SERVICES FROM MM DD YY TO MM DD YY

19. ADDITIONAL CLAIM INFORMATION (Designated by NUCC)

20. OUTSIDE LAB? ☐ YES ☐ NO — $ CHARGES

21. DIAGNOSIS OR NATURE OF ILLNESS OR INJURY Relate A-L to service line below (24E) — ICD Ind.

A. E11.22 B. C. D.
E. F. G. H.
I. J. K. L.

22. RESUBMISSION CODE — ORIGINAL REF. NO.

23. PRIOR AUTHORIZATION NUMBER

	24. A. DATE(S) OF SERVICE From MM	DD	YY	To MM	DD	YY	B. PLACE OF SERVICE	C. EMG	D. PROCEDURES, SERVICES, OR SUPPLIES (Explain Unusual Circumstances) CPT/HCPCS	MODIFIER	E. DIAGNOSIS POINTER	F. $ CHARGES		G. DAYS OR UNITS	H. EPSDT Family Plan	I. ID. QUAL.	J. RENDERING PROVIDER ID. #
1	01	14	XX	01	14	XX	11		99213		1	$125	00	1		NPI	11122233344
2																NPI	
3																NPI	
4																NPI	
5																NPI	
6																NPI	

25. FEDERAL TAX I.D. NUMBER: 098-76-5432 — SSN ☐ EIN ☑

26. PATIENT'S ACCOUNT NO.: RW125638

27. ACCEPT ASSIGNMENT? (For govt. claims, see back) ☑ YES ☐ NO

28. TOTAL CHARGE: $ 125 00

29. AMOUNT PAID: $ 0

30. Rsvd for NUCC Use

31. SIGNATURE OF PHYSICIAN OR SUPPLIER INCLUDING DEGREES OR CREDENTIALS (I certify that the statements on the reverse apply to this bill and are made a part thereof.)

Robert Wilson, MD — 01/14/XX

SIGNED — DATE

32. SERVICE FACILITY LOCATION INFORMATION
Feel Better Family Practice
101 Jack Place
New York, NY, 10001
(212) 555-1212
a. 22233344455 b.

33. BILLING PROVIDER INFO & PH # ( )
Robert Wilson, MD
101 Jack Place
New York, NY, 10001
(212) 555-1212
a. 11122233344 b.

PHYSICIAN OR SUPPLIER INFORMATION

NUCC Instruction Manual available at: www.nucc.org — *PLEASE PRINT OR TYPE* — APPROVED OMB-0938-1197 FORM 1500 (02-12)

FIGURE 15.7 Completed CMS-1500 Health Insurance Claim Form.

TABLE 15.2 Information Required for Completion of the CMS-1500 Health Insurance Claim Form

BLOCK	INFORMATION NEEDED
	Completed patient registration/intake form
	Photocopy of insurance card or cards (front and back)
	Encounter form
	Preauthorization or precertification number (when applicable)
Section 1: Carrier	
1	Type of insurance
Section 2: Patient and Insured Information	
1a	Insured's identification (ID) number (primary insurance)
2	Patient's full name
3	Patient's date of birth and gender
4	Insured's name (primary insurance)
5	Patient's address and telephone number • Permanent address (including apartment number if appropriate) • City, state, zip code • Telephone number
6	Patient's relationship to insured
7	Insured's address and telephone number • Permanent address (including apartment number if appropriate) • City, state, zip code • Telephone number
9	Other insured's name (secondary insurance)[a]
9a	Policy or group number (secondary insurance)[a]
9b	Secondary insured's date of birth and gender[a]
9c	Secondary insured's employer or school name[a]
9d	Secondary insured's insurance plan or program name[a]
10a-c	If patient's condition or illness is related to employment, auto accident, or some other type of accident, make sure information is obtained as outlined in Block 1
10d	Claim codes as designated by NUCC
11	Insured's policy, group, or FECA number (primary insurance)
11a	Primary insured's date of birth and gender
11b	Other claim ID designated by NUCC
11c	Primary insured's insurance plan or program name
11d	Determine whether the patient also is covered by a secondary health insurance plan
12	Confirm that the patient's release of information form has been signed, dated, and is in the patient's record
13	Confirm that the insured's authorization of benefits form has been signed, dated, and is in the patient's record
Section 3: Physician or Supplier Information	
14	Date current illness, injury, or pregnancy began
15	Determine whether patient has had the same or similar symptoms
16	From-To dates if patient was unable to work at current occupation
17	Name of ordering or referring provider
17a	Not required
17b	Ordering or referring provider's NPI
18	From-To dates if patient encounter included an inpatient hospital stay
19	Determine whether insurance carrier in carrier block and Block 1 requires any information to be entered in this field
20	Determine whether an outside laboratory was used; if so, enter charges billed to provider for outside lab services
21	ICD-10-CM code or codes for patient's condition, illness, or injury (maximum of twelve per claim)
22	Is Medicaid claim being resubmitted? If yes, provide reference number from original Medicaid claim submitted
23	If prior authorization and/or referral is required, provide authorization (approval) number from insurance payer (preauthorization or precertification number)
24A	From-To dates of service for current encounter
24B	Place of service (POS) code
24C	If an emergency, put a Y in this box
24D	CPT and/or HCPCS code CPT and/or HCPCS modifier(s) (maximum of four per charge line)
24E	Block 21 field or reference number (1, 2, 3 and/or 4)
24F	Total charge for CPT- or HCPCS-coded services listed in Block 24D • If more than 1 day or unit is indicated in Block 24G, multiply the charge for the service(s) coded in Block 24D by the number of days/units in Block 24G; enter the result in Block 24F
24G	Total number of days or units
24H	EPSDT or Family Plan code (Medicaid or AFDC)
24I	Qualifier ID code (if no NPI available)

TABLE 15.2 Information Required for Completion of the CMS-1500 Health Insurance Claim Form—*continued*

BLOCK	INFORMATION NEEDED
24J	Rendering (treating) provider's NPI—unshaded field PIN (if no NPI is available)—shaded field
25	Rendering provider's federal tax ID number (EIN or SSN)
26	Patient's account number with rendering provider
27	Determine whether contract or agreement between provider and insurance carrier allows provider to accept assignment
28	Total charges from Block 24F, lines 1–6
29	Amount paid by patient, insured, or other insurance
30	Balance due (if any amount paid is shown in Block 29)
31	Signature of provider performing service or procedure
32	Address of facility where services were rendered
32a	NPI number of service facility listed in Block 32
32b	Qualifier ID number and PIN of facility listed in Block 32 (if no NPI available)
33	Name, address, and phone number of performing (rendering) provider
33a	NPI of provider listed in Block 33
33b	Qualifier ID number and PIN of provider listed in Block 33 (if no NPI available)

[a]Only required if a secondary insurance exists and is to be submitted to the insurance carrier.
AFDC, Aid to Families with Dependent Children; *CPT,* Current Procedural Terminology coding system; *EIN,* employer identification number; *EPSDT,* Early and Periodic Screening, Diagnosis, and Treatment; *FECA,* Federal Employees Compensation Act; *HCPCS,* Health Care Common Procedural Coding System coding method; *ICD-10-CM,* International Classification of Diseases, Tenth Revision, Clinical Modification coding method; *NPI,* National Provider Identifier; *PIN,* personal identification number; *POS,* place of service.

Violations of the laws governing reimbursement may have the following results:

- Nonpayment of claims
- Civil monetary penalties (CMPs)
- Exclusion from the payer program
- Criminal and civil liability
- In extreme cases, jail time

These laws may be changed or updated. The person who is responsible for coding must pay close attention to detail and act as a sort of medical detective to prevent a case against a provider or clinic. The ICD-10-CM and CPT/HCPCS manuals are updated annually. New coding manuals have a few pages dedicated to the updates for that particular year. Accurate use of ICD-10-CM and CPT/HCPCS manuals is essential for the correct translation of the claim information in the health record into the correct codes. However, as models of providing healthcare change, they can present some challenges for accurate coding and billing procedures.

Guidelines for Reviewing Claims before Submission

The following guidelines can help ensure that clean insurance claims are submitted.

- Proofread the form or data entered into the electronic system carefully for accuracy and completeness.
- Make certain any necessary attachments are included with the completed form.
- Follow office policies and guidelines for claim review and signatures.
- Forward the original claim to the proper insurance carrier either by mail or electronically.
- Make sure the patient's and/or insured's name, address, ID, group, and/or policy number are identical to the information printed on the insurance card.
- Make sure the patient's birth date and gender are the same as in the medical record.
- Section 2, Patient and Insured Information **(Blocks 1–13)**: Complete these blocks accurately, according to the insurance carrier's guidelines.
- **Block 11:** Enter the policy, group or FECA number. If there is no group number, leave it blank.
- **Block 12:** Make sure the patient has authorized the release of information and that Block 12 has a handwritten signature, the words "Signature on File," or the acronym SOF.
- **Blocks 14–24J** (required fields for diagnosis and procedure): Make sure these blocks are completed accurately, according to NUCC or carrier-specific guidelines.
- Make sure the diagnosis is not missing or incomplete.
- Check that the diagnosis has been coded accurately, according to the ICD-10-CM coding manual and is linked to the treatment.
- List the fees for each charge individually; or, if more than 1 day or unit is entered in **Block 24G**, the fees must be computed correctly.
- **Blocks 17** and **17b:** If applicable, enter the referring provider's name and NPI number.
- **Block 25:** Double-check the provider's federal Social Security number (SSN) or employer identification number (EIN) to ensure accuracy.
- **Block 27** (Accept Assignment?): Put an X in the YES box if the provider is a PAR provider or has an agreement with the insurance company to accept assignment.
- **Block 31:** Check for the provider's signature, which must be on the form.
- **Block 24J** and **Block 33a:** Make sure the provider's NPI, corresponding to the insurance carrier being billed, has been entered in Block 24J and again in Block 33a.

Preventing Rejection of a Claim

It is important for the medical assistant to understand and comply with the specific guidelines for completing a CMS-1500 established by each insurance company. This prevents delays in reimbursement and denial of payment. The guidelines for Medicare, Medicaid, TRICARE, and workers' compensation can be found online at the websites of these healthcare insurers. Most practice management billing systems have built-in **claim scrubbers** that help in the process. If claims are sent electronically through a clearinghouse, claims auditing is done before the clearinghouse transmits the claim to the insurance company. Claims without errors of any type are called *clean claims*. Claims with incorrect, missing, or insufficient data are called *dirty claims*.

Communication with Providers about Third-Party Requirements

It can be challenging for a provider to keep up with the annual changes made by the government plans, private health insurance companies, and the coding updates. This is why healthcare providers trust their medical office staff to stay up to date on the various changes in the health insurance industry.

Some providers may be so focused on patient care that they feel uncomfortable with change. This may be the case with the encounter form/superbill used in patient care. A provider may feel comfortable using the same form, but over time, some codes may have changed or become obsolete, or new medical services offered may not be listed on the form.

A medical coder should tactfully discuss with the provider the benefits of using an updated encounter form. If the provider is still reluctant to change the form, even though it is outdated, the medical coder may suggest that the form will not be changed, just the codes on it. Adjust the encounter form to include an open text box for providers to add medical procedures that they perform occasionally.

When communicating with the provider about coding issues, you must always have a respectful attitude. The many changes occurring in medical coding and billing can be overwhelming and confusing for some providers. The approach of coding professionals should be to guide them patiently through these changes.

CRITICAL THINKING APPLICATION **15.4**

Being tactful means using good manners as you provide truthful, sensitive information or honest critical feedback to another person. Tactful behaviors include showing respect, discretion, compassion, honesty, diplomacy, and courtesy while you deliver a message. Tactful behaviors encompass nonverbal and verbal communication, including what you say, how you say it, and your body language during the communication. A critical element of being tactful is considering the other person's feelings and reactions as you deliver the information. When you use tactful behaviors, you demonstrate professionalism and preserve relationships by avoiding conflicts and finding common ground.

Many times the medical biller is the expert on the third-party requirements, and providers rely on the biller to help them understand the requirements. Being tactful with providers as you communicate third-party requirements is critical to your working relationship with the provider and is also important in the overall financial scope of the agency. It is crucial to assist the provider in a tactful manner, understanding his or her role in meeting third-party requirements.

Using the following case study, role-play with two peers how you would display tactful behaviors when communicating with medical providers about third-party requirements.

You are the medical biller for your clinic. The two providers have not been communicating with you about procedures that need prior authorization from the insurance companies. As a result, multiple claims are being denied, and the clinic has had to write off much of the cost. Today you are talking with the providers, explaining common procedures that require prior authorizations and the process of getting preauthorizations.

CLAIM FOLLOW-UP

The majority of claims are paid in a timely fashion without any issues, but some claims need some extra time and effort. Claims can become lost in either the healthcare organization's system or in the insurance company's system. Claims tracking is an important task used to follow up on those lost claims. Some claims can be rejected or denied. Why this occurs can be found on the EOB/RA. It is also important to review those documents and follow up on the claims that have been rejected or denied. The next section goes over how to track claims and follow up on rejected or denied claims.

Claims Tracking

The medical biller should keep track of every submitted claim to ensure timely reimbursement. Clearinghouses send a confirmation report after submission of a claim. The medical biller should always confirm that the claims submitted to the clearinghouse match the claims listed on the confirmation report. If direct billing is used, the medical biller must set up a system to track the claims that were submitted. Medical assistants should maintain this practice to ensure every claim is submitted correctly.

The claim submission confirmation report also indicates claims that were rejected because they were incomplete. These claims should be corrected and resubmitted electronically immediately. Often these claims are rejected for data entry errors. The medical biller should compare the patient's information in the practice management software to the information on the patient's registration form and scanned insurance card to ensure accuracy.

It typically takes 10 to 14 business days for insurance companies to process insurance claims electronically. If the insurance company has not responded after 30 days, the medical biller should inquire about the status of the claim. This can be done through the company's provider web portal or by calling the provider services number on the back of the patient's insurance ID card. To verify the claim status, you must provide the following information:

- Insured subscriber's member number and birth date
- Patient's name and birth date
- Date of service

With this information, the insurance company should be able to tell if the claim has been paid, is still in process, was denied, or was never received. The medical biller will use this information for the proper follow-up. This could involve a number of actions:

- Investigating the records at the clinic to see if the payment came in but was applied to the incorrect patient account.
- Researching the denial and resubmitting the claim.
- Determining why the claim was not received and resubmitting it.

The state insurance commission has standards that insurance companies must abide by, including claim processing times and payment guidelines. Medical assistants should keep the commission's contact information in the office medical billing manual as a reference in case a claim should be reported.

Explanation of Benefits/Remittance Advice

An explanation of benefits (EOB) is a document the insurance company sends to the patient. A remittance advice (RA) is that same information, but it is sent directly to the provider who submitted an insurance claim and often lists multiple patients. A remittance advice is usually sent electronically. If the patient has signed the assignment of benefits statement, the RA will come with a check, if it is in paper format, or a document indicating that funds were electronically transferred.

The healthcare facility cannot just deposit the check and disregard the EOB/RA, which provides detailed accounting for the submitted insurance claim. The EOB/RA breaks down each line-item charge from Block 24 on the CMS-1500 into the charged amount, the amount allowable, and the amount paid. Most EOB/RAs will also indicate how much was applied to the deductible, the patient's co-insurance amount, and if any services were denied (Figure 15.8 and Figure 15.9).

Reading an Explanation of Benefits/Remittance Advice

The EOB/RA contains essential information about the submitted health insurance claim:

- Patient's name
- Date of service
- Services provided, including the CPT/HCPCS codes
- Charged amount
- Covered or allowed amount
- Deductible amount
- Co-insurance amount
- Payment amount
- Reason codes to explain a denial or an adjustment to the payment amount

To properly apply payments to a patient's account, it is vital that the medical assistant understand all the elements of an EOB/RA. When interpreting the EOB/RA, review the following steps:

1. Verify that the EOB/RA applies to the correct patient by comparing the account number and date of service on the EOB/RA with the submitted claim.
2. Confirm that the EOB/RA shows the same charged amount as the submitted claim. In other words, the line items and charges should match. Sometimes the EOB/RA summarizes the entire claim in one charged amount. In this case, confirm that the total charged is the same as in the submitted claim.
3. Post the payment and adjusted amount per line item. In the practice management billing software, these are posted on the same line. The patient's responsibility, as determined by the primary insurance EOB/RA, is calculated using the following equation:

   Charged amount − Payment amount −
   Adjustment amount = Patient's responsibility

4. Once the patient's responsibility has been determined, check for a secondary insurance. If one is listed, submit a health insurance claim with the balance due determined by the primary insurance EOB/RA. If no secondary insurance is listed, the patient is billed for the balance due.
5. Review the *remark codes* on the EOB/RA for any additional messages or information about the claim. The remark codes area is where the insurance company indicates the conditions under which the claim was paid. For example, code 01 states that the claim amount allowed was established by the contract between the health insurance plan and the provider. Other remark codes give the reasons a claim was denied or rejected. Some remark codes indicate that the claim is pending, awaiting specific information.
6. All remark codes on pending or denied claims should be followed up immediately upon receipt of the EOB/RA to prevent further delay in payment for other claims.

There is no standard format for the EOB, so patients often have difficulty understanding them. One of the responsibilities of the medical biller is to explain the EOB to the patient. When patients understand why a claim was paid in a certain way, they are more willing to pay their share.

Explanation of benefits

Temple Insurance Company
1000 Alameda Blvd.
San Jose CA 98877
800-333-444-5555
800-333-444-6666 (FAX)

Insured's name: Kenneth Koziak
Temple member # J4235916P

Date: 09/20/20XX
Provider: Walden-Martin Family Medical Clinic
J.A. Martin NPI 1234567890
Claim no. 9885050333-XX
Check no. 2034422

Patient name: Kenneth Koziak
916 Maple St.
Anytown, AL 12345

Date of service	CPT code	Charge amount	Allowable charges	Applied to deductible	Copay	Total benefit	Reason code(s)
09/06/20XX	99205	132.28	125.00	0.00	0.00	100.00	42
09/06/20XX	82947	15.00	15.00	0.00	0.00	12.00	
09/06/20XX	86580	11.34	11.34	0.00	0.00	9.07	
Total		158.62	151.34	0.00	0.00	121.07	

Reason code: 42 charges exceed our fee schedule or maximum allowed amount

FIGURE 15.8 Sample Explanation of Benefits (EOB).

Temple Insurance Company
Remittance Advice

09/20/20XX

Walden-Martin Family Medical Clinic
1234 Anystreet
Anytown, AL 12345-0001

Patient name	Treatment dates	CPT code	Charge amount	Reason code	Covered amount	Deductible amount	Copay amount	Paid at	Payment amount
Koziak, Kenneth	09/06/20XX	99205	132.28	42	125.00	0.00	0.00	80%	100.00
	09/06/20XX	82947	15.00		15.00	0.00	0.00	80%	12.00
	09/06/20XX	86580	11.34		11.34	0.00	0.00	80%	9.07
	Totals		158.62		151.34				121.07
Slomkowski, Larry	09/07/20XX	99212	28.55		28.55	0.00	0.00	80%	22.84
	Totals		28.55		28.55				22.84
Vale, Julie	09/04/20XX	99203	70.92	42	69.23	0.00	0.00	80%	55.38
	09/04/20XX	71020	40.97	42	34.95	0.00	0.00	80%	27.96
	Totals		111.89		104.18				83.34

Reason code: 42 charges exceed our fee schedule or maximum allowed amount

Check no: 56390 $227.25

FIGURE 15.9 Sample Remittance Advice (RA).

Rejected Claims

The EOB/RA provides detailed information on rejected claims. A rejected claim contains one or more errors. All rejected claims have a code with a legend toward the bottom of the page. Here are some of the reasons claims are rejected:

- The time period for filing the claim expired (check the insurance plan's billing policies manual for details).
- Incorrect ICD-10-CM, CPT, and/or HCPCS codes or combinations of codes were entered.
- The insurer claims that the ICD-10-CM code and the CPT/HCPCS codes do not match—that is, the claim lacks **medical necessity**.
- More than one CPT/HCPCS code was filed on the same date of service, and they are mutually exclusive when billed together.
- The claim was submitted to the wrong insurance company.

Rejected claims should be resubmitted as soon as possible to prevent further delay in reimbursement.

Denied Claims

The EOB/RA will list the claims that have been denied, showing a zero payment. It is important the EOB/RA is reviewed to find those denied claims. A medical biller should recognize the reason codes that indicate that a claim has been denied and why.

The two main reasons for denial of payment are technical errors and insurance policy coverage issues. Technical errors include incorrect or incomplete information, data entry, and/or mathematical errors. Common reasons for denial and the process for correcting it include the following:

- The patient was not covered by the insurance plan on the date of service.
  Contact the patient to obtain the correct insurance plan information and submit the claim to that insurance plan.
- A listed procedure was not an insurance benefit.
  Contact the patient to make sure that she or he understands that the procedure was not covered by the person's insurance plan. This denial can be avoided by obtaining precertification/preauthorization.
- Preauthorization for the service was not obtained.
  Talk to the business office supervisor to determine if the patient can be billed for services or if an adjustment to the patient's account will need to be made.
- The service was deemed not to be a medical necessity.
  Review the documentation to determine if the correct diagnosis and procedure codes were submitted. If they were incorrect on the original claim, a new claim should be submitted with the corrected information.

After finding the denied claims on the EOB/RA, the medical biller should review the reason codes and make the appropriate changes to the claim to get it paid. If the patient was not covered by that plan at the time the service was provided, they should be contacted for updated insurance information and the claim should be submitted to the new carrier. If there is no insurance coverage, the patient should be billed for those services.

Medical Necessity. Insurance companies determine medical necessity based on the diagnostic and procedural codes submitted on the claim. The diagnostic code is the reason that the procedure was necessary. For example, if a claim submitted to the insurance company indicated that a bunionectomy was performed for tonsillitis, the insurer will deny the claim based on medical necessity. Procedure codes are linked to diagnostic codes in the claim. The health record must support the reason for each service provided.

If an insurance claim is denied for medical necessity, the medical assistant should review the claim information and the health record. If there is an error on the claim, such as the wrong diagnostic code on the encounter form, a new claim should be submitted.

TABLE 15.3 Comparing Patient Financial Responsibilities

PATIENT'S FINANCIAL RESPONSIBILITY	WHEN PATIENT PAYS	AMOUNT PATIENT PAYS
Copayment	At the time of medical service	Fixed amount, $10 to $75 per visit
Deductible	Before the insurance company will pay	Variable amount, $250 to $5000
Co-insurance	After the provider has been paid	Variable amount, up to 30%

If an insurance claim is denied for medical necessity and the medical assistant believes that it was coded correctly, an appeal letter should be sent to the insurance company. The appeal letter should identify the denied claim and include a statement from the provider detailing the medical reasoning for performing the procedure. Additional medical reports (e.g., laboratory reports, operative reports, and history and physical examination findings [H&P]) should be sent if they support the provider's treatment decision (Procedure 15.4).

THE PATIENT'S FINANCIAL RESPONSIBILITY

Most MCO health insurance contracts require patients to pay a copayment, which is collected at the time of service (Table 15.3). Copayments can range from $10 to $75 for office visits. They vary depending on whether the patient is seen by a PCP or specialist, in urgent care, or the emergency department. Office visits and prescription copayments do not count toward the yearly deductible. The medical assistant must make sure that the proper copayments are received and credited to patients' accounts.

A *deductible* is a set dollar amount the policyholder is responsible for each year before the insurance company begins to reimburse the healthcare provider. The deductible amount is stated in the insurance policy.

Co-insurance means that the insured and the insurance company share the cost of covered medical services after the deductible has been met. The insurance company and the patient split the cost of the services. An 80/20 split is very common, especially for traditional insurance. This means that after the yearly deductible has been met, the insurance company pays 80% of the fee, and the insured pays 20%. The patient's deductible or co-insurance responsibility is shown on the EOB.

To help patients understand their health insurance benefits, the medical assistant must be confident in defining the terms *copayment*, *co-insurance*, and *deductible* (Procedure 15.5).

The medical office can contact the insurance company on the patient's behalf to determine the amount of the deductible the patient has already paid in the calendar year. The process of precertification enables the healthcare provider to inform patients of how much the procedure will cost them.

Calculating the Co-insurance and Deductible

Consider this example: Mrs. Anita Jones' health insurance plan has a $500 annual deductible, after which the insurance company pays 95% of all charges. Mrs. Jones, therefore, has a 5% co-insurance expense, in addition to the deductible. Mrs. Jones has incurred a $10,000 charge for cardiac surgery performed by her provider.

	Column A	Column B
Total Charge	$10,000	$20,000
Deductible (paid by Mrs. Jones)	$500	$500
Coinsurance (5% paid by Mrs. Jones)	5% of $9500 (Total charge minus the deductible) = $475	5% of 19,500 (Total charge minus the deductible) = $975
Total amount paid by Mrs. Jones	$975	$1475
Total amount paid by insurance	95% of $9500 (Total charge minus the deductible) = $9025	95% of $19,500 (Total charge minus the deductible) = $18,525

FIGURE 15.10 Deductible and Co-insurance.

In Figure 15.10, Column A shows that Mrs. Jones paid the $500 deductible and 5% of $10,000 (i.e., an additional $475). The insurance company then paid the remaining balance of $9,025.

Also in Figure 15.10, Column B shows that if Mrs. Jones' cardiac surgery cost $20,000, her total out-of-pocket expense is now $1475, and the insurance company is responsible for paying the balance of $18,525.

Allowed Amount

Another factor to be considered when determining the patient's financial responsibility is whether or not the provider is a PAR provider. To become a participating provider in an insurance network, the provider must agree to accept the insurance plan's fee schedule as payment in full for services rendered. This means that if the provider's fee is higher than the plan's allowed amount, the difference should be adjusted. For example, a provider may charge $80 for a Level I office visit; however, the insurance plan's allowable amount may be only $60. Providers who are participating providers are obligated to adjust the difference between these two amounts—$20. The patient is not responsible for that $20. However, providers who are not participating providers can bill the patient for the $20 balance. Because contracts between insurance companies and providers vary greatly, it is important for the medical assistant to closely examine the EOB to ensure that the proper adjustments are made.

Let's look at how this would affect the example in Figure 15.10. If the allowable amount for Mrs. Jones' $10,000 cardiac surgery is $8500, the $1500 difference between the provider's charge and the allowed amount would be either written off or passed on to the patient. Figure 15.11 demonstrates the differences in the patient's responsibility and provider reimbursement.

CRITICAL THINKING APPLICATION 15.5

The providers in the practice where Ann works are not in-network for a preferred provider organization (PPO) that is often used in their geographic area. Many patients are confused when they have to pay a larger out-of-pocket fee for their medical services. How can Ann explain the reason for these higher fees to patients?

Discussing the Patient's Financial Responsibility

The *guarantor* is the person legally responsible for the entire bill. It is important that the patient and the guarantor understand what the financial responsibilities are for services provided. Some patients expect insurance to pay all costs simply because they are paying a premium. Often patients do not even read their insurance policies and have no idea what is and is not covered.

	PAR	NonPAR
Total Charge	$10,000	$10,000
Allowed amount	$8500	$8500
$1500 difference between charged amount and allowed amount	Written off as an adjustment	Billed to the patient
Deductible (paid by Mrs. Jones)	$500	$500
Coinsurance (paid by Mrs. Jones)	$8500 – $500 (deductible) × 5% = $400	$8500 – $500 (deductible) × 5% = $400
Total amount paid by Mrs. Jones	$900	$2400
Total amount paid by insurance	$7600	$7600

FIGURE 15.11 PAR vs. NonPar.

The medical assistant may need to educate patients about their policies and help them work with their insurance company to get answers to questions and make sure they are receiving all the benefits to which they are entitled. If problems come up with the insurance company, it is in the practice's best interest to actively assist the patient. The medical billing staff is usually more knowledgeable than the patient is about health insurance. Helping patients with issues can help ensure that the provider is compensated for his or her services.

Medical assistants gain knowledge about the insurance industry when they actively assist patients with their concerns. The more experience a medical assistant has in working with insurance, the more helpful that assistant can be to patients. As mentioned previously, medical assistants should keep a manual of medical billing policies and procedures for most of the insurance plans they handle; this can serve as an excellent source of guidance and suggestions for working with a particular payer.

Always be sure to obtain the guarantor's signature on an agreement to pay for services. Most patient information sheets have a section referring to the guarantor. A statement may be included that serves as an agreement to pay the costs of medical care. States have statutes that deal with guarantors, so be sure the office's policies comply with those laws. It is especially important to secure a written agreement to pay for services when the care will be long term or involves costly treatment or surgical procedures. Procedure 15.6 explains how to inform patients of their financial obligations for services rendered.

Showing Sensitivity When Discussing the Patient's Finances

Most patients use health insurance, but they do not always recognize that they will have financial obligations after the insurance plan pays its share. This is common among Medicare patients, who often feel they should have all their medical expenses paid because they have government insurance. It usually falls to the medical assistant to inform patients of their financial responsibilities (Procedure 15.7).

> **Advance Beneficiary Notice (ABN)**
>
> Medicare does not cover some healthcare services, so the **Advance Beneficiary Notice (ABN)** is presented to patients in these circumstances. The ABN provides an option for patients to pay the provider's fee in full to receive services that Medicare does not cover. Patients then decide whether they still want to receive the services from the provider and complete the information on the form (Figure 15.12).

Patients seeking medical care are not usually feeling like themselves because they may be suffering from pain and discomfort. As a result, their behavior may not be typical when the medical assistant suggests discussing their financial responsibilities.

Medical assistants should show patience and sensitivity when discussing a patient's financial obligations (Figure 15.13). Patients should never be harassed to make a payment or forced into payment arrangements. Medical assistants should always be courteous when discussing payments with patients. In addition, the medical practice should offer a variety of payment options to meet patients' needs, including credit card and online payment options.

CLOSING COMMENTS

Accurate insurance billing practices are essential for the financial success of every healthcare facility. Medical assistants are strong assets to the healthcare facility when they can submit claims electronically, manage denied and rejected claims, and discuss financial responsibilities with patients professionally. Medical assistants should always maintain a positive attitude toward patients and keep in mind that those who are ill or facing challenges are not always at their best and may not respond in a positive way when discussing their financial responsibilities.

Patient Coaching

Patients often do not have a strong understanding of health insurance. There are so many different options out there, and their policies can change often. By explaining just what deductibles, copayment, and co-insurance are, we can help our patients understand just what their financial responsibilities are, even when they have health insurance. We can also help smooth the way for a good relationship with our patients by making sure that they understand the payment policies. No one likes to be blindsided by a request for payment. By patiently explaining why a patient owes a balance, you can have a positive discussion about how to resolve that balance.

Legal and Ethical Issues

From time-to-time patients may ask for a reduced fee after the insurance has already paid. If the provider is a participating provider with the health insurance plan, then he or she is obligated to follow the terms of the contract. This includes collecting the patient's financial responsibility detailed in the EOB. The routine waiving of copays can be considered a fraudulent practice. The insurance plan can penalize the healthcare facility if a concerted effort is not made to collect the patient's co-insurance and deductible amounts, thus not following the terms of the participating provider's health insurance contract.

Patient-Centered Care

Most patients are unaware of their benefits and coverage through their insurance policies. The medical assistant should encourage patients to read the entire policy to become familiar with its limitations and exclusions. Inform patients that when they call the insurance company with questions, they should always write down the date, the time, and the name of the person with whom they spoke. Using email is helpful because a record of the correspondence can

A. Notifier: John Doe, MD, College Clinic, 4567 Broad Avenue, Woodland Hills, XY 12345 555-486-9002
B. Patient Name: Mary Judd **C. Identification Number:** 0920XX7291

Advance Beneficiary Notice of Noncoverage (ABN)

NOTE: If Medicare doesn't pay for **D.** B12 injections below, you may have to pay.
Medicare does not pay for everything, even some care that you or your health care provider have good reason to think you need. We expect Medicare may not pay for the **D.** B12 injections below.

D.	**E. Reason Medicare May Not Pay:**	**F. Estimated Cost**
B12 injections	Medicare does not usually pay for this injection or this many injections	$35.00

WHAT YOU NEED TO DO NOW:

- Read this notice, so you can make an informed decision about your care.
- Ask us any questions that you may have after you finish reading.
- Choose an option below about whether to receive the **D.** B12 injections listed above.
  Note: If you choose Option 1 or 2, we may help you to use any other insurance that you might have, but Medicare cannot require us to do this.

G. Options: **Check only one box. We cannot choose a box for you.**

☑ **OPTION 1.** I want the **D.** B12 injections listed above. You may ask to be paid now, but I also want Medicare billed for an official decision on payment, which is sent to me on a Medicare Summary Notice (MSN). I understand that if Medicare doesn't pay, I am responsible for payment, but **I can appeal to Medicare** by following the directions on the MSN. If Medicare does pay, you will refund any payments I made to you, less co-pays or deductibles.

☐ **OPTION 2.** I want the **D.** ____________ listed above, but do not bill Medicare. You may ask to be paid now as I am responsible for payment. **I cannot appeal if Medicare is not billed.**

☐ **OPTION 3.** I don't want the **D.** ____________ listed above. I understand with this choice I am **not** responsible for payment, and **I cannot appeal to see if Medicare would pay.**

H. Additional Information:

This notice gives our opinion, not an official Medicare decision. If you have other questions on this notice or Medicare billing, call **1-800-MEDICARE** (1-800-633-4227/**TTY:** 1-877-486-2048).
Signing below means that you have received and understand this notice. You also receive a copy.

I. Signature: Mary Judd	**J. Date:** March 20, 20XX

According to the Paperwork Reduction Act of 1995, no persons are required to respond to a collection of information unless it displays a valid OMB control number. The valid OMB control number for this information collection is 0938-0566. The time required to complete this information collection is estimated to average 7 minutes per response, including the time to review instructions, search existing data resources, gather the data needed, and complete and review the information collection. If you have comments concerning the accuracy of the time estimate or suggestions for improving this form, please write to: CMS, 7500 Security Boulevard, Attn: PRA Reports Clearance Officer, Baltimore, Maryland 21244-1850.

Form CMS-R-131 (03/11) Form Approved OMB No. 0938-0566

FIGURE 15.12 Advance Beneficiary Notice for Medicare patients. (From Fordney MT: *Insurance handbook for the medical office,* ed 14, St. Louis, 2017, Elsevier.)

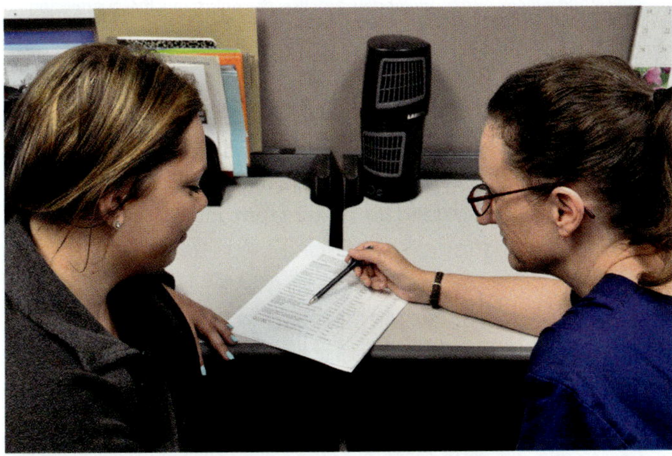

FIGURE 15.13 Medical assistants must show respect and sensitivity when discussing financial issues with patients.

easily be saved or printed. Making sure that patients have a general understanding of their health insurance coverage is well worth the effort.

Often patients do not dispute the decision or question the insurance company when a claim is rejected or not paid in the expected amount. Encourage them to call the company and question rejections if they do not understand why the claim was denied.

Professional Behaviors

Medical billers must have strong organizational skills. Not only are they responsible for submitting claims electronically in a timely manner, they must also manage claim denials and rejections. Denied and rejected claims need to be adjusted and rebilled for prompt payment. An organized medical biller ensures that all medical billing activities are worked on daily.

SUMMARY OF SCENARIO

Ann realizes that the best way to keep track of all the carriers is to keep an up-to-date manual that contains the addresses, phone numbers, and medical billing policies and procedures for each insurance plan the healthcare facility accepts. This manual can help prevent the rejection and denial of many claims because the claims will be submitted accurately the first time.

The medical assistant's understanding of how to calculate deductibles, co-insurance, and allowed amounts for procedures and services benefits both the provider and the patients. The provider's productivity, income, and losses can be easily tracked, and the patients can be educated regarding the exact amounts they are responsible for paying.

Ann also has learned the importance of being courteous to patients when discussing their financial obligations. She has learned how to use the Assignment of Financial Responsibility form to communicate what the patient owes in a clear, straightforward manner.

SUMMARY OF LEARNING OBJECTIVES

1. **Explain the medical billing process, including the types of information contained in the patient's billing record and managed care policies and procedures.**

   The revenue cycle of the medical billing process starts when a patient makes an appointment and is complete when payment has been received. Be sure to collect pertinent insurance billing information when the patient calls to schedule an appointment. Much of this information is on the patient registration form, which is completed when the patient comes to the medical office for the initial visit.

   Medical assistants should be aware that services provided to patients sponsored by a managed care organization (MCO) plan may not be reimbursed if the policies and procedures of the specific insurance plan are not followed. To submit accurate health insurance claims, medical assistants should establish office procedures for applying MCO policies and procedures.

   See Procedure 15.7 for instructions on how to show sensitivity when communicating with patients regarding third-party requirements and Procedure 15.2 for information on how to perform precertification with documentation.

2. **Examine how claims are submitted to third-party payers.**

   The medical assistant's medical billing tasks begin when the patient seeks medical services from the provider, usually when an appointment is made. Insurance billing and coding tasks typically completed by the medical assistant includes collecting accurate information and submitting a complete insurance claim.

   Medical billers should familiarize themselves with the claim submission policies and procedures of the health insurance plans commonly seen in their office. A medical assistant can successfully manage the requirements of the different insurance plans commonly seen in the practice by keeping an up-to-date manual containing the billing policies and procedures of these third-party payers. Electronic claims are insurance claims that are transmitted over the internet from the provider to the health insurance company. Most claims-processing software is designed to generate electronic claims.

   The medical assistant should follow an established list of guidelines for completing the CMS-1500 Health Insurance Claim Form, issued by the Centers for Medicare and Medicaid Services (CMS), which includes obtaining a signed assignment of benefits. The National Uniform Claim Committee (NUCC) is the best resource for claims completion. The CMS-1500 has 33 blocks; except for specific blocks that require information about the patient and the insured, the requirements for completing the form vary from payer to payer. Accuracy in completing the CMS-1500 is vital. The process for completing claim forms accurately is outlined in Procedure 15.3.

3. **Examine the impact of accurate coding.**

   Abuse in coding can be likened to actions that are contrary to ethical standards in the medical office. Unlike fraud, abuse is an inadvertent action that directly or indirectly results in an overpayment to the healthcare provider. Abuse is similar to fraud, except that it is unclear whether the unethical practice was committed deliberately. The term *intentional* is important in defining fraud and abuse and in deciphering whether the coding practices were ethical or not.

   It can be challenging for providers to keep up with the annual changes published by Medicare, private health insurance companies, and the ICD-10-CM code set updates. Staff meetings to review third-party requirements should be conducted regularly by the medical billing supervisor.

   Medical assistants should be respectful to the healthcare provider when discussing third-party requirements that demand more effort on the provider's part. An understanding and patient attitude goes a long way. Rejection and delay of claims cost the medical facility time and money. Proven methods of preventing rejection and delay should be established and followed; these may include reviewing electronic claims submission reports and following up on aging reports.

4. **Examine the methods for following up on claims.**

   It is important to track health insurance claims once they have been submitted electronically. A regular practice of confirming the submission of a claim with the health insurance plan or the clearinghouse is essential for prompt payment. If more than 2 weeks pass after a claim submission without a response from the insurance company, it is wise to follow up either through the online insurance provider web portal or by phone.

   The insurance company sends the explanation of benefits (EOB) form to the provider who submitted the insurance claim, along with a check or a document indicating that funds were transferred electronically. The EOB breaks down each line-item charge into the amount allowable, how much the insurance plan paid, and how much the patient is contracted to pay to the provider.

   The two main reasons for denial of payment are technical errors and insurance policy coverage issues. Technical errors include incorrect or incomplete information and typographic or mathematical errors.

   Accurate diagnosis codes must be submitted and linked to the medical procedure code reported to ensure correct reimbursement. The diagnosis code is the reason the medical procedure performed was nec-

SUMMARY OF LEARNING OBJECTIVES—cont'd

essary. If an insurance company denies a claim on the grounds that the medical treatment provided was not medically necessary, an appeal letter should be sent (see Procedure 15.4). The appeal letter should identify not only the denied claim in question but also include a statement from the provider detailing the medical reasoning for providing the billed treatment. Additional medical reports should be sent (e.g., lab reports, operative reports, the history and physical examination findings [H&P]) if these documents support the provider's decision to treat the patient.

5. **Explain a patient's financial obligations for services rendered.**
   Patients must understand that the guarantor is the person ultimately responsible for the entire bill. The insurance policy is a contract between an insurance company or MCO and the policyholder or a group of people (e.g., through an employer). The provider is not a party to this contract. Therefore, providers and their staff members are not responsible for pursuing an insurance payment for the benefit of the patient. However, it is in the best interest of the staff to actively assist the patient if problems occur in securing payment.

PROCEDURE 15.1 Perform Precertification with Documentation

TASK: Obtain precertification from a patient's insurance carrier for requested services or procedures.

SCENARIO: You are working with Dr. Julie Walden at Walden-Martin Family Medical Clinic. Erma Willis (DOB 12/09/19XX) is seen for excessive snoring, and Dr. Walden orders a sleep study. You need to complete a prior authorization/certification form for the sleep study, which will be conducted by Dr. Jim Sandman. You checked, and there is a signed release of information form.

INSURANCE INFORMATION	CLINIC AND PROVIDER INFORMATION
Aetna	Walden-Martin Family Medical Clinic
1234 Insurance Way	1234 Anystreet
Anytown, AL 112345-1234	Anytown, AL 12345
Member ID Number: EW8884910	Provider: Julie Walden, MD
Group Number: 66574W	Fax: 123-123-5678
	Phone: 123-123-1234
	Provider Contact Name: (your name)

Service Information

Place: Walden-Martin Family Medical Clinic
Service Requested: Sleep study
Starting Service Date: 1 week from today
Ending Service Date: 1 week from today
Service Frequency: Once
ICD-10-CM code: R06.83
CPT code: 95807
Not related to an injury or workers' compensation

EQUIPMENT and SUPPLIES

- *Paper method:* Patient's health record, prior authorization (precertification) request form, copy of patient's health insurance ID card, a pen
- *Electronic method:* Electronic health record system, such as SimChart for the Medical Office (SCMO)

PROCEDURAL STEPS

1. For the paper method, gather the health record, precertification/prior authorization request form, copy of the health insurance ID card, and a pen. For the electronic method, access the Simulation Playground in SCMO.
2. Using the health record, determine the service or procedure that requires precertification/preauthorization.
3. For the paper method, complete the precertification/prior authorization request form. For the electronic method, click on the Form Repository icon in SCMO. Select Prior Authorization Request from the left INFO PANEL. Use the Patient Search button at the bottom to find the patient. Complete the remaining fields of the form.
   PURPOSE: This provides information on the ordered procedure or service to the insurance company, which will notify the provider's representative if the procedure or service will be covered under the plan.
4. Proofread the completed form and make any revisions needed.
   PURPOSE: To ensure the accuracy of the information.
5. With the paper method, file the document in the health record after it has been faxed to the insurance carrier. With the electronic method, print and fax or electronically send the form to the insurance company and save the form to the patient's record.
   PURPOSE: Copies of all forms completed for the patient need to be maintained in the health record.

PROCEDURE 15.2 Generate an Insurance Claim

TASK: Accurately generate an insurance claim using NUCC guidelines.

SCENARIO: Mr. Walter Biller had an appointment with Dr. Walden on November 16, 20XX. He came in for an influenza vaccination, and while he was there, he wanted Dr. Walden to look at his ear because he was having problems hearing. His right ear canal was impacted with cerumen; the ear canal was irrigated, and the cerumen was removed during the visit.

PATIENT DEMOGRAPHICS	CLINIC AND PROVIDER INFORMATION
Walter B. Biller (patient and insured)	Walden-Martin Family Medical Clinic
87 Willoughby Lane	1234 Anystreet
Anytown, AL 12345-1234	Anytown, AL 12345
Phone: 123-237-3748	123-123-1234
DOB: 01/04/1970	POS–11 Office
SSN: 285-77-7796	Established patient of Julie Walden, MD
HIPAA form on file: Yes—March 19, 20XX	Federal Tax ID# 651249831
Signature on file: Yes—March 19, 20XX	NPI# 1467253823

Insurance Information

Account Number: 16611

Aetna

Policy/ID Number: CH8327753

Group Number: 33347H

Diagnosis	ICD-10-CM Code
Impacted cerumen, right ear	H61.21

SERVICE	CPT CODE	FEE
Est. minimal OV	99212	$24.00
Cerumen removal	69210	$46.00
Vaccine–Flu, 3 Y+	90658	$24.00
Preventive–Flu Administration	90471	$7.00

EQUIPMENT and SUPPLIES

- Patient's health record
- Copy of patient's insurance ID card or cards
- Patient registration/intake form
- Encounter form
- Insurance claims processing guidelines
- Electronic claims software such as SimChart for the Medical Office

PROCEDURAL STEPS

1. Gather the documents required to generate the claim.
2. Perform a patient search to locate the correct patient. Verify name and date of birth.
3. Ensure that all the demographic information has been entered into the practice management software accurately
   PURPOSE: The electronic claim will require the demographic information. If it has been entered inaccurately, the claim could be denied.
4. Select the correct encounter needed for the claim.
   PURPOSE: When the correct encounter is selected, the auto-populated areas of the claim will contain the correct information.
5. Review the auto-populated patient information and document any additional information needed. Save this information.
   PURPOSE: Accurate patient information is needed for the claim to be processed correctly.
6. Review the auto-populated provider information, and document any additional information that is needed. Save this information.
7. Review the auto-populated payer information and document any additional information that is needed. Save this information.
8. Review the patient claim information, including the diagnoses; if the condition is related to employment, auto accident, or other accident; disability information; release of information; assignment of benefits; and referring physician. Document any additional information needed. Save this information.
9. Verify or enter the date of service, CPT/HCPCS and POS codes, and link the diagnoses to the correct charge, modifiers, fees, and units. Save this information
10. Submit the claim.

PROCEDURE 15.3 Complete an Insurance Claim Form

TASK: Accurately complete a CMS-1500 Health Insurance Claim Form (see Figure 15.7) using NUCC guidelines.

SCENARIO: Kyle Reeves had an appointment with Dr. Walden on March 20, 20XX. He came in because he was experiencing extreme fatigue, fever, sore throat, and head and body aches. Upon examination, Dr. Walden also discovered swollen lymph nodes in the neck and armpits along with a swollen liver and spleen. She ordered a complete blood count (CBC), a mononucleosis test, and a urinalysis. The mononucleosis test came back positive.

PROCEDURE 15.3 Complete an Insurance Claim Form—*continued*

PATIENT DEMOGRAPHICS	CLINIC AND PROVIDER INFORMATION
Kyle T. Reeves (patient)	Walden-Martin Family Medical Clinic
8448 Washington Ave	1234 Anystreet
Anytown, AL 12345-1234	Anytown, AL 12345
Phone: 123-255-6499	123-123-1234
DOB: 01/01/2004	POS – 11 Office
SSN: 933-35-3754	Established patient of Julie Walden, MD
HIPAA form on file: Yes—March 19, 20XX	Federal Tax ID# 651249831
Signature on file: Yes—March 19, 20XX	NPI# 1467253823

Insurance Information

Account Number: 16611
Insured: Kim Reeves (mother)
Blue Cross Blue Shield
Policy/ID Number: K20568R
Group Number: 21548R

DIAGNOSIS:	ICD-10-CM CODE
Infectious mononucleosis	075

SERVICE	CPT CODE	FEE
Est. Expanded OV	99213	$43.00
CBC w/auto differential	85025	$35.00
Mononucleosis test	86663	$34.00
U/A, w/micro non-automated	81001	$27.00

EQUIPMENT and SUPPLIES

- Patient's health record
- Copy of patient's insurance ID card or cards
- Patient registration/intake form
- Encounter form
- Insurance claims processing guidelines
- Blank CMS-1500 Health Insurance Claim Form

PROCEDURAL STEPS

Almost all medical billing is done electronically through practice management billing software. The paper CMS-1500 Health Insurance Claim Form is provided only to help students practice and develop their medical billing skills.

Complete each block (as appropriate) of the CMS-1500 using the information provided.

1. Gather the documents required to complete the claim form.
2. Complete the claim form using a pen. Use capital letters. Do not use punctuation (commas or dollar signs) unless indicated in the insurance manual or guidelines. Use a hyphen to hyphenate last names.
3. Using the patient's health insurance ID card, determine the type of insurance and the insurance ID number. Enter this information into Blocks 1 and 1a.
   PURPOSE: After selecting the appropriate type of health insurance, the medical assistant can refer to the claims processing guidelines for that plan.
4. Using the ID card, the encounter form, and the registration/intake form, determine the patient's and insured individual's information. Accurately complete Blocks 2, 3, 5, 6, 9, and 10 a–c by entering the patient's information. Complete Blocks 4, 7, and 11 a–d with the insured's information.
   PURPOSE: By distinguishing between the patient and the insured, the medical biller can determine whether the insurer requires additional information for submission of an accurate claim.
5. Complete Blocks 12 and 13 by entering "signature on file" and the date. *Note:* The Assignment of Benefits form should have been signed by the patient or the insured at registration. Enter the dates in either the six (6)-digit format (MM/DD/YY) or the eight (8)-digit format (MM/DD/YYYY).
   PURPOSE: The medical practice must be authorized to release the service information on behalf of the patient or the insured to submit an insurance claim.
6. Accurately enter the physician or supplier information by completing Blocks 14 through 23. Use the eight (8)-digit format (MM/DD/YYYY) when needed.
7. Using the encounter form, complete Block 24 and the appropriate blocks from 24A through 24H. Note the following:
   - *Block 24A:* Enter the dates of service, both From and To. For ambulatory services, enter the same date in the FROM and TO fields. Enter a date for each procedure or service, or supply it in eight (8)-digit format (MM/DD/YYYY).
   - *Block 24F:* Enter the charge for the listed service or procedure. *Do not use commas when reporting dollar amounts.* The cents column is the small column to the right.
   - *Block 24G:* Enter the number of days or units. This block is usually used for multiple visits, units of supplies, anesthesia units or minutes, or oxygen volume. If only one service was performed, enter 1.
8. Complete Blocks 24I through 27 by entering information on the provider or the healthcare facility where the service was provided and the patient's account number. Check the correct box to indicate acceptance of assignment of benefits.
9. Complete Blocks 28 and 29 by entering the total charges, total amount paid, and total amount due. Complete Blocks 31 through 33a by entering the provider's and facility's information.
10. Review the claim for accuracy and completeness before submitting it. Correct any errors and provide any missing information.
    Note: Before sending the claim, make a copy of the form and file the copy in the patient's insurance claim file.
    PURPOSE: It is important to double-check the form for accuracy and for required information that has not been provided.

PROCEDURE 15.4 Use Medical Necessity Guidelines: Respond to a "Medical Necessity Denied" Claim

TASK: Resolve the insurance company's denial of a claim for medical necessity by completing an accurate claim form.

SCENARIO: You are working at the Walden-Martin Family Medical Clinic, 1234 Anystreet, Anytown, AL 12345 (phone: 123-123-1234). You receive a letter indicating that Medicare has denied the following claim for not being medically necessary.

Patient: Norma B. Washington
DOB: 08/07/19XX
Policy/ID Number: 847744144A
Date of Service: 06/13/20XX
ICD: G43.101 (Migraine)
CPT: J3420 (B-12 injection)
Provider: Julie Walden, MD

You do some research and find that this was the only information sent to Medicare for that encounter. The following information was the correct information for the encounter.

Patient: Norma B. Washington
DOB: 08/01/19XX
Date of Service: 06/15/20XX
ICD: G43.101 (Migraine) CPT: J1885 (Toradol 15 mg—$15.50) and 96372 (Injection, Ther/Proph/Diag—$25.00)
ICD: D51.0 (Vitamin B_{12} deficiency anemia) CPT: J3420 (B-12 injection—$24.00) and 96372 (Injection, Ther/Proph/Diag—$25.00)
To be billed to: Medicare, 1234 Insurance Road, Anytown, AL 12345-1234

EQUIPMENT and SUPPLIES

- *Paper method:* Patient's health record, copy of patient's insurance ID card or cards, patient registration form, encounter form, blank CMS-1500 Health Insurance Claim Form, pen
- *Electronic method:* SimChart for the Medical Office
- Insurance denial letter or scenario (presented earlier)

PROCEDURAL STEPS

1. Review the insurance denial letter (scenario) carefully. Compare the patient's information from the denial letter to the health record, claim, and encounter form. Look for errors in the patient's name and date of birth.
   PURPOSE: Errors in patient information can be a reason for denial.
2. Compare the insurance denial letter (scenario) to the health record, claim, and encounter form. Look for errors in the date of service, diagnosis, and procedure codes. The procedure must be medically necessary for the diagnosis indicated.
   PURPOSE: Errors related to the encounter must match for the claim to be accepted. The procedure codes must indicate an acceptable standard of treatment for the diagnosis listed. In some cases, the encounter form may contain a diagnosis that did not make it into the original claim form. Review the patient's health record to determine whether the procedure was medically necessary.
3. Complete a claim (either CMS-1500 or an electronic claim using SimChart) by entering the information about the carrier, patient, and insured.
4. Enter the information about the physician, procedures, and diagnosis. Make sure to include all the information from the encounter.
5. Proofread the claim form for accuracy before submitting the claim.

PROCEDURE 15.5 Assist a Patient in Understanding an Explanation of Benefits (EOB)

TASK: Explain an explanation of benefits (EOB) to a patient.

SCENARIO: Noemi Rodriguez has stopped by the WMFM Clinic with an explanation of benefits she recently received from her insurance company (shown here). She states that her policy has a $1000 deductible and 80/20 coinsurance. She doesn't understand why the insurance company didn't pay the bill in full, as she had services earlier in the year. She also is not clear on what she is financially responsible for.

WMFM Clinic is a participating provider with the Aetna Preferred Provider Plan that Ms. Rodriguez is part of.

Explanation of Benefits

Aetna
1234 Insurance Way
Anytown, AL 12345-1234
800-333-444-5555
800-333-444-6666 (FAX)

Insured's Name: Noemi Rodriguez
Policy ID # NR5006789

Date: 03/03/20XX

Patient's Name: Noemi Rodriguez
441 Hyacinth Way
Anytown, AL 12345

Provider: Walden-Martin Family Medical Clinic
J.A. Martin NPI 1234567890
Claim No. 9885050333-XX
Check No. 2034422

DATE OF SERVICE	CPT CODE	CHARGE AMOUNT	ALLOWABLE CHARGES	APPLIED TO DEDUCTIBLE	COPAY	TOTAL BENEFIT	REASON CODE(S)
01/14/20XX	99205	225.00	200.00	150.00	0.00	40.00	01/42
01/14/20XX	85025	35.00	30.00	0.00	0.00	24.00	42
01/14/20XX	82272	7.00	7.00	0.00	0.00	5.60	
01/14/20XX	80061	47.00	45.00	0.00	0.00	36.00	42
01/14/20XX	80076	39.00	32.50	0.00	0.00	26.00	42
01/14/20XX	80069	41.50	40.00	0.00	0.00	32.00	42
01/14/20XX	85652	16.00	16.00	0.00	0.00	12.80	
01/14/20XX	81001	27.00	25.00	0.00	0.00	20.00	42
Total		437.50	395.50	150.00	0.00	236.40	

Reason Code:
01 Deductible amount
42 Charges exceed our fee schedule or maximum allowed amount

DIRECTIONS: Explain to a peer (acting as Ms. Rodriguez) how the insurance company payment was determined, including an explanation of the allowed amount and her deductible. Also, explain how much of the charge amount Ms. Rodriguez is responsible for.

EQUIPMENT and SUPPLIES

- The explanation of benefits

PROCEDURAL STEPS

1. Review each of the columns found on the explanation of benefits. Have a clear understanding of how the insurance company came up with the patient's responsibility.
2. Determine if any amount has been applied to Ms. Rodriguez's deductible. Explain to Ms. Rodriguez how that impacts how much the insurance company will pay and her financial responsibility.
   PURPOSE: If the deductible amount is not met, the amount that the insurance company pays for services can be impacted, which in turn impacts the patient's financial responsibility.
3. Compare the charge amount for each service to the allowed amount. Explain to Ms. Rodriguez how the difference between those two is taken care of.
   PURPOSE: How the difference between the charged amount and the allowed amount is handled can impact the patient's financial responsibility.
4. Calculate what Ms. Rodriguez's financial responsibility is and explain to her how you came up with that amount.
5. Ask if the patient has any further questions.

PROCEDURE 15.6 Inform a Patient of Financial Obligations for Services Rendered

TASK: Inform the patient of his or her financial obligation and demonstrate professionalism and sensitivity when discussing the patient's billing record.

SCENARIO 1: Mr. Walter Biller arrives for his appointment. You need to check his eligibility for services and whether he has a copayment for today's visit. His insurance information is as follows: account number:16611; Aetna, Policy/ID Number: CH8327753; and Group Number: 33347H

SCENARIO 2: Christi Brown is meeting with you regarding the bill she received in the mail. She called to make the appointment and voiced her confusion about the bill. She stated that she thought her insurance covered everything. You check her record and see that she met her deductible and now needs to pay 20% of the billed amount. She owes $170.

DIRECTIONS: Role-play the scenarios with a peer. For the first scenario, the peer will be the insurance representative and then the patient. You will be the medical assistant. You need to be professional and sensitive when working with patients regarding payments. You also need to follow the clinic's policy.

EQUIPMENT and SUPPLIES

- Facility's payment policy
- Copy of patient's insurance card (or see the information in the scenario)
- Patient's account record (or see the information in the scenario)

PROCEDURAL STEPS

Scenario 1: Role-play with a peer who will be the insurance representative.

1. Contact the patient's insurance company and verify the patient's eligibility for services. Provide the representative with the patient's information. Find out if the patient has a copayment for today's visit. Document the information obtained.
   PURPOSE: Understanding the patient's financial responsibility from the insurance plan will help you explain the terms to the patient.

Scenario 1 update: You need to inform the patient that he owes a copayment for today's visit.

2. Inform the patient of his financial obligation of the copayment.

Scenario 1 update: He states he does not have the cash with him.

3. Inform the patient of the clinic policy regarding copayments and how the payment can be made.
4. Demonstrate sensitivity and professionalism when discussing the payment.

Scenario 2: Role-play with a peer who will be the patient.

5. Determine the amount the patient owes by reviewing the patient's account record. Inform the patient of the amount owed for services rendered.

Scenario 2 update: Patient states she does not have the money to pay the entire bill today.

6. Inform the patient of the clinic policy regarding overdue accounts and scheduling appointments. Provide the patient with options for the overdue amount based on the clinic policy.
7. Demonstrate sensitivity and professionalism when discussing the payment and the situation.

PROCEDURE 15.7 Show Sensitivity When Communicating with Patients Regarding Third-Party Requirements

TASKS: Communicate in an assertive, professional manner with a third-party representative. Demonstrate sensitivity through verbal and nonverbal communication when discussing third-party requirements with a patient. Display tactful behavior when communicating with a provider regarding third-party requirements.

SCENARIO: Ken Thomas (DOB 10/25/19XX) saw Jean Burke, NP, for his asthma today. He was prescribed a fluticasone inhaler, 220 mcg, and a refill on his Albuterol inhaler. When Ken stops at the checkout desk to make a follow-up appointment, he looks concerned. You inquire how you can help him, and he states that he is wondering if his new insurance will pick up the fluticasone inhaler. He further explains that he has used one in the past with great results, but he recently switched insurance plans and is finding that his new plan doesn't have the same coverage as his old plan.

ROLE-PLAY 1: You call the insurance company and discuss the coverage with the insurance carrier's representative. The representative tells you that the fluticasone inhaler is not covered. The representative gives you the names of two other inhalers that would be covered.

PROCEDURE 15.7 Show Sensitivity When Communicating with Patients Regarding Third-Party Requirements—*continued*

When you ask if the drug would be covered through the exceptions process, the representative indicates that the provider must send a letter indicating the drug is appropriate for the patient's condition because all other drugs covered by the plan have not been effective, or those drugs have side effects that may be harmful to the patient, or the patient is allergic to the other drugs.

ROLE-PLAY 2: You must explain to Ken, who is upset over his insurance coverage, that he would have to cover the $250 cost of the inhaler.

ROLE-PLAY 3: Ken explains he does not have $250 for the inhaler. He asks what else he should do. You mention the exception process, and Ken requests the provider to send a letter. You need to role-play notifying the provider of the third-party requirements.

DIRECTIONS: Role-play the scenarios with a peer. The peer will play the part of the insurance representative, the patient, and the provider. You need to be professional and assertive with the insurance representative. When working with the patient, you need to show sensitivity. When communicating with the provider, you need to be professional and tactful.

EQUIPMENT and SUPPLIES

- Copy of patient's health insurance ID card
- Prescription for new medication

PROCEDURAL STEPS

1. Obtain a copy of the patient's health insurance ID card and the prescription for the new medication.
   PURPOSE: Having the required documents will help you be more efficient as you perform the task.
2. Review the insurance card for coverage information and the phone number for providers.
   PURPOSE: You will need the phone number from the ID card to call the insurance company. You will also need to provide the insurance representative with the patient's information.
3. Using role-play 1, contact the insurance company and clearly state the patient's information, question, and the name of the new medication.
   PURPOSE: The insurance representative will need the patient's information and the question to assist you. As you provide the information, speaking clearly will help the listener understand what you are asking.
4. Demonstrate professionalism and verbal communication skills by stating a respectful, clear, and organized message, pronouncing medical terminology and medication names correctly.
5. Explain to the patient the message from the insurance representative using language that the patient can understand.
   PURPOSE: For the patient to understand your message, you need to use language that patients can understand.
6. Demonstrate sensitivity to the patient by paying attention and responding appropriately to his or her body language and verbal message.
   PURPOSE: Demonstrating sensitivity can be done through verbal messages and body language. Paying attention to the patient and responding appropriately to his or her message and nonverbal communication are important.
7. Demonstrate sensitivity to the patient by showing empathy and clarifying that you understand what the patient is stating. Give the patient your full attention during the conversation and reserve judgment.
8. Demonstrate sensitivity to the patient by using a pleasant, courteous tone of voice. Use body language to communicate respect (e.g., eye contact if culturally appropriate, keeping arms uncrossed and relaxed).
   PURPOSE: As the patient's frustration and anger increase, it is important to use a pleasant, courteous, and normal tone of voice. Keeping your body appearance relaxed (e.g., arms uncrossed, hands relaxed) will show the patient you are calm.
9. Demonstrate tactful behavior when explaining the third-party requirements to the provider.
   PURPOSE: Providing the patient with choices also shows the patient that you care.

PATIENT ACCOUNTS AND PRACTICE MANAGEMENT

16

SCENARIO

Laura Casper has been working in the back office at Walden-Martin Family Medical (WMFM) Clinic for the past 3 years. Her primary job has been working with patient accounts. She has recently also been asked to take on some of the accounts payable responsibilities. This will involve banking procedures and bill paying.

While working with patient accounts, Laura has become familiar with the billing cycle and collection procedures, and she is training new employees. It can be a complicated process, but Laura finds it challenging and enjoyable.

After the addition of the banking responsibilities to her work duties, Laura met with a bank representative. They discussed some time-efficient ways to bank with mobile depositing and online banking. Laura realizes that she still has much to learn about the daily financial duties in a healthcare facility, including working with the patient account management software, making daily deposits, reconciling bank statements, and many other banking responsibilities.

Laura wants to increase the value of the healthcare facility's bank accounts by looking for bank accounts that pay a higher interest rate and reducing the office's operational expenses. Laura also wants to encourage patients at the healthcare facility to use debit or credit cards, instead of checks, to pay for services because she knows that returned patient checks have created problems in the past.

While studying this chapter, think about the following questions:

- Why is it important to post charges, payments, and adjustments in a timely manner?
- What should you do when a patient wants to make payments on an outstanding patient account balance?
- What should you do when patient accounts are outstanding for more than 90 days after the date of service?
- How is online banking affecting banking in healthcare facilities?
- How can an office manager determine whether an employee can be trusted with banking procedures?
- What precautions should the healthcare facility take when accepting patient payments?
- Why is making daily deposits a good idea?
- How can the office manager reconcile the bank account, and why is this important?

LEARNING OBJECTIVES

1. Explain the components of accounts receivable in the healthcare facility.
2. Examine the various methods used for patient payments.
3. Examine successful collection techniques for patient accounts.
4. Explain the components of accounts payable in the healthcare facility.
5. Examine banking procedures as related to the ambulatory care setting.
6. Examine banking practices in today's business world.

VOCABULARY

assets All property available for the payment of debts.

belligerent (buh LIG er ent) Hostile and aggressive.

bookkeeping The process of recording financial transactions.

cash on hand The amount of money the healthcare facility has in the bank that can be withdrawn as cash.

counterfeit (KOWN ter fit) An imitation intended to be passed off fraudulently or deceptively as genuine; forgery.

defendant An individual or a business against which a lawsuit is filed.

discretionary income Money in a bank account that is not assigned to pay for any office expenses.

emancipated minor (ih MAN suh pay tid MIE ner) A minor who has been granted emancipation by the court; the minor can assume the rights and responsibilities of adulthood.

embezzlement (em BEZ ul ment) The misuse of funds for personal gain.

EMV chip technology Global technology which includes embedded microchips that store and protect cardholder data; also called *chip and PIN* and *chip and signature.*

executor An individual assigned to make financial decisions about the estate of a deceased patient.

explanation of benefits (EOB) A document sent by the insurance company to the provider and the patient explaining the allowed charge amount, the amount reimbursed for services, and the patient's financial responsibilities.

expletive (EK sple tiv) An oath or a swear word.

VOCABULARY—*continued*

Federal Reserve Bank The central bank of the United States. The Federal Reserve system consists of a seven-member Board of Governors with headquarters in Washington, D.C., and 12 Federal Reserve banks in major cities throughout the country.

fee schedule A list of fixed fees for services.

gross The amount earned before any tax deductions or adjustments.

guarantor The person legally responsible for the entire bill. This is usually the patient, but in the case of a minor it would be a parent or legal guardian.

incurred To come into or acquire.

indigent (IN di jent) Poor, needy, impoverished.

intangible (in TAN juh buhl) Something of value that cannot be touched physically.

interest Money the bank pays to the account holder, based on the account balance, for the privilege of using the money in the account.

negotiable instrument (ni GOH shee uh buhl) instrument A document guaranteeing payment of a specific amount of money to the payer named on the document.

net The amount someone is paid after taxes and other deductions have been subtracted.

patient account A running balance of all financial transactions for a specific patient.

pegboard system A manual bookkeeping system that uses a day sheet to record all financial transactions for the date of service and maintains patient account balances by using physical ledger cards.

plaintiff An individual or a party who brings the suit to court.

reconciliation (rek uh n sill ee AY shun) To bring into agreement.

salary A fixed compensation periodically paid to a person for regular work.

small claims court A special court established to handle small claims or debts without the services of lawyers.

tickler file A chronologic file used as a reminder that something must be dealt with on a certain date.

trustee The coordinator of financial resources assigned by the court during a bankruptcy case.

unsecured debt Debt that is not guaranteed by something of value; credit card debt is the most common type of unsecured debt.

INTRODUCTION

Managing the finances in a healthcare facility is an important task. Every patient encounter creates a financial transaction for the facility. Transactions generated by the patient encounter include a variety of charges, payments, and adjustments that need to be accounted for on a daily basis. Financial management is essential if the healthcare facility is to pay the business operating expenses. This includes maintaining **patient accounts** and performing collection activities and banking duties. If the expenses of operating the healthcare facility exceed the fees collected for services rendered, the business will be forced to close.

A medical assistant who works in the front office is responsible for posting charges, accepting and posting a variety of payments and adjustments, endorsing and depositing checks, writing checks for office expenses, and regularly reconciling bank and credit card statements. Mobile deposit allows healthcare facilities to deposit checks on the date payments are received because it is conveniently done in the office. The medical assistant will have to master basic math skills (e.g., addition and subtraction) for all banking functions.

The purpose of financial management is to ensure that the healthcare facility earns enough money to cover its operating expenses. The financial records of the healthcare facility should show the following: how much money was earned in a given period, how much money was collected, how much money is still owed, and the distribution of all operational expenses.

An accountant can prepare monthly and annual financial records from daily **bookkeeping** records. Periodic analyses of these reports result in improved business practices, improved time management, elimination of unprofitable services, and more efficient expense budgeting.

For medical assistants to be able to properly manage finances, it is crucial that they understand the difference between accounts receivable and accounts payable.

- *Accounts receivable* (A/R) is money that is expected but has not yet been received. The amount charged on the encounter form is an example of accounts receivable for the healthcare facility. When a payment is made on the patient's account, the received payment becomes **cash on hand**.
- *Accounts payable* (A/P) is the management of debt **incurred** and not yet paid. All invoices, statements, and operating expenses are included in accounts payable. When expenses have been paid, they are no longer categorized as accounts payable.

ACCOUNTS RECEIVABLE (A/R)

Accounts receivable refers to the money that is owed to the healthcare facility. The majority of this comes from patient accounts. It is important for a medical assistant to understand how the patient account system works. Most healthcare facilities use practice management software (PMS) for daily bookkeeping transactions. A/R transactions come from the encounter form. The charges documented on the encounter form are used to complete the health insurance claim form. *Payments* to the healthcare facility come as reimbursement from the insurance company or from a patient's payment. *Adjustments* are made to a patient's account when it is necessary to add or subtract an amount that is not a payment from the balance—for example, the difference between the provider's charged amount and the contracted insurance payment amount.

Patient Ledger

A patient account is created when the healthcare provider renders services. Charges are applied to the patient account when an *encounter form* (Figure 16.1) is completed during the office visit. The *ledger* is where all the procedures and charges for services rendered are listed.

STATE LIC.# C1503X
SOC. SEC. # 000-11-0000
PIN # ______

Walden-Martin Family Medical Clinic
1234 Anystreet, Anytown, AK 12345-1234

Phone: 555-486-9002

☐ Private ☒ Bluecross ☐ Ind. ☐ Medicare ☐ Medi-cal ☐ Hmo ☐ Ppo

Patient's last name	First	Account #:	Birthdate	Sex	Today's date
Thomas	Ken	11594111	10 / 25 / 19XX	☒ Male ☐ Female	09 / 17 / 20XX

Insurance company	Subscriber	Plan #	Sub. #	Group
Blue Cross Blue Shield	Ken Thomas		KT4496785	55124T

ASSIGNMENT: I hereby assign my insurance benefits to be paid directly to the undersigned physician. I am financially responsible for non-covered services.
SIGNED: Patient,
or parent, if minor Today's date 09 / 17 / 20XX

RELEASE: I hereby authorize the physician to release to my insurance carriers any information required to process this claim.
SIGNED: Patient,
or parent, if minor *Ken Thomas* Today's date 09 / 17 / 20XX

✓	DESCRIPTION	CODE		FEE
	OFFICE VISITS	NEW	EST.	
	Blood pressure check		99211	
	Level II	99202	99212	
	Level III	99203	99213	
X	Level IV	(99204)	99214	$175
	Level V	99205	99215	
	PREVENTIVE EXAMS	NEW	EST.	
	Age 65 and older	99387	99397	
	Age 40 - 64	99386	99396	
	Age 18 - 39	99385	99395	
	Age 12 - 17	99384	99394	
	Age 5 - 11	99383	99393	
	Age 1 - 4	99382	99392	
	Infant	99381	99391	
	Newborn ofc		99432	
	OB/NEWBORN CARE			
	OB package	59400		
	Post-partum visit N/C			
	LAB PROCEDURES			
	Urine dip	81000		
	UA qualitative	81005		
	Pregnancy urine	81025		
	Wet mount	87210		
	kOH prip	87220		
	Occult blood	82270		

✓	DESCRIPTION	CODE	FEE
	Venipuncture	36415	
	TB skin test	86580	
	Hematocrit	85013	
	Glucose finger stick	82948	
	IMMUNIZATIONS		
	Allergy inj. X1	95115	
	Allergy inj. X2	95117	
	Trigger pt. inj.	20552	
	Therapeutic inj.	96372	
	VACCINATION PRODUCTS		
	DPT	90701	
	DT	90702	
	Tetanus	90703	
	MMR	90707	
	OPV	90712	
	Polio inj.	90713	
	Flu	90662	
	Hemophilus B	90645	
	Hepatitis B vac.	90746	
	Pheumovax	90670	
	VACCINE ADMINISTRATION		
	Age: Through 18 yrs. (1st inj.)	90460	
	Age: Through 18 yrs. (ea. addt'l. inj.)	90461	
	Adult (1st inj.)	90471	
	Adult (ea. addt'l. inj.)	90472	

✓	DESCRIPTION	CODE	FEE
	OFFICE PROCEDURES		
	Anoscopy	46600	
	Ear lavage	69210	
	Spirometry	94010	
	Nebulizer Rx	94664	
	EKG	93000	
	SURGERY		
	Mole removal (1st)	17110	
	(2nd to 14th)	17003	
	Flat warts (1st - 14th)	07110	
	15 or more	17111	
	Biopsy, 1 lesion	11100	
	Addt'l. lesions	11101	
	Endometrial Bx	58100	
	Skin tags to 15	11200	
	Each addt'l. 10	11201	
	I & D abscess	10060	
	SUPPLIES/MISCELLANEOUS		
	Surgical tray	99070	
	Handling charge	99000	
	Special report	99080	
	DOCTOR'S NOTES:		

DIAGNOSES **ICD-10-CM**

___ Abdominal pain/unspec. . . R10.9
___ Absess . . . . L02._
___ Allergic reaction . . . . T78.40_
___ Alzheimer's disease G30
___ Anemia/unspec. D64.9
___ Angina/unspec. I20.9
___ Anorexia R63.0
___ Anxiety/unspec. F41.9
___ Apnea, sleep G47.30
___ Arrhythmia, cardiac I49.9
___ Arthritis, rheumatoid. M06.9
___ Asthma/unspec. J45.909
___ Atrial fibrillation. I48.0
___ B-12 deficiency. E53.8
___ Back pain, low M54.5
___ BPH N40
___ Bradycardia/unspec. R00.1
___ Broncitis, acute. . . . . J20._
___ Bronchitis, chronic. J42
___ Bursitis/unspec. M71.9
___ CA, breast . . . . C50._
___ CA, lung . . . . C34._
___ CA, prostate C61
___ Cellulitis . . . . L03._
___ Chest pain/unspec. R07.9
___ Cirrhosis, liver/unspec. . . . K74.60
___ Cold, common J00
___ Colitis/unspec. K51.90
___ Confusion R41.0
___ CHF. I50.9
___ Constipation K59.00
___ COPD J44.9
___ Cough R05
___ Crohn's disease/unspec. . . K50.90
___ CVA I63.9
___ Decubitus ulcer. . . . . L89._
___ Dehydration. E86.0
___ Dementia/unspec. F03
___ Depression, major/unsp. . . F32.9
___ Diab I, no complications . . E10.0
___ Diab II, no complications. . E11.9
___ w/kidney complic. . . . . . . E11.2_
___ w/ophthalmic compl. . . . . E11.3_
___ w/neurolog.compl. . . . . . E11.4_
___ w/circulatory cmpl. . . . . . E11.5_
___ Insulin use. Z79.4
___ Diarrhea/unspec. R19.7
___ Diverticulitix. K57.92
___ Diverticulosis. K57.90
___ Dizziness. R42
___ Dysuria R30.0
___ Edema/unspec. R60.9
___ Endocarditis I38
___ Esophageal reflux K21.0
___ Fatigue (lethargy) R53.83
___ FUO R50.9
___ Gastritis. K29.70
___ Gastroenteritis (colitis) . . . K52.9
___ G.I. bleed K92.2
___ Gout/unspec. M10.9
___ Headache R51
___ Health exam . . . . 200._
___ Hematuria/unspec. R31.9
___ Herpes simplex. B00.9
___ Herpes zoster. B02.9
___ Hiatal hernia K44.9
___ HTN (HBP) I10
___ Hyperlipidemia/unspec. . . E78.5
___ Hypothyroidism/unspec. . . E03.9
___ Impotentce. . . . . N52._
___ Influenza, respiratory J10.1
___ Insomnia. G47.0
___ IBS, diarrhea . . . . K58.
___ Lupus, systemic erythim. . M32.9
___ MI, acute. . . . . I21._
___ MI, old. I25.2
___ Migraine G43.9
___ Myalgia. M79.1
___ Neck pain M54.2
___ Neuropathy. G62.9
___ Nausea R11.1
_X_ Nausea/vomiting R11.0
___ Obesity/unspec. E66.9
___ Osteoarthritis (site). . . . . . M19._
___ Otitis media . . . . H66.9_
___ Parkinson's disease G20
___ Pharyngitis, acute. J02.9
___ Pleurisy R09.1
___ Pneumonia J18.9
___ Pneumonia, viral J12.9
___ Prostatitis/unspec. N41.9
___ PVD I73.9
___ Radiculopathy . . . . M54.1_
___ Rectal bleeding K62.5
___ Renal failure. N19
___ Sciatica. . . . . M54.3_
___ Shortness of breath R03.02
___ Sinusitis, chr./unspec. J32.9
___ Syncope R55
___ Tachycardia/unspec. R00.0
___ Tachy., supraventric I47.1
___ Tendinitis/unspec. M77.9
___ TIA G45.9
___ Ulcer, duodenal/unspec. . . K26.9
___ Ulcer, gastric/unspec. K25.9
___ Ulcer, peptic/unspec. K27.9
___ URI/unspec. J06.9
___ UTI N39.0
___ Vertigo R42
___ Weight gain R63.5
___ Weight loss R63.4

Diagnosis/additional description:

Doctor's signature/date
Dr. Martin 09-17-20XX

Return appointment information: -with whom (Self)/other
Days Wks. (Mos.) 1 month

PLEASE REMEMBER THAT PAYMENT IS YOUR OBLIGATION, REGARDLESS OF INSURANCE OR OTHER THIRD-PARTY INVOLVEMENT.

Rec'd. by:
☐ Cash
☐ Check
☐ Credit
______

Total today's fee	$175
Co-payment	$50
Amount rec'd. today	

FIGURE 16.1 Encounter form with charges. (Courtesy Bibber Systems, an InHealth Company, Petaluma, CA, 800-242-2376, www.bibbero.com.)

All transactions for professional services are posted to the patient's ledger daily. In this way, the ledger becomes the source for answering questions from patients about their financial obligations. The patient ledger should include all information related to collecting the balance due:

- Name and address of the guarantor
- Insurance identification information
- Home, work, and cell phone numbers
- Any special instructions for billing
- Emergency or alternative contact information

The ledger (Figure 16.2) provides a running balance, the result of all the different financial transactions performed in the account, including charges, payments, and adjustments. This same information can be found in the PMS in an electronic format.

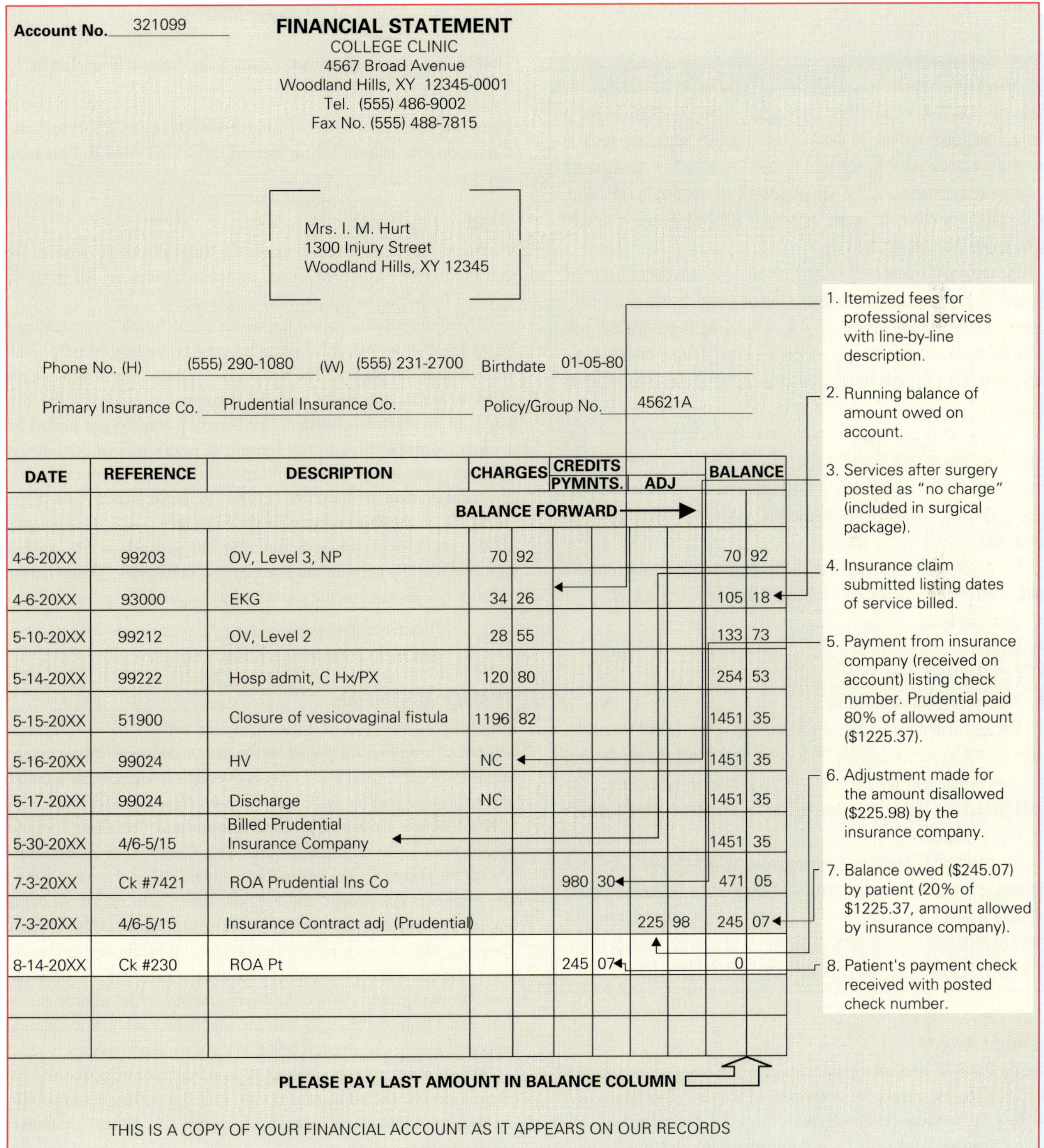

Account No. 321099

FINANCIAL STATEMENT
COLLEGE CLINIC
4567 Broad Avenue
Woodland Hills, XY 12345-0001
Tel. (555) 486-9002
Fax No. (555) 488-7815

Mrs. I. M. Hurt
1300 Injury Street
Woodland Hills, XY 12345

Phone No. (H) (555) 290-1080 (W) (555) 231-2700 Birthdate 01-05-80

Primary Insurance Co. Prudential Insurance Co. Policy/Group No. 45621A

DATE	REFERENCE	DESCRIPTION	CHARGES	CREDITS PYMNTS.	CREDITS ADJ	BALANCE
		BALANCE FORWARD →				
4-6-20XX	99203	OV, Level 3, NP	70 92			70 92
4-6-20XX	93000	EKG	34 26			105 18
5-10-20XX	99212	OV, Level 2	28 55			133 73
5-14-20XX	99222	Hosp admit, C Hx/PX	120 80			254 53
5-15-20XX	51900	Closure of vesicovaginal fistula	1196 82			1451 35
5-16-20XX	99024	HV	NC			1451 35
5-17-20XX	99024	Discharge	NC			1451 35
5-30-20XX	4/6-5/15	Billed Prudential Insurance Company				1451 35
7-3-20XX	Ck #7421	ROA Prudential Ins Co		980 30		471 05
7-3-20XX	4/6-5/15	Insurance Contract adj (Prudential)			225 98	245 07
8-14-20XX	Ck #230	ROA Pt		245 07		0

PLEASE PAY LAST AMOUNT IN BALANCE COLUMN

THIS IS A COPY OF YOUR FINANCIAL ACCOUNT AS IT APPEARS ON OUR RECORDS

1. Itemized fees for professional services with line-by-line description.
2. Running balance of amount owed on account.
3. Services after surgery posted as "no charge" (included in surgical package).
4. Insurance claim submitted listing dates of service billed.
5. Payment from insurance company (received on account) listing check number. Prudential paid 80% of allowed amount ($1225.37).
6. Adjustment made for the amount disallowed ($225.98) by the insurance company.
7. Balance owed ($245.07) by patient (20% of $1225.37, amount allowed by insurance company).
8. Patient's payment check received with posted check number.

FIGURE 16.2 Patient ledger. (From Fordney WT: *Insurance handbook for the medical office*, ed 14, St. Louis, 2017, Elsevier.)

The Patient Ledger and the Pegboard System

When a **pegboard system** is used (Figure 16.3), transactions are initiated before the patient goes to the exam room. The patient account ledger card is inserted under the first or next available receipt, and the first available writing line of the card is aligned with the carbonized strip on the receipt. Enter the receipt number and the date, enter the account balance in the space labeled *previous balance,* and then enter the patient's name. A copy of the receipt is detached and clipped to the patient's chart to be routed to the provider.

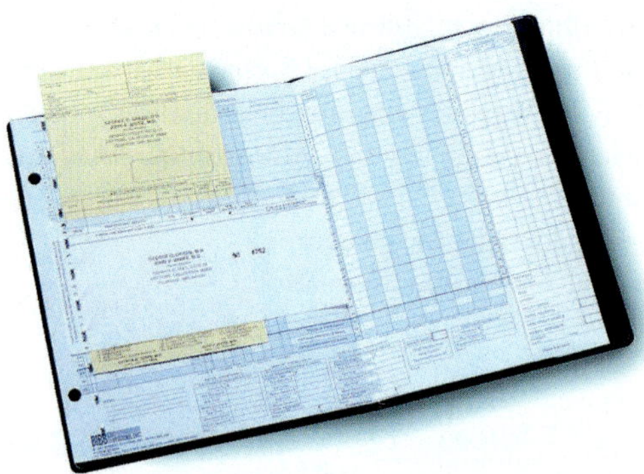

FIGURE 16.3 Pegboard billing system. (Courtesy Bibber Systems, an InHealth Company, Petaluma, CA, 800- 242-2376, www.bibbero.com.)

Manual Bookkeeping

Although we live in a technology-savvy world, some providers still use a manual pegboard system. In many cases, providers who have been in practice for many years do not want to invest in a practice management software system because of the cost associated with moving to PMS. Also, if the office computers go down, employees will have to use a manual system until the system is back up.

The medical assistant must be familiar with both manual and electronic patient account management systems. The pegboard system is the most popular manual system for this purpose. It is simple to operate and contains the same components as a computer system. Once a medical assistant learns the pegboard system, computer systems are much easier to understand.

The pegboard system gets its name from the board that is used. This board has a row of pegs along the side or top that holds the forms in place. The patient account ledger cards are perforated for alignment on the pegs (see Figure 16.3). All the forms used in any system must be compatible to be aligned perfectly on the board.

The pegboard system generates all the necessary financial records for each transaction (by writing once with carbonless forms) as follows:

- Encounter form
- Receipt
- Patient account ledger card
- Bookkeeping transaction entry

The system also may include a statement and bank deposit slip. It provides current accounts receivable totals and a daily record of bank deposits and cash on hand, in addition to the record of income and expenses. The need for separate posting to patient accounts is eliminated, and the chance for error is reduced.

The pegboard system allows the medical assistant to control cash, collections, and receivables and ensures that every cent is accounted for and properly entered. It provides a record of every patient, every charge, and every payment, plus a daily recap of earnings—a running record of receivables and an audited summary of cash—and requires little time.

Posting Charges

When a PMS is used, charges are entered into the ledger automatically from the encounter form after the office visit (Procedure 16.1). The fees for services rendered come from the **fee schedule**. Most practice management systems will automatically determine the fee based on the Current Procedural Terminology (CPT)/Healthcare Common Procedure Coding System (HCPCS) code and insurance company.

Posting Payments

Payments can be received by mail, electronically, or in person. They can come from a patient or an insurance company. All payments need to be posted to the patient's account.

Third-party payments are payments made by an insurance company. In other words, third-party payers pay the healthcare provider on behalf of the patient. The patient is one party, the healthcare provider is the second party, and the insurance company is the third party. In an electronic system, third-party payments are posted line by line, corresponding to the submitted health insurance claim. All payment amounts posted should match the total amount shown on the **explanation of benefits (EOB)** or remittance advice (Figure 16.4). Once the third party pays the insurance claim, the total owed to the provider becomes the amount charged minus the payment amount and the amount adjusted by the third party. The remaining balance is still owed to the provider by the patient:

Insurence payment amount + Adjustment amount
+ Patient responsibility = Total charged

Posting Adjustments

Adjustments are used to either credit or debit a patient's account. Credit adjustments are posted to the patient ledger when an amount needs to be subtracted from a patient's balance. An example would be when the provider's fee exceeds the amount allowed stated on the EOB. The difference between the billed amount and the allowed amount would need to be adjusted (written off). Credit adjustments should always be posted to the patient account record at the same time as the payment. The patient ledger should have a column for the adjustments. Remember, payments and credit adjustments are both credits; however, payments are money that is received in the healthcare facility, and credit adjustments simply reduce the balance that the patient owes on the account. When the payments and credit adjustments are subtracted from the charged amount, the balance is either the patient's responsibility or the amount billed to the secondary insurance.

Before posting to the next EOB line item, confirm that the payment amount, the adjusted amount, and the patient responsibility/secondary insurance balance exactly match the amounts calculated on the EOB.

Debit adjustments are posted to the patient ledger when an amount needs to be added to the patient's balance but is not a charge for services. An example would be if a check the patient had written to the healthcare facility were returned for nonsufficient funds. The amount had initially been credited to the account, but the healthcare facility never actually got the funds. A debit adjustment must be made to add the amount of the check back to the patient's balance (Figure 16.5).

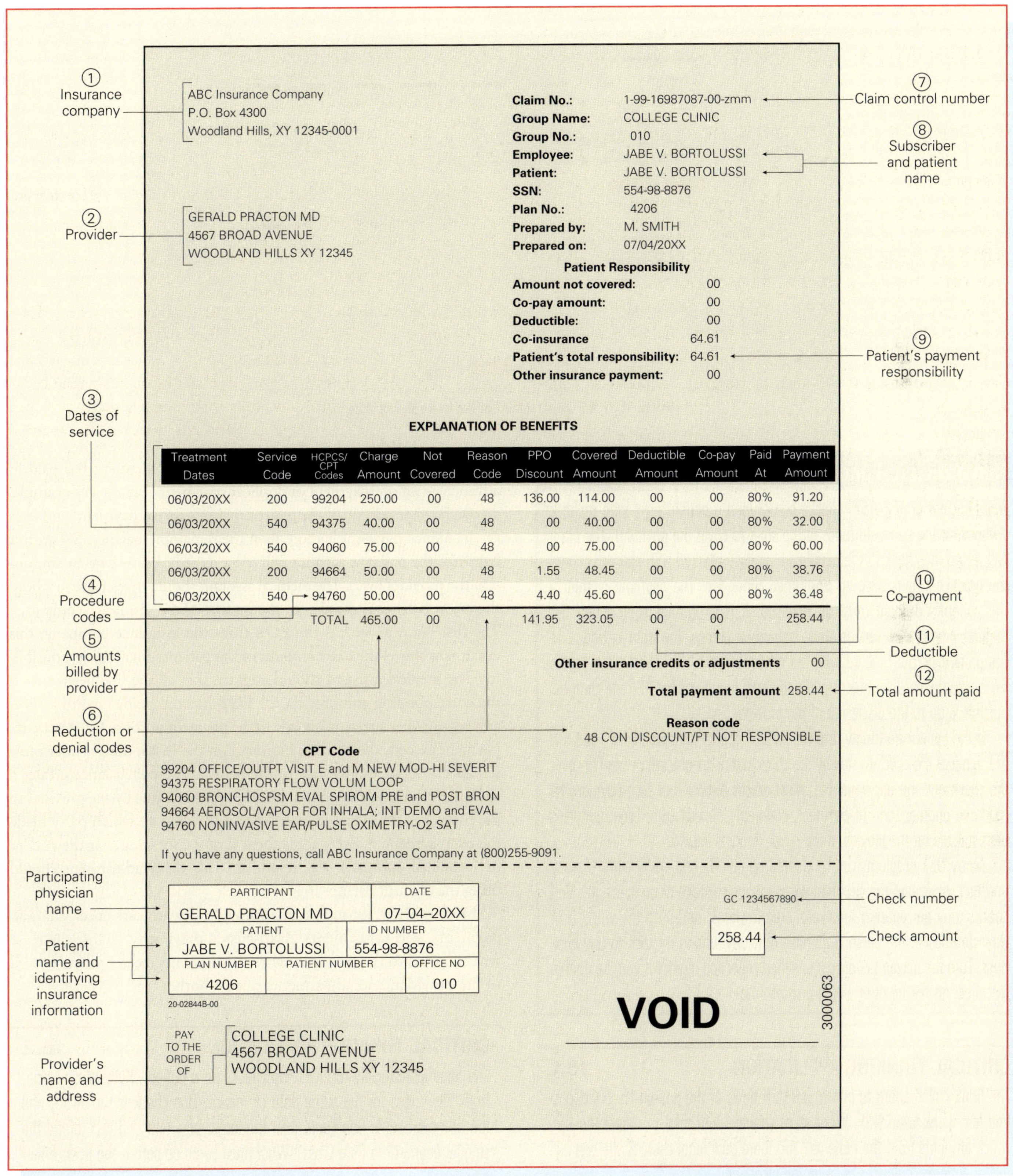

ABC Insurance Company
P.O. Box 4300
Woodland Hills, XY 12345-0001

GERALD PRACTON MD
4567 BROAD AVENUE
WOODLAND HILLS XY 12345

Claim No.: 1-99-16987087-00-zmm
Group Name: COLLEGE CLINIC
Group No.: 010
Employee: JABE V. BORTOLUSSI
Patient: JABE V. BORTOLUSSI
SSN: 554-98-8876
Plan No.: 4206
Prepared by: M. SMITH
Prepared on: 07/04/20XX

Patient Responsibility
Amount not covered: 00
Co-pay amount: 00
Deductible: 00
Co-insurance 64.61
Patient's total responsibility: 64.61
Other insurance payment: 00

EXPLANATION OF BENEFITS

Treatment Dates	Service Code	HCPCS/CPT Codes	Charge Amount	Not Covered	Reason Code	PPO Discount	Covered Amount	Deductible Amount	Co-pay Amount	Paid At	Payment Amount
06/03/20XX	200	99204	250.00	00	48	136.00	114.00	00	00	80%	91.20
06/03/20XX	540	94375	40.00	00	48	00	40.00	00	00	80%	32.00
06/03/20XX	540	94060	75.00	00	48	00	75.00	00	00	80%	60.00
06/03/20XX	200	94664	50.00	00	48	1.55	48.45	00	00	80%	38.76
06/03/20XX	540	94760	50.00	00	48	4.40	45.60	00	00	80%	36.48
		TOTAL	465.00	00		141.95	323.05	00	00		258.44

Other insurance credits or adjustments 00

Total payment amount 258.44

Reason code
48 CON DISCOUNT/PT NOT RESPONSIBLE

CPT Code
99204 OFFICE/OUTPT VISIT E and M NEW MOD-HI SEVERIT
94375 RESPIRATORY FLOW VOLUM LOOP
94060 BRONCHOSPSM EVAL SPIROM PRE and POST BRON
94664 AEROSOL/VAPOR FOR INHALA; INT DEMO and EVAL
94760 NONINVASIVE EAR/PULSE OXIMETRY-O2 SAT

If you have any questions, call ABC Insurance Company at (800)255-9091.

PARTICIPANT		DATE
GERALD PRACTON MD		07–04–20XX
PATIENT		ID NUMBER
JABE V. BORTOLUSSI		554-98-8876
PLAN NUMBER	PATIENT NUMBER	OFFICE NO
4206		010

20-02844B-00

GC 1234567890

258.44

VOID

3000063

PAY TO THE ORDER OF
COLLEGE CLINIC
4567 BROAD AVENUE
WOODLAND HILLS XY 12345

FIGURE 16.4 Explanation of benefits (EOB). (From Fordney MT: *Insurance handbook for the medical office*, ed 14, St. Louis, 2017, Elsevier.)

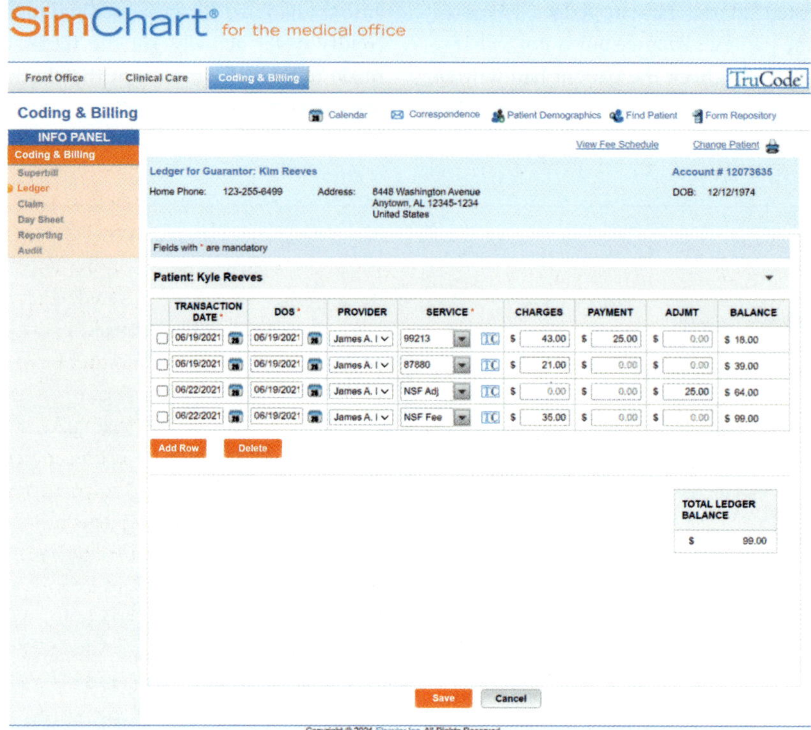

FIGURE 16.5 NSF Adjustments in SimChart for the Medical Office.

Nonsufficient Funds Checks (NSF)

Nonsufficient funds (NSF) checks occur when a patient pays with a check without having sufficient funds in the bank to cover the payment. The bank will return the check to the healthcare practice marked NSF and will charge the practice's bank account a returned check fee. The payment posted to the patient's account must be reversed. It is important to note that the original payment is not deleted; instead, a charge line item is added to the patient account record with the amount of the NSF check (see Figure 16.5). Many medical offices add additional line items for NSF fee charges, but this is up to the discretion of the provider.

If the healthcare facility receives an NSF check, call immediately and ask the signer of the check to stop by the office to pay the amount needed to cover the check and the additional fee. Most offices require that such payment be made by another form of payment, preferably a credit card. Legal remedies are available for the provider if the check remains unpaid.

Many NSF problems can be cleared up quickly and easily with courtesy and tact, assuming the situation was simply a mistake or an oversight. Bad checks may be reported to several organizations, and once the writer is in their databases, the person will have difficulty writing a check to any business. Turn the account over to a qualified collection agency if you are unable to collect on the account within a short time.

CRITICAL THINKING APPLICATION 16.1

The bank called Laura to inform her that three of the patient checks deposited last week were NSF. What steps should Laura take to collect the NSF check amounts from the patients? Are there additional charges she can add to the patients' balances to cover the inconvenience?

Credit Balances. A *credit balance* occurs when a patient has paid in advance, or an overpayment or duplicate payment is made. For example, an overpayment occurs if the patient makes a partial payment, and later the insurance payment is more than the remaining balance. When this happens, the patient's account will show a credit balance or an amount that the provider owes. The medical assistant should investigate to whom the credit balance is owed (i.e., the patient or the insurance company). The first place to look is the EOB from the insurance company; this document shows the exact amount of the patient's financial responsibility. The medical assistant should confirm that all the line items match the corresponding amounts on the EOB because many credit balances are created when an error is made in the payment posting. If the patient's payment exceeds the amount indicated on the EOB, the provider must send a check for the balance to the patient. A credit balance creates a *debit* in the patient's account or an amount that is due by the provider to the patient or the insurance company, depending on which party made the overpayment. A debit adjustment is done, showing that the patient or insurance company was refunded. This debit adjustment should bring the account balance to zero.

Most patient account management software can enter charges, payments, and adjustments. As discussed previously, charges increase what is owed to the provider, whereas payments reduce what is owed to the provider, and adjustments can do both.

CRITICAL THINKING APPLICATION 16.2

The healthcare facility receives two checks for a patient, Kelly Washington, from Blue Cross for the same date of service. One check is for $438, and the other is $534. Can Laura post the larger payment and just refund the smaller payment to Blue Cross? What must Laura do before she posts either payment?

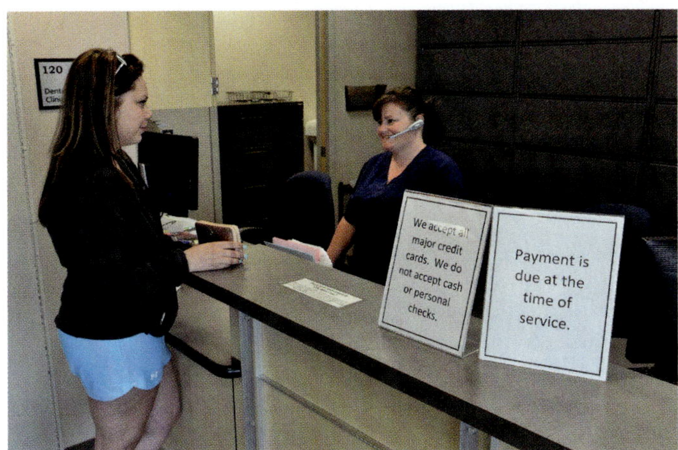

FIGURE 16.6 Most healthcare facilities display a sign informing patients that payments are due at the time of service.

CRITICAL THINKING APPLICATION **16.3**

Laura received a claim denial for a patient, Clara Martin, for the date of service 1/11/20XX. The denial stated that Ms. Martin was not covered on this date of service. Laura reviewed her notes in the patient's account and found the verification of eligibility that was done on 1/11/20XX for Clara Martin. What should Laura do to prepare to call the insurance company?

Payment at the Time of Service

For the most part, patients are expected to pay their copayment at the time of service unless previous arrangements have been made (Figure 16.6). Patients without health insurance should pay after the visit has been completed. When an appointment is made, patients should be informed that payment is expected at the time of service. That way, they are not surprised when asked for payment at the healthcare facility. The medical assistant may say, "Your charge for today is $25. Will that be cash, check, or credit or debit card?" If a patient asks to be billed, the medical assistant may say, "Our normal procedure is to pay at the time of service unless other arrangements are made in advance." Procedure 16.2 describes how to display sensitivity when requesting payment from patients.

Displaying Sensitivity When Requesting Payment

Informing patients of the amount they will be required to pay before the person arrives for the appointment can help with the payment process. Use tact and good judgment when collecting payments. Understand that it can be uncomfortable for the patient to talk about money. Requests for payment should be made in a private setting. Do not be embarrassed to ask for payment for the valuable services that have been provided. Give each patient individual attention and personal consideration; also, be courteous and show a sincere desire to help the patient with financial problems.

CRITICAL THINKING APPLICATION **16.4**

Adam Page comes to the front desk to pay his copay with a credit card. His card is declined. How can Laura handle the situation? What options could be offered to Mr. Page to make a payment at the time of service?

Payment Agreements

With the increase in high-deductible insurance plans, there has been an increase in the need for payment agreements. If the patient has an elective procedure, payment can be made before or at the time of service. If the procedure or therapy is expensive, the patient may need to spread the payments over time. Therefore, the medical assistant must explain to the patient the fees and the office credit policies. In most healthcare practices, the appropriate staff member sits down with the patient for a financial consultation before a payment arrangement contract is offered. The payment arrangement contract states the monthly payment, how many months it must be paid, the payment due date, whether interest will be charged, and the penalties of nonpayment. If the patient is going to be making more than four payments, the Truth in Lending Act comes into play.

Truth in Lending Act. It is considered an offer of credit when the healthcare facility allows the patient to make more than four payments on an outstanding balance. When offering credit options for patients, the healthcare facility should be in compliance with Regulation Z of the Truth in Lending Act (TILA). TILA is enforced by the Federal Trade Commission (FTC) and is part of the Consumer Credit Protection Act. TILA requires that individuals be provided certain information when credit is extended:

- The annual percentage rate (APR)
- The monthly interest rate
- The total costs to the borrower
- When payments are due
- The amount of any late payment charges and when they will be applied

If the healthcare facility and patient agree that payment will be made in more than four installments, the practice must provide a Federal Truth-in-Lending Disclosure Statement (Figure 16.7). This document should be in place even if no finance fees are charged. The statement is signed by the practice's representative and the patient.

Monthly Patient Account Statements

Healthcare facilities should send monthly statements for all patient accounts that have a balance due. A set schedule should be established for sending statements to patients. Sending them monthly is most common, but they can be sent every 2 weeks or even quarterly. When a monthly system is used, patient accounts are divided into equal segments, usually alphabetically. One segment is sent out each week of the month. This keeps an even flow of money into the healthcare facility. It can also spread-out patients' calls about their statements. Statements should be printed on clean, good-quality paper. Payment options, such as check, e-check, online payment, or credit card, should be presented clearly. The statement should provide itemized details on the following:

- Date of service
- Services provided
- Insurance payments and adjustments
- Patient payments, including copayments

Envelopes should be printed with "Address Service Requested" in the appropriate place to maintain up-to-date mailing lists. A self-addressed return envelope included with the statement is convenient for the patient and encourages prompt payment. The statement should also indicate how old the balance is, such as 30, 60, 90, 120, or >120 days. For accounts that are more than 60 days past due,

Walden-Martin Family Medical Clinic
1234 Anystreet
Anytown, AL 12345-1234
(123) 123-1234

DATE 2/2/20XX

FEDERAL TRUTH IN LENDING STATEMENT

For Professional Services Rendered

Responsible Party: Quinton Brown
4554 Browning Street
Anytown, AL 12345-1234

Patient: Quinton Brown

1. Total Cash Price:	3553.00
2. Down Payment Amount:	200.00
3. Unpaid Balance of Cash Price:	0.00
4. Amount Financed:	3353.00
5. Total Finance Charge:	0.00
6. Finance Charge Expressed as Annual Percentage Rate:	0.00
7. Total of all Payments (4 + 5):	3353.00
8. Deferred Payment Price (2 + 4 + 5):	3553.00

Total of ALL PAYMENTS (item 7 above) is payable to our office at the above address in 4 monthly installments. The first 3 installments are $1,000.00 each. The first installment is payable on 2/20/20XX and each subsequent payment is due at the beginning payment period until paid in full.

The amount estimated to be covered by insurance is $0.00. Insurance coverage is only an estimation. Guarantor is responsible for all treatment not covered by insurance.

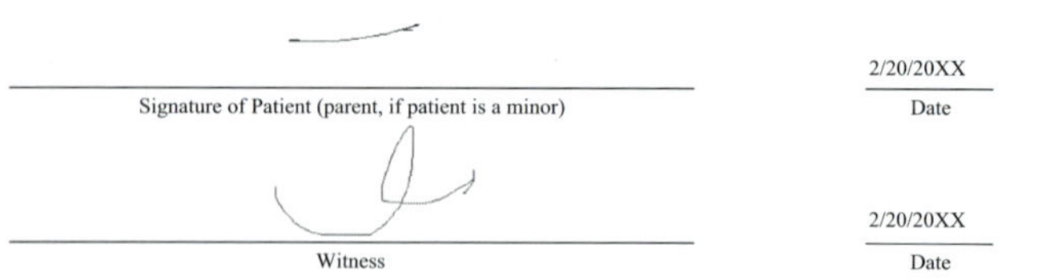

Signature of Patient (parent, if patient is a minor) — 2/20/20XX Date

Witness — 2/20/20XX Date

FIGURE 16.7 Federal Truth-in-Lending Disclosure Statement. (Courtesy of Patterson Office Supplies, Inc.)

some offices apply neon-colored stickers to emphasize the need to pay the balance as soon as possible and thus, avoid further collection activity.

Billing Minors

According to federal regulations, a minor cannot be held financially responsible for an account balance unless the individual is an **emancipated minor**. Bills for minors are usually addressed to the **guarantor**. If a bill is addressed to a minor, parents could take the stand that they are not responsible because they never received a statement.

If the parents are separated or divorced, the parent who brings the child in for treatment is responsible for payment. Whatever financial agreement exists between the parents is strictly their personal business and should not concern the healthcare practice. The responsible parent should be so informed from the first appointment.

If a minor appears in the office and requests treatment, you should determine if the person is legally emancipated. If they are, the minor will be financially responsible. Minors can be treated for certain conditions, such as sexually transmitted infections (STIs), pregnancy, and contraception, without parental consent. Each state has differences in the laws in these cases. Medical assistants must be familiar with their state laws and office policies to determine where the statement should be sent.

Medical Care for Those Who Cannot Pay

The medical profession traditionally has accepted the responsibility of providing medical care occasionally for individuals who are unable to pay for these services. There are government programs to help care for the medically **indigent**, but there are still patients who are not covered. In many instances, medical care for the indigent is available through social service agencies. Medical assistants should learn about local organizations and agencies that can aid patients in obtaining the necessary assistance. The provider can only provide medical services. Other agencies can help pay for hospitalization and arrange for and help pay for special therapy, rehabilitation, or medications.

Unfortunately, another segment of the population consists of uninsured or underinsured employees who are not eligible for public assistance, are not covered under a group policy, and cannot afford the high premiums for private medical insurance. Give special attention to helping these people arrange payment of their medical bills. If a provider knows in advance that a patient cannot pay for services and decides to still provide care, complete records must still be kept on the patient. The only difference in procedure is that an adjustment would be made to the account so that the balance would be zero.

Fees in Hardship Cases

Sometimes a healthcare practice is faced with the problem of deciding whether to reduce or cancel a fee in a hardship case. Before adjusting or canceling a fee, the provider or medical assistant should have a frank discussion with the patient about the financial situation. Find out whether the patient is entitled to or qualifies for medical assistance. If the patient's injuries are the result of a car accident, there may be medical insurance through the automobile policy. The patient may qualify for local or state public assistance, such as crime victim assistance. Maintain information about such agencies in the area and direct the patient to the appropriate one.

If the provider is aware of the hardship before services are provided, the fee can be discussed and payment arrangements made. The healthcare facility may suggest that a medically indigent patient seek care at a clinic that provides public assistance. A provider should be free to choose a form of charity and should not feel obligated to substantially reduce or cancel a fee when the circumstances are known in advance.

The provider and the patient may agree on a fee, but special circumstances may come up that create a hardship. If the provider agrees to reduce the fee, the patient should be told that the reduction will only occur after the adjusted amount is paid in full. For instance, if a fee of $500 is reduced to $350, the full amount of the $500 charge should appear on the ledger, and when $350 has been received, the remainder can be written off as an adjustment.

PITFALLS OF FEE ADJUSTMENTS

Problems can come up when providers begin to reduce their fees. Patients may begin to expect fees to be reduced in all circumstances. Patients may even doubt the competency of a provider who habitually reduces fees. Make fee reductions the exception rather than the norm.

Take great care in reducing the fee for the care of a patient who dies. This could be misinterpreted and result in a suit for malpractice. The family may suspect that the fee was reduced because the provider knowingly made an error.

PATIENT PAYMENT MANAGEMENT

Patients can make payments in a variety of ways. Each method has its own processes and precautions. Those processes and precautions are discussed in the next several sections.

Accepting Cash Payments

Some patients may prefer to pay in cash instead of by check, debit or credit card. Cash transactions can occur with little or no paperwork; therefore, an audit trail is harder to establish.

To prevent the mismanagement of cash, many healthcare facilities do not allow patients to pay cash for services. Healthcare facilities that have a no-cash payment policy should post a sign in the lobby to inform patients of this in advance. If a patient does not have a bank account, the medical staff can kindly refer the patient to a local money order dealer. Patients may see this as an inconvenience, but the medical assistant should explain that the policy is intended to protect the patient's account.

If the healthcare facility chooses to accept cash payments, keep in mind the following precautions:

- Make sure the cash is not **counterfeit**; use a marker or tool designed for this purpose to confirm its authenticity. If you suspect that the cash may be counterfeit, do not accept the payment and contact the local law enforcement office.
- Establish a checks-and-balance system in which the employee accepting cash must document cash payments on a register and in the patient's account to establish an audit trail.
- Inform patients that change cannot be made for larger bills.

Accepting Checks

Most payments sent through the mail are in the form of a personal check. Patients may also write a check when they are making a payment at the time of service. If it is the healthcare facility's policy to accept checks, then certain precautions need to be taken:

- Inspect the check carefully for the correct date, amount, and signature.
- Do not accept a check with corrections on it.
- Ask for a state-issued picture ID, and compare the signature on the ID to the check signature.
- Do not accept an out-of-town check, government check, payroll check, starter check, or an unnumbered check.
- Do not accept a third-party check. For example, Mrs. Richards, a patient, receives a check written to her by her neighbor for $30. Mrs. Richards brings the check to her visit with the provider and presents it to the clinic to pay her copayment. If the check is accepted and subsequently returned by the bank, obtaining reimbursement from the patient or the neighbor may be difficult. A check from the patient's health insurance carrier is the only exception.
- When accepting a postal money order for payment, make sure it has only one endorsement. Postal money orders with more than two endorsements will not be honored.
- Do not accept a check marked "Payment in Full" unless it does pay the account in full, up to and including the date on which it is received. If a check so marked is less than the amount due, you will be unable to collect the balance on the account once you have accepted and deposited such a check. It is illegal to cross out the words "Payment in Full."
- Do not accept a check written for more than the amount due; returning cash for the difference between the amount of the check and the amount owed is poor policy. If the check is not honored by the bank, your office not only suffers the loss of the amount of the check but also of the amount returned in cash.

CRITICAL THINKING APPLICATION 16.5

A new patient wants to pay for his services at the end of the office visit. The charge is $75. The patient writes a check for $100 and asks Laura for $25 in currency in return. How should Laura handle the situation?

Accepting Debit Cards

Most debit cards are connected to a checking account. When the debit card is used, the amount of the transaction is immediately withdrawn from the available balance in the account. A personal identification number (PIN) is assigned to the card for cash withdrawal and point-of-sale (POS) purchases. The cards usually have a MasterCard or Visa logo and can be used wherever they are accepted. In most situations, when there are not enough funds in the account to make a purchase, the card is declined unless the account has some type of overdraft protection. Substantial fees may be charged if the bank elects to pay the debit when the account has insufficient funds.

Currently, some banks decline debit card charges at the point of sale when an account has insufficient funds. They do not charge an insufficient funds fee toward the attempted purchase. Stay abreast of recent banking legislation, and always follow office policy when accepting debit cards as payment for medical services. The medical assistant may see various types of debit cards in the provider's office. Many states issue a debit card to individuals receiving child support payments or some types of state financial assistance.

Advantages of Using Debit Cards

Using debit cards for payment has many advantages:

1. Debit cards are both safe and convenient, particularly for making payments online.
2. Transactions are completed quickly.
3. The cards can be used either as debit or credit cards. For use as a debit card, the user must have a personal identification number (PIN). For use as a credit card, the user often must provide identification.
4. If stolen or lost, the debit card can be canceled quickly with minimum liability.
5. Receipts and statements provide a permanent, reliable record of disbursements for tax purposes.
6. The debit card statement provides a summary of receipts.
7. The cards can usually be used anywhere that accepts MasterCard or Visa.

Accepting Credit Cards

Credit cards are a common method of payment from patients. Drawbacks of credit card payments include the small processing fee deducted from the amount deposited into the healthcare facility's bank account. There is also an increased risk of fraud with credit cards.

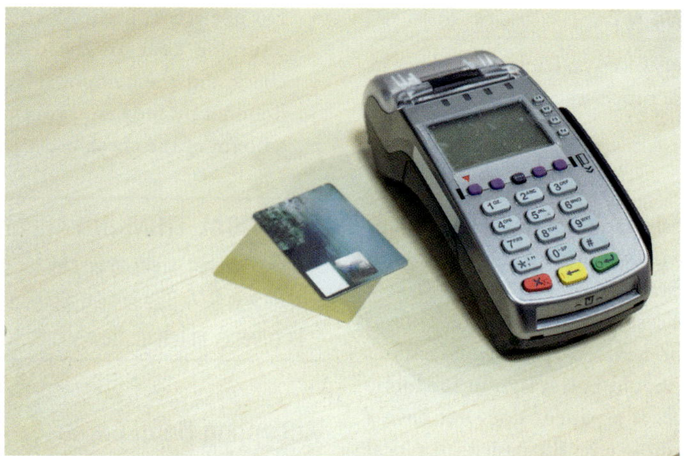

FIGURE 16.8 Card reader terminal with both EMV chip and magnetic strip readers.

To help reduce fraud, magnetic strip cards are being replaced with cards embedded with **EMV chip technology**. These chip cards offer advanced security for in-person payments, but the EMV chip cards require a special terminal to read the chips. If a healthcare facility accepts credit or debit cards, it is important to have a terminal that processes the EMV chip cards. Businesses that cannot process the chip cards may be liable for fraud losses to their customers.

Many credit card processing terminals can accept both credit cards and debit cards (Figure 16.8), and some can also process check payments electronically. Debit card transactions use a PIN but do not need a patient's signature. Credit card transactions do not need a PIN, but patients may need to sign.

Although using the credit card processing terminal incurs per-transaction charges, valuable time is saved because an office employee does not need to visit the bank branch to make the daily deposit. Credit card transactions also can reduce the chances of money mismanagement in the office, such as **embezzlement**.

Contactless Payment Systems

New technology, called *contactless payment systems,* allows payment with a phone or other device linked to a credit or debit card. With this type of system, the patient can simply tap her or his card on the device instead of swiping or inserting the card. If office policy allows this type of payment to be made, special equipment will be purchased to accommodate it.

Online Payment Options

Many offices choose to accept payment online. Patients can use their patient portal to make payments by debit or credit card, electronic check, or direct transfer. If your office uses this for payments, it should be noted in patients' bills so they know they have this option for payments.

Precautions for Accepting Credit and Debit Cards

Just as the medical assistant must take precautions when accepting checks, care must be taken when accepting a credit or debit card as payment for medical services. Make sure that the person presenting the card is the person to whom it was issued. Always ask for a state-issued ID. Compare the name and signature to the one on the credit card. Follow the healthcare facility's policy on verifying identity if the name on the state-issued ID does not match the name on the credit card. Some patients may use a prepaid credit card, which is purchased with cash and does not have the patient's name printed on it, to make payments on their accounts. These cards, if allowed by office policy, pay just like a normal credit card. If patients become belligerent when their credit card is denied, refer them to the office manager.

COLLECTION PROCEDURES

Most patients are more than willing and able to pay their responsibility for the services provided to them by the healthcare facility, but some cannot. There can be many reasons why someone is not able to pay the bill, and it can be the responsibility of the medical assistant to help determine the best way to collect the balance owed. The next sections examine the collection process.

When to Start Collection Procedures

Collection is the process of using all legal resources available to collect payment for past-due patient-account balances. Sometimes patients may have difficulty meeting all of their financial obligations. The patient may have lost a job or insurance coverage. An emergency could arise that depletes finances. When patients must choose between paying their medical bills and having electricity, the provider is often forced to wait for payment. Although a few patients absolutely refuse to pay for their medical care, most are honest and willing to pay but may need help with a payment plan. As discussed earlier, terms can be arranged for collecting payment in full when the office and the patient cooperate with each other. The medical assistant should attempt to work out a plan that the patient can abide by, and the patient should be expected to make promised payments. For those patients who do not pay their bills, further action is necessary.

Preparing Patient Accounts for Collection Activity

Sometimes it becomes necessary to aggressively attempt to collect the balances that patients owe. Collection procedures include telephone calls, collection reminders and letters, and personal interviews.

Before you begin collection action, it is essential to determine which accounts have a balance due and how old the account balance is. Some accounts are grouped together, or "aged," according to the dates of the last payment activity, whereas others are grouped according to the original date of service (Figure 16.9). Common account aging categories are as follows:

- Current
- 31–60 days
- 61–90 days
- 91–120 days
- >120 days

Most bills with balances less than 30 days old are probably waiting for the health insurance to pay, so no collection action is needed.

Patient Account Aging Report: Walden-Martin Family Medical Clinic

Starting Date: 9/1/20XX Ending Date: 9/30/20XX Report Date 9/30/20XX

Jacob Abraham (3406)			Last Payment: 7/12/20XX			15.00		
Guarantor: Self			Home: 954-233-9033			Work: NA		
Date	**Code**	**Billed**	**Current**	**31-60**	**61-90**	**91-120**	**>120**	**Total**
7/12/20XX	99201	45.00			45.00			45.00
7/12/20XX	Cash	(15.00)			(15.00)			(15.00)
Patient Total		30.00	0.00	0.00	30.00	0.00	0.00	30.00
Frank Bullock (3412)			Last Payment: 8/20/20XX			45.00		
Guarantor: Wife			Home 954-388-0196			Work: 954-233-5803		
Date	Code	Billed	**Current**	**31-60**	**61-90**	**91-120**	**>120**	**Total**
8/20/20XX	99205	195.00		195.00				195.00
8/20/20XX	Check	(45.00)		(45.00)				(45.00)
Patient Total		150.00	0.00	150.00	0.00	0.00	0.00	150.00
Cynthia Dearing (3433)			Last Payment: 7/25/20XX			10.00		
Guarantor: Self			Home: 953-518-2100			Work: 954-333-9003		
Date	**Code**	**Billed**	**Current**	**31-60**	**61-90**	**91-120**	>120	**Total**
6/12/20XX	99386	185.00				185.00		185.00
7/15/20XX	BCBS	(160.00)				(160.00)		(160.00)
7/25/20XX	Check	(10.00)				(10.00)		(10.00)
Patient Total		15.00	0.00	0.00	0.00	15.00	0.00	15.00
Kirsha Macken (3462)			Last Payment: 7/10/20XX			50.00		
Guarantor: Parent			Home: 954-736-7227			Work: FT Student		
Date	**Code**	**Billed**	**Current**	**31-60**	**61-90**	**91-120**	**>120**	**Total**
4/23/20XX	58900	230.00					230.00	230.00
4/23/20XX	Cash	(50.00)					(50.00)	(50.00)
7/10/20XX	99214	90.00		3309	90.00			90.00
7/10/20XX	90658	30.00			30.00			30.00
7/10/20XX	Cash	(50.00)			(50.00)			(50.00)
Patient Total		250.00	0.00	0.00	70.00	0.00	180.00	250.00
Larry Nerod (3501)			Last Payment: 6/22/20XX			15.00		
Guarantor: Self			Home: 953-736-7227			Work: 954-332-001		
Date	**Code**	**Billed**	**Current**	**31-60**	**61-90**	**91-120**	**>120**	**Total**
6/22/20XX	99204	140.00				140.00		140.00
6/22/20XX	CCard	(15.00)				(15.00)		(15.00)
Patient Total		125.00	0.00	0.00	0.00	125.00	0.00	125.00
Emanuel Perez (3513)			Last Payment: 7/12/20XX			46.00		
Guarantor: Self			Home: 956-303-2070			Work: 953-322-5500		
Date	**Code**	**Billed**	**Current**	**31-60**	**61-90**	**91-120**	**>120**	**Total**
7/12/20XX	68500	403.00			403.00			403.00
7/12/20XX	Check	(46.00)			(46.00)			(46.00)
Patient Total		357.00	0.00	0.00	357.00	0.00	0.00	357.00
Report Totals			0.00	150.00	457.00	140.00	180.00	927.00
Percent of Total			0.00%	16.18%	49.3%	15.10%	19.41%	100.00%

FIGURE 16.9 Sample aging report.

Patient account balances of more than 90 or 120 days old require a final demand letter before the account is turned over to a collection agency. Always allow the provider to review and approve the list of patient accounts being sent to a collection agency.

The medical assistant can use a variety of techniques to collect patient accounts, such as collection phone calls, collection letters, and skip tracing. Often more than one technique must be used to obtain payment. Always be courteous and kind when using all collection techniques.

Collection Telephone Calls

Whenever attempts are made to collect a debt, the Fair Debt Collection Practices Act must be kept in mind. A telephone call at the right time, with the right presentation, is more successful than notes, patient account statements, or collection letters. The personal contact call often prompts patients to mail in their payments or make payments over the phone with a credit card. If the staff does not have enough time to make calls, the collection letter is the next best approach. If collections are a serious problem, it may be worth an extra salary to hire a person to make the phone calls.

Fair Debt Collection Practices Act

In March 1978, the Fair Debt Collection Practices Act went into effect. It was designed to eliminate abusive, deceptive, and unfair debt collection practices. The act states that collection calls cannot be made in the following situations:

- At any time or place that is unusual or known to be inconvenient to the patient, before 8 a.m. or after 9 p.m.
- When the creditor is aware that the debtor is represented by an attorney with respect to the debt.
- To the patient's place of work if the patient's employer prohibits such contacts.
- If the patient has notified the debt collector in writing to cease further communication.

Always treat patients with the utmost respect on the telephone. Keep their financial records nearby in case they have questions about their bill; also, have their insurance company's phone number handy. Remember that some patients may not understand anything about insurance or third-party payers. Helping them to understand and acting as their advocate in getting as much reimbursement as possible can reduce the patient's share. Never simply insist that the insurance plan has paid and the patient's balance is due. This puts the patient in a negative mindset. Try using phrases such as the following:

- "Mrs. Diggs, it looks as if your insurance company paid late last month. You have co-insurance for your surgery that amounts to $450. Let me review some payment options to help make that as easy as possible for you to pay."
- "Mr. Hildebrand, we're showing that you have a balance due from your surgery. Your insurance has paid, and it looks as if you owe $700. We would be happy to help you by splitting that into two or three payments. When can I schedule that first payment for you?"
- "Mrs. Crumley, it seems that you have a balance due of $450 from your surgery, and I called to see whether I could help you budget that. For example, you could pay $50 this week and split the remaining $400 into two payments over the next 2 months."

Always abide by office policy when making payment arrangements in collection situations. Never be **belligerent** with a patient. If the conversation becomes heated, simply state that the person can call back when ready to discuss a solution for paying the account, say good-bye, and gently hang up the phone. Never listen to **expletives** or allow verbal abuse. Respectfully end the phone call by saying thank you and good-bye; do not slam down the phone.

Before a final demand for payment is made, a letter must be sent indicating that legal or collection proceedings will be started.

General Rules for Telephone Collections

What to do:

- Call the patient when it can be done privately.
- Call only between 8 a.m. and 9 p.m.
- Determine the identity of the person with whom you are speaking. If you ask, "Is this Mrs. Noble?" and she answers, "Yes," it could be the patient's mother-in-law or daughter-in-law, who may also be "Mrs. Noble." Use the person's full name. Include suffixes, such as "Thomas Melborn, III." This may sound too formal, but it helps to ensure that the correct person is on the phone.
- Be respectful. One can be friendly and professional at the same time.
- Ask the patient whether it is a convenient time to talk. Unless you have the attention of the patient, there is little to be gained by continuing. If you are told that it is an inopportune time, ask for a specific time to call back or get a promise that the patient will call the office at a specified time.
- After a brief greeting, state the purpose of the call. Make no apology for calling, but state the reason in a friendly, businesslike way. The provider expects payment, and the medical assistant is interested in helping the patient meet the financial obligation. Open the call with a phrase such as "This is Alice, Dr. Walden's medical assistant. I'm calling about your account." A well-placed pause at this point in the call sometimes gets an immediate response from the debtor with regard to the nonpayment.
- Assume a positive attitude. For example, convey the impression that the patient intended to pay, and it is only a matter of working out some suitable arrangements.
- Keep the conversation brief and to the point; do not make threats of any kind.
- Try to get a definite commitment—payment of a certain amount by a certain date.
- Follow up on promises made by the patient. This is best accomplished by using a **tickler file** or a note on the calendar. If the payment does not arrive by the promised date, remind the patient with another call. If the medical assistant fails to do this, the whole effort has been wasted.
- Document the call in the patient's record.

What *not* to do:

- Do not call between 9 p.m. and 8 a.m. To do so may be considered harassment.
- Do not make repeated telephone calls on the same day.
- Do not call the patient's place of work if the employer prohibits personal calls.
- If a call is placed to the patient at work and the person cannot take the call, leave a message asking the patient to "call Ms. Black

at 951-727-9238" without revealing the nature of the call—that is, do not state that the call is from "Dr. Walden's office" or "Dr. Walden's medical assistant."

- Refrain from showing any kind of hostility. An angry patient is a poorly paying patient. Insulted patients often do not pay at all.

Collection Letters

Some experts believe that a printed collection letter or reminder enclosed with a statement is more effective than a personal letter. The idea is that a patient may be embarrassed by a personal letter and feel that they have been singled out for attention. An impersonal printed message will probably encourage the patient to send a payment.

Letters that are friendly requests for an explanation of why payment has not been made are effective in most cases. These letters should indicate that the provider is sincerely interested in the patient's health and well-being and wants to help resolve the financial obligation. Invite the patient to the office to explain the reasons for nonpayment so that payment arrangements can be made. To lessen the patient's embarrassment, these letters can suggest that previous statements may have been overlooked.

When receiving these letters, most patients make some effort to explain their failure to make payment. Patients who are really having financial difficulties may be able to get some type of assistance. If it is a temporary financial problem, the provider and the patient may work together to come up with a satisfactory installment plan for payment.

The medical assistant is often given a free hand in designing collection patterns and composing collection letters. Many medical assistants compose a series of collection letters using example letters they have found effective. Such a series usually includes at least five letters in varying degrees of forcefulness.

Sometimes even a person with poor paying habits will pay, as long as they are treated with respect and consideration. The medical assistant should never go beyond the authority granted by the provider in pursuing collections. If questions come up about special collection problems, always check with the provider or office manager before proceeding. The provider and the medical assistant should agree on general collection policies, as outlined earlier in this chapter, and the policies should be followed. In all cases, when an account is to be assigned to a collection agency, make sure the provider is aware and approves.

In most healthcare facilities, medical assistants sign collection letters using their title, such as "Medical Assistant," below a typewritten signature. Do not list "Collections" below the name because the patient may assume that the account has been placed with a collection agency. Some providers want to sign these communications personally, but generally, the medical assistant who handles the patient accounts also signs the collection letters.

Personal Finance Interviews

Personal finance interviews with patients can sometimes be more effective than a whole series of collection letters. Oftentimes speaking with a patient face to face can result in a better understanding of the problem, and an agreement about future payment plans can be reached (Figure 16.10).

Occasionally a patient may undergo a long course of treatment and yet make no attempt to pay anything on the account. The patient may be waiting for the provider or the medical assistant to suggest that a payment be made. When it is known well in advance that the patient requires extensive treatment, the matter of payment should be discussed early in the course of treatment. The credit policy should be explained, and some agreement should be reached on a payment plan.

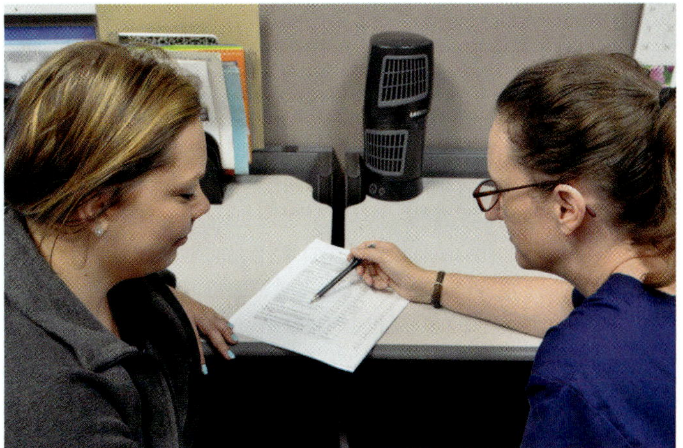

FIGURE 16.10 A face-to-face personal finance interview may motivate patients to take steps to settle their account balances.

Because medical services are far more **intangible** than any commercial service, collection efforts must not be delayed too long. Most responsible, sincere patients will call the provider's office after receiving a second statement and explain the delay in payment or ask for a payment plan. This is best accomplished in a private, personal interview.

If the account ultimately must be referred to a collection agency, find a good agency with a high recovery rate. All collection activity is costly. Know when to stop and call on the services of a professional agency.

Collection Situations

There are several unique collection situations that occur in the healthcare facility. Tracing skips, claims against estates, and bankruptcy are three of the challenging collection situations. How to handle those situations will be discussed in the following sections.

Tracing Skips

When a patient account statement is returned marked "Moved—no forwarding address," you may consider this account a skip. This could be an innocent error on the part of the patient, who may have forgotten to provide a forwarding address to the post office. The patient could also be attempting to avoid liability for debts. Whichever is the case, immediate action should be taken. Do not wait until the next billing cycle to attempt to trace the debtor.

The internet can be a valuable tool in tracing skips. You can use the online white pages to search for the patient's name. Patients might even be found on social networking sites, such as Facebook, and that information may provide clues about the person's whereabouts. Investigate the search results carefully, so that collection efforts are directed at the right person. If all attempts fail, turn the account over to a collection agency without delay. Do not keep a skip account too long because as time passes, the trail may become so cold that even collection experts won't be able to follow it.

Suggestions for Tracing Skips

- Review the patient's original office registration card.
- Call the telephone number listed in the patient account record. Occasionally a patient may move without leaving a forwarding address but will transfer the old telephone number.
- If you are unable to contact the individual by telephone, make a few discreet calls to the references listed on the registration card to get leads.
- Check the internet to find the names and telephone numbers of neighbors or the landlord and contact these people to obtain information about the debtor's whereabouts.
- Do not inform a third party that the patient owes money. Simply state that you are trying to locate or verify the location of the individual.
- Check the guarantor's place of employment for information. If the person is a specialist in a particular field of work, the local union or similar organizations may be contacted. Although they may not give you the person's current address, they will relay the message that you are attempting contact. Often people are prompted to pay if they think their employer may learn of their failure to pay.

Claims Against Estates

The patient account for a deceased patient may be handled a little differently from regular accounts. Courtesy dictates that a bill not be sent immediately but do not delay longer than 30 days. The **executor** will expect to receive the statements from all healthcare providers. Use the following format to address the statement:

- Estate of (name of patient)
- c/o (spouse, next of kin, or executor if known)
- Patient's last known address

A will generally is filed within 30 days of a death. The name of the executor usually can be obtained by sending a request to the Probate Department of the Superior Court, County Recorder's Office, in the county where the person lived. The time limits for filing an estate claim are determined by the state where the person resided.

An itemized statement should be sent to the executor of the estate by certified mail, return receipt requested. If no response is received in 10 days, contact the executor or the county clerk where the estate is being settled and obtain forms for filing a claim against the estate. This claim against the estate must be made within a certain time. This time frame varies from 2 to 36 months, depending on the state where it is filed.

The executor of the estate either accepts or rejects the claim. If it is accepted, the executor will send an acknowledgment of the debt. Payment can be delayed because of the legal complications involved in settling an estate. If the claim has been accepted, the provider eventually receives the payment. If the executor rejects the claim, file a claim against the executor according to state laws. The time limit in such cases starts with the date on the letter of rejection.

States have different time limits and statutes with regard to these issues. The medical assistant should contact the provider's attorney or the local court for the exact procedure to follow. Or, the provider may prefer to turn such matters over to legal counsel immediately.

Bankruptcy

Bankruptcy laws were passed to ensure equal distribution of the **assets** of an individual among the individual's creditors. These are federal laws that apply in all the states. When notified that a patient has declared bankruptcy, do not send statements, or make any attempt to collect on the account from the patient.

Chapter 7 bankruptcy is usually a "no asset" situation. Because the provider's charges are considered an **unsecured debt**, there is little purpose in pursuing collection. Chapter 13 is known as *wage-earner bankruptcy,* which means that the patient-debtor pays to a **trustee** a fixed amount agreed upon by the court. This money is passed on to the creditors. During this period, none of the creditors can attach the debtor's wages or otherwise attempt to collect the debt. However, the debts are paid in order, secured debts first. Consequently, the provider may never receive payment from a debtor who has filed for bankruptcy.

Using a Collection Agency

The medical assistant should try every means possible to collect on accounts before they become delinquent. An account should be sent to a collection agency as soon as all collection activities have been exhausted. If the patient has failed to respond to the final letter or has twice failed to send a promised payment, the account should be considered uncollectable. Skips should be sent immediately.

Even though the collection agency will keep 40% to 60% of the amount owed, waiting only reduces the chances of recovery by the professional collector. If the agency finds that the case deserves special consideration, it will ask the provider's advice before proceeding further.

The collection agency represents the healthcare facility. Therefore, the healthcare facility should ensure that its patients are treated with as much respect and dignity as possible throughout the collection process. There are many collection agencies. If one doesn't work out, prepare to switch to another that can better represent the healthcare practice.

A collection agency needs certain data to begin collection procedures on overdue accounts:

- Guarantor's full name
- Spouse's full name
- Last known address
- Full amount of the debt
- Date of the last entry (charge, payment, or adjustment) on the account
- Occupation of the debtor
- Employer's address and phone number

After an account has been sent to a collection agency, the healthcare facility can make no further collection attempts. Once the agency has begun its work, a number of guidelines and procedures should be followed:

- Send no more patient statements.
- The patient account should be closed for activity because the account was forwarded to a collection agency. The balance should be written off.
- Refer patients to the collection agency if they contact the office about the account.
- Promptly report any payments made directly to your office to the collection agency and pay the collection agency's fee.
- Call the agency if any information is obtained that will be of value in tracing or collecting the account.

CRITICAL THINKING APPLICATION **16.6**

Laura has had several complaints about the collection agency the office uses. Patients have called to report that the collectors are threatening and unprofessional. The collection agency's supervisor has been disrespectful to patients and has said that because they owe the money, the collection agency's job is to collect the account in whatever way necessary. How should the healthcare facility approach the collection agency about these complaints?

Posting Collection Agency Transactions

Collection agencies charge the healthcare practice different percentages of the amount owed to collect delinquent accounts; the agency with the cheapest fee is rarely the most effective. Agencies pay the *netback,* which is the amount of money paid to the practice after the agency has been paid its fee. The netback is the figure that should be considered when a collection agency is used, not simply the fee percentage. If a patient sends a payment after the account has been turned over to a collection agency, the payment must be recorded in the patient account record. Because the agency charges a fee for its collection efforts, the amount sent to the healthcare facility might be less than the actual payment amount. For instance, if the agency charges 40%, a $100 payment results in a $60 payment to the healthcare facility and the agency keeps $40. When the payment is posted, the patient account must credit the full amount paid to the collection agency. This would be done by posting a $60 payment and $40 adjustment (Figure 16.11; Procedure 16.3).

Small Claims Court

Many healthcare practices find **small claims court** a satisfactory, inexpensive means of collecting delinquent accounts. State law places a limit on the amount of debt for which relief may be sought in small claims court. This limit should be determined before the small claims court process is started.

Parties to small claims actions are not represented by an attorney at the hearing but may send another person to court on their behalf to produce records supporting the claim. Providers often send their medical assistants with the records of unpaid accounts to show the judge.

If the court awards a judgment for the amount owed, the **plaintiff** in small claims court may also recover the costs of the suit. For a very small investment in time and money, the provider who uses this method saves the time of a civil court action and eliminates attorneys' fees.

After being awarded a judgment, the healthcare practice must still collect the money. The only person in a small claims action who has the right of appeal is the **defendant**. An appeal by the defendant may have the judgment set aside. The plaintiff cannot file an appeal in a small claims action; the decision of the court is final.

The necessary papers for filing the action and full instructions on the course to follow may be obtained from the clerk of the local small claims court. It would be wise for medical assistants who have never appeared in court to attend once as spectators to preview the procedure; this should allow them to feel more at ease when appearing for the provider.

ACCOUNTS PAYABLE (A/P)

Accounts payable refers to the money that the healthcare facility owes others. A/P transactions also require bookkeeping entries. Writing checks and maintaining the checking account register are examples of A/P bookkeeping entries. Expenses are tracked by category (e.g., rent, clinical supplies, and administrative supplies). Managing

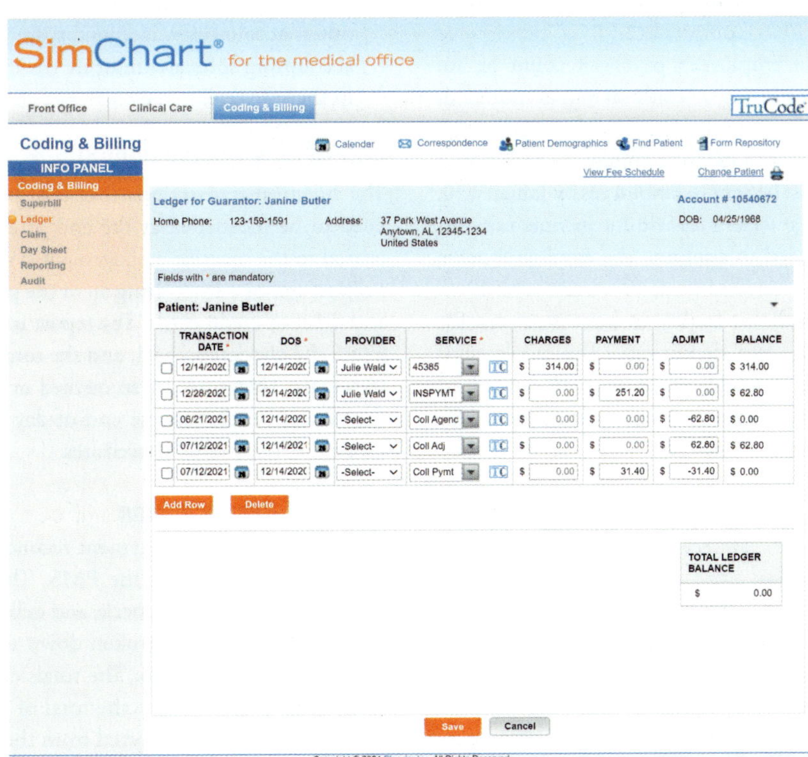

FIGURE 16.11 Posting a collection agency payment in SimChart for the medical office.

accounts payable may be the responsibility of the medical assistant. There are many aspects of accounts payable, which will be discussed in the next section.

Vendors

The healthcare facility would not be able to function without supplies and services from various vendors. These vendors provide the following:

- Office space
- Utilities
- Medical supplies
- Office supplies
- Cleaning supplies and services
- Parking lot plowing and maintenance

These vendors need to be paid for their service and supplies. They will supply an invoice, and it must be reviewed for accuracy before it is paid. It can be the medical assistant's responsibility to review the invoices and then process the payment.

Employee Payroll

A medical assistant is oftentimes responsible for processing employee payroll for the healthcare facility. Employees can be paid either on an hourly basis or with a **salary**. The **net** paycheck of a salaried employee will always be the same dollar amount. If the employee is paid hourly, the net paycheck will depend on how many hours the person worked during the pay period. The hourly rate is multiplied by the number of hours worked to determine these individuals' **gross** pay. In either situation, the gross amount earned is used to determine how much is withheld for taxes.

Each employee must complete a W-4 form, an Employee's Withholding Allowance Certification. This form indicates the person's tax status and how many allowances the individual is claiming. This information is used to determine how much money is withheld for income taxes.

Other deductions from an employee's paycheck could be for insurance premiums, retirement savings, health savings accounts, or flexible spending accounts.

All employers are required to provide their employees with a W-2 form on a yearly basis. This must be sent to employees by January 30. This form lists the amounts that were withheld for income tax purposes. This information is needed to compute the employee's taxes for the year.

It is important for the healthcare facility to keep exact records regarding payroll, withholding, and deductions. The employer is responsible for submitting the withheld tax amounts to the federal and state governments in a timely fashion. These are usually submitted on a quarterly basis (i.e., every 3 months).

BANKING PROCEDURES IN THE AMBULATORY CARE SETTING

Healthcare facilities use bank accounts to deposit funds (as cash, checks, debit cards, or credit card transactions) and pay their operational expenses by check or credit card. Accounting management software can simplify the banking transactions of healthcare facilities. This type of software is compatible with many online banking portals. That means that daily transactions can be downloaded directly into the accounting program. Attentive medical assistants who download daily can manage all account balances on a regular basis. Office expenses and invoices can be entered into the accounting management software as accounts payable, and payments can be scheduled for entered invoices. Checks to vendors can be printed at any time from the accounting software, documenting the transaction—and documented transactions make bank reconciliation a snap!

How to Write a Check

Checks are written in ink or produced using the software. Write or key the check by the following steps:

- Date the check using one of these formats: May 23, 20XX; 05/23/XX; or 5/23/XX.
- On the "Pay to the Order of" line, correctly write or key the person's name or the company's name.
- On the line with the dollar sign, write out the exact amount of the check starting next to the dollar sign (e.g., $135.00, not $135).
- On the line below the recipient's name, write out the amount, making sure to start at the left edge. The cents are written in a fraction. Draw a single line through the rest of the line to prevent any additions (e.g., One hundred thirty-five and 50/100————).
- On the Memo line, indicate the purpose of the payment (optional).
- The check needs to be signed to be valid. If the provider is signing the check, clip the invoice to the check and place it on the provider's desk for a signature. If you are responsible for signing checks, your name must be on the signature card on file at the bank. For checks over a certain amount, two signatures will be needed.
- If you make a mistake when writing the check, it cannot be altered by crossing out or changing anything that was written. You will need to void the check and rewrite another check. Write "VOID" on the stub and the check. File the voided check with other accounting documents for auditing purposes. If using accounting software, indicate the check number has been voided in the software.

End-of-Day Reconciliation

The financial transactions that take place in the healthcare facility need to be reconciled at the end of each day. When payments are posted to the practice management system, they can be tracked, and a report can be run showing all of the payments made by cash, check, and debit or credit cards. The report is then compared to the cash on hand, the checks received, and the totals from credit card processing terminals. They must be reconciled or matched. Preparing the bank deposit is also part of the end-of-day reconciliation. The following sections discuss those procedures.

Payment Reconciliation

To start the process of payment reconciliation, you must run a daily transaction report from the PMS. This report will provide a total dollar amount for cash, check, and debit/credit card payments. These reports can be further broken down to show which accounts those payments were posted to. The totals can be compared to the actual cash taken in for the day, the total of checks received, and the total debit/card payments reported from the credit card processing terminal. Figure 16.12 provides a template for cash reconciliation. The

Cash reconciliation template

Date:

Starting cash					Ending cash				
Denomination	X	Qty	=	Amount	Denomination	X	Qty	=	Amount
$20	X		=		$20	X		=	
$10	X		=		$10	X		=	
$5	X		=		$5	X		=	
$1	X		=		$1	X		=	
Quarters	X		=		Quarters	X		=	
Dimes	X		=		Dimes	X		=	
Nickels	X		=		Nickels	X		=	
Pennies	X		=		Pennies	X		=	
		Total		$			Total		$

Ending cash total – Starting cash total = Cash taken in

____________ – ____________ = ____________

Ending cash total   Starting cash total   Cash taken in

FIGURE 16.12 Cash reconciliation template.

ending cash total should match the cash total from the daily transaction report. The deposit slip total should match the check total from the daily transaction report. The credit card total from the credit card processing terminal should match the debit/credit card total from the daily transaction report. Comparing the reports will ensure that all the payment amounts have been entered correctly (Procedure 16.4).

Making Bank Deposits

The medical assistant should make daily bank deposits, which minimizes the risks of keeping large sums of money on hand and also makes the money available to pay expenses. Depositing checks daily is important for these reasons:

- Checks may have a restricted time payment or may be lost, misplaced, or stolen over time.
- A stop-payment order may be placed on a check, or it may be returned for insufficient funds.
- Prompt processing is a courtesy to the payer.

Prompt check processing ensures that the money is available for the healthcare facility to use or to be used to build interest.

The medical assistant must prepare a deposit slip (ticket) that accompanies the funds being deposited. The deposit slip, which can be paper or electronic, itemizes the cash or checks being deposited. It provides the information for the bank account into which the funds need to be deposited (Figure 16.13). All details of the daily deposit should be recorded in the accounting software program; each check should be entered separately. The check number, payer, and check amount should also be recorded in the accounting software program so that the deposit amount from the software matches the bank deposit record. Many banks will not credit deposits made after 3 p.m. until the following business day (see Procedure 16.4).

Another option for depositing checks is using a credit card terminal that electronically processes checks at the time of payment. Also, small healthcare facilities can snap a picture of the check and use the bank's app to do a mobile deposit. Facilities receiving a high volume of checks can use a mobile check scanner (Figure 16.14). Checks are scanned individually and documented as a bank transaction on the monthly statement. Mobile deposits can save staff time and do not require a deposit slip because the software (app) is linked to the bank account being used. When mobile deposits are used, the daily deposit amount must match the exact daily deposit amount in the accounting management software.

Check Endorsements

An endorsement is a signature plus any other writing on the back of a check by which the endorser transfers all rights in the check to another party. Endorsements are made with either a pen or rubber ink stamp. The medical assistant needs to endorse the back of the check in the box indicated. Regardless of how checks are deposited, they all need to be endorsed.

Types of Endorsements

Four principal types of endorsements can be used: blank, restrictive, special, and qualified (Table 16.1). Blank and restrictive endorsements (Figure 16.15) are most commonly used.

Methods of Endorsement

Any endorsement should exactly match the name on the Pay To line of the check. If the name of the payee is misspelled, the payee usually must endorse the check the way the name is spelled on the face, followed by the correctly spelled signature.

A stamp can be used to endorse checks from patients and other sources. As they arrive, these checks should be recorded in the ledger and immediately stamped with the restrictive endorsement "For Deposit Only." This is a safeguard that prevents the cashing of lost or stolen checks. Most banks accept routine stamp endorsements that are restricted to For Deposit Only if the customer is well known and maintains an established account.

A signature can also be used as an endorsement. Some insurance checks or drafts require a personal signature endorsement; a stamped endorsement is not acceptable. This is stated on the back of the check. In such cases, ask the payee to endorse the check, then stamp immediately below the signature the restrictive endorsement For Deposit Only.

Overdraft

When a depositor writes a check for more than the amount available in the account, the account is overdrawn. Issuing a check for more

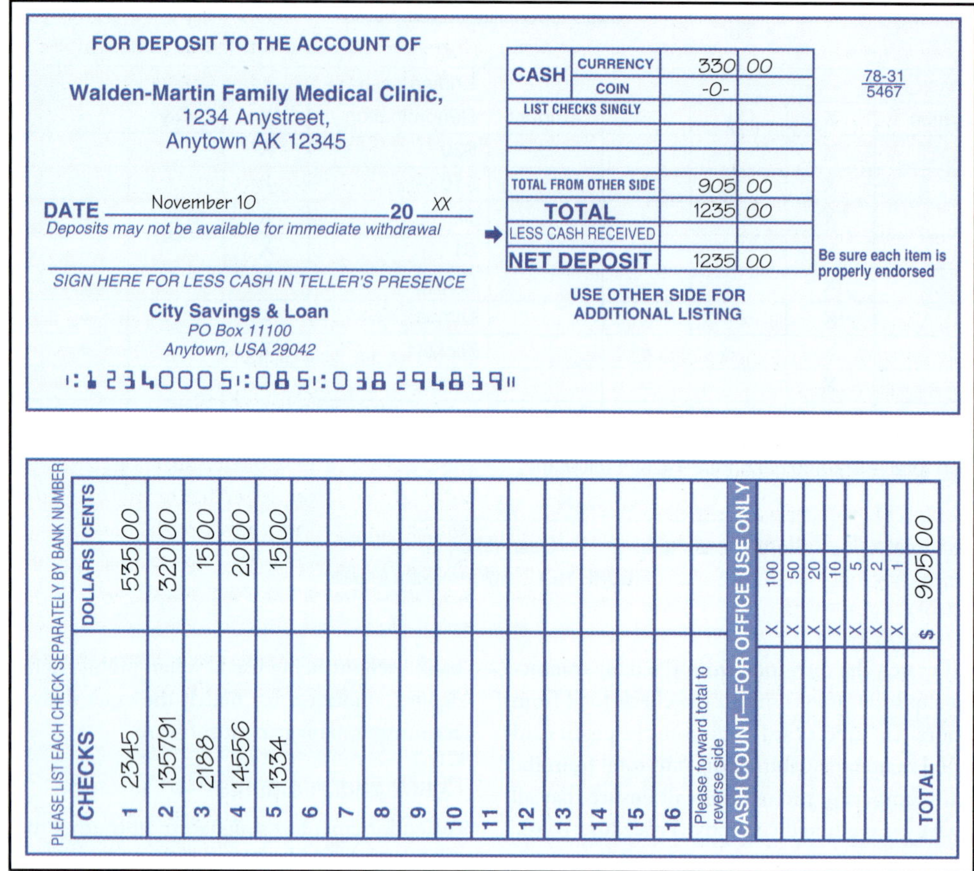

FOR DEPOSIT TO THE ACCOUNT OF

Walden-Martin Family Medical Clinic,
1234 Anystreet,
Anytown AK 12345

DATE November 10 20 XX
Deposits may not be available for immediate withdrawal

SIGN HERE FOR LESS CASH IN TELLER'S PRESENCE

City Savings & Loan
PO Box 11100
Anytown, USA 29042

⑆1234000 5⑆085⑆038 294839⑈

CASH	CURRENCY	330	00
	COIN	-0-	
LIST CHECKS SINGLY			
TOTAL FROM OTHER SIDE		905	00
TOTAL		1235	00
LESS CASH RECEIVED			
NET DEPOSIT		1235	00

78-31
5467

Be sure each item is properly endorsed

USE OTHER SIDE FOR ADDITIONAL LISTING

PLEASE LIST EACH CHECK SEPARATELY BY BANK NUMBER

CHECKS	DOLLARS	CENTS
1 2345	535	00
2 135791	320	00
3 2188	15	00
4 14556	20	00
5 1334	15	00
6		
7		
8		
9		
10		
11		
12		
13		
14		
15		
16		
Please forward total to reverse side		
TOTAL	$ 905	00

CASH COUNT—FOR OFFICE USE ONLY

X 100
X 50
X 20
X 10
X 5
X 2
X 1
$

FIGURE 16.13 Front and back of a deposit slip.

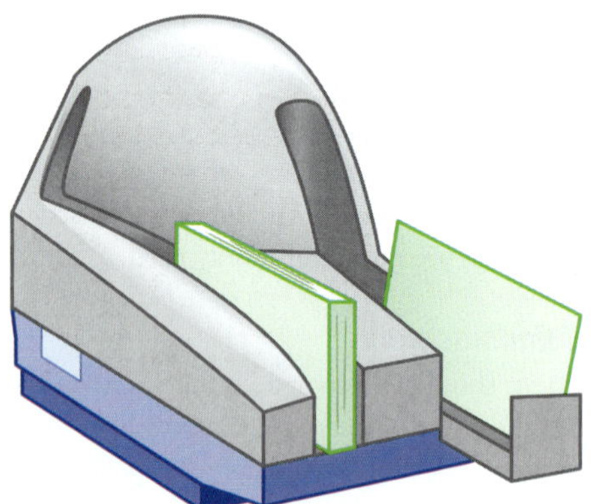

FIGURE 16.14 Mobile check scanner.

than the amount on deposit in the bank is illegal. Such a check is said to "bounce." Should this happen through error or oversight and a check is written by an established depositor, the bank may honor the check and notify the depositor that the account is overdrawn. If the bank pays or covers the check, it issues an overdraft on the depositor's account. Considerable fees ($20 to $40) normally are charged for an overdraft. If the bank does not cover the amount of the check, it will be returned as NSF.

Stop Payments

A depositor or check writer who wants to take back the check has the right to request that the bank stop payment on it. Stop-payment orders should be used only when absolutely necessary; as with overdrafts, most banks charge a fee for this service. There are several reasons for stop-payment requests:

- Loss of a check
- Disagreement about a purchase
- Disagreement about a payment

Bank Statements and Reconciliation

The bank creates a statement at the end of each month. The medical assistant can download the bank statement directly into the accounting management software, which has a **reconciliation** feature. The purpose of reconciliation is to start with the beginning balance, add all deposits, and subtract all checks and other debit transactions. This will then leave the ending statement balance. The ending balance should match the ending balance on the bank statement. If it does, the account has been reconciled. Bank statement reconciliation is used as an audit or to ensure that the bank is managing the funds in the account accurately. It can also help locate any errors made in the checking account register. Any errors on the bank statement should be immediately reported to the bank. Bank statements typically contain the following elements (Figures 16.16 and 16.17):

- Beginning balance
- Deposits made
- Checks paid (including images of all cleared checks)
- Transfer transactions
- Online payment transactions
- Bank charges
- Ending balance

TABLE 16.1 Types of Endorsements

TYPE	DESCRIPTION
Blank endorsement	The back of the check is signed with only the payee's name. This makes the check payable to the bearer. It is the simplest and most common type of endorsement on personal checks but should be used only when the check is to be cashed or deposited immediately.
Restrictive endorsement	Specifies the purpose of the endorsement (see Figure 16.15). It is used in preparing checks for deposit to the provider's checking account.
Special endorsement	Includes words specifying the person to whom the endorser makes the check payable. For instance, a check written to Helen Barker as the payee may be endorsed to the provider by writing on the back of the check as follows: Pay to the order of Theodore F. Wilson, M.D. Helen Barker The check is still negotiable but requires Dr. Wilson's signature or endorsement.
Qualified endorsement	The effect of the endorsement is qualified by disclaiming or destroying any future liability of the endorser. Usually the words "without recourse" are written above by an attorney who accepts a check on behalf of a client but who has no personal claim in the transaction.

Pay to the Order of
Midwest National Bank
Main Branch
For Deposit Only
ROBERT SPALDING
301-012697

FIGURE 16.15 Example of a restrictive endorsement.

What to Do When the Balances Do Not Match

When there are many transactions from check deposits and bill payment activities, it can be challenging to match the closing balance of the bank statement with the closing balance indicated in the accounting management software. Keeping accurate records of deposits and bill payment activities makes the bank reconciliation much smoother. All deposit copies should be maintained with a copy of the calculator tape totaling the day's deposit. Every online bill pay transaction should be recorded accurately in the accounting management system.

If you have carefully recorded every transaction and the balances still do not match, ask yourself the following questions:

- Is your math correct? Could a deposit, check, or online bill pay amount be transposed?
- Did you forget to include one of the outstanding checks?
- Did you fail to record a deposit, or did you record one twice?

Most banks ask to be notified within a reasonable time (e.g., 10 days) of any error found in the statement. The bank statement should be reconciled as soon as it is received. Most banks provide a form for reconciliation (bank statement reconciliation formula) on the last page of the bank statement:

Bank statement balance	$ ________
Minus outstanding checks	$ ________
Plus deposits not shown	$ ________
Corrected bank statement balance	$ ________
Checkbook balance	$ ________
Minus any bank charges	$ ________
Corrected checkbook balance	$ ________

If the two corrected balances agree, stop there. If they do not agree, subtract the lesser figure from the greater figure; the difference usually provides a clue to the error. For instance, if the shortage is $35, examine all the transactions for $35 on the statement and checkbook register and determine whether one of them has a posting error. Check the math and make sure all figures were added and subtracted correctly. Look at each figure and make sure none has been transposed. These tips usually catch the mistake.

Preventing Check Fraud in the Healthcare Facility

The National Check Fraud Center suggests the following steps to minimize the chance of check fraud in the healthcare facility:

- Check bank statements immediately after receiving them. If check fraud is not reported within 30 days of receipt of a monthly statement, the bank usually does not have to reimburse the loss.
- Make sure all extra checks, deposit slips, bank statements, and records are stored securely (e.g., locked in a file cabinet or a secure electronic folder).
- Bank statements and records should be maintained for up to 7 years and then shredded before disposal.

For more information on how to prevent check fraud or what to do if fraud occurs, consult the National Check Fraud Center's website at http://ckfraud.org.

Petty Cash

Petty cash is a small amount of money kept on hand for small, miscellaneous expenses, such as the following:

- Parking money for a conference
- Postage due
- Lunch for the provider
- Deliveries
- Minor office supplies

Although it is a small amount of money, records still need to be kept and expenses tracked. If an employee is being reimbursed for expenses, a receipt should be written out and the disbursement tracked in the petty cash log. Periodically the petty cash fund should be balanced, much like the checking account reconciliation.

If funds are running low in the petty cash fund, a check should be written, and the addition of the new funds noted on the petty cash register.

0621-402054

#821

N
2

Call (888) 555-2932
24 HOURS/DAY, 7 DAYS/WEEK
FOR ASSISTANCE WITH
YOUR ACCOUNT.

Page 1 of 2 — This statement covers: 6/22/2023 through 7/22/2023

Interest Checking 0621-402054

Summary

Previous balance	252.10
Deposits	68.74 +
Interest earned	.18 +
Withdrawals	109.55 –
Customer service calls	.00 –
Interlink/purchase fee	.00 –
Monthly checking fee and other charges	.00 –
▶ New balance	211.47

Minimum balance	142.55
Average balance	220.00
Annual percentage yield earned	.95%
Interest earned	2.23

Use your express card to make unlimited purchases at retailers displaying the interlink symbol (a $1 monthly fee may apply)
Try it today at Arco...Mobil...Lucky...Ralphs...Safeway and more!

Checks and withdrawals

Check	Date paid	Amount	Check	Date paid	Amount
202	7/05	15.05	203	7/15	94.50

Deposits

	Date posted	Balance
Customer deposit	7/22	68.74
interest payment this period	7/22	.18

Balance information

Date	Balance	Date	Balance	Date	Balance
6/22	252.10	7/05	237.05	7/15	142.55
				7/22	211.47

24 Hour Customer Service

Each account comes with 3 complimentary calls per statement period.
Calls to 24 hour customer service this statement period: 0

Interest information

From	Through	Interest rate	Annual percentage yield (APY)
6/22	7/22	1.00%	1.01%

Interest rate/APY as of 7/22/2023 if your balance is

$0–4,999	1.00%	1.01%
$5,000–$9,999	1.00%	1.01%
$10,000 and over	1.00%	1.01%

Call 1-800-555-2932 in California anytime for current rates.

Member FDIC

STATEMENT

FIGURE 16.16 Example of a regular checking account statement.

Paying Bills to Maximize Cash Flow

It is important to establish a systematic plan for paying bills. Some offices use an online bill-paying system and pay bills as soon as they are received. Some pay bills monthly. In establishing the procedure for accounts payable, a medical assistant should keep in mind that most vendors allow 30 days to pay. When each invoice is received, check the "terms," which are usually located at the top of the document. Sometimes a bill will be discounted if it is paid within a specified time, such as 10 days. Such discounts usually are indicated at the bottom of invoices or billing statements. If the terms say, "Net 30," this means the total amount of the bill is due within 30 days.

Remember to allow a certain number of days for mailing (2 to 5, depending on where the payment is sent). If the business checking account is an interest-bearing one, do not pay bills before their due date. This way, the funds in the account continue to earn interest until the check is cashed. Also, if the practice has a weekly service (e.g., a laundry or cleaning service) that bills several times a month, accumulate the invoices and issue only one check per month.

This worksheet is provided to help you balance your account

1. Go through your register and mark each check, withdrawal, Express ATM transaction, payment, deposit or other credit listed on this statement. Be sure that your register shows any interest paid into your account, and any service charges, automatic payments, or Express Transfers withdrawn from your account during this statement period.
2. Using the chart below, list any outstanding checks, Express ATM withdrawals, payments or any other withdrawals (including any from previous months) that are listed in your register but are not shown on this statement.
3. Balance your account by filling in the spaces below.

ITEMS OUTSTANDING		
NUMBER	AMOUNT	
TOTAL	$	

Enter

The new balance shown on this statement .... $______

Add

Any deposits listed in your register or transfers into your account which are not shown on this statement
$______
$______
$______
+$______

Total .... + $______

Calculate the subtotal .... $______

Subtract

The total outstanding checks and withdrawals from the chart at left .... – $______

Calculate the ending balance

This amount should be the same as the current balance shown in your check register .... $______

If you suspect errors or have questions about electronic transfers

If you believe there is an error on your statement or Express ATM receipt, or if you need more information about a transaction listed on this statement or an Express ATM receipt, please contact us immediately. We are available 24 hours a day, seven days a week to assist you. Please call the telephone number printed on the front of this statement. Or, you may write to us at United Trust Company, P.O. Box 327, Anytown, USA.

1. Tell us your name and account number or Express card number.
2. As clearly as you can, describe the error or the transfer you are unsure about, and explain why you believe there is an error or why you need more information.
3. Tell us the dollar amount of the suspected error.

You must report the suspected error to us no later than 60 days after we sent you the first statement on which the problem appeared. We will investigate your question and will correct any error promptly. If our investigation takes longer than 10 business days (or 20 days in the case of electronic purchases), we will temporarily credit your account for the amount you believe is in error, so that you may have use of the money until the investigation is completed.

FIGURE 16.17 Reverse side of a bank statement, which is used for reconciling a checking account.

Invoices and Statements

The vendor usually includes an *invoice* for payment with the delivery of the merchandise. An invoice describes the products delivered and shows the amount due. Always verify that the items listed on the packing slip and invoice are included in the delivery.

Invoices should be placed in a designated accounts payable folder until paid. The healthcare facility may make more than one purchase from the same vendor during the month and send only a single payment at the end of the month for all deliveries.

CRITICAL THINKING APPLICATION **16.7**

Laura does not recall ordering a certain item from the office supply company. However, it was included in her last shipment and was shown on the packing list. How can she determine whether the item was ordered?

Online Bill Pay

Online banking is a common practice for personal and business accounts. The healthcare facility can set up the account, so bills are paid automatically. This results in debiting the customer's account and crediting the merchant's account. This works well for those bills that occur every month or on a regular cycle, such as insurance premiums, rent payments, and utility bills. All banking transactions can be downloaded into an accounting management program for efficient money management. Online banking is also an excellent way to research the checks that have cleared the bank and compute accurate bank balances.

Direct Deposit

Direct deposit, also known as *electronic funds transfer* (EFT), is the electronic payment of payroll, money owed to vendors or business establishments, and payments from government agencies. Direct deposit payments are safe, secure, efficient, and less expensive than paper checks. Their greatest advantage is the cost savings: the US government pays $1.03 to issue each check payment but only $0.105 to issue a direct deposit. Electronic processing becomes more common each day, and business transactions are processed faster and more efficiently through electronic means.

BANKING IN TODAY'S BUSINESS WORLD

Banks can be used to centralize all financial transactions for a healthcare facility. The bank account tracks all deposits, withdrawals, and transfers. Monthly bank account balances can help healthcare facilities establish and maintain a monthly operational budget. Banks also provide opportunities to earn **interest** and invest for future financial gain. Overall, banks organize funds for the financial management of the healthcare facility.

Fees for banking services depend on the bank and services used (Table 16.2). The type of bank the medical practice will use is a decision made by the provider and the office manager, depending on the needs of the medical practice.

Although the **Federal Reserve Bank** (Figure 16.18) manages all banks in the United States, healthcare facilities can choose from a number of different types of banks with which to do business:

- *Retail banks:* Offer basic banking services to the public; these banks have hundreds of branches to provide easy consumer access.
- *Commercial banks:* Offer business banking services to businesses of all sizes; they are equipped to handle large volumes of check deposits and credit card transactions.
- *Credit unions:* Nonprofit banking institutions owned by members; credit unions use the funds deposited to make loans to their members, which enables them to offer loans at lower than market rates.
- *Online banks:* Offer basic banking services at competitive rates because all banking transactions are done online; there are no branch locations to visit.

The medical assistant will most likely manage only the bank accounts set up for the income and operating expenses of the healthcare facility.

Because of their large volume of bookkeeping transactions, many healthcare facilities use accounting management software. Most online banking systems allow for the download of bank account data. These software systems can be complicated to use, so the medical assistant should be in regular contact with the accountant chosen by the provider, who can answer questions when needed.

TABLE 16.2 Common Banking Fees

FEE	DESCRIPTION	AVERAGE FEE	WAIVABLE?
Account maintenance fee	Fee for using the bank account	$5–$25 per month	Some bank accounts waive monthly account maintenance fees if a specific balance is maintained in the account or if direct deposit is used.
Overdraft fee	Fee for the bank paying a check or debit when the balance is not in the account	$25–$40 per occurrence	Not usually. To avoid the fee in the future, tie the checking account with an overdraft account just in case the balance is low.
Returned deposit fee	Fee charged when a deposited check is returned from the drawer's account	$5–$10 per occurrence	Not usually. However, the practice can require the check drawer to cover this expense because the check did not clear.
Hard copy statement fee	Fee for the bank to send paper copies of bank statements	$5–$10 per statement	This fee can be avoided by downloading all electronic bank statements when they are released.
Nonsufficient funds (NSF) fee	Fee charged when a check is written against an account with not enough funds and the check is returned unpaid	$25–$40 per occurrence	Not usually. To avoid the fee in the future, tie the checking account with an overdraft account just in case the balance is low.
Transaction fee	Fee charged when too many transactions are made on a bank account	$.50–$1 per transaction	Online banking is usually free, but nowadays banks are charging fees to visit bank branches and to complete transactions with customer service over the phone.

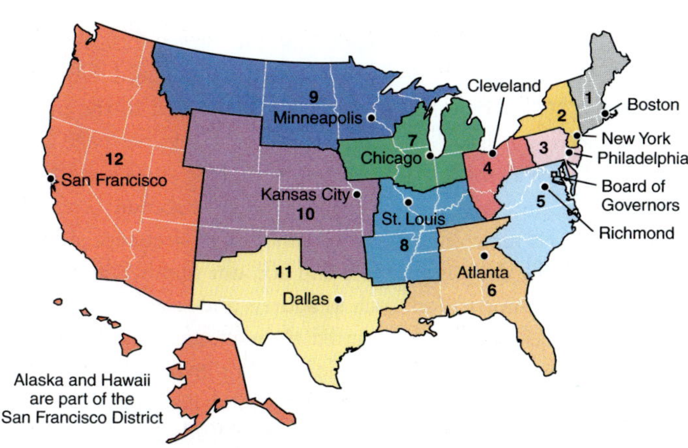

FIGURE 16.18 The 12 Federal Reserve districts.

The Federal Reserve

In 1913 Congress created the Federal Reserve Banking System. This was to provide the nation with a safer, more flexible, and stable monetary and financial system that consists of the following:

- A seven-member Board of Governors with headquarters in Washington, D.C.
- 12 Federal Reserve banks in major cities throughout the country (see Figure 16.18)

The Federal Reserve Bank monitors the movement of money, in the form of checks, from one bank account to another. Each check has the following:

- A routing number
- An account number

These numbers identify which Federal Reserve Bank jurisdiction, bank location, and specific bank accounts are used in each transaction.

For additional information on the Federal Reserve System and its regional banks, visit its website at www.federalreserve.gov.

Common Types of Bank Accounts

The healthcare facility will utilize several different types of bank accounts to manage its money. Each account serves a purpose for the cash flow and financial health of the organization. The most common types of bank accounts are discussed next.

Checking Accounts

By placing an amount of money in a bank, a depositor can set up a checking account. Simply stated, a checking account is a bank account from which checks can be written or debit cards used, and funds can be transferred to the payable party. Banks typically charge a monthly account maintenance fee. In addition, there may be fees associated with banking services, such as transferring funds to other banks or using the checking overdraft (see Table 16.2).

Savings Accounts

Money that is not needed for current expenses can be deposited into a savings account. In most cases, savings accounts earn a higher interest rate than checking accounts. Interest rates fluctuate with the financial market.

A standard savings account earns interest at the lowest prevailing rate and has no minimum balance requirement or check-writing privileges. However, penalties apply for withdrawing funds from a savings account more than six times per month. The provider may deposit a certain percentage of **discretionary income** into a savings account each month to earn interest. The money in a savings account can be transferred to a checking account when needed.

Money Market Savings Account

An insured money market savings account combines features of a checking and savings account. A minimum balance is required (anywhere from $500 to $5000). It earns interest at money market rates (usually a higher percentage rate than for a regular savings account), and it allows only a specified number of checks (frequently three) to be written per month. Such checks are usually written to transfer funds to a checking account. Some businesses transfer excess funds from the business checking account to a money market account over the weekend or over an extended holiday period to earn higher interest on the funds.

Signature Cards

When an account is opened at a bank branch, the account signer is required to provide a handwritten signature on a physical or electronic card, which is kept on file with the bank. If a check comes through and some suspicion arises that the depositor's signature has been forged, bank personnel compare the signature on the check with the original on the signature card.

The task of paying bills is often delegated to a responsible medical assistant. In this case, any staff members who have been authorized to sign the medical facility's checks must go to the bank and add their handwritten signatures to the signature card. Only those whose names appear on the signature card are authorized to sign checks, and the bank is responsible for verifying any questionable signatures.

Online Banking

Internet banking has changed the way financial institutions manage money. People once had to fight traffic and wait in line at crowded banks; now, they can bank from their offices any time of day. A healthcare facility's banking transactions, such as paying bills and transferring funds between accounts, can be done online. In addition, staff members have access to supply companies online and can easily review costs from the office instead of driving to numerous companies to compare prices.

Online banking is a means of performing banking services electronically via the internet. All banks and credit unions have this capability, and most of them offer both basic and advanced services. With basic services, a customer usually can do the following:

- Check account balances
- Transfer funds between accounts in the same bank
- Pay bills electronically and create checks
- Determine whether a check has cleared the bank
- Download account information
- View images of transactions

More advanced services include being able to deposit checks online.

A major concern with online banking is fraud. Concern that unauthorized users may gain access to the healthcare facility's account balances is valid. Some experts believe that online banking involves a slightly greater risk of fraud than conventional banking. Despite the disadvantages, studies show that internet banking is now mainstream.

Checks

A *check* is a bank draft or an order to pay a certain sum of money, on demand, to a specified person or entity. When a check is presented for payment, the *drawee* (the bank on which the check is drawn or written) pays the specified sum of money written on the face of the check to the *holder* (the person presenting the check for payment).

A check is considered a **negotiable instrument** if it meets the following requirements:

- Is written and signed by the *drawer* (the person who writes the check)
- Contains a promise or order to pay a sum of money
- Is payable on demand or at a fixed future date

To ensure that the amount is taken from the correct account number, the routing and account numbers are printed with magnetic ink on the bottom of the check. The check should have the amount written as a number and text to confirm the amount. Finally, the check must be signed and dated by the drawer of the account.

Routing and Account Numbers

A *routing transit number* (RTN) is a nine-digit code printed on the bottom left side of checks. An RTN is assigned to every banking institution under the Federal Reserve Banking System. It identifies the bank upon which the check was drawn. RTNs are also used for direct deposits and the transfer of funds between banks. The first two digits indicate the Federal Reserve district where the bank is located. The third digit indicates the specific district office. And the rest of the digits represent the individual accounts that belong to the bank.

Bank account numbers are assigned to each individual account. No two account numbers in the same financial institution can be the same. *Wire transfers* and *automated clearinghouse (ACH) transfers* use the routing and account numbers to transfer funds between exact accounts. Wire transfers are between two separate banking institutions in which both accounts are verified, so funds are available quickly. ACH transfers also involve two different banking institutions, but because both accounts are not verified, a few extra days are needed for funds to be available.

Types of Negotiable Instruments

The following are different types of negotiable instruments:

- Personal check
- Cashier's check
- Money order
- Business check
- Voucher check

Personal Check. A personal check is drawn by a bank against funds deposited to a personal account in another bank. Patients typically write these checks for copayments and other financial responsibilities.

Cashier's Check. A cashier's check is a bank's own check, drawn on itself and signed by the bank cashier or other authorized official. A cashier's check is obtained by paying the bank the amount of the check in cash. Many banks charge a fee for this service. Cashier's checks often are issued for a savings account customer who does not have a checking account.

Money Order. Money orders can be purchased at banks, some retail stores, and the US Postal Service. Money orders are often used to pay bills by mail when a person does not have a checking account. The maximum face value varies depending on the source. Cashier checks are preferable to money orders when larger amounts need to be paid.

Business Check. The checkbook most widely used in the professional office is a ledger-type book with three checks per page and a perforated stub at the left side of the check. The stubs serve as the checking account register, where the balance of the account is tracked. The checks and matching stubs are numbered in sequence and preprinted with the depositor's name and account number, along with any additional information, such as address and telephone number. Business checks can also be printed through accounting management software programs when vendors submit invoices. Today, most business checks can be prepared through online banking.

Voucher Check. A voucher check has a detachable voucher form or could be attached to an EOB. The voucher portion is used to itemize or specify the purpose for which the check was drawn. The voucher portion of the check is removed before the check is presented for deposit. The voucher is then used to post the payment in the patient account ledger (Figure 16.19).

How Checks Are Processed from One Bank to Another

Checks received by the drawee's bank are turned over daily to a regional banking clearinghouse, which clears each one. The identifying code numbers, printed on the face of the check with magnetic ink, enable this "clearing" process to be accomplished quickly and efficiently. Checks due from and to all banks outside a specific region are settled by electronic entries. The bank keeps the canceled checks, and an electronic copy of the check is returned to the *drawer* or the writer of the check. When the drawer needs proof of payment, a copy of the check can be requested from the bank, or the drawer can review monthly bank statements for printed copies of cleared checks. Check copies can also be obtained online through the banking portal.

Electronic Check

In an effort to prevent check fraud, many healthcare facilities accept only electronic checks. When the patient presents a personal check to the healthcare facility, the bottom of the check, which includes the routing and account numbers, is scanned. The funds are then automatically transferred from the patient's checking account and into the healthcare facility's account. Once the transaction has been approved, the paper check is returned to the patient with "VOID" printed across it to show that it has already been used. Electronic checks reduce the time involved in transferring funds from one account to another.

CLOSING COMMENTS

Patient accounts management and collections are critical responsibilities in the healthcare facility, and a responsible medical assistant is a great asset in this important area. Always maintain a positive attitude with patients when discussing financial matters. Remember that people who are ill or facing challenges are not always cordial, so they may not respond positively to a discussion of their patient account balances. Make every attempt to work with each patient to develop a financial plan for settling the account balance. The healthcare facility works hard to collect every dollar, so effective financial management is essential for practice success.

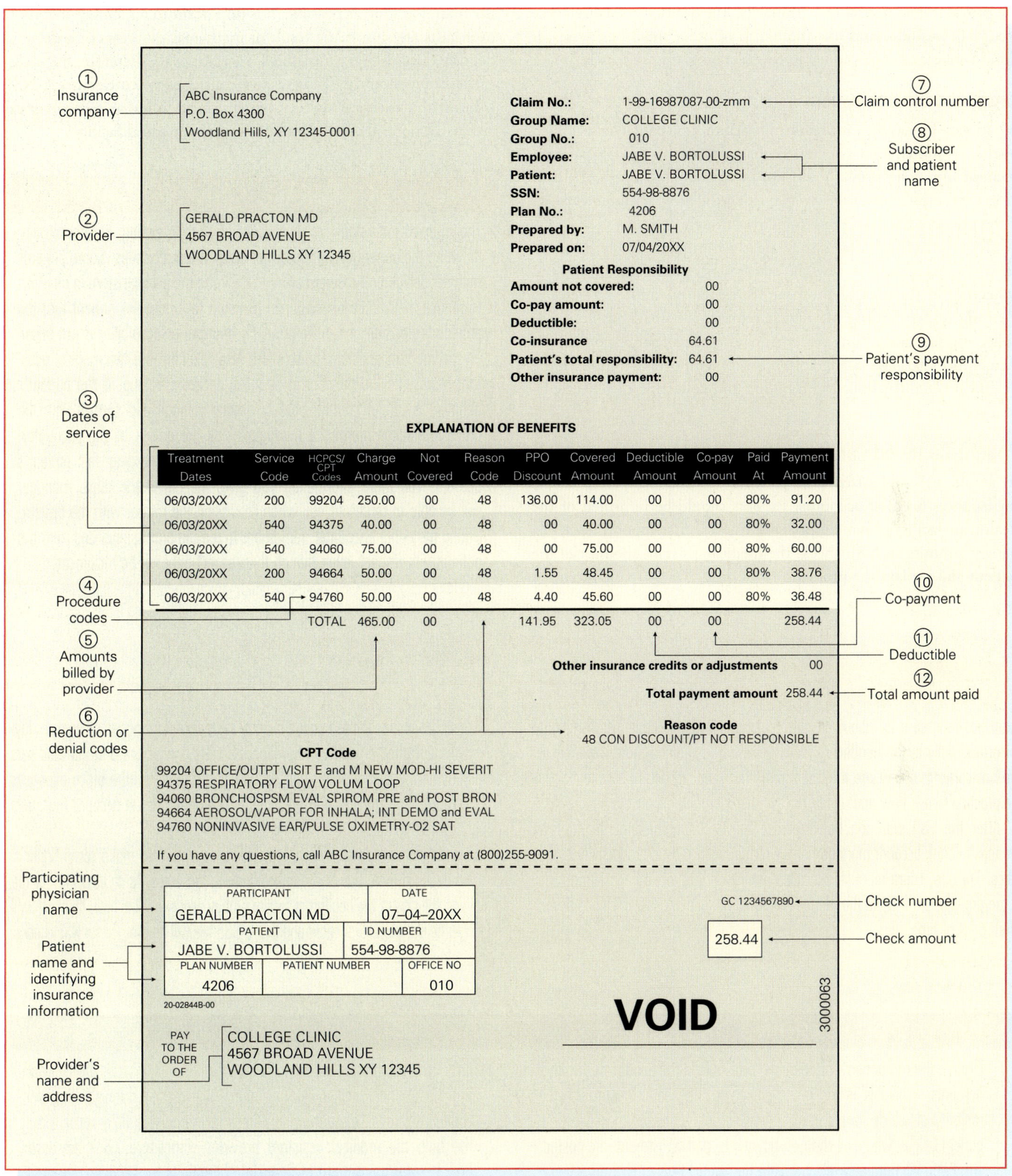

ABC Insurance Company
P.O. Box 4300
Woodland Hills, XY 12345-0001

Claim No.: 1-99-16987087-00-zmm
Group Name: COLLEGE CLINIC
Group No.: 010
Employee: JABE V. BORTOLUSSI
Patient: JABE V. BORTOLUSSI
SSN: 554-98-8876
Plan No.: 4206
Prepared by: M. SMITH
Prepared on: 07/04/20XX

GERALD PRACTON MD
4567 BROAD AVENUE
WOODLAND HILLS XY 12345

Patient Responsibility

Amount not covered: 00
Co-pay amount: 00
Deductible: 00
Co-insurance 64.61
Patient's total responsibility: 64.61
Other insurance payment: 00

EXPLANATION OF BENEFITS

Treatment Dates	Service Code	HCPCS/ CPT Codes	Charge Amount	Not Covered	Reason Code	PPO Discount	Covered Amount	Deductible Amount	Co-pay Amount	Paid At	Payment Amount
06/03/20XX	200	99204	250.00	00	48	136.00	114.00	00	00	80%	91.20
06/03/20XX	540	94375	40.00	00	48	00	40.00	00	00	80%	32.00
06/03/20XX	540	94060	75.00	00	48	00	75.00	00	00	80%	60.00
06/03/20XX	200	94664	50.00	00	48	1.55	48.45	00	00	80%	38.76
06/03/20XX	540	94760	50.00	00	48	4.40	45.60	00	00	80%	36.48
		TOTAL	465.00	00		141.95	323.05	00	00		258.44

Other insurance credits or adjustments 00

Total payment amount 258.44

Reason code
48 CON DISCOUNT/PT NOT RESPONSIBLE

CPT Code
99204 OFFICE/OUTPT VISIT E and M NEW MOD-HI SEVERIT
94375 RESPIRATORY FLOW VOLUM LOOP
94060 BRONCHOSPSM EVAL SPIROM PRE and POST BRON
94664 AEROSOL/VAPOR FOR INHALA; INT DEMO and EVAL
94760 NONINVASIVE EAR/PULSE OXIMETRY-O2 SAT

If you have any questions, call ABC Insurance Company at (800)255-9091.

PARTICIPANT	DATE
GERALD PRACTON MD	07–04–20XX

PATIENT	ID NUMBER
JABE V. BORTOLUSSI	554-98-8876

PLAN NUMBER	PATIENT NUMBER	OFFICE NO
4206		010

20-02844B-00

GC 1234567890

258.44

VOID

3000063

PAY TO THE ORDER OF
COLLEGE CLINIC
4567 BROAD AVENUE
WOODLAND HILLS XY 12345

FIGURE 16.19 Sample voucher check. (From Fordney MT: *Insurance handbook for the medical office*, ed 14, St. Louis, 2017, Elsevier.)

An equally important financial aspect for the healthcare facility is accounts payable. This must also be handled in an efficient manner. Being aware of the different banking options can help with depositing funds and paying bills. Making sure that there are policies in place for patient payment methods is crucial. Patients should also be made aware of those policies.

Patient Coaching

In some cases, patients may not fully appreciate all the costs involved in providing high-quality healthcare. The medical assistant may need to respectfully educate the patient about the basic costs associated with the services provided by the healthcare facility. Patients may not need a lengthy explanation, but they should be informed that the provider does not set fees arbitrarily. The healthcare facility office is a small business, and like thousands of other small businesses, it should collect enough money to cover its operating expenses.

Legal and Ethical Issues

A patient who has filed for bankruptcy cannot be contacted or billed further. Another legal concern is that a threat to send a patient's account into collections should not be made unless this is the provider's intention. Never tell a patient that the provider intends to act if the provider does not plan to follow through.

Because collection laws vary greatly from state to state, medical assistants should review the statutes pertaining to billing and collecting in the area of the healthcare facility's address. Develop a strong understanding of what is required of small businesses in collecting fees and billing patients for their financial responsibility. Remember that laws change often, so it is important to update the healthcare facility's policies on billing and collecting to reflect current statutes.

Patient-Centered Care

It should be emphasized that patients are financially responsible for balances on their accounts. Patients should be informed of the healthcare facility's payment policy at the very first appointment. If a patient submits an NSF check, the medical assistant should call the patient and explain the problem, requesting that the patient correct the matter as soon as possible. It is important to remember that most overdrafts are simply the result of mathematical errors or a delay in deposited funds being available for withdrawal. Therefore, the medical assistant should be patient and courteous when discussing NSF issues with patients. However, patients need to know that overdrafts are costly, not only to them but also to the medical facility.

Professional Behaviors

The medical assistant is responsible for coordinating communication between the patient and the provider about financial issues. Some patients may act belligerently toward or try to bully the medical assistant in an effort to reduce their financial obligation. Be sure to inform the patient that the provider's decision about the patient's financial responsibility is not based on the medical assistant's discretion. Also, explain that the medical assistant represents the provider in financial decision making. If the patient's behavior is out of control, politely excuse yourself and consult with the office manager. Inform the manager of all the details of the encounter, including the healthcare provider's instructions regarding the patient's account. The more information you give, the better the office manager will be able to represent you when discussing the matter with the patient. During the entire encounter, remember to remain professional and treat the patient with respect, even though that respect may not be reciprocated.

SUMMARY OF SCENARIO

Laura has learned a lot about the different types of bookkeeping transactions performed daily in the healthcare facility. As she has gained more experience, she has come to appreciate the important role of patient accounts collection in the practice's cash flow and ability to cover its operating expenses.

After the visit with the bank representative, Laura implemented a few changes in bank account management, which have increased productivity in the office. For one, Laura requested that the bank send a mobile deposit machine to the provider's office, so that deposits can be made in-house, which has saved Laura a lot of time.

Laura has also set up an online bill pay system and manages all invoice payments through the banking portal online. She sits down once a month and sets up all payments for the month. In this way, she can budget the office expenses for the month and transfer unused funds to a money market account that pays a higher interest rate.

Laura is working closely with the providers at WMFM to make some financial policy changes in the office to streamline banking processes. As of January 1 of the new year, the sign at the healthcare facility's lobby window will explain that cash will no longer be accepted for services and that a $35 fee will be charged for NSF checks.

SUMMARY OF LEARNING OBJECTIVES

1. **Explain the components of accounts receivable in the healthcare facility.**
Accounts receivable is the money owed to the healthcare facility, the majority of which comes from patient accounts. This is tracked on the patient ledger, where all charges, payments, and adjustments are posted. The PMS will automatically calculate the correct fees or charges when a CPT/HCPCS code is entered (see Procedure 16.1). All insurance payment amounts posted should also match the total amount paid on the EOB. The patient account record should have a column for the adjustment to be posted as a credit.

The medical assistant must believe that the provider and the facility have a right to charge for the services provided. Do not be embarrassed to ask for payment for the valuable services the clinician provides. When tact and good judgment are used during billing and collecting processes, patients appreciate the service they receive and the help the medical assistant provides. Procedure 16.2 discusses how to inform a patient of financial obligations for services rendered. Give each patient individual attention and personal consideration; also, be courteous and show a sincere desire to help the patient with financial problems.

If credit options are offered for patients, the healthcare facility should be in compliance with Regulation Z of the Truth in Lending Act (TILA). If an agreement exists between provider and patient that the healthcare

SUMMARY OF LEARNING OBJECTIVES—*continued*

facility will accept full payment in more than four installments, the healthcare facility must provide a Federal Truth in Lending Statement, even if no finance fees are charged, and it should be signed by the healthcare facility representative and the patient.

Patient account statements should be sent on a monthly basis. Having a set schedule for statements will keep an even flow of money coming into the healthcare facility. The statement should tell the patient the date of service, what services were provided, the charge for those services, insurance payments and adjustments, and patient payments.

2. **Examine the various methods used for patient payments.**
Although cash is an option for payment, many healthcare facilities refuse to accept cash from patients to prevent employees from being tempted to embezzle. In addition, cash cannot be deposited through mobile payment methods, and maintaining records for accepting cash can be difficult.

Checks are a common way for patients to pay for services. It is important to inspect the check carefully for the date, amount, and signature. A state-issued picture ID should be requested so that the image and signature can be compared. Third-party checks should not be accepted.

The advantages of debit cards include their safety and convenience, in addition to the availability of receipts and statements. The most important precaution in accepting credit cards is to verify the patient's identity by asking to see the person's state-issued ID. Patients must know the debit card's PIN, which is considered a verification of identity.

3. **Examine successful collection techniques for patient accounts.**
The medical assistant can use a variety of techniques to collect payments for patient accounts, such as collection phone calls, collection letters, and skip tracing. Often more than one technique must be used to obtain payment. Always be courteous and kind when using collection techniques. Personal finance interviews with patients sometimes can be more effective than a whole series of collection letters. By speaking with a patient face to face, the medical assistant can come to an understanding of the problem more quickly, and an agreement about future payment plans can be reached.

When a check is drawn on an account with insufficient funds, the bank returns the check to the healthcare facility marked "NSF" and charges the healthcare facility bank account a returned check fee. The payment posted to the patient's account must be reversed. Note that the original payment is not deleted; rather, a charge line item is added with the amount of the NSF check; the transaction description should read "NSF Date 02/23/20XX." Many medical offices include additional line items for NSF fee charges, but this is up to the discretion of the provider. Because collection agencies charge a fee for their collection efforts, the amount credited to the patient's account might be less than the actual payment amount. See Procedure 16.3.

4. **Explain the components of accounts payable in the healthcare facility.**
Vendors provide services and supplies to the healthcare facility. Payment for those services and supplies are part of accounts payable. This process includes reviewing the invoice for accuracy to ensure that the services or supplies were received before payment was sent.

When working with employee payroll, the medical assistant must understand the differences between salary, net pay, and gross pay in order to ensure that the proper amount for taxes is withheld. There are also a number of forms involved with employee payroll, including W-4 and W-2.

5. **Examine banking procedures as related to the ambulatory care setting.**
Banking procedures include withdrawals, deposits, writing checks, reconciling bank statements, paying bills, and other transactions, most of which can be done conveniently in the healthcare facility through online banking or accounting management software.

Writing checks is a routine and basically simple function; however, certain guidelines should be followed to prevent potential problems. The bank account should have a check signer on file with the bank, and correction fluid for errors should not be used on checks.

End-of-day reconciliation starts the process of getting funds to the bank. The reports generated from the PMS must match the amount of cash on hand, the total amount of the checks received, and the reports from the credit card processing terminals. If they do not match, the error must be tracked down and corrected before moving on to preparing the deposit for the bank.

Deposits should be made daily for these reasons: a stop-payment order may be placed; the check may be lost, misplaced, or stolen; delay may cause the check to be returned because of insufficient funds; the check may have a restricted time for cashing; prompt processing is a courtesy to the payer; and the accounts receivable may be inflated because payments have not been deposited daily. The process for preparing a bank deposit is outlined in Procedure 16.4.

Endorsements include (1) a blank endorsement, when the back of the check is signed with only the payee's name; (2) a restrictive endorsement, which specifies in which bank and which specific account the funds are to be deposited; (3) a special endorsement, which names a specific person on the back of the check as payee; and (4) a qualified endorsement, which disclaims future liability. This type of endorsement is used when the person who accepts the check has no personal claim in the transaction.

6. **Examine banking practices in today's business world.**
The bank accounts most commonly used by healthcare facilities are checking, savings, and money market accounts.

When an account is opened at a bank branch, the depositor is required to provide a handwritten signature on a physical or electronic card, which is kept on file with the bank. If a check comes through and some suspicion arises that the depositor's signature has been forged, bank personnel compare the signature on the check with the original on the signature card.

Online banking allows healthcare facilities to perform mobile deposits, thereby reducing the number of times a staff member visits the bank branch. Online banking also provides up-to-the-minute account balances, online bill pay, and easy account balance transfers so that the healthcare facility's manager can spend less time managing the bank account.

The different types of negotiable instruments used to transfer funds from one bank account and deposit them in another are the personal check, cashier's check, money order, business check, and voucher check.

PROCEDURE 16.1 Post Charges and Payments to a Patient's Account

TASK: Enter charges into the patient account record manually and electronically.

SCENARIO: Ken Thomas is a returning patient of Dr. Martin. He makes his $50 copayment at the time of the office visit.

EQUIPMENT and SUPPLIES

- Patient account ledger card
- SimChart for the medical office software
- Encounter form/superbill (Figure 16.1)
- Provider's fee schedule

PROCEDURAL STEPS

Posting Charges Manually

1. For new patients, create the patient account by entering the following information on a patient account ledger card:
   - Patient's full name, address, and at least two contact phone numbers
   - Date of birth (DOB)
   - Health insurance information, including the subscriber number, group number, and effective date
   - Subscriber's name and date of birth (if the subscriber is not the patient)

   PURPOSE: To keep all insurance and collection information available with the patient account record balance for reference.
2. For returning patients, review the account record to see whether a balance is due. If there is a balance, bring this to the patient's attention at the time of the appointment. Respectfully explain that the provider would appreciate a payment on the previous balance before seeing the patient. Use the following dialogue:

   Laura: Good morning, Ken. How are you feeling today?

   Ken: Not so good; I really need to see Dr. Martin again because my headaches have been getting worse.

   Laura: I'm sorry to hear that. Let's get you in to see the doctor right away. I can collect the $50 copayment for today's visit, and here is a statement for your previous balance of $214. How would you like to take care of that today?

   Ken: Oh, I didn't know about the previous balance. Can I just pay the copayment today?

   Laura: Dr. Martin would like at least half of this previous balance paid before seeing you today, please. I know that medical bills can pile up pretty quickly, but Dr. Martin would like to continue to provide you with quality care so you can feel back to yourself really soon.

   Ken: Yes, I know you're right. I need to keep coming to see Dr. Martin. I can pay half of the $214 today, along with the copayment.

   Laura: Thanks, I know Dr. Martin really appreciates you as a patient. Will that be a check or credit card?

   Ken: Credit card, please.

   Laura: Okay, here is the credit card receipt and a copy of the updated statement. By the way, I'd like to document on your patient account when you will be able to pay the rest of this statement amount.

   Ken: I'll pay the balance next month. Is that okay?

   Laura: I'll let Dr. Martin know and put a note in your account. Thanks. You'll be called in shortly.

   PURPOSE: To respectfully inform the patient of the financial obligation and the provider's intention to have the previous balance paid in full.

   After seeing the patient, the provider completes the encounter form, which includes all procedures and the associated fee schedule. Using the completed encounter form in Figure 16.1, enter the charges manually on the ledger card for the patient's account record. Total all the charges on the encounter form for the services rendered. Then subtract the copayment made from the total charges. The previous balance, if any, is added to this new total. Use the following worksheet to calculate the new balance. The new balance-due amount should be presented to the patient before the patient leaves the healthcare facility.

TOTAL CHARGES	$__________
Amount paid (copayment)	$__________
+ Previous balance (if any)	$__________
= New balance due	$__________

Posting Charges in SimChart for the Medical Office

1. After logging into SimChart, locate the established patient by clicking on Find Patient; enter the patient's name, verify the DOB, and click on the radio button. This will bring you to the Clinical Care tab. If no encounter is shown, create an encounter by clicking on Office Visit under Info Panel on the left, selecting a visit type, and clicking on Save. Once an encounter has been created, return to the Patient Dashboard and click on the Superbill link on the right (or click on the Coding and Billing tab). (See the Figure 16.1.)

PROCEDURE 16.1 Post Charges and Payments to a Patient's Account—*continued*

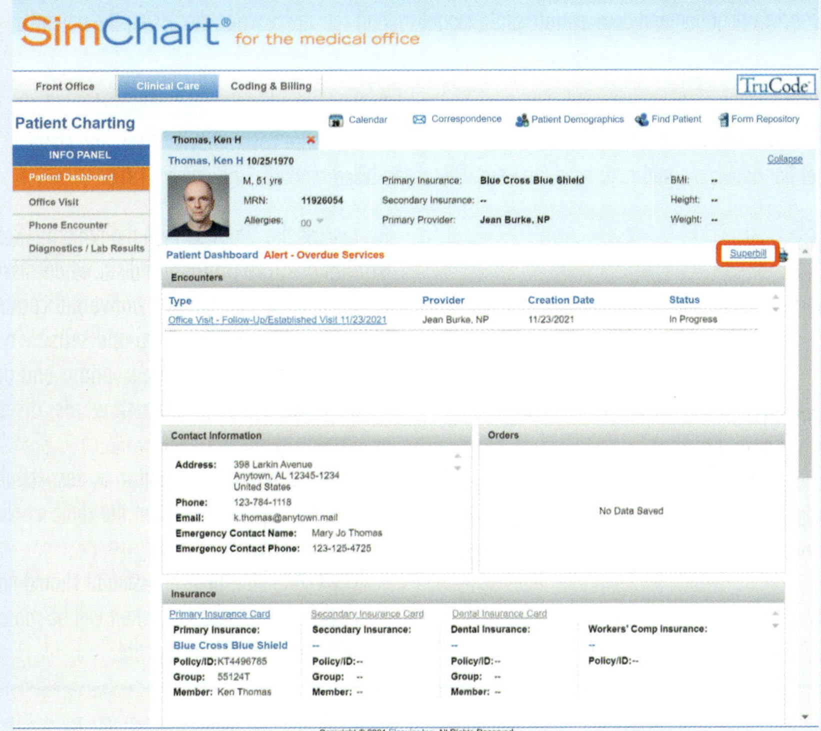

2. From the Superbill area, in the Encounters Not Coded section, click on the encounter (in blue) (Figure 16.2). On page 1 enter the diagnosis in the Diagnosis field, and document the services provided (additional services are found on pages 2 and 3 of the Superbill).

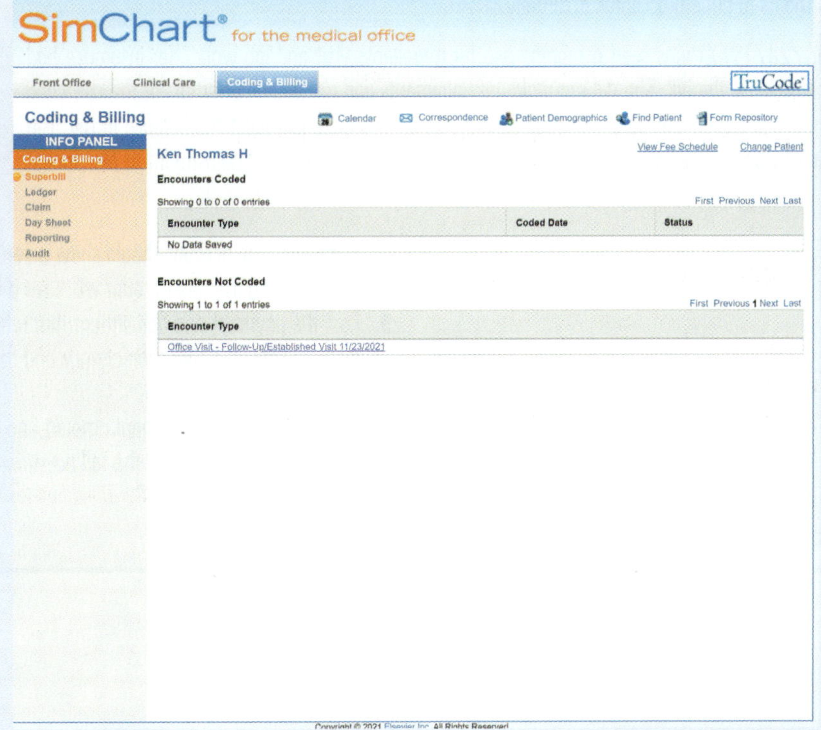

3. Complete the information needed on page 4 of the Superbill and submit.
4. Click on Ledger on the left, and search for your patient. Once your patient has been located, click on the arrow across from the name in the ledger.
5. Enter the payment received. The balance will be autocalculated for you.

PROCEDURE 16.2 Inform a Patient of Financial Obligations for Services Rendered

TASK: Inform a patient of the financial obligation and demonstrate professionalism and sensitivity when discussing the patient's billing record.

SCENARIO: During this role-play, Christi Brown is meeting with you regarding the bill she received in the mail. When she called to make the appointment, she voiced her confusion about the bill, stating she thought her insurance covered everything. You check her record and see that she has met her deductible and now needs to pay 20% of the billed amount. She owes $170.

EQUIPMENT and SUPPLIES

- Patient's account record
- Copy of patient's insurance card

PROCEDURAL STEPS

1. Determine the patient's financial responsibility under the insurance plan by reviewing the copy of the patient's insurance card.
   PURPOSE: Having an understanding of the patient's financial responsibility from the insurance plan will help you explain the terms to the patient.
2. Determine the amount the patient owes by reviewing the patient's account record.
   PURPOSE: It is important when working with a patient that you are familiar with the facts of the situation.
3. Discuss the situation with the patient. (Role-play the above scenario.)
4. Demonstrate professionalism when discussing the situation with the patient. Verbal and nonverbal communication should demonstrate patience, understanding, and sensitivity. The medical assistant should refrain from inappropriate and unprofessional behavior, including eye rolling, harsh words, disrespectful comments, and similar behaviors.
5. Demonstrate professionalism by respectfully providing the patient with payment options based on the clinic's policies and what the patient can pay on a monthly basis.
   PURPOSE: The medical assistant should not force or harass the patient into paying. The medical assistant will be more successful if the communication with the patient is respectful.

PROCEDURE 16.3 Post Payments and Adjustments to a Patient's Account

TASK: Post payments and adjustments to patient accounts accurately.

SCENARIO: Monique Jones (06/23/19XX) was seen 6 months ago for a wellness visit and lab work. Her insurance had lapsed, and she is completely responsible for the bill. She did not make any payments and resisted all attempts at the collection of the balance of $172. Her account was turned over to a collection agency, which was able to collect the balance in full. The collection agency retains 50% of what it collects as payment. Post the collection agency payment and adjustment to Ms. Jones' account.

EQUIPMENT and SUPPLIES

- Patient account ledger card, or SimChart for the medical office software

PROCEDURAL STEPS

1. Look up the ledger card for the patient account (or the patient ledger in SimChart). Confirm that you have the correct patient account.
   PURPOSE: All transactions need to be posted to the correct account.
2. Post an adjustment to reverse the adjustment done when the account was turned over to the collection agency.
   PURPOSE: The account should show a zero balance. If the reverse adjustment is not done, the account will have a credit balance.
3. Post the payment and adjustment that reflects the actual dollar amount received from the collection agency and the amount retained as payment (see the following figure).
   PURPOSE: Both the payment amount and adjustment must be posted to give the patient credit for the full payment sent to the collection agency.

PROCEDURE 16.4 End-of-Day Reconciliation

TASK: Complete the end-of-day reconciliation, including preparing a bank deposit for currency and checks.

SCENARIO: The following payments were received today at Walden-Martin Family Medical Clinic:

Cash

Reuven Ahmad: $25.00
Amma Patel: $15.00
Ken Thomas: $40.00
Maude Crawford: $25.00
Al Neviaser: $30.00

At the start of the day, the cash drawer had ten $1 bills, ten $5 bills, ten $10 bills, and ten $20 bills for a total of $360.00. At the end of the day, there is a total of $495.00.

Checks

Julia Berkley: #3456 for $89.00
Jana Green: #6954 for $136.00
Kyle Reeves: #9854 for $1366.65
Truong Tran: #8546 for $653.36
Quinton Brown: #9865 for $890.22

The healthcare facility's name is Walden-Martin Family Medical Clinic, account number 123-456-78910, and the bank is Clear Water Bank, Anytown, Anystate.

Credit Cards

Tai Yan: $150.00
Ella Rainwater: $300.00
Diego Miller: $75.00
Carl Bowden: $25.00
Noemi Rodriguez: $45.00

Daily Transaction Report

DATE	PATIENT	ACCOUNT	CASH	CHECK	DEBIT/ CREDIT
11/6/20XX	Reuven Ahmad	11872534	$25.00		
11/6/20XX	Amma Patel	12156063	$15.00		
11/6/20XX	Ken Thomas	11644627	$40.00		
11/6/20XX	Maude Crawford	12568850	$25.00		
11/6/20XX	Al Neviaser	11279412	$30.00		
11/6/20XX	Julia Berkley	12062515		$89.00	
11/6/20XX	Jana Green	10944532		$136.00	
11/6/20XX	Kyle Reeves	12073635		$1366.65	
11/6/20XX	Truong Tran	11726005		$650.36	
11/6/20XX	Quinton Brown	11272882		$890.22	
11/6/20XX	Tai Yan	12658901			$150.00
11/6/20XX	Ella Rainwater	11885104			$300.00
11/6/20XX	Diego Lupez	12530423			$75.00
11/6/20XX	Carl Bowden	11265329			$25.00
11/6/20XX	Noemi Rodriquez	11766543			$45.00
Total			$135.00	$3132.23	$595.00

EQUIPMENT and SUPPLIES

- Daily transaction report (see Scenario)
- Checks and currency for the deposit (see Scenario)
- Check for endorsement
- Calculator
- Paper method: bank deposit slip
- Electronic method: SimChart for the Medical Office (SCMO)

PROCEDURAL STEPS

Cash Reconciliation

1. Complete the Starting Cash portion of the Cash Reconciliation form (see Figure 16.12) using the information from the scenario.
   PURPOSE: This will provide the starting point for cash reconciliation.
2. Complete the Ending Cash portion of the Cash Reconciliation form using the information from the scenario.
   PURPOSE: This allows for the comparison of the Cash Reconciliation form and the Daily Transaction report.
3. Compare the Cash Taken In from the Cash Reconciliation form to the Cash total from the Daily Transaction Report. If the totals do not match, compare the individual transactions and determine where the error occurred.
   PURPOSE: To ensure that all cash transactions were posted to the PMS.

Debit/Credit Card Reconciliation

4. Compare the total from the Credit Card Processing terminal and the Debit/Credit Card total from the Daily Transaction Report. If the totals do not match, compare the individual transactions and determine where the error occurred.
   PURPOSE: To ensure that all debit/credit card transactions were posted to the PMS.

Check Reconciliation

5. Gather the documents to be used to prepare the bank deposit. For the electronic method, enter the Simulation Playground in SCMO. Click on the Form Repository icon. On the INFO PANEL, click on Office Forms and select Bank Deposit Slip.
6. Enter the date on the deposit slip.
7. Using the calculator, calculate the amount of currency to be deposited. Enter the amount in the CURRENCY line, completing the dollar and cent boxes.
8. Enter the total amount in the TOTAL CASH line.
9. For each check to be deposited, enter the check number, the dollars, and the cents. List each check on a separate line.

Continued

PROCEDURE 16.4 End-of-Day Reconciliation—*continued*

PURPOSE: The bank requires that each check be listed separately; this also helps when verifying the checks before the deposit.

10. Calculate the total to be deposited, and enter the number in the TOTAL FROM ATTACHED LIST box.
11. Enter the number of items deposited in the TOTAL ITEMS box.
12. Before completing the deposit slip, verify the check amounts listed and recalculate the totals. For the electronic method, click on SAVE.
    PURPOSE: It is crucial to verify the accuracy of check amounts and totals.
13. Place a restrictive endorsement on the check(s).
    PURPOSE: To prevent cashing of checks in case of loss or theft.
14. Compare the total from the Deposit Slip to the total for checks from the Daily Transaction Report. If the totals do not match, compare the individual transactions and determine where the error occurred.
    PURPOSE: To ensure that all check transactions were posted to the PMS.

ADVANCED ROLES IN ADMINISTRATION

17

SCENARIO

Kate Gilliam is the office manager for Walden-Martin Family Medical (WMFM) Clinic. The clinic has a full appointment schedule each day. Kate encourages the medical office staff to communicate and work as a cohesive team to meet the goal of providing exceptional care to the practice's patients. Kate knows that positive motivation will encourage the office team to meet this goal. At weekly staff meetings, employees are free to offer their suggestions on office procedures. Kate regularly consults her team members and always asks for their thoughts on how the office can function more effectively. She recognizes that employees need to feel that they are part of the team, and by implementing some of the procedures her team members suggest, she creates a forward-thinking and empowered work environment for the office staff.

Kate has been praised by the providers as a transformational manager because she has implemented new and efficient health information systems and technologies in the clinic. In addition, when an office position becomes vacant, Kate is careful about whomever she hires. She always checks at least three references per applicant and verifies each previous place of employment. She also always requests a background check, a credit check, a drug test, and a bond if the applicant is assigned to manage office money matters.

Kate trains each new employee herself, using the office's policies and procedures manual. She makes sure the employee knows that this manual also contains a detailed job description, so the employee knows the duties associated with the job. Kate regularly reviews employee performance and keeps checklists that reflect that new employees are trained accurately. All new employees are probationary until Kate evaluates them 90 days after they were hired. She works hard to improve the types of benefits offered to her team, to increase employee satisfaction and retention.

Kate makes sure all employees have the tools needed to do their jobs effectively. She also trains the team in ways to reduce expenses and waste in the medical office. Major office changes are presented to the entire staff, and although providers make the final decision, Kate seeks the suggestions of other employees. The cooperative attitude between management and employees of the healthcare facility provides a great atmosphere for teamwork, and Kate and the providers are pleased with the team-building atmosphere they have implemented.

While studying this chapter, think about the following questions:

- How friendly should office managers become with staff members?
- Why are checking references and performing a background check important when considering a new staff member?
- How should negative employee evaluations be handled?
- How can the office manager promote a teamwork atmosphere in the medical office?

LEARNING OBJECTIVES

1. Examine the qualities and responsibilities of a successful office manager in a healthcare facility.
2. Examine the responsibilities of a medical office manager.
3. Examine the skills necessary to be a successful medical office manager.
4. Examine the process for finding and hiring the right employee for the job.
5. Determine the needs for working with new and established employees.
6. Describe how office policies and procedures are different from personnel policies.
7. Examine the role of reports in the medical office.

VOCABULARY

cohesive (koh HEE siv) Sticking together tightly; exhibiting or producing cohesion.

compliant (kum PLIE unt) Obeying, obliging, or yielding.

consensus (kun SEN sus) General agreement

credential (kri DEN shul) Evidence of authority, status, rights, entitlement to privileges.

delegate To appoint a person as a representative.

disparaging (di SPAR a jing) Slighting; having a negative or degrading tone.

human resources file (HR file) Contains all documents related to an individual's employment.

VOCABULARY—*continued*

incentive Things that incite or spur to action; rewards or reasons for performing a task.
matrix (MAY triks) The environment where something is created or takes shape. A base on which to build.
mentor A steady employee whom a new staff member can approach with questions and concerns.
rapport (ra PORE) A relationship of harmony and accord between the patient and the healthcare professional.
retention A term referring to actions taken by management to keep good employees.
solvent (SOL vent) Able to pay all debts.

INTRODUCTION

The management of a professional healthcare facility can greatly influence the success of the business. Good management allows the provider to see and treat patients in a functional environment with the confidence that the business side of the facility is operating as it should be. A well-managed office is not something that just happens. Great effort and teamwork are necessary to ensure that the day-to-day activities are carried out efficiently, and the many details needing attention are handled urgently.

Although most medical assistants do not enter medical office management right after graduation, they can look forward to advancing their careers as they gain experience. The information in this chapter can help the medical assistant understand what it takes to become a good manager. Many of these traits can be developed as a new employee after graduation, such as punctuality, respect, and responsibility. Additionally, the medical assistant will learn the employment process from the office manager's point of view. This information is also valuable to a new medical assistant who is applying for a position. By studying office management, the medical assistant prepares for future management positions but also learns to see both the employee side and the manager side of the operating healthcare facility.

MEDICAL OFFICE MANAGEMENT

Medical assistants can be amazing office managers. They have a background in multiple areas of the healthcare organization, and that is a valuable asset. When a medical assistant makes the choice to move into a management position, there are some important factors to consider. This chapter focuses on the skills needed to become a successful office manager.

Choosing Healthcare Management as a Profession

There are many aspects to healthcare. Some people are attracted to the clinical side, with direct patient care. Some people are attracted to the administrative side, with some patient contact. What everyone who works in healthcare has in common is the desire to help others. There can be many different routes to becoming a manager in a healthcare setting. Some will pursue an educational route that is solely aimed at healthcare management, such as a degree in healthcare administration. Another educational route could include a degree in business administration. Yet another route could be a healthcare worker, such as a medical assistant or registered nurse, who has worked in the field for a period of time and has developed an interest in the management side of healthcare.

For those who come from a clinical care background, some additional education may be needed in the healthcare administration area. Those who come from more of a business background may need to call on others with clinical expertise in certain situations. For example, if there is a complaint about the care given to a patient by a certain provider, the manager with a business background may ask another provider or clinical staff member to review the care that was given.

Traits of a Successful Medical Office Manager

Successful medical office managers have excellent communication and organizational skills. These skills are very useful when you are working with patients, staff, and providers. A manager will have to deal with situations involving hiring and firing, disciplinary actions, and irate patients. The office manager is often the liaison between the staff and providers. If the staff has an issue with the provider or vice versa, the issue will come to the office manager, who will be expected to work toward a solution. Proper professional communication is needed in all aspects of managing a medical office.

It is necessary to have an understanding of budgeting and financial reports. Those with an educational background in management will have that knowledge. Someone moving into management may need to take some courses in those areas.

In addition, an office manager must possess good leadership skills. The office staff will look to the manager for direction and will follow the example set by the manager. When possible, the manager should seek out the opinions of the staff when a major decision is going to be made. That decision will likely impact how many people do their jobs and they would like to contribute to the decision-making process. If **consensus** is used to reach a decision, the staff will feel more invested in the decision. They will also feel more valued as employees and will develop a sense of loyalty to the organization.

Keeping the Management Relationship Professional

When people work together for an extended period of time, the relationship sometimes develops into a close friendship. This is a normal occurrence, but office managers must be careful about becoming too close to the employees. When the relationship is too friendly, reprimanding an employee when needed can be difficult. Some employees take advantage of a good relationship with the office manager and may begin to arrive late or call in sick more than usual. A healthy respect for each other must be maintained. The manager can have a good **rapport** with employees without becoming overly friendly, which is the best policy. Some facilities have strict rules about socializing with employees outside the work facility. It is advisable to keep the relationship on a professional level at all times.

CRITICAL THINKING APPLICATION **17.1**

The clinical medical assistants at WMFM usually celebrate payday by going out to eat after work every other Friday. After she has been on the job for about 6 months, they invite Kate to join them. Should she go with the employees? Why or why not?

Most offices plan parties for Christmas or at other times during the year. Are these good for employee morale, or should they be avoided?

OFFICE MANAGEMENT RESPONSIBILITIES

Having a background as a medical assistant is a good foundation for becoming a medical office manager, but as a manager, there are some areas where additional training will be necessary. The next section explores those areas that are not typically part of the medical-assistant role.

Personnel Management

There are many aspects to personnel management, including performance evaluation and salary review, maintaining employment records, and recruiting and selecting new staff members.

Performance evaluations typically occur on an annual basis. Salary review usually occurs at the same time, with a merit increase given if appropriate. Disciplinary actions are also part of the office manager's responsibilities. Performance evaluations and the disciplinary process will be discussed in more detail later in the chapter.

The performance evaluation is part of the employment record, but an office manager will also be responsible for employees' Social Security numbers, the number of tax exemptions claimed, wages, and the deductions associated with payroll. The employment record will also include **credential** documentation for the providers and staff—that is, making sure that licenses and certifications are kept up to date.

Financial Management

To keep the healthcare facility **solvent**, the office manager is responsible for tracking all of the income. This involves billing, collections (patient and insurance), and banking procedures. Having some accounting knowledge is helpful in this area.

Financial management planning involves setting guidelines and goals in the financial area, such as determining what expenses might be coming up in the near future and planning for bigger expenses, such as expanding the healthcare facility.

Scheduling

Several types of scheduling can occur in a healthcare facility. The most obvious is patient scheduling. Getting the **matrix** established (see Chapter 9) can be the responsibility of the office manager, working in conjunction with the provider, in addition to developing the scheduling policies and procedures. An office manager can also be responsible for setting the staff schedule. If these schedules are not handled properly, it can affect employee morale and patient satisfaction.

Facility and Equipment Management

Overseeing the inventory of equipment and supplies is part of the office manager's responsibilities. Having adequate supplies and equipment that works properly will help to ensure that things flow smoothly and efficiently. Making decisions about equipment replacement usually falls to the office manager. Arranging for the maintenance of the facility is also the responsibility of the office manager.

Risk Management

Risk management involves identifying, planning, and implementing strategies to minimize the provider's risk of a lawsuit. Creating policies and procedures is part of this process and will be discussed in more detail later in this chapter. Reviewing incident reports (see Chapter 4) to see if changes need to be made to procedures or facility management will also help with risk management. The office manager is very involved in this process.

OFFICE MANAGEMENT SKILLS

Certain skills are needed to be a successful medical office manager. Cultivating communication and listening skills along with motivation techniques will benefit anyone considering becoming a medical office manager. Those skills can be used when conducting staff meetings and helping to create a team environment.

Communication

Effective communication is a vital skill for anyone working in healthcare. An office manager will be communicating with employees, patients, vendors, insurance companies, and providers. This communication can happen in person or written format. Good office managers will be able to communicate professionally with anyone they come in contact with. Using the 5 Cs of good communication is an excellent place to start.

It is also important to keep in mind some basic communication guidelines:

- Speak slowly and clearly to ensure that your message is received and misunderstanding does not occur.
- Do not interrupt when someone is speaking. This can convey that what the speaker is saying is not important.
- Use a respectful tone of voice.
- Ask for feedback to ensure that the correct message was sent.

5 Cs of Good Communication

- *Clear:* Use words that accurately convey your meaning and are presented in a logical order.
- *Concise:* Get to the point, and do not wander off topic.
- *Consistent:* Provide the same message day-to-day so that people can rely on what you say.
- *Correct:* Use technical terms correctly. Make sure you do not make any grammatical or spelling errors.
- *Courteous:* Be friendly, open, and honest.

Active Listening

A large part of the communication process is actually listening. Active listening is discussed in Chapter 2 as it relates to working with patients, but the same concepts apply when working with staff, providers, vendors, and insurance companies. Active listening means that the listener is concentrating on what is being said and how it is being said. The words are important, but so is the nonverbal communication that accompanies them. Distractions should be eliminated so that you can really focus on what the person is saying. This may mean taking the individual somewhere other than your office, where the phone can ring, or others can interrupt. A conference room or an empty exam room can be used. The office manager should also be aware of who might overhear a conversation. The Health Insurance Portability and Accountability Act (HIPAA) considerations must be kept in mind. Whether the office manager is talking with an employee about an issue with a co-worker, a patient with a treatment concern, or a provider about a billing issue, active listening will help to ensure that all parties receive the correct message.

Characteristics of a Good Listener

- Remain nonjudgmental and neutral.
- Refrain from interrupting with a comment or question.
- Allow for periods of silence.
- Smile and nod your head to show you are listening to the message.
- Use appropriate eye contact, so the speaker is not intimidated.
- Lean slightly forward or sideways toward the speaker.
- Avoid distractions (e.g., fidgeting, looking at the clock, doodling).

CRITICAL THINKING APPLICATION **17.2**

A situation with an upset patient came up. The patient was visibly distressed and asked to speak with the office manager. What steps should Kate take to minimize distractions and protect the patient's privacy?

Time Management

Time management is a skill that is invaluable for an office manager. Not only are you responsible for getting your tasks done, but you need to make sure that the staff is also able to complete their tasks. Prioritization is the key to good time management.

Goal setting is the first step in prioritization. If you know what the goals are for the week, month, and year, you can then develop a plan to reach those goals. There will be goals for the healthcare facility, the staff, patient care, and personal goals. Determining the goals for the whole facility will govern some of the goals for the office manager and the staff. Once the goals have been defined, deciding how to achieve those goals will become the task.

Once the tasks have been defined, they can be prioritized. One way to prioritize is to use an ABC system. The most urgent or important task is given an A, less urgent or important tasks are given a B, and those that are the least urgent or important are given a C. Within those categories, the tasks can be ranked by importance, such as A1, A2, B1, B2, etc. (Figure 17.1). An office manager does not have to do all of the tasks; some can be **delegated** to others who are qualified to do them. The tasks can be tracked on a To-Do list that is kept either on paper or electronically. Another method for prioritization can be found in Chapter 1.

Monthly Planning

Keeping track of the activities that occur in the healthcare facility can be a daunting task. Laying out the office schedule for the month is one way to do that. Noting all of the providers' vacations and conferences, vendor meetings, and accountant meetings will help you stay on track and avoid double-booking.

The office manager is also in charge of approving staff vacations. By having a calendar in place that shows when everyone is on vacation, including the providers, the office manager can make sure the approval process moves forward more smoothly. Part of time management for the healthcare facility is making sure that there is adequate staff coverage at all times, keeping in mind that someone may call in sick or have a family emergency during that time.

Week of Nov. 7th

- [x] A1 - Place ad
- [ ] A2 - Arrange Dr. Walden's air transportation to convention
- [ ] A3 - Prepare agenda for staff meeting
- [ ]
- [x] B1 - Prepare performance appraisal for A. Weaver
- [ ] B2 - Set schedule matrix for next quarter
- [ ] B3 - Order supplies
- [ ]
- [ ] C1 - Reorganize supply cabinet
- [ ] C2 - Go through toys in reception area
- [ ]
- [ ]

FIGURE 17.1 ABC system of prioritization.

Staff Meetings

Staff meetings are a formal channel used to keep the office manager and other team members current and communicating on a regular basis. One of the most common complaints from office personnel is that they are unable to discuss problems with the providers. The solution to this problem may be to hold regular staff meetings, which may be scheduled as frequently as weekly but should be held no less often than quarterly. Some of the best ideas for improvement come from the staff; the expression and exchange of good ideas should be encouraged.

Set aside a specific time for regular meetings at an hour when most people can attend with the least disruption. The meetings need not be long or overly formal, but, to be effective, they must be planned and organized. There must be a leader, often the office manager, and someone should be appointed to take notes. All members of the staff should be encouraged to submit ideas for discussion.

Draw up a simple agenda listing the issues to be discussed, and prepare any supporting data needed for the meeting. The agenda can be distributed to the team members ahead of the meeting so that everyone can prepare and participate.

There are many kinds of staff meetings; they may be purely informational, problem-solving, or brainstorming meetings. They may be work sessions for updating manuals, training seminars, or whatever is necessary to the individual practice. Meetings also may be scheduled to discuss new ideas and any changes to in-office procedures. Some meetings are held simply to resolve specific problems. The staff meeting must not be allowed to deteriorate into gripe sessions. Individual complaints should be handled privately.

The meeting's agenda might be similar to that of any business meeting:

1. Reading of the last meeting's minutes
2. Discussion of any unfinished business
3. Discussion of any problems in the clinical area
4. Discussion of any problems in the administrative area
5. Discussion of any problems in common areas
6. Adjournment

Some providers like to combine the staff meeting with breakfast or lunch. The time or place is not important as long as it meets the needs of the practice. Meetings should be conducted democratically and without interruption. Meetings should be kept as brief as possible. Always follow up on the items discussed; otherwise, the only result will be frustration and a reluctance to discuss problems at future meetings. The status of action items from the staff meeting should be introduced in the next staff meeting as *minutes*.

Motivation

Managers have a great deal of influence over the staff they supervise. Successful managers must be interested in the people they work with on a daily basis. It is said that if we help others get what they want in life, then we usually also get what we want.

Successful managers learn that their employees should be encouraged to perform at optimum levels, and managers should be confident enough in their own skills to give credit to employees who develop ideas and concepts for the team. These managers know how to let their employees help them look good. A manager with a group of outstanding employees usually is looked upon as an effective leader.

Frederick Herzberg, known as the Father of Job Enrichment, stated, "Quality work that fosters job satisfaction and health enjoys top priority in industry all over the world." In his book, *The Motivation to Work,* Herzberg stated three points:

1. Jobs must be satisfying and motivate employees to grow and reach their full capabilities.
2. Employees who show greater ability should be given more responsibility.
3. If an employee is not able to achieve success in a specific role, a different employee who can grow and find motivation in the work should be placed in that position.

Effective medical office managers, or office team leaders, recognize those employees are more than static workers. Therefore, motivation is a key component in developing successful employees.

The Power of Motivation

A number of factors can motivate a person to reach a goal:

- Challenging work
- Money
- Recognition
- Satisfaction
- Freedom
- Fear
- Family
- Insecurity
- Competition
- Fulfillment
- Integrity
- Honor
- Reputation
- Responsibility
- Prestige
- Needs
- Love

Any of these motivators can prompt an employee to action. There are two general types of motivation. *Intrinsic motivation* is internal or originates within a person. Intrinsic motivation is long term and can be focused on a lifelong goal. *Extrinsic motivation* is external and more material in nature. Generally, extrinsic motivation is short lived and less satisfying than intrinsic motivation.

Use of Incentives and Employee Recognition

The staff of the provider's office should feel satisfied with the working conditions and atmosphere in the facility. The office manager plays a part in ensuring that this happens.

Incentives give employees reasons to perform over and above the level expected of them. An important element in incentive success is that management establishes clear and attainable goals. If the staff meets or exceeds a goal that has been set, the provider may elect to provide tickets to a sports or entertainment event for the entire staff. Some providers have an incentive program for outstanding patient account collection for a given period. These ideas provide a goal for the employees to work toward and an opportunity to expand their efforts as a team.

Incentives and employee recognition should reward employees for a job well done; also, they will motivate staff members to keep up the great work. Here are some sensible incentives and employee recognition opportunities:

- After an office accomplishment, take the staff out to lunch, order lunch into the office, or schedule a potluck lunch.
- Recognize an employee for exceptional work during a team meeting with a personalized certificate and modest award.
- Set aside a specific time to play office games, trivia, or bingo for modest prizes at the end of a workweek.
- Schedule a weekend activity, such as a company picnic, to which employees can invite their families.

Recognition is a strong method of improving employee morale and encouraging outstanding performance. Offering certificates for peak performance is a great way to motivate employees. For instance, the office manager may decide to award a certificate each month to the employee who provides the highest rated customer service. Patients could even be involved by allowing them to nominate employees for this honor. When an award is at stake, most employees enjoy participating and striving to accomplish the goals that have been set.

CRITICAL THINKING APPLICATION 17.3

Kate has noticed that the medical coding department has been running behind more than usual. As a result, health insurance reimbursements have been lagging. What can Kate do to motivate her employees?

Creating a Team Environment

Teamwork is critical in the medical profession. Communication improves when staff members collaborate as a team in the healthcare workplace, and improved communication can reduce medical errors and increase patient satisfaction. Therefore, the manager must promote an atmosphere where employees are willing to work together toward common goals. Morale in the office may be low because of recent changes in policies or procedures, changes in staff or management, recent terminations of employees, lack of business, or any number of other reasons. Some managers try to shield employees from negative information, but this practice can cause rumors to circulate and worsen morale.

One of the most effective ways to improve employee morale is to communicate openly and honestly. Regular staff meetings, emails, and memos are critical for good communication and the smooth operation of a healthcare facility (Figure 17.2). Communicating changes and developments that affect employees help to improve morale. Morale can also be improved by scheduling activities that involve the families of employees.

Recognize and Overcome Barriers to Communication

Effective communication is important to increase efficiency and improve teamwork. Recognizing barriers to communication in the workplace is critical to the health of the team. The following are five barriers that can occur in a healthcare agency. It is important for the medical assistant to recognize the barriers and help the team overcome them.

- *Physical separation barriers:* In large healthcare facilities, employees can be separated by departments or even by distance if they are in different buildings. Communicating via email can be difficult, and communication cues can be missed, leading to misinterpretation of the message. Using technology (e.g., videoconferencing and webcams) can help employees interact and strengthen communication.
- *Language barriers:* Our workplaces are becoming more diverse. Employees live and train in different areas, learning different communication styles and different words for the same thing. For instance, a surgical instrument may be known by several names as a result of providers training in different parts of the world. Supervisors who encourage awareness and acceptance of everyone's language and cultural differences will strengthen the team's communication.
- *Status barriers:* People may perceive that only those in higher-ranking positions in a healthcare organization are important. This can lead to communication barriers and malfunctioning teams. It is important for the supervisor to promote awareness and acceptance by emphasizing that everyone counts and every position on the team is important.
- *Gender difference barriers:* Males and females communicate differently, with females typically preferring a closer, more personal communication style than males. In some situations, the minority gender in an organization may not be as comfortable communicating with peers. It is important for the supervisor to ensure that all employees, regardless of gender, feel empowered to communicate openly with others.
- *Cultural diversity barriers:* Behaviors, words, and gestures have different meanings from one cultural group to another. How persons of different cultural groups communicate can also be different. For instance, some cultural groups do not believe in eye contact, whereas other groups may perceive a person to be lying or uncomfortable if eye contact is minimal. It is important for the supervisor to help the team embrace the cultural differences among the members and educating the team on the differences can promote understanding and cohesion.

FINDING THE RIGHT EMPLOYEE FOR THE JOB

The most important asset of any healthcare facility is a staff that genuinely cares for patients. From providers to the receptionist, all play a vital role in the quality of the healthcare delivered. Hiring staff members who can be molded into a **cohesive** team is not an easy task. Care should be taken to choose employees who have the necessary skills and the right personality for the ambulatory care facility.

Determining the Need for a New Employee and Getting the Word Out

When the need for a new employee arises, the office manager should discuss with the providers the type of employee needed and the job description for that individual. Ask what qualities the providers desire for the position and the tasks for which the

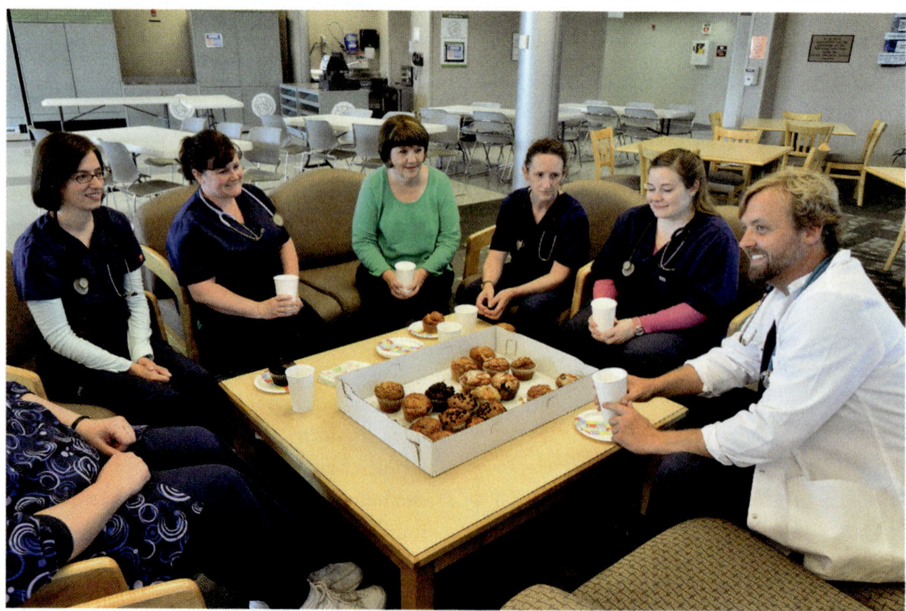

FIGURE 17.2 Communication is vital when building a team. Employees appreciate good communication with management. Sharing good and bad news openly with employees leads to fewer rumors and eases workers' concerns.

person will be responsible. Once the need has been established and the duties confirmed, the office manager can begin the recruiting process.

One of the most effective methods of finding new employees is allowing medical assistant students to complete their practicum at the healthcare facility. This provides an opportunity for the student to learn about the facility, staff, and providers, and for the supervisor to see how the student interacts with others. Even if no openings exist, supervisors can ask the students for a résumé to keep on file until a position opens up. Another effective method for finding new employees is advertising on local job boards. Larger facilities will post the job on their employment website and link to other job boards. Smaller agencies will usually advertise on local, free or low-cost job boards and in local newspapers.

When creating an online ad or a job posting on an employment website, the office manager should list the basic responsibilities and expectations for the position. Briefly describe the office, location, and the qualifications needed. Some offices also list a few of the benefits offered to attract applicants and may also disclose a salary range.

Job Description

A job description is a tool designed to inform job candidates about the duties they would be expected to perform. Well-written and detailed job descriptions list the essential functions of the job and reveal the chain of command the employee should follow when questions or concerns arise. These documents provide a good guideline for potential employees so that they will understand exactly what is expected of them and their responsibilities at work.

Job descriptions are essential in the search for the perfect candidate. They highlight the specific educational background and skill set needed to be successful in the position. A clear job description in the hiring process increases the chance that an applicant with the required skills will apply for the open position. If a job description is too vague, many unqualified applicants may apply, and sorting through all the applications to find the right person for the position will be difficult.

The job description should include a statement that says the employee must perform any additional duties assigned by the supervisor. With this statement in place, the employee cannot say, "That's not my job." All employees should be willing to pull together and assist with any tasks, but this statement gives added weight to assignments that are not specified in the written job description.

An effective manager understands the phrase "inspect what you expect." When duties are assigned, the manager should ensure that the tasks are completed correctly and in a timely manner. New employees should be monitored to make sure their delegated tasks are being done and done right. Without inspection, the manager cannot know whether the new employee is meeting expectations. Once employees have earned a degree of trust, inspecting their work is not as necessary as in the beginning. Some managers practice a skill called "management by walking around." By strolling through the areas where subordinates work, managers can observe and hear about issues that might be brewing, and at the same time, they can improve morale by offering encouragement and praise.

Job Description for a Medical Assistant

Medical assistants are qualified for a variety of tasks in the ambulatory care site. To fill any open medical assisting positions, the manager must determine which specific types of experience will meet the facility's needs. With experience, professional skills can develop in specific aspects of the medical assisting profession. The website www.monster.com provides the following general job description for medical assistants.

Medical Assistant's Job Responsibilities

- Helping patients through information, services, and assistance.

Medical Assistant's Job Duties

- Interviews patients to collect health data; records medical history and confirms purpose of the visit.
- Collects vital patient data by taking blood pressure, weight, and temperature; reports patient history summary.
- Secures patients' private information and preserves patient confidentiality according to HIPAA standards.
- Performs diagnostic and procedural coding, medical billing, and collection procedures for all patient accounts.
- Schedules patient appointments in the medical office and for surgery. Prepares the health record, pre-admit paperwork, and all required consent forms.
- Counsels patients on following provider's orders and answers patients' questions about follow-up care.
- Manages biohazard waste and infection control to protect patients and medical office staff.
- Works with the medical care team to create a safe, secure, and healthy work environment by following office policies and procedures.
- Maintains inventory for medical supplies in the office by taking stock, placing orders, and verifying receipts.
- Supports healthcare facility equipment maintenance by following operating instructions, troubleshooting equipment failure, conducting preventive maintenance, and calling for repairs.
- Displays exceptional customer service to all patients, regardless of age, race, gender, religion, or socioeconomic background.

Medical Assistant's Skills and Qualifications

- Customer service, clinical skills, written and verbal communication, infection control management, time management, scheduling, professionalism, confidentiality, working on a team.

Reviewing Applications

Depending on the situation, the manager may look at the applications as they come in or at the closing date. With today's technology, many agencies have applicants submit cover letters, résumés, and applications online, although some still use paper documents. The first step in reviewing résumés is to separate the applications that meet the minimal qualifications from those that do not. Typically, the minimal qualification includes successful completion of a medical assistant program or a medical assistant credential.

Applicants who meet the minimum qualifications are divided into three stacks: individuals to call for an interview; candidates, but not the strongest; and those who will not be called for an interview. Usually, the manager makes these decisions after reviewing the résumés. Those with related experience, strongly related skill sets (e.g., customer service), no unexplained employment gaps, and customized, error-free résumés and cover letters are more apt to be moved to the top of the pile.

Online Job Applications

Many healthcare facilities request job applicants to complete their employment applications online. The online job application portal is beneficial for the job applicant and the health facility. The health facility can provide specific details about the open medical assisting positions, including the job responsibilities, a brief description of the benefits package, and a description of the company, including its mission statement. For the healthcare facility employer, online medical assisting applicants can be filtered by individual professional experience, skills, certifications, and educational background. These portals allow employers to ask for more information specific to the job description; they can reduce the pool of applicants to just a few skilled candidates.

Once the applications have been reviewed, the office manager can return to the qualifying applications to determine which candidates to interview. Careful judgment and objectivity must be used to search for an employee suitable for the healthcare facility. The manager should review the final applications with the following questions in mind:

- Does the applicant's grammar meet the office's standards? Can the applicant write a business letter?
- Does the applicant have basic computer skills?
- Has the applicant been employed previously in an ambulatory care facility? What were some of the applicant's responsibilities? Is this experience in line with the job description of the open position?
- If the applicant was previously employed, how long was she or he in the last position? Why did the applicant leave?
- Does the applicant seem to accept and enjoy responsibility? Does the applicant have any professional goals that the medical office can train the individual to achieve?
- What is the applicant's formal education? Is she or he registered or certified?
- Is the applicant a member of a professional organization? Does the applicant attend meetings?

Arranging the Personal Interview

In many of the larger healthcare facilities, a human resources representative will conduct a prescreening interview, either over the phone or using technology such as Zoom. At this time, the representative can ask basic questions to gauge the applicant's interest. That information is then forwarded to the office manager. In other agencies, the office manager may conduct the prescreening interview to evaluate the person's telephone voice, attitude, and communication skills. In addition, the manager may want to ask several questions about the person's education, skills, and professional experience. Because the employee probably will speak with patients on the telephone, a qualified candidate should speak with ease. Those who perform well during the prescreening phone call should be scheduled for an interview.

CRITICAL THINKING APPLICATION 17.4

Kate was impressed with Carol Limpken's résumé and application, but when scheduling an interview on the telephone, she noticed that Carol's grammar was not as professional as Kate would like. Should this influence Kate's decision on whether to hire Carol? Why is speech such an important issue in a healthcare facility? Should Kate be concerned about a candidate's grammar and spelling errors on the résumé or application? Why or why not?

Set a time for the personal interview when the applicant can be given undivided attention. When an in-person interview is used, an applicant being considered for employment should have an opportunity to see the facility during a period of fairly normal activity. The candidate who is interviewed in a peaceful, quiet office may not be prepared for the activity on a normal working day.

Before interviewing any applicant, become thoroughly familiar with the federal, state, and local fair employment practice laws affecting hiring practices. The Equal Employment Opportunity Act of 1972 prohibits inquiries into an applicant's race, color, gender, religion, and national origin. Inquiries about medical history, arrest records, or previous drug use also are illegal. Office managers must research the laws that pertain to employment in their states or work with the human resources team, who are more familiar with these laws. It is important to develop a list of questions that will be asked of all interviewees. Creating a question list before the interviews helps to ensure no illegal questions are asked and that all interviewees are fairly evaluated (Table 17.1).

TABLE 17.1 Legal and Illegal Interview Questions

LEGAL QUESTIONS	ILLEGAL QUESTIONS
• Why did you leave your last job? • What are your strengths and weaknesses? • What motivates you to succeed? • What are some of your hobbies? • Are you willing to work more than 40 hours a week?	• How long have you been working? • When was the last time you used drugs? • Do you have any children? • What religion do you practice? • Are you married?

Laws Affecting Employment

Numerous laws affect the way employees are treated, from the interview through the end of employment. The office manager should be familiar with these laws and how they affect the practice.

Fair Labor Standards Act

- State standards for minimum wage and overtime pay; employees must be paid minimum wage and time and a half for overtime hours, as they apply
- Prohibits those under age 18 from performing certain kinds of work and restricts the hours of workers under age 16

Occupational Safety and Health Act

- Regulates conditions affecting employees' safety and health in the workplace

Workers' Compensation

- Regulates the benefits of employees who have been injured on the job
- Determines pay for employees who are not working because of an on-the-job injury

Family and Medical Leave Act

- Requires employers of 50 or more employees to offer up to 12 weeks of unpaid, job-protected leave to eligible employees for the birth of a child, an adoption, or a personal or family illness

Pregnancy Discrimination Act

- Forbids employers from refusing to hire a woman based on pregnancy, childbirth, or related medical conditions
- Requires employers to hold open a job for a pregnancy-related absence for the same length of time that a job would be held open for employees on sick or disability leave

Americans with Disabilities Act

- Prohibits discrimination against individuals with disabilities

Age Discrimination Act

- Prevents discrimination in hiring on the basis of age
- Prevents discrimination in promoting, discharging, and compensating employees

The Interview

The interview is usually conducted by the office manager or with a panel of employees. If a panel is being used, the members should meet before the interview to create a list of interview questions and discuss the flow of the interview. Each interviewee should be asked the same questions. Additional questions may be asked of individual candidates to clarify responses to the standard set of questions.

The interview typically starts with an introduction of the interviewers and a review of the job description. Usually, the first question (e.g., "Tell us about yourself") is meant to put the person at ease and get a summary of the person's professional and educational background. As the interview progresses, different types of questions will be asked to explore the person's past experiences and personality. Straightforward questions relate to the position duties. Behavioral questions are given to explore how the person behaved during a difficult past situation to anticipate how that candidate might handle future issues. Situational questions help the interviewers understand how the person would handle a hypothetical situation. The interviewers use the questions to explore the person's personality and past experiences and to gauge how the person might fit into the existing team.

After the questions are completed, the manager should allow the interviewee an opportunity to ask questions. Some interviews conclude with a discussion of the benefits and pay, but many times this occurs when the job is being offered to the applicant because the human resources representative is the best resource for this information. Last, the office manager should give the interviewee an idea of the next steps in the process and when the decision will be made. If the person hasn't completed an application form, it is important to have that completed before the person leaves. References should also be collected from the interviewee.

Once the applicant leaves, the interviewers should rate or summarize their impressions of the applicant, listing the strengths and weaknesses on the interview question form. Be objective and professional, and do not write **disparaging** information. The form will be kept on file in case of discrimination claims in hiring practices.

Usually, discussions of the candidate among the interview team are not encouraged until after all the interviews are completed. After all the interviews are conducted, the interviewers, as a group, should rank the candidates and finalize the top choices.

Follow-up Activities

Always carefully check all references and follow through on any leads for information. Contact all listed references. When speaking with a candidate's former employer, be sure to listen between the lines. Note the tone of the replies to the questions. Do not ask questions that might incriminate the person answering them. The following questions are effective as an introduction:

- When did (the applicant) work for you? For how long?
- What duties and responsibilities were assigned to the employee? Did the employee assume responsibility well?
- Did the employee work well in a team environment? Did any conflicts arise that we should know about?

Some employers provide information only on the date of hire, job title, and date of termination of the employment. However, if the employer states, "She worked in our office from May 2018 to July 2019 and is not eligible for rehire," the reasonable assumption is that the employee did not perform well. The tone of voice and emphasis on the word *not* should be clues that this person is probably not right for the job. Still, if all other references are glowing, call and ask the applicant about the facility that gave the negative response. There could be a reasonable explanation for what might have been a bad experience. Respect the company's policy and do not press for further information.

After the applicant list has been narrowed to two or three candidates whose references have been checked thoroughly, a second interview may be arranged. The providers may want to participate in these interviews.

Selecting the Right Applicant

Once the final interviews have been conducted, it is time to choose the best candidate. Never rely strictly on a gut instinct about a potential employee. Base hiring decisions on logical conclusions drawn from all contacts with the applicant, including the following:

- Grammar and enunciation
- Office manners and customer service skills

- Professional appearance
- Work history
- Match to required job skills
- Friendly, personable attitude

When a decision has been reached to hire someone, either a human resource representative or the office manager will contact the person. This is the most common time to discuss wages and benefits. The applicant may request 2 to 3 days to think over the offer. Make sure you have a firm date when the applicant will deliver a decision.

When the position is filled, the human resources representative or the office manager needs to contact all the applicants and explain the job has been filled. This notification can occur through email, a letter, or a phone call. Be courteous in the notification, and thank the individual for applying.

WORKING WITH NEW AND ESTABLISHED EMPLOYEES

The needs of a new employee can be different from the needs of an established employee, but both want the office manager to recognize their needs and then act to meet those needs. The following sections discuss how that can be done.

Documentation for New Employees

The office manager should develop a checklist of the documents needed for newly hired staff members and all the information that should be covered with the new employee at the start of the job. Basic new employee documentation often includes the following:

- HIPAA confidentiality statement
- Computer passwords and agreement statement
- Job application
- Form I-9 (Employment Eligibility Verification)
- W-4 Form (Employee's Withholding Allowance Certificate)
- Notice of workers' compensation coverage
- Consent for background check, drug testing, and search (if applicable)
- Acknowledgment of receipt of company handbook or policy manual
- Agreements regarding pay, wage deductions, benefits, schedule, work location, and so on
- Notices of at-will employment status
- Direct deposit application
- Occupational Safety and Health Administration (OSHA) compliance acknowledgment or checklist

All of these forms, once completed and signed, should be kept in the employee's personnel file. Other forms and documents may be necessary that vary from state to state and company to company. The Form I-9 (Employment Eligibility Verification) is required by the federal government (Figure 17.3). This form must be completed for all newly hired employees to verify their identification and authorization to work in the United States. The most current form is available at www.uscis.gov, along with training materials. The newly hired employee should complete the first section of the form and provide it to the human resource representative or office manager on the first day of work. The remaining information is completed by the representative or manager. Specific documents need to be shown to prove the person's identification and authorization to work in this country. A person who cannot provide the required documentation should not be allowed to remain as an employee.

Employees should also understand the *at-will employment* status. Under the at-will employment principle, the employer can terminate the employment at any time, for any reason/cause, and without notice. Unless the employer violated labor laws or the employee's rights, the employee has little recourse. Only a few states protect employees from termination without good cause. At-will employment also means that the employee can leave the employment at any time, but professionally it is important to give the employer the required notice.

Orientation and Training for New Employees

The hiring process does not end with hiring a new employee. Orientation and training help new employees understand what is expected and to develop to their full potential (Figure 17.4). A critical error made when bringing new staff members aboard is failing to provide them with a fair orientation and training period.

Some managers assign a **mentor** to assist the new employee during the initial probationary period. This type of buddy system is a good practice because the new person does not feel isolated and alone during the first few weeks on the job.

Acquaint the new employee with the following:

- Staff members and their names
- Physical environment and layout of the office
- Nature of the practice and specialty
- Types of patients seen in the office
- Office policies and procedures
- Employee benefits
- Short- and long-range expectations
- HIPAA and computer training

Types of Employee Benefits

- *Employer-sponsored health insurance:* The employer pays a percentage of the employee's health insurance premiums.
- *Dental and vision benefits:* The employer may offer dental and vision benefits for employees but may choose not to sponsor any of the premium.
- *Cafeteria plan:* A tax-free account in which employees can invest some of their paycheck and from which they can withdraw amounts for qualified health or child day-care expenses.
- *401k retirement account matching:* The employer matches the exact amount or a percentage of the investment the employee makes every pay period (2% to 3%) up to a specific amount ($1,500).
- *Life insurance:* The employer pays for a small life insurance policy (usually up to $15,000) for minimal after-death expenses.
- *Disability insurance:* A benefit employees pay for that pays them if they are disabled and unable to work.

All new employees should be required to familiarize themselves with important office policies and procedures by reviewing the policies and procedures manual. It is advisable for the manager to require the employee to sign a statement verifying that the manual has been read.

Department of Homeland Security
U.S. Citizenship and Immigration Services

Form I-9, Employment Eligibility Verification

Read instructions carefully before completing this form. The instructions must be available during completion of this form.

ANTI-DISCRIMINATION NOTICE: It is illegal to discriminate against work-authorized individuals. Employers CANNOT specify which document(s) they will accept from an employee. The refusal to hire an individual because the documents have a future expiration date may also constitute illegal discrimination.

Section 1. Employee Information and Verification *(To be completed and signed by employee at the time employment begins.)*

Print Name: Last | First | Middle Initial | Maiden Name

Address *(Street Name and Number)* | Apt. # | Date of Birth *(month/day/year)*

City | State | Zip Code | Social Security #

I am aware that federal law provides for imprisonment and/or fines for false statements or use of false documents in connection with the completion of this form.

I attest, under penalty of perjury, that I am (check one of the following):

☐ A citizen of the United States
☐ A noncitizen national of the United States (see instructions)
☐ A lawful permanent resident (Alien #) ______
☐ An alien authorized to work (Alien # or Admission #) ______
until (expiration date, if applicable - *month/day/year*)

Employee's Signature | Date *(month/day/year)*

Preparer and/or Translator Certification *(To be completed and signed if Section 1 is prepared by a person other than the employee.) I attest, under penalty of perjury, that I have assisted in the completion of this form and that to the best of my knowledge the information is true and correct.*

Preparer's/Translator's Signature | Print Name

Address *(Street Name and Number, City, State, Zip Code)* | Date *(month/day/year)*

Section 2. Employer Review and Verification *(To be completed and signed by employer. Examine one document from List A OR examine one document from List B and one from List C, as listed on the reverse of this form, and record the title, number, and expiration date, if any, of the document(s).)*

	List A	OR	List B	AND	List C
Document title:					
Issuing authority:					
Document #:					
Expiration Date *(if any)*:					
Document #:					
Expiration Date *(if any)*:					

CERTIFICATION: I attest, under penalty of perjury, that I have examined the document(s) presented by the above-named employee, that the above-listed document(s) appear to be genuine and to relate to the employee named, that the employee began employment on *(month/day/year)* ______ **and that to the best of my knowledge the employee is authorized to work in the United States. (State employment agencies may omit the date the employee began employment.)**

Signature of Employer or Authorized Representative | Print Name | Title

Business or Organization Name and Address *(Street Name and Number, City, State, Zip Code)* | Date *(month/day/year)*

Section 3. Updating and Reverification *(To be completed and signed by employer.)*

A. New Name *(if applicable)* | B. Date of Rehire *(month/day/year) (if applicable)*

C. If employee's previous grant of work authorization has expired, provide the information below for the document that establishes current employment authorization.

Document Title: ______ Document #: ______ Expiration Date *(if any)*: ______

I attest, under penalty of perjury, that to the best of my knowledge, this employee is authorized to work in the United States, and if the employee presented document(s), the document(s) I have examined appear to be genuine and to relate to the individual.

Signature of Employer or Authorized Representative | Date *(month/day/year)*

Form I-9 (Rev.) Y Page 4

FIGURE 17.3 The I-9 Form (Employment Eligibility Verification) is designed to help the employer gather the documents necessary to prove that an employee is eligible to work in the United States.

Continued

LISTS OF ACCEPTABLE DOCUMENTS

All documents must be unexpired

LIST A **Documents that Establish Both Identity and Employment Authorization**	OR	LIST B **Documents that Establish Identity**	AND	LIST C **Documents that Establish Employment Authorization**
1. U.S. Passport or U.S. Passport Card		**1.** Driver's license or ID card issued by a State or outlying possession of the United States provided it contains a photograph or information such as name, date of birth, gender, height, eye color, and address		**1.** Social Security Account Number card other than one that specifies on the face that the issuance of the card does not authorize employment in the United States
2. Permanent Resident Card or Alien Registration Receipt Card (Form I-551)		**2.** ID card issued by federal, state or local government agencies or entities, provided it contains a photograph or information such as name, date of birth, gender, height, eye color, and address		**2.** Certification of Birth Abroad issued by the Department of State (Form FS-545)
3. Foreign passport that contains a temporary I-551 stamp or temporary I-551 printed notation on a machine-readable immigrant visa		**3.** School ID card with a photograph		**3.** Certification of Report of Birth issued by the Department of State (Form DS-1350)
4. Employment Authorization Document that contains a photograph (Form I-766)		**4.** Voter's registration card		**4.** Original or certified copy of birth certificate issued by a State, county, municipal authority, or territory of the United States bearing an official seal
5. In the case of a nonimmigrant alien authorized to work for a specific employer incident to status, a foreign passport with Form I-94 or Form I-94A bearing the same name as the passport and containing an endorsement of the alien's nonimmigrant status, as long as the period of endorsement has not yet expired and the proposed employment is not in conflict with any restrictions or limitations identified on the form		**5.** U.S. Military card or draft record		**5.** Native American tribal document
6. Passport from the Federated States of Micronesia (FSM) or the Republic of the Marshall Islands (RMI) with Form I-94 or Form I-94A indicating nonimmigrant admission under the Compact of Free Association Between the United States and the FSM or RMI		**6.** Military dependent's ID card		**6.** U.S. Citizen ID Card (Form I-197)
		7. U.S. Coast Guard Merchant Mariner Card		**7.** Identification Card for Use of Resident Citizen in the United States (Form I-179)
		8. Native American tribal document		**8.** Employment authorization document issued by the Department of Homeland Security
		9. Driver's license issued by a Canadian government authority		
		For persons under age 18 who are unable to present a document listed above:		
		10. School record or report card		
		11. Clinic, doctor, or hospital record		
		12. Day-care or nursery school record		

Illustrations of many of these documents appear in Part 8 of the Handbook for Employers (M-274)

Form I-9 (Rev.) Y Page 5

FIGURE 17.3 cont'd

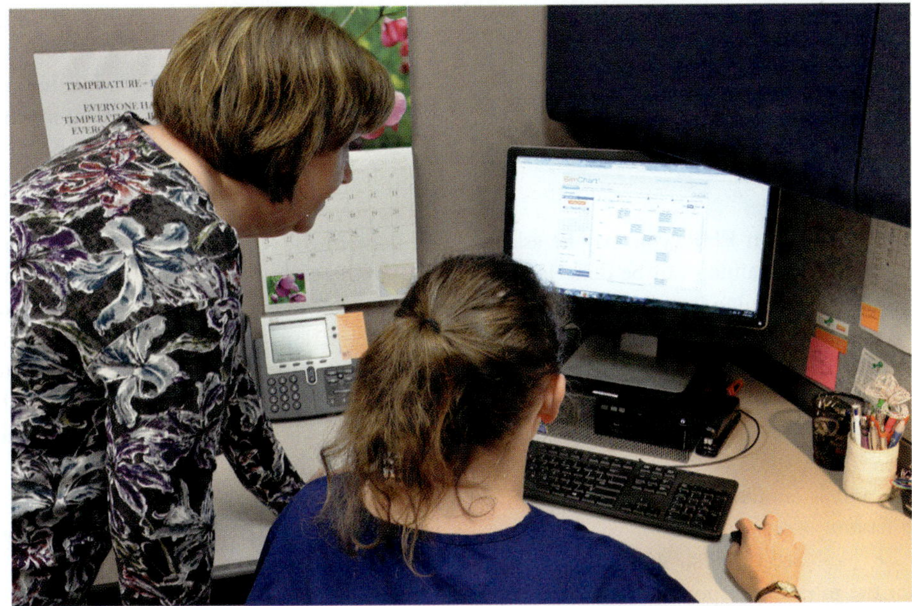

FIGURE 17.4 The training of successful employees begins with the job orientation.

Make sure the employee's file is complete before allowing the person to work even 1 hour. Also, make sure all federal and state regulations that apply to new employees have been met.

Training for All Employees

Ongoing training for all employees is important so that all employees have the ability to do their jobs correctly and efficiently. This may mean face-to-face training or virtual training. It is part of the office manager's role to ensure that these training sessions offer the employees what they need. The next sections discuss training as well as coaching and mentoring techniques.

Remote/Virtual Training and Support

With the adoption of an electronic health record (EHR) and as systems are updated, there will be a need for training and ongoing support for users. Oftentimes the training or support is done remotely or virtually. It is important to make sure that everyone has what they need to be able to access the training. Here are some things to consider before providing remote/virtual training:

- *Equipment needs*: Does everyone have the equipment needed for remote/virtual training, such as a camera and microphone?
- *Internet access:* Does everyone have reliable internet access so that they can be involved in the training?
- *Learning styles:* People learn differently, and effective training must keep in mind the different learning styles and have content that relates to those styles.
- *Protection from online intrusion:* All users must have adequate online security in order to protect all of the information that is being shared or accessed.

EHR Training and Documentation

Several different materials can be employed when training users on an EHR system. The EHR vendor may provide training manuals to explain the basics of the system, but each healthcare organization will want to develop a training manual that is specific to that specific organization. This manual should be available in both print and electronic format.

Many users find it helpful to have computer-based learning modules and online tutorials available, even after the initial training. These materials then become a resource for all users to refer to when a question comes up.

When looking to develop EHR training materials, several factors should be kept in mind:

- Needs assessment
  - Is the training needed?
  - Who needs it? How will they learn best?
- Design/development
  - How will the training be provided?
  - What level of training is needed?
  - What resources are needed and are available?
- Implementation/evaluation
  - New training can be done with just a few users who can then provide feedback. Make changes as needed before rolling out to all users.
  - Use surveys to gauge satisfaction and determine what changes might need to be made.

All training provided should be documented to stay compliant with state and federal regulations. This documentation should include who received the training, when the training was provided, and what the training involved. The human resources department typically keeps track of staff training, and it becomes part of the employment record.

EHR Software Reference Library. Electronic health records are used to provide the best possible care to patients. This involves making sure that providers have access to the most up-to-date information. Reference libraries within the EHR are where that information is located. This information can include resources on specific diagnoses and treatment recommendations, data about medications and their side effects, and guidelines for patient decision making. Another use of EHR reference libraries is in the clinical decision support systems

(CDSS). CDSS can analyze the data found in the EHR and provide prompts and reminders at the point of care. The EHR can let the healthcare professional know that patients need certain immunizations or preventive health services such as a mammogram or colonoscopy.

Coaching and Mentoring Techniques

As you gain experience working with an EHR, you may be asked to coach or mentor other users. This training can be done in several different ways. One strategy for training is to create a group of "super users." Super users are staff members who are well versed in how the EHR functions and are willing to work with others sharing helpful hints, tips, and techniques. It is helpful if each department has at least one super user per shift to be available for questions. Ideally, a super user has been trained to move through the EHR system quickly and efficiently and is familiar with the organization's workflow and patient population.

Another strategy is to use role-based training. With this training, the sessions are tailored for the roles and responsibilities of the user group and focus on their needs when using the EHR.

Process-based training involves helping the staff to understand the new workflows when a new EHR system is introduced or as updates to the current EHR system occur.

Procedure for Disseminating Updated Information

When there is new information regarding the EHR system that needs to get to users but does not require a full training session, this information can be sent out in an email or discussed at department meetings. However, the information is dispersed to users; it should be made clear how they can get answers to questions that might come up. If the information is given during a staff or department meeting, a super user should be the one to present the information and be available to answer questions.

Using Performance Evaluations Effectively

A new employee should be granted a probationary period. The traditional period is 60 to 90 days, but many employers believe that 2 weeks is sufficient to determine whether the employee will be able to learn and adapt to the position. Set a specific date for a performance evaluation covering the probationary period when the new employee is hired. This evaluation should not be squeezed in between patient visits or be given a token few minutes at the end of a day. Schedule a time that provides the opportunity to relax and talk. Tell the new employee how well expectations have been met and whether there are any deficiencies; then, give the employee an opportunity to ask questions. Sometimes employees fail to perform because they were never told what was expected. Although the probationary period does not always allow time to train an individual fully for a specific position, it is fair to assume that the potential for being a satisfactory employee can be judged at this time. Now is the time to talk about any problems and make suggestions for improvement. Sometimes the employee is released after an unsuccessful probationary period.

The formal performance appraisal usually occurs at the end of the probationary period and then at the hiring date anniversary. A typical appraisal includes feedback on teamwork, punctuality and attendance, motivation, accuracy with skills, customer service, professionalism, and potential continuing education and future goals. In many facilities, the appraisal relates to the pay increase the person will receive. Agencies do performance appraisals differently, yet one of the more common methods is for the supervisor to gather input from peers that work with the employee. The 360-degree evaluation is a process in which the supervisor, peers, and those who interact with the employee outside of the department provide feedback for the performance appraisal. If an employee works well with peers in the department yet is rude and unprofessional to employees in other areas of the facility, the 360-degree evaluation will provide that information. This evaluation process holds employees accountable for all their interactions in the facility.

When negative information is relayed to the employee during a performance appraisal, sandwich the negative comment between two positive ones whenever possible. For instance, tell the employee, "Jewel, you are a pro at greeting patients and making them feel at home. I would like to see you improve your time management skills, however, because I feel you are spending too much time with individual patients. I must confess that they feel a part of the clinic family. Let's work on some time management issues and keep making them feel so welcome!"

Managers also may use the "feel, felt, found" approach when talking with employees about their performance. For example, "Jewel, I feel the same way you do about patients taking up a lot of our time. I know there are some who want to talk with us for hours, and I have felt the pressure of wanting to make them feel comfortable but having so much to do, too. I have found that if I explain that I have a meeting or another patient to assist, they are very understanding and not offended. Perhaps you can try that approach, too."

No supervisor enjoys giving an evaluation (Figure 17.5) that is not a positive one. It is difficult to know exactly where to begin when the employee has not performed as expected or hoped. Perhaps the best way to open the conversation is to say, "Rebecca, your review today is not going to be a positive one. It seems that we do not have a meeting of the minds about your duties and our expectations of you. Let's talk about your performance and discuss whether this position is a good match for you." Having detailed documentation of performance issues leaves little room for argument and places the manager on the offensive. The employee may be apprehensive or even defensive at this point, but the phrasing will certainly command attention, and the discussion should produce either the motivation to improve or the clarity that termination is in order.

Fair Salaries and Raises

Medical office managers should recruit employees who want to remain with the office for a long time. There are always situations such as a part-time worker returning to college or a summer worker going back to school. However, good employee **retention** is the goal.

The practice must pay them a fair salary with regular raises to retain good employees if they perform as expected. The office manager can find information about salary comparisons on the internet. Periodically review job descriptions and salary analyses online to see whether the salary the medical facility offers is comparable to that for similar jobs in the area.

Merit raises are increases based on an employee's commendable performance. Cost-of-living increases are given when earned, usually after specific periods or annually, and are based on national statistics

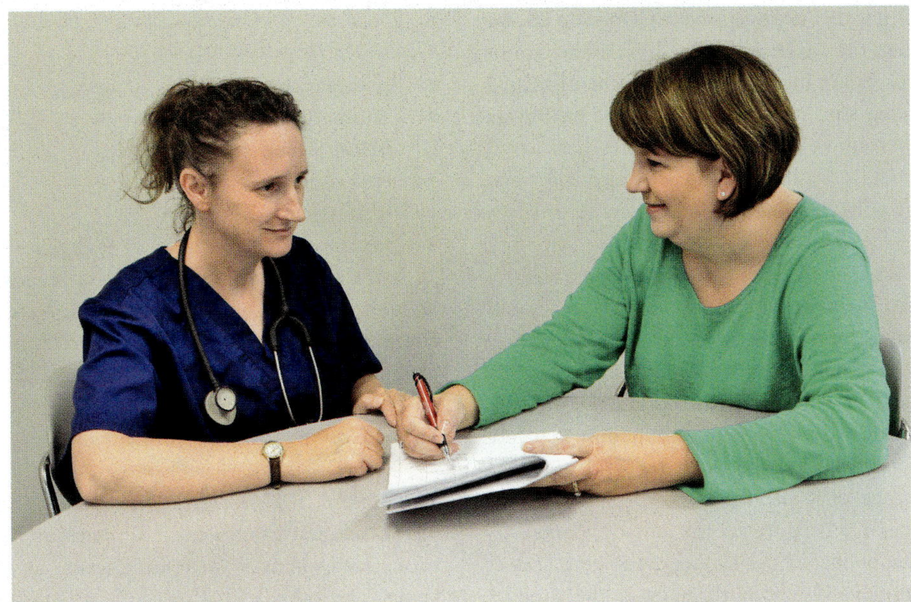

FIGURE 17.5 **Performance Evaluation and Development Plan.** Performance evaluations should be considered tools that help employees reach their personal goals and the goals of the organization.

and trends. An employee who is promoted should also be awarded a salary increase. When the office pays a fair salary for work done, the facility retains happy employees.

Problem Employees

Occasionally, employees do not perform at the expected level or demonstrate unprofessional behaviors. Counseling these employees to determine the source of their difficulties is the first step toward resolution. Many employees can be redirected to become productive staff members with a little patience and understanding on the manager's part. Employees who display a willingness to improve their attitude are worth the investment the office manager makes to help them succeed.

Many offices allow one verbal warning before written reprimands go into the employee's file. It is important that the manager document the specific times, dates, and descriptions of incidents, even issues such as tardiness. If the manager does not make a habit of writing a formal warning in the employee's **human resources file (HR file)**, there may be insufficient documentation of problems. The manager should never be in a position in which the termination of an employee cannot be justified through documentation.

CRITICAL THINKING APPLICATION 17.5

Kate has two employees who have never seemed to get along. One of the employees has a history of being vindictive and manipulative, but never in an obvious enough way for Kate to have sufficient proof to reprimand her in writing. One day, one of the employees comes to Kate's office to report that she saw the other employee, who has an exemplary record, taking drugs from the supply cabinet. How does Kate handle this situation? What steps should Kate take from here?

Terminating Employees

Terminating an employee is unpleasant at best, but if the ground rules are decided in advance, written into the office policies and procedures manual, and explained to all employees, the problem is partially solved. The policies must be applied equally and impartially to all employees. The providers of the healthcare facility will most probably make the final decision on dismissal, but it may be based on the recommendation of the office manager. Unless there are mitigating factors that suggest otherwise, the person who does the hiring should do the firing.

A probationary employee who does not prove satisfactory should be dismissed at the end of the probationary period, with tact and a full explanation of the reasons for dismissal. In all fairness, an individual should be told why the employment is ending and not be given weak excuses or untruths that do not help correct deficiencies. If the manager is not straightforward in giving the reason for dismissal, the employee will not have the opportunity to grow and improve future performance.

An employee who has been in service for some time and is not performing satisfactorily should be warned and given an explanation of the specific improvements expected. If a second chance does not produce improvement in performance or attitude, dismissal must follow. It should be done privately, with tact and consideration.

Most practice consultants believe that firing should come close to the end of the day and end of the workweek after all other employees have left and that the break should be clean and immediate. A dismissed employee should never be allowed to train or influence a replacement.

The exit meeting should be planned just as carefully as the employment interview. Be honest with the employee. Discuss both the employee's assets and liabilities and give the reasons for the termination. There is no need to dwell on the employee's deficiencies. These should have been thoroughly discussed at the warning interview, and the employee need only be told that the necessary improvements have not been made. Listen to the employee's feedback unless it becomes lengthy or abusive. This may reveal some important administrative problems that need correction.

After dismissing an employee, do not leave that person in the office unattended. Request the office keys and any other equipment in the employee's possession immediately before the dismissed employee leaves the building, and block all access to the healthcare facility's electronic health records (EHRs). Most states have strict payday laws that do not allow holding the final paycheck for any reason. Do not offer to give the employee a good reference unless it can be done sincerely.

If there is any indication that an employee may become abusive or violent once told about the termination, the supervisor should bring a representative from the human resources department or security to the final interview. It is possible that an employee can "snap" and suddenly become violent; however, more often, it is the warning flags raised by an employee's behavior before termination that justify care in the termination interview. Therefore, supervisors should always document any strange or suspicious employee behavior and any breach of office policy or procedures in the employee's personnel file, according to office policy. Documenting everything creates a clear picture of the employee's actions throughout the time of employment. Of course, the supervisor must be willing to confront an employee about negative actions in the workplace.

Some specific employee behaviors in the workplace, such as embezzlement, insubordination, and violation of patient confidentiality, are grounds for immediate dismissal without warning. These behaviors display a lack of respect for the healthcare facility and can lead to the mistreatment or endangerment of patients if the employee is not terminated immediately.

Occasionally an employee voluntarily leaves a position without giving a valid reason. The provider or office manager may want to follow up with a letter to the former employee to determine whether a problem prompted the resignation. The employee may reveal serious issues with other personnel or with the office that need to be addressed and corrected.

CRITICAL THINKING APPLICATION **17.6**

While Kate is explaining to a particularly poor employee why she plans to terminate her, the employee begins screaming and accusing Kate of discrimination and harassment. How should Kate handle this situation? What are Kate's options if the employee does not stop the inappropriate behavior?

POLICIES AND PROCEDURES

Within the medical office, many different policies and procedures are needed to ensure the smooth running of the facility. Personnel policies focus on the rules related to the employer-employee relationship, and office policies and procedures focus on the tasks that are completed within the medical office.

Personnel Policy Manual

Information about the employer-employee relationship is found in the personnel policy manual, sometimes referred to as the employee handbook. It spells out the healthcare facility's rules regarding issues such as the following:

- Health benefits
- Vacation time
- Sick leave
- Holidays
- Overtime
- Performance evaluations
- Termination of employment
- *Grievance* (complaint) process
- Dress code
- Office safety
- Employee's role in case of an emergency

Some agencies will give each new employee a copy of the personnel policy manual, and others keep a copy in a central location. More commonly, the manual will be found electronically on the agency's intranet. The personnel policy manual should be updated on a regular basis. This can easily be done when it is in an electronic format, but employees should be notified when an update occurs.

Workplace Sexual Harassment

The US Equal Employment Opportunity Commission states that sexual harassment is unwelcome sexual advances, requests for sexual favors, and other verbal or physical harassment of a sexual nature. Sexual harassment is against the law. Both the victim and the harasser can be either a woman or a man, and the victim and harasser can be of the same sex. The harasser can be the victim's supervisor, a supervisor in another area, a co-worker, or someone who is not an employee of the employer, such as a client or customer.

A medical office manager will need to make all employees aware of what conduct is considered sexual harassment. When an employee feels that she or he is being sexually harassed, the employee should report it to the supervisor or office manager. Once a report has been made, the manager must investigate the allegation. Actions must be taken to protect all employees because the healthcare facility is at risk for a lawsuit.

The office manager wants to ensure that the healthcare facility is a comfortable place for all employees to work without being the target of unwanted sexual advances. There are no laws against two employees dating each other, but it is a good idea to have a policy in place regarding supervisors dating subordinates. It can be hard to determine whether the subordinate felt pressured to date the supervisor in order to keep the job.

Employees should keep in mind that it can be considered sexual harassment to have an explicit calendar or poster. If another employee finds it offensive, that person can make a claim of sexual harassment. Some organizations will have a policy regarding office decorations.

Workplace Bullying

Workplace bullying is defined by the Workplace Bullying Institute as: repeated mistreatment of an employee by one or more employees; abusive conduct that is threatening, humiliating, or intimidating; work sabotage; or verbal abuse. The institute's 2017 survey showed that 19% of Americans are bullied, and 60.4 million people are affected by workplace bullying. Only 29% of those who are bullied report it. It is likely that these workers will leave their jobs to get away from the bullying. It is the office manager's responsibility to take all accusations seriously and also to create an environment in which employees will freely come to the manager when there is an issue, whether the person is the victim or a witness. It has to be made clear that bullying will not be tolerated.

Office Policies and Procedures

Office policies and procedures differ from personnel policies in that they provide direction on how to complete tasks within the healthcare facility.

Clinical Procedures

Clinical procedures will vary from one healthcare facility to another, depending on the type of facility. A family practice facility will have different procedures than a plastic surgery facility. All procedures should have a list of instruments and supplies needed, along with step-by-step instructions on how to complete the procedure. Having a standard procedure that everyone follows ensures consistency in patient care.

Administrative Procedures

Administrative procedures can also vary, depending on the type of medical practice, but they usually cover topics such as opening and closing the office, appointment scheduling, patient account processing, insurance claim processing, and eligibility verification.

Regulatory Compliance

It is important for an office manager in a healthcare facility to stay current with all changes in legislation at both the state and federal levels. This will ensure that the facility is working within the legal boundaries. There can be severe consequences when a healthcare facility is noncompliant.

Health Insurance Portability and Accountability Act (HIPAA)

The office manager is responsible for ensuring that the healthcare facility is **compliant** with all aspects of HIPAA (see Chapter 4). All employees should be trained in HIPAA compliance, such as protecting patient information. Violations of HIPAA can result in fines and possible jail time. The Office for Civil Rights (OCR) is responsible for enforcing the HIPAA Privacy and Security Rules. The fines were increased when the Health Information Technology for Economic and Clinical Health Act (HITECH) was enacted.

Health Information Technology for Economic and Clinical Health Act (HITECH)

HITECH includes provisions that allow for increased enforcement of the privacy and security of electronic transmission of health information. HITECH expanded on HIPAA by doing the following:

- Making business associates directly liable for compliance with HIPAA.
- Prohibiting the sale of protected health information (PHI) without the patient's authorization.
- Creating a tiered violation category: unknowing, reasonable cause, willful neglect–corrected, and willful neglected–uncorrected. Violation penalties range from $100 for each "unknowing" violation to $1.5 million per calendar year. The greater the violation, the greater the penalty amount. Individuals, healthcare agencies, and business associations could be penalized and fined.
- *Breach* notification requirements were increased. Individuals must be notified of the breach via mail or email. If the facility does not have up-to-date contact information for 10 or more patients, then a notice must be posted on the company's website for at least 90 days. If more than 500 individuals were impacted, then the media and the OCR secretary must be notified. A list of breaches reported is published on the OCR website (https://ocrportal.hhs.gov/ocr/breach/breach_report.jsf).

TABLE 17.2 HIPAA[a] Penalties

HIPAA VIOLATION	MINIMUM PENALTY	MAXIMUM PENALTY
Unknowing	$100 per violation, with an annual maximum of $25,000 for repeat violations	$50,000 per violation, with an annual maximum of $25,000
Reasonable cause	$1000 per violation, with an annual maximum of $100,000 for repeat violations	$50,000 per violation with an annual maximum of $100,000
Willful neglect but violation is corrected within the required time period	$10,000 per violation, with an annual maximum of $250,000 for repeat violations	$50,000 per violation, with an annual maximum of $250,000
Willful neglect and is not corrected within the required time period	$50,000 per violation, with an annual maximum of $1.5 million	$50,000 per violation, with an annual maximum of $1.5 million

[a]Health Insurance Portability and Accountability Act.

Table 17.2 describes the possible penalties that could be imposed by OCR.

On June 1, 2018, a $4.3 million fine was imposed on the University of Texas MD Anderson Cancer Center. There were three separate data breaches that involved the theft of an unencrypted laptop and the loss of two unencrypted thumb drives that contained unencrypted electronic protected health information (ePHI) of more than 33,500 individuals. HIPAA compliance should not be taken lightly.

You can see why compliance with HIPAA and HITECH is very important. It is one of the responsibilities of an office manager to make sure that the healthcare facility is completely compliant with all regulations.

Occupational Safety and Health Act

The Occupational Safety and Health Act of 1970 (OSH Act) was created and is enforced by the Occupational Safety and Health Administration (OSHA). OSHA sets workplace standards and inspects employers to ensure employee safety. The standards that apply to the healthcare setting include those related to bloodborne pathogens, hazard communication, occupational exposure to hazardous chemicals in laboratories, ionizing radiation, nonionizing radiation, and means of egress. Employers must be compliant with all of OSHA's regulations. More information on the OSHA standards can be found in Chapter 4. Employers with more than 10 employees are required to keep a record of serious work-related injuries and illnesses. Each year employers must post a summary of the injuries and illnesses recorded for the previous year. This tracking and reporting is the responsibility of the office manager.

GENERATING AND USING REPORTS

The office manager will be involved in generating and using reports to ensure that the healthcare facility is running as smoothly and efficiently as possible. This includes clinical and financial reports. These reports can help determine productivity and opportunities for improvement in policies and procedures. These reports can also be used for quality improvement measures. The following sections discuss the generation of reports and how they are used.

Methods of Generating Reports

The practice management software provides the ability to generate various types of reports, including reports regarding clinical services provided and financial reports. These reports can be used to ensure that patients are getting all of the care they need and the healthcare facility remains healthy financially.

Clinical Reports

Several clinical reports can be generated by the practice management software:

- Symptoms of disease/illness
  - Review of systems
- History information
  - Past medical history
  - Social history
  - Family history
- Medications
- Laboratory test results
- Imaging results

Federal regulations require that patients receive an encounter summary at the end of each visit. This summary includes the topics discussed, diagnoses, medications, and treatment plans, including upcoming appointments. This encounter summary is a report that pulls data from several different areas of the EHR.

Reports can also be generated to show what types of services are most often utilized, individual provider productivity, and what are the most common diagnoses for the patient population. These reports can help determine if the healthcare facility needs to make any changes to the services provided.

Financial Reports

A number of financial reports are used in a healthcare facility:

- *Daysheet:* This report compiles all the daily payments for service.
- *Billing/payment status:* This report contains information on insurance claims that have been billed, require modification, or have not been paid.
- *Aging report:* This report lists the accounts that have balances owing and how long they have been outstanding.
- *Production by provider:* This report lists the patients that each provider has seen, along with the services provided.
- *Procedure list:* This report lists procedures performed by the Current Procedural Terminology (CPT) code.
- *Production by insurance:* This report lists the payments made by each insurance company, along with any adjustments that were made.
- *Deposit:* This report lists all of the deposits made for a given date range and includes payments made by cash, credit card, or checks (paper and electronic).
- *Ledgers:* This report lists all of the activity done on an individual patient's account.

These reports are used to make many of the administrative decisions within a healthcare facility, including staffing needs, equipment purchases, and scheduling.

Data Validation Techniques and Procedures

The practice management system has the ability to flag errors and possible discrepancies. This could be the generation of an error report when information is uploaded from one system to another. The report requires someone to follow up, find the reason for the error, and then correct it. It could also be a pop-up message when a prescription is entered for a medication that the patient is allergic to.

The practice management system may also use claim scrubbers that evaluate the data entered for claim submission. The claim scrubber looks for missing data, data that does not match (a pap test for a male patient or an Evaluation & Management wellness visit code that does not match the age of the patient), wrong place of a service code, and so on. This would generate a report so the missing information can be entered or the incorrect information can be corrected before the claim is submitted. Claim payments will not be delayed due to a denied claim.

Auditing should be done on a regular basis. An internal audit can help to catch compliance issues before the regulatory agency finds them, thereby allowing the issues to be corrected before a fine can be issued. Audits can also identify where training may need to occur to correct the issue.

Whenever discrepancies within and among EHRs, practice management systems, or other software systems are discovered, they should be reported to the supervisor so that corrective action can be taken.

Data Mining and Extraction Methods

To generate the different types of reports used in a healthcare facility, data mining, and extraction of data are required. The practice management system can access all areas and pull the required information if we give it the right directions. Data mining is the process of extracting usable data from a larger set of raw data. An example would be if an organization wanted to know how many patients with type I diabetes mellitus were being seen. The practice management system could be told to search for the *International Classification of Diseases,* 10th Revision (ICD-10) code and come up with a list of patients. Filters could be used further to break down this data by provider, age group, or any other criteria needed.

Quality Improvement Measures

All healthcare facilities want to track the quality of care that their organization delivers and look for ways to improve the care given. Reports can be used to show what is being done well and what can be improved upon. By using data mining and filters, an organization can determine what patients are in need of preventive care and then use that report to contact those patients and set up the needed services. Reports can also be generated to see if the healthcare facility is being utilized to its fullest extent. This could result in better scheduling practices. Reports can be used for organizational and departmental goal setting by highlighting areas that need improvement.

Common Reporting Errors

EHRs provide a lot of data that can be used to generate any number of reports that can help with providing excellent patient care and quality improvement measures. Ensuring that the information provided in those reports is accurate is very important, as that information is being used to make decisions in the healthcare facility. Providing training for all users will help to ensure that the data is being entered appropriately. With the use of point-of-care and real-time documentation, information is less likely to be missed. Using standardized templates helps with the consistent collection of data. Software reference libraries and clinical vocabularies allow all users to access the most up-to-date information and incorporate it into their documentation. Along with the entering of data, there should be periodic reviews of the criteria used to create the report. Meeting the clinical or operational needs is the purpose of the report, so the correct criteria must be used to collect the right data.

These are the most common reporting errors:

1. *Supplying too much data:* Using proper data mining and filters can help eliminate this issue.
2. *Ignoring mistakes:* All data should be verified.
3. *Including unnecessary information:* Verifying the criteria is one way to ensure that users get the information they need.
4. *Not using standardized templates:* Templates can help ensure that the proper data is collected.

CLOSING COMMENTS

Medical assistants are not likely to go into office management immediately after graduation. The goal of this chapter is to introduce and discuss further professional opportunities in office management and the supervision of the healthcare facility staff. Successful office managers care about their employees and the vision for the healthcare facility. The areas of authority and responsibility must be clearly defined to prevent management problems. A detailed office policies and procedures manual helps the healthcare manager run an efficient facility.

Legal and Ethical Issues

Office managers must stay abreast of current employment laws and regulations for all the different agencies that govern the medical office. Joining a local office managers' association can help the manager keep the office up-to-date and in compliance. Periodic online checks of the websites of various organizations (e.g., OSHA) are a good way for the office manager to keep up with the most recent changes in policies and rules.

HIPAA compliance training should be required for all healthcare facilities. The facility's office manager should be knowledgeable not only about all HIPAA provisions, including those affecting the privacy and security of patient health information but also about the penalties associated with information breaches.

Patient-Centered Care

Office managers who diligently complete all of the responsibilities associated with their position ensure that patient care will be the best it can possibly be. A good office manager will make sure that the staff is more than competent and have the tools needed to provide that care. These managers will ensure that there are policies and procedures in place that will protect both the patients and the staff. A good office manager will look at the whole picture and take the appropriate actions to safeguard the healthcare facility by ensuring compliance with all state and federal regulations. Good office managers understand that if there are no patients, there is no need for the healthcare facility to exist; they take the appropriate measures to provide the means for patient-centered care.

Professional Behaviors

Managers who encourage their staff will create a strong team in the healthcare facility. By focusing on team building, office managers can accomplish more tasks efficiently, delegate some of their workload, and promote high-quality patient care. Office managers can become immersed in their daily office responsibilities; however, they must keep in mind that slacking off on staff training and team development meetings results in lower office productivity. Staff meetings should be scheduled in advance, and attendance should be mandatory.

SUMMARY OF SCENARIO

Kate has had a positive effect on her team at WMFM Clinic. She treats her employees well and is fair about administering office policies and procedures. Her staff appreciates her flexibility and professionalism as she manages the day-to-day operations of the facility. Kate treats her employees as team members and never speaks to them as if she were superior to them. She shares vital information with the staff so that they feel a part of the whole team, and she believes that even negative information should be relayed to the staff so that everyone is aware of the challenges the office faces. She makes strong hiring decisions and firmly believes in a good orientation and training program. Dr. Walden has placed a great deal of trust in Kate, and she has performed well, proving to be a reliable office manager.

Kate knows she should display a friendly attitude toward her staff members when it is appropriate to do so. She is kind and considerate and treats the staff as individuals. She does not fraternize with them but is open to having lunch with the staff at various times and participates in all casual office activities. She maintains a healthy distance so she can be an effective manager, but she listens to those who are experiencing difficulty and is compassionate about helping whenever possible.

Kate knows when hiring for a vacant position, she must be diligent in checking references so that she brings reliable, qualified individuals on board as staff members. Unless she receives acceptable references, she will not hire a medical assistant to become a part of her team. Once she hires someone, she conducts a thorough training program and takes special care to share the experience and skills of the new staff member with the rest of the team.

When Kate must give a negative employee evaluation, she states that fact at the beginning of the meeting. Although she is compassionate, she is able to point out a staff member's shortcomings in a detailed, fair way. She usually is willing to give an employee time to improve, but if the employee fails to perform, Kate does not hesitate to end the employment.

Kate leads a group of cooperative team members who function well together every day, and this results in an efficient office and a pleasant work environment.

SUMMARY OF LEARNING OBJECTIVES

1. **Examine the qualities and responsibilities of a successful office manager in a healthcare facility.**
The provider counts on the office manager to run the business aspects of the office so that the provider can focus on offering good patient care. A high degree of trust is placed in the office manager. A good office manager is fair and flexible. Good communication skills are necessary, as is attention to detail. The manager should care about the employees and have a sense of fairness. The ability to remain calm in a crisis is important, as is the use of good judgment and the ability to multitask. Successful medical office managers promote a positive team environment to facilitate cohesion.
2. **Examine the responsibilities of a medical office manager.**
The medical office manager has a variety of responsibilities. This includes managing the employees or personnel, ensuring that all of the documentation is current, and giving performance evaluations. Managing the finances in order to keep the healthcare facility solvent is another responsibility. The medical office manager is also responsible for creating and maintaining the patient appointment matrix and scheduling employees. Overseeing the inventory of equipment and supplies is also part of the medical office manager's responsibilities, as is ensuring that there are adequate supplies and equipment to keep the office running smoothly. Identifying and minimizing the risks to patients, employees, and the healthcare facility falls under risk management and is another responsibility of the medical office manager.
3. **Examine the skills necessary to be a successful medical office manager.**
The successful medical office manager understands the importance of effective communication. Using the 5 Cs of good communication and developing active listening skills will ensure that the communication with employees, patients, vendors, insurance companies, and providers is done in a professional manner.

   Medical office managers must have excellent time management skills so they can stay on track with their own duties and help staff members complete their tasks. Prioritization is the key to time management, and a manager will be setting goals for themselves, the staff, and the organization as a whole.

   Staff meetings are an opportunity to communicate with the staff of the healthcare facility. This will allow the staff to discuss any problems that have come up with the office manager and the providers. Issues to be discussed should be solicited from all employees, and then an agenda can be put together. Having an agenda will help to make sure that all concerns are addressed.

   Keeping employees motivated can be a challenge for any manager. Employees are motivated by various factors, including money, praise, insecurity, honor, prestige, needs, love, fear, satisfaction, and many others. An effective manager attempts to discover what motivates an employee to do a good job and uses that information to keep employees performing at optimum levels. Employees can also be motivated by incentives and recognition.

   Teamwork is critical in the medical profession. In the healthcare facility, the manager must promote an atmosphere in which employees are willing to work together toward common goals. Morale in the facility may be low because of recent changes in policies or procedures, changes in staff or management, recent terminations of employees, lack of business, or any number of other reasons. The wise manager takes steps to improve employee morale continuously, including scheduling frequent meetings and keeping employees abreast of changes and developments that affect them.
4. **Examine the process for finding and hiring the right employee for the job.**
From the providers to the receptionist, all play a vital role in the quality of healthcare delivered to patients. When hiring staff members, care should be taken to choose employees who have the necessary skills and the right personality for the ambulatory care facility.

   To fill an open medical assisting position, the manager must determine the specific experience that meets the facility's needs. Management should summarize the educational and skill sets needed to be successful at the position in the job description.

   Résumés and applications should be reviewed for accuracy and completeness. Gaps in employment dates should be explained fully, and the office manager should verify any references. Documents should be legible, and the information should be consistent and without oversights.

   The interviewer should be aware of various federal and state laws protecting the interviewee. Title VII of the Civil Rights Act of 1964, as amended by the Equal Employment Opportunity Act of 1972, prohibits inquiries into an applicant's race, color, gender, religion, and national origin. Inquiries about a person's medical history, arrest record, or previous drug use also are illegal. Most states have laws designed to protect the rights of job applicants, and these laws may impose additional restrictions. Office managers must research the laws that pertain to employment in their states.

   The first step in reviewing résumés includes separating applicants who meet the minimal qualifications from those who do not. Applicants with related experience, strongly related skill sets (e.g., customer service), no unexplained employment gaps, and customized, error-free résumés and cover letters will be considered for an interview.

   When the interview is over, the office manager or interview team should immediately take a few moments to rate or summarize the applicant's strengths and weaknesses. After all the interviews have been conducted, the team then rates the interviewees and identifies the top candidates. References are checked, and a second interview may occur before the final person has been selected.
5. **Determine the needs for working with new and established employees.**
The office manager should develop a checklist of the documentation needed for newly hired staff and all the information that should be covered with the new employee at the start of the job. Basic new employee documentation often includes a job application; Form I-9 (Employment Eligibility Verification); W-4 Form (Employee's Withholding Allowance Certificate); Notice of Workers Compensation coverage; consent for a background check and drug testing; acknowledgment of receipt of the company handbook or policy manual; agreements regarding pay, wage deductions, benefits, schedule, work location, and so on; notices of at-will employment status; acknowledgment of ethics statement; direct deposit application; and the Occupational Safety and Health Administration (OSHA) compliance acknowledgement or checklist. Orientation and training help new employees understand what is expected and develop to their full potential.

SUMMARY OF LEARNING OBJECTIVES—cont'd

All employees will need ongoing training to stay current in their field and with the changes made within the healthcare facility. The office manager is very much involved in making sure that training happens. Understanding how remote/virtual training can be used is part of that role. Finding those who are best at training others is another important part of that role.

When negative information is to be relayed to an employee during a performance appraisal, the office manager should sandwich the negative comment between two positive ones whenever possible. Counseling these employees to find the source of their difficulties is the first step toward resolution. Many employees can be redirected to become productive staff members with a little patience and understanding on the manager's part. The manager should have good documentation of the problems that led to the poor evaluation. An employee who has been in service for some time and is offering unsatisfactory performance should be warned and given an explanation of the specific improvements expected. If a second chance does not produce improvement in performance or attitude, dismissal must follow. It should be done privately, with tact and consideration.

To keep good employees, the practice must pay a fair salary with regular raises if the staff member performs as expected. The office manager can find information about salary comparisons on the internet. The manager should periodically review job descriptions and salary analyses online to see whether the salary the medical facility offers is comparable to those for similar jobs in the area.

6. **Describe how office policies and procedures are different from personnel policies.**

The personnel policy manual should include information regarding health benefits, vacation time, sick leave, holidays, overtime, performance evaluations, termination policies, grievance process, dress code, office safety, and the employee's role in case of an emergency.

The office policies and procedures provide direction on how to complete tasks within the healthcare facility. These policies and procedures cover clinical as well as administrative procedures.

The office manager must stay up-to-date with current changes in state and federal legislation. The office manager is also responsible for complying with all reporting that is required by that legislation. It is also important to make sure that the staff is trained in all of the requirements to remain in compliance.

7. **Examine the role of reports in the medical office.**

Generating and using reports is an important part of managing the medical office. These reports are essential to ensure that the office is running as smoothly and efficiently as possible. The EHR and practice management software together can provide a wealth of information. Reports on clinical activities can be used to show what services are being utilized most often, what patients are being seen for, and what services providers are frequently using. This information can be used to make decisions about what services should be continued or added. Financial reports are used to keep the healthcare facility financially sound.

Reports are also used to validate the data entered into the EHR and practice management software. Errors and possible discrepancies can be flagged and corrected before they impact the healthcare facility. Claim scrubber software is an example of using reports to validate data.

Reports can also be used for quality improvement. Using data mining and filters, the healthcare facility can determine patient needs, such as an annual physical, and then contact those patients to set that up. These types of reports can also be used to improve processes such as scheduling.

INTRODUCTION TO MEDICAL TERMINOLOGY AND ANATOMY 18

SCENARIO

Daniela Garcia is a part-time float receptionist at Walden-Martin Family Medical (WMFM) Clinic. Daniela has also recently started the medical assistant program at the local community college. She is currently taking a medical terminology course along with a human body and disease course.

As a float receptionist, she works in many different departments. Her job duties are consistent among the departments. She greets and checks in patients and also updates their information on the computer. The most challenging part of her new job is the medical terminology. The different diagnoses and procedures can get confusing. So she makes a list of new words that she hears. During her breaks, she looks up the words using an online medical dictionary. Audio pronunciation tools help her learn how to say the words. Daniela really enjoys working with the different departments because she continues to learn new information that is helping her in college.

While studying this chapter, think about the following questions:

- What are eponyms, abbreviations, acronyms, and symbols?
- What are prefixes, suffixes, roots, and combining vowels of medical terms?
- What are the functions, major organs, and combining terms for the body systems?
- What are the guidelines for building, defining, and pronouncing medical terms?
- What is the organization of the body?
- What terms are used to describe surface anatomy, directions, and positions of the body?
- What are the body cavities and abdominopelvic quadrants?
- What are predisposing factors and causes of disease?

LEARNING OBJECTIVES

1. Differentiate among eponyms, abbreviations, acronyms, symbols, and medical terminology word parts.
2. Explain the common combining forms used for the different body systems.
3. Explain the guidelines for building, defining, and pronouncing medical terms.
4. Explain the structural organization of the body from simple to complex.
5. Differentiate among the positional reference terms used for the body, including the anatomic position, planes, cavities, and abdominopelvic quadrants.
6. Explain the mechanisms in the body that maintain the acid-base balance.
7. Explain the basics of pathology, including the terminology, protection mechanisms, and predisposing factors.
8. Differentiate among the common causes of diseases.

VOCABULARY

acronym An abbreviation formed from the first letter of each word of a phrase and pronounced as a word.

anaplastic (an uh PLAS tic) A rapidly dividing cancer cell that has little to no similarity to normal cells.

antibodies (AN tih bod ees) Protein substances produced in the blood or tissues in response to a specific antigen that destroys or weakens the antigen. Part of the immune system.

antigens (an TIE jens) Substances that stimulate the production of an antibody when introduced into the body. Antigens include toxins, bacteria, viruses, and other foreign substances.

biopsy (BIE op see) Process of viewing living tissue that has been removed for the purpose of diagnosis or treatment.

chromosomes (KROH muh sohms) Rod-shaped structures found in the cell's nucleus; they contain genetic information.

cytoplasm (SYE toh plaz um) Jelly-like substance that surrounds the nucleus and fills the cells.

diaphragm A broad, dome-shaped muscle used for breathing that separates the thoracic and abdominopelvic cavities.

differentiated (dif uh REN shee ayt ed) Describes how malignant tissues or cells look like the normal tissues or cells they came from; poorly-differentiated means they do not look like the normal tissues or cells, and well-differentiated means they look like the normal tissues or cells.

endoscope A scope with a camera attached to a long, thin tube that can be inserted into the body.

eponym A word that comes from the name of a person, place, or thing associated with the word.

homeostasis (hoh mee uh STAY sis) The internal environment of the body that is compatible with life. A steady state that is created by all the body systems working together to provide a consistent and unvarying internal environment.

intercellular Located between cells.

VOCABULARY—*continued*

metastasize (MEH tas tuh sizes) To spread from one part of the body (the primary tumor) to another part of the body, forming a secondary tumor.
oncologist (on KOL uh jest) A specially trained doctor who diagnoses and treats cancer.
organelle Structures inside of the cell that has specific functions to maintain the cell.
pathogen A disease-causing organism.
pathologist (pa THOL uh jest) A physician specially trained in the nature and cause of disease.
pathology The study of disease.
peristalsis (per uh STAL sis) Wavelike motion.
physiology (fi zee ALL uh jee) The study of body functions.
plasma membrane Outer covering surrounding the cell that allows certain substances to enter the cell and blocks other substances. Can also be called the cell membrane.
toxins (TOK sins) Substances created by microorganisms, plants, or animals that are poisonous to humans.
vasoconstriction Contraction of the muscles, causing narrowing of the inside tube of the vessel.

INTRODUCTION

This chapter has two major focuses: medical terminology and general anatomy. Students are introduced to common word parts related to the different body systems. You will learn how to label, identify, and define medical terms. General anatomy concepts, directional terms, and diagnostic tests are also discussed. Having a mastery of medical terminology, basic anatomy terms and concepts, and disease terminology and testing will give you the tools to understand the language and procedures presented in each medical specialty.

MEDICAL TERMINOLOGY

To many healthcare students, the vocabulary used in the medical environment may seem like words in a foreign language. Medical terminology relates to anatomy, diseases, diagnostic tests, procedures, and so on. The vocabulary used is a combination of **eponyms**, abbreviations, **acronyms**, symbols, and medical terminology.

Eponyms

Diseases and medical instruments are just a few of the areas where eponyms are used. Eponyms in medicine have been developed to honor scientists and providers who have created an innovative device or researched a new disease. Eponyms must be memorized. Examples of eponyms include the following:

- Parkinson disease was named after James Parkinson.
- Graves disease was named after Dr. Robert James Graves.
- Hashimoto disease was named after Dr. Hakaru Hashimoto.
- Cushing disease was named after Dr. Harvey Cushing.
- The Jackson-Pratt drain, used in some surgical procedures, was named after its inventors, Dr. Fredrick Jackson and Dr. Richard Pratt.
- The Snellen eye chart was named after its inventor, Dr. Herman Snellen.

Abbreviations, Acronyms, and Symbols

An *abbreviation* is a shortened version of a word or phrase. The abbreviation can be derived from the letters in the word or from combining the first letter of each word. Here are some examples of medical abbreviations:

- BP: blood pressure
- CBC: complete blood count
- CC: chief complaint
- HTN: hypertension
- Ca: cancer
- HA: headache
- PT: physical therapy

Acronyms are also abbreviations that become pronounceable words. Here are some examples of acronyms:

- ACE: angiotensin-converting enzyme
- AIDS: acquired immunodeficiency syndrome
- ARDS: acute respiratory distress syndrome
- HIPAA: Health Insurance Portability and Accountability Act
- LASER: light amplification by stimulated emission of radiation
- RICE: rest, ice, compression, elevation
- SIDS: sudden infant death syndrome

A *symbol* is a picture that represents a word or phrase. Symbols were used more often with paper health records. Using symbols increases the speed of documentation and reduces the amount of paper required. The use of symbols has decreased with the use of electronic health records.

Throughout the textbook, abbreviations and acronyms are listed. It is important to learn these. Making and using flashcards to study these can be useful.

Most healthcare facilities have lists of approved abbreviations and symbols that healthcare professionals can use. Make sure to use only the approved abbreviations and symbols. Using unapproved abbreviations and symbols in messages and documentation may lead to confusion and patient care errors.

Symbols

$\bar{s}$ = without
$\bar{p}$ = after
$\bar{a}$ = before
↑ = increase
↓ = decrease
Δ = change
♀ = female
♂ = male

CRITICAL THINKING APPLICATION 18.1

Every day Daniela hears abbreviations and acronyms at her job. List a medical abbreviation and an acronym and provide the meanings for both.

Medical Terminology

Medical terms used in healthcare can be divided into two groups, depending on whether or not they are made of word parts. Medical terms not made up of word parts need to be memorized. Medical terms made up of word parts can be literally defined.

Medical term word parts have either a Greek or Latin origin. By knowing the meaning of the word parts, a person can easily create or define medical terms. Here are four common word parts:

- *Prefix*: A word part found at the beginning of the word. Prefixes modify the meaning of the word. In this textbook, prefixes are listed with a hyphen, such as "bi-" and "mal-."
- *Suffix*: A word part found at the end of the word. Suffixes follow a hyphen, such as "-is" and "-tic."
- *Root*: A word part that is the foundation of the term.
- *Combining vowel*: A vowel that links the root to the suffix or a root to a root. Typically, the combining vowel is an "o."

When the root is added to the combining vowel, the result is called a *combining form*. Combining forms can be given by stating the root word part followed by a slash and the vowel (e.g., oste/o and chol/e).

The following section discusses prefixes and suffixes. Combining forms are presented by the body systems.

Prefixes and Suffixes

The prefix is added to the beginning of the word. Not all medical terms have prefixes. Table 18.1 lists common prefixes and their

TABLE 18.1 Prefixes

PREFIX	MEANING	PREFIX	MEANING
a-, an-	without, no, not	intra-	within
ab-	away from	ipsi-	same
ad -	near, toward	macro-	very large
af-	toward	mal-	bad
ana-	up, apart	megalo-	large
ante-	before, forward, in front of	meta-	change, beyond
anti-	against	micro-	small
bi-	two, both	neo-	new
brady-	slow	par-	near, beside
con-	together, with	para-	near, abnormal, beside
contra-	opposite	per-	through
dia-	complete, through	peri-	surrounding, around
dys-	difficult, painful, abnormal, bad	poly-	many, much, excessive, frequent
ec-	outside, out	post-	after, behind
echo-	using ultrasonic waves	pre-	before, in front of
ef-	away from	pro-, pros-	forward, before
electro-	using electricity	quadri-	four
end-, endo-	in, inner, within	re-, retro-	behind, back
epi-	above, upon	sub-	under, less than
ex-	out	supra-	upward, above
extra-	outside of	syn-	together, with
hemi-	half	tachy-	fast
hyper-	excessive, too much, above	trans-	through, across
hypo-	deficit, too little, below	tri-	three
in-	into, in	ultra-	beyond
inter-	between	uni-	one

meanings. Some prefixes have more than one meaning. The prefix modifies the root by describing the following elements:

- Location or position: peri- (surrounding, around) and endo- (within, in, inner)
- Number: bi- (two, both) and tri- (three)
- State or problem: mal- (bad) and an- (without, no, not)
- Size: macro- (very large) and micro- (small)
- Speed or level: hyper- (above normal) and hypo- (below normal)

The suffix is added to the end of the word. Table 18.2 lists suffixes and their meanings.

COMBINING FORMS

A combining form contains both the root word part and the combining vowel. A combining form is linked to a root or a suffix.

Learning combining forms by body system can be helpful. The following sections describe the body systems and list the related combining forms. Table 18.3 provides the directional combining forms.

Cardiovascular System

The function of the cardiovascular system is to transport materials throughout the body using the blood. The blood transports oxygen and nutrients and collects wastes through the body. Components in the blood also fight infections and form clots. The cardiovascular system includes the heart, arteries, arterioles, veins, venules, and blood. Combining terms related to the cardiovascular system include the following:

- angi/o (vessel, blood vessel)
- aort/o (aorta)
- apic/o (apex)
- arteri/o (artery)

TABLE 18.2 Suffixes

TYPE	SUFFIX	MEANING
Adjective	-ac -al -ar -ary -eal -ent -ic -ior -ine -ous -tic	pertaining to
Body structure and function	-crine	secretion
	-dipsia	thirst
	-gen	to produce
	-is	structure
	-lapse	to fall, slide
	-partum	birth
	-phagia	to eat, swallow
	-phasia	to speak
	-plasm	formation
	-stasis	to stand, place, stop, control
	-tension	pressure
	-trophy	nourishment; development
	-um	structure, membrane

TYPE	SUFFIX	MEANING
Conditions and diseases	-algia	pain
	-ation	process, condition
	-cele	herniation
	-emia	blood condition
	-ia	diseased or abnormal condition
	-ism	condition, process
	-itis	inflammation
	-lysis	loosening, breakdown, separation, destruction
	-malacia	softening
	-megaly	enlargement
	-oma	tumor, mass
	-osis	abnormal condition
	-pathy	disease condition
	-plegia	paralysis
	-pnea	breathing
	-rrhagia	rapid flow of blood
	-rrhea	flow, discharge
	-sclerosis	abnormal condition of hardening
	-stenosis	abnormal condition of narrowing
	-thesis	to put, place (state of putting or placing)
	-uria	urine condition
	-y	process of, condition

TABLE 18.2 Suffixes—*continued*

TYPE	SUFFIX	MEANING	TYPE	SUFFIX	MEANING
Instruments/ recording	-graph	instrument to record		-plasty	surgical repair
	-gram	record or recording		-rrhaphy	suture repair
	-meter	instrument to measure		-scopic	pertaining to visual examination
	-scope	instrument to view		-scopy	process of visual examination
Noun ending	-icle -ole -ule	small or tiny structure		-section	to cut
				-stomy	surgical creation of artificial opening
Procedures	-cision	process of cutting		-tomy	incision, cut into
	-centesis	surgical puncture and aspiration of fluid		-tripsy	crushing
	-ectomy	surgical removal, excision, resection	Specialty	-ist	one who specializes
	-graphy	process of recording		-logist	one who specializes in the study of
	-metry	process of measuring			
	-opsy	process of viewing		-logy	study of
	-pexy	surgical fixation	Miscellaneous	-ad	toward

TABLE 18.3 Directional Combining Forms

COMBINING FORM	MEANING	COMBINING FORM	MEANING
anter/o	front	infer/o	downward
caud/o	tail	later/o	side
cephal/o	head	medi/o	middle
cubit/o	elbow	poplit/o	back of knee
dextr/o	right	poster/o	back
dist/o	far	proxim/o	near
dors/o	back	sinistr/o	left
fer/o	to carry	super/o	upward
front/o	front	ventr/o	belly
glute/o	buttocks		

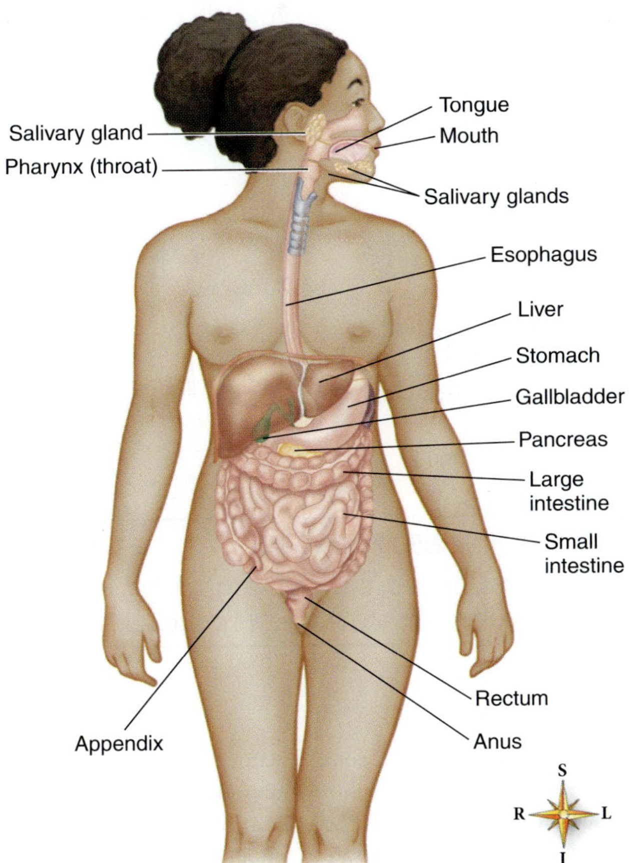

FIGURE 18.1 **Digestive System.** (From Patton KT, Thibodeau GA: *The human body in health and disease*, ed 7, St. Louis, 2018, Elsevier.)

- cardi/o, coron/o (heart)
- hemat/o (blood)
- phleb/o, ven/o (vein)
- plasm/o (plasma)
- valv/o (valve)
- ventricul/o (ventricle)

Gastrointestinal System

The gastrointestinal system, also called the digestive system, breaks down, digests, and absorbs nutrients. The digestive system includes the mouth, tongue, teeth, pharynx, esophagus, stomach, small intestine, large intestine, liver, gallbladder, pancreas, and appendix (Figure 18.1). Combining terms related to the digestive system include the following:

- abdomin/o (abdomen)
- an/o (anus)
- append/o, appendic/o (appendix)
- chol/e (gall, bile)
- col/o, colon/o (colon)
- corpor/o, som/o, somat/o (corporis, body)
- enter/o (small intestine)
- esophag/o (esophagus)
- gastr/o (stomach)
- gingiv/o (gum)
- hepat/o (liver)
- lumin/o (lumen)
- or/o, stomat/o (mouth)
- pancreat/o (pancreas)
- pharyng/o (pharynx)
- rect/o (rectum)

Endocrine System

The endocrine system produces hormones that circulate in the blood. These hormones go to target tissues, which stimulate a particular action. The endocrine system includes the pituitary gland, pineal gland, hypothalamus, thyroid gland, pancreas, adrenal cortex and medulla, parathyroid gland, thymus gland, ovaries, and testes. Combining terms related to the endocrine system include the following:

- adren/o (adrenal gland)
- hypophys/o (pituitary gland)
- oophor/o, ovari/o (ovary)
- orch/o, orchi/o (testis)
- pancreat/o (pancreas)
- parathyroid/o (parathyroid gland)
- pituitary/o (pituitary gland)
- thyroid/o (thyroid gland)

CRITICAL THINKING APPLICATION **18.2**

Using the prefixes, combining forms, and suffixes, create four words each for the cardiovascular, endocrine, and gastrointestinal systems.

Integumentary System

The integumentary system is a barrier that protects the body and acts as a sense organ. It helps to retain body fluids, protect against infection, and regulate body temperature. The integumentary system includes the skin, subcutaneous tissue, sweat and sebaceous glands, hair, nails, and sense receptors. Combining terms related to the integumentary system include the following:

- cutane/o, derm/o, dermat/o (skin)
- hidr/o (sweat)
- myc/o (fungus)
- necr/o (death—cells, body)
- onych/o, ungu/o (nail)
- pachy/o (thick)
- pil/o, trich/o (hair)
- seb/o (sebum, oil)
- xer/o (dry)

Lymphatic and Immune Systems

The lymphatic system maintains fluid balance. The immune system provides immunity to some diseases. Both systems protect the internal environment of the body. The lymphatic and immune systems include the lymph, lymph vessels, lymph nodes, thymus, tonsils, spleen, lymphocytes, and antibodies (Figure 18.2). Combining terms related to the lymphatic and immune systems include the following:

- lymph/o (lymph)
- lymphaden/o (lymph node)
- lymphangi/o (lymph vessel)
- myel/o (bone marrow, spinal cord)
- splen/o (spleen)
- thym/o (thymus)

Musculoskeletal System

The musculoskeletal system is made up of the muscular and skeletal systems. Since these two systems work so closely together, they are

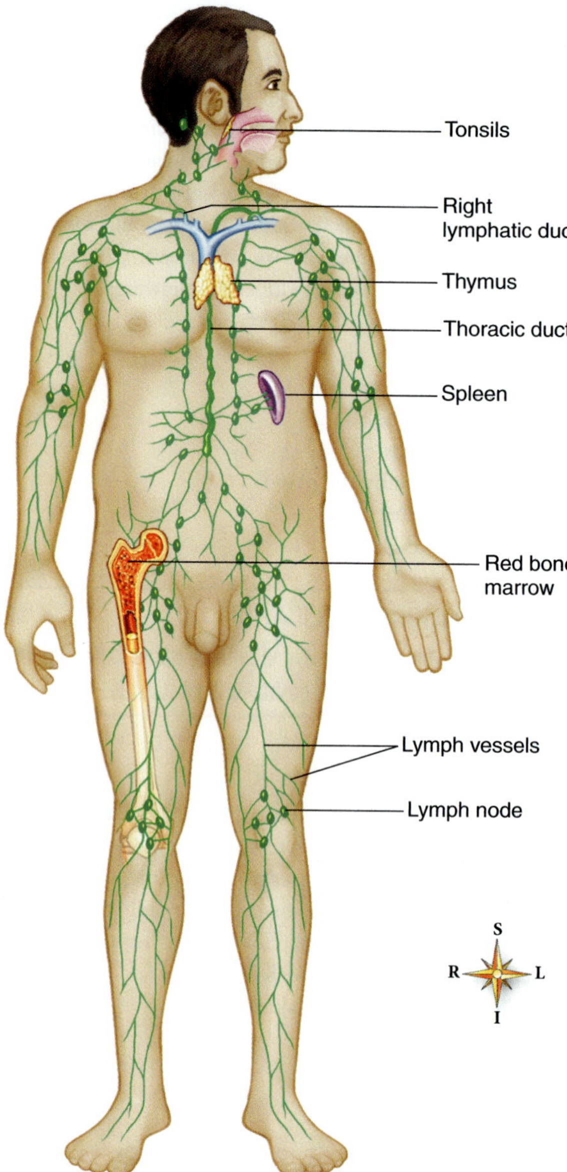

FIGURE 18.2 Lymphatic and Immune Systems. (From Patton KT, Thibodeau GA: *The human body in health and disease*, ed 7, St. Louis, 2018, Elsevier.)

commonly referred to as the musculoskeletal system. The muscular system is involved with heat production, and muscle contractions, tone, and posture. The muscular system includes the muscles. The skeletal system protects, supports, and provides a framework for organs in the boy. It helps with movement, development of new bone, regulation of blood calcium, and the formation of blood cells and platelets. The skeletal system includes the bones, joints, and supportive connective tissues, including ligaments, tendons, and cartilage. Combining terms related to the musculoskeletal system include the following:

- acromi/o (acromion)
- ankyl/o (stiff, bent)
- arthr/o (joint)
- carp/o (carpals)
- chondr/o (cartilage)
- cost/o (rib)
- cox/o (hip)
- crani/o (skull)
- digit/o (finger/toe)
- femor/o (thigh)
- ligament/o (ligament)
- lumb/o (lumbar)
- muscul/o, my/o, myos/o (muscle)
- oste/o (bone)
- patell/o, patell/a (kneecap)
- pelv/i, pelv/o (pelvis)
- pub/o (pubis)
- sacr/o (sacral)
- scapul/o (scapula)
- scoli/o (crooked, curved spine)
- stern/o (sternum)
- ten/o, tendin/o (tendon)
- thorac/o (chest)
- vertebr/o (vertebra)

CRITICAL THINKING APPLICATION 18.3

Using the prefixes, combining forms, and suffixes, create two words each for the integumentary, lymphatic, immune, and musculoskeletal systems.

Nervous System

The nervous system controls body structures to maintain **homeostasis.** It receives and processes information from other body structures. The nervous system includes the brain, spinal cord, neurons, neuroglial cells, peripheral nerves, and autonomic nerves. Combining terms related to the nervous system include the following:

- cerebell/o (cerebellum)
- cerebr/o (cerebrum)
- dur/o (dura mater)
- encephal/o (brain)
- gangli/o, ganglion/o (ganglion)
- gli/o (glia)
- mening/o, meningi/o (meninges)
- myel/o (spinal cord, bone marrow)
- neur/o (nerve)

Reproductive System

The reproductive system produces hormones and is involved with reproduction. The female reproductive system includes the ovaries, fallopian tubes, uterus, vagina, vulva, mammary glands, ovum, estrogen, and progesterone. The male reproductive system includes the epididymis vas deferens, prostate gland, testes, scrotum, penis, urethra, sperm, and testosterone. Combining terms related to the reproductive system include the following:

- cervic/o (cervix)
- colp/o, vagin/o (vagina)
- fund/o (fundus)
- mamm/o, mast/o (breast)
- men/o (menstruation)
- oophor/o, ovari/o (ovary)
- orch/o, orchi/o, orchid/o, test/o, testicul/o (testis)
- prostat/o (prostate gland)
- salping/o (fallopian tube)
- scrot/o (scrotum)
- umbilic/o (umbilical)
- uter/o, hyster/o, metri/o, metr/o (uterus)

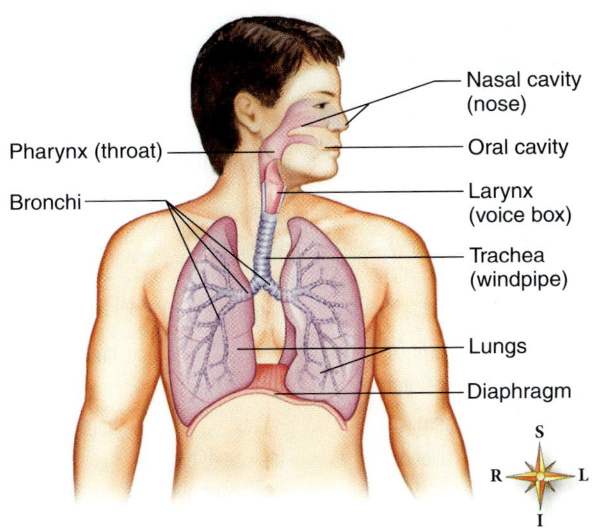

FIGURE 18.3 **Respiratory System.** (From Patton KT, Thibodeau GA: *The human body in health and disease*, ed 7, St. Louis, 2018, Elsevier.)

Respiratory System

The respiratory system delivers oxygen to the cells and removes carbon dioxide from the body. The respiratory system includes the nose, sinuses, pharynx, larynx, trachea, bronchi, lungs, bronchioles, and alveoli (Figure 18.3). Combining terms related to the respiratory system include the following:

- alveol/o (alveolus, air sac)
- bronch/o, bronchi/o (bronchial tube)
- cyan/o (blue)
- epiglott/o (epiglottis)
- laryng/o (larynx)
- nas/o, rhin/o (nose)
- pharyng/o (pharynx)
- phren/o (diaphragm)
- pneumon/o, pulmon/o, pneum/o (lung)
- sin/o, sinus/o (sinus)
- thorac/o, steth/o, pector/o (chest)
- trache/o (trachea)

CRITICAL THINKING APPLICATION 18.4

Using the prefixes, combining forms, and suffixes, create four words each for the nervous, reproductive, and respiratory systems.

Sensory System

The sensory system gathers information through the senses of vision, hearing, balance, taste, and smell. The sensory system consists of the eyes, ears, taste buds, olfactory receptors, and sensory receptors. Combining terms related to the sensory system include the following:

- audi/o (hearing)
- aur/i, aur/o (ear)
- blephar/o (eyelid)
- cochle/o (cochlea)
- conjunctiv/o (conjunctiva)
- corne/o (cornea)
- dipl/o (two, double)
- ir/o, irid/o (iris)
- myring/o (tympanic membrane, eardrum)
- ocul/o, ophthalm/o (eye)
- opt/o (vision)
- ot/o (ear)
- retin/o (retina)
- scler/o (sclera)
- vestibul/o (vestibule)

Urinary System

The urinary system eliminates nitrogenous waste and maintains the electrolyte, water, and acid-base balances. The urinary system includes the nephron unit, kidneys, ureters, bladder, and urethra. Combining forms related to the urinary system include the following:

- cyst/o, vesic/o (urinary bladder)
- glyc/o, glycos/o (sugar)
- hil/o (hilum)
- hydr/o (water)
- lith/o (stone)
- noct/i (night)
- nephr/o (kidney)
- olig/o (scanty)
- pyel/o (renal pelvis)
- ren/o (kidney)
- ureter/o (ureter)
- urethr/o (urethra)
- urin/o, ur/o (urinary)

CRITICAL THINKING APPLICATION 18.5

Using the prefixes, combining forms, and suffixes, create four words each for the urinary and sensory systems.

BUILDING, DEFINING, AND PRONOUNCING MEDICAL TERMS

For a person to successfully build, define, and pronounce medical terms, remembering key guidelines and processes can be helpful. The following sections discuss guidelines for building medical terms and the process for defining and pronouncing medical terms.

Building Medical Terms

When building a medical term, it is important to know when to use a combining vowel, how to order the combining forms, and how to spell singular and plural terms.

When building medical terms, remember these guidelines:

- When combining a root with a suffix,
  - If the suffix begins with a consonant, use a combining vowel between the root and the suffix.
  - If the suffix begins with a vowel, do not use a combining vowel. Furthermore, if the root ends in a vowel and the suffix starts with the same vowel, one of the vowels is dropped.
- When adding a root to a root, use a combining vowel. Figure 18.4 shows how cholangiopancreatography and pyloromyotomy are built. A combining vowel is used even if the second root begins with a vowel.
- Do not use a combining vowel between a prefix and a root (Figure 18.5).

See Table 18.4 for examples of building medical terms following these root-suffix guidelines.

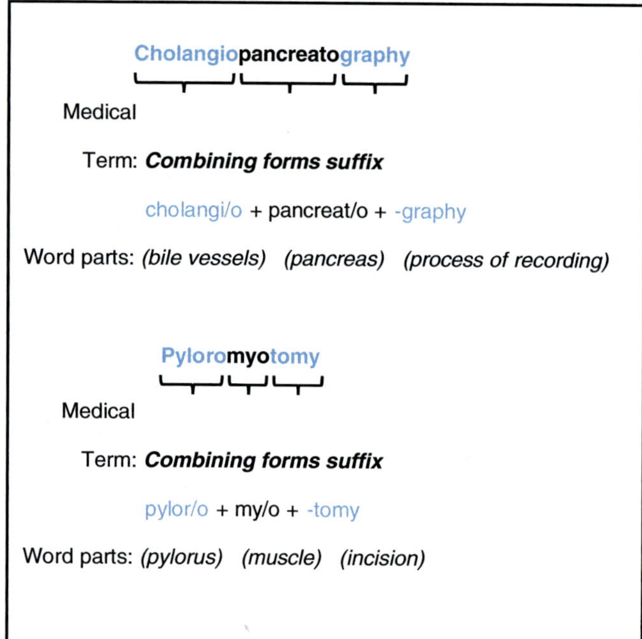

FIGURE 18.4 **Combining Roots.** (From Niedzwiecki, B: *Kinn's Medical Assisting Fundamentals*, ed 2, St. Louis, 2022, Elsevier.)

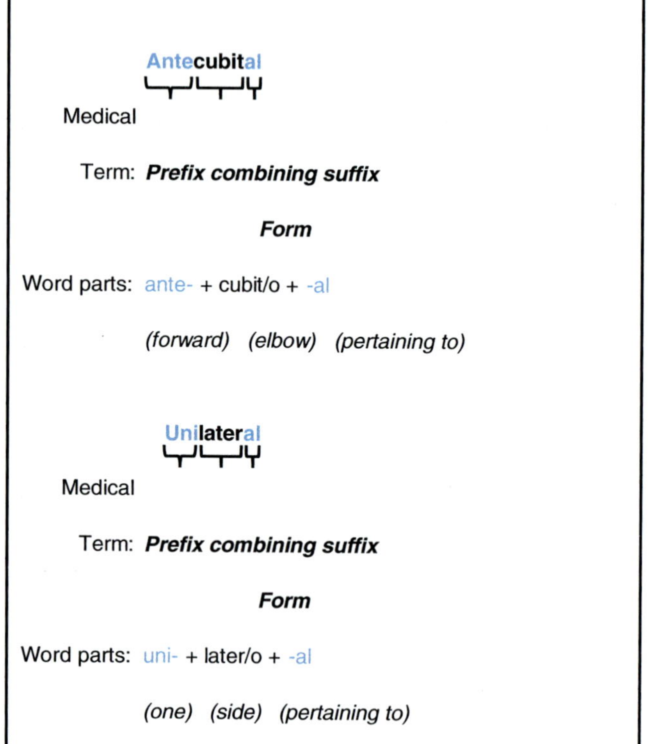

FIGURE 18.5 **Prefixes.** (From Niedzwiecki, B: *Kinn's Medical Assisting Fundamentals*, ed 2, St. Louis, 2022, Elsevier.)

Some medical terms have two or more combining forms. With some terms, the order of the combining forms follows the sequence of the procedure. For instance, when a proctosigmoidoscopy is performed, an **endoscope** is used. (Remember, -scopy means process of visual examination.) At the start of the procedure, the provider inserts the endoscope into the anus. The endoscope enters the rectum (proct/o) and then is advanced into the sigmoid colon (sigmoid/o).

TABLE 18.4 Use of a Combining Vowel

COMBINING VOWEL	COMBINING FORM (MEANING)	SUFFIX (MEANING)	MEDICAL TERM
When the suffix begins with a consonant, the combining vowel is used.	arteri/o (artery)	-sclerosis (abnormal condition of hardening)	arteriosclerosis
	neutr/o (neutral)	-phil (attraction)	neutrophil
	hem/o (blood)	-stasis (to stand, place, stop, control)	hemostasis
	thromb/o (clot, clotting)	-cyte (cell)	thrombocyte
When the suffix begins with a vowel, the combining vowel is not added.	sept/o (septum)	-al (pertaining to)	septal
	esophag/o (esophagus)	-eal (pertaining to)	esophageal
	ventricul/o (ventricle)	-ar (pertaining to)	ventricular
	coron/o (heart)	-ary (pertaining to)	coronary
When the suffix begins with a vowel and the root ends in the same vowel, one of the vowels is dropped.	arteri/o (artery)	-itis (inflammation)	arteritis
	cardi/o (heart)	-itis (inflammation)	carditis
	ovari/o (ovary)	-itis (inflammation)	ovaritis

Singular and Plural Terms

When singular Latin and Greek terms are changed to the plural forms, special rules apply. Table 18.5 shows how to change these terms to plural forms. When Latin terms that consist of a noun and an adjective are pluralized, both terms need to be pluralized. For example, *placenta previa* would become placentae *previae.*

It is also helpful to remember these English rules for pluralizing nouns:

- Most words can be made into the plural form by adding -s. For example, the plural form of *heart* is *hearts.*
- If the term ends in -s, -x, -ch, or -sh, add -es. For example, the plural form of *stitch* is *stitches.*
- If the term ends in -y after a consonant, drop the -y and add -ies. For example, the plural form of *artery* is *arteries.*
- If the term ends in -o after a consonant, add -nes. For example, the plural form of *comedo* is *comedones.*

There are some exceptions to these rules, and the spelling of those terms must be memorized.

TABLE 18.5 Changing Latin and Greek Terms to Plural Terms

SINGULAR TERM ENDS IN	CHANGE TO A PLURAL TERM	EXAMPLES	
		SINGULAR FORM	PLURAL FORM
-a	add e	bursa	bursae
-ax	change the x to a c and add es	thorax	thoraces
-ex -ix	drop -ex or -ix and add -ices	appendix	appendices
-is	drop -is and add -es	diagnosis	diagnoses
-ma	add -ta	fibroma	fibromata
-nx	change the x to a g and add es	larynx	larynges
-on	drop the -on and add -a	spermatozoon	spermatozoa
-um	drop -um and add -a	atrium	atria
-us	drop -us and add -i	bronchus	bronchi
-yx	change the x to a c and add es	calyx	calyces

CRITICAL THINKING APPLICATION 18.6

Using English rules for pluralizing nouns, list four (nonmedical) words that follow one of these rules.

Defining Medical Terms

When you encounter an unknown medical term, take the following steps to identify the meaning:

1. Divide the term into word parts. For example, divide *vasculitis* into word parts.
   vascul/itis
2. Label each word part and combining form.
   vascul/o -itis
   combining form, suffix
3. Define each word part.
   vascul/o -itis
   combining form – vessel; suffix – inflammation
4. Define the term. Start with the suffix definition. Then add the definition(s) for the rest of the word, starting at the beginning of the term.
   inflammation of the (blood) vessel

Pronouncing Unusual Letter Combinations

As a medical assistant, it is important to accurately pronounce medical terms. Some medical terms are easy to pronounce, whereas others are more difficult. Use the following tips when learning medical term pronunciations:

- Listen to the pronunciation. Many online medical dictionaries have pronunciation tools available.
- Break apart unfamiliar terms. Pronounce each section separately.
- Think about similar-looking terms and how they are pronounced.
- Focus on letter combinations that have different sounds (Table 18.6).
- Practice saying the terms out loud.

TABLE 18.6 Pronouncing Letter Combinations

LETTER COMBINATION	SOUND	EXAMPLE
C before the vowel e or i	S	cilia
G before the vowel e or i	J	gene
C before the vowels a, o, or u	K	cochlear
G before the vowels a, o, or u	G	gallbladder
eu	you	eustachian tube
ch	K	cholangiogram
ph	F	physiology
pn	N	pneumothorax
ps	S	psychosis
pt	T	ptosis
rh, rrh	R	rhinorrhagia
x-	Z	xenograft
cy	ss	cyanosis
qu	kw	quadrant

STRUCTURAL ORGANIZATION OF THE BODY

The remaining sections of the chapter focus on the basics of anatomy, physiology, and pathology. *Anatomy* is the study of how the body is shaped and structured. It includes the structures, levels of organization, and the relationships among different body parts. Later chapters will describe the anatomy, **physiology**, and **pathology** of each body system. Anatomy, physiology, and pathology information is used in many ways in clinical and administrative settings. From coding and billing to entering diagnostic orders, having a strong understanding of this information will help medical assistants perform their roles more efficiently.

When starting with the anatomy basics, we need to examine the makeup of the body. If we were to break apart the body, we would have many body systems. Examples include the digestive, cardiovascular, musculoskeletal, and respiratory systems. Each system is composed of different organs. For instance, the stomach and intestines are digestive system organs. Each organ is made up of combinations of tissues, and these tissues are composed of cells. So, when studying the organization of the body, it is easier to start at the level of cells and work up to the organism (human body) level.

Cells

The basic unit of life is the cell. Cells determine the functional and structural characteristics of the entire body. Cells are microscopic.

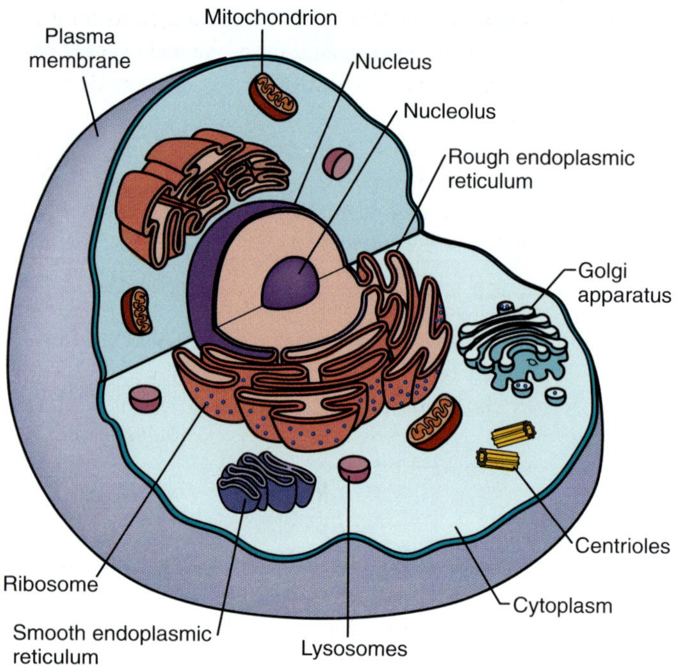

FIGURE 18.6 Cell structures.

They have a variety of shapes and perform a vast array of functions. A cell is covered by a **plasma membrane**. **Organelles** are suspended in the **cytoplasm** (Figure 18.6).

The following organelles can be found in the cell:

- *Ribosome:* Free-floating organelle that makes enzymes and proteins. Contains ribonucleic acid (RNA). Considered the cell's "protein factories."
- *Rough endoplasmic reticulum* (ER): Organelle that is a network of membranes; connects to the nucleus. Ribosomes are attached to the ER, causing the rough appearance. Involved with making protein.
- *Smooth endoplasmic reticulum* (ER): Tubelike organelle; role differs based on the type of cell. Roles may include storage of calcium and making steroids and lipids.
- *Golgi apparatus:* Organelle that processes and packages the proteins and lipids made by the cell. Considered to be the cell's "processing plant."
- *Lysosomes:* Organelles that contain enzymes and are involved with digesting nutrients and other substances in the cell. Considered to be the cell's "waste collectors."
- *Mitochondrion*: Organelle that produces the energy for the cell. Called the cell's "power plant."
- *Nucleus*: Control center of the cell; contains **chromosomes** that are made up of deoxyribonucleic acid (DNA), which carries genetic information.
- *Nucleolus:* Inside of the nucleus; produces ribosomes.
- *Centrioles*: Tubelike structures that help with cell division and the formation of the spindle fibers (a type of microtubule).

Cells can also have extensions or projections on the surface, including these:

- *Cilia:* Fine, hairlike extensions on the surface of the cell. Used to detect surroundings or chemicals.
- *Microvilli:* Small projections on the surface of the cell. This increases the surface area, which allows for additional absorption.
- *Flagellum:* Single long hairlike extension on the surface of the cell. Used to propel or move cell.

Cell Reproduction

Most human cells reproduce by mitosis. *Mitosis* is a process in which one cell splits into two identical daughter cells. The two cells are genetically identical to the parent cell. Prior to the mitosis process, the cell enters the interphase stage. During this stage, the genetic information, chromosomes, replicate. Each sister pair of chromosomes (called *chromatids*) are joined together until they are pulled apart later in the mitosis process. The point where the two chromatids are joined is called the *centromere*. The centromere is also the attachment point for spindle fibers, which will be involved in the mitosis process. The mitosis process consists of four phases:

- *Prophase*: The membrane around the nucleus starts to break down. Centrioles produce spindle fibers and start to move toward opposite sides of the cell.
- *Metaphase*: Each pair of chromatids lines up, and each chromatid is attached to a spindle fiber.
- *Anaphase*: Spindle fibers pull the sister chromatids apart.
- *Telophase*: The nucleus reforms around each set of chromosomes. The cell continues to separate into two daughter cells.

CRITICAL THINKING APPLICATION **18.7**

Daniela is learning about the cell structures in school. While on break one night, she talked to Bella. Bella just graduated and is now a certified medical assistant (CMA). Daniela mentioned she was learning about cell parts. Bella encouraged Daniela to associate the cell parts with things she might see in an old city. For instance, she stated, "The plasma membrane could be the walls around the city." What other associations could be made between the cell structures and a city?

Tissues

A *tissue* is a group of similar cells from the same source that together carry out a specific function. The microscopic study of body tissues is known as *histology*. All of the body tissues are grouped into four types:

1. *Epithelial tissue:* Acts as an internal or external covering for organs. Examples of epithelial tissue include the outer layer of the skin, glands, and linings of body cavities and organs. In epithelial tissue, the cells are packed so closely together that there is little to no **intercellular** material. Two types of epithelial tissue include simple and stratified. *Simple epithelium* is a single layer of the same-shaped cells. *Stratified epithelium* contains multiple layers of cells. Epithelial tissue is classified according to shape:
   - *Squamous*: Flat in appearance
   - *Cuboidal*: Square in appearance
   - *Columnar*: Long and narrow in appearance
   - *Transitional*: Varying shapes that can stretch
2. *Connective tissue:* Supports and binds other body tissues. Examples of connective tissue include bone, blood, fat, fibrous tissue, areolar tissue, and cartilage. Connective tissue is the most frequently occurring tissue in the body.
3. *Muscle tissue:* Produces movement. Classifications of muscle tissue include the following:
   - *Skeletal*: Voluntary muscles that appear *striated* or striped. Attached to bones and produce voluntary body movements when contracted.
   - *Cardiac*: Involuntary muscles that appear striated and form the heart muscle wall.

- *Smooth*: Involuntary nonstriated muscles. Line the blood vessel walls and hollow organs and cause **peristalsis** and **vasoconstriction**.

4. *Nervous tissue:* Includes cells that provide transmission of information to control a variety of functions. Nervous tissue controls the body's functions to maintain homeostasis. Nervous tissue is made up of *neurons* **(nerve cells)** and supportive structures called *neuroglial cells.*

Organs

An organ is a structure composed of two or more types of tissue. An organ may have one or more functions. For instance, the pancreas has two functions: it produces insulin and digestive enzymes. Organs are grouped within body systems. An organ may be part of one or more systems. For instance, the pancreas is part of the endocrine system and also part of the digestive system.

Body Systems

A body system is composed of several organs and their related structures. These structures work together to perform a specific function in the body. Body systems include the cardiovascular, respiratory, nervous, endocrine, gastrointestinal, integumentary, lymphatic, immune, muscular, skeletal, reproductive, sensory, and urinary systems.

Organism

The organism of the body is made up of many body systems. These work together to maintain a steady environment in the body called homeostasis. If the balance is off or if the environment moves out of the normal range, diseases can occur.

CRITICAL THINKING APPLICATION **18.8**

Bella's tip really helped Daniela with the cell structures. Now Daniela needs to remember the organization of the body in order from the simplest to the most complex. Bella encourages Daniela to create a phrase or word that will help her remember cells, tissues, organs, body systems, and organisms. What might be a way to remember these five items in order?

ANATOMIC POSITION, PLANES, CAVITIES, AND QUADRANTS

In healthcare, we use medical terminology to communicate a precise message to others. Earlier in the chapter, medical terminology word parts were discussed. Medical terminology also includes directional terms, planes, body cavities, and abdominopelvic quadrants and regions. All of these terms are used in healthcare to give precise descriptions and are based on a standard frame of reference, the anatomic position. The *anatomic position* means the body stands erect with the face forward, arms at the sides, palms forward, and toes pointed forward. Figure 18.7 shows the body in this position.

Body Planes

The body can be divided into planes using the anatomic position as another frame of reference. *Planes* are imaginary cuts or sections through the body. The use of plane terminology is common when discussing diagnostic imaging (e.g., computed tomography [CT] scan) of the body. Diagnostic imaging will be discussed in more detail later in the chapter. Planes include the coronal, midsagittal, and transverse planes:

- *Coronal plane* or *frontal plane:* Divides the body into front and back portions (Figure 18.8). The front of the body is referred to as the *anterior* or *ventral.* The back of the body is referred to as the *posterior* or *dorsal.*
- *Midsagittal plane* or *median plane:* Separates the body into equal right and left halves. The medial line starts at the top of the head (cranium) and continues down the body to between the legs to the ground. This is also referred to as the *midline* of the body. Closer to the midline is referred to as *medial,* and farther away from the midline is called *lateral.*
- *Transverse plane* or *horizontal plane:* Divides the body horizontally into upper and lower sections. The area above the plane is called *superior* (pertaining to upward) or *cephalad* (toward the head). The area below the plane is called *inferior* (pertaining to downward) or *caudad* (toward the tail).

Directional and Positional Terms

Besides the directional terms discussed in the prior section (e.g., anterior, posterior, superior), additional terms can be used to indicate a position on the patient. Here are some additional positional and directional terms:

- *Unilateral* pertains to one side; *bilateral* pertains to two sides.
- *Dextrad* means toward the right side, and *sinistrad* means toward the left side. Dextrad and sinistrad are opposites.
- *Afferent* pertains to carrying toward a structure. *Efferent* pertains to carrying away from a structure. For example, the afferent arteriole brings blood to the glomerulus; the efferent arteriole carries blood away from the glomerulus.
- *Ipsilateral* pertains to the same side. *Contralateral* pertains to the opposite side. For example, the right leg is ipsilateral to the right arm but contralateral to the left arm.
- *Superficial* is toward the surface of the body. *Deep* is away from the surface of the body. For example, the skin is superficial, whereas bones are deep in the body.
- *Proximal* pertains to near the origin or toward the trunk of the body. *Distal* pertains to far from the origin or farthest from the trunk of the body. For example, the toes are distal to the knee; the hip is proximal to the knee.
- Body positions refer to the physical orientation of the body. *Supine* means a person is lying face up, and *prone* is lying face down. Lying on one's side is called the *lateral* position.

CRITICAL THINKING APPLICATION **18.9**

Bella continues to help Daniela on breaks during work. Today, Daniela is learning directional terms. Bella encourages Daniela to repeat the term and definition as she points to that part of her body. How else might Daniela learn the directional terms and the opposite pairs?

Body Cavities

The body contains cavities or hollow areas that are filled with organs. The body is separated into the *dorsal* (posterior) and *ventral* (anterior) body cavities.

The dorsal body cavity protects nervous system organs and contains the following:

- *Cranial cavity:* Contains the brain; surrounded and protected by the cranium (skull).

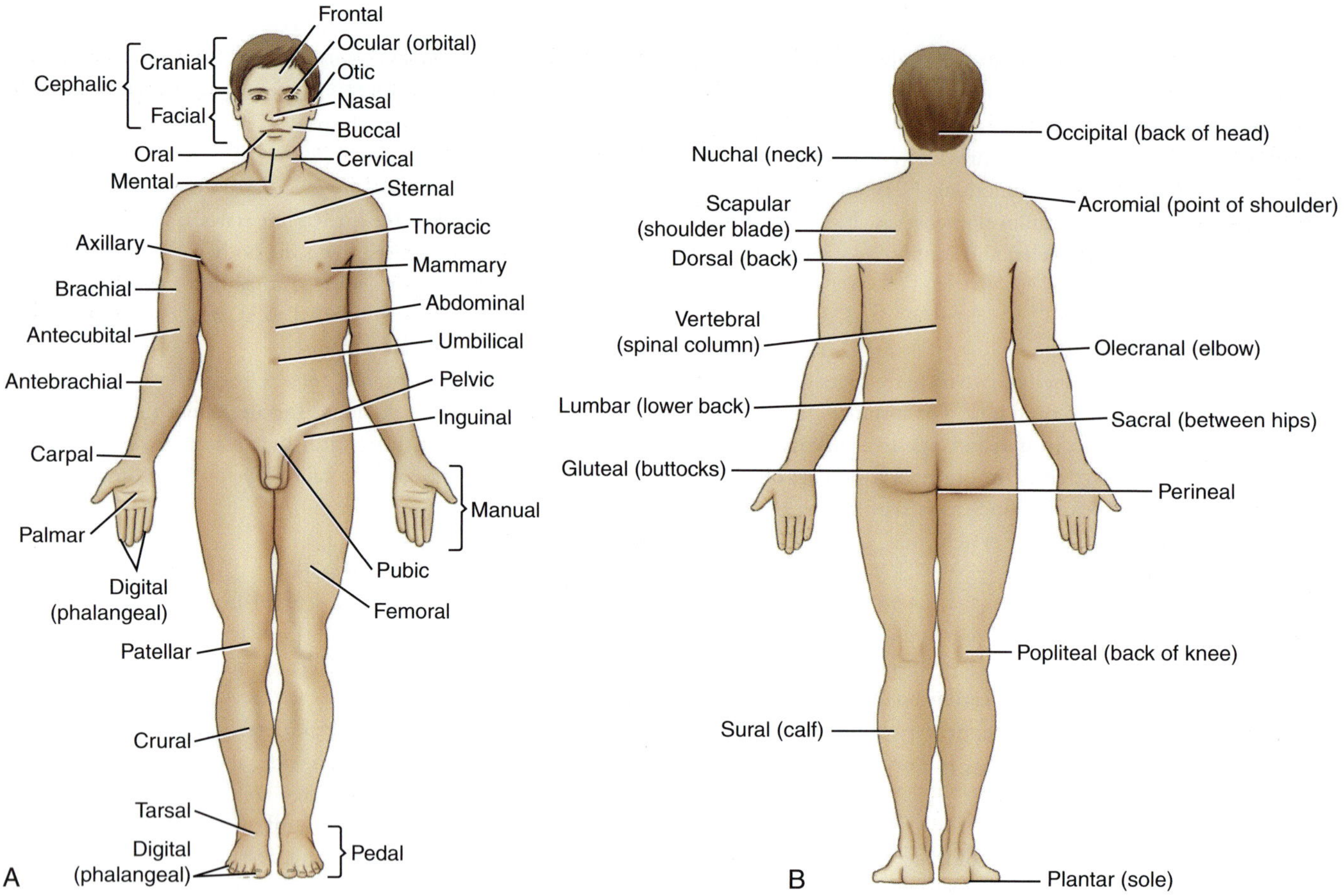

FIGURE 18.7 **(A)** Ventral surface anatomy. **(B)** Dorsal surface anatomy. (From Shiland B: *Mastering healthcare terminology*, ed 5, St. Louis, 2016, Elsevier.)

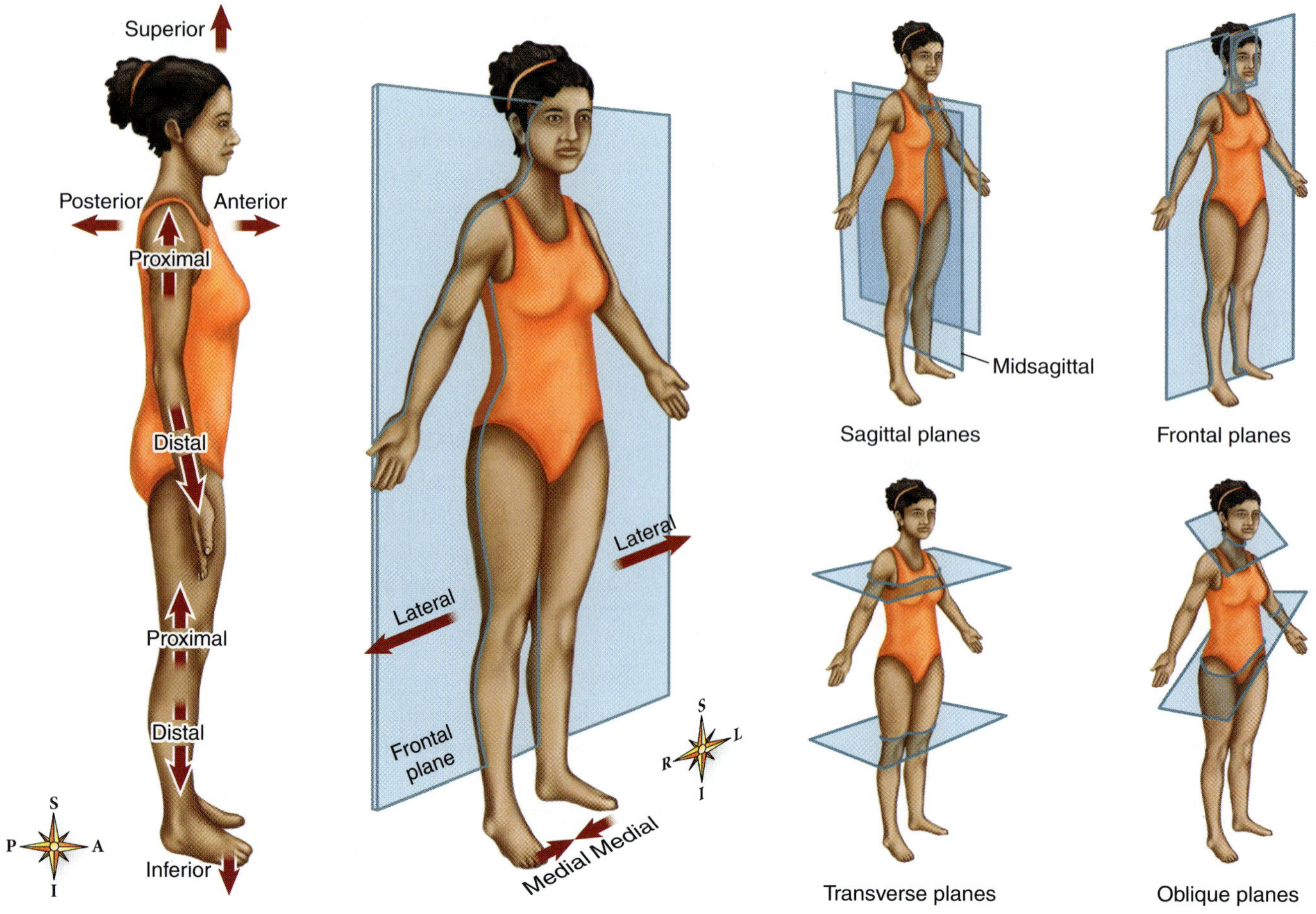

FIGURE 18.8 Body planes. (Patton KT, Thibodeau GA: *The human body in health and disease*, ed 7, St. Louis, 2018, Elsevier.)

- *Spinal cavity:* Contains the spinal cord; surrounded and protected by the vertebrae (bones of the spine).

The ventral body cavity consists of two cavities that are divided by the **diaphragm** (Figure 18.9):

- *Thoracic cavity:* Contains the heart, lungs, esophagus, and trachea (windpipe). Protected by the ribs, the sternum (breastbone), and the vertebrae (backbones).
- *Abdominopelvic cavity:* Can be divided as follows:
  - *Abdominal cavity:* Contains the abdominal organs (e.g., stomach, liver, gallbladder, intestines)
  - *Pelvic cavity:* Contains the urinary bladder and the reproductive organs

Abdominopelvic Quadrants and Regions

The abdominopelvic cavity is extensive. Either the four quadrants or the nine regions can be used to help describe a location in the abdominopelvic area. Descriptions that focus on the quadrants are simpler to understand and may be used with patients. The regions are more specific and are typically used by healthcare providers.

With the abdominopelvic quadrants, an imaginary line is drawn down the midline of the body. A horizontal line is drawn across the abdominopelvic cavity, intersecting at the naval (Figure 18.10). These quadrants are referred to as either right or left and upper or lower. Typically, abbreviations are used when documenting information about the patient. The four quadrants are as follows:

- *Right upper quadrant* (RUQ): Includes the right lobe of the liver, gallbladder, right kidney, small intestine (duodenum), large intestine (ascending and transverse colon), and head of the pancreas
- *Left upper quadrant* (LUQ): Includes the stomach, spleen, left lobe of the liver, pancreas, left kidney, and large intestine (transverse and descending colon)
- *Right lower quadrant* (RLQ): Includes the appendix, cecum, right ovary, right ureter, right spermatic cord, large intestine (ascending colon), and right kidney
- *Left lower quadrant* (LLQ): Includes the small intestine, large intestine (descending and sigmoid colon), left ovary, left ureter, left spermatic cord, and left kidney

The nine abdominopelvic regions lie over the abdominopelvic cavity. They provide a more specific location than the quadrants. The following table shows the abdominopelvic regions with the underlying organs (Figure 18.11).

RIGHT HYPOCHONDRIAC REGION	EPIGASTRIC REGION	LEFT HYPOCHONDRIAC REGION
Liver, gallbladder, right kidney	Kidneys, pancreas, liver, stomach	Stomach, liver, left kidney, spleen
RIGHT LUMBAR REGION	**UMBILICAL REGION**	**LEFT LUMBAR REGION**
Small intestine, large intestine (ascending colon), liver, right kidney	Small intestine, large intestine (transverse colon), pancreas, stomach	Small intestine, large intestine (descending colon), left kidney
RIGHT ILIAC REGION	**HYPOGASTRIC REGION**	**LEFT ILIAC REGION**
Appendix, small intestine, large intestine (cecum and ascending colon)	Small intestine, large intestine (sigmoid colon), bladder	Small intestine, large intestine (descending and sigmoid colon)

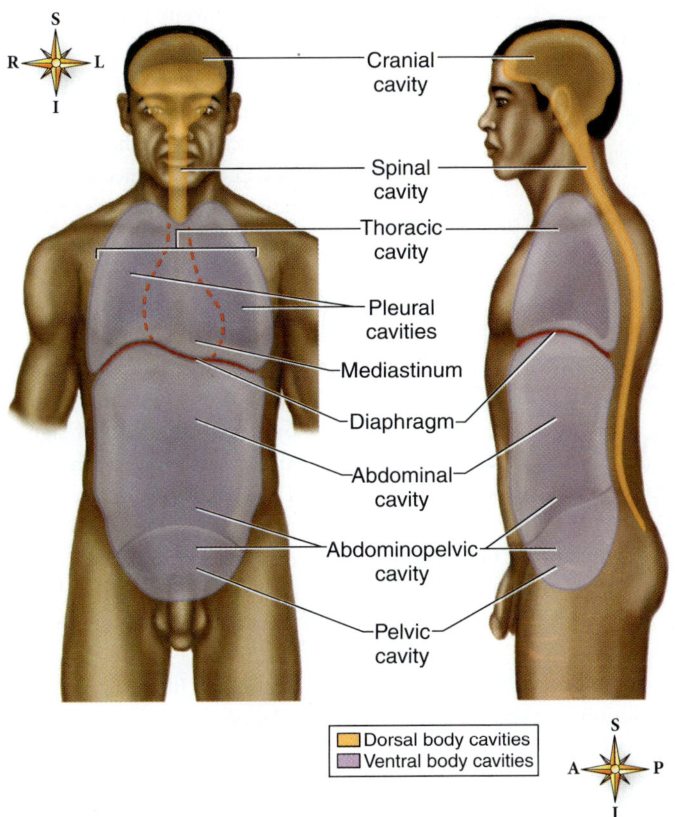

FIGURE 18.9 Body cavities. (Patton KT, Thibodeau GA: *The human body in health and disease*, ed 7, St. Louis, 2018, Elsevier.)

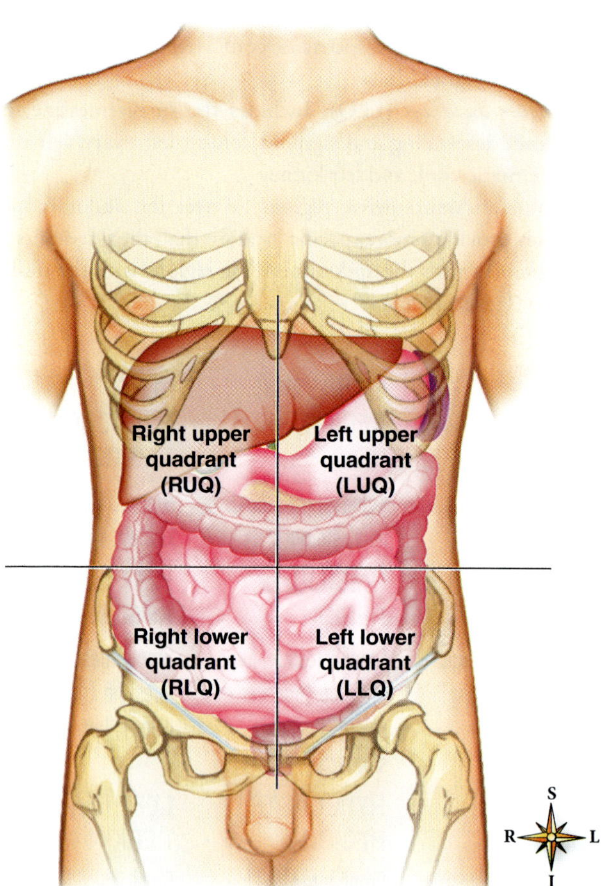

FIGURE 18.10 Abdominopelvic quadrants. (Patton KT, Thibodeau GA: *The human body in health and disease*, ed 7, St. Louis, 2018, Elsevier.)

CRITICAL THINKING APPLICATION 18.10

Tonight Bella is helping Daniela practice positional and directional terms with the regions. Bella asks Daniela these questions:

1. What regions are lateral to the umbilical region?
2. What regions are superior to the lumbar regions?
3. What region is medial to the hypochondriac regions and superior to the umbilical region?
4. What region is inferior to the umbilical region?
5. What regions are lateral to the sides of the hypogastric region?

What should Daniela's answers be to these questions?

ACID-BASE BALANCE IN THE BODY

The acid-base balance is a basic concept that the medical assistant needs to understand when learning about the physiology of the body. Knowing the normal pH range of the body and how the body adjusts to keep the pH within the normal range helps one to understand how homeostasis is maintained.

pH of the Body

The *pH* refers to the acid-base level of a solution on a scale of 1 to 14. A neutral pH is 7. An acidic solution has a pH under 7 and contains more hydrogen ions. A base or an alkaline solution has a pH over 7 and contains fewer hydrogen ions. To maintain homeostasis, the body attempts to keep the pH between 7.35 and 7.45. To maintain the acid-base range in the body, the concentration of hydrogen ions must remain constant. If the pH moves outside of this range, serious illness or even death can occur.

Factors That Change the Acid-Base Balance

The pH of our bodies can change based on the food we eat, the air we breathe, and the urine we excrete. To help maintain the pH range, the urinary system, the respiratory system, and chemical buffers must all work together. *Buffers* (e.g., bicarbonate) work to prevent changes in the pH. If there are more hydrogen ions, which will lower the pH, buffers will absorb some of the hydrogen ions. This will raise the pH. If the pH is too high, the buffers will "donate" hydrogen ions, bringing the pH down to the normal range.

The respiratory system regulates the carbon dioxide (CO_2) in our blood. CO_2 in the blood can combine with water to form the buffer bicarbonate. If a person *hyperventilates* (breathes rapidly), the CO_2 levels in the blood decrease, which also causes a decrease in the bicarbonate levels in the blood. This causes the pH of the body to rise.

The urinary system also has a role in the acid-base levels. The kidneys can absorb more base or more acid, depending on what the body needs for homeostasis. The kidneys can also produce bicarbonate if needed.

PATHOLOGY BASICS

Pathology is the study of diseases. In the ambulatory care setting, many patients' visits relate to the diagnosis or treatment of one or more disease processes. As a person ages, it is common to have more than one chronic illness. Understanding common diseases is important for medical assistants. The body system chapters that follow will cover the most common diseases affecting the system discussed. This chapter provides you with the basics to help you understand the concepts discussed in the future chapters. Common pathology terminology, protective mechanisms in the body, predisposing factors for disease, and causes of disease will be discussed.

Pathology Terminology

As you learn more about diseases, you will notice different terms used. Here is a list of terms commonly used when discussing pathology:

- *Disease*: A specific illness with a recognizable group of signs and symptoms and a clear cause (e.g., infection, environment)
- *Syndrome*: A group of signs and symptoms that occur together and are associated with a condition
- *Disorder*: A disruption of the function or structure of the body; many times, the words *disorder* and *disease* are used interchangeably in healthcare
- *Prevalence*: How often the disease occurs
- *Incidence*: Reflects the number of people newly diagnosed with the disease
- *Morbidity:* Illness
- *Mortality:* Death
- *Acute*: A severe, sudden onset of a disease

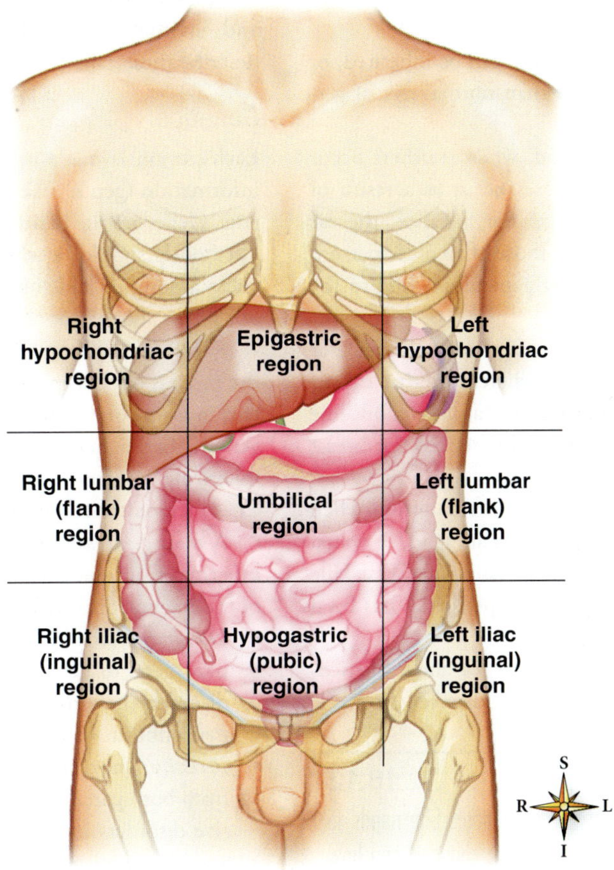

FIGURE 18.11 Abdominopelvic regions. (Patton KT, Thibodeau GA: The human body in health and disease, ed 7, St. Louis, 2018, Elsevier.)

- *Chronic*: A disease, disorder, or syndrome that lasts longer than 6 months
- *Prognosis*: A medical prediction of the outcome of the disease or disorder process
- *Prevention*: Methods to avoid getting the disease

The specialty chapters will discuss common diseases. For most of the diseases, the following sections will be discussed. It is important for the medical assistant to be familiar with the terminology used:

- *Etiology*: The cause of the disorder or disease.
- *Sign*: Something that is measured or observed by others; also called *objective data.* Examples of signs include redness, swelling or edema, blood pressure, and pulse.
- *Symptom*: Something that is only perceived by the patient; also called *subjective data.* Examples include pain, headache, dizziness, and nausea. Many times, *signs* and *symptoms* are used interchangeably, but there is a difference in their definitions.
- *Diagnostic procedures*: Tests and procedures that are used to help diagnose or monitor a condition.
- *Treatments*: Management of a disease or disorder; can include follow-up care and home treatments (e.g., medications, special diets, testing).

CRITICAL THINKING APPLICATION **18.11**

Daniela is struggling to remember the difference between signs and symptoms. What might be ways to remember these two terms? What are some examples of signs and symptoms?

Protection Mechanisms

The body has built-in mechanisms that protect against infection. The body's first line of defense includes chemical and physical barriers. Consider these examples:

- Skin forms a waterproof barrier.
- Tears and saliva contain an enzyme that breaks the cell wall of the **pathogen**.
- Mucus is a slick secretion produced in the respiratory, reproductive, and digestive systems. It protects the tissues and traps substances (e.g., bacteria, dust).
- Cilia are fine hairs that work closely with the mucus in the respiratory tract, trapping substances.
- Stomach acid is a very strong acid that kills bacteria, parasites, and other invaders that are swallowed.
- "Good" bacteria found on the skin and in the digestive system prevent "bad" bacteria from taking over.
- Urine flushes pathogens from the bladder and urethra.

If the structures are altered (e.g., a cut in the skin), pathogens can get into the body. When this happens, the second line of defense, the immune system, kicks in. White blood cells and the lymphatic system work together to protect the body.

Predisposing Factors

Predisposing factors are risk factors for disease. These factors make it more likely or increase the risk that the person may develop the disease or condition. Some predisposing factors can be changed to reduce the risk of developing a disease, whereas others cannot be changed. Predisposing factors include the following:

- *Hereditary or genetic factors*: Certain diseases can be inherited, or members of a family can have a higher-than-normal risk of getting a specific disease.
- *Age*: Certain diseases occur in childhood, whereas others occur more often in older adults. Some diseases occur as a result of changes in the body structures with age. For instance, the ear structures in an infant are different from those of an older person. Degenerative diseases occur in the older generations due to the wear and tear on the structures.
- *Sex*: Certain diseases occur more in one sex than the other. For instance, testicular cancer affects males, whereas uterine cancer affects females. Sometimes both sexes may get a disease, but one sex has a higher risk factor. Women are at higher risk for breast cancer than men.
- *Environmental factors*: Certain diseases are more common when a person has been exposed to pollutants in the air, land, or water. Though pesticides can reduce the risk of disease (e.g., West Nile virus disease and rabies), exposure to certain pesticides has been found to increase the risk of cancer.
- *Lifestyle*: Stress, poor diet, infrequent exercise, or abuse of nicotine, alcohol, or drugs can increase the risk for disease.

CRITICAL THINKING APPLICATION **18.12**

While on break at work, Daniela works on an assignment. She needs to determine which predisposing factors to disease can be changed and how they can be changed. What might be her answers?

CAUSES OF DISEASE

Disease can result from a change in homeostasis or can be the result of the body's response to a perceived threat. There are several common causes of diseases, including genetics, infectious pathogens, inflammatory processes, immunity, nutritional imbalance, trauma and environmental agents, and neoplasms. The following sections describe these causes.

Genetics

Each person is made up of 46 chromosomes, which carry genetic information (genes). We get 23 chromosomes from each of our parents. Genes are the basic units of heredity or the instructions on how our bodies should develop and function. Genes provide the differences among us and the similarities in families. From genes we get our physical appearance and our susceptibility to disease.

Recall that chromosomes are found in the cell's nucleus. During the process of conception and the cell division that follows, an extra chromosome or a change in the chromosome structure may occur. A genetic disease may result from a chromosomal error or the patient inheriting a defective gene from either parent. Types of genetic diseases include the monogenic and chromosomal disorders.

A *monogenic disorder* is caused by a single defective gene that is inherited from one or both parents. There are three main categories of monogenic disorders:

- *Dominant.* The child only needs to inherit one defective dominant gene to get the disease. Examples of autosomal dominant disorders include Huntington disease, Marfan syndrome, and neurofibromatosis type 1 (NFI).
- *Recessive.* The child would need to inherit a defective, recessive gene from both parents to get the disease. Examples of autosomal recessive disorders include cystic fibrosis, Tay-Sachs disease, sickle cell anemia, albinism (Figure 18.12), and phenylketonuria (PKU).
- *X-linked.* Sex determination is based on the father:
  - Dominant X-linked traits appear in a person who inherits one defective X chromosome. Fragile X syndrome (FXS) is an example of a dominant X-linked disorder. Both males and females are affected, but females usually have milder symptoms.

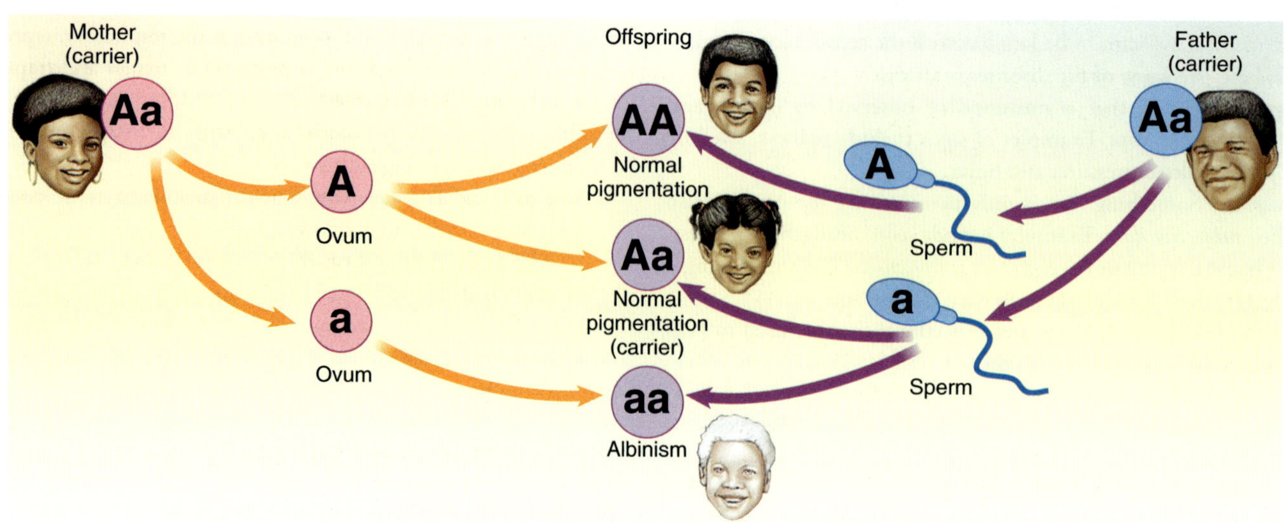

FIGURE 18.12 Inheritance of albinism. Albinism is a recessive trait, producing abnormalities only in those with two recessive genes (a). Presence of the dominant gene (A) prevents albinism. (From Patton KT, Thibodeau GA: *The Human Body in Health and Disease*, ed 7, St. Louis, 2018, Elsevier.)

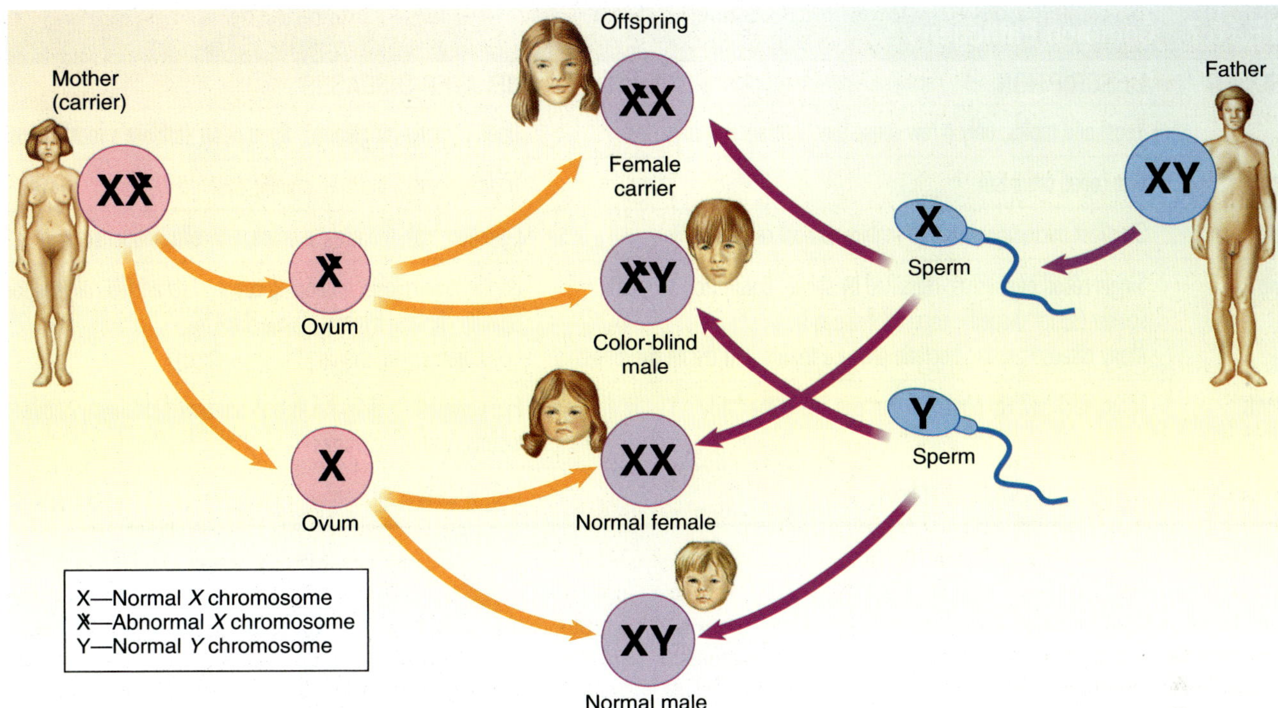

FIGURE 18.13 Sex-linked inheritance. Some forms of color blindness involve recessive X-linked genes. In this case, a female carrier of the abnormal gene can produce male children who are color blind. (From Patton KT, Thibodeau GA: *The human body in health and disease*, ed 7, St. Louis, 2018, Elsevier.)

- For recessive X-linked traits, the female would need two recessive X-linked genes to get the disorder. Because the male only has one X chromosome, inheriting one recessive X-linked gene will produce the recessive trait. Red-green color blindness and hemophilia A are examples of X-linked recessive conditions (Figure 18.13).

X and Y Chromosomes

The X and Y chromosomes are sex chromosomes. A biological female will have two X chromosomes, one from each parent. A biological male will have an X chromosome and a Y chromosome. The X chromosome comes from the mother and the Y chromosome from the father.

The X chromosome is about three times the size of the Y chromosome. The X chromosome contains more than 900 genes, also called *X-linked genes*. The Y chromosome only has about 55 genes, which are called *Y-linked genes*. These traits are only expressed in males.

With a *chromosomal disorder*, an abnormal number of chromosomes or a change in the chromosomal structure causes the disease. These are examples of chromosomal disorders:

- *Down syndrome:* The person has an extra chromosome.
- *Trisomy X syndrome:* The female has three X chromosomes.
- *Turner syndrome:* The female inherits only one copy of the X chromosome.

Infectious Pathogens

Many microorganisms are nonpathogenic, which means they do not cause disease. They can be found in our body, maintaining homeostasis. Other microorganisms are pathogenic, which means disease causing (Table 18.7). These pathogens enter our bodies through direct contact, indirect contact, or by vectors.

- *Direct contact*: A susceptible person comes in contact with an infected person, and the pathogen is spread via contact with blood, body fluids, and excretions (e.g., stool, urine, and saliva). Methods of direct contact include the following:
  - *Person to person*: Spread from sneezing, touching, and coughing. Tuberculosis and influenza are spread this way.
  - *Animal to person*: Spread from being bitten, scratched, or handling animal waste. Rabies is spread through this method.
  - *Mother to unborn child*: Varicella, herpes simplex viruses, and toxoplasmosis are just some of the diseases that are spread from an infected mother to the unborn child.
- *Indirect contact*: The pathogen is spread from contact with a contaminated object (e.g., water, food, drinking glass, airborne transmission). Escherichia coli and botulism are spread by indirect contact.
- *Vectors:* Most blood-sucking insects consume the disease-causing microorganism from one host and transmit it during a "meal" to another host. Mosquitoes are vectors for yellow fever, malaria, West Nile fever, and Zika virus. Ticks are vectors of Lyme disease, tick-borne encephalitis, and rickettsial diseases. Fleas are vectors for plague.

Disease Process

When a pathogen enters our body and starts to multiply, an infection occurs. Changes occur in our bodies, yet we do not feel any different. This is the *incubation period*. It starts at the time of exposure and ends when the signs and symptoms appear. The incubation period is different for each disease. For instance, strep throat has an incubation period of 2 to 5 days, whereas varicella (chickenpox) has

TABLE 18.7 Common Pathogens

PATHOGEN	DESCRIPTION	RELATED DISEASES
Fungi	Yeast and molds; only a few cause fungal disease or mycoses	Tinea corporis (ringworm), tinea pedis (athlete's foot), thrush
Protozoa	One-celled organism	Trichomoniasis, malaria, amebic dysentery
Viruses	Smallest microorganism that requires a host cell to multiply	Common cold, measles, mumps, varicella, influenza
Bacteria	Single-celled organisms; classified by shape: bacilli (rod shaped), spirilla (spiral shaped), cocci (dot shaped) Many disease-causing bacteria produce **toxins** that create the illness	Bacilli: tuberculosis, whooping cough, *Escherichia coli,* salmonella Spirilla: cholera, syphilis, Lyme disease Cocci: gonorrhea, meningitis, strep throat
Helminths	Large, multicellular parasites that can live in the body	Flatworms (including flukes and tapeworms), thorny-headed worms, and roundworms
Ectoparasite	A parasite that lives on the body	Lice, scabies

an incubation period of 14 to 16 days. As our body tissues become damaged from the infection, we start to see the signs and symptoms. This is when the disease occurs.

Some diseases are *noncommunicable*. They cannot be transmitted from one person to another. For instance, a person with tetanus cannot spread the disease to another person. Other diseases are *communicable*. These diseases are transmitted from one person to another. If a communicable disease is known to be easily transmitted, it is called a *contagious disease*. Strep throat, coronavirus disease (COVID-19), and influenza are examples of contagious diseases. For instance, people with strep throat are contagious from the start of the fever until they have been on the appropriate antibiotics for 24 hours. The period during which a disease can spread to another is called the *contagious period*. It is important for people in healthcare to understand the ways diseases are spread. Taking required precautions will minimize your risk of "catching something" from your patients.

CRITICAL THINKING APPLICATION **18.13**

At school, Daniela is learning about the transmission of pathogens. As a receptionist, she sees a lot of sick people stopping at her desk. She encourages those who cough to wear a mask. Hand sanitizer and tissues are also available. In light of disease transmission, why are these three items important in the prevention of disease?

Inflammatory Processes

The inflammatory response is the body's efficient way of protecting itself. Inflammation occurs when the tissues are injured. The injury could be the result of bacteria, trauma, heat, toxins, or other causes. The damaged cells release the chemicals histamine, prostaglandins, and bradykinin. These chemicals cause the following responses:

- Blood vessels at the site dilate. This causes more local blood flow. With the increase in blood flow, *erythema* (redness) and warmth occur in that area.
- Blood vessel walls allow more white blood cells and plasma to move out of the vessel into the surrounding tissues. The white blood cells work to protect the cells and clean up the dead tissue. The extra fluid from the blood causes *edema* (swelling), pain, and loss of movement. For instance, if an injury occurs in your finger joint area, the edema may be so great that it prevents you from moving your finger.

Five key signs of inflammation are erythema, edema, pain, warmth, and loss of function.

Even though the inflammatory process can be efficient, it can also be the cause of disease. *Autoinflammatory diseases* (e.g., familial Mediterranean fever) differ from autoimmune diseases, which will be described later in the chapter. Autoinflammatory diseases result from a genetic mutation that causes the inflammatory process to activate without a reason. The person may experience brief recurring attacks of pain and fevers, and blood work indicates systemic inflammation.

Immunity

Our immune system protects our bodies against potentially harmful substances. Our immune system "remembers" the **antigens** from diseases and responds with specific **antibodies**. The antibodies destroy or attempt to destroy the harmful substances. As with the autoinflammatory conditions, at times, the immune response can work against us. These malfunctions are classified as follows:

- *Allergies*: Reactions occur if a person is exposed to a food (e.g., milk, tree nuts, peanuts, eggs, soy, and wheat), pollen, dust mites, latex, mold, pet dander, inhalants, or other substances.
- *Autoimmunity*: The immune system does not recognize the body's own antigens and starts attacking itself. Rheumatoid arthritis, lupus, and psoriasis are examples of autoimmune disorders.
- *Immunodeficiency*: This is caused by a deficiency in one or more of the immune system's key players (e.g., white blood cells, such as the B cells and T cells). A person with immunodeficiency has impaired resistance to infections.

Nutritional Imbalance

Nutritional imbalances include too little or too much of a nutrient. Nutritional imbalances can affect growth, disease, and death. Causes of nutritional imbalances include the following:

- *Vitamin and mineral deficiencies*: Some of these deficiencies can be caused by alcoholism, disease, dietary deficiencies (and poverty), weight loss surgery, and metabolic disorders.
- *Vitamin and mineral excesses*: Vitamin excesses can occur when a person takes too much of a vitamin. The water-soluble vitamins (vitamins B and C) pass through the body fairly quickly. The fat-soluble vitamins (vitamins A, D, E, and K) can accumulate in the body. This can lead to toxic conditions. Mineral excess can be caused by diet, medication, or a metabolic error.
- *Obesity*: This is caused by eating too many calories, getting too little exercise, or having an endocrine or metabolic condition. Obesity can increase a person's risk for other diseases, including heart disease, diabetes, hypertension (high blood pressure), and stroke.
- *Starvation*: Eating too little food can result from disease or poverty.

Trauma and Environmental Agents

Trauma from auto accidents, violence, falls, and other events can cause disease. Common traumatic injuries include fractures, lacerated and ruptured organs, bleeding, neck and spinal injuries, and head injuries. Psychological trauma can also cause disorders.

Environmental changes, such as severe hot or cold temperatures and extremes of atmospheric pressures, can affect health. Poisonings, insect and animal bites, burns, electric shock, and near drownings can also cause diseases.

Neoplasms

When cells grow quicker than normal or do not die as fast as they should, an abnormal mass is created. This mass is called a *neoplasm* or *tumor*. Tumors can be *benign* (noncancerous) or *malignant* (cancerous). Table 18.8 shows the difference between benign and malignant tumors.

As the malignant cells grow, they can break through the *basement membrane*. This delicate membrane separates the epithelial cells from connective tissues. Once this occurs, the cancerous cells can invade blood and lymph vessels. The circulating fluid (blood, lymph fluid) can then carry the cancerous cells to another location in the body. Thus, cancerous cells from the *primary tumor* (original site) can metastasize to another location in the body, creating a *secondary tumor*.

TABLE 18.8 Differences between Benign and Malignant Tumors

CHARACTERISTIC	BENIGN TUMOR	MALIGNANT TUMOR
Cellular structure	Same as surrounding tissue	**Anaplastic** changes and poorly **differentiated**
Type of growth	Grows within a "shell" (encapsulated)	Infiltrates and **metastasizes**; spreads to distant site(s) in the body via the bloodstream or lymph system
Rate of growth	Usually slow; rarely fatal	May be slow, rapid, or very rapid; almost always fatal if left untreated
Destruction of localized tissue	None	Common; invades and takes over the surrounding tissue

If a provider suspects a patient may have cancer, a number of blood tests and imaging tests will be ordered. A **biopsy** may be performed. The surgeon may also take a biopsy of nearby lymph nodes so the tissue can be checked for malignant cells. Based on the diagnostic results, the **oncologist** or **pathologist** will grade and stage the cancer.

Classifications of Cancer

There are more than 100 different types of cancer. Cancers are classified based on the type of tissue from which they originate. The six major classifications are as follows:

- *Carcinoma*: A cancer of epithelial origin or cancer of the internal or external lining of the body. Carcinoma can originate from many areas of the body, including the skin, lungs, breast, colon, and prostate. Carcinomas make up about 80% to 90% of all cancer cases. Two major subtypes of carcinomas are these:
  - *Squamous cell carcinoma*: A cancer that originated from the squamous epithelium (Figure 18.14). One example is squamous cell carcinoma of the lung.
  - *Adenocarcinoma*: A cancer that starts in an organ or a gland. One example is gastric adenocarcinoma.
- *Sarcoma*: A cancer that starts in supportive and connective tissues (e.g., bones, tendons, cartilage, fat, and muscle). Examples include osteosarcoma, chondrosarcoma, hemangiosarcoma, mesothelioma, and glioma.
- *Myeloma*: A cancer that originated in the plasma cells (a type of white blood cells) in the bone marrow. An example is multiple myeloma.
- *Leukemia*: A cancer of the bone marrow. An example is acute myelocytic leukemia.
- *Lymphoma*: A cancer that originated in the lymphatic system. There are two types of lymphomas:
  - *Hodgkin lymphoma*: Diagnosed by the detection of Reed-Sternberg cells, a cell specific only to this disease
  - *Non-Hodgkin lymphoma*: All lymphomas other than Hodgkin lymphoma
- *Mixed types*: Cancer that has a combination of cells from within one classification or between two cancer classifications. Examples are teratocarcinoma and carcinosarcoma.

Grade

Grade refers to how abnormal the malignant cells look. If the malignant cells and tissues closely resemble normal cells and tissue, the tumor is called *well differentiated*. These are more slow-growing tumors. If the malignant cells and tissues do not look like normal cells and tissue, they are called *undifferentiated* or *poorly differentiated*. The microscopic look of the cell is graded using 1, 2, 3, or 4 to indicate the appearance. Grade 1 means well differentiated, or the cells and organization of the malignant tissue look close to that of normal tissue. Grade 2 means moderately differentiated, or the tissue does not look like normal tissue. The cells are also growing at a faster rate than normal. Grades 3 and 4 do not look like normal tissue and tend to spread quicker.

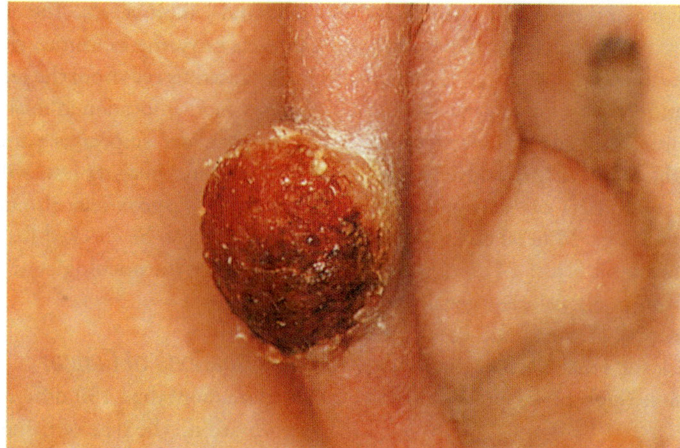

FIGURE 18.14 Squamous cell carcinoma on the ear. (From McCance KL, Huether SE: *Pathophysiology: the biologic basis for disease in adults and children*, ed 6, St. Louis, 2010, Mosby.)

TABLE 18.9 Stages of Cancer

STAGE	DEFINITION
In situ	Abnormal cells are present; no spreading has occurred.
Localized	Cancer cells are present; no spreading has occurred.
Regional	Cancer has spread to nearby lymph nodes, organs, or tissues.
Distant	Cancer has metastasized.
Unknown	Not enough information is available.

Stage

Stage refers to the extent of the cancer, including its size and whether it has spread. A cancer is referred to by this stage. Several staging systems are used, and various factors must be taken into consideration with staging systems:

- Location of the tumor
- Type of cell
- Size of the tumor
- Whether it has spread to nearby lymph nodes
- Whether it has spread to other locations in the body
- Tumor grade, or how abnormal the cells look compared with normal sizes and how quickly it grows and spreads

The following section describes the TNM staging system, which is widely used. Table 18.9 describes another type of staging system.

TNM Staging System. The letters T, N, and M are followed by a number or letter. X after T, N, or M indicates that it cannot be measured.

T refers to the size and extent of the primary tumor:

- T0: primary tumor cannot be found
- T1, T2, T3, and T4: refer to the size and extent of the primary tumor; the higher the number, the larger or more extensive the tumor

N refers to the number of nearby lymph nodes affected by the malignant cells:

- N0: no cancer in the nearby lymph nodes
- N1, N2, N3, and N4: refers to the location and number of nearby lymph nodes that have cancer; the higher the number, the more nodes are affected

M refers to whether the tumor has metastasized:

- M0: no metastasis has occurred
- M1: metastasis has occurred

Once TNM staging has been done, the three elements are combined for an overall stage.

- Stage 0: Abnormal cells are present; no spreading has occurred.
- Stages I, II and III: Malignancy is present. The number is greater for larger tumors and tumors that have spread to nearby tissues.
- Stage IV: Cancer has metastasized.

CLOSING COMMENTS

Patient Coaching

Putting medical terminology into understandable language is important for every patient. Many patients will benefit from having medical terms put into simpler, everyday language. Choose your words carefully. Describe body parts, systems, and procedures in language that is clear and understandable to your patient. Ask your patients to repeat instructions back to you so that you know that they are clear on all instructions. Listen to your patient and be open and willing to answer any questions that are within a medical assistant's scope of practice. Have written instructions available whenever possible.

Legal and Ethical Issues

Communication is key to providing the best possible patient care and serving the patient in an ethical manner. Using proper terminology, spelling, and pronunciation will help you inform your patients in a useful way. Being certain that your patients are clear on all instructions is vital. If patients do not receive clear instructions, they may make mistakes in preparing for diagnostic procedures, taking medication, or following treatment or therapy regimens. Clear communication is essential.

Patient-Centered Care

Understanding medical terminology, basic anatomy, and basic pathology allow the medical assistant to help patients in very real ways. The medical assistant can "translate medical terms into day-to-day language. Medical assistants who can describe procedures in everyday terms help their patients understand what will happen during a procedure and may put a patient's mind at ease. Knowing what to expect helps relieve the fear of the unknown.

Professional Behaviors

Having a good understanding of the structural organization of the body will help as you learn about each body system. Knowing how medical terminology relates to body organization, cavities, quadrants, regions, and planes is important for accurate communication. As a medical assistant, you will be communicating with providers and peers. Using correct medical terminology and having a strong understanding of the body systems will help you communicate effectively in the ambulatory care setting.

SUMMARY OF SCENARIO

Daniela continues in her position as a float receptionist. She is gaining a lot of experience in the Walden-Martin Family Medical Clinic. She is excited to be able to understand so many medical terms. When she comes across a new term, she is now able to decode it by breaking it down into word parts. With her knowledge of the most common prefixes and suffixes, she can get a general idea of what the term means even if she does not know the meaning of all the word parts. She can already see how she will be able to use her knowledge of medical terminology in other classes in her medical assistant program.

Bella continues to help Daniela study for her medical terminology and human body courses. Daniela really appreciates the study tips and reviewing assistance that Bella gives her. Some of her favorite ways to study these courses include the following:

- Making flashcards with the term or word part on one side and the definition on the other. Bella warned her to keep the definition short and simple. For nonmedical terminology, she learned more when she wrote her own definition. She realized the tests did not always use the exact words used in the textbook.
- Daniela realized that she learned better when she listened to the content. So she recorded herself going through her flashcards and review sheets. She found that if she stated the term or question and then paused, when she listened, she could fill in the blank before hearing the answer.
- Lastly, Daniela learned that she sometimes felt she knew the content but was not always sure until it came to the test. So she decided to test herself on the content during her study times to see what she really knew.

Daniela is very excited that she will soon complete her human body and disease course and medical terminology course. She is also excited to apply the study practices she is learning to her future medical assistant courses.

SUMMARY OF LEARNING OBJECTIVES

1. **Differentiate among eponyms, abbreviations, acronyms, symbols, and medical terminology word parts.**
   An eponym is a word that comes from the name of a person, place, or thing associated with the word. An *abbreviation* is a shortened version of a word or phrase. Acronyms are also abbreviations that become pronounceable words. A *symbol* is a picture that represents a word or phrase. Medical term word parts have either a Greek or Latin origin. Medical terms may be created from prefixes, suffixes, roots, and combining forms. Tables 18.1 and 18.2 provide lists of common prefixes and suffixes and their meanings.
2. **Explain the common combining forms used for the different body systems.**
   Many of the combining terms can be organized by body systems. Some of the related combining terms for each body system include the following:
   - Cardiovascular system: angi/o, cardi/o, hemat/o, and phleb/o
   - Digestive system: abdomin/o, chol/e, col/o, and hepat/o
   - Endocrine system: adren/o, ovari/o, pancreat/o, and thyroid/o
   - Integumentary system: cutane/o, derm/o, pil/o, and seb/o
   - Lymphatic and immune systems: lymph/o, myel/o, splen/o, and thym/o
   - Musculoskeletal system: arthr/o, cost/o, my/o, and ten/o
   - Nervous system: cerebell/o, cerebr/o, mening/o, and neur/o
   - Reproductive system: cervic/o, mamm/o, orch/o, and uter/o
   - Respiratory system: bronch/o, laryng/o, nas/o, and pneumon/o
   - Sensory system: audi/o, aur/o, ocul/o, and ot/o
   - Urinary system: cyst/o, ren/o, ureter/o, and urethr/o
3. **Explain the guidelines for building, defining, and pronouncing medical terms.**
   When combining a root with a suffix, if the suffix begins with a consonant, use a combining vowel between the root and the suffix. If the suffix begins with a vowel, do not use a combining vowel. Furthermore, if the root ends in a vowel and the suffix starts with the same vowel, one of the vowels is dropped. When adding a root to a root, use a combining vowel. Do not use a combining vowel between a prefix and a root. With some terms, the order of the combining forms follows the sequence of the procedure.

   When defining terms, start by dividing the term into word parts. Then label and define each word part. Define the term by starting with the suffix definition and then add the definitions for the rest of the word, starting at the beginning of the term.

   Table 18.6 provides a list of letter combinations that have different sounds.

Continued

SUMMARY OF LEARNING OBJECTIVES—*continued*

4. **Explain the structural organization of the body from simple to complex.**
   Anatomy is the study of how the body is shaped and structured. It includes the structures, levels of organization, and the relationships among different body parts. Physiology is the study of body functions.
   To summarize the structural organization of the body from simple to complex:
   - Cells are the most basic unit.
   - Tissues are groups of similar cells from the same source that carry out a specific function.
   - Organs are structures made up of two or more types of tissues.
   - Body systems are made up of several organs and their related structures.
   - An organism is made up of many body systems that work together for homeostasis in the body.
5. **Differentiate among the positional reference terms used for the body, including the anatomic position, planes, cavities, and abdominopelvic quadrants.**
   The anatomic position is a standard frame of reference. This means the body stands erect with the face forward, arms at the sides, palms forward, and toes pointed forward. Using the anatomic position, the body can be divided into planes as another frame of reference. Coronal plane or frontal plane: Divides the body into front and back portions. Midsagittal plane or median plane: Separates the body into equal right and left halves. Transverse plane or horizontal plane: Divides the body horizontally into upper and lower sections.
   The body contains cavities or hollow areas that are filled with organs. The body is separated into the dorsal (posterior) and ventral (anterior) body cavities. The dorsal body cavity is divided into the cranial and spinal cavities. The ventral body cavity consists of the thoracic cavity and the abdominopelvic cavity.
   With the abdominopelvic quadrants, an imaginary line is drawn down the midline of the body. A horizontal line is drawn across the abdominopelvic cavity, intersecting at the naval. These quadrants are referred to as either right or left and upper or lower. The nine abdominopelvic regions lie over the abdominopelvic cavity. They provide a more specific location than the quadrants.
6. **Explain the mechanisms in the body that maintain the acid-base balance.**
   The *pH* refers to the acid-base level of a solution on a scale of 1 to 14. A neutral pH is 7. An acidic solution has a pH under 7, and a base or an alkaline solution has a pH over 7. The body attempts to keep the pH between 7.35 and 7.45 to maintain homeostasis. The pH of our bodies can change based on the food we eat, the air we breathe, and the urine we excrete. To help maintain the pH range, the urinary system, the respiratory system, and chemical buffers must all work together.
7. **Explain the basics of pathology, including the terminology, protection mechanisms, and predisposing factors.**
   Pathology is the study of diseases. Pathology terminology includes the following terms: *disease, syndrome, disorder, prevalence, incidence, morbidity, mortality, acute, chronic, prognosis, prevention, etiology, sign, symptom, diagnostic procedures,* and *treatments.*
   Protection mechanisms are the body's built-in mechanisms that protect against infection. The body's first line of defense includes chemical and physical barriers.
   Predisposing factors are risk factors for disease. Predisposing factors include hereditary or genetic factors, age, sex, environmental factors, and lifestyle.
8. **Differentiate among the common causes of diseases.**
   There are several common causes of diseases, including genetics, infectious pathogens, inflammatory processes, immunity (allergies, autoimmunity, and immunodeficiency), nutritional imbalance, trauma and environmental agents, and neoplasms.

INFECTION CONTROL

19

SCENARIO

Rosa Lucia is a certified medical assistant working for Walden-Martin Family Medical (WMFM) Clinic. She is quite concerned about contracting an infectious disease while caring for her patients. Rosa learned about Standard Precautions while enrolled in her medical assisting program and now must implement that knowledge in the workplace. Two important factors in preventing the spread of infection are (1) understanding how to break the chain of infection and (2) recognizing the importance of correct and frequent hand washing.

While studying this chapter, think about the following questions:

- How can Rosa use her understanding of infection control to prevent the spread of infection?
- What is the significance of an exposure control plan at Walden-Martin Family Medical Clinic?
- What are the important details of the office's compliance with the guidelines established by the Occupational Safety and Health Administration (OSHA)?
- How can Rosa implement required infection control procedures at Walden-Martin Family Medical Clinic?

LEARNING OBJECTIVES

1. Apply the chain of infection process to healthcare.
2. Examine how the human body defends itself from infectious agents.
3. Analyze the differences among acute, chronic, latent, and opportunistic infections.
4. Examine the role of the Occupational Safety and Health Administration Standards in infection control.
5. Apply the concepts of medical and surgical asepsis to the healthcare setting.

VOCABULARY

antibodies Protein substances produced in the blood or tissues, in response to a specific antigen, that destroy or weaken the antigen; part of the immune system.

antiseptics (an ti SEP tiks) Substances that inhibit the growth of microorganisms on living tissue (e.g., alcohol and povidone-iodine solution [Betadine]); they are used to cleanse the skin, wounds, and so on.

autoimmune A disease in which the body produces antibodies that attack its own tissues and cells, leading to the deterioration of structure or function.

candidiasis (kan di DIE i sis) An infection caused by a yeast, Candida albicans, that typically affects the vaginal mucosa and skin.

communicable (kuh MYOO ni kuh buhl) Diseases spread from person to person, either by direct or nondirect contact (i.e., insects, examination tables).

defecation (def i KAY shun) The act of voiding waste from the bowels through the anus; the act of having a bowel movement.

degenerative (dih JEN er uh tiv) An illness resulting from the deterioration of tissues and organs.

disinfectant (dis in FEK tant) Any chemical agent used on nonliving objects to destroy or inhibit the growth of harmful organisms; not effective against bacterial spores.

fatigue (fuh TEEG) Extreme tiredness.

germicides (JUR muh sides) Agents that destroy pathogenic organisms.

hereditary (huh RED i ter ee) Passed from parents to offspring through the genes.

impervious (im PUR vee uhs) Not permitting penetration.

inanimate Not animate; lifeless.

ingested Taken, as food, into the body.

inhalation (in huh LAY shuhn) The act of breathing in.

interferon (in ter FEER on) A protein formed when a cell is exposed to a virus; the protein blocks viral action on the cell and protects against viral invasion.

malaise (ma LAYZ) A condition of general bodily weakness or discomfort.

noninvasive procedures Procedures that do not penetrate human tissue.

nosocomial infections (nos uh KOH mee uhl) Infections acquired in a healthcare setting.

parenteral (pa REN ter uhl) Taken into the body by any route other than the digestive tract (e.g., subcutaneous, intravenous, or intramuscular administration).

pathogenic Capable of producing disease.

VOCABULARY—*continued*

pyemia (pie EE mee uh) The presence of pus-forming organisms in the blood.

relapse The recurrence of the symptoms of a disease after apparent recovery.

remission The partial or complete disappearance of the clinical and subjective characteristics of a chronic or malignant disease.

spore A thick-walled, dormant form of bacteria that is very resistant to disinfection measures.

Standard Precautions A set of infection control practices used to prevent the transmission of diseases that can be acquired by contact with blood, body fluids, nonintact skin, and mucous membranes.

sterile (STER il) Free of all microorganisms, pathogenic and nonpathogenic.

tinea (TIN ee uh) Any fungal skin disease that results in scaling, itching, and inflammation; examples include ringworm and athlete's foot.

transmission The passage or spread of disease.

vectors Animals or insects (e.g., ticks, rodents, mosquitos) that transmit a pathogen.

INTRODUCTION

To gain an understanding of the importance of infection control, you must comprehend the concepts of disease transmission and the body's response to infection. One of the easiest ways to prevent the spread of disease is to wash your hands or use alcohol-based hand sanitizers. Every procedure must begin and end with hand hygiene practices. Making sure that **sterile** technique is used is another huge component of infection control. The fundamental concepts of this chapter should be used whenever you are faced with an infection control issue. The guidelines established by the Occupational Safety and Health Administration (OSHA) also have stated this. The guidelines in this chapter are basic to all clinical skills, and following them can reduce the transmission of disease organisms and lessen the severity of disease. These guidelines also may save a patient's or co-worker's life, or even your own.

CHAIN OF INFECTION

Disease is defined as a specific illness with a recognizable group of signs and symptoms and a clear cause (e.g., infection, environment). We recognize and categorize many types of diseases: **hereditary** (genetic), drug induced, **autoimmune**, **degenerative**, **communicable**, and infectious, to name only a few. Sometimes a specific disease may fit two or more categories.

Any disease caused by the growth of **pathogenic** microorganisms in the body falls into the category of *infectious diseases.* The entrance of a living microbe into the body is not a disease until the infected cell or individual shows harmful changes in structure, function, or biochemistry. In fact, a pathogen may be **ingested**, injected, or inhaled and never cause disease. However, an unaffected person can still transmit the infection to another person. In this case, we call the unaffected person a *carrier.*

Microorganisms are almost everywhere. We carry them on our skin, in our bodies, and on our clothing. They can be in ice, boiling water, the soil, and the air. The only places free of microorganisms are certain internal body organs and tissues and sterilized medical equipment and supplies. In the normal state, organs and tissues that do not connect with the outside by means of mucus-lined membranes are free of all living microorganisms.

Certain factors are required for an infectious disease to spread. These factors, or links, make up the chain of infection. Break the chain, and you break the infection process (Figure 19.1).

The chain of infection starts with the infectious agent. Infection cannot occur without the presence of an infectious microorganism. The best way for healthcare workers to prevent the spread of disease is to use infection control procedures, such as the following:

- Consistent hand washing
- Proper use of **antiseptics**
- Effective disinfection and sterilization methods

Infectious Agents

There are five types of potentially pathogenic agents or microorganisms: viruses, bacteria, fungi, protozoa, and helminths. Each of these will be discussed in the following sections.

Viruses

Viruses, the smallest of all pathogens, lead the list of important disease-causing agents. Viral particles insert their own deoxyribonucleic acid (DNA) or ribonucleic acid (RNA) into a host cell and then use the host cell to help reproduce more viral particles. Viral invasion may not cause immediate symptoms because host cells infected with viruses can produce a substance called **interferon**. This protects nearby cells. Interferon leaves the infected cell and acts somewhat like Paul Revere, warning neighboring cells that "a virus is coming!" The neighboring cells then produce antiviral proteins, which prevent the virus from replicating inside the cells, slowing or halting the infection.

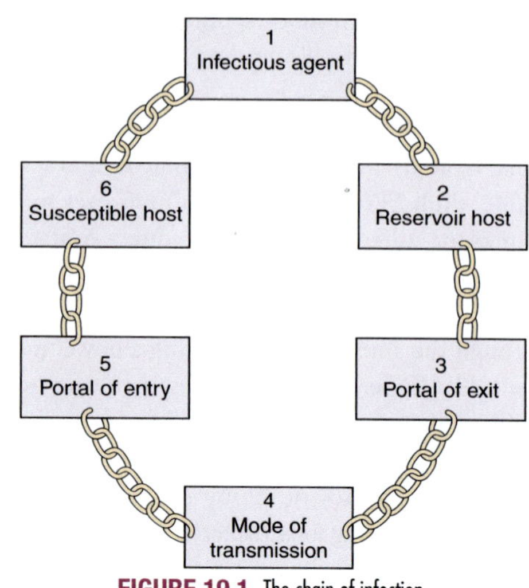

FIGURE 19.1 The chain of infection.

Antibiotics are unable to destroy viral invaders. The only way to destroy a viral invader is to destroy the host cell. Therefore, the treatment for viral infections typically focuses on relieving symptoms, or *palliative treatment,* and antiviral medications that slow the rate of viral replication. Interferon and antiviral agents may be prescribed, depending on the specific viral agent. Viral diseases include the following:

- Common cold
- COVID-19
- Influenza A and B
- Herpes
- Infectious hepatitis (e.g., hepatitis B and C)
- Acquired immunodeficiency syndrome (AIDS), which is caused by the human immunodeficiency virus (HIV)

COVID-19

COVID-19, also known as coronavirus disease, is caused by the SARS-CoV-2 virus. In 2020 COVID-19 was declared a pandemic as it rapidly spread worldwide. Most people who get COVID-19 experience mild to moderate respiratory symptoms. Anyone can get COVID-19 and have serious problems, but it especially impacts older people and those with underlying medical conditions like cardiovascular disease, diabetes, chronic respiratory disease, or cancer.

To prevent the spread of COVID-19, the Centers for Disease Control and Prevention (CDC) has provided the following recommendations:

- Get vaccinated.
- Wear a mask.
- Practice social distancing.
- Avoid crowds.
- Wash your hands often.
- Cover coughs and sneezes.
- Clean and disinfect.
- Monitor your health daily.

Antiviral Agents

- Acyclovir (Zovirax)
- Adefovir dipivoxil (Hepsera)
- Famciclovir (Famvir)
- Oseltamivir (Tamiflu)
- Penciclovir (Denavir)
- Valacyclovir hydrochloride (Valtrex)

Bacteria

Bacteria are tiny, simple cells that produce disease in a variety of ways. Pathogenic bacteria can secrete toxic substances that do the following:

- Damage human tissues
- Act as parasites inside human cells
- Grow on body surfaces, disrupting normal functions

Bacteria are classified according to their shape, or *morphology.* Some bacteria can produce resistant internal structures, called **spores**, that make treatment difficult. When bacteria invade the body, the patient can be treated in several ways. The most common approach is to use antibiotics to destroy the invader or inhibit its growth. We all have nonpathogenic bacteria that reside in various body systems. For example, a harmless form of *Escherichia coli (E. coli)* lives in the large intestine. These bacteria protect against disease by competing for nutrients, taking up space, and excreting waste. All of these actions discourage pathogens. Common diseases caused by bacteria include the following:

- Tuberculosis
- Urinary tract infections
- Pneumonia
- Strep throat
- Food poisoning
- Sexually transmitted infections

Bacteria Morphology

- Spherical
  - Coccus (singular), cocci (plural)
- Rod shaped
  - Bacillus (singular), bacilli (plural)
- Spiral shaped
  - Spirillum (singular), spirilla (plural)
  - Spirochete (singular), spirochetes (plural)
  - Vibrio (singular), vibrios (plural)

Cocci, diplococci

Bacillus

Diplobacillus

Spirochete

ANTIBIOTIC RESISTANCE

Antibiotic resistance is one of the world's most significant public health problems. Infectious microorganisms that once were easily treated with antibiotics are growing increasingly resistant to the actions of these drugs. The CDC reported that at least 2.8 million people in the United States become infected with antibiotic-resistant bacteria, and at least 35,000 people die each year as a direct result of these infections. Resistance occurs when an antibiotic is used inappropriately to treat an infection. This allows the pathologic organism to change or mutate in some way, which reduces or eliminates the effectiveness of the drug. The mutation can occur in the following situations:

- An antibiotic is prescribed when it is not needed (e.g., for a viral infection).
- The antibiotic is prescribed inaccurately (e.g., lower dosage, fewer days than recommended).
- The antibiotic is not taken as prescribed.

Although mutations are rare, overuse of antibiotics provides more opportunities for them to occur. Antibiotics should be used to treat bacterial infections; however, they are not effective against viral infections, such as the common cold, most sore throats, and the flu. Cautious use of antibiotics is the key to preventing the spread of resistance. The CDC makes the following recommendations for providers:

- Prescribe antibiotic therapy only when it will benefit the patient.
- Treat the patient with an antibiotic that is specific to the infecting pathogen.
- Prescribe the recommended dose and treatment duration of the medication.

CRITICAL THINKING APPLICATION **19.1**

Susie Chen, a 3-year-old patient, is being seen today. She has been complaining of a cough and nasal congestion. Susie's father does not understand why the pediatrician did not order an antibiotic for his daughter's viral infection. Rosa needs to reinforce the doctor's decision. How can she help the father understand the proper use of antibiotics?

Fungi

Fungi may be unicellular or multicellular; they include such organisms as mushrooms, molds, and yeasts. Many forms are pathogenic and can cause diseases, such as **candidiasis** and **tinea** infections. Fungi grow best in warm, moist environments. Treatment with antifungal agents includes the application of topical preparations (e.g., clotrimazole [Lotrimin]) for tinea infections, vaginal suppositories (e.g., miconazole [Monistat]) for candidiasis, and oral medications (e.g., fluconazole [Diflucan], ketoconazole [Nizoral], and terbinafine [Lamisil]). Fungal infections also are called *mycotic* infections.

Protozoa

Protozoa are unicellular parasites that can replicate and multiply rapidly once inside the host. Examples of diseases caused by protozoa include giardiasis, which is typically caused by the ingestion of water contaminated by feces, and malaria, in which *Plasmodium* organisms invade the blood system. Protozoal infections are frequently seen in tropical climates, which have large insect populations. These insects serve as **vectors** for many protozoal diseases. For example, the mosquito transmits the organisms that cause malaria. Protozoa and helminths (worms) are usually grouped together as parasites.

Helminths

Helminths are multicellular and include tapeworms, roundworms, and flatworms (flukes). Tapeworms live in the intestines of some animals and can be transferred to humans who eat undercooked meat from infected animals. Most parasitic roundworm eggs are found in the soil and enter the human body when a person picks them up on the hands and then transfers them to the mouth. Roundworms eventually migrate to human intestines and cause infection and disease. Hookworms are intestinal parasites that are spread if the infected person defecates outside in nature or if the feces is used as fertilizer. The eggs are deposited in the soil and mature into larvae. The larvae can penetrate the skin of humans who walk barefoot or ingest contaminated soil (e.g., dirt on fingers or food). Flatworms with an external sucker are referred to as *flukes*. Flukes are found in raw or improperly cooked fish.

Proper diagnosis and treatment are key to breaking the chain of infection at the infectious agent link. Providers also have to take caution to prevent antibiotic resistance.

Reservoir

The second link in the chain of infection is the reservoir. The most common reservoirs are people, insects, animals, water, food, and contaminated instruments and equipment. Most pathogens must gain entrance into a host, or else they die. The reservoir host supplies all of the conditions needed for microbial growth, allowing the microbes to multiply. The pathogen either causes infection in the host or, in the case of vector-borne diseases, exits the host in great enough numbers to cause disease in another host.

Sanitization, disinfection, and sterilization are key to breaking the chain of infection at the reservoir link. Pest control can also help with the insect and animal components.

Portal of Exit

The chain of infection continues with the means, or *portal*, of exit—that is, how the pathogen escapes the reservoir host through the mouth, eyes, intestines, reproductive tract, nose, ears, urinary tract or open wounds. The use of **Standard Precautions** (e.g., gloves, masks, proper wound care, correct disposal of contaminated products, and handwashing) helps control the ability of infectious material to spread from one host to another.

It is important to use proper hand hygiene and personal protective equipment to break the chain of infection at the portal of exit link. Taking measures to control the splatter of body fluids, whether it be a cough or sneeze or during a procedure, is another important way to break this link.

Mode of Transmission

After exiting the reservoir host, the organism needs to be a mode of **transmission**. Transmission is either direct or indirect. *Direct transmission* occurs from contact with an infected person, with discharges from an infected person (e.g., feces or urine), or with infected soil. Direct transmission includes droplet transmission. This refers to the droplets that come from sneezing, coughing, or even talking. Those droplets land on the next potential host. *Indirect transmission* refers to the transfer of microorganisms by suspended particles in the air, **inanimate** objects, or animals and insects. When microorganisms are suspended particles, this is considered airborne transmission. Transmission occurs through **inhalation** of the microorganisms. *Vectors* are animals or insects that harbor pathogens and can transmit them. Transmission can also occur through contaminated food or drink or contact with contaminated objects (called *fomites*). Proper sanitation of water and food; the use of sanitization, disinfection, and sterilization procedures; and the use of **germicides** (e.g., Wavicide and Cidex) all help to control the transmission of pathogens.

To break the chain of infection at the mode of transmission link, hand hygiene and personal protective equipment are, again, important factors, along with food safety, sanitization, disinfection, and sterilization.

Portal of Entry

The next link in the chain of infection is the means, or portal, of entry. This is how the transmitted pathogen enters a new host through the mouth, eyes, intestines, reproductive tract, nose, ears, urinary tract, or open wounds. As with the portal of exit, the use of Standard Precautions helps to prevent the infectious agent from entering the body.

It is important to use proper hand hygiene and personal protective equipment to break the chain of infection at the portal of entry link. Providing proper first aid and personal hygiene play a role in breaking this link.

Susceptible Host

The final link in the chain of infection is exposure of the pathogen to a susceptible host. If the host is *susceptible* (i.e., capable of supporting the growth of the infecting organism), the organism multiplies. Various factors contribute to a host's susceptibility:

- Genetic factors
- Quantity of organisms
- State of the individual's physical health
- Stress
- Poor health
- Poor nutrition
- Poor hygiene or crowded living conditions

If conditions are right, the organism reaches infectious levels, and the susceptible host can start the chain of infection all over again.

Immunizations and patient education play an important role in reducing that susceptibility to break the chain of infection at the susceptible host link.

CRITICAL THINKING APPLICATION 19.2

Tommy Anderson, a 5-year-old patient, is in the office because of an outbreak of impetigo. Rosa must apply the concepts of the chain of infection and infection control methods to teach Tommy and his mother how to prevent the spread of the infection to other members of the family. What procedures should she follow after Tommy's visit to prevent the spread of the infection to other patients, other staff members, and herself?

HOW DOES THE BODY DEFEND ITSELF?

After taking a look at the infection cycle, you may be asking yourself, why aren't we sick all the time? There are so many ways for infectious agents to impact our health. Well, the human body has a number of ways to defend itself, and in the following sections, you will see how that works.

First Line of Defense

The first line of defense against pathogenic invasion is made up of the body's physical and chemical barriers. An intact *integumentary system*, or skin, serves as a physical barrier to infection. Other anatomic defense mechanisms include the following:

- Tears
- Cilia
- Mucous membranes
- pH of body fluids
- **Defecation** and vomiting

Second Line of Defense

The body's second line of defense is nonspecific chemical and cellular responses. *Phagocytic* cells engulf and destroy the microbes. Inflammation occurs, bringing white blood cells to the area. The inflammatory response produces swelling, redness, heat, and pain.

The *inflammatory response* (Figure 19.2) starts when the body experiences trauma or is exposed to pathogens. To defend itself, the body starts certain responses to destroy and remove pathogenic organisms and their by-products. If this is not possible, it will limit the damage caused by the invading pathogen. This process results in the four classic symptoms of inflammation:

- *Erythema* (redness)
- *Edema* (swelling)
- Pain
- Heat

When the body is exposed to an infectious agent or a foreign substance, cellular damage occurs at the site. Inflammation mediators (i.e., *histamine*, *prostaglandins*, and *kinins*) are released, causing three different responses at the cellular level. All three actions are designed to increase the number of white blood cells (WBCs) at the injury site.

First, blood vessels at the site dilate, causing an increase in local blood flow, which results in redness (inflammation) and heat. Blood vessel walls become more *permeable*, which allows for the movement of WBCs through the vessel wall to the site. The WBCs begin to form a fibrous capsule around the site to protect surrounding cells from damage or infection. Blood plasma also filters out of the more permeable vessel walls, resulting in edema (swelling), which puts pressure on the nerves and causes pain. Finally, *chemotaxis* or the release of chemical agents, occurs, attracting even more WBCs to the site. The increased number of WBCs at the site results in phagocytosis. Destroyed pathogens, cells, and WBCs collect in the area and form a thick, white substance called *pus*. If the pathogenic invasion is too great for localized control, the infection may collect in the body's lymph nodes, where more WBCs are present to help fight the battle. This causes swollen glands, or *lymphadenopathy*. If the body is too weak or the number of pathogens is too great, the infection may spread to the bloodstream. A systemic infection, called *septicemia* or *blood poisoning*, may occur, which ultimately could affect the entire

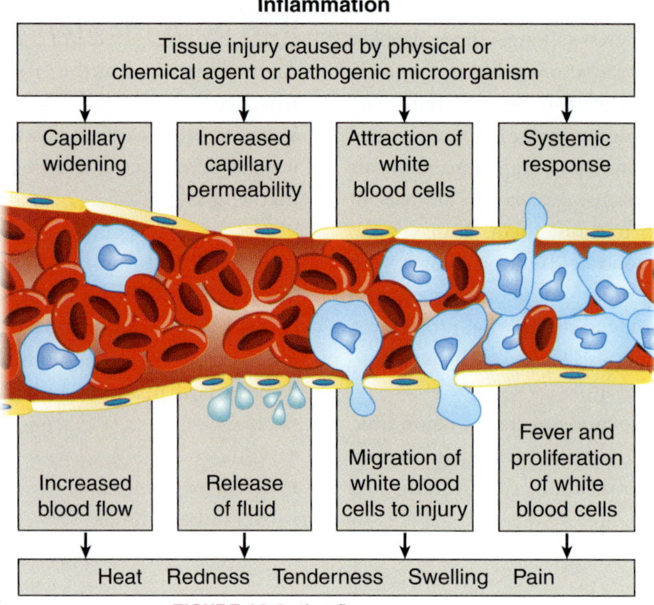

FIGURE 19.2 The inflammatory response.

body. Another term for septicemia is **pyemia**. Without appropriate medical intervention, death can occur from a systemic infection.

Third Line of Defense

The third line of defense involves specific immunity. The immune system responds by producing **antibodies** specifically designed to combat the presence of a foreign substance, or *antigen*. This process is called *humoral immunity* and is the responsibility of the body's B cells. Another immune system response involves T cells. This is called *cell-mediated immunity* and causes the destruction of pathogenic cells at the site of invasion or infection.

How Humoral Immunity Is Acquired

- There are two ways that antibodies can be acquired: actively or passively. These groups can be further categorized as artificial or natural.
- With actively acquired immunity, the body actively makes antibodies after exposure to the disease-causing organism. This could result from having the actual disease or from a vaccination.
- With passively acquired immunity, the body is given the antibodies without having to work for them. This could be the result of placental transfer, breastfeeding, or an injection of immunoglobulins.

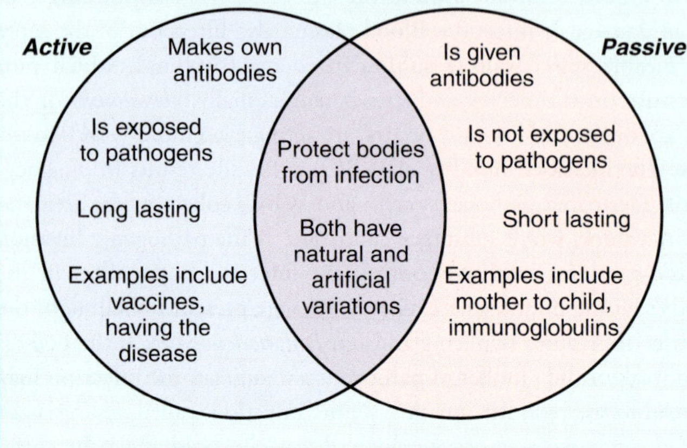

Immunizations trigger the development of antibodies. These antibodies mean that an individual is not susceptible to that disease even if she or he is exposed to the pathogen. However, some people do not develop immunity to diseases even after following immunization guidelines. The CDC has estimated that, depending on the vaccine, individuals do not develop immunity 1% to 5% of the time. The provider can check for immunity by ordering an antibody titer. A *titer* is a laboratory test that measures the level of antibodies in a blood sample. If a vaccine stimulated a person's immune system to create antibodies to a disease, the antibodies will be present in adequate amounts in the titer. If not, the provider decides whether another dose of the vaccine should be given to try to boost the person's immune response.

The Body's Natural Protective Mechanisms

The body has many levels of protection against the invasion of pathogenic microorganisms:

- Intact skin serves as a natural barrier to disease.
- Mucous membranes lining the openings of the body help protect underlying tissues and trap foreign substances.
- Tiny, hairlike projections, called *cilia*, line the respiratory tract and move in a coordinated upward motion to expel trapped foreign substances.
- Trapped substances can be expelled with sneezing and coughing before the organisms invade underlying tissue.
- Some body secretions, such as tears, have antimicrobial properties that help destroy invading pathogens.
- The natural pH of many of the body's organs discourages the growth of microbes. The acidic pH of urine, the vaginal mucosa, and the stomach helps prevent pathogenic invasion. The body's resident microbes create and maintain this environment.

CRITICAL THINKING APPLICATION 19.3

Rosa's next patient appears to have a localized inflammatory response to a splinter. What signs and symptoms should she expect the patient to show?

Rosa answers a telephone call from a patient who had surgery 3 days ago. The patient is concerned that the incision site is red, swollen, and hot. Is this a normal postoperative response? How might Rosa know whether the response is abnormal?

TYPES OF INFECTION

If an infectious agent does make it through and causes an infection, that infection can be classified in several different ways. The following sections discuss the different types of infections.

Acute Infection

An *acute infection* has a rapid onset of symptoms but lasts a relatively short time. This type of infection will go through the following stages:

- *Incubation:* The period of time between exposure to the pathogen and the appearance of the first symptoms. It can be from a few days to a few months. The incubation period for mononucleosis is 4 to 6 weeks.
- *Prodromal:* The short period of time when the first symptoms appear. With mononucleosis, the patient may have 1 to 2 weeks of **fatigue**, **malaise**, *myalgia*, and a low-grade fever.
- *Acute:* The disease is at its peak, and symptoms are fully developed. With mononucleosis, *pharyngitis*, *tonsillitis*, and *lymphadenopathy* are common symptoms.
- *Declining:* The symptoms of the disease start to subside. If patients have been prescribed antibiotics, this is when they may decide to stop taking them. It is important to stress to patients that they must take all of the medication. With mononucleosis, the declining stage can take several weeks or even months.
- *Convalescent:* In this stage, patients will regain their strength and return to a state of good health.

The prodromal stage of an acute infection is the time when the patient first shows vague, nonspecific symptoms of disease. For example, the person is not vomiting and does not have a fever, but the individual just does not feel well. In an acute viral infection, the host cell typically dies within hours or days. In most acute infections, such as the common cold, the body's defense mechanisms eliminate the virus within 2 to 3 weeks.

Chronic Infection

A *chronic infection* is one that persists for a long period of time, sometimes for life. In the case of chronic hepatitis B infection, patients are *asymptomatic,* or without symptoms. The virus is still detectable with blood tests and remains transmissible throughout the person's life. Hepatitis B infection is transmitted by blood or blood products and all body fluids. It is a serious health hazard to those who work in healthcare. All individuals employed in a healthcare setting should be immunized against hepatitis B. OSHA requires all employers to offer hepatitis B vaccination to their employees.

Latent Infection

A *latent infection* is a persistent infection in which the symptoms cycle through periods of **relapse** and **remission**. Cold sores and genital herpes are latent viral infections caused by the herpes simplex virus (HSV) types 1 and 2, respectively. The virus enters the body and causes the original lesion. It then lies dormant in nerve cells away from the surface until a certain trigger (illness with fever, sunburn, or stress) causes it to leave the nerve cell and seek the surface again. Once the virus reaches the superficial tissues, it becomes detectable for a short time and causes a new outbreak at the site. Another herpes virus, the varicella-zoster virus, causes chickenpox (varicella). This virus may lie dormant along a nerve pathway for years and later erupt as the painful disease shingles (herpes zoster).

Opportunistic Infections

Opportunistic infections are caused by organisms that are not typically pathogenic but cause disease under certain circumstances. A host with an impaired immune system response, such as individuals infected with HIV, is susceptible to opportunistic infections. Over time, the person's immune system becomes weakened, and diseases result that are not typically seen in patients with a healthy immune system, such as *Pneumocystis jiroveci* pneumonia and oral candidiasis. People without a compromised immune system can have an opportunistic infection.

OCCUPATIONAL SAFETY AND HEALTH ADMINISTRATION STANDARDS FOR THE HEALTHCARE SETTING

In 1987, in response to concern about the increasing prevalence of HIV and hepatitis B virus (HBV), the CDC recommended a new approach to potentially infectious materials, called *Universal Precautions.* The underlying concept of Universal Precautions is that because healthcare workers do not know whether a patient has an infectious organism, all blood and certain body fluids must be treated as if they contain infectious bloodborne pathogens. Therefore, precautions must be implemented for all patients, regardless of the information available about the person's individual health history. In turn, Universal Precautions protect patients from any bloodborne infection the healthcare worker may carry.

In 2001 OSHA developed the Bloodborne Pathogens Standard, which includes Universal Precautions. The goal of the Bloodborne Pathogens Standard is to safeguard all healthcare employees and their patients who are at risk of exposure to blood and other potentially infectious materials (OPIM). Items contaminated with any of the following potentially infectious materials require special handling:

- Body fluids
- Semen
- Vaginal secretions
- Cerebrospinal fluid (CSF)
- Synovial fluid
- Pleural fluid
- Pericardial fluid
- Peritoneal fluid
- Amniotic fluid
- Saliva in dental procedures
- Any body fluid that is visibly contaminated with blood
- All body fluids that are present in situations in which it is difficult or impossible to differentiate between body fluids
- Any unfixed tissue
- Any pathogenic microorganism

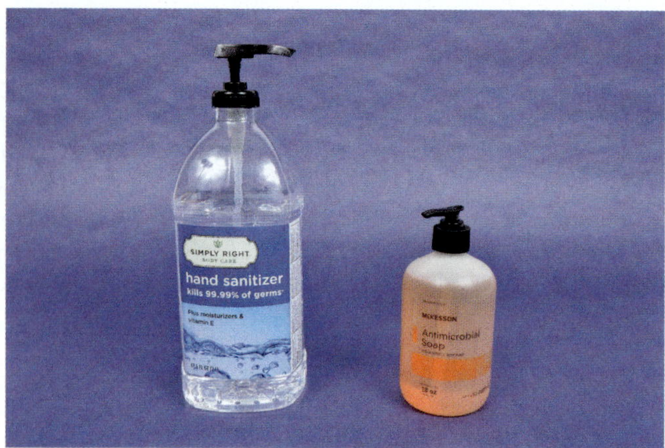

FIGURE 19.3 Alcohol-based hand sanitizer and soap.

Bloodborne Pathogens Standard

In 2000 Congress passed the Needlestick Safety and Prevention Act. This was in response to the CDC's concern about employees' risk when working with sharps. OSHA then amended the Bloodborne Pathogens Standard. Employers are required to keep a sharps injury log that describes the device involved in the incident and the details of how and where the incident occurred. Employers must also make available to employees effective sharps management devices, such as these:

- Syringes with self-sheathing needles
- Needles that retract after use
- Needleless intravenous (IV) systems

Parenteral exposure includes accidental needlesticks, occupation-related human bites, and exposure of nonintact skin (e.g., cuts and abrasions on the employee's hands) to OPIM. An employer who fails to comply with OSHA's Bloodborne Pathogens Standard could face a maximum penalty of $7000 for the first violation and up to $70,000 for repeated violations.

The Bloodborne Pathogens Standard also clarifies the use of washing or flushing of any exposed body area or mucous membrane immediately or as soon as possible after exposure to OPIM. This includes hand washing after the removal of gloves or other personal protective equipment.

Hands should be washed with soap and warm, running water when available. When running water is not available, alcohol-based hand sanitizers can be used. Studies have shown that correct use of alcohol-based hand sanitizers significantly reduces the number of microorganisms on the skin. It also takes less time than traditional hand washing and causes less irritation to the skin (Figure 19.3).

The CDC's recommendations for adequate hand hygiene are as follows:

- Visibly soiled hands should be washed for a minimum of 15 seconds with soap and warm, running water (see Procedure 19.2).
- Alcohol-based hand sanitizers that contain at least 60% alcohol should be used before and after contact with each patient and also after removing gloves to prevent cross-contamination among patients and healthcare workers (see Procedure 19.2).
- Use an alcohol-based hand sanitizer properly, applying the label-recommended amount to the palm of one hand and rubbing the hands together, covering all surfaces until the hands are dry.
- Artificial nails should not be worn; studies show that even after careful hand hygiene, healthcare workers with artificial nails have more pathogenic microbes under their nails and on their fingertips than workers with natural nails. Artificial nails also cause nail changes that contribute to the transmission of microbes.
- Natural nail tips should be no longer than one-fourth of an inch to prevent microbial growth under the nail.

The best way to reduce the risk of infection is to follow the Bloodborne Pathogens Standard. Healthcare workers must take adequate and consistent precautions to protect themselves and their patients. Figure 19.4 summarizes the Bloodborne Pathogens Standard. Healthcare facilities must establish specific policies and procedures for the management of an exposure incident (e.g., accidental needlestick) and the exposed employee.

Compliance Guidelines

The Bloodborne Pathogens Standard is for anyone working in the healthcare field. Only some of the regulations apply to the ambulatory care setting. Safety and infection control go beyond hand washing and knowledge of the disease cycle. The information presented here applies to the medical assisting profession.

Personal Protective Equipment

Personal protective equipment (PPE) should be used when contact with blood or OPIM is expected. PPE includes specialized clothing or equipment that prevents the healthcare worker from coming in contact with blood or OPIM. This prevents or minimizes the entry of infectious material into the body. Types of PPE used in the healthcare setting include gloves, gowns/aprons, shoe covers, laboratory coats, masks and respirators, protective eyewear, and face shields (Figure 19.5).

Gloves are the most commonly used PPE in a healthcare facility. Gloves must be worn if the medical assistant is at all likely to be involved in any of the following activities (Procedure 19.1):

- Touching a patient's blood, body fluids, mucous membranes, or skin that is not intact.
- Handling items and surfaces contaminated with blood and body fluids.
- Performing venipuncture, fingerstick/capillary puncture, injections, and other vascular procedures.
- Assisting with any surgical procedure. If a glove is torn during the procedure, the glove should be removed, the hands washed carefully, and new gloves put on as soon as possible.
- Handling, processing, and disposing of all blood and body fluid specimens.
- Cleaning and decontaminating spills of blood or other body fluids.

The same pair of gloves cannot be worn for the care of more than one patient; new disposable gloves must be used for each individual patient.

> **Safety Alert**
>
> Protective equipment contaminated with body fluids of any kind must be removed and placed in a designated area or biohazard waste container. The hands or any other exposed areas must be washed or flushed as soon as possible. Face shields that cover the mouth, nose, and eyes must be worn whenever splashes, sprays, or droplets are possible. Utility gloves may be reused if they are intact (i.e., have no cracks, tears, or punctures). All PPE must be removed before the medical assistant leaves the medical facility (Figure 19.6).

Requirements of Employers: OSHA Bloodborne Pathogens Standard

EXPOSURE CONTROL PLAN

Each medical office must develop a written exposure control plan (ECP). The purpose of an ECP is to identify tasks where there is the potential for exposure to blood and other potentially infectious materials.

- A timetable must be published indicating when and how communication of potential hazards will occur.
- The employer must offer employees the hepatitis B vaccine within 10 working days of employment (at no cost to the employee). If employees sign a form to refuse the vaccine, they can change their minds at no cost to the employee.
- The employer must document the steps that should be taken in case of an exposure incident, including a postexposure evaluation and follow-up, strict record keeping, implementation of engineering controls, provision for personal protective equipment, and general housekeeping standards. This plan must be posted in the medical office.
- There must also be written procedures for evaluating the circumstances of an exposure incident.
- Training records must be kept for 3 years.

ENGINEERING CONTROLS AND WORK PRACTICES

The employer must provide engineering controls or equipment and facilities that minimize the possibility of exposure. Examples of engineering controls include the following:

- Providing puncture-resistant containers for used sharps.
- Providing handwashing facilities that are readily accessible.
- Equipment for sanitizing, decontaminating, and sterilizing.

The employer must also enforce work practice controls. Work practice controls also minimize the possibility of exposure by making sure employees are using the proper techniques while working. Examples include the following:

- Enforcing proper handwashing or sanitizing procedures.
- Enforcing proper techniques for using and handling needles to prevent needlesticks.
- Enforcing proper techniques to minimize the splashing of blood.

PERSONAL PROTECTIVE EQUIPMENT

Employers must provide, and employees must use, personal protective equipment (PPE) when the possibility exists of exposure to blood or contaminated body fluids. This equipment must not allow blood or potentially infectious material to pass through to the employee's clothes, skin, eyes, or mouth. Examples of PPE include the following:

- Gowns
- Face shields
- Goggles
- Gloves

If an employee has an allergy to powder or latex, the employer must provide hypoallergenic or powderless gloves. The employee cannot be charged for PPEs.

EXPOSURE INCIDENT MANAGEMENT

An exposure incident is contact with blood or biohazard infectious material that occurs when doing one's job. When an exposure incident is reported, the employer must arrange for an immediate and confidential medical evaluation. The information and actions required are as follows:

- Documenting how the exposure occurred.
- Identifying and testing the "source" individual, if possible.
- Testing the employee's blood if consent is granted.
- Providing counseling.
- Evaluating, treating, and following up on any reported illness.

Medical records must be kept for each employee with occupational exposure for the duration of employment plus 30 years.

COMMUNICATION OF POTENTIAL HAZARDS TO EMPLOYEES

A medical assistant will be exposed to hazardous chemicals on the job. Most chemicals handled by assistants are not any more dangerous than those used in the home. In the workplace, however, exposure is likely to be greater, concentrations higher, and exposure time longer.

The "right to-know" law, OSHA's hazard communication standard, states that each employee has a right to know what chemicals he or she is working with in the workplace. The right-to-know law is intended to make the workplace safer by making certain that all information regarding chemical hazards is known to the employee. This information is supplied in the material safety data sheet (MSDS), a fact sheet about a chemical that includes the following information:

- Identification of the chemical
- Listing of the physical and health hazards
- Precautions for handling
- Identification of the chemical as a carcinogen
- First-aid procedures
- Name, address, and telephone number of manufacturer

Many SDS information sheets can be obtained in repositories on the Internet. An SDS should be updated at least every 3 years. Employers must ensure that all products have an up-to-date SDS when they enter the workplace.

Potential hazards are also communicated with labels and color. Any containers with biohazard waste must be orange (or reddish orange) and display the biohazard symbol. These labels and colors alert employees to the risk of possible exposure.

FIGURE 19.4 Requirements of Employers: OSHA Bloodborne Pathogens Standard. (Occupational Safety and Health Administration, www.osha.gov.)

CRITICAL THINKING APPLICATION 19.4

Rosa is caring for an injured 3-year-old child with an open wound on his right knee. She puts on disposable gloves to clean the wound, and the mother demands to know why. How can she explain her actions?

Environmental Protection

Environmental protection refers to minimizing the risk of injury by isolating or removing any physical or mechanical health hazard in the workplace. Every medical assistant must adhere to these safety rules:

- Read warning labels on biohazard waste containers and equipment.
- Minimize splashing or spraying of OPIM. Blood that splatters onto exposed areas of the skin or mucous membranes is a proven mode of HBV transmission.
- Bandage any breaks or lesions on your hands before gloving.
- If any body surface is exposed to potentially infectious material, scrub the area with soap and warm, running water as soon as possible after the exposure.
- If your eyes come in contact with body fluids, continuously flush them with water as soon as possible for a minimum of 15 minutes using an eyewash unit. A stationary unit connected to warm, running water is the best method for properly flushing potentially infectious material out of the eyes.

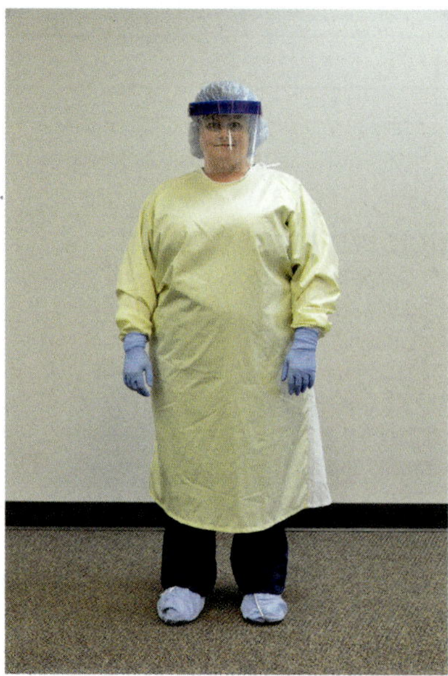

FIGURE 19.5 Personal protective equipment.

- Contaminated needles and other sharps should never be recapped, bent, broken, or resheathed; needle units must have protective safety devices to cover the contaminated needle after injection.
- Contaminated sharp instruments, such as operating scissors, should not be processed in a way that requires employees to reach into containers to grasp them.
- Immediately after use, dispose of syringes and needles, scalpel blades, and other disposable sharp items in a labeled, leakproof, puncture-resistant biohazard container. The container must be located as close as possible to the area where the item is used.
- All specimens must be placed in a container that prevents leakage during collection, handling, processing, storage, transport, and shipping. Avoid contaminating the outside of the container or the label with the specimen substance. The container must have a biohazard label to alert others that it holds potentially infectious material. Gloves should be worn throughout this procedure.
- Equipment requiring repair that has been contaminated with blood or body fluids should be decontaminated before being repaired in the office or transported for repair. There is no

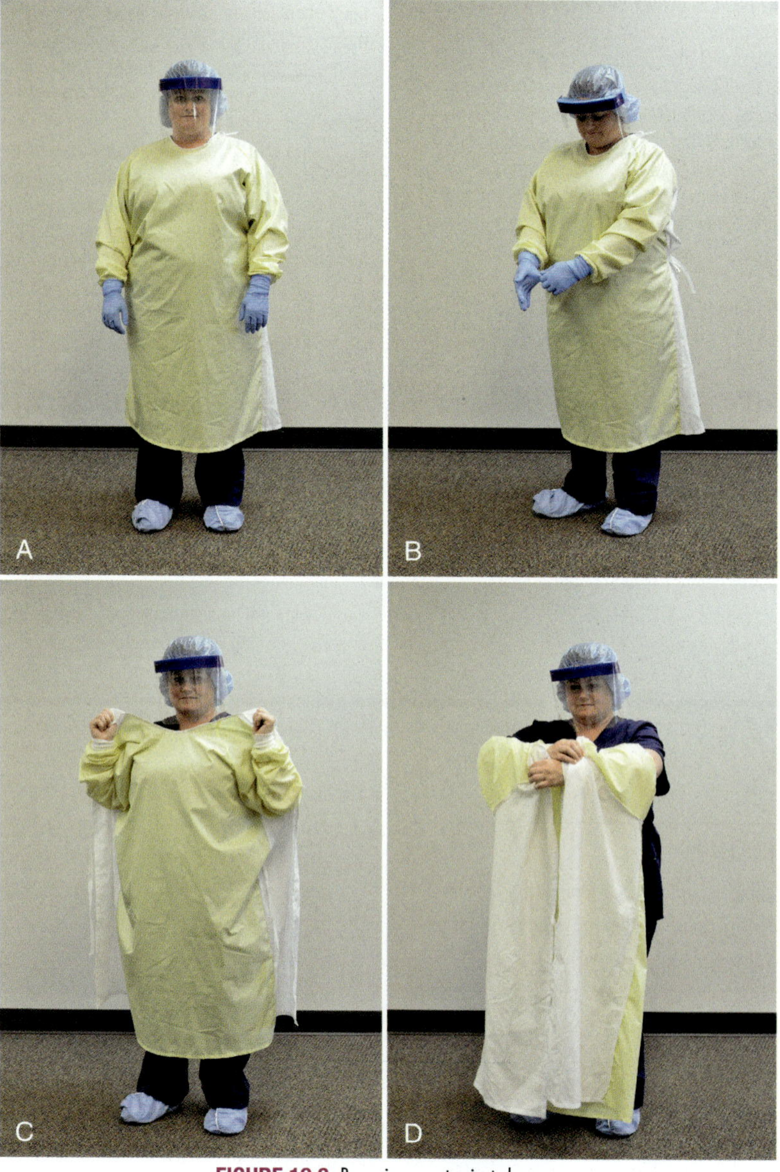

FIGURE 19.6 Removing a contaminated gown.

documented evidence of HIV transmission from contaminated environmental surfaces, but surface contamination is a proven mode of transmission of HBV.

- Smoking, eating, drinking, applying cosmetics or lip balm, and handling contact lenses are prohibited in work areas where there is a reasonable likelihood of contamination by pathogens.
- Food and beverages cannot be kept in refrigerators, freezers, or cabinets or on countertops where infectious materials could be present.

Housekeeping Controls

The Bloodborne Pathogens Standard requires certain housekeeping measures to ensure a sanitary work area. A schedule must be posted for the cleaning and decontaminating of each work area where exposures could occur. Documentation of these procedures must include information about the surface cleaned, the type of waste encountered, and procedures performed in the designated area.

- After accidental spills of blood or body fluids, at the end of each procedure and each shift, work surfaces must be immediately cleaned and then disinfected with a **disinfectant** registered with the Environmental Protection Agency (EPA).
- All reusable containers must be disinfected and decontaminated on a routine basis.
- Sharps containers must be kept as close as possible to the work area. Never attempt to reach inside a sharps container, and do not overfill them. Replace containers on a routine basis and be certain that the lid is closed securely before preparing them for biohazard waste disposal.
- Never pick up spilled material or broken glassware with your hands. Brooms, brushes, dustpans, and pickup tongs or forceps should be used. The material should be placed immediately into an **impervious** biohazard waste container at the spill site (Figure 19.7). Use an absorbent, professional biohazard spill preparation as directed to decontaminate the site.
- Handle soiled linen as little as possible, and always wear gloves or other protective equipment during disposal. Linens soiled with blood or body fluids should be double-bagged and transported in labeled, leakproof biohazard bags.
- Contaminated materials and infectious waste must be handled with extreme caution to prevent exposure. Biohazard waste must be collected in impermeable, red polyethylene or polypropylene biohazard-labeled bags or containers and sealed (Figure 19.8).

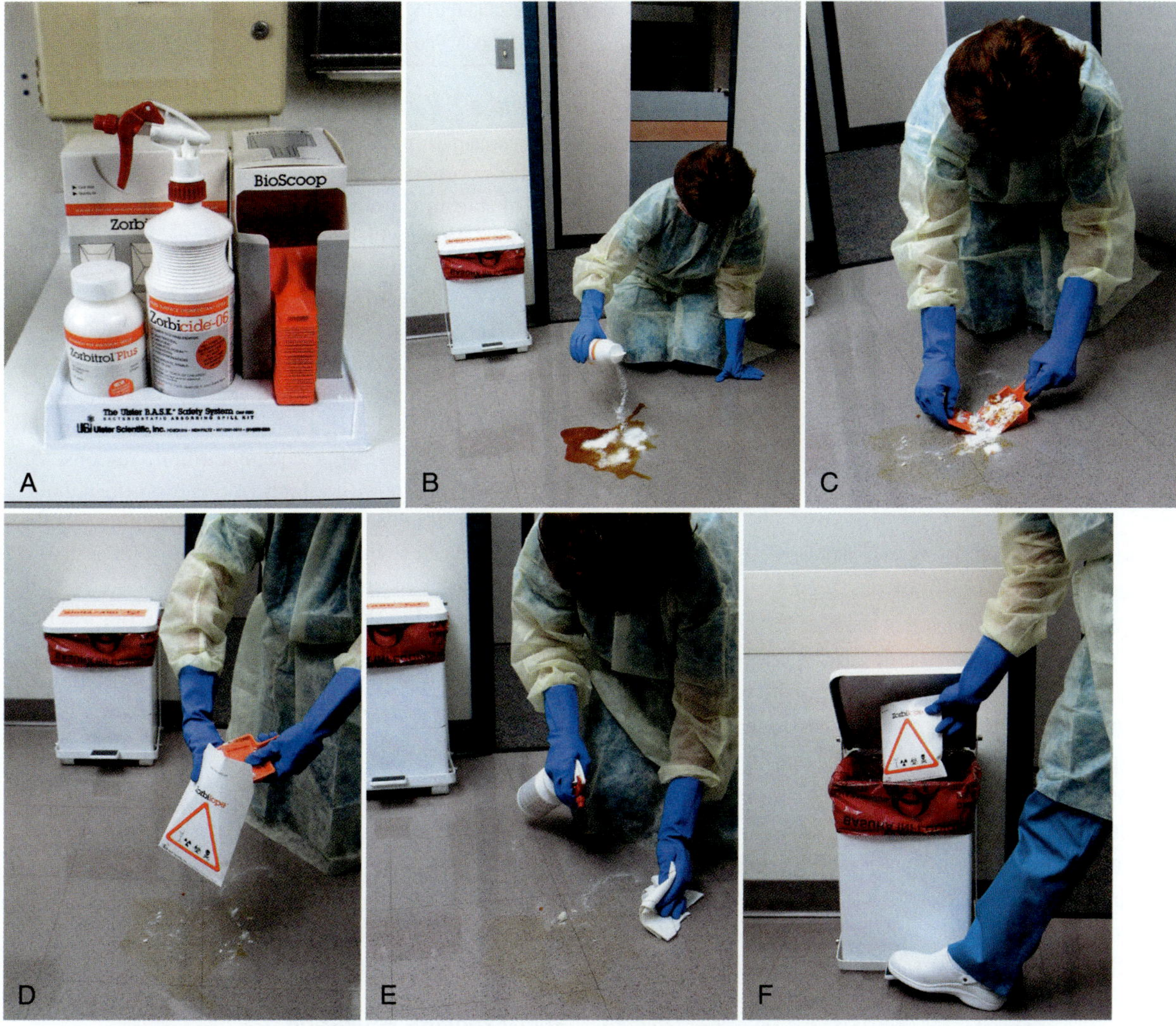

FIGURE 19.7 Cleaning up spilled material. **(A)** Clean-up kit with printed instructions. **(B)** Sprinkle congealing powder over the spill. **(C)** Scoop up the spill. **(D)** Place the contents in a biohazard bag. **(E)** Wipe the area thoroughly with a germicide. **(F)** Place all contaminated material in a biohazard bag or container.

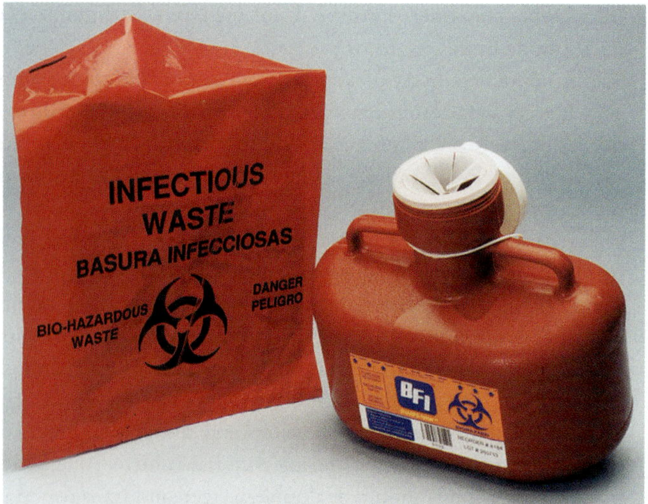

FIGURE 19.8 Biohazard bag and biohazard sharps container.

This waste must be disposed of in accordance with all federal, state, and local regulations. Disposal methods include treatment by heat, incineration, steam sterilization, chemical treatment, or other equivalent methods that will render the waste inactive before it is placed in a landfill.

Protocols for Disposal of Biological Chemical Materials

The Medical Waste Tracking Act set the standards for governmental regulation of medical waste; however, that law expired in 1991. The states were then given responsibility for regulating the disposal of medical waste. Each state varies in its degree of regulation, ranging from no regulation to strict rules. The following are some examples of regulations covering the disposal of hazardous materials:

- Biomedical waste should be collected in containers that are leakproof and strong enough to prevent breakage during handling; the containers must be labeled with the biohazard symbol.
- Workers who handle biomedical waste should observe Standard Precautions.
- Biological waste containers and boxes should not be held in the healthcare facility for longer than 30 days.
- Sharps are instruments intended to cut or penetrate the skin; they include lancets, scalpel blades, needles, and syringe/needle combinations. Sharps must be placed in red, hard plastic sharps boxes after use; sharps boxes should be closed when three-fourths full.
- Boxes for disposal of chemicals should be labeled with the chemicals' names and any other pertinent data; they must be adequately sealed to prevent breakage or leakage.
- Each healthcare facility must hire a biomedical waste disposal service whose employees are trained to collect and haul away biomedical waste in special containers (usually cardboard boxes or reusable plastic bins) for treatment at a facility designed to handle biomedical waste.

The cost to the healthcare facility for biomedical waste disposal is typically based on the weight of the contaminated items collected (i.e., the weight of filled sharps containers, biohazard boxes, and bags).

Hepatitis B Vaccine Declination

I understand that due to my occupational exposure to blood or other potentially infectious materials, I may be at risk of acquiring hepatitis B virus (HBV) infection. I have been given the opportunity to be vaccinated with hepatitis B vaccine at no charge to myself. However, I decline hepatitis B vaccination at this time. I understand that by declining this vaccine, I continue to be at risk of acquiring hepatitis B, a serious disease. If in the future I continue to have occupational exposure to blood or other potentially infectious materials and I want to be vaccinated with hepatitis B vaccine, I can receive the vaccination series at no charge to me.

Name: ____________________ Date: __________

FIGURE 19.9 Sample hepatitis B declination form. (Occupational Safety and Health Administration. www.osha.gov/SLTC/etools/hospital/hazards/bbp/declination.html.)

19.5 CRITICAL THINKING APPLICATION

Your office manager asks you to prepare a fact sheet for your co-workers that summarizes the details of OSHA's Bloodborne Pathogens Standard. What should you include?

Hepatitis B Vaccination

HBV vaccination must be available free of charge to all employees at risk for occupational exposure to bloodborne pathogens within 10 days of starting employment. The vaccine is given by intramuscular injection. There will be a two- or three-dose series depending on which vaccine brand is used. Boosters for the hepatitis B immunization are not currently recommended. However, if they are recommended in the future, boosters must be made available to eligible employees without cost.

After the completion of the hepatitis B vaccine series, more than 90% of healthy adults and more than 95% of infants, children, and adolescents develop adequate antibody responses. Despite this, healthcare workers with a high risk of exposure should have a titer drawn after completing the series to determine whether they have antibodies against the disease. Antibody testing should be done 1 to 2 months after completion of the vaccine series. If the employee did not respond to the first series, or if the series was not completed, revaccination with a second three-dose series is recommended. If antibodies still do not develop, no further vaccination is given.

Employees have the right to decline hepatitis B immunization, but they are required to sign a declination form (Figure 19.9) that is kept on file as a record of their refusal. The statement can be signed only after the employee has received training about the following:

- Hepatitis B and the hepatitis B vaccination
- Safety, route of administration, and benefits of vaccination

In addition, the employee must be informed that the vaccine will be administered free of charge. Employees who change their minds may receive the vaccine at a future date free of charge.

Post-Exposure Follow-up

If an employee is exposed through an accidental needlestick, a human bite, exposure to broken skin, or from a splash or splatter onto mucous membranes, such as the eyes, certain procedures must be followed. The following specific steps should be taken after exposure to contaminated waste:

- Immediately or as soon as possible after exposure, the worker should wash or flush the exposed area.
- The exposure incident must be immediately reported to the supervisor.
- The employee must immediately receive a confidential medical evaluation. The provider caring for the exposed employee must receive written details of the exposure incident, including the route and circumstances surrounding the incident. All documentation related to the exposure must do the following:
  - Remain confidential.
  - Not be disclosed to any individual without the employee's express written permission.
  - Be kept for at least the duration of the worker's employment plus 30 years.
- An incident report must be filed that documents the details surrounding the exposure incident, the route or type of exposure, and the identity, if known, of the source individual. The source individual is the person, living or dead, whose blood or potentially infectious material was the source of the occupational exposure.
- The source individual is screened for HBV, hepatitis C virus (HCV), and HIV. Depending on state regulations, consent may or may not be required from the source individual to perform the screening. If consent is required but not given, the employer must document that consent was not received from the source individual. If screening is done, OSHA requires that the employee be informed of the results of the source individual's tests.
- The exposed employee is tested for HBV, HCV, and HIV if consent is given to determine whether the employee already has one of these infectious diseases. If the employee refuses the tests but blood is drawn, the sample must be stored for 90 days for the worker to decide whether screening is wanted.
- If the employee has not been vaccinated against HBV, vaccination is offered.
- The injured employee must receive a copy of the healthcare provider's written opinion within 15 days of completion of the evaluation.
- The exposed employee must receive health counseling about the risk of illness or other adverse outcomes of exposure and the potential for and consequences of transmission of the disease to family, patients, and others.

Healthcare students are at risk for bloodborne pathogen exposure and should follow all OSHA guidelines designed to protect individuals from exposure. A complete, unabridged copy of OSHA's Bloodborne Pathogens Standard may be obtained at the OSHA website (www.osha.gov).

The CDC has developed a checklist that ambulatory care facilities can use to systematically assess employee adherence to infection prevention and ensure that the facility has policies and procedures in place and has adequate supplies available to prevent infections at the site. If the answer to any of the questions is no, the facility must do all it can to correct the problems with either staff or supplies (Table 19.1).

TABLE 19.1 Modified CDC Infection Prevention Checklist[a]

FACILITY POLICIES	PRACTICE PERFORMED		IF ANSWER IS NO, DOCUMENT PLAN FOR REMEDIATION
1. Administrative Policies and Facility Practices			
a. Written infection prevention policies and procedures are available, current, and based on evidence-based guidelines, regulations, or standards.	Yes	No	
b. Infection prevention policies and procedures are reassessed at least annually or according to state or federal requirements and updated if appropriate.	Yes	No	
c. At least one individual trained in infection prevention is employed by or regularly available to the facility.	Yes	No	
d. Supplies necessary for adherence to Standard Precautions are readily available.	Yes	No	
e. Healthcare personnel for whom contact with blood or other potentially infectious material is anticipated are trained in the Occupational Safety and Health Administration (OSHA) Bloodborne Pathogens Standard upon hire and at least annually.	Yes	No	
f. The facility maintains a log of needlesticks, sharps injuries, and other employee exposure events.	Yes	No	
g. Following an exposure event, postexposure evaluation and follow-up, including prophylaxis as appropriate, are available at no cost to the employee.	Yes	No	
h. Hepatitis B vaccination is available at no cost to all employees at risk of occupational exposure.	Yes	No	
i. Postvaccination screening for hepatitis B surface antibodies is conducted.	Yes	No	

Continued

TABLE 19.1 Modified CDC Infection Prevention Checklist[a]—*continued*

FACILITY POLICIES	PRACTICE PERFORMED		IF ANSWER IS NO, DOCUMENT PLAN FOR REMEDIATION
j. All personnel are offered annual influenza vaccination at no cost.	Yes	No	
k. All personnel with potential exposure to tuberculosis (TB) are screened for TB upon hire and annually (if negative).	Yes	No	
2. Surveillance and Disease Reporting			
a. Updated list of reportable diseases is readily available to all personnel.	Yes	No	
3. Hand Hygiene			
a. Facility provides training and supplies necessary for adherence to hand hygiene.	Yes	No	
4. Personal Protective Equipment (PPE)			
a. Facility provides training and supplies for appropriate PPE.	Yes	No	
b. Impermeable gowns are worn during procedures in which contact with blood or body fluids is anticipated.	Yes	No	
c. PPE is removed and discarded prior to leaving the exam room.	Yes	No	
d. Hand hygiene is performed immediately after removal of PPE.	Yes	No	
5. Environmental Cleaning			
a. Policies and procedures exist for routine cleaning and disinfection of environmental surfaces.	Yes	No	
b. Cleaning procedures are periodically monitored and assessed to ensure that they are consistently and correctly performed.	Yes	No	
c. The facility has a policy/procedure for decontamination of spills of blood or other body fluids.	Yes	No	

[a]The complete checklist is available at the Centers for Disease Control and Prevention (CDC) website for Infection Prevention in Outpatient Settings.
Modified from the Occupational Safety and Health Administration, www.cdc.gov/HAI/settings/outpatient/checklist/outpatient-care-checklist.html.

Risk of Infection after an Occupational Exposure

Hepatitis B Virus (HBV)

Healthcare workers who have received the hepatitis B vaccine and have developed immunity to the virus are at virtually no risk for infection. For an unvaccinated person, the risk from a single needlestick or a cut exposure to HBV-infected blood ranges from 6% to 30%.

Hepatitis C Virus (HCV)

The estimated risk for infection after a needlestick or cut exposure to HCV-infected blood is approximately 1.8%. The risk after a blood splash is unknown but is believed to be very small.

Human Immunodeficiency Virus (HIV)

The average risk for HIV infection after a needlestick or cut exposure to HIV-infected blood is about 0.3%; the risk after exposure to the eye, nose, or mouth is near zero; the risk after exposure of the skin to HIV-infected blood is estimated to be less than 0.1%.

From the Occupational Safety and Health Administration, www.cdc.gov/hiv/workplace/healthcareworkers.html.

19.6 CRITICAL THINKING APPLICATION

Rosa's office has been especially busy today. While administering an injection to a frightened 6-year-old child, a co-worker accidentally sticks herself with the needle. She tells Rosa about the incident, but she does not know what to do next. What steps should be taken to manage the situation?

ASEPTIC TECHNIQUES: PREVENTING DISEASE TRANSMISSION

Asepsis means free from infection or infectious material. *Medical asepsis* is defined as the destruction of disease-causing organisms. By using the principles of medical asepsis, we can prevent the spread of disease. The goal is to eliminate or minimize pathogens by following OSHA's Bloodborne Pathogens Standard and disinfecting objects as soon as possible after contamination. This creates a healthcare environment as free of pathogens as possible.

Surgical asepsis is the destruction of all organisms. This technique is used for any procedure that enters the body's skin or tissues, such as surgery or injections. Anytime the skin or a mucous membrane is punctured, pierced, or incised, surgical aseptic techniques are practiced. Everything that comes in contact with the patient should be sterile:

- Gowns
- Drapes
- Instruments
- Gloves

Minor surgery, urinary catheterization, injections, and some specimen collections, such as blood collection and biopsies, are performed using surgical aseptic technique.

Because skin cannot be sterilized, the goal of hand hygiene is to reduce the number of microorganisms. Hand washing uses mechanical friction, soap, and warm, running water. Alcohol-based hand sanitizers are also effective in reducing the number of microorganisms. The alcohol kills the microorganisms. If the hands are visibly soiled, hand washing should be done.

Normally, two types of microorganisms are found on the skin: normal *resident flora* and *transient flora*. Normal resident flora lives harmlessly on the skin. Transient flora includes bacteria, viruses, and other organisms picked up on the hands. Resident flora is firmly attached to the skin, whereas transient flora is not. This means that transient flora is easily removed by thorough hand hygiene, preventing the transfer to patients.

The most effective barrier against infection is intact skin. If the skin and mucous membranes are intact, medical asepsis can be used for most **noninvasive procedures**, such as pelvic and proctologic examinations. Instruments and objects used in medical aseptic procedures must be sanitized and disinfected or sterilized before being used on another patient. Medical aseptic procedures may include the use of gowns and masks, but these are not sterile and are worn to protect the healthcare worker more than the patient. Many healthcare facilities are providing masks for patients to use if they present with productive cough, fever, and other influenza-like symptoms. In addition to masks, hand sanitizer stations are provided. Both of these measures can help prevent the spread of disease.

Another practical application of medical aseptic technique is to set up work areas in the medical office's laboratory. One side of the laboratory is the "clean" side, where only noninfectious procedures are performed. The other side is the "dirty" side, where potentially infectious materials are processed or cleaned.

Hand Hygiene

Hand hygiene can be accomplished in two different ways. If the hands are visibly soiled, they must be washed using a medical aseptic technique. If the hands are not visibly soiled, alcohol-based hand sanitizer can be used. Hand hygiene, using the correct technique, must be done before and after each patient is examined or treated and also when stipulated by the Bloodborne Pathogens Standard.

When you wash your hands for the first time in the morning, spend at least 1 minute on the scrub. For subsequent hand washing, the CDC recommends 15 seconds. Each office sink should be equipped with a liquid soap dispenser. A water-soluble lotion may be rubbed into the hands after they have been washed and dried. Dry, cracked, chapped skin is no longer intact and can provide a means of entry for microorganisms.

Proper handwashing depends on two factors: running water and friction. The water should be warm. Water that is too hot or too cold causes the skin to become chapped. Friction is the firm rubbing of all surfaces of the hands and wrists. Remember that your fingers have four sides, and fingernails have two sides. For medical aseptic hand washing, all jewelry except a plain wedding band is removed. A wristwatch may be left on if it can be moved up on the forearm away from the wrist area. The hands are washed under running water with the fingertips pointing downward. Soap and friction are applied to the hands and wrists. The water is allowed to wash debris away from the wrists and down toward the fingertips (Procedure 19.2).

When you use an alcohol-based hand sanitizer, it should take 20 to 30 seconds to rub all of it into the skin. Be sure to cover all surfaces and continue rubbing it in until your hands are dry (see Procedure 19.2). Evidence suggests that hand hygiene with an alcohol-based hand sanitizer is more effective at reducing **nosocomial infections** than plain hand washing. Antimicrobial-impregnated wipes (e.g., towelettes) are not a substitute for an alcohol-based hand sanitizer or soap.

Remember, the goal of hand hygiene is to protect yourself from infection and prevent cross-contamination from one patient to another.

When to Use Hand Hygiene

Medical aseptic hand washing or alcohol-based hand sanitizer should be used in the following situations:

- After you finish with one patient and before you attend to another patient
- After you finish handling one specimen and before you handle another specimen
- After you use toilet facilities
- Whenever you touch something that causes your hands to become contaminated
- When you arrive at work and before you leave the facility
- After removing gloves
- Before and after eating

According to the CDC, proper hand hygiene must be performed in the following instances, even if disposable gloves are worn:

- Before and after contact with the patient or his or her immediate care environment
- Before performing an aseptic task (e.g., giving an injection, drawing blood)
- After contact with blood, body fluids, or contaminated surfaces
- When hands move from a contaminated body site to a clean body site during patient care

Sanitization

Sanitization is the cleaning process that reduces the number of microorganisms to a safe level. You must carefully clean instruments and other items used in the healthcare facility before proceeding with disinfection or sterilization. This cleansing process removes debris such as blood and other body fluids from instruments or equipment. This debris can protect the microorganisms from disinfection or sterilization (Procedure 19.3).

The medical assistant should always wear gloves while performing sanitization. Thick utility gloves will help protect your hands when you work with instruments that have sharp or pointed edges. Gloves prevent possible personal contamination with OPIM that may be present on the articles being cleaned. The procedure should be completed immediately after the use of the instruments. A separate workroom, or the "dirty" side of the utility room, is used to prevent cross-contamination of clean instruments and equipment. If sanitization cannot be done immediately, rinse the used items under cold water immediately after the procedure and place them in a detergent solution. Never allow blood or other substances to dry on an instrument.

When you are ready to sanitize instruments, rinse each instrument in cold running water. Sharp instruments should be kept separate from the other instruments. Metal instruments may damage the cutting edges, and sharp instruments may damage other instruments or injure you. Clean all sharp instruments at the same time when you can concentrate on preventing injury. Open all hinges, and scrub serrations and ratchets with a small scrub brush or toothbrush. Rinse the instruments in hot water and then carefully check that they are in proper working order before they are disinfected or sterilized. The items should be hand dried with a towel to prevent spotting and allowed to air dry before further processing.

Sanitization is a very important step, and it cannot be overlooked or done carelessly. The use of disposable instruments minimizes the need for sanitization, disinfection, and sterilization.

Ultrasonic Sanitization

Sound waves can be used to sanitize instruments. The instruments are placed in an ultrasonic bath of cleaner and water. Sound waves cause the solution to vibrate, which loosens the materials attached to the instruments. Ultrasonic cleaners are beneficial because they do not damage even the most delicate instruments, and workers do not run the risk of an accidental sharps injury.

Disinfection

Disinfection is the process of killing pathogenic organisms or of rendering them inactive. It is not always effective against spores, tuberculosis bacilli, and certain viruses. Some disinfectant chemicals can kill microbes within a short time, but they are usually hard on instruments. Some chemicals, such as Cidex, are effective enough to kill all organisms, but the usual immersion time is 10 hours or longer. For exam tables and countertop surfaces, there are two common disinfectants: hydrogen peroxide and bleach. Both are low cost and effective.

Many other types of disinfecting agents are available for instruments and equipment. It is important to follow the manufacturer's guidelines on the following factors:

- How to use each product properly
- Advantages and disadvantages
- Possible sources of error

Levels of Disinfectants

The CDC defines three levels of disinfectants:

- Low-level disinfectants can kill most vegetative bacteria, some fungi, and some viruses. They are used for exam tables and countertops. Example: hydrogen peroxide.
- Intermediate-level disinfectants can kill mycobacteria, vegetative bacteria, most viruses, and most fungi, but they do not kill spores. They are used for noncritical items, such as stethoscopes and percussion hammers. Example: isopropyl alcohol.
- High-level disinfectants will kill all microorganisms except large numbers of bacterial spores. They are used for semicritical items, such as a flexible fiberoptic *sigmoidoscope*. Example: Cidex OPA.

Here are common errors that can cause chemicals to lose their effectiveness:

- Instruments are not thoroughly sanitized. Attached organic matter inhibits or prevents the action of the disinfectant. No chemical can kill unless it reaches all instrument surfaces; therefore, complete sanitization is absolutely necessary.
- The disinfectant solution is left in an open container, and evaporation changes its concentration.
- Solutions are not changed after the recommended period for use has expired.
- Solutions are not prepared properly or are not mixed properly before use.
- The manufacturer's recommended temperature for use and storage is not maintained.

Chemical disinfectants cannot be used on skin or tissues because they can damage them. Therefore antiseptics, such as alcohol, are used on the skin to reduce the number of pathogens. Alcohol is the most widely used antiseptic, but studies indicate that it is not as effective as other products in inhibiting the growth and reproduction of microorganisms on the skin's surface. Other antiseptic chemicals, such as povidone-iodine solution (Betadine), are effective antimicrobial agents that are safe to use on a patient's skin.

Sterilization

Sterilization is essential for surgical asepsis. Sterilization can be achieved with moist heat, dry heat, ultraviolet light, ionizing radiation, gas, or chemicals. Medical facilities typically use the autoclave method, which uses moist heat. Steam under pressure in the autoclave offers an excellent method of sterilization because it kills all pathogens and spores. You will learn more about surgical asepsis and the sterilization process in Chapter 24.

19.7 CRITICAL THINKING APPLICATION

Rosa is responsible for the orientation of the new medical assistant in the office's sanitization and disinfection procedures. Outline the important concepts and methods of each one.

Role of the Medical Assistant in Asepsis

Asepsis is one of the few procedures that will directly affect the health of the patient, the provider, and the staff. The spread of pathogens in the ambulatory care setting can be controlled only through the effective, consistent application of the Bloodborne Pathogens Standard and by proper sanitization, disinfection, and sterilization of supplies, equipment, and work surfaces.

The medical assistant must develop the skills needed for performing aseptic procedures properly. It is important that these techniques be done on such a routine basis that they become an unbreakable habit. The use of disposable items is highly recommended for infection control purposes. However, when disposable equipment is used, the assistant must follow recommended disposal guidelines to ensure infection control.

CLOSING COMMENTS

Patient Coaching

The medical assistant should take every opportunity to educate patients about the infection process and ways to prevent the transmission of disease. The best time to instruct a patient in aseptic techniques that can be used at home is while performing the aseptic procedure. Consider these examples:

- While washing your hands, explain to the patient that this routine is particularly important for patients who are very young or old or who get sick frequently. Instruct the patient that the hands should be washed before and after meals, after sneezing, coughing, or blowing the nose, after using the restroom, before and after changing a dressing, and after changing an infant's diaper.
- Advise the patient to carry an alcohol-based hand sanitizer and use it as indicated throughout the day.
- Explain to the patient that coughing or sneezing into a bent elbow is an effective method for preventing the spread of disease.
- Instruct the patient on the differences between sterile and clean dressings and bandages. Demonstrate each step in changing a dressing properly and explain how to dispose of contaminated items.

A medical assistant can help patients live healthier lives in many ways. For example, here are a few more suggestions for teaching the patient about asepsis and infection control:

- Set up an information table in the waiting room with take-home pamphlets and literature.
- Mail, email, or post on the healthcare facility's website a periodic newsletter to patients about infection control, especially during flu season.
- Demonstrate and explain aseptic procedures to patients and family members, inviting them to participate.

Legal and Ethical Issues

Medical asepsis and infection control in ambulatory care practices give rise to numerous legal and ethical concerns. Personal discipline is the primary concern in medical asepsis. Typically, the medical assistant is alone when performing an aseptic procedure; therefore, if contamination occurs, the medical assistant is the only one who knows. If contamination should occur, the medical assistant must start over again with clean supplies.

A primary reason for performing aseptic procedures completely and effectively is to prevent the development of nosocomial infections in susceptible patients. These infections, which are acquired in the healthcare environment, can be especially dangerous for older or debilitated patients. Ignorance of the various aseptic techniques or carelessness can be dangerous and is inexcusable before the law.

Professional Behaviors

One of the medical assistant's main responsibilities is to perform sanitization, disinfection, and sterilization procedures with precision and total effectiveness. There is no room for compromise. These procedures have a huge impact on infection control. Patients should have absolute confidence that they are being treated in an aseptic atmosphere and under aseptic conditions. This assurance is just as important for the protection of the provider and staff as it is for the patient. Allowing the provider to assume, incorrectly, that the required aseptic techniques were used to prepare for a procedure and allowing him or her to use contaminated equipment on a patient, may result in a malpractice lawsuit. Honesty on the part of the medical assistant builds self-respect and contributes to professional achievement.

SUMMARY OF SCENARIO

Implementing Standard Precautions throughout daily practice is crucial to the welfare and protection of both the patient and the healthcare worker. Rosa must be sure to wash her hands routinely or to use an alcohol-based hand sanitizer. She also must familiarize herself with the office's exposure control plan, follow OSHA's Bloodborne Pathogens Standard, use PPE when needed, follow environmental protection guidelines, use appropriate procedures for cleaning up contaminated spills and other housekeeping controls, and understand post-exposure follow-up if an accidental exposure occurs. In addition, Rosa must follow guidelines for the sanitization, disinfection, and sterilization of appropriate instruments and equipment.

SUMMARY OF LEARNING OBJECTIVES

1. **Apply the chain of infection process to healthcare.**
   The chain of infection is the way infectious disease is spread. It begins with the infectious agent and moves to the host, the means or portal of exit from the host, the mode of transmission, and the means or portal of entry into a new host. It ends with the presence of the infection in a susceptible host. At least one of these links must be broken to stop the spread of infection.

   Pathogenic microorganisms include viruses, bacteria, protozoa, fungi, and helminths. Viruses, the smallest of all pathogens, lead the list of important disease-causing agents. Viral particles insert their own deoxyribonucleic acid (DNA) or ribonucleic acid (RNA) into a host cell and then use the host cell to help reproduce more viral particles. Viral infections cannot be treated with antibiotics because they are parasites within a cell. Bacteria are tiny, simple cells that produce disease by secreting

Continued

SUMMARY OF LEARNING OBJECTIVES—*continued*

toxins, act as parasites inside human cells, or grow on body surfaces, disrupting normal human functions. Bacteria are classified according to their shape. Bacterial infections can be treated with antibiotics. Protozoa are unicellular parasites that can replicate and multiply rapidly once inside the host. They are frequently carried by insects that serve as vectors for the disease. Fungi may be unicellular or multicellular; they include molds and yeasts and cause tinea infections. Helminths are multicellular and include tapeworms, roundworms, and flatworms (flukes).

2. **Examine how the human body defends itself from infectious agents.**
The first line of defense is the body's physical and chemical barriers. An intact integumentary system is our greatest physical barrier. Chemical barriers include tears and the pH of our body fluids.

The second line of defense involves nonspecific chemical and cellular responses, including the inflammatory response. The inflammatory response is one aspect of the body's ability to defend itself against infection. It involves the body's reaction to the introduction of a foreign substance or an antigen, an increase in blood flow to the site, and the release of inflammatory mediators that attract white blood cells to the site. White blood cells isolate and destroy the source of inflammation.

The third line of defense involves specific immunity or humoral immunity. Humoral immunity creates specific antibodies to combat antigens through the action of B cells. The immune system also reacts at the cellular level with T-cell activity in cell-mediated immunity by causing the destruction of pathogenic cells at the site of invasion.

3. **Analyze the differences among acute, chronic, latent, and opportunistic infections.**
Acute diseases have a rapid onset and short duration. Chronic diseases are present over a long period, perhaps a lifetime. Latent diseases cycle through relapse and remission phases. Opportunistic infections are caused by organisms that are not typically pathogenic but that occur in hosts with an impaired or weakened immune system response, such as individuals with HIV.

4. **Examine the role of the Occupational Safety and Health Administration Standards in infection control.**
In 1987 the Centers for Disease Control and Prevention (CDC) developed Universal Precautions to protect healthcare workers and patients. In 2001 Occupational Safety and Health Administration (OSHA) developed the Bloodborne Pathogens Standard, which includes Universal Precautions. The goal of the Bloodborne Pathogens Standard is to protect all healthcare employees and their patients. The Bloodborne Pathogens Standard identified Other Potentially Infectious Materials (OPIM) and specified that they are treated as if they were infected with pathogens. Potentially infectious body fluids include cerebrospinal fluid; mucus; synovial, pleural, pericardial, peritoneal, and amniotic fluids; blood; vaginal and seminal secretions; saliva; and human tissue.

OSHA requires incorporation of a site-based Exposure Control Plan into facility management procedures. The plan must be revised annually and available for employees to review. It must reflect current safety technology, identify employees at risk for exposure, and contain specifics about protection from bloodborne pathogens, including PPE, training, hepatitis B immunization, exposure, follow-up, record keeping, and the labeling and disposal of all biohazard waste. The OSHA Compliance Guidelines include barrier protection devices, environmental protection, housekeeping controls, hepatitis B immunization, and post-exposure follow-up.

OSHA also requires post-exposure evaluation and follow-up. This includes cleaning of the site and having exposed individuals report to their supervisor immediately. A medical assessment is performed immediately. Testing the source individual's and the worker's blood is performed if possible and if consent is given. Health counseling is provided. Strict confidentiality of all medical records is maintained.

5. **Apply the concepts of medical and surgical asepsis to the healthcare setting.**
Medical asepsis is the removal or destruction of pathogens. Medical aseptic techniques are used to reduce the number of microorganisms as much as possible. For proper handwashing, refer to Procedure 19.2. Surgical asepsis is the destruction of all microorganisms. Surgical asepsis is used when the patient's skin or mucous membranes are disrupted.

Sanitization is the medically aseptic technique for cleaning contaminated articles or surfaces to reduce the number of microorganisms (refer to Procedure 19.3). Disinfection, also medical asepsis, involves the use of physical or chemical means to destroy pathogens or their components on inanimate surfaces or objects. Sterilization, surgical asepsis, removes all living microorganisms.

Asepsis is important to the health of the patient, the provider, and the staff. The medical assistant must develop the necessary skills, in addition to a firm grasp of the principles involved, to perform aseptic procedures properly.

PROCEDURE 19.1 Remove Contaminated Gloves and Discard Biohazard Material

TASK: Minimize exposure to pathogens by aseptically removing and discarding contaminated gloves.

EQUIPMENT and SUPPLIES

- Disposable gloves
- Biohazard waste container with labeled red biohazard bag

PROCEDURAL STEPS

1. With the dominant hand, grasp the glove of the opposite hand near the palm and begin removing the first glove (see the following figure). The arms should be held away from the body with the hands pointed down.

PROCEDURE 19.1 Remove Contaminated Gloves and Discard Biohazard Material—*continued*

PURPOSE: Holding the hands down and away from the body helps prevent possible contamination.

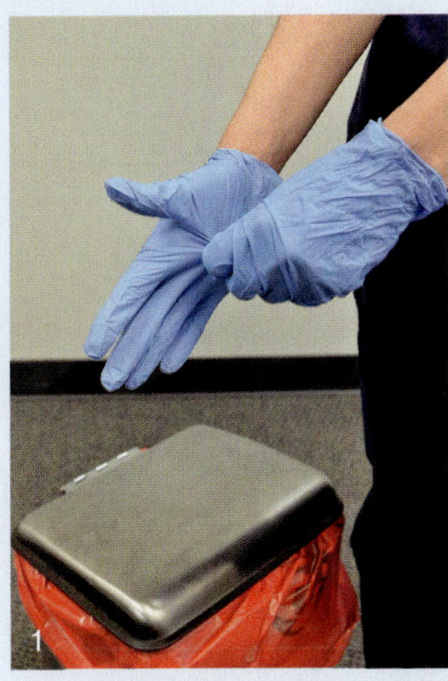

2. Pull the glove inside out (see the following figure). After removal, ball it into the palm of the remaining gloved hand.
PURPOSE: Taking off the glove inside out prevents transmission of pathogens to another surface.

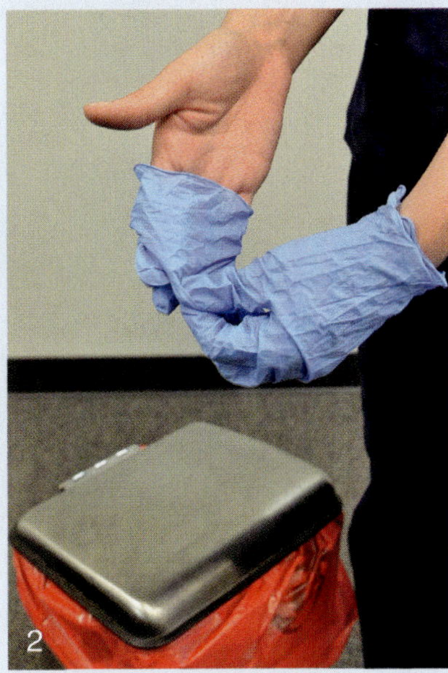

3. Insert two fingers of the ungloved hand between the edge of the cuff of the other contaminated glove and the hand (see the following figure).

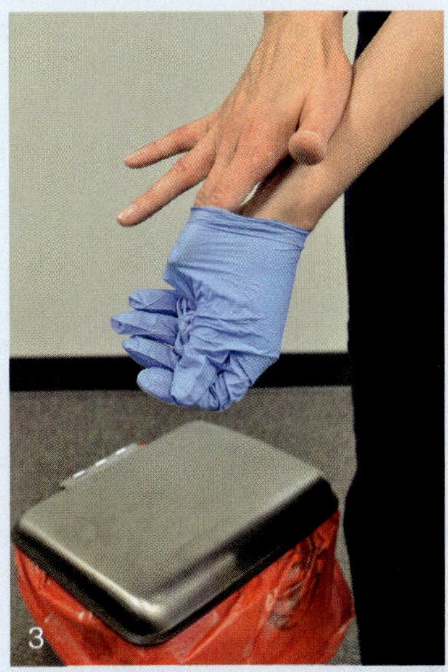

4. Push the glove down the hand, inside out, over the contaminated glove being held, leaving the contaminated side of both gloves on the inside.
PURPOSE: This technique protects the wearer from the contaminated surfaces of both gloves.
5. Properly dispose of the inside-out contaminated gloves in a biohazard waste container (see the following figure).
PURPOSE: To prevent the spread of infection.

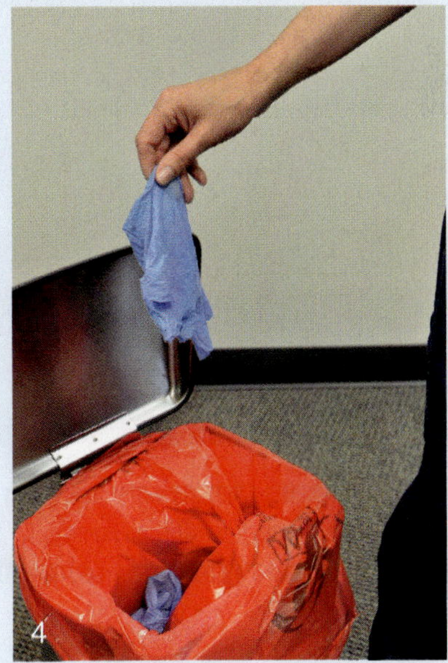

6. Perform a medical aseptic hand wash as described in Procedure 19.2, or sanitize the hands with an alcohol-based sanitizer.
PURPOSE: To minimize the number of pathogens on the hands, thereby reducing the number of transient flora and the risk of transmission of pathogens.

PROCEDURE 19.2 Perform Hand Hygiene

TASK: Minimize the number of pathogens on the hands, thus reducing the risk of transmission of pathogens.

EQUIPMENT and SUPPLIES

- Sink with warm running water
- Liquid soap in a dispenser (bar soap is not acceptable)
- Disposable nail brush or orange stick
- Paper towels in a dispenser
- Water-based lotion
- Covered waste container with foot pedal
- Alcohol-based hand sanitizer

PROCEDURAL STEPS

Medical Aseptic Hand Washing

1. Remove all jewelry except your wristwatch, if it can be pulled up above your wrist, and a plain wedding ring.
   PURPOSE: Jewelry can harbor microorganisms.
2. Turn on the faucet and regulate the water temperature to lukewarm.
   PURPOSE: Water that is too hot can cause the skin to become dry and chapped.
3. Wet your hands, apply soap, and lather using a circular motion with friction while holding your fingertips downward (see the following figure). Rub well between your fingers. If this is the first hand wash of the day, use a nail brush or an orange stick and clean under every fingernail. Inspect your nails thoroughly.
   PURPOSE: Friction removes soil and contaminants from the hands and wrists.

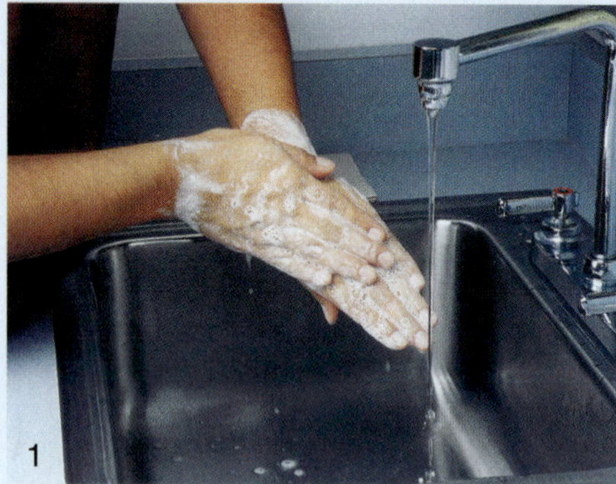

4. Rinse well, holding your hands so that the water flows from your wrists downward to your fingertips (see the following figure).
   PURPOSE: Soil and contaminants will wash off the skin and down the drain.

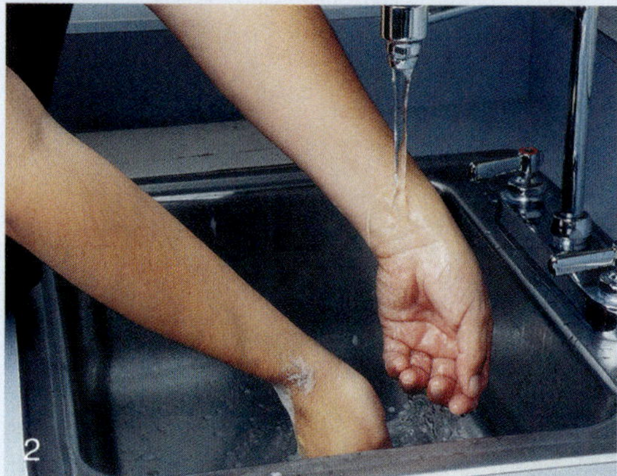

5. If this is the first hand wash of the day or if your hands are obviously contaminated, wet your hands again and repeat the scrubbing procedure using a vigorous, circular motion over the wrists and hands for at least 1 to 2 minutes.
   PURPOSE: Time is required for friction and motion to eliminate all possible soil and contaminants.
6. Rinse your hands a second time, keeping the fingers lower than your wrists.
   PURPOSE: To ensure removal of all transient flora.
7. Dry your hands with paper towels. Do not touch the paper towel dispenser as you obtain towels (see the following figure).
   PURPOSE: Touching the dispenser contaminates your hands, and you will need to start over.

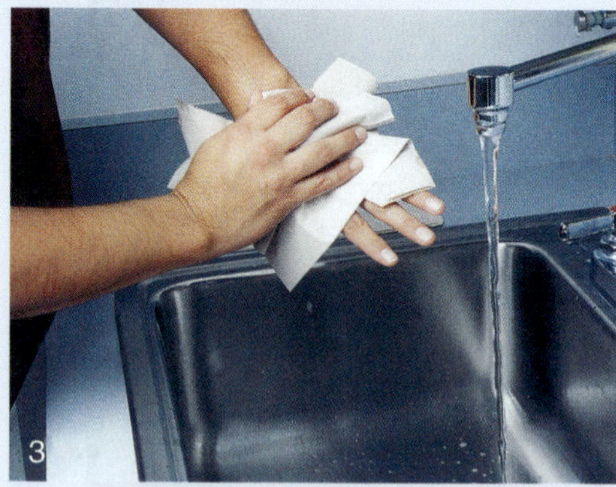

8. If the faucets are not foot operated, turn them off with a dry paper towel (see the following figure).
   PURPOSE: The faucet is dirty and will contaminate your clean hands.

PROCEDURE 19.2 Perform Hand Hygiene—*continued*

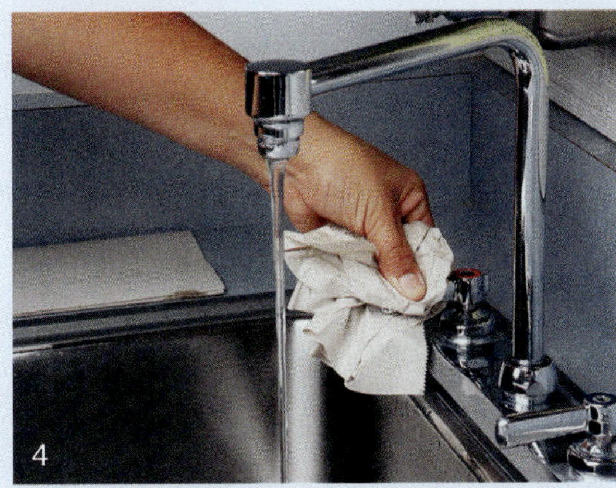

4

9. After you finish drying your hands and turning off the faucets, discard used towels in a covered waste container.
PURPOSE: Always discard contaminated waste in a covered waste container immediately to eliminate the source of infection.

10. If needed, apply a water-based antibacterial hand lotion to prevent chapped or dry skin.
PURPOSE: Chapped skin eliminates the first line of defense against infectious organisms.

11. Repeat the procedure as indicated throughout the day.
PURPOSE: To eliminate contaminants and prevent the transmission of pathogens to yourself and others.

APPLYING AN ALCOHOL-BASED HAND SANITIZER

1. Inspect your hands to ensure they are not visibly soiled.
PURPOSE: If the hands are visibly soiled, then the medical aseptic hand wash should be performed.

2. Remove your watch or push it up on your arm; remove rings.
PURPOSE: Watches and rings can harbor microorganisms.

3. Apply alcohol-based hand sanitizer to the palm of one hand: gel or lotion (dime sized), foam (walnut sized).
PURPOSE: Using too much alcohol-based hand sanitizer can be drying to the skin. Dry skin cracks and chaps, creating portals of entry for microorganisms.

4. Thoroughly spread sanitizer over all surfaces of both hands, including around and under the fingernails.
PURPOSE: All surfaces need to be exposed to the alcohol-based hand sanitizer to effectively kill all microorganisms.

5. Rub your hands until dry (20 to 30 seconds).

PROCEDURE 19.3 Sanitize Soiled Instruments

TASK: Remove all contaminated matter from instruments in preparation for disinfection or sterilization while following Standard Precautions and wearing appropriate personal protective equipment (PPE).

EQUIPMENT and SUPPLIES

- Sink with cold and hot running water
- Sanitizing agent or low-sudsing soap with enzymatic action
- Decontaminated utility gloves that show no signs of deterioration
- Chin-length face shield or goggles and face mask if contamination with bloodborne pathogens is possible
- Impermeable gown
- Disposable brush
- Disposable paper towels
- Utility gloves
- Disinfectant cleaner prepared according to manufacturer's directions
- Covered waste container with foot pedal
- Biohazard waste container with labeled red biohazard bag

PROCEDURAL STEPS

1. Put on an impermeable gown and face shield or goggles and mask if the potential for splashing of infectious material exists (see the following figure).
PURPOSE: To provide personal protection against potentially infectious matter.

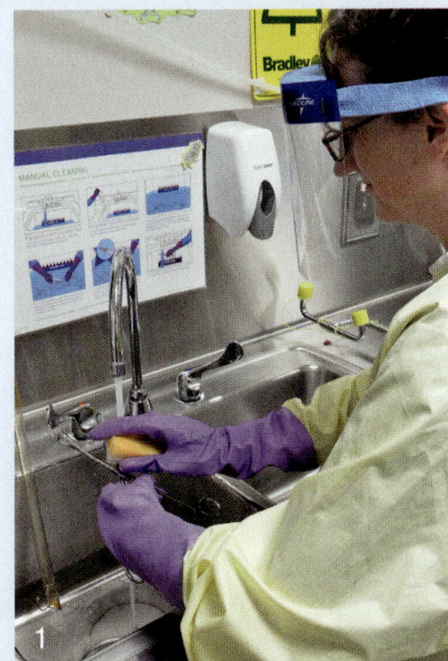

1

Continued

PROCEDURE 19.3 Sanitize Soiled Instruments —*continued*

2. Put on utility gloves.
   PURPOSE: To provide personal protection against potentially infectious matter and sharp instruments.
3. Separate the sharp instruments from other instruments to be sanitized.
   PURPOSE: To prevent possible self-injury and exposure to infectious matter.
4. Rinse the instruments under cold running water.
   PURPOSE: To help remove debris and body fluids.
5. Open hinged instruments, and scrub all grooves, crevices, and serrations with a disposable brush (see the following figure).
   PURPOSE: Microorganisms can hide under contaminants and may not be destroyed by the disinfection process.

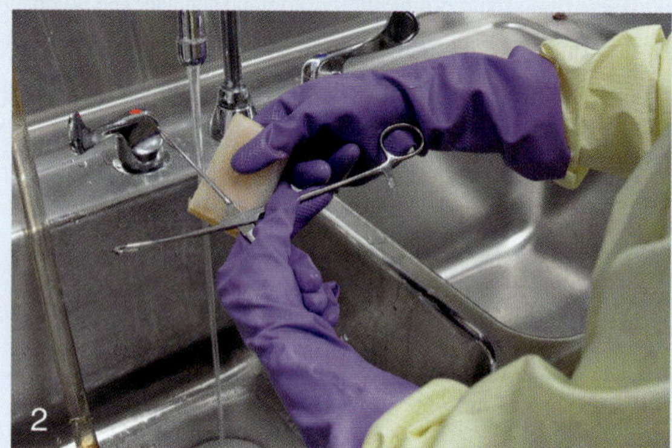

6. Rinse well with hot water.
   PURPOSE: Hot water removes all soap and contaminant residue.
7. Towel-dry all instruments thoroughly and dispose of contaminated towels and disposable brush in a biohazard waste container. Do not touch the paper towel dispenser as you are obtaining towels.
   PURPOSE: All contaminated material must be discarded in a labeled biohazard container or a labeled red biohazard bag. Touching the dispenser with the utility gloves contaminates the dispenser. Wet instruments can rust or become dull.
8. Remove the utility gloves and wash your hands according to Procedure 19.2.
   PURPOSE: To remove any contaminants.
9. Towel-dry your hands and put on gloves. Decontaminate the utility gloves and work surfaces using a disinfectant cleaner.
   PURPOSE: To prevent personal exposure to contaminants. All equipment and working surfaces should be cleaned and decontaminated with a disinfectant to prevent transmission of infectious organisms.
10. Dispose of the contaminated towels in a covered waste container.
    PURPOSE: All contaminated material must be disposed of in a labeled biohazard container or a labeled red biohazard bag.
11. Place sanitized instruments in a designated area for disinfection or sterilization.
    PURPOSE: Sanitized instruments must be removed from the cleaning area to prevent possible cross-contamination.
12. Remove the gloves according to Procedure 19.1. Dispose of the gloves in a biohazard waste container. Sanitize the hands.
    PURPOSE: To prevent the spread of infectious organisms and remove any possible contaminants.

20 VITAL SIGNS

SCENARIO

Carlos Ricci is a certified medical assistant (CMA) who has met the requirements of the American Association of Medical Assistants (AAMA). He works at Walden-Martin Family Medical (WMFM) Clinic. Carlos graduated from a medical assistant program 3 years ago and now enjoys the variety of patients and the patient contact involved in working on the clinical side of WMFM Clinic. One of Carlos' primary responsibilities is to accurately measure and record each patient's vital signs before the patient is seen. Over the past 3 years, he has come to understand the importance of taking accurate vital sign measurements and accurately documenting those results.

While studying this chapter, think about the following questions:

- What factors might alter a patient's vital signs?
- What methods could be used to gather and record a patient's temperature, pulse, respiration, blood pressure, height, weight, and body mass index (BMI)?
- What are the current guidelines for diagnosing and treating hypertension?

LEARNING OBJECTIVES

1. Examine the process for taking an accurate body temperature.
2. Examine the process for taking an accurate pulse rate.
3. Examine the process for taking an accurate respiration rate.
4. Examine the process for taking an accurate blood pressure reading.
5. Examine the process for measuring oxygen saturation.
6. Examine the process for obtaining anthropometric measurements.

VOCABULARY

apnea (AP nee ah) Abnormal, periodic cessation of breathing.

arteriosclerosis (ar teer ee oh sklah ROH sis) Thickening, decreased elasticity, and calcification of arterial walls.

auscultated (AW skuhl tay ted) Listening to the sounds within the body with a stethoscope.

bounding Describes a pulse that feels full because of the increased power of cardiac contraction or as a result of increased blood volume.

bradycardia (brad ee KAHR dee uh) A slow heartbeat; a pulse below 60 beats per minute.

bradypnea (brad IP nee ah) Abnormally slow breathing.

calibrated (KAL uh bray ted) Determined by or checked against a standard (as in readings).

cerumen (si ROO muhn) A waxy secretion in the ear canal; commonly called ear wax.

Cheyne-Stokes respiration Deep, rapid breathing followed by a period of apnea.

chronic obstructive pulmonary disease (COPD) A progressive, irreversible lung condition that results in diminished lung capacity.

diurnal (die UR nl) variation Fluctuations that occur during each day.

dyspnea (DISP nee ah) Difficult or painful breathing.

essential hypertension Elevated blood pressure of unknown cause that develops for no apparent reason; sometimes called primary hypertension.

febrile (FEB ruhl) Pertaining to an elevated body temperature.

fluctuate (FLUHK choo ayt) To shift back and forth.

homeostasis (hoh mee oh STAY sis) The internal environment of the body that is compatible with life. A steady state that is created by all the body systems working together to provide a consistent and unvarying internal environment.

hyperpnea (hie PURP nee ah) Excessively deep breathing.

hyperventilation (hie pur ven ti LAY shun) Abnormally increased breathing.

hypotension Blood pressure that is below normal (systolic pressure below 90 mm Hg and diastolic pressure below 50 mm Hg).

idiopathic (id ee uh PATH ik) Of unknown cause.

intermittent pulse A pulse in which beats occasionally are skipped.

larynx (LAR inks) The voice box.

lymphedema (lim fuh DEE mah) A condition in which extra lymph fluid builds up in tissues and causes swelling. It may occur in an arm or leg if lymph vessels are blocked, damaged, or removed by surgery.

malaise (ma LAYZ) A condition of general bodily weakness or discomfort, often marking the onset of a disease.

VOCABULARY—*continued*

myocardium (mie oh KAR dee um) The middle layer, and thickest layer, of the heart; composed of cardiac muscles.
occlude To close, shut, or stop up.
orthopnea (or THOP nee ah) A condition of difficult breathing unless in an upright position.
orthostatic (postural) hypotension A temporary fall in blood pressure when a person rapidly changes from a recumbent position to a standing position.
otitis externa Inflammation or infection of the external auditory canal; commonly called swimmer's ear.
peripheral (puh RIF er uhl) Refers to an area outside of or away from an organ or structure.
pulse deficit A condition in which the radial pulse is less than the apical pulse; it may indicate a peripheral vascular abnormality.
pulse pressure The difference between the systolic and diastolic blood pressures (30 to 50 mm Hg is considered normal).
pyrexia (pie REK see ah) A febrile condition or fever.
rales (rayls) An abnormal lung sound heard on auscultation, characterized by discontinuous bubbling noises.
rhonchi (RON kie) An abnormal rumbling sound heard during auscultation, caused by airways blocked by secretions or muscle contractions.
sinus arrhythmia An irregular heartbeat that originates in the sinoatrial node (pacemaker).
stertorous (STUR ter uhs) Heavy, as related to snoring.
syncope (SING kuh pee) Fainting; a brief lapse in consciousness.
tachycardia (tak i KAHR dee ah) A rapid but regular heart rate; one that exceeds 100 beats per minute.
tachypnea (tack ip NEE ah) Rapid, shallow breathing.
thready Describes a pulse that is thin and feeble.
vertigo (VUR tih goh) Dizziness; an abnormal sensation of movement when there is none.
wheezing (WHEE zing) Whistling sound made during breathing.

INTRODUCTION

Almost every patient who visits the healthcare facility will have some vital signs measured. These signs are the body's indicators of internal **homeostasis** and the patient's general state of health. Medical assistants are often responsible for obtaining these measurements. It is crucial that they have confidence in the theory and practical applications of vital sign measurements. A medical assistant who understands the principles of and reasons for these measurements is a valuable asset to any healthcare facility.

Accuracy is essential. A change in one or more of the patient's vital signs may indicate a change in general health. Variations may suggest the presence or disappearance of a disease process. This may lead to changes in the treatment plan. Taking vital signs is a task that requires consistent attention to accuracy and detail. These findings are necessary to come up with a correct diagnosis. Vital signs should never be measured in an indifferent or a casual manner. In addition to performing measurements accurately, you must take care when documenting the findings in the patient's health record.

The *vital signs* are the patient's temperature, pulse, respiration, and blood pressure. These four signs are abbreviated *TPR* and *BP* and may be referred to as *cardinal signs*. Many organizations consider pulse oximetry, SpO_2, a vital sign also. The medical assistant must understand the significance of the vital signs and must measure and record them accurately. *Anthropometric measurements* are not considered vital signs but are usually obtained at the same time as vital signs. These measurements include height, weight, body mass index (BMI), and other body measurements, such as fat composition.

Vital signs are influenced by many factors, both physical and emotional. A patient may have had a hot or cold beverage just before the examination or may be anxious or fearful about what the provider may find. For example, consider that a patient has been asked to return for a repeat Papanicolaou (Pap) test because the first one showed the presence of suspicious cells. The medical assistant measures the patient's blood pressure and finds it significantly elevated compared with previous readings. The patient may be anxious and concerned about the test results. The elevated blood pressure readings likely reflect her anxiety.

What impact would it have on a temperature reading if a patient could not find a parking place and had to walk four blocks to the office, knowing he would be late for his appointment? If you said it would be elevated, you are right. Certainly, this patient's metabolism would increase because of the physical exercise. As a result, his temperature would be elevated, along with his pulse, respirations, and blood pressure. The medical assistant should give the patient some time to recover from his sprint to the office before taking any vital sign measurements.

Vital signs are often altered if the patient is in pain. Pay attention to nonverbal signs that might indicate discomfort or pain, especially if the patient's blood pressure, pulse, and respirations are elevated. In addition, many patients are uneasy about being seen by the provider. This may alter vital signs. The medical assistant must help the patient relax before taking any readings. Measurements sometimes must be obtained a second time after the patient is more calm or comfortable. For a better picture of the patient's vital signs, the medical assistant may be asked to take the vital signs twice: at the beginning of the visit and just before the patient leaves the examination room.

TEMPERATURE

Body temperature is defined as the balance between heat lost and heat produced by the body. It is measured in degrees Fahrenheit (F) or Celsius (C). The process of chemical and physical change in the body that produces heat is called *metabolism*. Body temperature is a result of this process. The core body temperature is maintained within a normal range by the *hypothalamus*.

Factors That May Influence Temperature

The average body temperature varies from person to person and is different for each person at different times throughout the day. In a healthy adult, this **diurnal variation** ranges from 97.7° to 99.5°F (36.5° to 37.5°C); the average daily temperature is 98.6°F (37°C). Some sources say the average daily temperature has been decreasing, with one study showing that adults' average temperature today is 97.8°F (36.6°C). Body temperature is lowest in the morning and highest in the late afternoon. Factors that may affect body temperature include the following:

- *Age:* The body temperature of infants and young children fluctuates more rapidly in response to external environmental temperatures. Aging adults lose the insulation of subcutaneous fat and thermoregulatory control.
- *Stress and physical activity:* Both exercise and emotional stress can increase the metabolic rate, causing an elevation in temperature.
- *Gender:* Hormone secretions result in fluctuations of the core body temperature in women throughout the menstrual cycle.
- *External factors:* Smoking, drinking hot fluids, and chewing gum can temporarily elevate an oral temperature. Environmental factors also can change body temperature. Cold weather tends to reduce body temperature, and hot weather tends to increase it.

In illness, an individual's metabolic activity increases. This causes an increase in internal heat production, which in turn raises the body temperature. The increase in body temperature is thought to be the body's defensive reaction because heat inhibits the growth of some bacteria and viruses.

When a fever is present, superficial blood vessels (those near the surface of the skin) constrict. The small papillary muscles at the base of hair follicles also constrict, creating "goose bumps." Chills and shivering may follow, producing internal heat. As this process repeats itself, more heat is produced, and the body temperature rises above the normal range. When more heat is lost than produced, the opposite effect occurs, and body temperature drops below the normal range.

Fever

Infection, either bacterial or viral, is the most common cause of fever in both children and adults. Infants do not usually develop **febrile** illnesses during the first 3 months of life; if one is present, it usually is very serious. However, fever, or **pyrexia**, is common in young children and accounts for an estimated 30% of office visits. Fevers are classified according to the 24-hour pattern they follow. The three most common patterns are as follows (Figure 20.1):

- *Continuous fever* rises and falls only slightly during a 24-hour period. The temperature consistently remains above the patient's average normal temperature range and **fluctuates** less than 3 degrees.
- *Intermittent fever* comes and goes, alternating between elevated and normal levels.
- *Remittent fever* fluctuates considerably (i.e., by more than 3 degrees) and never returns to the normal range.

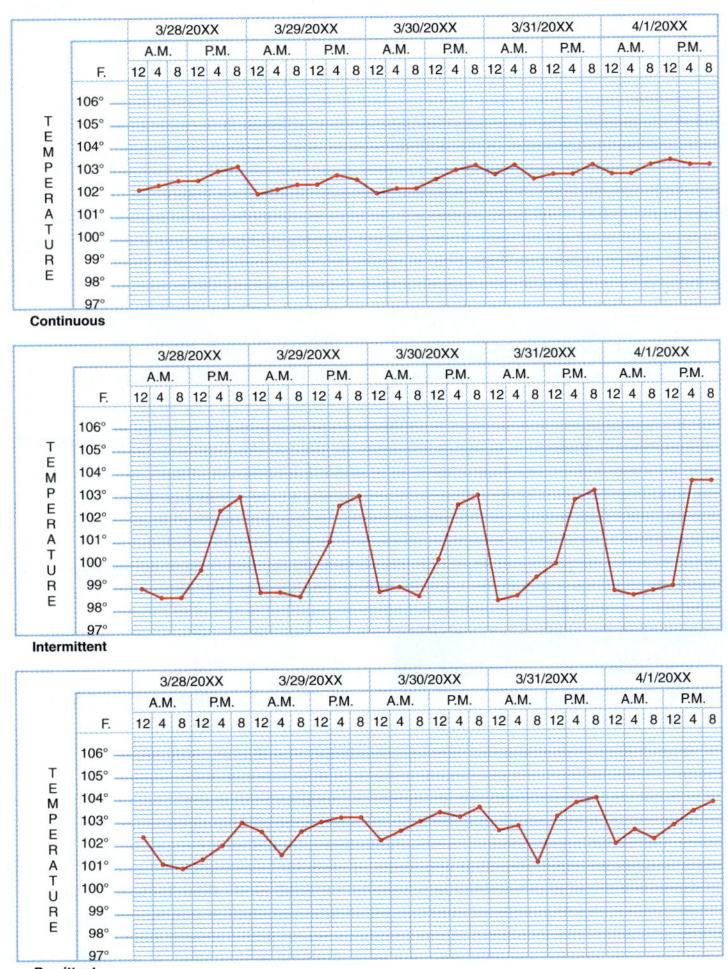

FIGURE 20.1 Fever Patterns.

Variation in the patient's average body temperature range may be the first warning of an illness or a change in the patient's current condition. Patients with fever usually have the following indicators:

- Loss of appetite (*anorexia*)
- Headache
- Thirst
- Flushed face
- Hot skin
- General **malaise**

Some patients experience an acute onset of chills and shivering, followed by an increase in body temperature. A possible serious complication in young children with high fevers is a febrile seizure. Medication to reduce the fever, or *antipyretic* drugs (e.g., acetaminophen or ibuprofen), should be taken as instructed to prevent dangerous spikes in temperature. A rectal, temporal, or aural (ear) temperature over 100.4°F (38°C), an oral temperature over 100°F (37.8°C), and an axillary temperature over 99°F (37.2°C) are all considered a fever.

Sites

Several types of thermometers and various sites can be used to take temperature readings. A digital thermometer is placed under the tongue, in the armpit, or the rectum; a tympanic thermometer is inserted into the ear, and a temporal artery thermometer is moved across the forehead. Temperatures can be read in either Fahrenheit or Celsius. Most thermometers will convert from one scale to the other. Average temperature values for adults are shown in Table 20.1.

Converting Temperatures

There are many options for converting temperatures between the Fahrenheit and Celsius scales. Most electronic health records (EHRs) will do the conversion when the temperature is entered. There also are online options. If you need to do the conversion manually, the following formulas will help you out.

FAHRENHEIT TO CELSIUS	CELSIUS TO FAHRENHEIT
°C = (°F − 32) ÷ 1.8	°F = (°C × 1.8) + 32
Example: 101°F	Example: 39°C
°C = (101–32) ÷ 1.8	°F = (39 × 1.8) + 32
°C = 69 ÷ 1.8	°F = 70.2 + 32
°C = 38.3	°F = 102.2

TABLE 20.1 Average Adult Temperatures

SITE	FAHRENHEIT	CELSIUS
Axillary	97.6°	36.4°
Oral	98.6°	37°
Tympanic	99.6°	37.6°
Rectal	99.6°	37.6°
Temporal artery	99.6°	37.6°

CRITICAL THINKING APPLICATION 20.1

Using the correct formula, convert the following temperatures from one system to the other:

1. 99°F = _________ °C
2. 102°F = _________ °C
3. 38°C = _________ °F
4. 39.5°C = _________ °F

There are a number of factors to consider when determining which site should be used.

Age	Birth–3 months: rectal or temporal artery 3 months–4 years: rectal, axillary, temporal artery; after the age of 6 months, a tympanic thermometer may be used 4 years or older: oral, axillary, tympanic, temporal artery, rectal
Condition	Mouth breathing: oral is not an option Ear infection or occlusion: tympanic is not an option Diarrhea: rectal is not an option Open wound or rash on forehead: temporal artery is not an option
State of consciousness	If unconscious: oral not an option
Thermometers available in the facility	May only have one or two types of thermometers available
Healthcare facility procedures	Based on patient's condition or provider's preference

When an oral temperature is obtained, you do not have to indicate the site when documenting the reading in the patient's health record. If you use an alternate site, you should document the following identifiers after recording the temperature:

- (T) for tympanic
- (A) for axillary
- (R) for rectal
- (TA) for temporal artery
- (IFR) for infrared

For example, T: 99.4°F (T) clarifies that an alternate site, tympanic, was used.

Axillary temperatures (A) and temporal artery temperatures (TA) are approximately 1°F (0.6°C) lower than oral readings because axillary readings are not taken in an enclosed body cavity. Tympanic and rectal temperatures are approximately 1°F (0.6°C) higher than oral readings. The actual reading from the thermometer should be documented with the correct abbreviation for the site.

The oral site is not typically used with young children. This site requires the patient to hold the thermometer under the tongue and keep the mouth closed, a task that can be difficult for children younger than age 3. A rectal temperature is most often used for infants. It is important to use the proper technique to avoid damaging the rectal tissue (see Procedure 20.3). However, most pediatricians prefer that infants' temperatures be taken with a temporal artery thermometer (Procedure 20.1) because it is more comfortable for the baby, less invasive, and eliminates the possible complication of a perforated rectum.

When taken correctly, the tympanic (ear/aural) temperature (T) is an accurate measure because it records the temperature of the blood closest to the hypothalamus. However, research on the temporal artery (TA) thermometer indicates that this method is more accurate than tympanic measurement for identifying elevated temperatures in infants. Pediatricians, therefore, may prefer TA temperatures in infants suspected of having a fever. The TA thermometer also records accurate temperature readings in all age groups. The tympanic method is still considered a fast, accurate, and noninvasive way of recording temperatures for older children and adults.

For patients younger than 3 years and those unable to hold a thermometer properly in their mouth during the procedure, a tympanic or temporal artery thermometer can be used; if not, a less accurate axillary temperature can be obtained.

CRITICAL THINKING APPLICATION 20.2

The mother of a 3-year-old calls the office to report that her child had an axillary temperature of 101°F at 9 o'clock this morning. The schedule is full today, so Carlos has to decide whether the child should be seen today or first thing tomorrow. When should Carlos schedule the appointment? What is the significance of the axillary temperature reading?

Measuring Temperature

As mentioned previously, there is a number of different thermometers for taking a temperature. It is important to understand each of the thermometers and when they should or should not be used. The healthcare facility may have more than one type of thermometer available, and the medical assistant should be familiar with each of them.

Types of Thermometers and Their Uses

The temporal artery thermometer has become the most commonly used thermometer in healthcare, but other methods are still used. All of the thermometers are discussed in the following sections.

Temporal Artery Thermometer. The temporal artery thermometer uses an infrared beam to assess the temperature of the blood flowing through the temporal artery of the forehead, where the artery lies about 1 mm below the skin (Figure 20.2). Because the artery is so close to the skin, it provides good surface heat conduction, allowing the thermometer to obtain a fast, accurate, and noninvasive measurement of body temperature. To perform the procedure, place the probe in the center of the forehead, halfway between the eyebrows and the hairline. Bangs should be pushed back off the forehead (this method cannot be used if bandages cover the area). Depress the button on the scanner and gently stroke the probe across the forehead toward the hairline (at the temples), keeping the probe flat on the patient's skin. As the scanner moves across the forehead, repeated temperature measurements are taken, and the highest measurement is recorded; keeping the button depressed, lift the scanner from the temporal area and lightly place the probe behind the earlobe. Release the button and remove the probe. Recording an accurate temperature takes about 3 seconds (see Procedure 20.1). Depending on the facility's infection control procedures, disposable covers can be used on the scanner, or it can be cleaned between patients with an alcohol wipe.

Tympanic Thermometer. The tympanic membrane of the ear can be used for quick, accurate, and safe assessment of a patient's temperature. It shares the blood supply with the hypothalamus, which is the brain's temperature regulator. The ear canal is a protected cavity. This means factors such as an open mouth, hot or cold drinks, or even a stuffy nose do not affect aural temperature.

The tympanic thermometer system consists of a handheld unit equipped with a tympanic probe, which is covered with a disposable probe cover (Figure 20.3). When the probe is placed into the ear canal, it gently seals the external opening of the canal, and the sensor detects the infrared energy produced by the tympanic membrane. This signal is digitized by the thermometer and shown on the display screen. Accurate readings are obtained in less than 2 seconds (see Procedure 20.2). The tympanic thermometer is popular due to the speed of obtaining the temperature and the comfort it affords the patient. This site should not be used if the patient is complaining of pain in both ears when the ear is touched. The patient may

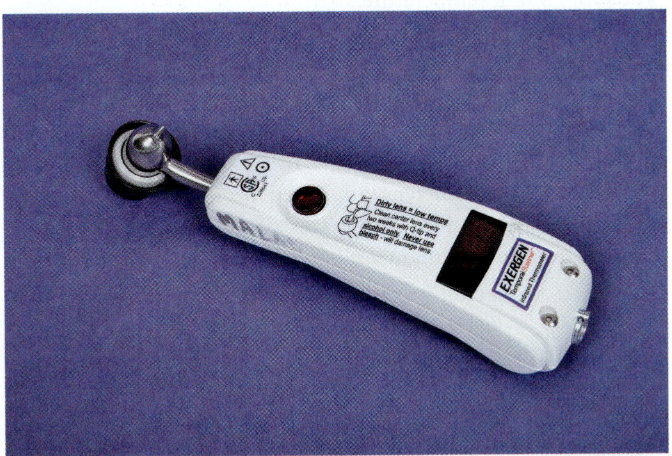

FIGURE 20.2 Temporal Artery Thermometer.

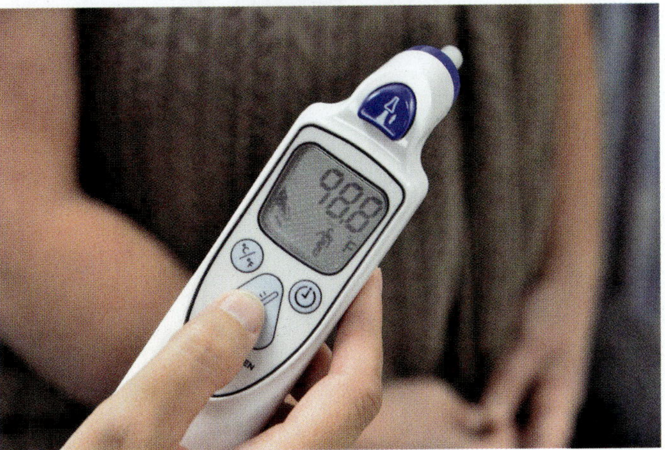

FIGURE 20.3 Tympanic Thermometer.

have bilateral **otitis externa**, making the procedure uncomfortable. In addition, if the patient has a history of or has impacted **cerumen** in both ears, do not use a tympanic thermometer because the reading may be inaccurate.

Insert the probe into the ear canal far enough to seal the opening without applying pressure. To expose the tympanic membrane in children younger than age 3, gently pull the earlobe down and back; for patients older than age 3, gently pull the pinna (top of the ear) up and back.

Digital Thermometer. Digital thermometers are battery operated. Disposable covers fit snugly over the probes and are easily and quickly removed by pushing in the colored end of the probe. The instrument sounds a beep when the process is complete (in 10 to 60 seconds), and the reading appears on a screen on the face of the instrument. Because the only part of the instrument that comes in contact with the patient is the probe, which is covered, the risk of cross-infection is greatly reduced (Figure 20.4).

When using a digital thermometer to take an oral temperature (Procedure 20.3), it is important to ask if the patient has recently had anything to eat, drink, or smoke. These factors may artificially alter the patient's temperature. Wait for 10 to 15 minutes before taking an oral temperature if those factors have occurred. In addition, the patient must be able to hold the thermometer under the tongue with the lips tightly sealed around the probe if an accurate oral reading is to be obtained. Be sure to use the blue probe for an oral temperature.

A digital thermometer with a blue probe can also be used for an axillary temperature (Procedure 20.4). It is important to make sure that there is a tight seal around the probe. This can be done by holding the patient's arm snugly across the chest. Remember, this site is considered the least accurate.

A digital thermometer with a red probe is used for rectal temperatures (Procedure 20.5). This site is used most often for infants. To take an infant's temperature rectally, lubricate the probe tip (most facilities use a lubricating product, such as K-Y Jelly), hold the baby securely with the legs elevated, and insert the probe approximately 1 inch; hold the probe carefully and continue to secure the infant's legs throughout the procedure to prevent rectal damage.

The digital unit or individual digital thermometers should be routinely cleaned with disinfectant. When ejecting the probe cover, be careful not to contaminate the probe or the processing unit. The probe cover should be deposited directly into a waste container. If a chance exists that a patient's body fluids touched the unit, wipe it with disinfectant before returning it to the storage area.

Infrared Thermometer. An infrared thermometer provides a touchless way to obtain a temperature and can easily be used on patients of all ages (Figure 20.5). The sensor picks up the infrared radiation the body produces.

To use this thermometer, hold it a few centimeters away from the center of the forehead, just above the eyebrows (Procedure 20.6). See the manufacturer's instructions for the specific placement. It only takes a few seconds to obtain the reading.

These thermometers are often used to screen for fever, especially for large groups of people. If the infrared thermometer indicates a fever, it is often confirmed using another type of thermometer.

CRITICAL THINKING APPLICATION **20.3**

How should the medical assistant adapt temperature-taking techniques for the following patients?

- A patient who talks continuously with the thermometer in his mouth
- A 7-year-old patient with bilateral otitis externa
- A 3-month-old patient when a temporal artery thermometer is available
- A 46-year-old patient with a severe asthma attack
- A 72-year-old patient with bilateral impacted cerumen
- A 28-year-old patient who has just smoked a cigarette

PULSE

A patient's pulse rate reflects the palpable beat of the arteries throughout the body as they expand in response to the contraction of the heart. With every beat, the heart pumps an amount of blood, known as the *stroke volume,* into the aorta. Arteries branch off the aorta as it travels down through the center of the abdomen, transferring the pulse beat throughout the body. To measure the

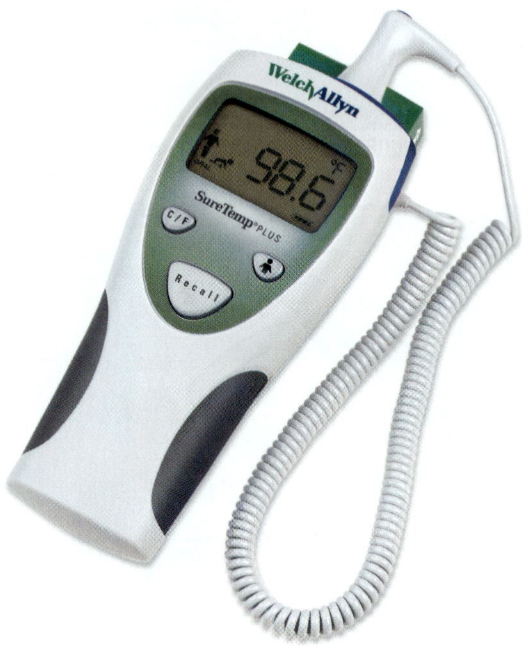

FIGURE 20.4 Digital Thermometer. (Courtesy Welch Allyn.)

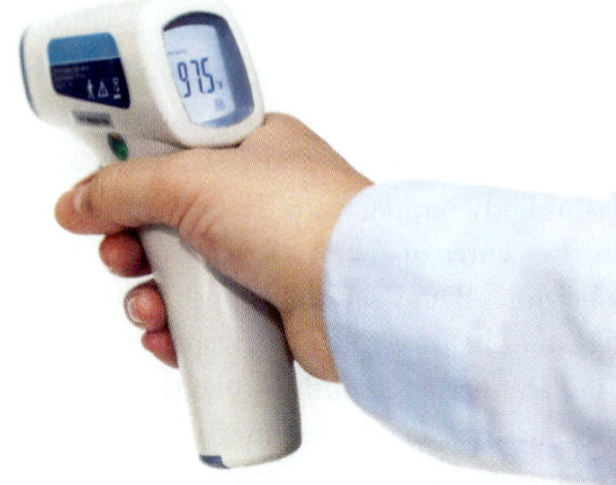

FIGURE 20.5 Infrared Thermometer. (From i/Stock.com/guvendemir.)

pulse, an artery is used that is close to the body surface and can be pushed against a bone. Palpating a **peripheral** pulse gives the rate, rhythm, and volume of the heartbeat and local information about the condition of the artery used.

Factors That May Influence Pulse Rate

Many factors can influence the pulse rate. The most common factors are as follows:

- *Age:* Infants have a higher pulse rate than adults.
- *Gender:* Women tend to have a faster pulse rate than men.
- *Fitness and activity levels:* Physical fitness can lower the pulse rate. Physical activity can temporarily raise the pulse rate.
- *Smoking:* Can increase the pulse rate.
- *Cardiovascular disease:* Can increase the pulse rate.
- *Thyroid disease:* An overactive thyroid gland can increase the pulse rate.
- *Caffeine use:* Can increase the pulse rate.
- *Emotions:* Strong emotions, either positive or negative, can increase the pulse rate.
- *Medications:* Certain medications are used specifically to raise or lower the pulse rate; some may do that as a side effect of the medication.

Pulse Sites

A pulse rate may be counted anywhere an artery is near the surface of the body, and the vessel can be pressed against a bone. The most common pulse sites are the temporal, carotid, brachial, radial, femoral, popliteal, and dorsalis pedis arteries (Figure 20.6). The apical pulse is taken by listening with a stethoscope.

The *temporal* pulse is located in the temple area of the skull, parallel and lateral to the eyes (Figure 20.7). It is seldom used as a pulse site but may be used as a pressure point to help control bleeding from a head injury.

The *carotid* artery is located between the **larynx** and the *sternocleidomastoid* muscle in the front and to the side of the neck (Figure 20.8). It is most frequently used in emergencies and to check the pulse during cardiopulmonary resuscitation (CPR). It can be felt by pushing the muscle to the side and pressing against the larynx.

The *brachial* pulse is felt at the inner (*antecubital*) aspect of the elbow. This is the artery that is felt and listened to when blood pressure is measured (Figure 20.9). It also can be felt in the groove between the biceps and triceps muscles on the inner surface of the middle-upper arm. This is the pulse that is checked on infants and young children receiving CPR.

The *radial* artery is the most commonly used site for counting the pulse rate. It is found on the thumb side of the wrist, 1 inch below the base of the thumb (Figure 20.10).

The *femoral* pulse is located at the site where the femoral artery passes through the groin (see Figure 20.6). The examiner must press deeply below the *inguinal* ligament to palpate this pulse.

The *popliteal* pulse is found at the back of the leg behind the knee (see Figure 20.6). Palpation of this pulse requires the patient to be in a recumbent position with the knee slightly flexed. The popliteal artery is deep and difficult to feel. It is palpated and monitored with a stethoscope when a leg blood pressure reading is necessary. The provider checks blood flow through the popliteal artery if a circulatory system problem, such as a blood clot, is suspected in the lower leg.

The *dorsalis pedis* (pedal) artery is felt across the arch of the foot, just slightly lateral to the midline, beside the extensor tendon of the great toe. This pulse may be congenitally absent in some patients. Because a good pulse rate at this site is an indicator of normal lower limb circulation and arterial sufficiency, the provider checks the pedal pulses in patients with peripheral vascular problems, such as patients with diabetes mellitus.

The *apical* heart rate, or the heartbeat at the apex of the heart, is heard with a stethoscope. It is used for infants and young children because the radial pulse is difficult to palpate in young patients. Apical rates are also recorded on adult patients who have irregular or difficult-to-feel radial pulses to ensure an accurate heart rate reading. An apical count may be requested if the patient is taking cardiac

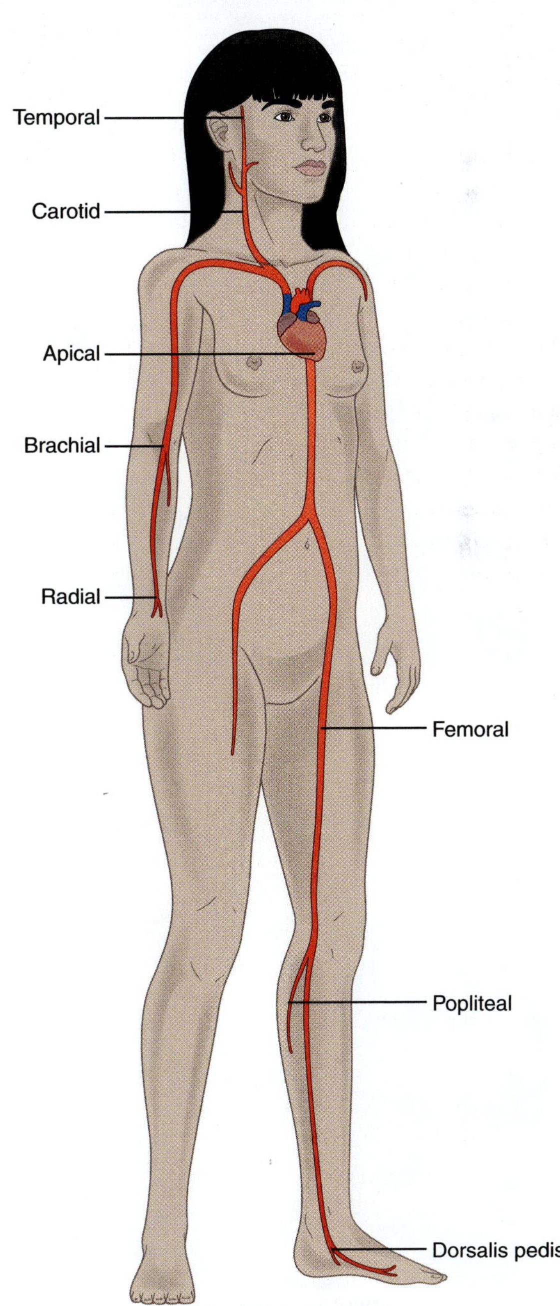

FIGURE 20.6 Pulse Sites.

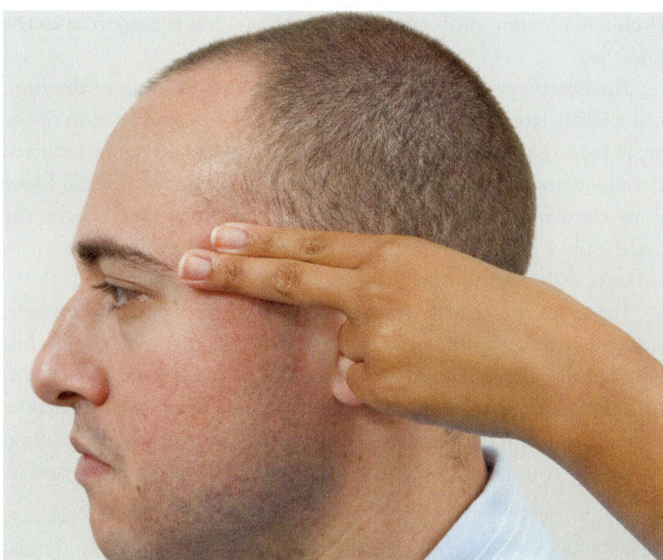

FIGURE 20.7 Temporal Pulse.

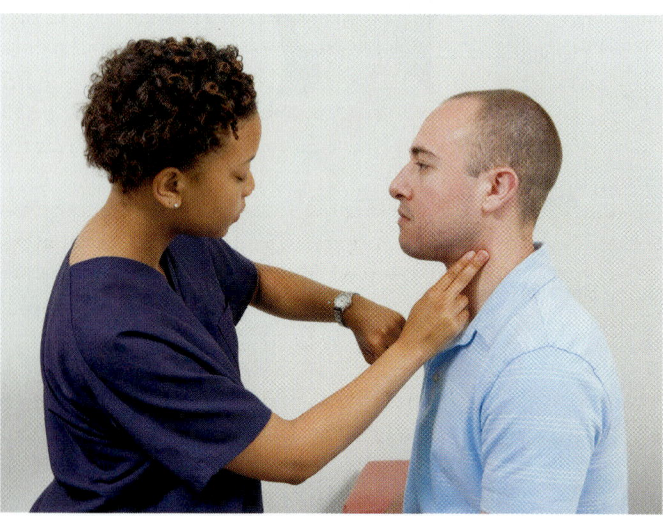

FIGURE 20.8 Carotid Pulse.

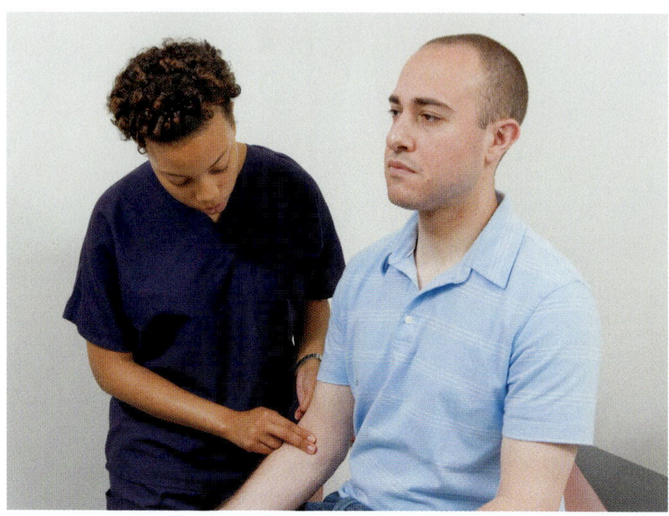

FIGURE 20.9 Brachial Pulse.

drugs or has **bradycardia** or **tachycardia**. To determine the presence of a **pulse deficit**, the provider may listen to the apical beat while the medical assistant counts the pulse at another site (usually the radial pulse). The stethoscope is placed at the apex of the heart. For infants and young children, the stethoscope would be placed at the left fourth intercostal space and midclavicular line—that is, between the fourth and fifth ribs on a line with the midpoint of the left clavicle intercostal. For older children, the stethoscope would be placed at the fifth intercostal space and the midclavicular line. The pulse should be counted for 1 full minute and documented with (AP) beside the recorded count (Procedure 20.7).

Measuring the Pulse Rate

When measuring the pulse rate, the medical assistant must be aware of the characteristics of the pulse and use the proper technique for the various sites to ensure an accurate measurement. The following sections explain the best process for measuring the pulse rate.

Characteristics of a Pulse

Rate, rhythm, and volume are the factors assessed when taking a pulse. These characteristics vary with the size and elasticity of the artery and the strength and regularity of the heart's contractions. A patient's pulse can reveal valuable information about the cardiovascular system.

Rate. The pulse rate is a measure of the number of beats felt from the movement of blood through an artery. When the heart contracts, blood is pumped into the arteries. The pressure throughout the arteries increases, and the arteries expand. When the heart relaxes, little blood is moving through the arteries, and arterial pressure decreases. Each contraction and relaxation of the heart muscle is a beat. The resulting expansion and relaxation of the arteries create a pulsation. This is the pulse rate. Normally, the beat (rate) and the pulse rate are the same. The rate of the pulse is the number of beats (pulsations) that occur in 1 minute.

Table 20.2 lists the normal pulse ranges for various age groups of patients.

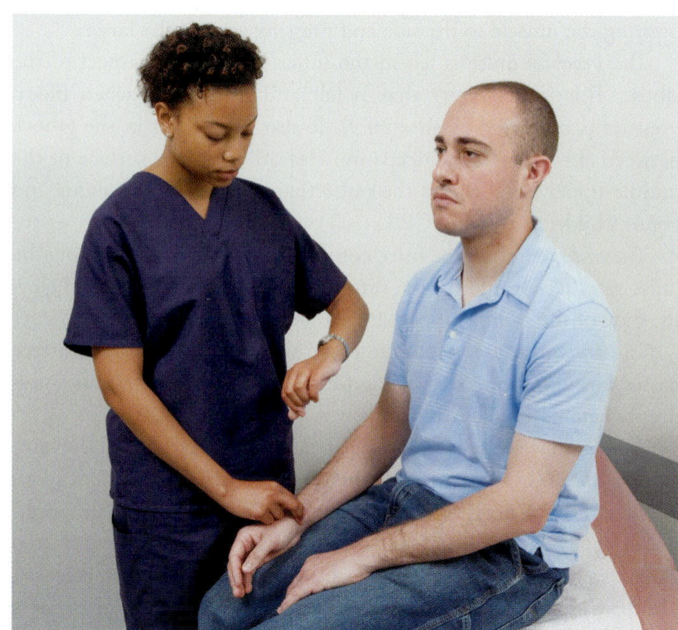

FIGURE 20.10 Radial Pulse.

Rhythm. The pulse rhythm is the time between pulse beats. A normal rhythm pattern has an even tempo, which indicates that the intervals between the beats are of equal duration. An abnormal rhythm, or arrhythmia, is described according to the rhythm pattern detected. An **intermittent pulse** may occur in healthy individuals during exercise or after drinking a beverage containing caffeine. A common irregularity found in children and young adults is a **sinus arrhythmia.** The heart rate varies with the respiratory cycle, speeding up with inspiration and slowing to normal with expiration. If beats are frequently skipped, or the beats are markedly irregular, the provider should be advised because this may indicate heart disease. If an irregular rhythm is detected, the pulse should be counted for a full minute to ensure accuracy. A note also should be made that the patient's pulse was irregular—for example, "P: 86 irregular."

Volume. The volume (*pulse amplitude*) reflects the strength of the heart when it contracts. Volume can be assessed by feeling the strength of the pulse as blood flows through the vessel. The force of each pulse beat is described as **bounding** or full, strong or normal, or **thready** or weak. The force of the heartbeat and the condition of the arterial wall (whether hard or soft) influence the volume of the pulse beat. The pulse may vary only in intensity and, otherwise, may be perfectly regular. This condition also can indicate heart disease. The pulse volume is recorded using a three-point scale.

TABLE 20.2 Approximate Age-Related Pulse Rates

AGE	RANGE (BEATS/MIN)	AVERAGE
Newborn	120–160	140
1–2 years	80–140	120
3–6 years	75–120	100
7–11 years	75–110	95
Adolescence to adulthood	60–100	80

Three-Point Scale for Measuring Pulse Volume

3+	Full, bounding pulse	Pulsation is very strong and does not disappear with moderate pressure.
2+	Normal pulse	Pulsation is easily felt but disappears with moderate pressure.
1+	Weak, thready pulse	Pulsation is not easily felt and disappears with slight pressure.

Radial and Apical Pulse Rates

To record an accurate radial pulse, you must have the patient in a comfortable position with the artery to be used at the same level as or lower than the heart (Procedure 20.8). The limb should be well supported and relaxed. The patient may be lying down or sitting. As with all palpated pulse readings, the pads of the first two or three fingers are placed over the artery. Never use your thumb to determine the pulse rate. The thumb has its own pulse, and you may confuse your pulse rate with the patient's rate. Push the radial artery against the bone until the strongest pulsation is felt. Both you and the patient should be in a relaxed position. Too much pressure **occludes** the artery, and too little pressure prevents the detection of irregularities or all the beats. The pulse should be counted for 1 full minute. A 30-second interval may be used once you become proficient at performing the skill. In either case, you should document the number of beats in 1 minute.

While counting the rate, you must also be aware of the rhythm and volume. Variations from normal should be noted, such as an arrhythmia or a pulse that is thready or bounding. Some pulses are more difficult to feel than others, and finding the correct pressure to be used for each patient and site requires repeated practice and experience.

For an apical pulse, the patient can be sitting or lying down. Place the stethoscope at the junction of the fifth intercostal space and the midclavicular line on the left side of the patient's chest (Figure 20.11). You will hear a lubb-dubb sound. Each lubb-dubb sound is one heartbeat. The apical pulse should always be **auscultated**

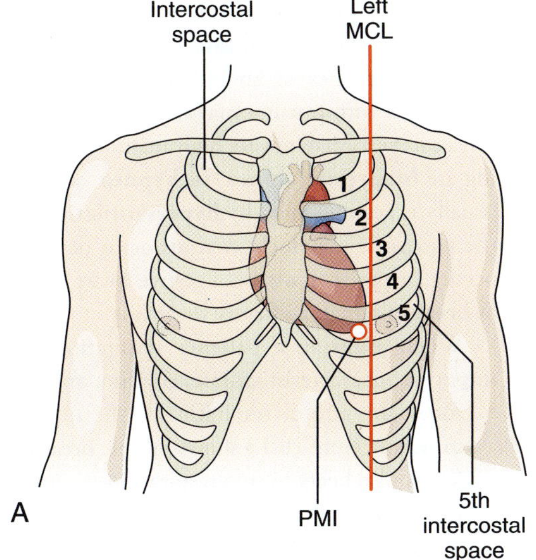

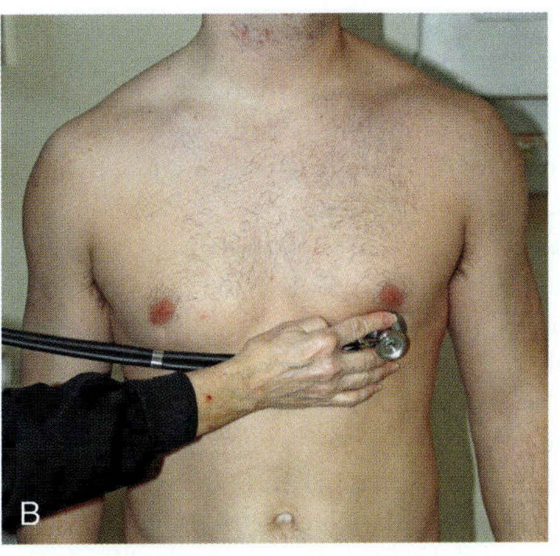

FIGURE 20.11 Apical pulse. (From Cooper K, Gosnell K: *Foundations of nursing*, ed 8, St. Louis, 2019, Elsevier.)

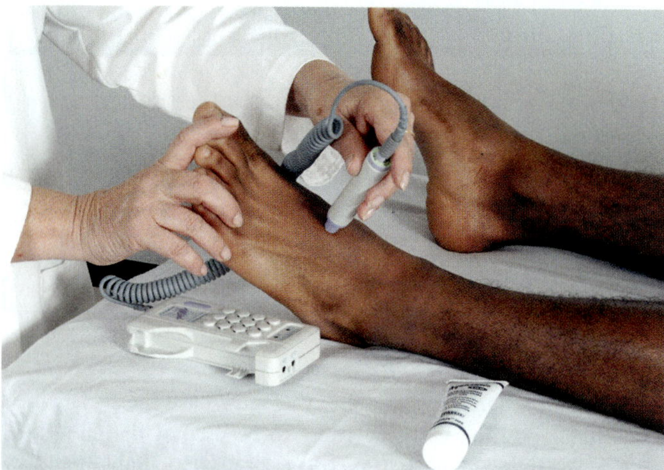

FIGURE 20.12 Doppler ultrasound unit measuring the pedal pulse. (From Jarvis C: *Physical examination and health assessment*, ed 7, St. Louis, 2016, Saunders.)

for a full minute to detect any irregularities in rate and rhythm. Remember, one reason you would decide to take an apical pulse on an adult patient is that you noted irregularities in the heart rate when palpating the radial pulse. Therefore, you should listen to an apical pulse for a full minute to make sure you are accurately counting the number of beats per minute. If the pulse rate is counted at any site other than the radial artery, the rate should be documented along with a notation of the site used.

CRITICAL THINKING APPLICATION **20.4**

Mrs. Arnez has a documented thready pulse. What site should Carlos use to measure the pulse? Why should he take the pulse for a full minute?

Femoral, Popliteal, and Pedal Pulses

Pulses in the lower extremities may be difficult to find and equally difficult to feel or hear. A Doppler unit, an ultrasound unit that magnifies the pulsation, may be used to locate and count these pulses accurately (Figure 20.12). A Doppler unit is battery operated and can be attached to a stethoscope so that only the provider can hear the beat, or it can be set so that both the provider and the patient can hear the pulsations.

RESPIRATION

Respiration allows for the exchange of oxygen and carbon dioxide with the atmosphere, the blood, and the body cells. Oxygen is taken into the body to be used for life-sustaining body processes, and carbon dioxide is released as a waste product.

One complete *inhalation* and *exhalation* is called a *respiration.* During the inhalation phase, the diaphragm contracts and drops down. The *intercostal* muscles pull the ribs up and outward; this causes the lungs to expand and fill with air. During the exhalation phase, the diaphragm returns to its normal, elevated position and the intercostal muscles relax; this causes the lungs to expel the waste air out of the body.

Both internal and external respirations occur. *External respiration* is the exchange of oxygen and carbon dioxide in the lungs. *Internal respiration* occurs at the cellular level. Oxygen in the bloodstream is transferred into the cells and used with sugars and fatty acids to produce energy. Carbon dioxide is released as a waste product and transported back to the lungs for exhalation.

The respiratory center in the medulla oblongata is sensitive to changes in blood oxygen and carbon dioxide levels. When carbon dioxide levels rise, the respiratory control center sends a message that triggers breathing. Respiration is controlled by the involuntary nervous system. This means that we breathe automatically. Because respiration can be controlled to a certain extent, it also is a voluntary function. However, breathing is ultimately under the control of the medulla oblongata. This is why we can hold our breath only for a short period of time. Once cells become oxygen starved, a stimulus is sent to the respiratory muscles (the diaphragm, and intercostal muscles) and breathing begins involuntarily.

Factors that May Influence Respiration

Pulse rate and respiratory rate are closely linked. The factors that influence pulse rate can also influence the respiratory rate:

- *Age:* Infants have a higher respiratory rate than adults.
- *Fitness and activity levels:* Physical fitness can lower the respiratory rate. Physical activity can temporarily raise the respiratory rate.
- *Smoking:* Can increase the respiratory rate.
- *Respiratory disease:* Diseases such as asthma, pneumonia, and **chronic obstructive pulmonary disease (COPD)** can increase the respiratory rate. Sleep apnea may decrease the respiratory rate.
- *Cardiovascular disease:* If the heart is not pumping efficiently to get the oxygen to the organs, the respiratory rate may increase.
- *Emotions:* Anxiety or fear can increase the respiratory rate. Depression may decrease the respiratory rate.
- *Medications:* Certain medications are used specifically to raise or lower the pulse rate; some may do that as a side effect of the medication.

Measuring the Respiration Rate

As with measuring the pulse rate, when measuring the respiratory rate, the medical assistant must be aware of the characteristics of the respirations. The following sections explain the best process for measuring the respiratory rate.

Characteristics of Respirations

Normally, a person's breathing is relaxed, automatic, and silent. However, respiratory disease or chronic conditions can influence the characteristics of an individual's respiration. **Dyspnea** occurs in patients with pneumonia, asthma, or COPD. It also occurs after physical exertion or at very high altitudes. Other alterations in breathing are **bradypnea**, **apnea**, **tachypnea**, and **hyperpnea**. Hyperpnea usually is accompanied by **hyperventilation** and often occurs when the patient is extremely anxious or in pain. **Orthopnea** frequently occurs in patients with congestive heart failure (CHF) or COPD. **Wheezing** signals difficulty breathing in patients with asthma.

When assessing a patient's respirations, you must note three important characteristics: rate, rhythm, and depth:

- *Rate:* The rate of respiration is the number of respirations per minute. Figure 20.13 shows sample breathing patterns. A ratio of four pulse beats to one respiration is typical. As a rule, both the pulse and respiratory rates respond to exercise or emotional upset. Table 20.3 lists normal respiratory ranges for patients in various age groups.

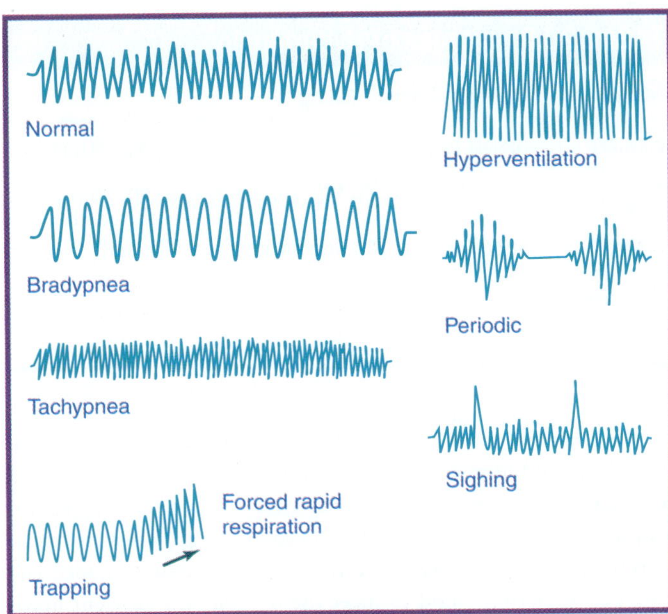

FIGURE 20.13 Breathing Patterns.

TABLE 20.3 Approximate Age-Related Respiration Ranges

AGE	RANGE (BREATHS/MIN)	AVERAGE
Newborn	30–50	40
1–3 years	20–30	25
4–6 years	18–26	22
7–11 years	16–22	19
Adolescence to adulthood	12–20	16

- *Rhythm:* Refers to the breathing pattern, the space between each breath. A regular breathing pattern is normal in adults; however, the breathing pattern for infants varies. Automatic interruptions, such as sighing, are also considered normal. The terms *regular* or *irregular* are used to document rhythm.
- *Depth:* The depth of respiration is the amount of air inhaled and exhaled. When a patient is at rest, normal respirations have a consistent depth, which can be noted as you watch the rise and fall of the chest. Rapid, shallow breathing at rest occurs with some diseases, such as asthma and emphysema. An alteration in the depth and sometimes rate of breathing is also seen in **Cheyne-Stokes respirations**. The terms *normal, deep, shallow,* and *gasping* should be used to document depth.

Normally, no noticeable breath sounds occur during the breathing process, except during snoring. Noticeable breath sounds are a sign of certain diseases, such as pneumonia, asthma, and pulmonary edema. After listening to breath sounds with a stethoscope, the provider can describe the characteristics of breath sounds by using specific terminology (e.g., **rales**, **rhonchi**, or **stertorous** breathing).

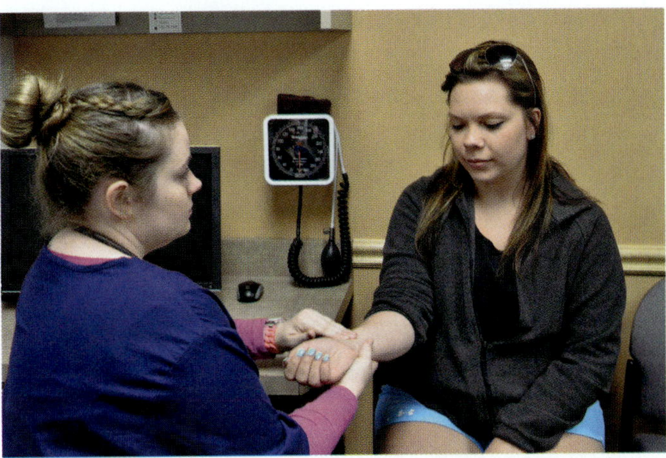

FIGURE 20.14 Hand position when counting respirations. The hands should be left in place as if still counting the patient's pulse.

When an individual cannot breathe enough oxygen to supply all body cells with oxygenated blood, normal skin coloring, particularly around the mouth and the nail beds, changes to a bluish, dusky color. This coloration, which indicates an increased level of carbon dioxide in the blood, is called *cyanosis.* The patient also may have other signs and symptoms, such as **vertigo**, chest pain (*angina*), and numbness in the fingers and toes.

Counting Respirations

Because most people can control their breathing to a certain extent, do not mention that you will be counting the person's respirations (see Procedure 20.8). Patients may self-consciously alter their breathing rate when they know they are being watched. Count the respirations while appearing to count the radial pulse. Keep your eyes alternately on the patient's chest and your watch while you count the pulse rate; then, without removing your fingers from the pulse site, determine the respiratory rate (Figure 20.14). If the patient is lying down, the arm on which you are taking the radial pulse may be crossed over the chest so that respirations can be felt with the rise and fall of the chest. Another way of observing respiration is to watch the movement of the patient's shoulders with each inspiration. Count the respirations for 30 seconds and multiply the number by 2. Do not use the 15-second interval because this count can vary by a factor of ±4, which is significant when dealing with such a small number. Note any variation or irregularity in the rhythm or depth. Record the respirations in the health record.

CRITICAL THINKING APPLICATION 20.5

Tina Anderson, a 36-year-old patient who is obese, is wearing a heavy knit sweater, and Carlos needs to obtain a respiratory count. What could he do to obtain an accurate measurement of Tina's respiratory rate?

BLOOD PRESSURE

A BP reading reflects the pressure of the blood against the walls of the arteries. Each time the ventricles contract, blood is pushed out of the

TABLE 20.4 Approximate Age-Related Blood Pressure Ranges

	RANGE	
AGE	SYSTOLIC	DIASTOLIC
Newborn	60–96	30–62
1–3 years	78–112	48–78
4–6 years	78–112	50–79
7–11 years	85–114	52–79
Adolescent	94–119	58–79
Adult	100–119	60–79

heart and into the aorta, exerting pressure on the walls of the arteries. There are actually two BP readings:

- The *systolic* pressure is the highest-pressure level that occurs when the heart is contracting and is the first sound heard.
- The *diastolic* pressure is the lowest pressure level when the heart is relaxed and is the last sound heard.

Systole (heart contraction) and diastole (heart relaxation) together make up the cardiac cycle. The difference between systolic and diastolic pressure is the **pulse pressure**.

Blood pressure is read in millimeters of mercury, abbreviated *mm Hg*. However, you need not include the abbreviation when documenting the reading in the patient's health record. BP is recorded as a fraction, with the systolic reading serving as the numerator (top) and the diastolic reading serving as the denominator (bottom) (e.g., 130/80). Table 20.4 lists normal BP ranges for patients of various age groups.

Factors That May Influence Blood Pressure

Factors that determine blood pressure include the following:

- Blood volume
- Peripheral resistance created by blood *viscosity* (the thickness of the blood)
- Vessel elasticity
- Condition of the heart muscle and arterial walls

Volume is the amount of blood in the arteries. An increased blood volume raises BP, and a decreased blood volume lowers BP. With extensive bleeding, or hemorrhage, the blood volume drops, and so does the BP.

The *peripheral resistance* of blood vessels refers to the lumen (the diameter of the vessel) and the amount of blood flowing through it. The smaller the lumen, the greater the resistance to blood flow. BP is higher with a small or reduced-size lumen and lower with a large lumen. Vessels affected by fatty cholesterol deposits (*atherosclerotic plaque*) become narrower over time. This results in smaller vessel lumens and, therefore, higher blood pressure.

Vessel elasticity is the ability of an artery to expand and contract to supply the body with a steady flow of blood. With advancing age, certain lifestyle factors, or the presence of **arteriosclerosis**, vessel elasticity may decrease. This causes the arterial walls to become firm and resistant, increasing the BP.

TABLE 20.5 Stages of Hypertension

Normal	Less than 120–80 mm Hg
Elevated	Systolic between 120–129 *and* diastolic less than 80 mm Hg
Stage 1	Systolic between 130–139 *or* diastolic between 80–89 mm Hg
Stage 2	Systolic at least 140 *or* diastolic at least 90 mm Hg
Hypertensive crisis	Systolic over 180 *and/or* diastolic over 120

The condition of the **myocardium** is a primary determinant of the volume of blood flowing through the body. A strong, forceful contraction empties the heart and tends to keep the BP within normal limits. If the myocardium becomes weak, pressure in the vessels begins to increase in an attempt to maintain an adequate level of circulating blood to meet the oxygen and nutrient needs of the body.

Evaluating the Blood Pressure

The American Heart Association (AHA) guidelines for the diagnosis and management of hypertension include five categories for diagnostic and treatment purposes (Table 20.5). The goal of the AHA recommendations is to reduce the number of people who die each year from hypertension-related illnesses, such as coronary artery disease, heart attack, heart failure, kidney disease, and stroke.

Hypertension can occur in children or adults, but individuals of African American descent, middle-aged and older adults, patients with diabetes mellitus, and those with kidney disease are at greatest risk. Hypertension has been called the silent killer because it frequently has no symptoms. Individuals may go for long periods without knowing they have a problem. Hypertension often is discovered during treatment for another problem.

Signs and Symptoms of Hypertension

- Blurred vision
- Vertigo
- Fatigue
- Flushing
- Angina
- Dyspnea
- Headache
- Nosebleeds (*epistaxis*)

Essential hypertension is the most common type of hypertension. It is **idiopathic** but is associated with obesity, a high blood level of sodium, elevated cholesterol levels, family history, and race (African Americans, Native Americans, Mexican Americans, Native Hawaiians, and some Asian Americans).

When there is a concern about a patient's BP, the individual is often asked to track it. These readings should be taken about the same time of day and by the same person using the same-size cuff and the same arm. *Secondary hypertension* is caused by another underlying pathologic condition, such as renal disease, complications of pregnancy, endocrine imbalance, or brain injury.

Temporary hypertension may occur with stress, pain, exercise, and exhaustion. Many patients experience "white coat syndrome"; their BP becomes elevated in the medical environment but is normal when they are away from the healthcare facility.

If a patient's BP is persistently in the prehypertension range at two or more office visits over time, essential hypertension is diagnosed. If the patient's BP is elevated initially, it should be checked again after the patient has been allowed to sit comfortably for at least 2 minutes. Check the BP in both arms with a cuff that is the proper size. If the readings are different, the provider uses the higher value for diagnostic purposes. All of the readings must be documented in the patient's record.

Metabolic Syndrome

Metabolic syndrome occurs when a patient has at least three of the five following conditions:

- Abdominal obesity
- Elevated blood pressure
- Elevated fasting plasma glucose
- High serum triglycerides
- Low high-density lipoprotein (LDL) levels

Metabolic syndrome is associated with an increased risk of developing cardiovascular disease and type 2 diabetes. It is estimated that one-quarter of adults in the United States have metabolic syndrome.

Treatment guidelines for hypertension have four basic aspects:

1. Individuals with prehypertension should be diagnosed and encouraged to make lifestyle changes before they require treatment or move into the hypertensive category. The AHA recommends limiting one's intake of salt and eating a diet rich in potassium, calcium, magnesium, and protein while reducing total fat intake, especially saturated fat. Individuals with prehypertension also should restrict their alcohol intake, engage in regular physical activity, and lose weight if necessary to maintain a healthy BMI range. Many times, just losing 10% of a person's weight lowers the blood pressure.
2. In people older than 50 years of age, the systolic reading is more important than the diastolic reading. Individuals over 50 should be treated if they have a systolic pressure of 140 mm Hg or higher, regardless of their diastolic blood pressure. Medical treatment at this age can reduce the development of cardiac and kidney disease later in life.
3. Most patients with hypertension require two or more medications to achieve desired blood pressure levels. The goal of treatment is to maintain blood pressure below 140/90 mm Hg or below 130/80 mm Hg in patients with diabetes or kidney disease. Patients should be treated with both a diuretic, to help the body excrete excess amounts of fluid and sodium, and an antihypertensive medication.
4. A patient-centered treatment approach should be implemented to motivate patients and maintain compliance with hypertension management. The medical assistant can play an active role in establishing a therapeutic relationship with the patient by providing ongoing education and support to ensure compliance with provider-recommended treatment. Using community resources, such as local dietitian referrals, may also help patients comply with treatment.

Hypotension is an abnormally low blood pressure, which may be caused by emotional or traumatic shock, hemorrhage, central nervous system (CNS) disorders, and chronic wasting diseases. Persistent readings of 90/60 mm Hg or lower usually are considered hypotensive. **Orthostatic (postural) hypotension** can cause patients to experience vertigo or **syncope**. Some medications can cause orthostatic hypotension.

CRITICAL THINKING APPLICATION 20.6

Mr. Samuel Long, a 43-year-old patient, recently was diagnosed with essential hypertension. What should Carlos discuss with Mr. Long to emphasize the dangers of his disease and teach him about lifestyle modifications that he must make to improve his health? Are any community resources available that might help Mr. Long and his family to effectively manage his disease?

Measuring Blood Pressure

The instrument used to measure blood pressure is called a *sphygmomanometer,* or blood pressure cuff. It consists of an inflatable cuff, an inflation bulb with a control valve, and a pressure gauge. The blood pressure mechanism consists of an aneroid dial attached to an inflatable cuff (Figure 20.15A); the device may be handheld, wall mounted, or a floor model (Figure 20.15B). Some systems have a trigger-style air release valve; these can be pumped up, and then the air is slowly released simply by pushing the trigger (Figure 20.16). With the more traditional sphygmomanometers, the valve must be unscrewed.

Sphygmomanometers are delicately **calibrated** instruments that must be handled carefully. They should be recalibrated regularly and checked for accuracy by the medical assistant or a medical supply dealer. The needle on the aneroid dial sphygmomanometer should rest within the small square or circle at the bottom of the dial. If the sphygmomanometer is not correctly calibrated, the patient's blood pressure reading will be inaccurate.

The sphygmomanometer must be used with a stethoscope. The goal of the procedure is to use the inflatable cuff to stop the circulation through an artery. The stethoscope is placed over the artery just below the cuff. As the cuff is slowly deflated to allow the blood to flow again, cardiac cycle sounds are heard through the stethoscope, and readings are taken when the first (systolic) and last (diastolic) sounds are heard (Procedure 20.9).

To obtain a correct blood pressure reading, the cuff used must be the proper size. The systolic and diastolic blood pressures can be lowered by as much as 5 mm Hg if the cuff is one size larger than appropriate; the blood pressure can be elevated by up to 6 mm Hg if the cuff is one size smaller. The inflatable part (the bladder) of a cuff of the correct size should cover about 80% of the circumference of the upper arm. To help with this, most blood pressure cuffs have predetermined markings on the internal side (the side placed on the patient's arm); as long as the cuff is secured within these lines, it should be the accurate size (Figure 20.17). Table 20.6 describes the various sizes of blood pressure cuffs available.

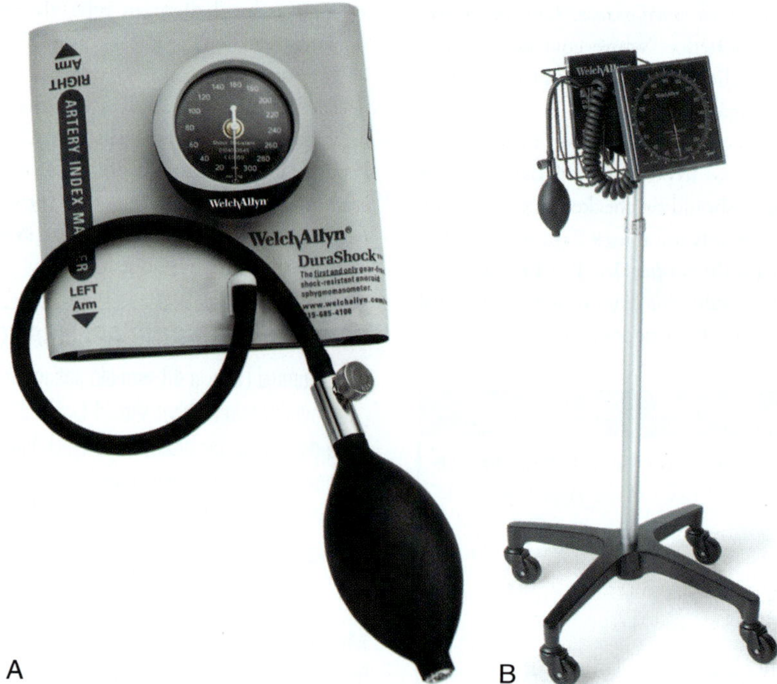

FIGURE 20.15 **(A)** Aneroid dial system with an inflatable cuff. **(B)** Aneroid floor model with a large, slanted face.

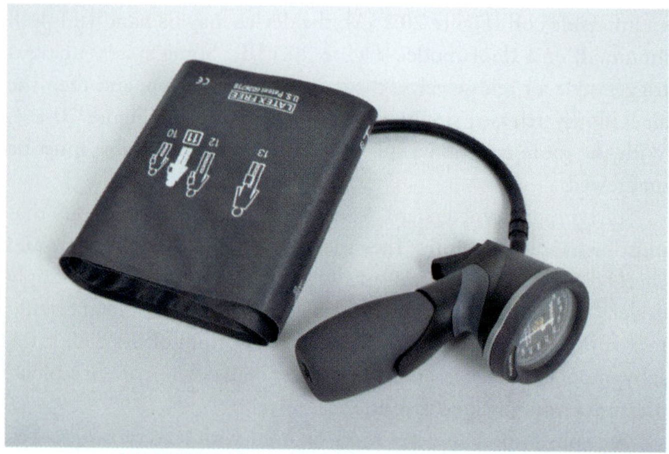

FIGURE 20.16 Trigger-release aneroid blood pressure valve.

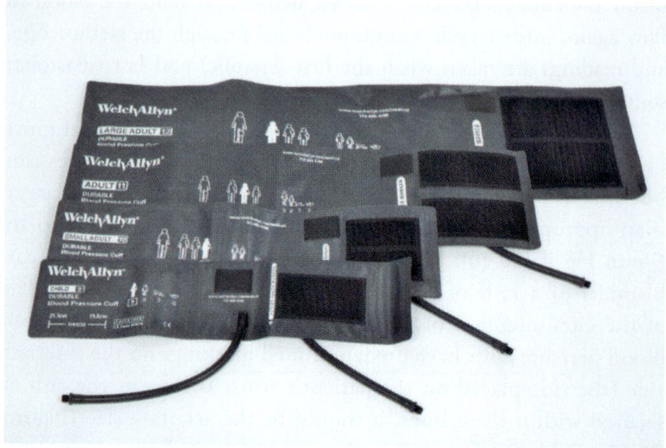

FIGURE 20.17 Variety of blood pressure cuff sizes.

When placed on the patient's arm, the cuff should cover two-thirds of the distance from the elbow to the shoulder. The lower edge of the cuff should be 2 to 3 cm (about 2 finger widths, or 1 inch) above the elbow or antecubital space to allow plenty of room to place the stethoscope without touching the cuff. If the stethoscope touches the cuff during the blood pressure reading, the sound of the deflating cuff may interfere with your ability to hear the correct reading. The patient's sleeve must be above the antecubital space; if the sleeve is tight, ask the patient to remove the arm from the sleeve. This is done for two reasons: tight clothing can restrict normal blood flow in the brachial artery, altering the blood pressure, and placing the stethoscope over clothing makes it difficult to hear blood pressure sounds. Provide a patient gown if needed to maintain the patient's privacy.

Blood pressure cuffs and stethoscopes are available in drug and retail stores for patients to use to measure their own blood pressure at home. These units can be aneroid, electronic, or computerized sphygmomanometers (Figure 20.18). If you have patients who are monitoring their pressure at home, be sure they understand the mechanics of obtaining an accurate reading. It is best to have the patient bring the equipment to the office and demonstrate its use. While the patient is showing you the home equipment, you will have an ideal opportunity to check technique and calibration and answer any questions the patient may have about the use of the equipment. This is also a good opportunity to reinforce treatment plans, such as medication, diet, and exercise. It is helpful for a patient who is monitoring blood pressure readings at home to keep a log and review it with the provider during visits to help detect blood pressure variations during normal daily activities.

Some providers will want the BP taken on the leg when a patient has undergone a bilateral mastectomy with lymph node removal or has an arteriovenous shunt (used for dialysis). This is to reduce the risk of **lymphedema**. If a patient has had a mastectomy on one side, the opposite side can be used for BP. When using the leg, the BP can be taken at either the thigh or ankle. When using the thigh, a cuff designed for the thigh should be used, and the popliteal artery would be auscultated. For the ankle, a regular cuff could be used, and the posterior tibial artery would be auscultated. It can be difficult to hear Korotkoff sounds at the posterior tibial artery, and a Doppler may need to be used. For either location, the patient should be supine (lying down) so that the leg is at the same level as the heart. The cuff should encompass 80% of the circumference of either the thigh or the ankle.

Effects of Body Position on Blood Pressure Measurement

Blood pressure is usually taken with the patient in either the sitting or the supine position. However, the diastolic pressure can be as much as 5 mm Hg higher when patients sit than when they are supine. In addition, if the patient's back is not supported and there is some muscle tension in the body (as occurs when the patient is seated on an examination table rather than in a chair), the diastolic pressure may be increased by 6 mm Hg. If patients cross their legs during the reading, the systolic pressure may be raised by 2 to 8 mm Hg. The position of the patient's arm can also have a major influence when the blood pressure is measured. If the upper arm is below the level of the right atrium (e.g., dangling at the patient's side), the reading is artificially elevated; if the arm is above the heart level, the reading is lowered. Or if the patient holds up the arm, muscular tension will raise the pressure. The arm should be placed at the level of the heart on a table next to an exam room chair or resting on the arm of the chair to avoid these issues (Figure 20.19). Patients should also have their feet flat on the floor. Having the legs crossed at the knee can raise the blood pressure.

If a patient has a full bladder, it can artificially raise the pressure up to 10 points. Ask patients if they need to use the restroom before taking vital signs.

TABLE 20.6 Blood Pressure Cuff Sizes

	ARM CIRCUMFERENCE	
CUFF	CENTIMETERS	INCHES
Small adult	22–26	9
Adult	27–34	Up to 13
Large adult	35–44	14–17
Adult thigh	45–52	18–20

Common Causes of Errors in Blood Pressure Readings

- The limb used for measurement is above the level of the heart.
- The bladder in the cuff is not completely deflated before a reading is started or retaken.
- The pressure in the cuff is released too rapidly.
- The patient is nervous, uncomfortable, or anxious (may cause a reading to be higher than the patient's actual blood pressure).
- The patient consumed caffeine or smoked cigarettes within 30 minutes of the blood pressure measurement.
- The cuff was applied improperly.
- The cuff is too large, too small, too loose, or too tight.
- The cuff was not placed around the arm smoothly.
- The bladder is not centered over the artery, or the bladder bulges out from the cover.
- There was a failure to wait 1 to 2 minutes between measurements.
- Instruments are defective:
    - Air leaks in the valve
    - Air leaks in the bladder
    - Aneroid needle not calibrated to zero

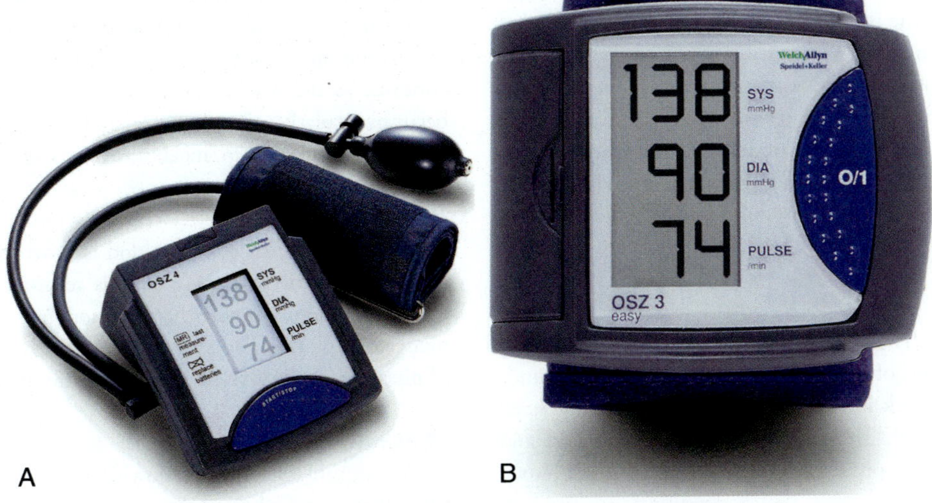

FIGURE 20.18 Personal blood pressure systems. **(A)** Digital arm cuff. **(B)** Digital wrist cuff.

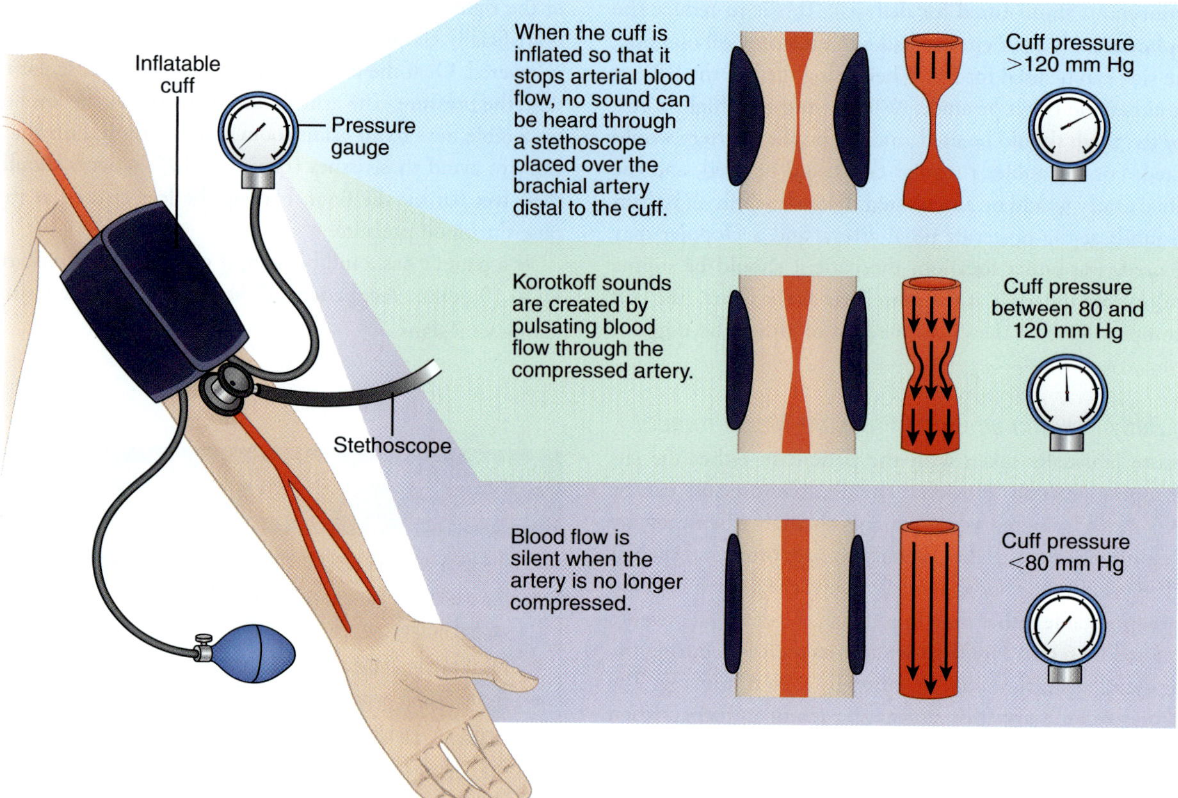

FIGURE 20.19 The science of taking a blood pressure.

Palpatory Method

The systolic pressure may be checked by feeling the radial pulse rather than hearing it with the stethoscope. Place the cuff in the usual position and palpate the radial pulse, noting rate and rhythm. Inflate the cuff until the pulse disappears, then add 30 mm Hg more of inflation to get above the systolic pressure. Do not remove your fingers from the pulse or change the pressure of your fingers. Carefully watch the gauge while slowly releasing the pressure in the cuff, and wait until you feel the first pulse beat. Note the reading on the gauge and document the first pulse felt as the systolic pressure. For example, if you first felt the radial pulse return at 102 mm Hg, the palpated blood pressure is recorded as 102/P, with P indicating that the systolic reading was palpated. The diastolic and Korotkoff phases cannot be determined by this method. This method can be very useful in times of a medical emergency, such as shock, when the patient's blood pressure cannot be auscultated. The palpatory method can be used to determine how far you need to pump the cuff to hear that first beat. This is useful for a new patient.

Korotkoff Sounds

Korotkoff sounds are the sounds heard during auscultation of blood pressure. Vibrations of the arterial wall produce these sounds when the blood surges back into the vessel after being compressed by the blood pressure cuff. The sounds were first discovered and classified into five distinct phases by Russian neurologist Nikolai Korotkoff.

Phase I

Phase I is the first sound heard as the cuff deflates. The blood is resurging into the patient's artery and can be heard clearly as a sharp, tapping sound. Note the gauge reading when this first sound is heard. Record this as the systolic blood pressure.

Phase II

As the cuff deflates, even more blood flows through the artery. The movement of the blood makes a swishing sound. If you did not follow proper procedure in inflating the cuff, you might not hear these sounds because of their soft quality. Occasionally blood pressure sounds completely disappear during this phase. Loss of the sounds, followed by their reappearance later, is called the *auscultatory gap*. The silence may continue as the needle falls another 30 mm Hg. Auscultatory gaps occur particularly in hypertension and certain types of heart disease, so if you notice such a gap, make sure to report it to the provider.

Phase III

In phase III, a great deal of blood is moving down into the artery. The distinct, sharp tapping sounds return and continue rhythmically. If you do not inflate the cuff enough, you will miss the first two phases completely, and you will incorrectly interpret the beginning of phase III as the systolic blood pressure (phase I).

Phase IV

At this point, the blood is flowing easily. The sound changes to a soft tapping, which becomes muffled and begins to grow fainter.

Occasionally these sounds continue to zero. This may occur in children, in patients of any age after exercise or with a fever, or in a pregnant patient with anemia. The AHA recommends that the beginning of phase IV be recorded as the diastolic reading for a child. Some providers call the change at phase IV the fading sound and want it recorded between systolic and diastolic recordings (e.g., 120/84/70, with 84 representing the gauge reading when the sounds of phase III have ended and those of phase IV are beginning). Other providers consider phase IV the true diastolic pressure.

Phase V

All sounds disappear in this phase. Note the gauge reading when the last sound is heard. Record this as the diastolic pressure.

CRITICAL THINKING APPLICATION 20.7

Vital signs are documented in a paper record in this order: temperature (T), pulse (P), and respiration (R). Blood pressure is recorded after TPR. Depending on the EHR system, they may be ordered differently. Correctly document the following vital signs:

1. Oral temperature 101.2°F; apical pulse 90, regular rhythm; respirations 22, regular rhythm, shallow volume; and orthostatic blood pressure in the right arm is 138/88 supine in the right arm and 110/70 standing in the right arm
2. Tympanic temperature 36.8°F; radial pulse 66, irregular rhythm, normal volume; respirations 18, regular rhythm, normal volume; and bilateral blood pressure 128/76 in the left arm, sitting and 132/80 in the right arm, sitting
3. Temporal artery temperature 102.4°F; apical pulse 102, irregular rhythm; respirations 27, regular rhythm, normal volume

OXYGEN SATURATION

Pulse oximetry is a noninvasive method of evaluating both the pulse rate and the oxygen saturation of the blood. It may also be referred to as saturation of peripheral oxygen (SpO_2). Many ambulatory settings use pulse oximeters to assess a patient's oxygenation status in disorders such as pneumonia, bronchitis, emphysema, or asthma.

Factors That May Affect the Measurement of Oxygen Saturation

Several factors can impact oxygen saturation measurements:

- *Poor circulation:* If the blood is not reaching the fingertips, the measurement will be low.
- *Skin temperature:* Cold skin can have less blood flow than warm skin, resulting in a low measurement.
- *Tobacco use:* The use of tobacco can cause a low measurement.
- *Fingernail polish:* Nail polish, especially darker colors, affect the infrared light passing through the finger to the sensor on the other side.

Measuring Oxygen Saturation

To perform this procedure, the medical assistant clips a probe on the patient's earlobe or finger (Figure 20.20). Fingernail polish must be removed before the clip is applied. If the patient has artificial nails, the earlobe should be used. A beam of infrared light passes through the tissue, and the amount of light absorbed by oxygenated hemoglobin is measured. This is displayed on the digital screen as a percentage. At the same time, the light measures the patient's pulse rate, which also is shown on the screen. A normal pulse oximetry reading is 95% or higher. Treatment, such as oxygen or bronchodilator therapies, usually is started when readings are at 90% to 92% or lower (Procedure 20.10).

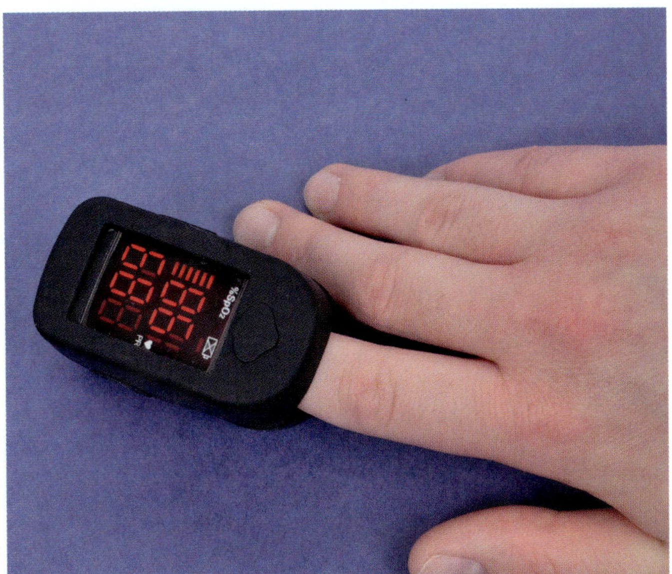

FIGURE 20.20 Pulse Oximeter.

ANTHROPOMETRIC MEASUREMENTS

Anthropometry is the science that deals with the measurement of the size, weight, and proportions of the human body. These measurements often are included in the initial recording of vital signs and before the provider performs a physical examination or a well-baby check. Because they are indicators of the patient's state of health and well-being, height and weight measurements and the associated body mass index are discussed as aspects of the vital signs.

Measuring Weight

A patient's weight and height can be helpful in diagnosis, and the medical assistant must obtain these readings with accuracy and empathy (see Procedure 20.10). In many healthcare facilities, weight and height are measured routinely as the patient is taken to the examination room. To safeguard patient confidentiality, the scale should be located in a private area where other people cannot see the patient's weight. Safeguard the patient's confidentiality by not repeating the measurement out loud. Others nearby might hear this private patient information. If this is the patient's first visit, anthropometric measurements are recorded in the history database and used as reference information during future visits as needed.

Weight can be a sensitive issue for many patients. Maintain a professional attitude when obtaining a patient's weight. Make sure heavy items are removed from pockets and that the patient is not holding a purse. Shoes should also be removed. If patients have difficulty with balance or stability, assist them onto the scale and help them balance themselves. A scale with built-in handrails is ideal for patients who are unable to maintain their balance. If the facility does not have this type of scale, a walker can be placed over the scale for the patient to

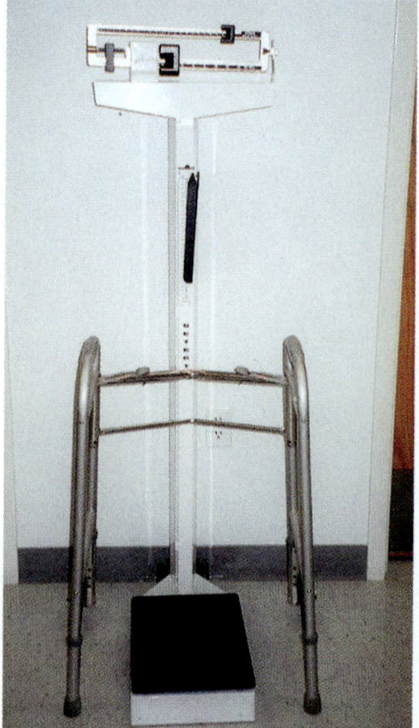

FIGURE 20.21 A walker is placed over the scale to aid the patient's balance.

use as hand support when getting on or off or maintaining balance while on the scale (Figure 20.21).

If the provider prescribes weight measurement at home, make sure the patient understands the importance of getting weighed at the same time each day in clothing of similar weight. Body weight may vary considerably from early morning to late afternoon, so it is usually best if the patient is weighed in the morning. If it is important for the patient to be weighed each day, be sure you remind the patient to document each weight and notify the clinic, as directed, if there are major shifts.

Certain medical specialties and specific medical problems may require continuous monitoring of weight. Hormone disorders (e.g., diabetes), growth patterns (seen in children), and eating disorders (e.g., obesity, bulimia) require accurate weight checks as part of every medical visit. In addition, pregnant patients must have their weight monitored to make sure they are gaining weight, but also as a precaution against too much weight gain, which may indicate fluid retention. Patients with cardiovascular disorders who tend to retain fluid should have their weight checked each time they are seen in the office. Many healthcare facilities document weight in kilograms, but most Americans understand the pound measurements better. When weight must be converted from one to the other, you can use formulas or an online-conversion calculator. EHR systems do the conversion automatically.

WEIGHT CONVERSION FORMULAS

Convert Kilograms to Pounds

1 kg = 2.2 lb

Multiply the number of kilograms by 2.2.

Example: A patient weighs 68 kg: 68 × 2.2 = 149.6 lb

Convert Pounds to Kilograms

1 lb = 0.45 kg

Multiply the number of pounds by 0.45 or divide the number of pounds by 2.2 kg.

Example: A patient weighs 120 lb: 120 × 0.45 = 54 kg, or 120 ÷ 2.2 = 54.5 kg.

CRITICAL THINKING APPLICATION **20.8**

- A patient weighs 87 kg. How many pounds does he weigh?
- A patient weighs 148 lb. How many kilograms does she weigh?

Measuring Height

Height can be measured in inches or centimeters. Measurement is easily accomplished by having the patient stand against a parallel bar attached to a wall ruler or on the scale and moving the bar to the top of the patient's head. Have the patient step away from the scale while holding the bar in position and read the measurement. Height can be measured in either inches or centimeters, depending on the provider's preference. Height is usually measured annually for adult patients, and if measured in inches, it is documented in feet and inches. If an adult patient has certain medical conditions, such as osteoporosis, height may be measured at each visit. Length measurements used in pediatrics and pediatric BMIs are discussed in Chapter 44.

Accurate height or length measurements are particularly important for children. The provider also may request routine height screening for patients diagnosed with osteoporosis because these patients may lose height over time.

Body Mass Index (BMI)

To determine how healthy an adult patient's weight is, the provider may ask the medical assistant to calculate the patient's BMI. The BMI is the relationship of weight to height that mathematically correlates the patient's measurements with health risks. It is a more accurate predictor of weight-related diseases than traditional height-weight charts because it provides a good estimate of the degree of body fat.

A patient's BMI can be calculated by dividing the weight in pounds by the height in inches squared and then multiplying by 703: BMI = Weight (lb) ÷ Height (inches) ÷ Height (inches) × 703. If using the metric system, you would divide the weight in kilograms by the square of the height in meters: BMI = Weight (kg) ÷ Height (m^2). However, to determine the BMI, clinics can use a wheel device that compares the patient's height to weight, an online BMI calculator, or a BMI chart. This is not necessary with EHR systems because the program automatically calculates the BMI after the patient's height and weight have been documented.

Individuals with a BMI of 19 to 22 are thought to live the longest. Death rates are significantly higher for people with a BMI of 25 or above. If the BMI indicates that the patient is overweight or obese, dietary modifications may be needed. The provider makes this decision after evaluating all of the patient's data.

CRITICAL THINKING APPLICATION **20.9**

Mrs. Johnson is being seen at WMFM Clinic for the first time. In what order should Carlos take her vital signs and her anthropometric measurements? Should blood pressure be measured in both arms, with the patient both sitting and standing? If so, what is the rationale?

CLOSING COMMENTS

We started this chapter with a discussion of TPR and then moved on to discuss BP and SpO_2. We ended with a discussion of weight, height, and BMI.

A medical assistant should be familiar with the different sites for taking a temperature and the different thermometers used. Using the correct site and thermometer will ensure that a proper temperature is obtained.

Pulse and respiration are often measured at the same time. This way, patients are unaware that you are watching them breathe. Until you are proficient at taking a radial pulse, it should be counted for a full minute. An apical pulse is done using a stethoscope. You will hear two sounds, lubb-dubb. Each lubb-dubb is one beat.

When you take blood pressure, it is important to use a cuff that is the correct size and have it positioned correctly over the brachial artery. By taking a palpated systolic blood pressure first, you can be certain that you do not miss the first Korotkoff sounds.

Pulse oximetry is often done when there is a question about a patient's ability to transport enough oxygen. A finger or earlobe can be used for this procedure. If a finger is used, it should be free of fingernail polish.

Weight and height are anthropometric measurements that are typically taken at a healthcare facility. Weight is usually taken at every visit. Height is usually measured annually for adults unless the patient has a specific medical condition. These measurements should be taken in a private location for the comfort of the patient. Accurate weight and height measurements are crucial for an accurate BMI calculation. Many providers use the BMI to counsel patients about lifestyle changes.

Patient-Centered Care

Measuring and documenting vital signs are a crucial part of the medical assistant's responsibilities. We must keep in mind that the results can cause the patient anxiety and concern. For example, it is important that you are sensitive to the concerns of a patient who is struggling to maintain a healthy blood pressure. A patient who is having difficulty maintaining or losing weight may be quite apprehensive, embarrassed, or even depressed about weight results. Being aware of concerns and showing sensitivity to needs regarding the patient's vital signs are part of being a medical assistant.

Professional Behaviors

Taking accurate vital signs and anthropometric measurements is an important aspect of a medical assistant's responsibilities. These measurements give the provider a strong indication of the patient's overall health. Being confident in the process of obtaining these measurements is crucial. Taking vital signs will become second nature over time, but a medical assistant must always take care to be as accurate as possible. It is also important to remember that patients may be concerned about those measurements. Practicing empathy and good listening skills are also part of being a good medical assistant.

SUMMARY OF SCENARIO

Carlos recognizes the significance of obtaining and documenting each patient's vital signs and anthropometric measurements. The providers at WMFM Clinic rely on Carlos to provide this information accurately. Carlos has never let these procedures become routine. He is always focused on the task because vital signs are an important reflection of a person's health status.

Carlos knows that a number of factors can alter a patient's vital signs, including the external environment, smoking, drinking hot beverages, exercise, and anxiety and pain. Carlos evaluates patient factors such as age, gender, level of compliance, and the presence of disease to determine the best method of accurately measuring vital signs. In addition, Carlos is sensitive to the need to safeguard the patient's privacy. When he was first hired by WMFM Clinic, he was concerned about privacy and confidentiality when he discovered that the patient scale was in the hall next to the waiting room. After he discussed this with the office manager, the scale was moved to an examination room so that patients could be weighed in privacy.

Carlos attended a workshop last year on the AHA guidelines for the diagnosis and treatment of hypertension, and he is prepared to explain those recommendations to patients. He recognizes his role in motivating patients diagnosed with prehypertension to stick with recommended lifestyle changes and follow the provider's treatment protocol.

SUMMARY OF LEARNING OBJECTIVES

1. **Examine the process for taking an accurate body temperature.**
   Multiple factors can affect body temperature, including the external environment, age, stress, physical exercise, gender, and illness. Fevers typically follow one of three different patterns: continuous, intermittent, or remittent.

   Body temperature can be taken at various sites on the body, including the temporal artery, as well as via tympanic, oral, axillary, and rectal routes. The site to be used can be impacted by age, condition, state of consciousness, thermometers available, and healthcare facility procedures. A medical assistant should be familiar with how to use each type of thermometer.

   The patient's temperature can be measured at the temporal artery using a temporal artery scanner, in the ear using an aural thermometer, and orally and in the axillary region with a digital thermometer. The axillary temperature is approximately 1°F (0.6°C) lower than an accurate oral reading because the reading is not taken in an enclosed body cavity. The tympanic temperature is accurate because it records the temperature of the blood closest to the hypothalamus. The temporal artery scanner is considered most accurate for infants. An infrared thermometer is often used for scanning large groups of people.

Continued

SUMMARY OF LEARNING OBJECTIVES—*continued*

After the temperature reading is documented, (TA) is recorded for a temporal artery reading, (T) for a tympanic reading, (A) for an axillary reading, (R) for a rectal reading, and (IFR) for an infrared reading, to clarify the site. Procedures 20.1 through 20.6 explain how to take and record patient temperatures using a variety of thermometers.

2. **Examine the process for taking an accurate pulse rate.**
Infants and children typically have a faster pulse than adults; as aging progresses, the pulse rate declines. As a rule, both the pulse and respiratory rates respond to exercise or emotional upset. (See Table 20.2 for approximate age-related pulse ranges.)

The pulse *rate* reflects the number of times the heart contracts in 1 minute. The pulse *volume* is the amount of force placed on the arterial walls when the heart beats; the *rhythm* of the pulse is the length of time between beats. Monitor and record the pulse rate, noting whether the rhythm is regular or arrhythmic and the volume is bounding, normal, or thready.

The most common sites used to feel the pulse are the temporal, carotid, apical, brachial, radial, femoral, popliteal, and dorsalis pedis arteries. (Procedures 20.7 and 20.8 present the specifics on recording apical and radial pulses.)

3. **Examine the process for taking an accurate respiration rate.**
As noted when discussing pulse rate, both the pulse and the respiratory rate, as a rule, respond to exercise and emotional upset. Table 20.3 presents a list of normal respiratory rates for patients in various age groups.

Count the number of respirations for 30 seconds and then multiply by 2. This should be done immediately after taking the patient's pulse while still holding the pulse point and without warning the patient because being aware that breaths are being counted may cause the patient to inadvertently alter the respiratory rate. (See Procedure 20.8.)

4. **Examine the process for taking an accurate blood pressure reading.**
Physiologic factors that affect blood pressure include the amount or volume of blood in circulation; the condition of the blood vessels, including the presence of atherosclerosis or arteriosclerosis; the degree of blood viscosity; and the condition of the myocardium. Table 20.4 lists the normal blood pressure ranges for patients of various age groups.

The cause of essential hypertension is unknown; it is diagnosed when a patient has a systolic reading higher than 140 mm Hg or a diastolic reading higher than 90 mm Hg. Secondary hypertension is caused by an underlying condition, such as renal disease, pregnancy, or a congenital heart defect.

The guidelines of the American Heart Association (AHA) for the diagnosis and management of hypertension include a prehypertension category. Table 20.5 identifies the categories of normal, elevated, stage 1 hypertension, stage 2 hypertension, and hypertensive crisis. The goal of the AHA recommendations is to reduce the number of people who die each year from hypertension-related illnesses. Treatment includes a combination of weight management, sodium reduction, lifestyle changes, and the use of two or more antihypertensive and diuretic medications.

The proper cuff size must be used to obtain a correct blood pressure reading. To make sure the size is correct, the inflatable part (bladder) should cover about 80% of the circumference of the upper arm. (Table 20.6 presents the various sizes of blood pressure cuffs available.)

The Korotkoff phases are the categories of sounds heard during blood pressure measurement. These sounds are produced by vibrations of the arterial wall when the blood surges back into the vessel after being compressed by the blood pressure cuff. Phase I is the first sound heard as the cuff deflates and is the systolic reading; phase II is the swishing sound made by the movement of blood through the artery, although an auscultatory gap may occur in which sounds completely disappear; phase III involves distinct, sharp tapping sounds made as the blood rushes through the artery; in phase IV, the sound changes to a soft tapping, which becomes muffled and begins to grow fainter; and in phase V, sound completely disappears. The last sound heard is the diastolic reading.

A sphygmomanometer is used with a stethoscope to hear the systolic over diastolic sounds. (Procedure 20.9 outlines the method for performing this skill.)

5. **Examine the process for measuring oxygen saturation.**
Pulse oximetry measures the oxygen saturation of the blood in the peripheral blood vessels. If a patient has pneumonia, bronchitis, emphysema, or asthma, pulse oximetry will likely be performed. Procedure 20.10 describes the process for performing pulse oximetry.

6. **Examine the process for obtaining anthropometric measurements.**
A patient's height and weight are anthropometric measurements that are recorded during the initial patient visit and periodically after that, depending on the patient's needs and the provider's preference. The scale should be kept in a private location. Variations in weight may indicate physical or emotional disorders, including diabetes, congestive heart failure, hormone abnormalities, depression, and eating disorders. (Procedure 20.11 describes the techniques for weighing a patient; the body mass index [BMI] is determined as indicated.)

To convert kilograms (kg) to pounds (lb), multiply the number of kilograms by 2.2. To convert pounds to kilograms, divide the number of pounds by 2.2 kg or multiply the number of pounds by 0.45 kg.

PROCEDURE 20.1 Accurately Measure and Record a Temperature Using a Temporal Artery Thermometer

TASK: Accurately measure and record a patient's temperature using a temporal artery thermometer.

EQUIPMENT and SUPPLIES

- Patient's record
- Professional temporal artery thermometer with probe covers
- Alcohol wipes
- Waste container

PROCEDURAL STEPS

1. Wash hands or use hand sanitizer.
   PURPOSE: To ensure infection control.
2. Gather the necessary equipment and supplies.
3. Greet the patient. Identify yourself. Verify the patient's identity with full name and date of birth. Explain the procedure to be performed in a manner that the patient understands. Answer any questions the patient may have about the procedure.
   PURPOSE: Identification of the patient prevents errors, and explanations are a means of gaining implied consent and patient cooperation.
4. Remove the protective cap on the probe. Depending on the facility's infection control procedures, disposable covers can be used on the scanner, or it can be cleaned by lightly wiping the surface with an alcohol wipe.
   PURPOSE: To ensure infection control.
5. Push the patient's hair up off the forehead to expose the site. Gently place the probe on the patient's forehead, halfway between the edge of the eyebrows and the hairline, at the center of the face (just above the nose).
   PURPOSE: This places the probe directly over the temporal artery.
6. Depress and hold the SCAN button, and lightly glide the probe sideways across the patient's forehead to the hairline just above the ear (see the following figure). As you move the sensor across the forehead, you will hear a beep, and a red light will flash.
   PURPOSE: This verifies that the scanner is recording temperatures as it moves across the surface of the temporal artery.

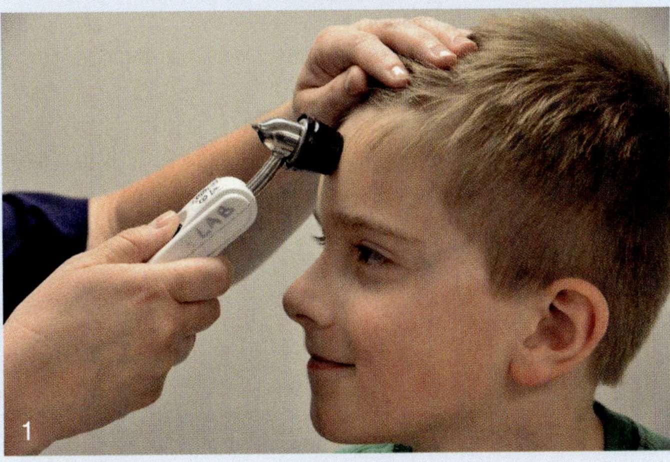

1

7. Keep the button depressed, lift the thermometer, and place the probe behind the ear lobe (see the following figure). The thermometer may continue to beep, indicating that the temperature is rising.
   PURPOSE: To continue scanning the temporal artery until the highest temperature is recorded on the thermometer.

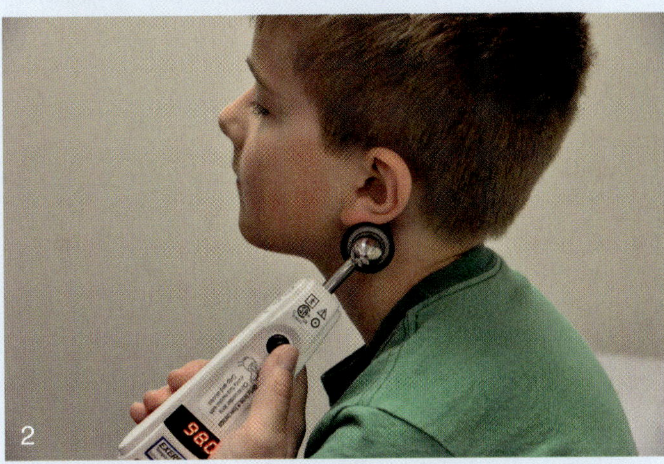
2

8. When scanning is complete, release the button and lift the probe. Note the temperature recorded on the digital display. The scanner automatically turns off 15 to 30 seconds after the release of the button.
9. If a probe cover was used, eject it directly into a waste container. Disinfect the thermometer if indicated and replace the protective cap.
   PURPOSE: To ensure infection control. Depending on the facility's infection control procedures, disposable covers can be used on the scanner, or it can be cleaned between patients with a disinfectant wipe.
10. Wash hands or use hand sanitizer.
11. Document the reading in the patient's medical record (e.g., T: 101.6°F [TA]).
    PURPOSE: Procedures that are not recorded are considered not done.

Documentation Example

8/1/20XX 11:20 a.m. T: 101.6°F (TA) ———— C. Ricci, CMA (AAMA)

PROCEDURE 20.2 Accurately Measure and Record a Temperature Using a Tympanic Thermometer

TASK: Accurately measure and record a patient's temperature using a tympanic thermometer.

EQUIPMENT and SUPPLIES

- Patient's record
- Tympanic thermometer
- Disposable probe covers
- Alcohol wipes
- Waste container

PROCEDURAL STEPS

1. Wash hands or use hand sanitizer.
   PURPOSE: To ensure infection control.
2. Gather the necessary equipment and supplies.
3. Greet the patient. Identify yourself. Verify the patient's identity with full name and date of birth. Explain the procedure to be performed in a manner that the patient understands. Answer any questions the patient may have about the procedure.
   PURPOSE: Identification of the patient prevents errors, and explanations are a means of gaining implied consent and patient cooperation.
4. Clean the probe with an alcohol wipe if indicated. Place a disposable cover on the probe (see the following figure).
   PURPOSE: To ensure a clean surface and prevent cross-contamination.

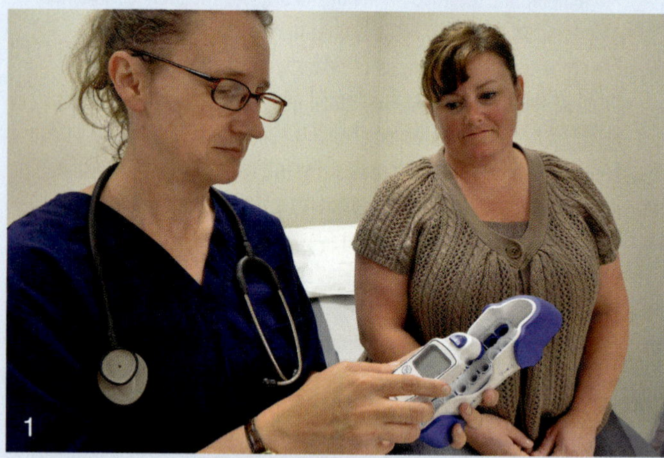
1

5. Insert the probe into the ear canal far enough to seal the opening. Do not apply pressure. For children younger than age 3, gently pull the earlobe down and back (see the first of the following figures); for patients older than age 3, gently pull the top of the ear (pinna) up and back (see the second of the following figures).
   PURPOSE: The external ear must be pulled gently to open the external auditory canal and expose the tympanic membrane for an accurate reading.

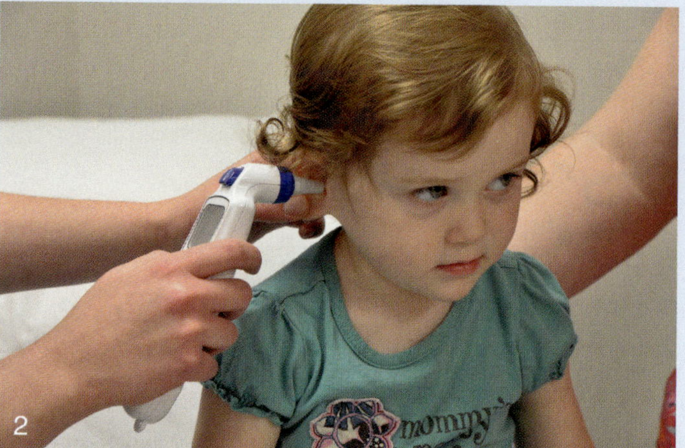
2

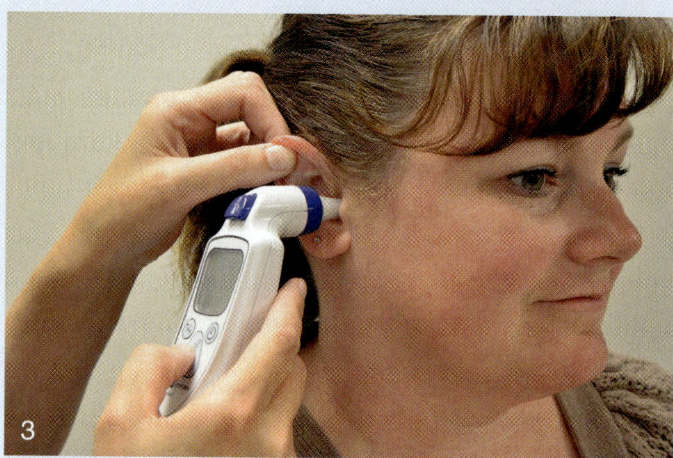
3

6. Press the button on the probe as directed. The temperature will appear on the display screen in 1 to 2 seconds.
7. Remove the probe, note the reading, and discard the probe cover into a waste container without touching it.
   PURPOSE: The probe cover is contaminated and must be discarded in a waste container.
8. Wash hands or use hand sanitizer and disinfect the equipment if indicated. See the manufacturer's manual for cleaning the probe tip. Many recommend cleaning the probe lens with alcohol wipes.
   PURPOSE: To ensure infection control.
9. Document the reading in the patient's medical record (e.g., T: 98.6°F [T]).
   PURPOSE: Procedures that are not recorded are considered not done.

Documentation Example

7/11/20xx 2:20 p.m. T: 101.2°F (T) ———— C. Ricci, CMA (AAMA)

PROCEDURE 20.3 Accurately Measure and Record an Oral Temperature Using a Digital Thermometer

TASK: Accurately measure and record a patient's oral temperature using a digital thermometer.

EQUIPMENT and SUPPLIES

- Patient's record
- Digital thermometer and probe cover
- Waste container

PROCEDURAL STEPS

1. Wash hands or use hand sanitizer.
   PURPOSE: To ensure infection control.
2. Assemble the needed equipment and supplies.
3. Greet the patient. Identify yourself. Verify the patient's identity with full name and date of birth. Explain the procedure to be performed in a manner that the patient understands. Answer any questions the patient may have about the procedure. Make sure the patient has not eaten, consumed any hot or cold fluids, smoked, or exercised during the 15 minutes before the temperature is measured.
   PURPOSE: Identification of the patient prevents errors, and explanations are a means of gaining implied consent and patient cooperation. The temperature will be inaccurate if hot or cold food or fluids have been consumed or if the patient has exercised within 15 minutes.
4. Prepare the probe for use as described in the directions (see the following figure). Make sure probe covers are always used.
   PURPOSE: To ensure infection control.

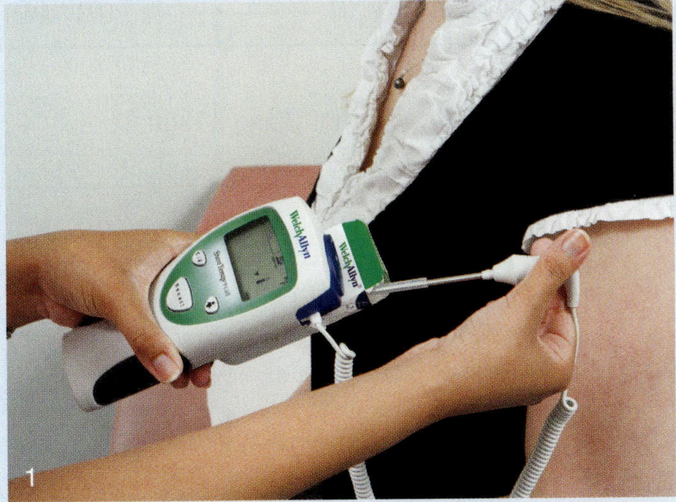

5. Place the probe under the patient's tongue (see the following figure) and instruct the patient to close the mouth tightly without biting down on the thermometer. Help the patient by holding the probe end, or the patient can hold the probe end if that is more comfortable.
   PURPOSE: Air seeping into the mouth interferes with an accurate body temperature reading.

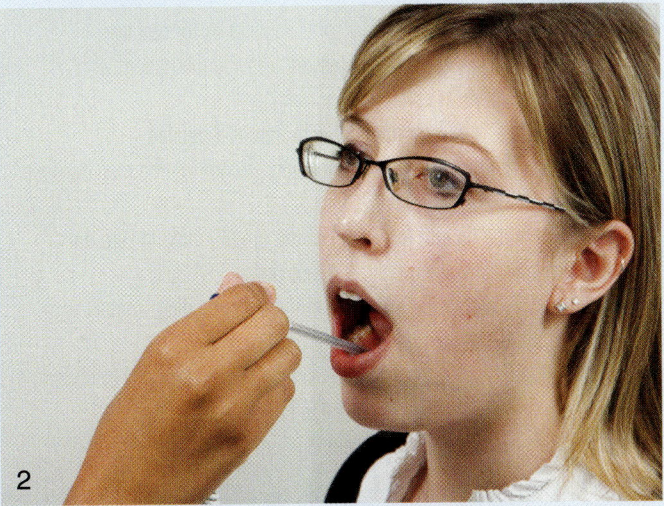

6. When a beep is heard, remove the probe from the patient's mouth and immediately eject the probe cover into an appropriate waste container.
   PURPOSE: The probe cover is contaminated and must be discarded in a waste container.
7. Note the reading on the display screen of the thermometer.
8. Document the reading in the patient's medical record (e.g., T: 97.7°F).
   PURPOSE: Procedures that are not documented are considered not done.
9. Wash hands or use hand sanitizer and disinfect the equipment as indicated.
   PURPOSE: To observe infection control measures and Standard Precautions.

Documentation Example

6/29/20XX 10:05 a.m. T: 97.7ºF ————— C. Ricci, CMA (AAMA)

PROCEDURE 20.4 Accurately Measure and Record an Axillary Temperature Using a Digital Thermometer

TASK: Accurately measure and record a patient's axillary temperature using a digital thermometer.

EQUIPMENT and SUPPLIES

- Patient's record
- Digital thermometer and probe cover
- Supply of tissues
- Patient gown as needed
- Waste container

PROCEDURAL STEPS

1. Wash hands or use hand sanitizer.
   PURPOSE: To ensure infection control.
2. Gather the needed equipment and supplies.

Continued

PROCEDURE 20.4 Accurately Measure and Record an Axillary Temperature Using a Digital Thermometer—*continued*

3. Greet the patient. Identify yourself. Verify the patient's identity with full name and date of birth. Explain the procedure to be performed in a manner that the patient understands. Answer any questions the patient may have about the procedure.
   PURPOSE: Identification of the patient prevents errors, and explanations are a means of gaining implied consent and patient cooperation.
4. Prepare the thermometer in the same manner as for oral use.
5. Expose the axillary region. If necessary, provide the patient with a gown for privacy.
6. Pat the patient's axillary area dry with tissues if needed.
   PURPOSE: To ensure an accurate reading. Do not rub the area because this may cause an elevated reading.
7. Place the probe tip into the center of the armpit, making sure the thermometer is touching only skin, not clothing.
   PURPOSE: To obtain the most accurate axillary reading; contact with clothing alters the reading.
8. Instruct the patient to hold the arm snugly across the chest or abdomen until the thermometer beeps (see the following figure).
   PURPOSE: To prevent air from leaking in and interfering with the temperature reading.

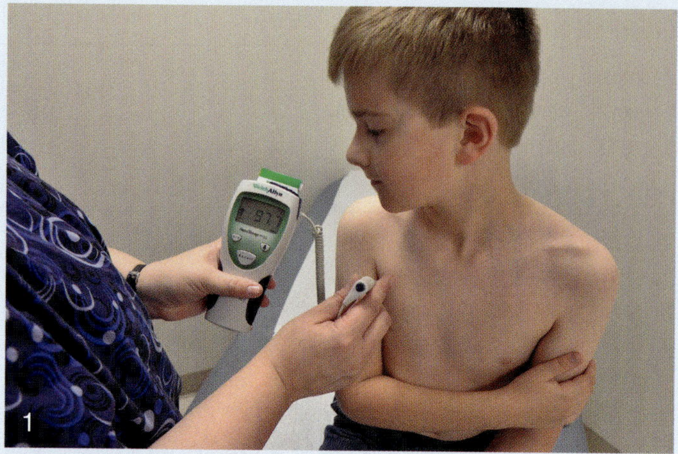

9. Remove the thermometer, note the digital reading, and dispose of the cover in the waste container.
10. Disinfect the thermometer if indicated.
    PURPOSE: To ensure infection control.
11. Wash hands or use hand sanitizer.
12. Document the reading in the patient's medical record (e.g., T: 97.6°F [A]).
    PURPOSE: Procedures that are not recorded are considered not done.

Documentation Example

6/29/20XX 10:05 a.m. T: 98.2°F (A) ———— C. Ricci, CMA (AAMA)

PROCEDURE 20.5 Accurately Measure and Record a Rectal Temperature of an Infant Using a Digital Thermometer

Task: Accurately measure and record a patient's rectal temperature using a digital thermometer.

EQUIPMENT and SUPPLIES

- Patient's record
- Digital thermometer and probe cover
- Disposable gloves
- Waste container

PROCEDURAL STEPS

1. Wash hands or use hand sanitizer.
   PURPOSE: To ensure infection control.
2. Assemble the needed equipment and supplies. Make sure that the red probe is used.
3. Greet the patient. Identify yourself. Verify the patient's identity with full name and date of birth. Explain the procedure to be performed in a manner that the patient's parent or caregiver understands. Answer any questions about the procedure.
   PURPOSE: Identification of the patient prevents errors, and explanations are a means of gaining implied consent and cooperation.
4. Have the parent or caregiver undress the infant.
5. Put on disposable gloves.
   PURPOSE: To ensure infection control.
6. Prepare the probe for use as described in the directions. Make sure probe covers are always used. Lubricate 2 inches of the probe.
   PURPOSE: To ensure infection control.
7. Gently insert the thermometer probe ½ inch for infants (this would change to ⅝ inch for children and 1 inch for adults). Remain with the patient at all times and hold the thermometer in place until a beep is heard.
8. Remove the probe and immediately eject the probe cover into an appropriate waste container.
   PURPOSE: The probe cover is contaminated and must be discarded in a waste container.
9. Note the reading on the display screen of the thermometer.
10. Remove soiled gloves and discard them into an appropriate waste container.
11. Wash hands or use hand sanitizer, and disinfect the equipment as indicated.
    PURPOSE: To observe infection control measures and Standard Precautions.
12. Document the reading in the patient's medical record.
    PURPOSE: Procedures that are not documented are considered not done.

Documentation Example

6/29/20XX 2:10 p.m. T: 100.7°F (R) ———— C. Ricci, CMA (AAMA)

PROCEDURE 20.6 Accurately Measure and Record a Temperature Using an Infrared Thermometer

TASK: Accurately measure and record a patient's temperature using an infrared thermometer.

EQUIPMENT and SUPPLIES

- Patient's record
- Infrared thermometer
- Alcohol wipes

PROCEDURAL STEPS

1. Wash hands or use hand sanitizer.
   PURPOSE: To ensure infection control.
2. Gather the necessary equipment and supplies.
3. Greet the patient. Identify yourself. Verify the patient's identity with full name and date of birth. Explain the procedure to be performed in a manner that the patient understands. Answer any questions the patient may have about the procedure.
   PURPOSE: Identification of the patient prevents errors, and explanations are a means of gaining implied consent and patient cooperation.
4. Check the sensor. If dirty, gently wipe the sensor with an alcohol wipe and allow to dry.
   PURPOSE: To ensure a clean surface and prevent cross-contamination.
5. Set the measurement mode to Body.
6. From a distance of 3 to 5 cm, aim the thermometer at the patient's forehead and depress the button until you hear one beep.
7. Read the temperature from the display screen.
8. Wash hands or use hand sanitizer and disinfect the equipment if indicated. See the manufacturer's manual for cleaning the sensor. Many recommend cleaning the sensor with alcohol wipes.
   PURPOSE: To ensure infection control.
9. Document the reading in the patient's medical record (e.g., T: 98.6°F [IFR]).
   PURPOSE: Procedures that are not recorded are considered not done.

Documentation Example

7/11/20xx 2:20 p.m. T: 98.6°F (IFR) ———— C. Ricci, CMA (AAMA)

PROCEDURE 20.7 Accurately Measure and Record an Apical Pulse

TASK: Accurately measure and record the patient's apical heart rate.

EQUIPMENT and SUPPLIES

- Patient's record
- Watch with a second hand
- Patient gown as needed
- Stethoscope
- Alcohol wipes

PROCEDURAL STEPS

1. Wash hands or use hand sanitizer and clean the stethoscope earpieces and diaphragm with alcohol wipes.
   PURPOSE: To ensure infection control and to follow Standard Precautions.
2. Greet the patient. Identify yourself. Verify the patient's identity with full name and date of birth. Explain the procedure to be performed in a manner that the patient understands. Answer any questions the patient may have about the procedure.
   PURPOSE: Identification of the patient prevents errors, and explanations are a means of gaining implied consent and patient cooperation.
3. If necessary, assist the patient in disrobing from the waist up, and provide the patient with a gown that opens in the front.
   PURPOSE: To expose the chest and provide privacy and warmth.
4. Assist the patient into the sitting or supine position.
   PURPOSE: To allow easier access to the apical site at the apex of the heart.
5. Hold the stethoscope's diaphragm against the palm of your hand for a few seconds.
   PURPOSE: To warm the diaphragm, promoting patient comfort.
6. Place the stethoscope at the left midclavicular line at the fifth intercostal space over the apex of the heart (see the following figures). Do not touch the bell end of the stethoscope.
   PURPOSE: This is the point of maximum contractile strength, where the heartbeat can be heard best. Touching the bell end of the stethoscope may interfere with the sound.

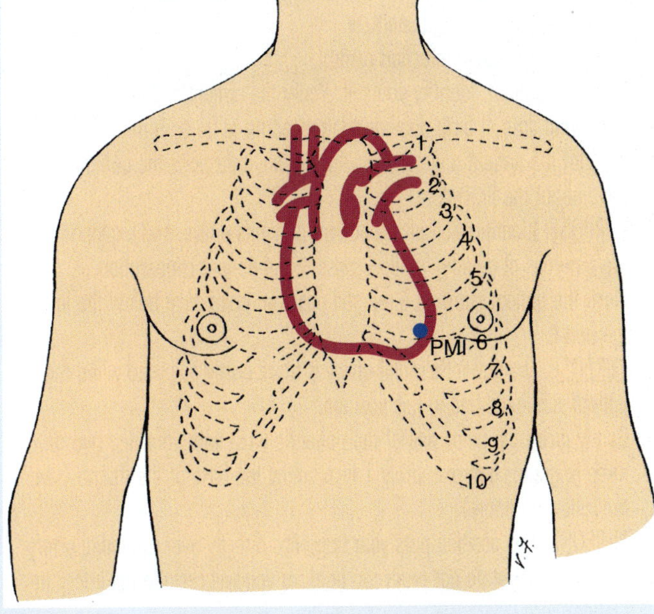

1

Continued

PROCEDURE 20.7 Accurately Measure and Record an Apical Pulse—*continued*

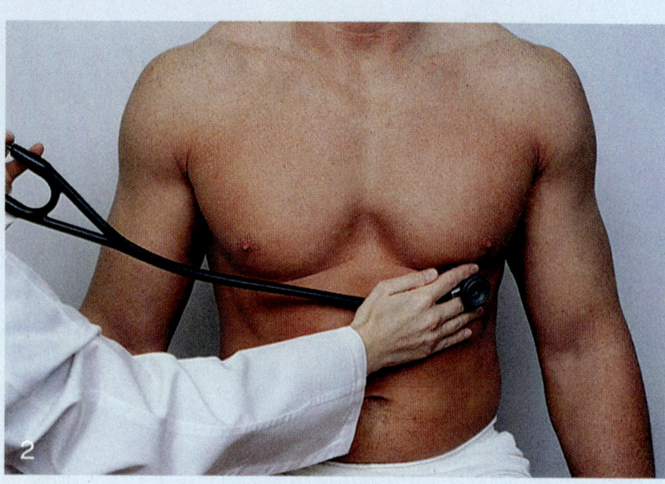

7. Listen carefully to the heartbeat. Count the pulse for 1 full minute. Note any irregularities in rhythm and volume.
   PURPOSE: The apical pulse is always measured for 1 full minute to obtain the most accurate reading.
8. Help the patient to sit up and dress.
9. Disinfect the stethoscope with an alcohol wipe.
   PURPOSE: To ensure infection control.
10. Wash hands or use hand sanitizer.
11. Document the reading in the patient's medical record (e.g., AP: 96), and record any arrhythmias.

Documentation Example

3/3/20XX 4:10 p.m. AP: 93 irregular ————————————
———————————————— C. Ricci, CMA (AAMA)

PROCEDURE 20.8 Accurately Measure and Record the Patient's Radial Pulse and Respiratory Rate

TASK: Accurately measure and document a patient's radial pulse rate, rhythm, and volume and respiratory rate, rhythm, and depth.

Note: Respirations should be assessed immediately after the radial pulse while the medical assistant appears to take the pulse, so that the patient does not artificially alter breathing patterns.

EQUIPMENT and SUPPLIES

- Patient's record
- Watch with a second hand

PROCEDURAL STEPS

1. Wash hands or use hand sanitizer.
   PURPOSE: To ensure infection control.
2. Greet the patient. Identify yourself. Verify the patient's identity with full name and date of birth. Explain the procedure to be performed in a manner that the patient understands. Answer any questions the patient may have about the procedure.
   PURPOSE: Identification of the patient prevents errors, and explanations are a means of gaining implied consent and patient cooperation.
3. Place the patient's arm in a relaxed position, palm at or below the level of the heart.
   PURPOSE: The patient's radial artery is more easily palpated when the patient is relaxed and in this position.
4. Gently grasp the palm side of the patient's wrist with your first two or three fingertips approximately 1 inch below the base of the thumb (see the following figure).
   PURPOSE: This position puts your fingertips directly over the radial artery. Press firmly (but do not press too hard, or you will occlude the artery and feel nothing).

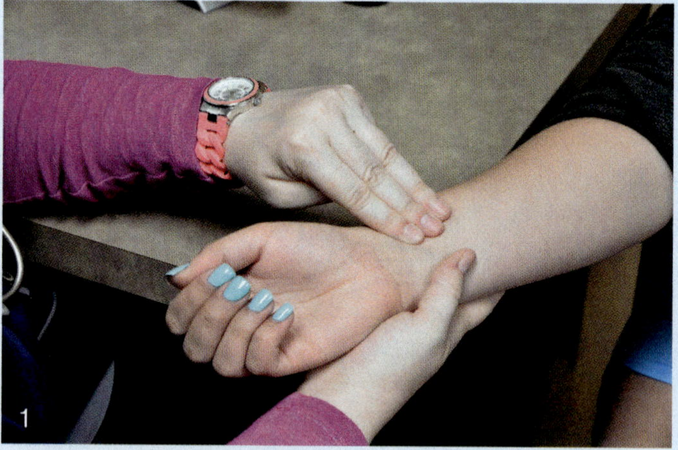

5. Count the beats for 1 full minute using a watch with a second hand.
   PURPOSE: Counting for 1 full minute allows you to obtain an accurate count, including any irregularities in rhythm and volume. Once you become more adept at taking a pulse, you can reduce this to 30 seconds and multiply that number by 2 to record the patient's heart rate.
6. While counting the beats, also assess the rhythm and volume of the patient's pulse.
7. While continuing to hold the patient's arm in the same position used to count the radial pulse, observe the rise and fall of the patient's chest

PROCEDURE 20.8 Accurately Measure and Record the Patient's Radial Pulse and Respiratory Rate—*continued*

(see Figure 20.14). If you have difficulty noticing the patient's breathing, place the arm across the chest to detect movement.
PURPOSE: The respiratory count may be altered if the patient is aware that you are counting; placing the arm across the chest allows you to feel or see the rise and fall of the chest wall as the patient takes breaths.

8. Inhalation and exhalation make up one complete breathing cycle or respiration. Count the respirations for 30 seconds and multiply by 2.
PURPOSE: Counting for 30 seconds allows you to obtain an accurate count and determine any irregularities in rhythm or depth, or unusual breathing patterns. If respirations are abnormal in any way, count for 1 full minute.
9. While counting, also assess the rhythm and depth of the patient's respirations.
10. Release the patient's wrist.
11. Wash hands or use hand sanitizer.
PURPOSE: To ensure infection control.
12. Document both the radial pulse and respiration counts in the patient's health record. In a paper record, the pulse is recorded immediately after the temperature and respiration after the pulse recording (e.g., P: 72, regular, thready R: 18, regular, normal).
PURPOSE: Procedures that are not recorded are considered not done.

Documentation Example

5/6/20XX 8:35 a.m. P: 72 regular, 1+ R: 18, regular, normal
________________________ C. Ricci, CMA (AAMA)

PROCEDURE 20.9 Accurately Measure and Record a Patient's Blood Pressure

TASK: Accurately measure and record a blood pressure measurement.

EQUIPMENT and SUPPLIES

- Patient's record
- Sphygmomanometer
- Stethoscope
- Antiseptic wipes/alcohol wipes

PROCEDURAL STEPS

1. Wash hands or use hand sanitizer.
PURPOSE: To ensure infection control.
2. Assemble the equipment and supplies needed. Clean the earpieces and diaphragm of the stethoscope with alcohol wipes.
PURPOSE: For infection control and to follow Standard Precautions.
3. Greet the patient. Identify yourself. Verify the patient's identity with full name and date of birth. Explain the procedure to be performed in a manner that the patient understands. Answer any questions the patient may have about the procedure.
PURPOSE: Identification of the patient prevents errors, and explanations are a means of gaining implied consent and patient cooperation.
4. Select the appropriate arm for application of the cuff (no mastectomy on that side, no injury or disease). If the patient has had a bilateral mastectomy, the blood pressure should be taken using a large thigh cuff with the stethoscope over the popliteal artery.
PURPOSE: The pressure of the cuff temporarily interferes with circulation to the limb.
CAUTION: If a female patient has had a mastectomy, the blood pressure should never be taken on the affected side. Compressing the arm may cause complications. If she has had a bilateral mastectomy, another site, such as the popliteal artery, must be used, which requires the use of a thigh cuff.
5. Seat the patient in a comfortable position with the legs uncrossed and the arm resting, palm up, at heart level on the arm of a chair or a table next to where the patient is seated.
PURPOSE: To expose the brachial artery; also, to promote patient relaxation and ensure a true reading. Crossed legs may increase the blood pressure, and positioning the arm above heart level may cause an inaccurate reading.
6. Roll the sleeve to about 5 inches above the elbow, or have the patient remove the arm from the sleeve.
PURPOSE: Tight clothing prevents an accurate reading.
7. Select the correct cuff size.
PURPOSE: An incorrect cuff size prevents accurate measurement of blood pressure. The cuff should fit comfortably around the patient's arm, and the bladder should be located over the brachial artery between the lines designated on the cuff. Pediatric, normal adult, and large adult cuff sizes should be available. Thigh cuffs may be needed for obese patients.
8. Palpate the brachial artery at the antecubital space in both arms. If one arm has a stronger pulse, use that arm. If the pulses are equal, select the right arm.
PURPOSE: A stronger pulse is easier to measure; the right arm is the universal arm of choice.
9. Center the cuff bladder over the brachial artery with the connecting tube away from the patient's body and the tube to the bulb close to the body (see the following figure).
PURPOSE: Pressure must be applied directly over the artery for an accurate reading. The cuff and its tubing should not touch the stethoscope. Noise from the tubing can interfere with a correct reading.

Continued

PROCEDURE 20.9 Accurately Measure and Record a Patient's Blood Pressure—*continued*

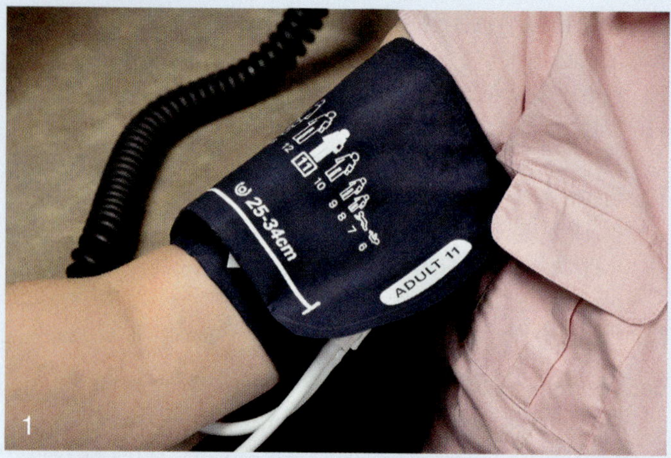

1

10. Place the lower edge of the cuff about 1 inch above the palpable brachial pulse, normally located in the natural crease of the inner elbow and wrap it snugly and smoothly.
PURPOSE: To help ensure an accurate reading. The cuff should be high enough on the arm that the stethoscope does not touch it, and the cuff sounds do not interfere with listening to the blood pressure sounds. A loose cuff results in an inaccurate reading.
11. Position the gauge of the sphygmomanometer so that it is easily seen.
PURPOSE: An aneroid gauge should show the needle within the zero mark.
12. Palpate the radial pulse, tighten the screw valve on the air pump, and inflate the cuff until the pulse can no longer be felt. Make a note of the point on the gauge where the pulse could no longer be felt. Mentally add 30 mm Hg to the reading. Deflate the cuff and wait 15 seconds.
PURPOSE: The point where the radial pulse is no longer felt provides an estimate of the systolic pressure. Pumping the cuff above that level ensures that phase I of the Korotkoff sounds will be heard.
13. Insert the earpieces of the stethoscope turned forward into the ear canals.
PURPOSE: With the earpieces in this position, the openings follow the anatomic line of the ear canal and the blood pressure will be accurately heard.
14. Place the stethoscope's diaphragm over the palpated brachial artery for an adult patient or the bell for a pediatric patient. Press firmly enough to obtain a seal but not so tightly that the artery is constricted. Only touch the edges of the stethoscope head.
PURPOSE: Forming a seal around the head of the stethoscope aids in listening for blood pressure sounds. Placing your fingers directly over the stethoscope head will cause interference with the sound.
15. Close the valve and squeeze the bulb to inflate the cuff, rapidly but smoothly, to 30 mm Hg above the palpated systolic level, which was previously determined (see the following figure).

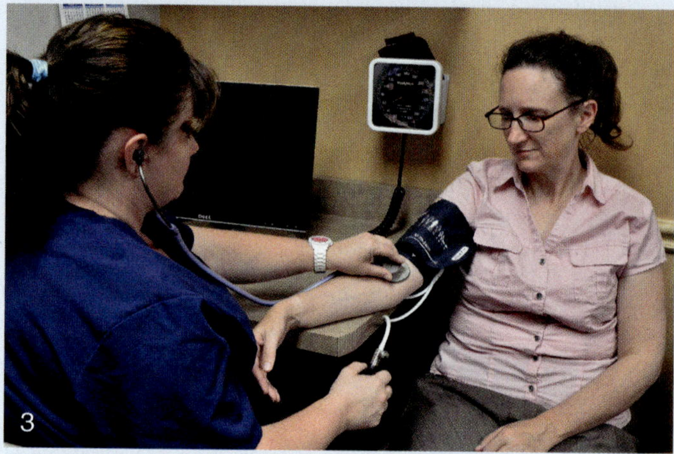

3

16. Open the valve slightly and deflate the cuff at a constant rate of 2 to 3 mm Hg per heartbeat.
PURPOSE: Careful, slow release allows you to listen to all sounds.
17. Listen throughout the entire deflation; note the point on the gauge at which you hear the first sound (systolic), the last sound (diastolic), and until the sounds have stopped for at least 10 mm Hg.
18. Do not reinflate the cuff once the air has been released. Wait 30 to 60 seconds to repeat the procedure if needed.
PURPOSE: Not allowing the blood to refill in the brachial artery results in inaccurate readings.
19. Remove the cuff from the patient's arm.
20. Remove the stethoscope from your ears, and document the systolic and diastolic readings and the arm used as BP systolic/diastolic (e.g., BP: 120/80 R arm).
Note: It is recommended that the blood pressure be checked and documented in each arm during the initial assessment of the patient and then bilaterally periodically after that for patients with hypertension.
PURPOSE: Procedures that are not recorded are considered not done.
21. Clean the earpieces and the head of the stethoscope with an alcohol wipe, and return both the cuff and the stethoscope to storage.
22. Wash hands or use hand sanitizer.
PURPOSE: To ensure infection control.

Documentation Example

5/19/20XX 11:00 a.m. BP: 124/82, Ⓛarm sitting ——————————
—————————————————— C. Ricci, CMA (AAMA)

PROCEDURE 20.10 Accurately Measure and Record Oxygen Saturation

TASK: Accurately measure and record the adequacy of oxygen levels (or oxygen saturation) in the blood using a pulse oximeter.

EQUIPMENT and SUPPLIES

- Patient's health record
- Pulse oximeter and probe of the appropriate size

PROCEDURAL STEPS

1. Wash hands or use hand sanitizer.
   PURPOSE: Standard Precautions must be followed to prevent the spread of disease.
2. Assemble the equipment.
3. Greet the patient. Identify yourself. Verify the patient's identity with full name and date of birth. Explain the procedure to be performed in a manner that the patient understands. Answer any questions the patient may have about the procedure.
   PURPOSE: An informed patient is more cooperative.
4. Turn on the monitor and attach the probe to the finger (preferred) or earlobe, so it is flush with the skin.
5. The light-emitting diode (LED) should be placed on top of the nail. If the patient is wearing nail polish or has artificial nails, these may have to be removed to get a strong pulse signal.
   PURPOSE: To measure the pulse and oxygen saturation level.
6. Sanitize the patient probe and the external portion of the monitor with an aseptic cleaner.
   PURPOSE: To follow Standard Precautions.
7. Wash hands or use hand sanitizer.
   PURPOSE: To ensure infection control.
8. Document the oxygen saturation percentage and pulse in the patient's health record. Include the date, time, and if the patient is receiving supplemental oxygen, record the amount in liters.
   PURPOSE: Procedures that are not documented are considered not done.

PROCEDURE 20.11 Accurately Measure and Record a Patient's Weight and Height

TASK: Accurately measure and record the weight and height of a patient as part of the physical assessment procedure.
Note: Make sure the scale is located in an area away from traffic to maintain the patient's privacy.

EQUIPMENT and SUPPLIES

- Balance beam scale with a measuring bar
- Paper towel
- Patient record

PROCEDURAL STEPS

1. Wash hands or use hand sanitizer.
   PURPOSE: To ensure infection control.
2. Greet the patient. Identify yourself. Verify the patient's identity with full name and date of birth. Explain the procedure to be performed in a manner that the patient understands. Answer any questions the patient may have about the procedure.
   PURPOSE: Identification of the patient prevents errors, and explanations are a means of gaining implied consent and patient cooperation.
3. Have the patient remove shoes. Place a paper towel on the scale platform. Check that the balance bar pointer floats in the middle of the balance frame when all weights are at zero.
   PURPOSE: A floating pointer indicates that the scale is properly adjusted and in balance.
4. Help the patient onto the scale. Make sure the patient has removed any heavy objects from pockets and is not holding anything such as a jacket or purse.
5. Move the large weight into the groove closest to the patient's estimated weight. The grooves are calibrated in 50-lb increments. If you choose a groove that is more than the patient's weight, the pointer will immediately tilt to the bottom of the balance frame. You then must move it back one groove (see the following figure).

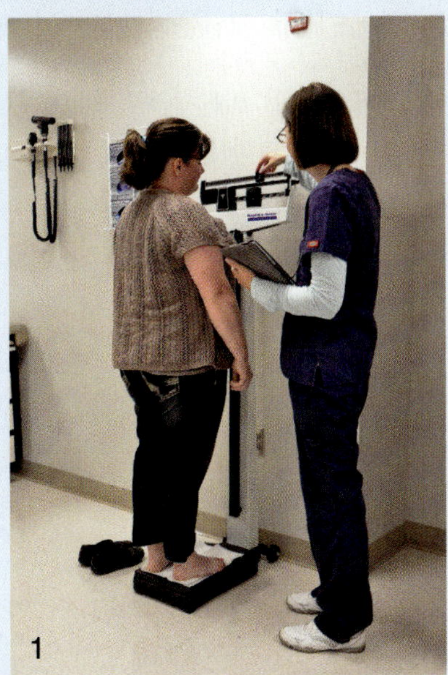

6. While the patient is standing still, slide the small upper weight to the right along the pound markers until the pointer balances in the middle of the balance frame.
   PURPOSE: The pointer floats between the bottom and the top of the frame when both lower and upper weights together balance the scale with the patient's weight.

Continued

PROCEDURE 20.11 Accurately Measure and Record a Patient's Weight and Height—*continued*

7. Leave the weights in place.
8. Ask the patient to step off the scale and move the height bar to a point above the patient's height. Extend the bar and ask the patient step back on the scale. On some scales, the patient may need to face away from the scale.
9. Adjust the height bar so that it just touches the top of the patient's head (see the following figure).

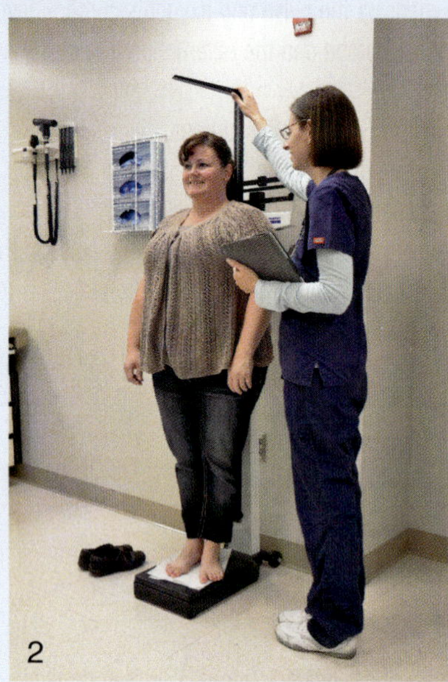

10. Leave the elevation bar set.
    PURPOSE: To maintain the height recording while protecting the patient from possible injury.
11. Assist the patient off the scale. Make sure all items that were removed for weighing are given back to the patient.
12. Read the weight scale. Add the numbers at the markers of the large and small weights and document the total to the nearest quarter of a pound in the patient's health record (e.g., Wt: 136½ lb).
13. Read the height. Read the marker at the movable point of the ruler and document the measurement to the nearest quarter of an inch on the patient's medical record (e.g., Ht: 5′ 6½″) (see the following figure).

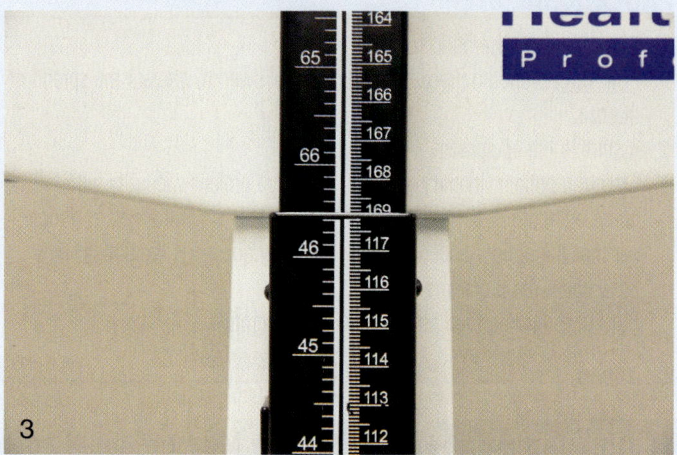

14. Use the patient's weight and height to determine the BMI if the EHR program does not do it automatically.
15. Return the weights and the measuring bar to zero.
16. Remove the paper towel and dispose of it in the waste container. Wash hands or use hand sanitizer.
17. Document the results in the patient's health record.
    PURPOSE: Procedures that are not documented are considered not done.

Documentation Example

5/26/20XX 11:07 a.m. Wt: 136½ lb, Ht: 5′6½″ ——————————
—————————————— C. Ricci, CMA (AAMA)

PHYSICAL EXAMINATION

21

SCENARIO

Chris Isaacson, a certified medical assistant (CMA) who has met the requirements of the American Association of Medical Assistants (AAMA), works for Walden-Martin Family Medical (WMFM) Clinic. He is responsible for initial patient interviews, taking medical histories, and documentation. Chris struggles with gathering the information needed from some patients. They do not always respond openly and honestly. Chris is also responsible for assisting with physical examinations. His duties include preparing and maintaining the examination room and equipment, getting the patient ready for specific physical examinations, and gowning, draping and positioning the patient as needed. Because Chris assists with examinations, he must be familiar with the physical examination procedure and the order in which the provider needs various pieces of medical equipment. Throughout the physical examination process, Chris needs to be aware of proper body mechanics.

While studying this chapter, think about the following questions:

- How can Chris learn to develop helping relationships so that the patient's medical history is as comprehensive as possible?
- Would it help if Chris displayed greater sensitivity to diverse populations?
- Would using active listening techniques and attending to the patient's nonverbal behaviors better enable Chris to develop therapeutic communications skills?
- How can Chris's supervisor help him become a better communicator and demonstrate comprehensive and accurate documentation in patients' health records?
- What equipment does Chris need to gather to make sure the examination goes smoothly and without interruption before the provider enters the examination room?
- What examination and treatment positions should Chris be familiar with, and when should the various positions be used?
- What measures can Chris take to protect himself from injury when lifting heavy items or assisting with the transfer of patients?

LEARNING OBJECTIVES

1. Examine how to collect the history information and the components of the patient's health history.
2. Discuss how to successfully understand and communicate with patients and display sensitivity to diverse populations.
3. Examine the patient interview, both in person and via telehealth.
4. Explain patient assessment and documentation.
5. Examine the medical assistant's role in preparing for the physical examination.
6. Examine the medical assistant's role in assisting with the physical examination.

VOCABULARY

auscultate (AW skuhl tayt) To listen with a stethoscope.

bruit (broot) An abnormal sound or murmur heard on auscultation of an organ, vessel (e.g., carotid artery), or gland.

chief complaint A statement in the patient's own words that describes the reason for the visit.

chronologic (kron ih LOJ ic) Arranged in the order of time.

clarification (klar i fi KAY shuhn) Allows the listener to get additional information.

clubbing Abnormal enlargement of the distal phalanges (fingers and toes) associated with cyanotic heart disease or advanced chronic pulmonary disease.

colonoscopy (kohl uh NOS kuh pee) A procedure in which a fiberoptic scope is used to examine the large intestine.

congruence (kun GROO uhns) Agreement; the state that occurs when the verbal expression of the message matches the sender's nonverbal body language.

correlate (CORE uh layt) To establish an orderly relationship or connection.

demographic (dem uh GRAF ik) Statistical data of a population. In healthcare, this includes the patient's name, address, date of birth, employment, and other details.

electrocardiogram (ECG, EKG) A record or recording of electrical impulses of the heart produced by an electrocardiograph.

emphysema (em fuh ZEE mah) Thinning and eventual destruction of the alveoli; usually accompanies chronic bronchitis.

VOCABULARY—*continued*

extension The process of stretching out; increasing the angle of a joint.

familial (fah MIL ee uhl) Occurring in or affecting members of a family more than would be expected by chance.

flexion The process of decreasing the angle of a joint.

gait The manner or style of walking.

history of present illness (HPI) Describes the signs and symptoms from the time of onset.

holistic (hoh LIS tik) Considering the patient as a whole; includes the physical, emotional, social, economic, and spiritual needs of the person.

inconspicuous (in kuhn SPIK yoo uhs) Not noticeable or prominent.

judicious (joo DISH uhs) Using good judgment; being discreet, sensible.

manipulation Movement or exercise of a body part by means of an externally applied force.

murmur An abnormal sound heard during auscultation of the heart that may or may not have a pathologic origin; it is associated with valve disease or a congenital heart defect.

nodules (NOD jools) Small lumps, lesions, or swellings that are felt when the skin is palpated.

palpation (pal PAY shuhn) The use of touch during the physical examination to assess the size, consistency, and location of certain body parts.

patient portal A secure online website that gives patients 24-hour access to personal health information using a username and password.

perineal (pair ih NEE uhl) Pertaining to the area between the vaginal opening and the rectum (perineum).

peripheral neuropathy (puh RIF er uhl noo ROP uh thee) A problem with the function of the nerves outside the spinal cord; symptoms include weakness, burning pain, and loss of reflexes; a frequent complication of diabetes mellitus.

rapport (ra POR) A relationship of harmony and accord between the patient and the healthcare professional.

sclera (SKLER uh) The white part of the eye that forms the orbit.

signs Objective findings determined by a clinician, such as a fever, hypertension, or rash.

symmetry (SIM ih tree) Similarity in size, form, and arrangement of parts on opposite sides of the body.

symptoms Subjective complaints reported by the patient, such as pain or nausea.

transillumination (trans ih LOO muh nay shun) Inspection of a cavity or organ by passing light through its walls.

trauma (TRAW muh) A physical injury or wound caused by external force or violence.

turgor (TUR ger) Referring to normal skin tension; the resistance of the skin to being grasped between the fingers and released. Turgor decreases with dehydration and increases with edema.

INTRODUCTION

Medical assistants are directly involved in gathering information from patients about their health. It is important to remember that a healthy state is more than the absence of disease. The assessment process should be a reflection of the entire patient, not just a report about signs and symptoms. Individual lifestyles and environmental factors can cause disease and should be considered when information is gathered about the patient's **chief complaint**. For example, patients who smoke or work in stressful occupations may be more prone to hypertension. Health professionals should consider all patient factors when gathering information about the patient's health status. The method of analyzing all factors that may contribute to the development of disease is based on a **holistic** perspective. Holistic patient care recognizes that illness is the result of many factors, not just physical ones.

As the first step in treating a disease process, the provider must determine the patient's medical diagnosis. A *differential diagnosis* considers which one of several diseases may be producing the patient's symptoms. The possible causes for a set of symptoms are considered in order to arrive at a diagnosis. For example, if a patient presents with moderate to severe knee pain, the provider might consider causes such as an injury or arthritis. A differential diagnosis is based on information gathered from the patient about symptoms, contributing family, personal, and social histories, and a complete physical examination. Multiple causes are not ruled out in a differential diagnosis because patients can be sick with more than one thing at once. Once all possible factors have been considered, the provider comes up with a working diagnosis and begins treatment. A working diagnosis is also called a *clinical diagnosis*. The clinical diagnosis is arrived at after taking a detailed history and doing a comprehensive physical examination, but before any laboratory tests or x-rays, diagnostic testing is done. For the patient with knee pain, after gathering detailed patient information and conducting a comprehensive physical examination, the provider decides that the clinical diagnosis is arthritic changes in the joint. The provider orders x-rays and a magnetic resonance image (MRI) of the knee to confirm the clinical diagnosis. The final diagnosis is determined after all diagnostic studies are completed.

However, patient care does not start with the physical examination; it begins when the patient first contacts the office. Even before the examination, the medical assistant has the opportunity to interact with the patient to ensure comfort during the process and that all of the necessary information is obtained.

Interviewing patients, assisting with examinations, and preparing documentation are important responsibilities for a medical assistant. You must know the components of a medical history and the techniques for interviewing patients to help the provider diagnose and treat the patient. The more complete the medical history, the better the provider will be able to treat the patient.

A medical assistant must also know how to best assist the provider during the physical examination. Understanding what supplies and instruments are needed will make the visit go more smoothly for both the patient and the provider. During a complete physical exam, the patient is placed in various positions to facilitate examination. It is often the medical assistant's responsibility to assist the patient into the correct position and drape him or her for modesty.

HEALTH HISTORY

Health history information is crucial to providing the best possible care to patients. Without knowing what has gone on in the past, it will be harder for the provider to determine the most appropriate course of action. Often, the medical assistant is responsible for collecting the health information initially. It is important to fully understand the forms used to collect this information and the components of a comprehensive health history.

Collecting the History Information

A new patient is asked to complete a health history form. This form is useful for diagnosing and treating the patient. This self-history also allows the patient to be more involved in the process. The form may be mailed to the patient's home before the appointment or may be completed in the office during the first visit. Some healthcare facilities use electronic forms. These can be emailed to the patient before the first appointment and incorporated into the patient's electronic health record (EHR) when the completed form is emailed back. The patient may also be able to complete the form online through a **patient portal**. If a paper form is used, it can be scanned into the patient's EHR after it is completed.

If you are responsible for taking a portion of the medical history, conduct the interview in a private area, free of distractions and where others cannot overhear anything. Patients will not talk freely where they may be overheard or interrupted. Legally and ethically, the patient has the right to privacy, and access to the patient's health record is permitted only for healthcare workers directly involved in the patient's care or individuals the patient has specified on his or her Health Insurance Portability and Accountability Act (HIPAA) complaint records release form.

Listen to the patient. Do not express surprise or displeasure at any of the patient's statements. Remember, you are not there to pass judgment but collect medical data. The medical assistant should document the information in an organized manner, exactly as given by the patient, without opinion or interpretation. The documentation should include the following:

- Purpose of the patient's visit, written as the chief complaint (CC)
- Patient's vital signs (VS)
- Height and weight
- Pain; documented using a scale of 1 to 10, with 1 being the least amount of pain and 10 being the greatest amount
- In some facilities, the provider takes the medical history during the patient's initial visit. The provider **correlates** the physical findings in the examination with the information in the history. The complete medical history and the physical examination are the starting point and foundation of all patient-provider contacts. EHR systems directly incorporate the patient's history and physical examination data into the health record (Figure 21.1).

Components of the Health History

Health history forms vary depending on the provider's preference, the practice specialty, and the EHR system used in the facility. The most commonly used health history forms include these components:

- *Database:* The record of the patient's **demographic** information, history, physical examination, and initial laboratory findings. As new information is added, it becomes part of this database.
- *Chief complaint (CC):* The purpose of the patient's visit. Generally, this is documented in the patient's own words.

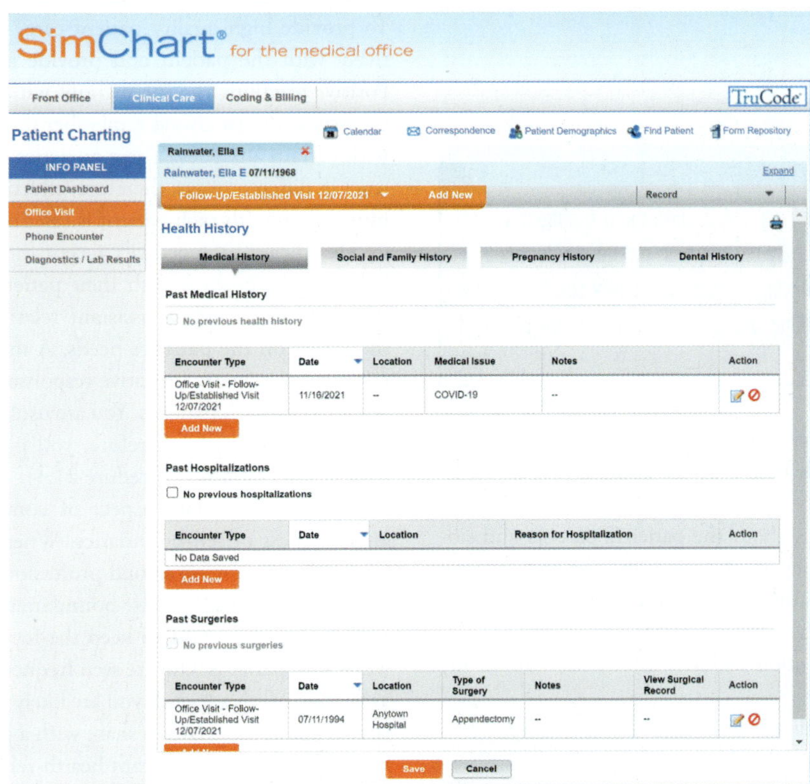

FIGURE 21.1 Example of an electronic health record (EHR) system.

- **History of present illness (HPI)**: The medical assistant should gather as much information about the health problem as possible and document it concisely in **chronological** order. The documentation should include the following descriptions:

  - *Location:* What area of the body is the current condition located in? (Have the patient point to the area.)
  - *Quality:* How would the patient describe the condition? If there is pain, is it sharp, dull, ache, intense, cramp, nagging, burning?
  - *Severity:* What is the severity of pain? (Pain is usually documented using a scale of 1 to 10 with 10, being the worst.)
  - *Duration:* How long has the condition been going on?
  - *Timing:* How long does it last when it occurs?
  - *Context:* What was the patient doing when she or he first noticed the condition?
  - *Modifying factors:* What makes it better or worse? Does it occur while standing, sitting, laying down, sleeping, or while eating? Does anything help (like Tylenol)?
  - *Associated signs and symptoms:* What other signs and symptoms occur with the condition (such as headache with blurred vision, back pain with numbness and tingling down the leg, or frequency and urgency with urination)?

- *Past history (PH)* or *past medical history (PMH):* A summary of the patient's previous health. It includes dates and details about the patient:
  - Usual childhood diseases (UCD or UCHD)
  - Major illnesses
  - Surgeries
  - Allergies
  - Accidents
  - Immunization record

Allergy Documentation

Each medical practice has a policy on how to document a patient's allergies. In a paper record, they typically are noted in red ink or identified by a colored sticker so that all healthcare workers can easily see them. EHR systems have methods for including allergy information on all pertinent screens in the patient's record.

The patient's medication history should include a record of currently prescribed drugs and frequently used over-the-counter (OTC) medications, including supplements.

- *Family history* (FH): Details about the patient's parents and siblings and their health; if they are deceased, the age and cause of death. This information is important because certain diseases and disorders have **familial** or hereditary tendencies.
- *Social history* (SH): This section includes information about the patient's lifestyle:
  - Whether the patient feels safe at home
  - Use of tobacco, alcohol, or recreational drugs
  - Sleeping and exercise habits
  - Typical diet
  - Education and occupation
- *Dental care history:* This section includes information about whether the patient sees a dentist regularly and what, if any, dental issues the patient has.
- For female patients, woman's last menstrual period (LMP), pregnancy history, and method of birth control if sexually active.
- It may be important to note the patient's cultural and religious background because these factors could influence certain lifestyle and dietary choices. This information helps the provider plan treatment for the patient or determine causative factors for disease. It also provides a holistic picture of the patient's health. To meet the requirements of Meaningful Use (see Chapter 10), providers are required to collect information on allergies, patient history, safety at home, and alcohol use.
- *Systems review* (SR) or *review of systems* (ROS): These questions provide a guide to the patient's general health and help detect conditions other than those covered under the present illness. Often a patient may think certain health problems are irrelevant and fail to mention them. However, these problems may help the provider determine the cause of the disorder currently being explored. A systems review is obtained through a logical sequence of questions about the state of health of body systems, beginning with the head and proceeding downward (Figure 21.2). The provider typically completes this medical history section while conducting the physical examination.

UNDERSTANDING AND COMMUNICATING WITH PATIENTS

To provide high-quality patient care, we must communicate effectively with the patient and provide a warm, caring environment. Positive reactions and interactions with the patient are vital. A medical assistant must always remember that each patient is an individual with certain anxieties. These anxieties often cause people to act and react in different ways; therefore, effective verbal and nonverbal communication with each patient is essential.

Healthcare professionals accept the responsibility of developing helping relationships with their patients. The interpersonal nature of the patient–medical assistant relationship means that the focus should be on the patient's needs. A medical assistant can bring out either a positive or a negative response simply by the way they treat and interact with patients. You are usually the first person the patient communicates with; therefore, you play a vital role in therapeutic patient interactions (Procedure 21.1).

Another important aspect of communicating with patients is an awareness of self-boundaries. When working in healthcare, it is important to develop a solid professional relationship with patients. By establishing realistic self-boundaries, that relationship can be protected. It is important to keep the focus on the patient. When you work with patients who are seen frequently, it is easy to think of them as friends. With a friend, you are likely to share personal information that is not appropriate to share with a patient. Patients may feel that they cannot share important health-related information because you

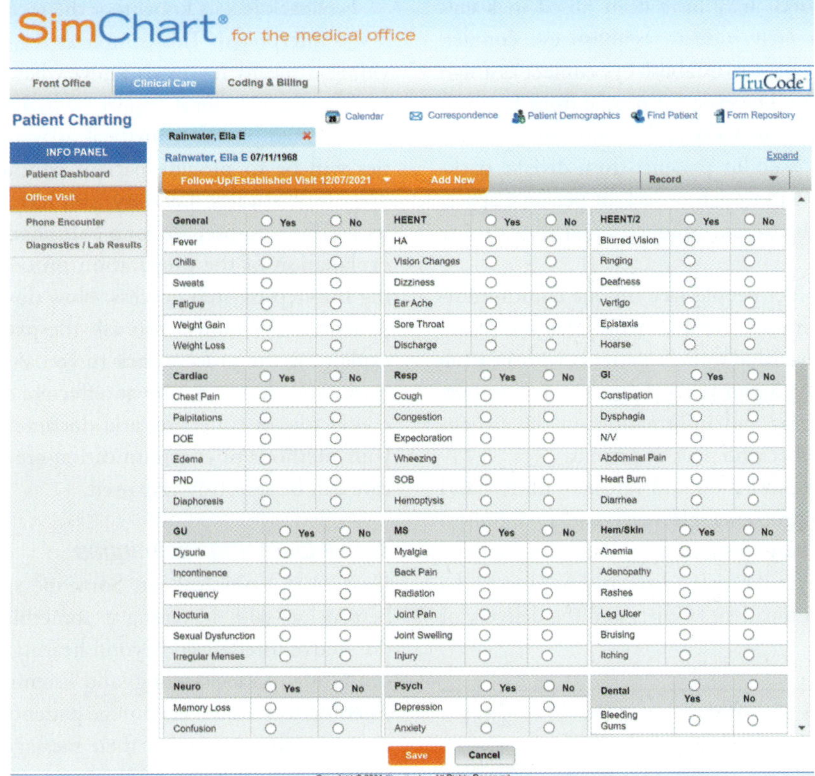

FIGURE 21.2 Example of review of systems (ROS) questions in an electronic health record.

are their friend, and it would be embarrassing to share that information with a friend.

Self-boundaries can also be thought of as professional boundaries. You need to treat patients with respect and keep the relationship professional. Be friendly to patients and always keep the focus on the patient.

Sensitivity to Diverse Patient Groups

Most healthcare facilities have a diverse patient population. The diversity could be based on race, age, culture, religion, or physical qualities, such as being deaf or hard of hearing. Whatever the origin of the diversity, practicing respectful patient care is extremely important. *Empathy* is the key to creating a caring, therapeutic environment. Empathy is different from sympathy. A medical assistant who is empathetic respects the patient's individuality and attempts to see the person's health problem through their eyes. The medical assistant also recognizes the effect of all holistic factors on the patient's well-being. Empathetic sensitivity to diversity requires you to examine your own values, beliefs, and actions; you cannot treat all patients with care and respect until you first recognize and evaluate personal biases. We think and act a certain way for many reasons. The first step in understanding the process is to evaluate your individual value system. Why do you have certain attitudes or beliefs about the worth of individuals or things?

Many factors influence the development of a value system. Value systems begin as learned beliefs and behaviors. Families and cultural influences shape the way we respond to a diverse society. Other factors that influence reactions include socioeconomic and educational backgrounds. To develop therapeutic relationships, you must recognize your own value system to determine whether it could affect how you interact with patients. Preconceived ideas about people because of their race, religion, income level, ethnic origin, sexual orientation, or gender can act as barriers to the development of a therapeutic relationship. You cannot treat your patients empathetically unless you can connect with them in some way. Personal biases or prejudices are huge barriers to developing therapeutic relationships (Figure 21.3).

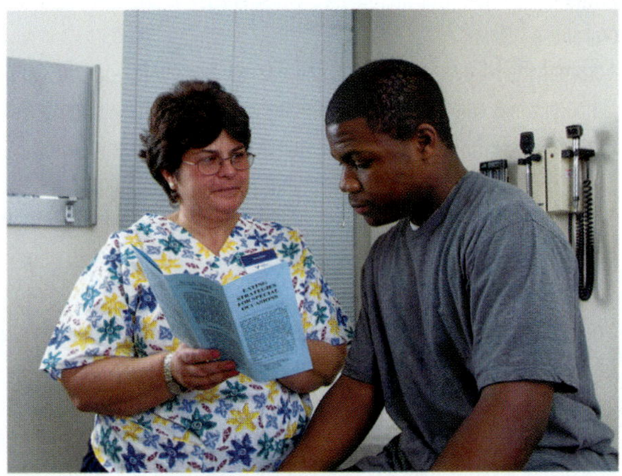

FIGURE 21.3 Respectful patientcare.

Regardless of the type of healthcare facility you work in, you will care for a wide variety of patients. The medical assistant should take the initiative to learn about the cultures represented in the healthcare practice. Some points to consider about diverse groups include the following:

- Patients of Asian backgrounds may have been raised in a culture that considers it extremely rude to establish eye contact. Americans view an unwillingness to establish eye contact as a sign of distrust or embarrassment; however, for people from Japan or China, lack of eye contact may be a way of demonstrating respect.
- Personal space may be an issue for patients from diverse backgrounds. If uncomfortable with touch or lack of personal space, attempt to accommodate the patient as much as possible during the office visit.
- Research has shown that older people face unique communication problems in the healthcare environment. The healthcare facility should have tools available to help patients with hearing or vision issues. When caring for an aging individual, it is important to focus patient teaching and information on the patient rather than the family member who may be present.
- Patients may use their religious beliefs and values to understand and cope with their health problems. However, using religion to guide healthcare decisions may result in a conflict with the provider's recommendations. Healthcare workers may need to find a balance between respect for a patient's beliefs and the delivery of high-quality healthcare.

CRITICAL THINKING APPLICATION **21.1**

Honestly evaluate your personal biases. What do you find unacceptable in people? Do you prejudge others based on their affiliation with a particular group or because of a certain lifestyle decision? Do these biases create barriers to the development of therapeutic relationships? If so, how can you get beyond these barriers?

Consider the following scenarios and discuss them with your classmates:

- While you are conducting a patient interview, the patient informs you that he has tested positive for the human immunodeficiency virus (HIV). Do you think this will affect your therapeutic relationship?
- You are responsible for recording an in-depth interview with a homeless person with very poor hygiene. Will this cause a problem with your professional manner?
- Your office manager tells you that an inmate of the county prison is being brought in this afternoon for an examination. Do you think his status will affect your interaction with the patient?
- You are attempting to interview a 20-year-old patient who brought her two young children with her to the office today. She is a single mother pregnant with her third child and receives public assistance. What do you think? Will you have difficulty being empathetic?

Therapeutic Techniques

Communication is an interactive process involving the sender of the message, the receiver, and feedback. Feedback is a crucial component of confirming that the message is received. The message can be sent by a number of methods:

- Face-to-face communication
- Telephone
- Email
- Letter
- Video conferencing

Feedback lets us know that the receiver got the message and how it was interpreted. This completes the communication cycle by providing a means for us to know what message the patient received exactly and whether it requires **clarification**.

For example, as a medical assistant, one of your responsibilities will be to provide patient education on how to prepare for diagnostic studies. Let's say, you have to explain to an older adult patient how to prepare for a **colonoscopy**. You provided a detailed explanation of the preparation procedure and a handout explaining the step-by-step process. How do you really know whether the patient understands? You ask the patient to provide feedback by explaining the process back to you. As a member of the healthcare team, you must become an effective communicator. You will play a vital role in collecting and documenting patient information. If your methods of communication are faulty, the quality of patient care can be seriously impaired.

Active Listening Techniques

Hearing is a physical act. Someone speaks, and we hear what the person has said. Listening is something we consciously choose to do. Active listeners go beyond hearing the patient's message to concentrating, understanding, and listening to the main points. Active listening techniques encourage patients to expand on and clarify the content and meaning of their messages. These techniques are very useful communication tools when a patient is agitated or upset. They help the medical assistant clarify the important details of the patient's chief complaint.

Three processes are involved in active listening: restatement, reflection, and clarification. *Restatement* is paraphrasing or repeating the patient's statements with phrases such as "My understanding of what you are saying is …" or "You are telling me the problem is …"

Reflection involves repeating the main idea of the conversation while also identifying the sender's *feelings*. For example, if the mother of a young patient is expressing frustration about her child's behavior, a reflective statement identifies that feeling with the response, "It sounds like you are frustrated about …" Or, if a patient who has been newly diagnosed with insulin-dependent diabetes shows anxiety about administering injections, an appropriate reflective statement recognizes the patient's feelings: "You appear anxious about …" Reflective statements clearly demonstrate to patients that you are not only listening to their words, you also are concerned and are attending to their feelings.

Clarification seeks to summarize or simplify the sender's thoughts and feelings and resolve any confusion in the message. Questions or statements that begin with, "Give me an example of …" or "Explain to me about …" or "So what you're saying is …" help patients to focus on the chief complaint and give you the opportunity to clear up any misconceptions before documenting patient information.

Listening is not a passive role in the communication process; it is active and demanding. You cannot be preoccupied with your own needs, or you will miss something important. For the duration of the patient interview, no one is more important than this particular patient. Listen to the way things are said, the tone of the patient's voice, and even to what the patient may not be saying out loud but is saying very clearly with body language (see Procedure 21.2).

Nonverbal Communication

Experts say that more than 90% of communication is nonverbal. Much of what we communicate to our patients is conveyed through body language. Our nonverbal actions, such as gestures, facial expressions, and mannerisms, are learned behaviors that are greatly influenced by our family and cultural backgrounds. The body naturally expresses our true feelings.

Most of the negative messages communicated through body language are unintentional. While conducting patient interviews, it is important to remember that nonverbal communication can seriously affect the therapeutic process.

The purpose of observing nonverbal communication is to become aware of the message conveyed by these behaviors rather than the words. This enables you to adapt your behavior to these feelings. You can deliberately select your response, either verbal or nonverbal, to have a favorable effect on others. The favorable effect may consist of the following:

- Providing emotional support
- Conveying that you care
- Defusing the patient's fear or anger
- Providing an invitation to release pent-up feelings by talking about the situation that aroused the feelings

Table 21.1 lists some nonverbal behaviors by patients that may indicate anxiety, frustration, or fear.

Helpful Listening Guidelines

- Listen to the main points in the discussion.
- Respond to both verbal and nonverbal messages.
- Be patient and nonjudgmental.
- Do not interrupt.
- Never intimidate the patient.
- Use active listening techniques: restatement, reflection, and clarification.

Your tone of voice can put a patient at ease. Your facial expression and the ease and confidence of your movements demonstrate a sincere interest in the patient. Therapeutic use of space and touch is also important for sending nonverbal messages to your patients. You should establish eye contact, sit in a relaxed but attentive position, and avoid using furniture as a barrier between you and the patient. Give the patient your undivided attention and let your body language inform each patient that you are interested in his or her medical problems (Figure 21.4 and Procedure 21.2).

The key to successful patient interaction is **congruence** between verbal and nonverbal messages. Although choosing the correct words is important, less than 10% of the message received is verbal; therefore, to be seen as honest and sensitive to the needs of your patients, you must be aware of your nonverbal behavior patterns. The nonverbal message the patient receives from the medical assistant's listening behavior should be, "You are a person of worth, and I am interested in you as a unique individual."

TABLE 21.1 Observations of Nonverbal Communication in Patients

AREA	OBSERVATION	INDICATION
Breathing patterns	Rapid respirations, sighing, shallow thoracic breathing	Anxiety, boredom, pain
Eye patterns	No eye contact, side-to-side movement, looking down at the hands	Anxiety, distrust, embarrassment
Hands	Tapping fingers, cracking knuckles, continuous movement, sweaty palms	Anxiety, worry, fear
Arm placement	Folded across chest, wrapped around abdomen	Anxiety, worry, fear, pain
Leg placement	Tension, crossed or tucked under, tapping foot, continuous movement	Frustration, anger

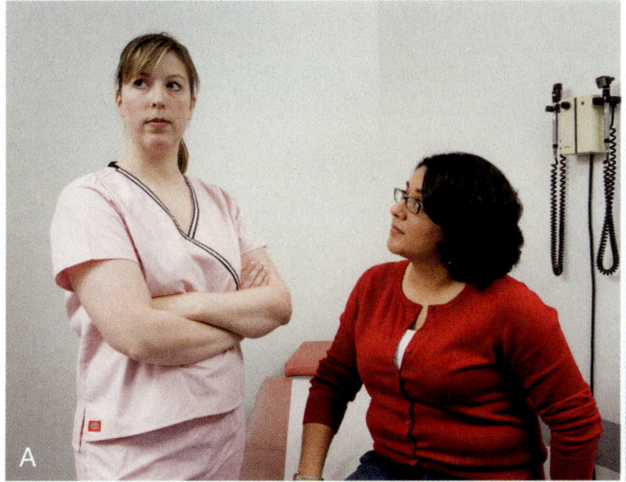

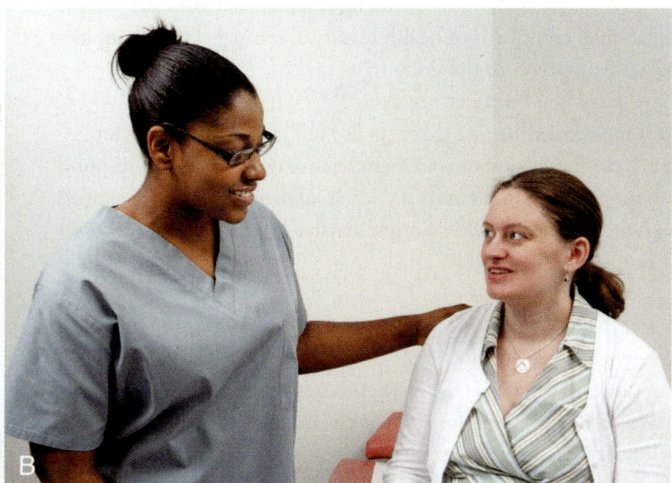

FIGURE 21.4 (A) Ineffective nonverbal language. **(B)** Therapeutic nonverbal language.

Nonverbal Language Behaviors

Nonverbal behavior—your body language—can have either a positive or a negative effect on patient interactions. Positive nonverbal behaviors enhance the patient's experience in the healthcare setting. Communication experts recommend the following:

- When gathering a health history, lean toward the patient to show interest.
- Face the patient squarely and at eye level to make the process more comfortable and demonstrate sensitivity and empathy.
- Eye contact is essential for therapeutic communication unless the patient is from a culture that discourages this.
- A closed posture (crossed arms or legs) may indicate disinterest.
- Be sensitive to the patient's personal space when possible. Maintain a comfortable distance from the patient, at least an arm's length, when conducting the interview.
- Be careful with body gestures, such as hand and arm movements. Gestures, such as nodding your head when the patient talks, can display interest, but too much body movement can be distracting.
- Your tone of voice should reflect your interest in the patient. Speaking too quietly or too loudly can detract from therapeutic communication.
- Continually observe the patient's body language during the interview; watch for signs of confusion, boredom, worry, and so on so that you can respond appropriately.
- Documenting in an EHR can distract both the medical assistant and the patient. Remind yourself to look at the patient frequently and use encouraging body language to maintain a personal interaction.

Open-Ended Questions or Statements

An *open-ended question* or statement asks for general information or states the topic to be discussed, but only in general terms. This communication tool is used in various ways:

- To begin the interview
- To introduce a new section of questions
- Whenever the person introduces a new topic

It is an effective method of gathering more details from the patient about the chief complaint or health history. Consider these examples:

"What brings you to the doctor?"

"How have you been getting along?"

"You mentioned having dizzy spells. Tell me more about that."

This type of question or statement encourages patients to respond in a manner they find comfortable. It allows patients to express themselves fully and provide comprehensive information about their chief complaint.

Closed-Ended Questions

Direct, or *closed-ended questions*, ask for specific information. This form of questioning limits the answer to one or two words—in many cases, yes or no. Use this form of questioning when you need confirmation of specific facts, such as when asking about past health problems. Here are some examples:

"Do you have a headache?"

"What is your birth date?"

"Have you ever broken a bone?"

Communication across the Life Span

The key to effectively communicating with patients is using an age-specific approach. Given the age and developmental level of your patient, how can you best interact with the person and with significant family members?

For example, Tasha, a 2-year-old patient, is scheduled for a physical examination. How can you best interact with her and her father to ensure that the history phase of the visit is complete and accurate? Therapeutic use of nonverbal language is essential to interacting with children of all ages. Getting down on the child's level, establishing eye contact, and using a gentle but firm voice are ways of gaining the child's confidence and cooperation. Children fear the unknown, so explaining all procedures with language that the child understands is important. At the same time, the medical assistant must communicate with the child's caregivers so that they can contribute to the intake process (Figure 21.5). The following are some important guidelines for obtaining the health history of a child:

- Make sure the environment is safe and attractive.
- Do not keep children and their caregivers waiting any longer than necessary because children become anxious and distracted quickly.
- Do not offer a choice unless the child can truly make one. If part of the treatment requires an injection, asking the child whether she would like her shot now is most likely to get an automatic "No!" However, giving her a choice of stickers after the injection is appropriate.
- Praising the child during the examination reduces anxiety and boosts self-esteem. When possible, direct questions to the child so that he or she feels like part of the process.
- Permitting the child to manipulate the equipment may help relieve anxiety and create a feeling of inclusion during the examination. If possible, use your imagination and make a game of the assessment or the procedure.
- A typical defense mechanism seen in sick or anxious children is regression. The child may refuse to leave the mother's lap or may want to hold a favorite toy during the procedure as a comfort

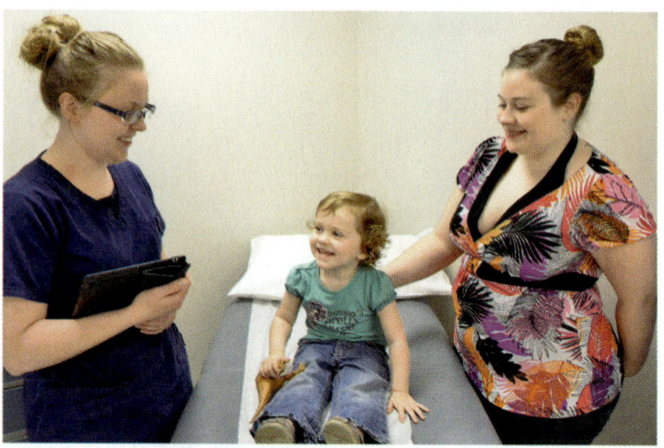

FIGURE 21.5 Interacting with a parent and child.

measure. Look for signs of anxiety, such as thumb sucking or rocking during the assessment and encourage caregivers to be involved in the process to help make the child feel as safe as possible.
- Listen to parents' concerns and respond truthfully to questions (Figure 21.6).

Older children may also have difficulty during the health visit (Figure 21.7). To help school-aged children gain a sense of control, allow them to make certain decisions about treatment. For example, Heather, a 13-year-old patient with diabetes, could be given the choice of having her father present during the visit. Or, if she requires an insulin injection, she could choose the site of the injection or perhaps administer the medication herself. This gives the medical assistant an opportunity to observe her technique and allows Heather to exert her independence.

Privacy is an important issue to consider with older children, especially adolescents. During the physical examination, respect privacy by keeping body exposure to a minimum and adequately preparing the child for procedures and positions. In addition, older children want to know what is going on during the examination, what to expect, and what the findings mean; therefore, keeping them informed in a language they can understand is important. Teen patients should always be encouraged to ask questions, which should be answered as completely and clearly as possible. It is important to keep in mind developmental stages when communicating with children. Refer to Chapter 2 for more information on Erickson's Stages of Psychosocial Development. Take every opportunity to teach your patients about their disease and to share information about significant wellness factors, regardless of their age.

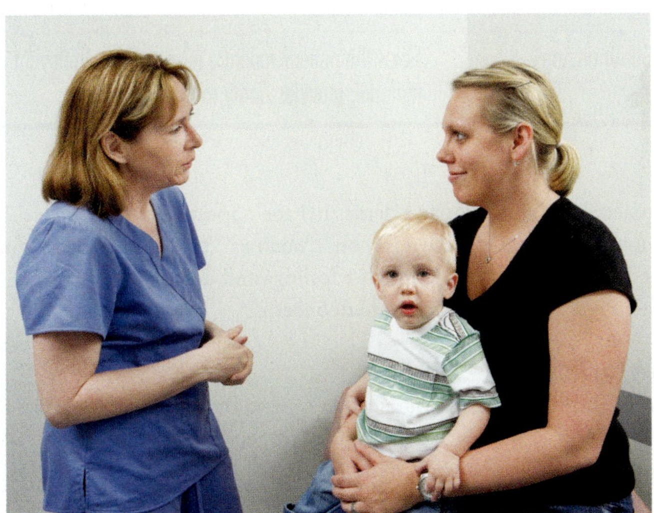

FIGURE 21.6 Responding to parental concerns.

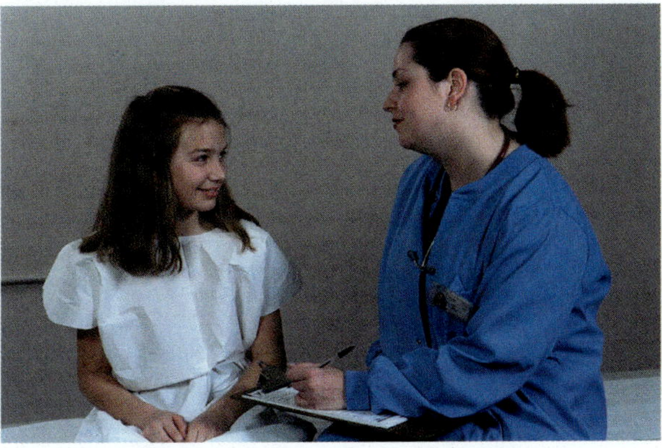

FIGURE 21.7 Interacting with a school-aged child.

Patient education is extremely important when interacting with adult patients. Using language that the adult patient understands and involving the patient in treatment decisions as much as possible are essential to developing a helping relationship with your older patients. Adults are bombarded by multiple responsibilities, which means that stress-related health problems are not unusual in these patients. Get to know your adult patients and emphasize preventive healthcare when possible.

INTERVIEWING THE PATIENT

The *interview*, or gathering the patient's medical history, is the first and most important part of data collection. The medical history identifies the patient's health strengths and problems and is a bridge to the next step in data collection, which is the physical examination performed by the provider. At this point, the patient knows everything about his or her health status, and you know nothing. Your interview skills help collect the necessary information and build **rapport** for a successful working relationship.

Consider the interview to be a type of contract between you and your patient. The contract consists of spoken and unspoken language and addresses what the patient needs and expects from the healthcare visit. The patient interview consists of three stages: the initiation or introduction, the body, and the closing.

Preparing the Appropriate Environment

- *Ensure privacy:* Ensure the room you use is unoccupied for the entire time allowed for the interview. The patient needs to feel sure that no one can overhear the conversation or interrupt.
- *Prevent interruptions:* Inform your co-workers of the interview and ask them not to interrupt you during this time. You need to concentrate on the patient and establish rapport. An interruption can destroy in seconds what you have spent many minutes building up.
- *Prepare comfortable surroundings:* Conducting the interview in comfortable surroundings reduces the patient's anxiety. Keep the distance between you and the patient at arm's length. Arrange chairs so that you and the patient are comfortably seated at eye level, and the desk or table does not act as a barrier between you.
- *Take* **judicious** *notes:* Note-taking should be kept to a minimum while you try to focus your attention on the person. Note-taking during the interview has disadvantages, such as breaking eye contact and shifting your attention away from the patient, which diminishes the patient's sense of importance. However, it is important to write down pertinent details as you are interviewing because you may forget important facts if you do not note them at the time of the discussion. With experience, you will develop a personal type of shorthand that you can use during the interview process. If using an EHR medical history template, efficiently open screens and choose the appropriate data while maintaining eye contact and using active listening techniques periodically throughout the interview.

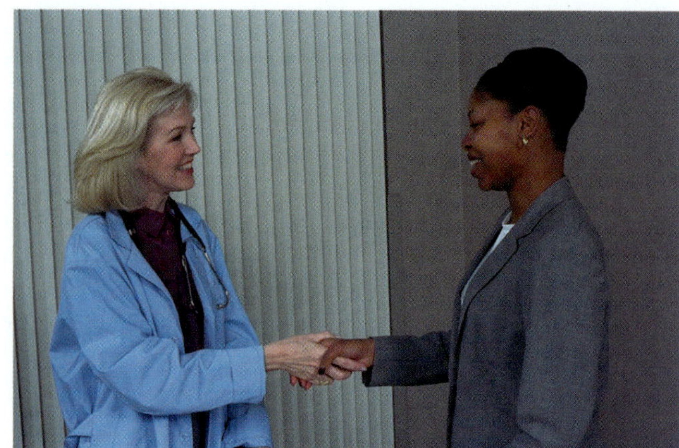

FIGURE 21.8 Greeting the patient.

The initiation of the interview is the time to introduce yourself, identify the patient, and determine the purpose of the interview (Figure 21.8). If you are nervous about how to begin, remember to keep it short. The patient probably is nervous, too, and is anxious to get started. Address the patient by his or her last name and give the reason for the interview—for example, "Mr. Coleman, my name is Stacey, and I am a certified medical assistant who works with Dr. Perez. I have some questions to ask you about your health history."

After the brief introduction, move on to the body of the interview. This is when you use various therapeutic communication techniques to determine the following:

- The reason the patient is seeking healthcare
- The patient's perception of the problem
- The characteristics of the problem
- The patient's expectations of care

During this time, use active listening skills, meaningful silence, congruent verbal and nonverbal communication, and a combination of open- and closed-ended statements and questions to gather the details of the patient's history and current health problem (Table 21.2).

Conclude the interview by summarizing the results of your interaction. The closing of the interview should clarify the patient's chief complaint, the purpose of the visit, and the patient's expectations of care. This is the patient's opportunity to add any additional details or explain further the characteristics of the health problem.

TABLE 21.2 Therapeutic Communication Techniques

TECHNIQUE	VALUE
Open-ended questions and statements	Encourage the patient to respond in more detail
Direct or closed-ended questions	Ask for specific information; usual reply is yes or no
Active listening	Nonverbally communicates your interest in the patient
Silence	Nonverbally communicates your acceptance of the patient and willingness to wait until the patient is ready to answer
Establishing guidelines	Informs the patient of what to expect during the interview
Acknowledgment	Shows the importance of the patient's role and respect for autonomy
Restating	Checks your interpretation of the patient's message for validation
Reflecting	Shows the patient your acknowledgment of his or her feelings
Summarizing	Helps the patient separate relevant from irrelevant material; provides clarity to the interview

Interview Barriers

To conduct an effective patient interview, you should be aware of the potential barriers to collecting all the necessary information. By being aware of these barriers, you can make sure that you are removing as many as possible and are providing a safe environment for your patient to share information. The most common barriers are discussed in the following sections.

Providing Unwarranted Assurance

Mrs. Miller says to you, "I know this lump is going to turn out to be cancer." The typical reply is almost automatic: "Don't worry, I'm sure everything will be fine." This type of answer indicates that her anxiety is insignificant and denies her the opportunity to further discuss her fears. A reflective response, such as "You sound really worried about …" acknowledges her feelings and demonstrates empathy and a willingness to listen to her concerns.

Giving Advice

Mrs. Thompson has just finished talking to the provider. She looks at you and says, "Dr. Rowe says I need surgery to get rid of these gallstones. I just don't know. What would you do?" If you tell her how you would handle the situation, you may have shifted the accountability for decision-making from her to you, and she has not worked out her own solution. Does this woman really want to know what you would do? Probably not. You could respond to her question by saying, "Based on what the doctor told you, what do you think you should do?" or "Do you need further information to make your decision?" If the patient continues to question the provider's recommendations, the medical assistant should encourage further discussion with the provider.

Using Medical Terminology

You must adjust your vocabulary to fit the patient. The more the patient understands what is happening and how to manage the problem, the better the outcome. Misinterpreted communication is the most common error in patient care. One of the biggest problems for the patient is understanding medical terminology. Closely observe the patient's body language while she or he is receiving instructions or patient education. If the patient shows signs of not understanding the procedure, ask the patient to repeat the information or instructions back to you. This return demonstration form of providing feedback ensures that the patient completely understands what is happening. It also allows the medical assistant the opportunity to clarify any misconceptions.

Leading Questions

During the interview, you ask the patient, "You don't smoke, do you?" By asking questions in this manner, you indicate the preferred answer. Telling you that he or she does smoke would surely meet with your disapproval. Keep your questions positive. A better way of asking would be, "Have you ever smoked?" or "Do you use tobacco?"

Talking Too Much

Some medical assistants associate helpfulness with verbal overload. The patient may let the interviewer talk at the expense of his or her own need to explain what is wrong. Always remember, when interviewing a patient, you should listen more than you talk. Pay close attention to the patient's body language to make sure you give the patient ample opportunity to discuss the health problem.

Defense Mechanisms

Many individuals respond to anxiety-provoking situations by automatically relying on defense mechanisms. Defense mechanisms are used consciously or unconsciously to block an emotionally painful experience. It is understandable that patients facing a traumatic diagnosis or a difficult treatment feel the need to protect themselves from the reality of the situation. Ensuring compliance with treatment becomes an issue if the patient is in denial, projecting feelings onto the healthcare worker, or repressing the need for treatment or diagnostic follow-up. The medical assistant must be sensitive to patients' use of defense mechanisms. Consistently applying therapeutic communication techniques to interactions with patients will help to overcome the defense mechanisms.

CRITICAL THINKING APPLICATION **21.2**

Mr. Gonzales, a 48-year-old patient, recently diagnosed with hypertension, did not show up today for his follow-up appointment. Chris calls to find out why he failed to keep the appointment, and the patient tells Chris he forgot to come, even though an appointment reminder call was made yesterday. He also tells Chris he has not been taking his medicine and does not understand why it is so important for him and his wife to meet with the dietitian. Is this patient using defense mechanisms? How should Chris respond? What communication skills might promote a therapeutic relationship?

Telehealth

We have seen a significant increase in the use of telehealth for the remote care of patients. Telehealth can be used in several different ways:

- *Store-and-forward telehealth* involves the transmission of medical data to providers. This could include laboratory reports, health history, x-ray images, and demographic information.
- *Remote patient monitoring (RPM)* allows the patient to remain at home and transmit data like blood pressure (BP), glucose levels, ECG activity, and weight.

Types of Defense Mechanisms

Patients may use defense mechanisms to protect themselves from a situation they cannot manage psychologically. Defense mechanisms may hide a variety of thoughts or feelings: anger, fear, sadness, despair, or helplessness. A patient who uses defense mechanisms can be difficult to deal with. If apprised of the patient's need for psychological protection, the medical assistant may be able to find a way to provide care for the patient while maintaining a therapeutic relationship. For example, Mrs. Alicia Simone, a 48-year-old patient, has just been told she has breast cancer. The following are defense mechanisms she might display to protect herself from the psychological reality of her disease:

- *Denial:* The patient completely rejects the information. Example: "I couldn't possibly have breast cancer. You must be mistaken."
- *Suppression:* The patient is consciously aware of the information or feeling but refuses to admit it. Example: "I don't think the test is accurate. My mammograms are always normal."
- *Reaction formation:* The patient expresses her feelings as the opposite of what she really feels. Example: If she is angry at the medical assistant for insisting that a biopsy be scheduled, she may express the opposite emotion—"I appreciate your trying to help me, but I just can't come to the hospital that day."
- *Projection:* The patient accuses someone else of having feelings that she has. Example: If the patient is angry about the diagnosis, she may say to the medical assistant, "You don't have to lose your temper about this," even though the medical assistant's demeanor is completely professional.
- *Rationalization:* The patient comes up with various explanations to justify her response. Example: "I think the results are wrong. I didn't follow the directions for the tests like I should have, and besides, there's no history of breast cancer in my family."
- *Undoing:* The patient tries to reverse a negative feeling by doing something that indicates the opposite feeling. Example: If the patient feels angry and violated about the diagnosis, but she finds those feelings unacceptable, she may say, "Don't worry, dear, I'm not upset with you for telling me about this."
- *Regression:* The patient reverts to an old, usually immature behavior to vent her feelings. Example: Perhaps instead of discussing the diagnosis and the need for treatment, she just storms out of the office. Or she may say, "I can't possibly schedule a procedure without discussing this with my mother."
- *Sublimation:* The patient redirects her negative feelings into a socially-productive activity. Example: Mrs. Simone eventually becomes an active member of a local support group for women recovering from breast cancer.

- *Virtual visits or telehealth services* provide real-time, face-to-face interaction between patient and provider through audio and video technology, usually through the healthcare facility's patient portal.

The most common way for medical assistants to be involved in telehealth is with virtual health. They can assist the patient in making sure that they have the technology needed to participate in an interactive session with their provider. They may also contact the patient at the appointed time and update the patient information, including demographics, health history, medications, and allergies in the electronic health record. When this is completed, the medical assistant will connect the patient with the provider. This may involve placing the patient in a virtual waiting room until the provider is available (Procedure 21.3).

During a telemedicine visit, supervision over a medical assistant assisting a healthcare practitioner with the telemedicine visit can be provided through interactive audio and video telemedicine technology (Figure 21.9).

CRITICAL THINKING APPLICATION **21.3**

Toby Anderson, a 52-year-old, was recently diagnosed with hypertension and prescribed Lotensin twice a day for treatment. He is being seen today for a follow-up measurement of his blood pressure. Mr. Anderson is 45 pounds overweight and was given information about a reduced-calorie, low-sodium diet 1 month ago, but he has not lost any weight. He tells Chris that he has been having side effects from the medication. He is sitting with his arms across his chest, tapping his foot and occasionally cracking his knuckles.

Communication factors Chris should consider include the following:

- What nonverbal language is Mr. Anderson using, and how should Chris interpret it?
- Mr. Anderson tells Chris he is not following "that crazy diet" and never will. What therapeutic communication skills can Chris use to get more information from Mr. Anderson and reinforce the provider's recommendations?
- During the discussion, Mr. Anderson tells Chris he stopped taking the Lotensin because of the side effects. What communication techniques and therapeutic body language can Chris use to emphasize the need for Mr. Anderson to take his medicine as prescribed?

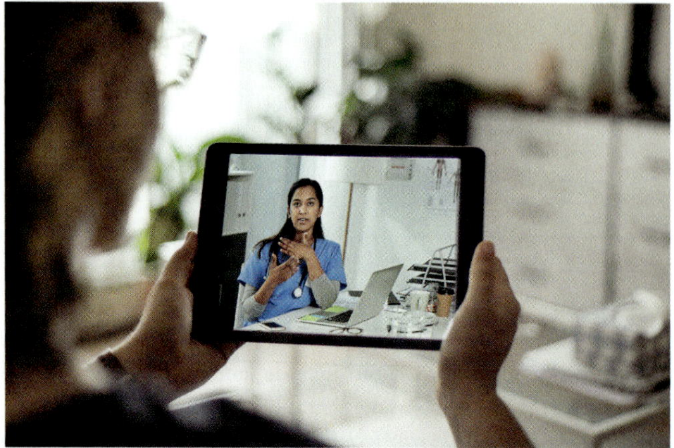

FIGURE 21.9 Medical assistant participating in interactive telehealth services. (From iStock_AJ_Watt.)

PATIENT ASSESSMENT AND DOCUMENTATION

After the interview is complete, the patient is escorted to an examination room and prepared for the physical examination. During the examination, the healthcare provider methodically checks all the body's systems. For each system, the provider mentally compares the system with established norms. Normal and abnormal findings are documented in the patient's health record. The physical examination typically starts with the head and progresses downward to the feet. However, the order may vary depending on the provider's specialty.

Signs and Symptoms

All the signs and symptoms are documented in the health record. To better understand the examination procedure, the medical assistant must know the difference between a sign and a symptom.

Subjective findings, or **symptoms**, are perceptible only to the patient; they are what the patient feels and can be interpreted only by the patient. For example, only the patient experiences and can describe his or her discomfort, pain, nausea, or dizziness. Symptoms of the greatest significance in identifying a disease are called *cardinal symptoms*. For example, crushing chest pain and difficulty breathing are cardinal symptoms of a possible heart attack.

Assessing Pain

Pain is difficult to assess. We typically rely on the patient's report of symptoms to determine his or her level of pain. Some questions you can ask to evaluate the patient's perception of pain are as follows:

- Where is the pain located? Is it associated with any particular movement?
- Can you describe how it feels? Is it constant or intermittent? Does anything relieve the pain?
- When was the onset of the pain? Did something cause the pain to start?
- Are you taking any medication to relieve the pain? What is it, and how often are you taking it? Is it effective? When was your last dose?
- Does pain affect your daily activities?
- On a scale of 1 to 10, with 10 being the highest pain level, where would you rate your pain (Figure 21.10)?

Objective findings, or **signs**, can be observed or measured by the provider or medical assistant. They are the indicators of health or disease that a provider detects when examining a patient. The provider feels, sees, hears, or measures the signs that often are associated with a certain disease or abnormal condition. For example, a mass that a provider palpates, or feels, in the patient's abdomen is an objective finding and a sign of an abnormal condition. In addition, objective data can be measured and recorded, and repeat measurements can be taken to confirm the presence of or changes in the sign. The patient's temperature, pulse, respiration, and blood pressure are objective signs the medical assistant measures and regularly records.

Documentation

Various methods can be used for documentation, depending on the healthcare provider's preference or the facility's EHR system. However, certain documentation procedures have been standardized to meet the legal requirements for maintaining medical records accurately and concisely. Complete, accurate documentation is one of the primary responsibilities of a medical assistant.

Documentation Guidelines

- Check the name on the record and make sure the documented information is recorded on the correct form in the correct patient's health record or, with an EHR system, that the correct information is recorded using the correct system prompts. Confirm the patient's identity by checking the patient's birth date.
- The month, day, and year must precede the entry; many facilities also require the time of the documentation.
- All unusual complaints, symptoms, or reactions must be noted in detail. Include complete information about the onset (when the problem started), duration (how long episodes last), and frequency (how often episodes occur) of each reported sign and symptom.
  Example: Pt reports night cough, which started 2 days ago, lasts approximately 10 minutes and occurs 3–4 times per night.
- Describe objective data, such as the presence of a wound, using correct anatomic medical terminology.
  Example: Observed wound on left distal anterior leg approximately 2 cm long and 1 cm wide.
- If the patient reports pain, record the quality and intensity of the pain using a pain scale of 1 to 10.
  Example: Pt c/o dull pain at wound site, a 4 on a scale of 1–10.
- If the comments are entered in the patient's own words, enclose them in quotation marks.
  Example: Pt states, "I fell against a stone foundation while cutting the grass and slashed my leg."
- Document the complete medication history, including both prescription and OTC medications taken on a regular basis, the last dose taken of the medication, its effectiveness, and any other pertinent details.
  Example: Pt reports taking 2 ibuprofen tablets for pain with moderate relief; last dose taken 45 minutes ago.
- Record details about the previous history of the current CC.
  Example: Pt reports having a similar cough 3 weeks ago.
- When entering information in the medical record, sign the entry, including the appropriate initials after your name (e.g., CMA).
- Learn to be observant and to note anything that seems pertinent.
- Use accurate abbreviations, symbols, and terminology (Table 21.3).
- Review your documentation immediately after completion to detect errors while the information is fresh in your mind.
- The electronic record system will automatically track any corrections made to the original documentation entry.
- If documenting in a paper record:
  - Do all charting in black ink except for noting allergies in red ink; never use pencil.
  - Write in a clear, legible manner.

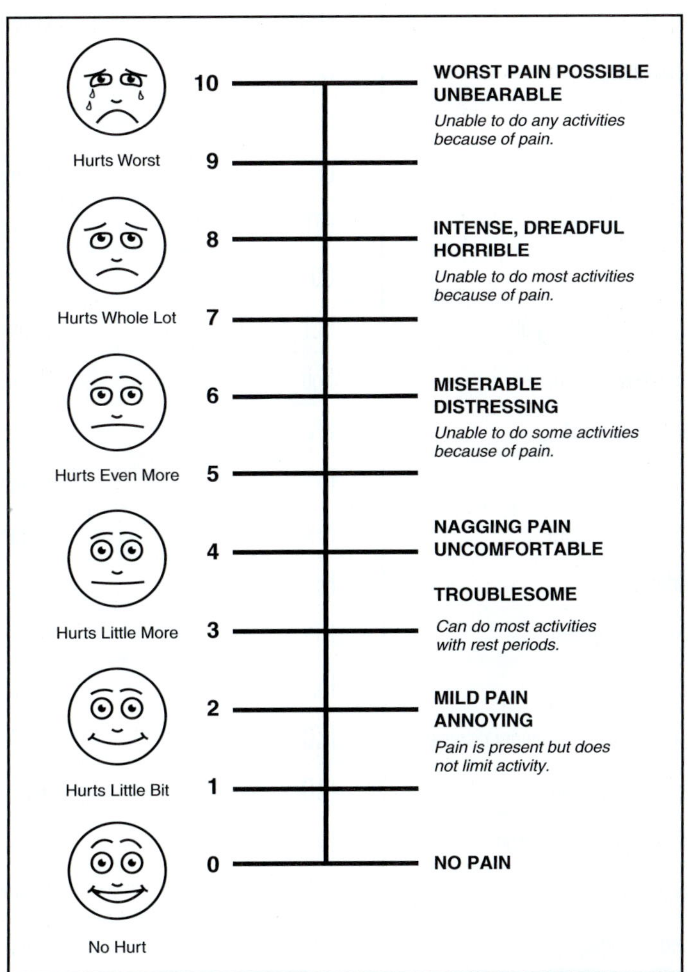

FIGURE 21.10 Wong-Baker faces pain scale.

TABLE 21.3 Medical Abbreviations

ABBREVIATION	DEFINITION	ABBREVIATION	DEFINITION
abd	Abdomen	CVA	Cerebrovascular accident
ABG	Arterial blood gases	CXR	Chest x-ray
ac	Before eating	DAT	Diet as tolerated
ACLS	Advanced cardiac life support	dc	Discontinue
ad lib	As desired	D&C	Dilation and curettage
AFP	Alpha-fetoprotein	DDx	Differential diagnosis
AKA	Above the knee amputation	DM	Diabetes mellitus
ASAP	As soon as possible	DNR	Do not resuscitate
ASHD	Atherosclerotic heart disease	DVT	Deep vein thrombosis
BE	Barium enema	Dx	Diagnosis
bid	Twice a day	ECG	Electrocardiogram
BM	Bowel movement	EENT	Eyes, ears, nose, throat
BMR	Basal metabolic rate	FBS	Fasting blood sugar
BOM	Bilateral otitis media	f/u	Follow up
BP	Blood pressure	FUO	Fever of unknown origin
BUN	Blood urea nitrogen	fx	Fracture
bx	Biopsy	GC	Gonorrhea
c̄	With	GI	Gastrointestinal
C&S	Culture and sensitivity	GTT	Glucose tolerance test
CA	Cancer	GU	Genitourinary
CABG	Coronary artery bypass graft	HCT	Hematocrit
CAD	Coronary artery disease	Hgb	Hemoglobin
CBC	Complete blood count	HIV	Human immunodeficiency virus
CC	Chief complaint	h/o	History of
CHF	Congestive heart failure	HPI	History of present illness
CHO	Carbohydrate	hs	At bedtime or hour of sleep
CNS	Central nervous system	HTN	Hypertension
c/o	Complains of	Hx	History
COPD	Chronic obstructive pulmonary disease	I&D	Incision and drainage
CPK	Creatinine phosphokinase	I&O	Intake and output
CPR	Cardiopulmonary resuscitation	IG	Immunoglobulin
CSF	Cerebrospinal fluid	lytes	Electrolytes
CT	Computed tomography	MI	Myocardial infarction

TABLE 21.3 Medical Abbreviations—*continued*

ABBREVIATION	DEFINITION	ABBREVIATION	DEFINITION
NG	Nasogastric	R/T	Related to
NKA	No known allergies	Rx	Treatment
NPO	Nothing by mouth	s̄	Without
N/V	Nausea and vomiting	SOB	Shortness of breath
p̄	After	s/s	Signs and symptoms
PE	Pulmonary embolism	STI	Sexually transmitted infection
prn	As needed	STAT	Immediately
pt	Patient	Sx	Symptoms
PE	Physical examination	Tx	Treatment
PT	Physical therapy	UA	Urinalysis
q	Every	URI	Upper respiratory infection
RBC	Red blood cells	UTI	Urinary tract infection
R/O	Rule out	VS	Vital signs
ROM	Range of motion	WNL	Within normal limits

- Do not leave any blank spaces on the paper record, and do not skip lines between documentation entries.
- Never scribble, erase, or use whiteout on an error. For legal purposes, it is crucial that the corrected error be readable.
- Correct the error by drawing one line through it. Write "error" above the corrected word or words and date and initial the correction. Then write in the correction.
- If details are omitted, add information by documenting after the last entry. Record "late entry," include date and time of note, and document the omitted information.

PHYSICAL EXAMINATION

The purpose of a physical examination is to determine the patient's overall state of well-being. All major organs and body systems are checked during a physical examination. As the entire body is examined, the provider interprets the findings. By the time the examination has been completed, the provider has formed an initial diagnosis of the patient's condition. Laboratory and other diagnostic tests are often ordered to supplement the provider's clinical diagnosis. The results of these tests are used to do the following:

- Refine the patient's diagnosis
- Help the provider plan or revise treatment for the patient
- Evaluate and maintain current drug therapy
- Determine the patient's progress

Before the examination, the medical assistant has the opportunity to make sure the patient feels comfortable during the examination process and that all the necessary medical information has been obtained. The medical assistant's duties include preparing and maintaining the examination room and equipment, preparing the patient, and assisting the provider during the physical examination.

Preparing the Examination Room

The medical assistant is responsible for making sure the examination room is ready for any procedure that might be performed during the physical examination. The area should be as comfortable as possible for the patient and free of any potential dangers, such as contaminated equipment or unlocked drug cabinets. You should prepare the examination room as follows:

- Check the area at the beginning of each day and between patients to ensure it is completely stocked with equipment and supplies and that all equipment is functioning properly. You must understand how to take care of and operate all equipment and instruments, and you should refer to operation manuals supplied by manufacturers as needed.
- Regularly check expiration dates on all packages and supplies; discard expired materials.
- Make sure the room is private, well lit, and at a comfortable temperature for the patient during the physical examination.
- Clean and disinfect the area daily and between patients to prevent the spread of infection and to ensure patients' comfort. When the patient leaves the room, discard the used exam table paper. Using disinfectant wipes, clean the table and any other potentially contaminated surface. When the table dries, replace the exam table paper.
- Arrange drapes, gowns, and all other patient supplies before the patient enters the room so that they are ready for use.

- To save time, prepare the instruments and equipment needed for the examination, arranging them for easy access before the provider enters the room.
- Make sure the examination room has all materials required for observing Standard Precautions, including gloves, a sink with soap, paper towels, biohazard waste containers, sharps containers, and impervious gowns and face guards. Sharps containers are replaced when they are two-thirds full, as indicated by Standard Precautions.

Assisting the Patient

Getting the patient ready for the examination includes taking care of paperwork before the patient enters the examination room and performing related clinical skills:

- Make sure the health record is complete and that any needed consent forms have been signed; document current medications and allergies; identify any medications that need refills. Medical assistants are not responsible for obtaining informed consent, but they should review the paperwork to ensure that the provider has reviewed the informed consent forms and that the patient signed the forms.
- Introduce yourself, verify the patient's identity, and use the patient's preferred name, making sure to show respect at all times. Pay close attention to the nonverbal language cues to make sure the patient understands what to expect.
- Obtain specimens (e.g., urine, blood) if the provider has preordered them or if this practice is part of the office policy.
- Measure and record the patient's height, weight, body mass index (BMI), and vital signs.
- Conduct the initial investigation into the reason for the visit and explain the examination procedure to the patient. Be prepared to answer the patient's questions and ease any fears. If needed, refer the patient's questions to the provider.
- Ask whether the patient needs to empty her or his bladder before the examination because a full bladder may interfere with the examination and can be uncomfortable for the patient.
- Help the patient physically prepare for the examination. Explain to the patient what clothing should be removed and what direction to put on the gown (open to the front or the back, depending on the type of examination); provide a drape to ensure the patient's privacy and help as needed.
- Assist the patient in and out of various examination positions as needed.
- Throughout this sequence of events, explain what is happening and consistently maintain the patient's privacy and confidentiality.
- Help the patient with dressing as needed after the examination.

Assisting the Provider

The medical assistant should be prepared to help the provider complete the physical examination as comprehensively and efficiently as possible. During the examination, the provider may expect the medical assistant to do the following:

- Hand the provider instruments and equipment as requested and provide supplies as needed.
- Alter the position of the light source to better illuminate the area being examined and turn lights on and off during specific phases of the examination.
- Position and drape the patient during different phases of the examination.
- Assist in collecting and properly labeling specimens such as urine, Pap test specimens, and throat cultures.
- Conduct any diagnostic tests preordered by the provider, including hearing and vision screenings.
- Conduct follow-up diagnostic procedures as ordered, including an **electrocardiogram (ECG, EKG)**, urinalysis, and phlebotomy.
- Document patient data in the health record, completing all forms required.
- Schedule post-examination diagnostic procedures, such as mammography, x-ray examination, or colonoscopy.

Supplies and Instruments Needed for the Physical Examination

The instruments typically used during the physical examination are shown in Figure 21.11. They enable the provider to see, feel, inspect, and listen to parts of the body. All equipment must be in good working order, properly disinfected, and readily available for the provider's use during the examination. The instruments most frequently used for a physical examination are described in Table 21.4. Physical examinations are typically performed from the head to the feet; the instruments are listed in the order the provider typically would request them.

ASSISTING WITH THE PHYSICAL EXAMINATION

During the actual physical examination, the medical assistant can be responsible for several different aspects of patient care. Throughout the examination, the patient may need to be placed in a number of different positions. To protect the patient's modesty, you should use the proper draping technique for each position. To protect yourself and your patient, you should also use proper body mechanics. It is important to have an understanding of the different methods of examination and the examination sequence. All elements of assisting with the physical examination are discussed in the following sections.

Positioning and Draping the Patient for the Physical Examination

Various patient positions are used to facilitate a physical examination. The medical assistant instructs the patient and assists the patient into these positions, ensuring as much ease and modesty as possible. The medical assistant may also help the patient maintain the position during the examination with as little discomfort as possible. Do not place a patient into a position that is uncomfortable or that compromises the patient's privacy until it is necessary to complete that part of the examination. Never leave the patient's side if the position could result in a fall.

Draping the patient with a sheet protects the individual from embarrassment and keeps the patient warm. However, the sheet must be positioned so that it allows complete visibility for the examiner and does not interfere with the examination. During the general examination, each part of the body is exposed one portion at a time. For gynecologic and rectal examinations, the sheet is positioned on the diagonal across the patient, or in a diamond shape, to provide maximum comfort for the patient while allowing the provider to perform the examination.

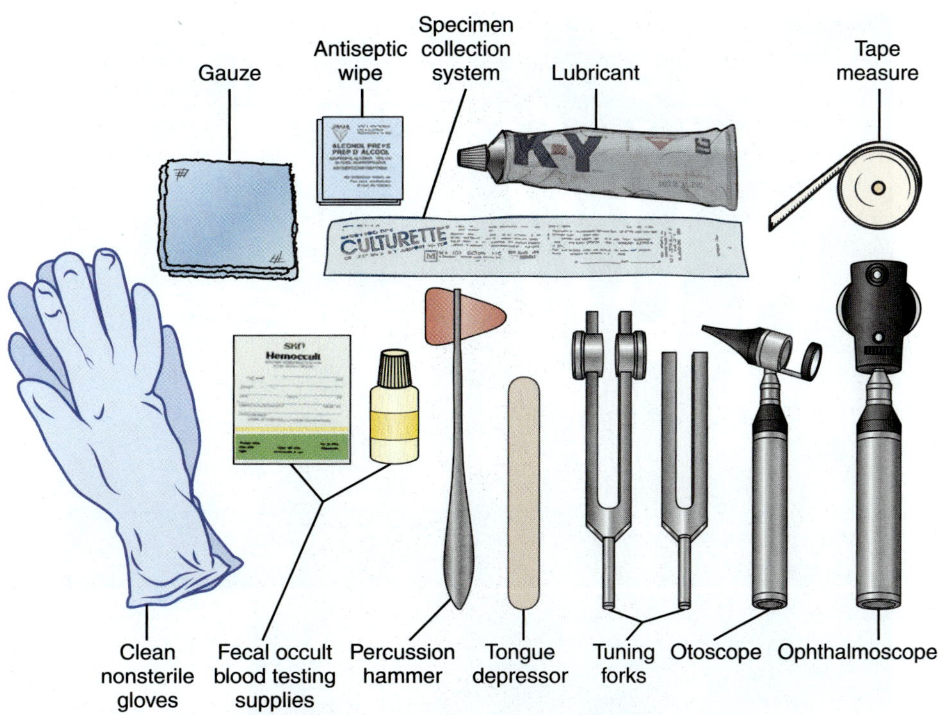

FIGURE 21.11 Instruments for the physical examination.

TABLE 21.4 Instruments Needed for the Physical Examination

INSTRUMENT	USE
Ophthalmoscope	To inspect the inner structures of the eye. It consists of a stainless-steel handle containing batteries and an attached head, which has a light, magnifying lenses, and an opening through which the eye is viewed.
Tongue depressor	A flat, wooden blade used to hold down the tongue when the throat is examined.
Otoscope	To examine the external auditory canal and tympanic membrane. It has a stainless-steel handle containing batteries or is part of a wall-mounted electrical unit. The head of the otoscope has a light that is focused through a magnifying lens; it should be covered with a disposable ear speculum. The light also may be used to illuminate the nasal passages and throat.
Tuning fork	Aluminum, fork-shaped instrument that consists of a handle and two prongs (Figure 21.12). The prongs produce a humming sound when the provider strikes them against his or her hand. Tuning forks are available in different sizes, and each size produces a different pitch level. A tuning fork is used to check the patient's auditory acuity and to test bone vibration. A tuning fork can also be used to test for diabetic **peripheral neuropathy**.
Tape measure	A flexible ribbon ruler that is usually printed in inches and feet on one side and in centimeters and meters on the reverse side. Measurements may be used to assess length and head circumference in infants, wound size, etc.
Stethoscope	A listening device used when certain areas of the body are auscultated, particularly the heart and lungs. This instrument is available in many shapes and sizes. All have two earpieces that are connected to flexible rubber or vinyl tubing (Figure 21.13). At the distal end of the tubing is a diaphragm or bell (many have both); when it is placed securely on the patient's skin, it enables the provider to hear internal body sounds.
Reflex hammer	Sometimes called a percussion hammer. This stainless-steel instrument has a hard rubber head that is used to strike the tendons of the knee and elbow to test the neurologic reflexes.
Gloves	Gloves protect the healthcare worker and the patient from microorganisms. According to Standard Precautions, gloves must be worn whenever the potential exists for contact with any body fluid, broken skin or wounds, or contaminated items.
Additional supplies	Gauze, cotton balls, cotton-tipped applicators, disposable tissues, specimen containers, fecal occult blood test cards, Pap test supplies for female patients, lubricating jelly for vaginal and rectal examinations, and laboratory request forms should be easily accessible during the examination.

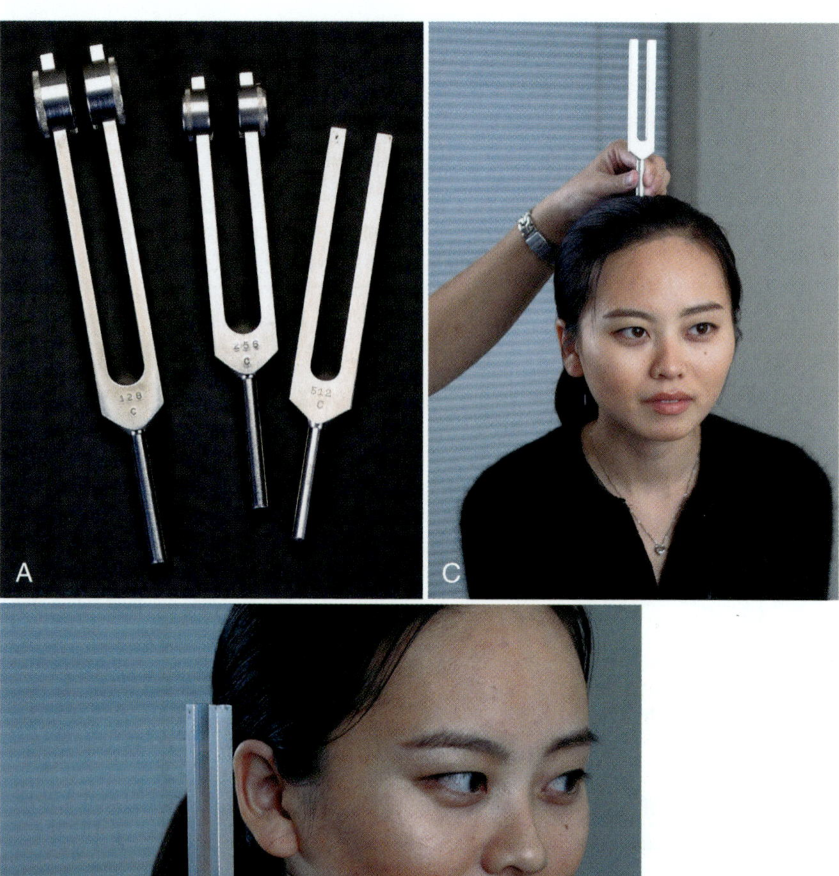

FIGURE 21.12 Tuning forks.

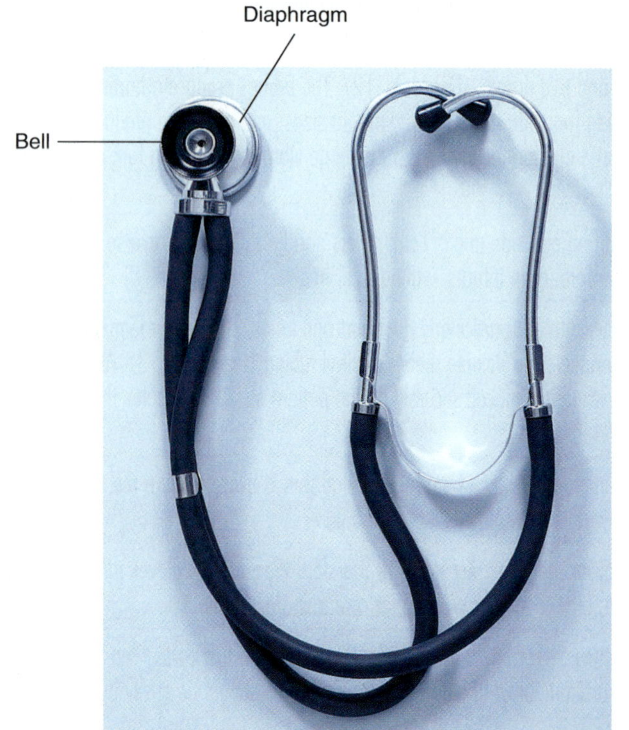

FIGURE 21.13 Stethoscope. (Modified from Ball JW, et al: *Seidel's guide to physical examination*, ed 8, St. Louis, 2015,Mosby.)

The following sections describe a number of the positions used during medical examinations.

Fowler Position

In the Fowler position, the patient sits on the examination table with the head of the table elevated 90 degrees. This position is useful for examinations and treatments of the head, neck, and chest and for patients who have difficulty breathing while lying down. Drape placement varies depending on the type of physical examination done and the need to maintain the patient's modesty (Procedure 21.4).

Semi-Fowler Position

The semi-Fowler position is a modification of the Fowler position. The head of the table is positioned at a 45-degree angle instead of at a full 90-degree angle. This position is useful for postoperative examinations, patients with breathing disorders, and patients suffering from head **trauma** or pain (see Procedure 21.4). The drape or gown should cover the entire patient from the nipple line down.

Supine (Horizontal Recumbent) Position

In the supine position, the patient lies flat with the face upward and the lower legs supported by the table extension (Procedure 21.5). This position is used to examine the front of the body, including the heart, breasts, and abdominal organs. The patient's gown should open down the front, and the drape should be placed over any exposed area that is not being examined.

Dorsal Recumbent Position

In the dorsal recumbent position, the patient lies face upward, with the weight distributed primarily to the surface of the back. This is accomplished by flexing the knees so that the feet are flat on the table. This position relieves muscle tension in the abdomen and may be used for examination or inspection of the rectal, vaginal, and **perineal** areas. It may also be used if the patient experiences back discomfort when lying supine. This position can be used for digital examination of the vagina and rectum, but it is not used if an instrument such as a speculum is needed. it is important to keep the patient completely draped, with the drape in a diamond shape, to ensure the patient's privacy, until the provider is present (see Procedure 21.5).

Lithotomy Position

The patient should not be placed in the *lithotomy* position until the provider is in the examination room and is ready for this part of the examination. Place the patient on his or her back with the knees sharply flexed and the arms at the sides or folded over the chest; have the patient slide the buttocks down to the bottom edge of the table. Support the feet in stirrups placed wide apart and somewhat away from the table, with the stirrup arms extended to match the length of the patient's legs. If the heels are too close to the buttocks, the possibility of leg cramps increases, and it is more difficult for the patient to relax the abdominal muscles. Make sure the stirrups are locked in place. Place a drape diagonally over the patient's abdomen and knees. The drape must be long enough to cover the knees and touch the ankles and wide enough to prevent the sides of the thighs from being exposed. The provider lifts the drape away from the pubic area when the examination begins (Procedure 21.6). The lithotomy position is used primarily for vaginal examinations that require the use of a speculum and for Pap tests.

Left Lateral Position

The patient is placed on the left side; the left arm and shoulder are drawn back behind the body so that the body's weight is predominantly on the chest. The right arm is flexed upward for support. The left leg is slightly flexed, and the buttocks are pulled to the edge of the table. The right leg is sharply flexed upward. The drape extends diagonally from under the arms to below the knees. The provider can raise a small portion of the sheet from the back of the patient to expose the rectum sufficiently. The remaining portion of the sheet covers the patient's chest area and thighs. This position is used for rectal examinations, for instillation of rectal medication, and for some perineal and pelvic examinations (Procedure 21.7).

Prone Position

In the prone position, the patient lies face down on the table on the ventral surface of the body. This is the opposite of the supine position and is another of the recumbent positions. The drape should cover from the middle of the back to below the knees, with the gown opening in the back (Procedure 21.8). This position is used to examine the back and for certain surgical procedures.

Knee-Chest Position

For the knee-chest position, the patient rests on the knees, and the chest with the head turned to one side. The arms can be placed under the head for support and comfort, or they can be bent and placed at the sides of the table near the head. The thighs are perpendicular to the table and slightly separated. The buttocks extend up into the air, and the back should be straight. The patient will need assistance to assume the knee-chest position correctly. Most patients have difficulty maintaining this position, so they should not be placed into it until it is required. The medical assistant must remain next to the patient for assistance and support the entire time the knee-chest position is needed. If the correct knee-chest position cannot be obtained, the patient may need to be placed in a knee-elbow position. This position puts less strain on the patient and is easier to maintain. These positions are used for proctologic examination and for sigmoid, rectal, and occasionally vaginal examinations. The patient's gown should open in the back, and a fenestrated (opening) drape or a single sheet should be draped diagonally over the patient's back at the sacral area (Procedure 21.9).

CRITICAL THINKING APPLICATION **21.4**

Determine the correct patient position and method of gowning and draping for the following examinations:

- Insertion of a rectal suppository
- Annual Papanicolaou (Pap) test
- Examination of the back
- Patient with dyspnea
- Breast examination

Principles of Body Mechanics

Medical assistants should consistently use proper body mechanics throughout the work environment when sitting or standing, lifting, or carrying objects, pushing or pulling, or transferring patients. Without consistent application of correct anatomic alignment, injuries, especially lower back injuries, easily occur.

Proper body alignment begins with good posture. Maintaining posture requires a combination of muscle efforts. Good posture keeps the spine balanced and aligned while a person is sitting or standing. A person in good body alignment can maintain balance without undue strain on the musculoskeletal system.

When reaching for an object, avoid twisting or turning; instead, move the feet to face the object needed; this prevents undue strain on the lumbar region. Do not cross the legs while sitting because this interferes with circulation to the legs and feet. When sitting, keep the popliteal area (behind the knees) free of the edge of the chair. Pressure in this area interferes with circulation and may damage nerves behind the knees. Do a mental check of your posture regularly. Hold the head erect, the face forward and the chin slightly up, the abdominal muscles contracted up and in, the shoulders relaxed and back, the feet pointed forward and slightly apart, and the weight evenly distributed to both legs, with the knees slightly bent. Always be alert for poor body mechanics that may cause injury (Figures 21.14 and 21.15).

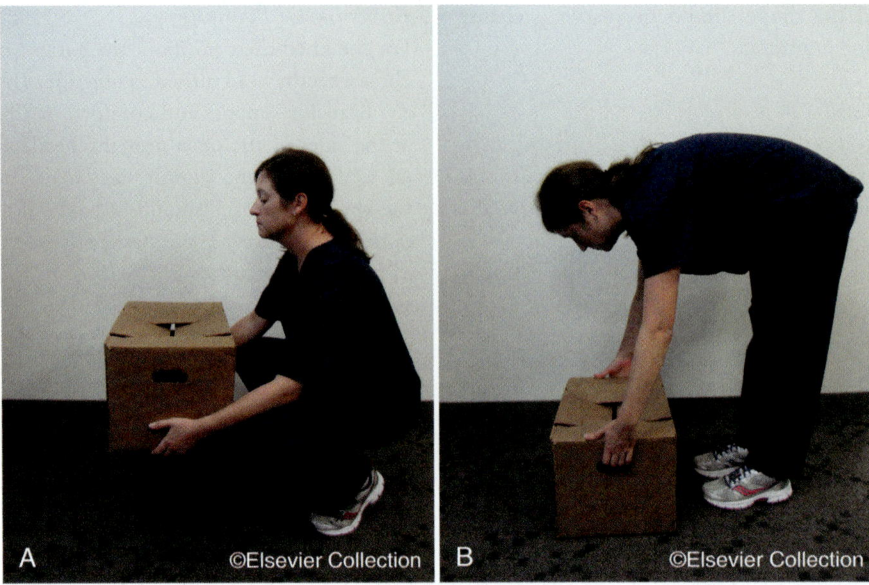

FIGURE 21.14 **(A)** Proper lifting technique. **(B)** Improper lifting technique.

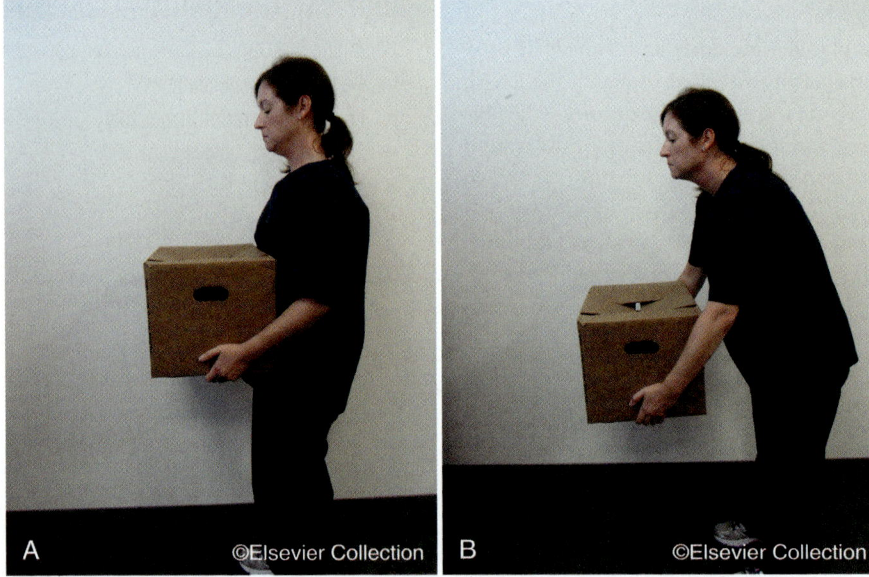

FIGURE 21.15 **(A)** Carrying an item close to the body. **(B)** Improper carrying technique.

Safe Lifting Techniques

- Always get help if the load is too heavy.
- Maintain correct body alignment, with the legs spread apart for a broad base of support.
- Do not reach for items; clear barriers out of the way and get as close as possible to what needs to be lifted.
- Bend at the knees with the feet shoulder-width apart and keep the back straight. Use the major muscle groups of the arms and legs rather than the weaker ones of the back to help lift a heavy item (see Figure 21.14).

Transferring a Patient

Patients may need assistance moving from a chair to the examination table or back again. Patients can be transferred in multiple ways, but all should focus on correct body mechanics. If the patient is in a wheelchair, move the chair at a 45-degree angle toward the footrest that extends from the bottom of the exam table (Figure 21.16), lock the wheels, and lift the footrests of the wheelchair out of the way. Explain the procedure to the patient and ask for his or her assistance.

If one side of the patient is weaker than the other, always provide support on the weak side. Support the patient close to your body on the strong side, with one hand under the axillary region and the other either grasping the patient's hand or holding the forearm. When bending, always bend at the knees and maintain the back's three natural curves, allowing the leg muscles to help in lifting. Give the patient a signal and lift as the patient assists. Help the patient step up onto the footrest with the strong leg first, then pivot. Ease the patient down onto the table, bending your knees while keeping your back aligned. Make sure the patient is comfortable and safely positioned on the table.

Use a gait belt as needed to help transfer patients, prevent injury to yourself, and safeguard patients from falling. A gait belt is a safety device that is used to help transfer a patient from a wheelchair to the

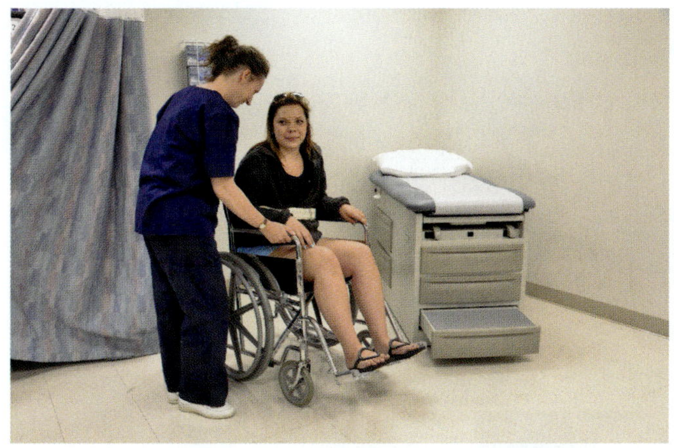

FIGURE 21.16 Wheelchair at a 45-degree angle at the end of the exam table.

exam table or to help a patient walk. The gait belt helps you support the patient while keeping your body in proper alignment to prevent back injuries. A gait belt should be used if the patient is weak and at risk of falling. Follow these steps to use a gait belt:

- Place the belt around the individual's waist over clothing with the buckle in front.
- Insert the belt through the teeth of the buckle and pull it tight to lock it.
- The belt should be tight, with just enough room to place your fingers under it.
- Grip the belt tightly, bend your knees and keep your back straight.
- Ask the patient to assist you; then lift using your arm and leg muscles.
- Avoid twisting or turning as you help the patient stand.
- Keep your body close to the patient with your knees in front of his or hers at all times to stabilize the patient and prevent falls.
- Complete the transfer without bending or twisting your body; encourage the patient to bear as much weight as possible and gently sit down on the table.
- After transferring the patient, remove the gait belt for the provider's examination and replace it to help transfer the patient back to the wheelchair after the provider is finished.
- If the patient should start to fall during a transfer, do not try to stop the fall because you may be injured; use the gait belt to help guide the patient to the floor as gently as possible.

You may need to remain with the patient until the examination has been completed to ensure his or her safety. If the provider prefers that the patient is in a supine position, place one arm across the patient's shoulders and the other under the knees and smoothly lower the patient's upper body to the table while raising the legs. Use the same pivoting techniques with proper body mechanics to help transfer the patient from the examination table back to the locked wheelchair. If the patient must hold onto you, have the person hold your waist or shoulders, not your neck (Procedure 21.10).

Methods of Examination

Examinations are performed as both a routine confirmation of wellness and a means of diagnosing disease. Healthcare providers use six methods to examine the human body:

- Inspection
- Palpation
- Percussion
- Auscultation
- Mensuration
- Manipulation

All six are part of a complete physical examination.

Inspection

During the *inspection*, the examiner uses observation to detect significant physical features or objective data. This method of examination ranges from focusing on the patient's general appearance (general state of health, including posture, mannerisms, and grooming) to more detailed observations, including body contour, **gait**, **symmetry**, visible injuries and deformities, tremors, rashes, and color changes. Inspection will be done before palpation or percussion so that there will be no changes made to the appearance of the skin.

Palpation

In **palpation**, the examiner uses the sense of touch (Figure 21.17A). A part of the body is felt with the hand to determine its condition or the condition of an underlying organ. Palpation may involve touching the skin or performing a firmer exploration of the abdomen for underlying masses. With this technique, the provider is assessing the following:

- Temperature
- Vibration
- Consistency
- Form
- Size
- Rigidity
- Elasticity
- Moisture
- Texture
- Position
- Contour

Palpation is performed with one hand, both hands (bimanual), one finger (digital), the fingertips, or the palmar aspect of the hand. A pelvic examination is done bimanually, whereas an anal examination is performed digitally. Do not confuse palpation with *palpitation*, which is a throbbing pulsation felt in the chest.

Percussion

Percussion involves tapping or striking the body, usually with the fingers or a small hammer. This will cause sounds, vibratory sensations, or involuntary reactions. Percussion can help to determine the position, size, and density of an underlying organ or cavity. The examiner both hears and feels the effect of percussion. It is helpful in determining the amount of air or solid matter in an underlying organ or cavity. The two basic methods of percussion are direct percussion and indirect percussion. *Direct percussion* is performed by striking the body with a finger or a reflex hammer. With *indirect percussion*, which is used more frequently, the provider places his or her hand on the area and then strikes the placed hand with a finger of the other hand (Figure 21.17B). Both a sound and a sense of vibration are evident. The examiner assesses the sound in terms of pitch, quality, duration, and resonance.

Auscultation

For *auscultation*, the provider uses a stethoscope to listen to sounds from the body. Auscultation is a complex method of examination

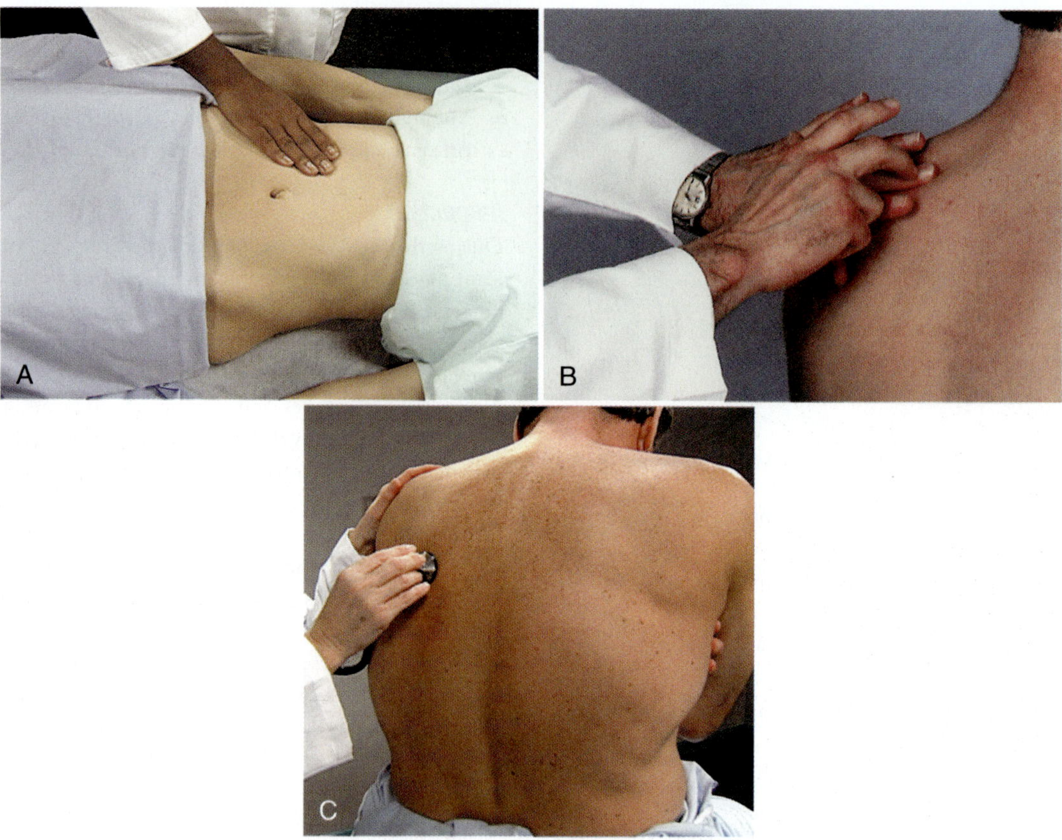

FIGURE 21.17 **(A)** Demonstration of palpation. **(B)** Demonstration of percussion. **(C)** Demonstration of auscultation. (From Ball JW, et al: *Seidel's guide to physical examination,* ed 8, St. Louis, 2015, Mosby.)

because the provider must distinguish between a normal sound and an abnormal sound (Figure 21.17C). It is particularly useful for evaluating sounds originating in the lungs, heart, and abdomen, such as a **murmur**, a **bruit**, and bowel sounds.

Mensuration

Mensuration is the process of measuring. Measurements that are recorded include the following:

- Height and weight
- Size and depth of a wound
- Extent of **flexion** or **extension** of an extremity
- Size of the uterus during pregnancy
- Pressure of a grip
- Length and diameter of an extremity

Measurements are taken with a flexible tape measure, a circular wound measurement device (Figure 21.18), or a specialized piece of equipment (e.g., a goniometer, which is used to measure joint angles) and usually are recorded in centimeters.

Manipulation

Manipulation is the passive movement of a joint to determine the range of extension or flexion of a part of the body. Insurance and industrial reports often request this information in detail. For example, a patient involved in a work-related accident that caused joint damage may have to perform assisted range-of-motion (ROM) exercises to the joint, with subsequent joint flexion and extension measurements to demonstrate improvement or lack thereof.

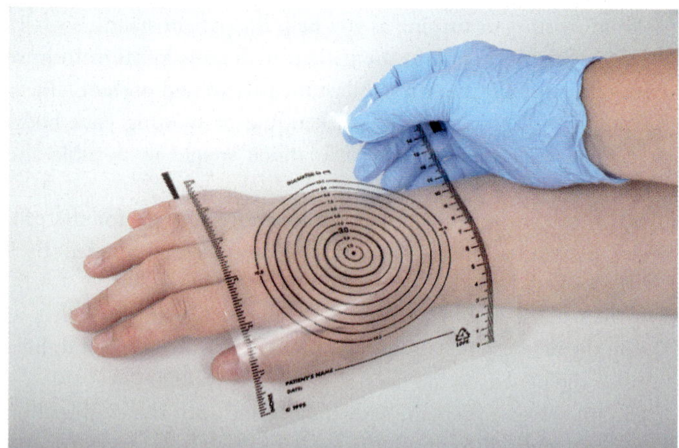

FIGURE 21.18 Circular wound measurement device.

Examination Sequence

The physical examination sequence is fairly standard; however, variations may occur, depending on the provider's specialty, the reason for the examination, and the provider's preference. Patients are more cooperative and less anxious if they understand what is expected of them. Start by giving the patient a brief explanation of the examination process. Many healthcare facilities provide the option for patients to have a chaperone present during physical examinations. Assemble all supplies and instruments needed for the examination before the provider enters the room. As the provider proceeds with the examination, make sure the patient remains unexposed by adjusting the drape and gown as needed. During the examination, the medical assistant assists by handing the provider the correct instruments and needed supplies. When the provider begins the examination, the medical assistant should keep conversation to a minimum and remain **inconspicuous**.

The examination usually starts with the patient seated at the end of the exam table or in the Fowler position if the patient needs support. If the provider uses reflected light, the light source should be behind the patient's right shoulder. If illuminated instruments are used, standard overhead lights are sufficient. Take care not to shine a light directly into the patient's eyes; this can be done by turning on lights while they are directed away from the patient and carefully moving the light toward the area.

Chaperones During Physical Examinations

It is becoming common for chaperones to be present during physical examinations. Having a third person in the exam room provides protection for both the patient and the provider. A medical assistant may be asked to be a chaperone.

A chaperone can reassure the patient about the professional character of the healthcare facility. The patient has the right to refuse to have a chaperone present in the room, but most are accepting. When the chaperone is another health professional, such as a medical assistant, she or he can serve two purposes: as a chaperone and as an assistant to the provider.

If a healthcare facility is going to have chaperones present, there should be a written policy that describes the role of the chaperone. This policy should allow for a private conversation between the patient and the provider.

General Appearance

The provider starts the physical examination by observing the patient's appearance, using an inspection technique. The general appearance explains whether the patient appears well and in good health (e.g., note whether the patient appears disoriented or in distress, well-nourished or undernourished, and answers questions with ease or confusion).

The patient's gait often provides important information. The patient may limp, walk with the feet wide apart, have a shuffle step, or have difficulty maintaining his or her balance. Posture is also checked for indications of pain, stiffness, or difficulty with limb movement. The provider notes body build and proportions. Any *gross* (immediately obvious) deformities are recorded. Sometimes abnormalities in height or body proportion may be caused by hormonal imbalances. If the medical assistant notices any of these or the patient reports any complaints, these should be documented in the patient's health record, along with the vital signs, before the provider begins the examination.

Speech

Speech may reveal a pathologic condition. Some basic speech defects include *aphonia,* the inability to speak because of loss of the voice, which is commonly seen with severe *laryngitis* or overuse of the voice; *aphasia,* the loss of expression by speech or writing because of an injury or disease of the brain; and *dysphasia,* lack of coordination and failure to arrange words in proper order, usually caused by a brain lesion. With *motor aphasia,* patients know what they want to say but cannot use muscles properly to speak; for example, this may be noted as slurred or incoherent speech that might occur after a cerebrovascular accident (CVA). In *sensory aphasia,* patients pronounce words easily but use them inaccurately, as in jumbled speech. Speech is also assessed in well-child checkups. A delay in speech development can indicate an issue (e.g., a neurologic deficit or possible autism spectrum disorder) and the need for a referral.

Skin

The skin's condition can be a reflection of the patient's nutritional status and hydration level. If dehydration is suspected, skin **turgor** is checked by pinching the skin on the posterior surface of the hands. The tissue is observed to see how quickly it returns to its normal location. A delay indicates a decrease in tissue fluid, confirming the diagnosis of dehydration. Extreme dryness, scaling, extended time for wound healing, or frequent breaks in the skin may indicate systemic disease.

Fingernails and toenails often give some indication of a person's health. Brittle, grooved, or lined nails may indicate local infection or systemic disease. **Clubbing** of the fingertips is associated with some congenital heart or lung diseases. Spooning of the nail is seen in some patients with severe iron-deficiency anemia. *Beau lines*, deep grooved horizontal lines, appear after an acute illness but grow out and disappear. The provider may refer a patient with skin disorders to a dermatologist for diagnosis and treatment.

Head

Once the provider makes the overall observations of the patient's general condition, the physical examination typically begins with the head and face and moves downward to the feet. The face reflects the patient's state and tells the provider a great deal about how the patient handles stress and illness. The skull, scalp, and face are palpated for size, shape, and symmetry. The distribution or lack of hair and hair texture may indicate hormonal changes. Excessive hair, especially facial hair in females, indicates a hormonal imbalance. As the head is palpated, the provider assesses possible **nodules**, masses, or signs of trauma.

Eyes

The pupils are checked for reaction by shining a light into one eye at a time. If the pupils constrict equally and smoothly to a light stimulus, the provider documents "PERRLA" (which means the pupils are equal, round, react to light, and accommodation). The **sclera** is checked for color, which ranges from white to pale yellow. If the eye is inflamed, it will be evident in the sclera. A sclera with a yellow tone indicates liver disease. Movements of the eyes are tested by having the patient follow the provider's finger. If eye movement is within average range, "extraocular movement (EOM) intact" is documented. The *ophthalmoscope* is used to examine the interior of the eye, including the retina and intraocular vessels. Some diseases, such as diabetes mellitus and hypertension, damage the blood vessels of the retina.

Ears

The ears are examined with an otoscope covered with a disposable speculum. The external ear is checked first for inflammation of the external auditory canal or *cerumen* (earwax). The *tympanic membrane* (eardrum) is examined and should appear pearly gray. Scars on the eardrum are frequently the result of earlier, chronic ear infections or perforations. The color of the eardrum is important to the diagnosis because it may indicate fluids such as blood or pus behind the eardrum in the middle ear. The patient may be asked to swallow several times to allow observation of movement of the tympanic membrane, which occurs because of pressure changes in the eustachian tube. The eustachian tube equalizes air pressure between the middle ear and the throat. The ability of the tympanic membrane to move is crucial to the hearing process.

Nose and Sinuses

The mucosa of the nasal cavity is examined for color and texture. The sinuses cannot be seen, but the frontal and maxillary sinuses may be examined by firm palpation over the area and by **transillumination**. When disorders of the eyes, ears, nose, and throat are observed, and the provider believes that the condition warrants the attention of a specialist, the patient is referred to an ophthalmologist or an otorhinolaryngologist (ear, nose, and throat specialist).

Mouth and Throat

The mouth, or oral cavity, is usually thought of in terms of oral hygiene and dental care. Dental hygiene includes the condition of the teeth, how the patient cares for the teeth and gums, and whether the teeth of the upper and lower jaws meet properly (occlude) for chewing. Healthy gums are pale pink, glossy, and smooth and do not bleed when pressure from a tongue depressor is applied. The palatine tonsils are usually visible. The provider may use a tongue depressor and a piece of gauze to grasp the tongue to examine it carefully. The floor of the mouth is examined by both inspection and palpation for enlarged lymph nodes, salivary gland function, and ulcerations. The insides of the cheeks and the gum line are also examined for any abnormal marks or color. The provider may use the otoscope light to help with the examination.

Neck

The neck is examined for ROM by having the patient move the head in various directions. The thyroid gland is given special attention for symmetry, size, and texture. The provider manually palpates the thyroid area while the patient swallows several times because this action elevates the thyroid lobes. The carotid artery is palpated and **auscultate**d for possible bruits. The lymph nodes are palpated. *Lymphadenopathy* (enlargement of the lymph nodes) can occur if the patient has an infection of the face, head, or neck.

Chest

While the patient is still in the sitting position, the chest, heart, and lungs are examined. The chest is examined for symmetric expansion. A tape measure may be used, especially if variation exists between the upper and lower chest expansion. A patient with a history of **emphysema** may have a barrel-shaped chest. The provider may use percussion to determine the density of lung tissues.

Placing a stethoscope on the patient's back, the examiner auscultates lung sounds. The patient is asked to take deep, regular breaths. This may produce slight dizziness, but the patient should be assured that it is only the result of the deep respirations and will rapidly pass. The provider notes the types of respirations and the presence of lung sounds in all lobes.

Because considerable concentration is required to interpret heart sounds, the provider must have complete silence when listening to the patient's heart. In patients with heart disease, the provider may spend an extended time listening to heart sounds. If lung or heart abnormalities are found, the provider typically orders further diagnostic tests, including blood analysis, x-ray evaluation, and an ECG. Once the results of these studies have been analyzed, the provider may refer the patient to a *cardiologist* for treatment of a heart condition, or a *pulmonologist* or a respiratory care specialist for treatment of a breathing disorder.

Abdomen

For the abdominal part of the examination, the patient is lowered to the dorsal recumbent or supine position, and the drape is lowered to the pubic hairline. The gown is raised to just under the breasts. The patient's arms may be placed at the side or the hands crossed over the chest or under the head. Relaxation of the abdominal muscles is needed for the abdominal examination. To assist in this goal and to promote patient comfort, a small pillow can be placed under the head and knees. The provider auscultates the abdomen in all quadrants to confirm the presence of complete bowel sounds and palpates the abdomen for any abnormalities. The provider also may use percussion to determine the density, position, and size of underlying abdominal organs.

Reflexes

The patient's reflexes are checked with the patient sitting, in the Fowler position, or supine. While the patient is sitting, the biceps are checked with the patient's arm flexed and supported by the examiner. The knee jerk (patellar reflex) and the ankle jerk (Achilles reflex) are checked using tapotement (a tapping or percussing movement) with either the fingers or the reflex hammer. The plantar reflexes (Babinski reflex and Chaddock reflex) are tested with the patient in an upright or a supine position.

Breasts and Testicles

Careful breast examination is part of the physical examination for every female, even if she is asymptomatic. The breasts are examined by inspection and by palpation with the patient in the supine position. The arm on the side that is being examined is bent and tucked under the head. Breast cancer is the most common malignancy in women, and early detection is the key to successful treatment. This is a good opportunity to discuss and reinforce the consistent use of monthly breast self-examination (BSE). For male patients who have reached puberty or are 14 years of age or older, the provider performs a testicular examination. The testicular self-examination (TSE) is an important self-examination for all males to perform each month because testicular carcinoma is a major health risk that has a high cure rate if discovered early.

CRITICAL THINKING APPLICATION 21.5

Alice Greenbaum, a 68-year-old patient of Dr. Walden, is scheduled for an annual physical examination, including a breast check and Pap test. Mrs. Greenbaum appears anxious and asks Chris whether the gynecologic examination is necessary. How should Chris answer this patient? What might help ease the patient's fears and prepare her for the examination?

Rectum

The rectal examination usually follows the abdominal examination or may be part of the examination of the genitalia. Preserving the patient's comfort and dignity is vital. For this part of the examination, the provider needs gloves and water-soluble lubricating jelly (e.g., K-Y Jelly). The examination light should be directed at the perineal area during the examination.

Fecal occult blood test specimens are often collected during the digital rectal examination. If this is a procedure the provider performs, be sure to include the necessary collection folder with the examination equipment. Patients diagnosed with gastrointestinal (GI) disorders may be referred to a gastroenterologist. Procedure 21.11 presents the steps for assisting with the physical examination.

CLOSING COMMENTS

Medical assistants play a vital role in the physical examination process. Having good communication skills helps in all aspects of the physical examination. Being familiar with the supplies needed and making sure they are available in the examination room makes the process more efficient. Using good body mechanics helps to protect you and your patient. Using what you have learned in this chapter will help to make you a valued medical assistant.

Patient Coaching

The physical examination process is an excellent time for the medical assistant to assess the need for patient education. This assessment should be performed to identify the best ways to meet the patient's needs. When identifying these needs, consider the following:

- The information the patient needs to know
- How to convey the information so that the patient understands it
- How the patient will use the information
- Whether any community resources are available that might help the patient understand and learn more about health problems or treatment protocols

Develop a plan to teach the patient. Think about the different modalities available, such as pamphlets, pictures, DVDs, demonstrations, websites, and community resources. The more interesting the information, the more fun it is to teach the patient and the more enjoyment the patient will get out of learning. Many facilities keep patient education files that contain handouts on a wide range of health issues. The medical assistant should always review teaching plans with the provider and follow the provider's direction in patient education.

Legal and Ethical Issues

The medical history is a confidential record that can be shared only with healthcare personnel directly involved in the patient's care. Data provided to you by the patient or that you read in the patient's health record is confidential; you must not share any of this information with anyone. The consequences for disclosing private information to individuals not involved in the patient's care can be very serious and can result in the loss of your job, court-imposed fines, and even imprisonment.

In addition to maintaining patient confidentiality, consistently implementing correct documentation procedures is crucial for medical practices. The medical record is considered a legal document, and court cases can be won or lost based on the clarity and completeness of staff documentation. It is essential that medical assistants document all patient information in a factual, nonjudgmental manner.

Patient-Centered Care

The ability to communicate effectively is crucial to the role of the professional medical assistant and allows for excellent customer service. Effective communication includes the use of all of the therapeutic tools discussed in this chapter. The professional medical assistant should do the following:

- Watch for nonverbal behaviors to verify congruence between what the patient states verbally and demonstrates via body language.
- Modify communication methods as needed to meet the needs of a diverse patient population.
- Use restatement, reflection, and clarification to gather pertinent and comprehensive patient information.
- Use electronic communication appropriately and effectively.

Professional Behaviors

Courteous and respectful care is the hallmark of professional medical assistant behavior. Many times, the physical examination process requires patients to expose very private parts of their bodies, which can make them feel quite uncomfortable. Safeguarding the patient's privacy as much as possible with adequate gowning and draping helps prevent undue exposure and embarrassment for patients during the examination process. Treating patients with thoughtful consideration goes a long way in making them feel more comfortable with physical examination procedures.

SUMMARY OF SCENARIO

Chris has met with the office supervisor and reviewed essential techniques for gathering patient information. Therapeutic communication includes demonstrating respectful patient care, using active listening skills, observing nonverbal behaviors, and using a combination of open- and closed-ended questions to gather the best possible detail about the patient's chief complaint. The supervisor gave Chris a variety of information on meeting the needs of a diverse patient population and also gave him suggestions on how to develop empathetic, helping relationships with patients.

Chris has also taken responsibility for ensuring that exam rooms are fully supplied and equipment is in working order. He is able to place patients in all of the appropriate positions during the examination and run the vision and screening tests ordered by the providers. He is also aware of using correct body mechanics when working at a healthcare facility.

SUMMARY OF LEARNING OBJECTIVES

1. **Examine how to collect the history information and the components of the patient's health history.**
The medical history consists of the patient's database, past medical history, and family and social histories, in addition to the review of systems. A new patient should fill out a health history form, either online through a patient portal, electronically, or on paper.

2. **Discuss how to successfully understand and communicate with patients and display sensitivity to diverse populations.**
Developing a professional helping relationship with patients is the responsibility of all healthcare workers. The helping relationship involves consistent application of respectful patient care that recognizes the impact of a patient's anxieties on interactions and responses to treatment. (See Procedure 21.1.)

   Sensitivity to diverse populations includes using empathetic communications and an awareness of the impact of individual value systems and personal prejudices on patient interactions.

   The linear communication model illustrates communication as an interactive process between the sender and the receiver of the message, with feedback as a crucial part of the process. Active listening techniques, including restatement, reflection, and clarification, help the medical assistant go beyond hearing the message to actually listening and appropriately responding to the patient's main point. (Refer to Procedure 21.1.)

   Approximately 90% of patient interactions occur through nonverbal language. The key to successful patient interaction is congruence between verbal and nonverbal messages. (Refer to Procedure 21.2 and Table 21.1.)

   Open-ended questions ask for general information and should be used to begin the interview, to introduce a new section of questions, or wherever the person introduces a new topic. Closed-ended questions are more direct and limit the answer to one or two words, typically yes or no.

   Therapeutic communication techniques vary according to the patient's age and developmental stage. A medical assistant should be aware of how to interact most effectively with various age groups, including young children, adolescents, adults, older patients, and family members. Age-specific interview styles enable clear communication between the health professional and the patient.

3. **Examine the patient interview, both in person and via telehealth.**
The interview should be considered a contract between you and your patient. Ask a variety of open- and closed-ended questions and conclude the interview by summarizing the results of your interactions.

   Certain communication styles can be misleading or can restrict the patient's response. The medical assistant must be careful to avoid using such faulty techniques as inappropriately providing reassurance, giving advice, using medical terminology without clarification, asking leading questions, and talking too much. These behaviors interfere with the process of gathering complete data during the interview and are obstacles to developing rapport with the patient.

   Patients use defense mechanisms to protect themselves in emotionally challenging situations. A medical assistant must consistently apply nonjudgmental therapeutic communication skills to maintain professional relationships.

   The patient interview is divided into the introduction, the body, and the summary, or closing. Throughout the interview, the medical assistant should use professional interviewing techniques, such as empathetic patient care, sensitivity to patient diversity, active listening skills, appropriate nonverbal communication, attention to the interview environment, avoidance of communication barriers, and the framing of questions and statements in an open or closed manner, depending on the information needed and the patient's communication behaviors.

   Medical assistants can also interview patients during an interactive telehealth visit. They will often gather the patient health history information and changes in demographics, update the electronic health record (EHR), and then connect the patient to the provider. Refer to Procedure 21.3.

4. **Explain patient assessment and documentation.**
Subjective findings are symptoms; they are perceptible only to the patient. *Objective findings* are *signs;* they can be observed or measured by the provider or medical assistant.

   The ability to document accurately and completely is an essential skill for all medical assistants. Documentation should describe the patient's chief complaint, identify all pertinent signs and symptoms, and demonstrate correct use of medical terminology with appropriate abbreviations. Any error in the health record must be corrected according to legally approved methods.

5. **Examine the medical assistant's role in preparing for the physical examination.**
Before the examination, the medical assistant can interact with the patient to ensure comfort during the examination process and that all necessary health information has been obtained. The medical assistant's duties include preparing and maintaining the examination room and equipment, preparing the patient by conducting the initial interview and measuring vital signs, assisting the provider with positioning and draping, and providing instruments and supplies as needed during the physical examination.

   Instruments and supplies typically used in a physical examination include an ophthalmoscope, otoscope, tongue depressor, reflex hammer, various tuning forks, stethoscope, sphygmomanometer, thermometer, tape measure, scale, examination light, disposable gloves, biohazard container, specimen bottles, laboratory requisitions, fecal occult blood test supplies, patient gown, drapes, and lubricating gel.

6. **Examine the medical assistant's role in assisting with the physical examination.**
The patient should be instructed on whether to wear the gown open in the front or the back, depending on the type of examination being done. The position assumed by the patient during the examination depends on the part of the body to be examined or the procedure to be done.

   Possible patient positions include *Fowler's position,* in which the patient sits straight up, and *semi-Fowler's position,* in which the patient's torso is elevated 45 degrees; the *dorsal recumbent position,* in which the patient lies on the back with the legs bent; the *supine position,* in which the patient lies flat on the back; the *lithotomy position,* in which the patient's buttocks are at the bottom of the table and the legs are positioned in stirrups; the *prone position,* in which the patient lies on the stomach; *left lateral position,* in which the patient lies on the left side with the limbs flexed so that the weight of the body is tilted forward; and the *knee-chest position,* in which the patient is on the knees with the buttocks elevated and the weight of the body tilted downward toward the chest. Draping requires constant attention to maintaining the patient's privacy throughout the examination while assisting the provider with exposure of the area being examined. The general rule is to cover all exposed body parts until the point in the examination when the provider must evaluate that particular area. Procedures 21.4 through 21.9 outline the steps for positioning and draping patients.

SUMMARY OF LEARNING OBJECTIVES—*continued*

Proper body alignment begins with good posture. When reaching for an object, avoid twisting or turning; instead, move the feet to face the object needed. Do not cross the legs while sitting, and keep the popliteal area free of the edge of the chair. Hold the head erect, the face forward, and the chin slightly up; the abdominal muscles contracted up and in; the shoulders relaxed and back; the feet pointed forward and slightly apart; and the weight evenly distributed to both legs, with the knees slightly bent.

Good body mechanics principles include maintaining balanced posture, bending the knees while maintaining the back's three natural curves, and using leg muscles to help lift. Move the wheelchair close to the examination table, lock the wheels, and lift the footrests of the wheelchair out of the way. Provide patient support close to your body on the patient's strong side. Place the wheelchair at a 45-degree angle next to the footrest at the end of the table, and with one hand under the axillary region and the other grasping the patient, help the patient step up onto the footrest with the strong leg; then help the patient pivot into a sitting position on the table. Use a gait belt as needed to assist in patient transfer. (Refer to Procedure 21.10.)

The examiner uses *inspection* to detect significant physical features, such as the patient's general appearance. With *palpation*, the sense of touch is used to feel the brachial pulse before a blood pressure reading is taken. *Percussion* involves tapping or striking the body to elicit sounds or vibratory sensations, as in percussion of the chest to detect fluid in the lungs. A stethoscope is used to *auscultate* or listen to the lungs and heart. *Mensuration* is the process of measuring the patient's height and weight. *Manipulation* is the passive, assisted movement of a joint to determine the range of extension or flexion.

The examination sequence depends on the type of examination and the provider's preference. The provider typically begins the examination by noting the patient's general health appearance, nutrition status, speech, breath odor, skin condition, and reflexes. The physical examination begins at the head and proceeds down through the body. Any abnormalities are noted and may be further investigated with diagnostic tools after the examination has been completed.

Prepare the examination room and the patient; complete the initial patient interview and measure and record vital signs; gather the needed equipment and place it in the order of use; gown and drape the patient as needed; provide patient instruction and check for understanding throughout the process; assist during the examination by handing the provider instruments, managing changes in lighting, collecting samples as ordered, and conducting diagnostic procedures as ordered; assist the patient when the examination is complete, including helping the patient dress, scheduling further diagnostic tests as ordered, and answering the patient's questions. Complete the documentation, disinfect the examination room and equipment, and restock supplies to ready the room for the next patient. Procedure 21.11 presents the steps for assisting with the physical examination.

PROCEDURE 21.1 Obtain and Document Patient Information

TASK: Use restatement, reflection, and clarification to obtain patient information and document patient care accurately.

EQUIPMENT and SUPPLIES

- History form or EHR system with the patient history window opened
- If using a paper form, a red pen for recording the patient's allergies and a black pen to meet legal documentation guidelines
- Quiet, private area

DIRECTIONS: Complete this procedure with another student playing the role of the patient. To make the experience more realistic, choose a student you know very little about. To maintain privacy, the student does not have to share any confidential information.

PROCEDURAL STEPS

1. Greet the patient. Identify yourself. Verify the patient's identity with full name and date of birth. Explain your role.
   PURPOSE: To make the patient feel comfortable and at ease.
2. Take the patient to a quiet, private area for the interview and explain why the information is needed.
   PURPOSE: A quiet, private area is necessary to protect confidentiality and prevent interruptions. An informed patient is more cooperative and, therefore, more likely to provide useful information.
3. Complete the history form using therapeutic communication techniques, including restatement, reflection, and clarification. Make sure all medical terminology is adequately explained. A self-history may have been mailed to the patient before the visit. If so, review the self-history for completeness.
   PURPOSE: Therapeutic communication techniques help the medical assistant gather complete information; the self-history is designed to save time and involve the patient in the process.
4. Speak in a pleasant, distinct manner, remembering to maintain eye contact with your patient.
   PURPOSE: Positive nonverbal behaviors create a friendly, caring atmosphere.
5. Remain sensitive to the diverse needs of your patient throughout the interview process.
   PURPOSE: Incorporate awareness of your personal biases into treating all patients with respect despite their diverse backgrounds.
6. Record the following statistical information:
   - Patient's full name, including middle initial
   - Address, including apartment number and zip code
   - Marital status
   - Sex (gender)
   - Age and date of birth
   - Telephone numbers for home, cell, and work

PROCEDURE 21.1 Obtain and Document Patient Information—*continued*

- Insurance information, if not already available
- Employer's name, address, and telephone number

7. Record the following medical history:
   - Chief complaint
   - Present illness
   - Past history
   - Family history
   - Social history

   PURPOSE: The provider needs this information to make an accurate assessment and diagnosis. The provider usually completes the review of systems (ROS) during the preexamination interview.
8. Ask about allergies to drugs and any other substances and record any allergies in red ink on every page of the history form, on the front of the patient record, and each progress note page; in the EHR, enter allergy information where designated.
   PURPOSE: The presence of an allergy may alter medication and treatment procedures.
9. If using a paper form, record all information legibly and neatly, and spell words correctly. Print rather than writing in cursive. Do not erase, scribble, or use whiteout. Do not leave any blank spaces or skip lines between documentation entries. If you make an error, draw a single line through the error, write "error" above it, add the correction, and initial and date the entry. If recording the information in the patient's EHR, accurately locate each box; errors in the EHR should be corrected and are automatically tracked within the system.
   PURPOSE: To maintain a medical record that is understandable and defensible in a court of law.
10. Thank the patient for cooperating and direct him or her back to the reception area.
11. Review the record for errors before passing it to the provider or exiting the EHR health history area.
12. Protect the integrity of the health record and the confidentiality of patient information. Safeguards mandated by the Health Insurance Portability and Accountability Act (HIPAA) include the following:
    - Passwords to secure access to all EHRs
    - Computer monitor shields to protect patient information if data is left on the screen
    - Turning monitors away from patient traffic areas to prevent accidental release of information
    - Securing all medical records

    PURPOSE: Patient information may be legally and ethically shared only with a member of the healthcare team who is directly providing care to the patient.

PROCEDURE 21.2 Respond to Nonverbal Communication

TASK: Observe the patient and respond appropriately to nonverbal communication.

SCENARIO: Monique Jones is a new patient with the chief complaint (CC) of intermittent abdominal pain with alternating diarrhea and constipation. Ms. Jones has experienced this discomfort for several months and appears frustrated. She sits on the end of the exam table with her arms wrapped around her abdomen. She sighs frequently and refuses to maintain eye contact. What is her nonverbal behavior telling you, and how can you establish therapeutic communication with this patient?

EQUIPMENT and SUPPLIES

- Patient's record

DIRECTIONS: Complete this procedure with another student playing the role of the patient. To make the experience more realistic, choose a student you know very little about. To maintain privacy, the student does not have to share any confidential information.

PROCEDURAL STEPS

1. Greet the patient. Identify yourself. Verify the patient's identity with full name and date of birth. Explain your role.
   PURPOSE: To make the patient feel comfortable and at ease.
2. Ask the patient the purpose of her visit and the onset, duration, and frequency of her symptoms. Pay close attention to her body language to determine whether what she is telling you is congruent with her body language.
   PURPOSE: Nonverbal language naturally expresses the patient's true feelings. Closely observing body language will help you reach more accurate conclusions about the patient's information.
3. Use restatement, reflection, and clarification to gather as much information as possible about the patient's CC. Make sure all medical terminology is adequately explained.
   PURPOSE: Therapeutic communication techniques help the medical assistant gather complete information; using feedback techniques and making sure the patient understands medical terms can help relieve anxiety.
4. Speak in a pleasant, distinct manner, remembering to maintain eye contact with your patient.
   PURPOSE: Positive nonverbal behaviors create a friendly, caring atmosphere. Remain sensitive to the diverse needs of your patient throughout the interview process.
5. Continue to observe nonverbal patient behaviors and select the appropriate verbal response to demonstrate your sensitivity to her discomfort, frustration, and anxiety.PURPOSE: Displaying sensitivity to and awareness of the patient's nonverbal body language demonstrates your concern for the patient and can help defuse the patient's concerns.

PROCEDURE 21.3 Participate in a Telehealth Interaction with a Patient

TASK: Using interactive technology, participate in a telehealth interaction with a patient.

SCENARIO: Dr. Perez has been using interactive telehealth visits to follow up with certain patients. She has asked you to update the patient demographics and health history information prior to Dr. Perez joining the visit.

The patient is Jana Green (DOB 05/01/19XX). Mrs. Green was seen 2 weeks ago by Dr. Perez at WMFM Clinic and was diagnosed with rheumatoid arthritis. Dr. Perez prescribed hydroxychloroquine and prednisone at that time and wanted a follow-up visit with Mrs. Green to see how she was tolerating the medication. At that visit, she mentioned that it was getting harder for her to come into the office as she and her husband no longer drove. Dr. Perez offered the option of an interactive telehealth visit that would utilize the WMFM Clinic patient portal. Mrs. Green is quite familiar with the portal and thought that would be a wonderful option for this visit. It was confirmed that Mrs. Green had the appropriate equipment to access the portal for a telehealth visit. Today is the day for this visit.

DIRECTIONS: Using the scenario, role-play the medical assistant's interaction with Mrs. Green via a virtual environment. Verify her address, phone number, and insurance information. Review her allergies and medication list. The partner (patient) should make up any information required.

EQUIPMENT and SUPPLIES

- Patient's record
- Access to a virtual environment such as Zoom

PROCEDURAL STEPS

1. Login into the virtual environment and connect with your patient. Make sure that you are not on mute and that your patient can hear and see you.
   PURPOSE: The equipment must be working properly for the interactive telehealth encounter can occur.
2. Greet the patient. Identify yourself. Verify the patient's identity with full name and date of birth. Explain what will happen during the medical assistant's portion of the interactive telehealth visit. Demonstrate respect for the patient. Be sincere, courteous, polite, and welcoming.
   PURPOSE: It is important that the patient feel comfortable in the virtual environment.
3. Using appropriate closed and open-ended questions, verify the patient's demographic information. Document any changes in the patient's health record.
   PURPOSE: The medical assistant must gather certain information before the provider sees the patient.
4. Using appropriate closed and open-ended questions and statements, review the patient's allergies. Document any changes in the patient's health record.
5. Using appropriate closed and open-ended questions and statements, review the patient's medication list. Document any changes in the patient's health record.
6. Using appropriate closed and open-ended questions and statements, obtain information about the patient's health, family, and social history. Document any changes in the patient's health record.
7. Thank the patient for her or his time and ask if the patient has any questions about the next stage of the interactive telehealth visit.
   PURPOSE: It is important that the patient feels confident with the technology being used for the visit.

PROCEDURE 21.4 Fowler and Semi-Fowler Positions

TASK: Position and drape the patient for examinations of the head, neck, and chest, or position and drape patients who have difficulty breathing when lying flat.

EQUIPMENT and SUPPLIES

- Patient's record
- Examination table
- Table paper
- Patient gown
- Drape
- Disinfectant wipes
- Gloves

PROCEDURAL STEPS

1. Wash hands or use hand sanitizer.
   PURPOSE: Hand sanitization is an important step for infection control.
2. Greet the patient. Identify yourself. Verify the patient's identity with full name and date of birth. Explain the procedure to be performed in a manner that the patient understands. Answer any questions the patient may have about the procedure.
   PURPOSE: To promote the patient's understanding and cooperation during the examination.
3. Give the patient a gown. Explain what clothing must be removed for the examination being done and whether the gown should open in the front or the back. Provide assistance as needed. Give the patient privacy while changing. Knock on the examination room door before reentering to ensure the patient has completed undressing and gowning.
4. For the Fowler position, elevate the head of the bed 90 degrees. Patients who feel more comfortable can sit at the end of the table. Extend the footrest as needed for patient comfort. The patient may be more comfortable in the semi-Fowler position. In this modification of the Fowler position, the head of the table is elevated 45 degrees. The semi-Fowler position

Continued

PROCEDURE 21.4 Fowler and Semi-Fowler Positions—*continued*

may be used for postoperative follow-up or for patients with a fever, head injury, or pain. It also is a comfortable, supportive position for patients with breathing disorders (see Figure 1).

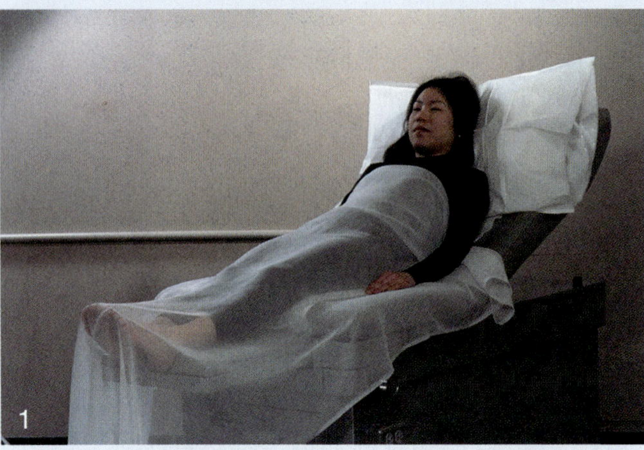

5. Drape the patient according to the type of examination and the required patient exposure.
   PURPOSE: Draping the patient provides warmth and privacy while giving the provider access to the examination site.
6. After the examination has been completed, assist the patient as needed to get off the table and get dressed.
7. Put on gloves and use disinfectant wipes to clean the exam table and all potentially contaminated surfaces. Dispose of used gloves and examination table paper according to facility policies. Pull clean paper over the table.
   PURPOSE: To ensure infection control and prevent the transmission of pathogens from one patient to another.
8. Wash hands or use hand sanitizer.
9. Follow up with the provider's orders regarding scheduling diagnostic studies, collecting specimens, or scheduling future appointments.

PROCEDURE 21.5 Supine (Horizontal Recumbent) and Dorsal Recumbent Positions

TASK: Position and drape the patient for examinations of the abdomen, heart, and breasts in the horizontal recumbent (supine) position and exams of the rectal, vaginal, and perineal areas in the dorsal recumbent position.

EQUIPMENT and SUPPLIES

- Patient's record
- Examination table
- Table paper
- Patient gown
- Drape
- Disinfectant wipes
- Gloves

PROCEDURAL STEPS

1. Wash hands or use hand sanitizer.
   PURPOSE: Hand sanitization is an important step for infection control.
2. Greet the patient. Identify yourself. Verify the patient's identity with full name and date of birth. Explain the procedure to be performed in a manner that the patient understands. Answer any questions the patient may have about the procedure.
   PURPOSE: To promote the patient's understanding and cooperation during the examination.
3. Give the patient a gown. Explain the clothing that must be removed for the examination being done and whether the gown should open in the front or back. Provide assistance as needed. For the horizontal recumbent position, the gown should be open in the front. Give the patient privacy while changing. Knock on the examination room door before reentering to ensure the patient has completed undressing and gowning.
4. Do not place the patient in the necessary positions until the provider is ready for that part of the examination.
   PURPOSE: To ensure the patient's privacy, comfort, and modesty.
5. Pull out the table extension that supports the patient's legs. For the horizontal recumbent (supine) position, help the patient lie flat on the table with the face upward (see Figure 1). For the dorsal recumbent position, have the patient lie flat on their back and flex their knees so the feet are flat on the table (see Figure 2). If needed, help the patient move down toward the foot of the table for the examination.

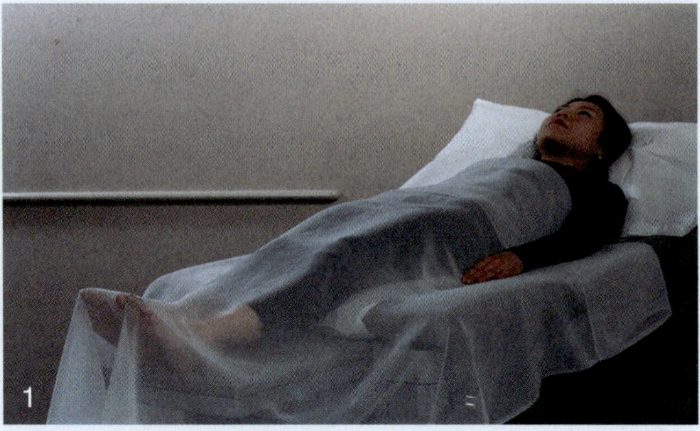

PROCEDURE 21.5 Supine (Horizontal Recumbent) and Dorsal Recumbent Positions—*continued*

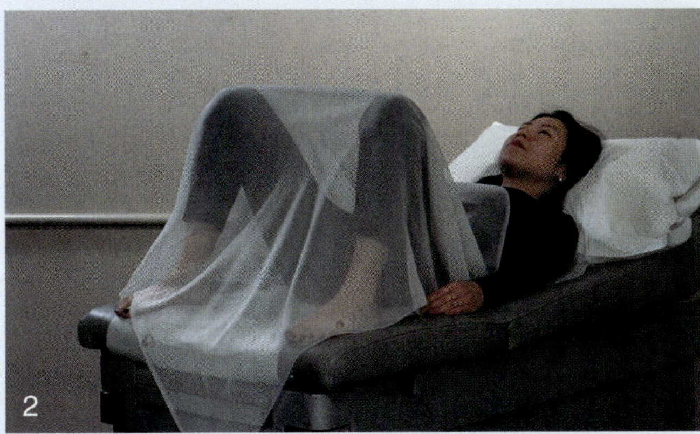

6. Drape the patient from nipple line to feet in the supine position and diagonally with the point of the drape between the feet for the dorsal recumbent position.
   PURPOSE: Draping the patient provides warmth and privacy while giving the provider access to the examination site.
7. After the examination has been completed, assist the patient as needed to get off the table and get dressed.
8. Put on gloves and use disinfectant wipes to clean the exam table and all potentially contaminated surfaces. Dispose of used gloves and examination table paper according to facility policies. Pull clean paper over the table.
   PURPOSE: To ensure infection control and prevent the transmission of pathogens from one patient to another.
9. Wash hands or use hand sanitizer.
10. Follow up with the provider's orders regarding scheduling diagnostic studies, collection of specimens, or scheduling future appointments.

PROCEDURE 21.6 Lithotomy Position

TASK: Position and drape the patient primarily for vaginal and pelvic examinations and Pap tests.

EQUIPMENT and SUPPLIES

- Patient's record
- Examination table
- Table paper
- Patient gown
- Drape
- Disinfectant wipes
- Gloves

PROCEDURAL STEPS

1. Wash hands or use hand sanitizer.
   PURPOSE: Hand sanitization is an important step for infection control.
2. Greet the patient. Identify yourself. Verify the patient's identity with full name and date of birth. Explain the procedure to be performed in a manner that the patient understands. Answer any questions the patient may have about the procedure.
   PURPOSE: To promote the patient's understanding and cooperation during the examination.
3. Give the patient a gown. Instruct the patient to undress from the waist down with the gown open in the back. If the provider is also doing a breast examination, the patient should undress completely and put on the gown so that it opens in the front. Provide assistance as needed. Give the patient privacy while changing. Knock on the examination room door before reentering to make sure the patient has completed undressing and gowning.
4. Do not place the patient in the lithotomy position until the provider is ready for that part of the examination.
   PURPOSE: To promote the patient's privacy, comfort, and safety.
5. Pull out the table extension that supports the patient's legs and help the patient lie face upward on the table. Pull out the stirrups, adjust their extension length for the patient's comfort, and lock them in place.
6. Reinsert the table extension, and have the patient move toward the foot of the table with her buttocks on the bottom table edge. Gently place the patient's legs in the stirrups, checking for comfort. Some offices may stock cloth or paper stirrup covers to protect the patient and make the position more comfortable. The patient's arms can be placed alongside the body or across the chest (see Figure 1).

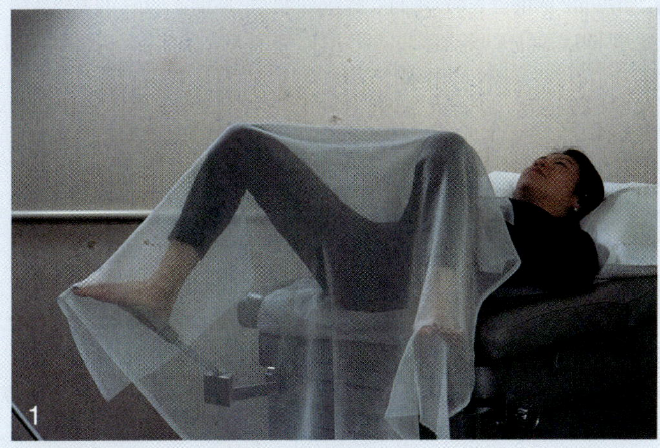

7. Drape the patient diagonally, with the point of the drape between the feet. The drape should be large enough to cover the patient from the nipple line to the ankles and wide enough that the patient's thighs are not exposed.

PROCEDURE 21.6 Lithotomy Position—*continued*

PURPOSE: To provide warmth and privacy for the patient while giving the provider access to the examination site.

8. After the examination has been completed, assist the patient as needed to get off the table and get dressed.
9. Put on gloves and use disinfectant wipes to clean the exam table and all potentially contaminated surfaces. Dispose of used gloves and examination table paper according to facility policies. Pull clean paper over the table.
   PURPOSE: To ensure infection control and prevent the transmission of pathogens from one patient to another.
10. Wash hands or use hand sanitizer.
11. Follow up with the provider's orders regarding scheduling diagnostic studies, collecting specimens, or scheduling future appointments.

PROCEDURE 21.7 Left Lateral Position

TASK: Position and drape the patient for examination of the rectum, instillation of rectal medication, perineal examination, and some pelvic examinations.

EQUIPMENT and SUPPLIES

- Patient's record
- Examination table
- Patient gown
- Table paper
- Drape
- Disinfectant wipes
- Gloves

PROCEDURAL STEPS

1. Wash hands or use hand sanitizer.
   PURPOSE: Hand sanitization is an important step for infection control.
2. Greet the patient. Identify yourself. Verify the patient's identity with full name and date of birth. Explain the procedure to be performed in a manner that the patient understands. Answer any questions the patient may have about the procedure.
   PURPOSE: To promote the patient's understanding and cooperation during the examination.
3. Give the patient a gown, and explain what clothing must be removed for the examination being done. Tell the patient that the gown should open in the back. Provide assistance as needed. Give the patient privacy while changing. Knock on the examination room door before reentering to make sure the patient has completed undressing and gowning.
4. Do not place the patient in the left lateral position until the provider is ready for that part of the examination.
   PURPOSE: To promote the patient's privacy, comfort, and safety.
5. Help the patient turn onto the left side; the left arm and shoulder should be drawn back behind the body so that the patient is tilted onto the chest. Flex the right arm upward for support, slightly flex the left leg, and sharply flex the right leg upward. Help the patient move the buttocks to the side edge of the table (see Figure 1).

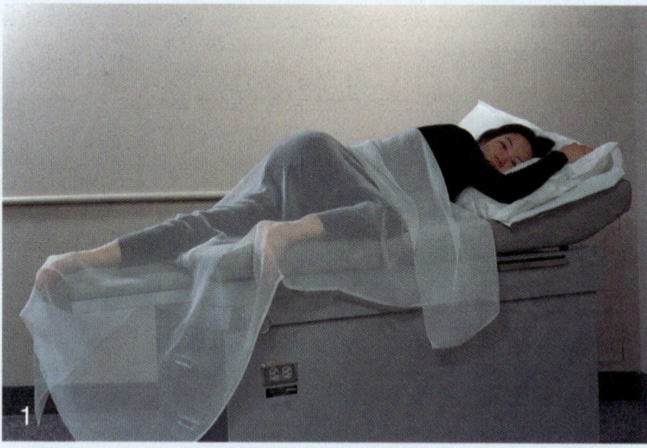
1

6. Drape the patient over an exposed area that is not included in the examination. The drape should cover from the shoulders to the feet so that the patient is not exposed accidentally.
   PURPOSE: Draping the patient provides warmth and privacy while giving the provider access to the examination site.
7. After the examination has been completed, assist the patient as needed to get off the table and get dressed.
8. Put on gloves and use disinfectant wipes to clean the exam table and all potentially contaminated surfaces. Dispose of used gloves and examination table paper according to facility policies. Pull clean paper over the table.
   PURPOSE: To ensure infection control and prevent the transmission of pathogens from one patient to another.
9. Wash hands or use hand sanitizer.
10. Follow up with the provider's orders regarding scheduling diagnostic studies, collecting specimens, or scheduling future appointments.

PROCEDURE 21.8 Prone Position

TASK: Position and drape the patient for examination of the back and for certain surgical procedures.

EQUIPMENT and SUPPLIES

- Patient's record
- Examination table
- Patient gown
- Table paper
- Drape
- Disinfectant wipes
- Gloves

PROCEDURAL STEPS

1. Wash hands or use hand sanitizer.
   PURPOSE: Hand sanitization is an important step for infection control.
2. Greet the patient. Identify yourself. Verify the patient's identity with full name and date of birth. Explain the procedure to be performed in a manner that the patient understands. Answer any questions the patient may have about the procedure.
   PURPOSE: To promote the patient's understanding and cooperation during the examination.
3. Give the patient a gown and explain what clothing must be removed for the examination being done. Tell the patient that the gown should open in the back. Provide assistance as needed. Give the patient privacy while changing. Knock on the examination room door before reentering to make sure the patient has completed undressing and gowning.
4. Do not place the patient in the prone position until the provider is ready for that part of the examination.
   PURPOSE: To promote the patient's privacy, comfort, and safety.
5. Pull out the table extension, and help the patient lie down on his or her stomach (see Figure 1).

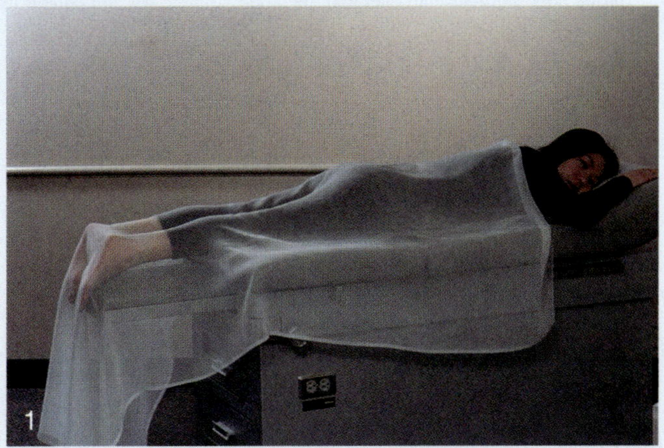

6. Drape the patient over any exposed area that is not included in the examination. For female patients, the drape should be large enough to cover from the breasts to the feet so that the patient is not accidently exposed if she is asked to roll over.
   PURPOSE: Draping the patient provides warmth and privacy while giving the provider access to the examination site.
7. After the examination has been completed, assist the patient as needed to get off the table and get dressed.
8. Put on gloves and use disinfectant wipes to clean the exam table and all potentially contaminated surfaces. Dispose of used gloves and examination table paper according to facility policies. Pull clean paper over the table.
   PURPOSE: To ensure infection control and prevent the transmission of pathogens from one patient to another.
9. Wash hands or use hand sanitizer.
10. Follow up with the provider's orders regarding scheduling diagnostic studies, collecting specimens, or scheduling future appointments.

PROCEDURE 21.9 Knee-Chest Position

TASK: Position and drape the patient for examinations of the back and rectum and for certain surgical procedures.

EQUIPMENT and SUPPLIES

- Patient's record
- Examination table
- Table paper
- Patient gown
- Drape
- Disinfectant wipes
- Gloves

PROCEDURAL STEPS

1. Wash hands or use hand sanitizer.
   PURPOSE: Hand sanitization is an important step for infection control.
2. Greet the patient. Identify yourself. Verify the patient's identity with full name and date of birth. Explain the procedure to be performed in a manner that the patient understands. Answer any questions the patient may have about the procedure.
   PURPOSE: To promote the patient's understanding and cooperation during the examination.
3. Give the patient a gown and explain what clothing must be removed for the examination being done. Tell the patient that the gown should open in the back. Provide assistance as needed. Give the patient privacy while changing. Knock on the examination room door before reentering to make sure the patient has completed undressing and gowning.
4. Do not place the patient in the knee-chest position until the provider is ready for that part of the examination.
   PURPOSE: To promote the patient's privacy, comfort, and safety.

Continued

PROCEDURE 21.9 Knee-Chest Position—*continued*

5. Pull out the table extension if necessary. Help the patient lie down on his or her back and then turn over into the prone position. Ask the patient to move up onto the knees, spread the knees apart, and lean forward onto the head so that the buttocks are raised. Tell the patient to keep the back straight and turn the face to either side. The patient should rest his or her weight on the chest and shoulders (see Figure 1).

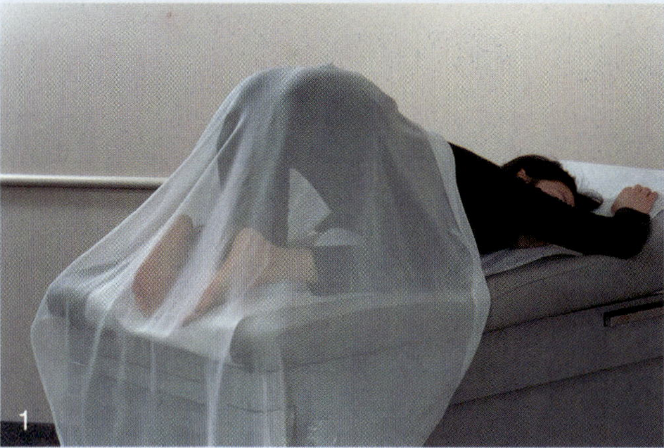

6. If the patient has difficulty maintaining this position, an alternative is to place weight on bent elbows with the head off the table.
7. Drape the patient diagonally in a diamond shape, with the point of the diamond dropping below the buttocks. Make sure the drape is large enough to prevent exposure of the patient.
   PURPOSE: Draping the patient provides warmth and privacy while giving the provider access to the examination site.
8. After the examination has been completed, assist the patient as needed to get off the table and get dressed.
9. Put on gloves and use disinfectant wipes to clean the exam table and all potentially contaminated surfaces. Dispose of used gloves and examination table paper according to facility policies. Pull clean paper over the table.
   PURPOSE: To ensure infection control and prevent the transmission of pathogens from one patient to another.
10. Wash hands or use hand sanitizer.
11. Follow up with the provider's orders regarding scheduling diagnostic studies, collecting specimens, or scheduling future appointments.

PROCEDURE 21.10 Use Proper Body Mechanics

TASK: Safely transfer a patient from a wheelchair to an examination table using proper body mechanics.

EQUIPMENT and SUPPLIES

- Patient's record
- Wheelchair
- Examination table with pull-out footrest
- Gait belt

PROCEDURAL STEPS

1. Wash hands or use hand sanitizer.
   PURPOSE: Hand sanitization is an important step for infection control.
2. Greet the patient. Identify yourself. Verify the patient's identity with full name and date of birth. Explain the procedure to be performed in a manner that the patient understands. Determine how much assistance the patient will need to transfer from the wheelchair to the examination table. Do not proceed if you think you will need additional help.
   PURPOSE: To promote the patient's cooperation during the transfer and prevent personal injury.
3. Place the wheelchair at a 45-degree angle toward the footrest at the base of the examination table (see Figure 21.17).
4. Lock the brakes on the wheelchair and move the footrests of the wheelchair out of the way (see Figure 1).
   PURPOSE: Never transfer a patient into or out of a wheelchair until the brakes are locked on both sides of the chair.

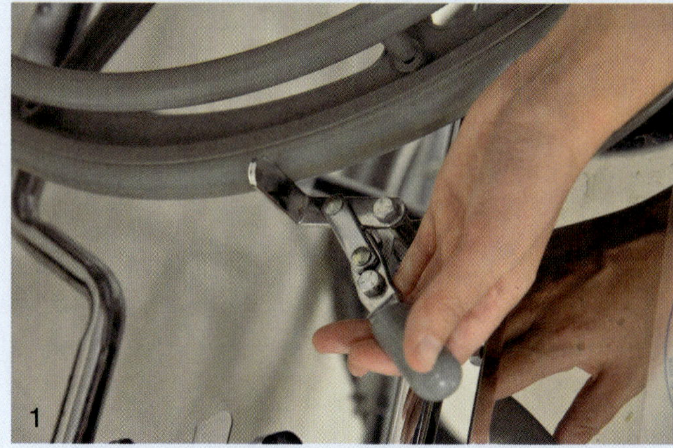

5. Place the gait belt around the patient's waist over clothing with the buckle in front. Insert the belt through the teeth of the buckle and pull it tight to lock it. The belt should be tight, with just enough room to place your fingers under it.

PROCEDURE 21.10 Use Proper Body Mechanics—*continued*

6. Request that the patient place both feet flat on the floor with the hands on the armrests.
   PURPOSE: This position helps you grasp the gait belt; the patient can use the wheelchair armrests to help push herself or himself into an upright position, and feet flat on the floor help with patient stability.
7. Stand directly in front of the patient with your feet apart, back straight, and knees bent (see Figure 2).
   PURPOSE: This position helps you maintain good body mechanics during the transfer.

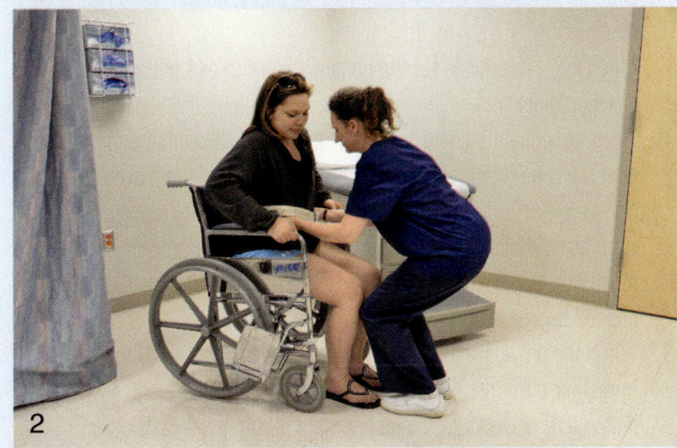

8. Slide your fingers under the gait belt on opposite sides of the patient's waist.
9. Instruct the patient at the count of 3 to push off from the armrests while you at the same time grasp the gait belt and, using your leg muscles, straighten your knees so that the patient is in a standing position.
   PURPOSE: This position allows the patient to assist as much as possible while you are using the large muscles of your legs to help lift the patient.
10. Ask the patient to step up onto the footrest at the bottom of the exam table and assist the person in pivoting and sitting down on the examination table. Remove the gait belt until the provider has completed the examination (see Figure 3).

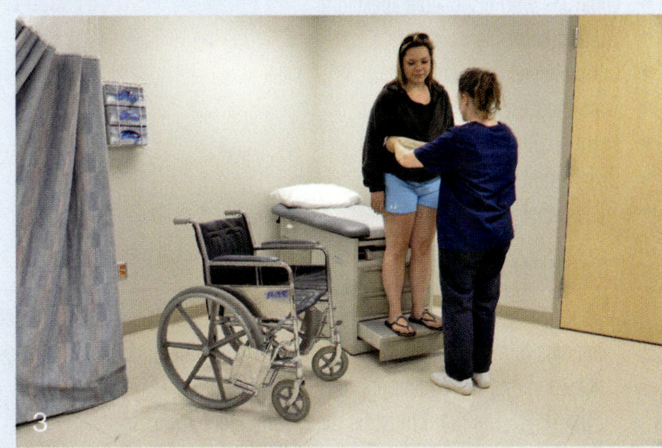

11. After the examination is complete, place the wheelchair at an angle next to the exam table and lock the wheels. Replace the gait belt. Make sure the patient is positioned at the edge of the table.
    PURPOSE: To prepare for transfer back to the wheelchair.
12. Place yourself directly in front of the patient with your back straight and your knees bent. Slide your fingers under the gait belt on opposite sides of the patient's waist.
13. Grasp the gait belt on both sides at the waist. Instruct the patient at the count of 3 to push off from the examination table and, using your leg muscles, straighten your knees so that the patient is in a standing position on the footrest of the examination table.
14. Maintaining your hold on the gait belt, ask the patient to step down. Pivot the person so that she or he can slowly sit in the wheelchair; at the same time, bend your knees but keep your back straight.
15. Remove the gait belt. Replace the wheelchair footrests and unlock the brakes on the wheelchair.

PROCEDURE 21.11 Assist the Provider with a Patient Exam

TASK: Aid the provider in the examination of a patient by preparing the patient and the necessary equipment and ensuring the patient's safety and comfort during the examination.

EQUIPMENT and SUPPLIES

- Patient's record
- Stethoscope
- Gauze
- Ophthalmoscope
- Penlight
- Scale with height measurement bar
- Tuning fork
- Tongue depressor
- Biohazard waste container
- Cotton balls
- Examination light
- Laboratory request forms
- Percussion hammer
- Specimen bottles and laboratory requisitions
- Lubricating gel
- Gloves
- Patient gown

Continued

PROCEDURE 21.11 Assist the Provider with a Patient Exam—*continued*

- Sphygmomanometer
- Drapes
- Otoscope with disposable speculum
- Thermometer
- Cotton-tipped applicators
- Tape measure
- Fecal occult blood test supplies
- Disinfectant wipes
- Table paper

PROCEDURAL STEPS

1. Check the examination room at the beginning of each day and between patients to make sure it is completely stocked with equipment and supplies and that the equipment functions properly.
   PURPOSE: The room must be ready for patient services.
2. Regularly check expiration dates on all packages and supplies and discard expired materials.
   PURPOSE: To ensure the patient's safety.
3. Prepare the examining room before and between patients according to acceptable medical rules of asepsis.
   PURPOSE: The room must be aseptically clean to prevent the spread of infection.
4. Wash hands or use hand sanitizer.
   PURPOSE: Hand sanitization is an important step for infection control.
5. Locate the instruments for the procedure. Set them out in order of use within reach of the provider and cover them until the provider enters the examination room.
   PURPOSE: To promote time management and ensure that all needed equipment and supplies are ready.
6. Greet and identify the patient, introduce yourself and determine whether the patient understands the procedure. If the patient does not, explain what to expect. Refer any unanswered questions to the provider.
   PURPOSE: To promote the patient's understanding and cooperation during the examination.
7. Review the medical history with the patient and investigate the purpose of the visit. Review current medications and document any changes or prescription refills needed. Document the interview results.
   PURPOSE: To verify that all information is current and complete.
8. Measure and record the patient's vital signs, height, weight, and body mass index (BMI). Instruct the patient on how to collect a urine specimen, if ordered, and hand the patient a properly labeled specimen container. Obtain blood samples for any tests ordered.
   PURPOSE: To gather data needed before the examination begins.
9. Hand the patient a gown and drape. Explain what clothes should be removed for the examination and whether the gown should open in the front or the back. Help the patient with undressing as needed (most patients prefer to undress in privacy). Knock on the door before reentering the room to protect the patient's privacy.
   PURPOSE: To assist the patient in preparing for the examination and safeguard the patient's privacy, comfort, and safety.
10. Assist the patient as needed in sitting at the foot of the examination table; place the drape over the patient's lap and legs. If the patient is an older adult, confused, or feeling faint or dizzy, do not leave him or her alone.
    PURPOSE: To provide for the patient's warmth and privacy and prevent a fall or injury.
11. Place the patient's paper health record in the designated area, or make sure the computer is ready for the provider to log in and access the patient's electronic health record (EHR). Be careful to safeguard patient confidentiality during this step of the procedure.
12. Assist during the examination by handing the provider instruments as needed and positioning and draping the patient.
13. When the provider has completed the examination, allow the patient to rest for a moment, then help the patient from the table. Assist with dressing, if necessary. Use proper body mechanics if assistance in transfer is needed.
    PURPOSE: To ensure the patient's stability and safety and protect yourself from injury.
14. Return to the patient and ask whether he or she has any questions. Give the patient any final instructions and schedule tests as ordered by the provider or the next appointment.
    PURPOSE: To clarify instructions, eliminate any misunderstandings and allow the patient to discuss any concerns. If the patient's misunderstandings or concerns are beyond your scope of experience or skill, arrange for the provider to speak with the patient again.
15. Put on gloves and dispose of used supplies and linens in designated biohazard waste containers. Dispose of exam table paper. Use disinfectant wipes to clean the examination table and any other potentially contaminated surface. Disinfect all equipment.
    PURPOSE: To prevent cross-contamination with any potentially infectious materials.
16. Remove the gloves, discard them in the biohazard waste container, and wash hands or use hand sanitizer.
    PURPOSE: To ensure infection control.
17. Cover the exam table with fresh paper, replace used supplies, and prepare the room for the next patient.

PATIENT COACHING

22

SCENARIO

Suzanne Peterson, a certified medical assistant (CMA) through the American Association of Medical Assistants (AAMA), has worked for Walden-Martin Family Medicine (WMFM) Clinic for 5 years. Her favorite part of her job is coaching patients on health topics, diagnostic tests, and treatment plans. Her patients know they can contact Suzanne if they have questions between appointments. Suzanne answers the questions she can and talks with the providers for other questions. She feels that it is very important for patients to understand how to self-manage their conditions and to know when to contact their providers.

Over the years, Suzanne has seen the role of the medical assistant expand. She has learned the importance of screening patients during the initial interview. The information that she enters into the electronic health record is then used to collect data on how well the clinic provides patient care. She has also learned the importance of patient care coordinators. She hopes WMFM Clinic implements a care coordinator program soon.

While studying this chapter, think about the following questions:

- What are basic concepts of teaching and learning? What are the domains of learning? How can a medical assistant adapt coaching to patients?
- What are types of disease prevention coaching?
- What are types of health maintenance coaching?
- What coaching should a medical assistant do for common diagnostic tests?
- What coaching can be done for treatment plans?
- What is the medical assistant's role in coordination of care, navigation, and community resource referrals?

LEARNING OBJECTIVES

1. Examine factors that influence health choices, including grief reactions and health belief and practices.
2. Differentiate among the three domains of learning, including barriers to learning, strategies for adapting to barriers, and tips for improving learning.
3. Examine the medical assistant's role with coaching, including areas of coaching and adapting coaching for the individual.
4. Examine how to adapt coaching based on the patient's developmental level.
5. Differentiate among the coaching strategies to use for different types of communication barriers.
6. Examine how cultural beliefs and practices influence health beliefs and practices.
7. Examine the teaching-learning process.
8. Demonstrate coaching on disease prevention, including cough etiquette, sexually transmitted infection prevention, and the cessation of tobacco and nicotine use.
9. Demonstrate coaching on self-exams for health maintenance and wellness.
10. Demonstrate coaching on screenings for health maintenance and wellness.
11. Examine the coaching provided by the medical assistant regarding diagnostic tests and treatment plans.
12. Examine the role of care coordination in ambulatory care.

VOCABULARY

adherence (ad HEER ehns) The act of sticking to something.
anhedonia (an hee DOE nee ah) The inability to feel or experience pleasure during a pleasurable activity.
cessation (se SAY shuhn) Bringing to an end.
compliance (kuhm PLIE ahns) The act of following through on a request or demand. Patient compliance sounds negative; thus, patient adherence is now being used.
patient navigator A person who identifies patients' barriers, works closely with the healthcare team and patients, and guides the patients through the healthcare system; may also be called a patient advocate.

INTRODUCTION

Healthcare is changing, and the role of the medical assistant is changing, too. Consider some of the current challenges in healthcare:

- Pressure to reduce costs
- Shorter primary care provider visits, yet an increased need for data collection to incorporate patient interviews and outcome measurements (e.g., test results)
- Patients leaving the facility without understanding what they were told
- An unwillingness on the part of patients to adhere to treatment plans (e.g., not taking medication or not taking it correctly or choosing not to make lifestyle changes that would improve their health)

Many experts have researched ways to meet these challenges. Several studies have examined patient medication **adherence** or **compliance**. *Medication adherence* means patients are taking the right dose at the right times as prescribed by the provider. Research has shown that medication adherence with chronic diseases is low. This leads to the progression of the disease and more medical visits for the patient. Ultimately, nonadherence to medication is increasing the cost of healthcare.

Why is it that patients do not take their medications correctly? This question has been a focus of many studies, and some common reasons have been determined:

- Forgetfulness and confusion on how to take it
- Side effects and cost of the medication
- Feeling it is not helping

Research has shown that many patients are confused after seeing their providers. Patients do not always understand the treatment plan designed to manage their conditions. Confusion about medication and home care is prevalent. Many patients are not able to manage their disease adequately between provider visits; thus, their condition worsens. To solve this problem, ambulatory care facilities are moving toward coaching and care coordination.

Before learning the areas of coaching, we must first explore factors that influence making health changes and the ways a person learns. The remaining sections of the chapter address the medical assistant's role with coaching, adapting coaching to the individual, and, lastly, care coordination.

MAKING CHANGES FOR HEALTH

Often, healthcare professionals see patients who do not comply with the treatment plan. They may not take the prescribed medication, or maybe they do not make the recommended lifestyle changes. If the diagnosis is life threatening or life changing, grief and loss can occur. Other times, patients may not perceive the change as necessary. The following sections examine theories that may explain why patients do not comply with the treatment plan.

Stages of Grief

Elisabeth Kübler-Ross studied people's reactions to death and dying. She found that people experienced similar stages. Over the years, these stages have been applied to grief and loss. When a patient and the family get a life-threatening or life-changing diagnosis, they can feel grief and loss. People go through the stages of grief in their own way and at their own pace (Table 22.1). This process can take weeks to months. Patients may not be open to making the recommended changes. Healthcare professionals may view this as the patient not wanting to comply with the treatment plan. Sometimes a patient must accept a diagnosis before compliance occurs. It is important for the medical assistant to be supportive, use empathy when communicating with patients, and adapt interactions to help with the stages of grief.

CRITICAL THINKING APPLICATION 22.1

Suzanne has seen many patients dealing with grief. Why might a patient who is grieving not adhere to a treatment plan?

TABLE 22.1 Stages of Grief and Dying

STAGE	DESCRIPTION	ADAPTIVE INTERACTIONS
Denial	Refuses to accept the fact (i.e., diagnosis or prognosis). May refuse to discuss the diagnosis. May not remember the health coaching. Denial is a defense mechanism that allows the person to ignore what is happening.	Provide handouts that explain the disease and treatment. Encourage family members to offer support for the treatment. Provide online and community resources (i.e., support groups).
Anger	Anger can be directed at oneself or others. Anger can surface at unrelated times and be directed toward unrelated issues.	Use therapeutic communication techniques (e.g., reflection) to acknowledge the patient's feelings about the issue. Recognize the real cause of the anger.
Bargaining	Attempts to bargain with the higher power the person believes in (e.g., God). Sometimes the patient will bargain with the provider to make lifestyle changes at a later time.	Work with the healthcare team regarding the bargaining requests. Help provide opportunities for the patient to make decisions.
Depression	Feels sadness, fear, and uncertainty. People may grieve the loss of their health or independence. They may dread the change that is occurring.	Encourage the use of community and healthcare resources to ease the change process for the patient and family members.
Acceptance	Has come to terms with the situation.	Provide coaching on aspects of the disease and self-care management.

Health Belief Model

The health belief model helps explain what factors influence a person's health beliefs and practices. The first part of this model deals with a person's perception of their chance of developing a disease. Consider these examples:

- Jess is in her 20s and has lost her mother, sister, and grandmother to breast cancer. She feels her chance of developing breast cancer is significant.
- Sam has an older brother with heart disease that is being managed by medication, diet, and exercise. Sam blames the disease on his brother's stressful job. Sam does not have a stressful job, so he feels he will not get heart disease. Even though Sam receives education on a heart-healthy lifestyle, he ignores the information.

The second part of this model deals with a person's perception of the severity of the disease. A person's perception is influenced by a number of factors:

- Personal factors (e.g., age, sex, race, employment)
- Social factors (e.g., peers, personality, family)
- Perceived threats of the disease
- Cues to action (e.g., mass media campaigns; social media; advice from family, friends, and healthcare providers and professionals)

In the prior examples, Jess has lost three family members to breast cancer. She perceives breast cancer as being a severe disease. Sam, on the other hand, may not perceive the severity of heart disease because his brother's heart disease is being managed.

The third part of the model focuses on whether the person will take preventive action. A person weighs the benefits of and barriers to taking the preventive actions. For example, Jess may decide to have a double mastectomy as a preventive strategy. For many, it may seem severe, but for Jess, she is willing to take such preventive action. Sam, on the other hand, may not see the benefit of following a heart-healthy lifestyle. He may feel that he must give up his current lifestyle and make changes.

It is important to remember this model when coaching patients on preventive actions. Start with identifying if the person perceives they are at risk for a disease. Exploring the patient's beliefs and educating the patient on the facts, in addition to getting rid of the myths, can be helpful. Discussing the severity of the disease or what the disease can lead to is the next important step. Finally, offering the patient help in eliminating or diminishing the barriers and helping the person see the benefits of the preventive action are important.

CRITICAL THINKING APPLICATION **22.2**

Suzanne has had patients state they do not want to give up their lifestyle and follow the provider's recommendations for better health. How might a medical assistant address this issue with a patient?

DOMAINS OF LEARNING

Learning is the process of gaining new knowledge or skills through instruction, experience, or study. We learn new information in three different ways or domains: cognitive, psychomotor, and affective. These domains are discussed in the coming sections.

Cognitive Domain

The *cognitive domain* of learning involves the mental processes of recall, application, and evaluation. We learn new information by listening to what is said and reading written words. Many experts believe we have three ways to store memories:

- *Sensory stage*: For a memory to be created, we must pick up something from our senses (e.g., touch, hearing, sight). Our senses are constantly picking up perceptions. Many will be forgotten in a split second. We will pay attention to just a few, and they will move to the short-term memory. The deciding factor between what is forgotten and what moves into the short-term memory is based on its importance to us.
- *Short-term memory*: This is our temporary working memory. If nothing is done with the memory, it will fade within 30 seconds. The short-term memory can only handle about seven units of information at once. By chunking information into meaningful units or attaching it to something we already know, we can increase the amount in our short-term memory.
- *Long-term memory*: The more we use short-term memories, the quicker they enter our long-term memory. We can add endless memories to our long-term memory, but without use (recall), those memories can fade.

Table 22.2 provides strategies to use for the cognitive domain. The *barriers,* or reasons learning does not occur effectively, are also listed. These barriers are important for the medical assistant to limit if possible.

Tips for Improving Learning

Our goal for patient education is to put the information into patients' long-term memory. Not everything we tell the patient will be picked up and remembered. We hope the important information will be. The following tips can be used to help patients remember critical information.

- *Present the information at an appropriate level for the patient:* Most studies show that patient education literature should be at a sixth-grade reading level. According to the US National Library of Medicine's website (https://medlineplus.gov), patient educational materials should be between a seventh- and eighth-grade reading level. If the patient's primary language is not English, a lower reading level is needed.
- *Build on the patient's prior knowledge about the topic:* Start by finding out what the patient knows about the topic. Clarify any inaccurate information, and then provide new information that builds on the existing knowledge.
- *Present information in small chunks in a clear, well-organized manner:* Do not overwhelm the patient; keep to the facts and keep it simple. For complex topics, meeting with the patient over several days may help the patient to retain the information.
- *Provide the information in two different ways*: For example, discuss the information with the patient and then provide a written handout.
- *Tell the patient, "This is important to remember," and repeat important information several times during the session.* Be aware that if everything is "important to remember," nothing will be remembered. Do not overuse this strategy.
- *Have the patient "teach back" the information you provided*: This allows you to check what the patient recalls and if it is accurate. Teaching back also enhances the patient's ability to remember the information.

Psychomotor Domain

The *psychomotor domain* is the "doing" domain. We learn new skills and procedures by watching demonstrations and assisting with

TABLE 22.2 Strategies to Use and Barriers for the Three Domains of Learning

	DOMAIN		
	COGNITIVE	**PSYCHOMOTOR**	**AFFECTIVE**
Involves	Learning new concepts and information	Learning new skill or procedure	A change in attitude or emotions that will influence the person's behavior
Teaching strategies to use	Discussion, written information, online videos, computer instruction	Demonstration and return demonstration	Discussion, role-play, and simulations
Barriers to learning	Memory or cognition issues; language barriers	Tremors and paralysis; sensory limitations (e.g., visual impairment, hearing impairment)	Anxiety, denial, pain, fatigue, or stress; cultural customs; previous experience; poor coping skills
Strategies for adapting to barriers	Keep it simple; provide easy-to-read handouts; use an interpreter and provide handouts in the patient's primary language if possible	Use adaptive equipment, such as a magnifying glass and a magnifier for syringes	Provide analgesics as ordered by the provider, help to minimize barriers, provide home instructions, and include additional family member(s) if possible

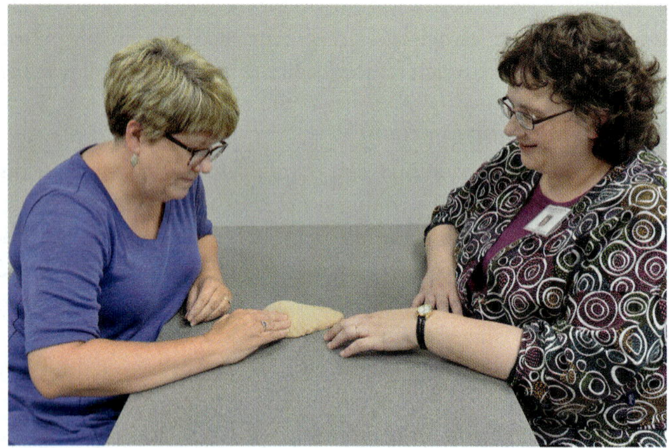

FIGURE 22.1 Having a patient do a return demonstration or "teach back" the skill allows the medical assistant to check the patient's knowledge and skills for accuracy.

something. Many people would prefer to attempt a skill versus reading about it or discussing it. They learn best through the psychomotor domain. Table 22.2 provides some barriers to the psychomotor domain.

Tips for Improving Learning

Here are some tips to help patients remember critical information:

- Provide written step-by-step directions for the patient to follow and then take home.
- Give timely feedback on the person's performance.
- Have the patient teach back the skill or do a return demonstration to check for accuracy (Figure 22.1).
- Repeated practice doing the skill helps with recall and retention of the steps.
- Make sure to use the equipment and supplies the patient will be using at home.

Affective Domain

The *affective domain* is the "feeling" domain. It includes our feelings, emotions, values, and attitudes. Our emotions and values are very important. They affect our motivation, confidence, and priorities. When our personal values conflict with the new information presented, a barrier to learning can occur. Pain is another example of an affective barrier. If you are instructing a patient on wound care and they are in pain, they may not remember what you said. Additional barriers to the affective domain are listed in Table 22.2.

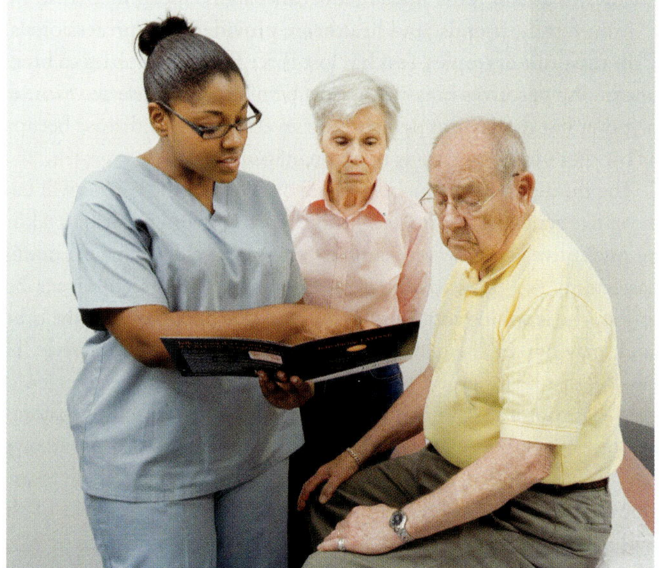

FIGURE 22.2 Teaching the family member along with the patient can provide the patient with more support.

Tips for Improving Learning

Here are some tips to help patients remember critical information:

- Make sure that you address (as much as you can) any affective domain barriers prior to educating a patient.
- If another family member has accompanied the patient, it can be helpful to instruct both the patient and the family member (Figure 22.2).
- Written home instructions should also be given.

THE MEDICAL ASSISTANT'S ROLE IN COACHING

Coaching provides patients with the skills, knowledge, support, and confidence needed to manage their disease between provider visits.

One study found that coaching by medical assistants increased the patients' compliance with medication regimens and lifestyle changes. Coaching is extremely valuable for patients.

Areas of Health Coaching

The medical assistant can assist a provider by coaching patients in many areas.

- *Disease prevention*: Provide patients with information on preventing the disease or the spread of disease. Medical assistants can provide information on respiratory hygiene, recommended vaccines, and nicotine **cessation**.
- *Health maintenance*: Provide patients with information on routine screenings and show patients how to do self-exams (e.g., foot, breast, and oral self-exams).
- *Diagnostic tests*: Instruct patients prior to diagnostic tests. This can include special preparation (e.g., fasting and bowel cleansing preparations).
- *Treatment plans*: Instruct patients on home care and follow-up as ordered by the provider. Research has shown that coaching can help patients understand information from the visit. It can ensure patients understand how they need to proceed and addresses any concerns before patients leave the facility. Coaching educates patients on self-management of diseases, thus increasing compliance with the treatment plans.

Specific information on these coaching topics will be discussed later in the chapter.

Coaching on Community Resources

Besides the four areas of health coaching discussed in the prior section, medical assistants can coach patients on community resources. By listening to patients and asking questions, the medical assistant can identify patients' unique needs. Patients have many needs that affect their health. For instance, if a patient has a limited income, does the patient purchase the prescribed medication or food? Community resources exist to address many needs, including low-cost medications, food banks, transportation, medical supplies, assisted living, and so on. Additional information on community resources will be discussed later in the chapter.

Adapting Coaching for Specific Needs

When you coach patients, it is important to recognize that they are individuals. Patients have unique concerns and barriers to learning. One way of presenting new information to a patient may not work for another patient.

Patients have unique concerns that can include personal, family, social, financial, and culture-related issues. By closely working with the patient, the medical assistant can provide emotional support and create a bond with the patient. This bond helps the patient feel comfortable. With encouragement, the patient may be more willing to call the medical assistant with questions and concerns between visits.

When coaching a patient, the medical assistant must consider the barriers to learning. Strategies used to coach a person with hearing impairments are different than strategies used for a person with visual impairments. The following sections examine strategies to use with different developmental levels and communication issues. Lastly, cultural differences that influence health practices and teaching are described.

ADAPTING COACHING FOR THE DEVELOPMENTAL LEVEL

As we grow and develop, our thought processes and behaviors change. We learn differently. We can understand more complex concepts than when we were younger. It is important for the medical assistant to consider the person's developmental level when coaching. For instance, young children are concrete thinkers. What you say is what they believe you will do. For example, if you say, "I am going to take your blood pressure," a 2-year-old child would have no idea what you are going to do. If you say, "I am going to give your arm a hug," then the child may have a better understanding of what you are going to do. Coaching techniques you use for teens will be different from those you use with older adults. Also, referencing materials as you talk can be helpful to the patient.

Erikson's psychosocial developmental stages can be useful when considering the developmental level of patients (Table 22.3). Understanding the goal of each stage can help a medical assistant to coach patients in that age group.

Working with Infants, Toddlers, and Preschoolers

When working with infants, the medical assistant should use a calm, soothing voice and hold the child securely. It is important to involve the parents and guardians as much as possible. The medical assistant should attempt to keep the infant's routines consistent as much as possible. For instance, if it is time for the infant to eat, allow the child to eat unless eating/drinking is restricted for a medical reason.

When working with toddlers, use simple, familiar words. The medical assistant should allow the child to handle equipment and make choices. Coaching can be adapted for this age group by using play to teach a toddler.

With preschoolers, use familiar words and simple explanations and demonstrations. The medical assistant should allow the child to handle equipment and make choices. When explaining a procedure to a preschooler, explain it as the child would sense it (e.g., how it feels and looks).

Working with School-Age Children and Adolescents

When working with school-age children, the medical assistant should use engaging, simple tools to communicate information. This would include videos, gaming software, and pamphlets. The medical assistant should encourage discussion and questions and allow the child to make choices. Coaching should be adapted to use concrete terms (with pictures and diagrams) when explaining procedures.

Providing privacy and independence is critical for adolescents. The medical assistant should promote responsible decision making and an honest discussion about lifestyle issues, such as vaping and drinking alcohol. When discussing procedures with adolescents, address how a procedure might affect the adolescent's appearance. The medical assistant should encourage discussion and questions when coaching adolescents.

Working with Adults

When working with adults in young adulthood or middle adulthood, it is important to identify their motivating factors. What is motivating the patient to learn the content? The medical assistant should find out what the person knows about the topic and correct any inaccuracies. Once this foundation has been established, the medical assistant can

TABLE 22.3 Erikson's Psychosocial Development Stages

DEVELOPMENT STAGE	AGE RANGE	GOALS OF STAGE
Trust versus mistrust	Infancy (0–1.5 years old)	Must develop trust, with the ability to mistrust should the need arise.
Autonomy versus shame and doubt	Toddler (1.5–3 years old)	Must explore and manipulate things in their "world" to develop autonomy and self-esteem.
Initiative versus guilt	Preschooler (3–6 years old)	Encourage to try new activities. Must assume responsibilities and learn new skills. Will make child feel purposeful and increase self-esteem.
Industry versus inferiority	School age (6–12 years old)	Must seek to finish tasks. Recognition for accomplishments is important.
Identity versus role confusion	Adolescence (12–18 years old)	To know who you are as a person and how you fit into the world around you. Creates a meaningful self-image.
Intimacy versus isolation	Young adulthood (18–25 years old)	Can vary. Develops friendships; takes on commitments.
Generativity versus stagnation	Middle adulthood (25–60 years old)	Achieve a balance between the concern for the next generation (having a family) and being self-absorbed.
Ego integrity versus despair	Late adulthood (60 years old or older)	Reflect on one's life and come to terms with it instead of regretting the past.

build on the prior information. The medical assistant must listen to the adult's concerns and provide resources as needed.

When working with patients in their late adulthood, the medical assistant must communicate with dignity and respect. Using simpler language and speaking clearly can help if the patient has communication barriers, such as impaired hearing. The medical assistant must allow time for the adult to respond. As with younger adults, it is important to find out what the person knows about the topic, correct any inaccuracies, and then build on their knowledge. The medical assistant must listen to the adult's concerns and provide resources as needed.

CRITICAL THINKING APPLICATION 22.3

In the family practice environment, Suzanne sees patients of all ages. Explain why the methods she uses with 2-year-old children should differ from those she uses when working with teens. What strategies could she use when coaching both populations?

ADAPTING COACHING FOR COMMUNICATION BARRIERS

Coaching patients with communication barriers can be a challenging process. Hearing, vision, and language barriers are common in healthcare. It is estimated that 2% of people in the United States have a visual impairment, 3% have a hearing impairment, and 9% have limited English proficiency. It is important to overcome these barriers when coaching patients.

For healthcare agencies accepting federal funds, the Civil Rights Act requires that all patients have equal access to services. People with vision, hearing, or speech impairments use different ways to communicate. The Americans with Disability Act requires effective communication with patients who have impairments. This may mean offering a qualified medical interpreter or other interpretation services free of charge. Large-print materials and written instructions are also required. Translated written materials are needed for non-English-speaking patients.

The following sections provide tips for communicating with patients. It is important to listen to patients concerning what works best for them.

Patients Who Have Impaired Vision

When you work with patients who have impaired vision, it is important to ensure the room has adequate light. Position the patient so they do not have to look directly toward the light source. Make sure the patient is wearing glasses or contacts if needed. When teaching a patient with impaired vision, the following points are important:

- Consider the impact of color contrast and glare on the materials used. Use a large black and white font (larger than 14 points) or an electronic copy that can be enlarged. Use bold markers for handwritten information.
- Ask the patient how they prefer the information. Provide the patient with large-print directions or brochures.
- Have adaptive equipment available or information on resources for such equipment. For instance, you need to show a patient how to draw up insulin using a syringe. Having a syringe magnifier can help the patient see the calibration markings on the syringe (Figure 22.3).
- Face the patient directly. Make eye contact, if culturally appropriate. Use a normal tone of voice.
- Note that gestures and other nonverbal cues are not as helpful with visual impairments.
- Encourage the patient to use their own magnification aids.

Patients Who Have Impaired Hearing

When teaching a patient with impaired hearing, the following points are important:

- Face the person when speaking.
- Determine if the person has better hearing in one ear than the other. Position yourself so your voice is close to the better-hearing side.

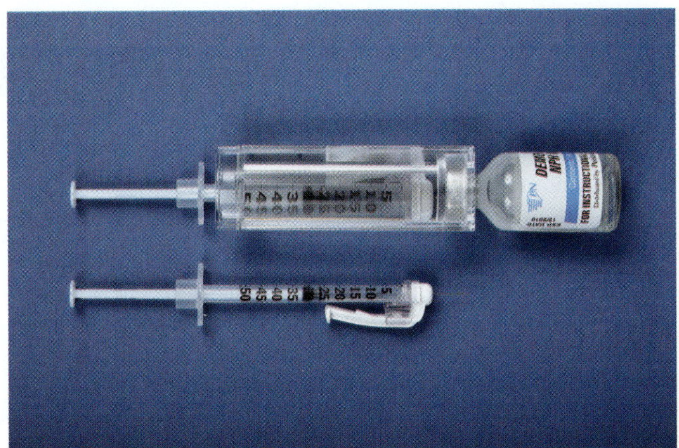

FIGURE 22.3 Syringe magnifiers are used by people with visual impairments. The magnifiers increase the size of the calibration markings on the syringes.

- If the patient has a hearing aid, encourage them to use it.
- Use a low-pitched voice, and speak clearly, slowly, and distinctly. Pause between sentences or phrases. Speak naturally; do not shout. Limit medical terms.
- Say the person's name before you begin a conversation.
- Keep your hands away from your face when talking.
- Speak louder if you are wearing a mask.
- If an interpreter is present, look at the patient, not the interpreter.
- Limit extra noises in the environment.
- Attempt to rephrase or find a different way to say something if the patient has difficulty understanding a phrase.
- Provide important information in writing.
- Have the person repeat back important information.

Patients Who Have Language Barriers

When teaching a patient who has a language barrier, these points are important:

- Address the patient by their last name (e.g., Mrs. Martinez, Mr. Nguyen).
- Be respectful and courteous.
- Use simple phrases. If medical terminology must be used, make sure to define it for patients.
- Use an interpreter or an interpretation service. Focus on the patient and not on the interpreter.
- Use translated materials.
- Note that pictures and models can be helpful during the coaching session.

CULTURAL DIVERSITY

Culture is the set of behaviors, ideas, and customs shared by a specific group of people that distinguishes the members from other people. Some characteristics of a culture group may include its language, religious beliefs, geographic origin, ethnicity, history, sexual orientation, and socioeconomic class. Culture can be learned from prior generations and passed on to future generations. It is dynamic and evolving. Our culture frames and shapes how we feel about our health and the world around us.

Factors Affected by Culture

A person's culture will affect a number of factors that healthcare professionals should consider:

- Role of the family and community: Who makes the healthcare decisions? Who pays for the healthcare? Who needs to be present during healthcare discussions?
- Religion: What are the beliefs about illness? Will the person's religious beliefs affect adherence to the treatment?
- Views on health, wellness, death, and dying
- Views on complementary therapies (e.g., chiropractic care, massage) and alternative therapies (other practices used in place of conventional medicine)
- Views on gender roles and relationships
- Beliefs related to food, diet, illness, and health
- Beliefs regarding sexuality, fertility, and childbirth

Similar Cultural Practices

In the United States, disease conditions are seen as more of a scientific situation. Science plays a major role in medicine. Many other cultures take more of a holistic approach. A *holistic approach* focuses on the interrelationship among the physical, mental, social, and spiritual aspects of a person's life. A holistic approach is broader than a scientific approach to health and illness.

Many cultures have similar practices:

- *Coining and spooning*: Rubbing a silver coin or spoon vigorously on the skin. These practices leave red marks on the skin. Do not confuse the marks with signs of abuse.
- *Cupping*: Applying suction to the skin, which can leave marks. Do not confuse these marks with signs of abuse.
- *Acupressure*: Applying firm pressure on specific points on the body.
- *Acupuncture*: Inserting fine needles into acupuncture points (specific sites on the body).

It is important to remember that not every member of the same culture has the same health beliefs. Differences are typically seen between the generations. The healthcare professional should not assume patients have specific health beliefs. However, being aware of possible cultural beliefs and practices of a group is important. It can help the medical assistant ask related questions to identify a patient's beliefs and practices.

Cultural Differences

The following are generalized cultural differences for a variety of cultures. It is important to remember the generalizations but realize that they will not apply to each person of that culture.

- African Americans
  - Extended family and church play important roles.
  - May have a key family member who must be consulted on healthcare decisions.
  - Older members may look at their health as being up to God's will, although younger members seek health screening and treatments as needed.
- Cambodians
  - Good health means the person is balanced; belief in the balance of hot and cold.
  - Illness may be seen as punishment for sins in a past life.

- Typically use traditional healing practices before seeking conventional medicine. May use herbs, cupping, coining, acupuncture, and acupressure.
- They may not be interested in preventive care and screenings.

- Chinese
  - May use acupuncture, massage, and herbs, seeking care from traditional practitioners for less severe illnesses.
  - Respectful of elders, teachers, and healthcare professionals. It may affect how a person interacts and discusses health topics with the healthcare professional. The person may not ask questions or discuss concerns.
- Hispanics/Latinos
  - May have strong family and religious beliefs. Family is respected and plays an important role. May view an illness as God's will.
  - May use home remedies or follow folk healer's advice over conventional medicine.
  - Sickness is caused by a person having too much heat or cold. Foods and herbs are used to bring back the balance. (Heat and cold are not temperature related.) Cold diseases have more unseen symptoms, such as a chest cold and an earache. Hot diseases have more visible symptoms, such as vomiting, fever, and sore throat.
  - Males often answer questions and give consent. Make sure to address the patient also. Friendliness and respectfulness are very important.
- Hmong
  - Lack words in native language for medical terms and some body organs.
  - May seek care from folk medicine doctors and shamans.
  - Herbs, massage, coining or spooning, and cupping can be used.
  - Accessories may be worn around wrists, necks, or ankles for health or religious reasons.
  - Respecting older family members is very important. Often oldest male in the family is the decision maker. Extended family is very important.
  - Eye contact is considered rude.
  - Touching the head of a child is not accepted. The head is considered sacred.
- Native Americans
  - May place a lot of value in family and spiritual beliefs.
  - State of health occurs when living in total harmony with nature. Illness is the imbalance between the person and nature.
  - May use a traditional tribal medicine person.
  - Often avoid direct eye contact out of respect and concern for the loss of one's soul.
- Russians
  - May view healthcare with some mistrust, based on past experience.
  - May not be used to asking questions and participating in a discussion with a provider.
  - Some practice home remedies and bonki. *Bonki* is practiced by pressing glass cups against the person's shoulders to ease the symptoms. Bruising can occur, which should not be confused with abuse.
  - Family likes to receive news about patient's condition and prognosis and may not give bad news to the patient. This lessens the person's anxieties and promotes calmness.
- Somalis
  - Believe that individuals do not prevent illness, which is only done through prayer and living a life according to their religion.
  - Use traditional spiritual healers.
  - May not take medication if they feel healthy.
  - Healthcare decisions are made by the family, and the father gives consent for procedures.
  - Male and female circumcisions are performed; being uncircumcised means the person is unclean.
- Vietnamese
  - Illness is often explained by mystical beliefs.
  - Health is the balance between the hot and cold poles that govern bodily functions.
  - Use alternative therapies, such as acupuncture, coining, spooning, and cupping.

CRITICAL THINKING APPLICATION 22.4

In the family practice environment, Suzanne sees patients from a variety of cultures. If you worked in a similar place, what would you do if you noticed red circles on a child's back but were unsure what caused those circles?

TEACHING-LEARNING PROCESS

Teaching opportunities vary greatly in ambulatory care. Sometimes a patient wants to know what a certain medication is for. Other times, the medical assistant needs to coach a patient on a diagnostic test.

Always take a moment to look over any information you provide to patients. Make sure you know the content before you review it with the patient. Providing information that conflicts with the handout will confuse the patient.

The medical assistant should start the coaching process by finding out what the patient knows about the topic. A simple way to do this is by asking a few questions, such as "Have you had an ultrasound before? If so, what do you remember about it?" This helps the medical assistant identify what the patient knows. From there, the medical assistant can begin teaching.

Steps of the Teaching-Learning Process

When coaching patients, it is important to follow these steps to ensure the coaching is relevant to the patient's needs:

1. *Identify the patient's educational needs:* What does the patient need to learn? What are the patient's motivations and concerns? What is the patient's learning style? It is important to identify the patient's learning goals or the main reason for learning the content.
2. *Identify barriers to learning*: It is important to identify barriers to learning and to use strategies to overcome those barriers. Be sure to consider the patient's individual needs (e.g., primary language, developmental level, barriers to learning). Teaching aids, such as brochures, online resources, models, health-related apps, and drawings, can be helpful to overcome certain barriers. For patients with lower reading levels or English as a second language, using more pictures can be helpful. Using different teaching strategies can also reduce barriers to learning. For skills, demonstration, and role-play

with demonstration are effective strategies. Discussion, videos, and internet sites can be helpful for teaching about a disease, diagnostic tests, or treatment.

3. *Coach the patient on the topic*: It is important to start with the basics and build from there. Keep the information simple, focused, and appropriate for the individual patient. Reinforce important information. If teaching a skill, make sure to have the equipment available that the patient will use at home. This will promote the patient's comfort with the task.
4. *Evaluate the patient's learning*: After teaching important points, have the patient summarize what you stated. Keeping patients involved will help them retain more information. Throughout the teaching session, make sure to ask patients for feedback to determine whether they understand what you are discussing. Instead of just saying, "Do you understand?" ask specific questions to evaluate the patient's learning, such as "What are four symptoms of low blood sugar?" Summarize the important points at the end of the teaching session. Answer any questions the patient may have. Identify areas in which the patient needs more information. If there will be more than one session, summarize what will occur during the next meeting
5. *Document the coaching*: It is important to document the content taught to the patient, how the patient responded, evidence that the patient learned the content, handouts given, and any plans for follow-up. Make sure to include the provider's name and any adaptations you made to individualize the teaching/learning experience. Evidence may include statements such as "Pt safely and accurately walked 20 feet using the walker" or "Pt stated six signs and symptoms of hypoglycemia."

Guidelines for Patient Education Materials

The following are some guidelines for medical assistants who are responsible for developing or ordering educational supplies:

- The material should be written in lay language at a sixth- to eighth-grade level to promote understanding.
- Good pictures can help patients understand the information.
- Information should be well organized and clearly described.
- All material should be checked for accuracy. (Providers will want to approve the information ahead of time.)
- Handouts should be attractive and professional.
- Copies should be available in languages other than English when possible and in large print for visually impaired clients.
- Disease information literature from medical and pharmaceutical companies that includes advertising of their products should not be used. (This type of information can create confusion if the patient is not using the product advertised.)

COACHING ON DISEASE PREVENTION

Medical assistants coach patients of all ages on disease prevention. It is important to help patients understand ways to prevent diseases in their lives. Common disease prevention coaching by age group includes the following:

- School-age children: Teaching about hand washing.
- Teens and adults: Teaching about ways to prevent sexually transmitted infections (STIs) and the risks of using cigarettes, smokeless tobacco, and e-cigarettes.
- All age groups: Teaching about respiratory hygiene/cough etiquette. Coaching patients and parents on the vaccines recommended for that specific age (Procedure 22.1). Childhood immunization schedules can be found on the website for the Centers for Disease Control and Prevention (CDC), www.cdc.gov/vaccines/schedules/downloads/child/0-18yrs-child-combined-schedule.pdf. Common adult vaccines usually include the following:
  - Influenza yearly.
  - Tetanus and diphtheria (Td) every 10 years and substitute tetanus, diphtheria, and acellular pertussis vaccine (Tdap) once.
  - Recombinant zoster vaccine (RZV), Shingrix, two doses for adults age 50 or older.
  - 13-Valent pneumococcal conjugate vaccine (PCV13), one dose usually after age 65 unless given before based on the patient's health.
  - 23-Valent pneumococcal polysaccharide vaccine (PPSV23 or PPSV), one to two doses, depending on the patient's health

Additional vaccines can be given based on the situation (e.g., traveling or job related); adulthood immunization schedules can be found on the CDC's website, www.cdc.gov/vaccines/schedules/downloads/adult/adult-combined-schedule.pdf.

Respiratory Hygiene/Cough Etiquette

It is important for everyone to be aware of respiratory hygiene/cough etiquette. The Centers for Disease Control and Prevention (CDC) encourages the use of respiratory hygiene/cough etiquette to prevent the transmission of all respiratory infections:

- Cover your mouth and nose with a tissue when coughing or sneezing.
- Discard the tissue in the nearest waste container.
- Wash your hands or use an alcohol-based hand sanitizer.

Sexually Transmitted Infections

Teaching teens and adults how to prevent STIs is important.

- *Abstinence* (not having any type of sex) is the most reliable way to prevent STIs.
- Long-term mutual monogamy (an agreement to be sexually active with just one person) with an uninfected partner is also a reliable way to prevent STIs.
- Reducing the number of partners reduces the risk. All partners need to be tested.
- Use latex condoms, although they are not 100% effective.
- Avoid sharing underwear and towels.
- Wash after intercourse.
- Avoid anyone with a genital rash, sore, discharge, or other symptoms.
- Get vaccinated for hepatitis B and human papillomavirus (HPV).

CRITICAL THINKING APPLICATION **22.5**

Suzanne works with teens. List ways to prevent STIs.

Tobacco and Nicotine Delivery Products

Teaching children, teens, and adults about the health risks associated with tobacco and nicotine delivery products is important. Often manufacturers of such products market to children and teens, making the products look attractive.

Local resources and prescriptive medications are available if a person wants to quit using these products. Websites (e.g., https://smokefree.gov) and quitlines are also available (e.g., the National Cancer Institute Smoking Quitline: 1-877-44U-QUIT).

Tobacco Products and Health Issues

The leaves of the tobacco plant are dried and fermented before they are used in tobacco products. Nicotine, an addictive chemical, is found in tobacco. Tobacco can come in several types of products:

- Smoked tobacco: cigarettes, cigars, bidis, and kreteks. Loose tobacco can be smoked in a pipe or hookah (water pipe).
- Smokeless tobacco: chewing tobacco, moist snuff, snus, and moist powder tobacco

The nicotine is readily absorbed into the blood. Nicotine triggers the release of epinephrine (adrenaline), which stimulates the central nervous system. The blood pressure, breathing rate, and heart rate increase. Nicotine also increases the level of dopamine in the brain. Increased levels of dopamine help a person feel happy, motivated, focused, and alert. Thus, the action of nicotine makes quitting hard.

Hookahs. Hookahs, also called narghile, argileh, shisha, hubble-bubble, and goza, are water pipes that are used to smoke specially made flavored tobacco. A typical hookah has a head, a metal body, a water bowl, and a flexible hose with a mouthpiece. Usually, hookah smoking occurs in a group, and users share the mouthpiece.

Hookah smoking has many of the same health risks as cigarette smoking. Both products deliver nicotine. The charcoal used to heat the tobacco in a hookah produces high levels of carbon monoxide, metals, and cancer-causing chemicals. Hookah use can cause lung, bladder, and oral cancers. Smoke inhalation is greater with the typical hookah used compared to smoking a cigarette; thus, there is a greater absorption of the toxic substances compared to cigarette smoking.

Hazards of Tobacco Smoke. Even though nicotine is addicting, the severe health risks are related to the other chemicals in tobacco smoke. Tobacco smoke contains more than 7000 chemicals, of which 250 are harmful, and at least 69 can cause cancer. One in five deaths is related to smoking. According to the CDC, smokers are more likely to develop heart disease, lung cancer, and strokes. Smoking can cause problems in all parts of the body, and quitting has numerous health advantages, which are discussed in length in Chapter 41.

Secondhand smoke causes lung cancer, strokes, low-birth-weight babies, and heart disease. Children exposed to secondhand smoke have increased risks of sudden infant death syndrome (SIDS), ear infections, bronchitis, pneumonia, colds, and asthma. *Thirdhand smoke* is the residue or chemicals from the smoke that gets on skin, clothing, furniture, carpeting, and so on. This can be harmful to little children and animals that spend time on the floor. This residue—and its chemicals—can be breathed in and ingested. They can be transferred from the carpet, clothing, and so on to hands and then into a person's mouth.

Hazards of Smokeless Tobacco Products. The CDC reports that at least 28 cancer-causing chemicals have been found in smokeless tobacco (e.g., chew and dip). Smokeless tobacco can cause cancer of the mouth, pancreas, and esophagus.

Electronic Cigarettes

Electronic cigarettes are known as e-cigarettes, e-cigs, e-hookahs, mods, vape pens, tank systems, electronic nicotine delivery systems (ENDS), or vapor cigarettes (Figure 22.4). These devices are battery operated or rechargeable. Manufacturers create these products to look like or to be concealed in everyday devices. Examples include pens, USB drives, vaping hoodies, backpacks, phone cases, and smartwatches.

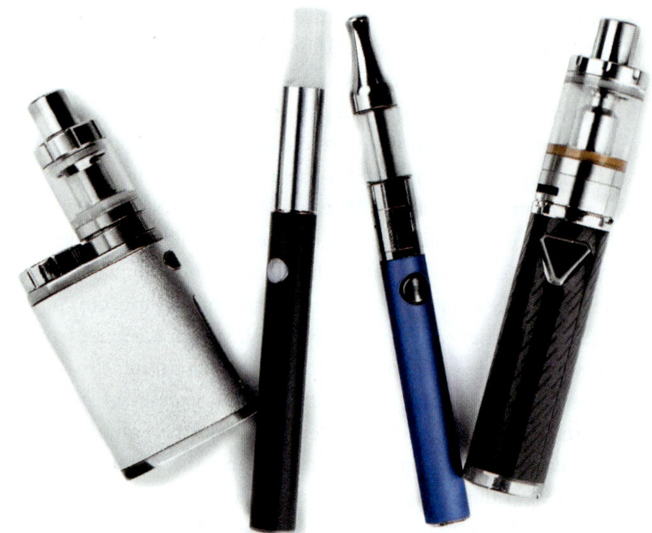

FIGURE 22.4 Electronic cigarettes or vaping devices. (Courtesy iStock.com/MakcouD.)

E-cigs use a liquid that contains nicotine, flavorings, and other chemicals. The liquid is heated, creating an aerosol. The user inhales the aerosol. The air exhaled contains the aerosol and can also be breathed in by bystanders. According to the CDC, the e-cig aerosol can contain the following:

- Flavorings such as diacetyl, which is linked to a serious lung disease
- Volatile organic compounds
- Cancer-causing chemicals
- Heavy metals (e.g., nickel, lead, and tin)
- Marijuana and other drugs

E-cig aerosol contains fewer harmful chemicals when compared to the smoke from tobacco products, but the aerosol contains causer-causing chemicals and tiny particles that can reach deep into the lungs. Nicotine salts (nic salts) are also used in e-cigs and allow high levels of nicotine to be inhaled. E-cigs are highly addictive, and the nicotine can harm brain development in children and adults. Nicotine is also dangerous for pregnant women and their developing babies in utero.

COACHING ON SELF-EXAMS FOR HEALTH MAINTENANCE AND WELLNESS

Often with health maintenance and wellness, the provider establishes standing orders for specific education to be given based on the patient's history or age. When the medical assistant rooms a patient, a health history is obtained, and screening questions are asked. Based on the patient's answers, the medical assistant may need to provide coaching on specific topics per the provider's standing orders. For instance, a patient states they smoke one pack of cigarettes daily. The provider's standing order for smokers requires the medical assistant to provide information on the hazards of tobacco use and resources for quitting.

Another example would be a patient who is turning 45. Because colon cancer screenings typically start at age 45, the provider's standing order would be to provide this information to the patient.

The following sections discuss self-exams that can be taught to patients. The purpose of self-exams is to identify changes in one's body. Sometimes these changes can be the first sign of a disease. Self-exams are typically done monthly. To help maintain a person's health, the early diagnosis of a disease such as cancer is important.

Breast and Testicular Self-Exams

Breast cancer can affect both females and males, though males are at a lower risk. Breast cancer is the second most common cancer in females after skin cancer. The risk of breast cancer increases with age. About one in eight women will have invasive breast cancer. Typically, the survival rate is higher the earlier the cancer is diagnosed.

According to the American Cancer Society, males at any age can develop testicular cancer. About 50% of those diagnosed are between 20 and 34 years of age. It is estimated that 1 in 263 males will get testicular cancer.

Breast Self-Exams

It is important for all women to know what is normal with their breasts. Any abnormality should be reported to their provider. Warning signs of breast cancer include the following:

- Change in the skin (redness, warmth, darkening of the color, dimpling, puckering)
- Lump or hard area inside the breast or in the axilla area
- Change in the size or shape of the breast
- Change in the nipple (inverted or pulling in appearance, rash, sore, or drainage)
- Pain that does not go away

According to the American Cancer Society, research has not shown a benefit from patient or provider breast exams when women are also getting mammograms. It is recommended for women with an average risk of breast cancer to have yearly mammograms between ages 45 and 54. Mammograms are optional before age 45 and should be done every two years after 55. It is important for all women to know what is normal with their breasts. Any abnormality should be reported to their provider. Some providers still recommend a monthly breast self-exam (BSE) to be done after the menses (discussed in Chapter 43).

Testicular Self-Exam

If testicular cancer is found early (before it has spread), there is a good chance of a cure. The American Cancer Society recommends that providers perform a testicular exam as part of a routine physical exam. Some providers recommend that after puberty (around age 15), males should do a monthly testicular self-exam (TSE) after a shower (discussed in Chapter 42).

Skin Self-Exam

Skin cancer is the most common type of cancer in the United States. The three most common types of skin cancer are basal cell, squamous cell, and melanoma. Basal cell and squamous cell carcinomas are curable. Melanoma is more dangerous and can cause death. These three types of skin cancers are caused by overexposure to ultraviolet (UV) light. UV exposure comes from the sun, tanning beds, and sun lamps. UV rays are an invisible kind of radiation that penetrates and changes skin cells.

Certain people have a greater risk than others for skin cancer. Risk factors for skin cancer include the following:

- Skin that is lighter than normal skin color; burns, freckles, or reddens easily; becomes painful in the sun
- Family or personal history of skin cancer
- History of sunburns (especially early in life) or indoor tanning
- Exposure to the sun through work or play
- Green or blue eyes
- Red or blond hair
- Certain types and a large number of moles

ABCDE Rule

Experts recommend monthly skin self-exams. It is important to watch for changes in moles. To remember how moles may change, use the ABCDE rule:

- **A**symmetry: One half of the mole does not match the other half.
- **B**order: The edges of the mole are blurred or irregular.
- **C**olor: The mole is not the same color throughout and has shades of tan, brown, black, red, white, or blue.
- **D**iameter: The mole is larger than 6 mm, about the size of a pencil eraser or pea, but it could be smaller.
- **E**volving: The mole changes over time.

Any change in moles, including the size, shape, color, elevation, or symptom (e.g., bleeding, itching, or crusting), should be reported immediately (Figure 22.5).

When doing the monthly skin check, start at the scalp and work toward the soles of the feet. Use mirrors to examine the back of the ears and the back. Many people miss mole changes on the back of their ears. When examining hands and feet, make sure to check between the fingers and toes and check the nail beds. Check all skin surfaces. Document the location of the moles and their appearances. Any changes seen or suspicious-looking moles should be reported to the provider immediately.

Oral Cancer Self-Exam

Oral cancer includes cancer of the lips, tongue, throat, salivary glands, pharynx, larynx, and sinuses. Here are some facts about oral cancer:

- Men get oral cancer twice as often as women.
- Using tobacco, drinking alcohol, or having oral HPV are risk factors for oral cancer.
- About 25% of those with oral cancer had no risks.
- Most oral cancers occur after age 40.

It is estimated that more than 40,000 new cases of oral cancer are diagnosed yearly, with almost 9000 related deaths. Early detection is important for oral cancer. Signs and symptoms of oral cancer include the following:

- White or red patches in the mouth or on the gums, tongue, or lips
- Numbness or pain in the mouth; pain with chewing or talking
- Long-term hoarseness or sore throat
- Swelling in the jaw area or constant earache
- Bleeding in the mouth or a long-term sore
- Feeling of a lump or something stuck in the throat

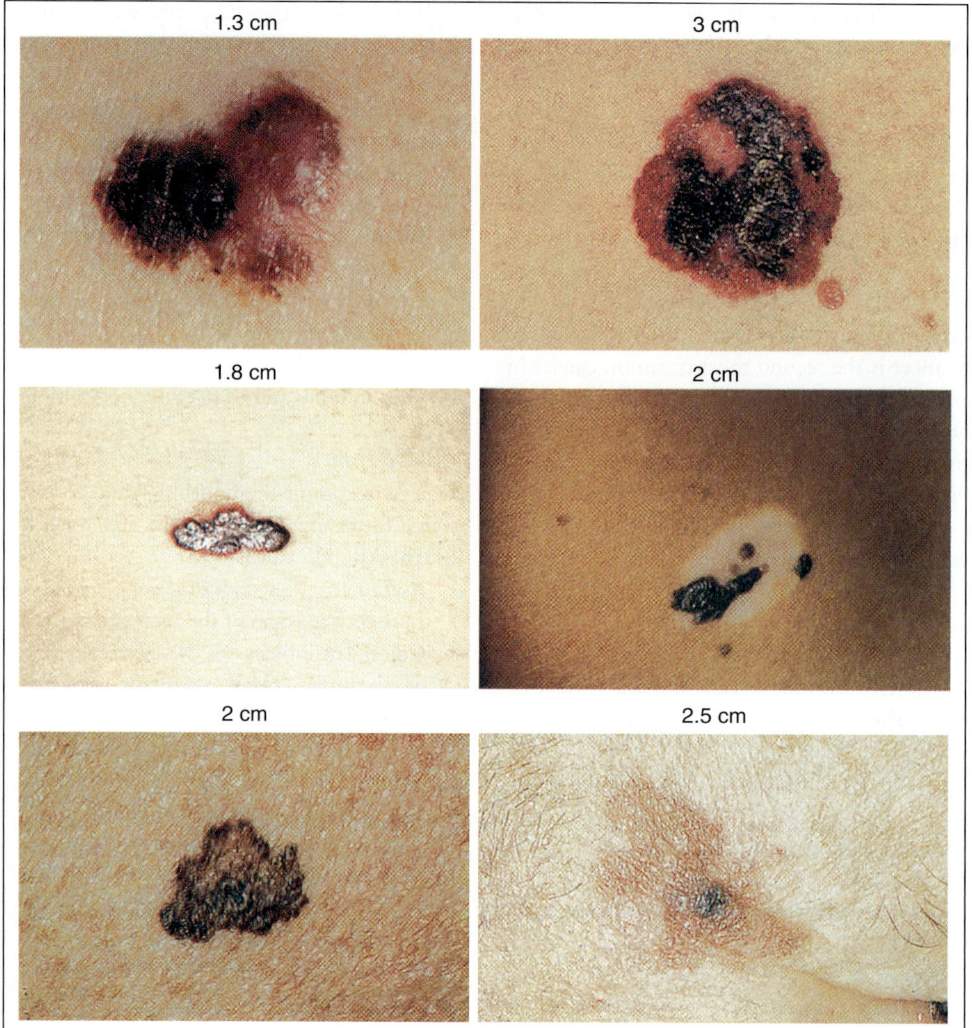

FIGURE 22.5 Malignant melanomas. Note the presence of the ABCDE characteristics. (From Rothrock J: *Alexander's care of the patient in surgery*, ed 14, St. Louis, 2011, Mosby.)

Steps for an Oral Cancer Self-Exam

Oral cancer screening is routinely done by the dentist and should occur every 6 months. It is important for people to do a monthly oral cancer self-exam. Any changes in appearance or sores that do not heal should be reported to the dentist immediately. According to the American Dental Hygienists Association, an oral cancer self-exam consists of looking for lumps and color changes and then feeling for lumps and swelling. To do an oral cancer self-exam, follow these steps:

1. Check the head and neck for lumps, bumps, or swelling. Is one side of the face larger than the other?
2. Check the skin on the face for changes. Is there a color change? Are there sores, moles, or growths?
3. Check for any lumps or tenderness in the neck.
4. Check the upper and lower lip for sores and color changes. After the visual inspection, feel for any changes in texture or lumps.
5. Check the inner cheek for any color changes (red, white, or dark patches). Then palpate the cheeks with a thumb on the outside and a finger inside. Are any lumps found?
6. Check the roof of the mouth for lumps and color changes. Feel for any lumps.
7. Check the floor of the mouth, using your tongue, for any lumps; also, check for color changes. Examine all angles. Feel the tongue with a finger for any lumps or tenderness.

COACHING ON SCREENINGS FOR HEALTH MAINTENANCE AND WELLNESS

The following sections discuss regular screenings, one-time screenings, and additional screenings the medical assistant may need to do while obtaining the patient's health information.

Regular Screening

Medical assistants in primary care typically need to talk with patients about the recommended regular screenings for different diseases. Suggested times for screenings are based on an adult with an average risk. If a patient has family members with the disease, that person may have a higher-than-normal risk. This means the patient may need to be screened earlier and more often than other adults. Regular preventive screenings are summarized by age in Table 22.4 and include the following:

TABLE 22.4 Preventive Recommendations

	AGE 18–39	AGE 45–64	AGE 65+
Blood Pressure	Age 18–39: Every 3–5 years; Age 40–44: Annually	Annually	
Bone Density (Females)			Every 2 years
Cholesterol	Every 4–6 years		
Fall Risk Screening			Annually
Fecal Stool Tests (gFOBT, FIT)		Age 45–75: Annually Age 75+: Individual decision	
Stool DNA Test (Cologuard)		Age 45–75: Every 3 years Age 75+: Individual decision	
Colonoscopy		Age 45–75: Every 10 years Age 75+: Individual decision	
Dental Exam	Annually		
Dilated Eye Exam		Age 60+: Every 2 years	
Lung Cancer Screening		Age 55–80 who meet the criteria: Annual low-dose computed tomography (LDCT)	
Mammogram (Females)	Age 40–44: Annually (optional)	Age 45–54: Annually Age 55+: Every 2 years	
Pap Test	Age 21–29: Every 3 years; age 30–65: every 3 years or if having an HPV test then every 5 years		Individual decision
Prostate Cancer (DRE or PSA test)		Age 50–69: Individual decision	
Diabetes Mellitus Type 2	Every 3 years or more frequently if patient has hypertension or obesity		

DRE, Digital rectal exam; *FIT*, fecal immunochemical test; *gFOBT*, guaiac fecal occult blood test; *HPV*, human papilloma virus; *PSA*, prostate-specific antigen.
From Healthfinder.gov, https://healthfinder.gov/HealthTopics/Category/doctor-visits; and American Cancer Society, www.cancer.org.

- *Blood pressure*: Patients at higher risk include African Americans, those who are overweight, and those with previously higher than normal blood pressure readings.
- *Bone density*: This screening provides information on the strength of the patient's bones and if the patient has osteoporosis. Women have a higher risk than men, and it increases with age.
- *Cholesterol*: Adults with a family history of high cholesterol levels or who have high cholesterol need more frequent testing.
- *Colorectal cancer screening*: The American Cancer Society recommends regular screening starting at age 45. Other organizations recommend starting regular screenings at age 50. Screening can either be stool based or visual exams (see Table 22.4).
- *Dental exam*: The American Dental Association recommends a dental exam and cleaning yearly. Dental health can affect the overall health of the body.
- *Dilated eye exam*: It is important to have a dilated eye exam if a person has a risk of eye disease (e.g., glaucoma). The CDC recommends dilated eye exams for the following individuals:
  - Patients with diabetes (recommended annually)
  - African American patients age 40 or older (recommended every 2 years)
  - Patients older than 60 years of age (recommended every 2 years)
  - Patients with a family history of glaucoma (recommended every 2 years)
- *Lung cancer screening*: Patients who are 55 to 80 years old, have a history of heavy smoking, and are currently smoking or quit in the previous 15 years should be screened for lung cancer. (Heavy smoking means smoking one pack of cigarettes a day for 30 years or two packs for 15 years.)
- *Mammogram*: This x-ray of the breasts helps to identify breast cancer. See Table 22.4 for the American Cancer Society recommendations. Mammogram screening recommendations vary by organization.
- *Pap test*: This test is used to identify cervical cancer.
- *Prostate cancer*: Risk factors include being 50 years old or older, being African American, exposure to Agent Orange, and having a father, brother, or son who had prostate cancer. No specific test exists for prostate cancer. The digital rectal exam (DRE) and the

prostate-specific antigen (PSA) test are used. The provider may offer either test after age 50. Frequency is based on the patient's history.

- *Blood glucose test*: Adults should be screened for type 2 diabetes mellitus every 3 years or more often, depending on their medical history.

Fall Risk Screening and Assessment

STEADI (Stopping Elderly Accidents, Deaths & Injuries) is a program established by the CDC to help screen, assess, and intervene when older adults are at risk for falls. The CDC and the American Geriatric Society recommend yearly fall risk screening for adults age 65 or older. If the screening shows the person is at risk, it is recommended that the patient have a fall assessment. According to the CDC, the following factors can cause falls:

- Advanced age, fear of falling, and poor vision
- Previous falls, muscle weakness, and gait and balance problems
- Postural hypotension
- Chronic conditions, such as arthritis, stroke, incontinence, Parkinson disease, dementia, and diabetes mellitus
- Poor stair design and lack of handrails
- Lack of bathroom grab bars
- Dim lighting or glare
- Objects in the walkway, tripping hazards, and slippery or uneven surfaces
- Improper use of assistive devices

The medical assistant can help screen patients by using screening tools available from the CDC or asking the following questions:

- Do you feel unsteady when standing or walking?
- Do you worry about falling?
- Have you fallen in the past year? If so, how many times? Were you injured?

More information on the STEADI program is available on the CDC's website: https://www.cdc.gov/steadi/.

CRITICAL THINKING APPLICATION **22.6**

Suzanne has seen more providers ordering the fecal immunochemical test (FIT) over the guaiac fecal occult blood test. What are the advantages of the FIT test?

One-Time Screenings

The medical assistant may also need to coach patients on one-time screening as indicated by the provider. People are recommended to have the following screenings at least once unless a person's risk is greater than average:

- *Abdominal aortic aneurysm*: Males between 65 and 75 years of age who have smoked at one time in their lives should receive this screening. This population has the highest risk of having an abdominal aortic aneurysm (AAA).
- *Human immunodeficiency virus (HIV) screen*: People 15 to 65 years old need to get an HIV blood test at least once in their lifetime. All pregnant women need to be tested. People with a high risk for HIV should have testing annually, if not more often. High-risk factors include multiple sexual partners, sexual partners who have or may have HIV, and those who use illegal injectable drugs.
- *Hepatitis C*: This condition is passed through blood from an infected person. A person with risk factors should be tested. The following are risk factors for hepatitis C:
  - Born between 1945 and 1965
  - History of a blood transfusion or organ transplantation before 1992
  - Use of injected illegal drugs
  - Chronic liver disease, HIV, or acquired immunodeficiency syndrome (AIDS)

Additional Screenings

When rooming patients, medical assistants have to perform different screenings. Either the patient's age or responses will trigger the need for the screening. Screenings have increased throughout the years. This is due to increased data collection requirements and focusing on prevention and quality patient care. The following are common screenings:

- *Alcohol misuse screening*: Drinking in moderation means that females have no more than one drink a day and males have no more than two drinks per day. (An alcoholic drink is classified as a 12-ounce [oz] bottle of beer, a 5-oz glass of wine, or a 1.5-oz shot of liquor.) Drinking more than the recommended daily amount may lead to health issues.
- *Nicotine or tobacco screening*: Various tools are used. Tools typically focus on whether or not tobacco products are used, how much is used per day, the history of use, and quitting behaviors (e.g., strategies used in the past or thoughts of quitting).
- *Drug abuse screening*: Various tools are used. Tools focus on prescription drug use for nonmedical reasons and illegal drug use. Tools usually identify any history of or recent drug abuse. Here are some common signs of drug abuse:
  - Poor hygiene; changes in eating and sleeping patterns
  - A loss of interest in favorite things
  - Being very energetic, talking fast, being very sociable
  - Being tired, sad, nervous, agitated, and in a bad mood
  - Missing school, work, or appointments
  - Spending money excessively
  - Slowed reaction time, paranoid thinking
- *Intimate partner violence screening*: This screening covers domestic abuse. It is important to remember that both males and females can be victims of domestic abuse. Many psychological and health problems come from violence, including substance abuse, obesity, depression, brain trauma, pregnancy complications, and chronic pain. Intimate partner violence includes controlling behaviors, physical abuse, sexual abuse, and emotional or verbal abuse.
- *Elderly safety screening*: These screening tools focus on how safe the older person feels at home and screen for abuse and neglect. Table 22.5 provides types and symptoms of elder abuse and neglect.
- *Neurological Status Exam*: This screening tool is used to test the patient's cognitive functions and provides a baseline of neurologic information for the provider. Part of the exam also requires gathering information from the patient's caregiver. (See Chapter 37 for more information on the neurological status exam.)
- *Functional status screening*: Several tools are available for primary care providers to use for older patients. By using a functional

TABLE 22.5 Elder Abuse and Neglect

TYPES	SIGNS
Physical abuse	Fractures, rope marks, cuts, bruising, dislocations, broken glasses, giving too little or too much medication, bleeding, and sudden changes in the person's personality or behavior
Sexual abuse	Unexplained sexually transmitted infections, bruising in the genital region, and reports from the older person
Emotional abuse	Not communicating, withdrawn, agitated, and symptoms that mimic dementia
Neglect	Malnutrition, dehydration, lack of proper living conditions, and failing to treat health problems
Abandonment	Leaving the person in a public place
Financial abuse	Stealing from the older person, forging signatures on financial transactions, and any other illegal action that represents a financial loss for the older person

status screening tool, the provider obtains information on the patient, such as the following:
- Physical functions with daily activities (e.g., grooming, bathing, walking, and eating)
- Psychological health (e.g., mood and anxiety)
- Role function (e.g., employed or volunteer)
- Social function (e.g., interacting with others or isolating self)

- *Depression screening*: Several tools are used to screen for depression. The screening tools ask questions related to moods, thoughts, and feelings. The number of questions will vary depending on the tools. For instance, the Patient Health Questionnaire–2 (PHQ-2) asks two questions that focus on the frequency of depressed mood and **anhedonia** over the previous 2 weeks. If the patient screens positive, then the Patient Health Questionnaire–9 (PHQ-9) is given to see if the patient meets the criteria for a depressive disorder (Figure 22.6). (The first two questions of the PHQ-9 are the two questions on the PHQ-2 tool.)
- *Peripheral neuropathy screening*: Screening questions focus on loss of feeling or a "pins and needles" sensation in the feet and hands. Besides asking the patient screening questions, the medical assistant may also need to do a monofilament foot test and coach the patient on foot care. Proper foot care can help to limit foot sores and identify suspicious areas sooner. (See Chapter 39 for more information on peripheral neuropathy screening and proper foot care instructions.)

COACHING ON DIAGNOSTIC TESTS AND TREATMENT PLANS

The provider can direct the medical assistant to provide coaching on diagnostic tests and treatment plans. The following sections describe coaching the medical assistant can do regarding diagnostic tests and treatment plans.

Coaching on Diagnostic Tests

It is important for the medical assistant to provide the necessary teaching for diagnostic and laboratory tests ordered for patients. For tests to be completed, the patient needs to be prepared. Some tests require fasting, whereas others do not. The medical assistant needs to provide answers to these questions:
- What is the test?
- Where does the patient need to go for the test? When is the test scheduled?
- Does the test require fasting? If so, for how long? If no foods or beverages can be consumed, does this include water?
- Should patients continue or stop taking their medications? This may require a discussion with the provider.

It is important to give patients the correct answers. Tables 22.6 and 22.7 provide information on common procedures and medical laboratory tests. Remember, patient preparation may vary based on the facility.

CRITICAL THINKING APPLICATION 22.7

Sometimes Suzanne has a patient who refuses to follow the preparation steps for a diagnostic test. How might you handle this situation?

Coaching on Treatment Plans

Many facilities have the medical assistants meet with the patients after the providers finish their examination. The medical assistants review the treatment plan with the patients. They answer any questions, explore any issues the patients may have, and provide additional instructions. As mentioned, this type of coaching has been shown to increase patients' adherence to the treatment plans. Additionally, it provides patients with a lifeline should they have questions or concerns at home.

Medical assistants coach patients on treatments to do at home, such as these:
- Taking medications
- Monitoring the blood pressure
- Caring for casts and splints, applying hot or cold therapy, and using assistive devices (discussed in Chapter 36)
- Testing blood glucose levels and coagulation using home monitors (discussed in Chapter 49)

Medication Administration at Home

It is important for patients to know how to take medications at home. Here are some helpful questions:
- When should the patient take the medications, and how should they take them?
- Do the medications need to be taken on an empty stomach?
- Can they be taken with the other medications?
- Do they need to be taken at bedtime?

Some patients are on a lot of medications. It is important that the medications are taken correctly. When updating the patient's current medication list, the medical assistant commonly finds discrepancies. For example, the patient may be taking the medication differently from how it was ordered. Any discrepancy found needs to be communicated to the provider.

The medical assistant may coach the patient on the proper ways to take medication. Sometimes the medical assistant may need to help

PATIENT HEALTH QUESTIONNAIRE-9 (PHQ-9)

Over the last 2 weeks, how often have you been bothered by any of the following problems? *(Use "✓" to indicate your answer)*	**Not at all**	**Several days**	**More than half the days**	**Nearly every day**
1. Little interest or pleasure in doing things	0	1	2	3
2. Feeling down, depressed, or hopeless	0	1	2	3
3. Trouble falling or staying asleep, or sleeping too much	0	1	2	3
4. Feeling tired or having little energy	0	1	2	3
5. Poor appetite or overeating	0	1	2	3
6. Feeling bad about yourself — or that you are a failure or have let yourself or your family down	0	1	2	3
7. Trouble concentrating on things, such as reading the newspaper or watching television	0	1	2	3
8. Moving or speaking so slowly that other people could have noticed? Or the opposite — being so fidgety or restless that you have been moving around a lot more than usual	0	1	2	3
9. Thoughts that you would be better off dead or of hurting yourself in some way	0	1	2	3

FOR OFFICE CODING __0__ + ______ + ______ + ______

=Total Score: ______

If you checked off any problems, how difficult have these problems made it for you to do your work, take care of things at home, or get along with other people?

Not difficult at all	Somewhat difficult	Very difficult	Extremely difficult
☐	☐	☐	☐

FIGURE 22.6 Example of a depression screening tool: Patient Health Questionnaire–9 (PHQ-9).

TABLE 22.6 Common Patient Instructions for Common Procedures

PROCEDURES	DESCRIPTION	COMMON PATIENT INSTRUCTIONS
X-ray	X-ray particles pass through the body, and an image is recorded. Many different types of x-rays.	Provide overview of test and why it is being done. X-rays are painless, although some body positions may be uncomfortable. • Patients may be asked to hold the breath during the procedure to get a clear x-ray. • Screen for pregnancy.
Computed tomography scan (CT scan, CAT scan)	Uses x-rays to create pictures of cross sections of the body. Several types of CT scans exist; each may have different preparations. Patient will lie on a narrow table that slides into the center of the CT scanner. The x-ray beam will rotate around the patient, creating separate images (slices) of the body.	Provide overview of test and why it is being done. May require an intravenous (IV) or oral contrast medium. If so, • Check allergies (contrast medium and iodine). • Check if patient has kidney disease or is on dialysis. • Nothing by mouth (NPO) for 4–6 hours before test. • Address if medications need to be stopped. • IV contrast medium may cause a slight burning feeling and a metallic taste in the mouth; flushing can occur.
Bone density scan (also called dual-energy x-ray absorptiometry [DEXA] scan)	Uses a low-dose x-ray test that measures calcium and other minerals in the bone. The measurement shows the strength and thickness of the bones and is used to diagnose osteoporosis.	Provide overview of test and why it is being done. • Patient must stop taking calcium supplements 24 to 48 hours before the test. • Patient should avoid wearing metal jewelry or clothes with metal buttons or buckles. • Patient must lie still in a supine position on a table. The scanning machine will pass over the lower spine and hip. A photon generator will pass beneath the patient. The two images are combined, and a computer image is created.

TABLE 22.6 Common Patient Instructions for Common Procedures—*continued*

PROCEDURES	DESCRIPTION	COMMON PATIENT INSTRUCTIONS
Magnetic resonance imaging (MRI)	Uses powerful magnets and radio waves to create images of the body. Does not use radiation. Several types of MRIs exist; may have different preparations. Patient will lie on a table. The machine makes loud noises. No metal is allowed in the room.	Provide overview of test and why it is being done. May require contrast (see CT scan contrast medium information). • May require being NPO for 4–6 hours • Must identify if patient is claustrophobic (afraid of or anxious about closed spaces). • Due to strong magnets, must screen for artificial heart valves, brain aneurysm clips, heart pacemaker or defibrillator, cochlear (inner ear) implants, recent artificial joint, vascular stents, or history of working with metal. • Must remove all metal from patient, including removable dental work (e.g., plates).
Mammography	An x-ray picture of the breasts used to find tumors. The breast will be compressed on a flat surface for the x-ray.	Provide overview of test and why it is being done. • Do not use any perfume, deodorant, powders, or ointments on the arms or breast on the day of the test; may interfere with the results of the x-ray. • Undress from the waist up and remove all jewelry from the neck and chest area. • Screen for pregnancy, breastfeeding, or if the patient has had a breast biopsy.
Positron emission tomography (PET) scan	Imaging test that uses an IV radioactive substance (tracer) to identify disease in the organs and tissues. Patient will lie on a table that slides into the tunnel-shaped PET scanner.	Provide overview of test and why it is being done. • May require patient to be NPO for 4–6 hours (with exception of water) before the scan. • Medications may be held (check with the provider). IV tracer will be given, which may cause a sharp sting. Afterward the patient needs to rest for 1 hour. During the test, the patient must lie still to prevent blurry images. • Screen for claustrophobia, pregnancy, and allergies to contrast medium and iodine.
Ultrasound (US)	Uses high-frequency sound waves to create the image of the organs and structures.	Provide overview of test and why it is being done. May require special preparation based on the type of US done. • Patient will need to expose the area. • A clear, water-based gel is applied to the skin, and a transducer (handheld probe) moves over the area.
Electroencephalogram (EEG)	Detects electrical activity in the brain using the electrodes that are placed on the scalp.	Provide overview of test and why it is being done. • Avoid caffeine. • Wash hair the night before or the day of the test. Do not use conditioner.
Colonoscopy	An endoscope is inserted through the anus and used to visualize the colon.	Provide overview of test and why it is being done. • Clear liquid diet day before and NPO day of test. • Colon prep as ordered. • Sedation is usually given. Patient may feel cramping or the urge to have a stool when the air is pumped into the colon.

patients find ways to remember to take medications. Many patients use medication boxes that they, a family member, or a pharmacy set up. The boxes typically are arranged for 7 days a week with one or more boxes per day (Figure 22.7). The medications are placed in each box based on the administration time. Some have boxes for morning, noon, and night medications.

If patients are receiving injections at home, they will need to know how to safely dispose of the needles. Patients can dispose of needles in biohazardous sharps containers. These containers are available at local pharmacies and medical supply stores. An internet search can identify local sites that take biohazardous sharps containers from patients. Some drug companies have mail-back programs for specific medications. (For more information, visit https://safeneedledisposal.org.)

Discarding Medications. It is important to encourage patients to discard expired, unwanted, or unused medications. This will help prevent misuse and theft. To get rid of controlled substances, take the medications in their original prescription bottles to a medicine take-back facility. Usually, Drug Enforcement Administration (DEA) representatives are available to take control of the controlled substances. Another option is to contact a DEA-authorized collector. The DEA's website has more information on both programs (https://www.deadiversion.usdoj.gov/).

If these programs are not available, some medications are labeled with specific disposal instructions. Many times, the label recommends flushing controlled substances down the sink or toilet. The website for the Food and Drug Administration (FDA) contains a complete list of medications that can be discarded by flushing (www.fda.gov).

TABLE 22.7 Patient Instructions for Common Medical Laboratory Tests

TEST	USE	COMMON PATIENT PREPARATION
Creatinine	Used to monitor kidney health and disease.	May need to fast overnight. May need to refrain from eating meat for a period of time, because it could increase the creatinine level.
Guaiac fecal occult blood test (gFOBT)	Fecal specimen exam to detect occult or hidden blood, which may indicate gastrointestinal (GI) bleeding. Intestinal bleeding may be an indicator of colon cancer.	Seven days prior to the test: • Stop taking aspirin and nonsteroidal antiinflammatory medications (e.g., ibuprofen, naproxen, and indomethacin). • Do not take vitamin C supplements. Three days before the test: • Do not eat red meat or raw fruits or vegetables (e.g., horseradish, turnips, broccoli, melons, and radishes). • Stool samples are collected over several days, and cards are prepared and sent to the laboratory.
Fecal immunochemical test (FIT)	Fecal specimen exam to detect human hemoglobin protein, which may indicate GI bleeding.	No preparation required. Stool sample is collected by the patient and sent to the laboratory.
Cologuard stool DNA test (FIT-DNA)	Used to detect blood in the stool. Computer analysis looks at the DNA in the stool, checking for cancer and precancerous cells.	No preparation required. Stool sample is collected by the patient and returned to a specific medical laboratory for testing.
Glucose tests	Used to determine the blood glucose level.	For a fasting glucose test, the patient needs to be NPO (nothing by mouth, except for water) for at least 8 hours. Other glucose tests may require fasting and eating at specific times.
Lipid profile	Used to monitor cholesterol levels and treatment.	May require NPO (except for water) prior to the test.
Pap test	Used to screen for cervical cancers and some uterine or vaginal infections.	Do not schedule the test during the menstrual period. For 2 days prior to test: • Refrain from sexual intercourse. • Do not douche or use vaginal medications or spermicidal products.

• Tetanus and diphtheria (Td) every 10 years and substitute tetanus, diphtheria, and acellular pertussis vaccine (Tdap) once.

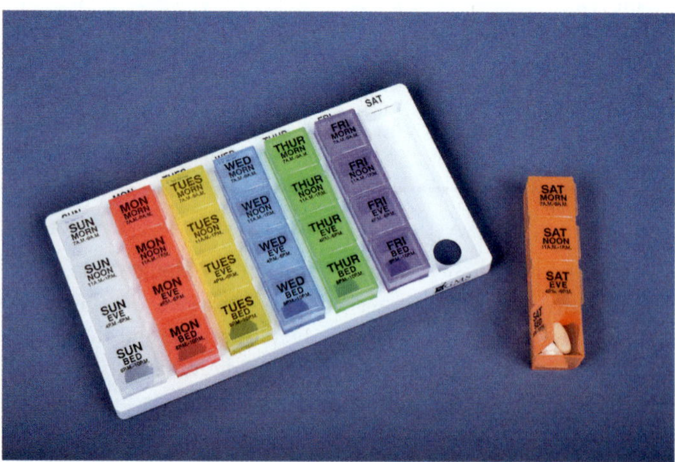

FIGURE 22.7 Daily medication boxes can help patients remember to take their medications.

If the label does not indicate flushing, then mix the medications in an unpalatable substance (dirt, used coffee grounds, or kitty litter). Place the mixture in a plastic bag. Seal and discard it in the household trash. Make sure all personal information and the prescription number have been scratched out on empty pill bottles.

Remote Blood Pressure Monitoring

Remote blood pressure (BP) monitoring can be done by using ambulatory monitors or having patients check their blood pressure using home monitoring machines.

Ambulatory blood pressure monitors can be used to check patients' blood pressures throughout the day. Typically, patients wear the monitor for up to 2 days. The blood pressure is automatically taken and recorded. The provider reviews the patient's blood pressure readings to check for elevated readings over the course of the day.

A variety of manual cuffs and automatic blood pressure monitors are available in stores for patients to purchase for home BP monitoring. Patients should check to see if their insurance covers the cost of the machine.

The American Heart Association (www.heart.org) recommends patients purchase validated automatic home monitors. The blood pressure monitors should be for the upper arm because they are more reliable than the wrist blood pressure monitors. Blood pressure monitors that transmit readings to providers or store blood pressure readings in the memory are recommended. Providers can review these readings to check the effectiveness of the blood pressure management strategies.

Obtaining an Accurate Blood Pressure Reading. When the medical assistant instructs patients how to take their blood pressure reading at home, it can be helpful to have patients bring in their monitors. The medical assistant can check the patient's technique and verify the accuracy of the blood pressure measurement. The patient should be encouraged to bring the machine into the facility every 6 to 12 months to check the accuracy of the reading.

Patients should be coached on the importance of relaxing for at least 5 minutes before taking the reading. Avoiding caffeine, exercise, and smoking for 30 minutes prior to the reading is recommended. They should use the same arm for the reading. The arm must rest 1 to 2 minutes between readings if repeated measurements are taken. These patients should check their BP at various times throughout the day. The medical assistant should also review the patient's position and other factors that impact the accuracy of the reading. Seven additional actions must be taken to obtain an accurate blood pressure reading:

1. *Empty a full bladder*: If the patient has a full bladder and needs to use the restroom, this should be done prior to taking the blood pressure. Dealing with a full bladder can add 10 mm Hg to the BP reading.
2. *Use the correct cuff size*: Using a cuff that is too small can add 2 to 10 mm Hg, and a cuff that is too large can decrease the reading by 5 mm Hg.
3. *Support the back and feet*: The person should be sitting in a chair with the back supported. The feet should be flat on the floor or on a footstool. An unsupported back, slouching, or dangling feet can increase the BP reading by 6 mm Hg.
4. *Keep legs uncrossed*: Large veins in the legs can be squeezed when legs are crossed. This can increase the BP reading by 2 to 8 mm Hg.
5. *Support the arm at heart level*: The arm should be supported on a table or counter, so the BP cuff is at heart level. The arm should be relaxed. The hand should not be clenched. An unsupported arm can increase the BP reading by 10 mm Hg.
6. *Place the cuff on a bare arm*: Have the patient roll up the sleeve or remove the arm from the sleeve. The clothing above the cuff should not be tight because this can restrict the blood flow and alter the BP reading. Placing the cuff over clothing can elevate the BP reading by 5 to 50 mm Hg.
7. *Refrain from engaging in a conversation*: Talking and active listening during the reading can increase the BP reading by 10 mm Hg.

CARE COORDINATION

Care coordination provides personalized patient- and family-centered care in a team-based environment. Care coordination presents numerous advantages:

- Offers greater efficiency in providing patient care
- Reduces costs
- Provides better patient care
- Allows for individualized patient guidance and services
- Encourages patients to focus on goals and self-management
- Reduces hospital emergency department visits and readmissions
- Ensures the patient's needs and preferences for healthcare services are met

Care Coordinator's Role

The care coordinator communicates between the patient and the healthcare team. Care coordinators ensure that patients get timely care and do not fall through the cracks. In the ambulatory care setting, care coordination can be set up in different ways. It has been shown to be successful in primary and specialty care areas. There are a number of overall goals:

- Help patients understand why and what services are needed
- Schedule and sequence appointments
- Provide instructions and directions to patients
- Ensure that test results are available to the providers during patient appointments
- Communicate the patient's needs and concerns to providers

A **patient navigator** (also called a *patient advocate*) has been described as a type of care coordinator. The navigator program was established at the Harlem Hospital Center in 1990. The goal was to assist cancer patients in accessing quality healthcare. Based on the success of patient navigators, the Patient Navigator, Outreach, and Chronic Disease Prevention Act of 2005 funded additional positions. Today, patient navigators typically guide chronically ill patients through the healthcare system. They identify patients' financial, cultural, physical, and emotional barriers. Then, they work closely with the healthcare team and the patients to ensure that barriers are eliminated and patients get timely care.

Medical Assistant's Role as a Care Coordinator

In the ambulatory care setting, medical assistants can be care coordinators. A person must have strong interpersonal skills to be successful as a care coordinator. The medical assistant must listen to the patient and family to identify their needs and concerns. The care coordinator must be compassionate yet provide firm guidance to patients who are difficult.

To contribute to care coordination, a medical assistant might do the following:

- Interview patients to identify their needs and barriers to wellness and healthcare.
- Provide patients with resources based on their needs and barriers.
- Schedule and sequence appointments.
- Make sure the required information is communicated to and from specialty departments.

- Assist with reducing language barriers by identifying bilingual providers and translators.
- Discuss special needs patients have with their healthcare team.
- Identify community resources:
  - Transportation and medical equipment
  - Adult daycare, assisted living, and long-term care
  - Educational programs and support groups
  - Low-cost medication programs
  - Low-cost preventive screening and immunizations

Procedure 22.2 describes the process of creating a current list of community resources and referring patients or family members.

CLOSING COMMENTS

It is an exciting time to become a medical assistant. The medical assistant's role is changing to meet healthcare needs. Studies have shown that medical assistants play an important role in coaching and helping patients comply with treatment and lifestyle changes. It is important for the medical assistant to coach patients in a manner that helps them understand and retain the information. By adapting the coaching methods to the patient's communication barriers, developmental stage, and cultural practices, the medical assistant can help the patient complete the treatment plan.

Patient Coaching

The focus of patient-centered care is to have patients make decisions about their healthcare. Patients need to be given information on such topics as diseases, tests, and treatments to make such decisions. Patient education materials are used to help patients learn more about different topics. With the advances in technology, patient education materials are no longer available just on paper. Apps can help providers explain procedures and diseases to patients. YouTube links and other websites provide videos and information on diseases, procedures, and treatments.

When you use patient education materials from apps and online sites, it is important to use only provider-approved sites. The information must be current and from a reputable source. The following are possible online websites for patient education materials:

- National Institutes of Health (NIH) from the US Department of Health and Human Services (https://www.nih.gov/health-information)
- Centers for Disease Control and Prevention (CDC) (https://www.cdc.gov/)
- MedlinePlus from the US National Library of Medicine (https://medlineplus.gov)
- American Diabetes Association (ADA) (https://www.diabetes.org/)
- American Heart Association (AHA) (https://www.heart.org/)
- Drugs.com (https://www.drugs.com/)
- Mayo Clinic (https://www.mayoclinic.org/)
- Cleveland Clinic (https://my.clevelandclinic.org/health)
- Familydoctor.org from the American Academy of Family Physicians (https://familydoctor.org)

Legal and Ethical Issues

After coaching a patient on a topic, it is important for the medical assistant to document the teaching. The medical assistant should indicate what the provider ordered for coaching, materials used, and general topics taught. The medical assistant should also document an evaluation statement regarding the learning.

Evaluating a patient's learning can be done through several methods, including asking the patient questions regarding the content or having the patient teach back the skill or content. The purpose of the evaluation is to determine if the patient accurately understood the information or skill. The evaluation method and the patient's response should be documented in the medical record for legal purposes.

Patient-Centered Care

Just by design, care coordination helps provide patients with individual assistance. Patients who feel well cared for and comfortable talking with their healthcare team stay with their provider. It is estimated that care coordination will increase in popularity in the coming years. This model of care will also promote exceptional customer service in healthcare.

Professional Behaviors

When coaching patients, the medical assistant must observe the patient's nonverbal and verbal communication. It is important for the medical assistant to listen to the patient and be open to questions from the patient. If the medical assistant does not know the answers to questions or if the questions are outside the medical assistant's scope of practice, the provider should be notified.

SUMMARY OF SCENARIO

During Suzanne's yearly review with her supervisor, she mentioned that she was interested in becoming a care coordinator. She and the supervisor discussed how the program might assist the providers and patients. Suzanne agreed to research the role and bring a proposal to her supervisor in the coming weeks. The supervisor would then take it to the provider meeting and discuss the care model with all of the WMFM Clinic providers. Both are excited to pursue new changes in the practice and continue to provide patients with the best possible care.

SUMMARY OF LEARNING OBJECTIVES

1. **Examine factors that influence health choices, including grief reactions and health beliefs and practices.**
The stages of grief include denial (refusal to accept the fact), anger at oneself or others, attempts to bargain, depression, and acceptance. Table 22.1 describes adaptive interactions for each stage.
The first part of the health belief model deals with a person's perception of the chance of developing a disease. The second part of this model deals with a person's perception of the severity of the disease. The third part of the model focuses on whether the person will take preventive action. A person weighs the benefits and barriers of taking the preventive actions.
2. **Differentiate among the three domains of learning, including barriers to learning, strategies for adapting to barriers, and tips for improving learning.**
We learn new information in three different ways or *domains:* cognitive, psychomotor, and affective. The *cognitive domain* of learning involves mental processes of recall, application, and evaluation. The *psychomotor domain* is the "doing" domain. We learn new skills and procedures by watching demonstrations and assisting with something. The *affective domain* is the "feeling" domain. It includes our feelings, emotions, values, and attitudes. Our emotions and values are very important.
3. **Examine the medical assistant's role with coaching, including areas of coaching and adapting coaching for the individual.**
The medical assistant can help the provider by coaching patients on disease prevention, health maintenance, diagnostic tests, and treatment plans. The medical assistant can also help provide community resources to patients.
The medical assistant must consider patients' unique concerns and barriers to learning, including hearing and visual impairments.
4. **Examine how to adapt coaching based on the patient's developmental level.**
It is important for the medical assistant to consider the barriers to learning and possible ways to help the patient overcome those barriers. It is also important for the medical assistant to remember the patient's developmental level. Erikson's psychosocial developmental stages are described in Table 22.3. Understanding the goal of each stage can help a medical assistant to coach patients in that age group.
5. **Differentiate among the coaching strategies to use for different types of communication barriers.**
For healthcare agencies accepting federal funds, the Civil Rights Act requires that all patients have equal access to services. People with vision, hearing, or speech impairments use different ways to communicate, and the Americans with Disability Act requires effective communication with patients who have impairments. The medical assistant may also need to adapt to communication barriers, including impaired vision and hearing and language barriers. Review the related sections in the chapter for more information on each of these areas.
6. **Examine how cultural beliefs and practices influence health beliefs and practices.**
Culture is the set of behaviors, ideas, and customs shared by a specific group of people that distinguishes the members of that group from other people. Factors affected by a person's culture that healthcare professionals should consider include the following:
   - Role of the family, community, and religion
   - Views on health, wellness, death, dying, complementary therapies, gender roles, and relationships
   - Beliefs related to food, diet, illness, health, sexuality, fertility, and childbirth

   Learning about cultural differences can help the medical assistant ask related questions to identify a patient's beliefs and practices.
7. **Examine the teaching-learning process.**
The medical assistant should start the coaching process by finding out what the patient knows about the topic. From there, the medical assistant can begin teaching. For lengthy coaching situations, the medical assistant should plan ahead so that the time is used efficiently. Using the teaching-learning process requires the following steps:
   - Assessing the patient's learning needs
   - Determining teaching priorities
   - Planning the teaching process
   - Implementing the teaching process
   - Evaluating the patient's learning
   - Documenting the teaching-learning process
8. **Demonstrate coaching on disease prevention, including cough etiquette, sexually transmitted infection prevention, and the cessation of tobacco and nicotine use.**
Medical assistants coach patients of all ages on disease prevention. These topics can include hand washing and cough etiquette, the prevention of sexually transmitted infections, the risks of tobacco and nicotine products, and vaccines recommended for specific age groups.
9. **Demonstrate coaching on self-exams for health maintenance and wellness.**
Often with health maintenance and wellness, the provider establishes standing orders for specific education to be given based on the patient's history or age. Based on the patient's answers to the health history and screening questions, the medical assistant may need to provide coaching on specific topics per the provider's standing orders. The medical assistant can provide coaching on self-exams, including breast, testicular, skin, and oral cancer.
10. **Demonstrate coaching on screenings for health maintenance and wellness.**
Besides self-exams, the medical assistant can provide coaching on regular screenings, on-time screenings, and additional screenings, such as tobacco screening and alcohol misuse screening. Many types of screening can be done. Refer to the sections for additional details.
11. **Examine the coaching provided by the medical assistant regarding diagnostic tests and treatment plans.**
It is important for the medical assistant to provide the necessary teaching for diagnostic and laboratory tests ordered for patients. For tests to be completed, the patient needs to be prepared.

Continued

SUMMARY OF LEARNING OBJECTIVES—*continued*

Many facilities have the medical assistants meet with the patients after the providers finish examining the patient. The medical assistants review the treatment plan with the patients. They answer any questions, explore any issues the patients may have, and provide additional instructions. The provider may ask the medical assistant to coach the patient on medication administration and blood pressure monitoring at home.

12. **Examine the role of care coordination in ambulatory care.**
Care coordination provides personalized patient- and family-centered care in a team-based environment. The care coordinator communicates between the patient and healthcare team. A patient navigator (also called a *patient advocate*) has been described as a type of care coordinator. Patient navigators typically guide chronically ill patients through the healthcare system. They identify patients' financial, cultural, physical, and emotional barriers. Then they work closely with the healthcare team and the patients to ensure barriers are eliminated and patients get timely care. Procedure 22.2 describes the process of creating a current list of community resources and referring patients or family members.

PROCEDURE 22.1 Coach a Patient on Disease Prevention

TASKS: Coach on the recommended vaccinations for the patient's age. Adapt the coaching for any communication barrier and the patient's developmental life stage. Document the coaching in the patient's health record.

SCENARIO: You are working with Dr. David Kahn. You need to room Charles Johnson (date of birth [DOB] 03/03/19XX), and his record indicates he has not been seen in several years. Charles has significant hearing loss, and he communicates by signing. His wife interprets for him. You look at his health record and see that he is due for influenza, tetanus and diphtheria (Td), and recombinant zoster (shingles) vaccines. Per the provider's standing order, you need to coach adult patients on potential vaccines they are due for during the initial rooming process.

DIRECTIONS: Role-play this scenario with two peers, who will play Charles and his wife. You are the medical assistant.

EQUIPMENT and SUPPLIES

- Vaccine Information Statements (VIS) (available at https://www.immunize.org/vis/)
- Patient's health record

PROCEDURAL STEPS

1. Wash hands or use hand sanitizer.
<u>PURPOSE</u>: Hand sanitization is an important step for infection control.
2. Greet the patient. Identify yourself. Verify the patient's identity with full name and date of birth. Explain what you will be doing.
<u>PURPOSE</u>: It is important to identify the patient in two different ways to ensure that you have the correct patient. Explaining the procedure can make the patient feel more comfortable and reduces anxiety.
3. Arrange the chairs so the patient can see both you and the person signing. Speak slowly. Pause as needed to allow the person who is signing to finish with the last statement. Look at the patient when communicating.
<u>PURPOSE</u>: The medical assistant must focus on the patient and not the person signing or the interpreter. Speaking slowly and pausing allows the person to sign what you are saying.
4. Use simpler language when talking. Speak clearly and respectfully while maintaining the patient's dignity. Allow time for the patient to respond. Listen to the patient's concerns. Use active listening skills and appropriate eye contact. Focus on the patient and avoid distractions.
<u>PURPOSE</u>: When working with older patients, it is important to treat them with respect and dignity. Listening is important.
5. Ask the patient if he has received vaccines somewhere else over the past few years.
<u>PURPOSE</u>: It is important to verify that the health record is accurate.

Scenario update: The patient has not seen any healthcare providers over the past few years. The only vaccines he has received were given at this facility.

6. Describe the vaccines that are due. Use the VIS for each vaccine as you coach the patient on the purpose of the vaccine.
<u>PURPOSE</u>: The VIS is written for patients and describes the vaccine, disease(s) it prevents, and adverse reactions (side effects).

Scenario update: The patient knows the shingles vaccine is not covered and costs more than $200. He refuses the shingles vaccine, and he does not believe in getting the influenza vaccine. He is interested in getting the Td vaccine.

7. Ask the patient which vaccines he is interested in getting. If he refuses, be respectful of his choice. Any reason he gives for the refusal should be communicated to the provider.
<u>PURPOSE</u>: Patients have the right to refuse. Any treatment refused must be communicated to the provider.
8. Document the coaching in the patient's health record. Include the provider's name, what was taught, how the patient responded, and any vaccines refused.
<u>PURPOSE</u>: It is important to document the procedure in the health record to show it was done.

Documentation Example

07/16/20XX 1305 Per Dr. Kahn's order, instructed pt on the recombinant zoster vaccine (RZV), influenza, and Td vaccines. Pt stated he was not interested in the influenza vaccine or the RZV. He also stated his insurance wouldn't cover the RZV, and he didn't have the money to pay for it. He is interested in receiving the Td vaccine. Reviewed the Td VIS (07/15/20XX) with the patient. Pt stated he understood and would call if he had any issues. Due to pt's hearing impairment, pt's wife interpreted for pt during the visit. ————————————————— Suzanne Peterson, CMA (AAMA)

PROCEDURE 22.2 Develop a List of Community Resources and Facilitate Referrals

TASKS: As a patient navigator, develop a current list of community resources that meet the patient's healthcare needs. Discuss the resources with the patient and facilitate referrals to the chosen resources.

SCENARIO 1: Robert Caudill (DOB 10/31/19XX) was just diagnosed with dementia. He currently lives with his daughter, Ruby, who works full time. Ruby is feeling overwhelmed with being his only caregiver and realizes that she needs to find someone to care for her father while she is working.

SCENARIO 2: Leslie Green (DOB 08/03/20XX) just tested positive for pregnancy. She does not feel that she has a support system to help her make decisions.

SCENARIO 3: Ella Rainwater's husband of 30 years died suddenly 1 month ago. Ella (DOB 07/11/19XX) stated that she feels alone and has no one to talk to. Her daughter feels that Ella needs the support of others who have gone through the same thing.

DIRECTIONS: The instructor will assign each student a scenario. For steps 1 and 2, research resources for the scenario. For the remaining steps, role-play the scenario with two peers.

EQUIPMENT and SUPPLIES

- Computer (with internet) or a telephone book
- Paper and pen
- Community Resource Referral Form or other referral forms
- Patient's health record

PROCEDURAL STEPS

1. Using the assigned scenario, identify the possible types of community resources that would assist the patient or family. Identify three different types of resources (e.g., medical equipment, support group) that would meet the patient's needs.
   PURPOSE: A variety of community resources are available for patients and families who are dealing with chronic illnesses and death. Such resources range from daycare, meals, transportation, medical equipment, assisted living, and support groups, to reduced costs for medications.
2. Using the internet or the phone book, identify two local options for each of the three kinds of resources (i.e., find two assisted living resources, two medical equipment suppliers, and so on). Make a list of six resources for the patient and family. Include the following:
   - Organization's name
   - Address and contact information
   - Summary of the services provided
   - Cost and other relevant information

   PURPOSE: As the patient navigator or care coordinator, it is important for you to provide patients and families with the contact information for various community resources. This information can help the family find the best solution for the situation.

Scenario update: Role-play the scenario indicated by the instructor.

3. Provide the patient or family member with a list of six resources. Describe the services offered and any costs.
4. Allow the patient or family member time to review the services. Answer any questions.
   PURPOSE: It is important that the patient and family members understand the services available.
5. Use professional, tactful verbal and nonverbal communication as you work with the patient or family member.
   PURPOSE: Patients and family members are more apt to respond positively to assistance if the medical assistant's communication is professional, empathetic, and tactful. Talking down to patients or acting superior are unprofessional behaviors that negatively affect the working relationship with patients.
6. Role-play making the community referrals. Have the patient or family member decide on two or more services they are interested in. Complete the referral document. Have the patient provide any additional information required on the form. Call the community resource agency and provide the referral information to the representative (a peer).
   Note: Some community referrals (e.g., support groups) will require the patient to make contact and not the healthcare professional.
   PURPOSE: Many organizations use the referral document to capture the patient's preferences and help process the referral.
7. Document the patient education and the referrals in the health record.
   PURPOSE: It is important to document all patient interactions and referrals in the health record.

NUTRITION AND HEALTH PROMOTION

23

SCENARIO

Kayla Smith, registered medical assistant (RMA), has been working at Walden-Martin Family Medical (WMFM) Clinic for 4 years. She enjoys working with the patients and the providers. Her supervisor is impressed with Kayla's motivation, patient care skills, and attention to detail. Kayla was asked to mentor Tim Brown, a medical assistant student from a local college.

Tim has finished his courses and is now completing his practicum at the clinic. Tim has an interest in nutrition because his mother is a registered dietitian. He is eager to see how Kayla works with patients who have dietary changes. He hopes he will have the opportunity to observe her and then assist with the teaching process before doing it by himself.

While studying this chapter, think about the following questions:

- Why are carbohydrates, fat, protein, minerals/electrolytes, vitamins, fiber, and water important to the body?
- What are the special dietary needs of those with diabetes, cardiovascular disease, hypertension, cancer, and lactose sensitivity?
- What are the special dietary needs of a person with allergies and celiac disease?
- How should a medical assistant coach patients regarding special dietary needs?
- How can a medical assistant show awareness of a patient's concerns regarding a dietary change?

LEARNING OBJECTIVES

1. Explain metabolism, including the phases and the variables that affect metabolism.
2. Examine carbohydrates, including action in the body and types of carbohydrates.
3. Examine proteins, including action in the body and types of amino acids.
4. Examine fats, including action in the body and types of fats.
5. Examine the role of minerals, vitamins, antioxidants, and water in the body.
6. Explain the key recommendations of the dietary guidelines.
7. Interpret a food label.
8. Differentiate among clear liquid, full liquid, soft, and high- and low-fiber diets.
9. Differentiate among diets with nutrient modifications, including changes related to calories, carbohydrates, sodium, fat, cholesterol, and protein.
10. Examine common food allergies, intolerances, and related diets.
11. Differentiate the nutritional needs for various populations, including for those who are pregnant, those who are lactating, those from different age groups, and those with disease conditions.
12. Demonstrate how to instruct patients on dietary changes while showing sensitivity and understanding to the patient's concerns.

VOCABULARY

amino acids (ah MEE noe) Found in protein-containing foods and released during the digestion process in the intestines; carried by the blood to cells, where they are used to make proteins. Used for growth, maintenance, and repair of cells; they also transport nutrients.

anaphylaxis (an ah fah LAK sis) A rapidly progressing, life-threatening allergic reaction; characterized by hives, swelling of the mouth and airway, difficulty breathing, wheezing, and loss of consciousness.

antioxidant (an tee OK si dahnt) Synthetic or natural substance found in food and supplements; may prevent or delay some types of cell damage.

coaching Providing information in a supportive environment that allows people to grow, change, or improve their situation

enriched Nutrients are added back into a food after they were lost during food processing.

enzymes (EN zimes) Special proteins that speed up chemical reactions in the body.

fatty acids Result when fats are broken down; used by the body for energy and tissue development.

fortified The addition of one or more substances to a food to increase its nutrient density.

glucagon (GLOO kah gon) A hormone produced by the alpha cells in the pancreas; works in the liver to release glycogen and thereby prevent dangerously low blood glucose levels.

glucose Results when carbohydrates are broken down; main sugar found in the blood and used as the main source of energy in the body.

VOCABULARY—*continued*

insulin (IN suh lin) A hormone produced by the beta cells in the pancreas; moves glucose into the cells so it can be used for energy.

kwashiorkor (kwah shee ORE kore) A severe protein deficiency syndrome that leads to edema, pigmentation changes of the skin and hair, impaired growth and development, abdominal distension, and liver changes. Typically seen in infants and children.

metabolism (me TAB oh lizm) The chemical process that occurs within a living organism to maintain life; the process the body uses to obtain or make energy from the food eaten.

recommended dietary allowance (RDA) The average daily food intake needed to meet the nutrient requirements of most healthy people.

registered dietitian (die eh TISH an) A credentialed healthcare professional who is trained in nutrition and is able to apply the information to the dietary needs of healthy and ill patients.

regular diet The food and drink a person typically consumes when there are no dietary limitations.

INTRODUCTION

Nutrition is a field of study that examines the substances in food that help us grow and stay healthy. Nutrition can also be defined as the intake of food for the body's dietary needs. It is important to eat a healthy and balanced diet. *Nutrients* are the chemicals in food that the body uses for energy, growth, and development. Nutrients include water, protein, carbohydrate, fat, vitamins, and minerals.

A medical assistant helps the provider by coaching patients on dietary changes. It is important to be aware of nutrients and the different types of diets commonly ordered in the ambulatory care environment. This chapter discusses metabolism and the nutrients essential for growth and development. Dietary requirements, along with medically ordered diets, are also discussed.

METABOLISM

Metabolism is the process the body uses to obtain or make energy from the food eaten. The following sections discuss the phases of metabolism and the variables that affect metabolism.

Phases of Metabolism

Metabolism has two phases:

- *Catabolism*: The process of breaking down molecules into smaller molecules, resulting in energy being released
- *Anabolism*: The process of smaller molecules being used to build larger molecules with the use of energy

For example, you eat a piece of chocolate candy with peanuts. It is broken down by **enzymes** in the intestines. The enzymes break down the proteins into **amino acids**, the fats into **fatty acids**, and the complex *carbohydrates* into simple sugars (e.g., **glucose**). These substances are absorbed by the blood and brought to the cells. In the cells, other enzymes catabolize, or break down, these substances, and energy is released. The energy released can be used or stored by the body. The small molecules created from catabolism are used to create larger molecules as the body repairs tissues and performs other functions. This process requires energy and is called *anabolism*. Every action of the body, involuntary or voluntary, requires energy.

Many times, metabolism is thought of as what influences our bodies to gain or lose weight. This is where calories come in. A *calorie* is a unit that measures how much energy is in a particular food. People use calories or energy at different rates. Some people eat a lot of food and do not put on any weight, whereas others feel they look at food and gain weight. The number of calories a person burns each day is affected by the following factors:

- How much the person exercises
- The amount of fat and muscle on the person's body
- The person's *basal metabolic rate* (BMR), or the rate the body burns calories while the person is at rest

Basal Metabolic Rate

The BMR can play a role in a person's tendency to gain weight. For example, two people eat and exercise the same amount, but they have two different BMRs. The person with the lower BMR would have a greater tendency to gain more weight. Remember, the body stores unused calories as fat.

A number of variables will affect the BMR:

- *Genetics*: Some people are born with a higher metabolism.
- *Sex*: Males have a higher density of lean muscle mass with a lower body fat percentage. This causes a higher BMR.
- *Age*: BMR decreases with age.
- *Weight*: The heavier an individual, the higher the BMR.
- *Body surface area*: This relates to a person's height and weight. The larger the body surface area, the higher the BMR.
- *Body fat percentage*: The lower a person's body fat percentage, the higher the BMR.
- *Diet*: Starvation and low-calorie diets can reduce the BMR.
- *Body temperature*: A higher body temperature results in an increased BMR.
- *External temperature*: The colder the external temperature, the more the body has to provide additional heat to maintain the body's temperature. This increases the BMR.
- *Thyroxin*: Produced by the thyroid gland, thyroxin can increase the BMR.
- *Exercise and lean muscle tissue*: Exercise will create lean muscle tissue, which increases the BMR.
- *Drugs*: Certain drugs (e.g., caffeine) can increase the BMR.

Nutrients

Nutrients in the food we eat have many roles in our body, including regulating metabolic processes. Nutrients can be classified into two different groups. *Essential nutrients* cannot be made by the body and must be in the food eaten. *Nonessential nutrients* are created by the body and do not need to be in food. For example, vitamin D is created from sun exposure on the skin, so it does not need to be consumed. Foods can also be described as follows:

- *Nutrient rich* (also called *nutrient dense*): Foods high in nutrients (e.g., vitamins, minerals, complex carbohydrates, healthy fats, and lean protein) and low in calories.
- *Non–nutrient rich*: Foods lacking vitamins, minerals, and fiber. They provide "empty calories" and can cause people to gain weight. The following sections will examine nutrients important in our diet.

CARBOHYDRATES

Carbohydrates are nutrients found in our diet. About 45% to 65% of our daily calories should come from carbohydrates. Carbohydrates are used for energy and to regulate protein and fat metabolism. This nutrient encompasses a broad range of simple sugars, starches, and fiber.

Simple Sugars

There are many types of simple sugars. Nutrient-rich foods containing simple sugars include the following:

- Fruits and vegetables, which contain fructose and glucose
- Milk and milk products, which contain lactose

Non–nutrient-rich foods and food additives containing simple sugars include desserts (cookies, cakes), candy, soda, syrups (including regular and high-fructose corn syrups), white sugar (sucrose), honey, and molasses.

During digestion, most sugars (except lactose from milk) break down into fructose and glucose. Lactose breaks down into glucose and galactose. Simple sugars are rapidly absorbed and quickly raise blood glucose levels. They provide a quick source of energy.

Starches

Starches are called *complex carbohydrates*. Food sources of complex carbohydrates include the following:

- *Nutrient-rich starches*: Legumes (e.g., split peas, beans [kidney, black, garbanzo, and pinto]), starchy vegetables (e.g., corn, green peas, and potatoes), and whole grains (e.g., oats, barley, quinoa, seeds, and brown rice)
- *Non–nutrient-rich starches*: White bread, crackers, and white rice

Complex carbohydrates are digested in the intestine before being absorbed. They break down into simple sugars and become a source of energy. The glucose from the simple sugars and starches raises the blood glucose level. With the help of **insulin**, glucose is moved out of the bloodstream and into cells; it is then used for energy. Some glucose is stored in the liver and muscles as *glycogen*. The body uses the stored glycogen in between meals and during strenuous exercise. As the blood glucose levels start to drop, **glucagon** works in the liver to release the stored glycogen. Glycogen is released back into the blood and raises the blood glucose level.

It is important to remember that excessive carbohydrates can be converted into fat. The following are smart carbohydrate dietary choices:

- Eat a variety of whole grains, fruits, vegetables, legumes, and low-fat or nonfat dairy products.
- At least half of all grains eaten should be whole grains.
- Limit processed foods in your diet, especially those with added sugar, salt, and fat.
- Eat **enriched** refined grains, if eating refined grains.

Whole Grains and Refined Grains

Foods made from wheat, oats, cornmeal, rice, and barley are grain products. Grains are divided into whole grains and refined grains:

- *Whole grains*: Use the entire grain kernel (e.g., bran, germ, and endosperm); they include whole-wheat flour, cracked wheat (bulgur), whole cornmeal, oatmeal, and brown rice.
- *Refined grains*: Are milled, and the bran and germ are removed to create a finer texture and longer shelf life. Examples include white flour, degermed cornmeal, white rice, and white bread. During the milling process, dietary fiber, iron, and many B vitamins are removed. For this reason, most refined grains are *enriched*. This means certain B vitamins and iron are added back to the grains. Fiber is not added back into the product.

Glycemic Index

The *glycemic index* (GI) is a numeric index used to indicate how much a carbohydrate food raises the blood glucose level. The foods are ranked from 0 to 100. Carbohydrates that are rapidly digested, absorbed, and considerably raise the blood glucose level are considered high-GI foods (≥70). Low-GI foods (≤55) produce a smaller change in the blood glucose level. The goal is to eat more low=GI foods to reduce the risk of type 2 diabetes mellitus and heart disease. Low-GI foods can also help maintain weight loss. Table 23.1 provides examples of the GI values of some common foods.

Fiber

Fiber is different from simple sugars and starches. It cannot be digested by the body, and thus, it does not raise the blood glucose level. Fiber helps a person feel full and can help with weight management. There are two types of fiber: soluble fiber and insoluble fiber.

Soluble fiber dissolves in water and forms a gel-like substance. Soluble fiber softens the stool. It lowers the blood glucose level by slowing sugar absorption. Soluble fiber lowers the low-density lipoprotein (or bad cholesterol) level by binding to fatty acids. Examples of soluble fiber foods include the following:

- *Nutrient-rich*: Legumes, oats, barley, fruits (e.g., avocados, apples, and citrus fruits), and carrots
- *Non–nutrient-rich*: Processed and refined goods

Insoluble fiber bulks up the stool and helps to prevent constipation. Examples of insoluble fiber include the following:

- *Nutrient-rich:* Whole grains (whole wheat and brown rice), vegetables (corn, broccoli, green beans, cauliflower, and potatoes with skins), nuts and seeds, popcorn, and prunes

TABLE 23.1 Glycemic Index (GI) for Foods

PER SERVING	GI	PER SERVING	GI
Bagel, white frozen	72	Skim milk	32
Bread, whole wheat	71	Apple	39
Tortilla, wheat	30	Banana	62
Gatorade	78	Watermelon	72
Instant oatmeal	83	Peanuts	7

- *Non–nutrient-rich:* Processed and refined goods

Fiber supplements are usually taken to reduce constipation. They can help a person be "regular." The active ingredient in the supplements can vary between natural and synthetic soluble fiber. Consider the following:

- *Metamucil* contains *psyllium husk*, a natural substance that contains about 70% soluble fiber and 30% insoluble fiber.
- Citrucel contains *methylcellulose*, a semisynthetic soluble fiber.
- Fibercon contains calcium *polycarbophil*, a synthetic soluble fiber.

It is important to drink plenty of water when taking fiber supplements. Some fiber supplements have been shown to lower blood pressure, blood glucose, and the risk of heart disease.

CRITICAL THINKING APPLICATION 23.1

Kayla wants to help Tim review carbohydrates. She asks him to list two foods from each category: simple sugars, starches, and fiber. What foods would you list?

PROTEIN

Protein is a nutrient in our diet. About 10% to 35% of our daily calories should come from protein. The following sections examine the role of protein in the body and the types of amino acids.

Role of Protein in the Body

Proteins are broken down into amino acids. Amino acids can be used as a source of energy in the absence of carbohydrates. Amino acids are also used to make proteins to help the body:

- Break down food (e.g., enzymes)
- Grow and repair body tissues (e.g., connective tissue, hair, nails, muscles)
- Perform other functions (e.g., those related to hemoglobin, antibodies, and hormones)

Proteins and amino acids are considered the building blocks of life. The body needs several amino acids in large enough amounts to maintain good health. Protein malnutrition is seen around the world and can lead to **kwashiorkor**. A lack of dietary protein can cause growth failure, loss of muscle mass, anemia, edema and potbelly, skin depigmentation and hair loss, weakening of the circulatory and respiratory systems, decreased immunity, and death.

Amino Acids

Amino acids are classified into three groups:

- *Essential amino acids*: Cannot be made by the body, thus must come from food eaten throughout the day
- *Nonessential amino acids*: Can be made by the body from essential amino acids or in the normal breakdown of proteins
- *Conditional amino acids*: Usually not essential except in times of illness and stress

Foods that have all the essential amino acids to support the body are called *complete proteins*. Foods that are considered complete proteins are fish, meat, poultry, dairy products, quinoa seeds, buckwheat, chia seeds, and eggs. Foods that do not contain all the essential amino acids are called *incomplete proteins*. Nuts, legumes, grains, and vegetables are examples of incomplete proteins.

Smart protein choices include the following:

- Choose lean or low-fat meat and poultry.
- Eat seafood rich in omega-3 fatty acids, such as salmon, trout, herring, Pacific oysters, and Atlantic and Pacific mackerel.
- Limit processed meats (e.g., ham, sausage, and deli meats), which contain added salt (sodium).
- Eat unsalted nuts and seeds to keep sodium intake low.

Omega-3 Fatty Acids

Omega-3 fatty acids are a group of polyunsaturated fatty acids found in fish (e.g., salmon, herring, halibut, and mackerel) and some nuts and seeds. These fatty acids play a role in reducing blood cholesterol, heart disease risk, inflammation, and depression. Omega-3 fatty acids also increase the effectiveness of anti-inflammatory and antidepressant drugs.

CRITICAL THINKING APPLICATION 23.2

Kayla wants to help Tim review proteins. She asks him to list six foods that contain proteins. What foods would you list?

FAT

Fat is an important nutrient in our diet. Fats provide 9 calories per gram, whereas carbohydrates and proteins provide only 4 calories per gram. About 20% to 35% of our daily calories should come from fats and less than 10% from saturated fatty acids.

Role of Fats in the Body

The body has many uses for fat:

- A source of energy. If glucose is not available for energy, the body will break down fat stores for energy. The process forms ketones, which can be seen in the urine and blood.
- Healthy skin and hair.
- Vitamin absorption. Vitamins A, D, E, and K are fat soluble.
- Insulation (cushion) for organs and to keep the body warm.
- Brain development, controlling inflammation, and blood clotting. Linoleic and linolenic acid, which are essential fatty acids, are used for these processes.

Fat is required in the diet. Table 23.2 describes the types of fats found in foods. Diets low in fats can cause cold sensitivity, increased infections, and amenorrhea in women. Long-term fat deficiency can lead to metabolic problems and fat-soluble vitamin deficiency.

Triglycerides

Triglycerides are another type of fat (lipid) in the body. Our livers make triglycerides from the calories we do not use. Triglycerides are also found in foods. Triglycerides are stored in the fat cells and have the following characteristics:

- Used for energy when carbohydrates are limited
- Absorb vitamins and other nutrients
- Contain essential fatty acids, which are important for growth and development

A person's triglyceride level is usually checked with their cholesterol levels. High triglyceride levels increase one's risk for heart disease and stroke. There are other reasons for high triglyceride levels, including poorly controlled type 2 diabetes mellitus, liver disease, kidney disease, and hypothyroidism.

TABLE 23.2 Types of Fats

TYPE	DESCRIPTION	IMPACT ON CHOLESTEROL	FOUND IN
Saturated fats	Solid at room temperature	Increase the LDL level	Butter, cheese, whole milk, ice cream, cream, fatty meats; processed coconut oil, palm oil
Unsaturated fats	Liquid at room temperature; two kinds: monounsaturated and polyunsaturated	Decrease the LDL level	Monounsaturated: olive and canola oil Polyunsaturated: safflower, sunflower, corn, and soy oil
Trans fatty acids	Also called *hydrogenated fats* and *trans fats*; created when hydrogen is added to vegetable oils during food manufacturing	Increase LDL and decrease HDL levels	Foods made with hydrogenated and partially hydrogenated oils; margarine, commercially prepared baked goods

HDL, High-density lipoprotein; *LDL*, low-density lipoprotein.

Here are the best ways to lower triglyceride levels:

- Cut back on calories and lose weight.
- Avoid sugary and refined food; choose monounsaturated fats over saturated fats.
- Limit the amount of alcohol consumed and exercise daily.
- Take medications that can be ordered to help reduce the triglyceride level.

Cholesterol

Cholesterol, a type of lipid, is a waxy, fatlike substance. It is used to make hormones, vitamin D, bile acids, and cell membranes. Cholesterol is created in the liver, and dietary cholesterol is found in animal-based foods (e.g., egg yolks, meat, shellfish, and cheese). Cholesterol is carried in the blood by the following lipoproteins:

- *High-density lipoprotein (HDL):* Considered "good" cholesterol. It helps move the cholesterol from the tissues to the liver. The liver helps remove cholesterol from the body. A low level of HDL increases the risk of heart disease.
- *Low-density lipoprotein (LDL):* Considered "bad" cholesterol. It moves cholesterol to tissues, including arteries. Most of the cholesterol in the blood is LDL. The higher the LDL level in the blood, the greater the risk for heart disease. LDL can be lowered through diet, exercise, and medications. Eating unsaturated fats can also help lower the LDL level.

CRITICAL THINKING APPLICATION 23.3

Kayla wants to help Tim review the three types of fats. She asks him to describe unsaturated fats, saturated fats, and trans-fatty acids. How would you describe them?

OTHER DIETARY NUTRIENTS

Besides carbohydrates, proteins, and fats, our bodies need other dietary nutrients. Minerals, vitamins, antioxidants, and water have unique roles in the body.

Minerals and Electrolytes

Minerals are naturally occurring inorganic substances (e.g., iron, zinc, and calcium). Minerals needed by the body are divided into two categories: major and trace. *Major minerals*, or *macrominerals*, are needed in larger amounts. *Trace minerals*, or *microminerals*, are needed in smaller amounts in the body.

Electrolytes are minerals in the body fluid that have an electrical charge. They are found in the blood, urine, and other body fluids. Electrolytes come from the foods we eat and fluids we drink (Table 23.3). Too little or too much water in the body, vomiting, diarrhea, sweating, and kidney problems can change our electrolyte levels. A provider will order laboratory tests to measure a patient's electrolyte levels.

CRITICAL THINKING APPLICATION 23.4

Kayla asks Tim how he would explain the difference between minerals and electrolytes. How would you respond?

Vitamins

Vitamins are organic substances that the body needs in very small amounts for specific roles. There are 13 vitamins required by the body. It is important to get the **recommended dietary allowance (RDA)** of each vitamin. A deficit of a vitamin can lead to disease.

Vitamins are either water soluble or fat soluble (Table 23.4). Water-soluble vitamins dissolve in water. These include the B vitamins and vitamin C. Any unused water-soluble vitamins leave the body through the urine. Vitamin B_{12} is an exception because the liver stores the vitamin for years. Water-soluble vitamins need to be taken in daily. Fat-soluble vitamins are vitamins A, D, E, and K. These vitamins are absorbed more easily with the presence of fat in the diet. Fat-soluable vitamins are stored in the fatty tissue and liver in the body.

Function of Dietary Supplements

Dietary supplements are oral products that contain a "dietary ingredient." This ingredient can include a vitamin, mineral, amino acid, herb, or another substance that can supplement a person's diet. Dietary supplements come in many forms, including tablets, powders, energy bars, and liquids. Federal law does not require a dietary supplement to be proven safe or the claim to be truthful before it appears on the market. The Food and Drug Administration (FDA) monitors the safety of such products after they are on the market.

The function of dietary supplements is to provide nutrients that are not obtained in the foods we eat and drink. Consider these uses of dietary supplements:

- Calcium and vitamin D for bone health and low vitamin D levels
- Folic acid in pregnancy to prevent spina bifida
- Iron for low iron levels
- Fiber for constipation

TABLE 23.3 Examples of Major and Trace Minerals

CATEGORY	MINERAL	ROLE IN THE BODY	FOUND IN
Major minerals (*macrominerals*)	Calcium	For healthy teeth and bones; muscle and nerve function, blood clotting, blood pressure regulation, immune system health	Milk products, canned fish (e.g., salmon), **fortified** soy milk, greens (e.g., broccoli), legumes
	Potassium	For proper muscle and nerve function, fluid balance	Milk, fresh fruits and vegetables, whole grains, legumes, meats
	Sodium	For proper muscle and nerve function, fluid balance	Table salt, processed foods, condiments
	Chloride	For proper fluid balance; stomach acid	Table salt, processed foods, tomatoes, celery, and olives
	Phosphorus	For healthy teeth and bones; important in the acid-base balance system	Meat, poultry, fish, eggs, milk, processed foods, soda pop
	Sulfur	Found in body proteins	Meats, poultry, fish, eggs, legumes, nuts
	Magnesium	Needed to make proteins; for muscle and nerve function and immune system health	Nuts, legumes, seeds, seafood, chocolate, and leafy green vegetables
Trace minerals (*microminerals*)	Iron	Part of hemoglobin found in the red blood cell, used for energy metabolism	Meats, fish, poultry, shellfish, egg yolks, legumes, dark leafy greens, iron-enriched or fortified foods
	Zinc	Used for making proteins, taste perception, wound healing, immune system health, production of sperm, normal growth	Vegetables, poultry, fish, meats
	Iodine	Found in thyroid hormone, which is involved with metabolism, growth, and development	Seafood, iodized salt, milk products
	Selenium	**Antioxidant**	Seafood, grains, and meats
	Fluoride	Involved with healthy teeth and bones	Fish, tea, and drinking water
	Chromium	Used in the metabolism of carbohydrates and fats; also aids in insulin action and glucose metabolism	Brewer's yeast, beef, liver, eggs, chicken, wheat germ, potatoes
	Copper	Helps to form red blood cells; involved with keeping the blood vessels, nerves, immune system, and bones healthy; aids in iron absorption	Shellfish, whole grains, beans, nuts, liver, dark leafy greens, dried fruits, yeast, and cocoa

TABLE 23.4 Fat- and Water-Soluble Vitamins

VITAMIN	RECOMMENDED DIETARY ALLOWANCE FOR ADULTS	ROLE IN THE BODY	FOUND IN	DEFICIENCY CAUSES	TOXIC?
Fat-Soluble Vitamins					
Vitamin A	700–900 mcg retinol activity equivalents (RAEs)	Antioxidant; helps form and maintain healthy teeth, bones, mucus membranes, soft tissue, and skin	Dark-colored fruits and leafy vegetables, egg yolks, fortified milk products, liver, beef, fish	Night blindness	Yes, can cause liver toxicity
Vitamin D	15–20 mcg (600–800 International Unit)	Bone growth; made by the body after being in the sun	Fatty fish (e.g., salmon, herring), fish liver oils, fortified cereals, fortified milk products	Bone pain, muscle weakness	Yes, *hypercalcemia* (elevated blood calcium levels) and kidney problems

Continued

TABLE 23.4 Fat- and Water-Soluble Vitamins—*continued*

VITAMIN	RECOMMENDED DIETARY ALLOWANCE FOR ADULTS	ROLE IN THE BODY	FOUND IN	DEFICIENCY CAUSES	TOXIC?
Vitamin E (tocopherol)	15 mg	Antioxidant; helps form red blood cells and helps the body use vitamin K	Avocados, dark green and dark leafy vegetables (e.g., spinach, broccoli, and asparagus); safflower, corn, and sunflower oil; papaya, mango, wheat germ, seeds, nuts	Hemolytic anemia, neurologic deficits	Yes, hemorrhagic toxicity can occur with supplement use
Vitamin K	90–120 mcg	Blood clotting; made in the intestine	Cabbage, cauliflower, cereals, dark green and dark leafy vegetables, fish, liver, eggs, beef	Bleeding	No toxic effects reported
Water-Soluble Vitamins					
Thiamine (vitamin B_1)	1.1–1.2 mg	Used for nervous system, muscle function, and carbohydrate metabolism	Egg, enriched flour, lean meats, legumes, nuts, seeds, organ meats, peas, whole grains	Beriberi usually in alcoholics	No toxic effects reported
Riboflavin (vitamin B_2)	1.1–1.3 mg	Works with other B vitamins; important for growth and red blood cell production	Milk, mushrooms, spinach, almonds, lamb	Riboflavin deficiency	No toxic effects reported
Niacin (vitamin B_3)	14–16 mg NE (niacin equivalents)	Used in digestive process and skin and nerve functions; treats low-HDL and high-LDL cholesterol and triglyceride levels	Avocados, eggs, enriched breads and cereals, lean meats, fish, poultry, legumes, nuts, and potatoes	Pellagra, digestive issues	Niacin-containing supplements should be taken as provider indicates
Pantothenic acid (vitamin B_5)	5 mg	Involved with metabolism and hormone and cholesterol production; needed for growth	Avocados, broccoli, egg yolks, legumes, milk, yeast, organ meats, potatoes, and whole grains	Vitamin B_5 deficiency	No toxic effects reported
Pyridoxine (vitamin B_6)	1.3–1.7 mg	Helps form red blood cells and maintain brain function; also used for protein metabolism	Avocados, bananas, legumes, meat, nuts, poultry, and whole grains	Cracks around mouth, depression, rash	No toxic effects reported
Biotin (vitamin B_7)	25–30 mcg	Used for fat and carbohydrate metabolism; also used in the production of hormones and cholesterol	Chocolate, legumes, milk, nuts, organ meats (e.g., liver, kidney) pork, egg yolk, and yeast	Hair loss, cheilitis, glossitis	No toxic effects reported
Folate (vitamin B_9, folic acid)	400 mcg DFE (dietary folate equivalents)	Works with vitamin B_{12} to help form blood cells; important in pregnancy to prevent spina bifida	Asparagus, broccoli, beets, brewer's yeast, legumes, enriched breads and cereals, green leafy vegetables, oranges, peanut butter	Anemia, diarrhea	Caution with high doses, limited data on toxicity
Cobalamin (vitamin B_{12})	2.4 mcg	Important for protein metabolism, the formation of red blood cells, and the maintenance of the central nervous system	Meat, eggs, fortified foods, milk products, organ meats, poultry, and shellfish	Pernicious anemia, confusion	No toxic effects reported
Vitamin C (ascorbic acid)	75–90 mg	Antioxidant; promotes healthy gums and teeth; helps absorb iron; maintains healthy tissue and promotes wound healing	Citrus fruits, tomatoes, broccoli, cabbage, cauliflower, potatoes, spinach, strawberries	Scurvy	Kidney stones, excess iron absorption, gastrointestinal disturbances

HDL, High-density lipoprotein; *LDL,* low-density lipoprotein; *mcg,* micrograms; *mg,* milligrams.
Some information was obtained from the Vitamins Food and Nutrition Board, Institute of Medicine, National Academies, www.nal.usda.gov/sites/default/files/fnic_uploads//DRI_Vitamins.pdf.

Before patients start a dietary supplement, it is important that they talk with the provider. Some medications may interact with dietary supplements. Some dietary supplements may work against medications. For instance, taking vitamin K promotes blood clotting, and Coumadin (warfarin) delays blood clotting.

CRITICAL THINKING APPLICATION 23.5

Kayla and Tim are reviewing vitamins that patients commonly take. Tim asks Kayla to explain the difference between water-soluble and fat-soluble vitamins. How would you explain the difference?

Free Radicals and Antioxidants

Free radical molecules, or *free radicals,* are natural by-products of normal metabolic processes. A free radical is an atom that has one or more unpaired electrons, causing it to be especially reactive. The free radical seeks out and takes electrons from other molecules. This usually causes damage to the other molecules.

The production of free radicals in the body can increase due to a number of lifestyle and environmental factors:

- Tobacco smoke and alcohol consumption
- Eating fried foods
- Exposure to toxins (e.g., pesticides) and air pollution
- Stress and excessive exercise

Free radicals play an important role in many cellular processes. They are involved in the inflammation process. Excessive free radicals can affect our health by attacking cells' deoxyribonucleic acid (DNA) and blood vessels, causing aging and illness. This increases the risk for cardiovascular disease, strokes, arthritis, cataracts, and other degenerative diseases.

Antioxidants protect cells from free radicals and limit the damage free radicals can do to the cells. Antioxidants are powerful and beneficial for us. Antioxidants include vitamins A, C, and E, beta-carotene, lycopene, lutein, and selenium.

Water

Drinking water every day is important for a person's health. Water is the basis for the fluids in the body. It makes up more than two-thirds of the body's weight. Without water, we would become dehydrated and die within a few days. All cells and organs need water to function and survive. Water plays important roles in the body:

- Keeps the body temperature normal with perspiration
- Lubricates organs and cushions joints (e.g., saliva, fluid around joints)
- Helps to prevent and relieve constipation by moving food through the intestines
- Protects the spinal cord, brain, and other sensitive tissues
- Gets rid of waste products in the body through urine, sweat, and stools

Our need for water increases in hot weather, when we are more active, or when we have a fever, diarrhea, or vomiting. The recommended daily intake of water for healthy men is about 13 cups; the recommendation for healthy women is 9 cups. The individual need for water is based on a person's weight, age, activity level, and certain medical conditions.

Water and Diseases

Some patients are placed on fluid restrictions. This means they can only have a certain amount of fluids a day. The provider will indicate the maximum amount of fluids to be consumed daily. It is important to limit fluids that act as a diuretic (e.g., alcohol and caffeinated beverages) because they pull fluid from the body and increase the risk of dehydration. Several conditions may require fluid restrictions:

- Heart problems, including congestive heart failure
- Kidney problems, such as those that might affect patients on dialysis and those with end-stage renal disease
- Adrenal insufficiency and corticosteroid treatment

Some diseases and conditions require more fluids/water to be consumed. People with postural orthostatic tachycardia syndrome (POTS) need to drink at least 2 to 3 liters of water a day to maintain their blood pressure. Other conditions, such as diabetes insipidus, diabetes mellitus, and Addison disease, may cause patients to excrete more urine, thus putting them more at risk for dehydration.

FOOD GUIDES AND DIETARY GUIDELINES

For over a century, the US Department of Agriculture (USDA) has provided food guides to the public. Some of the more recent guides include the following:

- 1992: Food Guide Pyramid, which showed the five basic food groups arranged in a pyramid. The lower part of the pyramid consisted of the food groups that made up the majority of the daily diet. People were to eat less of the food groups at the top of the pyramid.
- 2005: MyPyramid Food Guidance System, which continued with the pyramid design but added physical activity and oils.
- 2011: MyPlate was introduced and later updated with the 2020 Dietary Guidelines for Americans.

MyPlate

MyPlate focuses on making healthy food choices because everything eaten matters (Figure 23.1). Some key messages are included with these dietary guidelines:

- Fill half the plate with fruits and vegetables. Focus on whole fruits and vary the types of vegetables.
- Make half of the grains eaten each day whole grains.
- Vary the types of proteins eaten.
- Move to low-fat or fat-free milk and yogurt.
- Choose foods and beverages with less added salt, sugars, and saturated fats.

MyPlate consists of five food groups, along with oil (Table 23.5). Oil contains required nutrients, so the USDA addresses it. Oil is usually consumed in nuts, fish, cooking oil, and salad dressing. Most children need 3 to 6 teaspoons, and adults need 5 to 7 teaspoons daily, depending on sex and age.

The MyPlate website (https://www.myplate.gov/) offers numerous online resources for individuals and professionals. Tip sheets, food plans, and other resources provide additional information. MyPlate is very flexible for cultural foods.

Dietary Guidelines

The USDA publishes Dietary Guidelines every 5 years. These guidelines are for individuals 2 years or older. The focus is on disease

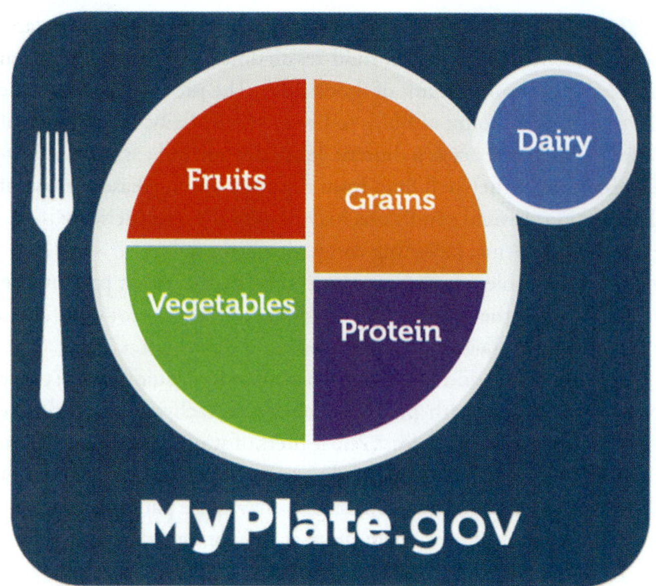

FIGURE 23.1 Choose MyPlate. (From the US Department of Agriculture, www.myplate.gov.)

prevention and health promotion. The current dietary guidelines focus on overall eating patterns, health, and the risk of chronic disease.

Key recommendations from the 2020–2025 Dietary Guidelines for Americans include those listed with MyPlate, in addition to the following:

- Added sugars: Limit to less than 10% of calories per day starting at age 2. Avoid for infants and toddlers
- Saturated fat: Limit to less than 10% of calories per day starting at age 2. Examples of saturated fats include butter, whole milk, fatty meats, coconut oil, and palm oil.
- Sodium: Limit to less than 2300 milligrams (mg) per day for those age 14 and older.
- Alcoholic beverages: Men should limit intake to two drinks or less per day. Women should limit intake to one drink or less per day.
- Pay attention to portion sizes.
- Food choices should be rich in nutrients.

FOOD LABELS

Knowing how to read a food label is important when making healthy food selections. The food label contains the nutritional information

TABLE 23.5 Food Groups with Serving Amounts for MyPlate

		RECOMMENDED DAILY AMOUNTS[a]			
FOOD GROUP	WHAT COUNTS?	CHILDREN 2–8 YR	CHILDREN 9–18 YR	WOMEN 19–51+ YR	MEN 19–51+ YR
Dairy	*1-cup equivalent:* 1 cup milk, yogurt, soymilk, almond milk, or coconut milk 1½ ounce (oz) natural cheese 2 oz processed cheese	2–2½ cups	3 cups	3 cups	3 cups
Proteins	*1-oz equivalent:* 1 oz meat, poultry, or fish ¼ cup cooked beans 1 egg 1 tablespoon peanut butter ½ oz nuts or seeds	2–4 oz	5–6½ oz	5–5½ oz	5½–6½ oz
Vegetables	*1-cup equivalent:* 1 cup raw or cooked vegetables or vegetable juice 2 cups raw leafy greens	½ cup	2–3 cups	2–2½ cups	2½–3 cups
Fruits	*1-cup equivalent:* 1 cup fruit or 100% fruit juice ½ cup dried fruit	1–1½ cups	1½–2 cups	1½–2 cups	2 cups
Grains	*1-oz equivalent:* 1 slice of bread 1 cup dry cereal ½ cup cooked rice, pasta, or cereal (at least half should be whole grains)	3–5 oz	5–8 oz	5–6 oz	6–8 oz

[a]Amount required is based on sex, age, and the amount of exercise. Ranges are indicated above; for more specific information, go to www.myplate.gov.

and the ingredient list. The government has required food manufacturers to include certain information on the food label. The amounts for "Trans Fat" and "Added Sugars" are some of the newer additions to the food label.

Reading a Food Label

Food labels provide nutritional facts. This information is presented in both the quantity (e.g., grams [g] or mg) and as a percentage. The percentage reflects the % Daily Value (DV). This is the percentage of the nutrient in a single serving in terms of the daily recommended amount based on a 2000-calorie diet. You will see this description at the bottom of the list of nutrition facts. Remember, if you are eating fewer than 2000 calories daily, these percentages will be different for you.

When reading the nutrition facts (Figure 23.2), start at the top and work down:

- Check the calories per serving. If you eat the entire container and it consists of two servings, you need to double the calories.
- Check the amount of fat. Limit the saturated fat intake and avoid trans fats.
- The amounts listed for cholesterol, sodium, total carbohydrates, and added sugars are also numbers to consider. Choose foods with low amounts of these nutrients.
- Examine the dietary fiber, protein, vitamin D, calcium, iron, and potassium. Make sure you are getting enough of these beneficial nutrients.

Nutrition Facts

2 servings per container
Serving size 1 1/2 cup (208g)

Amount per serving
Calories 240

	% Daily Value*
Total Fat 4g	**5%**
Saturated Fat 1.5g	**8%**
Trans Fat 0g	
Cholesterol 5mg	**2%**
Sodium 430mg	**19%**
Total Carbohydrate 46g	**17%**
Dietary Fiber 7g	**25%**
Total Sugars 4g	
Includes 2g Added Sugars	**4%**
Protein 11g	
Vitamin D 2mcg	10%
Calcium 260mg	20%
Iron 6mg	35%
Potassium 240mg	6%

* The % Daily Value (DV) tells you how much a nutrient in a serving of food contributes to a daily diet. 2,000 calories a day is used for general nutrition advice.

FIGURE 23.2 Nutrition facts. (From the US Food and Drug Administration, www.fda.gov/Food/IngredientsPackagingLabeling/LabelingNutrition/ucm537159.htm.)

Ingredient Lists

Ingredient lists on foods are also important to understand (Figure 23.3). The ingredients are listed in descending order, starting with the one that weighs the most and ending with the one that weighs the least. There are several reasons a person may look at the ingredient list:

- *To look for trans fats:* Even if the nutrition information indicates 0 grams of trans fats, the product may still contain less than 0.5 gram of trans fats per serving. Look for ingredients such as "hydrogenated" or "partially hydrogenated oil." This indicates the presence of trans fats. So even if the nutrition information indicates 0 grams of trans fats, you may quickly reach your daily limit if you eat more than one serving.
- *To avoid certain ingredients:* Some people try to avoid ingredients such as high-fructose corn syrup and certain food colorings.
- *To identify allergens:* More than 160 foods have been found to be allergens. The government has identified eight allergens—milk, eggs, fish, crustacean shellfish, tree nuts, peanuts, wheat, and soybeans—that make up about 90% of all food allergy reactions. Laws regulating food labeling require manufacturers to indicate if any of the top allergens are in the food product. Advisory statements, such as "May contain peanuts" or "Made in a factory that also processes tree nuts," are optional and not required by law. (More information on allergens will be presented later in the chapter.)

PRESCRIBED DIETS WITH CONSISTENCY MODIFICATIONS

Patients may need to change their diet for a variety of reasons, including preparation for a procedure, dental or oral problems, or illness. When the provider orders a specific test or a particular diet, the medical assistant may need to coach the patient on the new diet. As with other instances of **coaching**, it is important for the medical assistant to provide the patient with a reference handout to take home. This will help guide the patient on the dietary changes. Learning about different medically ordered diets is important for the medical assistant.

Clear Liquid Diet

A clear liquid diet is made up of foods and beverages that are liquid at room temperature. Clear means you need to see through the liquids. Here are some of the foods included in a clear liquid diet:

- Water, tea, coffee, sports drinks, and clear soda
- Popsicles and juice without pulp
- Soup broth and gelatin (e.g., Jell-O)

Food Label #1	Food Label #2
Ingredients: Semolina (wheat), durum flour (wheat), eggs, partially hydrogenated oil, niacin, ferrous sulfate, thiamin mononitrate, riboflavin. **Contains: Wheat, eggs. Manufactured in a facility that uses tree nuts and eggs.**	**Ingredients:** Grapes, corn syrup, high-fructose corn syrup, fruit pectin, and citric acid.

FIGURE 23.3 Ingredient list on food labels.

Clear liquid diets are ordered for only a short time because they do not contain adequate nutrition. A clear liquid diet may be used when a person experiences diarrhea, vomiting, or nausea. It is commonly ordered after surgery and as part of the preparation for intestinal procedures. If a person is undergoing an intestinal procedure, red or pink clear liquids are not allowed because they could be mistaken for blood in the intestine.

Full Liquid Diet

A full liquid diet is made up of foods and beverages that are liquid at room temperature. Unlike the clear liquid diet, the full liquid diet includes milk products. These foods are included in a full liquid diet :

- Clear liquids (see previous section, Clear Liquid Diet)
- Strained creamy soups
- Milk, milkshakes, pudding, plain yogurt, custard, and ice cream
- Liquid supplements
- Sugar, honey, syrups, butter, margarine

Some providers will allow cooked, refined cereals (e.g., cream of rice), baby food, strained meats, and potatoes pureed in soup on a full liquid diet. This diet is a step above a clear liquid diet and below a **regular diet**.

Full liquid diets are ordered for only a short time because they do not contain adequate nutrition. A full liquid diet may be used before or after surgery, as part of the preparation for tests or procedures, and if a person has difficulty chewing or swallowing.

CRITICAL THINKING APPLICATION **23.6**

Kayla and Tim are working with Janine Butler. Janine needs to undergo an intestinal procedure and needs to be on clear liquids for 2 days. Janine states, "I was on a full liquid diet last year for a procedure. What is the difference between a clear liquid diet and a full liquid diet?" How would you answer this question?

Soft and Mechanical Soft Diets

A soft diet is a transition between a liquid diet and a regular diet. The foods on this diet are soft in texture, low in fiber, and easy for a person to digest. These foods are included in a soft diet:

- Grains: soft breads, crackers, white rice, pasta
- Fruits and vegetables: soft cooked, canned (no skin)
- Milk products: milk, yogurt, cottage cheese, ice cream, pudding
- Protein: tender meat, poultry, and fish; eggs, tofu, smooth peanut butter

The soft diet eliminates foods that are hard to chew and swallow:

- Raw fruits and vegetables
- Chewy or crispy breads
- Tough meats, broccoli, cauliflower, nuts, and seeds
- Fried, greasy foods
- Highly seasoned or spicy foods

This diet is used for patients recovering from surgery or a lengthy illness. It can also be used for people with chewing or swallowing problems due to illness or dental issues.

Mechanical soft diets consist of foods that have been prepared for easier chewing and swallowing using household tools (e.g., grinder, blender, and knife). Typically, there are no limitations (e.g., spicy, gassy, and fried foods) to mechanical soft diets. Mechanical soft diets are used for the following groups:

- Those recovering from head, neck, or mouth surgery
- Those who have difficulty swallowing (*dysphagia*), poor-fitting dentures, or no teeth
- Those who are too ill to chew

High- and Low-Fiber Diets

A prior section of the chapter discussed fiber as a carbohydrate. The provider may order a low-fiber or restricted-fiber diet. This type of diet limits the types of vegetables, grains, and fruits eaten. Limiting fiber and food residue (e.g., peels, nuts, and seeds) makes stools smaller and lessens irritation on the intestinal lining. There are several possible reasons for one to go on a low-fiber diet:

- Narrowing of the intestine due to a tumor
- A flare-up of an intestinal disease (e.g., irritable bowel syndrome, Crohn disease, and diverticulitis)
- After intestinal surgery
- Prior to an intestinal procedure (e.g., radiation and colonoscopy)

The provider can also order a high-fiber diet. This diet adds more bulk to the stools. High-fiber diets are used for a variety of reasons:

- Reducing constipation and possibly lowering the risk of hemorrhoids
- Lowering cholesterol levels
- Controlling blood glucose levels
- Weight loss

Bland Diet

A bland diet includes foods that are soft and low in fiber. This diet eliminates foods that are spicy, fried, or raw and beverages that contain caffeine or alcohol. Citrus juices and foods may also be eliminated. The foods included in a bland diet are similar to those incorporated into a soft diet. A bland diet is ordered to help treat gastroesophageal reflux disease (GERD), ulcers, nausea and vomiting, diarrhea, and gas. It can also be used after stomach or intestinal surgery.

PRESCRIBED DIETS WITH NUTRIENT MODIFICATIONS

Patients with various conditions, such as hypertension, obesity, and renal disease, require dietary changes. If the dietary change is also a lifestyle change, the provider may refer the patient to a **registered dietitian**. The registered dietitian can provide in-depth coaching and counseling on dietary changes.

Weight Control Diet

When trying to achieve or maintain a healthy weight, a person needs to find the balance between the number of calories eaten and the number used. Extra calories eaten and not used will result in a weight gain. For people to lose 1 to 2 pounds per week, they need to reduce their caloric intake by 500 to 1000 calories a day or increase their exercise to burn more calories. Identifying the calories consumed is an important step in achieving a healthy weight. Food diaries, apps, and trackers are available to help gauge food intake and activity.

Patients trying to achieve a healthy weight should follow these nutritional tips:

- Commit to a lifestyle change. Identify resources for information and support.
- Track foods eaten and beverages drunk, along with physical exercise.

- Set realistic goals, knowing that slips will occur.
- Eat healthy meals. They should be low in saturated fat, trans fat, cholesterol, salt, and added sugar. Eat lean meats, fish, poultry, beans, eggs, and nuts. Include fruits (especially whole fruits), vegetables, whole grains, and fat-free or low-fat milk products.
- Control portion sizes. *Portion size* is the amount of food we eat. *Serving size* is a standard measurement of food (e.g., 1 cup or 1 ounce [oz]). Many foods that come as a single portion actually contain multiple servings. For instance, a serving size of potato chips is 1 oz. The 3-oz potato chip bag is a single portion, but three servings. Another example is bread. You use two pieces of bread for a sandwich (portion size), but a serving is one slice. Most people overestimate serving sizes. It is best to measure the food or use a quick estimate method (Table 23.6).

Portion Size and Obesity

In some cases, portion sizes and serving sizes are the same. Over the years, many portion sizes have changed. Some experts attribute the growing obesity epidemic in the United States to this change. In the 1950s, the dinner plate was 9 inches in diameter; today, it is 11 to 12 inches. Some restaurants use even larger plates. With the plate change, the average portion of food also has increased. Restaurants have increased the amount of food they serve, and more Americans are eating out. With the increase in portions, *portion distortion* is occurring. The size of restaurant portions is causing Americans to rethink what the "normal" portions of food should be. Here are some examples of portion changes since the 1990s:

- Bagels have increased by 3 inches and added 210 calories.
- Muffins have increased by 3.5 ounces (oz) and added 290 calories.
- Cheeseburgers have increased in size and added almost 260 calories.
- Soda size has increased by 13.5 oz and added almost 170 calories.

As these examples show, the increase in portion sizes has led to an increase in the number of calories. Remember, the calories consumed and not used turn into fat. (Information from the National Heart, Lung, and Blood Institute, www.nhlbi.nih.gov/health/educational/wecan/eat-right/distortion.htm.)

TABLE 23.6 Quick Methods to Estimate Portion Size

AMOUNT OF FOOD	APPROXIMATE SIZE
3 ounces (oz) chicken and lean beef	Deck of cards
1 medium potato	A computer mouse
½ cup cooked pasta	Tennis ball
1 oz of cheese	Two dice
1 medium-sized fruit	Tennis ball
1 cup fruit or cooked vegetables	Baseball
1 oz of nuts	Handful
1 oz of chips or pretzels	Two handfuls (13–16 chips)
1 cup	Woman's fist
1 tablespoon (T.)	First joint of thumb
1 teaspoon (tsp.)	Fingertip

CRITICAL THINKING APPLICATION 23.7

Kayla and Tim are working with Amma Patel. Kayla is explaining the weight control diet that Dr. Perez ordered for her. They are discussing serving size and portions. Amma states she is confused by the difference. How might you explain the difference between these two concepts? Provide an example for Amma.

Obesity

According to the Centers for Disease Control and Prevention (CDC), about 42.4% of adults were obese in 2017–2018, which was up from 10 years earlier. Obesity-related diseases (e.g., heart disease, type 2 diabetes, stroke, and certain types of cancer) are some of the leading causes of death in the United States.

Childhood obesity remained stable over that time period and affects about 18.5% of children. According to the CDC, about 13.7 million children and adolescents are obese. The prevalence of childhood obesity is higher in children after age 6 than in earlier years of life.

People are considered overweight or obese when they weigh more than what is considered a healthy weight for their height. The body mass index (BMI) is a screening tool for obesity. If a person's BMI is higher than 25 but lower than 30, that person is considered to be overweight; someone with a BMI of 30 or higher is considered to be obese.

Treatment for obesity includes the following:

- *Dietary changes*: Cutting calories, making healthier choices, restricting certain foods, and meal replacements.
- *Exercise and activity*: Exercising 150 to 300 minutes a week.
- *Behavior changes*: Trying to eliminate the obstacles to managing weight (e.g., high-risk situations). Recording diet and exercise patterns. Counseling and support groups can be helpful.
- *Prescription weight-loss medications* (Table 23.7).
- *Vagal nerve blockade*: An implanted device sends electrical impulses to the vagus nerve, telling the brain when the stomach is empty or full.
- *Weight-loss surgery*: Also called *bariatric surgery,* it helps the person feel fuller sooner. Here are some common weight-loss surgeries:
    - *Gastric bypass surgery*: A small pouch is created at the top of the stomach, and the rest of the stomach is stapled shut. The small intestine is cut, and the surgeon attaches the jejunum to a small hole in the pouch. With the smaller intestine, patients may have issues with iron and calcium absorption. Vitamin B_{12} supplements must be taken.
    - *Laparoscopic adjustable gastric* band (LAGB) surgery: A band is placed on the upper part of the stomach, creating a small pouch that helps restrict food. A small port is implanted below the skin, and fluid can be injected into the band to adjust the size of the pouch outlet.
    - *Gastric sleeve surgery*: A small pouch is created in the stomach, and about 67% of the stomach is removed. The person feels full sooner.

Diabetic Eating Plans

People with diabetes mellitus need to monitor their carbohydrate intake. Remember that carbohydrates are broken down into glucose

TABLE 23.7 Weight Loss Medications

MEDICATION	CLASS	ACTION	COMMON SIDE EFFECTS
Orlistat (Xenical, Alli)	Lipase inhibitors	Prevents some of the fat consumed from being absorbed in the intestines	Oily spotting, loose stools, difficulty controlling stools, stomach pain, headache
Phentermine and topiramate (Qsymia)	Anorectic (phentermine), anticonvulsants (topiramate)	Reduces appetite and causes a person to feel fuller longer after eating	Headache, dizziness, numbness and burning in hands and feet, decreased sensation, excessive tiredness, dry mouth, thirst
Naltrexone and bupropion (Contrave)	Opiate antagonist (naltrexone), antidepressant (bupropion)	Reduces hunger and helps control cravings	Drowsiness, anxiety, dry mouth, headache, stomach pain, vomiting, loss of appetite, excessive sweating, constipation
Liraglutide (Saxenda, Victoza)	Incretin mimetics	Helps the pancreas release the right amount of insulin when the blood glucose is high	Headache, constipation, heartburn, cough, tiredness, difficulty urinating

in the body. Insulin moves the glucose from the blood into the cells. For people with diabetes, the body either does not make enough insulin or does not respond to the insulin produced. As a result, their blood glucose levels are high. In the absence of insulin, the body metabolizes fat and uses ketones for energy. Ketones build up in the body. (Too many ketones can lead to ketoacidosis, a life-threatening condition.) See Chapter 39 for more information on the treatments for type 1 and type 2 diabetes.

Over the years, several different diabetic eating plans have been created for people with diabetes mellitus. You may hear of patients being on diet plans, such as the exchange list system. This diet plan grouped similar foods with the same amount of carbohydrates, protein, fat, and calories. Each food item had a measurement (e.g., 1 cup) to indicate how much could be eaten for that exchange. Three main groups were given in the plan: carbohydrate, meat, and fat.

The American Diabetes Association (www.diabetes.org) encourages the following diabetes meal plans: the glycemic index approach, the Create Your Plate method, and carb counting. The GI was explained earlier in this chapter. Eating lower-GI foods helps one to maintain a more stable blood glucose level.

The Create Your Plate method uses a 9-inch dinner plate (Figure 23.4). To follow this meal plan, a person would do the following:

- Fill half of the plate with nonstarchy vegetables (e.g., beans, broccoli, carrots, salad greens, and peppers).
- Split the remaining unfilled side of the plate in half. Fill one half with a protein (e.g., lean meat, poultry, and fish) and fill the other half with a grain or a starchy vegetable (e.g., brown rice, potatoes, squash, green peas, and corn).
- Complete the meal with a serving of fruit, a serving of dairy (a milk product), and a nonsweetened beverage.

Carb counting, or carbohydrate counting, is another meal planning tool used by people with diabetes mellitus. Using this method, a person keeps track of the amount of carbohydrates eaten each day. Carbohydrates are measured in grams. This system may give some people better control of their diabetes, but adapting to this system is a learning process. The person needs to identify which foods contain carbohydrates and how to estimate the number of grams. The total grams are calculated over the day. Some people with type 1 diabetes may need to adjust the amount of insulin they take for a specific meal based on the amount of carbohydrates they will consume.

Low-Sodium Diet

Sodium is essential to our bodies because it helps to regulate fluid balance. The Food and Drug Administration (FDA) recommends that healthy adults consume no more than 2300 mg of sodium per day. Patients with high blood pressure, heart disease, or kidney disease are usually on reduced-sodium diets. Excessive sodium in a person's diet can lead to increased blood pressure, thus increasing the risk for heart disease and stroke.

If a patient is on a reduced-sodium diet, the provider will usually refer that person to a registered dietitian. The dietitian will help educate the individual on the sources of sodium. The following foods are high in sodium:

- Processed meats (e.g., deli meats, bacon, frankfurters, and sausage)
- Frozen dinners and ready-to-eat cereals
- Canned foods (e.g., soups, vegetables, and vegetable juice)
- Salted nuts and peanut butter, chips and pretzels, salted crackers
- Buttermilk, cheese, and processed cheese products
- Quick breads and instant cakes and puddings
- Prepackaged mixes for potatoes, rice, and pasta
- Olives, pickles, sauerkraut, pickled vegetables, and spaghetti sauce
- Soy sauce, seasoning salt, marinades, ketchup, mustard, and salad dressings

Typically, alternative lower-sodium foods are discussed. Reading labels is also an important skill for those on reduced-sodium diets.

Dietary Approaches to Stop Hypertension

Dietary Approaches to Stop Hypertension (DASH) is a flexible eating plan recommended for those with hypertension and cardiovascular disease. The goal of the plan is to reduce blood pressure and LDL and triglyceride levels. Here are some of the foods included in the DASH eating plan:

- Fruits and vegetables
- Low-fat or fat-free dairy foods
- Whole grains
- Poultry and fish
- Beans, nuts, and vegetable oils
- Foods high in potassium, calcium, magnesium, protein, and fiber
- Foods low in salt (sodium)

These foods are prohibited or limited on the DASH eating plan:

- Foods high in saturated fat, total fat, and cholesterol

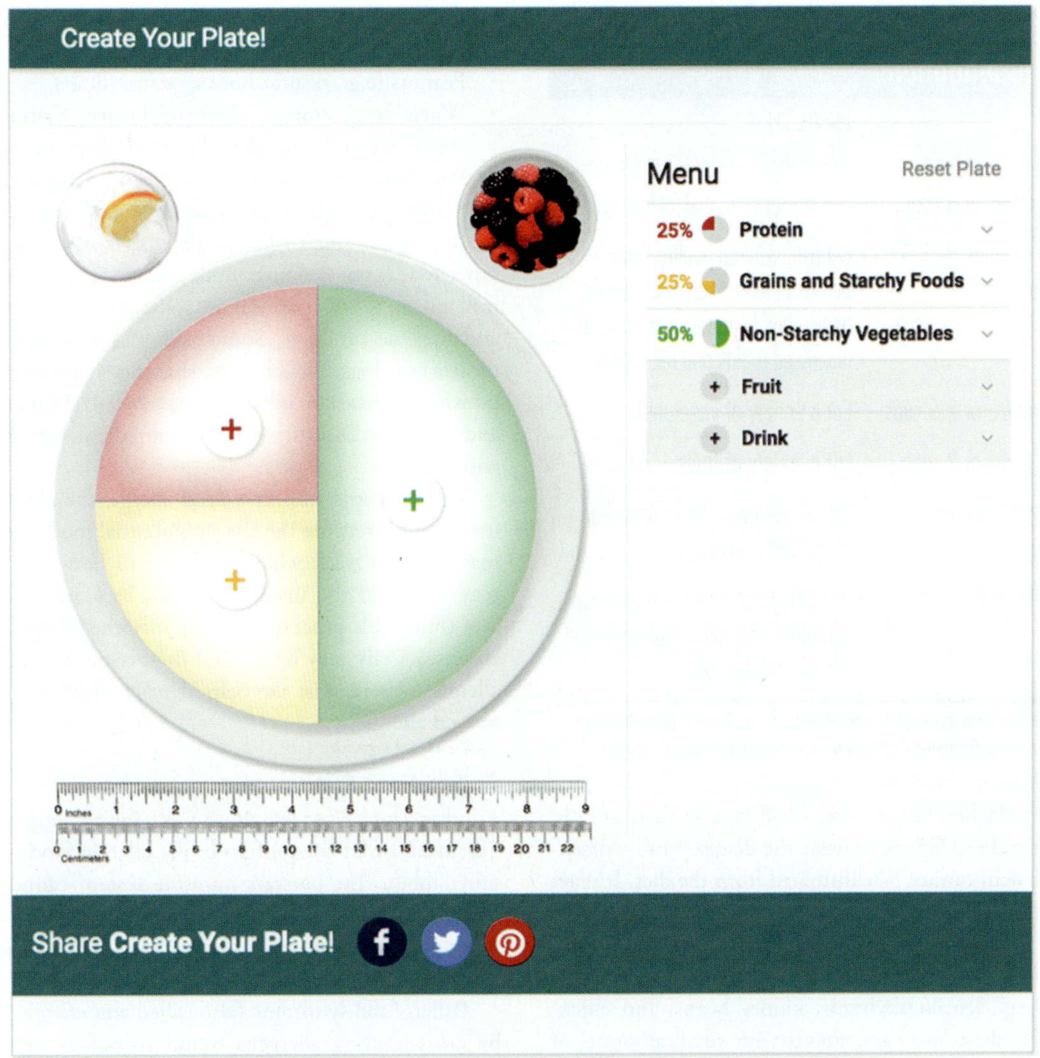

FIGURE 23.4 Create Your Plate! method recommended by the American Diabetes Association.

- Red meats
- Sugar-sweetened beverages and sweets
- High-salt (sodium) foods
- Full-fat dairy foods
- Tropical oils (coconut, kernel, and palm oil)

CRITICAL THINKING APPLICATION 23.8

Kayla and Tim are working with Al Neviaser, who has hypertension. Dr. Martin has ordered the DASH eating plan instructions for Mr. Neviaser. Tim explains to Mr. Neviaser that high-salt foods make the blood "salty," and more water is needed in the bloodstream to bring the "salty" level down. The extra water in the blood increases the blood pressure. Mr. Neviaser asks which foods he should stay away from. Give 10 foods that are high in salt (sodium).

Heart-Healthy Diet

The diet and lifestyle recommendations of the American Heart Association (AHA) closely resemble the DASH diet and the MyPlate guidelines. The AHA incorporates a focus on exercise, along with a healthy diet. The following are the AHA's recommendations:

- Limit sugary drinks, sweets, fatty meats, and salty or highly processed foods.
- Read labels and select products with the lowest amounts of sodium, added sugar, and saturated fats. Eat fewer than 2400 mg of sodium a day to lower blood pressure. Sodium can be reduced to 1500 or 1000 mg per day to lower the blood pressure even further.
- Be physically active. Balance the calories you burn during exercise with the calories you consume to maintain your weight. Include 150 minutes of moderate physical activity or 75 minutes of vigorous physical activity or a combination of both each week. Break up exercise into 10-minute sessions if needed. To lower blood pressure or cholesterol, 40 minutes of aerobic exercise of moderate to vigorous intensity three to four times a week is recommended.
- Drink alcohol in moderation. Women should have only one drink, and men should have only two drinks per day.

Table 23.8 lists the adult servings for each food group. These are based on a 2000-calorie per day diet.

Low-Protein Diet

The body uses protein for tissue repair, growth, healing, and the ability to fight infection. When protein is broken down in the body, the waste products (e.g., urea and ammonia) are eliminated in the urine. People with liver and kidney disease are often prescribed a low-protein diet. They limit or restrict foods that contain high amounts of protein. Their bodies cannot clear the protein waste products. They

TABLE 23.8 American Heart Association's Eating Healthy Recommendations

FOOD GROUP	DAILY AMOUNTS	HEALTHY RECOMMENDATIONS
Dairy	3 servings, or 3 cups	Use low-fat (1%) and fat-free options.
Proteins	1–2 servings, or 5.5 ounces (oz)	Eat fish, skinless poultry, lean and extra lean meat, nuts, seeds, beans, and legumes; limit fatty or processed meats and red meats.
Vegetables	5 servings, or 2.5 cups	Eat a variety of vegetables.
Fruits	4 servings, or 2 cups	Eat a variety of fruits.
Grains	3–6 servings, or 3–6 oz	Eat whole grains for at least half of the daily servings.
Oils	3 tablespoons	Use polyunsaturated and monounsaturated oils; avoid hydrogenated oils and tropical oils.

Information from the American Heart Association, www.heart.org/en/healthy-living/healthy-eating/eat-smart/nutrition-basics/what-is-a-healthy-diet-recommended-serving-infographic.

can have nausea, headaches, fatigue, and a bad taste in their mouth. Eating a low-protein diet helps to prevent the disease from worsening. Remember, protein cannot be eliminated from the diet. It plays an essential role in the body.

Foods high in protein include milk products (e.g., yogurt and cheese), peanut butter, nuts (e.g., almonds, pistachios, and cashews), quinoa, legumes (e.g., lentils, soybeans, kidney beans, and chickpeas), meat, fish, poultry, and eggs. Foods with small amounts of protein include vegetables and starches (e.g., bread, cereals, and pasta). Fruits, sugars, and fats have trace amounts of protein.

DIETS FOR ALLERGIES AND INTOLERANCES

A food allergy occurs when the immune system overreacts to a protein in the food. The immune system makes IgE antibodies in response to the protein. This causes the person to quickly experience allergy symptoms. Symptoms may include itching, hives, nausea and vomiting, diarrhea, difficulty breathing (e.g., tightness in the throat or chest, coughing, wheezing), or **anaphylaxis.**

With a *food intolerance*, the body cannot digest, metabolize, or absorb certain nutrients. Lactose and gluten intolerance are the most common types of food intolerances. *Food sensitivities* are less severe than food intolerance. Typically, people can consume foods they are sensitive to in moderation. Food sensitivities can resolve over time.

Elimination Diet and Food Allergies

Nine of the most common food allergens can be hiding in ingredient lists under other names. Some examples are listed here:

- Milk (e.g., cream, casein, ghee, galactose, lactalbumin, lactose, and whey)
- Eggs (e.g., albumin, eggnog, ovalbumin, and ovomucin)
- Fish (e.g., cod, bass, flounder)
- Crustacean shellfish (e.g., crab, lobster, shrimp)
- Tree nuts (e.g., almonds, cashews, filberts, hazelnuts, marzipan, nut meal)
- Peanuts (e.g., peanut butter, peanut flour)
- Wheat (e.g., emmer, einkorn, durum, Kamut, modified wheat starch, wheat bran, wheat flour, wheat germ)
- Soybeans (e.g., edamame, miso, soya, tempeh, tofu)
- Sesame (a hidden ingredient in "spices" and "natural flavors")

It is important to realize that parts of these foods are used in other foods. For instance, milk proteins (e.g., whey and casein) and milk sugar *(lactose)* appear in some surprising foods, medications, and hygiene products. Some examples include chicken broth, deli meats, hot dogs, French fries, shampoos and conditioners, and dry powder medication inhalers (e.g., Advair Diskus, Flovent Diskus, and Serevent Diskus). Reading ingredient lists is critical for those with allergies.

When people suspect a food allergy, the *elimination diet* can be used. People remove the allergy-potential foods from their diet. They may need to track what they eat and how they feel. Slowly, they may then add the suspicious foods back into their diet, one food at a time. This process helps identify the allergen. In some cases, a cross-reactivity may occur, and the person will have additional food allergies. An allergist can help identify additional food and environmental allergies.

Pollen-Food Syndrome

Another issue faced by those with food allergies is *cross-reactivity.* This means that the protein in the allergic food is similar to that in other foods. The person's immune system cannot tell the proteins apart and thus reacts to similar foods. Cross-reactivity can occur with foods and nonfood items. For instance, a person with a latex allergy could also be allergic to avocados, bananas, chestnuts, and kiwi.

Pollen-food syndrome (also called *oral allergy syndrome*) is caused by cross-reacting allergens found in pollens, raw foods, and tree nuts. Symptoms include itchy mouth and ears, scratchy throat, and swollen lips, mouth, tongue, and throat. Typically, the symptoms disappear when the food is out of the mouth. Some common cross-reactions include the following:

- *Ragweed pollen:* Cucumber, banana, melons, potatoes, and zucchini
- *Grass pollen:* Celery, melons, oranges, peaches, and tomatoes
- *Birch pollen:* Pitted fruit (e.g., plum, pear, peach, and apple), kiwi, carrot, celery, almond, and hazelnut

Alpha-gal Syndrome

Alpha-gal syndrome or allergy is an allergy to the alpha-gal sugar molecule found in mammals (except for people, apes, and monkeys). The alpha-gal sugar molecule can also be found in products made from mammals, including gelatin, some vaccines and medications, cosmetics, and milk products.

It is believed that the Lone Star tick carries this disease from animals to humans. Most cases occur in the southeastern and midwestern United States and infect adults over age 50. Younger adults and children can also have it. Here are some symptoms of alpha-gal syndrome:

- Rash, hives, difficulty breathing, and wheezing
- Swelling of the lips, face, throat, and tongue
- Drop in blood pressure, dizziness, and faintness
- Nausea, vomiting, severe stomach pain

Symptoms can be life threatening and commonly appear 3 to 6 hours after exposure (eating meat or using products). A skin test or a blood test can be used to diagnose alpha-gal syndrome. Treatment consists of avoiding foods and products that cause the reaction.

Celiac Disease

People with celiac disease are put on a gluten-free diet. (See Chapter 34 for additional information on celiac disease.) Gluten is a protein found in a number of food sources:

- Barley and malt products (e.g., flavoring and vinegar)
- Rye
- Triticale (wheat and rye crossbred hybrid)
- Wheat (e.g., durum flour, farina, graham flour, spelt, semolina, and Kamut)

Gluten is commonly found in bread, cereals, pasta, cakes, cookies, and other foods. It causes inflammation in the small intestine of people with celiac disease. Removing gluten from the diet helps to control the symptoms.

The FDA regulates the gluten-free food labeling claim. This is a voluntary claim that manufacturers may opt to use. If they use the label, they are accountable for using the claim in a truthful way.

Lactose Intolerance Diet

Lactose intolerance or lactose sensitivity are not allergies. Lactose is the main sugar found in dairy products. Lactose is broken down by lactase, an enzyme created by the small intestine. If a person's small intestine does not produce enough lactase, the lactose moves into the large intestine. The bacteria in the large intestine break down the lactose, causing bloating, cramps, diarrhea, nausea, and gas. Treatment for lactose intolerance or sensitivity involves avoiding milk products or using an oral enzyme replacement supplement.

NUTRITIONAL NEEDS FOR VARIOUS POPULATIONS

Nutritional needs change throughout life. Our needs for calories, vitamins, minerals, and protein change as we grow and develop. With pregnancy and breastfeeding, the needs increase. With disease conditions, the needs change. We have already discussed different diets and conditions treated with those eating plans. Table 23.9 describes the nutritional needs by age group.

Pregnancy and Lactation

During pregnancy, it is important to eat a healthy diet. The first trimester can be difficult with nutrition. Depending on the mother's morning sickness, eating a balanced diet can be tricky. Many providers recommend eating small, frequent meals to combat morning sickness. Dry crackers and toast are also encouraged. Eating low-odor protein foods can also help. Avoiding triggers such as spicy foods and certain smells are important in managing morning sickness.

Providers usually recommend a daily prenatal vitamin and mineral supplement to ensure adequate folic acid and prevent spina bifida. Consuming alcohol during pregnancy is not recommended. Despite the saying "eating for two," the daily caloric intake only needs to increase by 340 calories for the second trimester and about 450 calories for the third trimester.

Women who are pregnant or breastfeeding should avoid eating raw fish or fish high in mercury. Two to three servings of seafood per week are recommended during pregnancy and when breastfeeding. According to the FDA, examples of the best choices of seafood to eat include salmon, cod, tilapia, catfish, haddock, lobster, perch, squid, trout, shrimp, and light canned tuna. Mercury, which can be toxic to the nervous system, can be found in higher levels in marlin, orange roughy, bigeye tuna, swordfish, shark, king mackerel, and tilefish from the Gulf of Mexico. Consumption of locally caught fish and white albacore tuna intake should be limited to no more than 6 ounces per week.

With lactation, or breastfeeding, the mother needs to eat a healthy diet, and a vitamin supplement may be recommended. It is important to get adequate vitamins and minerals, which are passed to the baby in the breast milk. The mother also needs to drink additional water to

TABLE 23.9 Nutritional Needs by Age Group

AGE	NUTRITIONAL NEEDS
Infancy to 2 years	• Birth to 6 months of age: Breast milk or formula is given. If an infant cannot tolerate milk-based formulas, other types of formulas are available, including soy formula. Some formulas are available by prescription only. • Six months of age: The child is started on soft, pureed solid foods. Usually, infant cereals, fruits, and vegetables are first introduced. • One year of age: The child is transitioned to whole milk, and pureed foods are gradually replaced with easy-to-eat foods. It is important to offer foods from each food group.
2 to 12 years	• Age 2: Children should eat several dairy products, fruits, vegetables, meats, breads, pasta, cereals, and beans. • As children grow and develop, more foods can be added to their diet. Portion sizes also grow.
12 to adulthood	• Adolescents experience rapid growth periods, which require more energy. Teens may need encouragement to consume dairy products (e.g., milk) instead of soda. The growth spurts require calcium for strong bones. • Females who have started menstruating should eat foods high in iron to replace the iron lost in menstrual blood.

Older adults	• As a person grows older, the metabolism decreases, and caloric needs also decrease.
	• Special nutritional concerns of the older adult include the following:
	  • Difficulty chewing and swallowing, which can be related to poor-fitting dentures
	  • Decrease in eating due to changes in the senses (e.g., taste, smell)
	  • Lack of a well-balanced diet (e.g., limited income, loneliness, and lack of initiative to cook for oneself)

maintain her milk volume. During the first 6 months of breastfeeding, the mother should consume about 330 extra calories and 400 extra calories during the remaining 6 months of the first year.

Eating Disorders

Treatment for eating disorders includes psychological, behavioral, and nutritional therapies. (See Chapter 38 for additional information on eating disorders.) Some patients with eating disorders have medical complications from malnutrition. Dietary needs for people with eating disorders are aimed at correcting nutritional imbalances and restoring their weight. Nutritional plans focus on consuming a wide and balanced range of foods. Eating regularly spaced meals is also important.

Epilepsy

Some patients with epilepsy follow a ketogenic diet. This diet consists of very low-carbohydrate, high-fat, and adequate protein foods. Some people have also used this type of diet to lose weight. Without carbohydrates, the body metabolizes fat, and the ketones are used for energy. It is important to monitor kidney function when a person is on a ketogenic diet.

HIV and AIDS

When a person has HIV infection or AIDS, it is important to eat a well-balanced diet. Making sure the immune system is nutritionally supported is critical. People with AIDS can struggle with several issues, including nausea, diarrhea, constipation, and poor appetite. The provider may order medications to help with the nausea. Drinking extra fluids will help with both diarrhea and constipation issues. Restricting milk products with diarrhea and increasing fiber intake with constipation can help. A poor appetite can cause weight and nutrient loss. Frequent small meals, nutritional supplements (e.g., Ensure), and light exercise may help. A provider may encourage a daily vitamin and mineral supplement. With unintended weight loss, additional "healthy" calories should be added to the diet.

Cancer

Patients undergoing radiation and chemotherapy can experience issues that affect eating. The treatments can harm fast-growing cells in the lining of the mouth, lips, and intestinal tract. Patients may have mouth sores that cause pain and swallowing problems. Taste and smell changes can occur. The treatments can cause appetite changes, diarrhea or constipation, fatigue, dry mouth, nausea, vomiting, and weight gain or loss. Good nutrition is critical for people to regain their strength and heal after the treatments. A registered dietitian is commonly involved with the team of healthcare professionals caring for patients undergoing treatment. Nutritional tips for patients undergoing cancer treatments include the following:

- Eat a soft, bland diet.
- Eat six to eight small meals a day instead of three meals. Attempt to eat high-calorie, high-protein snacks (e.g., hard-cooked eggs, peanut butter, nuts, supplements, trail mix, and canned chicken).
- Take only sips of liquids during meals. Drink most liquids between meals. Drink 8 to 10 cups of liquid a day to prevent constipation. Water, prune juice, and warm liquids are helpful.
- To reduce mouth dryness and sores, limit caffeine and alcohol; keep the mouth clean using water or a mild mouth rinse; avoid tart, acidic or salty foods; eat lukewarm, cold, soft, and creamy foods; and use anesthetic rinses prior to eating.
- Avoid foods with strong odors and those that are overly sweet, spicy, greasy, or fried.
- Eat small bites and chew the food well. Eat dry foods (e.g., crackers, toast).
- In addition, use a straw or a small spoon and puree food as needed. Suck on hard candies and ice chips to soothe the mouth and prevent mouth dryness.

CRITICAL THINKING APPLICATION 23.9

Kayla and Tim are working with Noemi Rodriguez, who is currently undergoing chemotherapy. She was not able to see her oncologist today, and she had a very sore mouth after the last treatment. List some nutritional tips for patients undergoing cancer treatments.

INSTRUCTING PATIENTS ON DIETARY CHANGES

When a patient needs a dietary change, the provider will give the order to the medical assistant. The provider will tell the medical assistant what type of diet the patient needs to be on. If the diet is only for a short period of time, the provider will indicate the time period. Sometimes the dietary change is related to a procedure. The provider will order the diagnostic procedure, and the medical assistant should be knowledgeable about the dietary changes required for that procedure.

Before meeting with the patient for coaching, it is important for the medical assistant to gather any brochures or information needed. Remember, it is a good idea to send the patient home with written instructions on dietary changes. If the patient does not understand English, use an interpreter service, and make sure brochures are in the patient's primary language.

Lastly, before meeting with the patient, the medical assistant should look over the brochure. It is important to be knowledgeable about the content you are explaining to the patient. Reading the brochure aloud as a way of instructing the patient is not professional. The patient may feel you do not know what you are talking about.

When a medical assistant instructs a patient on a dietary change, it is important to know why people eat what they do and to understand how cultural dietary traditions relate to illness, as described in the following section. The following section also reviews the communication techniques and nonverbal behaviors that can show awareness of a patient's concerns. Procedure 23.1 details the process of coaching a patient regarding a dietary change.

Showing Awareness of a Patient's Concerns

Being aware means being alert and understanding what you are perceiving. When working with patients, identify the patient's concerns. After you become aware of the patient's concerns, you can show that you are aware. It is important to be accurate in your perception of the patient's concerns. If your perceptions are incorrect, you could speak or behave in a way that is insensitive to the patient.

Chapter 2 discusses therapeutic communication techniques. Let's review a few ways a medical assistant can show awareness of the patient's concerns:

- *Reflection*: The medical assistant puts words to the patient's emotional reaction, which acknowledges the person's feelings; for example, "It sounds like you are unsure of this new way of eating."
- *Restatement or paraphrasing*: The medical assistant rewords or rephrases a patient's statement to check the meaning and interpretation. This shows you are listening and understanding the patient. You might say, for example, "What I am hearing is that you really like your family traditions for holiday meals."
- *Summarizing*: This allows the medical assistant to recap and review what was said; for example, "If I understand how you feel about this new eating plan..."

Remember that a medical assistant can also show awareness by using positive and open nonverbal behaviors. These nonverbal behaviors could be used when working with a patient on a dietary change:

- *Position:* The medical assistant should be at the level of the other person and angled toward the patient. For example, if the patient is sitting, then the medical assistant should be sitting also.
- *Arms and posture*: The medical assistant should be poised with their arms to the side. This is an open, positive nonverbal behavior that shows interest in the other person.
- *Facial expression*: The medical assistant should be smiling. Refrain from rolling your eyes, yawning, or frowning. These can be perceived as being bored or rude.
- *Gestures and touch*: The medical assistant should use small gestures and an appropriately light touch on the hand of the patient, depending on the situation.
- *Mannerisms*: The medical assistant should focus on the patient. It is not appropriate to look at your watch, phone, or the clock. This gives the patient the feeling you are bored or impatient.

Factors That Can Affect a Person's Diet

When you work with patients regarding a dietary change, it is important to understand the factors that can affect what they eat:

- *Cost*: How much money we have affects what foods we purchase. It can be expensive to purchase fresh fruits and vegetables, fish, and lean cuts of meat. Less expensive options are available, but they may not have the same taste or appeal.
- *Convenience*: With busy lifestyles, people sometimes choose what is easiest and quickest. This usually includes eating out or take-home meals.
- *Background*: Our background can influence the foods we eat. Some cultures have healthier diets than others. It can be helpful for people to modify cultural dishes by cutting the salt, fat, and sugar without giving up the taste.
- *Emotional comfort*: Some people may eat when they are happy or when they are sad. Usually, under these conditions, the food choices are not the healthiest. Some people stop eating when they are emotional.
- *Routine*: People eat what they always eat out of habit, personal preference, and availability. People may also eat with certain activities, like viewing a sports event, driving, or watching television. These habits are difficult to break.

It is important for the medical assistant to get to know what the patient is eating and why. This helps when coaching a patient on a dietary change. For instance, knowing your patient has a limited food budget is helpful when coaching them on healthier choices. You might be able to share ideas on healthy foods that are less costly or places to shop that are cheaper.

Cultural Diets

Medical assistants should be familiar with the diets of the various cultural groups in the area where they are practicing. This information can be helpful when coaching patients on specific diets ordered by the provider. Here is some general cultural diet information:

- Asian diets include whole grains (e.g., millet and rice), fruits, vegetables, legumes, nuts, and seeds. Fats are derived largely from vegetable oils (peanut or sesame oils). Dairy products are not traditionally eaten. Protein sources include broiled or stir-fried fish and seafood, egg whites, tofu, and nuts.
- Latin American diets include food from plant sources at each meal. This can include maize (corn), potatoes, fruits, vegetables, whole grains, beans, and nuts. Poultry, fish, and dairy are typically consumed daily. Meat and eggs are eaten weekly.
- Mediterranean diets include whole grains, fresh fruits and vegetables, and all types of legumes (e.g., beans, lentils, and peas) daily. Olive oil is used. Fish, poultry, and eggs are consumed weekly and meat monthly.
- Mexican diets include corn or flour tortillas, cabbage, legumes, squash, tomatoes, corn, and potatoes daily. Cheeses are eaten, but milk is not regularly consumed. Protein sources typically are fish, beef, poultry, lamb, and many types of beans.

CLOSING COMMENTS

Patient Coaching

Good nutrition is important for a person's health and well-being. For many people, changing their diet can be difficult and uncomfortable. It is important for the medical assistant to be sensitive to the change that the patient is asking about. Educating the patient about the benefits of making a dietary change may make the transition easier. Compliance with the diet increases if the person meets certain conditions:

- Can modify special foods and not give them up completely
- Has support from family and friends
- Can slowly transition to the new diet, though this might not always be possible

The medical assistant is an important team member when there is a need to help patients transition to a new diet. It is important for the medical assistant to be familiar with the dietary changes required for common procedures and diagnoses.

Legal and Ethical Issues

After the medical assistant coaches a patient on a dietary change, it is important to document the teaching in the health record. The documentation should reflect the provider ordering the teaching, the general topics taught, and how the patient's learning was evaluated. If the medical assistant provided the patient with written materials, this should also be noted in the documentation.

Patient-Centered Care

As medical assistants work with patients from various cultures, it is important for them to know more about those cultures. Many cultures have dietary traditions that influence how they respond to illness. In some cultures, food is considered a cure for illness. For instance, in the Mexican culture, when people are sick, they are out of balance in that they have too much heat or cold. To correct this balance, the person needs to eat foods of the opposite quality. It is important to be sensitive to these cultural practices. If the dietary change conflicts with the cultural practice, it is important to talk with the provider. A referral to a registered dietitian may provide the patient with extra support and information.

Professional Behaviors

When you work with patients who are making dietary changes, it is important to be respectful of the patient. It is easy to tell a patient what to eat and what not to eat, but that might not be the best way to approach the situation. A medical assistant may want to start by finding out the patient's favorite foods. What foods does the patient typically eat at meals? Are any health beliefs related to that food? Learning about the patient's diet can help the medical assistant coach the patient.

If the medical assistant feels the patient needs additional dietary support, talking with the provider is important. The provider can refer the patient to a registered dietitian for additional assistance.

SUMMARY OF SCENARIO

Tim really enjoyed working with Kayla for his practicum. He learned a lot from her as she worked with patients. His favorite part of the experience was the patient education, in which he was able to observe and participate. Kayla also learned from Tim during the experience. Because of his interest in nutrition, Tim was able to share with Kayla what he knew about current dietary trends.

Tim hopes to obtain a job as a medical assistant in a practice like the one where he did his practicum. He feels that the family practice environment will allow him to use many of the skills he learned in school. He will also have a lot of experience talking to patients about dietary changes.

SUMMARY OF LEARNING OBJECTIVES

1. **Explain metabolism, including the phases and the variables that affect metabolism.**
   Metabolism is the process the body uses to obtain or make energy from the food eaten. Catabolism and anabolism are the two phases of metabolism. Variables that affect the basal metabolic rate (BMR) include genetics, sex, age, weight, body surface area, body fat percentage, diet, body temperature, thyroxin, exercise, lean muscle tissue, and drugs.
2. **Examine carbohydrates, including their action in the body and types of carbohydrates.**
   Carbohydrates are used for energy and to regulate protein and fat metabolism. Simple sugars, starches, and fiber are carbohydrates. Desserts, milk products, bread, and fruits are some examples of carbohydrates.
3. **Examine proteins, including action in the body and types of amino acids.**
   Proteins break down into amino acids; both are considered building blocks for the body. Essential amino acids must come from food eaten, whereas nonessential amino acids are made in the body. Meat, poultry, dairy products, eggs, and nuts are sources of protein.
4. **Examine fats, including action in the body and types of fats.**
   Fat provides a source of energy when carbohydrates are not available. Saturated fats are solid at room temperature and should be limited in the diet. Unsaturated fats are liquid at room temperature. Monounsaturated and polyunsaturated fats are two types of unsaturated fats. Trans fatty acids or trans fats are created during the food manufacturing process and are considered unhealthy.
5. **Examine the role of minerals, vitamins, antioxidants, and water in the body.**
   - Minerals in the body are called electrolytes. Some examples include calcium, potassium, sodium, sulfur, iron, and iodine. Table 23.3 describes the role of electrolytes in the body.
   - Vitamins can be either fat or water soluble. Vitamins A, D, E, and K are fat soluble, and B vitamins and vitamin C are water soluble. A deficit of a vitamin can lead to a disease. Table 23.4 describes the role of vitamins in the body.
   - Antioxidants protect cells from free radicals and limit the damage free radicals can do to the cells.
   - Water is the basis for the fluids in the body. Our bodies need water to function and survive.
6. **Explain the key recommendations of the dietary guidelines.**
   The US Department of Agriculture publishes Dietary Guidelines every 5 years. The guidelines are for individuals 2 years or older. Key recommendations from the 2020–2025 Dietary Guidelines for Americans include those listed with the MyPlate regimen, in addition to the following:
   - Added sugars: Limit to less than 10% of calories per day starting at age 2. Avoid for infants and toddlers
   - Saturated fat: Limit to less than 10% of calories per day starting at age 2.

SUMMARY OF LEARNING OBJECTIVES—*continued*

- Sodium: Limit to less than 2300 mg per day for those age 14 and older.
- Alcoholic beverages: Men should limit intake to two drinks or less per day. Women should limit intake to one drink or less per day.
- Pay attention to portion sizes.
- Food choices should be rich in nutrients.

7. **Interpret a food label.**
Food labels provide nutritional facts. This information is presented in both the quantity (e.g., grams [g] or milligrams [mg]) and as a percentage. The percentage reflects the % Daily Value (DV). This is the percentage of the nutrient in a single serving in terms of the daily recommended amount, based on a 2000-calorie diet. Refer to the section in the chapter for additional steps to take when reading food labels.
8. **Differentiate among clear liquid, full liquid, soft, and high- and low-fiber diets.**
   - Clear liquid diet: Made up of foods and beverages that become liquid at room temperature.
   - Full liquid diet: Made up of clear liquids and milk products.
   - Soft and mechanical soft diet: Made up of foods soft in texture, low in fiber, and easy to digest. Mechanical soft diets are prepared for easier chewing.
   - High- and low-fiber diets: Limit or add fiber to the diet. A high-fiber diet helps with constipation and weight loss. Low-fiber diets are used during a flare-up of an intestinal disease.
   - Bland diet: Consists of foods that are soft and low in fiber and eliminates foods that are spicy, fried, and raw. Citrus foods, caffeine, and alcohol are eliminated.
9. **Differentiate among diets with nutrient modifications, including changes related to calories, carbohydrates, sodium, fat, cholesterol, and protein.**
   - Weight control diet: Can help people lose or maintain weight. Control of portion sizes is very important on the weight control diet.
   - Diabetic eating plans: Used for people with diabetes who need to monitor their carbohydrate intake. There are several diabetic eating plans, including the glycemic index approach, the "Create Your Plate" method, and carb counting.
   - Low-sodium diet: Helps to lower the blood pressure and used to address kidney disease. Dietary Approaches to Stop Hypertension (DASH) is used for hypertension and cardiovascular disease.
   - Heart-healthy diet: Consists of limiting sugary, salty, and highly processed foods. Limiting the consumption of saturated fats, trans fats, and added sugar is also important.
   - Low-protein diet: Used for people with liver and kidney disease.
10. **Examine common food allergies, intolerances, and related diets.**
A food allergy occurs when the immune system overreacts to a protein in the food. With a food intolerance, the body cannot digest, metabolize or absorb certain nutrients. Food sensitivity is less severe than food intolerance. Common diets for allergies and intolerances include the following:
    - Elimination diet: Removes suspicious allergens from the diet. Slowly they are reintroduced to find the allergens.
    - Gluten-free diet: Used for people with celiac disease. Wheat, barley, and rye foods are removed from the diet.
    - Lactose-intolerance diet: Involves avoiding milk products or using oral enzyme replacement supplements.
11. **Differentiate the nutritional needs of various populations, including those who are pregnant, those who are lactating, those from different age groups, and those with disease conditions.**
    - Table 23.9 describes the nutritional needs by age group.
    - Pregnancy and lactation: A healthy diet is recommended, along with a daily prenatal vitamin and mineral supplement. Consuming alcohol during pregnancy is not recommended. The daily caloric intake only needs to increase by 340 calories for the second trimester and about 450 calories for the third trimester. Women who are pregnant or breastfeeding should avoid eating raw fish or fish high in mercury.
    - Epilepsy: Some patients with epilepsy follow a ketogenic diet. This diet consists of very low-carbohydrate, high-fat, and adequate protein foods.
    - HIV and AIDS: It is important to eat a well-balanced diet. The provider may order medications to help with nausea. Drinking extra fluids will help with both diarrhea and constipation issues. Restricting milk products while experiencing diarrhea and increasing fiber intake when constipated can help. Frequent small meals, nutritional supplements (e.g., Ensure), and light exercise may help. A provider may encourage a daily vitamin and mineral supplement.
    - Cancer: Many patients undergoing cancer treatment may have changes in their appetite. Good nutrition is critical for people to regain their strength and heal after the treatments. Refer to the Cancer section for more nutritional tips for patients undergoing cancer treatment.
12. **Demonstrate how to instruct patients on dietary changes while showing sensitivity and understanding to the patient's concerns.**
When a medical assistant instructs a patient on a dietary change, it is important to know why people eat what they do and understand how cultural dietary traditions relate to illness. When working with patients regarding a dietary change, it is important to understand the factors that can affect what we eat: cost, convenience, background, emotional comfort, and routine. It is important for the medical assistant to get to know what the patient is eating and why. This helps when the medical assistant is coaching a patient on a dietary change. Procedure 23.1 details the process of coaching a patient regarding a dietary change.

PROCEDURE 23.1 Instruct a Patient on a Dietary Change

TASK: Instruct a patient regarding a dietary change related to the patient's special dietary needs. Show empathy for the patient's concerns regarding the dietary change. Document in the patient's health record.

SCENARIO: You are working with Dr. Angela Perez, a family practice provider. She just finished seeing Al Neviaser (date of birth [DOB] 6/21/19XX). Dr. Perez orders that the patient be given instructions on a heart-healthy diet.

DIRECTIONS: Role-play the scenario with a peer. You are the medical assistant, and the peer is the patient.

EQUIPMENT and SUPPLIES

- Patient's health record
- Heart-healthy diet brochure

PROCEDURAL STEPS

1. Assemble supplies needed for the provider's order. Ensure that the patient can read and understand the written materials. Verify the order if you have any questions.
   PURPOSE: Using written materials is helpful when instructing a patient on a dietary change.
2. Greet the patient. Identify yourself. Verify the patient's identity with the full name and date of birth. Explain the order from the provider. Answer any questions the patient may have.
   PURPOSE: It is important to identify the patient in two different ways to ensure that you have the correct patient. Explaining the order can make the patient feel more comfortable and reduces anxiety.
3. Position yourself at the same level as the patient. Angle yourself toward the patient. Have a poised position.
   PURPOSE: This position shows positive nonverbal behaviors to the patient. Being at the same level as the patient and angling toward the patient show openness.
4. Accurately instruct the patient on the new diet. Use the written materials as you discuss the new eating plan.
   PURPOSE: The information taught to the patient should match what is in the written materials. Any inaccuracies will confuse the patient.
5. Use words that the patient can understand. Refrain from jargon and medical terminology. Use professional verbal and nonverbal communication.
   PURPOSE: Jargon and medical terminology can confuse patients. Unprofessional nonverbal behaviors, such as rolling your eyes, checking the clock, or yawning, are disrespectful to the patient.
   Scenario update: After going over the heart-healthy eating plan, Mr. Neviaser states he is not sure this diet is for him. He likes his red meat and does not like to eat fish. He does not have a lot of money to buy expensive fresh fruits and vegetables.
6. Demonstrate empathy by listening to the patient and learning about their experiences and concerns. Use therapeutic communication techniques and positive nonverbal behaviors, including appropriate eye contact. Show your support and respect.
   PURPOSE: By using therapeutic communication techniques, the medical assistant can demonstrate empathy and respect.
7. Based on the patient's concerns, provide food alternatives that meet the eating plan requirements.
   PURPOSE: The medical assistant can show awareness of the patient's concerns by providing alternative food choices that would meet the patient's requirements.
8. Evaluate the patient's understanding of the teaching by asking the patient to summarize the eating plan or describe a day's worth of meals. Answer any questions the patient may have.
   PURPOSE: It is important to check the patient's understanding of what was taught. Having the patient provide information back to the medical assistant is a better evaluation of understanding than asking, "Do you understand?"
9. Document the instruction in the patient's health record. Include the order, instruction given, written materials provided, and the patient's feedback.
   PURPOSE: Documentation indicates that the patient was provided with the instruction.

Documentation Example

11/04/20XX 0923 Per Dr. Perez's order, the pt and his wife were instructed on a heart-healthy diet. Pt indicated he did not eat fish and was concerned about the cost of fresh foods. Alternative healthy proteins and inexpensive food options were discussed with the patient. The pt and his wife were able to describe a day's worth of heart-healthy meals. Pt was encouraged to call with any additional questions. ———————————— Kayla Smith, RMA

SURGICAL SUPPLIES AND INSTRUMENTS

24

SCENARIO

Tom Anderson, a certified medical assistant (CMA) who has met the requirements of the American Association of Medical Assistants (AAMA), works for Walden-Martin Family Medical (WMFM) Clinic. Tom enjoys assisting with the minor surgical procedures performed in the office. Tom is also responsible for maintaining stock supplies in the minor surgery room, including solutions and medications, and for cleaning, maintaining, and inspecting the surgical instruments. Because no procedures are scheduled for today, Tom plans to compile an inventory of supplies and equipment and perform routine maintenance activities.

While studying this chapter, think about the following questions:

- What solutions and medications should be available in the surgical area of a medical office?
- What are the typical instruments used in minor surgical procedures?
- How are surgical instruments identified and classified?
- How should surgical instruments be cared for and handled before, during, and after a surgical procedure?
- What types of sutures and needles are used in minor surgical procedures?

LEARNING OBJECTIVES

1. Examine the minor surgery room and the solutions and medications used for a minor surgical procedure.
2. Differentiate the surgical instruments used in a minor surgical procedure.
3. Examine the drapes, sutures, and other closure material used in a minor surgical procedure.
4. Examine surgical asepsis and the preparation of surgical instruments.

VOCABULARY

abscess Localized collection of pus, which may be under the skin or deep in the body, that causes tissue destruction.

anesthetic (an ehs THET ik) An agent that causes partial or complete loss of sensation.

cannula (KAN yuh la) A rigid tube that surrounds a blunt trocar or a sharp, pointed trocar, which is inserted into the body; when the trocar is withdrawn, fluid may escape from the body through the cannula, depending on the insertion site.

caustic (KAW stik) Capable of burning, corroding, or destroying living tissue.

curettage (kyoo reh TAHZH) The act of scraping a body cavity with a surgical instrument, such as a curette.

dilation (die LAY shuhn) The opening or widening of the circumference of a body orifice with a dilating instrument.

diluent (DIL yoo uhnt) A liquid substance that dilutes or lessens the strength of a solution or mixture; it is added to vials of powdered medications to create a solution of the drug for injection.

dissect To cut or separate tissue with a cutting instrument or scissors.

fornix (FORE niks) A recess in the upper part of the vagina caused by protrusion of the cervix into the vaginal wall.

impervious (im PUR vee uhs) Not permitting penetration.

infection Invasion of body tissues by microorganisms, which then multiply and damage tissues.

obturator (OB tuh rayt oar) A metal rod with a smooth, rounded tip that is placed in hollow instruments to reduce injury to body tissues during insertion.

patency (PAT en see) Open condition of a body cavity or canal.

pathogen A disease-causing organism.

permeable (PUR mee uh buhl) Allowing for penetration.

spore A thick-walled, dormant form of bacteria that is very resistant to disinfection measures.

stylus (STIE luhs) A metal probe that is inserted into or passed through a catheter, needle, or tube used for clearing purposes or to facilitate passage into a body orifice.

transient (TRAN zee uhnt) Not lasting, enduring, or permanent; transitory.

vasoconstriction (vay zoh kuhn STRIK shuhn) Contraction of the muscles causing the narrowing of the inside tube of the vessel.

INTRODUCTION

Office surgery is restricted to the management of minor problems and injuries. The medical assistant is expected to prepare the patient and the sterile field, assist the provider as needed, take care of the patient after the procedure, properly disinfect the area, and document appropriately. Some medical assistants are employed in outpatient surgical facilities and are expected to assist with procedures that once were performed in hospitals. Although these more difficult operations may involve complete gowning and gloving with surgical masks and caps, the two surgical chapters in this text limit discussion and descriptions to the routines necessary to prepare for and assist in minor surgery only. This chapter includes a discussion of surgical supplies and instruments, the care and handling of instruments, the different types of surgical sutures and needles, and sterilization procedures. The next chapter explores preparation of the sterile field, specific minor surgical procedures, and care of the patient.

PREPARING FOR MINOR SURGERY

It is important to have an understanding of how the minor surgery room is set up and what solutions and medications should be available during a minor surgical procedure. Being prepared for all possible needs ensures that the procedure will go as smoothly as possible. It is often the medical assistant's responsibility to prepare the minor surgery room, including checking that all solutions and medications are available. The following sections discuss the minor surgery room and the solutions and medications needed.

Minor Surgery Room

When minor surgery is routinely performed, a minor surgery room that is separate from the other examining rooms may be used. Recovery rooms and family waiting areas may also be available and are common in the larger surgery centers. The minor surgery room in a provider's office, often called the *procedure room,* should be near a workroom with a sink and an autoclave. In some facilities, the sink and autoclave will be located in the procedure room. Cabinets with countertops serve as a side or back table during surgical procedures. Regardless of the setup, it should be easy to disinfect the area, and it should remain uncluttered to allow for easy access to the patient and necessary supplies.

Surgical supplies, wound care equipment, medications, and biopsy containers are stored in the cabinets. The exam table should be easy to adjust. In addition, the room should have bright lighting, a Mayo stand for instruments, vital signs equipment, and possibly an electrocardiograph (ECG) machine as part of the standard equipment (Figure 24.1).

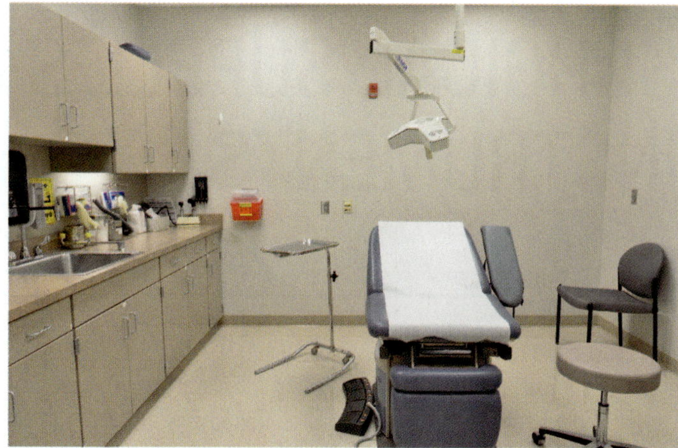

FIGURE 24.1 Typical surgical procedure room in an ambulatory care setting.

Surgical Solutions and Medications

Procedure room supplies include the standard solutions and medications used in minor surgery and dressing changes. Although the solutions and medications listed here are basic, every healthcare facility has preferred items and methods of applying them. The medical assistant is responsible for their care and for maintaining up-to-date supplies.

Sterile water is kept in two forms. Multiple-dose or single-use vials are used as a **diluent** for medications. Larger containers of sterile water are for irrigating wounds or rinsing instruments that have been in a chemical disinfectant solution.

Sterile normal saline solution is also stocked in two sizes. The small vial is used for injection (e.g., 0.9% Sodium Chloride Injection USP single-dose vials, Bacteriostatic 0.9% Sodium Chloride Injection USP multiple-dose vials). A larger plastic container of sterile saline (e.g., 0.9% Sodium Chloride Irrigation USP) is used for cleaning, rinsing, and irrigating wounds. These commercially prepared products are ordered from a medical supply company.

Before surgery, the surgical site on the patient must be disinfected with an antiseptic skin cleansing preparation. This will reduce the number of **pathogens**. Although it is not possible to remove all microorganisms from the skin, using an antiseptic cleanser will remove most of the **transient** and pathogenic microorganisms; resident flora will also be reduced. Research indicates that chlorhexidine gluconate products (Hibiclens) and povidone-iodine (Betadine) are safe and effective antiseptics.

The provider's hands and those of the medical assistant should be scrubbed to reduce the chances of wound contamination, even though the hands will be covered by sterile gloves. Surgical scrub preparations should perform the following functions:

- Be effective against bacterial **spores**
- Work to reduce transient bacteria
- Show evidence of persistent activity on the skin
- Work despite the presence of organic matter, such as blood or wound drainage

Research has shown that using a hand sanitizer can be as effective as an extensive surgical scrub.

Even minor surgical procedures require the use of **anesthetics**, which either are injected locally at the site of the procedure or may be applied topically to the skin. For patients who find injections of a local anesthetic painful or traumatic, the provider may first apply a topical anesthetic. Topical anesthetics come in many forms, including sprays, gels, lotions, swabs, and foams. After the topical anesthetic has time to take effect, the provider injects the local anesthetic around the surgical area.

Another topical anesthetic is an ethyl chloride spray, a vapocoolant that controls pain associated with minor surgical procedures (e.g., lancing boils, incision, and drainage of small **abscesses**) by causing freezing of the affected area. Because ethyl chloride is highly flammable, it should never be used in the presence of electrical cauterizing equipment. In addition, petroleum jelly must be applied to the surrounding areas to protect them from the cooling action of the spray. Ethyl chloride spray has a short duration of action, so all equipment must be prepared, and the provider must be ready to perform the procedure before the spray is applied.

Local anesthetics are injected into the subcutaneous tissue. These produce a temporary numbing at the site of injection by blocking the generation and conduction of nerve impulses. Many types of local anesthetics are available, but all share the same suffix, *-caine,* such as lidocaine (Xylocaine), procaine (Novocain), chloroprocaine (Nesacaine), and bupivacaine (Sensorcaine). Local anesthetics are purchased in multiple-dose vials of 30 to 50 mL and various strengths, such as 0.5%, 1%, and 2%. They begin acting relatively quickly, within 5 to 15 minutes; the duration of action depends on the type of anesthetic, but they usually last 1 to 3 hours. When highly vascular areas are involved, local anesthetics containing epinephrine may be used. Epinephrine causes **vasoconstriction** at the site, which keeps the anesthetic in the tissues longer, prolonging its effect. It also minimizes bleeding. However, epinephrine is not used in areas where decreased circulation may cause problems with healing, such as fingertips or toes.

All tissues removed or biopsied are sent to the pathology laboratory for analysis. A 10% formalin solution is typically used to preserve excised tissue for specimens. Specimen bottles are purchased with preservatives included and should be part of the supplies prepared for a surgical procedure if a biopsy is to be done. The provider places the specimen in the container. The medical assistant is responsible for accurately labeling the container with the following information:

- Patient's name and date of birth
- Medical history number
- Date of collection
- Type of specimen

Sometimes the provider may want to use topical silver nitrate ($AgNO_3$) solution or coated applicator sticks to stop localized bleeding, such as with *epistaxis* (nosebleed) or capillary bleeding at the site of a wound. The applicators must be kept in lightproof containers. The applicator sticks are convenient for use in the mouth or nose.

Additional Surgical Supplies

- Sterilized gauze squares or strips saturated with petroleum jelly or petrolatum—used to pack wounds
- Surgical sponges—used to absorb blood and protect tissues during surgery
- Syringes and needles—used to inject local anesthetics and irrigate wounds
- Sterile dressing and bandaging materials

CRITICAL THINKING APPLICATION 24.1

Tom is ready to do an inventory of supplies in the minor surgery room. What solutions, medications, and miscellaneous supplies should he make sure are on hand for the busy surgical schedule planned for next week?

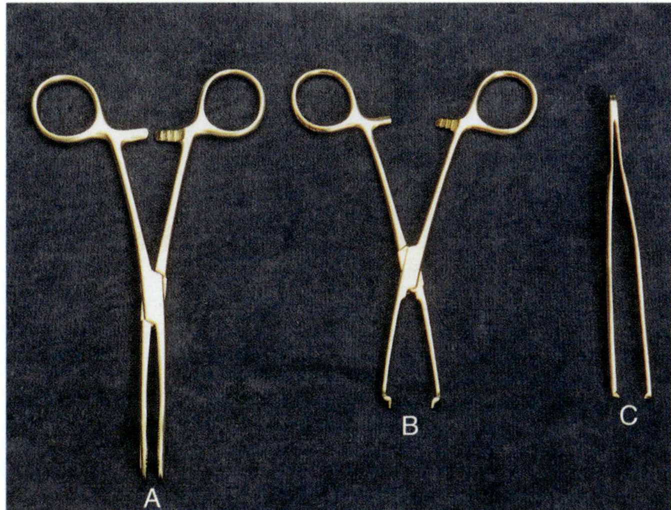

FIGURE 24.2 **(A)** and **(B)** Ring-handle forceps. **(C)** Spring-handle thumb forceps.

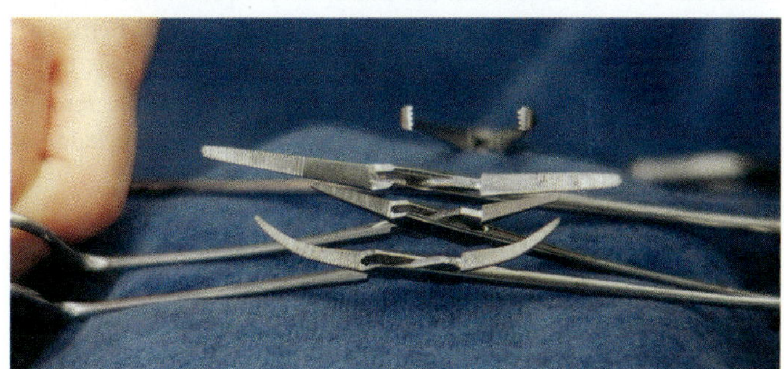

FIGURE 24.3 Instruments with serrations.

SURGICAL INSTRUMENTS

The medical assistant must know which instruments are used for each procedure and should be able to identify and understand the function of the surgical instruments that the provider prefers. Instruments have clearly identifiable parts and can be visually differentiated from one another. The basic components are the handle, the closing mechanism, and the part that comes in contact with the patient, commonly called the *jaws.* Many instruments can have either straight or curved tips, depending on the operator's preference and the task to be performed.

Instruments have either ring handles (finger rings) (Figure 24.2A–B) or spring handles (Figure 24.2C)*;* these sometimes are called *thumb-handled* or *thumb grasp* instruments. Scissors are an example of a ring-handled instrument; forceps (tweezers) have spring handles. Some instruments have a hinge-type mechanism called a *box lock.*

Ratchets resemble gears and are located just below or next to the ring handle (see Figure 24.2A–B). They are used to lock an instrument into position. Most ratchets can be closed at three or more positions, depending on the thickness of the tissue or materials being grasped.

The inner surfaces of the jaws on some instruments have ridged teeth, called *serrations*; both ring-handled and thumb-type instruments may have them. These serrations may be crisscross, horizontal, or lengthwise (Figure 24.3). Serrations prevent small blood vessels and tissue from slipping out of the jaws of the instrument.

Instrument tips or jaws may be plain tipped or toothed (Figure 24.4A–B). Tissue forceps usually are toothed instruments and are identified by the number of intermeshing teeth (e.g., 1 × 2, 2 × 3, 3 × 4). Allis tissue forceps (Figure 24.4C) are used to grasp delicate, soft tissues, so the teeth are finer, shallower, and more rounded. Other forceps have teeth that are sharper and deeper. Still, others have sharp, hooklike, single or double teeth, such as a tenaculum (see Figure 24.12C). Toothed instruments commonly have ratchets for locking into towels or human tissues. Instrument tips may be either straight or curved, depending on their use.

An instrument can be named for its use (e.g., splinter forceps, for removing splinters) or after the person or people who developed it (e.g., Foerster sponge forceps). Many general instruments are identified by the part of the body on which they are used (e.g., rectal speculum and nasal speculum).

Thousands of surgical instruments have multiple names. The same instrument may have two or three different names, depending on the provider identifying it or the part of the country in which the practice is located. For example, a request for a clamp or forceps might be made when the provider wants a Kelly hemostat. It is important to learn the provider's preferred terminology. Learn to recognize the distinctive parts of instruments and the reasons for each part, and you will quickly build a working knowledge of hundreds of instruments.

Classifications of Surgical Instruments

Surgical instruments are generally classified according to their use, and most belong to one of four groups:

- Cutting and dissecting
- Grasping and clamping
- Retracting
- Probing and dilating

Cutting and Dissecting Instruments

Cutting and dissecting instruments, which are used for cutting, incising, scraping, punching, and puncturing, include scissors (Table 24.1), scalpels, chisels, elevators, curettes, punches, drills, and needles. Instruments with a sharp blade or surface can cut, scrape, or **dissect** (Figures 24.5 and 24.6).

Most scalpels used in minor procedures are disposable (Figure 24.7), with different handle sizes and types of blades already attached to the handles. However, stainless steel, reusable scalpel handles can also be used. A variety of blades can be used, which must be attached to the handle using forceps and sterile technique. After the procedure, the handles are sterilized, and the blades are discarded in a sharps container. Once used, disposable scalpel/blade units are also discarded in a sharps container.

TABLE 24.1 Scissors

INSTRUMENT	DESCRIPTION
Lister bandage scissors	• Blunt probe tip • Easily inserted under bandages with relative safety • Used to remove bandages and dressings
Operating scissors	• 5 to 6 inches long • Curved or straight blade tips • Used to cut and dissect tissue
Suture scissors	• Blade has beak or hook to slide under sutures • Used to remove sutures

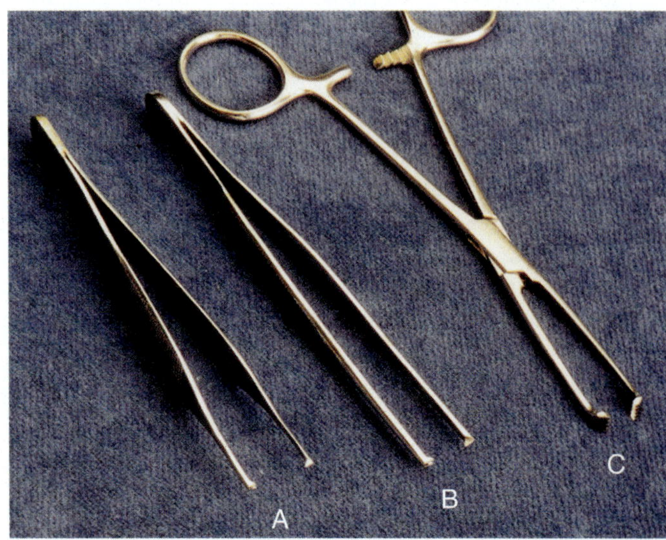

FIGURE 24.4 **(A)** and **(B)** Toothed jaws. **(C)** Teeth of Allis tissue forceps.

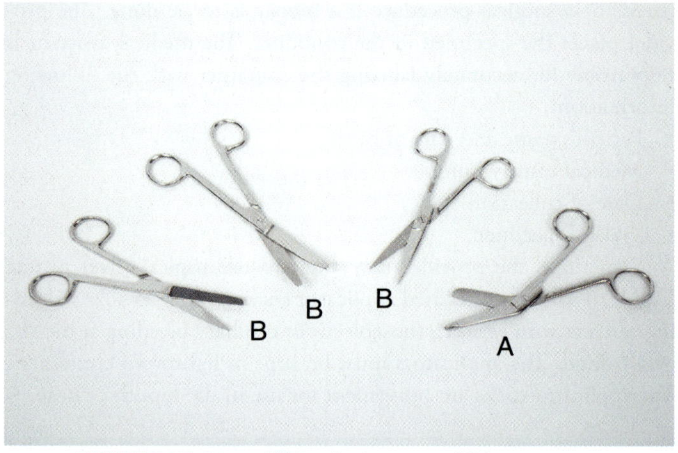

FIGURE 24.5 Scissors. **(A)** Lister bandage scissors. **(B)** Operating scissors.

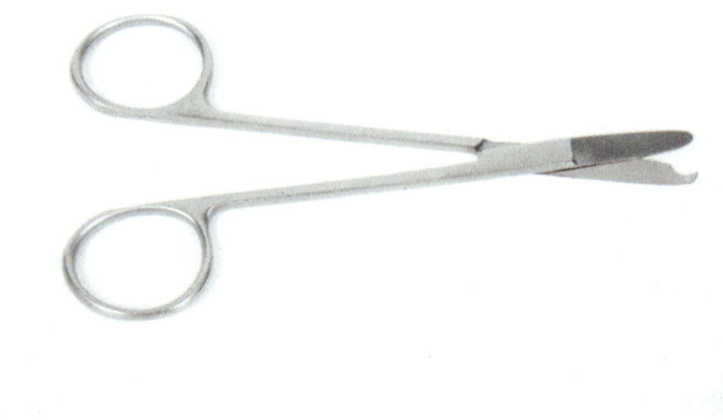

FIGURE 24.6 Suture scissors.

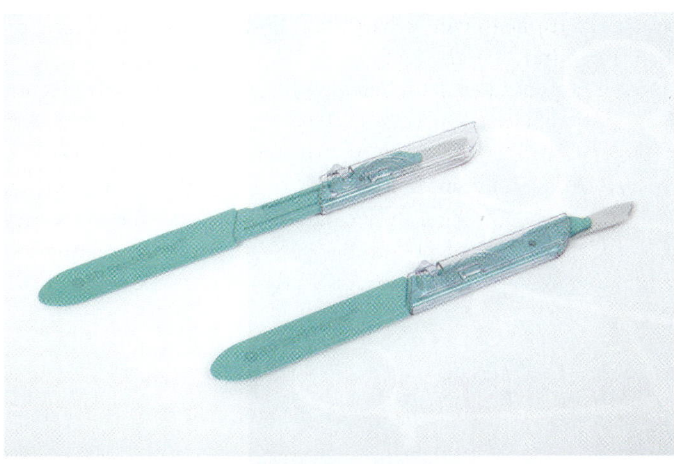

FIGURE 24.7 Disposable scalpels.

- *Handles:* No. 3 is the standard handle; No. 3L and No. 7 are used in deeper cavities.
- *Blades:* No. 15 is commonly used; Nos. 10, 11, and 12 are used for specialty incisions.

Grasping and Clamping Instruments

Clamping instruments are used for many different tasks. Many have a sharp tooth or teeth and are used to retract, hold, and manipulate fascia. The most common clamping instruments are hemostats, which originally were designed to stop bleeding or to clamp severed blood vessels. Some clamping instruments are used to grasp other instruments or sterilized materials. Sometimes hemostats and other clamping instruments are used interchangeably. Table 24.2 lists the most common grasping and clamping instruments (Figures 24.8 to 24.12).

TABLE 24.2 Grasping and Clamping Instruments

INSTRUMENT	DESCRIPTION
Hemostatic forceps	• Jaws may be fully or partly serrated, without teeth • May be curved or straight • Used to clamp small vessels or hold tissue • Mosquito forceps (4 inches) are smaller and used for very small vessels • Kelly forceps (6 to 7 inches) are larger
Needle holder	• 4 to 7 inches long • Jaws are shorter and stronger than hemostat jaws • Jaws may be serrated or may have a groove in the center • Used to grasp a suture needle firmly
Splinter forceps	• Design and construction vary • Fine tip for foreign object retrieval
Plain thumb (dressing) forceps	• Manufactured in lengths from 4 to 12 inches • Varying types of serrated jaws but no teeth • Used to insert packing into or remove objects from deep cavities
Towel clamp	• Various lengths from 3 to 6½ inches • May have sharp or atraumatic (dull-edged) tips • Used to hold drapes in place during surgery
Allis tissue forceps	• Available in different lengths and jaw widths • Used to grasp tissue, muscle, or skin surrounding a wound
Toothed tissue forceps	• Manufactured in 4- to 18-inch lengths • Pincher grip • Used to grasp tissue, muscle, or skin surrounding a wound
Foerster sponge forceps	• Used to hold gauze squares to sponge the surgical site • Used as transfer forceps to arrange items on a sterile tray • Straight or curved, with or without serrations
Bozeman sponge forceps	• Designed to hold sponges or dressings • Capable of reaching the cervix through the vagina • Used to swab the area or apply medication
Tenaculum forceps	• Very sharp, pointed tips • Used to hold tissue (e.g., the cervix) while a tissue specimen is obtained or to lift the cervix so that the **fornix** can be seen

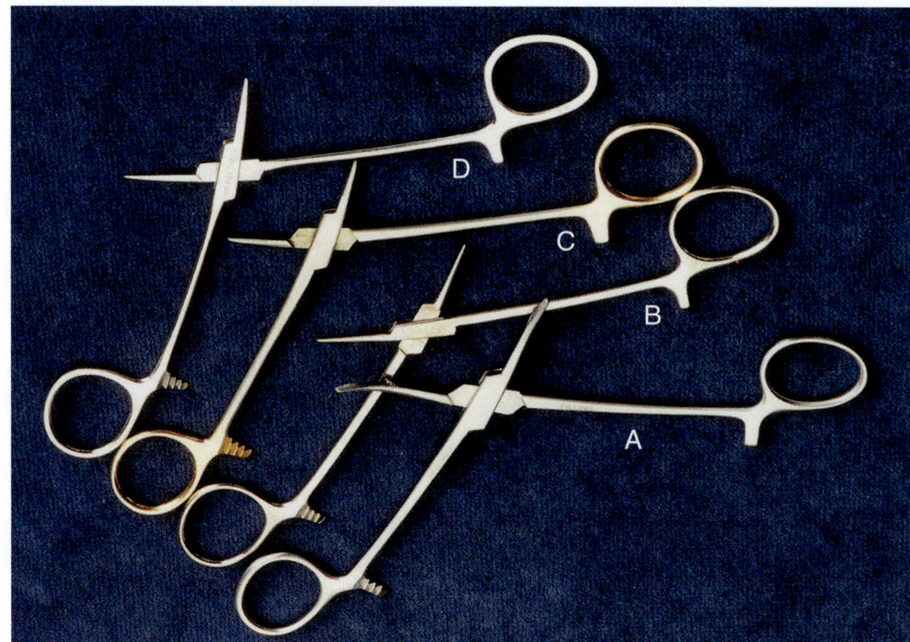

FIGURE 24.8 **(A)** Kelly hemostatic forceps. **(B)** Mosquito hemostatic forceps. **(C)** Needle holder. **(D)** Smooth-tip needle holder.

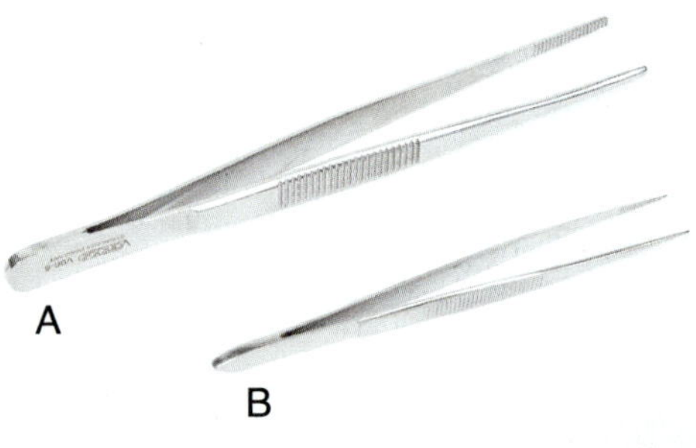

FIGURE 24.9 **(A)** Plain-thumb (dressing) forceps. **(B)** Splinter forceps.

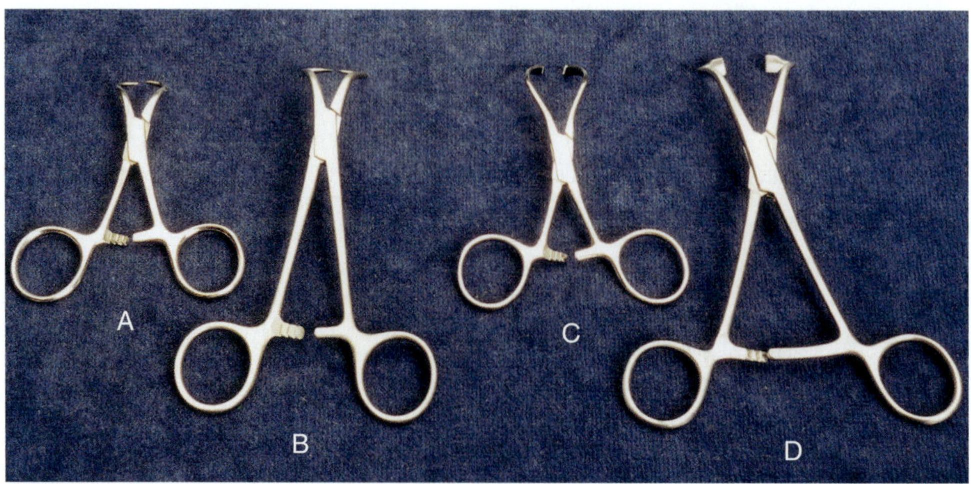

FIGURE 24.10 **(A)** Small sharp towel forceps. **(B)** Large sharp towel forceps. **(C)** Small atraumatic towel forceps. **(D)** Large atraumatic towel forceps.

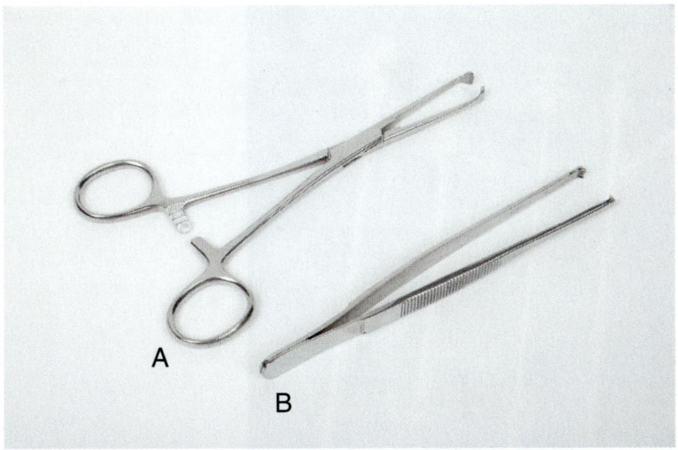

FIGURE 24.11 **(A)** Allis tissue forceps. **(B)** Toothed tissue forceps.

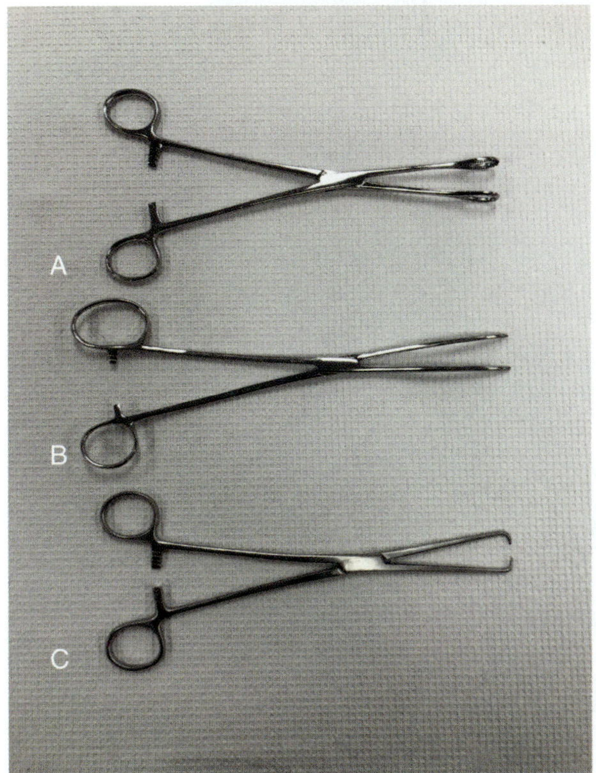

FIGURE 24.12 **(A)** Foerster sponge forceps. **(B)** Bozeman sponge forceps. **(C)** Tenaculum forceps.

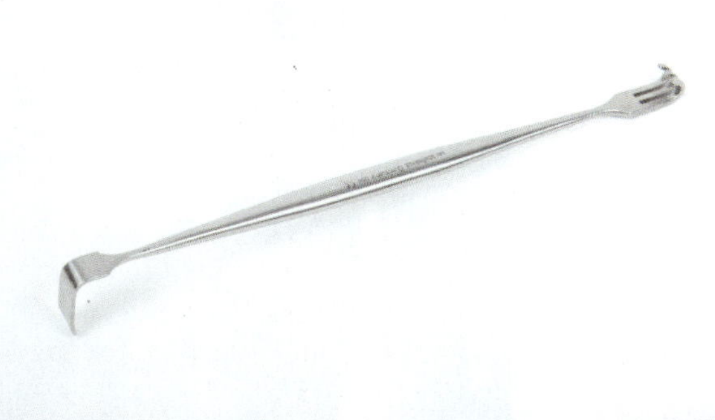

FIGURE 24.13 Senn retractor.

TABLE 24.3 Probes and Dilators

INSTRUMENT	DESCRIPTION
Probes	• Lengths range from 4 to 12 inches; available with or without bulbous tip • May be smooth or may have a grooved director • Used to find foreign bodies embedded in dermal tissue or muscle or to trace a wound tract
Trocars and **obturators**	• Available in various sizes • Consist of a sharply pointed **stylus** (obturator) contained in a **cannula** • Used to withdraw fluids from cavities or for draining and irrigating with a catheter
Specula	• Most common dilator used • Valves are spread apart, dilating the opening • Used to open or distend a body orifice or cavity • The most common of these is the vaginal speculum used during gynecologic examinations (see Figure 24.16C); vaginal specula can be stainless steel (reusable) or plastic (disposable) and can also have a light source for illumination

Retractors

Retracting instruments hold tissue away from the surgical wound (incision). Depending on the provider's preference, handheld skin hooks and Senn retractors (Figure 24.13*)* are used to retract during most minor surgical procedures. They have the following characteristics:

- The flat end is a blunt retractor.
- The three-prong end may be sharp or dull.
- They are used to retract small incisions or secure a skin edge for suturing.

Probes and Dilators

Probes and dilators are used both for surgery and for examinations. Probes can be used to search for a foreign body in a wound or to enter a fistula. Dilators are used to stretch a cavity or opening for examination or before inserting another instrument to obtain a tissue specimen. Table 24.3 lists the most common probes and dilators (Figures 24.14 and 24.15).

Specialty Instruments

Although all instruments fall into the same four categories as the surgical instruments just discussed, the following instruments are organized into specialty groupings. Presenting the instruments in this manner makes it easy to see how they relate to particular examinations. In addition to recognizing the name and use of each instrument, the medical assistant must organize and set out the instruments needed for each particular examination in what is called a *tray setup*.

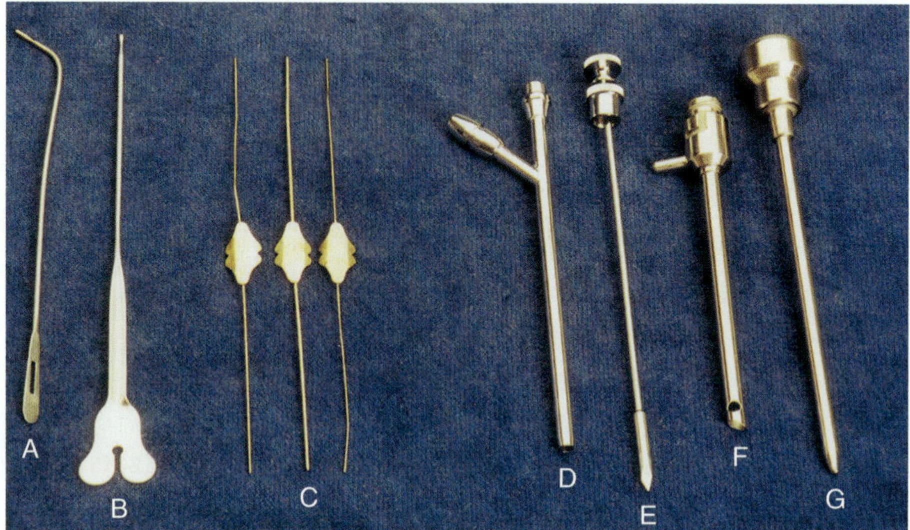

FIGURE 24.14 **(A)** Probe. **(B)** Grooved dilator. **(C)** Lacrimal duct probes. **(D)** Double-ended cannula. **(E)** Sharp trocar. **(F)** Canula. **(G)** Blunt-tip obturator.

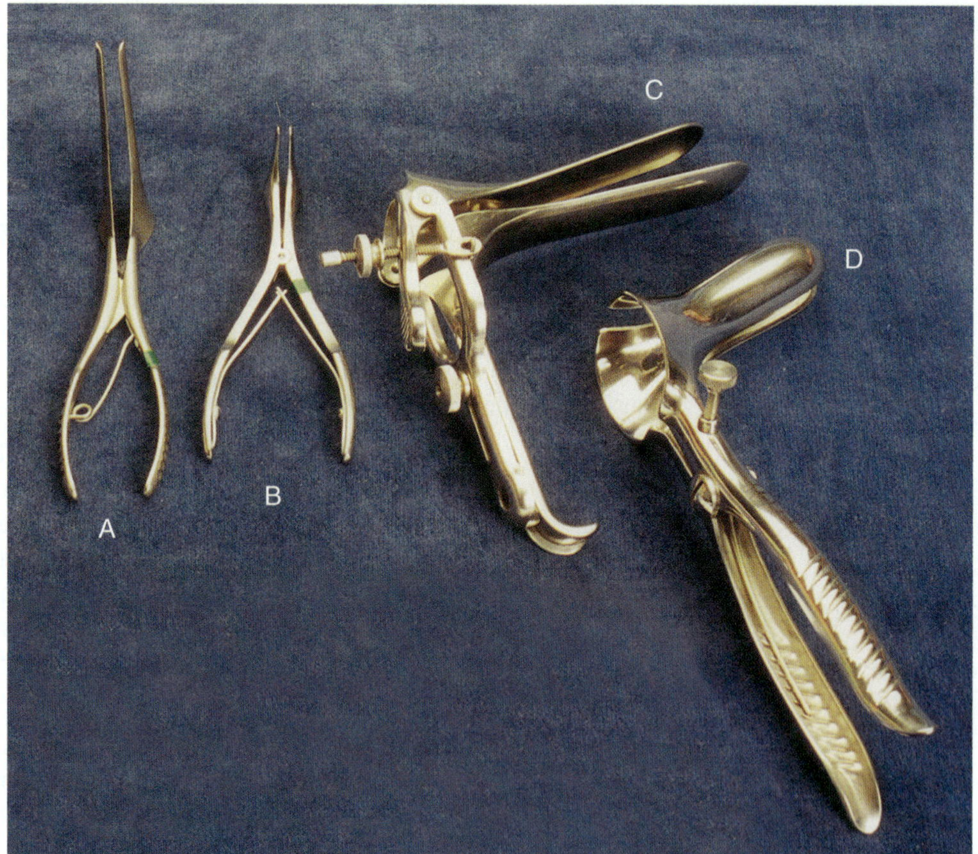

FIGURE 24.15 **(A)** Long nasal speculum. **(B)** Short nasal speculum. **(C)** Graves vaginal speculum. **(D)** Anal speculum, self-retaining.

Gynecologic Instruments

Table 24.4 describes the common gynecologic instruments used in an office setting (Figures 24.16 and 24.17).

Ophthalmologic and Otolaryngologic Instruments

Table 24.5 describes the common ophthalmologic and otolaryngologic instruments used in an office setting (Figures 24.18 and 24.19).

Biopsy Instruments

Table 24.6 describes the common biopsy instruments used in an office setting (Figure 24.20).

Genitourinary Instruments

Table 24.7 describes the common genitourinary instruments used in an office setting (Figure 24.21).

TABLE 24.4 Gynecologic Instruments

INSTRUMENT	DESCRIPTION
Placenta forceps	• Used to remove tissue from the uterus
Endocervical curette	• Smaller than the uterine curette • Used in the same way as the uterine curette
Uterine curette	• Available in several sizes • Hollow and spoon shaped; used for scraping • Used to remove polyps, secretions, and bits of placental tissue
Schroeder uterine vulsellum forceps	• Very sharp, pointed tips • Used to hold tissue (e.g., the cervix) while a tissue specimen is obtained or to lift the cervix so that the fornix can be seen
Hegar uterine dilators	• Available in sets • Double or single ended • Used to dilate the cervix for **dilation** and **curettage**
Uterine sounds	• Used to check the **patency** of the cervical os or the urethral meatus

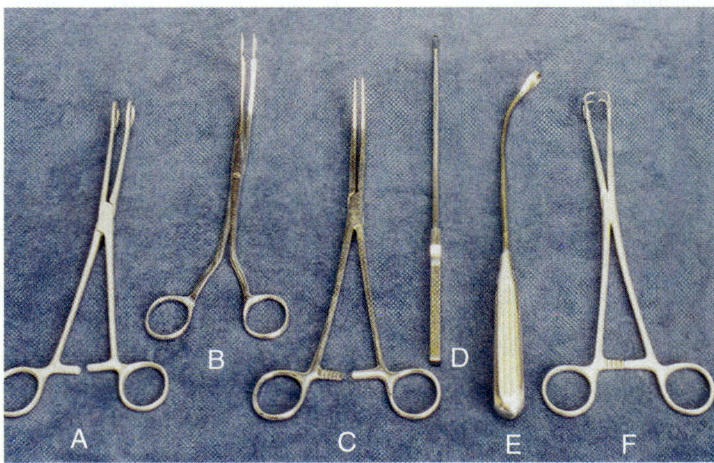

FIGURE 24.16 **(A)** Foerster sponge forceps. **(B)** Placenta forceps. **(C)** Bozeman uterine dressing forceps. **(D)** Endocervical curette. **(E)** Uterine curette. **(F)** Schroeder uterine vulsellum forceps.

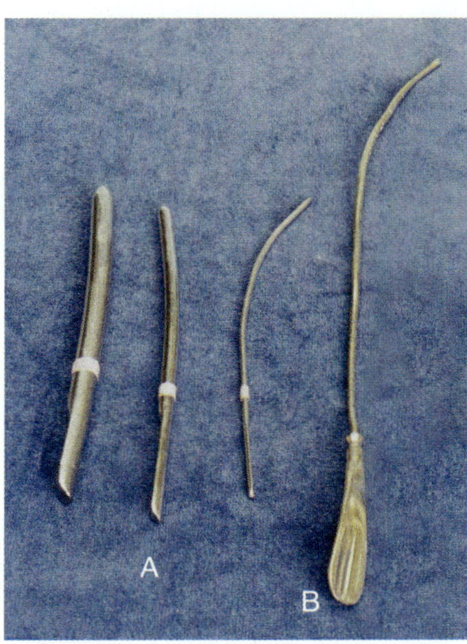

FIGURE 24.17 **(A)** Uterine dilators. **(B)** Uterine sounds.

DRAPES, SUTURES, AND OTHER CLOSURE MATERIAL

Drapes are used during a minor surgical procedure for a variety of reasons. They can provide a sterile field around the surgical site and also provide modesty for the patient. Sutures and other closure materials are used when a surgical incision or other wound needs to be closed. The following sections \ discuss drapes and closure materials.

Drapes

Disposable surgical drapes are available in several materials and sizes. These typically have an opening (*fenestrated*) for the operative site (Figure 24.22). The drape is placed over the operative area using sterile technique after the patient's skin preparation has been completed. If a fenestrated drape is not available, multiple nonfenestrated drapes can be used to create a sterile field around the surgical site.

Sutures

The word *suture* is used as both a noun and a verb. As a noun, it refers to a surgical stitch or the material used to close a wound. As a verb,

TABLE 24.5 Ophthalmologic and Otolaryngologic Instruments

INSTRUMENT	DESCRIPTION
Krause nasal snare	• Wire loop at the tip that can be tightened • Used to remove polyps from the nares
Metal tongue depressor	• Used to depress the tongue for oral examinations
Hartmann "alligator" ear forceps	• 3-inch shaft; made in a variety of styles • Action of the jaw similar to that of an alligator's jaws • Used to remove foreign bodies or polyps
Laryngeal mirror	• Made in various sizes • May have a nonfogging surface • Used for examination of the larynx and postnasal area
Ivan laryngeal metal applicator	• 6 to 9 inches long with curved end for use in throat or postnasal areas • Holds cotton in place with its roughened end; used to swab or sponge throat or postnasal tissue • Used to remove foreign bodies embedded in the pharynx
"Buck" ear curette	• Manufactured in various sizes • Available as disposable curettes in many different sizes • Has a stainless steel loop at the end • Made with sharp or blunt scraper ends • Used to remove foreign matter from the ear canals
Sharp ear dissector	• Used to remove debris from the ear canal
Wilde ear forceps	• Angled, with serrated tips • Provides easier access to the ear canal and nasal cavities • Used for packing after ear or nasal procedures • Can be used to remove foreign bodies

it refers to the act of stitching. The primary purpose of a suture is to hold the edges of a wound together until natural healing occurs.

A suture may also be used as a *ligature.* This is a strand of suture material used to tie off a blood vessel or strangulate tissue. If a ligature is used to tie off an internal tubular structure, it must last permanently or long enough for the structure itself to disintegrate. The ideal suture material has certain characteristics:

- Easy to handle and makes a secure knot
- Does not cause a localized tissue reaction and is nonallergenic
- Has adequate strength without cutting through tissue
- Can be sterilized

The provider will request a certain type of suture based on the specific properties of the suture material, such as rate of absorption, size of the suture, and type of needle. Both natural and synthetic suture materials are available. Sutures may be classified as either absorbable or nonabsorbable. Many suture materials are available, each having its advantages and disadvantages. Suture materials commonly used in minor surgical procedures are described in the following paragraphs (Figure 24.23).

Absorbable Sutures

Absorbable sutures are dissolved by the body's enzymes during the healing process. They are used when deep incisions or lacerations require inner layers of sutures to close the wound. Absorbable suture material is also used in areas where suture removal is difficult (e.g., oral surgery). Catgut (sheep, cattle, or pig intestine) was once the absorbable suture material of choice, but it has largely been replaced in recent years by synthetic absorbable suture material (e.g., Vicryl). Other synthetic absorbable suture materials include Dexon, polydioxanone (PDS), and Maxon. These materials remain stable longer than natural catgut (up to 11 weeks), allowing the wound to completely heal before absorption occurs.

Nonabsorbable Sutures

Nonabsorbable suture material is left in place until healing is complete. It frequently is used in minor surgical procedures performed in the medical office because most of the suturing required is superficial. It can be used in areas where sutures can be easily removed after healing has taken place. Silk is a common nonabsorbable suture material because it is strong and easy to tie. It is treated with a coating to prevent tissue drag and flaking. Polyester fiber sutures (e.g., Dacron and Prolene) are among the strongest nonabsorbable sutures, along with surgical steel. These fine filaments are braided and have great strength. Nylon suture is strong and has a high degree of elasticity. It is used primarily for skin closure. Due to its elasticity and stiffness, many knots must be used because they tend to untie if placed incorrectly.

Suture Sizing and Packaging

Suture material is available in a variety of diameters and lengths. The diameter of the suture strand determines its size; the smaller gauges are numbered below 0 (pronounced *aught*), and the larger gauges are identified with numbers above 0. For instance, 2-0 suture is thinner than size 0, which is thinner than size 2. The sizes from 6-0 to 2-0 are used most frequently in the medical office. The length of the suture material may vary, with strands precut in 18-, 24-, 54-, and 60-inch lengths.

Suture Sizes[a]

SUTURE SIZE	DIAMETER
6-0	0.07 mm
5-0	0.10 mm
4-0	0.15 mm
3-0	0.20 mm
2-0	0.30 mm
0	0.35 mm
1	0.40 mm
2	0.50 mm

[a] Sutures are sized according to the US Pharmacopoeia (USP) scale.

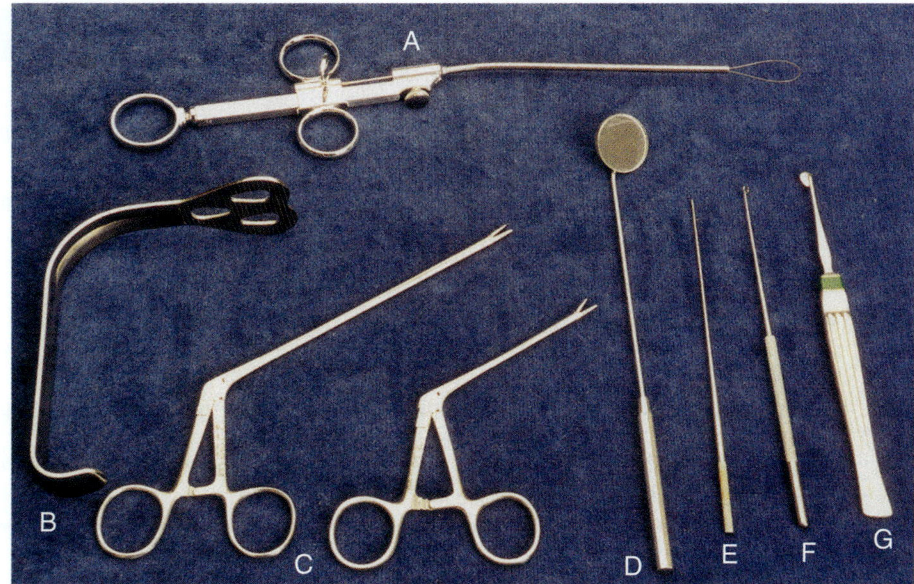

FIGURE 24.18 **(A)** Krause nasal snare. **(B)** Metal tongue depressor. **(C)** Long and short alligator forceps. **(D)** Laryngeal mirror. **(E)** Ivan metal applicator. **(F)** "Buck" ear curette. **(G)** Sharp ear dissector.

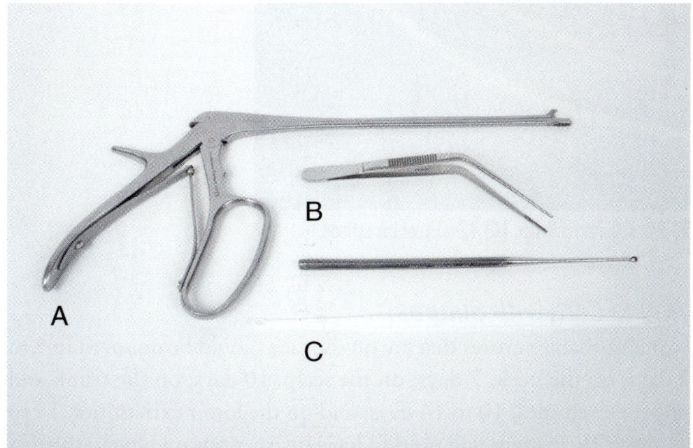

FIGURE 24.19 **(A)** Rectal biopsy punch. **(B)** Wilde ear forceps. **(C)** Ear curette.

TABLE 24.6 Biopsy Instruments

INSTRUMENT	DESCRIPTION
Cervical biopsy forceps	• Available with or without teeth • Used to obtain cervical specimens for diagnostic examination
Rectal biopsy punch	• Available in different lengths and styles • Manufactured with interchangeable stems • Used through a proctoscope or sigmoidoscope
Silverman biopsy needle	• Manufactured with a split cannula • Stylus is removed, and cannula is inserted to retrieve the specimen • Needle biopsy can eliminate the need for surgical incision

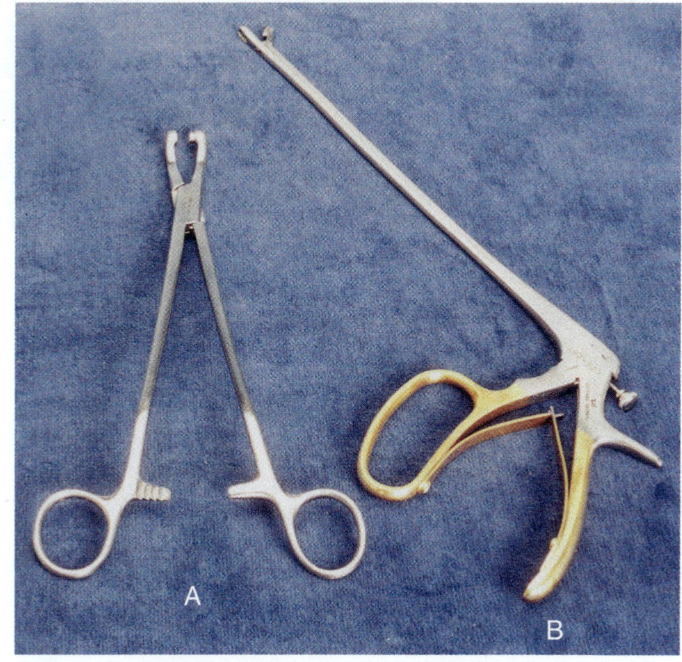

FIGURE 24.20 **(A)** Cervical biopsy forceps. **(B)** Rectal biopsy punch.

Needles. Surgical needles are chosen according to the area in which they are to be used and the depth and width of the desired suture. They are classified according to shape, which may be straight or curved. Most sutures are applied with curved needles because they allow the provider to penetrate the surface and then come up on the other side. The sharper the curve of the needle, the deeper the provider can pass it into the tissue. The point of a needle can be a taper or a cutting edge. A taper is used on delicate tissues. The cutting-edge needle is used on the skin. It lacerates the skin as the needle is passed through. This is advantageous for tougher tissues, such as connective tissue.

TABLE 24.7 Genitourinary Instruments

INSTRUMENT	DESCRIPTION
Foley catheter with inflated balloon	• Manufactured in sizes 8 to 32 French with a double rubber lining toward the tip (each French unit is equal to 1.32 mm; the higher the number, the larger the lumen) • After insertion, sterile solution is injected into the inner lining (inflating the balloon) to hold it in the bladder • Used as an indwelling catheter
Red Robinson catheter	• Soft rubber urethral catheter in sizes 8 to 32 French • Inserted temporarily into the bladder for drainage or to obtain a specimen
Coudé-tip catheter	• Slightly curved catheter tip • Designed to allow it to navigate past obstructions in the urinary tract, such as a swollen prostate in men
12-mL Luer-Lok syringe	• Typically used to inject sterile saline into a catheter to inflate the balloon at the tip of an indwelling catheter • Used for injecting amounts greater than 5 mL

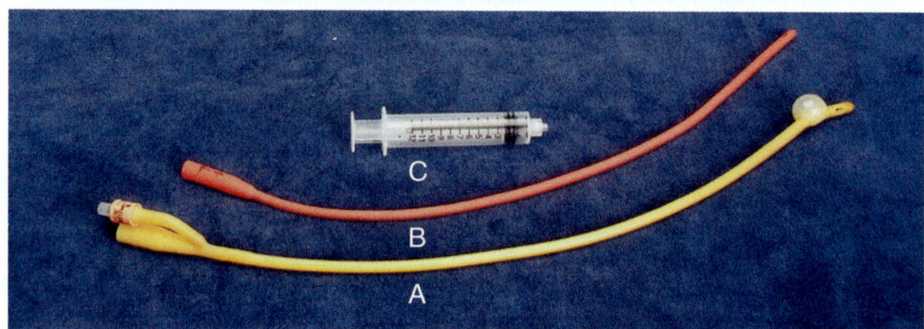

FIGURE 24.21 **(A)** Foley catheter with inflated balloon. **(B)** Red Robinson catheter. **(C)** 12-mL Luer-Lok syringe.

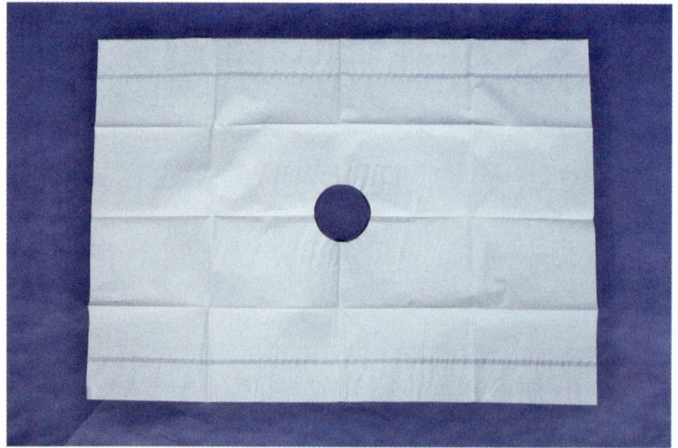

FIGURE 24.22 Fenestrated drape.

Needles are manufactured with the suture material attached, or *swaged,* to the needle. These atraumatic needles do not have an eyelet and cause the least amount of trauma as they are passed through the tissue. Manufacturers package suture strands with the suture needle attached in peel-apart sterile, disposable packages. These may be obtained as single, individually packed, or multipack sutures in a variety of needle types and sizes with a wide range of suture materials and lengths. The most common needle type for minor skin repair is the curved, cutting-edge, swaged needle (Figure 24.24).

Wound Care with Sutures

Nonabsorbable sutures that are on the face should be removed in 5 to 7 days, on the neck, 7 days; on the scalp, 10 days; on the trunk and upper extremities, 10 to 14 days; and on the lower extremities, 14 to 21 days. The patient will need to have instructions on how to care for the site while the sutures are still in place. Those instructions should include the following guidelines:

- Keep the area clean and dry for the first 24 to 48 hours after the sutures have been placed.
- After 24 to 48 hours, gently wash around the site one to two times daily with cool water and soap. Do not wash or rub the sutures directly.
- Dab the site dry. Do not rub the area, and avoid using the towel directly on the stitches.
- If there was a bandage, replace it with a new clean bandage and antibiotic ointment if instructed to do so.
- Return for suture removal as directed by the provider.

Other Closure Materials

Surgical staples can also be used for skin closure. They are made of stainless steel or titanium and are available in different sizes. Surgical staples usually remain in place for 7 to 14 days. They are applied (Figure 24.25) and removed (Figure 24.26) with specific staple instruments. Care for a surgical site closed with surgical staples is the same as the care for a site closed with sutures.

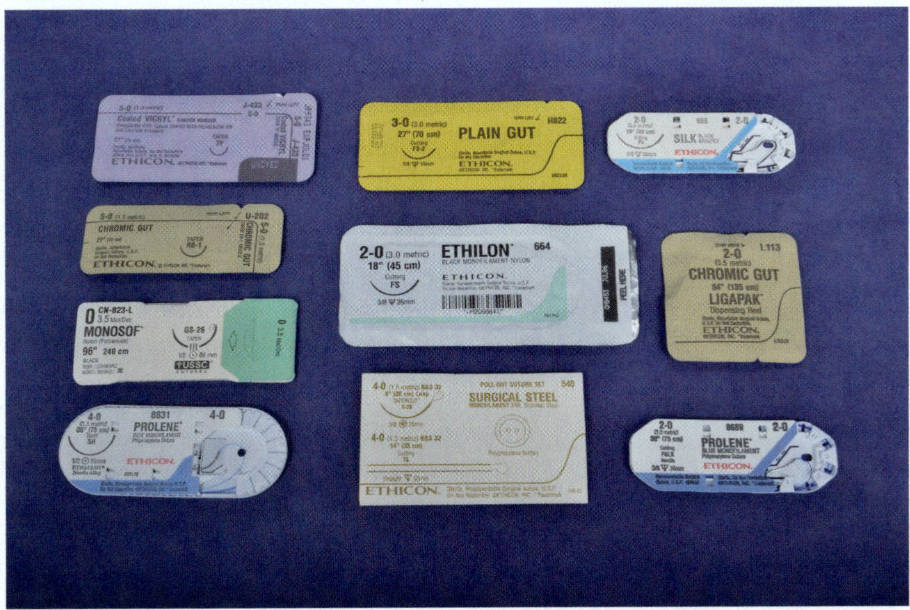

FIGURE 24.23 Suture packets labeled according to size, type, length, and type of needle point and shape.

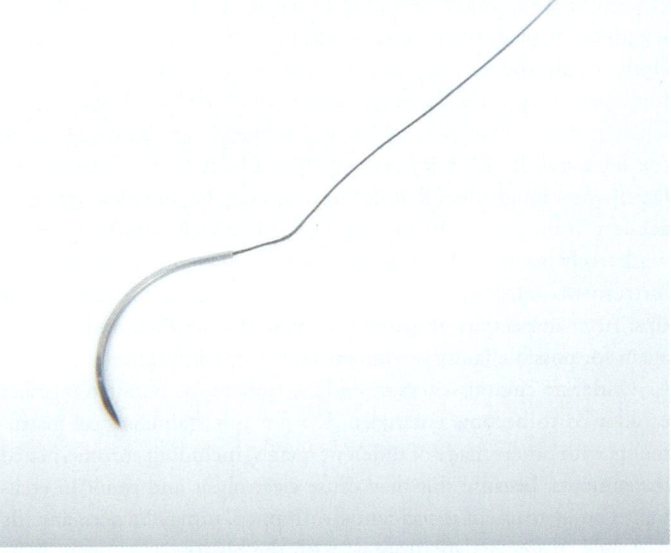

FIGURE 24.24 Swaged suture needle.

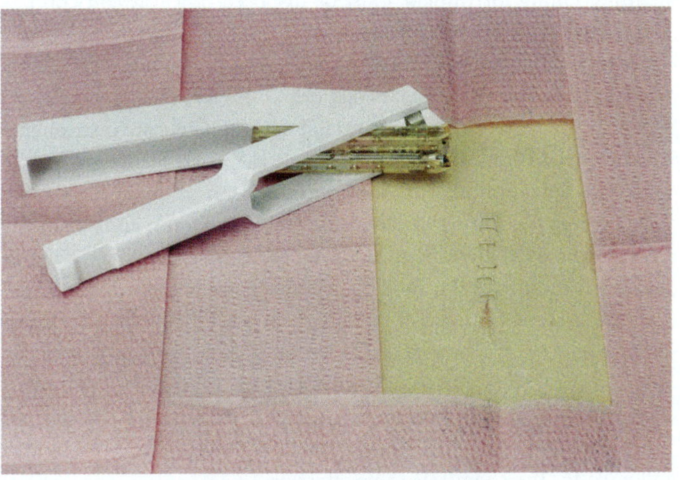

FIGURE 24.25 Disposable skin stapler.

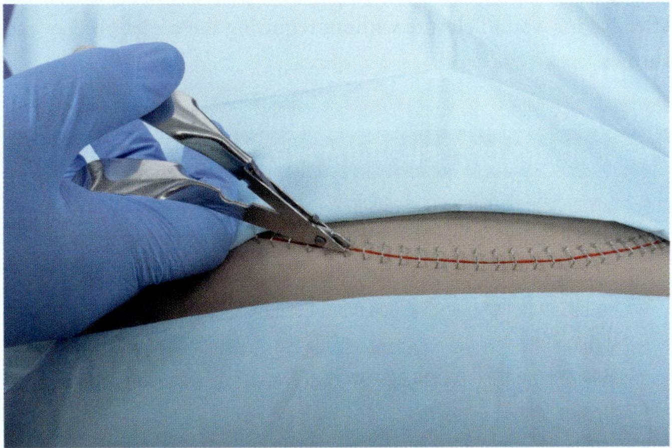

FIGURE 24.26 Surgical staple remover.

Another technique for wound closure is the use of adhesive skin closure strips, which are self-adhesive tapes that are placed over the wound, pulling the wound edges together. Using a tincture of benzoin prior to the application of adhesive skin closure strips can help them remain in place longer. A tincture of benzoin is applied parallel to the edges of the wound. Care should be taken so that it does not go into the wound because it can cause burning pain. The compound becomes tacky, and the adhesive skin strips stay on longer. Adhesive skin strips can be used to support a wound if there is potential tension at the site or for superficial wounds. Frequently, small, clean lacerations may be closed with adhesive skin strips (Figure 24.27). These strips reduce the chance of infection and do not leave suture scars. Adhesive skin strips are used on areas of the body that are protected from movement and stress. They often are used on the face. A medical assistant can place adhesive skin strips as ordered by the provider. They are placed on the wound in the same sequence and at the same intervals as interrupted sutures and are left in place until they fall off or the wound heals. The patient can wash or shower with them in place but should take care to pat dry with a clean towel instead of rubbing.

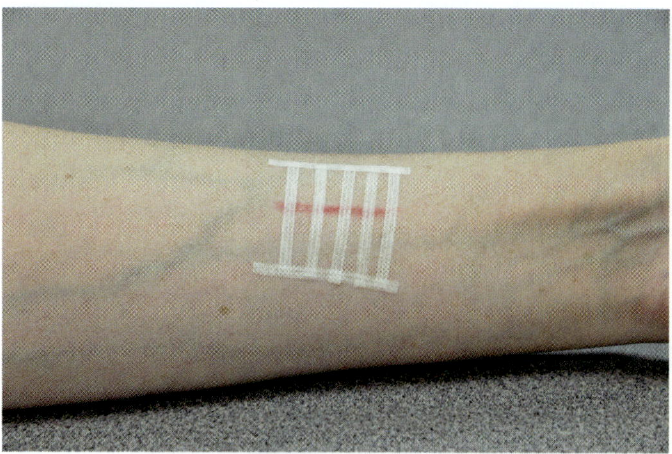

FIGURE 24.27 Wound closed with adhesive skin closures.

Tissue adhesives, similar to glue, can also be used for superficial wounds. Examples of tissue adhesives are Histoacryl, Dermabond, and SurgiSeal. Tissue adhesives form a strong bond across wound edges, allowing normal healing to occur below. Skin adhesives are also an alternative to sutures. They are frequently used for the closure of facial lacerations, especially in pediatric patients, because they are effective for wound closure without requiring the use of needles and sutures.

Advantages of Tissue Adhesive

- Saves time during wound repair
- Creates a flexible, water-resistant protective coating for the wound
- Eliminates the need for suture removal
- Results in better cosmetic outcomes because there is no scarring from suture entry
- May also be used on larger wounds for which subcutaneous sutures are needed
- Especially helpful for use on pediatric patients or individuals who are afraid of needles

SURGICAL ASEPSIS AND PREPARATION OF SURGICAL INSTRUMENTS

Asepsis is the condition of being free of **infection** or infectious material. *Medical asepsis* is the reduction of microorganisms and the prevention of the transfer of microorganisms. This creates an environment that is clean but not *sterile* (i.e., free of microorganisms). The principles of medical asepsis are implemented to prevent reinfection of a patient and cross-infection of another patient or medical personnel. To prevent cross-contamination, potential microorganisms and pathogens must be isolated by following standard blood and body fluid precautions and by sanitizing, disinfecting, or sterilizing objects as soon as possible after they become contaminated.

Surgical asepsis is the complete destruction of microorganisms. This technique is mandatory for any procedure that invades the body's skin or tissues, such as surgery. In surgical asepsis, everything that comes in contact with the surgical site must be sterile, including surgical gowns, drapes, instruments, and the gloved hands of the surgeon and surgical assistants. Any time the skin or a mucous membrane is punctured or pierced, as in venipunctures or injections, surgical aseptic techniques must be practiced. Urinary catheterizations, biopsies, and dressing changes on open wounds are performed using sterile technique. The next section discusses how to prepare instruments to be used in surgically aseptic procedures.

Care and Handling of Instruments

Because instruments are expensive, and the success of the procedure depends on their quality, the medical assistant must properly care for each instrument to maximize its life and ensure that every part is in safe working order.

Instruments that are not disposable are made of fine-grade stainless steel. The term *stainless* usually is taken too literally. Although stainless steel does resist rust and keeps a fine edge and tip longer, even the best stainless steel may develop water spots and stains. Proper hardness and flexibility are important. Inexpensive instruments that are chrome plated may be too brittle or too soft. In addition, mistreatment of chrome-plated instruments can cause tiny breaks in the finish that may become a source of contamination or may tear the provider's gloves.

All instruments should be carefully examined when they are purchased. Scissors should be tested to see whether they shear the full length of the blades completely to the tip. If the scissors cut a piece of cloth cleanly and do not chew at any point, even at the tip, they are functioning correctly. Teeth and serrations should be checked to see whether they intermesh completely and whether the jaws are even on the sides and tip. Each instrument should be felt over its entire surface for any rough areas that may tear or snag the provider's gloves or act as a future source of contamination. Box locks and hinges must work freely but should not be too loose. Thumb- and spring-handled instruments must have the correct tension and meet evenly at the tips. After inspection, instruments should be sanitized and checked again for possible faulty workmanship before sterilization.

Under no circumstances should instruments be bundled together or allowed to become entangled. Do not mix stainless steel instruments with others made of different metals, including chrome-plated instruments, because this may cause electrolysis and result in etching. If an instrument is accidentally dropped, it may be permanently damaged. If scissors are dropped with the blades partly open, there may be a nick at the point where the blades cross. Any damaged or malfunctioning instrument must be disposed of to prevent complications during a surgical procedure.

After a surgical procedure, contaminated instruments should be placed in a basin of disinfectant solution. Heavier instruments should be on the bottom of the basin and lighter, more delicate instruments on top. Always unlock each instrument before immersing it in the chemical decontaminant to permit sanitization of the entire surface area. Never allow blood or other substances to dry on an instrument because they will be difficult to remove. If immediate sanitization and disinfection are not possible, the instruments should be rinsed well and placed in a cold-water solution with a blood solvent and mild detergent. It is best to use a detergent with a neutral pH, is low sudsing, and can be rinsed off easily. The manufacturer's recommendations for the correct dilution and time of immersion of the various sanitizing agents, disinfectants, and blood solvents must be strictly followed for the chemicals to be effective.

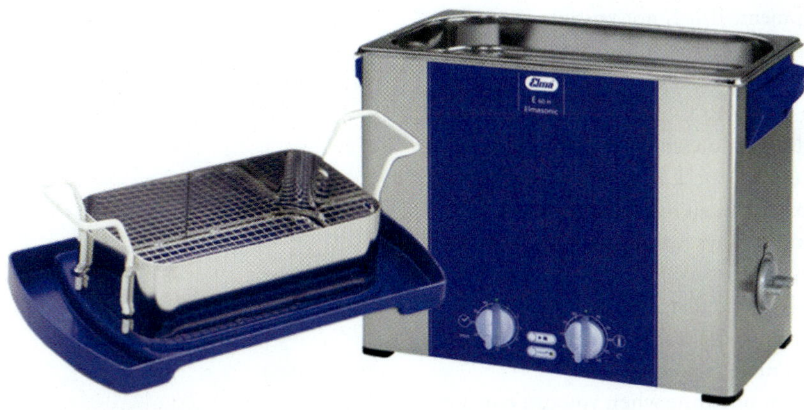

FIGURE 24.28 Elmasonic E ultrasonic cleaner unit. (Courtesy Tovatech, South Orange, NJ.)

When the surgical procedure is completed, the receiving basin for instruments should be transferred from the surgical area to the disinfection and sterilization room. It is important to remove used instruments from the patient's view as soon as possible. After sanitization is complete, instruments should be rinsed thoroughly and either washed by hand or washed mechanically using an ultrasonic device. Some delicate instruments, such as microsurgical and lensed instruments, should be washed by hand with a mild, low-sudsing, neutral-pH detergent solution and a soft brush.

All instruments should be cleaned while submerged to prevent the airborne spread of microorganisms. Throughout the sanitization process, the medical assistant should wear heavy utility gloves to prevent possible exposure to contaminants. Some clinical policies require the medical assistant to wear disposable gloves under utility gloves for added protection from contaminants. Instruments then should be rinsed, dried with a lint-free cloth, and inspected for proper functioning before they are packed for sterilization.

Mechanical washing, such as with an ultrasonic device, can be used for most instruments and is an especially good method for sanitizing sharp instruments to prevent injuries (Figure 24.28). In an ultrasonic cleaning unit, the instruments are immersed in a cleaning solution, and the device produces sound waves that clean contaminants from the instruments' surfaces. Some units then rinse and dry the instruments, leaving them ready for the sterilization process. However, manufacturers' guidelines should be followed for rubber and plastic materials.

After sanitization and inspection, the instruments are ready for the sterilization process. Commercially prepared, disposable packs are available for most minor surgical procedures. They save time and eliminate the need for sanitization, disinfection, and sterilization of reusable stainless-steel instruments, but they may also be too costly for individual practices.

CRITICAL THINKING APPLICATION **24.2**

Tom is preparing instruments and supply packs for specific procedures performed by Dr. Martin. One of the packs he is preparing for the autoclave is for removal of a nasal polyp. Based on your understanding of typical and specialty instruments and supplies, what items should Tom include in the instrument pack?

Sterilization

Before an instrument or piece of equipment can be used in a surgical procedure, it must first be sanitized and then sterilized to remove all forms of microorganisms. It is essential that you understand the concepts of sanitization and disinfection before learning sterilization methods. Written sanitization, disinfection, and sterilization procedures should be in place for each workplace.

Utility Room

An area should be set aside to ensure proper sterilization for surgical aseptic procedures. The area should be divided into two sections, one dirty and one clean. The dirty section is used for receiving contaminated instruments and other materials at the end of surgical procedures. This area should have a sink, receiving basins, proper sanitizing and disinfecting agents, brushes, utility gloves, autoclave wrapping paper or cloth, autoclave envelopes and tape, sterilizer indicators, and gloves. Designated biohazard waste containers are needed for gloves worn when handling contaminated items. Personal protective equipment (PPE) for sanitization, disinfection, and autoclave procedures includes the following:

- Fluid-resistant gloves to prevent contact with contaminants
- A laboratory coat or impervious gown, if needed, to protect against splashes
- A face shield or goggles if a splash hazard exists
- Heat-resistant autoclave gloves for unloading

The clean section of the utility room should be reserved for receiving the sterile items after they have been removed from the autoclave. Clear, clean plastic bags in which to store sterile packs may be kept in the clean area. Both areas should be spotless and well organized.

Instruments and other items used in ambulatory surgery, examination, or treatment must be carefully cleaned before proceeding with the steps of disinfection or sterilization. *Sanitization* is the cleansing process that removes organic material and reduces the number of microorganisms to a safe level. This cleansing process removes debris, such as blood and other body fluids, from instruments or equipment. Sanitization should be completed immediately after instruments are used. This should occur in a separate workroom or area or on the "dirty" side of the utility room to prevent cross-contamination of clean instruments and equipment. If it is not possible to sanitize instruments immediately after a procedure, they should be rinsed under cold water immediately and placed in a low-sudsing, rust-inhibiting, enzyme-containing detergent solution. Blood and debris must be removed so that later disinfection with chemicals or sterilization can penetrate all the instruments' surfaces. Never allow blood or other substances to coagulate or dry on an instrument.

The medical assistant should always wear utility gloves while performing sanitization to prevent possible personal contamination with potentially infectious body fluids that may be present. When you are ready to sanitize instruments, drain the soaking solution and rinse each instrument in cold, running water.

Clean all sharp instruments at one time when you can concentrate on preventing injury to yourself. Open all hinges and scrub serrations and ratchets with a small scrub brush or toothbrush. Rinse the instruments in hot water, and then carefully check that they are in proper working order before they are disinfected or sterilized. Generally, these instruments are left out to air dry, but they may be hand dried with a microfiber towel to prevent spotting. Follow facility policy as to how instruments should be dried.

Disinfection is the process of killing pathogenic organisms or rendering them inactive. Many types of disinfecting agents are available, and they have varying degrees of effectiveness. It is important to follow the manufacturer's guidelines on how to use each product properly and understand its advantages and disadvantages and possible sources of error. Disinfectants are used on equipment that cannot be sterilized (e.g., blood pressure cuffs and stethoscopes), on countertops and other physical surfaces in the healthcare facility, and for soaking instruments and equipment before sterilization. It is important to wear proper protective equipment when using disinfectants because they are generally strong enough to damage human tissue and will often leave burns if allowed prolonged contact with the skin.

CRITICAL THINKING APPLICATION **24.3**

The office manager tells Tom he needs to review the office policy and procedures manual on sanitization, disinfection, and sterilization methods. Why is this important to accomplish before Tom starts performing sterilization procedures? What information in this manual would be most important to Tom as he starts this new position? Why?

Autoclave

Sterilization can be achieved with moist heat, dry heat, ultraviolet or ionizing radiation, gas, or chemicals. Medical facilities typically use the autoclave method, which uses moist heat and pressure to achieve sterilization. Steam under pressure in the autoclave (Figure 24.29) is an excellent method of sterilization because it kills all pathogens and spores.

Pressurized steam is fast, convenient, and dependable. The pressure allows for heat higher than the boiling point. Steam from a pot of boiling water on a stove is about 212°F (100°C). We know that spores can survive temperatures of up to 240°F (115°C) for 4 hours. In an autoclave, the steam is contained within a chamber and is under

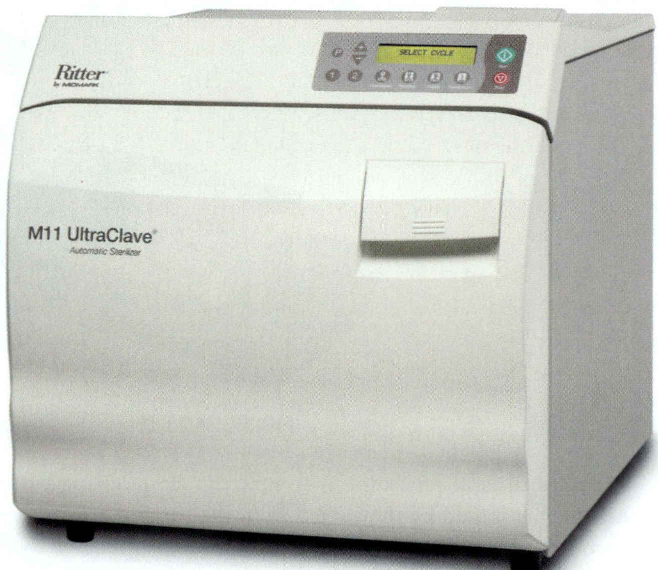

FIGURE 24.29 Steam autoclave. (Courtesy Midmark Corp., Dayton, OH.)

15 pounds per square inch (psi) of pressure. This pressure allows the steam to reach 250°F (121°C). No organism can last at that temperature for more than 15 minutes. When steam enters the autoclave chamber, it simultaneously heats and wets the object, coagulating the proteins present in all living organisms. When the cycle is complete and the chamber has cooled, the steam condenses and explodes the cells of microorganisms, thus destroying them. The steam moisture must come in contact with all surfaces being sterilized to be effective. Steam under pressure is capable of much faster penetration of fabrics and textiles than dry heat, but its use has definite limitations if the proper techniques are not followed.

The recommended temperature for sterilization in an autoclave is 250° to 255°F (121° to 123°C). Follow the guidelines that come with the autoclave; in general, unwrapped items are sterilized for 20 minutes, small wrapped items for 30 minutes, and large or tightly wrapped items for 40 minutes. Processing time starts *after* the autoclave reaches normal operating conditions of 250°F (121°C) and 15 pounds per square inch (psi) pressure. There are different autoclave cycles for different materials; ambulatory care facilities do not autoclave liquids or dressing material, so the most used cycle will be the gravity cycle, which is used to sterilize stainless steel instruments. In the *gravity ("fast exhaust") cycle,* the autoclave fills with steam and is held at a set temperature for a set period. When the cycle is complete, a valve opens, and the chamber rapidly returns to atmospheric pressure. Drying time may be added to the end of the cycle.

Incorrect operation of an autoclave may result in superheated steam. If steam is brought to too high a temperature, it is literally dried out, and the advantage of a higher heat is diminished. Wet steam is another cause of incomplete sterilization. Wet steam results from failing to preheat the chamber, which causes excessive condensation in the interior of the chamber. Condensation is necessary, but too much prevents the sterilization process from being completed properly. It can be compared with taking a hot shower in a cold bathroom, which results in heavily steamed mirrors, walls, and towels. If packs become too saturated to dry during the drying cycle, they pick up and absorb bacteria from the air or any surface on which they are placed after removal from the autoclave. Placing cold instruments in a hot chamber also increases condensation. Other causes of wet steam include opening the door too wide at the end of the cycle or allowing a rush of cold air into the chamber. Overfilling the water reservoir may produce this same effect (Table 24.8).

The main cause of incomplete sterilization in the autoclave is the presence of residual air. Without the complete elimination of air, an adequately high temperature cannot be reached. Air and steam do not mix. Because air is heavier than steam, it pools wherever possible. One-tenth of 1% (0.1%) of residual air trapped around an instrument prevents complete sterilization. This is especially dangerous in older autoclaves that do not have a chamber thermometer separate from the pressure gauge. Adequate chamber pressure does not guarantee a proper chamber temperature. Table 24.9 provides tips for improving autoclave techniques.

Wrapping Materials. Maintaining the sterility of the autoclaved package depends completely on the wrapper and method of wrapping (Procedure 24.1). The wrapping material must be **permeable** to steam but **impervious** to contaminants. Acceptable wrapping materials for autoclaving should allow the steam to penetrate and prevent pathogens from entering during storage and handling. A wrapper should not be used if it is torn or has a hole in it.

The types of wrapping material used for instruments that are to be autoclaved are disposable double-ply autoclave paper and peel-apart polypropylene bags (Figure 24.30). Multiple layers of autoclave paper are recommended to maintain the integrity of

TABLE 24.8 Common Factors Influencing the Effectiveness of Sterilization

CAUSES	POTENTIAL PROBLEM
Improper sanitization of instruments	Protein and salt debris may prevent direct contact with pressurized steam and heat in the autoclave.
Improper packaging	Prevents penetration of the sterilizing agent; packing material may melt.
Wrong packaging material for the method of sterilization Excessive packaging material	Reduces penetration of the steam and heat.
Improper loading of the sterilizer Overloading	Increases heat-up time and decreases penetration of pressurized steam and heat to the center of the sterilizer load.
No separation between packages, even without overloading	May prevent or reduce thorough contact of the sterilizing agent with all the items in the chamber.
Improper timing and temperature Incorrect operation of the sterilizer	Insufficient time at proper temperature to kill organisms.

Adapted from The Centers for Disease Control and Prevention (CDC): Infection Control, hwww.cdc.gov/infectioncontrol/guidelines/disinfection/sterilization/sterilizing-practices.html.

TABLE 24.9 Tips for Improving Autoclave Techniques

PROBLEM	CAUSES	CORRECTION
Damp autoclave paper	Clogged chamber drain; items removed from chamber too soon after cycle; improper loading	Remove strainer; free openings of lint. Allow items to remain in sterilizer an additional 15 min with door slightly open. Place packs on edge; arrange for least possible resistance to flow of steam and air.
Stained autoclave paper	Dirty chamber	Clean chamber with mild detergent solution; never use strong abrasives, such as steel wool; rinse thoroughly after cleaning.
Corroded instruments	Poor sanitization; residual soil; exposure to hard chemicals (e.g., iodine, salt, and acids); inferior instruments	Improve sanitization process; do not allow soil to dry on instruments—sanitize first. Do not expose instruments to hard chemicals; if exposure occurs, rinse immediately. Use only top-quality instruments.
Spotted or stained instruments	Mineral deposits on instruments; residual detergents from cleaning; mineral deposits from tap water	Wash with soft soap and detergent with good wetting properties. Rinse instruments thoroughly with distilled water.
Instruments with soft hinges or joints	Corrosion or soil in joint; instrument parts out of alignment	Clean with warm, weak acid solutions (e.g., 10% nitric acid solution); rinse thoroughly. Have instrument realigned by qualified instrument repair professional.
Steam leakage	Worn gasket; door closed improperly	Replace gasket; reopen door and shut carefully; have serviced if unable to close door properly.
Chamber door does not open	Vacuum in chamber (check chamber pressure gauge)	Turn on controls to start steam pressure; wait until equalized, then vent and open door.

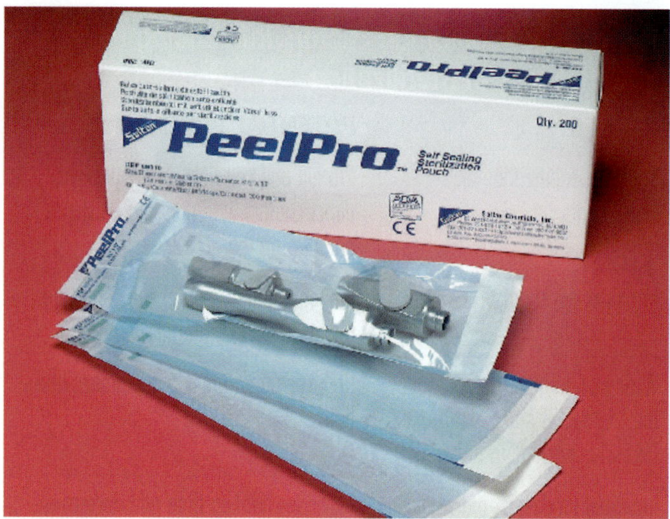

FIGURE 24.30 Sterilization pouches with sterilization indicators on the outside and inside of the envelope. The puncture-resistant, tinted plastic front is safety sealed to an autoclave paper backing. (Courtesy Practicon Dental, Greenville, NC.)

sterilization during handling and storage of autoclaved instrument packs. Double-layered autoclave paper provides multiple layers of protection; this shields surgical instruments from contamination and saves time because wrapping is done only once.

CRITICAL THINKING APPLICATION **24.4**

Tom is processing instruments and trays when he notices that one of his co-workers never places gauze squares around the tips of sharp instruments before wrapping a pack. He also notices that not all of the packs are labeled properly. What is the significance of Tom's observation? How should he handle this situation? Why?

Wrapping Instruments. The method used to wrap instruments for autoclave sterilization must allow the pack to be opened without becoming contaminated. The rules for protecting package contents include the following:

- Discard autoclave paper that is torn or has holes.
- Wrap all hinged instruments in the open position to allow full steam penetration of the joint.
- Place a gauze square around the tips of sharp instruments to prevent them from piercing the wrapping material.
- If a number of instruments are to be placed on a stainless-steel tray for wrapping, first, place a double-folded towel on the tray, and then position the instruments. This helps to protect them.
- Polypropylene is a plastic capable of withstanding autoclaving, but it is resistant to heat transfer. Therefore, materials in a polypropylene pan take longer to autoclave than the same materials in a stainless-steel pan.
- When using sterilizing bags, insert the handles of the instruments into the end of the bag to be opened first to ensure that the grasping end of the instrument can be reached easily when the bag is opened.
- When using two-ply autoclave paper, use specialized autoclave tape to seal the package.

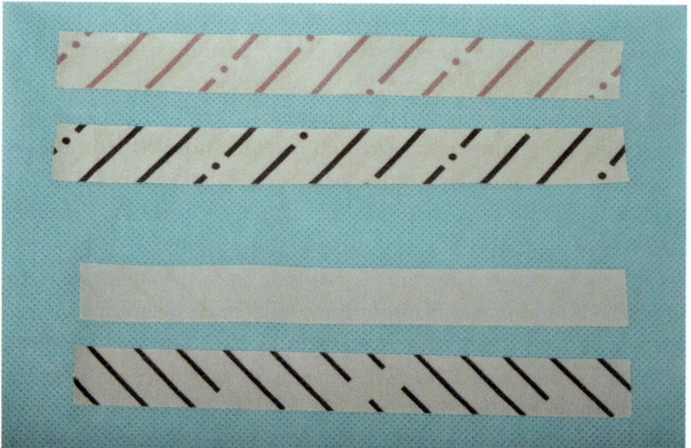

FIGURE 24.31 Autoclave tape.

- Label each pack according to the instrument contents and sterilization date, and write your initials. Use a permanent marker; never use a ballpoint pen.

Whether you are wrapping one item or many items together on a tray as a surgical pack, the procedure is the same; be sure the wrapper is large enough to cover the items to be sterilized.

Sterilization Indicators. Sterilization is achieved only when steam reaches the optimum temperature for a designated length of time and has penetrated to the center of the articles. Sterilization indicators must be used routinely to determine whether all microorganisms have been destroyed. The two basic types of sterilization indicators are chemical indicators (e.g., autoclave tape) and biological indicators.

Autoclave tape, a commonly used sterilization indicator, contains a chemical dye that changes color when exposed to steam (Figure 24.31). The tape is not an absolute indication that the proper sterilization time, temperature, and steam have been maintained. It merely indicates that a high temperature was reached while the article was in the autoclave. The tape strip must completely change color (colors vary by manufacturer) or reveal the word *autoclaved* to show effective operation. The main function of autoclave tape, besides holding the wrapping material together, is to verify at a glance that the package was autoclaved. Other chemical indicators are placed inside the instrument packages to verify steam and heat penetration of the wrapping. Some instruments are autoclaved unwrapped, such as stainless-steel vaginal specula. A chemical indicator should be placed in the autoclave with unwrapped instruments in an area most difficult for steam to access, such as under the tray or between the instruments.

The healthcare facility should have a policy for how frequently the autoclave is tested using biologic sterilization indicators. The Centers for Disease Control and Prevention (CDC) recommends that this procedure should be performed weekly. Spore strip indicators have been replaced by rapid-readout biologic indicators that use ampules of *Bacillus stearothermophilus,* which are destroyed at 250°F (121°C). The ampule is placed in the center of the largest pack that is autoclaved in the facility to determine the accuracy of the autoclave and autoclave procedures in destroying all microbes. On completion of the cycle, the ampule is sent to a laboratory for analysis of any type of microbial growth. If tests show that microbes are present in the sample, then a report is sent to the facility notifying it that the autoclave, or possibly its sterilization procedures, are not effective in achieving sterilization. Results from the biologic indicator testing must be documented. Failed tests must be investigated and the causes resolved.

Quality Assurance Records for Office Sterilization. Every office should have specific protocols for quality assurance evaluations of the autoclave, including regular maintenance. This is done at specified intervals, depending on the volume and frequency of autoclave use. A log must be kept of the type of control test done, when it was performed, and the testing results. If the testing results indicate that sterilization was inadequate, a report must be made and filed. The report should identify the nature of the problem and how and when it was corrected. The report also should contain proof of correction by indicating the date and time of a first, subsequent, and successful sterilization run.

Loading the Autoclave. Prepare all packs and arrange the load in a way that allows maximum circulation of steam and heat (Procedure 24.2). Articles should be resting on their edges and should not be crowded. Placing the packs in stainless steel racks prevents the packing of the autoclave too tightly. Instruments may be autoclaved unwrapped if they do not need to be sterile when used later. For example, although vaginal specula do not need to be sterilized for use (the vagina is a body cavity that is naturally open to the external environment), they must be sanitized and sterilized to prevent cross-contamination among patients. They can be placed unwrapped on a perforated stainless-steel tray in the autoclave and then stored in a clean area for future use.

Unloading Guidelines. When the autoclave's sterilization cycle is complete, the pressure should be released according to the manufacturer's guidelines. Once the pressure gauge reads "0," the medical assistant should stand behind the door and, with heat-resistant gloves, open the door approximately one-quarter of an inch. Allow the load to dry for at least 15 minutes (this time varies according to the type of autoclave and the size of the load). Packs can act as a sponge, attracting outside moisture and microorganisms. Touching a wet pack allows microorganisms on your hands to penetrate the wrappings, making the contents of the pack nonsterile. Dry, wrapped packs may be removed with clean, dry hands, but it is safer to wear heat-resistant gloves to reduce the possibility of burns from the hot instruments inside the packs. If possible, allow all packs to cool in the autoclave with the door open. Place the packs on a dry, dust-free surface inside an enclosed cupboard or drawer for storage. Do not place the packs on cold surfaces because hot packs may cause condensation, and moisture will contaminate the contents.

Guidelines for Unloading an Autoclave

- Stand behind the door when opening it to prevent accidental steam burns.
- Slowly open the door only a crack, allowing the items to cool for 15 to 20 minutes before removing them.
- If for any reason the integrity of the sterilization process is in question, the load should be considered contaminated and autoclaved again. Reasons for concern include the following:
  - If a load fails to convert a sterilization indicator strip (autoclave tape), this indicates that the autoclave is not working properly.
  - If loads were processed after a biologic test, this indicates that the autoclave is not working properly.

Shelf Life of Sterilized Packs. The CDC no longer identifies specific time limits for the shelf life of sterilized packs. The general recommendation is that as long as the sterilized items are stored so that the packaging material remains intact and undamaged, then the pack is considered sterile. All sterile packs should be stored on dry, dust-free, covered shelves or in drawers. Some facilities continue to date every sterilized package and use shelf-life practices, such as first in, first out; other facilities have switched to event-related practices. With event-related practices, items remain sterile until some event causes contamination (e.g., a pack becomes wet or packing material is torn). The quality of the packaging material, storage conditions, and how much the packs are handled all affect the possibility of contamination. Therefore, sterile packs should be inspected before they are used to verify the integrity of the wrapping material. Any package that is wet, torn, dropped on the floor, or damaged in any way should be sanitized, disinfected, wrapped in new autoclave paper, or placed in new autoclave pouches, and autoclaved again.

CRITICAL THINKING APPLICATION 24.5

Tom discovers a number of packages of paper-wrapped sterile instruments that appear to have water marks on them. The indicator tape shows that they have been autoclaved. What should he do with these packs? Why?

Chemical Sterilization

In the medical office, chemical sterilization is used for instruments that cannot be exposed to the high temperatures of steam sterilization. The sterilizing chemical solution must be mixed exactly according to the instructions on the bottle. The solution must be marked with the date of preparation and expiration. Materials to be sterilized must be submerged in this chemical bath with a closed lid for 8 hours or longer. Items are removed with sterile forceps and must be rinsed with water to remove all traces of the chemical before the items are used on a patient. You must avoid skin contact with the sterilizing solution because it is very **caustic**.

The use of chemicals for sterilization is not very practical in the ambulatory facility. The instruments or equipment cannot be wrapped during processing in the liquid chemical. Once they are removed from the liquid, they are no longer considered sterile. In addition, because of the caustic nature of the chemicals, instruments must be rinsed with water after removal from the chemical fluid. This water is typically not sterile. However, high-level chemical disinfectants do have a place in healthcare. They can be used on instruments (e.g., endoscopes) that would be damaged by autoclaving. Because of the limitations of using liquid chemicals for sterilization, their use should be restricted to reprocessing critical devices that are heat sensitive and incompatible with other sterilization methods.

CLOSING COMMENTS

Assisting with a minor surgical procedure can be an exciting role a medical assistant. Having an understanding of the minor surgery room, the solutions and medications used, the instruments and supplies needed, and how to maintain surgical asepsis will make you a valuable asset.

Patient Coaching

Patients may have questions about the instruments the provider will use, and the medical assistant can help allay patients' fears by answering these questions. Explaining how the patient will be prepared for the procedure, how the procedure will be performed, and what to expect afterward helps make the procedure go more smoothly and encourages the patient to follow the provider's advice and orders.

Legal and Ethical Issues

It is important for patient health that medical assistants ensure that all instruments used in procedures are sterile. The sterilization process begins with sanitization. No shortcuts should be taken when prepping instruments for sterilization. It might be easier to overlook the damaged sterilization pack but using instruments from that pack could lead to an infection, which in turn could lead to a lawsuit.

Professional Behaviors

Performing medical assistant duties responsibly and accurately is crucial in the surgical area of the ambulatory care setting. The provider relies on the medical assistant to have the appropriate supplies and instruments available before a procedure begins. To achieve this goal, the medical assistant must have a working knowledge of the typical instruments and supplies used in the facility, in addition to an understanding of the types of instruments needed for each procedure. Medical assistants must make sure tasks are completed according to the facility's policies and procedures so they are able to assist the provider and protect the patient.

SUMMARY OF SCENARIO

Tom has worked for the providers at Walden-Martin Family Medical Clinic for 2 years and is familiar with their preferences in surgical solutions, local anesthetics, and suture materials, in addition to the typical instruments used in the practice. He also has worked hard to update the policies and procedures manual to include standards for instrument care so that other medical assistants in the office will know how instruments should be sanitized, disinfected, inspected, and prepared for the autoclave. Tom realizes he needs to continue his education in surgical procedures and takes advantage of professional workshops on the topic. Tom consistently attempts to stay up to date on surgical advances and the medications and instruments used at WMFM.

SUMMARY OF LEARNING OBJECTIVES

1. **Examine the minor surgery room and the solutions and medications used for a minor surgical procedure.**
   The minor surgery room may be a separate room, or an examination room may be used. If it is a separate room, it should be near the workroom with a sink and an autoclave. This room should also contain supplies, wound care equipment, and biopsy containers. The exam table should be easy to adjust, and the room should have bright lighting.
   Solutions used in minor surgery include sterile water for mixing with medications or rinsing instruments; sterile saline for injection or wound irrigation; antiseptic skin cleansers (e.g., Hibiclens and Betadine) for site preparation; and local anesthetics, including topical applications, in addition to lidocaine, Nesacaine, or Sensorcaine injectables. These local anesthetics may come packaged with or without epinephrine. The provider also may use topical silver nitrate to control local bleeding.
2. **Differentiate the surgical instruments used in a minor surgical procedure.**
   Surgical instruments are classified according to their use as cutting, grasping, retracting, probing, or dilating tools. The components of the instruments include the type of handle, the closing mechanism, and the jaws. Instrument tips may be either straight or curved and toothed or not toothed. The instruments used in minor surgical procedures depend on the type of procedure and the provider's preference. Specialty instruments are used in specialty practices (e.g., gynecology, ophthalmology, otolaryngology) and for particular procedures (e.g., biopsies). Refer to Tables 24.1 through 24.7.
3. **Examine the drapes, sutures, and other closure material used in a minor surgical procedure.**
   Surgical drapes come in various sizes and materials. They are placed over the operative area after the skin preparation has been completed. There is typically an opening (fenestrated) for the operative site.
   Suture material is available as absorbable (for internal sutures) and nonabsorbable (for skin closure). Dexon, PDS, and Maxon are popular absorbable materials; nonabsorbable sutures can be made of silk or nylon, or staples can be used. Tissue adhesives, similar to glue, can also be used for superficial wounds. Suture materials range in size from smaller gauges (i.e., below 0 [aught] for finer tissues) to thicker gauges (above 0) and are available in various lengths. Surgical needles are either straight or curved. Most needles are manufactured with swaged suture material.
4. **Examine surgical asepsis and the preparation of surgical instruments.**
   Surgical asepsis is the complete destruction of microorganisms and is mandatory for any procedure that invades the body's skin or tissues. Anything that comes in contact with the surgical site must be sterile. Surgical asepsis is also necessary when performing venipunctures, injections, urinary catheterizations, biopsies, and dressing changes.
   Surgical instruments are expensive and must be cared for properly to maintain function and maximize durability. Instruments must be examined when purchased for proper working order and possible faults with mechanisms. Stainless steel instruments should be kept separate from other metal types. Each instrument must be cleaned according to the manufacturer's guidelines, unlocked, and disinfected immediately after use. Most instruments can be cleaned with an ultrasonic washer, which helps prevent injuries.
   After the minor surgical procedure is complete, the instruments and equipment used must be sanitized and disinfected before being sterilized. After sanitization and disinfection, the instruments must be prepared for sterilization using appropriate wrapping materials (see Procedure 24.1).
   The autoclave is the most common way of sterilizing instruments in a medical office. This process uses steam under pressure to ensure the destruction of all microorganisms. Items must be loaded and unloaded correctly to achieve and maintain sterility (see Procedure 24.2).

PROCEDURE 24.1 Wrap Instruments and Supplies for Sterilization in an Autoclave

TASK: Place dry, inspected, and sanitized supplies and instruments inside appropriate wrapping materials for sterilization and storage without contamination.

EQUIPMENT and SUPPLIES

- Dry, inspected, and sanitized instruments
- Double-ply autoclave paper
- Autoclave tape
- Sterilization strip
- Waterproof, felt-tipped pen
- Gloves (if part of office policy)

PROCEDURAL STEPS

1. Wash or sanitize your hands. Collect and assemble already inspected, sanitized instruments to be wrapped. Gloves may be worn.
2. Place the double-ply autoclave paper on a clean, flat surface.
3. Place the instruments diagonally at the approximate center of the double-ply autoclave paper. Make sure the size of the square is large enough for the items (see the following figure).
   PURPOSE: Each of the four corners must fold over and completely cover the instruments, with a few extra inches of overlap for folding.

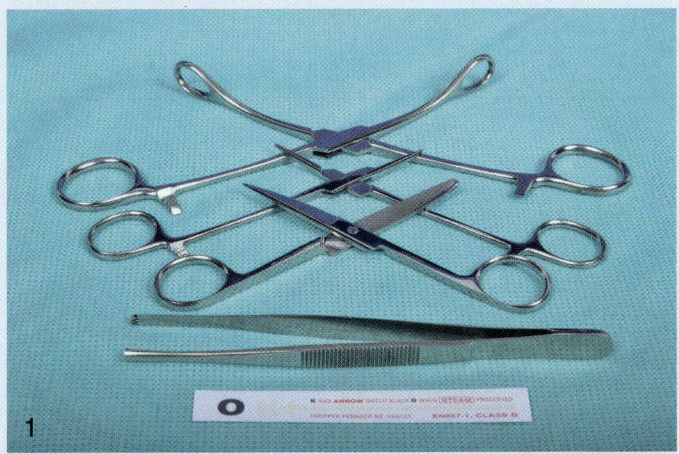

4. Open any hinged instruments. If the instrument is sharp, its teeth or tip should be shielded with cotton or gauze.
   PURPOSE: To prevent puncture of the package or injury to the operator.
5. Place a sterilization strip in the center of the pack to check for sterilization standards.
   PURPOSE: To ensure that the autoclave is reaching effective levels of heat and pressure to destroy all microorganisms.
6. Bring up the bottom corner of the wrap, and fold back a portion of it.
   PURPOSE: This folded-back flap is the only part of each wrapper corner that can be touched when a sterile package is opened (see the following figure).

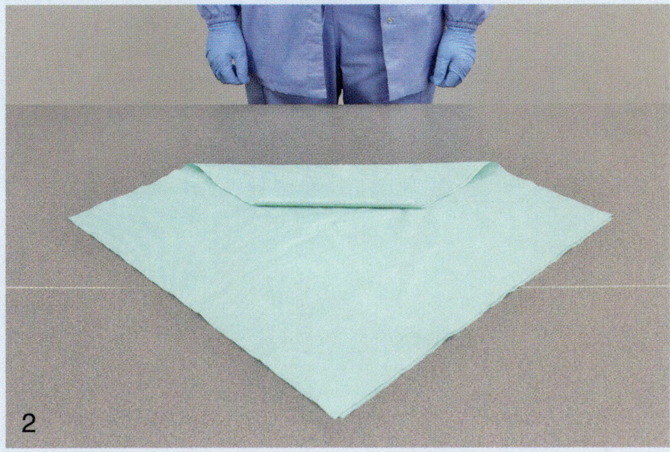

7. Repeat the previous step with each corner, making sure to turn back a portion each time (see the following figures).

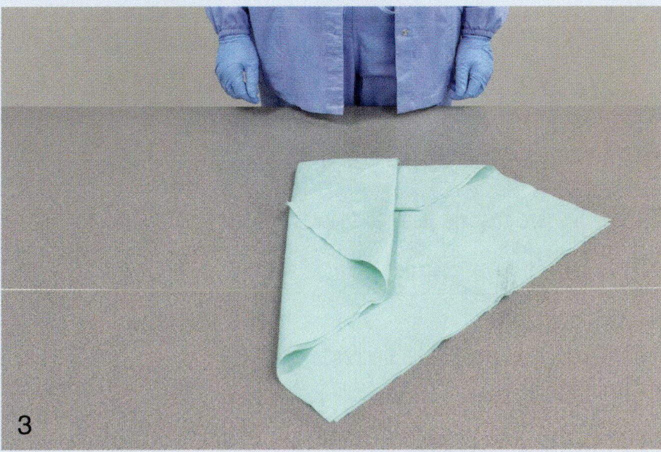

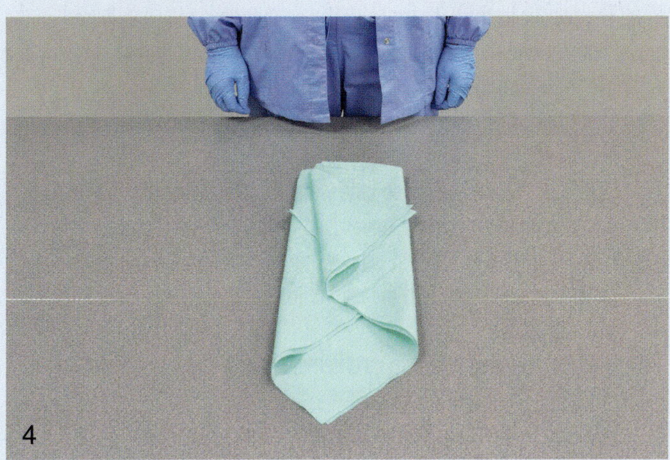

Continued

PROCEDURE 24.1 Wrap Instruments and Supplies for Sterilization in an Autoclave—*continued*

8. Fold the last flap over (see the following figure).

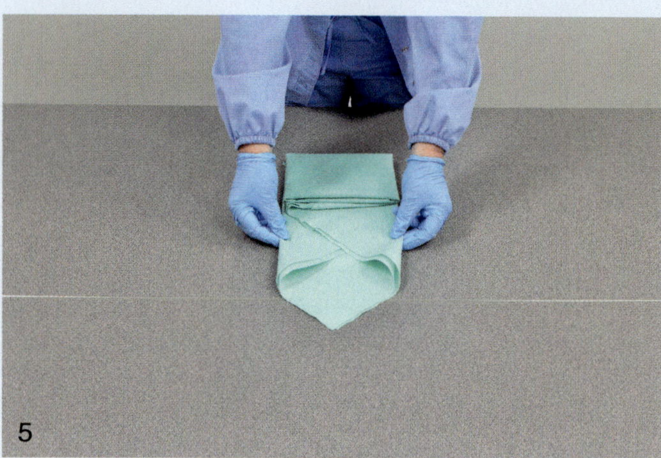

9. Secure with autoclave tape (see the following figure), and label the package with the date, including the year, contents, and your initials.
   PURPOSE: So staff members will know what is in the pack, when it was autoclaved, and who performed the task.

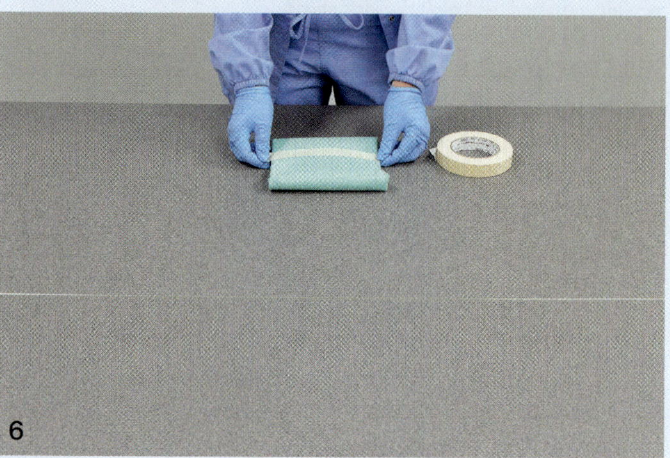

PROCEDURE 24.2 Operate the Autoclave

TASK: Sterilize properly prepared supplies and instruments using the autoclave.

EQUIPMENT and SUPPLIES

- Autoclave
- Wrapped items ready to be sterilized
- Heat-resistant gloves

PROCEDURAL STEPS

Note: The specific instructions for operating an autoclave may vary based on the model number and manufacturer. Refer to the instructions that accompany the autoclave to be sure the appropriate steps are followed.

1. Check the water level in the reservoir and add distilled water as necessary.
   PURPOSE: Too much or too little water may alter the effectiveness of the equipment. Tap water leaves lime deposits in the chamber.
2. Turn the control to "Fill" to allow water to flow into the chamber. The water flows until you turn the control to its next position. Do not let the water overflow.
3. Load the chamber with wrapped items, spacing them for maximum circulation and penetration.
   PURPOSE: To ensure sterilization of all items.
4. Close and seal the door.
   PURPOSE: The door must be closed, or the heated water in the chamber evaporates.
5. Turn the control setting to "On" or "Autoclave" to start the cycle.
6. Watch the gauges until the temperature gauge reaches at least 250°F (121°C) and the pressure gauge reaches 15 pounds.
   PURPOSE: The proper temperature and pressure must be reached before sterilization can begin.
7. Set the timer for the desired time.
8. At the end of the timed cycle, turn the control setting to "Vent."
   PURPOSE: This releases steam and pressure. The water at the bottom of the chamber drains back into the reservoir. Newer autoclaves automatically perform this step.
9. Wait for the pressure gauge to reach zero.
10. Standing behind the autoclave door, carefully open the chamber door one-quarter of an inch.
    PURPOSE: To allow steam to escape faster. Be careful to prevent accidental burns.
11. Leave the autoclave control at "Vent" to continue releasing heat.
    PURPOSE: To dry the items faster.
12. Allow complete drying of all articles.
13. Using heat-resistant gloves, remove the items from the chamber and place the sterilized packages on dry, covered shelves or open the autoclave door and allow the items to cool completely before removal and storage.
14. Turn the control knob to "Off," and keep the door slightly ajar.
    PURPOSE: To allow the inside of the autoclave to dry completely.

ASSISTING WITH SURGICAL PROCEDURES

25

SCENARIO

Callie Casper, a certified medical assistant (CMA) who has met the requirements of the American Association of Medical Assistants (AAMA), works for the Walden-Martin Family Medical (WMFM) Clinic. Callie was hired to work as an administrative medical assistant at the front desk, but one of the clinical medical assistants unexpectedly quit, and the office manager has offered Callie the position. Callie is excited about this opportunity, especially the chance to work with Dr. Angela Perez, but she is also concerned about her skill level in sterile procedures. At least she is familiar with a number of the patients, most of the staff, and the types of outpatient surgeries performed in the facility. Surgical asepsis and assisting with surgery were her favorite topics when she was in her medical assisting program. However, before she can assist with surgeries, Callie must demonstrate her ability to set up a sterile field without contaminating the site. She also must show that she can perform wound care skills, including applying sterile dressings and changing bandages.

While studying this chapter, think about the following questions:

- What are common surgical procedures performed in an ambulatory care facility?
- What is the medical assistant's role in preparing the patient, equipment, and room for a surgical procedure?
- What crucial steps must Callie follow to set up and maintain a sterile field?
- What techniques must Callie follow to prepare for and assist with a surgical procedure?
- Why is it important that Callie understand and be prepared to answer patients' questions about the process of wound healing?
- What bandaging techniques should Callie be prepared to perform?

LEARNING OBJECTIVES

1. Examine the basic types of minor surgical procedures performed in the ambulatory care setting.
2. Examine the preparation needed for surgical procedures.
3. Examine the role of the medical assistant when assisting with surgical procedures.
4. Examine the wound healing process and how wounds should be cared for.

VOCABULARY

approximated (uh PROK si may ted) Near, close together.

cicatrix (SIK uh triks) Early scar tissue that appears pale, contracted, and firm.

hemostasis (hee muh STAY sis) The stoppage of bleeding.

plume Vapor, smoke, and particle debris produced by laser procedures.

vigilance (VIJ uh lahns) Keen watchfulness to detect danger.

INTRODUCTION

Common surgical procedures that are routinely performed in the primary care facility include suturing, cyst removal, incision and drainage (I&D) of abscesses, and collection of biopsy specimens. The medical assistant should be proficient in the following skills:

- Explaining each of these procedures to the patient
- Preparing the patient and the room
- Assisting the provider with the surgery
- Applying a sterile dressing and bandage after the procedure is finished

Each surgical procedure requires appropriate skin preparation and draping with a *fenestrated* drape. This is a surgical drape with an opening in the center. The size of the opening depends on the size of the surgical field. The opening is placed directly over the surgical site after the site has been prepared (or "prepped," as it is called in healthcare practice). A minor surgery tray is opened, and a sterile field is created on a Mayo stand. Sutures, scalpels, and any other instruments needed are added to the field according to the provider's preference. An injectable or a spray local anesthetic should also be ready for the provider's use, with the needed injection supplies.

After achieving suitable local anesthesia, the provider opens the skin with an incision. If a cyst is being removed, the provider dissects around it and usually tries to "deliver" it from the wound intact. If the procedure is an I&D, foul matter will start oozing from the wound immediately after the skin is incised. The wound is drained completely and flushed with copious amounts of sterile saline solution. If the procedure is a biopsy, a small amount of tissue or fluid is removed and placed in a specimen container with preservative. The specimen container must be carefully labeled with the appropriate patient information, the date, and specifics about the specimen type and location. It is then sent to the laboratory, where it is examined microscopically for changes or abnormalities.

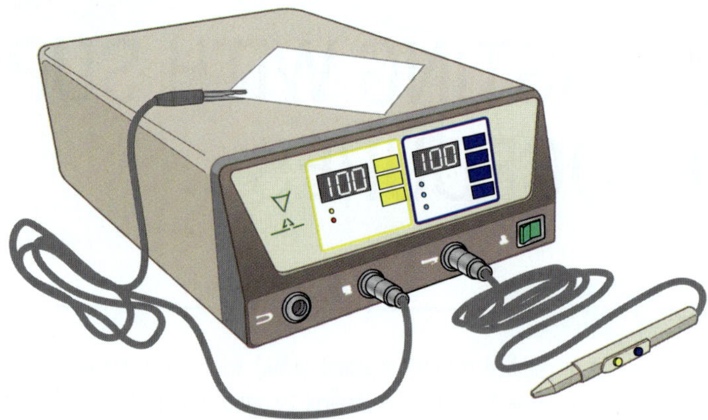

FIGURE 25.1 Electrosurgical unit.

SURGICAL PROCEDURES

As a medical assistant helping with minor surgical procedures, it is important for you to have an understanding of the basic types of procedures performed in the ambulatory care setting. With that understanding, you will be able to help the provider give the patient the best possible care. The following sections examine those basic types of procedures.

Electrosurgery

Electrosurgery is also known as *electrocautery.* An electrosurgical unit (ESU) uses high-frequency current to cut through tissue and coagulate blood vessels. A small probe with an electric current running through it is used to *cauterize* (i.e., burn or destroy) the tissue. This process seals blood vessels, minimizing cellular oozing and bleeding. Electrosurgery may be used to destroy granulations and small polyps or take a tissue sample for pathology examination. The loop electrosurgical excision procedure (LEEP) uses a wire loop heated by an electric current to remove cells and tissue as part of the diagnosis and treatment of abnormal or cancerous conditions of the uterine cervix.

Necessary components are the ESU's power source, the grounding cable and pad, and the active electrode (i.e., a pencil-like instrument with a tip and cord). The grounding pad is a gel-covered adhesive electrode that provides a safe return path for the electrosurgical current. Electrode tips are disposable and are used according to the type of procedure performed. The two most commonly used tips are the needle and flat designs.

Important Tips about the Grounding Pad

- Carefully inspect the pad, cable, and skin before the procedure.
- Place the pad close to the operative site.
- The pad must be tight against the patient's skin.
- Apply the pad to a fleshy area, such as the thigh.
- Do not place the pad over a bony area.
- Do not place the pad over body hair.
- Do not place the pad over metal implants or a pacemaker.
- Carefully inspect the pad site on the skin after the procedure for signs of burns.

Holding the pencil-like instrument, the provider touches the tissue with the tip and activates the electric current with a switch on the instrument. The electric current is delivered to the tissues, and tissue is vaporized at the site of contact, or a specimen can be removed for pathology (Figure 25.1).

Laser Surgery

Laser is an acronym for *l*ight *a*mplification by *s*timulated *e*mission of *r*adiation. Because a laser beam is so small and precise, it can be used to safely treat specific tissue with minimal damage to surrounding tissues and limited scar formation. Lasers were first used in medicine to treat diseases of the retina, and they now are used for many procedures:

- Excision of lesions
- Cauterization of blood vessels
- Removal of warts or moles
- Cosmetic surgical procedures

Several types of lasers are used, including the carbon dioxide, yttrium-aluminum-garnet (YAG), and pulsed dye lasers. Each laser has a specific use. The color of the laser light beam is directly related to the type of surgery performed.

A medical assistant must be specially trained in lasers before assisting with laser surgery. Laser equipment requires careful handling, care, and maintenance. Laser light destroys tissue and can harm the patient, the provider, and you if handled improperly. The medical assistant should complete a full laser safety program before assisting in laser procedures. Once trained, the medical assistant's role during laser surgery includes a number of duties:

- Protecting the patient's eyes from the potential damaging light of the laser
- Observing the surgical field through safety goggles for possible contamination
- Keeping wet sponges ready
- Removing any flammable items from the laser's path
- Assisting with suctioning of the **plume** to maintain a clear visual field
- Providing a basin of sterile normal saline solution and a filled irrigating syringe
- Watching each application of the laser beam and anticipating the need for protective supplies, special equipment, or instruments

Microsurgery

Microsurgery involves the use of an operating microscope to perform delicate surgical procedures. One of its major uses is in ophthalmologic surgery. It also is used in otologic, rhinologic and sinus,

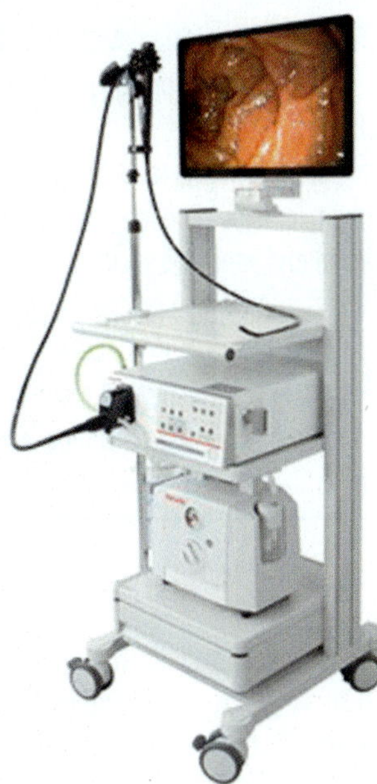

FIGURE 25.2 Flexible colonoscope with monitor and video recorder. (Courtesy Omnia Health.)

laryngologic, neurosurgical, microvascular, gynecologic, and genitourinary procedures. A medical assistant must acquire a basic knowledge of the operation and care of a microscope before becoming qualified to assist in these types of procedures.

The basic components of an operating microscope are the light source, eyepieces (also called the *oculars*), lenses, and cord. Accessory pieces include assistant and observer lenses, cameras, video recorders, television monitors, and printers. These are all valuable for documentation and teaching purposes. Disposable sterile drapes and handle covers are used on the microscope during surgical procedures.

Surgical microscopes are expensive, delicate instruments that require extreme care in handling and cleaning. All lenses and cords should be carefully inspected before and after each use.

Endoscopic Procedures

An endoscope is a medical device consisting of a miniature camera mounted on a flexible tube with an optical system and a light source used to examine the area inside an organ or a cavity. Many types of endoscopes are used, and they are named according to the organs or areas they are used to explore, such as the urinary bladder, bronchus, larynx, colon (Figure 25.2), stomach, uterus, abdomen, and various joints. Small instruments can be used to take samples of suspicious tissues through the endoscope.

Direct visualization with an endoscope is used for diagnostic purposes or to perform surgical procedures. Endoscopes may be rigid (e.g., laparoscope or hysteroscope), semirigid, or flexible (e.g., colonoscopes, bronchoscopes, gastroscopes). All are delicate and expensive, and they require extreme care in handling to protect them from damage.

Accessory equipment used with endoscopes includes fiberoptic light cables and light source, irrigators for solution instillation and suction, and a camera, monitor, printer, and video recorder. The fiberoptic light cable consists of hundreds of glass fibers. It is important to protect it from being bent, dropped, kinked, squashed, or smashed. The light source can become very hot and must be kept out of contact with the patient, the provider, the staff, and any flammable material, such as surgical draping. All equipment must be checked before and after use. Always follow the manufacturer's recommendations for the use, care, and maintenance of equipment. Endoscopic instruments would be damaged by the high temperature and steam under pressure in autoclaves. Special care must be taken in sanitizing and using high-level disinfectants after each procedure to destroy pathogenic organisms and prevent cross-contamination to subsequent patients.

Cryosurgery

Cryosurgery involves the use of a very low-temperature probe to destroy tissue by freezing it on contact. The probe's temperature is usually below 4°F (−20°C). This cold temperature is achieved by circulating liquid nitrogen through the tip of the probe. A local anesthetic is usually administered before cryosurgery. Cryosurgery is used to treat cancers of the skin and warts. In many situations, cryosurgery is less invasive than traditional surgery and, therefore, generally has fewer associated complications. Cryosurgery is often performed in an ambulatory setting or an outpatient surgery center.

Joint Aspiration and Therapeutic Injections

A *joint aspiration*, also known as an arthrocentesis, can easily be done in the provider's office. This procedure involves the removal of fluid from a joint, most commonly from the knee. This may be done to reduce swelling from an injury or infection. It may also be done to help diagnose arthritis or other conditions of the joint. A therapeutic injection involves injecting medication, such as corticosteroids, into the joint to relieve pain. For both a joint aspiration and therapeutic injection, sterile technique is used, and ultrasound is usually used to help guide the needle within the joint. If an aspiration is done, a sample of the fluid removed will be examined under the microscope to help determine the cause of the accumulation of fluid in the joint. After either of these procedures, the patient should remain sitting for several minutes to make sure that they are not dizzy.

PREPARATION FOR SURGICAL PROCEDURES

For a procedure to go smoothly, things must be prepared well. If patients do not understand what they are required to do before the procedure, the procedure may have to be postponed. If the room is not properly prepared, the procedure may be delayed, upsetting the provider and patient. The following sections discuss the proper preparation of the patient and the procedure room.

Preparation of the Patient

Whether minor surgery is performed because of an unforeseen accident or is a planned, elective procedure, the patient needs both psychological and physical support. A patient facing a surgical procedure may be concerned about pain, disfigurement, and the possible diagnosis. An injured patient may feel anxious about medical bills or possible loss of employment. Because surgery is a frightening experience, the medical assistant must take the time, both preoperatively and at the time of surgery, to help the patient deal with fears and anxieties. The best way to help is to make sure that the patient understands the details of the procedure, all questions are answered by the provider, and the patient has the opportunity to talk about the procedure and voice any concerns.

Questions should be answered directly, but you should answer only the questions that are within your scope of knowledge and the policies of the office. If you cannot answer a question, assure the patient that you will relay it to the provider before the procedure and then be sure to do so. What may seem like a minor or unimportant question to you may be a frightening concern to the patient. The minor surgery room can be intimidating, so unless the patient is sedated, try to make conversation with him or her while you prepare for the provider's arrival.

Preoperative preparation may include the following:

- Blood and urine tests
- Completion of a consent form
- Gathering of the current history concerning any recent illnesses
- Medications and allergies

Patient preparations before surgery may include a shave prep, cleansing enemas, food intake restrictions, special bathing, and the administration of a sedative medication. On the day of surgery, the patient is instructed to empty the bladder and undress and gown as requested. The vital signs are recorded in preparation for the procedure.

Preoperative Instructions

When office surgery is planned, certain procedures are followed before the appointment, such as these:

- Having the necessary consent forms ready to sign
- Giving the patient the necessary preoperative instructions, such as medications to be used and special skin-cleansing instructions
- Telling the patient to bring a relative or friend to drive him or her home after the surgery
- Instructing the patient to leave jewelry and other valuables at home
- Calling the patient the day before the scheduled surgery to confirm any special instructions

Informed Consent

The provider must have the patient's written informed consent before the sedating medication is given and surgery begins (Figure 25.3). To sign an informed consent form permitting the provider to legally

WALDEN-MARTIN
FAMILY MEDICAL CLINIC
1234 ANYSTREET | ANYTOWN, ANYSTATE 12345
PHONE 123-123-1234 | FAX 123-123-5678

General Procedure Consent

Patient Name: ____________________ **Date:** ______________

The doctor has discussed with you your condition and the recommended surgical or medical procedures to be performed. This discussion was intended to ensure that you had the opportunity to receive the information necessary to make a reasoned and informed decision whether or not to consent to the procedure. This document is written confirmation of the discussion and contains some of the more significant medical information discussed.

1. Based on this discussion, I understand the following condition may exist in my case:

2. I understand the procedure proposed for treating or diagnosing my condition is:

3. I have been informed of the purpose and reasonable expected benefits of the proposed procedure, the possibility of success or failure, major problems of recuperation, the reasonably anticipated consequences if the procedure is not performed, and the available alternatives.

4. I understand that all surgical and therapeutic procedures involve some risks including pain, scarring, bleeding, and infection.

5. I am aware that in the practice of medicine, other unexpected risks or complications not discussed may or may not further acknowledge that no guarantees or promises have been made to me concerning the results of any procedures. Although the benefits are judged to outweigh the risks, should any complications occur, any one of them could be permanent. I hereby voluntarily give my authority and consent to the doctor to perform the proposed procedure described above.

6. I have been given the opportunity to ask questions about my condition, alternative forms or treatment, risk treatment, the procedure to be used, and the risks and hazards involved. I believe I have sufficient information to give this informed consent.

I understand and I have read and fully understand the contents of this form, that the disclosures referred to above were made to me, and that all blanks and statements requiring insertion or completion were filled in before I signed my name below.

Patient Signature: ____________________ **Date:** ______________

If a patient is a minor or unable to give consent, signature of person authorized to consent for patient: ____________________

Relationship to Patient: ____________________

FIGURE 25.3 Informed Consent Form. (From Niedzwiecki B: *Kinn's Medical Assisting* Fundamentals, ed 5, St. Louis, 2022, Elsevier.)

perform the surgery, the patient must understand certain details about the procedure:

- What procedure will be performed
- Why it should be done
- The potential risks and benefits of the surgery
- Alternative treatments (including no treatment)
- Possible risks of any alternative treatment

This legal requirement is not met simply by having the patient sign a consent form; a discussion must occur, during which the provider gives the patient or the patient's legal representative enough information to enable the person to decide whether to proceed with the proposed surgical treatment. After this discussion, the patient either consents to or refuses the surgery. The patient then signs or refuses to sign the consent form. The discussion must be fully documented in the patient's health record. A copy of the signed form must also be included in the patient's record. Sometimes the patient will sign the form directly on the electronic record. Treatment may not exceed the scope of the consent form.

The patient must not be under the influence of any sedative medication at the time he or she signs the consent form. An interpreter must be used if the patient does not understand English. This condition must *never* be violated.

CRITICAL THINKING APPLICATION **25.1**

Callie is preparing a patient for a biopsy of a suspected cancer of the skin. The consent form has been signed and is in the chart. While Callie is chatting with the patient during completion of the final setup for the procedure, it becomes clear the patient thinks she is having a "skin tag" removed from her back. What action should Callie take, if any? What is the significance of what the patient said in this situation?

Positioning

Have the patient disrobe sufficiently to expose the surgical site completely so that accidental contamination does not occur during the procedure. Clothing may also act as a tourniquet or make applying a proper dressing or bandage difficult. In addition, the patient's clothing may be stained by the skin prep solution or may interfere with adequate site preparation.

The patient needs to be positioned as comfortably as possible for the procedure. An uncomfortable position can be held for only a limited time, and the patient may have to move, perhaps in the middle of a procedure, if you have not ensured his or her comfort from the beginning. When deciding on the correct position, consider where you and the provider will stand or sit, where the instruments will be placed, and where other needed equipment will be located. If the patient has an open wound, wear gloves to assist the patient into position. If there is active and profuse bleeding, wear an impermeable gown and gloves. If there is a danger of blood and body fluid contamination to your face or eyes, wear a face shield.

Skin Preparation

The human skin is a reservoir of bacteria, but it cannot be sterilized without the risk of damaging cells and tissues. The goal of adequate skin preparation for a surgical procedure is to reduce the number of transient floras so that any transfer of harmful organisms at the incision site is limited. Cleansing the patient's skin before surgery with surgical soap and an antiseptic and shaving the area if needed is called a *skin prep* (Procedure 25.1). Sometimes the patient may be instructed to repeatedly cleanse the surgical area with bacteriostatic or antiseptic soap several days before the surgery. Disposable skin prep trays and electric razors should be available in the ambulatory facility.

Preparation of the Room

If you are to assist in a minor surgical procedure, study the provider's care preferences, review the procedure, and note the materials needed. Next, prepare the room and gather the supplies to be used. Sterile supplies are opened just before the procedure. Opened materials that have been exposed longer than 1 hour, usually because of a delay, are considered nonsterile. Supplies should not be placed where they can be knocked over or dropped. Wrapped sterile supplies that fall to the floor must not be used. Make sure the patient and family members understand that they should not approach or touch the sterile field.

ASSISTING WITH SURGICAL PROCEDURES

Surgery performed in a medical office is restricted to the management of minor problems and injuries. The medical assistant is expected to assist with preparing the patient and setting up the sterile field. The following procedures must be used without exception when assisting with minor surgery. Individual facilities may have specific guidelines for some of these procedures; however, the theory behind sterile technique is universal, regardless of where you work.

Sterile Technique

Accurately performing surgical aseptic technique requires a great deal of concentration and planning of all movements and procedural steps. The procedures covered in this chapter are for minor surgery, but they are the same techniques used during major surgery. To develop a sound knowledge of sterility and sterile technique, use the following memory aid: *Everything sterile is white, and everything that is not sterile is black. There is no gray!* Sterile surfaces must *never* come in contact with nonsterile surfaces. If this occurs, the sterile surface immediately is considered contaminated or nonsterile. Constant **vigilance** and absolute honesty are essential for maintaining sterile techniques. When a sterile surface comes in contact with a nonsterile item, this is called a *break* in sterility or a *break* in the sterile field. During any procedure, everything must stop at this point, and the break must be corrected immediately. This usually means the assistant must start over again at the very beginning of the procedure. Any break could lead to serious wound contamination, postoperative infection, and even death.

Before assisting with minor surgery, the medical assistant must perform a series of procedures to ensure surgical asepsis (Procedures 25.2 to 25.5). These skills must be learned, practiced, and followed precisely to establish and maintain the sterile environment required during a surgical procedure. Surgical asepsis directly affects the health and well-being of the patient, the provider, and the office staff and must be practiced without fail.

CRITICAL THINKING APPLICATION 25.2

After completing a surgical scrub before assisting with a minor surgical procedure, Callie realizes that she forgot to lay out the practitioner's sterile glove package. She opens the storage cabinet and quickly adds this to the collection of sterile supplies. Can she now put on her sterile gloves? Why or why not?

Sterile Field

A sterile field is any sterile surface on which sterile items are placed. In the ambulatory facility, a sterile field most often is set up on a Mayo stand (Figure 25.4). In surgery, a sterile field is created by draping sterile towels (either disposable or from autoclaved packs) over a Mayo stand or table. The surgical site on the patient's skin is prepared and then covered with sterile towels or drapes so that it also becomes a sterile field.

Hands and hair are two of the greatest sources of contamination when a sterile field is set up. With practice, you will get to know what may be touched with your hands and what must be touched only with sterile gloved hands. Hair that falls freely over the shoulders and forward gives off a cloud of bacteria with every movement. It must always be secured back and up, not touching the shoulders.

RULES FOR MAINTAINING A STERILE FIELD

- Talking should be kept to a minimum because air currents carry bacteria.
- Sterile team members should always face one another.
- Always keep the sterile field in your view. If you turn your back on a sterile field or lose sight of it, it is considered contaminated.
- Nonsterile body parts (e.g., hands or elbows) and items should never cross over the sterile field.
- Tables and trays are sterile only at table level; anything that falls below the edge of the Mayo tray is considered contaminated. A 1-inch border around the edge of the tray is considered contaminated, so anything placed on the tray within that 1-inch border is contaminated.
- Consider a sterile barrier contaminated if it has been wet, cut, or torn.
- Packages placed on a clean surface are contaminated on the outside, but the inside of the sterilized package may be used as a sterile field.
- Keep sterile gloved hands above waist level at all times; do not let hands drop below the waist.
- Never remove and then replace any item in the field (e.g., using sterile forceps to cleanse a wound), or the field is contaminated.
- The inside of a sterile package remains so if the package is peeled open properly; it should be opened the entire way, and the contents then tossed onto the field without crossing over the sterile area; a two-person transfer can be used, where one person opens the sterile supplies and another, wearing sterile gloves, removes the contents from the package and places them on the sterile tray.
- If a sterile package falls to the floor, it must be discarded.
- If you are in doubt about the sterility of anything, consider it contaminated.

Assisting the Provider during Surgery

The provider ultimately is responsible for the patient. The medical assistant is responsible for ensuring that everything the assistant and

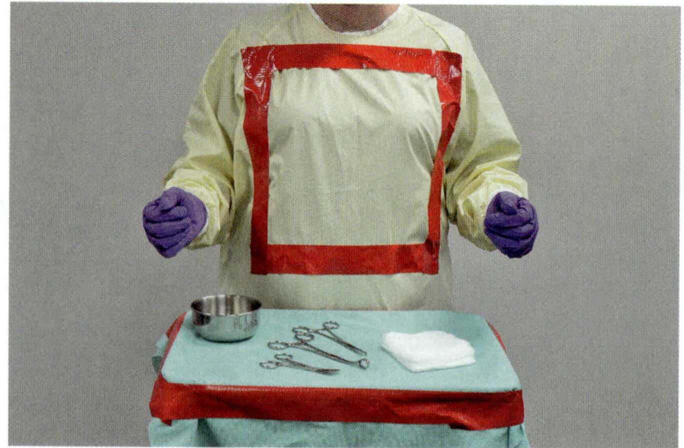

FIGURE 25.4 Sterile field *(red outline).*

the provider will use in caring for the surgical patient is accounted for, ready for use, and prepared in a safe and sterile manner (Procedure 25.6). Every team has preferences about the sequence it follows during routine minor surgery. Once a routine has been established, it should be followed in every case. Sample setups for various types of minor surgery are provided in Table 25.1.

The medical assistant sorts and places the scalpels, hemostats, scissors, tissue forceps, and retractors on the sterile field according to their sequence and frequency of use. Scalpels and sharp instruments should be conspicuously placed so that they do not accidentally injure a team member. The provider enters the room after scrubbing and then puts on gloves. The provider drapes the patient with towels or a fenestrated drape as the medical assistant hands him or her the drapes, one at a time. Once the site has been draped, the Mayo stand with the sterile field is positioned below the site, and the medical assistant stands opposite the provider over the patient, ready to help as needed.

Passing Instruments

During a procedure, the medical assistant must protect the sterile field from contamination. Notify the provider if a break in sterile technique occurs, dispose of soiled sponges in the biohazard waste container, and anticipate the provider's need for instruments. The provider may request instruments or may use hand signals. As the team works together over time, the provider may not need to give any signals because the assistant will be able to anticipate the instrument needed next during the procedure.

Instrumentation is logical; if the practitioner requests a suture, scissors will be needed next to cut the suture strand. In the case of sudden hemorrhage from a bleeding vessel, the provider will need an appropriately sized hemostat. While gaining experience, the assistant watches, listens, and learns to judge what will be needed or performed next. While wearing sterile gloves, pass instruments with a firm, purposeful motion so that the provider does not have to look up. Wait until you feel the provider grasp the instrument so that it does not drop onto the patient or the floor. Be careful that you and the provider are protected from injury. Pass the scalpel with the blade down and present the handle to the provider. Hold all instruments by their tips and pass the handle ends into the provider's palm or fingers (Figure 25.5).

TABLE 25.1 Setups for Minor Surgeries

PROCEDURE	SIDE COUNTER	STERILE FIELD	COMMENTS	POSTOPERATIVE CARE
Suture repair	Local anesthetic, dressings and bandages, splints or guards, tape, drape, gloves, sterile normal saline solution	Syringe and needle, hemostats (three), scissors, sponges, suture material and needle, tissue forceps or skin hook, needle holder	If a patient arrives with a pressure dressing over a laceration, follow Standard Precautions. Do not remove the pressure dressing until the provider is ready to suture. If the patient's pressure cloth must be removed, have ample sterile dressings ready to apply immediately. Ask the patient the approximate length, depth, and exact location of the laceration. Follow the provider's directions regarding cleansing of the wound.	Clean lacerations in a moderately protected area; may not require a dressing. The patient is instructed to keep the area clean and dry. Some lacerations may be closed with wound closure strips or a topical skin adhesive.
Needle biopsy	Specimen container with prepackaged fixative or preserving solution, laboratory form and label, local anesthetic, gloves	Biopsy needle, syringe and needle, sponges	A biopsy is the examination of tissue removed from the living body. Biopsies usually are done to determine whether a growth is malignant or benign; however, a biopsy may be done as a diagnostic aid when treating other diseases or infections. A needle biopsy may be done by aspiration with a needle and syringe or with a special biopsy needle. The specimen then is sent to a pathologist for either a cytologic or a histologic examination.	Usually no special dressing is required after a needle biopsy. An adhesive bandage strip (e.g., Band-Aid) often is sufficient.
Cyst removal	Local anesthetic, disinfectant (skin prep), laboratory form, dressing (size depends on site), gloves, drape, specimen container with prepackaged fixative or preserving solution	Kelly hemostats (two straight and two curved), dressing forceps (two), suture and needle, scissors, dissector (provider's choice), skin hook, syringe and needle, disposable scalpel with No. 11 or No. 15 blade, tissue forceps (two), Allis forceps, needle holder, sponges	A sebaceous cyst is a benign retention cyst of a sebaceous gland containing fatty substance from the gland. The cyst is attached to the skin and moves freely over the underlying tissue. For cosmetic reasons the provider makes the incision on the natural skin crease lines if possible.	See suture repair, earlier, or apply a small sterile dressing, depending on the size of the incision.

CRITICAL THINKING APPLICATION **25.3**

In passing the scalpel to the provider while assisting with an incision and drainage (I&D), Callie feels the blade slice through her glove. She quickly and secretly looks at it and notices a tiny nick in her glove. Because this is a "dirty" procedure, she decides to say nothing and continues assisting with the procedure. Is her reasoning sound here? What is the best approach to handling this situation? Why?

Specimen Collection

If a specimen is collected during a procedure, it is placed in a sterile specimen cup or basin. Do not remove the specimen from the sterile field until the provider gives the order. The provider may want to examine the specimen again during the procedure. After the procedure has been completed, place the specimen in an appropriate container, label it, and send it to the laboratory for analysis.

Completing the Surgical Procedure

At the conclusion of the procedure, the provider begins wound closure. The techniques and methods of tissue closure vary; all of them cannot be described or illustrated here. The two basic methods of suturing are the continuous running suture (Figure 25.6A) and the interrupted suture (Figure 25.6B), where each knot is placed and tied one at a time, so that if one breaks, the others keep the wound closure intact. The interrupted technique is used for most skin closures in a medical office.

The provider may prefer that the medical assistant place the needle in a needle holder and pass it, handle first. When the wound is closed, you may assist by cutting the suture and sponging the site. If an interrupted suture method is used, the first suture is placed at the midpoint of the incision. Then each side of the first suture is mentally divided in half again, and the next two sutures are placed at each of these midpoints. The rest of the sutures are placed using

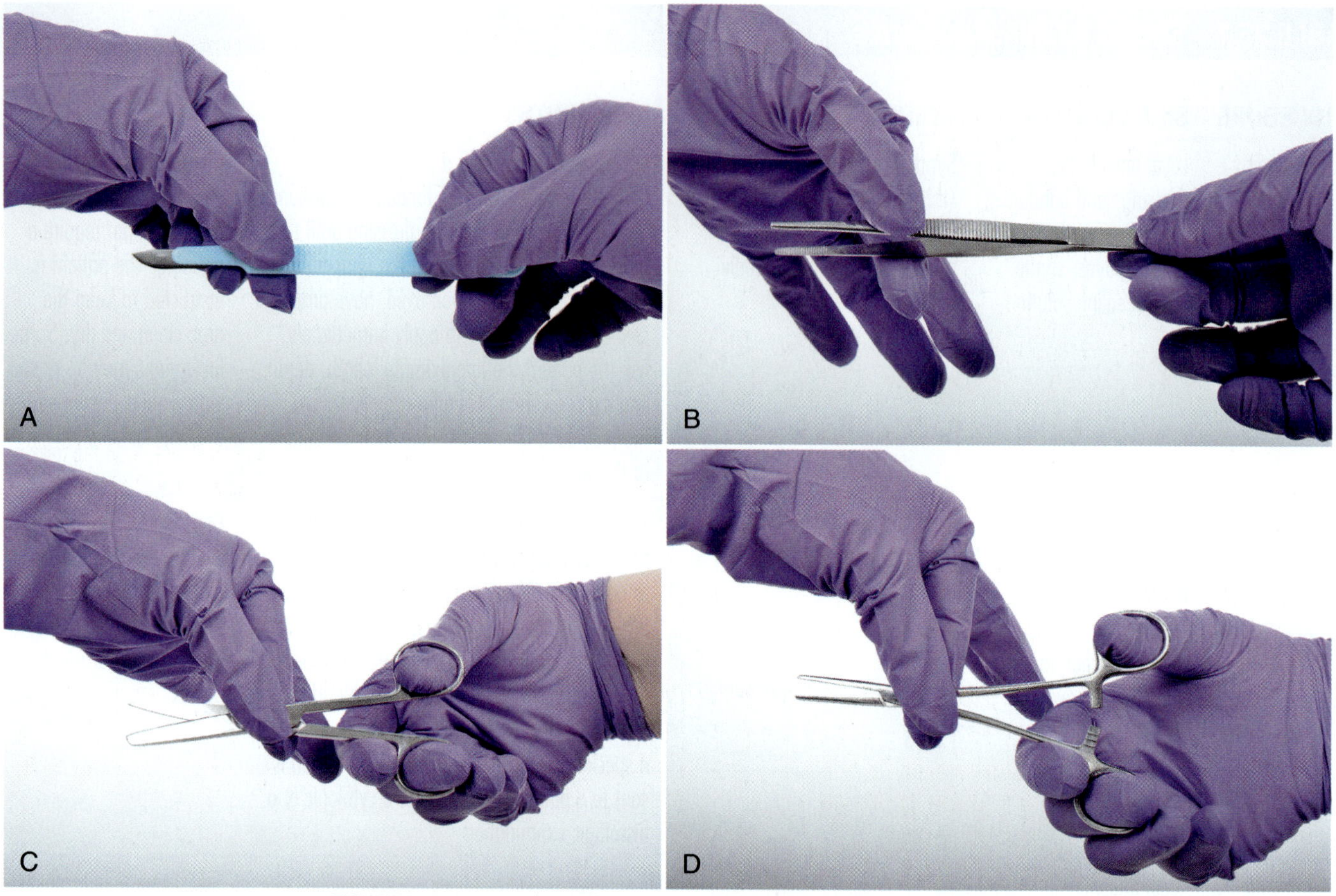

FIGURE 25.5 Passing sterile surgical instruments. **(A)** Scalpel. **(B)** Forceps. **(C)** Scissors. **(D)** Clamp.

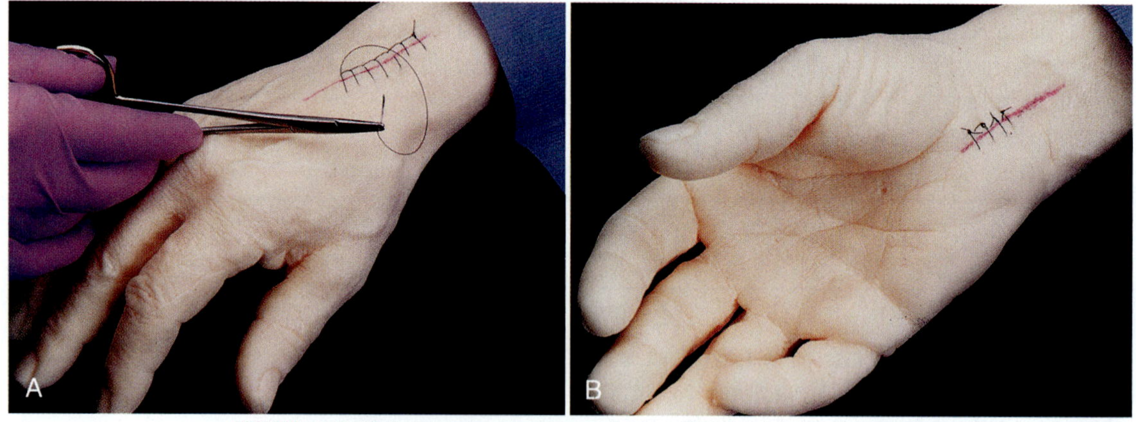

FIGURE 25.6 **(A)** Continuous (i.e., running) suture placement. **(B)** Interrupted suture placement.

the same technique until the wound edges have been completely **approximated**. The provider may also choose to close a wound with surgical staples.

After the skin closure, the blood and iodine should be gently removed and the area blotted dry using sterile dry sponges. Care must be taken not to disturb the wound edges or sutures. Next, a sterile dressing is placed over the incision (Procedure 25.7), and a bandage is applied to support the dressing.

Postoperative Responsibilities

After caring for the patient, the medical assistant clears the sterile field, following Standard Precautions. Wear gloves until all contaminated materials have been properly removed and handled. Place disposable equipment and supplies in biohazard waste containers or sharps containers. The room should be checked for any blood spills or other contamination and disinfected appropriately. After completing this process, remove the contaminated gloves and sanitize your hands.

Single-Assistant Preparation for Minor Surgery

1. Sanitize your hands and gather all supplies:
   - *Sterile side (Mayo tray):* Two towel packs, skin prep pack, patient drape pack, instrument pack, miscellaneous pack or packs, three glove packs, face shields, impermeable gowns
   - *Nonsterile side (side counter):* Syringes, suture material, anesthetic solutions, additional sponges, sterile dressings, bandages, transfer forceps, waste basin, sharps and biohazard waste containers, nonsterile gloves, face shields, and impermeable gowns
2. Verify that the informed consent has been signed and is in the patient's health record.
3. Identify the patient, and escort him or her into the room.
4. Greet and converse with the patient.
5. Position the patient on the table.
6. Sanitize your hands.
7. Open the first towel pack.
8. Open the skin prep pack.
9. Pour the soap and antiseptic solutions.
10. Expose the site to be prepped.
11. Put on gloves and arrange prep items within the sterile field.
12. Place sterile towels at skin scrub boundaries using sterile technique.
13. Prep the patient's skin.
14. Discard skin prep materials in appropriate sharps/biohazard containers.
15. Discard gloves: sanitize your hands, following the guidelines for a surgical hand scrub (see Procedure 25.2) if this procedure is part of the policy of the provider or the facility.
16. Open the table drape pack on the Mayo stand to create a sterile field.
17. Open the instrument pack or packs and transfer the instruments to the sterile field. Add the sterile syringe unit.
18. Add sterile items as requested. The provider joins you and converses with the patient.
19. Open the provider's glove pack (the provider now puts on gloves).
20. Open the patient drape pack (the provider now drapes the surgical site).
21. Cleanse and hold up the anesthetic vial for the provider to withdraw the anesthetic with the sterile syringe (the provider now administers the anesthetic).
22. Repeat the surgical hand wash; reglove with a new glove pack.
23. Arrange the sterile field instruments and other materials for safety and in sequence; check the condition of each instrument.
24. Open the suture/needle pack per the provider's choice; load the first suture into the needle holder, grasping the needle in the third of the needle closest to where it joins the suture.
25. Place two gauze squares at the site.
26. Assist with the procedure:[a]
   - *For the provider:* Pass the instruments, maintain the field, anticipate his or her needs, and cut sutures.
   - *For the patient:* Retract tissue, sponge blood from the wound, apply the sterile bandage, and care for the specimen.
27. Help the patient sit up and dress if needed, and monitor vital signs as instructed.
28. Record and prepare specimens.
29. Sanitize and disinfect the room; clear materials and discard in biohazard waste containers.
30. Document the procedure in the patient's health record.
31. Help the patient prepare to leave the office.
32. Sanitize, disinfect, and sterilize the equipment at the first available time.

[a] By law, the assistant may not clamp tissues, place sutures, or alter body tissues in any way.

Wear gloves while disinfecting the room, including the table, Mayo stand, side and back tables, any other equipment in the room, and the floor. Used instruments must be sanitized, disinfected, and resterilized for future use.

The provider and the medical assistant both document the surgical procedure in the patient's health record.

Postoperative Instructions and Care

The patient should be given time to rest after the surgery. If a sedative was administered, make sure the patient has recovered sufficiently to avoid injury after the surgery or during the trip home. If the patient was given a topical or local anesthetic, explain to him or her that the anesthesia effect will wear off and that some discomfort may be felt at the operative site. Check with the provider to determine if pain medication needs to be prescribed. If medication has been prescribed, review the purpose of the medication and the directions for its use with the patient and his or her companion. Make a follow-up appointment before the patient leaves the office.

Postoperative care extends for the total recovery period, not just for the time of immediate care before the patient leaves the office. Most medical assistants are responsible for teaching patients to care for themselves at home after surgery. A postoperative patient may have trouble comprehending or remembering instructions. All instructions should be given to the patient in writing. They should be simple and easily understood by both the patient and caregivers. These instructions can be preprinted forms for each type of surgery or a general form with checked boxes for particular postoperative instructions that apply specifically to the individual patient (Figure 25.7).

Warning Signs

Explain to the patient the importance of calling the office if any questions come up or changes occur that cause the person concern. If the patient does not call within the next 24 hours, you should call the patient. Many patients tend to "ride it out" or say they did not want to disturb you. Never allow the postoperative patient to leave the office without the provider's knowledge and approval. Tell patients to call the office immediately if they note redness around the operative site, bleeding from the wound, fever, swelling, or increasing or severe pain. The wound should be kept clean and dry, and the patient should be taught how to change the dressing if needed.

Follow-Up

If the healing process is long or the wound becomes infected, the patient may return for follow-up care. If the wound requires a new

POSTOP INSTRUCTIONS FOR ______________________________

☐ Elevate your arm.
☐ Elevate your leg.
☐ Limit food intake to ______________________________.
☐ Limit activity to ______________________________.
☐ Do not bathe or shower.
☐ Sponge bath only.
☐ Change dressing as instructed.
☐ Call the office for fever, redness, pain, swelling, or bleeding.
☐ Take ______________ every 4 hours as needed for pain.
☐ Return to school/work in ________ days.
☐ Call the office tomorrow before ________ p.m.
☐ Your next appointment is on M T W Th F S __________ at ______.

FIGURE 25.7 An example of preprinted postoperative patient instructions.

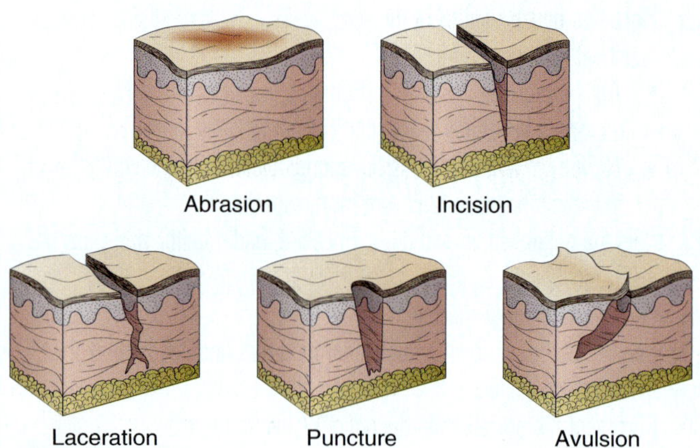

FIGURE 25.8 Five types of open wounds. (From Cooper K, Gosnell K: *Foundations of Nursing,* ed5, 2019, Elsevier)

dressing, follow Standard Precautions; wear gloves and other protective barriers as appropriate. If at any time you determine that the wound may be infected, stop and have the provider examine it. Generally, no bandaging material should be reused, including elastic bandage wraps.

Tape applied directly to a patient's skin is not a good dressing immobilizer. If tape is used, always keep it to a minimum. If tape is holding a dressing in place, always remove it by pulling toward the wound. If it is adhering to a hairy area of the body, lift the outer tape edge with one hand and slowly and gently separate the underlying hair and skin from the tape with the thumb of your other hand. Peel the skin from the bandage, not the bandage from the skin. Never rapidly rip tape from the body because this may injure the skin. If the tape is not irritating to the patient, it may be advisable to leave the tape in place until total healing has taken place.

When the wound has healed, the provider may ask the medical assistant to remove the patient's sutures or staples. The patient must return to the facility to have the sutures/staples removed (Procedure 25.8). When removing sutures or staples, it is important for medical assistants to alert the provider to any concerns they have with the wound healing and to document the procedure.

WOUND CARE

A wound can be intentional (e.g., from a surgical incision) or accidental, and it may be open or closed (Figure 25.8). An open wound has an outward opening; the skin is broken, exposing the underlying tissues. A closed or nonpenetrating wound does not have an outward opening, but the underlying tissues are damaged, as in a hematoma, contusion, or bruise. Closed wounds usually are the result of some type of blunt trauma to the body. An aseptic (i.e., clean) wound is not infected with pathogens. Septic wounds are infected with pathogens.

Open wounds may be classified according to the appearance of their openings. An incised wound has a clean edge and is made with a cutting instrument. An incised wound may be the result of surgery, an accident, or a knife wound. A lacerated wound has torn or mangled tissues and is made by a dull or blunt instrument. A penetrating or puncture wound is caused by a sharp, slender object, such as a needle or an ice pick, passing through the skin into the underlying tissues. A perforated wound is a penetrating wound that passes through to a body organ or cavity, such as a gunshot wound.

Wound Healing

All wounds go through a healing or repair process that has four phases. **Hemostasis** is the first phase. Blood vessels contract to control hemorrhage, and blood platelets form a network that acts as a glue to plug the wound. After a cascade of chemical reactions, fibrin is released into the wound and clotting begins. Fibrin continues to collect red blood cells (RBCs), and the clot dries into a scab.

The second, or inflammatory, phase focuses on destroying bacteria and removing debris. Special white blood cells (WBCs), called *macrophages,* arrive to clear away bacteria and dead tissue. Within 1 to 4 days, the fibrin threads contract and pull the edges of the wound together under the scab. During this phase, edema, *erythema* (redness), heat, and pain can occur.

The third phase, *proliferation,* encompasses wound healing and new growth; this lasts 5 to 20 days. During this phase, the tissues repair themselves. New cells form, and the wound continues to contract and seal. If the wound is a clean surgical incision, complete contraction usually occurs and a **cicatrix** forms.

The final phase, the *remodeling* phase, extends from day 21 onward. Clean, shallow wounds may contract in the first two stages; large or mangled wounds require the time and cellular activity of this third phase to build a bridge of new tissue to close the gap of the wound. The cells produce a fibrous protein substance called *collagen* (i.e., connective tissue) that gives the wounded tissues strength and forms scar tissue. Scar tissue is not true skin; it usually is very strong, but it lacks the elasticity of normal skin tissue. There is no blood supply or nerves in scar tissue.

Several factors influence the healing process. People who are young, in good general health, and have adequate nutrition heal more rapidly. Adequate protection and rest of the injured area also enhance the healing process. Destruction or reinjury during the second phase can delay healing and increase scarring. Wounds are susceptible to infection because the normal skin barrier is broken. If debris is present in a wound as the result of the breakdown of various cellular components, this dead (i.e., necrotic) tissue acts as a culture medium for bacterial growth. Suppuration (i.e., pus) contains necrotic tissue, bacteria, dead WBCs, and other products of tissue breakdown. Necrotic tissue must be removed; debris removal is called *debridement,* which may occur naturally or may be performed surgically.

Sometimes the provider may prefer no dressing or bandage on small wounds. This is called *open wound healing.* There are some advantages to open wound healing:

- Air can circulate freely around the wound.
- The wound is not irritated or rubbed by a dressing.
- The wound stays dry, which inhibits bacterial growth, reducing the chance of infection.
- Sutures stay dry and hold together better.
- Any preexisting infection remains localized and is not spread by the dressing or bandage.

Dressings

A dressing is a sterile covering placed over a wound for the following purposes:

- Protecting the wound from injury and contamination
- Maintaining constant pressure to minimize bleeding and swelling
- Holding the wound edges together
- Absorbing drainage and secretions

A dressing usually consists of a strip of lubricated mesh gauze, a nonstick Telfa pad, or a clear dressing placed over a sutured wound. Gauze may be placed over nonadhering material, depending on the provider's preference. Body cavities or wounds that need to remain open for a time are dressed with long, thin packing material that often is impregnated with an antiseptic or a lubricant; this sometimes is called *packing.* A good dressing must be effective, comfortable, and remain in place. If the dressing covers a hairless area, it may be anchored with tape, but no tape should touch the wound.

When changing a patient's dressing, the medical assistant should examine it for any drainage (exudate). There are five different types of exudates to look for:

- *Sanguineous:* Thick consistency, bright red blood
- *Serous:* Thin watery consistency, clear or yellowish appearance due to serum and white blood cells
- *Serosanguineous:* Consistency is thinner than sanguineous and thicker than serous; pink appearance due to the presence of red blood cells and serum
- *Purulent:* Can have a very thick consistency; yellow, green or brown in color due to the presence of white blood cells, dead cell debris, and dead bacteria. Indicates infection.
- *Seropurulent:* Consistency is thinner than purulent due to the presence of serum; cloudy pink, gray, yellow, tan, brown, green or white in color. This also indicates infection.

IMPLICATIONS FOR FAILURE TO COMPLY WITH CENTER FOR DISEASE CONTROL (CDC) REGULATIONS IN HEALTHCARE SETTINGS

Standard precautions were developed by the Centers for Disease Control and Prevention (CDC) and are regulated by the Occupational Safety and Health Administration (OSHA). These precautions are used for all patient care. The goal is to protect patients and healthcare workers. Standard precautions include the following practices:

- Perform hand hygiene
- Use personal protective equipment whenever there is an expectation of possible exposure to infectious material
- Follow respiratory hygiene/cough etiquette principles
- Properly handle and properly clean and disinfect patient care equipment and instruments/devices
- Follow safe injection practices
- Ensure healthcare worker safety, including proper handling of needles and other sharps

Failure to comply with this CDC regulation can result in loss of infection control for both the patient and healthcare worker, injury to the patient or healthcare worker, possible litigation from the patient or healthcare worker, and fines from OSHA.

Bandages

Bandages hold dressings in place and also help maintain even pressure, support the affected part, and help protect the wound from injury and contamination. Bandages can be gauze, cloth, or elastic cloth rolls and are bound by clips, tape, or ties. Dressings and bandages frequently appear easy and simple to apply; however, special skill is required to use different types of bandaging techniques. Bandages that are too loose fall off, whereas those that are too tight may compromise circulation and further harm the patient.

Plain roller gauze is seldom used. It is difficult to handle, has no elasticity, and tends to bind. It also tends to slip because it does not adhere to itself. Wrinkled crepe–type roller bandages (e.g., Kling) are preferred because they easily conform to various shapes of the body and adhere to themselves (Figure 25.9A). If the bandage is to cover a wound, it should always be applied over a sterile dressing.

Plain elastic cloth bandages or elastic roller cloth bandages with adhesive backing (e.g., Ace) (Figure 25.9B) make flexible, secure covers. When an elastic roller bandage is applied as a pressure bandage, especially to the lower limbs, it is essential to keep the bandage consistent in spacing and tension to ensure even pressure. Even, gentle pressure stimulates circulation and healing. Uneven pressure causes constriction points that can create pressure sores, ulcers, or edema. Roller bandages are usually applied from the distal to the proximal part of the area because they are more even and snug if wrapped from a smaller to a larger circumference. Elevate the limb while you are bandaging and work with the roller facing upward, close to the patient's skin. Elastic bandages are excellent for bandaging the hand and wrist and the foot and ankle.

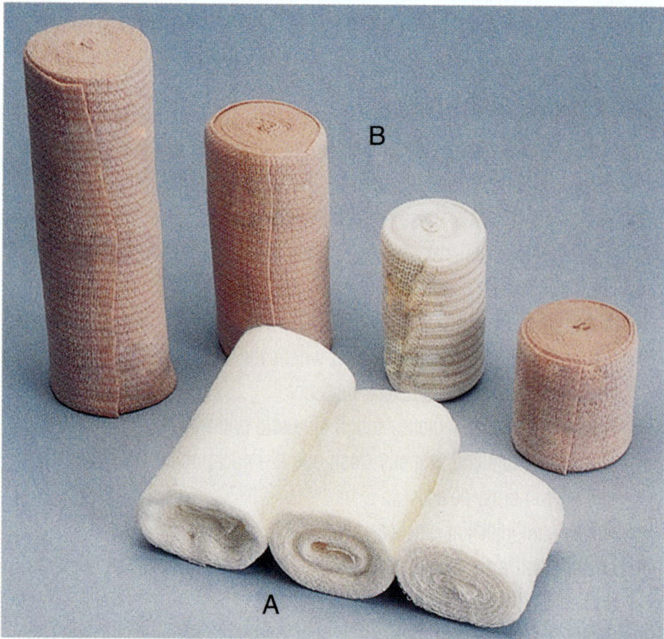

FIGURE 25.9 (A) Wrinkled crepe-type roller bandages (e.g., Kling). **(B)** Elastic roller bandages (e.g., Ace).

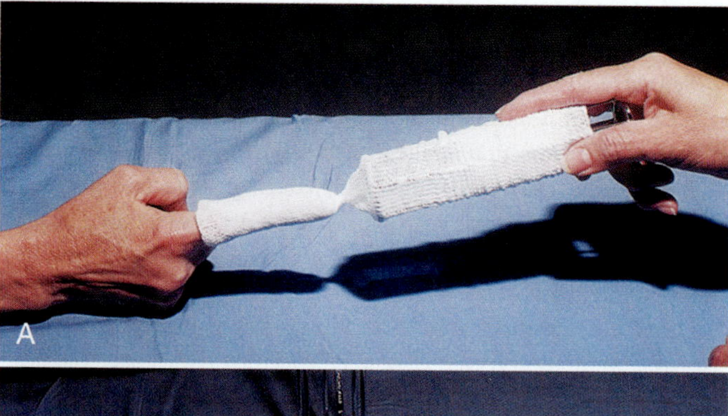

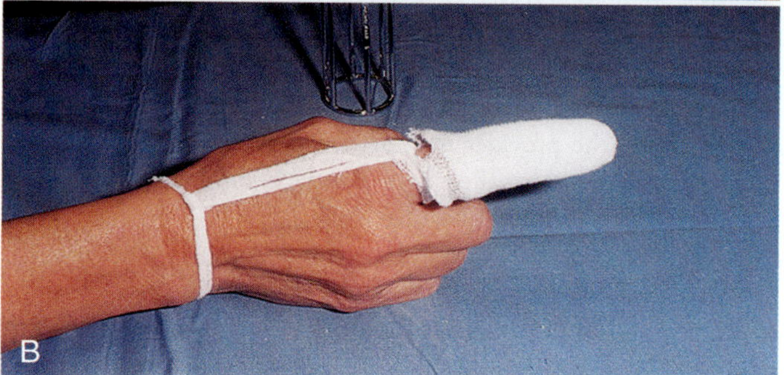

FIGURE 25.10 (A) Tube gauze is applied with even tension and is twisted at the fingertip before the next layer is applied. **(B)** A tube gauze bandage has been applied and secured by tying at the wrist.

Remember: CMST When Bandaging

When applying bandages, you should assess the following:

- **C**olor: Should be the same as the opposite extremity; report any bluish or white fingers or toes.
- **M**ovement: Should be able to move fingers/toes.
- **S**ensation: Should be able to feel fingers/toes; report any numbness.
- **T**emperature: Should be the same as the opposite extremity; report any cool/cold fingers/toes.

A seamless tubular gauze bandage, with or without elastic, is a superior material for covering round, narrow surfaces such as fingers or toes. It can be used as a dressing if the gauze material is sterile; it can also be used as a bandage. A tubular gauze bandage is applied with a cagelike applicator (Figure 25.10). Work with the open circle of the applicator toward the patient. Hold the applicator in the dominant hand and control the tension flow with your fingers as the applicator is gradually rotated and the material slides off. Tubular dressing may be applied with or without slight pressure. Beyond the tip of the bandaged part, give the applicator a full half-turn, place the applicator again over the part, and repeat the process, being careful not to create a tourniquet effect when you reverse the applicator. When the desired thickness of the bandage is reached, cut the gauze and anchor the final gauze application with tape or by tying it at the wrist.

CLOSING COMMENTS

Assisting with minor surgery can be challenging and rewarding. There are many things to remember, but the key piece is to always maintain sterile technique. Whether it is handling instruments, setting up trays, or assisting the provider, sterile technique must be followed to protect our patients.

Patient Coaching

The best time for a medical assistant to instruct the patient in aseptic techniques to be used at home is during an aseptic procedure. Patient education includes the purpose and importance of handwashing; using disposable tissues to cover the nose and mouth when coughing or sneezing and properly disposing of used tissues; the differences between sterile and clean dressings and bandages; and step-by-step instructions on how to change a dressing properly and dispose of contaminated items.

Legal and Ethical Issues

Many minor surgical procedures previously performed in the hospital are now being done in a medical office, surgery center, or clinic. As insurance companies continue to recognize the cost-effectiveness of performing minor surgical procedures in these settings, the role of the medical assistant continues to expand.

Patients should have absolute assurance that they are being taken care of in an aseptic atmosphere and under the most stringent aseptic conditions. This assurance is just as important for the protection of the office staff as it is for the patient. Allowing the provider to assume the correct aseptic techniques have been used in the preparation of equipment and allowing him or her to use contaminated equipment on a patient can result in claims of malpractice and charges of battery. Absolute, uncompromising honesty on the part of the assistant builds self-respect and contributes to professional achievement and satisfaction.

To have a good understanding of the subject, you must become familiar with the various techniques of sanitization, disinfection, and sterilization. Ignorance or carelessness can be dangerous and is inexcusable before the law.

The medical assistant must know what procedure is scheduled and whether the patient has been informed about the procedure. In the surgical setting, the medical assistant must realize the full extent of his or her role as the patient's advocate and the physician's agent.

Confirm that the provider has explained the procedure to the patient and that the patient fully understands all aspects of the procedure to be performed. This means that when patients sign the informed consent for surgery, they are fully informed. Legal action can result if complications arise because of failure to complete consent forms. The surgical procedure is expedited when the patient is given instructions and knows what to expect. Increasing the patient's understanding ensures greater compliance with presurgical preparations, and the patient is more likely to follow instructions and advice after surgery.

The medical assistant must practice perfect aseptic technique. A break in technique may invite infection and possible legal action. It is the medical assistant's duty to protect the patient. A major responsibility of the medical assistant is to adhere strictly to aseptic technique and to correct immediately any break in technique.

Patient-Centered Care

A medical assistant's duty may include calling the patient the day before surgery to confirm the scheduled surgical procedure and appointment time. Explaining the procedure and what to expect during and after surgery prepares the patient and helps calm the person's fears or concerns. Lying still during surgery is important, and eating a light meal the night before should be encouraged. Bathing before coming to the office reduces the number of bacteria on the skin, and the patient should wear comfortable, loose clothing. Sometimes during general conversation, the medical assistant can pick up hints of concerns the patient may have and direct the conversation into a discussion of these concerns.

Patients should be informed that they may need someone to accompany them home. A bandage is applied after surgery, and it must be kept clean and dry. The patient may have some pain, and the provider will probably prescribe some type of analgesic. After the procedure is complete, make sure the patient makes an appointment for a return visit and examination. Patients should also be encouraged to call the office immediately if they suspect an infection or have a sudden increase in pain at the surgical site.

Professional Behaviors

Accountability is a crucial part of the medical assistant's professional responsibilities. An accountable individual recognizes if an error has been committed and does everything possible to correct his or her mistake. Personal accountability and discipline are the primary concerns in surgical asepsis. Often the assistant is alone when performing a surgical aseptic procedure; if contamination occurs, no one may know except the medical assistant. If there is any doubt about the sterility of the surgical field, instruments, or supplies, or if sterile technique is broken in any way, it is the assistant's responsibility to begin the procedure again. There is no room for compromise.

SUMMARY OF SCENARIO

Callie is finding her clinical medical assisting position at the Walden-Martin Family Medical Clinic to be rewarding, exciting, and challenging. She enjoys coming to work every day and has learned all aspects of her position much more quickly than most of her peers. Callie frequently reads the latest information on new developments in the practice of minor surgery. Her concern for her patients' well-being makes her stand out, and the providers constantly get positive comments on her level of professionalism.

Callie has made a few errors in sterile technique since starting the clinical assistant position, but she has learned from each situation and has never covered up a mistake. Whenever she realized that she did not follow procedure, she discussed the issue with her supervisor and Dr. Perez. In this way, errors can be corrected, if possible, and she most likely will not make the same or similar mistakes again.

Callie is a team player who consistently tries to anticipate the needs of the provider and patient both before and during surgery. Her cooperative, supportive manner is appreciated by everyone on the clinical staff.

SUMMARY OF LEARNING OBJECTIVES

1. **Examine the basic types of minor surgical procedures performed in the ambulatory care setting.**
   Typical minor surgical procedures include incision and drainage (I&D) of a cyst; electrosurgery, which uses a high-frequency current to cut through tissue and coagulate blood vessels; laser surgery, which uses tiny light beams to safely treat specific tissues with minimal damage to surrounding tissues and limited scar formation; microsurgery, which involves the use of an operating microscope to perform delicate surgical procedures; endoscopic procedures, which use a fiberoptic instrument with a miniature camera mounted on a flexible tube to examine the area within an organ or cavity and which are named according to the organs or areas they explore; and cryosurgery, which is the use of extreme cold to destroy tissues such as warts and skin lesions.
2. **Examine the preparation needed for surgical procedures.**
   The medical assistant is responsible for preparing the patient for surgery, performing the physician's preoperative orders, confirming that the patient has signed an informed consent form, making sure all the patient's questions and concerns have been addressed, assisting with positioning the patient, performing skin preparation if ordered, and preparing the room for the procedure.

Continued

SUMMARY OF LEARNING OBJECTIVES—*continued*

Refer to Procedure 25.1 for the steps to follow when performing a skin prep for surgery.

A surgical hand scrub is done to lower the number of transient floras on the practitioner's hands and reduce the risk of wound contamination (see Procedure 25.2).

3. **Examine the role of the medical assistant when assisting with surgical procedures.**
Sterile surfaces must never come in contact with nonsterile surfaces. If this occurs, the sterile surface immediately is considered contaminated. The rules for maintaining a sterile field include (1) keep talking to a minimum, (2) maintain sight of the sterile field, and (3) never cross over the sterile field. Anything that falls below the edge of the Mayo tray and within a 1-inch border surrounding the tray is considered contaminated. A sterile barrier that is wet, cut, or torn is contaminated. Sterile gloved hands must be kept above waist level at all times. An item is never removed from and then again put into the field. A sterile package should be opened the entire way and the contents tossed onto the field without crossing over the sterile area. If a sterile package falls to the floor, it must be discarded. If any doubt exists about sterility, the field must be considered contaminated, and the process must start all over again.
   - Put on sterile gloves without contaminating them. Refer to Procedure 25.3.
   - Open a sterile pack and create a sterile field. Refer to Procedure 25.4.
   - Transfer sterile instruments and pour solutions into a sterile field. Refer to Procedure 25.4.
   - Perform a two-person sterile tray setup. Refer to Procedure 25.5.

   The physician is responsible for the patient; however, the medical assistant is responsible for ensuring that everything the assistant and the physician will use in caring for the surgical patient is accounted for, ready to use, and prepared in a safe and sterile manner. Refer to Procedures 25.6 and 25.7.

   If medication is prescribed, review the purpose of the medication and directions for its use with the patient and his or her companion, and make a follow-up appointment. The patient should be taught to care for himself or herself at home after surgery and receive both verbal and written instructions. Explain to the patient the importance of calling the office if any questions arise or if he or she notes redness around the operative site, bleeding from the wound, fever, swelling, or increasing or severe pain. If the patient does not call within the next 24 hours, the medical assistant should call the patient.

   Refer to Procedure 25.8 for the steps to follow when removing sutures and surgical staples.
4. **Examine the wound healing process and how wounds should be cared for.**
All wounds go through a healing or repair process that has three phases. The lag phase occurs first when the blood vessels contract to control hemorrhage, platelets form a fibrin network, and a clot dries into a scab. Proliferation is a new growth period during which tissues repair themselves. During the final, or remodeling, phase, a bridge of new tissue is built to close the gap of the wound. Collagen gives the wounded tissues strength and forms scar tissue. Wounds are classified by the way they repair themselves: either by first intention, with clean, straight edges that heal quickly, or by granulation (or second intention), as occurs in tissues that are severely damaged and are left open or fail to close.

   Refer to Procedure 25.7 to properly apply dressings and bandages to surgical sites. Refer to Procedure 25.8 to properly apply an elastic support bandage.

PROCEDURE 25.1 Perform Skin Prep for Surgery

TASK: Prepare the patient's skin and remove hair from the surgical site to reduce the risk of wound contamination.

EQUIPMENT and SUPPLIES

Disposable skin prep kit, or collect the following:
- Gauze
- Cotton-tipped applicators
- Soap
- Gloves
- Electric clippers
- Two small bowls
- Antiseptic or antiseptic swabs (e.g., Betadine swabs)
- Sterile normal saline solution
- Optional: cotton balls, nail pick, scrub brush
- Sterile drape
- Biohazard waste/sharps containers
- Patient's record

PROCEDURAL STEPS

1. Wash hands or use hand sanitizer.
PURPOSE: To follow Standard Precautions.
2. Greet the patient. Identify yourself. Verify the patient's identity with full name and date of birth. Explain the procedure to be performed in a manner that the patient understands. Answer any questions the patient may have about the procedure.
PURPOSE: To ensure cooperation and demonstrate awareness of possible patient concerns.
3. Ask the patient to remove any clothing that might interfere with exposure of the site and provide a gown if needed.
4. Assist the patient into the proper position for site exposure. Provide a drape if necessary to protect the patient's privacy.
5. Expose the site. Use a light if necessary.

PROCEDURE 25.1 Perform Skin Prep for Surgery— *continued*

6. If hair is present, the area may need to be shaved. Put on gloves and shave the required area with electric clippers.
   PURPOSE: Hair should be removed before any invasive procedure to limit the potential for infection; follow Standard Precautions regarding sharps.
7. While wearing gloves, open the skin prep pack and add the soap to the two bowls.
8. Start at the incision site and begin washing with the soap on a gauze sponge in a circular motion, moving from the center to the edges of the area to be scrubbed (see the following figure).
   PURPOSE: A circular motion from inside to outside drags contaminants away from the incision site.

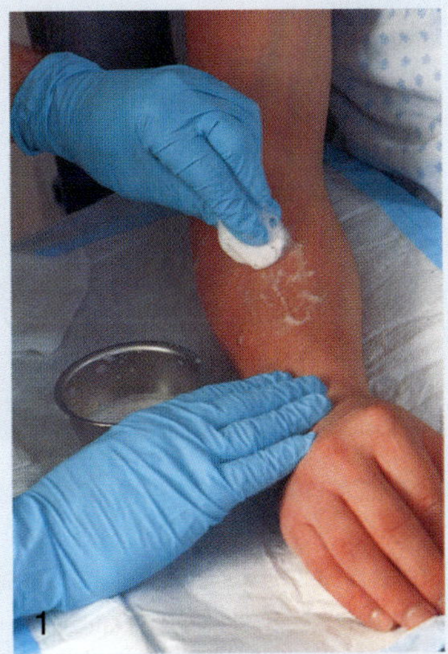

9. After one complete wipe, discard the sponge and begin again with a new sponge soaked in the antiseptic solution.
   PURPOSE: After one circular sweep, the sponge is contaminated with skin bacteria and debris.
10. Repeat the process, using sufficient friction, for 5 minutes (or follow office policy for the length of time required for a particular prep).
11. Rinse the area with sterile normal saline solution (see the following figure).

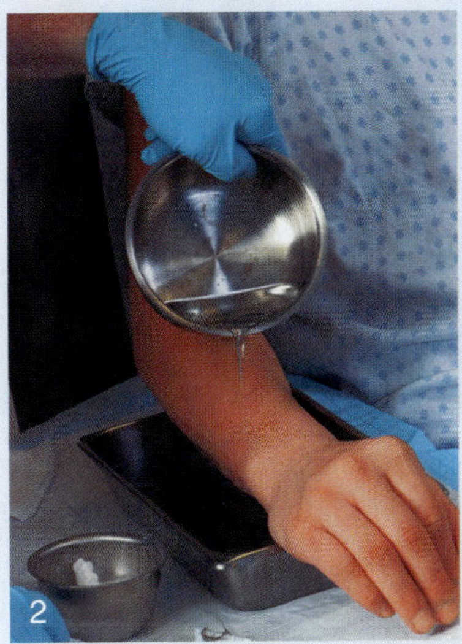

12. Dry the area using the same circular technique with dry sponges. The area may be dried by blotting with a sterile towel.
13. Paint on the antiseptic with the cotton-tipped applicators or gauze sponges, using the same circular technique and never returning to an area that has already been painted.
14. Place a sterile drape or towel over the area.
15. Answer all the patient's questions to relieve anxiety about the upcoming surgical procedure.
16. Document completion of the skin prep in the patient's health record.

PROCEDURE 25.2 Perform a Surgical Hand Scrub

TASK: Scrub the hands with surgical soap, using friction, running water, and a disposable sterile brush to sanitize the skin before assisting with any procedure that requires surgical asepsis.

EQUIPMENT and SUPPLIES

- Sink with foot, knee, or arm control for running water
- Surgical soap in a dispenser
- Towels (sterile towels if indicated by office policy)
- Nail file or orange stick
- Sterile disposable brush

PROCEDURAL STEPS

1. Remove all jewelry.
   PURPOSE: Jewelry harbors bacteria and is not permitted in surgical asepsis.
2. Roll long sleeves above the elbows.
3. Inspect your fingernails for length and your hands for skin breaks.
4. Turn on the faucet and regulate the water to a comfortable temperature, being careful to stand away from the sink to prevent contamination of clothing from contact with the sink or countertop.
5. Keep your hands upright and held at or above waist level (see the following figure).
   PURPOSE: Water running from the unscrubbed area above the elbow to the hands can carry bacteria back onto the hands. All areas below the waist are considered contaminated during all surgical procedures.

Continued

PROCEDURE 25.2 Perform a Surgical Hand Scrub—*continued*

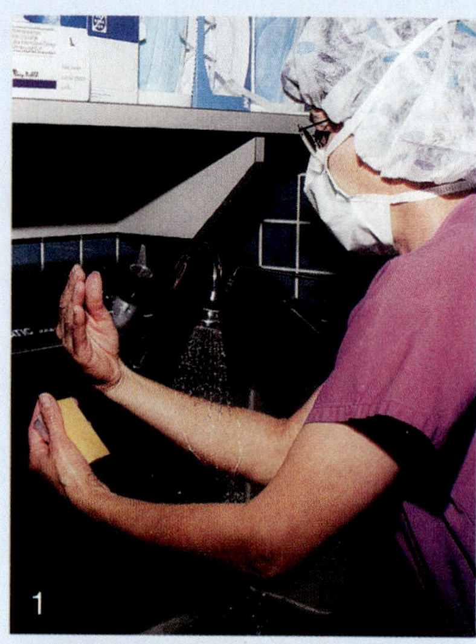
1

6. Clean your fingernails with a file, discard it (in most situations, you will drop the file into the sink and discard it later to prevent contamination by lowering your hands or touching a waste receptacle), and rinse your hands under the faucet without touching the faucet or the inside of the sink basin (see the following figure).

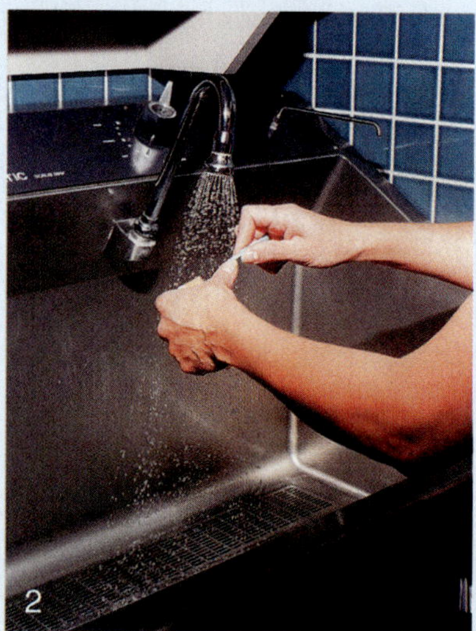
2

7. Allow the water to run over your hands from the fingertips to the elbows without moving the arm back and forth under the water.
   PURPOSE: Water running from the elbow to the hands can carry bacteria back onto the hands.
8. Apply surgical soap from the dispenser to the sterile brush (or use a prepared disposable brush) and start the scrub by scrubbing the palm of the hand in a circular fashion.
9. Continue from the palm to the base of the thumb, then move on to the other fingers, scrubbing from the base, along each side, and across the nail, holding the fingertips upward and remembering to rub between the fingers (see the following figure). After the fingers have been completely scrubbed, clean the posterior surface of the hand in a circular fashion and then proceed to the wrist. The scrub process should take at least 5 minutes for each hand and arm.
   PURPOSE: The surfaces of the fingers have four sides that all need to be thoroughly cleaned.

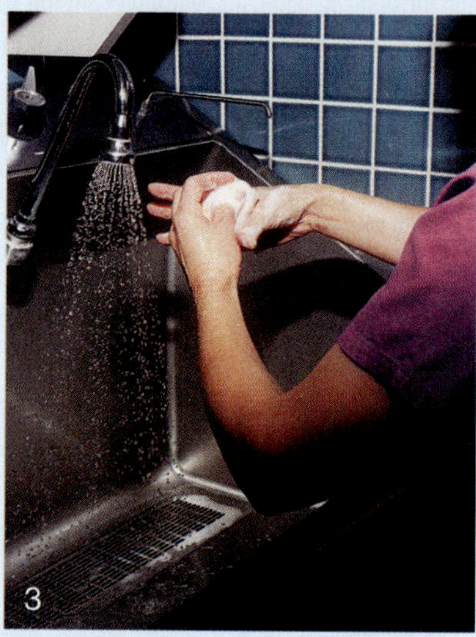
3

10. Do not return to a clean area after you have moved to the next part of the hand.
    PURPOSE: Once an area has been scrubbed, it is considered surgically clean, and rubbing that area again contaminates it.
11. Wash the wrists and forearms in a circular fashion around the arm while holding your hands above waist level (see the following figure).

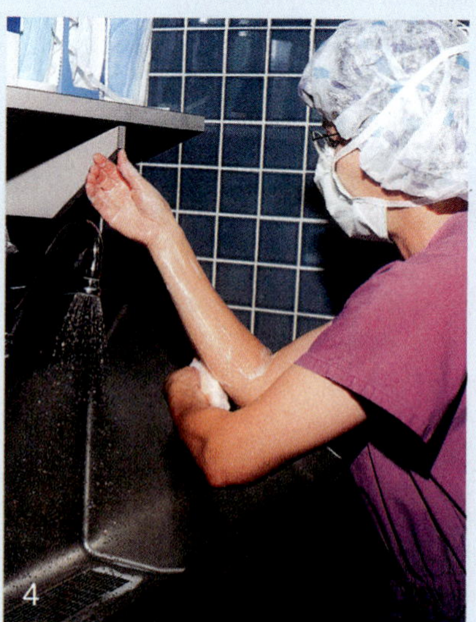
4

PROCEDURE 25.2 Perform a Surgical Hand Scrub—*continued*

12. Rinse the arms and forearms from the fingertips upward, holding the fingers up, without touching the faucet or the inside of the sink basin (see the following figure).
PURPOSE: Keep the fingers higher than the rest of the arm to prevent contamination from water running down from the elbow. Touching the dirty faucet or basin causes contamination.

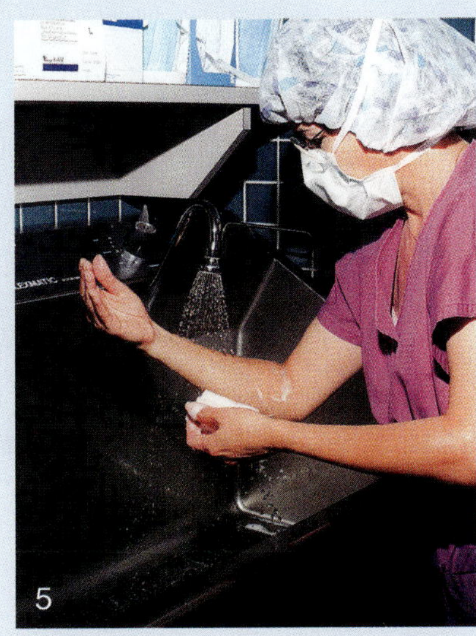

13. Apply more solution without touching any dirty surface, and repeat the scrub on the other side, remembering to wash and use friction between each finger with a firm, circular motion.
14. Scrub all surfaces, being careful not to abrade your skin. The second hand and arm should take at least 5 minutes.
15. Rinse thoroughly, keeping your hands up and above waist level. Discard the scrub brush without lowering the arms below the waist (see the following figures).

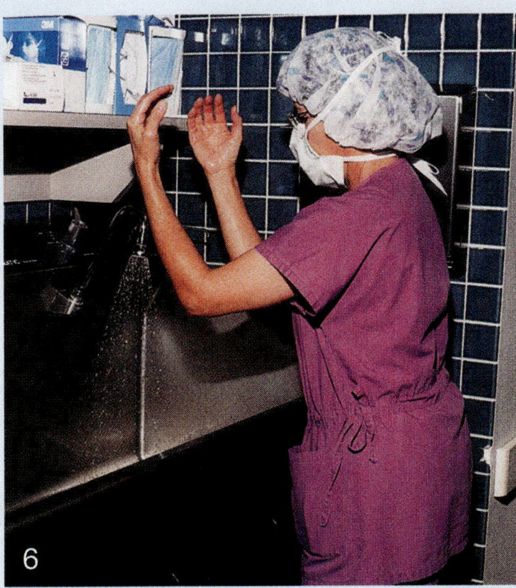

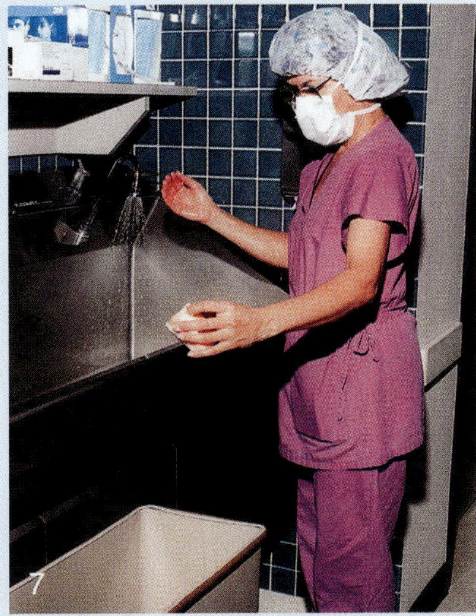

16. Turn off the faucet with the foot, knee, or forearm lever, if available.
PURPOSE: To prevent clean hands from touching the contaminated faucet handles.
17. Dry your hands with a sterile towel, being careful to keep the fingers pointing upward and your hands above the waist. Do not rub back and forth, dragging contaminants from the dirtier area of the upper arm down toward the hands (see the following figures). Use the opposite end of the towel for the other hand.
PURPOSE: To keep your clean hands from touching the part of the towel that comes in contact with your forearms, which are not as clean as your hands. If you are to gown and glove for a procedure, you must use a sterile towel.

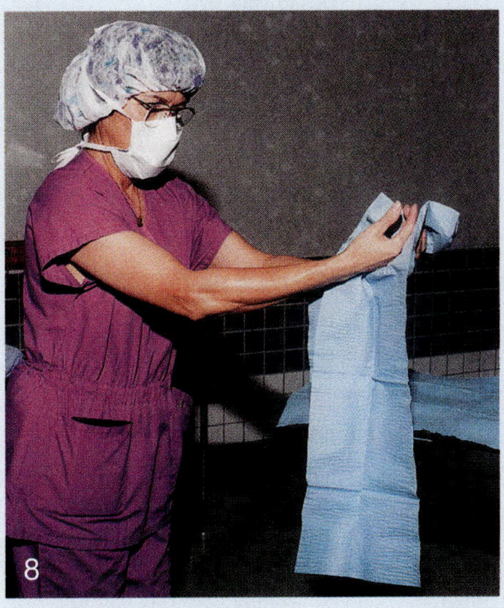

Continued

PROCEDURE 25.2 Perform a Surgical Hand Scrub—*continued*

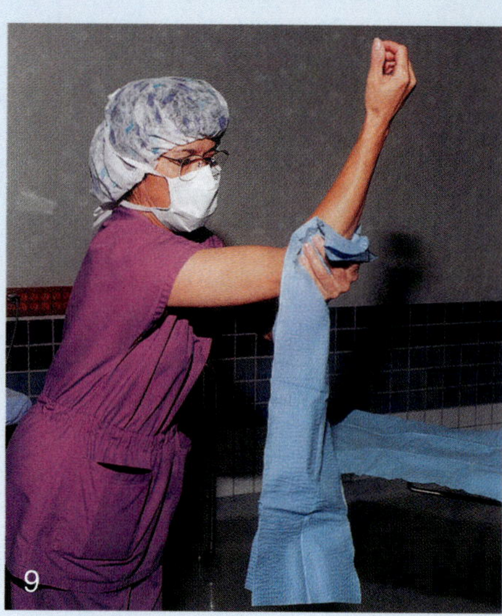

9

18. Using a patting motion, continue to dry the forearms. Discard the towel and keep your hands up and above waist level (see the following figure).

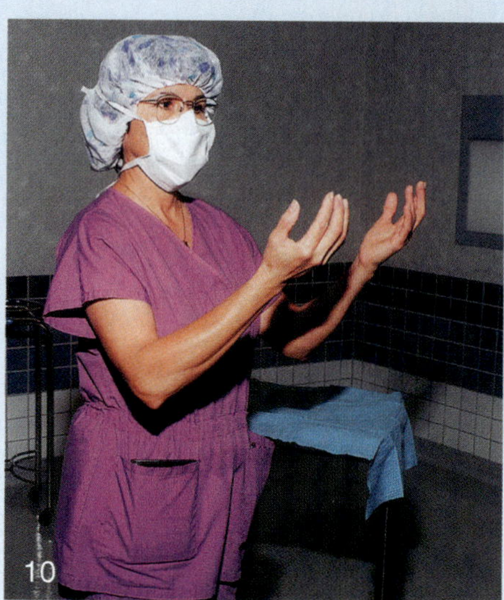

10

PROCEDURE 25.3 Put on Sterile Gloves

TASK: Put on sterile gloves correctly before performing sterile procedures.

EQUIPMENT and SUPPLIES

- Pair of packaged sterile gloves in your size

PROCEDURAL STEPS

1. Perform the surgical hand scrub as explained in Procedure 25.2 before putting on sterile gloves.
2. Open the glove pack, being careful not to cross over the open area in the middle of the pack. Remember, a 1-inch area around the perimeter of the glove wrapper is considered not sterile.
   PURPOSE: The open glove pack is a sterile field.
3. Glove your dominant hand first.
   PURPOSE: This sets up your dominant hand to do the more difficult step, which is to put on the second glove.
4. With your nondominant hand, pick up the glove for your dominant hand with your thumb and forefinger, grabbing the edge of the folded cuff closest to you, which is the inside of the glove, being careful not to cross over the other sterile glove (see the following figure).
   PURPOSE: The inside of the glove will be next to your skin and is considered not sterile.

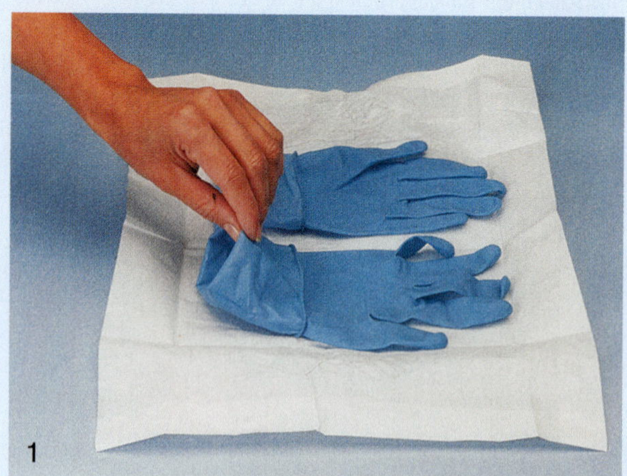

1

5. Lift the glove up and away from the sterile package.
   PURPOSE: To prevent accidental contamination from touching the glove on the 1-inch area around the perimeter of the glove wrapper.
6. Hold your hands up and away from your body and the sterile field (containing the other glove). Slide the dominant hand into the glove (see the following figure).

PROCEDURE 25.3 Put on Sterile Gloves—*continued*

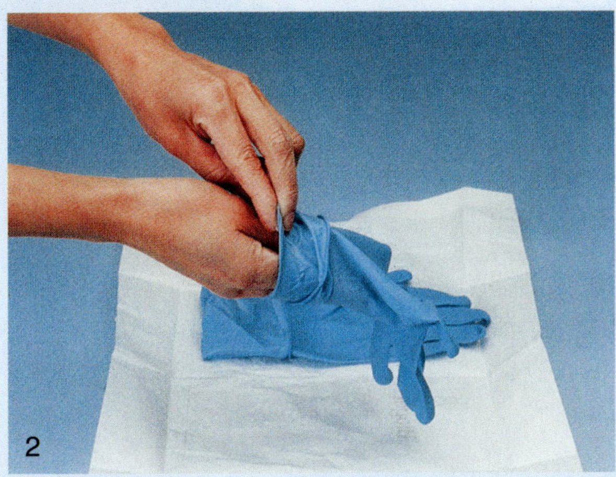

7. Leave the cuff folded (see the following figure).
PURPOSE: You will unfold the cuff later.

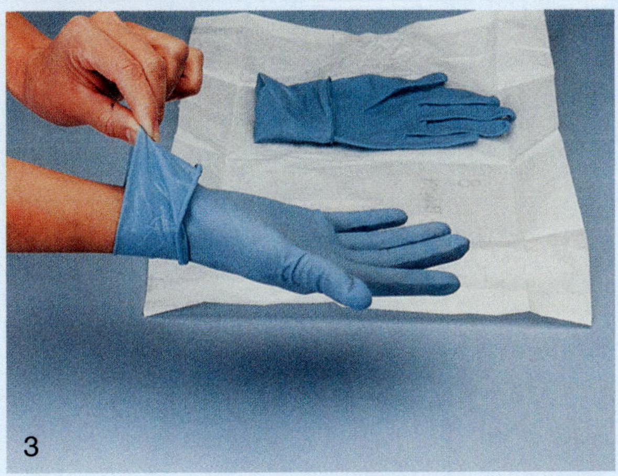

8. With your gloved dominant hand, pick up the second glove by slipping your gloved fingers into the cuff, extending the thumb up and away from the glove (thumbs up position), so that your gloved fingers touch only the outside of the second glove (see the following figure).
PURPOSE: Sterile surfaces must always touch sterile surfaces.

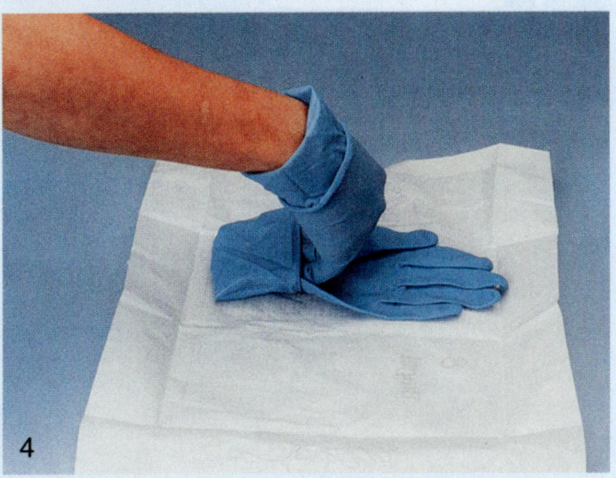

9. Slide your nondominant hand into the glove without touching the exterior of the glove or any part of the gloved hand (see the following figures).

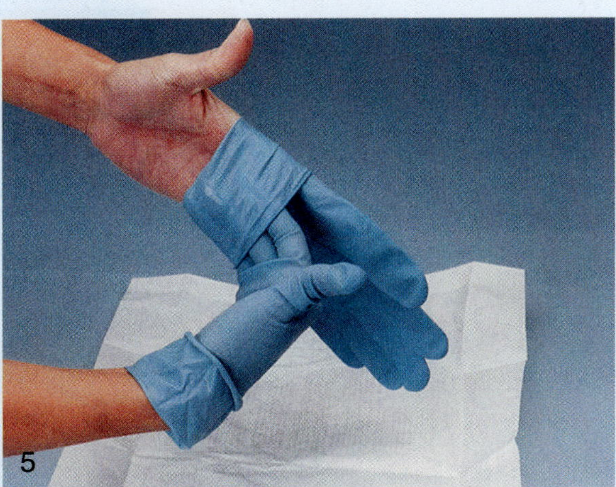

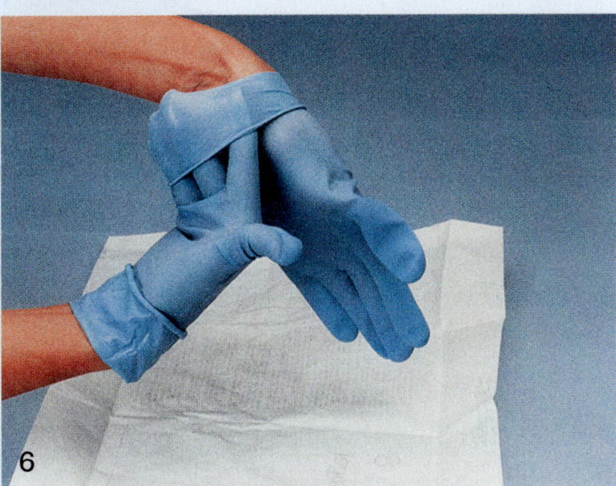

10. Still holding your hands away from you, unroll the cuff by slipping the fingers into the cuff and gently pulling up and out. Do not touch your bare arm or the internal surface of the glove with any part of the sterile glove (see the following figure).

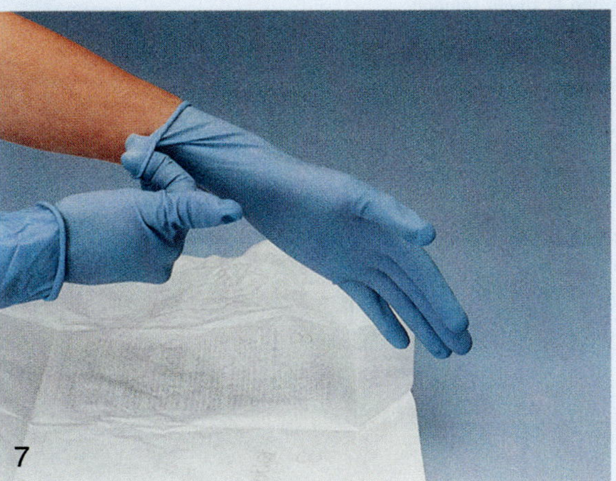

Continued

PROCEDURE 25.3 Put on Sterile Gloves—*continued*

11. Now, slip your gloved fingers up under the first cuff and unroll it, using the same technique (see the following figure).

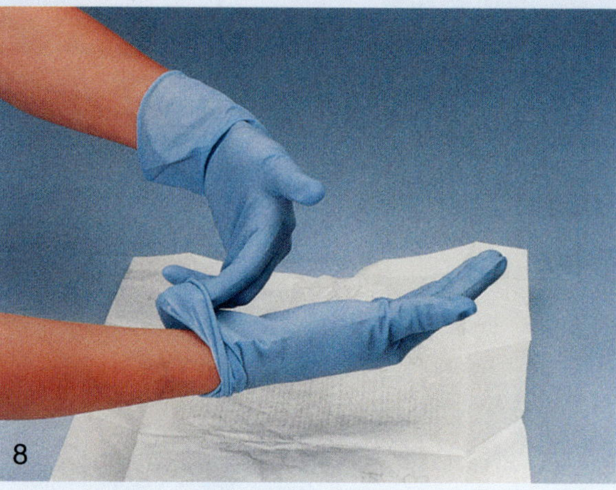

PROCEDURE 25.4 Prepare a Sterile Field, Use Transfer Forceps, and Pour a Sterile Solution Into a Sterile Field

TASKS: Open a sterile instrument pack using correct aseptic technique and create a sterile field; move sterile items on a sterile field or transfer sterile items to a gloved team member; pour a sterile solution into a sterile stainless steel bowl or container sitting at the edge of a sterile field.

EQUIPMENT and SUPPLIES

- A sterile instrument pack wrapped with autoclave paper that, when opened, will serve as a sterile table drape or field
- Mayo stand or countertop
- Disinfectant and gauze sponges or disinfectant wipes
- Sterile item to move or transfer
- Sterile wrapped transfer forceps
- Bottle of sterile solution
- Sterile bowl or container
- Sink or waste receptacle

PROCEDURAL STEPS

1. Check that the Mayo stand or countertop is dust free and clean. If it is not, disinfect and allow to air-dry.
   PURPOSE: Although some areas cannot be sterile, steps must be taken to keep contamination to a minimum; moisture on a tray contaminates the pack.
2. Wash your hands or use hand sanitizer and make sure they are completely dry. If you will be assisting with a surgical procedure immediately after opening the sterile pack, perform the surgical hand scrub as explained in Procedure 25.2.
   PURPOSE: To reduce the number of transient floras on your hands and forearms; moisture on your hands contaminates the pack.
3. Gather supplies. Check the label of the ordered solution. Check the solution name and the expiration date.
4. If using an autoclaved pack, check the indicator tape for a color change.
   PURPOSE: Autoclave indicator tape changes color after the sterile processing cycle.
5. Open the outside cover (see the following figure). Position the package so that the outer envelope flap is at the top and the tab facing you.
   PURPOSE: This positions the pack for correct opening so that you do not have to cross over the sterile pack to open it.

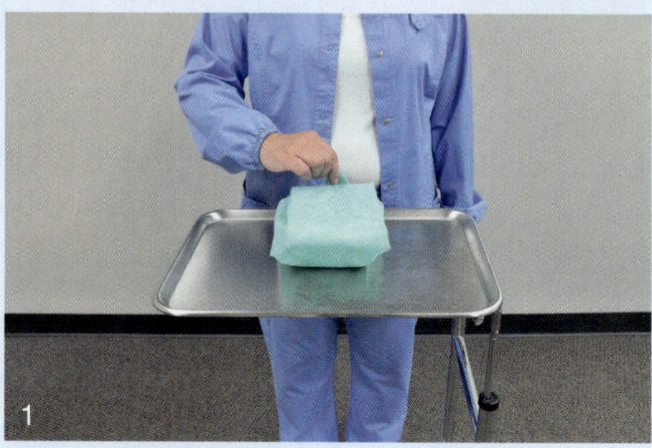

PROCEDURE 25.4 Prepare a Sterile Field, Use Transfer Forceps, and Pour a Sterile Solution Into a Sterile Field—*continued*

6. Open the outermost flap (see the following figure). Next, open the first flap away from you. You can cross over the uncovered portion of the Mayo stand because it is not sterile. Do not cross over the pack.

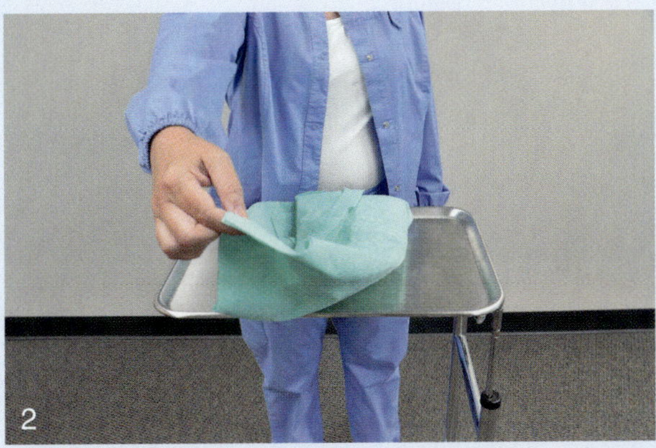

2

7. Open the second corner, pulling to the side (see the following figure).
   PURPOSE: To prevent contamination of the sterile field.

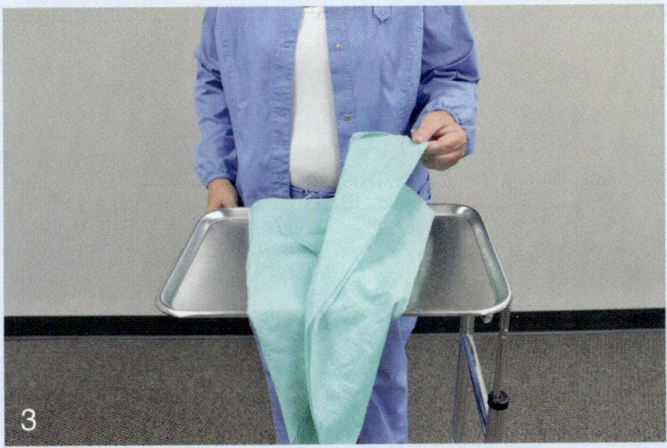

3

8. Be careful to lift the flaps by touching only the small, folded-back tab and without touching or crossing over the inner surface of the pack or its contents. Open the remaining two corners of the pack (see the following figure).

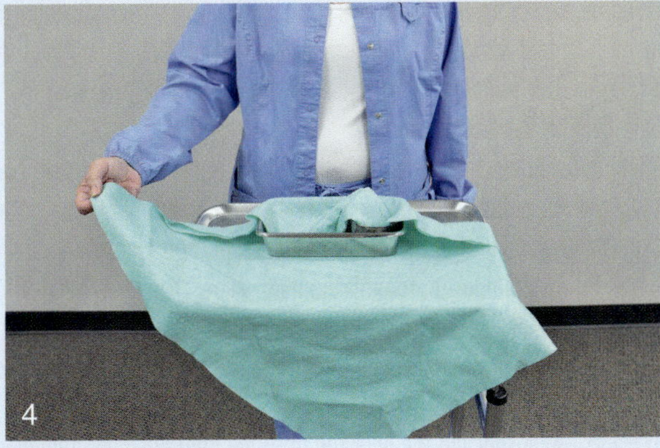

4

9. You now have a sterile drape as a sterile field from which to work and for the distribution of additional sterile supplies and instruments (see the following figure).

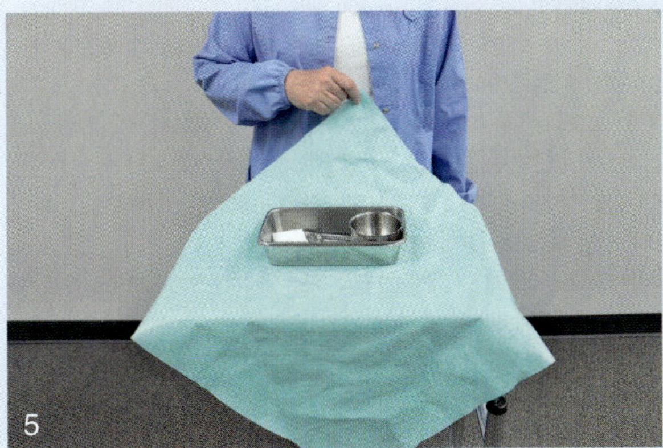

5

10. Open a package containing sterile transfer forceps (see the following figure). Using sterile technique, handle the sterile forceps by the ring handle only. Always point the forceps tips down.
    PURPOSE: If the tips are turned upward, any solution encountered will run onto the nonsterile area and then back down over the sterile end when the tips are turned down again, thus contaminating the forceps.

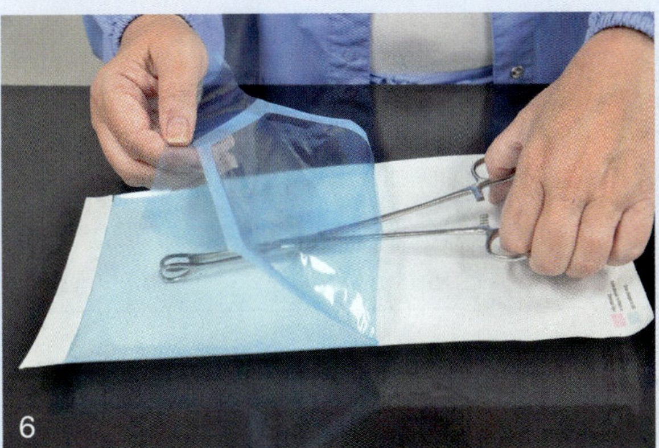

6

11. Grasp an item on the sterile field with the sterile forceps, points down, and move it to its proper position for the procedure, making sure not to cross the sterile field with the hand or contaminated end of the forceps (see the following figure).

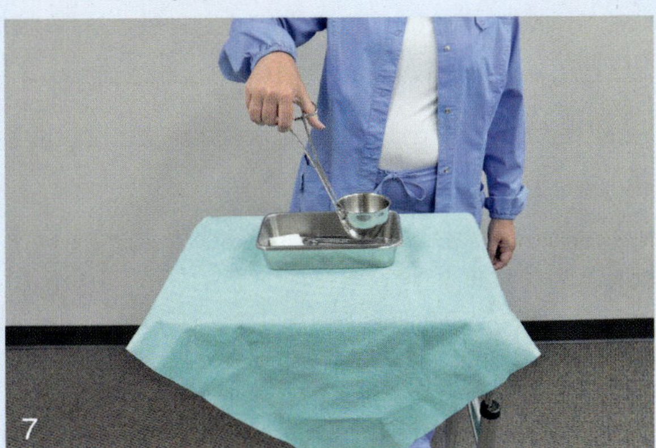

7

Continued

PROCEDURE 25.4 Prepare a Sterile Field, Use Transfer Forceps, and Pour a Sterile Solution Into a Sterile Field—*continued*

12. Set the forceps aside after one-time use.
 Note: The sterile bowl should be placed, using sterile transfer forceps, near one edge of the field and the perimeter of the 1-inch barrier.
13. Check the label of the ordered solution when first obtaining the solution.
 PURPOSE: Always perform the three label checks before administering any solution or medication.
14. Check the label of the solution for the second time. Place your hand over the label and lift the bottle.
 Note: If the container has a double cap, set the outer cap on the counter, inside up, and then proceed.
15. Lift the lid of the bottle straight up and then slightly to one side; hold the lid in your nondominant hand facing downward.
 PURPOSE: Air currents carry contaminants that could settle on the inside of the lid.
16. Pour away from the label without allowing any part of the bottle to touch the bowl and without crossing over the sterile field (see the following figure).
 PURPOSE: Spills down the side of the bottle can stain the label or make it unreadable. The bottle exterior is not sterile, so it cannot pass over the sterile field.

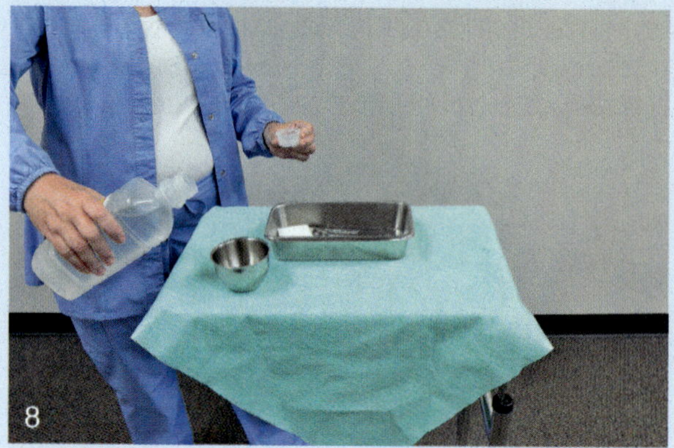

17. Tilt the bottle up to stop the pouring while it is still over the bowl.
 PURPOSE: Solutions spilled on the sterile field may contaminate the field.
18. Check the label of the solution for the third time. Replace the cap (or caps) off to the side, away from the sterile field, being careful not to touch and, therefore, contaminate the internal surface of the lid.

PROCEDURE 25.5 Two-Person Sterile Tray Setup

TASK: Perform a sterile tray setup for a cyst removal.

EQUIPMENT and SUPPLIES

- Sterile drape
- Sterile gloves
- In a sealed autoclave pouch: needle holder, operating scissors, tissue forceps, hemostatic forceps
- Suture material with needle
- Sterile 4 × 4s
- Disposable scalpel

Note: This procedure involves two people. One person will act as the nonsterile person, and the other will have on sterile gloves and place the items on the sterile tray.

PROCEDURAL STEPS

Nonsterile Person

1. Check that the Mayo stand or countertop is dust free and clean. If it is not, disinfect and allow to air-dry.
 PURPOSE: Although some areas cannot be sterile, steps must be taken to keep contamination to a minimum; moisture on a tray contaminates the pack.
2. Wash your hands or use hand sanitizer and make sure they are completely dry. If you will be assisting with a surgical procedure immediately after opening the sterile pack, perform the surgical hand scrub as explained in Procedure 25.2.
 PURPOSE: To reduce the number of transient floras on your hands and forearms; moisture on your hands contaminates the pack.
3. Place the package containing the sterile drape on a flat surface near the Mayo stand/tray. Check the integrity of the outer package. Open the package without touching the barrier field.
4. Pick up the barrier field by the corner as you move away from the table and allow it to unfold without touching anything else. Drape over the Mayo stand.
 PURPOSE: This maintains the sterility of the barrier field, creating the sterile field on the Mayo stand.
5. Inspect the sterile pack for holes and tears; discard if seen and start over. Slowly pull the sides of the peel pack of sterile 4 × 4s away from each other. Maintain control of the item inside the package by opening only enough for a sterile person to grab the item. Allow the sterile person to take the 4 × 4s. Inspect the package for holes, tears, and indicators before the sterile person places the item on the sterile field. Inspect and discard the wrapper.
 PURPOSE: By inspecting the package after the item has been removed, you can ensure that it is truly sterile.

PROCEDURE 25.5 Two-Person Sterile Tray Setup—*continued*

6. Slowly pull the sides of the peel pack of sutures away from each other. Maintain control of the item inside the package by opening only far enough for the sterile person to grab the item. Allow the sterile person to take the suture package. Inspect the package for holes, tears, and indicators before the sterile person places the item on the sterile field. Inspect and discard the wrapper.
7. Slowly pull the sides of the peel pack of a scalpel away from each other. Maintain control of the item inside the package by opening only far enough for the sterile person to grab the item. Allow the sterile person to take the scalpel. Inspect the package for holes, tears, and indicators before the sterile person places the item on the sterile field. Inspect and discard the wrapper.
8. Slowly pull the sides of the peel pack of instruments away from each other. Maintain control of the items inside the package by opening only far enough for the sterile person to grab the items. Allow the sterile person to take all of the instruments. Inspect the package for holes, tears, and indicators before the sterile person places the items on the sterile field. Inspect and discard the wrapper.

Sterile Person

1. Wash your hands or use hand sanitizer and make sure they are completely dry. If you will be assisting with a surgical procedure immediately after opening the sterile pack, perform the surgical hand scrub as explained in Procedure 25.2.
   PURPOSE: To reduce the number of transient floras on your hands and forearms; moisture on your hands contaminates the pack.
2. Put on sterile gloves as explained in Procedure 25.3.
3. Remove an item from a peel pack and maintain sterile technique.
4. After the nonsterile person has indicated that the peel pack has not been compromised, place the item on the sterile tray. Repeat for all items. Arrange items on the sterile tray.
5. Maintain the sterility of the sterile field and sterile supplies.

PROCEDURE 25.6 Assist with Minor Surgery

TASKS: Maintain the sterile field, and pass instruments in a prescribed sequence during a surgical procedure that involves making a surgical incision and removing a growth.

EQUIPMENT and SUPPLIES

- Open patient drape pack on the side counter
- Mayo stand covered with a sterile drape
- Packaged sterile gloves (two pairs)
- Needle and syringe for local anesthetic medication
- Vial of local anesthetic medication
- Sterile drape
- Disposable scalpel with No. 15 blade
- Tissue forceps
- Skin retractor
- Three hemostats
- Needle holder
- Supply of sterile gauze sponges
- Biohazard waste container
- Sharps container
- Needle with suture material
- Specimen cup
- Laboratory requisitions
- Patient's record

PROCEDURAL STEPS

1. Prep the patient's skin with surgical soap and antiseptic solution as explained in Procedure 25.1. Explain the prep procedure to the patient.
   PURPOSE: To ensure infection control and demonstrate awareness of possible patient concerns.
2. Perform the surgical hand scrub as explained in Procedure 25.2.
3. Instruct and prepare the patient for the procedure. Explain what will occur, what the patient should do during the procedure, how long the procedure will take, and what the patient will sense (e.g., feel, smell). Set up the sterile field with instruments and supplies (see the following figure).

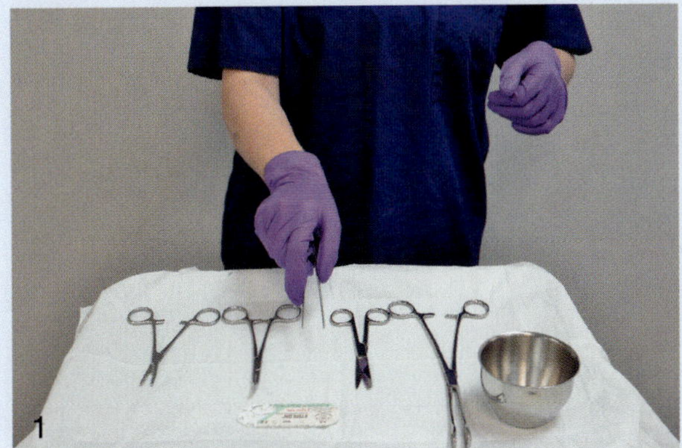
1

4. Position the Mayo stand near the patient and the operative site, making sure the patient understands not to touch the sterile field (see the following figure).

Continued

PURPOSE: To prevent contamination of supplies and provide easy access for the provider.

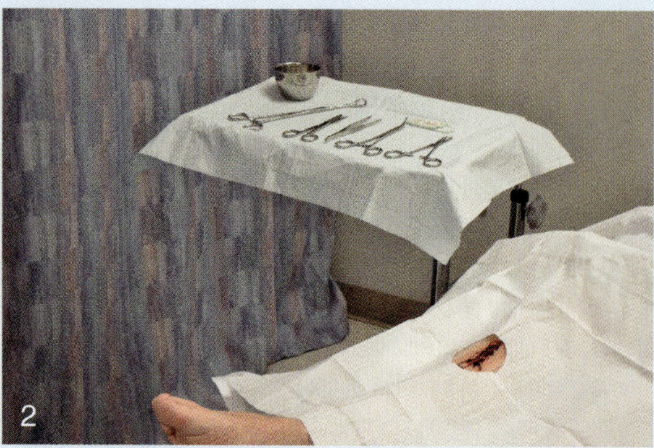
2

5. Put on sterile gloves using surgical technique.
6. Grasp the patient drape by holding one edge or corner in each hand (see the following figure).

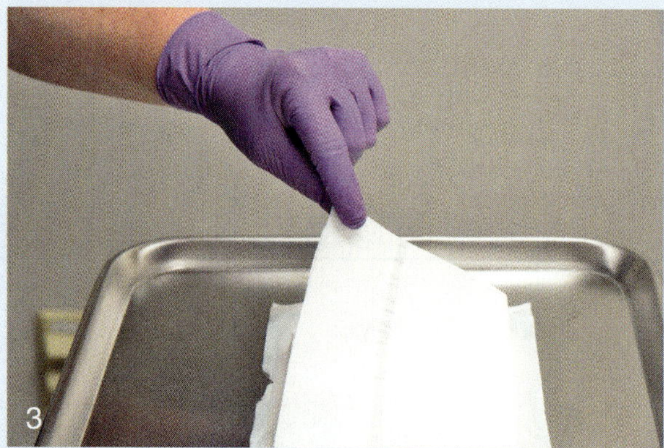
3

7. Drape the surgical site without touching any part of the patient or the operating area with your gloved hands.
8. If the provider requests medication, such as a local anesthetic, a second circulating assistant holds the vial of local anesthetic so that the provider can read the label. The provider withdraws the desired amount using sterile technique (see the following figure).
   PURPOSE: The vial of local anesthetic medication must be held by the second assistant away from the sterile field to prevent crossing over the field with a nonsterile item. The medication label must be checked before a medication is dispensed or administered.

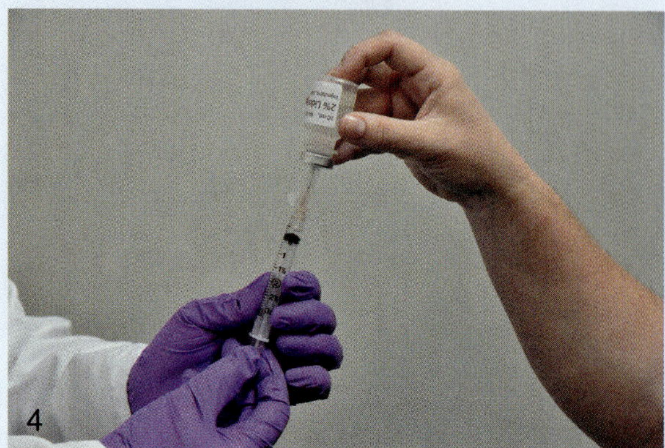
4

9. The provider injects the local anesthetic and waits a few minutes for it to take effect.
10. Position yourself across from the practitioner. Arrange the sterile field. Check the placement location on the Mayo stand (see the following figure).

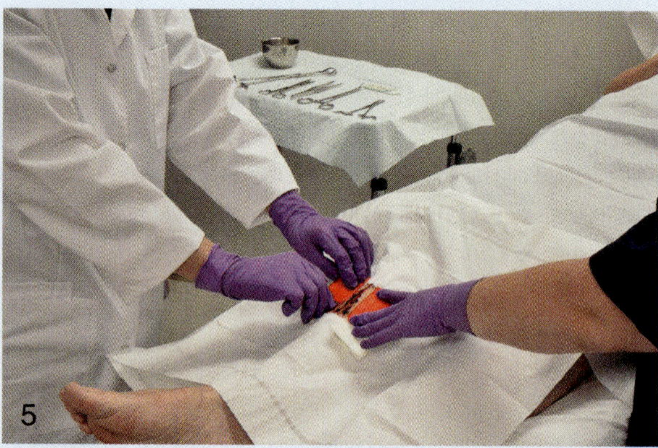
5

11. Keep all sharp equipment conspicuously placed on the sterile field.
    PURPOSE: Sharp instruments that are not clearly visible may injure a team member.
12. Pass the scalpel, blade down and handle first, to the provider, or the provider will reach for it. The provider will take the scalpel with the thumb and forefinger in the position ready for use (see the following figure).
    PURPOSE: To protect the practitioner and yourself from injury.

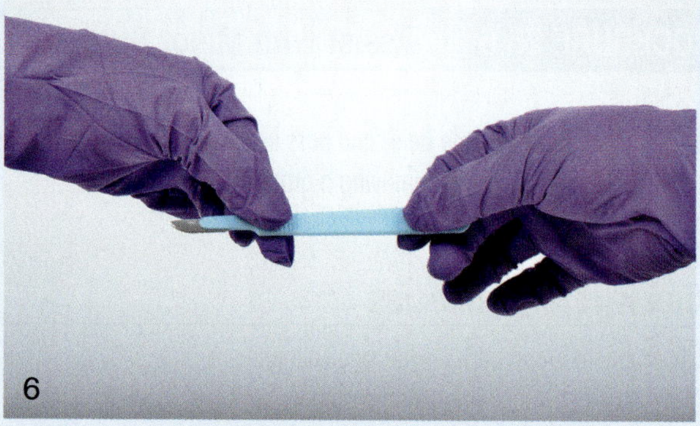
6

13. Pick up a tissue forceps by the tips and pass it to the provider to grasp a piece of the tissue to be excised (see the following figure).

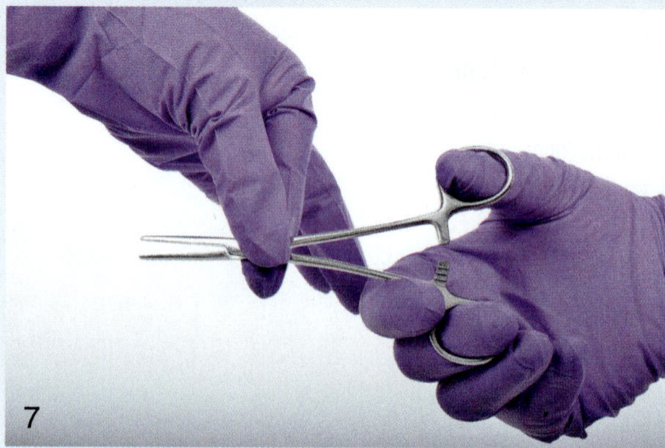
7

14. Dispose of soiled sponges in the biohazard waste container, being careful to keep your hands above your waist and avoid touching any nonsterile items.
15. Hold clean sponges in your hand to pat or sponge the wound as needed.
16. Safely position the specimen (if any) where it will not be disturbed in a sterile container on the sterile field.
17. If there is a bleeding vessel or a hemostat is requested, pass the hemostat in the manner described in step 13.

PROCEDURE 25.6 Assist with Minor Surgery—*continued*

18. Continue to sponge blood from the wound site.
19. Retract the wound edge, as needed, with a skin retractor.
20. Continue to monitor the sterile field and assist the provider as needed.
21. Pass the needle and suture material to close the wound, and apply a sterile dressing as requested (see the following figure).

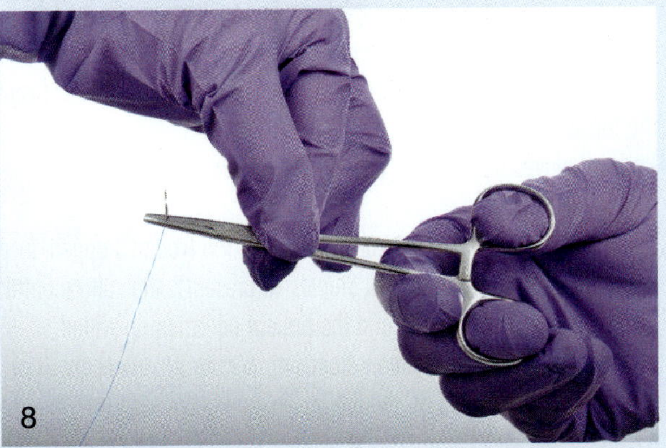

22. Monitor the patient and provide assistance as needed.
23. When the provider is finished, clean the surgical site using sterile technique.
24. Collect the specimen using Standard Precautions, place it in a labeled specimen cup, and send it to the laboratory with the proper requisitions.
25. Wash your hands or use hand sanitizer. Document the procedure, wound condition, and patient education on wound care.

PROCEDURE 25.7 Apply a Sterile Dressing

TASKS: Perform a dressing change. Apply a sterile dressing while maintaining aseptic technique. Instruct and prepare the patient for the procedure. Explain the rationale for the procedure.

PROVIDER'S ORDER: Change dressing and apply a sterile dressing. Culture wound drainage.

SCENARIO: Dr. Walden ordered a dressing change. You are to apply a sterile dressing after you obtain a culture of the wound drainage. As you are beginning the procedure, the patient asks you questions regarding personal protective equipment (PPE) and the reason for the wound culture. You need to explain the rationale for wearing PPE and why a wound culture is obtained.

DIRECTIONS: Role-play the scenario with a peer. The peer will be the patient, and you are the medical assistant. After the role-play, the rest of the procedure is done on a mannequin.

EQUIPMENT and SUPPLIES

- Gloves
- Biohazard waste container
- Sterile water or hydrogen peroxide (optional)
- Disposable ruler
- Culture swab
- Lab requisition, label, and plastic specimen bag for transport
- Sterile gloves
- Antiseptic swabs
- Sterile dressing and ABD pad
- Tape
- Mannequin with a wound
- Patient's record

PROCEDURAL STEPS

1. Wash your hands or use hand sanitizer. Assemble supplies on the Mayo stand/tray and place a biohazard waste container within easy reach.
   PURPOSE: To follow Standard Precautions.
2. Greet the patient. Identify yourself. Verify the patient's identity with full name and date of birth. Verify the patient's allergies.
3. Instruct and prepare the patient for the procedure. Explain the procedure to be performed in a manner that the patient understands. Explain what will occur, what the patient should do during the procedure, how long the procedure will take, and what the patient will sense (e.g., feel, smell). Answer any questions the patient may have about the procedure.
   PURPOSE: To ensure cooperation and demonstrate awareness of possible patient concerns.
   Scenario update: The patient questions why you need to change gloves so much during the procedure. She also asks why the wound culture needs to be done.
4. Based on the patient's comments, explain the reason for changing your gloves during the procedure and for the wound culture.
   PURPOSE: Demonstrates empathy and appropriate nonverbal communication while addressing the patient's questions and concerns.
   Scenario update: The rest of the steps are done on a mannequin.
5. Put on gloves. Loosen tape on the old bandage from the edges to the middle, toward the wound. Remove bandage and dressing, one at a

Continued

PROCEDURE 25.7 Apply a Sterile Dressing—*continued*

time. If the dressing is stuck, use a small amount of sterile water or hydrogen peroxide to loosen it.

PURPOSE: To follow Standard Precautions.

6. Check for drainage on the dressing and bandage. Note the color of the drainage. Measure any drainage using a disposable ruler, then discard everything in the biohazard waste container.
7. Assess the wound. If present, count the sutures or staples. Check if they are intact. Check the wound for signs of infection.
8. If the wound is open or redness or drainage is present, do the following:
   a. Culture the wound using a sterile swab (if ordered). The swab should be moved across the wound in a zig-zag motion from margin to margin. The swab should only touch the wound. Place in a culture transfer tube. Squeeze the tube to release formalin to preserve the specimen.
   b. Concisely and accurately report the relevant information (any issues with the wound or wound closures) to the provider. Ask the provider to check the wound before redressing.
9. Remove gloves and place them in a biohazard waste container.
10. Wash your hands or use hand sanitizer.
11. Open and arrange sterile supplies in the order they will be used. Apply the principles of sterile technique.
12. Put on sterile gloves. State that the nondominant hand will be nonsterile and the dominant hand will be sterile.
13. With the nondominant hand, pick up the antiseptic swab container. With the dominant hand, grasp an antiseptic swab without touching the package. Clean from the center of the wound to the edge; use one roll of the swab and discard it in the waste container. Start with a new swab where you left off with the previous swab. Continue until all the exudate is removed.

    PURPOSE: By cleaning from the center of the wound to the edge, you prevent contamination of the open wound.
14. With the dominant hand, remove the sterile dressing without touching the package. Place the sterile dressing material over the wound and cover the wound completely.
15. With the dominant hand, place an ABD pad over the dressing as a bandage.
16. Remove and discard the sterile gloves. Secure the bandage with tape.
17. Provide patient education as needed for wound care.
18. Complete the lab requisition for the culture. Put on gloves. Label the culture tube and place it in the plastic specimen bag for transport to the lab.
19. Clean up the area. Discard all biohazard waste in biohazard waste containers. Discard all other waste in the regular waste containers. Disinfect the tables.
20. Remove gloves and dispose of them appropriately. Wash hands or use hand sanitizer.
21. Using the patient's health record, document the wound's appearance, the number of intact sutures or staples (if present), the culture obtained, the wound care performed, and the patient education provided.
22. In the following written response section, discuss the implications of failing to comply with CDC regulations in healthcare settings.

Documentation Example

10/12/20XX 2:15 p.m.: Dressing change completed to wound on mid-forearm. Area slightly inflamed, mod amt serosanguineous drainage noted. Site cleansed and sterile dressing applied. Pt instructed on home wound care and to notify provider if drainage changes, inflammation increases, or fever occurs. ——————— Callie Casper, CMA (AAMA)

WRITTEN RESPONSE QUESTIONS

You fail to wear gloves when changing a patient's dressing. During the procedure, you get blood on your hands. Discuss the implications of failing to comply with CDC regulations in healthcare settings. Answer the following questions:

1. How might your action (i.e., not wearing gloves) affect the patient's health and safety?
2. How might your action (i.e., not wearing gloves) affect your health and safety?

PROCEDURE 25.8 Remove Sutures or Surgical Staples

TASK: Remove sutures or surgical staples from a healed incision using sterile technique without injuring the closed wound.

EQUIPMENT and SUPPLIES

Sterile suture removal kit containing the following:

- Suture removal scissors
- Gauze
- Thumb dressing forceps
- Wound closure strips or adhesive bandage strips (e.g., Band-Aids)
- Skin antiseptic swabs (e.g., Betadine swabs)
- Surgical staple remover with 4 × 4-inch gauze
- Biohazard waste/sharps container
- Sterile gloves
- Patient's record

PROCEDURAL STEPS

1. Wash your hands or use hand sanitizer. Assemble the necessary supplies.
2. Greet the patient. Identify yourself. Verify the patient's identity with full name and date of birth. Explain the procedure to be performed in a manner

PROCEDURE 25.8 Remove Sutures or Surgical Staples—*continued*

that the patient understands. Answer any questions the patient may have about the procedure. Instruct the person to lie or sit still during the procedure.
PURPOSE: To ensure cooperation during the procedure.

3. Position the patient comfortably and support the sutured area.
4. Place dry towels under the site.
5. Check the incision line to make sure the wound edges are approximated and there are no signs of infection, such as inflammation, edema, or drainage.
   PURPOSE: Sutures or staples should not be removed unless the site is completely healed with the wound edges together; infection at the site will interfere with the healing process; removing sutures or staples before the site is completely healed may result in the wound edges separating.
6. Put on gloves. Using antiseptic swabs, cleanse the wound to remove exudate and destroy microorganisms around the sutures or staples. Clean the site from the inside out, starting at the top of the wound and working your way down. Use a new swab if the step must be repeated. Remove gloves and discard.
   PURPOSE: Dried exudate on sutures or staples may make removing them without traumatizing the wound more difficult. Cleansing the wound reduces the possibility of wound infection.
7. Open the suture or staple removal pack while maintaining the sterility of the contents.
8. Place sterile gauze next to the wound site.
   PURPOSE: To receive the removed sutures or staples.
9. Put on sterile gloves.
10. Remove the sutures or staples.

To Remove Sutures

a. Grasp the knot of the suture with the dressing forceps without pulling.
b. Cut the suture at skin level.
c. Lift, do not pull, the suture toward the incision and out with the dressing forceps.
d. Place the suture on the sterile gauze sponge and check that the entire suture strand has been removed.

PURPOSE: Suture fragments left in a wound could cause irritation or infection and may prolong the healing process.

e. If any bleeding occurs, blot the area with a sterile gauze sponge before continuing.
f. Continue in the same manner until all sutures have been removed.

To Remove Staples

a. Gently place the bottom jaw of the staple remover under the first staple (see the following figure).

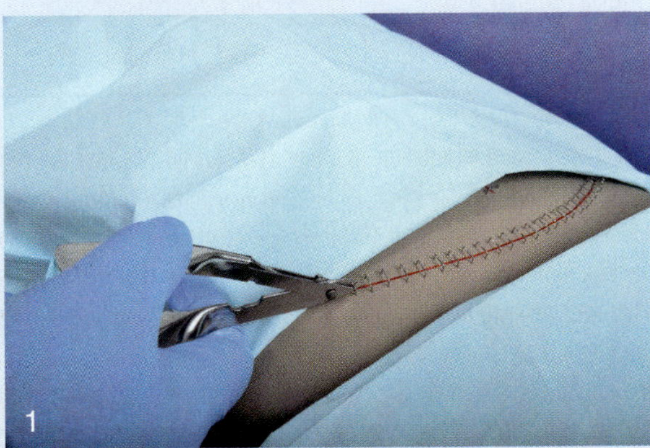

b. Tightly squeeze the staple handles together.
c. Carefully tilt the staple remover upward until the staple lifts out of the wound.
d. Place the removed staple on a 4 × 4-inch gauze square.
e. Continue the process until all staples have been removed.

11. Remove the gauze holding the sutures or staples. Dispose of the sutures in the biohazard waste container. Dispose of the staples in the biohazard sharps container.
12. The provider may apply or may have you apply wound closure strips or an adhesive bandage strip for added support, strength, and protection.
13. Instruct the patient to keep the wound edges clean and dry and not to place excessive strain on the area.
14. Document the procedure, wound condition, number of sutures or staples removed, whether a dressing or bandage was applied, and the instructions on wound care given to the patient.
    PURPOSE: A procedure that is not documented was not done.

Documentation Example

07/30/20XX 10:20 a.m.: Pt in for suture removal. The edges of the wound are well approximated with 5 intact sutures. There is no sign of infection. The site was cleaned with Betadine, and 5 sutures were removed. Pt instructed on home wound care and to notify provider if drainage changes, inflammation increases, or fever occurs ——————————
—————————————— Callie Casper, CMA (AAMA)

PRINCIPLES OF ELECTROCARDIOGRAPHY 26

SCENARIO

Renee Thomas, a certified medical assistant (CMA) who has met the requirements of the American Association of Medical Assistants (AAMA), is working at Walden-Martin Family Medical (WMFM) Clinic. According to her manager, over the time that she has been at WMFM Clinic, she has excelled. Because of Renee's professionalism and attention to detail, her manager, Sue, has asked her to mentor a new employee, Eva Ning.

Eva Ning, a registered medical assistant (RMA), just graduated from a local medical assistant program. She really enjoyed the hands-on learning with the skills. During her clinical experience for school, she worked in a cardiology department for 6 weeks and enjoyed the experience. Now that she has graduated, she looks forward to learning on the job.

Eva and Renee will spend a month with each provider. This month they are working with Dr. David Kahn, who sees many older patients. Renee tells Eva that they will be doing a lot of cardiac tests and treatments. Eva looks forward to learning from Renee and Dr. Kahn.

While studying this chapter, think about the following questions:

- What are the components of an ECG tracing?
- Where are the electrodes placed on the body for a 12-lead ECG?
- How can a medical assistant obtain a clear ECG?
- What are the different types of artifacts? Why does each type of artifact occur? What can the medical assistant do to prevent the artifact?
- What are other types of ECG tests?

LEARNING OBJECTIVES

1. Examine the structure of the heart, along with the blood flow through the heart.
2. Examine the heart's conduction system.
3. Analyze the components of an ECG tracing of the cardiac cycle.
4. Examine the three types of leads in a 12-lead ECG.
5. Examine ECG supplies, including the paper and electrodes.
6. Examine the features, settings, and maintenance of electrocardiographs (ECG machines).
7. Examine the medical assistant's role in obtaining an ECG tracing.
8. Analyze artifact, including the appearance, cause, and corrective action.
9. Examine how to evaluate an ECG tracing.
10. Differentiate between an exercise stress test and a nuclear stress test.
11. Differentiate among types of remote ECG monitoring.

VOCABULARY

arrhythmia (ah RITH mee ah) An abnormal heart rate or rhythm.

artifact A substance, structure, or event that does not naturally occur in a situation. Examples include interference, or electrical "garbage" on an ECG, or crystals, lint, or contamination of a staining technique.

bipolar Having two poles or electrical charges.

caliper A pocket-sized tool used for measuring the height and width of the ECG waves and intervals.

dextrocardia (dek stro KAHR dee ah) The condition in which the heart is located on the right side of the chest, and the apex is pointing to the right.

echocardiography (ECHO) (eck oh KAR dee ah gruh fee) The use of ultrasonic waves directed through the heart to study the structure and motion of the heart. The visual record produced is called an echocardiogram.

electrocardiogram (ECG, EKG) (ee leck troh KAR dee ah gram) A record or recording of electrical impulses of the heart as produced by an electrocardiograph.

electrodes Adhesive patches that conduct electricity from the body to the ECG machine wires.

ion (AHY ons) An electrically charged atom, or the smallest component of an element.

unipolar Having one pole or electrical charge.

INTRODUCTION

Heart disease is the leading cause of death in the United States. Medical assistants in primary and specialty areas often care for patients with heart disorders and must do the following:

- Understand the cardiovascular system
- Recognize early symptoms of potential disorders
- Coach patients on cardiac tests and treatments ordered by providers
- Accurately perform cardiac tests
- Identify and troubleshoot problems when performing tests

The heart is a complex organ. Electrical impulses move through the heart, and the cells react by contracting. The contracting cells result in contraction of the chambers. The contractions cause the blood to move through the heart and out to the arteries. Both the electrical and mechanical activities of the heart can be assessed to monitor the heart's function. When a provider needs to assess the electrical activity of the heart, an **electrocardiogram** is commonly ordered.

Electrocardiography is a painless test. **Electrodes** are placed on the body, and wires connect the electrodes to the ECG machine *(electrocardiograph).* Electrical impulses from the heart make their way to the surface of the skin. Think of what occurs when you throw a rock into a lake. Waves are created, and they eventually make their way to the shore. The electricity from the heart eventually makes its way to the surface of the skin. The electrodes pick up the electricity, and the electricity moves into the machine. The electrocardiograph creates a record of the impulses, which is called an *electrocardiogram* (ECG, EKG).

A medical assistant performs the electrocardiography. The provider reads and interprets the ECG to identify any abnormalities in the electrical conduction in the heart. It is important for the medical assistant to do the following:

- Know the normal function of the heart
- Perform the procedure accurately
- Identify problems during the ECG procedure and take appropriate actions

This chapter discusses ECGs. The chapter begins with a review of the cardiovascular system. The components of the ECG and the process of obtaining an ECG follow the review.

HEART STRUCTURE

The heart is divided into four chambers. Two atrial chambers receive blood from the body. Two ventricular chambers pump blood out to the body. The septum divides the right and left sides of the heart.

The tricuspid valve is found between the right atrium and the right ventricle (Figure 26.1). The pulmonary valve is between the right ventricle and the pulmonary artery. The bicuspid, or mitral, valve is found between the left atrium and left ventricle. The aortic valve is between the left ventricle and the aorta. When the valves open, blood moves to the next chamber or out of the heart through the arteries. The mechanical action of the heart and valves can be assessed by **echocardiography** (ECHO).

Heart Wall Structure

The heart wall has three layers: the epicardium, the myocardium, and the endocardium. Cardiac muscle fibers in the myocardium

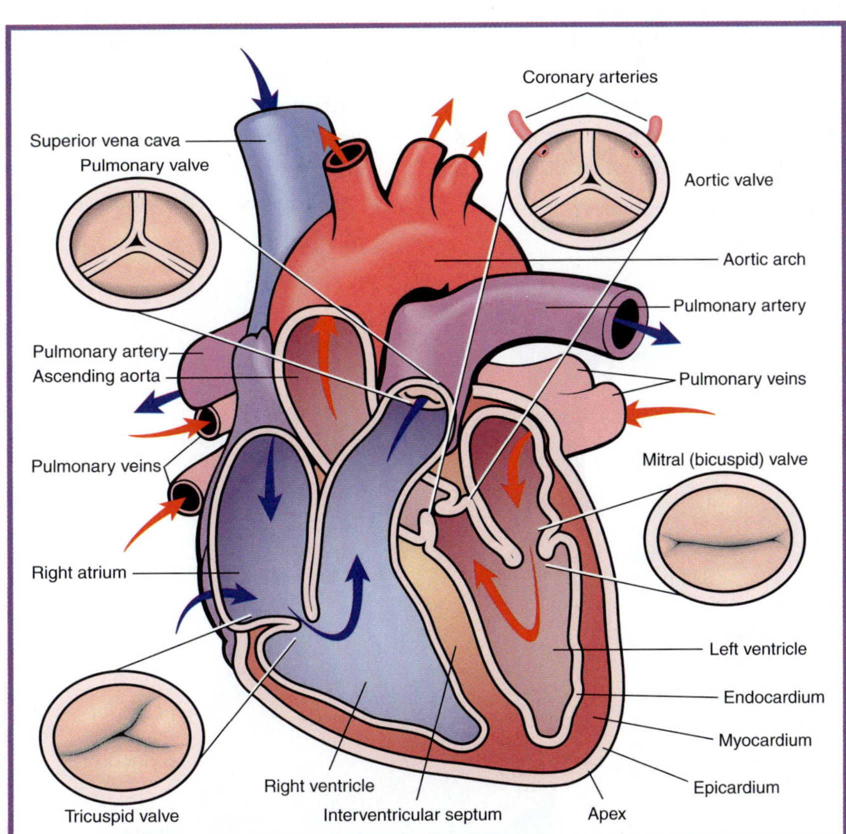

FIGURE 26.1 Chambers and valves of the heart. (From Damjanov I: *Pathology for the health-related professions,* ed 4, St. Louis, 2012, Saunders.)

are electrically linked together, forming one unit. A myocardial cell forms a strong connection to the next cells through special junctions called *intercalated discs*. These discs allow electricity to flow freely from one cell to the next. The intercalated discs are responsible for the cell-to-cell communication that is required for coordinated muscle contraction. The intercalated discs help the muscle fibers form one unit that contracts all at once instead of a little at a time. The one-unit approach is important because the atria and ventricles need to contract in an appropriately timed and coordinated effort.

Blood Flow

The right atrium receives deoxygenated blood from these structures:

- Superior vena cava (blood comes from the head, neck, chest, and upper extremities)
- Inferior vena cava (blood comes from the abdomen, pelvis, and lower extremities)
- Coronary sinus (blood from the coronary veins in the heart muscle)

When the right atrial chamber contracts, the tricuspid valve (atrioventricular [AV] valve) opens. Blood empties from the right atrium into the right ventricle. When the ventricles contract, the deoxygenated blood in the right ventricle passes through the opened pulmonary valve (semilunar [SL] valve) and moves into the pulmonary artery. The pulmonary artery brings the blood to the lungs. In the lungs, the blood picks up oxygen (O_2) and gives up carbon dioxide (CO_2). The pulmonary vein brings the oxygenated blood back to the left atrium. When the left atrial chamber contracts, the blood is pushed past the opened mitral (or bicuspid) valve (AV valve). The blood empties into the left ventricle. When the ventricles contract, the blood in the left ventricle moves through the opened aortic valve (SL valve) and into the aorta. The aorta transports oxygenated blood to the body. The first arteries to split off the aorta are the left and right coronary arteries. These arteries bring the oxygenated blood to the heart muscles.

A complete heartbeat, or *cardiac cycle*, can be divided into diastole and systole phases. During the *diastole phase*, the heart is at rest, and the atria fill with blood. The *systole phase* occurs when the heart is contracting.

CRITICAL THINKING APPLICATION **26.1**

Renee wants to help Eva review the cardiovascular structures before they see their first patient of the day. She asks Eva to describe the blood flow through the heart, starting with the superior vena cava and the inferior vena cava. Describe the blood flow.

HEART'S CONDUCTION SYSTEM

The electrical cells make up the conduction system of the heart. These cells are found throughout the myocardium. They can respond to and transmit electrical impulses to neighboring cells. The following sections review the conduction system and the cardiac cell cycles. Understanding the anatomy and physiology of the heart helps when learning electrocardiography.

Conduction Pathway

The conduction system is composed of five structures (Figure 26.2).

- *Sinoatrial (SA) node:* The SA node is called the "pacemaker of the heart." It is located in the posterior superior wall of the right atrium. The cardiac cells in the SA node generate the impulse. An impulse from the SA node starts each heartbeat. When the SA node discharges the impulse, it travels in many directions through the heart muscle. Nearby atrial cardiac cells slowly pick up the impulse. The impulse also moves quickly across special bands of tissue called *intermodal tracts*. The *Bachmann bundle*, a specialized intermodal tract, takes the impulse to the left atrium. Other intermodal tracts take the impulse quickly to the AV node.
- *Atrioventricular (AV) node*: The AV node is located at the base of the interatrial septum. When the impulse reaches the AV node, it moves very slowly through the node. This slowdown allows the atrial chambers to finish contracting, moving the blood into the ventricular chambers.
- *Bundle of His* (or *AV bundle*): The bundle of His is located in the upper interventricular septum. When the impulse leaves the AV node, it moves to the bundle of His.

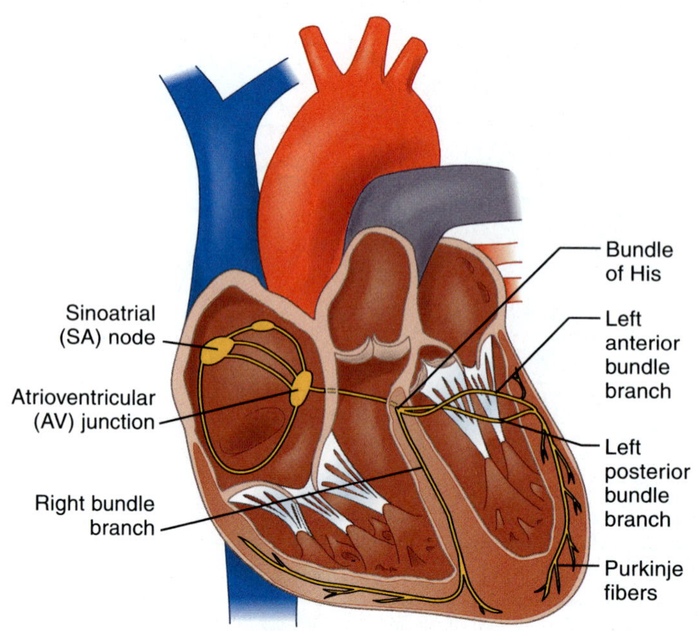

FIGURE 26.2 Cardiac conduction system.

- *Right and left bundle branches*: The bundle branches are located in the lower interventricular septum. After the impulse passes through the bundle of His, it enters the right and left bundle branches. The right bundle branch brings the impulse to the right ventricle. The left bundle branch brings the impulse to the left ventricle.
- *Purkinje fibers*: The bundle branches split into many Purkinje fibers. The Purkinje fibers transmit the impulse quickly and efficiently to the ventricular cardiac cells. This helps the ventricular chambers to contract.

States of Cardiac Cells

The cardiac cells cycle through three states, or steps, in the same sequence for each impulse.

- *Polarized state*: Before the impulse hits the cardiac cell, the cell is in the resting state, or resting potential. The inside of the cardiac cell is negatively charged. Outside of the cell is positively charged. There is no electrical activity seen on the ECG tracing during the polarized state.
- *Depolarized state*: When the impulse hits the cardiac cell, large numbers of positively charged sodium **ions** move into the cell. A small number of potassium ions move outside the cell. The movement of sodium and potassium changes the cell's charge to positive. The change, also called *action potential*, allows the impulse to move through the cell. *Depolarization* (when the impulse hits the cell) causes electrical activity on the ECG tracing.
- *Repolarized state*: After the impulse passes over the cell, the sodium and potassium ions move back to their original locations. This causes the cell's charge to change back to a negative charge. This recovery phase is called the *repolarized state*. Electrical activity (less than the depolarized state) can be recorded during the repolarized state.

Remember that the impulse occurs first and very soon after the contraction starts. These are two distinct activities, yet they appear to be close together. The electrical activity from the depolarized state and repolarized state is recorded on the ECG tracing. The contractions are mechanical actions and are not recorded on the ECG tracing. An echocardiogram (ECHO) can be used to gather information on the mechanical action of the heart, such as the valves opening and closing.

CRITICAL THINKING APPLICATION **26.2**

Renee, knowing they have ECGs scheduled for today, asks Eva to list the conduction system structures in order and briefly describe polarization, depolarization, and repolarization. List the conduction system structures in order, and then describe polarization, depolarization, and repolarization.

ECG TRACING OF THE CARDIAC CYCLE

The medical assistant performs the ECG procedure. The ECG is read or interpreted by the provider. It is important for the medical assistant to understand the components of the ECG tracing. A medical assistant must be able to identify **artifact** in the recording. If artifact is seen, corrective action needs to be taken to get a clear ECG tracing. The medical assistant will also need to know how to identify life-threatening rhythms. When these are seen, it is important that the medical assistants get immediate help. Artifact and life-threatening rhythms are discussed later in the chapter.

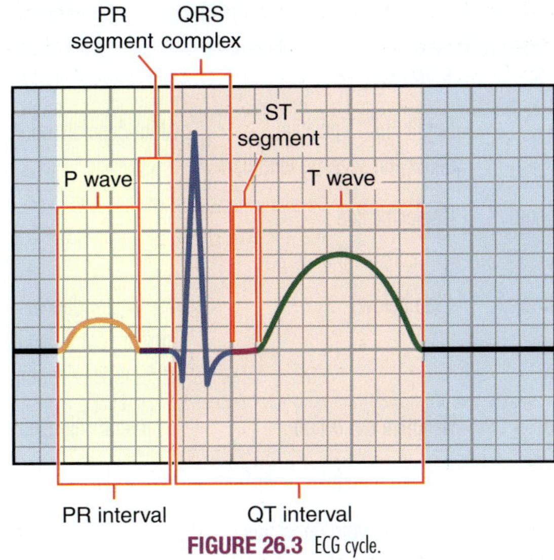

FIGURE 26.3 ECG cycle.

ECG Terminology

It is important to understand the common terminology used to comprehend the ECG tracing:

- *Isoelectric line*: A straight line that is also called the *baseline*. It represents a period of time with no electrical activity.
- *Deflection*: Any movement away from the baseline in the tracing. The deflections reflect the heart's electrical flow. Upward movement is called a *positive deflection*. Downward movement is a *negative deflection*.
- *Wave*: A deflection from the baseline.
- *Complex*: A form made up of many waves (e.g., QRS complex).
- *Segment*: A part of a line between two points (e.g., the ST segment starts at the end of the S wave and ends at the start of the T wave).
- *Interval*: A period of time between two points or events. During an interval, many waves can occur.

Each deflection in the ECG tracing corresponds to a part of the cardiac cycle. The ECG cycle consists of waveforms that are labeled P, Q, R, S, T, and U (Figure 26.3). The Q, R, and S waves are usually grouped together and are referred to as the *QRS complex*. The next section explores each part of the ECG in more detail.

ECG Waves and Segments

The *P wave* is the first deflection in the tracing. It is created from the electrical impulses moving through the right and left atria. The P wave appears as a small, rounded hill. The first part of the P wave reflects the impulse moving from the SA node to the AV node in the right atrium. The second part of the P wave reflects the impulse in the left atrial chamber. Electricity given off when the atrial cells are depolarized creates the P wave. Thus, the P wave represents *atrial depolarization*. During the P wave, the atrial chambers contract and the blood moves into the ventricles (Table 26.1).

The *PR segment* follows the P wave and appears as an isoelectric line. The electrical impulse moves slowly through the AV node. This electricity is not picked up on the ECG tracing. The PR segment is the time between the end of the *atrial depolarization* and the start

TABLE 26.1 Summary of ECG Waves and Segments

WAVES	APPEARANCE	SUMMARIZED	CONDUCTION SYSTEM	MECHANICAL ACTION
P wave	Small "hill" (positive deflection seen on lead II)	Atrial depolarization	Impulse moves from the SA node (pacemaker) to the AV node.	Atrial chambers contract; blood moves into the ventricles.
PR segment	Isoelectric line		Impulse moves slowly through AV node; electricity is not picked up on tracing.	
QRS complex	(See below)	Ventricular depolarization; interventricular septal depolarization; and atrial repolarization (hidden)	AV node to the bundle of His to the right and left bundle branches to the Purkinje fibers.	Ventricular chambers contract, pushing blood out of the heart.
Q wave	Negative deflection	Interventricular septal depolarization		
R wave	Positive triangular deflection	Ventricular depolarization; atrial repolarization (hidden)		
S wave	Any downward deflection following the R wave			
ST segment	Isoelectric line			
T wave	Positive deflection (upright and rounded in lead II)	Ventricular repolarization		
U wave	Usually not seen	Purkinje fibers are repolarized		

AV, Atrioventricular; *SA*, sinoatrial.

of the ventricular depolarization. During the PR segment, the atrial chambers finish contracting.

The *QRS complex* is the next wave in the tracing. The impulse moves from the AV node through the remaining conduction system structures. The electricity given off from the impulse moving down the septum and around the outer walls of the ventricles creates the QRS complex. The electricity from the activity in the ventricles masks the repolarization electricity given off from the atrial cells as they recover. The QRS complex activity can be summarized as *ventricular depolarization* and *atrial repolarization.* During the QRS complex, the ventricles start contracting, and the blood moves into the arteries.

Each wave in the QRS complex is different. The Q wave is a negative deflection and represents *interventricular septal depolarization.* The large, triangular-shaped R wave reflects the depolarization of most of the ventricular walls. The S wave is the final depolarization of the ventricular walls. Not all of these three waves may be seen. The positive and negative deflections of these waves can be different in the 12 leads, or pictures, of the ECG.

The *ST segment* follows the last wave in the QRS complex and ends at the start of the T wave. The *J point* is the point where the QRS complex ends, and the ST segment starts. The ST segment is an isoelectric line. There is no electrical activity in the heart during this segment. (Remember, the impulse moving through the conduction system finished in the QRS complex.) During the ST segment, the ventricles finish contracting.

Repolarization causes electrical activity that creates the remaining waves. The T wave follows the ST segment and appears as a smooth, rounded, asymmetric waveform. The electrical activity from *ventricular repolarization* creates the T wave.

The U wave may follow the T wave, but in many cases, it is not seen. The U wave is created from the repolarization of the Purkinje fibers. A U wave may also appear if the patient has hypercalcemia, hypokalemia, or digoxin toxicity.

CRITICAL THINKING APPLICATION 26.3

Before doing the ECGs scheduled for today, Renee reviews the waveforms with Eva. She asks Eva the following questions regarding the ECG tracing:

- What shows atrial depolarization?
- What shows ventricular depolarization?
- What shows ventricular repolarization?

ECG Intervals

An *interval* is a period of time from a start point to an end point. It is not a wave. If you need to define what occurs during an interval, you will simply summarize the activities that happen for each wave and segment during the interval period of time.

The PR interval starts at the beginning of the P wave and ends at the start of the Q wave. It represents atrial depolarization. The QT interval starts at the beginning of the Q wave and extends to the end of the T wave. During the QT interval, the atrial chambers move from repolarization to the polarized state. The ventricular chambers depolarize and then move into the repolarized state.

CRITICAL THINKING APPLICATION 26.4

Eva is confused about the PR interval and the QT interval. How might Renee describe these two intervals?

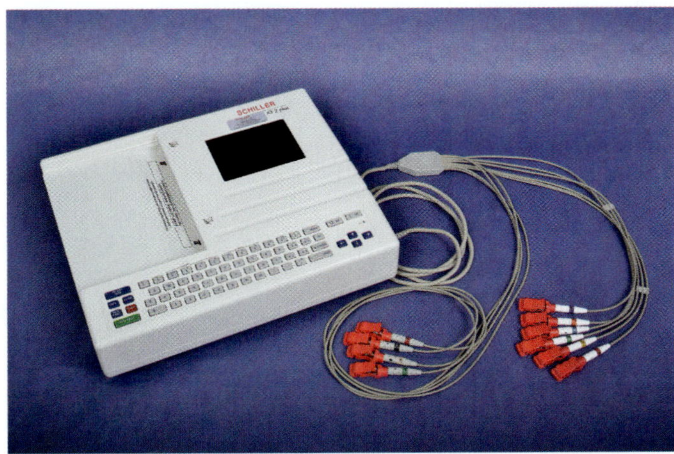

FIGURE 26.4 ECG machine.

12-LEAD ECG

One of the most common ECG procedures in the ambulatory care setting is a resting 12-lead ECG. The medical assistant is responsible for the following:

- Assembling the supplies and equipment needed
- Preparing the patient for the test
- Performing the test

Before the medical assistant finishes the procedure, the ECG tracing must be examined for artifact. If any artifact is present on the tracing, the medical assistant must problem-solve the situation. Ultimately, the goal is to give the provider a clear ECG.

For a resting 12-lead ECG, the patient rests on the exam table. Ten electrodes are placed on the body. Lead wires attach to the electrodes and connect to the ECG machine (electrocardiograph). The 10 electrodes and lead wires pick up the electrical impulse from the surface of the body and carry it to the ECG machine (Figure 26.4). The machine creates the ECG tracing.

A more in-depth discussion of electrode placement and artifact are presented later in the chapter. For now, it is important to have an idea of where the electrodes are placed on the body. An electrode is placed on each of the arms and legs. The right leg electrode is considered the ground electrode and is required for a clear ECG tracing. Six electrodes are placed on the chest.

Using the 10 electrodes and lead wires, the ECG machine creates 12 images, or pictures, which are called *leads*. Each lead picture looks different. Think of a photographer moving around a person, taking 12 pictures. Each picture looks different because of the change in the photographer's angle. For each lead, the picture is created differently. It is important for the medical assistant to know what electrodes and lead wires create the leads when troubleshooting unclear tracings. The three types of leads—bipolar, augmented, and precordial—are discussed in the following sections.

> **CRITICAL THINKING APPLICATION 26.5**
>
> Robert Caudill is scheduled for an ECG today. When he arrives, Eva discusses the procedure. Robert asks what "12 lead" stands for. How would you answer his question?

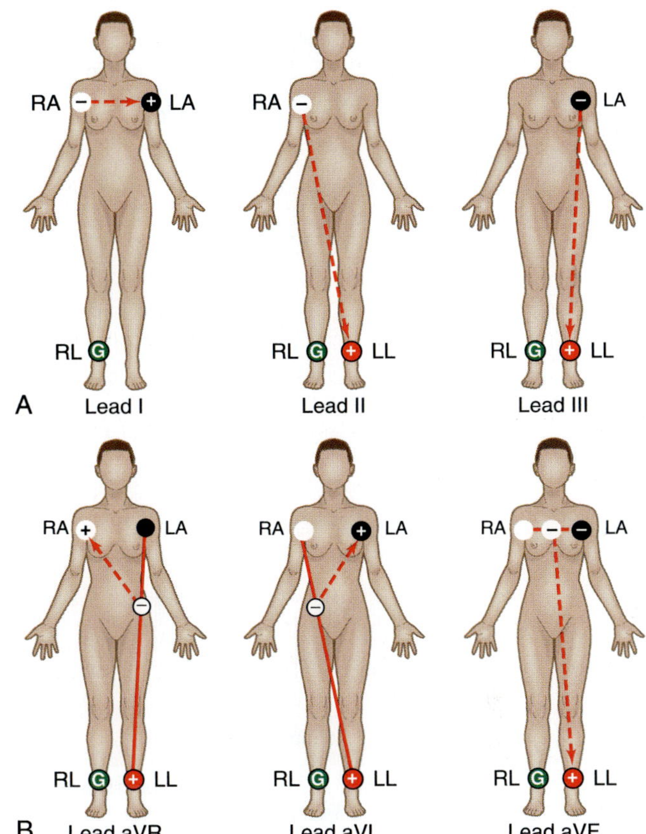

FIGURE 26.5 **(A)** Bipolar, or standard, leads (right arm [RA], left arm [LA], right leg [RL], and left leg [LL]). **(B)** Augmented leads (augmented Vector Right [aVR], augmented Vector Left [aVL], and augmented Vector Foot [aVF]).

Bipolar (or Standard) Leads

The **bipolar** or standard leads are named leads I, II, and III. They use the arm electrodes and the left leg electrode to create pictures of the vertical (or frontal) plane of the heart. (Remember, the right electrode is used as a ground and is important for all leads.)

The bipolar leads are created from a measurement of current traveling from a negative pole to the positive pole (Figure 26.5A):

- Lead I: Right arm (RA) to left arm (LA)
- Lead II: Right arm (RA) to left leg (LL)
- Lead III: Left leg (LL) to left arm (LA)

If you join the end points (positive poles) of these three leads, you get a triangle. This triangle is known as the *Einthoven triangle*.

It is important to know which two electrodes create each lead when troubleshooting problems with the ECG tracing. If a lead has artifact, the medical assistant must check the two electrodes and the lead wires that create the lead.

> **CRITICAL THINKING APPLICATION 26.6**
>
> As Eva and Renee perform an ECG, they find artifact on a few leads. For the following leads, which electrodes should be checked in each situation?
>
> - Lead II is unclear.
> - Leads I and III are unclear.
> - Leads II and III are unclear.

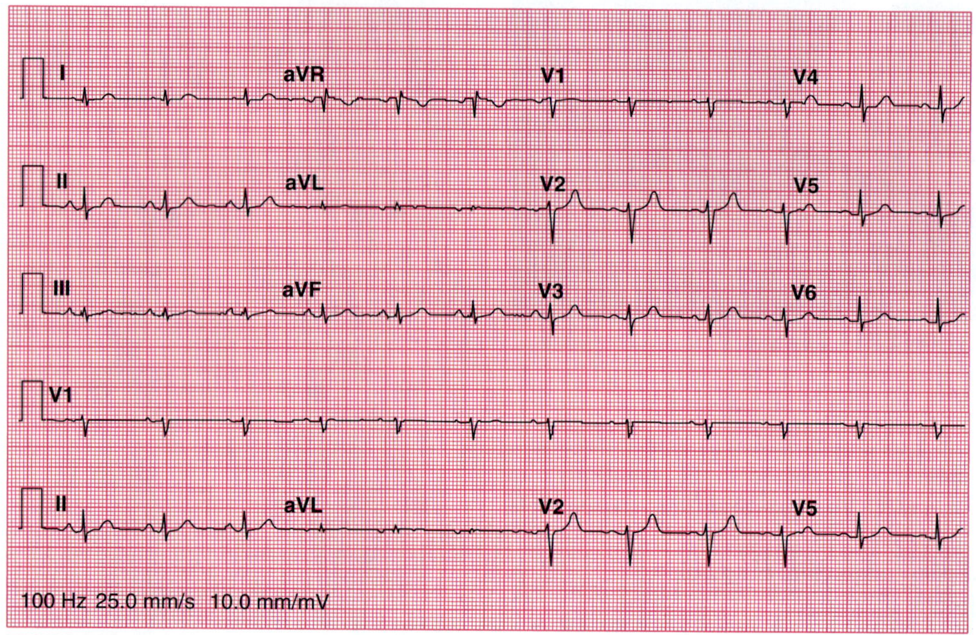

FIGURE 26.6 A 12-lead ECG showing a normal sinus rhythm. (From Phalen T, Aehlert BJ: *The 12-lead ECG in acute coronary syndromes,* ed 3, St. Louis, 2012, Mosby.)

Augmented Leads

Augmented vector (aV) leads, commonly referred to as augmented leads, provide information on the vertical (frontal) plane of the heart (see Figure 26.5B). These **unipolar** leads are *augmented,* or increased in size, on the tracing. Augmented leads use the right arm (RA), left arm (LA), and left leg (LL) electrodes.

Each augmented lead uses all three extremity electrodes (RA, LA, and LL) to create the picture. Midpoint between two of the electrodes is the negative pole. The current is measured as it moves from the negative pole to the positive pole.

- Lead aVR (augmented Vector Right) records current traveling between the right arm and the central point between the left arm and left leg.
- Lead aVL (augmented Vector Left) records current traveling between the left arm and the central point between the right arm and left leg.
- Lead aVF (augmented Vector Foot) records current traveling between the left leg electrode and the central point between the left and right arms.

If the medical assistant identifies artifact on the aVR lead, all three electrodes and lead wires should be checked. (Check the RA, LA, and LL electrode and lead wires.)

Chest (or Precordial) Leads

The chest (precordial) leads are also unipolar leads. Each is a positive pole. The precordial leads provide information on the horizontal (front to back) plane of the heart. The six precordial leads are labeled V_1, V_2, V_3, V_4, V_5, and V_6 (Figure 26.6).

The six leads are numbered the same as the precordial lead wires (i.e., V_1 through V_6). If one of the leads is unclear, the medical assistant should refer to the related lead wire and electrode. For instance, with artifact on V_4, the medical assistant will check the V_4 electrode and lead wire.

ECG SUPPLIES

The medical assistant needs to be familiar with the supplies used for ECGs. It is important to monitor the expiration dates of ECG supplies. Using expired supplies can cause unclear ECG tracings.

Thermal ECG Paper

ECG machines with printers use special ECG paper. The paper can be either Z-fold paper or 8.25 × 11-inch paper. A special heat-sensitive coating on the paper allows the tracing to be "burned" onto the paper. Here are some tips for handling the ECG paper:

- Store in a dry, cool, dark location.
- Do not expose to heat, bright light, or an ultraviolet (UV) light source.
- Do not expose to alcohol, adhesives, cleaners, or solvents.
- Do not store with vinyl, shrink wrap, or plastics.

The ECG paper is universally created with small and large boxes. The small box is 1 × 1 mm, and the large box is 5 × 5 mm. The large box is made up of 25 small boxes (five rows and five columns) (Figure 26.7). It has a thicker border than the small boxes. When the provider analyzes the tracing, the height and the width of the waveforms are measured with a **caliper** (Figure 26.8). The small and large boxes can help in the interpreting process.

The vertical lines measure the amplitude, or *voltage,* of the waveforms. Each small box is 0.1 mV (millivolt), and each large box is 0.5 mV. To determine the amplitude, count the small boxes vertically, starting at the baseline, to the highest/lowest point of the wave.

The horizontal lines measure the time. When the paper speed *(chart speed)* is set at 25 mm/second, each small box is 0.04 second, and each large box equals 0.2 second. To determine the width and time of the waveform, count the small boxes horizontally from the start to the finish of the wave. Multiply the number of small boxes by 0.04 to find the time.

Electrodes

Electrodes are single-use disposable adhesive tabs that are placed on the skin. The skin is a poor conductor of electricity. The electrodes contain an electrolyte gel that helps pick up the electrical impulses. As the impulses make their way to the surface of the body, the electrolyte gel helps to conduct the impulses into the lead wires. For a resting 12-lead ECG, the most common type of electrode is the tab variety (Figure 26.9A). The snap electrode is used more often for exercise stress tests and in hospital settings (Figure 26.9B).

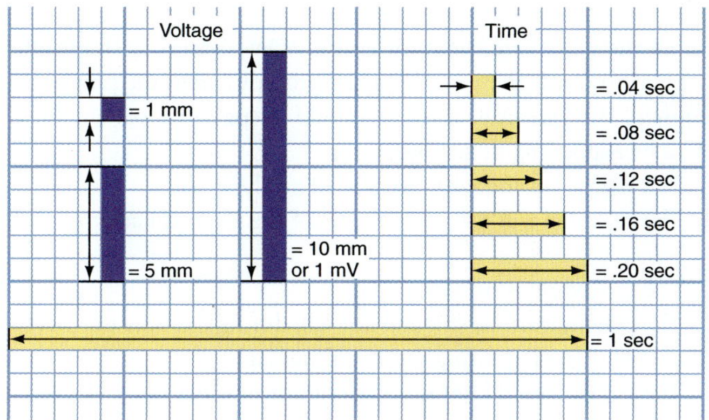

FIGURE 26.7 ECG paper.

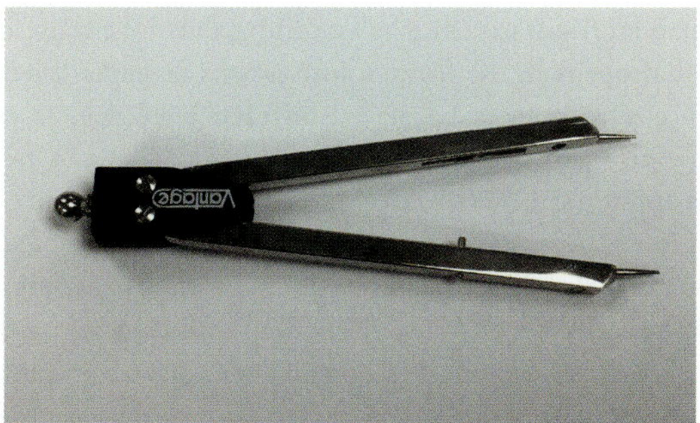

FIGURE 26.8 Caliper.

It is important to check the expiration date of the electrodes. If they are expired, the gel may be dried out, and the conduction will be poor. Many operators' manuals for ECG machines recommend not mixing different manufacturers' electrodes.

ELECTROCARDIOGRAPH

The lead wires may have a snap or a clip (also called an *alligator clip*; *patient end adaptor*) that attaches to the electrode. The lead wires merge into the patient cable that takes the electrical impulses to the electrocardiograph (ECG machine). In the machine, the impulses pass through an amplifier, which magnifies the impulses. A digital converter changes the analog signal into a digital signal. The digital signal can be printed off on special ECG paper, which is discussed in the next section.

Features

The features of ECG machines can vary greatly. The two types of ECG devices in ambulatory healthcare facilities include the box model and computer-based models. The box model ECG machine usually has an LCD screen. The computer-based ECG may have a touch screen and stress testing features. The software can be preloaded onto its own computer, or the facility can purchase software to be added to any laptop computer. These additional features are commonly seen in both types of ECG devices:

- Interpretive software: Assists providers with reading the tracing
- Bluetooth or Wi-Fi capacity: Allows the ECG to be sent to providers and printers and to be uploaded into an electronic health record (EHR)
- Thermal printers
- Spirometer

Settings and Calibration

ECG machines have settings that can be useful for obtaining a tracing. Many machines have filters to block disturbances. Filters can help to create a clearer tracing. Refer to the operators' manual when changing settings. Table 26.2 presents common settings. It is important to indicate on the tracing if any of the default settings were changed. Changes to the default settings will affect how the provider measures and interprets the tracing.

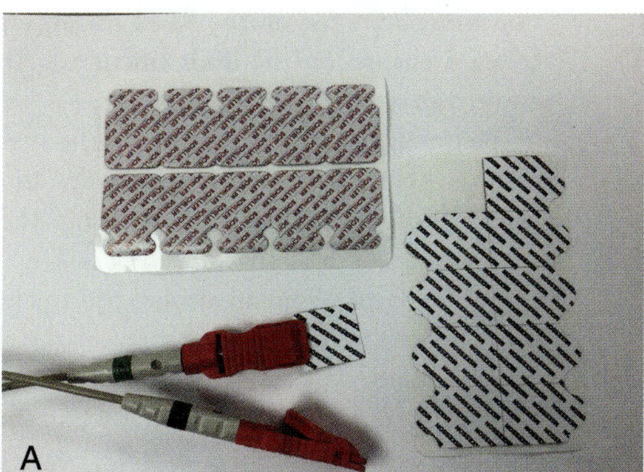

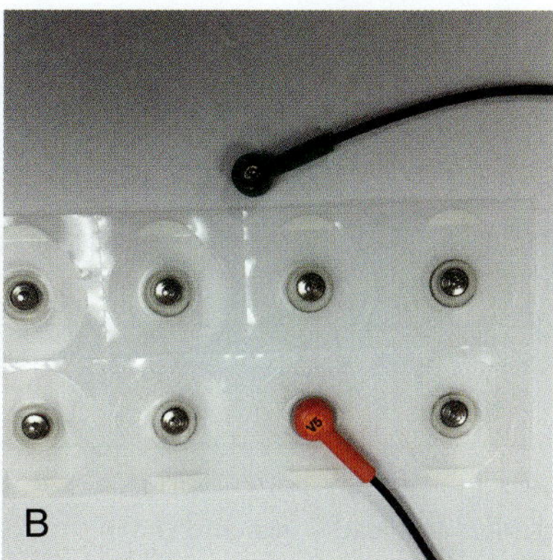

FIGURE 26.9 (A) The appearance of tab electrodes can vary, depending on the manufacturer. Alligator clips on the lead wires attach to the tab electrodes. **(B)** Snap electrodes use the snap adaptors on the lead wires.

TABLE 26.2 Common ECG Settings

SETTING	DESCRIPTION	NORMAL DEFAULT	REASON TO CHANGE SETTING
Chart speed	Regulates the speed of the paper during the recording. *Example:* 25 mm/s means 25 millimeters (25 small blocks) of tracing is printed in 1 second.	25 mm/s (second)	*For a very fast rate*: Increase speed to 50 mm/s to get more defined waveforms. *For a very slow rate*: Reduce rate to 5 or 10 mm/s to capture more waveforms on the paper.
Gain or sensitivity	Regulates the height (amplitude) of the tracing. *Example:* 10 mm/mV means 1 mV (millivolt) of electricity causes the recorder to move up 10 millimeters (10 small blocks).	10 mm/mV	*For very short waveforms:* Increase to 20 mm/mV, which doubles the height of the waves. *For very tall waveforms:* Reduce to 5 mm/mV, which reduces the wave height by half.

Most ECG machines automatically complete a self-test when the machine is turned on. Typically, the self-test examines the battery and the memory. Like many machines used in the healthcare setting, the ECG machine needs to be calibrated daily or per the facility's policy. The calibration results should be documented on the log flow sheet.

When ECG machines are calibrated, the *sensitivity* (also called *gain*) should be checked. The machines usually print a calibration marking either at the beginning or the end of the tracing. This marking is called the *standardization mark*. If the machine is set at 10 mm/mV, the standardization mark will be an upward rectangle that is 10 small boxes tall. If the gain is doubled, then the standardization mark also will be doubled in size (Figure 26.10).

Maintenance

After the ECG is obtained and the patient has left, the medical assistant must clean the room and the electrocardiograph. Maintenance of the machine includes these steps:

- Clean the lead wires as indicated in the users' guide. The lead wires are not disposable.
- Handle the lead wires and patient cable with care. They should be stored in a loose coil. Tight coils or bending of the wires and cable can result in breakage of the fine wires inside the unit. This will cause artifact on the ECG and requires replacement of the cable.
- Clean the tracing stylus and the machine casing as indicated in the users' guide.

CRITICAL THINKING APPLICATION **26.7**

The next day, Eva prepares to do an ECG on Charles Johnson. She turns on the machine to see if it has been set up correctly. She notes the following:

- Chart speed: 10 mm/s
- Gain: 10 mm/mV

Which of these settings is normal, and which needs to be changed prior to the next ECG?

ECG PROCEDURE

The medical assistant must prepare the patient prior to the ECG procedure, apply the electrodes and lead wires, and coach the patient just before taking the ECG tracing. Providing coaching prior to the procedure helps to decrease the patient's anxiety.

Patient Preparation

Before the procedure begins, it is always important for the medical assistant to coach the patient on the procedure and the preparation required. The medical assistant should prepare the patient for an ECG by explaining these points:

- Ten electrodes and wires are placed on the body.
- The machine will take 12 pictures of the electrical activity of the heart.
- The procedure is painless.
- The patient must be still and not talk during the time the pictures are being made (during the actual tracing).
- The patient should not use a cell phone or other electronic device during the procedure.
- The provider will need to look at the ECG pictures, and then the patient will be notified of the results. (Remember, the medical assistant cannot tell the patient if it is normal or abnormal.)

The patient needs to remove all clothing above the waist and wear a gown that opens in the front. Cloth gowns or paper capes can be used. An electrode must be placed on each lower leg, so tights or pantyhose also must be removed. Socks and pants can be moved to allow application of the electrodes, so they can usually stay on (Procedure 26.1).

The patient should be in the supine position on the exam table. A pillow can be placed under the patient's head. The patient's legs and arms need to be supported on the table. It is important for the patient to be relaxed and comfortable during the procedure. If the patient has chest pain or problems breathing, the head of the exam table may be elevated. Any change of position from the supine position must be noted on the ECG tracing. Any position change can create a change on the leads (pictures). The provider needs to be aware of it when reading the tracing.

Before placing the electrodes on the skin, it is important to prepare the skin. This helps the electrodes adhere and minimizes artifact, thus producing an accurate tracing. There are several techniques used to prepare the skin:

- Wipe the area with an alcohol pad to clean it. This helps remove sweat and lotion that may prevent the electrodes from adhering to the skin.
- Use a razor to shave chest hair. Obtain the patient's verbal consent before shaving the chest.
- Gently abrade the skin using a gauze sponge, special gel, or special fine sandpaper tape (Figure 26.11).

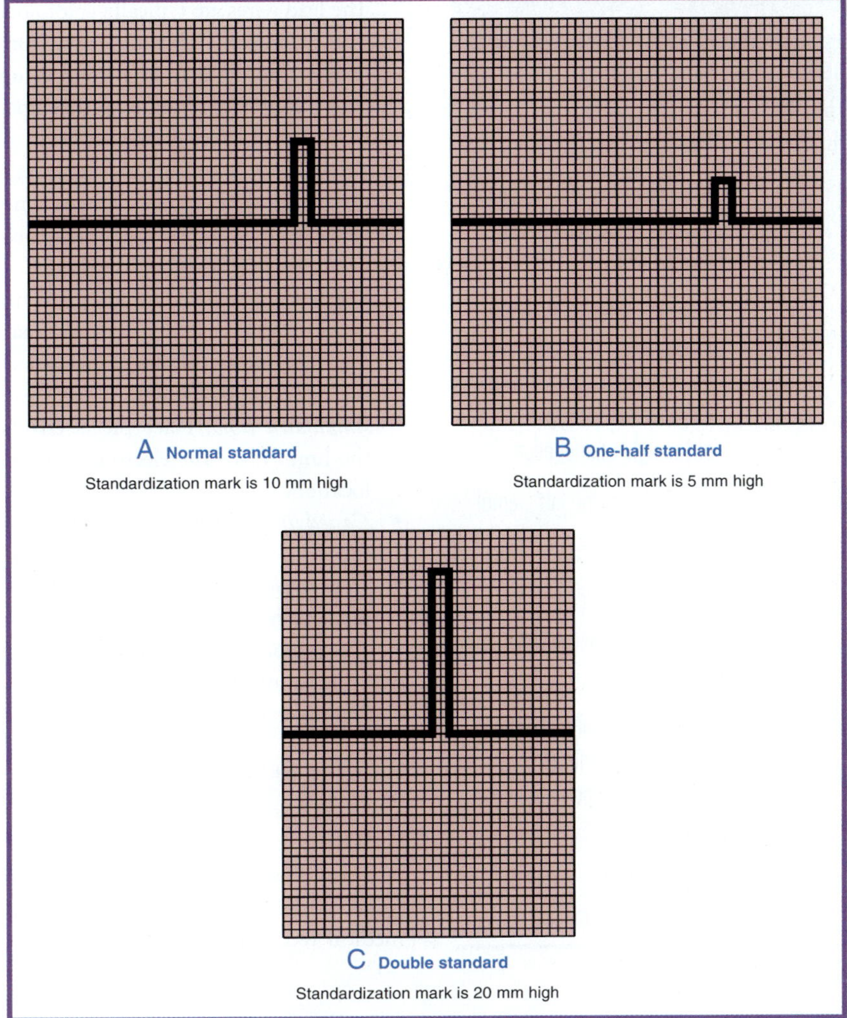

FIGURE 26.10 Sensitivity standards.

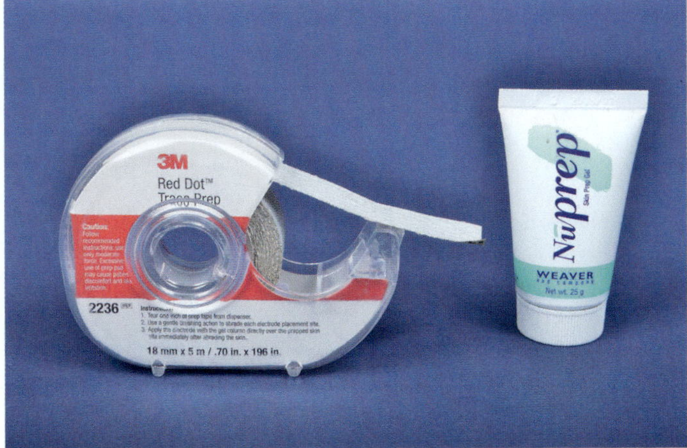

FIGURE 26.11 Special fine sandpaper tape and Nuprep skin prep gel are used to abrade the skin. This provides a better ECG tracing.

Applying Electrodes and Lead Wires

Apply electrodes to both arms and legs. The electrodes on the lower legs should be placed on the inner side, just above the ankles. If tab electrodes are used, have the tabs on the leg electrodes point toward the center of the person. All the other tabs can be facing the feet.

The placement of the arm electrodes may vary depending on the ECG machine and manufacturer. For instance, many Schiller ECG machines indicate that the electrodes should be placed just above the wrists. Other machines indicate placement on the upper arms. Check the users' guide for correct placement of the arm electrodes. Table 26.3 describes where to place the electrodes on the limbs and the chest (Figure 26.12).

TABLE 26.3 Electrode and Lead Wire Placement

ELECTRODE	LEAD WIRE ABBREVIATION AND COLOR	PLACEMENT
Right arm	RA (white)	Just above the wrist or upper arm, as indicated in the users' guide
Left arm	LA (black)	
Right leg	RL (green)	Inner lower leg, just above the ankle
Left leg	LL (red)	
Chest V_1	V1 (red)	Fourth intercostal space (ICS) at the right sternal edge
Chest V_2	V2 (yellow)	Fourth ICS at the left sternal edge
Chest V_3	V3 (green)	Midway between V_2 and V_4
Chest V_4	V4 (blue)	Fifth ICS on the midclavicular line
Chest V_5	V5 (orange)	Same horizontal plane as V_4 at the left anterior axillary line or the midpoint between V_4 and V_6
Chest V_6	V6 (purple)	Same horizontal plane as V_4 at the midaxillary line

The lead wires are typically color coded and include an abbreviation on each wire. Colors may vary from manufacturer to manufacturer. It is important to know and to use the abbreviations. One of the most common errors is to mix up the right and left limb lead wires. This can cause abnormal leads (pictures) and result in additional patient workup before the mistake is discovered. It is important to always double-check the placement of the lead wires.

In some cases, the electrodes may need to be placed in alternative locations, such as with the following:

- **Dextrocardia**: Place the chest electrodes on the right side of the chest using the same intercostal spacing and landmarks. Switch the right and left limb lead wires (e.g., LA would be attached to the right arm electrode).
- *Amputated limb*: Place the electrode on the remaining part of the limb. Place the electrode on the opposite limb in the same location.
- *Casted limb*: Place the electrode above the cast on the limb. Place the electrode on the opposite limb in the same location.
- *New surgical incision or wound*: Place the electrodes near the correct area but not on the incision or wound.

It is important to note on the ECG tracing any electrode placement deviation from the normal location. The provider reading the tracing needs to take the placement into consideration.

Running the ECG Tracing

Once the lead wires are attached to the electrodes, the medical assistant enters the patient information into the ECG machine. In some facilities, this may be done prior to bringing the patient into the room for the ECG. Typically, the patient's name, date of birth, and medical record number are entered. Facilities will have additional

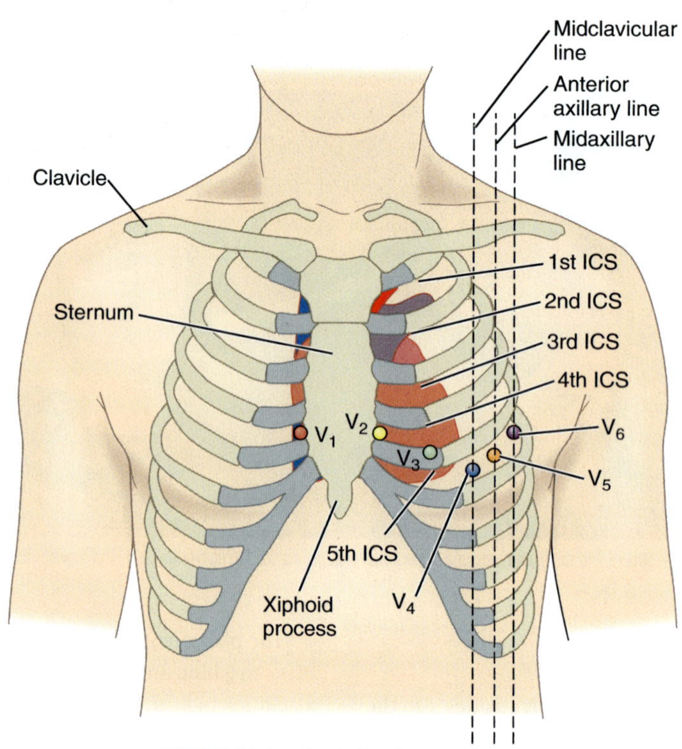

FIGURE 26.12 Chest leads. *ICS,* Intercostal space.

information that they require to be entered, such as the ordering provider's name and the provider reading the ECG.

After the information is entered, the medical assistant should remind the patient to remain still and not talk during the procedure. It usually takes a minute or less for the tracing to be created with a multichannel machine. Talking and movement will create artifact. Use a blanket to cover the patient who is cold.

Prior to running the tracing, double-check that all the electrodes are attached, and the lead wires are in the correct location. If the ECG machine has a screen, check the digital picture of the leads. Are they clear (without artifact)? If not, is the filter(s) on? Are the leads (pictures) an equal distance from each other? Is the baseline horizontal, or is it moving up and down like a roller coaster? Do not run the tracing until it is clear, and the baseline is horizontal. Problem-solve and fix the issue before running the tracing or redo the tracing if it was printed. Additional problem-solving strategies are discussed later in this chapter. Once the tracing looks good on the screen, print it.

Single- and Multiple-Channel ECG Machines

ECG machines can be single-channel or multichannel. In *single-channel* models, the machine contains one amplifier channel and one recording stylet. The single-channel machines record one lead (picture) at a time. The medical assistant must manually switch to the next lead until the procedure is done. When these machines are used, the process of recording a tracing takes up to 3 to 5 minutes. Single-channel machines can use paper rolls or Z-fold paper. These small strips of paper need to be mounted.

Multichannel machines monitor all 12 leads. This model has several stylets that allow for four groups of three leads to be traced every few seconds. With some machines, a fourth stylet traces one lead for the entire width of the page. Typically, the multichannel machines print the tracing on 8.25 × 11-inch or Z-fold paper.

Finishing the ECG Procedure

If the ambulatory care facility uses an EHR system and the ECG machine interfaces with the EHR software, then the medical assistant should follow the procedure and upload the tracing to the patient's health record. The provider will read the tracing once it is uploaded.

The provider must read the ECG before it is filed in the paper medical record. If the tracing was done on small strips of ECG paper, the strips need to be mounted per the facility's procedures. Special 8.5 × 10-inch paper with adhesive strips is used to stick the ECG tracing strips. Once the strips are mounted, they can be given to the provider to read. If the ECG prints on 8.5 × 10-inch paper, it does not need to be mounted. It can be given to the provider immediately.

CRITICAL THINKING APPLICATION **26.8**

The clinic uses an ECG machine that uploads the ECGs into patients' electronic health records. Based on what you have learned so far in your courses, why is this useful and efficient?

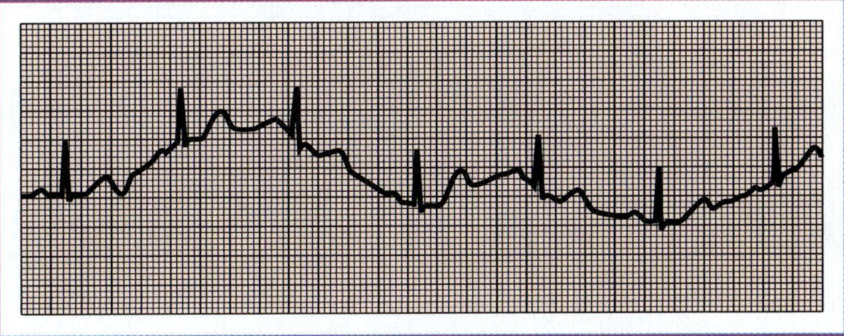

FIGURE 26.13 Wandering baseline artifact.

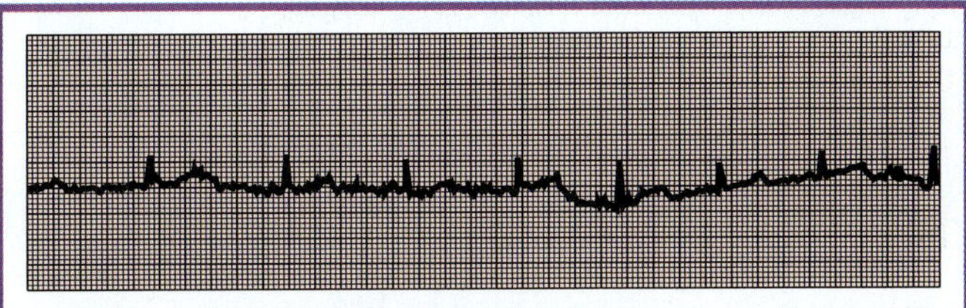

FIGURE 26.14 Somatic tremor artifact.

TROUBLESHOOTING ARTIFACT

Artifact is signal distortion or unwanted, erratic movement of the stylus caused by outside interference. The medical assistant needs to identify the type of artifact and then take actions to prevent the artifact. The leads can be viewed on the screen or after printing the ECG tracing. Carefully look for artifact. The following sections discuss the appearance and causes of the common types of artifact and ways to prevent them.

Wandering Baseline

Wandering baseline artifact is an upward and downward movement of the waveform (Figure 26.13). The isoelectric lines shift locations. This artifact can be the result of the following:

- *Poor skin preparation*: The patient has oily skin or used lotion. The electrodes are falling off.
- *Old electrodes*: The electrodes are dirty or expired, or the gel on the electrodes is dried.
- *Placement of electrodes*: The electrodes are placed on bony areas.
- *Movement*: The movement of breathing can also be the cause of this artifact.

The medical assistant should take these steps:

- Clean the skin with alcohol and allow it to dry. Slightly abrade the skin with a gauze pad or fine sandpaper tape to help the electrodes stick to the skin.
- Replace the electrode with a new one. Ensure the electrodes are not expired and the gel is not dried.
- Make sure all electrodes and lead wires are firmly attached.
- Make sure the baseline filter is turned on (if it is a feature of the machine).

Somatic Tremor

Somatic tremor artifact, also called *muscle artifact*, appears as jagged peaks with irregular heights and spacing (Figure 26.14). There are several causes:

- *Involuntary movement*: Tremors from disease conditions (e.g., Parkinson disease), shivering due to coldness

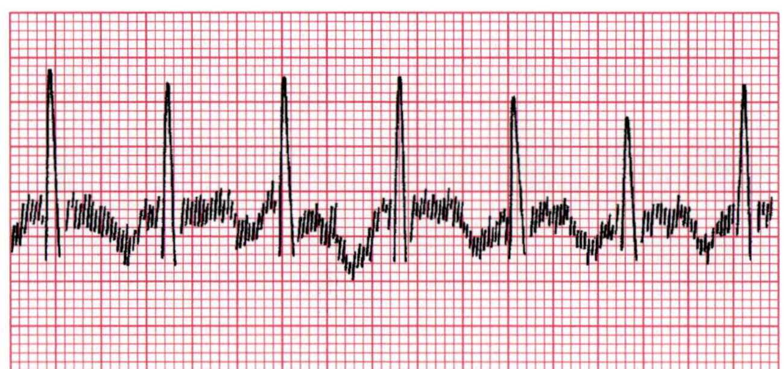

FIGURE 26.15 AC interference artifact. (From Urden L, Stacy K, Lough M: *Thelan's critical care nursing: diagnosis and management*, ed 7, St. Louis, 2014, Mosby.)

- *Voluntary movement*: Talking, chewing gum, supporting arms or legs because the table is too small for the person

The medical assistant should take the following steps:
- Help the patient relax. Cover the patient with a blanket if cold.
- Remind the patient not to move or talk during the tracing.
- Watch for a pattern with involuntary movements. Take the tracing when the movements lessen.
- Use a larger exam table for the procedure.
- If the machine has a muscle tremor filter, make sure it is turned on.

AC Interference

Alternating current (AC) interference artifact, also called *60-cycle interference artifact,* appears as a series of small spikes that creates a thick-looking tracing (Figure 26.15). Electrical interference causes AC interference artifact. Electrical interference arises due to a number of factors:
- There are too many electrical devices in the area.
- The patient cable and lead wires are wrapped closely together.
- An electrical cord is under the exam table, and an electrical outlet is improperly grounded.
- A cell phone in a patient's pocket or a smartwatch may also cause interference.

The medical assistant should do the following:
- Unplug the ECG machine.
- Unplug or remove nearby electrical devices (e.g., laptops, pagers, cell phones).
- Separate the lead wires so they do not overlap.
- Move the table away from the wall or move to another room for the procedure.
- Ensure that no cell phones are near the procedure area.

Interrupted Baseline

Interrupted baseline artifact (also called *intermittent signal artifact*) occurs when the tracing looks normal at the beginning but then disappears or goes all over when the electrical connection is interrupted (Figure 26.16). When the electrical connection is interrupted, interrupted baseline artifact occurs. The electrical connection is interrupted when a cable or lead wire becomes loose or a cable, clip, or lead wire is broken. If the lead wire or electrode falls off, an isoelectric line will appear on the tracing.

The medical assistant should do the following:
- Check that all electrodes and lead wires are attached.
- If a broken wire is suspected, be prepared to supply a new cable.

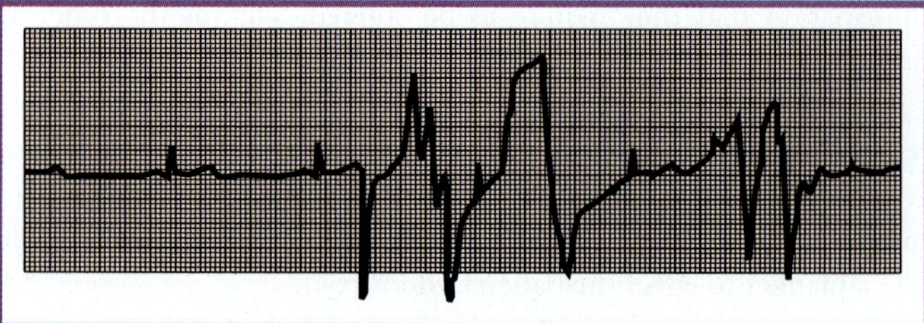

FIGURE 26.16 Interrupted baseline artifact.

TABLE 26.4 Sequence Method

NUMBER OF LARGE (5-MM) BOXES BETWEEN R WAVES	HEART RATE
1	300
2	150
3	100
4	75
5	60
6	50
7	43
8	37

CRITICAL THINKING APPLICATION 26.9

While Eva is performing Charles Johnson's 12-lead ECG, she notices that the tracing line looks thick. On closer inspection, she finds that there are small, spiked lines that make the tracing look like a thick line. What is occurring? How might Eva troubleshoot the problem?

EVALUATING AN ECG TRACING

The provider reads the ECG, but the medical assistant must be able to determine abnormal rates and rhythms that might be life threatening. This section discusses how to determine the heart rate, evaluate the ECG tracing, and identify abnormal rhythms.

Rate

Many machines indicate the heart rate. The medical assistant can also calculate the rate from the ECG tracing. Numerous methods can be used to calculate a regular heart rate when the paper speed (chart speed) is 25 mm/second:
- *Six-second method*: Count the number of P waves in a 6-second strip (30 large boxes) and multiply by 10 (least accurate method).
- *1500 method*: Count the number of small boxes between two R waves or the two P waves. Divide the number into 1500.
- *Sequence method*: Count the number of large boxes between the R waves. By memorizing the numbers in Table 26.4, you will have a quick method to calculate the heart rate.

TABLE 26.5 Analyzing an ECG Tracing

TRACING FEATURE	NORMAL	QUESTIONS TO ADDRESS	TIMING (HORIZONTAL–LENGTH)
P wave	Largest in lead II Upright in all leads except aVR Voltage (vertical height): less than 2.5 small boxes (0.25 millivolts)	• Is there one P wave before each QRS complex? • Is each P wave a positive deflection? • Are all the P waves similar in size and shape? • Is there more than one P wave per cardiac cycle?	>0.11 seconds
PR interval	From start of P wave to start of QRS complex	• Are the PR intervals the same size throughout the tracing?	0.12–0.2 seconds
QRS complex	Largest in lead II compared to leads III and I	• Is there a QRS complex without a previous P wave?	0.06–0.12 seconds
ST segment	On the baseline	• Is the ST segment lower or higher than the baseline? (Could be an indication of infarction or ischemia.)	Not usually measured
QT interval	From start of Q wave to end of T wave	• Are the QT intervals the same size throughout the tracing?	0.40 seconds

Analyzing an ECG Tracing

For most medical assistants, their job description states that they need to be able to perform ECGs. Some medical assistants may work as ECG technicians. In this position, they may need to analyze an ECG tracing.

The ECG rhythm strip (lead II view) is evaluated from left to right. The following should be assessed:

- *Rate:* What is the rate?
- *Rhythm:* Is it regular or irregular? An irregular rhythm on an ECG tracing will have time differences between cardiac cycles. With a regular rhythm, each cardiac cycle occurs the same length of time apart.
- *Appearance of the segments, waves, and intervals:* Table 26.5 lists questions to consider when analyzing a tracing.

Identifying an Abnormal Rhythm

When performing an ECG, the medical assistant must identify if the patient has an **arrhythmia** that requires immediate care by the provider. If the medical assistant identifies a life-threatening arrhythmia, it is important to keep the patient hooked up to the ECG machine and to get the provider immediately.

Sinus Arrhythmias

A sinus rhythm is considered normal (Figure 26.6). The electrical activity begins in the SA node and goes through the rest of the conduction system. Atrial and ventricular depolarizations occur. With sinus arrhythmias, the electrical pathway is normal. The rate or rhythm of the heartbeat is altered. The alteration may result from the SA node firing too slowly or too quickly.

- *Sinus bradycardia*: The adult heart rate is below 60 beats per minute. This is a normal finding in well-conditioned athletes. It is abnormal in other individuals.
- *Sinus tachycardia*: The adult heart rate is above 100 beats per minute. This is normal in a person doing aerobic exercise. It is abnormal in a resting individual.

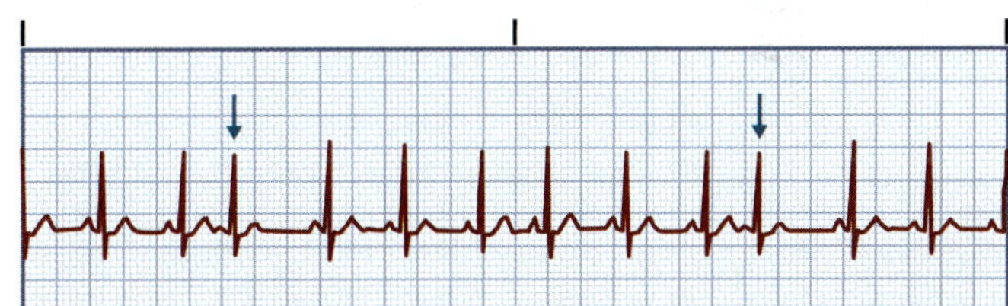

FIGURE 26.17 Premature atrial contractions (arrows). (From Harding, M: *Lewis's medical-surgical nursing: assessment and management of clinical problems*, ed 11, St. Louis, 2020, Elsevier.)

Atrial Arrhythmias

Atrial arrhythmias occur when there is a problem with the SA node starting the impulse. They can also occur due to a conduction problem in the atria.

- *Premature atrial contractions (PACs)*: Occur when the atria contract sooner than they should. The P wave can be abnormally shaped, or an extra P wave can be seen (Figure 26.17). PACs can be seen in people who smoke or consume large amounts of caffeine. An occasional PAC is not abnormal. More than six PACs in a minute is considered abnormal.
- *Atrial flutter*: Occurs when the atria contract faster than the ventricles (up to 300 beats per minute) (Figure 26.18). They become out of sync with the ventricles. Extra P waves are seen with regular QRS complexes. Atrial flutter can be caused by alcohol and stimulants (cocaine, caffeine, diet pills, and cold medications). It can also be caused by coronary heart disease, hypertension, cardiomyopathy, heart valve diseases, hyperthyroidism, obstructive pulmonary disease, and pulmonary embolism diseases. Atrial flutter is reversed with medication to slow the heart or with cardioversion (electrical shock).

Heart Block

A heart block occurs when there is a disruption or slowing of the electrical impulse through the heart. Heart block can be congenital or acquired. Heart disease, surgery, or medications can cause acquired

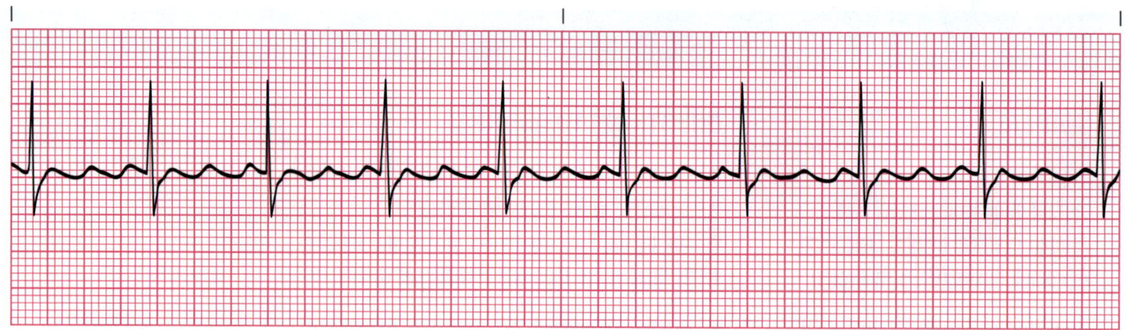

FIGURE 26.18 Atrial flutter. (Modified from Atwood S, Stanton C, Storey Davenport J: *Introduction to basic cardiac dysrhythmias,* ed 4, St. Louis, 2009, Mosby/JEMS.)

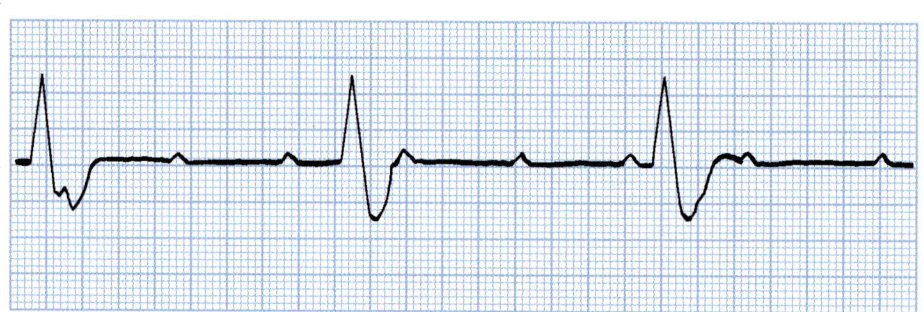

FIGURE 26.19 Complete third-degree atrioventricular block. Note that there is no relationship between P waves and QRS complexes because the atria and ventricles are depolarizing independently. (From Banasik, J: *Pathophysiology,* ed 7, St. Louis, 2022, Elsevier.)

heart block. There are three types of heart block, with third-degree heart block being the most severe:

- *First-degree heart block*: The impulse slows as it moves from the atria to the ventricles. This creates a longer PR segment. First-degree heart block may not cause symptoms. It may not require treatment.
- *Second-degree heart block*: The impulse slows or is blocked as it moves into the ventricles. When blocked, there is no QRS complex after the P wave, and the ventricles do not contract. When the impulse slows, the PR segment is longer. This arrhythmia requires a pacemaker to help maintain the heart rate. Pacemakers are discussed in a later section of this chapter.
- *Third-degree heart block*: The impulse does not reach the ventricles. As a backup system, special ventricular cells create an impulse that causes the ventricles to contract. On the ECG tracing, the P wave is faster than normal, and the QRS complex is not coordinated with the P wave (Figure 26.19). This is a life-threatening arrhythmia and requires emergency treatment and a pacemaker.

Ventricular Arrhythmias

Ventricular arrhythmias are abnormalities in the ventricles. Most of the ventricular arrhythmias discussed are life-threatening rhythms:

- *Premature ventricular contractions (PVCs)*: Occur when the ventricles contract sooner than they should. An impulse originating in the ventricles creates this abnormality. The QRS complex appears before a P wave. The P wave can also be absent. The T wave can be abnormally shaped, and a widened QRS complex can be seen (Figure 26.20A–B). PVCs can be caused by tobacco, alcohol, epinephrine, and anxiety. They can also be caused by hypertension, coronary artery disease, and lung disease. Infrequent PVCs can be normal. More than six PVCs in a minute is abnormal and can lead to a life-threatening condition.

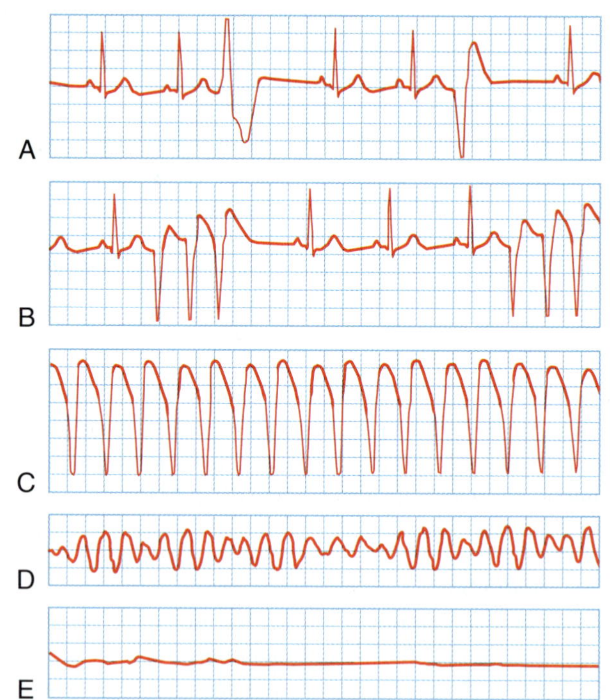

FIGURE 26.20 **(A)** Premature ventricular contraction (PVC). **(B)** Three PVCs in a row. **(C)** Ventricular tachycardia (V-tach). **(D)** Ventricular fibrillation (V-fib). **(E)** Asystole.

- *Ventricular tachycardia (V-tach)*: Occurs when the ventricles beat at a rapid rate (up to 250 beats per minute). It may be seen with multiple PVCs in a row. It may be a short run of fast beats or may last longer than 30 seconds (Figure 26.20C). V-tach is a life-threatening condition. If it is not reversed with drugs or cardioversion, it can become ventricular fibrillation.

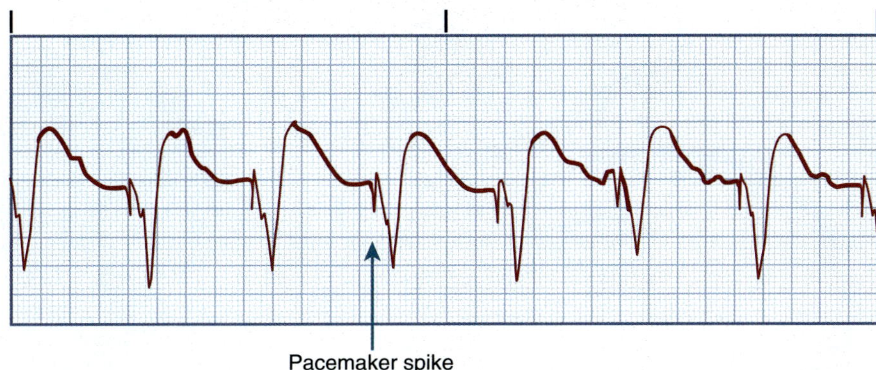

FIGURE 26.21 Pacemaker rhythm strip. (From Lewis S, et al: *Medical-surgical nursing*, ed 9, St. Louis, 2014, Mosby.)

- *Ventricular fibrillation (V-fib)*: Occurs when the ventricles quiver uncontrollably (Figure 26.20D). They are essentially ineffective at pumping any blood. The patient has no pulse, is not breathing, and is unresponsive. This is the most critical, life-threatening arrhythmia. Cardioversion with a defibrillator is necessary to restore normal function of the electrical conduction system.
- *Asystole*: Results in the absence of a heartbeat. A flat line appears on the tracing (Figure 26.20E).

Implantable Device Rhythms

Implantable devices (e.g., pacemaker and implantable cardioverter-defibrillator) create abnormal waveforms on the ECG tracing. A pacemaker is used to treat some types of arrhythmias. It uses low-energy electrical pulses to assist the heart in beating at a normal rate. Pacemakers can change the ECG tracing. Figure 26.21 shows a pacemaker rhythm strip. There are two types of pacemakers:

- *Temporary pacemaker*: Used in an emergency until the permanent pacemaker can be placed; also used for temporary conditions (e.g., heart attack and medication overdose).
- *Permanent pacemaker:* Surgically inserted into the chest or abdomen. Patients can use technology (e.g., smartphones) to transmit their pacemaker data to their provider.

An implantable cardioverter-defibrillator (ICD) can provide low-energy electrical pulses and high-energy pulses (Figure 26.22). The high-energy pulses can treat life-threatening arrhythmias. ICDs are surgically implanted in the chest or abdomen. The ICD is programmed to meet the needs of the patient. Some ICD functions can be checked using technology such as pacemakers. ICD batteries can last 5 to 7 years.

STRESS TESTING

Besides the 12-lead resting ECG, an ECG can be obtained during exercise and nuclear stress tests. The following sections examine exercise stress tests and nuclear stress tests.

Exercise Stress Test

An exercise stress test records the ECG while the patient is exercising. The patient either walks on a treadmill with an incline or uses an exercise bike (Figure 26.23). During the test, a continual ECG is recorded, and the blood pressure is monitored.

The test may be ordered for these reasons:

- The patient is starting an exercise program.
- The patient has angina that is getting worse.
- To evaluate the patient's heart after an angioplasty or bypass surgery.
- To evaluate heart rhythm changes with the stress of exercise.

Preparation for the test includes the following:

- The patient should wear clothes and shoes for exercising.
- The provider will indicate what daily medications should be taken prior to the test.
- The patient should not take a dose of Viagra, Cialis, or Levitra for erectile dysfunction 48 hours before a stress test.
- The patient should not smoke or consume caffeine or alcohol 3 hours before the test.
- The patient signs a consent form prior to the test.

Here is what occurs during the test:

- Electrodes and lead wires will be placed on the patient. A blood pressure cuff will be applied to the patient's arm.
- The patient will begin to exercise slowly, and gradually the exercise difficulty will increase.
- The provider should always be present during the test. If the patient has chest discomfort, dizziness, palpitations, or shortness of breath, the test will stop. Emergency supplies or a crash cart should be kept nearby in case of an emergency.

Nuclear Stress Test

The nuclear stress test shows the blood flow into the heart muscle during rest and activity. A radioactive substance (e.g., thallium or sestamibi) is injected into a vein using an intravenous line (IV). After the patient has rested for 15 to 45 minutes, a gamma camera is used to take images of the blood flow in the heart. Then the person either exercises or is given a vasodilating medication to dilate the coronary arteries. The radioactive substance is again injected, and the person rests. After the required rest period, the gamma camera is used to take additional images of the blood flow through the coronary vessels. Throughout the test, the blood pressure and ECG are monitored.

REMOTE ECG MONITORING

With the advances in technology, several types of remote ECG monitoring can be used for patient care. The following sections discuss types of remote ECG monitoring that can be used.

Holter Monitor

A Holter monitor is used to monitor the heart over a 24- to 48-hour period while patients go about their normal activities. Sometimes patients experience a heart issue that cannot be picked up on a resting 12-lead ECG. Having a longer monitoring period can capture the abnormalities.

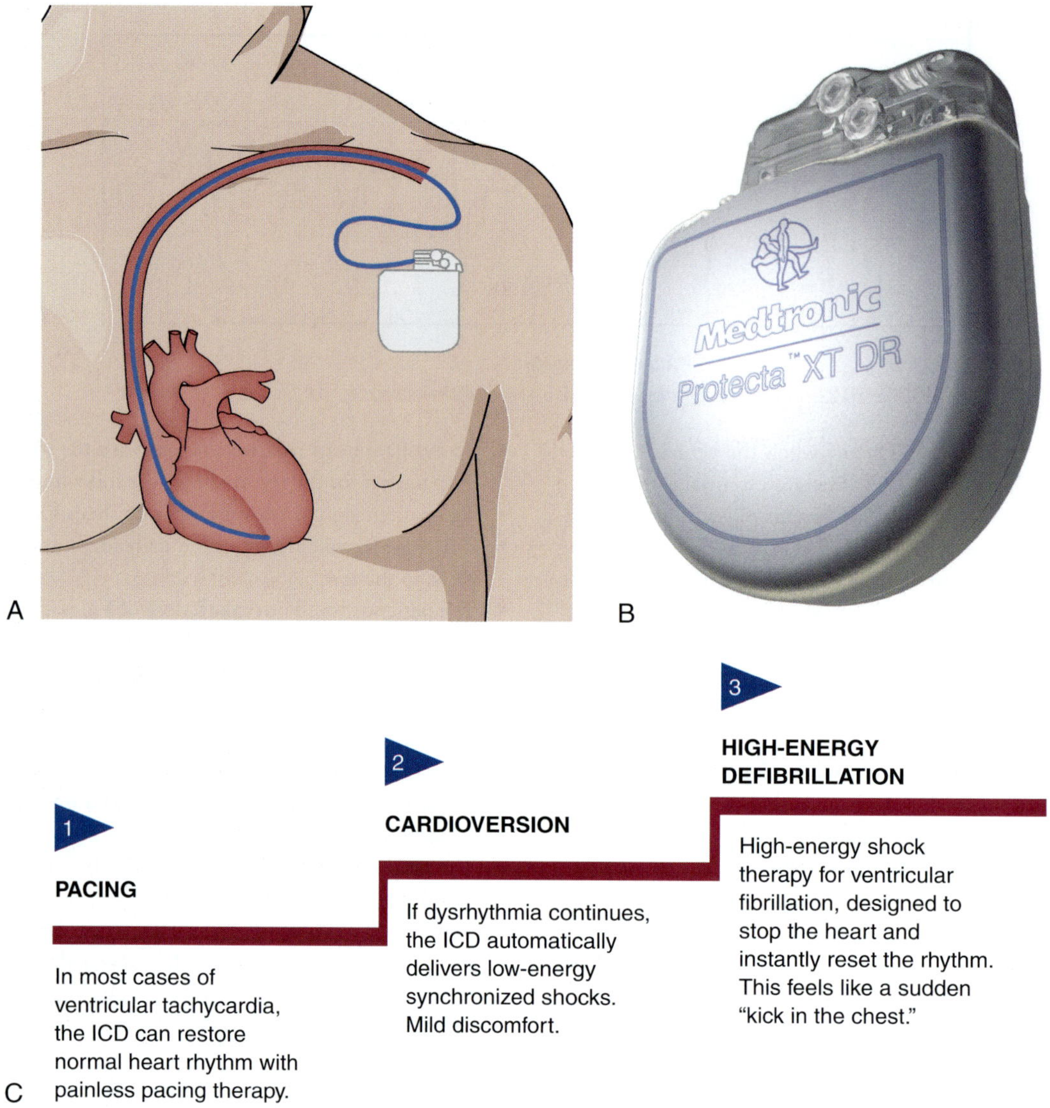

A

B

Medtronic
Protecta™ XT DR

C

1 **PACING**

In most cases of ventricular tachycardia, the ICD can restore normal heart rhythm with painless pacing therapy.

2 **CARDIOVERSION**

If dysrhythmia continues, the ICD automatically delivers low-energy synchronized shocks. Mild discomfort.

3 **HIGH-ENERGY DEFIBRILLATION**

High-energy shock therapy for ventricular fibrillation, designed to stop the heart and instantly reset the rhythm. This feels like a sudden "kick in the chest."

FIGURE 26.22 Implanted cardioverter-defibrillator (ICD). (From Urden L, Stacy K, Lough M: *Thelan's critical care nursing: diagnosis and management,* ed 7, St. Louis, 2014, Mosby.)

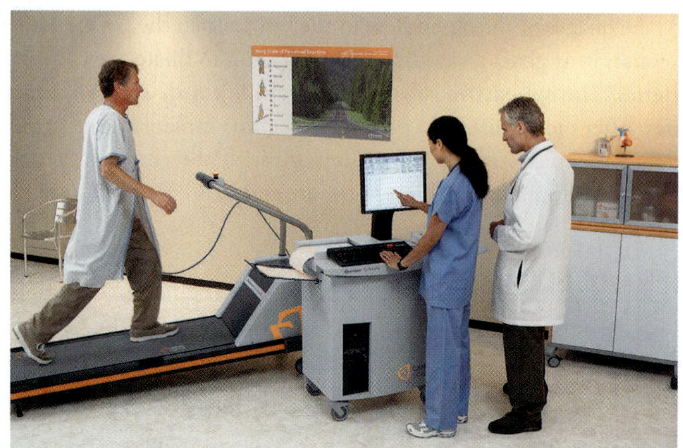

FIGURE 26.23 Exercise stress test. (From Pagana, K, Pagana, T, Pagana, T: *Mosby's manual of diagnostic and laboratory tests,* ed 7, St. Louis, 2022, Elsevier.)

When placing electrodes for a Holter monitor, consult the users' guide. There are many configurations for electrode placement. Different monitors use varying numbers of electrodes. Holter monitors typically use three to seven chest electrodes. As with the resting 12-lead ECG, lead wires attach the electrodes to the small Holter monitor. The monitor runs on batteries and is small enough to fit into a pocket.

The following are patient education points for a Holter monitor test:

- Wear the monitor continuously. The monitor will be removed during your appointment in 24 to 48 hours.
- While wearing the Holter monitor, avoid metal detectors, large magnets, high-voltage areas, x-rays, and electric blankets. Do not get the monitor wet (e.g., no bathing, showering, or swimming).
- Keep a detailed journal of the symptoms experienced. These symptoms could include chest pain, shortness of breath, palpitations or changes in the heartbeat, dizziness, or fainting. Document the date, time, symptoms experienced, and the activity being done at

the time. (Many facilities provide patients with a journal for the documentation.)
- During the return visit, the provider will look at the tracing for abnormalities. The journal of timed activities will help the provider identify what is occurring.
- The patient is instructed on what to do if the electrodes or lead wires fall off.
- The patient is instructed on who to contact with questions or if problems occur.

Procedure 26.2 describes the steps to follow when applying a Holter monitor to a patient.

Cardiac Event Recorder

The cardiac event recorder is a portable, battery-powered ECG device. The recorder is activated by the patient when symptoms occur, and it records the ECG. Patients may wear a cardiac event recorder for 30 days. When symptoms occur only occasionally, it is difficult to capture the abnormality on a resting 12-lead ECG or a Holter monitor. The patient may also be asked to keep a journal, as with the Holter monitor. With the cardiac event recorder, patients go about their daily activities. The monitor can be removed during bathing and showering or swimming.

When patients experience symptoms, they push the recorder's activation button. An ECG is recorded and stored. The ECG can be sent to the provider via a phone or other technology. A provider will review the tracing. If there is an emergency, the patient will be called and told to go to the nearest emergency department.

There are two types of cardiac event recorders:
- *Looping memory monitor* (also called a *cardiac loop recorder*): A pager-sized monitor that connects to two chest electrodes by wires. The monitor continuously records the ECG. When the memory is full, it overwrites from the beginning (i.e., continues the loop of recording). When a patient has symptoms, they activate the monitor. The ECG from prior to, during, and for a short while after the event is stored. It does not overwrite the stored ECGs.
- *Symptom event monitor* (also called a *post-event monitor*): Can be a handheld device or worn on the wrist. When symptoms are felt, the patient activates the monitor and places it on the chest. Small metal disks on the back of the monitor act as electrodes. The current ECG is recorded and stored. Unlike the looping memory monitor, the symptom event monitor cannot record and store the ECG prior to the symptoms.

Implantable Loop Recorder

The implantable *loop recorder* (also called a *loop recorder implant*) is a small recorder (under 2 inches) that looks like a flash drive. It is surgically implanted just under the skin in the upper left chest. It can be implanted in an ambulatory care facility.

Often the device is used for patients who have episodes of fainting, seizures, and palpitations, and other ECG tests have not been able to detect the abnormality. It also catches infrequent arrhythmias that can be missed with traditional ECG monitoring.

The device continuously records the ECG for 2 to 3 years. It records the ECG if the heart rate falls below or rises above the preset limits (set by the provider). The patient can also record the ECG if symptoms are experienced. The provider can download the saved ECG data at the next appointment.

Transtelephonic Monitoring

A *transtelephonic monitor* (TTM) is a small device that records a patient's ECG when the patient pushes the activation button. The TTM has four electrodes on the back of the device that can record a single lead. The ECG data is sent via phone to the base station at the provider's office. The signal is converted to a readable tracing that can be displayed on a monitor or printed out. There are two types of TTMs:
- *TTM with internal memory*: The ECG is recorded and stored when the patient pushes a button. The data can be transmitted by phone to the provider. This type of TTM is used for patients with infrequent arrhythmias.
- *TTM with no internal memory*: The TTM is placed over the heart, and the phone receiver is placed over the TTM. Once the activation button is pushed, the TTM records and immediately sends the live ECG to the provider via the phone line. The data is not saved on the device. This type of TTM is used for patients with pacemakers and internal cardioverter-defibrillators. It allows the provider to monitor the patient remotely.

Portable Handheld ECG Monitors

There are a variety of portable handheld ECG monitors on the market. Many produce a single lead. The ECG data can then be transferred to other devices using software, Bluetooth, smartphones, or USB ports. These devices are marketed to be used at home. A person can use the device and save ECG tracings. The tracings can then be reviewed by the person's provider at the next visit. The machines work differently, some having several electrode options. Finger contact, chest contact (bare skin just below the nipple), and regular chest electrodes can be used to create an ECG tracing.

CRITICAL THINKING APPLICATION 26.10

Monique Jones is Eva's last patient before lunch. As Eva is gathering Ms. Jones' history, Ms. Jones mentions that she has heart palpitations. She had heard about ECG monitors that could be used at home. She was able to order one off the internet and capture her palpitation spell. She is here today to show the doctor her monitor results. Eva has never heard of such a thing. How might she respond to the patient?

CLOSING COMMENTS

Patient Coaching

For any cardiac procedures that patients need to undergo, it is important for the medical assistant to coach the patient on the required preparation. The medical assistant should instruct the patient about what to expect during the test and then explain any follow-up required. Explaining procedures to patients can reduce the stress and confusion they experience.

Legal and Ethical Issues

When a medical assistant is performing an ECG, it is important that the electrodes and lead wires are placed on the patient correctly. If the arm lead wires are reversed, the P, QRS, and T waves are negative deflections in lead I. If the leg lead wires are reversed, Lead III is inverted, and the P wave is larger in lead I compared to lead II. Normally, the P wave is larger in lead II. Taking an ECG when the lead wires are reversed can lead to more cardiac testing and additional provider visits. The medical assistant has a professional responsibility to perform ECGs accurately so that the patient receives the best possible care.

Patient-Centered Care

When a patient is undergoing cardiac testing to rule out or rule in a heart condition, it can be a stressful experience. It is important for the medical assistant to be sensitive to the patient's concerns and feelings. Questions from the patient and family members should be addressed, and any questions outside the medical assistant's scope of practice should be directed to the provider.

The medical assistant should provide patients with clear directions on the cardiac procedure being done. After the procedure, the medical assistant should let patients know who will contact them about the test results. If possible, give patients a timeline so that they will know when to anticipate the notification.

Professional Behaviors

Many times, patients may think that the medical assistant can read ECGs. They may ask the medical assistant if everything looks all right or if the ECG is normal. It is outside of the medical assistant's scope of practice to read ECGs. This is the role of the provider. The medical assistant should explain to the patient that the provider will read the ECG, and the patient will be informed of the results. The medical assistant should take care not to add false hope comments, such as "I am sure the ECG will be normal." These types of comments may give the patient a false impression of the results, and the medical assistant's behavior is unprofessional.

SUMMARY OF SCENARIO

Renee is enjoying working with Eva. They have seen many different cardiac tests while working with Dr. Kahn's patients. If Renee does not have the answers to Eva's questions about cardiac tests, she looks up the information. She finds herself learning new information as a result.

Eva is really enjoying working with Renee and Dr. Kahn. She is feeling so much better performing ECGs. Her understanding of the ECG tracing and how to resolve artifact has greatly improved. She also feels more confident when performing cardiac testing. She is hoping to be able to work with Dr. Kahn in the future because she enjoys doing ECGs so much.

SUMMARY OF LEARNING OBJECTIVES

1. **Examine the structure of the heart, along with the blood flow through the heart.**
   The heart is divided into four chambers. Two atrial chambers receive the blood from the body. Two ventricular chambers pump blood out to the body. The septum divides the right and left sides of the heart. The tricuspid valve is found between the right atrium and the right ventricle. The pulmonary valve is between the right ventricle and the pulmonary artery. The bicuspid or mitral valve is found between the left atrium and left ventricle. The aortic valve is between the left ventricle and the aorta. When the valves open, blood moves to the next chamber or out of the heart through the arteries.
2. **Examine the heart's conduction system.**
   The conduction system is made up of the sinoatrial (SA) node, atrioventricular (AV) node, bundle of His, right and left bundle branches, and the Purkinje fibers. The cardiac cells cycle through the following states:
   - *Polarized state:* Resting phase
   - *Depolarized state:* The impulse hits the cardiac cell
   - *Repolarized state:* Recovery phase
3. **Analyze the components of the ECG tracing of the cardiac cycle.**
   Common ECG terminology includes isoelectric line, deflection, wave, complex, segment, and interval. The components of the ECG tracing are as follows:
   - *P wave:* Shows atrial depolarization; atrial chambers contract, and the blood is pushed to the ventricles
   - *PR segment:* Isoelectric line; allows the atria to finish contracting
   - *QRS complex:* Shows ventricular depolarization; atrial repolarization also occurs during this time, though it is hidden; the ventricles contract, pushing blood out of the heart
   - *ST segment:* Isoelectric line; allows the ventricles to finish contracting
   - *T wave:* Ventricular repolarization and atrial polarization

   The *PR interval* starts at the beginning of the P wave and ends at the start of the Q wave. It represents atrial depolarization. The *QT interval* starts at the beginning of the Q wave and extends to the end of the T wave. During the QT interval, the atrial chambers move from repolarization to the polarized state. The ventricular chambers depolarize and then move into the repolarized state.
4. **Examine the three types of leads in a 12-lead ECG.**
   For a resting 12-lead ECG, three leads are bipolar, three are augmented, and the remaining six are precordial. The bipolar leads are created from a measurement of current traveling from a negative pole to the positive pole:
   - *Lead I:* Right arm (RA) to left arm (LA)
   - *Lead II:* Right arm (RA) to left leg (LL)
   - *Lead III:* Left leg (LL) to left arm (LA)

SUMMARY OF LEARNING OBJECTIVES—*continued*

Each augmented lead uses all three extremity electrodes (RA, LA, and LL) to create the picture. Midpoint between two of the electrodes is the negative pole. The precordial leads provide information on the horizontal (front to back) plane of the heart. The six precordial leads are labeled V_1, V_2, V_3, V_4, V_5, and V_6.

5. **Examine ECG supplies, including the paper and electrodes.**
   ECG machines with printers use special ECG paper. A special heat-sensitive coating on the paper allows the tracing to be "burned" onto the paper. The ECG paper is universally created with small and large boxes. The small box is 1 × 1 mm, and the large box is 5 × 5 mm. The vertical lines measure the amplitude, or *voltage*, of the waveforms. The horizontal lines measure the time.

   Tab or snap electrodes are single-use disposable adhesive tabs that are placed on the skin. The electrodes contain an electrolyte gel that helps pick up the electrical impulses.
6. **Examine the features, settings, and maintenance of electrocardiographs (ECG machines).**
   Box and computer-based ECG models are used in ambulatory care. Features vary by ECG machines. The chart speed regulates the speed of the paper during the recording, and the normal default is 25 mm/s. The gain or sensitivity regulates the height (amplitude) of the tracing, and the normal default is 10 mm/mV. If the ECG machine is set at the defaults, the standardization mark will be an upward rectangle that is 10 small boxes tall.

   The medical assistant should maintain the machine by cleaning the lead wires, tracing stylus, and machine casing as indicated in the users' guide.
7. **Examine the medical assistant's role in obtaining an ECG tracing.**
   The medical assistant must prepare the patient for the procedure. This includes coaching the patient on the procedure, changing clothing, and arranging the patient's position during the procedure. The medical assistant must prepare the skin and apply the electrodes and lead wires. Just prior to obtaining the tracing, the medical assistant should coach the patient not to talk and to relax. The tracing can be uploaded to the electronic health record (EHR) or mounted if done on small strips of ECG paper,
8. **Analyze artifact, including the appearance, cause, and corrective action.**
   - *Wandering baseline* **artifact is an upward and downward movement of the waveform. The medical assistant should clean the skin, replace the electrode with a new one, make sure all electrodes and lead wires are firmly attached, and turn on the baseline filter.**
   - *Somatic tremor* **artifact appears as jagged peaks with irregular heights and spacing. The medical assistant should help the patient relax and encourage no talking or moving during the procedure.**
   - *Alternating current (AC) interference* **artifact appears as a series of small spikes that creates a thick-looking tracing. The medical assistant should unplug the ECG machine and other electrical devices. The lead wires should not overlap, and no cell phones should be near the patient.**
   - *Interrupted baseline* **artifact (also called** *intermittent signal artifact*) **occurs when the tracing looks normal at the beginning, but then it disappears or goes all over when the electrical connection is interrupted. The medical assistant should check that all electrodes and lead wires are attached.**
9. **Examine how to evaluate an ECG tracing.**
   A sinus rhythm is considered normal. Alterations of the sinus rhythm include sinus bradycardia and sinus tachycardia. Atrial arrhythmias occur when there is a problem with the SA node starting the impulse. Atrial arrhythmias include premature atrial contractions (PACs) and atrial flutter. A heart block occurs when there is a disruption or slowing of the electrical impulse through the heart. Ventricular arrhythmias are abnormalities in the ventricles and include premature ventricular contractions (PVCs), V-tach, V-fib, and asystole.
10. **Differentiate between an exercise stress test and a nuclear stress test.**
    An exercise stress test records the ECG while the patient is exercising. The patient either walks on a treadmill with an incline or uses an exercise bike. The nuclear stress test shows the blood flow into the heart muscle during rest and activity. A radioactive substance (e.g., thallium or sestamibi) is injected into a vein using an intravenous line (IV), and a gamma camera is used to take images of the blood flow through the heart and coronary arteries.
11. **Differentiate among types of remote ECG monitoring.**
    A Holter monitor is used to monitor the heart over a 24- to 48-hour period while patients go about their normal activities. The cardiac event recorder is a portable, battery-powered ECG device that is activated by the patient when symptoms occur, and it records the ECG. The implantable *loop recorder* is a small recorder that is surgically implanted just under the skin in the upper left chest. A *transtelephonic monitor* (TTM) is a small device with four electrodes on the back that records a single lead when the patient pushes the activation button. There are a variety of portable handheld ECG monitors that are used for home use. The ECG data can then be transferred to other devices using software, Bluetooth, smartphones, or USB ports and provided to the provider.

PROCEDURE 26.1 Perform Electrocardiography

TASKS: Perform electrocardiography. Document the procedure in the patient's health record. Show empathy regarding the patient's concerns and incorporate critical thinking skills when performing patient care.

EQUIPMENT and SUPPLIES

- ECG machine
- Disposable electrodes
- ECG paper
- Alcohol pads
- Razor (optional)
- Gauze pads (optional)
- Patient gown or paper cape
- Tissue
- Disinfecting wipes
- Gloves
- Waste container
- Patient's health record

PROCEDURAL STEPS

1. Wash your hands or use hand sanitizer.
   PURPOSE: Hand sanitization is an important step for infection control.
2. Assemble equipment and supplies needed for the ECG procedure. Plug in and turn on the ECG machine. Verify that the standardization and chart/paper speed are correct.
   PURPOSE: Having the equipment ready reduces the patient's wait time.
3. Greet the patient. Identify yourself. Verify the patient's identity with full name and date of birth. Make sure the patient's information matches the order and the record. Explain the procedure in a manner that the patient understands. Answer any questions the patient may have about the procedure.
   PURPOSE: It is important to identify the patient in two different ways to ensure that you have the correct patient. Explaining the procedure can make the patient feel more comfortable and reduces anxiety.
   Scenario update: The patient states that she is really worried that something is wrong with her heart. She states that she is nervous about having an ECG.
4. Demonstrate empathy by listening to the patient and learning about their experiences and concerns. Use therapeutic communication techniques and positive nonverbal behaviors, including appropriate eye contact. Position yourself at the same level as the patient. Show your support and respect.
   PURPOSE: Using therapeutic communication techniques can show patients you hear their concerns. It also always helps the medical assistant to clarify the patient's concerns.
5. Ask the patient to remove all clothing from the waist up, including undergarments, and put on the gown/cape so that the opening is in the front. Ask if the patient needs assistance. If so, provide help. If not, leave the room and allow the patient time to change. When reentering the room, provide a courtesy knock on the door.
   PURPOSE: The patient needs to be undressed from the waist up for you to place the electrodes. Patients require privacy to change.
6. Assist the patient into a comfortable supine position on the exam table. Provide support for the legs and arms.
   PURPOSE: To reduce artifact on the tracing, the patient must be comfortable, and the extremities need to be supported.
7. Identify the locations for the ECG electrodes on the chest. Prepare the skin. If the patient has a hairy chest, get the person's permission prior to shaving the areas (optional). Wipe each spot with alcohol and allow it to dry. Fold the gauze pad over your index finger and briskly rub the site to abrade the skin (optional) (Figure 1).
   PURPOSE: The alcohol will prepare the skin and help the electrode to adhere to the skin.

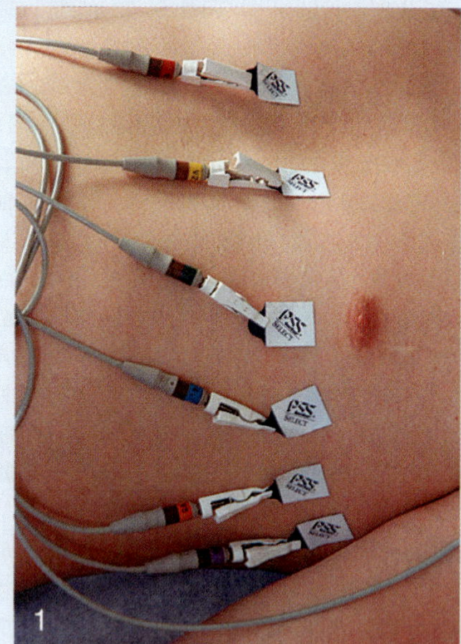

8. Correctly apply the six chest electrodes. If tab electrodes are used, the tabs should be pointed toward the waist.
   PURPOSE: Having the tabs face the core of the body will reduce the tension on the lead wires when they are attached.

PROCEDURE 26.1 Perform Electrocardiography—*continued*

9. Identify the locations for the ECG electrodes on the extremities. Refer to the users' guide for arm electrode position if needed. Wipe each spot with alcohol and allow it to dry. Correctly apply the four limb electrodes to nonbony areas. If using tab electrodes, the lower leg tabs should point toward the waist. The arm/wrist tabs should be pointed toward the fingers.
   PURPOSE: The alcohol will prepare the skin and help the electrode to adhere to the skin.
10. Attach the correct lead wire to each of the electrodes. The wires should follow the natural contour of the body and not overlap.
    PURPOSE: Overlapping wires can cause artifact.
11. Enter the patient's data into the ECG machine. Identify any changes with the default settings, electrode position, or patient's position.
    PURPOSE: The ECG tracing needs to be labeled with the patient's identifying information. The provider must be aware of any changes in the procedure. Electrode position changes, chart/paper speed, and so on can change the appearance of the tracing.
12. Double-check that the lead wires are in the correct position and attached to the electrodes. Make sure each electrode is attached to the skin. Take any corrective action necessary.
    PURPOSE: The lead wires and electrodes must be in the correct spot and attached for the tracing to be accurate.
13. Instruct the patient to lie still and not talk during the tracing. Tell the patient how long the tracing will take.
    PURPOSE: Talking and moving during the tracing will create artifact.
14. Verify that the filters are on. Check the leads on the screen or monitor. Based on what you observe, use critical thinking skills, and take any corrective action necessary. Run the tracing when the leads look clear and without artifact.
    PURPOSE: The filters will minimize the artifact. Checking the appearance of the leads helps to determine if corrective action is needed to minimize artifact.
15. Check the tracing for clarity, artifact, and abnormal life-threatening rhythms. Based on what you observe, use critical thinking skills, and take any corrective action necessary.
    PURPOSE: The provider will need a clear tracing. Life-threatening rhythms need to be identified, and the provider needs to be told immediately.
16. Disconnect the lead wires and remove the electrodes. Wipe any residue from the patient's skin. Wash your hands or use hand sanitizer. Instruct the patient to get dressed. Ask if the patient needs assistance. If so, help the patient to dress.
    PURPOSE: The medical assistant must be the one to remove the wires and electrodes.
17. Provide the patient with information about following up with the provider. Complete any necessary actions with the ECG (e.g., upload to the electronic health record, mount, and route to the provider).
    PURPOSE: After tests, patients will want to know what the results are. The provider will need to read the tracing before any results are given to the patient.
18. Document accurately in the patient's health record. Indicate the name of the provider ordering the test, what test was performed, how the patient tolerated the test, and what you did with the ECG tracing. You can also add any instructions you provided to the patient regarding follow-up.
    PURPOSE: Indicating who ordered the test and what was done is important for insurance reimbursement and legal reasons.
    Scenario update: Perform routine machine maintenance by adding paper to the ECG machine or printer.
19. Review the users' guide on how to change the paper. Gather the new ream or roll of ECG paper.
    PURPOSE: The users' guide will indicate how the paper should be added to the machine.
20. Open the machine. Remove the remaining paper and add the new paper per the steps in the guide.
    PURPOSE: It is important to remove the last few sheets of the old paper to make room for the new ream.
21. Put on gloves and disinfect the lead wires per the users' guide. Disinfect the exam table. Clean up the work area. Remove your gloves and dispose of them in the waste container. Wash your hands or use hand sanitizer.
    PURPOSE: For infection control purposes, it is important to disinfect the lead wires and exam table between each use.

Documentation Example

08/06/20XX 1423 Per Dr. James Martin's order, a resting 12-lead ECG was performed. Pt tolerated the procedure well. Pt was instructed to call the clinic tomorrow for the ECG results. The ECG tracing was routed to Dr. Martin
________________________ Eva Ning, RMA

PROCEDURE 26.2 Apply a Holter Monitor

TASKS: Apply a Holter monitor, and coach a patient on the procedure. Document the procedure in the patient's health record

EQUIPMENT AND SUPPLIES

- Holter monitor, new batteries, flash memory card (if required), carrying case, and operator's manual
- Disposable electrodes
- Razor (optional)
- Sharps container
- Alcohol pads
- Gauze pads (optional)
- Cloth nonallergenic tape (optional)
- Journal
- Waste container
- Patient's health record

PROCEDURAL STEPS

1. Wash your hands or use hand sanitizer.
   PURPOSE: Hand sanitization is an important step for infection control.
2. Assemble the equipment and supplies needed for the procedure. Insert a flash memory card if required. Insert new batteries into the monitor (Figure 1). Consult the users' guide for the required number and placement of electrodes.
   PURPOSE: Having the equipment ready reduces the patient's wait time. New batteries will ensure accurate functioning.

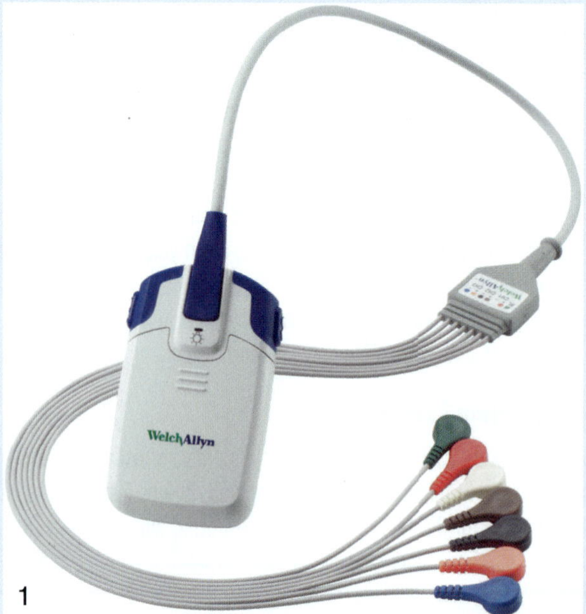

1

3. Greet the patient. Identify yourself. Verify the patient's identity with full name and date of birth. Make sure the patient's information matches the order and the record. Explain the procedure in a manner that the patient understands. Answer any questions the patient may have about the procedure.
   PURPOSE: It is important to identify the patient in two different ways to ensure that you have the correct patient. Explaining the procedure can make the patient feel more comfortable and reduces anxiety.
4. Ask the patient to remove clothing from the waist up and to sit at the end of the exam table. Ask if the patient needs assistance. If so, help. If not, leave the room and allow the patient time to change. When reentering the room, provide a courtesy knock on the door.
   PURPOSE: The patient needs to be undressed from the waist up for you to place the electrodes. Patients require privacy to change.
5. Identify the locations for the electrodes and prepare the skin for the electrodes. Shave the area if the patient has a hairy chest. Wipe the area with the alcohol pad and allow it to dry. Fold the gauze pad over your index finger, and briskly rub the site to abrade the skin.
   PURPOSE: These techniques help the electrodes to better adhere to the skin, which creates a better tracing.
6. Snap the lead wire onto the electrode. Apply the electrodes to the sites as indicated by the manufacturer. Press firmly, and make sure the entire electrode adheres completely to the skin (Figure 2).
   PURPOSE: Secure electrode attachment is necessary to produce an accurate tracing.

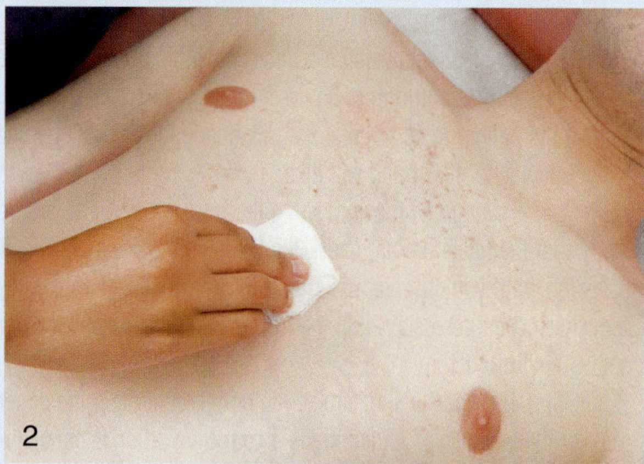
2

7. Loop and tape down the wires on the chest.
   PURPOSE: The tape will hold the wires in place and reduce the tension on the electrodes.
8. Attach the patient cable to the monitor if required. Turn on the recorder and set as indicated by the manufacturer. Enter the patient data as indicated.
   PURPOSE: Each manufacturer will have directions for operating the monitor.
9. Have the patient get dressed. Assist as needed.
   PURPOSE: Some patients may require assistance when hooked up to the monitor.
10. Coach the patient about making journal entries while wearing the monitor (Figure 3). Provide the required patient education.
    PURPOSE: It is important for patients to keep a diary of what they are doing. The provider will check the ECG for abnormalities and then check what the patient was doing during the event.

PROCEDURE 26.2 Apply a Holter Monitor—*continued*

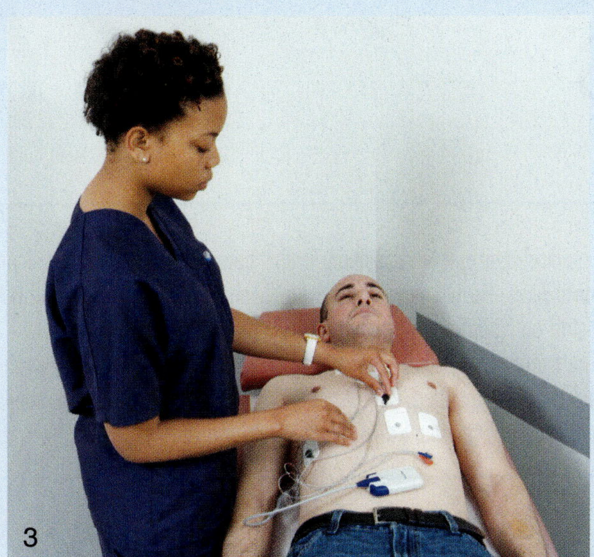
3

11. Assist the patient in scheduling a return appointment in 24 hours. Provide the patient with contact information should a question arise.
    PURPOSE: The patient will need to return in 24 hours for the monitor to be removed. Providing contact information will reduce the patient's anxiety.
12. Document accurately in the patient's health record. Indicate the name of the provider ordering the test, the procedure done, the patient education provided, and the return appointment.
    PURPOSE: Indicating who ordered the test and what was done is important for insurance reimbursement and for legal reasons.

Documentation Example

08/06/20XX 1423 Per Dr. James Martin's order, a Holter monitor was applied. Pt was instructed on how to complete the diary, and a contact number was provided in case pt has additional questions. Pt verbalized what he was to write in the diary. Appointment was made for 08/07/20XX to remove the monitor. ——————————— Eva Ning, RMA

Courtesy Welch Allyn, Skaneateles Falls, NY.

MEDICAL EMERGENCIES

27

SCENARIO

Gabe Garcia, a certified medical assistant (CMA) who has met the requirements of the American Association of Medical Assistants (AAMA), has worked for Walden-Martin Family Medical (WMFM) Clinic for 7 years. He was hired right after he completed his medical assistant program. Gabe has learned a lot through the years. He has impressed his supervisor with his dedication, attention to detail, punctuality, and patient care skills. Gabe was just promoted to a medical assistant lead position. In this new position, Gabe has additional responsibilities. He will now oversee the crash carts in the clinic, and he will train staff on emergency procedures.

The current emergency procedures need to be revised, and the crash cart procedures need updating. Gabe is excited to take over his new responsibilities. He looks forward to what he will learn in this new role.

While studying this chapter, think about the following questions:

- How are emergencies handled in ambulatory care settings?
- What are common emergency equipment and supplies found in the ambulatory care settings?
- What are the first aid actions for cold and heat illnesses, burns, poisonings, anaphylaxis, bites, and foreign bodies in the eye?
- What are the first aid actions for diabetic emergencies?
- What are the first aid actions for musculoskeletal emergencies?
- What are the first aid actions for neurologic emergencies, including vertigo, concussion, seizure, and stroke?
- What are the first aid actions for respiratory emergencies, including hyperventilation, asthmatic attack, and choking?
- What are the first aid actions for cardiovascular emergencies, including syncope, bleeding, shock, and heart attack?

LEARNING OBJECTIVES

1. Examine types of emergencies, along with the screening and triage process that occurs in ambulatory care.
2. Examine the team members' roles and the importance of documentation in code situations.
3. Differentiate among the equipment and supplies used in code situations.
4. Differentiate among first aid procedures for temperature-related emergencies.
5. Differentiate among the types of environmental emergencies and the related first aid procedures.
6. Differentiate between hypoglycemic and hyperglycemic medical emergencies, including signs, symptoms, and treatments.
7. Examine screening questions and first aid procedures for musculoskeletal emergencies.
8. Differentiate among neurologic emergencies, including signs, symptoms, and first aid procedures.
9. Differentiate among respiratory emergencies, including signs, symptoms, and first aid procedures.
10. Differentiate among cardiovascular emergencies, including signs, symptoms, and first aid procedures.

VOCABULARY

Ambu bag A self-refilling bag-valve-mask unit used for artificial respiration that is effective for ventilating and oxygenating intubated patients. Acronym for *artificial manual breathing unit*.

basic life support (BLS) A number of emergency procedures needed to ensure a person's immediate survival. Procedures include cardiopulmonary resuscitation, controlling bleeding, treatment of shock and poisoning, stabilization of injuries, and basic first aid.

cardiopulmonary resuscitation (CPR) (ri sus i TAY shun) The application of manual chest compressions and ventilations (also called rescue breathing) to patients who are not breathing or do not have a pulse; a part of basic life support.

code A term used in healthcare settings to indicate an emergency situation and to summon the trained team to the scene

endotracheal tube (ET) (en doe TRAY kee al) A catheter that is inserted into the trachea through the mouth; provides a patent airway.

intraosseous (in tra OS ee us) Within bone; route for delivery of fluids and medications through a needle inserted into the marrow of certain bones (e.g., humerus, tibia, and femur).

VOCABULARY—*continued*

nasopharyngeal airway tube (NPA) (nae zoe fah RIN jee ahl) A soft, flexible tube that is inserted in the nose and provides a patent airway; also known as a nasal trumpet.

necrosis (neh KROH sis) Tissue death.

patent (PAY tent) Open.

pocket face mask A device used to deliver a rescue breath.

pruritus (proo RIE tuss) Itching.

recovery position A position on the person's side that helps to keep the airway open and clear.

rescue breathing Life-saving maneuver to resuscitate a person who has stopped breathing. The rescuer forces air into the victim's lungs at intervals by exhaling into the victim's mouth, nose, or stoma from a laryngectomy.

retractions (re TRAK shuns) The sucking in of tissues between the intercostal spaces and neck due to respiratory distress; classic sign of severe asthma.

standard of care The level and type of care an ordinary, prudent healthcare professional with the same training and experience in a similar practice would have provided under a similar situation.

triage (tree AHZH) To sort out and classify the injured; used in the military and emergency settings to determine the priority of a patient to be treated.

triaging flow map A written flow map to make triage decisions; based on answers to questions, the person moves through the map until a triage decision is made.

vasoconstriction Contraction of the muscles, causing narrowing of the inside tube of the vessel.

INTRODUCTION

Emergencies happen everywhere. As a medical assistant, it is important for you to know how to handle emergencies because you may need to respond to one:

- *Outside of your job, in the community:* You may be one of the first people on the scene and need to provide first aid to the victims.
- *In the healthcare setting:* You may need to provide first aid as the provider assesses the injured person. Additional treatments, such as oxygen and medications, are provided in the healthcare setting.
- *Over the phone:* You may need to obtain information from someone involved in an emergency and provide first aid coaching. The medical assistant asks screening questions and provides the information to the provider. The provider instructs the medical assistant what to tell the caller.

This chapter starts by discussing emergencies in the healthcare setting and the medical assistant's role. Next, common emergency medical equipment, supplies, and medications are explained. Lastly, emergency conditions are described, along with the first aid procedures to perform.

EMERGENCIES IN HEALTHCARE SETTINGS

Emergencies can happen at any time in the ambulatory care facility. If medical assistants are responsible for screening patients, they should be trained on the procedures established by the providers and supervisors. The following sections discuss types of emergencies that can occur in ambulatory care, along with the screening and triage processes that are typically used.

Types of Emergencies

In the ambulatory care setting, many different types of emergencies can occur. Some of the more common emergencies include the following:

- A patient who is being seen and treated has a life-threatening occurrence (e.g., an allergic reaction to a medication).
- A person (e.g., employee, visitor, or patient) has an accident or health issue that results in an emergency.
- A *walk-in patient* (a patient without an appointment) comes to the facility with a critical health issue.
- An individual calls about an emergency.

How these are handled can differ greatly among ambulatory care facilities. How emergencies are handled is determined by the following factors:

- Facility's size and distance from emergency medical services
- Available equipment and supplies
- Providers' training and scope of practice
- Number and type of clinical care employees (medical assistants, licensed practical nurses, and registered nurses) and their scopes of practice

Some facilities only have minimal staff, whereas others have specific employees who respond to emergencies.

Screening and Triaging Emergencies

In small facilities, the medical assistant may be responsible for screening emergency calls and walk-in patients. These medical assistants must follow the facility's screening protocols. They cannot assess the patient or give advice. The information collected must be reported to the provider. The provider tells the medical assistant what should be done. Examples of screening questions are provided later in the chapter.

In larger facilities, registered nurses (sometimes called **triage** nurses) gather information from walk-in patients and emergency calls. Using a **triaging flow map** or triaging software, the nurse identifies how quickly the patient needs to be seen and where the patient needs to be seen (Figure 27.1).

Sometimes patients come to the ambulatory healthcare setting with life-threatening conditions. The provider sees these patients immediately and assesses their conditions. The provider will order 911 to be called if needed. Treatment is provided as the team waits for the emergency responders to transport the patient to the emergency department. The following sections explain the first aid given for different types of emergencies.

CRITICAL THINKING APPLICATION 27.1

Gabe knows that there are times when medical assistants need to screen phone calls. This can be intimidating for new medical assistants. What procedures would Gabe put in place to help medical assistants screen emergency calls accurately yet minimize their feelings of intimidation?

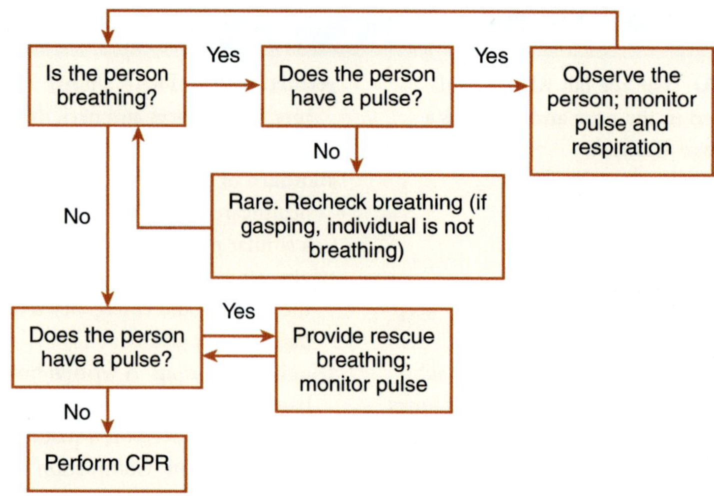

FIGURE 27.1 Example of a flow map. Similar flow maps can be used when triaging or treating emergencies.

ROLES AND DOCUMENTATION IN CODE SITUATIONS

Every employee in a healthcare setting should know how to get help in an emergency. This process will vary. Healthcare facilities use special phrases for emergencies. For instance, "**Code** Blue Urgent Care" may indicate an emergency is occurring in Urgent Care. Sometimes the code words indicate the age of the person. For instance, "Code Pink Family Practice" may mean that an emergency is occurring in Family Practice, and "pink" indicates a child.

Role of Team Members

Once the call goes out for help, staff members respond to the scene. In small settings, most members of the staff may be needed. In large facilities, only certain staff members respond. Usually, medical assistants, licensed practical nurses (LPNs), registered nurses (RNs), and providers attend the emergency. In codes, **basic life support** is provided. Possible roles for each team member include the following:

- *Provider*: Assesses the patient, orders treatments and procedures, performs advanced procedures, may administer intravenous (IV) medications, and indicates when 911 needs to be called.
- *Nurse*: RNs may administer IV medications and fluids. LPNs may do the same if permitted by the state's scope of practice. RNs and LPNs assist with treatments and procedures, perform **cardiopulmonary resuscitation (CPR)**, call 911, and document the code activities as they occur.
- *Clinical medical assistant*: Assists with treatments and procedures, performs CPR, documents the code activities as they occur, and calls 911. They may hand supplies to staff members and assist with caring for the family (moving them to a private area away from the emergency).
- *Administrative medical assistant*: Performs CPR and hands supplies to the staff (in small agencies), calls 911, escorts the emergency responders to the patient, and assists with caring for the family.

Importance of Documentation

In a code situation, it is important for at least one team member to document everything that occurs. This is a stressful job because many things occur during an emergency. There are several reasons why accurate documentation is critical:

- The information is used during the code. For instance, CPR was started, and the team member documented "1413 CPR initiated." As the code progresses, the provider may want to know when the CPR was started.
- Emergency responders will need to know what occurred during the code. (What medications were given? When were they given? How much was given?)
- The documentation will provide evidence that the **standard of care** was met in the treatments given to the patient. Many lawsuits have originated from emergencies. The lawyers review the documentation. They look for delays in emergency care and a lack of appropriate treatment. Complete and accurate documentation may make a difference between a lawsuit surviving or being dismissed in favor of the healthcare team.

If you are new to codes and, if given the option, perform a role other than documenting. Observe what occurs during a code as you complete your task. Study the code documentation form during noncode times. As you become more comfortable with codes, assist the documenter if you can. A second pair of eyes is always helpful. Lastly, become the documenter and have a seasoned team member assist you.

CRITICAL THINKING APPLICATION **27.2**

Currently, the clinic does not have a procedure for documentation during code situations. The provider documents after the emergency. Gabe would like to discuss using a standard code form for all emergencies. A team member would be responsible for documentation during the code. Discuss the pros and cons of documenting during the code.

EMERGENCY EQUIPMENT AND SUPPLIES

The emergency supplies available at healthcare facilities will vary based on the size and location of the facility. Some practices have a small box that contains a few supplies and medications. Other practices place many crash carts throughout the building (Figure 27.2). A *crash cart* is a rolling supply cart that contains emergency equipment.

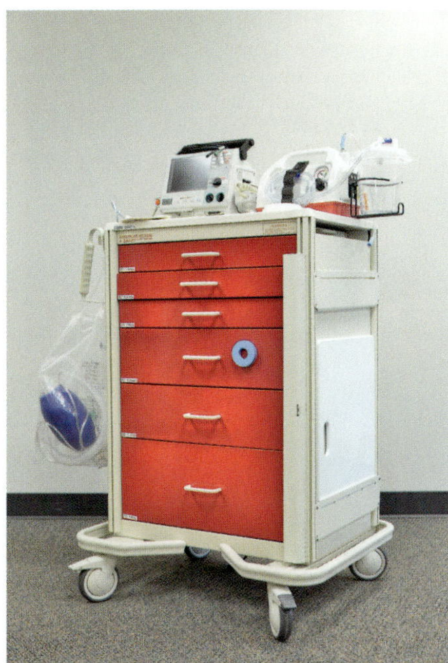

FIGURE 27.2 Crash carts are used in an emergency. The drawers should be labeled to allow speedy retrieval of supplies.

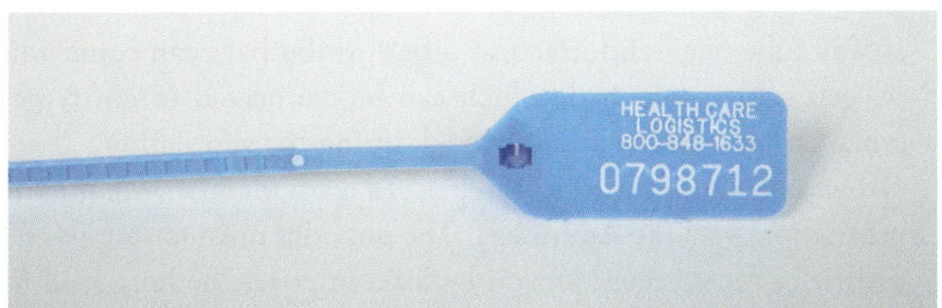

FIGURE 27.3 A plastic lock is placed on the inventoried crash cart. The number is written on the inventory form for tracking purposes. These locks are easy to break in emergencies.

The crash cart should be checked monthly. This can be done by the supervisor or by two qualified employees (e.g., medical assistants, LPNs, or RNs). Expiration dates on the supplies are checked. Old supplies are replaced with new supplies. All the equipment and supplies are inventoried. When the inventory is completed, a plastic lock (or locking tag) is placed on the cart (Figure 27.3). The crash cart is used only in emergencies. You should never break the lock and use something from the crash cart unless it is an emergency. The plastic locks should be kept safe and used only when the cart is inventoried monthly or after an emergency. Many of the locks are numbered, and the number is written on the inventory document. Keeping the locks safe minimizes the number of people going into the crash cart for nonemergency reasons.

This section focuses on the equipment and supplies typically found on a crash cart. The medical assistant should be familiar with the supplies and their location on the crash cart.

Oxygen and Airway Supplies

Oxygen and airway supplies are common items found on crash carts. **Pocket face masks** and other barrier devices for **rescue breathing** may be found on the crash cart (Figure 27.4A). If the patient needs oxygen, the provider will order oxygen to be applied via a mask or a nasal canula. (Refer to Chapter 41 for additional information on oxygen delivery systems.)

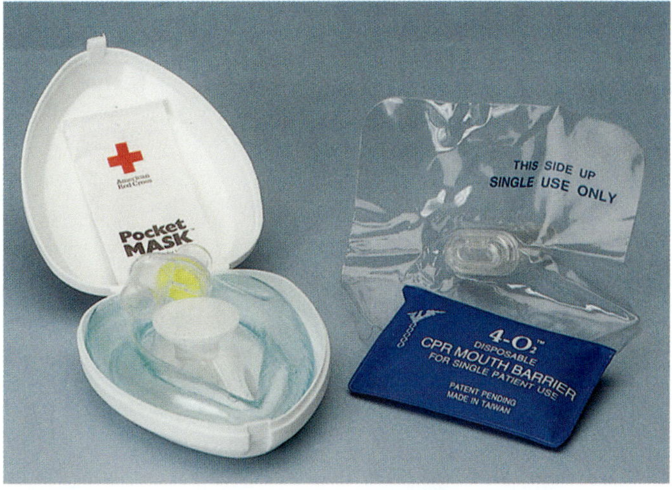

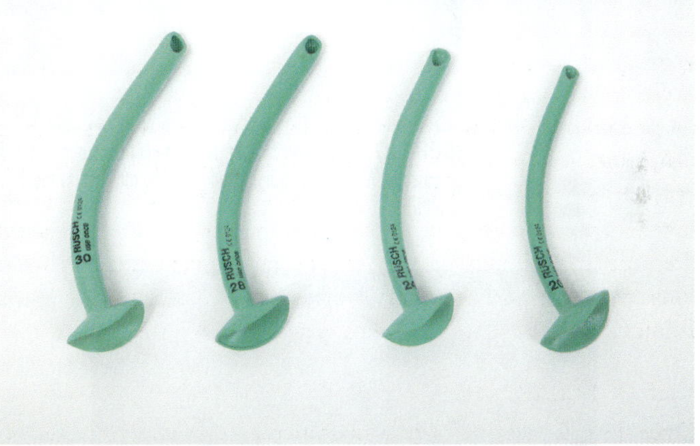

FIGURE 27.4 **(A)** Rescue breathing mouth barriers. **(B)** Nasopharyngeal airways come in a variety of sizes.

If the patient has difficulty breathing or if an airway constriction may be occurring, the provider will insert a **nasopharyngeal airway (NPA) tube** or an **endotracheal (ET) tube** to create a **patent** airway (Figure 27.4B). Providers also use the following to maintain airways:

- *Esophageal tracheal tubes*, which are placed in the trachea or esophagus
- *Laryngeal mask airways*, which are inserted through the mouth and advanced to the hypopharynx
- *Laryngeal tubes*, which are also inserted through the mouth and placed in the hypopharynx

Endotracheal Tube Intubation

The medical assistant should be aware of the equipment required during an ET tube intubation. During an endotracheal intubation, the provider will need the following:

- *Laryngoscope* with either a curved (MacIntosh) or a straight (Miller) blade. The sizes of blades are indicated on the side or back of the blade (Figure 27.5A). The medical assistant must hand the laryngoscope with the blade attached to the provider (Figure 27.5B).
- *ET tube* in the appropriate size. Cuffed ET tubes come in a variety of sizes for adults and older children (e.g., 7.5, 8, and 8.5). Uncuffed ET tubes come in a variety of sizes for children (e.g., 2.5, 3, and 3.5) (Figure 27.6A). A syringe is used to inflate the cuff with air once it is in place.

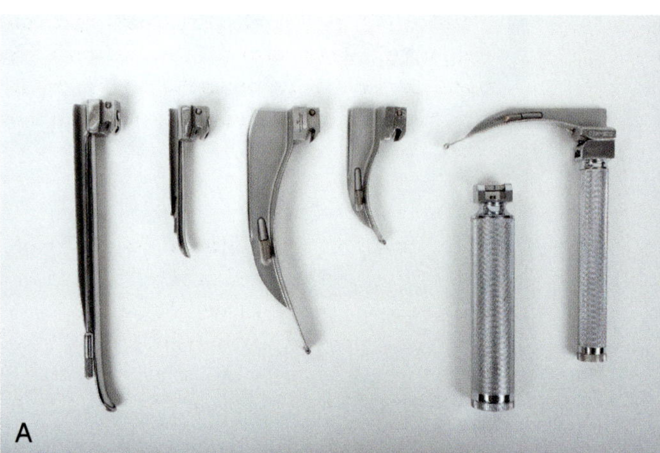

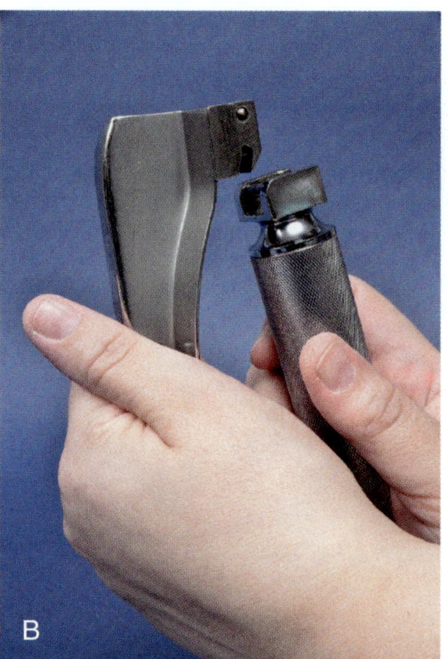

FIGURE 27.5 (A) *Left to right:* Two different sizes of straight blades and curved blades; adult laryngoscope handle and an assembled pediatric laryngoscope. A curved or straight blade must be attached to the laryngoscope handle. **(B)** To attach the blade, hold the blade parallel to the handle and attach.

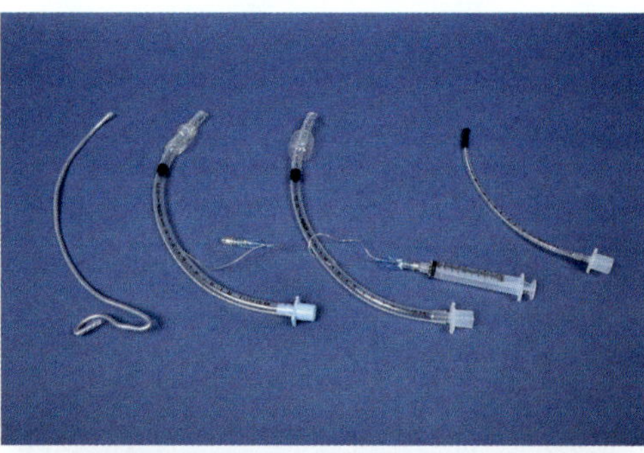

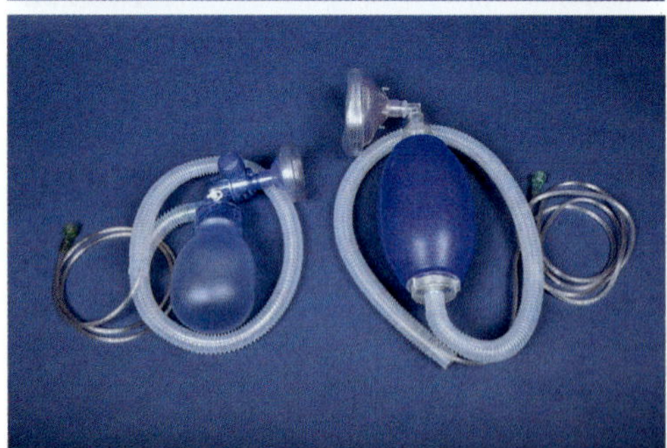

FIGURE 27.6 (A) *Left to right:* A stylet is threaded into the endotracheal (ET) tube to help maintain the tube's curve. ET tubes for adults are cuffed (or have a balloon that is inflated using a syringe). ET tubes for children are uncuffed *(far right picture)*. ET tubes come in a variety of sizes. **(B)** *Left to right:* Pediatric and adult Ambu bags. An Ambu bag can cover the mouth or can be attached to an airway tube (e.g., endotracheal tube). Ambu bags can come with oxygen tubing attached. The tubing can be connected to an oxygen tank. Oxygen can be administered during the ventilation.

- *Stylet* is a metal or flexible plastic wire inserted into the ET tube to create a firm, curved tube (see Figure 27.6A). After the ET tube is in place, the stylet is removed.
- **Ambu bag**, which is attached to the ET tube and used to administer room air or oxygen (Figure 27.6B). An Ambu bag, which is a bag-valve-mask unit, can cover the mouth or be attached to an airway tube (e.g., endotracheal tube). Ambu bags can come with oxygen tubing attached, which can be connected to an oxygen tank. Oxygen can be administered during the ventilation.
- *Stethoscope.* Once the tube is in place, a team member will provide ventilation with the Ambu bag. The provider must ensure the ET tube is in the correct location by listening over the lung field for air movement. If the ET tube is in the wrong location, the abdomen will become bloated with air; the patient is not being ventilated. (A provider will usually state that breath sounds are heard bilaterally. This is important to document on the code form. This verifies the ET tube is in the correct location.)

CRITICAL THINKING APPLICATION **27.3**

Gabe has decided that the crash carts must be inventoried monthly. He will have two medical assistants inventory each cart. Gabe feels it is important that all medical assistants have an opportunity to inventory the crash cart at least every 4 months. Why would this be important for the medical assistants? Besides checking expiration dates, what else could they do to increase their skills and knowledge for emergencies?

Defibrillator

A *defibrillator* is a device that delivers an electrical shock to the heart muscle in an attempt to restore a normal heartbeat. The defibrillator's shock causes the heart to momentarily stop. When it restarts, the hope is the heart will beat at a normal rhythm. The quicker a defibrillator can be used, the better the person's chances of survival.

Typically, a defibrillator or an automated external defibrillator (AED) is used in healthcare facilities.

- A defibrillator consists of two handheld paddles that are placed on gel pads located on the patient's chest (Figure 27.7A). Gel

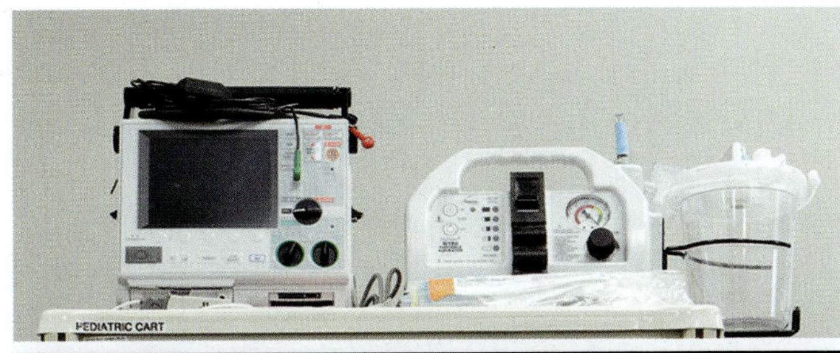

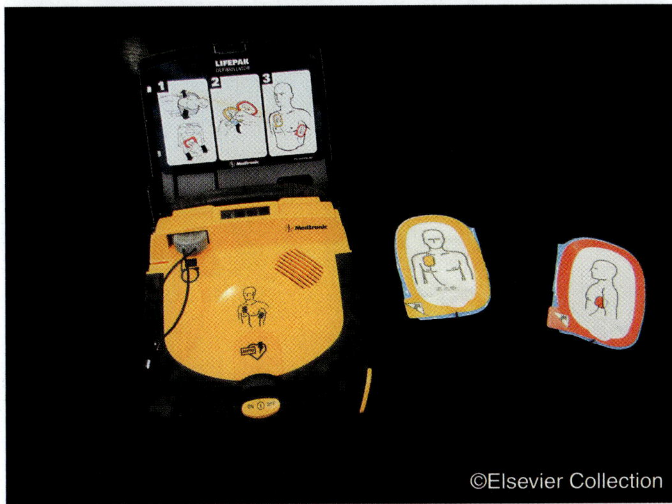

FIGURE 27.7 **(A)** *Left to right:* The defibrillator usually sits on top of the crash cart. Other equipment, such as a suction machine, can also be found on the top of the crash cart. **(B)** Automated external defibrillator.

pads are required to prevent burns. They provide better electricity conduction from the paddles to the patient. The provider indicates how many joules at which to set the machine, and someone announces "All clear" to ensure no one is touching the patient. The provider pushes the button to give the shock.

- An *automated external defibrillator* is a portable, lightweight machine (Figure 27.7B). Sticky pads that contain electrodes (sensors) are attached to the patient's chest. The AED checks the heart rate and determines if a shock is required. If a shock is needed, the AED gives audible directions to the user to administer a shock.

Medications

The medications in crash carts can vary. Common medications used in emergencies are listed in Table 27.1. Most crash carts and emergency supply boxes include IV supplies. An IV line is usually inserted into the patient's hand, wrist, or arm. If an IV line cannot be inserted, the provider may insert an **intraosseous** needle that can be used to give IV fluids and medications (Figure 27.8). The intraosseous needle can be inserted into the humerus, tibia, femur, sternum, or iliac crest. The provider must be specially trained to insert the intraosseous needle.

Administering IV medications is outside the scope of practice for the medical assistant. In many states, inserting an IV line and giving IV fluids are also outside the medical assistant's scope of practice. The medical assistant may help by getting the required supplies and documenting what was given.

TABLE 27.1 Common Medications Used in Emergencies

MEDICATION	ACTION	USED FOR
Amiodarone (Cordarone, Pacerone)	Slows the heart rate and allows blood to fill the ventricular chambers	Ventricular tachycardia, ventricular fibrillation
Atropine	Increases the heart rate	Bradycardia
Calcium Chloride	Increases the calcium levels in the serum	Hyperkalemia and *hypocalcemia* (too little calcium in the blood)
Diazepam (Valium)	Affects the chemicals in the brain	Seizures, agitation
Diphenhydramine (Benadryl)	Antihistamine that reduces the effects of histamine	Allergic reactions, second-line drug for anaphylaxis (used after epinephrine has been given)
Dopamine (Intropin)	Increases the stimulation of the heart muscle	Hypotension, heart failure
Epinephrine (Adrenalin)	Increases the stimulation of the heart muscle; vasoconstrictor and bronchial relaxant	Anaphylaxis, cardiac arrest, severe asthma, bronchospasms
Glucagon	Hormone that stimulates the liver to release glucose into the blood	*Hypoglycemia* (too low glucose in the blood)
Lidocaine	Helps to restore the regular heart rhythm	Ventricular arrhythmias
Magnesium	Electrolyte that helps maintain a normal heart rhythm	Arrhythmias
Naloxone (Evzio, Narcan)	Blocks or reverses the opioid medication effects	Opioid (narcotic) overdose
nitroglycerin	Vasodilator	Congestive heart failure, angina
Sodium bicarbonate	Reduces the pH of the serum	Metabolic acidosis, *hyperkalemia* (excessive potassium in the blood)

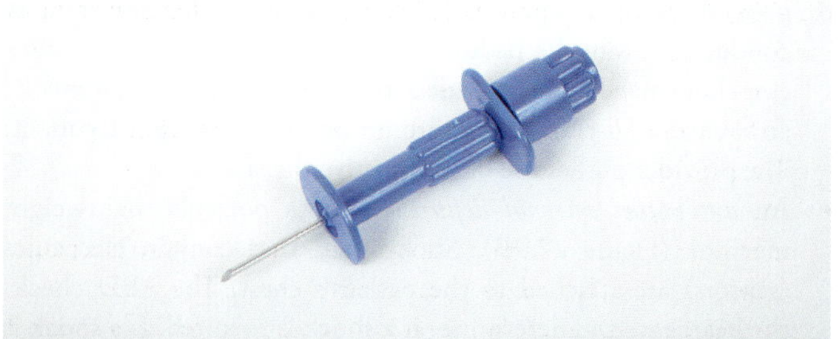

FIGURE 27.8 An intraosseous needle may be used to give IV fluids and medications in an emergency.

Other Supplies

Various other supplies can be found in the crash cart. Some items not already mentioned include the following:

- Personal protective equipment (PPE), such as gloves, a sharps disposal container, and a pocket face mask
- *Algorithms*, or step-by-step instructions, for reference
- Clipboard with documents for charting the code
- Backboard, which is placed under the patient to provide a firm surface for compressions
- Extra batteries for the laryngoscope

Pediatric Supplies

In the 1980s, James Broselow, a family practice doctor working in an emergency department, came up with an idea for simplifying how to determine pediatric medication doses administered during emergencies. Medications for children are based on weight. Rescue personnel spent critical moments during emergencies calculating medication doses for children. Broselow's idea was to measure the child's length and come up with a suggested dose. After much research, the Broselow tape was created (Figure 27.9A).

A healthcare professional measures a child using the tape. The tape is placed from the top of the head to the child's heel. The length is measured as a specific color (Figure 27.9B). Based on the "color" of the child, the tape lists common medication dosages and emergency equipment sizes that should be used for that size of child. This system has sped up the response time for treating children during emergencies. It eliminates the use of reference guides and calculators for medication dosages.

Many ambulatory care settings that routinely see sick children use the Broselow tape. In addition to the tape, pediatric crash carts (e.g., Broselow ColorCode Cart) have been created (Figure 27.10). Each color on the tape has a matching drawer. Each drawer contains the right-sized equipment for that size of the child.

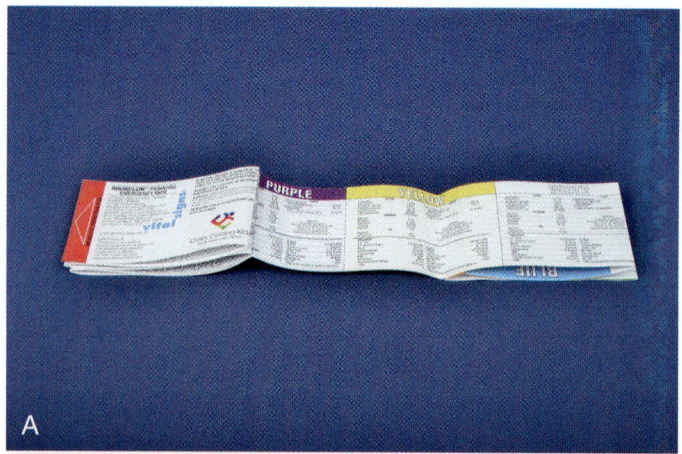

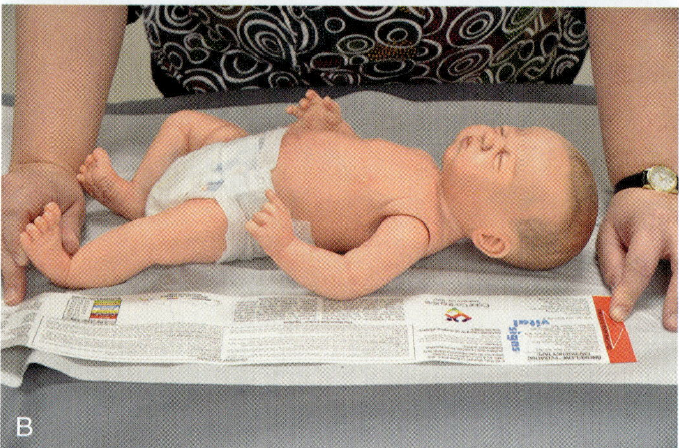

FIGURE 27.9 **(A)** Broselow tape. **(B)** Measure the child with the Broselow tape. Measure from the head to the heel and identify the color by the child's heel. This is the color to use during the emergency.

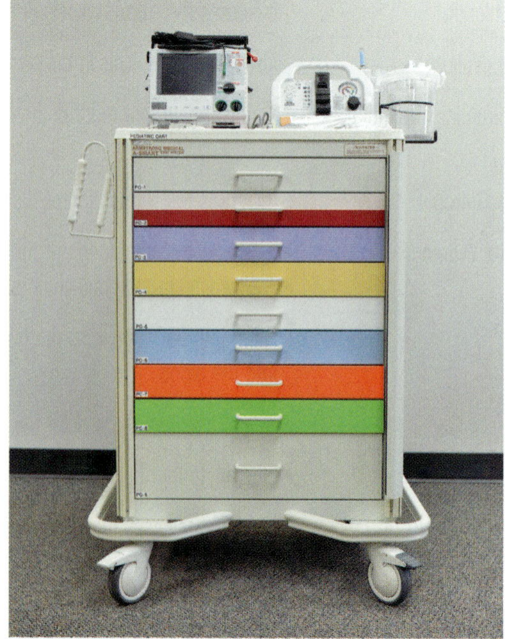

FIGURE 27.10 Each drawer in the Broselow ColorCode Cart is color coded.

TEMPERATURE-RELATED EMERGENCIES

Overexposure to hot or cold temperatures can cause mild to life-threatening issues. Environmental temperatures affect the body's temperature.

Cold-Related Conditions

Cold-related conditions include frostbite and hypothermia. In cold weather, our bodies tend to lose heat faster than we can produce it. This results in a lowered body temperature. Uncovered skin can result in injuries faster than covered skin. It does not take long for frostbite to occur. For instance, with a 10 mile per hour (mph) wind speed and a temperature of −5°F (−20.6°C), a person can get frostbite within 30 minutes. With the same wind speed and a temperature of −25°F (−31.7°C), a person can get frostbite within 5 minutes. There are a number of risk factors for cold-related conditions:

- Smoking or taking a beta-blocker medication (e.g., atenolol)
- Having diabetes or poor blood circulation
- High winds, wet clothes
- Dehydration and exhaustion

Possible screening questions for cold-related conditions include the following:

- What is the person's age?
- How long was the person exposed to the cold temperature?
- What symptoms does the person have? What color is the exposed skin?
- What is the person's medical history?

Frostbite

Frostbite occurs when the skin and body tissues are exposed to cold temperatures. Susceptible areas include cheeks, nose, ears, fingers, toes, and chin. Frostbite is caused by exposure to cold temperatures. The person may experience a pins-and-needles sensation followed by numbness in the frostbitten area. The skin is hard, pale, and cold; blisters may occur. The affected area may ache or lack feeling. First aid procedures include the following:

- Move the person to a warmer location.
- Remove all wet clothing and cover the person with warm, dry clothing.
- Observe for signs of hypothermia.
- Seek medical care; if it is not available, then rewarm the area by soaking it in warm water (104°F to 108°F [40°C to 42.2°C]) for 20 to 30 minutes. Do not rub the area. Apply a sterile dressing to the area.
- Give the person a warm drink to replace lost fluids; do not give alcohol.

Hypothermia

With hypothermia, the core body temperature drops below 95°F (35°C). In severe hypothermia, the body temperature drops below 82°F (27.8°C), causing a life-threatening condition and arrhythmias. Hypothermia is caused by exposure to cold temperatures or immersion in cold water for a long period of time. A person with hypothermia may experience slurred speech and slow, shallow breathing and weak pulse. Additional signs and symptoms include clumsiness, drowsiness, confusion, and a loss of consciousness. With infants, the skin may be bright red and cold. Here are the first aid procedures to follow in cases of hypothermia:

- Move the person to a warmer location.
- Remove all wet clothing, and cover the person with warm, dry clothing.
- Seek medical care.
- Give the person a warm drink to replace lost fluids; do not give alcohol.

Warming a patient with hypothermia too quickly can also lead to cardiac issues and additional tissue damage. Because of this, the emergency department gradually warms all patients with hypothermia.

Heat-Related Conditions

Heat-related conditions include heat cramps, exhaustion, and stroke. Heat injuries occur most often on hot, humid days and are caused by prolonged heat exposure. With high humidity, sweat, which cools the skin, does not evaporate as quickly. Risk factors for heat injuries include the following:

- Age (older adults and children age 4 and younger)
- Dehydration, heart disease, and poor blood circulation
- Fever and sunburn
- Mental illness
- Using alcohol and taking certain prescription drugs, such as antidepressants, anticonvulsants, antipsychotics, and diuretics

Consider these possible screening questions for heat-related conditions:

- What is the person's age?
- How long was the person exposed to the hot temperature?
- What symptoms does the person have? Is the person sweating? What does the skin look like? Is the person alert or confused?

It is important to treat heat-related illnesses immediately. An untreated condition can progress to become a more severe situation. An effective way to lower the person's temperature is to apply cool, wet cloths and then fan the moist skin. This will lower the person's body temperature through the evaporation process.

Heat Cramps

Heat cramps are a mild heat-related illness that causes muscle pain and spasms in the abdomen, arms, or legs, due to electrolyte imbalance. It usually occurs with strenuous activities or in those who sweat a lot. First-aid measures are as follows:

- Have the person rest for several hours in a cool place.
- Have the person drink cool electrolyte (sports) beverages to replace electrolytes lost.

Heat Exhaustion

Heat exhaustion is a milder form of a heat-related illness. It is caused by exposure to high temperatures and inadequate fluid and electrolyte replacement. A person with heat exhaustion may experience the following:

- Heavy sweating, muscle cramps, nausea, and vomiting
- Pale, cool, moist skin
- Fast, weak pulse and fast, shallow respirations
- Tiredness, weakness, dizziness, headache, and fainting

First aid procedures for heat exhaustion include the following:

- Move the person to a shady or air-conditioned area and encourage the person to rest.
- Have the person drink cool sports beverages.
- Do not give the person caffeinated or alcoholic beverages to drink.
- Have the person take a cool shower or sponge bath.

Heat Stroke

Heat stroke is a serious heat-related illness. The body is unable to sweat and thus cannot cool down. The body temperature is higher than 103°F (39°C). The skin is red, hot, and dry. The person may have a rapid, strong pulse. Dizziness, a throbbing headache, nausea, confusion, and eventually loss of consciousness can occur.

First aid procedures include the following:

- Move the person to a shady or air-conditioned area.
- Spray or sponge down the person with cool water.
- Seek medical attention immediately.

CRITICAL THINKING APPLICATION 27.4

Describe first aid procedures for the three types of heat-related conditions.

TABLE 27.2 Types of Burns

CONDITION	FIRST-DEGREE BURN	SECOND-DEGREE BURN	THIRD-DEGREE BURN	FOURTH-DEGREE BURN
Also known as	Superficial burn	Partial-thickness burn	Full-thickness burn	Deep full-thickness burn *(not universally accepted)*
Description	Damage to the epidermis	Damage to the epidermis and part of the dermis	Damage to the epidermis, dermis, and subcutaneous tissue	Damage beyond the subcutaneous tissue into the muscle and bone (not universally accepted)
Signs and symptoms	Redness (*erythema*), tenderness, physical sensitivity; no scar development	Redness, blisters, and pain; possible scar development	No pain because nerve endings are destroyed; skin appears deep red, pale gray, brown, or black; scar formation is likely	
First aid procedures	For minor burns: For unbroken skin, soak in cool water (not ice water) for at least 5 minutes. Cover with sterile dressing. (For second-degree burns 3 inches or larger or located on the hands, feet, groin, buttock, or over a joint, treat as major burn.)		For major burns: Seek immediate medical attention (call 911). Do not remove burned clothing stuck to skin. Monitor breathing. Perform rescue breathing or cardiopulmonary resuscitation (CPR) as needed. Raise burned body part above the heart level. Separate burned fingers or toes with a dry, sterile dressing.	

OTHER ENVIRONMENTAL EMERGENCIES

Besides temperature-related conditions, other conditions can be considered environmental emergencies. Environmental emergencies arise from exposure to a harmful environmental agent rather than a traumatic injury or medical condition already present in the patient. For instance, a bite from certain reptiles can cause death if not treated immediately. A flying piece of metal in a factory can cause blindness. Many environment-related emergencies are severe enough that the affected person seeks medical care.

Burns

Heat, freezing-cold temperatures, chemicals, sunlight, radiation, and electricity can cause burns to the body tissues. Hot liquids, fires, and flammable products are the most common causes of burns. Breathing in smoke can cause inhalation injuries.

Here are some possible screening questions for situations involving burns:

- What occurred? What caused the burn?
- Where was the person burned?
- What symptoms does the person have? What does the person's skin look like?
- If the burn affects the face or chest, is the person experiencing any breathing issues?

Table 27.2 describes the different degrees of burns. Providers estimate the percent of total burn surface area (%TBSA) by using the Rule of Nines diagram (Figure 27.11). Table 27.3 shows the difference between the Rule of Nines for an adult and an infant.

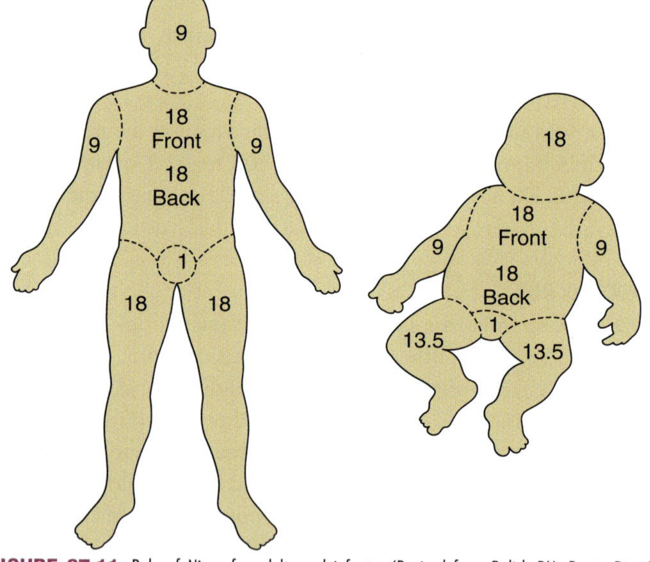

FIGURE 27.11 Rule of Nines for adults and infants. (Revised from Bolick BN, Reuter-Rice K, Madden MA, Severin PN: *Pediatric acute care: a guide for interprofessional practice,* ed 2, St. Louis, 2021, Elsevier.)

Poisonings

Poison can enter the body through swallowing, inhaling, injecting, or absorbing it through the skin. Here are some common poisons:

- Medications (prescription or over the counter) taken in high doses
- Overdoses of illegal drugs
- Household products, such as laundry detergent, furniture polish, and cleaning products
- Indoor and outdoor plants
- Pesticides and fertilizers
- Metals, such as mercury and lead

The American Association of Poison Control Centers is a national poison resource with 55 centers throughout the country. This resource is available online (https://poisonhelp.org) and via a hotline (1-800-222-1222). Medical assistants should have the phone number and website available for reference. If the medical assistant receives a call regarding a poisoning, the call must be handled according to the facility's protocols. Many times, the medical assistant must contact Poison

TABLE 27.3 Rule of Nines for Adults and Infants

AREA BURNED	ADULT	INFANT
Head and neck	9%	18%
Front of torso	18%	18%
Back	18%	18%
Arm, hand, and shoulder	9% (LA) 9% (RA)	9% (LA) 9% (RA)
Leg and foot	18% (LL) 18% (RL)	13.5% (LL) 13.5% (RL)
Genital	1%	1%
Total	100%	100%

LA, Left arm; *RA,* right arm; *LL,* left leg; *RL,* right leg.

Control while keeping the patient on the phone. The medical assistant then relays the information from Poison Control to the patient.

Signs and symptoms of poisoning can develop over time. They can also vary based on the poison. Symptoms include the following:

- Bluish lips, cough, and difficulty breathing
- Heart palpitations and chest pain
- Nausea, vomiting, and abdominal pain
- Numbness, tingling, dizziness, weakness, double vision, drowsiness, irritability, and headache
- Unusual odor
- Confusion, seizures, stupor, and unconsciousness

First Aid Procedures

First aid includes checking and monitoring the person's airway, breathing, and pulse. If required, rescue breathing and CPR are provided. Call 911 for medical help. If the person vomits, clear the airway. Monitor the person until help arrives. If poisoning is suspected, it is important to identify the toxin and the amount taken.

Do not have the person vomit unless you are instructed to by the Poison Control staff. If the person has swallowed a corrosive substance, it will cause additional injury as it is vomited. In this type of situation, a tube must be passed into the stomach to remove the substance. This is usually done in the emergency department.

Poisoning Facts

- Children younger than 6 years of age make up about half of the poisoning exposures reported.
- Children ages 1 to 2 have the greatest risk of poisoning.
- Cosmetics and personal care products, followed by cleaning products, are the most common substances involved in childhood poison exposures.
- About 22% of adult poisonings and 48% of teen poisonings are suspected suicides.
- Analgesics, followed by sedative/hypnotics/antipsychotic medications, are the top substances in adult poisonings.

From Poison Control, www.poison.org/poison-statistics-national.

CRITICAL THINKING APPLICATION 27.5

Where might Gabe post the Poison Control numbers around the clinic? Describe places where this number will be useful.

Chemical Exposures

Chemical exposures can cause burns or be absorbed through the skin or lungs. Information on treatments for chemical exposures can be obtained from a product's Safety Data Sheet (SDS) or by contacting the Poison Control Center.

Follow the information for first aid from the SDS or the Poison Control Center. Typical first aid for chemical exposures involves the following:

- Removing the person from the source of exposure while protecting yourself from exposure. If the chemical is on the person's clothing, the clothing should be removed.
- If the chemical is airborne or the exposure is affecting the lungs, bring the person to fresh air.
- For chemical exposures to the eye, flush the eye with cool water for 15 minutes while protecting the other eye from accidental exposure.

For patients with symptoms of shock, trouble breathing, or burns, call 911 so that the person can be seen in the emergency department. While waiting for help, provide rescue breathing or CPR as needed.

Anaphylaxis

Anaphylaxis is a severe allergic reaction that can be life threatening. These are the most common causes of allergens:

- Animal dander
- Insect bites and stings (especially bee stings)
- Medicines
- Plants and pollens
- Foods: Eggs, fish, milk, tree nuts (hazelnuts, walnuts, almonds, Brazil nuts), peanuts (groundnuts), shellfish (crab, mussels, shrimp), soy, sesame, and wheat

Anaphylaxis signs and symptoms include the following:

- Anxiety, warm feeling, and flushing
- Shortness of breath (SOB), *dyspnea* (difficulty breathing), wheezing, and cough
- Throat tightening, difficulty swallowing
- Pain or cramping, vomiting, and diarrhea
- Palpitations, dizziness, shock, and loss of consciousness

Allergic reactions that affect breathing are life threatening.

First Aid Procedures and Treatment

Here are the first aid procedures for severe allergic reactions:

- Do the 3 Cs: *C*heck the scene for safety. *C*all 911. *C*are for the victim.
- Give epinephrine (e.g., EpiPen) if the person has it available (Figure 27.12).
- Stay with the individual and try to keep the person calm.
- If the person has a bee sting, scrape the stinger off the skin if it is visible. Use a fingernail or credit card to scrape it. Do not use tweezers, which can squeeze the stinger, releasing more venom.
- Monitor the individual's airway, breathing, and pulse. Perform rescue breathing or CPR if needed.

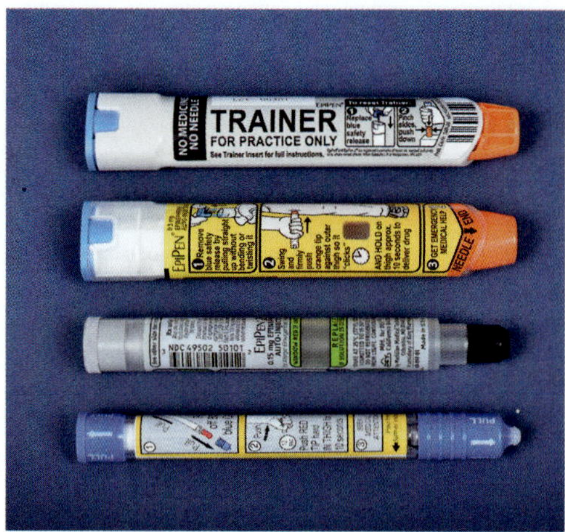

FIGURE 27.12 *Top to bottom:* Trainer that comes with the EpiPen, adult EpiPen, EpiPen Jr., and a generic adult epinephrine pen.

- Have the person lie flat and raise the feet 12 inches. Keep the person warm. This will help to prevent shock.

In the ambulatory care facility, if the medical assistant suspects the patient is starting to have an allergic reaction, she or he should immediately notify the provider. The provider will order epinephrine and oxygen to be administered. Research has shown that epinephrine administered intramuscularly (IM) into the vastus lateralis absorbs quicker than that given IM in the deltoid or subcutaneously in the arm. If ordered, repeat every 5 to 10 minutes. Do not administer repeated injections in the same site because **vasoconstriction** may cause tissue **necrosis**. Here is the typical dose of epinephrine injectable solution (1 mg/mL) for anaphylaxis:

- Children and adults (66 lb [30 kg] or more): 0.3 to 0.5 mg (0.3–0.5 mL)
- Children (under 66 lb [30 kg]): 0.01 mg/kg (0.01 mL/kg) with a maximum dose per injection of 0.3 mL

The 3 Cs Are Important When Responding to Emergencies

If you are the first to arrive at the scene of an emergency, it is important to follow the 3 Cs:

- Check the scene of the emergency. Is it safe for you? Are there any toxic or electric hazards? What occurred? How many victims are involved? Where did it occur (so you can tell the 911 dispatcher)?
- Call 911 or the local emergency number. Provide all the details you know.
- Care for the victims if it is safe to do so.

Always make sure you are safe before you assist others. If it is not safe for you, wait for the emergency responders to arrive.

Insect Bites and Stings

Insect bites and stings can cause immediate skin reactions, including pain, burning, erythema, numbness, swelling, and **pruritus**. In some cases, the venom can cause severe illness and death. Some people have anaphylactic reactions to stings and bites (e.g., bee stings). Anaphylaxis symptoms were addressed in the prior section.

Screening Questions

If the medical assistant receives a phone call regarding a bite or sting, it is important to gather additional information for the provider by asking questions, such as the following:

- What bit you?
- Do you have any allergies?
- How does the wound look? Describe the wound to me.
- Are you having any problems breathing? Any wheezing, shortness of breath, or difficulty breathing?
- Is there any swelling in the mouth or lips?

First Aid Procedures

First aid for severe reactions includes all the steps indicated in the anaphylaxis section. Additional steps include removing any nearby constricting items, such as rings and clothing. The affected area may swell, and constricting items can cause additional problems. First aid for mild reactions includes the following:

- Move to a safe location.
- Remove the stinger if it is visible.
- Wash the affected area with soap and water.
- To reduce pain and swelling, apply a cool cloth and elevate the extremity.
- For pain, apply hydrocortisone or lidocaine cream to the area. An over-the-counter pain reliever can also be taken.
- Calamine lotion or a similar product can be applied to the area to reduce the pruritus.

Patients may also call for advice on removing ticks. Ticks can spread diseases, including Rocky Mountain spotted fever, Powassan virus, Babesia infection, Lyme disease, and ehrlichiosis. If a person has a tick embedded, it needs to be removed. Wear gloves and use pointed, fine-tipped tweezers. Get as close to the head as possible. Do not squeeze the abdomen because it may inject secretions into the person's body. Slowly pull the head out. Do not twist. Do not burn it or use petroleum jelly or nail polish. Once the tick is removed, place it in a container of rubbing alcohol to kill it. Clean the site with antiseptic soap and water. Apply an antibiotic ointment. Monitor the site for infections or other complications.

CRITICAL THINKING APPLICATION **27.6**

Gabe realized that there were no patient education pamphlets in the exam rooms. He would like to talk with his supervisor about getting brochure racks for each room. His thought was to include home emergencies/first aid procedures for patients. If you were Gabe, describe the talking points you could make to your supervisor in favor of placing patient education materials in the exam rooms.

Animal Bites

Patients who have animal bites will typically seek care or call their providers.

Screening Questions

It is important for the medical assistant to ask some screening questions before talking with the provider:

- What type of animal bit you? Do you know the animal? If so, are the shots up to date?

- How does the wound look? Is it bleeding, dirty, or deep? Was it a puncture wound?
- Have you had the rabies vaccine series?
- When was your last tetanus vaccine?

First Aid and Treatment

Frequently, the bites are caused by domestic pets (e.g., dogs and cats). First aid for minor bites that only break the skin includes washing the area with soap and water. Then the person should apply over-the-counter antibiotic cream and cover the area with a clean bandage.

It is important to seek medical attention in the following situations:

- *For fang punctures*: For instance, cat bites. Bacteria are left deep in the puncture wound. Initially, the wound may not look bad, but in a few hours, the entire area could be hot and swollen.
- *For bleeding wounds*: Apply pressure with a clean cloth or bandage and seek help.
- *For dirty or deep wounds*: The person may require a tetanus vaccine booster if the last injection was given 5 or more years earlier.
- *For wounds that look infected*: The wound may look swollen, red, painful, or oozing.
- *For questions about the rabies risk*: Any wild or domestic mammal can get rabies and pass it on to people. Animals commonly seen with rabies include raccoons, skunks, bats, woodchucks (groundhogs), foxes, coyotes, cats, dogs, and cattle.

In the ambulatory care facility, the wound is examined, cleaned, and bandaged. The medical assistant should gather information on the patient's last tetanus booster. A tetanus immunization may be given. If there is a chance of rabies exposure, the provider will discuss the treatment options. Treatment for rabies can be costly, and the treatment time window is narrow. Table 27.4 describes the medications that can be given as treatment.

Foreign Body in the Eye

It is common for people with "something in the eye" to call or visit an ambulatory healthcare facility. This condition is known as a foreign body in the eye.

First aid for a foreign body in the eye is eye irrigation. Washing your hands before starting is important. The eye should be flushed with clean, warm water or saline eye drops. Saline eye drops will be less irritating than water. If the foreign body cannot be removed through irrigation, the person should seek immediate medical care. It is important not to rub the eye, which may cause further damage.

In the ambulatory care facility, the medical assistant needs to ask the patient how the injury occurred. Further irrigation may be ordered after the provider examines the patient. It is important to check the date of the patient's last tetanus booster. The provider may order an updated tetanus booster, along with additional treatments.

DIABETIC EMERGENCIES

Diabetic emergencies occur when the person's blood glucose level is too low or too high. When a person eats carbohydrates (starches and sugars [e.g., bread, candy]), the blood glucose level rises. Insulin from the pancreas or insulin injections help bring down the blood glucose level. Insulin is the only thing that moves the glucose out of the blood and into the cells, where it is used for energy. Without enough insulin, the blood glucose level rises. With too much insulin, the blood glucose level drops.

If the blood glucose gets too high (*hyperglycemia*) or too low (*hypoglycemia*), the person can go into a diabetic coma. Permanent brain damage and death can occur. If you encounter an unresponsive person, check to see if the individual has a medical alert bracelet or necklace. (Some individuals have tattoos instead of wearing medical alert jewelry.) The medical alert information may provide clues to what is occurring.

Diabetic Ketoacidosis

Diabetic ketoacidosis (DKA) is severe hyperglycemia. DKA is caused by an imbalance between insulin and blood glucose. Too much glucose is in the blood because the individual did one or more of the following:

- Took too little insulin
- Ate too many carbohydrates
- Is ill, has an infection, trauma, or surgery
- Used an illegal drug (e.g., cocaine, ecstasy)

Here are some signs and symptoms of hyperglycemia:

- Very dry mouth, thirst, and frequent urination
- Nausea, vomiting, hunger, and stomach pain
- Fatigue, rapid pulse, and shortness of breath

Signs of diabetic ketoacidosis include a fruity odor on the breath, diabetic coma, and death.

TABLE 27.4 Rabies Postexposure Treatment for Nonimmunized Individuals

MEDICATION	PURPOSE	ADMINISTRATION
Rabies immune globulin (RIG)	Antibodies specifically for rabies. Provides rapid (immediate) passive immune protection against rabies.	Dose based on weight. Administer only once between day 0 (day of the bite) and day 7. Provider injects RIG around the bite wound if present. The remaining volume of RIG is administered intramuscularly (IM) in the vastus lateralis or deltoid muscle (most distant from the wound). *If required, live-virus vaccines (varicella, measles) must be either given with or spaced out 4 months after RIG.*
Rabies vaccine	Helps to provide long-term active immune protection against rabies.	Administer 1 mL IM in the deltoid muscle for adults and the vastus lateralis for children. Administer one dose on days 0, 3, 7, and 14. A fifth dose may be recommended on day 28 for immunocompromised individuals.

First Aid Procedures

First aid for hyperglycemia includes the following:

- Call 911, and get medical help. Monitor the airway and pulse. Perform rescue breathing and CPR as needed.
- The patient will need IV fluids, insulin, and monitoring to bring down the blood glucose level.

Insulin Shock

Insulin shock, also called insulin reaction, is severe hypoglycemia (low blood glucose). Insulin shock occurs when there is an imbalance between insulin and blood glucose. Too little glucose is in the blood because the individual did one or more of the following:

- Took too much insulin
- Ate too few carbohydrates
- Engaged in too much physical activity
- Drank alcohol (may occur up to 2 days after drinking)

Here are some signs and symptoms of hypoglycemia:

- Double or blurry vision
- Fast pulse, palpitations
- Irritable, aggressive, nervous, headache, and unclear thinking
- Shaking, tired, hungry, sweaty, and cold skin

Severe hypoglycemia can cause disorientation, seizures, shock, incautiousness, diabetic coma, and death.

First Aid Procedures

First aid for hypoglycemia includes the following:

- Test the blood glucose level if possible.
- If the individual is conscious and able to swallow: Give 4 ounces of fruit juice or regular (not diet) soda or three glucose tablets. Test the blood glucose every 15 minutes. If the blood glucose is under 70, give additional glucose. Continue until the glucose level is 70 or above (Procedure 27.1).
- If the individual is unconscious: Place the patient in the **recovery position**. Call 911, and get medical help. Monitor the airway and pulse. Perform rescue breathing and CPR as needed. For an unconscious adult patient, glucagon 1 mL is given subcutaneously or IM (Figure 27.13). Repeat the dose in 15 minutes if the patient is unconscious. (Children younger than 6 years of age get 0.5 mL.) Monitor the blood glucose. Once the patient is alert and able to swallow, give additional food (e.g., a sandwich).

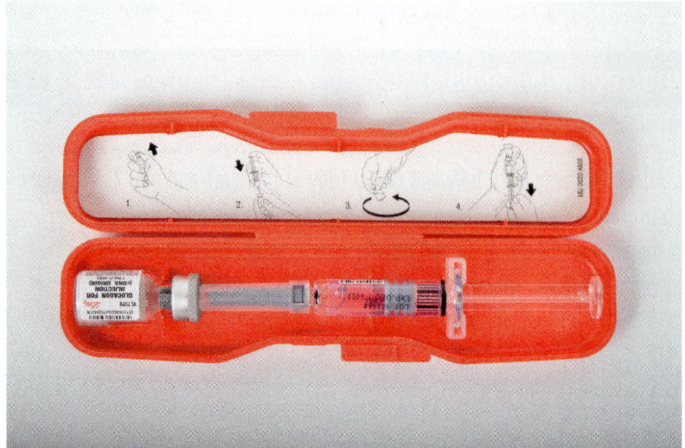

FIGURE 27.13 Glucagon is given to unconscious patients with diabetes. This hormone stimulates the liver to release glucose into the bloodstream, thus increasing the blood glucose level.

How to Place a Person in the Recovery Position

- Kneel at the person's side. Straighten the person's arms and legs.
- Take the person's arm next to you and extend it out and above the person's head.
- Extend the person's arm farthest from you across their chest. Place the hand next to the person's cheek (Figure 27.14A). It will support the person's head.
- Take the leg farthest from you and bend the leg at the knee (Figure 27.14B).
- You want to roll the person as one unit in case of head, neck, or spinal injuries. To do this, support the person's head and neck; gently take the bent knee and carefully roll the person toward you and onto the side (Figure 27.14C).
- Make sure the person is steady and cannot roll.
- Support the head with the person's hand. Ensure the airway is opened and clear.

MUSCULOSKELETAL EMERGENCIES

Without a diagnosis, it is hard to tell if an injury is a strain, sprain, fracture, or dislocation. It is always important to treat the injury as a fracture until the provider diagnoses it. A few symptoms will indicate if the injury is more severe (e.g., dislocation):

- The person has difficulty moving the extremity normally or is not able to do so.
- The extremity is deformed.
- Bone is exposed through the skin.
- There is heavy bleeding.

Screening Questions

Many times, patients will contact their provider regarding musculoskeletal injuries. The medical assistant should screen the patient and relay the information to the provider. Here are some possible screening questions for musculoskeletal emergencies:

- What happened?
- What does the injured body part look like? Is it deformed? Is it bleeding?
- Can the person move the injured part? Is there pain?
- How does the skin look over and near the injury?

First Aid Procedures and Treatment

If a person has any symptoms of a severe injury or an injury related to major trauma, call 911 and get medical help. Additional first aid involves the following steps:

- *If the person is going into shock*: Make sure the person is lying down with the head slightly lower than the abdomen and elevate the legs. Monitor the person's breathing and pulse rate. Provide rescue breathing and CPR if needed.
- *For bleeding*: Apply pressure to the wound with a clean cloth or sterile bandage.
- *Immobilize the injured area*: Do not push the bone back. Do not move the area affected by the injury. Apply a splint beyond the joint above and the joint below the injury (Figure 27.15 A and B).

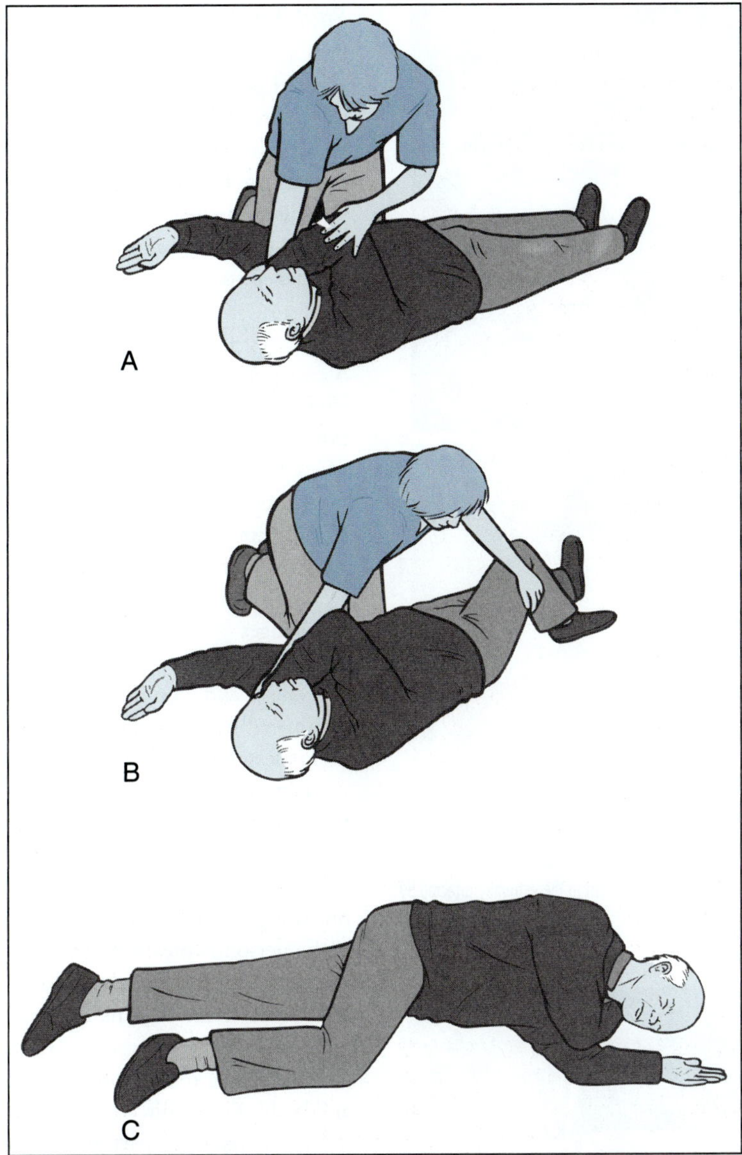

FIGURE 27.14 Recovery position. **(A)** Extend the person's arm farthest from you across their chest. Place the hand next to the person's cheek. **(B)** Take the leg farthest from you and bend the leg at the knee. **(C)** Support the person's head and neck; gently take the bent knee and carefully roll the person toward you and onto the side. (From Harrison R, Daly L: *A nurse's survival guide to acute medical emergencies,* ed 3, St. Louis, 2019, Elsevier.)

- *To limit swelling*: Apply a cold pack to the area. Make sure to cover the cold pack with a towel. Do not apply the cold pack directly on the skin (Figure 27.16).
- To splint an extremity, the person should do the following:
  - Splint the body part in the position it is in. Do not attempt to readjust the area or straighten it.
  - Use a commercial splint or create a splint. Use sticks, a board, or rolled-up magazines, newspaper, or clothing as a splint.
  - Make sure the splint extends below and above the injury.
  - Secure the splint with ties (e.g., belt, cloth strips).
  - Check the injured area for swelling, paleness, or numbness, which may indicate the ties are too tight. Loosen ties if needed.

Typically, the provider will need to examine the patient; then, an x-ray will be taken before a final diagnosis is made. Depending on the diagnosis, the medical assistant may need to help apply a splint, cast, sling, or another device. Good patient education is required. The medical assistant should coach the patient on checking the circulation of the affected extremity. Coaching the patient on how to handle the protective device (e.g., cast, splint) while doing basic hygiene activities (e.g., showering) is important. Typically, musculoskeletal injuries require **r**est, **i**ce, **c**ompression, and **e**levation (RICE).

NEUROLOGIC EMERGENCIES

Neurologic emergencies can range from minor conditions, such as dizziness, to serious conditions, such as stroke. The medical assistant should know how to handle neurologic emergencies.

Vertigo and Dizziness

Vertigo is a false sensation that you or your environment is spinning or moving. *Peripheral vertigo* is caused by a problem in the inner ear (i.e., vestibular labyrinth, semicircular canals, and vestibular nerve).

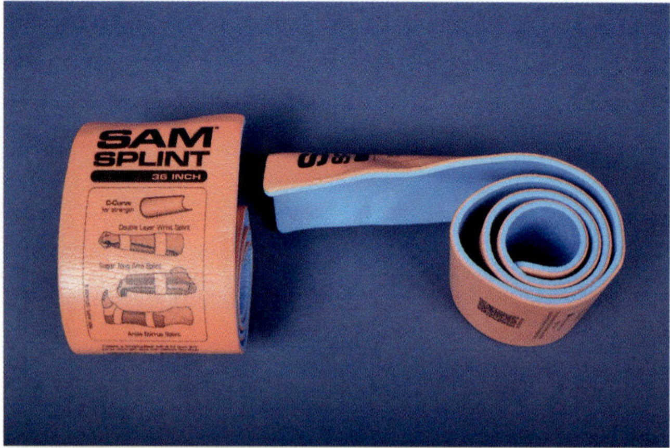

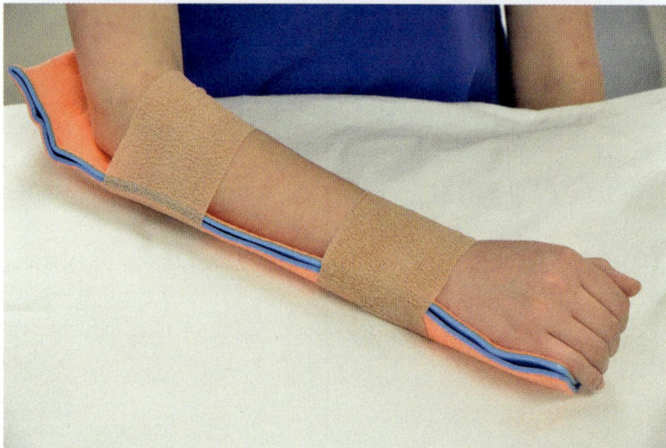

FIGURE 27.15 **(A)** SAM Splint is a reusable splint that can conform to the extremity affected by the injury. **(B)** Splint beyond the joint, above and below the injury.

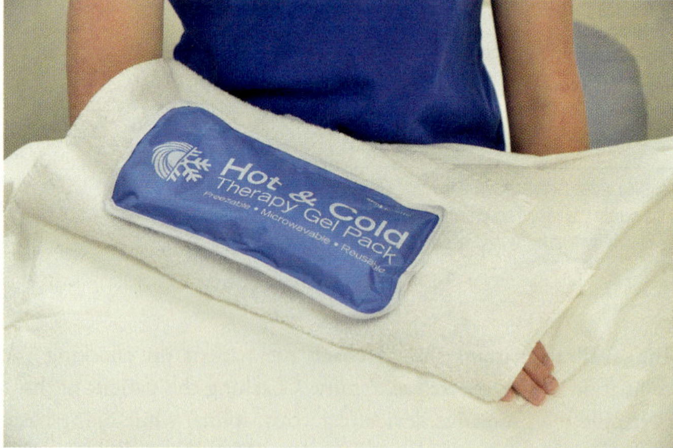

FIGURE 27.16 Place a towel between the cold pack and the skin.

This issue affects the sense of balance. *Central vertigo* is caused by a brainstem or cerebellum disorder. It can be caused by certain drugs (e.g., aspirin, anticonvulsants, and alcohol), migraines, multiple sclerosis, stroke, and tumors.

With dizziness, people may feel light-headed or lose their balance. Many people get dizzy if they move too quickly from a sitting or lying position to a standing position. Their blood pressure drops, causing dizziness. People may feel as if they will pass out. Usually, dizziness resolves on its own, but it could be a symptom of another disorder.

First Aid Procedures

First aid for vertigo and dizziness involves sitting or lying down. The affected person should gradually resume activities when the episode passes. In addition, the person should avoid sudden position changes and bright lights and should drink more fluids. The patient should contact the provider if any of the following apply:

- This is the first episode of vertigo or dizziness.
- The episodes are increasing in number.
- The episodes are getting worse.

Concussion

A *concussion* is a traumatic brain injury caused by a blow to the head. Violently shaking the head can also cause a concussion. Concussions can occur with sports injuries, falls, physical assaults, and traffic accidents. Concussion symptoms may be slow to develop and could last for weeks. Here are some signs and symptoms:

- Head pressure or headache
- Temporary loss of consciousness right after the incident
- Confusion, amnesia, disorientation, irritability, and personality changes
- Dizziness and ringing in the ears
- Nausea and vomiting; taste and smell issues
- Slurred speech and delayed response to questions
- Listlessness, tiredness, sleep disturbances, and concentration and memory problems
- Loss of balance and unsteady gait (walk)

First aid for moderate to severe head injuries involves immediately calling 911. Monitor the person until help arrives. Check the breathing and pulse. Provide rescue breathing and CPR as needed. If the person is breathing and has a pulse, treat the condition like a spinal injury. Stabilize the head and neck by placing your hands on both sides of the person's head. Prevent any movement of the head and keep the head in line with the spine until help arrives. If the person vomits, roll the person to the side, and move the head, neck, and body as one unit. Moderate to severe head injuries are often seen in the emergency department.

Screening Questions

Patients will call or come to ambulatory care facilities if they have a possible concussion or a mild head injury (Procedure 27.2). Here are some possible screening questions:

- What happened?
- Did the person lose consciousness? If so, for how long?
- Was there any bleeding? Any vomiting?
- How is the person doing?
- Are the pupils dilated, or is one larger than the other?
- Does the person remember what happened? Is the person confused or slurring their speech?

First Aid Procedures and Treatment

For mild head injuries, usually, a person should seek medical treatment if these occur:

- Loss of consciousness lasting longer than 30 seconds after the initial injury
- Repeated vomiting
- Worsening headache
- Changes in behavior or coordination (irritable, stumbling, or falling)

- Changes in orientation and speech (disoriented, confused, or slurred speech)
- Neurologic changes (seizures, visual disturbance, recurrent dizziness, difficulty with concentration, and one pupil larger than the other or both pupils dilated)

The patient may need to undergo radiologic testing to check for skull fractures and internal bleeding. If there are no fractures, the provider will educate the patient about other symptoms that would require follow-up and postconcussion care. Athletes need to refrain from playing sports until the concussion symptoms are gone. Another hit on the head can cause additional damage.

CRITICAL THINKING APPLICATION 27.7

Gabe has a 12-year-old son who plays middle school football. Before the season started, Gabe and his wife had to sign an acknowledgment form discussing concussions. What are the benefits of informing parents of school athletes about concussion symptoms?

Seizures

A seizure is a sudden increase of electrical activity in one or more parts of the brain. Epilepsy is a disorder that causes recurring seizures. Seizures are classified based on how the abnormal brain activity begins. There are three major classifications of seizures:

- *Generalized onset seizure*: Affects both sides of the brain at the same time. Includes several types of seizures, such as tonic-clonic and absent. Symptoms may include jerking, rigid or twitching muscles, and staring spells.
- *Focal onset seizure*: Affects one area of the brain. This type of seizure used to be called a partial seizure. There are two subgroups of focal onset seizures:
  - *Aware seizure*: The person is awake and alert during the seizure.
  - *Impaired awareness seizure*: The person is confused during the seizure. This type of seizure was known as a complex partial seizure.
- *Unknown onset seizure*: When the start of the seizure was not witnessed.

In most situations, seizures last 30 seconds to 2 minutes. Usually, they do not cause lasting issues. It is a medical emergency if the seizure lasts longer than 5 minutes or if a person has multiple seizures without becoming conscious between them.

Screening Questions

Parents commonly call when their child has had a seizure. According to the facility's protocol, the medical assistant may need to ask some screening questions and relay the information to the provider. Here are some possible screening questions for musculoskeletal emergencies:

- What did the patient do during the seizure? How long was the seizure?
- Did the person lose consciousness?
- How is the patient now after the seizure?

First Aid Procedures

If a person has a seizure in the healthcare facility, the medical assistant must notify the provider immediately (Procedure 27.3). First aid for seizures focuses on the safety of the individual:

- Move the person to the floor and place the patient in the recovery position. Gently raise the chin to tilt the head back slightly to open the airway. Monitor the person's breathing and pulse. Perform rescue breathing after the seizure has stopped if the patient does not resume breathing. Provide CPR if needed.
- Protect the patient from harm. Clear the area of anything hard or sharp. Place a soft, folded towel under the head.
- Do not place anything in the patient's mouth.
- Remove any glasses and loosen any constrictive clothing around the neck (e.g., ties).
- Time the length of the seizure. Call 911 if the seizure lasts longer than 5 minutes.
- Stay with the person until the person is fully awake and alert.

Cerebrovascular Accident

A cerebrovascular accident (CVA), also called a *stroke,* is a medical emergency. There are three types of strokes:

- *Ischemic stroke*: Occurs when the arterial blood flow to part of the brain is blocked. The brain cells start to die after a few minutes. This is the most common type of stroke. There are two common types of ischemic stroke:
  - *Thrombotic stroke*: A blood clot forms in an artery, blocking the blood flow to part of the brain.
  - *Embolic stroke*: A blood clot or other debris forms elsewhere in the body and moves into the brain arteries, blocking the blood flow.
- *Hemorrhagic stroke*: Occurs when an artery in the brain leaks or ruptures. The leaked blood puts pressure on the surrounding brain cells, causing damage. There are two causes of hemorrhagic stroke:
  - *Intracerebral hemorrhage*: The most common type of stroke; occurs when a cerebral aneurysm ruptures.
  - *Subarachnoid hemorrhage*: Bleeding occurs in the subarachnoid space, usually as a result of small aneurysms.
- *Transient ischemic attack* (TIA): Also called a "mini-stroke" because it lasts for only a few minutes. The blood supply to a part of the brain is briefly blocked. Symptoms are similar to stroke symptoms but do not last as long (e.g., 1 to 24 hours).

The symptoms of a CVA relate to the part of the brain affected. The individual may not have all the symptoms. Possible symptoms of CVAs include the following:

- Confusion or mental changes; sudden severe headache
- Speech problems (difficulty forming words, difficult to understand, or using words that do not make sense)
- Numbness of the face, arm, or leg, usually on one side of the body
- Problem seeing in one or both eyes; facial drooping
- Trouble walking, lack of coordination or balance, or arm weakness

First Aid Procedures

First aid for stroke-type symptoms involves getting help (calling 911) immediately. The emergency department (ED) is the best place for a patient to go. There is a small window of time during which clot-dissolving medications (e.g., a tissue plasminogen activator) can be given to help the body break down the clot that is blocking the artery. If a bleeding artery has caused the stroke, the ED providers can detect this on radiologic studies.

If a patient comes to the ambulatory care facility with strokelike symptoms, it is important for the provider to see the patient immediately. Be ready to call 911 when the provider orders you to do so. Also, monitor the patient's vital signs for changes.

Fast

The American Stroke Association promotes FAST to spot stroke signs and encourages calling 911:

F: Face drooping. Is one side of the face drooping or numb? Ask the person to smile to see if the smile is uneven or drooping on one side.

A: Arm weakness. Is one arm weak or numb? Raise both arms and watch for an arm to drift downward.

S: Speech difficulty. Is the person slurring their words? Is the person having problems speaking? Do the words not make sense, or are they hard to understand? Give the person a simple sentence to say and see if it is repeated correctly.

T: Time to call 911. If the person is showing any of these symptoms, call 911 immediately. Let the emergency responders know you think it might be a stroke. Watch the person's respiration rate and pulse rate. Do not give the person anything to eat or drink. Have the person sit upright if possible.

American Stroke Association, www.stroke.org/en/about-stroke/stroke-symptoms.

RESPIRATORY EMERGENCIES

Respiratory emergencies can create a number of different signs and symptoms. Consider these examples:

- *Skin:* Unusually moist, flushed, pale, bluish, or ashen
- *Respirations:* Slow, rapid, deep, or shallow; trouble breathing or no breathing
- *Audible breathing sounds:* Gasping, gurgling, high-pitched noises (e.g., whistling sound), wheezing
- *Patient complaints:* Shortness of breath, dizziness, light-headedness, chest pain, tingling in the extremities, a sense of fearfulness

It is important to get help immediately with respiratory emergencies. After calling 911, help the conscious individual into a comfortable position, and monitor the respirations and pulse. Be ready to provide rescue breathing and CPR if required.

Common respiratory emergencies are discussed in the following sections. It is important for the medical assistant to recognize when a patient is having a respiratory emergency and get help immediately.

Hyperventilation

Hyperventilation, or overbreathing, is rapid and deep breathing. This leads to a low carbon dioxide level in the blood. This gas imbalance creates symptoms that can mimic those of a heart attack, thus increasing the person's anxiety, in addition to the hyperventilation. Hyperventilation can have the following symptoms:

- Dry mouth, belching, and bloating
- Light-headedness, weakness, dizziness, and difficulty concentrating
- Shortness of breath, breathlessness, chest pain, and heart palpitations
- Muscle spasms; numbness and tingling in the arms or around the mouth

Hyperventilation can be caused by many things, including panic attacks, stress, anxiety, bleeding, heart attack, drugs, and infections.

First Aid Procedures

First aid treatments focus on raising the carbon dioxide level in the blood. This can be done by relaxing and using pursed-lip breathing or slowly blowing out through the lips. A person should seek medical care if the hyperventilation episodes get worse. After diagnosing the condition, the provider may have the patient breathe slowly into a paper bag. This helps to restore the carbon dioxide and oxygen balance in the blood.

Asthmatic Attack

Asthma affects the airway and the lungs. During an asthma attack, the airway constricts, reducing the air moving into and out of the lungs. Mucus clogs up the airway, making airflow more difficult. Asthma causes wheezing, breathlessness, chest tightness, and coughing. Typically, asthma attacks occur at night or in the early morning hours.

Screening Questions

If a patient or family member calls about an asthma attack, it is important to gather information quickly and talk with the provider. Here are some possible questions to ask:

- What symptoms is the person experiencing?
- Was medication given? What was the medication, and how much was administered?
- Did the medication ease the symptoms?
- Is the person having severe respiratory distress (e.g., unable to talk, blue lips, or **retractions**)? (This would be a medical emergency, and calling 911 is critical.)

First Aid Procedures

In the ambulatory healthcare setting, an asthma attack is an emergency. The provider needs to see the patient immediately. First aid actions for an asthma attack include these:

- Helping the person into a comfortable sitting position. Usually, sitting upright allows for easier breathing.
- Giving short-acting inhalers (e.g., albuterol), which will lessen the asthma attack within minutes.
- Monitoring the pulse oximetry and vital signs.

Choking

Choking can occur in all age groups. Most choking cases relate to swallowing large pieces of food or doing an activity (e.g., running) while eating. Other causes are denture-related issues and eating too fast. Children under age 5 tend to choke on candy, grapes, and large pieces of food. They are also more likely to put nonfood items in their mouth. Plastic, balloon pieces, coins, and buttons are extremely dangerous to children. Objects smaller than 1.75 inches (the diameter of a golf ball) can be caught in the throat and cause choking.

Any object caught in the throat is considered a foreign body obstruction. Here are some signs of a partial airway obstruction:

- Can still speak; forceful or weak coughing
- Labored, noisy, or gasping breathing

- Panicked appearance, extreme anxiety, or agitation

Signs of a total airway obstruction include these:

- Clutching the throat with one or both hands
- Unable to breathe, cry, cough, or speak
- Bluish skin color (e.g., lips)

Do not give the person any liquids until the obstruction is cleared.

First Aid Procedures

First aid for an adult or child over 1 year of age for choking includes asking people if they are choking. If the person is forcefully coughing, stand by and see if the person can clear the airway without assistance. Procedure 27.4 describes the abdominal thrusts used on a conscious adult with a total airway obstruction. If a person is pregnant or obese, wrap your arms around the person's chest. Place your fist in the middle of the breastbone between the nipples. Give firm, backward thrusts.

First aid for a conscious choking infant includes the following:

- Do the 3 Cs after gaining consent from the parent or guardian; check the scene, have someone call 911, and care for the infant. (If you are alone and have a cell phone, call 911. If you are alone without a cell phone, it is recommended that you attempt to clear the airway or provide rescue breathing or CPR for 1 minute to children younger than 8 years of age before calling 911. Most cardiopulmonary arrests in young children are related to airway issues.)
- Hold the child with the head below the chest for the entire procedure. This allows gravity to help move the obstruction. Support the chin with your hand and the infant's body with your arm.
- With the child facing downward, give five back blows between the shoulder blades with the heel of your hand (Figure 27.17A).
- Flip the infant, and place two or three fingers below the nipple line on the chest. Give five chest thrusts (Figure 27.17B).
- Do a mouth check and insert a finger only to pull a loose object out. Doing a finger sweep is not recommended because it can push the item in farther.
- Continue until the object is out or the child becomes unconscious. If the child is unconscious, place the child on a hard surface and begin CPR, starting with chest compressions. Make sure 911 was called.

CARDIOVASCULAR EMERGENCIES

Cardiovascular emergencies can be common in ambulatory care. Between patients calling with concerns or patients having cardiovascular concerns, the medical assistant needs to be aware of cardiovascular emergencies.

Syncope

Syncope means fainting, passing out, or having a temporary loss of consciousness. When people are about to faint, they may feel dizzy, nauseous, or light-headed. The skin may be cold and clammy. People may experience a "black out" or "white out" in their visual field. Muscle control is lost. Fainting occurs when the blood pressure drops suddenly, and the blood flow to the brain is reduced. Shock has a number of possible causes:

- Being dehydrated or too hot.
- Using alcohol.
- Standing up too quickly.
- A drop in blood glucose.
- Using certain medications, such as diuretics, antihistamines, levodopa, calcium antagonists, angiotensin-converting enzyme (ACE) inhibitors, nitrates, antipsychotics, and narcotics.
- Having a heart condition.
- Having a neurologic condition, such as Parkinson disease, postural orthostatic tachycardia syndrome (POTS), and diabetic neuropathy.
- Vasovagal syncope caused by emotional stress, trauma, pain, reaction to the sight of blood, or prolonged standing.
- Carotid sinus syncope caused by constriction of the carotid artery in the neck. The constriction can occur with turning the head, shaving, or wearing tight clothing around the neck.
- Situational syncope, which occurs during defecation, urination, and coughing.

First Aid Procedures

First aid actions for people who feel faint include having them sit and place their head between their knees (Figure 27.18A). For people who faint, position them on their back. Check their airway and make sure it is clear. Check for a pulse. If the pulse is not present, start CPR.

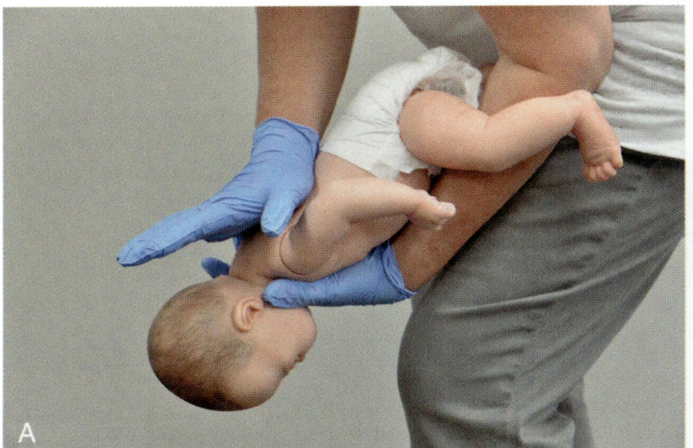

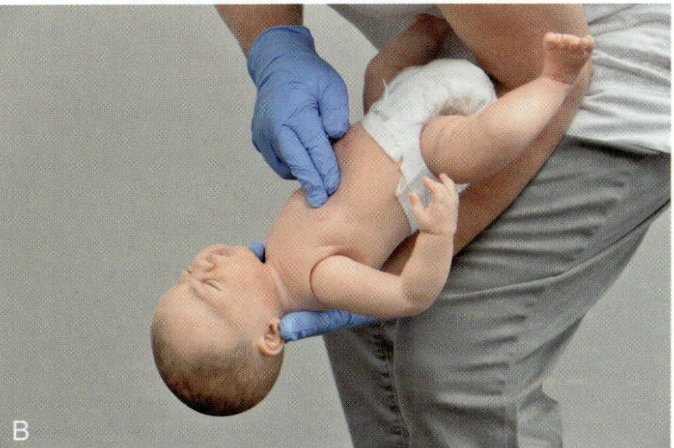

FIGURE 27.17 (A) Support the infant with your arm and thigh while giving back blows. **(B)** Chest thrusts are administered in the same position as for cardiac compressions.

Here are some additional first aid actions:

- Loosen any constrictive clothing.
- Raise the legs above the heart level (about 12 inches) (Figure 27.18B).
- Get help/call 911 if the person does not regain consciousness within 1 minute.

Bleeding

Bleeding can occur with and without trauma. First aid for bleeding involves stopping the bleeding and calling for help (Procedure 27.5). Nosebleeds are common in certain people. If a nosebleed is experienced, have the person sit upright and lean forward to prevent the swallowing of blood. Pinch the nostrils for 5 to 10 minutes, which helps to stop the bleeding. Continue to pinch the nostrils until the bleeding stops. The individual should refrain from blowing the nose for several hours to prevent rebleeding.

In the ambulatory care facility, always wear gloves and the required PPE before assisting patients. Follow these steps to stop the bleeding:

- For bleeding wounds, remove any obvious debris. Do not remove any large objects embedded in the wound.
- Place a sterile gauze or clean cloth over the wound and press firmly to control the bleeding. Do not put direct pressure over an embedded object, an eye, or displaced organs.
- For severe bleeding, help the person lie down and cover them with a blanket. This will keep the person warm and conserve body heat.
- If the bleeding seeps through the gauze, apply another layer on top of the initial gauze. Do not move the initial gauze.
- To slow the bleeding or if the bleeding is spurting from an artery, follow these steps:
  - Elevate the bleeding extremity above the heart level.
  - Hold direct pressure over the site.
  - If the bleeding does not stop with the elevation and direct pressure, apply pressure to the artery above the wound by pushing the artery against a bone. Continue to apply direct pressure on the wound.
  - To see if the bleeding has stopped, slowly lift your fingers from the pressure point over the artery. Check to see if the wound is still bleeding. If so, continue to apply pressure.
  - Do not hold pressure at the pressure point for longer than 5 minutes after the bleeding stops.

Shock

Shock occurs when the body is not getting enough blood flow. The vital organs (e.g., heart, brain) do not get enough oxygen and nutrients for the cells to function properly and survive. Organ damage can occur. Shock is a life-threatening condition. There are many types of shock, such as these:

- *Cardiogenic shock*: Due to heart muscle damage caused by a myocardial infarction (also known as MI or heart attack); the heart cannot pump enough blood to the other organs.
- *Hypovolemic shock*: Due to heavy bleeding (i.e., accident or internal bleeding) or dehydration; blood volume is too low to provide nutrients and oxygen to the organs.
- *Anaphylactic shock*: Caused by a severe allergic reaction (anaphylaxis); blood pressure drops, and the airway narrows. Not enough blood gets to the vital organs, and the narrowed airway prevents adequate oxygenation.
- *Septic shock*: Caused by a severe infection (severe sepsis) that affects the functioning of vital organs (e.g., heart, brain, kidneys). The blood pressure falls, and major organs can fail.
- *Neurogenic shock*: Due to a central nervous system injury (e.g., spinal cord injury). Leads to vasodilation (not enough blood can return to the heart) and low blood pressure.

Here are some possible signs and symptoms of shock:

- Anxiety, agitation, dizziness, feeling faint, light-headedness, confusion, and unconsciousness
- *Cyanosis* (blue lips, fingernails) and shallow respirations
- Chest pain and a rapid, weak pulse
- Moist skin and *diaphoresis* (profuse sweating)
- Poor or no urine output

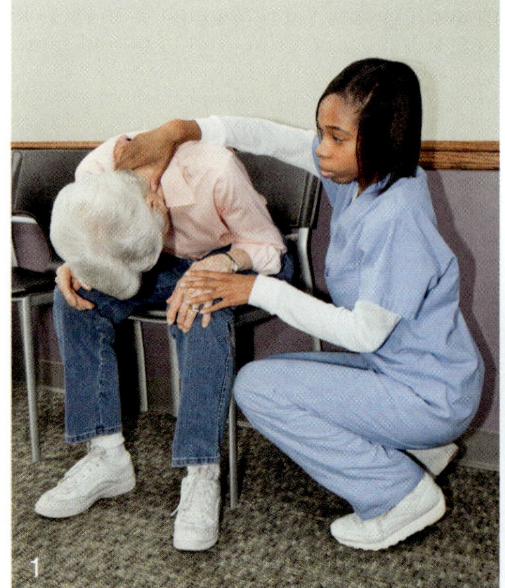

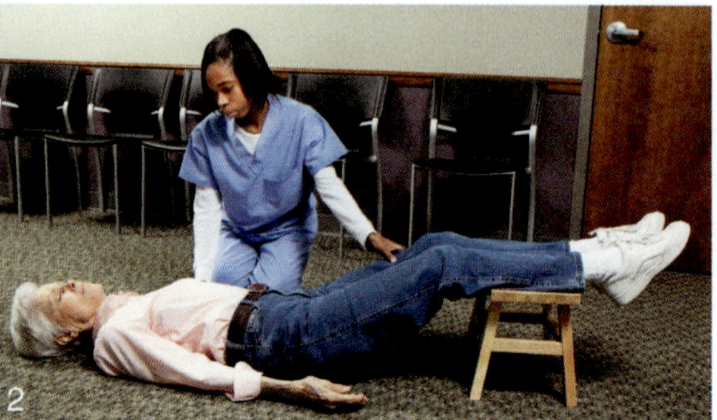

FIGURE 27.18 **(A)** Placing the head between the legs helps to reduce the faint feeling. **(B)** Elevate the legs about 12 inches using pillows, blankets, or a small stool.

First Aid Procedures and Treatment

Shock requires immediate treatment for the person to have a chance of survival. First aid actions for shock include calling 911 immediately. Check the person for responsiveness. Monitor the airway, breathing, and pulse. If needed, perform rescue breathing and CPR. If the person is breathing and has a pulse, monitor the vital signs at least every 5 minutes. If the person does not have any injuries to the head, neck, back, or legs, raise the legs 12 inches. This helps the blood to move back to the vital organs of the body. If the person has pain with raising the legs, keep them flat. Make sure the person's head is flat. Loosen clothing and provide the appropriate first aid for the person's injuries (Procedure 27.6).

If a person goes into shock in the ambulatory healthcare facility, the provider will order that 911 be contacted. Oxygen and IV fluids are given. The vital signs are monitored, and the person's legs are elevated. Based on the medications available and the person's blood pressure, the provider may give IV medications that will increase the blood pressure. The goals are to keep the blood pressure high enough to sustain life and get the patient to the emergency department as quickly as possible.

Myocardial Infarction

Myocardial infarction (MI) is more commonly known as a heart attack. Coronary arteries that bring blood to the heart muscle are blocked by a clot or narrowed by plaque. When the blood flow to an area of the heart is limited or stopped, the heart cells die, and an MI occurs. Chest pain (angina pectoris), cold sweats, and heartburn are the most common symptoms. Chest pain can be described as mild or severe; sharp, burning, heaviness, squeezing, pressure; and constant or intermittent (comes and goes). Additional symptoms include the following:

- Upper body discomfort or pain in one or both arms, shoulders, neck, jaw, upper part of the abdomen, or back
- Arrhythmia, palpitations, tiredness without a reason, nausea, and vomiting
- Shortness of breath with activity or rest, cold sweats, dizziness, and light-headedness
- Back pain in women

First Aid Procedures and Treatment

First aid for a heart attack includes these measures:

- Have the person sit down and rest. Keep the individual calm, and loosen any tight clothing on the chest and neck area.
- Have the person take nitroglycerin if prescribed.
- Call 911 within 5 minutes of the onset of pain.
- Have the person chew an aspirin (if not allergic).
- Monitor the person's respirations and pulse. Perform rescue breathing and CPR if needed (Figures 27.19 to 27.20, Table 27.5, and Procedure 27.7).

If a patient arrives at the ambulatory care facility with chest pain or other MI-type symptoms, immediately take the patient to a procedure or exam room. Notify the provider at once. Usually, the provider will give these orders:

- Give the person one aspirin, to be chewed, and nitroglycerin administered sublingually.
- Call 911.
- Obtain vital signs, pulse oximetry, and an electrocardiogram (ECG), and administer oxygen while waiting for the ambulance.

The goals are to limit the damage to the heart muscle and transport the patient to the emergency department.

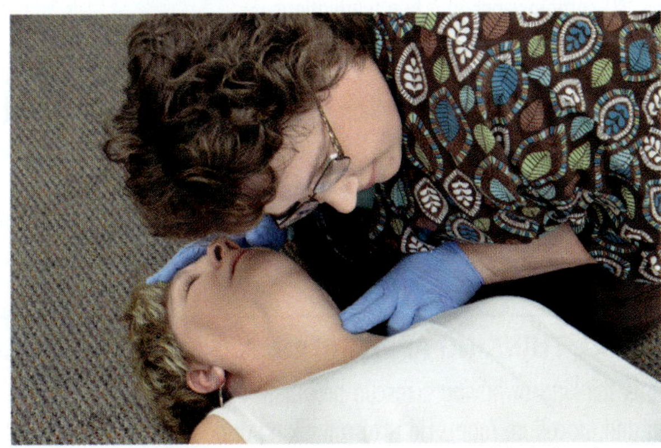

FIGURE 27.19 Use the head-tilt position to open an adult's airway while checking the carotid pulse.

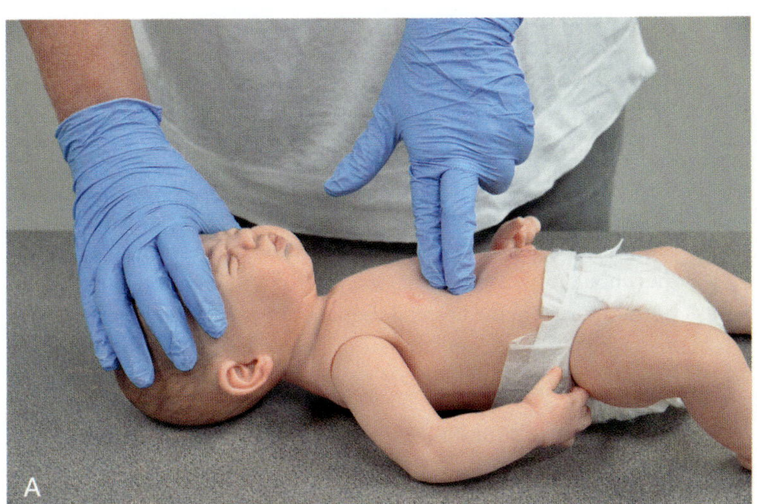

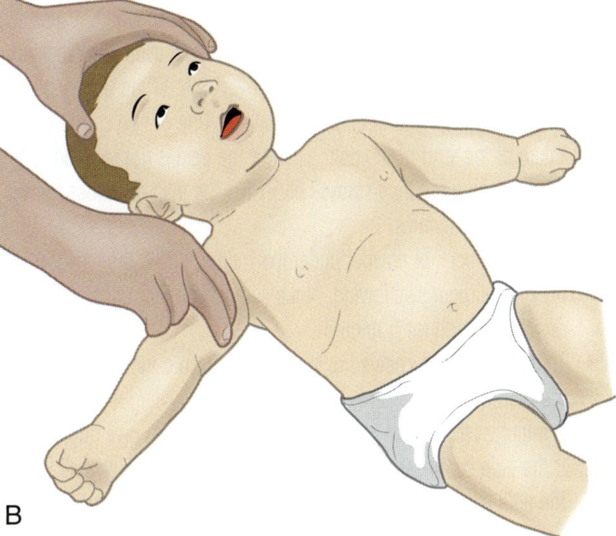

FIGURE 27.20 **(A)** Open an infant's airway by tilting the head to a neutral position. For chest compressions, place two fingers below the nipple line. **(B)** In an infant, check for a brachial pulse.

TABLE 27.5 Summary of Rescue Breathing and Cardiopulmonary Resuscitation Differences

	ADULT	CHILD	INFANT
Age	8+ years old	1–8 years old	Less than 1 year
Check Responsiveness	Shout, "Are you all right?"		Tap the foot.
Open Airway	Use head-tilt, or if spinal injury is suspected, use the jaw thrust without head extension (see Figure 27.19).	Tilt head slightly past the neutral position.	Tilt head to the neutral position (see Figure 27.20A).
Assess Pulse	Feel for a carotid pulse near the middle of the throat (see Figure 27.19).	Feel for the carotid pulse. If pulse is less than 60 beats/minute with signs poor perfusion (such as skin color changes), start CPR.	Feel for a brachial pulse on the inside upper arm (see Figure 27.20B).
Give Rescue Breathing (Ventilation) Only	One rescue breath every 5–6 seconds. About 10–12 breaths per minute. Deliver each breath for 1 second.	One breath every 2–3 seconds or about 20–30 breaths per minute.	
Chest Compression Hand Position	Heel of a hand is placed on the lower part of the chest (below the nipple line), and the other hand is placed on top, so it overlaps the first hand.		Place two fingers just below the nipple line (see Figure 27.20A).
Compressions	2–2.4 inches deep; 100 per minute.	2 inches deep; 100–120 per minute.	1.5 inches deep with two fingers; 100–120 per minute.
Compression to ventilation ratio	One or two rescuers: 15 compressions and two ventilations.	One rescuer: 30 compressions and two ventilations. Two rescuers: 15 compressions and two ventilations.	
Automated External Defibrillator (AED) Pads	Use only adult pads. Place one pad on the upper right chest and the second on the left side of the chest.	Use pediatric pads for children younger than 8 years; if not available, use adult pads. If pads touch, place one on the back between the shoulder blades.	Use pediatric pads; if not available, use adult pads. Place one pad on the chest and the other on the back.

Nitroglycerin and Angina

Nitroglycerin is used for angina (chest pain). It dilates the coronary arteries, allowing more blood to move into the heart muscle. Nitroglycerin can be given as an oral spray, a sublingual (SL) powder, or sublingual tablets.

- Do not shake the spray. Prime (or release a test spray) 5 to 10 times for new bottles, up to 5 times for bottles not used within 3 months, and 1 to 2 times for bottles that have not been used in more than 6 weeks. Prime the bottles away from everyone. When administering the dose, spray onto or under the tongue. One or two sprays can be taken at the start of the pain. Then, if the pain is not relieved in 5 minutes, give the third spray. Call 911 if the pain continues for an additional 5 minutes.
- Empty the pack of powder under the tongue. Allow the powder to dissolve without swallowing. Make sure the patient does not eat or rinse the mouth for 5 minutes.
- Tablets cannot be chewed or swallowed. Place a tablet under the tongue and let it dissolve. Usually, it starts providing relief within 1 to 5 minutes. If the pain is not relieved in 5 minutes, give another tablet. If the pain continues after 5 minutes, give a third tablet. Call 911 if the pain is not relieved 5 minutes after taking the third tablet. (Do not give more than three tablets within 15 minutes.)

Nitroglycerin works fast. The patient may feel dizzy, light-headed, or faint after taking the medication.

CRITICAL THINKING APPLICATION 27.8

Gabe is thinking of having a rescue breathing mouth barrier in each exam room and procedure room. He is also thinking of adding one to each of the first aid kits located in other parts of the clinic. Why is it important to make mouth barrier devices more available in the clinic?

CLOSING COMMENTS

Patient Coaching

Many ambulatory care facilities coach patients on what types of emergencies can be addressed in their facilities and what conditions need to be addressed in emergency departments. People seeking care in emergency departments for possible strokes, heart attacks, and similar conditions will receive timely care, whereas such services in the ambulatory care facilities are limited and require the patient to be transported to the hospital. Educating patients through voice mail messages, websites, and flyers can help the public understand the limitations of ambulatory care services.

Legal and Ethical Issues

Lawsuits related to care provided during emergencies in healthcare settings are prevalent. Ambulatory care facilities need to have procedures in place to handle emergencies. Staff members need to be trained in handling emergencies. Many agencies have mock codes to help prepare staff. These are training events that allow staff members to practice their skills. Often after mock events, the supervisors assess how the training went. They identify processes and procedures that need refinement and additional training.

Another method of improving processes comes after a real-life code situation. Usually, a few days after a code, the staff involved will gather to debrief or discuss what occurred. They will usually talk about the following:

- How the code progressed, from the time the patient had symptoms to the time the patient was transported to the emergency department
- What went well and what went not so smoothly
- Where more training is needed

These debriefings are extremely important after an emergency situation.

Patient-Centered Care

Medical emergencies are scary for patients and their families. We may be focused on providing emergency care, but we need to remember to communicate with the patient. Being sensitive to what patients are feeling is important. Remember to explain what you are doing. Ask the patients how they are doing.

Families of patients are often forgotten. In emergencies, often, the family is moved to another room to allow more room for those helping with the code. It is helpful for the family to have a staff person wait with them. If this is not possible, a staff person needs to report to the family and provide updates. It is important to remember that the rules of the Health Insurance Portability and Accountability Act (HIPAA) still apply in emergency situations.

Professional Behaviors

Code situations can be anxiety inducing and stressful for staff members. It is important to talk through what occurred, taking confidentiality into account. Besides talking, it is critical to manage one's stress by maintaining a healthy diet and getting adequate sleep and exercise.

An employee assistance program (EAP) is also helpful after stressful code situations. An EAP is a work-based program designed to help employees resolve issues. These issues can be personal (e.g., financial, marital, or involving substance abuse) or professional (e.g., communication issues with co-workers and stress-related issues). The EAP services are confidential and designed to help the employee's work performance. EAP counselors help employees to deal with the aftereffects of an emergency.

SUMMARY OF SCENARIO

Gabe has been in his new position for only 2 weeks. Already he has a list of concerns and possible solutions he wants to address with his supervisor. Gabe also wants to discuss forming an emergency response team. This team would respond when a code is called throughout the building.

He hopes to begin quarterly mock codes within the next 3 months. He wants to rotate the types of emergencies addressed by the mock codes. Gabe hopes that with additional training and more exposure to emergency supplies, the medical assistants will feel more comfortable with emergencies.

SUMMARY OF LEARNING OBJECTIVES

1. **Examine types of emergencies, along with the screening and triage process that occurs in ambulatory care.**
   Some of the more common emergencies include a person being treated for a life-threatening occurrence, a person who has an accident or health issue, a walk-in patient with a critical health issue, and an individual who calls regarding an emergency. In some facilities, medical assistants must screen phone calls and walk-in patients using screening protocols. Larger facilities have registered nurses that triage patients.
2. **Examine the team members' roles and the importance of documentation in code situations.**
   Healthcare facilities use special phrases for emergencies. Once the call goes out for help, staff members respond to the scene. In small settings, most members of the staff may be needed. In large facilities, only certain staff members respond. Usually, medical assistants, licensed practical nurses (LPNs), registered nurses (RNs), and providers attend the emergency. Documentation of the code situation is critical during the experience for emergency responders and provides evidence that the standard of care was met.
3. **Differentiate among the equipment and supplies used in code situations.**
   The emergency supplies available at healthcare facilities will vary based on the size and location of the facility. Some practices have a small box that contains a few supplies and medications. Other practices place many crash carts throughout the building. Equipment and supplies include the following:
   - Oxygen, airway supplies (includes endotracheal tube intubation supplies and equipment), a defibrillator or an automated external defibrillator (AED)
   - Medications and IV supplies
   - Other supplies include personal protective equipment, a sharps disposal container, a pocket face mask, algorithms, a clipboard with documents for charting the code, a backboard, and extra batteries for the laryngoscope
   - Pediatric supplies
4. **Differentiate among first aid procedures for temperature-related emergencies.**
   Cold-related conditions include frostbite and hypothermia. The person may experience a pins-and-needles sensation followed by numbness in the frostbitten area. The skin is hard, pale, and cold; blisters may occur. With hypothermia, the core body temperature drops below 95°F (35°C). First aid for both cold-related conditions was discussed, and hypothermia requires immediate medical attention.
   Heat-related conditions include heat cramps, exhaustion, and stroke. Heat cramps are a mild heat-related illness that causes muscle pain and

Continued

SUMMARY OF LEARNING OBJECTIVES—*continued*

spasms due to electrolyte imbalance. Heat exhaustion is a milder form of a heat-related illness. Heat stroke is a serious heat-related illness. The body is unable to sweat and thus cannot cool down. First aid differs for these three conditions, with heat stroke requiring immediate medical attention.

5. **Differentiate among the types of environmental emergencies and the related first aid procedures.**
   In addition to temperature-related conditions, environmental emergencies include burns, poisonings, chemical exposures, anaphylaxis, insect bites and stings, animal bites, and foreign body in the eye:
   - Minor burns can be treated at home; however, people with major burns need to seek immediate medical attention.
   - First aid for severe allergic reactions and severe reactions related to bites and stings includes giving epinephrine and monitoring the patient's airway, breathing, and pulse.
   - First aid for poisonings includes monitoring the patient's airway, breathing, and pulse. Call 911. The Poison Control staff can be a resource for poisonings and chemical exposures.
   - First aid for a foreign body in the eye is to try to irrigate it out. Flush the eye with clean, warm water or with saline eye drops. Saline eye drops will be less irritating than water. If the foreign body cannot be removed through irrigation, the person should seek immediate medical care.
6. **Differentiate between hypoglycemic and hyperglycemic medical emergencies, including signs, symptoms, and treatments.**
   First aid for hyperglycemia and diabetic ketoacidosis includes the following:
   - Call 911 and get medical help. Monitor the airway and pulse. Perform rescue breathing and CPR as needed.
   - The patient will need IV fluids, insulin, and monitoring to bring down the blood glucose level.

   First aid for hypoglycemia and insulin shock includes the following:
   - Test blood glucose if possible.
   - If the individual is conscious and able to swallow: Give 4 oz. of fruit juice or regular (nondiet) soda or three glucose tablets. Test blood glucose every 15 minutes. If the blood glucose is under 70, give additional glucose. Continue until the glucose level is 70 or above (see Procedure 27.1).
   - If the individual is unconscious: Place the patient in the recovery position. Call 911 and get medical help. Monitor the airway and pulse. Perform rescue breathing and CPR as needed. For an unconscious adult patient, administer glucagon 1 mL, given subcutaneously or IM.
7. **Examine screening questions and first aid procedures for musculoskeletal emergencies.**
   Screening questions include finding out what occurred, how the injured body part looks, and if the patient can move the injured part. First aid involves the following:
   - Call 911 for major injuries.
   - Other first aid actions include applying pressure for bleeding, immobilizing the injury, and applying a cold pack to minimize swelling.
   - If in shock, make sure the person is lying down with the head slightly lower than the abdomen and elevate the legs. Monitor the person's breathing and pulse rate. Provide rescue breathing and CPR if needed.
8. **Differentiate among neurologic emergencies, including signs, symptoms, and first aid procedures.**
   Types of neurologic emergencies include vertigo, concussion, seizures, and cerebrovascular accident (stroke). First aid involves the following:
   - For vertigo and dizziness, help the person to sit or recline.
   - For moderate to severe head injuries, call 911 immediately. Monitor the person until help arrives. Provide rescue breathing and CPR as needed. If the person is breathing and has a pulse, treat the condition like a spinal injury. Stabilize the head and neck by placing your hands on both sides of the person's head.
   - For seizures, keep the person safe. Move the person to the floor and into the recovery position.
   - For stroke-type symptoms, call 911 and monitor the patient until help arrives.
9. **Differentiate among respiratory emergencies, including signs, symptoms, and first aid procedures.**
   Hyperventilation, asthmatic attack, and choking are respiratory medical emergencies. First aid for these conditions includes the following:
   - For hyperventilation, encourage the person to relax and use pursed-lip breathing or slowly blow out through the lips.
   - For an asthmatic attack, help the person into a sitting position, give short-acting inhalers, and monitor the pulse oximetry and vital signs.
   - For choking, monitor a patient who has a partial obstruction. Procedure 27.4 discusses first aid for a complete choking.
10. **Differentiate among cardiovascular emergencies, including signs, symptoms, and first aid procedures.**
    Cardiovascular emergencies include syncope, bleeding, shock, and myocardial infarction. First aid for these conditions includes the following:
    - For syncope, Have the person sit and place the head between the knees. For people who have fainted, position them on their back and monitor their airway and pulse.
    - For bleeding, depending on the type of wound, different actions may be taken. Sterile gauze should be placed over the wound. If the bleeding seeps through, additional gauze should be added. Refer to Procedure 27.5 for first aid steps for a patient with a bleeding wound, fracture, or syncope.
    - For shock, call 911 immediately. Check the person for responsiveness. Monitor the airway, breathing, and pulse. If needed, perform rescue breathing and CPR. If the person is breathing and has a pulse, monitor the vital signs at least every 5 minutes. If the person does not have any injuries to the head, neck, back, or legs, raise the legs 12 inches.
    - For myocardial infarction, call 911. The person should take nitroglycerin, if available. If there are no allergies to it, a person can chew an aspirin. Monitor the person and perform CPR or rescue breathing if needed. Refer to Procedure 27.7 for the steps to provide rescue breathing and CPR and for using an automated external defibrillator (AED).

PROCEDURE 27.1 Provide First Aid for a Patient with an Environmental Emergency and Insulin Shock

TASK: Provide first aid to an individual with a dog bite and hypoglycemia.

BACKGROUND INFORMATION: For someone with hypoglycemic symptoms, test the blood glucose level. If the blood glucose is under 70 and the patient is conscious and able to swallow, give 4 ounces of fruit juice or regular soda or three glucose tablets. Test the blood glucose in 15 minutes. Continue with these steps until the glucose level is 70 or above.

SCENARIO: You are working with Dr. Martin, a family practice provider. Maude Crawford (date of birth [DOB] 12/22/19XX) is being seen for a dog bite on her left arm. The wound is still bleeding.

DIRECTIONS: Role-play the scenario with a peer. The peer will be the patient, and you will be the medical assistant.

EQUIPMENT and SUPPLIES

- Gloves and sterile gauze
- Sugary drink (4-oz fruit juice or regular soda) or three glucose tablets
- Patient's health record

PROCEDURAL STEPS

1. Wash your hands or use hand sanitizer.
   PURPOSE: Hand sanitization is an important step for infection control.
2. Greet the patient. Identify yourself. Verify the patient's identity with full name and date of birth.
   PURPOSE: It is important to identify the patient in two different ways to ensure that you have the correct patient.
3. Apply gloves. Place sterile gauze over the wound, and apply direct pressure to control the bleeding.
4. Identify when the patient had her last tetanus booster.
   Scenario update: Mrs. Crawford has diabetes and states that she thinks she has low blood sugar. She has blurry vision, tremors, and a headache. She asks you for something to eat. According to the facility's policy, you check her blood glucose level, and it is 48 mg/dL.
5. Obtain a sugary drink or glucose tablets. Indicate how much to give to the patient.
   PURPOSE: Consuming a sugary food or drink will help to increase the blood glucose.
   Scenario update: After 15 minutes, her blood glucose level is 59 mg/dL. You notify the provider while a co-worker stays with the patient.
6. Describe follow-up care for the patient. (See the background information.)
   PURPOSE: A blood glucose test should be done to find out how low the patient's level is. After 15 minutes of her eating/drinking the sugary food, the glucose test should be done. If her level is below 70 mg/dL, give her additional sugary food/drink and repeat the glucose test in 15 minutes. Continue until the blood glucose level is 70 or higher.
   Scenario update: After 15 minutes, her blood glucose level is 82 mg/dL. You notify the provider.
7. Document the situation in the patient's health record. Include the blood glucose levels, your actions, the provider who was notified, and the patient's response.

Documentation Example

10/04/20XX 1023 Sterile gauze and pressure applied to wound on her left arm. Pt c/o blurry vision, tremors, and a headache. She stated she thought she had low blood sugar. Four oz. of orange juice given to pt. After 15 minutes, her blood glucose was 59 mg/dL. Dr. Martin notified and ordered additional orange juice and to recheck blood glucose until 70 mg/dL or more. Four oz. of orange juice given, and after 15 minutes, her blood glucose was 82 mg/dL. Provider notified. ———————————— Gabe Garcia, CMA (AAMA)

PROCEDURE 27.2 Incorporate Critical Thinking Skills When Performing Patient Assessment

TASKS: Use critical thinking skills while performing a patient assessment regarding a neurologic emergency.

SCENARIO: You are working with Dr. Martin, a family practice provider. Maude Crawford's daughter calls concerned about her mother. The daughter states that Maude Crawford (DOB 12/22/19XX) fell and hit her head.

DIRECTIONS: Role-play the scenario with a peer. The peer will be the daughter, and you will be the medical assistant. The peer can make up information regarding the scenario. Your instructor will be the provider.

WMFM: NEUROLOGIC EMERGENCY PHONE PROTOCOL

Obtain the patient's name, date of birth, signs/symptoms, and the history of the situation. After the call, document the situation, symptoms, and action in the patient's health record.

If a patient reports the following neurologic concerns, send the patient to the emergency department via the ambulance immediately:

- Seizure or seizure-like symptoms lasting 3 or more minutes
- Passing out or fainting; dizziness or weakness that does not go away

PROCEDURE 27.2 Incorporate Critical Thinking Skills When Performing Patient Assessment—*continued*

- Sudden or unusual headache that starts suddenly
- Unable to see or speak, sudden confusion
- Neck or spine injury
- Injuries that cause loss of feeling or inability to move
- Head injury with passing out, fainting, or confusion
- Facial drooping or sudden speech difficulties or visual problems

If a patient reports the following concerns, schedule a visit for the same day. If no appointments are available, consult the triage nurse or the provider regarding the situation:

- Headache/migraine
- Nonemergent neurologic concerns, such as muscle stiffness or rigidity that is progressively getting worse, insomnia, or a history of blurry or double vision

EQUIPMENT and SUPPLIES

- Patient's health record
- Paper and pen
- Emergency Phone Protocol for clinic

PROCEDURAL STEPS

1. Obtain the patient's name and date of birth.
   PURPOSE: Obtaining the patient's information is important for any patient-related phone call.
2. Using critical thinking skills, ask appropriate questions to obtain information about the patient's condition. Write down the patient's issues or concerns or the situation.
   PURPOSE: Writing down the information will help when you discuss the situation with the provider and document the call. Thoughtful questions about the situation and the patient's condition must be asked to gather the appropriate information.
   Scenario update: The daughter stated that Maude was "knocked out" for about a minute. She has been acting differently since the fall. You need to follow the Neurological Emergency Phone Protocol.
3. Complete the protocol and determine what actions to take using critical thinking skills.
   PURPOSE: Protocols are approved and signed by the providers. They need to be followed by the staff.
4. Instruct the caller on what should be done based on the protocol. Talk with the provider if needed.
   PURPOSE: The caller needs clear directions on what to do.
5. Document the call in the patient's health record. Include the caller's name, the patient's condition (e.g., signs, symptoms, and concerns), the name of the protocol used, the information given to the caller, and the provider who was notified.
   PURPOSE: Legally, it is important to document all patient interactions.

PROCEDURE 27.3 Provide First Aid for a Patient with a Stroke and Seizure Activity

TASKS: Provide first aid to an individual having a stroke and seizure activity. Document care in the health record.

SCENARIO: You are working with Dr. Martin, a family practice provider. Walter Biller (DOB 1/4/19XX) arrives for his appointment.

DIRECTIONS: Role-play the scenario with a peer. The peer will be the patient, and you will be the medical assistant.

EQUIPMENT and SUPPLIES

- Watch, stethoscope, and sphygmomanometer
- Folded towel, blanket, or coat
- Patient's health record
- Gloves and other personal protective equipment (as required)

PROCEDURAL STEPS

1. Wash your hands or use hand sanitizer.
   PURPOSE: Hand sanitization is an important step for infection control.
2. Greet the patient. Identify yourself. Verify the patient's identity with full name and date of birth.
   PURPOSE: It is important to identify the patient in two different ways to ensure that you have the correct patient.
   Scenario update: As you room Mr. Biller, you notice that he seems to be dragging his left leg when walking, the left side of his face is drooping, and he states his left arm is weak. You suspect that he might be having a stroke. He asks for a drink of water when you get to the exam room.
3. You call for help and assist the patient onto the examination table. Place the patient in the recovery position with the head slightly raised.
4. Monitor the patient's airway. Obtain the patient vital signs.
5. Speak calmly to the patient. Do not give the patient anything to drink.
   PURPOSE: The patient may be at risk of choking.
   Scenario update: While you are waiting for the provider, Mr. Biller starts to jerk his arms, and he becomes unresponsive.
6. Keep the patient in the recovery position. Note the time when the seizure started. Gently raise the chin to tilt the head back slightly to open the airway. Yell for help if help has not arrived.
   PURPOSE: The recovery position will help open up the person's airway. Yelling for help in the ambulatory care facility is reserved for emergencies.
7. Continue to monitor his pulse rate and respiration rate. Put on gloves and other personal protective equipment as needed.
   PURPOSE: Wearing personal protective equipment will protect you if the patient vomits or becomes incontinent of urine or stool during the seizure.

PROCEDURE 27.3 Provide First Aid for a Patient with a Stroke and Seizure Activity—*continued*

8. Clear any hard or sharp items away from the patient. Place a soft, folded towel, blanket, or coat under the patient's head.
   PURPOSE: It is important to protect the patient from harm.
9. Remove the patient's glasses (if on), and loosen any constrictive clothing around the neck. Stay with the person until he is fully awake and continue to monitor the respiration and pulse rates.
10. Document the first aid measures you provided in the order they occurred. In addition, document the seizure activity you witnessed, the length of the episode, and the provider notified.
    PURPOSE: Specifying the care provided, along with details of the seizure activity, will help the provider.

Documentation Example

10/05/20XX 1423 Patient appeared to be dragging his left leg when walking, the left side of his face was drooping, and he stated his left arm was weak. Pt was placed in the recovery position on the examination table. Provider was called. Patient started to jerk his arms, and he became unresponsive. P: 86 regular, 1+; R: 18 regular, normal. Dr. Martin arrived. Pt's clothing was loosened. The seizure activity lasted for 4.5 minutes. ———

——— Gabe Garcia, CMA (AAMA)

PROCEDURE 27.4 Provide First Aid for a Choking Patient

TASKS: Provide first aid to a conscious adult who is choking. Document it in the health record.

SCENARIO: You are working with Dr. Martin, a family practice provider. As you return from lunch, you notice that an adult visitor is having an issue. It appears that she had been eating fast food, and now she is holding her neck with both hands. She appears to be panicking.

DIRECTIONS: Role-play the scenario with a peer. The peer will be the visitor, and you will be the medical assistant.

EQUIPMENT and SUPPLIES

- Patient's health record
- Gloves
- Mannequin

PROCEDURAL STEPS

1. Approach the person and ask, "Are you choking?"
   PURPOSE: If the person can speak and is coughing forcefully, then let her cough and try to dislodge the obstruction. If the person is not able to speak, then assist the patient.
   Scenario update: She nods her head yes but cannot speak. She is standing.
2. Yell for help. Put on gloves if available. Stand behind the victim with your feet slightly apart. Reach your arms around the person's waist.
   PURPOSE: With an obstructed airway, the person may lose consciousness at any time. The rescuer must be prepared to safely lower the unconscious individual to the floor. If the person in distress is a child, the rescuer may need to kneel when providing assistance.
3. Make a fist and place it just above the person's navel. Make sure your thumb side is next to the person. Grasp the fist tightly with your other hand (Figure 1).
   PURPOSE: Correct hand position is important as you do abdominal thrusts.

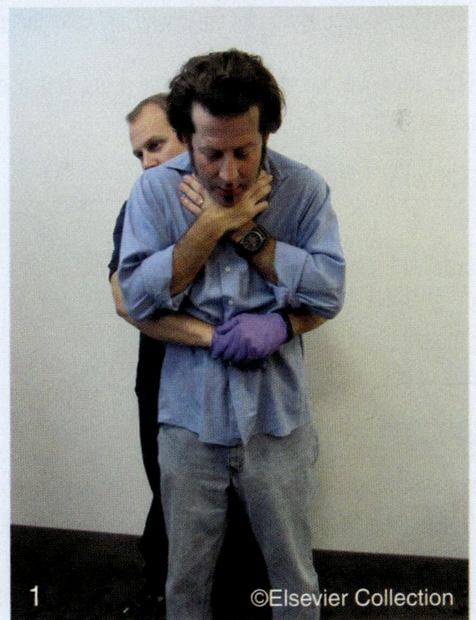
1 ©Elsevier Collection

Scenario update: The next steps must be done on a mannequin.

4. With the correct hand position, make quick upward and inward thrusts with your fist. Do five abdominal thrusts before doing back blows.
   PURPOSE: The fist should be placed in the soft tissue of the abdomen to avoid injury to the sternum or rib cage. If the person is supine, straddle and face the person's head. Push your grasped fist upward and inward.

Continued

PROCEDURE 27.4 Provide First Aid for a Choking Patient—*continued*

5. Stand behind the person and wrap one arm around the person's upper body. Position the person so that the person is bent forward with the chest parallel to the ground.
   PURPOSE: This position helps objects to dislodge.
6. Use the heel of your other hand to give a firm blow between the shoulder blades. Check to see if the object dislodges. If not, continue by giving another four back blows.
   PURPOSE: Back blows can help dislodge the item.
7. Continue to give five abdominal thrusts followed by five back blows until the object is dislodged or the person loses consciousness.
   PURPOSE: Repeated abdominal thrusts and back blows can help dislodge the item.
   Note: If the person faints or loses consciousness, lower the person to the floor. Call 911 (or the local emergency number) or have someone else call. Begin CPR, starting with chest compressions. Check to see if the item is in the airway. Remove it only if it is loose.
   Scenario update: After two sets of abdominal thrusts and back blows, the woman coughs out a piece of food. She can now talk.
8. Arrange for the person to be seen by the provider. Document the first aid measures you provided in the order that they occurred.
   PURPOSE: Specifying the care provided, along with details of the situation, will present the provider with a full picture of what happened.

Documentation Example

10/06/20XX 1223 Pt was found in reception room with her hands on her throat. She appeared to be panicky. She could not speak but indicated with a nod of her head that she was choking. After being given two sets of back blows and abdominal thrusts, she was able to cough out some undigested food. R: 22 regular, normal. Pt is alert. She agreed to see Dr. Martin immediately.
———————————— Gabe Garcia, CMA (AAMA)

PROCEDURE 27.5 Provide First Aid for a Patient with a Bleeding Wound, Fracture, or Syncope

TASKS: Provide first aid to an individual with a suspected fracture, a bleeding wound, and syncope. Document the first aid you provide.

SCENARIO: You are returning from lunch and see a person fall at the entrance of the healthcare facility. He is an older man and complains of pain in his right lower arm. His arm looks deformed and is bleeding. You call for help. A provider comes, and co-workers bring supplies. The provider tells you to care for the wound and splint the arm before moving the individual. You have a co-worker helping you.

DIRECTIONS: Role-play the situation with two peers. One peer will be the patient, and the other peer will be a coworker. You will be the medical assistant.

EQUIPMENT and SUPPLIES

- Gloves
- Sterile gauze
- Bandage
- Splinting material (e.g., SAM Splint)
- Coban wrap or gauze roll

PROCEDURAL STEPS

1. Wash your hands or use hand sanitizer if possible. Identify yourself to the patient. Obtain the patient's name and date of birth as you put on gloves.
   PURPOSE: It is important to wear gloves when working with a wound. Obtaining the patient's name is important because the patient will be seen, and you need to document the first aid provided.
2. Using sterile gauze, apply direct pressure over the wound to stop the bleeding. Make sure to immobilize the injured arm as you apply pressure. If possible, elevate the arm to help slow the bleeding. If the blood seeps through the gauze, apply another layer of gauze on the initial one. Continue with direct pressure until the bleeding stops.
   PURPOSE: Applying pressure and elevating the arm will slow the bleeding.
3. Once the bleeding has stopped, cover the dressing with a bandage. Remember to immobilize the injured arm as you work.
   PURPOSE: It is important to cover the wound with a bandage in case the bleeding restarts. Immobilizing a suspected arm is important until the splint can be applied.
   Scenario update: As you apply the bandage to the injured arm, the patient states he does not feel good. He says he feels dizzy and thinks he is going to pass out. Your peer takes over by supporting his arm, and the man faints. He is still breathing and has a pulse.
4. Position the patient on his back. Continue to check his respiration and pulse rates.
   PURPOSE: If the patient is not breathing or does not have a pulse, administer rescue breathing and begin CPR.
5. Loosen any constrictive clothing around the neck and chest. Raise the legs above the heart level (about 12 inches).
   PURPOSE: Raising the legs allows the blood to return to the vital organs.
   Scenario update: After a few minutes, he starts to come around. He jokes that blood makes him faint. As he is lying on his back talking with you, you need to splint his injured arm.
6. Use the splint material and shape it to the injured arm. Do not straighten the arm. Apply the splint beyond the joint above and the joint below the injury.
   PURPOSE: It is important to keep the arm in the same position until the provider examines the arm and x-rays are taken.
7. Use Coban or a gauze roll to secure the splint in place. Encourage the patient to hold the injured arm against his chest as he moves.
   PURPOSE: If the patient can hold the arm, this will reduce the pain.

PROCEDURE 27.5 Provide First Aid for a Patient with a Bleeding Wound, Fracture, or Syncope—*continued*

8. Document the first aid measures you provided in the order they occurred. Note that the provider was at the scene.
   PURPOSE: Specifying the care provided, along with details of the seizure activity, will help the provider.

Documentation Example

10/07/20XX 1215 Pt fell at the clinic entrance. He c/o pain in his lower right arm. Dr. Martin ordered wound care and splinting of the arm before moving the pt. Using sterile gauze, applied direct pressure over the wound until the bleeding stopped. Wound was covered with a bandage while arm was manually immobilized. Pt stated he felt dizzy and fainted. P: 68 regular, 1+; R: 16 irregular, normal. Pt was positioned on his back with his feet elevated. Within a few minutes patient came to and started talking. SAM Splint applied to right arm and Coban applied to hold the splint. Pt held arm while transferring into wheelchair. Pt to see Dr. Martin immediately. ——————————————— Gabe Garcia, CMA (AAMA)

PROCEDURE 27.6 Provide First Aid for a Patient in Shock

TASKS: Provide first aid to an individual who is in shock. Document the first aid you provide.

SCENARIO: You are working with Dr. Julie Walden. The administrative medical assistant at the reception desk notifies you that Robert Caudill (DOB 10/31/19XX) is here and looks very ill. You bring the patient and his wife immediately back to the procedure room because it is the only available room. He asks to move to the exam table, and you assist him as he transfers to the table. You obtain his vital signs: P: 92, irregular, 1+; R: 26, regular, shallow; BP 72/48 RA, lying; and T: 103.2°F.

DIRECTIONS: Role-play the scenario with two peers. One peer will be the patient, and the other will be the wife. You will be the medical assistant.

EQUIPMENT and SUPPLIES

- Stethoscope
- Watch
- Pen
- Sphygmomanometer (blood pressure cuff)
- Pillows, blankets, or small stool to help elevate the feet
- Exam table

PROCEDURAL STEPS

1. Call for help. Monitor the patient's breathing and pulse until the provider arrives.
   PURPOSE: It is important to have the provider see the patient immediately.
   Situation update: The provider examines the patient and suspects septic shock. You administer 2 L of oxygen per nasal canula as the provider ordered. The triage RN inserts an IV and administers IV fluids. The provider directs another medical assistant to call 911.
2. Raise the patient's legs 12 inches.
   PURPOSE: Raising the person's legs helps the blood return to the heart. Some tables will allow you to elevate the foot section. If this is not possible, use things such as pillows, blankets, or a small stool.
3. Make sure the patient's head is flat on the bed.
   PURPOSE: This helps the blood to flow to the head.
4. Loosen the person's clothing. Make sure the clothing does not restrict the neck and chest area.
   PURPOSE: Tight clothing can affect the breathing.
5. Obtain a pulse rate, respiration rate, and blood pressure. Continue to monitor the patient's airway, pulse rate, and respiration rate.
   PURPOSE: Monitor the patient's vital signs. If the person is not breathing, provide rescue breathing. If the person has no pulse, start CPR.
6. While monitoring the patient, speak calmly with him. Use a gentle tone of voice. Demonstrate calming body language (e.g., do not appear scared, rushed, or out of control).
   PURPOSE: It is important to keep the patient calm during the crisis. Anxiety can be a symptom of shock.
7. Talk calmly with the patient's wife and explain what is occurring. Answer any questions the wife may have.
   PURPOSE: In an emergency, it is important to keep the family in the room updated on what is occurring. Depending on the emergency, sometimes a staff person will take the family members to another room.
8. Document the first aid measures you provided in the order they occurred. Indicate which provider examined the patient. In addition, document the administration of oxygen and the vital signs obtained.
   PURPOSE: Specifying the care provided, along with the vital signs, will help the provider and the emergency responders.

Documentation Example 1

10/07/20XX 1525 P: 92 irregular, 1+; R: 26 regular, shallow; BP: 72/48 RA lying; T: 103.2°F (TA). Notified Dr. Walden. Pt resting on table with his wife at his side. ——————— Gabe Garcia, CMA (AAMA)

Documentation Example 2

10/07/20XX 1535 Administered 8 L of oxygen per mask per Dr. Walden's order. Raised legs about 12 inches, and head is flat. P: 98 irregular, 1+; R: 32 regular, shallow; BP: 70/42 RA lying. ——————————————— Gabe Garcia, CMA (AAMA)

PROCEDURE 27.7 Provide Rescue Breathing, Cardiopulmonary Resuscitation (CPR), and Automated External Defibrillator (AED)

TASKS: Perform rescue breathing and CPR. Use the AED machine.

SCENARIO: You are in the healthcare facility parking lot and find a person on the ground. No one is around.

DIRECTIONS: Role-play the scenario with a peer. Your peer will be the person on the ground. You will be the medical assistant.

EQUIPMENT and SUPPLIES

- AED machine with adult pads
- Barrier ventilation device
- Mannequin
- Gloves (if available)

PROCEDURAL STEPS

1. Check the scene for safety. Is it safe to approach and provide help to the victim?
   PURPOSE: It is important to look for toxic or electrical hazards. Also, look for other hazards that make the scene unsafe for you. If you find something, call 911 and wait for the emergency responders.
2. Check the person's response. Tap the individual on the shoulder and shout, "Are you all right?" Pause for a few moments for a response.
   PURPOSE: If the patient is responsive, the individual will talk, moan, move, or do something that indicates responsiveness.
   Scenario update: There is no response from the individual. A bystander comes up, and you direct that person to find an AED machine.
3. Call 911 and answer the questions from the dispatcher.
   PURPOSE: The dispatcher needs to know what is occurring and where the emergency is located.
4. Put on gloves if available. Roll the person over if the person is face down. Roll the person as an entire unit, supporting the head, neck, and back. Open the airway and assess the respiration and pulse for 10 seconds.
   Note: Occasional gasping is not considered breathing.
   a. *Person is breathing and has a pulse:* Monitor the person until the emergency responders arrive. If needed and if no head, neck, or spinal injury is suspected, place the patient in the recovery position.
   b. *Person is not breathing and has a pulse:* Give one breath every 5 to 6 seconds. Check the pulse every 2 minutes. If pulse remains, continue with rescue breathing. If pulse is absent, start CPR.
   c. *Person is not breathing and has no pulse:* Give CPR, starting with compressions. Give 15 compressions and two breaths.

   PURPOSE: Before you initiate rescue breathing or CPR, you need to know if the person is breathing or has a pulse.
   Scenario update: The individual has a weak pulse and is not breathing. (Use a mannequin for the following steps.)
5. Use a barrier device if available. Pinch the person's nose and give each rescue breath over 1 second. Watch for the chest to rise. Give the appropriate number of ventilations for the person's age (see Table 27.5). Continue to monitor the pulse as you give rescue breaths.
   Note: If the person has been choking, look in the mouth before giving a rescue breath. If you see the object, sweep it out with your finger. You can also provide nose ventilation if the mouth is injured. Stoma ventilation must be done if the person has a stoma (in the throat area).
   PURPOSE: Adults get a rescue breath every 5 to 6 seconds. Children and infants get one every 2 to 3 seconds. If the chest does not rise, reposition and open the airway.
   Scenario update: When you check the pulse again, there is no pulse.
6. Place your hands in the correct location on the chest (Figure 1). Bring your shoulders directly over the victim's sternum as you compress downward. Keep your elbows locked (Figure 2).
   PURPOSE: The correct position will allow you to do the compressions at the necessary depth.

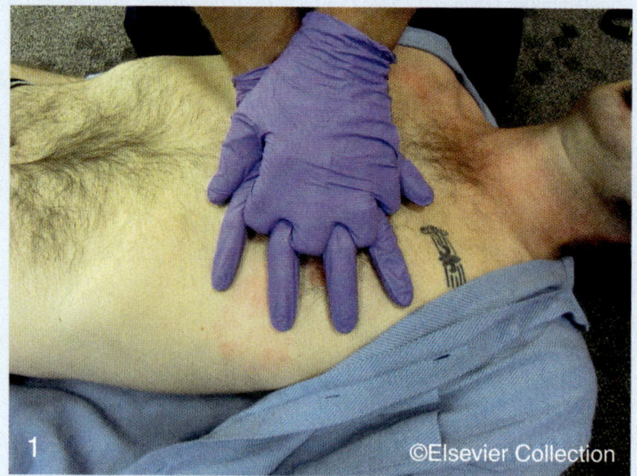
1 ©Elsevier Collection

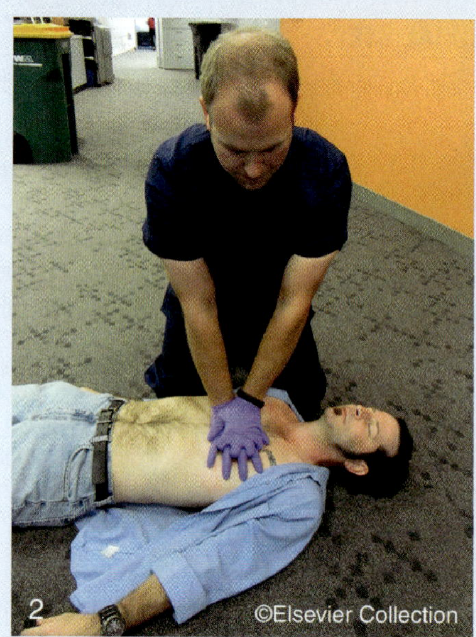
2 ©Elsevier Collection

7. Give 15 compressions at the appropriate depth (see Table 27.5). Give two ventilations and watch for the chest to rise. Continue with the cycle. Give approximately 100 compressions per minute to an adult.

PROCEDURE 27.7 Provide Rescue Breathing, Cardiopulmonary Resuscitation (CPR), and Automated External Defibrillator (AED)—*continued*

PURPOSE: The appropriate depth is required to help compress the chambers of the heart. It is important to continue to provide ventilations and compressions until you are too exhausted, the person is breathing, an AED arrives, or emergency responders arrive.

Scenario update: After two cycles, a bystander brings an AED but does not know how to use it. The bystander also does not know CPR. You need to stop the CPR and use the AED.

8. Turn on the AED and follow the directions. Attach the AED pads to the individual's bare, dry chest (see Table 27.5 and Figure 3). Attach the pads to the machine if required.
   Note: Make sure to remove any medication patches and medication residue from the chest before applying the pads.
   PURPOSE: The pads need to be placed on the bare, dry chest for the AED to work correctly.

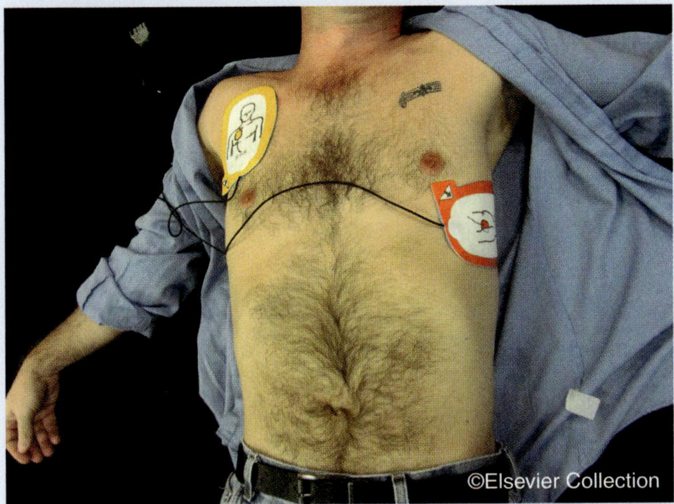

9. Have everyone stand back from the patient by announcing, "Stand clear." Push the analyze button and allow the machine to analyze the heartbeat.
   PURPOSE: "Stand clear" tells everyone not to touch the patient during this step.
10. Follow the prompts on the AED machine.
    a. *Shock advised:* Announce, "Stand clear," and make sure no one is touching the individual. Press the shock button. After the shock, do CPR for 2 minutes, starting with compressions. Continue following the prompts until the emergency responders arrive.
    b. *Shock not advised:* Continue doing CPR for 2 minutes, starting with compressions. Continue following the prompts until the emergency responders arrive.

    PURPOSE: The AED will prompt you as to what to do next.

PRINCIPLES OF PHARMACOLOGY 28

SCENARIO

Gabe Garcia, a certified medical assistant (CMA) who has met the requirements of the American Association of Medical Assistants (AAMA), has worked for Walden-Martin Family Medical (WMFM) Clinic for 7 years. He was hired right after he completed his medical assistant program. Gabe was asked to be Mark Allen's mentor for practicum. Mark has just completed all of his medical assistant courses at the local college and now needs 160 hours of practicum. He is excited to be working with Gabe.

Gabe works with several of the WMFM Clinic providers. He spends 1 to 2 hours a day working with prescription refills. Gabe also rooms patients, obtains their vital signs and history, and assists with injections. Mark will have a lot of great experiences with Gabe.

While studying this chapter, think about the following questions:

- What are the sources and uses of drugs?
- What is pharmacokinetics?
- How does drug legislation affect the medical assistant practice?
- What are the four names of a drug?
- What information is contained in the different sections of the drug reference information?
- How does a medical assistant prepare prescriptions for the provider to sign?

LEARNING OBJECTIVES

1. Analyze the sources and uses of drugs.
2. Distinguish among the phases of pharmacokinetics.
3. Examine drug actions, including influencing factors, therapeutic effects, and adverse reactions.
4. Examine drug legislation that impacts the ambulatory care setting.
5. Examine how healthcare professionals must comply with the Controlled Substance Act.
6. Differentiate between brand and generic drugs.
7. Examine the information available in drug references.
8. Differentiate among the types of solid, semisolid, and liquid medication forms.
9. Differentiate among the types of medication orders.
10. Examine prescriptions, including the parts, the information required, and the medical assistant's role in preparing prescriptions.

VOCABULARY

addiction A disease that occurs when a person cannot stop or limit the use of a drug, even after negative consequences have been experienced.

analgesic (an ahl JEE zik) A drug that reduces or eliminates pain.

antiarrhythmic (an tee ah RITH mik) A drug that prevents or alleviates heart arrhythmias.

antibiotic (an ti bie OT ik) A drug that destroys or inhibits the growth of bacteria.

anticoagulant (an tee koe AG yuh lant) A substance (i.e., medication or chemical) that prevents the clotting of blood.

anticonvulsant (an tee kahn VUL sahnt) A drug used to prevent or treat seizures.

antihistamine (an tee HIS tah meen) A drug that counteracts the effects of histamine.

anti-inflammatory (an tee in FLAM ah tor ee) A medication that prevents or reduces inflammation.

antimalarial (an tee mah LAR ee ahl) A drug used to treat or prevent malaria.

antiseptic (an ti SEP tik) A substance that inhibits the growth of microorganisms on living tissue (e.g., alcohol and povidone-iodine solution [Betadine]).

controlled substances A behavior-altering or addictive drug or chemical substance whose possession and use are prohibited by or regulated under the federal Controlled Substances Act.

form Physical characteristics of a medication (e.g., tablet and suspension).

metabolites (muh TAB uh lites) By-products of drug metabolism

National Provider Identifier (NPI) An identifier assigned by the Centers for Medicare and Medicaid Services (CMS) that classifies the healthcare provider by license and medical specialties.

VOCABULARY—*continued*

psychiatrists Medical doctors who have been specially trained to diagnose and treat patients with mental, emotional, and behavioral conditions.

reconciling Comparing a document with another document to ensure that they are consistent.

side effects Unpleasant effects of a drug in addition to the desired or therapeutic effect.

therapeutic range The blood concentrations of a medication that are high enough to produce the drug's therapeutic effect.

toxicity The harmful and deadly effect of a medication that can develop due to the buildup of medication or by-products in the body.

INTRODUCTION

Pharmacology is the study of the properties, actions, and uses of drugs. A *drug* is a chemical substance used to cure, treat, prevent, or diagnose disease. In the ambulatory care setting, medical assistants deal with medication, from history taking to administering medications. Medical assistants must have a general understanding of the classification of drugs. They need to know how to pronounce the medication names. They must know how to give medications, the dosage to give, and typical **side effects**. New medications are continually being developed and released for patient treatment. Thus, medical assistants must stay updated on medications.

PHARMACOLOGY BASICS

Medications have been around for a long time. The first medications came from natural products found in our ancestors' living environment. Today, with advancing technology, most medications are created in a laboratory setting. These sources and others will be explained, along with the uses of medications.

In addition, this section presents a basic description of how medication enters, moves through, and exits the body. This knowledge will help the medical assistant identify patients who may be at risk for medication issues because of their age or a disease process.

Sources of Drugs

Drugs are either created from natural sources or made synthetically in a laboratory. Plants, animals, minerals, and microbiologic sources are natural sources of drugs.

Natural Sources of Drugs

Plants are the oldest source of drugs. Our ancestors found that different plants helped with different symptoms. Leaves, bark, stems, roots, and fruits have been used in medicinal preparations through the years. Some examples of medicinal plant sources include the following:

- Digitalis, an **antiarrhythmic** medication, comes from the purple foxglove flower.
- Nicotine comes from tobacco leaves.
- Quinidine, an **antimalarial** medication, comes from the bark of the cinchona tree.

Animals are also a source of medications. Natural substances are extracted from animal tissues and organs. *Heparin*, an **anticoagulant**, comes from pig intestines. Lanolin is found in topical preparations used to protect the skin. It comes from the sebaceous glands of sheep. Other medications are developed with lactose and gelatin, which are from animals.

Minerals and microbiologic substances are other natural sources of medications. Examples of mineral use include the following:

- Iron is used to treat iron-deficiency anemia.
- Iodine is an **antiseptic**.
- Zinc is used as a supplement and is found in topical pastes for wounds.

One microbiologic source is *Penicillium chrysogenum*. This is a fungus that creates penicillin.

Synthetic Sources of Drugs

Many medications originated in nature but have been recreated in the laboratory setting. For instance, insulin initially came from cattle and pigs. Many people developed allergies to the insulin. Now synthetic insulin is widely used. Biotechnology and genetic engineering techniques are continually being used to create new medications. With the help of technological advances, individualized medications are also being produced. (Individualized medications are discussed later in the chapter.) Synthetic medications are cheaper to produce because they are created in mass volumes. The quality of synthetic medications can also be controlled.

Uses of Drugs

When you are studying medications, it is important to identify the uses of drugs. Why are they being prescribed? What do they do in the body? Some medications may have more than one use. There are eight common uses of drugs:

- *Prevention*: Drugs used to prevent diseases. For example, vaccines are given, and the body creates antibodies to protect against specific diseases.
- *Treatment*: Drugs that relieve the symptoms while the body fights off the disease. For example, acetaminophen, an *antipyretic* medication, brings down a fever while the body fights off a viral infection.
- *Diagnosis*: Drugs used to diagnose or monitor a condition. For example, a contrast medium (radiopaque dye) is given to highlight organs on x-rays.
- *Cure*: Drugs that eliminate the disease. For example, amoxicillin, an **antibiotic**, is used to cure strep throat.
- *Contraceptive*: Drugs used to prevent pregnancy. For example, Depo-Provera is an injectable contraceptive medication.
- *Health maintenance*: Medications used to maintain or enhance health. Vitamins and minerals are examples.
- *Palliation*: Drugs that do not cure or treat the disease but improve the quality of life. For example, morphine, an **analgesic**, is commonly used by patients with cancer.

- *Replacement*: Drugs used to increase the blood levels of naturally occurring substances in the body. For example, levothyroxine is used for patients with hypothyroidism.

CRITICAL THINKING APPLICATION **28.1**

Gabe and Mark are discussing the basics of pharmacology and the eight common uses of medications. Gabe asks Mark which use would include taking an **antihistamine** for allergy symptoms. How would you answer this question?

PHARMACOKINETICS

Pharmacokinetics is the study of drug absorption, distribution, metabolism, and excretion in the body. Through pharmacokinetics, we understand when a medication starts to work in the body. We know how it moves through the body and what organs metabolize and excrete the drug from the body. Some of the patients you will be working with will have greater risks of side effects and **toxicity**. Understanding the basics of pharmacokinetics will help you identify those at greater risk for problems.

Absorption

Drugs can be administered in many ways. *Route* is the means by which a drug enters the body. Where a drug enters the body is considered the *site of administration. Absorption* is the movement of a drug from the site of administration to the bloodstream. The following are commonly used routes:

- *Oral* (po, PO): Taken by mouth
- *Sublingual* (SL): Placed under the tongue to dissolve
- *Buccal*: Placed between the cheek and the gums to dissolve and absorb quickly
- *Intramuscular* (IM): Injected into the muscle
- *Subcutaneous* (SUBQ): Injected just below the skin; moves into the capillaries or the lymphatic vessels and is brought to the bloodstream
- *Intravenous* (IV): Injected directly into the bloodstream

Factors Influencing Absorption

The rate of absorption is influenced by the following factors:

- *Route*: Oral medications need to pass through the gastrointestinal (GI) tract. This takes time. IV medications are directly administered into the bloodstream and have virtually no absorption time. They start working faster than drugs given by other routes.
- *Blood flow to the absorption area*: The greater the number of blood vessels, the quicker the absorption. Medication given by the sublingual and buccal routes is absorbed quickly into the bloodstream. These sites are rich in blood vessels. IM medications absorb quicker than SUBQ medications. The muscle tissue has more blood vessels than the subcutaneous tissue.
- *Ability of the medication to be absorbed*: Liquid medications are easier to absorb than solid medications. Solid medications need to be broken down before they absorb. Acidic medications are absorbed in the stomach. Base (or alkaline) medications are absorbed in the intestines.
- *Conditions at the site of the absorption*: Some medications must be taken with food, which can slow the absorption of the medication. Typically, medications taken on an empty stomach can be absorbed faster. The intestines provide more surface area than the stomach for the absorption of medications.

Distribution

Once the drug is absorbed into the blood, it rapidly circulates through the body (unless it must go through the liver). During this time, the drug is brought to the body tissues. The movement of absorbed drugs from the blood to the body tissues is called *distribution*. The speed of the drug's movement from the blood to the tissues varies greatly. Some drugs bind with proteins in the blood and move slowly into tissues. Some drugs accumulate in certain tissues. These tissues act as *reservoirs*, slowly releasing the drug into the bloodstream and keeping the blood levels from decreasing too rapidly. This process prolongs the effect of the drug. Circulation issues (e.g., peripheral artery disease) can also slow the distribution of medication.

For the medication to move into certain organs, it must be able to pass through the tissues. The blood-brain barrier allows only certain fat-soluble medications to pass into the cerebrospinal fluid and the brain. In comparison, the placental membrane allows most drugs to pass through from the mother to the baby in utero. Therefore, only certain medications are prescribed during pregnancy.

Routes Affect the Dose

Oral medications are absorbed in the stomach or the intestines. The blood containing the absorbed digestive nutrients and drugs passes through the hepatic portal vein and the liver before it circulates to the rest of the body. In the liver, some of the drugs are chemically altered. Some of the active drugs are lost during this first pass through the liver. This reduces the amount of drugs in the circulating blood that can be used.

For instance, a person is having an allergic reaction and needs Benadryl. If the drug is to be taken orally, the person takes 50 mg. If it is to be given intravenously, 10 mg may be given. This is because all 10 mg gets into the bloodstream, whereas some of the 50 mg is lost as it passes through the liver before circulating through the body. It is important for a medical assistant to realize that doses (e.g., 10 mg) may vary based on the route used to give the medication.

Metabolism

Metabolism is a series of chemical processes whereby enzymes change drugs in the body. Metabolism is necessary so that medications can be cleared from the body. Active forms of drugs may be converted into water-soluble compounds, which are eventually excreted.

Most drug metabolism occurs in the liver. Younger children, older adults, and those with liver disease may have problems metabolizing medications. These populations could be at risk for drug toxicity. The dose of medication is adjusted for at-risk populations to prevent toxicity.

Prodrugs

Prodrugs are medications that are administered in an inactive form. Through the normal metabolic processes, the medication is changed into an active form of a drug. The liver and the intestines are sites that can convert prodrugs to active forms of drugs. For instance, sulfasalazine (Azulfidine) is an **anti-inflammatory** drug that is used to treat ulcerative colitis. It is also a prodrug because it is ingested in an inactive form. Bacteria in the colon change the drug into an active drug that the body will use.

Excretion

Excretion is the movement of **metabolites** out of the body. Most drugs are excreted through the large intestine and kidneys. The large intestine excretes the undigested drug products in the stool. The kidneys excrete metabolites in the urine. Clinical Laboratory Improvement Amendments (CLIA)–waived urine drug screening tests can detect certain metabolites.

Drugs can also be excreted in breast milk. This is critical information to have when a mother is breastfeeding her baby. As with pregnancy, only a limited number of drugs are safe with breastfeeding. Most drug references indicate if medications pass into the breast milk. Other ways drugs can be excreted are through sweat, exhaled air, and saliva.

Young children, older adults, and those with kidney disease are at risk for the buildup of metabolic drug by-products in the body. These populations are at greater risk for symptoms of toxicity.

DRUG ACTION

Drugs are chemicals that can cause changes in the cells. There are four main drug actions:

- *Depressing*: Slows down the cell's activity. For example, narcotic medications reduce the activity in the brain's respiratory center. This action slows the respiration rate.
- *Stimulating*: Increases the cell's activity. For instance, caffeine increases brain activity.
- *Destroying*: Kills cells or disrupts parts of cells. For example, chemotherapy medications destroy cancer cells.
- *Replacing substances*: Substances required by the body can be given as medications. For instance, patients with type 1 diabetes mellitus take insulin.

Factors Influencing Drug Action

One might think that a drug works the same for everyone. This is not so. Personal characteristics can cause minor differences in how a drug works from one person to another. Many factors influence drug action:

- *Age*: Infants and older adults have problems metabolizing and excreting medications. Their liver and kidneys are less effective. This can lead to possible drug accumulation and toxicity.
- *Body size*: A person's size affects the amount of drug needed. Children's dosages are calculated based on body weight. Thinner people require less medication than heavier people.
- *Sex*: Women have a higher proportion of body fat. Hormonal differences can affect metabolism. Women can react differently to some medications compared to men.
- *Genetics*: Genetic makeup can affect how a person responds to drugs. (This is discussed in more depth in the Pharmacogenomics section.)
- *Diseases*: Poor circulation, liver disease, and kidney disease can alter drug action.
- *Diet*: Certain foods can affect a drug's action. For instance, milk products can diminish the effects of tetracycline, an *antibiotic.*
- *Drug dosage, route, and timing of administration*: The greater the amount of drug taken, the greater the effect will be. The route will also affect drug action. Drugs are absorbed, distributed, and metabolized differently based on the administration route. Some drugs work better when taken with food, whereas others do not.
- *Mental state*: People with positive attitudes tend to do better than those with negative attitudes.
- *Environmental temperature*: In hot weather, heat relaxes blood vessels. This can speed up the distribution of medication, thus speeding up the drug's action.

Pharmacogenomics

Most medications are dosed as "one size fits all." Each person's genetic makeup affects how that person responds to medications. *Pharmacogenomics* or *pharmacogenetics* is the study of how genetic factors influence a person's metabolic response to a specific medication. Pharmacogenomics testing usually requires a small blood or saliva sample. The sample is analyzed to determine if a specific medication will be an effective treatment for an individual. Testing can determine the best dose of medication and if the person could have serious adverse reactions (unexpected or life-threatening reactions) to the medication. A different test is required for each medication. Pharmacogenomics is largely used in cancer treatments, but it is becoming more common in other areas of medicine.

Therapeutic Effects

Medications can have local or systemic effects. Medication effects that are seen at the site of administration are *local effects*. Medication effects that are seen throughout the body are *systemic effects*. Each medication has one or more *therapeutic effects,* or desired effects. This is the intended action of the medication. For instance, the therapeutic effect of a pain reliever is to reduce pain.

Sometimes multiple doses are needed to achieve the therapeutic effect. Other times just one dose of medication can achieve the therapeutic effect. The provider may prescribe a higher initial dose for some medications, called a *loading dose.* This helps to quickly increase the medication level in the blood. A loading dose helps the person achieve the **therapeutic range** sooner. A *maintenance dose* is the amount of medication needed to keep the blood levels within the therapeutic range. If the blood levels go beyond the therapeutic range, the person can experience signs and symptoms of toxicity. This is considered a toxic dose of medication. A lethal dose is the amount of medication that could kill a person.

CRITICAL THINKING APPLICATION **28.2**

Gabe and Mark are discussing therapeutic effect and loading dose. Gabe shares that patients sometimes get confused about how much medication to take when they are given two amounts, a loading dose and the regular amount. How might a healthcare professional instruct a patient who needs to take a loading dose?

Adverse Reactions

Most of the time, when a medication is correctly administered, the therapeutic effect occurs. However, sometimes issues arise, and the person has problems with the medication. The person can experience an unexpected or life-threatening reaction called an *adverse reaction.* Table 28.1 lists common adverse reactions.

TABLE 28.1 Common Adverse Reactions

ADVERSE REACTION	DESCRIPTION
Allergy	Drug allergy occurs when a person develops antibodies against a specific drug. When the drug is taken, the antibodies attack the antigens from the drug. Tissues are damaged during this process, and histamines are released. Histamines cause the allergic reactions.
Anaphylaxis	Extreme hypersensitivity to a specific drug (antigen) can cause life-threatening symptoms, including swelling of the mouth and airway, difficulty breathing (*dyspnea*), wheezing, loss of consciousness, and death.
Idiosyncrasy	A peculiar response to a certain drug. For instance, Benadryl causes drowsiness. However, when it is given to children, they often get extremely agitated.
Cumulative effect	For medications taken routinely, often the prior dose is not completely metabolized and excreted before the next dose is given. This can lead to a buildup of medication or by-products that can produce toxic effects.
Toxicity	The harmful and possibly deadly effects of a medication that can develop due to the buildup of medication or by-products in the body. People with liver or kidney disease, young children, older adults, and those who overdose are at risk for toxicity.
Drug interactions	When two or more drugs are taken, sometimes a drug-drug interaction can occur. The interactions can be helpful or harmful. Three types of drug interactions can occur: • *Antagonism*: One drug reduces or blocks the effect of another drug. For example, naloxone is given for narcotic overdosage. • *Synergism*: The combined effect of two drugs used together is greater than the sum of each drug's effect (e.g., 1 + 1 > 2). Example of a harmful interaction: Alcohol has a synergistic effect on antidepressants. • *Potentiation*: A type of synergism; one drug increases the effect of the second drug. With L-dopa and carbidopa, one drug has no effect but increases the effect of the other drug (e.g., 0 + 1 > 1).
Tolerance	The need for a larger dose to get the same therapeutic or desired effect. Tolerance can be seen when narcotic pain medications are taken with **anticonvulsants**.
Drug dependence	Strong psychological or physical need to take a certain drug. Withdrawal symptoms can be experienced when a person stops using a drug. Drug dependence can occur with or without **addiction.**

Many experts and drug reference information will include side effects with adverse reactions. They may divide these into mild, moderate, and severe reactions. The side effects usually fall into the mild category. Severe adverse reactions are those that can cause disability, hospitalization, death, or birth defects.

Other reference information separates adverse reactions/events and side effects. Adverse reactions or events would be those that are life-threatening and may cause disability or birth defects. Side effects would be unpleasant effects of the drug, in addition to the desired or therapeutic effect. They can be harmless or may cause injury. The most common side effects include symptoms of GI distress, such as nausea, vomiting, constipation, and diarrhea.

DRUG LEGISLATION AND THE AMBULATORY CARE SETTING

In the ambulatory care environment, medications can be prescribed, administered, and dispensed.

- *Prescribe* means to order medication as a treatment for a condition. Doctors (MDs [including **psychiatrists**], doctors of osteopathic medicine [DOs], and dentists) and advanced practice professionals, including physician assistants (PAs), nurse practitioners (NPs), and certified nurse-midwives (CNMs), can prescribe medications. State prescribing laws can vary for advanced practice professionals.
- *Administer* means to give a prescribed dose of medication to a patient. Medical assistants, nurses, and providers can administer medications. State laws related to medication administration by medical assistants can vary.
- *Dispense* means to give a supply of medication that the patient will take later. In most scenarios, pharmacists dispense medications.

Federal and state legislation governs these three activities. The following sections will discuss these laws, the agencies responsible for overseeing the laws, and the laws' effect on medical assistants.

CRITICAL THINKING APPLICATION 28.3

At WMFM Clinic, pharmaceutical representatives drop off sample medications that are given to patients. Usually, the provider will give a few days' worth of samples to a patient to ensure the patient is tolerating the medication. Patients who have no issues can then have the prescription filled. Mark sees the provider bag up a few samples and attach directions to the bag. The provider gives the bag to Gabe and asks him to give it to the patient. Mark asks Gabe, "Who is dispensing the medication?" How would you answer this question?

Food, Drug, and Cosmetic Act

The Food, Drug, and Cosmetic Act of 1938 is enforced by the Food and Drug Administration (FDA). The FDA is a federal agency in the Department of Health and Human Services (HHS). The FDA is responsible for the safety, effectiveness, security, and quality of drugs, cosmetics, and food. The FDA oversees a number of areas:

- *Foods*: Dietary supplements, bottled water, food additives, infant formula, and other food products
- *Drugs*: Prescription drugs (brand name and generic) and nonprescription (over-the-counter [OTC]) drugs
- *Biologics*: Vaccines, blood, and blood products
- *Medical devices*: Medical equipment (from simple [tongue depressor] to complex [heart pacemaker]), dental devices, and surgical implants

Manufacturers must submit applications for new products to the FDA. Manufacturers must provide adequate data to show the safety and effectiveness of the product. The FDA must determine if drugs, devices, and products are safe and effective. Once this is determined, then the product is released to the general public.

FDA Adverse Event Reporting System

The FDA monitors the safety of products released to the market. The FDA Adverse Event Reporting System (FAERS) is a computerized database that helps the FDA monitor drugs. It contains reports of adverse events reported to the FDA. MedWatch is the FDA's reporting program. It provides information on products overseen by the FDA. MedWatch is available to healthcare professionals (www.fda.gov/safety/medwatch-fda-safety-information-and-adverse-event-reporting-program).

If the FDA determines a medication is unsafe, it will recall the medication. The medical assistant should remove any recalled medications from the stock and sample cabinets. (*Sample medications* come from pharmaceutical companies and are used for patients.) Concerned patients may contact their providers. The provider will determine what action to take for each patient.

Controlled Substances Act

The Controlled Substances Act (CSA), Title II of the Comprehensive Drug Abuse Prevention and Control Act of 1970, is a federal law. The Drug Enforcement Agency (DEA) is a federal law enforcement agency under the US Department of Justice. The DEA enforces the CSA. The DEA oversees the manufacturing, importation, possession, use, and distribution of legal (or prescription) **controlled substances**. The DEA also handles illegal controlled substances, which cannot legally be manufactured, purchased, or sold in the United States.

Under the CSA, controlled substances are divided into five schedules. These schedules are arranged from the greatest to the least abuse potential (Table 28.2). State statutes also address procedures related to scheduled medications. It is important for the medical assistant to know the schedule of commonly ordered medications. Some controlled substance prescriptions are handled differently. This is discussed later in the chapter.

COMPLIANCE WITH THE CONTROLLED SUBSTANCE ACT

Providers prescribing controlled substances need a DEA registration number. Each provider has a unique number. The DEA number is good for 3 years. The medical assistant may need to assist the provider in renewing or obtaining a DEA number. This can be done at the DEA website at www.deadiversion.usdoj.gov. Additional state

TABLE 28.2 Schedule of Controlled Substances

SCHEDULE	PSYCHOLOGICAL AND PHYSICAL DEPENDENCE	EXAMPLES
I	Highest potential for abuse; drugs with no currently accepted medical use	Heroin, lysergic acid diethylamide (LSD), ecstasy
II/IIN (2/2N)	High level of abuse; can lead to severe psychological or physical dependence	Schedule II narcotics: hydromorphone (Dilaudid), methadone (Dolophine), oxycodone (OxyContin, Percocet), fentanyl (Duragesic), codeine, morphine Schedule IIN stimulants: dextroamphetamine and amphetamine (Adderall), methamphetamine (Desoxyn), methylphenidate (Concerta, Ritalin LA)
III/IIIN (3/3N)	Moderate to low physical dependence or high psychological dependence	Schedule III narcotics: acetaminophen with codeine (Tylenol #2 or #3), buprenorphine Schedule IIIN non-narcotics: benzphetamine (Didrex), ketamine, anabolic steroids (e.g., Depo-Testosterone)
IV (4)	Low potential for abuse relative to substances in Schedule III	Schedule IV substances: alprazolam (Xanax), carisoprodol (Soma), clonazepam (Klonopin), diazepam (Valium), lorazepam (Ativan), temazepam (Restoril)
V (5)	Lowest potential for abuse relative to substances listed in Schedule IV; contains limited quantities of certain narcotics	Schedule V substances: Robitussin AC, ezogabine (Potiga)

requirements may need to be met before a provider can prescribe controlled substances.

Controlled substances have a paper trail. This record starts with the manufacturer and ends when the medication is dispensed or administered. In some healthcare facilities, the in-house pharmacy handles the controlled substances that are administered. The provider gives the medical assistant a prescription for a patient. The medical assistant gives the pharmacist the prescription and, in return, gets the medication. (Please note that some state laws do not allow medical assistants to administer controlled substances.) In this scenario, the pharmacist is responsible for managing the paperwork for the controlled substances.

In healthcare facilities without pharmacies, providers must take the responsibility of ordering controlled substances from the manufacturer. The medical assistant must help the provider comply with the Controlled Substance Act. The following sections discuss common compliance activities.

Storage

All controlled substances must be adequately safeguarded. They need to be kept in a locked cabinet or safe of substantial construction. Keys should be placed in a locked area accessible only to authorized persons. Store controlled substances in a different location than non-narcotic medications. Additional storage guidelines apply to all medications:

- Make sure all medications are kept in their original containers.
- Store medications in a cool, dry location. Keep medications away from light, heat, or moisture. Refer to package inserts for specific storage information.
- Do not combine or repackage medications with different lot numbers or expiration dates.
- Keep stock medications (purchased by department) separated from sample medications (given by pharmaceutical manufacturers for patients).
- Keep medications out of exam rooms. Lock medication cabinets at the end of the day.

Inventory Records

It is important to keep an ongoing log of controlled substances received from manufacturers and administered to patients. Medications are tracked by the manufacturer, lot number, and expiration date. This information is found on the package. When a patient needs a controlled substance, the medical assistant must complete the log. The log typically requires the following data:

- The medication information (name, dose, lot number, and expiration date)
- The ordering provider's name
- Information on the patient receiving the medication (name, date of birth, address, health record number, and so on)
- The name or initials of the healthcare professional administering the medication

The log must be kept separate from the patient's health record. The medication must also be documented in the patient's health record after it is administered.

Periodic **reconciling** of the log with the actual inventory count is important to identify missing medications. An inventory of all controlled substances must be done at least annually unless required more often by law. Some states have special requirements for the inventory. It is important for the medical assistant to be knowledgeable about the special state requirements. The controlled substance inventory and log records need to be kept for 2 years. The records may be inspected by individuals authorized by the state attorney general.

Drug Destruction

Expired controlled substances are returned to the place from where they were received. For example, controlled substances that were sent by the manufacturer must be returned to the manufacturer, along with the required paperwork.

Sometimes a controlled substance must be destroyed in the healthcare facility, such as in the following situations:

- Only part of the medication is used for the patient; the extra amount must be destroyed.
- The patient refuses the medication after it has been opened and prepared.
- The medication is accidentally contaminated before it can be administered.

In these situations, the controlled substance must be destroyed in the presence of two authorized persons (e.g., medical assistants, nurses). An entry on the waste log must be made. This information must include the date; the drug's name, strength, and quantity; the reason for destruction; and the signatures of both persons.

Discarding Medications in the Healthcare Facility

Discard medication that is expired, contaminated, unlabeled, or opened and not used. Some healthcare facilities have medication discarding programs to prevent medications from entering the city's water supply. Remember, if the medication is a controlled substance, two authorized employees must sign a waste log before the medication is discarded. Both employees must witness the disposal.

To discard medication, follow these steps if the facility has no other procedures in place:

- Return expired controlled substances to the place they were received from (e.g., manufacturer), accompanied by the proper paperwork.
- Flush liquids down the sink.
- Flush pills down the toilet.
- Mix powdered medications with water and flush them down the toilet.
- Flush fluid from syringes down the sink and discard the syringe in a biohazardous sharps container.

Theft and Diversion Reporting

Diversion of controlled substances means using the medication for personal reasons. If a medical assistant identifies that controlled substances are missing, it is important to notify the provider and supervisor. Many states and the DEA require any theft or loss to be reported to them within a given period. A report must be completed and filed by the deadline.

Medical Assistant's Role in Preventing Drug Abuse

By following these guidelines, the medical assistant can help prevent drug abuse:

- Carefully monitor patients who repeatedly call for prescription refills of controlled substances. Be aware that some patients will give aliases (false names).
- Request health records from other facilities for patients who report previous prescriptions for scheduled drugs.
- If the facility uses paper prescription pads, keep blank pads in a locked cabinet. They should be stored away from patient treatment areas.
- Never use prescription pads for notepads. Never use preprinted or presigned forms.
- Secure computers used for electronic health record (EHR) documentation to prevent patient access to prescription generation.
- Keep only a limited supply of controlled substances on hand.
- Keep accurate, complete records of controlled substances administered. Patients' records should contain information on prescribed and administered controlled substances.

BRAND AND GENERIC DRUGS

The following sections discuss the four drug names, along with the difference between a brand-name drug and a generic drug. When the medical assistant updates a patient's medication record and assists with preparing prescriptions, knowing trade and generic medication names is critical in preventing errors.

Drug Names

A single drug may have up to four names: chemical, generic, official, and brand. Not all drugs will have four names, but ibuprofen is an example of a drug that does.

- *Chemical name*: Represents the drug's exact chemical formula. For example, the chemical name of ibuprofen is 2-(4-isobutylphenyl) propanoic acid.
- *Generic name*: Assigned by the US Adopted Names (USAN) Council. Similar medications are given similar-sounding generic names. All drugs need to have the generic name on the packaging. For example, ibuprofen is a generic name.
- *Official name*: Used to list the medication in the *United States Pharmacopeia and the National Formulary* (USP–NF). This book provides the standards (e.g., strength, purity, and so on) for drugs in the United States. In many cases, the official name is the same as the generic name. For example, ibuprofen is also the drug's official name.
- *Brand name* or *trade name*: The manufacturer assigns and registers the medication name. No other company can use that name. Usually, the brand name begins with a capital letter and is followed by the registered sign (®). For example, brand names of ibuprofen include Advil and Motrin.

Generic versus Brand Medications

If you ever walk through the pain medication aisle at a local store, you will see many bottles of ibuprofen products. Generally, the more expensive products are name brands, and the less expensive products are generic.

The company that initially created the medication will market it using a brand name. That company has sole rights to manufacture the medication until the patent expires. During this time, it is not uncommon for the price to be higher. The manufacturer may have spent years developing the medication before it went to market. Once the patent expires, other companies may create their own version of the medication. Some will market the medication under a brand name, and others will use generic names.

Inactive and Active Ingredients

When a company creates a medication, the company determines the appearance of the medication (e.g., color, size, and shape). It also comes up with the *inactive ingredients* or additives. This might be a color, sweetener, flavor, fillers, binders, and so on. For the active ingredient of the medication (e.g., ibuprofen), the company must comply with the regulations of the Food and Drug Administration (FDA). The active ingredient must be of the same quality, purity, and amount as any other FDA-approved ibuprofen product of the same strength.

Most people do not notice a difference between generic and brand-name medications. Other people do notice a difference. Their bodies may react to the inactive ingredients differently. This can affect their treatment for certain conditions. The provider can indicate if a generic medication can be used for prescriptions. This is important to keep in mind if you are assisting a provider by preparing prescriptions.

CRITICAL THINKING APPLICATION 28.4

Mark and Gabe are working with Janine Butler, a patient being seen for hypertension. While they are reviewing Janine's current medications list, she asks them what the difference is between generic and brand-name medications. How might you answer this question?

DRUG REFERENCE INFORMATION

A medical assistant is obligated to become familiar with the drugs that are most frequently prescribed in the department. It is essential to know their indications, adverse reactions, administration routes, dosage, and storage. Using drug reference information can help the medical assistant learn about drugs. In the ambulatory care environment, drug reference information is available in both print and digital forms.

With each drug (including drug samples and stock medications), the manufacturer includes a package insert. The package insert provides information about the medication, side effects, administration techniques, dosages, storage, and so on.

Drug handbooks provide condensed, more common information on the drugs. Many of these books are organized by the generic names of drugs.

The *Prescribers' Digital Reference* (PDR) has replaced the *Physician's Desk Reference*. This digital product contains a comprehensive collection of package insert information. The PDR is available as an app and is also integrated with electronic health records. More information can be found on the PDR website (www.pdr.net).

The digital drug reference information has a huge advantage over print information. Digital information can be updated more quickly and easily than print information. The market for digital drug information has grown over the years. Digital drug reference information is available online, through apps, and with electronic health records.

- Online drug reference information is available from many sites. It is important for the medical assistant to use reliable websites. Government websites (e.g., https://medlineplus.gov/ and www.fda.gov) contain updated, reliable information. Sites that patients use may contain older information and can include medications that are not available in the United States.
- When selecting an app for drug reference information, be sure it is routinely updated. Read the reviews and research the company providing the information. Only use reputable apps for drug reference information.
- Many EHR software programs incorporate drug reference information. This makes it easy for healthcare professionals to look up drug information.

Drug Classification

Drugs are grouped by classification or class. It is important for a medical assistant to be aware of the class of drugs. Patients will often ask what a specific medication is for, and the medical assistant can provide that information. Table 28.3 provides a list of classifications of medications with descriptions.

TABLE 28.3 Examples of Medication Classifications

CLASSIFICATION	DESCRIPTION
Analgesic	Relieves pain
Anesthetic	Produces local or general anesthesia
Antacid	Neutralizes stomach acid
Anti-Alzheimer	Treats dementia (Alzheimer disease)
Antianxiety	Reduces anxiety and tension
Antiarrhythmic	Treats heart arrhythmias
Antibiotic	Treats bacterial infections
Anticholinergic	Reduces smooth muscle spasms
Anticoagulant	Reduces blood clotting ability
Anticonvulsant	Reduces the frequency and severity of seizures
Antidepressant	Treats depression
Antiemetic	Reduces nausea and vomiting
Antifungal	Treats fungal infections
Antigout	Reduces the uric acid in the body
Antihistamine	Relieves allergies by blocking the histamine action
Antihyperglycemic	Reduces the blood glucose level
Antihypertensive	Lowers blood pressure
Anti-inflammatory	Reduces inflammation
Antimigraine	Treats or prevents migraine headaches
Antineoplastic	Slows or stops the growth of cancer cells
Antiplatelet	Prevents the function of platelets (formation of clots)
Antipsychotic	Alters the chemical actions in the brain
Antitussive	Suppresses coughs
Antiviral	Treats viral infections
Bronchodilator	Relaxes the smooth muscles of the bronchi
Cholesterol-lowering agent	Reduces low-density lipoprotein and triglycerides in the blood while increasing the high-density lipoprotein
Contraceptive	Inhibits conception (prevents pregnancy)
Corticosteroid	Reduces inflammation
Decongestant	Relieves nasal and sinus congestion
Diuretic	Increases urinary output and lowers blood pressure
Electrolyte	Maintains normal electrolyte level and proper functioning of the body systems
Erectile dysfunction agent	Facilitates an erection
Expectorant	Thins bronchial secretions, making it easier to cough up the mucus
Hematopoietic	Promotes blood cell production
Hemostatic	Clots blood
Hormone replacement	Replaces hormones or compensates for hormone deficiencies
Laxative	Promotes stools
Leukotriene receptor antagonist	Blocks the action of substances that cause asthma and allergic rhinitis
Miotic	Drains excessive fluid from the eye; used for glaucoma
Muscle relaxant	Reduces pain
Mydriatic	Dilates the pupil; used for ophthalmic procedures
Osteoporosis agent	Promotes bone mineral density; used to treat osteoporosis
Proton-pump inhibitor	Reduces the acid produced in the stomach
Sedative-hypnotic	Slows brain activity, allowing sleep
Stimulant	Stimulates the brain and body, makes the person more alert
Tumor necrosis factor (TNF) inhibitor	Blocks the action of TNF, preventing inflammation in autoimmune disorders

Drug Terminology

Regardless of how drug reference information is obtained, it is important for the medical assistant to understand the terminology. The following terminology is typically found in drug reference information:

- *Names*: Usually, the generic name is listed with the trade names. Some references may indicate if the trade name found is in the United States or Canada.
- *Description*: Describes the medication and its general use.
- *Boxed warning*: Also referred to as a *black box warning*. It addresses serious or life-threatening risks. This information also appears on the drug's label.
- *Dosage*: Specifies the route, dose, and timing of the medication; usually corresponds to an indication (disease or condition). May provide information on doses for different age ranges. *Maximum dosage* indicates the greatest amount of medication a person should have within a 24-hour period.
- *Indications*: Conditions or diseases for which the drug is used.
- *Dosage considerations*: Indicates recommended changes in dosages for special populations (e.g., patients with hepatic impairment, renal impairment).
- *How supplied*: Lists the **form** (e.g., chewable tablets, capsules) and the strength (e.g., 250 mg).
- *Administration*: Provides information on how the medication should be administered. Includes important administration techniques, such as information on shaking the medication, if it needs to be taken with food, and so on.
- *Action*: How the drug provides therapeutic results in the body or the use of the drug.
- *Adverse reactions*: Also called *side effects* in some information. This section describes known undesirable experiences associated with the medication. Reactions may be divided into severe (life threatening, serious reactions), moderate, and mild.
- *Interactions*: Includes medications, foods, and beverages that interact with the medication. These products may either increase or reduce the medication level in the blood. They may also increase the risk of adverse reactions if taken together with the drug.
- *Contraindications*: Reasons or conditions that make administration of the drug improper or undesirable. For example, aspirin is contraindicated in patients with GI bleeding.
- *Precautions*: Indicates necessary actions or special care that needs to be taken when the patient is on the medication. May include information on laboratory tests, special populations (children and geriatric), pregnancy, breastfeeding, and so on. (More information is discussed in the following section.)
- *Pharmacokinetics*: Provides information on the absorption, distribution, metabolism, and excretion of the medication. Information on when the drug is at its highest level in the body or when it starts working may be included. The following terms are important for understanding the pharmacokinetics of a drug:
  - *Biological half-life*: The time it takes half of the drug to be metabolized or eliminated by normal biological processes
  - *Onset*: The time it takes for the drug to produce a response
  - *Peak*: The time it takes for the drug to reach its greatest effective concentration in the blood
  - *Duration*: The time during which the drug is present in the blood at great enough levels to produce a response

Table 28.4 provides drug information on the top commonly prescribed medications. Please use drug reference information for additional information on these products.

Pregnancy and Lactation Labeling Rule

Since 1979 the Food and Drug Administration (FDA) has enforced the use of pregnancy risk categories. The A, B, C, D, and X categories indicate the risk to the baby in utero. In 2015 the Pregnancy and

TABLE 28.4 Information on Commonly Prescribed Medications

GENERIC NAME	BRAND/TRADE NAME(S)	CLASS/ SCHEDULE	MEDICATION INFORMATION
tamsulosin	Flomax	Alpha blocker	*Indication:* Benign prostatic hyperplasia (BPH) *Desired effects/action:* Relaxes prostate and bladder muscles *Side effects:* Diarrhea, back pain, weakness, sleepiness, facial pain *Adverse reactions:* Painful erection lasting for hours, rash, itching, hives
hydrocodone/ acetaminophen	Vicodin, Norco, Lortab	Analgesics (narcotic [opioids])/ Schedule 2	*Indication:* Moderate to severe pain *Desired effects/action:* Changes the way the brain and nervous system respond to pain *Side effects:* Gastrointestinal (GI) intolerance, difficulty urinating, anxiety, fuzzy thinking *Adverse reactions:* Slowed breathing, chest tightness
oxycodone	OxyContin	Analgesics (narcotic [opioids])/ Schedule 2	*Indication:* Moderate to severe pain *Desired effects/action:* Changes the way the brain and nervous system respond to pain *Side effects:* GI intolerance, flushing, headache, mood changes *Adverse reactions:* Slowed breathing, angina, hypersensitivity, seizures
tramadol	Conzip	Analgesics (narcotic [opioids])/ Schedule 2	*Indication:* Moderate to severe pain *Desired effects/action:* Changes the way the brain and nervous system respond to pain *Side effects:* GI intolerance, insomnia, change in mood, dry mouth *Adverse reactions:* Hallucination, agitation, hypersensitivity, arrhythmias

TABLE 28.4 Information on Commonly Prescribed Medications—*continued*

GENERIC NAME	BRAND/TRADE NAME(S)	CLASS/ SCHEDULE	MEDICATION INFORMATION
alprazolam	Xanax	Antianxiety (benzodiazepines)/ Schedule 4	*Indications:* Anxiety and panic disorders *Desired effects/action:* Reduces abnormal excitement in the brain *Side effects:* drowsiness, headache, dizziness, GI intolerance, dry mouth, weight changes *Adverse reactions:* Seizures, jaundice, depression, memory problems
clonazepam	Klonopin	Antianxiety (benzodiazepines)/ Schedule 4	*Indications:* Seizures, panic attacks *Desired effects/action:* Reduces abnormal excitement in the brain *Side effects:* Drowsiness, coordination problems, joint pain, blurred vision, changes in sex drive *Adverse reaction:* Hypersensitivity
amoxicillin	Amoxil, Moxtag	Antibiotics (Penicillin)	*Indication:* Bacterial infection (e.g., pneumonia, gonorrhea, ear, and throat) *Desired effects/action:* Stops bacterial growth *Side effect:* GI intolerance *Adverse reactions:* Hypersensitivity, seizures, jaundice
warfarin	Coumadin, Jantoven	Anticoagulants	*Indication:* Prevents blood clots from forming *Desired effects/action:* Reduces clotting ability of the blood *Side effects:* GI intolerance, loss of hair, chills *Adverse reactions:* Hypersensitivity, infection, angina, jaundice, bleeding
gabapentin	Neurontin, Horizant	Anticonvulsants	*Indications:* Seizures, postherpetic neuralgia, restless legs syndrome (RLS) *Desired effects/action:* Reduces abnormal excitement in the brain; reduces seizures *Side effects:* Drowsiness, blurred vision, anxiety, memory problems, weakness, GI intolerance *Adverse reactions:* Hypersensitivity, seizures
bupropion	Wellbutrin, Zyban	Antidepressant (atypical) and antismoking agent	*Indications*: Depression, seasonal affective disorder (SAD), smoking cessation *Desired effects/action:* Increases certain types of activity in the brain *Side effects:* Drowsiness, insomnia, dry mouth, stomach pain, weight loss *Adverse reactions*: Blisters, dyspnea, chest pain, seizures, hallucinations
duloxetine	Cymbalta	Antidepressant (selective serotonin and norepinephrine reuptake inhibitors [SNRIs])	*Indications:* Major depressive disorder, generalized anxiety disorder, diabetic peripheral neuropathy, fibromyalgia, chronic pain *Desired effects/action:* Increases the amounts of serotonin and norepinephrine in the brain; helps to maintain mental balance and stop pain signals in the brain *Side effect:* Orthostatic hypotension *Adverse reactions:* Suicidal thoughts, hepatotoxicity, seizures, glaucoma, hyponatremia
venlafaxine	(no brand names)	Antidepressant (selective serotonin and norepinephrine reuptake inhibitors [SNRIs])	*Indications:* Depression, generalized anxiety disorder (GAD), social anxiety disorder, panic disorder *Desired effects/action:* Increases serotonin in the brain *Side effects:* Drowsiness, weakness, headache, nightmares, dry mouth *Adverse reactions:* Chest pain, seizures, arrhythmias, bleeding, problems with coordination
citalopram	Celexa	Antidepressant (selective serotonin reuptake inhibitors [SSRIs])	*Indication:* Depression *Desired effects/action:* Increases the amount of serotonin in the brain; helps to maintain mental balance *Side effects:* GI intolerance, frequent urination, weakness, joint pain, weight loss *Adverse reactions:* Angina, shortness of breath, arrhythmias, hallucinating, coma, hypersensitivity, confusion, seizures, suicidal thoughts

Continued

TABLE 28.4 Information on Commonly Prescribed Medications—*continued*

GENERIC NAME	BRAND/TRADE NAME(S)	CLASS/ SCHEDULE	MEDICATION INFORMATION
escitalopram	Lexapro	Antidepressant (selective serotonin reuptake inhibitors [SSRIs])	*Indications:* Depression, generalized anxiety disorder (GAD) *Desired effects/action:* Increases the amount of serotonin in the brain; helps to maintain mental balance *Side effects:* GI intolerance, increased sweating, change in sex drive, flu-like symptoms *Adverse reactions:* Unusual excitement, hallucinations, confusion, arrhythmias, severe muscle stiffness, suicidal thoughts
fluoxetine	Prozac, Rapiflux	Antidepressant (selective serotonin reuptake inhibitors [SSRIs])	*Indications:* Depression, obsessive-compulsive disorder (OCD), panic attacks *Desired effects/action:* Increases serotonin in the brain *Side effects:* Nervousness, anxiety, insomnia, diarrhea, heartburn *Adverse reactions:* Joint pain, dyspnea, seizures, abnormal bleeding
sertraline	Zoloft	Antidepressant (selective serotonin reuptake inhibitors [SSRIs])	*Indications:* Depression, OCD, panic attacks, posttraumatic stress disorder (PTSD) *Desired effects/action:* Increases the amount of serotonin in the brain; helps to maintain mental balance *Side effects:* GI intolerance, weight changes, insomnia, change in sex drive, excessive sweating *Adverse reactions:* Seizures, abnormal bleeding, arrhythmias, hypersensitivity, suicidal thoughts
trazodone	Oleptro	Antidepressant (serotonin modulators)	*Indication:* Depression *Desired effects/action:* Increases the amount of serotonin; helps to maintain mental balance *Side effects:* GI intolerance, weakness, headache, confusion, sweating, decreased coordination *Adverse reactions:* Angina, fainting, seizures, coma, arrhythmias, suicidal thoughts
allopurinol	Aloprim, Zyloprim	Antigout (xanthine oxidase inhibitors)	*Indication:* Gout *Desired effects/action:* Reduces uric acid production *Side effects:* Upset stomach, diarrhea, drowsiness *Adverse reactions:* Dysuria, eye irritation, hematuria
glipizide	Glucotrol	Antihyperglycemics	*Indication:* Type 2 diabetes mellitus *Desired effects/action:* Lowers blood glucose by causing increased insulin production and usage *Side effects:* Flatus, diarrhea, dizziness, shaking, feeling jittery *Adverse reactions:* Jaundice, dark urine, light-colored stools, bleeding
metformin	Glucophage, Fortamet, Glumetza, Riomet	Antihyperglycemics	*Indication:* Type 2 diabetes mellitus *Desired effects/action:* Reduces glucose absorption and increases body's response to insulin; controls the blood glucose level *Side effects:* GI intolerance, metallic taste in the mouth, flushing of the skin, nail changes *Adverse reactions:* Angina, rash
losartan	Cozaar	Antihypertensive (angiotensin II receptor antagonists)	*Indications:* Hypertension, heart failure *Desired effects/action:* Lowers the blood pressure *Side effects:* Headache, dizziness, diarrhea, muscle cramps and pain, nasal congestion, cough, upper respiratory infection, sinusitis *Adverse reactions:* Chest pain, difficulty swallowing, dyspnea, hoarseness
lisinopril	(no brand names)	Antihypertensive (angiotensin-converting enzyme [ACE] inhibitors)	*Indications:* hypertension, heart failure *Desired effects/action:* Causes vasodilation, reducing the blood pressure *Side effects:* Cough, dizziness, tiredness, GI intolerance, rash *Adverse reactions:* Angina, light-headedness, dyspnea, difficulty swallowing, hypersensitivity

TABLE 28.4 Information on Commonly Prescribed Medications—*continued*

GENERIC NAME	BRAND/TRADE NAME(S)	CLASS/ SCHEDULE	MEDICATION INFORMATION
atenolol	Tenormin	Antihypertensive (beta-blockers)	*Indications:* Hypertension, angina *Desired effects/action:* Relaxes blood vessels and slows the heart rate, thus improving blood flow, and reduces blood pressure *Side effects:* Dizziness, tiredness, depression, GI intolerance *Adverse reactions:* Shortness of breath, swelling of legs and hands, weight gain, fainting
metoprolol	Lopressor, Toprol XL	Antihypertensive (beta-blockers)	*Indications:* Hypertension, angina *Desired effects/action:* Relaxes blood vessels and slows the heart rate, thus improving blood flow, and reduces blood pressure *Side effects:* Dizziness, tiredness, depression, GI intolerance *Adverse reactions:* Hypersensitivity, weight gain, arrhythmias
carvedilol	Coreg	Antihypertensive (beta-blockers)	*Indications:* Heart failure, hypertension *Desired effects/action:* Relaxes blood vessels and slows the heart rate, thus improving blood flow, and reduces blood pressure *Side effects:* Hyperglycemia, tiredness, weakness, dizziness, visual changes, joint pain, insomnia *Adverse reactions:* Shortness of breath, swelling of arms and legs, arrhythmias
propranolol	Inderal LA, Inderal XL	Antihypertensive (beta-blockers)	*Indications:* Hypertension, arrhythmias *Desired effects/action:* Relaxes blood vessels, slows heart rate *Side effects:* Dizziness, light-headedness, tiredness, diarrhea, constipation *Adverse reactions:* Weight gain, arrhythmias, feeling faint, swelling of face and throat
amlodipine	Norvasc	Antihypertensive (calcium channel blockers)	*Indications:* Hypertension, angina *Desired effects/action:* Relaxes the vessels so the heart does not have to pump as hard *Side effects:* GI intolerance, headache, swelling of legs and arms, tiredness, flushing *Adverse reactions:* More frequent or severe angina, fainting, arrhythmias
meloxicam	Mobic	Anti-inflammatories (nonsteroidal anti-inflammatory drugs [NSAIDs])	*Indications:* Osteoarthritis, rheumatoid arthritis *Desired effects/action:* Reduces pain, tenderness, swelling, and stiffness *Side effects:* Diarrhea, constipation, flatus, sore throat *Adverse reactions:* Dyspnea, hives, blisters, tachycardia, jaundice
clopidogrel	Plavix	Antiplatelets	*Indication:* Used to prevent clots after a stroke, heart attack, or severe angina *Desired effects/action:* Prevents platelets from collecting and forming clots *Side effects:* Excessive tiredness, GI intolerance, nosebleed, dizziness *Adverse reaction:* Hypersensitivity, bloody and tarry stools, coffee grounds–looking emesis, blood in urine, visual changes
albuterol	Ventolin HFA, Proventil HFA, Proair	Bronchodilators	*Indication:* Bronchospasm (e.g., asthma) *Desired effects/action:* Relaxes bronchial muscles and increases airflow to lungs *Side effects:* Headache, dizziness, insomnia, cough, sore throat, nausea, vomiting, dry mouth *Adverse reactions:* Paradoxical bronchospasm, cardiovascular effects, hypersensitivity, hypokalemia
atorvastatin	Lipitor	Cholesterol-lowering agent	*Indications:* Hyperlipidemia, hypertriglyceridemia *Desired effects/action:* Slows production of cholesterol in the body; reduces low-density lipoprotein (LDL) and triglycerides; increases high-density lipoprotein (HDL) *Side effects:* GI intolerance, joint pain, memory loss, confusion *Adverse reactions:* Muscle pain, lack of energy, angina, weakness, hypersensitivity, dark-colored urine, jaundice

Continued

TABLE 28.4 Information on Commonly Prescribed Medications—*continued*

GENERIC NAME	BRAND/TRADE NAME(S)	CLASS/ SCHEDULE	MEDICATION INFORMATION
pravastatin	Pravachol	Cholesterol-lowering agent	*Indications:* Heart disease, hyperlipidemia, hypertriglyceridemia *Desired effects/action:* Slows cholesterol production *Side effects:* Heartburn, headache, memory loss, confusion *Adverse reactions:* Jaundice, extreme tiredness, dark-colored urine, unusual bleeding
rosuvastatin	Crestor, Ezallor	Cholesterol-lowering agent	*Indications:* Hyperlipidemia, hypertriglyceridemia *Desired effects/action:* Slows production of cholesterol in the body; reduces LDL and triglycerides; increases HDL *Side effects:* Headache, depression, muscle and joint pain, insomnia, GI intolerance *Adverse reactions:* Muscle damage leading to acute renal failure and liver damage
simvastatin	Zocor, Flolipid	Cholesterol-lowering agent	*Indications:* Hyperlipidemia, hypertriglyceridemia *Desired effects/action:* Slows production of cholesterol in the body; reduces LDL and triglycerides; increases HDL *Side effects:* GI intolerance, memory loss, confusion, headache *Adverse reactions:* Muscle pain, dark red urine, lack of energy, jaundice, hypersensitivity
ethinyl estradiol and norethindrone	Loestrin, Leena, Microgestin	Contraceptive (oral)	*Indication:* Prevent pregnancy *Desired effects/action:* Estrogen and progestin prevent ovulation and pregnancy from developing *Side effects:* Headache, bloating, swelling, weight changes, breast tenderness *Adverse reactions:* Severe abdominal pain, dark urine, jaundice, heavy vaginal bleeding
fluticasone	Flonase allergy relief nasal spray, Flovent HFA, Flovent Diskus	Corticosteroid (nasal and inhaled)	*Indications:* Hay fever, allergies (nasal spray); asthma (inhaled) *Desired effects/action:* Reduces inflammation and allergy reaction *Side effects:* Headache, dryness in mouth, hoarseness, or deepened voice *Adverse reactions:* Reduced bone marrow density, immunosuppression, adrenal suppression, glaucoma, cataracts, hypersensitivity in individuals with milk allergy (Diskus)
prednisone	Sterapred	Corticosteroids (oral)	*Indications:* Severe allergic reaction, multiple sclerosis, lupus, and some types of arthritis *Desired effects/action*: Increases the levels of corticosteroid; reduces swelling and redness *Side effects*: Headache, dizziness, insomnia, personality and mood changes, slowed healing *Adverse reactions:* Vision problems, seizures, arrhythmias, confusion
furosemide	Lasix	Diuretics	*Indication:* Hypertension *Desired effects/action:* Causes the kidneys to increase the excretion of water and salt *Side effects:* Frequent urination, blurred vision, headache, constipation, diarrhea *Adverse reactions:* Ringing in the ears, loss of hearing, blisters, jaundice, hypersensitivity
hydrochloro-thiazide	Microzide, Oretic	Diuretics	*Indication:* Hypertension *Desired effects/action:* Causes the kidneys to increase the excretion of water and salt *Side effects:* Frequent urination, diarrhea, loss of appetite, headache, hair loss *Adverse reactions:* Joint pain, unusual bleeding, hypersensitivity, visual change
potassium	K-Tab, K-Dur, Micro-K	Electrolyte	*Indication:* Mineral supplement needed for certain diseases and medications (e.g., diuretic) *Desired effects/action:* Proper functioning of the body systems *Side effect:* GI intolerance *Adverse reactions:* Confusion, listlessness, gray skin, black stools

TABLE 28.4 Information on Commonly Prescribed Medications—*continued*

GENERIC NAME	BRAND/TRADE NAME(S)	CLASS/ SCHEDULE	MEDICATION INFORMATION
insulin glargine	Lantus, Toujeo	Hormone replacement (insulin, long acting)	*Indications:* Type 1 and type 2 diabetes mellitus *Desired effects/action:* Replaces insulin in the body *Side effects:* Redness and swelling at injection site, fever, cough, sore throat *Adverse reactions:* Tachycardia, hoarseness, sweating, wheezing
levothyroxine	Synthroid, Levoxyl	Hormone replacement (thyroid hormone)	*Indications:* Hypothyroidism, pituitary thyroid-stimulating hormone (TSH) suppression *Desired effects/action:* Replacement hormone; regulates body's energy and metabolism *Side effects:* Reversible hair loss, dry skin, GI intolerance, headache, nervousness *Adverse reactions:* Cardiac arrhythmias, angina, myocardial infarction, heart failure
montelukast	Singulair	Leukotriene receptor antagonists	*Indications:* Asthma, exercise-induced bronchospasms *Desired effects/action:* Blocks the action of substances that cause asthma and allergic rhinitis *Side effects:* Headache, dizziness, heartburn, stomach pain, tiredness *Adverse reactions:* Hypersensitivity, numbness in arms and legs, swelling of the sinuses
cyclobenzaprine	Amrix	Muscle relaxant	*Indications:* Painful musculoskeletal conditions (e.g., strains, sprains, muscle injuries) *Desired effects/action:* Works on the brain and nervous system to allow muscle relaxation *Side effects:* GI intolerance, extreme tiredness, dry mouth *Adverse reactions:* Hypersensitivity, angina
omeprazole	Prilosec	Proton-pump inhibitors	Indications: Gastroesophageal reflux disease (GERD), ulcers, Helicobacter pylori (H. pylori) infection *Desired effects/action:* Reduces stomach acid *Side effects:* GI intolerance, headache *Adverse reactions:* Hypersensitivity, dizziness, arrhythmias, muscle spasm
pantoprazole	Protonix	Proton-pump inhibitors	*Indications:* GERD and esophagitis *Desired effects/action:* Reduces the amount of acid made in the stomach *Side effects:* Headache, nausea, vomiting, flatus, joint pain, diarrhea, dizziness *Adverse reactions:* Blistering, hives, dyspnea, difficulty swallowing, severe diarrhea
zolpidem	Ambien, Edluar, Zolpimist	Sedative-hypnotics/ Schedule 4	*Indication:* Insomnia *Desired effects/action:* Slows activity in the brain, allowing sleep *Side effects:* Drowsiness, headache, dizziness, drugged feeling, unsteady walking, GI intolerance *Adverse reactions:* Jaundice, hypersensitivity, light-colored stools, angina, blurred vision
dextroamphe-tamine and amphetamine	Adderall	Stimulants/ Schedule 2	*Indications:* Attention deficit hyperactivity disorder (ADHD), narcolepsy *Desired effects/action:* Changes the amount of certain substances in the brain *Side effects:* Stomach pain, nausea, tachycardia, insomnia, weight loss *Adverse reactions:* Agitation, hallucination, mania, blurred vision, depression
methylphenidate	Concerta, Ritalin LA	Stimulants/ Schedule 2	*Indications:* ADHD, narcolepsy *Desired effects/action:* Changes certain substances in the brain, allowing a person to concentrate and focus *Side effects:* Nervousness, insomnia, GI intolerance, restlessness, muscle tightness *Adverse reactions:* Angina, arrhythmias, seizure, blurred vision
ergocalciferol	Drisdol, Vitamin D_2	Vitamin D	*Indication:* Hypoparathyroidism *Desired effects/action:* Helps the body use more calcium found in foods or supplements *Side effects:* Pale skin, tiredness *Adverse reactions:* Feeling tired, drowsiness, muscle aches, stiffness

Lactation Labeling Rule (PLLR) replaced the pregnancy risk letter categories with more comprehensive information. The goal is to supply the provider and patient with pregnancy and lactation information. This information can be used when discussing the risks versus the benefits of a medication. The FDA created the new system to help with patient-specific counseling and informed decision making for pregnant and breastfeeding mothers who need medication therapies. The system consists of three subcategories with detailed information about the following:

- *Pregnancy*: Includes information on the risks during pregnancy for the mother and baby, in addition to data on the risk of adverse developmental outcomes
- *Lactation*: Includes information on the presence of the drug in breast milk, the effects on a breastfed child, and the impact on milk production
- *Females and males of reproductive potential*: Includes information about when pregnancy testing or contraception is required during drug therapy and data that suggests drug-associated fertility effects

CRITICAL THINKING APPLICATION 28.5

Gabe mentions to Mark that he learned that the FDA had changed the pregnancy risk categories. Mark had not heard about this. Gabe further explains why. Describe how the changes provide more information to providers and patients.

FORMS OF MEDICATIONS

The form refers to the physical characteristics of the medication. Forms can be grouped into solids, semisolids, and liquids. Solid and semisolid medications are commonly prescribed and found in OTC products.

Solid Medication Forms

Examples of solid medication forms include the following:

- *Tablet*: Solid formed by compressed powdered medication; may be coated. Can come in various sizes and shapes (Figure 28.1).
- *Chewable tablet*: Designed to be chewed prior to swallowing—for example, a chewable vitamin.
- *Caplet*: Coated, oval medication tablet.
- *Capsule*: Medication in a hard or soft gelatin shell.
- *Scored tablet*: A notched tablet, which can be split into half with a pill cutter or splitter (Figure 28.2).
- *Enteric-coated tablets* or *capsules*: Coated to pass through the acidic environment of the stomach. Breaks down in the base environment of the intestines. These tablets should not be crushed, cut, or chewed because the protective property will be lost.
- *Buffered*: A solid medication containing the active medication and an antacid. The antacid neutralizes the stomach acid and thereby reduces stomach irritation. One example is buffered aspirin.
- *Fast-dissolving tablet* or *film strip*: Also called *oral disintegrating tablets*. Solid form of medicine that is placed on the tongue (or by the cheek [buccal]) and breaks down rapidly in the presence of saliva. Examples include Fasprin and acetaminophen.
- *Extended-release tablet* or *capsule*: Designed to break down over time. These tablets should not be crushed, cut, or chewed because doing so may cause an overdose. Many acronyms are used (Table 28.5)—for example, Calan SR.
- *Effervescent tablet*: Contains an acid substance and carbonate or bicarbonate. When placed in water, it releases carbon dioxide, creating a carbonated drink. K-Lyte Effervescent Tablets are one example.
- *Lozenge* (*troche*): Flat, round form containing active medication and a sweetened flavoring; dissolves on the tongue. Used for local treatment of the mouth and throat. A cough drop is one example.
- *Powder*: Nonpotent powdered medication that must be mixed with a liquid before it can be taken. MiraLAX is an example.

Some forms of medications can be crushed, whereas others cannot. Over the past few years, the FDA has approved new drug delivery systems or drug forms. This has provided additional options to those who cannot swallow pills. It is common for patients or parents to have concerns about swallowing pills.

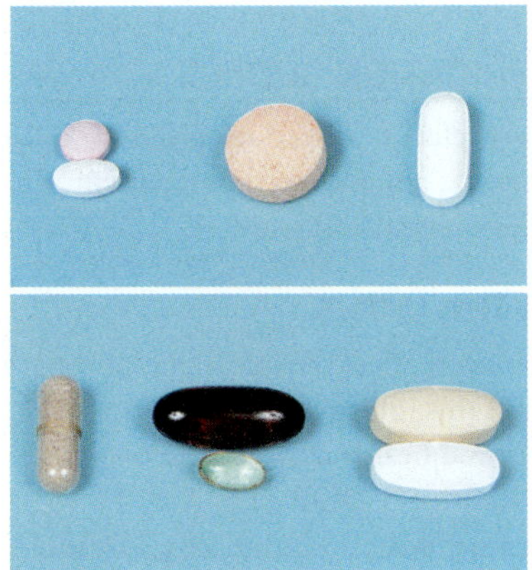

FIGURE 28.1 *Left to right:* Top row: Tablets, chewable, and caplet. Bottom row: Hard-shelled capsule, soft-shelled capsules, and scored caplets.

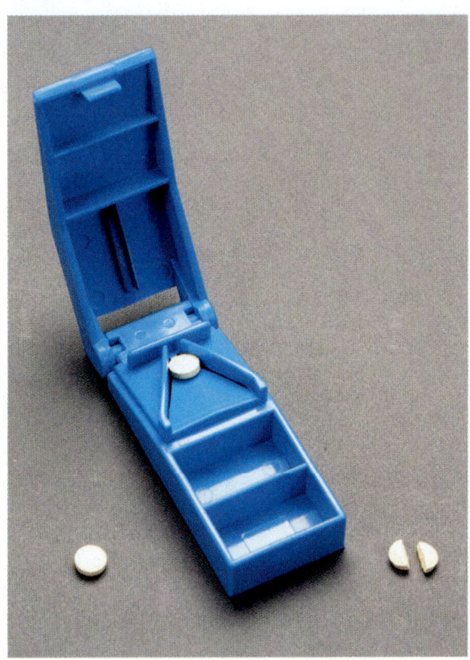

FIGURE 28.2 Pill cutter or splitter.

CRITICAL THINKING APPLICATION **28.6**

What is an advantage of the fast-dissolving tablet or film strip? For what populations would this form be beneficial?

Semisolid Medication Forms

Examples of semisolid medication forms include the following:

- *Ointment* and *paste*: Semisolid, greasy drug preparations that are applied to the skin, rectum, or nasal mucosa. Pastes are thicker and less penetrating than ointments. One example is Nystatin Ointment.
- *Cream*: Semisolid drug preparation made of active medication, oil, and water. One example is Nystatin Cream.
- *Suppository* and *pessary*: Active medication mixed in an oil base (e.g., cocoa butter). These medications are solid at room temperature but melt at body temperature. Suppositories are typically shaped like a small bullet and are used in the rectum, urethra, or vagina. Pessaries are vaginal suppositories. An example is the Dulcolax suppository.

Liquid Medication Forms

Liquid medications have various uses. They can be swallowed, rubbed on the skin, or instilled in the nose, eyes, or ears. Liquid medications are easily taken by children, older adults, and those with swallowing problems. With liquid medications, the active medication is mixed with water, alcohol, or both.

If the active medication dissolves in the liquid, the medication is a *solution*. The following are examples of solutions:

- *Tincture*: Very potent solution of alcohol or alcohol and water and the active medicine—for example, an iodine tincture.
- *Fluid extract*: Alcoholic plant source extractions; very concentrated and more potent than tinctures—for example, belladonna fluid extract.
- *Spirit*: An alcoholic solution with substances that easily evaporate—for example, aromatic ammonia spirit.
- *Elixir*: Clear sweetened liquid preparation that contains alcohol—for example, digoxin elixir.
- *Syrup*: A sugar and water solution that contains flavoring and medicinal substance—for example, cough syrup (some syrups contain alcohol).

If the active medication does not dissolve and becomes suspended in the liquid, it is called a *suspension*. Over time the suspended drug will settle to the bottom of the container. It is important to shake suspensions before pouring the medication. The following are examples of suspensions:

- *Emulsion*: A suspension of oil and water—for example, ophthalmic cyclosporine.
- *Gel* and *magma*: Suspensions consisting of minerals and water. Gels are semisolids and contain finer particles than magmas. The minerals settle out with standing. Shake before using. One example is milk of magnesia.
- *Liniment*: A suspension that is rubbed on the skin; used to reduce pain and stiffness—for example, Ben-Gay.
- *Lotion*: A water-based suspension that is applied to the skin—for example, calamine lotion.
- *Aerosol*: A suspension of medication in a gas, usually used for respiratory or sinus conditions—for example, an albuterol metered-dose inhaler.

TABLE 28.5 Examples of Acronyms for Slow-Release Tablets

ACRONYM	DEFINITION
CD	controlled delivery
CR	controlled release
DR	delayed release
ER	extended release
LA	long acting
SA	sustained action
SR	sustained release
TD	time delay
TR	time release
XL	extended release
XR	extended release

Alcohol in Medications

Several forms of liquid medications contain alcohol. This is a concern for patients who are recovering alcoholics or have other health issues, such as diabetes. An internet search can provide lists of medications with their alcohol content. The drug reference information also provides information on the ingredients.

If a patient mentions being a recovering alcoholic, it is important for the medical assistant first to acknowledge the person's accomplishment. Then the medical assistant should communicate the information to the provider. This may make a difference in what medication the provider gives to the patient. Giving a patient medication with alcohol may be harmful to the patient's success and health.

CRITICAL THINKING APPLICATION **28.7**

What forms of medication would not be helpful to people who are recovering from alcoholism?

TYPES OF MEDICATION ORDERS

A *medication order* refers to directions given by a provider for a specific medication to be administered to a patient. The following sections discuss types of medication orders.

Verbal and Written Orders

The medical assistant receives the information from the provider. The provider must give this information:

- Patient's name and health record number or date of birth (DOB) (e.g., Nancy Rodriguez DOB 11/04/1971)
- Medication name, dose, and route (e.g., Tylenol 1 g po)

The provider can give the order over the phone or in person. This type of order is called a *verbal order*. It is important for the medical assistant to write down the order and read it back to the provider. This process ensures the order was heard and recorded correctly. The provider can also give the medical assistant a *written order*. Usually, these are written on a prescription pad or in an electronic message. A written order only needs clarification from the provider if the medical assistant cannot read the order or has a question.

Types of Orders

In addition to describing how medication orders are given to the medical assistant, they can be described by the type of order. The following are five types of medication orders:

- *Routine order*: Medication taken at a regular interval until it is canceled or expired. (Most non-narcotic routine orders expire in 12 months.) Examples would be "Vitamin B_{12} 100 mcg IM monthly" and "Synthroid 75 mcg qam po."
- *Standing order*: An order that applies to all patients who meet specific criteria. For departments, usually, all providers agree collectively on standing orders and sign the order—for instance, "For patients 18 years or older, with no allergy to acetaminophen and who have a temperature of 103°F or higher: give acetaminophen 650 mg po × 1 dose."
- *PRN order*: Medication that is given on an "as needed" basis for specific signs and symptoms. (It is important to indicate these symptoms when documenting the administered medication in the patient's health record.) One example would be "Acetaminophen 325 mg, 2 tabs po q4–6h prn pain."
- *Single order* or *one-time order*: Medication is administered one time—for example, "Acetaminophen 650 mg po × 1 dose."
- *Stat order*: Medication is administered one time right now—for example, "EpiPen 0.3 mg IM stat."

PRESCRIPTIONS

A *prescription* is a written order by a provider to the pharmacist. It tells the pharmacist what medication and how much should be dispensed to the patient. There are four parts to a prescription: superscription, inscription, signature, and subscription. Figure 28.3 describes the four parts of a prescription.

Medical Assistant's Role

In some ambulatory care facilities, there are scenarios in which medical assistants prepare prescriptions for providers to sign:

- A patient may request refills while the medical assistant is rooming the patient. The medical assistant may prepare the prescriptions, so the provider just needs to sign for the refills.
- A patient may call the department and request a refill on a medication. Using a medication refill protocol, the medical assistant needs to see if the patient can get a refill (Figure 28.4). If the patient can, then the medical assistant prepares the prescription and has the provider sign it.

The prescription must be written in ink or be computer generated. A medical assistant can prepare prescriptions for the provider to sign. The provider is responsible for ensuring the prescription meets federal and state laws and regulations. All prescriptions need to include this information:

- Date of issue (when it was written)
- Patient information (name and address are required, date of birth is helpful)
- Provider's full name and address
- Drug name (e.g., amoxicillin)
- Drug strength (e.g., 500 mg)
- Dosage form (e.g., tablets)

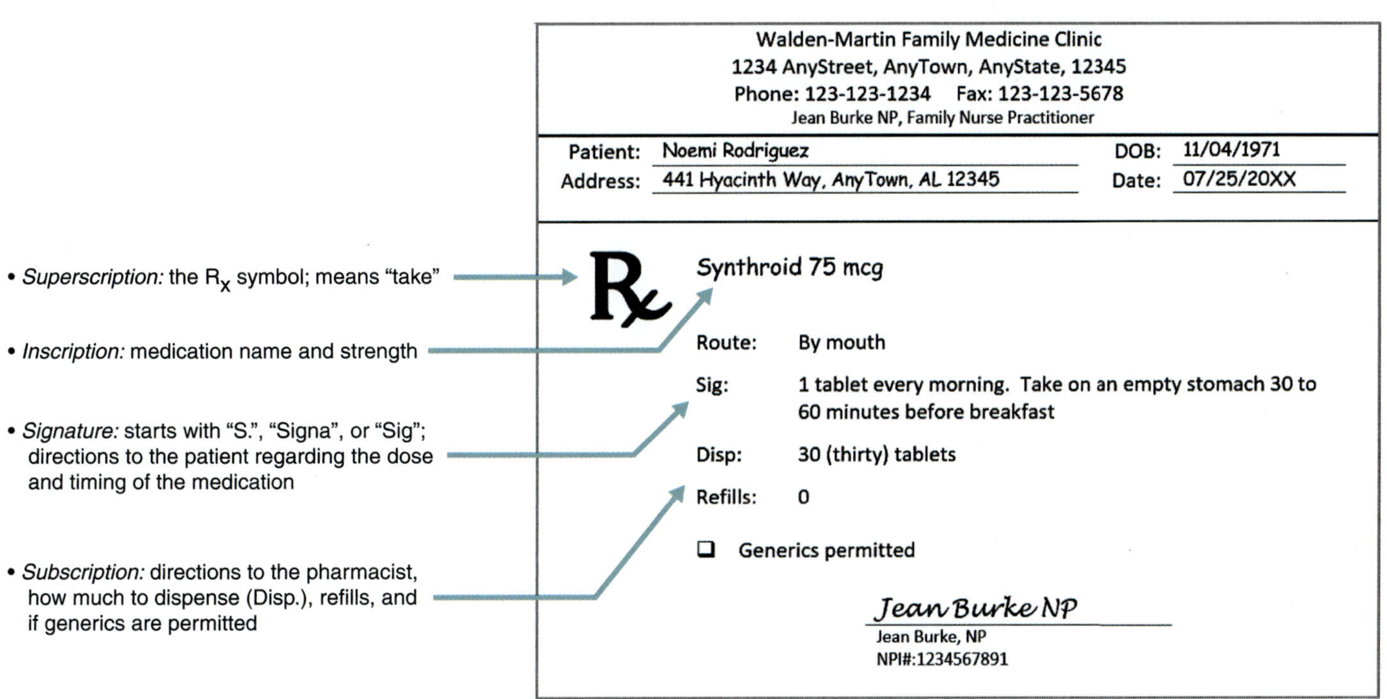

FIGURE 28.3 Parts of a prescription.

Prescription Refill Protocol
Walden-Martin Family Medical Clinic

Description: A certified medical assistant (CMA) can refill current hypertensive medications that fall within the guidelines of this protocol.

Step 1	Step 2	
For medications to be refilled, the following points need to be addressed.	**Qualifying Medications**	**Prescription Refill**
• Has the person seen the provider within the past year? • Is the prescription for a hypertensive, hyperlipidemia, or hyperthyroidism medication a current prescription? • Is the person free of concerns or complications due to the medication? • Is it time for a refill? (The medical assistant must verify that it is time for a refill.) If the answers to the above questions are all YES, then proceed to Step 2. If any of the answers to the above questions are NO, then schedule the person for an appointment with the provider.	amlodipine amlodipine/benazepril atenolol atenolol/chlorthalidone benazepril captopril diltiazem enalapril felodipine fosinopril irbesartan isradiprine lisinopril losartan nifedipine quinapril ramipril	Extend the current prescription for 6 months. Instruct patient that in 6 months: • A visit to the provider will be required • Blood pressure reading will be required • Lab work may be required

FIGURE 28.4 Example of a prescription refill protocol. The medical assistant uses a protocol to determine what action to take with prescription refill requests.

- Quantity prescribed (e.g., 14 [fourteen]); writing out the number prevents people from altering the prescription, which is especially important with controlled substances
- Directions for use (e.g., Take 1 tablet q12h)
- Number of refills (e.g., Refills 0)
- **National Provider Identifier (NPI)** and signature of provider (a manual signature is required for controlled substances)
- Must indicate if a generic is acceptable

If an electronic prescription is sent to the pharmacy and a paper copy is given to the patient, the copy should indicate that it is a copy ("Copy only—not valid for dispensing"). Procedure 28.1 indicates how to prepare prescriptions using a prescription refill procedure. Only facility-approved abbreviations should be used when preparing prescriptions and documenting the patients' health records. Table 28.6 provides commonly approved abbreviations.

Once the prescriptions are prepared, they need to be given to the provider to sign. Either the provider or the medical assistant needs to document the refills in the patient's health record. The facility's policy will indicate who is responsible for the documentation.

Controlled Substance Prescriptions

For security reasons, the provider's DEA number should be used only on controlled substance prescriptions. It is not appropriate for the number to appear on non-narcotic prescriptions. The NPI is a national number that is unique to the provider. This number is found on prescriptions and may be used for tracking or treatment identification purposes.

The medical assistant needs to be aware of the special requirements for controlled substances. It is important for the medical assistant to stay updated on which frequently prescribed medications are controlled substances. Table 28.7 describes common requirements for scheduled substances.

CRITICAL THINKING APPLICATION 28.8

Mark and Gabe are working on prescription refills. A patient who has just started taking a Schedule 2 medication calls in for a refill. He says he is not happy that there were no refills on his original prescription. How might Gabe handle this type of call? What could he say to help the patient understand the situation?

CLOSING COMMENTS

Patient Coaching

OTC medications and herbal supplements can affect medication treatment. It is important for the medical assistant to obtain a list of the patient's current prescription and OTC medications, in addition to herbal supplements (Tables 28.8 and 28.9). Some patients may hesitate or may not want to share this information. They may not realize that OTC medications and herbal supplements can interfere with prescription medications. It is important for medical assistants to be professional and respectful when dealing with these situations. If they coach patients that sometimes the OTC medications and herbal supplements react with prescription medications, patients may be more willing to share information on what they take.

Legal and Ethical Issues

The magnitude of opioid abuse has increased dramatically, and it is currently considered a crisis. According to the Centers for Diseases Control and Prevention (CDC) (www.cdc.gov), more than 93,000 drug overdose deaths occurred in the United States in 2020. This equates to about 255 deaths daily from drug overdoses. Synthetic opioid overdoses increased during this period compared to the prior year. With the frequency of opioid abuse, prescribing guidelines are changing. Many ambulatory care facilities have adopted procedures for specific controlled substance prescriptions. Before patients can

TABLE 28.6 Commonly Approved Abbreviations

ABBREVIATIONS RELATED TO	ABBREVIATIONS	MEANING
Medication route	SUBQ	subcutaneous
	ID	intradermal
	IM	intramuscular
	IV	intravenous
	NAS	nasal
	po, PO	by mouth
Medication form	tinct	tincture
	ung.	ointment
	sol, soln	solution
	cap	capsule
	tab(s)	tablet(s)
Measurements	C	Celsius
	F	Fahrenheit
	m	meter
	cm	centimeter
	mm	millimeter
	kg	kilogram
	g	gram
	mg	milligram
	mcg	microgram
	L	liter
	mL	milliliter
	gr	grain
	gtt(s)	drop(s)
	lb	pound
	fl oz	Fluid ounce
	oz	ounce
	pt	pint
	qt	quart
	Tbs, tbsp	tablespoon
	tsp	teaspoon
Timing	ac	before meals
	pc	after meals
	ad lib	as desired
	d	day
	AM, a.m.	morning
	PM, p.m.	afternoon
	noc, noct	night
	h, hr	hour
	min	minute
	p̄	after
	prn	as needed
	qh	every hour
	q(2,3,4,6,8)h	every (2, 3, 4, 6, 8) hours; (q2h = every 2 hours)
	qid	four times a day
	tid	three times a day
	bid	twice a day
	qam	every morning
	stat, STAT	immediately
Medications	ASA	aspirin
	Fe	iron
	K	potassium
	MOM	milk of magnesia
	NS	normal saline
	NSAID	nonsteroidal anti-inflammatory drug
	OTC	over the counter (drugs)
	PPD	purified protein derivative (tuberculin skin test)
Miscellaneous	a̅a̅	of each (used in prescriptions)
	aq	water
	c̄	with
	med	medicine
	NKA	no known allergies
	NKDA	no known drug allergies
	NPO	nothing by mouth
	Pt, pt	patient
	qs	quantity sufficient
	Rx	Take
	Sig	give the following directions
	s̄	without
	VO	verbal order
	x	times

get these prescriptions, they need to have a urine drug test. The urine drug test helps providers assess what drugs patients have taken. Providers expect the results to show the drug prescribed, but they check for other prescribed controlled substances and illicit drugs. In many cases, if the drug test shows evidence of illicit drug use or prescription-controlled substances not prescribed by the provider, the patient is referred for substance abuse counseling and treatment.

The CDC has published the document Guidelines for Prescribing Opioids for Chronic Pain (available at www.cdc.gov/drugoverdose/pdf/Guidelines_Factsheet-a.pdf). These guidelines help support providers who are working with patients with chronic pain. The provider may have the medical assistant coach patients on home care treatments. Opioids are not first-line or routine therapy for chronic pain. The medical assistant may need to coach the patient on the importance of using nonpharmacologic therapy and nonopioid pharmacologic therapy for chronic pain. For patients who receive opioid prescriptions, frequent follow-up is needed for the provider to evaluate the benefit and risks of the drug.

TABLE 28.7 Special Requirements for Controlled Substances

SCHEDULE	PRESCRIPTION SPECIFICS
I	Drugs with no currently accepted medical use.
II/IIN (2)	Written prescription manually signed by the provider or an electronic prescription that meets all Drug Enforcement Administration (DEA) requirements for electronic prescriptions for controlled substances. No refills. In some cases the prescription can be faxed to the pharmacy. The medication cannot be dispensed until the original prescription is given to the pharmacy.
III/IIIN and IV (3, 4)	Call-in prescriptions, written prescriptions, and electronic prescriptions are allowed. Faxed prescriptions must be manually signed by the provider prior to faxing. Prescription good for 6 months. No more than five refills are allowed.
V (5)	Phoned prescriptions, written prescriptions, e-prescriptions, and faxed prescriptions allowed. Prescription is good for 12 months (as with non-narcotic prescriptions). Refill quantity is up to the provider.

Patient-Centered Care

Most healthcare facilities require that patients receive a printout of their current medications at the end of each visit. When patients are taking several medications, it is important for the medical assistant to encourage these patients to carry a current medications list in their wallet or purse. This can be helpful in an emergency or when the patient needs to see a different provider.

Professional Behaviors

When working with prescription refills, it is important for the medical assistant to process the refill in a timely fashion. If the medical assistant procrastinates and does not process refills, then patients may not have their medications when they need them. Some medications need to be taken daily. If a dose is skipped, the patient may have serious consequences.

It is also important for the medical assistant to honor what that patient was told. If the patient is told the medication will be sent to a pharmacy by a specific time, it is important for the medical assistant to ensure this is done. If the medication is held up for some reason, the medical assistant should notify the patient about the delay.

TABLE 28.8 Common Over-the-Counter (OTC) Medications

GENERIC NAME	BRAND/TRADE NAME(S)	CLASS/SCHEDULE	MEDICATION INFORMATION
acetaminophen	Tylenol	Analgesics and antipyretics	*Indications:* Pain, fever *Desired effects/action:* Pain reliever and fever reducer *Side effects:* Nausea, vomiting *Adverse reactions:* Jaundice, stomach pain
diphenhydramine	Benadryl	Antihistamine	*Indications:* Hay fever, allergies, insomnia, motion sickness *Desired effects/action:* Blocks the action of histamine in the body *Side effects:* Dry mouth, dizziness, weakness, excitement (in children), constipation, nervousness *Adverse reactions:* Visual problems, difficulty urinating, painful urination
ibuprofen	Advil, Motrin, Midol	Anti-inflammatory drugs (nonsteroidal [NSAIDs])	*Indications:* Osteoarthritis, rheumatoid arthritis, fever, pain *Desired effects/action:* Stops the body's production of substances that cause pain, fever, and inflammation *Side effects:* Gastrointestinal (GI) intolerance, ringing in the ears *Adverse reactions:* Weight gain, hypersensitivity, hoarseness, jaundice, bloody urine, stiff neck

TABLE 28.8 Common Over-the-Counter (OTC) Medications—*continued*

GENERIC NAME	BRAND/TRADE NAME(S)	CLASS/SCHEDULE	MEDICATION INFORMATION
naproxen	Aleve, Naprosyn	Anti-inflammatory drugs (nonsteroidal [NSAIDs])	*Indications:* Osteoarthritis, rheumatoid arthritis, fever, pain *Desired effects/action:* Stops the body's production of substances that cause pain, fever, and inflammation *Side effects:* GI intolerance, ringing in the ears *Adverse reactions:* Weight gain, hypersensitivity, hoarseness, jaundice, bloody urine, stiff neck
dextromethorphan	(Many DM cough and cold formulas)	Antitussives	*Indication:* Cough *Desired effects/action:* Reduces coughs *Side effects:* Drowsiness, restlessness, light-headedness, stomach pain, dizziness *Adverse reaction:* Hives
pseudoephedrine	Sudafed	Decongestant	*Indications:* Colds, hay fever, sinus congestion *Desired effects/action:* Relieves nasal and sinus congestion *Side effects:* Restlessness, nausea, vomiting, weakness, headache *Adverse reactions:* Hypertension, vasospasm, arrhythmia, cerebrovascular accident
aspirin (ASA)	Bufferin, Ecotrin, (many brand names)	Salicylates	*Indications:* Arthritis, fever, pain, heart attack prevention *Desired effects/action:* Relieves pain, fevers; increases clotting time *Side effects:* Nausea, stomach pain, heartburn, drowsiness, ringing in the ears *Adverse reactions:* Visual changes, tachycardia, wheezing, back pain, confusion

TABLE 28.9 Commonly Used Herbal Supplements

NAME	USES	SIDE EFFECTS AND CAUTIONS
Acai	Weight loss and antiaging; antioxidant.	Little scientific information about the safety of acai; no scientific evidence to support use for any health-related purpose; might affect magnetic resonance imaging (MRI) results.
Aloe vera	Aloe gel is used for burns, frostbite, psoriasis, and cold sores. It can also be taken orally for osteoarthritis, bowel diseases, and fever.	Topical use of aloe gel is likely to be safe. More studies are needed to determine the safety of oral preparations. People with diabetes should be cautioned against using aloe because it may lower blood glucose levels.
Black cohosh	Relieve symptoms of menopause; treat menstrual irregularities and premenstrual syndrome; induce labor.	Headaches, gastric complaints, heaviness in the legs, weight problems; safety unknown for pregnant women or those with breast cancer.
Echinacea	Treat or prevent colds, flu, and other infections; believed to stimulate the immune system.	Most studies indicate echinacea does not appear to prevent colds or other infections; some people experience allergic reactions, including rashes, increased asthma, and anaphylaxis; gastrointestinal (GI) side effects.
Flaxseed	Flaxseed and flaxseed oil are used for constipation, diabetes, high cholesterol levels, cancer, and other conditions.	Few reported side effects; contains soluble fiber and is an effective laxative; both flaxseed and flaxseed oil can cause diarrhea. It is not recommended during pregnancy.
Garlic	Treat high cholesterol, heart disease, hypertension; prevent certain types of cancer, including stomach and colon cancer.	Some evidence indicates garlic can slightly lower blood cholesterol levels and may slow development of atherosclerosis; side effects include breath and body odor, heartburn, GI upset, and allergic reactions; acts as a mild anticoagulant (similar to aspirin); may increase the risk of bleeding; interferes with effectiveness of saquinavir, a drug used to treat human immunodeficiency virus (HIV) infection.

Continued

TABLE 28.9 Commonly Used Herbal Supplements—*continued*

NAME	USES	SIDE EFFECTS AND CAUTIONS
Ginger	Alleviate nausea associated with postoperative state, motion sickness, chemotherapy, and pregnancy; used for rheumatoid arthritis, osteoarthritis, and joint and muscle pain.	Short-term use can safely relieve pregnancy-related nausea and vomiting; also may help with chemotherapy nausea and vomiting. Side effects most often reported are gas, bloating, heartburn, and nausea.
Asian ginseng	Support overall health and boost immune system; improve mental and physical performance; treat erectile dysfunction, hepatitis C, and menopause symptoms; lower blood glucose and control blood pressure.	Limited information available, more studies needed. May affect blood glucose levels and blood pressure; thus, patients should discuss this with their provider. May interact with certain medications such as anticoagulants.
Ginkgo biloba	No conclusive evidence that it helps any health condition.	Side effects may include headache, stomach upset, and allergic skin reactions. Ginkgo may increase the risk of bleeding with pregnancy and in those taking anticoagulants.
Green tea	Improve mental alertness, relieve digestive symptoms and headaches, promote weight loss; may have protective effects against heart disease and cancer.	Safe in moderate amounts; possible complications include liver problems with concentrated green tea extracts but not when used as a beverage. A specific green tea extract ointment is a prescription drug used for treating genital warts.
St. John's wort	Treat mental disorders and nerve pain; kidney and lung diseases, insomnia, and wounds.	Some scientific evidence shows it helps treat mild to moderate depression; not effective in treating major depression. Side effects include photophobia (increased sensitivity to sunlight), anxiety, dry mouth, dizziness, GI symptoms, fatigue, headache, and sexual dysfunction. Can cause life-threatening reactions with certain medications. Drugs that can be affected include the following: • Antidepressants • Birth control pills • Cyclosporine (prevents rejection of transplants) • Digoxin (heart medication) • Some HIV and cancer medications • Warfarin and related anticoagulants

Modified from the National Center for Complementary and Alternative Medicine, https://nccih.nih.gov/health/herbsataglance.htm.

SUMMARY OF SCENARIO

Mark is enjoying working with Gabe. He is amazed at how much Gabe knows about medications that the providers commonly prescribe. Mark feels that he will never be as fluent with the medications as Gabe is. He even mentioned this to Gabe. His mentor laughed and said he felt the same way during his own practicum. Over the years, he has used drug reference materials to help him learn about medications. He has made it a practice to look up medications he does not know. This helped him to become more fluent. He assured Mark that if he was willing to read up on medications, he, too, would become fluent with them.

Mark is looking forward to administering medications with Gabe. Now that he understands how to use the drug reference materials, he will be working hard to learn about the medications he encounters.

SUMMARY OF LEARNING OBJECTIVES

1. **Analyze the sources and uses of drugs.**
   Drugs are either created from natural sources or made synthetically in a laboratory. Plants, animals, minerals, and microbiologic sources are natural sources of drugs. There are eight common uses of drugs: prevention, treatment, diagnosis, cure, contraceptive, health maintenance, palliative, and replacement.
2. **Distinguish among the phases of pharmacokinetics.**
   Pharmacokinetics is the study of drug absorption, distribution, metabolism, and excretion in the body. Absorption is the movement of a drug from the site of administration to the bloodstream. The movement of absorbed drugs from the blood to the body tissues is called *distribution*. Metabolism is a series of chemical processes whereby enzymes change drugs in the body. Excretion is the movement of the metabolites out of the body.
3. **Examine drug actions, including influencing factors, therapeutic effects, and adverse reactions.**
   Drugs are chemicals that can cause changes in the cells. Four main drug actions are: depressing, stimulating, destroying, and replacing substances. This chapter discussed the factors that influence drug action, including age, body size, sex, genetics, diseases, diet, drug dosage, route, the timing of administration, mental state, and environmental temperature. Each medication has one or more therapeutic effects or desired effects. This is the intended action of the medication. The person can experience an unexpected or life-threatening reaction called an adverse reaction. Table 28.1 lists common adverse reactions.
4. **Examine drug legislation that impacts the ambulatory care setting.**
   The Food, Drug, and Cosmetic Act is enforced by the Food and Drug Administration (FDA). The FDA is responsible for the safety, effectiveness, security, and quality of drugs, cosmetics, and food. The Controlled Substances Act (CSA), Title II of the Comprehensive Drug Abuse Prevention and Control Act of 1970, is a federal law. The Drug Enforcement Agency (DEA) enforces the CSA. The DEA oversees the manufacturing, importation, possession, use, and distribution of illegal and legally controlled substances.
5. **Examine how healthcare professionals must comply with the Controlled Substance Act.**
   Healthcare professionals comply with the Controlled Substance Act by the following activities:
   - Providers prescribing controlled substances need a DEA registration number. Each provider has a unique number. The DEA number is good for 3 years.
   - All controlled substances must be adequately safeguarded. They need to be kept in a locked cabinet or safe of substantial construction. Keys should be placed in a locked area accessible only to authorized persons.
   - The inventory log must be completed when receiving orders of controlled substances from manufacturers and when administering them to patients.
   - Periodic reconciling of the log with the actual inventory count is important to identify missing medications. Logs need to be kept for 2 years.
   - Controlled substances must be destroyed in the presence of two authorized persons, and an entry must be made in the waste log.
   - The medical assistant must notify the provider and supervisor if controlled substances are missing.
6. **Differentiate between brand and generic drugs.**
   There are four types of drug names:
   - *Chemical name*: Represents the drug's exact chemical formula
   - *Generic name*: Assigned by the US Adopted Names (USAN) Council
   - *Official name*: Used to list the medication in the United States Pharmacopeia and the National Formulary (USP–NF)
   - *Brand name*: Also called the *trade name*, used by one manufacturer
7. **Examine the information available in drug references.**
   Print drug references include package inserts and drug handbooks. Digital drug references include apps, products integrated with electronic health records, and online websites.

   Table 28.3 provides a list of classifications of medications with descriptions. Table 28.4 lists commonly prescribed medications and information on each, including the generic name, brand/trade name, class, schedule, indication, desired action, side effects, and adverse reactions.

   The following terminology is typically found in drug reference information: names, description, boxed warning, dosage, indication, dosage considerations, contraindications, precautions, adverse reactions, interactions, action, biological half-life, peak, and duration. Refer to that section for definitions of these terms.
8. **Differentiate among the types of solid, semisolid, and liquid medication forms.**
   The form is the physical characteristics of the medication. Forms of medications include the following:
   - *Solid* medication forms: Examples include tablet, chewable tablet, caplet, capsule, scored tablet, and enteric-coated tablet.
   - *Semisolid* medication forms: Examples include ointment, paste, cream, suppository, and pessary.
   - *Liquid* medication forms: Examples include solutions and suspensions.
     - *Solution*: Examples include tincture, fluid extract, spirit, elixir, and syrup.
     - *Suspension*: Examples include emulsion, gel, magma, liniment, lotion, and aerosol.
9. **Differentiate among the types of medication orders.**
   The provider can give the order over the phone or in person; this type of order is called a *verbal order*. The provider can also give the medical assistant a *written order* using a prescription pad or an electronic message. Besides describing medication orders by how they are given to the medical assistant, they can also be described by the type of order. Five types of medication orders are as follows:
   - *Routine order*: Medication is taken at regular intervals until it is canceled or expired.
   - *Standing order*: Order applies to all patients who meet specific criteria.
   - *PRN order*: Medication is given on an "as needed" basis for specific signs and symptoms.

SUMMARY OF LEARNING OBJECTIVES—*continued*

- *Single order* or *one-time order*: Medication is administered one time.
- *Stat order*: Medication is administered one time right now.

10. **Examine prescriptions, including the parts, the information required, and the medical assistant's role in preparing prescriptions.**
    There are four parts to a prescription: superscription, inscription, signature, and subscription. Figure 28.3 describes the four parts of a prescription. All prescriptions need to include the date of issue; patient information; provider's full name and address; drug name, strength, and dosage form; quantity prescribed; directions for use; number of refills; National Provider Identifier (NPI); and if a generic is acceptable. Procedure 28.1 describes how to prepare prescriptions using a prescription refill procedure. Table 28.5 provides commonly approved abbreviations regarding route, medication form, measurements, timing, and medications.

PROCEDURE 28.1 Prepare a Prescription

TASKS: Prepare a prescription using a prescription refill protocol. Use approved abbreviations.

SCENARIO: You receive a call from Noemi Rodriguez (DOB 11/04/19XX). She is requesting refills on three of her prescriptions from Jean Burke, NP. She saw Jean Burke 10 months ago. Noemi has no known allergies (NKA). She is doing well with the prescriptions and has no concerns. You determine it is time for refills. Her prescriptions include Coumadin 5 mg, 1 tablet orally daily; Tenormin 50 mg, 1 tablet orally daily; and Plendil 5 mg, 1 tablet orally daily.

EQUIPMENT and SUPPLIES

- SimChart for the Medical Office (SCMO) or paper prescriptions and a pen
- Prescription refill protocol (see Figure 28.4)
- Drug reference book or online resource

PROCEDURAL STEPS

1. Using the scenario, look up the generic medication names using the drug reference book or online resource.
   PURPOSE: Generic names are typically used in healthcare facilities, though patients may give the brand name.
2. Read the prescription refill protocol. Compare the generic names to the list of medications given. Identify medications that meet the protocol.
   PURPOSE: All the criteria need to be met for the medical assistant to prepare prescriptions using the prescription refill protocol.
3. Prepare prescriptions for refill per the protocol using SCMO or paper prescriptions.
   - *Using SCMO:* Search for the patient. Verify the date of birth before selecting the patient. On the INFO PANEL, select Phone Encounter. Complete the fields on the Create New Encounter window and save. Check the box beside the No known allergy statement on the allergy screen and save. Select Order Entry from the Record dropdown list and select Add in the Out-of-office section (see the following figure).
   - *Using paper prescriptions:* Add in the patient's complete name, date of birth, and address.

   PURPOSE: Most agencies using electronic health records require medical assistants to update the allergy screen when preparing refills. Prescriptions require the patient's name and address. If the DOB is available, add this to the prescription. An electronic health record will automatically add this information when it sends the prescription to the pharmacy.

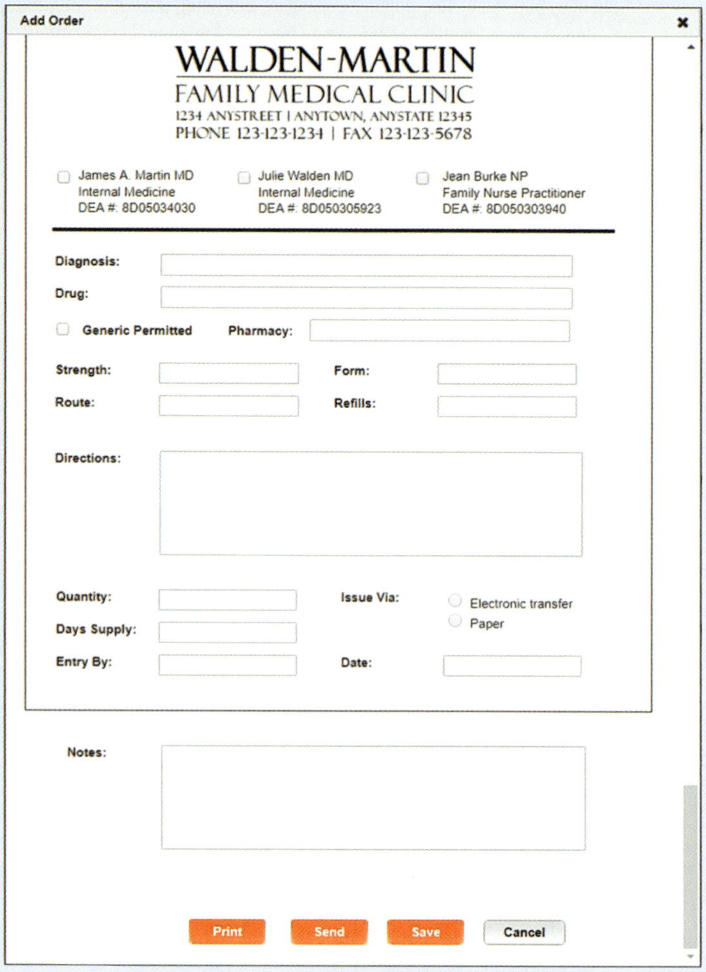

Add Order

WALDEN-MARTIN
FAMILY MEDICAL CLINIC
1234 ANYSTREET | ANYTOWN, ANYSTATE 12345
PHONE 123-123-1234 | FAX 123-123-5678

James A. Martin MD, Internal Medicine, DEA #: 8D05034030
Julie Walden MD, Internal Medicine, DEA #: 8D050305923
Jean Burke NP, Family Nurse Practitioner, DEA #: 8D050303940

Diagnosis:
Drug:
Generic Permitted
Pharmacy:
Strength:
Form:
Route:
Refills:
Directions:
Quantity:
Issue Via: Electronic transfer / Paper
Days Supply:
Entry By:
Date:
Notes:

Print | Send | Save | Cancel

PROCEDURE 28.1 Prepare a Prescription—*continued*

4. Using the information in the scenario, complete the prescription information on either the paper prescription or in the SCMO fields. Use only approved abbreviations.
   PURPOSE: All information is required on the prescription for it to be accepted by the pharmacist and filled for the patient.
5. Complete any additional prescriptions as needed by the prescription refill protocol.
   PURPOSE: The patient requested refills on the medications indicated. Any medications that can be refilled should have prescriptions prepared for the provider.
6. Review the prescriptions for any errors. Void the prescription and redo it if needed.
   PURPOSE: It is important to prepare accurate prescriptions. Any errors need to be fixed before giving the prescriptions to the provider.
   Note: After the provider signs the prescriptions, depending on the facility's policy, the medical assistant may need to document the refill in the health record. This cannot be done until the provider approves the prescriptions.

29 PHARMACOLOGY MATH

SCENARIO

Gabe Garcia, CMA (AAMA), has worked for Walden Martin Family Medical (WMFM) Clinic for 3 years. During his first year at WMFM Clinic, Gabe worked almost exclusively with a family practice provider who cared for older patients. Once the provider retired, Gabe switched providers. He is now working with both children and adult patients. He finds himself administering more injections when working with children than he does when working with adults.

Gabe was asked to be Mark Allen's mentor for his clinical experience. Mark has just completed all of his medical assistant courses at the local college and now needs 160 hours of clinical experience. He is excited to be working with Gabe. This week, Gabe will be working with Mark to review reading syringes and applying the math used for medication calculations.

While studying this chapter, think about the following questions:

- What are the parts of a drug label?
- What are the basic units of measure in the household and metric systems?
- How can a person convert amounts between different measurement systems?
- How can a temperature be converted between Fahrenheit and Celsius?
- How are medication doses calculated?
- How does a person read the calibration markings on syringes?

LEARNING OBJECTIVES

1. Examine the information on drug labels.
2. Examine how to solve basic math problems involving fractions, decimals, and percentages.
3. Examine math basics for medication calculations, including healthcare rules for numbers, rounding numbers, and the value of Roman numerals.
4. Examine the apothecary, household, and metric measurement systems.
5. Demonstrate how to convert between Fahrenheit and Celsius temperatures.
6. Calculate the number of tablets needed for an entire course of treatment and the number needed for a dose.
7. Calculate liquid medication doses.
8. Calculate a medication dose using a solution.
9. Calculate a pediatric dose of medication.
10. Determine the amount of medication in various types of syringes.

VOCABULARY

dosage May also be referred to as dose; the quantity of medication to be administered at one time.

exclusivity (ik skloo SIV i tee) The sole right to market an approved medication granted by the Food and Drug Administration (FDA); may occur with the patent.

minim (MIN im) An apothecary unit of measurement for liquid; approximately equal to one drop.

patent (PAT ent) A grant from the government that gives a creator (or manufacturer) of an invention the sole right to produce, use, and sell the product for a set period of time.

place value The numeric value that a digit has based on its position in a number.

product The number obtained by multiplying two or more numbers together.

scored tablet A tablet with a groove on the surface, used for splitting it in half.

unit-dose packaging A packaging method for drugs; holds a specified quantity of medication in a single-use container (e.g., syringe, blister pack).

INTRODUCTION

Medical assistants are responsible for being absolutely certain that the medication they prepare and administer to a patient is exactly what the provider ordered. Although drugs often are delivered by the pharmacy or supplied by pharmaceutical representatives in **unit-dose packaging**, the dosage ordered may differ from the dosage on hand. In this case, the medical assistant must be prepared to calculate the correct dose accurately before dispensing and administering the medication. There is never a margin of error in drug calculations; even a minor mistake may result in serious complications for the patient. The medical assistant, therefore, must take meticulous care in calculating all drug dosages.

DRUG LABELS

A drug label contains a lot of information. Some of the information is used when verifying the right medication and calculating the drug dose. Other information may be used when documenting medication. The following sections discuss the information found on drug labels.

Label Information for Drug Administration

When the medical assistant prepares medications, it is important to compare the medication's name and strength with the provider's order. The first step in safely calculating a drug **dosage** is to accurately read the label of the drug on hand to determine whether the provider's order and the packaged drug are in the same system of measurement. The label shows the following information:

- *Trade* or *brand name*: The manufacturer's name for the drug (e.g., Cardizem) (Figure 29.1). The brand name is capitalized and typically in bold print. The brand name is copyright protected; therefore, it is followed by an ® symbol that indicates the US government has granted a Federal Registration Certificate for the drug.
- *Generic name*: The drug name used by all manufacturers who make that specific medication (e.g., diltiazem HCl, cephalexin) (see Figure 29.1). The name is printed in lowercase letters and usually appears under the brand name in smaller print. If the **patent** and **exclusivity** have expired, only a generic name may be present on the label.
- *Strength*: The amount of drug in the unit dose (e.g., 200 mg, 180 mg/5 mL). In Figure 29.1, each tablet of Cardizem is 120 mg.

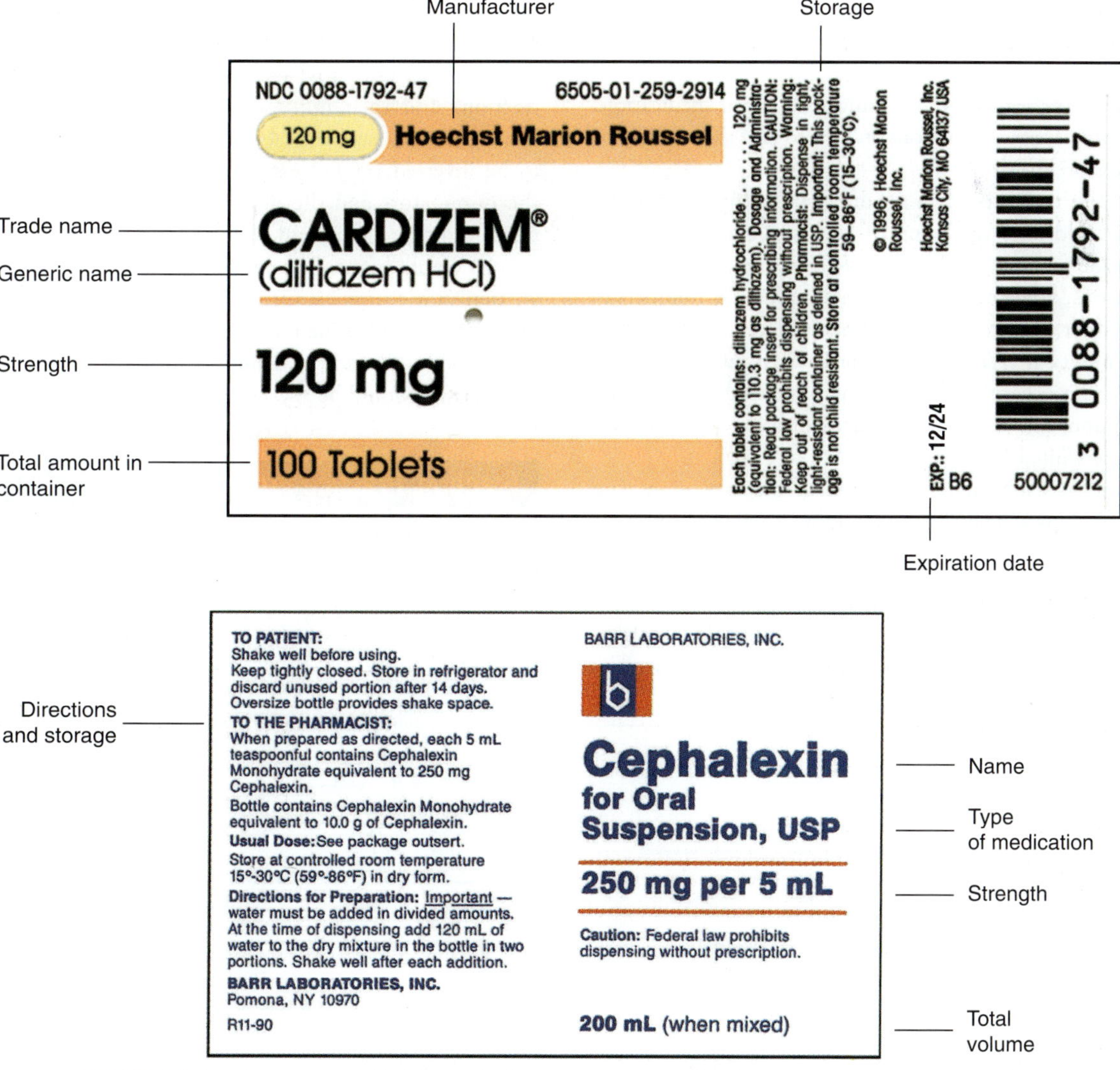

FIGURE 29.1 Drug labels. (From Brown M, Mulholland JM: *Drug calculations: process and problems for clinical practice*, ed 9, St. Louis, 2012, Mosby.)

Cephalexin is a suspension (liquid), and the strength or unit dose is 250 mg (of powdered medication) per 5 mL (of liquid).

- *Total amount* or *total volume*: Both liquid and solid medication labels indicate the amount of medication in the container.

Patents and Exclusivity

A patent is granted on a drug for 20 years from the date of filing for the patent. Patents are granted at any point in time during the development of a drug.

Exclusivity is granted by the Food and Drug Administration (FDA) to give exclusive marketing rights to the manufacturers of the drug when it earns FDA approval. This exclusive marketing right can vary from 3 to 5 years. If a medication has been on the market longer than 20 years or after the exclusive rights to the drug have expired, the generic name may be the only one listed (e.g., meperidine instead of Demerol or diazepam rather than Valium).

Additional Information on Drug Labels

Besides the information mentioned in the prior section, the drug label contains additional information that is useful to the medical assistant. Additional information found on the drug label includes the following:

- *Manufacturer*: The name of the manufacturer of the medication.
- *Directions and storage*: Instructions on how to take the medication and how to store the drug.
- *Expiration date*: Indicates when the drug can no longer be used.
- *Lot number*: Indicates the batch of drug the medication came from. The lot number is important to document when giving immunizations. Some agencies may require that lot numbers be documented for all medications administered.
- *National Drug Code (NDC)*: A unique 10-digit number indicating the product. The NDC is required by federal law to be on all prescription and nonprescription medication packages and inserts in the United States.

The medical assistant should also look at the expiration date. Preparing medications will be discussed in more detail in Chapter 30.

CRITICAL THINKING APPLICATION **29.1**

Gabe and Mark are discussing the labels on vaccines. Mark asks Gabe why the lot numbers are important on vaccine vials. How would you answer this question?

MATH BASICS

When working with math in healthcare, you need to thoroughly understand the addition, subtraction, multiplication, and division of fractions and decimals, the relationship between decimals and fractions, and how they are converted from one to the other.

Fractions

When you divide a whole unit into parts, you can create a fraction with a part. For instance, you cut a tablet into 2 parts; each part is 1/2. If you cut a pizza into 8 slices, each slice is $^1/_8$. The top number in a fraction is the *numerator*, and the bottom number is the *denominator*.

Proper and Improper Fractions

In a *proper fraction*, the numerator is smaller than the denominator, such as $^3/_4$. In *improper fractions*, the numerator is equal to or greater than the denominator, such as $^6/_5$ and $^5/_5$. Improper fractions can be converted into whole numbers by dividing the numerator by the denominator. For example, if you had an improper fraction of 12/3, you would divide the numerator by the denominator, or 12 ÷ 3 = 4. Some improper fractions can be simplified. For example, 12/5 would be 12 ÷ 5 = $2^2/_5$, which is considered a mixed number. A mixed number is a whole number with a proper fraction.

Multiplying and Dividing Fractions

When multiplying fractions, you multiply the two numerators and the two denominators. Then you reduce the answer into the simplest form. Let us use this problem: 1/6 × 2/4. The two numerators are multiplied (1 × 2), and the two denominators are multiplied (6 × 4). The answer would be $^2/_{24}$. Now we must reduce the fraction to its lowest terms. Two is the largest number that will divide equally into 2 and 24. Therefore, divide the numerator by 2 (2 ÷ 2 = 1) and the denominator by 2 (24 ÷ 2 = 12). Thus, the final answer would be $^1/_{12}$.

To divide fractions, you must invert the *divisor* (the second fraction) and then multiply the numerators and denominators. Let us use this problem: $^3/_5 \div {}^3/_2$. The divisor is $^3/_2$, which needs to be inverted ($^2/_3$). Next, we rewrite the problem and multiply the numerators and the denominators: $^3/_5 \times {}^2/_3$. Multiplying the numerators (3 × 2) would be 6, and multiplying the denominators (5 × 3) would be 15. The answer would be $^6/_{15}$, but it needs to be written in the simplest form. Three is the largest number that will divide equally into the 6 and 15. Therefore, divide the numerator by 3 (6 ÷ 3 = 2) and the denominator by 3 (15 ÷ 3 = 5). Thus, the final answer would be $^2/_5$.

Fraction: Practice Problems

Directions: Convert the improper fractions to mixed numbers. Write the answer in its simplest form.

1. 22/3 = ______ 2. 17/12 = ______ 3. 52/20 = ______
4. 25/7 = ______ 5. 15/4 = ______ 6. 62/30 = ______

Directions: Solve these problems, and write the answer in its simplest form.

7. 1/3 × 2/3 = ______ 8. 2/5 × 6/4 = ______
9. 4/5 × 6/8 = ______ 10. 2/3 ÷ 5/6 = ______
11. 12/3 ÷ 4/7 = ______ 12. 1/3 ÷ 2/3 = ______

Decimals

A decimal is similar to a fraction, but it is expressed in units of tenths (0.1), hundredths (0.01), and thousandths (0.001). To perform drug calculations, fractions first must be converted into decimals. To convert a fraction into a decimal, simply divide the numerator by the denominator.

For example, if a dose of medication is $^{2}/_{5}$ mL, the provider's order would be written in the decimal equivalent. To perform this math, you may need to add zeroes after the decimal point at the end of the numerator. The problem would be written: 2 ÷ 5. The answer would be 0.4 mL.

Decimal: Practice Problems

Directions: Convert the fractions to decimals.

2. 3/5 = ______ 3. 6/10 = ______ 4. 2/10 = ______
5. 5/2 = ______ 6. 4/5 = ______ 7. 5/100 = ______

Percentage

A *percentage* is a number expressed as part of 100.

- To convert a decimal to a percent, multiply the decimal by 100. Then add a percent sign (%). Another way to convert the decimal is to move the decimal point two spaces to the right and add a percent sign (%).
- To convert a fraction to a percent, divide the numerator by the denominator. Multiply the answer by 100 and add a percent sign. Here are some examples:
  0.25 = $^{25}/_{100}$ = 25%
  0.5 = $^{5}/_{10}$ = 50%
  0.75 = $^{75}/_{100}$ = 75%
  0.055 = $^{55}/_{1000}$ = 5.5%

Percentage: Practice Problems

Directions: Convert the decimals to percentages.

1. 0.3 = ______ 2. 1.03 = ______ 3. 0.04 = ______
4. 0.52 = ______ 5. 0.6 = ______ 6. 0.32 = ______

MATH BASICS FOR MEDICATIONS

All medical assistants should be able to convert between units of measure. It is also important to be able to accurately calculate medication dosages. This section discusses different types of math problems that a medical assistant should be able to solve. Please note that in some states, calculating medical dosages may be outside the legal scope of practice for medical assistants. State laws vary.

The following sections present guidelines for writing and calculating dosages. The medical assistant should always verify answers for dose calculations with a co-worker or the provider.

Healthcare Rules When Writing Numbers

With medications, it is important to be accurate in calculating and documenting amounts. There are four rules to follow when writing medication dosages in healthcare:

1. Follow the number with the correct abbreviation for the unit of measure. Leave a space between the number and the abbreviation. Do not use a period with the abbreviations.
   Correct examples: 2 mg and 10 mL
   Incorrect examples: mg.2 and 10mL
2. Write a fraction of a dose as a decimal.
   Correct examples: 0.2 mg and 0.5 mg
   Incorrect examples: $^{1}/_{5}$ mg and 1/2 mg
3. If the dose is less than 1, place a zero to the left of the decimal point. This reduces the risk of misreading the dose as a whole number.
   Correct examples: 0.75 mcg and 0.2 mL
   Incorrect examples: .75 mcg and .2 mL
4. Do not place a decimal point and a zero after a whole number. This can be easily misread, and the patient would be given an overdose of medication.
   Correct examples: 2 mL and 5 mL
   Incorrect examples: 2.0 mL and 5.0 mL

Rounding Numbers

When you calculate answers, sometimes the number needs to be rounded. The following steps describe the process for rounding a number.

1. Find the **place value** where you want to end up. (Most answers in this chapter will be rounded to the nearest tenth, or one place after the decimal point.)

HUNDREDS	TENS	ONES	TENTHS	HUNDREDTHS	THOUSANDTHS
7	5	1	.3	5	7

2. Look at the number to the right of the place value. If the number is
   - *4 or below,* drop the number(s) to the right of the place value
   - *5 or above,* add 1 to the rounded place value and drop the number(s) to the right of the place value

Let us practice rounding to the nearest tenth using the following examples:

- First example: 569.365. In this example, 3 sits in the tenth-place value. The number to the right of the 3 is a 6. This means we need to add 1 to the 3, and then we can drop the 6 and 5. The answer is 569.4.
- Second example: 339.926. In this example, 9 sits in the tenth-place value. The number to the right of the 9 is a 2. This means we just need to drop the 2 and 6. The answer is 339.9.

Rounding: Practice Problems

Directions: Round the following numbers to the nearest tenth. Write out as you would for a medication dose with a zero before the decimal point if the answer is less than 1 and no trailing zeros.

1. 2.467 = ______ 2. .358 = ______ 3. .98 = ______
4. 4.65 = ______ 5. 45.234 = ______ 6. 7.788 = ______

Roman Numerals

Sometimes a number might be written using Roman numerals. It is good for a medical assistant to be familiar with the following Roman numerals. In healthcare, you will see them written in lowercase letters. Sometimes a line may be written above the Roman numeral.

I = 1	vi = 6	$\overline{ss}$ = 1/2 or 0.5	Examples:
ii = 2	vii = 7	(for "$\overline{ss}$": write out	1. vss = 51/2or 5.5
iii = 3	viii = 8	"one-half" in	2. $\overline{\text{iii}}$ss = 31/2 or 3.5
iv = 4	ix = 9	documentation notes	
v = 5	x = 10	to avoid errors)	

CRITICAL THINKING APPLICATION **29.2**

Mark is confused by the numbers 5 and 10 in the Roman numeral system. Come up with a way to remember the difference between these two and share it with a classmate.

MEASUREMENT SYSTEMS

In healthcare, both the household and metric systems are used. For instance, we weigh patients in pounds and tell a mother to give her son 1 teaspoon of medication before meals. Using the metric system is more accurate. The provider will use a child's weight in kilograms (kg) to calculate a medication dosage. The pharmacist will show the mother that 1 teaspoon is 5 mL on the oral syringe. The oral syringe and plastic medicine cup are more accurate for measuring medications than the spoons used in the kitchen.

Apothecary System

The apothecary system is the oldest measuring system for medications. Dry medications were measured based on a grain (gr), which equaled the weight of one grain of wheat. For liquid measurements, the basic unit of volume is a **minim**. When writing numbers and abbreviations for the apothecary system, the abbreviation is written before the lowercase Roman numeral (e.g., gr v). Fractions are used for portions less than a full unit (e.g., gr ¼). Half of a unit can be expressed as ss (e.g., gr vss). The apothecary system has been replaced by the metric system. Medications should be calculated based on the metric system.

Household System

Sometimes we need to work within the household system as we solve problems. Other times we need to use both the metric and household measurement systems. The following are common household measurement abbreviations.

gtt, gtts	drop, drops
tsp	teaspoon
Tbs or tbsp	tablespoon
fl oz	fluid ounce
oz	ounce
qt	quart
pt	pint
lb	pound

Household and Metric Equivalents

The following table shows the household and metric equivalents for weights and liquids. Some find remembering the following equivalents to be helpful: 1 oz = 2 Tbs = 6 tsp = 30 mL.

WEIGHT	LIQUIDS
2.2 lb = 1 kg	3 tsp = 1 Tbs
16 oz = 1 lb	1 tsp = 60 gtt
	1 oz = 30 mL
	1 tsp = 5 mL
	1 Tbs = 15 mL
	1 oz = 2 Tbs
	1 oz = 6 tsp

Converting between Household and Metric Equivalents

There are many ways to set up problems when converting between household and metric equivalents. The proportion method is one of the easiest techniques. In the proportion method, the cross-**products** are equal. This approach is easy if you remember three things:

1. Keep the information separate. The problem information is on one side of the equal sign, and the equivalent information is on the other side.
2. Keep the labels in the same place. The labels should be in the exact same location on both sides of the equal sign.
3. Cross-multiply in the direction of the two numbers, then divide by the remaining number. You have your answer.

The following steps show how to solve household and metric problems.

Problem: 20 Tbs = __________ mL

Solution for problem:

Step 1: Turn the problem into a fraction. It does not matter which number is the *numerator* (top number in a fraction) and which is the *denominator* (bottom number in a fraction); keep the label with the number. Use *x* for the unknown number.

PROBLEM

$$\frac{20\ \text{Tbs}}{x\ \text{mL}}$$

Step 2: Add an equal sign and make a fraction on the opposite side. Fill in the labels. The labels need to be in identical locations on both sides of the equal sign.

PROBLEM		EQUIVALENT
$\frac{20\ \text{Tbs}}{x\ \text{mL}}$	=	$\frac{\_\_\_\_\ \text{Tbs}}{\text{mL}}$

Step 3: Using the Household and Metric Equivalents box, find the equivalent for Tbs and tsp. Fill in the numbers in the equivalent fraction. Make sure to put the right number in front of the correct label.

PROBLEM		EQUIVALENT
$\frac{20\ \text{Tbs}}{x\ \text{mL}}$	=	$\frac{1\ \text{Tbs}}{15\ \text{mL}}$

Step 4: Now solve for the unknown.

Using a calculator: Multiply in the diagonal direction of the two numbers (20 × 15), and then divide by the number in the other direction (1); the answer is *x*.

PROBLEM	EQUIVALENT
$\frac{20\text{ Tbs}}{x\text{ mL}}$ =	$\frac{1\text{ Tbs}}{15\text{ mL}}$

$20 \times 15 = 300 \div 1 = 300$

To solve without a calculator: Solve for x by cross-multiplying.

Cross-multiply the fractions: $20 \times 15 = 1x$

Solve for x: $300 = 1x$

Simplify for x: $\frac{300}{1} = \frac{1x}{1}$

$300 = x$

Answer: 300 mL – Always make sure to label your answer.

Household and Metric: Practice Problems

Directions: Solve the following problems. Round your answers to the nearest tenth.

1. 11 oz = ______ lb 2. 90 mL = ______ oz 3. 8 tsp = ______ mL
4. 20 Tbs = ______ mL 5. 5.5 oz = ______ Tbs 6. 4 oz = ______ tsp
7. 23 lb = ______ kg 8. 28 kg = ______ lb 9. 56 oz = ______ lb

Metric System

The metric system is commonly used in healthcare. We use it when measuring medications and wounds. A medical assistant should know how to use the metric system. Note these standards when using the metric system:

- Weight is measured in *grams* (g).
- Volume is measured in *liters* (L).
- Length is measured in *meters* (m).

Gram, liter, and meter are called *root words*. *Prefixes* are added to the front of root words to indicate the size of the unit. Figure 29.2 lists the prefixes that can be added to the root words. Table 29.1

Size of the unit of measure	Prefixes	Size	Or another way to look at it!	
LARGE	Kilo (k)	1000 base units	1 kilo = 1000 base units	Larger than the base unit
	BASE UNITS [Meter (distance), Liter (volume) or Gram (mass or weight)]			
↓	Centi (c)	0.01 base unit	100 centi = 1 base unit	Smaller than the base unit
	Milli (m)	0.001 base unit	1000 milli = 1 base unit	
SMALL	Micro (mc)	0.000001 base unit	1,000,000 micro = 1 base unit	

FIGURE 29.2 Prefixes of metric measurement.

TABLE 29.1 Metric Measurements and Equivalents Used in Healthcare

	VOLUME	LENGTH	WEIGHT
Units of Measure with Abbreviations	Liter (L) Milliliter (mL or ml) [Note: 1 cc = 1 mL Cubic centimeter (cc)]	Meter (m) Centimeter (cm) Millimeter (mm)	Gram (g) Kilogram (kg) Milligram (mg) Microgram (mcg)
Equivalents Commonly Used	1 L = 1000 mL 1 L = 1000 cc 1 mL = 1 cc (*To avoid errors in documentation, use mL instead of cc.*)	1 m = 100 cm 1 m = 1000 mm 1 cm = 10 mm	1 g = 1000 mg 1 g = 1,000,000 mcg 1 kg = 1000 g 1 mg = 1000 mcg

provides the metric measurements and equivalents commonly used in healthcare.

Solving Metric Problems

Remember that a person cannot convert from base unit to base unit (i.e., gram to liter or meter to gram). A person can only convert within a base unit (i.e., centimeter to millimeter). Figure 29.3 provides a memory tool for solving metric problems. There are many ways to do so. The following steps show how to solve metric problems.

Problem: 17 g = _______ mg

Solution for problem

Step 1: Turn the problem into a fraction. It does not matter which number is the numerator and which is the denominator, just keep the label with the number. Use *x* for the unknown number.

PROBLEM

$$\frac{17\text{ g}}{x\text{ mg}}$$

Step 2: Add an equal sign and make a fraction on the opposite side. Fill in the labels. The labels need to be in identical locations on both sides of the equal sign.

PROBLEM		EQUIVALENT
$\frac{17\text{ g}}{x\text{ mg}}$	=	$\frac{\text{g}}{\text{mg}}$

Step 3: Using Table 29.1, find the equivalent for gram (g) and milligram (mg). Fill in the numbers in the equivalent fraction. Make sure to put the right number in front of the correct label.

PROBLEM	EQUIVALENT
$\frac{17\text{ g}}{x\text{ mg}}$ =	$\frac{1\text{ g}}{1000\text{ mg}}$

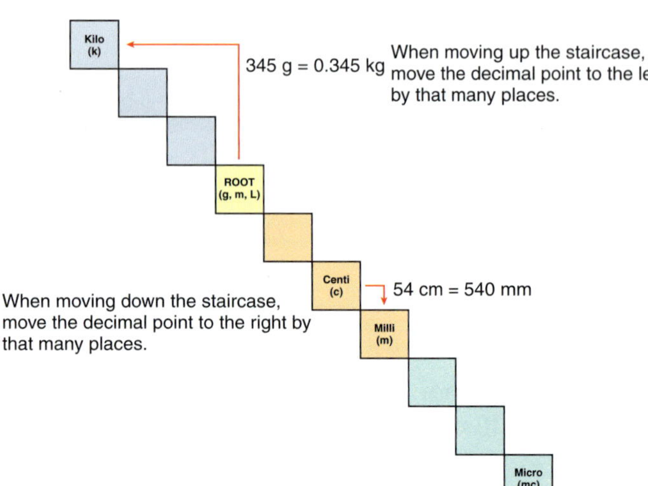

FIGURE 29.3 Memory tool for solving metric problems.

Step 4: Now solve for the unknown.

Using a calculator: Multiply in the diagonal direction of the two numbers (17 × 1000) and then divide by the number in the other direction (1); the answer is *x*.

PROBLEM	EQUIVALENT
$\frac{17\text{ g}}{x\text{ mg}}$ =	$\frac{1\text{ g}}{1000\text{ mg}}$

$17 \times 1000 = 17{,}000 \div 1 = 17{,}000$ mg

To solve without a calculator: Multiply diagonally and solve for *x*.

$$17 \times 1000 = 1x$$
$$17{,}000 = 1x$$
$$\frac{17{,}000}{1} = \frac{1x}{1}$$
$$17{,}000 = x$$

Answer: 17,000 mg. Always make sure to label your answer.

Metric: Practice Problems

Directions: Solve the following problems.

1. 235 mL = ______ L	2. 2.13 L = ______ mL
3. 1.2 g = ______ mg	4. 500 mg = ______ g
5. 20 mm = ______ cm	6. 410 cm = ______ m

CRITICAL THINKING APPLICATION 29.3

What unit of measure (e.g., liter, meter, or gram) would be used to measure the following?

1. Volume of urine
2. Length and width of a wound
3. Weight of a child

TEMPERATURE CONVERSION

Fahrenheit (°F) and Celsius (°C) are used in healthcare. A medical assistant should be able to convert between these two units of measure. To remember the steps for temperature conversion, use the memory tool presented in Figure 29.4.

Converting from Fahrenheit to Celsius

The following steps show how to convert a Fahrenheit temperature to a Celsius temperature.

Problem: 102°F = __________ °C

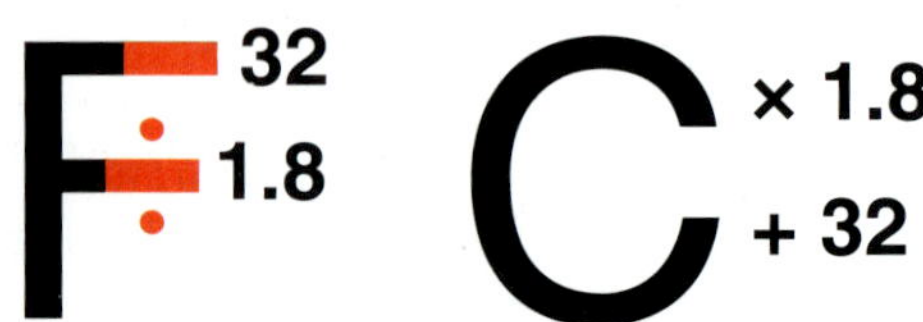

FIGURE 29.4 Memory tool for temperature conversions.

Solution for problem

Step 1: Subtract 32 from the Fahrenheit temperature.

102 – 32 = 70

Step 2: Divide the answer by 1.8 and round to the nearest tenth.

70 ÷ 1.8 = 38.88889

Answer: 38.9°C

Converting from Celsius to Fahrenheit

The following steps show how to convert a Celsius temperature to a Fahrenheit temperature.

Problem: 25°C = __________ °F

Solution for problem

Step 1: Multiply the Celsius temperature by 1.8

25 × 1.8 = 45

Step 2: Add 32 to the answer.

45 + 32 = 77

Answer: 77°F

Temperature Conversion: Practice Problems

Directions: Solve the following problems. Round your answers to the nearest tenth.

1. 93.3°F = ____ °C 2. 42.9°F = ____ °C 3. 53°F = ____ °C
4. 103°C = ____ °F 5. 39.9°C = ____ °F 6. 88.2°C = ____ °F

SOLID MEDICATION DOSES

Often the medical assistant must use the drug order or the drug label and calculate the number of tablets needed. The following two sections describe how to calculate the number of tablets needed for two different scenarios—for the entire course of treatment and for a dose.

Number of Tablets Needed for Entire Course

It is important for the medical assistant to be able to calculate how many tablets a patient needs for an entire course of treatment. This section describes how to calculate the number of tablets needed for the entire course of treatment.

It is not uncommon for patients to call the provider to request enough medication for a trip. The same steps can be used if you need to calculate the number of tablets needed for a specific period of time.

Figure 29.5 shows a medication order. The first part shows the name of the medication, along with the tablet size (strength of each tablet). The last part of the order shows the following:

- How many tablets to take *(dose)* (e.g., 1 tab [tablet])
- How many times to take the medication during the day (e.g., tid [three times a day])
- The route (e.g., po [oral])
- How long to take the medication (e.g., 10 days)

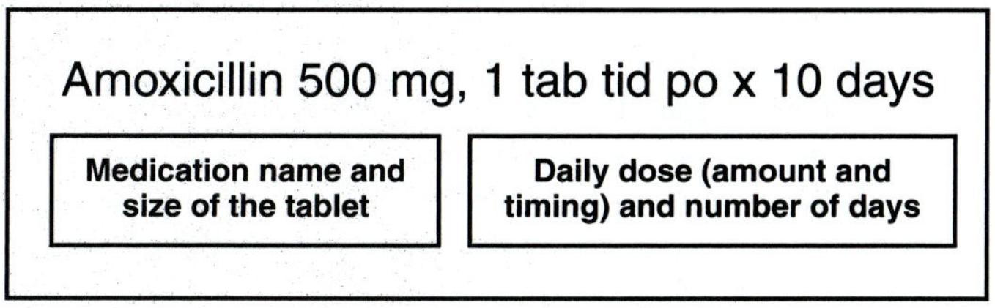

Amoxicillin 500 mg, 1 tab tid po x 10 days

Medication name and size of the tablet

Daily dose (amount and timing) and number of days

FIGURE 29.5 Medication order.

The following steps show how to calculate the number of tablets needed for the entire course of medication.

Problem: Amoxicillin 500 mg, 1 tab tid po × 10 days. How many tablets would the patient need for the entire course of medication?

Solution for problem

Step 1: Figure out the number of tablets per dose. (Use the abbreviation list if you need to. One tab equals 1 tablet.)

Step 2: Figure out the number of tablets taken throughout the day. Do this by multiplying the number of tablets per dose (1 tablet) by the number of times the medication is taken during the day (tid means 3 times a day).

1 tablet per dose × 3 times a day = 3 tablets per day

Step 3: Figure out the number of tablets needed. Multiply the number of tablets per day by the number of days.

3 tablets per day × 10 days = 30 tablets needed

Answer: 30 tablets needed

Number of Tablets Needed for the Entire Course: Practice Problems

Directions: Calculate the number of tablets the patient will need for the entire course.

1. Prescription: XYZ medication 200 mg, 5 tabs tid × 6 days.
2. Prescription: XYZ medication 250 mg, 3 tabs qid × 14 days.
3. Prescription: XYZ medication 50 mg, 4 tabs bid × 10 days.
4. Prescription: XYZ medication 70 mg, 4 tabs tid × 13 days.
5. Prescription: XYZ medication 120 mg, 3 tabs tid × 12 days.

Number of Tablets per Dose

It is common for the provider to give medication orders without a tablet amount. For instance, the provider orders "Tylenol 975 mg po." The medical assistant must figure out how many tablets to give the patient for each dose. To start, figure out the number of milligrams in each tablet, which will be indicated on the stock medication label. Once the tablet size is identified, the medical assistant can calculate the number of tablets required.

Using the Proportion Method

The following steps show how to calculate the number of tablets needed for the dose (Procedure 29.1).

Problem: Order: Tylenol 975 mg po. Stock: Tylenol 325 mg per tablet. How many tablets should be given?

Solution for problem

Step 1: Put the stock information into a fraction on one side. It does not matter the location of the numbers. Make sure to add the labels. (Remember: 325 mg per tablet means 325 mg in each tablet.)

STOCK

$$\frac{325 \text{ mg}}{1 \text{ tab}}$$

Step 2: Add an equal sign and make a fraction on the opposite side. Fill in the labels. The labels need to be in identical locations on both sides of the equal sign.

STOCK **ORDER**

$$\frac{325\text{ mg}}{1\text{ tab}} = \frac{\text{mg}}{\text{tab}}$$

Step 3: Fill in the order information. You do not know the number of tablets, so that is the unknown (*x*).

STOCK **ORDER**

$$\frac{325\text{ mg}}{1\text{ tab}} = \frac{975\text{ mg}}{x\text{ tab}}$$

Step 4: Now solve for the unknown.

Using a calculator: Multiply in the diagonal direction of the two numbers (1 × 975), and then divide by the number in the other direction (325); the answer is *x*.

STOCK **ORDER**

$$\frac{325\text{ mg}}{1\text{ tab}} = \frac{975\text{ mg}}{x\text{ tab}}$$

$$1 \times 975 = 975 \div 325 = 3$$

To solve without a calculator: Multiply diagonally and solve for *x*.

$$1 \times 975 = 325x$$
$$975 = 325x$$
$$\frac{975}{325} = \frac{325x}{325}$$
$$3 = x$$

Answer: 3 tablets

It is important to double-check your answers. If the order is larger than the stock tablet, then you will be giving more than 1 tablet. If the order is smaller than the stock tablet amount, then you will be giving less than a tablet.

Using the Formula Method

The formula method can also be used for this type of problem. The following steps show how to solve the problem using the formula method.

Problem: Order: Tylenol 975 mg po. Stock: Tylenol 325 mg per tablet. How many tablets should be given?

The set up for the formula method is the following:

$$\frac{\text{D (desired [order])}}{\text{H (on hand)}} \times \text{V (vehicle [tablet or liquid])}$$

Step 1: D (desired) is 975 mg. H (on hand) is 325 mg. V (vehicle) is 1 tablet. Put the values into the formula method.

$$\frac{975\text{ mg}}{325\text{ mg}} \times \text{V (vehicle [tablet or liquid])}$$

Step 2: Multiply 975 by 1 and then divide the answer (975) by 325 to figure out the tablet amount.

$$\frac{975\text{ mg}}{325\text{ mg}} \times 1\text{ tablet} = \frac{975}{325}$$

Answer: 3 tablets

Number of Tablets per Dose: Practice Problems

Directions: Calculate the number of tablets to give the patient.

1. Order: ABC 120 mg po; stock: ABC 80 mg po **scored tablet.**
2. Order: ABC 150 mg po; stock: ABC 30 mg po scored tablet.
3. Order: ABC 105 mg po; stock: ABC 30 mg po scored tablet.
4. Order: ABC 65 mg po; stock: ABC 130 mg po scored tablet.
5. Order: ABC 210 mg po; stock: ABC 70 mg po scored tablet.

LIQUID MEDICATION DOSES

When preparing a liquid medication, you will see two different units of measure on the bottle label. These two units are the weight of the powdered medications and the volume of liquid. The units typically used include the following:

- Weight of the powdered medication: units, g, mg, or mcg
- Volume of liquid: cc or mL

For instance, a bottle label states, "50 mg/2 mL." This means there are 50 mg of powdered medication in every 2 mL of liquid. If you want 50 mg of medication, then you would need to give 2 mL of liquid. Another example is 1500 mg/mL. This means there are 1500 mg of powdered medicine in each milliliter of liquid. Remember that sometimes 1 mL is indicated by just "mL."

Liquid Medication Dose with Matching Labels

If the unit label of the ordered medication is the same as the stock medication, then the units are considered to match. For instance, in the following problem, the ordered medication dose label is shown in milligrams (mg). The stock medication is 1300 mg/2 mL. The powdered medication label (mg) matches the label on the order.

Using the Proportion Method

The following steps show how to calculate the amount of medication needed for a dose when the labels match (see Procedure 29.1).

Problem: Order: ABC medication 1500 mg. Stock: ABC medication 1300 mg/2 mL. How much medication (in mL) should be given?

Solution for problem

Set up the problem: Make sure the label information is on the stock side of the equation. The order is on the opposite side. Remember labels need to be in the same location on both sides of the equal sign.

Step 1: Put the stock information into a fraction. It does not matter the location of the numbers. Make sure to add the labels.

STOCK

$$\frac{1300\text{ mg}}{2\text{ mL}}$$

Step 2: Put the order information on the other side. Make sure the labels are in the exact same location.

STOCK		**ORDER**
$\frac{1300\text{ mg}}{2\text{ mL}}$	=	$\frac{1500\text{ mg}}{x\text{ mL}}$

Step 3: Now solve for the unknown.

Using a calculator: Multiply in the diagonal direction of the two numbers (2 × 1500), then divide by the number in the other direction (1300). Round your answer to the nearest tenth.

STOCK		**ORDER**
$\frac{1300\text{ mg}}{2\text{ mL}}$	=	$\frac{1500\text{ mg}}{x\text{ mL}}$

$$2 \times 1500 = 3000 \div 1300 = 2.3\text{ mL}$$

To solve without a calculator: Multiply diagonally and solve for *x*. Round your answer to the nearest tenth.

$$1300x = 1500 \times 2$$
$$1300x = 3000$$
$$\frac{1300x}{1300} = \frac{3000}{1300}$$
$$x = 2.3\text{ mL}$$

Answer: 2.3 mL

Using the Formula Method

The following steps show how to calculate the liquid medication dose with matching labels using the formula method.

Problem: Order: ABC medication 1500 mg. Stock: ABC medication 1300 mg/2 mL. How much medication (in mL) should be given? The setup for the formula method is the following:

$$\frac{\text{D (desired)}}{\text{H (on hand)}} \times \text{V (vehicle [tablet or liquid])}$$

Step 1: D (desired) is 1500 mg. H (on hand) is 1300 mg. V (vehicle) is 2 mL. Put the values into the formula method.

$$\frac{1500\text{ mg}}{1300\text{ mg}} \times 2\text{ mL}$$

Step 2: Multiply 1500 by 2 and then divide the answer (3000) by 1300 to figure out the amount. Round the answer to the nearest tenth.

$$\frac{1500\text{ mg}}{1300\text{ mg}} \times 2\text{ mL} = \frac{3000}{1300}$$

Answer: 2.3 mL

> **Liquid Medication Dose with Matching Labels: Practice Problems**
>
> *Directions:* Calculate how many milliliters to give the patient. Round your answers to the nearest tenth.
> 1. Order: ABC 3200 units; Stock: ABC 2800 units/mL.
> 2. Order: ABC 230 units; Stock: ABC 120 units/mL.
> 3. Order: ABC 10 mg; Stock: ABC 25 mg/3 mL.
> 4. Order: ABC 45 mg; Stock: ABC 125 mg/mL.
> 5. Order: ABC 120 mg; Stock: ABC 280 mg/mL.
> 6. Order: ABC 500 mg; Stock: ABC 1200 mg/2 mL.

Liquid Medication Dose with Nonmatching Labels

Sometimes the stock medication's unit of measure does not directly match the order's unit of measure. For instance, the provider may want "ABC 500 mg" to be given. The stock vial indicates "1 g/mL." This might be confusing. The first step is to identify if there is a shared base unit between the order and the stock medication. In this example, they share the same base unit—gram. The second step is to change one of the shared unit labels (e.g., mg and gram) to match the other label. Remember that two of the labels need to match before you can solve the problem. Once the labels match, then the problem can be solved like the problems in the prior section.

The following steps show how to calculate the amount of medication needed for a dose when the labels do not match.

Problem: Order: ABC medication 1.5 g. Stock: ABC medication 1300 mg/2 mL. How much medication (in mL) should be given?

Solution for problem

Step 1: Identify the two similar base unit labels. In this example, they are 1.5 g and 1300 mg. Essentially, a person could either convert the grams to milligrams or convert the milligrams to grams. This example shows how to convert from grams to milligrams (1.5 g = ____ mg). Set up the problem and solve it.

PROBLEM		**EQUIVALENT**
$\frac{1.5\text{ g}}{x\text{ mg}}$	=	$\frac{1\text{ g}}{1000\text{ mg}}$

$$1.5 \times 1000 = 1500 \div 1 = 1500\text{ mg}$$

Answer: 1500 mg (If it helps, cross out the 1.5 g and write in 1500 mg.)

Step 2: Put the stock information into a fraction. The location of the numbers does not matter. Make sure to add the labels.

STOCK

$$\frac{1300\text{ mg}}{2\text{ mL}}$$

Step 3: Put the order information on the other side. Make sure the labels are in the exact same location.

STOCK		**ORDER**
$\frac{1300\text{ mg}}{2\text{ mL}}$	=	$\frac{1500\text{ mg}}{x\text{ mL}}$

Step 4: Now solve for the unknown.

Using a calculator: Multiply in the diagonal direction of the two numbers (2 × 1500), then divide by the number in the other direction (1300). Round your answer to the nearest tenth.

STOCK		ORDER
$\frac{1300 \text{ mg}}{2 \text{ mL}}$	=	$\frac{1500 \text{ mg}}{x \text{ mL}}$

$$2 \times 1500 = 3000 \div 1300 = 2.3 \text{ mL}$$

To solve without a calculator: Multiply diagonally and solve for *x*. Round your answer to the nearest tenth.

$$1300x = 1500 \times 2$$
$$1300x = 3000$$
$$\frac{1300x}{1300} = \frac{3000}{1300}$$
$$x = 2.3 \text{ mL}$$

Answer: 2.3 mL

Liquid Medication Dose with Nonmatching Labels: Practice Problems

Directions: Calculate how many milliliters to give the patient. Round your answers to the nearest tenth.

1. Order: ABC 2500 mg; Stock: ABC 2.8 g/2 mL.
2. Order: ABC 1800 mg; Stock: ABC 2 g/mL.
3. Order: ABC 1.2 g; Stock: ABC 2500 mg/2 mL.
4. Order: ABC 450 mg; Stock: ABC 1.2 g/2 mL.
5. Order: ABC 420 mg; Stock: ABC 1 g/2 mL.
6. Order: ABC 750 mg; Stock: ABC 1.2 g/2 mL.
7. Order: ABC 650 mg; Stock: ABC 1.8 g/3 mL.
8. Order: ABC 400 mg; Stock: ABC 3 g/2 mL.

SOLUTIONS

In the ambulatory care environment, many anesthetics used for minor surgeries come in a solution. When comparing solutions, the medical assistant should be able to recognize the weaker and stronger solutions. The following sections discuss solutions and how to calculate a dose using a solution.

The Makeup of a Solution

For instance, a provider asks you to get the strongest Xylocaine vial in the cabinet. You see a 1% and a 2% vial. What does this mean?

When the manufacturer made the medication, the recipe called for powdered drug to be mixed with a liquid:

- A 1% solution means 1000 mg of powdered drug is mixed in 100 mL of liquid.
- A 2% solution means 2000 mg of powdered drug is mixed in 100 mL of liquid.

(The 100 mL of liquid always remains, regardless of the number in front of the percentage sign.) Going back to the provider's request, you would give the provider the 2% vial because it is the strongest solution (or contains the most powdered drug).

Solution Dose

If a medical assistant needs to calculate a dose of medication using a stock solution vial, the process is similar to that used for the prior problems. The initial step would require the medical assistant to change the percent into a fraction. For example, the fraction for a 5% solution would be 5000 mg/100 mL. The remaining steps would be the same as for the previous problems.

The following steps show how to calculate the amount of medication needed for a dose when using a solution.

Problem: Order: ABC medication 20 mg. Stock: ABC medication 2% solution. How much medication (in mL) should be given?

Solution for problem

Step 1: Change the 2% into a fraction. *Tip:* Take the number before the percentage sign. Add 3 zeros and mg after it. Then put it over 100 mL.

$$2\% = \frac{2000 \text{ mg}}{100 \text{ mL}}$$

Step 2: Use the fraction created in step 1 as the stock medication.

STOCK
$\frac{2000 \text{ mg}}{100 \text{ mL}}$

Step 3: Put the order information on the other side. Make sure the labels are in the exact same location.

STOCK		ORDER
$\frac{2000 \text{ mg}}{100 \text{ mL}}$	=	$\frac{20 \text{ mg}}{x \text{ mL}}$

Step 4: Now solve for the unknown.

Using a calculator: Multiply in the diagonal direction of the two numbers (100 × 20), then divide by the number in the other direction (2000). Round your answer to the nearest tenth.

STOCK		ORDER
$\frac{2000 \text{ mg}}{100 \text{ mL}}$	=	$\frac{20 \text{ mg}}{x \text{ mL}}$

$$100 \times 20 = 2000 \div 2000 = 1 \text{ mL}$$

To solve without a calculator: Multiply diagonally and solve for *x*. Round your answer to the nearest tenth.

$$2000x = 100 \times 20$$
$$2000x = 2000$$
$$\frac{2000x}{2000} = \frac{2000}{2000}$$
$$x = 1 \text{ mL}$$

Answer: 1 mL

Solution Dose: Practice Problems

Directions: Calculate how many milliliters to give the patient. Round your answers to the nearest tenth.

1. ABC 60 mg. Stock: ABC 4% solution.
2. ABC 80 mg. Stock: ABC 10% solution.
3. ABC 30 mg. Stock: ABC 4% solution.
4. ABC 70 mg. Stock: ABC 5% solution.
5. ABC 120 mg. Stock: ABC 11% solution.
6. ABC 50 mg. Stock: ABC 6% solution.

PEDIATRIC DOSE

As with all medication calculations, it is important to be accurate for the safety of the patient. It is recommended that two people calculate a dose to be sure of the accuracy. Know the facility's policies and procedures regarding the calculation of pediatric doses because variations may be seen.

Steps to Calculate a Pediatric Dose

Medication dosages for children are typically based on the child's weight. For this type of problem, the medical assistant needs the child's weight, the drug order, and the information on the stock medication label. For instance, a child's weight is 33 pounds (lb), the drug order is ABC medication 0.1 mg/kg, and the stock medication label states "ABC medication 1 mg/mL." Notice that the child's weight is in pounds, and the order is 0.1 mg per every kilogram of weight. The unit of measure for weight is different, one being pounds and the other kilograms.

The following are the steps to calculate a pediatric dose:

Step 1: Convert the patient's weight to kilograms. This goes back to converting between the household and metric systems, which was discussed earlier in the chapter.

Step 2: Calculate the number of milligrams of medication the child needs. Imagine this scenario: A person tells you that you can have two chocolate bars for each kilogram you weigh. How would you figure it out? A simple way is to multiply the number of kilograms you weigh by 2 (68 × 2 = 136 bars). You can use this same method to calculate the medication order—multiply the kilograms by the order.

Step 3: Calculate the liquid medication dose or the number of milliliters you will give. An example of this step was shown in the Liquid Medication Dose with Matching Labels section.

Calculating the Amount of Medication

The following steps show how to calculate the amount of medication for a pediatric patient (see Procedure 29.1). You can modify the steps and use the formula method if you like.

Problem: Patient's weight: 33 lb. Order: ABC medication 0.1 mg/kg. Stock: ABC medication 1 mg/mL. How much medication (in mL) should be given?

Solution for problem

Tip on solving the problem: There are three main steps to this problem. When you complete a step, round two places beyond your answer. For instance, if your answer is to be in tenths, then during the problem, round to the thousandth (3 places after the decimal). This will ensure accuracy in the answer.

Step 1: Convert the patient's weight into kg. This can be done several ways. Use your favorite method or follow the example and solve for the unknown.

Problem: 33 lb = ______ kg

PROBLEM		EQUIVALENT
$\frac{33 \text{ lb}}{x \text{ kg}}$	=	$\frac{2.2 \text{ lb}}{1 \text{ kg}}$

Using a calculator: Multiply in the diagonal direction of the two numbers (33 × 1), then divide by the number in the other direction (2.2). Round your answer to the nearest thousandth (if needed).

To solve without a calculator: Multiply diagonally and solve for *x*. Round your answer to the nearest thousandth (if needed).

$$33 \times 1 = 2.2x$$
$$33 = 2.2x$$
$$\frac{33}{2.2} = \frac{2.2x}{2.2}$$
$$15 = x$$

Step 2: Calculate the number of mg of medication needed. Again, there are several ways. The easiest is to multiply the weight by the order (15 kg × 0.1 mg), or you can set it up like the example and solve it. Because this is in the middle of the problem, round to the nearest thousandth (if needed).

ORDER		WEIGHT
$\frac{0.1 \text{ mg}}{1 \text{ kg}}$	=	$\frac{x \text{ mg}}{15 \text{ kg}}$

$$0.1 \times 15 = 1.5 \div 1 = 1.5 \text{ mg}$$

Updated order: ABC medication 1.5 mg

Step 3: Calculate the liquid medication dose. Put the stock information into a fraction. Put the order information on the other side. Make sure the labels are in the exact same location.

STOCK		ORDER
$\frac{1 \text{ mg}}{1 \text{ mL}}$	=	$\frac{1.5 \text{ mg}}{x \text{ mL}}$

Using a calculator: Multiply in the diagonal direction of the two numbers (1.5 × 1), then divide by the number in the other direction (1). Round your answer to the nearest tenth (if needed).

To solve without a calculator: Multiply diagonally and solve for *x*. Round your answer to the nearest tenth (if needed).

$$1x = 1 \times 1.5$$
$$1x = 1.5$$
$$\frac{1x}{1} = \frac{1.5}{1}$$
$$x = 1.5 \text{ mL}$$

Answer: 1.5 mL

Pediatric Dose: Practice Problems

Directions: Calculate how many milliliters to give the patient. Round to the nearest thousandth while solving, then round your answer to the nearest tenth.

1. Patient's weight: 40 lb; Order: ABC medication 0.3 mg/kg; Stock: ABC medication 2 mg/mL.
2. Patient's weight: 58 lb; Order: ABC medication 0.8 mg/kg; Stock: ABC medication 60 mg/2 mL.
3. Patient's weight: 145 lb; Order: ABC medication 2 mg/kg; Stock: ABC medication 80 mg/mL.
4. Patient's weight: 31 lb; Order: ABC medication 0.3 mg/kg; Stock: ABC medication 2 mg/mL.
5. Patient's weight: 60 lb; Order: ABC medication 0.8 mg/kg; Stock: ABC medication 50 mg/2 mL.
6. Patient's weight: 86 lb; Order: ABC medication 1.5 mg/kg; Stock: ABC medication 80 mg/2 mL.

Using Drug Labels

Now that you have learned how to calculate medications, use the labels to identify how the medication comes and the amount of medication to give the patient.

1. Order: Crestor 20 mg po daily. Available drug (Figure 29.6):
   How does the medication come?
   How many tablets would you give?
2. Order: Amoxicillin 875 mg po. Available drug (Figure 29.7):
   How does the medication come?
   How many milliliters would you give?
3. Order: Cefaclor 262 mg po. Available drug (Figure 29.8):
   How does the medication come?
   How many milliliters much would you give?
4. Order: Cefprozil 75 mg po. Available drug (Figure 29.9):
   How does the medication come?
   How many milliliters would you give?

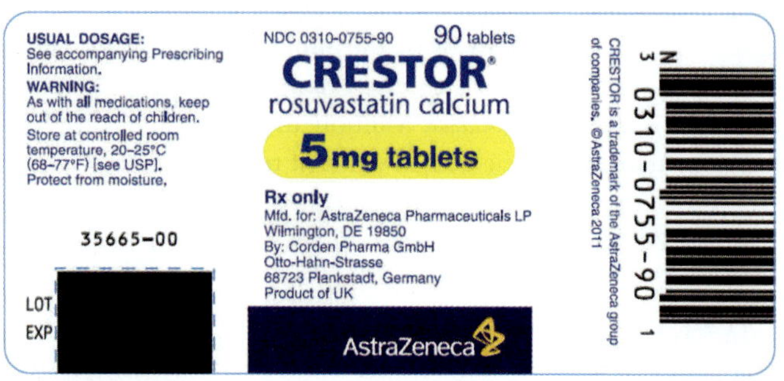

FIGURE 29.6 Crestor 5 mg tabs. (From Kee JL, Marshall SM: *Clinical calculations*, ed 8, St. Louis, 2017, Elsevier.)

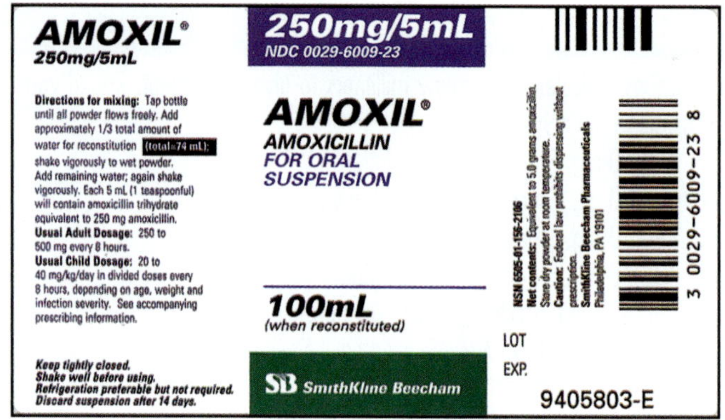

FIGURE 29.7 Amoxil 250 mL/5 mL. (From Kee JL, Marshall SM: *Clinical calculations*, ed 8, St. Louis, 2017, Elsevier.)

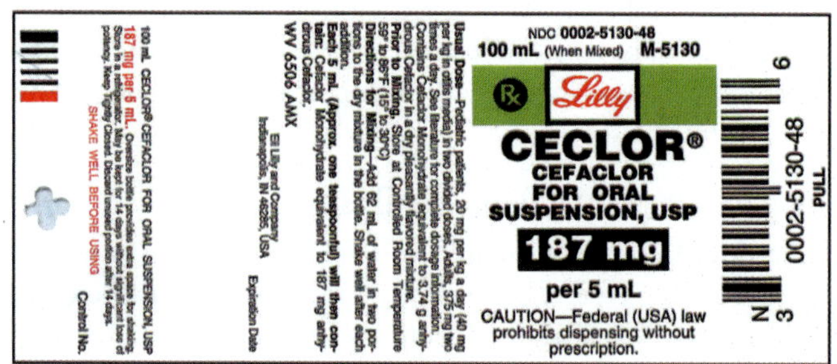

FIGURE 29.8 Ceclor 187 mg/5 mL. (From Kee JL, Marshall SM: *Clinical calculations*, ed 8, St. Louis, 2017, Elsevier.)

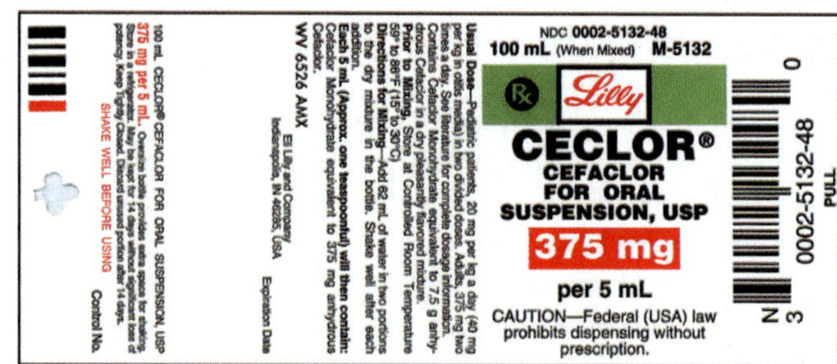

FIGURE 29.9 Cefzil 125 mg/5 mL. (From Kee JL, Marshall SM: *Clinical calculations*, ed 8, St. Louis, 2017, Elsevier.)

READING SYRINGES

For the safety of patients, it is important that medical assistants be accurate when measuring medications in syringes. Syringes have calibrations printed on the barrel. These markings are used when measuring the medication prior to administration. The calibration markings include longer or darker lines and shorter lines. The first step in reading a syringe is to identify the amount of each calibration line. With many types of syringes, a person should count the number of lines for 1 mL or 0.1 mL, depending on the syringe.

When you use a syringe, the rubber stopper on the plunger indicates the amount in the syringe. Some rubber stoppers are pointed (Figure 29.10A), and others are flat (Figure 29.10B). The top of the rubber stopper that touches the barrel is used for measuring. That part of the rubber stopper should be right on the correct calibration mark. The red arrow indicates this location on both rubber stoppers.

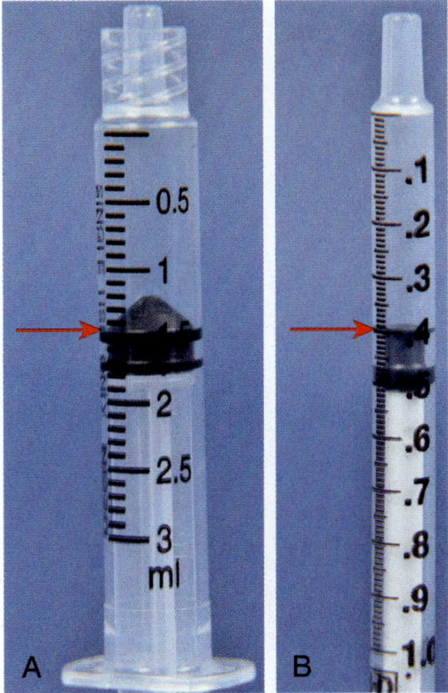

FIGURE 29.10 **(A)** The rubber stopper is pointed. **(B)** The rubber stopper is flat.

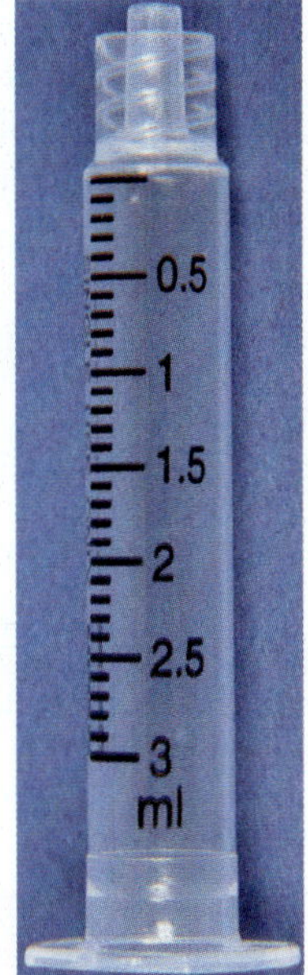

FIGURE 29.11 A 3-mL syringe.

Reading a 3-mL Syringe

Figure 29.11 shows a 3-mL syringe, the most commonly used syringe in ambulatory care. The maximum amount that the syringe can hold is indicated at the bottom of the syringe. To identify what each line is worth, count the lines for 1 mL. For this syringe, there are 10 lines for 1 mL, which means each line is equal to 0.1 mL. Medication amounts to the nearest tenth (one place after the decimal point) can be measured using this syringe.

Reading a 10-mL Syringe

Figure 29.12 shows a 10-mL syringe. The calibration markings on this syringe are the same as on most 5-, 6-, 10- and 12-mL syringes. For this syringe, there are 5 lines for 1 mL, which means each line is equal to 0.2 mL. Syringes with this type of calibration can only measure medication ordered in even numbers (e.g., 1.2 mL, 2 mL, 3.6 mL).

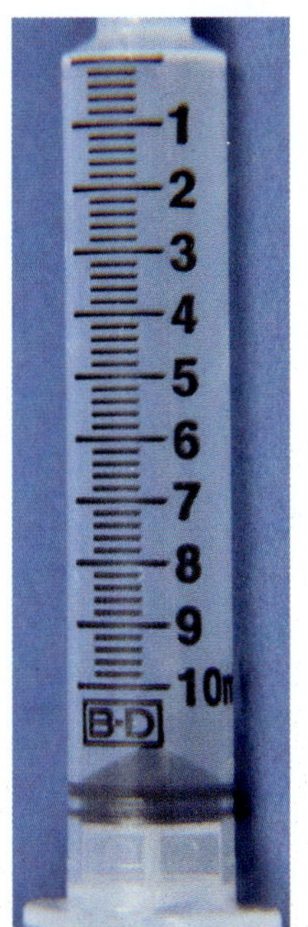

FIGURE 29.12 A 10-mL syringe.

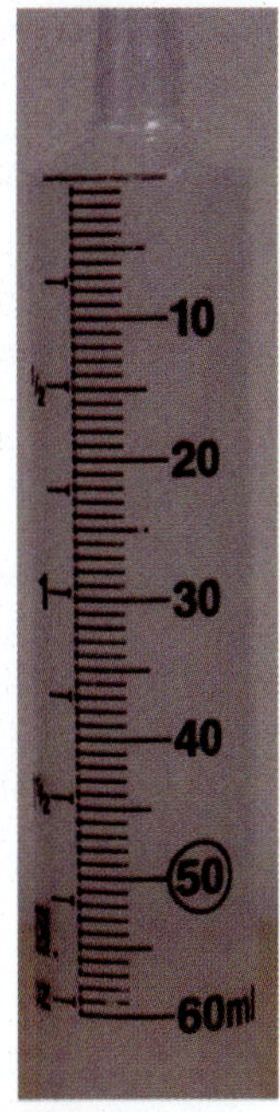

FIGURE 29.13 A 60-mL syringe.

Reading a 60-mL Syringe

Figure 29.13 shows a 60-mL syringe. The calibration markings are different with this type of syringe. Unlike prior syringes, the numbers labeled are in increments of 5 (e.g., 5, 10, 15). Each line is equal to 1 mL. Syringes with this type of calibration can only measure whole number amounts (e.g., 5, 9, 11). This type of syringe may be used in ambulatory care for irrigation.

Reading a 1-mL Syringe

Figure 29.14 shows a 1-mL syringe. The numbers on this syringe are tenths (e.g., .1, .2). For this syringe, there are 10 lines for 0.1 mL, which means each line is equal to 0.01 mL. Syringes with this type of calibration can measure to the hundredth place (e.g., 0.08, 0.09, 0.15). The most common use of these syringes is for tuberculin (TB) skin tests.

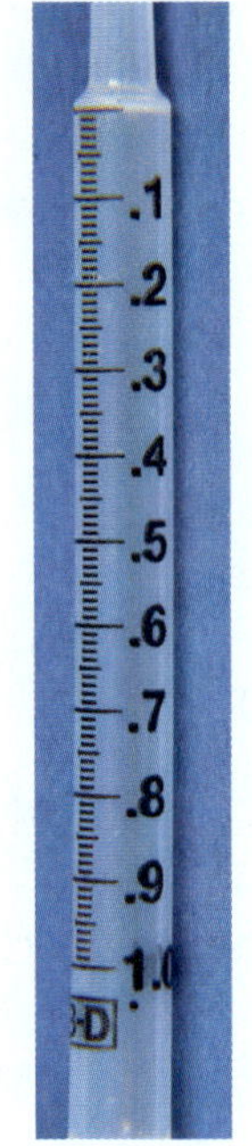

FIGURE 29.14 A 1-mL syringe.

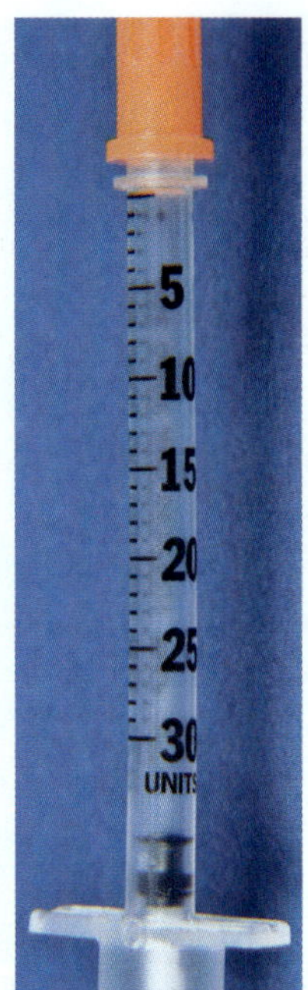

FIGURE 29.15 U-100 insulin syringe.

If a medication order indicates that 0.14 mL is to be given, the medical assistant should find the calibration marking for 0.1. A trick is to think of 0.1 as 0.10. The next small line would be 0.11, then 0.12, and so on. If a medication order indicates that 0.04 mL is to be given, the medical assistant should find the large line at the top of the syringe. This would be 0, and the next little line would be considered 0.01, followed by 0.02, and so on.

Reading an Insulin Syringe

Figure 29.15 shows an insulin syringe. Insulin is measured in units. The calibration markings on this type of insulin syringe are similar to those of the 60-mL syringe. The numbers labeled are in increments of 5 (e.g., 5, 10, 15). Each line is equal to 1 unit. Syringes with this type of calibration can only measure whole number amounts (e.g., 5, 9, 11). This type of syringe may be used in ambulatory care for U-100 insulin administration.

CLOSING COMMENTS

Patient Coaching

In some cases, the medical assistant needs to teach patients and parents how to read oral medical syringes. These syringes are used to draw up and administer oral medications, usually to young children. When coaching a patient or a parent on using an oral syringe to measure medications, it is important for the medical assistant to refer to the provider's order. If the order states 1 teaspoon, the medical assistant should coach the person that this is the same as 5 mL. Prior to finishing the coaching session, the medical assistant should have the patient or parent draw up (with air) the dose ordered to determine if the person understands the procedure.

Legal and Ethical Issues

Not all states allow medical assistants to calculate medication dosages. It is important for the medical assistant to review the state's scope of practice laws. Some agencies may also have policies and procedures for calculating medication dosages. The medical assistant must follow both the state's scope of practice laws and the agency's policies and procedures.

Professional Behaviors

If a medical assistant needs to calculate a medication dosage, it is important to have another qualified staff person recheck the calculations. If a medical assistant forgets how to calculate a medical dosage or has questions regarding the procedure, the medical assistant must talk with the provider for clarification.

SUMMARY OF SCENARIO

Mark is enjoying working with Gabe. Mark was able to review the different types of commonly used math problems in ambulatory care. Besides working on calculations, Mark and Gabe reviewed syringes. The WMFM Clinic carries 1-mL and 3-mL syringes for medication administration, 5-mL and 10-mL syringes for medication mixing procedures, and 60-mL syringes for wound irrigation procedures. A small box of insulin syringes is also available in case a patient needs insulin administration directions. It took Mark a couple of days to get comfortable measuring medications using the various syringes, but he realized that being accurate when measuring medications is critical to patients' safety.

SUMMARY OF LEARNING OBJECTIVES

1. **Examine the information on drug labels.**
   The label shows the following information: brand name, generic name, strength, total amount or total volume, manufacturer, directions and storage, expiration date, lot number, and the National Drug Code. When preparing medications, the name, strength, and expiration date are important.
2. **Examine how to solve basic math problems involving fractions, decimals, and percentages.**
   When multiplying fractions, you multiply the two numerators and the two denominators. Then you reduce the answer into the simplest form. To divide fractions, you must invert the divisor (the second fraction) and then multiply the numerators and denominators.

   Fractions first must be converted into decimals to perform drug calculations. To convert a fraction into a decimal, divide the numerator by the denominator.

   A percentage is a number expressed as part of 100. Decimal numbers can be converted to percentages by multiplying the number by 100 and adding a percent sign (%). To convert a fraction to a percentage, divide the numerator by the denominator. Multiply the answer by 100 and add a percent sign.
3. **Examine math basics for medication calculations, including healthcare rules for numbers, rounding numbers, and the value of Roman numerals.**
   Important healthcare rules when writing numbers include the following:
   - Follow the number with the correct abbreviation for the unit of measure. Leave a space between the number and the abbreviation. Do not use a period with the abbreviations.
   - Write a fraction of a dose as a decimal.
   - If the dose is less than 1, place a zero to the left of the decimal point.
   - Do not place a decimal point and a zero after a whole number.

   When rounding, remember the following:
   - 4 or below: Drop the number(s) to the right of the place value.
   - 5 or above: Add 1 to the rounded place value and drop the number(s) to the right of the place value.
4. **Examine the apothecary, household, and metric measurement systems.**
   The apothecary system is the oldest measuring system for medications.

   The apothecary system has been replaced by the metric system. Medications should be calculated based on the metric system.

   The Household and Metric Equivalents box shows the equivalents between the two systems. Using the proportion method, a person can calculate between household and metric equivalents.

   The metric system is commonly used in healthcare. Weight is measured in grams (g). Volume is measured in liters (L). Length is measured in meters (m). Table 29.1 provides the metric measurements and equivalents commonly used in healthcare.
5. **Demonstrate how to convert between Fahrenheit and Celsius temperatures.**
   When converting from a Fahrenheit temperature to a Celsius temperature, subtract 32 from the Fahrenheit temperature. Then divide the answer by 1.8 and round the answer to the nearest tenth. When converting from a Celsius temperature to a Fahrenheit temperature, multiply the Celsius temperature by 1.8. Add 32 to the answer and then round the answer to the nearest tenth.
6. **Calculate the number of tablets needed for an entire course of treatment and the number needed for a dose.**
   To calculate the number of tablets needed for the entire course of medication, use the following steps:
   - Figure out the number of tablets per dose.
   - Figure out the number of tablets taken throughout the day. Do this by multiplying the number of tablets per dose by the number of times the medication is taken during the day.
   - Figure out the number of tablets needed. Multiply the number of tablets per day by the number of days.

   The proportion method can be used to calculate the number of tablets per dose. Put the stock information into a fraction on one side and the order information on the opposite side. Then solve for the unknown.
7. **Calculate liquid medication doses.**
   When calculating a liquid medication dose with matching labels, the proportion method can be used. Put the stock medication on one side and the order medication on the other. Solve for the unknown and round the answer to the nearest tenth.

   When calculating a liquid medication dose with nonmatching labels, start by identifying the two similar base unit labels. Calculate the equivalent so you have two matching labels. Then solve as described above.
8. **Calculate a medication dose using a solution.**
   The first step is to convert the solution percent into a fraction. If using a 2% solution, the fraction would be 2000 mg/100 mL. The proportion method can be used by putting the stock medication fraction on one side and the order on the other. Solve for the unknown, then round the answer to the nearest tenth.
9. **Calculate a pediatric dose of medication.**
   The following are the steps to calculate a pediatric dose.
   - Convert the patient's weight to kilograms.
   - Calculate the number of milligrams of medication the child needs.
   - Calculate the liquid medication dose or the number of milliliters you will give.
10. **Determine the amount of medication in various types of syringes.**
    When reading syringes, the first step is to identify how much each calibration line is worth.
    - If there are 10 lines per 1 mL, each line is equal to 0.1 mL.
    - If there are 5 lines per 1 mL, each line is equal to 0.2 mL.
    - If there are 10 lines per 0.1 mL, each line is equal to 0.01 mL.
    - Insulin syringes calibration lines are usually measured in 1-unit increments.

PROCEDURE 29.1 Calculate Medication Dosages

TASK: Calculate dosages for oral medication, injectable medication, and dosages for children.

ORDERS:

- Order 1: Dr. Martin orders ABC medication 135 mg. Stock bottle reads: 45 mg scored tablets.
- Order 2: Dr. Martin orders ABC medication 650 mg. Stock bottle reads: 1300 mg scored tablets.
- Order 3: Dr. Martin orders XYZ medication 430 mg IM. Stock vial reads: 1000 mg/2 mL.
- Order 4: Dr. Martin orders XYZ medication 680 mg IM. Stock vial reads: 1200 mg/mL.
- Order 5: Dr. Martin orders MNO medication 3 mg/kg IM. Child weighs 53 pounds. Stock vial reads: 125 mg/mL.
- Order 6: Dr. Martin orders MNO medication 5 mg/kg IM. Child weighs 71 pounds. Stock vial reads: 225 mg/mL.

EQUIPMENT and SUPPLIES

- Provider's order
- Paper and pencil
- Calculator (optional per instructor)

PROCEDURE STEPS

1. Using order 1, calculate the number of tablets to give the patient. Label your answer.
   PURPOSE: It is important to label your answer to avoid any mistakes in the dosage.
2. Using order 2, calculate the number of tablets to give the patient. Label your answer.
3. Using order 3, calculate the amount in milliliters to give the patient. Round your answer to the nearest tenth. Label your answer.
   PURPOSE: Most injections are measured in tenths of a milliliter.
4. Using order 4, calculate the amount in milliliters to give the patient. Round your answer to the nearest tenth. Label your answer.
5. Using order 5, calculate the amount in milliliters to give the patient. Round your answer to the nearest tenth. Label your answer.
   Note: When working through the problem, round your answer two places beyond your answer. In this situation, round your answer as you work to the thousandth place (or three places after the decimal point).
6. Using order 6, calculate the amount in milliliters to give the patient. Round your answer to the nearest tenth. Label your answer.
7. Double-check your answers to ensure the correct dose will be given.
   PURPOSE: When calculating medications, it is important to recheck the work to ensure your answer is correct.

ADMINISTERING MEDICATIONS 30

SCENARIO

Gabe Garcia, CMA (AAMA), has worked for the Walden-Martin Family Medical (WMFM) Clinic for 7 years. He is currently Mark Allen's mentor for practicum. Mark has been working with Gabe for a couple of days. He has learned how Gabe handles prescriptions from the providers. As Mark advances in his practicum, he will be working with Gabe to administer medications to patients. Mark enjoyed practicing injections on his peers in school and looks forward to improving his skills during practicum.

While studying this chapter, think about the following questions:

- What are the nine rights of medication administration? Why are they important?
- What forms and routes of medications are commonly used in the ambulatory care setting?
- How are oral medications given in the ambulatory care setting?
- How should a medical assistant uncap and recap needles? How should needles be switched?
- How are parenteral medications prepared?
- Why is tuberculin testing done? What is the procedure for tuberculin testing? What is two-step testing?
- What are administration techniques for intradermal, subcutaneous, and intramuscular injections?
- How does a medical assistant locate the sites for intradermal, subcutaneous, and intramuscular injections?
- How does a medical assistant administer intradermal, subcutaneous, and intramuscular injections?

LEARNING OBJECTIVES

1. Differentiate among the nine rights of medication administration.
2. Examine the medical assistant's role in administering vaccines.
3. Differentiate among the routes of medication.
4. Examine the needles and syringes used for parenteral medication administration.
5. Demonstrate how to assemble needles and syringes, along with uncapping, recapping, and switching needles.
6. Demonstrate preparing parenteral medications using an ampule, prefilled sterile cartridge, vials, powdered medication, and insulin.
7. Examine the medical assistant's role in parenteral medication preparation, including site and patient preparation.
8. Demonstrate how to administer and read an intradermal tuberculin skin test.
9. Demonstrate how to administer a subcutaneous injection.
10. Demonstrate how to administer an intramuscular injection.

VOCABULARY

aspirate (AS pi rayt) To withdraw fluid using suction.

diluent (DIL yoo ent) A liquid substance that dilutes or lessens the strength of a solution or mixture.

form Physical characteristics of a medication (e.g., tablet, suspension).

gauge The inner measurement of a hollow space in a needle.

induration The hardening of a normally soft tissue.

local Affecting the area where applied.

precipitate (pri SIP i tayt) Solid particles that settle out of a liquid.

reconstituted (ree KON sti toot ed) A dried substance (powder) that has been restored to a fluid form, so it can be injected.

route The means by which a drug enters the body.

systemic Affecting the entire body.

viscosity (vis KOS i tee) Resistance to flow; the thicker the liquid, the higher the viscosity.

wheal A raised mark on the skin.

INTRODUCTION

Chapter 28 discussed the basics of pharmacology, and Chapter 29 discussed pharmacology-related math problems. You will use these skills when administering medications. This chapter discusses administration safety techniques, along with medication **forms** and **routes**. The techniques of preparing and administering medications will be the primary focus.

NINE RIGHTS OF MEDICATION ADMINISTRATION

Throughout this chapter, administration procedures for various routes will be given. Before learning how to give medications, it is important to understand medication safety rights. Over the years, the guidelines have grown to include additional steps to address patient education and the right to refuse a medication.

Each time you prepare and give medication, it is important that you follow the nine rights of medication administration. These rights are designed to help you look at the details and avoid making errors during the procedure (Figure 30.1).

Right Medication

An order or a prescription from a provider is required before a medication can be given. As discussed in a prior chapter, orders can be written or verbal. For all verbal orders, make sure to write down the order and read it back to the provider. This helps to ensure the accuracy of the order. The order requires several elements, including the medication's name and form.

With the order in hand, the medical assistant must prepare the medication. This requires finding the correct medication. Use drug reference information if you are not familiar with the medication listed on the order. Sometimes the provider will give a brand name, but the stock medication will indicate only a generic name. Make sure you have the correct medication, which includes the correct form (e.g., tablet, suppository, suspension).

You will need to check the medication order against the label three times during the preparation process to ensure that you have the correct name and form of medication. You check the label in the following situations:

- When you get the medication from the storage area (e.g., cabinet, freezer, or refrigerator)
- Before preparing the medication
- Before you return the medication to the storage area

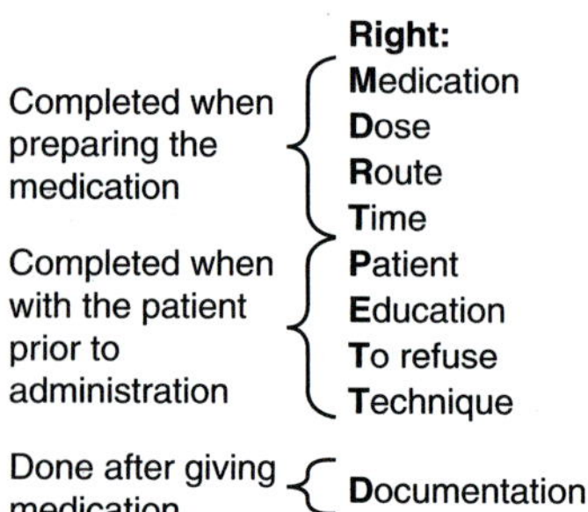

Mnemonic: **M**aybe **D**ogs **R**eally **T**alk, **PET**s **T**ruly **D**o.

FIGURE 30.1 Mnemonic for the nine rights of medication administration.

It is important that you do an activity between each check. For instance, after you do the first check, assemble the supplies you need to prepare the medication. Then do the second check. As you clean up your area, you do the third check. Too often, we reach for something based on the color, size, or location of the object. We may look at the label and think we see what we want to see. Checking the label three times, with activities between, helps to ensure that you have the right medication.

Right Dose

The dose of medication is on the order. The provider may have written the order in two different ways, even though the amount is the same. For example, both of these orders give the patient 1000 mg:

- Acetaminophen 500 mg, 2 tabs po × 1 dose
- Acetaminophen 1000 mg po × 1 dose

The first order shows the tablet strength (e.g., 500 mg) and the number of tablets (e.g., 2) to give. If the stock medication comes in 500-mg tablets, the medical assistant has no calculations to do. The second order just shows the number of milligrams to give (e.g., 1000 mg). The medical assistant would need to calculate how many tablets to give. (This procedure was discussed in Chapter 29.)

Right Route

Besides checking the label for the name and form of the mediation, it is also important to check the route. The route is the means by which a drug enters the body. The route of the medication must match the provider's order. The route should be checked along with the name and form, three times before the medication is given.

Right Time

Medications need to be given at the right time. For most medication orders, the time is part of the order. Some orders are STAT, whereas others are every month. Vaccines are a little different, and this will be described later in the chapter.

Right Patient

Before you administer the medication, it is important to correctly identify the patient. Ask patients or parents/guardians to state their full name and date of birth. Some agencies require patients to spell their last names. Verify the information against the order and the patient's health record. All three must match. Any differences must be resolved before the medication is given.

In some agencies, patients are given identification bracelets that are scanned before medication is given. The medication is also scanned. An automatic entry is made in the electronic health record (EHR). This is a common practice in hospitals and is starting to be used in ambulatory care facilities. The identification process with bracelets still requires asking the patient's name and date of birth. The information is checked against the bracelet and the order.

CRITICAL THINKING APPLICATION 30.1

Gabe is introducing Mark to the facility's medication procedures. Gabe encourages Mark to have the patients give their complete name and date of birth. He also tells Mark it is a good idea to have the patients spell their last names. Why is spelling the last name an important safety check?

Right Education

Before administering the medication to the patient, the medical assistant must do the following:

1. Give the patient the name of the medication and who ordered it. For example, "Dr. Martin ordered acetaminophen for your fever."
2. Explain the desired effect or action of the medication. For example, "The acetaminophen will bring down your fever."
3. Describe common side effects of the medication. For example, "The acetaminophen may cause nausea, rash, and a headache."
4. Verify the patient's allergies.

If the patient is receiving certain vaccines, a Vaccine Information Statement (VIS) must be given to the patient. VIS will be discussed later in this chapter.

CRITICAL THINKING APPLICATION **30.2**

Part of the WMFM Clinic's policy is to explain to patients what was ordered and why they are getting it. Why is it important to tell patients the name of a medication or procedure and the reason it has been prescribed? How might this add to patient-centered care?

Right to Refuse

The patient or the person legally responsible for the patient (e.g., parent, guardian) has a right to refuse any medication. If a patient refuses the medication, the medical assistant should respect the patient's wishes. Do not pressure the patient. Notify the provider that the ordered medication was refused and specify the reason if it was shared. Document the refusal of the medication and identify the provider who was informed. The provider will talk with the patient regarding other options.

Right Technique

When administering the medication, the medical assistant must give it in the right way. This may include an assessment before the medication is administered. Examples of the right technique include the following:

- Obtain vital signs before giving a specific medication. For instance, digoxin must be withheld if an adult's pulse is under 60.
- Obtain information about the patient's pain level before giving an analgesic medication. The medical assistant can ask the patient to rate the pain using a 0 to 10 scale. Zero is no pain, and 10 is the worst pain ever. Another pain assessment tool is the Wong-Baker FACES Pain Rating Scale, which is discussed in Chapter 44. The medical assistant should explain the scale to patients. Then patients can indicate how they feel. This scale works well for children.
- Some medications must be taken with food and others with a full glass of water. Medications that need to be taken on an empty stomach need to be taken 1 hour before meals or 2 hours after meals.

Information regarding the techniques to use when administering the medication can be found in the drug reference information.

Right Documentation

After giving a medication, the medical assistant must document it in the patient's health record. If the medication is not documented, it will appear to others as though it were not given. The documentation will vary based on what the patient received. Some documentation is done in narrative form, whereas vaccines are documented on paper or electronic vaccination forms. Elements that should be in the documentation include the following:

- Provider ordering the medication
- Assessment done (e.g., vital signs or pain level)
- Allergies
- Coaching/instructions given to patient (includes the edition date of the VIS for vaccine teaching)
- Name of medication (e.g., acetaminophen)
- Dose given (e.g., 650 mg)
- Route given (e.g., po)
- Lot number, expiration date, and manufacturer (usually only required for vaccines and controlled substances)
- How the patient tolerated the medication
- Additional information as needed (e.g., patient is resting on exam table)
- Signature if the note is handwritten (an EHR uses automatic signatures for documentation entries)

ADMINISTERING VACCINES

In many states, medical assistants administer vaccines, especially in primary care departments. A medical assistant must understand the types of vaccines and the special procedures involved when administering vaccines. The following sections discuss the types of vaccines and the importance of the Vaccine Information Statements.

Types of Vaccines

There are several types of vaccines:

- *Inactivated vaccines*: The microorganism is dead. Examples of inactivated vaccines include hepatitis A, (injectable) influenza, (injectable) polio, and rabies.
- *Live-attenuated vaccines:* The microorganism is alive but *attenuated* (weakened) in the laboratory. Examples of live virus vaccines include MMR (measles-mumps-rubella), smallpox, varicella (chickenpox), and yellow fever. Live virus vaccines need to be kept cool. Patients may not receive a live-virus vaccine in the following circumstances:
  - They were vaccinated with another live-virus vaccine less than 28 days earlier.
  - They are pregnant or may become pregnant in the next month.
  - They are immunocompromised (e.g., cancer, leukemia, human immunodeficiency virus [HIV] infection).
  - They are receiving chemotherapy or high-dose steroid therapy.
  - They recently received a blood transfusion, immune (gamma) globulin, or antiviral medication.
- *Messenger RNA (mRNA) vaccines:* According to the Centers for Disease Control and Prevention (CDC), the mRNA vaccines cause the cells to make a protein that triggers the immune response, which then causes antibodies to be produced. These antibodies protect the body when it is exposed to the disease.

The mRNA COVID-19 vaccines are examples of this type of vaccine.

- *Subunit, recombinant, polysaccharide, and conjugate vaccines:* Use specific pieces of the microorganism, which creates a very strong immune response. Examples of these types of vaccines include Hib (Haemophilus influenzae type b), hepatitis B, HPV (human papillomavirus), pertussis, pneumococcal, meningococcal, and shingles (Shingrix). These vaccines can be used by people with weakened immune systems. HPV is contraindicated with pregnancy.
- *Toxoid vaccines:* Use the toxin made by the microorganism. Examples of toxoid vaccines include diphtheria and tetanus.
- *Viral vector vaccines*: Use a modified version of a different virus as a vector to deliver protection. The COVID-19 vaccine is an example of this type of vaccine.

Vaccines to Prevent COVID-19

In December 2020, the US Food and Drug Administration (FDA) issued an Emergency Use Authorization (EUA) to permit the emergency use of two unapproved messenger RNA (mRNA) vaccines to prevent COVID-19. In 2021, the FDA issued an EUA for the Janssen vaccine. Since then, the mRNA vaccines have received the FDA approval.

Pfizer-BioNTech COVID-19 Vaccine (COMIRNATY): The primary series for this mRNA vaccine consists of 2 intramuscular (IM) doses in the deltoid, spaced 3 to 8 weeks apart. Boosters may be recommended. The vials should be protected from direct sunlight and ultraviolet light. The vaccine will be an off-white suspension.

Moderna COVID-19 Vaccine (Spikevax): The primary series for this mRNA vaccine consists of 2 IM doses in the deltoid, spaced 4 to 8 weeks apart. Boosters may be recommended. The suspension is whitish in color.

Janssen COVID-19 Vaccine: The vaccine is available in some situations per the CDC. This viral vector vaccine is given as a single intramuscular dose. Protect the vials from light. The vaccine is clear, colorless to slightly yellow.

Do not use if the vaccine is discolored or contains particulate matter. According to the CDC, there is a rare risk of myocarditis and pericarditis associated with mRNA COVID-19 vaccination and thrombosis with thrombocytopenia syndrome with the Janssen vaccine. See package inserts for more information on storage, administration, dosage, contraindications, and adverse effects of the vaccine. Clinical research continues with these vaccines. For the latest developments, see the COVID vaccine information on the CDC (https://www.cdc.gov) and the FDA (https://www.fda.gov) websites.

Types of Diphtheria, Tetanus, and Pertussis Vaccines

There are many types of diphtheria, tetanus, and pertussis (also called *whooping cough*) vaccines. Diphtheria is abbreviated with a D, tetanus with a T, and acellular pertussis (aP). Types of vaccines include the following:

- **DT**: Generic vaccine available
- **Td**: Tenivac and generic vaccines available
- **DTaP**: Daptacel, Infanrix, Kinrix, Pediarix, Pentacel, Quadracel, and Vaxelis are trade names of the available vaccines
- **Tdap**: Adacel and Boostrix are available vaccines

The uppercase letter indicates that the vaccine contains a full-strength dose of that vaccine. A lowercase letter indicates a smaller dose of that vaccine. For example, Td contains a full-strength dose of the tetanus vaccine and a smaller dose of the diphtheria vaccine. It is important how you write or type the name of the medication in the patient's health record.

Timing of Vaccines

Timing for vaccines may not be written on the provider's order, but the medical assistant should ensure that it is the correct time for a vaccine to be given. The timing of a vaccine is based on the patient's vaccination history and the person's age. Using immunization schedules or the immunization tables in EHRs, the medical assistant can determine what vaccines are due. The immunization schedule indicates the person's age and the timing between doses. If a vaccination is administered too early or before the patient reaches a specific age, the patient may need to be revaccinated.

The provider will postpone vaccinations when patients have a moderate or severe acute illness. Specific vaccines are not given if a person has had a severe allergic reaction to a vaccine component, to latex, or to a prior dose.

Consult the CDC website for information on vaccine schedules and catch-up schedules (www.cdc.gov/vaccines/index.html). The CDC also offers a free app that provides vaccine information.

Vaccine Information Statements

The VIS can be displayed on a computer screen or as a laminated copy that the patient can read prior to the administration of the vaccine. Copies of the VIS can be given to the patient or parent/guardian to take home. The provider must offer the information; however, the patient or parent/guardian has the right to decline to take the document. If the patient cannot read, the medical assistant should review the VIS with the patient. VISs can be downloaded in about 40 different languages for patients who do not speak English.

Besides giving the patient or parent/guardian the VIS prior to the vaccination, the medical assistant must document the vaccine name, dose, route, and site along with the following in the patient's health record:

- The edition date of the VIS. This is found on the back of the document in the bottom right corner. Make sure to have the latest edition of the VIS.
- The date the VIS was provided and the date the vaccine was administered (usually, the two are done on the same day).
- The office address, name, and title of the person who administered the vaccine.
- The vaccine's manufacturer and lot number.

ROUTES OF MEDICATION

For drug administration, the route is how a drug enters the body. As discussed in a prior chapter, the dose of medication can differ based on the route. The following sections discuss common routes of medication. There are many other routes that are not commonly used in the ambulatory care environment.

Oral Route

Medications taken by the oral (po) route are those we take by mouth (Procedure 30.1). Special administration techniques may be required for oral medications. These may include the following:

- Oral medications that coat the mouth or throat should not be immediately followed with water.
- Oral medications that require water for swallowing call for more than a sip. Some medications require a glass of water after taking the medication.
- A straw should be used for liquid medications that stain the teeth.
- Liquid medications should be measured only with a plastic medication cup or an oral medication syringe. Household measuring devices, such as spoons, are not accurate.

It is important to notify the provider if the patient is unable to take the medication due to nausea, vomiting, or problems swallowing. Do not attempt to see if the patient can swallow the pill. It is better to talk with the provider if the patient is concerned. Some medications can be crushed safely, whereas others cannot.

Crushing Medications

Children, older adults, and others may have problems swallowing solid medications. Crushing medications is sometimes an option. The medication should be placed in a small amount of food or liquid (e.g., pudding or jam). It is important to eat or drink all the food or liquid to get the entire dose of medication.

Solid medications typically have an unpleasant taste. It is important to share with parents that children sometimes shy away from foods with an unpleasant taste. For instance, if a parent mixes the medication with the milk in a bottle, the baby may not want to drink the milk. This can be a problem if the baby drinks only milk.

Medications that cannot be crushed include the following:

- *Slow- or extended-release tablets*: Crushing, chewing, or cutting the tablet can cause a person to get the dose faster than they should, resulting in an overdose.
- *Enteric-coated tablets*: Crushing, chewing, or cutting the tablet causes the protective nature of the coating to be lost. The person could have more stomach distress.

CRITICAL THINKING APPLICATION 30.3

Gabe and Mark are working with Charles Johnson, who has a temperature of 103.4°F (39.7°C). The provider orders acetaminophen 500 mg, 2 tabs po for the patient. Mr. Johnson tells Gabe and Mark that he cannot swallow pills. Can they give him liquid acetaminophen, or must they talk with the provider first about the situation?

Sublingual and Buccal Routes

Sublingual (SL) medications are placed under the tongue. *Buccal* medications are placed between the cheek and the gums. Both mucous membrane areas are rich in blood vessels. The medication is absorbed rapidly into the bloodstream. Special administration techniques may be required for SL and buccal medications. These may include the following:

- Do not eat or smoke prior to taking SL and buccal medications.
- Do not chew or swallow SL or buccal medications.
- Water can be taken prior to the medication to wet the mouth. No liquids can be taken until the medication has dissolved.
- Alternate cheeks used for buccal medication to avoid mucosal irritation.

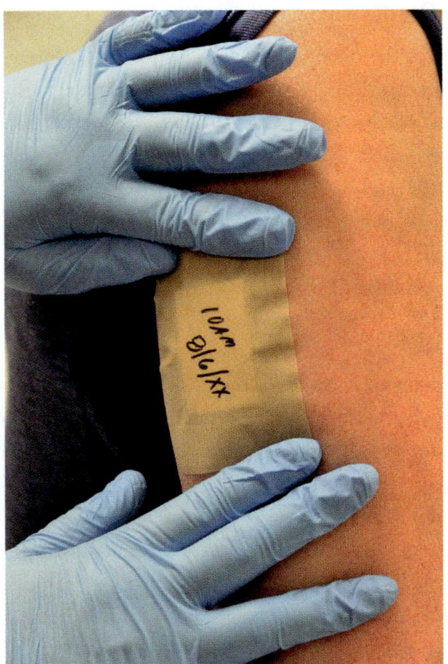

FIGURE 30.2 Transdermal patch.

Transdermal Route

Transdermal medications are placed on the skin and absorbed into the bloodstream. Transdermal medications are different from topical medications, which provide a **local** action. Transdermal medications provide a **systemic** action. The transdermal drug delivery system uses patches that adhere to the skin (Figure 30.2). Medication in the patch is slowly absorbed through the skin. Depending on the medication, the patch may be worn for a part of a day to many days.

When replacing a patch or teaching a patient to use transdermal patches, follow these steps:

1. Write the date and time on the new patch.
2. Wear gloves if changing a patch on another person.
3. Remove the old patch. Fold the sticky sides together and discard. If the old patch is not removed, the person may be at risk for an overdose.
4. Remove any residual medication from the skin using a tissue.
5. Decide where to apply the new patch. Select a different location. Depending on the medication, it may be on the shoulder, back, upper arm, lower abdomen, or hip. Clean and dry the new site.
6. Remove the protective liner on the patch. Do not use torn patches. Do not touch the sticky side of the patch.
7. Place the patch's sticky side on the skin. Press down on the patch to ensure it adheres to the skin. Make sure the patch is smooth, without folds.

Inhalation Route

Medications for the nose, throat, and lungs can be inhaled. The small particles of medication are aerosolized in a fine mist. The medication is inhaled and reaches the mucous membrane or alveoli in the lungs, where it is absorbed. Metered-dose inhalers (MDIs) and nebulizers are common devices for inhaled drugs. Many nebulized medications come in a premixed solution. If the medication is not premixed, normal saline is usually recommended to dilute the medication. (Chapter 41 discusses MDIs and nebulizers.)

Topical Route

Applying a drug to a mucous membrane or the skin is considered use of the *topical route*. Absorption through the mucous membrane is usually faster than through the skin. Topical medications provide a local effect.

Many times, when a drug is ordered to be applied "topically," it means that it should be applied to the skin. Topical drugs may also be administered by other routes. The provider will indicate a more specific route, such as rectal, vaginal, ophthalmic, nasal, or optic, for these medications.

When the medical assistant applies a topical medication to a patient's skin, it is important to do the following:

- Wear gloves.
- Use a sterile applicator (tongue blade or swab) to remove medication from the container. A new sterile applicator must be used each time to keep the container sterile.
- Rub creams gently into the skin, pat lotions onto the skin, and apply ointment using a sterile applicator.
- Liniments must be rubbed into the skin.
- For topical aerosol sprays, hold the bottle 3 to 6 inches from the skin and spray.

Vaginal Route

The vaginal route is used to insert suppositories, tablets, creams, and foams into the vagina. Typically, vaginal medications are used to treat local infections. Most medications can be inserted using the accompanying applicator. If no applicator is available, the patient should insert medications as is done with suppositories, using a finger. Usually, the medication must be inserted about 3 to 4 inches.

Vaginal instillation is most effective if the patient remains lying down after administration to prevent leakage. Many medications are intended to be used at bedtime. The patient may need to wear a pad to absorb drainage.

Rectal Route

Rectal medications are inserted into the rectum. Suppositories and enemas are the most common forms of rectal medications (Figure 30.3). The medication is absorbed slowly and irregularly through the rectal mucous membrane. This route is useful when a patient cannot tolerate oral medications or if the patient is constipated. It is important for the medical assistant to remind patients to give both the enema and suppository time to work before using the bathroom.

Sometimes a medical assistant needs to teach a patient about inserting suppositories. It is helpful for the patient to know what supplies are needed and where the supplies can be purchased. Supplies required include the suppository, gloves, and water-soluble jelly (KY jelly). Encourage the patient to review the storage directions for the suppositories. The following tips are helpful for inserting a suppository:

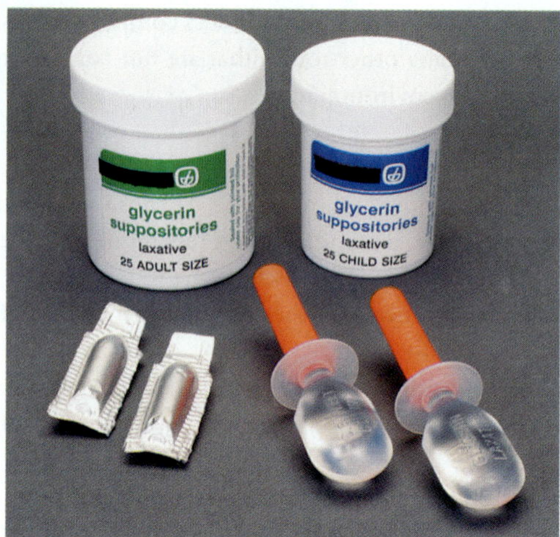

FIGURE 30.3 Rectal suppositories and enemas.

- Remove the wrapping from the suppository.
- Lubricate the pointed part of the suppository with water-soluble jelly.
- Be in the side-lying position, with the knee drawn up toward the chest.
- Carefully insert the suppository pointed side first.
- For adults and older children: Use the gloved index finger to push the medication in. Both vaginal and rectal suppositories should be inserted about 3 to 4 inches. Have the person slowly breathe to help with the discomfort.
- For small children: Use the gloved little finger to insert the medication. Rectal suppositories should be advanced about 2 inches.

CRITICAL THINKING APPLICATION 30.4

Gabe and Mark are working with Jana Green. She needs to have an intestinal procedure performed. To prepare, she needs to give herself an enema at home prior to the procedure. Why is it important for Gabe and Mark to provide her with information on how to do the procedure and where to purchase the supplies?

Nasal Route

Drugs given via the nasal route are breathed in through the nose. The medication is absorbed through the nasal mucous membrane. The medication can have local or systemic effects. If the medical assistant is administering the nasal medication, it is important to wear gloves. Patients should blow their noses prior to receiving the medication. They should sit in an upright position. The patient should sniff when the medication is given. Intranasal medications should be charted as "intranasal."

Ocular Route

Medication may be *instilled* (poured drop by drop) into the eye to treat an infection, soothe irritation, anesthetize the eye, or dilate the pupils before examination or treatment. Ophthalmic medications are available in different forms. Liquid drops usually are supplied in small squeeze bottles. The tip allows one drop at a time to be administered. Other bottles may have a dropper that is used to administer the medication. Eye ointments come in small, metal or plastic tubes. The tip allows a small ribbon of ointment to be administered along the inner lower eyelid margin.

When instilling eye medications, avoid injuring the eye. Do not touch the eye with the tip or applicator. Always keep the tip or applicator sterile. If it gets contaminated, discard the container. See Chapter 31 for more information on eye medication instillation.

Otic Route

Ear conditions can cause pain and make hearing difficult. Medication may be instilled into the ear to treat infection or inflammation or to soften cerumen. It is important to ensure that the ear drops get into the external canal. See Chapter 31 for more information on ear instillation.

Irrigation Route

Irrigation is also a route of administration. *Irrigation* means to bathe or flush open wounds or body cavities. Irrigation can be used to remove foreign bodies or debris. It can also be used to bathe the area with medication. Wound, eye, and ear irrigations are commonly seen in ambulatory care settings. (Chapter 31 discusses eye and ear irrigations.)

Eye irrigation is done to remove foreign bodies or to flush irritants (e.g., chemicals) from the eye. Irrigation of the external auditory canal will do the following:

- Remove excessive or impacted cerumen
- Remove a foreign body (contraindicated if the item will absorb fluid [e.g., bean, pea, or corn kernel])
- Treat the inflamed ear with an antiseptic solution

CRITICAL THINKING APPLICATION **30.5**

Aaron Jackson comes in with a dried pea stuck in his ear. Mark is excited to do an ear irrigation, but Gabe tells Mark that the provider may not order irrigation. Why might irrigation not be ordered for foreign bodies that can absorb fluid?

Parenteral Route

The *parenteral route* involves administration by infusion, injection, or implantation. In the ambulatory care environment, injections and infusions are common. Vaccine administration in primary care settings (e.g., family practice and internal medicine) is a frequent duty of medical assistants. Types of injections performed by medical assistants include the following:

- *Intramuscular* (IM): Administration within a muscle
- *Subcutaneous* (SUBQ): Administration beneath the skin
- *Intradermal* (ID): Administration within the dermis

The rest of the chapter will focus on the parenteral route. The following topics are discussed: injection supplies, medication preparation, site location, and medication administration. Chapter 51 discusses intravenous (IV) infusions and the role of the medical assistant. An *intravenous infusion* means fluid and medications are administered into a vein.

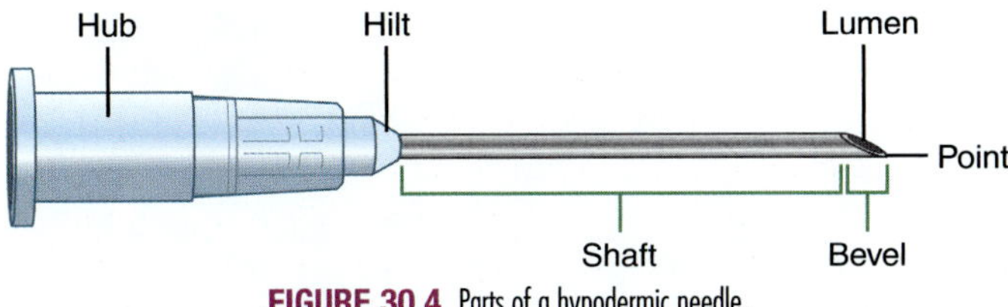

FIGURE 30.4 Parts of a hypodermic needle.

NEEDLES AND SYRINGES

When administering injectable medication, the medical assistant must use the correct needle and syringe. Using the correct technique to uncap, recap, and switch needles is important for infection control. The following sections discuss needles, syringes, and the correct techniques to use when working with them.

Hypodermic Needles

A hypodermic needle attaches to a hypodermic syringe. Hypodermic needles come with syringes or are packaged separately. The entire needle needs to remain sterile for the injection. It is important for the medical assistant to know the parts of the needle (Figure 30.4). The parts of a hypodermic needle include the following:

- *Hub*: Attaches or screws onto the syringe
- *Hilt*: Where the needle attaches
- *Bevel*: Slanted end of the shaft
- *Lumen*: Hollow space inside the needle; the size is indicated by the *gauge* number

Gauge and Length

Each needle has two measurements: the gauge (G) and the length. The lumen size is indicated by the gauge and is given a numeric value. The higher the gauge number, the smaller the lumen. The thickness of the needle wall increases along with the lumen size. This means that an 18 G needle makes a larger hole than a 25 G needle. The 18 G needle has a thicker wall than the 25 G needle. As the gauge number increases, the needles bend more easily. Thicker-walled needles (smaller gauge numbers) are used for deeper injections. Thinner-walled needles (larger gauge numbers) are used for more superficial injections.

The medication's **viscosity** is also an important factor when selecting the gauge of the needle. A medication with a syrupy thickness (high viscosity) would be harder to push out of a needle compared with a medication as thin as water. Using a wider lumen needle (smaller gauge number) would be better for thicker medications. Using a finer lumen needle (a larger gauge number) would be more appropriate for watery medications.

The needle length refers to the length of the shaft. The needle length used is dependent on the type of injection given and the size of the patient. The length of the needle for an intradermal injection is smaller than that used for an intramuscular injection. The length of an intramuscular injection needle for a 300-pound person would be longer than that for a 100-pound person. Knowing the length and gauge required for an injection are important information for the medical assistant.

Safety Needles

Due to the Needlestick Safety and Prevention Act, safety needles are common in the ambulatory care setting. Safety needles are designed

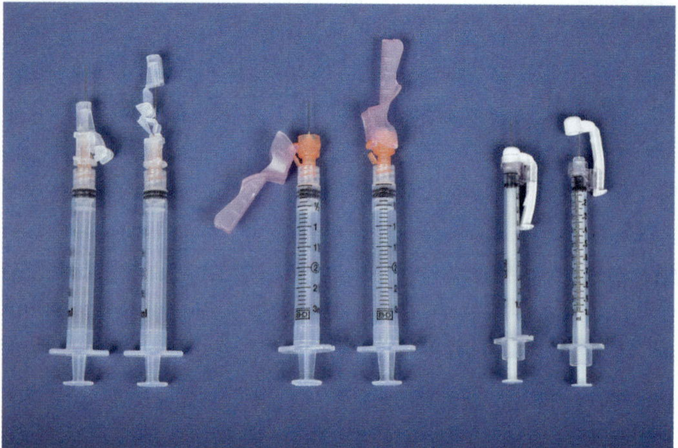

FIGURE 30.5 Protective sheaths and hinged needle shields must be activated by the healthcare professional. Each type of needle is shown before the injection and after the safety device has been activated.

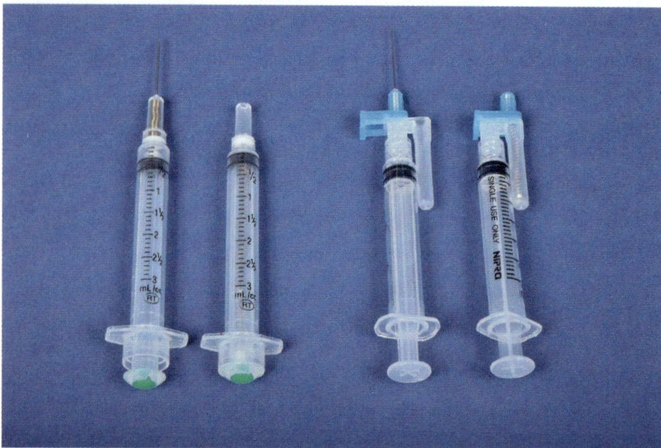

FIGURE 30.6 With retractable needles, the needle is retracted into the syringe or another chamber. Each type of needle is shown before the injection and after the needle has been retracted.

to reduce the risk of needlesticks after an injection. A *passive safety needle* is designed so that the needle is automatically covered after the injection. Passive safety needles are currently used with insulin pens (e.g., the BD AutoShield Duo pen needle). An *active safety needle* requires the healthcare professional to activate the safety device. These are most common for injections. Current active safety needles fall into two groups:

- *Protective sheaths and hinged needle shields*: The safety device is a sleeve over the syringe barrel or a hinged needle shield (Figure 30.5). These devices are moved over the needle after the injection. Once they are in place, the needle cannot be uncovered. The risk of needlesticks decreases if the safety device is activated with the hand holding the syringe.
- *Retractable needles*: After the injection, the healthcare professional activates a device that retracts the needle either into the syringe or into another chamber (Figure 30.6).

Hypodermic Syringes

Hypodermic syringes attach to needles and hold the medication for the injection. They come in many sizes (e.g., 1, 3, 5, 6, 10, and 12 mL), but usually, the facility only stocks three or four sizes (Figure 30.7). Figure 30.8 shows the parts of the syringe. Syringes can have either a Luer-Lok tip or a slip tip (Figure 30.9). Calibration marks

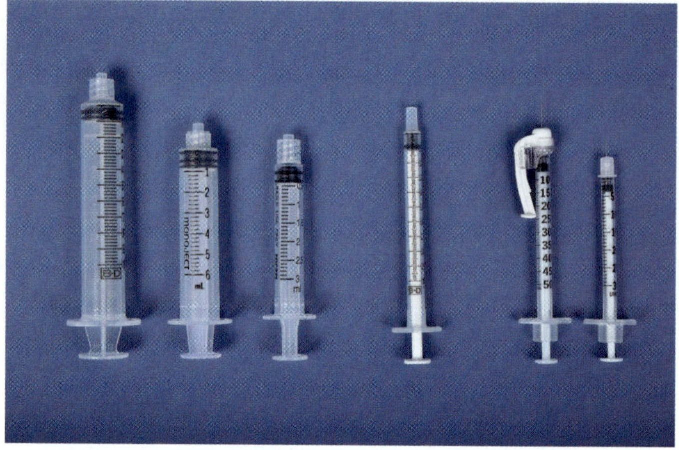

FIGURE 30.7 Syringes come in various sizes. Some come with the needles attached.

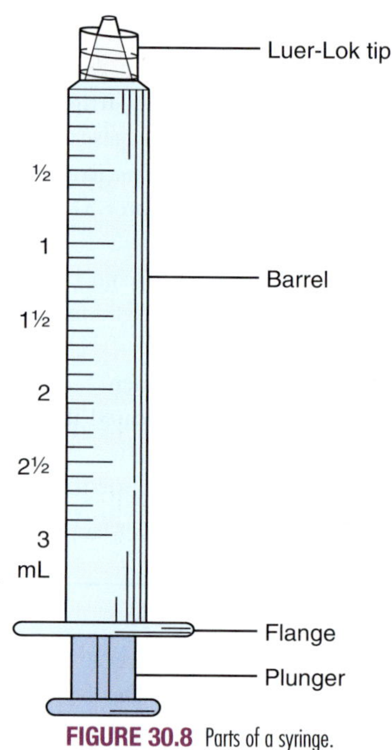

FIGURE 30.8 Parts of a syringe.

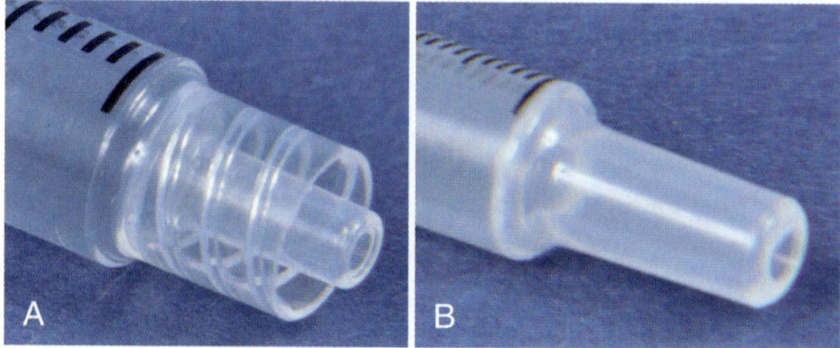

FIGURE 30.9 **(A)** Luer-Lok. **(B)** Slip tip.

are on the barrel of the syringe. It is important for the medical assistant to be able to read medication amounts in syringes.

WORKING WITH THE NEEDLE AND SYRINGE

Syringes come packaged in different ways:

- A syringe can be packaged without a needle. A needle must be added to the syringe when giving an injection.

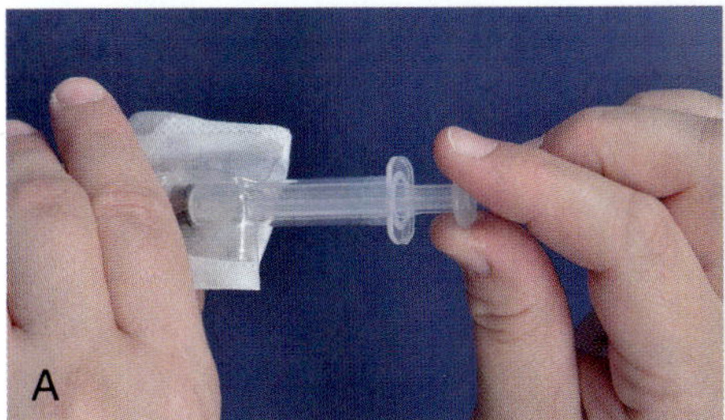

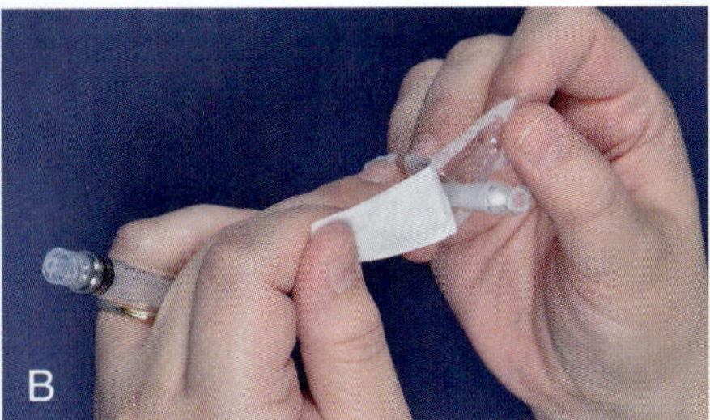

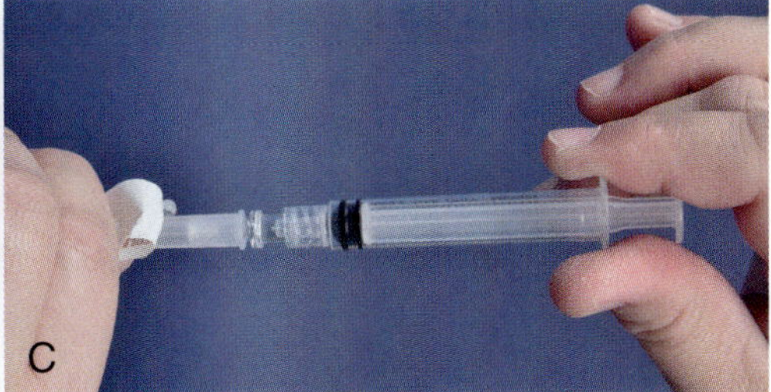

FIGURE 30.10 **(A)** When removing the syringe from the packaging, just touch the flange or barrel. **(B)** Place the syringe between your fingers with the tip face away from your fingers. Then open the needle package. **(C)** Hold down the packaging flaps to prevent contamination of the needle. Attach the syringe.

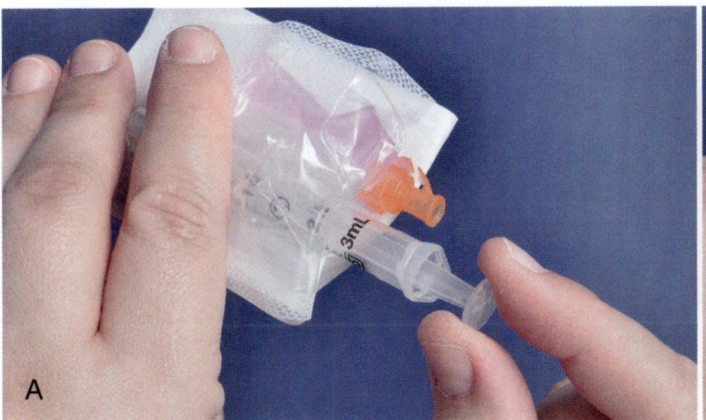

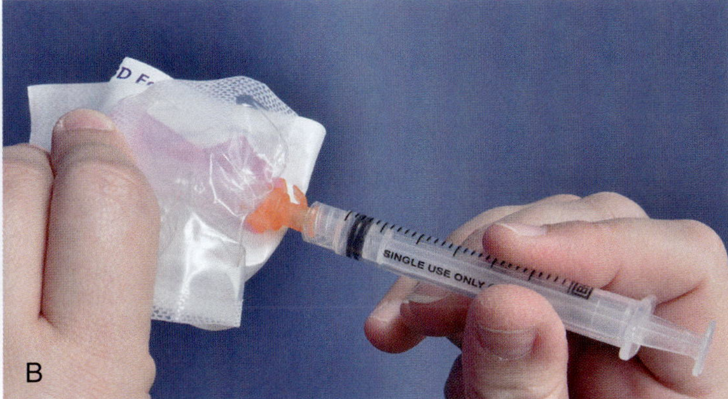

FIGURE 30.11 **(A)** Remove the syringe without touching the needle. **(B)** Continue to hold down the packaging flaps, and attach the needle to the syringe.

- A syringe may be packaged with a needle that is not attached. The unit must be assembled.
- A syringe and needle unit may come preassembled. Always tighten the needle on the syringe before using the unit.

The needle and syringe can be assembled with clean, ungloved hands.

When a syringe is packaged by itself, first open the syringe. When removing the syringe from the packaging, it is important not to touch the syringe tip to anything (Figure 30.10A). The tip needs to remain sterile because it attaches to the needle. The syringe should be held until the needle is attached. As you are holding the syringe between your middle and ring fingers, use your thumbs and index fingers to open the needle package (Figure 30.10B). It is important to hold down the packaging flaps to prevent contamination of the needle. Attach the syringe to the needle and lift the needle out of the package (Figure 30.10C). The needle and syringe unit can be placed on the counter. The needle cover should remain on to protect the sterility of the needle.

When the needle and syringe are packaged together but not assembled, carefully open the packaging. Hold down the packaging flaps. Angle the contents so the syringe can be grasped without going over or touching the needle (Figure 30.11A). Remove the syringe, then attach it to the needle (Figure 30.11B). Remove the needle from the packaging. Once the syringe and needle are assembled, the unit can be placed on the counter.

When working with the plunger, only touch the section that remains outside of the syringe when the plunger is completely pushed in (Figure 30.12). Touching the plunger that goes inside the barrel could potentially contaminate the medication.

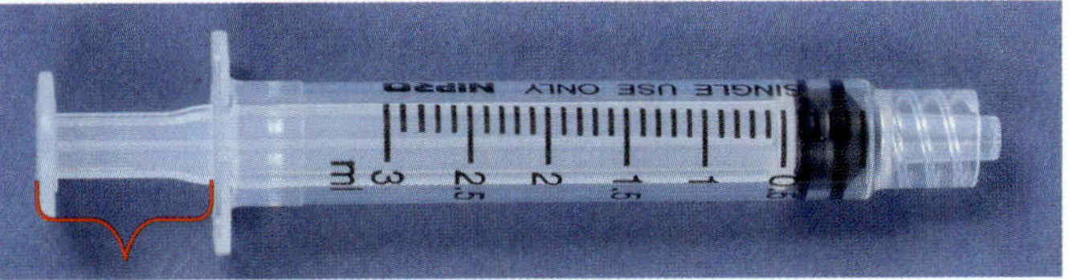

FIGURE 30.12 Touch only the part of the plunger that is outside of the barrel.

Uncapping and Recapping Needles

Never recap a needle that has been used on a patient. Needles can be recapped until they are used on a patient. As you prepare medication, you will need to uncap and recap the needle. It is important to maintain the sterility of the needle. If there is any doubt, consider the needle contaminated and replace it with a new one.

- *To uncap*: Hold the cover between the fingers and thumb of your nondominant hand. Hold the syringe with the fingers and thumb of your dominant hand. Pull your hands apart horizontally (side to side) in a smooth continuous motion (Figure 30.13A).
- *To recap*: Use the one-handed scoop technique. Place the cover on a firm, flat surface. If the cover rolls, place a finger of your nondominant hand at the far end of the cover. This will keep the cover in place. Carefully insert the needle into the cover. If the needle touches the outside surface of the cover or any other surface, it is contaminated and must be replaced. Scoop up the cover and secure the cover onto the needle (Figure 30.13B).

Switching Needles

When switching needles, it is important not to give yourself a needlestick and to protect the sterility of the new needle. Several methods

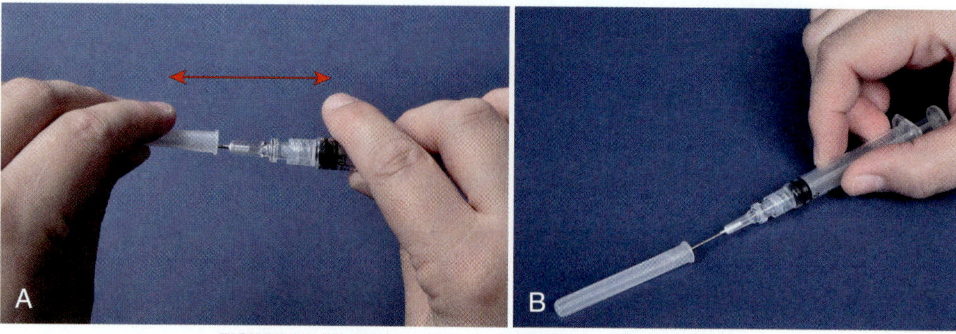

FIGURE 30.13 **(A)** Uncapping a needle. **(B)** One-handed scoop technique.

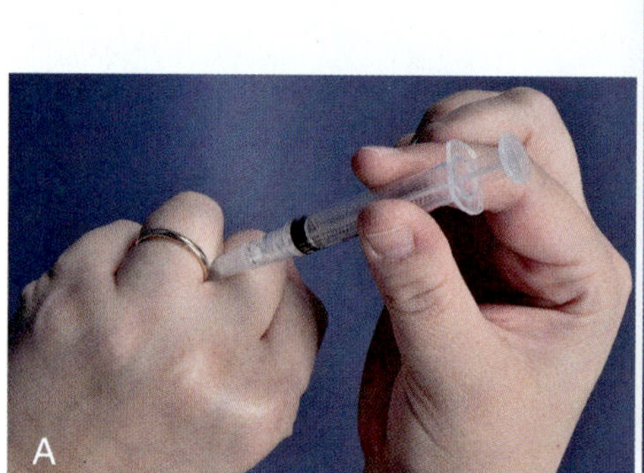

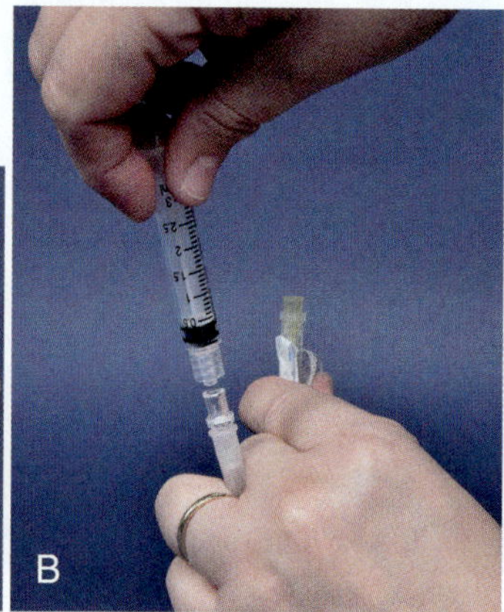

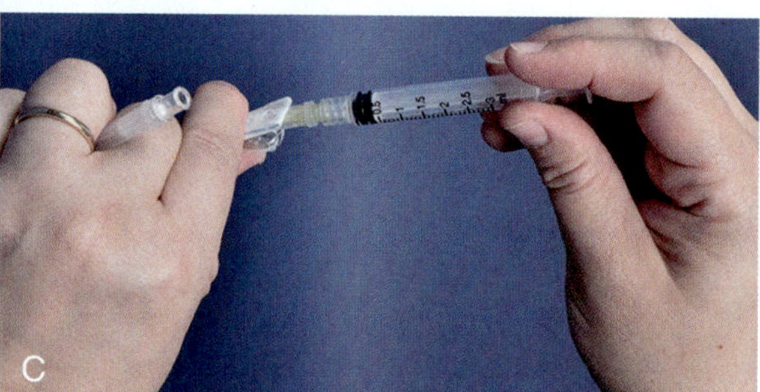

FIGURE 30.14 **(A)** Place the syringe unit between the fingers of your nondominant hand, and firmly grasp the covered needle. **(B)** Hold the old covered needle securely as you detach it from the syringe. **(C)** Attach the new needle while holding the old needle between your fingers.

are used to switch needles. One method includes opening the new needle package. Hold the packaging flaps down with the index finger and thumb of your nondominant hand. With your dominant hand, place the syringe with the covered needle between the middle and ring fingers of your nondominant hand (Figure 30.14A). Firmly grasp the covered needle in your palm. The syringe should be above the top of your hand. With your dominant hand, remove the syringe from the old needle and attach it to the new needle (Figure 30.14B–C). Your nondominant hand should be holding both needles the entire time. Discard the old needle into the biohazardous sharps container.

PREPARING PARENTERAL MEDICATION

As with all medication preparation, it is important to be in a well-lit room and free from distraction. The medical assistant must be focused on the procedure to reduce the risk of errors. For all parenteral medications, do the following:

- If the medication looks abnormal in color or clarity, discard it.
- Some medications will have **precipitate** at the bottom of the vial. If this is normal for that medication, make sure to mix it prior to withdrawing the medication. If the precipitate is abnormal, a chemical reaction may have occurred. The vial needs to be discarded.
- If the medication has expired, discard it.
- If the medication is no longer sterile, discard it.

Using an Ampule

Ampules contain a single dose of medication. They may contain more than the patient needs. The extra medication is wasted. Medications in ampules react to other substances and require the all-glass environment to remain stable. An ampule has a prescored neck, which is snapped off during the preparation process. An ampule opener or breaker is a safety device used to snap off the top of the ampule (Figure 30.15). A filter needle on a syringe is used to **aspirate** the medication into the syringe. This needle has a small filter that catches glass particles before they enter the syringe barrel. The filter needle must be removed before the injection is given to the patient. Procedure 30.2 describes the steps required to prepare medication from an ampule.

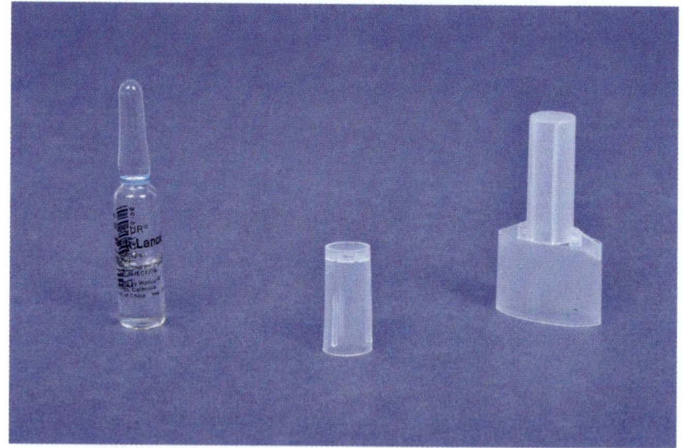

FIGURE 30.15 An ampule with two different ampule openers/breakers.

Using a Prefilled Sterile Cartridge

A prefilled, sterile cartridge comes filled with a single dose of medication. It is not uncommon for the medication in the syringe to be more than what the provider ordered. The cartridge may come with

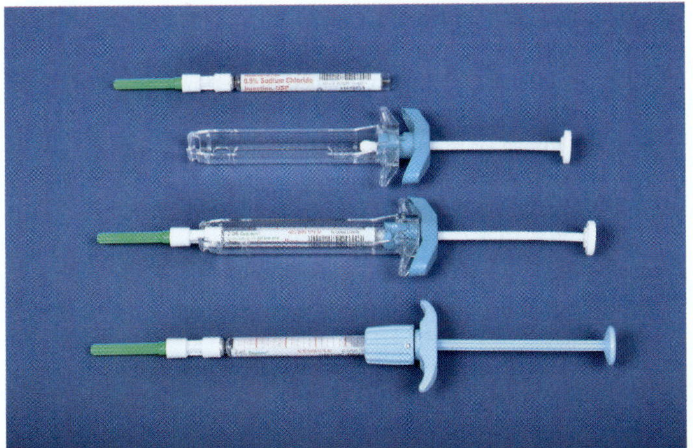

FIGURE 30.16 Top to bottom: Prefilled syringe, Carpuject holder, prefilled syringe in a Carpuject holder, and a prefilled syringe in a Tubex cartridge holder.

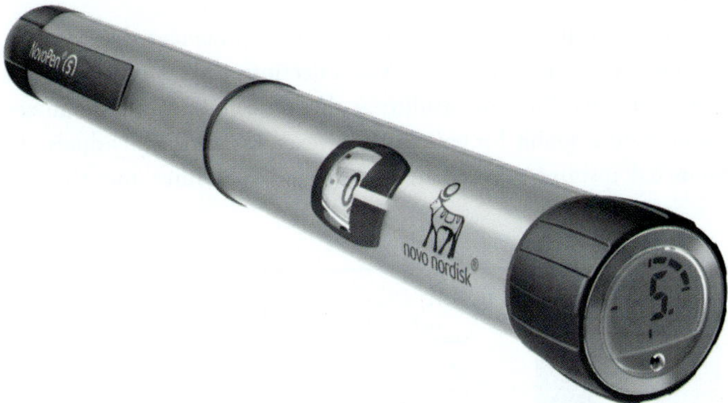

FIGURE 30.17 NovoPens use insulin cartridges. Patients change the cartridges and retain the pen.

or without a needle. A safety needle can be attached to the Luer-Lok on the prefilled cartridge. A reusable cartridge holder (e.g., Carpuject or Tubex) is needed to dispense the medication (Figure 30.16). The medical assistant must assemble the cartridge and the reusable cartridge holder prior to administering the medication. Procedure 30.3 describes how to use a Carpuject holder and prepare the medication.

Specialty Syringe Units

Specialty syringe units are designed so that patients can administer their own medication. Different types of syringe units are available. Figure 30.17 shows an insulin pen. The dose of insulin required can be set by the dial. The patient needs to change the needle with each dose. Insulin pens cannot be shared between patients.

The EpiPen and other epinephrine pens are automatic injector systems (Figure 30.18). The pens are dosed for adults or children. People at risk for anaphylactic reactions (e.g., from food allergens, bee stings) should carry epinephrine pens to prevent a fatal reaction. Simulators can accompany some of the injector systems. These are useful when teaching patients how to give their own injections.

Using a Vial

A vial is a plastic or glass container with a rubber stopper that is covered by a cap. Vials contain powdered or liquid medications. Liquid medication is more common. The liquid can be a parenteral medication, sterile *normal saline* (0.9% sodium chloride), or sterile water. Vials come in single dose or multidose (Figure 30.19). Single-dose or

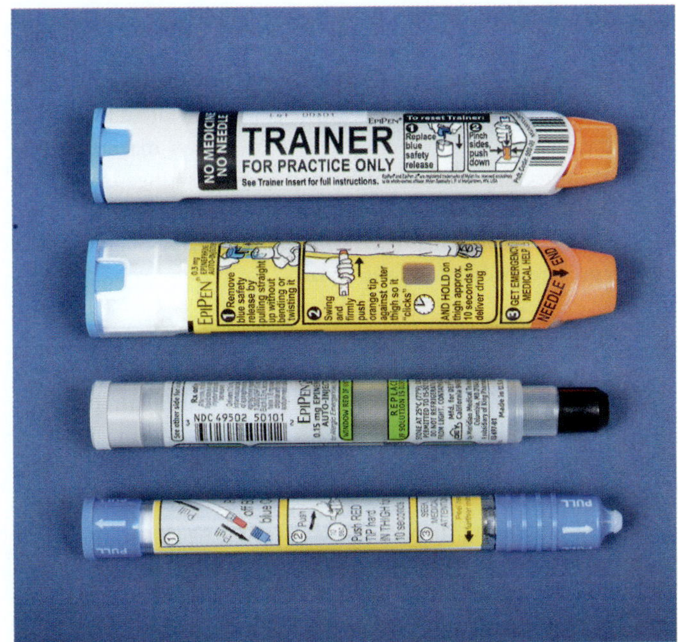

FIGURE 30.18 *Top to bottom:* EpiPen trainer, EpiPen for older children and adults, EpiPen Jr for children, and a generic epinephrine pen.

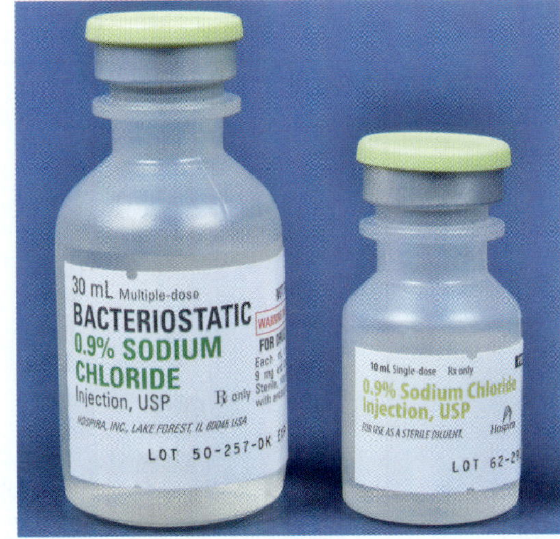

FIGURE 30.19 Multidose and single-dose vials.

single-use vials are only good for a single patient and a single injection procedure. If the vial needs to be entered more than once for a single patient as part of a single procedure, then a new needle and syringe must be used. Discard the vial after the procedure. Single-dose vials do not contain any ingredients that would prohibit microorganism growth. Thus, they are only good for a single use.

Multidose vials contain many doses of medication. The label will clearly state that the vial is a multidose vial. These vials contain an antimicrobial preservative that prevents the growth of bacteria. The preservative does not help protect the fluid against viruses and other sources of contamination if safe injection practices are not followed. When multidose vials are opened (the cap is removed or the stopper is punctured), they are only good for 28 days (unless the manufacturer states otherwise). The new expiration date should be written on the label. If the manufacturer's expiration date comes sooner than 28 days, then the earlier date must be used.

Each time the multidose vial is entered, the rubber stopper must be disinfected, and a sterile needle and syringe must be used. The vial is under pressure. You need to add air into the vial before you draw out the amount of liquid you need. The amount of air added should equal the amount of liquid you draw out. Always make sure you have the correct amount of medication in your syringe before you withdraw the needle. Never inject unneeded medication back into the vial once the needle has been removed. Procedure 30.4 describes how to prepare medication from a vial.

Reconstituting Powdered Medication

As previously mentioned, vials can contain powdered medication. A powdered medication needs to be mixed with a **diluent.** Typically, sterile normal saline or sterile water is used as a diluent, although other medications may also be used (according to the provider's order and the manufacturer's directions). The most common powdered medications in primary care are live-virus vaccines. These need to be **reconstituted** (Procedure 30.5).

If the vial is a multidose vial, it is important to write the expiration date on the label. The expiration dates for reconstituted medications will vary. See the manufacturer's insert for the length of time that the medication will remain stable after reconstitution. Besides the expiration date, include your initials and the fluid that was used to reconstitute the medication. These three pieces of information need to be on the multidose label.

There are four major steps in reconstituting powdered medication and withdrawing a dose of the medication (Figure 30.20):

- *Step 1:* Remove air from the powdered medication vial and put air into the diluent vial.
- *Step 2:* Withdraw liquid from the diluent vial and add it to the powdered medication vial.
- *Step 3:* Mix the liquid with the powdered medication.
- *Step 4:* Add in air and withdraw the dose needed.

CRITICAL THINKING APPLICATION 30.6

Mark struggles to remember the steps to reconstitute powdered medication. What are the steps?

Mixing Insulins

Patients with diabetes may use insulin to help manage their disease. Taking insulin requires about four injections a day. Some patients may need two different insulins at the same time. Many premixed insulins are available for patients. However, for some individuals, the premixed insulins are not an option, and they must mix the two

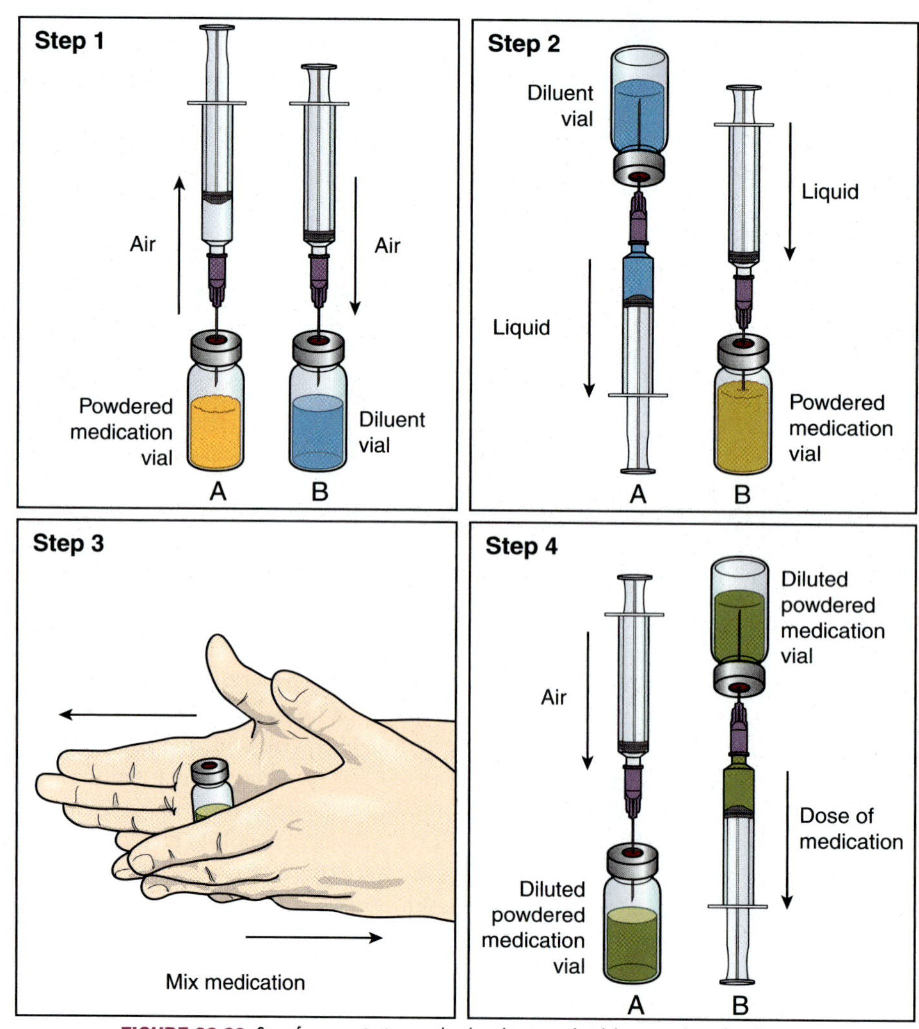

FIGURE 30.20 Steps for reconstituting powdered medication and withdrawing a dose of medication.

insulins in one syringe. During this combination process, it is important that the vials do not become contaminated with another type of insulin. If by chance contamination occurs, it is better for the rapid-acting or short-acting insulin (Regular insulin) to be mixed in the intermediate-acting insulin vial (e.g., NPH insulin). This means that Regular insulin must be drawn up in the syringe first, and then NPH is added (Figure 30.21). Procedure 30.6 describes the steps for mixing two insulins in one syringe.

Depending on state laws and facility policies, administering insulin may be within the medical assistant's scope of practice. Understanding how to mix two insulins in the same syringe is important. Not all insulins can be mixed. Use drug reference information to ensure that the two insulins ordered can be mixed.

As discussed earlier, insulin is measured in units. Special insulin syringes are available to measure small or large insulin dosages. Insulin is typically stored in the refrigerator and should be warmed to room temperature prior to administration. Cloudy insulins (e.g., NPH) are suspensions and need to be mixed before drawing up the insulin. Mix cloudy insulins by gently rolling the vial between your hands. Clear insulin (e.g., Regular insulin) does not need to be mixed or rolled in your hand.

Patients receiving insulin must rotate their injection sites. This prevents tissue damage and absorption issues with the insulin. It might be helpful for patients to mark the site of the last injection with a spot bandage or a piece of tape. The easiest way to rotate sites is to give subsequent injections in a circular pattern around the first injection site in a specific location. The goal is to avoid using the same location again for another month.

CRITICAL THINKING APPLICATION 30.7

Mark struggles to remember the order for drawing up insulin. What might be a few good ways to remember the process of drawing up two insulins in the same syringe?

GIVING PARENTERAL MEDICATIONS

Some medications can be given by several routes. Other medications can only be given by injection. Parenteral medication administration has several advantages:

- It is useful when the patient has gastrointestinal distress or is unconscious.
- It offers good absorption compared with other routes, such as the oral route.
- The *onset* (time medication starts working) is more rapid than with other routes.
- Some types of parenteral medications have a longer *duration time* (time the medication works in the body).

Pain with the injection and a risk of infection due to the injection are disadvantages of parenteral medications. Another disadvantage is an unpredictable absorption rate for those with poor circulation (e.g., patients with peripheral artery disease, diabetes, obesity, or Raynaud disease).

When it comes to giving injections, you will gain confidence, and it will become easy over time. Always do the following:

- Follow the nine rights of medication administration.
- Check the medication's label against the order three times.
- Know about the medication you are giving. (What is it, why is it being ordered, how is it given, and what are the common side effects?)
- Label all syringes with the name of the medication they contain.
- Follow medical asepsis and the Bloodborne Pathogens Standard established by the Occupational Safety and Health Administration (OSHA).
- Ensure that the needle is not directed at your hand holding the patient when giving an injection. Slight movement may cause a needlestick.

Following these guidelines will help you perform injections safely and protect your patient from medication errors.

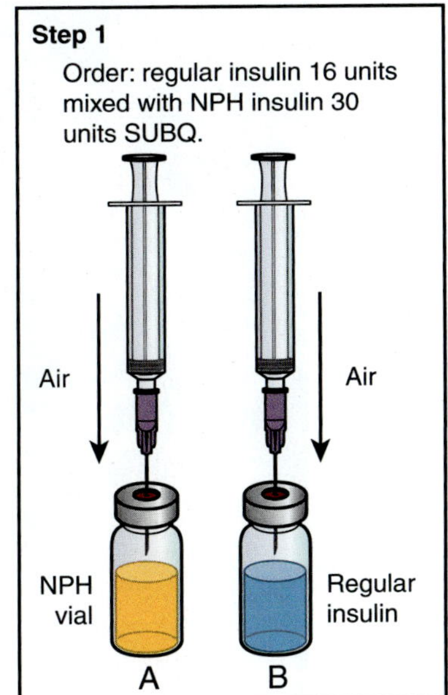

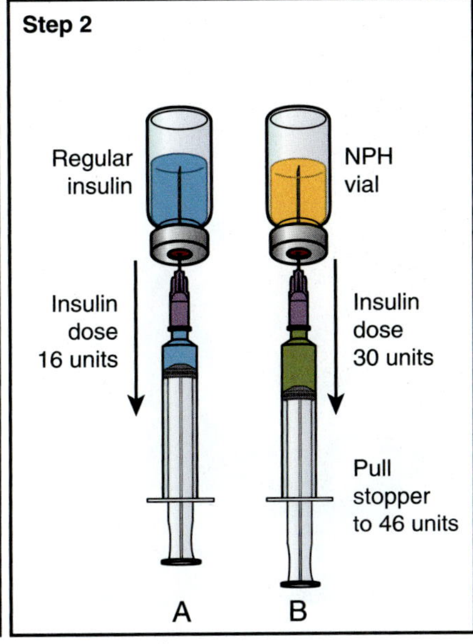

FIGURE 30.21 Mixing two insulins.

Guidelines for Parenteral Medications

Prepare and store medications in a separate area, away from the exam rooms. Medications can be prepared without the use of gloves. Ensure that all needles are tightly covered and placed on a tray when carrying them to the exam room. Never transport medication in your pockets. Bring only one patient's medication at a time to avoid confusion and error.

Follow these guidelines when selecting an injection site:

- Never give an injection near bones or blood vessels.
- Avoid scar tissue, a change in skin pigmentation or texture, or abnormal growth (e.g., mole or wart).
- Avoid abrasions, lesions, wounds, bruises, and edematous areas.
- Select a site that is large enough to hold the amount of medication injected.
- Avoid sites recently used (within the last month).

According to the Immunization Action Coalition (www.immunize.org), it is safe to give SUBQ and IM vaccines into a tattoo. However, it is not a good idea to inject into a newly tattooed area. If you must inject into a tattooed area, attempt to use a lighter pigmented area. All injections pose the risk of a reaction or an infection at the injection site. Dark pigments may mask a reaction or an infection.

Reducing Pain and Anxiety

To minimize pain with injections, insert SUBQ and IM needles swiftly. Inject the medication at the rate of 10 seconds per 1 mL to avoid unnecessary discomfort. Remove the needle quickly, using the same angle as for entry.

Various techniques can be used to reduce a patient's pain and anxiety about injections:

- Give a sugar-coated pacifier or sugar water (must be ordered by the provider), which helps soothe children under the age of 1 after injections.
- Apply a topical anesthetic skin refrigerant (e.g., Pain Ease), which works immediately (Figure 30.22).
- Apply a topical anesthetic (e.g., EMLA cream) at the injection site, which works in about 30 to 40 minutes.
- Talk with the patient to distract them from the procedure.
- Have patients move their toes or fingers on the extremity receiving the IM injection. (Have a patient "play the piano" with their fingers when giving a deltoid injection.)
- Administer the most painful injection last.
- Use products that provide cold and vibration sensations (e.g., Buzzy), which overwhelm the nerves affected by the injection (Figure 30.23).

CRITICAL THINKING APPLICATION **30.8**

Gabe talks with Mark about distractions to use when giving IM injections. He mentions having patients wiggle their toes or move their fingers when an injection is given on that extremity. He explains that he tells the patient about the movement prior to starting the injection. Gabe reminds the patient when he is aspirating, just prior to injecting the medication. What might be the benefit of reminding the patient when aspirating?

Special Situations

Even if the procedure was done correctly, sometimes things can go wrong. It is important for the medical assistant to know what to do in those situations.

If a needle breaks during an injection or separates from the syringe, pull out the needle if it is visible. Discard the needle in the biohazardous sharps container. If the needle breaks off and is not visible, mark the spot with a pen and yell for help. If the injection was given in the arm, place a tourniquet above the spot to prevent the needle from moving in the body. Notify the provider immediately.

With intramuscular injections, sometimes the bone can be hit during the procedure. If this occurs, pull the needle out about one-quarter inch and give the medication.

With any medication, a patient can experience an anaphylactic reaction. *Anaphylaxis* is a severe allergic reaction that can be life-threatening. Having the patient wait 15 minutes after an injection allows you to monitor for unusual symptoms. Symptoms include the following:

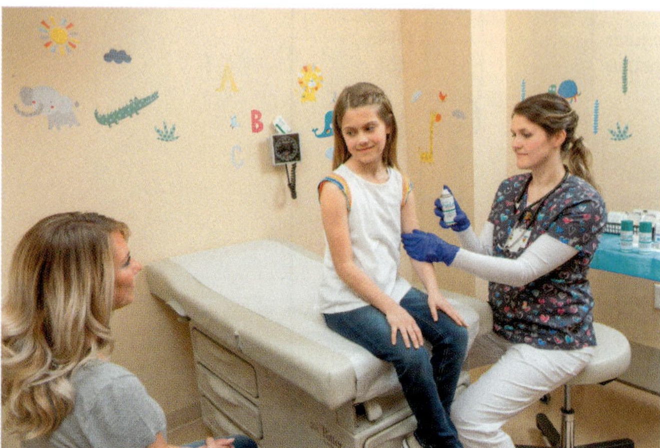

FIGURE 30.22 Topical anesthetic skin refrigerant spray. (Courtesy Gebauer-Tri-Point-Medical, Cleveland, OH.)

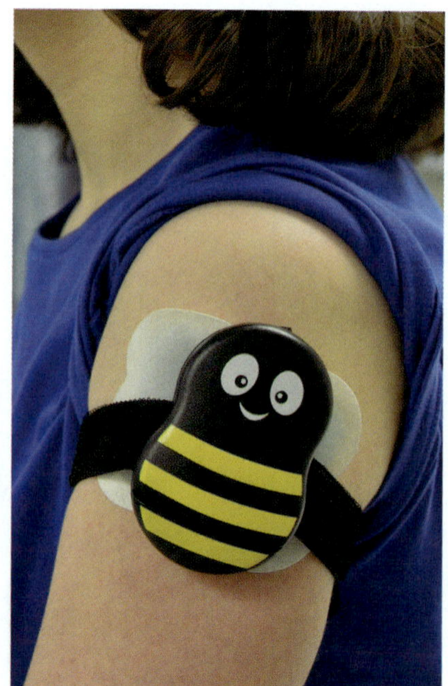

FIGURE 30.23 Buzzy helps reduce pain naturally by overwhelming the nerves with vibration and cold sensations.

- Warm feeling, flushing, throat tightening, difficulty swallowing, cough
- Shortness of breath, *dyspnea* (difficulty breathing), wheezing
- Anxiety, loss of consciousness, shock
- Pain or cramping, vomiting, diarrhea, palpitations, dizziness

If the patient is experiencing any unusual symptoms, it is important to tell the provider immediately. The first-line medication for anaphylaxis is epinephrine.

INTRADERMAL TUBERCULIN TESTING

Intradermal (ID) injections are given just under the epidermis (Figure 30.24). Because the drug is dispersed in an area where many nerves are present, it causes momentary burning or stinging. Small amounts of medication are injected. Figure 30.25 show sites recommended for intradermal injections. Table 30.1 contains a summary of intradermal injection information. In ambulatory care, intradermal injections may be given for the Mantoux tuberculin skin test (TST) and allergy testing. (Allergy testing is described in Chapter 33.)

Two types of tuberculin tests have been approved by the FDA: the skin test and the blood test. The TST is used to determine whether a patient is infected with *Mycobacterium tuberculosis*. It is important for the medical assistant to be knowledgeable about and skilled at administering and reading the test.

Tuberculin Skin Testing

The TST can be given to most patients, including infants, pregnant women, patients infected with the human immunodeficiency virus (HIV), and those vaccinated with bacillus Calmette-Guérin (BCG). Patients with a history of BCG vaccination may have a positive reaction to the TST. If a patient mentions a history of receiving BCG vaccine, it is important for the medical assistant to inform the

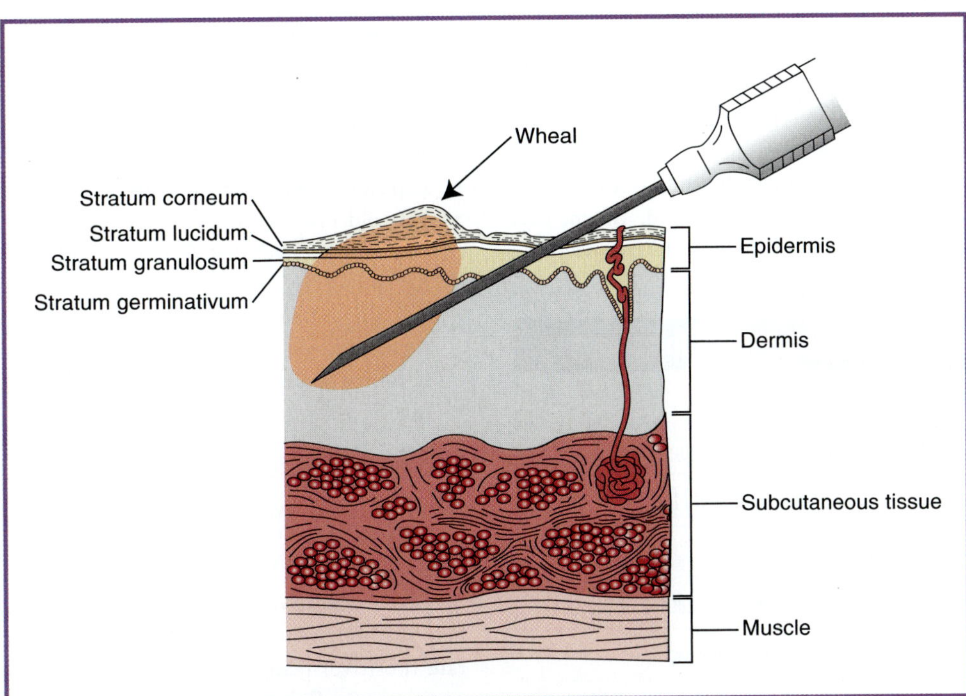

FIGURE 30.24 The intradermal (ID) injection is administered just under the epidermis.

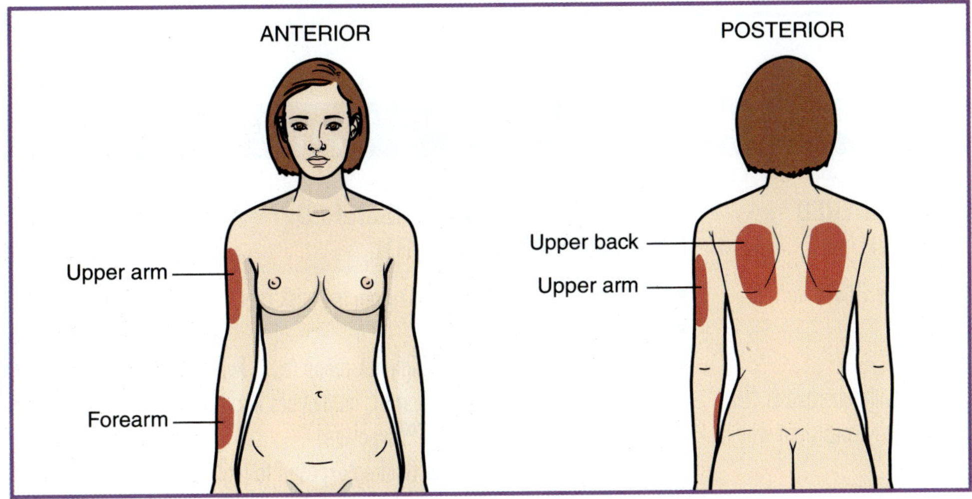

FIGURE 30.25 Sites recommended for intradermal injections.

provider before performing the skin test. The provider may opt to have the patient undergo the blood test instead.

The TST is contraindicated in patients who had the following:

- A severe reaction to a past TST (e.g., necrosis, ulcers, blisters, or anaphylaxis)
- A history of a positive TST result
- A live-virus vaccine less than 4 to 6 weeks earlier (A TST and a live-virus vaccine can be given on the same day, or the TST can be given 4 to 6 weeks after the vaccine.)

Tuberculin Skin Test Procedure and Reading

To perform the TST, tuberculin purified protein derivative (PPD) 0.1 mL is given ID into the inner surface of the forearm (Procedure 30.7). A tuberculin syringe and needle, with the bevel facing upward, are used to slowly inject the PPD, creating a tense, pale **wheal.** The wheal must measure 6 to 10 mm in diameter, or the test must be repeated.

The patient returns within 48 to 72 hours to have the test read. Reading before or after this time invalidates the results. When reading the test, palpate the site to check for a raised, hardened area, called an **induration**. If an induration is felt, measure the raised area across the forearm (perpendicular to the bone). The *erythema* (redness) is not measured. The diameter of the induration is read in millimeters (mm) and must be noted in the health record. The medical assistant can never state whether the test result is positive or negative.

TABLE 30.1 Summary of Intradermal Injections

Syringe used	1 mL (tuberculin syringe)
Needle size	¼ to ½ inch; 25–27 gauge
Angle of entry	5 to 15 degrees with bevel facing upward
Maximum volume	0.1 mL
Common sites	Forearm, upper arm, and middle of the back
Additional sites	Separate by at least 2 inches
Patient position	Sitting with arm extended if using forearm
Administration	Pull skin taut at injection site

The provider uses the test results and the patient history to determine if the patient has tuberculosis (TB). A TST reading between 5 and 15 mm can be positive for different populations. Table 30.2 describes the different populations.

Incorrect Tuberculin Skin Test Readings

At times, the TST reading may be incorrect. A *false-positive reaction* means the person reacted to the test even though no *M. tuberculosis* is present. Reasons for false-positive reactions with TST include the following:

- Lung infection with nontuberculous mycobacteria (NTM). This organism is found in the water and soil and is inhaled.
- Previous vaccination with BCG vaccine. Many foreign-born patients from countries with a high risk of TB may have received BCG abroad. The BCG vaccine has been approved by the FDA, but it is used in very limited situations.
- Incorrect administration or reading of the TST.

A *false-negative reaction* means the person may not have reacted to the test, even though the patient is infected with *M. tuberculosis*. Reasons for false-negative results with TST include the following:

- Weakened immune system
- Exposure to TB infection within the previous 8 to 10 weeks
- Very old TB infection
- Patient is younger than 6 months old
- Recently received a live-virus vaccine (e.g., measles, yellow fever, chickenpox), or had a viral infection (e.g., influenza), or received corticosteroids or immunosuppressive medications (a false reaction may occur up to 5 to 6 weeks afterward)
- Incorrect administration or reading of TST

Two-Step Testing

In some patients who have had a TB infection, the body forgets to react to the TST. This can occur if the infection was many years before. The initial TST may be negative, and the person may have a false-negative reaction. Receiving a second TST can help the body remember the infection, thus causing a more accurate (positive) reading. This is called the *booster effect* or *booster phenomenon*. The second TST can be done 1 to 3 weeks after the initial test was read.

New residents in long-term care facilities (e.g., nursing homes) usually have a two-step TST done. Healthcare students and

TABLE 30.2 Tuberculin Skin Reaction Categories

INDURATION ≥5 MM CONSIDERED POSITIVE IN PATIENTS WITH	INDURATION ≥10 MM CONSIDERED POSITIVE IN PATIENTS WITH	INDURATION ≥15 MM CONSIDERED POSITIVE IN PATIENTS WITH
• Human immunodeficiency virus (HIV) infection • Organ transplant • Immunosuppression • Recent contact with a person with tuberculosis (TB) • Fibrotic changes on a chest x-ray consistent with prior TB	• Recent immigrants (<5 years) from high-risk areas • Injection drug users • People living or working in high-risk areas (e.g., living in a group setting [jail, nursing home], employees in a clinical position with a high risk of TB exposure) • Children <4 years of age or children exposed to high-risk adults	• No known risk for TB

From Centers for Disease Control and Prevention (CDC), www.cdc.gov/tb/publications/factsheets/testing/skintesting.htm.

professionals also need to have a two-step TST. Once the two-step TST has been completed, they need yearly TSTs. If the time since the last TST exceeds 1 year, they may need to complete another two-step TST. Figure 30.26 shows what occurs if the initial test result is positive or negative.

Tuberculin Blood Tests

The FDA has approved two tuberculin blood tests: the the QuantiFERON-TB Gold Plus (QFT-Plus) test and the T-SPOT.TB test. If a patient has had the BCG vaccine or is unable to return for the skin test reading, the blood test is preferred. The blood test replaces the skin test. A healthcare professional or student only needs one blood test initially, unlike the two-step skin test. After the initial test, a yearly skin or tuberculin blood test is required.

After the medical assistant draws a patient's blood, it is sent to the laboratory for analysis. The error rate with a blood test is much lower than with the palpated, measured reading of the TST. The next step will depend on whether the TB blood test result is positive or negative:

- *Positive*: The person has been infected with TB. The provider will order additional tests to determine if the person has a latent TB infection or TB disease. (See Chapter 41 for more information on these two diseases.)
- *Negative*: It is unlikely the person has TB.

CRITICAL THINKING APPLICATION 30.9

Gabe and Mark are working with Julia Berkley, who has come in for a physical prior to starting college. She is going into the healthcare field, and her paperwork indicates that she needs a two-step TB skin test. Julia asks what this means. How might you explain a two-step TB skin test?

SUBCUTANEOUS INJECTIONS

Subcutaneous (SUBQ) injections involve placing medication into the subcutaneous layer under the dermis (Figure 30.27). The subcutaneous layer has fewer blood vessels than the muscles do. The medication absorbs more slowly in the subcutaneous layer compared with

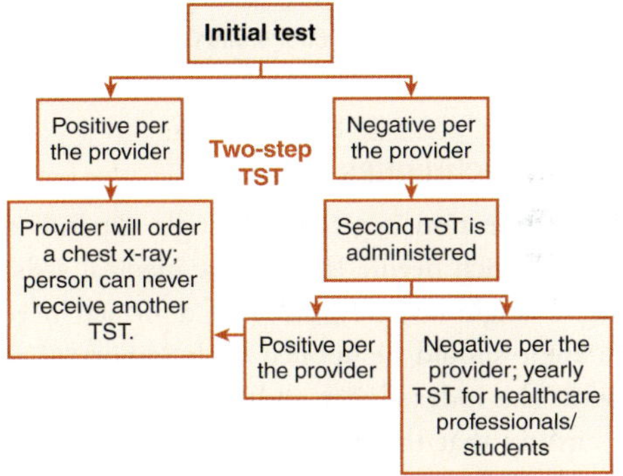

FIGURE 30.26 The process with two-step TST

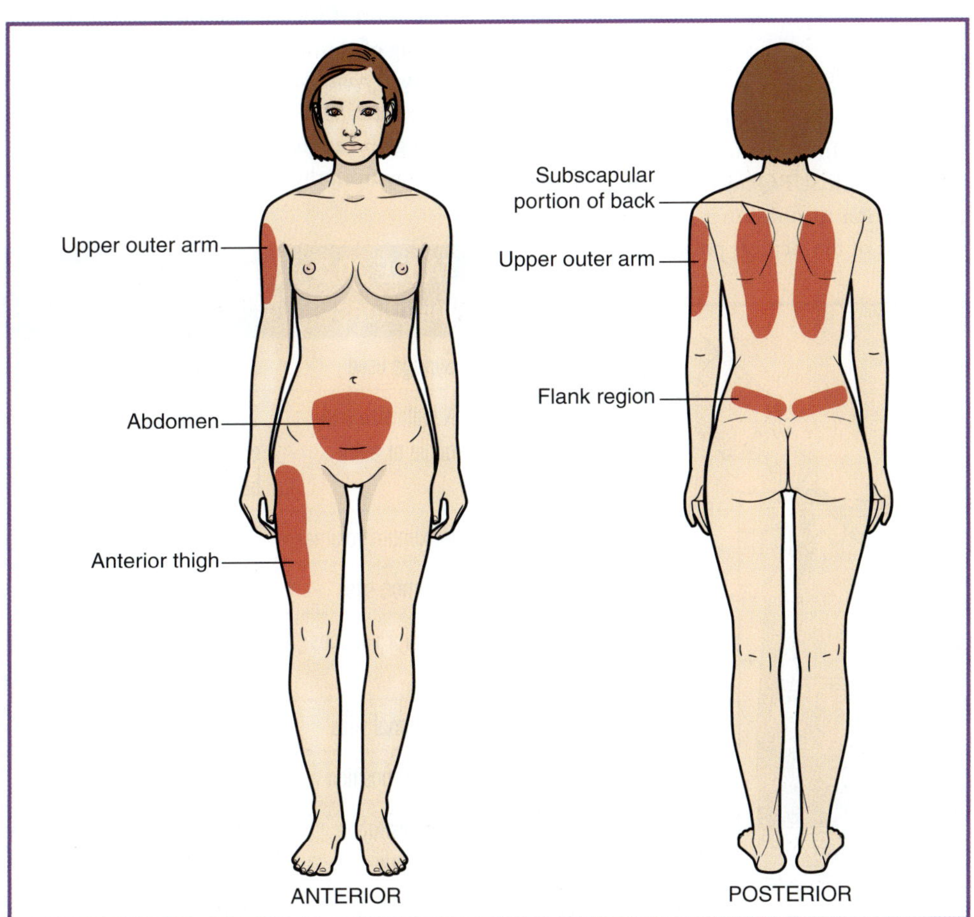

FIGURE 30.27 The subcutaneous (SUBQ) injection sites commonly used include the outer posterior aspect of the upper arm, the lower abdomen, and the anterior aspect of the thigh. The subscapular portion of the back and the flank region are other SUBQ sites.

medications injected into the muscles. The patient may complain of discomfort or pain with a subcutaneous injection. Subcutaneous tissue contains pain receptors.

Common medications given via the subcutaneous route include several vaccines (e.g., MMR, varicella, and polio), enoxaparin (Lovenox), heparin, and insulin.

> **Abbreviations for Subcutaneous Injections**
>
> There have been many abbreviations for subcutaneous injections over the years. Some may still be used in practice, although they are not recommended. The Institute for Safe Medication Practices (ISMP) discourages the use of SC, SQ, and sub q. Healthcare professionals should use SUBQ or *subcutaneously*. For more information, refer to the ISMP website at www.ismp.org/recommendations/error-prone-abbreviations-list.

Administration Techniques

When a SUBQ injection is given, the angle depends on the needle length. If a ⅝-inch needle is used, the medical assistant should use a 45-degree angle (Figure 30.28). If a ½-inch needle is used, a 90-degree angle should be applied. It is important to pinch up the tissue with the index finger and thumb of the nondominant hand. This ensures that the injection is given into the subcutaneous tissue. Table 30.3 contains a summary of subcutaneous injection information.

Aspiration

Aspiration is used to check if the needle is in a blood vessel. This is done once before the medication is given. (The aspiration technique will be discussed in detail in the Intramuscular Injections section, presented later in the chapter.) With SUBQ injections, the aspiration should be done if the medication manufacturer recommends it. It should also be done if it is part of the facility's policy.

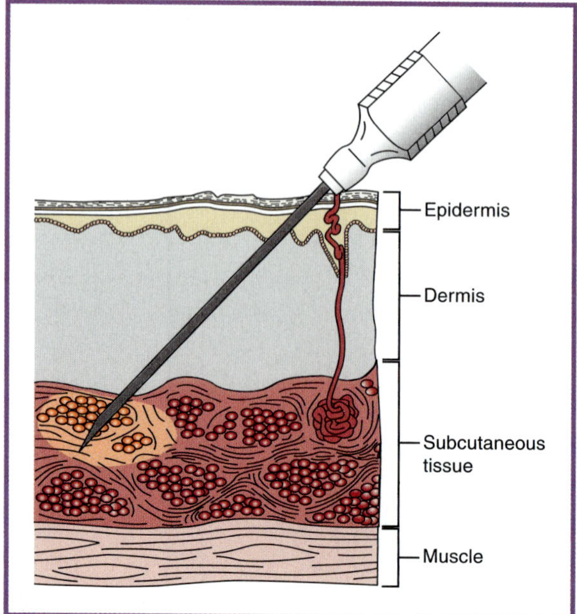

FIGURE 30.28 The subcutaneous (SUBQ) injection is administered in the subcutaneous layer. This method is used for small amounts of nonirritating medications in aqueous solution.

Insulin is not aspirated. SUBQ immunizations do not need to be aspirated, as recommended by the CDC. Anticoagulants, such as enoxaparin and heparin, are administered in the abdomen. They are not aspirated, as specified by the manufacturers.

> **SPECIAL CONSIDERATIONS WHEN GIVING ENOXAPARIN**
>
> When administering enoxaparin (Lovenox), follow these instructions:
>
> 1. Make sure the drug is clear and colorless or pale yellow.
> 2. Do not push any air or drug out of the syringe before giving the injection unless your healthcare provider tells you to. The air allows the medication to enter slower, reducing the risk of bruising.
> 3. Using your finger and thumb, pinch a fold of skin 1 to 2 inches away from the umbilicus in the lower abdomen. Push the entire needle into the skin. Press down on the syringe plunger and inject the medication. Hold the pinched skin the entire time during the injection. Remove the needle. Do not rub or massage the site after the injection.

Subcutaneous Sites

Typically, three SUBQ sites are used in ambulatory care:

- *Abdominal site*: Have the patient remove the clothing in that area. Provide a drape sheet if needed to protect the patient's modesty. The site is located below the costal margins to the iliac crests. Stay 2 inches away from the umbilicus. It is important to stay away from the waistline and any scars. The patient may have more discomfort if the injection is given at the waistline due to the rubbing of clothing.
- *Outer posterior aspect of the upper arm*: Expose the arm. The outer posterior site extends from 3 inches above the elbow to about 3 fingerbreadths below the acromion process. It is important to stay away from the shoulder area.

TABLE 30.3 Summary of Subcutaneous (SUBQ) Injections

Syringe used	3 mL most common; 1 mL could be used
Needle size and angle of entry	23–27 gauge; ½ inch with a 90-degree angle of entry or ⅝ inch with a 45-degree angle of entry; the bevel position does not matter
Maximum volume	0.5–1.5 mL (0.5 mL in children)
Common sites	Abdomen, anterior thigh, and upper outer arm
Sites for vaccines	<1 year of age: anterior thigh >1 year of age: upper outer arm or anterior thigh
Additional sites	Separate sites by 1 inch
Patient position	Sitting
Administration technique	Pinch site. If 2 inches of tissue can be pinched, insert the needle at a 90-degree angle. If 1 inch of tissue can be pinched, insert the needle at a 45-degree angle. Rotate sites.

- *Anterior aspect of the thigh*: Place one hand above the knee and the other hand below the greater trochanter. The site is the middle one-third of the thigh. The site extends from the front midline to the back midline, wrapping around the outer thigh. Usually, only the middle one-third—from the front midline to the outer thigh—is used. Injections are not done on the back of the leg because sitting would irritate the injection site.

Procedure 30.8 describes the steps to follow when giving a subcutaneous injection.

INTRAMUSCULAR INJECTIONS

Intramuscular injections involve placing medication into the muscle (Figure 30.29). There are more blood vessels in the muscles; thus, absorption is faster than in the subcutaneous layer. For medications given by IM injection, *aqueous* (watery) medications should be given with a higher gauge needle than that used for oil-based medications. Table 30.4 contains a summary of intramuscular injection information. Common medications given via the intramuscular route include the following:

- Several vaccines (e.g., hepatitis A and B, tetanus-diphtheria (Td) or with pertussis (TDaP), influenza, and meningococcal)
- Antibiotics and medroxyprogesterone (Depo-Provera)

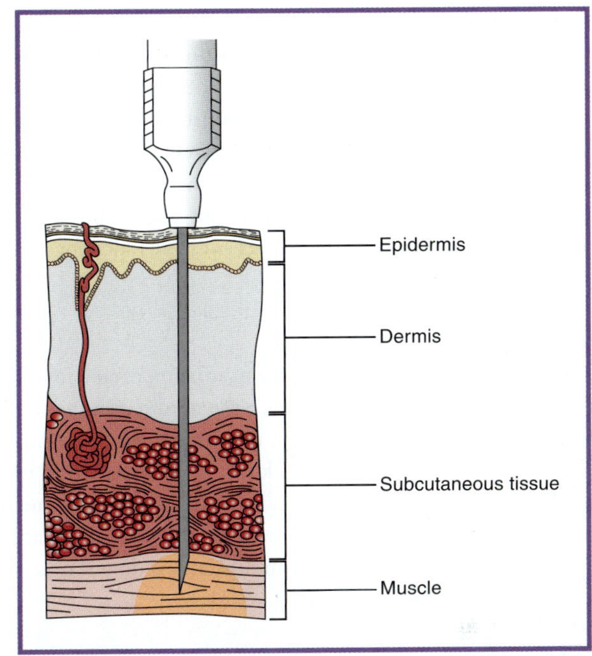

FIGURE 30.29 Anatomic illustration of the intramuscular (IM) injection. Note that the needle is inserted at a 90-degree angle, which deposits the medication into the large central part of the muscle.

TABLE 30.4 Summary of Intramuscular (IM) Injections

	DELTOID	VASTUS LATERALIS	VENTROGLUTEAL
Syringe Used	3 mL		
Needle Length (Determined by the Patient's Size)	1–11 yr: ⅝ –1 inch Adults: ⅝ –1½ inch ***By Weight:*** <130 lb: ⅝ inch 130–152 lb: 1 inch Females 152–200 lb/males 152–260 lb: 1 –1½ inch Females >200 lb/males >260 lb: 1½ inch	Birth-28 days: ⅝ inch 1–12 mo: 1 inch 1–18 yr: 1½ inch 18+ yr: 1 –1½ inch	Birth–28 days: ⅝ inch 1 mo–12 yr: 1 inch 12+ yr: 1–1½ inch
Needle Gauge (G) (Determined by the Medication)	22–25 G	Children: 22–25 G Adults: oil-base: 18–21 G; aqueous: 20–25 G	
Angle of Entry	90 degrees (bevel does not matter)		
Maximum Volume	1 mL for teens and adults	Birth–1 yr: 1 mL 1–11 yr: 2 mL 12+ yr: 3 mL	
Sites for Vaccines Per CDC	1–3 yr: Only if muscle mass is adequate 3+ yr: Can be used	Birth–1 yr: Required 1–3 yr: Preferred 3+ yr: Can be used	
Additional Sites	Separate sites by 1 inch		
Patient/Position	Sitting	Sitting, supine	Side lying
Administration Technique	Stretch the skin over the injection site; use a 90-degree angle of entry		
Possible Complications	Necrosis, hematoma, ecchymosis (bruising), abscess, pain, and vascular and nerve injuries		

Administration Techniques

As with all injections, it is important to do the procedure safely. The medical assistant must identify the correct site and follow the guidelines for medical asepsis. When administering an IM injection, it is important to use a 90-degree angle for entry. The skin should be flattened or stretched over the site with the nondominant hand. Administration techniques for IM injections consist of being safe, minimizing pain, and finding the correct site. The following sections address these three goals.

Aspiration

When giving an intramuscular injection, it is important to aspirate prior to injecting the medication. Once the needle is in the site, the medical assistant should pull back on the plunger for 5 seconds and check the barrel of the syringe. A lack of blood in the barrel means the needle is not in a blood vessel, so it is safe to inject the medication. If blood appears in the barrel, remove the needle, discard the syringe, and restart the procedure. Immunizations do not need to be aspirated, according to the CDC.

Air Lock Technique

When an IM injection is given, the air lock technique can be used. Remove the bubbles in the syringe and measure the exact amount of medication needed. Once these steps have been done, add 0.2 to 0.5 mL of air into the syringe. This is known as the *air lock technique*. When the IM injection is given, the medication is pushed in first, followed by the air. When the needle is withdrawn, the air creates a "lock," keeping the medication in the muscle. The air fills in the needle hole. The air lock prevents the irritating medication from tracking back up the tissues to the skin, creating pain for the patient.

Z-Track Technique

The Z-track technique is another injection method that can reduce pain and discomfort for the patient. Like the air lock technique, this method prevents the medication from tracking back through the subcutaneous tissue. The medication is sealed in the muscle, thus minimizing discomfort for the patient.

The Z-track technique should be used for irritating medications. The ventrogluteal site is the recommended site for injections of irritating medications. For the Z-track technique, the skin is pulled laterally with the medical assistant's nondominant hand. The site is cleansed, and the injection is given (Figure 30.30A–B). As the needle is withdrawn, the skin is released (Figure 30.30C).

Intramuscular Sites

When giving an intramuscular injection, certain sites are used for different ages of patients. For instance, the deltoid site is not used for infants. Certain medications can only be given in specific sites. For example, medroxyprogesterone (Depo-Provera) intramuscular injection can be given in the deltoid and ventrogluteal sites. Knowing how to locate the intramuscular sites is critical when giving intramuscular injections.

Deltoid Site

The deltoid is a triangular-shaped muscle located near the shoulder and upper arm (Figure 30.31). This muscle site is used to give a small volume of aqueous medications, such as vitamin B_{12} and vaccines. The CDC recommends this site be used when vaccines are given to teens and adults. To find the site, expose the upper arm. Make sure the sleeve does not act as a tourniquet. If the sleeve is tight, have the patient slip the arm out of the shirt.

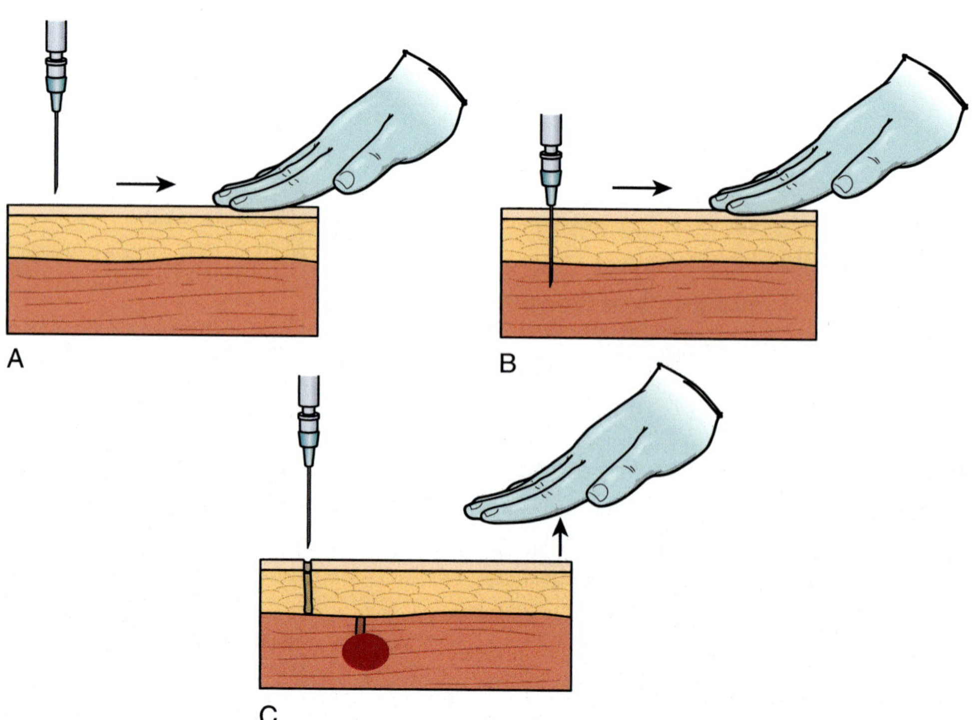

FIGURE 30.30 Z-track technique. **(A)** Displace and then cleanse the skin. **(B)** Inject the medication. **(C)** Release the skin and pull the needle out at the same time. The medication is locked in the muscle.

Palpate the acromion process. Place a finger on the acromion process and then 2 fingers below that. The top of the site is 1 to 2 inches (or 2 fingerbreadths) below the acromion process. The bottom of the site is at the anterior axillary fold (top of the axilla). The injection site should be somewhere between the top and the bottom of the site. Once the medical assistant finds the site, it is a good idea to have the patient lift their arm. The medical assistant can find the bulk (biggest part) of the deltoid muscle. The injection should be given into the bulk of the deltoid muscle.

Vastus Lateralis Site

The vastus lateralis site is used on patients from birth through adulthood. This site uses a thick, well-developed muscle. The CDC recommends this site until the deltoid muscle is the appropriate size for vaccines (after the patient is 1 year or older). Have patients remove the clothing over the thigh. Remember to give patients a drape sheet to protect their modesty during the procedure.

To find the site, you will need to create a rectangle. Think about dividing the thigh into three sections. With adults, each of your hands will cover one-third of the thigh. Place one hand above the knee and the other hand below the greater trochanter (Figure 30.32A). This creates the top and bottom borders of the rectangle (or the vastus lateralis site). The middle one-third is used for the injection site. Next, find the midline of the thigh (remember, the midline creates equal right and left sides). That is the inner border of your rectangle. The final border is created by the midline of the outer thigh (i.e., it creates equal front and back sections of the thigh). Once the site is identified, the medical assistant should have the patient slightly lift the thigh. This allows the medical assistant to see if the injection site is in the bulk of the muscle, which is the goal (Figure 30.32B). Procedure 30.9 describes the procedure for giving an intramuscular injection.

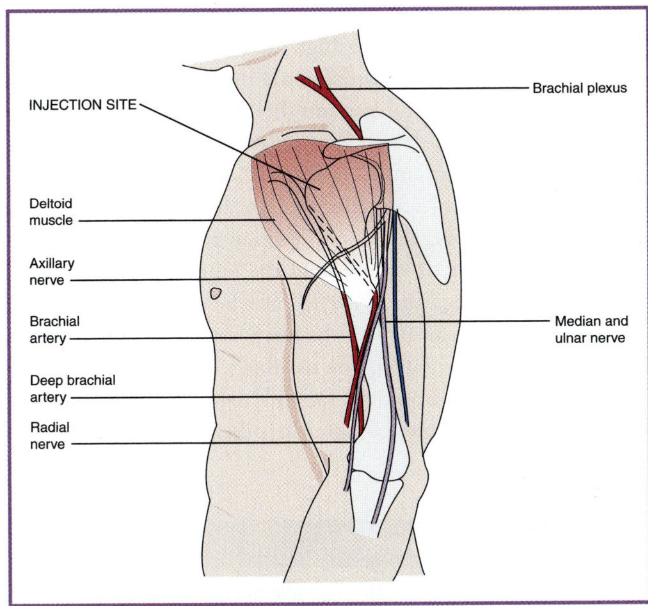

FIGURE 30.31 Deltoid site.

Ventrogluteal Site

The ventrogluteal site is an excellent site for oil-based medications and irritating medications. This site is being used more often because the dorsogluteal site is no longer a recommended site for IM injections due to the risk of injury. It is important to have patients remove clothing from this area to administer an injection in the ventrogluteal site. Offering a drape sheet to protect their modesty is important. For this injection, the patient needs to be in a side-lying position.

The most complex part of using the ventrogluteal site is to ensure that the correct hand is used to find the site. Remember to use the hand opposite the injection site. For instance, if the injection site is on the patient's left side, then use your right hand. Follow these steps to find the site:

1. Place the palm of your hand on the patient's greater trochanter.
2. Your fingers need to point toward the patient's head and your thumb to the patient's groin. (If your thumb is facing the patient's backside, you are using the wrong hand!)

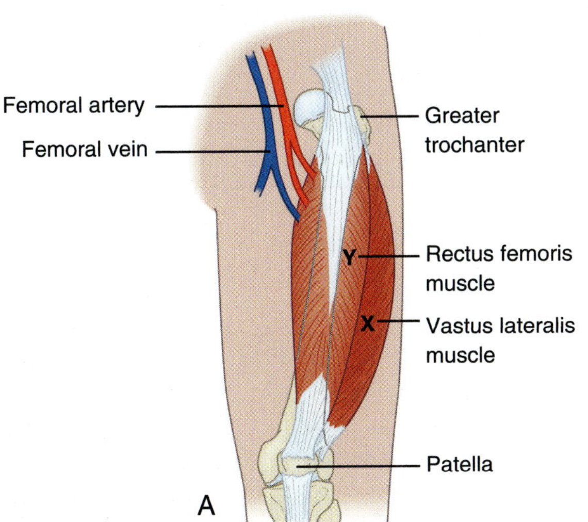

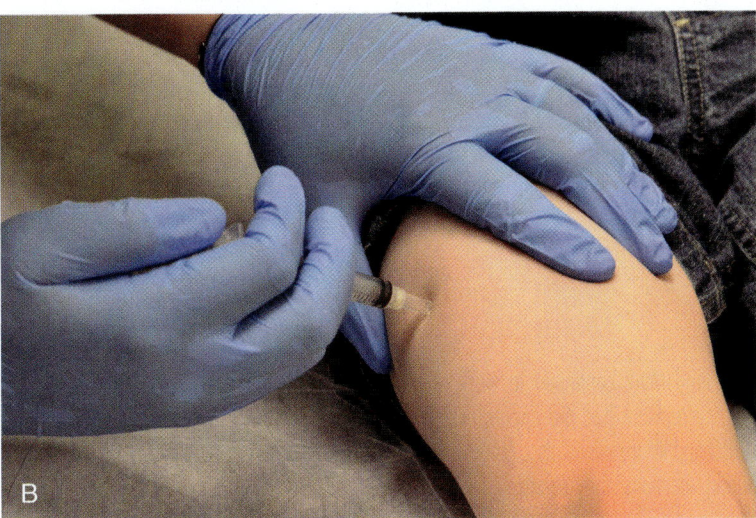

FIGURE 30.32 **(A)** Vastus lateralis site. The vastus lateralis muscle is typically used in ambulatory care. The rectus femoris muscle is used more by patients for intramuscular (IM) injections than by healthcare professionals. **(B)** The vastus lateralis is the recommended site for IM injections in infants and young children.

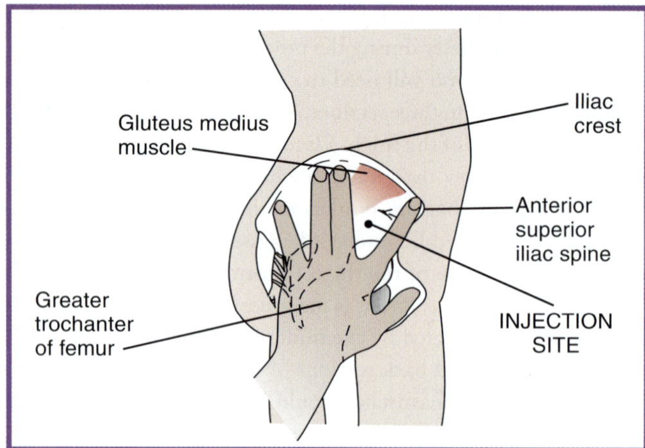

FIGURE 30.33 Ventrogluteal site.

3. Place your index finger on the anterior superior iliac spine. If your fingers are short or if the patient is tall, point your index finger toward the anterior superior iliac spine.
4. Move your middle finger back along the iliac crest toward the patient's buttock (Figure 30.33).

The positioning of your index and middle fingers forms a triangle. The injection point is at the center of the triangle. Remember, if you are giving an irritating medication, use the Z-track method to reduce pain. Procedure 30.10 describes the steps of the Z-track technique.

CLOSING COMMENTS

It is important to remember that medications can cause serious harm to patients. It is critical to pay attention to the details when you prepare and administer medications. Preventing errors and providing superior patient care are goals each time medication is given. Administering medication is an important responsibility for healthcare professionals.

Patient Coaching

When administering medications, the medical assistant must be aware that several forms of liquid medications contain alcohol. This is a concern for patients who are recovering alcoholics or have other health issues, such as diabetes.

The medical assistant may need to teach patients about what types of medications contain alcohol. An internet search can provide lists of medications with their alcohol content. Such online drug references also provide information on the ingredients.

If a patient mentions being a recovering alcoholic or addict, it is important for the medical assistant first to acknowledge the person's accomplishment. Then the medical assistant should communicate the information to the provider. This may make a difference in what medication the provider gives to the patient.

Legal and Ethical Issues

The medical assistant's scope of practice regarding injections differs across the nation. It is important for medical assistants to know their scope of practice in their state. Agencies may also have limitations on what medical assistants can do. For instance, if a scope of practice in the state allows medical assistants to give injections, but the agency does not allow it, medical assistants must abide by the agency's policies and procedures.

Patient-Centered Care

For injections given to small children, the subcutaneous (SUBQ) and intramuscular (IM) sites in the thigh are in the same location. It is helpful to have the parent/guardian hold the child's upper body and hands (however, the medical assistant should anticipate that the adult may not hold securely). If another staff member is available, having them hold the lower extremities is helpful. Many times, children may need more than one injection. For this scenario, it is helpful to have two medical assistants each give an injection at the same time.

The medical assistant should hold the joint above the injection site and the lower leg. The lower leg can be carefully bent off the table. The lower leg can be held between the side of the table and the medical assistant's body. If you use this technique, be careful not to hurt the child's leg. Injections for children need to be done using the one-handed technique because the other hand is holding near the site.

Professional Behaviors

The medical assistant has an important role in administering medications. Paying attention to details is critical. If a medication error occurs, the medical assistant must act immediately to notify the provider. The provider will identify what steps need to be taken. The medical assistant needs to also complete an incident report. (Incident reports are discussed in Chapter 4.) The supervisor needs to also be notified. In most cases, the supervisor will ensure that the patient is not charged for the medication given in error. The supervisor may also need to complete a state or federal report on the medication error.

SUMMARY OF SCENARIO

Gabe and Mark continued to work together for the remaining weeks of the practicum. Mark had the opportunity to give several TSTs. He was able to do SUBQ and IM injections also. Mark learned the importance of distracting patients during injections; they seemed to tolerate the injection much better.

One of the other medical assistants had a medication error. The medication was given to the wrong patient. This error really impressed upon Mark the importance of the nine rights of medication administration. He is adamant that he will never forget to follow each right each time he gives medications. He does not want to deal with a medication error.

SUMMARY OF LEARNING OBJECTIVES

1. **Differentiate among the nine rights of medication administration.**
Each time you prepare and give medication, it is important that you follow the nine rights of medication administration. These rights include the right medication, right dose, right route, right time, right patient, right education, right to refuse, right technique, and right documentation.
2. **Examine the medical assistant's role in administering vaccines.**
There are several types of vaccines, including inactivated, live-attenuated, messenger RNA, toxoid, viral vector, and subunit, recombinant, polysaccharide, and conjugate vaccines.
The medical assistant should ensure that it is the correct time for a vaccine to be given. The timing of a vaccine is based on the patient's vaccination history and the person's age.
The patient can read the Vaccine Information Statement (VIS) before the administration of the vaccine. Besides documenting the vaccine administered, the medical assistant must document the edition date of the VIS and the date when the VIS was provided, along with the date the vaccine was given, the office contact information, the title of the person giving the vaccine, and the vaccine manufacturer and lot number.
3. **Differentiate among the routes of medication.**
Medications taken by the oral route (po) are medications we take by mouth. *Sublingual* (SL) medications are placed under the tongue. *Buccal* medications are placed between the cheek and the gums. *Transdermal* medications are placed on the skin and absorbed into the bloodstream. Medications for the nose, throat, and lungs can be *inhaled.* Applying a drug to a mucous membrane or skin is considered use of the *topical* route. Vaginal medications are inserted into the vagina, and rectal medications are inserted into the rectum. Nasal medications are administered into the nose. Ocular medications are given in the eyes, and otic medications are administered into the ear. *Irrigation* means to bathe or flush open wounds or body cavities. The *parenteral* route involves administration by infusion, injection, or implantation.
4. **Examine the needles and syringes used for parenteral medication administration.**
The parts of a hypodermic needle include the following:
   - Hub: Attaches or screws onto the syringe.
   - Hilt: Where the needle attaches.
   - Bevel: Slanted end of the shaft.
   - Lumen: Hollow space inside the needle. The lumen size is indicated by the gauge and is given a numeric value.

   The length of the needle refers to the length of the shaft. The parts of a hypodermic syringe include the Luer-Lok tip, barrel, flange, and plunger.
5. **Demonstrate how to assemble needles and syringes, along with uncapping, recapping, and switching needles.**
The needle and syringe unit can be placed on the counter after it is assembled. The needle cover should remain on to protect the sterility of the needle.
Never recap a needle that has been used on a patient. Needles can be recapped until they are used on a patient. It is important to maintain the sterility of the needle. If there is any doubt, consider the needle contaminated and replace it with a new one. To uncap needles, pull your hands apart horizontally as one hand holds the cap and the other hand is on the syringe. To recap needles, use the one-handed scoop technique.
6. **Demonstrate preparing parenteral medications using an ampule, prefilled sterile cartridge, vials, powdered medication, and insulin.**
This chapter described several procedures for preparing parenteral medications. See the following procedures for more information on preparing parenteral medications:
KC: CHECKED
   - Procedure 30.2, Prepare Medication from an Ampule
   - Procedure 30.3, Prepare Medication Using a Prefilled Sterile Cartridge
   - Procedure 30.4, Prepare Medication from a Vial
   - Procedure 30.5, Reconstitute Powdered Medication
   - Procedure 30.6, Mix Two Insulins in One Syringe
7. **Examine the medical assistant's role in parenteral medication preparation, including site and patient preparation.**
Prepare and store medications in a separate area, away from the exam rooms. Medications can be prepared without the use of gloves. Ensure that all needles are tightly covered and placed on a tray when carrying them to the exam room.
When selecting the site, never give an injection near a bone or blood vessel. Avoid scar tissue, abnormal growths, abrasions, wounds, and edematous areas. Select a site that is large enough to hold the amount of medication injected.
Use various techniques to help the patient relax and to reduce the patient's anxiety. Inject the medication at a rate of 1 mL per 10 seconds.
If the needle breaks during the injection, pull out the needle if it is visible. If the needle is not visible, mark the spot and yell for help. Place a tourniquet about the spot if the injection was given in the arm. If a bone is hit when giving an intramuscular injection, pull the needle out one-quarter inch and give the medication. If the patient is experiencing any unusual symptoms, it is important to tell the provider immediately.
8. **Demonstrate how to administer and read an intradermal tuberculin skin test.**
Procedure 30.7 discusses how to administer an intradermal injection. A tuberculin skin test is one of the most common intradermal injections given by medical assistants. Table 30.1 provides a summary of intradermal injections.
The tuberculin skin test (TST) is contraindicated in patients who had a severe reaction to a past TST, a history of a positive TST result, or had a live-virus vaccine less than 4 to 6 weeks earlier. To perform the TST, tuberculin purified protein derivative (PPD) 0.1 mL is given intradermally into the inner surface of the forearm. The patient returns within 48 to 72 hours to have the test read. If a second TST needs to be done, it can be done 1 to 3 weeks after the initial test was read.
9. **Demonstrate how to administer a subcutaneous injection.**
Procedure 30.8 discusses how to administer a subcutaneous injection. Table 30.3 provides a summary of subcutaneous injections.
10. **Demonstrate how to administer an intramuscular injection.**
Procedure 30.9 discusses how to administer an intramuscular injection, and Procedure 30.10 describes how to give an IM injection using the Z-track technique. Table 30.4 provides a summary of intramuscular injections.

PROCEDURE 30.1 Administer Oral Medications

TASKS: Calculate the dose to give. Prepare a liquid and a solid medication and administer medications to a patient. Document medication administration.

EQUIPMENT and SUPPLIES

- Provider's orders
- Patient health record
- Drug reference information
- Liquid medication and a solid medication
- Paper cup
- Plastic medication cup
- Marker
- Medication tray
- Glass of water

ORDER: Diltiazem 240 mg po and Cephalexin Oral Suspension 375 mg po

PROCEDURAL STEPS

1. Using the drug reference information and the orders, review the information on the medications.
   PURPOSE: The medical assistant must know about the medication that is being given.
2. Using the orders and the labels in Figure 1, calculate the amount of medication you need to give. Verify the right doses with the instructor. Verify if it is the right time for the order if that applies.
   PURPOSE: The orders do not specify the number of tablets or the amount of liquid (mL) to be given. The medical assistant must calculate both. It is important to check your answer with a peer in the workplace before preparing the medication. This ensures that the right dose is being given.

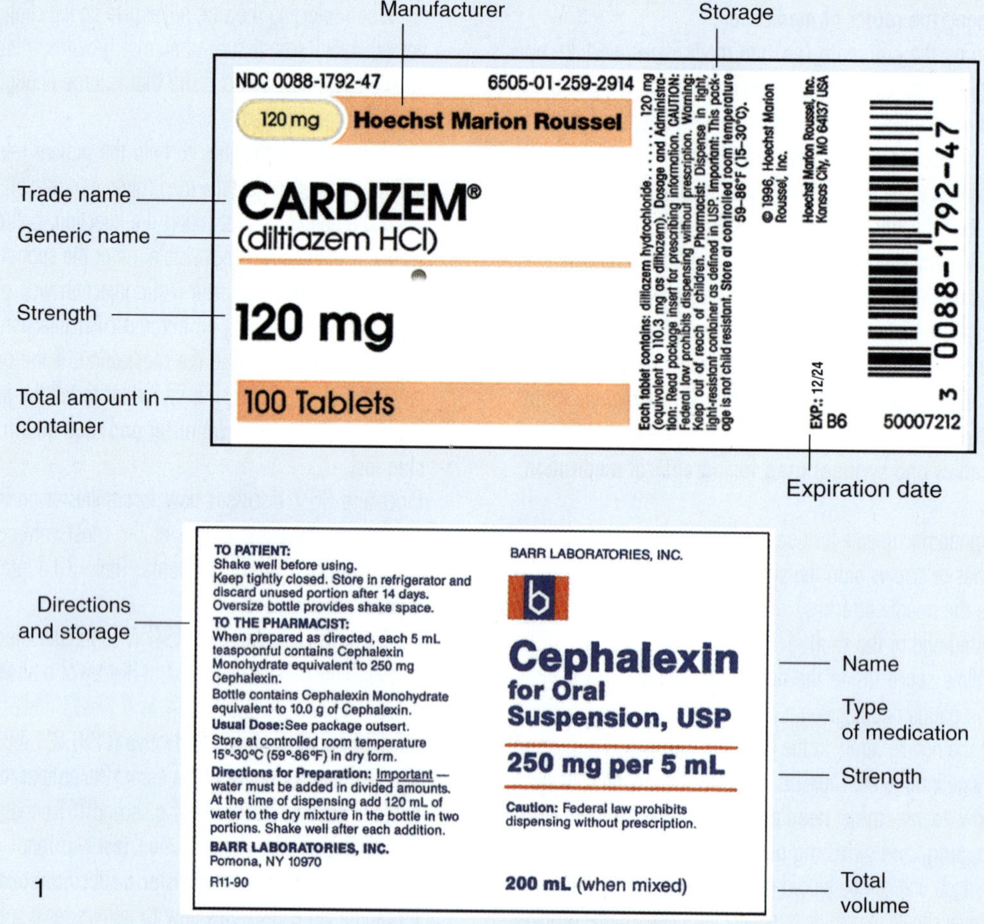

1

PROCEDURE 30.1 Administer Oral Medications—*continued*

3. Wash your hands or use hand sanitizer. Select the right medications from the storage area. Check each medication label against the order. Check for the right name, form, and route. Check the expiration date to make sure the drug has not expired.
   PURPOSE: It is important to do the first check of the label when getting medications from the cabinet. Do not administer expired medications.
4. Assemble the supplies required to prepare the medications. Using the marker, write the medication name and dose on the appropriate cups (Figure 2).
   PURPOSE: The paper cup will be used for the tablets, and the plastic cup will be used for the liquid. Make sure not to write over the measurement markings on the plastic cup. Labeling the cups is a safety measure. All medications prepared need to be labeled. Writing an assessment reminder on the cup is optional and can be helpful when the medical assistant needs to do an assessment (e.g., blood pressure) prior to the administration.

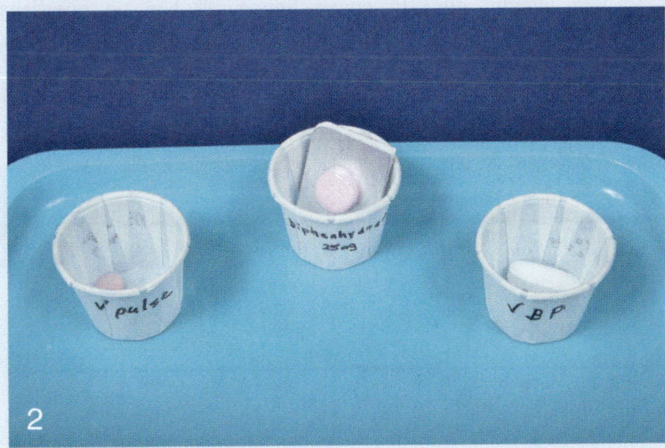

2

5. Perform the second medication check. Check each medication label against the order. Check for the right name, form, and route.
   PURPOSE: It is important to check the label a second time before pouring the medications into the cups.
6. For the solid medication: Remove the cover of the container and hold it so the inside is facing up. Carefully pour the correct number of tablets into the cover. If you pour too many into the cover, pour the extra tablets back into the bottle. When you have the correct number of tablets in the cover, pour them from the cover into the paper cup. Place the cover on the container. Make sure not to contaminate the inside of the container or the cover.
   PURPOSE: Inside the medication container and the cover are sterile. You can pour the tablets back and forth between these two sites until you have the correct number of tablets in the cover. Once you pour the tablets into the paper cup, they are no longer sterile. They cannot be put back into the sterile medication container. If using *unit dose* (individually packaged tablets [blister packs]), tear off the number of tablets needed and place them in the paper cup. Do not open until you are with the patient. If the patient refuses the medication, the unopened unit dose medications can be returned to the original box.
7. For the liquid medication:
   a. Place the plastic medication cup on a high, even surface. Uncover the bottle and place the cover on the counter, making sure the inside is facing up. Place your palm over the medication label. Position yourself so you are eye level with the medication cup (Figure 3).
   PURPOSE: The cup needs to be on an even surface. Read the amount at eye level to ensure the accuracy of the measurement. Palming the label keeps the label clean as you pour the medication.

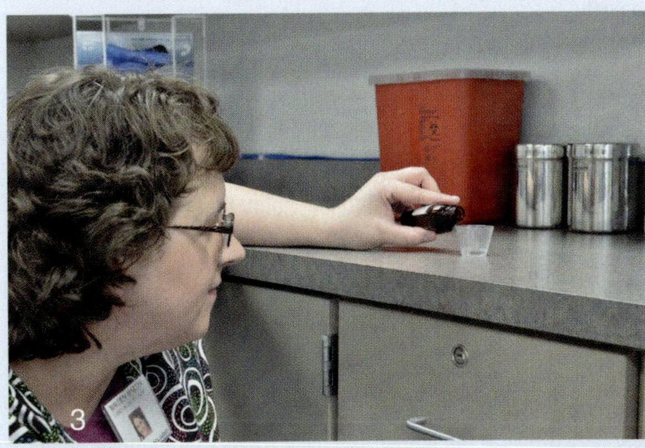

3

   b. Pour the medication into the cup until the lowest point of the meniscus is at the measurement needed (Figure 4).
   PURPOSE: When liquid is poured into a container, it is higher at the edges than in the middle. This is called the *meniscus*. The liquid must be measured at the lowest point of the meniscus.

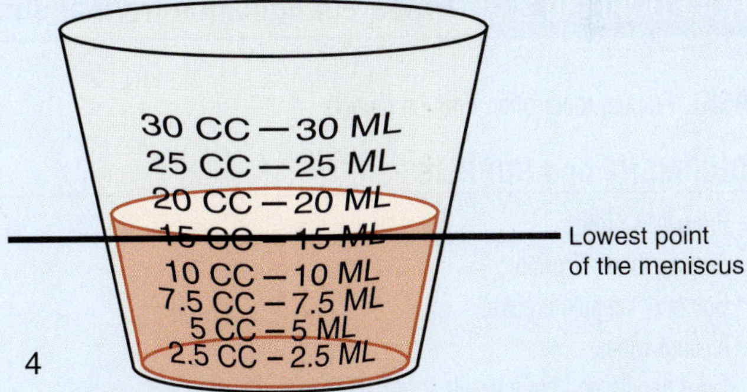

4

   c. If too much medication is poured into the cup, flush the extra down the sink. Replace the cover on the bottle without contaminating the inside of the cover or bottle.
   PURPOSE: Any extra medication in the cup cannot be poured back into the sterile medication bottle. The medication in the bottle and the inside cover need to remain sterile.
8. Place the medication cups on the medication tray. Clean up the area.
   PURPOSE: It is important for the medical assistant to clean up the work area.
9. Perform the third medication check. Check each medication label against the order. Check for the right name, form, and route. Verify that the amount of medication in each cup is correct according to the order.
   PURPOSE: It is important to check the label a third time before placing the medications back into the cabinet.

Continued

PROCEDURE 30.1 Administer Oral Medications—*continued*

10. Prior to entering the exam room, knock on the door and wait a moment. Greet the patient. Identify yourself. Verify the patient's identity with full name and date of birth. Make sure the patient's information matches the order and the record. Explain what you are going to do.
PURPOSE: It is important to identify the patient in two different ways to ensure that you have the correct patient. Explaining the procedure can make the patient feel more comfortable and reduces anxiety.

11. Provide the right education to the patient. Explain the medication ordered, the desired effect, and common side effects, and identify the provider who ordered it. Answer any questions the patient may have. Use language the patient can understand. Ask if the patient has any allergies. If the patient refuses the medication, notify the provider.
PURPOSE: The patient needs to be aware of what you are giving, the action, the side effects, and who ordered it. It is also important to double-check the patient's allergies before administering the medication.

12. Perform the right technique. Do any assessments required prior to giving the medication. If the patient can have water with the medication, have water available.
PURPOSE: Some medications require assessments prior to administration.

13. Allow patients to take the medication in their hands or to use the cup. Stay with the patient until the medication has been taken.
PURPOSE: The medical assistant needs to ensure that the medication is taken.

14. Document the procedure in the health record. Include assessments done; allergies; teaching or instructions provided; the name of the provider who ordered the medication; the medication's name, dose, and route; and how the patient tolerated the medication. For vaccines and controlled substances, add the lot number, the expiration date, and the manufacturer's number.
PURPOSE: The medications given need to be documented to indicate that they were given.

Documentation Example

10/30/20XX 0936 BP 162/92 left arm, sitting, adult cuff. NKA. Per Dr. Martin's order, administered diltiazem 120 mg, 2 tabs po and cephalexin suspension 250 mg/5 mL, 375 mg po. Medication action and side effects discussed with patient prior to administration. Pt had no questions and verbalized understanding. Pt tolerated the medications without problems.
———————— Gabe Garcia CMA (AAMA)

(From Brown M, Mulholland JM: Drug calculations: process and problems for clinical practice, ed 9, St. Louis, 2012, Mosby.)

PROCEDURE 30.2 Prepare Medication from an Ampule

TASK: Prepare medication from an ampule.

EQUIPMENT and SUPPLIES

- Provider's order
- Ampule of medication
- Gauze or ampule breaker
- Alcohol wipes
- Filter needle and hypodermic safety needle
- 3-mL syringe
- Biohazard sharps container
- Waste container
- Drug reference information
- Marker

ORDER: 0.9% Sodium chloride 0.7 mL IM

PROCEDURAL STEPS

1. Wash your hands or use hand sanitizer. Using the drug reference information and the order, review the information on the medication if needed. Clarify any questions you have with the provider.
PURPOSE: Hand sanitization is an important step for infection control. It is important to be knowledgeable about the medication you are giving.

2. Select the right medication from the storage area. Check the medication label against the order. Check for the right name, form, and route. Check the expiration date to make sure the drug has not expired. Verify the right dose and the right time.
PURPOSE: It is important to do the first check of the label when getting medications from the cabinet. Do not administer expired medications.

3. Assemble the supplies required for the procedure.
PURPOSE: Remember to split up the three medication checks with activities between each check.

4. Perform the second medication check. Check the medication label against the order. Check for the right name, form, dose, and route.
PURPOSE: It is important to check the label a second time before continuing with the procedure.

5. Attach the filter needle to the syringe without contaminating the unit. Using a marker, label the syringe with the medication name.
PURPOSE: You will use the filter needle first during the procedure.

6. Gently tap the medication from the head of the ampule or hold the ampule securely, upright in your hand (Figure 1). Quickly move your hand downward. After all the medication has drained into the body of the ampule, wipe the neck with an alcohol wipe.

PROCEDURE 30.2 Prepare Medication from an Ampule—*continued*

PURPOSE: Any medication left in the head will be lost after it is snapped off. Tapping or quickly bringing the ampule down will drain the medication into the body.

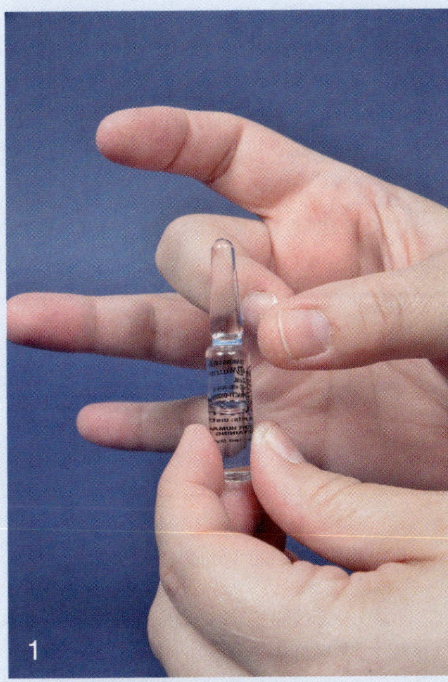

1

7. Place the ampule breaker over the head of the ampule (following the directions from the manufacturer) or wrap the neck with gauze (Figures 2–4). Hold the body with your nondominant hand. With your dominant hand, firmly hold the head (or breaker) between your first two fingers and thumb. Quickly snap off the head of the ampule, making sure it breaks away from your body and others.
PURPOSE: It is important to protect your fingers from the broken glass.

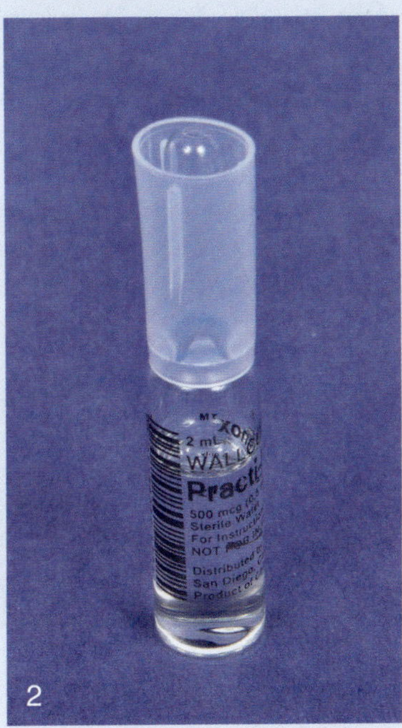

2

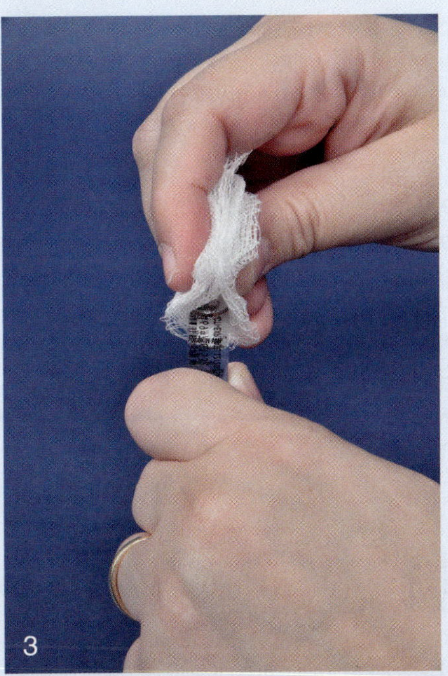

3

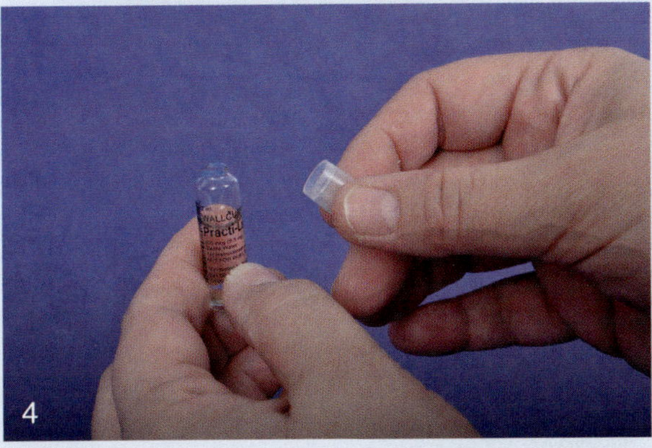

4

8. Discard the breaker or gauze with the ampule head in a biohazardous sharps container.
PURPOSE: It is important to discard the head immediately to protect yourself.

9. Place the ampule on a flat surface. Uncover the filter needle and insert the needle into the ampule without contaminating the needle. Keeping the bevel in the medication, pull the plunger upward, aspirating the medication into the syringe. Tilt the ampule as you remove all the medication.
PURPOSE: Keeping the bevel in the medication will prevent air from being aspirated into the syringe.

10. Recap the needle using the one-handed scoop technique. Perform the third medication check. Check the medication label against the order. Check for the right name, form, and route. Discard the ampule in the biohazardous sharps container.
PURPOSE: It is important to check the label a third time before seeing the patient.

Continued

PROCEDURE 30.2 Prepare Medication from an Ampule—*continued*

11. Remove the filter needle and attach a new needle without contaminating the unit. Discard the filter needle in the biohazardous sharps container.
    PURPOSE: The filter needle needs to be removed before the injection is given.
12. Hold the syringe in a vertical position with the uncapped needle pointed upward. Tap the barrel carefully with the fingertips or a pen to move the air bubbles up to the top of the barrel. Once all the air bubbles are at the top, push the plunger slowly to the correct calibration marking for the ordered dose. Recap the needle.
    PURPOSE: The air needs to be at the top of the syringe before you measure the correct amount of medication.
13. Double-check the dose of medication measured against the order. Make sure no air bubbles are in the syringe.
    PURPOSE: Air bubbles take up space. If air bubbles are present, the correct dose will not be given.
14. Maintain sterility of the medication and the needle throughout the procedure.
    PURPOSE: The needle and medication need to be sterile for the injection.
15. Clean up the work area. Packaging and other waste should be discarded in the waste container.
    PURPOSE: It is professional to clean up after yourself. Never fill a biohazardous sharps container with uncontaminated waste (e.g., packaging).

PROCEDURE 30.3 Prepare Medication Using a Prefilled Sterile Cartridge

TASKS: Prepare medication using a prefilled sterile cartridge. Discard a prefilled sterile cartridge while keeping the reusable holder.

EQUIPMENT and SUPPLIES

- Provider's order
- Prefilled sterile cartridge
- Hypodermic safety needle (if needed)
- Carpuject cartridge holder
- Biohazard sharps container
- Waste container
- Drug reference information

ORDER: 0.9% Sodium chloride 1.6 mL IM

PROCEDURAL STEPS

1. Wash your hands or use hand sanitizer. Using the drug reference information and the order, review the information on the medication if needed. Clarify any questions you have with the provider.
   PURPOSE: Hand sanitization is an important step for infection control. It is important to be knowledgeable about the medication you are giving.
2. Select the right medication from the storage area. Check the medication label against the order. Check for the right name, form, and route. Check the expiration date to make sure the drug has not expired. Verify the right dose and the right time.
   PURPOSE: It is important to do the first check of the label when getting the medication from the cabinet. Do not administer expired medications.
3. Assemble the supplies required for the procedure.
   PURPOSE: Remember to split up the three medication checks with activities between each check.
4. Perform the second medication check. Check the medication label against the order. Check for the right name, form, dose, and route.
   PURPOSE: It is important to check the label a second time before continuing with the procedure.
5. Break the seal. With one hand on the needle cover and the other on the barrel of the prefilled cartridge, move your hands together until you hear a pop. If needed, remove the cover on the cartridge and attach a covered safety needle.
   PURPOSE: The seal needs to be broken before the cartridge is used.
6. Hold the Carpuject holder so the opening (for the barrel) is facing up. Pull the plunger rod out until it clicks. Turn the blue lock until it clicks. This should increase the space between the blue lock and the flange (Figure 1).
   PURPOSE: The Carpuject holder needs to be opened before the cartridge can be placed in it.

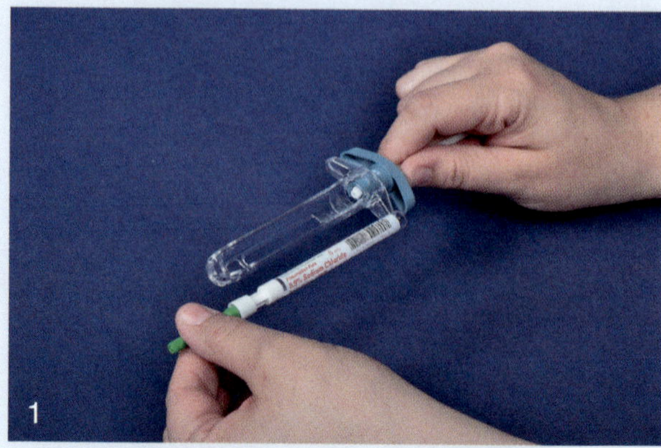
1

PROCEDURE 30.3 Prepare Medication Using a Prefilled Sterile Cartridge—*continued*

7. Insert the cartridge into the Carpuject holder (Figure 2). To secure the cartridge, turn the blue lock on the Carpuject holder until it clicks. The space between the blue lock and the flange should decrease. Turn the white plunger rod until it screws onto the rubber stopper (Figure 3).
   PURPOSE: The cartridge must be secured in the Carpuject holder.

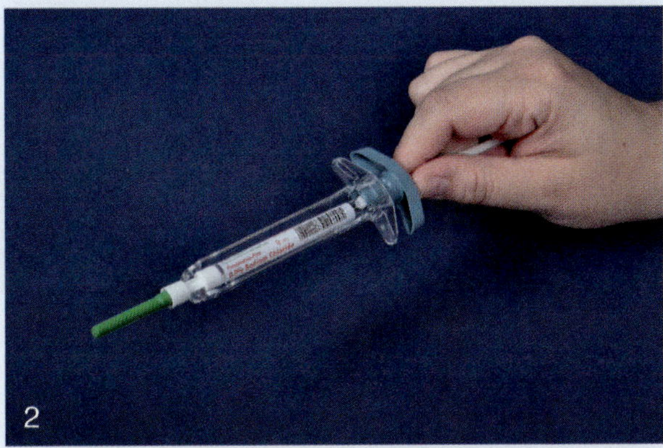
2

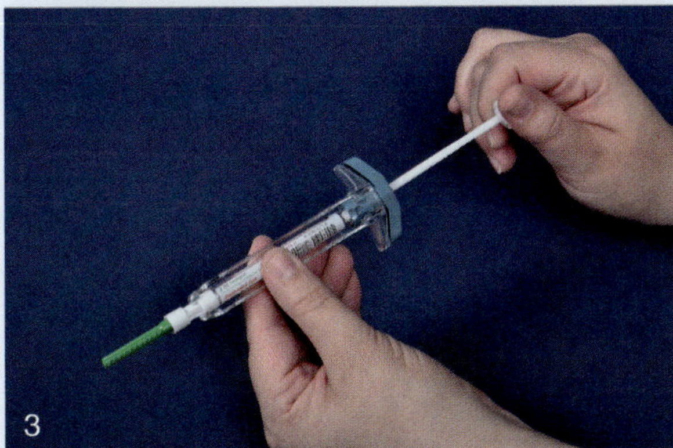
3

8. Remove the cover. Hold the syringe unit in a vertical position with the uncapped needle or tip pointed upward. Tap the barrel carefully with the fingertips or a pen to move the air bubbles up to the top of the barrel. Once all the air bubbles are at the top, push the plunger slowly to the correct calibration marking for the ordered dose.
   PURPOSE: The air needs to be at the top of the syringe before you measure the correct amount of medication.
9. Recap the needle using the one-handed scoop technique. Perform the third medication check. Check the medication label against the order. Check for the right name, form, and route.
   PURPOSE: It is important to check the label a third time before seeing the patient.
10. Double-check the dose of medication measured against the order. Make sure no air bubbles are in the syringe.
    PURPOSE: Air bubbles take up space. If air bubbles are present, the correct dose will not be given.
11. Maintain sterility of the medication and the needle throughout the procedure.
    PURPOSE: The needle and medication need to be sterile for the injection.
12. After giving the injection, unscrew the plunger rod and pull it out until it clicks. Turn the blue lock until it clicks. The space between the blue lock and the flange should increase in size.
    PURPOSE: The Carpuject holder needs to be opened to remove the used cartridge.
13. Carefully invert the Carpuject holder over a biohazardous sharps container to discard the cartridge (Figure 4). Hold the Carpuject holder firmly so it does not end up in the sharps container.
    PURPOSE: Only the cartridge should be discarded.

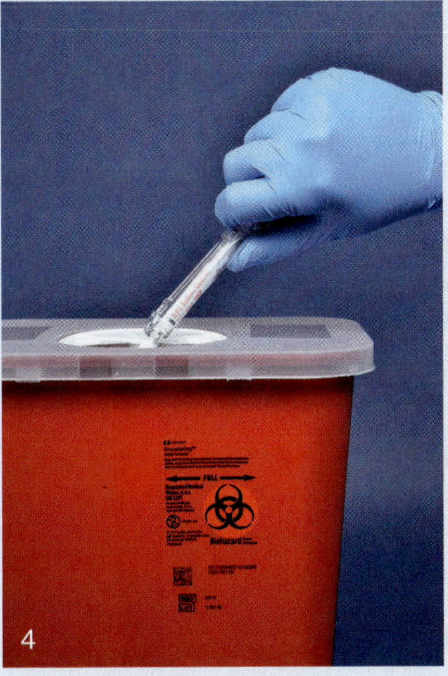
4

14. Disinfect the Carpuject holder. Clean up the work area. Waste should be put in the waste container.
    PURPOSE: Disinfection is an important step for infection control.

PROCEDURE 30.4 Prepare Medication from a Vial

TASK: Prepare medication from a vial.

EQUIPMENT and SUPPLIES

- Provider's order
- Vial of medication
- Alcohol wipes
- Hypodermic safety needle and 3-mL syringe or needle/syringe unit
- Biohazard sharps container
- Waste container
- Drug reference information
- Marker

ORDER: 0.9% Sodium chloride 1.2 mL IM

PROCEDURAL STEPS

1. Wash your hands or use hand sanitizer. Using the drug reference information and the order, review the information on the medication if needed. Clarify any questions you have with the provider.
   PURPOSE: Hand sanitization is an important step for infection control. It is important to be knowledgeable about the medication you are giving.
2. Select the right medication from the storage area. Check the medication label against the order. Check for the right name, form, and route. Check the expiration date to make sure the drug has not expired. Verify the right dose and the right time.
   PURPOSE: It is important to do the first check of the label when getting medications from the cabinet. Do not administer expired medications.
3. Assemble the supplies required for the procedure.
   PURPOSE: Remember to split up the three medication checks with activities between each check.
4. Perform the second medication check. Check the medication label against the order. Check for the right name, form, dose, and route.
   PURPOSE: It is important to check the label a second time before continuing with the procedure.
5. Open the syringe and needle. Tighten the preassembled syringe and needle unit or attach the needle to the syringe. Using a marker, label the syringe with the medication name.
   PURPOSE: Labeling the medication is critical for medication safety.
6. Mix the medication by rolling it with your hands if needed (Figure 1). Remove the cap on the vial (if present). Clean the rubber stopper with an alcohol wipe (Figure 2). Let the stopper dry.
   PURPOSE: The rubber stopper must be disinfected each time you enter the vial with a needle.

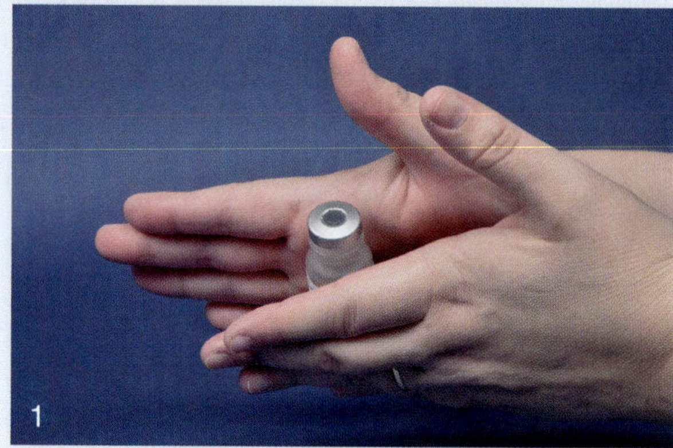

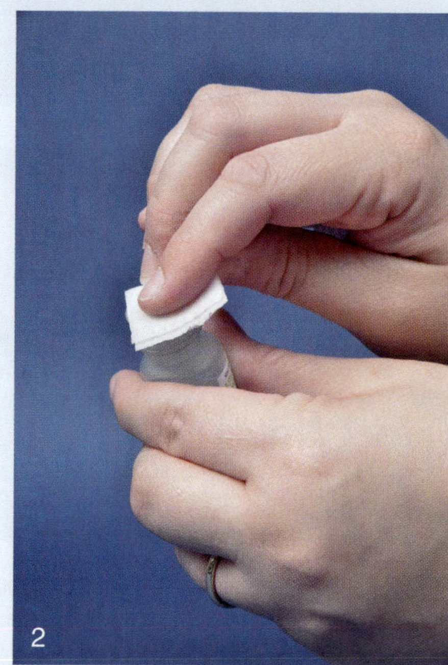

7. With the syringe in a vertical position, pull the syringe plunger down. Draw up an amount of air equal to the amount of medication ordered.
   PURPOSE: The vial is under pressure. When fluid is taken out, air must be added in. Not enough replaced air makes it difficult to withdraw the medication. Too much air causes the pressure to increase in the vial. The extra pressure causes the medication to be forced into the syringe without the plunger being pulled.
8. Hold the vial firmly against a flat surface. Insert the needle into the center of the dried rubber stopper. Inject the aspirated air above the fluid in the vial (Figure 3).
   PURPOSE: Adding the air into the fluid will increase the bubbles.

PROCEDURE 30.4 Prepare Medication from a Vial—*continued*

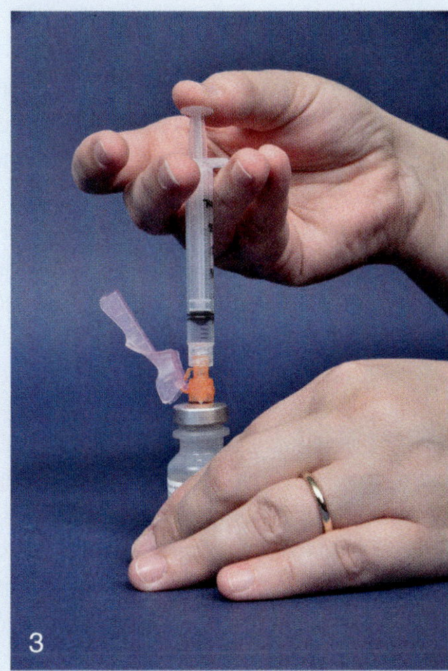

9. With the palm of your nondominant hand facing upward, grasp the vial between your middle and index fingers. Keeping the syringe unit in the vial, pick up and invert them. Use your thumb and the ring and little fingers of your nondominant hand to stabilize the syringe in the vial (Figure 4).
   PURPOSE: It is important to stabilize the syringe so the needle does not bend.

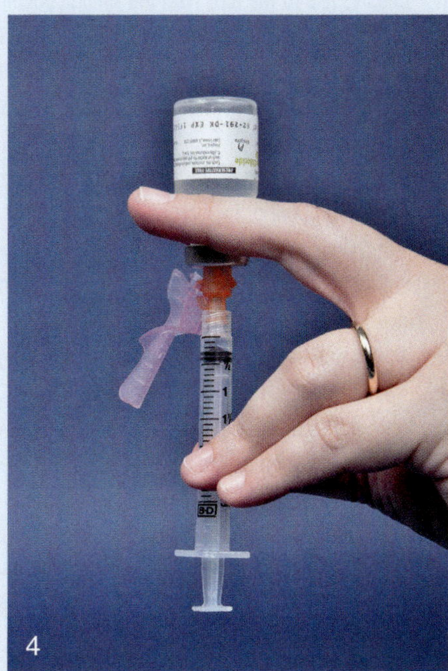

10. With the syringe at eye level, pull the plunger down using your dominant hand. Fill the syringe with more medication than what was ordered (Figure 5).
    PURPOSE: Air bubbles will need to be ejected back into the vial. The extra medication helps with this process.

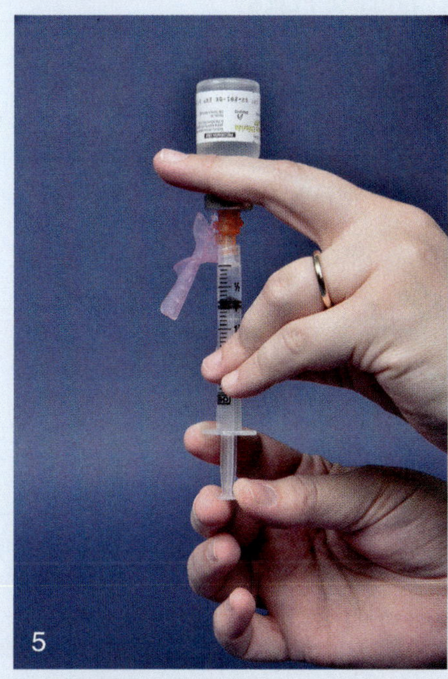

11. Continue to hold the vial/needle/syringe unit in a vertical position (with the needle pointing upward) with your nondominant hand. With your dominant hand, either use your fingers or a pen to tap the bubbles to the top of the barrel.
    PURPOSE: Bubbles rise to the top. With the syringe pointing straight up, the bubbles tend to move to the top of the barrel near the needle.
12. Once all the air bubbles are at the top, push the plunger slowly to the correct calibration marking for the ordered dose.
    PURPOSE: The air needs to be at the top of the syringe before you measure the correct amount of medication.
13. Double-check that no air bubbles are in the syringe and the right dose was measured. If everything is correct, remove the vial from the syringe/needle unit.
    PURPOSE: Air bubbles take up space. If air bubbles are present, the correct dose will not be given.
14. Use the one-handed scoop technique to cover the needle. Perform the third medication check. Check each medication label against the order. Check for the right name, form, and route.
    PURPOSE: It is important to check the label a third time before seeing the patient.
15. Maintain sterility of the medication and the needle throughout the procedure.
    PURPOSE: The needle and medication need to be sterile for the injection.
16. Clean up the work area.
    PURPOSE: It is professional to clean up after yourself.

PROCEDURE 30.5 Reconstitute Powdered Medication

TASKS: Reconstitute powdered medication and prepare the dose of medication.

EQUIPMENT and SUPPLIES

- Provider's order
- Vial of powdered medication
- Vial of diluent
- Alcohol wipes
- Two hypodermic syringes (a 3 mL and a larger syringe)
- Two hypodermic safety needles
- Biohazard sharps container
- Waste container
- Drug reference information
- Marker

ORDER: (Powdered medication name) 0.5 mL IM

PROCEDURAL STEPS

1. Wash your hands or use hand sanitizer. Using the drug reference information and the order, review the information on the medication if needed. Clarify any questions you have with the provider.
   PURPOSE: Hand sanitization is an important step for infection control. It is important to be knowledgeable about the medication you are giving.
2. Select the right medication from the storage area. Check the medication label against the order. Check for the right name, form, and route. Check the expiration date to make sure the vials have not expired. Verify the right dose and the right time. Read the medication label to determine the correct diluent. Obtain the diluent and check the name, route, and expiration date.
   PURPOSE: It is important to do the first check of the label when getting the medications from the cabinet. The label of the powdered medication will indicate the diluent to use. The diluent label must also be checked.
3. Assemble the supplies required for the procedure. If needed, calculate the dose of medication required.
   PURPOSE: Remember to split up the three medication checks with activities between each check.
4. Perform the second medication check. Check the medication labels against the order and directions for reconstituting the powder. Check for the right name, form, and route.
   PURPOSE: It is important to check the label a second time before continuing with the procedure.
5. Open and assemble the syringes and needles. Using a marker, label the 3-mL syringe with the medication name.
   PURPOSE: It is important to keep the needle sterile. If contamination occurs, discard the equipment and start over.
6. Remove the caps on the vials. Clean the rubber stoppers with an alcohol wipe. Let the stoppers dry.
   PURPOSE: The rubber stopper must be disinfected each time you enter the vial with a needle.
7. With the powdered medication vial on a firm surface, insert the needle of the largest volume syringe unit. Make sure the tip stays out of the powder. Pull back on the plunger and withdraw air equal to the amount of diluent that must be added. Pull the needle/syringe out of the stopper.
   PURPOSE: The vial is under pressure. When liquid is put in, the same volume of air must be removed to keep the pressure equal.
8. Using the syringe with the aspirated air (equal to the amount of diluent needed), insert the needle into the center of the dried rubber stopper of the diluent vial. Push the air into the vial, but do not force the air into the vial. Make sure the needle is not in the fluid.
   PURPOSE: Adding the air into the fluid will increase the bubbles. Forcing the air into the vial may cause the vial to have too much pressure.
9. With the palm of your nondominant hand facing upward, grasp the vial between your middle and index fingers. Keeping the syringe unit in the vial, pick up and invert them. Use your thumb and the ring and little fingers of your nondominant hand to stabilize the syringe in the vial. Pull down on the plunger until you have more diluent than you need.
   PURPOSE: It is important to stabilize the syringe so the needle does not bend.
10. Continue to hold the vial/needle/syringe unit in a vertical position (with the needle pointing upward) with your nondominant hand. With your dominant hand, either use your fingers or a pen to tap the bubbles to the top of the barrel.
    PURPOSE: Bubbles rise to the top. With the syringe pointing straight up, the bubbles tend to move to the top of the barrel near the needle.
11. Once all the air bubbles are at the top, push the plunger slowly to the correct calibration marking for the ordered dose. Keep the syringe at eye level.
    PURPOSE: The air needs to be at the top of the syringe before you measure the correct amount of medication.
12. Double-check that no air bubbles are in the syringe and the right dose was measured. If everything is correct, remove the vial from the syringe/needle unit.
    PURPOSE: Air bubbles take up space. If air bubbles are present, the correct dose will not be given.
13. Using an alcohol wipe, clean the rubber stopper of the powdered medication vial. With the vial flat on a hard surface, insert the needle into the dried stopper. Push the diluent into the vial. If resistance is met, take your finger off the plunger and allow air to fill in the syringe. Gradually work all the diluent into the vial. Withdraw the needle from the vial and discard the needle and syringe in the biohazardous sharps container.
    PURPOSE: Forcing the diluent into the vial may cause the vial to "explode" at the weakest point.
14. Gently mix the vial by rolling it in your palms. Mix the medication until all the powder is dissolved.
    PURPOSE: The powder needs to be totally dissolved so the correct dose is given.

PROCEDURE 30.5 Reconstitute Powdered Medication—*continued*

15. Clean the rubber stopper of the powdered medication vial with an alcohol wipe. Let the stopper dry. With the second syringe in a vertical position, pull the syringe plunger down. Draw up an amount of air equal to the amount of medication ordered.
PURPOSE: Think of this step as starting over. Air needs to be inserted into the diluted powder vial to draw up the correct amount of medication.

16. Hold the vial firmly against a flat surface. Insert the needle into the center of the dried rubber stopper. Inject the aspirated air above the fluid in the vial.
PURPOSE: Adding the air into the fluid will increase the bubbles.

17. With the palm of your nondominant hand facing upward, grasp the vial between your middle and index fingers. Keeping the syringe unit in the vial, pick up and invert them. Use your thumb and the ring and little fingers of your nondominant hand to stabilize the syringe in the vial.
PURPOSE: It is important to stabilize the syringe, so the needle does not bend.

18. With the syringe at eye level, pull the plunger down using your dominant hand. Fill the syringe with more medication than what was ordered.
PURPOSE: Air bubbles will need to be ejected back into the vial. The extra medication helps with this process.

19. Continue to hold the vial/needle/syringe unit in a vertical position (with the needle pointing upward) with your nondominant hand. With your dominant hand, either use your fingers or a pen to tap the bubbles to the top of the barrel.
PURPOSE: Bubbles rise to the top. With the syringe pointing straight up, the bubbles tend to move to the top of the barrel near the needle.

20. Once all the air bubbles are at the top, push the plunger slowly to the correct calibration marking for the ordered dose.
PURPOSE: The air needs to be at the top of the syringe before you measure the correct amount of medication.

21. Double-check that no air bubbles are in the syringe and the right dose was measured. If everything is correct, remove the vial from the syringe/needle unit.
PURPOSE: Air bubbles take up space. If air bubbles are present, the correct dose will not be given.

22. Use the one-handed scoop technique to cover the needle. Perform the third medication check. Check each medication label against the order. Check for the right name, form, and route.
PURPOSE: It is important to check the label a third time before seeing the patient.

23. Maintain sterility of the medication and the needle throughout the procedure.
PURPOSE: The needle and medication need to be sterile for the injection.

24. If the medication is in a multidose vial, label the vial with the expiration date, diluent added, and your initials. Clean up the work area. Put the packaging and other waste in the waste container. Discard the vial(s) in the biohazardous waste container.
PURPOSE: It is professional to clean up after yourself.

PROCEDURE 30.6 Mix Two Insulins in One Syringe

TASK: Mix two types of insulins in one syringe.

EQUIPMENT and SUPPLIES

- Provider's order
- Regular insulin vial
- NPH insulin vial
- Alcohol wipes
- U100 insulin needle and syringe unit
- Biohazard sharps container
- Waste container
- Drug reference information
- Marker

ORDER: Regular insulin 16 units mixed with NPH insulin 30 units SUBQ

PROCEDURAL STEPS

1. Wash your hands or use hand sanitizer. Using the drug reference information and the order, review the information on the medication if needed. Clarify any questions you have with the provider.
PURPOSE: Hand sanitization is an important step for infection control. It is important to be knowledgeable about the medication you are giving.

2. Select the right medications from the storage area. Check the medication labels against the order. Check for the right name, form, and route. Check the expiration date to make sure the vials have not expired. Verify the right dose and the right time.
PURPOSE: It is important to do the first check of the label when getting the medications from the cabinet.

Continued

PROCEDURE 30.6 Mix Two Insulins in One Syringe—*continued*

3. Assemble the supplies required for the procedure. If the insulin is cold, roll the vials in your hands to warm the medication.
   PURPOSE: Remember to split up the three medication checks with activities between each check.
4. Perform the second medication check. Check the medication labels against the order. Check for the right name, form, and route.
   PURPOSE: It is important to check the label a second time before continuing with the procedure.
5. Open and assemble the syringe and needle. Using a marker, label the syringe with the medication name. Mix the NPH insulin by rolling the vial in your hands. If present, remove the metal or plastic caps on the vials. Clean the rubber stoppers with an alcohol wipe. Let the stoppers dry.
   PURPOSE: The rubber stopper must be disinfected each time you enter the vials with a needle.
6. With the syringe in a vertical position, pull the syringe plunger down. Draw up an amount of air equal to the amount of NPH insulin ordered. With the NPH vial on a firm surface, insert the needle into the rubber stopper. Inject the air into the NPH vial, keeping the needle tip out of the medication. Withdraw the needle from the stopper.
   PURPOSE: The vial is under pressure. Adding air is required before removing medication.
7. With the syringe in a vertical position, pull the syringe plunger down. Draw up an amount of air equal to the amount of Regular insulin ordered. With the Regular vial on a firm surface, insert the needle into the rubber stopper. Inject the air into the Regular vial, keeping the needle tip out of the medication.
   PURPOSE: The vial is under pressure. Adding air is required before removing medication.
8. With the palm of your nondominant hand facing upward, grasp the vial between your middle and index fingers. Keeping the syringe unit in the vial, pick up and invert them. Use your thumb, ring, and little fingers of your nondominant hand to stabilize the syringe in the vial. Pull down on the plunger until you have more Regular insulin than you need.
   PURPOSE: It is important to stabilize the syringe, so the needle does not bend.
9. Continue to hold the vial/needle/syringe unit in a vertical position (with the needle pointing upward) with your nondominant hand. With your dominant hand, either use your fingers or a pen to tap the bubbles to the top of the barrel.
   PURPOSE: Bubbles rise to the top. With the syringe pointing straight up, the bubbles tend to move to the top of the barrel near the needle.
10. Once all the air bubbles are at the top, push the plunger slowly to the correct calibration marking for the ordered dose. Keep the syringe at eye level.
    PURPOSE: The air needs to be at the top of the syringe before you measure the correct amount of medication.
11. Double-check that no air bubbles are in the syringe and the right dose was measured. If everything is correct, remove the vial from the syringe/needle unit.
    PURPOSE: Air bubbles take up space. If air bubbles are present, the correct dose will not be given.
12. Using an alcohol wipe, wipe the rubber stopper of the NPH vial. Calculate the total amount of insulin that needs to be given.
    PURPOSE: This total represents the calibration marking where the rubber stopper of the plunger needs to be pulled down when withdrawing the NPH insulin.
13. With the NPH vial flat on a hard surface, insert the needle into the dried stopper. With the palm of your nondominant hand facing upward, grasp the vial between your middle and index fingers. Keeping the syringe unit in the vial, pick up and invert them. Use your thumb and the ring and little fingers of your nondominant hand to stabilize the syringe in the vial. Pull down on the plunger until the rubber stopper reaches the calibration mark required. Do not withdraw any extra NPH insulin.
    PURPOSE: If any additional NPH insulin is drawn up, the syringe must be discarded in the biohazardous sharps container. No insulin can be injected into the NPH vial.
14. Double-check that no air bubbles are in the syringe and the right dose was measured. If everything is correct, remove the vial from the syringe/needle unit.
    PURPOSE: Air bubbles take up space. If air bubbles are present, discard the syringe and start over.
15. Use the one-handed scoop technique to cover the needle. Perform the third medication check. Check each medication label against the order. Check for the right name, form, and route.
    PURPOSE: It is important to check the label a third time before seeing the patient.
16. Maintain sterility of the medication and the needle throughout the procedure.
    PURPOSE: The needle and medication need to be sterile for the injection.
17. Clean up the work area. Put the packaging and other waste in the waste container. Place the insulin vials back in their storage location.
    PURPOSE: It is professional to clean up after yourself.

PROCEDURE 30.7 Administer an Intradermal Injection

TASKS: Prepare medication from a vial, administer an intradermal injection, read the tuberculin skin test, and document it in the health record.

EQUIPMENT and SUPPLIES

- Provider's order
- Patient's health record
- Vial of medication
- Alcohol wipes
- 1-mL syringe with a ¼- to ½-inch, 25- to 27-gauge safety needle
- Bandage (if per facility's policy)
- Medication tray
- Biohazard sharps container
- Waste container
- Drug reference information
- Gloves
- Marker and pen
- Millimeter ruler

ORDER: Tuberculin purified protein derivative (PPD) (5 tuberculin units) 0.1 mL ID

PROCEDURAL STEPS

1. Draw medication up from a vial (see Procedure 30.4).
2. Prior to entering the exam room, knock on the door and wait a moment. Greet the patient. Identify yourself. Verify the patient's identity with full name and date of birth. Make sure the patient's information matches the order and the record. Explain what you are going to do.
   PURPOSE: It is important to identify the patient in two different ways to ensure that you have the correct patient. Explaining the procedure can make the patient feel more comfortable and reduces anxiety.
3. Provide the right education to the patient. Explain the medication ordered, the desired effect and common side effects; also identify the provider who ordered it. Answer any questions the patient may have. Use language the patient can understand. Ask if the patient has any allergies. If the patient refuses the medication, notify the provider.
   PURPOSE: The patient needs to be aware of what you are giving, its action and side effects, and who ordered it. It is also important to double-check the patient's allergies before administering the medication.
4. Perform the right technique. Ask the patient the following questions:
   - Can you return in 48 to 72 hours for the reading?
   - Have you ever had BCG?
   - Have you ever had a TB skin test? If yes, did you have a reaction to it?

PURPOSE: These questions are important to determine if the patient should get the test or if the medical assistant should talk with the provider.

5. Use hand sanitizer and put on gloves.
   PURPOSE: Hand sanitization is an important step for infection control.
6. Have the patient extend a forearm. With the palm facing upward, identify an appropriate site for the injection. The site should be 2 to 4 inches below the elbow. Loosen the cap on the needle, but still protect the needle from contamination. Open the alcohol wipes.
   PURPOSE: The site should be free from veins, scars, wounds, abrasions, and so on. If the person has a reaction, having the site away from the elbow does not limit its motion. Loosening the cap prior to starting allows you to remove the cap with one hand during the procedure.
7. Place your nondominant hand to the side of the site, pulling the skin taut (Figure 1). *Option:* Place your nondominant hand on the back of the patient's forearm, pulling the skin taut (Figure 2).
   PURPOSE: The skin needs to be taut to insert the needle.

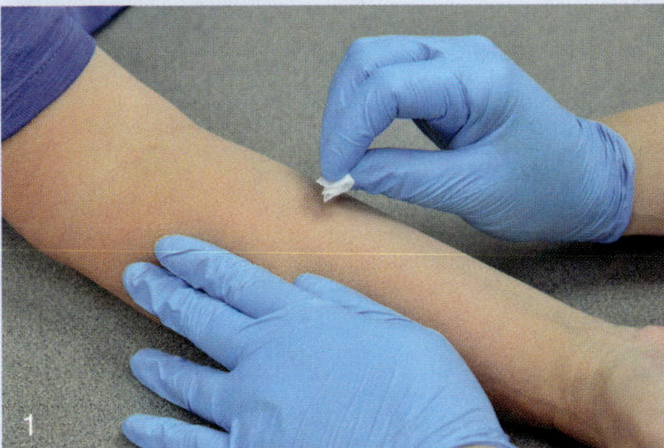
1

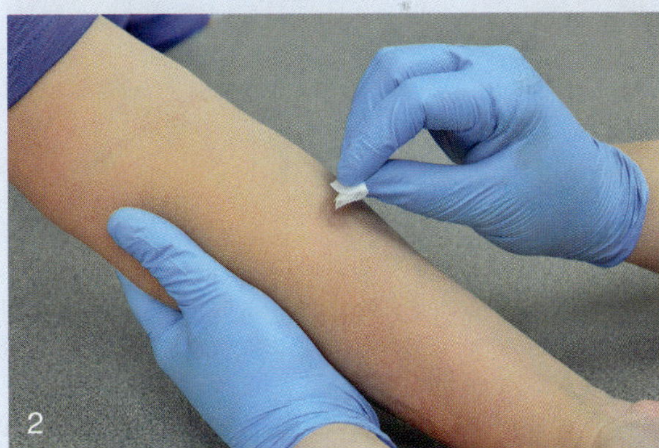
2

8. Cleanse the site with an alcohol wipe using a circular motion. Move from the center outward, using some friction to help clean the site. Create about a 2-inch circle at the site. Let the site dry while continuing to hold the area.
   PURPOSE: Cleaning from the inside to the outside prevents contamination of the cleaned area. Avoid waving over or blowing on the alcohol, which contaminates the site.
9. Pick up the syringe and tip it to remove the cover. Grasp the syringe in your dominant hand, using your thumb and index finger. Make sure to have no fingers under the syringe. Ensure that the bevel is up.
   PURPOSE: The syringe needs to be lowered to the skin after it has been inserted. Having fingers under the syringe changes the angle and can affect the administration.

Continued

PROCEDURE 30.7 Administer an Intradermal Injection—*continued*

10. At a 5- to 15-degree angle, slowly insert the needle until the bevel is covered with skin (Figure 3). Carefully lower the syringe to the skin and hold it steady with your dominant hand (Figure 4).
PURPOSE: If a greater angle is used or if more of the needle is inserted, the injection may be given deeper than it should be. Holding the syringe against the skin helps support it during the injection.

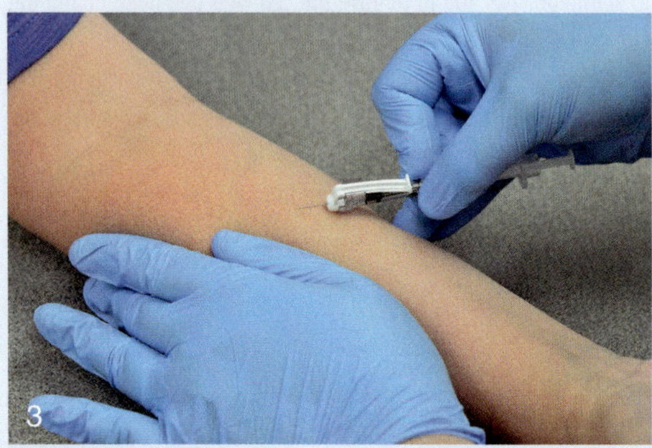
3

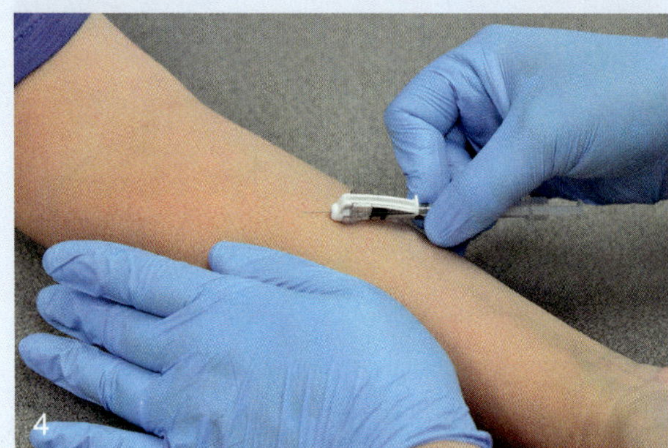
4

11. Carefully move your nondominant hand to the plunger. Slowly and steadily inject the medication by pressing on the plunger (Figure 5). If a 6- to 10-mm wheal does not appear, repeat the test at least 2 inches from the site (Figure 6).
PURPOSE: Any movement of the needle/syringe can dislodge the needle from the site.

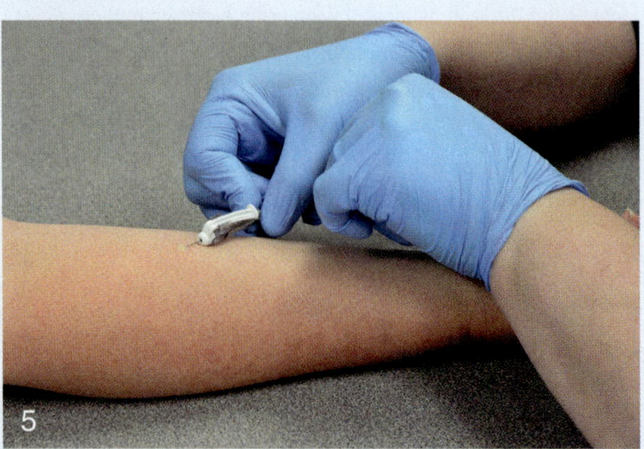
5

12. Double-check the barrel of the syringe to make sure all the medication was administered. Withdraw the needle. Activate the needle's safety device with one hand.
PURPOSE: It is important to administer all the medication. Using more than one hand to activate the safety device increases the risk for needlestick injuries.

13. Discard the needle/syringe in a biohazardous sharps container. Make sure to put the needle in first.
PURPOSE: Safely discarding the needle/syringe will help prevent needlestick injuries.

14. Do not massage the area. Per the facility's policy, if the person has a light-colored shirt with long sleeves, offer a bandage. Place the bandage on very loosely to just absorb any blood from the site.
PURPOSE: It is very important that the bandage not be put on snugly because some of the medication could be lost at the site. If a bandage is used, it needs to be loosely applied. Some agencies will not allow the use of a bandage.

15. Observe the patient for any adverse reactions. Clean up the area. Discard the waste in the waste container. Sanitize your hands.
PURPOSE: It is important to monitor the patient and clean up the work area.

16. Document the procedure in the health record. Include assessments done, allergies, teaching or instructions provided; the medication name, dose, and route; the name of the provider who ordered the medication; and how the patient tolerated the medication. Also include the manufacturer, the lot number, and the expiration date of the vial.
PURPOSE: Medications given need to be documented to indicate they were given.
Scenario update: The patient returns for the reading.

17. Check the health record to identify the location of the test. Greet the patient. Identify yourself. Verify the patient's identity with full name and date of birth. Make sure the patient's information matches the order and the record. Explain what you are going to do.
PURPOSE: It is important to identify the patient in two different ways to ensure that you have the correct patient. Explaining the procedure can make the patient feel more comfortable and reduces anxiety.

18. Palpate the site for an induration. If an induration is felt, ask patients if you can write on their arms. Using a ballpoint pen, draw a line toward the induration from the outer edge of the arm. Repeat on the other side (Figure 7). *Option:* Palpate the induration to find the edge and then mark it with a pen. Repeat on the other side. Using a millimeter ruler, accurately measure the distance between the two points.
PURPOSE: The ballpoint pen will stop at the edge of the induration. This provides you with two visible points to measure the size of the induration.

PROCEDURE 30.7 Administer an Intradermal Injection—*continued*

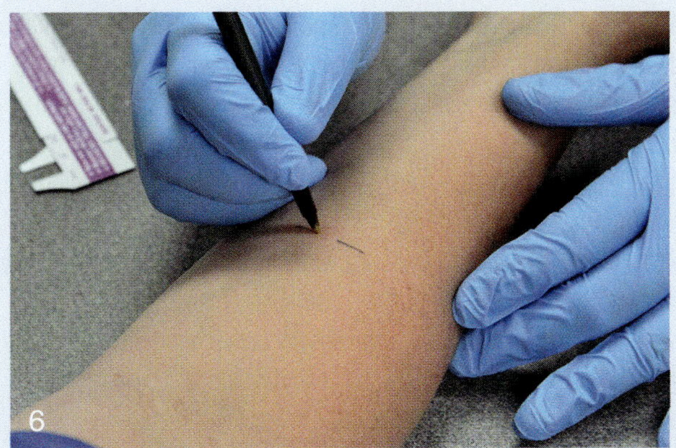

19. Document the reading in the patient's health record. Include the reason for the patient's visit, the test site, the size of the induration in millimeters, and the name of the provider who was notified.

PURPOSE: The medical assistant must document the size of the induration if one is present. If no induration is present, then document 0 mm. The provider will determine if the test is negative or positive.

Documentation Example 1

11/1/20XX 0805 NKA. No prior history of TST. Per Dr. Martin's order, administered: Tuberculin purified protein derivative (PPD) 0.1 mL (5 tuberculin units) ID left forearm. (Vial: ABC Manufacturer, Lot#1345, Expires 10/20XX). Pt tolerated test without a problem. Test side effects discussed with pt prior to administration. Pt instructed to return between 48 and 72 hours, and follow-up appointment was made. Pt had no questions and verbalized understanding of instructions. —————————— Gabe Garcia CMA (AAMA)

Documentation Example 2

11/3/20XX 1005 Pt returned for TST reading. Left forearm induration measured 4 mm. Dr. Martin was notified. —————————— Gabe Garcia CMA (AAMA)

PROCEDURE 30.8 Administer a Subcutaneous Injection

TASKS: Prepare medication from a vial, administer a subcutaneous injection, and document the medication administration in the health record.

SCENARIO: Dr. Martin orders polio vaccine (IPV) 0.5 mL SUBQ for Johnny Parker (DOB 06/15/20XX). (Vial information: ABC Manufacturer, Lot #1234, expires 1 year from today.)

EQUIPMENT and SUPPLIES

- Provider's order
- Patient's health record
- Vial of medication
- Alcohol wipes
- 3-mL syringe with a ½-inch or ⅝-inch, 23- to 27-gauge safety needle
- Gauze
- Bandage
- Medication tray
- Biohazard sharps container
- Waste container
- Drug reference information
- VIS for polio vaccine (IPV) (optional)
- Gloves
- Marker

ORDER: Polio vaccine (IPV) 0.5 mL SUBQ

PROCEDURAL STEPS

1. Draw the medication up from a vial (see Procedure 30.4).
2. *(Peer will play the parent.)* Prior to entering the exam room, knock on the door and wait a moment. Greet the parent/patient. Identify yourself. Verify the patient's identity with full name and date of birth. Make sure the patient's information matches the order and the record. Explain what you are going to do.
   PURPOSE: It is important to identify the patient in two different ways to ensure that you have the correct patient. Explaining the procedure can make the patient feel more comfortable and reduces anxiety.
3. Provide the right education to the parent/patient. Explain the medication ordered, the desired effect, and common side effects; also identify the provider who ordered it. Answer any questions the parent/patient may have. Use language the parent/patient can understand. Ask if the patient has any allergies. If the parent/patient refuses the medication, notify the provider.
   PURPOSE: The patient needs to be aware of what you are giving, its action and side effects, and who ordered it. It is also important to double-check the patient's allergies before administering the medication.
4. Use hand sanitizer and put on gloves.
   PURPOSE: Hand sanitization is an important step for infection control.
5. Loosen the cap on the needle, but still protect the needle from contamination. Open the alcohol wipes. Have gauze and a bandage available.
   PURPOSE: Loosening the cap prior to starting allows you to remove the cap with one hand during the procedure. You should never remove the cap with your teeth.

Continued

PROCEDURE 30.8 Administer a Subcutaneous Injection—*continued*

6. *(Peer will play the patient.)* Find the injection site.
PURPOSE: It is important to find the correct location for the injection.

7. Cleanse the site with an alcohol wipe using a circular motion (Figure 1). Move from the center outward, using some friction to help clean the site. Create about a 2-inch circle at the site. Let the site dry. Avoid waving over or blowing on the alcohol, which contaminates the site.
PURPOSE: Cleaning from the inside to the outside prevents contamination of the cleaned area.

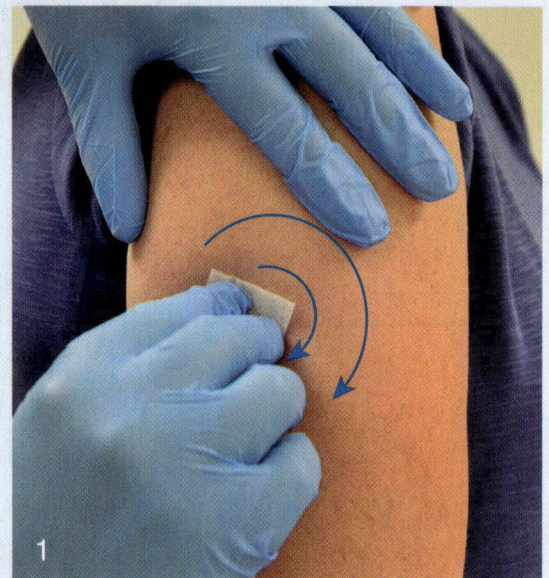

8. Perform the right technique. Place a gauze between the index and middle fingers of your nondominant hand. With that hand, use your index finger and thumb to pinch up at the cleansed area.
PURPOSE: The site needs to be pinched for a SUBQ injection.

9. Pick up the syringe and tip it to remove the cover. Hold the syringe between the thumb and index finger of your dominant hand (Figure 2). Quickly and smoothly insert the needle into the site at a 45- or 90-degree angle, depending on the needle size. Insert the entire needle. Make sure the needle tip is not pointed toward your nondominant hand.
PURPOSE: Ensuring that the tip is not pointed toward your hand will lessen the needlestick risk. Aspiration for SUBQ injections is based on the facility's policy and the recommendation from the manufacturer.

10. *One-handed option:* Continue to pinch the site. Securely grasp the syringe between the fingers of your dominant hand. With your dominant hand, aspirate if required, and then push the plunger to inject the medication. *Two-handed option:* Release the pinch, and with the nondominant hand, aspirate if required, then push the plunger to inject the medication.
PURPOSE: Follow the facility's policy on whether to use the one- or two-handed option.

11. Inject the medication at a rate of 1 mL over 10 seconds. Ensure that all the medication has been injected before pulling out the needle at the same angle used for entry. Release the pinch if using the one-handed option.
PURPOSE: Injecting the medication too slowly or too quickly can be uncomfortable for the patient.

12. Activate the needle's safety device with one hand while using the other hand to cover the site with gauze. Gently apply pressure at the site to stop any bleeding. Apply a bandage if the patient requests it.
PURPOSE: Ask if the patient would like a bandage if the site has stopped bleeding. Remember that some bandages may contain latex, which can be an allergen for some people. Some people may be allergic to the adhesive.

13. Discard the needle/syringe in a biohazardous sharps container. Make sure the needle goes into the sharps container first.
PURPOSE: Safely discarding the needle/syringe will help prevent needlestick injuries.

14. Observe the patient for any adverse reactions. Clean up the area. Discard the waste in the waste container. Sanitize your hands.
PURPOSE: It is important to monitor the patient and clean up the work area.

15. Document the procedure in the health record. Include assessments done, allergies, teaching or instructions provided; the name of the provider who ordered the medication; the medication's name, dose, and route; and how the patient tolerated the medication. Also include the manufacturer, the lot number, and the expiration date for vaccines and controlled substances. Figure 3 shows the documentation using an electronic health record.
PURPOSE: Medications given need to be documented to indicate they were given.

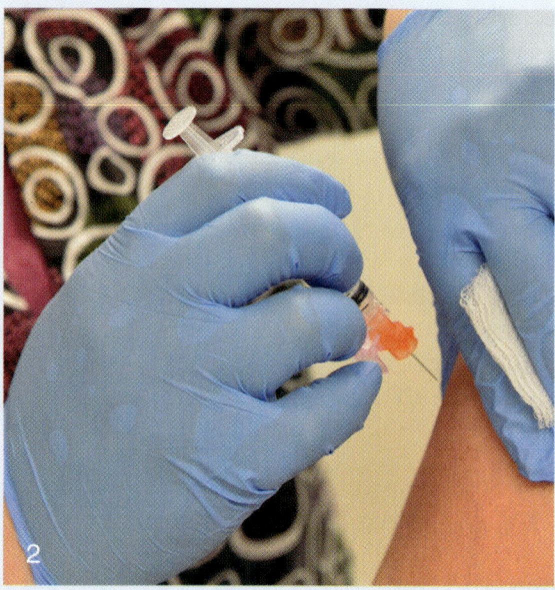

PROCEDURE 30.8 Administer a Subcutaneous Injection—*continued*

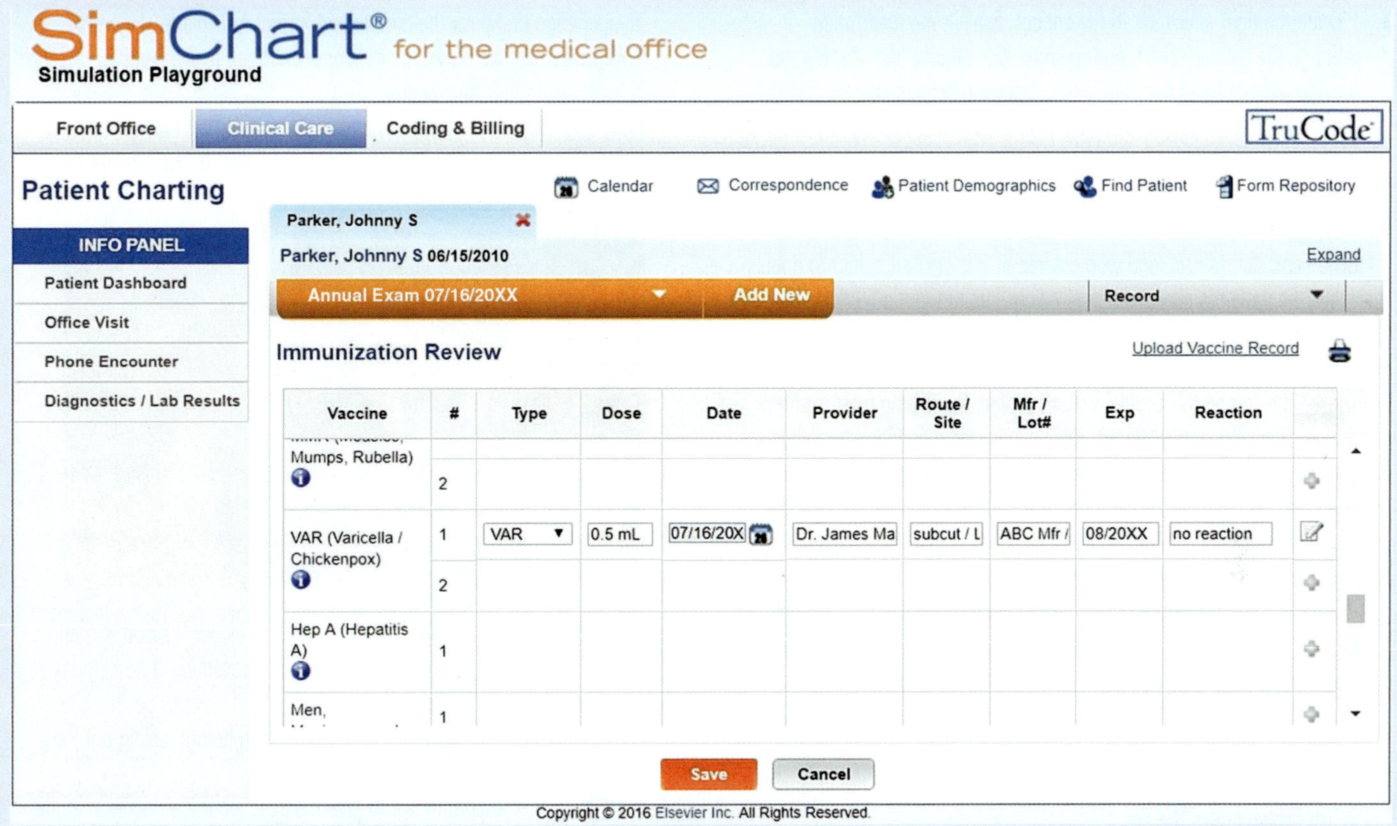

PROCEDURE 30.9 Administer an Intramuscular Injection

TASKS: Prepare medication from a vial, administer an intramuscular injection, and document the medication administration in the health record.

SCENARIO: Dr. Martin ordered influenza vaccine (IIV) 0.5 mL IM for Erma Willis (DOB 12/09/19XX). (Vial information: MN Manufacturer, Lot #7845, expires 1 year from today.)

EQUIPMENT and SUPPLIES

- Provider's order
- Patient's health record
- Vial of medication
- Alcohol wipes
- 3-mL syringe
- 22–25 gauge, ⅝- to 1½-inch safety needle
- Gauze
- Bandage
- Medication tray
- Biohazard sharps container
- Waste container
- Drug reference information
- VIS for influenza vaccine (optional)
- Gloves
- Marker

ORDER: Influenza vaccine (IIV) 0.5 mL IM.

PROCEDURAL STEPS

1. Draw medication up from a vial (see Procedure 30.4).
2. Prior to entering the exam room, knock on the door and wait a moment. Greet the patient. Identify yourself. Verify the patient's identity with full name and date of birth. Make sure the patient's information matches the order and the record. Explain what you are going to do.
   PURPOSE: It is important to identify the patient in two different ways to ensure that you have the correct patient. Explaining the procedure can make the patient feel more comfortable and reduces anxiety.

Continued

PROCEDURE 30.9 Administer an Intramuscular Injection—*continued*

3. Provide the right education to the patient. Explain the medication ordered, the desired effect, and common side effects; also identify the provider who ordered the medication. Answer any questions the patient may have. Use language the patient can understand. Ask if the patient has any allergies. If the patient refuses the medication, notify the provider.
   PURPOSE: The patient needs to be aware of what you are giving, its action and side effects, and who ordered it. It is also important to double-check the patient's allergies before administering the medication.
4. Use hand sanitizer and put on gloves.
   PURPOSE: Hand sanitization is an important step for infection control.
5. Loosen the cap on the needle, but still protect the needle from contamination. Open the alcohol wipes. Have gauze and a bandage available.
   PURPOSE: Loosening the cap prior to starting allows you to remove the cap with one hand during the procedure. You should never remove the cap with your teeth.
6. Find the site using the landmarks.
   PURPOSE: It is important to find the correct location for the injection.
7. Cleanse the site with an alcohol wipe using a circular motion. Move from the center outward, using some friction to help clean the site. Create about a 2-inch circle at the site. Let the site dry.
   PURPOSE: Cleaning from the inside to the outside prevents contamination of the cleaned area. Avoid waving over or blowing on the alcohol, which contaminates the site.
8. Perform the right technique. Place a gauze between the index and middle fingers of your nondominant hand. With that hand, stretch or flatten the site. Hold the site.
   PURPOSE: The site needs to be flattened or stretched for an intramuscular injection.
9. Pick up the syringe and tip it to remove the cover. Hold the syringe like a dart with your dominant hand (Figure 1). Quickly and smoothly insert the needle into the site at a 90-degree angle. Insert the entire needle.
   PURPOSE: Inserting the needle quickly is important to minimize pain.

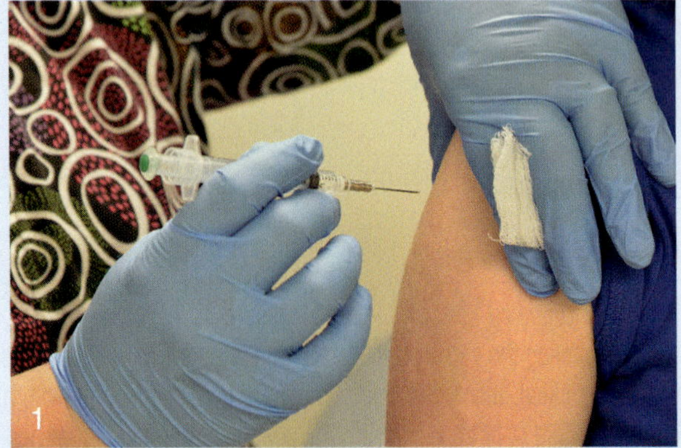

1

10. *One-handed option:* Continue to hold the site. Securely grasp the syringe between the fingers of your dominant hand. Place your thumb under the plunger edge and push the plunger out farther to aspirate (Figure 2).
    Two-handed option: Move the nondominant hand to the plunger. Pull the plunger out farther to aspirate.
    PURPOSE: It is important to aspirate before giving an IM injection. Follow the facility's policy on whether to use the one- or two-handed option.

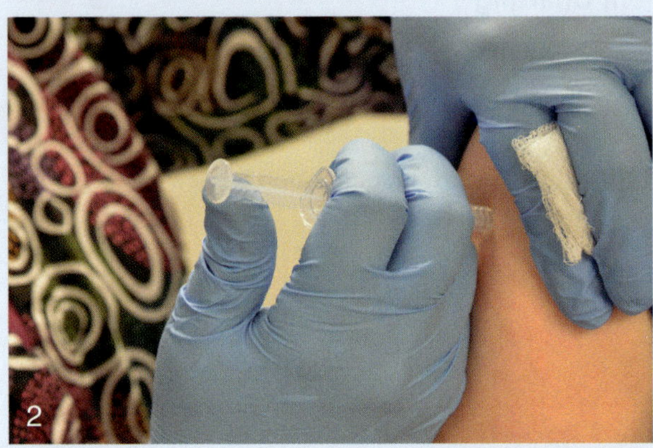

2

11. Aspirate for 5 seconds and check the barrel for blood. If blood is seen, pull out the needle and discard it. Restart the procedure. If no blood is seen, inject the medication at a rate of about 10 seconds per milliliter. Ensure that all the medication has been injected before pulling out the needle at the same angle used for entry.
    PURPOSE: It is important not to give the injection if the needle is in the bloodstream.
12. Activate the needle's safety device with one hand while using the other hand to cover the site with gauze. Gently apply pressure at the site to stop any bleeding. Apply a bandage if the patient requests it.
    PURPOSE: Ask if the patient would like a bandage if the site has stopped bleeding. Remember that some bandages may contain latex, which can be an allergen for some people. Some people may be allergic to the adhesive.
13. Discard the needle/syringe in a biohazardous sharps container. Make sure to put the needle in first.
    PURPOSE: Safely discarding the needle/syringe will help prevent needlestick injuries.
14. Observe the patient for any adverse reactions. Clean up the area. Discard the waste in the waste container. Sanitize your hands.
    PURPOSE: It is important to monitor the patient and clean up the work area.
15. Document the procedure in the health record. Include assessments done, allergies, teaching or instructions provided; the name of the provider who ordered the medication; the medication's name, dose, and route; and how the patient tolerated the medication. Also include the manufacturer, lot number, and expiration date for vaccines and controlled substances. Figure 3 shows the documentation using an electronic health record.
    PURPOSE: Medications given need to be documented to indicate they were given.

PROCEDURE 30.9 Administer an Intramuscular Injection—*continued*

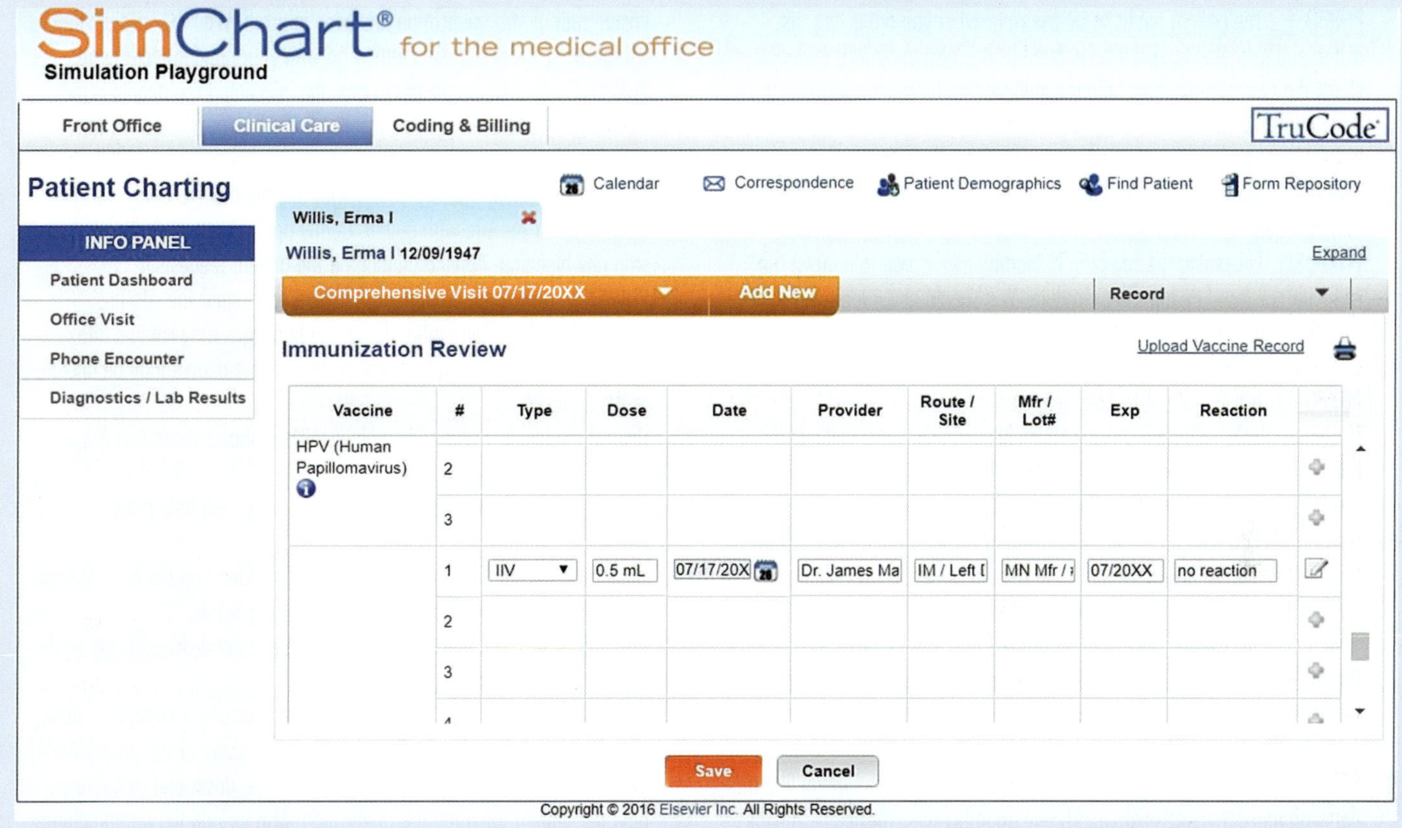

PROCEDURE 30.10 Administer an Intramuscular Injection Using the Z-Track Technique

TASKS: Prepare medication from a vial, administer an intramuscular injection, and document the medication administration in the health record.

SCENARIO: Dr. Martin orders Iron Dextran 0.5 mL IM for Erma Willis (DOB 12/09/19XX). (Vial information: FE Manufacturer, Lot #625, expires 1 year from today.)

EQUIPMENT and SUPPLIES

- Provider's order
- Patient's health record
- Vial of medication
- Alcohol wipes
- 3-mL syringe
- 18–21 gauge, 1- to 1½-inch needle
- Gauze
- Bandage
- Medication tray
- Biohazard sharps container
- Waste container
- Drug reference information
- Gloves
- Marker

PROCEDURAL STEPS

1. Draw medication up from a vial (see Procedure 30.4).
2. Prior to entering the exam room, knock on the door and wait a moment. Greet the patient. Identify yourself. Verify the patient's identity with full name and date of birth. Make sure the patient's information matches the order and the record. Explain what you are going to do.
   PURPOSE: It is important to identify the patient in two different ways to ensure that you have the correct patient. Explaining the procedure can make the patient feel more comfortable and reduces anxiety.
3. Provide the right education to the patient. Explain the medication ordered, the desired effect, and common side effects; also identify the provider who ordered the medication. Answer any questions the patient may have. Use language the patient can understand. Ask if the patient has any allergies. If the patient refuses the medication, notify the provider.

Continued

PROCEDURE 30.10 Administer an Intramuscular Injection Using the Z-Track Technique—*continued*

PURPOSE: The patient needs to be aware of what you are giving, its action and side effects, and who ordered it. It is also important to double-check the patient's allergies before administering the medication.

4. Use hand sanitizer and put on gloves.
   PURPOSE: Hand sanitization is an important step for infection control.
5. Loosen the cap on the needle, but still protect the needle from contamination. Open the alcohol wipes. Have gauze and a bandage available.
   PURPOSE: Loosening the cap prior to starting allows you to remove the cap with one hand during the procedure. You should never remove the cap with your teeth.
6. Find the site using the landmarks.
   PURPOSE: It is important to find the correct site.
7. Perform the right technique. Place a gauze between the index and middle fingers of your nondominant hand. With that hand, displace the tissue.
   PURPOSE: The tissue needs to be displaced before you cleanse the site.
8. Cleanse the site with an alcohol wipe using a circular motion. Move from the center outward, using some friction to help clean the site. Create about a 2-inch circle at the site. Let the site dry while continuing to hold the area.
   PURPOSE: Cleaning from the inside to the outside prevents contamination of the cleaned area. Avoid waving over or blowing on the alcohol, which contaminates the site.
9. Pick up the syringe and tip it to remove the cover. Hold the syringe like a dart with your dominant hand. Quickly and smoothly insert the needle into the site at a 90-degree angle. Insert the entire needle.
   PURPOSE: Inserting the needle quickly is important to minimize pain.
10. Continue to hold the site. Securely grasp the syringe between the fingers of your dominant hand. Place your thumb under the plunger edge and push the plunger out farther to aspirate.
    PURPOSE: It is important to aspirate before giving an IM injection. Follow the facility's policy on whether to use the one- or two-handed option.
11. Aspirate for 5 seconds and check the barrel for blood. If blood is seen, pull out the needle and discard it. Restart the procedure. If no blood is seen, inject the medication at a rate of about 10 seconds per mL. Ensure that all the medication has been injected. Wait 10 seconds before withdrawing the needle and letting go with your nondominant hand.
    PURPOSE: It is important not to give the injection if the needle is in the bloodstream. Waiting 10 seconds allows the medication to start absorbing.
12. Activate the needle's safety device with one hand while using the other hand to cover the site with gauze. Gently apply pressure at the site to stop any bleeding. Apply a bandage if the patient requests it.
    PURPOSE: Ask if the patient would like a bandage if the site has stopped bleeding. Remember that some bandages may contain latex, which can be an allergen for some people. Some people may be allergic to the adhesive.
13. Discard the needle/syringe in a biohazardous sharps container. Make sure to put the needle in first.
    PURPOSE: Safely discarding the needle/syringe will help prevent needlestick injuries.
14. Observe the patient for any adverse reactions. Clean up the area. Discard the waste in the waste container. Sanitize your hands.
    PURPOSE: It is important to monitor the patient and clean up the work area.
15. Document the procedure in the health record. Include assessments done, allergies, teaching or instructions provided; the name of the provider who ordered the medication; the medication's name, dose, and route; and how the patient tolerated the medication. Also include the manufacturer, lot number, and expiration date for vaccines and controlled substances.
    PURPOSE: Medications given need to be documented to indicate they were given.

Documentation Example

11/1/20XX 1420 NKA. Per Dr. Martin's order, administered Iron Dextran 0.5 mL IM in left ventrogluteal site using Z-track method. Pt stated she had pain initially but is feeling better. Side effects were discussed with pt prior to administration. Pt had no questions and verbalized understanding of instructions.
———————————————— Gabe Garcia CMA (AAMA)

OPHTHALMOLOGY AND OTOLARYNGOLOGY

31

SCENARIO

Kim Tau, a certified medical assistant (CMA) through the American Association of Medical Assistants (AAMA), has worked at Walden-Martin Family Medical (WMFM) Clinic for several years. Kim has always enjoyed working with ophthalmology and otolaryngology patients. Amy Ling was recently hired at WMFM, and Kim's supervisor asked her to help orient Amy to the practice. Amy recently graduated from a medical assistant program and is familiar with basic eye and ear procedures, but she has many questions about her responsibilities at the clinic. Amy will be responsible for performing initial Snellen and Ishihara screening examinations on new patients and assisting the ophthalmologist and the optician in the practice. She also must become proficient in conducting audiometry screening tests on pediatric patients, performing ear irrigations, and administering otic medications. Kim recognizes that it is important for Amy to be able to perform these skills with accuracy and confidence; however, she also must develop a sensitivity to the communication and education needs of patients with eye and ear disorders.

While studying this chapter, think about the following questions:

- What is the basic anatomy and physiology of the eye and the ear?
- What are the major types of refractive errors?
- Which eye and ear disorders does Amy need to be familiar with on a routine basis?
- How is a Snellen test performed?
- What important steps should Amy follow when performing eye and ear irrigations and medication applications?
- How is an examination with an audiometer conducted?
- How should Kim prepare Amy to care for patients with sensory loss?

LEARNING OBJECTIVES

1. Examine the anatomy and physiology of the eye.
2. Examine the anatomy and physiology of the ear.
3. Analyze the life span changes that occur in the eyes and ears.
4. Examine the diseases and disorders of the eye, including the signs, symptoms, etiology, diagnostic procedures, and treatments.
5. Examine the diseases and disorders of the ear, including the signs, symptoms, etiology, diagnostic procedures, and treatments.
6. Examine the medical assistant's role in examinations, diagnostic procedures, and treatments for conditions of the eye and ear.

VOCABULARY

accommodation Adjustment of the eye that allows a person to see various sizes of objects at different distances.

amblyopia (am blee OH pee ah) Dull or dim vision, with no apparent organic defect.

audible (AW di buhl) Capable of being heard.

audiologist (aw dee OL uh jist) Allied healthcare professional who specializes in the evaluation of hearing function, detection of hearing impairment, and determination of the anatomic site of impairment.

auditory cortex The region of the cerebral cortex that receives auditory data.

biconvex (bie KON veks) Has two outward curving surfaces on a lens.

binocular (buh NOK yuh ler) Involving, relating, or seeing with both eyes.

dynamic (die NAM ik) **equilibrium** Relating to balance when moving at an angle or rotating.

equilibrium (ee kwi LIB ree uhm) A state of rest or balance due to the equal action of opposing forces.

evert (ih VURT) To turn the eyelid inside out; the provider typically does this to inspect the area for foreign bodies.

gonioscopy (goh nee AH skuh pee) Used to diagnose glaucoma and inspect ocular movement.

hertz (hurts) The unit of measurement used in hearing examinations; a wave frequency equal to one cycle per second.

medulla oblongata (muh DUHL uh ob lawng GAH tah) The lowest part of the brain, continuous with the top of the spinal cord.

miotic (my OT ik) Any substance or medication that causes constriction of the pupil.

otosclerosis (oh tuh skleh ROH sis) The ossicles of the middle ear (malleolus, incus, and stapes) become fused and act as a single unit instead of as individual bones.

ototoxic (oh tuh TOK sik) A medicine or substance capable of damaging cranial nerve VIII or the organs of hearing and balance.

VOCABULARY—*continued*

photophobia (foh toh FOH bee ah) Extreme sensitivity to light.
presbyopia (pres bee oh pee- uh) Farsightedness due to ciliary weakness and loss of elasticity in the lens.
psoriasis (suh RIE i sis) A usually chronic, recurrent skin disease marked by bright red patches covered with silvery scales.
seborrhea (seb uh REE ah) An excessive discharge of sebum from the sebaceous glands, forming greasy scales or crusty areas on the body.
sensorineural (sen suh ree NOOR uhl) Involving the sensory nerves, especially as they affect hearing.
serous (SEER uhs) A thin, watery serum-like drainage.
static equilibrium (STAT ik) Relating to balance when moving in a straight line.
suppurative (SUHP yuh ruh tiv) Characterized by the formation or discharge of pus.
thalamus (THAL uh muhs) The middle part of the brain through which sensory impulses pass to reach the cerebral cortex.
tinnitus (TIN it uhs) A noise sensation of ringing heard in one or both ears.
tonometer (toh NOM i ter) An instrument used to measure intraocular pressure.
vascular (VAS kyuh ler) Having (blood) vessels that conduct or circulate liquids (blood).
vertigo (VUR ti goh) Dizziness; abnormal sensations of movement when there is none.

INTRODUCTION

A medical assistant is responsible for performing a wide variety of procedures in an ophthalmologic or otorhinolaryngologic practice. First, the medical assistant must be familiar with the normal anatomy and physiology of the eyes, ears, nose, and throat. With an understanding of how these specialty sensory organs function, the medical assistant can master the skills needed to become a valuable asset to providers who specialize in the treatment of eye and ear disorders.

Ophthalmology is the science of the eye and its disorders and diseases. A physician who specializes in the diagnosis and treatment of disorders and diseases of the eye is an *ophthalmologist.* An ophthalmologist is a licensed medical physician who can diagnose eye disorders, prescribe medication, conduct eye screenings, prescribe glasses or contact lenses, and perform optic surgery. An *optometrist* is not a medical doctor, but this individual is licensed and has earned a degree as a doctor of optometry (OD). An optometrist can perform eye examinations, diagnose vision problems and eye diseases, prescribe ophthalmic medications, and treat visual defects through corrective lenses and eye exercises. *Opticians* are trained to fill prescriptions written by ophthalmologists and optometrists for corrective lenses by grinding the lenses and dispensing eyewear.

Otorhinolaryngology is the medical specialty that deals with the ear, nose, and throat. It frequently is referred to as *otolaryngology* or even as a single specialty of otology or laryngology. Usually, the specialty otorhinolaryngology is referred to simply as *ear, nose, and throat* (ENT). An otolaryngologist is a licensed medical physician who is trained in the medical and surgical management and treatment of patients with diseases and disorders of the ear, nose, throat, and related structures of the head and neck.

ANATOMY AND PHYSIOLOGY OF THE EYE

The eye can be divided into the *ocular adnexa,* the structures that surround and support the function of the eyeball, and the structures of the eye itself. The anatomy of the ocular adnexa and the eyeball will be discussed in the following sections.

Ocular Adnexa

Each of our eyes is encased in a protective, bony socket called the *orbit.* Our **binocular** vision sends two slightly different images to the brain that produce depth of vision. Within the orbit, a cushion of fatty tissue protects the eyeball. Only about one-sixth of the eye is outside the orbit. The eyelid helps protect the eye from trauma. The eyebrows help keep irritants out of the eyes. The eyelashes line the margins of the eyelids and help trap foreign particles (Figure 31.1).

The *conjunctiva* is a thin mucous membrane that lines the eyelid. It covers the outside of the eyeball except for the most central portion. The *cornea* covers the center of the eye. The mucus secreted from the conjunctiva helps keep the eye moist. The eye blinks about every 2 to 3 seconds. The meibomian glands are located along the edge of the eyelids near the lashes. These glands secrete an oil that is part of the eye's tears. This oil helps prevent tears from drying up too quickly, creating dry eyes. Blinking causes the *lacrimal gland,* located in the superior outer portion of the upper eyelid to secrete tears. Tears move across the eyes, cleansing and moistening the surface of the eye. Tears drain into the lacrimal canals in the medial corner

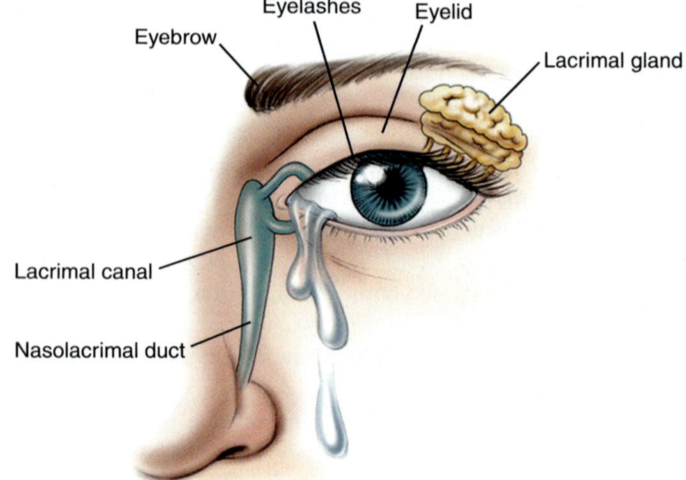

FIGURE 31.1 Ocular adnexa. (From Herlihy B, Maebius NK: *The human body in health and illness,* ed 4, Philadelphia, 2011, Saunders.)

of the eye. The tears then drain into the nasal cavity through the *nasolacrimal* duct. This is why, when a person cries, the excess tears ultimately empty into the nose, producing a watery nasal discharge.

Eyeball

The eyeball consists of three layers. The outermost layer is made up of the white, opaque *sclera* (SKLAYR a) and the transparent cornea. The sclera is a tough, fibrous lining that protects the entire eyeball lying within the orbit. It is also known as the white of the eye. The transparent cornea covers the exposed one-sixth of the eyeball. The cornea acts like a window that allows light to enter the eye. The cornea also *refracts,* or bends the direction of light rays, after they enter the eye (Figure 31.2).

The middle layer is made up of the *choroid*, the *iris*, and the *ciliary body.* The iris is the colored portion of the eye. It is doughnut shaped, with an opening in the center called the *pupil.* The iris contains muscles that regulate the size of the pupil depending on the intensity of light. It becomes smaller in bright light and opens wider in dim light. The ciliary body contains both the ciliary muscle, which regulates the shape of the lens and the ciliary processes, which secrete *aqueous humor*. The choroid is the posterior portion of the middle layer of the eye. It is the eye's **vascular** layer. It contains many blood vessels that supply nutrients to the outer layers of the *retina*. The choroid also has a brown pigment that absorbs excess light rays that could interfere with vision.

The inner layer of the eye includes the retina in the posterior portion and the lens in the anterior portion. The delicate tissue of the retina is composed of light-sensitive neurons called rods and cones. *Rods* are highly sensitive to light and can function in dim light. *Cones* function in bright light and detect color. Rods and cones convert light into nerve impulses. These impulses travel through the optic nerve to the brain, where they are converted into images.

The lens is a transparent, **biconvex** body that helps focus light after it passes through the cornea. The lens and the ciliary body divide the eye into two cavities. The posterior cavity, which is between the lens and the retina, contains the transparent, gel-like *vitreous humor*. The vitreous humor maintains the shape of the posterior eyeball. The anterior cavity, between the cornea and the lens, is filled with aqueous humor, which is continuously produced by the ciliary processes. Aqueous humor helps maintain normal pressure within the eye and provides nutrients to the lens and the cornea (Figure 31.2).

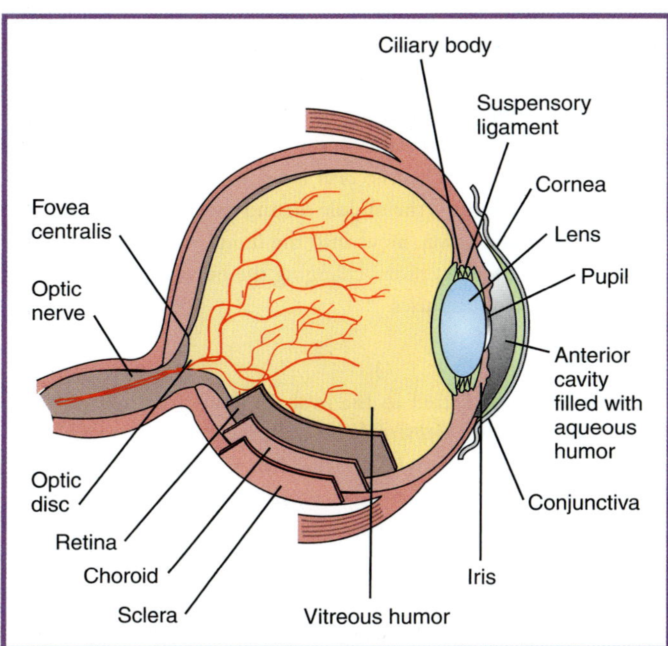

FIGURE 31.2 Anatomy of the eye.

> **CRITICAL THINKING APPLICATION 31.1**
>
> To help Amy become familiar with the terminology used in ophthalmology, Kim asks her to describe the three layers of the eyeball. How would you respond?

Physiology of the Eye

Vision requires light and depends on the proper functioning of all parts of the eye (Table 31.1). A visual impulse begins with the passage of light through the cornea, where the light is refracted; it then passes through the aqueous humor and the pupil into the lens. The ciliary muscle adjusts the curvature of the lens to again refract the light rays so that they pass into the retina, triggering the photoreceptor cells

TABLE 31.1 Functions of the Major Parts of the Eye

STRUCTURE	FUNCTION
Sclera	External protection
Cornea	Light refraction
Choroid	Blood supply
Iris	Light absorption and regulation of pupil width
Ciliary body	Secretion of vitreous fluid; changes the shape of the lens
Lens	Light refraction
Retinal layer	Light receptor that transforms optic signals into nerve impulses
Rods	Distinguish light from dark and perceive shape and movement
Cones	Color vision
Central fovea	Area of sharpest vision
Macula lutea	Center of the retina; contains the fovea centralis, the area of most highly acute vision
External ocular muscles	Move the eyeball
Optic nerve	One of a pair of nerves that transmit visual stimuli to (cranial nerve II) the brain
Lacrimal glands	Produce tears
Eyelid	Protects eye

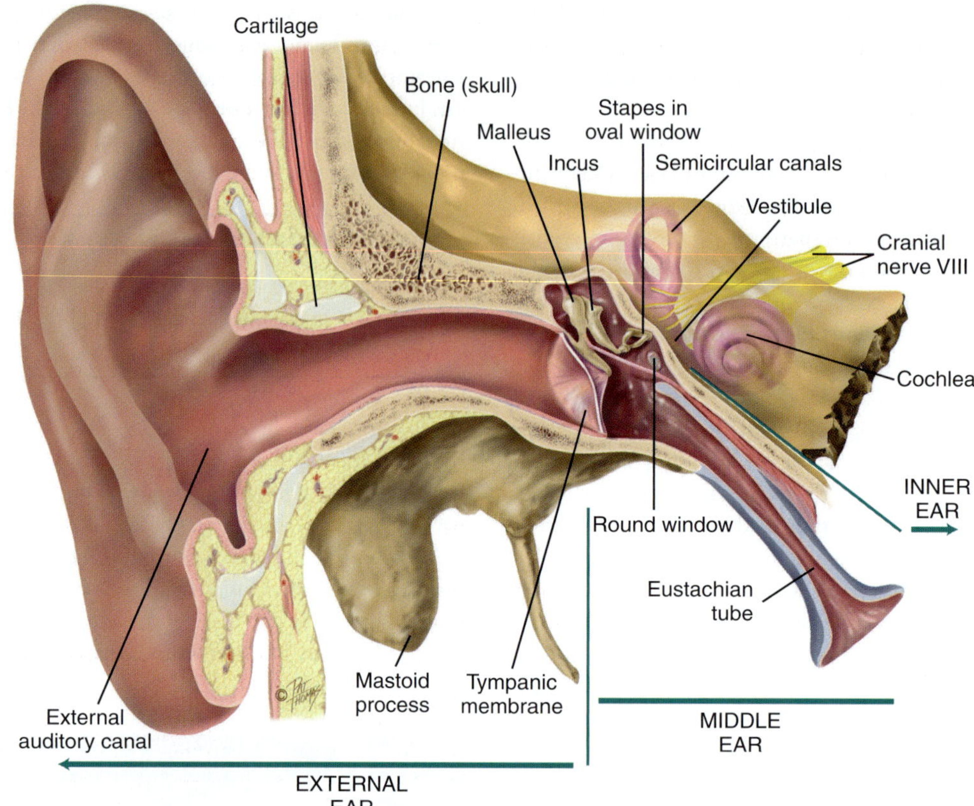

FIGURE 31.3 Anatomy of the ear. (From Jarvis C: *Physical examination and health assessment*, ed 7, Philadelphia, 2016, Saunders.)

of the rods and cones. At this point, the light energy is converted into an electrical impulse, which is sent through the optic nerve to the visual cortex of the occipital lobe of the brain; there, the light impulse is interpreted, and a picture is created.

ANATOMY AND PHYSIOLOGY OF THE EAR

The visible portion of the ear is only a small part of the actual organ of hearing. Most of the sensory structure lies hidden in the *temporal* bone of the skull. The ear is divided into the outer, middle, and inner ear (Figure 31.3). The anatomy of the ear is discussed in the following sections.

Outer (External) Ear

The outer ear consists of the *auricle*, or *pinna*. This is the fleshy part of the ear that can be seen on the side of the head. The next structure is the external *auditory canal*, the tube that extends from the auricle into the *tympanic membrane* (eardrum).

The auricle collects sound waves and sends them into the auditory canal. The skin that lines the auditory canal contains numerous hair follicles and many nerve endings. Earwax, or *cerumen*, is secreted by modified sweat glands within the external auditory canal. Both the hair and the waxy cerumen help prevent foreign objects from reaching the eardrum. The canal has a slightly curved shape and is approximately 1 inch (2.5 cm) long.

Middle Ear

The middle ear is an air-filled cavity that contains three tiny bones called the *ossicles*: malleus, incus, and stapes. Tiny ligaments link these three tiny bones to form a bridge from the tympanic membrane to the inner ear. The ossicles transmit sound to the inner ear through the movement of the stapes. Within the middle ear is an opening for the *eustachian tube*. This is a connection between the ears and the throat. This connection helps equalize pressure within the middle ear. Without equalized pressure in the ear, hearing would not be possible.

The tympanic membrane is a thin, disc-shaped tissue that seals off the outer ear from the middle ear. Sound waves conducted through the external auditory canal hit the tympanic membrane and cause it to vibrate. The vibrations are picked up by the three ossicles and are changed from air-conducted sound waves to bone-conducted sound waves. The ossicles transmit the bone-conducted sound waves through the middle ear to the *oval window*. The oval window is a membrane that connects the middle ear and the inner ear. At the oval window, the sound waves move into the fluids of the inner ear. The fluid motion excites receptors, changing the bone-conducted sound into **sensorineural** impulses.

Inner Ear

Once sound is conducted to the oval window, it is transmitted to a structure called the *labyrinth*, or the inner ear. The inner ear is divided into the *cochlea* and the *semicircular canals*, which are joined by the *vestibule*. The semicircular canals and vestibule function to maintain **equilibrium**. The cochlea is responsible for the sense of hearing.

The *organ of Corti*, which contains the receptors for sound, is located within the cochlea. It is made up of hairlike sensory cells surrounded by sensory nerve fibers that form the cochlear branch of the eighth cranial nerve. Sound impulses cause the hairs to bend and rub against the nerve fibers, which initiate stimuli to travel through the cochlear nerve into the brain for sound interpretation.

The semicircular canals are responsible for evaluating the position of the head in relation to the pull of gravity. The three canals are positioned at right angles to one another on different planes. When the head turns rapidly, these fluid-filled canals must rapidly adjust and send the information to the central nervous system (CNS). The CNS then interprets the information and initiates the desired response to maintain balance. The semicircular canals detect **dynamic equilibrium**. Within the vestibule, two saclike structures function to establish the body's **static equilibrium**. With repetitive or excessive stimulation to the equilibrium receptors, some people become nauseated and may vomit. This condition is known as *motion sensitivity* or *motion sickness.*

Physiology of the Ear

Hearing starts with the sound waves reaching the tympanic membrane. Those sound waves cause the tympanic membrane to vibrate, which causes the ossicles to transmit the waves to the oval window. It is at the inner ear that the sensorineural impulses reach the cochlea.

The organ of Corti contains the receptors for sound and is located within the cochlea of the inner ear. Sound impulses cause the hairlike sensory cells of the cochlea to bend and rub against the nerve fibers. The movement initiates an auditory impulse, which travels through the cochlear nerve onto the eighth cranial nerve. The eighth cranial nerve transmits the auditory impulse to the **medulla oblongata**. The impulses then travel to the **thalamus** and on to the **auditory cortex** of the temporal lobe of the brain. The brain then interprets the auditory impulse into **audible** sound and speech patterns.

LIFE SPAN CHANGES

As we age, changes occur in the functioning of the eyes and ears, and diseases and disorders of the eyes and ears may develop. The following sections discuss some of those changes.

Changes in Children

Infants have to learn to see. When they are born, they have to learn to focus their eyes, use them together, and move them accurately. By about 3 months of age, a baby will be able to follow moving objects and reach for things. By the age of 2, eye-hand coordination and depth perception should be well developed. The American Academy of Ophthalmology recommends that vision screenings begin between the ages of 3 to 5 years. The function of the eyes is assessed from birth forward.

In children, the most prevalent disorder of the eyes is conjunctivitis (commonly known as pinkeye), which accounts for a large number of pediatric visits. Because it is highly contagious, entire classrooms may be infected due to one student's infection. Most newborns receive erythromycin shortly after birth. This has significantly reduced the number of cases of ophthalmia neonatorum conjunctivitis, which is usually due to gonorrhea or chlamydial infection.

One of the biggest changes within the ear for children is in the eustachian tube. This structure connects the middle ear to the throat, and in young children, it is shorter and more horizontal than in adults. This can lead to more ear infections in young children.

Unlike vision, an infant does not need to learn to hear, but regular hearing tests begin when one is a newborn. If all is well with that screening, the next screening should occur at school age, unless the parent suspects there is an issue with the child's hearing.

Few babies are born with a hearing loss. The Universal Newborn Hearing Screening (UNHS) test is a means to detect deafness in infancy. Once an infant has been diagnosed, the parents can plan for future treatments and determine how to best handle the condition.

Changes in Older Adults

As we age, there are changes to the eye that can impact vision. **Presbyopia** is the most common. Other conditions will be discussed later in this chapter.

Age-related macular degeneration (ARMD) and cataracts are the most common causes of blindness in older adults. Although there are several successful procedures to treat cataracts, currently, there are no treatments to cure ARMD. Diabetic retinopathy is the most common cause of blindness, but it may also occur much earlier in life. Presbyopia is a visual disorder that usually accompanies aging and results in farsightedness.

Hearing loss is also common as we age. This is referred to as *presbycusis.* Hearing loss can truly impact the quality of life for many people. They may decide that it is just too hard to be in large groups of people and have to continually ask people to repeat themselves. Hearing aids may help with this hearing loss and provide some improvement in that quality of life.

EYE DISEASES AND DISORDERS

The following sections discuss the common diseases and disorders of the eye, including the signs, symptoms, etiology, diagnostic procedures, and treatments.

Refractive Errors

Four major types of refractive errors result when the eye is unable to focus light effectively on the retina. *Refraction* is the ability of the lens of the eye to bend parallel light rays coming into the eye so that the rays are focused simultaneously on the retina. An *error of refraction* means that the light rays are not refracted or bent properly and consequently do not focus correctly on the retina. Defects in the shape of the eyeball can cause a refractive error. Most refractive errors can be corrected with corrective lenses, contacts, or surgery (Figure 31.4).

Hyperopia (Farsightedness)

When light enters the eye and focuses behind the retina, a person has *hyperopia.* This disorder occurs when the eyeball is too short from the anterior to the posterior wall. An individual with hyperopia has difficulty seeing objects that are close, at reading or working level. A convex corrective lens helps the eye's internal lens place objects directly on the retina and creates a sharp, detailed image, or refractive surgery may be done to correct the shape of the lens.

Myopia (Nearsightedness)

Myopia occurs when light rays entering the eye focus in front of the retina, causing objects at a distance to appear blurry and dull. Objects viewed at reading or working level are seen clearly. This disorder causes the eyeball to become elongated from the anterior to the

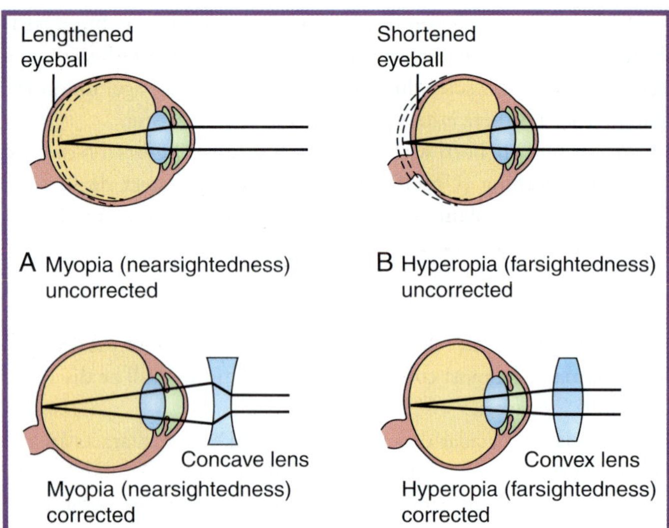

FIGURE 31.4 Errors in refraction. **(A)** Myopia. **(B)** Hyperopia.

posterior wall, and images cannot be sharpened by the internal lens of the eye. A concave corrective lens is used to focus the light rays on the retina, or surgery can be done to change the shape of the cornea. However, the surgery is performed only on adults who have had a stable eye prescription for at least 1 year.

Presbyopia

As people age, the lens of the eye becomes less flexible, and the ciliary muscles weaken; consequently, changing the point of focus from distant to near becomes difficult. This is called presbyopia. The condition results in difficulty seeing at reading level. A combination corrective lens, known as a *bifocal lens* or *progressive lens correction,* is used to focus both distal and proximal objects directly on the retina. Presbyopia actually starts at approximately age 10, but most people do not report an alteration in vision until their early 40s. Conductive keratoplasty is a laser surgical procedure used to treat presbyopia.

Astigmatism

Astigmatism occurs when light rays entering the eye are focused irregularly. This usually occurs because the cornea or the lens is not a smooth sphere but rather has an irregular shape. Ophthalmologists describe the lens as being shaped like a football rather than a sphere, such as a basketball. This causes light rays to be unevenly or diffusely focused on the retina, resulting in blurred vision. It is like attempting to focus on objects seen through a wavy piece of window glass. Astigmatism can be corrected with glasses, contacts, or surgery. Surgical correction attempts to reshape the cornea into a more spherical or uniformly curved surface.

Signs and Symptoms of Refractive Errors

Refractive errors in vision can lead to squinting, frequent rubbing of the eyes, and headaches. The individual notices blurred vision, fading of words at reading level, or both. Some refractive errors are familial in nature.

Treatment of Refractive Errors

Eyeglasses and contact lenses are the traditional treatments for visual acuity problems caused by refractive errors. However, problems with the shape of the lens can be corrected surgically. Surgery is performed on an outpatient basis and requires only a short stay in the facility. Medical assistants employed in an outpatient eye surgery facility must be trained to fulfill this specialized role.

Surgical Correction of Refractive Errors

Most types of health insurance do not cover surgery for refractive corrections. On average, each eye costs $1500 to $3000. The following are some of the surgical procedures performed to correct refractive errors:

- *Photorefractive keratectomy (PRK):* The first surgical procedure developed to reshape the cornea with a laser. The same type of laser is used for PRK and LASIK. The major difference between the two types of surgery is how the middle layer of the cornea is exposed before it is vaporized with the laser. In PRK, the top layer of the cornea (the epithelium) is scraped away to expose the stromal layer underneath. In LASIK, a flap is cut in the stromal layer.
- *Laser-assisted in situ keratomileusis (LASIK):* LASIK uses an excimer laser to reshape the central cornea to treat myopia, hyperopia, and astigmatism. A thin, hinged flap of the cornea is created, the flap is lifted, and the exposed surface of the cornea is reshaped. After the corneal curvature has been corrected, the flap is replaced, and the area heals without stitches.
- *Laser-assisted epithelium keratomileusis (LASEK):* In LASEK surgery, the surface epithelial cells of the eye are softened with an alcohol solution, allowing the epithelial layer to be rolled back and the cornea to be exposed. A laser is then used to reshape the cornea and treat myopia, hyperopia, and astigmatism. The epithelial flap is returned to its original position, and a contact lens is placed on the cornea as a bandage for several days to aid healing and reduce pain.
- *Conductive keratoplasty (CK):* CK uses heat created by a laser to reshape the cornea. Heat is applied to the cornea's outer edge to tighten and steepen the cornea. CK is used in patients older than 40 years of age who need correction for hyperopia, presbyopia, and myopia. The procedure causes little or no discomfort and improves vision almost instantly. The corneal changes are not permanent, and retreatment may be required.

CRITICAL THINKING APPLICATION 31.2

Amy is assisting Dr. Martin with visual acuity examinations. He asks her whether she understands the causes of refractive errors. Amy has difficulty explaining why refractive errors occur, so she tells Dr. Martin she will research the topic and get back to him. What have you learned about the different refractive disorders and why they occur?

Strabismus

Strabismus is failure of the eyes to track together, which means that both eyes do not look in the same direction at the same time. Adults can develop strabismus because of a condition or disease elsewhere in the body, such as diabetes mellitus, muscular dystrophy, or hypertension, or as the result of a head injury. In children, strabismus is caused by weakness in the muscles that control eye movement. If the condition appears in infancy or childhood, it is most commonly associated with **amblyopia**. Treatment involves having the child wear a patch over the unaffected eye so that the muscles of the "lazy" eye are strengthened or administering atropine eyedrops to the unaffected eye to medically decrease visual acuity in the "sound" eye, thereby forcing the amblyopic eye to compensate. It was once standard therapy that an eye patch would be worn up to 6 hours per day, but getting young children to comply with this treatment is very challenging. In children with moderate amblyopia, research shows that patching daily for 2 hours is as effective as patching for 6 hours daily, and daily atropine is as effective as daily patching. Children older than 7 years may still benefit from patching or atropine, particularly if they have not previously received treatment for amblyopia. Amblyopia recurs in 25% of children after patching is discontinued; however, slowly reducing the amount of time the patch is worn each day at the end of treatment reduces the risk of recurrence. The main symptom in all age groups is *diplopia* (double vision).

Nystagmus

A constant, involuntary movement of one or both eyes are called *nystagmus.* The eye can move in any direction, and the movement is accompanied by blurred vision. A child may be born with the problem (congenital nystagmus), or the condition may be acquired as a result of a brain tumor, an inner ear lesion, multiple sclerosis, or substance abuse. Nystagmus is caused by an abnormal function in the part of the brain that controls eye movements. Congenital nystagmus is more common than acquired nystagmus, is usually milder, does not worsen over time, and is not associated with any other disorder. A patient with signs and symptoms of nystagmus should initially have a neurologic evaluation to determine the cause of the disorder, with treatment based on those findings. However, congenital nystagmus has no cure. Affected individuals typically are not aware of the eye movements, but they may have a decrease in visual acuity that can be corrected with surgery or corrective lenses.

Infections of the Eye

Many acute disorders of the eye are seen in the ophthalmologist's office. These include the following:

- *Hordeolum* (sty): A localized, purulent infection of a sebaceous gland of the eyelid. The area is inflamed, swollen, and painful. The infection usually is caused by staphylococci, and it is treated with warm compresses and topical or systemic antibiotics.
- *Chalazion:* A small cyst that results from blockage of a meibomian gland (sebaceous gland) and lubricates the posterior margin of each eyelid. The cyst can become infected, inflamed, swollen, and painful. It may disappear spontaneously or may need to be removed surgically.
- *Keratitis*: Inflammation of the cornea that results in superficial ulcerations. It can be caused by the herpes simplex virus, bacteria, or fungi, or it may develop as a result of corneal trauma (e.g., intense light). Symptoms include inflammation, tearing, pain, and **photophobia**. The condition is treated with ophthalmic ointments, eye drops, and use of an eye patch.
- *Conjunctivitis*: Inflammation of the conjunctiva caused by irritation, allergy, or bacterial infection. Bacterial conjunctivitis (pinkeye) is highly contagious and produces a purulent discharge. Symptoms include inflammation, swelling and itching of the sclera, photophobia, and tearing. Bacterial infections are treated with antibiotic ophthalmic preparations.
- *Blepharitis:* Inflammation of the glands and lash follicles along the margins of the eyelids that may be caused by staphylococcal infection, allergies, or irritation. Symptoms include itching and inflammation along the eyelash margins; the condition is treated with antibiotic ophthalmic ointment.

Disorders of the Eyeball

The following sections discuss the common disorders of the eyeball, including the signs, symptoms, etiology, diagnostic procedures, and treatments.

Corneal Abrasion

The cornea, the transparent outer covering of the eye, is prone to abrasion because of its location. Symptoms of corneal abrasion include pain, inflammation, tearing, and photophobia. The abrasion is usually caused by a foreign body in the eye or by direct trauma, such as from poorly fitting or dirty contact lenses. A corneal ulcer may form and become infected.

Diagnosis is based on the patient's signs and symptoms, but it can be confirmed with the instillation of fluorescein stain (Figure 31.5). After instillation of the stain, the provider uses a cobalt blue filtered light to visualize the abrasion, which appears green (Figure 31.6). If the abrasion is caused by a foreign body, it must be removed first; the eye can then be treated with antibiotic ophthalmic ointment to prevent infection. Although patching the affected eye has been recommended in the past, studies now show that patching does not reduce the patient's pain and may actually prolong healing time. Corneal abrasions are quite painful, so the patient may be prescribed topical nonsteroidal anti-inflammatory ophthalmic drops, such as diclofenac (Voltaren) and ketorolac tromethamine (Acular), in addition to oral analgesics. Most corneal abrasions heal in 24 to 72 hours, but the patient should be aware that symptoms can worsen if the affected eye is exposed to bright light, if excessive blinking occurs, or if the patient rubs the injured surface of the cornea against the inside of the eyelid. Because the patient may develop a secondary infection from the corneal injury, topical antibiotics, including ciprofloxacin

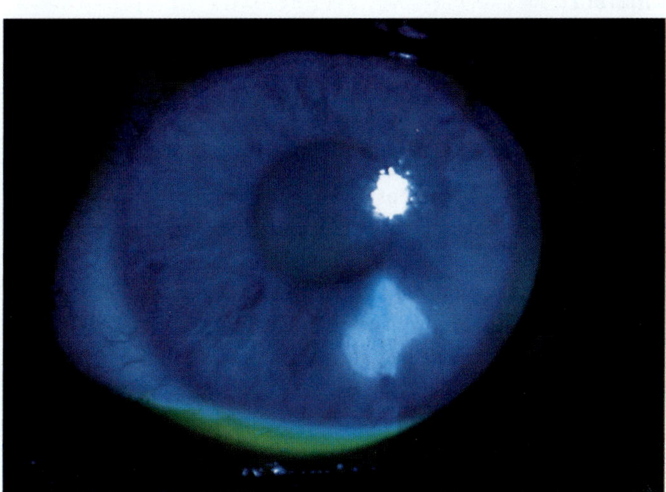

FIGURE 31.5 Corneal abrasion stained with fluorescein.

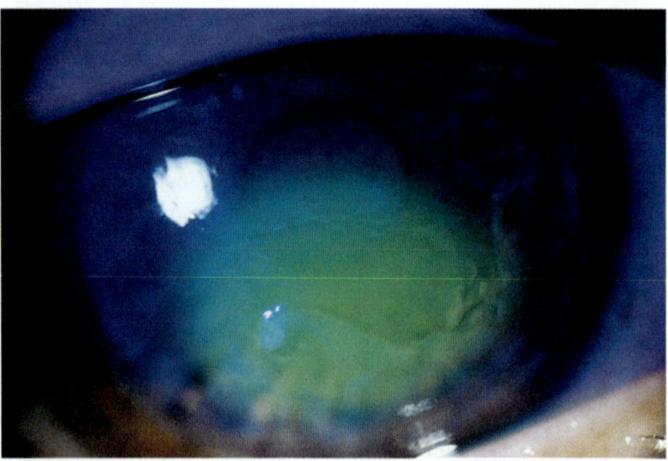

FIGURE 31.6 Corneal abrasion stained with fluorescein and highlighted by cobalt blue light.

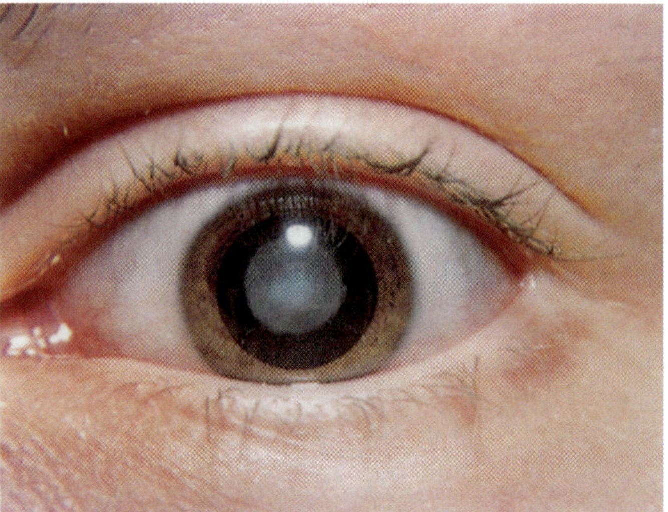

FIGURE 31.7 Cataract. (From Black JM, Hawks JH, Keene A: *Medical surgical nursing: clinical management for positive outcomes*, ed 8, Philadelphia, 2009, Saunders.)

0.3% (Ciloxan) ointment or drops and gentamicin 0.3% ointment or drops may be prescribed. Patients with contact lenses may be prescribed oral antibiotics and should not wear their contacts until the abrasion has healed and the course of antibiotics has been completed.

Cataract

A cataract is a cloudy or opaque area in the normally clear lens of the eye that blocks the passage of light into the retina, causing impaired vision. This condition may result from injury to the eye, exposure to extreme heat or radiation, or inherited factors. However, most cataracts develop slowly and progressively as a result of the natural aging deterioration of the lens of the eye and typically occur after age 60. With advanced cataracts, the pupil of the eye appears white or gray (Figure 31.7).

A cataract scatters the light as it passes through the lens, preventing a sharply defined image from reaching the retina resulting in blurred and dimmed vision. The patient may need a brighter reading light or must hold objects closer to the eyes for better viewing. Continued clouding of the lens may cause diplopia. The patient also needs frequent changes of eyeglass prescriptions. Patients with cataracts report difficulty with *night vision* (nyctalopia), seeing halo images around lights, and increased sensitivity to glare. If left untreated, cataracts ultimately can lead to blindness.

When the patient's vision becomes distorted or appears to be deteriorating, the ophthalmologist performs a *slit lamp* procedure, in which the structures at the front of the eye are examined using a combination of a low-power microscope and a high-intensity light that shines into the eye as a slit beam.

The symptoms of early cataracts may be improved with new eyeglasses, brighter lighting, and antiglare sunglasses. If these measures do not help, surgical removal of the lens is the only effective treatment. This is performed as an outpatient procedure in a clinic or hospital. After the eye has been anesthetized, the inner portions of the lens (the nucleus and the cortex) are removed. The provider may use an extracapsular extraction, in which the cataract is removed in one piece, or phacoemulsification, in which an ultrasonic probe is used to break up the cataract and the pieces are aspirated before an artificial intraocular lens (IOL) is implanted. The incision may be closed with fine sutures, or it may be sutureless and self-sealing. The procedure usually takes 15 minutes, and the patient typically can leave the facility after 1 hour. Patients should be aware that they will not be able to drive until cleared by the ophthalmologist and that they may need help at home until their vision is clear.

The patient is seen in the office the day after surgery and as frequently as needed for the next month. Vision gradually improves until it stabilizes, usually within 2 to 6 weeks; the patient then is fitted with new corrective lenses to match the improved vision.

Glaucoma

One of the most common and serious ocular disorders is a group of diseases known as *glaucoma.* Glaucoma is characterized by increased intraocular pressure (IOP), which damages the optic nerve and causes blindness if left untreated. It rarely occurs in people younger than age 40 and usually is seen in individuals older than age 60. The cause is unknown, but a hereditary tendency toward development of the most common forms has been noted. Glaucoma is responsible for approximately 12% of all cases of blindness. After cataracts (which are typically age related and can be resolved surgically), glaucoma is the leading cause of blindness among African Americans. It is estimated that more than 3 million Americans have glaucoma, but only half of those know they have it.

The ciliary body constantly produces aqueous humor, which should circulate freely between the anterior and posterior chambers of the eye and eventually empty into the general circulation. A healthy eye is filled with fluid in an amount carefully regulated to maintain the shape of the eyeball. In chronic open-angle glaucoma, the channels that drain the fluid malfunction, and over time aqueous humor builds up, resulting in increased pressure, which affects the blood supply to the retina and the optic nerve. With acute closed-angle glaucoma, the opening of the drainage system narrows or closes completely, causing a sudden increase in IOP.

Patients can have chronic open-angle glaucoma for a long time before symptoms occur. Early detection through regular ophthalmic examinations that include IOP measurements is crucial to prevent permanent vision loss. The need to change eyeglass prescriptions frequently, loss of peripheral vision (often called "tunnel vision"), mild headaches, and impaired adaptation to the dark are some of the signs and symptoms that may be seen with chronic glaucoma. Acute closed-angle glaucoma has more obvious symptoms; the patient complains of severe pain, headaches, inflammation, photophobia, and seeing halos around lights. If left untreated, acute glaucoma can cause permanent blindness in a matter of days.

Screening for glaucoma is conducted during a complete eye examination. The ophthalmologist first uses a **tonometer** with a slit lamp to measure IOP. The air puff tonometer records the degree of indentation of the cornea from a puff of pressurized air without touching the eye. An applanation tonometer records the pressure needed to indent the cornea when the instrument is applied to the front surface of the eye. *Electronic tonometry* is the most recently developed technique. The ophthalmologist gently places the rounded tip of a tool that looks like a pen directly on the cornea, with results evident on a small computer panel. **Gonioscopy** can also be used to examine the aqueous fluid drainage system and determine whether the glaucoma is the open- or closed-angle type. In addition, an ophthalmoscopic examination can identify cupping of the optic disc, which indicates atrophy of the optic nerve.

Diagnosis and immediate treatment for early-stage, open-angle glaucoma can delay the progression of the disease. Open-angle glaucoma can be relieved with **miotic** and beta-blocker eye drops. The combinations of drugs used to treat glaucoma can vary considerably. Miotic medications increase the outflow of aqueous humor, and beta-blockers reduce the production of aqueous humor. It is imperative that the patient use prescribed eye drops and take oral medications daily to prevent further damage to the optic nerve. Laser surgery may be performed to create an opening or build a new channel for drainage of the aqueous humor. The goal of treatment in any type of glaucoma is to diagnose the disease early and effectively treat its progression because any loss of sight that has occurred as the result of increased IOP cannot be regained. In closed-angle glaucoma, medications to lower IOP are prescribed so that surgery can be performed to create a channel in which aqueous fluid can circulate. This is a medical emergency because the pressure must be relieved within a few hours or permanent vision damage occurs.

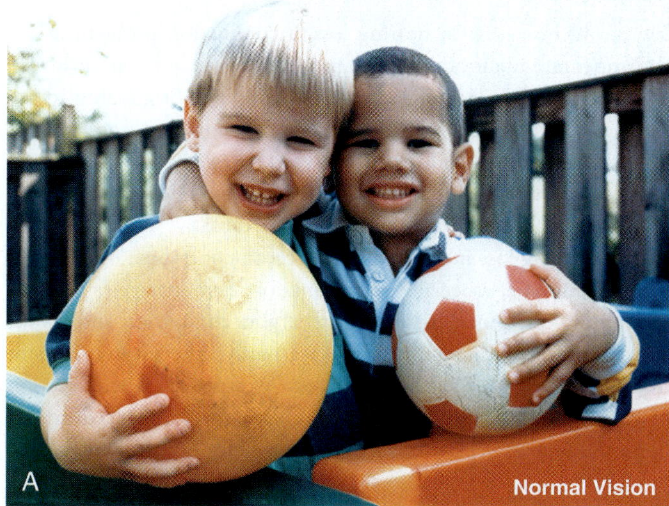

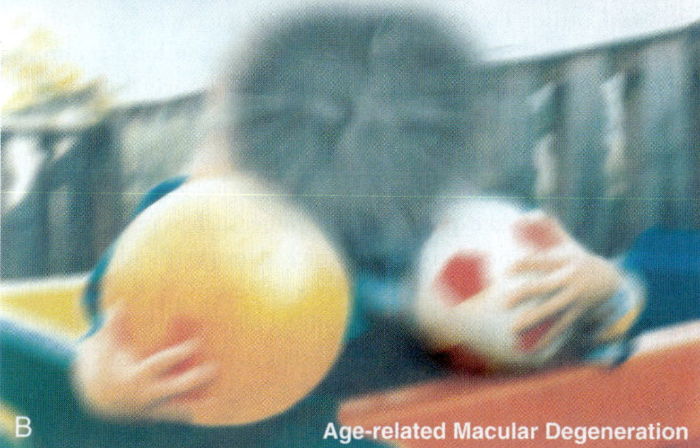

FIGURE 31.8 Visual field for a patient with macular degeneration. (From the National Eye Institute: Age-related macular degeneration: what you should know, National Institutes of Health, Bethesda, MD.)

Diabetic Retinopathy

Diabetic retinopathy is a complication of diabetes mellitus. The blood vessels of the retina become damaged from *hyperglycemia*, causing blockages in the small blood vessels and a decrease in the blood flow to the retina. New blood vessels form but don't develop properly and can leak easily. In the early stages of the disease, there are not many symptoms, but over time the patient may develop spots or dark strings floating in their vision, blurred or fluctuating vision, dark or empty areas in their vision, and vision loss. A comprehensive eye examination can diagnose diabetic retinopathy. Fluorescein angiography and optical coherence tomography may also be used. Treatment is focused on slowing or stopping the progression of the disease. For advanced diabetic retinopathy injection of endothelial growth factor inhibitors can be done to decrease the fluid buildup and to help stop the growth of new blood vessels. Photocoagulation, a laser treatment, can be done to slow or stop the leakage of blood and fluid in the eye. Another type of laser treatment, panretinal photocoagulation, also known as scatter laser treatment, can shrink the vessels. Vitrectomy, a tiny incision in the eye, can be done to remove blood from the middle of the eye and scar tissue.

Macular Degeneration

The *macula lutea*, the part of the retina near the optic nerve, defines the center of the field of vision. Macular degeneration is a progressive deterioration of the macula lutea, which causes loss of central vision; the patient can see only the edges of the visual field (Figure 31.8). The condition affects more than 11 million Americans and is a leading cause of blindness in those older than 50.

Two types of macular degeneration can occur. The dry form accounts for most cases; it is painless and develops slowly, affecting sharp vision over time so that reading and other activities that require fine, detailed vision become impossible. Wet macular degeneration causes 90% of all severe vision losses from the disease and has an acute onset and rapid progression. Dry macular degeneration is caused by the breakdown of light-sensitive cells in the region of the macula; the wet form is seen when new blood vessels behind the retina form and leak blood and fluid into the macula. The condition is age related, but additional risk factors include cigarette smoking, obesity, family history, cardiovascular disease, elevated blood cholesterol levels, light eye color, and excessive sun exposure. The disease has no known cure, but research indicates that antioxidants, including beta carotene and vitamins C and E with zinc and copper, may prevent the condition or help treat the disease in people who have intermediate macular degeneration.

EAR DISEASES AND DISORDERS

The following sections discuss the common diseases and disorders of the ear, including the signs, symptoms, etiology, diagnostic procedures, and treatments.

Hearing Loss

Two problems result in hearing loss, a conduction problem and a sensorineural impairment. Some individuals have both conditions.

Conductive hearing loss is caused by a problem originating in the external or middle ear that prevents sound vibrations from passing through the external auditory canal, limits the vibration of the tympanic membrane, or interferes with the passage of bone-conducted sound in the middle ear. Some common causative factors in conductive hearing loss include impacted cerumen; trauma to the tympanic membrane, especially scar formation; hemorrhage or fluid in the middle ear; **otosclerosis**; and recurrent chronic ear infections. Patients with conductive hearing loss receive the greatest benefit from a hearing aid. If the hearing loss is caused by a malfunction or congenital abnormality of the ossicles, a surgical procedure can be performed to replace the damaged ossicles with manufactured models.

A *sensorineural hearing loss* results from an abnormality of the organ of Corti or the auditory nerve. Viral infection (e.g., rubella, influenza, herpes) can result in hearing loss, as can head trauma or certain **ototoxic** medications. The first sign of ototoxic drug complications usually is **tinnitus**. This sometimes occurs with high doses of aspirin, certain antibiotics (erythromycin and vancomycin), and chemotherapeutic agents. A sensorineural hearing loss also can occur because of prolonged exposure to loud noise, such as repetitive noise in the workplace, or loud music, which damages the delicate cilia lining the organ of Corti.

Presbycusis, the hearing loss that affects older adults, is caused by a reduction in the number of receptor cells in the organ of Corti and is also classified as a sensorineural loss. Children can be born with a congenital hearing deficit or deafness because of an intrauterine infection, such as measles (rubella) (Figure 31.9).

If the sensorineural hearing loss cannot be improved by hearing aids, an option is surgical insertion of cochlear implants. These are complex devices that use electrical impulses to stimulate the auditory nerve, which carries the current to the brain to be interpreted as sound. Cochlear implants bypass damaged portions of the ear and directly stimulate the auditory nerve. These implants do not create normal hearing but provide increased sound for a person with profound or complete hearing loss.

Mixed hearing loss is a combination of conductive and sensory deafness. This type of loss can result from tumors, toxic levels of certain medications, hereditary factors, and stroke.

Otitis

There are two common types of otitis. The first affects the external ear canal and is called *otitis externa* or swimmer's ear. Otitis externa may be caused by dermatologic conditions, such as **seborrhea** or **psoriasis**, trauma to the canal, or continuous use of earplugs or earphones. Swimmers frequently have otitis externa because water collects in the ears and mixes with cerumen to form an ideal culture medium for bacteria and fungus. Patients with otitis externa complain of severe pain and have inflammation and swelling of the external auditory canal, hearing loss, and possibly purulent (containing pus) or **serous** drainage. The inflammation is treated with antibiotic or steroid eardrops, and the canal must be kept clean and dry, or the condition can become chronic.

Otitis media is an inflammation of the normally air-filled middle ear that results in a collection of fluid behind the tympanic membrane. Otitis media can be serous (otitis media with effusion [OME]) or **suppurative**. Serous otitis media occurs because of a buildup of clear fluid in the middle ear; patients complain of a full feeling and some hearing loss. In suppurative otitis media, purulent fluid is present in the middle ear, and the patient has fever, pain, and hearing loss. Otitis media often is associated with an upper respiratory tract infection caused by a virus or an allergic reaction that results in swelling and inflammation of the sinuses and eustachian tubes. A child's eustachian tube is shorter, narrower, and more horizontal than that of an adult. The small size and decreased angle

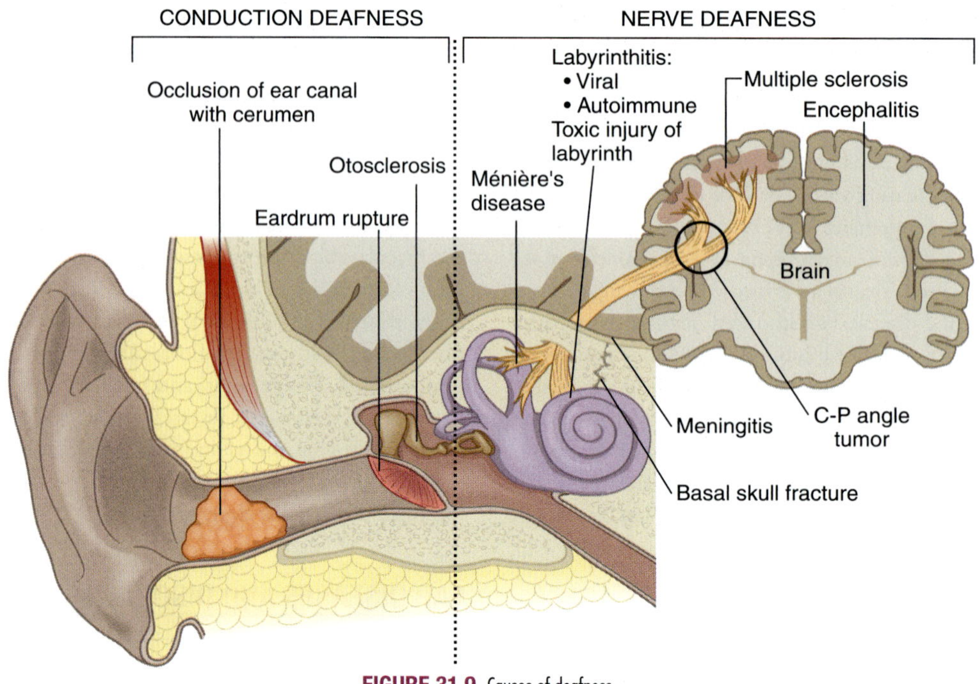

FIGURE 31.9 Causes of deafness.

for drainage increases the chance that inflammation will block the tube and cause fluid to collect in the middle ear, which not only is uncomfortable but also interferes with the conduction hearing process (Figure 31.10).

Risk Factors for Otitis Media

Factors That Cannot Be Controlled

- Sex (male)
- Age (infants and younger children [6 to 18 months])
- Premature birth
- Family history
- Siblings with infections
- Seasonal factors (most common during cold and flu season), seasonal allergies
- Underlying disease (cleft palate, Down syndrome, asthma, allergies)
- Ethnicity (Native American and Alaskan Inuit because of the shape of the eustachian tubes)
- Cochlear implants

Factors That Can Be Controlled

The following behaviors can lower a child's risk for otitis media:

- Limit exposure to large-group child care settings.
- Do not expose the child to second-hand smoke.
- Hold the child upright during bottle feeding.
- Do not use pacifiers beyond 6 months, which may increase the risk.
- Wash hands frequently to prevent the spread of colds and flu.
- Have the child immunized with the pneumococcal conjugate vaccine (Prevnar) and the flu vaccine.

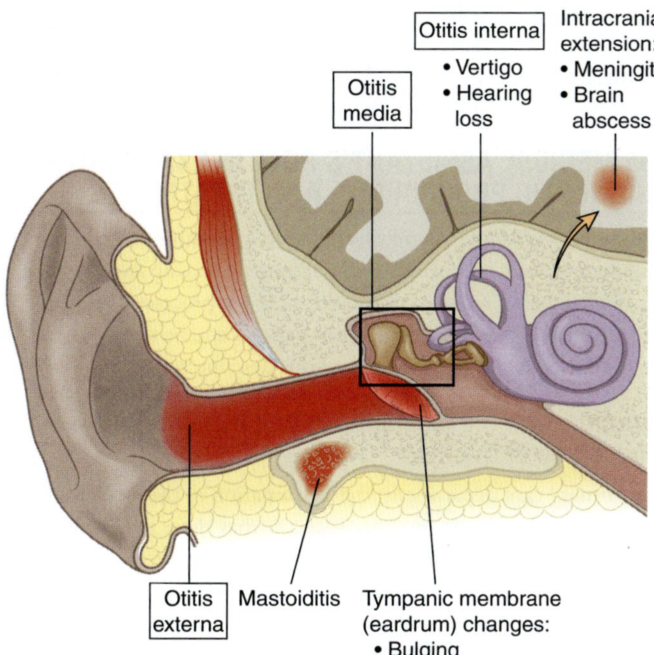

FIGURE 31.10 Inflammation and infection of the ear and surrounding tissues.

An otoscopic examination reveals that the normally pearly gray tympanic membrane is inflamed (bright pink or red) and bulging (Figure 31.11). Areas of fluid or pus may be visible through the membrane. A *tympanogram* may be done to determine the air pressure of the middle ear and the mobility of the tympanic membrane. During a tympanogram test, a small earphone is placed into the ear canal, and the air pressure is gently changed. This test is helpful in showing whether an ear infection or fluid is present in the middle ear (Figure 31.12). A tympanic membrane responding normally to an increase in air pressure will move, resulting in a peaked tympanogram. If fluid or pus in the middle ear is putting pressure on the tympanic membrane, the membrane moves only slightly or not at all, resulting in a slight peak or a flat tympanogram recording.

Treatment of otitis media may be a conservative "watch and wait" approach. However, if a fever and pronounced pain are present, the individual may be given antibiotics and told to take over-the-counter analgesics such as acetaminophen or ibuprofen. If this condition becomes chronic, the provider may recommend a *myringotomy,* which is the creation of a surgical incision in the tympanic membrane to drain the fluid, followed by the insertion of a tympanostomy tube to continually drain the middle ear of fluid. This may be necessary to prevent permanent hearing loss caused by damage to the ossicles (Figure 31.13).

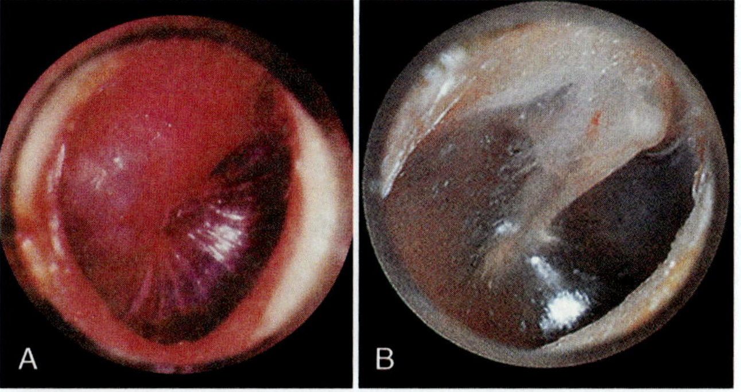

FIGURE 31.11 **(A)** Tympanic membrane with otitis media. **(B)** Normal tympanic membrane. (From LaFleur Brooks M: *Exploring medical language*, ed 9, St. Louis, 2014, Mosby.)

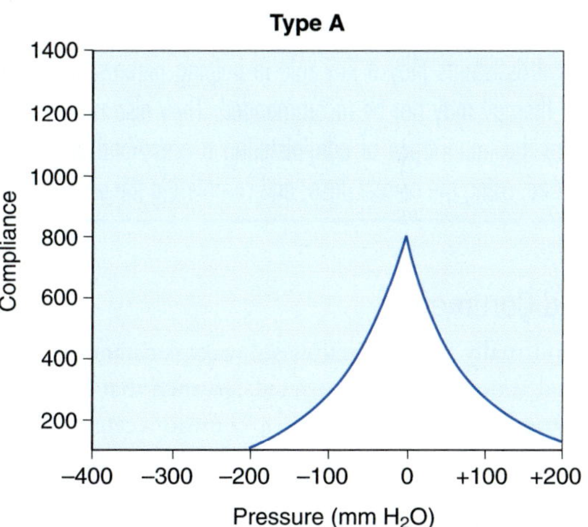

FIGURE 31.12 A normal tympanogram shows a peak at normal pressure (0). An ear with fluid produces a flat tympanogram.

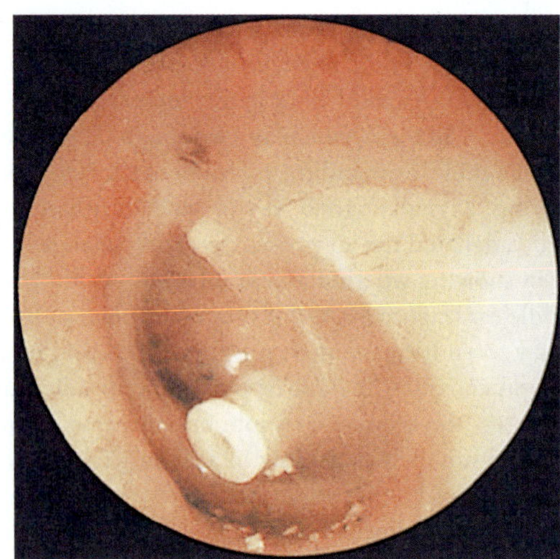

FIGURE 31.13 Tympanic membrane with a tympanostomy tube. (From Frazier MS, Drzymkowski JW: *Essentials of human diseases and conditions*, ed 5, St. Louis, 2013, Saunders.)

Recommendations for Treating Otitis Media

The development of drug-resistant strains of bacteria due to overprescribed antibiotics is a growing concern. The American Academy of Pediatrics recommends the following for the treatment of otitis media:

- Treatment with antibiotics should be delayed, giving the child's immune system a chance to fight the infection by itself. This delay should last 24 hours in children 6 to 24 months old and 72 hours for older children. Approximately 61% of children improve within 24 hours, regardless of whether they are treated. If the child's condition does not improve, an appropriate antibiotic can be prescribed.
- The child typically improves within 48 to 72 hours, but the parent should understand how important it is to complete the antibiotic medication as ordered to prevent the infection from recurring.
- The provider may decide to treat otitis media with a short course of antibiotics (i.e., 5 days) but at a higher dose. The drugs of choice include amoxicillin (Amoxil), azithromycin (Zithromax), and cefuroxime (Rocephin).
- Antibiotics will not help if otitis is caused by a virus. The child should be observed for possible complications, and analgesics should be administered for pain control. Viral otitis media typically resolves within 7 to 14 days.

Medical assistants play a key role in helping parents understand why antibiotic therapy may not be recommended. They also must educate parents about the importance of administering a prescribed antibiotic at the time ordered, using the correct dose, and completing the entire prescription.

Impacted Cerumen

Cerumen normally is a soft, yellowish, waxy substance that lubricates the external auditory canal. Impacted cerumen that has been pushed up tightly against the eardrum is a common cause of conductive hearing loss because sound vibrations cannot pass through the cerumen to initiate movement of the tympanic membrane. Individuals with psoriasis, abnormally narrow ear canals, or an excessive amount of hair growing in the ear canals are more prone to this condition. Excessive secretion of cerumen can gradually cause hearing loss, tinnitus, a feeling of fullness, and *otalgia* (ear pain).

An otoscopic examination quickly reveals this problem. If impacted cerumen is found, it must be removed. This can be done by softening the wax with oily drops, such as carbamide peroxide (Debrox), and then irrigating the ear with warm water until the plug is removed. Because this condition can recur, the patient may need to schedule periodic examinations. If the patient is experiencing hearing loss because of the impaction, it is immediately remedied with the removal of the cerumen.

Ménière Disease

Ménière disease is a disorder of the inner ear. It is characterized by **vertigo**, tinnitus, progressive hearing loss, and sometimes a feeling of pressure or fullness in the ear. It usually only affects one ear. The cause of Ménière disease is not well understood. The inner ear of persons with this condition seems to have an abnormal amount of fluid (endolymph). What causes the excess fluid is not known. Research indicates the following possible causes: abnormal anatomy of the inner ear, genetic predisposition, possible autoimmune condition, head trauma, or migraines.

Ménière disease causes swelling and edema in an endolymphatic sac of the semicircular canals, along with an overproduction or collection of excess endolymph. When an acute attack occurs, the patient may experience nausea, vomiting, and problems with balance. These attacks can last a few hours to several days, and they may increase in severity over time. Although the cause of this problem is unknown, Ménière disease is a chronic, progressive condition that triggers episodes of recurring attacks of vertigo, tinnitus, a sensation of pressure in the affected ear, and advancing hearing loss.

During active periods of the disease, the patient is treated symptomatically with medications for nausea and vomiting. A salt-restricted diet, diuretics, and antihistamines may be prescribed to control edema in the labyrinth of the inner ear. Surgical destruction of the affected labyrinth is an option. Although this relieves symptoms, it may also result in permanent deafness if the cochlea is damaged.

THE MEDICAL ASSISTANT'S ROLE IN EXAMINATION, DIAGNOSTIC PROCEDURES, AND TREATMENTS

As a medical assistant, you may be involved in assisting with the examination, diagnostic procedures, and treatments. Having an understanding of what will be required of you during those processes will help you provide the best possible care for your patients and be the best assistant for your provider. The following sections describe your role.

Assisting with the Examination and Diagnostic Procedures of the Eye

In a primary care department, the examination of the eye is a screening examination. If the provider suspects that there may be an issue with a patient's eyes, the patient will likely be sent to an ophthalmologist for further evaluation and treatment. There are several screening diagnostic procedures that a medical assistant can administer when directed to do so by the provider. The following sections discuss how the medical assistant is involved in the examination and diagnostic procedures of the eye.

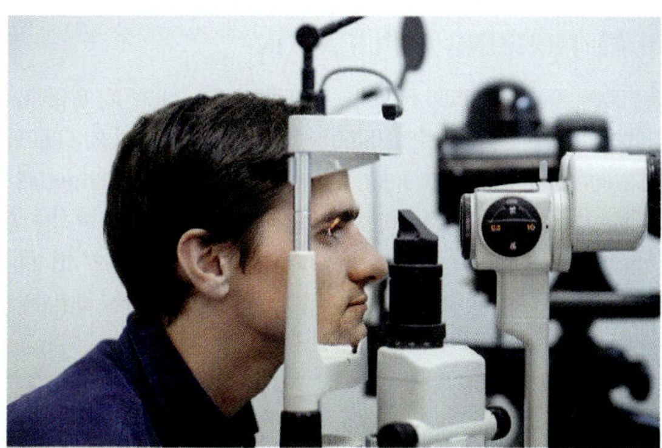

FIGURE 31.14 Slit-lamp examination. A high intensity beam of light is projected through a narrow slit and a cross section of the illuminated part of the eye is examined through a magnifying lens. (From Leonard, P: *Building a medical vocabulary*, ed 11, Philadelphia, 2021, Saunders.)

Assisting with the Examination of the Eye

A complete examination of the eye is technical and requires expensive equipment and the expertise of an ophthalmologist or optometrist. However, a primary care provider performs some basic examinations and treatments of the eye. The ophthalmoscope is used to examine the interior of the eye. It projects a bright, narrow beam of light through the lens and illuminates the interior parts of the eye and retina. It is helpful for detecting disorders of the eyes and certain systemic disorders, such as capillary changes that occur with diabetes mellitus.

The eyelids are examined for edema, which may be the result of nephrosis, heart failure, allergy, or thyroid deficiency. *Blepharoptosis,* also called *ptosis,* is drooping of the upper eyelid that can be caused by a disorder of the third cranial nerve, muscular weakness as seen in muscular dystrophy, or myasthenia gravis.

The pupils of the eyes are normally round and equal. Normal pupils constrict rapidly in response to light. This is demonstrated by shining a bright, pinpoint light into one eye from the side of the patient's head. The pupil of an illuminated eye constricts, and the pupil of the other eye constricts equally. This test is called *light and* **accommodation** (L&A). The eyes of an older patient do not accommodate as well as those of a younger person. Each eye is checked this way. The patient is then asked to look at the provider's finger as it is moved directly toward the patient's nose to check for eye coordination. If the pupils are equal and round, respond normally to light, and adjust and focus on objects at different distances in a reasonable length of time, the provider charts the acronym PERRLA (which stands for "pupils, equal, round, reactive to, light [and], accommodation").

PERRLA

P Pupils
E Equal
R Round
R Reactive to
L Light (and)
A Accommodation

Special techniques used in the ophthalmologist's office include examinations performed with a slit lamp biomicroscope (Figure 31.14). This device is used to view fine details in the anterior segments of the eye. It may be used to view a foreign body because it gives a well-illuminated and highly magnified view of the area. For this examination,

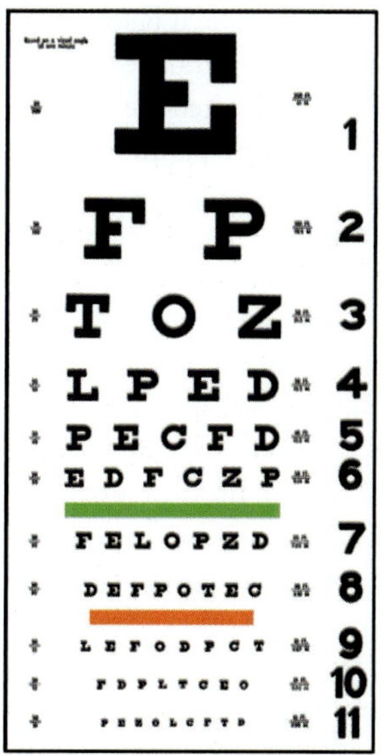

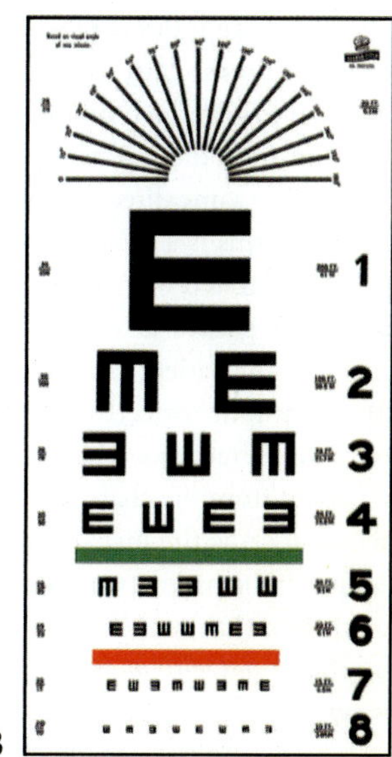

FIGURE 31.15 (A) Snellen visual acuity chart. **(B)** Tumbling E chart. (From Wilson SF, Giddens GF: *Health assessment for nursing practice*, ed 5 St. Louis, 2013, Elsevier.)

the provider first orders the administration of a *mydriatic* eye drop to dilate the pupil and enhance the visualization of eye structures.

A patient with *exophthalmia* (abnormal protrusion of the eye, possibly resulting from an overactive thyroid or a tumor behind the eyeball) is checked with an exophthalmometer. This instrument measures how far the eye protrudes beyond the edge of the eye socket and helps determine the level of tissue swelling and enlargement behind the eye.

Distance Visual Acuity

Determining distance visual acuity frequently is part of a complete physical examination (see Procedure 31.1). It is widely used in schools and industry and is the best single test available for vision screening. Many cases of myopia, astigmatism, and hyperopia have been detected with this routine test. The chart most commonly used is the Snellen alphabetical chart (Figure 31.15A). This chart displays various letters of the alphabet, which the patient must identify in ever smaller font sizes. Patients with limited knowledge of the English alphabet can be tested with the E chart (Figure 31.15B). In addition, a chart that uses pictures and symbols is available. This chart is used for young children or individuals who do not know the alphabet. To avoid patient confusion over the E chart or the symbol chart, the medical assistant should review the charts with patients first to make sure they know how to demonstrate the E visualized or the meaning of each picture or symbol. The symbol on the top line of the chart can be read at 200 feet by people with normal vision. In each of the succeeding rows, from the top down, the size of the symbols is reduced so that a person with normal vision can see them at distances of 100, 70, 50, 40, 30, and 20 feet consecutively.

The patient must not be allowed to study the chart before taking the test. The room or hall should be long enough that the 20-foot distance can be marked off accurately and without interruptions from patient and staff traffic. The chart should be hung at the patient's eye level and illuminated with maximum light, without glare on the chart. Most adults do not need the standard Snellen chart explained, but if the E chart is used, an explanation must be given as to how the E's are to be read. The patient may point up or down or right or left toward the part of the letter that is open. If the E chart is to be used for a child, practice with an index card with a large E drawn on it before the child is tested. Turn the card in different directions to simulate the position of the "fingers" of the E on the chart and give children the opportunity to demonstrate the direction of the E fingers by pointing their own fingers in the same direction (Figure 31.16).

Because this is a gross screening of distance visual acuity, the eyes are typically tested with corrective lenses; therefore, the patient should not remove glasses or contact lenses unless the provider requests it. Indicate in the patient's health record whether the assessment was done with or without corrective lenses. Record the results of each eye separately and as fractions. The numerator (top number) is the distance of the patient from the chart (always 20 feet), and the denominator (bottom number) is the lowest line read satisfactorily by the patient. For example, if the patient reads the 20 line at 20 feet, the fraction 20/20 is recorded for that eye. *The last line the patient can read without squinting or straining and with no more than two mistakes is the line recorded in the patient's record for that eye.* The medical assistant should document the outcomes of the test, specifying the results for each eye and both eyes. The Joint Commission no longer recommends using medical abbreviations for the eyes and ears because they are frequently confused or misinterpreted; therefore, the medical assistant must now document right eye, left eye, and both eyes.

Interpreting Snellen Results

- The patient always stands 20 feet from the chart.
- Each result is a record of how well the patient can see compared with normal vision.
- Example: A patient with a 20/40 reading can see that line correctly standing at 20 feet, but an individual with normal vision can see the same line correctly at 40 feet, so the patient's vision is not as acute as someone with normal vision.
- Example: A patient with a 20/15 reading can see that line accurately standing at 20 feet, but a person with normal vision must stand at 15 feet to have the same vision, meaning the patient's vision is better than someone with normal vision.

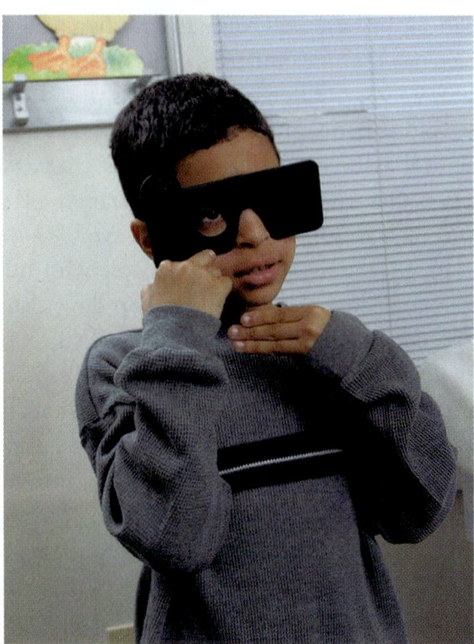

FIGURE 31.16 Visual acuity test with the E chart.

CRITICAL THINKING APPLICATION 31.3

Susie Anthony, a 19-year-old patient, is being seen today for a general eye examination. The provider orders a routine Snellen test, and Kim administers it. Susie wears contacts. With her right eye, she reads without errors to the 20/25 line; however, she squints and makes three errors at the 20/20 line. With her left eye, Susie makes two mistakes at the 20/30 line; with both eyes, she reads the 20/25 without errors. How should Kim document this procedure?

Near Visual Acuity

Near visual acuity can be tested with the near vision acuity chart (Figure 31.17). This test is given to screen for presbyopia or hyperopia. If the patient wears corrective lenses, they should be worn during the test. The size of the type on the card varies from a 66-point font (newspaper headlines) to a 3-point font (medicine bottle labels). The test should be given in a well-lit room, with the patient holding the card approximately 14 to 16 inches away. As with the Snellen examination, the near visual acuity test is given for each eye, starting with the right eye. The eye not being tested should be covered with an occluder but left open. The patient should be monitored for indications of difficulty, such as squinting or tearing. The patient reads the card, starting at the top until reaching the smallest print that can be read. The medical assistant should document the number at which the patient had no more than two errors for each eye and the two eyes together, whether corrective lenses were worn, and any signs of eyestrain.

Ishihara Color Vision Test

Defects in color vision are classified as congenital or acquired. Congenital defects are caused by an inherited color vision defect and are found most often in males. Acquired defects are caused by eye injury or disease. The Ishihara test is a simple, convenient, and accurate procedure that detects total color blindness, in addition to the red-green blindness prevalent in congenital blindness (see Procedure 31.2). The test assesses the perception of primary colors and shades of colors.

The test booklet contains polychromatic plates made of colored dots in numeric patterns. The numbers are one color, and the background dots are a different color. Patients with average visual acuity can read the number within the dot matrix without difficulty. Patients with color vision defects are unable to read the number, or they see a totally different number. A section of plates is included that contains colored line trails through a background of dots. These plates are designed to be used with children and adults who are unable to read numbers. In this situation, the patient uses a finger to follow the dotted trail through the picture.

The test should be administered in a quiet room that is well illuminated by sunlight, not by artificial lighting. If this cannot be done, the best situation possible is created by adjusting lights to resemble the effect of natural daylight. The test uses 14 color plates. The basic test consists of plates 1 through 11. Plates 12 through 14 are used if the patient appears to be having difficulty with red-green differentiation. The medical assistant records the number of plates read correctly. If the score is 10 or higher, the patient is within the average range. If the score is 7 or lower, the patient is suspected of having a color deficiency, and the ophthalmologist performs additional assessment tests using more precise color vision testing equipment.

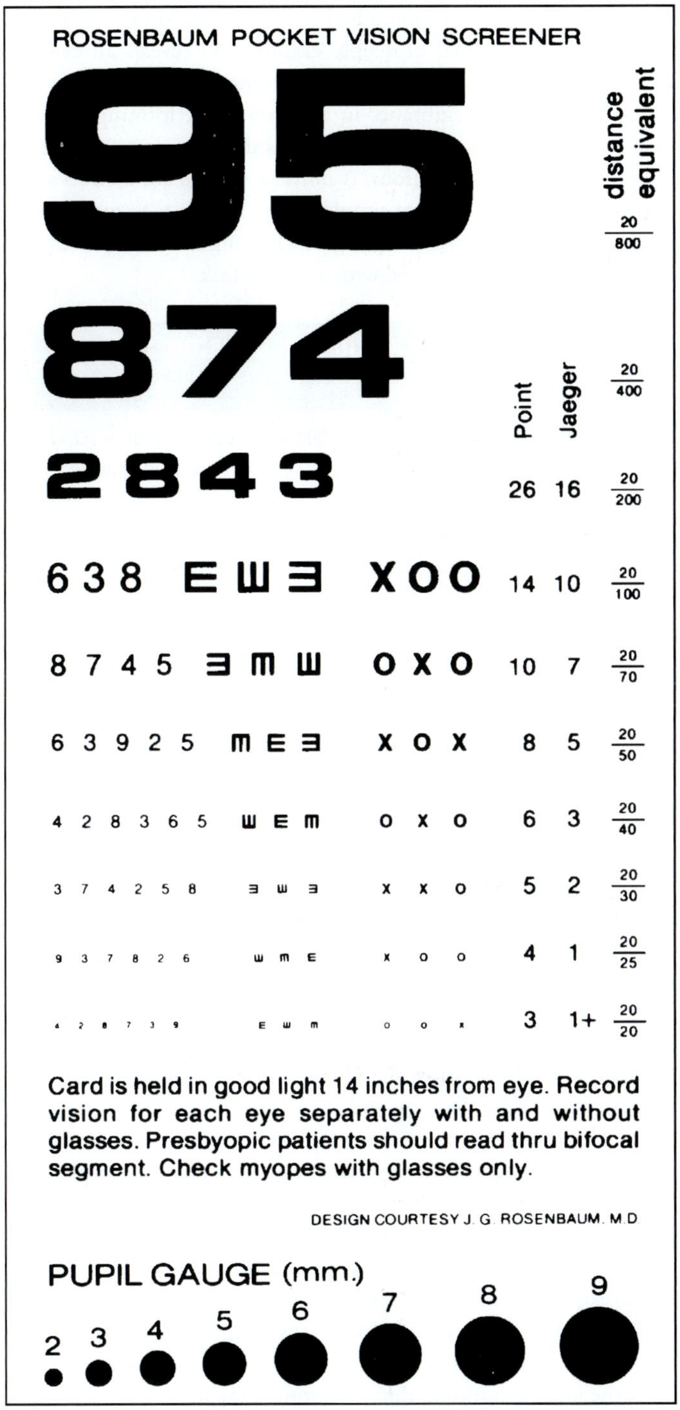

FIGURE 31.17 Near vision acuity chart.

Assisting with Treatments of the Eye

Patients with ophthalmology conditions are prescribed a variety of medications. The following are some of the more common classifications of medications used for this specialty:

- *Topical antibiotic ointments*: Used to treat bacterial infections
- *Anti-inflammatory agents*: Used to reduce inflammation
- *Anti-infectives*: Used to treat viral infections

Refer to Table 31.2 for information on the classification, including indications for use, desired effect, side effects, adverse reactions, and generic and trade names. Medical assistants should be familiar with medications that are prescribed to patients.

Eye Irrigation

The eye is irrigated to relieve inflammation, remove drainage, dilute chemicals, or wash away foreign bodies. Sterile technique and equipment must be used to prevent contamination (see Procedure 31.3). Follow the procedure as ordered, making sure the patient is comfortable. Record the treatment in the patient's health record immediately after it has been determined. Remember, if it is not recorded, it has not been done.

Foreign bodies in the eye are very irritating and may cause considerable pain. Most foreign bodies are superficial and can be removed easily. Occasionally, a foreign particle may be deeply embedded, requiring eye surgery. Notify the provider immediately if a patient comes into the office with something in their eye.

The first objective of the provider's examination is inspection. The patient is asked to look to either side and up and down so that the anterior surface of the eye can be inspected. For the provider to fully inspect under the upper lid, the patient must cooperate by looking downward while the provider **everts** the upper lid using a cotton-tipped applicator. While the lid is maintained in an everted position, any foreign materials may be rinsed away with sterile water or saline solution. If the provider's order is for you to remove the foreign body, do so with irrigation only. If this technique is unsuccessful, cover both of the patient's eyes with a gauze dressing and notify your supervisor immediately. The eyes track each other, so to prevent movement in the affected eye, both eyes must be covered to prevent possible eye trauma.

Safety Alert

Never attempt to remove a foreign body from the cornea using a cotton-tipped applicator. Scratches to the cornea may result, causing scar formation and impaired vision.

TABLE 31.2 Medication Classifications

Classification	Description	Examples
Antivirals	Indications for use: Treat viral infections, including oral and genital herpes, influenza, and HIV. Desired effects: Inhibit the growth or reduce the spread of viral cells. Side effects and adverse reactions: Confusion, diarrhea, headache, kidney disease, urticaria, vomiting.	Oseltamivir (Tamiflu) Acyclovir (Zovirax)
Mydriatics	• Indications for use: Ophthalmic procedures. • Desired effect: Dilate the pupil; some cause paralysis of the ciliary muscle. • Side effects and adverse reactions: Stinging, burning, dry mouth, urine retention.	• Atropine (Isopto Atropine) • Cyclopentolate (Cyclogyl, Pentolair)

CRITICAL THINKING APPLICATION 31.4

The provider tells Kim to irrigate the left eye of a 22-year-old patient to remove a foreign body. She is to irrigate the eye with normal sterile saline solution until clear. How should Kim document this procedure?

Instillation of Eye Medication

Medication may be instilled into the eye to treat an infection, soothe an eye irritation, anesthetize the eye, or dilate the pupils before examination or treatment (Procedure 31.4). Ophthalmic medications are available in several forms. Liquid drops usually are supplied in small squeeze bottles with tips that allow one drop at a time to be dispensed, or the bottle may contain a dropper with a small rubber attachment used to dispense the medication by drops. Eye ointments are dispensed in small metal or plastic tubes with an ophthalmic tip that allows them to be dispensed in a small ribbon of ointment directly into the bottom eyelid.

Safety Alert

Whatever the medication, the dispenser should never touch the eye while the prescribed amount of medication is administered. This can traumatize the eye and can contaminate the medication applicator. If the tip of the dispenser touches any surface, dispose of it in a biohazard waste container because it is contaminated.

Assisting with Examination and Diagnostic Procedures of the Ear

As with examination and diagnostic procedures of the eye, the medical assistant can be involved in the examination and diagnostic procedures of the ear. These examinations and diagnostic procedures will likely be screening in nature with a referral to an otolaryngologist if needed.

The following sections discuss how the medical assistant is involved in the examination and diagnostic procedures of the eye.

Assisting with the Examination of the Ear

An ear examination involves viewing the external auditory canal with an otoscope covered by an ear speculum (Figure 31.18). Disposable plastic speculum covers should be used each time to prevent disease transmission. A normal otoscopic examination reveals an external auditory canal with a small amount of cerumen and a pearly gray and concave tympanic membrane. In addition to performing the otoscopic examination, the provider palpates the area around the pinna for abnormalities or sensations. A number of tests are used to assess hearing acuity, ranging from simple tuning fork tests to quantitative and qualitative audiometric testing. If a hearing loss is suspected, the next test usually is performed with a tuning fork.

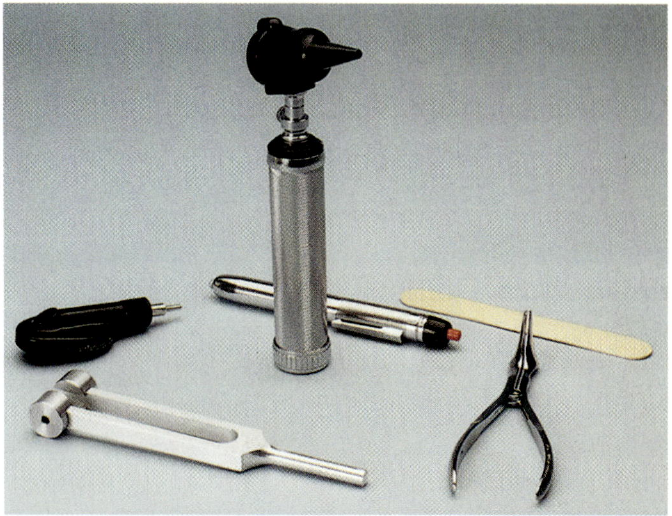

FIGURE 31.18 Instruments used in an otoscopic examination.

Useful Questions for Gathering a History of Ear Problems

- Are you experiencing nausea, vomiting, dizziness, ear pain, fever, headache, upper respiratory infection, ringing of the ears, drainage, loss of balance, or hearing loss?
- What are the onset, duration, and frequency of symptoms?
- Have you taken any medication for the symptoms? If so, what medication? Has it helped?
- Do you have the problem in both ears?
- Are you experiencing pain? On a scale of 1 to 10, with 10 being the worst pain, how would you rate the pain? Is it localized or radiating, in one ear or both?
- Has anything you have tried relieved the symptoms?

Tuning Fork Testing

Tuning fork tests measure hearing by air conduction and bone conduction. Remember that in bone conduction, the sound vibrates through the cranial bones to the inner ear. Tuning forks are available in different sizes, each with a different frequency. The most commonly used tuning fork is the 512 **hertz** (Hz), which means that it vibrates 512 cycles per second, the level of normal speech patterns. To activate the fork, the provider holds it by the stem and strikes the tines softly on the palm of the hand. Striking the tines too forcefully creates a tone that is too loud for diagnostic use. The two tests used to evaluate hearing are the Weber and Rinne tests. Both of these procedures are commonly used to evaluate conductive and sensory losses.

The Weber test is used if the patient reports that hearing is better in one ear than in the other. The vibrating fork is placed in the center of the top of the head, and the patient is asked in which ear the tone is louder or if the tone is the same in both ears. Because the patient hears the tone by bone conduction through the head, a normal result is hearing the sound equally in both ears.

The Rinne test is designed to compare air conduction sound with bone conduction sound. In this test, the stem of the vibrating fork is placed on the patient's mastoid process, and the patient is instructed to raise a hand when the sound disappears. The fork is quickly inverted so that the vibrating tines are approximately 1 inch in front of the external ear canal. If hearing is normal, the patient should still hear a sound. In normal hearing, the sound is heard twice as long by air conduction as by bone conduction.

Audiometric Testing

An audiometric test may be done in an otology or a family practice and is performed by medical assistants who have received additional training. Audiometry measures the lowest intensity of sound an individual can hear (Figure 31.19). The patient, frequently a child, is assisted in placing headphones over the ears.

Newer machines give the operator the choice of performing a traditional manual hearing test or an automated one. In the automatic mode, the patient is prompted through the earphones to press a hand button upon hearing a tone. The advantages of automated machines are that voice prompts are available in multiple languages, and the test requires less time to complete. The medical assistant can watch the progress of the test on the audiometer's LCD screen. Whether the test is delivered manually or with an automated model, each ear is tested by delivering a single frequency at a specific intensity, starting with low-frequency tones and going up to very high frequencies. The patient is asked to signal when the sound is heard. The results are printed on a graph, called an *audiogram,* or the medical assistant charts the results on a graph sheet (Procedure 31.5). Adults with normal hearing can hear tone frequencies below 25 decibels, and children with normal hearing can hear those below 15.

If initial screening indicates a hearing deficit, the provider may recommend an appointment with an **audiologist** for an audiometric evaluation. The evaluation consists of a battery of tests that assesses the level of hearing impairment and provides valuable information as to how the patient may be helped. The first test evaluates speech comprehension and assesses the patient's ability to follow verbal instructions. Once this evaluation is complete, the patient is placed in a soundproof booth with earphones over the ears. From this point on, the audiologist speaks to the patient and conducts all testing through the earphones. The assessment includes testing the frequency, intensity, and audibility of sound. This process takes approximately 1 hour.

Assisting with Treatments of the Ear

A medical assistant may be involved in providing treatments for diseases or disorders of the ear. The following sections discuss two of the most common treatments for the ear.

Ear Irrigation

Irrigation of the ear is done to remove excessive or impacted cerumen, remove a foreign body, or treat the inflamed ear with an antiseptic solution (Procedure 31.6). A medical assistant with the proper training and competency may perform the ear irrigation procedure when ordered by the provider. To prevent discomfort for the patient, it is important to administer the irrigating solution with the applicator tilted up toward the top of the external canal, so that the solution is not directed at the tympanic membrane. Some discomforts the patient may experience during ear irrigation include vertigo, coughing, or a tickle in the back of the throat. Perform the procedure as prescribed, making sure the patient is comfortable. Always document the treatment and its results immediately after completion.

CRITICAL THINKING APPLICATION 31.5

Kim is instructed to perform a bilateral ear irrigation on a 68-year-old patient with impacted cerumen. Before the procedure, she uses an otoscope to check the auditory canal and sees a large amount of dark brown cerumen in the right ear, completely covering the tympanic membrane. The left ear has a moderate amount of golden-brown cerumen covering the bottom half of the tympanic membrane. After the procedure, both membranes were visible, and the patient tolerated the procedure without complaints. How should Kim document the procedure?

Instillation of Ear Medications

Medication ordered for ear instillation is given to soften impacted cerumen, relieve pain, or as an antibiotic drop for an infectious pathogen (Procedure 31.7). Patients with ear conditions may be in considerable pain and have difficulty hearing, which makes health teaching a challenge. Wait until after the procedure has been completed and the patient is more comfortable to reinforce healthy behaviors.

CLOSING COMMENTS

Patient Coaching

Patients with vision or hearing impairment face serious challenges. For these patients, the medical assistant must use good listening

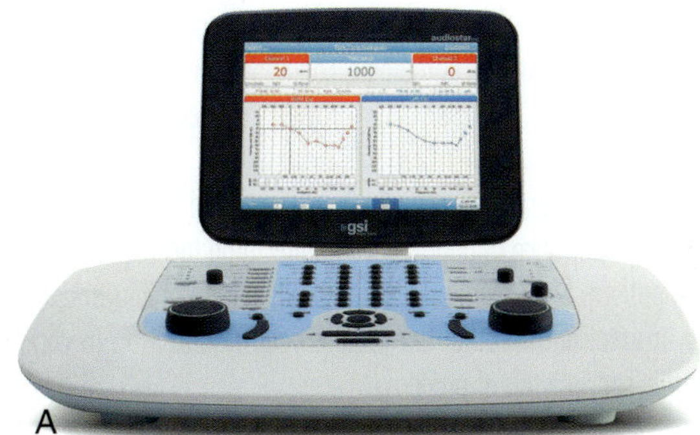

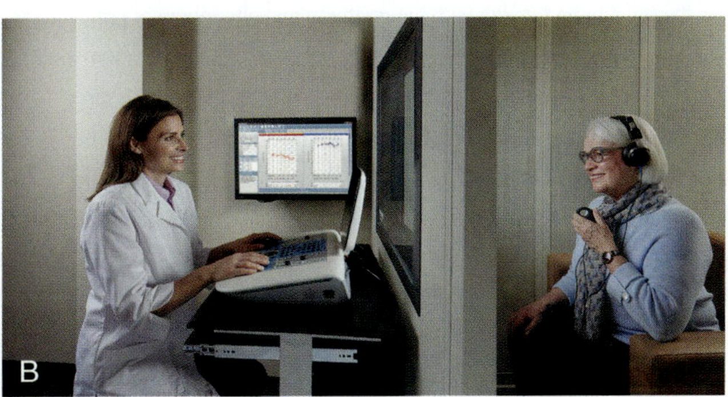

FIGURE 31.19 (A) Audiometer. **(B)** The patient signals when he hears a sound. (Courtesy GSI Grason-Stadler.)

skills, appropriate nonverbal methods, and touch to communicate empathy and understanding. Teaching may have to be adapted to meet the special needs of these patients. A person with a vision loss benefits from large-print forms and handouts, increased lighting, and verbal rather than written instructions to reinforce learning. For an individual with a hearing deficit, printed instructions, demonstrations of how to manage treatments, or even sign language interpretation should be available to ensure accurate communication. Including family members in the patient's treatment plan and offering referrals to appropriate community or professional resources may be very beneficial to a patient with sensory loss. Each patient must be assessed individually to determine the type of adaptation needed.

An important part of patient coaching for those administering eye medications at home is stressing the need to maintain the sterility of the medication. Patients and family members must be taught how to apply the medication while preventing trauma to the eye and contamination of the applicator. Patients administering ear treatments also must understand how to instill the medication.

Legal and Ethical Issues

The Americans with Disabilities Act (ADA) was passed in 1990, and amendments were added in 2008. The Americans with Disabilities Act Amendments (ADAA) prohibit discrimination based on disability. An individual with a disability is defined by the ADAA as a person who has a physical or mental impairment that substantially limits one or more major life activities, a person who has a history or record of such an impairment, or a person who is perceived by others as having such an impairment. Public facilities, including ambulatory care facilities and other healthcare buildings, must comply with ADAA requirements for physical accommodations. Public medical facilities must provide individuals with disabilities access to communication devices if they have a problem with vision, hearing, reading, or comprehension. Additional details can be found at www.ada.gov/nprm_adaaa/adaaa-nprm-qa.htm.

Patient-Centered Care

Diminished sight or hearing may render a patient seriously impaired. To prevent accidents and office injuries, always ask sight- or hearing-impaired patients whether they require assistance. When you escort the patient to an examination room, offer your arm and tell the patient the approximate distance you will be walking. If the patient is to have an examination that involves local anesthesia or eye drops that dilate the pupil, be sure the patient has recovered, has sunglasses, and that someone is available to drive the patient home before allowing them to leave the facility. Never assume that the patient is capable of leaving alone. If the patient insists on leaving before the designated recovery time, inform the provider and record the time and circumstances surrounding the event in the patient's health record.

Professional Behaviors

Patients with vision and hearing problems require an extra level of professional courtesy and respectfulness. Imagine what it would be like if you could not see clearly or if you had difficulty understanding what your provider was saying to you. How would you like a family member who has sensory difficulties to be treated when visiting the provider? Focus on how you can adapt the facility's environment to accommodate the needs of these patients. Is there adequate lighting? Are patient education materials available that have been adapted for individuals with vision impairment? How can you most effectively and respectfully communicate with a patient who has hearing loss? Many times, just the act of empathy—imagining yourself in the place of the patient—can help you treat patients with the respect and courtesy they deserve.

SUMMARY OF SCENARIO

After observing Kim and asking many questions, Amy is beginning to understand her special responsibilities in the ophthalmology and otorhinolaryngology areas. She recognizes the need to be familiar with the anatomy and physiology of both the eye and the ear, in addition to the importance of being able to perform specialty-related skills, such as irrigations, medication instillations, and diagnostic procedures. Amy has become quite proficient at performing Snellen and Ishihara screening examinations and accurately documenting the results. Kim has taught her to use the audiometer and assisted her with the first few screenings, so she is now ready to do hearing tests on her own.

Although she learned about eye and ear medications in her medical assistant program, Amy found that instilling these medications in an actual patient is different from working on mannequins and classmates. Kim has reinforced the skills she learned in her program, continually emphasizing infection control procedures and reinforcing patient education information. Amy realizes that she needs to understand the pathologic conditions that can occur in the sensory organs so that she can assist the provider as needed and answer patients' questions.

After working with patients who have vision and hearing deficits, Amy understands the importance of adapting communication techniques to meet the needs of each patient. She has decided to take advantage of educational opportunities at the hospital and through her professional organization to continue to learn about this special area of practice.

SUMMARY OF LEARNING OBJECTIVES

1. **Examine the anatomy and physiology of the eye.**
The anatomy of the eye begins with the outer covering, the conjunctiva, and three layers of tissue: sclera, choroid, and retina. The retina is where light rays are converted into nervous energy for interpretation by the brain.
Vision begins with the passage of light through the cornea, where it is refracted. The light rays then pass through the aqueous humor and pupil into the lens. The ciliary muscle adjusts the curvature of the lens to again refract the light rays so that they pass into the retina, triggering the photoreceptor cells of the rods and cones. Light energy is converted into an electrical impulse that is sent through the optic nerve to the brain, where interpretation occurs. Table 31.1 shows how vision requires light and depends on the proper functioning of all parts of the eye.
2. **Examine the anatomy and physiology of the ear.**
The anatomy of the ear begins with the outer ear, specifically the auricle. The next area is the middle ear, where sound is transmitted via the ossicles to the inner ear. The inner ear is divided into the cochlea and the semicircular canals. Sound is then transmitted to the eighth cranial nerve and on to the brain.
The external ear consists of the auricle, or pinna, and the external auditory canal, which transmits sound waves to the tympanic membrane. The middle ear is an air-filled cavity that contains the ossicles. The sound vibration passes through the tympanic membrane, causing the ossicles to vibrate. This bone-conducted vibration passes through the oval window into the inner ear. The organ of Corti, in the cochlea of the inner ear, converts sound waves into nervous energy, which is sent to the brain for interpretation. The semicircular canals in the inner ear maintain equilibrium.
3. **Analyze the life span changes that occur in the eyes and ears.**
Infants must learn how to use their eyes to be able to see clearly. This happens during the first few years of life. By 2 years of age, eye-hand coordination and depth perception should be well developed. Routine vision screenings should begin between the ages of 3 to 5 years.
The most prevalent eye disorder in children is conjunctivitis. It is highly contagious, and all efforts to contain it should be taken.
The eustachian tube undergoes an important change as the child grows older as it lengthens, and the angle from the middle ear to the throat changes and reduces the chance of ear infections in children.
A hearing test is done on a newborn, and if that screening is normal, the next screening will occur at school age.
Older adults will see changes in their vision, referred to as presbyopia. Age-related macular degeneration is another common disorder in older adults and affects the visual field.
Hearing loss is also common in older adults. There is a concern about how this impacts the quality of life. Hearing aids can help with hearing loss and provide some improvement in the quality of life.
4. **Examine the diseases and disorders of the eye, including the signs, symptoms, etiology, diagnostic procedures, and treatments.**
Refractive errors include hyperopia, myopia, presbyopia, and astigmatism. All are caused by a problem with bending light so that it can be accurately focused on the retina. These conditions usually are caused by defects in the shape of the eyeball and can be corrected with glasses, contacts, or surgery.
Eye disorders can range from problems with eye movement, as in strabismus and nystagmus, to infections of the eye, including hordeolum, chalazion, keratitis, conjunctivitis, and blepharitis. Disorders of the eyeball include corneal abrasions, cataracts, glaucoma, and macular degeneration.
5. **Examine the diseases and disorders of the ear, including the signs, symptoms, etiology, diagnostic procedures, and treatments.**
Conductive hearing loss is caused by a problem that originates in the external or middle ear and prevents sound vibrations from passing through the external auditory canal, limiting tympanic membrane vibrations or interfering with the passage of bone-conducted sound in the middle ear. A sensorineural hearing loss results from damage to the organ of Corti or the auditory nerve and prevents vibrations from being converted into nervous stimuli.
Otitis externa is an inflammation of the auditory canal, and otitis media is an inflammation of the normally air-filled middle ear, resulting in the collection of serous or suppurative fluid behind the tympanic membrane. Impacted cerumen is a common cause of conductive hearing loss. Ménière disease is a chronic, progressive condition that affects the labyrinth and causes recurring attacks of vertigo, in addition to tinnitus, a sensation of pressure in the affected ear and advancing hearing loss.
6. **Examine the medical assistant's role in examinations, diagnostic procedures, and treatments for conditions of the eye and ear.**
Diagnostic procedures for the eye begin with a visual examination of the eye with an ophthalmoscope. Next, the eyelids are examined for abnormalities, and the pupils are tested for PERRLA (pupils, equal, round, reactive to, light [and], accommodation). More advanced techniques include using a slit lamp to view the fine details of the eye and an exophthalmometer to measure the distance of the eyeball from the orbit. Distance visual acuity typically is assessed with a Snellen chart; near visual acuity is tested with a near vision acuity chart. A patient can be tested for a color vision defect with the Ishihara test.
Procedure 31.1 explains the Snellen evaluation.
Procedure 31.2 outlines the color acuity examination.
Eye irrigation relieves inflammation, removes drainage, dilutes chemicals, or washes away foreign bodies. Sterile technique and equipment must be used to prevent contamination. Medication may be instilled into the eye to treat an infection, soothe an eye irritation, anesthetize the eye, or dilate the pupils before examination or treatment. Procedure 31.3 describes the method for eye irrigation, and Procedure 31.4 explains how to administer eye medications.
An ear examination involves viewing the external auditory canal with an otoscope covered by an ear speculum. If hearing loss is suspected, the next test is usually performed with a tuning fork. Be sure to ask questions about symptoms (including onset, frequency, and duration), medications, if the problem is in both ears, and if pain is present.
The ear exam begins with an otoscopic examination. It can include various tuning fork tests to detect conductive or sensorineural hearing deficits and more advanced audiometric testing. Procedure 31.5 explains the audiometry examination.
The ear may be irrigated to remove excess or impacted cerumen, remove a foreign body, or treat the inflamed ear with an antiseptic solution. Medication is instilled into the ear to soften impacted cerumen, relieve pain, or treat an infectious pathogen. Procedure 31.6 describes how to perform an ear irrigation. Procedure 31.7 explains how to administer otic drugs.

PROCEDURE 31.1 Measure Distance Visual Acuity

TASK: Determine the patient's degree of visual clarity at a measured distance of 20 feet using the Snellen chart.

EQUIPMENT and SUPPLIES

- Patient's health record
- Provider's order
- Snellen eye chart
- Disposable eye occluder or an alcohol wipe to clean the occluder before use
- Pen or pencil and paper

PROCEDURAL STEPS

1. Wash hands or use hand sanitizer.
   PURPOSE: Hand sanitization is an important step for infection control.
2. Prepare the area. Make sure the room is well lit and that a distance marker is 20 feet from the chart.
3. Greet the patient. Identify yourself. Verify the patient's identity with full name and date of birth. Explain the procedure to be performed in a manner that the patient understands. Answer any questions the patient may have about the procedure. Instruct the patient not to squint during the test because this temporarily improves vision. The patient should not have an opportunity to study the chart before the test is given. If the patient wears corrective lenses, they should be worn during the test.
   PURPOSE: Explanations help gain the patient's cooperation and alleviate apprehension.
4. Assist the patient into a standing or sitting position at the 20-foot marker.
   PURPOSE: Twenty feet is the standard testing distance.
5. Check that the Snellen chart is positioned at the patient's eye level.
6. If the occluder is not disposable, disinfect it before the procedure starts. Then, instruct the patient to cover the left eye with the occluder and to keep both eyes open throughout the test to prevent squinting (Figure 1).
   PURPOSE: Traditionally, the right eye is tested first.

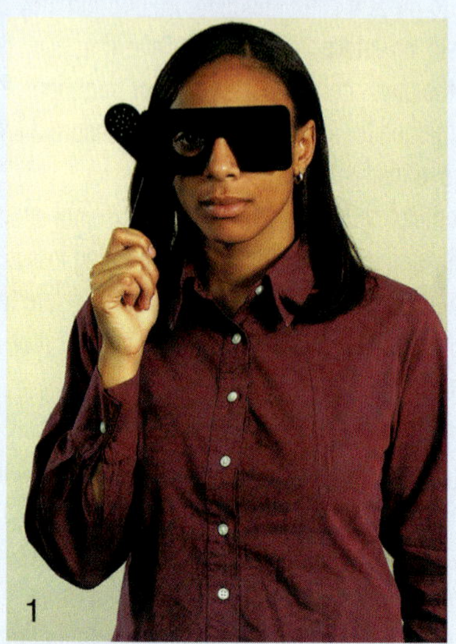
1

7. Stand beside the chart and point to each row as the patient reads it aloud, starting with the 20/70 row (Figure 2).
   PURPOSE: Starting with larger letters gives the patient confidence and allows for accommodation of vision.

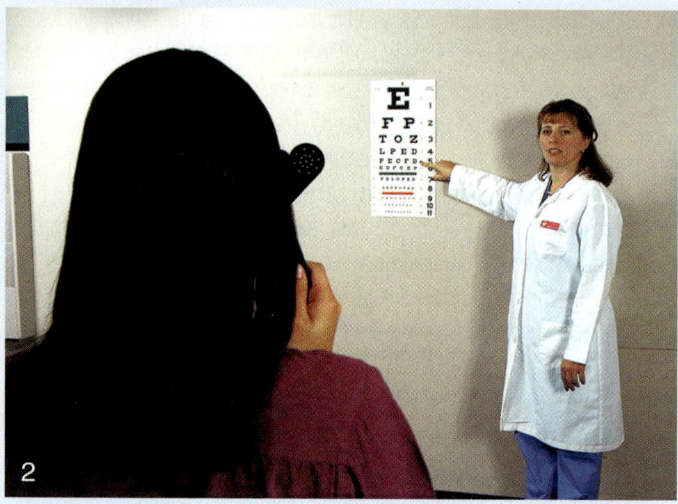

2

8. Proceed down the rows of the chart until the smallest row the patient can read with a maximum of two errors is reached. If one or two letters are missed, the outcome is recorded with a minus sign and the number of errors (e.g., 20/40–2). If more than two errors are made, the previous line should be documented.
9. Record any of the patient's reactions while reading the chart.
   PURPOSE: Reactions such as squinting, leaning, tearing, or blinking may indicate that the patient is having difficulty with the test.
10. Repeat the procedure with the left eye, covering the right eye.
11. Repeat the procedure with both eyes uncovered.
12. Disinfect the occluder if it is not disposable. Wash hands or use hand sanitizer.
    PURPOSE: To follow infection control procedures.
13. Document the procedure in the patient's record, including the date and time, visual acuity results, and any reactions by the patient. Also, record whether corrective lenses were worn.
    PURPOSE: Procedures that are not recorded are considered not done.

Documentation Exercise

The medical assistant conducted a Snellen exam on Carlene Anderson, who wears contacts. The results were right eye 20/60; left eye 20/30, but she missed one letter at the 20/30 line; both eyes 20/40. Carlene did not squint or strain during the exam.

Correct Documentation

8/01/20XX 2:20 p.m. DVA completed c̄ Snellen chart. Right eye 20/60, left eye 20/30–1, both eyes 20/40 c̄ corrective lenses. No squinting noted.
———————————— Kim Tau, CMA, (AAMA)

PROCEDURE 31.2 Assess Color Acuity Using the Ishihara Test

TASK: Assess a patient's color acuity correctly and record the results.

EQUIPMENT and SUPPLIES

- Patient's health record
- Provider's order
- Room with natural light if possible
- Ishihara color plate book
- Pen, pencil, and paper
- Watch with a second hand

PROCEDURAL STEPS

1. Assemble the equipment and prepare the room for testing. The room should be quiet and illuminated with natural light.
   PURPOSE: Natural light is needed to test colors correctly.
2. Greet the patient. Identify yourself. Verify the patient's identity with full name and date of birth. Explain the procedure to be performed in a manner that the patient understands. Answer any questions the patient may have about the procedure. Use a practice card during the explanation, and make sure it is understood that the patient has 3 seconds to identify each plate.
   PURPOSE: These steps help to make sure you have the right patient. Also, an informed patient is a cooperative patient. The first plate is a practice plate and is designed to be read correctly.
3. Hold up the first plate at a right angle to the patient's line of vision and 30 inches from the patient. Be sure both of the patient's eyes are kept open during the test (Figure 1).

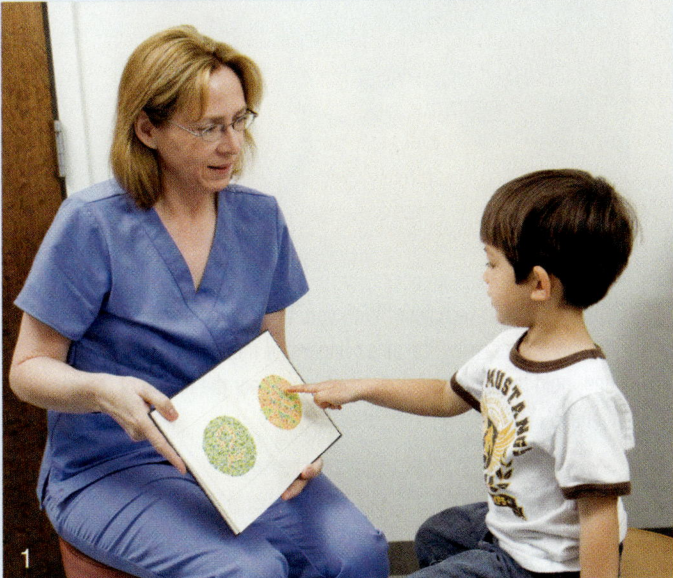
1

4. Ask the patient to tell you the number on the plate. Record the plate number and the patient's answer (Figure 2).

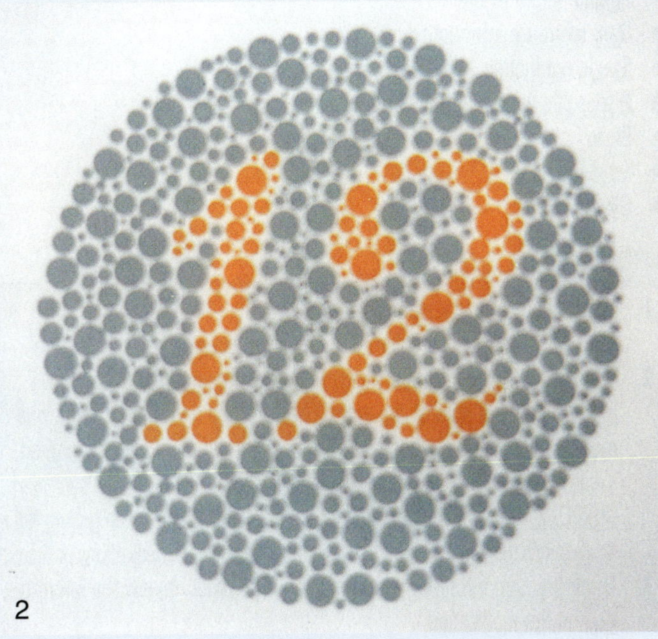
2

5. Continue this sequence until all 11 plates have been read. If the patient cannot identify the number on the plate, place an X in the record for that plate number. Your record should look like this:

Plate 1 = pass, Plate 2 = pass, Plate 3 = X, Plate 4 = pass, and so on

6. Include any unusual symptoms in your record, such as eye rubbing, squinting, or excessive blinking.
7. Place the book back in its cardboard sleeve and return it to its storage space.
   PURPOSE: The Ishihara color plates must be stored in a closed position away from external light to protect the colors.
8. Document the procedure in the patient's health record, including the date and time, the testing results, and any patient symptoms shown during the test.
   PURPOSE: Procedures that are not recorded are considered not done.

PROCEDURE 31.3 Irrigate a Patient's Eye

TASK: Irrigate a patient's eye and document patient care.

EQUIPMENT and SUPPLIES

- Provider's order
- Patient health record
- Drug reference information
- Sterile ophthalmic irrigation solution and supplies
- Disposable waterproof pad and towels
- Basin
- Sterile gauze
- Gloves

PROCEDURAL STEPS

1. Wash hands or use hand sanitizer.
   PURPOSE: Hand sanitization is an important step for infection control.
2. Select the right medication (fluid) from the storage area. Check the medication label against the order. Check for the right name, form, and route. Check the expiration date to make sure the fluid has not expired. Verify the right dose and the right time.
   PURPOSE: It is important to do the first check of the label when getting the medications from the cabinet. Do not administer expired medications or fluids.
3. Using the drug reference information and the order, review the information on the medication.
   PURPOSE: The medical assistant must know about the medication being given.
4. Perform the second medication check. Check the medication label against the order. Check for the right name, form, and route.
   PURPOSE: It is important to check the label a second time before continuing with the procedure.
5. Assemble the supplies required for the procedure.
   PURPOSE: You need to have the supplies ready before going to the exam room.
6. Perform the third medication check. Check each medication label against the order. Check for the right name, form, and route.
   PURPOSE: It is important to check the label a third time before seeing the patient.
7. Prior to entering the exam room, knock on the door and wait a moment. Greet the patient. Identify yourself. Verify the patient's identity with full name and date of birth. Make sure the patient's information matches the order and the record. Explain what you are going to do.
   PURPOSE: It is important to identify the patient in two different ways to ensure that you have the correct patient. Explaining the procedure can make the patient feel more comfortable and reduces anxiety.
8. Provide the right education to the patient. Explain the procedure ordered, the name of the provider ordering the procedure, the desired effect, and common side effects. Answer any questions the patient may have. Use language the patient can understand. Ask if the patient has any allergies. If the patient refuses the procedure, respectfully ask the patient the reason and notify the provider.
   PURPOSE: The patient needs to be aware of what you are giving, the action, side effects, and who ordered it. It is also important to double-check the patient's allergies before starting the procedure.
9. Using room temperature fluid, set up the equipment. If using an intravenous (IV) bag, prime or run fluid through the tubing. If using a prepackaged solution, remove the cover. If using a bulb syringe, pour the required fluid into a basin. Remember to palm the label. Draw the solution into the bulb syringe.
   PURPOSE: Having the fluid ready for the irrigation is important before you hold the eye open.
10. Assist the patient into a sitting or supine position. Have the patient remove glasses or contact lenses. Ask the patient to turn the head toward the side of the affected eye. Place the disposable waterproof pad over the patient's neck and shoulder. Place or have the patient hold the drainage basin next to the affected eye.
    PURPOSE: Protecting the unaffected eye from the solution is important so it does not also get contaminated. The basin will collect the irrigation fluid from the eye.
11. Put on gloves. Moisten a gauze pad with the irrigation fluid. Using the gauze, clean the eyelid from the inner to outer canthus (Figure 1). Discard the gauze after each wipe.
    PURPOSE: Debris on the eyelid must be removed before the irrigation can be done.

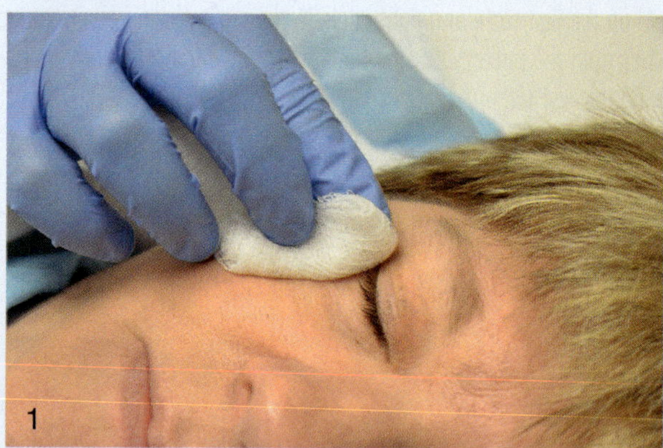

12. Perform the right technique. With your nondominant hand, separate and hold the eyelids using the index finger and thumb. With the dominant hand, hold the irrigation equipment on or near the bridge of the nose (Figure 2).

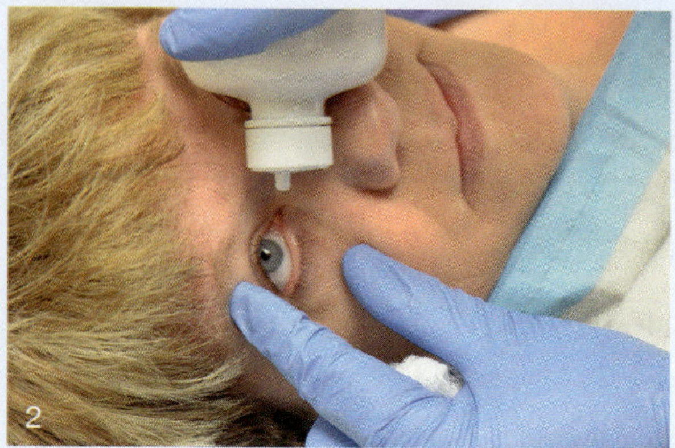

PROCEDURE 31.3 Irrigate a Patient's Eye—*continued*

PURPOSE: Using the nose to help steady the irrigation will help to maintain a steady flow of fluid going into the eye.

13. Direct the solution toward the lower conjunctiva of the inner canthus. Allow a steady flow of solution to slowly flush the eye from the inner to the outer canthus. Do not touch the tip of the irrigation equipment to the eye.
    PURPOSE: Touching the eye with the irrigation equipment could lead to an eye injury.
14. Continue until the ordered amount of fluid has flushed the eye. Dry the eyelid with sterile gauze, moving from the inner to the outer canthus.
    PURPOSE: It is important to follow the exact order of the provider.
15. Help the patient into a comfortable position. Clean up the area. Remove gloves, and wash hands or use hand sanitizer.
    PURPOSE: It is important that the patient is comfortable.
16. Document the procedure in the health record. Include allergies, teaching or instructions provided, the name of the provider ordering the irrigation, the fluid used for the irrigation, the amount used, the site, and how the patient tolerated the procedure.
    PURPOSE: The irrigation performed needs to be documented to indicate that it was done.

PROCEDURE 31.4 Instill an Eye Medication

TASK: Instill an eyedrop or ointment and document medication administration.

EQUIPMENT and SUPPLIES

- Provider's order
- Patient health record
- Drug reference information
- Sterile ophthalmic eyedrops or ointment
- Sterile gauze
- Gloves

PROCEDURAL STEPS

1. Wash hands or use hand sanitizer.
   PURPOSE: Hand sanitization is an important step for infection control.
2. Select the right medication from the storage area. Check the medication label against the order. Check for the right name, form, and route. Check the expiration date to make sure the drug has not expired. Verify the right dose and the right time.
   PURPOSE: It is important to do the first check of the label when getting the medications from the cabinet. Do not administer expired medications.
3. Using the drug reference information and the order, review the information on the medication.
   PURPOSE: The medical assistant must know about the medication being given.
4. Perform the second medication check. Check the medication label against the order. Check for the right name, form, and route.
   PURPOSE: It is important to check the label a second time before continuing with the procedure.
5. Assemble the supplies required for the procedure.
   PURPOSE: You need to have the supplies ready before going to the exam room.
6. Perform the third medication check. Check each medication label against the order. Check for the right name, form, and route.
   PURPOSE: It is important to check the label a third time before seeing the patient.
7. Prior to entering the exam room, knock on the door and wait a moment. Greet the patient. Identify yourself. Verify the patient's identity with full name and date of birth. Make sure the patient's information matches the order and the record. Explain what you are going to do.
   PURPOSE: It is important to identify the patient in two different ways to ensure that you have the correct patient. Explaining the procedure can make the patient feel more comfortable and reduces anxiety.
8. Provide the right education to the patient. Explain the medication ordered, identify the provider ordering the medication, describe the desired effect, and note the common side effects. Answer any questions the patient may have. Use language the patient can understand. Ask if the patient has any allergies. If the patient refuses the medication, notify the provider.
   PURPOSE: The patient needs to be aware of what you are giving, the action, side effects, and who ordered it. It is also important to double-check the patient's allergies before administering the medication.
9. Assist the patient into a sitting or supine position. Ask the patient to tilt the head backward and look up.
   PURPOSE: These positions allow the medical assistant to instill the medication.
10. Put on gloves. If crusting or drainage is present on the eyelid, gently wash the area from the inner to the outer canthus. Dry the area.
    PURPOSE: Gloves are used for infection control purposes. Washing and drying the eye prepares the area for the medication.
11. Perform the right technique. With your nondominant hand holding a sterile gauze, pull the lower conjunctival sac downward, creating a pocket for the medication (Figure 1). Instruct the patient to look up.

Continued

PROCEDURE 31.4 Instill an Eye Medication—*continued*

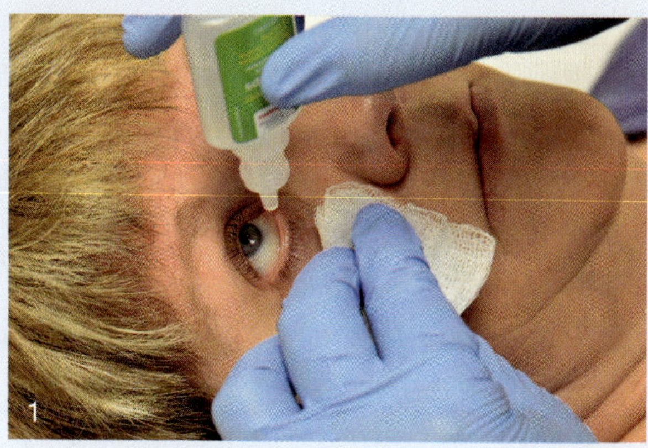

a. For the eyedrops: With your dominant hand, hold the bottle or the dropper ¾ inch away from the conjunctival sac. Drop the required number of drops into the eye (Figure 1). If the drop misses the eye or the patient blinks, wipe the liquid on the skin and repeat the drop. Have the person keep the eye closed for 2 to 3 minutes after the administration of the drop. Have the person gently press against the inner corner of the eye and nose bone for 2 to 3 minutes.

PURPOSE: Pressing in the corner after the drops keeps the medication from draining into the tear ducts and nose. This decreases the systemic effects of the medication.

b. For eye ointment: With the dominant hand, hold the ointment container above the lower lid. Working from the inner to the outer canthus, apply a small strip (about ½ inch of ointment along the inner lower lid margin) (Figure 2). Have the patient close the eye for 1 to 2 minutes to allow the medication to be absorbed. Wipe any extra ointment from the eyelid.

PURPOSE: Rubbing the eyelid after administering the ointment helps spread the medication over the eye.

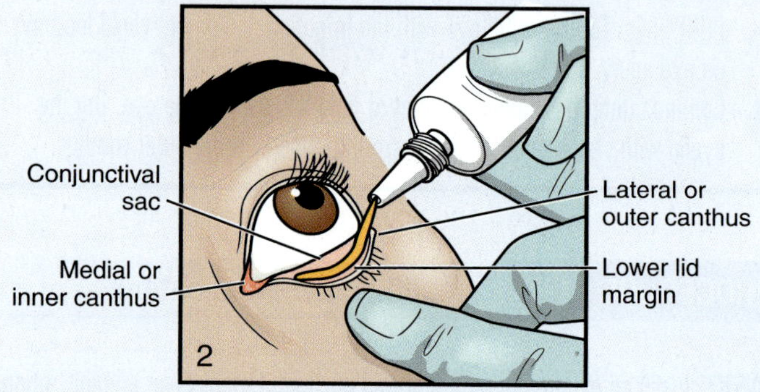

12. Help the patient into a comfortable position. Clean up the area. Remove gloves, and wash hands or use hand sanitizer.
    PURPOSE: It is important that the patient is comfortable.
13. Document the procedure in the health record. Include allergies; teaching or instructions provided; the name of the provider ordering the medication; the medication name, dose, and route; and how the patient tolerated the medication.
    PURPOSE: The medication needs to be documented to indicate it was given.

PROCEDURE 31.5 Measure Hearing Acuity with an Audiometer

TASK: Perform audiometric testing of hearing acuity.

EQUIPMENT and SUPPLIES

- Patient's health record
- Provider's order
- Audiometer with adjustable headphones and graph paper
- Quiet area

PROCEDURAL STEPS

1. Wash hands or use hand sanitizer, assemble the equipment, and bring the patient into a quiet area.
   PURPOSE: The testing room should be free of distractions and noise, so the patient can concentrate completely on the hearing evaluation.
2. Greet the patient. Identify yourself. Verify the patient's identity with full name and date of birth. Explain the procedure to be performed in a manner that the patient understands. Answer any questions the patient may have about the procedure.
   PURPOSE: These steps help to make sure you have the right patient. Also, explanations help gain the patient's cooperation and ease apprehension.
3. Explain that the audiometer measures whether the patient can hear various sound wave frequencies through the headphones. Each ear is tested separately. When a frequency is heard, the patient should raise a hand or push the button to signal the medical assistant.
   PURPOSE: Patient education is needed for compliance with the examination.
4. Place the headphones over the patient's ears, making sure they are adjusted for comfort.

PROCEDURE 31.5 Measure Hearing Acuity with an Audiometer—*continued*

5. The audiometer tests each ear separately, starting at a low frequency. If the machine does not automatically record the results, the medical assistant documents the patient's response to the frequencies on a graph or audiogram. Results for the left ear are marked with an X, and those for the right ear are marked with an O (Figure 1). More advanced machines automatically record the results. The medical assistant must have specialized training to conduct this test.

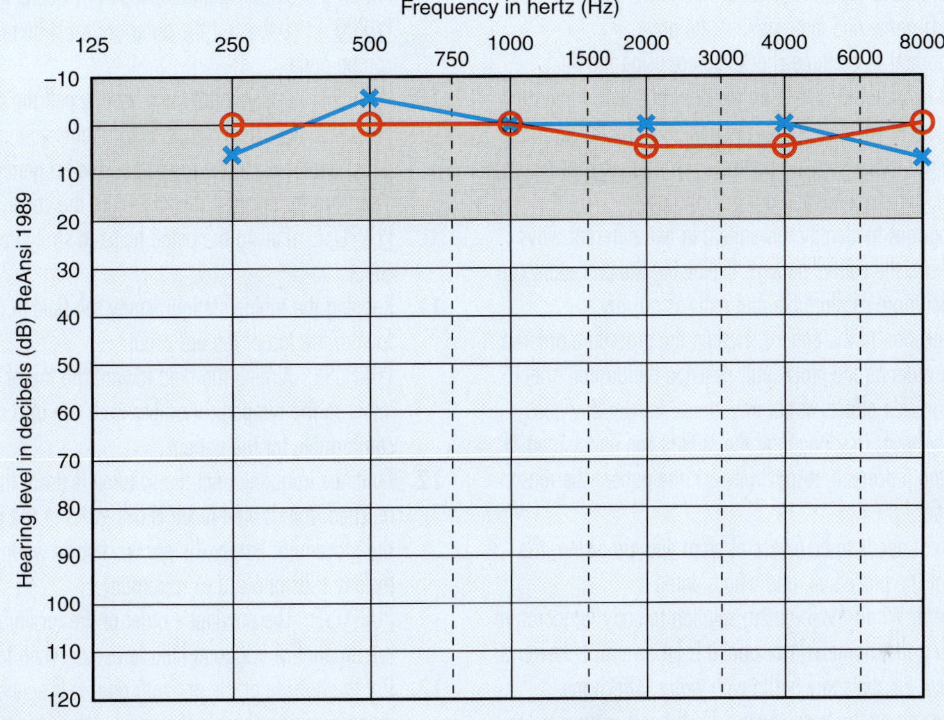

6. Frequencies are increased gradually to test the patient's ability to hear. Each response by the patient is documented.
7. After one ear has been tested, the other ear is then tested, and the results are documented.
8. The results are given to the provider for interpretation or downloaded into the patient's electronic health record for the provider to review.
9. The equipment is sanitized and disinfected according to the manufacturer's guidelines.
10. Wash hands or use hand sanitizer.

PROCEDURE 31.6 Irrigate a Patient's Ear

TASK: Irrigate a patient's ear and document patient care.

EQUIPMENT and SUPPLIES

- Provider's order
- Patient health record
- Ear washbasin
- Elephant ear wash system (or other ear wash system)
- Disposable waterproof pad and towels
- Thermometer (optional)
- Otoscope and disposable speculum (optional)
- Gauze
- Gloves
- Waste container

ORDER

Irrigate left ear with warm sterile water.

PROCEDURAL STEPS

1. Read the order. Wash hands or use hand sanitizer.
   PURPOSE: Hand sanitization is an important step for infection control.
2. Select the right medication (fluid) from the storage area. Check the medication label against the order. Check for the right name and route; check the expiration date.
   PURPOSE: It is important to do the first check of the label when getting the medications from the cabinet.

Continued

PROCEDURE 31.6 Irrigate a Patient's Ear—*continued*

3. Assemble the supplies required for the procedure. Perform the second medication check. Check the medication (fluid) name and route against the order.
   PURPOSE: You need to have the supplies ready before going to the exam room.
4. Clean up the work area and perform the third medication check. Check the medication (fluid) name and route against the order.
   PURPOSE: It is important to do three checks before using the fluid.
5. Prior to entering the exam room, knock on the door and wait a moment. Greet the patient. Identify yourself. Verify the patient's identity with full name and date of birth. Make sure the patient's information matches the order and the record. Explain what you are going to do.
   PURPOSE: It is important to identify the patient in two different ways to ensure that you have the correct patient. Explaining the procedure can make the patient feel more comfortable and reduces anxiety.
6. Provide the right education to the patient. Explain the procedure ordered, identify the provider ordering the procedure, describe the desired effect, and note the common side effects of ear irrigations. Answer any questions the patient may have. Use language the patient can understand. If the patient refuses the procedure, respectfully ask the patient the reason and notify the provider.
   PURPOSE: The patient needs to be aware of what you are giving, the action, side effects of the procedure, and who ordered it.
7. Prepare the equipment. Warm the irrigating solution to body temperature (98.6°F [check with a thermometer]) or until it is lukewarm. Lukewarm is neither hot nor cold. Fill the spray bottle with water. Attach the disposal tip to the nozzle on the hose (Figure 1). If another type of ear wash system is being used, prepare the equipment and the water.
   PURPOSE: It is important to have the fluid ready for the irrigation before holding the ear.

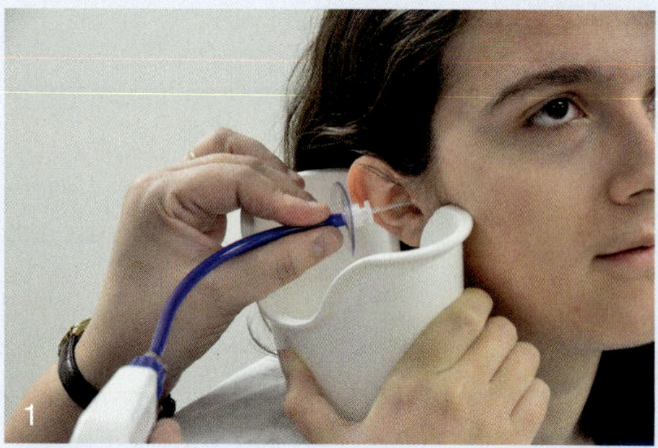
1

8. Assist the patient into a sitting position. Wrap a waterproof pad around the person's shoulder, protecting the clothing. Have a towel available for the patient if needed. Have the patient tilt the head toward the affected ear. Have the patient hold the ear washbasin under the affected ear.
   PURPOSE: It is important to protect the patient's clothing from the irrigating fluid.
9. Put on gloves. Using gauze, wipe any debris from the outer ear.
   PURPOSE: Debris on the outer ear must be removed before the irrigation can be done.
10. With your nondominant hand, gently pull the pinna up and back if the patient is older than age 3. For patients younger than 3, pull the pinna down and back. Insert the disposable tip gently into the ear. Do not insert too far because it could injure the canal.
    PURPOSE: Pulling the pinna helps to straighten the external auditory canal.
11. Keeping the tubing straight, spray the fluid in the ear canal. Aim the fluid toward the top of the ear canal.
    PURPOSE: Aiming the fluid toward the top of the canal helps prevent injury to the tympanic membrane. It can also make the procedure more comfortable for the patient.
12. Continue irrigating until the solution is used, the maximum time has been reached, the desired result is achieved, or the patient has problems with the procedure. Empty the ear washbasin when it fills. Observe the fluid for any substances (i.e., cerumen).
    PURPOSE: The provider's order or the facility's procedures will indicate the amount of irrigation fluid to use or when to stop the irrigation.
13. Dry the outside of the ear with gauze. If agency procedure indicates, use an otoscope to observe the canal. Attach the speculum to the otoscope. Straighten the ear canal by pulling in the appropriate direction on the pinna. Gently insert the otoscope. Observe the canal.
    PURPOSE: Observing the canal helps you check the results of the irrigation.
14. Place a clean, absorbent towel on the examination table. Have the patient rest quietly with the head turned to the irrigated side while you wait for the provider to return to check the affected ear.
    PURPOSE: Allows the fluid in the canal to drain out.
15. Clean up the work area. Remove your gloves and dispose of them in the waste container. Wash hands or use hand sanitizer.
    PURPOSE: Hand sanitization is an important step for infection control.
16. Document the procedure in the health record. Include teaching or instructions provided, the name of the provider ordering the irrigation, the fluid used for the irrigation, the amount used, the site, and how the patient tolerated the procedure.
    PURPOSE: The irrigation performed needs to be documented to indicate that it was done.

PROCEDURE 31.7 Instill Eardrops

TASK: Instill eardrops, and document medication administration.

EQUIPMENT and SUPPLIES

- Provider's order
- Patient health record
- Drug reference information
- Otic drops
- Gauze
- Gloves

PROCEDURAL STEPS

1. Wash hands or use hand sanitizer.
   PURPOSE: Hand sanitization is an important step for infection control.
2. Select the right medication from the storage area. Check the medication label against the order. Check for the right name, form, and route. Check the expiration date to make sure the drug has not expired. Verify the right dose and the right time.
   PURPOSE: It is important to do the first check of the label when getting the medications from the cabinet. Do not administer expired medications.
3. Using the drug reference information and the order, review the information on the medication.
   PURPOSE: The medical assistant must know about the medication being given.
4. Perform the second medication check. Check the medication label against the order. Check for the right name, form, and route.
   PURPOSE: It is important to do the second check of the label before continuing with the procedure.
5. Assemble the supplies required for the procedure.
   PURPOSE: You need to have the supplies ready before going to the exam room.
6. Perform the third medication check. Check each medication label against the order. Check for the right name, form, and route.
   PURPOSE: It is important to do the third check of the label before seeing the patient.
7. Prior to entering the exam room, knock on the door and wait a moment. Greet the patient. Identify yourself. Verify the patient's identity with full name and date of birth. Make sure the patient's information matches the order and the record. Explain what you are going to do.
   PURPOSE: It is important to identify the patient in two different ways to ensure that you have the correct patient. Explaining the procedure can make the patient feel more comfortable and reduces anxiety.
8. Provide the right education to the patient. Explain the medication ordered, identify the provider ordering the medication, describe the desired effect, and note the common side effects. Answer any questions the patient may have. Use language the patient can understand. Ask if the patient has any allergies. If the patient refuses the medication, respectfully ask the patient the reason and notify the provider.
   PURPOSE: The patient needs to be aware of what you are giving, the action, side effects, and who ordered it. It is also important to double-check the patient's allergies before administering the medication.
9. Assist the patient into a sitting or side-lying position on the unaffected side.
   PURPOSE: These positions allow the medical assistant to instill the medication.
10. Warm the medication bottle with your hands if needed. The drops should be at room temperature. Shake the medication if needed. Put on gloves.
    PURPOSE: If the drops are either too hot or too cold, the patient may experience nausea and vertigo. Gloves are used for infection control purposes.
11. Perform the right technique. Have the patient tilt the head so the affected ear is upward. If cerumen or drainage is blocking the canal, gently remove it with a cotton-tipped application.
    PURPOSE: The canal must be open to instill the drops.
12. With your nondominant hand, gently pull the pinna up and back if the patient is older than age 3. This straightens the external auditory canal. For patients younger than 3, pull the pinna down and back.
    PURPOSE: Straightening the canal allows the medication to flow down it.
13. Remove the cover of the bottle. Hold the dropper firmly in your dominant hand. Place the tip of the dropper about ½ inch above the ear canal (Figure 1). Be sure not to contaminate the dropper by touching it to the patient. Carefully drop the required number of drops in the patient's ear. Replace the cover.
    PURPOSE: If the bottle tip gets contaminated, it needs to be discarded.

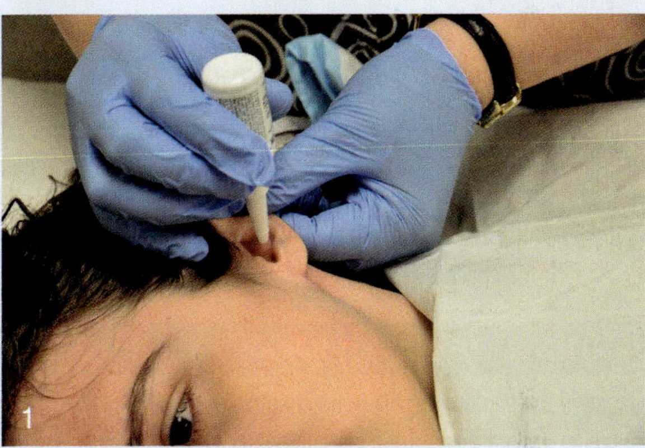

14. Have the patient keep the ear facing up for 3 to 5 minutes, depending on the medication (Figure 2).
    PURPOSE: Allows the medication to move throughout the canal.

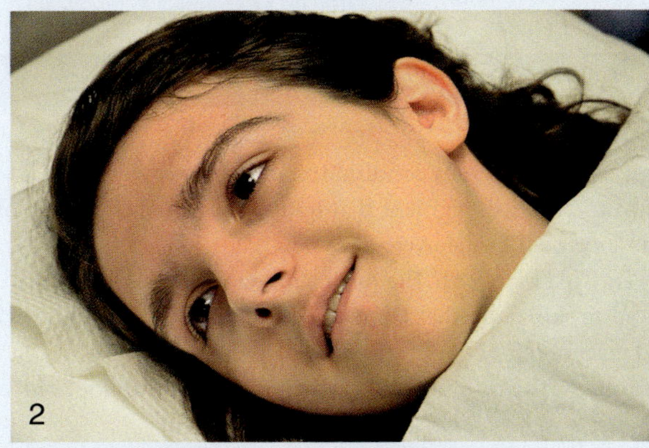

15. Help the patient into a comfortable position. Clean up the area. Remove and dispose of gloves in the waste container. Wash hands or use hand sanitizer.
    PURPOSE: It is important that the patient is comfortable.
16. Document the procedure in the health record. Include allergies; teaching or instructions provided; the name of the provider ordering the medication; the medication name, dose, and route; and how the patient tolerated the medication.
    PURPOSE: The medication needs to be documented to indicate it was given.

DERMATOLOGY

32

SCENARIO

Mai Vang is a medical assistant who has been working at the Walden Martin Family Medical (WMFM) Clinic for 2 years. She really wanted to work in a family practice clinic so she could see patients of varying ages and medical conditions. Mai has noticed that skin conditions are a frequent reason for patient visits. When she was in high school, she visited her physician to get help for an acne breakout that would not go away. She remembers feeling self-conscious about the condition, so she tries to be especially sensitive to patients with skin diseases and disorders. There is a new patient on the schedule today, Casey Hernandez, and the scheduler indicates that the visit is to discuss possible treatments for acne. Mai understands that she needs to be familiar with common diseases and disorders that affect the skin, be ready to assist with dermatologic procedures, and be prepared to reinforce patient education about the treatment and prevention of dermatologic conditions.

While studying this chapter, think about the following questions:

- What are the basic anatomy and physiology of the integumentary system?
- What are common diseases and disorders that affect the integumentary system?
- How can Mai determine the difference between the levels of burn injuries?
- Why is it important that Mai understand the concepts of staging and grading malignant tumors?
- What are the primary malignancies of the skin?
- What dermatologic procedures should Mai be prepared to assist with in a dermatology practice?

LEARNING OBJECTIVES

1. Examine the anatomy of the integumentary system.
2. Examine the functions of the integumentary system.
3. Analyze the life span changes that occur in the integumentary system.
4. Examine the diseases and disorders of the integumentary system, including the signs, symptoms, etiology, diagnostic procedures, and treatments.
5. Examine carcinomas of the integumentary system, including the signs, symptoms, diagnostic procedures, and treatments.
6. Examine the medical assistant's role in assisting with examinations, diagnostic procedures, and treatments for integumentary system conditions.

VOCABULARY

basal Bottom layer.

benign A noncancerous condition; not malignant, harmless.

bilirubin A reddish pigment that results from the breakdown of red blood cells in the liver.

collagen (KAH lah jen) The most abundant structural protein found in skin and other connective tissues. It provides strength and cushioning to many parts of the body.

cryosurgery The technique of exposing tissue to extreme cold to produce a well-defined area of cell destruction.

ecchymosis (ek i MOH sis) Discoloration of the skin caused by the escape of blood into the tissues from ruptured blood vessels; typically caused by bruising.

elastin (ee LAS tin) A highly elastic protein in connective tissue that allows tissues to resume their shape after stretching or contracting. It is found abundantly in the dermis of the skin.

epithelial cells (ep i THEE lee al) Form cellular sheets that cover surfaces, both inside and outside the body. Epithelial cells are closely packed, take on different shapes, and strongly stick to each other.

excoriated (ik SKOHR ee ay ted) To strip off or remove the skin from an area.

glomerulonephritis (gloh mer yuh loh neh FRIE tis) Kidney disease affecting the capillaries of the nephron (glomeruli); characterized by albuminuria, edema, and hypertension.

hyperplasia (hahy per PLEY zhee uh) Enlargement due to an abnormal multiplication of cells.

jaundice A yellow discoloration of the skin and mucous membranes caused by deposits of bile.

leukoderma Lack of skin pigmentation, especially in patches.

malignant A descriptive term for things or conditions that threaten life or well-being. Malignant is the opposite of benign.

VOCABULARY—*continued*

melanocytes (meh LAN oh sites) Cells of the stratum germinativum that produce a brownish pigment called melanin. Melanin gives us our skin color.

opaque (oh PAYK) Not transparent; cloudy or murky.

pathogen A disease-causing organism.

petechiae (peh TEEK kee ah) Very small, round hemorrhage in the skin or mucous membrane.

pores Tiny openings in the surface of the skin that allow gases, liquids, or microscopic particles to pass.

strata Naturally or artificially formed layers of material, usually multiple layers.

synthesis (SIN theh sis) Formation of a chemical compound from simpler compounds or elements.

INTRODUCTION

The skin is the largest organ of the human body. In an average-size adult, it covers a total area of about 20 square feet. Forming the outer boundary of the body, the skin performs several essential functions: it acts as a barrier to protect vital internal organs from infection and injury, helps to dissipate heat and regulate body temperature, and synthesizes vitamin D when exposed to ultraviolet (UV) light. In addition, various sensory receptors present throughout the skin enable it to respond to such sensations as heat, cold, pain, and pressure.

The specialty of dermatology deals with the skin and its accessory structures: hair, nails, and sweat glands, and the subcutaneous tissue that lies beneath the skin. A physician who specializes in dermatology is called a *dermatologist.*

ANATOMY OF THE INTEGUMENTARY SYSTEM

The most important function of the skin (or integument) is protecting the body from disease. The skin provides a physical barrier that is our first line of defense against **pathogens**. It is the largest organ of the body, and, in addition to physically protecting the body, it also helps to do the following:

- Regulate the body temperature
- Provide information about the environment through sensory activity
- Assist in the **synthesis** of vitamin D
- Eliminate waste products from the body

The skin functions together with accessory structures that include the hair, nails, *sebaceous* glands or oil glands, and *sudoriferous* glands or sweat glands. Any damage or injury to the skin has the potential to lessen its ability to carry out these functions, which can lead to disease.

The skin is considered a *cutaneous membrane,* made up of **epithelial cells** that cover the entire body. The skin is composed of two layers: the *epidermis,* which forms the outermost layer, and the *dermis,* which forms the inner layer (Figure 32.1). The dermis is attached to a layer of connective tissue called the *subcutaneous* layer, or hypodermis, which is mainly composed of fat or *adipose* tissue.

Epidermis

The epidermis is the top layer of the skin and is composed of several different **strata** of epithelial tissue. This type of tissue covers many of

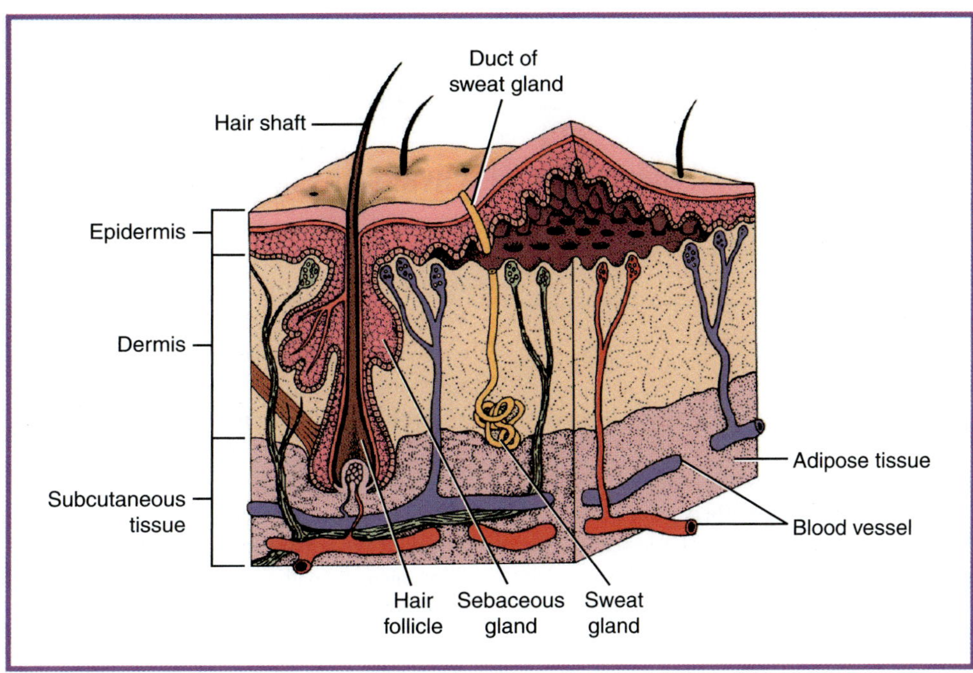

FIGURE 32.1 Diagram of the skin.

the external and internal surfaces of the body and has a microscopic scaly appearance.

The epidermis is *avascular*, which means it contains no blood vessels. New skin cells are formed in the **basal** layer of the epidermis, called the *stratum germinativum*. This layer is also where *melanin*, which is a pigment, is produced by **melanocytes**. When the skin is exposed to ultraviolet (UV) light, the melanocytes secrete more melanin. Birthmarks, age spots, and freckles result from clumps of melanin. Individuals have different skin colors because of varying numbers of melanocytes in the stratum germinativum of the skin.

New cells produced in the stratum germinativum move upward toward the top layer, the *stratum corneum*. During the transition from the basal layer to the upper layer, the cell's cytoplasm is replaced with *keratin*. Once this process is complete, the cells are called *keratinocytes*. Keratin is a hard protein material that enhances the skin by making it waterproof, abrasion resistant, and able to retain moisture in the body. These properties add to the protective nature of the skin.

A variety of microorganisms are normally found on the skin. These organisms are referred to as *normal flora*. Healthcare workers are taught to wash their hands or use hand sanitizer before and after each procedure. Good hand hygiene helps prevent the spread of microorganisms, reduces the likelihood of transferring possible pathogens, and decreases the risk of skin infections for our patients.

Dermal-Epidermal Junction

The *dermal-epidermal junction* is where the two layers of the skin meet. The top layer of the dermis contains *dermal papillae*, which are peglike projections that help fasten the dermis and epidermis together. This unique junction not only uses dermal papillae to create a bond but also uses a specialized gel that acts as a glue to keep the two layers of the skin connected.

If the dermal-epidermal junction is damaged by a burn, irritation, abrasion, or friction, a blister may occur. If the dermal-epidermal junction is destroyed, the skin will fall apart. If this happens in a small area, the body can heal the damage. If a large area of the junction is destroyed, it results in an overwhelming infection that could be serious and possibly fatal.

CRITICAL THINKING APPLICATION **32.1**

Yesterday Mai wore a new pair of shoes to work and developed a little blister on the heel of her right foot. What skin layers are affected by the formation of a blister? How should Mai properly care for her blister over the next few days?

Dermis

The *dermis* is the thick, underlying layer of the skin that is composed of vascular connective tissue arranged in two layers. The dermis gives the skin strength and stretch that the epidermis does not possess. The thin upper layer of the dermis is composed of fibers made from loose connective tissue, **collagen**, and some **elastin**. The lower, thicker layer of the dermis is composed of dense collagen. Collagen gives the skin toughness, and elastin fibers help the skin stretch and have flexibility. Distributed throughout the dermis are hair follicles, sweat glands, and old glands.

There are two types of sweat glands: *eccrine* and *apocrine*. Eccrine sweat glands are dispersed throughout the body and help maintain a constant body temperature by releasing sweat through **pores** in the skin. Apocrine sweat glands open into hair follicles and are concentrated in the axillae (armpits), scalp, face, and the pigmented skin around the genitals. Apocrine sweat glands release a fatty sweat in response to stress. They enlarge and become more active at puberty.

The dermis contains many small blood vessels that supply the skin with nutrients and oxygen and take away waste products and carbon dioxide. Sensory receptors for the nervous system (pain, temperature, and pressure) are also located in the dermis.

Subcutaneous Tissue

The subcutaneous tissue is not a layer of the skin. It lies below the dermis and creates a connection between the skin and the structures that are below the skin, such as muscle or bone. Subcutaneous tissue is made up of loose connective tissue and adipose (fat) tissue. This tissue is not rigid but rather movable and pliable. The subcutaneous tissue can slip over underlying structures. Without subcutaneous tissue, our skin would tear with movement.

The subcutaneous tissue provides insulation for the body and serves as a calorie reserve in the adipose tissue. It also contains blood vessels, nerves, and the base of hair follicles. Subcutaneous tissue is distributed unevenly, and as the body ages, it thins. This can make administering injections or drawing blood on older adult patients more challenging. Also, the loss of subcutaneous tissue makes it more difficult for older adults to regulate body temperature; they are hotter when temperatures rise and colder when temperatures drop. Aging skin can be fragile and easily traumatized or damaged. The medical assistant must be careful to avoid injuring the skin of older patients.

CRITICAL THINKING APPLICATION **32.2**

Mai goes to the waiting area and calls back Casey Hernandez. She introduces herself and shows Casey back to the exam room. After vital signs are completed, Mai asks Casey the reason for her visit. Casey looks down and is a bit shy as she talks. Mai notices that the palms of Casey's hands are sweaty. What types of glands produce sweat in the integumentary system? Where are they concentrated in the body?

PHYSIOLOGY OF THE INTEGUMENTARY SYSTEM

The five functions of the integumentary system are listed and discussed next:

- Protection
- Sensory organ activity
- Temperature regulation
- Excretion
- Synthesis of vitamin D

Protection

The skin protects the internal organs by providing a flexible, waterproof barrier to the outside environment. It is part of the first line of defense from microbial pathogens, toxic chemicals, and physical tears, cuts, and abrasions. The keratin in our skin cells protects us from excessive fluid loss and dehydration. Finally, the melanin in the epidermis of the skin protects the body from damaging UV light. Skin is so amazing!

Sensory Organ Activity

The skin has many sensory receptors scattered throughout the tissue. Sensory receptors can feel pain, pressure, heat, and cold. These receptors send messages to the brain that allow us to respond to the environment and make appropriate changes to keep ourselves from harm.

Temperature Regulation

The skin is a very good thermoregulator. When we are cold, it constricts blood vessels close to the skin's surface. This preserves body heat and lessens the heat loss to the surrounding environment. When we are hot, it can produce sweat that evaporates and cools us off. Because of the extensive blood supply to the skin, the body can help regulate and maintain a consistent body temperature. This is all part of homeostasis.

Excretion

The body can regulate the amount of sweat produced and the chemical content of the sweat. When we sweat, we lose water, electrolytes, and small amounts of other waste products. The integumentary system can excrete substances through the skin to help maintain the necessary chemical balance in the body as a whole.

Synthesis of Vitamin D

The *synthesis* of vitamin D is a vital function of the body, and it all starts in the skin. When skin is exposed to the sun's ultraviolet rays, it manufactures a vitamin D precursor molecule. The molecule is carried to the liver and kidneys by way of the blood. The precursor molecule is then converted to the active form of vitamin D that the body can use. Research has uncovered many body functions affected by vitamin D, a few of which are as follows:

- Proper absorption of calcium
- Maintaining normal calcium and phosphorus levels in the blood; calcium helps maintain strong bones, proper blood clotting, muscle function, and immunity
- Protection against osteoporosis, high blood pressure, and some forms of cancer
- Preventing consistently low vitamin D levels, which can put a person at a higher risk for developing multiple sclerosis, heart disease, osteoporosis, and depression

LIFE SPAN CHANGES

Across the life span, many changes occur that affect the integumentary system. The following sections discuss those changes.

Changes in Children

While a baby is in utero, a protective coating forms on the baby's skin. This is called *vernix* and is a white, creamy biofilm that protects the baby's skin from the amniotic fluid in the last trimester of the pregnancy. *Lanugo*, a special type of body hair, serves as an anchor to hold the vernix to the skin.

The skin of a newborn is thinner than the skin of an adult, and the skin of a preterm infant is even less than that of a full-term newborn. This can lead to increased fluid and heat loss and can result in electrolyte imbalance, reduced thermoregulation, and increased infection risk.

Children routinely appear at physician offices with skin disorders. Some of the most common are impetigo, acne, seborrheic dermatitis, cellulitis, and pediculosis. Although none of these are serious disorders, impetigo and pediculosis are highly contagious. Also seen are the different degrees of burns, usually accidental but potentially life threatening.

Changes in Older Adults

Older patients have a completely different set of diagnoses. The disorders categorized as those related to cornification, especially corns and calluses, are seen routinely in medical offices. These masses or thickenings of the skin are formed as a defensive response to constant friction, usually within shoes. Pressure sores (also called *bedsores* or *decubitus ulcers*) are seen most often in bedridden patients whose skin may already be atrophied and thin. Eczema, cellulitis, and fungal infections are also common complaints. The last category of skin disorders often seen in older adults are skin cancers. Although younger patients with skin cancers are often seen, older patients have had a longer time to be exposed to the sun and develop malignancies.

DISEASES AND DISORDERS OF THE INTEGUMENTARY SYSTEM

Diseases of the integumentary system are varied in appearance and cause. Figure 32.2 shows examples of many common lesions of the skin. Many factors can cause skin diseases, such as bacterial, fungal, viral, and parasitic infections. Here are some of the common signs and symptoms seen in patients with skin diseases and disorders:

- Skin discoloration or redness
- Itching, weeping, or bleeding lesions
- Blisters, macules, papules (see Figure 32.2 for examples)
- Scaly or flaky skin surface
- New or changing lesions

The underlying cause will vary and likely dictate the type of treatment needed.

A skin *lesion* is any visible, localized abnormality of skin tissue. It can be described as either primary or secondary. Primary lesions are early skin changes that have not yet undergone natural evolution or change caused by manipulation. Secondary lesions are the result of natural evolution or the manipulation of a primary lesion (see Figure 32.2).

CRITICAL THINKING APPLICATION 32.3

Jean Burke, a nurse practitioner, comes into the exam room and greets Casey. Jean sits down, and she and Casey talk about the reason for Casey's visit, which is her acne, and what improvements Casey would like to see in her skin. Jean mentions that she had issues with acne as a teenager and assures Casey that they will develop a plan together. What type of lesions could Casey have with acne? Review Figure 32.2, and share your thoughts with the class.

Skin Lesions

Skin lesions can be caused by a systemic problem, such as an allergic reaction to a medication, or they may develop from a localized infection. When communicating with the provider and documenting in the patient's health record, always use correct medical terminology to describe skin lesions, such as "The patient reports a widespread maculopapular rash across the anterior trunk" rather than "The patient has a red, raised rash on his stomach."

PRIMARY LESIONS

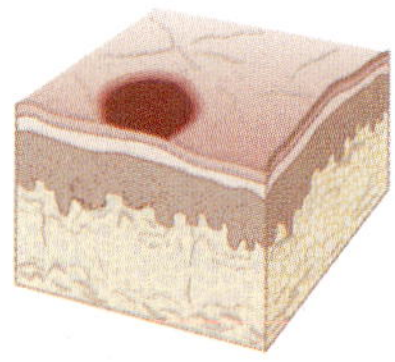

MACULE
Flat area of color change (no elevation or depression)

Example: Freckles

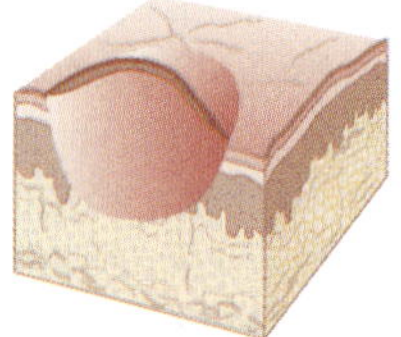

PAPULE
Solid elevation less than 0.5 cm in diameter

Example: Allergic eczema

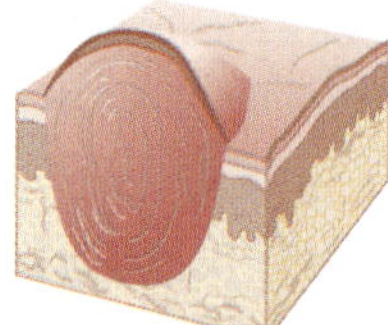

NODULE
Solid elevation 0.5 to 1 cm in diameter. Extends deeper into dermis than papule

Example: Mole

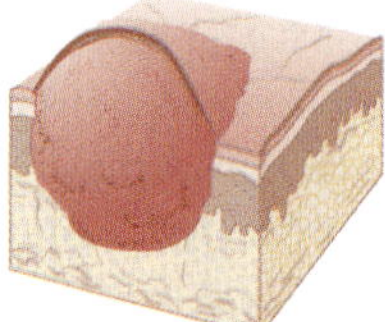

TUMOR
Solid mass—larger than 1 cm

Example: Squamous cell carcinoma

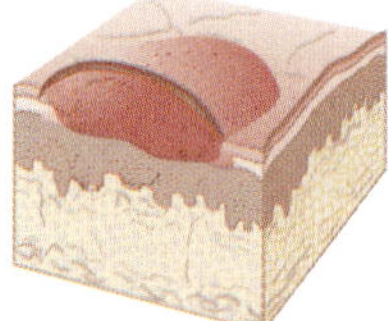

PLAQUE
Flat elevated surface found on skin or mucous membrane

Example: Thrush

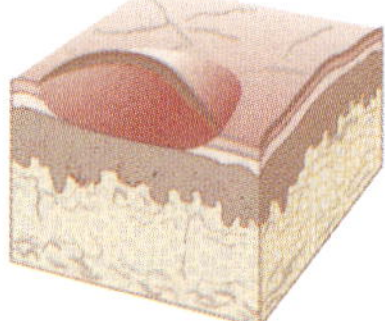

WHEAL
Type of plaque. Result is transient edema in dermis

Example: Intradermal skin test

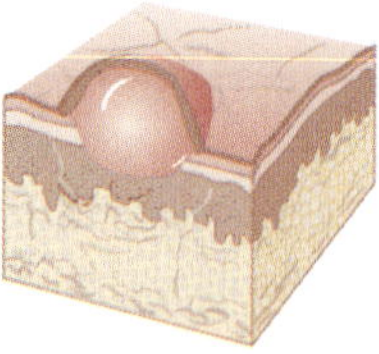

VESICLE
Small blister—fluid within or under epidermis

Example: Herpesvirus infection

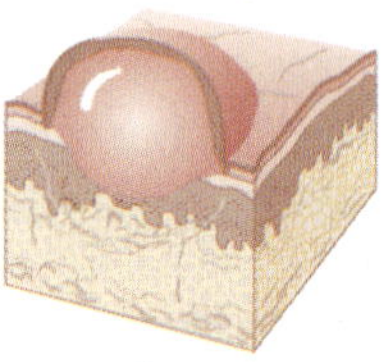

BULLA
Large blister (greater than 0.5 cm)

Example: Burn

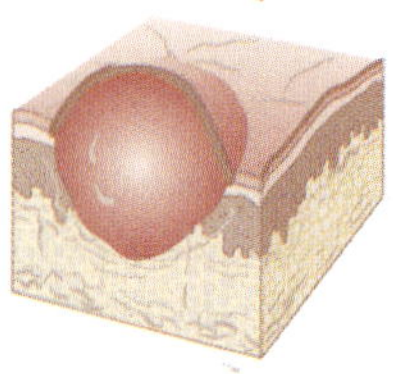

PUSTULE
Vesicle filled with pus

Example: Acne

SECONDARY LESIONS

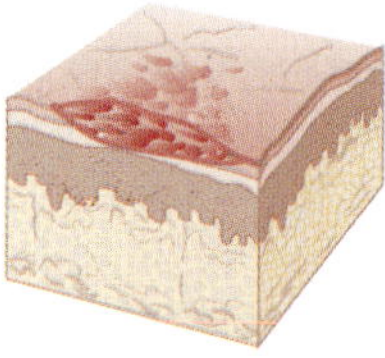

SCALES
Flakes of cornified skin layer

Example: Psoriasis

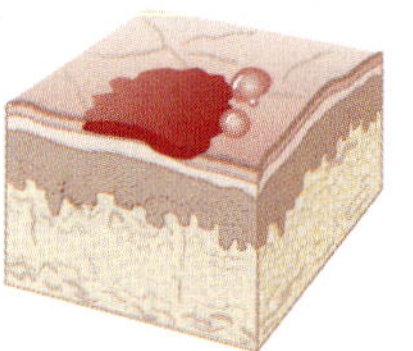

CRUST
Dried exudate on skin

Example: Impetigo

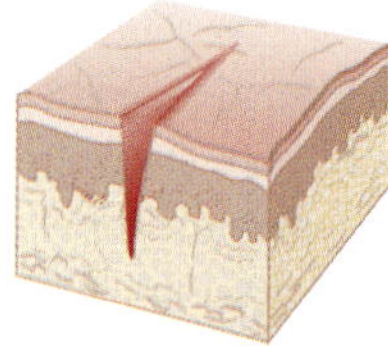

FISSURE
Cracks in skin

Example: Athlete's foot

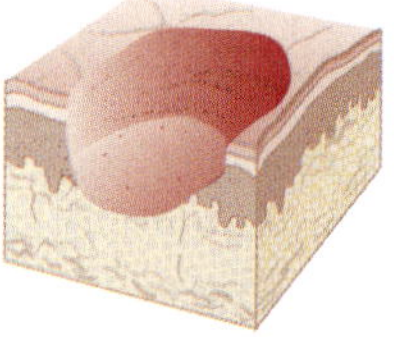

ULCER
Area of destruction of entire epidermis

Example: Decubitus (pressure sore)

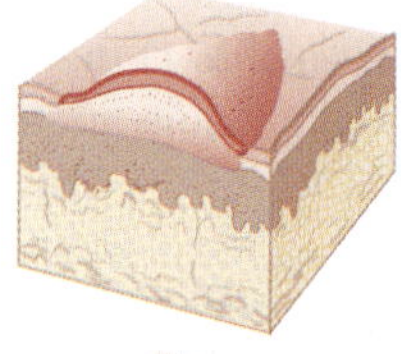

SCAR
Excess collagen production after injury

Example: Surgical healing

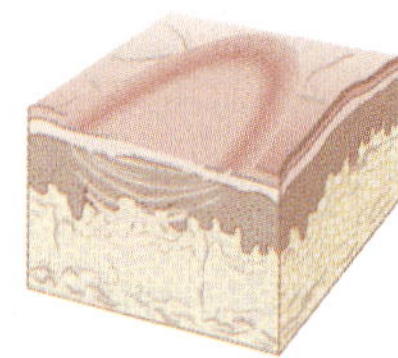
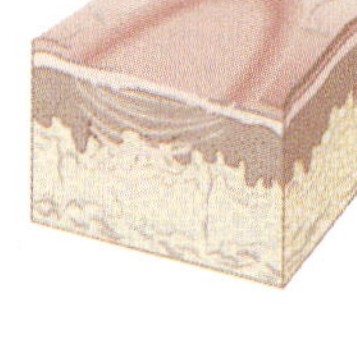

ATROPHY
Loss of some portion of the skin

Example: Paralysis

FIGURE 32.2 Different types of skin lesions.

When you gather details from the patient about the characteristics of lesions, here are some of the elements you should consider:

- Describe the color, elevation, and texture of the lesion.
- Does the patient have any pain or *pruritus* (itching)? If pruritus is present, is the area **excoriated** or inflamed?
- Is any drainage present? If so, what are its characteristics?
- What is the exact anatomic location of the lesion? Have changes occurred over time?

Primary lesions are those that appear immediately. Macules, papules, plaques, nodules, cysts, wheals, and pustules are all primary lesions. *Secondary lesions* are the result of alterations in a primary lesion. Examples of secondary lesions include scales, crusts, fissures, erosions, ulcerations, and scars (see Figure 32.2). For instance, vesicles (blisters) from a partial-thickness burn are primary lesions, but if the blisters break and ulcerations form, healing ends in a scar. Ulcerations and scars are secondary lesions.

Infections

Infections of the integumentary system can be caused by many different pathogens. When working with patients in this specialty, it is important to have an understanding of the different types of infections. These infections are discussed in the following sections.

Bacterial Infections

When working in dermatology, a medical assistant should be familiar with the common bacterial infections that are found in the integumentary system. The following sections discuss those bacterial infections.

Impetigo. Impetigo is a common, superficial infection caused by *Streptococcus sp.* or *Staphylococcus aureus* that usually affects children. Initially, impetigo looks like small vesicles on the face (especially around the nose and mouth) that quickly enlarge and rupture, excreting a honey-colored exudate. The exudate forms crusty lesions, and beneath the crust, the area is inflamed and moist (Figure 32.3). Pruritus accompanies the infection, and scratching helps spread the lesions at the site. Impetigo is contagious, and bacteria are transmitted by direct contact with the drainage, whether this occurs at other sites or with other children through the sharing of toys and physical contact. Consistent handwashing is required to help break the chain of infection. It is also important to keep personal items that may be contaminated, such as washcloths, linens, and drinking glasses, away from other members of the family. If the areas of infection are limited, topical treatment with an antibiotic ointment may be effective. However, impetigo caused by streptococci may result in **glomerulonephritis**; more involved infections may require treatment with oral antibiotics.

Acne Vulgaris. Acne vulgaris is a skin condition that occurs when a hair follicle becomes plugged with oil and dead skin cells (Figure 32.4). Acne is most common on the face, but it can occur on other sites of the body, such as the neck, chest, shoulders, and back. Acne is most common during adolescence, but it can occur at any age. Because acne can cause scarring, it is best treated as early as possible to minimize scars and emotional distress.

The main causes of acne include excess oil production, pores clogged with dead skin cells and oil, and bacterial infections. Once a pore is clogged, bacteria trapped in the pore multiply and cause inflammation. Risk factors for acne include age (adolescents are most prone due to hormonal changes), medications (corticosteroids, androgens, oral contraceptives, and lithium), stress, and diet (a diet that is high in dairy products and simple carbohydrates, such as refined sugars, processed foods, and sweets, can make acne worse). The signs and symptoms of acne can vary in severity. Common symptoms include the following:

- Whiteheads and blackheads
- Papules and pustules
- Large, solid, painful nodules
- Painful, pus-filled lumps beneath the skin's surface, known as *cystic acne*

There are many treatments used for acne, from simple over-the-counter (OTC) lotions to more extensive use of medications, antibiotics, and dermatologic procedures:

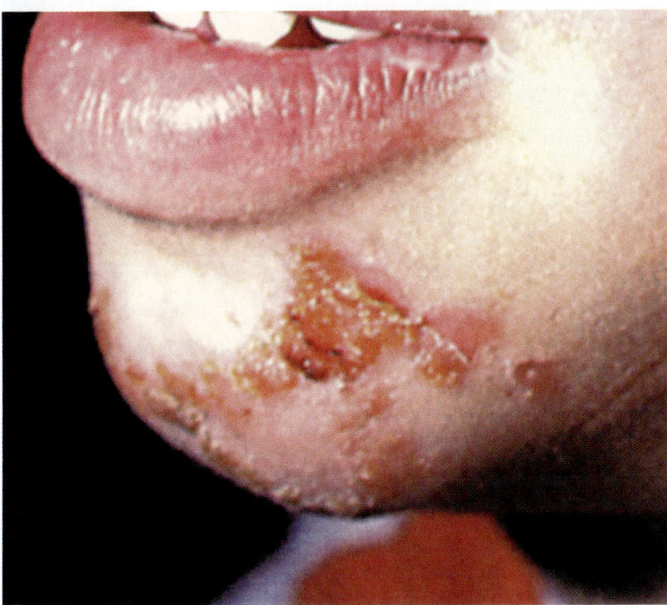

FIGURE 32.3 Impetigo. (From Marks J, Miller J: *Lookingbill and Marks' principles of dermatology*, ed 5, Philadelphia, 2014, Saunders.)

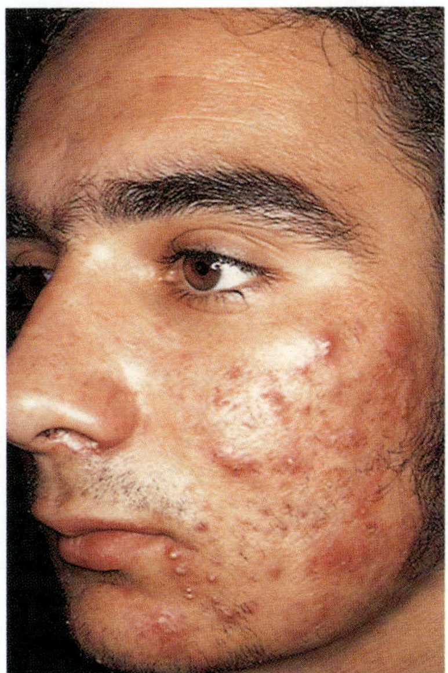

FIGURE 32.4 Acne. (From Paller A, Mancini A: *Hurwitz clinical pediatric dermatology: a textbook of skin disorders in childhood and adolescence*, ed 4, Philadelphia, 2011, Saunders.)

- Common medications include topical prescription-strength benzoyl peroxide, antibiotics, retinoids, and oral contraceptives.
- Common dermatologic procedures include light therapy, chemical peels, extraction of whiteheads and blackheads by a provider, and steroid injections.
- Common dietary changes recommended include reducing or eliminating dairy products, refined sugar, and simple carbohydrate foods. Examples include juice, soda, sweets, pasta, and bread.
- More extensive treatments include dermabrasion, laser resurfacing, and minor skin surgery to repair areas of damage or excessive scarring.

Acne often requires extended treatment and follow-up, depending on the severity of the condition.

Rosacea. Rosacea is a chronic disease seen most frequently in women between the ages of 30 and 60. It causes inflammation and pustule formation and begins as frequent flushing across the nose, forehead, cheeks, and chin.

As the condition progresses, capillaries of the face dilate and are visible across affected areas as small, red, edematous lines; these are accompanied by eye inflammation and photosensitivity. Over time, the face appears red, eye inflammation is more apparent, and painful nodules and pustules form. Men with rosacea may develop *rhinophyma*, a large, inflamed, bulbous nose caused by **hyperplasia** of sebaceous nasal tissue (Figure 32.5). Individuals with rosacea eventually may develop an obvious thickening of the skin across the forehead, nose, cheeks, and chin.

The condition is treated with topical antibiotics and, as symptoms progress, with oral antibiotics, such as doxycycline (Oracea), which helps reduce the number of pimples and bumps on the face; however, it may not reduce the redness and flushing.

Furuncles and Carbuncles. A *furuncle*, or boil, is a localized staphylococcal infection that begins as inflammation of a hair follicle (folliculitis) or skin gland. The affected area is raised, inflamed, and painful and eventually may produce purulent drainage. A carbuncle is a collection of furuncles that have joined to form a large, infected area that may drain through multiple sites or form an abscess. Both infections are treated with oral antibiotics, frequent cleansing of the area, application of an antibiotic ointment and, in some cases, surgical incision and drainage of the purulent material.

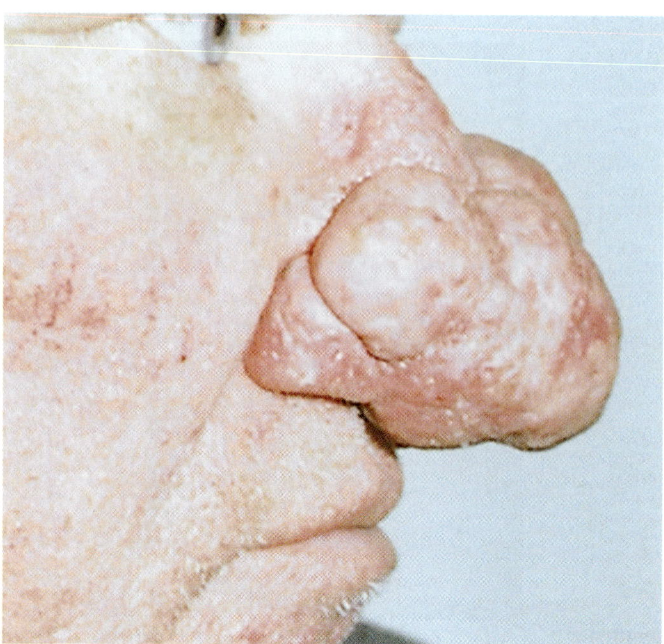

FIGURE 32.5 Rhinophyma. (Courtesy Michael O. Murphy, MD.)

Cellulitis. *Cellulitis* is an acute infection of the skin and subcutaneous tissue caused by staphylococci or streptococci. It begins from a small cut or as a result of a skin injury or develops at the site of a furuncle or an ulcer. The area surrounding the site becomes inflamed, edematous, and painful, with red streaks along the lymph vessels that lead from the infection. The condition is treated with oral antibiotics. Warm compresses applied locally aid healing, and analgesics may be needed to relieve discomfort. It is important that patients with cellulitis are treated appropriately because a systemic infection can develop if the lymph glands become involved.

Fungal Infections (Dermatophytoses)

Fungal, or mycotic, infections, such as *tinea pedis* (athlete's foot) (Figure 32.6A), *tinea cruris* (jock itch), and *tinea corporis* (ringworm) (Figure 32.6B), are extremely common. These pathogens infect hair follicles or the nails, causing almost no inflammation in

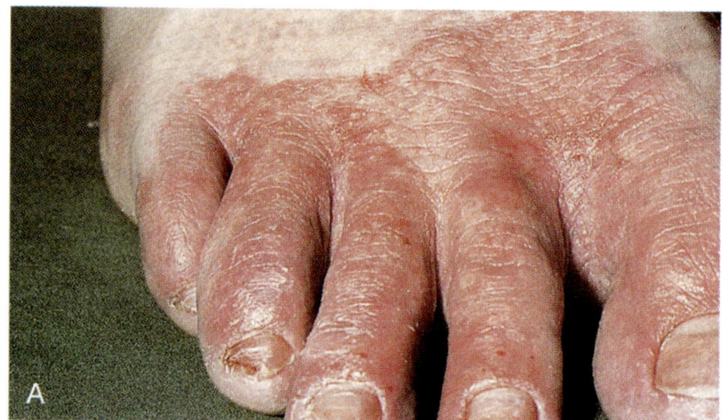

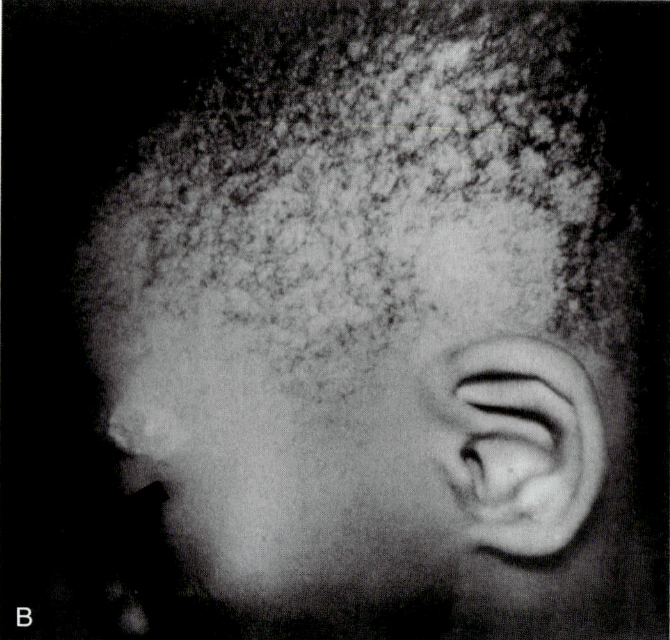

FIGURE 32.6 Fungal infections. **(A)** Tinea pedis. **(B)** Tinea corporis. (A, from Gawkrodger D: *Dermatology*, ed 5, New York, 2012, Churchill Livingstone; B, from Mahon CR, et al: *Textbook of diagnostic microbiology*, ed 5, Philadelphia, 2015, Saunders.)

the underlying skin. The fungus invades the skin where it has been damaged or is consistently moist. All of these lesions are pruritic and characterized by a distinct border with scaling areas that have a clear center. Secondary bacterial infections may occur with excoriation.

The provider typically diagnoses a fungal infection by noting how the skin looks and the patient's complaints of pruritus. The skin may be scraped to obtain cells for examination under a microscope, and sometimes the provider may order a skin culture, in which a suspicious area is swabbed or scraped using sterile technique. The sample is sent to the laboratory for analysis. Treatment consists of topical antifungal agents, such as clotrimazole (Lotrimin), ketoconazole (Nizoral), econazole, or nystatin (Mycostatin). Antibiotics may be necessary if a secondary infection occurs. Because mycotic infections thrive in dark, moist areas, the patient should be advised to keep the site clean and dry and to wear loose clothing if possible. All types of dermatophytoses can become chronic infections if not managed carefully.

Tinea unguium, or *onychomycosis* (Figure 32.7), is a fungal infection of the toenails and fingernails. Unlike athlete's foot, which occurs on the skin's surface, nail fungus lives in the nail bed and the nail plate. The nail provides the fungus with an extremely well-protected place to live, which is why nail fungus may be especially difficult to treat. The primary sign of nail fungus is the appearance of the nail, which turns yellow, white, or **opaque**. The texture also changes, and the nail becomes thick and brittle. If the fungus has been present for a long time, the nail can become twisted or distorted. The most effective treatment for nail fungus is oral terbinafine hydrochloride (Lamisil) or itraconazole (Sporanox); both inhibit the production of fungal cells. However, the drug must be taken for 6 weeks to treat fungal infection of a fingernail and for 12 weeks for infection of a toenail; treatment carries the risk of liver complications.

Viral Infections

Infections in the integumentary system can also be caused by viruses. The following sections discuss the common viral infections of the integumentary system.

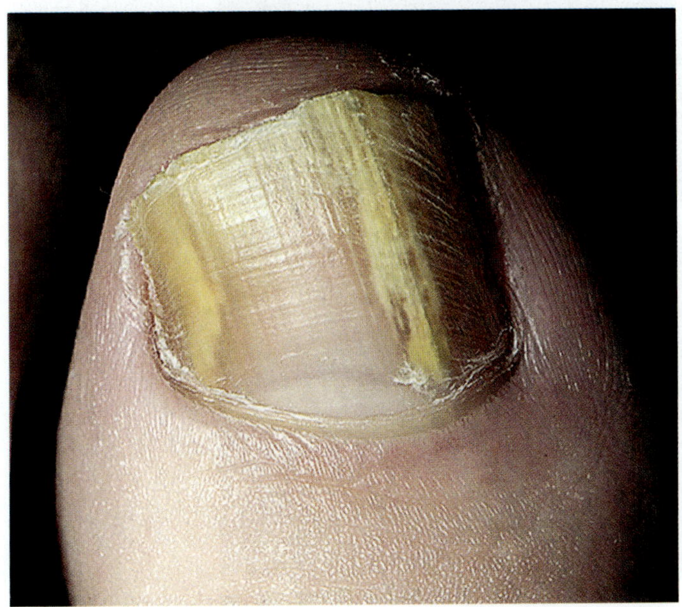

FIGURE 32.7 Tinea unguium. (From Habif TP: *Clinical dermatology*, ed 5, St. Louis, 2010, Mosby.)

Warts. Warts, or verrucae, are caused by the human papillomavirus (HPV). Infection with HPV results in hyperplasia of the epidermis and a raised, cauliflower-like appearance. Verrucae can develop anywhere, but the most common sites are the fingers and the soles (plantar warts). Most warts resolve over time, but they can be treated with topical chemicals, excised surgically, vaporized with lasers, or removed with **cryosurgery**.

Herpes Simplex (Cold Sores). Cold sores, or fever blisters, are caused by herpes simplex virus type 1 (HSV-1). The initial infection may be asymptomatic or may cause painful ulcers along the gum lines of the mouth or on the lips. After the primary infection, the virus remains dormant in the trigeminal nerve and can be reactivated by exposure to the sun or cold, by the presence of another infection such as an upper respiratory infection, or when the patient is under stress. The patient reports a feeling of burning, tingling, or numbness before the eruption of vesicles. The blisters heal in 2 to 3 weeks, but the process may be sped up by the use of topical antiviral drugs, such as acyclovir (Zovirax), docosanol (Abreva), or penciclovir cream (Denavir), or with oral antivirals, including famciclovir (Famvir), acyclovir, or valacyclovir (Valtrex). If started at the first indications of a cold sore, antiviral medications can limit the duration and severity of the outbreak.

Parasites

Parasitic infestations of the skin can occur at any age. They are spread in group settings, such as among families or childcare groups, school classes, nursing homes, prisons, and dormitories. The two most common types of skin parasites seen are scabies (itch mites) and pediculosis (lice). Both parasites infect the skin and cause itching. Both parasites can be treated, and the infection resolved.

Scabies is caused by the itch mite *Sarcoptes scabiei.* This little mite burrows under the skin, causing intense itching (Figure 32.8).

Pediculosis is caused by lice that populate three specific areas of the body (Figure 32.9). A person can have head lice (*Pediculus capitis),* body lice *(Pediculus corporis),* or pubic lice or crabs *(Pthirus pubis).* Lice crawl but cannot fly or hop.

Both itch mites and lice can move from person to person through close physical contact and sharing of inanimate objects or *fomites,* such as combs, brushes, clothes, and bedding.

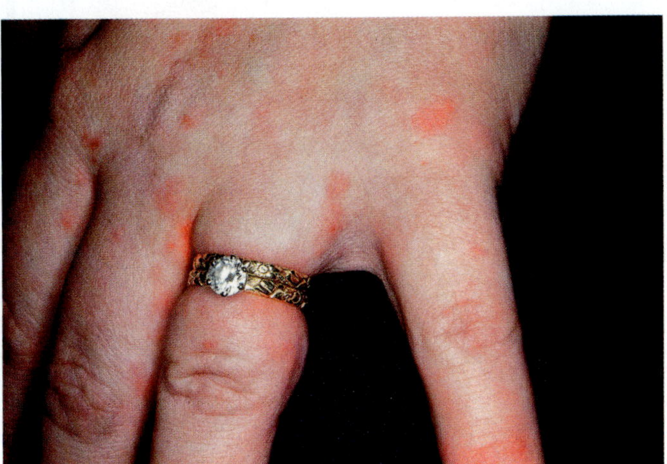

FIGURE 32.8 Scabies rash of the hand. (From James WD, et al: *Andrews' diseases of the skin*, ed 11, Philadelphia, 2011, Saunders.)

The signs and symptoms of scabies and pediculosis are similar:

- Intense itching
- Tickling feeling as parasites move hair on the skin
- Lice: small red bumps on the skin and nits (eggs) on the body, facial, or pubic hair
- Scabies: little burrows or tunnels can be seen under the skin; frequently in areas of the skin that fold, such as between fingers and toes, around the waist, in the armpits, and on knees and elbows

Diagnosis of lice infestation is often done with a magnifying lens to see the lice and nits on hair. A Wood's light, which produces UV light, can also be used to detect the nits. They look pale blue. For scabies, physical examination involves looking for characteristic burrows under the skin. The provider may scrape the skin and examine it under the microscope to look for eggs. Prescription shampoo, body wash, and lotion can be used to kill the parasites on the head, hair, and body. The lice and mites are generally killed quickly, but the patient must follow all instructions to make sure eggs are also killed. There may be some itching after the parasites are killed, but that does not necessarily indicate a continued infection. Women who are pregnant and the parents of infants should consult their provider before applying antiparasitic products. They are strong chemicals that may cause complications for the very young and pregnant women.

In addition to properly washing the hair and body, all clothing, bedding, personal items, and furniture should also be cleaned with hot, soapy water. If all the eggs are not removed, reinfections can occur.

Inflammatory Skin Disorders

Inflammatory skin disorders are the most common problem with the integumentary system. These disorders can be either acute or chronic. The patient usually has some itching and redness from these disorders. The following sections discuss the common inflammatory skin disorders.

Seborrheic Dermatitis

Seborrheic dermatitis is one of the most common chronic inflammatory conditions of the sebaceous glands. It alters the amount and quality of the sebum, resulting in dry or moist, greasy-appearing scales and yellowish crusts on the scalp, eyebrows, eyelids, and sides of the nose (Figure 32.10A), behind the ears, and in the middle of the chest. The condition has many different forms, including cradle cap in infants (Figure 32.10B) and dandruff in adults. Seborrheic dermatitis of the scalp can be treated with tar- or sulfur-based shampoos; inflammations of the skin usually are treated with topical corticosteroids, such as generic triamcinolone diacetate or betamethasone valerate, or fluocinolone acetonide (Synalar). Seborrheic keratosis (age spots) is characterized by **benign**, slightly raised, tan to black lesions that occur with aging.

Contact Dermatitis

Contact dermatitis is an acute inflammatory response to a skin irritant or exposure to a substance that causes an allergic reaction (Figure 32.11). An individual who is allergic to latex gloves or who has been exposed to poison ivy shows the signs and symptoms of contact dermatitis. The individual complains of redness (*erythema*), edema, pruritus, and vesicles. The patient should be encouraged to wash the affected area immediately after exposure to remove the irritant. Medical treatment includes the application of a corticosteroid cream or the use of oral corticosteroid medications (e.g., prednisone, methylprednisolone [Medrol]) if the symptoms are severe.

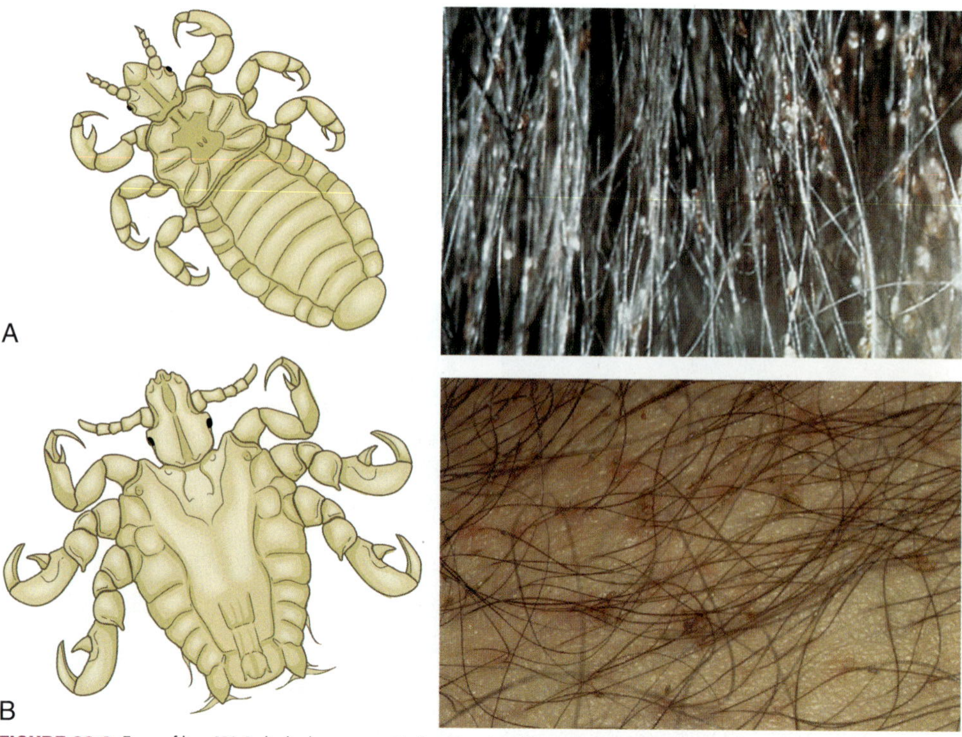

FIGURE 32.9 Types of lice. **(A)** *Pediculus humanus* capitis (head louse) and lice in the hair. **(B)** *Phthirus pubis* (pubic or crab louse) and pubic lice rash. (A, from Lissauer T, et al: *Illustrated textbook of paediatrics*, ed 4, London, 2012, Mosby; B, from Long SS, et al: *Principles and practice of pediatric infectious diseases*, ed 4, Philadelphia, 2012, Saunders.)

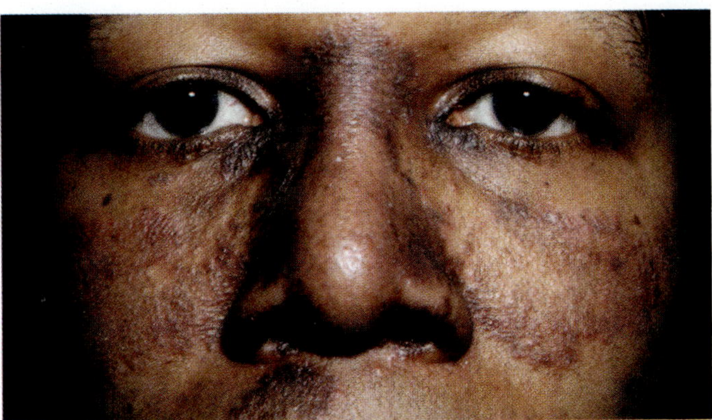

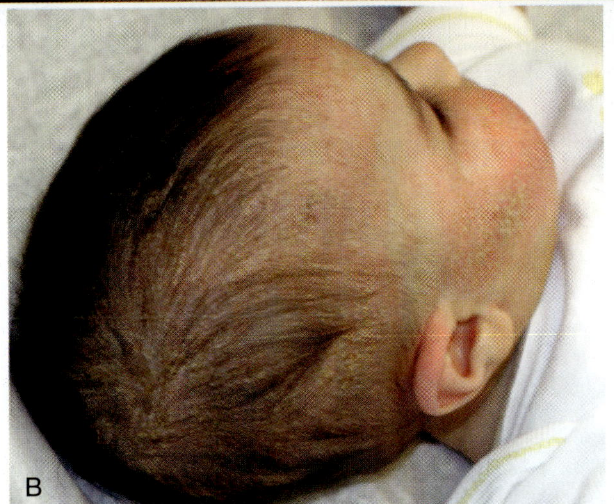

FIGURE 32.10 Seborrheic dermatitis. **(A)** Sides of the nose. **(B)** Cradle cap. (A, from Micheletti RG, et al: *Andrews' diseases of the skin clinical atlas*, ed 2, St. Louis, 2023, Elsevier; B, from Mercdante KJ, Kliegman RM: *Nelson essentials of pediatrics*, ed 8, Philadelphia, 2019, Elsevier.)

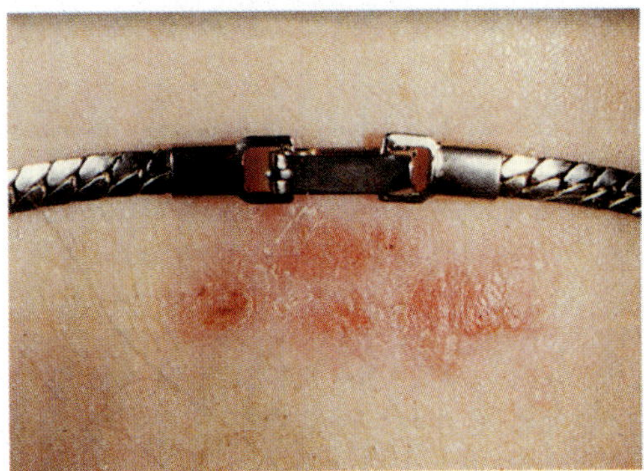

FIGURE 32.11 Nickel contact dermatitis. The location and distribution of the rash are often helpful in determining the cause of a contact dermatitis. In this case, wrist lesions were triggered by the nickel in her bracelet clasp. (From McIntire SC, et al: *Zitelli and Davis' atlas of pediatric physical diagnosis*, St. Louis, ed 8, 2023, Elsevier.)

Eczema (Atopic Dermatitis)

Eczema, also known as *atopic dermatitis*, is a group of conditions that make the skin irritated, inflamed, red, and itchy (Fig 32.12). It is more common in children but can occur at any age. Eczema is a chronic condition that may become worse occasionally and then subside. Eczema is a group of conditions with an inherited tendency. It is often seen in combination with asthma or hay fever. Most children who develop eczema outgrow it by their 10th birthday. Some adults continue to have symptoms throughout their lifetime. The disease can often be controlled with proper treatment.

The cause of eczema is unknown, but it is more common in families with a history of allergies and asthma. Flare-ups can occur in response to specific substances, conditions, or triggers. Temperature, exposure to certain chemicals, fabric texture, pet dander, and stress are all examples of possible irritants. Some of the common signs and symptoms of eczema include itchy skin; rash on the face, back of the knees, hands, wrists, or feet; and a dry, thickened, or scaly appearance of the skin that starts out pink or red but can turn brownish with time.

A pediatrician, dermatologist, or primary care provider will observe the rash and ask specific questions about the signs and symptoms. Sometimes the provider will perform allergy tests to try to pinpoint a specific trigger or irritant. Most frequently, observation and the patient history are sufficient to diagnose eczema. The treatment of eczema is focused on relieving itching and preventing scratching of the skin, which can lead to infection. Using a provider-recommended lotion or cream to keep the skin moist is the most common treatment. Applying topical treatments when the skin is damp (i.e., after a bath or shower) may help the skin to retain moisture. Cold compresses and 1% hydrocortisone cream are also common treatments.

If over-the-counter (OTC) remedies are not providing relief, creams and ointments that contain corticosteroids can be prescribed to lessen inflammation of the skin. Antibiotics may also be prescribed if an area becomes infected after vigorous itching. Additional treatments include antihistamines and ultraviolet (UV) light therapy. For patients with moderate to unresponsive eczema, cyclosporine or topical immunomodulators (TIMs) may be prescribed to help prevent flare-ups.

Autoimmune Skin Disorders

Some of the common skin disorders are autoimmune disorders. *Autoimmune disorders* occur when the immune system mistakenly attacks the body. There are several autoimmune disorders that affect the skin. The common autoimmune disorders of the skin are discussed in the following sections.

Psoriasis

Psoriasis is an autoimmune disease that affects the life cycle of skin cells. Psoriasis causes skin cells to build up rapidly on the surface of the skin. The extra skin cells form thick, silvery scales and itchy, dry, red patches that are sometimes painful. There may be times when symptoms get better, alternating with times when the psoriasis worsens.

Psoriasis is caused by a malfunction in the immune cells called T lymphocytes (T cells). T lymphocytes normally travel through the body looking for pathogens (bacteria and viruses) to destroy. But in people who have psoriasis, the T lymphocytes attack healthy skin cells. This T-cell overactivity causes the skin to produce too many new skin cells and the immune system to produce too many T cells.

It is unclear why the immune system of people with psoriasis acts this way. It can become a vicious circle of rapid skin cell production, which leads to the characteristic psoriasis plaques. Anyone can develop psoriasis, but risk factors include a family history of psoriasis, stress, a history of recurring streptococcal infections, obesity, and smoking. Signs and symptoms of psoriasis can vary, but plaques have a characteristic appearance:

- Red patches of skin covered in silvery scales
- Dry, cracked skin that may bleed and small patches of scaly spots

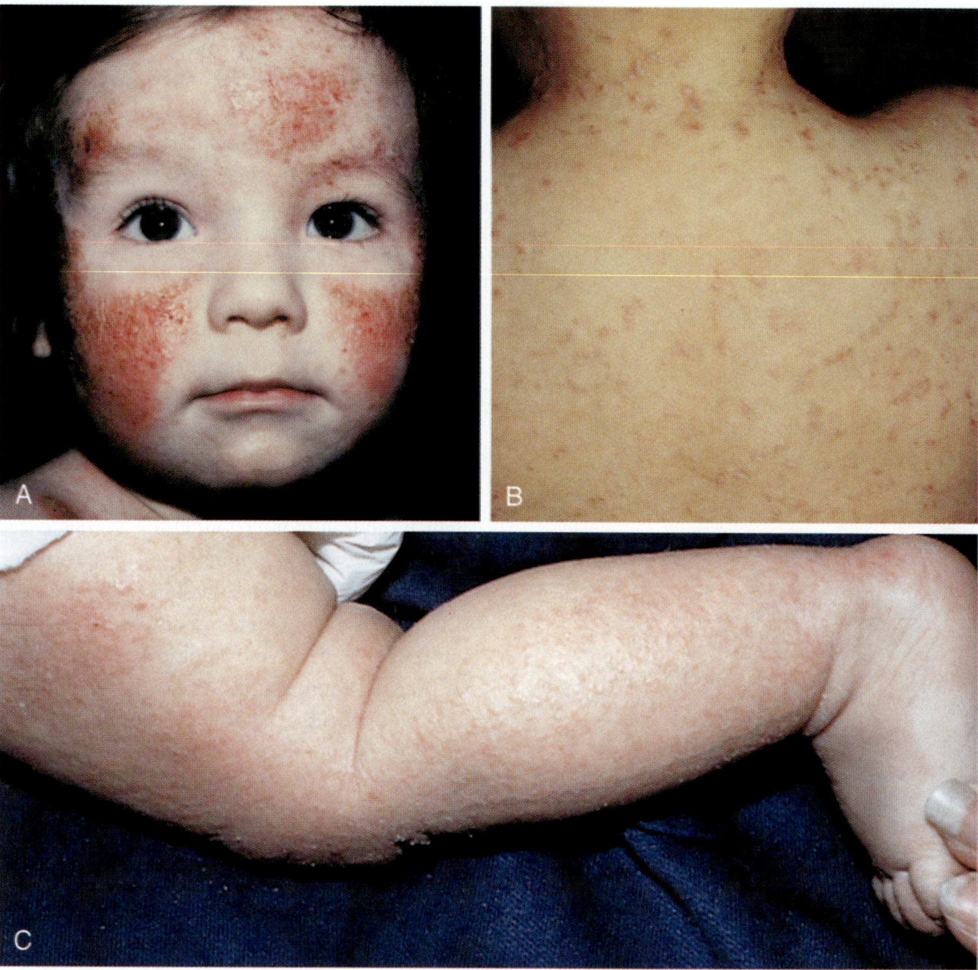

FIGURE 32.12 Infantile atopic dermatitis or eczema. **(A)** This infant has an acute, weeping dermatitis on the cheeks and forehead. **(B and C)** Involvement of the trunk and the extremities, with erythema, scaling, and crusting, is evident. Usually the diaper area is the only portion of the skin surface that is spared. (A, from McIntire SC, et al: *Zitelli and Davis' atlas of pediatric physical diagnosis,* ed 8, St. Louis, 2023, Elsevier; B and C, from Fireman P, Slavin RG: *Atlas of allergies,* New York, 1991, Gower.)

- Itching, burning, and pain in and around plaques
- Thick, pitted, or ridged finger and toenails
- Swollen and stiff joints

Some people may only have a few spots of psoriasis; others may have large skin eruptions that may cover large areas of the body. Psoriasis may erupt, then get better, and continue this cycle for years.

Some of the most common forms of psoriasis are plaque, nail, scalp, and psoriatic arthritis, which also affects the joints (Figure 32.13).

Discoid Lupus Erythematosus

Discoid lupus erythematosus (DLE) is the most common form of chronic cutaneous lupus. It is a chronic autoimmune disease of the skin that presents as sores with inflammation and scarring favoring the face, ears, and scalp (sun-exposed areas) and, at times, other body areas. The sores are usually coin-shaped red lesions with inflamed patches with a scaly or crusty appearance. These lesions can cause disfiguring scars. If the lesions are on the scalp, there may be permanent hair loss after the lesions have healed (Figure 32.14).

Diagnosis is made with a physical examination with a complete history and laboratory evaluation. Patients with cutaneous lupus may not have any abnormal laboratory test results. A skin biopsy of a lesion may be done. Discoid lupus is very photosensitive, so prevention of sun exposure is very important. Treatments include using sunscreen and avoiding sun exposure; corticosteroid creams or ointments may be used in conjunction with injections.

Burns

Burns are injuries to tissues that result from exposure to thermal, chemical, electrical, or radioactive agents. They are classified into four different degrees of severity, depending on the layers of the skin that are damaged. Burns that are second degree or higher should be further categorized according to the "rule of nines." The rule of nines regarding burns divides the body into percentages that are, for the most part, multiples of nine: the head and neck equal 9%, each upper limb 9%, each lower limb 18%, the front of the torso 18%, back of the torso 18%, and the genital area 1% (Figure 32.15). Figure 32.16 illustrates the different degrees of burns.

Because burns are injuries, the cause is trauma of some kind. Many risk factors could be included in this discussion, but particular caution should be exercised when participating in activities that involve fire, chemicals, or electrical hazards. Proper safety equipment should always be available and ready to use when burns are a possibility.

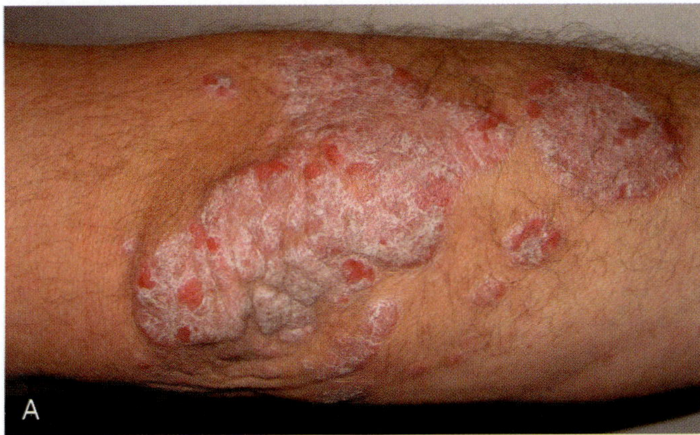

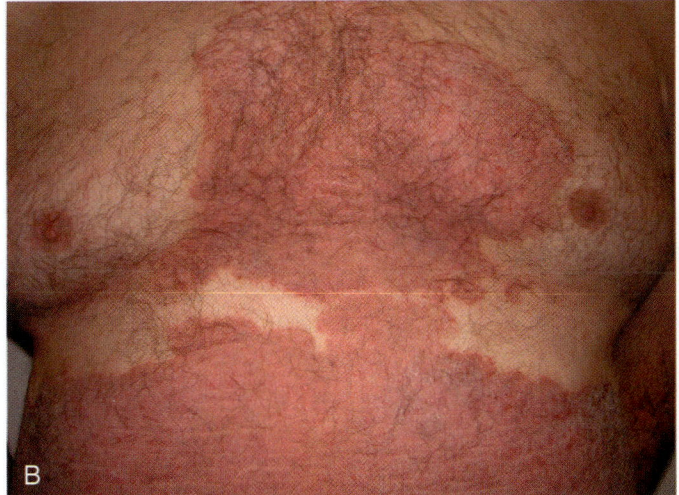

FIGURE 32.13 Psoriasis. (From Marks J, Miller J: *Lookingbill and Marks' principles of dermatology*, ed 5, Philadelphia, 2014, Saunders.)

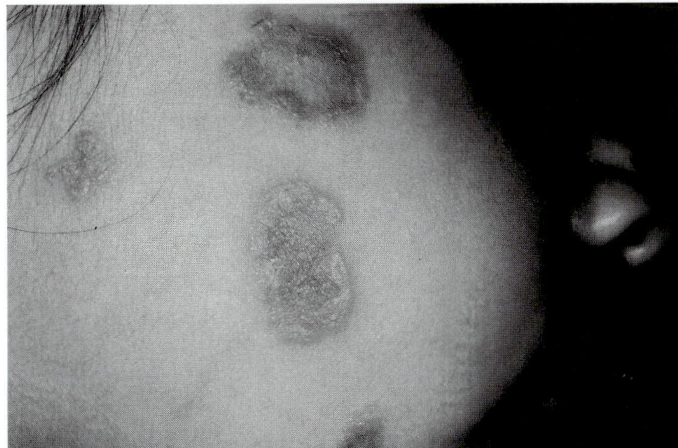

FIGURE 32.14 Discoid lupus erythematosus (DLE). This young girl showed well-circumscribed, elevated, indurated, red to purplish annular plaques of DLE. (From Paller AS, Mancini AJ: *Hurwitz clinical pediatric dermatology, a textbook of skin disorders of childhood and adolescence,* ed 5, Philadelphia, 2016, Elsevier.)

The categories of burns are as follows:

- *First-degree burn (superficial burn):* A burn in which only the first layer of the skin, the epidermis, is damaged. It is characterized by redness (*erythema*), tenderness, and physical sensitivity (*hyperesthesia*), with no scar development.

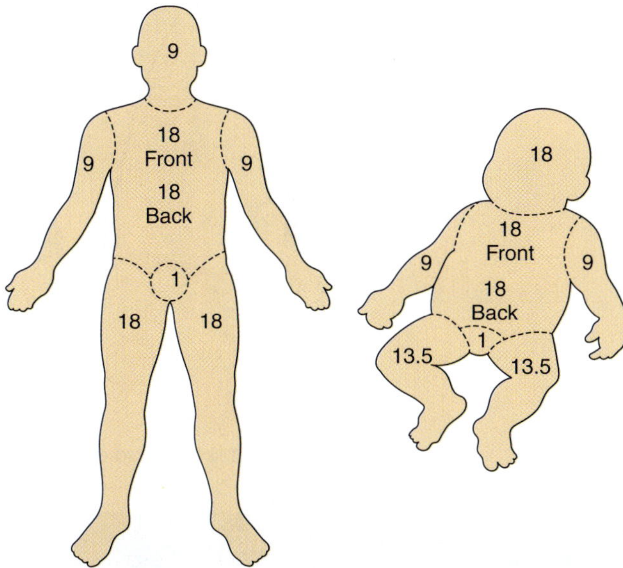

FIGURE 32.15 Rule of nines for adults and infants. (Revised from Bolick BN, et al: *Pediatric acute care: a guide for interprofessional practice,* ed 2, St. Louis, 2021, Elsevier.)

- *Second-degree burn (partial-thickness burn):* A burn in which only the first and second layers of the skin (the epidermis and part of the dermis) are affected. If the burn extends to the papillary level, it is classified as a *superficial partial-thickness burn.* If it extends farther to the reticular layer, it is classified as a *deep partial-thickness burn.* This type of burn is characterized by redness, blisters, and pain, with possible scar development.
- *Third-degree burn (full-thickness burn):* A burn that damages the epidermis, dermis, and subcutaneous tissue. Pain is not present because the nerve endings in the skin have been destroyed. The skin may appear deep red, pale gray, brown, or black. Scar formation is likely.
- *Fourth-degree burn (deep full-thickness burn):* Although not a universally accepted category, some burn specialists use this category to describe a rare burn that extends beyond the subcutaneous tissue into the muscle and bone.

Burns may not uniformly affect an injured area, so determining the depth of a burn and the extent of tissue damage is important. Burns are treated differently depending on the depth of damage. Treatment is based on the category of burn.

The American Burn Association defines a severe burn as a burn that affects 25% of the total body surface area or any burn involving the eyes, ears, face, hands, feet, or groin. With a severe burn, the patient may require additional testing, such as laboratory tests, x-rays, or other diagnostics. The treatment of burns listed in Table 32.1 is based on the category of burn.

Cold Injuries

Cold injuries usually are less severe than burns, but prolonged exposure to cold temperatures can result in infection, gangrene, amputation and, in severe cases, death. Frostbite is caused by exposure to subfreezing temperatures. Damage occurs at the level of the capillaries, which become permanently dilated and unable to regulate local blood flow. Signs and symptoms of superficial frostbite include burning, tingling, numbness, and a white or grayish color of the skin. With deep frostbite, blisters form, and the area is hard, mottled, edematous, and blue or gray after thawing.

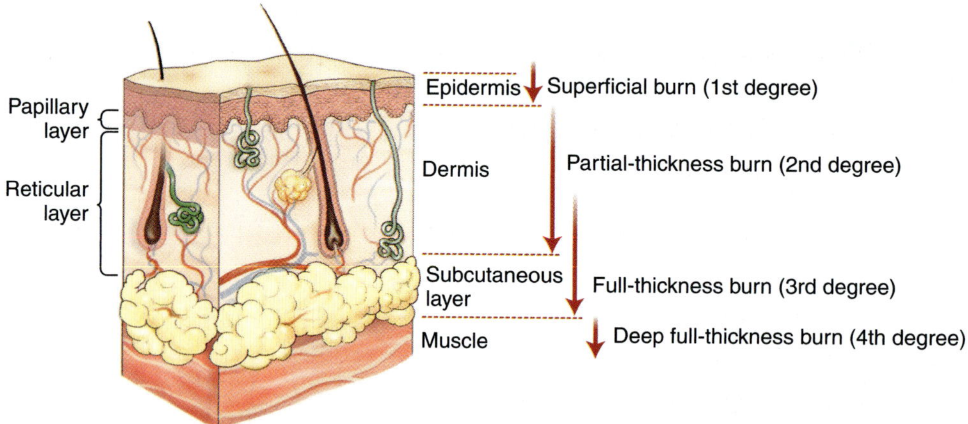

FIGURE 32.16 Burn category tissue involvement. (From Shiland B: *Mastering healthcare terminology*, ed 5, St. Louis, 2016, Elsevier.)

TABLE 32.1 Treatment of Burns

	FIRST-DEGREE BURN	SECOND-DEGREE BURN	THIRD- AND FOURTH-DEGREE BURNS[a]
Treatment, nondrug	• Cool to cold water to immerse the affected area	Rinse burned skin with cool water until the pain stops, 10–30 minutes; additional cool compresses as needed • Do not break open blisters • Bandage the area if blisters are broken to prevent infection • Wrap area loosely; do not put pressure on the area • If the burn is on an arm or a leg, keep the area raised to reduce swelling	• Cover the affected area with sterile gauze or a clean cloth, depending on the size of the burn, until medical help arrives • Do not open blisters or remove clothing stuck to the burned area • Elevate body part if possible
Treatment, medications	• Analgesics for pain	• Analgesics for pain	• Pain medications consistent with pain needs; analgesics, opioids • Antibiotics
Surgical intervention	• None	• None	• Will often require skin grafts to close the wound and heal the affected area; plastic surgery and muscle/bone surgical restoration may be required; if bone and muscle are destroyed, amputation of affected areas may be necessary and prosthetics may be required
Other treatments	Topical over-the-counter burn cream, aloe vera gel used to promote healing and limit scarring	Depending on the severity of the burn and tissue damage, the following services may be needed: • Physical therapy • Occupational therapy • Pain management • Counseling to deal with emotional issues during and after recovery	
Follow-up treatments	Seek medical attention if area looks infected or is not healing	Seek medical attention *immediately* if blistered area looks infected or is not healing	Ongoing depending on the extent of tissue damage

[a]This category of burn needs immediate and ongoing medical attention.

The extent of the injury is determined by visual examination and the history of the exposure. Treatment consists of warming the area with immersion in warm water (100°F to 106°F [38°C to 41° C]). The affected site should never be rubbed because this increases cellular destruction. The person's vital signs should be monitored, and the provider's orders should be followed explicitly.

TABLE 32.2 Additional Diseases and Disorders of the Integumentary System

DISEASE/DISORDER	DESCRIPTION
Albinism	Complete lack of melanin production by existing melanocytes, resulting in pale skin, white hair, and pink iris of the eye.
Callus	Common painless thickening of the stratum corneum at locations of external pressure or friction.
Candidiasis	Yeast infection in moist, creased areas of the skin (armpits, inner thighs, underneath pendulous breasts) and mucous membranes; also called *moniliasis.*
Decubitus ulcers	Also called *bedsore* or *pressure ulcer.* Injuries to the skin and underlying tissue from prolonged pressure to the skin. Most common on skin that covers bony areas of the body, such as heels, ankles, hips, tailbone, elbows, and shoulders.
Hyperhidrosis	Excessive perspiration. Possible causes include hyperthyroidism, menopause, hot temperatures, emotional situations, and infection.
Hypertrichosis	Also known as *hirsutism.* Abnormally hairy.
Kaposi sarcoma (KS)	A rare reddish purple skin cancer. Seen frequently in patients with acquired immunodeficiency syndrome (AIDS) and other immunocompromised conditions. Causative agent is human herpes virus-8 (HHV8).
Scleroderma	An autoimmune disease. Local condition affects the skin. Systemic condition also affects internal organs. Demonstrates a chronic hardening and contraction of the skin or connective tissue. (See Chapter 33 for additional information on autoimmune diseases.)
Systemic lupus erythematosus (SLE)	An autoimmune disease. Can affect many systems or organs of the body, including skin, joints, kidneys, brain, lungs, and heart. (See Chapter 33 for additional information on autoimmune diseases.)
Urticaria	Also called *hives.* May be caused by an allergic reaction to specific foods or personal care products. Raised, round, red welts on the skin. Accompanied by intense itching.
Vitiligo	An autoimmune disease. Skin appears to have random areas with little or no pigment. Unknown etiology (Figure 32.20).

Additional Diseases and Disorders of the Integumentary System

We have covered some of the more common diseases and disorders of the integumentary system, but there are many others. Table 32.2 lists additional diseases and disorders, along with a brief description.

CARCINOMAS OF THE SKIN

Skin cancer is the abnormal, **malignant** growth of skin cells. Skin that is exposed to the sun is at higher risk for developing skin cancer, but skin cancer can also occur on skin not ordinarily exposed to sunlight.

There are three major types of skin cancer:

- Basal cell carcinoma
- Squamous cell carcinoma
- Melanoma, often called *malignant melanoma*

Skin cancer starts with mutations that occur in the DNA of skin cells. The mutations cause the cells to grow out of control and form cancer cells. Skin cancer begins in the epidermis.

Skin cancer can happen in three different types of cells in the epidermis:

- *Squamous cells* lie just below the outer surface of the skin.
- *Basal cells* produce new skin cells and are located beneath the squamous cells.
- *Melanocytes* produce melanin, the pigment that gives skin its normal color. They are located in the lower part of the epidermis.

These cancers are thought to be caused by exposure to UV rays of the sun. UV rays can damage DNA in the skin's cells, which starts a mutation. However, not all cancers develop in areas of the body exposed to the sun; it is still unknown what other specific factors influence the start of a malignant mutation. Additional risk factors for skin cancer include fair skin with blond or red hair, light-colored eyes, and skin that freckles or sunburns easily; a history of sunburns that have blistered; moles that look irregular and are generally larger than normal moles; and a family history of skin cancer (if one parent or a sibling has had skin cancer, there may be an increased risk of the disease).

Basal Cell Carcinoma

Basal cell carcinoma most frequently appears on sun-exposed areas (Figure 32.17) and may appear as follows:

- A pearly or waxy bump
- A flat, flesh-colored or brown scarlike lesion

Squamous Cell Carcinoma

Squamous cell carcinoma most frequently appears on sun-exposed areas (Figure 32.18) and may appear as follows:

- A firm, red nodule
- A flat lesion with a scaly, crusted surface

Melanoma

Melanoma can develop anywhere on the body (Figure 32.19). It can start in normal-looking skin or an existing mole. Skin that has not been exposed to sunlight can still develop melanoma. Melanoma can affect people of any skin color. People with darker skin can develop

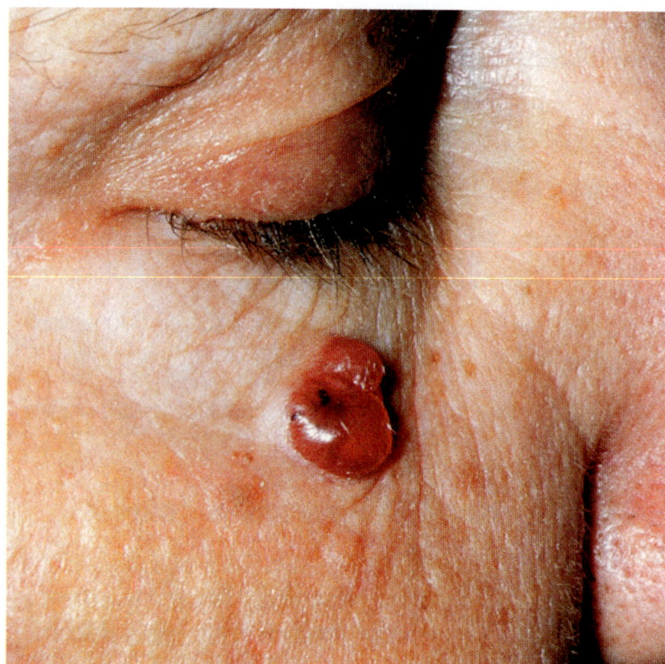

FIGURE 32.17 Basal cell carcinoma. (From James WD, et al: *Andrews' diseases of the skin*, ed 11, Philadelphia, 2011, Saunders.)

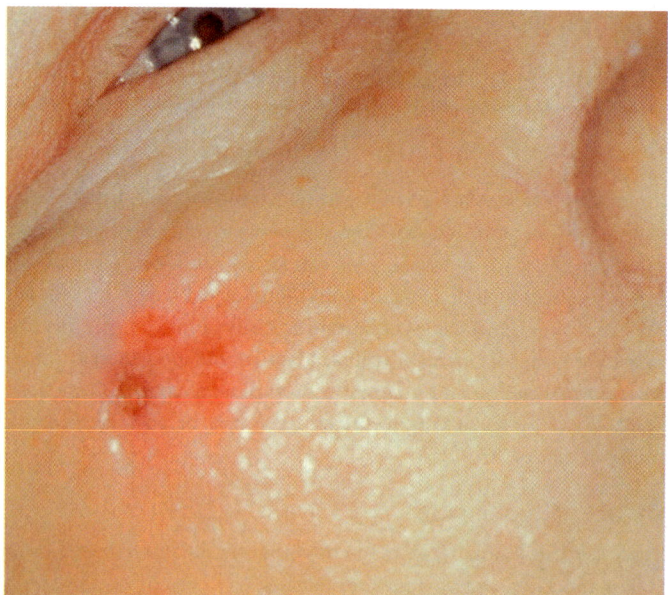

FIGURE 32.18 Squamous cell carcinoma. (From Pfenninger JL, Fowler GC: *Pfenninger and Fowler's procedures for primary care*, ed 3, Philadelphia, 2011, Saunders.)

melanoma on the palms of their hands or the soles of their feet, or even under fingernails or toenails. Melanoma may appear as follows:

- A large brownish spot with darker speckles
- A mole that changes in color, size, or feel or that bleeds
- A small lesion with an irregular border and portions that appear red, white, blue, or blue-black
- Dark lesions on the palms of the hands, soles of the feet, fingertips, or toes

To diagnose any type of skin cancer, the provider will do the following:

- Examine the skin and look for changes that are likely to be skin cancer.

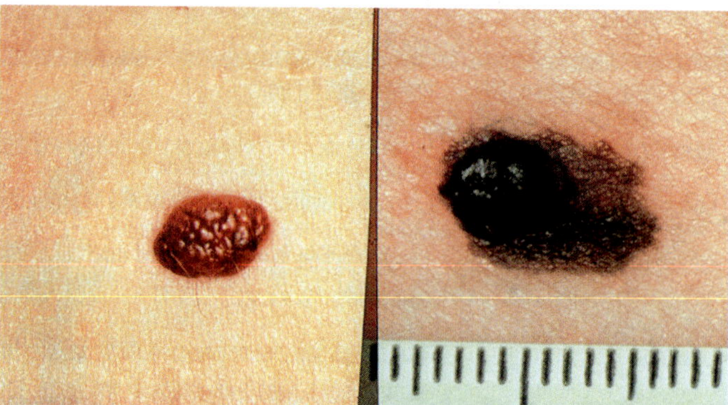

FIGURE 32.19 Pigmented skin lesions. *Left,* Benign pigmented nevus (mole). *Right,* Malignant melanoma. (Courtesy National Cancer Institute, Bethesda, MD.)

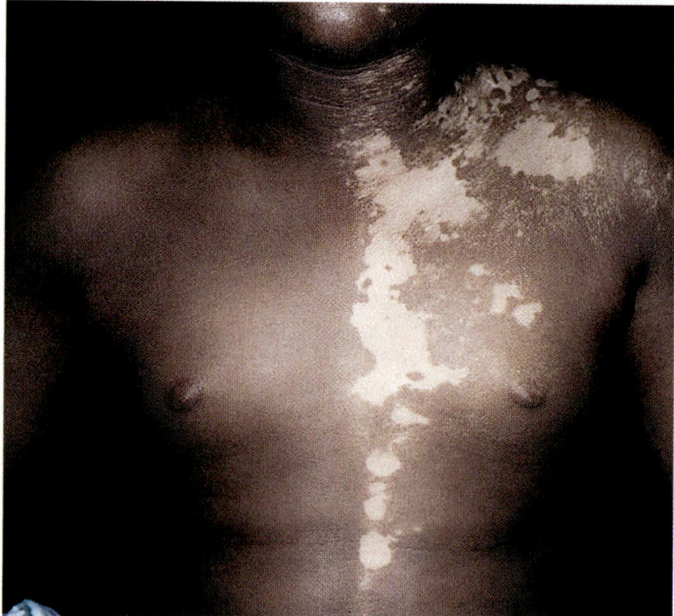

FIGURE 32.20 Vitiligo. (From Shiland B: *Mastering healthcare terminology*, ed 5, St. Louis, 2016, Elsevier.)

- If abnormal areas of the skin are found, a skin biopsy will be performed. A biopsy will determine whether skin cancer is present and what type of cancer it is.
- Additional tests may be done to determine the extent or stage of the skin cancer. These tests might include the following:
  - Imaging tests to examine nearby lymph nodes for signs of cancer.
  - Removal of a nearby lymph node that will be tested for signs of cancer and staged; a skin cancer's stage helps determine which treatment options will be most effective.

Treatment for skin cancer varies greatly, depending on the type of skin cancer and its stage. Early detection and treatment are always the best options for any type of skin cancer, but that is not always possible.

Common treatments for basal cell and squamous cell carcinomas include the following:

- Mohs micrographic surgery
- Excisional surgery
- Topical medications and photodynamic therapy (PDT)
- Electrosurgery, cryosurgery, or laser surgery

Treatment for melanoma varies greatly, depending on the location and stage of the cancer. Treatment ranges from minor localized surgery to major surgery, radiation, and chemotherapy.

CRITICAL THINKING APPLICATION 32.4

After Jean Burke and Casey go over the proposed treatment plan, Jean takes out a brochure on skin cancer. She shows the brochure to Casey and reminds her of how important her skin is. Even though Casey is young, precautions taken now could help prevent skin cancer in her future. List five preventive measures that she can take now in order to protect her skin from cancer. Share with the class.

THE MEDICAL ASSISTANT'S ROLE IN EXAMINATIONS, DIAGNOSTIC PROCEDURES, AND TREATMENTS

The integumentary system can reflect both internal and external reactions, disease processes. The skin holds information about the body's circulation, nutritional status, and signs of systemic diseases. It also acts as a mirror, reflecting aging changes that occur in all organs of the body. For many people, self-esteem is linked to a youthful appearance, and dermatologic conditions may be very threatening to feelings of self-worth. As you prepare patients for a dermatologic examination, allow them to express their anxieties. The conditions that most frequently bring a patient to the dermatologist's office are cosmetic disfigurements caused by a skin disease, pain and pruritus, and interference with sensations or movements.

Assisting with the Examination

During a dermatologic examination, the provider inspects the entire body, beginning with the scalp and continuing to the soles, including the genital area. Inspection of the skin is followed by a detailed examination of suspicious areas through palpation, diascopy, and special tests. A *diascope* is a glass plate held firmly against the skin to permit observation of changes produced in underlying areas when pressure is applied. Inspection may include using a magnifying lens and a bright light to closely examine a suspicious lesion or growth. Dermatologists frequently ask medical assistants to take photographs of moles or to document specific measurements and locations of suspicious lesions. These are placed in the health record for comparison when the patient returns for follow-up visits.

In the physical examination, concerns about the integumentary system include abnormal colorings, such as cyanosis, pallor, vitiligo, erythema, **leukoderma**, or excessive brown patches. **Jaundice** may indicate an increase in the level of **bilirubin** in the blood. Lesions, ulcers, and bruises may be the result of pathologic conditions. Localized red or purple discoloration may be caused by vascular neoplasms, birthmarks, or subcutaneous hemorrhages (**petechiae** and **ecchymosis**). Palpation helps confirm the findings of the inspection. Therefore, inspection and palpation are interrelated in confirming the diagnosis of an integumentary system disorder. Palpated findings may include the skin's texture or elasticity or the presence of edema or a neoplasm.

Gowning and draping a patient for a skin examination depends on the area to be examined. Remember to expose the area adequately but also to protect the patient's privacy. Try to make the patient as comfortable as possible and offer support when it is needed.

Assisting with Diagnostic Procedures

The medical assistant is often involved in assisting with diagnostic procedures of the integumentary system. It is important to remain professional during these interactions. The following sections describe the medical assistant's role in helping with those diagnostic procedures.

Tissue Biopsy

Three methods are used to obtain a small piece of tissue for examination under a microscope. In an *excision biopsy,* such as the removal of a mole, the entire lesion may be removed for analysis. A *punch biopsy* involves the removal of a small section from a designated location in the lesion; the center usually is the optimum site. If the lesion is on the surface of the skin (e.g., a mole), this is done with a scalpel-like circular punch instrument (Figure 32.21); in other cases, a large-gauge needle and syringe unit are used to aspirate cells and fluid from a suspicious area (e.g., a breast biopsy). A *shave biopsy* is performed with a scalpel or razor by cutting or shaving off the growth or lesion for a thin specimen of the combined epidermis and upper dermis cells. This method is used to biopsy a possible squamous cell carcinoma lesion. The medical assistant may help the provider perform these biopsy procedures.

The medical assistant should follow these steps to assist with a tissue biopsy:

1. Assemble the necessary supplies for the procedure.
2. Prepare the patient with proper gowning, draping, and positioning, and make sure the patient understands the procedure.

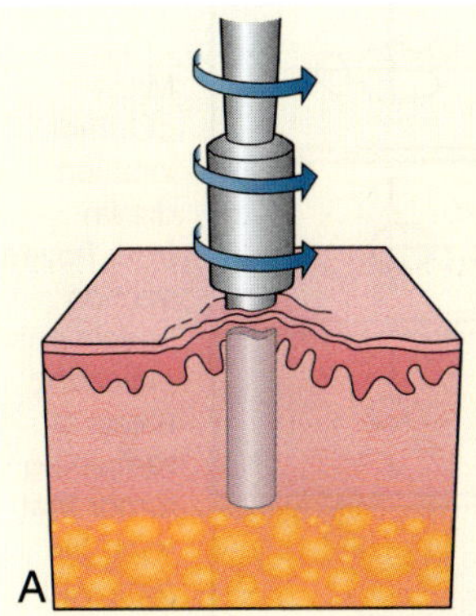

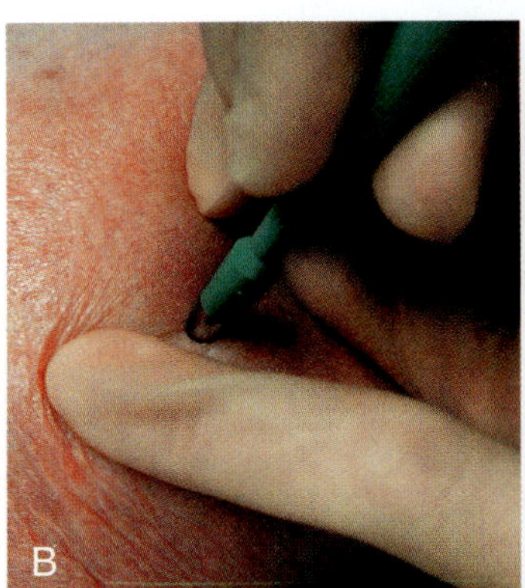

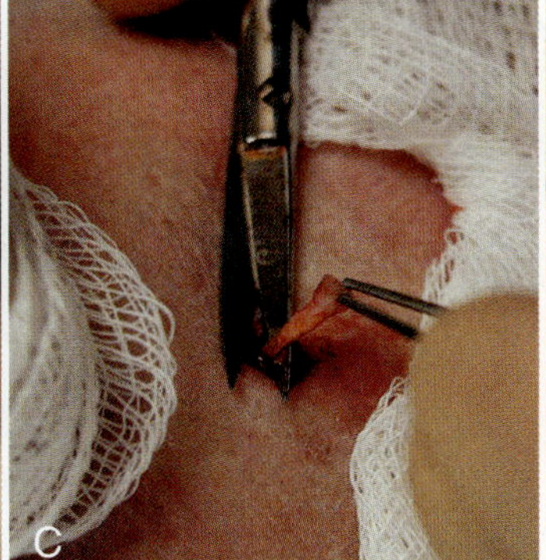

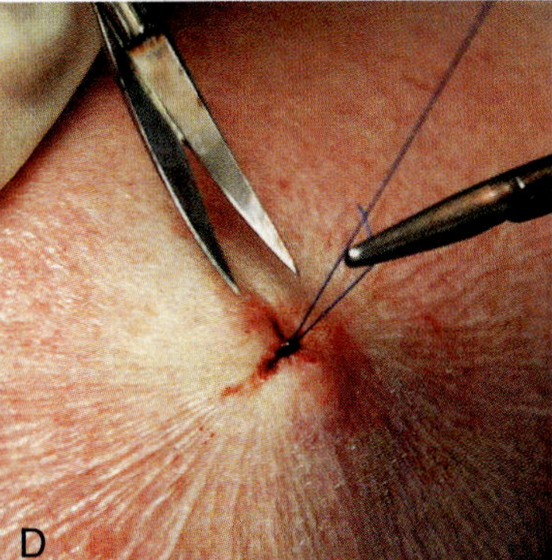

FIGURE 32.21 **(A)** Punch biopsy. **(B)** Punch biopsy instrument rotated into the skin. **(C)** Cutting the base of the specimen. **(D)** Closure of the biopsy wound with a simple epidermal stitch. (Modified from Bolognia J: *Dermatology*, ed 2, Edinburgh, 2008, Mosby.)

3. Confirm that the provider has obtained the patient's informed consent.
4. Prepare the site of the biopsy according to office protocol.
5. Assist the provider as needed, using appropriate personal protective equipment according to Standard Precautions.
6. Label the sample container and prepare it for transport to the testing laboratory. Remember to include laboratory request forms.
7. Clean the procedure area, properly dispose of all waste materials, and disinfect and sterilize equipment used in the procedure.
8. Sanitize your hands and document the procedure, including the patient education provided on biopsy site care.

Assisting with Treatments

When working in dermatology, the medical assistant is often involved in assisting with the treatment of various integumentary conditions. The following sections discuss that role.

Burns

The treatment of burns will vary depending on the severity of the burn. Burns can be treated with medications, along with nonsurgical and surgical interventions. First-degree burns can be treated by immersing the affected area in cool to cold water and providing analgesics for pain. Topical OTC burn cream or aloe vera gel can be used to promote healing and limit scarring. Second-degree burns can be rinsed with cool water until the pain stops (10 to 30 minutes), and then additional cool compresses can be applied as needed. It is important to leave blisters intact. If a blister breaks open, the area should be bandaged to prevent infection. Elevating the limb can help to reduce the swelling. The same OTC creams suggested for first-degree burns can be used for second-degree burns. Both first- and second-degree burns can be treated at home, but the patient should seek medical attention if the area looks infected or is not healing. Third- and fourth-degree burns need immediate and ongoing medical attention. The area should be covered with sterile gauze or a clean cloth until medical intervention is obtained. Clothing stuck to the burned area should not be removed except by medical personnel. Pain medications may be prescribed, including analgesics or opioids. Antibiotics also will likely be prescribed. Third- and fourth-degree burns will often require skin grafts to close the wound. Treatment for these burns is an ongoing process.

Mohs Surgery

Mohs surgery is done to remove skin cancer lesions. The procedure involves repeated removal and microscopic examination of the layers of a lesion until no cancerous cells are seen (Figure 32.22). As with any surgical procedure, sterile technique must be maintained.

Psoralen Plus Ultraviolet A (PUVA) Therapy

A psoralen topical medication plus ultraviolet A (PUVA) therapy is used to treat a number of different skin diseases and is commonly used for psoriasis. The psoralen lotion or gel is applied to the affected area for 10 minutes to treat small areas before exposure to UVA.

Appearance Modification Procedures

The medical assistant may also provide help in procedures that can modify a patient's appearance.

Chemical Peel (Chemoexfoliation). Topical agents are used in chemical peels to minimize or remove minor skin features, such as acne scars, hyperpigmentation, and fine wrinkles. Agents used for chemical peels include tretinoin cream with 0.05% to 0.1% concentration (Retin-A) and a number of different acidic preparations. During

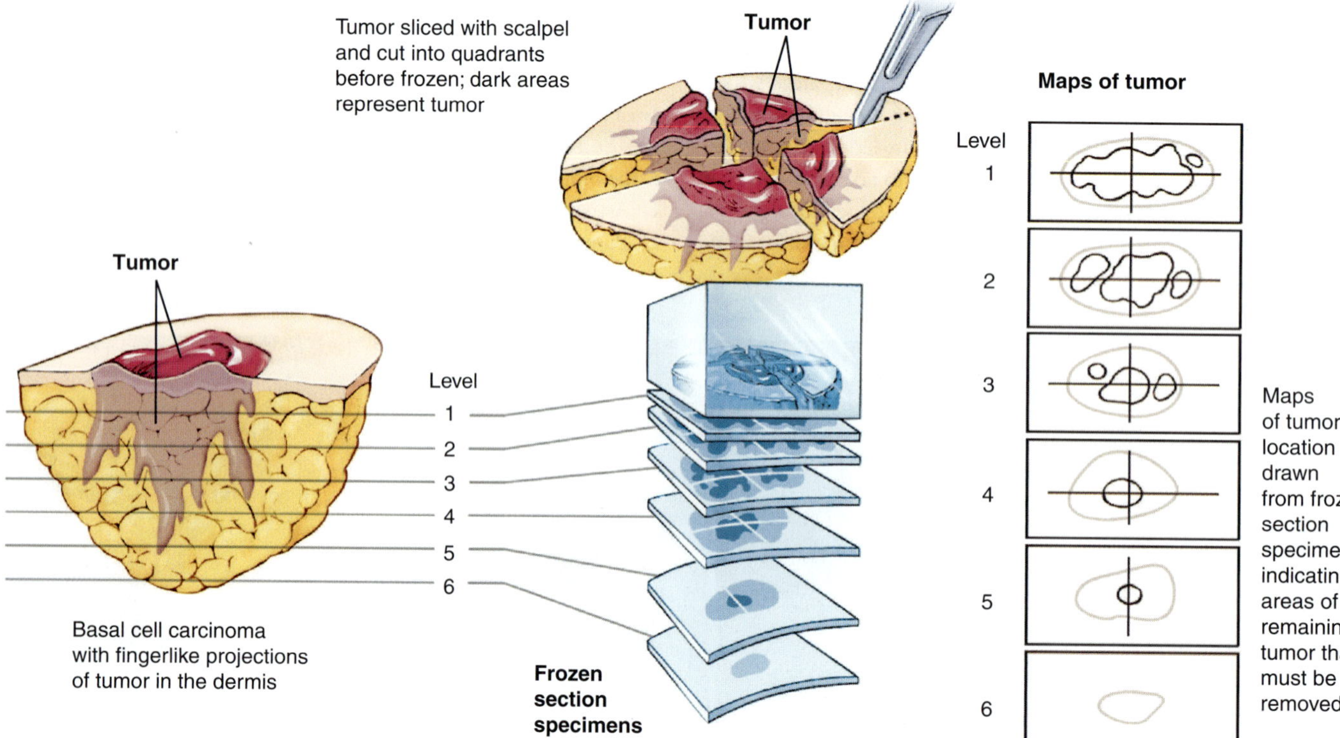

FIGURE 32.22 Mohs surgery. (From Shiland B: *Mastering healthcare terminology*, ed 5, St. Louis, 2016, Elsevier.)

application, care must be taken to prevent the solution from entering the eyes. The use of chemical exfoliating agents may cause the skin to appear inflamed and dry, with crusting and edema. The patient may complain of stinging and burning at the beginning of the treatment regimen. The patient should avoid sun exposure for the length of treatment and should use a sunscreen with a minimum SPF of 15 because photophobia (light sensitivity) is a typical side effect of treatment.

Dermabrasion. A dermabrader is a handheld device that mechanically evens the layers of dermal tissue. It is effective in the treatment of scars from acne vulgaris. Topical anesthetics (e.g., ethyl chloride) or locally injected anesthetics are used for the procedure. Besides the dermabrader, the dermatologist may use a variety of wire brushes, abrasive discs, or other devices to smooth scar tissue. Standard Precautions must be followed, including the use of face and eye guards, to prevent aerosol or splatter contamination from the site. The patient should be educated about wound care, signs of infection, and the presence of photophobia for 6 to 12 months after the procedure.

Laser Resurfacing (Photothermolysis). Laser therapy may be used to address fine lines and wrinkles, pigmented areas, shallow scars, and tattoo removal. Typically, the patient is instructed to prepare the site 3 to 6 weeks before the procedure with tretinoin (Retin-A), alpha-hydroxy solutions, or bleaches. Laser procedures are performed with the patient under local, regional, or general anesthesia. During the procedure, it is extremely important the patient and all personnel wear the type of eye protection recommended by the laser manufacturer. After the procedure, cool packs are applied to help reduce swelling, and topical antibiotic ointment is used to prevent infection. The treated area appears inflamed and edematous and can take up to 2 weeks to heal; it can take as long as 6 months for the inflammation to fade.

Botox Injections. Botox is a strong neurotoxin (a substance toxic to nerves) produced by *Clostridium botulinum,* a bacterium that causes food poisoning. Two strains of the botulism bacterium are used in dermatologic procedures for appearance modification. Botox treatments involve injection of the substance around the eyes, mouth, and forehead. The toxin interferes with nerve stimulation, which temporarily paralyzes the muscles of the face that cause wrinkles to form. It also smooths out the skin and makes it look younger and fresher. The effects are short term, so treatments must be repeated every 3 to 4 months, and some patients complain of an inability to show facial expression because of muscle paralysis.

CLOSING COMMENTS

Patient Coaching

When working with dermatology patients, it is important to make them aware of the possible risks of skin cancer. The American Cancer Society has developed the acronym ABCDE to evaluate moles, birthmarks, or any skin changes. This is a great tool for patients. Any of these warning signs should be reported to the provider immediately. Early detection and self-examination are crucial to cancer survival.

- **A**symmetry: one area of the mole is changing
- **B**orders: moles are becoming irregular
- **C**olors: changes or uneven pigmentation
- **D**iameter: increasing size more than 6 mm or one-fourth of an inch
- **E**levation: a mole that once was flat against the skin is now raised and elevated.

Legal and Ethical Issues

While working in dermatology, you will hear many patients express concern about skin disorders. Allow patients to express their concerns. Use therapeutic listening techniques but be careful when offering encouragement about the course and outcome of treatment. The improvement made with the treatment of a skin disorder may be slow and gradual. Keep encouragement on a positive level. Help the patient recognize small improvements, but remember that it is the provider's role to explain potential treatment outcomes. Making promises about outcomes could lead to a lawsuit.

Patient-Centered Care

The medical assistant must develop the ability to interact therapeutically with patients, families, co-workers, and other members of the healthcare team. When interacting with patients in a dermatology practice, the medical assistant needs to be especially sensitive to the patient's nonverbal behaviors and emotions. Many of the conditions seen in a dermatology practice affect how patients look and view themselves. Sensitivity to the importance of appearance, especially when skin conditions or treatments might alter a patient's appearance, is a crucial trait for healthcare professionals working in a dermatology practice.

Professional Behaviors

Patients with dermatologic issues are often embarrassed by the appearance or location of those issues. As a medical assistant working in dermatology, it is important to remain professional. To help put patients at ease, be sure to protect their privacy by using proper draping techniques to expose only the necessary areas and keep the exposure time to a minimum. Maintaining a calm and empathetic demeanor will help your patient feel more comfortable discussing and revealing the problem areas.

SUMMARY OF SCENARIO

Casey is back at WMFM Clinic for her follow-up visit. In the past 2 months, she has followed the treatment plan and is happy to show Mai and Jean Burke the improvements that have taken place. Her acne has improved greatly. She is pleased with the results and glad that she decided to visit WMFM Clinic about her skin issues. Casey also thanks Mai and Jean for being understanding on her first visit. How did Mai and Jean help Casey on her first visit? List three things that they did to help make Casey's experience positive.

SUMMARY OF LEARNING OBJECTIVES

1. **Examine the anatomy of the integumentary system.**
   The skin is made up of three layers: the epidermis, which is the thin, uppermost layer; the dermis, the thicker layer beneath, which makes up approximately 90% of the skin mass; and the subcutaneous layer, which consists primarily of fatty or adipose tissue.
2. **Examine the functions of the integumentary system.**
   The five functions of the integumentary system are protection, sensory organ activity, temperature regulation, excretion, and synthesis of vitamin D.
3. **Analyze the life span changes that occur in the integumentary system.**
   The most common skin disorders seen in children include impetigo, acne, seborrheic dermatitis, cellulitis, and pediculosis. Accidental burns are also a common occurrence in this age group.

   With older patients, disorders related to cornification are some of the most common skin disorders seen. For patients who are bedridden, pressure ulcers are also common. Skin cancers often develop in this age group due to having had a longer time exposed to the sun.
4. **Examine the diseases and disorders of the integumentary system, including the signs, symptoms, etiology, diagnostic procedures, and treatments.**
   Figure 32.2 shows different types of skin lesions. The diagnosis of skin lesions is based on the color, elevation, and texture of the lesion, whether pruritus, excoriation, pain, or drainage is present, and whether the lesion is a primary or secondary growth.

   Integumentary system infections include bacterial infections, such as impetigo, acne vulgaris, furuncles, carbuncles, and cellulitis; fungal infections, including a variety of tinea growths; viral infections, which cause warts and herpes simplex; and scabies or lice infestations.

   Inflammatory and autoimmune integumentary system disorders include a variety of seborrheic dermatitis inflammations, contact dermatitis, eczema, and the autoimmune disorders psoriasis, systemic lupus erythematosus, and scleroderma.

   Burns are classified as superficial, partial-thickness, or full-thickness wounds, depending on the depth of the wound. The most important concern in the treatment of burns is the prevention of infection. Cold injuries usually are less severe than burns, but prolonged exposure can result in infection, gangrene, amputation, and death.
5. **Examine carcinomas of the integumentary system, including the signs, symptoms, diagnostic procedures, and treatments.**
   Three cancerous lesions of the skin can occur: basal cell carcinoma, which is very slow growing and the most frequently seen form of skin cancer; squamous cell carcinoma, which grows rapidly and is more serious because it has a tendency to metastasize; and melanomas, which are pigmented lesions that are asymmetric, have irregular borders, and usually are larger than 6 mm. Treatment depends on the type of lesion, the level of invasion, and the location. The provider may surgically remove the tumor or may destroy it with cryosurgery, electrodesiccation, laser treatment, the application of chemotherapeutic agents, or Mohs surgery.

   The ABCDE rule includes examination of the site for any of the following: *a*symmetry, irregular *b*order, *c*hange in color, increase in *d*iameter, and *e*levation. If a mole displays any of these characteristics, a dermatologist should check it immediately.
6. **Examine the medical assistant's role in assisting with examinations, diagnostic procedures, and treatments for integumentary system conditions.**
   During a dermatologic examination, the dermatologist frequently asks the medical assistant to take photographs of moles or to document specific measurements and locations of suspicious lesions.

   Dermatologic procedures that can be performed in ambulatory care practices include performing a biopsy or procedure to remove a cancerous area and appearance modification procedures, including chemical peels, dermabrasion, laser resurfacing, and Botox injections.

ALLERGY AND INFECTIOUS DISEASE

33

SCENARIO

Julia Shaw, a certified medical assistant (CMA) who has met the requirements of the American Association of Medical Assistants (AAMA), is working at Walden-Martin Family Medical (WMFM) Clinic. She is working with Dr. Angela Perez today. Julia enjoys the family practice setting and likes the variety that she sees each day in terms of the patients' ages and medical conditions. Today, Dr. Perez and Julia will see a patient who is new to the clinic. The rest of their appointments are with existing patients. Each day is different. Each day is busy. Each day brings patients who need help and encouragement. Julia is a people person. Helping patients is Julia's passion.

While studying this chapter, think about the following questions:

- What are the structures related to the immune and lymphatic systems? What are the functions of the lymphatic and immune systems?
- What are the common pathologic conditions of the immune and lymphatic systems? What medical terms must you know in order to identify and explain these patient disorders?
- What diagnostic and treatment procedures are typically ordered for patients with immune and lymphatic disease?
- What are the medical assistant's primary responsibilities for working with patients with immune and lymphatic problems?
- What clinical skills are required in this specialty practice?

LEARNING OBJECTIVES

1. Examine the anatomy of the immune and lymphatic systems.
2. Examine the physiology of the immune and lymphatic systems.
3. Analyze the life span changes that occur in the immune and lymphatic systems.
4. Examine the diseases and disorders of the immune system.
5. Examine the diseases and disorders of the lymphatic system.
6. Examine the medical assistant's role in examinations, diagnostic procedures, and treatments for the immune and lymphatic systems.

VOCABULARY

antibody A protein substance produced in the blood or tissues in response to a specific antigen that destroys or weakens the antigen. Part of the immune system.

antigen A substance that stimulates the production of an antibody when introduced into the body. Antigens include toxins, bacteria, viruses, and other foreign substances.

cytoplasm The cell substance that fills the area between the nucleus and the cell membrane. It contains the organelles of the cell.

debris (duh BREE) The remains of anything broken down or destroyed; ruins, rubble.

differentiate (dif uh REN shee ayt) To distinguish one thing from another. To make a distinction between items.

enzymes (EN ziemz) Special proteins that speed up a chemical reaction in the body.

homeostasis (hoh mee uh STAY sis) The internal environment of the body that is compatible with life. A steady state that is created by all the body systems working together to provide a consistent and unvarying internal environment.

inflammation (in fluh MAY shuhn) A pathology characterized by redness, swelling, pain, tenderness, heat, and disturbed function of an area of the body. Especially a reaction of tissues to injury.

intact (in TAKT) Complete or whole. Not altered; unbroken.

lymph (limf) A clear, yellowish fluid containing white blood cells in a liquid similar to plasma. The fluid comes from the tissues of the body and is moved through the lymphatic vessels and the bloodstream.

lymphocyte (LIM fuh site) A type of white blood cell that has a large, round nucleus that is surrounded by a thin layer of agranular cytoplasm.

macrophages (MACK roh fay jehs) Large white blood cells that live in the tissues. They engulf foreign particles, microorganisms, and cell debris.

microbiome (mIE kroh BIE ohm) The total collection of microorganisms and their genetic material present on or in the human body or a specific site in the human body.

microorganisms Any living organisms of microscopic size. Examples include bacteria, protozoa, fungi, parasites, and helminths. Some definitions include viruses, which are not alive.

VOCABULARY—*continued*

monocyte (MON uh site) An agranulocyte that engulfs foreign particles, microorganisms, and cell debris.

pandemic A disease that is prevalent throughout an entire country, continent, or the whole world.

pathogens (PATH uh jehns) Disease-causing organisms.

permeable (PUR mee ah buhl) A substance or structure that can be passed through, especially by liquids or gases.

Peyer patches (PAYH urh PACH ehz) Small masses of lymphatic tissue found mostly in the ileum of the small intestine. They are an important part of the immune system because they monitor intestinal bacteria populations and prevent the growth of pathogenic bacteria in the intestines.

reflexes Movements or processes caused by a reflex response; a reflex is an automatic response that does not require thought.

replication The production of exact copies of a complex molecule, such as DNA.

stem cells Undifferentiated cells that can become specialized cells in the body.

vasoconstriction (vas oh kuhn STRIK shuhn) A contraction of muscles that causes narrowing of the inside tube of a vessel.

viability (vie a BIL ih tee) The ability to live.

INTRODUCTION

When working with allergies and infectious diseases it is important to be familiar with the lymphatic and immune systems. They are two different systems; however, they cooperate and work together to maintain **homeostasis**. They also defend the body from foreign pathogens, which can cause infectious diseases. The cells, tissues, and organs of the lymphatic and immune systems are almost the same. But the two systems help the body in very different ways. The lymphatic system can be described as mostly structural. It is the physical component of the two systems. The immune system can be described as mostly functional. The cells of the immune system work to keep the body safe from **pathogens**. These two systems together make up an amazingly complex and efficient means of maintaining the body's health.

The lymphatic system is responsible for a number of functions with the help of the immune system. Lymphatic functions include cleansing the cellular environment, returning proteins and tissue fluids to the blood, providing a pathway for the absorption of fats into the bloodstream, and defending the body against disease.

Immunology is the healthcare specialty that deals with many immune- and lymphatic-related diseases and disorders. An *immunologist* is a specialist involved in the diagnosis, treatment, and prevention of disorders of the immune and lymphatic systems.

Other healthcare specialists who work with the diseases and disorders of the lymphatic and immune systems are cardiologists, otolaryngologists, allergists, rheumatologists, endocrinologists, pulmonologists, and nephrologists.

ANATOMY OF THE IMMUNE AND LYMPHATIC SYSTEMS

The immune and lymphatic systems are composed of many structures that allow these two systems to function and protect the body. The immune system involves white blood cells to help protect against pathogens. The following sections discuss the anatomy and physiology of the immune and lymphatic systems.

Anatomy of the Immune System

Two very important cells in the immune system, **monocytes** and **lymphocytes**, pass from the bloodstream through the blood capillary walls into the spaces between the cells in body tissue. When they pass into the lymph that surrounds cells, they perform their protective functions. Monocytes are in the blood, but once they are in the lymph, they are called **macrophages**. These cells destroy pathogens and collect **debris** from damaged cells. Lymphocytes are much more complicated. They are essential to the immune response, so they are discussed in a later section of this chapter.

Cells of the Immune System

The *immune system* is composed of organs, tissues, cells, and chemical messengers. The components of the immune system interact to protect the body from external invaders and the body's own internally altered cells. The chemical messengers are *cytokines*. They are secreted by cells of the immune system that direct immune cellular interactions. Most of the cells involved in the lymphatic and immune systems are white blood cells (WBCs). A quick review of white blood cells may help in the discussion of the immune system.

Granular White Blood Cells. The three types of granular WBCs are *neutrophils*, *eosinophils*, and *basophils*. They are characterized by their heavily granulated **cytoplasm** and segmented nuclei. Neutrophils are aggressively *phagocytic*—that is, they engulf and destroy invading pathogens. Eosinophils are involved in allergies. Basophils play a part in inflammation.

Unlike red blood cells (RBCs), WBCs are found in both the bloodstream and the tissues. During **inflammation**, the blood carries neutrophils through blood vessels to the site of injury. Capillary walls become more **permeable**, and the granular cells squeeze through to the site of infection. Once at the site of infection or injury, the neutrophils engulf the invading microorganism. The collection of WBCs, dead WBCs, bacteria, and tissue cells creates *pus* at the site of infection.

CRITICAL THINKING APPLICATION 33.1

Julia needs to change a dressing on a patient's infected wound today. Robert Harrison has an abrasion that became infected. It is red and a little swollen, and there is pus at the margins of the wound.

What is pus? Write down a definition in your own words, and be ready to share it with the class.

Agranular White Blood Cells. The two types of agranular leukocytes are *monocytes* and *lymphocytes*. They have a clear cytoplasm (no granules) and a solid nucleus. Monocytes are large and become *macrophages* when they enter tissues. Macrophages are also aggressively phagocytic cells that engulf pathogens and debris. Lymphocytes are small cells that have a big job! They are responsible for much of the work in specific immunity. Lymphocytes are further classified into T lymphocytes and B lymphocytes, depending on their function in the immune response. B lymphocytes and T lymphocytes do not look different. But they function differently. B and T lymphocytes are also called *B cells* and *T cells*.

Anatomy of Lymph System

Lymph, or interstitial fluid, flows through the lymphatic system (Figure 33.1), which is composed of these structures:

- Lymph vessels, lymph nodes, lymph glands, and lymphoid tissue
- Lymph organs: the tonsils, adenoids, vermiform appendix, spleen, thymus gland, and **Peyer patches**

Lymph moves in one direction. This prevents pathogens from flowing through the entire body. The system filters out the **microorganisms** as the lymph passes through various capillaries, vessels, and nodes.

PHYSIOLOGY OF THE IMMUNE AND LYMPHATIC SYSTEMS

The best way to understand the immune system is to learn about the body's various levels of defense. The goal of foreign pathogens is to enter the body, reproduce, and damage healthy tissue. The immune system's primary function is to **differentiate** what is "self" from what is "foreign" and then destroy anything that is foreign. The immune system wants to stop pathogens from causing harm. Figure 33.2 illustrates the levels of defense in the immune system. The two outside circles represent *nonspecific immunity* (also known as *innate immunity*) and its two levels of defense. The inner circle represents the various mechanisms of *specific immunity* (also known as *adaptive immunity*). These can be natural or acquired. Most pathogens can be contained by the first two lines of nonspecific defense. However, some pathogens get past nonspecific defenses. These pathogens are met with the third line of defense, or specific immunity.

Nonspecific Immunity

The term *nonspecific immunity* refers to the many ways the body protects itself from pathogens without having to "recognize" them. The first line of defense in nonspecific immunity consists of the following methods of protection.

- *Physical:* Examples include **intact** skin and mucous membranes. These are physical barriers to pathogens. The skin protects the inside of the body from the outside environment. The sticky mucous membranes at many body openings trap pathogens.
- **Reflexes**: Examples include coughing, sneezing, vomiting, and diarrhea. These actions help get rid of pathogens by forcing them back out of the body.

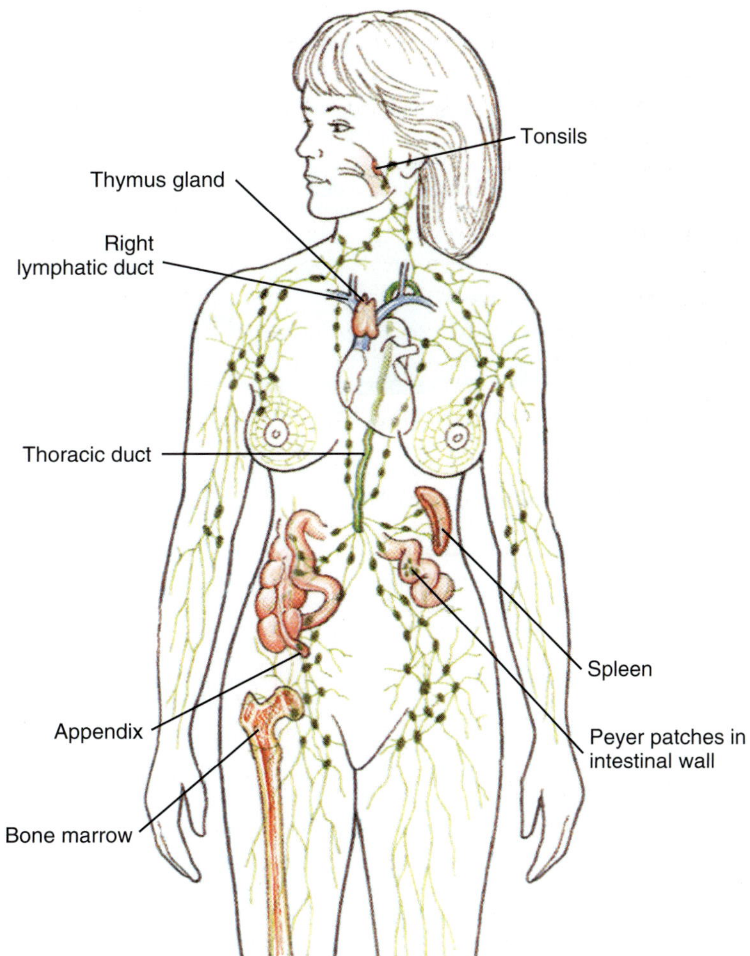

FIGURE 33.1 Organs of the lymphatic and immune systems. (From Shiland B: *Mastering healthcare terminology*, ed 5, St. Louis, 2015, Elsevier.)

- *Chemical:* Examples include tears, saliva, and perspiration. These have a slightly acidic pH, which discourages pathogens from entering the body. All these fluids also help wash the pathogens away. In addition, stomach acids and **enzymes** try to kill pathogens.

CRITICAL THINKING APPLICATION 33.2

What are the three methods of protection in the first line of defense? Write all three down, and briefly describe each one in your own words. Share your answers with your classmates.

The second line of defense in nonspecific immunity goes to work if the pathogens make it past the first line of defense. The second line of defense uses cellular and chemical responses to destroy the pathogen. The following are the protective measures of the second line of defense:

- *Phagocytosis*: The process of cells engulfing and destroying invaders. Pathogens that make it past the first line of defense and enter the bloodstream may be consumed by neutrophils, monocytes, or macrophages.
- *Inflammation*: A protective response to irritation or injury. Signs and symptoms of inflammation include heat, swelling, redness, and pain. This process causes immediate **vasoconstriction**, followed by an increase in vascular permeability. These conditions provide a good environment for healing. If caused by a pathogen, the inflammation is called an *infection.*
- *Pyrexia*: The medical term for fever. When an infection is present, fever helps protect the infected area. Fever increases the action of phagocytes and reduces the **viability** of certain pathogens. Most pathogens love normal body temperature, so when a fever is present, the environment gets too hot, and they cannot function as they should.
- *Protective proteins* are part of the second line of defense. These include *interferons*, which disrupt viral **replication** and limit a virus's ability to damage cells. *Complement* is a group of proteins made in the liver that is involved in blood clotting and blood **antigen-antibody** interactions. Complement proteins are inactive in the blood until they encounter bacteria. Meeting bacteria activates complement, enabling it to *lyse* (destroy) the organisms.
- *Natural killer* (NK) cells are the last cell type involved in the second line of defense. They are derived from **stem cells** in the bone marrow, concentrated in the liver and lungs, and involved in nonspecific immunity and inflammation. NK cells are also capable of destroying targeted cells, such as tumor cells and virus-infected cells. They are *not* phagocytic cells. This special kind of lymphocyte acts nonspecifically to kill cells that have been infected by certain viruses and cancer cells.

Figure 33.3 presents an overview of nonspecific immunity.

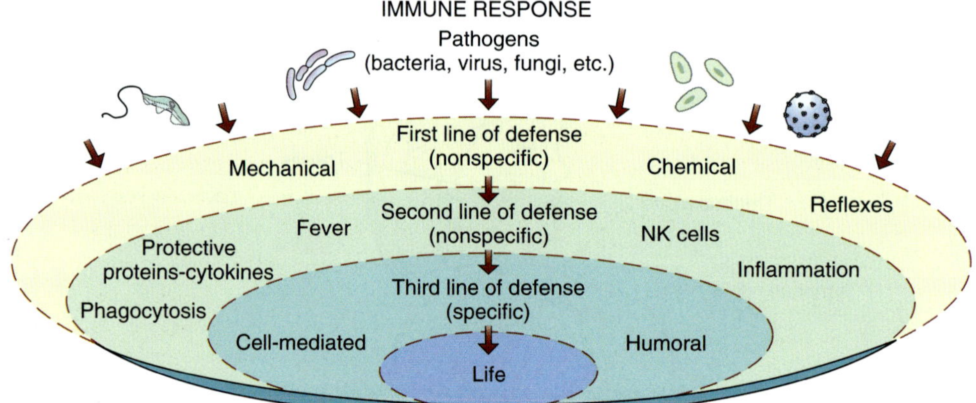

FIGURE 33.2 Immune system levels of defense. (From Shiland B: *Mastering healthcare terminology*, ed 5, St. Louis, 2015, Elsevier.)

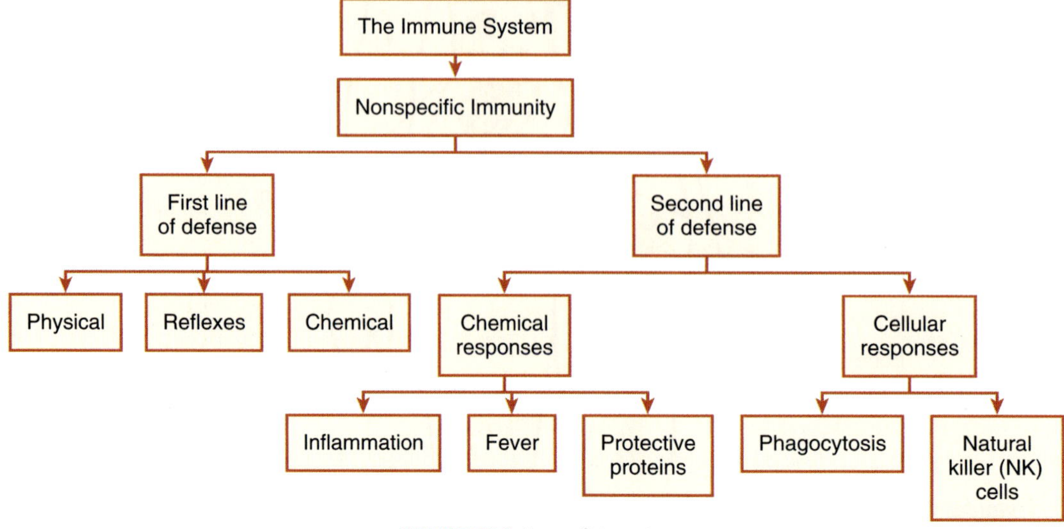

FIGURE 33.3 Nonspecific immunity.

CRITICAL THINKING APPLICATION **33.3**

Review the second line of defense in nonspecific immunity. What are the five different chemical or cellular responses discussed in this text? Briefly describe each of the five protective measures. Can you name the characteristic signs and symptoms of inflammation? Write down your answers and share them with the class.

Specific Immunity

Specific immunity is different from nonspecific immunity in several ways:

- Specific immunity means that the immune response is generated against one specific antigen. The response will not be effective against any other antigens.
- Specific immunity counts on the immune cells to identify antigens and recognize them if they encounter them again. An antigen can be an infectious agent from outside the body (*exogenous*), or it can be a malignant or tumor cell inside the body (*endogenous*). Both types of antigens are foreign, something that is not normal to the immune system.
- Specific immunity prepares a specific response (antibody production) to that unique antigen.
- Specific immunity intensifies with repeated challenges by the same antigen. When the body encounters a known antigen, it can respond more efficiently and react to the antigen quickly.
- Specific immunity may be either genetic or acquired. Genetic immunity is an inherited ability to resist certain diseases because of one's species, race, gender, or individual genetic makeup.

Antibodies belong to a group of proteins called *immunoglobulins* (Igs). There are five distinct classes of immunoglobulins: IgG, IgM, IgE, IgA, and IgD. Each class of immunoglobulin responds to different types of immune challenges, or antigens.

Specific immunity has two different methods of destroying pathogens: humoral immunity and cell-mediated immunity.

Humoral Immunity

Humoral immunity, also known as *antibody-mediated immunity*, involves the production of antibodies. B cells are formed from stem cells in the bone marrow. They then migrate to lymph organs (e.g., lymph nodes, spleen), where they multiply and live. B cells are the most important cell in humoral immunity, but T cells and macrophages are also involved in the process. When an antibody combines with an antigen, an antibody-antigen complex is formed.

Antibodies are protein molecules that specifically attach to antigens. They can neutralize toxins or destroy viruses directly. They can combine with larger antigens (e.g., bacteria) to form antibody-antigen complexes. These complexes signal neutrophils to come and destroy them. Neutrophils engulf the complexes and destroy the antigen.

Antibodies can protect the body in many ways. They circulate in the plasma and are present in secretions (i.e., tears, saliva, colostrum), ready to attach to unsuspecting antigens. However, there is one thing antibodies are unable to do—they cannot enter a cell. That can be a problem because sometimes antigens go inside host cells. When that happens, antibodies cannot destroy the antigen. This is when cell-mediated immunity takes over.

Cell-Mediated Immunity

T cells are formed from stem cells in bone marrow. They then migrate to the thymus, where they mature and learn their role in the immune system. They are the most important cell in cell-mediated immunity. T cells do *not* produce antibodies, but they can help antibodies do their job. T cells are very effective against intracellular pathogens (antigens). When an antigen enters a cell, T cells help expose the antigen so that antibodies can destroy it. There are different types of T cells that have different roles in cell-mediated immunity.

Different Types of T Cells

Four main types of T cells work in specific immunity. Look at the following list and see how important T cells are to immunity in general.

1. *T helper cells* (T_H), also known as $CD4^+$ T cells. They help in B-cell activation and activation of cytotoxic T cells.
2. *Cytotoxic T cells* (T_C), also known as $CD8^+$ cells. They destroy virus-infected cells and tumor cells. They also can cause damage to or rejection of organ transplants. In addition, they can cause autoimmune diseases.
3. *Memory T cells* rapidly proliferate if the body is reexposed to the antigen.
4. *Regulatory T cells* (T_{reg}), also known as *suppressor T cells*. They help shut down the immune response when the antigen has been destroyed.

Cell-mediated immunity is particularly well suited to destroying viruses. Viruses must be inside a host cell to reproduce. Cytotoxic T cells destroy a virus once it gets inside a cell. Cell-mediated immunity helps stop the spread of viral infections within the body. Another job of cell-mediated immunity is to recognize and destroy cancer cells or tumor cells. Even though these cells are part of a person's body, they are not normal. They have changed and are now harming the body. Cell-mediated immunity recognizes malignant changes in cells. It works to destroy them before they cause disease (cancer) or tumors.

Figure 33.4 presents an overview of specific immunity.

Types of Acquired Immunity

Immunity is one way our body protects us from infectious diseases. Acquired immunity is classified as active or passive. *Active immunity* requires the body to respond to an antigen and produce antibodies for protection. *Passive immunity* does not require the body to do anything. In passive immunity, premade antibodies are given to a person. This occurs through transmission from the mother to the fetus or infant or through an injection of immune globulin. The immune system is not required to make anything.

Active immunity and passive immunity are each categorized as natural immunity or artificial immunity. All four types of acquired immunity describe ways the body has acquired antibodies to specific diseases. Figure 33.5 helps to explain acquired immunity.

CRITICAL THINKING APPLICATION **33.4**

T cells provide a very important function in the immune system. List two ways that T cells help to protect the body from foreign antigens. Share your thoughts with the class.

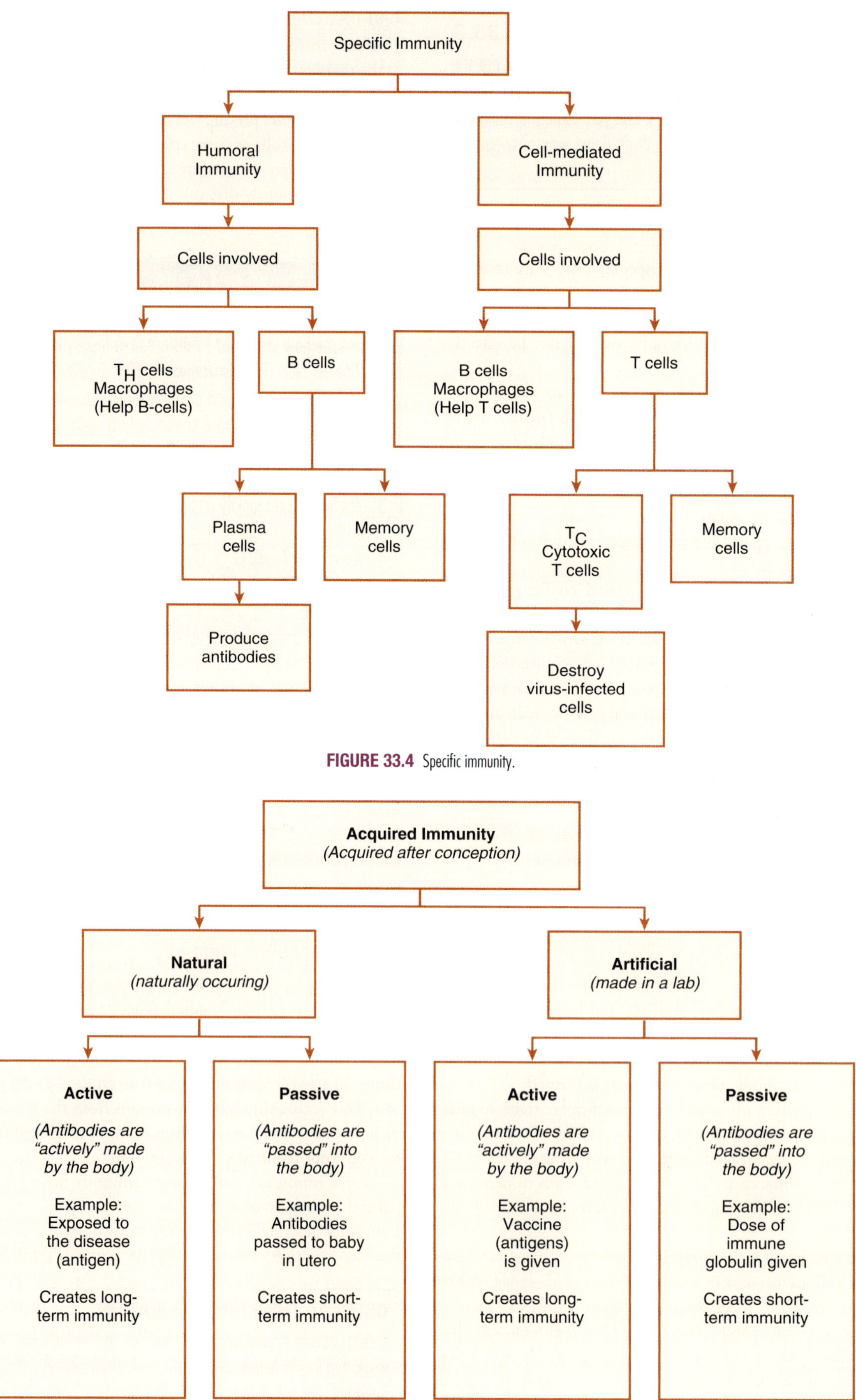

FIGURE 33.4 Specific immunity.

FIGURE 33.5 Acquired immunity.

Allergies

The immune system is quite remarkable. When it works well, it keeps our bodies from harm. When it doesn't work properly, the immune system can harm the body. *Allergies* are an example of the immune system overreacting. Allergies are also known as hypersensitivity reactions.

Hypersensitivity is defined as an immune response that causes tissue damage in the host. It is an excessive response to a stimulus or foreign agent. A hypersensitivity reaction does not occur the first time an antigen is encountered. It is when the person encounters the antigen for a second or subsequent exposure that the reaction develops.

An allergic reaction is a type I hypersensitivity reaction (Table 33.1). It is the body responding to an allergic trigger called an *allergen*. Allergens are harmless environmental substances, but in an allergic reaction, the body overreacts to their presence.

When the body responds to an allergen, immune cells release *histamines, kinins,* and other inflammatory substances. This causes the characteristic allergy symptoms: runny nose, watery eyes, and possibly a rash or hives. Sometimes drugs called *antihistamines* are used to alleviate allergy symptoms.

If an allergic reaction is severe, it can cause a dangerous condition called *anaphylactic shock* (see Chapter 27). This can be a life-threatening condition. People who know they are highly allergic to a substance should carry an EpiPen to treat an anaphylactic reaction.

To learn more about the specific emergency care that should be provided during an anaphylactic reaction, see Chapter 27.

TABLE 33.1 Hypersensitivity Reactions

TYPE	REACTIONS	EXAMPLES
Type I—immediate hypersensitivity; also called an *allergic reaction*	Reactions may be local (runny nose, itching eyes). Reactions can also be systemic (swelling of the airway and tongue). Anaphylaxis is the systemic form of immediate hypersensitivity. It can be fatal.	Food allergies, insect venom allergies (bee and wasp stings), latex allergies
Type II	Antibodies to cell surface antigens are produced.	Hemolytic disease of the newborn (HDN), blood bank transfusion reactions
Type III	Antibody-antigen complexes are deposited in tissues of the body.	Organ damage with systemic lupus erythematosus (SLE), glomerulonephritis, rheumatic fever, rheumatoid arthritis
Type IV, also known as delayed hypersensitivity	Allergic reaction appears 24 to 48 hours after exposure to an antigen.	Poison ivy rash, tuberculosis (TB) skin tests, organ transplant rejection

CRITICAL THINKING APPLICATION 33.5

- What type of hypersensitivity is hemolytic disease of the newborn (HDN)?
- What type of hypersensitivity is anaphylaxis?
- What type of hypersensitivity is delayed hypersensitivity?

CRITICAL THINKING APPLICATION 33.6

Rich and Jan Dallman have an appointment to see Dr. Perez today. They both want to get the shingles vaccine. Julia prepares their vaccinations and then sits down with Rich and Jan to go over the Vaccine Information Statement (VIS), which discusses the vaccine. What type of immunity is a vaccination, active or passive?

LIFE SPAN CHANGES

As we age, there are changes that can occur with both the immune system and the lymphatic system. Some of those changes are discussed in the following sections.

Changes in Children

Some antibodies are passed from mother to baby, which provides some protection when they are born. More antibodies are passed to the baby through colostrum and breast milk. These passively acquired antibodies will protect for a short time. It will take some time for the immune and lymphatic systems to fully develop. Babies produce their own antibodies when they are exposed to a pathogen, whether by having the disease or getting a vaccination.

Childhood disorders of the lymphatic and immune systems include the following:

- Hypersensitivities or allergies to foods, pollen, or pet dander
- Childhood leukemias or lymphomas
- The development of autoimmune disease in late adolescence

Changes in Adults

As we age, there is a reduction in the production of the B and T cells in the bone marrow and thymus. There is also a diminished function of the mature lymphocytes in the lymph tissue. This results in a lesser response to challenges to the immune system than when we were younger.

Unlike children, adults and seniors will have a host of diagnoses from this chapter in their health records. Autoimmune diseases are most common in young adulthood to middle age. Cancers of these systems also appear in significant numbers. Non-Hodgkin's lymphoma and acute myelogenous leukemia (AML) account for thousands of hospitalizations every year. Multiple myeloma is most frequently diagnosed after age 60.

DISEASES AND DISORDERS OF THE IMMUNE SYSTEM

Diseases of the immune system are diverse and have many causes but often have common signs and symptoms such as fatigue, joint pain, swollen joints, low-grade fever, skin changes, and weight loss. Many factors can be associated with immune system diseases, disorders, and infections. These diseases can involve the cells, tissues, and organs of the immune system.

Autoimmune Diseases and Disorders

Recall that the goal of the immune system is to protect the body from foreign pathogens and prevent infectious diseases. The immune system normally can distinguish *self* from *foreign*. However, in autoimmune diseases, something goes wrong in the immune system—it begins to attack healthy *self* cells.

According to the National Institutes of Health website MedlinePlus (https://medlineplus.gov), there are more than 80 different autoimmune diseases. The common factor among all autoimmune diseases is that a person's own immune system attacks healthy tissues. No matter what the symptoms are, the underlying cause of the disease is an immune system that is not working properly.

The cause of autoimmune diseases is a mystery. There are many theories about how the immune system becomes confused. The following is a brief list of suspected causes:

- A viral or bacterial infection that triggers the immune system to attack healthy cells
- Exposure over time to toxins (e.g., chemicals, pesticides, and food additives)
- A weakness in a person's immune system brought on by stress, past infections, and hormone fluctuations
- An imbalance in the intestinal **microbiome**
- Existing allergies (another type of immune system overreaction)

Many scientists think that a combination of all these possible causes influences a person's risk of developing an autoimmune disease. Autoimmune diseases are an area of intense scientific research because more people are being diagnosed with autoimmune conditions. Risk factors for being diagnosed with an autoimmune disease include female gender, especially between the ages of 15 and 45, and African, Hispanic, or Native American race.

Common Autoimmune Diseases

- Rheumatoid arthritis
- Inflammatory bowel disease (IBD)
- Type 1 diabetes mellitus
- Psoriasis
- Myasthenia gravis
- Systemic lupus erythematosus (SLE)
- Multiple sclerosis (MS)
- Guillain-Barré syndrome
- Grave's disease
- Hashimoto's thyroiditis

Autoimmune diseases vary in their signs and symptoms, depending on the cells or tissues affected in the body. Some common signs and symptoms seem to affect a number of different autoimmune conditions. They include skin changes (discolorations, rashes, or lesions), joint pain, fatigue/malaise, low-grade fever, and general ill-feeling. Commonly affected cells or tissues include joints, muscles, skin, blood vessels and red blood cells, connective tissue, and endocrine glands (i.e., thyroid, pancreas).

To diagnose an autoimmune condition, the provider takes a complete history and performs a thorough physical examination. Laboratory and diagnostic testing procedures vary depending on the patient's signs and symptoms. For most suspected autoimmune conditions, some or all of the following laboratory tests may be ordered:

- *Antinuclear antibody test* (ANA): A blood test that looks for the presence of antibodies to the nucleus or the organelles of the nucleus. A serum sample is used for this type of test.
- *Autoantibody test*: A blood/serum test that looks for autoantibodies.
- *Complete blood cell count* (CBC): A blood test. See Chapter 40 and Chapter 49 for more information. Some Clinical Laboratory Improvement Amendments (CLIA)-waived tests are available.
- *Comprehensive metabolic panel* (CMP): A blood test. See Chapter 40 and Chapter 49 for more information. Some CLIA-waived tests are available.
- *C-reactive protein* (CRP): A blood test that measures CRP. CRP is elevated in people with inflammation. Some CLIA-waived tests are available.
- *Erythrocyte sedimentation rate* (ESR): A whole blood test. People with inflammation have elevated values. Some CLIA-waived tests are available.
- *Urinalysis*: See Chapter 47 for more information. Some CLIA-waived tests are available.

Imaging tests, such as joint and bone x-rays, magnetic resonance imaging (MRI), and ultrasound scans, in addition to tissue biopsies, may be ordered. Information on each of these procedures can be found in Chapter 18.

Treatments will vary depending on the signs and symptoms of the condition. However, common goals of treatment for most autoimmune conditions include diminishing the signs and symptoms of the condition and/or reducing their occurrence, controlling the autoimmune process, and maintaining the body's ability to fight disease and infections.

Treatments may include physical therapy, blood transfusions (if the condition affects blood cells), a modified diet (to reduce inflammation and boost the immune system with nutrient-dense foods), stress reduction, adequate sleep, regular exercise, and smoking cessation.

Medications may include nonsteroidal anti-inflammatory drugs (NSAIDs) (e.g., ibuprofen), corticosteroids, supplementation to replace substances lacking in the body (examples include thyroid hormones, insulin, vitamin B_{12}, and vitamin D), and immunosuppressive drugs to reduce the body's immune response (examples include prednisone, cyclosporine [Neoral], and adalimumab [Humira]).

Some alternative therapies that may bring symptom relief include yoga, massage therapy, and relaxation therapy. Special diets may also be used to help reduce inflammation or remove specific types of proteins from the diet (e.g., gluten-free diet, grain-free diet, and the elimination of sugar and natural/artificial sweeteners).

Sjogren's Syndrome

Sjogren's syndrome is an autoimmune disorder that affects the glands that make tears and saliva but can also damage other parts of the body, such as the following:

- Joints
- Thyroid
- Kidneys
- Liver
- Lungs
- Skin
- Nerves

The cause of Sjogren's syndrome is unknown. Genetics play a part and can put some people at higher risk, but there is also a triggering mechanism, such as an infection with a particular virus or bacteria. Risk factors include being female, over the age of 40, or having a rheumatic disease like rheumatoid arthritis or systemic lupus erythematosus (SLE).

This disease can be difficult to diagnose as the signs and symptoms are similar to other diseases and can vary from patient to patient. Blood tests will likely be done to look at the levels of the different types of blood cells, presence of antibodies common to Sjogren's syndrome, evidence of inflammatory conditions, and indications of the problems with the liver and kidneys. Eye tests will be done to measure the dryness of the eyes. A biopsy of the lip may be done to detect clusters of inflammatory cells.

There is no cure for Sjogren's syndrome. Treatment is focused on managing the signs and symptoms. The dry eyes and dry mouth may be helped with over-the-counter eyedrops and sipping water more frequently. Some patients may need prescription medications. Patients should not smoke as this can irritate and dry out the mouth. Sugarless gum or citrus-flavored hard candies can stimulate saliva flow.

Systemic Lupus Erythematosus

SLE is another autoimmune disease that can attack many different body systems, including joints, skin, kidneys, blood cells, the brain, and the heart and lungs. SLE is more common in women, can occur at any age, and is more common in African Americans, Hispanics, and Asian Americans.

The cause of SLE is unknown, but, like Sjogren's syndrome, genetics can play a part. Environmental factors seem to provide a trigger for SLE. Potential triggers include sunlight, infections, and certain medications.

The most common signs and symptoms include the following:

- Fatigue
- Fever
- Joint pain, stiffness, and swelling
- Skin lesions that appear or worsen with sun exposure
- Butterfly-shaped rash on the face that covers the cheeks and bridge of the nose; or rashes elsewhere (Figure 33.6)
- Dry eyes
- Shortness of breath
- Chest pain
- Headaches, confusion, and memory loss
- Fingers and toes that turn white or blue when exposed to cold or stress

As with Sjogren's syndrome, diagnosing SLE can be difficult. The signs and symptoms can change over time and overlap with many other disorders. Blood tests will likely include a complete blood count (CBC), an evaluation of the erythrocyte sedimentation rate, kidney and liver assessments, and an antinuclear antibody (ANA) test. A urinalysis is also done.

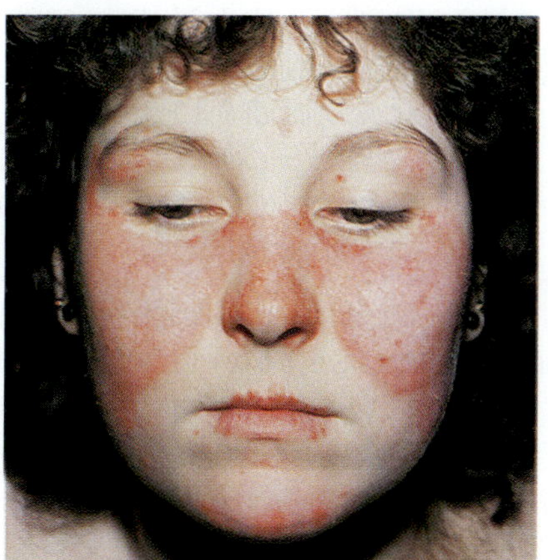

FIGURE 33.6 Systemic lupus erythematosus flare. The classic butterfly rash occurs over the nose and cheek area. (From Habif TP, Campbell JL Jr, Chapman MS, et al: *Skin disease: diagnosis and treatment,* ed 3, St. Louis, 2011, Saunders.)

Treatment of SLE depends on the patient's signs and symptoms. Medications that might be used include nonsteroidal anti-inflammatory drugs (NSAIDs), antimalarial drugs, corticosteroids, immunosuppressants, and biologics.

HIV/AIDS

Acquired immunodeficiency syndrome (AIDS) is a chronic condition caused by the human immunodeficiency virus (HIV). HIV attacks the immune system of its host and specifically damages the $CD4^+$ T lymphocytes (helper T cells). HIV impairs the immune system's ability to fight infectious agents that can cause disease.

Currently, HIV/AIDS can be treated but not cured; without proper and consistent treatment, it is a life-threatening disease. The treatment for HIV/AIDS that is available now slows the progression of the disease and allows a person to live a relatively normal life.

HIV is the causative agent of AIDS. HIV is a bloodborne virus that can be transmitted through sexual contact, through a sharps exposure (e.g., needlestick), or from mother to child during pregnancy or childbirth.

Risk factors for acquiring HIV include having unprotected sex, using intravenous drugs (especially if sharing needles), and having another sexually transmitted infection (STI). Being an uncircumcised man increases your risk of acquiring HIV if any of the other risk factors also exist.

A primary HIV infection occurs when a person is first exposed to the virus. Signs and symptoms of primary HIV include flulike symptoms, swollen lymph nodes (especially in the neck), diarrhea, and weight loss.

After the initial infection with HIV, the virus becomes *latent* (shows no signs or symptoms). During this time, the person will test positive on an HIV blood test, but will not show signs or symptoms of the infection. HIV can remain latent for 18 months to 10 years. If an HIV-positive person is not treated with antiviral drugs, HIV will change from a latent infection to an active one, and it will progress to AIDS.

Signs and symptoms of AIDS include chronic and persistent diarrhea, recurring fevers, night sweats, profound fatigue, weight loss, skin rashes, continual white patches or lesions on the tongue or in the mouth, and repeated opportunistic infections.

Most individuals infected with HIV take about 12 weeks to produce anti-HIV antibodies. The diagnosis of HIV is made by testing a blood sample or a saliva sample for anti-HIV antibodies. Newer generation testing can also detect a protein made by the HIV virus shortly after infection, thus providing a quicker diagnosis. CLIA-waived kits are available for home use, but their results should be confirmed by laboratory tests. Confirmatory tests include the enzyme-linked immunosorbent assay (ELISA) and Western blot testing.

As mentioned, HIV/AIDS currently can be treated but not cured, and without proper and consistent treatment, it is a life-threatening disease. The goal of treatment is to slow the disease progression and allow the person to live a relatively normal life. A regimen of antiviral medications is available to control the virus. There are a number of different drug classes that can be used to control HIV. Most providers recommend using three drugs from at least two different drug classes. This helps to keep the virus from becoming resistant to a single drug. All HIV drugs block the virus from entering the $CD4^+$ T lymphocytes but in different ways.

Infectious Diseases

Infectious diseases are those caused by organisms such as bacteria, viruses, fungi, or parasites. As healthcare professionals, we know that many of our patients seek treatment for infectious diseases of all sorts. The next several sections discuss common infectious diseases.

Viral Hepatitis

Hepatitis is an inflammation of the liver. Inflammation can damage the liver and cause impaired liver function. There are many causes for hepatitis in general, but this material will specifically cover hepatitis that has a viral cause. Viral hepatitis is an infectious disease that, in most cases, can be prevented. Viral hepatitis can be caused by five main viral strains: A, B, C, D, and E. Hepatitis A and hepatitis E are both transmitted primarily through fecal-oral contact. Hepatitis B, hepatitis C, and hepatitis D are transmitted as bloodborne pathogens. Table 33.2 provides detailed information on viral hepatitis.

TABLE 33.2 Viral Hepatitis

	HEPATITIS A (HAV) AND E (HEV)	HEPATITIS B (HBV), C (HCV), AND D (HVD)
Etiology and Risk Factors	• Person-to-person transmission through fecal-oral contamination. • Ingesting something that has been contaminated with the feces of an infected person. Ingesting contaminated food or water. Undercooked foods that are contaminated; examples include raw shellfish, vegetables, and fruits. • Sexual/intimate contact with an infected person.	• Person-to-person transmission through activities that involve *percutaneous* (through the skin) or mucosal contact with infected blood or body fluids (semen, saliva). Sex with an infected partner. Injection drug use that involves sharing needles, syringes, or drug-preparation equipment. Birth to an infected mother. Needlesticks or sharp instrument exposure. • Sharing personal items such as razors or toothbrushes with an infected person.
Signs and symptoms	• Children younger than 6 years are frequently asymptomatic; older children and adults are frequently symptomatic. • If symptoms occur, they can include fever, fatigue, loss of appetite, nausea, vomiting, abdominal pain, dark urine, jaundice, joint pain, and clay-colored feces.	• Children younger than 5 years and newly infected immunosuppressed adults are frequently symptomatic. • Among children older than 5 years, only about 30% to 50% are symptomatic.
Diagnostic Procedures	• A provider will perform a history and physical exam; if there is any indication of hepatitis, blood testing will most likely be done. For hepatitis A, B, C, and D, specific antibody testing is done to confirm the presence and type of hepatitis. • There is no reliable antibody testing for hepatitis E; the history, physical exam, recent travel, and signs and symptoms are used to diagnose hepatitis E.	
Treatment	• Lots of rest. Eat and drink tiny amounts at one time to cope with nausea. Do not drink alcohol, and consult the provider about any existing medications that may affect the liver; this includes over-the-counter medications. • For hepatitis A and E, treatment is generally supportive	• *Hepatitis B or D—acute infection*: treatment is supportive. • *Hepatitis B or D—chronic infection:* antiviral medications to prevent liver damage or liver cancer. • *Hepatitis C—acute infection:* treated aggressively with antiviral medications to minimize the possibility of developing chronic hepatitis C. • *Hepatitis C—chronic infection:* treated with antiviral medications to minimize the possibility of liver damage, cirrhosis, liver cancer, or organ failure.
Comments ***With any type of viral hepatitis, serious complications can occur, including liver failure or death; liver failure requires liver transplantation.***	• Hepatitis E is endemic in areas of Africa, the Middle East, Asia, and Mexico; if pregnant, consult the provider for travel recommendations.	• Hepatitis D is only possible as a co-infection with hepatitis B; if a co-infection occurs, it can develop into a superinfection; a superinfection can cause liver failure and death. To prevent hepatitis D, vaccinate against hepatitis B.

Information summarized from the Centers for Disease Control and Prevention, www.cdc.gov/hepatitis/index.htm.

Sexually Transmitted Infections

STIs can be seen in any individual who is sexually active. Signs and symptoms of STIs can be vague or nondescript. So anyone who is sexually active should be tested for STIs, especially if they have engaged in any high-risk behavior. Tables 33.3 and 33.4 give an overview of commonly encountered STIs. For additional information on STIs, please visit www.cdc.gov/std/default.htm.

Coronavirus 2019 (COVID-19)

COVID-19 was discovered in December of 2019 in Wuhan, China. It quickly became a **pandemic**. It is caused by the SARS-CoV-2 virus and most often causes respiratory symptoms similar to a cold, flu, or pneumonia. This virus can also attack other parts of the body, and it has gone through several mutations. These mutations or variants are still SARS-CoV-2 but may act differently. Some are more contagious, more severe, or resistant to the treatments that have been developed.

The common signs and symptoms include the following:

- Fever or chills
- Cough
- Shortness of breath or difficulty breathing
- New loss of taste or smell
- Sore throat
- Congestion or runny nose
- Fatigue
- Muscle or body aches
- Headache
- Nausea or vomiting
- Diarrhea

Most people have mild symptoms, but some people become very ill. Those most at risk are older adults and those with underlying conditions such as the following:

- Cancer
- Chronic kidney disease
- Chronic liver disease
- Chronic lung disease
- Diabetes (type 1 or type 2)
- Heart conditions
- Immunocompromised state
- Overweight or obesity
- Pregnancy
- Sickle cell disease or thalassemia
- Organ or blood stem cell transplant
- Stroke
- Substance abuse disorders
- Tuberculosis

At the time of writing this there are three vaccines available for COVID-19:

TABLE 33.3 Bacterial/Protozoal Sexually Transmitted Infections

FEATURE	CHLAMYDIA	GONORRHEA	SYPHILIS	TRICHOMONIASIS
Etiology	*Chlamydia trachomatis* (bacterium)	*Neisseria gonorrhoeae* (bacterium)	*Treponema pallidum* (spirochete bacteria)	*Trichomonas vaginalis* (protozoon)
Signs and symptoms—male	• May be asymptomatic • Dysuria • Itching and thin, watery discharge from penis • Testicular pain	• Dysuria and urinary frequency • Thick, cloudy, or bloody discharge from penis	• Painless lesion (chancre) • Serous discharge from chancre • Lymphadenopathy	• Asymptomatic • Itching or irritation inside penis • Burning after urination or ejaculation • Some discharge from penis
Signs and symptoms—female	• Asymptomatic • Dysuria • Urinary frequency • Abdominal pain • Increased vaginal discharge	• Dysuria • Urinary frequency • Abdominal pain • Increased vaginal discharge	• Painless lesion (chancre) • Serous discharge from chancre • Lymphadenopathy	• Asymptomatic • Urinary frequency, urgency • Dysuria • Frothy, yellow-green vaginal discharge • Pruritus
Diagnostic procedures	• Testing a first-catch urine specimen (male) • Collecting swab specimens from the endocervix or vagina (female) • Nucleic acid amplification test (NAAT)	• Urethral swab (male) • Endocervical swab or vaginal swab (female) • Urine specimen (both male and female) • NAAT • Gram stain for symptomatic males	• Rapid plasma regain (RPR), Venereal Disease Research Laboratory (VDRL), fluorescent treponemal antibody absorption (FTA-ABS)	• NAAT • Wet mount preparation of the vaginal discharge examined under a microscope • Culture of discharge • Retest 3 months after treatment
Treatment, medications	Curable with antibiotic therapy; single dose of azithromycin or 1 week of doxycycline	Curable with antibiotic therapy; ceftriaxone, azithromycin, or doxycycline	Penicillin G; if patient is allergic to penicillin, doxycycline or tetracycline	Single dose of metronidazole or tinidazole; partner must be treated

TABLE 33.4 Viral Sexually Transmitted Infections

FEATURE	GENITAL HERPES	GENITAL WARTS	HIV/AIDS
Etiology	Herpes simplex virus-2 (HSV-2)	Human papillomavirus (HPV)	Human immunodeficiency virus (HIV)
Signs and symptoms – male Signs and symptoms – female	Painful genital vesicles and ulcers; erythema and pruritus; tingling or shooting pain 1–2 days before outbreak; cycle through episodes	Elevated papillomas on external genitalia; single or cluster of warts	Flulike symptoms, also referred to as *acute retroviral syndrome* (ARS) or *primary HIV infection:* Fever Swollen glands Sore throat Rash, muscle and joint aches and pains Headache
Diagnostic procedures		Examination and possible biopsy of warts	Enzyme-linked immunosorbent assay (ELISA); if positive, a Western blot test to confirm Saliva test Viral load test
Treatment, medications	No cure, but antiviral therapy during episodes shortens duration of lesions; acyclovir, famciclovir, valacyclovir	Topical medications; podofilox solution, imiquimod cream, cryosurgery, electrocautery	Antiretroviral (ART) medications: non-nucleoside reverse transcriptase inhibitors, nucleoside reverse transcriptase inhibitors, protease inhibitors, fusion inhibitors, integrase inhibitors

	PFIZER-BIONTECH	PFIZER-BIONTECH	MODERNA	MODERNA	JOHNSON & JOHNSON'S JANSSEN
Recommended Age	6 mo - >5 years old	5+ years old	6 mo - 17 years old	18+ years old	18+ years old
Primary Series	3 doses; 1st and 2nd doses 3-8 weeks apart, 3rd dose at least 8 weeks after 2nd dose	2 doses Given 3 weeks apart	2 doses given 4-8 weeks apart	2 doses Given 4 weeks apart	1 dose
Booster Dose	Not authorized	Children ages 5-11; at least 5 months after last dose of primary series. Everyone ages 18 years and older 1st booster at least 5 months after last dose of primary series. Adults ages 50 years and older; 2nd booster at least 4 months after 1st booster	Not authorized	Everyone ages 18 years and older at least 5 months after the last dose of primary series. Adults ages 50 years or older; 2nd booster at least 4 months after 1st booster	Everyone ages 18 years and older 1st booster with Pfizer-BioNTech or Modera at least 2 months after primary dose of Johnson & Johnson Janssen vaccine, 2nd booster of Pfizer-BioNTech or Moderna at least 4 months after 1st booster
Fully Vaccinated	2 weeks after 3rd dose	2 weeks after 2nd dose	2 weeks after 2nd dose	2 weeks after 2nd dose	2 weeks after 1st dose

From the Centers for Disease Control and Prevention, https://www.cdc.gov/coronavirus/2019-ncov/vaccines/stay-up-to-date.html#recommendations.

In October of 2020, the Food and Drug Administration (FDA) approved remdesivir (Veklury), an antiviral drug, to treat COVID-19. This medication modestly improved recovery time for patients with COVID-19 that needed hospitalization. Several other drugs are being developed and tested.

Infectious Mononucleosis

Infectious mononucleosis is also known as mono or the kissing disease. It is commonly acquired as a child or an adolescent. Most children do not show signs and symptoms, or they are very mild. People who acquire the disease in late childhood, adolescence, or young adulthood usually have signs and symptoms. It is generally a mild, self-limiting viral infection, but it can have serious complications, such as hepatosplenomegaly. Mono is passed from person to person via saliva—that's why it can be passed by kissing. It can also be passed by sneezing, coughing, or by sharing eating or drinking utensils.

Although other viruses can cause infectious mononucleosis, the Epstein-Barr virus (EBV), a type of herpes virus, is by far the most common. Most adults have antibodies to EBV by the end of their 20s. A person is considered immune and cannot have mono again once antibodies develop. Although the disease is usually mild, some people can develop complications and may become very sick.

Risk factors for acquiring mono include activities that involve contact with someone who has an active infection—for example, kissing, sharing food and drink, and sharing eating utensils or toothbrushes. EBV has an incubation period of 4 to 6 weeks for adolescents and young adults.

Signs and symptoms of infectious mononucleosis may include fatigue, fever, swollen lymph nodes in the neck and armpits, sore throat, swollen tonsils (may obstruct breathing or cause wheezing), headache, skin rash, swollen upper abdomen, and soft-swollen spleen. Signs and symptoms usually subside within 2 to 4 weeks. Fatigue and enlargement of the lymph nodes and spleen may last 4 to 6 weeks.

Complications of mono may include an enlarged spleen and pain in the left upper abdomen (the spleen could rupture if left untreated), hepatitis, jaundice, anemia, and thrombocytopenia. Rarely, complications may include myocarditis, meningitis, encephalitis, and Guillain-Barré syndrome. Severe complications can occur in someone who is immune compromised, such as a person with HIV/AIDS or on immunosuppressive drugs.

Diagnostic procedures include the history and physical exam (to look for swollen lymph nodes, liver, and spleen; fever; and sore throat); blood tests, including a Monospot to detect antibodies to EBV; and a CBC and differential to look for an elevated WBC count and atypical lymphocytes in the blood (Figure 33.7).

Treatment for mono is supportive care—it is a viral infection. Antibiotics are not necessary and are not useful for viral infections. Lots of rest, fluids (especially water), over-the-counter (OTC) pain- or fever-reducing medications (not aspirin), and a healthy diet are the best treatments for mono. Within 2 to 4 weeks, the virus should run its course, and most people recover completely.

One more important treatment for mono is to limit activities while symptoms remain. Staying away from school or work, getting extra rest,

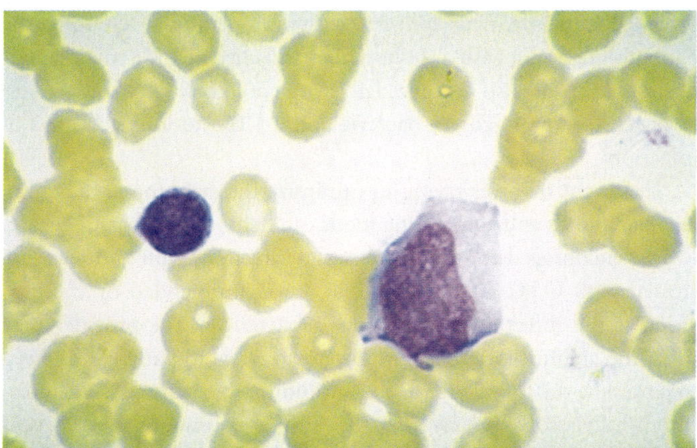

FIGURE 33.7 Atypical lymphocytes. (From Thibodeau GA, Patton KT: *Anatomy and physiology*, ed 7, St. Louis, 2010, Mosby.)

and limiting physical activities and sports are recommended. The provider should give the patient permission to resume a normal schedule.

Treating the complications of infectious mononucleosis may include these measures:

- Sometimes streptococcal throat infections can occur secondary to mono. Antibiotics should be used to treat streptococcal infections.
- If hepatosplenomegaly occurs, the person should seek medical attention. Sometimes corticosteroids are given to reduce the inflammation of the liver and spleen.

DISEASES AND DISORDERS OF THE LYMPHATIC SYSTEM

Diseases of the lymphatic system can appear to be similar to those of the immune system, as these two systems are closely related. The following sections examine the common diseases and disorders of the lymphatic system.

Lymphoma: Hodgkin's and Non-Hodgkin's

Lymphoma is a cancer of the lymphatic and immune systems. Lymphocytes, a type of white blood cell, mutate and reproduce rapidly in lymphoma. The overproduced, diseased lymphocytes crowd out healthy WBCs. This causes the patient to be more susceptible to infections.

There are two main types of lymphoma:

- Hodgkin's lymphoma: Also called *Hodgkin disease.* It is characterized by the presence of Reed-Sternberg cells in the blood. This type of cell is specific to Hodgkin's lymphoma.
- Non-Hodgkin's lymphoma: A collection of all other lymphatic cancers that are not Hodgkin's lymphoma; this is the more common of the two types.

The cause of lymphoma is not well understood or obvious in most cases. There isn't a direct link to any one event, chemical exposure, or genetic mutation that can predict the development of lymphoma. However, some factors may increase a person's risk of developing this type of cancer.

Risk factors for developing Hodgkin's lymphoma include a family history of lymphoma, being 15 to 30 years old or over age 55, being male, and having had an Epstein-Barr (EBV) infection (infectious mononucleosis [mono]).

Risk factors for developing non-Hodgkin's lymphoma include being over age 60; being on immunosuppressive therapy or medications; and having had certain infections, such as EBV, HIV, or *Helicobacter pylori*, which causes stomach and intestinal ulcers.

Signs and symptoms of both Hodgkin's lymphoma and non-Hodgkin's lymphoma include painless swelling of lymph nodes (especially in the neck, armpits, or groin), fatigue, fever, chills, night sweats, and unexplained weight loss. Additional symptoms more common with non-Hodgkin's lymphoma are abdominal swelling or pain, trouble breathing, coughing, or chest pain.

For both types of lymphoma, the diagnostic process is the same. The provider will perform a physical exam, specifically looking for enlarged and nontender lymph nodes, liver, and spleen. Blood and urine tests will be done to rule out other possible disease conditions and infections. Blood tests would likely include a CBC and differential and a CMP. Urinalysis also is likely. Imaging tests may include x-rays, computed tomography (CT), MRI, or positron emission tomography (PET) scans. A lymph node, tissue, or bone marrow biopsy may also be done. The provider can make an accurate diagnosis about the type of lymphoma present and the stage of the disease by using information obtained in a biopsy. Staging cancer is important because it affects the treatment plan the provider will recommend.

Treatment depends on the type and stage of the lymphoma. Not all lymphomas are treated. For instance, some slowly progressing types of non-Hodgkin's lymphoma are monitored and may not be treated. Depending on the type and stage of the lymphoma, treatment may include chemotherapy, radiation therapy, and stem cell transplantation (bone marrow transplantation). A stem cell transplant is used to replace diseased bone marrow with healthy stem cells. Stem cells can then repopulate the bone marrow with healthy cells. Also, biologic drugs may be used to enhance the patient's immune system, helping it to destroy lymphoma cells.

Multiple Myeloma

Multiple myeloma is a cancer of the white blood cells called *plasma cells*. Plasma cells are a type of B lymphocyte that produce antibodies to help fight infection. In multiple myeloma, plasma cells reproduce so much that they crowd out healthy blood cells. The malignant plasma cells don't produce antibodies. Instead, they produce an abnormal protein (M protein) that can cause kidney damage.

This condition is called multiple myeloma because the tumors are found in many or multiple bones. If it occurs in only one bone or area, the tumor is referred to as a plasmacytoma.

The cause of multiple myeloma is unknown, or *idiopathic*. But for most people, multiple myeloma starts as monoclonal gammopathy of undetermined significance (MGUS). People with MGUS also produce M protein, but at such a low level, it does not harm the body. Risk factors for developing multiple myeloma include being over the age of 60, male gender (blacks are more likely to develop multiple myeloma than whites), and a history of MGUS. This makes developing multiple myeloma more likely.

Signs and symptoms of multiple myeloma may be subtle at first. There may be no symptoms at all in the beginning. Noticeable signs and symptoms include bone pain, especially in the spine, chest, or hips; anemia; loss of kidney function; excessive thirst; nausea; loss of appetite; weight loss; constipation; fatigue; frequent infections; weakness or numbness in the legs; and mental confusion.

Tests that may be used to help diagnose multiple myeloma include blood tests, which may include a CBC and differential, tests for the presence of M protein, and a CMP (includes kidney and liver function tests); urinalysis (M proteins in the urine are called *Bence Jones proteins*); a bone marrow biopsy; and examination of cells. Imaging tests may include x-ray, MRI, CT, and PET scans. At diagnosis, multiple myeloma will be staged, and a treatment plan will be based on the staged diagnosis.

Treatment for asymptomatic multiple myeloma, MGUS, may not be needed. The provider will want to watch the condition and run periodic blood and urine tests to monitor signs of activity. Treatment for multiple myeloma includes targeted cancer therapy (designed to target specific weaknesses in myeloma cancer cells to kill the cells), biologic therapy, chemotherapy, radiation therapy, and possibly stem cell transplantation.

Lymphedema

Lymphedema is when there is an accumulation of protein-rich fluid that accumulates in the tissue, causing swelling, usually in the arms or legs. This fluid is usually drained by the lymphatic system. The lymph vessels could be compromised by infection, cancer, scar tissue from radiation therapy, or surgical removal of the lymph nodes.

Signs and symptoms of lymphedema include the following:

- Swelling of all or part of the arm or leg
- A feeling of heaviness or tightness
- Restricted range of motion
- Recurring infections
- Hardening and thickening of the skin (fibrosis)

Diagnosis of lymphedema may be made based on the presenting signs and symptoms if the patient is at risk for developing lymphedema. If that is not the case, an MRI, CT, or ultrasound may be done to see if there are obstructions in the lymphatic system.

There is no cure for lymphedema, and treatment focuses on reducing the swelling. Compression bandages or compression garments may be used to encourage lymph fluid drainage. A sequential pneumatic compression sleeve is connected to a pump that intermittently inflates the sleeve using pressure to help move the lymph fluid away from the fingers and toes. There are several surgical procedures that can help, including lymph node transplants, development of new drainage paths, and removal of fibrous tissue that has become hardened.

Tonsillitis

Tonsillitis is the inflammation of the tonsils found at the back of the throat. Most cases of tonsillitis are caused by common viruses. Bacteria can also cause tonsillitis, with Streptococcus pyogenes (group A Streptococcus) being the most common. These bacteria also cause strep throat.

Signs and symptoms of tonsillitis include these:

- Red, swollen tonsils
- Sore throat
- Difficult or painful swallowing
- Fever
- Enlarged, tender lymph glands in the neck
- White or yellow coating or patches on the tonsils
- Scratchy, muffled or throaty voice
- Bad breath
- Stomachache
- Neck pain or stiff neck
- Headache

The throat, nose, and ears will be examined to look for the infection. Palpating the neck for swollen lymph glands, listening to the patient's breathing with a stethoscope, and checking for enlargement of the spleen will also be done. Lab work could include a throat swab to check for streptococcal bacteria and a CBC to look for signs of infection.

Treatment involves trying to minimize the symptoms. Providing adequate fluids and comforting foods can help soothe the sore throat. Rest is encouraged to help combat the infection. Pain and fever are treated with OTC medications that are recommended by the provider. If the infection is caused by a bacterium, the provider may prescribe an antibiotic. It is important to stress to patients the need to complete the full course of the antibiotics to ensure that the infection is fully resolved. A *tonsillectomy*, surgery to remove the tonsils, is performed when tonsillitis frequently recurs, with chronic tonsillitis, or when bacterial tonsillitis does not respond to antibiotic therapy.

THE MEDICAL ASSISTANT'S ROLE IN EXAMINATION, DIAGNOSTIC PROCEDURES, AND TREATMENTS

As a medical assistant, you may be involved in assisting with examination, diagnostic procedures, and treatments. Having an understanding of what is required of you during those processes will help you provide the best possible care for your patients and become the best assistant for your provider. The following sections describe the medical assistant's role.

Assisting with the Examination and Diagnostic Procedures

When working with patients who have infectious diseases, it is important to protect yourself and other patients in the healthcare facility. A patient who has made an appointment to be seen for a cough or other respiratory issue may be asked to put on a mask when checking in for the appointment. This will help to protect the other patients in the reception area. Hand sanitizer is often available in the reception area so that patients can use it after they have sneezed, coughed, or wiped their noses.

Many healthcare facilities will also have the medical assistant wear a mask when working with patients with potentially infectious diseases, especially respiratory infections. A simple explanation that you are wearing the mask as a precaution will help to make the patient feel more comfortable with the situation.

Preparing a patient for an infectious disease examination includes having the patient disrobe appropriately, depending on which body system is involved. For allergy testing, the patient usually must disrobe to the waist, and the gown is open in the back.

An important part of any examination is taking a health history. When working with a patient who has a potential infectious disease, the medical assistant should gather the history of the present illness (HPI) information and review the past medical history (PMH).

When working with a patient with potential allergies, it is important to ask what the reaction to the allergen was. The reaction can indicate whether the patient has an allergy or a sensitivity. With a true allergy, there is an immune system response that can affect many organs in the body (e.g., difficulty breathing or hives). Allergies can be severe or even life threatening. With a *sensitivity,* there is no immune system response, but there is an exaggeration of a normal side effect. This could range from digestive issues to neurologic issues. Figure 33.8 is an example of how allergies would be documented in the electronic health record. Table 33.5 lists common allergens.

Assisting with Diagnostic Procedures

The medical assistant is often involved in assisting with diagnostic procedures of the immune system. It is important to remain professional during these interactions. The following sections describe the medical assistant's role in assisting with those diagnostic procedures.

Testing for Allergies. Skin testing to detect allergies requires a percutaneous application or intradermal injection of a small amount of antigen (or groups of antigens) and later examination of the test sites for a visible reaction. The larger the localized skin reaction, the more profound the patient's allergic response to the tested allergen.

A percutaneous, or scratch, test may be performed on the forearm, upper arm, or back. The back is favored in young children because of the large area of skin available. It also is easier to immobilize the

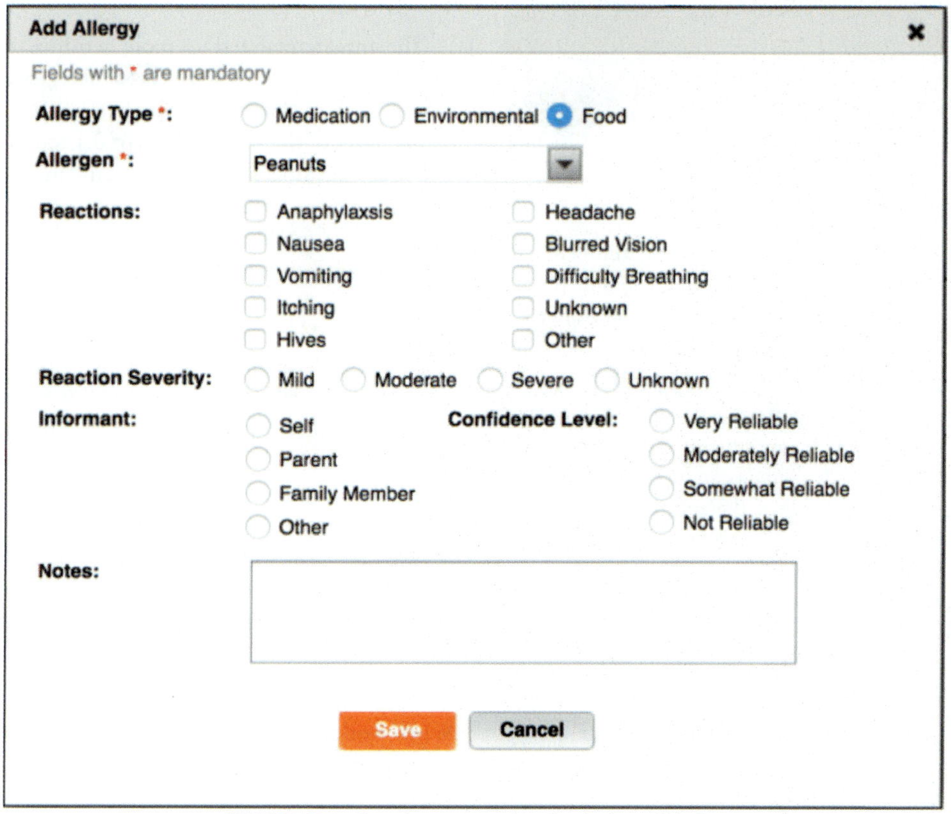

Add Allergy ×

Fields with * are mandatory

Allergy Type *: Medication | Environmental | Food (selected)

Allergen *: Peanuts

Reactions: Anaphylaxsis, Nausea, Vomiting, Itching, Hives, Headache, Blurred Vision, Difficulty Breathing, Unknown, Other

Reaction Severity: Mild | Moderate | Severe | Unknown

Informant: Self, Parent, Family Member, Other

Confidence Level: Very Reliable, Moderately Reliable, Somewhat Reliable, Not Reliable

Notes:

Save | Cancel

FIGURE 33.8 Allergy documentation in SimChart for the Medical Office.

TABLE 33.5 Common Medication, Environmental, and Food Allergens

MEDICATION	ENVIRONMENTAL	FOOD
Penicillin and related antibiotics	Dust mites	Eggs
Sulfonamides (antibiotics)	Pollen	Peanuts
Anticonvulsants	Pet dander	Tree nuts
Nonsteroidal anti-inflammatory drugs (NSAIDS)	Mold	Wheat
Chemotherapy drugs	Cigarette smoke	Shellfish

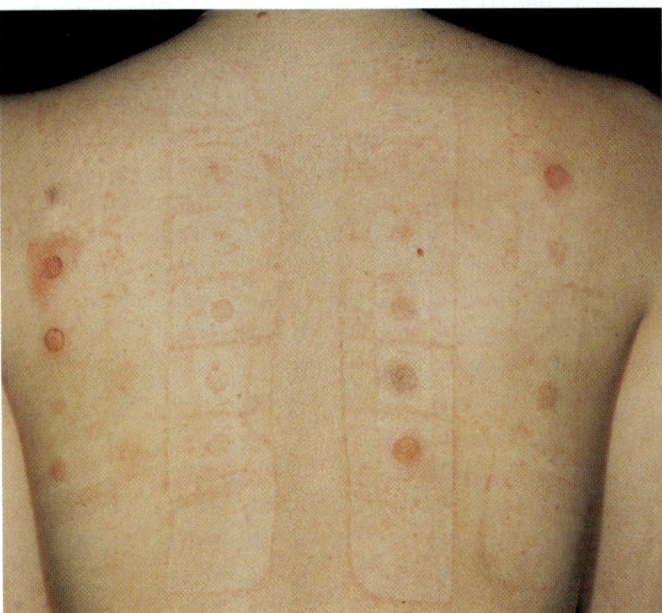

FIGURE 33.9 Results of allergy testing. (From Habif TP: *Clinical dermatology,* ed 5, St. Louis, 2010, Mosby.)

child in this position. The skin surface is labeled or numbered in rows 1½ to 2 inches apart, and a small amount of allergen is placed on the skin, which is then scratched or pricked to place the allergen just under the skin surface. Many allergists use a plastic device that is dipped into the designated allergens and lightly pressed into the skin so that the prick and allergen deposition occur at the same time. Seventy or more tests may be done at one time. It is essential to follow a pattern so that the site of each allergen can be easily identified. The first step should be to number all of the sites before applying the allergen. This type of allergy testing is used for allergic rhinitis, asthma, and detection of food allergies.

A reaction usually occurs within 10 to 30 minutes of exposure to the allergen. If the reaction is positive, a wheal (hive) forms at the site of the scratch (Figure 33.9). Interpretation of the test result should always be based on a comparison of this reaction with that of the control, which is a scratch with a plain fluid free of any allergy-producing extract.

After 15 minutes, the medical assistant measures the erythema (redness) and the wheal at each site. If a strong reaction occurs, the allergen extract should be carefully wiped off to prevent any further exposure. Frequently, large or significant reactions are accompanied by local itching. Patients should remain in the office for at least 30 minutes after completion of the test in case a delayed systemic allergic response occurs.

A patch test uses an allergen that is applied to a patch that is placed on the skin. Patch testing helps detect delayed allergic reactions associated with contact dermatitis. The patches are placed on the arms or back and must remain in place for 48 hours. The patient needs to avoid bathing and activities that cause heavy sweating. The patches are removed at a subsequent office visit. Skin irritation at the patch site indicates an allergy to that particular substance.

Five Guidelines for Allergen Skin Testing

- The patient should stop taking all antihistamines or allergy medications 3 to 10 days before testing to prevent false-negative results. The patient should stop taking certain medications as directed by their provider for 3-10 days prior to the test. This may include prescription antihistamines, over-the-counter antihistamines, tricyclic antidepressants, and certain heartburn medications.
- Recommended sites for injection or application of the allergen are the anterior forearm, the upper arm, and the back.
- Allergen sites must be specifically labeled and spaced approximately 1½ to 2 inches apart.
- If the patient shows signs of anaphylaxis, notify the provider immediately and prepare emergency supplies. Allergy testing should be performed only when the provider is onsite.
- Skin testing may cause a mild systemic allergic response, resulting in rhinitis, wheezing, and sneezing. The patient should contact the provider if a more severe reaction occurs.

The intradermal test is more sensitive than the percutaneous test and usually is used to diagnose allergies to penicillin and insect venom, such as from bee stings. Extracts are injected into the intradermal layer of the skin in doses of 0.1 to 0.2 mL. This method also is used for the tuberculin (purified protein derivative [PPD]) test and the Valley Fever coccidioidomycosis test. When intradermal injections are used for allergy testing, 10 to 15 allergens may be tested at one time on each arm. The reaction time is identical to that of the scratch test; however, the antigen is more dilute.

The radioallergosorbent test (RAST) measures the level of antibodies created when a sample of the patient's blood is mixed with allergens in the laboratory. The RAST is easier to perform than skin testing because it requires a single venipuncture. Although skin testing remains the preferred method of diagnosing hypersensitivity, the RAST may be indicated when the patient cannot stop antihistamine medications, when a skin disorder makes accurate interpretation of skin test results difficult, or when skin test results are negative, but the patient's signs and symptoms support further investigation. RAST blood tests are primarily used to identify food allergies.

Assisting with Treatments

When working with patients who have diseases and disorders of the immune and lymphatic systems, the medical assistant often assists with the treatment of the various conditions within those systems. The following sections discuss that role.

Treatment of Allergies

The classic treatment of allergies is to encourage the patient to avoid known or suspected allergens. Unfortunately, this is not always possible, so the provider may prescribe antihistamine medications, such as levocetirizine (Xyzal), for the relief of allergy symptoms. Over-the-counter antihistamines include Allegra, Zyrtec, and Claritin. Another option is using immunotherapy, a series of injections in which minute doses of known allergens are administered subcutaneously over time to desensitize the patient's immune system and ultimately develop a resistance to the immune response. This usually requires weekly or bimonthly injections over several years. Some patients are cured, whereas others have only a minor reduction in allergic symptoms. Immunotherapy is controversial because it is an expensive, invasive, and potentially dangerous treatment with unpredictable results. It is recommended only for patients with severe allergic symptoms that are not relieved by antihistamine medications.

If you are responsible for administering allergen injections, you must take great care to dispense the correct dose of each allergen; administer each subcutaneous injection at a separate site; accurately document the procedure and the exact location of each injection; record any local or systemic reactions; and observe the patient for at least 20 to 30 minutes after the injections to detect possible systemic allergic responses, including urticaria (hives), wheezing, or hypotension. If the patient shows any localized or systemic reactions, the provider should be notified.

CLOSING COMMENTS

Patient Coaching

We know that proper hand hygiene plays a key role in preventing the spread of infectious diseases. Often our patients are not aware that hand hygiene is considered to be the most important element of infection control. Coaching our patients on the when and how of hand washing can help keep everyone healthier. According to the recommendations of the Centers for Disease Control and Prevention (CDC), you should wash your hands at the following times:

- Before, during, and after preparing food
- Before eating food
- Before and after caring for someone who is sick
- Before and after treating a cut or wound
- After using the toilet
- After changing diapers or cleaning up a child who has used the toilet
- After blowing your nose, coughing, or sneezing
- After touching an animal, animal feed, or animal waste
- After handling pet food or pet treats
- After touching garbage

Washing your hands with soap and water is recommended, but if that is not available, an alcohol-based hand sanitizer with at least 60% alcohol can be used. When washing with soap and water, the hands should be scrubbed for at least 20 seconds. Be sure to lather the backs of your hands, between your fingers, and under your nails.

Legal and Ethical Issues

By law, diseases considered of great public health importance must be reported. Some diseases must be reported at the federal level to the CDC; others must be reported at the state level. Most states will have a "reportable diseases" list. Many of those diseases are also on the federal list.

It is important for medical assistants to know which diseases need to be reported for the state in which they are working. See Chapter 4 for more information on required reporting.

Patient-Centered Care

Part of providing care for patients with sexually transmitted infections is education on the ways to prevent those infections. This education must be presented in a nonjudgmental way. Abstinence, limiting the number of sex partners, and using male and female condoms and cervical diaphragms (for cervical gonorrhea, chlamydia, and trichomoniasis) are all ways to reduce the risk of contracting a sexually transmitted infection.

Professional Behaviors

When you have a strong work ethic, it becomes hard to stay home when you are sick. You may say to yourself, "I'm not that sick," "We are shorthanded already," "I don't want to put more work on my co-workers' shoulders," and so on. If you are sick, it is best for everyone for you to stay at home and get better. The quicker you get better, the quicker you will be back at work, giving 100% again. It is also better for your co-workers and patients if you stay home rather than risk spreading your illness to others. Many of your patients are at the healthcare facility because they are already ill. You risk exposing them to another illness if you go to work when you are sick. If you have a fever or have been vomiting, it is best to stay home.

SUMMARY OF SCENARIO

Julia has had a busy day with many different conditions being presented. She has helped with allergy testing, and after working with Dr. Perez, she has a better understanding of what causes allergies and how allergies are diagnosed. Julia is discovering that the immune system is complex, and she plans to take some continuing education courses to better understand it.

Julia has always recognized the importance of preventing the spread of disease, and she has had the opportunity today to educate patients. Proper hand hygiene can go a long way toward keeping people healthy.

SUMMARY OF LEARNING OBJECTIVES

1. **Examine the anatomy of the immune and lymphatic systems.**
The lymphatic system is made up of lymph vessels, lymph nodes, lymph glands, and lymphoid tissue. Lymph organs include the tonsils, adenoids, vermiform appendix, spleen, thymus gland, and Peyer patches.

   Within the immune system, there are two very important cells, monocytes and lymphocytes. These cells move from the bloodstream into the lymph to perform their protective functions. The granular white blood cells play an important role in the immune system protection function.
2. **Examine the physiology of the immune and lymphatic systems.**
Nonspecific immunity uses physical methods of protection, along with reflexes and chemical methods, as the first line of defense. Phagocytosis, inflammation, pyrexia, protective proteins, and natural killer cells are all involved in the second line of defense.

   Specific immunity is another way that the body protects itself from infectious diseases. It is called specific immunity because the response is directed at one specific antigen. Specific immunity involves the development of antibodies. Humoral immunity and cell-mediated immunity are both parts of specific immunity.

   Allergies are also known as hypersensitivity reactions. A hypersensitivity reaction does not occur the first time an antigen is encountered. When the body responds to an allergen, immune cells release *histamines, kinins,* and other inflammatory substances. This causes the characteristic allergy symptoms: runny nose, watery eyes, and possibly a rash or hives. Sometimes drugs called *antihistamines* are used to alleviate allergy symptoms.

   Active immunity requires the body to produce antibodies in response to the presence of an antigen. Passive immunity does not require the body to do anything because the premade antibodies are given to the person.
3. **Analyze the life span changes that occur in the immune and lymphatic systems.**
Babies can acquire some immunity from the mother before birth and some from the colostrum and breast milk. Longer lasting immunity can be acquired by having the disease or getting a vaccination.

   With older adults, we see a reduction in the production of the B and T cells in the bone marrow and thymus. This results in a lesser response to immune system challenges.
4. **Examine the diseases and disorders of the immune system.**
In autoimmune diseases and disorders, the body attacks healthy self-cells rather than foreign antigens. The cause of autoimmune diseases is unknown, but there are several suspected causes, including an infection that triggers the immune system to attack healthy cells, exposure over time to toxins, a weakness in a person's immune system, an imbalance in the intestinal microbiome, or existing allergies.

   Signs and symptoms vary depending on the cells or tissues involved. The common signs and symptoms include skin changes, joint pain, fatigue/malaise, and a low-grade fever.

   A thorough history and physical examination, along with various blood tests, are used to help diagnose autoimmune diseases and disorders.

   Treatments vary depending on the cells or tissues involved but could include physical therapy, blood transfusions, modified diet, stress reduction, NSAIDs, prescription corticosteroids, and immunosuppressive drugs.

   The human immunodeficiency virus is the virus that causes HIV/AIDS. It attacks the immune system and impairs its ability to fight infectious agents. AIDS is the last stage of an HIV infection.

   Signs and symptoms of AIDS include chronic and persistent diarrhea, recurring fevers, night sweats, profound fatigue, weight loss, skin rashes, continual white patches or lesions on the tongue or in the mouth, and repeated opportunistic infections.

   HIV can be diagnosed using a CLIA-waived test and then confirmed with ELISA or Western blot testing.

   There is no cure for HIV, but treatment includes a regimen of antiviral medication. Treatment should also include eating healthy, nutrient-rich food, getting adequate sleep, exercise, relaxation, and staying up to date on immunizations.

   COVID-19, caused by the SARS-Cov-2 virus, quickly became a pandemic in 2020. This virus oftentimes causes respiratory symptoms similar to a cold, flu, or pneumonia. This virus continues to mutate, and those variants can be more contagious, more severe, or resistant to the treatments that have been developed. Infectious diseases are those caused by organisms such as bacteria, viruses, fungi, or parasites. Hepatitis is an inflammation of the liver. Sexually transmitted infections may be seen in any individual who is sexually active. Strep throat is a bacterial infection caused by *Streptococcus pyogenes.* Influenza is a viral respiratory infection that is referred to as the flu. Respiratory syncytial virus (RSV) produces upper respiratory "cold" symptoms. Infectious mononucleosis is a generally mild viral infection, but it can have serious complications.
5. **Examine the diseases and disorders of the lymphatic system.**
Hodgkin's and non-Hodgkin's are the two main types of lymphoma. The cause of lymphomas is not completely understood. Risk factors include a family history of lymphoma, being 15 to 30 years old or over age 55, being male, and having had an Epstein-Barr infection.

   Signs and symptoms include painless swelling of lymph nodes, fatigue, fever, chills, night sweats, and unexplained weight loss. With non-Hodgkin's lymphoma, there could be abdominal swelling and/or pain, trouble breathing, coughing, or chest pain.

   A physical examination, along with blood and urine tests, will be done to diagnose Hodgkin's or non-Hodgkin's lymphoma. The provider may order imaging tests and a biopsy of lymph nodes, tissue, or bone marrow.

   Treatment depends on the type and stage of the lymphoma. Some types of non-Hodgkin's lymphoma may just be monitored. Hodgkin's lymphoma may be treated with chemotherapy, radiation therapy, or stem cell transplantation.

   The cause of multiple myeloma is unknown. Risk factors include being over the age of 60, male gender, and a history of MGUS; blacks are more likely to develop multiple myeloma than whites.

   Signs and symptoms can be very subtle at first, but when noticeable could include bone pain, especially in the spine, chest, or hips; anemia; loss of kidney function; excessive thirst; nausea; loss of appetite; weight

SUMMARY OF LEARNING OBJECTIVES—*continued*

loss; constipation; fatigue; frequent infections; weakness or numbness in the legs; and mental confusion.

Blood tests, including a CBC and differential; tests for the presence of M protein; a comprehensive metabolic panel (CMP), which includes kidney and liver function tests, along with urinalysis; and bone marrow biopsy and examination of cells are used to help diagnose multiple myeloma. Imaging tests may include x-ray, MRI, CT, and PET scans. At diagnosis, multiple myeloma will be staged, and a treatment plan will be based on the staged diagnosis.

Often the provider will watch the condition and run periodic blood and urine tests to monitor asymptomatic multiple myeloma. Treatment for multiple myeloma includes targeted cancer therapy (designed to target specific weaknesses in myeloma cancer cells to kill the cells), biologic therapy, chemotherapy, radiation therapy, and possibly stem cell transplantation.

Lymphedema occurs when there is an issue with lymph vessels that allows the protein-rich fluid to accumulate in the tissue, causing swelling. The lymph vessels could be compromised by infection, cancer, scar tissue from radiation therapy, or surgical removal of the lymph nodes. Compression bandages or garments are used to encourage the drainage of fluid from the affected areas.

Tonsillitis is the inflammation of the tonsils found at the back of the throat. This inflammation can cause enlargement of the tonsils resulting in a sore throat, difficult or painful swallowing, or a scratchy, muffled, or throaty voice. The patient may also have a fever, enlarged tender lymph glands in the neck, white or yellow patches on the tonsils, bad breath, stomachache, and a headache. The inflammation can be caused by either a virus or bacteria. The provider will order tests to determine the cause, and then a treatment plan can be developed. Whether it is viral or bacterial, several things can be done to reduce the symptoms; these include adequate fluid, the use of OTC medications to treat the pain and fever, and sufficient rest.

6. **Examine the medical assistant's role in examinations, diagnostic procedures, and treatments for the immune and lymphatic systems.**
The medical assistant must help where needed but also protect himself or herself by wearing a mask. Preparing a patient for an infectious disease examination includes having the patient disrobe appropriately, depending on which body system is involved. For allergy testing, the patient usually must disrobe to the waist, and the gown is open in the back.

Skin testing for allergies can be done with a percutaneous patch, intradermal test, or radioallergosorbent test. These tests can help determine just what the patient is allergic to so that a treatment plan can be designed.

Diagnostic procedures for respiratory infections include many CLIA-waived tests.

Treatments for allergies include encouraging patients to avoid the known or suspected allergen, but if that is not possible, medications may be recommended. Another option is immunotherapy to desensitize the patient's immune system.

Treatments for respiratory infections could include the use of antibiotics for bacterial infections. For both bacterial and viral infections, the provider may recommend over-the-counter medication for fever and plenty of fluids to prevent dehydration.

GASTROENTEROLOGY

34

SCENARIO

Keith Williams, CMA (AAMA) (certified medical assistant through the American Association of Medical Assistants), has been newly hired as a medical assistant at the Walden-Martin Family Medical (WMFM) Clinic. He just graduated from the local community college last semester after returning to school to study for a second career. Now, at age 49, he has accepted a job at WMFM Clinic. Keith's supervisor has asked him to assist the gastroenterology outreach team, which comes to WMFM Clinic twice a week.

Keith is excited about his new duties yet realizes that he needs to review the digestive system and related diseases. He decides to spend the next week reviewing the anatomy, physiology, and pathology related to the digestive system, along with the diagnostic procedures and commonly ordered treatments.

While studying this chapter, think about the following questions:

- What structures are in the gastrointestinal system?
- What are the functions of the gastrointestinal system?
- What are commonly diagnosed gastrointestinal diseases and disorders? What are the etiologies, signs and symptoms, diagnostic processes, and treatment?
- What are the medical assistant's primary responsibilities when working with patients who have gastrointestinal diseases and disorders?

LEARNING OBJECTIVES

1. Examine the anatomy of the gastrointestinal tract.
2. Examine the anatomy of the accessory organs.
3. Differentiate between digestion, absorption, and excretion.
4. Analyze the life span changes to the gastrointestinal system.
5. Examine the diseases and disorders of the mouth, including the signs, symptoms, etiology, diagnostic procedures, and treatments.
6. Examine the diseases and disorders of the esophagus and stomach, including the signs, symptoms, etiology, diagnostic procedures, and treatments.
7. Examine the diseases and disorders of the intestines, including the signs, symptoms, etiology, diagnostic procedures, and treatments.
8. Examine the diseases and disorders of the accessory organs, including the signs, symptoms, etiology, diagnostic procedures, and treatments.
9. Examine the cancers of the gastrointestinal system, including the signs, symptoms, etiology, diagnostic procedures, and treatments.
10. Examine the medical assistant's role in examinations, diagnostic procedures, and treatments for gastrointestinal diseases and disorders.

VOCABULARY

anastomosis (ah nas tih MOH sis) The surgical connection of separate or severed tubular hollow organs to form a continuous channel.

cholecystitis Inflammation of the gallbladder.

colostomy (koh LOS tuh mee) A surgical procedure in which the large intestine is brought through the abdominal wall, creating either a temporary or a permanent opening (stoma) to allow stool to pass out of the body.

dysphagia Difficulty swallowing.

emulsifies (ee MUL sih fyez) When a substance suspends tiny droplets of one liquid in a second liquid. By creating an emulsion, you can mix two liquids that usually do not mix well, such as oil and water.

endocrine A glandular secretion that is released into the blood or lymph directly (does not go through a duct).

enema Fluid introduced into the rectum for a therapeutic or diagnostic purpose.

epiglottis (ep i GLOT is) A lidlike structure over the glottis that prevents food and liquids from entering the trachea when swallowing occurs.

exocrine A glandular secretion released through a duct.

fissure A crack, cleft, or narrow opening.

hemolytic uremic syndrome A kidney disorder that can occur after a digestive infection with Escherichia coli, shigella, or salmonella; red blood cells are destroyed and block the kidneys' filtering system, causing acute kidney failure.

incarcerated Confined or trapped.

intrinsic factor Secreted by the parietal cells of the stomach; necessary for the absorption of vitamin B_{12} to prevent pernicious anemia.

VOCABULARY—*continued*

lumen The cavity, channel, or open space within a tube or tubular organ.

mucous membrane A mucus-producing membrane that lines tracts and structures of the body (e.g., GI tract, respiratory tract); also called mucosa.

occult Hidden or unseen.

peristalsis (payr i STAHL sis) Wave-like movement from alternate circulate contraction and relaxation of a tubular structure (e.g., intestine), which propels the content forward.

plaque Sticky substance made of mucus, food particles, and bacteria that builds up on the exposed part of the tooth.

polyp A growth or mass protruding from a mucous membrane (e.g., nose, bladder, intestine).

rebound pain Pain felt when the pressure on the abdomen is released.

referred pain Pain that is felt at a site in the body at a distance from the cause (e.g., the injury or diseased part).

resection Surgical removal of all or part of an organ.

rugae (ROO gah) Folds in the wall of an organ; when an organ (e.g., stomach, bladder, uterus) fills or needs to expand, the rugae unfold.

sphincter (SFINGK ter) A circular muscle that either constricts and closes the opening or relaxes and allows substances to pass through the opening.

stoma (STOH mah) A temporary or permanent surgically created opening used for drainage (i.e., urine, stool).

strangulation Constriction of a tubular structure, such as an intestine or vessel, leading to a lack of blood supply to the tissues

Zollinger-Ellison syndrome Rare condition that causes tumors to form in the pancreas or duodenum. Tumors secrete large amounts of gastrin, which causes an increase in acid production.

INTRODUCTION

Gastroenterology is the healthcare specialty that deals with most digestive diseases and disorders. A *gastroenterologist* is a specialist involved in the diagnosis, treatment, and prevention of disorders of the digestive organs and liver. A *proctologist* is a subspecialist who treats disorders of the rectum and anus. *Hepatology* is a subspecialty that deals with liver disorders. A *hepatologist* is a specialist who focuses only on the liver.

Gastrointestinal system disorders are common in the ambulatory care facility. Besides the gastroenterology department, patients with digestive concerns are seen in primary care, pediatrics, internal medicine, and urgent care settings.

The gastrointestinal (GI) system is also called the digestive system. It is made up of the gastrointestinal tract and the accessory organs, which are discussed in the following sections.

CRITICAL THINKING APPLICATION **34.1**

As Keith starts to review the anatomy of the digestive system, he tries to remember the major and accessory organs. List the major organs and accessory organs of the gastrointestinal system.

ANATOMY OF THE GASTROINTESTINAL TRACT

The gastrointestinal tract is also called the *digestive tract* and the *alimentary canal.* It consists of a large, muscular tube that, with the help of hormones and enzymes, digests food. The GI tract starts at the mouth and extends to the anus. It includes the mouth, pharynx (throat), esophagus, stomach, small intestine, and large intestine. Each of these structures is discussed in depth.

Mouth

The cheeks, lips, tongue, hard palate, and soft palate form the mouth (also called the *oral cavity* or *buccal cavity*) (Figure 34.1A). The roof of the mouth is created by the anterior hard palate and the posterior soft palate. The uvula is a fleshy structure that hangs above the throat, at the back of the soft palate. Adults have 32 permanent teeth that are set in the gums (also called *gingivae*). Saliva from the salivary glands helps to lubricate the food, making it easier to swallow (Figure 34.1B). The salivary glands will be discussed later in the chapter.

Pharynx

When food or liquid is swallowed, it moves into the pharynx (FAIR inks), or throat. The pharynx is divided into three sections:

- *Nasopharynx*: Located behind the nasal cavity
- *Oropharynx*: Located behind the mouth; part of the respiratory and digestive systems
- *Laryngopharynx*: Located between the **epiglottis** and the esophagus

Esophagus

The esophagus connects the pharynx to the stomach (Figure 34.2). This muscular tube runs behind the trachea and the heart. The esophagus is lined with a **mucous membrane** that secretes mucus, helping the mass of food, or bolus, pass into the stomach. **Peristalsis**, or the muscular contractions of the esophagus, helps to move the food into the stomach.

A **sphincter** is located at the top and bottom of the esophagus. When the upper esophageal sphincter (UES) constricts, it prevents air from entering the esophagus. The lower esophageal sphincter (LES), or the cardiac sphincter, is located between the esophagus and the stomach. When the LES constricts, it prevents the stomach contents from moving up the esophagus. When a person swallows, the LES relaxes, allowing the bolus to move into the stomach.

Stomach

The stomach serves as a reservoir for food. The stomach is divided into three sections:

- *Fundus*: Top of the stomach, sits just below the diaphragm
- *Body:* Main part of the stomach
- *Pylorus*: Bottom of the stomach, between the body and the small intestine

The stomach wall contains **rugae**, which, when unfolded, allow for greater expansion of the stomach size.

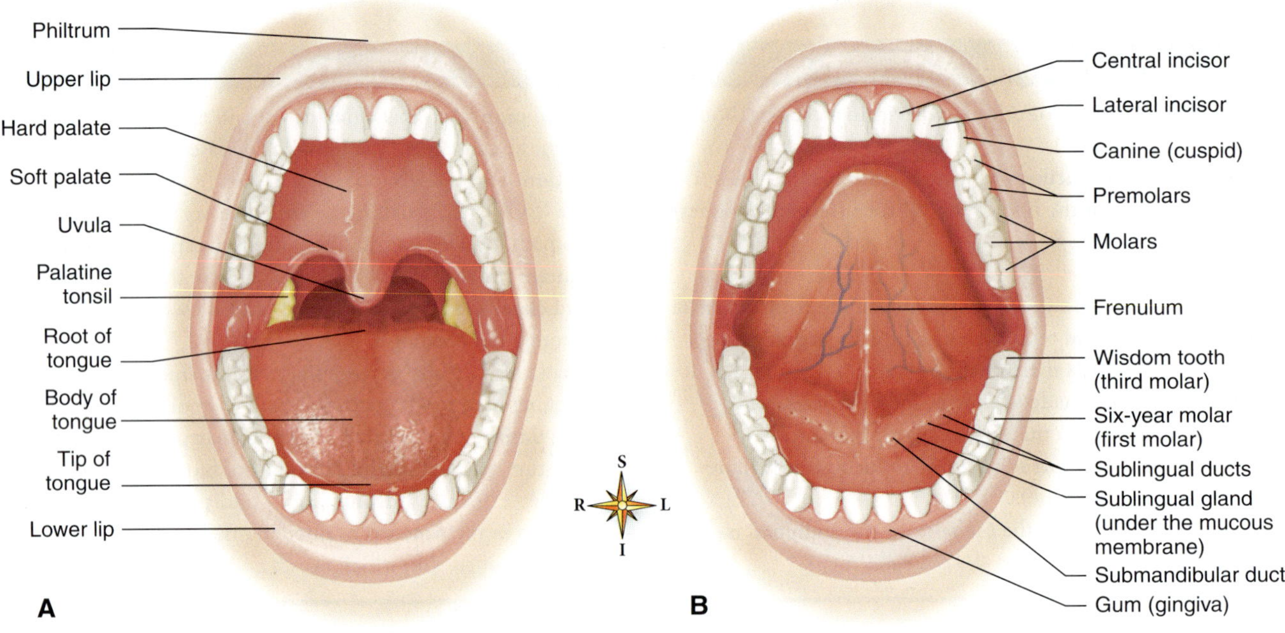

FIGURE 34.1 Mouth. **(A)** Mouth cavity showing the hard and soft palates, tongue surface, and uvula. **(B)** Undersurface of tongue showing the frenulum, sublingual gland, and opening of sublingual duct. GI, Gastrointestinal. (From Patton KT, Thibodeau GA: *The human body in health and disease*, ed 7, St. Louis, 2018, Elsevier.)

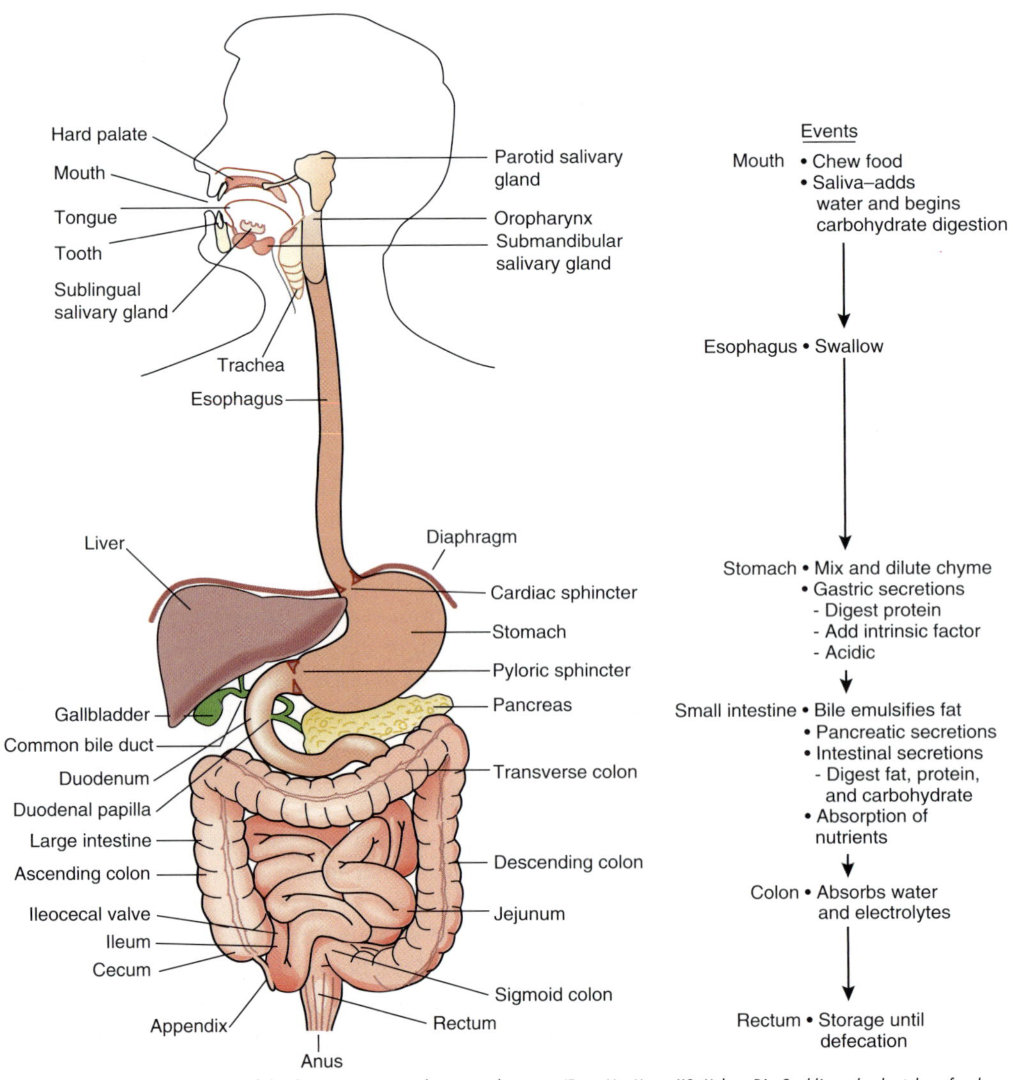

FIGURE 34.2 The anatomy of the digestive system and associated events. (From VanMeter KC, Hubert RJ: *Gould's pathophysiology for the health professions*, ed 5, Philadelphia, 2015, Saunders.)

Tiny glands in the mucous membrane lining of the stomach produce digestive enzymes, **intrinsic factor,** hydrochloric acid, mucus, and bicarbonate. These make up the gastric juice. Gastric juice is continually being made, but the amount made at certain times varies. Certain things trigger more gastric juice to be made, including thoughts of eating, the smell of food, and the presence of food in the mouth and stomach. The smooth muscles in the stomach provide churning and mixing action, which helps combine the gastric juice with the food ingested, creating a mixture called *chyme.* A continuous coating of mucus protects the stomach and the rest of the digestive system from the acidic nature of chyme and gastric juices.

Besides being a food reservoir and secreting gastric juices, the stomach has additional roles:

- Producing *gastrin,* a hormone that regulates the digestive functions
- Producing *ghrelin,* which increases the appetite
- Protecting the body by killing disease-causing bacteria in food
- Absorbing alcohol, some water, certain drugs, and some fatty acids

The pyloric sphincter is located between the pylorus and the small intestine and regulates the passage of food into the small intestine (Figure 34.3). When the pyloric sphincter relaxes, the chyme empties out of the stomach and into the small intestine.

CRITICAL THINKING APPLICATION 34.2

Keith tries to remember the roles of the stomach as he prepares for his day with the gastroenterologist. List the roles of the stomach.

Small Intestine

The small intestine has about a 1-inch **lumen** and is about 20 feet long. It loops around and fills most of the abdominal cavity. The small intestine is made up of three parts:

- *Duodenum*: Smallest part of the small intestine; connected to the stomach by the pyloric sphincter.
- *Jejunum*: Second largest part of the small intestine; connected to the duodenum and the ileum.
- *Ileum*: Largest part of the small intestine; connects to the jejunum and the large intestine. It joins the cecum at the ileocecal valve.

The lining of the small intestine has *plicae* (folds), which contain small projections called *villi.* The villi are covered by *microvilli* (epithelial cells that have a brushlike shape). The villi and microvilli increase the surface area of the small intestine and make absorption of nutrients more efficient. Each villus contains a *lacteal* (lymph vessel) that absorbs lipids (fats) and fat-soluble vitamins. The blood capillary absorbs glucose and amino acids (Figure 34.4).

Each of the three sections of the small intestine has important roles:

- *Duodenum:* Receives chyme from the stomach. Pancreatic enzymes, bile from the liver, and bicarbonate mix with the chyme. Pancreatic enzymes break down chyme. Bile helps break down and absorb fat. Bicarbonate neutralizes the acid from the stomach.
- *Jejunum:* Contains larger villi; thus, absorption is the primary function of this section. Sugars, fatty acids, and amino acids are absorbed.
- *Ileum:* Limited absorption occurs in this section. Bile acids and vitamin B_{12} are most often absorbed for reuse in the body.

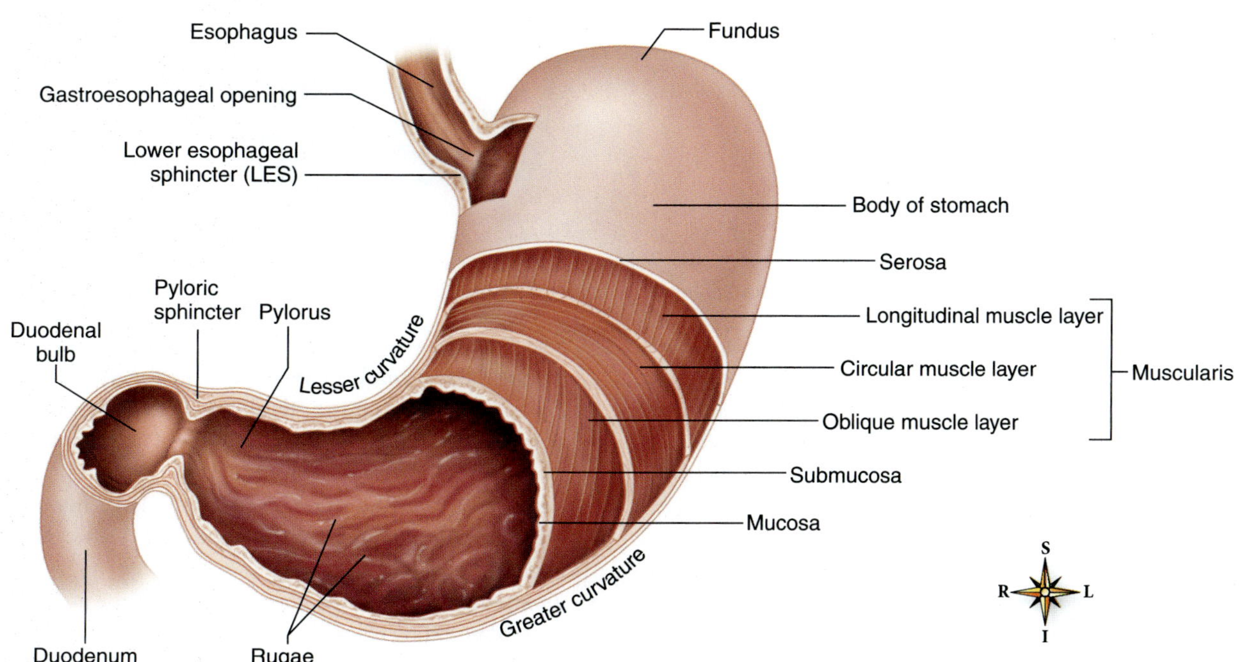

FIGURE 34.3 Stomach. A portion of the anterior wall has been cut away to reveal the three muscle layers of the stomach wall. Notice that the mucosa lining the stomach forms folds called rugae. (From Patton KT, Thibodeau GA: *The Human body in health and disease*, ed 7, St. Louis, 2018, Elsevier.)

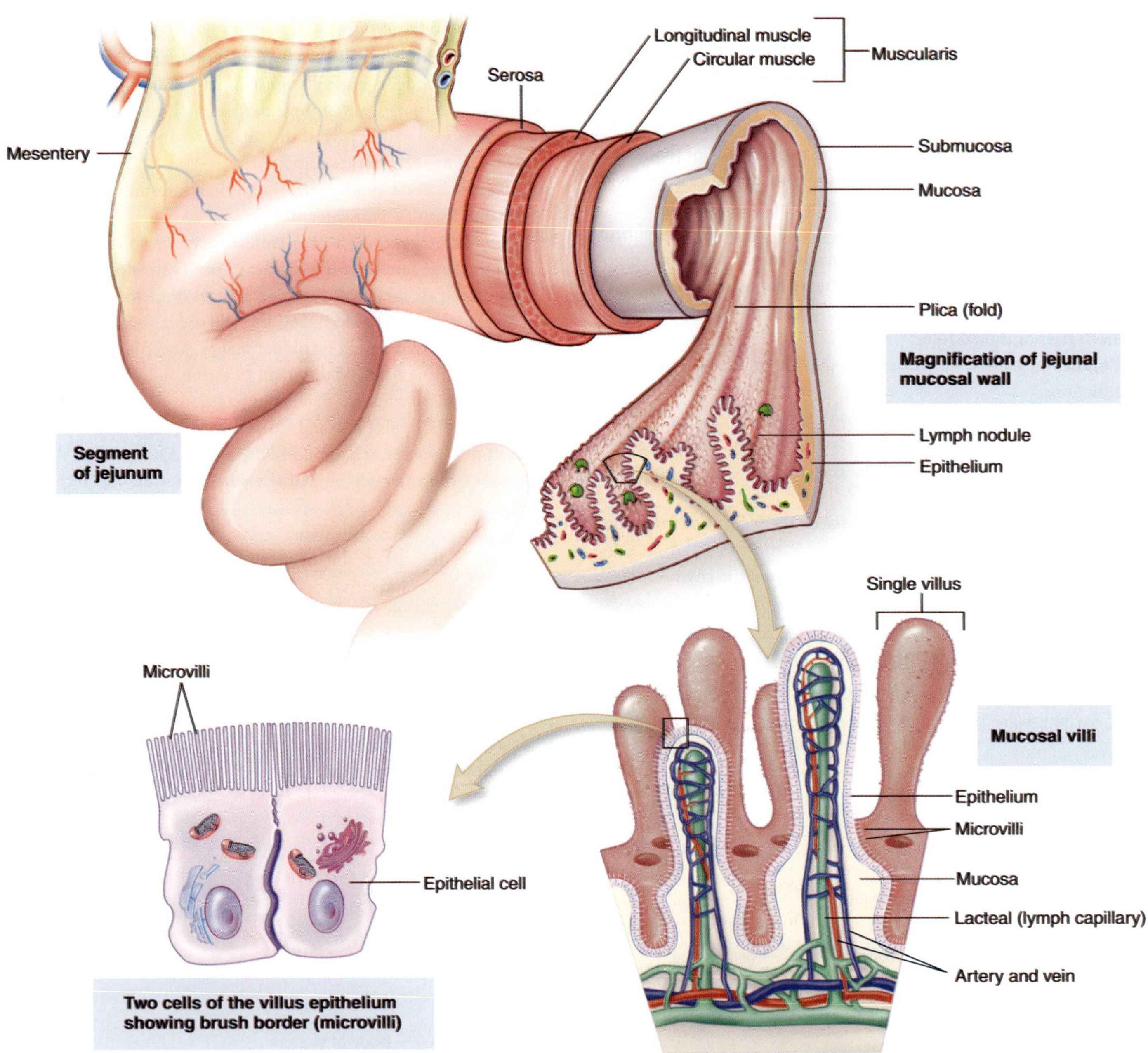

FIGURE 34.4 Small intestine. Note the four tissue coats or layers and the presence of villi and microvilli, which increases the area available for absorption. (From Patton KT, Thibodeau GA: *The human body in health and disease*, ed 7, St. Louis, 2018, Elsevier.)

Chyme from the stomach empties into the duodenum. Peristalsis moves the chyme through the duodenum, jejunum, and the ileum. The ileocecal valve is found between the ileum (of the small intestine) and the cecum (of the large intestine). The ileocecal valve controls the passage of chyme into the cecum and prevents the backflow of chyme into the small intestine.

Large Intestine

The large intestine or colon has about a 3-inch lumen and is about 5 feet long. The large intestine is made up of these six sections:

- *Cecum*: A 2- to 3-inch pouch or tubelike structure in the lower right abdomen that is considered the first section of the large intestine. The main roles of the cecum include receiving chyme from the small intestine and absorbing fluids and salts. Mucus is also mixed with the chyme in the cecum. Attached to the cecum is the vermiform appendix. The function of the appendix is not entirely known, though research suggests that it harbors "good bacteria," which will repopulate the intestines after an illness.
- *Ascending colon:* The second part of the large intestine, which extends vertically from the cecum to just below the liver (see Figure 34.2).
- *Transverse colon:* Extends horizontally from the ascending colon to the descending colon.
- *Descending colon:* Extends vertically on the left side of the abdomen from the transverse colon to the sigmoid colon.
- *Sigmoid colon:* Forms an S-shaped curve; attaches to the descending colon and the rectum.

- *Rectum:* Stores the stool until defecation, or a bowel movement (BM), occurs, and the stool is released through the anus.

The watery waste products move from the small intestine into the large intestine. The primary functions of the large intestine include the following:

- Reabsorbing water and electrolytes: The large intestine has no villi for nutrient absorption but can reabsorb water and electrolytes (e.g., sodium and potassium). The longer the stool is in the colon, the more water is absorbed. The quicker the stool passes through the large intestine, the more water it contains.
- Making vitamin K: The bacteria in the large intestine make vitamin K, which is used for blood coagulation, bone mineralization, and cardiovascular health.
- Eliminating waste products from the body.

Bacteria in the Colon

The bacteria in the colon can help with the digestion of some materials. This digestive process can cause gas to be formed, and when it is released through the anus, it is called *flatus*. The bacteria in the colon produce vitamin K and biotin (vitamin B_7).

The majority of the colon bacteria are nonpathogenic. The bacteria colonized in the colon (also called *gut flora* or *microbiota*) are important for our maturation, immune system development, and metabolism. Cardiovascular disease, metabolic diseases (e.g., diabetes and obesity), and inflammatory bowel disease are some diseases that have been associated with changes in the intestinal bacteria. Antibiotic therapy can also change the delicate microbiota balance in the gut.

Usually, the microbiota prevents *Clostridium difficile* colonization. With some antibiotic therapies, *C. difficile* may be allowed to grow, causing intestinal inflammation, diarrhea, and, in some cases, death. *C. difficile* is spread by the fecal-oral route and is shed in the stool of infected patients. The *C. difficile* spores have a long survival and are difficult to kill. They are not destroyed by alcohol-based hand sanitizers. *C. difficile* infections are treated with antibiotics, and the risk of reinfection is high.

CRITICAL THINKING APPLICATION **34.3**

Keith is reviewing the anatomy of the GI tract. List the sections of the small and large intestines in order.

ANATOMY OF THE ACCESSORY ORGANS

Accessory organs have a role in digestive activities, though they are not part of the gastrointestinal tract. Accessory organs include the salivary glands, liver, gallbladder, and pancreas. These structures secrete fluids into the GI tract, aiding in digestion. Each of these accessory organs will be discussed in the following sections.

Salivary Glands

Three pairs of salivary glands are found in the mouth. The *parotid glands* are near the ear in the cheeks. The *submandibular glands* are on the floor of the mouth, and the *sublingual glands* are under the tongue. These glands produce and secrete saliva, which mixes with the food eaten. Saliva not only moistens the food but also aids in the breakdown and swallowing of food. Saliva contains salivary amylase, an enzyme that will be discussed later in the chapter.

Liver

The liver is one of the largest organs in the body and is located just below the diaphragm, in the right hypochondriac and epigastric regions (see Figure 34.2). The liver is divided into two major lobes and two smaller lobes.

The hepatic artery brings oxygenated blood to the liver. The hepatic portal vein brings blood from the digestive tract, which can contain nutrients, medications, alcohol, and toxic substances. These substances are filtered from the blood and are processed, stored, changed, detoxified, and returned to the blood or eliminated in the stool. Besides these roles, the liver has additional important functions:

- Producing plasma proteins (e.g., albumin and blood clotting factors).
- Breaking down old or damaged blood cells.
- Breaking down proteins and fats and producing energy.
- Producing up to a liter of bile a day. Bile contains bilirubin (a breakdown product of red blood cells), bile acids or salts, cholesterol, water, salts (e.g., sodium, potassium), and metals (e.g., copper). Bile is stored in the gallbladder until it is secreted into the duodenum. Bile breaks down fats into fatty acids.
- Removing extra minerals (e.g., iron and copper), vitamins (B_{12}, A, D, and K), and glucose from the blood and storing them in the liver. The liver releases them into the blood when needed. (For instance, the liver stores extra glucose as glycogen. When the blood glucose level decreases, the liver breaks down the glycogen and releases the glucose into the blood.)
- Manufacturing triglycerides and cholesterol.

CRITICAL THINKING APPLICATION **34.4**

Keith is amazed at all of the activities that occur in the liver. List at least four roles of the liver.

Gallbladder

The gallbladder (GB) is found in a small area on the underside of the liver (see Figure 34.2). The gallbladder stores and concentrates bile. The bile is made by the liver and then flows through the common bile duct to smaller ducts before going into the gallbladder, where it is stored. When a person eats, the gallbladder contracts and squeezes the bile through the bile duct and into the common bile duct before emptying into the duodenum. If gallbladder emptying is delayed (as in pregnancy), gallstone formation can occur.

Pancreas

The pancreas is a gland found behind the stomach and in front of the spine (see Figure 34.2). It is about 6 to 10 inches long. The pancreas has two main roles:

- **Exocrine** function: About 95% of the pancreas is made up of exocrine tissue that produces digestive enzymes. These enzymes are released into the duodenum.

- **Endocrine** function: About 5% of the pancreas is made up of endocrine cells, called *islets of Langerhans,* which make hormones (e.g., insulin) that regulate blood sugar and pancreatic secretions. (See Chapter 39 for additional details.)

The pancreatic enzymes created in the exocrine tissue include trypsin, chymotrypsin, amylase, and lipase. When food enters the stomach, pancreatic enzymes and sodium bicarbonate are released into the main pancreatic duct. This duct joins the common bile duct to form the ampulla of Vater (also called the *hepatopancreatic duct* or *ampulla*), which is located at the duodenum.

PHYSIOLOGY OF THE GASTROINTESTINAL SYSTEM

The role of the digestive system is to provide nutrients to the cells of the body. Four processes occur in the digestive system:

- *Ingestion:* The intake of food and liquids into the body
- *Digestion:* The breakdown of food into chemical substances
- *Absorption:* The passage of substances and liquids through the lining of the GI tract into the body fluids and tissues
- *Excretion:* The elimination of indigestible materials and waste products of metabolism

The following sections focus on the digestion, absorption, and elimination processes in the body.

CRITICAL THINKING APPLICATION 34.5

Summarize the four processes that occur in the GI system.

Digestion

Once food is ingested, it must be digested for absorption to occur. Two digestive processes happen to break down food into chemical substances:

- *Mechanical digestion:* The breakdown of food into smaller particles. This process starts in the mouth as the food is being chewed. The smooth muscles in the stomach provide the churning and mixing action, which also aids in the breakdown of the food.
- *Chemical digestion:* The smaller particles of food are broken down into small molecules that can be absorbed.

Chemical Digestion

Chemical digestion starts in the mouth. During *mastication* (the process of chewing), saliva moistens and aids in the breakdown and swallowing (*deglutition*) of food. Saliva contains an enzyme called *salivary amylase,* which starts to break down complex carbohydrates.

In the stomach, hydrochloric acid softens and breaks down proteins and other foods. The pH of hydrochloric acid also kills many pathogens (e.g., bacteria) that are consumed. Pepsin, an enzyme found in the gastric juices, breaks down proteins into amino acids.

Hydrochloric acid, amino acids, or fatty acids in the stomach or duodenum stimulate the small intestine to secrete cholecystokinin (CCK), a hormone. CCK causes the gallbladder to contract and release bile into the duodenum through the common bile duct. Bile from the liver is also secreted in the duodenum and **emulsifies** fats. CCK also increases secretion of pancreatic juices, which contain the following enzymes:

- *Trypsin* and chymotrypsin: Break down proteins into amino acids
- *Amylase:* Breaks down carbohydrates into sugars
- *Lipase:* Breaks down fats into fatty acids and glycerol

Pancreatic juices also contain sodium bicarbonate, which helps to neutralize the acidity of the chyme in the duodenum.

In the small intestine, *brush-border enzymes* (sucrase, lactase, and maltase) are found in the microvilli. These enzymes help with the final breakdown of carbohydrates:

- *Sucrase:* Breaks down sucrose (or cane sugar) into glucose and fructose.
- *Lactase:* Breaks down lactose (found in milk) into galactose and glucose.
- *Maltase:* Breaks down maltose (from starches) into glucose.

CRITICAL THINKING APPLICATION 34.6

Summarize the chemical digestion of carbohydrates, proteins, and fats.

Absorption and Excretion

Once chemical digestion is complete, small nutrient molecules move from the small intestines into the bloodstream through the process of absorption. As mentioned earlier, the villi and microvilli in the small intestine increase the surface area, which makes the absorption of nutrients more efficient. The lacteal in the villus absorbs lipids, and the capillary absorbs glucose and amino acids. Chemical digestion and nutrient absorption are completed by the time chyme leaves the small intestine.

As chyme moves through the large intestine, water and electrolytes are reabsorbed to prevent dehydration. The consistency of chyme changes to a soft-formed solid, called *feces,* which is excreted. The composition of feces is water, bacteria, undigested carbohydrates, fiber, and some protein and fat.

LIFE SPAN CHANGES OF THE GASTROINTESTINAL SYSTEM

Throughout life, changes occur in both the GI tract and the accessory organs. The following sections discuss the changes that occur with age and pregnancy.

Changes with the GI Tract

At birth, the baby's digestive system is not fully mature. The infant does not have teeth to help break down food. Salivary secretions (which start starch breakdown) are insufficient until about 6 months of age. Pancreatic amylase levels may not be sufficient until 12 to 18 months of age. Bile salts and lipase levels are not sufficient until 6 to 9 months of age.

During pregnancy, progesterone (a hormone) causes the smooth muscles to relax. This causes less peristalsis in the digestive system, thus slowing digestion. Gallbladder emptying may be delayed, leading to gallstone formation. Morning sickness, constipation, and heartburn can result from digestive system changes.

With age, the stomach cannot accommodate as much food because of decreased elasticity. The stomach empties more slowly. The lactase levels also decrease with age, leading to lactose intolerance (milk products). Bacterial overgrowth (excessive growth of certain intestinal bacteria) is more common with age and leads to bloating, weight loss, and pain. Bacterial overgrowth can also lead to reduced absorption of certain nutrients (e.g., iron, calcium, and vitamin B_{12}). With aging, constipation is more common and can be caused by many factors, including the following:

- Slowing of fecal contents through the large intestine, allowing for more water absorption
- Increased use of drugs that can cause constipation
- Decreased physical activity and fluid intake

Changes with the Accessory Organs

Age-related changes can be seen with the accessory organs. A decrease of salivary flow is not related to age, although it is common in older adults. It is related to diseases, medications, and head and neck radiation therapy (used for cancers). The pancreas decreases in weight as some tissue is replaced with scar tissue, although these changes do not affect the organ's ability to produce digestive enzymes and sodium bicarbonate. With age, the liver gets smaller, and blood flow decreases. Liver function test results, however, are unchanged. Metabolism of many substances decreases, which affects drug metabolism; thus, older adults may experience dose-related side effects. The production and flow of bile decrease with age, leading to more gallstones.

> **Common Signs and Symptoms of Gastrointestinal Disorders**
>
> - Constipation, diarrhea, *hematochezia* (bloody stool), and *melena* (black, tarry stools)
> - *Pyrosis* (heartburn), *dyspepsia* (indigestion), and *flatus* (gas)
> - *Halitosis* (bad-smelling breath)
> - Nausea, vomiting, and *hematemesis* (vomiting of blood)
> - *Jaundice* (yellowing of the skin and whites of the eyes caused by elevated bilirubin levels)

MOUTH DISEASES AND DISORDERS

Disorders can impact the structures of the mouth, including the gums, hard and soft palate, tissues, tongue, teeth, and lips.

Orofacial Clefts

Orofacial clefts are one of the most common birth defects in the United States. Orofacial clefts include the following congenital disorders:

- *Cleft lip:* An opening in the upper lip caused by the lip tissues not completely joining before birth.
- *Cleft palate:* The tissue that makes up the palate (roof of the mouth) does not completely join before birth. The hard palate makes up the front section, and the soft palate makes up the back section. Cleft palate can affect one or both palates.

Children can have a cleft lip, a cleft palate, or both (Figure 34.5). Children with clefts can have problems with feeding, speaking, hearing, and ear infections.

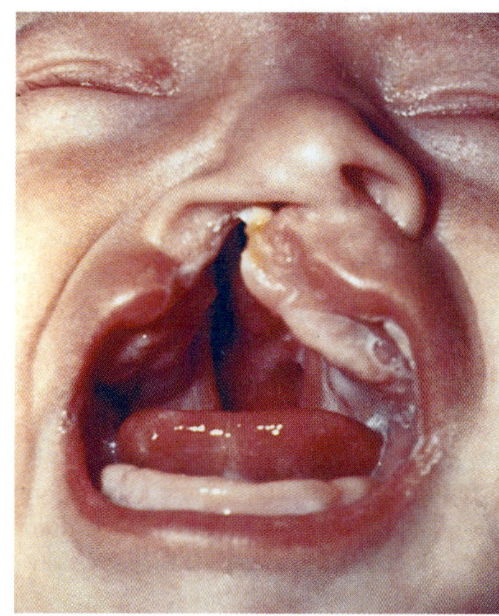

FIGURE 34.5 Cleft lip and cleft palate. (Zitelli BJ, Davis HW: *Atlas of pediatric physical diagnosis*, ed 4, St. Louis, 2002, Mosby.)

In most cases, the etiology is unknown, but researchers believe it involves genetics and environmental factors. Research studies have shown that women who smoke, have diabetes, or use certain medications (e.g., valproic acid) during pregnancy have an increased risk of having a baby with an orofacial cleft. The signs of an orofacial cleft are visible at birth. The child may have a split in the lip or the roof of the mouth. The cleft can affect one or both sides of the face.

The provider will identify the cleft right after birth. Sometimes the cleft is detected during a prenatal ultrasound. Treatment involves surgery to improve the child's ability to eat, speak, and hear. A team of specialists is involved with the treatment of the related complications.

Additional Mouth Diseases and Disorders

Additional diseases and disorders of the mouth include the following:

- *Cavities:* Also called *tooth decay* or *dental caries*; **plaque** on the tooth creates the decay.
- *Gingivitis:* An inflammatory disease of the gums that causes redness, swelling, and bleeding. Part of the early stages of periodontal disease; caused by plaque depositing on the tooth for a short amount of time.
- *Herpetic stomatitis:* Inflammation of the mouth caused by the herpes simplex virus (also known as a *fever blister* or a *cold sore*).
- *Leukoplakia:* A condition of white patches on the lips and buccal mucosa often associated with tobacco use.
- *Periodontal disease:* Infection and inflammation in the mouth that destroys the gums, periodontal ligaments, and bone that support the teeth.
- *Thrush:* A yeast infection of the mouth and tongue. Risk factors include older age, infants, poor health, a compromised immune system (e.g., infection with the human immunodeficiency virus [HIV], acquired immunodeficiency syndrome [AIDS], chemotherapy), and taking antibiotics.

ESOPHAGEAL AND STOMACH DISEASES AND DISORDERS

Certain esophageal and stomach diseases and disorders can occur in early childhood, whereas others affect older people. The following sections describe common esophageal and stomach diseases and disorders.

Gastroesophageal Reflux Disease

Gastroesophageal reflux (GER) occurs when the stomach contents back up into the esophagus, causing acid reflux or heartburn. Gastroesophageal reflux disease (GERD) is more serious and longer lasting than GER. GERD can occur in adults and infants. The presentation in infants is different from that in adults.

The cause of GERD is a weakened or abnormal lower esophageal sphincter. The sphincter may relax when it should not, causing stomach contents to back up into the esophagus. The risk for GERD and GER in adults increases with pregnancy, being overweight, certain medications, and smoking. The most common symptom of GERD in adults is heartburn. Other common GERD symptoms in adults include bad breath, nausea, vomiting, chest pain, upper abdominal pain, respiratory problems, and erosion of the teeth.

A provider will do a history and physical examination. Diagnostic procedures include an upper endoscopy, esophageal manometry, ambulatory acid probe test, and an upper-digestive system x-ray. Treatment is based on the severity of the symptoms and can include lifestyle changes, medications, or surgery. Usually, patients are encouraged to reduce their intake of foods and drinks that make the symptoms worse.

GER and GERD in Infants

Infants can have gastroesophageal reflux (GER) and gastroesophageal reflux disease (GERD). The cause of GER and GERD in infants is an immature (not fully developed) lower esophageal sphincter. The sphincter becomes weak or relaxed, and stomach contents back up into the esophagus.

The main sign of GERD in infants is spitting up more than normal. Additional signs include the following:

- Arching of the back during or right after feedings
- Colic, coughing, trouble breathing, wheezing, gagging, and projectile or forceful vomiting
- Poor feeding and refusal to feed
- Poor growth and weight gain; malnutrition

Treatment for GERD focuses on feeding changes and medications. Rice cereal may be added to the milk. Holding the baby upright for 30 minutes after feeding and avoiding overfeeding the child may be encouraged. H_2 blockers or proton-pump inhibitors may be given to reduce acid production. Surgery may be recommended in severe cases. Most infant GERD resolves by 9 to 18 months of age.

CRITICAL THINKING APPLICATION **34.7**

What are the similarities and differences between the presentation of GERD in adults and that in infants?

Hiatal Hernia

A hiatal hernia occurs when a section of the upper stomach pushes through an opening of the diaphragm into the chest (Figure 34.6).

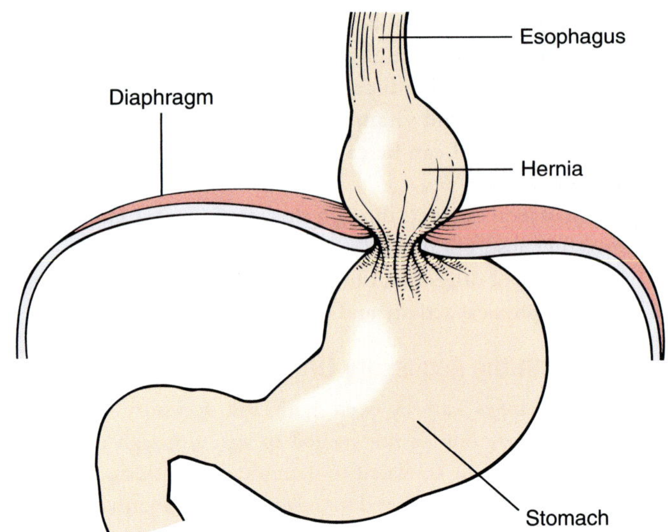

FIGURE 34.6 Hiatal hernia. (Frazier MS, Drzymkowski JW: *Essentials of human diseases and conditions*, ed 4, Philadelphia, 2008, Saunders.)

The cause is unknown. The risk of hiatal hernias increases with age, obesity, and smoking. Often people over 50 years of age experience this condition. The signs and symptoms include chest pain, heartburn, and difficulty swallowing.

The provider will order an upper GI (UGI) series (also called a *barium swallow*) and an esophagogastroduodenoscopy (EGD) to help diagnose the condition. The goal of treatment is to relieve symptoms and prevent complications. Treatment includes medications for acid reflux and surgery to repair the hernia. The person should avoid alcohol and use medications with care.

Peptic Ulcers

Peptic ulcers are also known as duodenal, gastric, and stomach ulcers. A peptic ulcer is a sore or breakdown in the lining of the stomach or duodenum. Gastric ulcers occur in the stomach, and duodenal ulcers occur in the first section of the small intestine.

The most common etiology for peptic ulcers is an infection of the stomach by *Helicobacter pylori (H. pylori)* bacteria. The risk for peptic ulcers may increase with drinking too much alcohol, regular use of aspirin or nonsteroidal anti-inflammatory drugs (NSAIDs) (e.g., ibuprofen and naproxen), using cigarettes and chewing tobacco, radiation treatments, and stress. **Zollinger-Ellison syndrome** can also cause peptic ulcers. Signs and symptoms include upper abdominal pain at night or when the stomach is empty (1 to 3 hours after a meal). Additional symptoms include nausea, melena, chest pain, fatigue, vomiting and hematemesis, and weight loss.

After a physical exam, the provider may order an upper GI (UGI) endoscopy or a UGI series to visibly examine the lining of the esophagus, stomach, and duodenum (Figure 34.7). Testing for *H. pylori* requires a biopsy of the stomach lining or a urea breath test. A stool **occult** blood test and a hemoglobin test may also be done. Treatment is based on the reasons for the ulcer. If *H. pylori* bacteria are present, the patient may need to take medication, such as antibiotics and an H_2 blocker or a proton-pump inhibitor (PPI) (e.g., omeprazole [Prilosec], lansoprazole [Prevacid], or esomeprazole [Nexium]). Additional ulcer treatment may include a lining protectant, such as sucralfate.

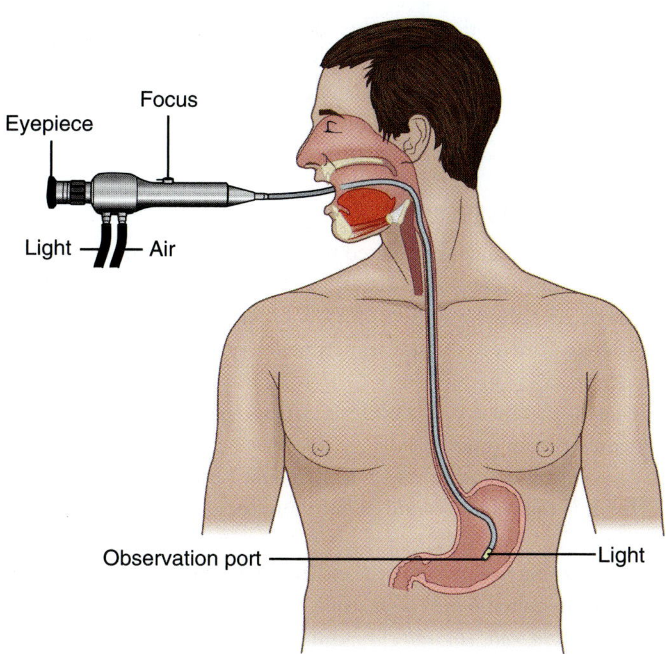

FIGURE 34.7 Upper gastrointestinal endoscopy.

Pyloric Stenosis

Pyloric stenosis is the narrowing of the pylorus, the muscular opening between the stomach and the small intestine. It occurs more often in males than females and in infants younger than 6 months.

The exact etiology is unknown, but there is a genetic link. Other risk factors include taking certain antibiotics, hyperacidity in the duodenum, and diseases such as type 1 diabetes mellitus. Vomiting is the most common sign. It can occur after feedings, may be *projectile* (forceful), and usually starts around 3 weeks of age. Other signs and symptoms include weight loss, constant hunger, dehydration, burping, abdominal pain, and a wavelike motion of the abdomen just before vomiting. Upon physical exam, the provider may feel an olive-sized mass in the upper abdomen.

The provider will order an abdominal ultrasound and possibly a UGI series to detect the stenosis, in addition to blood tests to identify electrolyte imbalances. Treatment depends on the severity of the stenosis and may include surgery to widen the pylorus (*pyloromyotomy*). If surgery cannot be done, an endoscope is inserted in the upper GI tract, and a balloon is inflated to widen the pylorus. Medications or a feeding tube may also be used to relax the pylorus.

Additional Esophageal and Stomach Diseases and Disorders

The following are additional diseases and disorders of the esophagus:

- *Achalasia:* The lower esophageal sphincter does not relax. Also, the esophageal peristalsis is reduced. Both factors delay the emptying of the food from the esophagus.
- *Barrett esophagus:* Caused by GERD; the lining of the esophagus changes to resemble the lining of the intestines; this can lead to a potentially fatal condition called *esophageal adenocarcinoma.*
- *Esophageal atresia:* The esophagus ends in a blind pouch and does not connect to the stomach.
- *Esophageal varices:* Enlarged veins in the esophagus, usually associated with severe liver disease; the veins can leak or rupture, causing life-threatening bleeding.

Additional diseases and disorders of the stomach include the following:

- *Cyclic vomiting syndrome* (CVS): Causes sudden, repeated episodes of severe nausea and vomiting; vomiting episodes usually occur at the same time each day and last for about the same amount of time.
- *Dumping syndrome:* Rapid gastric emptying; occurs when foods (most commonly carbohydrates) empty too quickly into the duodenum; can occur after bypass surgery or other types of bariatric surgeries for weight loss.
- *Gastritis:* Inflammation of the stomach lining; caused by bacteria, pain relievers, and alcohol.
- *Gastroparesis:* Stomach motility is slowed, causing delayed gastric emptying; can be caused by certain medications (e.g., opioids, antidepressants, and antihypertensives).
- *Hypochlorhydria:* Deficiency in the hydrochloric acid in the stomach, which can lead to improper digestion, lack of nutrient absorption, infections, and other health issues.

INTESTINAL DISEASES AND DISORDERS

Many intestinal diseases and disorders occur in adults, but some conditions affect children. The following sections describe common diseases and disorders of the intestine.

Acute Appendicitis

Appendicitis is an inflammation of the appendix. Commonly, it occurs between the ages of 10 and 30, though it can occur at any age.

The etiology is a blockage in the appendix that can increase pressure, affect blood flow, and cause inflammation. If the blockage is not treated, the appendix can burst and cause *peritonitis* (inflammation of the peritoneum), a life-threatening condition. The pain usually begins near the umbilicus and then moves to the lower right side of the abdomen. **Rebound pain** can occur with peritonitis. Additional signs and symptoms include low fever, abdominal bloating, anorexia, nausea, vomiting, constipation, diarrhea, and an inability to pass gas.

After the physical exam, blood and urine laboratory tests will be performed to rule out other conditions. A complete blood count (CBC) will show an elevated white blood cell count. Imaging tests (e.g., x-ray, computed tomography [CT] scan, and abdominal ultrasound [US]) will be done to confirm appendicitis or rule out other conditions. Treatments consist of antibiotics and an appendectomy. Laparoscopic surgery will result in a few small incisions. If a laparotomy is done, the incision may be 2 to 4 inches long. If the appendix bursts and an abscess forms, surgery may be delayed while the abscess is drained.

Celiac Disease

Celiac disease, also called *gluten-sensitive enteropathy* or *celiac sprue,* is a digestive and autoimmune disorder. When people with this disease eat foods with gluten, their immune system damages their small intestine. Gluten, a protein, is found in barley, rye, wheat, spelt, and triticale. It can also be found in other products, including vitamins and supplements, toothpaste, lip balm, and hair and skin products.

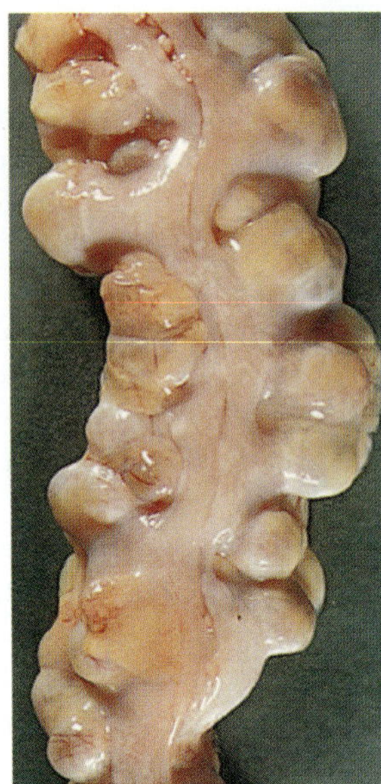

FIGURE 34.8 Diverticulitis. (From Damjanov I: *Pathology: a color atlas*, St. Louis, 2000, Mosby.)

Celiac disease is a genetic autoimmune disorder. The signs and symptoms of celiac disease can vary depending on the age of the person:

- Young children: Abdominal pain, vomiting, diarrhea, bloating, and constipation; irritability, emotional withdrawal, or very dependent behavior; failure to gain weight and grow; and obesity.
- Teenagers: Diarrhea, constipation, delayed puberty, hair loss, slowed growth, and short height.
- Adults: Diarrhea, constipation, fatigue, bone or joint pain, depression, anxiety, irritability, missed menstrual periods, anemia, and osteoporosis.
- Celiac disease can also cause lactose intolerance, anemia, dermatitis herpetiformis (an itchy, blistering skin condition), and canker sores in the mouth.

The provider will perform a history and physical exam. Blood tests and an intestinal biopsy may be ordered. Treatment consists of a gluten-free diet. Foods that are safe to eat include rice, oats, corn, quinoa, millet, and buckwheat.

Diverticulitis

Diverticula are small marble-sized pouches that form in the large intestine (Figure 34.8). The pouches protrude through the weakened walls of the large intestine. These pouches are common after age 40 and usually do not cause symptoms unless they become inflamed or infected. When the diverticula become inflamed or infected, the condition is called *diverticulitis.*

When a diverticulum tears, inflammation and infection can occur. Risk factors include aging, obesity, smoking cigarettes, lack of exercise, a low-fiber diet, and a high saturated fat diet. Medications such as steroids, opioids, and NSAIDs can also increase the risk. Signs and symptoms of diverticulitis include constant lower left abdomen pain and tenderness, nausea, vomiting, diarrhea, constipation, and fever.

After a physical exam, the provider will order imaging and medical laboratory tests. Blood and urine tests are used to rule out infection, pregnancy, and liver disease. A CT scan can identify the inflamed pouches, thus confirming the diagnosis. Treatment depends on the symptoms. Antibiotics, over-the-counter (OTC) analgesics, and a liquid diet may be recommended. With severe attacks, intravenous (IV) antibiotics are given, and abscesses, if present, are drained. A primary bowel **resection** or a bowel resection with a **colostomy** may be done.

Foodborne Illnesses

Eating or drinking contaminated food can result in a food-borne illness. Typically, food-borne diseases and disorders are acute illnesses, which occur suddenly and last for a short time. Most people recover without treatments, though sometimes more serious complications can occur.

Many different types of bacteria, viruses, parasites, and chemicals can contaminate food:

- *Salmonella:* Found in raw or undercooked meat, poultry, and seafood. It can also be found in dairy products, eggshells, and inside eggs.
- *Shigella:* Bacterium that spreads to others from one infected person's unwashed hands after using the bathroom.
- *Escherichia coli (E. coli):* Found in raw or undercooked hamburger, unpasteurized milk and fruit juices, and fresh produce.
- *Listeria monocytogenes:* Found in raw and undercooked meats, unpasteurized milk, deli meats, soft cheeses, and hot dogs.
- *Clostridium botulinum:* Found in improperly canned foods and smoked and salted fish.
- *Norovirus:* Found in foods prepared by infectious food handlers; can cause inflammation of the intestines and stomach.
- *Hepatitis A:* A virus spread through food or drinks contaminated with a small amount of stool from an infected person.
- *Trichinella spiralis:* A roundworm parasite found in raw or undercooked pork or wild game.

Common signs and symptoms include vomiting, diarrhea, abdominal pain, chills, and fever. Symptoms may last for a few hours to a few days. Complications can lead to dehydration, **hemolytic uremic syndrome,** and other disorders, such as reactive arthritis and irritable bowel syndrome.

After a physical exam, the provider may order a stool culture and blood work. Treatment consists of replacing lost fluids and electrolytes. Over-the-counter antidiarrheal medications such as loperamide (Imodium) and bismuth subsalicylate (Pepto-Bismol, Kaopectate) can help decrease diarrhea in adults. These medications should not be used if the person has bloody diarrhea, which could be a sign of a parasitic or bacterial infection.

Hemorrhoids

Hemorrhoids are swollen and inflamed veins. External hemorrhoids are located around the anus, and internal hemorrhoids affect the lining of the anus and the lower rectum. About 50% of those over 50 years of age have hemorrhoids.

Hemorrhoids can be caused by straining during a bowel movement, pregnancy, aging, chronic constipation, and diarrhea. The most common symptom of internal hemorrhoids is bright red bleeding, which usually goes away within a few days. Anal itching can occur with external hemorrhoids.

During the physical exam, the provider will check the anal area and perform a digital rectal exam. An anoscope, a proctoscope, or a sigmoidoscope may be used to examine the lower part of the large

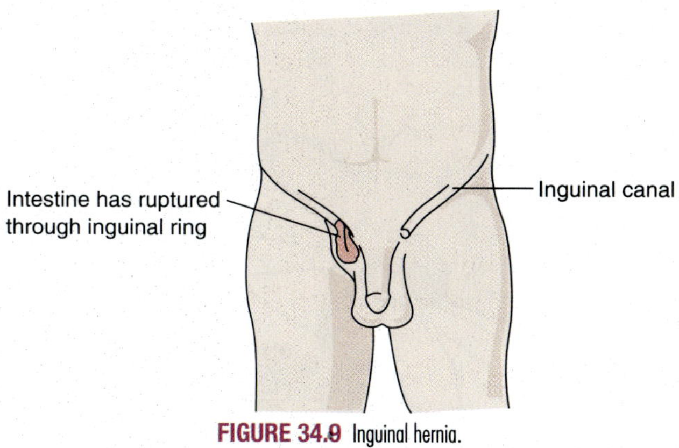

FIGURE 34.9 Inguinal hernia.

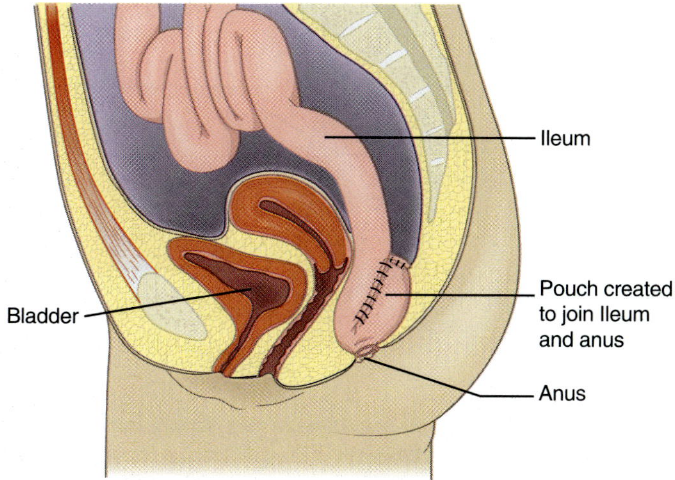

FIGURE 34.10 Ileal pouch–anal anastomosis (IPAA).

intestine and rectum. Home treatment includes a high-fiber diet, topical treatments (e.g., hydrocortisone, analgesic), sitz baths (soaking in a warm bath), cold packs, oral analgesics, and keeping the area clean.

Hernia

A hernia is a common disorder that occurs when part of an internal organ (e.g., intestine) bulges through a weak area in the muscles. The hiatal hernia was already discussed in a prior section. Other types include the following:

- *Femoral hernia*: A bulge below the groin, in the upper thigh. More common in women.
- *Inguinal hernia*: Most common type of hernia. A bulge forms in the groin and may extend into the scrotum.
- *Umbilical hernia*: The muscle around the umbilicus does not close at birth, and a bulge forms.

Inguinal Hernia

An inguinal hernia occurs when tissue (e.g., part of the intestine) protrudes through a weak spot in the abdominal muscles (Figure 34.9). Sometimes people can gently push the hernia back into the abdomen, but other times the hernia may become trapped (**incarcerated**), and blood flow may be cut off to the tissue (**strangulation**), causing tissue death. This can be a life-threatening complication if it is not treated.

For some inguinal hernias, the etiology is unknown. Other times, straining, strenuous activities, pregnancy, or chronic coughing may cause it. Signs and symptoms include bulging on the side of the pubic bone, burning or aching at the bulge, and groin heaviness, pain, or pressure.

The provider will do a physical examination. The patient may be asked to stand and cough, which makes the inguinal hernia more prominent. A CT or magnetic resonance imaging (MRI) scan may be ordered if the hernia is not felt. For a small hernia that is asymptomatic, the provider may just wait and monitor it. Painful or enlarged hernias are treated with surgery (either an open hernia repair or a laparoscopic repair).

Inflammatory Bowel Disease

Inflammatory bowel disease (IBD), an autoimmune disorder, includes two chronic diseases that cause inflammation of the digestive tract:

- *Ulcerative colitis:* Usually starts in the rectum and spreads into the large intestine. Damaged areas are in patches along the intestine. The inflammation may affect many layers of the GI tract wall.
- *Crohn disease:* Can affect any part of the GI tract but most often affects the ileum. Damage appears in patches next to healthy tissue. The inflammation affects several layers of the GI tract walls.

The etiology of IBD is unknown, but it is the result of a defective immune system. IBD has a genetic component, and environmental triggers cause inflammation of the digestive tract. Common signs and symptoms of IBD include persistent diarrhea, abdominal pain, blood in the stool, weight loss, and fatigue.

After the medical history and physical exam, the provider will order imaging tests and endoscopy exams. Stool samples are tested to rule out other conditions. Treatment consists of corticosteroids, immunomodulators, and biologics. Severe IBD may require surgery to remove the damaged GI tract. Common surgical procedures include colectomy, proctocolectomy, proctocolectomy with ileal pouch-anal **anastomosis** (IPAA), and ileostomy (Figure 34.10).

Intestinal Obstructions

Intestinal obstructions are also called *bowel obstructions.* The obstruction can be either partial or complete and prevents stool or food from moving through the intestine. A complete intestinal obstruction is a medical emergency.

The obstruction can be related to a mechanical cause, such as adhesions, hernias, volvulus, impacted feces, and cancers. A nonmechanical obstruction, also called *ileus* or *paralytic ileus*, occurs because peristalsis stops. A paralytic ileus can be caused by infections, certain medications (e.g., narcotics), an electrolyte imbalance, a decrease in intestinal blood flow, or abdominal surgery. Signs and symptoms include severe abdominal pain, cramping, bloating, nausea, vomiting, swelling of the abdomen, loud bowel sounds, inability to pass flatus (gas), and constipation.

Tests to diagnose an intestinal obstruction can include an abdominal CT scan, an abdominal x-ray, a lower gastrointestinal (LGI) series, and an upper gastrointestinal (UGI) series. Treatment includes hospitalization and a *nasogastric tube* (a tube passed from the nose to the stomach), which is used to relieve abdominal contents and swelling. A bowel resection surgery may be required if the

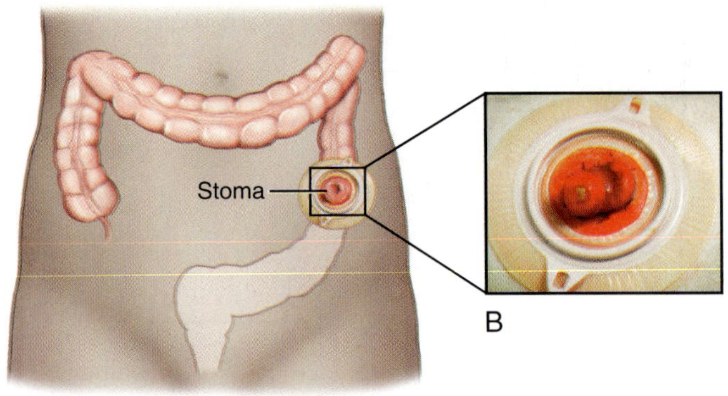

FIGURE 34.11 **(A)** Colostomy. **(B)** The inset shows the stoma. (Potter PA, Perry AG: *Fundamentals of nursing*, ed 7, St. Louis, 2011, Mosby.)

obstruction continues. A temporary or permanent colostomy may be done (Figure 34.11).

Irritable Bowel Syndrome

Irritable bowel syndrome (IBS) is a disorder of the large intestine, although it does not cause harm to the colon. IBS is a common disorder, affecting females twice as often as males. People younger than age 45 often have IBS.

There is no known cause of IBS. Factors that may lead to IBS include changes in peristalsis, severe infection, early life stress, and changes in the intestinal microbes. Stress can increase the symptoms of IBS. The signs and symptoms include abdominal cramping, bloating, constipation, and diarrhea. Sometimes people go back and forth between diarrhea and constipation.

There is no specific test for IBS. The provider may do a colonoscopy, an upper endoscopy, x-ray, or CT scan to rule out other diseases. Treatment for IBS includes dietary changes, stress management, medications, and probiotics.

Additional Intestinal Diseases and Disorders

The following list presents additional intestinal diseases and disorders:

- *Anal fissure:* A small tear (**fissure**) in the anal mucosa that causes pain.
- *Anorectal abscess:* A collection of pus in the anal and rectal area caused by a blocked gland, an anal fissure, trauma, or a sexually transmitted infection (STI). Deep rectal abscesses can be caused by intestinal disorders such as Crohn disease.
- *Bowel incontinence*: Accidental passage of a stool; also called accidental bowel leakage.
- *Fistula:* An abnormal connection between body parts, commonly developing between different organs, such as the bowel and vagina; can be caused by injuries, infections, complications from surgery, and diseases, such as Crohn disease and ulcerative colitis.
- *Gastroenteritis:* Inflammation of the intestinal lining; caused by a virus, bacteria, or parasites. Viral gastroenteritis is a very common illness.
- *Hirschsprung disease:* Congenital disorder caused by malformed intestinal nerves; also called congenital megacolon. Leads to severe constipation and intestinal obstructions.
- *Intestinal ischemia* and *infarction:* Occur when there is a partial or complete blockage in the arteries supplying the intestines. Can cause damage or death to the intestinal tissues.

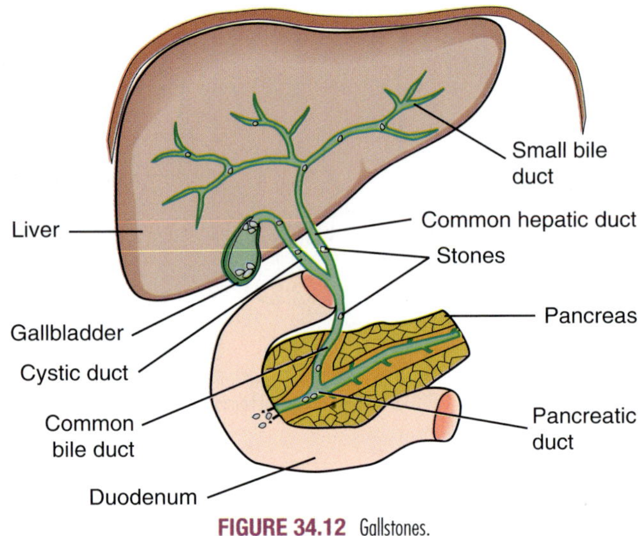

FIGURE 34.12 Gallstones.

- *Intestinal volvulus:* Occurs when the intestine twists around itself and the supporting mesentery, leading to an obstruction.
- *Intussusception:* Occurs when part of the intestine slides onto another portion of the intestine. It can cause an intestinal blockage. The blood supply may be constricted, leading to intestinal tissue death.
- *Small intestinal bacterial overgrowth* (SIBO): Caused when a large number of bacteria grow in the small intestine, which may use up important nutrients needed by the body, leading to malnourishment.

DISEASES AND DISORDERS OF THE ACCESSORY ORGANS

A number of diseases and disorders affect the accessory organs: the salivary glands, liver, gallbladder, and pancreas. The following sections describe common diseases and disorders of the accessory organs.

Cholelithiasis

Cholelithiasis (or gallstones) occurs when the substances in the bile harden and form stones (Figure 34.12). The stones can be small, like a piece of rice, or large, like a walnut. Cholesterol gallstones are the most common type and usually contain undissolved cholesterol. Pigment gallstones are darker black and occur when the bile contains too much bilirubin.

It is unclear why gallstones form, but it may be related to the bile containing too much cholesterol or bilirubin. They may also form if the gallbladder does not empty completely, causing the bile to become concentrated. Females, Native Americans, Mexican Americans, and people over age 40 are at higher risk for gallstones. Additional risk factors include the following:

- Eating a high-fat, high-cholesterol, or low-fiber diet
- Being overweight or obese; losing weight very quickly
- Having diabetes, leukemia, sickle cell anemia, or liver disease
- Having a family history of gallstones
- Taking estrogen-containing medication

If signs and symptoms are present, they may include nausea, vomiting, and **referred pain.** The person may have pain in the upper

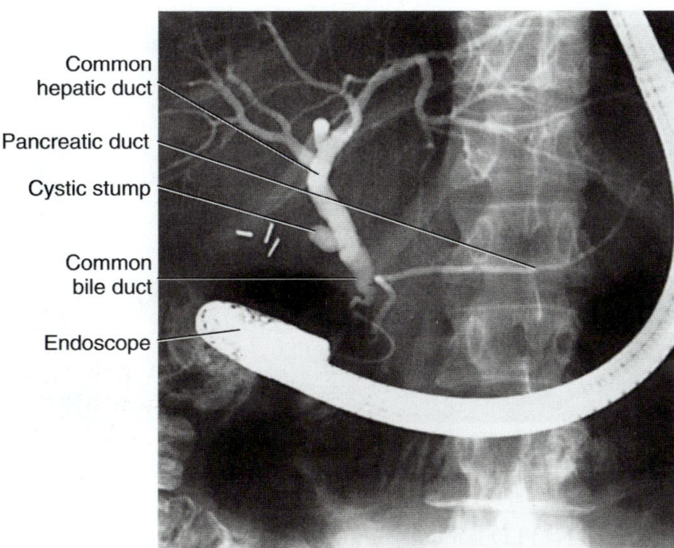

FIGURE 34.13 Endoscopic retrograde cholangiopancreatography (ERCP). (From Frank ED, Long BW, Smith BJ: *Merrill's atlas of radiographic positions and radiologic procedures*, ed 12, St. Louis, 2012, Mosby.)

back, right shoulder, upper right abdomen, or below the sternum. Many of these symptoms are similar to a heart attack; thus they can be scary for the patient.

After a physical exam, a gallbladder radionuclide scan, MRI, or endoscopic retrograde cholangiopancreatography (ERCP) may be done. Treatment is based on the intensity of the symptoms. A cholecystectomy may be done. Gallstones can be removed during the ERCP (Figure 34.13). Patients who cannot undergo surgery may take medications to dissolve the gallstone, although it may take months or years to work.

CRITICAL THINKING APPLICATION 34.8

Keith is rooming a female patient who works as an office assistant. She has had upper back and right shoulder pain, nausea, and vomiting for 2 days. The patient states that she has lost 50 pounds in the past 3 months. She is on oral contraceptives and acetaminophen for pain as needed. After examining the patient, Dr. Martin wants her to have an MRI for possible gallstones. What risk factors does this patient have for gallstones? What signs and symptoms does she have that are related to gallstones?

Cirrhosis

Cirrhosis is a chronic liver disease. The liver cells are damaged and are replaced with scar tissue (Figure 34.14). The scar tissue reduces the liver's ability to function, and over time the liver fails.

Diseases such as alcoholic liver disease, nonalcoholic fatty liver disease, and chronic hepatitis B and C cause cirrhosis. The signs and symptoms of cirrhosis may not appear until the liver is significantly damaged. Cirrhosis can cause nosebleeds, abdominal swelling, hypertension, kidney failure, jaundice, severe itching, gallstones, varices in the stomach and esophagus, and increased sensitivity to medications. Cirrhosis, like other liver diseases, can cause ascites, a buildup of fluid in the space between the organs and the abdominal lining.

Besides a medical history and physical exam, liver function tests, imaging tests, and a liver biopsy may be done. There is no cure for cirrhosis. Treatment of the underlying disease causing cirrhosis can help to slow liver destruction.

Hepatitis

Hepatitis is an inflammation of the liver. It can affect the functioning of the liver. Hepatitis can be an acute or chronic infection, depending on the type. There are different types of hepatitis, including alcoholic, toxic, autoimmune, and viral. With viral hepatitis, there are five main types of hepatitis: A, B, C, D, and E. In the United States, hepatitis A, B, and C are the most common. Vaccines to prevent hepatitis A and B are available.

Hepatitis is caused by alcohol use, toxins, certain medications and conditions, and viruses:

- *Alcoholic hepatitis*: Caused by heavy alcohol use.
- *Toxic hepatitis*: Caused by certain chemicals, medications, supplements, or poisons.
- *Autoimmune hepatitis*: A chronic type of hepatitis caused by the body's immune system attacking the liver.
- *Viral hepatitis*: Hepatitis A virus (HAV) and hepatitis E virus (HEV) are spread from ingestion of food or drink contaminated by infected fecal matter. Hepatitis B virus (HBV), hepatitis C virus (HCV), and hepatitis D virus (HDV) are spread through contact with blood, semen, and other body fluids from an infected person. These viruses can also be passed from an infected mother to her baby during birth.

The signs and symptoms include fatigue, nausea, vomiting, anorexia, abdominal pain, clay-colored stools, dark urine, low-grade fever, joint pain, jaundice, and intense itching.

Besides a medical history and physical exam, the provider will order blood tests to diagnose hepatitis. Imaging tests may also be ordered. Screening for hepatitis C is recommended for adults ages 18 to 79. Treatment depends on the type of hepatitis. Chronic hepatitis may cause liver failure or liver cancer. A liver transplant may be needed. Treatment for hepatitis A and E includes bed rest and fluids. Supportive care is given with hepatitis D. Hepatitis B and C are treated with rest, interferon, and antiviral medications. Antiviral medications for hepatitis B include adefovir, entecavir, lamivudine, telbivudine, and tenofovir.

CRITICAL THINKING APPLICATION 34.9

Summarize how hepatitis A, B, C, D, and E are transmitted. What strategies can be taken to prevent the transmission of each type?

Jaundice in the Newborn

Jaundice in newborns can be life threatening. Jaundice is a condition caused by high levels of bilirubin in the blood. Bilirubin is a yellow to orange pigment that results when heme (from red blood cells) is broken down.

The cause of jaundice in newborns is *hyperbilirubinemia* (excess bilirubin). During the first days of life, red blood cells are produced and broken down at a faster rate compared to adults. In infants, the bilirubin can build up in the blood because the liver is not mature enough to get rid of it. Additional disorders that may cause jaundice

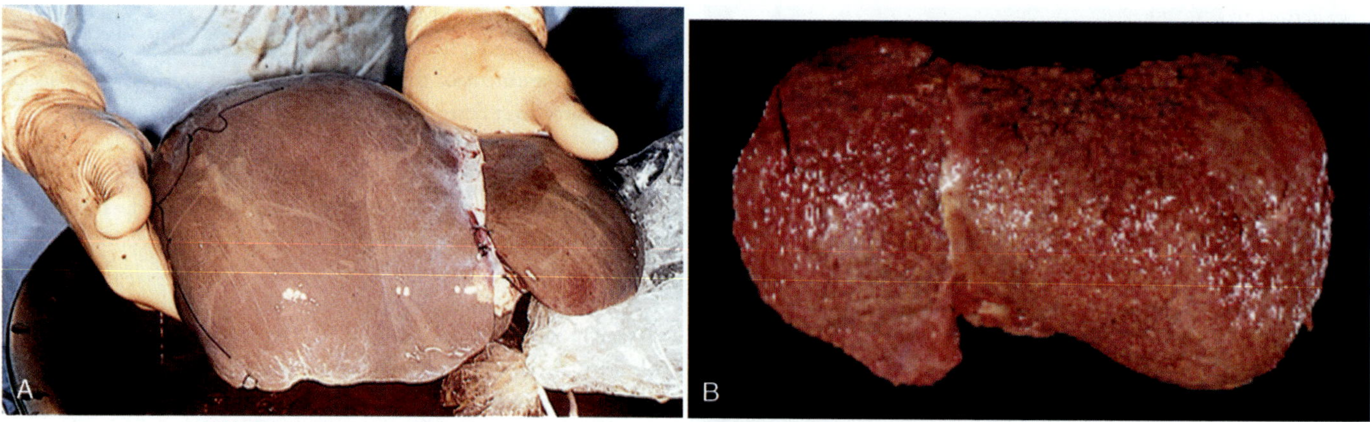

FIGURE 34.14 **(A)** Normal liver. **(B)** Cirrhosis of the liver. (A, from Mahan LK, Escott-Stump S: *Krause's food and nutrition therapy*, ed 12, Philadelphia, 2008, Saunders/Elsevier. B, from Damjanov I: Pathology: *A color atlas*, St. Louis, 2000, Mosby.)

in newborns include hemorrhage, infection, incompatibility between the mother's blood and the baby's blood, liver malfunction, red blood cell abnormality, and an enzyme deficiency. The risk for jaundice also increases with premature birth, significant bruising during birth, and breastfeeding. Signs and symptoms of jaundice include yellowish coloring of the skin and sclera, listlessness, poor feeding and weight loss, and high-pitched cries.

High levels of bilirubin can lead to severe complications in newborns. Acute bilirubin encephalopathy occurs when the bilirubin passes into the baby's brain. Signs and symptoms include listlessness, difficulty waking, high-pitched crying, fever, backward arching of the neck and back, poor sucking, and poor feeding. *Kernicterus* occurs if acute encephalopathy causes permanent brain damage. Signs of kernicterus include involuntary and uncontrolled movements, a permanent upward gaze, and hearing loss.

The provider will do a physical exam and then order a blood test to measure the bilirubin level. Treatment may consist of these measures:

- *Phototherapy:* The infant is placed under a lamp that emits blue-green spectrum light, which changes the structure of the bilirubin molecule. The change allows the bilirubin to be excreted in the urine and stool. Light therapy can also be done using a light-emitting mattress or pad. The baby wears only a diaper and protective eye patches.
- *Intravenous immunoglobulin* (IVIg): Used for blood incompatibility–related jaundice. The immunoglobulin reduces the levels of antibodies and may reduce the jaundice.
- *Exchange transfusion of blood:* Used for severe jaundice.

Nonalcoholic Fatty Liver Disease

Nonalcoholic fatty liver disease (NAFLD) causes a buildup of fat in the liver, unrelated to drinking alcohol.

The cause of NAFLD is unclear. The risks for NAFLD include obesity, prediabetes, type 2 diabetes, high cholesterol and triglycerides, and high blood pressure. Additional risks include rapid weight loss, gastric bypass surgery, bowel disease, and medications (e.g., calcium channel blockers and some chemotherapy drugs). A person with NAFLD may experience fatigue and upper right abdominal pain. If the person has liver damage, then weakness, loss of appetite, nausea, jaundice, itching, leg and abdominal swelling, GI bleeding, and mental confusion may be experienced.

Often NAFLD is found during routine blood tests. The provider may order additional laboratory tests, including a CBC, prothrombin time, and blood albumin level. US, MRI, a CT scan, and a liver biopsy may also be done. Treatment is focused on healthy choices, including losing weight, healthy eating, being physically active, and not drinking alcohol.

Pancreatitis

Pancreatitis is an inflammation of the pancreas. The digestive enzymes start to break down the pancreas. If treated, acute pancreatitis may last a few days, but chronic pancreatitis worsens over time, and permanent damage occurs.

Gallstones commonly cause acute pancreatitis, and patients may have severe upper abdominal pain radiating to the back, a rapid pulse, nausea, and vomiting. Heavy alcohol use, cystic fibrosis, some inherited and autoimmune diseases, and certain medications can lead to chronic pancreatitis. Signs and symptoms of chronic pancreatitis include nausea, vomiting, weight loss, and oily stools.

Besides a medical history and physical exam, lab and imaging tests are used to diagnose pancreatitis. Treatment includes hospitalization, IV fluids, analgesics, antibiotics, and nutritional support (e.g., low-fat diet, enteral feeding).

Additional Diseases and Disorders of the Accessory Organs

The following diseases and disorders are related to the accessory organs.

- *Acute* **cholecystitis:** A sudden inflammation and swelling of the gallbladder, which causes severe abdominal pain; can be caused when a gallstone blocks the cystic duct, causing irritation and pressure in the gallbladder.
- *Mumps:* Caused by a viral infection, which leads to painful swelling of the salivary glands.
- *Primary biliary cirrhosis:* Chronic liver disease causing the bile ducts to be inflamed and damaged, leading to the buildup of bile in the liver.
- *Hemochromatosis:* Causes too much iron to build up in the body, especially in the liver, heart, and pancreas, which damages the organs and causes a bronze or gray skin color.

- *Sialoliths:* The buildup of crystallized saliva deposits blocks the flow of saliva, causing pain and swelling; also called *salivary stones.*
- *Sialadenitis:* A bacterial infection of a salivary gland, usually related to blockage of the duct; can cause a painful lump in the gland, severe pain, high fever, and foul-tasting pus in the mouth.

GASTROINTESTINAL SYSTEM CANCERS

Cancer can affect any part of the GI system. The cause of cancer is a mutation of the cells, which leads to a tumor. To diagnose cancer, the provider will do a physical exam, endoscopy procedures, imaging tests, blood work, and a biopsy. Treatment consists of surgery, radiation therapy, and chemotherapy. Targeted therapy, which uses medications that attack only the cancer cells, can be used for some types of GI system cancers.

The risk factors, signs, and symptoms can vary for the different types of cancer. These are discussed in the following sections.

Oral Cavity, Pharyngeal, and Laryngeal Cancers

Oral cavity, pharyngeal, and laryngeal cancers can form in any of the tissues in the mouth and throat. Males are more likely than females to have oral cavity or pharyngeal cancer.

Using alcohol and tobacco products (e.g., cigarettes, betel quid, and gutka) can increase the risk of these cancers. A personal history of oral or throat cancer, human papillomavirus (HPV) infection, or Epstein-Barr virus can also increase the risk. The signs and symptoms depend on the type of cancer:

- *Oral cancer:* White or red patches, bleeding, or a continuous sore in the mouth, loose teeth, pain with swallowing, earache, and a lump in the neck
- *Throat cancer* (pharyngeal and laryngeal cancers): Continuous sore throat, lump in the neck, ear pain, ringing in the ear, and problems swallowing

Besides a history and physical exam, the provider may order a biopsy of the mouth lesion. A UGI endoscopy and imaging tests, such as CT scans, are used for throat cancer. Treatment consists of the following:

- Surgical removal of the tumor, a laryngectomy, or a pharyngectomy
- *Targeted therapy,* which uses medications that attack only the cancer cells
- Radiation therapy and chemotherapy

Stomach Cancer

About 65% of stomach cancer cases occur in adults over age 65. Diagnosing stomach cancer in its early stages can be difficult because the symptoms (e.g., indigestion and stomach discomfort) can be caused by many other conditions.

Males have a greater risk of stomach cancer. A personal history of *H. pylori* infection or stomach inflammation is also a risk factor, along with a family history of stomach cancer. The risk of stomach cancer increases with cigarette smoking and often consuming smoked, pickled, or salted foods. Besides indigestion and stomach discomfort, other signs and symptoms include bloody stools, vomiting, weight loss, jaundice, and difficulty swallowing.

Besides a history and physical exam, the provider will order UGI endoscopy and imaging tests (e.g., CT scan and UGI series). Treatment consists of the following:

- Surgical removal of the tumor, subtotal gastrectomy (with an anastomosis), or total gastrectomy (Figure 34.15)
- Radiation therapy, chemotherapy, and targeted drug therapies

Pancreatic Cancer

Pancreatic cancer is difficult to diagnose in its early stages because the symptoms are vague and may go unnoticed. This type of cancer spreads quickly, and because the condition usually is diagnosed in the later stages of the disease, it can be difficult to treat.

Risk factors for pancreatic cancer include smoking, long-term diabetes mellitus, chronic pancreatitis, and certain hereditary disorders. Signs and symptoms include jaundice, abdominal and back pain, weight loss, and fatigue.

Besides a history and physical exam, the provider will order an endoscopic ultrasound and imaging tests (e.g., CT scan, MRI, positron emission tomography [PET]). Blood tests and biopsies may also be done. Treatment consists of the surgical removal of the tumor, a partial or total pancreatectomy, radiation therapy, and chemotherapy.

Liver Cancer

Liver cancer can either be *primary* (the initial site) or *metastatic* (spread to the liver from the initial site elsewhere in the body). Primary liver cancer may be difficult to treat if it is diagnosed in an advanced stage.

Risk factors for primary liver cancer include a personal history of hepatitis B or C, cirrhosis, obesity, diabetes, hemochromatosis, and heavy alcohol use. Signs and symptoms include jaundice, right

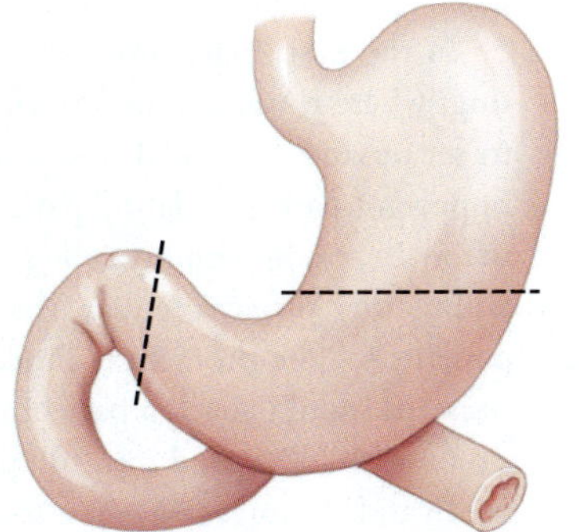
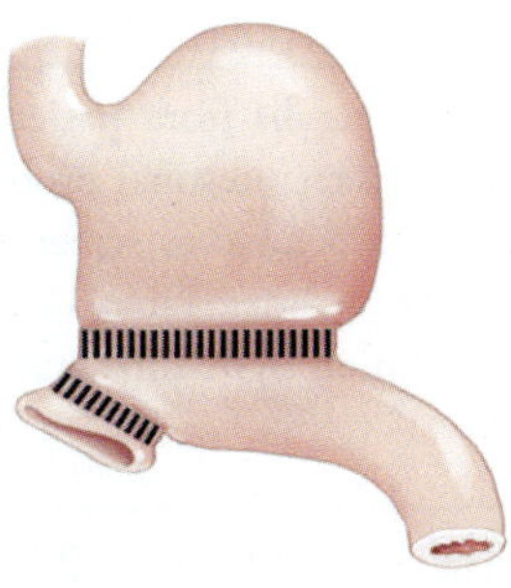

FIGURE 34.15 Anastomosis. Part of the stomach has been cut out, and the duodenum has been anastomosed to the remaining stomach. (From Frank ED, Long BW, Smith BJ: *Merrill's atlas of radiographic positions and radiologic procedures,* ed 12, St. Louis, 2012, Mosby.)

abdominal pain, and a lump in the right abdomen. The symptoms may not appear until the cancer is in an advanced stage.

Besides a history and physical exam, the provider will order blood tests, imaging tests (e.g., CT scan, MRI, and US), and a biopsy. Treatment consists of the following:

- Surgical removal of the tumor or liver transplantation
- Localized treatments, including heating or freezing cancer cells, injecting alcohol or chemotherapy into the tumor or placing radiation beads into the liver
- Radiation therapy, chemotherapy, targeted drug therapies, and immunotherapy

Small Intestinal Cancer

Small intestinal or small bowel cancer can also be called *duodenal, ileal,* and *jejunal cancer.* Adenocarcinoma is the most common form of small intestine cancer.

Risk factors for small intestine cancer include eating a high-fat diet or having a personal history of Crohn disease, colonic **polyps,** or celiac disease. Signs and symptoms include abdominal pain, weight loss, bloody stools, and a lump in the abdomen.

Besides a history and physical exam, the provider will order blood tests, imaging tests (e.g., CT scan, MRI, PET, LGI series, and US), and endoscopic procedures (e.g., upper endoscopy and capsule endoscopy). Treatment consists of surgery, chemotherapy, targeted drug therapies, and immunotherapy.

Colorectal Cancer

Colorectal cancer is also called *colon cancer* and *rectal cancer.* It affects both males and females. Screening is recommended to start at age 45 for those with an average risk.

Risk factors for colorectal cancer include being over 50 years of age, smoking tobacco, and eating a high-fat diet. A family history of colorectal cancer, ulcerative colitis, or Crohn disease also increases the risk. A person with colorectal cancer may experience diarrhea, constipation, bloody stools, cramps, bloating, flatus (gas), nausea, vomiting, fatigue, or weight loss.

Besides a history and physical exam, the provider will order a colonoscopy and biopsy. A carcinoembryonic antigen (CEA) blood test may also be done. CEA is sometimes produced by colon cancers. Treatment consists of the following:

- Surgical removal of the tumor or polyp (*polypectomy*) or colectomy
- Radiation therapy, chemotherapy, targeted drug therapies, and immunotherapy

THE MEDICAL ASSISTANT'S ROLE IN EXAMINATIONS, DIAGNOSTIC PROCEDURES, AND TREATMENTS

Many times, the medical assistant may get calls from patients or parents of patients who are experiencing gastrointestinal problems. It is important for the medical assistant to be able to screen these phone calls and gather information for the provider. Table 34.1 provides possible screening questions for common signs and symptoms (Procedure 34.1).

CRITICAL THINKING APPLICATION 34.10

List three screening questions for each of these symptoms a patient has vomiting, abdominal pain, and diarrhea.

Assisting with the Examination

When a patient describes and points to the location of the pain, the medical assistant must know the underlying organs that may be involved. Record the abdominal quadrant or region in which the pain is located so the provider can immediately assess this area when the examination begins. (See Chapter 18 for a discussion on the abdominopelvic quadrants and regions.)

The provider's inspection of the abdomen begins with noting any change in skin color, such as jaundice. *Striae* (silver stretch marks), *petechiae* (small, purple hemorrhagic spots), scars, and visible masses may be seen. The contour of the abdomen may be flat, rounded, or bulging in localized areas.

The provider uses palpation and percussion to evaluate the entire abdominal area. If present for the examination, the medical assistant should remove the drape from the area to be examined and redrape the patient once this segment of the examination is completed. In addition, the provider may want the medical assistant to document findings as the examination progresses. If the provider wants to examine the anal area, have the patient turn onto the left side and assist the patient into the Sims position. As this is done, make sure the patient remains draped. After the patient is in the Sims position, adjust the drape on an angle so that it can be easily lifted for the final part of the examination.

A digital rectal examination (DRE) may be done to identify abnormalities in the rectum (see Chapter 42). To do the DRE, the provider inserts a gloved, lubricated finger into the rectum to feel for abnormalities in the prostate, bladder, and so on. The provider may use an anoscope to examine the anal area. For this exam, a short speculum is inserted into the anal canal and lower rectum. This allows for the detection of hemorrhoids, **polyps**, fissures, fistulas, and abscesses.

Assisting with Diagnostic Procedures

Many tests and procedures are used to help diagnose gastrointestinal diseases and disorders. Table 34.2 describes common diagnostic procedures. The medical assistant should be familiar with the description of these tests and the patient preparation required. Table 34.3 describes medical laboratory tests for gastrointestinal diseases and disorders. (Refer to Chapter 50 for stool-based tests.)

Colonoscopy

A colonoscopy is a procedure in which the provider uses a colonoscope to look into the rectum and colon. The visual inspection of the colon and rectum allows the provider to see irritation, swelling, ulcers, polyps, and potentially cancerous areas.

In the past, many providers did colonoscopies in the office setting, where it was important for the medical assistant to know how to set up and assist with the procedures. Today, anesthesia plays an important part in sedating patients for the procedure. This is one of the main reasons colonoscopies are now usually done in a hospital or ambulatory surgical center. The medical assistant's role is preparing patients for the procedure. Procedure 34.2 describes how a medical assistant should coach a patient on the procedure.

As with all procedures, the patient needs to be informed of any medication changes or when to not take medications. The provider will determine when the patient needs to stop taking any blood-thinning prescriptions and over-the-counter medications. If the patient is on diabetic, antihypertensive, or heart medications, the provider will

TABLE 34.1 Examples of Screening Questions for Common Complaints

SIGNS AND SYMPTOMS	EXAMPLES OF SCREENING QUESTIONS
Dysphagia	• Is there pain when you swallow? If so, what does the pain feel like? (For instance, is there burning pain?) • Does it feel like a blockage, or something stuck in your throat?
Vomiting	• When did the vomiting start? How often does it occur? • What is the color of the vomit? • Is there anything that alleviates the vomiting? Is there anything that makes it worse?
Abdominal pain	• When did the pain start? • Where is the pain located? What does the pain feel like? (For instance, is it burning, cramping, sharp, or dull?) • Is the pain constant, or is it intermittent? • How severe is the pain? (Use the 0–10 pain scale.) • Does anything relieve the pain? Does anything increase the pain?
Diarrhea	• How many stools do you have in a day? • Is there blood, pus, or mucus in the stool? • What color is the stool? • Is there anything that increases the diarrhea? Is there anything that decreases the diarrhea? • Do you have cramping with the diarrhea? Do you have a stool incontinence?
Constipation	• When did it start? When was your last stool? • Have you tried any over-the-counter medications? If so, did it help?

TABLE 34.2 Diagnostic Procedures for Gastrointestinal Diseases and Disorders

PROCEDURE	DESCRIPTION	PATIENT COACHING
Endoscopy		
Capsule endoscopy	Pill-sized video camera is swallowed, which allows examination of the small intestine. Used to detect bleeding, polyps, inflammatory bowel disease, ulcers, and tumors in the small intestine.	• Food and drink restrictions for 12 hours before the procedure; screen for pacemaker, defibrillator, history of abdominal surgery or intestinal obstructions, and inflammatory bowel disease. • Patient wears a small recording device that receives pictures from the camera. The capsule is excreted.
Colonoscopy	An endoscope is inserted through the anus. Used to visualize the large intestine. Polyps can be removed during the procedure.	• Usually, clear liquids the day before the test. No red liquids allowed. Laxatives or **enema**(s) are used to clean the bowel. May have food and fluid restrictions prior to the test. • During the test, air is instilled into the colon. The provider will examine the colon and may take biopsies.
Flexible sigmoidoscopy	A sigmoidoscope is inserted into the rectum, sigmoid colon, and descending colon. Used to diagnose inflammatory diseases, ulcers, polyps, and cancer.	
Endoscopic retrograde cholangiopancreatography (ERCP)	An endoscope is inserted into the mouth and passed through the stomach and duodenum before it is inserted into the bile ducts. Used to treat stones, tumors, or narrowed areas of the ducts. Can obtain biopsies with this procedure.	• Food and drink restrictions for 8 hours before the procedure. Aspirin and other blood thinners may need to be stopped several days before the procedure. • During the test, the patient is sedated. After the test, the patient may feel bloated due to the air introduced into the stomach.

Continued

TABLE 34.2 Diagnostic Procedures for Gastrointestinal Diseases and Disorders—*continued*

PROCEDURE	DESCRIPTION	PATIENT COACHING
Endoscopic ultrasound (EUS)	An endoscope is inserted either into the mouth or rectum. Sound waves are sent out the end of the tube and bounce off the organs. Ultrasound pictures are created on the computer that receives these waves. A thin needle can be passed through the endoscope to take a sample or biopsy.	• Bowel preparation, including laxatives, enema, and a liquid diet may be used to prepare the patient. Food and drink restrictions for 6–8 hours before the procedure. Blood thinners may be stopped several days prior to the procedure. • During the procedure, the patient is given medication to help relax them.
Esophagogastroduodenoscopy (EGD) (also called an upper endoscopy)	An endoscope is inserted into the mouth and passed through the stomach and duodenum. Biopsies can be taken.	• Iron, aspirin, Pepto Bismol, and non-steroidal anti-inflammatories drugs (NSAIDS) are stopped days before the procedure. Food and drink restrictions for 6–8 hours before the procedure.
Proctoscopy	Inspection of the rectum with a proctoscope.	• Bowel preparation, including laxatives, enema, and a liquid diet may be used to prepare the patient. Food and drink restrictions are usually used before the procedure. • The patient may experience cramping during the procedure.
Upper gastrointestinal (UGI) endoscopy	Fiberoptic view of the esophagus and stomach. Used to diagnose GERD, ulcers, cancer, Barrett esophagus, celiac disease, strictures, and blockages.	• Food and fluid restrictions for 8 hours before the test. A consent form must be signed. • An IV sedative is given. Back of the throat is sprayed with a local anesthetic to reduce gag reflex as tube is passed. The patient must avoid driving after the test.
Imaging Procedures		
Abdominal computed tomography (CT) scan	Used to help detect diseases of the digestive system.	• May have food and fluid restrictions prior to the test. Oral or IV contrast may be given. • The patient cannot move during the test and at some points may be asked to hold their breath.
Abdominal Ultrasound (US)	Used to produce a picture of the abdominal organs (e.g., liver, gallbladder, bile ducts, and pancreas). Used to diagnose liver disease, gallstones, pancreatic tumor, abscess, or inflammation.	• Food and drink restrictions for 8–12 hours before the procedure. • During the test, the sonography will spread gel on the patient's abdomen. The transducer is pressed gently on the abdomen.
Computed tomography (CT) colonography, or virtual colonoscopy	A small tube is inserted into the rectum. The lower colon is inflated with gas. CT images are taken of the colon and rectum.	• Usually, clear liquids the day before the test. No red liquids allowed. Laxatives or enema(s) are used to clean the bowel. May have food and fluid restrictions prior to the test. • During the test, air is instilled into the colon. The provider will examine the colon and may take biopsies.
Gallbladder radionuclide scan	Nuclear scan of the liver, gallbladder, and bile ducts. Used to diagnose cholecystitis, bile duct obstructions, and liver disorders. Also known as cholescintigraphy, hepatobiliary iminodiacetic acid (HIDA) scan, and hepatobiliary scintigraphy.	• Food and drink restrictions for 4–6 hours before the procedure. • A radioactive tracer is given IV. The patient must lie face up on the table under the scanner. Images are taken every 5–15 minutes.

TABLE 34.2 Diagnostic Procedures for Gastrointestinal Diseases and Disorders—*continued*

PROCEDURE	DESCRIPTION	PATIENT COACHING
Lower gastrointestinal (LGI) series	X-ray evaluation of large intestine after instillation of a barium sulfate enema. Used to diagnose colorectal cancer or inflammatory disease of the colon. It can also detect polyps, diverticula, or obstructions. Also known as a barium enema.	• Requires a clear liquid diet for 1–3 days before the test. The patient may need to take laxatives or enemas prior to the test. The intestine needs to be clear for the test. The medical assistant should screen for allergies. A consent form may need to be signed. • An enema is given and may cause fullness, cramping, and general discomfort. The patient may need to change positions during the test. After the test, the patient may have white-colored stools for 24–72 hours. A mild laxative or enema may be given to help the barium pass.
Upper gastrointestinal (UGI) series (also called a barium swallow)	X-ray evaluation of the esophagus, stomach, and duodenum after the patient drinks barium sulfate. Used to diagnose swallowing issues, esophageal disorders, hiatal hernia, ulcers, tumors, and GERD.	• May need to eat a low-fiber diet 2 or 3 days before the test. Food, liquids, and smoking restricted prior to the test. Must remove all jewelry. A consent form may be signed. • The patient needs to drink the barium during the test. After the test, the patient may have white-colored stools for 24–72 hours. A mild laxative or enema may be given to help the barium pass.

GERD, gastroesophageal reflux disease.

TABLE 34.3 Medical Laboratory Tests for Gastrointestinal Diseases and Disorders

TEST	DESCRIPTION
Comprehensive metabolic panel	Includes glucose, electrolytes, liver function, and kidney function tests. Some CLIA-waived tests are available.
C-reactive protein (CRP)	The CRP increases with inflammation in the body. May be used as an inflammation marker test for IBD. Some CLIA-waived tests are available.
Fecal immunochemical test (FIT)	Also called the immunochemical fecal occult blood test (iFOBT). Stool test that detects human hemoglobin from the large intestine.
Guaiac fecal occult blood test (gFOBT)	A test that detects occult blood in a stool smear; a CLIA-waived test.
Helicobacter pylori testing	Includes blood test, breath test, and stool tests, all of which can be used to detect H. pylori. Some CLIA-waived tests are available.
Hepatitis virus panel	Series of blood tests used to detect current or past infection with hepatitis A, B, and C.
Liver function tests	Also called hepatic function panel and liver panel. Measures proteins, enzymes, and other substances. Examples of tests included in this panel include albumin, total protein, liver enzymes (alanine transaminase [ALT], aspartate transaminase [AST], alkaline phosphatase [ALP], and gamma-glutamyl transpeptidase [GGT]), bilirubin, and prothrombin time. Some CLIA-waived tests available.
Multitargeted stool DNA test (MT-sDNA)	Stool test that screens for DNA markers (cancer and precancerous cells) and the presence of occult hemoglobin.
Ova and parasite examination (O&P)	A microscopic exam that looks for parasites and eggs (ova) in a stool specimen.
Stool culture	Also called fecal culture. A stool exam to test for the presence of pathogenic bacteria in the feces.
Total bilirubin	A blood test or urine test used to measure the level of bilirubin. Some CLIA-waived tests available.

CLIA, Clinical Laboratory Improvement Amendments; DNA, deoxyribonucleic acid; IBD, irritable bowel disease.

TABLE 34.4 Common Treatments Used for Gastrointestinal Diseases and Disorders

PROCEDURE	DESCRIPTION
Appendectomy	Surgical removal of the appendix
Cholecystectomy	Surgical removal of the gallbladder
Colectomy	Surgical removal of the colon
Colostomy	Surgical redirection of the bowel to a **stoma**
Gastrectomy	Surgical removal of part of the stomach (subtotal gastrectomy) or all of the stomach (total gastrectomy)
Hemorrhoidectomy	Surgical removal of hemorrhoids
Herniorrhaphy	Surgical repair of a hernia
Ileostomy	The end of the ileum is brought to the surface of the abdomen through a stoma, allowing waste to drain from the body
Laparoscopic surgery	Surgical procedure using a laparoscope; several small incisions are made in the abdominal wall
Laryngectomy	Surgical removal of all or part of the larynx (voice box)
Pancreatectomy	Surgical removal of part or all of the pancreas
Pharyngectomy	Surgical removal of all or part of the pharynx (throat)
Proctocolectomy	Surgical removal of the rectum and part or all of the colon
Proctocolectomy with ileal pouch–anal **anastomosis** (IPAA)	Requires multiple surgeries; a proctocolectomy is done, but the anus and anal sphincter muscles remain; a pouch is created with the ileum when it is connected to the anus
Pyloromyotomy	Often a laparoscopy surgery done to cut through part of the pyloric muscle of the pyloric valve

determine how these should be handled. The medical assistant needs to communicate these instructions to the patient.

Assisting with Treatments

Table 34.4 describes common treatments for gastrointestinal diseases and disorders. Patients can also be prescribed a variety of medications. The following are some of the more common classifications of medications:

- *Antacid:* Used to treat gastric hyperacidity
- *Antidiarrheal*: Used to treat diarrhea
- *Antiemetic:* Used to prevent and relieve nausea, vomiting, and motion sickness
- *Laxative:* Used to increase and hasten bowel evacuation
- *Proton-pump inhibitor*: Used to treat gastroesophageal reflux disease (GERD) and ulcers

Refer to Table 34.5 for information on the medication classification, including indications for use, desired effect, side effects, adverse reactions, and generic and trade names. Medical assistants should be familiar with medications that are prescribed to patients.

CLOSING COMMENTS

Patient Coaching

After the medical assistant coaches a patient on a topic, it is important for the medical assistant to evaluate the patient's learning. The medical assistant should encourage the patient to "teach back" the preparation instructions or information so that she or he can evaluate whether the patient has an accurate understanding of the directions. Any errors or misunderstandings can be clarified. The patient should have a copy of directions or information to take home.

Legal and Ethical Issues

The medical assistant's responsibility is to assist the provider and act as the patient's advocate. All information discussed between the patient and the provider and all testing procedures ordered and done must remain confidential. Confidentiality and trust are closely linked, and these two issues form the basis of a sound patient-provider relationship. The medical assistant is an important part of that relationship and can strengthen it through ethical, professional conduct.

Patient-Centered Care

When coaching patients about diagnostic procedures, it is important for the medical assistant to give the patient a list of supplies (e.g., laxatives, enemas) required for the preparation. Patients may even need directions on where to purchase the supplies. The medical assistant should encourage the patient to call if there are questions or concerns to complete the preparation directions. If the patient is not completely prepared, the procedure may not be able to be done and may need to be rescheduled.

TABLE 34.5 Medication Classifications

CLASSIFICATION	INFORMATION	GENERIC NAME (TRADE NAME)
Antacid	• Indications for use: Treats gastric hyperacidity. • Desired effect: Neutralizes stomach acid. • Side effects and adverse reactions: GI distress, increased urination, metallic taste.	• Calcium carbonate (Os-Cal 500, Rolaids, Tums)
Antidiarrheal	• Indications for use: Controls acute diarrhea and chronic diarrhea related to inflammatory bowel disease. • Desired effects: Decreases the amount of fluids and electrolytes in the bowel and slows down the peristalsis. Some decrease intestinal inflammation. • Side effects and adverse reactions: Constipation, fatigue, bloody stools, stomach pain or swelling, rash.	• Loperamide (Imodium) • Bismuth subsalicylate (Pepto-Bismol, Kaopectate, Bismusal)
Antiemetic	• Indications for use: Prevents and relieves nausea and vomiting; treats motion sickness. • Desired effect: Acts on hypothalamic center in the brain to reduce or prevent nausea and vomiting. • Side effects and adverse reactions: Dry mouth, sedation, drowsiness, diarrhea, blurred vision.	• Ondansetron (Zofran, Zuplenz)
Laxative	• Indications for use: Increases and hastens bowel evacuation (defecation). • Desired effect: Increases activity in the large intestine, promoting stools. • Side effects and adverse reactions: Nausea, bloating, flatulence, cramping.	• Bisacodyl (Dulcolax) • Psyllium (Fiberall, Genfiber, Konsyl, Metamucil)
Proton-pump inhibitor	• Indications for use: Treats gastroesophageal reflux disease (GERD) and ulcers. • Desired effect: Decreases the amount of acid produced in the stomach. • Side effects and adverse reactions: Confusion, drowsiness, arrhythmias, sweating, flushing.	• Omeprazole (Prilosec) • Pantoprazole (Protonix) • Esomeprazole (Nexium)

Professional Behaviors

Diagnostic procedures and treatment protocols, especially medications, are constantly changing. The professional medical assistant must be committed to lifelong learning to keep up with the rapid changes in the medical field. Maintaining a current understanding of the human body, the disease process, and how specific GI system diseases are diagnosed and treated requires a willingness to learn and adapt over time. This commitment to lifelong learning is a crucial part of becoming a professional medical assistant.

SUMMARY OF SCENARIO

Keith has learned a lot from the gastroenterology outreach team. He was able to shadow at the hospital to see several diagnostic procedures. Keith realizes that he will be continually learning with the team. He looks forward to learning more about digestive diseases, diagnostic procedures, and treatments. With everything he has seen to this point, he feels excited about his medical assistant career.

SUMMARY OF LEARNING OBJECTIVES

1. **Examine the anatomy of the gastrointestinal tract.**
The gastrointestinal tract consists of a large, muscular tube that, with the help of hormones and enzymes, digests food. The GI tract includes the mouth, pharynx (throat), esophagus, stomach, small intestine, and large intestine. The small intestine is made up of the duodenum, jejunum, and ileum. The large intestine is made up of the cecum, ascending colon, transverse colon, descending colon, sigmoid colon, and rectum.
2. **Examine the anatomy of the accessory organs.**
The accessory organs include the salivary glands, gallbladder, liver, and pancreas. These structures secrete fluids into the GI tract, aiding in digestion.
3. **Differentiate among digestion, absorption, and excretion.**
After food is ingested, the following three processes occur:
   - *Digestion*: The breakdown of food into chemical substances.
   - *Absorption*: The passage of substances and liquids through the lining of the GI tract into the body fluids and tissues.
   - *Excretion:* The elimination of indigestible materials and waste products of metabolism.

   The chemical digestion of carbohydrates, proteins, and fats occurs.
   - *Carbohydrates*: Saliva contains an enzyme called *salivary amylase*, which starts to break down complex carbohydrates. Pancreatic juices contain *amylase*, which breaks down carbohydrates into sugars. In the small intestine, brush-border enzymes (*sucrase*, *lactase*, and *maltase*) are found in the microvilli and help with the final breakdown of carbohydrates.
   - *Proteins*: In the stomach, hydrochloric acid softens and breaks down proteins and other foods. Pepsin, an enzyme found in the gastric juices, breaks down proteins into polypeptides. Pancreatic juices contain trypsin and chymotrypsin, which break down proteins into amino acids.
   - *Fats:* Bile from the liver is also secreted in the duodenum and emulsifies fats. Pancreatic juices contain *lipase*, which breaks down fats into fatty acids and glycerol.
4. **Analyze the life span changes to the gastrointestinal system.**
Changes in the GI system occur during the first years of life. During pregnancy, progesterone causes the smooth muscles to relax, which affects the digestive system. With age, the stomach empties slower. Aging does not affect nutrient absorption. Constipation is more common with aging.
5. **Examine the diseases and disorders of the mouth, including the signs, symptoms, etiology, diagnostic procedures, and treatments.**
Diseases and disorders of the mouth include orofacial clefts (cleft lips and cleft palates), cavities, gingivitis, herpetic stomatitis, leukoplakia, periodontal disease, and thrush. Refer to this chapter for more information on these diseases and disorders.
6. **Examine the diseases and disorders of the esophagus and stomach, including the signs, symptoms, etiology, diagnostic procedures, and treatments.**
Diseases and disorders of the esophagus and stomach include gastroesophageal reflux disease, hiatal hernia, peptic ulcers, pyloric stenosis, achalasia, Barrett esophagus, esophageal atresia, esophageal varices, cyclic vomiting syndrome, dumping syndrome, gastritis, gastroparesis, and hypochlorhydria. Refer to this chapter for more information on these diseases and disorders.
7. **Examine the diseases and disorders of the intestines, including the signs, symptoms, etiology, diagnostic procedures, and treatments.**
Diseases and disorders of the intestines include acute appendicitis, celiac disease, diverticulitis, foodborne illnesses, hemorrhoids, hernias, inflammatory bowel disease (e.g., ulcerative colitis and Crohn disease), intestinal obstructions, irritable bowel syndrome, anal fissure, anorectal abscess, bowel incontinence, fistula, gastroenteritis, Hirschsprung's disease, intestinal ischemia and infarction, intestinal volvulus, intussusception, and small intestinal bacterial overgrowth. Refer to this chapter for more information on these diseases and disorders.
8. **Examine the diseases and disorders of the accessory organs, including the signs, symptoms, etiology, diagnostic procedures, and treatments.**
Diseases and disorders of the accessory organs include cholelithiasis, cirrhosis, hepatitis, jaundice in newborns, nonalcoholic fatty liver disease, pancreatitis, acute cholecystitis, mumps, primary biliary cirrhosis, hemochromatosis, sialoliths, and sialadenitis. Refer to this chapter for more information on these diseases and disorders.
9. **Examine the cancers of the gastrointestinal system, including the signs, symptoms, etiology, diagnostic procedures, and treatments.**
Cancers of the gastrointestinal system include cancers of the oral cavity, pharyngeal and laryngeal cancers, stomach cancer, pancreatic cancer, liver cancer, small intestinal cancer, and colorectal cancer. Refer to this chapter for more information on these cancers.
10. **Examine the medical assistant's role in examinations, diagnostic procedures, and treatments for gastrointestinal diseases and disorders.**
When a patient describes and points to the location of the pain, the medical assistant must know the underlying organs that may be involved. Table 34.1 provides possible screening questions for common signs and symptoms.

    Table 34.2 discusses the diagnostic procedures for gastrointestinal diseases and disorders, along with the patient coaching for the procedure. Table 34.3 describes the medical laboratory tests for gastrointestinal diseases and disorders, which includes a comprehensive metabolic panel, C-reactive protein test, fecal immunochemical test, guaiac fecal occult blood test, *H. pylori* test, hepatitis liver panel, liver function tests, multitargeted stool DNA test, ova and parasite examination, stool culture, and total bilirubin.

    Common treatments used for gastrointestinal diseases and disorders are described in Table 34.4. The more common classifications of medications used for GI conditions include antacids, antidiarrheal, antiemetics, laxatives, and proton-pump inhibitors.

PROCEDURE 34.1 Use Critical Thinking When Performing Patient Screening

TASKS: Incorporate critical thinking skills when performing patient assessment. Document the patient's history and chief complaint.

SCENARIO 1: You work at Walden-Martin Family Medical (WMFM) Clinic. A patient calls and states that they have had nausea, vomiting, diarrhea, and abdominal pain for 3 days. You need to gather the patient's information before talking with the provider, per the facility's policy.

SCENARIO 2: You work at WMFM clinic. A patient calls and states that they have had vomiting and constipation for 4 days. You need to gather the patient's information before talking with the provider, per the facility's policy.

DIRECTIONS: Role-play the scenario with a peer, who is the patient. Your instructor is the provider.

EQUIPMENT and SUPPLIES

- Phone log and pen
- Patient's health record
- Phone

PROCEDURAL STEPS

1. Answer the telephone by the third ring, speaking directly into the mouthpiece or headset. Speak distinctly, using a pleasant tone and expression, at a moderate rate, and with sufficient volume.
   PURPOSE: Answering promptly conveys interest in the caller. Proper positioning of the mouthpiece or headset allows for an audible tone.
2. Greet the caller, identify the facility and yourself, and offer to help the caller.
   PURPOSE: Giving the facility's name, in addition to the name of the staff member to whom the patient is speaking, lets the patient knows the correct number has been reached.
3. Verify the identity of the caller and the date of birth; access the patient's record. Note the patient's phone number in case you are disconnected.
   PURPOSE: To have the patient's health record ready for reference about the health history and recent care.
4. Determine the caller's needs using therapeutic communication skills.
   PURPOSE: To gather comprehensive information about the caller's complaint and communicate empathetically about the caller's needs.
5. Upon learning the patient's complaint, use critical thinking skills and ask appropriate questions to obtain information about the patient's condition for the provider. Identify the onset, frequency, and duration of the complaint. If related to pain, identify the exact location, quality (e.g., sharp, dull, stabbing), and rating (using a 0–10 pain scale). Identify significant history and factors that increase or decrease the complaint.
   PURPOSE: Gathering relevant information helps the provider form an opinion on the patient's care.
   Scenario update: You know the provider is available, and the patient is willing to be put on hold as you talk with the provider.
6. Discuss the patient's information with the provider. Present the information in an accurate, logical method.
   PURPOSE: Presenting the patient's information in a logical manner helps eliminate confusion and misunderstanding.
7. Upon returning to the phone, give the patient the information from the provider. Conclude the phone call.
8. Document the patient interaction, including the patient's medical history, the provider notified, and the information relayed to the patient.
   PURPOSE: For legal reasons, it is important to document all patient interactions.

PROCEDURE 34.2 Coach a Patient on Preparing for a Colonoscopy

TASKS: Coach a patient on the colonoscopy preparation. Document the coaching in the health record.

SCENARIO: You work at WMFM Clinic. You are working with Dr. David Kahn, who has asked you to coach Charles Johnson (DOB 03/03/19XX) on the colonoscopy patient instructions. Dr. Kahn wants Charles to take his antihypertensive medication the morning of the procedure, 1 hour after finishing the preparation solution.

The ambulatory surgical center requires that Charles not eat or drink anything starting at midnight on the day of the procedure. He needs to arrive 90 minutes before the procedure, which is scheduled for 11 a.m. He will be receiving IV sedation during the procedure and will need a driver to take him home.

Continued

PROCEDURE 34.2 Coach a Patient on Health Maintenance: Colonoscopy—*continued*

PATIENT INSTRUCTIONS

Purpose of the colonoscopy:

- To detect abnormal changes in the large intestine and rectum.

Dietary preparations:

- Two days before the procedure: Do not take fiber supplements or eat foods high in fiber (e.g., nuts, seeds, whole grains, and raw or cooked fruits and vegetables).
- One day before the procedure: Do not eat solid foods; just drink clear liquids (e.g., broth, gelatin, coffee, tea, clear juice, popsicles, and sports drinks). Do not drink red liquids or eat red gelatin. Do not drink or eat dairy products or alcohol.
- On the day of the procedure: Do not eat solid foods or drink liquids other than the preparation solution from midnight onward.

Colon cleansing:

- Split the preparation solution (e.g., GoLYTELY, Colyte) and take half the evening before the procedure. Take the rest of the solution in the morning. The solution must be completed at least 2 hours before the procedure.
- Usually, within 1 hour of starting the preparation solution, liquid stools can occur and continue until 2 hours after completing the solution. Chills, headaches, cramping, weakness, nausea, vomiting, and bloating can occur when taking the solution. Drinking the preparation more slowly can reduce severe vomiting and cramping.

During the test:

- Sedation is usually given. You will be lying on your side on the exam table.
- The colonoscope will be inserted into your rectum. Air or carbon dioxide is pumped into the intestine to help the provider see the lining of the colon. This can cause some cramping.
- The procedure takes about 30 to 60 minutes.

After the test:

- You will need to recover about an hour after the test.
- Do not drive. Plan to have someone bring you home.

Directions: Role-play the scenario with a peer, who is the patient. Your instructor is the provider. Make up the location, date, and time of the procedure.

EQUIPMENT and SUPPLIES

- Patient instructions
- Patient's health record

PROCEDURAL STEPS

1. Wash hands or use hand sanitizer.
   PURPOSE: Hand sanitization is an important step for infection control.
2. Greet the patient. Identify yourself. Verify the patient's identity with full name and date of birth. Explain what you will be doing in a manner that the patient understands. Answer any questions the patient may have.
   PURPOSE: It is important to identify the patient in two different ways to ensure that you have the correct patient. Explaining the procedure can make the patient feel more comfortable and reduces anxiety.
3. Use simple language when talking. Speak clearly. Communicate with dignity and respect. Allow time for the patient to respond. Listen to the patient's concerns.
   PURPOSE: As with all patients, it is important to treat older patients with respect and dignity. Listening is important.
4. Ask if the patient has ever had a colonoscopy. If so, ask what the patient remembers about it.
   PURPOSE: It is important to find out what the patient already knows about the topic.
5. Discuss the purpose of the colonoscopy and the preparation involved. Refer to the written instructions that the patient will be taking home.
   PURPOSE: Referring to the written directions that will be sent home with the patient helps eliminate confusion.
6. Explain what the patient should expect during and after the procedure.
   PURPOSE: Explaining what to expect during and after the procedure will reduce the patient's anxiety about the procedure.
7. Ask the patient to teach back the preparation to you. Clarify any misconceptions or inaccuracies. Answer any questions the patient may have. Give a phone number to call the patient has questions.
   PURPOSE: Using the teach-back method to evaluate the patient's understanding will help identify any misunderstandings the patient may have.
8. Let the patient know when to anticipate the results. Also, give the patient the appointment information for the procedure, including the location, date, and time.
   PURPOSE: Letting patients know when to expect test results helps alleviate confusion and anxiety.
9. Document the coaching in the patient's health record. Include the provider's name, what was taught, how the patient responded, and any written directions (including appointment information) sent home with the patient.
   PURPOSE: It is important to document the procedure in the health record to show it was done.

Documentation Example

08/14/20XX 1105 Per Dr. Kahn's order, instructed pt on the colonoscopy preparation. Patient taught back the instructions accurately. Gave the patient the "Colonoscopy Patient Directions" booklet. Pt was notified of appointment on 08/25/20XX at 11 a.m. at AnyTown Surgical Center. ————————————————— Keith Williams, CMA (AAMA)

ORTHOPEDICS AND RHEUMATOLOGY

35

SCENARIO

Suzanne Peterson, CMA (AAMA) works with Dr. Kahn at the Walden-Martin Family Medical (WMFM) Clinic. Dr. Kahn hired Suzanne right out of school as a new graduate. She has seen a lot in her 20 years as a medical assistant. Many aspects of her day have changed from when she first started as a CMA, but one thing that has not changed is her love for helping patients.

Suzanne was approached by representatives of the local medical assistant program to serve as the adviser for a student who is about to begin her clinical experience. Today, Marissa, the medical assistant student, is starting her clinical experience at WMFM Clinic. Suzanne will be her mentor for the entire 6 weeks. Suzanne is excited but a bit overwhelmed by the thought of guiding a student. She remembers how nervous she was during her practicum experience. She knows she can give Marissa a lot of great experiences.

Their first patient is Walter Biller, who is in his late 40s, is in good general health, is near his ideal weight, and has no chronic conditions. He saw Dr. Kahn a few weeks ago when he experienced worsening pain in his hands and knees. He had been planting in his garden and noticed the next day that he had more pain and stiffness in his hands than usual. Bending down on his hands and knees in the garden was not as easy as it used to be. Dr. Kahn performed a physical exam and ordered lab tests. He asked Walter to make a follow-up appointment to go over the results. Today Walter is back at the clinic, and Suzanne is ready to room him for his appointment.

While studying this chapter, think about the following questions:

- What structures are in the skeletal system and muscular system?
- What are the functions of the skeletal system and muscular system?
- What are commonly diagnosed musculoskeletal diseases and disorders?
- What are the etiologies, signs and symptoms, diagnostic measures, and treatments for the commonly diagnosed musculoskeletal diseases and disorders?

LEARNING OBJECTIVES

1. Examine the anatomy of the axial skeleton and the appendicular skeleton.
2. Examine the physiology of the skeletal system.
3. Examine the anatomy of the muscular system.
4. Examine the physiology of the muscular system.
5. Analyze the life span changes that occur in the musculoskeletal system.
6. Examine skeletal diseases and disorders, including the signs, symptoms, etiology, diagnostic procedures, and treatments.
7. Examine arthritic joint diseases and disorders, including the signs, symptoms, etiology, diagnostic procedures, and treatments.
8. Examine nonarthritic joint diseases and disorders, including the signs, symptoms, etiology, diagnostic procedures, and treatments.
9. Examine muscular diseases and disorders, including the signs, symptoms, etiology, diagnostic procedures, and treatments.
10. Examine the medical assistant's role in examinations, diagnostic procedures, and treatments.

VOCABULARY

acetylcholinesterase (ah SEET l KOE leh nes teeh RASE) An enzyme that destroys acetylcholine and counteracts its action.

adenosine triphosphate (ATP) A high-energy molecule found in every cell that supplies large amounts of energy for various biochemical processes.

aerobic Occurring in the presence of oxygen

anaerobic Occurring without the presence of oxygen

analgesic (an ahl JEE zik) A drug that reduces or eliminates pain.

anticonvulsant (an tee kuhn VUL sahnt) A drug used to prevent or treat seizures.

aponeurosis A tough, fibrous connective tissue that attaches muscles to muscles.

autoimmune An immune response against a person's own tissues, cells, or cell parts, as in autoimmune disease, leads to the deterioration of tissue.

biopsy (BIE op see) Removal of tissue or cells for examination by a pathologist.

callus Hard bony tissue that forms at the ends of fractured bones during the healing process.

cartilage (KAR tih lij) Flexible connective tissue that covers the ends of many bones at the joint.

compact bone Consists of tightly packed osteons; denser and heavier compared to spongy bone.

VOCABULARY—*continued*

fasciculations (fah SIK yeh LAE shuhns) Involuntary muscle tremors and fine movements.

hematopoiesis (hee mah toh poh EE sis) The formation of the blood cells and platelets.

homeostasis The internal environment of the body that is compatible with life. A steady state that is created by all the body systems working together to provide a consistent and unvarying internal environment.

immunosuppressant A drug used to suppress the immune system.

ligaments (LIH gah ments) Supportive connective tissue that connects bones at a joint.

neurotransmitters Chemicals that help a nerve cell communicate with another nerve cell or muscle.

permeability (pur mee ah BIL i tee) A quality or characteristic of a material that allows another substance to pass through it.

process A prominence or projection on a bone.

psoriasis (sah RIE ah sis) A usually chronic, recurrent skin disease marked by bright red patches covered with silvery scales.

red bone marrow Soft, gelatinous tissue that consists of blood stem cells that can become white or red blood cells or platelets. Found at the center of most bones.

remission The partial or complete disappearance of the clinical and subjective characteristics of a chronic or malignant disease.

respiration A metabolic process by which cells break down substances (e.g., carbohydrates, amino acids, and fats) to produce adenosine triphosphate (ATP).

spongy bone Lighter and less dense than compact bone; also called cancellous bone. Usually found at the ends of bones and contains red bone marrow.

synapse (SIN aps) A point of communication between two cells.

tendons (TEN duns) Connective tissue that attaches muscles to bone.

vertebrae (VUR teh bray) A series of small, irregularly shaped bones that form the spine. Each vertebra has several projections, joint surfaces, areas for muscle attachment, and a hole where the spinal cord passes.

INTRODUCTION

Orthopedics is the healthcare specialty that deals with most skeletal disorders and associated muscle, joint, and **ligament** conditions. An *orthopedist* is a physician who is specially trained to diagnose and treat skeletal system disorders. Some orthopedists specialize in certain areas of the body, such as hand, ankle, and foot injuries. An *orthopedic surgeon* is a specially trained physician who medically, surgically, and physically treats musculoskeletal disorders. *Podiatry* is the branch of medicine that deals with the diagnosis, treatment, and prevention of foot disorders. A *podiatrist* is a physician who specializes in treating the foot and ankle.

Rheumatology is a specialty that deals with disorders of connective tissue, including bone and **cartilage**. Rheumatology also deals with many diseases that are classified as **autoimmune** disorders. A *rheumatologist* is a physician who specializes in internal medicine and rheumatology. A rheumatologist treats patients with diseases of joints, muscles, bones, and **tendons**.

Musculoskeletal system diseases and disorders are common in an ambulatory care facility. When they are not seen in the orthopedic department, patients with musculoskeletal concerns are seen in primary care and urgent care settings.

Musculoskeletal System

The musculoskeletal system (MS) consists of bones, joints, muscles, and supportive connective tissues (cartilage, tendons, and ligaments). The musculoskeletal system is responsible for the following functions:

- Body movement
- Protection, support, and framework for the organ systems of the body
- Storage for important minerals such as calcium and phosphorus
- Continually forming new blood cells by the process of **hematopoiesis**, which occurs in the **red bone marrow** inside some bones. Red blood cells, white blood cells, and platelets are all made in the bone marrow.

In this chapter, the discussion of the anatomy, physiology, and pathology of the musculoskeletal system is divided into the skeletal system and the muscular system.

ANATOMY OF THE SKELETAL SYSTEM

Human bones appear in a variety of shapes and sizes that suit their function in the body. Bones generally are categorized by shape:

- *Flat bones* protect internal organs. Examples include the cranium, ribs, and sternum.
- *Short bones* provide stability with their cube shape. Examples include carpals and tarsals.
- *Long bones* support weight and help with movement. Examples include the humerus, radius, femur, and tibia.
- *Irregular bones* have an irregular shape and help protect internal organs. The **vertebrae** are an example of irregular bones.
- *Sesamoid bones* are embedded in the tendons and help protect the tendons. The patella is the largest sesamoid bone in the body.

The human skeleton is composed of more than 200 bones. Bones are divided into two categories: the axial skeleton and the appendicular skeleton (Figure 35.1).

Axial Skeleton

The axial skeleton is composed of 80 bones:

- The skull is made up of the following structures:
    - *Cranium*, which encloses and protects the brain. The eight bones that make up the cranium include the frontal, parietal (2), temporal (2), occipital, sphenoid, and ethmoid bones.
    - *Facial bones*, which include the mandible and vomer bone, and two each of the following bones: nasal, zygomatic, lacrimal, palatine, inferior nasal conchae, and maxillary (also called the maxilla or upper jawbone)
- *Ossicles*, or the three small bones of the middle ear that transmit sound vibrations from the eardrum to the inner ear. The small bones include the malleus (hammer), incus (anvil), and stapes (stirrup).

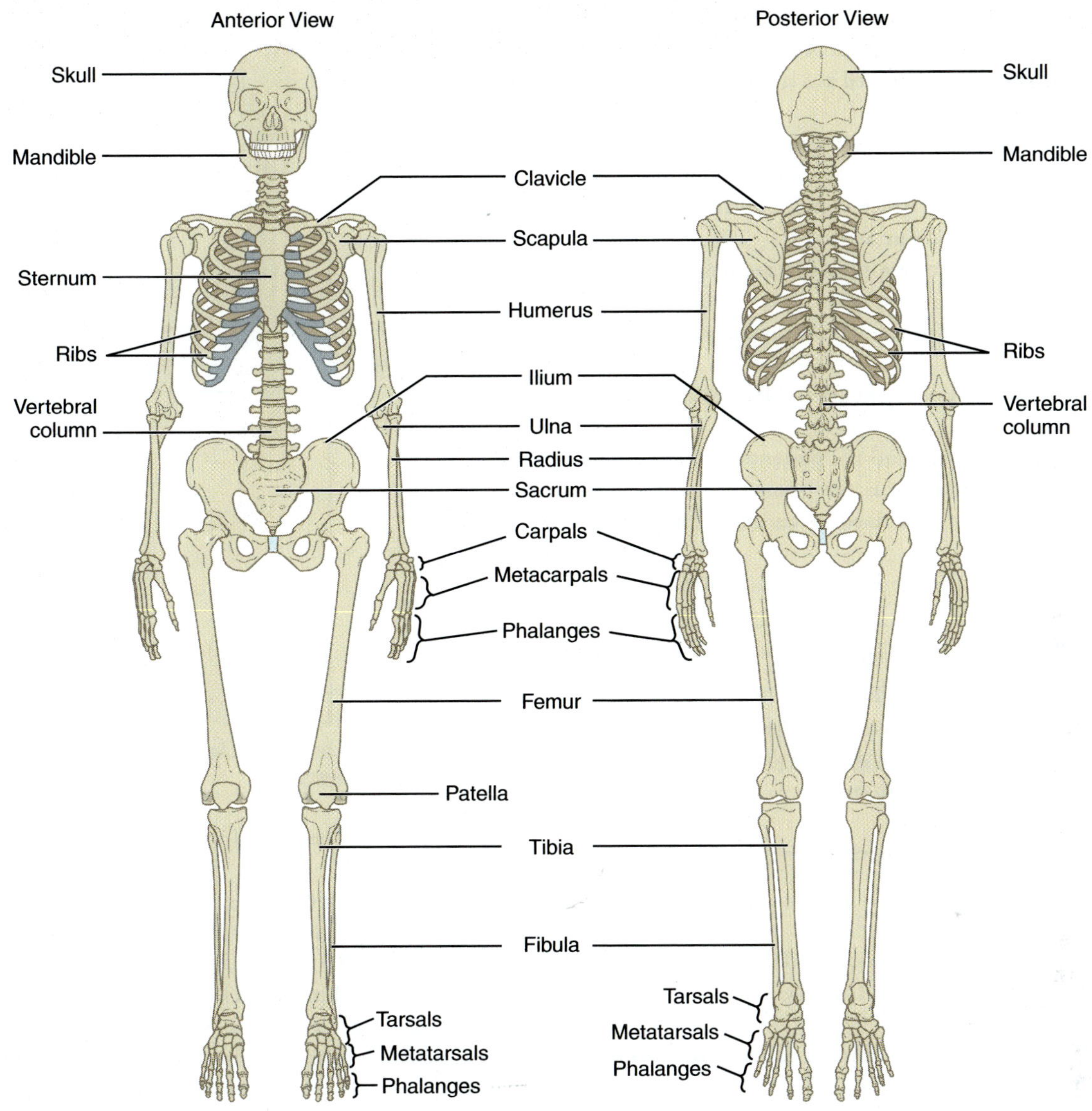

FIGURE 35.1 Axial skeletal bones *(outside columns)* and appendicular skeletal bones *(middle column)*.

- The *hyoid bone*, in the neck above the larynx, is the attachment point for the extrinsic tongue muscle and other mouth muscles.
- The *spinal* or *vertebral column* is divided into five regions: cervical, thoracic, lumbar, sacral, and coccygeal. The spinal column is composed of 26 **vertebrae.** Soft disks filled with a jelly-like substance are between the vertebrae to cushion and keep them in place.
- The rib cage is made up of these structures:
  - *Sternum* (breastbone), which is made up of the manubrium, body, and xiphoid **process.**
  - Seven pairs of *true ribs,* which attach to the sternum by costal cartilage.
  - Five pairs of *false ribs.* The first three pairs of false ribs attach to the seventh rib and indirectly to the sternum by costal cartilage. The last two pairs of false ribs are called *floating ribs* because they are not attached in the front of the body.

The ribs, thoracic vertebral column, and sternum form the thorax.

Appendicular Skeleton

The appendicular skeleton is composed of 126 bones. It can be divided into the upper and lower extremities.

The upper extremities are made up of these structures:

- *Clavicle* (collarbone).
- *Scapula* (shoulder blade); the *acromion process* is the lateral tip of the scapula. The acromion process is used as a landmark when injections are given in the deltoid muscle.
- *Humerus* (upper arm bone).
- *Radius* and *ulna* (lower arm bones). The radius is the bone on the thumb side, and the ulna is the little finger side of the forearm.
- *Carpals* (wrist bones), *metacarpals* (in the palm of the hand), and the *phalanges* (finger bones).

The lower extremities are made up of these structures:

- Pelvic girdle (coxal bone), which includes the *ilium*, *ischium*, and *pubis.* The male pelvis is deep and narrow. The female pelvis is broad and shallow. The pelvic inlet is wider to accommodate the birth of the baby.

- *Femur* (thigh bone), which is the longest and heaviest bone in the body. The *greater trochanter* is a protrusion near the neck of the femur. The greater trochanter is used as a landmark when ventrogluteal injections are given.
- *Patella* (kneecap), which is the largest sesamoid bone.
- *Tibia* (shin bone) and *fibula* (lower leg bone). The tibia is larger and stronger than the fibula, which is on the outer side of the leg. The protrusions on the ankle are as follows:
  - *Medial malleolus*, part of the tibia and located on the inner side of the ankle
  - *Posterior malleolus*, part of the tibia and located on the back of the ankle
  - *Lateral malleolus*, part of the fibula and located on the outer side of the ankle
- *Tarsals*, which form the heel and the posterior side of the foot. The tarsals include the calcaneus (heel bone), talus, navicular, cuboid, medial cuneiform, intermediate cuneiform, and the lateral cuneiform.
- *Metatarsals* (feet bones) and the *phalanges* (toe bones).

CRITICAL THINKING APPLICATION **35.1**

Suzanne is thinking about Walter as she prepares the exam room for his appointment. Walter's hands and knees are bothering him. The hands and knees are both a part of the appendicular skeleton. She thought for a moment and quickly named the major structures in the appendicular and axial skeleton. Can you name them?

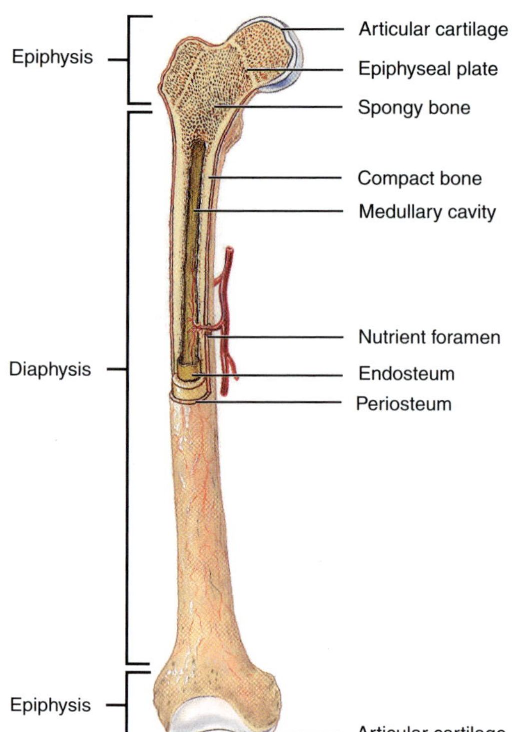

FIGURE 35.2 Long bone features. (From Applegate E: *The anatomy and physiology learning system*, ed 4, St. Louis, 2011, Saunders.)

Anatomy of Long Bones

The outer covering of a long bone is called the *periosteum,* and the inner lining is called the *endosteum*. The long bone is composed of the following parts:

- *Diaphysis:* The long shaft, which is made of hard, **compact bone** (Figure 35.2).
- *Medullary cavity:* The hollow space inside the diaphysis. *Yellow bone marrow* is found in the medullary cavity. Yellow bone marrow is a soft, gelatinous tissue that consists mostly of fat cells and a small amount of primitive blood cells.
- *Epiphysis:* The end of the long bone, which is made of **spongy bone.** The epiphysis is covered with articular cartilage and is attached by ligaments to the epiphysis of another bone, forming a joint. Articular cartilage reduces the stress of weight bearing and the friction of movement. The thickness of the cartilage depends largely on the amount of stress placed on a particular joint.
- *Metaphysis:* The narrow strip between the diaphysis and epiphysis. The metaphysis contains the *epiphyseal plates* (also called *growth plates*). This is where bone growth normally occurs.

Compact bone is made up of structural units called *osteons.* Osteons are composed of *osteocytes* (bone cells) and calcified matrix. The matrix stores phosphorus and calcium for the body to use. The *nutrient foramina* are small passageways that contain blood vessels that supply osteocytes with nutrients.

Joints

Bones are connected to each other at junctions known as *joints (articulations).* The range through which a joint can extend and flex is called its *range of motion* (ROM). Joints can be classified by their ROM:

- *Synarthroses*: Immovable (no ROM) joints held together by fibrous cartilaginous tissue. An example of this joint is the suture lines of the skull.
- *Amphiarthroses*: Limited ROM joints, which are joined together by cartilage that is slightly movable. Examples of these joints include the vertebrae and the pubic bones of the pelvic girdle.
- *Diarthroses* (or *synovial joints*): Full ROM joints. Examples include the hinge joints in the knee and the ball-and-socket joint in the hip. The following section will provide more details on diarthrotic joints.

CRITICAL THINKING APPLICATION **35.2**

As Dr. Kahn examines Walter's hands, he has Walter open and close his hands, wiggle his fingers, grip tightly around two of Dr. Kahn's fingers, and move his wrist. Throughout the exam, Dr. Kahn watches Walter's hands and wrists. Dr. Kahn is looking at the ROM in Walter's hands. Describe in your own words what the acronym ROM means. List the three joint types (based on ROM), and give one example of each.

Diarthrotic Joints

Many of the diarthroses, or synovial joints, have *bursae.* Bursae are sacs of *synovial fluid* located between the bones of the joint and the tendons that hold the muscles in place. Bursae help cushion and support the joints when they move. Synovial joints also have joint capsules that enclose the ends of the bones (Figure 35.3). A synovial membrane lines the joint capsules. This membrane secretes synovial fluid that lubricates the joint. Joints also have cartilage that covers

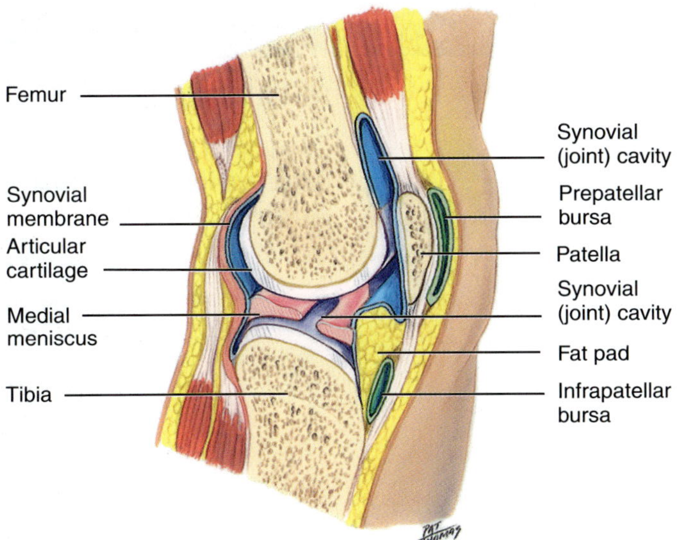

FIGURE 35.3 Sagittal section of the knee joint. (From Applegate E: *The anatomy and physiology learning system*, ed 4, St. Louis, 2011, Saunders.)

and protects the bone. The *meniscus* consists of crescent-shaped cartilage in the knee joint that also cushions the joint. Ligaments are strong bands of white, fibrous connective tissue that connect one bone to another at the joints.

There are six classifications of *diarthroses* (or synovial joints). Each type has its own unique movement.

- *Hinge joint:* Permits flexion and extension (Table 35.1). Examples include the elbow, knee, and finger joints.
- *Pivot joint:* Permits rotation. Examples of pivot joints include the joint found between the atlas and the axis (first and second cervical vertebrae) and the joint between the ulna and radius.
- *Saddle joint:* Allows for flexion, extension, and other movements. An example is the thumb crossing over the palm of the hand.
- *Condyloid joint*: Permits flexion, extension, and circular motion. An example would be the movement of the atlas.
- *Ball-and-socket joint:* Allows free movement (rotation). Examples include the shoulder and hip joints.
- *Gliding joint*: Allows a bone to slide over another bone. This occurs in the wrist and between the vertebrae.

PHYSIOLOGY OF THE SKELETAL SYSTEM

The skeletal system has several important roles in the body:

- Protecting, supporting, and providing a framework for organ systems of the body
- Helping with movement
- Developing new bone
- Regulating the blood calcium level
- *Hematopoiesis*, the formation of blood cells and platelets

The last three roles will be addressed in more depth in the following sections.

Development of New Bone

Between the periosteum and the endosteum, the osteoclasts and osteoblasts continuously remodel bones. The *osteoclasts* are bone cells that break down bone. The *osteoblasts*, bone-forming cells, make the bones strong, durable, and able to heal. Because bones have a good blood supply, they easily heal after trauma or a break (*fracture*).

When a fracture occurs, a protective blood clot and **callus** form at the break. During the healing process, new bone cells start to grow on both sides of the break. Eventually, the new bone from both sides meets, closing the fracture, and the callus is absorbed.

Regulation of the Blood Calcium Level

About 98% of the body's calcium is stored in the bones. Calcium is moved between the blood and bones through the work of the osteoblasts and osteoclasts. It is removed from the blood as the osteoblasts form new bone. This lowers the blood calcium level. When the osteoclasts break down bone, calcium is released into the blood, thus increasing the blood calcium level.

Two hormones work to maintain the blood calcium level. The *parathyroid hormone* from the parathyroid gland increases the activity of the osteoclasts when the blood calcium level is decreased. *Calcitonin*, which is produced in the thyroid, helps lower the blood calcium level. Calcitonin promotes bone formation by the osteoblasts and inhibits the bone breakdown by the osteoclasts.

Hematopoiesis

Spongy bone is found at the center of most bones. It is less dense than compact bone and has a network of open spaces that contain red bone marrow. The red bone marrow is a soft, gelatinous tissue that consists of blood stem cells. These stem cells can become white or red blood cells or platelets.

ANATOMY OF THE MUSCULAR SYSTEM

Muscles attach to bones and are found in internal organs and blood vessels. They create movement throughout the body. Not only do muscles help create movement of the arms and legs, but they also assist with many internal processes, including breathing, digestion, and the circulation of blood.

Types of Muscles

Muscle tissue is composed of muscle cells (also called *muscle fibers* or *myocytes*). There are three types of muscle tissue in the body: skeletal, smooth, and cardiac. Each type has unique functions.

Skeletal Muscles

Skeletal muscles have multiple nuclei and striations that give them a striped appearance (Figure 35.4A). Special fibers allow them to shorten (contract) and lengthen (relax), which creates movement. Skeletal muscles are voluntary, meaning we have control of them. They are found as follows:

- Attached to the bones of the skeleton by tendons. This allows for movement of the bones at the joints and enables the body to maintain posture.
- In the upper section of the esophagus to help with swallowing.
- In the eye to allow for eye movements.
- In the urinary and digestive systems. Sphincter muscles allow for the voluntary passage of urine and stool.

TABLE 35.1 Types of Body Movement

MOVEMENT	DEFINITION OR EXAMPLE
Flexion 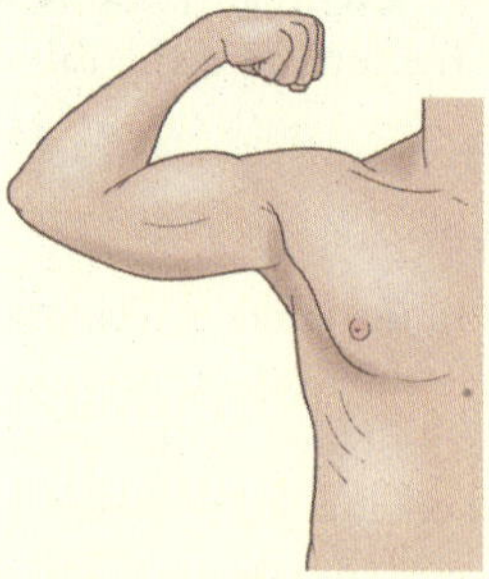	Reduces the angle of the joint and brings the two bones closer together
Extension 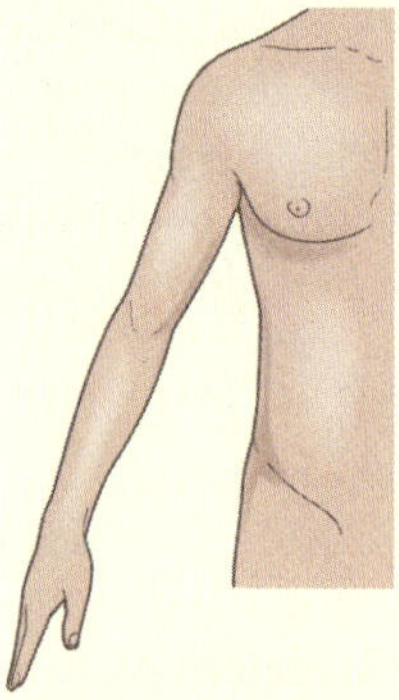	The opposite of flexion; increases the angle or distance between two bones or parts of the body
Hyperextension 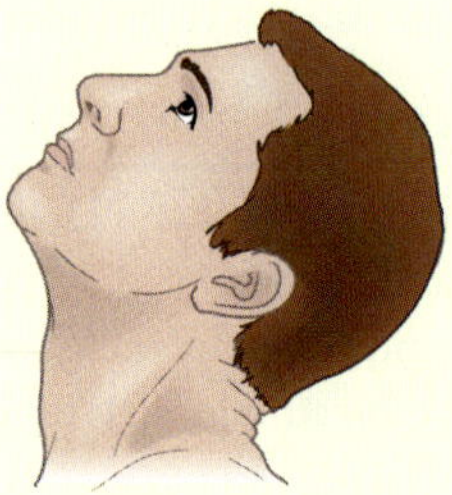	Extension 180 degrees (e.g., the neck is extended backward or the toes are pointed downward)
Abduction 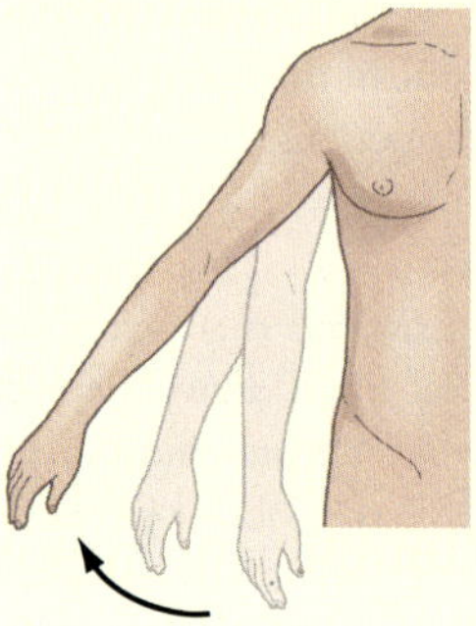	Moving the body part away from the midline or median plane of the body
Adduction 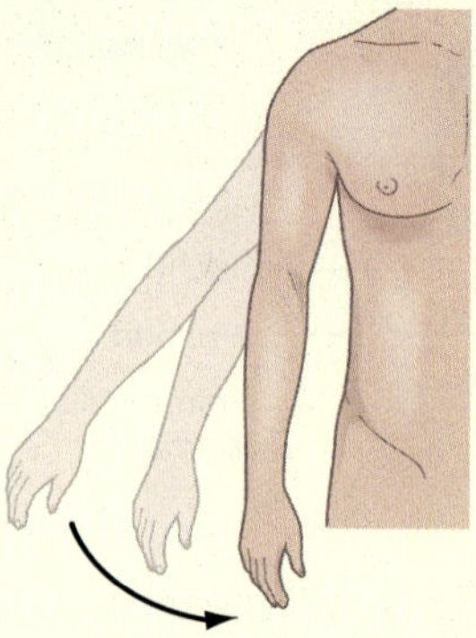	The opposite of abduction; moving the body part toward the midline of the body
Rotation 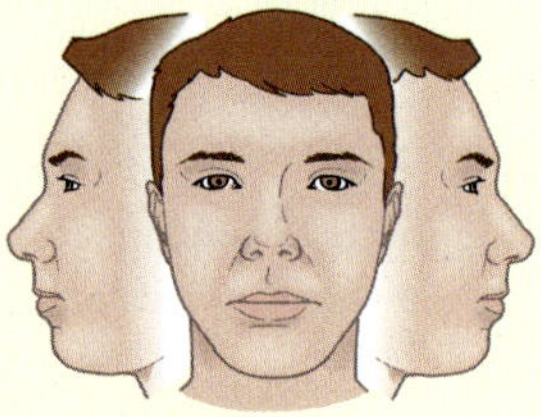	Moving a bone around its central axis; common in ball-and-socket joints
Circumduction 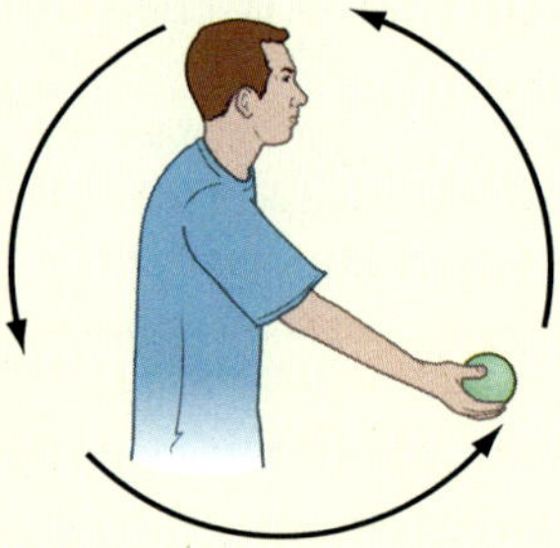	Circular movement of a limb; a combination of abduction, adduction, extension, and flexion
Dorsiflexion 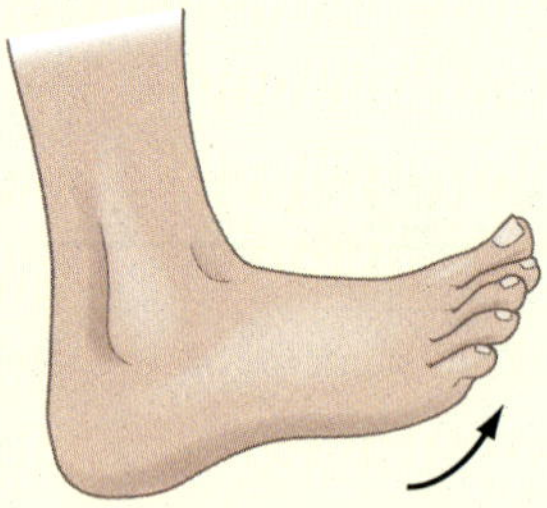	Moving the instep of the foot up and dorsally, reducing the angle between the foot and the leg

TABLE 35.1 Types of Body Movement—*Cont'd*

MOVEMENT	DEFINITION OR EXAMPLE	MOVEMENT	DEFINITION OR EXAMPLE
Plantar flexion	A toe-down movement of the foot at the ankle; increases the angle of the joint	Inversion	The opposite of eversion; turning the sole of the foot medially, or inward
Eversion	Turning the sole of the foot laterally, or outward	Pronation	Rotation of the forearm that turns the palm of the hand downward, or posteriorly
		Supination	The opposite of pronation; rotation of the forearm that turns the palm of the hand upward, or anteriorly

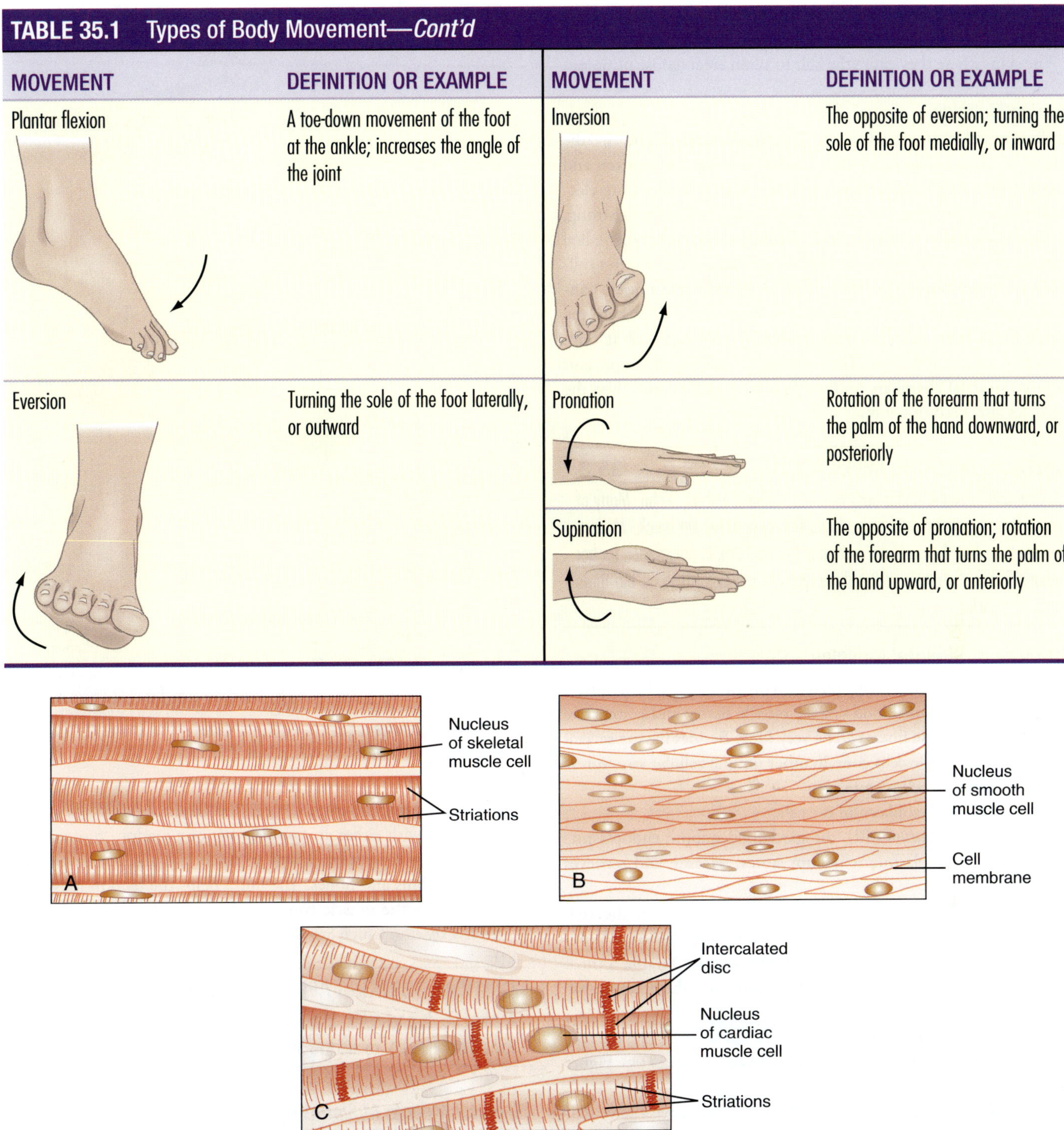

FIGURE 35.4 **(A)** Skeletal muscle. **(B)** Smooth muscle. **(C)** Cardiac muscle. (From Applegate E: *The anatomy and physiology learning system,* ed 4, St. Louis, 2011, Saunders.)

Smooth Muscles

Smooth muscles are nonstriated and have a single nucleus (Figure 35.4B). They are involuntary muscles, which means we cannot control smooth muscles. Smooth muscles contract in response to hormones or **neurotransmitters** (e.g., acetylcholine and norepinephrine).

Smooth muscles are found in the following locations:

- The hollow organ walls of the urinary, reproductive, and digestive systems. Smooth muscles in the urinary bladder, uterus, stomach, and intestines help with movement. These visceral smooth muscles can simulate each other to contract, creating a wavelike motion called *peristalsis.* This motion helps substances through tubelike organs. Peristalsis can be seen in the esophagus, intestines, and fallopian tubes.
- The respiratory system organ walls, where they regulate the airflow into the lungs.
- The walls of the blood vessels and large lymphatic vessels. The smooth muscles change the diameter of the vessels, helping the blood and lymph to circulate.

- The eyes, where they change the size of the iris and shape of the lens.
- The skin, where they cause the hair to stand erect (goose pimples).

Cardiac Muscles

Cardiac muscles are involuntary, striated muscles found in the walls of the heart (Figure 35.4C). Cardiac muscles can shorten and lengthen their fibers for contraction. Cardiac muscle fibers are electrically linked, forming one unit. A myocardial cell forms a strong, electrical connection to the next cells through special junctions called *intercalated discs*. The intercalated discs are responsible for the cell-to-cell communication that is required for coordinated muscle contraction and relaxation of the heart. The intercalated discs help the muscle fibers form one unit that contracts and relaxes all at once instead of a little at a time. The "one unit" approach is important because the atrial chambers need to contract together, and then the ventricles also need to contract at the same time.

CRITICAL THINKING APPLICATION 35.3

Marissa and Suzanne had a busy morning working with Dr. Kahn. Many of their morning patients had musculoskeletal symptoms. On break, Marissa decides to review the muscular system in her textbook in preparation for her national exam. She reviews the three types of muscles. Describe the three types of muscles.

Structure of Skeletal Muscles

An entire skeletal muscle is considered an organ. Each skeletal muscle consists of nerve tissue, blood vessels, muscle tissue, and connective tissue. Skeletal muscle fibers can be very long. Besides having several nuclei, skeletal muscle cells contain other unique cellular structures:

- *Sarcolemma*, the cell membrane.
- *Sarcoplasm*, the cytoplasm in the cell.
- *Sarcoplasmic reticulum* (SR), the specialized smooth endoplasmic reticulum. Sarcoplasmic reticulum stores, releases, and retrieves calcium ions.
- *Myofibrils*, which are proteins that run the length of the cell. Myofibrils are made up of connecting *sarcomeres,* the basic functioning unit of a muscle. The sarcomere contains *myosin,* a thick myofilament, and *actin,* a thin myofilament, which create the striated appearance (Figure 35.5).

A tough fibrous connective tissue called *fascia* covers the muscle. The muscle also contains three layers of connective tissues (see Figure 35.5):

- The *endomysium* is a thin inner layer of connective tissue that wraps around individual muscle fibers or cells. The endomysium contains extracellular fluid and nutrients to help maintain muscle fiber.
- The *perimysium* is the middle layer of connective tissue. Individual muscle fibers are bundled together into *fascicles.* Each fascicle is covered with perimysium. Separate fascicles can be triggered for specific movements; thus, the entire muscle organ does not need to respond.
- The *epimysium,* a dense irregular connective tissue, is the outer layer. All of the fascicles are bundled together and covered with epimysium. The epimysium allows the muscle to maintain its structure during contraction yet move independently in the body.

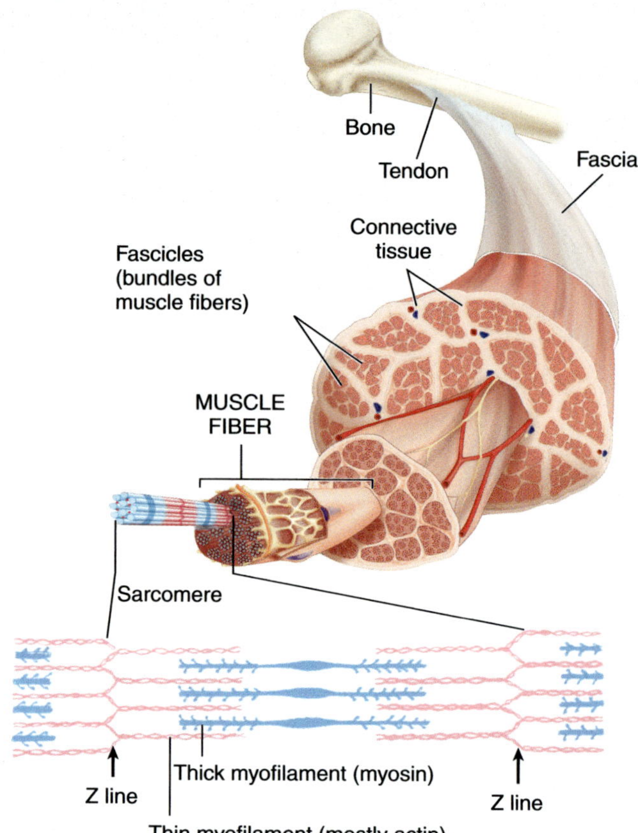

FIGURE 35.5 Structure of skeletal muscle. Each muscle organ has many muscle fibers, each containing many bundles of thick and thin myofilaments. The diagrams show the overlapping thick and thin filaments arranged to form adjacent segments called sarcomeres. (From Patton KT, Thibodeau GA: *The human body in health and disease*, ed 7, St. Louis, 2018, Elsevier.)

- The three layers of connective tissue extend beyond the muscle and mesh with either an **aponeurosis** or a tendon. *Bursae* (small sacs filled with synovial fluid) lie under the tendons or between some tendons and bones. The bursa helps the tendon move over the bone as the muscle contracts. Some tendons are enclosed in *tendon sheaths*, which are lubricated with synovial fluid.

CRITICAL THINKING APPLICATION 35.4

Marissa needs a refresher on the skeletal muscle structure. The muscle contains three layers of connective tissue. Describe each of these layers.

Skeletal Muscle Movement

Most skeletal muscles attach to two bones and stretch across a joint. During a movement, one of the bones is considered to be *stationary* since it does not move. The other bone is the movable bone. The muscle's attachment to the stationary bone is called its *origin*, and the attachment to the movable bone is called its *insertion*. The body of the muscle sits between the origin and insertion (Figure 35.6).

Many skeletal muscles work in pairs or groups, using antagonistic muscle movement for smooth movements. This means muscles contract while other muscles relax. The *prime mover* (or *agonist*) is the muscle responsible for the majority of the movement. The muscles that help the prime mover are called *synergists*. The synergists contract at the same time as the prime mover and stabilize the joint. This

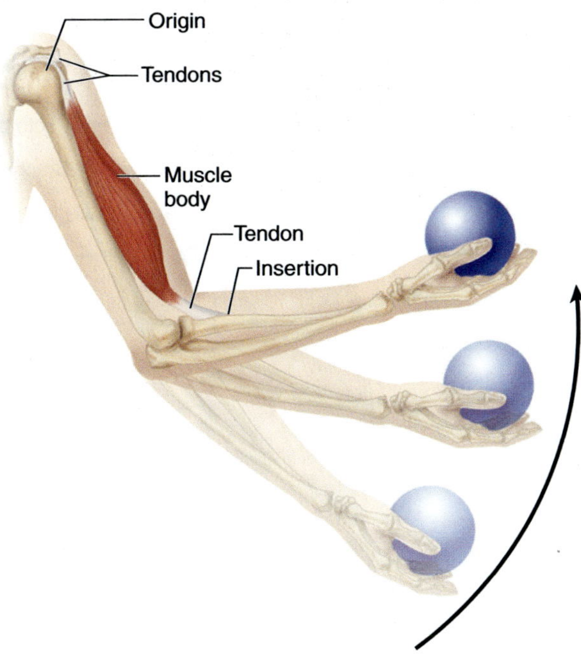

FIGURE 35.6 Attachments of a skeletal muscle. A muscle originates at a relatively stable part of the skeleton (origin) and inserts at the skeletal part that is moved when the muscle contracts (insertion). (From Patton KT, Thibodeau GA: *The human body in health and disease*, ed 7, St. Louis, 2018, Elsevier.)

allows the prime mover muscle to work smoothly. The *antagonist* is the muscle that produces the opposite movement, relaxation. When the antagonist muscle contracts, the prime mover and its synergists produce an opposite movement.

Names of Skeletal Muscles

The names of skeletal muscles are often based on the characteristics of the muscle. Some of the characteristics include size, shape, direction of muscle fibers, number of origins, location, action, and the points of the origin and insertion.

The muscles of the head and neck include (Figure 35.7) the following:

- *Frontal*: Raises the eyebrows
- *Orbicularis oculi*: Closes the eyes
- *Orbicularis oris*: Draws the lips together
- *Zygomaticus*: Elevates the corners of the mouth and lips
- *Buccinator*: Flattens the cheeks, used for whistling and blowing, aids in chewing
- *Temporal* and *masseter*: Close the jaw
- *Sternocleidomastoid*: Rotates and flexes the head and neck
- *Trapezius*: Extends the head and neck; moves or stabilizes the scapula

The muscles of the upper extremities include the following:

- *Pectoralis major*: Flexes and helps adduct the upper arm
- *Latissimus dorsi*: Extends and helps adduct the upper arm
- *Deltoid*: Abducts upper arm
- *Biceps brachii*: Flexes elbow
- *Triceps brachii*: Extends elbow

The muscles of the abdomen include the following:

- *External oblique, internal oblique, and transversus abdominis:* Compress the abdomen
- *Rectus abdominis:* Flexes the abdomen
- *Diaphragm:* Expands the chest cavity during inspiration

The muscles of the lower extremities include the following:

- *Iliopsoas*: Flexes the thigh or trunk
- *Sartorius*: Flexes the thigh and rotates the leg
- *Gluteus maximus*: Extends the thigh
- *Adductor group (adductor longus, adductor gracilis, and adductor pectineus):* Adducts the thigh
- *Hamstring group (semimembranosus, semitendinosus, and biceps femoris):* Flexes the knee
- *Quadriceps group (rectus femoris, vastus lateralis, vastus intermedius, and vastus medialis):* Extends the knee
- *Tibialis anterior*: Dorsiflexes ankle
- *Gastrocnemius* and *soleus*: Plantar flexes the ankle
- *Fibularis group (fibularis longus, fibularis brevis, and fibularis tertius):* Everts (turns outward) and plantar flexes the ankle

PHYSIOLOGY OF THE MUSCULAR SYSTEM

Muscle tissues have four characteristics in common:

- *Excitability*: Ability to react to a stimulus
- *Contractility*: Ability to shorten in response to a stimulus
- *Extensibility*: Ability to be extended in response to a stimulus
- *Elasticity*: Quality of being elastic

Primary Functions

The muscular system has four primary functions:

1. *Muscle contractions provide muscle tone and posture.* This function will be discussed in the following section.
2. *Maintains the body temperature*: A by-product of the energy (**acetylcholinesterase**, or ATP) used for muscle contraction is heat

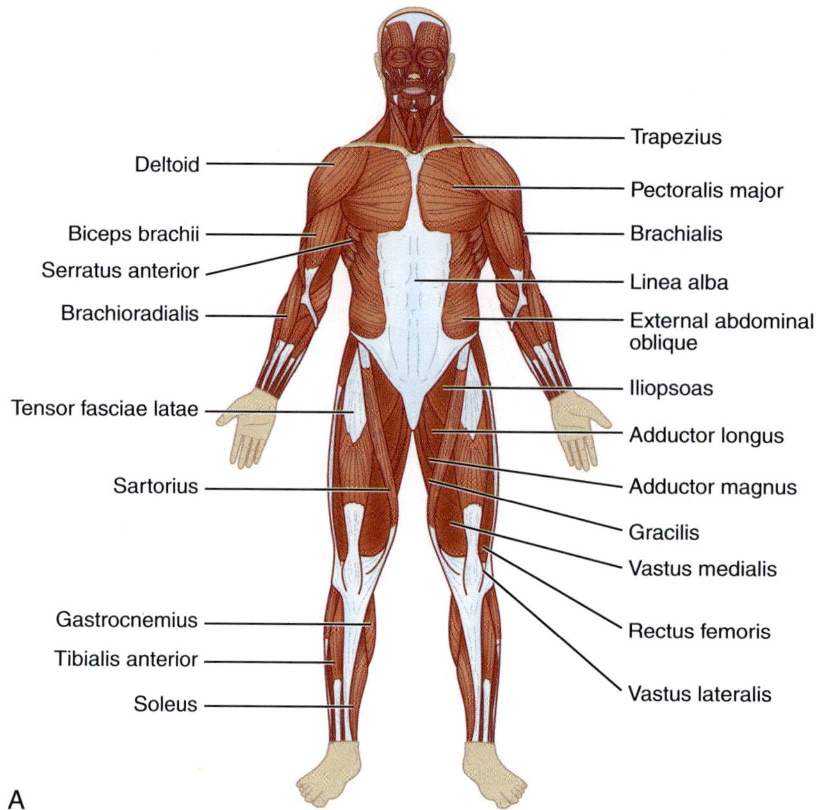

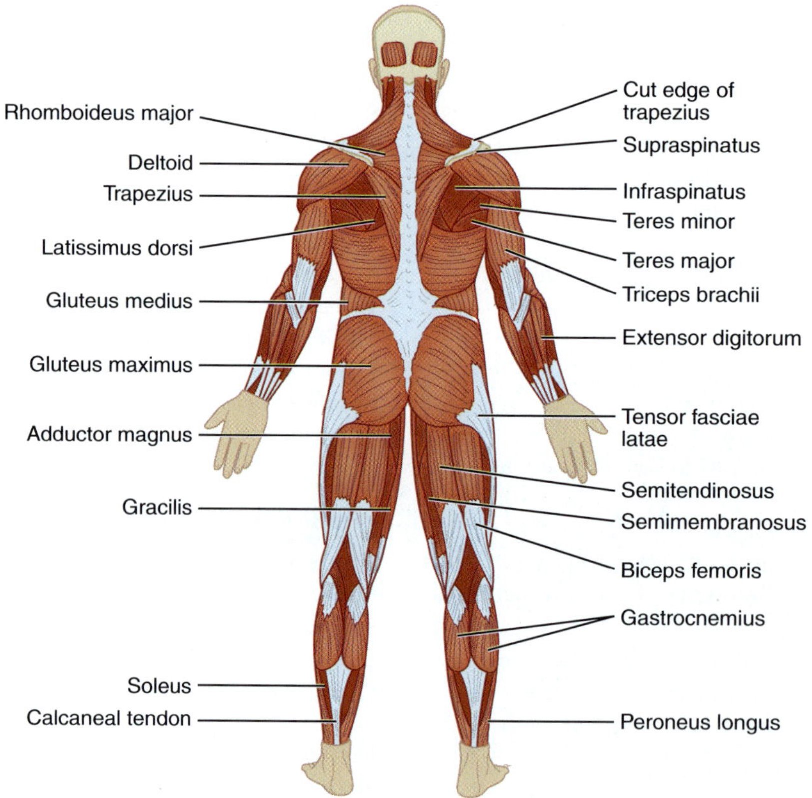

FIGURE 35.7 Muscles of the body. **(A)** Anterior view. **(B)** Posterior view.

production. All types of muscle contractions produce heat, with the skeletal muscles providing the most heat. About 85% of body heat comes from muscle contractions. When a person is cold, shivering (contractions of random skeletal muscles) produces heat. This helps maintain the body temperature.

3. *Provides joint stability:* Muscles and tendons stabilize joints during movement and at rest. The tendons extend over the joint, stabilizing the joint. Joint stability depends on the strength and coordination of joint muscles. Muscle weakness can lead to joint instability.
4. *Controls passageways in the body: Sphincters* are ringlike muscles that open and close body structures, regulating the flow of substances. Involuntary sphincters are found in the digestive tract, urethra, and the iris of the eye. The outer anal sphincter and urethral sphincter are voluntary and allow for a bowel movement and the passage of urine. These two sphincters are made of skeletal muscles.

Muscle Contractions

Before a skeletal muscle can contract, it must be stimulated by an impulse that comes from the brain or spinal cord. The impulse moves away from the brain toward the muscle via a nerve cell called a *motor neuron*. The point of contact between the nerve ending and the muscle fiber is called a *neuromuscular junction* (NMJ), a type of **synapse**. At the synapse, there is a very small gap called a *synaptic cleft*. Neurotransmitters are released by the motor neuron in response to a nerve impulse.

For example, acetylcholine (ACh), a neurotransmitter, must travel across the synaptic cleft to continue the stimulus and generate a muscle contraction. The released ACh triggers a change in the **permeability** of the individual muscle fiber. Then, sodium ions flow into the fibers, causing calcium ions to be released from their storage area in the muscle fiber. When calcium is released, the thin actin fibers slide between the thick myosin fibers, causing the muscle to shorten or *contract*. Muscles need calcium and energy in the form of **adenosine triphosphate (ATP)** to contract. The muscle will relax once the ACh is inactivated by **acetylcholinesterase**, and the calcium ions are sent back to their storage areas of the muscle.

Muscle Fatigue

When you start exercising, your muscles feel strong. After repeating the same movements without rest, the muscles start to feel weaker, the strength decreases, and the ability to contract may be lost. This is called *muscle fatigue*.

For muscles to contract, they need ATP, which is produced through **anaerobic respiration** with oxygen and glucose. If insufficient oxygen is available at the site for use, energy will be created through **anaerobic** respiration. A by-product of **anaerobic** respiration is lactic acid. As the lactic acid builds up in the muscle, it changes the pH of the muscle tissue. This causes a burning sensation in the muscle and leads to fatigue. As the person slows the activity, the breathing depth and rate remain at a high level. Extra oxygen is required (by increased respirations) until the lactic acid has been oxidized. The extra amount of oxygen required to rid the muscles of lactic acid is called *oxygen debt*. This is an example of **homeostasis.** The extra oxygen helps return the energy and oxygen reserves to the normal resting level.

Muscle Tone and Posture. Even when we are not actively moving, our muscles are in a state of partial contraction called *muscle tone*. Nerve impulses help maintain muscle tone, so muscles are ready to act when needed. Muscle tone is an important factor in proper posture. When sitting or standing, the *posture* (or the position of the body) is maintained by skeletal muscles. Muscle tone works against gravity to keep the body in a stationary position.

Types of Muscle Contractions. Besides muscle tone and posture, there are four other types of muscle contractions:

- *Twitch*: A quick, fine movement of a small area of muscles in response to a stimulus.
- *Tetanic*: Sustained and steady contraction response to a stimulus. Muscles can shorten, lengthen, or remain a constant length during a tetanic contraction. Lifting a heavy object with one hand is an example of a tetanic contraction. Tetanic contractions can occur with isotonic and isometric contractions.
- *Isotonic*: Muscle contraction that usually produces movement at a joint. The muscle usually shortens and thickens (bulges), and a task is done. Examples include walking, running, lifting weight, and twisting (Figure 35.8).
- *Isometric*: Muscle contraction usually does not produce movement. There is no change in muscle length, but there is an increase in muscle tension. Examples include pushing against an immovable object, pushing against a wall, and pushing the palms together—there is no movement, but there is an increase in muscle tension.

CRITICAL THINKING APPLICATION 35.5

Walter tells Dr. Kahn about his love of gardening. He loves being outdoors and feeling the dirt on his hands. Dr. Kahn palpates the sore muscle on Walter's forearm and asks about the gardening activities that make the pain worse. Walter replies, "The activities that hurt the most are digging, pulling weeds, and pushing dirt in around the small plants." Which of these three actions are an isotonic contraction of the muscle, and which are isometric?

LIFE SPAN CHANGES

Over the life span, changes occur in both the skeletal and muscular systems. The following sections discuss the changes that occur.

Skeletal System Changes

When the skeleton is developing prior to birth, cartilage and fibrous structures are present. Over time, these structures are replaced with bone matrix, and the bones change size due to the continual remodeling process of the bone cells.

During childhood, bones grow rapidly. The prime time to build bone mass or density is from childhood to young adulthood. Bone density can increase through a calcium-rich diet and regular weight-bearing exercise. Poor nutrition, inactivity, smoking, and excessive alcohol intake can reduce bone density.

The following are common skeletal system changes that occur with age:

- Bones lose calcium and other minerals, which reduces bone mass or density. Bone density starts to decrease around age 30 to 40 in both males and females. It accelerates in women after menopause. The loss of bone density makes the bones more brittle, leading to osteoporosis and fractures.

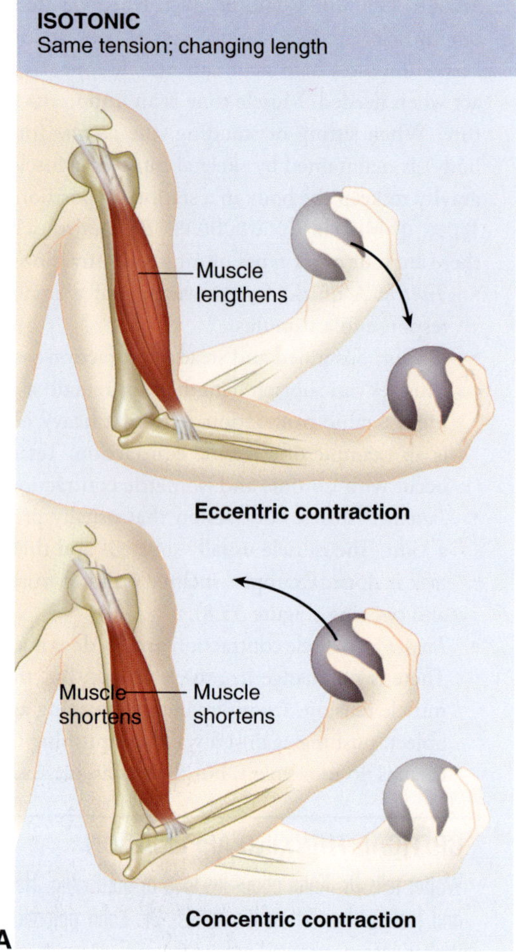

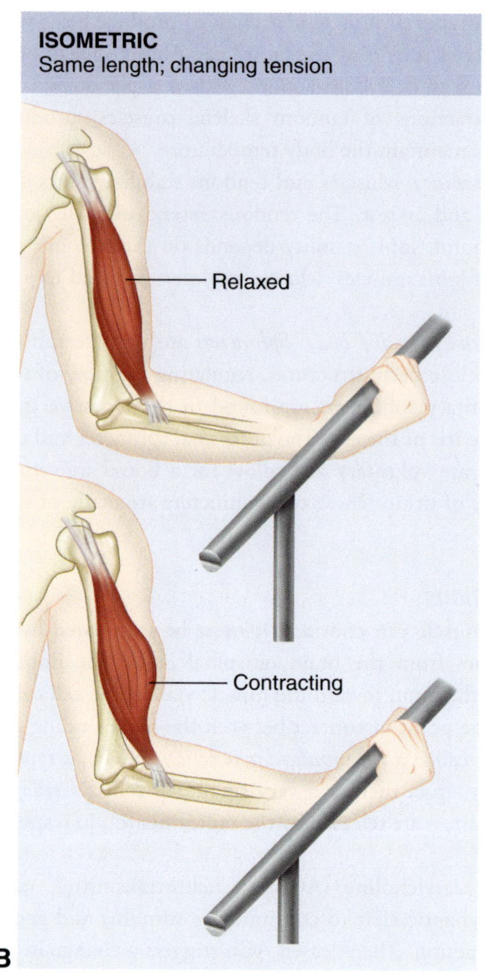

FIGURE 35.8 Types of muscle contraction. **(A)** In isotonic contraction, the muscle changes length, producing movement by either eccentric contraction (muscle lengthens) or concentric contraction (muscle shortens). **(B)** In isometric contraction, the muscle pulls forcefully against a load but does not shorten. (From Patton KT, Thibodeau GA: *The human body in health and disease*, ed 7, St. Louis, 2018, Elsevier.)

- The disks between the vertebrae wear and tear with age. They can dehydrate, and the cartilage can stiffen, causing the disk to bulge.
- Loss of height from the compression and curving of the spinal column occurs, which can cause a more stooped posture.
- Joints become stiffer and less flexible. Synovial fluid decreases, and cartilage may wear away, causing degenerative changes. This can lead to inflammation, stiffness, pain, and deformities.

Muscular System Changes

Men can see muscle changes in their 20s, whereas women are usually in their 40s when changes become obvious. With age, muscle tissue is replaced more slowly and may be replaced with tough, fibrous tissue. This makes the extremities look thin and bony. Muscles have less of an ability to contract. Lean body mass decreases. With the muscle mass changes, older people experience a loss of strength and endurance. They can experience fatigue and reduced activity tolerance. **Fasciculations** are more common with age. People who are unable to move an extremity may get muscle contractures.

SKELETAL SYSTEM DISEASES AND DISORDERS

The skeleton, muscles, and joints together work as a unit to move the body. Diseases and disorders of the musculoskeletal system often affect the ability to move with ease. Here are some common signs and symptoms of musculoskeletal disorders:

- Inflammation
- Pain or swelling in the joints or bones
- Temporary loss of function or loss of normal mobility

The following sections describe in detail some of the more common diseases seen in the ambulatory care setting. Conditions affecting the skeletal system, joints, and muscular system will be described.

Fractures

A *fracture* is a broken bone. With an *open* (or *compound*) fracture, the skin is broken above the fracture (Figure 35.9A). With a *closed* (or *simple*) fracture, the skin is not broken, and no wound is visible (Figure 35.9B). Fractures can also be classified by the type of damage to the bone:

- *Incomplete*: The fracture line does not go across the entire cross section of the bone.
- *Complete*: The fracture line goes across the entire cross section of the bone (Figure 35.9C).
- *Displaced*: The bone fragments are not in alignment.
- *Nondisplaced*: The bone fragments remain in alignment.
- *Comminuted*: The bone breaks into three or more fragments.

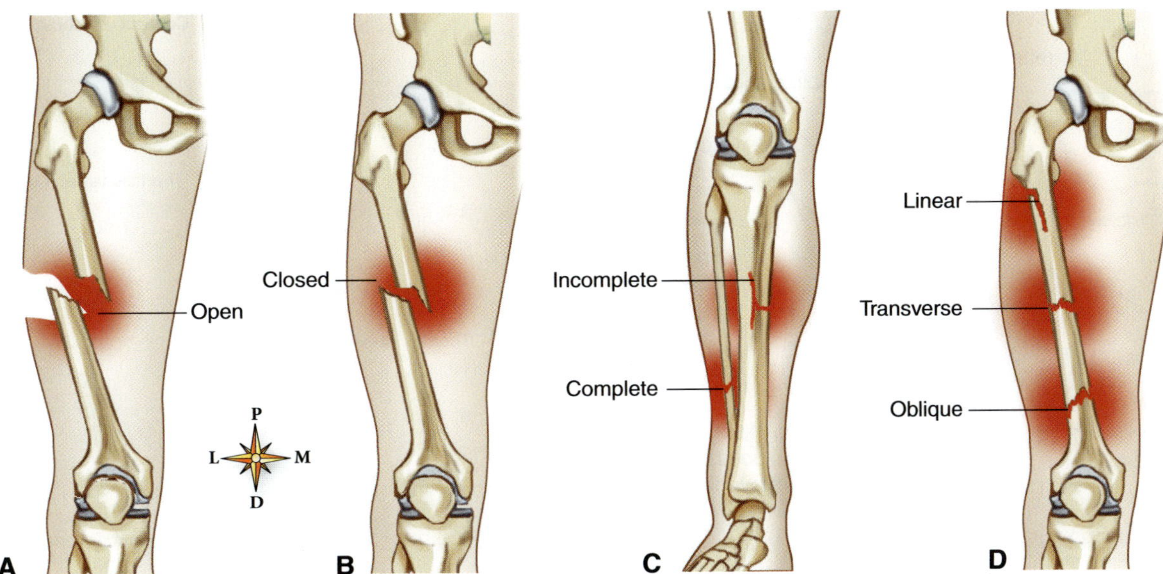

FIGURE 35.9 Bone fractures. **(A)** Open. **(B)** Closed. **(C)** Incomplete and complete. **(D)** Linear, transverse, and oblique. (From Patton KT, Thibodeau GA: *The human body in health and disease*, ed 7, St. Louis, 2018, Elsevier.)

- *Compression*: The fracture results in the bone (e.g., vertebrae) collapsing.
- *Greenstick*: The bone breaks on one side and is bent but still intact on the other side; commonly seen in children.
- *Impacted*: The bone fragments are driven into each other.
- *Linear* or *longitudinal*: The fracture line runs along the length of the bone (Figure 35.9D).
- *Oblique*: The fracture runs at an oblique angle across the bone.
- *Pathologic* (or *spontaneous*): The fracture is due to weakening of the bone structure by a pathologic condition.
- *Spiral*: The fracture line resembles a spiral; caused by the bone being twisted.
- *Transverse*: The fracture runs perpendicular across the bone.

Fractures can occur from trauma, overuse, or diseases. A *pathologic fracture* results from an underlying disease, such as osteoporosis or cancer. Signs and symptoms of a fracture include pain, swelling, bruising, numbness or tingling, deformity, and difficulty using or inability to use the affected area. Bleeding at the site of the break will also occur with compound fractures.

Most commonly, the provider will order an x-ray, but a bone scan, computed tomography (CT) scan, or magnetic resonance imaging (MRI) may also be used as a diagnostic test for some types of fractures. Depending on the type of fracture, treatment may include a cast, splint, or brace to immobilize the area. Surgery will be done if the bones are not aligned. During an open reduction and internal fixation (ORIF) surgery, the surgeon *reduces* (repositions and aligns) the bones and uses *internal fixators* (special metal devices [rods, screws, plates]) to hold the bones in place during the healing process (Figure 35.10). Sometimes, external fixators and traction are used to hold the bones in place. Medications may also be prescribed depending on the severity of the fracture. The provider may order **analgesics** for the pain, anti-inflammatory drugs, and muscle relaxants. Fractures may take several weeks to months to heal. Crutches or other assistive devices may be used for lower extremity fractures. A sling is used for an upper extremity fracture. Physical therapy may be ordered once the fracture is healed to strengthen the extremity.

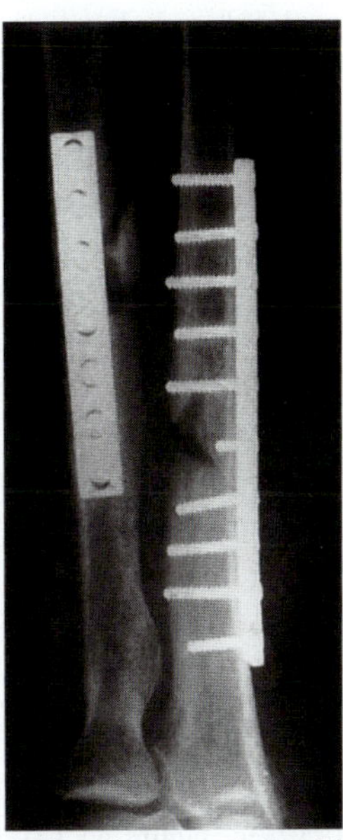

FIGURE 35.10 Orthopedic hardware from open reduction of fractures of the radius and ulna. (From Mettler MA: *Essentials of radiology*, ed 3, Philadelphia, 2004, Saunders.)

CRITICAL THINKING APPLICATION 35.6

A patient comes into the clinic hopping on one foot and holding the other in the air. She thinks she broke her ankle when she stepped off the curb wrong and fell. What tests will Dr. Kahn most likely order? Why?

Herniated Disk

When one of the soft disks between the vertebrae has a crack, some of the jelly-like substance can leak out (Figure 35.11). This is called a *ruptured, slipped,* or *herniated* disk. The leaking jelly-like substance can lead to inflammation and compression of the local nerve.

The disks can degenerate with age. Middle-aged and older men are more at risk for a herniated disk. Typically, herniation occurs with strenuous activities, but it can also occur with lifting heavy objects,

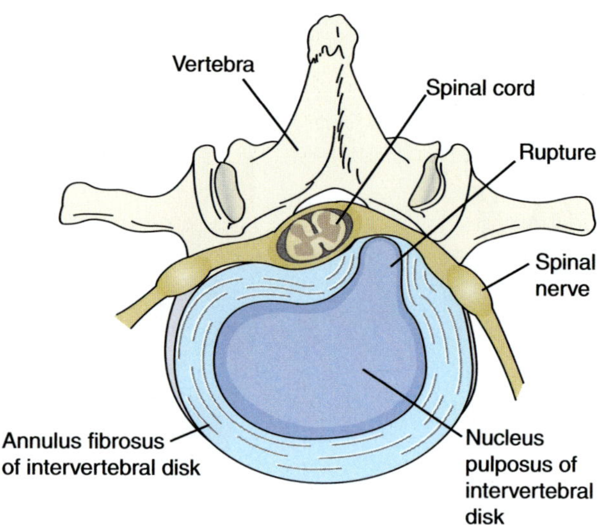

FIGURE 35.11 Herniation of a vertebral disk.

obesity, repetitive movements involving the lower back, long periods of sitting or standing, inactivity, and smoking. Signs and symptoms of a lower back herniated disk include *sciatica* (pain and numbness from the hip down to the foot), back pain, and weakness. The pain usually starts slowly and gets worse with standing or sitting. A herniated disk in the neck may cause pain and numbness from the shoulder down to the fingers.

The provider will check the patient's reflexes and muscle strength. The provider may order diagnostic tests (e.g., myelogram and electromyography [EMG]) and imaging procedures (e.g., spine MRI, spine CT, and spine x-ray). The following are common treatments:

- Medications (e.g., nonsteroidal anti-inflammatory drugs [NSAIDs], narcotics, and muscle relaxants) to help reduce the pain, inflammation, and muscle spasms
- Rest and physical therapy
- Surgery to remove the herniation if the symptoms remain unchanged

Usually, the condition improves in 4 to 6 weeks.

Lordosis, Kyphosis, and Scoliosis

The spine has normal curves (Figure 35.12). Abnormal curvatures of the spine deprive the body of important features related to spinal strength, balance, and posture. The three most common curvatures are as follows:

- *Lordosis* (swayback): An exaggerated forward curve in the lumbar region, which makes the buttock appear larger (Figure 35.13A)
- *Kyphosis* (hunchback): An exaggerated curve in the thoracic region (Figure 35.13B)
- *Scoliosis*: An abnormal side-to-side (S or C) curvature that could be in both the thoracic and lumbar regions of the back (Figure 35.13C)

Lordosis is caused by genetic and congenital conditions (e.g., muscular dystrophy, spondylolisthesis). Kyphosis can occur at any age, but it more commonly occurs in adults due to degenerative diseases of the spine, fractures, and injury. Kyphosis can also be caused by Paget disease, muscular dystrophy, scoliosis, and tumors. Many times, scoliosis occurs in children from age 10 to early teens, and the cause is unknown. Abnormalities in any of the spinal curves can

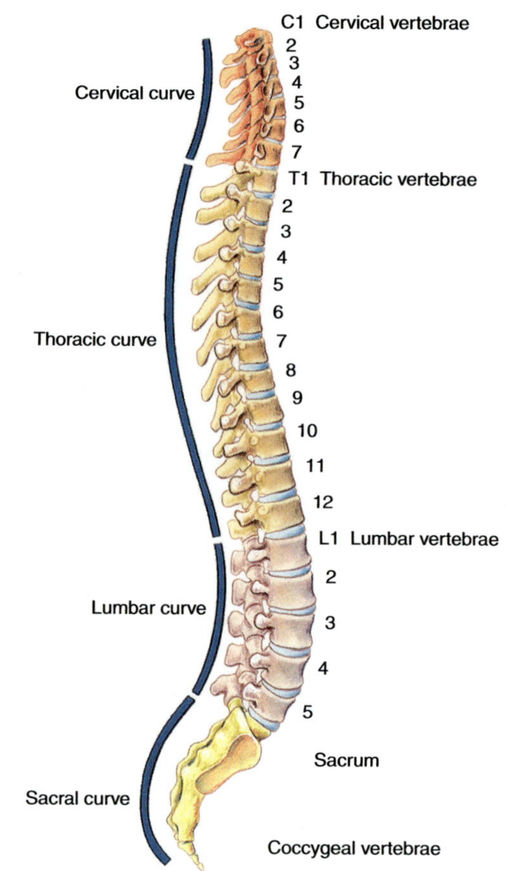

FIGURE 35.12 Normal curves of the spine. (From Applegate E: *The anatomy and physiology learning system*, ed 4, St. Louis, 2011, Saunders.)

cause pain and fatigue in the lower back and legs. Lordosis can also cause pain that may affect mobility. Mild kyphosis may cause few symptoms, but severe kyphosis can cause back pain, stiffness, and an abnormally curved spine. Scoliosis can cause uneven shoulders and waist. One shoulder blade may be more prominent, and one hip may be higher than the other.

The provider will perform a physical exam of the spine and a neurologic exam. A spinal x-ray, an MRI, and CT scan are also used as diagnostic tools. The treatment depends on the severity of the curve and the patient's age and condition. Treatments include physical therapy, medications (analgesics, NSAIDs, steroids, and muscle relaxants), spinal fusion surgery, and a back brace; surgical placement of metal stabilizing rods may be needed for scoliosis. In most cases, with treatment, the prognosis is good.

Osteomalacia and Rickets

Osteomalacia is the softening of bones due to the lack of vitamin D. Vitamin D helps the body absorb calcium. Calcium is needed for strong bones. Osteomalacia occurs in adults and children; in children, this disease is called *rickets*.

Osteomalacia and rickets are caused by a lack of vitamin D, which can be related to an absorption issue (e.g., after gastric bypass surgery) or a lack of dietary intake. Osteomalacia can also be related to kidney failure, liver disease, and certain medications (e.g., **anticonvulsants**). Signs and symptoms include bone fractures without related injuries, muscle weakness, and widespread bone pain, usually in the hips.

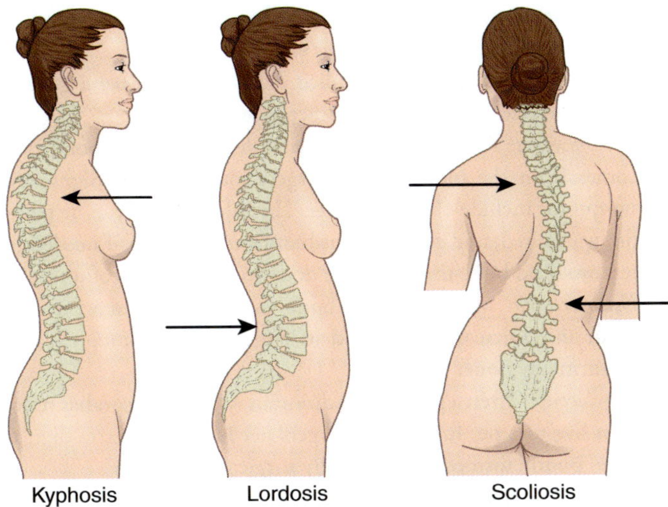

FIGURE 35.13 Spinal curve abnormalities.

The provider will order blood tests to check the vitamin D level, along with creatinine, electrolytes (e.g., calcium, phosphate), alkaline phosphatase, and parathyroid hormone levels. Bone x-rays, a bone density test, and a bone **biopsy** may be done. Treatment involves oral supplements of vitamin D, calcium, and phosphorus. Sunlight for vitamin D production is also recommended. With early treatment, the prognosis for rickets in children is excellent. The prognosis for osteomalacia is good if the vitamin D deficiency is addressed.

Osteoporosis

Osteoporosis is a condition that causes bones to become brittle and weak. Healthy bone is constantly being broken down and remodeled. When a person has osteoporosis, bones are being broken down more quickly than new bone can be created. This leads to weak bones that are easily fractured, especially in the wrist, hip, and spine.

As people age, bone mass is lost faster than it can be produced, leading to osteoporosis. Increased risks for osteoporosis include menopause, family history, small body frame, white or Asian descent, hormonal imbalance, dietary deficiencies (low calcium intake), long-term corticosteroid use, celiac disease, kidney or liver disease, cancer, and some autoimmune conditions. A sedentary lifestyle, tobacco use, and excessive alcohol consumption are also risk factors for osteoporosis. Early osteoporosis is asymptomatic, but as the bones become weaker, back pain, height loss, stooped posture, and fractures can occur.

A bone density test is the only diagnostic tool for osteoporosis. This low-level x-ray determines the mineral content of the bone. The following treatments are used for osteoporosis:

- Weight-bearing exercises to maintain bone density
- Modifying risk factors to prevent falls
- Appropriate calcium and vitamin D intake from food or supplements
- Medications, such as bisphosphonates and hormone replacement therapy (estrogen)

Osteoporosis is a chronic condition that can be managed but does progress with age.

Healthy, Strong Bones

Peak bone mass is usually achieved around age 30. After that time, a little more bone is lost through remodeling than what is gained. This leads to a decrease in bone mass or density. For good bone health, it is important to do the following:

- Eat a diet rich in calcium. Good sources of calcium include dairy products, canned salmon with bones, soy products (e.g., tofu), broccoli and kale, and almonds.
- Take in adequate amounts of vitamin D. Vitamin D helps the body absorb dietary phosphorus and calcium. Good dietary sources of vitamin D include oily fish (e.g., trout, tuna, salmon), mushrooms, eggs, and fortified cereals and milk. Sunlight also helps in the body's production of vitamin D.
- Limit tobacco and alcohol use. Tobacco use can lead to weak bones. Drinking more than one alcoholic drink per day for women and two for men can increase bone density loss.
- Do weight-bearing exercises. Weight-bearing exercises, such as jogging, climbing stairs, and walking, help build strong bones and slow bone loss.

CRITICAL THINKING APPLICATION 35.7

Mrs. Viola Carson, a 78-year-old patient, is being seen in the office today for follow-up after hip replacement surgery. Mrs. Carson fractured her hip in a simple fall at the grocery store. Why would the physician suspect she has osteoporosis? What treatment might be recommended to prevent further fractures in this patient?

Spinal Stenosis

Spinal stenosis is the narrowing of the spine. The stenosis puts pressure on the nerves and spinal cord. Usually, spinal stenosis occurs in people over age 50, but it can affect younger people with spinal injuries. *Cervical stenosis* causes narrowing of the cervical spine in the neck. *Lumbar stenosis* causes narrowing of the lumbar spine in the lower back.

Causes of spinal stenosis include overgrowth of bone, herniated disks, tumors, spinal injury, and thickening of ligaments. Cervical spinal stenosis causes numbness, tingling, and weakness in the extremities. Neck pain, difficulty walking, and bowel and bladder incontinence can occur. With lumbar spinal stenosis, a person can experience weakness, tingling, numbness, cramping, and pain in the legs and feet. It can also cause back pain.

After an exam, the provider may order x-rays, an MRI, and a CT scan. Sometimes a CT myelogram is done. With a CT myelogram, a contrast dye is injected, which outlines the spinal cord and nerves, showing abnormalities. Spinal stenosis can be treated with surgery, analgesics, physical therapy, and steroid injections.

Paget Disease

Paget disease is also called *osteitis deformans*. Paget disease causes abnormal bone destruction and regrowth. The new bone is larger but weaker, leading to deformities. Often the bones in the arms, legs, spine, skull, pelvis, and collarbones are involved.

The etiology is unknown. It may be related to genetic factors or a viral infection. Most patients experience no symptoms. If symptoms occur, the person may experience bone pain, joint stiffness and pain, and fractures. Deformities, such as an enlarged skull and bowing of the legs, can occur. A person can experience a reduction in height, kyphosis, and spinal stenosis. Hearing loss can also occur.

After an examination, the provider may order a bone scan and x-rays. Laboratory tests such as alkaline phosphatase (ALP), bone-specific isoenzyme, and serum calcium may be performed. Not all patients with Paget disease need to be treated. Patients with deformities and other symptoms may be treated with medications to reduce bone remodelings, such as bisphosphonates and calcitonin. For lumbar spinal stenosis due to a thickened ligament, *percutaneous image-guided lumbar decompression* (PILD) can be done. For this procedure, needle-like instruments are used to remove parts of the thickened ligament, thus widening the narrowed spinal canal.

Plantar Fasciitis

The plantar fascia is a tough fibrous tissue that connects the toes to the heel on the bottom of the feet, creating the arch of the foot. *Plantar fasciitis* occurs when the plantar fascia becomes inflamed or swollen from being overstretched or overused. Plantar fasciitis is one of the most common foot issues.

People with flat feet or high arches are at risk for plantar fasciitis. Other risk factors include running long distances, obesity, wearing shoes with poor arch support, and having a tight Achilles tendon. Signs and symptoms include foot pain immediately in the morning, after standing, sitting, or intense exercise, and when climbing stairs. The pain can be on the bottom of the foot or along the sole of the foot. Mild foot swelling, redness, or stiffness can also be seen.

The provider will do an examination. A foot x-ray may be ordered to rule out other issues. Treatment involves over-the-counter analgesics, heel and foot stretches, and good arch supports in shoes. Severe cases may require immobilization, custom-made shoe inserts, steroid injections in the heel, and surgery. Plantar fasciitis usually resolves with treatment.

Additional Skeletal System Disorders

There are many skeletal disorders. The following are some examples:

- *Amputation*: The removal of a leg, foot, toes, fingers, or arm as a result of a trauma, accident, poor blood flow to the extremity, uncontrolled or worsening infection, tumor, or severe frostbite or burn. Risks of amputations include blood clots, bleeding, infection, poor surgical wound healing, and phantom sensations. After a limb is removed, a person may feel that the limb is still there. This can include experiencing numbness, hot or cold sensations, and pain (called *phantom pain*) in the limb that is no longer there. Depending on the type of amputation, many amputees use an artificial limb. Recovering from an amputation may require physical therapy, treatment with medicine, or counseling to help deal with sadness, anger, and frustration.
- *Chondrosarcoma*: A rare type of cancer that begins in bones or soft tissue near the bones.
- *Ewing sarcoma*: A rare type of cancer that starts in the bone or soft tissue near the bone. More common in children and teenagers.
- *Fibrous dysplasia*: Abnormal fibrous tissue replaces bone, leading to weak bones.
- *Mastoiditis*: Infection of the mastoid bone, commonly related to middle ear infections *(acute otitis media)*.
- *Osteogenesis imperfecta*: Also called *brittle bone disease;* a genetic condition that causes bones to fracture easily.
- *Osteomyelitis*: A bacterial or fungal infection of the bone that comes from the bloodstream, surgery, or an injury. Signs and symptoms include chills and fever. The infected area can be painful, warm, red, and swollen. Antibiotics and surgery, if needed to remove dead bone tissue, can be done to treat the infection.
- *Osteosarcoma*: Most common bone cancer in children but can occur in adults; usually found in large bones, although it can occur in any bone.
- *Polydactyly*: Often a genetic condition in which a person has more than five toes per foot or five fingers per hand. The extra digit is often poorly formed and is usually surgically removed.
- *Spina bifida occulta*: Mildest form of spina bifida; no spinal nerves are involved, but one or more vertebrae are malformed; no signs or symptoms may be present. The only indication may be an abnormal cluster of hair, a small dimple, or a birthmark on the infant's back.
- *Spondylolisthesis*: A forward displacement of a vertebra over the one below it; usually occurs in the lumbar or sacral area; can be related to a birth defect or acute trauma.
- *Syndactyly*: The digits (fingers and toes) are fused together or are webbed together. Most commonly seen with the second and third toes.
- *Talipes (clubfoot)*: Most common congenital disorder of the legs; one foot or both feet are turned inward and downward; the calf and foot may be slightly smaller; treatment depends on the severity and can include stretching, casting, braces, and surgery.

ARTHRITIC JOINT DISEASES AND DISORDERS

Arthritis is a term that refers to any inflammatory joint condition. More than 54 million Americans have some form of arthritis. Arthritis is the leading cause of work disabilities in the United States. About 50% of arthritic cases are in those 65 years or older, though arthritis can occur at any age.

Arthritis can be caused by autoimmunity, infection, injury, and genetic conditions. The following sections discuss common arthritic conditions.

Osteoarthritis

Osteoarthritis (OA), also called *degenerative joint disease* (DJD), is the most common form of arthritis. OA can occur in any joint but most often affects the hands, hips, spine, and knees.

Osteoarthritis occurs when the cartilage at the end of the bones wears down, causing the bones to rub together, leading to permanent damage to the joint. Risk factors include genetics, being female, obesity, age, and injury to the joint. The signs and symptoms develop gradually and worsen over time. OA can cause pain, tenderness, stiffness, and swelling in joints, reducing the range of motion (Figure 35.14A). Bone spurs may form around the affected joint.

The provider will examine the affected joints and check the range of motion. X-rays, MRI, joint fluid analysis, and blood tests may be ordered to check for joint damage and rule out other types of arthritis. Treatment is focused on slowing the progression by maintaining a

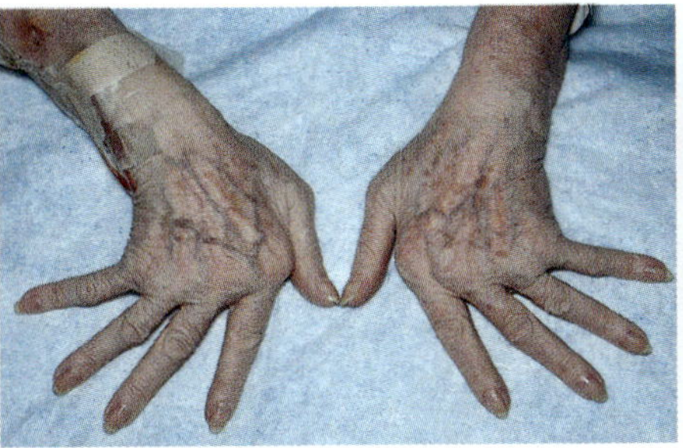
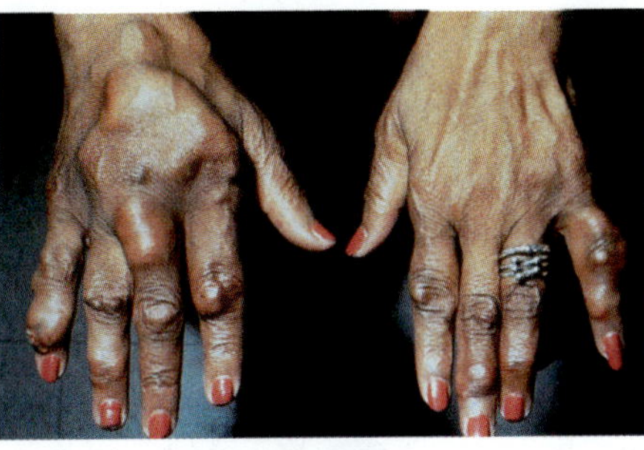

FIGURE 35.14 Types of arthritis. **(A)** Osteoarthritis. Note the presence of nodes in the proximal interphalangeal joints (Bouchard nodes) and distal interphalangeal joints (Heberden nodes). **(B)** Rheumatoid arthritis. Note the marked ulnar (elbow-like) deviation of the wrists. **(C)** Gouty arthritis. Note the tophi (stones) containing sodium urate crystals. (From Swartz MH: *Textbook of physical diagnosis*, ed 6, Philadelphia, 2010, Saunders.)

healthy weight, and limiting pain with the use of analgesics, NSAIDs, and duloxetine (Cymbalta). Additional interventions include physical therapy, occupational therapy, and cortisone injections in the joint to relieve pain. Joint replacement surgery (arthroplasty), such as a total hip or knee replacement, may also be done. The prognosis is good with surgery.

CRITICAL THINKING APPLICATION 35.8

An 80-year-old male patient with arthritis comes into the office complaining of severe pain in his knees, hips, and lower back. The pain makes it impossible for him to get up onto the examination table. What should Suzanne do? Is this patient required to get onto the examination table? Why or why not?

Rheumatoid Arthritis

Rheumatoid arthritis (RA) is an autoimmune and inflammatory disease. RA often starts in middle age and is common in older adults. A person can have the disease for a short time, or episodes may come and go. The severe form of RA is chronic.

With this autoimmune disease, the immune system attacks the healthy cells, causing inflammation in the joints, eyes, lungs, and mouth. Usually, it affects the wrist, finger, and knee joints. The lining of the joints becomes inflamed, causing damage to the joint tissue. Older adults and females are at most risk for RA, though women who have breastfed have a decreased risk. Other risk factors include genetics, cigarette use, and obesity. Signs and symptoms of RA include pain, achiness, stiffness, swelling, and tenderness in more than one joint (Figure 35.14B). Weight loss, fever, weakness, and fatigue can occur. Early stages of RA can be difficult to diagnose because the symptoms are similar to those of other joint diseases.

During the examination, the provider will check the reflexes, muscle strength, and the joints for signs of inflammation (e.g., swelling, redness, and warmth). Imaging tests (x-rays, MRI, and ultrasound [US]) may be done, along with blood tests, including the erythrocyte sedimentation rate (ESR), C-reactive protein (CRP), rheumatoid factor (RF), and anti–cyclin citrullinated peptide (anti-CCP) antibodies. There is no cure for RA, but recent research has shown that early use of disease-modifying antirheumatic drugs (DMARDs) can increase the chances of **remission.**

Gout

Gout (also called *gouty arthritis*) is a common form of inflammatory arthritis (Figure 35.14C). Gout can be acute or chronic, and attacks can last longer as time progresses.

The etiology is a buildup of uric acid in the body (Figure 35.15). Uric acid results from the breakdown of purines in foods (e.g., liver, dried peas and beans, and anchovies). The risk factors for gout include being male, a family history of gout, obesity, drinking alcohol, and eating too many purine-rich foods. Certain medications (e.g., diuretics, aspirin, niacin, and levodopa) may also increase the risk of gout. The signs and symptoms of gout include swollen, red, warm, and stiff joints. The great (big) toe is the most common site for gout, though it can affect the heel, ankle, knee, elbow, wrist, and fingers (see Figure 35.14C).

To diagnose gout, the provider will do a physical examination and order an x-ray and lab tests. The provider may take a sample of fluid from the inflamed joint area to look for uric acid crystals. Pseudogout has a similar presentation, but it is caused by calcium phosphate.

Treatment includes the following:

- NSAIDs can reduce pain and swelling.
- Corticosteroids (e.g., prednisone) can reduce inflammation.
- Colchicine (Colcrys, Gloperba) should be taken within the first 12 hours of the attack.

Full recovery may take up to 14 days. For additional treatments or to prevent future attacks by reducing the uric acid level in the blood, the person may need to take allopurinol, febuxostat, probenecid, or pegloticase. Patients are also encouraged to control their weight, limit alcohol intake, and reduce their dietary intake of meats and fish rich in purines.

Juvenile Arthritis

Juvenile arthritis (JA) is a generic phrase for autoimmune, inflammatory, or rheumatic conditions that affect children under 16 years of age. Juvenile idiopathic arthritis (JIA) is the most common form of JA. Other types of JA include these:

- *Juvenile dermatomyositis (JDM):* Causes weakness and a rash on the eyelids and knuckles
- *Juvenile systemic lupus erythematosus:* An autoimmune disease that affects the kidneys, blood, skin, and joints
- *Juvenile scleroderma:* Causes skin to tighten and harden
- *Kawasaki disease:* Causes rash, swollen lymph nodes, fever, inflammation of blood vessels, and heart damage

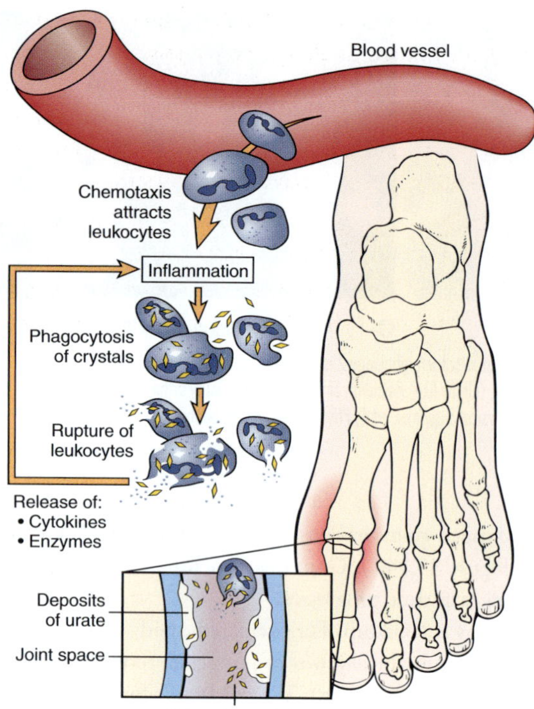

FIGURE 35.15 Gout is characterized by deposits of uric acid crystals in the connective tissue. The inflammation most often affects the joint of the big toe. (From Damjanov I: *Pathology for the health-related professions*, ed 4, St. Louis, 2012, Saunders.)

There is no known cause of JA. For some types of JA, there may be a genetic predisposition for the condition. Signs and symptoms of JA depend on the specific condition. Most JA conditions cause pain, swelling, redness, and warmth in the joints. Some JA conditions may also cause issues with the eyes, muscles, digestive system, and the skin.

The provider will perform an examination and order lab work, though no specific blood test diagnoses JA. The goal of the treatment is to provide the child with the best quality of life; therefore, pain control and reducing inflammation are important. A combination of medications, physical therapy, and nutrition therapy may be used.

Lyme Disease and Arthritis

Lyme disease is the most common tick-borne infectious disease in the United States. Lyme disease can cause flu-like symptoms and a rash (Figure 35.16A). If the infection is not treated, about 60% of people develop Lyme arthritis.

Lyme disease is caused by the bacterium *Borrelia burgdorferi* and, rarely, *Borrelia mayonii* in the United States. Infected deer and western black-legged ticks transmit the bacteria that cause Lyme disease (Figure 35.16B). This bacterial infection is prevalent in Wisconsin, Minnesota, California, and between Virginia and Maine. Exposure to grassy and heavily wooded areas increases the risk of coming in contact with infected ticks. Early signs and symptoms of Lyme disease include flu-like symptoms (fever, chills, achiness, fatigue, swollen lymph nodes, and headache) and a rash *(erythema migrans)*. The rash appears about 70% to 80% of the time, usually starting 3 to 30 days after the bite. The rash begins at the bite site and slowly expands over the skin, reaching up to 12 inches or more. It can appear as a bull's-eye or target.

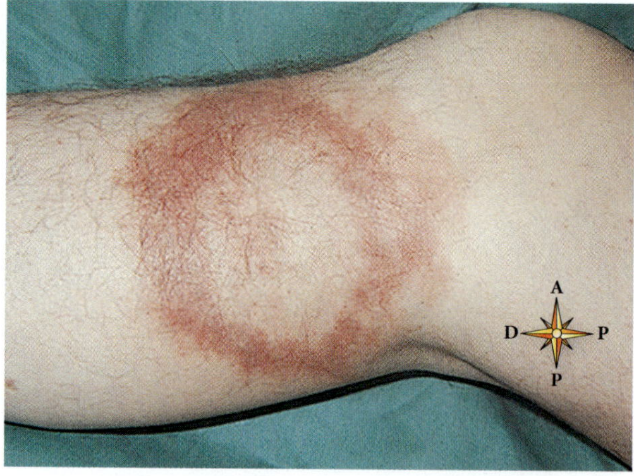

A

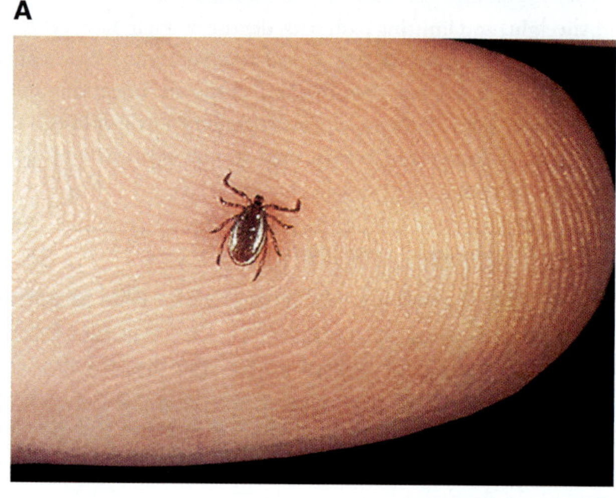

B

FIGURE 35.16 Lyme disease. **(A)** Circular, expanding rash resembling a bull's-eye target caused by the spirochete bacteria Borrelia burgdorferi. **(B)** Deer tick, vector for transmission of Lyme disease. (A: From Callen JP, Paller AS, Greer KE, et al: *Color atlas of dermatology*, ed 2, Philadelphia, 2000, WB Saunders; B: From Habif TP: *Clinical dermatology*, ed 5, St. Louis, 2010, Mosby.)

If left untreated, Lyme disease can cause arthritis, severe joint pain, meningitis, Bell palsy, facial palsy (affecting both sides of the face), numbness and weakness in the extremities, heart palpitations (Lyme carditis), short-term memory issues, and eye inflammation.

After an examination, the provider will order an enzyme immunoassay (EIA) or immunofluorescence assay (IFA) blood test. If the results are positive or equivocal, further testing with IgM and/or IgG Western blot will be done. The lab test results are more reliable if a person has been infected for several weeks. Treatment includes antibiotics, such as amoxicillin, cefuroxime, and doxycycline. Some people may have post-treatment Lyme disease syndrome, which will resolve in time.

Patient Education for Lyme Disease

According to the Centers for Disease Control and Prevention (CDC), patient education for Lyme disease includes the following instructions:

- Minimize the risk for ticks in your yard by clearing tall grass, leaves, and brush.
- Treat clothing, boots, and camping gear with 0.5% permethrin.

- Use Environmental Protection Agency (EPA)–registered insect repellents. They contain DEET, picaridin, IR3535, Oil of Lemon Eucalyptus, para-menthane-diol (PMD), or 2-undecanone. You can also use the information found at the EPA website, www.epa.gov/insect-repellents/find-repellent-right-you.
- Wear pants tucked into socks and long-sleeved shirts when walking in wooded or grassy areas.
- Walk in the center of trails and avoid wooded and high-grass areas.
- Deer ticks are no bigger than the head of a pin. After you come indoors, check your entire body and your clothing, gear, and animals for ticks. Showering within 2 hours of potential exposure can reduce the chances of Lyme disease.
- If a person has a tick embedded, it needs to be removed. Wear gloves if possible. Use fine-tipped pointed tweezers. Get as close to the head as possible. Do not squeeze the abdomen because it may inject secretions into the person's body. Pull upward with steady pressure to pull out the head. Once the tick is removed, place it in a container of rubbing alcohol to kill it. Clean the site with antiseptic soap and water. Apply an antibiotic ointment. Monitor the site for infection or other complications.
- If you develop a rash or fever within several weeks of removing a tick, see your healthcare provider. Be sure to tell the provider about your recent tick bite and when the bite occurred.
- Do not assume you are immune. Lyme disease can occur in the same person more than once.

Additional Arthritic Joint Disorders

There are several other arthritic conditions:

- *Ankylosing spondylitis*: A type of hereditary inflammatory arthritis affecting the back and spine, usually occurring between 17 and 35 years of age. Causes low back pain and stiffness, especially at night and in the morning.
- *Infectious arthritis*: Also called septic arthritis. Arthritis is caused by a joint bacterial (Staphylococcus aureus), viral, or fungal infections. Causes pain, swelling in a joint, fever and chills.
- *Patellofemoral arthritis*: The articular cartilage on the underside of the patella wears down and becomes inflamed and causes pain in the front of the knee. It makes kneeling, squatting, and taking the stairs difficult. Caused by dysplasia and patellar fracture.
- *Psoriatic arthritis*: A chronic autoimmune disease that can occur with **psoriasis**. The etiology is unknown. It causes joint pain and stiffness, fatigue, swelling of hands and feet, skin rashes, and eye problems.

NONARTHRITIC JOINT DISEASES AND DISORDERS

Besides arthritis, other conditions impact the joint and a person's ability to move. The following sections describe nonarthritic joint diseases and disorders.

Bursitis

Bursitis is the inflammation of the bursa. It usually affects the hip, buttock, knee, calf, and shoulder.

Bursitis is common after age 40. It occurs with the overuse or repetitive use of a joint. Injuries can also cause bursitis. Stress and inflammation from other conditions, such as gout and thyroid disorders, can increase the risk for bursitis. Pain is the most common symptom. Joint stiffness, swelling, and redness can also occur.

After an examination, the provider may order an x-ray, MRI, and ultrasound to rule out other conditions. Treatment consists of rest, splinting, heat and cold therapy, medications (NSAIDs, analgesics, and corticosteroid injection), and physical therapy.

CRITICAL THINKING APPLICATION 35.9

Suzanne has been a runner for years, but recently she was diagnosed with bursitis in her knees. Explain how Suzanne's running may have contributed to this condition.

Carpal Tunnel Syndrome

Carpal tunnel syndrome results when the median nerve becomes compressed at the wrist. The carpal tunnel is a narrow passageway located on the palm side of the wrist that is surrounded by bones and ligaments. This tunnel protects the median nerve to the hand and the nine tendons that bend the fingers.

The etiology includes repetitive motions, trauma, injury to the wrist, and conditions such as thyroid disease and rheumatoid arthritis. Females are more likely to have carpal tunnel syndrome than males. Signs and symptoms start gradually, with tingling, burning, or numbness of the thumb and fingers, except for the little finger. Symptoms can come and go initially but can worsen and become more persistent with time. Without treatment, a person can lose grip strength and feeling in the fingertips.

The provider will examine the arm and wrist. X-rays and an electromyogram may be done. Treatments include limiting repetitive tasks, cold therapy, a wrist splint, NSAIDs, and corticosteroid injections. Surgery may be performed to relieve pressure on the median nerve. With treatment, the prognosis is good.

Dislocation and Subluxation

A *dislocation* (or *luxation*) occurs when a bone has been completely displaced from the joint (Figure 35.17). A ***subluxation*** is a partial or incomplete dislocation of the joint. The most common site of joint dislocation in children is the elbow, whereas, in an adult, it is the shoulder. Other joints that can be dislocated include the ankle, knee, hip, jaw, toe, or finger.

The etiology of dislocations is related to sports and trauma (e.g., a blow or fall), which forces the joint out of position. The larger the joint, the greater the force needed for dislocation. Some people have a hereditary risk because their ligaments are looser, making them more prone to injury. Signs and symptoms include pain and swelling in the joint area and the inability to move the extremity. Many times, a visual distortion in the joint area is seen.

A dislocated joint is an emergency and requires immobilization and application of a cold pack as first aid. Once the provider examines the joint, an x-ray may be ordered. Treatment depends on the severity of the injury and the joint involved. The joint needs to be manipulated back into position. Additional complications may require surgical intervention. Once the joint is back into its normal position, the area may be immobilized in a splint or sling to heal. NSAIDs to reduce inflammation and pain may be ordered. Once a joint has been dislocated, there is a greater risk of dislocating it in the future.

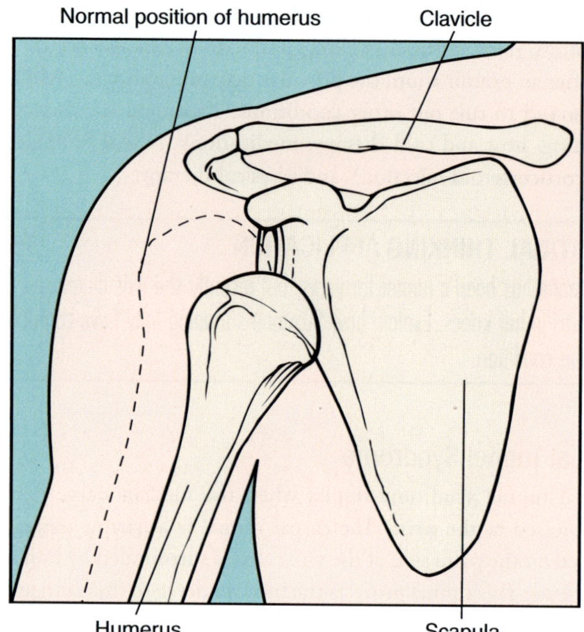

FIGURE 35.17 Dislocation (luxation) of the shoulder. (From Frazier MS, Drzymkowski JW: *Essentials of human diseases and conditions*, ed 3, Philadelphia, 2004, Saunders.)

CRITICAL THINKING APPLICATION **35.10**

A patient comes into the office from her weekly softball game. After sliding into home plate, she was immediately unable to move her right arm, and she says she has a lot of pain in her right shoulder. What steps should Suzanne take to help this patient?

Hallux Valgus

Hallux valgus, also called a *bunion*, is a progressive condition. A bunion is an abnormal enlargement of the first metatarsophalangeal (MTP) joint of the great toe, caused by inflammation of the synovial bursa. Extra bone and a fluid-filled sac at the base of the big toe cause a bump to appear. Over time, the enlargement can cause lateral displacement of the toe.

Bunions can be genetic. Some people have abnormalities with their feet bones that increase the likelihood of bunions. Wearing narrow-toed, high-heeled shoes can lead to bunion development. Females are more likely to have bunions than males. A person can experience a hard bump and pain in the large toe joint. The large toe may bend toward and cross over the second toe.

After the exam, the provider will usually order a foot x-ray. Many times, the x-ray shows an abnormal angle of the big toe. As the bunion starts to develop, patients are encouraged to wear wide-toed shoes. Soft pads and toe spacers can be used to protect the bunion and separate the toes. The provider may recommend a *bunionectomy* to realign the toe and remove the medial *eminence* (protrusion) of the metatarsal bone. It is important to keep a bunion from worsening. Surgery may help in some cases.

Hip Dysplasia

Hip dysplasia is an abnormality of the hip joint in which the femoral head does not fit in the acetabulum as it should. When people are born with this condition, it is called developmental *dysplasia of the hip* or *congenital hip dislocation.*

About 1 in every 1000 infants is born with hip dysplasia. Firstborn children and females are more at risk for hip dysplasia. Hip dysplasia can be caused by genetics. It can also result if the baby's position in the womb puts pressure on the hip. Signs and symptoms can include hip pain, a loose or unstable hip joint, limping, and unequal leg lengths. People with mild hip dysplasia may not have symptoms until their teen to young adult years.

Providers screen for hip dysplasia in infants by checking for it shortly after birth and during well-child exams. X-rays, ultrasound, and CT scans may also be used to confirm the diagnosis. The goal of treatment is to manage the pain and protect the hip joint. A brace may be used for an infant younger than age 6 months. Physical therapy can help strengthen the joint and increase flexibility. In most cases, the provider will perform surgery to repair or replace the hip socket. Surgery usually corrects the dysplasia.

Patellofemoral Syndrome

Patellofemoral syndrome is also called *chondromalacia patella* and "runner's knee." It causes pain at the front of the knee around the patella. It is more common in adolescents, young adults, and women.

Patellofemoral pain syndrome can be caused by overuse of the knee joint, muscle weakness, and trauma to the patella. Dull, achy knee pain at the front of the knee is the primary symptom. The pain increases when running, kneeling, squatting, or doing stairs.

After an examination, the provider might order an x-ray, CT, and MRI of the knee. Arthroscopy may also be done. Treatment consists of rest, avoiding climbing stairs and kneeling, and over the counter (OTC) analgesics. Additional treatments may include physical therapy, supportive braces, and cold therapy. For severe cases, surgical realignment procedures may be done. With treatment, the prognosis is good.

Sprain

A *sprain* is a stretched or torn ligament. A sprain can be graded to indicate the severity:

- Grade I for a stretched ligament
- Grade II for a partial tear
- Grade III for a complete tear of the ligament

Sprains of the ankle and wrist are the most common. A sprain is different from a strain, which is a stretched or torn tendon or muscle.

Sprains occur when a person overextends or tears a ligament when stressing a joint. Sprains can occur with sports injuries, falls, and walking on uneven surfaces. Signs and symptoms of sprains include pain, swelling, and difficulty moving the affected muscle. With sprains, a popping sound may be heard at the time of the injury, and bruising may occur later.

During the examination, the provider will check the affected area and the range of motion. X-rays and an MRI may be ordered to rule out other injuries. Treatment includes *r*est, *i*ce (cold applications), *c*ompression (elastic wraps), and *e*levation (RICE) to help minimize the swelling. NSAIDs and analgesics may be taken. With severe sprains, a brace or splint may be used to immobilize the area. Surgery may be done to repair a torn ligament. With treatment, the prognosis is good. Stretching, warming up, and cooling down exercises are important to prevent sprains.

Additional Joint Disorders

There are many joint disorders. The following are some examples:

- *Adhesive capsulitis*: Also known as a *frozen shoulder;* the movement in the shoulder is limited due to inflammation of the shoulder joint capsule.
- *Collateral ligament injury*: The medial collateral ligament (MCL) runs along the inside of the knee, and the lateral collateral ligament (LCL) runs along the outside of the knee. When one or both ligaments are stretched or torn, the knee becomes unstable.
- *Contracture*: Occurs when the normal tissue is replaced with a nonstretchy, fiber-like tissue. This can affect the skin, muscles, ligaments, and tendons. The affected joint can have a limited range of motion. Contracture can be related to disorders (e.g., cerebral palsy, stroke), nerve damage, scarring, or reduced use of the joint.
- *Cruciate ligament injury*: The anterior cruciate ligament (ACL) is in the middle of the knee and works with the posterior cruciate ligament (PCL). When one or both ligaments are stretched or torn, the knee becomes unstable.
- *Cubital tunnel syndrome*: Pressure or stretching of the ulnar nerve causes numbness and tingling of the ring and small fingers, forearm pain, and hand weakness.
- *Dupuytren contracture*: A thickening and shortening of the palmar fascia in the hand results in the contracture of one or more fingers.
- *Hammertoe*: An abnormal bend in the middle joint of the second, third, or fourth toe.
- *Temporomandibular joint disorder* (TMD): Causes difficulty chewing and pain and tenderness in the jaw.
- *Torn meniscus*: The meniscus in the knee joint tears, causing pain, swelling, and locking of the knee.

MUSCULAR SYSTEM DISEASES AND DISORDERS

Diseases and disorders of the muscular system often involve other body systems, including the skeletal and nervous systems. Common signs and symptoms of muscular disorders include the following:

- Swelling in the joints and muscles
- *Malaise* (generalized weakness or discomfort)
- *Myalgia* (muscle pain), *myositis* (inflammation of a muscle), and muscle tenderness
- Temporary loss of function or loss of normal mobility

The following sections address common muscular system disorders.

Compartment Syndrome

Compartment syndrome is a serious condition that can occur after a traumatic injury. Increased pressure is applied to muscle compartments, leading to muscle and nerve damage.

Fascia separates groups of muscles. Inside each fascial layer is a compartment space that contains muscle tissue, nerves, and blood vessels. Swelling in the compartment space will lead to increased pressure in the area because the fascia does not expand. Increased pressure can cause an interruption in the blood flow to the area, leading to muscle death.

Acute compartment syndrome can be caused by a fracture, bruised muscle, severe sprain, or a crushing injury. This condition can also occur if a cast or bandage is too tight. Chronic compartment syndrome is caused by repetitive activities, such as running. Compartment syndrome can cause pale skin, swelling, severe pain, and inability to move the extremity. The person may experience a decrease in sensation, numbness, tingling, or weakness in the extremity.

After an exam, the provider may need to measure the compartment's pressure. A needle attached to a pressure meter is inserted into the compartment. Treatment includes immediate surgery (*fasciotomy*) to prevent permanent damage. An incision is made in the fascia and muscle to relieve the pressure. With prompt treatment, the prognosis is good. If treatment is delayed, permanent muscle loss and nerve injury can occur.

Fibromyalgia

Fibromyalgia causes muscle pain, fatigue, and "tender points" on the legs, hips, back, arms, shoulders, and neck. It is estimated that 10 million people in the United States have fibromyalgia. Women develop fibromyalgia more often than men. Usually, the diagnosis occurs before age 50.

The etiology is unknown. Research indicates that trauma, infection, or injury may change how the central nervous system (CNS) responds to pain, leading to chronic pain. The signs and symptoms of fibromyalgia include widespread muscle pain, burning, aching, stiffness, or soreness. Additional symptoms include fatigue, sleep disturbances, mood and concentration problems, anxiety, headache, abdominal pain, bloating, constipation, diarrhea, bladder spasms, dizziness, numbness or tingling in the hands and feet, and tender points around the body.

The provider will perform an examination and rule out other conditions. With no diagnostic tests for fibromyalgia, the provider may use these results:

- Widespread Pain Index (WPI) score, which evaluates 19 areas of the body for pain
- Symptom Severity (SS) score, on which the patient scores specific fibromyalgia symptoms, including cognitive issues, fatigue, headache, and dizziness

The treatment is focused on minimizing the pain and fatigue experienced through the use of medications (e.g., pregabalin, duloxetine, and milnacipran), exercise, biofeedback, and acupuncture.

Muscular Dystrophy

Muscular dystrophy (MD) is a collection of more than 30 inherited diseases that cause muscle weakness and muscle loss. Some of these diseases affect children, whereas others appear in middle-aged adults.

About half of the people with MD have Duchenne muscular dystrophy (DMD), which is the most common form of MD. DMD is usually diagnosed in boys between the ages of 3 and 5. This fast-progressing condition usually causes weakness in the arms and legs, leading to trouble walking. It is usually diagnosed by the age of 3. Boys are affected much more frequently than girls.

Muscular dystrophy may be congenital or caused by a genetic mutation that disrupts the body's ability to make muscle-protecting proteins. The signs, symptoms, onset, and affected muscle groups depend on the specific disease, though the main sign of MD is progressive muscle weakness. The signs and symptoms of Duchenne muscular dystrophy include frequent falls, trouble running and moving from lying to sitting position, muscle pain and stiffness, and learning disabilities.

After the examination, the provider may order a creatine kinase (CK) blood test. Without trauma, high levels of CK suggest muscle disease, such as MD. Additional diagnostic tests include electromyography, genetic testing, and a muscle biopsy. Treatments can help improve quality of life, help people remain mobile for as long as possible, and reduce or prevent bone and spinal complications. Treatments include corticosteroids, heart medication, range of motion and stretching exercises, braces, and assistive devices (e.g., walkers, wheelchairs). There is no cure for muscular dystrophy.

Myalgic Encephalomyelitis

Myalgic encephalomyelitis (ME), also called *chronic fatigue syndrome* (CFS), is a disabling, complex illness. People who have ME are not able to do their normal activities.

ME is most common in people between the ages of 40 and 60, though it can affect anyone. Women are affected by it more often than men. The cause of ME is unknown, but it has been associated with viral infections. Myalgic encephalomyelitis can cause the following conditions:

- Greatly diminished ability to do activities that the person could do prior to the illness.
- Severe fatigue not relieved by sleep or rest.
- Sleep problems, either falling asleep or staying asleep.
- Problems with memory or thinking. Brain fog is common.
- Irregular heartbeat, shortness of breath, and orthostatic intolerance. The person may become dizzy, weak, faint, or lightheaded upon standing or sitting upright.
- Digestive issues and allergies and sensitivities to foods and other products.
- Chills, night sweats, joint pain, and muscle weakness.

The provider may do a complete physical and mental status examination. Blood, urine, and other tests may be ordered to rule out other conditions. Treatment includes the management of symptoms. There is no cure for myalgic encephalomyelitis.

Myasthenia Gravis

Myasthenia gravis affects the voluntary muscles, causing weakness and fatigue with activity, which improves with rest. Myasthenia gravis is most common in men older than 60 and women younger than 40 years of age.

The etiology is an **autoimmune** neuromuscular disease. The body produces antibodies that block the muscle cells from responding to neurotransmitters from nerve cells. Myasthenia gravis causes muscle weakness, leading to issues with breathing, chewing, swallowing, talking, climbing stairs, lifting objects, and maintaining a steady gaze. Additional symptoms include drooping eyelids, facial paralysis, fatigue, hoarseness, and double vision.

After a detailed neurologic examination, the provider will order imaging tests (CT or MRI), pulmonary function tests, and electromyography (EMG). With myasthenia gravis, the person will have a positive result on an acetylcholine receptor antibody blood test. The treatment is focused on increasing periods of **remission.** Lifestyle changes are encouraged, including resting, using eye patches, and avoiding stress and heat exposure, which can make symptoms worse. Medications such as neostigmine and pyridostigmine can help with the neuromuscular communication process. **Immunosuppressants** (e.g., prednisone, azathioprine, cyclosporine, and mycophenolate) may also be used. There is no cure for myasthenia gravis.

Strain

A *strain* is a tear, partial tear, overuse, or overstretching of a muscle or tendon. A strain can occur suddenly or over time. Hamstring and back muscle strains are common.

Acute strains occur when falling, jumping, or lifting heavy objects. Chronic strains occur with repetitive muscle movements, usually related to one's job or during a sports activity. Poor condition, fatigue, failing to do warm-up exercises, environmental conditions (e.g., ice), and poor equipment are risk factors for strains. Signs and symptoms of strains include pain, swelling, and difficulty moving the affected muscle. With strains, muscle spasms may be felt.

During the examination, the provider will check the affected area and the range of motion. X-rays and MRI scans may be ordered to rule out other injuries. Treatment includes *r*est, *i*ce (cold applications), *c*ompression (elastic wraps), and *e*levation (RICE) to help minimize the swelling. Nonsteroidal anti-inflammatory drugs (NSAIDs) and analgesics may be taken. With severe strains, a brace or splint may be used to immobilize the area. Surgery may be done to repair a ruptured muscle. With treatment, the prognosis is good.

CRITICAL THINKING APPLICATION **35.11**

Marissa overhears Dr. Kahn telling a patient to remember RICE for a strain. What does RICE stand for? Why is it used?

Tendinitis

Tendinitis is the inflammation of a tendon. It causes severe swelling of the tendon. Tendinitis occurs after repeated injury to a joint, such as the wrist or ankle. Some of the most common forms are named after the sports that increase their risk:

- *Tennis elbow* (lateral epicondylitis): Causes pain in the forearm and wrist
- *Golfer's elbow* (medial epicondylitis): Causes pain in the inner forearm and numbness or tingling in the fingers
- *Pitcher's shoulder, swimmer's shoulder, tennis shoulder* (rotator cuff tendinitis, impingement syndrome): Causes pain and swelling in the front of the shoulder, a clicking sound when raising the arm, and loss of mobility
- *Jumper's knee* (patellar tendinitis): Pain occurs with bending or straightening of the leg

Tendinitis causes pain, tenderness, inflammation in the joint area, and a limited range of motion.

The provider will do an examination. In most cases, x-rays and other imaging procedures are not required unless the problem continues. Treatment consists of rest, splinting, heat and cold therapy, medications (NSAIDs, analgesics, and corticosteroid injections), and physical therapy.

Tetanus

Tetanus, also called "lockjaw," is a serious condition that can lead to a medical emergency. Getting the tetanus vaccine can help prevent tetanus.

Tetanus is caused by *Clostridium tetani* bacteria. The spores from the *Clostridium tetani* bacteria are found in the soil, dust, manure, and saliva. Often, the spores enter the body through an injury, such as a deep cut, puncture wound, or eye injury. Once the spores enter the body, they develop into bacteria. Tetanus can cause painful muscle stiffness throughout the body, jaw cramping, headaches, seizures, fever, sweating, and vital sign changes (e.g., blood pressure and pulse). A person can have trouble opening her or his mouth and swallowing.

The provider performs an exam. No diagnostic tests exist to confirm tetanus. Treatment includes hospitalization, human tetanus immune globulin (TIG), medications to manage the muscle spasms, tetanus vaccine, and antibiotics. The more severe the case of tetanus, the poorer the prognosis. For those that survive tetanus, recovery may take up to 4 months.

Torticollis

Torticollis occurs when the neck muscles spasm. This causes the head to tilt, lean forward or backward, or be rotated.

Torticollis can be genetic. In infants, it can be caused by birth trauma or a spinal abnormality. In adults, it can be caused by poor posture, insufficient head support while sleeping, or neck injury or infection. Torticollis causes neck spasms, tremors, headache, neck pain, and swelling and stiffness of the neck muscles. The range of motion for the head can be limited. One shoulder may be higher than the other shoulder.

After an examination, the provider may order an x-ray or CT scan. Treatment for torticollis present at birth involves passive stretching of the shortened neck muscle. Depending on the cause, treatment may involve heat and cold therapy, physical therapy, Botox injections, and surgery if other treatments fail.

Additional Muscular System Disorders

There are several other muscular system diseases:

- *Botulism*: A rare but serious disease caused by *Clostridium botulinum,* which enters the body through contaminated food (e.g., honey, home-preserved/canned foods). The toxins cause muscle paralysis, leading to visual changes, slurred speech, and difficulty swallowing and breathing.
- *Congenital myopathies:* Rare congenital diseases that cause a lack of muscle tone and muscle weakness, cramps, and contractions, along with delayed motor skills, facial weakness, and drooping eyelids.
- *Dermatomyositis* (DM): Affects people of all ages and is most common in women. Symptoms start with a rash on the face, chest, or extremities, followed by muscle weakness.
- *Endocrine myopathies:* Caused by abnormal thyroid gland activity; they lead to weakness, atrophy, stiffness, cramps, and slowed reflexes.
- *Ganglion cyst*: A benign round or oval lump that develops in the wrist, hand, ankle, or foot. The cyst is filled with a jelly-like fluid and develops along the tendons or joints. These cysts are painless unless they put pressure on a nearby nerve. Then, the person may experience tenderness, weakness, numbness, tingling, or pain in the affected area.
- *Muscle atrophy*: The loss or wasting of muscle tissue. *Physiologic atrophy* occurs when muscles are not used enough, muscle tissue is lost. People who are bedridden or have conditions that cause limited movement (e.g., casts, strokes) are at risk for muscle atrophy. *Pathologic atrophy* is seen with starvation, long-term corticosteroid use, and aging. *Neurogenic atrophy* is caused by an injury (e.g., spinal cord injury) or disease of a nerve that connects with a muscle (e.g., amyotrophic lateral sclerosis and polio).
- *Myositis*: Inflammation of the muscles caused by an injury, infection, or an autoimmune disease.
- *Myotonia congenita*: A congenital condition that causes a delay in muscle relaxation after contraction. Early symptoms include difficulty swallowing, shortness of breath, falls, and difficulty opening the eyes. After the person starts moving, the muscles relax, and the movements become normal.
- *Sarcopenia*: Causes progressive skeletal muscle loss due to age; this causes a decrease in muscle strength.
- *Shin splints*: Cause pain in the front of the lower leg due to overuse of the leg muscles, tendons, or tibia. They are the result of inflammation of the bone tissue, tendons, and muscles around the tibia.

THE MEDICAL ASSISTANT'S ROLE IN THE EXAMINATION, DIAGNOSTIC PROCEDURES, AND TREATMENTS

Musculoskeletal disorders are common in primary care, urgent care, orthopedics, and rheumatology departments. Medical assistants help the provider with examinations, diagnostic procedures, and treatments. Chapter 36 provides additional information on the medical assistant's role in examinations, diagnostic procedures, and treatments.

Assisting with the Examination and Diagnostic Procedures

During the exam, the provider may use inspection, palpation, range-of-motion (ROM) testing, and muscle testing to examine the major skeletal muscles and joints. Many times, the unaffected side is examined first and compared to the affected side. The provider may compare the size, position, and strength of the extremities. Depending on the concern, the provider may also perform a *gait analysis*, which means the provider observes the patient walking. Gait abnormalities may be the cause or the result of different musculoskeletal conditions.

If medical assistants are in the room for the exam, they may be responsible for taking notes, keeping the patient draped properly, and assisting by handing equipment to the provider. Always keep patient safety in mind, especially when the patient is transferring onto and off of the exam table and changing positions.

The medical assistant assists with diagnostic procedures by scheduling and preparing patients for procedures and laboratory tests. Chapter 36 describes common diagnostic procedures for the musculoskeletal system. Table 35.2 lists common laboratory tests used for musculoskeletal conditions.

CRITICAL THINKING APPLICATION **35.12**

As Dr. Kahn finishes his exam with Walter, he asks Suzanne to join them as they discuss Walter's test results. Dr. Kahn ordered an RF test, Lyme disease antibody test, ESR, and C-reactive protein (CRP) through the clinical laboratory. What information will each of the lab tests give Dr. Kahn?

TABLE 35.2 Medical Laboratory Tests for Musculoskeletal Diseases and Disorders

TEST	DEFINITION
Acetylcholine receptor (AChR) antibody test	Blood test that measures the AChR antibodies, which are produced by the immune system. AChR antibodies mistakenly attack the protein, AChR, found on voluntary (skeletal) muscles.
C-reactive protein (CRP)	Blood test; some are CLIA-waived tests. CRP is produced by the liver and increases with inflammation. The CRP is a nonspecific indicator of inflammation.
Creatine kinase (CK) or creatine phosphokinase (CPK)	Blood test that measures the CK, which is an enzyme that increases with damage or disease of the skeletal muscle, heart, or brain.
Erythrocyte sedimentation rate (ESR)	CLIA-waived blood test. Measures how quickly the red blood cells (RBCs) in a blood sample settle to the bottom of the test tube. The quicker they settle, the more it indicates inflammation in the body. The ESR is a nonspecific indicator of inflammation.
Lyme disease blood antibodies	Blood or cerebrospinal fluid test; some are CLIA-waived tests. Also called Lyme Antibodies IgM/IgG by Western Blot. Tests looks for antibodies to Borrelia, which causes Lyme disease.
Rheumatoid factor (RF)	Blood test; some are CLIA-waived tests. Looks for RF present in the blood.

Assisting with Treatments

Musculoskeletal conditions are treated with a variety of procedures, devices, and medications. (Chapter 36 discusses immobilization therapies, additional therapies, and assistive devices that are used for musculoskeletal disorders.) Table 35.3 lists common procedures used to treat musculoskeletal conditions.

The following are some of the more common classifications of medications used for musculoskeletal conditions:

- *Analgesic*: Relieves pain
- *Anticonvulsant and mood stabilizer*: Used to prevent seizures and to treat neuromuscular disorders and epilepsy
- *Antigout*: Treats gout
- *Anti-inflammatory*: Reduces the inflammation in the body and is used to treat injuries and inflammatory conditions, such as arthritis, strains, and tendinitis
- *Corticosteroid*: Reduces the inflammation in the body and is used to treat chronic inflammatory diseases (e.g., arthritis)
- *Muscle relaxant*: Works on the central nervous system (CNS) to relax muscles, which treats conditions such as sprains and muscle injuries
- *Osteoporosis agent*: Promotes bone mineral density and reverses the progression of osteoporosis
- *Tumor necrosis factor (TNF) inhibitor:* Treats autoimmune disorders (e.g., rheumatoid arthritis)

Refer to Table 35.4 for information on the medication classification, including indications for use, desired effect, side effects, adverse reactions, and generic and trade names. Medical assistants should be familiar with medications that are prescribed to patients.

CLOSING COMMENTS

Patient Coaching

An informed patient is better prepared to continue with home care. Skeletal conditions, particularly arthritis, can be so painful and debilitating that these patients may be easy prey for miracle drug promotions. It is important for you to recognize the need for patient education about the condition and work diligently with the patient and family to encourage participation in effective care programs. When you work with the provider and the physical therapist in helping the patient, you become an important member of the healthcare team. This type of involvement leads to patient satisfaction, personal satisfaction, and a sense of achievement for the medical assistant.

Legal and Ethical Issues

When performing a procedure on a patient, it is important to follow these guidelines:

- You must have a written order from the provider.
- You must follow the procedure precisely as it is ordered, without variation.
- Never advise the patient without permission.
- Make sure you know what instructions the provider gave the patient and reinforce them.
- If you have any concerns about a procedure, discuss them with the provider privately before proceeding.
- Do not perform a procedure if you are uncomfortable; get someone to help you.

Always remember that you are the assistant, and this is the provider's patient. The provider is ultimately responsible for every aspect of the patient's care. Always stay within the legal and ethical guidelines of the medical assisting profession in your state.

Patient-Centered Care

Patients with musculoskeletal diseases may be on several medications to manage the disease and pain. The medical assistant should ensure the patient is taking the medication as prescribed. It is important to ask questions regarding the side effects of medications and pain levels in order to identify any issues the patient may be having. The information gathered from the patient should be reported to the provider. The goal is to give patients the highest quality of life.

Professional Behaviors

Musculoskeletal injuries and disorders are commonplace in the ambulatory care setting. For this reason, patients may ask for your advice on how to manage their health problems. Remember that as the medical assistant, you should never diagnose or recommend treatment for a patient. That is the provider's responsibility. Responding professionally to inquiries and offering provider-approved educational materials and websites can be very helpful. Respectful and courteous behavior should be standard practice for medical assistants when they interact with patients and their families.

TABLE 35.3 Common Treatments Used for Musculoskeletal Diseases and Disorders

PROCEDURE	DESCRIPTION
Arthrocentesis	Surgical procedure that involves a puncture of the joint and removal (aspiration) of fluid.
Bunionectomy	Surgical removal of a bunion.
Fasciotomy	Surgical procedure that involves opening the muscle compartment to reduce the pressure and restore blood flow.
Fixation device	Used to keep fractured bones stabilized and in alignment. • External fixation (EF) device: Screws are placed into the bone above and below the fracture. The external fixation device is attached to the screws outside the skin. • Internal fixation (IF) device: Rods, screws, or plates are surgically inserted into the bones to stabilize the bones.
Meniscectomy	Surgical removal of a meniscus.
Myorrhaphy	Surgical suturing of a muscle.
Prosthesis	An artificial body part, such as a leg, to replace a missing part.
Reduction	Alignment and immobilization of; there are two types: • Open reduction (OR): Requires a surgical incision for the repair. • Closed reduction (CR): Does not require a surgical incision.
Tenomyoplasty	Surgical procedure to repair a tendon and muscle.
Total or partial joint replacement/arthroplasty	Surgical removal of part or all of the joint and insertion of artificial plastic or metal joint parts. Partial joint replacement means only part of the joint structures are replaced. With a total joint replacement, all of the joint structures are replaced. Minimally invasive replacement surgery involves less cutting of the tissue. Here are some examples: • Patellofemoral replacement: Type of partial knee replacement. • Total elbow replacement: The damaged part of the humerus and ulna are replaced with artificial components. • Total hip replacement (THR): The damaged femoral head and the acetabulum are replaced with artificial components. Also known as hip arthroplasty. • Total knee replacement (TKR): Replaces the knee joint. Also known as knee arthroplasty. • Total shoulder replacement: Replaces the shoulder joint. Also known as shoulder arthroplasty.
Traction	Treatment of a dislocation; process of pulling the bone into correct alignment.

TABLE 35.4 Medication Classifications

CLASSIFICATION	INFORMATION	GENERIC NAME (TRADE NAME)
Analgesic	*Indications for use:* Relieves pain *Desired effects:* Reduces the sensory function of the brain; blocks pain receptors *Side effects and adverse reactions: Nonnarcotic:* Gastrointestinal (GI) distress, liver and kidney disorders, and tinnitus *Narcotic:* hypotension, decreased respirations, agitation, blurred vision, confusion, constipation, sedation, restlessness	***Nonnarcotic over the counter (OTCs):*** • Aspirin (Ecotrin, Bayer Aspirin, Bufferin) • Acetaminophen (Tylenol, Tempra) • Ibuprofen (Advil, Motrin) ***Narcotic (opioids):*** • Oxycodone (OxyContin) • Hydrocodone with acetaminophen (Lortab, Norco, Vicodin) • Oxycodone with acetaminophen (Percocet, Oxycet, Roxicet) • Tramadol (Conzip)

Continued

TABLE 35.4 Medication Classifications—*cont'd*

CLASSIFICATION	INFORMATION	GENERIC NAME (TRADE NAME)
Anticonvulsant and mood stabilizer	*Indications for use:* Treats epilepsy, trigeminal neuralgia, mania and mixed episodes (mania and depression) with bipolar disorder *Desired effects:* Reduces the frequency and severity of seizures by reducing excessive stimulation of the brain *Side effects and adverse reactions:* Sedation, vertigo, visual disturbances, GI disturbances, liver complications	• Carbamazepine (Tegretol, Equetro) • Lamotrigine (Lamictal) • Topiramate (Topamax) • Valproic acid (Depakene, Depakote) • Gabapentin (Neurontin, Horizant)
Antigout	*Indications for use:* Treats gout *Desired effects:* Reduce the uric acid in the body *Side effects and adverse reactions:* GI distress, eye irritation, itching, rash, blood in urine	• Allopurinol (Zyloprim, Aloprim) • Febuxostat (Uloric)
Anti-inflammatory	*Indications for use:* Treats arthritis and other inflammatory disorders (e.g., allergic rhinitis) *Desired effect:* Reduces inflammation *Side effects and adverse reactions:* GI distress, GI bleeding, hepatitis, drowsiness, tinnitus, irregular heart rate, kidney disorders	***Nonsteroidal anti-inflammatory drugs (NSAIDs):*** • Ibuprofen (Advil, Motrin, Midol) • Naproxen (Naprosyn) • Meloxicam (Mobic) ***Steroidal:*** • *See Corticosteroids (oral)*
Corticosteroid (oral)	*Indications for use:* Treats chronic inflammatory diseases (e.g., arthritis) and acute conditions (e.g., poison ivy, asthma) *Desired effects:* Reduces inflammation *Side effects and adverse reactions:* Headache, mood changes, difficulty falling asleep or staying asleep, increased sweating, vision problems, depression, and weight gain	• Prednisone (Prednisone Intensol, Sterapred) • Prednisolone (Flo-Pred, Orapred, Pediapred) • Methylprednisolone (Medrol)
Muscle relaxant	*Indications for use:* Treats painful musculoskeletal conditions (e.g., strains, sprains, muscle injuries) *Desired effect:* Works on the central nervous system (CNS) to relax muscles, which decreases pain *Side effects and adverse reactions:* Drowsiness, clumsiness, tachycardia, GI intolerance, difficulty breathing, fever, weakness, burning in the eyes, seizures	• Carisoprodol (Soma) • Cyclobenzaprine (Amrix)
Osteoporosis agent	*Indications for use:* Promotes bone mineral density and reverse progression of osteoporosis *Desired effects:* Inhibits bone reabsorption or promotes the use of calcium *Side effects and adverse reactions:* GI disorders, esophageal irritation	• Alendronate (Fosamax, Binosto) • Risedronate (Actonel, Atelvia) • Ibandronate (Boniva) • Raloxifene (Evista)
Tumor-necrosis factor (TNF) inhibitor	*Indications for use:* Treats autoimmune disorders (e.g., rheumatoid arthritis) *Desired effect:* Blocks the action of TNF, preventing inflammation *Side effects and adverse reactions:* GI distress, weakness, seizures, bleeding	• Infliximab (Remicade) • Etanercept (Enbrel)

SUMMARY OF SCENARIO

Dr. Kahn, Suzanne, and Walter wrap up the appointment. Dr. Kahn has recommended that Walter garden for shorter stretches of time, use a knee cushion when weeding, and take acetaminophen when he needs pain relief. Degenerative joint disease is manageable, and with a few changes to Walter's gardening routine, the prognosis is good.

Suzanne walks Walter out to the lobby. As she returns to the exam room, she reflects back on her 20 years as a medical assistant and is very happy with the choice she made so many years ago.

SUMMARY OF LEARNING OBJECTIVES

1. **Examine the anatomy of the axial skeleton and the appendicular skeleton.**
The musculoskeletal system (MS) consists of bones, joints, muscles, and supportive connective tissues (cartilage, tendons, and ligaments). The human skeleton is composed of more than 200 bones. Bones are divided into two categories: the axial skeleton and the appendicular skeleton. The axial skeletal is made up of the skull, rib cage, spinal column, and hyoid bone. The appendicular skeleton is made up of the shoulders, arms, wrists, pelvic girdle—hip bones, legs, and ankle/feet bones.
2. **Examine the physiology of the skeletal system.**
The skeletal system protects, supports, and provides a framework for the organ systems of the body. The skeletal system helps with movement and developing new bone. The osteoclasts are bone cells that break down bone. The osteoblasts, bone-forming cells, make the bones strong, durable, and able to heal. Calcium is moved between the blood and bones through the work of the osteoblasts and osteoclasts. It is removed from the blood as the osteoblasts form new bone. This lowers the blood calcium level. When the osteoclasts break down bone, calcium is released into the blood, thus increasing the blood calcium level. Spongy bone has a network of open spaces that contain red bone marrow, which consists of blood stem cells. These stem cells can become white or red blood cells or platelets.
3. **Examine the anatomy of the muscular system.**
There are three types of muscles:
   - Skeletal muscles have multiple nuclei and striations that give them a striped appearance. Special fibers allow them to shorten (contract) and lengthen (relax), which creates movement. Skeletal muscles are voluntary, meaning we have control of them. They are found attached to bones, in the upper section of the esophagus, in the eye, and the urinary and digestive system sphincter muscles.
   - Smooth muscles are nonstriated and have a single nucleus. They are involuntary muscles, which means we cannot control smooth muscles. Smooth muscles are found in the hollow organ walls, the eye, and the skin.
   - Cardiac muscles are involuntary, striated muscles found in the walls of the heart. Cardiac muscles can shorten and lengthen their fibers for contraction. Cardiac muscle fibers are electrically linked, forming one unit. A myocardial cell forms a strong, electrical connection to the next cells through special junctions called *intercalated discs*.
4. **Examine the physiology of the muscular system.**
The muscular system has four primary functions:
   - Allows for muscle contractions, which provide muscle tone and posture
   - Maintains the body temperature.
   - Provides joint stability.
   - Controls passageways in the body.
5. **Analyze the life span changes that occur in the musculoskeletal system.**
During childhood, bones grow rapidly. The prime time to build bone mass or density is from childhood to young adulthood. Bone density can increase as a result of a calcium-rich diet and regular weight-bearing exercise. With age, bones lose calcium and other minerals. The disks between the vertebrae wear and tear with age. Height can be lost from the compression and curving of the spinal column. Joints become stiffer and less flexible. With age, muscle tissue is replaced more slowly and may be replaced with tough, fibrous tissue.
6. **Examine skeletal diseases and disorders, including the signs, symptoms, etiology, diagnostic procedures, and treatments.**
Common signs and symptoms of musculoskeletal disorders are as follows:
   - Inflammation
   - Pain or swelling in the joints or bones
   - Temporary loss of function or loss of normal mobility

   This chapter discussed fractures, herniated disk, lordosis, kyphosis, scoliosis, osteomalacia, rickets, osteoporosis, spinal stenosis, Paget disease, and plantar fasciitis. Refer to the disease sections for more information on the signs, symptoms, etiology, diagnostic procedures, and treatments.
7. **Examine arthritic joint diseases and disorders, including the signs, symptoms, etiology, diagnostic procedures, and treatments.**
Arthritis can be caused by autoimmunity, infection, injury, and genetic conditions. Osteoarthritis, rheumatoid arthritis, gout, juvenile arthritis, Lyme disease, and arthritis are discussed in this chapter. Refer to the individual disease sections for more information on the signs, symptoms, etiology, diagnostic procedures, and treatments.
8. **Examine nonarthritic joint diseases and disorders, including the signs, symptoms, etiology, diagnostic procedures, and treatments.**
Nonarthritic joint disorders discussed in this chapter include bursitis, carpal tunnel syndrome, dislocation, subluxation, hallux valgus, hip dysplasia, patellofemoral syndrome, and sprain. Refer to the individual disease sections for more information on the signs, symptoms, etiology, diagnostic procedures, and treatments.
9. **Examine muscular diseases and disorders, including the signs, symptoms, etiology, diagnostic procedures, and treatments.**
Muscular system disorders discussed in the chapter include compartment syndrome, fibromyalgia, muscular dystrophy, myalgic encephalomyelitis, myasthenia gravis, strain, tendinitis, tetanus, and torticollis. Refer to the individual disease sections for more information on the signs, symptoms, etiology, diagnostic procedures, and treatments.
10. **Examine the medical assistant's role in examinations, diagnostic procedures, and treatments.**
If medical assistants are in the room for the exam, they may be responsible for taking notes, keeping the patient draped properly, and assisting by handing equipment to the provider. The medical assistant helps with diagnostic procedures by scheduling and preparing patients for procedures and laboratory tests. Table 35.2 lists common laboratory tests used for musculoskeletal conditions.

    Table 35.3 provides a list of procedures that are used to treat musculoskeletal conditions. Medication classifications used for musculoskeletal diseases include analgesics, anticonvulsants, antigout drugs, anti-inflammatories, corticosteroids, muscle relaxants, osteoporosis agents, and tumor necrosis factor (TNF) inhibitors.

PHYSICAL MEDICINE AND REHABILITATION

36

SCENARIO

Tim Paul, CMA (AAMA), has worked for Walden-Martin Family Medical (WMFM) Clinic for 2 years. Prior to being hired, Tim completed the medical assistant program at the local college. For his practicum, he spent part of the experience in family medicine and the remaining 100 hours in a local physical medicine and rehabilitation clinic. Tim enjoyed both experiences and realized he would eventually like to work in a physical medicine and rehabilitation clinic. He wanted to start his career in family medicine and to get comfortable with all of the various skills he learned in school.

One of the most interesting things Tim learned in practicum was how to remove a cast. Most people new to the experience were anxious about the procedure. Tim and his mentor took time to reassure the patients and showed them the equipment that they would use. Most of the patients were surprised to learn that the cast saw did not have a sharp blade. That helped to reduce their anxieties.

While studying this chapter, think about the following questions:

- What diagnostic procedures are related to orthopedic conditions?
- How do you apply a sling?
- What coaching is required for patients with casts?
- What is the action of cold and heat therapies?
- What coaching is required to help patients with assistive devices?

LEARNING OBJECTIVES

1. Examine how the medical assistant can help the provider with the examination.
2. Examine the medical assistant's role in diagnostic procedures.
3. Differentiate among various types of immobilization treatments, including the purpose of the treatment and the medical assistant's role.
4. Differentiate between cold and heat therapies, including the purpose of the treatment and the medical assistant's role.
5. Differentiate among the uses of various physical therapy treatments.
6. Examine the medical assistant's role in helping patients with assistive devices.
7. Examine complementary therapies used for musculoskeletal conditions.

VOCABULARY

analgesic (an ahl JEE zik) A drug that reduces or eliminates pain.

anticoagulant (an tee koe AG yoo lant) A substance (i.e., medication or chemical) that prevents the clotting of blood.

cartilage (KAR tih lij) Flexible connective tissue that covers the ends of many bones at the joint.

compartment syndrome A serious condition that involves increased pressure, usually in the muscles; it leads to compromised blood flow and muscle and nerve damage.

crepitation (krep i TAY shun) A dry, crackling sound or sensation.

dynamometer (die nah MOM eh ter) An instrument used for measuring the degree of muscle power or force.

electrodes Adhesive patches that conduct electricity from the body to machine wires (e.g., electrocardiograph [ECG] and transcutaneous electrical nerve stimulation [TENS] unit).

gait The manner or style of walking.

goniometer (go nee OHM eh ter) A calibrated device designed to measure the arc, angle, or range of motion of a joint.

ligaments (LIH gah ments) Supportive connective tissue that connects bones at a joint.

modalities (moe DAL i tees) Therapeutic treatments for a disorder.

stoma A temporary or permanent surgically created opening used for drainage (i.e., urine, stool).

tendons (TEN duns) Connective tissue that attaches muscles to bone.

tripod position The standing position when using crutches; crutch tips are 4 to 6 inches to the side and front of each foot.

vasoconstriction (vay zoe kuhn STRIK shuhn) Contraction of the muscles that causes a narrowing of the inside tube of the blood vessel.

INTRODUCTION

Physical medicine and rehabilitation (PM&R) is also called *physiatry* or *rehabilitation medicine.* PM&R uses therapies and physical agents (e.g., heat, electricity, and light) to diagnose, prevent, and treat disorders. This area of medicine is focused on improving and restoring a patient's ability and quality of life when the person has physical impairments. Such disabilities include conditions that impact the nervous, muscular, and skeletal systems. The goals of PM&R are to do the following:

- Help the patient become as independent as possible with *activities of daily living* (e.g., grooming, walking, eating)
- Improve the person's quality of life (e.g., reduce pain, increase a person's ability to do activities)

A *physiatrist* is a physician who specializes in physical medicine and rehabilitation. A physiatrist diagnoses and prescribes treatments and therapies for the patient. As the patient undergoes rehabilitation, the physiatrist manages the patient's medical conditions. A physiatrist works closely with several therapies:

- *Physical therapy* (PT) focuses on improving a person's movement, strength, and mobility through the use of stretches, exercises, and other physical activities. A physical therapist works with patients to help them learn to walk with assistive devices, such as walkers and canes.
- *Occupational therapy* (OT) focuses on improving a person's ability to perform activities of daily living, such as bathing, grooming, toileting, and eating. OT is focused on a patient's fine and gross motor skills.
- *Speech therapy* is involved with the diagnosis and treatment of patients with swallowing and communication (speech and language) difficulties.

Often medical assistants are hired to assist physiatrists with patient care. Medical assistants in other areas of ambulatory care also work with patients who have conditions that affect movement and mobility. Coaching patients on how to use a sling, cold therapy, or assistive devices, such as crutches, is common in urgent care, orthopedics, and primary care settings. This chapter addresses the medical assistant's role in assisting with the examination and treatments of conditions related to rehabilitation.

ASSISTING WITH THE EXAMINATION

When a patient arrives for an examination, the medical assistant obtains the patient's vital signs and medical history. Allergies and medication lists are updated. The following sections describe the medical assistant's role in preparing the patient for the examination and assisting the patient during the examination.

Preparing for the Examination

When the medical assistant gathers a medical history on patients with a musculoskeletal concern, it is important to ask about the symptoms, the pain level, and the effect on the patient's life. When discussing the symptoms, the medical assistant should obtain information about the onset and what reduces or increases the symptoms. The medical assistant can ask the patient to rate the pain using a 0 to 10 scale. Zero is no pain, and 10 is the worst pain ever. Another pain assessment tool is the Wong-Baker FACES Pain Rating Scale, which is described in Chapter 21. The medical assistant should explain the scale to patients, and then patients can state how they feel. This scale works well for children. The healthcare facility may also require a functional assessment to be done, which gathers information on the patient's mobility and ability to do activities of daily living (ADLs) (e.g., toileting, bathing, grooming, and eating).

Assisting Patients

When you work with a patient who has an injury, assist the patient into a comfortable position and offer a pillow or folded blanket to support the extremity. For recent injuries, if ordered by the provider, apply a cold application to the injured area. (This procedure will be discussed later in the chapter.)

Patients may have limited mobility because of pain. The medical assistant may need to help patients change into the examination gown. Explain clearly what is happening and what the patient can expect.

CRITICAL THINKING APPLICATION 36.1

What is the advantage of using a pain scale when patients are experiencing pain?

ASSISTING WITH DIAGNOSTIC PROCEDURES

The medical assistant helps with diagnostic procedures by scheduling and preparing patients for procedures. If tests require restrictions of food or fluids, the medical assistant should address the following points with the patient after talking with the provider:

- Can the patient have water prior to the test?
- Which medications should the patient take prior to the test, or when can the patient resume the current medications?

Table 36.1 describes common diagnostic procedures used for musculoskeletal conditions. The medical assistant may need to screen the patient for specific allergies, medications, and so on prior to scheduling the procedure. For some procedures, a signed consent form is required. Patients should be notified of what they will experience during the procedure and any follow-up care required after the test.

Range-of-Motion Measurement

Often orthopedic injuries severely affect the normal range of motion (ROM) of a joint. The *range of motion* is the normal movement allowed by the joint. Testing the ROM of specific joints is an objective measure of both the seriousness of an injury and the recovery progress. The joint may be evaluated with active and passive ROM. To determine the *active ROM* of a joint, the patient is asked to move the joint as far as possible. To evaluate *passive ROM,* the provider moves the joint as far as possible.

A **goniometer** is the most common tool used to measure the ROM of a joint. Goniometers have calibration markings to indicate the measurement. A goniometer has two arms that are fixed together with a hinge joint at one end (Figure 36.1A). Each of the arms is lined up with a bone on each side of the joint being tested (Figure 36.1B). The degrees of motion are indicated on a scale on the hinged center of the nondigital instrument or on the digital display of the digital goniometer. All ROMs are measured in degrees. Usually, pain, tenderness, or **crepitation** is also noted during the procedure.

TABLE 36.1 Diagnostic Procedures for Musculoskeletal Conditions

PROCEDURE	DESCRIPTION	PATIENT PREPARATION
Arthrogram	Provides visualization of the soft tissues in the joint (e.g., **tendons**, **ligaments**, **cartilage**). A series of x-rays is taken of a joint after a contrast medium (e.g., dye) is injected into the joint.	Screen for pregnancy, **anticoagulant** use, and for allergy to contrast medium (iodine) or other medications used. Have patient sign a consent form. Patient may feel a sting when the medication is given. After the test, mild pain and swelling in the joint area may occur. Ice and **analgesics** are typically ordered.
Bone scan	Imaging test used to diagnose bone disease, tumor, or cancer. A small amount of radiotracer is injected into the vein and collects in the bones and organs. A camera slowly scans the body and takes pictures of the radiotracer that collects in the bones.	Screen for pregnancy. Patient should not take any medication with bismuth (e.g., Pepto-Bismol) for 4 days before the test. Have the patient remove all metal items (e.g., jewelry). A small amount of pain is felt when the needle is inserted. The scan is painless. Depending on the condition, an initial scan may be done as the radiotracer is injected and then another in 3 to 4 hours after the radiotracer has collected in the bone.
Computed tomography (CT, CT scan)	Used to detect fractures, tumors, and other abnormalities. This imaging test takes cross-sectional pictures of the body. Contrast medium may be used.	Screen for pregnancy and for allergy to contrast medium (iodine). Patient should not eat or drink for 4 to 6 hours prior to the test if a contrast medium is used. Have the patient remove all metal items (e.g., jewelry) and put on a gown. When the contrast medium is given, the person may feel some burning and flushing and may have a metallic taste in the mouth.
Dual-energy x-ray absorptiometry (DEXA) scan	A bone density test used to measure the calcium and other minerals in the bone. Central DEXA requires the scanner to pass over the spine and hip. Peripheral DEXA measures the bone density in the wrist, fingers, legs, or heels.	Screen for pregnancy. Patient should not take calcium supplements for 24 hours before the test. Have the patient remove all metal items (e.g., jewelry). Test is painless. The test results are reported as a T-score (compares the bone density to that of a healthy woman) and Z-score (compares the bone density to other people of the same age, gender, and race).
Electromyography (EMG)	Checks the nerves and muscles. Thin needle electrodes are inserted through the skin into the muscle to pick up the electrical activity in the muscle.	Screen for anticoagulant use. No special preparation is required. The person may feel a little pain when the needles are inserted. The site may be tender or bruised for a few days after the test.
Myelogram	Uses fluoroscopy and contrast medium to evaluate the spinal cord and related structures.	Screen patient for pregnancy and allergy to iodine contrast medium. Anticoagulants should be stopped several days before the test. Patient may have food and liquid restrictions prior to the test. Patient will feel a brief sting when the medication is given. The table is moved into different positions as the images are taken.
Nerve conduction velocity (NCV)	Used with an EMG to test the speed of electrical signals through a nerve. Electrodes are placed on the skin. Each electrode gives off a mild electrical impulse that stimulates the nerve.	Screen the patient for a cardiac defibrillator or pacemaker. Patient should not wear lotion, perfume, or moisturizer. The impulse will feel like a small electric shock.

CRITICAL THINKING APPLICATION 36.2

How can Tim best assist Dr. Kahn in testing upper extremity ROM in a new patient? What equipment should Tim have ready? What patient position would best facilitate this examination? Why?

Muscle Strength Evaluation

During the ROM evaluation, the provider also assesses each muscle group for strength. Normal muscle strength allows for complete voluntary ROM despite resistance. This resistance can be gravity, as when rising from a sitting to a standing position, or physical, as in pulling, pushing, or lifting an object. Muscle strength is bilaterally equal in normal conditions.

Hand grip strength can be measured with a **dynamometer** (Figure 36.2A). Digital and nondigital dynamometers are available. A dynamometer provides an objective measurement of hand grip strength. The patient holds the dynamometer in the hand being tested. Typically, the arm is at the side of the patient with the elbow bent at 90 degrees. Various arm and hand positions may be used for different assessments. If a dynamometer is not available, a blood pressure cuff can be used (Figure 36.2B). Follow these steps to assess the hand strength:

1. Roll up an aneroid blood pressure cuff, and have the patient hold it in one hand.
2. Inflate the cuff to 20 mm Hg of pressure, and lock the valve.
3. Ask the patient to squeeze the cuff as tightly as possible.

4. Note the increase in pressure on the dial (a normal grip registers above 150 mm Hg).
5. Record the hand tested and the results of the test.
6. Repeat on the other hand.

ASSISTING WITH IMMOBILIZATION TREATMENTS

There is a wide range of immobilization treatments used for patients with musculoskeletal conditions and rehabilitation. The following sections describe devices that provide varying degrees of immobilization to the affected extremity. The medical assistant needs to be familiar with how to apply the devices and the required coaching for patients.

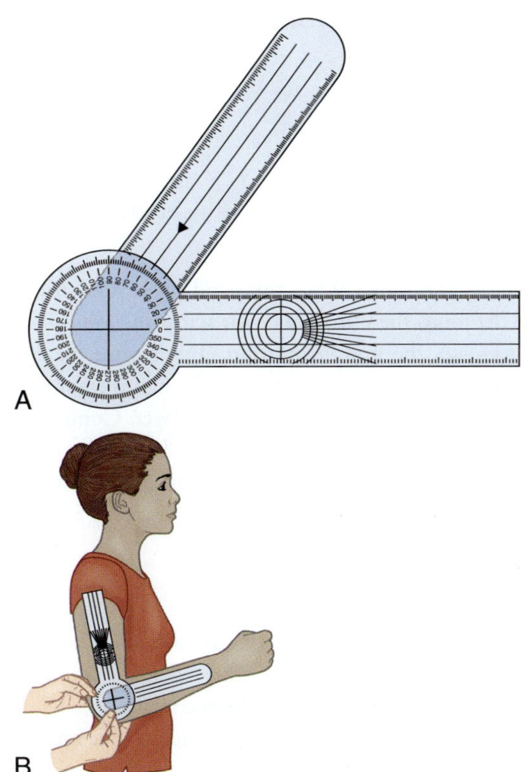

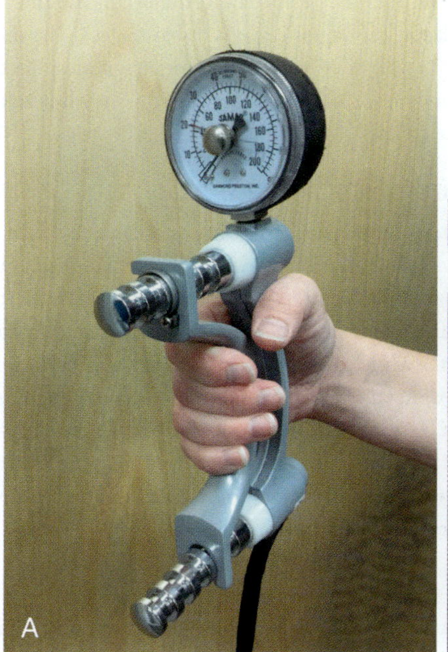

FIGURE 36.1 **(A)** Goniometer. **(B)** Correct position of the goniometer on the arm.

Elastic Bandages

An elastic bandage, a roller bandage, is sometimes called an ACE wrap, ACE bandage, and compression wrap. Besides being used as a bandage over a wound, an elastic bandage is used to limit swelling (edema) in the injured or operative extremity. Commonly, elastic bandages are used for sprains and can restrict movement and provide support to an extremity. Special skill is required to apply elastic bandages properly. Different wrap techniques can be used when applying the elastic bandage. Bandages that are too loose fall off, and those that are too tight can compromise circulation and further harm the patient. It takes practice and attention in order to apply bandages correctly.

Bandaging Techniques

Before beginning the bandaging process, the medical assistant must select the correct size bandage if it is not indicated by the provider. Usually for older teens and adults, a 2-inch-wide elastic bandage is used for the hand; a 3-inch-wide bandage is used for the forearm, arm, and lower leg; and a 4 to 6-inch-wide bandage is used for the thigh. The extremity should be clean and dry. During the bandaging process, the body part should be positioned in a normal resting position (position of function). As the bandage is applied, ensure it is smooth and free of wrinkles.

Start the wrapping at the distal end of the extremity, moving proximally. Leave the fingers or toes exposed for circulation checks. Check the circulation below the bandage. Loosen the bandage if the circulation is impaired.

Several bandaging techniques can be used:

- *Anchor technique*: Can be used at the beginning of the bandaging procedure to secure the elastic bandage. To start, place the end of the bandage at an angle on the extremity, then wrap the bandage around the limb twice. The angled corner edge of the bandage forms a small triangle. Fold the corner edge over the second turn

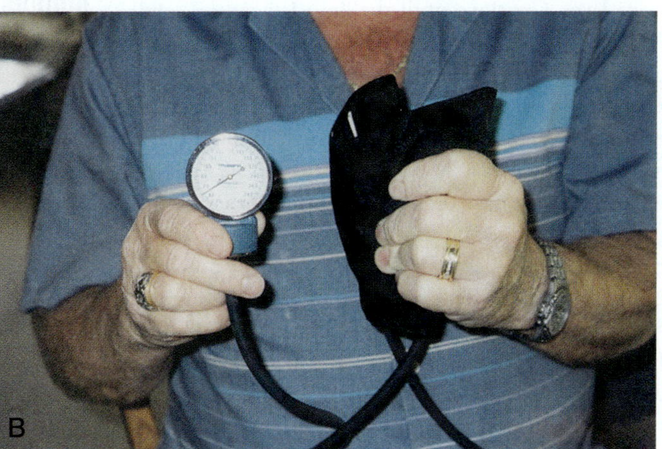

FIGURE 36.2 **(A)** Dynamometer. **(B)** Assessing grip strength using a blood pressure cuff.

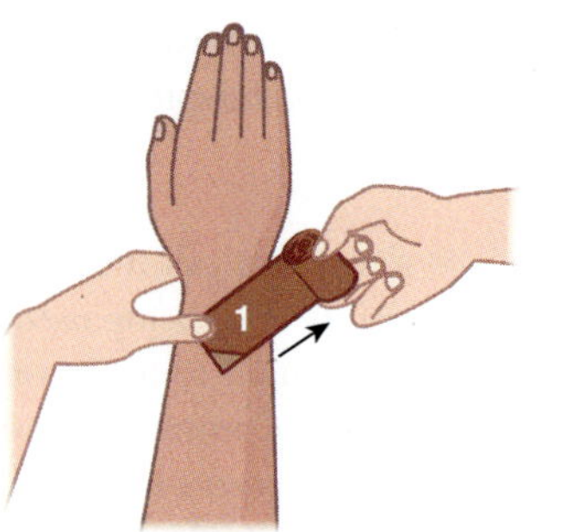

1. Place the end of the roller bandage on a slant.

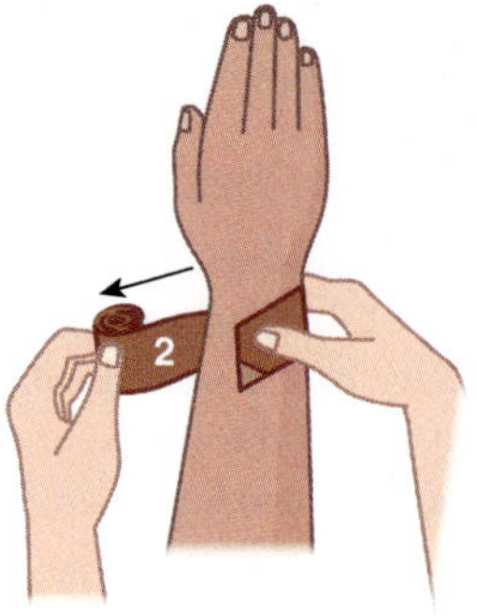

2. Encircle the part while allowing the corner of the bandage to extend.

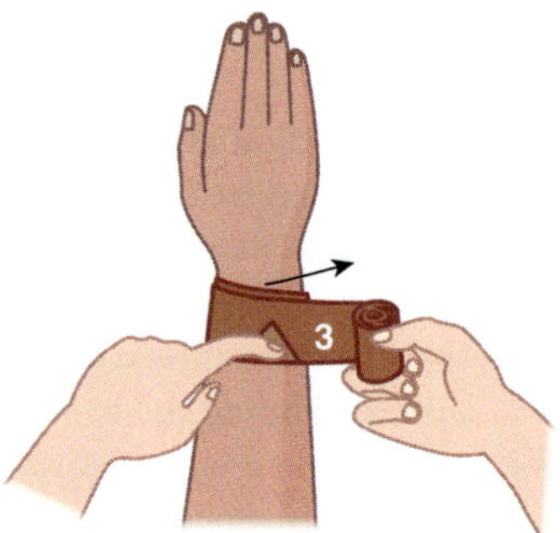

3. Turn down the corner of the bandage.

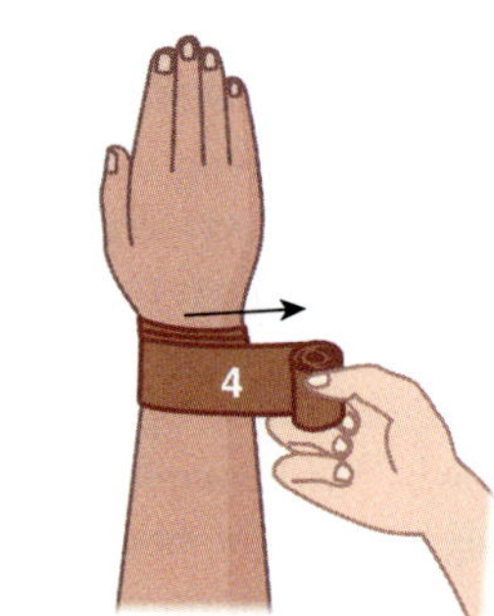

4. Make another circular turn around the part.

FIGURE 36.3 The anchor technique can be used at the beginning of the bandaging procedure, before other techniques are used.

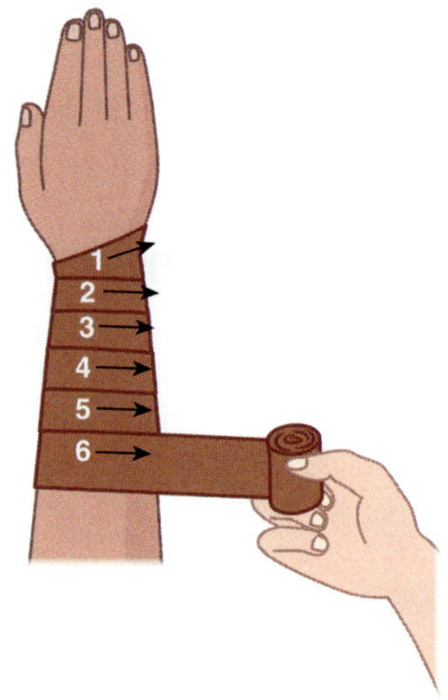

FIGURE 36.4 The spiral technique is used on arms and legs. It is not used over the ankle or elbow.

and cover the corner as you wrap the bandage around the limb the third time. This will anchor the bandage (Figure 36.3).

- *Circular technique*: Can be used at the beginning of the bandaging procedure in place of the anchor technique and is most commonly used at the end of the procedure to secure the bandage before applying tape, clips, or the Velcro. Roll the elastic bandage over the affected area in a circular motion. The second and subsequent layers should overlap the previous layer completely.
- *Spiral technique*: Is used to cover the arm or leg. Start by using an anchor or circular technique. Then wrap the limb in a spiral manner with the new layer of wrapping covering about one-third of the previous layer. Continue until the limb is wrapped, and complete the procedure with a circular technique before securing the bandage (Figure 36.4).
- *Spiral reverse technique*: Is used to cover the arm or leg. Start by using an anchor or circular technique. Then use the spiral technique for four turns, then reverse the spiral turn. Place a finger on the top edge of the bandage on the extremity and then direct the bandage downward so it folds onto itself. The upper edge of the bandage should be parallel to the lower edge of the previous turn, and overlap it by two-thirds of the width. Continue until the limb is wrapped, and complete the procedure with a circular technique before securing the bandage (Figure 36.5).
- *Figure-eight technique*: Is used to support and limit joint movement. Start with the anchor or circular technique. Next, wrap the bandage below the joint, then bring the bandage up diagonally and across the joint. Wrap the bandage around the extremity above the joint, then bring it down across the joint diagonally so that it crosses the upward portion. This creates the figure-eight appearance. Continue to wrap using the figure-eight method and overlapping two-thirds of the previous layer. Continue until the joint is wrapped, and complete the procedure with a circular technique before securing the bandage (Figure 36.6, Procedure 36.1).

Figure 36.7 shows two techniques for wrapping an amputation stump.

Splints

Splints are temporarily applied to immobilize joints and bones after injury or surgery. The splint can be adjusted as the swelling changes. It provides partial protection while the site heals.

A splint consists of a strip of rigid material that immobilizes an extremity. Custom-designed and ready-made splints are used in the ambulatory care environment. Custom-designed splints commonly use a strip of fiberglass as the rigid material. The fiberglass is held in place by elastic bandages (e.g., ACE bandages). The medical assistant can help the provider apply custom-designed splints. Ready-made splints usually have Velcro straps, which help when taking off or putting on the splints.

Immobilizers, Braces, and Ankle Boots

Immobilizers, braces, and ankle boots are usually used after an injury or surgery. Often the terms *immobilizer* and *brace* are used interchangeably, but they are different. An *immobilizer* keeps the joint from moving (Figure 36.8). A *brace* provides stability and protection to the joint while allowing the joint to still function. Some knee braces have metal hinges that allow the knee to bend and straighten.

An *ankle boot* (also called a *moon boot* or *walker boot*) is a rigid, removable boot. It is used to protect and stabilize the ankle and lower leg after an injury or surgery. These boots can be used for partial, full, or non–weight-bearing extremities.

Slings

A *sling* is a device used to support and immobilize an injured part of the body, such as the arm, wrist, or shoulder. A sling is often used to

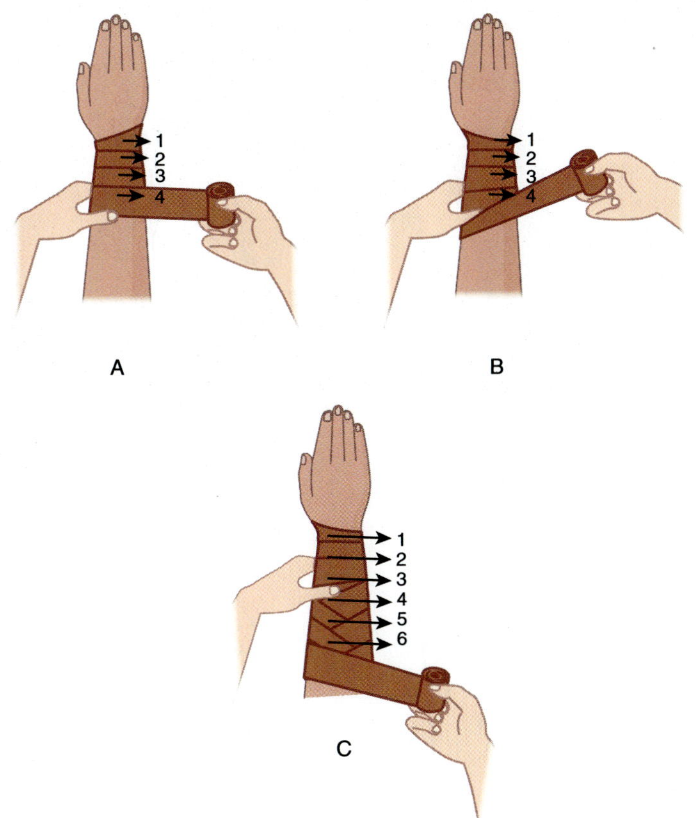

FIGURE 36.5 The spiral reverse technique creates a V-shaped fold that allows the bandage to fit the curves of the extremity. It is more often used with nonelastic bandages.

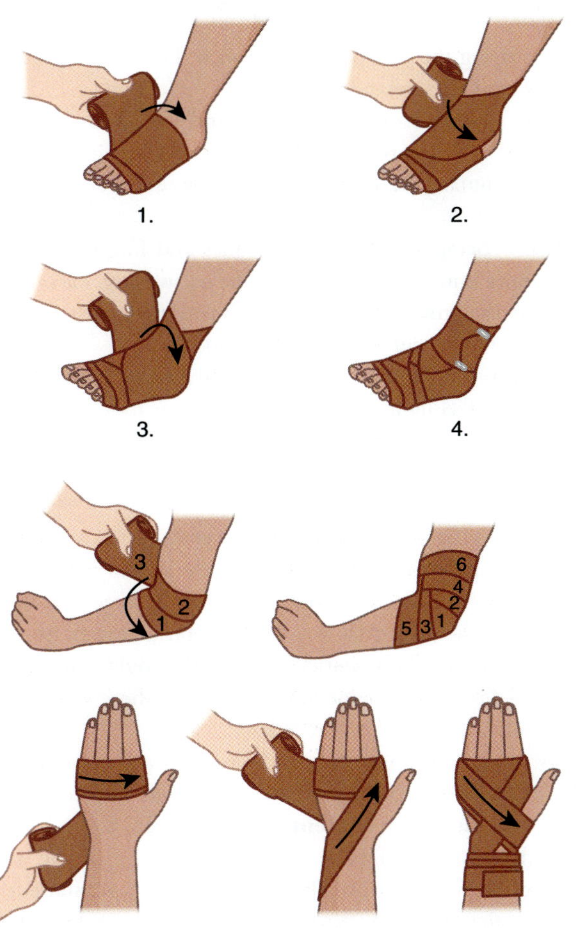

FIGURE 36.6 The figure-eight technique is used to bandage the hand, elbow, foot, ankle, and knee.

help support the arm if a person has an arm casted (Procedure 36.2). A sling can help keep the hand elevated to reduce swelling in the hand and fingers. Slings come in adult and pediatric sizes.

If the sling is too loose, it may place stress and strain on the arm. The elbow should be kept at a 90-degree angle. If the sling is too tight, it can compromise or restrict circulation. The patient may have numbness, tingling, or swelling in the hand. The fingers and hand may be blue and cool to the touch.

Casts

Casts are applied to immobilize joints and bones after injury or surgery and provide additional protection. Casts are made from fiberglass or plaster. Fiberglass casts can be colorful, lightweight, durable, and porous. X-rays penetrate fiberglass casts better than plaster casts. Thus, fiberglass casts do not need to be removed for x-rays. Plaster casts are cheaper and easier to shape. The medical assistant can help the provider apply the cast.

Casts applied in ambulatory care facilities are usually either long or short casts:

- A *short arm cast* extends from the palm to just before the elbow.
- A *long arm cast* extends from the palm to the mid-upper arm.
- A *short leg cast* extends from the foot to just before the kneecap (patella).
- A *long leg cast* extends from the foot to the mid-thigh.

Extremity casts do not cover the fingers or toes because it is important to check circulation.

During the fiberglass cast application, the medical assistant assembles the supplies and assists the provider with the application (Procedure 36.3).

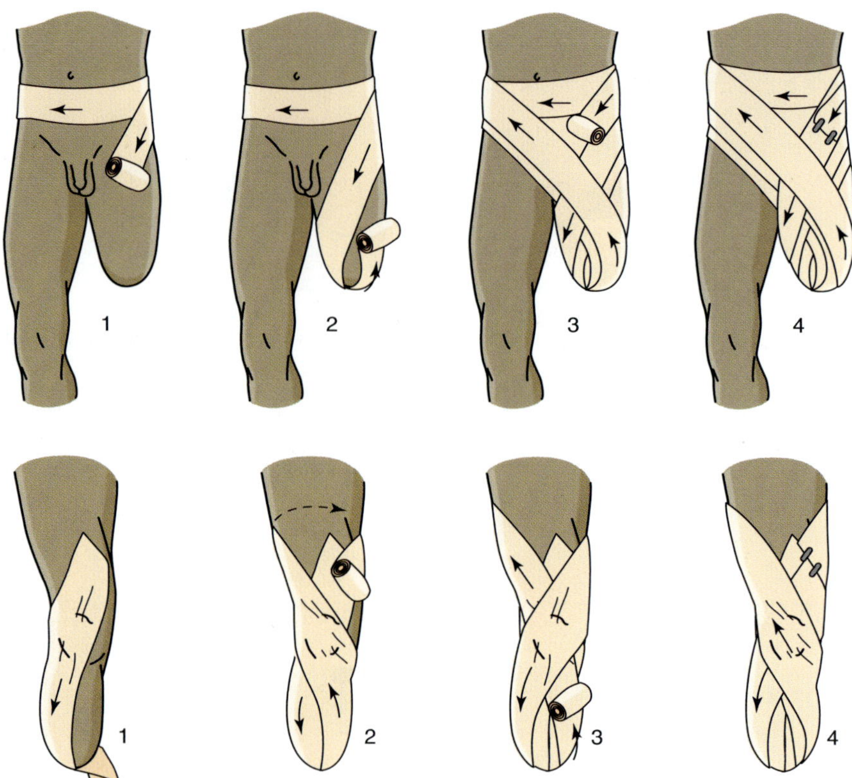

FIGURE 36.7 Bandaging amputation stumps. Start from outer thigh moving down to cover the amputated region, crossing it over the inner thigh, and repeat the process to form layers. *Top,* Correct method for bandaging a midthigh amputation stump. Note that the bandage must be anchored around the patient's waist. *Bottom,* Correct method for bandaging a midcalf amputation stump. Note that the bandage need not be anchored around the patient's waist. (From Monahan F, et al: *Phipps' medical-surgical nursing: health and illness perspectives,* ed 8, St. Louis, 2006, Mosby.)

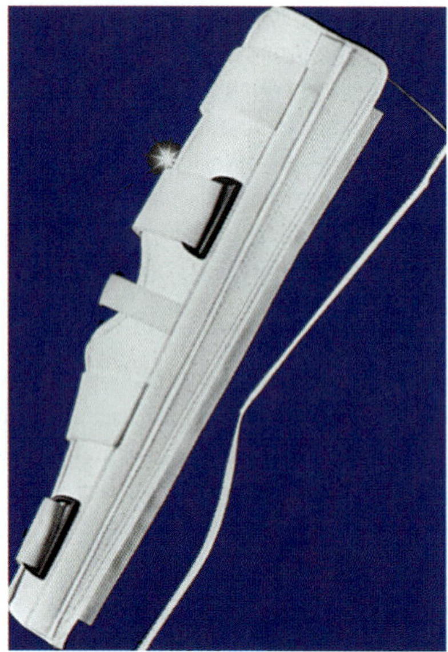

FIGURE 36.8 Knee immobilizer. (From Maher AB, Salmond SW, Pellino T, editors: *Orthopaedic nursing,* ed 3, Philadelphia, 2002, Saunders.)

CRITICAL THINKING APPLICATION 36.3

Describe the advantages of a fiberglass cast over a plaster cast.

Patient Coaching on CMST

The medical assistant needs to provide cast care instructions to patients. It is important to teach patients about checking the CMST and comparing the casted extremity with the unaffected extremity. Here is what CMST stands for:

- ***Color***: The color of the extremity and nail beds should match those of the opposite extremity. It should be pink. The patient should contact the provider if the toes or fingers are bluish or pale.
- ***Motion***: Being able to move the toes and fingers of the casted extremity is normal. There should be no swelling. Patients should contact the provider if they are unable to move the toes or fingers or if swelling occurs in the fingers and toes.
- ***Sensation***: Normal sensation should be intact. The person should be able to feel light touch on the fingers or toes. Patients should contact the provider if they notice any of the following:
  - An increased pain, burning, stinging, or numbness in the toes or fingers
  - A "sleeping" or pins-and-needles sensation
  - An inability to feel light touch on the toes or fingers
- ***Temperature***: The temperature of the toes or fingers on the casted extremity should match that of the opposite extremity. The fingers or toes should be warm. The patient should contact the provider if the fingers or toes are cooler than those of the opposite extremity.

Any suspicious abnormal findings should be reported to the provider immediately. If the extremity swells too much for the size of the cast, **compartment syndrome** can occur. The swelling of the casted extremity can cause damage to the muscles, blood vessels, and nerves. The damage can be permanent if not treated.

CRITICAL THINKING APPLICATION 36.4

In your own words, how would you explain CMST to a patient, including the signs and symptoms to report to the provider?

Patient Coaching on Cast Care

It is important for the patient to learn how to care for the cast and the extremity:

- Elevate and place dry cold packs on the casted extremity as indicated by the provider. Usually, this is done for the first 24 hours after an injury.
- Continue to move the fingers or toes, which helps to return the blood to the heart and to reduce the swelling.
- Keep the cast clean and dry. Contact the provider if the cast becomes smelly, moldy, or if drainage is noted.
- Cover the cast with a plastic bag prior to bathing or showering. If the fiberglass cast gets wet, use a hair dryer on a cool setting to dry it.
- Avoid putting weight or pressure on the cast.
- Do not put anything inside the cast, including sharp objects, powder, or lotion.
- A metal file can be used to smooth down rough sections of a fiberglass cast. Pad the rough areas to protect the skin.
- A sling can be used to support a casted arm.

Removing Casts

The medical assistant can remove casts in the ambulatory care facility (Procedure 36.4). During the removal procedure, the medical assistant should provide adequate support for the extremity. Once the cast is off, the extremity should be washed with a mild soap and warm water, then dried. Skin lotion can be applied. This might be done in the ambulatory care facility or can be done at home.

The medical assistant must coach the patient prior to the cast removal that the extremity may look different. The skin may be dry and flaky. The extremity may be smaller and weaker than the other side. The patient may have some discomfort in the bones and joints that were immobilized. Sometimes patients will need physical therapy to help regain strength and movement in the affected side.

ASSISTING WITH COLD AND HEAT THERAPIES

Cold and heat therapeutic **modalities** or treatments are used for orthopedic injuries and infections. The applications can be as follows:

- *Dry*: No moisture is left on the skin. Dry applications tend to pull moisture out of the skin.
- *Moist*: Moisture is left on the skin. Moist applications tend to increase tissue elasticity and allow heat or cold to penetrate deeper into the tissues.

When using heat or cold applications, the medical assistant should ask the patient if it feels too hot or too cold. The medical assistant should monitor the area being treated. Some patients are at higher risk for tissue injury with heat or cold applications:

- Younger children because of their thinner skin
- Older adults due to their reduced sensitivity to pain
- People with impaired circulation (e.g., those with peripheral vascular diseases and diabetes mellitus)
- People with altered sensitivity (e.g., those who are confused or have neurologic disorders, including diabetic neuropathy and spinal cord damage)
- Those for whom the application is placed on an open wound, broken skin, or **stoma** (this tissue is more sensitive)
- Those for whom the application is placed on edematous or scarred areas (scars and edema reduce sensitivity)

Patient Education for Cold and Heat Applications

- Know what supplies are required and where they can be purchased.
- Use a protective covering between the skin and the application.
- Never fall asleep with an application on the skin.
- Never place an application over metal jewelry.
- Know the length of time for each application, the number of times a day ordered, and the number of days for treatment.
- Heat and cold therapy should be applied for 15 to 20 minutes. Additional time can harm the tissues.
- After the session, remove the application. Allow the skin to return to its normal temperature before applying again.
- Prolonged erythema or paleness, pain, swelling, and blisters should be reported to the provider.

Cold Therapy

Cold therapy is typically used for sprains, strains, fractures, joint injuries, shin splints, and other injuries. In some facilities, it is a common practice to provide a cold pack to a patient who comes in with a recent injury.

A cold application causes **vasoconstriction**, which reduces blood flow to the area. As a result, tissue metabolism decreases, less oxygen is used, and less swelling occurs. The nerve endings in the area become numb. The blood viscosity increases, which can cause clotting. Cold therapy helps to reduce pain and inflammation and prevents edema (swelling) in the injured area. Table 36.2 describes common types of cold applications. Procedure 36.5 describes how to apply a cold pack.

Heat Therapy

Heat therapy can be used to relieve the following conditions:

- Acute pain (e.g., back and menstrual) and chronic pain (e.g., arthritis)
- Sinus congestion
- Infection (e.g., localized abscesses)

Heat therapy can help with muscle relaxation. It can produce local vasodilation, which increases circulation. The increased blood supply to a local area helps to absorb the extra fluid (from edema). Table 36.3 discusses the types of hot applications. Additional types of heat therapy will be discussed. Procedure 36.6 describes how to apply a hot pack.

Paraffin Bath Therapy

Paraffin provides deep heat therapy. The heat can reduce pain and tenderness. It has been found to maintain muscle strength and increase mobility. Paraffin therapy is a common treatment for arthritis and other conditions that cause pain and stiffness.

TABLE 36.2 Types of Cold Applications

TYPE	DRY OR MOIST	DESCRIPTION
Cold compress	Moist	Washcloth or other soft cloth is dampened with a cold solution (e.g., water) and applied to the skin.
Chemical cold pack	Dry	Comes in a variety of sizes. Stored at room temperature. Contains inner areas of a dry chemical and water. When activated, the water and chemical mix creates coldness.
Ice bag	Dry	A bag with cubes or pieces of ice.
Gel pack	Dry	Aqueous gel that freezes. Reusable. Stored in freezer.
Bead pack	Dry	Little beads of gel conform to the site even when frozen. Similar to a frozen bag of peas. Reusable. Stored in freezer.

TABLE 36.3 Types of Hot Applications

TYPE	DRY OR MOIST	DESCRIPTION
Hot soak/ whirlpool bath (Hydrotherapy)	Moist	Part of the body is submerged in warm water or a warm medicated solution. Should be warmed to 105°F to 110°F (40.6°C to 43.3°F).
Hot compress	Moist	Washcloth or other soft cloth is dampened with a hot solution (e.g., water) and applied to the skin.
Heating pad	Dry	Electric pad that warms. Inspect for safety purposes.
Chemical hot pack	Dry	Comes in a variety of sizes. Stored at room temperature. Contains inner areas of a dry chemical and water. When activated, the water and chemical mix, creating heat for a period of time.
Gel pack	Dry	Aqueous gel that can be microwaved. Reusable.
Bead pack	Dry	Little beads of gel that can be microwaved. Reusable.

A paraffin bath uses melted paraffin and mineral oil warmed to about 125°F (51.7°C). The patient bathes a foot or hand in the bath. Once the extremity is coated, the patient should lift it out and let it dry for a few seconds (Figure 36.9). This process is repeated until the patient has 10 to 12 layers of wax built up on the extremity. The foot or hand is wrapped in plastic and then in a towel to retain the moisture and heat. After 20 minutes, it is unwrapped, and the wax is removed.

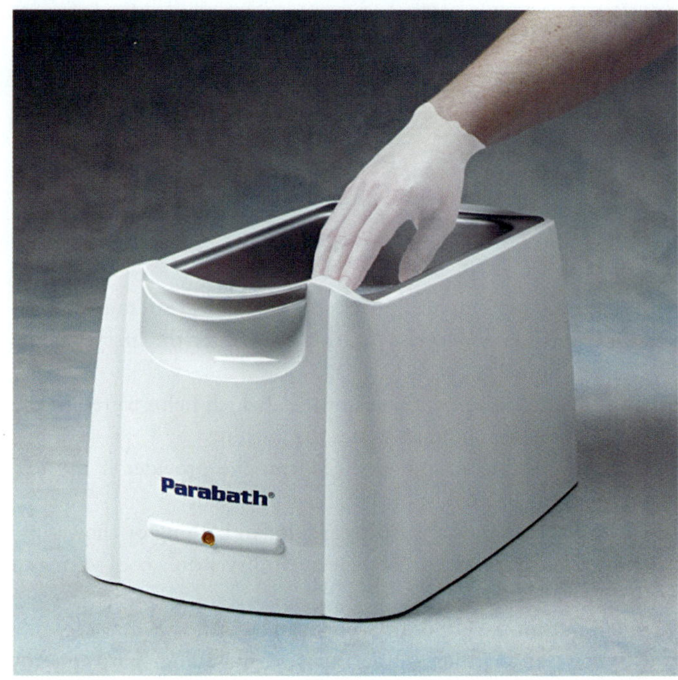

FIGURE 36.9 A paraffin bath is especially helpful for relieving pain in patients with arthritis.

Heat Lamp Therapy

Two commonly used heat lamp therapies are red light therapy and near infrared light therapy. Red light therapy is used to treat skin conditions. Near infrared light therapy penetrates deeper, killing pathogens, healing tissue, improving circulation, and relieving pain.

PHYSICAL THERAPY TREATMENTS

Different physical therapy treatments can be used to help treat musculoskeletal conditions. The medical assistant should be familiar with the treatments.

Ultrasound Therapy

Ultrasound therapy has been used for a long time to treat pain and promote healing. The ultrasound transducer head produces sound waves. Ultrasound gel is applied to the skin. As the transducer head is moved over the skin, the gel helps with the transmission of sound waves into the soft tissue. There are two main types of ultrasound therapy: thermal and mechanical. The main difference between these types is the speed at which the sound waves penetrate the soft tissue. Ultrasound therapy must be done by a trained therapist. This treatment is often provided in chiropractic, sports medicine, physical therapy, and occupational therapy facilities.

RICE Therapy

For orthopedic injuries, RICE is commonly ordered as a treatment, usually for the first 48 to 72 hours. After 72 hours, moist heat is prescribed. Here is what RICE stands for:

- ***Rest***: Reduce activities for a period of time. Crutches can help an injured leg/ankle rest.

- *Ice*: Apply a cold pack to the injured area for 15 to 20 minutes, four to eight times daily.
- *Compression*: Use elastic bandage (e.g., ACE Wrap) or splints to reduce swelling. It is important to monitor the CMST of a wrapped extremity.
- *Elevation*: Elevate the injured extremity higher than the level of the heart to reduce swelling.

CRITICAL THINKING APPLICATION **36.5**

In your own words, how would you explain RICE to a patient?

Exercise Therapy

Often patients are encouraged to exercise to maintain their strength and joint mobility. Patients recovering from surgery (e.g., orthopedic, cardiac) may need to see a physical therapist or an occupational therapist. These therapists work with patients to help them regain their mobility and strength. Isometric, isotonic, and range-of-motion exercises are encouraged to maintain strength, flexibility, and mobility.

Isometric contractions do not change the muscle length, but they do increase the muscle tension. Isometric exercises help to maintain a person's strength. *Isotonic* contractions cause muscles to shorten and thicken and cause movement at a joint. Isotonic exercises help restore movement after an injury and relieve stiffness and pain. ROM exercises help to maintain flexibility and joint mobility and reduce stiffness. *Active ROM exercises* are done by the patient, whereas *passive ROM exercises* are done by a caregiver or therapist. For patients who have had a stroke or other trauma that affects movement, daily ROM exercises are critical to prevent joints from freezing up. Frozen joints have limited to no movement.

CRITICAL THINKING APPLICATION **36.6**

In your own words, describe isometric, isotonic, active ROM exercises, and passive ROM exercises.

Electrical Muscle Stimulation

A transcutaneous electrical nerve stimulation (TENS) unit is used for pain relief (Figure 36.10). **Electrodes** are placed on the skin in specific locations. The adjustable low-voltage machine sends electrical current through disposable gel electrodes into the skin. The current stimulates specific nerves, producing a tingling or massaging sensation that reduces pain. TENS units have been used for passive exercise of muscles when a patient cannot exercise the extremity (e.g., due to injury or stroke). The electrical stimulation can prevent atrophy of normal muscles. TENS units are also used to treat the pain from muscle, joint, or other orthopedic conditions.

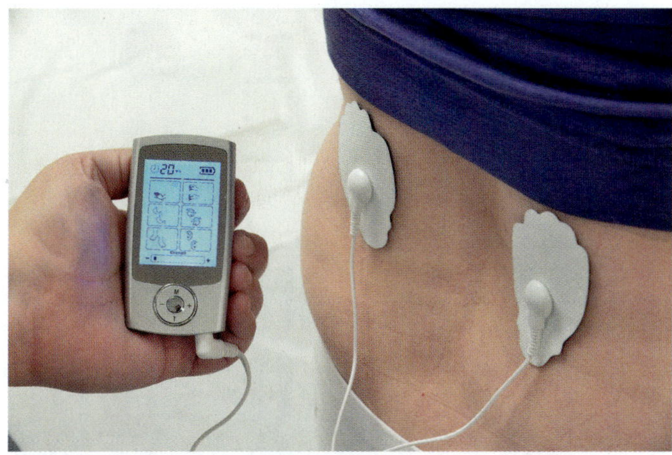

FIGURE 36.10 Application of a transcutaneous electrical nerve stimulation (TENS) unit.

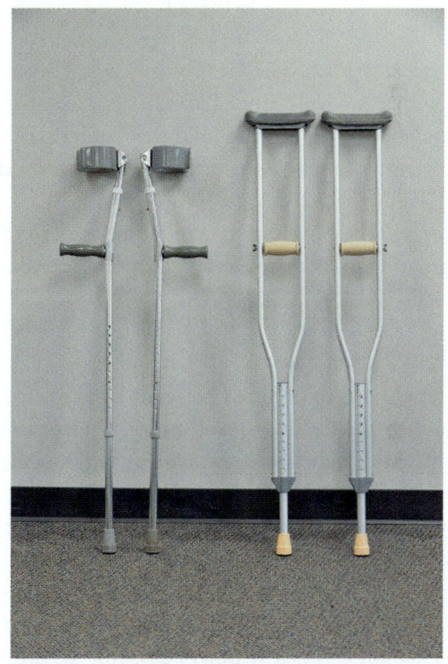

FIGURE 36.11 Forearm crutches *(left)* and axillary crutches *(right)*.

ASSISTING WITH ASSISTIVE DEVICES

An assistive device is used to help a person perform a specific task, such as walking. Crutches, walkers, canes, and wheelchairs are considered assistive devices. Many times, these assistive devices can be purchased at pharmacies and medical supply stores. The medical assistant should know how to adjust the device to fit the patient. Medical assistants may also coach patients on the proper use of the assistive device. Improper use of assistive devices can lead to falls and injuries.

Crutches

Crutches are used to help a person walk. Crutches can be made out of aluminum or wood and can be adjusted for the patient. The more common crutches are as follows:

- *Axillary crutches*: Most common type; used when recovering from a foot, ankle, or leg injury or surgery (Figure 36.11).
- *Forearm crutches*: Also called *Lofstrand* or *elbow crutches;* require more upper body strength. An open elbow cuff fits around the patient's forearm (see Figure 36.11). These crutches help with proper posture and body mechanics.
- *Extension crutches*: Also called *Canadian crutches.* These combine the underarm crutch with an elbow cuff, which provides extra support for the patient.

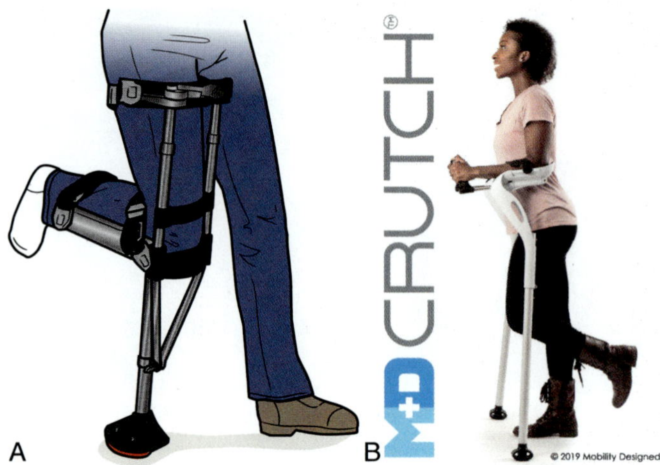

FIGURE 36.12 **(A)** Hands-free crutch. **(B)** M+D crutches by Mobility Designed, Inc. (Courtesy of Mobility Designed, Inc.)

- *Platform crutches*: Also called *triceps crutches*. They have padded armrests with handgrips. These crutches are used when patients cannot straighten their arms to hold the handgrip of the crutch.
- *Hands-free crutch*: Straps to the thigh, and a platform supports the lower leg (Figure 36.12A).
- *M+D crutches*: The hinged arm cradles the strap to the forearms, thus eliminating pressure in the axillae, wrists, and hands (Figure 36.12B).

Fitting Axillary Crutches

Axillary crutches need to be fitted correctly to allow for good body mechanics and to reduce the risk of injury. *Crutch palsy* can occur with poorly fitted crutches or if the patient rests on the top of the crutches while walking. The axillary nerves can be temporarily or permanently damaged. This can cause loss of hand strength and weakening of the wrist and forearm muscles.

When you fit axillary crutches, the patient must be wearing shoes. Have the patient stand straight up. Fit the crutches so they are 1 to 1½ inches (about 2 finger widths) below the armpit. The crutch should be about 4 to 6 inches to the side and front of each foot. Handgrips must be near the wrist and even with the top of the hip line. When the hands are on the handgrip, the elbow should be bent 15 to 30 degrees.

Limitations with Crutches

Providers will indicate the type of crutch, along with any limitations. Common limitations with crutches include the following:

- *Weight bearing as tolerated*: Patients can place more than half of their body weight on their "bad," or affected, extremity if it is not painful.
- *Partial weight bearing*: The provider will indicate how much weight can be placed on the affected extremity.
- *Toe-touch weight bearing*: Patients can touch the ground with their toes on the affected side. The toe-touch helps with balance. No weight bearing is allowed on the affected extremity.
- *Non–weight bearing*: Patients cannot put weight on their affected extremity. This type of limitation would require the three-point crutch **gait**.

Crutch Gaits

There are several crutch gaits that a medical assistant should know. The provider may also specify the gait the patient should use. The gait depends on whether the patient can put weight on the affected extremity. The following are common gaits:

- *Two-point crutch gait*: Mimics normal walking. The patient must be able to put some weight on both legs. From the **tripod position** (starting position) use this sequence: Move the right crutch with left foot forward and then move the left crutch with the right foot forward. There are two individual movements with this gait. Repeat this pattern (Figure 36.13A).
- *Four-point crutch gait*: Must be able to put some weight on both legs. This gait is slower, but safer for those with generalized weakness. From the tripod position, use this sequence: Move the right crutch forward, then move the left foot forward, next move the left crutch forward, and lastly bring the right foot forward. There are four individual movements with this gait. Repeat this pattern (Figure 36.13B).
- *Three-point crutch gait*: Used when partial weight bearing or non–weight bearing is indicated. From the tripod position, use this sequence: Move both crutches and the affected leg forward, then move the "good," or unaffected, leg forward. Repeat this pattern (Figure 36.13C and Procedure 36.7).
- *Swing to crutch gait*: Must be able to put some weight on both legs. From the tripod position, use this sequence: Move both crutches forward, then swing the body so the feet are even with the line of the crutches. Repeat this pattern.
- *Swing-through crutch gait*: Must be able to put some weight on both legs. From the tripod position, use this sequence: Move both crutches forward, then swing the body so the feet land in front of the line of the crutches. Repeat this pattern (Figure 36.13D).

CRITICAL THINKING APPLICATION **36.7**

Describe how a person would perform each of the five crutch gaits. Which gait(s) would be used for toe-touch weight bearing? Partial weight bearing? Non—weight bearing?

Walkers

Some patients use walkers after surgery. Many older adults use walkers for help with balance and support. Walkers provide more support than canes. A walker's wide base helps stabilize the gait of the patient and can support up to 50% of the body weight. Walkers have a metal frame and can easily be adjusted to fit an individual. They are lightweight, and several types can fold flat for storage and travel. Several types of walkers are available:

- *Hemi-walker*: Also called a *one-hand walker*. These walkers are used by patients who can only grasp the walker with one hand due to a stroke or arm/hand amputation (Figure 36.14).
- *Standard walker*: A very common walker; it has four nonskid, rubber-tipped legs (see Figure 36.14). A person needs to pick up the walker with every completed step. Sometimes tennis balls are inserted over the feet to help to move the walker easily across the floor.

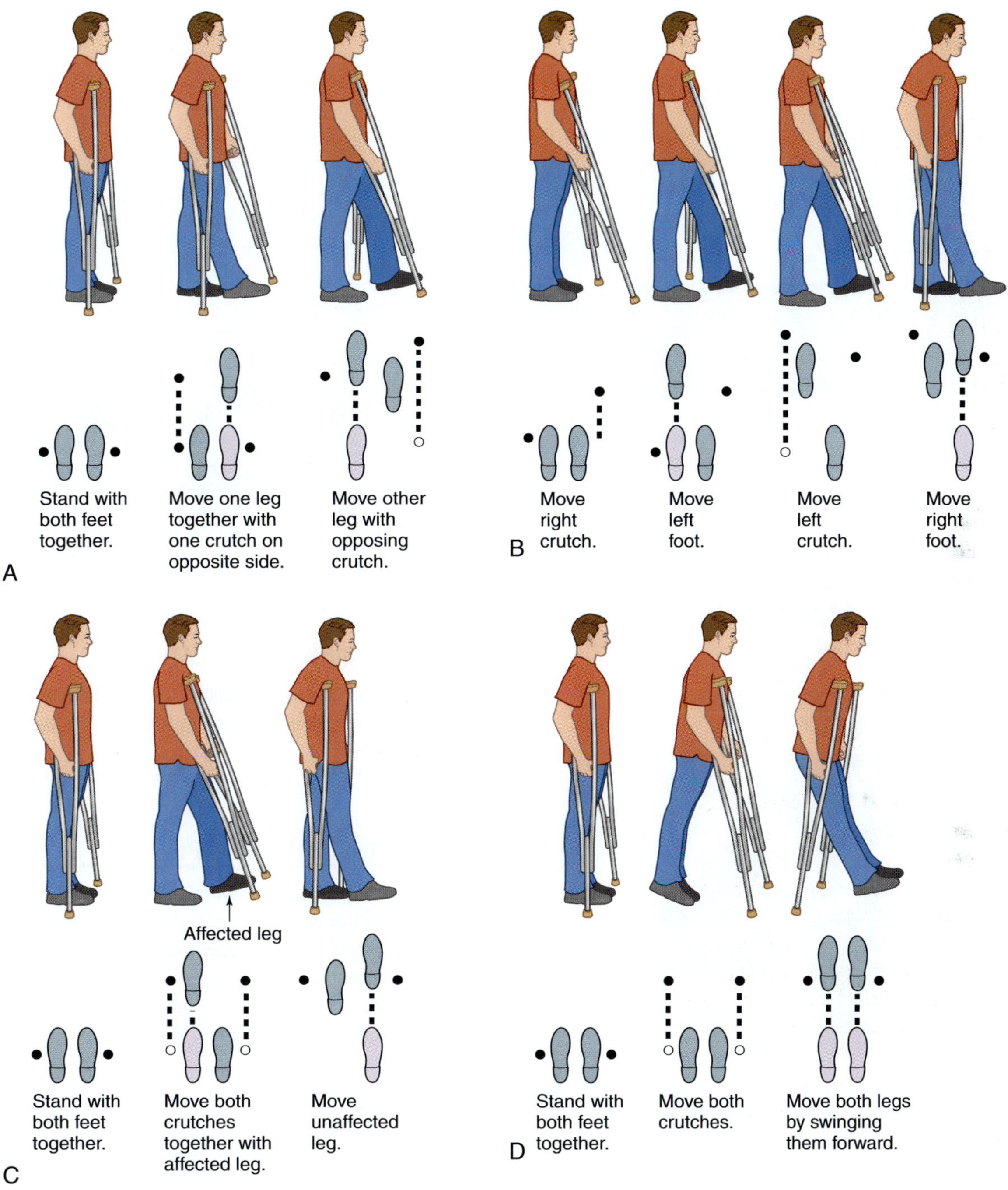

FIGURE 36.13 Crutch gaits. **(A)** Two-point crutch gait. **(B)** Four-point crutch gait. **(C)** Three-point crutch gait. **(D)** Swing-through gait.

- *Two-wheel walker*: Resembles the standard walker, but the front two legs have wheels. This type of walker is for those who need some help but not constant weight-bearing help (see Figure 36.14).
- *Three-wheel walker* and *four-wheel walker*: Also called a *Rollator.* Each leg has a wheel, and many Rollators have brakes by the handles. Some models have a seat and a basket. These walkers are for people who do not need to lean on a walker for balance.
- *Knee walker*: A foot-propelled scooter that has a platform to rest the knee and lower leg (Figure 36.15). This is commonly used instead of axillary crutches for leg or foot conditions.

When you fit a walker, the patient must be wearing shoes. Have the patient step into the walker and relax the arms at the sides of the body. The top of the walker grip should be near the crease in the wrist and even with the top of the hip line. With the shoulders relaxed and the hands on the grips, the elbows should be bent 15 degrees. Procedure 36.8 discusses fitting a walker and coaching a patient to use a walker.

Canes

A cane can provide extra assistance for a person who has a minor balance or stability problem. There are two basic types of canes but several different grips or handles. Here are the basic types of canes:

- Single-tipped cane: Provides minimal assistance with walking (Figure 36.16).
- Four-tipped cane: Also called a *quad cane.* It provides greater stability for patients than the single-tipped cane (see Figure 36.16).

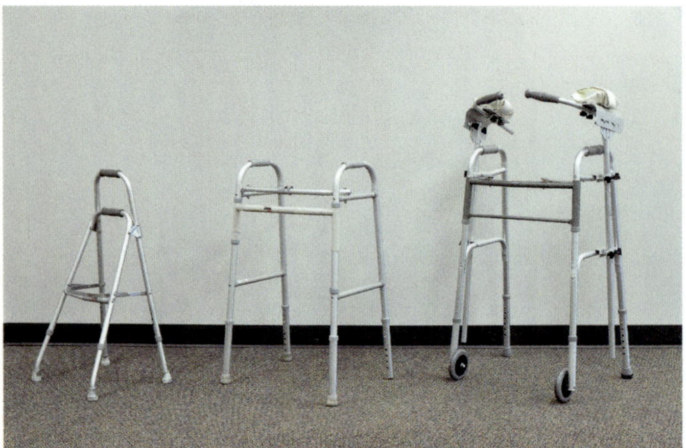

FIGURE 36.14 *Left to right:* Hemi walker, regular walker, and a two-wheel walker with a platform walker attachment. The platform attachment is designed for a patient who has limited strength and cannot grip the walker. An adjustable strap secures the patient's forearm onto the padded section of the attachment.

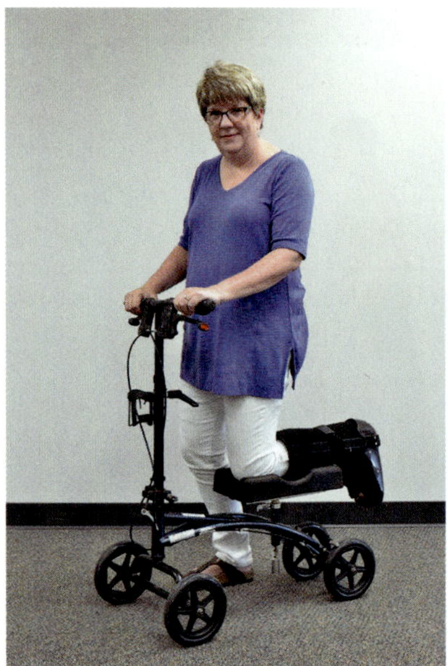

FIGURE 36.15 Knee walker.

When you measure a cane, the patient must be wearing shoes and have the arms relaxed at the sides of the body. The top of the cane should be near the crease in the wrist. With the shoulders relaxed and the hand on the cane, the elbow should be bent 15 degrees. Procedure 36.9 discusses measuring a cane and coaching a patient to use a cane. Tingling, numbness, or pain in the hand and fingers may indicate the handle is not appropriate for the person.

Wheelchairs

Wheelchairs provide mobility for patients who cannot walk or who are able to walk only short distances. With a regular wheelchair, the patient uses arm muscles for mobility. Motorized wheelchairs are also available. The patient is referred to a medical equipment store, where the appropriate wheelchair is fitted to the individual. It is important to encourage the patient to always lock the wheels before transferring into and out of a wheelchair.

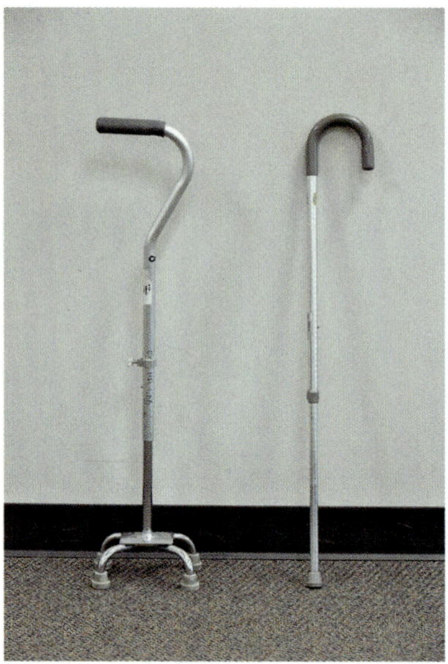

FIGURE 36.16 Four-tipped cane *(left)* and single-tipped cane *(right)*.

CRITICAL THINKING APPLICATION 36.8

Put the assistive devices (wheelchair, cane, crutches, and walker) in order from the device that gives the most assistance to the device that gives the least assistance.

COMPLEMENTARY THERAPIES

Complementary therapies are used together with conventional medicine. For instance, massage and chiropractic care are considered complementary therapies. Sometimes people will use the term *alternative,* but that means the therapy is being used instead of conventional medicine. Most patients using complementary therapies will also see their healthcare provider.

Massage Therapy

Massage therapy ranges from light stroking to deep rubbing. With massage therapy, pressure is applied to a person's skin and muscles. Studies have shown that massage reduces stress, pain, and muscle tension. Massage is performed by massage therapists, who are specially trained in the procedures. There are several types of massage:

- *Deep massage*: Used to help with muscle damage from injuries. Slower, more forceful massage is done to the muscles and connective tissues (e.g., tendons and ligaments).
- *Swedish massage*: Used to relax a person. Involves a gentle massage of long strokes and deep circular movements that can energize the individual.
- *Sports massage*: Used on athletes to help prevent or treat injuries. The technique is similar to Swedish massage.
- *Trigger point massage*: Used to help with muscle damage from injury or overuse. Involves a focused massage on tight muscles.

Chiropractic Care

Chiropractic care focuses on the relationship between the spine and the function of the body. The goal is to correct alignment problems and thereby alleviate pain, improve function, and support the body's natural ability to heal itself. Spinal manipulation has been shown to be beneficial for low back pain, headaches, neck pain, whiplash-associated disorders, and upper and lower extremity joint conditions.

Chiropractic doctors have at least 4 years of additional training beyond a bachelor's degree. The training includes both classroom and direct patient care. The doctors must pass the national licensing exam. State law regulates their practice, and many state boards require continuing education to maintain the license.

Acupressure and Acupuncture

Both acupressure and acupuncture have been practiced for thousands of years. *Acupressure* involves applying firm pressure to specific points on the body. *Acupuncture* involves inserting fine needles into acupuncture points (specific sites on the body). The needles may be removed quickly or left in for longer periods of time. Acupressure and acupuncture are used to treat a wide range of symptoms, including pain, nausea, neuropathy, anxiety, depression, and sleep disturbance.

CLOSING COMMENTS

Patient Coaching

When patients are using assistive devices, falls can occur. The medical assistant should teach patients how to prevent falls when using assistive devices. These instructions should include the following:

- Wear shoes with rubber or nonskid soles.
- Remove items in the walkway that can cause falls (e.g., throw or loose rugs, cords, and clutter). Small indoor animals may also cause falls if they are near the person's feet.
- Make sure that floors are clean and dry.
- When attempting to sit, back up until the seat touches the back of the legs. With a free hand, grab the seat or armrest and lower yourself into the chair or onto the toilet.
- To stand, scoot forward in the chair and use the free hand to push up from the seat to stand up. Make sure to get your balance before moving.
- Consider adding handrails inside the tub and by the toilet.

Legal and Ethical Issues

Working with patients who have musculoskeletal conditions may require assisting with assessments and performing procedures that directly involve the patient's recovery plan. Many of the procedures in this chapter are not the basic procedures you will be required to perform when you are first hired as a medical assistant. All of these techniques involve additional on-the-job training and practice. Before performing any of the described procedures, you should check with your local and state medical assistant organizations about the laws in your state. Whenever you perform the procedures and techniques described in this chapter, you are responsible for doing them correctly.

Patient-Centered Care

With muscular system disorders, a patient may experience limited mobility or have pain with moving. One of the ways to provide patient-centered care is to furnish the patient with information on safety at home. Patients using assistive devices such as crutches or canes should wear shoes with nonskid soles. Throw rugs, cords, and toys should be removed from walkways. Adaptive ideas for safely bathing and grooming are important for patients to know. Providing patients with helpful tips on home care is important for the patient's safety.

Professional Behaviors

Pain and limited mobility resulting from muscular disorders can affect a person's behavior. A patient may be short tempered or have limited patience. The medical assistant must remember to talk calmly and remain composed, even if the patient is not. Treating a patient with respect and listening to the person's concerns helps the patient to feel respected.

SUMMARY OF SCENARIO

Within the next few years, Tim hopes a full-time clinical medical assistant position is posted at the physical medicine and rehabilitation clinic where he did his practicum. In the meantime, Tim enjoys assisting the WMFM Clinic providers. With the wide variety of patients seen at WMFM Clinic, Tim knows he will learn a lot about patient care, diseases, and treatments. This information will be helpful when, hopefully, he moves into the physical medicine and rehabilitation clinic in the future.

SUMMARY OF LEARNING OBJECTIVES

1. **Examine how the medical assistant can help the provider with the examination.**
   When the medical assistant gathers a medical history on patients with a musculoskeletal concern, it is important to ask about the symptoms, the pain level, and the effect of the condition on the person's life.
2. **Examine the medical assistant's role in diagnostic procedures.**
   The medical assistant should ensure that the patient knows how to prepare for procedures, including food, fluid, and medication restrictions. Table 36.1 describes common diagnostic procedures for musculoskeletal disorders. The medical assistant may be involved in range-of-motion (ROM) measurements and muscle strength evaluations. A goniometer is used to measure the ROM of a joint. A dynamometer may be used to provide an objective measurement of hand grip strength.
3. **Differentiate among various types of immobilization treatments, including the purpose of the treatment and the medical assistant's role.**
   An *elastic bandage* is used for a variety of conditions. The medical assistant is typically the person applying the bandage to the patient's extremity. Several bandaging techniques can be used. A *splint* is temporarily applied to immobilize joints and bones after injury or surgery. The splint can be adjusted as the swelling changes. An *immobilizer* keeps the joint from moving. A *brace* provides stability and protection to the joint while allowing the joint to still function. An *ankle boot* is a rigid, removable boot that is used to protect and stabilize the ankle and lower leg after an injury or surgery. A *sling* is a device used to support and immobilize an injured part of the body, such as the arm, wrist, or shoulder. *Casts* are applied to immobilize joints and bones after injury or surgery and provide additional protection.

   The medical assistant should instruct the patient on the purpose of the device. If the device can be removed for periods of time, the medical assistant must coach the patient on how to apply and remove the device. Coaching regarding color, movement, sensation, and temperature (CMST) is important to ensure adequate circulation to the affected extremity. For patients with casts, learning how to handle the cast is important.
4. **Differentiate between cold and heat therapies, including the purpose of the treatment and the medical assistant's role.**
   Cold and heat modalities can be either dry or moist applications. *Cold therapy* is typically used for sprains, strains, fractures, joint injuries, shin splints, and other injuries. Cold therapy helps to reduce pain and inflammation and prevents edema (swelling) in the injured area. *Heat therapy* is used to relieve pain, sinus congestion, and infection. It can relax muscles and produce local vasodilation. Heat therapy can reduce edema. Paraffin baths and heat lamp therapy are examples of heat therapy.
5. **Differentiate among the uses of various physical therapy treatments.**
   Different physical therapy treatments can be used to help treat musculoskeletal conditions:
   - *Ultrasound therapy*: Used to treat pain and promote healing. There are two main types of ultrasound therapy: thermal and mechanical. The main difference between these types is the speed at which the sound waves penetrate the soft tissue.
   - *RICE therapy*: Used for the first 48 to 72 hours after an injury. RICE stands for rest, ice, compression, and elevation. After 72 hours, moist heat is prescribed. Isometric and isotonic exercises help patients maintain their strength and joint mobility.
   - *Exercise therapy*: Isotonic exercises help restore movement after an injury and relieve stiffness and pain. ROM exercises help to maintain flexibility and joint mobility and reduce stiffness. Active ROM exercises are done by the patient, whereas passive ROM exercises are done by a caregiver or therapist.
   - *Transcutaneous electrical nerve stimulation (TENS) unit*: Used for pain relief.
6. **Examine the medical assistant's role in helping patients with assistive devices.**
   Assistive devices are used to help a person perform a specific task, such as walking. This chapter discussed the different types of crutches, how to fit crutches, and the different crutch gaits. Walkers are used to help with balance and support. Several types of walkers are available for patients. Canes are used for minor balance or stability problems. Canes can be single tipped or four tipped. The handles or grips can vary. Wheelchairs provide mobility when a patient cannot walk.
7. **Examine complementary therapies used for musculoskeletal conditions.**
   Complementary therapies are used together with conventional medicine. Complementary therapies include the following:
   - *Massage:* Ranges from light stroking to deep rubbing. Pressure is applied to a person's skin and muscles. Types include deep, Swedish, sports, and trigger point massages.
   - *Chiropractic care:* The goal is to correct alignment problems and thereby alleviate pain, improve function, and support the body's natural ability to heal itself.
   - *Acupressure:* Involves applying firm pressure on specific points on the body.
   - *Acupuncture:* Involves inserting fine needles into acupuncture points.

PROCEDURE 36.1 Apply Elastic Bandages

TASKS: Apply elastic bandages to the forearm using the spiral technique and to the ankle using a figure-eight technique. Document the procedure.

EQUIPMENT and SUPPLIES

- Patient's health record
- Two 3-inch elastic bandages with clip or Velcro closures
- Provider's order

PROVIDER'S ORDER

Apply an elastic bandage to the right arm and right ankle.

PROCEDURAL STEPS

1. Wash hands or use hand sanitizer. Read the provider's order. Assemble the necessary supplies.
   PURPOSE: For infection control. A provider's order is required to gather a urine specimen by a straight catheterization.
2. Greet the patient. Identify yourself. Verify the patient's identity with full name and date of birth. Explain the procedure to be performed in a manner that the patient understands. Answer any questions the patient may have on the procedure.
   PURPOSE: It is important to answer the patient's questions before starting a procedure.
3. Hold the roll so the bandage can be rolled away from you. Using the patient's arm, perform an anchor or circular technique at the distal end.
   PURPOSE: This secures the elastic bandage.
4. Keep the roll close to the patient, and keep it facing upward. With each successive turn, overlap the previous bandage turn by one-third. Maintain even tension and spacing as you continue to apply the bandage up the forearm. The bandage should be smooth. Finish with the circular technique, and then secure the bandage with clips, tape, or Velcro.
   PURPOSE: To maintain even, light pressure over the entire area.
5. Hold the roll so the bandage can be rolled away from you. Using the patient's ankle, perform a circular or anchor technique at the starting point near the most distal part of the foot (near the toes).
   Note: The patient's ankle should be at a 90-degree angle. Make sure the end of the bandage is not on the bottom of the foot, which would cause discomfort.
   PURPOSE: Performing a circular turn at the starting point helps to anchor the bandage.
6. Keep the roll close to the patient, and keep it facing upward. Slowly circle the bandage around the arch of the foot and then around the ankle. With each successive turn, overlap two-thirds of the previous bandage layer. Maintain even tension and spacing as you continue to apply the bandage on the foot and up the ankle. The bandage should be smooth.
   PURPOSE: To maintain even, light pressure over the entire area.
7. Continue until the joint is wrapped, and complete the procedure with a circular technique before securing the bandage with clips, Velcro, or tape.
8. Check the nail beds for cyanosis; ask the patient whether the bandages are comfortable or feel too tight. Check the pulse on the wrapped extremities, if available. Have the patient move the fingers and toes on the wrapped extremities.
   PURPOSE: To ensure that the bandage is not acting as a tourniquet if applied too tightly.
9. Document the procedure in the patient's health record. Include the name of the provider ordering the bandage, the procedure done, how the patient tolerated the procedure, and instructions given to the patient.
   PURPOSE: The procedure is not completed until it is recorded, dated, and signed.

Documentation Example

10/18/20XX 9:10 a.m. Per Dr. Walden's order, an elastic bandage using a spiral wrap technique was applied to the right forearm, and an elastic bandage using a figure-eight wrap technique was applied to the right foot and ankle. Patient denied that the bandage was too tight. Fingers warm to touch. Explained to patient how to replace bandage if needed and how to check for good circulation in the fingers and toes. Patient verbalized understanding of the information and described signs of poor circulation. ———————————— Tim Paul, CMA (AAMA)

PROCEDURE 36.2 Apply a Sling

TASKS: Apply a sling to a patient's arm. Document the procedure in the patient's health record.

SCENARIO: Dr. Kahn orders a commercial sling to be applied to a patient's left arm.

EQUIPMENT and SUPPLIES

- Adult-sized sling
- Provider's order
- Patient's health record

PROCEDURAL STEPS

1. Wash hands or use hand sanitizer.
   PURPOSE: Hand sanitization is an important step for infection control.
2. Read the provider's order. Assemble the equipment. Make sure to have the correct-sized sling for the patient.
   PURPOSE: It is important to know the provider's order before starting the procedure.
3. Greet the patient. Identify yourself. Verify the patient's identity with full name and date of birth. Explain the procedure to be performed in a manner that the patient understands. Answer any questions the patient may have about the procedure.

Continued

PROCEDURE 36.2 Apply a Sling—*continued*

PURPOSE: It is important to identify the patient in two different ways to ensure that you have the correct patient. Explaining the procedure can make the patient feel more comfortable and reduces anxiety.

4. Gently place the arm and elbow in the sling. Support the arm on both sides of the injury. Make sure the sling fits comfortably around the elbow. The patient's hand should come to the end of the sling.
   PURPOSE: Having the correct-sized sling will help prevent complications. The sling should not be so snug that it is uncomfortable. The hand should be supported by the sling. If the hand hangs down at the wrist, the sling is too small for the patient.
5. Position the strap behind the elbow, and pull the strap around the back of the neck. Make sure the strap does not rub against or cut into the skin on the neck. Secure the strap to the loops on the sling near the hand.
   PURPOSE: The strap should be comfortably positioned around the patient's neck and shoulder.
6. Adjust the straps so the hand and forearm are elevated to the level of the elbow.
   PURPOSE: This prevents swelling in the hand and wrist.
7. Check the CMST of the fingers. Ask the patient if the fingers feel numb or asleep.
   PURPOSE: If the circulation is compromised, CMST will indicate a problem, such as numb, blue, and cold fingers.
8. Document the procedure in the patient's health record. Include the provider's name, the order, what was taught, and how the patient responded.
   PURPOSE: It is important to document the procedure in the health record to show it was done.

Documentation Example

07/20/20XX 1505 Per Dr. Kahn's order, applied a commercial sling to the pt's left arm. Left hand and fingers elevated. CMST normal. Pt's questions were answered. Pt was encouraged to call the department with any additional questions or concerns. ———————————— Tim Paul, CMA (AAMA)

PROCEDURE 36.3 Assist with Application of a Cast

TASKS: Assist the provider in applying a fiberglass cast. Document the procedure in the patient's health record.

SCENARIO: You are working with Dr. David Kahn, and he needs to apply a fiberglass cast on the left lower leg of Johnny Parker (DOB 06/15/20XX). You will assist the provider.

EQUIPMENT and SUPPLIES

- Patient's health record
- Rolls of fiberglass
- Basin for casting material
- Bandage
- Stockinette
- Gloves
- Sheet wadding and/or spongy padding
- Stand to support foot (lower extremity)
- Tape
- Scissors
- 2–3 Towels
- Water
- Cast care instructions (optional)

PROCEDURAL STEPS

1. Wash hands or use hand sanitizer. Assemble the necessary equipment.
   PURPOSE: Hand sanitization is an important step for infection control.
2. Greet the patient. Identify yourself. Verify the patient's identity with full name and date of birth. Explain the procedure to be performed in a manner that the patient understands. Answer any questions the patient may have about the procedure.
   PURPOSE: It is important to identify the patient in two different ways to ensure that you have the correct patient. Explaining the procedure can make the patient feel more comfortable and reduces anxiety.
3. Seat the patient comfortably, as directed by the provider. If the cast is being applied to the lower extremity, the toes must be supported by a stand.
   PURPOSE: The amount of ankle flexion can be controlled by supporting the toes so that the patient can more easily maintain the desired position without fatigue.
4. Clean the area that the cast will cover. Note any objective signs and ask about subjective symptoms (chart them at the end of the procedure).
   PURPOSE: The condition of the area under the cast must be noted before the cast is applied so that it can be compared with the site when the cast is removed. Clean the area with a mild soap solution or as directed. Dry thoroughly.
5. Cut the stockinette to fit the area the cast will cover. Apply the stockinette smoothly to the area. Leave 1 or 2 inches of excess stockinette above and below the cast area to finish the cast (see the first of the following figures). Excess stockinette may be cut away where wrinkles form, such as at the front of the ankle (see the second of the following figures).
   PURPOSE: The stockinette will help protect the skin. The stockinette must lie smoothly and cannot be too bulky or wrinkled because this may cause a pressure wound.

PROCEDURE 36.3 Assist with Application of a Cast—*continued*

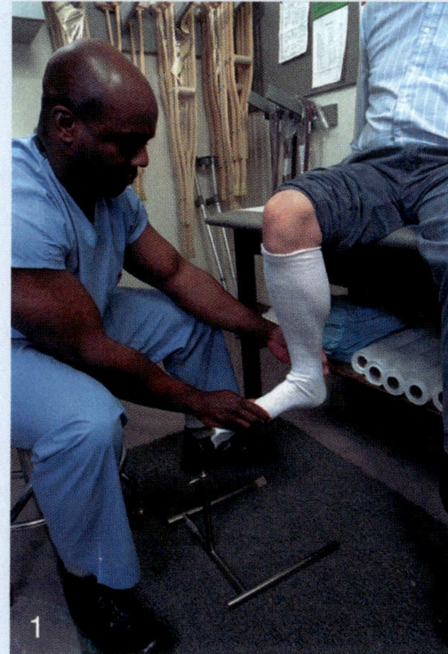

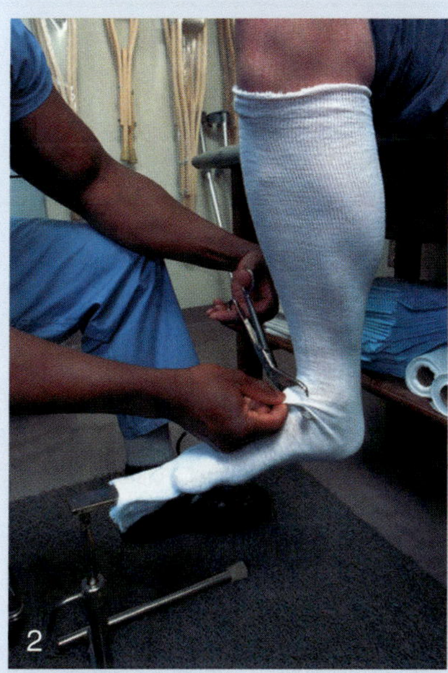

6. Apply sheet wadding along the length of the cast using a spiral bandage turn. Extra padding may be used over bony prominences, such as the bones of the elbow or ankle.
   PURPOSE: Padding the cast helps reduce pressure against bony prominences, which could cause skin breakdown.
7. Put on gloves. With lukewarm water in the basin, wet the fiberglass tape as directed by the provider (see the following figure).
   PURPOSE: Immersing the roll of fiberglass tape in water begins the chemical reaction that will cause the cast to harden. The cast can be shaped while wet and will harden in the shape that is formed.

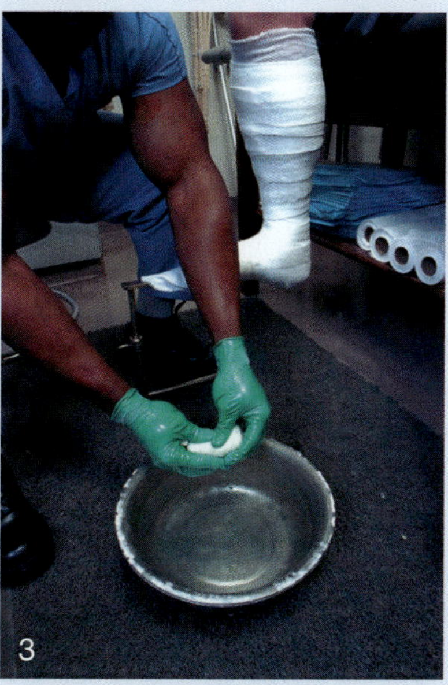

8. Assist as directed as the provider applies the inner layer of fiberglass tape. A length of 1 to 2 inches of stockinette is rolled over the inner layer of the cast to form a smooth edge when the outer layer is applied.
9. As directed by the provider, help to open and apply an outer layer of fiberglass tape (shown in the first of the following figures as blue).
10. Help shape the cast as directed. All contours must be smooth (see the second of the following figures).
    PURPOSE: If flat or dented areas develop on the cast, they may cause pressure on the skin below.

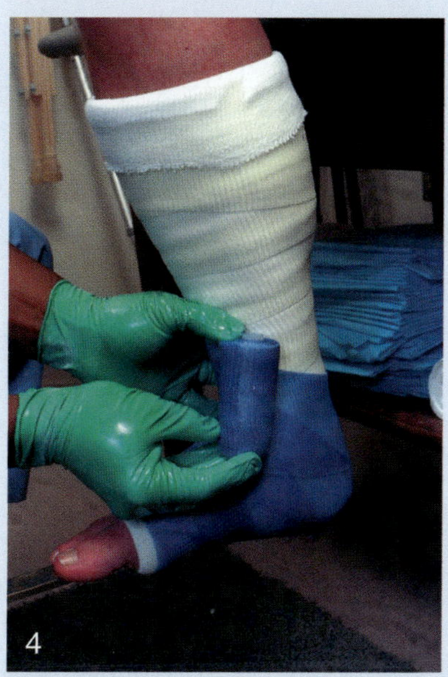

Continued

PROCEDURE 36.3 Assist with Application of a Cast—*continued*

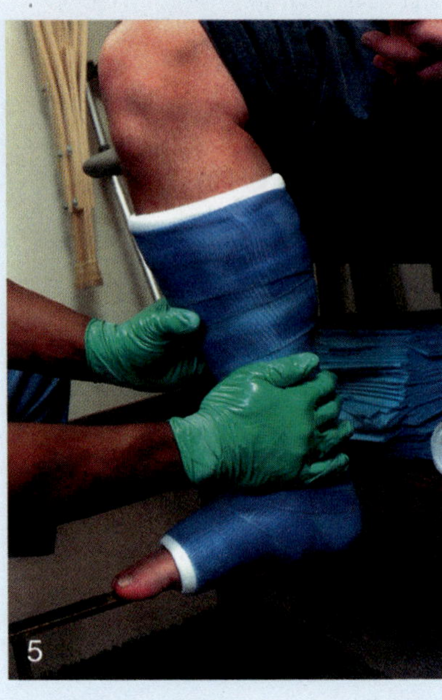

11. Discard the water and excess materials. Remove your gloves. Wash hands or use hand sanitizer.
12. Reassure the patient, review cast care verbally, and provide written instructions (optional).
13. Document the procedure in the patient's health record. Include the provider's name, the procedure, what was taught, and how the patient responded.
    PURPOSE: It is important to document the procedure in the health record to show it was done.

Documentation Example

07/19/20XX 1005 Assisted Dr. Kahn with fiberglass cast application to left leg. Skin under cast dry and intact. Pt and mother given verbal and written cast care instructions. No questions. Instructed mother to call provider if there is numbness, tingling, swelling of toes, or blue discoloration. Reinforced the need for elevation and ice per Dr. Kahn's order. ————————————

———————————————————— Tim Paul, CMA (AAMA)

PROCEDURE 36.4 Assist with Cast Removal

TASKS: Remove a cast. Document the procedure in the patient's health record.

SCENARIO: You are working with Dr. David Kahn, and he orders removal of the lower left leg cast on Johnny Parker (DOB 06/15/20XX).

EQUIPMENT and SUPPLIES

- Patient's health record
- Cast cutter
- Cast spreader
- Large bandage scissors
- Basin of warm water
- Mild soap
- Towel
- Skin lotion

PROCEDURAL STEPS

1. Wash hands or use hand sanitizer. Assemble the necessary equipment.
   PURPOSE: Hand sanitization is an important step for infection control.
2. Greet the patient. Identify yourself. Verify the patient's identity with full name and date of birth. Explain the procedure to be performed in a manner that the patient understands. Answer any questions the patient may have about the procedure.
   PURPOSE: It is important to identify the patient in two different ways to ensure that you have the correct patient. Explaining the procedure can make the patient feel more comfortable and reduces anxiety.
3. Provide adequate support for the limb throughout the procedure. Using the cast cutter, make a cut on the medial and lateral sides of the long axis of the cast (see the following figure).
   PURPOSE: To ensure the patient's comfort.

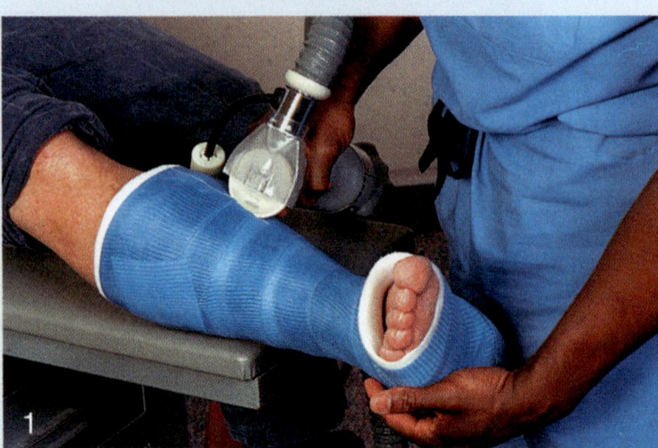

4. Use the cast spreader to pry apart the two halves (see the following figure). Carefully remove the two parts of the cast. Use the large bandage scissors to cut away the stockinette and padding remaining.
   PURPOSE: A cast spreader is needed to pry apart the cast.

PROCEDURE 36.4 Assist with Cast Removal—*continued*

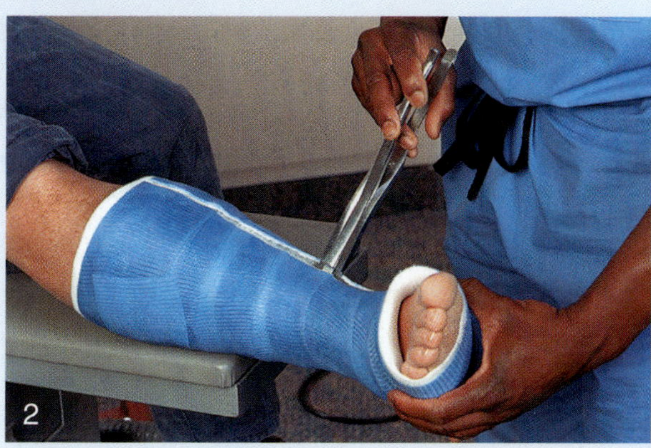

5. Gently wash the area that was covered by the cast with mild soap and warm water. Dry the area and apply a gentle skin lotion.
   PURPOSE: To ensure the patient's comfort.
6. Give the patient appropriate instructions about exercising and using the limb, as directed by the provider.
   PURPOSE: To enhance continued healing, restore lost strength, and prevent injury.
7. Clean up the area. Wash hands or use hand sanitizer.
8. Document the procedure in the patient's health record. Include the provider's name, the procedure, what was taught, and how the patient responded.
   PURPOSE: It is important to document the procedure in the health record to show it was done.

Documentation Example

9/10/20XX 1205 Dr. Kahn ordered the left leg fiberglass cast to be removed. Cast removed, skin washed and dried. Lotion applied. Pt and mother instructed on appropriate exercises to do per the provider's order. Questions answered. Encouraged patient's mother to call with concerns. ——————————————————Tim Paul, CMA (AAMA)

PROCEDURE 36.5 Apply a Cold Pack

TASKS: Apply a cold pack (chemical, gel, or bead) to a body area to reduce pain and prevent further swelling per treatment plan. Document the procedure in the patient's health record.

SCENARIO: You are working with Dr. David Kahn. Johnny Parker (DOB 06/15/20XX) arrives holding his arm and crying. Another medical assistant brings the patient and parent to the exam room. The medical assistant comes out and updates you on Johnny. His parent states that Johnny fell off his bike an hour ago and has since been complaining of pain in his right wrist. The providers in the department have a standing order to apply a cold pack to orthopedic injuries if the patient does not arrive with one in place. The medical assistant asks you to apply the cold pack as he completes the vital signs and medical history on Johnny.

EQUIPMENT and SUPPLIES

- Cold pack (chemical, gel, or bead)
- Towel or another type of protective covering for the cold pack
- Provider's order or standing order for orthopedic injuries
- Patient's health record

PROCEDURAL STEPS

1. Wash hands or use hand sanitizer.
   PURPOSE: Hand sanitization is an important step for infection control.
2. Read the standing order or the provider's order. Assemble the equipment. If using a chemical cold pack, activate the pack by squeezing it.
   PURPOSE: It is important to know the provider's order or the standing order before starting the procedure.
3. Greet the patient. Identify yourself. Verify the patient's identity with full name and date of birth. Explain the procedure to be performed in a manner that the patient understands. Answer any questions the patient may have about the procedure.
   PURPOSE: It is important to identify the patient in two different ways to ensure that you have the correct patient. Explaining the procedure can make the patient feel more comfortable and reduces anxiety.
4. Cover the cold pack with a towel or protective covering.
   PURPOSE: The cold pack must never be put directly on the skin. Place a towel or protective covering between the cold pack and the skin to prevent injuries.
5. Position the cold pack over the injured area (see the following figure).
   PURPOSE: Some patients like to place the cold pack themselves on the injured area.

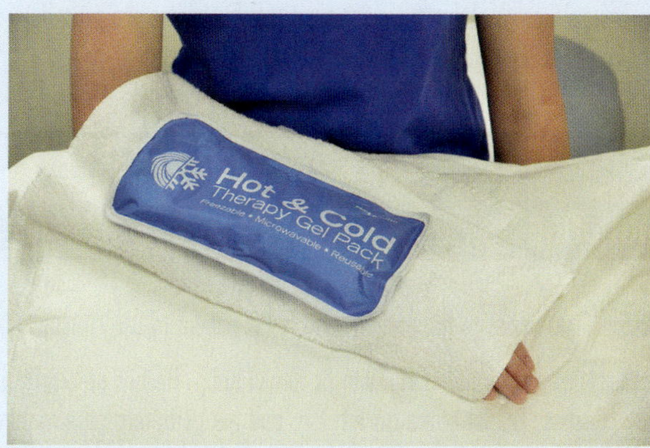

6. Coach the patient on the use of a cold pack. Advise the patient to leave the cold pack in place for 15 to 20 minutes or until the area feels numb, whichever comes first.
   PURPOSE: Cold applications are typically applied for 15 to 20 minutes or per the provider's order.
7. Document the procedure in the patient's health record. Include the provider's name, the order, what was taught, and how the patient responded.
   PURPOSE: It is important to document the procedure in the health record to show it was done.

Continued

PROCEDURE 36.5 Apply a Cold Pack—*continued*

Documentation Example

07/19/20XX 1505 Pt arrived holding right wrist and complaining of pain. Parent stated that he fell off his bike about 1 hour ago. Per Dr. Kahn's standing order, applied cold pack to pt's right wrist. Instructed pt and parent to keep the cold pack (covered with a towel) on the wrist for 15–20 minutes. Parent stated she would remove it at that time. ———————————— Tim Paul, CMA (AAMA)

PROCEDURE 36.6 Apply a Hot Pack

TASKS: Apply a hot pack (chemical, gel, or bead) to an infected wound. Document the procedure in the patient's health record.

SCENARIO: Dr. Kahn orders a hot pack to be applied to an infected wound for 15 minutes. He also orders coaching for the patient to continue the treatment at home four times a day for the next 3 days.

EQUIPMENT and SUPPLIES

- Hot pack (chemical, gel, or bead)
- Towel or another type of protective covering for the hot pack
- Provider's order
- Patient's health record

PROCEDURAL STEPS

1. Wash hands or use hand sanitizer.
   PURPOSE: Hand sanitization is an important step for infection control.
2. Read the provider's order. Assemble the equipment. If using a chemical hot pack, activate the pack by squeezing it. If the pack needs to be warmed, follow the manufacturer's directions.
   PURPOSE: It is important to know the provider's order or the standing order before starting the procedure.
3. Greet the patient. Identify yourself. Verify the patient's identity with full name and date of birth. Explain the procedure to be performed in a manner that the patient understands. Answer any questions the patient may have about the procedure.
   PURPOSE: It is important to identify the patient in two different ways to ensure that you have the correct patient. Explaining the procedure can make the patient feel more comfortable and reduces anxiety.
4. Cover the hot pack with a towel or protective covering.
   PURPOSE: The hot pack must never be put directly on the skin. Place a towel or protective covering between the hot pack and the skin to prevent injuries.
5. Position the hot pack over the covered wound.
   PURPOSE: Some patients like to place the hot pack themselves on the area.
6. Coach the patient on the use of a hot pack. Advise the patient to leave the hot pack in place for 15 to 20 minutes per the provider's order or until the area feels warm, whichever comes first.
   PURPOSE: Hot applications are typically applied for 15 to 20 minutes or per the provider's order.
7. Wash hands or use hand sanitizer.
8. Document the procedure in the patient's health record. Include the provider's name, the order, what was taught, and how the patient responded
   PURPOSE: It is important to document the procedure in the health record to show it was done.

Documentation Example

07/21/20XX 1505 Per Dr. Kahn's order, applied hot pack to pt's left lower arm. Instructed pt to keep the hot pack (covered with a towel) on the wound for 15 minutes. Instructed patient how to apply a hot pack at home. Instructed patient to apply a hot pack for 15 minutes, four times a day for the next 3 days. Pt's questions were answered. Pt was encouraged to call the department with any additional questions or concerns. ———————————— Tim Paul, CMA (AAMA)

PROCEDURE 36.7 Coach a Patient in the Use of Axillary Crutches

TASKS: Fit crutches to the patient. Coach the patient to use crutches. Document your teaching in the patient's health record.

SCENARIO: You are working with Dr. David Kahn. He has ordered you to teach Daniel Miller (DOB 3/21/20XX) how to use axillary crutches. Daniel broke his left leg, and his treatment plan requires that he not bear weight on the left leg for 6 weeks. Daniel's bedroom is on the second floor, so he has to learn how to use crutches on the stairs also.

EQUIPMENT and SUPPLIES

- Axillary crutches
- Handout on crutch walking (optional)
- Provider's order
- Patient's health record

PROCEDURAL STEPS

1. Wash hands or use hand sanitizer.
   PURPOSE: Hand sanitization is an important step for infection control.
2. Read the provider's order. Assemble the equipment.
   PURPOSE: It is important to know the provider's order before starting the procedure.
3. Greet the patient. Identify yourself. Verify the patient's identity with full name and date of birth. Explain the procedure to be performed in a manner that the patient understands. Answer any questions the patient may have about the procedure.

PROCEDURE 36.7 Coach a Patient in the Use of Axillary Crutches—*continued*

PURPOSE: It is important to identify the patient in two different ways to ensure that you have the correct patient. Explaining the procedure can make the patient feel more comfortable and reduces anxiety.

4. Ensure the patient is wearing shoes and ask the patient to stand up straight. Assist as needed. Fit the crutches to the patient so they are 1 to 1½ inches (about 2 finger widths) below the armpit (Figure 1). The crutch should be about 4 to 6 inches to the side and front of each foot.
   PURPOSE: Pressure in the axilla can cause crutch palsy. Adjust the length of the crutches as needed.

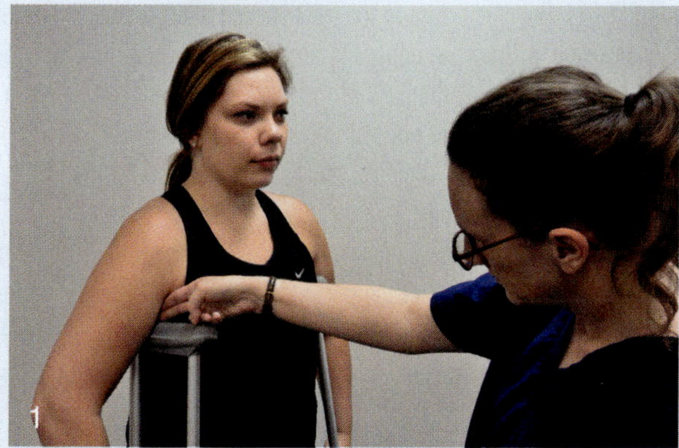
1

5. Adjust the handgrips so they are near the patient's wrist and even with the top of the hip line. This should allow for a 15- to 30-degree bend in the elbow when the patient's hands are on the handgrip.
   PURPOSE: This position allows for the most strength with the hands.
6. Instruct the patient to keep the injured leg as relaxed as possible. The knee should be slightly bent, and the patient should look forward when walking. Instruct the patient not to bear weight on the axilla.
   PURPOSE: For a child, it is important to keep your language simple and to demonstrate what you are saying.
7. Have the patient start in the tripod position and then move the crutches about 12 inches in front of the body (or less for a child).
   PURPOSE: When doing the three-point crutch gait, placing the crutches in front of the body is the first step.
8. Have the patient put the weight on the crutches and move the body forward. Finish the step by having the patient swing the "good," or unaffected, leg forward. Do not place weight on the "bad" or affected leg. Continue with these steps.
   PURPOSE: Placing weight on the affected extremity may harm the leg.
9. *To sit down:* Instruct the patient to do the following: Back up to the chair, toilet, or bed until the seat touches the back of the legs. Move the "bad," or affected, leg forward, balancing on the "good," or unaffected, leg. Hold both crutches on the side with the "bad," or affected, leg. Use the free hand to grab the seat or armrest. Slowly sit down.
   PURPOSE: Backing up until the seat touches the back of the legs is important to prevent falls.
10. *To stand up:* Instruct the patient to do the following: Move toward the front of the seat and move the "bad," or affected, leg forward. Hold both crutches on the side with the "bad," or affected, leg. Use the free hand to push up from the seat to stand up. Balance on the "good," or unaffected, leg while placing a crutch in each hand. Balance is needed before moving.
    PURPOSE: If the person is unstable, the risk of falling is greater. Stand still until balance is achieved.
11. *To go up the stairs:* Instruct the patient to do the following: Step up with the "good," or unaffected, leg first. Then bring the crutches up, one in each arm. Finally, place weight on the "good," or unaffected, leg and bring the "bad," or affected, leg up.
    PURPOSE: It is important to go up the stairs, starting with the "good," or unaffected, leg.
12. *To go down the stairs:* Instruct the patient to do the following: With a crutch in each hand, place the crutches on the first step. Then move the "bad," or affected, leg forward and down. Lastly, follow with the "good," or unaffected, leg.
    PURPOSE: When going down the stairs, the crutches and then the "bad," or affected, leg come first.
13. Instruct the patient and family on ways to prevent falls. Wash hands or use hand sanitizer.
    PURPOSE: It is important to also educate the patient on how to prevent falls.
14. Document the patient education in the patient's health record. Include the provider's name, the order, what was taught, how the patient responded, how the patient did the demonstration, and any handouts provided.
    PURPOSE: It is important to document the patient education in the health record to show it was done.

Documentation Example

07/21/20XX 1423 Per Dr. Kahn's order, pt fitted with crutches and taught with his mother on the three-point crutch gait. They were told of the non–weight-bearing limitation on the left leg × 6 wk. Pt was able to correctly walk 20 feet using the three-point gait. He was able to walk up and down the stairs safely with crutches. Pt was also taught to sit down and get up from a chair. Pt demonstrated the techniques correctly. Pt's mother was given the crutch booklet. All their questions were answered, and the mother was given a follow-up number for additional questions. ———————————————— Tim Paul, CMA (AAMA)

PROCEDURE 36.8 Coach a Patient in the Use of a Walker

TASKS: Fit a standard walker to a patient. Coach the patient to use a standard walker. Document your teaching in the patient's health record.

SCENARIO: You are working with Dr. David Kahn. He has ordered you to teach Jana Green (DOB 5/1/19XX) how to use a standard walker. Jana needs the walker for extra stability.

EQUIPMENT and SUPPLIES

- Standard walker
- Walker handout (optional)
- Provider's order
- Patient's health record

PROCEDURAL STEPS

1. Wash hands or use hand sanitizer.
   PURPOSE: Hand sanitization is an important step for infection control.
2. Read the provider's order. Assemble the equipment.
   PURPOSE: It is important to know the provider's order before starting the procedure.
3. Greet the patient. Identify yourself. Verify the patient's identity with full name and date of birth. Explain the procedure to be performed in a manner that the patient understands. Answer any questions the patient may have about the procedure.
   PURPOSE: It is important to identify the patient in two different ways to ensure that you have the correct patient. Explaining the procedure can make the patient feel more comfortable and reduces anxiety.
4. Ensure the patient is wearing shoes and ask the patient to step into the walker. The top of the walker grip should be even with the top of the hip line and near the crease in the wrist when the arms are at the side of the body. Adjust as needed. Keeping the shoulders relaxed and the hands on the grips will ensure the elbows are bent at a 15-degree angle (see the following figure).
   PURPOSE: For body mechanics, it is important to have the walker adjusted to fit the person. Using a walker that is too tall or too short can cause stress on the upper shoulders and back. A person should not lean over to walk because this increases the risk of falls.

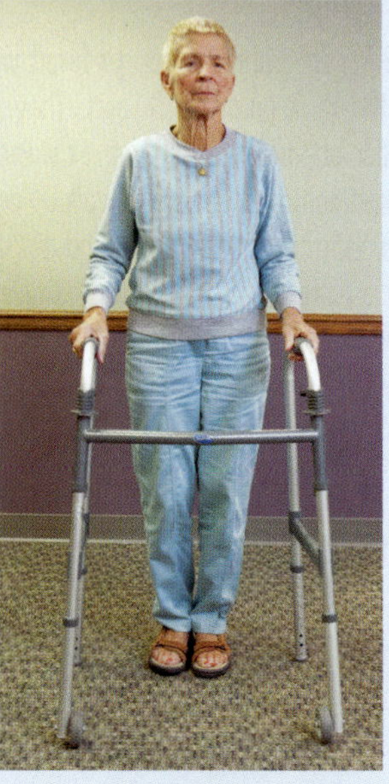

5. Have the patient place the walker one step ahead of the body. Instruct the patient to use the "bad," or affected, leg to step into the walker. The patient should not touch the front bar with the leg. Have the patient step forward with the other leg to complete the step. The patient will continue with this pattern while holding up the head and looking forward.
   PURPOSE: Being too close to the front bar can affect the patient's stability.
6. *To sit down:* Instruct the patient to back up to the chair, toilet, or bed until the seat touches the back of the legs. The patient can then use one hand to grab the seat or armrest and slowly sit down.
   PURPOSE: Backing up until the seat touches the back of the legs is important to prevent falls.
7. *To stand up:* Instruct the patient to move toward the front of the seat. Have the walker in front of the person. Have the patient use one hand to push up from the seat to stand up and then place hands on the walker. Remind patients to make sure they have their balance before moving.
   PURPOSE: If the person is unstable, the risk of falling is greater. It is important to stand still until balance is achieved.
8. Instruct the patient on ways to prevent falls. The walker should never be used on stairs or an escalator. If the patient will be using a bag on the front of the walker, instruct the patient to make sure not to overload it. Make sure to place all four legs of the walker on the ground before moving into the walker. Wash hands or use hand sanitizer.
   PURPOSE: It is important to educate the patient on how to prevent falls. Too much weight in the front of the walker may cause it to tilt and the patient to fall.
9. Document the patient education in the patient's health record. Include the provider's name, the order, what was taught, how the patient responded, how the patient did the demonstration, and any handouts provided.
   PURPOSE: It is important to document the patient education in the health record to show it was done.

Documentation Example

07/21/20XX 1423 Per Dr. Kahn's order, patient was fitted with a walker and instructed how to use it. Pt was able to walk using the walker correctly. Pt was also able to sit and stand while using the walker. Pt demonstrated techniques correctly and safely. Coached patient on safety issues with the walker and how to reduce the risk of falls. Pt was able to verbalize four ways to prevent falls when using the walker. All of the pt's questions were answered. Pt was given the walker booklet to take home. ————————————————— Tim Paul, CMA (AAMA)

PROCEDURE 36.9 Coach a Patient in the Use of a Cane

TASKS: Fit a cane to a patient. Coach the patient to use a cane. Document your teaching in the patient's health record.

SCENARIO: You are working with Dr. David Kahn. He has ordered you to teach Ella Rainwater (DOB 7/11/19XX) how to use a cane. Ella has left-side weakness.

EQUIPMENT and SUPPLIES

- Cane
- Handout on cane walking (optional)
- Provider's order
- Patient's health record

PROCEDURAL STEPS

1. Wash hands or use hand sanitizer.
   PURPOSE: Hand sanitization is an important step for infection control.
2. Read the provider's order. Assemble the equipment.
   PURPOSE: It is important to know the provider's order before starting the procedure.
3. Greet the patient. Identify yourself. Verify the patient's identity with full name and date of birth. Explain the procedure to be performed in a manner that the patient understands. Answer any questions the patient may have about the procedure.
   PURPOSE: It is important to identify the patient in two different ways to ensure that you have the correct patient. Explaining the procedure can make the patient feel more comfortable and reduces anxiety.
4. Ensure the patient is wearing shoes. The top of the cane should be near the crease in the wrist when the arms are at the side of the body. Adjust as needed. With the patient's shoulders relaxed and hand on the cane, ensure the elbows are bent at a 15-degree angle.
   PURPOSE: For body mechanics, it is important to have the cane fitted correctly.
5. Instruct the patient to hold the cane on the "good," or unaffected, side. The patient should take a step moving the "bad," or affected, leg and the cane forward at the same time and then step forward with the "good" leg. Instruct the patient to lean on the cane as needed.
   PURPOSE: The cane is held on the "good," or unaffected, side so it can provide added support to the opposite leg.
6. *To sit down:* Instruct the patient to back up to the chair, toilet, or bed until the seat touches the back of the legs. The patient can then use a hand to grab the seat or armrest and slowly sit down.
   PURPOSE: Backing up until the seat touches the back of the legs is important to prevent falls.
7. *To stand up:* Instruct the patient to move toward the front of the seat and move the "bad," or affected, leg forward. The patient can then use a hand to push up from the seat to stand up. Remind patients to make sure to get their balance before moving.
   PURPOSE: If the person is unstable, the risk of falling is greater. Instruct the patient to stand still until balance is achieved.
8. *To go up the stairs:* Instruct the patient to step up with the "good," or unaffected, leg first while holding onto the rail. Then the patient should bring up the "bad," or affected, leg to the same step. If there is no handrail, the cane and the "bad" leg should be placed on the stair at the same time.
   PURPOSE: It is important to go up the stairs, starting with the "good" or unaffected leg.
9. *To go down the stairs:* Instruct the patient to hold onto the rail and move the "bad," or affected, leg down first. Then the patient should place the "good," or unaffected, leg on the same step as the "bad" leg. When there is no handrail, instruct the patient to place the cane on the lower step, then place the "bad," or affected, leg, and lastly place the "good," or unaffected, leg next to the "bad," or affected, leg.
   PURPOSE: When going down the stairs, the cane and then the "bad" leg come down first, followed by the "good" leg.
10. Instruct the patient on ways to prevent falls. Wash hands or use hand sanitizer.
    PURPOSE: It is important to also educate the patient on how to prevent falls.
11. Document the patient education in the patient's health record. Include the provider's name, the order, what was taught, how the patient responded, how the patient did the demonstration, and any handouts provided.
    PURPOSE: It is important to document the patient education in the health record to show it was done.

Documentation Example

07/25/20XX 1105 Per Dr. Kahn's order, pt was fitted with a cane and was instructed on walking with a cane, doing stairs, and sitting/standing. Pt was able to walk about 30 feet with a cane correctly. Pt was able to safely walk up and down and sit/stand while using the cane. Pt's questions were answered. Pt was given the Using a Cane booklet. ——————————— Tim Paul, CMA (AAMA)

NEUROLOGY 37

SCENARIO

Nancy Gehir, CMA (AAMA), is a medical assistant at Walden-Martin Family Medical (WMFM) Clinic. She was hired at WMFM Clinic shortly after passing her CMA exam. She has recently accepted a position to help the outreach providers. Outreach providers deliver specialty services that are not offered at WMFM Clinic.

Nancy will be assisting the neurology providers, who come to the clinic weekly to see patients. Prior to starting with neurology, Nancy spent some time reviewing her anatomy textbook and researching common diseases. Today, she is helping Dr. Arzt and Tammy Tamar, a nurse practitioner.

While studying this chapter, think about the following questions:

- What structures are in the nervous system?
- What are the functions of the nervous system?
- What are commonly diagnosed neurologic diseases and disorders? What are the etiologies, signs and symptoms, diagnostic processes, and treatments?
- What are the medical assistant's primary responsibilities when working with patients who have neurologic diseases and disorders?

LEARNING OBJECTIVES

1. Differentiate among the structures of the central nervous system.
2. Differentiate among the structures of the peripheral nervous system.
3. Differentiate among the cells of the nervous system.
4. Examine the physiology of the nervous system.
5. Examine neurodegenerative diseases and disorders, including the signs, symptoms, etiology, diagnostic procedures, and treatments.
6. Examine functional diseases and disorders, including the signs, symptoms, etiology, diagnostic procedures, and treatments.
7. Examine infections that impact the nervous system, including the signs, symptoms, etiology, diagnostic procedures, and treatments.
8. Examine structural diseases and disorders that impact the nervous system, including the signs, symptoms, etiology, diagnostic procedures, and treatments.
9. Examine injuries that impact the nervous system, including the signs, symptoms, etiology, diagnostic procedures, and treatments.
10. Examine congenital diseases and disorders that impact the nervous system, including the signs, symptoms, etiology, diagnostic procedures, and treatments.
11. Examine vascular diseases and disorders that impact the nervous system, including the signs, symptoms, etiology, diagnostic procedures, and treatments.
12. Examine the medical assistant's role in examinations, diagnostic procedures, and treatments for neurologic diseases and disorders.

VOCABULARY

afferent (AF er uhnt) Pertaining to carrying toward a structure.

amygdala (ah MIG dah lah) A small mass of gray matter found in each temporal lobe of the cerebrum involved with memories, emotions, and activating the fight-or-flight response; part of the limbic system.

amyloid plaques Masses or clumps of proteins that form between neurons and disrupt cellular function.

analgesic (an ahl JEE zik) A drug that reduces or eliminates pain.

aneurysm (AN yeh rizm) An abnormal blood-filled sac formed by a localized dilation of the wall of a vein, artery, or heart.

aphasia (ah FAY zhah) Partial or complete loss of the ability to articulate ideas or understand written or spoken language.

ataxia Loss of the ability to coordinate muscular movement.

autoimmune An immune response against a person's own tissues, cells, or cell parts, as in autoimmune disease, leading to the deterioration of tissue.

axon (AK son) A long extension of a nerve fiber that conducts the impulse away from the nerve cell body; white matter.

biomarkers Detectable cellular indicators used as a marker for a substance or disease process.

cataplexy (KAT ah PLEK see) A sudden loss of muscle strength and tone associated with an emotional stimulus.

choroid plexus (KOR oid PLEK sus) A network of capillaries found in the lateral ventricles and the third and fourth ventricles that secrete cerebrospinal fluid.

VOCABULARY—*continued*

coma A state of deep, often prolonged unconsciousness, usually the result of a head injury, neurologic disease, intoxication, or metabolic abnormalities.

concussion A type of traumatic brain injury resulting from a hit to the head or body that causes the brain to move rapidly back and forth.

efferent (EF er uhnt) Pertaining to carrying away from a structure.

evoked potential test A nerve response test that uses electrodes, which are placed on the scalp to measure brain reaction to a stimulus.

fissure (FISH er) A groove that divides an organ into lobes or parts.

fontanel (fon tah NEL) A soft membranous gap between the incompletely formed cranial bones of an infant; also called a soft spot.

foramen magnum (for AY men MAG num) A large opening in the base of the skull. It forms a passageway for the spinal cord.

Glasgow Coma Scale A scale used to measure the level of consciousness and severity of a head injury; the ability to open the eyes, verbal response, and motor response are evaluated, and the score is determined based on the findings.

gray matter Nerve tissue that lacks the insulation that causes a white appearance to other nerves; thus, gray matter looks gray.

gyri (JIE rie) Folds or convolutions on the surface of the cerebral hemisphere, which increase the gray matter surface area. Gyrus (JIE rus) is the singular form.

hallucination (hah LOO si nae shun) A sensory experience (e.g., a smell, sound, sight, touch, or taste) involving something that is not present.

hematoma A localized collection of blood, usually clotted, caused by a break in a blood vessel wall.

hippocampus (hip oh KAM pus) A ridge in the floor of the lateral ventricle; composed of gray matter. Involved with the limbic system and with creating and filing new memories.

homeostasis (hoh mee oh STAY sis) The internal environment of the body that is compatible with life. A steady state that is created by all the body systems working together to provide a consistent and unvarying internal environment.

hydrocephalus (hi droe SEF ah luhs) An abnormal accumulation of cerebrospinal fluid that causes enlargement of the skull and compression of the brain.

limbic system Consists of several structures, including the amygdala, hippocampus, and hypothalamus; plays an important role in behavior, memories, and emotions.

meninges (meh NIN jeez) A protective covering around the brain and spinal cord.

myelin sheath (MIE uh lin sheeth) A protective insulation that covers the axons and helps with the transmission of nerve impulses.

neuralgia (noo RAL jah) Sharp, spasm-like pain in a nerve or along the course of one or more nerves.

neurofibrillary tangles Abnormal structures composed of twisted protein fibers within nerve cells.

neurotransmitter A chemical that helps a nerve cell communicate with another nerve cell or muscle.

paralysis A loss of muscle function or sensation causing the inability to move or use a body part.

pineal gland A small organ in the brain that secretes melatonin, a hormone that regulates the sleep/awake cycle.

shaken baby syndrome A condition resulting from internal head injuries that occur when a baby or young child is violently shaken.

sulci (SUL sie) Grooves or depressions on the surface of the brain between the gyri. Sulcus (SUL kus) is the singular form.

syncope Loss of consciousness and postural tone caused by diminished blood flow to the brain.

target tissue The destination, or intended tissue, in the nervous impulse (e.g., a muscle).

tract A system of tissues (e.g., neuronal axons) or organs (e.g., intestines) that function together.

INTRODUCTION

Neurology is the healthcare specialty that deals with the diseases and disorders of the nervous system. A *neurologist* is a specialist involved in the diagnosis, treatment, and prevention of nervous system diseases and disorders. A *neurosurgeon* is a surgeon who operates on the nervous system as treatment for a neurologic disorder.

Besides the neurology department, patients with nervous system concerns can be seen in primary and urgent care departments. The medical assistant may help the provider with the examination and screening questions.

Nervous System Structures

The main structures of the nervous system include the brain, spinal cord, and nerves. Various other sense organs, besides the nerves, exist throughout the body, such as the eyes. The nervous system is made up of nerve cells, or *neurons*. (Neurons are discussed in the Physiology of the Nervous System section.)

The nervous system is divided as follows:

- *Central nervous system* (CNS), which is composed of the brain and the spinal cord.
- *Peripheral nervous system* (PNS), which is made up of all the nervous tissue outside of the CNS, including the 12 pairs of cranial nerves and 31 pairs of spinal nerves. The PNS can be further divided:
  - *Somatic nervous system*, which is voluntary. It collects information and returns instructions to the skin, voluntary muscles, and joints.
  - *Autonomic nervous system* (ANS), which is involuntary. It collects information and returns instructions to involuntary structures (e.g., involuntary muscles, glands, organs).

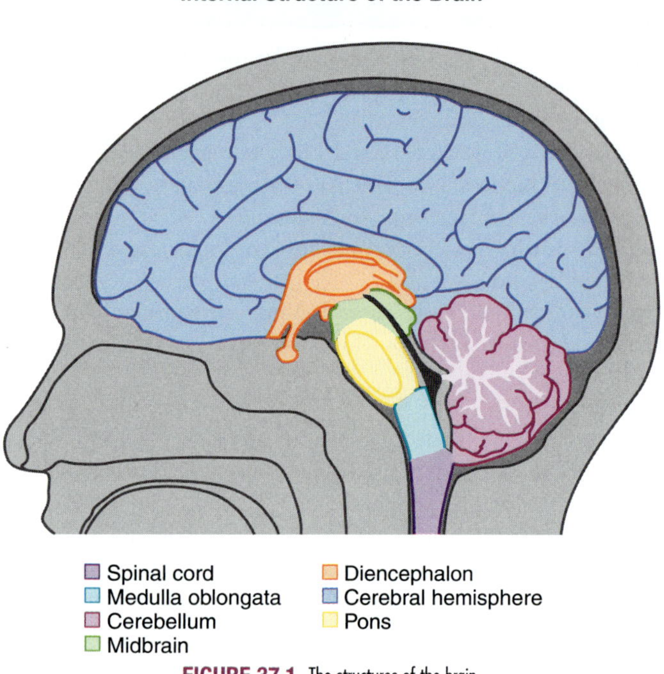

FIGURE 37.1 The structures of the brain.

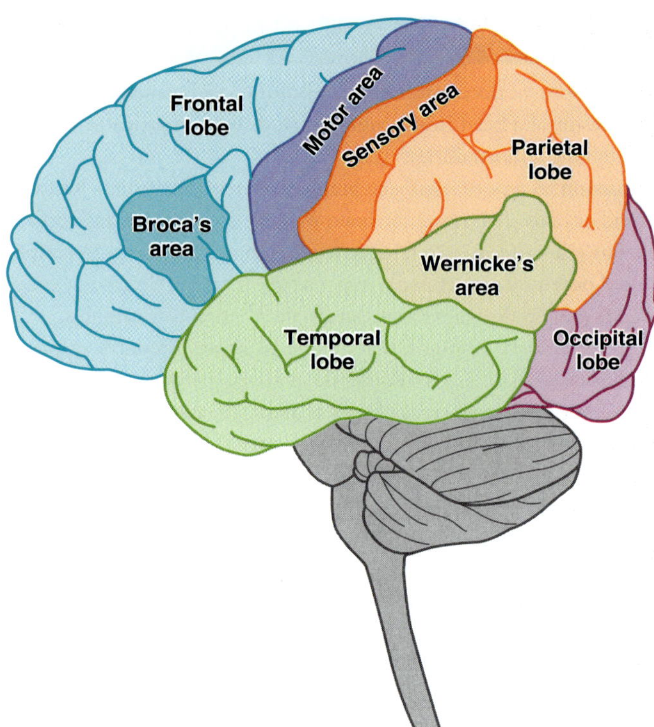

FIGURE 37.2 The lobes of the cerebrum.

CENTRAL NERVOUS SYSTEM

The central nervous system is composed of the brain and spinal cord. The following sections examine the brain and spinal cord.

Brain

The brain, enclosed in the skull, is one of the most complex organs of the body. It is divided into the cerebrum, cerebellum, diencephalon, and brainstem (Figure 37.1).

Cerebrum

The cerebrum is the largest portion of the brain and is divided into two hemispheres by a deep **fissure**. The right hemisphere controls artistic functions, such as drawing, rhythm, and picture memory. The left hemisphere controls verbal functions, such as reading, writing, speaking, and mathematic calculations. The hemispheres are connected by the *corpus callosum*, a bundle of nerve tissue that facilitates communication between the two sides of the brain. If the corpus callosum only partially develops or is absent, the person is diagnosed with *corpus callosum agenesis*.

Most of the signals between the brain and body cross over. This means that the left cerebral hemisphere primarily controls the right side of the body, and the right hemisphere primarily controls the left side of the body. For instance, if a person has a stroke affecting the right hemisphere, the symptoms will be seen on the left side of the body.

The surfaces of the hemispheres are covered by **gray matter**, or the *cerebral cortex*. The cerebral cortex is a thin layer ranging from 1 to 4.5 mm in thickness. Most of the information processing in the brain takes place in the cerebral cortex. **Gyri** add more surface area, thus increasing the amount of information that can be processed. **Sulci** are also visible in the cerebral cortex.

Lobes. Each cerebral hemisphere is further divided into four sections, called *lobes*. These are the functions of the lobes:

- *Frontal lobes*: Lie directly behind the forehead. These lobes are responsible for personality, intelligence, concentration, self-awareness, problem-solving, short-term memory, planning, and judgment. In the back of the frontal lobe is a *motor area* that controls the voluntary movements on the opposite side of the body. The *Broca area*, found in the left frontal lobe, is involved with speech (e.g., moving thoughts into words when speaking and writing) (Figure 37.2). When damage occurs in the Broca area (e.g., stroke or head injury), **aphasia** can occur.
- *Parietal lobes*: Found behind the frontal lobes. These lobes are involved with reading and interpreting visual, auditory, motor, sensory, and memory signals, along with spatial and visual perceptions. The *sensory areas*, found near the motor area of the frontal lobe, receive information from the body regarding touch, pain, and temperature (see Figure 37.2). Reading and math skills are also functions of the parietal lobe.
- *Occipital lobes*: Found at the back of the brain. These lobes handle images from the eyes and connect the information with stored image memories. Damage to or a lack of these lobes can cause blindness.
- *Temporal lobes*: Found in front of the occipital lobes on the right and left sides of the brain. The top of each temporal lobe receives information from the ears, and the underside of the lobe forms and retrieves sound-related memories. The *Wernicke area*, found in the left temporal lobe, is important for language comprehension and speech (see Figure 37.2). The temporal lobes are also responsible for processing memories and sensations of taste, touch, sight, and sounds. The **amygdala** is found in each temporal lobe and is involved with the **limbic system.**

Cerebellum

The cerebellum is located below the occipital lobe of the cerebrum. It is also covered by the cortex. The cerebellum gathers input from other parts of the brain and spinal cord to provide accurate timing for coordinated smooth movements. The cerebellum coordinates the equilibrium or balance, posture, and muscle coordination. Damage to the cerebellum caused by a stroke can cause nausea, dizziness, and balance and coordination issues.

Diencephalon

The diencephalon is located just above the brainstem and is almost surrounded by the cerebral hemispheres. It serves as a relay station for sensory input neurons and other parts of the brain. It plays an important role in the functioning of the CNS, endocrine system, and limbic system. The diencephalon is composed of the posterior pituitary gland and the **pineal gland,** which are part of the endocrine system. The diencephalon also includes two other parts:

- *Thalamus*: Processes information going to and from the body and the cerebrum.
- *Hypothalamus*: Controls body temperature, hunger, and thirst; part of the limbic system.

A **tract** of nerve cells connects the thalamus and hypothalamus to the **hippocampus**. The hippocampus works with memories, sending memories to cerebral hemispheres for storage (long-term memories) and then retrieving them when needed.

CRITICAL THINKING APPLICATION 37.1

Nancy has roomed Elaine. While Nancy is taking her medical history, Elaine mentions that she feels unsteady from time to time and loses her balance a few times. What part of the brain is involved in maintaining balance?

Brainstem

The brainstem connects the cerebral hemispheres to the spinal cord. It controls the flow of information from the body to the brain. The brainstem is composed of these structures:

- *Midbrain*: Connects the hemispheres of the cerebrum with the pons. It serves as a relay center for auditory, visual, and motor information. It also contains centers to regulate pupillary reflexes and eye movements.
- *Pons*: Serves as a bridge between the medulla oblongata and the cerebrum and helps regulate respiration.
- *Medulla oblongata*: Lowest part of the brainstem. It contains vital centers of life (e.g., cardiac, respiratory, and vasomotor centers) that regulate the heart rate, respiration, and the diameter of blood vessels, which affect the blood pressure. Nonvital centers also are found in the medulla oblongata, including centers that regulate coughing, sneezing, hiccupping, vomiting, and swallowing. Some medications work to quiet these centers.

Spinal Cord

The spinal cord is a bundle of nervous tissue. It extends from the medulla oblongata to about the second lumbar vertebra (Figure 37.3). The spinal cord passes through the **foramen magnum** in the skull and is protected by the vertebrae. It is covered by **meninges**. The spinal cord is composed of the cell bodies of motor neurons (gray matter) and the myelin-covered **axons**. Thirty-one pairs of spinal nerves extend from the spinal cord. Each nerve stimulates a specific organ or area of the body. The spinal cord carries messages between the spinal nerves and the brain. This can slow with age.

Meninges

Meninges are a protective covering around the brain and spinal cord. They are composed of three membranes (Figure 37.4):

- *Dura mater*: Outer layer of meninges; made up of a tough white fibrous connective tissue. The space below the dura mater is called the *subdural space*, which contains tiny blood vessels.
- *Arachnoid mater:* Middle layer of meninges; made up of a thin layer of threadlike strands resembling a cobweb. The space below the arachnoid is called the *subarachnoid space,* which is filled with cerebrospinal fluid (CSF) and blood vessels.
- *Pia mater:* Innermost layer of meninges; a thin, highly vascular membrane that is tightly bound to the surface of the spinal cord and brain.

The ventricular system in the brain is made up of four connected *ventricles* (spaces or cavities). CSF originates in the **choroid plexus** in the ventricles. CSF is a clear fluid that resembles water, and it has three roles:

- Cushions the brain and spinal cord
- Removes waste products from cerebral metabolism
- Supplies nutrients to the nervous system tissues

CSF flows through the ventricles, exits into the cisterns at the base of the brain, and moves around the brain and spinal cord. Eventually, CSF is reabsorbed into the bloodstream. The balance between CSFs production and absorption is critical. Excessive amounts of CSF result in an abnormal widening of the ventricles, which can put pressure on the brain tissue and lead to **hydrocephalus.**

PERIPHERAL NERVOUS SYSTEM

The peripheral nervous system is made up of the nerves that exit the brain or spinal cord. Cranial and spinal nerves are part of the peripheral nervous system.

Cranial Nerves

The peripheral nerves exiting the brain directly through the skull are called *cranial nerves.* Cranial nerves originate from the underside of the brain and relay information to and from the sensory organs and muscles of the face and neck (Table 37.1). Cranial nerves have a motor function, sensory function, or both.

Spinal Nerves

The *spinal nerves* exit the spinal canal through spaces between the vertebrae. Spinal nerves closely mimic the organization of the vertebrae and provide stimulation to the rest of the body. If the nerve fibers from several spinal nerves form a network, it is called a *plexus.* Spinal nerves are named by their vertebrae location (e.g., cervical, thoracic) and by number. Spinal nerves carry information to and from the brain through the spinal cord.

Dermatomes are skin surface areas supplied by a single **afferent** spinal nerve. These areas are so specific that the body can be mapped by dermatomes (Figure 37.5). Shingles, for example, appears on specific dermatomes based on which nerve the virus has infected.

CRITICAL THINKING APPLICATION 37.2

Using the mnemonic "On Old Olympus Towering Top A Fine Vocal German Viewed Some Hops," lists the cranial nerves in order.

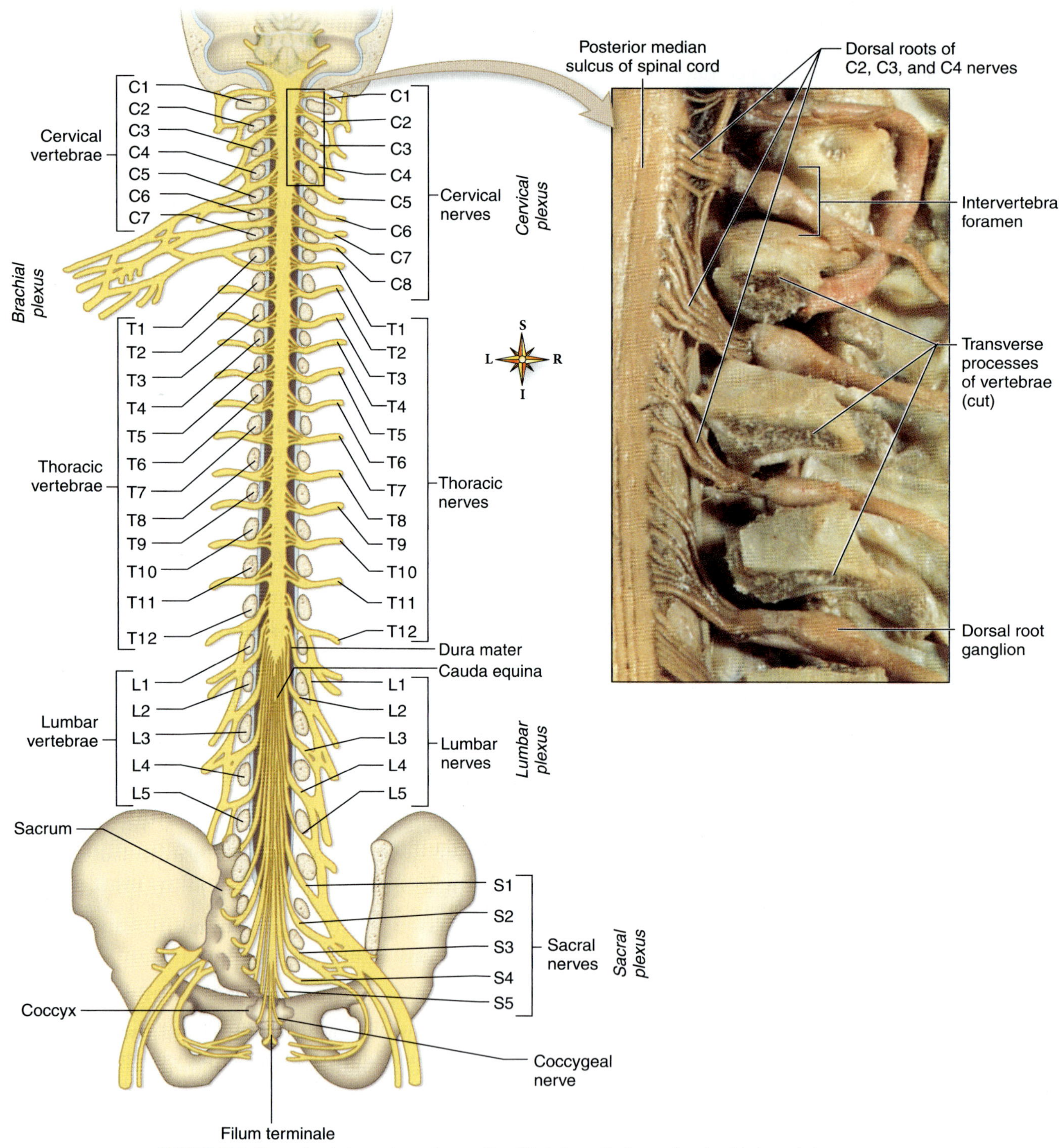

FIGURE 37.3 The spinal cord, showing the spinal nerves. (From Vidic B, Suarez FR: *Photographic atlas of the human body*, St. Louis, 1984, Mosby.)

CELLS OF THE NERVOUS SYSTEM

The nervous system is made up of two types of cells:

- *Neurons:* Also called *parenchymal cells*, which carry out the work of the nervous system.
- *Neuroglia*: Also called *stromal cells* or *glia*. These cells provide a supportive function for the neurons.

Neurons

The nervous system is composed of nerve cells, or *neurons.* Neurons are composed of a cell body, dendrites, and an axon. The *dendrites* are short projections from the cell body. They pick up electrical impulses, often from other neurons, and send the signals to the cell body. The impulse is then passed to the axon, which is a long extension off the

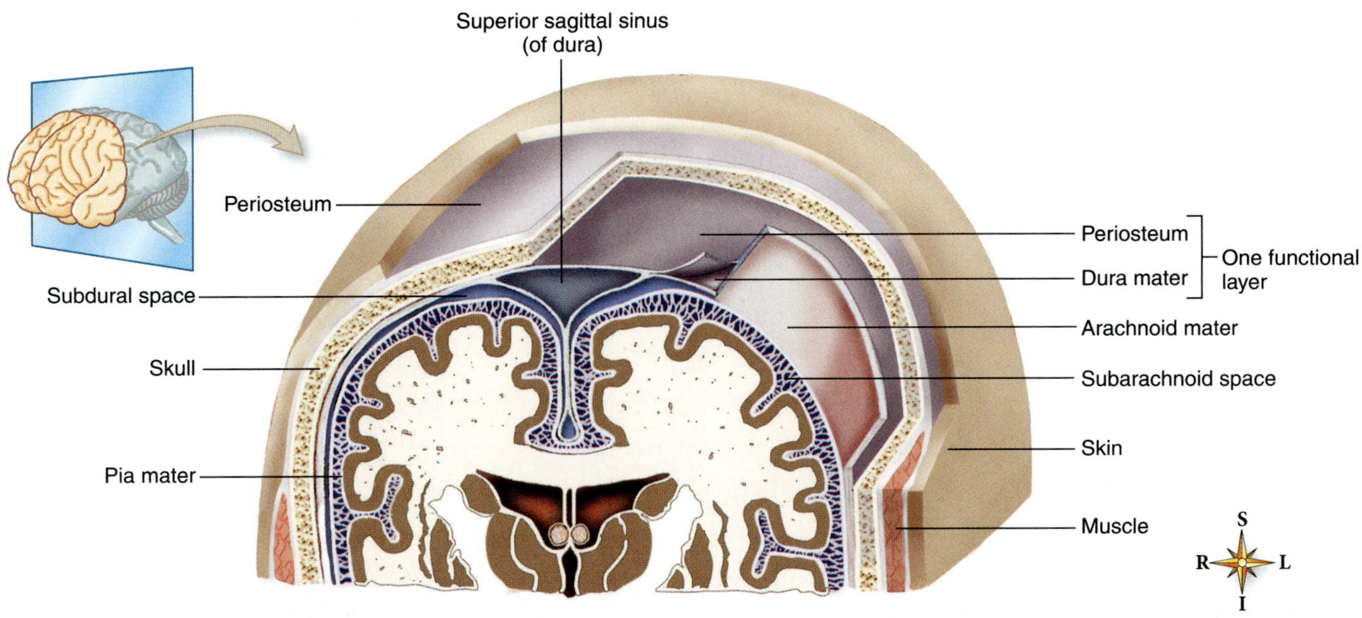

FIGURE 37.4 Protective coverings of the brain. (Modified from Patton K, Thibodeau G: *Anatomy and physiology,* ed 9, St. Louis, 2016, Mosby.)

TABLE 37.1 Cranial Nerves

NUMBER	NAME	FUNCTION	HOW IT IS TESTED
I	Olfactory	Sensory function: Smell	Identifying familiar odors while the eyes are closed.
II	Optic	Sensory function: Vision	A visual acuity test may be given. A light may be shined in the eyes.
III	Oculomotor	Sensory and motor functions: Eye movement, pupil constriction and accommodation	The pupil is examined using a light. The patient may be asked to follow the light with the eyes without moving the head.
IV	Trochlear	Motor function: Eye movement	Testing to see if the eyes can follow a moving light, as described for cranial nerve III.
V	Trigeminal	Sensory and motor functions: Muscles for chewing, general sensations from the anterior half of the head, including the face and meninges	The provider may feel the face in different locations and have the patient clench the teeth.
VI	Abducens	Motor function: Eye movement	Testing to see if the eyes can follow a moving light, as described for cranial nerve III.
VII	Facial	Sensory and motor functions: Muscles used for facial expressions; tearing, salivation, and taste	Patient may be asked to identify common tastes, puff cheeks, smile, wrinkle forehead, and close eyes tightly.
VIII	Vestibulocochlear	Sensory function: Hearing and equilibrium	Assessed using a hearing acuity test.
IX	Glossopharyngeal	Sensory and motor functions: Swallowing and taste	Gag reflex is tested with a tongue blade.
X	Vagus	Sensory and motor functions: Breathing, speech, sweating, regulating heartbeat, stimulating muscles of the gastric region	Patient is asked to say "ahh," swallow, and talk (voice quality assessed). Gag reflex is tested with a tongue blade.
XI	Spinal accessory	Motor function: Shoulder and head movements	Assessed by turning the head from side to side against mild resistance and shrugging the shoulders.
XII	Hypoglossal	Motor function: Tongue movements	Assessed by sticking out and moving the tongue from side to side.

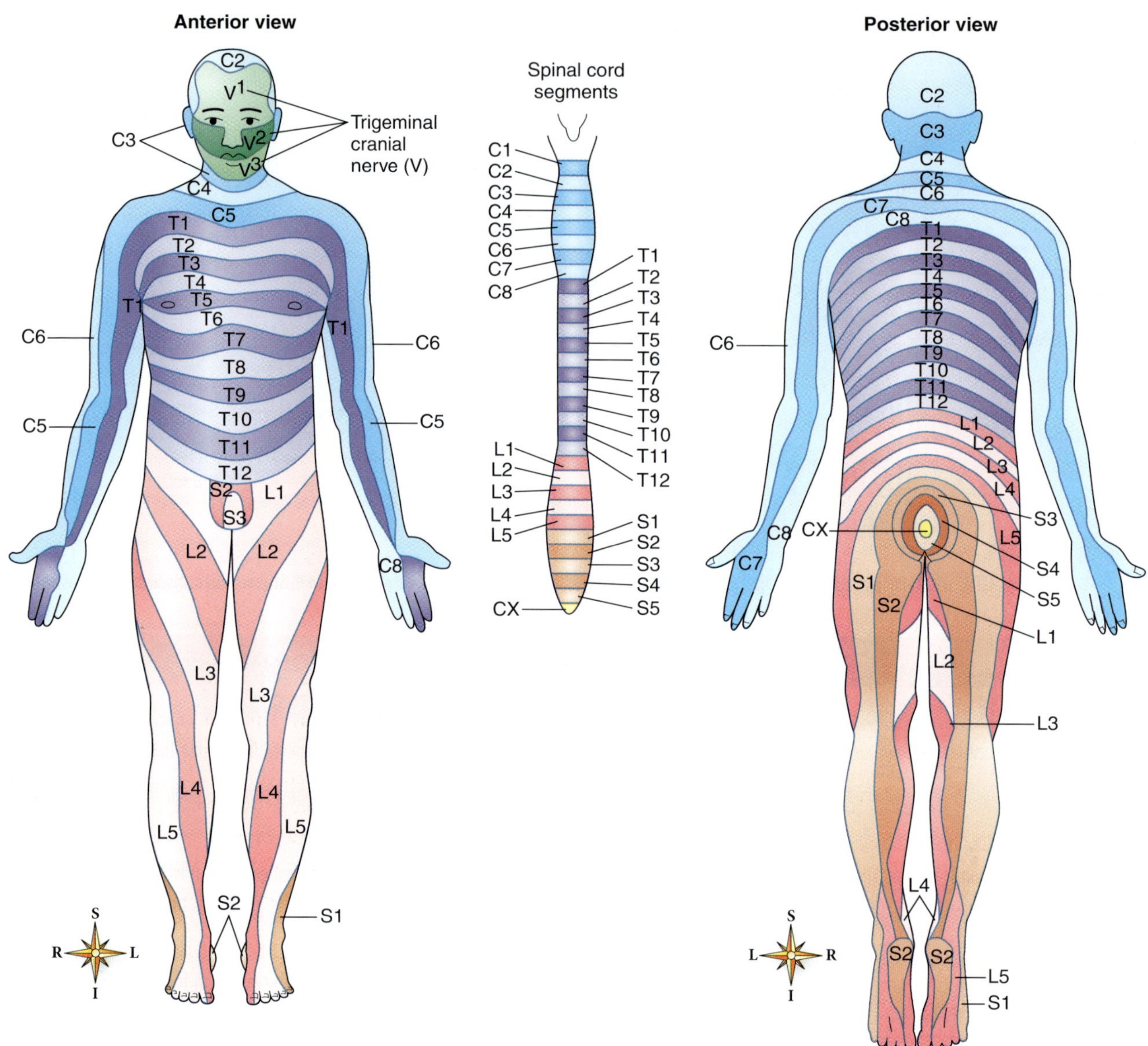

FIGURE 37.5 Map of the dermatomes. (From Patton K, Thibodeau G: *The human body in health & disease*, ed 7, St. Louis, 2018, Mosby.)

cell body. Some axons can be over 3 feet long. The axon transmits the impulse to other dendrites, glands, or muscles.

Neuroglia

Neuroglial cells care for and support neurons throughout the body. These specialized cells perform specific functions within the nervous system. There are several types of neuroglia, including the following:

- *Schwann cells:* Form the **myelin sheath**, which covers the axons of peripheral nerves.
- *Astrocytes:* Help form the *blood-brain barrier* (BBB), which closely regulates what substances enter the brain tissue. Oxygen, water, and glucose molecules easily pass into the brain. Many chemicals and drugs are prevented from moving into brain tissue.
- *Microglia*: Found in the CNS. If brain tissue is inflamed or damaged, microglia engulf and destroy microorganisms or debris.
- *Oligodendrocytes:* Found in the CNS; they myelinate the CNS axons and help hold nerve fibers together.

CRITICAL THINKING APPLICATION **37.3**

What type of cell produces the myelin sheath that surrounds some nerve axons?

PHYSIOLOGY OF THE NERVOUS SYSTEM

The *nervous system* is a complex system that plays a major role in **homeostasis**. The nervous system works in partnership with the endocrine system to help the body respond to its internal and external environments. This effort is responsible for communication and control throughout the body. There are three main functions of the nervous system:

- Collecting information about the external and internal environments (sensing)
- Processing this information and making decisions about action (interpreting)
- Directing the body to put into action the decisions made (acting)

For example, the sensory function begins with a *stimulus* (e.g., the uncomfortable pinch of a tight shoe). That information travels to the brain, where it is *interpreted*. The return message is sent to *react to the stimulus* (e.g., remove the shoe).

The basic flow of information in the nervous system includes the following:

- *Afferent* or *sensory neurons*, which collect stimuli received from receptors. Receptors are found throughout the body (e.g., skin, eyes, nose, tongue, and internal organs). Pain receptors are also found throughout the body. The afferent neurons carry the stimuli from the receptors to the CNS (e.g., brain and spinal cord).

- The brain and spinal cord process the information and direct the necessary response. The central nervous system contains *interneurons*, nerve cells, that connect sensory and motor neurons.
- The response from the CNS is sent via the **efferent** or *motor neurons.* The efferent neurons carry the response to an organ, gland, or muscle. The efferent neurons that direct the skeletal muscles are part of the somatic nervous system. The efferent neurons that direct internal organs to contract and secrete are part of the autonomic nervous system.

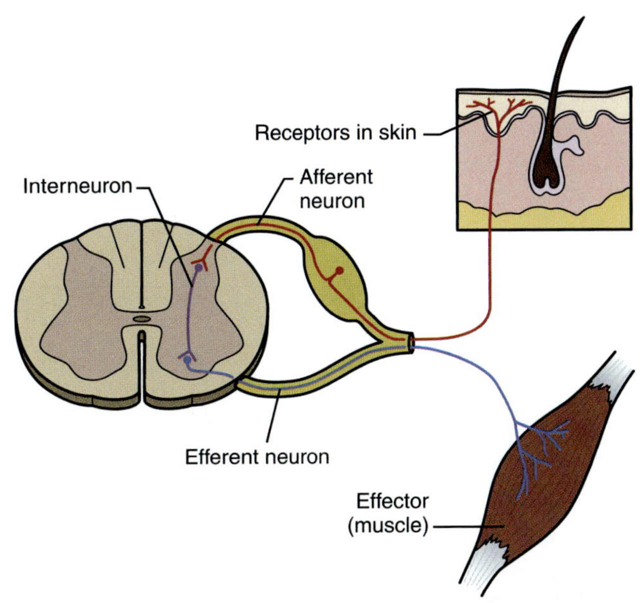

FIGURE 37.6 Three-neuron arc. (From Niedzwiecki B: *Kinn's medical assisting fundamentals: administrative and clinical competencies with anatomy & physiology*, ed 2, St. Louis, 2022, Elsevier.)

Peripheral Nervous System

The peripheral nervous system consists of voluntary and involuntary nerves. The PNS can be divided into the *somatic nervous system* (voluntary nervous system) and the *autonomic nervous system* (involuntary nervous system). The autonomic nervous system can be further divided into the sympathetic nervous system and the parasympathetic nervous system.

Somatic Nervous System

The somatic nervous system is the part of the peripheral nervous system that sends motor impulses to the skeletal muscles. The somatic nervous system transmits signals from the CNS to the skeletal muscles and the sense receptors (vision, hearing, and touch). It is associated with the voluntary control of body movements and is also involved with involuntary reflex arcs.

Reflex Arc. A *reflex* is an involuntary, almost instantaneous movement in response to a specific stimulus. A reflex arc is the route followed by nerve impulses in the production of a reflex act. The stimulus is picked up by the receptors. The impulse is carried by the afferent neuron to the central nervous system (brain or spinal cord). The efferent neuron carries the message from the central nervous system to the effector organ, where the response occurs.

A *three-neuron arc* consists of sensory neurons, interneurons, and motor neurons (Figure 37.6). A *two-neuron arc* is the simplest reflex arc. It does not require the brain to cause a response. The two-neuron arc consists of just sensory neurons and motor neurons. The knee-jerk reflex, also called the *patellar reflex,* is an example of the two-neuron arc. A sharp tap on the patellar tendon below the patella results in a sudden kicking movement of the lower leg. The tap on the tendon (the stimulus) is picked up by receptors. The impulse is carried by the afferent neuron (part of the femoral nerve) to the spinal cord. The response from the spinal cord is sent back by the efferent neuron to the thigh muscles. The muscles contract and the kick occurs.

Autonomic Nervous System

The autonomic nervous system consists of nerves that conduct impulses from the brainstem or spinal cord to cardiac and smooth muscle tissue and glands. The ANS controls the muscles in blood vessel walls, organs, and glands. It regulates involuntary functions such as breathing, heart rate, sweating, circulation, and digestion.

The motor portion of this system is further divided into the sympathetic and parasympathetic nervous systems. These two opposing systems help maintain homeostasis throughout the body (Figure 37.7).

Sympathetic Nervous System. The *sympathetic nervous system* can produce a fight-or-flight response. This part of the nervous system helps the individual respond to perceived stress. It speeds up the heart rate, raises blood glucose levels, raises blood pressure, slows the digestive system, and widens the bronchioles, allowing more oxygen to enter the body quickly. It also stimulates the adrenal glands to increase their secretions.

Parasympathetic Nervous System. The *parasympathetic nervous system* does the opposite of the sympathetic nervous system. It slows the heart rate, lowers blood pressure, increases digestive functions, and reduces adrenal and sweat gland activity.

Action Potential

Neurons carry information from one cell to another by creating and spreading electronic impulses. An *action potential* is a self-propagating wave of electrical impulse that travels along the surface of a neuron membrane. An action potential proceeds in the following steps:

1. A stimulus (e.g., pressure, temperature, sound wave) starts an impulse.
2. The resting nerve cell has a slightly positive charge (due to sodium ions) on the outside of the cell membrane and a negative charge inside the cell. This state is called *polarization.*
3. When a section of the membrane is stimulated, the positively charged ions on the outside of the cell enter the nerve cell. This changes the outside charge to a negative charge. This state is called *depolarization.*
4. Almost immediately after the impulse passes, the positively charged ions move outside the nerve cells again. This returns the outside charge to a positive charge. This state is called *repolarization.*

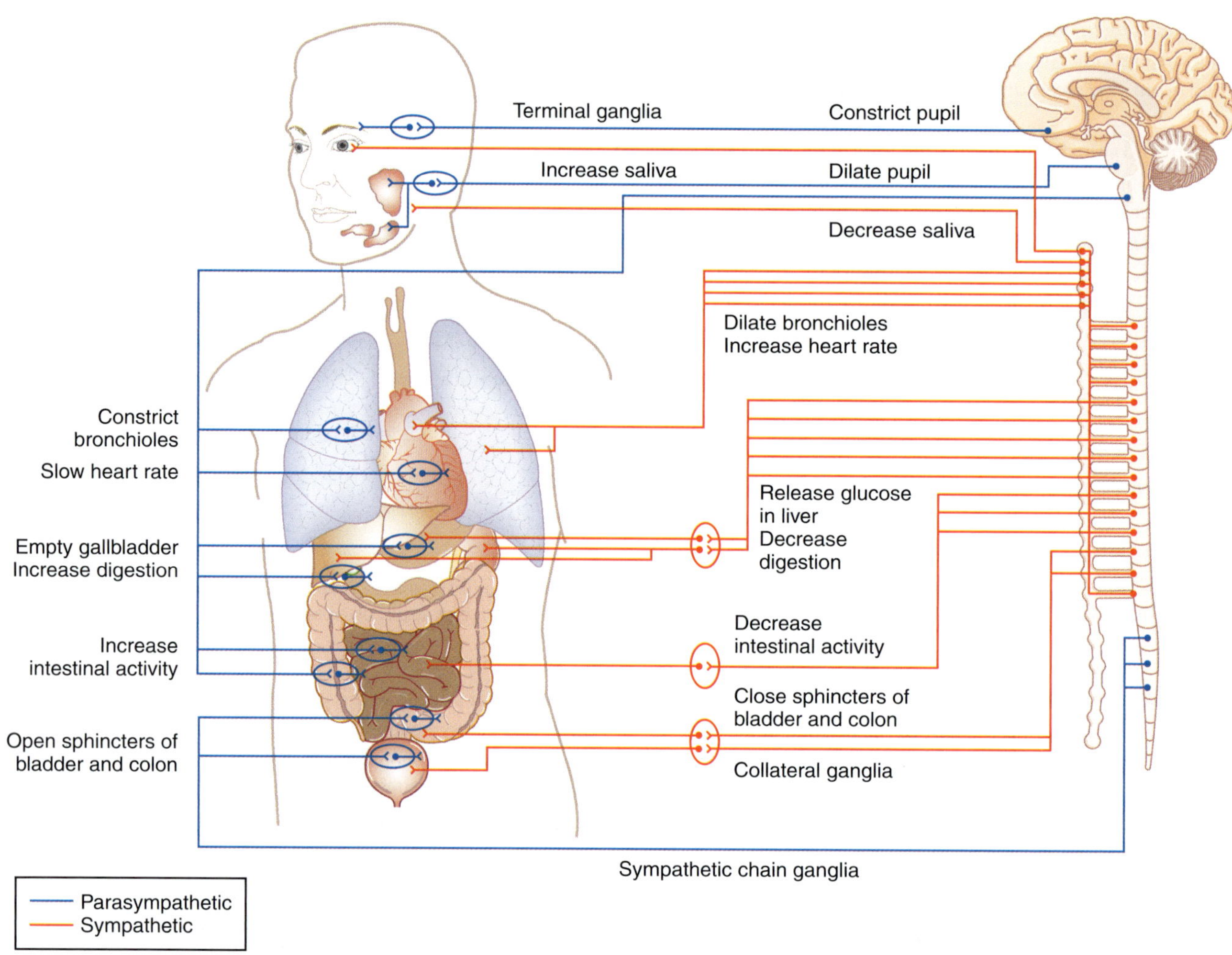

FIGURE 37.7 Structure and function of the autonomic nervous system. (From Applegate E: *The anatomy and physiology learning system,* ed 4, St. Louis, 2011, Saunders.)

5. Once everything changes back, the cell is at rest again, and the cycle continues.

The transfer of the action potential begins as the electrical impulse travels down an axon. It becomes a chemical impulse while moving across the *synapse,* the gap between the neurons. The transfer of impulses from the end of one neuron to the dendrites of another is enhanced by chemical **neurotransmitters** found in the synapse (Figure 37.8). Examples of neurotransmitters include epinephrine, norepinephrine, dopamine, serotonin, endorphins, and enkephalins.

Neurotransmitters bind to specific receptor sites on the dendrites of the next neuron or the **target tissue.** Messages move throughout the entire nervous system in this manner. Impulses in the neuron are electrical; the impulses become chemical as a neurotransmitter is released at each synapse. The action potentials become electrical again as they are picked up by the next dendrites of another neuron or by the target tissue. Changes in the number of available neurotransmitters can cause different conditions.

CRITICAL THINKING APPLICATION 37.4

It is important to know the differences between the sympathetic and parasympathetic nervous systems. List three characteristics of each, and compare your list with that of a classmate. Do your lists agree?

Life Span Changes in the Neurologic System

Infants are born with an immature nervous system. Over the first few years of life, the process of myelination continues, causing an increase in the child's brain size. As the child matures, learning and thinking processes become more complex. During adulthood, brain function is stable.

As a person ages, the nervous system changes. The brain and spinal cord lose nerve cells. Nerve cells break down in the brain, and waste products accumulate, which can cause plaques and neurofibrillary tangles to form. Nerve impulses become slower. This causes a slower reaction time, and tasks may take longer to perform. Reflexes can also be reduced. Slowing of thought, thinking, and memory is a normal part of aging.

NEURODEGENERATIVE DISEASES AND DISORDERS

Neurodegenerative diseases affect a person's ability to move, talk, and breathe. These diseases can also affect a person's balance and heart function. The etiology may be genetic, related to a medical condition (e.g., tumor, stroke), or caused by a virus or toxin. With some diseases, the etiology is unknown.

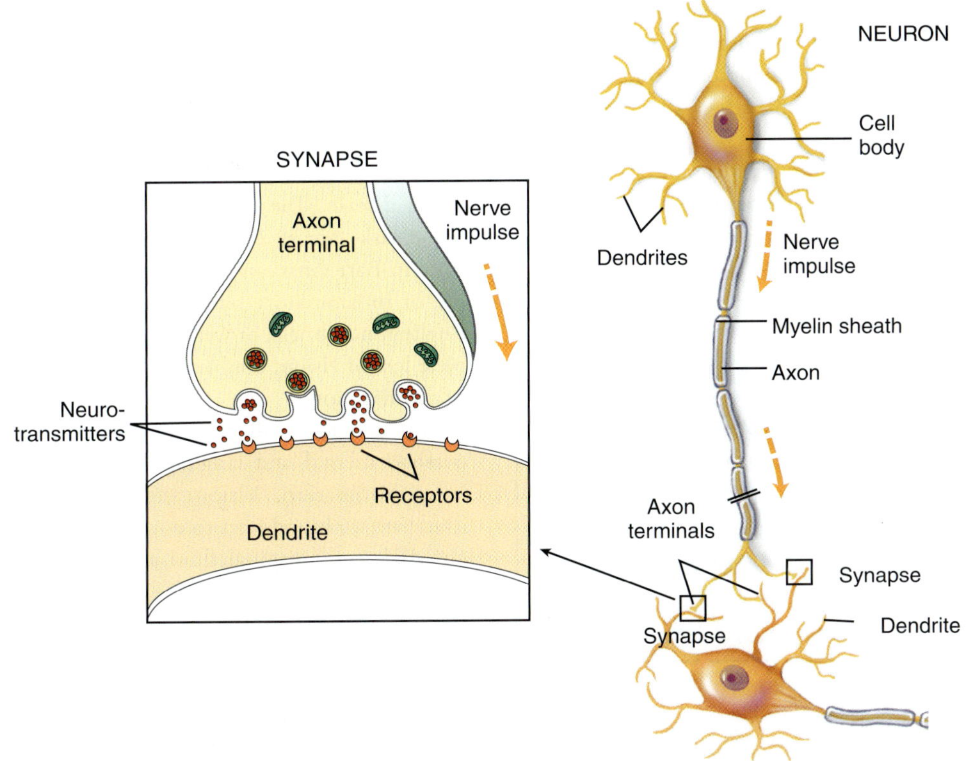

FIGURE 37.8 Neuron and synapse *(inset)*. (From Shiland B: *Mastering healthcare terminology*, ed 5, St. Louis, 2016, Mosby.)

Neurologic Diseases and Disorders

Common signs and symptoms of neurologic diseases and disorders include the following:

- **Neuralgia**, *paresthesia* (feelings of prickling, burning, or numbness)
- Lack of coordination, muscle rigidity, *spasms* (involuntary muscle contractions, such as stuttering and tics), seizures, and *tremors* (rhythmic, purposeless muscle movements)
- Recurrent headache, amnesia *(memory loss)*, difficulty speaking or finding the right word, slurred speech
- Loss of sight or double vision
- Confusion, disorientation, or loss of consciousness

Amyotrophic Lateral Sclerosis

Amyotrophic lateral sclerosis (ALS), or Lou Gehrig disease, is a progressive neurologic disorder that attacks the motor neurons in the brain and spinal cord. ALS usually affects adults between 40 and 60 years of age.

There is no known *etiology* (cause) for ALS, though there is a genetic component to the disease in up to 10% of the cases. Early signs and symptoms include mild muscle problems, including trouble walking, running, writing, swallowing *(dysphagia)*, and speaking. The muscle weakness starts in the hands and feet and spreads throughout the body, leading to an inability to move the legs and arms. Eventually, the person has difficulty eating, speaking, and breathing. Some people experience memory issues and dementia.

The provider will do an examination that will show abnormal reflexes, weakness, twitching, and difficulty moving. Tests may be done to rule out other conditions, including blood tests, computed tomography (CT), magnetic resonance imaging (MRI), electromyography, and lumbar puncture. Breathing tests may be done to assess the lung muscles. Riluzole (Rilutek) may be prescribed to slow symptoms, and other medications may be given to help with the symptoms. Physical therapy and assistive devices (e.g., wheelchair, braces) may be used. A feeding tube may help with the nutritional status. Assistance with breathing may also be needed. There is no cure for ALS.

Alzheimer Disease

Alzheimer disease (AD) is a degenerative disease of the brain. It is characterized by disorientation, memory failure, speech disturbance, and a loss of mental capacity. It is the most common cause of dementia. AD causes an increased amount of microscopic **neurofibrillary tangles** and **amyloid plaques** in the cerebral cortex and the loss of neurons.

Usually, AD begins after age 60, and the risk increases with age. The risk also increases if family members have AD. Researchers feel that AD is caused by a combination of lifestyle, genetics, and environmental factors that affect the brain. Some research suggests a link between herpes simplex virus type 1 and AD. The causes are not fully understood. The signs and symptoms of AD begin slowly; initially, there is difficulty remembering recent activities or the names of people the person knows. AD affects thinking, reasoning, making judgments and decisions, memory, performing familiar tasks, personality, and behavior. Over time, the symptoms worsen, affecting a person's ability to speak, read, write, or remember family members. Personality changes, aggression, and wandering away from home can occur.

The provider will do a medical history and physical exam. There is no specific test for AD. Neurologic tests, CT, MRI, positron emission tomography (PET), psychiatric evaluation, and cognitive and neuropsychological tests may be done. Laboratory tests are done to rule out other conditions. A lumbar puncture may be done, and the cerebrospinal fluid may be examined for **biomarkers** that indicate AD. Current treatments may only keep symptoms from worsening for a limited time; no cure is available. The following medications can be used to treat cognitive symptoms:

- Cholinesterase inhibitors: Boost the acetylcholine in the brain, which is depleted with AD. Common medications include donepezil (Aricept), rivastigmine (Exelon), and galantamine (Razadyne).
- Memantine (Namenda) is used for moderate to severe AD.

Dementia

Several diseases and disorders, such as a stroke or Alzheimer disease (AD), cause dementia, though dementia is not a disease. It is a name for a group of symptoms that affect the brain. Symptoms of dementia include being unable to do normal activities of living (e.g., eating, dressing, grooming), solve problems, and control emotions. To be diagnosed with dementia, a person needs to have at least two or more problems with brain function (e.g., memory, language). AD is the leading cause of dementia.

Huntington Disease

Huntington disease (HD), also called *Huntington chorea*, is a progressive neurodegenerative disorder. There are two forms of HD:

- Early-onset HD: Begins during childhood or in the teen years; affects a small number of people.
- Adult-onset HD: Symptoms usually start in the 30s or 40s; most common form of HD.

Usually, people with HD die within 15 to 20 years.

HD is caused by a genetic defect. If the gene is inherited from one parent, the child has a 50% chance of getting the disease. As the gene is passed through families, the disease develops at an earlier age. Behavior issues are usually seen first, including behavioral disturbances, **hallucinations**, moodiness, irritability, restlessness, psychosis, and paranoia. Abnormal movements can also occur, including facial grimacing, jerky movements, slow and uncontrolled movements, or a prancing gait. Dementia also occurs and affects the memory and speech.

The provider will do an examination and order additional tests, including psychological testing, head CT or MRI, and a PET scan of the brain. There is no cure for HD. The goal of the treatment is to slow the symptoms. Medications such as dopamine blockers help reduce abnormal movements and behaviors, and amantadine may help control extra movements.

Multiple Sclerosis

Multiple sclerosis (MS) is an **autoimmune** neurodegenerative disorder that affects the brain and spinal cord. The myelin sheath is damaged, leading to slowed or blocked messages to the brain. MS often occurs between the ages of 20 to 40 and affects females more than males. The disease can be mild, but some people may not be able to write, walk, or speak. There are four types of MS:

- *Clinically isolated syndrome (CIS)*: A person has an MS-like episode but does not meet the criteria for an MS diagnosis.
- *Relapsing-remitting MS (RRMS)*: Most common form; a person experiences relapses of the neurologic symptoms, followed by periods of partial or complete remission (recovery).
- *Secondary progressive MS (SPMS)*: Follows the initial relapsing-remitting course; most people will eventually have worsening symptoms.
- *Primary progressive MS (PPMS)*: Symptoms worsen from the onset. The person does not experience early relapses or remissions.

The etiology is unknown, though the disorder is an autoimmune disease. The immune system destroys the myelin sheath. Some risk factors include a family history, infection with the Epstein-Barr virus, and a history of thyroid disease, type 1 diabetes, or inflammatory bowel disease. Signs and symptoms include tingling, numbness, or weakness in the extremities, partial or complete loss of vision, double vision, slurred speech, fatigue, and lack of coordination.

The provider will perform an examination and evaluate the person's mental and language functions, along with movement and coordination. Vision and other senses will be evaluated. There are no blood tests to diagnose MS. The provider may order an MRI, cerebrospinal fluid analysis, and an **evoked potential test.** There is no cure for MS, though the goal of treatment is to slow the progression of the disease and speed up recovery time from attacks. Corticosteroid medications may be given to reduce nerve inflammation. Ocrelizumab (Ocrevus) may be used in some cases of MS.

Parkinson Disease

Parkinson disease (PD) is a progressive neurodegenerative disorder that affects movement. With PD, the dopamine-producing neurons in the brain gradually die. The dopamine levels decrease in the brain, leading to the symptoms. PD usually begins around age 60 and is more common in males.

The cause of PD is unknown, but genetics and environmental triggers (e.g., exposure to certain toxins) can increase the risk of the disease. Signs and symptoms of PD include the following:

- Tremors and *pill-rolling tremors* (thumb and forefinger are rubbed back and forth)
- *Bradykinesia* (slow movement), shuffling gait, rigid muscles, impaired balance and posture, stooping, and writing changes
- Loss of automatic movements (e.g., blinking, smiling), *masked face* (facial appearance of depression or anger), and speech changes (e.g., slurring, soft voice)
- Loss of sense of smell, trouble sleeping, dizziness, and constipation
- Excessive sweating or very little sweating, and drooling

There are no specific tests for PD. The provider will do a neurologic examination, and with the history of symptoms, the diagnosis can be made. Additional tests may be done to rule out other diseases. The following medications can be used to manage the symptoms:

- Carbidopa-levodopa (Sinemet): Used to increase the dopamine in the brain.
- Dopamine agonist: Used to mimic dopamine's effect in the brain. Examples include pramipexole (Mirapex), ropinirole (Requip), and rotigotine (Neupro).
- MAO-B inhibitors: Prevent the breakdown of dopamine. Examples include safinamide (Xadago) and selegiline (Eldepryl, Zelapar).

Deep brain stimulation (DBS) may also be done. This treatment requires a generator to be implanted, and electrodes from it send impulses to the brain, which decrease the symptoms.

Restless Legs Syndrome

Restless legs syndrome (RLS) is also known as *restless legs syndrome/Willis-Ekbom disease* (RLS/WED). RLS causes a creeping, tingling, or burning sensation in the legs when the person is lying down or sitting. Moving the legs helps reduce the sensations for a short period of time. RLS can affect a person's quality of sleep. Most people with RLS also have periodic limb movement disorder (PLMD), which causes the legs or arms to twitch or jerk uncontrollably in sleep. RLS can occur at any age and can worsen with age.

In many situations, there is no known cause for RLS. For some people, RLS is caused by a condition (e.g., pregnancy, anemia) or a medication. Caffeine, alcohol, and tobacco can worsen the symptoms. Researchers believe that RLS may be related to a dopamine imbalance in the brain. There also may be a genetic cause if the condition appears before age 40. Associated risk factors for RLS include peripheral neuropathy, iron deficiency, kidney failure, and spinal cord lesions. The signs and symptoms include abnormal sensations in the legs and feet that begin after rest (often at night) and decrease with movement. The abnormal sensations can be described as itching, electric, aching, throbbing, pulling, crawling, or creeping. The symptoms may disappear for a while and then come back.

Besides an examination, the provider may order blood tests and a sleep study. Treatments include exercise and massage of the legs, stress reduction activities, and decreased caffeine and tobacco use. Medication therapy may include iron for anemia and medications to increase the dopamine in the brain, including ropinirole (Requip), pramipexole (Mirapex), and rotigotine (Neupro). Opioids and anticonvulsants, such as gabapentin (Neurontin, Horizant), pregabalin (Lyrica), and clonazepam (Klonopin), may be used. RLS is a lifelong condition with no cure.

Other Neurodegenerative Diseases and Disorders

The following are additional neurodegenerative diseases and disorders:

- *Friedreich ataxia*: An inherited disease that causes damage to the spinal cord and nerves. Signs and symptoms are seen as early as 5 years of age. The person can experience **ataxia,** difficulty walking, muscle weakness, scoliosis, heart palpitations, involuntary eye movements, and speech issues. There is no cure for this disease. Treatments may include assistive devices (e.g., wheelchair), braces, physical therapy, and surgery.
- *Frontotemporal dementia* (also called *Pick disease*): A rare condition that can start by age 20. Pick bodies and cells (abnormal proteins) are found in the damaged neurons. Behavior changes, speech difficulty, and problems thinking occur and slowly get worse. There is no specific treatment, but medications may be used to help with mood swings.
- *Lewy body disease* (also called *dementia with Lewy bodies*): Lewy bodies (abnormal structures) build up in the brain. Signs and symptoms include decreased alertness, hallucinations, muscle stiffness, confusion, and loss of memory. This disease is one of the more common causes of dementia. There is no cure; treatments help with symptoms.
- *Tay-Sachs disease*: An inherited disease that progressively destroys the neurons in the brain and spinal cord. With the most common form, signs and symptoms are seen in infancy. The infant's motor skills (e.g., sitting, crawling, and rolling) are affected. As the disease progresses, the child can experience seizures, vision and hearing loss, intellectual disability, and **paralysis.**
- *Vascular dementia*: The second most common cause of dementia for people over age 65. This disease is caused by small strokes over time. Signs and symptoms include difficulty performing tasks, language issues, misplacing items, sleep pattern changes, hallucinations, poor judgment, and memory issues. The goal is to control symptoms because there is no treatment.

CRITICAL THINKING APPLICATION 37.5

Nancy is trying to remember the different neurologic diseases. Summarize the following neurodegenerative diseases discussed:

- Amyotrophic lateral sclerosis
- Alzheimer disease
- Huntington disease
- Multiple sclerosis
- Parkinson disease

FUNCTIONAL DISEASES AND DISORDERS OF THE NERVOUS SYSTEM

Functional diseases and disorders impact the function of the neurologic system. The most common functional diseases and disorders include headaches, migraines, seizures, and epilepsy.

Cluster Headaches

Cluster headaches occur in cyclical patterns or clusters. The person may awaken in the middle of the night with a headache on one side of the head.

The etiology is unknown, but there may be an increase in the release of histamine or serotonin that causes the pain. The signs and symptoms include a severe, sudden, one-sided headache with tearing of the eyes, droopy eyelids, and stuffy nose. The onset commonly occurs 2 to 3 hours after falling asleep.

The provider will do a physical examination and may order an MRI to rule out other conditions. Often medications such as sumatriptan (Imitrex), dihydroergotamine (DHE), and **analgesics** may be ordered. Breathing in 100% pure oxygen may also help to reduce the headaches. The cluster of headaches may last for weeks to months, and then a remission period follows.

Tension Headaches

Tension headaches are the most common type of headaches. Tension headaches occur when the neck and scalp muscles become tense. Stress, depression, anxiety, and head injuries may be the most common causes. The person may experience a dull, aching headache and feelings of tightness and pressure in the forehead area to the back of the head.

After taking a history, the provider may order a CT scan or MRI. Usually, the patient manages the pain with home treatments, such as over-the-counter (OTC) analgesics. Muscle relaxants and antidepressants may also be used.

Migraines

Migraines are recurring headaches that can affect children through adults. The causes of migraines may include stress, anxiety, hormone changes, strong smells, and bright lights. Many times, migraines progress through four stages:

- *Prodrome* (1 to 2 days before): May cause mood changes, food cravings, neck stiffness, increased thirst, and constipation.
- *Aura* (may occur before or during the migraine): May cause visual, sensory, motor, or verbal disturbances. Examples include hearing noises, difficulty speaking, vision loss, and jerking.
- *Attack* (may last up to 72 hours): May cause throbbing pain on one or both sides of the head; sensitivity to light, noise, and smells; nausea and vomiting, blurred vision, and lightheadedness.
- *Postdrome* (up to 24 hours after): May cause confusion, moodiness, dizziness, weakness, and sensitivity to noise and light.

The provider will do physical and neurologic examinations. Treatment consists of rest, fluids, and medications, such as sumatriptan (Imitrex), dihydroergotamine (DHE), and analgesics.

Seizure Disorders

A *seizure* (or *convulsion*) is a sudden increase of electrical activity in one or more parts of the brain. The seizures are classified based on how the abnormal brain activity begins.

- *Generalized onset seizure* (was called generalized seizure): Affects both sides of the brain.
- *Focal onset seizure* (was called partial seizure): Affects one area of the brain.
- *Unknown onset seizure*: How it affects the brain is unknown.

Some seizures may start as a focal onset and then spread to both sides of the brain, like clonic and atonic seizures. There are many types of seizures, and the more common types are listed in Table 37.2.

Seizures can be caused by medications, high fevers, head injuries, diseases, and illegal drugs. The signs and symptoms of the different seizure classifications are listed in Table 37.2. Most seizures do not cause harm, but if they last longer than 5 minutes or the person has repeated seizures without waking up between them, it is a medical emergency.

The provider will do a neurologic exam and may order blood tests to check for conditions associated with seizures (e.g., infections). Additional tests may include neuropsychological tests, an electroencephalogram (EEG), CT, MRI, PET, and a single-photon emission computed tomography (SPECT) scan. Depending on the type of seizure, antiseizure medication may be used.

CRITICAL THINKING APPLICATION 37.6

Nancy is attempting to remember the three classifications of seizures. What might be ways that she can remember them?

TABLE 37.2 Seizure Classification

NEW GROUPS	NEW CLASSIFICATION (OLDER NAME)	DESCRIPTION	SYMPTOMS
Generalized onset	*Tonic-clonic* (Grand mal)	Loses consciousness. Tonic phase (rigid muscles) comes first, followed by clonic phase (jerking rapidly). May be incontinent of stool and urine. Lasts 1–3 minutes; sleepy and confused after seizure.	Motor: Sustained jerking *(clonic)*, weak muscles *(atonic)*, rigid muscles *(tonic)*, brief twitching (*myoclonus*), and spasms Nonmotor: Staring spells, twitching
	Focal to bilateral tonic-clonic (Secondarily generalized)	Starts in one area of the brain and spreads to involve both sides. Usually lasts 1–3 minutes.	
	Absent (Petit mal)	Lapse of awareness of the environment; more common in children.	
	Atypical absence	Will stare but may be able to respond; begin and end gradually. May fall. Can last 5–30 seconds.	
Focal onset	*Focal aware* (Simple partial)	Awake and alert during seizure; lasts less than 2 minutes.	Motor: Clonic, atonic, tonic, myoclonus, spasms, automatic movements (e.g., lip smacking, clapping, chewing)
	Focal impaired awareness (Complex partial)	Confused during seizure; lasts 1–2 minutes. Aura may occur.	Nonmotor: Changes in emotions, thinking, heart palpitations, goose bumps, lack of movement
	Atonic	Can begin as a focal seizure and then spread to both sides of the brain, becoming a generalized seizure). Lasts less than 15 seconds.	Loss of muscle tone, head or body may go limp; head may drop
Unknown onset/ unknown		When seizure began is not known, or seizure was not witnessed.	Motor: Tonic-clonic, spasms Nonmotor: No movements, stares

From the Centers for Disease Control and Prevention (CDC), www.cdc.gov/epilepsy/communications/features/seizures.htm; and the Epilepsy Foundation, www.epilepsy.com/learn/types-seizures.

Epilepsy

Epilepsy is a disorder that causes recurring seizures. A person must have at least two unprovoked seizures before epilepsy is diagnosed. The type of seizure is classified either as generalized or focal. Epilepsy can affect anyone at any age, ethnic background, or sex. Children can outgrow epilepsy.

There are several causes of epilepsy, including genetics, brain injury, abnormal development, and illness. Many times, the cause is not known. Signs and symptoms vary based on the type of seizure and can include confusion, staring, uncontrolled jerking, and loss of consciousness (see Table 37.2). *Status epilepticus*, an emergency condition, occurs when a seizure lasts longer than 10 minutes or if the person has three or more seizures without regaining consciousness between them.

The provider will do a neurologic examination and may order the tests listed in the Seizure Disorder section. Treatments include antiseizure medications, a ketogenic diet (eating foods high in fats and low in carbohydrates), vagus nerve stimulation, and deep brain stimulation (from a surgically implanted generator and electrodes). If medications fail to control the seizures, surgery can be done to remove the portion of the brain causing the seizures.

Other Functional Diseases and Disorders

Additional functional diseases and disorders include the following:

- *Functional neurologic disorder (FND)* (also called *conversion disorder* and *functional movement disorder*): A neurologic disorder that affects the transmission of signals from the nervous system and the body. The cause is unknown. Symptoms include motor dysfunction (e.g., limb weakness, paralysis, spasms, problems walking), dysphagia, sensory dysfunction (e.g., numbness, loss of vision), **syncope**, and seizures.
- *Narcolepsy*: A chronic neurologic disorder that affects the brain's ability to control the sleep-wake cycle, thus causing extreme daytime sleepiness, **cataplexy**, hallucinations, and sleep paralysis. Narcolepsy can be genetic and also an autoimmune disease.
- *Sciatica*: Occurs when the sciatic nerve can become compressed by a herniated disk, spinal stenosis, or a bone spur on the vertebrae. This condition causes burning or stabbing pain that radiates along the path of the sciatic nerve. The person can have pain and numbness in the lower back, hip, buttock, and leg on one side of the body.
- *Tourette syndrome (TS):* A neurologic disorder that causes tics and can be seen as early as 3 years of age. *Tics* are repetitive, involuntary movements and vocalizations. *Simple motor tics* involve a small number of muscle groups and cause sudden, brief, repetitive movements, such as eye blinking, facial grimacing, shoulder shrugging, and head jerking. *Complex motor tics* involve several muscle groups and movements (e.g., grimacing, shrugging, and jerking). *Simple vocal tics* involve sounds made by moving air through the mouth or nose, causing barking, hissing, sniffing, grunting, or throat-clearing. *Complex vocal tics* may include repeating phrases, words, or sentences. People may repeat their own phrases, another person's words, or obscene words. Tics can worsen with emotion (e.g., excitement and anxiety).

INFECTIONS

Infections, such as encephalitis and meningitis, can also impact the nervous system. The following sections discuss these infections, along with shingles.

Encephalitis

Encephalitis is the inflammation of the brain. There are several types of encephalitis:

- *Japanese encephalitis*: Mosquito-transmitted viral infection that occurs in Asia and the western Pacific. Travelers can be vaccinated for the prevention of this disease.
- *La Crosse encephalitis*: Mosquito-transmitted viral infection that occurs in the upper Midwestern, mid-Atlantic, and southeastern states.
- *Saint Louis encephalitis*: Mosquito-transmitted viral infection that occurs in the eastern and central states.

Encephalitis can be caused by a viral or bacterial infection. With a mild case, a person may have flu-like symptoms. With a severe case, a person may experience a severe headache, drowsiness, vomiting, confusion, seizures, and a sudden fever. Babies may constantly cry, not eat well, and have body stiffness and bulging **fontanels**.

After a physical and neurologic examination, the provider may order a cerebrospinal fluid analysis, which requires a lumbar puncture. Blood laboratory tests and CT may also be done. Severe cases require hospitalization and intravenous (IV) medications to treat the infection and reduce brain inflammation. Milder bacterial infections require oral antibiotics. Physical, speech, and occupational therapies may be required for some patients after other symptoms have resolved.

Meningitis

Meningitis is the inflammation of the meninges surrounding the brain and spinal cord. Viral meningitis, the most common form, is caused by a viral infection that affects the nose or mouth and travels to the brain. Bacterial meningitis, usually caused by pneumococcal or meningococcal infections, starts with a cold-like infection and can be deadly. The meningitis vaccine can help prevent certain types of bacterial infections that cause meningitis.

Meningitis can be caused by a viral, bacterial, or fungal infection. There is also a noninfectious meningitis and cancer-related meningitis. The symptoms may include a sudden high fever, severe headache, stiff neck, nausea, and vomiting. Bacterial meningitis can cause hearing loss, brain damage, and a stroke.

After a physical exam and a neurologic examination, the provider will order blood tests (e.g., blood culture), imaging tests, and a lumbar puncture to obtain a cerebrospinal fluid specimen for analysis. With bacterial meningitis, the patient usually receives IV antibiotics to treat the infection and corticosteroids to reduce the inflammation. With viral meningitis, bed rest, fluids, and OTC analgesics are usually prescribed. Antifungal medications will be given for a fungal meningitis. The underlying cause of meningitis also needs to be treated.

Shingles

Herpes zoster, also known as *shingles*, affects about 33% of all adults. Anyone who has had chickenpox can get shingles, including children.

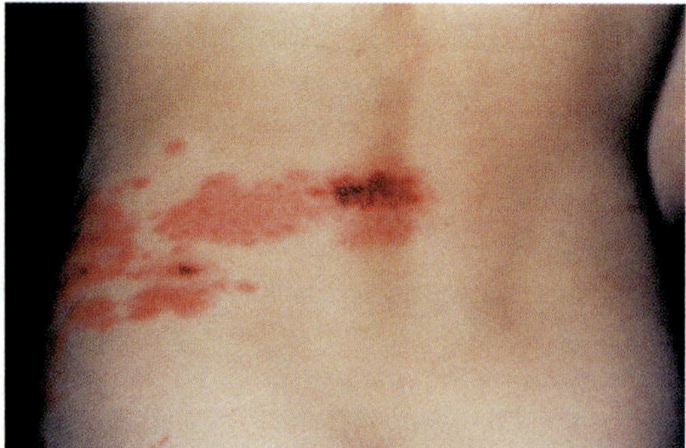

FIGURE 37.9 Herpes zoster (shingles).

Typically, if a person gets shingles, it only occurs once, but there have been cases in which it has developed more than once. Vaccines are available to help prevent shingles.

Shingles is caused by the varicella-zoster virus, the same virus that causes chickenpox. After a person has chickenpox, the virus remains inactive in the body. It can reactivate for unknown reasons and cause shingles. The beginning symptoms include tingling, pain, or itchiness on one side of the body or face, usually on the torso. This can occur 1 to 5 days before a rash with fluid-filled blisters develops (Figure 37.9). The person is contagious to others who have not had chickenpox until the blisters scab over, in about 10 days. The rash clears up within 1 month. The person may also have fever, chills, headache, and nausea. Shingles can cause postherpetic neuralgia, vision loss, encephalitis, and facial paralysis.

The provider will do a history and physical examination to diagnose shingles. There is no cure, but antiviral medications may be ordered to help reduce complications and hasten recovery. Depending on the pain, the provider may also order anticonvulsants, antidepressants, or analgesics.

STRUCTURAL DISEASES AND DISORDERS

Structural diseases and disorders of the nervous system include Bell's palsy, Guillain-Barré syndrome, and trigeminal neuralgia. These diseases and disorders are discussed in this section.

Bell's Palsy

Bell's palsy is the most common cause of facial paralysis. The symptoms typically affect one side of the face and are at their worst about 48 hours after the onset. The exact cause is unknown. The facial nerve becomes swollen and inflamed. The risk of Bell's palsy increases with pregnancy, diabetes, or an upper respiratory viral infection. The signs and symptoms include facial twitching, weakness, and paralysis; drooping of the eyelid or corner of the mouth; dry eyes or excessive tearing; drooling, dry mouth, and a diminished ability to taste (Figure 37.10).

The provider will do a medical history and a physical examination. No other tests are usually ordered. Usually, symptoms resolve within 2 weeks, but it may take 3 to 6 months to return to normal function. Some mild cases do not require treatment, whereas others may be treated with antiviral and corticosteroid medications. Protecting the eye from injury is important; thus eye drops for lubrication and a patch for protection may be used.

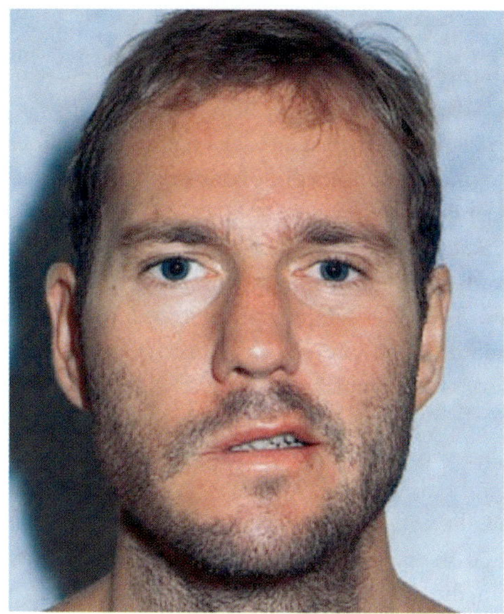

FIGURE 37.10 Bell's palsy (right sided).

Guillain-Barré Syndrome

Guillain-Barré syndrome is a rare autoimmune disorder in which the immune system attacks the peripheral nervous system. The etiology is unknown, but the disorder may be triggered by surgery, an infection, or vaccination. Weakness and tingling start in the legs and spread through the body, making the person almost paralyzed. The disease is life-threatening, and the person may require a respirator to breathe. It may take several weeks before the symptoms improve, and recovery can take up to a few years.

After the physical examination, the provider may order electromyography, nerve conduction studies, and a lumbar puncture. This disorder is difficult to diagnose. Treatment is aimed at relieving the symptoms and supporting breathing if needed.

Trigeminal Neuralgia

Trigeminal neuralgia (TN) is also called *tic douloureux*. TN is a chronic pain condition that affects the trigeminal nerve (cranial nerve V).

A blood vessel or tumor pressing on the trigeminal nerve can cause trigeminal neuralgia. People with multiple sclerosis can also experience TN. This condition is more common in people over age 50 and in females than males. Pain is felt in the cheek, lips, gums, or chin on one side of the face. Pain can vary from sudden, severe, and stabbing to constant, aching, and burning. The pain can be widespread or just in a small area. Activities such as shaving, eating, and talking can trigger intense flashes of pain. The symptoms can stop for a period of time but will come back with greater intensity.

The provider will perform a physical examination and neurologic examination. An MRI may also be ordered. Treatment may include analgesics, anticonvulsants, and antidepressants. Surgical procedures may also be done. A *rhizotomy* is a surgical procedure that damages nerve fibers to block pain. This procedure may cause sensory loss and facial numbness. Trigeminal neuralgia is a debilitating disorder.

Other Structural Diseases and Disorders

The following are additional structural diseases and disorders.

- *Astrocytoma*: A malignant tumor of nervous tissue composed of astrocytes. This type of tumor can spread widely throughout the brain, making it hard to surgically remove.
- *Medulloblastoma*: A fast-growing brain tumor composed of medulloblasts, seen in children and adolescents.
- *Meningioma*: A common malignant tumor that begins in the meninges. The risk increases with age, and this tumor is more common in females.
- *Neuroblastoma*: A rare malignant tumor of the sympathetic nervous system seen in young children.

INJURIES

Injuries are common reasons for neurologic conditions. The CDC estimates 1.5 million Americans sustain a traumatic brain injury (TBI) each year. Besides TBI, spinal cord injuries and peripheral neuropathy cause injuries to the nervous system.

Traumatic Brain Injury

Traumatic brain injury (TBI) is an acquired brain injury. TBIs can occur as a result of falls, motor vehicle accidents, violence (e.g., **shaken baby syndrome,** gunshot wounds), sports injuries, and service in military combat zones. A **concussion** is a mild form of a TBI and is the most common type of sports injury. A *contusion* is bruising or swelling of the brain that occurs when small cerebral blood vessels bleed into brain tissue.

TBI can occur as a result of a violent jolt or blow to the head or body or when something pierces the skull (e.g., a bullet) and injures the brain tissue. Symptoms of TBI may not appear for weeks after the injury. TBI can be mild, moderate, severe, or life threatening, depending on the brain damage.

- Mild TBI symptoms include headache, neck pain, nausea, ringing in the ear, dizziness, lightheadedness, blurred vision, tiredness, dazed feeling, mood changes, and trouble concentrating or remembering. Children experience irritability and changes in eating.
- Moderate or severe TBI symptoms are similar. The headache is constant and gets worse. The person may experience repeated vomiting, seizures, inability to awaken, dilation of one or both pupils, slurred speech, agitation, loss of coordination, and weakness in the extremities. Children may also be inconsolable and refuse to eat.

For severe injuries, emergency personnel will use the **Glasgow Coma Scale** to assess the patient. In the hospital, imaging tests (CT and MRI), along with intracranial pressure monitoring, will be done. In the ambulatory care facility, the provider will obtain information on the injury and perform physical and neurologic examinations. CT or MRI may be ordered to check for skull fractures. For mild TBIs, treatment consists of rest and OTC analgesics. For moderate to severe TBIs, medications are given to reduce the brain swelling and prevent more damage. Surgery may be done to remove **hematomas,** repair skull fractures, stop bleeding in the brain, and relieve pressure (by removing a portion of the skull). Various rehabilitation specialists may be involved during the recovery phase.

Shaken Baby Syndrome

Shaken baby syndrome (SBS) is the leading cause of child abuse deaths. There are more than 1300 cases a year in the United States, and about a quarter of the children die. SBS occurs when a child is violently shaken, or the head strikes against a hard surface (e.g., wall, counter, floor). Crying is the leading trigger for the violence that leads to SBS, and most babies are less than 6 months old when it occurs.

Signs and symptoms of SBS include lethargy, extreme irritability, bruises, rigidity, difficulty breathing, bulging fontanels, inability to focus the eyes or track movement, unequal pupil size, seizures, and poor feeding.

About 80% of the children who survive SBS have lifelong disabilities, including blindness, seizures, hearing loss, developmental delays (e.g., speech, learning, memory, attention), cerebral palsy, and severe mental retardation.

According to the National Center on Shaken Baby Syndrome (www.dontshake.org), the Period of PURPLE Crying program is an evidence-based shaken baby syndrome prevention program that helps caregivers understand crying in infants and helps to prevent SBS. The letters in PURPLE describe important information for parents and caregivers.

Peak of crying: Crying may increase weekly until 2 months of age.
Unexpected: The child may cry off and on, though the parent/caregiver may not know why.
Resists soothing: The child may not stop crying regardless of what the parent/caregiver does.
Painlike face: The facial appearance may indicate that the child is in pain, though that may not be the situation.
Long lasting: The child can cry more than 5 hours a day.
Evening: Crying may increase in the late afternoon or evening.

Spinal Cord Injury

Spinal cord injuries occur when a blow, gunshot, or stabbing fractures or dislocates the vertebrae, and the bone pieces cut into the cord or press on the nerves. This is a medical emergency. Common causes include motor vehicle accidents, falls, acts of violence, alcohol, and diseases. Spinal cord injuries can fall into the following categories:

- *Complete*: No signals can be sent below the level of the injury, and the person is paralyzed below the injury.
- *Incomplete*: Some signals can be sent below the injury, and thus the person has some movement and sensation below the injury.

Initially, the person may experience extreme back or neck pain, bowel or bladder incontinence, difficulty breathing, and paralysis.

- *Quadriplegia* (or *tetraplegia*): The spinal cord injury affects the arms, hands, trunk, legs, and pelvic organs (e.g., bowel, bladder, and sexual functions).
- *Paraplegia*: The spinal cord injury affects some or all of the trunk, legs, and pelvic organs.

The emergency providers will perform physical and neurologic examinations. Imaging studies (x-ray, myelogram, MRI, and CT) will be done. Treatments include surgery, traction, corticosteroids, and rehabilitation (e.g., physical and occupational therapies).

Peripheral Neuropathy

Peripheral neuropathy occurs as a result of damage to the peripheral nervous system. More than 100 types of peripheral neuropathy have been identified, each with its own symptoms. Diabetic neuropathy is one of the most common forms.

The cause of peripheral neuropathy may be inherited, acquired, or unknown (called *idiopathic*). Acquired peripheral neuropathy can be caused by the following:

- *Physical injury:* Related to trauma (accidents, sports-related activities, surgical procedures, and falls) or stress from repetitive activities.
- *Diseases:* Related to metabolic and endocrine diseases (e.g., diabetes mellitus), small vessel disease (e.g., vasculitis), autoimmune diseases (e.g., lupus, rheumatoid arthritis), kidney disorders, cancer, and infections (Lyme disease).
- *Exposure to toxins:* Includes medications, environmental and industrial toxins, and heavy alcohol consumption.

Signs and symptoms include tingling and numbness, paresthesia, weakness, increased sensitivity to stimuli, burning pain, muscle wasting, paralysis, and organ dysfunction. With diabetic neuropathy, pain and numbness are felt in both legs, with gradual progression up the legs. Eventually, the person may feel pain and numbness in the fingers, hands, and arms.

The provider will do physical and neurologic examinations. Additional tests will be done, including nerve conduction velocity (NCV), electromyography (EMG), MRI, and nerve and skin biopsies. Treatment addresses the underlying causes and symptom management. Medications such as antidepressants, anticonvulsants, antiarrhythmics, narcotics, and nonsteroidal anti-inflammatory drugs (NSAIDs) may ease the neuropathic pain.

CRITICAL THINKING APPLICATION 37.7

Nancy's last patient of the day has severe neuropathy in both her hands and feet. The patient states that she can't feel much with her hands. After rooming the patient, Nancy thinks about her own life and what it might be like if she could not feel much in her hands and feet. How might that affect a person's life? What complications might occur?

CONGENITAL DISEASES AND DISORDERS

Congenital diseases and disorders include a wide range of structural and functional abnormalities present at birth. Many congenital diseases and disorders impact the nervous system. The following sections examine common congenital diseases and disorders that involve the nervous system.

Fetal Alcohol Spectrum Disorders

Fetal alcohol spectrum disorders (FASDs) are a group of conditions that occur in a person whose mother drank alcohol during the pregnancy. The physical and mental deficiencies will last for life. The disorders include the following:

- *Fetal alcohol syndrome* (FAS), which is at the farthest end of the spectrum, is the most complex disorder. People can experience the signs and symptoms indicated in the following section. People with FAS have a difficult time with school and getting along with others.
- *Alcohol-related neurodevelopmental disorder* (ARND), which affects learning and behavior.
- *Alcohol-related birth defects* (ARBD), which cause problems with the heart, kidneys, bones, and hearing.

These disorders are caused by alcohol consumption by the mother during the pregnancy. The alcohol in the mother's bloodstream crosses the placenta. Alcohol can interfere with oxygen and nutrient delivery in the growing baby. It can also harm the development of tissues and organs. The signs and symptoms depend on the amount of alcohol consumed during the pregnancy and the time during the pregnancy it was consumed. Here are the common signs and symptoms:

- Poor memory, hyperactive behavior, difficulty with attention and math concepts
- Speech and language delays, learning and intellectual disabilities
- Poor reasoning and judgment skills
- Vision or hearing problems
- Babies may experience low body weight, sleeping and sucking problems
- Poor coordination, small head size, shorter-than-average height, abnormal facial features (e.g., smooth ridge between the nose and upper lip)
- Heart, kidney, or bone problems

Knowing at delivery that the mother drank alcohol during the pregnancy can help with early diagnosis. At birth, a thorough assessment will be done. The provider will assess for issues during childhood. The child will be screened for cognitive, learning, and language development delays. Health issues, along with social and behavioral problems, will also be monitored. There is no cure for FASDs. Early intervention can help reduce some of the effects. Not drinking alcohol during pregnancy is the only way to prevent FASDs.

Spina Bifida

Spina bifida is a neural tube defect that occurs when the spinal column does not close during the first month of pregnancy. Spina bifida can cause damage to the nerves and spinal cord. Pregnant females are encouraged to take folic acid during pregnancy to reduce the risk of spina bifida. The cause is unknown. There are four types of spina bifida:

- *Spina bifida occulta*: Mildest form; no spinal nerves are involved, but one or more vertebrae are malformed. No signs or symptoms may be present. The only indication may be an abnormal cluster of hair, a small dimple, or birthmark on the infant's back (Figure 37.11).
- *Closed neural tube defect*: Includes a malformation of the fat, bone, or meninges associated with the spinal cord. Symptoms

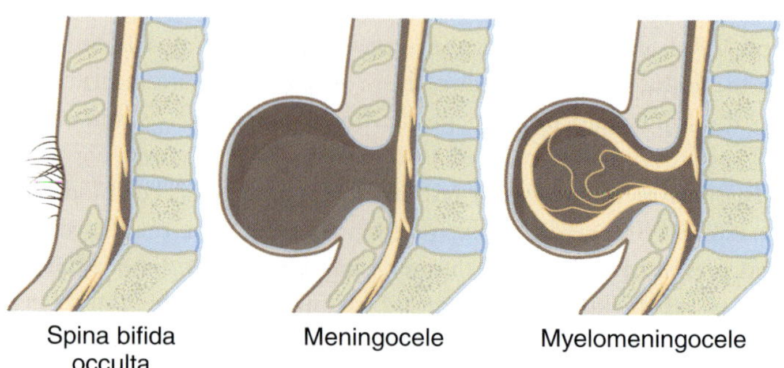

FIGURE 37.11 Types of spina bifida.

range from no symptoms to incomplete paralysis with bowel and urinary dysfunction.

- *Meningocele*: The meninges protrude through an abnormal vertebral opening, creating a sac. The sac is filled with fluid. Symptoms range from no symptoms to complete paralysis with bowel and bladder dysfunction.
- *Myelomeningocele*: The most serious type because the spinal canal is open along several vertebrae. A sac containing fluid, part of the spinal cord, and nerves comes through the opening in the infant's back. This type can cause partial or complete paralysis below the opening. The child may have weakness or paralysis of the legs, bowel and bladder incontinence, lack of feeling in the legs, and an increase in cerebrospinal fluid.

During pregnancy, the mother can take a maternal serum alpha-fetoprotein (MSAFP) test (also known as the *Triple Test* and *Quad Screen*). If abnormally high amounts of alpha-fetoprotein (AFP) are found, it suggests that the baby has a neural tube defect (e.g., spina bifida). The accuracy of the MSAFP test is not perfect. Even though abnormally high levels of AFP are found, the baby may be normal. With negative test results, there is still a small risk of spina bifida. Amniocentesis can also be done if the MSAFP test result comes back abnormal. Most of the time, ultrasound can detect the two most severe types of spina bifida during pregnancy.

Prenatal surgery for spina bifida can occur around 26 weeks of pregnancy. The child may have fewer disabilities if the spinal cord is repaired at that time. Surgery can also occur after birth. Additional treatments focus on the complications that occur, including leg weakness, bowel or bladder problems, and hydrocephalus (Figure 37.12).

Shunt System

Hydrocephalus can be treated with a surgical placement of a shunt system. The shunt system drains the extra cerebrospinal fluid (CSF) from the ventricles in the brain into another part of the body (e.g., abdomen), where it is absorbed into the bloodstream. The ventriculoperitoneal shunt is one of the more common shunts (Figure 37.13).

The shunt system consists of the following parts:

- An inflow *catheter* (a tube) with a pressure-sensitive valve. When the pressure reaches a certain level, the valve opens, allowing CSF to drain into the catheter.
- A valve mechanism that regulates the pressure levels. Usually, this device is implanted under the skin on the top of the head or behind the ear.
- An outflow catheter, which drains the CSF into another part of the body.

A shunt system needs to be replaced as the person ages or when it gets blocked. Increased intracranial pressure (ICP) is a sign that the shunt system is not functioning correctly. A person may experience a headache, nausea and vomiting, confusion, double vision, and decreased mental abilities with ICP.

Other Congenital Diseases and Disorders

The following are additional structural diseases and disorders.

- *Anencephaly*: The infant is born without parts of the brain. The remaining part of the brain may not be covered by the cranium or skin.
- *Cerebral palsy* (CP): A group of nonprogressive disorders caused by abnormal brain development or brain injury, resulting in muscle weakness or problems with using the muscles. CP can affect people's ability to move and maintain their posture and balance. Signs and symptoms usually appear during infancy or the preschool years. The child can have abnormal reflexes, floppiness or rigidity of the extremities, abnormal posture, involuntary movements, and an unsteady *gait* (manner or style of walking). CP is classified by the main type of movement disorder involved: *spasticity* (stiff muscles), *dyskinesia* (uncontrollable movements), and ataxia.
- *Down syndrome* (also called *trisomy 21*): The most common chromosomal condition in the United States. It is a condition in which a person is born with an extra copy of chromosome 21. The complications from Down syndrome range in severity and can include intellectual disabilities, dementia, heart disease, hearing, and visual issues, thyroid disease, and musculoskeletal complications (e.g., poor muscle tone).
- *Encephalocele*: A saclike protrusion of the brain and the meninges. Results when the neural tube does not completely close during pregnancy, and the protrusion commonly occurs at the back and top of the head or between the forehead and nose (Figure 37.14).
- *Microcephaly*: A small head size compared to the rest of the body. Often reflects poor brain development and is usually associated with cognitive impairments.
- *Tuberous sclerosis*: A rare genetic disease that causes benign tumors to grow in major organs (e.g., heart, brain, liver, and skin). Symptoms depend on the location of the tumors and may include seizures, intellectual disabilities, and kidney problems.

VASCULAR DISEASES AND DISORDERS

Vascular diseases and disorders that affect the nervous system tend to affect the brain. These can include **aneurysms** and hemorrhages, which can lead to strokes.

Cerebrovascular Accident

A cerebrovascular accident (CVA), also called a *stroke*, is the fifth leading cause of death in the United States and a major cause of serious disability. Strokes can occur at any age but usually occur in older adults. A stroke is a medical emergency. There are three types of strokes:

- *Ischemic stroke*: Occurs when the arterial blood flow to part of the brain is blocked. The brain cells start to die after a few minutes. This is the most common type of stroke. There are two common types of ischemic stroke:
  - *Thrombotic stroke*: A blood clot forms in an artery, blocking the blood to part of the brain.
  - *Embolic stroke*: A blood clot or other debris forms elsewhere in the body and moves into the brain arteries, blocking the blood flow.
- *Hemorrhagic stroke*: Occurs when an artery in the brain leaks or ruptures. The leaked blood puts pressure on the surrounding brain cells, causing damage. High blood pressure and aneurysms can cause hemorrhagic strokes. There are two types of hemorrhagic stroke:
  - *Intracerebral hemorrhage*: The most common type; occurs when a cerebral aneurysm ruptures.
  - *Subarachnoid hemorrhage*: Bleeding occurs in the subarachnoid space, usually caused by small aneurysms.

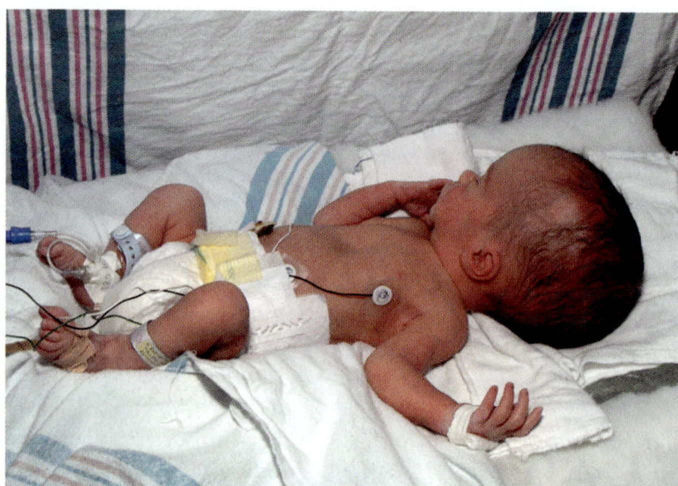

FIGURE 37.12 Hydrocephalus. (From Kliegman R, Stanton BF, St. Geme JW, et al: *Nelson textbook of pediatrics*, ed 19, St. Louis, 2011, Saunders.)

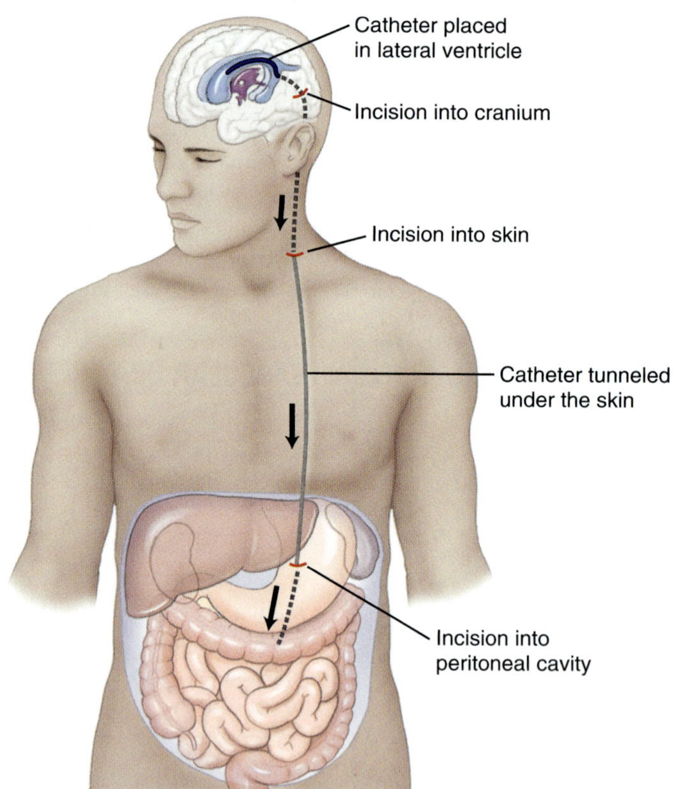

FIGURE 37.13 Ventriculoperitoneal shunt. (From Shiland B: *Mastering healthcare terminology*, ed 5, St. Louis, 2015, Elsevier.)

- *Transient ischemic attack (TIA)*: Also called a "ministroke" because it lasts for only a few minutes. The blood supply to a part of the brain is briefly blocked. Symptoms are similar to stroke symptoms but do not last as long (e.g., 1 to 24 hours).

Risk factors for CVAs include the following:

- Family history of stroke
- Cardiovascular disease, hypertension, and high cholesterol
- Diabetes
- Cigarette smoking, heavy or binge drinking, and use of illicit drugs (e.g., cocaine and methamphetamines)
- Being overweight and physical inactivity

The symptoms of a CVA relate to the part of the brain affected. The individual may not have all the symptoms:

- Confusion or mental changes
- Speech difficulty (trouble forming words, difficult to understand, or using words that do not make sense)
- Numbness of the face, arm, or leg, usually on one side of the body
- Problem seeing in one or both eyes
- Trouble walking, lack of coordination or balance, or arm weakness
- Sudden, severe headache
- Facial drooping

- *Hemiparesis* (weakness on one side of the body) and *hemiplegia* (one-sided paralysis)

The emergency department providers will perform physical and neurologic examinations. Blood tests and imaging tests (CT, MRI, and cerebral angiogram) will indicate the type of stroke. The type of stroke determines the treatment:

- Ischemic strokes are treated with clot-dissolving medications (e.g., a tissue plasminogen activator) that help the body break down the clot that is blocking the artery. The clot can also be removed by surgery if needed.
- Hemorrhagic strokes are treated with antihypertensives and surgical repair of the vessel. If the person is taking an anticoagulant or antiplatelet medication, medications to reverse the effects may be given.
- TIAs are treated with antihypertensive, anticoagulant, and antiplatelet medications. The goal is to prevent a future stroke.

Additional treatments address the life-changing complications of a stroke. Physical, occupational, and speech therapies may be used to help with disabilities.

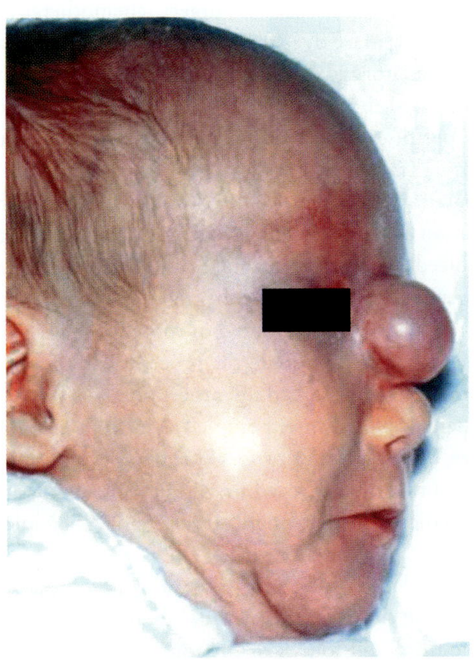

FIGURE 37.14 Encephalocele. (From Lesperance MM: *Cummings pediatric otolaryngology*, ed 2, St. Louis, 2022, Elsevier.)

CRITICAL THINKING APPLICATION 37.8

A patient had a stroke in the right side of her brain that affected her left arm and hand. What types of daily activities (e.g., bathing, grooming, eating) might she struggle with if she is left-hand dominant? What if she is right-hand dominant?

Hematoma

The most common cranial hematomas include these:

- *Epidural hematoma*: A collection of blood between the skull and the dura mater (Figure 37.15).
- *Subdural hematoma*: A collection of blood between the dura mater and the arachnoid mater, which causes pressure on the brain.
- *Intraparenchymal* or *intracerebral hematoma*: A collection of blood pools in the brain.

The pressure outside the brain increases the *intracranial pressure* (ICP) (the pressure in the skull). With increased ICP, both the nervous system and blood vessel tissues are under pressure, which can be life-threatening. Thus, a cranial hematoma is a medical emergency.

Head trauma is the most common cause of hematomas. An intraparenchymal hematoma can also be caused by a leaking aneurysm, high blood pressure, or a tumor. These conditions can cause blood to leak into the brain. The following are signs and symptoms of an epidural hematoma:

- Confusion, dizziness, altered level of alertness, or drowsiness
- Enlarged pupil, severe headache
- Loss of consciousness, followed by alertness, and then deterioration of alertness
- Nausea and vomiting
- Weakness in part of the body

Imaging procedures are the best method to determine the location and size of the hematoma. Imaging procedures used include a head CT scan, MRI, and angiogram to diagnose blood vessel conditions. The treatment goals include controlling symptoms and minimizing permanent damage. Emergency surgery to remove the hematoma (craniotomy), surgery to reduce the ICP, and life support measures are done. Medications to prevent seizures and to help reduce the ICP are also given.

THE MEDICAL ASSISTANT'S ROLE IN EXAMINATIONS, DIAGNOSTIC PROCEDURES, AND TREATMENTS

Neurologic diseases are common in primary care and urgent care departments, as well as in neurology and neurosurgery departments.

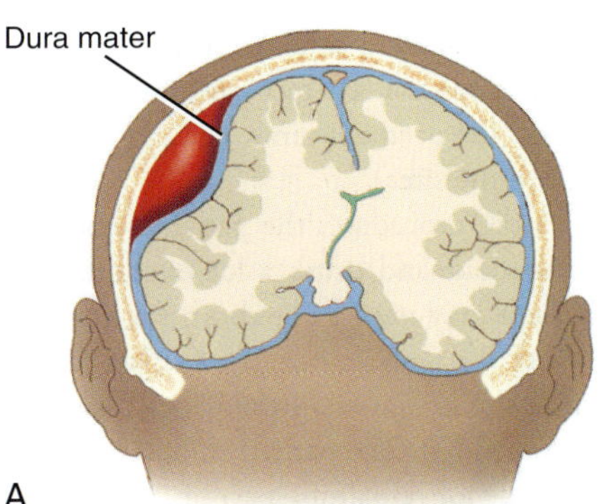

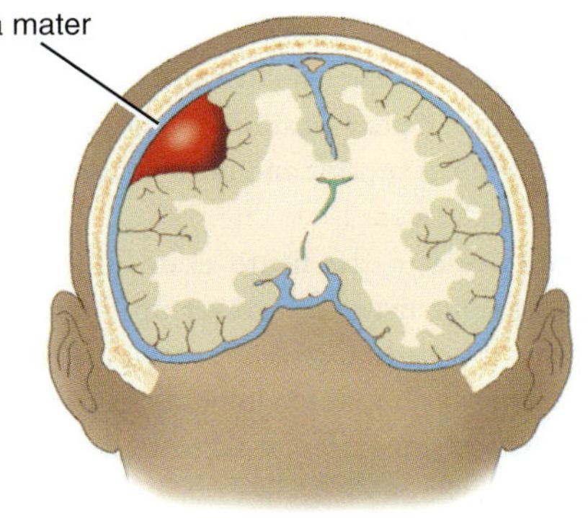

FIGURE 37.15 (A) Epidural hematoma. **(B)** Subdural hematoma. (From Damjanov I: *Pathology: a color atlas*, St. Louis, 2000, Mosby)

Medical assistants help the provider with the examination, diagnostic procedures, and treatments.

Assisting with the Examination

As with other physical examinations, a careful history presents the provider with valuable clues for diagnosing neurologic diseases. Such clues may include a record of seizures, syncope, *diplopia* (double vision), incontinence, or any previously mentioned subjective symptoms. The patient's general health often complicates a neurologic diagnosis.

Neurologic Examination

As part of the medical history, the provider may ask a medical assistant to give and score a neurologic status exam (if this is within the medical assistant's scope of practice for that state and agency). This exam tests the patient's cognitive functions and provides a baseline of neurologic information for the provider (Figure 37.16; also see Procedure 37.1). Part of the exam also requires gathering information from the patient's caregiver.

The provider will do a neurologic examination, also called a neuro exam, to evaluate the functioning of the patient's nervous system. During the examination, the provider may determine the effect of the symptoms on the patient's emotional status, intellectual performance, cognitive ability, and general behavior (see Procedure 37.2). Grooming and mannerisms are carefully observed, as is the patient's ability to communicate effectively, including the appropriate use of speech, language, and writing skills. The exam may assess many areas:

- *Mental status:* The patient's level of awareness of person, place, and time are assessed. "Person" is assessed by asking the person's name. "Place" is assessed by asking where the patient is. "Time" is assessed with questions related to what year or day it is. If the patient provides the correct answers, providers may document "Alert and oriented," "Alert and oriented to person, place, and time," or "A&O×3."
- *Functioning of the cranial nerves*: Table 37.1 describes how the nerves are assessed.
- *Motor function, balance, and coordination:* To assess these areas, the patient needs to do the following:
  - Push or pull against the provider's hand with each extremity
  - Walk following a line on the floor
  - Stand with the eyes closed
  - Touch the nose with the eyes closed
- *Sensory function:* The provider may test the patient's ability to feel sensations by using sharp, dull, or light touches, in addition to hot, cold, and vibrating items.
- *Reflexes (children and adults):* Using a reflex hammer, the provider will tap the extremities in different locations to check the reflexes (Figure 37.17). If the reflex is present and normal, a small movement of the extremity will occur.

The medical assistant's role in the neuro exam differs among facilities. The medical assistant may need to set up for the exam. Some providers may have the medical assistant remain in the room and assist by handing them supplies and helping the patient change positions. The medical assistant may also be asked to document the provider's findings during the exam.

Assisting with Diagnostic Procedures

The medical assistant helps with diagnostic procedures by scheduling and preparing patients for procedures. If tests require restrictions on food or fluids, the medical assistant should address the following points with the patient after talking with the provider:

- Can the patient have water prior to the test?
- Which medications should the patient take prior to the test, or when can the patient resume the current medications?

Table 37.3 describes common diagnostic procedures used for neurologic diseases. The medical assistant may need to screen the patient for specific allergies, medications, and so on prior to the scheduling of the procedure. For some procedures, a signed consent form is required. The patient should be notified of what will be experienced during the procedure and any follow-up care required after the test. The following sections describe the lumbar puncture and the electroencephalography procedures in more detail.

Lumbar Puncture

A lumbar puncture (LP), also known as a spinal tap, is done to collect a small amount of CSF, to measure the pressure of the CSF, and to inject medication into the spinal cord structures. These medications may include spinal anesthetic for surgery, chemotherapy for cancer treatment, and contrast dye (for x-ray procedures, such as myelography). In ambulatory care, the most frequent reason for an LP is to obtain a sample of the CSF. The CSF is analyzed to help confirm or rule out many diseases, including meningitis, encephalitis, cancer, and dementia (Table 37.4).

In preparation for the procedure, the patient should be asked if any medication or herbal products have been taken that may increase the risk of bleeding (e.g., anticoagulant and antiplatelet medications, garlic, ginger, St. John's wort, and ginseng). The patient may be restricted from eating or drinking 3 or more hours prior to the procedure. The provider will explain the procedure to the patient, and a consent form is signed prior to the procedure.

The patient is placed in either a left side-lying position with the knees drawn up to the chest or in a sitting position leaning forward on a stable surface (see Procedure 37.3). For an infant or young child, the medical assistant might need to hold the child in a side-lying position during the procedure.

The site is cleansed with an antiseptic, and a local anesthetic is injected to numb the area. The provider then inserts a hollow needle between the third and fourth or the fourth and fifth lumbar vertebrae and advances it into the subarachnoid space (Figure 37.18). The CSF flows out of the needle into the sterile collection tubes. Usually, 1 to 2 mL of fluid is needed in each tube. When multiple tubes are required, a total of 10 to 15 mL of CSF is typically collected. The tubes need to be numbered in the order that they are collected. The needle is removed, and a bandage or small dressing is applied to the site.

After the procedure, the patient typically needs to lie down for about an hour and drink a lot of fluid. If more CSF is removed, the patient may need to lie down for a longer period of time. Prior to leaving the ambulatory care facility, the provider will check the insertion site and assess if the patient has any issues (e.g., problems moving the legs). The patient should not drive and will need to rest at home the for remaining part of the day.

WALDEN–MARTIN
FAMILY MEDICAL CLINIC
1234 ANYSTREET | ANYTOWN, ANYSTATE 12345
PHONE 123-123-1234 | FAX 123-123-5678

Instructor: Becky Swisher

Neurologic Status Exam

The Neurologic Status Examination tests the individual's sense of cognitive functions and quickly allows the provider to screen for cognitive impairment and/or loss. In addition to testing language recall and motor skills, the NSE also allows you to test an individual's orientation to time, detail, and attention.

There are five sections. Each section of the test involves relating a series of questions or commands to a patient; the patient should receive one point for each correct answer. Conduct the test without interruptions in a well-lit, private exam room. Instruct the patient to listen carefully and answer each question as accurately as possible. In the event that there is a caregiver accompanying the patient, ask the Caregiver Questions and record the responses (these are not part of the final score).

Read each question once and document the patient's response. Do not time the patient's answers or duration of the test overall; once completed, score the test immediately. To do so, add only the number of correct responses. The individual can receive a maximum score of 10 points; a score below 4 indicates cognitive impairment.

Patient Name: ______________________ **Date of Birth:** ______________________
Performed By: ______________________ **Date:** ______________________

Caregiver Questions (if available): (Yes, No, Not Aware)

Name of Caregiver: ______________________	**Yes**	**No**	**Not Aware**
• Does the patient have difficulty remembering recent events or conversions?	☐	☐	☐
• Does the patient have difficulty performing activities of daily living (bath, driving, cooking, etc.)	☐	☐	☐
• Have you noticed changes to speech patterns?	☐	☐	☐

Patient Interview

Sequencing:

Read the following statement to the patient three consecutive times: **"Drive the red car to Washington Street."** Then ask patient to restate the sentence; you will ask the patient to recall the statement later in the test.

	Yes	**No**
The patient was able to repeat the exact statement to you.	☐	☐

Total: __________

Time Orientation:

Ask the patient the following questions:

	Correct	**Incorrect**
• What is today's date?	☐	☐
• What season is it?	☐	☐
• What is the day of the week?	☐	☐

Total: __________

Drawing:

Give the individual a piece of paper and ask him/her to copy a design of the two intersecting shapes. One point is awarded for correctly copying the shapes. All angles on both figures must be present, and the figures must have one overlapping angle.

Correct	**Incorrect**
☐	☐

Total: __________

Information:

Ask the patient the following questions:

	Correct	**Incorrect**
• Who is president of the United States?	☐	☐
• How many stars are on the American flag?	☐	☐

Total: __________

Recall:

Ask the patient to restate the sentence that you asked him/her at the beginning of the procedure. One point is given for repeating each of the following words.

	Correct	**Incorrect**
• Drive	☐	☐
• Red car	☐	☐
• Washington Street	☐	☐

Total: __________

Total Exam Score: __________

FIGURE 37.16 Neurologic Status Exam Form.

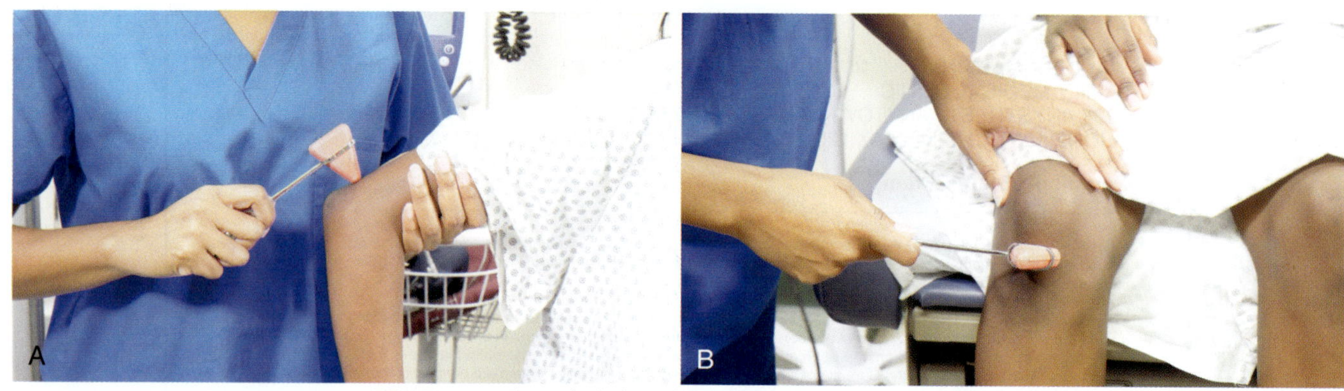

FIGURE 37.17 The provider checks **(A)** the triceps reflex and **(B)** the quadriceps reflex.

TABLE 37.3 Diagnostic Procedures for Neurologic Diseases and Disorders

PROCEDURE	DESCRIPTION	PATIENT PREPARATION
Cerebral angiography	Used to see how the blood flows through the brain. A person must lie on the x-ray table without moving. The head is held still. A local anesthetic is given in the groin area, and a catheter is threaded through an artery in the groin until it reaches the neck. X-ray is used to help guide the process. A dye is injected and highlights the blood flow through the brain.	Screen for bleeding problems or taking anticoagulants, allergy to contrast dye, pregnancy, or kidney function problems. The patient may not eat or drink for 4 to 8 hours prior to the test. The patient may feel a brief discomfort during the anesthetic injection and the threading of the catheter. The contrast dye may cause a warming or burning feeling on the face and head.
Cerebral spinal fluid analysis	CSF is analyzed to determine any abnormalities. The specimen is gathered by a lumbar puncture (spinal tap) performed by a provider. An anesthetic will be given. A needle is inserted, and the fluid is collected. The CSF is then sent to the laboratory for testing.	Screen for bleeding problems or taking anticoagulants. A consent form must be signed. The patient may be put in an uncomfortable position during the test and will need to hold the position through the procedure. The patient may feel a sting when the anesthetic is injected.
Electromyography (EMG)	Used to test the health of nerves and muscles. A fine needle with an electrode is inserted into the muscle. The electrode picks up the electrical activity from the muscle during activity and at rest. The activity is recorded.	Screen if taking an anticoagulant. Patient should avoid using creams and lotions on the day of the test. The patient should have normal body temperature because a lowered temperature can affect the test. The patient may feel the insertion of the needles. After the test, the muscle may be tender. The patient may have bruising for a few days.
Nerve conduction velocity (NCV) test	Usually done with EMG. Done to test the speed of electrical signals as they move through a nerve. Electrode patches are placed on the skin over nerves and give off a mild electrical impulse. The electrical activity is recorded by other electrodes.	Screen if the patient has a cardiac defibrillator or pacemaker. Patient should avoid any lotions, sunscreen, perfume, or moisturizer on the test day. The patient may feel the impulse and have some discomfort.
Nerve biopsy	The removal of a small piece of the nerve for examination. After applying an analgesic, the provider makes a small surgical incision and removes a piece of the nerve from the ankle, forearm, or rib area.	There is no special preparation. The patient may feel the injection of the local anesthetic medication. The biopsy site will be sore for a few days after the test.

Lumbar punctures may cause a number of conditions:

- Post-lumbar puncture headaches due to CSF leaking into nearby tissues. The patient may experience nausea, vomiting, and dizziness. Usually, the headaches resolve after lying down. These headaches may last for a week or more after the procedure.
- Bleeding at the site or into the epidural space.
- Brainstem herniation.
- Back discomfort, tenderness, or pain in the lower back. Pain may radiate down the back of the legs.

The patient should notify the provider of any abnormalities, including numbness and tingling in the legs, draining or pain at the injection site, an increase in the number or intensity of headaches, and inability to urinate.

Electroencephalography

Electroencephalography (EEG) is used to record the brain wave activity of a patient. An EEG may be done to rule out or confirm seizure activity, AD, psychosis, and narcolepsy, a sleep disorder.

TABLE 37.4 Typical Laboratory Values for Cerebrospinal Fluid

	NORMAL CSF	ABNORMAL CSF AND RELATED CONDITIONS
Pressure (mm H_2O)	70–180	*Increased:* Increased intracranial pressure *Decreased:* Spinal cord tumor, fainting, diabetic **coma**, and shock
Appearance	Clear, colorless	*Cloudy:* Infection, elevated white blood cells or protein *Bloody or red:* Bleeding *Brown, orange, or yellow:* Increased protein or previous bleeding
Glucose (mg/dL)	50–80	*Increased:* Hyperglycemia (high blood glucose) *Decreased:* Hypoglycemia (low blood glucose), bacterial or fungal infection (e.g., bacterial meningitis), tuberculosis
Protein (mg/dL)	15–60	*Increased:* Blood in the CSF, diabetes, polyneuritis, injury, inflammation, infection, or tumor *Decreased:* Rapid CSF production
Blood Cells	0–5 White blood cells (WBCs) 0 Red blood cells (RBCs)	*Increase in WBCs:* Meningitis, acute infection, tumor, abscess, stroke, multiple sclerosis *Increase in RBCs:* Traumatic lumbar puncture, bleeding into the CSF

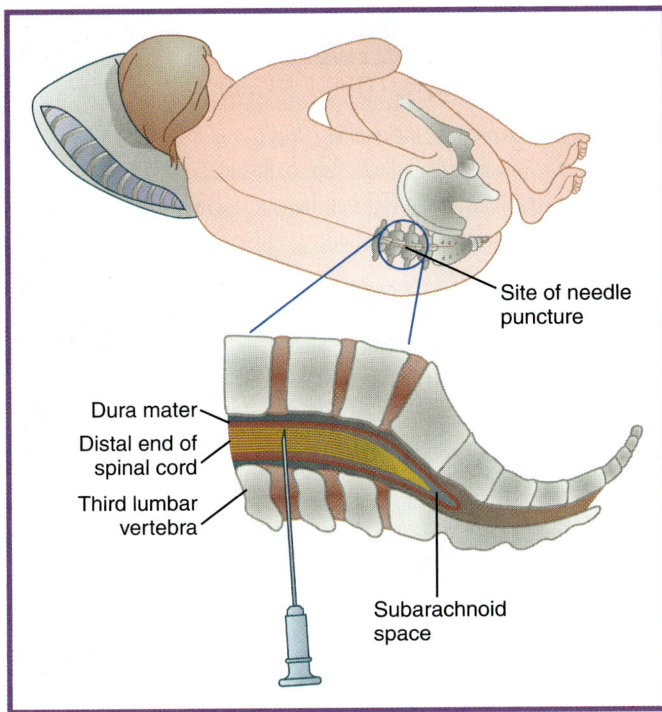

FIGURE 37.18 Lumbar puncture.

The medical assistant should coach the patient on the preparations for an EEG (see Procedure 37.4). In preparation for the procedure, patients should wash their hair the evening before or the morning of the procedure. They should not use any conditioner or hair care products (e.g., gels, hairspray). Using hair care products can interfere with the electrodes adhering to the scalp. Providers may have patients hold (not take) certain medications before the test if they may interfere with the EEG. Patients should avoid consuming any caffeine on the day of the test. If the EEG requires patients to sleep during the test, providers may encourage them to limit their sleep to 4 or 5 hours the night before.

TABLE 37.5 Common Treatments Used for Nervous System Diseases and Disorders

PROCEDURE	DESCRIPTION
Craniectomy	Surgical removal of a portion of the cranium.
Craniotomy	Surgical incision into the skull.
Neurectomy	Surgical removal of part or all of a nerve.
Neuroplasty	Surgery of the nerve.
Ventriculoperitoneal shunt	A catheter is inserted into the brain and drains extra fluid from the brain ventricles into the abdominal cavity.

During the procedure, the patient will be relaxing in a bed or reclining chair. The technician will apply 16 to 25 electrodes to the scalp, either with a cap or paste. The wires from the electrodes bring the electrical impulses to the computer. The electrical activity in the brain is then recorded. The technician will record brain activity while the patient is at rest or asleep and with activities and stimuli (e.g., bright flashing light). The test takes between 45 minutes and 2 hours.

Once the test is done, the electrodes are removed, and the paste is removed with warm water. If the patient was given a sedative, no driving is allowed after the test. Mild skin irritation may occur for a few hours after the test. The patient should be informed of when to restart medications and when to anticipate the test results.

Assisting with Treatments

Patients with neurologic diseases may be treated with surgical procedures (Table 37.5), or they may be prescribed a variety of medications. The following are some of the more common classifications of medications:

- *Analgesic*: Relieves pain.
- *Anesthetic*: Produces *local anesthesia* (no loss of consciousness).

- *Anti-Alzheimer*: Used to treat AD by increasing naturally occurring substances, such as acetylcholine, in the brain.
- *Anticonvulsant*: Reduces the frequency and severity of seizures by reducing excessive stimulation of the brain.
- *Antidepressant*: Used to treat depression, anxiety, and other neurologic disorders.
- *Antimigraine*: Alters circulation to the brain and is used to treat migraine headaches.
- *Corticosteroid*: Used to treat chronic inflammatory and some autoimmune diseases (e.g., multiple sclerosis).

Refer to Table 37.6 for information on the medication classification, including indication for use, desired effect, side effects, adverse reactions, and generic and trade names. Medical assistants should be familiar with medications that are prescribed to patients.

CLOSING COMMENTS

Patient Coaching

Patients often need to take medications daily or several times a day with neurologic diseases and disorders. Because of the symptoms of the disease, remembering can be difficult for some patients. The medical assistant may need to help patients figure out strategies to remember to take their medications. The following methods can be used:

- Placing medications near the kitchen table if they need to be taken with food. (Always remember to keep medications out of the reach of children.)
- Getting into a routine and always taking the medications after doing a specific task (e.g., feeding the pet, brushing teeth, taking a shower).
- Using an alarm on a phone, clock, or app to remind the patient about medication times.
- Having a family member call to check if the medication was taken.
- Crossing out the day on the calendar after taking the medication.
- Using weekly pill boxes. Some pharmacies will help set up pill boxes; otherwise, have a family member help set it up weekly if needed.

The medical assistant should also provide the patient with directions in writing about what to do if the medication was missed.

TABLE 37.6 Medication Classifications

CLASSIFICATION	INFORMATION	GENERIC NAME (TRADE NAME)
Analgesic	Indications for use: Relieves pain. Desired effects: Reduces the sensory function of the brain; blocks pain receptors. Side effects and adverse reactions: *Nonnarcotic:* GI distress, liver and kidney disorders, and tinnitus. *Narcotic:* hypotension, decreased respirations, agitation, blurred vision, confusion, constipation, sedation, restlessness.	*Nonnarcotic over-the-counter (OTCs):* • Aspirin (Ecotrin, Bayer Aspirin, Bufferin) • Acetaminophen (Tylenol, Tempra) (APAP) • Ibuprofen (Advil, Motrin) *Narcotic (opioids):* • Oxycodone (OxyContin) • Hydrocodone with acetaminophen (Lortab, Norco, Vicodin) • Oxycodone with acetaminophen (Percocet, Oxycet, Roxicet) • Tramadol (Qdolo, Conzip)
Anesthetic	Indications for use: Produces local anesthesia (no loss of consciousness) or general anesthesia (loss of consciousness). Desired effects: Produces insensibility to pain or the sensation of pain; blocks nerve impulses to the brain, resulting in unconsciousness. Side effects and adverse reactions: Hypotension, cardiopulmonary depression, sedation, nausea, vomiting, headaches.	*Local:* • Lidocaine (Xylocaine) *General:* • Midazolam (Versed)
Anti-Alzheimer	Indications for use: Treats Alzheimer disease Desired effect: Treats dementia by increasing naturally occurring substances in the brain. Side effects and adverse reactions: GI distress, frequent urination, muscle cramps, confusion, bradycardia, angina, bloody vomit, or stools.	• Donepezil (Aricept) • Memantine (Namenda)
Anticonvulsant and mood stabilizer	Indications for use: Treats epilepsy, trigeminal neuralgia, mania, and mixed episodes (mania and depression) with bipolar disorder Desired effects: Reduces the frequency and severity of seizures by reducing excessive stimulation of the brain. Side effects and adverse reactions: Sedation, vertigo, visual disturbances, GI disturbances, liver complications.	• Carbamazepine (Tegretol, Equetro) • Lamotrigine (Lamictal) • Topiramate (Topamax) • Valproic acid (Depakene, Depakote) • Gabapentin (Neurontin, Horizant)

TABLE 37.6 Medication Classifications—*continued*

CLASSIFICATION	INFORMATION	GENERIC NAME (TRADE NAME)
Antidepressant	Indications for use: Treats depression, anxiety, and other neurologic disorders. Desired effect: Treats depression. Side effects and adverse reactions: Anorexia, anxiety, sexual dysfunction, fatigue, drowsiness, vertigo, weight gain, confusion, blurred vision.	*Selective serotonin reuptake inhibitors (SSRIs):* • Fluoxetine (Prozac, Rapiflux, Sarafem, Selfemra) • Citalopram (Celexa) • Escitalopram (Lexapro) • Sertraline (Zoloft) *Serotonin and norepinephrine reuptake inhibitors (SNRIs):* • Venlafaxine • Duloxetine (Cymbalta) *Atypical antidepressants:* • Bupropion (Wellbutrin, Zyban) *Serotonin modulators:* • Trazodone (Oleptro) *Tricyclic antidepressants:* • Amitriptyline *Monamine oxidase inhibitors (MAOIs):* • Phenelzine (Nardil)
Antimigraine	Indications for use: Treats or prevents migraine headaches. Desired effect: Alters circulation to the brain. Side effects and adverse reactions: Confusion, psychomotor slowing, difficulty concentrating, memory problems, rare but serious cardiac events.	• Sumatriptan (Imitrex) • Zolmitriptan (Zomig)
Corticosteroid (oral)	Indications for use: Treats chronic inflammatory diseases (e.g., arthritis) and acute conditions (e.g., poison ivy, asthma). Desired effects: Reduces inflammation. Side effects and adverse reactions: Headache, mood changes, difficulty falling asleep or staying asleep, increased sweating, vision problems, depression, and weight gain.	• Prednisone (Prednisone Intensol, Sterapred) • Prednisolone (Flo-Pred, Orapred, Pediapred) • Methylprednisolone (Depo-Medrol, Solu-Medrol, Medrol)

Legal and Ethical Issues

In neurology, you will be faced with a variety of behaviors and personality changes that frequently are a part of neurologic diseases and disorders. Often a patient is not aware of these changes and may act as though nothing is wrong. It is important for the medical assistant to remember to treat the patient with respect. All patient information, including pictures, audio recordings, and so on, is confidential. The medical assistant must also remember not to repeat information (gossip) to peers about the patient's actions and behaviors. Only staff members immediately involved with the patient have a right to the information required for their care of the patient.

Patient-Centered Care

Providing patient-centered care extends to the caregiver of the patient. In many situations, the caregiver is the patient's spouse or significant other; sometimes, it may be an adult child. With many chronic neurologic diseases, the patient may require a caregiver to assist with daily care (e.g., toileting, bathing, grooming), meal preparation, shopping, medical appointments, and so on. As the condition worsens, more burdens fall on the caregiver. Providing 24/7 care to a loved one is physically and emotionally stressful. With behavioral differences and increasing dependency, relationship roles may change, and the stress can affect the caregiver's health.

The medical assistant needs to recognize the importance of the caregiver in the patient's life. The caregiver's concerns are important, as are the patient's concerns. The medical assistant may need to provide the caregiver with emotional encouragement and resources for additional assistance, including in-home services, adult day care, support groups, and medical equipment.

Professional Behaviors

When you work with patients with dementia, communicating with them can be challenging. The medical assistant should remember the following:

- Speak clearly and use short sentences.
- Make eye contact.
- Give the patient time to respond. Do not pressure the person into giving a response.
- Allow patients to speak for themselves.
- Keep the tone of your voice friendly and positive. Remain calm.
- Do not patronize or ridicule the patient.

SUMMARY OF SCENARIO

Nancy had a very busy day with the outreach neurologic services providers. One of the most interesting parts of Nancy's day was talking with a patient's wife. The patient had a stroke, and his wife shared with Nancy the different types of adaptive equipment available. Nancy learned that there were different kinds of walkers, shower chairs and tub benches, raised toilet seats with handles, dressing devices, grooming aids, kitchen utensils (e.g., rocker knives, cutting boards with suction cups), and specially shaped utensils. Many of the devices were designed to be used with one hand. Nancy was impressed with the variety of adaptive equipment available.

During the day, Nancy felt a little overwhelmed by the complexity of neurologic tests and the different types of test orders. She realizes that she needs to research more about neurologic diseases and diagnostic tests before she assists the outreach providers next week. She enjoyed working with the patients and their caregivers and looks forward to getting to know them in the coming months.

SUMMARY OF LEARNING OBJECTIVES

1. **Differentiate among the structures of the central nervous system.**
   The central nervous system is composed of the brain and spinal cord, which are covered by meninges. The brain is made up of the following parts:
   - Cerebrum: Composed of the frontal, parietal, occipital, and temporal lobes
   - Cerebellum
   - Diencephalon: Composed of the thalamus and hypothalamus
   - Brainstem: Composed of the midbrain, pons, and the medulla oblongata

   The spinal cord passes through the foramen magnum in the skull and is protected by the vertebrae. It is covered by meninges.
2. **Differentiate among the structures of the peripheral nervous system.**
   The peripheral nervous system is composed of the following:
   - Cranial nerves, which exit the brain and have motor function, sensory function, or both. See Table 37.1.
   - Spinal nerves, which exit the spinal cord. Spinal nerves are named by their vertebrae location (e.g., cervical, thoracic) and by number.
3. **Differentiate among the cells of the nervous system.**
   The nervous system is composed of two types of cells: neurons and neuroglia. Neurons are made of a cell body, dendrites, and an axon. A stimulus starts an impulse. During polarization, the resting nerve cell has a slightly positive charge on the outside of the cell membrane and a negative charge inside the cell. When a section of the membrane is stimulated, the positively charged ions on the outside of the cell enter the nerve cell. This changes the outside charge to a negative charge. This state is called *depolarization.* Almost immediately after the impulse passes, the positively charged ions move outside the nerve cells again almost immediately after the impulse passes. This returns the outside charge to a positive charge. This state is called *repolarization.* Once everything changes back, the cell is at rest again, and the cycle continues.
4. **Examine the physiology of the nervous system.**
   There are three main functions of the nervous system:
   - Collecting information about the external and internal environments (sensing)
   - Processing this information and making decisions about action (interpreting)
   - Directing the body to put into action the decisions made (acting)

   The peripheral nervous system can be divided into the *somatic nervous system* (voluntary nervous system) and the *autonomic nervous system* (involuntary nervous system). The autonomic nervous system consists of nerves that regulate involuntary function. The ANS is an automatic system that regulates body functions such as breathing, heart rate, sweating, circulation, and digestion. It also controls the actions of muscles in blood vessel walls, organs, and glands. The motor portion of this system is further divided into the sympathetic and the parasympathetic nervous systems.

   The *sympathetic nervous system* can produce a fight or flight response. This part of the nervous system helps the individual respond to perceived stress. It speeds up the heart rate, raises blood glucose levels, raises blood pressure, slows the digestive system, and widens the bronchioles, allowing more oxygen to enter the body quickly. The *parasympathetic nervous system* does the opposite of what the sympathetic nervous system does. It slows the heart rate, lowers blood pressure, increases digestive functions, and reduces adrenal and sweat gland activity.
5. **Examine neurodegenerative diseases and disorders, including the signs, symptoms, etiology, diagnostic procedures, and treatments.**
   Neurodegenerative diseases affect a person's ability to move, talk, and breathe. These diseases can also affect a person's balance and heart function. Neurodegenerative diseases include the following:
   - *Amyotrophic lateral sclerosis* (ALS), or Lou Gehrig disease, a progressive neurologic disorder that attacks the motor neurons in the brain and spinal cord.
   - *Alzheimer disease* (AD), the most common reason for dementia. It damages and kills brain cells.
   - *Huntington disease* (HD), also called *Huntington chorea,* a progressive neurodegenerative disorder.
   - *Multiple sclerosis* (MS), an autoimmune neurodegenerative disorder that affects the brain and spinal cord.
   - *Parkinson disease* (PD), a progressive neurodegenerative disorder that affects movement.
   - *Restless legs syndrome* (RLS): Causes a creeping, tingling, or burning sensation in the legs when the person is lying down or sitting.
6. **Examine functional diseases and disorders, including the signs, symptoms, etiology, diagnostic procedures, and treatments.**

SUMMARY OF LEARNING OBJECTIVES—*continued*

Functional diseases and disorders impact the function of the neurologic system. The most common functional diseases and disorders include headaches, migraines, seizures, and epilepsy. There are three classifications of seizures:

- *Generalized onset*: Affects both sides of the brain. Includes tonic-clonic seizures, which cause loss of consciousness, and absence seizures, which cause lapses of awareness of the environment.
- *Focal onset*: Affects one area of the brain. Includes focal aware seizures and focal impaired awareness seizures.
- *Unknown onset*: Seizure that was not witnessed or the beginning of the seizure was unknown.

7. **Examine infections that impact the nervous system, including the signs, symptoms, etiology, diagnostic procedures, and treatments.**

Encephalitis is inflammation of the brain and can be caused by a viral or bacterial infection. In mild cases, a person may have flu-like symptoms. With severe cases, a person may experience a severe headache, drowsiness, vomiting, confusion, seizures, and a sudden fever.

Meningitis is inflammation of the meninges surrounding the brain and spinal cord. Viral meningitis, the most common form, is caused by a viral infection of the nose or mouth that travels to the brain. Bacterial meningitis, usually caused by pneumococcal infections or meningococcal infections, starts with a cold-like infection but can be deadly.

Shingles, also called herpes zoster, begins with tingling, pain, or itchiness on one side of the body or face, usually on the torso. This can occur 1 to 5 days before a rash with fluid-filled blisters develops.

8. **Examine structural diseases and disorders that impact the nervous system, including the signs, symptoms, etiology, diagnostic procedures, and treatments.**

Structural diseases and disorders of the nervous system include the following:

- *Bell's palsy*: The most common cause of facial paralysis. The symptoms typically only affect one side of the face and are at their worst about 48 hours after the onset.
- *Guillain-Barré syndrome*: A rare autoimmune disorder in which the immune system attacks the peripheral nervous system.
- *Trigeminal neuralgia*: A chronic pain condition that affects the trigeminal nerve.

9. **Examine injuries that impact the nervous system, including the signs, symptoms, etiology, diagnostic procedures, and treatments.**

Injuries that impact the nervous system include the following:

- *Traumatic brain injury* (TBI): An acquired brain injury that can occur as a result of falls, motor vehicle accidents, violence, sports injuries, and work in military combat zones.
- *Spinal cord injuries*: Occur when a blow, gunshot, or stabbing fractures or dislocates the vertebrae and the bone pieces cut into the cord or press on the nerves.
- *Peripheral neuropathy*: Occurs as a result of damage to the peripheral nervous system.

10. **Examine congenital diseases and disorders that impact the nervous system, including the signs, symptoms, etiology, diagnostic procedures, and treatments.**

Congenital diseases and disorders include a wide range of structural and functional abnormalities present at birth. Congenital diseases and disorders that impact the nervous system include the following:

- *Fetal alcohol spectrum disorders:* A group of conditions that occur to a person whose mother drank alcohol during the pregnancy. The physical and mental deficiencies will last for life.
- *Spina bifida:* A neural tube defect that occurs when the spinal column does not close during the first month of pregnancy.

11. **Examine vascular diseases and disorders that impact the nervous system, including the signs, symptoms, etiology, diagnostic procedures, and treatments.**

Vascular diseases and disorders that affect the nervous system tend to affect the brain. These can include aneurysms and hemorrhages, which can lead to cerebrovascular accidents (CVA), also called a *stroke*. There are three types of strokes:

- *Ischemic stroke*: Occurs when the arterial blood flow to part of the brain is blocked. Two common types of ischemic strokes are thrombotic and embolic strokes. Ischemic strokes are treated with clot-dissolving medications.
- *Hemorrhagic stroke*: Occurs when an artery in the brain leaks or ruptures. Two types of hemorrhagic strokes are intracerebral and subarachnoid strokes. Hemorrhagic strokes are treated with antihypertensives and surgical repair of the vessel.
- *Transient ischemic attack (TIA)*: Also called a "mini-stroke" because it lasts for only a few minutes. The blood supply to a part of the brain is briefly blocked. TIAs are treated with antihypertensive, anticoagulant, and antiplatelet medications.

12. **Examine the medical assistant's role in examinations, diagnostic procedures, and treatments for neurologic diseases and disorders.**

As part of the medical history, the provider may ask a medical assistant to give and score a neurologic status exam. The medical assistant may also assist the provider during a neurologic examination. During the examination, the provider may determine the effect of the symptoms on the patient's emotional status, intellectual performance, cognitive ability, and general behavior.

The medical assistant helps by scheduling and preparing patients for the diagnostic procedures. The medical assistant may help during a lumbar puncture by holding the patient and monitoring them after the procedure. The medical assistant can coach a patient on the preparation for an EEG.

Some neurologic conditions can be treated with surgical procedures (see Table 37.5). Patients with neurologic diseases and disorders can also be prescribed a variety of medications.

PROCEDURE 37.1 Perform a Neurologic Status Exam

TASKS: Administer and score the neurologic status exam.

SCENARIO: Dr. David Kahn has ordered a neurologic status exam form to be completed on Robert Caudill (DOB 10/31/19XX). Mr. Caudill is accompanied by his caregiver.

DIRECTIONS: Role-play this scenario with two other peers. One will play the patient, and the other will be the caregiver.

EQUIPMENT and SUPPLIES

- Patient's health record
- Order for the neurologic status exam
- Neurologic Status Exam Form (see Figure 37.11) or SimChart for the Medical Office (SCMO).

PROCEDURAL STEPS

1. Wash hands or use hand sanitizer.
   PURPOSE: Hand sanitization is an important step for infection control.
2. *SCMO:* Click on the Form Repository and select the Neurologic Status Exam on the INFO PANEL. Read the form. *Paper form:* Read the directions for the test.
   PURPOSE: The directions need to be followed to complete the test accurately. Know the directions before completing the exam with the patient.
3. Greet the patient. Identify yourself. Verify the patient's identity with full name and date of birth. Explain the procedure to be performed in a manner that the patient understands. Answer any questions the patient may have about the procedure.
   PURPOSE: It is important to identify the patient in two different ways to ensure that you have the correct patient. Explaining the procedure can make the patient feel more comfortable and reduces anxiety.
4. *SCMO:* Click on Patient Search. Select the patient and verify the DOB. Click Select, and the patient's name and DOB will autofill into the form field. Key in the information for the performed by and the date fields.
   Paper form: Complete the following information on the exam form: patient name, date of birth, performed by, and date.
   PURPOSE: The patient information needs to be completed on the form. Your name and the date also need to be completed.
5. Ask for the caregiver's name and clearly ask the caregiver related questions from the form. Accurately document the information obtained.
   PURPOSE: The caregiver's information is important for the completion of the exam.
6. Perform the patient interview, following the directions on the form. Clearly provide the patient with the directions and the questions. Accurately document the information obtained from the patient.
   PURPOSE: Accurately documenting the information is critical for the accuracy of the exam.
7. Accurately score the test as indicated by the directions.
   SCMO: Key the scores in the total fields. Save the form when completed.
   Paper form: Write the scores on the total line. Give the completed form to the provider.
   PURPOSE: The score is important because the provider will use it for diagnostic purposes.

PROCEDURE 37.2 Assist with the Neurologic Exam

TASKS: Set up for a neurologic exam and prepare a patient for the procedure. Assist the provider and the patient during the neurologic exam.

EQUIPMENT and SUPPLIES

- Patient's health record
- Patient gown
- Drape
- Otoscope
- Ophthalmoscope
- Percussion hammer
- Disposable pinwheel or other disposable sharps per provider
- Penlight
- Tuning fork
- Cotton ball
- Tongue depressor
- Small vials of warm, cold, sweet, and salty liquids
- Small vials of substances with distinct odors (e.g., spices, coffee, vanilla)
- Gloves
- Disinfecting wipes
- Biohazard sharps container
- Waste container

PROCEDURAL STEPS

1. Wash hands or use hand sanitizer.
   PURPOSE: Hand sanitization is an important step for infection control.
2. Assemble supplies and equipment in the exam room.
   PURPOSE: Having all the supplies and equipment for the procedure is important.
3. Greet the patient. Identify yourself. Verify the patient's identity with full

PROCEDURE 37.2 Assist with the Neurologic Exam—*continued*

name and date of birth. Explain the procedure to be performed in a manner that the patient understands. Answer any questions the patient may have about the procedure.
PURPOSE: It is important to identify the patient in two different ways to ensure that you have the correct patient. Explaining the procedure can make the patient feel more comfortable and reduces anxiety.

4. Instruct the patient to change into the gown. The opening should be in the back. Ask the patient if assistance is needed. If so, help. If not, leave the room and allow the patient time to change. When reentering the room, provide a courtesy knock on the door.
   PURPOSE: The patient needs to undress for the procedure. Patients require privacy to change.
5. During the examination, be prepared to assist the patient in changing positions as necessary. Have the necessary examination instruments ready for the provider at the appropriate time during the examination. Record all results from the examination as indicated by the provider.
   PURPOSE: Assisting the patient and provider helps to facilitate a thorough, accurate neurologic examination.
6. After the exam, put on gloves and clean the exam room. Discard sharps in the biohazard sharps container. Discard other waste in the appropriate waste containers. Disinfect equipment and surfaces (e.g., exam table). Remove gloves and discard.
   PURPOSE: Disinfecting equipment and surfaces is an important step for infection control.
7. Wash hands or use hand sanitizer.

PROCEDURE 37.3 Assist with a Lumbar Puncture

TASKS: Set up for a lumbar puncture and prepare a patient for the procedure. Assist the provider during the lumbar puncture procedure. Document the procedure in the patient's health record.

EQUIPMENT and SUPPLIES

- Patient's health record
- Patient gown
- Drape
- Local anesthetic vial
- Syringe and needle
- Alcohol wipes
- Sterile, disposable lumbar puncture kit with specimen tubes
- Mayo stand
- Permanent marker or printed patient labels
- Laboratory requisition and specimen transport bag
- Gloves
- Biohazard waste container
- Biohazard sharps container
- Waste container
- Consent form
- Lumbar puncture instructions (optional)

PROCEDURAL STEPS

1. Wash hands or use hand sanitizer.
   PURPOSE: Hand sanitization is an important step for infection control.
2. Assemble supplies and equipment in the treatment room.
   PURPOSE: Having all the supplies and equipment for the procedure is important.
3. Greet the patient. Identify yourself. Verify the patient's identity with full name and date of birth. Explain the procedure to be performed in a manner that the patient understands. Answer any questions the patient may have about the procedure. Encourage the patient to use the restroom before the procedure.
   PURPOSE: It is important to identify the patient in two different ways to ensure that you have the correct patient. Explaining the procedure can make the patient feel more comfortable and reduces anxiety.
4. Check to make sure the consent form was signed. If the consent was not signed, ask if the patient has any questions. If there are no questions, explain the consent form and have the patient sign the form. If the patient has questions, let the provider know.
   PURPOSE: A signed consent form is needed for the procedure. If the patient has questions, the consent form cannot be signed. The provider should be notified so the questions can be answered.
5. Instruct the patient to change into the gown. The opening should be in the back. Ask the patient if assistance is needed. If so, help. If not, leave the room and allow the patient time to change. When reentering the room, provide a courtesy knock on the door.
   PURPOSE: The patient needs to be undressed for the procedure. Patients require privacy to change.
6. Assist the patient into a left side-lying position with the knees drawn up to the chest or into a sitting position leaning forward on a stable surface. Support the patient's head with a pillow as necessary and provide a pillow for between their knees if needed.
   PURPOSE: To give the provider the easiest access to the lumbar region while making the patient as comfortable as possible.
7. Prepare the skin preparation for the provider to use. Open the sterile disposable lumbar puncture kit on a Mayo stand. Without contaminating the supplies, add a sterile needle and sterile syringe to the sterile field.
   PURPOSE: The sterile kit should be opened as close to the start of the procedure as possible to prevent contamination.
8. If needed, help the patient remain in the proper position. Use the drape to cover the patient. Give verbal encouragement to the patient during the procedure.

PROCEDURE 37.3 Assist with a Lumbar Puncture—*continued*

PURPOSE: Encouraging the patient throughout the procedure helps to provide support.

9. Assist the provider as needed during the procedure. When the provider is ready for the anesthetic, wipe the top of the vial with alcohol. Show the label to the provider, and then hold the vial upside down as the provider withdraws the medication needed.
   PURPOSE: To maintain sterile technique and expedite the procedure.
10. Attach the printed labels to the specimen tubes or, using the permanent marker, label the specimens #1, #2, #3, and so on in the order in which they are collected.
    PURPOSE: Different tests are done on different tubes. The accuracy of these tests depends on the tube on which they are performed.
11. Complete the laboratory requisition form and prepare the CSF specimens for transport to the laboratory.
    PURPOSE: To ensure that all the necessary tests are ordered correctly.
12. Put on gloves. Discard the needle/syringe in a biohazard sharps container. Make sure to put the needle in first. Clean up the area. Discard the waste in the appropriate waste container. Remove gloves and discard.
    PURPOSE: Sharps should be discarded as soon as possible after the procedure is over.
13. Wash hands or use hand sanitizer.
14. Monitor the patient and give liquids as directed by the provider. When the patient is ready to leave, instruct the patient to get dressed. Ask the patient if assistance is needed. If so, help. If not, leave the room and allow the patient time to change.
    PURPOSE: The patient needs to be watched after the procedure. The provider should be notified of any concerns or questions.
15. After the patient leaves, put on gloves and clean the room. Disinfect surfaces and discard waste. Remove gloves and discard.
    PURPOSE: Disinfecting surfaces is an important step for infection control.
16. Wash hands or use hand sanitizer.
17. Document the procedure in the patient's health record. Include the provider's name, the samples obtained, how the patient tolerated the procedure, and any instructions given.
    PURPOSE: A procedure is not complete until it has been documented accurately in the patient's health record.

Documentation Example

9/15/20XX 1402 Pt had no questions regarding procedure. Consent signed for the lumbar puncture, which was performed by Dr. Kahn. Four vials of 2 mL each of CSF were collected, labeled, and sent to the lab. Pt laid flat on exam table for 60 minutes after procedure. No drainage noted on dressing. Pt has no c/o discomfort. VS: P: 86 regular, 2+; R: 20 regular, normal; BP 132/68 left arm, sitting. Patient was instructed to avoid strenuous activity for the rest of the day, to drink plenty of fluids, and to contact the provider if she gets a headache. The Lumbar Puncture instruction sheet was given to the patient. Pt had no questions.
————————————— Nancy Gehir, CMA (AAMA)

PROCEDURE 37.4 Coach a Patient for an Electroencephalogram

TASKS: Coach a patient on the preparation needed for an electroencephalogram. Document the instruction in the patient's health record.

ORDER: Provide EEG instructions

Patient instructions

Purpose of the EEG:

- An EEG is done to check for changes in the brain activity and can be helpful when diagnosing different disorders.

Patient preparation:

- Avoid caffeine on the day of the test.
- Take daily medications unless the provider indicates to hold medications until after the test.
- Wash hair the night before or the morning of the test, but do not use conditioners or any other hair care products.
- If you are to sleep through the EEG test, stay up later the night before the test or avoid sleeping.

During the test:

- Electrodes (patches with wires) will be attached to your head either with adhesive or by using a special cap.
- There will be little or no discomfort during the test.
- The technician may ask you questions during the test.

After the test:

- The technician will remove the electrodes.
- If sedation was used, you cannot drive after the test and for the rest of the day. Plan to have someone bring you home. Rest for the remaining part of the day.

PROCEDURE 37.4 Coach a Patient for an Electroencephalogram—*continued*

DIRECTIONS: Role-play the scenario with a peer, who is the patient. Your instructor is the provider. Make up the location, date, and time of the procedure.

EQUIPMENT and SUPPLIES

- Patient's health record
- Patient instructions for EEG

PROCEDURAL STEPS

1. Wash hands or use hand sanitizer.
   PURPOSE: Hand sanitization is an important step for infection control.
2. Greet the patient. Identify yourself. Verify the patient's identity with full name and date of birth. Explain what you will be doing in a manner that the patient understands. Answer any questions the patient may have.
   PURPOSE: It is important to identify the patient in two different ways to ensure that you have the correct patient. Explaining the procedure can make the patient feel more comfortable and reduces anxiety.
3. Explain the purpose of an EEG.
   PURPOSE: The patient needs to understand why the EEG is being done.
4. Explain how the patient should prepare for the test.
   PURPOSE: Appropriate preparations are needed for quality test results.
5. Explain what the patient should expect during and after the test.
   PURPOSE: Explaining what to expect during and after the procedure will reduce the patient's anxiety about the procedure.
6. Ask the patient to teach back the preparation to you. Clarify any misconceptions or inaccuracies. Answer any questions the patient may have. Give the patient a phone number to call if he has questions.
   PURPOSE: Using the teach-back method to evaluate the patient's understanding will help identify any misunderstandings the patient may have.
7. Let the patient know when to anticipate the results from the EEG. Also, give the patient the appointment information for the EEG, including the location, date, and time.
   PURPOSE: Letting patients know when to expect test results helps to alleviate confusion and anxiety.
8. Document the teaching in the patient's health record. Include the provider's name, what was taught, how the patient responded, and any written directions (including appointment information) sent home with the patient.
   PURPOSE: A procedure is not complete until it has been documented accurately in the patient's health record.

Documentation Example

9/12/20XX 1508 Per Dr. Kahn's order, EEG instructions were given to the pt. Pt's questions were answered. Patient taught back the instructions accurately. Patient was given the "Having an EEG" booklet. Pt was notified of appointment on 9/20/20XX at 9 a.m. at AnyTown Neurology Clinic
———————————— Nancy Gehir, CMA (AAMA)

38 BEHAVIORAL HEALTH

SCENARIO

Mike Brewer, CMA (AAMA), is a medical assistant at Walden-Martin Family Medical (WMFM) Clinic. He has been with the clinic for 2 years. Mike currently assists outreach providers who come to WMFM Clinic to provide services for patients. Recently, Mike has been working with the outreach behavioral health providers. During his medical assistant training, Mike learned about different behavioral health diseases and disorders but never felt he wanted to go into that specialty. Over the past 2 years at WMFM Clinic, he has realized that no matter what position he holds, he works with patients who have behavioral health disorders, depression being the most common. He is looking forward to learning more about behavioral health disorders as he continues to help the outreach providers.

While studying this chapter, think about the following questions:

- What are the titles of the different healthcare professionals who work in behavioral health?
- What is the importance of the DSM-5 in behavioral health?
- What are early warning signs of behavioral health diseases and disorders?
- What are common behavioral health diseases and disorders, including the signs, symptoms, etiology, diagnostic procedures, and treatments?
- What are common substance use disorders, including the signs, symptoms, diagnostic procedures, and treatments?

LEARNING OBJECTIVES

1. Examine the types of behavioral health professionals and their use of the *Diagnostic and Statistical Manual of Mental Disorders.*
2. Examine common signs, symptoms, and etiologies of behavioral health diseases and disorders over the life span.
3. Differentiate among various anxiety disorders, including the signs, symptoms, etiology, diagnostic procedures, and treatments.
4. Differentiate among various forms of depression and other mood disorders, including the signs, symptoms, etiology, diagnostic procedures, and treatments.
5. Differentiate among various behavioral disorders, including the signs, symptoms, etiology, diagnostic procedures, and treatments.
6. Differentiate among various eating disorders, including the signs, symptoms, etiology, diagnostic procedures, and treatments.
7. Differentiate among autism spectrum disorder, dissociative disorder, personality disorder, post-traumatic stress disorder, and schizophrenia.
8. Differentiate between substance use disorders and other addictions.
9. Examine the etiology, warning signs, protective factors, and treatments for suicidal behavior.
10. Examine the medical assistant's role in behavioral health examinations.
11. Examine the medical assistant's role regarding behavioral health diagnostic procedures.
12. Examine the medical assistant's role regarding treatments used for behavioral health diseases and disorders.

VOCABULARY

amnesia (am NEE zhah) Memory loss.

amygdala (ah MIG dah lah) A small mass of gray matter found in each temporal lobe of the cerebrum and involved with memories, emotions, and activating the fight-or-flight response; part of the limbic system.

coma A state of deep, often prolonged unconsciousness, usually the result of a head injury, neurologic disease, intoxication, or metabolic abnormalities.

delusion (de LOO zhun) Unshakable belief in something that is untrue; may be accompanied by hallucinations and/or paranoia.

depersonalization Alternative perception of the self; a person's own reality is lost. People feel they are not in control of their own actions or speech.

derealization Loss of sensation of the reality of one's surroundings.

euphoria (yoo FOR ee ah) An exaggerated sense of physical and mental well-being.

hallucination (hah loo si NAY shun) A sensory experience (e.g., a smell, sound, sight, touch, or taste) involving something that is not present.

VOCABULARY—*continued*

mania (MAY nee ah) Abnormally elated mental state; the person may have feelings of euphoria, lack of inhibitions, sleeplessness, talkativeness, risk-taking behaviors, and irritability.

morbidity (more BID i tee) The rate of a disease in a population.

mortality (more TAL i tee) The relative frequency of deaths in a specific population.

orientation An awareness of one's environment, with reference to people, place, and time.

paranoia An unfounded or excessive suspicion of the motives of others.

psychotherapy (sie KOE ther ah pee) The treatment of behavioral health disorders through the use of psychological techniques, which encourage communication of conflicts and insights into the person's problems. The goals of this treatment include symptom relief, changes in behavior leading to improved social and vocational function, and personality growth.

psychotherapy notes Patient-provider details from private, group, or family therapy, including what the patient stated and the provider's analysis of the statements and situation.

INTRODUCTION

Many times, healthcare students hear about behavioral health and quickly decide whether or not they are interested in that specialty. In today's healthcare environment, many healthcare professionals, including medical assistants, are involved with behavioral health issues, regardless of where they work. The number of people in the United States with a behavioral health disorder has been increasing over the years. It is estimated that 1 in 5 adults in the United States has a behavioral health condition. According to the Centers for Disease Control and Prevention (CDC), 100,306 people died from a drug overdose in the United States in 12 months ending in April 2021. The majority of those deaths were related to a prescription or illicit opioid.

This chapter begins by describing behavioral health specialists and locations where patients are treated. Information on specific behavioral health, substance use disorder, and addiction disorders will follow. The chapter concludes with information on behavioral health diagnostic procedures and treatments.

BEHAVIORAL HEALTH

According to the CDC, *mental health* encompasses our psychological, emotional, and social welfare. Our mental health influences how we behave, feel, think, handle stress, interact with others, and make choices. Over the years, the field of mental health has changed and grown. *Psychiatry* is the healthcare specialty that studies the brain and its effects on the body. Today, the phrase *behavioral health* refers to mental health, substance use, and associated physical disorders.

The following sections discuss the types of behavioral health professionals and the importance of the *Diagnostic and Statistical Manual of Mental Disorders*. Both topics are important for medical assistants, regardless of where they practice. Many patients seen in primary care also are seen by behavioral health professionals.

Behavioral Health Professionals

Psychotherapist is a general term for a healthcare professional who treats people with behavioral health conditions. This term is used for psychiatrists, psychologists, social workers, and so on. In behavioral health departments, there are people with many different credentials. Having a basic understanding of behavioral health professionals is important. The following are some of the more common behavioral health professionals:

- *Psychiatrist*: Trained as a medical doctor and has had 4 years of residency training in psychiatry, usually in a hospital setting. A psychiatrist assesses the mental and physical conditions related to psychological disorders. A psychiatrist treats patients with psychological disorders and can prescribe medications.
- *Psychologist*: Studied personality development, psychological problems, and how to diagnose mental and emotional disorders; must obtain a PhD or PsyD doctoral degree. Primarily focuses on providing **psychotherapy** and performing psychological testing. Most psychologists cannot prescribe medications.
- *Social worker*: Has a similar educational background as a psychologist but cannot provide psychological testing. The social worker provides psychotherapy. Depending on the state licensure, social workers may have different titles: licensed clinical social worker (LCSW), licensed independent clinical social worker (LICSW), and licensed social worker (LSW).
- *Cognitive behavioral therapist*: Specializes in cognitive behavioral therapy and helping people change the way they think and behave in order to help manage their condition (e.g., depression, relationship issues).
- *Psychiatric nurse*: A registered nurse who has advanced training (e.g., master's or doctoral degree) in assessing and treating behavioral health issues.
- *Substance use (or addiction) therapist* or *counselor*: Has specialized training to treat patients with substance use disorders and other addictions.
- *Mental health therapist* or *counselor*: Trained to treat patients with behavioral health disorders (e.g., depression, anxiety).

In many states, most of these healthcare professionals need a license to practice. There are some exceptions. Some states allow unlicensed behavioral health professionals to provide treatment to patients, but their billing capacity is limited. State laws dictate the licensing and credential requirements for behavioral health professionals.

Patients with behavioral health conditions may be seen in community mental health clinics or private practice clinics. When patients are a threat to themselves or others, they may be admitted to hospitals until their behavioral health conditions stabilize. Specialty inpatient settings for people with eating disorders and addictions are also available.

CRITICAL THINKING APPLICATION 38.1

A patient asks Mike to explain the difference between a psychiatrist and a psychologist. If you were asked this question, how would you respond?

Diagnostic and Statistical Manual of Mental Disorders

The *Diagnostic and Statistical Manual of Mental Disorders* (DSM) is used by behavioral health professionals in the United States and other countries. The first DSM was published in 1952, and subsequent versions have been published since then; the latest is the DSM-5. The DSM provides descriptions, signs, symptoms, and other criteria for diagnosing behavioral health disorders. It provides a common language that is used in the behavioral health environment.

The DSM-5 contains the International Classification of Disease (ICD) codes required for insurance reimbursement and monitoring **morbidity** and **mortality** statistics. In other words, the ICD codes allow researchers to gather information on how often the disorder occurs and how many deaths are attributed to the disease.

CRITICAL THINKING APPLICATION 38.2

Where have you seen or heard morbidity and mortality statistics? Explain your answer.

BEHAVIORAL HEALTH DISEASES AND DISORDERS

Behavioral health diseases and disorders cause changes in the mood, behavior, or thoughts of an individual. These disorders can affect how a person functions on a day-to-day basis, at work, school, and at home.

Biological factors (e.g., genetics), life experiences, and a family history of behavioral health problems can contribute to behavioral health problems. It is important for a person to seek help immediately if signs of behavioral health disorders exist.

The following sections discuss the common signs and symptoms of behavioral health diseases and disorders, along with concerns across the life span.

Common Signs and Symptoms

Common signs and symptoms of behavioral health diseases and disorders include the following:

- Withdrawing from others, isolating oneself
- Eating or sleeping too little or too much
- Having no or low amounts of energy
- Feeling helpless, hopeless, numb, or as if nothing matters
- Having unexplained pains and aches
- Smoking, drinking alcohol, or using drugs more than usual
- Feeling unusually forgetful, on edge, angry, worried, scared, confused, or upset
- Having persistent thoughts or memories stuck in one's head
- Thinking of harming oneself or others
- Inability to function or perform daily activities
- Hearing voices or believing things that are not true

Behavioral Health Diseases and Disorders across a Life Span

Behavioral health problems are very common. Research has shown that 1 out of 7 children in the United States from ages 2 to 8 have been diagnosed with a mental, developmental, or behavioral disorder. Many times, the related factors included poverty, neighborhood concerns, parents with behavioral health issues, and childcare problems that affected the parent's job. Other studies have found that about half of all behavioral health disorders affect a person before the age of 14, and 75% of disorders begin before age 24. Less than 20% of children with a diagnosed behavioral health problem receive the treatment they need.

Behavioral health disorders in children cause changes in the way children learn, behave, or handle their emotions. This can cause problems getting through their days. Common disorders in childhood include anxiety, depression, oppositional defiant disorder, conduct disorder, attention deficit hyperactivity disorder (ADHD), obsessive-compulsive disorder (OCD), and post-traumatic stress disorder (PTSD). Substance use and suicides are occurring in growing numbers.

The National Alliance on Mental Illness (www.nami.org) states that about 1 in 5 adults experience a behavioral health disorder every year. About 4% of the adult population in the United States lives with a serious behavioral health condition (e.g., bipolar disorder, major depression, and schizophrenia). In 2018, about 20.3 million adults in the United States had a substance use disorder. With older adults who have been diagnosed with heart disease, diabetes, and a stroke, research has shown that depression is more prevalent. Depression can complicate treatment and change a person's quality of life.

ANXIETY DISORDERS

Having periodic anxiety about a problem or an important decision is normal. With an anxiety disorder, the anxious feeling is a constant companion, and it gets worse with time. The anxiety interferes with daily living—for instance, school, work, and relationships.

The risk factors for anxiety disorders include shyness in childhood, being divorced or widowed, exposure to stressful life events, a family history of anxiety disorder, and a parental history of behavioral health disorder. The following sections discuss the different types of anxiety disorders.

Generalized Anxiety Disorder

With generalized anxiety disorder (GAD), a person has many different worries. The person finds it difficult to control the anxiety. GAD is a common disorder that can affect a person at any age. GAD occurs more often in females than in males.

The cause of GAD is unknown, but genetics may be a factor. Stress also contributes to the development of GAD. The main symptom of GAD is excessive worrying for over 6 months about multiple issues without a clear reason. Other signs and symptoms of GAD include restlessness, fatigue, irritability, difficulty concentrating, difficulty stopping or controlling anxiety, muscle tension, and sleep problems.

There is no test to diagnose GAD. A physical exam and laboratory tests may be done to rule out other conditions. The provider will ask questions regarding the symptoms of GAD prior to making the diagnosis. The goal of treatment is to help the person feel and function better. Treatment includes psychotherapy. The most effective and common type of talk therapy is cognitive behavioral therapy (CBT). With CBT, a person learns to identify stressors, gain control of panic-causing thoughts, manage stress, and to relax. Medications such as antidepressants and sedative-hypnotics may be prescribed.

Obsessive-Compulsive and Related Disorders

Obsessive-compulsive disorder (OCD) causes a person to have frequent, upsetting thoughts (*obsessions*). Examples of obsessions include fear of germs or of being hurt. Then, to control the thoughts, the person has an overwhelming urge to repeat certain behaviors (*compulsion*). Examples of compulsions include hand washing, counting, rechecking things (e.g., locked doors), or cleaning. The obsessions and compulsions affect the person's daily life.

The cause of OCD is not completely understood, but it may relate to changes in brain function, genetics, and environmental factors. Risk factors include a family history of OCD, other behavioral health disorders (e.g., depression, substance use), or a traumatic event. The symptoms start gradually and may increase in severity over time. Signs and symptoms of OCD include the following:

- Fear of touching items others touched
- The need for items to be in a certain position, organized, and orderly
- Doubts about locking the door or turning off an appliance, causing continual rechecking
- Avoidance of events that trigger the obsessions
- Frequent hand washing, even to the point that the skin is raw
- Silently repeating a prayer or phrase

The provider will do a physical exam, laboratory tests (e.g., blood work, thyroid tests), and a psychological evaluation. Treatment consists of psychotherapy (e.g., cognitive behavioral therapy and exposure and response prevention) and antidepressants.

Hoarding Disorder

Hoarding disorder (HD) is the persistent difficulty of getting rid of personal possessions. People with HD feel they need to save items and are distressed at the thought of discarding them or having them touched or moved without their permission. Sometimes the thoughts center around "hurting the feelings" of the item if it is discarded. Others hold onto their possessions because they may come in handy someday, or, if discarded, the memories attached to the object may be lost. As a result, people with HD have cluttered living areas that can become a significant public health burden and safety issue. It is estimated that up to 5% of the population has HD.

The cause of hoarding disorder is unknown. Risk factors include being indecisive, a family history of hoarding disorder, and stressful life events. A person with hoarding disorder may excessively acquire items that are not needed and have difficulty throwing out items. A person may feel the need to save items. People with hoarding disorder can be indecisive and perfectionists. They can also use avoidance and procrastination.

The behavioral health provider will perform a psychological evaluation. The provider may also review pictures of the patient's living conditions and talk with family members. Treatment consists of cognitive behavioral therapy. Medications can be ordered if the patient has anxiety or depression.

CRITICAL THINKING APPLICATION 38.3

List three safety issues related to hoarding and share them with your class.

Panic Disorder

Panic disorder causes recurrent, unexpected panic attacks, or sudden feelings of terror without real dangers being present. A person experiencing a panic attack is very frightened and feels a loss of control.

The cause of panic disorder is unknown, but genetics, major stress, sensitivity to stress, and certain changes in brain function may play a factor. A person having a panic attack may experience a sense of impending doom, abdominal cramping, nausea, dizziness, lightheadedness, and numbness. Sweating, trembling, chills, hot flashes, chest pain, and a rapid and pounding heart rate can also occur. The signs and symptoms can mimic those of a heart attack, which can also increase the person's anxiety.

After performing a physical exam and ordering laboratory tests to rule out other conditions, the provider will do a psychological evaluation. The DSM-5 criteria for panic disorder include the following:

- Having frequent, unexpected panic attacks.
- One attack is followed by 1 month or more of constant worry about having another attack.
- The panic attack is not related to substance use, medications, or other medical or behavioral health conditions.

Treatment for panic disorder is similar to that for GAD; psychotherapy and medications can be helpful.

Phobias

A phobia is a type of anxiety disorder in which a person has a strong, irrational fear of something that causes little to no danger. There are many types of phobias (Table 38.1). Phobias typically start in childhood and continue into adulthood.

TABLE 38.1 Examples of Phobias

TYPE	FEAR OF…
Acrophobia	Heights
Agoraphobia	open spaces
Algophobia	Pain
Aquaphobia	Water
Arachnophobia	Spiders
Aviophobia	Flying
Belonephobia	Needles
Brontophobia	Thunder
Cancerophobia	Cancer
Chionophobia	Snow
Claustrophobia	Closed spaces
Cyberphobia	Computers
Dentophobia	Dentist or dental procedures
Glossophobia	Speaking in front of an audience
Hemophobia	Blood or injury
Kleptophobia	Stealing
Nosophobia	Disease
Ochlophobia	Crowds

Phobias can be caused by negative experiences, genetics, changes in brain function, and the environment. A phobia can cause panic, persistent and unreasonable fear, an increase in the heart rate, shortness of breath (SOB), trembling, and a strong desire to get away. A phobia can interfere with a person's daily life.

The provider will do a physical exam and gather a medical history. Often, treatment includes psychotherapy, exposure therapy, and medication.

Social Anxiety Disorder

With social anxiety disorder, people have a persistent and irrational fear of social situations. People avoid situations in which they feel others will judge them. They may avoid attending social gatherings, eating and drinking in public, meeting new people, and public speaking. They may also avoid using public restrooms. This disorder affects a person's ability to go to school, function at work, and have relationships. The disorder may begin in a person's teenage years. Males and females are equally affected by this disorder.

The cause of social anxiety disorder may be related to overprotective parents or limited social opportunities. Other possible causes include genetics, learning behaviors established early on in life, and an overactive **amygdala** in the brain, which increases the fear response. Social anxiety disorder causes blushing, an increased heart rate, trembling, sweating, nausea, dizziness, lightheadedness, SOB, and muscle tension. Elevated afternoon cortisol levels have also been reported.

After a physical exam and laboratory tests to rule out other conditions, the provider will do a psychological evaluation. The DSM-5 criteria for social anxiety disorder include the following:

- Persistent, intense anxiety or fear related to social situations in which one perceives others will be judgmental
- Avoidance of such social situations
- Excessive anxiety that interferes with daily life
- Fear or anxiety that is not related to substance use or a medical or behavioral health disorder

Treatment for social anxiety disorder includes psychotherapy and medications:

- Antidepressants: Selective serotonin reuptake inhibitors (SSRIs) and serotonin and norepinephrine reuptake inhibitors (SNRIs)
- Antianxiety medications, including benzodiazepines
- Beta-blockers

DEPRESSION AND OTHER MOOD DISORDERS

Depression is the second leading behavioral health condition and can happen at any age. The symptoms affect how a person acts, thinks, feels, and handles their daily life. Depression must be present for at least 2 weeks for a diagnosis to be given.

Depression

There are several types of depression:

- *Persistent depressive disorder*: Also called *dysthymia*; depression that lasts for at least 2 years.
- *Postpartum depression*: Occurs after giving birth. The person has feelings of extreme sadness, exhaustion, and anxiety. These feelings interfere with daily life and caring for the new baby.
- *Psychotic depression*: Episodes of psychosis occur with severe depression. The person experiences **delusions** and **hallucinations**.
- *Seasonal affective disorder:* Depression occurs during the winter months when there is less sunlight. The depression usually lifts in the spring. During the winter, the person may experience increased sleepiness, weight gain, and social withdrawal.

The cause of depression is not known, but many factors may be involved, including changes in the brain and the functioning of neurotransmitters, hormone changes, and genetics. Risk factors include age (from teens to 30-year-olds), being female, low self-esteem, a stressful event, a family history (of depression, bipolar disorder, alcoholism, or suicide), substance use, chronic medical or behavioral health illness, and certain medications. Depression can have a number of consequences:

- Feeling sad, very tired, hopeless, irritable, anxious, or guilty
- Loss of interest in favorite activities (e.g., hobbies)
- Pain, headaches, cramps, digestive issues, anorexia, and overeating
- Thoughts of death or suicide

The provider will do a physical exam, possibly laboratory tests (e.g., complete blood count, thyroid function tests), and radiology tests (Figure 38.1). A psychiatric evaluation will also be completed to gather more information on the patient's symptoms, thoughts, feelings, and behaviors. Psychotherapy and medications are the most common treatments for depression. Common medication categories used for depression include antidepressants (selective serotonin reuptake inhibitors [SSRIs], serotonin and norepinephrine reuptake inhibitors [SNRI]s, tricyclic, and atypical) and monoamine oxidase inhibitors (MAOIs).

CRITICAL THINKING APPLICATION 38.4

Mike rooms Mrs. Johnson, who states she has not been sleeping well since her husband died 10 days ago. She states she has not been feeling hungry and is always tired. If you encountered a patient like Mrs. Johnson, how would you respond?

Bipolar Disorder

Bipolar disorder causes people to go from **mania** to depression. They cycle through highs and lows in their moods, with periods of normal moods. Bipolar disorder usually starts in the late teens to early adult years and lasts a lifetime.

The cause of bipolar disorder is unclear. There is a genetic link to the disorder, and abnormal brain structure and function may also be related. Bipolar disorder causes the following:

- Mania and hypomania: **Euphoria** and energetic feelings, decreased need for sleep, distractibility, poor decision making, and an exaggerated sense of well-being
- Major depression episode: Insomnia or sleeping too much, fatigue, feelings of worthlessness, suicidal thoughts, feelings of no pleasure, and weight gain or loss
- Moods affect relationships, school, or job performance, and even cause suicide

The provider will do a physical exam and a psychiatric assessment. Patients may be asked to chart their moods. Treatments include lifelong treatments, psychotherapy, and support groups. Medications

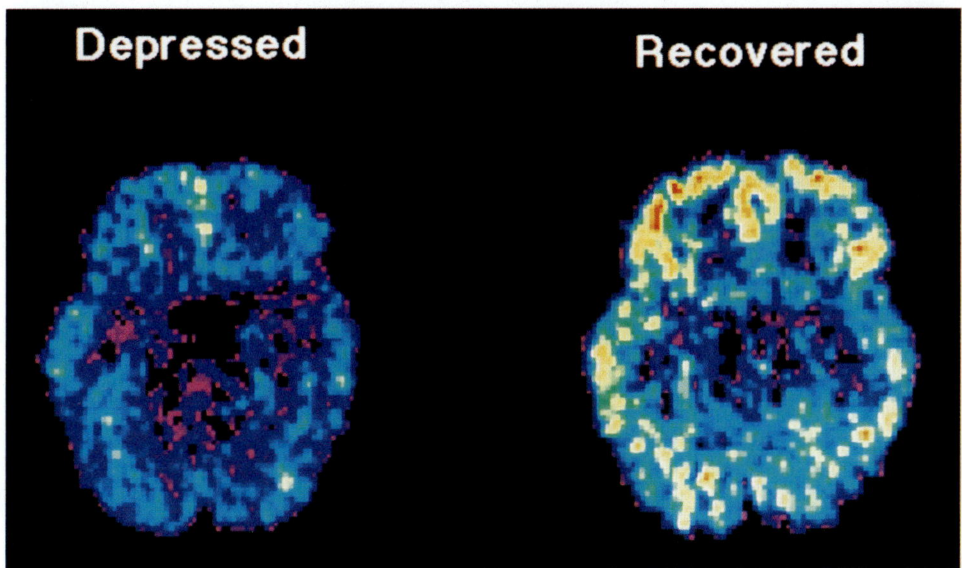

FIGURE 38.1 PET scans of an individual's brain when depressed *(left)* and after recovery through treatment with medication *(right)*. Several brain areas, particularly the prefrontal cortex *(at top)*, show diminished activity *(darker colors)* during depression. (From Fortinash KM: *Psychiatric mental health nursing*, ed 4, St. Louis, 2008, Mosby.)

can also be prescribed and include anticonvulsants and mood stabilizers, antidepressants, anxiolytics, and antipsychotics.

BEHAVIORAL DISORDERS

Behavioral disorders in children involve a pattern of disruptive behaviors that cause issues at home, in school, and social situations. According to the diagnostic criteria, the disruptive behaviors must have lasted at least 6 months. Behavioral disorders may involve defiant behavior, impulsiveness, hyperactivity, inattention, drug use, and criminal activity. Behavioral disorders include the following:

- Attention deficit hyperactivity disorder (ADHD)
- Oppositional defiant disorder (ODD)
- Conduct disorder (CD)

ODD and CD are also considered disruptive behavior disorders. Disruptive behavior disorder involves uncooperative or hostile action patterns of behavior. The person may have temper tantrums, argue, demonstrate cruel and defiant behaviors, and fight with others. People with disruptive behavioral disorders have problems controlling their emotions and actions, leading to issues at school and home.

Attention Deficit Hyperactivity Disorder

ADHD is a chronic condition that affects children and can continue into adulthood. With ADHD, a person is not able to focus or control behaviors, may be overactive, or any combination of these characteristics. ADHD and ADD (attention deficit disorder) are often used interchangeably, but the correct term is ADHD. Typically, symptoms begin before age 12, yet some have seen it in the toddler years. This disorder is more prevalent in males than in females.

The cause of ADHD is unknown, but possible factors include genetics, environmental factors (e.g., lead exposure), and developmental factors. Many conditions can co-exist with ADHD, including learning disabilities, anxiety, depression, bipolar disorder, and Tourette syndrome. ADHD has the following results:

- *Inattention*: Fails to pay close attention, has problems staying focused, appears not to listen, has difficulty following directions, has trouble with organizational skills, and is easily distracted.
- *Hyperactivity and impulsivity*: Fidgets, constantly moving, talking too much, difficulty waiting for their turn, and problems doing quiet activities.

Males may be more hyperactive, whereas females may be quietly inattentive. According to the diagnostic criteria, the symptoms can range from mild to severe and must last for at least 6 months, affecting school and home life. There are three subtypes of ADHD based on the symptoms: predominantly inattentive, predominantly hyperactive-impulsive, and combined (a mix of both).

There is no specific test for ADHD. The provider will do a physical exam, including vision and hearing, and ask the parents and teachers questions. Treatments for ADHD include behavioral therapy to help manage the symptoms and provide coping skills. Medications can also be prescribed:

- Stimulants: Methylphenidate (Ritalin LA, Concerta, Methylin) and amphetamine (Adzenys ER, Dyanavel XR, Evekeo). Stimulants provide a calming effect by increasing the dopamine in the brain, which helps with attention and motivation.
- Nonstimulants: Atomoxetine (Strattera), guanfacine (Intuniv, Tenex), and clonidine (Catapres, Kapvay).

Conduct Disorder

With conduct disorder (CD), the person demonstrates disruptive and violent behaviors. The person hurts others and destroys property. Children with CD can have behavior problems that last into adulthood. Symptoms usually start during the preteen and teen years, though they can be seen in preschool. The disorder is more common in males.

There is no single cause for CD. Having a parent with a behavioral disorder, exposure to neglect, abuse, or violence, and a high emotional reactivity can be risk factors. Conduct disorder causes:

- Aggression toward animals and people: Includes bullying, threatening, starting fights, using weapons, forcing others into sexual activity, stealing from others, and physical cruelty to people or animals.
- Destruction of property, such as setting fires.
- Deceit or theft: Includes lying to get things, breaking in and stealing items, and shoplifting.

- Serious violations of rules: Includes running away from home overnight at least twice, or once without returning for a long time, and truancy.

There is no specific test for CD, so the provider will do a complete medical history. Treatment is based on the individual's need and addresses co-existing diseases. Common intervention programs include parent training, behavioral family therapy, skills-based interventions, anger management, and coping skills.

Oppositional Defiant Disorder

With oppositional defiant disorder (ODD), the child or teen demonstrates ongoing hostility to parents, friends, and teachers. ODD usually is diagnosed during preschool or childhood. There is no single cause for ODD. Having a parent with a behavioral disorder, exposure to neglect, abuse, or violence, and a high emotional reactivity can be risk factors. Depression and anxiety can co-exist with ODD. Oppositional defiant disorder can cause ongoing hostility, defying rules, holding grudges, and rebel-like behaviors. These symptoms interfere with school and home life. There are three types of ODD:

- *Angry and irritable mood*: Annoyed by others easily, loses one's temper, and has rage outbursts
- *Argumentative and defiant behaviors*: Argues with those in authority, defies rules, purposely annoys others, and blames others
- *Vindictiveness*: Being cruel, nasty, vengeful, and mean

There is no specific test for ODD, so the provider will do a complete medical history. Treatment is based on the individual's need and addresses co-existing diseases. Common intervention programs include parent training, behavioral family therapy, and skills-based interventions, which teach the patient how to reduce behavior problems and appropriately interact with peers. Anger management and coping skills are also part of the intervention.

EATING DISORDERS

Eating disorders affect both sexes, but the occurrence of eating disorders in females is 2.5 times greater than it is in males. Eating disorders typically appear during the teen years or young adulthood, but they can start earlier or later in life.

Eating disorders are real, treatable illnesses. They typically co-exist with other illnesses, including substance use, anxiety disorders, and depression. Eating disorders, especially anorexia, can be life threatening without treatment.

Anorexia Nervosa

Anorexia nervosa causes people to lose more weight than is healthy. Individuals with this disorder have an intense fear of gaining weight (Figure 38.2). Often it starts during the preteen to teen years. It is more prevalent in females.

The etiology is unknown. Genetics, hormones, and social attitudes may play a role in developing anorexia nervosa. This condition has the following risk factors:

- A history of anxiety disorder or eating problems as a child
- Worry about weight and shape of the body and a negative self-image
- An exaggerated focus on rules and trying to be perfect

Signs and symptoms of anorexia nervosa include the following:

- Being underweight, an intense fear of gaining weight, and a very distorted body image

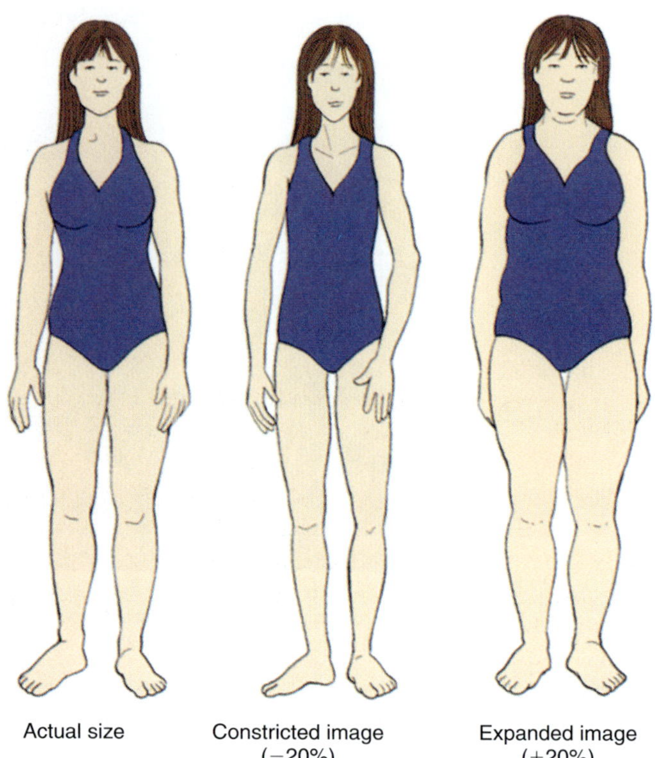

FIGURE 38.2 The perception of body shape and size can be evaluated with the use of special computer drawing programs. These programs allow a subject to distort (increase or decrease) the width of an actual picture of a person's body by as much as 20%. Individuals with anorexia consistently adjusted their own body picture to a size 20% larger than its true form. This suggests that they have a major problem with the perception of self-image. (From Stuart GW, Laraia MT: *Principles and practice of psychiatric nursing*, ed 9, St. Louis, 2009, Mosby.)

- Severely limiting the amount of food eaten and refusing to eat around others
- Exercising all the time
- Going to the bathroom right after meals, vomiting secretly after eating
- Using diuretics, laxatives, or diet pills
- Blotchy or dry yellow skin covered with fine hair and a dry mouth
- Confused, poor memory or judgment, slow thinking, depression
- Extreme sensitivity to cold
- Osteoporosis, wasting away of muscle, and loss of body fat

The provider will order extensive laboratory tests to look at thyroid, liver, and kidney function. An electrocardiogram and bone density test may also be ordered. Many healthcare facilities have patients with eating disorders get on the scale backward, so they cannot see their weight (Figure 38.3). Treatment focuses on helping these patients recognize they have an illness. Many types of treatments are available, including psychotherapy (e.g., cognitive behavioral therapy, group therapy, and family therapy) and support groups. Compliance with treatment is difficult, and it is common for the disease to return.

Binge Eating Disorder

Binge eating disorder, also called compulsive overeating, is the most common eating disorder in the United States. It occurs when people regularly eat unusually large amounts of food in a short amount of time. They feel out of control and unable to manage what or how much they eat. A person may have a binge eating disorder if this behavior occurs weekly for 3 months. It affects young women and middle-aged men.

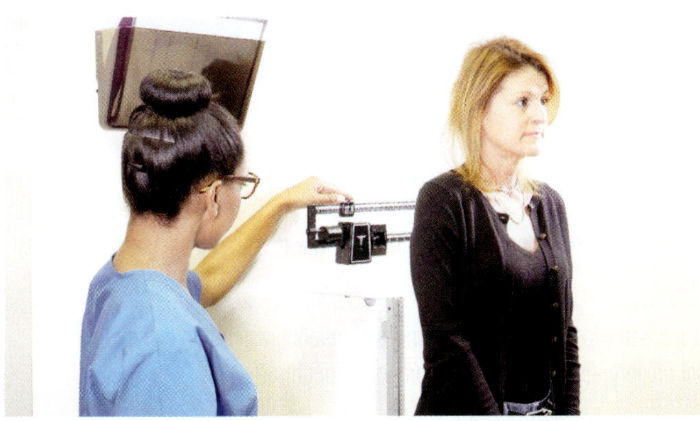

FIGURE 38.3 Weighing a patient backward. The medical assistant should help, if needed, as the patient steps on and off the scale.

The exact cause is unknown. Genetics, depression, stress, unhealthy dieting, and changes in brain chemicals may be factors in the condition. Here are the signs and symptoms of binge eating disorder:

- Eating quickly and eating until uncomfortably full
- Eating when not hungry
- Eating huge amounts of food over a very short period of time
- Eating in secret
- Feeling disgusted, ashamed, or depressed about one's eating patterns
- Frequent dieting

A physical exam and a psychological evaluation will be done. Blood and urine tests (e.g., cholesterol, blood glucose) may be done to evaluate the consequences of binge eating. Treatment may consist of behavioral weight-loss programs and psychotherapy (e.g., cognitive behavioral therapy, interpersonal psychotherapy, and dialectical behavior therapy). Medications may also be used, including lisdexamfetamine (Vyvanse), topiramate (Topamax, Qudexy XR, Trokendi XR), and antidepressants.

Bulimia Nervosa

Bulimia nervosa, or bulimia, causes overeating that leads to purging and can be a life-threatening disorder. Self-induced vomiting, laxatives, weight-loss supplements, and enemas may be used to prevent weight gain. Bulimia may also occur with anorexia nervosa. More females than males have bulimia. It is more common in teens and young women.

The etiology is unknown. Genetics, hormones, and social attitudes may play a role in the development of bulimia. Here are the signs and symptoms of bulimia nervosa:

- Broken blood vessels in the eyes (this occurs from the strain of vomiting)
- Dry mouth and a pouchlike look to the cheeks
- Rashes and pimples
- Small cuts and calluses on the tops of fingers (from inducing vomiting)
- Dehydration and electrolyte imbalance

Other people may notice the following behaviors:

- Excessive exercising
- Eating large amounts of food or buying large amounts of food that disappear right away
- Trips to the bathroom after meals
- Discarded boxes from laxatives, diet pills, and emetics to induce vomiting, or diuretics

The provider will do a physical exam and urine and blood tests. Treatment is usually on an outpatient basis unless the individual has a co-existing diagnosis. Support groups, counseling, and medications can be helpful.

Other Eating Disorders

Additional eating disorders to be aware of are as follows:

- *Pica*: Eating of nonfood materials, such as paper, ice, clay, or dirt. Seen in children and during pregnancy. May be caused by a lack of certain nutrients that produce unusual cravings.
- *Rumination disorder*: A condition in which a person regurgitates food from the stomach and rechews the food.
- *Avoidant/restrictive food intake disorder (ARFID)*: Similar to anorexia because it limits the amount of food consumed, but with ARIFD, the person is not stressed about body shape or size. When the condition occurs in children, the child does not consume enough calories to grow and develop. Previously called selective eating disorder.

CRITICAL THINKING APPLICATION 38.5

Describe the three types of eating disorders in your own words.

OTHER BEHAVIORAL HEALTH DISEASES AND DISORDERS

The following sections discuss common behavioral health diseases and disorders, including autism spectrum disorder, dissociative disorder, personality disorder, post-traumatic stress disorder, and schizophrenia.

Autism Spectrum Disorder

Autism spectrum disorder (ASD) is a developmental disorder with symptoms that appear by age 2. The child has difficulty interacting and communicating with others. The communication issues and behaviors, such as repetitive behaviors and limited interests, affect the person's ability to function at school and home. There can be a wide range of symptoms and severity; thus, it is known as a "spectrum" disorder. Prior diagnoses, such as Asperger syndrome, are now included in ASD.

The exact cause of ASD is unknown, but research suggests that a person's genetics, with environmental influences, can affect development, leading to ASD. Risk factors for ASD include having a family member with ASD, older parents, certain genetic conditions, and a low birth weight.

Autism spectrum disorder can cause:

- Social communication and interaction behavior issues: Little to no eye contact, not listening to others, failing to respond when being called, difficulty with holding a conversation, talks at length about a favorite topic without realizing others are not interested, body language does not match the verbal message, and having a singsong or flat, robotlike tone of voice.
- Restrictive and repetitive behaviors: Repeating certain behaviors or words, intense interest in certain topics (e.g., numbers, details, facts), getting upset with routine changes, and more or less sensitivity to light, noise, clothing, or temperature.

Often people with ASD have sleeping issues. They may be strong auditory and visual learners who excel in art, music, science, or math. They may remember information for long periods of time and can learn information in detail.

The American Academy of Pediatrics recommends screening children for developmental delays during the 9-month, 18-month, and

TABLE 38.2 Types of Personality Disorders

CLUSTER	TYPES	DESCRIPTION
Cluster A personality disorders	Paranoid personality disorder	Unjustified beliefs that others are trying to do harm to the person. Very suspicious, untrusting, angry, and hostile. May feel that their partner is unfaithful.
	Schizoid personality disorder	Avoidance of social activities and interacting with other people. The person may be seen as a loner and may not show emotion.
	Schizotypal personality disorder	Odd, peculiar, and unusual behaviors; flat or inappropriate emotional responses; belief in special powers, excessive social anxiety, and suspicious or paranoid thoughts.
Cluster B personality disorders	Antisocial personality disorder	No regard for others; persistent lying, and impulsive and aggressive behaviors.
	Borderline personality disorder	Intense relationships, distorted self-image, impulsivity, and extreme emotions (e.g., intense fear of abandonment, anger, mood swings). Usually begins in early adulthood and may get better with age.
	Histrionic personality disorder	Seeks constant attention. Very dramatic, emotional, and opinionated.
	Narcissistic personality disorder	Inflated ego, an excessive need for attention, lacks empathy for others, has troubled relationships and a very fragile self-esteem.
Cluster C personality disorders	Avoidance personality disorder	Too sensitive to criticism; feels inadequate; avoids interpersonal contact or is extremely shy/ withdrawn during social activities.
	Dependent personality disorder	Very clinging and dependent on another person. Fears being left alone. Lacks self-confidence.
	Obsessive-compulsive personality disorder	Preoccupied with rules, organization/orderliness, and details. Wants to control everything (e.g., tasks, situations, people, events).

24- or 30-month well-child visit. ASD screening tools are available. Children suspected of having ASD are referred for additional evaluation by a healthcare team specializing in diagnosing ASD. Treatment may consist of medication and behavioral, educational, and psychological therapies. These therapies focus on teaching the person skills to live independently, including social, communication, and language skills.

Dissociative Disorders

Dissociative disorders cause a person to involuntarily escape from reality. A person may have a disconnection between memories, thoughts, actions, identity, and surroundings. Dissociative disorder can cause a variety of conditions, such as **amnesia** and alternative identities. Here are some common dissociative disorders:

- *Dissociative amnesia:* Memory loss without an explained medical condition. No recollection of self, events, and familiar people. May involve confused wandering away from home (*dissociative fugue*). May last for hours to years.
- *Dissociative identity disorder:* Formerly known as multiple personality disorder. People may feel two or more people "in their head" as if they have alternative identities. Each identity may have a name, history, and unique personality.
- *Depersonalization-derealization disorder*: Episodic or long-term sense of detachment with **depersonalization** and **derealization**. People feel they are an outside observer of their thoughts, actions, and sensations. They also feel as if they are detached from their surroundings

Dissociative disorders develop as a coping mechanism due to trauma (e.g., abuse, war, and natural disasters). A risk factor includes experiencing long-term sexual, physical, or emotional abuse during childhood. Dissociative disorders can cause a number of conditions:

- Amnesia and an unclear sense of identity
- A sense of being detached from oneself
- A distorted or unreal perception of others
- Significant stress and inability to cope
- Behavioral health issues, such as depression and anxiety

The provider will do a physical exam and a psychiatric evaluation. Treatment consists of psychotherapy and medications (e.g., antidepressants, antianxiety drugs, and antipsychotics).

Personality Disorders

Personality disorders include a group of conditions that involve long-term patterns of unhealthy and inflexible thoughts and behaviors that affect relationships and work. Personality disorders cause people to have difficulty dealing with stress and problems. Personality disorders are grouped by clusters (Table 38.2):

- *Cluster A personality disorders:* Cause odd, eccentric thinking and behaviors
- *Cluster B personality disorders:* Cause dramatic, overly emotional thinking and behaviors
- *Cluster C personality disorders:* Cause anxiety, fearful thinking and behaviors

The etiology of personality disorders is unknown, but childhood experiences and genetics may play a role in the disorders. The signs and symptoms can range from mild to severe and vary based on the type of disorder. People with a personality disorder may feel they do not have a problem and blame others for their problems.

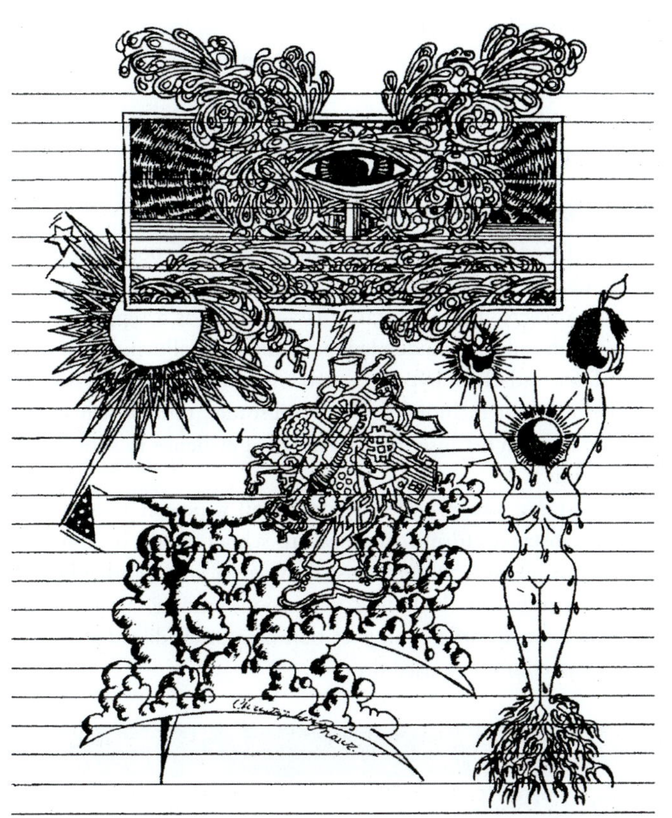

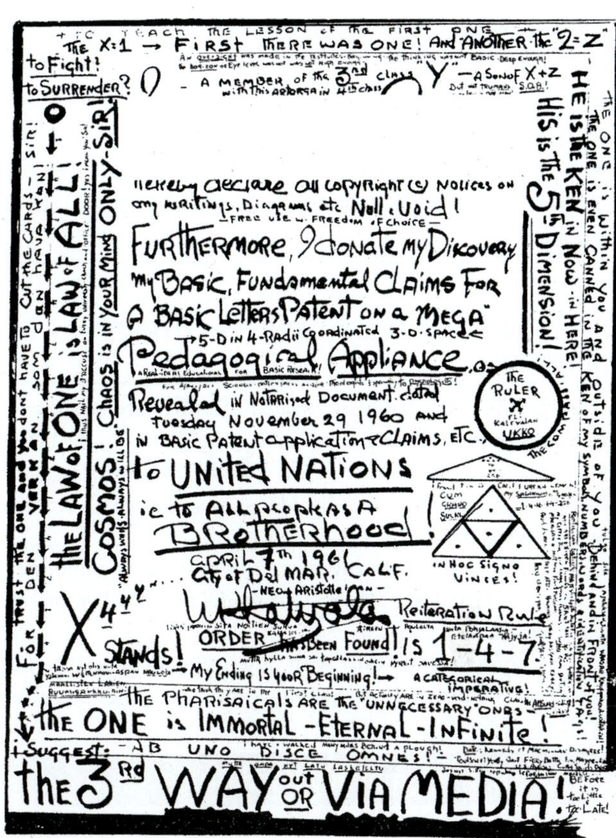

FIGURE 38.4 **(A)** Drawing by a delusional patient with schizophrenia. **(B)** This drawing by a patient with schizophrenia demonstrates thought disorder. (From Stuart GW, Laraia MT: *Principles and practice of psychiatric nursing*, ed 9, St. Louis, 2009, Mosby.)

The provider will do a physical exam and a psychiatric evaluation. Treatments involve psychotherapy and medications (e.g., antidepressants, mood stabilizers, antipsychotic medications, and antianxiety medications).

Post-Traumatic Stress Disorder

Post-traumatic stress disorder (PTSD) is a condition that occurs after a person experiences or witnesses a traumatic or terrifying event. The symptoms of PTSD can vary over time and from person to person. Anyone can develop PTSD, from children to war veterans to people who have experienced the death of a loved one, physical or sexual assault, an accident, or a natural disaster. Females are more likely to have PTSD than males.

The cause of PTSD is experiencing a stressful, terrifying event. It is unknown why some develop the disorder, and others do not. Here are some signs and symptoms of PTSD:

- *Intrusive memories*: Reliving the trauma (flashbacks); nightmares and recurrent distressful memories
- *Negative changes*: Negative thoughts, hopelessness, and difficulty maintaining close relationships
- *Changes in reactions*: Being easily frightened, self-destructive activities (drinking, drugs), trouble concentrating and sleeping, and aggressive behaviors
- *Avoidance*: Avoiding places, people, and things that remind one of the situations; not talking about the event

The provider will do a physical exam and a psychological evaluation. Treatment is focused on helping the person to regain a sense of control. Psychotherapy, including cognitive therapy, eye movement desensitization and reprocessing (EMDR), and exposure therapy, may be prescribed. Antidepressants and antianxiety medications may be prescribed.

Schizophrenia

Schizophrenia causes disruptions in thought processes, perceptions, emotional responsiveness, and social interactions (Figure 38.4). Schizophrenia is usually diagnosed in the late teen years to the early 30s. The symptoms tend to occur earlier for males than females. Schizophrenia is a debilitating disorder, and about half of those with it also have another behavioral health disorder.

The cause of schizophrenia is unknown, but, as with many other conditions, it is believed that a combination of brain chemistry, environmental factors, and genetics play a role in developing the disease. Schizophrenia can have the following characteristics:

- Delusions, hallucinations, and disorganized thinking and speech
- Abnormal motor behavior and lack of response (no eye contact, lack of facial expression)
- Neglect of personal hygiene
- Teens are more likely to withdraw and have insomnia

The provider will do a physical exam and may order a magnetic resonance imaging (MRI) or computed tomography (CT) scan to rule out other conditions. A psychiatric evaluation will be done. Treatment is lifelong and includes psychosocial therapy and antipsychotic medications. Hospitalization is required if the person experiences severe or life-threatening symptoms.

CRITICAL THINKING APPLICATION **38.6**

Mike rooms Mr. James, who states he is seeing little green men coming out of the wall. If you encountered a patient like Mr. James, how would you respond?

SUBSTANCE USE DISORDERS AND OTHER ADDICTIONS

In the DSM-5, substance use-related disorders are addressed with addictive disorders. Research has shown similarities in the biology of addictions to that of substance use disorders. Comparing gambling disorder with substance use disorder shows that they share the following characteristics:

- There is an urge or craving state prior to using or gambling.
- The activity reduces anxiety and results in a positive mood state ("a high").
- The disorder can co-exist with other types of substance use disorders. For instance, many with gambling addictions also have a substance use disorder. Many with one type of substance use disorder also have another type.
- Similar abnormal functioning in the brain's cortex has been found in both.

The following sections discuss substance use disorders, alcohol use disorders, and other addictions.

Substance Use Disorders

In the DSM-5, substance use disorder includes both substance use and substance dependence. Substance use disorder is measured from mild to severe. Each substance is addressed as a separate disorder. These substances include alcohol, cannabis, hallucinogens, opioids, inhalants, sedatives, hypnotics, anxiolytics, tobacco, and stimulants. Caffeine is not included in the use disorder, though it may be in a future revision because there is sufficient evidence to support such a condition.

Substance use disorder occurs when a person uses alcohol or other substances (drugs) that lead to school, work, or home issues. Many people with substance use disorders also have other behavioral health conditions, including depression, anxiety, attention deficit hyperactivity disorder, and post-traumatic stress disorder. Table 38.3 describes commonly used drugs.

TABLE 38.3 Commonly Used Drugs

DRUG	STREET NAMES	COMMON FORM/WAYS TAKEN	POSSIBLE HEALTH EFFECTS	WITHDRAWAL SYMPTOMS
Ayahuasca	Aya, Yage, Hoasca	Brewed as tea/swallowed	Strong hallucinations, increases in heart rate (HR), hypertension (HTN), gastric burning.	Unknown
CNS depressants	*(Barbiturates, pentobarbital)* Barbs, Red Birds, Yellow Jackets, Yellows	Pill, capsule, liquid/swallowed, injected	Drowsiness, slurred speech, poor concentration, confusion, dizziness, problems with movement and memory, lowered blood pressure (BP), slowed breathing.	Must be discussed with a healthcare provider; barbiturate withdrawal can cause a serious abstinence syndrome that may even include seizures.
	(Benzodiazepines) Candy, Downers, Sleeping pills, Tranks	Pill, capsule, liquid/swallowed, snorted		
	(Sleep medications) Mexican Valium, R2, Roche, Roofies, Roofinol, Rope, Rophies	Pill, capsule, liquid/swallowed, snorted		
Cocaine	Blow, Bump, C, Candy, Charlie, Coke, Crack, Flake, Rock, Snow, Toot	White powder, whitish rock crystal/swallowed, snorted, smoked	Enlarged pupils, increased HR, HTN, abdominal pain, euphoria, increased energy; violent behavior, panic attacks, **paranoia**, stroke, seizure, **coma**.	Depression, tiredness, increased appetite, insomnia, vivid unpleasant dreams, slowed thinking and movement, restlessness.
Dextromethorphan (over-the-counter DM products)	Robotripping, Robo, Triple C	Syrup, capsule/swallowed	Slurred speech, increase HR, HTN, dizziness.	Unknown
Dimethyltryptamine	DMT, Dimitri	White or yellow crystalline powder/smoked, injected	Intense visual hallucinations, depersonalization, and altered perception, HTN, increased HR, agitation, seizures, dilated pupils.	Unknown

TABLE 38.3 Commonly Used Drugs—continued

DRUG	STREET NAMES	COMMON FORM/WAYS TAKEN	POSSIBLE HEALTH EFFECTS	WITHDRAWAL SYMPTOMS
Gamma Hydroxybutyrate (GHB)	Home Boy, G, Georgia, Goop, Grievous Bodily Harm, Liquid Ecstasy, Liquid X, Soap, Scoop	Colorless, liquid, white powder/swallowed, often combined with alcohol and other beverages	Euphoria, drowsiness, vomiting, confusion, memory loss, unconsciousness, slowed HR, seizures, coma, death.	Insomnia, anxiety, tremors, sweating, increased HR and BP, psychotic thoughts.
Heroin	Brown Sugar, China White, Dope, H, Horse, Junk, Skag, Skunk, Smack, White Horse	White or brownish powder, or black sticky substance known as "black tar heroin"/injected, smoked, snorted	Euphoria, slowed HR, constipation and stomach cramps, liver or kidney disease, pneumonia.	Restlessness, muscle and bone pain, insomnia, diarrhea, vomiting, cold flashes with goose bumps ("cold turkey").
Inhalants	Poppers, Snappers, Whippets, Laughing gas	Paint thinners, lighter fluid, permanent markers, glue, spray paint, and other types of aerosol products/Inhaled through the nose or mouth	Confusion, slurred speech, lack of coordination, hallucination, headaches, heart failure, seizures, coma, death, liver, and kidney damage.	Nausea, tremors, irritability, problems sleeping, and mood changes
Ketamine	*(Anesthetic in veterinary practice)* Cat Valium, K, Special K, Vitamin K	Liquid, white powder/injected, snorted, smoked, swallowed	Problems with attention, learning, and memory; hallucinations, sedation, HTN, very slowed breathing; kidney problems.	Unknown
Khat	Abyssinian tea, African salad, Catha, Chat, Kat, Oat	Fresh or dried leaves/chewed or brewed as a tea	Euphoria, increased alertness, depression, loss of appetite, fine tremors, heart attack.	Depression, nightmares, hypotension, decreased energy
Kratom	Herbal speedball, Biak-biak, Ketum, Kahuam, Ithang, Thom	Fresh or dried leaves, liquid, gum/chewed, eaten with other foods, smoked	Increased energy, alertness, sedation, euphoria, decreased pain, hallucinations.	Muscle aches, insomnia, hostility, jerky movements, aggression
Lysergic acid diethylamide (LSD)	Acid, Blotter, Blue Heaven, Cubes, Microdot, Yellow Sunshine	Tablet; capsule; clear liquid; small, tainted decorated absorbent paper squares/swallowed, absorbed through mouth tissues	Rapid emotional swings; HTN, increased HR, tremors, enlarged pupils, visual disturbances, paranoia, mood swings.	Unknown
Marijuana (Cannabis)	Blunt, Bud, Dope, Ganja, Grass, Green, Herb, Joint, Mary Jane, Pot, Reefer, Sinsemilla, Skunk, Smoke, Trees, Weed; Hashish: Boom, Gangster, Hash, Hemp	Greenish gray mixture of dried, shredded leaves, stems, seeds, and/or flowers; resin (hashish) or sticky, black liquid (hash oil)/smoked, eaten (mixed in food or brewed as tea)	Enhanced sensory perception and euphoria, drowsiness, slowed reaction time; problems with balance and coordination; HTN, anxiety, chronic cough.	Irritability, trouble sleeping, decreased appetite, anxiety
MDMA (Ecstasy/Molly)	Adam, Clarity, Eve, Lover's Speed, Peace, Uppers	Colorful tablets, capsules, powder, liquid/swallowed, snorted	Lowered inhibitions, increase in heart rate and blood pressure, kidney failure, death.	Fatigue, loss of appetite, depression, problems concentrating
Mescaline (Peyote)	Buttons, Cactus, Mesc	Fresh or dried buttons, capsule/swallowed	Enhanced perception and feeling, euphoria, hallucinations, HTN, sweating, problems with movement.	Unknown
Methamphetamine	Crank, Chalk, Crystal, Fire, Glass, Go Fast, Ice, Meth, Speed	White powder or pill, shiny blue-white rocks/swallowed, snorted, smoked, injected	Increased wakefulness, increase HR, HTN, paranoia, hallucinations, delusions, dental problems.	Depression, anxiety, tiredness

Continued

TABLE 38.3 Commonly Used Drugs—continued

DRUG	STREET NAMES	COMMON FORM/WAYS TAKEN	POSSIBLE HEALTH EFFECTS	WITHDRAWAL SYMPTOMS
Loperamide (Imodium)	None	Table, capsule, liquid/ swallowed	High doses cause euphoria, lessen drug craving, kidney failure, loss of consciousness.	Severe anxiety, vomiting, and diarrhea
Phencyclidine (PCP, or "angel dust")	Angel Dust, Boat, Hog, Love Boat, Peace Pill	White or colored powder, tablet, or capsule; clear liquid/ injected, snorted, swallowed, smoked	Delusions, hallucinations, paranoia, anxiety, HTN, sweating, drooling, loss of balance, seizures, coma, and death.	Headaches, increased appetite, sleepiness, depression
Prescription opioids	Captain, Cody, Lean, Schoolboy, Purple (multiple names depending on medication)	Varies: tablet, capsule, liquid/ swallowed, injected, snorted	Pain relief, drowsiness, euphoria, slowed breathing, death.	Restlessness, pain, insomnia, cold flashes with goose bumps ("cold turkey"), leg movements
Psilocybin	Little Smoke, Magic Mushrooms, Purple Passion, Shrooms	Fresh or dried mushrooms with long, slender stems topped by caps with dark gills/swallowed	Hallucinations, altered perceptions, inability to tell fantasy from reality, panic, problems with movement, enlarged pupils, drowsiness.	Unknown
Rohypnol (Flunitrazepam)	*(Similar to Xanax and Valium)* Date rape drug, Mind Eraser, Mexican Valium, Roach (multiple names)	Tablet/swallowed	Drowsiness, amnesia; impaired reaction time, motor coordination, mental functioning, and judgment; confusion; slurred speech.	Headache, extreme anxiety, restlessness, confusion, irritability; hallucinations; delirium; convulsions; seizures; or shock
Salvia	Magic mint, Maria Pastora, Sally-D, Shepherdess's Herb	Fresh or dried leaves/smoked, chewed, brewed as tea	Intense hallucination, altered perceptions, mood swings, sweating.	Unknown
Tobacco	Multiple brands	Cigarettes, cigars, bidis, hookahs, smokeless tobacco (snuff, spit tobacco, chew)/ smoked, snorted, chewed, vaporized	Increased HR, HTN, risk of lung and oral cancer, chronic bronchitis; emphysema; heart disease; leukemia; cataracts; pneumonia.	Irritability, attention and sleep problems, depression, increased appetite

From the National Institute of Drug Abuse, www.drugabuse.gov/drugs-abuse.

The exact cause of substance use disorders is unknown, but genetics, drug action, peer pressure, anxiety, depression, emotional distress, and stress can all be factors. Substance use disorders can cause the following:

- Confusion, violence, and hostility
- Making excuses to use drugs, lack of control over use, and need for regular/daily use
- Continuing drug use even when work, family, and health are affected
- Missing work or school
- Secretive behaviors related to drugs
- Neglecting to eat or to care for one's appearance

To diagnose substance use, urine and blood drug tests (toxicology screens) are done. Treatment starts by recognizing the problem. Substances may either be slowly withdrawn or stopped abruptly. Hospitalization or residential treatment programs address withdrawal symptoms and behaviors. Medications may be given for some withdrawal symptoms. Support groups are helpful.

Alcohol Use Disorder

Alcohol use disorder (AUD) is a chronic relapsing brain disease that includes a compulsion to use alcohol, loss of control over alcohol intake, and a negative emotional state when abstaining from alcohol. Many people are not aware of what a standard drink means. According to the National Institute of Drug Abuse (NIAAA) (www.niaaa.nih.gov), one "standard" drink is about 14 grams of pure alcohol. This can be found in the following forms:

- 12 fluid oz of regular beer (about 5% alcohol)
- 8–9 fluid oz of malt liquor (about 7% alcohol)
- 5 fluid oz of table wine (about 12% alcohol)

- 1.5 fluid oz of distilled spirits (gin, rum, tequila, vodka, and whiskey) (about 40% alcohol)

According to the NIAAA, in 2019, about 15 million people in the United States had AUD, including 414,000 children under the age of 18. AUD can range from mild to severe. AUD can include periods of alcohol intoxication and symptoms of withdrawal.

Psychological, genetic, social, and environmental factors can play a role in how alcohol affects one's body and behavior. Alcohol intoxication signs include inappropriate behavior, unstable moods, impaired judgment, slurred speech, impaired memory, poor coordination, and blackouts. Here are some signs and symptoms of AUD:

- Being unable to limit the amount of alcohol consumed
- Wanting to cut back on drinking or making unsuccessful attempts to do so
- Spending significant time obtaining alcohol, drinking, and recovering
- Having the effects of alcohol affect one's work, school, or home life
- Being unable to stop drinking even if it is causing problems in one's life
- Using alcohol in situations in which it is not safe (e.g., driving, boating, swimming)
- Feeling as if one needs more alcohol to get the same effect
- Drinking to avoid withdrawal symptoms

Alcohol has many effects on the body:

- Changes in mood and behavior; makes it harder to think clearly and move with coordination
- High blood pressure, stroke, arrhythmias (irregular heartbeat), and cardiomyopathy
- Liver inflammation, fatty liver, alcoholic hepatitis, fibrosis, and cirrhosis
- Pancreatitis
- Cancer of the mouth, esophagus, throat, liver, and breast
- A weakened immune system

The provider will do a physical exam, urine and blood tests, imaging tests, and a psychological evaluation. Treatment includes medically managed detoxification and withdrawal in an inpatient setting. Sedating medications may be required to help manage the withdrawal symptoms, which can last 2 to 7 days. Treatment also consists of psychological counseling, behavior change techniques, support groups, lifelong support, and medications, including the following:

- Naltrexone (ReVia, Vivitrol), which blocks the "feel good" part of alcohol and reduces the urge to drink
- Acamprosate (Campral), which helps reduce the cravings
- Disulfiram (Antabuse), which helps prevent drinking by causing flushing, nausea, vomiting, and headaches if alcohol is consumed

Other Addictions

Several addictions have been recognized by the behavioral health professionals. The following are examples of addictions, though they are not all currently recognized as disorders in the ICD and DSM-5.

- *Exercise addiction*: This is a compulsive disorder that causes people to feel the uncontrollable need to exercise excessively; it can lead to illness or injury. This addiction can co-exist with anorexia nervosa or bulimia nervosa.
- *Gambling addiction*: With this disorder, people cannot control their gambling, and it affects their financial, social, recreational, familial, and occupational functioning. With gambling, dopamine is released in the brain (about 10 times the normal amount), causing a "feel good" sensation.
- *Gaming addiction*: With this serious disorder, a person excessively plays video games, which disturbs normal life activities, including school, work, and hygiene.
- *Internet addiction*: With this disorder, people have tremendous anxiety if they are forced to be without the internet (e.g., their phones, tablets, computers). They have an excessive preoccupation or behaviors related to computer use and internet access. Excessive internet usage has been associated with other behavioral health and psychosocial conditions, including social isolation, impaired social skills, ADHD, depression, and suicidal ideation.
- *Shopping addiction*: It is known by many names, including compulsive spending or compulsive buying disorder. The person has an intense preoccupation with buying and shopping and an uncontrollable urge to do these activities, even if negative consequences exist. It is estimated that about 6% of the adults in the United States have a shopping addiction.

In future editions of the ICD and DSM, more addictions may be added. Currently, gambling is the only addictive disorder listed in the DSM-5.

SUICIDAL BEHAVIOR

Suicide is death caused by a self-inflicted injury with an intent to die as a result of the behavior. A *suicide attempt* is a nonfatal, self-directed, potentially harmful behavior with an intent to die as a result of the behavior. The attempt may not cause an injury. *Suicidal ideation* refers to thinking about, considering, or planning suicide.

Suicide is a leading cause of death in the US, with almost 46,000 deaths in 2020. More than 1.2 million Americans attempt suicide, and on average, 130 die by suicide each day. Suicide is the third leading cause of death of those between ages 10 and 24, and it is the ninth leading cause of death of those between ages 35 and 64.

Etiology and Warning Signs

The three most common methods of suicide are firearms, suffocation, and poisoning. Certain factors increase the risk of suicide. Ninety percent of those who die by suicide have a mental disorder at the time, including depression, bipolar disorder, and schizophrenia. Additional risk factors include previous suicide attempts, a family history of suicide, substance use, incarceration, a low level of job satisfaction, and being the victim of bullying. Those with the highest risk for suicide include males, people over age 45, Caucasians, American Indians, and Alaskan Natives. Veterans and other military personnel also have a higher risk of suicide. People with suicidal ideation are often overwhelmed with hopelessness and sadness.

The following are warning signs and symptoms of suicidal behavior:

- Looking for a way to kill oneself
- Talking about killing oneself or wanting to die; feelings of hopelessness, feeling trapped or in unbearable pain; having no reason to live or the feeling of being a burden on others
- Increased use of drugs or alcohol
- Social withdrawal and isolation; a sense of agitation, feelings of rage, anxiousness, and behaving recklessly
- Sleeping too much or too little
- Extreme mood swings

If someone is showing some of these signs or symptoms, it is important to get help for the person. The National Suicide Prevention Lifeline is 1-800-273-TALK (8255).

The provider will do a physical exam and possibly lab tests to rule out other conditions. The provider will ask the patient in-depth questions about mental and physical health conditions and alcohol, drug, and prescriptive medication use.

Protective Factors and Treatments

Protective factors help prevent suicidal thoughts and behaviors. The following are considered protective factors: effective clinical care for behavioral health conditions and physical and substance use disorders; easy access to care; family and community support; support from ongoing medical and behavioral healthcare relationships; and skills in problem solving, conflict resolution, and nonviolent ways of handling disputes. Treatment for suicide attempts includes treating any behavioral health disorders. Medications and psychotherapy (e.g., cognitive behavior therapy) may also be used.

THE MEDICAL ASSISTANT'S ROLE REGARDING BEHAVIORAL HEALTH EXAMINATIONS

Medical assistants working in behavioral health facilities may perform administrative duties, such as scheduling appointments, working with patients' health records, and handling telephone calls. Medical assistants may also perform clinical duties for the psychiatrist, which are described in the following sections.

Assisting with the Examination

Prior to the patient seeing the provider, the medical assistant rooms the patient. The provider may require the medical assistant to obtain and document the patient's vital signs, weight, and medical history. The medical assistant may need to prepare prescription refills for the provider to complete and sign.

Weighing Patients

When treating patients who have been diagnosed with eating disorders, many times, the psychiatrist will want the patient to be weighed. When the medical assistant obtains the weight, it is important to have patients empty their pockets and remove shoes and extra clothing. This will help ensure the accuracy of the patient's weight because the weight is an important sign in the treatment plan. Many healthcare facilities have patients with eating disorders get on the scale backward, so they cannot see their weight (see Figure 38.4). They are not told what their weight is. If people gain weight, they may feel "fat," and it may not be helpful for their treatment. Providers will share the weight with the patient if they feel it is appropriate for the patient's treatment.

CRITICAL THINKING APPLICATION **38.7**

Mike weighs Alexis White, who is being treated for anorexia. He has her step backward on the scale and does not allow her to see the weight. She asks him repeatedly to tell her the weight. If you encountered a patient like Alexis, how would you handle the situation?

THE MEDICAL ASSISTANT'S ROLE REGARDING BEHAVIORAL HEALTH DIAGNOSTIC PROCEDURES

Some behavioral health facilities may have the medical assistant help with specimen collection and testing (e.g., venipuncture, urine drug test). Most of the diagnostic testing is done by psychologists who perform psychological testing. The medical assistant should have a basic understanding of mental status testing and other psychological testing.

Mental Status Testing

Mental status testing (also called *neurocognitive testing*) assesses a person's ability to think. Providers can identify cognitive impairments. The testing involves the provider asking the patient a series of questions. Common tests include the Mini-Mental State Examination (MMSE), Folstein test, and the Montreal Cognitive Assessment.

The provider assesses cognitive functioning by examining the following aspects:

- *Short- and long-term memory*: Questions relate to recent and past events. The person may be asked to remember something and, in 5 minutes, will need to recall what was remembered.
- *Attention span and concentration*: Can the person complete a thought and solve problems? The provider may ask the patient to count by fives or sevens.
- **Orientation**: Does the person know their name, age, and job? Does the person know the day, time, date, and season?
- *Language and communication skills*: Questions will examine the person's ability to form clear ideas. The patient may be asked to read or write a sentence.
- *Judgment and intelligence*: The person is given a scenario and asked to solve it.

The provider's general observations are formed by assessing the physical appearance, behavior, motor activity, mood, and affect. For the physical appearance, behavior, and motor activity, the provider checks the appropriateness of clothing, grooming, posture, facial expression, and eye contact. Does the stated age match the apparent physical appearance? Is the person friendly, withdrawn, shy, hostile, irritable, relaxed, or cooperative? For the mood and affect, the provider asks the patient to give information on their emotional state or mood. The provider observes the patient's emotional state through body movements and facial expressions. The provider observes the person's *affect* or external expression of emotion. The provider uses the body language and the facial features to detect expressions of emotion. The following are types of affects:

- *Restricted or constricted affect*: A small reduction in the intensity of the affect.
- *Blunted affect*: A severe reduction in the intensity of the affect; much less emotion is shown compared to the restricted affect.
- *Flat affect*: A lack of emotional expression in both the face and the body language.
- *Labile affect*: Rapidly changing emotions that are unrelated to external events.
- *Inappropriate affect*: The emotional expressions are incongruent with the situation or the person's verbal message.

Psychological Testing

Many psychological tests are used to help diagnose behavioral health diseases and disorders. Tests are available to examine the following:

- *Intellectual functioning*: There are a variety of tests available, including the *Wechsler Adult Intelligence Scale (WAIS)*, which measures the verbal intelligent quotient (IQ), performance IQ, and full-scale IQ. It is used for people 16 years of age or older. Other versions of the Wechsler can be used for younger children.

- *Academic achievement*: General tests along with specific tests for math, oral and written language, and reading are available. *The Boehm Test of Basic Concepts* is an example of a test in this category. It tests a child's understanding of basic positional concepts. Using pictures, the child must select the correct one when given cues such as "over," "least," and "left."
- *Psychological process*: A variety of tests are available based on the person's age. For instance, the *Bender Visual Motor Gestalt Test* is used to evaluate a person's visual-motor maturity. It is used to screen for developmental delays and can be used to assess for neurologic issues and brain damage. This test is used for people 5 years or older.
- *Adaptive behavior*: These tests are used to evaluate a person's learning difficulties, ADHD, or other impairments related to speech, language, hearing, and motor skills. This is an example.
- *Personality and attitudes*: A variety of tests are available:
  - *Draw-a-Person (DAP) Test:* An analysis to measure nonverbal intelligence and screen for behavioral or emotional disorders in children.
  - *Minnesota Multiphasic Personality Inventory (MMPI):* A widely used and researched personality assessment. It is used to diagnose behavioral health disorders, to screen for certain high-risk jobs, and as part of criminal defense and custody issues in legal cases.
  - *Thematic Apperception Test (TAT):* A test in which patients are asked to make up stories about the pictures on cards they are shown. This may provide information about a patient's thoughts, attitudes, and emotional responses.

THE MEDICAL ASSISTANT'S ROLE REGARDING BEHAVIORAL HEALTH TREATMENTS

Medical assistants working in behavioral health must know the medication classifications typically used for conditions and the common types of psychotherapies used. The following sections discuss these treatments.

Medications

Patients with behavioral health diseases and disorders are prescribed a variety of medications. The following are some of the more common classifications of medications for behavioral health disorders:

- *Antianxiety*: Used to reduce anxiety, produce calmness, and release muscle tension
- *Anticonvulsant and mood stabilizer*: Used to treat mania and mixed episodes (mania and depression) with bipolar disorder
- *Antidepressant*: Used to treat depression, anxiety, and other behavioral health disorders
- *Antipsychotic*: Used to treat schizophrenia and bipolar disorder
- *Sedative-hypnotic*: Used to treat insomnia
- *Stimulant*: Used to treat ADHD

Refer to Table 38.4 for information on the medication classification, including a drug's indication for use, desired effect, side effects, adverse reactions, and generic and trade names. Medical assistants should be familiar with medications that are prescribed to patients.

Psychotherapy

Many behavior health diseases and disorders are treated with psychotherapy. Psychotherapy is commonly referred to as "talk therapy." It is a general term used for a variety of treatment techniques that help a person identify and change troubling behaviors, thoughts, or emotions. Behavioral health therapists are trained in several types of psychotherapy. Based on the person and the disorder being treated, the therapist may use one or more types of psychotherapy:

- *Cognitive behavioral therapy (CBT)*: A scientifically proven treatment that produces changes in behavior by helping the person face fears, role-play situations, and learn problem-solving skills to cope with difficult issues. It is used for many behavioral health disorders, including depression, anxiety disorders, substance use disorders, and eating disorders.
- *Dialectical behavioral therapy (DBT)*: This evidence-based CBT approach is used for individuals who are diagnosed with personality disorders, are suicidal, or engage in self-harm behaviors. DBT

TABLE 38.4 Medication Classifications

CLASSIFICATION	INFORMATION	GENERIC NAME (TRADE NAME)
Antianxiety	Indications for use: Produces calmness and relaxes muscle tension; sedation. Desired effects: Reduces anxiety and tension. Types: SSRI, SNRIs, tricyclic antidepressants (see antidepressants), and benzodiazepines. Side effects and adverse reactions: Drowsiness, weakness, blurred vision, GI distress, hypersensitivity, jaundice, arrhythmias.	*Benzodiazepines*: • lorazepam (Ativan, Lorazepam Intensol) • alprazolam (Xanax) • clonazepam (Klonopin)
Anticonvulsant and mood stabilizer	Indications for use: Treats epilepsy, trigeminal neuralgia, mania, and mixed episodes (mania and depression) with bipolar disorder Desired effects: Reduces the frequency and severity of seizures by reducing excessive stimulation of the brain. Side effects and adverse reactions: Sedation, vertigo, visual disturbances, GI disturbances, liver complications.	• carbamazepine (Tegretol, Equetro, Carbatrol) • lamotrigine (Lamictal) • topiramate (Topamax, Qudexy XR) • valproic acid (Depakene, Depakote) • gabapentin (Neurontin, Horizant, Gralise)

TABLE 38.4 Medication Classifications—continued

CLASSIFICATION	INFORMATION	GENERIC NAME (TRADE NAME)
Antidepressant	Indications for use: Treats depression, anxiety, and other neurologic disorders. Desired effect: Treats depression. Side effects and adverse reactions: Anorexia, anxiety, sexual dysfunction, fatigue, drowsiness, vertigo, weight gain, confusion, blurred vision.	*Selective serotonin reuptake inhibitors (SSRIs):* • fluoxetine (Prozac, Rapiflux, Sarafem, Selfemra) • citalopram (Celexa) • escitalopram (Lexapro) • sertraline (Zoloft) *Serotonin and norepinephrine reuptake inhibitors (SNRIs):* • venlafaxine • duloxetine (Cymbalta) *Atypical antidepressants:* • bupropion (Wellbutrin, Zyban) *Serotonin modulators:* • trazodone (Oleptro) *Tricyclic antidepressants:* • amitriptyline *Monamine oxidase inhibitors (MAOIs):* • phenelzine (Nardil)
Antipsychotic	Indications for use: Treats the symptoms of schizophrenia and bipolar disorder. Desired effect: Alters chemical actions in the brain. Side effects and adverse reactions: GI distress, hypotension, electrocardiographic (ECG) changes, vertigo, sedation, headache, photosensitivity.	*Typical antipsychotics:* • haloperidol • chlorpromazine *Atypical antipsychotics:* • olanzapine (Zyprexa) • lurasidone (Latuda) • aripiprazole (Abilify) • risperidone (Risperdal) • quetiapine (Seroquel)
Sedative-hypnotic	Indications for use: Treats insomnia; obtain sedation (lower doses). Desired effects: Slows activity in the brain to allow sleep. Side effects and adverse reactions: Daytime sedation, confusion, dry mouth, hypersensitivity.	• eszopiclone (Lunesta) • temazepam (Restoril) • zolpidem (Ambien, Edluar, Zolpimist)
Stimulant	Indications for use: Treats attention deficit/hyperactivity disorder (ADHD) and narcolepsy. Desired effects: Stimulates the brain and body; making the messages move faster between the brain and the body. The person becomes more alert and physically active. Side effects and adverse reactions: arrhythmias, aggression, memory loss, flushing, hypertension, restlessness, fainting.	• atomoxetine (Strattera) • methylphenidate (Concerta, Methylin, Ritalin LA)

focuses on behavioral change, problem solving, and the regulation of emotions in a manner that is socially acceptable.

- *Exposure therapy*: A type of CBT that is used to help people process their traumatic experiences or feared situations. The person revisits and recounts the memories, which gradually helps the person emotionally process the experience or situation. The person may start by thinking about the object or situation, then progress to looking at pictures of it, getting near it, and then touching it or experiencing it for short periods of time.
- *Eye movement desensitization and reprocessing (EMDR)*: Used to process and resolve traumatic memories (e.g., PTSD). During the therapy, the person concentrates on the memory while focusing on controlled stimuli (e.g., eye movements or sounds). The patient discusses any new thoughts that occur and continues until the memory is no longer distressing.
- *Interpersonal psychotherapy (IPT)*: Used to treat behavioral health disorders, such as eating disorders and major depression, by helping the person understand the relationship between symptoms and social interactions, thus improving social skills and functioning.
- *Play therapy*: Used for children who are experiencing behavioral, emotional, social, or relational disorders. The child is able to express feelings and thoughts using play and the therapeutic relationship.

- *Psychodynamic therapy*: Used to treat depression, addictions, social anxiety disorder, and eating disorders. It focuses on helping the patient recognize, express, and overcome negative feelings and repressed emotions so that the person's interpersonal experiences and relationships improve.

CLOSING COMMENTS

Patient Coaching

In the behavioral health environment, the medical assistant has an important role in coaching patients on their medications. Patients should be aware of the following details:

- When and how to take the medication
- What to do if the medication is forgotten
- What side effects may occur
- When to contact the provider

Compliance can be an issue with medications in behavioral health. Patients who are experiencing issues may stop the medication. This may increase the signs and symptoms of the disorder. For some disorders, this can be a life-threatening complication. Sometimes hospitalization is required until medications can stabilize the situation.

Legal and Ethical Issues

Under the Health Insurance Portability and Accountability Act (HIPAA), **psychotherapy notes** are treated with higher levels of confidentiality than other health records. Psychotherapy notes need to be stored separately from the patient health record. They are not released with other health records and must be specifically indicated by the patient to be released.

If an electronic health record system is used, access to the psychotherapy notes must be limited to the behavioral health staff that require the notes for their job. Additional information from the visit is not held at a higher level of confidentiality and includes prescriptions, session times, types and frequency of treatments, and results of clinical tests.

Like HIPAA, many federal and state laws address the confidentiality of drug and substance abuse information. These laws require these patient health records to be held at a higher level of confidentiality.

Patient-Centered Care

In behavioral health, patient-centered care not only includes the patient but may also include the family. Behavioral health professionals need to develop a strong professional, therapeutic relationship with patients. This relationship provides the emotional support that helps patients feel accepted so that they are willing to share their concerns, thoughts, and feelings with behavioral health professionals.

Often families play an important part in the management and treatment of behavioral health disorders. Some of these disorders may come from issues related to family relationships. Other times, the family needs to provide emotional support to assist the patient through treatment. Depending on the situation and the patient, family members may be brought into the therapy to ultimately help the patient through the situation or effectively manage the disorder.

Inappropriate comments to the patient or about the patient to others are unprofessional and should not happen. Remember, all information about the patient is confidential.

Professional Behaviors

Medical assistants working outside the behavioral health department will often come in contact with patients who have behavioral health disorders. It is important for medical assistants to remain professional in their nonverbal and verbal communication. If patients make inappropriate or nonsensical statements, seem "off" in their affect, or demonstrate other unusual behaviors, the medical assistant should relay the information to the provider.

SUMMARY OF SCENARIO

Mike has learned a lot about the policies and procedures used by the behavioral health staff. At first, he was uncomfortable working with patients who were experiencing signs and symptoms of behavioral health disorders. To his surprise, Mike has found that working with patients in the behavioral health environment is interesting and rewarding. Because Mike had learned about these conditions in school, he was nervous and did not know how he would deal with such situations. However, Mike is professional and feels he has provided excellent patient-centered care. Mike realizes he still has a lot more to learn because there are more than 200 behavioral health disorders and many substance-use disorders. He looks forward to spending more time with the behavioral health staff.

SUMMARY OF LEARNING OBJECTIVES

1. **Examine the types of behavioral health professionals and their use of the *Diagnostic and Statistical Manual of Mental Disorders*.**
   Common behavioral health professionals include psychiatrists, psychologists, social workers, cognitive behavioral therapists (CBTs), psychiatric nurses, substance abuse (or addiction) therapists or counselors, and mental health therapists or counselors. In many states, most of these healthcare professionals need a license to practice, and they all have different degrees of training and specialties.

   The *Diagnostic and Statistical Manual of Mental Disorders* (DSM) provides descriptions, signs, symptoms, and other criteria for diagnosing behavioral health disorders. The DSM-5 contains the International Classification of Disease (ICD) codes required for insurance reimbursement and monitoring morbidity and mortality statistics.
2. **Explain common signs, symptoms, and etiologies of behavioral health diseases and disorders over the life span.**

Continued

SUMMARY OF LEARNING OBJECTIVES—*continued*

Behavioral health disorders are conditions that cause changes in the mood, behavior, or thoughts of an individual. Common etiologies include biological factors, life experiences, and a family history of behavioral health problems. A variety of common signs and symptoms exist.

3. **Differentiate among various anxiety disorders, including the signs, symptoms, etiology, diagnostic procedures, and treatments.**
With an anxiety disorder, the anxious feeling is a constant companion, and it gets worse with time. The anxiety interferes with daily living—for instance, school, work, and relationships. Anxiety disorders discussed in this chapter included generalized anxiety disorder, obsessive-compulsive disorder, hoarding disorder, panic disorder, phobia, and social anxiety disorder.
4. **Differentiate among various forms of depression and other mood disorders, including the signs, symptoms, etiology, diagnostic procedures, and treatments.**
Depression is the second leading behavioral health condition and can happen at any age. The symptoms affect how a person acts, thinks, feels, and handles daily life. Types of depression and mood disorders discussed include persistent depressive disorder, postpartum depression, psychotic depression, seasonal affective disorder, and bipolar disorder.
5. **Differentiate among various behavioral disorders, including the signs, symptoms, etiology, diagnostic procedures, and treatments.**
Behavioral disorders in children involve a pattern of disruptive behaviors for at least 6 months that cause issues at home, in school, and in social situations. Behavioral disorders include attention deficit hyperactivity disorder (ADHD), oppositional defiant disorder (ODD), and conduct disorder (CD).
6. **Differentiate among various eating disorders, including the signs, symptoms, etiology, diagnostic procedures, and treatments.**
Eating disorders affect both sexes and can co-exist with other illnesses. Eating disorders discussed include anorexia nervosa, binge eating disorder, bulimia nervosa, pica, rumination disorder, and avoidant/restrictive food intake disorder (ARFID).
7. **Differentiate among autism spectrum disorder, dissociative disorder, personality disorder, post-traumatic stress disorder, and schizophrenia.**
Autism spectrum disorder (ASD) is a developmental disorder where the person has difficulty interacting and communicating with others. There can be a wide range of symptoms and severity.
Dissociative disorders cause a person to involuntarily escape from reality. Dissociative disorder can cause a variety of conditions, such as amnesia and alternative identities. Examples of dissociative disorders include dissociative amnesia, dissociative identity disorder, and depersonalization-derealization disorder.
Personality disorders include a group of conditions that involve long-term patterns of unhealthy and inflexible thoughts and behaviors that affect relationships and work. Personality disorders are grouped into clusters A, B, and C.
Post-traumatic stress disorder (PTSD) is a condition that occurs after a person experiences or witnesses a traumatic or terrifying event, such as war, assault, an accident, or a natural disaster. The symptoms of PTSD can vary over time and from person to person.
Schizophrenia, a debilitating disorder, causes disruptions in thought processes, perceptions, emotional responsiveness, and social interactions. It is usually diagnosed in the late teen years to the early 30s. Schizophrenia can co-exist with another behavioral health disorder.
8. **Differentiate between substance use disorders and other addictions.**
Substance use disorder includes both substance use and substance dependence. Substance use disorder is measured from mild to severe and includes drug and alcohol use. Other types of addictions—exercise, gambling, gaming, internet use, and shopping—were also summarized.
9. **Examine the etiology, warning signs, protective factors, and treatments for suicidal behavior.**
Suicide is death caused by a self-inflicted injury with an intent to die as a result of the behavior. A *suicide attempt* is a nonfatal, self-directed, potentially harmful behavior with an intent to die due to the behavior. The attempt may not cause an injury. *Suicidal ideation* refers to thinking about, considering, or planning suicide.
10. **Examine the medical assistant's role regarding behavioral health examinations.**
Medical assistants room patients and obtain vital signs and medical histories. If a patient was diagnosed with an eating disorder, the provider might have the medical assistant weigh the patient backward and not notify the patient of the weight. Preparing prescription refills is also part of the medical assistant's role in some facilities.
11. **Examine the medical assistant's role regarding behavioral health diagnostic procedures.**
Some behavioral health facilities may have the medical assistant help with specimen collection and testing (e.g., venipuncture, urine drug test). Behavioral health diagnostic testing is done by the psychologist, and the medical assistant should have an understanding of the tests. Mental status testing (also called neurocognitive testing) assesses a person's ability to think, and providers can identify cognitive impairments. There are several types of psychological testing used to diagnose behavioral health disorders.
12. **Examine the medical assistant's role with treatments used for behavioral health diseases and disorders.**
The most common treatments for behavioral health disorders include medications and psychotherapy. The medications used for behavioral health disorders include antianxiety, anticonvulsants and mood stabilizers, antidepressants, antipsychotics, sedative-hypnotics, and stimulants. Psychotherapy is commonly referred to as *talk therapy*. Behavioral health therapists are trained in several types of psychotherapy.

39 ENDOCRINOLOGY

SCENARIO

Cecilia Cukier, CMA (AAMA), has worked at Walden-Martin Family Medical (WMFM) Clinic for 3 years. She enjoys working with the primary care providers. Working with patients who have diabetes mellitus has been a special interest of hers since her medical assistant practicum in college. When a position was posted to work with the outreach endocrinology team, which came from a clinic 50 miles away, Cecilia applied for the position. She was accepted and now will be working 2 days a week with the endocrinology team, which sees WMFM Clinic patients. During the remaining 3 days, Cecilia will continue to work with the primary care team.

Cecilia is excited to start working with the endocrinology team and patients. She has decided to review the anatomy, physiology, and pathology of the endocrine system in preparation for her new duties.

While studying this chapter, think about the following questions:

- What structures are in the endocrine system?
- What are the functions of the endocrine system?
- What are commonly diagnosed endocrine diseases and disorders? What are the etiologies, signs and symptoms, diagnostic processes, and treatments?
- What are the medical assistant's primary responsibilities when working with patients with endocrine diseases and disorders?

LEARNING OBJECTIVES

1. Examine the connection between the endocrine and nervous systems.
2. Differentiate between the hormones of the anterior lobe and those of the posterior lobe of the pituitary gland.
3. Differentiate between the hormones of the thyroid and those of parathyroid glands.
4. Differentiate between the hormones of the adrenal cortex and those of the adrenal medulla.
5. Differentiate among the hormones of the pancreas, thymus gland, gonads, and pineal gland.
6. Examine the physiology of the endocrine system.
7. Examine pituitary gland diseases and disorders, including the signs, symptoms, etiology, diagnostic procedures, and treatments.
8. Examine thyroid gland and parathyroid gland diseases and disorders, including the signs, symptoms, etiology, diagnostic procedures, and treatments.
9. Examine adrenal gland diseases and disorders, including the signs, symptoms, etiology, diagnostic procedures, and treatments.
10. Examine pancreatic diseases and disorders, including the signs, symptoms, etiology, diagnostic procedures, and treatments.
11. Examine the medical assistant's role in examinations, diagnostic procedures, and treatments for endocrine diseases and disorders.

VOCABULARY

calcium A naturally occurring element that is necessary for many body functions, including strong bones and teeth, proper blood clotting, nerve conduction, and muscle contractions.

cataract Clouding of the lens, leading to decreased vision.

diabetic retinopathy (die ah BET ik reh tin OP ah thee) Damages the blood vessels in the retina, leading to loss of vision and eventual blindness.

diffuse To spread, scatter, disperse, or move.

electrolyte (ee LEK troe lite) A chemical substance that separates into ions in solution (water) and is capable of conducting an electric current. Electrolytes found in body fluids include sodium, potassium, calcium, magnesium, chloride, bicarbonate, and phosphate.

exocrine A glandular secretion released through a duct.

fatty acids Result when fats are broken down; used by the body for energy and tissue development.

glaucoma (glou KOE mah) Increase in the fluid pressure in the eye; can lead to blindness if not treated.

homeostasis (hoe mee oh STAY sis) The internal environment of the body that is compatible with life. A steady state that is created by all the body systems working together to provide a consistent and unvarying internal environment.

libido Sexual drive or instinct.

mediastinum (mee dee AH sti nuhm) The space in the thoracic cavity that lies between the lungs, containing the heart, trachea, and esophagus.

VOCABULARY—*continued*

negative feedback loop A process in which a change from the normal ranges causes a response that opposes or decreases the change, thus helping maintain homeostasis.

nucleus A specialized organelle of a cell that is encased in a membrane and directs growth, metabolism, and reproduction of the cell.

organelle A structure within a cell that performs a specific function.

positive feedback loop A process in which a change causes a response that enhances that change.

preeclampsia (pree ih KLAMP see ah) A form of toxemia during pregnancy, characterized by high blood pressure, fluid retention, and protein in the urine. May progress to eclampsia.

receptors Structures or sites on or in a cell that bind with substances such as hormones, antigens, or drugs.

target cell A cell selectively affected by a specific agent, such as a drug, hormone, or virus.

water deprivation test A test to measure the amount and concentration of urine produced when water is withheld from a patient for a period of time.

INTRODUCTION

Endocrinology is the healthcare specialty that deals with endocrine disorders. These disorders relate to endocrine glands, hormones, and hormonal effects on the body. An *endocrinologist* is a specialist involved in the diagnosis, treatment, and prevention of endocrine disorders.

Besides being seen in the endocrine department, patients with endocrine concerns are typically seen in primary and urgent care departments. Medical assistants should have a strong understanding of common endocrinology diseases, diagnostic tests, and treatments.

NEUROENDOCRINE SYSTEM

The endocrine system is composed of ductless glands throughout the body. Endocrine glands release hormones directly into the bloodstream, and the blood transports them to **target cells.** The hormones act as messengers to the target cells, telling the cells to alter their functions to help maintain **homeostasis** in the body. Hormones function as the body's chemical messengers, transferring information from one group of cells to another. They control metabolism, growth, mood, sexual maturity, reproduction, and water and **electrolyte** balance. Hormone levels vary and can be affected by outside factors, such as illness and stress. Figure 39.1 shows the endocrine glands and their locations.

Maintaining Homeostasis

The nervous system and the endocrine system can work alone or together. Working jointly, as a neuroendocrine system, they perform communication functions and maintain homeostasis. The brain sends out signals to and continually receives feedback from the endocrine system. The nervous system communicates quickly through nerve impulses and delivers rapid responses to maintain homeostasis. The endocrine system communicates slowly through hormones, which maintain homeostasis for a longer period of time. The body needs both systems working together through communication to maintain homeostasis.

Hypothalamus

The *hypothalamus,* located in the middle of the brain, is the major connection for the neuroendocrine system. It plays an important role in controlling the endocrine system. When the hypothalamus detects rising levels of a target organ's hormones, it sends a signal to the pituitary gland to release or prevent pituitary hormone production.

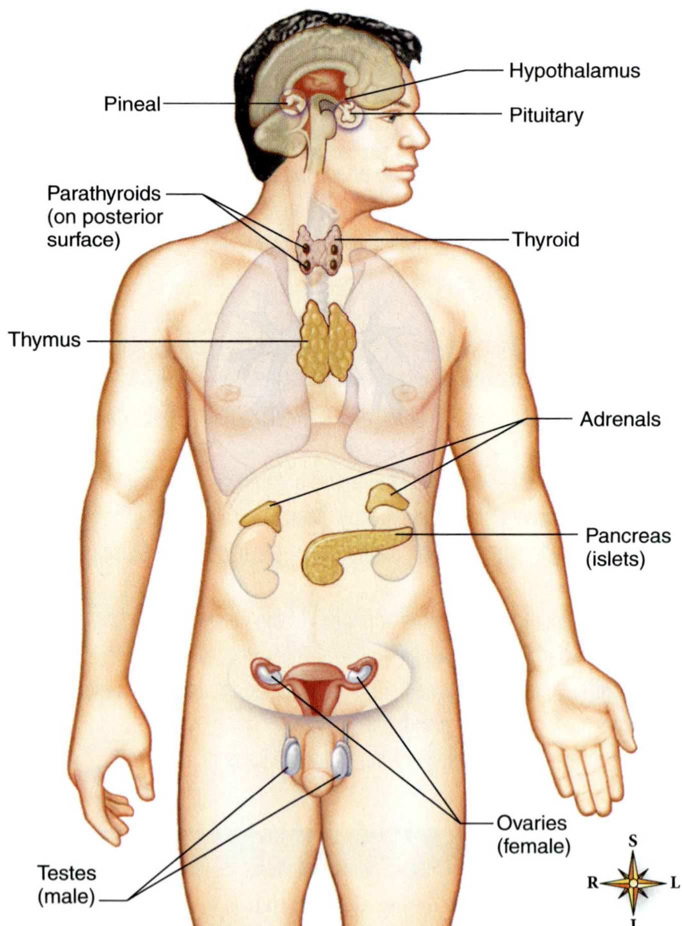

FIGURE 39.1 Location of the endocrine glands. (From Patton KT, Thibodeau GA: *Anatomy and physiology*, ed 9, St. Louis, 2016, Mosby.)

The hypothalamus is also responsible for the production of antidiuretic hormone (ADH) and oxytocin. These two hormones are produced by the hypothalamus and stored and secreted by the posterior lobe of the pituitary gland. They will be discussed in more detail in the next section.

ANATOMY OF THE PITUITARY GLAND

The *pituitary gland* is also known as the *hypophysis.* The pituitary gland is a pea-sized gland connected to the hypothalamus by the *infundibulum,* a small stalk of tissue. The hormones from the

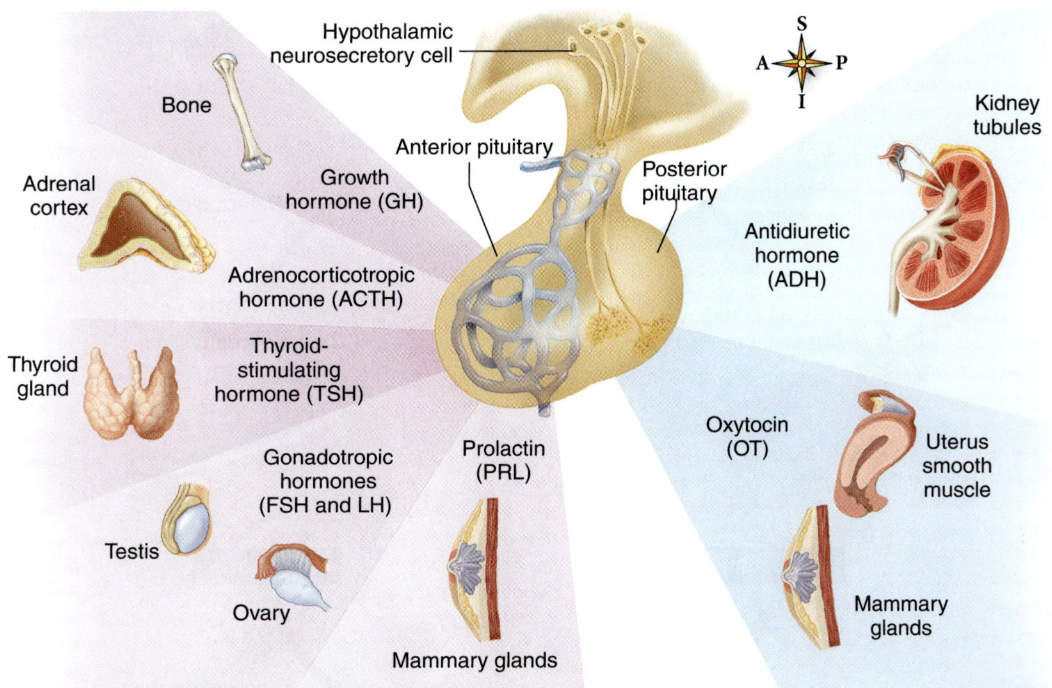

FIGURE 39.2 Anterior and posterior pituitary hormones and the target organs. (From Patton KT, Thibodeau GA: *The human body in health and disease*, ed 6, St. Louis, 2014, Mosby.)

pituitary control the other endocrine glands; thus, the pituitary gland is called the "master gland." The pituitary gland is composed of two lobes. The anterior and posterior lobes act as separate glands, each having its own function.

Anterior Lobe of the Pituitary Gland

The anterior lobe, also known as the *adenohypophysis*, produces and secretes these hormones (Figure 39.2):

- *Adrenocorticotropic hormone* (ACTH): Causes the adrenal cortex to produce and release steroids (e.g., cortisol).
- *Follicle-stimulating hormone* (FSH): Stimulates the development of ova (eggs) through ovulation in females and stimulates the seminiferous tubules to produce sperm in males.
- *Growth hormone* (GH): Stimulates growth of the long bones and muscles in children and teens. Growth hormone is also involved with glucose metabolism in the body. Growth hormone is also called *somatotropin* or *somatotropic hormone* (STH).
- *Luteinizing hormone* (LH): In females, it stimulates the ovaries to produce estrogen, ova to mature, and the production of progesterone. LH also initiates ovulation and signals the corpus luteum to develop. In men, it stimulates interstitial cells in the testes to develop and secrete testosterone. Thus, in men, LH is also called *interstitial cell–stimulating hormone* (ICSH).
- *Prolactin (PRL)*: Stimulates breast tissue development and milk production toward the end of pregnancy and after childbirth.
- *Thyroid-stimulating hormone (TSH)*: Stimulates the thyroid gland to release T_3 and T_4. (More information about the thyroid will be presented later in the chapter.)

Posterior Lobe of the Pituitary Gland

The posterior lobe, also known as the *neurohypophysis*, is composed of nervous tissue. It does not produce hormones but stores hormones produced by the hypothalamus. The hormones are transported from the hypothalamus to the posterior lobe directly through the infundibulum. The posterior lobe stores the hormones until it gets a signal from the hypothalamus to release them into the bloodstream. The blood then carries the hormones to the target organ (see Figure 39.2). Two hormones are released by the posterior lobe:

- *Antidiuretic hormone* (ADH): Also called *vasopressin.* Stimulates contraction of the blood vessels, raising the blood pressure. It also stimulates the kidney tubules to reabsorb water, which concentrates the urine.
- *Oxytocin* (OT): During the delivery of a child, OT is released and stimulates the uterine muscles to contract. This is an example of a **positive feedback loop** (Figure 39.3). OT also helps release breast milk by stimulating the contraction of the muscles surrounding the mammary ducts.

CRITICAL THINKING APPLICATION **39.1**

Cecilia is struggling to remember the hormones secreted by the posterior and anterior lobes of the pituitary gland. What might be some helpful ways to remember the hormones from this gland?

ANATOMY OF THE THYROID AND PARATHYROID GLANDS

The thyroid gland and the parathyroid glands are located in the neck. Both glands have very unique functions. The following sections discuss these glands.

Thyroid Gland

The thyroid gland is a butterfly-shaped gland in the neck above the collarbone. The thyroid produces, stores, and secretes the following:

- *Triiodothyronine* (T_3): Regulates metabolism and increases the basal metabolic rate.
- *Thyroxine* (T_4): Regulates metabolism and increases the basal metabolic rate. It also supports the activities of growth hormones.

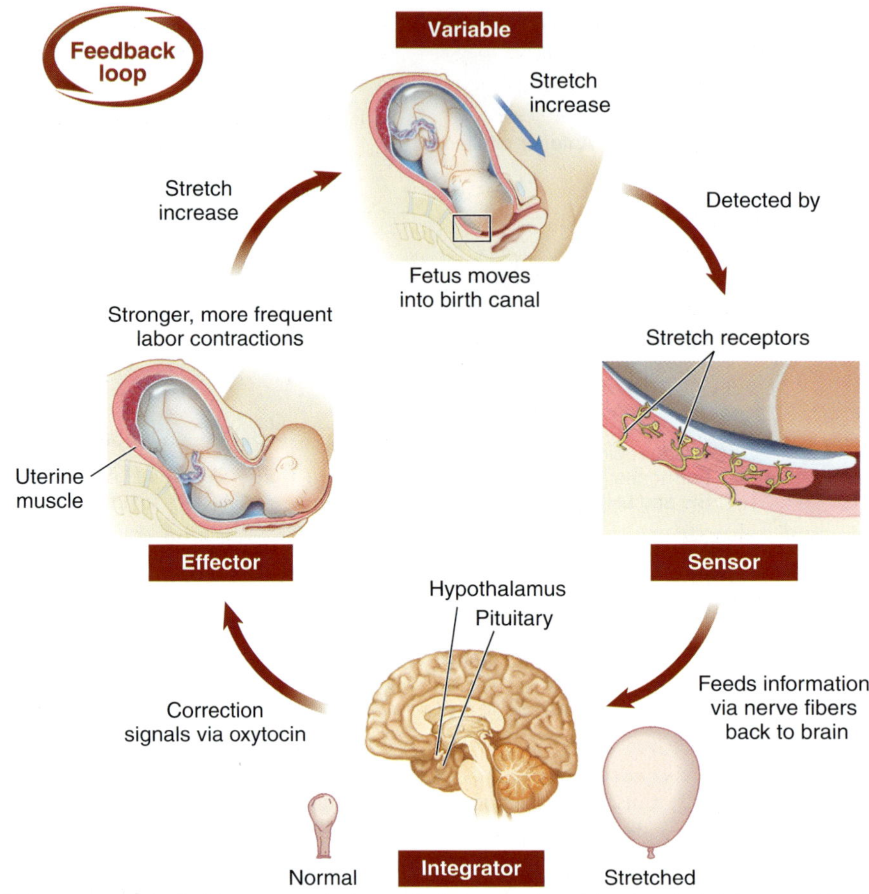

FIGURE 39.3 Positive feedback loop. An example of positive feedback occurs when a baby is born. As the baby is pushed from the womb *(uterus)* into the birth canal *(vagina)*, stretch receptors detect the movement of the baby. Stretch information is fed back to the brain, triggering the pituitary gland to secrete a hormone called *oxytocin* (OT). OT travels through the bloodstream to the uterus, where it stimulates stronger contractions. Stronger contractions push the baby farther along the birth canal, thereby increasing stretch and stimulating the release of more OT. Uterine contractions quickly get stronger and stronger until the baby is pushed out of the body, and the positive feedback loop is broken. OT also can be injected therapeutically by a physician to stimulate labor contractions. (From Patton KT, Thibodeau GA: *The human body in health and disease*, ed 7, St. Louis, 2018, Elsevier.)

- *Calcitonin*: Regulates calcium and phosphate levels in the blood. It works against the parathyroid hormone action. Calcitonin helps lower blood **calcium** levels by inhibiting osteoclast activity. By inhibiting the breakdown of bone, it helps to retain calcium in the bones. Calcitonin also works in the kidney by reducing the resorption of calcium, thus also lowering the blood calcium level.

When thyroid hormone levels decrease in the body, the hypothalamus secretes TSH-releasing hormone. This hormone "tells" the anterior lobe of the pituitary gland to produce TSH, which stimulates the thyroid to produce hormones. Iodine from our diet is absorbed in the blood and carried to the thyroid gland. Iodine is required to produce T_3 and T_4.

Increasing the Basal Metabolic Rate

T_3 and T_4 hormones increase the **basal metabolic rate,** which has the following functions:

- Causes an increase in the body temperature and pulse rate; it also creates a stronger heartbeat.
- Helps the brain mature in children and promotes growth.
- Improves concentration and faster reflexes.
- Uses more energy (calories).

Parathyroid Glands

The parathyroid glands are four pea-sized glands located on the back side of the thyroid gland. They secrete *parathyroid hormone* (PTH), which helps regulate calcium and phosphorus levels in the body. When the blood calcium level decreases, PTH is secreted, causing calcium to be released from bone. The released calcium is absorbed in the blood, which increases the blood calcium levels.

A balance needs to be maintained. If too much PTH is secreted, hyperparathyroidism occurs, causing bones to lose calcium and the blood calcium level to rise. If too little PTH is secreted, hypoparathyroidism occurs. The blood calcium level decreases, and the blood phosphorus level increases.

ANATOMY OF THE ADRENAL GLANDS

The adrenal glands are located on the top of each kidney. The outer part of the gland is the *adrenal cortex*, and the inner part is called the *adrenal medulla*.

Adrenal Cortex

The adrenal cortex produces cortical hormones, also called *steroids*. As a group, these three hormones are called corticosteroids:

- *Mineralocorticoids*: Regulate the electrolytes in the body. Aldosterone, the most important mineralocorticoid, regulates the sodium and water balance in the body through the reabsorption of sodium and water in the kidneys. As the sodium is reabsorbed into the blood, hydrogen or potassium is excreted into the urine.
- *Glucocorticoids*: Regulate protein, fat, and carbohydrate metabolism. They also hasten the breakdown of proteins into amino acids, which are converted to glucose in the liver. This process increases the blood glucose level. Norepinephrine and epinephrine need glucocorticoids to constrict blood vessels, which increases blood pressure. Glucocorticoids also have anti-inflammatory properties. The main glucocorticoid secreted is cortisol (also called *hydrocortisone*). Cortisone and corticosterone are produced in lesser amounts. Stress can also increase the number of glucocorticoids secreted.
- *Gonadocorticoids*: Small amounts of male sex hormones (androgens) are secreted and responsible for some of the secondary sexual characteristics (e.g., pubic and axillary hair) in both males and females during puberty.

The hypothalamus and the anterior lobe of the pituitary gland (through the secretion of ACTH) regulate the corticosteroids secreted by the adrenal cortex.

CRITICAL THINKING APPLICATION 39.2

The actions of mineralocorticoids and glucocorticoids confuse Cecilia. Summarize the actions of these two corticosteroids.

Adrenal Medulla

The hypothalamus, with the help of the sympathetic nervous system, stimulates the adrenal medulla to secrete these nonsteroid hormones:

- *Epinephrine* (adrenaline): Secreted in response to physical or mental stress, providing the fight-or-flight response. It increases the heart rate and strength of the contractions, blood pressure, and blood glucose level. It also relaxes the smooth muscles in the bronchioles. These changes allow more glucose and oxygenated blood to get to the cells for the fight-or-flight response.
- *Norepinephrine* (noradrenalin): Also secreted in times of stress. It increases the blood glucose level, heart rate, and the force of the heart's contractions; in addition, it causes vasoconstriction, thus raising the blood pressure.

ANATOMY OF OTHER ENDOCRINE GLANDS

Additional endocrine glands include the pancreas, thymus gland, gonads, and pineal gland. The following sections describe these glands.

Pancreas

The *pancreas* is located inferior and posterior to the stomach. It has both endocrine and **exocrine** functions. As already discussed, an endocrine gland releases hormones into the blood, whereas an exocrine gland releases secretions through ducts. The pancreas releases digestive enzymes into the small intestine through pancreatic ducts.

The pancreas contains *pancreatic islets* or *islets of Langerhans*, which produce hormones. The pancreas produces several hormones:

- *Glucagon*: Secreted by the alpha islet cells. It raises the blood glucose level in two different ways. It stimulates the stored glycogen in the liver to be converted into glucose. It also stimulates amino and **fatty acids** in the liver to be converted into glucose. The glucose is absorbed by the bloodstream, which increases the blood glucose level.
- *Insulin*: Secreted by the beta islet cells. Normally after a meal, the blood glucose level is elevated. This triggers the pancreas to release insulin. Insulin helps move the blood glucose from the blood to the cells. This lowers the blood glucose level. This is an example of a **negative feedback loop** (Figure 39.4).
- *Somatostatin*: Secreted by the delta islet cells; it regulates the other pancreatic hormones and inhibits the secretion of growth hormones.
- *Ghrelin* (GHRL): Secreted by the epsilon islet cells. Research has found that GHRL works in the brain to regulate body weight, glucose metabolism, and food intake. Multiple additional actions of ghrelin have been reported in research studies, including its involvement with learning, memory, intestinal peristalsis, gastric acid secretion, sleep/wake rhythm (circadian rhythms), reward-seeking behavior, and taste sensation.

Thymus Gland

The *thymus gland* is in the **mediastinum** behind the sternum (breastbone) and secretes *thymosin* and *thymopoietin* hormones. These hormones stimulate the production and maturity of T cells, a type of lymphocyte (white blood cell). T cells have an important role in immunity.

Gonads

The *gonads* are considered the primary sex organs. The male gonads are the testes, and the female gonads are the ovaries. Both types of gonads produce hormones:

- Testes: Secrete *testosterone*, which stimulates the development of male secondary sexual characteristics (e.g., voice changes, growth of facial and pubic hair). Testosterone also promotes sperm production and muscle development.
- Ovaries: Produce *estrogen* and *progesterone*. Estrogen stimulates the development of breasts and other female secondary sexual characteristics. Progesterone helps maintain a pregnancy. Both estrogen and progesterone are important in the menstrual cycle.

Pineal Gland

The pineal gland is located deep within the brain and secretes the hormone melatonin. Melatonin helps regulate waking and sleeping patterns and may affect seasonal reactions to the availability of sunlight.

PHYSIOLOGY OF THE ENDOCRINE SYSTEM

The physiology of the endocrine system involves hormone regulation, target cells, hormone action, and prostaglandins. These topics are discussed in depth in the following sections.

Mechanisms of Hormone Regulation

The goal of hormone regulation is to maintain homeostasis. Nervous system stimulation, endocrine control, and feedback systems regulate hormone secretion. The following examples demonstrate these three mechanisms:

- *Nervous system regulation*: During a stressful event, the adrenal medulla releases adrenaline (epinephrine) in response to stimulation from the sympathetic nervous system.

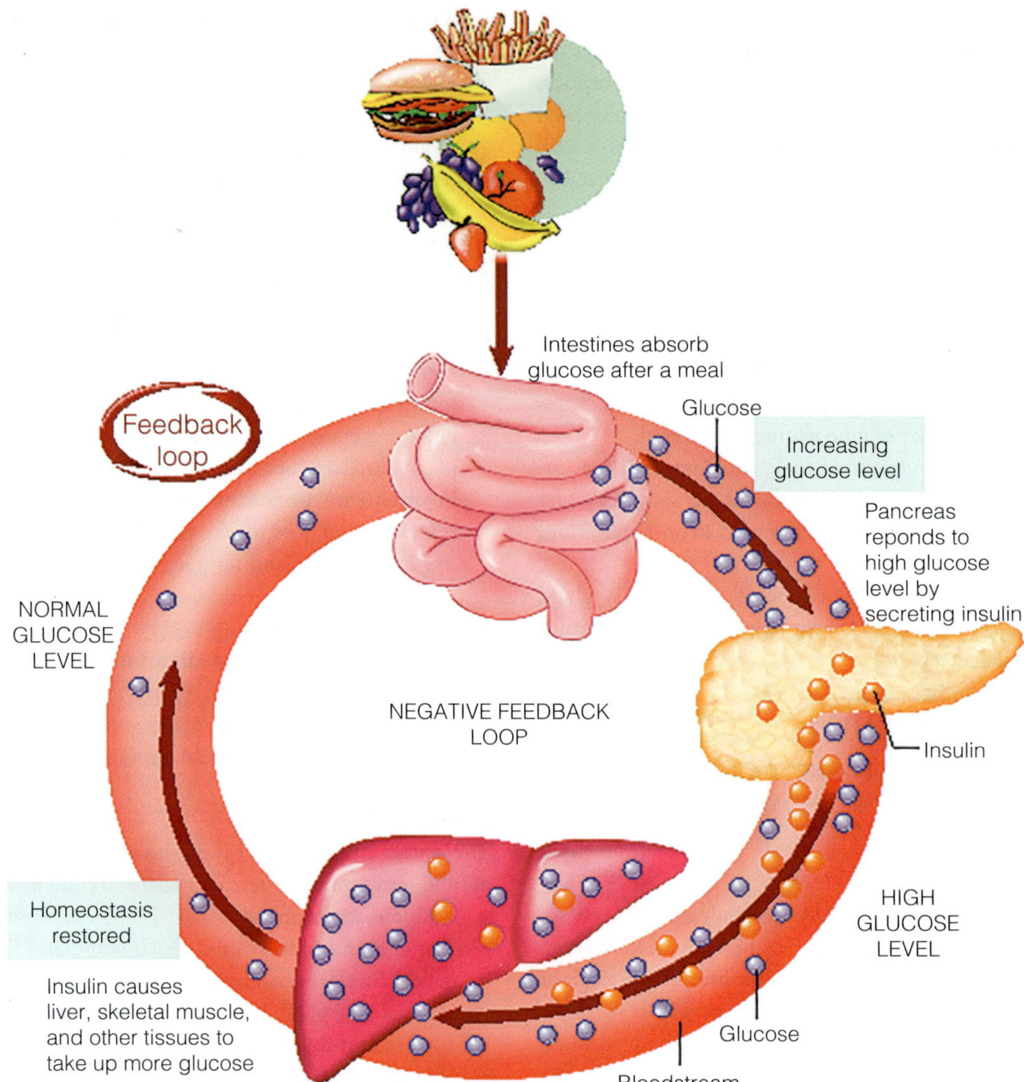

FIGURE 39.4 Negative feedback loop. The secretion of most hormones is regulated by negative feedback mechanisms that tend to reverse any deviations from normal. In this example, an increase in blood glucose triggers the secretion of insulin. Because insulin promotes glucose uptake by cells, the blood glucose level is restored to its lower, normal level. (From Patton KT, Thibodeau GA: *The human body in health and disease*, ed 7, St. Louis, 2018, Elsevier.)

- *Endocrine control regulation*: TSH from the anterior pituitary stimulates the thyroid to secrete T_3 and T_4. (A hormone from one gland stimulates another gland to secrete a hormone.)
- *Feedback system regulation*: A negative feedback loop system example: If the calcium blood level falls below normal, the parathyroid glands are stimulated to release PTH. PTH increases blood calcium levels by stimulating the absorption of calcium from the intestines or by chemically breaking down bone to release stored calcium into the blood. The change in the blood calcium level is detected by the parathyroid gland, which then stops production of PTH. (An imbalance activates the endocrine gland, which acts to correct the imbalance by stopping the hormone secretion process.)

Target Cells

Each hormone released into the bloodstream has specific target cells for action. The target cells have **receptors** that attract only certain hormones. The cell membrane only lets selected hormones pass into the cell and affect cellular action.

Hormone Action

There are two categories of hormones: nonsteroid hormones and steroid hormones. All hormones are messengers, but how they deliver their message is where they differ. Both types of hormones maintain homeostasis.

Nonsteroid hormones are made up of protein or amino acids. This type of hormone attaches to a target cell membrane. Another molecule takes the message from the nonsteroid hormone and carries it to the target cell **nucleus** or **organelle,** which puts the message into action in the cell.

Steroid hormones are small *lipid-soluble* (fat-soluble) molecules that attach to a target cell membrane and then pass directly into the target cell. Once inside the target cell, steroid hormones travel to and enter the nucleus. They bind to a receptor site, which creates a hormone–receptor site complex. This complex communicates its message with deoxyribonucleic acid (DNA) in the nucleus, and the DNA tells the cell how to put the hormone's message into action.

Prostaglandins

Prostaglandins (PGs), also known as *tissue hormones,* are substances found in many body tissues. PGs are produced in tissues and **diffuse** only a short distance to affect cells in their local area. They help regulate processes such as respiration, blood pressure, digestive system secretions, and reproductive functions. They are powerful molecules that are made locally and act locally.

Life Span Changes

Changes in hormone levels vary with age. Some increase and others decrease. The following hormones decrease with age:

- *Estrogen*: In females, the declining level leads to menopause.
- *Testosterone*: In males, levels gradually decrease.
- *Growth hormone*.
- *Melatonin*: Older adults may experience a loss of the normal sleep/wake cycles.

Cortisol, insulin, and thyroid hormone usually remain unchanged or slightly decrease with age. Norepinephrine, epinephrine, parathyroid hormone, follicle-stimulating hormone, and luteinizing hormone may increase with age.

Common Signs and Symptoms of Endocrine Conditions

Many diseases affect the endocrine system. Most of the pathology of the endocrine system is the result of either hyper- (excessive) or hypo- (deficient) hormonal secretion. Here are the common signs and symptoms of endocrine conditions:

- *Exophthalmia*, a noticeable protrusion of the eyeball
- *Glucosuria*, the presence of glucose in the urine
- *Goiter*, the swelling of the neck and visible enlargement of the thyroid gland
- *Hirsutism*, excessive facial or body hair growth in women
- *Hypocalcemia*, a low blood calcium level
- *Hypoglycemia*, a low blood glucose (sugar) level
- *Ketoacidosis*, the presence of ketones in the blood that cause metabolic acidosis (a pH imbalance due to too much acid)
- *Ketonuria*, the presence of ketones in the urine
- *Polydipsia*, excessive thirst
- *Polyphagia*, excessive eating
- *Polyuria*, excessive urine volume

PITUITARY GLAND DISORDERS AND DISORDERS

Anterior pituitary gland dysfunction can lead to several diseases and disorders. Hypersecretion of growth hormone causes acromegaly and gigantism, whereas hyposecretion causes dwarfism. Hypersecretion of prolactin causes prolactinoma. Women with hyposecretion of prolactin are unable to maintain breast milk production. Hyposecretion of all the anterior pituitary hormones causes panhypopituitarism.

Posterior pituitary gland hypersecretion of ADH causes syndrome of inappropriate antidiuretic hormone (SIADH), and hyposecretion causes diabetes insipidus. The following sections discuss the more common pituitary diseases.

Acromegaly

Acromegaly is a rare condition in which there is too much growth hormone in the body. It is seen after normal bone growth has stopped (end of puberty).

Acromegaly is caused when the pituitary gland makes too much growth hormone. Usually, a benign tumor in the pituitary gland releases too much GH. Acromegaly can cause the following:

- Excessive sweating and body odor
- Decrease in muscle strength, carpal tunnel syndrome, and joint pain and swelling
- Large bones of the face, jaw, feet, and hands (Figure 39.5)
- Hirsutism, high blood pressure, and weight gain
- Decreased peripheral vision, headache, hoarseness, and sleep apnea

After a medical history and physical, the provider will order laboratory tests, including those used to analyze blood glucose, growth hormone and growth hormone suppression, insulin-like growth factor 1, and prolactin. A magnetic resonance imaging (MRI) scan of the brain and a spinal x-ray may be ordered, along with an echocardiogram, colonoscopy, and sleep study. Treatment consists of surgery to remove the tumor, radiation, and medication to block the GH production. Follow-up visits are usually required to ensure that acromegaly does not come back.

Gigantism

Gigantism is a rare condition in which there is too much growth hormone in the body during childhood.

Gigantism is caused when the pituitary gland makes too much growth hormone. Usually, a benign tumor of the pituitary gland releases too much GH. Gigantism can also be caused by rare genetic diseases. The child will grow extremely large for his or her age (Figure 39.6). Additional signs and symptoms include the following:

- Delayed puberty and irregular periods (menstruation)
- Double vision, difficulty with peripheral vision, and voice changes
- Large hands and feet, thickening of facial features, and prominent forehead and jaw
- Joint pain, weakness, and gaps between teeth
- Increased sweating and headaches

After an examination, the provider will order laboratory tests, such as the following:

- Insulin-like growth factor -1 (IGF-1) level, growth hormone levels, and oral glucose tolerance test (OGTT)
- Cortisol and prolactin
- Estradiol (type of estrogen) for girls and testosterone for boys
- GH suppression test and thyroid hormone

A computed tomography (CT) or MRI scan of the head may also be done. Surgery can cure many cases. If the tumor cannot be completely removed, medications that suppress the GH release can be given.

Dwarfism

Dwarfism is also known as "short stature," and someone with this condition may be referred to as a "little person." The person has a short stature or an adult height of under 4 feet 10 inches (58 inches)

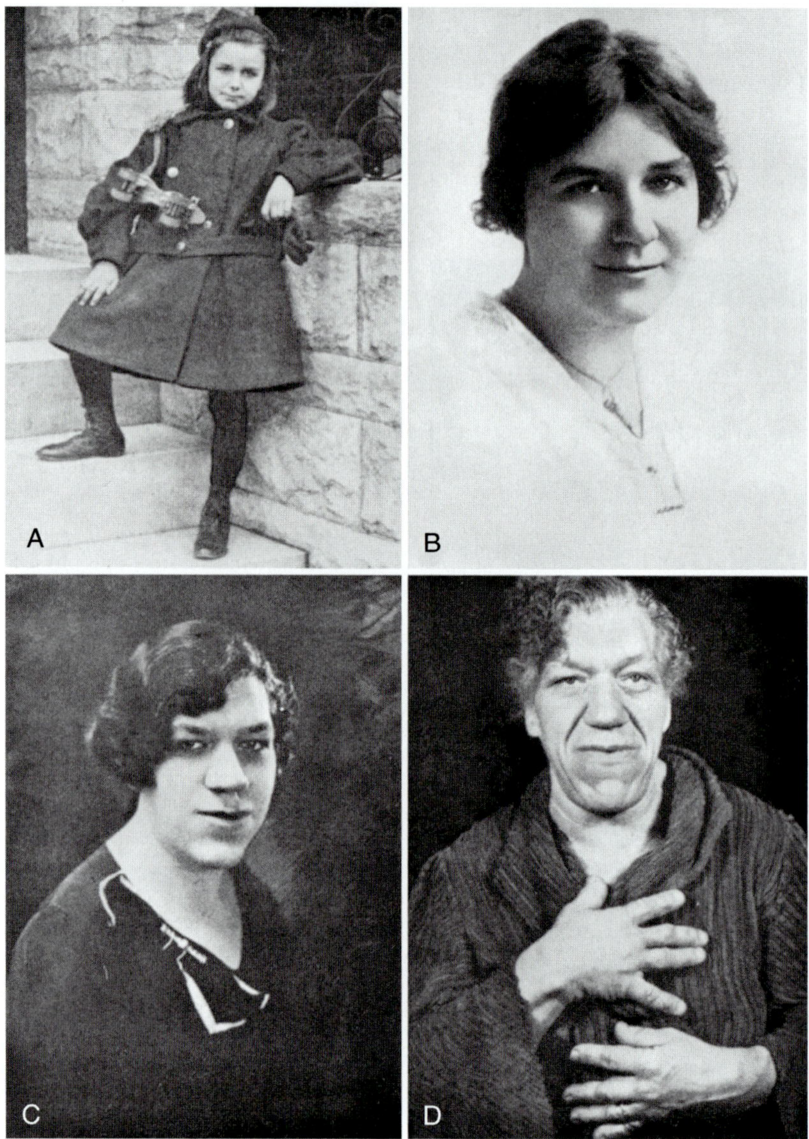

FIGURE 39.5 Progression of acromegaly. **(A)** Patient at age 9. **(B)** Patient at age 16, with possible early features of acromegaly. **(C)** Patient at age 33, with well-established acromegaly. **(D)** Patient at age 52, end-stage acromegaly. (From Clinical Pathological Conference, *Am J Med* 20:133, 1956.)

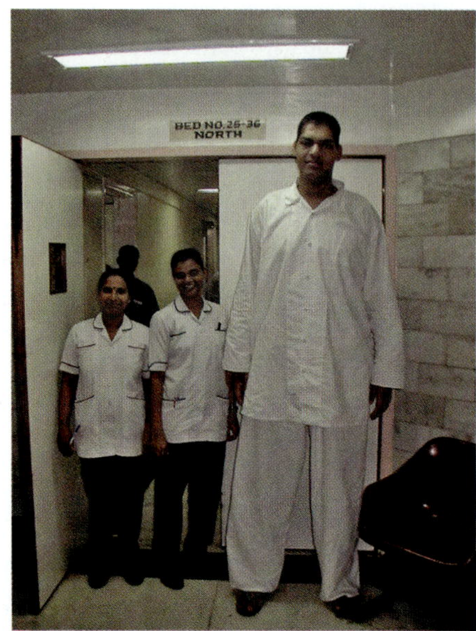

FIGURE 39.6 Gigantism. (From Sainani GS, Joshi VR, Sainani RG: *Manual of clinical & practical medicine*, New Delhi, 2010, Elsevier India.)

(Figure 39.7). Dwarfism does not affect intelligence. It can occur in families with average-height parents. There are two types of dwarfism:

- *Disproportionate dwarfism,* which occurs when some parts of the body are small, whereas others are average or above-average size.
- *Proportionate dwarfism,* which occurs when the parts of the body are proportionate. Usually, medical conditions in early childhood that limit growth and development cause proportionate dwarfism.

Most types of dwarfism are caused by a genetic mutation. There are more than 300 different conditions that cause dwarfism, with achondroplasia being the most common. Achondroplasia, a genetic condition, causes the arms and legs to be short compared to the head and trunk. Metabolism problems, hormones, kidney disease, and other genetic conditions can also cause dwarfism. Besides a short stature, the signs and symptoms vary based on the condition causing the dwarfism. People with disproportionate dwarfism may have the following characteristics:

- Short fingers, arms, and legs; limited mobility at the elbows; bowed legs; and swayed lower back
- Average-size trunk
- Disproportionately large head with a prominent forehead

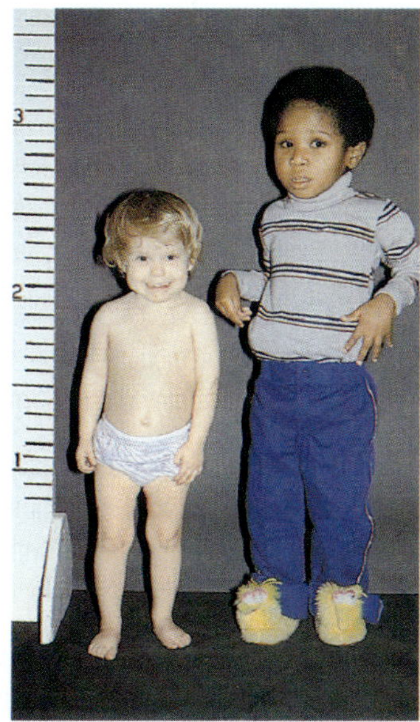

FIGURE 39.7 The normal 3-year-old boy is in the 50th percentile for height. The short 3-year-old girl exhibits the characteristic "kewpie doll" appearance, suggesting a diagnosis of growth hormone deficiency (GHD). (From Zitelli BJ, Davis HW: *Atlas of pediatric physical diagnosis,* ed 5, St. Louis, 2007, Mosby.)

People with proportionate dwarfism have a height below the third percentile on growth charts. Their growth rate is slower than expected for their age. Sexual development is delayed or absent during the teen years.

Dwarfism can be diagnosed during pregnancy or early in life as the child's growth slows. Measurements and appearance, along with imaging technology (e.g., x-rays), genetic testing, and hormone tests, are used. Treatment is focused on maximizing functioning and independence. Most treatments do not increase the stature but rather correct problems caused by complications. For some patients, growth hormone therapy can be given to help increase stature. Daily injections may be needed for several years until the child stops growing.

Diabetes Insipidus

Diabetes insipidus (DI) is caused by a hyposecretion of ADH. The hypothalamus does not produce enough of the hormone, or the posterior pituitary gland does not release a sufficient amount of it.

There are several types of DI, and the causes vary, including genetics, a tumor, trauma, or pituitary gland surgery. Diabetes insipidus can also occur if there is an inadequate response to ADH in the renal tubules of the nephrons due to kidney disease or certain medications. The signs and symptoms usually have an acute onset and include the following:

- Polydipsia, polyuria, *nocturia* (frequent urination at night), and very dilute urine
- Trouble sleeping, fussiness, and irritability
- Fever, vomiting, diarrhea, and *hypotension* (low blood pressure)
- Delayed growth and weight loss in children

Complications, such as *hypernatremia* (abnormally high blood sodium level), severe dehydration, electrolyte imbalance, and hypotension may occur.

The provider will do a physical exam and may order laboratory tests, including a urinalysis and blood tests. A **water deprivation test** and imaging tests can also be done. Diabetes insipidus can be fatal if not adequately treated. Treatment focuses on the cause of the condition. Medications such as a synthetic ADH hormone (desmopressin [DDAVP]) and diuretics may be given.

Additional Pituitary Gland Disorders

Additional pituitary gland diseases include the following:

- *Prolactinoma*: A benign tumor of the pituitary gland that causes the hypersecretion of prolactin. Women have abnormal lactation and abnormal menstrual cycles. Men experience impotence.
- *Panhypopituitarism*: Caused by the hyposecretion of all anterior pituitary hormones, which results from the destruction or deficiency of the entire anterior lobe. It is most common in women. It causes hypotension, weight loss, weakness, and loss of **libido.**
- *Syndrome of inappropriate antidiuretic hormone* (SIADH): Caused by the hypersecretion of ADH. SIADH causes an inability to produce and secrete diluted urine. Water retention, *hyponatremia* (a low blood sodium level), and weight gain are seen.

CRITICAL THINKING APPLICATION **39.3**

Cecilia is working with Landon, who was just diagnosed with diabetes insipidus. Landon's mother asks Cecilia how often he would need to take insulin. How would you address this question? Could you, as a medical assistant, correct the mother's misconception about diabetes insipidus?

THYROID GLAND AND PARATHYROID GLAND DISEASES AND DISORDERS

Hypersecretion and hyposecretion of the hormones from the thyroid and parathyroid glands cause diseases and disorders. The following sections examine thyroid and parathyroid diseases and disorders.

Thyroid Diseases

Thyroid diseases cause hypersecretion or hyposecretion of thyroid hormone. Table 39.1 describes thyroid diseases. Hyperthyroidism and hypothyroidism are described in depth in the following sections.

Hyperthyroidism

Hyperthyroidism occurs when too much thyroid hormone is produced. Hyperthyroidism is more common in women, people with other thyroid conditions, and those over 60 years of age.

The most common cause of hyperthyroidism is Graves disease, and additional causes include thyroid nodules, pituitary disorders and tumors, and thyroiditis (see Table 39.1). Risk factors include a family history of thyroid disorders and having an existing autoimmune disease. Hyperthyroidism can cause the following conditions:

- Fatigue, muscle weakness, sensitivity to heat, and increased sweating
- More frequent bowel movements and weight loss, even with adequate food intake and an increased appetite
- Difficulty sleeping, restlessness, irritability, nervousness, and anxiety
- Rapid heart rate, irregular heart rate, and palpitations
- Goiter and exophthalmia (Figures 39.8 and 39.9)
- Changes in the menstrual cycle
- *Thyrotoxicosis* (thyroid storm), a life-threatening condition that causes elevated vital signs (e.g., temperature, pulse, respiration, and blood pressure)

TABLE 39.1 Diseases That Cause Hyperthyroidism and Hypothyroidism

DISEASE	THYROID FUNCTION	DESCRIPTION
Simple goiter	Hyperthyroidism or hypothyroidism	Simple enlargement of the thyroid gland, causing swelling in the neck. Usually not malignant. Can be caused by iodine deficiency, immune disorders, infections, medications, and other thyroid conditions. More common in people over age 40, women, and those with a family history of goiters. Depending on the symptoms, may be treated with potassium iodide or thyroid hormone.
Thyroid nodule	Hyperthyroidism or hypothyroidism	A growth in the thyroid gland. Can be benign or malignant. More common in women. Causes neck enlargement, pain, hoarseness, and problems swallowing. Treatment may consist of monitoring, surgery, and thyroid hormone if hypothyroidism is occurring.
Thyroiditis	Hyperthyroidism or hypothyroidism	Inflammation of the thyroid. There are several types of thyroiditis. Can be an autoimmune condition or caused by a virus, bacteria, or medication. For several types, the patient may start with hyperthyroidism symptoms and then have hypothyroidism symptoms. Treatment depends on the symptoms and type.
Thyroid carcinoma	Hyperthyroidism or hypothyroidism	The most common types of thyroid carcinoma are follicular and papillary. Both have high 5-year survival rates. Women are three times more at risk for thyroid cancer. Causes a hard, painless lump in the thyroid gland. May cause hoarseness and enlargement of the neck. Treatment depends on the type of cancer; may include surgery, chemotherapy, radiation, and thyroid hormone.
Graves' disease	Hyperthyroidism	Autoimmune disease that results in hypersecretion of the thyroid hormone. Most common cause of hyperthyroidism. Causes heat intolerance, heart palpitations (pounding heart in chest), weight loss, and nervousness. Can cause Graves' eye disease or Graves' ophthalmopathy (e.g., bulging of the eyes [exophthalmia], double vision, light sensitivity, and irritation).
Cretinism	Hypothyroidism	Occurs during infancy and childhood. Leads to low metabolic rate, stunted growth and sexual development, and cognitive deficits. Treated with thyroid hormone.
Myxedema	Hypothyroidism	Occurs during adolescence and adulthood. Symptoms include menorrhagia; dry, scaly skin with no perspiration; weakness; fatigue; bloating; facial puffiness; cold intolerance; and cognition issues. Treated with thyroid hormone.
Hashimoto thyroiditis	Hypothyroidism	A chronic autoimmune disease that attacks the thyroid gland. Often occurs in middle-aged females. Occurs slowly, leading to difficulty thinking, dry skin, goiter, fatigue, hair loss, cold intolerance, mild weight gain, and irregular periods. Treatment may include thyroid medication.

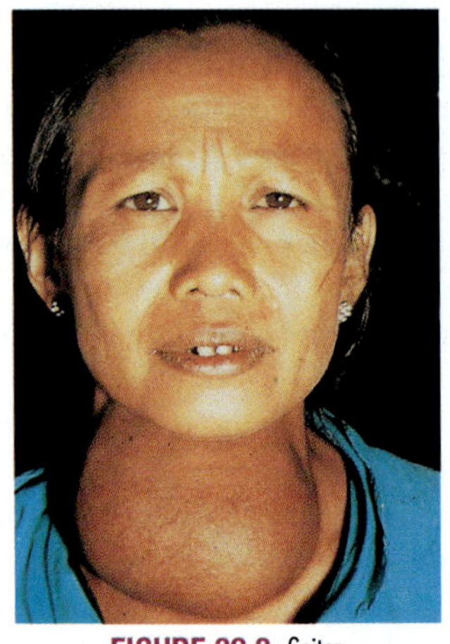

FIGURE 39.8 Goiter.

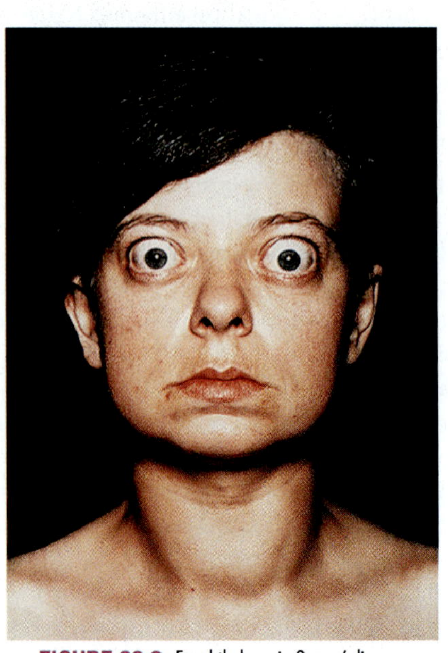

FIGURE 39.9 Exophthalmos in Graves' disease.

After performing a physical exam, the provider may order thyroid function tests and a radioactive iodine uptake (RAIU) scan. Treatment includes radioactive iodine therapy to shrink the thyroid, antithyroid medication (e.g., methimazole [Tapazole]), and a thyroidectomy.

Hypothyroidism

Hypothyroidism occurs when too little thyroid hormone is produced. Hypothyroidism occurs after thyroidectomy and radiation therapy. Table 39.1 describes additional conditions that cause hypothyroidism. Risk factors for hypothyroidism include having a history of an autoimmune disease, a family history of hypothyroidism, or pregnancy in the past 6 months. Another risk factor is being a female over 60 years of age. The signs and symptoms related to the metabolism slowing down and may include the following:

- Fatigue, muscle weakness, tenderness, aches, and stiffness
- Constipation and weight gain
- Dry skin, sensitivity to cold, and thinning hair
- Slowed heart rate, hoarseness, and depression
- Elevated blood cholesterol

After the provider performs the physical exam, thyroid function tests and a thyroid ultrasound may be done. Treatment requires taking lifelong synthetic thyroid hormone (e.g., levothyroxine [Synthroid]).

CRITICAL THINKING APPLICATION 39.4

Cecilia is working with a patient who has been diagnosed with hypothyroidism. What are the signs and symptoms of hypothyroidism? What treatments are usually prescribed?

Parathyroid Gland Diseases

Hyperparathyroidism occurs when there is hypersecretion of parathyroid hormone, and *hypoparathyroidism* occurs when there is hyposecretion of the hormone.

Hyperparathyroidism

Hyperparathyroidism is a relatively common disorder. It occurs when one or more of the four parathyroid glands oversecrete PTH. Hyperparathyroidism causes excessive bone resorption, and the calcium from the bones causes *hypercalcemia* (abnormally high blood calcium level).

Primary hyperparathyroidism occurs as a result of an adenoma or hyperplasia of one of the four glands, causing an increase in PTH secretion. Secondary hyperparathyroidism occurs with renal disease, which causes hypocalcemia and low vitamin D levels that trigger PTH secretion. The signs and symptoms are related to hypercalcemia and include the following:

- Muscle pain, atrophy, and weakness
- Gastrointestinal pain, nausea, vomiting, and anorexia
- Cardiac arrhythmias, renal calculi, bone tenderness, and fractures

After the physical exam, the provider may order blood tests (e.g., calcium, phosphorus) and imaging tests (e.g., x-ray studies, bone density tests, radioimmunoassay studies). Treatment depends on the cause. Minimally invasive surgery may be done to remove a tumor or gland(s). When hyperplasia occurs, all but half of a gland can be removed. For secondary hyperparathyroidism, the underlying cause is treated. Medications may be prescribed to help increase calcium excretion by the kidneys.

CRITICAL THINKING APPLICATION 39.5

Cecilia is rooming Mr. Jones, who came with his wife, Sally. Over the past few months, he has been depressed, forgetful, and weak. At times he has experienced abdominal pain and joint pain. His primary care provider diagnosed him with hyperparathyroidism, and today he came to see the specialist. Mr. Jones had never heard about the parathyroid gland, and he asked Cecilia about it. How would you explain the parathyroid gland to a patient?

Hypoparathyroidism

Hypoparathyroidism occurs when there is hyposecretion of parathyroid hormone. This reduction of PTH causes hypocalcemia to occur.

Hypoparathyroidism results from injury or damage to the parathyroid glands. Damage and destruction of the glands can result from cancer, radiation, and surgery (e.g., thyroidectomy). The signs and symptoms relate to the hypocalcemia and can include the following:

- Numbness and tingling, spasms, and twitching in the hands and feet
- Confusion and irritability
- *Tetany* (continuous muscle spasms), laryngospasm, arrhythmias, respiratory paralysis, and death

The provider will perform a physical exam and order blood tests (e.g., calcium, phosphate), an electrocardiogram, and imaging tests (e.g., radioimmunoassay studies). Lifelong treatment includes calcium and vitamin D supplements and a high-calcium diet.

ADRENAL GLAND DISEASES AND DISORDERS

Hyposecretion of cortisol from the adrenal gland causes Addison disease. Hypersecretion of cortisol causes Cushing syndrome. The following sections discuss these conditions.

Addison Disease

Addison disease is a malfunction of the adrenal cortex, leading to adrenal insufficiency (hyposecretion) of cortisol. Addison disease affects adults ages 30 to 50, though it can occur at any age. Addison disease can be acute or chronic. Acute Addison disease may be called Addisonian crisis, a condition marked by life-threatening symptoms. A crisis can be brought on by stressful situations, infections, minor illnesses, or surgery.

The causes of Addison disease include an autoimmune reaction, tuberculosis, and damage to or disease of the adrenal glands or pituitary gland. Acute Addison disease can cause the following responses:

- Pain in the lower back, abdomen, and legs
- Severe vomiting and diarrhea, dehydration, and low blood pressure
- Loss of consciousness
- *Hyperkalemia* (an abnormally high blood potassium level) and hyponatremia

Chronic Addison disease may occur over weeks to months. It can cause the following:

- Irritability, extreme fatigue, weight loss, lack of appetite, and a craving for salt

- Darkening of the skin and buccal membranes (*hyperpigmentation*) (Figure 39.10)
- Hypotension, fainting, nausea, diarrhea, and vomiting
- Hypoglycemia
- Muscle pain, depression, and loss of body hair

After a physical exam, the provider may order blood tests (e.g., cortisol, sodium, potassium, and ACTH), imaging tests, and an ACTH stimulation test. The ACTH stimulation test measures the blood cortisol level before and after an injection of synthetic ACTH. If the adrenal gland is damaged, cortisol levels will still be low or absent after ACTH stimulation. Addisonian crisis treatment requires the immediate administration of an intravenous saline and dextrose solution with corticosteroids. Other treatments involve corticosteroids to replace cortisol and aldosterone and dietary changes (e.g., a diet high in carbohydrates and protein; adequate sodium and fluids).

Cushing Disease

Cushing disease is a malfunction of the cortex of the adrenal gland, causing increased levels of cortisol.

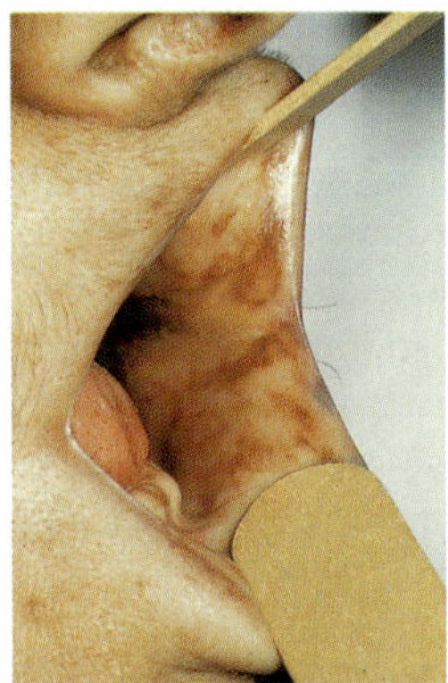

FIGURE 39.10 Hyperpigmentation caused by Addison disease. (From Thibodeau GA, Patton KT: *The human body in health and disease*, ed 5. St. Louis, 2010, Mosby.)

Cushing disease has the following causes:

- A benign pituitary tumor
- An adrenal adenoma (benign adrenal cortex tumor), a tumor that secretes ACTH
- Taking long-term corticosteroids for another medical condition (e.g., organ transplantation, severe asthma, or rheumatoid arthritis)

Cushing disease can cause the following:

- High blood pressure
- Weight gain, especially in the abdomen, upper back, face (moon face), and between the shoulder blades (buffalo hump) (Figure 39.11)
- Pink or purple stretch marks on the abdomen, thighs, breasts, and arms
- Fragile, thin skin that bruises easily
- Infections, slow-healing wounds, and acne
- Severe fatigue, muscle weakness, and headaches
- Depression, anxiety, irritability, loss of emotional control, and difficulty thinking clearly
- Slowed or impaired growth in children
- Decreased libido and infertility in men
- Thicker or more noticeable facial and body hair (*hirsutism* or *hypertrichosis*) in women (Figure 39.12)

After obtaining a medical history and performing a physical exam, the provider may order a number of tests:

- Blood, saliva, and urine tests to measure cortisol levels
- An ACTH stimulation test
- Imaging tests

Treatment is focused on the cause of the disorder and may include medications to control cortisol levels, radiation therapy to shrink the tumor, or surgery to remove the tumor.

CRITICAL THINKING APPLICATION 39.6

Describe the difference between Cushing disease and Addison disease.

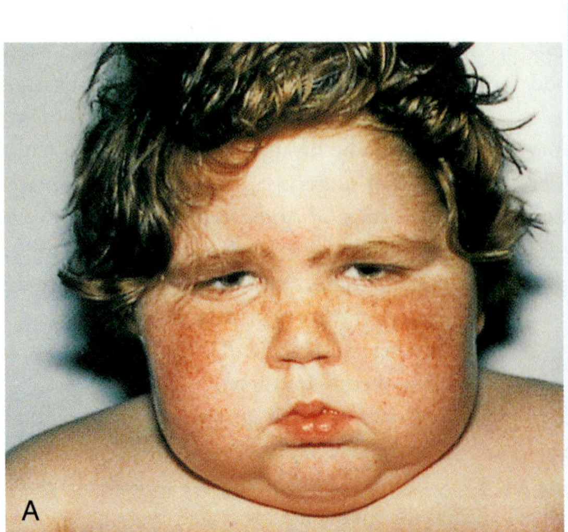

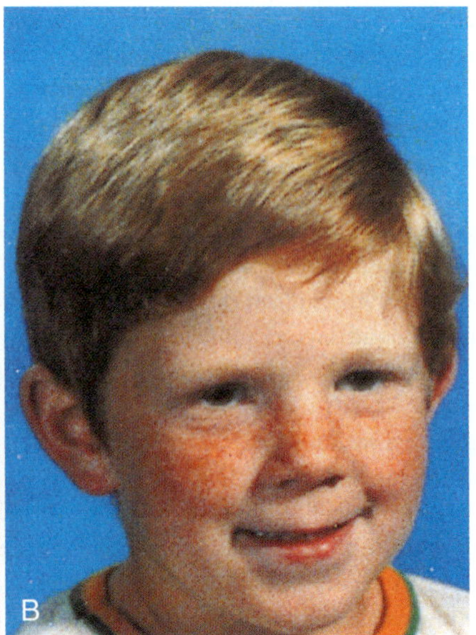

FIGURE 39.11 Cushing disease. **(A)** First diagnosed. **(B)** After 4 months of treatment. (From Shiland B: *Mastering healthcare terminology*, ed 5, St. Louis, 2016, Elsevier.)

Additional Adrenal Gland Diseases and Disorders

Additional adrenal gland diseases include these:

- *Adrenocortical carcinoma*: A malignant adrenal tumor that starts in the adrenal cortex.
- *Congenital adrenal hyperplasia* (CAH): A genetic disorder that causes the body to make a decreased amount of cortisol. Usually, people with CAH also have other hormone imbalances.
- *Pheochromocytoma*: A type of paraganglioma tumor that develops in the adrenal medulla and produces adrenaline, causing high blood levels of epinephrine.

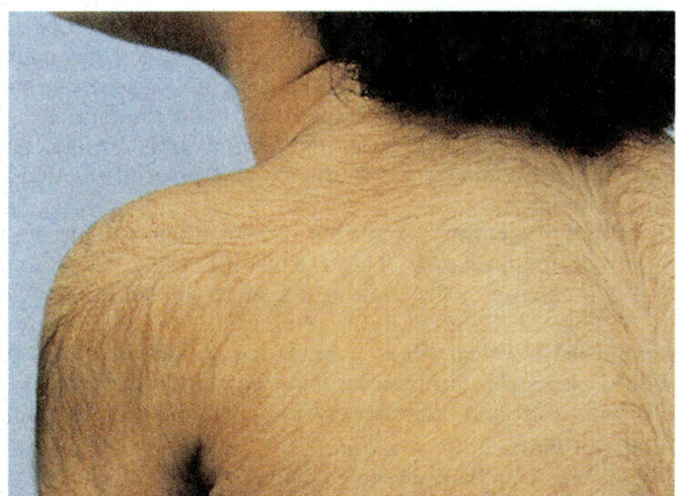

FIGURE 39.12 Hirsutism. (From *Mosby's medical, nursing, and allied health dictionary*, ed 8, St. Louis, 2009, Mosby.)

PANCREATIC DISEASES AND DISORDERS

Diabetes mellitus (DM) is the most common pancreatic disease. The following sections discuss type 1, type 2, and gestational diabetes.

Diabetes Mellitus

DM is a group of metabolic disorders characterized by an inadequate production of insulin, a resistance to insulin, or a combination of both. Table 39.2 describes type 1 DM, type 2 DM, and latent autoimmune diabetes in adults (LADA, sometimes called type 1.5 DM). (Gestational diabetes will be discussed in a separate section.)

The exact cause of DM is unknown. Type 1 DM and LADA are autoimmune conditions. The immune system destroys the beta islet cells of the pancreas. See Table 39.2 for risk factors for the different types of diabetes.

Signs and symptoms relate to hyperglycemia. With type 1 DM, the hyperglycemia can occur suddenly, whereas with type 2 DM and LADA it can be gradual. Hyperglycemia signs and symptoms include polydipsia, polyuria, polyphagia, weight loss, fatigue, blurred vision, frequent infections, and slow-healing wounds.

After a medical history and physical exam, the provider will order laboratory tests. The following diagnostic results suggest diabetes:

- Glycated hemoglobin (A_{1C}) test, 6.5% or greater on two separate samples
- Fasting blood glucose test, 126 mg/dL or greater on two separate samples
- Oral glucose tolerance test, greater than 200 mg/dL for the 2-hour level
- Random blood glucose test, no matter when the person ate last, 200 mg/dL or greater and diabetes symptoms

See Table 39.2 for the treatments for each type of DM.

TABLE 39.2 Types of Diabetes Mellitus

	TYPE 1 DIABETES MELLITUS	TYPE 2 DIABETES MELLITUS	LATENT AUTOIMMUNE DIABETES IN ADULTS
Onset	Occurs at any age, though it is often diagnosed between childhood and the young adult years.	More common in older adults, but with the rise in obesity, children and younger adults are also diagnosed with it.	Usually seen in adults over 30 years of age.
Use of Insulin/ Function of the Pancreas	The pancreas produces very little or no insulin.	Insulin resistance occurs, or the pancreas does not make enough insulin to meet the body's needs, leading to hyperglycemia.	The pancreas slowly stops producing adequate insulin.
Risk Factors	Family history of type 1 diabetes mellitus (DM), genetics, age (peaks between ages 4 to 7 and then again between ages 10 to 14). Possible viral or environmental exposure.	Obesity, extra fat carried in the abdominal area, inactivity, family history of type 2 DM, race (greater risk if Native American, Asian American, Hispanic, or African American), greater risk if over 45 years of age or with a history of prediabetes, gestational diabetes, or polycystic ovarian syndrome.	May have a family history of diabetes; obesity, physical inactivity, alcohol consumption, and smoking.
Treatment	Insulin injections, regular exercise, frequent blood glucose monitoring, and dietary changes, including carbohydrate, fat, and protein counting.	Healthy eating, regular exercise, weight loss if obese, medications (e.g., antihyperglycemics, insulin), and glucose monitoring. Bariatric surgery if body mass index (BMI) is 35 or greater.	Initially managed with diet, weight loss if needed, exercise, and oral medication. Insulin injections will be needed months to years after the patient is diagnosed.

Hyperglycemia

With a fasting blood glucose test, the normal level is 70 to 99 mg/dL. *Hyperglycemia* occurs when the blood glucose level is elevated or above the normal limit. Blood glucose levels increase due to the following:

- Eating too many carbohydrates without enough insulin
- An infection, injury, or surgery, regardless of the amount of carbohydrates eaten
- Missing an insulin injection

Usually during an illness, people with type 1 diabetes mellitus have a special diabetic management plan to follow, which may include extra insulin and increased blood glucose monitoring.

CRITICAL THINKING APPLICATION **39.7**

Summarize the difference between type 1 and type 2 diabetes mellitus.

Complications of Diabetes Mellitus

According to the Centers for Disease Control and Prevention (CDC; www.cdc.gov), since the early 2000s, the number of people with DM has tripled. During that same time span, the top complications of DM—heart attack and stroke-have decreased because of the advances in DM education and care. The complications of diabetes mellitus develop over time. Two factors increase the risk of complications: the longer a person has DM and the more uncontrolled the blood glucose is.

Diabetes affects the entire body. The following list provides a snapshot of possible complications of diabetes mellitus:

- *Cardiovascular disease*: People with DM have twice the risk of having a heart attack and stroke compared to people without diabetes mellitus. Diabetes increases the risk for coronary artery disease with *angina* (chest pain) and *atherosclerosis* (narrowing of the arteries).
- *Blindness and eye conditions*: **Diabetic retinopathy**, **glaucoma**, and **cataracts** can lead to vision loss. Early prevention and screening can prevent blindness with diabetic retinopathy. It is recommended that people with diabetes have their eyes checked every 4 to 6 months.
- *Neuropathy*: One of the most common complications of DM is nerve damage affecting the digestive system, reproductive system, cardiovascular system, and the extremities. Capillaries help nourish the nerves in the body, but hyperglycemia can damage the capillary walls, thus also causing nerve damage. Damage to the nerves in the gastrointestinal (GI) system can cause nausea, vomiting, constipation, or diarrhea. Men can have erectile dysfunction. A person with neuropathy can experience burning, tingling, pain, and numbness in the fingers and toes, which gradually move up the extremities. If left untreated, a loss of feeling in the extremities may occur, which can affect functioning.
- *Poor healing of wounds*: Diabetes also makes a person more susceptible to bacterial and fungal skin infections. With the lack of feeling in the extremities, the person is more at risk for foot sores, blisters, and cuts. Left untreated, they can become infected, which increases the blood glucose levels. This affects the healing process, which may lead to amputations to stop the spread of infection.
- *Kidney disease*: Hyperglycemia also damages the tiny blood vessels (glomeruli) in the kidney, leading to chronic kidney disease (CKD). Untreated CKD leads to kidney failure, which requires dialysis or a kidney transplantation.
- *Dementia*: Type 2 diabetes increases a person's risk of dementia-related disorders (e.g., Alzheimer disease).
- *Depression*: Is common in patients with type 1 and type 2 DM.
- *Periodontal disease*: Gum infections and tooth loss can occur, which also increases hyperglycemia. It is recommended that patients with diabetes have dental cleanings and exams twice a year.

CRITICAL THINKING APPLICATION **39.8**

Cecilia is rooming Susie Westwood, who has had type 2 DM for 4 years. Cecilia asks Susie when she last had her eyes checked and had a dental exam. Susie could not remember and asked Cecilia why that was important. How would you answer Susie?

Gestational Diabetes

Gestational diabetes develops during pregnancy. Hyperglycemia can affect the health of the pregnancy and the baby. Usually, after the pregnancy, gestational diabetes resolves, though there is a greater risk for type 2 DM.

The exact cause is unknown, though hormones produced by the placenta impair the action of insulin, leading to hyperglycemia. Risk factors include being older than age 25, having a family history of type 2 DM, having a personal history of prediabetes, being overweight, and race (risk is greater if one is Native American, Asian, Hispanic, or African American). There are no signs or symptoms of gestational diabetes.

A routine oral glucose tolerance test is usually done during weeks 24 to 28 of pregnancy. Treatment for gestational diabetes includes eating a healthy diet, monitoring blood glucose levels, regular exercise, insulin injections, and closer follow-up for both the patient and the baby.

Complications of Gestational Diabetes

Complications of gestational diabetes can include issues with the baby and the mother. The following complications can affect the baby:

- Excessive growth in utero: The extra glucose in the mother's blood passes into the baby's bloodstream, causing the baby's pancreas to make extra insulin. This causes extra weight to be added to the baby, thus increasing the likelihood the child may need to be delivered by a C-section.
- Death: If the mother does not get treated for gestational diabetes, the risk of death for the baby during pregnancy or after birth increases.
- Hypoglycemia shortly after birth: With the extra insulin production in utero, the baby may be at risk for hypoglycemia shortly after birth.

- Risk of developing obesity and type 2 DM later in life.

For the mother, complications include **preeclampsia** and C-section delivery. She is at a greater risk for gestational diabetes with future pregnancies and having type 2 DM later in life.

Diabetic Ketoacidosis

Diabetic ketoacidosis (DKA) is a life-threatening hyperglycemic condition more commonly seen in people with type 1 DM and LADA.

DKA occurs when there is not enough insulin in the body, which helps the blood glucose move to the cells. Because the cells need energy, the body starts rapidly breaking down fats, which leads to a buildup of ketones in the blood and urine, causing ketoacidosis. DKA can cause the following:

- Decreased alertness and headache
- Nausea, vomiting, abdominal pain, and dry mouth
- Muscle aches or stiffness, dry skin, and flushed face
- Frequent urination or thirst lasting for 1 or more days
- Fruity-smelling breath

Laboratory tests include blood glucose, urine, and blood ketones. A basic metabolic panel (which includes electrolytes [e.g., sodium and potassium] levels) may also be done. The goals of treatment are to correct the hyperglycemic level, replace lost fluids, and correct any electrolyte imbalances. Treatment usually consists of insulin, intravenous (IV) fluids, and frequent glucose and electrolyte monitoring. Sometimes, DKA treatment can be done in an ambulatory care facility; other times patients will be transported to the local emergency department for care.

Hypoglycemia

Hypoglycemia means low blood glucose (below 70 mg/dL). Hypoglycemia is commonly seen with DM but also can be seen with other conditions.

Hypoglycemia in DM usually occurs due to a medication side effect. A person takes too much insulin or oral medication for the amount of carbohydrates consumed, thus dropping the blood glucose level. Early hypoglycemia can cause irregular heart rhythm, pale skin, sweating, shakiness, and fatigue. The person may experience irritability, hunger, a tingling sensation around the mouth, and crying out while sleeping. As hypoglycemia worsens (the blood glucose level drops more), a person may experience behaviors that may be similar to being intoxicated:

- Visual disturbances and blurred vision
- Clumsy movements and seizures
- Confusion, abnormal behavior (e.g., incoherent speech, slurring words, inability to complete routine tasks), and loss of consciousness

Immediate treatment is required and involves increasing the blood glucose level. If people are alert and can swallow, they should follow the 15/15 rule. For an unconscious adult patient or child over age 6, glucagon 1 mL should be given subcutaneously or intramuscularly (IM) to treat hypoglycemia. This dose should be repeated in 15 minutes if the patient is still unconscious. Children younger than 6 years of age should receive glucagon 0.5 mL. The blood glucose should be monitored, and once the person is alert and able to swallow, additional food should be given.

15/15 Rule

People should eat 15 grams of fast-acting carbohydrates, then wait 15 minutes before retesting their blood glucose level. This cycle should be followed until the blood glucose level returns to normal. At that time, the person should eat a small, balanced snack that contains both a protein and a carbohydrate if the next meal is more than 2 hours away. Examples of 15 grams of fast-acting carbohydrate include the following:

- 3 glucose tablets
- 4 ounces or ½ cup of fruit juice or regular soda (not diet soda)
- 6 to 7 hard candies
- 1 tablespoon of sugar

Additional Pancreatic Diseases and Disorders

Additional pancreatic diseases and disorders include the following:

- *Hyperinsulinism*: Hypersecretion of insulin; seen in some newborns of diabetic mothers. Causes severe hypoglycemia.
- *Islet cell carcinoma*: Also called *pancreatic cancer;* fourth leading cause of cancer death in the United States. Treated with a Whipple procedure (pancreatoduodenectomy).
- *Prediabetes*: Condition in which the blood glucose level is higher than normal but not high enough for a diagnosis of type 2 diabetes.

THE MEDICAL ASSISTANT'S ROLE IN EXAMINATIONS, DIAGNOSTIC PROCEDURES, AND TREATMENTS

Endocrine diseases and disorders are common in primary care and endocrinology departments. Medical assistants help the provider with examinations, diagnostic procedures, and treatments.

Assisting with the Examination

When the medical assistant is rooming a patient, it is important to accurately measure the vital signs and obtain the medical history. Encouraging the patient to voice any concerns or issues is vital. The medical assistant may be required to ask specific screening questions. Peripheral neuropathy screening questions for patients with DM may include the following:

- Do you have tingling, burning, numbness, cramps, or sharp pains in your hands and feet?
- Do you have a reduced ability to feel temperatures or pain in your hands and feet?
- Are your hands or feet more sensitive to touch?
- Do your hands or feet feel weaker?
- Do you have any problems with loss of balance or coordination?
- Do you have any sores, blisters, or any concerns with your feet?

When completing the medication section of the medical history, the medical assistant must verify the medication name, the dose amount, and the number of doses taken each day. Sometimes the information in the health record is different from what the patient is really doing. Having accurate information in the health record helps the provider evaluate the complete picture of the patient's health.

During the physical exam, the provider often needs to examine the patient's feet for any abnormalities. The medical assistant should assist the patient in removing shoes and socks as needed. For infection control purposes, the patient's bare feet should never touch the floor. The medical assistant should place a piece of paper towel or some other barrier between the patient's feet and the floor.

Peripheral Neuropathy Screening

Many providers have medical assistants perform peripheral neuropathy screening by doing the monofilament foot exam. This is commonly done for diabetic patients but needs to be done for any patient experiencing peripheral neuropathy symptoms. Procedure 39.1 describes the monofilament foot exam procedure.

Assisting with Diagnostic Procedures

Tables 39.3 to 39.4 provide information about common diagnostic procedures and medical laboratory tests done for endocrine conditions. The medical assistant may be responsible for coaching patients on diagnostic procedures done in other departments. As with other diagnostic procedures, the medical assistant should coach the patient regarding the following:

- Patient preparation (e.g., dietary restrictions and medications to hold)
- Location and time of the test
- What to expect during the procedure
- Any follow-up required after the procedure

Assisting with Treatments

Some endocrine disorders are treated with surgery (Table 39.5). Many endocrine disorders are treated with medications. The following are some of the more common classifications of medications:

TABLE 39.3 Diagnostic Procedures for Endocrine System Diseases and Disorders

PROCEDURE	DESCRIPTION	PATIENT PREPARATION
Thyroid ultrasound	Ultrasound of the thyroid gland. Used to check for nodules and other abnormalities in the gland.	Patient is asked to remove jewelry and clothing around the neck. The sonographer will apply warm gel to the neck and gently press a transducer along the neck.
Thyroid scan	Uses a radioactive iodine tracer to examine the thyroid gland. The patient swallows a pill with the radioactive iodine. The scan is done 4 to 6 hours later as the iodine collects in the thyroid. Often done with the radioactive iodine uptake test.	Screen the patient for allergies (e.g., iodine, shellfish), diarrhea, and history of CT scans using iodine in the past 2 weeks. The patient must remove jewelry, dentures, and other metal products. During the scan, the patient must remain still.
Radioactive iodine uptake (RAIU) scan	Uses a radioactive iodine tracer to measure the uptake of iodine in the thyroid. As with the thyroid scan, the patient swallows a radioactive iodine pill. A scan is done 4 to 6 hours after the pill is taken and then again 24 hours later. Often done along with the thyroid scan.	Screen the patient for allergies (e.g., iodine, shellfish), diarrhea, and a history of CT scans using iodine in the past 2 weeks. The patient must remove jewelry, dentures, and other metal products. During the scan, the patient must remain still.

TABLE 39.4 Medical Laboratory Tests for Endocrine System Diseases and Disorders

Test	Description
HbA_{1C} test	Also called A_{1C} and hemoglobin A_{1C} test. Measures the average blood glucose level over the past 3 months. Some CLIA-waived tests are available. • Normal level: <5.7%, • Indicates prediabetes: 5.7–6.4% • Indicates diabetes: >6.5% ADA's formula for HbA_{1C} conversion to estimated average glucose (eAG) in mm/dl: $28.7 \times HbA_{1C} - 46.7 = eAG$
Calcium blood test	Measures the calcium level in the blood. Total calcium test measures the calcium attached to specific proteins in the blood. Ionized calcium test measures the calcium unattached to proteins in the blood.
Fasting blood glucose (FBG) test	Measures the glucose level in the blood after fasting. Some CLIA-waived tests are available. • Normal level: 70–99 mg/dL • Indicates prediabetes: 100–125 mg/dL • Indicates diabetes: >126 mg/dL
Urine glucose test	Measures the amount of glucose in the urine sample. Some CLIA-waived tests are available. May also be part of a urinalysis.
Urine ketone test	Measures the amount of ketones in the urine sample. Ketones are produced when fat is used for energy instead of glucose. Some CLIA-waived tests are available.
Serum ketone test	Measures the level of ketones in the blood.

TABLE 39.4 Medical Laboratory Tests for Endocrine System Diseases and Disorders—continued	
Oral glucose tolerance test (OGTT)	Blood test to measure the body's response to a concentrated glucose solution. Patient fasts for 8 to 12 hours and then drinks 75 or 100 grams of glucose. Blood may be drawn and tested prior to the drink and then every 30 to 60 minutes for up to 2 to 3 hours after taking the glucose. Nonpregnant levels: • Normal level: fasting 60–100 mg/dL; 1 hr <200 mg/dL; 2 hr <140 mg/dL • Indicates prediabetes: 2 hr 140–200 mg/dL • Indicates diabetes: >200 mg/dL
Random blood glucose test	Measures the glucose level in the blood without fasting. A glucometer (a handheld instrument) may be used at home or in the ambulatory care environment. Some CLIA-waived tests are available. • Normal level: <125 mg/dL • Indicates diabetes: >200 mg/dL
Thyroid antibody test	Measures the thyroid antibodies in the blood. Used to diagnose autoimmune thyroid disorders.
Thyroid function tests (TFTs)	Measures the levels of TSH, T_3, and T_4 in the blood. Used to evaluate the thyroid function. Some CLIA-waived tests are available.
Thyroid-stimulating hormone (TSH)	Blood test that measures the thyroid-stimulating hormone. TSH stimulates the thyroid to make T_3 and T_4. When the thyroid does not, the pituitary continues to release TSH. High levels of TSH may indicate hypothyroidism. Low blood levels of TSH may indicate hyperthyroidism. Some CLIA-waived tests are available.
Triiodothyronine (T_3) test	A blood test that measures the triiodothyronine level. Bound T_3 is attached to proteins and stored for later use. Free T_3 is the active form of T_3. Tests are available to measure free T_3 and total T_3 (bound plus unbound) in the blood.
Thyroxine (T_4) test	A blood test that measures the thyroxine levels. As with T_3, there is bound T_4 and free T_4. Free T_4 is the thyroxine that can enter the body tissues. This test is preferred for checking thyroid function.

CLIA, Clinical Laboratory Improvement Amendments. ADA, American Diabetes Association.
Formula from the American Diabetes Association, https://professional.diabetes.org/sites/professional.diabetes.org/files/media/average_glucose_flyer.pdf.

TABLE 39.5 Common Treatments Used for Endocrine System Diseases and Disorders

PROCEDURES	DESCRIPTION
Adrenalectomy	Surgical removal of one or both of the adrenal glands
Hypophysectomy	Surgical removal of the pituitary gland
Pancreatectomy	Surgical removal of part or all of the pancreas
Parathyroidectomy	Surgical removal of one or more of the parathyroid glands
Thyroidectomy	Surgical removal of part or all of the thyroid gland

- *Antihyperglycemic*: Used to manage diabetes mellitus
- *Hormone replacement*: Used to maintain adequate hormone levels
  - *Estrogen*: Used for menopause
  - *Estrogen and progestin*: Used for menopause
  - *Insulin*: Used to treat type 1 and type 2 diabetes mellitus
  - *Thyroid hormone*: Used for hypothyroidism
  - *Vasopressin*: Used for diabetes insipidus

Refer to Table 39.6, Medication Classifications, for information on drug classification, including indication for use, desired effect, side effects, adverse reactions, and generic and trade names. Medical assistants should be familiar with medications that are prescribed to patients.

In the ambulatory care facility, when a patient is prescribed insulin for the first time, the medical assistant may need to do some coaching if the patient is not seeing a diabetic educator immediately. If it is within the scope of practice for the medical assistant, the following topics should be addressed with the patient:

- How to draw up and give an insulin injection (discussed in Chapter 30)
- Signs and symptoms of hyperglycemia and hypoglycemia
- Immediate treatments for hyperglycemia and hypoglycemia
- How to use a glucometer to monitor blood glucose levels (discussed in Chapter 49)
- When to contact the provider or seek additional care
- Storage of supplies and how to discard used needles

Insulin

Insulin is used to treat type 1 and, in some cases, type 2 diabetes mellitus. Most commonly, insulin is injected subcutaneously several times a day. Table 39.7 describes the different types of insulins. The *onset* is the length of time before the insulin begins to work. The *peak* is the period when the insulin is most effective. The *duration* is the length of time the insulin exerts an effect on the body.

Many people take two types of insulin a day. Premixed insulins available in the United States include the following:

- *Premixed—Intermediate- and rapid-acting*: 75% insulin lispro protamine, 25% insulin lispro (Humalog Mix 75/25); 50% insulin lispro protamine, 50% insulin lispro (Humalog Mix 50/50); and 70% insulin aspart protamine, 30% insulin aspart (NovoLog Mix 70/30)

TABLE 39.6 Medication Classifications

CLASSIFICATION	INFORMATION	GENERIC NAME (TRADE NAME)
Antihyperglycemics (noninsulin)	Indications for use: Manages diabetes mellitus. Desired effect: Reduces blood glucose level. Side effects and adverse reactions: GI irritation, fatigue, hypoglycemia, vertigo; possible hypersensitivity reaction	*Oral (type 2):* • Rosiglitazone (Avandia) • Sitagliptin (Januvia) • Glipizide (Glucotrol) • Glyburide (DiaBeta, Glynase) • Metformin (Glucophage, Fortamet, Glumetza, Riomet) *Injectable (type 2):* • Exenatide (Byetta, Bydureon) • Dulaglutide (Trulicity) *Injectable (used with other type 1 or 2 medications):* • Pramlintide (SymlinPen 60)
Hormone replacement—*Estrogen*	Indications for use: Maintains adequate hormone levels. Desired effects: Replaces hormones or compensate for hormone deficiency. Side effects and adverse reactions: Hot flashes, decreased sex drive, nausea, vomiting.	• Estrogen (Estrace, Ortho-est, Premarin)
Hormone replacement—*Estrogen and progestin*	Indications for use: Maintains adequate hormone levels. Desired effects: Replaces hormones or compensate for hormone deficiency. Side effects and adverse reactions: Double vision, depression, unusual bleeding, acne, swelling of the hands and feet, nervousness, brown or black skin patches	• Conjugated estrogens and medroxyprogesterone (Premphase, Prempro) • Ethinyl estradiol and norethindrone (Jinteli, FemHRT) • Estradiol and norethindrone (Activella, Mimvey)
Hormone replacement—*Insulin*	Indications for use: Treats type 1 and type 2 diabetes mellitus Desired effects: Lowers the blood glucose level. Side effects and adverse reactions: Shortness of breath, blurred vision, tachycardia, sweating, weakness, muscle cramps, arrhythmias, and other hypoglycemic symptoms	*Rapid-Acting Insulin:* • Insulin aspart (NovoLog, Novolog Mix 70/30, Fiasp) • Insulin glulisine (Apidra) • Insulin lispro (Humalog, Admelog) *Short-Acting Insulin:* • Regular insulin (Humulin R, Novolin R) *Intermediate-Acting Insulin:* • NPH human insulin (Humulin N, Novolin N) *Long-Acting Insulins:* • Insulin degludec (Tresiba) • Insulin detemir (Levemir) • Insulin glargine (Basaglar, Lantus, Toujeo) *Ultra-Long-Acting Insulin:* • Insulin glargine U-300 (Toujeo 300 units/mL)
Hormone replacement—*Thyroid hormone*	Indications for use: Maintains adequate hormone levels. Desired effects: Replaces hormones or compensate for hormone deficiency. Side effects and adverse reactions: Weight loss, tremor, headache, chest pain, arrhythmias	• Levothyroxine (Synthroid, Levoxyl, Unithroid)
Hormone replacement—*Vasopressin*	Indications for use: Maintains adequate hormone levels. Desired effects: Replaces hormones or compensate for hormone deficiency. Side effects and adverse reactions: Restlessness, seizures, hallucinations, slowed reflexes, tiredness	• Desmopressin (DDAVP)

TABLE 39.7 Types of Insulin

TYPE	GENERIC NAME (BRAND NAME)	ONSET	PEAK	DURATION	FORM/ ADMINISTRATION
Rapid-acting	Insulin glulisine (Apidra), insulin lispro (Humalog, Admelog), insulin aspart (NovoLog, Fiasp)	About 15 min	About 1 hr	2–4 hr	Clear liquid/Take 5–15 min before meal
Rapid-acting inhaled	(Afrezza)	About 15 min	About 1 hr	2.5–3 hr	White powder/Take at start of meal
Short-acting	Regular human insulin (Humulin R, Novolin R)	About 30 min	2–3 hr	3–6 hr	Clear/Take 30–45 min before meal
Intermediate-acting	NPH human insulin (Humulin N, Novolin N)	2–4 hr	6–8 hr	12–18 hr	Cloudy/Take 30 min before meal
Long-acting	Insulin glargine (Basaglar, Lantus, Toujeo), insulin detemir (Levemir), insulin degludec (Tresiba)	2–4 hr	Does not apply	Up to 24 hr +	Clear/Does not need to be taken with meal
Ultra-long-acting	Insulin glargine U-300 (Toujeo)	6 hr	Does not apply	Up to 36 hr	Clear/Does not need to be taken with meal

From the Food and Drug Administration, www.fda.gov/consumers/free-publications-women/insulin; and the American Diabetes Association, www.diabetes.org/healthy-living/medication-treatments/insulin-other-injectables/insulin-basics.

- *Premixed—Intermediate- and short-acting*: 70% NPH, 30% regular insulin (Novolin 70/30, Humulin 70/30)
- *Premixed—Long- and rapid-acting*: 70% insulin degludec, 30% insulin aspart (Ryzodeg 70/30)

Insulin can be given in the following ways:

- *Syringe and vial*: Insulin is drawn up in the syringe, and then the injection is given. Adaptive equipment is available to help patients see the calibration lines on the syringe.
- *Insulin pump*: This is a computerized device that administers insulin through a needle-tipped catheter attached to tubing and the medication container. The needle can be inserted in several locations, including the abdomen, outer thigh, back of the arm, hip, and buttock. The pump is programmed to deliver a *basal rate*, or the continuous infusion of a small dose of insulin over a 24-hour period. The person can also set the pump to deliver extra insulin to cover the carbohydrates being consumed. This method more closely resembles the body's normal surge of insulin and is designed to maintain blood glucose levels consistently within normal limits.
- *Injector pen*: An injection device that is preloaded with insulin cartridges for easy use (Figure 39.13). Insulin pens are disposable or refillable and easily portable and therefore can be used by patients with diabetes when they are away from home.
- *Inhaler*: A cartridge containing the insulin is loaded into the inhaler. The person breathes in the insulin.

CRITICAL THINKING APPLICATION 39.9

Explain why it is important for patients who take insulin to be aware of the onset, peak, and duration of the insulin.

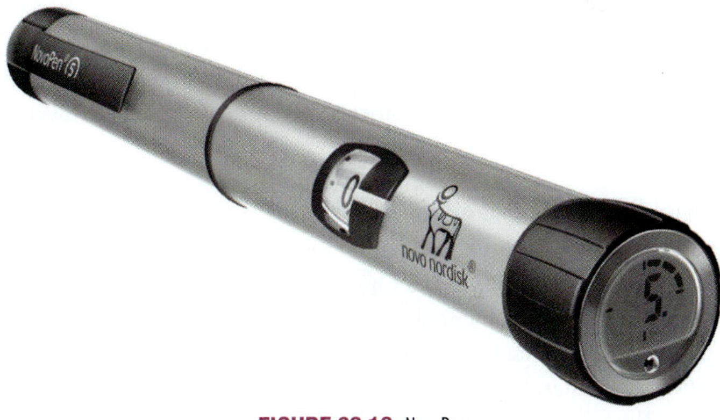

FIGURE 39.13 NovoPen.

Insulin Strengths. U-100 is the most common insulin strength in the United States. U-100 means that 100 units of insulin are dissolved or suspended in each milliliter (mL) of fluid. Additional insulin strengths are more concentrated.

- Humalog KwikPen contains 200 units of insulin per mL (U-200 insulin).
- Insulin glargine U-300 (Toujeo) contains 300 units of insulin in each mL of fluid or three times the amount of insulin compared to U-100 insulin.
- Humulin R U-500 contains 500 units of insulin in each mL of fluid or five times the amount of insulin compared to U-100 insulin.

More concentrated forms of insulin require additional patient education and special equipment (e.g., syringes or pens) to prevent insulin overdoses.

Storage of Insulin. Most insulin manufacturers recommend that insulin should be stored in the refrigerator. Because injecting cold insulin is uncomfortable, usually, the vial being used is stored at room temperature. An insulin vial stored at room temperature will last for about 1 month. It is important to keep insulin away from extreme heat or cold (e.g., freezer, direct sunlight, or in the glove compartment of a vehicle).

Afrezza, the inhaled insulin, should be stored in the refrigerator in the original closed container. Before using, the cartridge should warm at room temperature for 10 minutes. At room temperature, unopened medication packs are good for 10 days. Once the pack is opened, the cartridges are good for 3 days. The inhaler can be used for up to 15 days before it must be discarded.

CLOSING COMMENTS

Patient Coaching

The medical assistant can coach the patient on proper foot care. It is important for patients to check their feet daily and also to care for their feet daily. The following points should be reinforced with patients who have neuropathy:

- Check your shoes for damaged areas or stones before putting them on. Wear good-fitting shoes at all times to protect your feet.
- Check your feet when taking off your shoes. Look at all sides of your feet and between the toes. Check for redness, blisters, swelling, sores, and so forth.
- Keep your toenails trimmed to a proper length.
- Wash your feet every day with lukewarm water and soap. Dry well with a soft towel. Use lotion, lanolin, or oil on dry skin, but do not put it between the toes because this could cause an infection.
- Seek medical care immediately for foot sores.
- Avoid putting pressure on areas with nerve damage for long periods of time.
- Use an elbow instead of the toes or hands to check the bathwater temperature.

Legal and Ethical Issues

Pathophysiology of the endocrine system can have far-reaching effects on the body's ability to function. Patient education interventions should be documented completely to establish legal proof of the information shared with the patient. Never just assume that the patient understands the disease process and treatment recommendations. The following suggestions can help ensure the patient's welfare and promote risk management.

- Advise patients that a MedicAlert bracelet with their diagnosis and medication information is an important safeguard.
- Patients must take medication as prescribed, following the directions for dosage, route of administration, and storage; they also must be alert for possible side effects.
- Patients newly diagnosed with diabetes should not drive until glycemic control has stabilized. These patients also should be warned about possible visual impairment from the disease.
- Remember that you are always representing your profession and employer, and respond to each situation accordingly.
- Ask for assistance or further information if you feel unprepared to perform a procedure or give accurate information.

Patient-Centered Care

Providing patients and families with information, education, and emotional support is part of providing patient-centered care. When working with patients with endocrinology disorders, especially diabetes mellitus, the medical assistant has an important role in connecting patients with additional resources. These can include local support groups, medication discount programs, and websites, including the following:

- American Diabetes Association: www.diabetes.org
- Centers for Disease Control and Prevention: www.cdc.gov
- National Institutes of Health: Genetic and Rare Diseases Information Center: https://rarediseases.info.nih.gov
- US National Library of Medicine: MedlinePlus: https://medlineplus.gov

Professional Behaviors

An important part of becoming a professional medical assistant is a commitment to lifelong learning. This chapter focused on the details of diabetes mellitus because it is the most common endocrine system disease and also one of the most serious. Regardless of where you work as a medical assistant, you will end up caring for patients with diabetes and interacting with their families on some level. Diabetes researchers are constantly discovering more information about the disease: how it is diagnosed, the best treatment methods, and the pathophysiology of possible complications. You must commit to continual learning about diabetes so that you are best prepared to care for patients with this life-threatening disorder.

SUMMARY OF SCENARIO

Cecilia enjoyed working with the endocrinology team and patients. She was able to observe the diabetic nurse educator work with a newly diagnosed patient. The amount of information newly diagnosed diabetic patients need to learn to manage their disease is incredible. All of the information was not given to the patient during the first visit. The nurse educator explained that over the coming weeks, the patient would get the information. During the first visit, the patient needed to learn how to administer insulin, test blood glucose levels, and learn about hypoglycemia and hyperglycemia. These topics were most critical at this stage.

Later in the day, Cecilia observed the dietitian working with a patient with type 2 DM. The patient stated he enjoyed his beer, snack foods, and sweets and really did not want to give them up. Cecilia was impressed by how the dietitian worked with the patient so that eventually, the patient was willing to cut back on some of his "not so healthy" habits. Cecilia's experiences reinforced her belief that she had made the right decision by volunteering to work with the endocrinology team.

SUMMARY OF LEARNING OBJECTIVES

1. **Examine the connection between the endocrine and nervous systems.**
The endocrine system is composed of ductless glands throughout the body. The hypothalamus, located in the middle of the brain, is the major connection between the nervous and endocrine systems and controls the endocrine system. When it detects rising levels of a target organ's hormones, it sends a signal to the pituitary gland to release or prevent pituitary hormone production.
2. **Differentiate between the hormones of the anterior lobe and those of the posterior lobe of the pituitary gland.**
The pituitary gland is connected to the hypothalamus and is composed of two lobes that act as separate glands, the anterior lobe and the posterior lobe. Hormones from the anterior lobe include adrenocorticotropic hormone, follicle-stimulating hormone, growth hormone, luteinizing hormone, prolactin, and thyroid-stimulating hormone. Hormones from the posterior lobe of the pituitary gland include antidiuretic hormone and oxytocin.
3. **Differentiate between the hormones of the thyroid and those of the parathyroid glands.**
The thyroid gland is a butterfly-shaped gland in the neck above the collarbone. Thyroid gland hormones include triiodothyronine, thyroxine, and calcitonin. The parathyroid glands are four pea-sized glands located on the thyroid gland. The parathyroid hormone comes from the parathyroid gland.
4. **Differentiate between the hormones of the adrenal cortex and those of the adrenal medulla.**
The adrenal glands are located on the top of each kidney. The outer part of the gland is the adrenal cortex; the inner part is called the *adrenal medulla*. Adrenal cortex hormones include mineralocorticoids, glucocorticoids, and gonadocorticoids. Adrenal medulla hormones include epinephrine and norepinephrine.
5. **Differentiate among the hormones of the pancreas, thymus gland, gonads, and pineal gland.**
The pancreas is located inferior and posterior to the stomach. The pancreas hormones are glucagon, insulin, somatostatin, and ghrelin. The thymus gland is in the mediastinum behind the sternum (breastbone) and secretes thymosin and thymopoietin hormones. The male gonads are the testes and secrete testosterone. The female gonads are the ovaries, which secrete estrogen and progesterone. The pineal gland is located deep within the brain and secretes melatonin.
6. **Examine the physiology of the endocrine system.**
The goal of hormone regulation is to maintain homeostasis. Nervous system stimulation, endocrine control, and feedback systems regulate hormone secretion. Each hormone released into the bloodstream has specific target cells for action. The target cells have receptors that attract only certain hormones. The cell membrane only lets selected hormones pass into the cell and affect cellular action.

   There are two categories of hormones, nonsteroid hormones and steroid hormones. Nonsteroid hormones attach to a target cell membrane. Another molecule takes the message from the nonsteroid hormone and carries it to the target cell nucleus or organelle, which then puts the message into action in the cell. Steroid hormones attach to a target cell membrane, then pass directly into the target cell, and bind to receptor sites. This complex communicates its message with DNA in the nucleus, and the DNA tells the cell how to put the hormone's message into action.

   Prostaglandins are produced in tissues and diffuse only a short distance to affect cells in their local area. They help regulate processes such as respiration, blood pressure, digestive system secretions, and reproductive functions.
7. **Examine pituitary gland diseases and disorders, including the signs, symptoms, etiology, diagnostic procedures, and treatments.**
Anterior pituitary gland disorders include the following:
   - Acromegaly and gigantism, which are caused by hypersecretion of growth hormone.
   - Dwarfism, which is caused by hyposecretion of growth hormone.
   - Prolactinoma, which is caused by hypersecretion of prolactin.
   - Panhypopituitarism, which is caused by hyposecretion of all the anterior pituitary hormones.

   Posterior pituitary gland hypersecretion of antidiuretic hormone (ADH) causes syndrome of inappropriate antidiuretic hormone (SIADH), and hyposecretion causes diabetes insipidus.
8. **Examine thyroid gland and parathyroid gland diseases and disorders, including the signs, symptoms, etiology, diagnostic procedures, and treatments.**
Hyperthyroidism occurs when too much thyroid hormone is produced. Hypothyroidism occurs when too little thyroid hormone is produced. Hyperparathyroidism occurs when there is hypersecretion of parathyroid hormone, and hypoparathyroidism occurs when there is hyposecretion of the hormone.
9. **Examine adrenal gland diseases and disorders, including the signs, symptoms, etiology, diagnostic procedures, and treatments.**
Hyposecretion of cortisol from the adrenal gland causes Addison disease. Hypersecretion of cortisol causes Cushing syndrome.
10. **Examine pancreatic diseases and disorders, including the signs, symptoms, etiology, diagnostic procedures, and treatments.**
Diabetes mellitus (DM) is the most common pancreatic disease. DM is a group of metabolic disorders characterized by an inadequate production of insulin, a resistance to insulin, or a combination of both. Types of DM include type 1, type 2, latent autoimmune diabetes in adults, and gestational diabetes.

    Diabetic ketoacidosis (DKA) is a life-threatening hyperglycemic condition that is more commonly seen with type 1 DM and latent autoimmune diabetes in adults (LADA). *Hypoglycemia* means low blood glucose (below 70 mg/dL). Hypoglycemia is commonly seen with DM but also can be seen with other conditions.
11. **Examine the medical assistant's role in examinations, diagnostic procedures, and treatments for endocrine diseases and disorders.**

    During an endocrinology examination, a medical assistant may be required to ask specific screening questions. When completing the medication section of the medical history, the medical assistant must verify the medication name, dose amount, and number of doses taken daily.

    During the physical exam, the medical assistant should assist the patient in removing shoes and socks as needed. Many providers have medical assistants perform peripheral neuropathy screening by doing a monofilament foot exam.

    Tables 39.3 and 39.4 provide information on the common diagnostic procedures and medical laboratory tests done for endocrine conditions. Some endocrine disorders are surgically treated (see Table 39.5). Many endocrine disorders are treated with medications (see Table 39.6).

PROCEDURE 39.1 Perform a Monofilament Foot Exam

TASKS: Perform a monofilament foot exam to screen for peripheral neuropathy. Provide health maintenance coaching by giving the patient foot care instructions. Document test results in the patient's health record.

EQUIPMENT and SUPPLIES

- 10 g monofilament tool
- Gloves
- Paper towel
- Provider's order or standing order
- Patient's health record

PROCEDURAL STEPS

1. Wash hands or use hand sanitizer.
   PURPOSE: Hand sanitization is an important step for infection control.
2. Read the provider's order. Assemble the equipment.
   PURPOSE: It is important to know the provider's order before starting the procedure.
3. Greet the patient. Identify yourself. Verify the patient's identity with full name and date of birth. Explain the procedure to be performed in a manner that the patient understands. Answer any questions the patient may have about the procedure.
   PURPOSE: It is important to identify the patient in two different ways to ensure that you have the correct patient. Explaining the procedure can make the patient feel more comfortable and reduces anxiety.
4. Ask the patient to remove socks and shoes and rest the feet on the paper towel. The paper towel should be placed under the person's feet, either on the floor or on the exam table step.
   PURPOSE: This prepares the patient for the test.
5. Using your hand, demonstrate that the monofilament is flexible and not sharp. Also, demonstrate the monofilament on the patient's hand. Put gloves on.
   PURPOSE: This alleviates the patient's anxiety. Demonstrating on the patient's hand allows the patient to know how it feels.
6. Instruct patients to close their eyes. Tell patients to say "yes" when they feel the monofilament on the foot.
   PURPOSE: The patient's eyes must be closed for this test to be accurate.
7. Start with the great toe and place the monofilament perpendicular to the skin. Press the monofilament until it bends, hold for 1 second, and release (Figure 1). Pause to give the patient an opportunity to confirm it was felt. A confirmation is a positive or normal response. The test result is abnormal if the patient cannot feel in one area.
   PURPOSE: It is important to hold the monofilament for 1 second for accurate results.

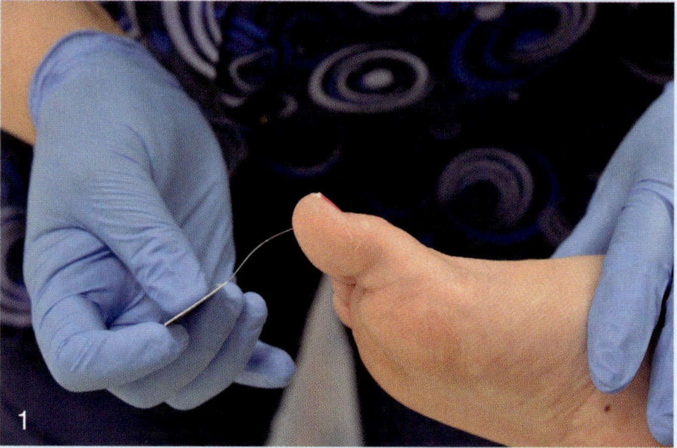
1

8. Do not cue the patient if no confirmation is given. Just move to the next location. Randomly test 9 to 12 locations on the anterior and posterior side of each foot or as the provider indicates (Figure 2). If a patient does not feel the site, check it three times randomly. Make sure to space out testing times (e.g., the time between each check).
   PURPOSE: If the test is done in a rhythmic way, the patient may confirm the feeling without really feeling the test.

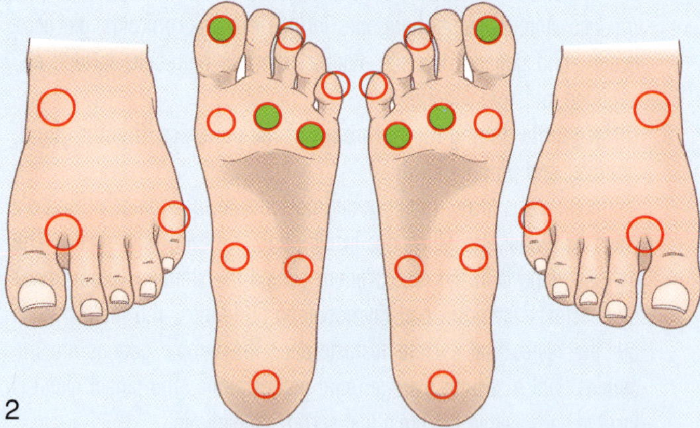
2

9. Discard supplies in the waste container. Remove gloves and wash hands.
   PURPOSE: Washing hands is important for infection control.
10. Coach the patient on proper foot care to prevent sores. Include when to check the feet, what to look for, and how to care for the feet daily. Suspicious areas need to be watched carefully and reported to the provider if they do not return to normal.
    PURPOSE: Careful monitoring can help prevent serious foot sores.

PROCEDURE 39.1 Perform a Monofilament Foot Exam—*continued*

11. Document the test results in the patient's health record. Include the provider's name, the order, and the results of the test. For the test, the first number indicates the total number of sites felt, and the last number indicates the total times done. Indicate all sites where the patient did not feel the test. If the provider indicates specific areas to test, documentation should reflect these areas. Include any teaching done.
    PURPOSE: It is important to document the patient education in the health record to show it was done.

Documentation Example

07/19/20XX 1625 Per Dr. Kahn's order, performed a monofilament exam on both feet. Right foot 9/12 and left foot 12/12. Right posterior great toe 0/3. Pt coached on foot care. Stressed daily foot care and inspections. Pt listed the daily foot care required. Pt indicated what and where on his feet he needs to examine daily. All the pt's questions were answered. The "Feet Guide for Neuropathy" brochure was given to the patient. ————————————

———————————————— Cecilia Cukier, CMA (AAMA)

CARDIOLOGY

40

SCENARIO

Rebecca White is a certified medical assistant (CMA) at Walden-Martin Family Medical (WMFM) Clinic. She was hired 8 months ago. She works with several family practice providers at the clinic. Many of the patients she works with have cardiovascular diseases. High blood pressure, or hypertension, seems to be the most common cardiovascular disease seen in her patients.

During her first few months at the clinic, Rebecca spent a lot of time learning about cardiovascular diseases, diagnostic procedures, and treatments. She found out that learning about the cardiovascular system takes time, but she is proud of how much she has learned over the months.

Rebecca's supervisor approached her and asked her to mentor a medical assistant student, Lizzy, for her clinical experience. Rebecca is excited about the opportunity, but she is a bit nervous teaching someone else about her job.

While studying this chapter, think about the following questions:

- What structures are in the cardiovascular system?
- What are the functions of the cardiovascular system?
- What are commonly diagnosed cardiovascular system diseases and disorders? What are the etiologies, signs and symptoms, diagnostic processes, and treatment?
- What are the medical assistant's primary responsibilities when working with patients who have cardiovascular system diseases and disorders?

LEARNING OBJECTIVES

1. Examine the anatomy of the cardiovascular system.
2. Differentiate among the pulmonary, systemic, coronary, hepatic portal, and fetal circulations.
3. Examine the anatomy of the blood.
4. Examine the physiology of the conduction system.
5. Examine the physiology of the blood, including coagulation and the factors that affect the blood pressure.
6. Analyze the life span changes to the cardiovascular system.
7. Examine heart diseases and disorders, including the signs, symptoms, etiology, diagnostic procedures, and treatments.
8. Examine blood vessel diseases and disorders, including the signs, symptoms, etiology, diagnostic procedures, and treatments.
9. Examine blood pressure-related diseases and disorders, including the signs, symptoms, etiology, diagnostic procedures, and treatments.
10. Examine blood diseases and disorders, including the signs, symptoms, etiology, diagnostic procedures, and treatments.
11. Examine the medical assistant's role in assisting with examinations, diagnostic procedures, and treatments for cardiology diseases and disorders.

VOCABULARY

anaphylaxis A rapidly progressing, life-threatening allergic reaction; characterized by hives, swelling of the mouth and airway, difficulty breathing, wheezing, and loss of consciousness.

antibodies Proteins produced by cells in the immune system in response to a specific antigen. Work to destroy or weaken a specific antigen.

antigens Substances (usually proteins) on the surface of cells, viruses, bacteria, fungi, and nonliving substances, including drugs, chemicals, toxins, and foreign particles (e.g., wood splinters).

arteriosclerosis A disease in which the arterial walls become thickened and lose their elasticity.

atheroma (ath uh ROH mah) A waxy lesion made up of cholesterol, fat, calcium, cells, and other substances, that builds up on the inner wall of an artery.

bilirubin (bil i ROO bin) A reddish yellow pigment that results from the breakdown of red blood cells in the liver.

cardiac defibrillator An external or implantable device that provides an electric shock to the heart to restore a normal sinus rhythm.

constrict To contract or shrink.

cytoplasm A jelly-like substance that surrounds the nucleus and fills the cells. Organelles (structures in the cell) are suspended in the cytoplasm.

deoxygenated Oxygen deficient; oxygen was removed.

ectopic pregnancy A pregnancy in which the fertilized egg implants outside the uterus (e.g., fallopian tubes).
electrocardiography The recording of electrical impulses of the heart as wave deflections on an instrument called an electrocardiograph. The record, or recording, is called an electrocardiogram.
embolus (EM boh lus) An air bubble, blood clot, or foreign body that travels through the bloodstream and blocks a blood vessel.
enzymes Special proteins that speed up a chemical reaction in the body.
filamentous (fil ah MEN tuhs) Composed of or containing filaments or strands of a substance.
glucose A simple sugar that is absorbed by the intestines and found in the blood. It is used by cells for energy, and the extra is stored in the liver as glycogen.
hematopoiesis The formation of blood cells.
incompetent valves Valves that do not close completely and allow blood to leak backward into the prior chamber; also called "leaky valves."
infarction (in FARK shuhn) Tissue death.
insufficiency Also called regurgitation or incompetence; the valve does not close completely, and blood leaks backward across the valve into the prior chamber.
mediastinum (mee dee uh STY num) The space in the thoracic cavity that lies between the lungs, containing the heart, trachea, and esophagus.
orthostatic (postural) hypotension A temporary fall in blood pressure that occurs when a person rapidly changes from a recumbent position to a standing position.
pitting edema Excessive fluid in the intercellular spaces in the tissue; when external pressure (e.g., socks, finger pressure) is relieved, a depression is seen in the tissue.
polycythemia (pol ee sie THEE mee ah) A condition caused by an abnormally large number of red blood cells (RBCs) in the blood.
purpura A condition characterized by hemorrhages in the tissues, causing the appearance of purplish spots.
solvent A liquid that can dissolve other substances.
stem cells Undifferentiated cells that can become specialized cells in the body.
stenosis (sten OH sis) Occurs when the heart valve flaps are stiff or fused together, thus narrowing the valve.
syncope (SING kuh pee) Fainting or loss of consciousness and postural tone caused by diminished blood flow to the brain.
thrombus (THRAHM bus) A blood clot that blocks the flow of blood.
valvulitis An inflammatory condition of a valve that results in valve stenosis and obstructed blood flow; caused most commonly by rheumatic fever, bacterial endocarditis, or syphilis.
viscosity Resistance to flow; the thicker the liquid, the higher the viscosity.
whole blood Plasma and the formed elements of blood in a free-flowing liquid form.

INTRODUCTION

Cardiology is the healthcare specialty that deals with cardiovascular diseases and disorders. A *cardiologist* is a physician who specializes in internal medicine and cardiology. A cardiologist treats patients with cardiovascular system diseases and disorders.

Vascular surgeons are medical doctors who specialize in vascular diseases. They diagnose and treat artery and vein conditions in every part of the body except for the brain and the heart. *Cardiothoracic surgeons* are medical doctors who specialize in surgical procedures involving the lungs, heart, esophagus, and other organs in the chest. They can also be called *cardiac surgeons, cardiovascular surgeons,* and *general thoracic surgeons.*

Hematology is the branch of medicine that focuses on the diagnosis and treatment of diseases related to blood and blood-forming organs. A *hematologist* is a physician who specializes in internal medicine and hematology. A hematologist treats patients with blood, bone marrow, vascular system, lymph gland, and spleen disorders.

Cardiology-related tests are common in the ambulatory care setting. Patients with cardiovascular diseases are seen in primary care, urgent care, and specialty departments. Patients seen for other conditions may also have cardiovascular diseases. Medical assistants may need to coach patients on cardiovascular procedures. Having a strong understanding of the cardiovascular system and common diseases is important for medical assistants.

ANATOMY OF THE CARDIOVASCULAR SYSTEM

The cardiovascular system is also called the *circulatory system.* The cardiovascular system brings oxygen (O_2), nutrients, water, and other substances (e.g., salts and hormones) to the body's cells. It also carries waste products away from the cells to be excreted. These waste products include metabolic waste and carbon dioxide (CO_2).

The cardiovascular system is a closed system that includes the following structures:

- Blood vessels, consisting of arteries, arterioles, capillaries, venules, and veins that act as pipes to carry the blood around the body
- A heart, which pumps the blood
- Blood, which contains the nutrients for the cells and the waste products to be excreted

Cellular injury and death of the cells will occur if the system malfunctions and critical substances are withheld from the cells.

Blood Vessels

Blood vessels create a pipeline for blood to move out to the body and back to the heart. Blood vessels differ in their role, structure, and size:

- *Arteries*: Strong, stretchy, thick-walled vessels that carry blood from the heart. They are made to withstand the pressure of the blood being pumped out from the heart. Arteries are involved in maintaining blood pressure (Figure 40.1).

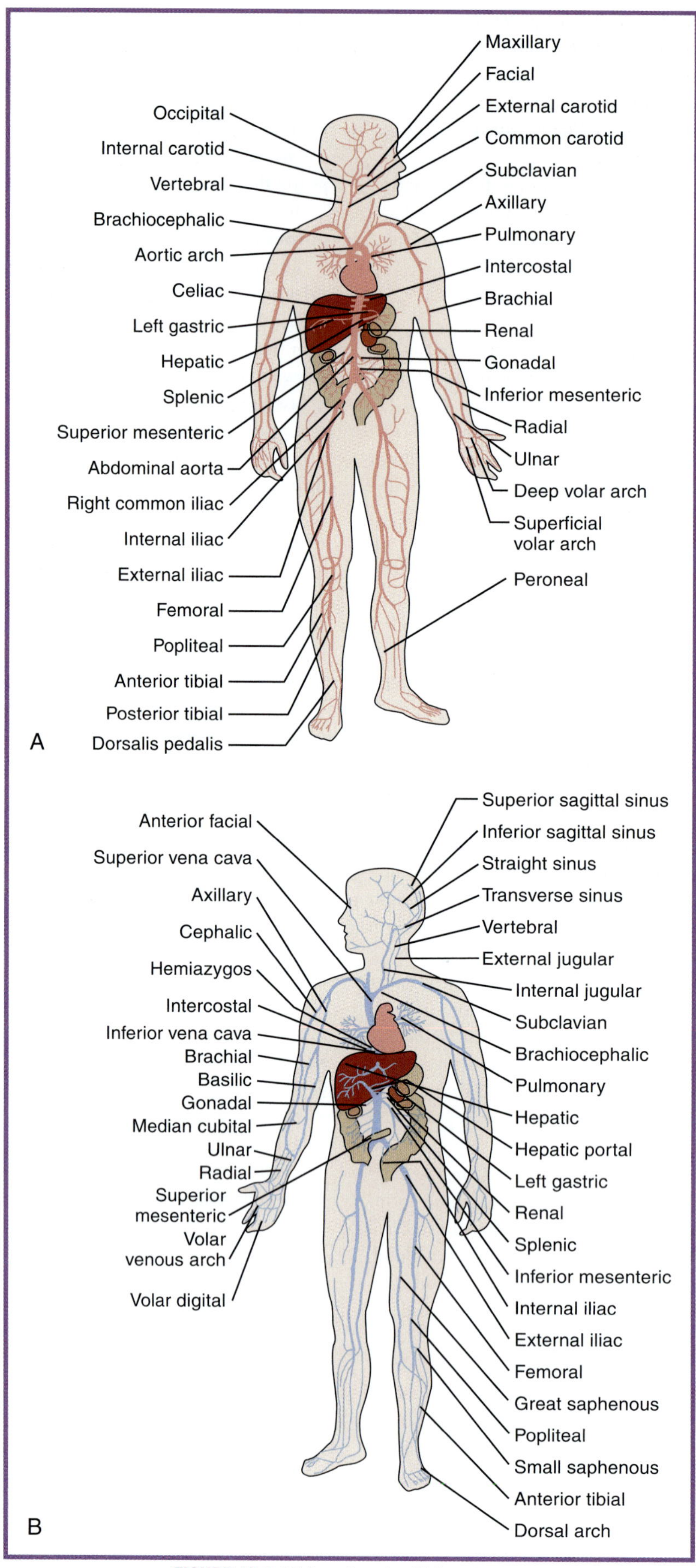

FIGURE 40.1 **(A)** Systemic arteries. **(B)** Systemic veins.

- *Arterioles*: Smaller arteries that move blood to the capillaries and are also involved with maintaining blood pressure.
- *Capillaries*: Thin-walled vessels that allow for the exchange of oxygen, nutrients, waste products, and other substances between the blood and cells. The diameter of the capillaries is so thin that only one blood cell can pass through at a time.
- *Venules*: Vessels that collect blood from capillaries and begin the return journey to the heart.
- *Veins*: Vessels that collect blood from the venules and return blood to the heart. Medium to large veins have valves, which help keep blood moving in one direction. The skeletal muscle contractions help move the blood toward the heart. Vessel walls are thinner and less rigid than arteries (see Figure 40.1 and Table 40.1). Veins hold about 70% of the blood supply at any one time.

The Heart

The heart, which is the size of a fist, is a complex muscular organ that pumps blood around the body. It is located in the **mediastinum** of the thoracic cavity, slightly left of the midline. The *apex* (pointed tip) of the heart rests just above the diaphragm. The area of the chest wall anterior to the heart and lower thorax is referred to as the *precordium*.

Heart Chambers

The heart has two sets of chambers. The two upper chambers are called *atria*. The atria are small chambers with thin walls. The right atrium receives blood from the body, and the left atrium receives blood from the lungs. The two larger, lower chambers with thick muscular walls are called the right and left *ventricles* (Figure 40.2). They pump blood to the body and the lungs.

The *septum* is the thick muscular wall that divides the heart into right and left sections. The *interatrial septum* separates the left and right atria, and the *interventricular septum* divides the right and left ventricles.

TABLE 40.1 Comparison of the Walls of the Arteries and Veins

LAYERS OF THE WALLS	ARTERIES	VEINS
Tunica intima (inner layer)	Contains epithelium and elastic-like fibers	Some contain valves to prevent backflow of blood
Tunica media (middle layer)	Thick layer of smooth muscles regulated by the autonomic nervous system that constricts or dilates vessels to maintain blood pressure	Contains smooth muscles; thin layer
Tunica externa (outer layer)	Made of connective tissue	Thickest layer and made of connective tissue

Heart Wall

The heart wall is composed of three layers:

- *Endocardium*: The inner thin endothelial layer that lines the chambers and valves.
- *Myocardium*: The middle and thickest layer of the heart, composed of cardiac muscles.
- *Epicardium* or *visceral pericardium*: The outer layer that covers the heart. A space separates the epicardium from the *parietal pericardium*, which loosely covers the heart like a sac. The two layers of pericardium are serous membranes. As the heart beats, the two layers rub against each other, and the moisture between the layers reduces the amount of friction.

Heart Valves

The heart has valves between the chambers and the arteries. The valves allow the blood to flow in one direction. Valves are *competent* if they open and close properly, letting through or holding back an expected amount of blood. The heart has two sets of valves: atrioventricular (AV) valves and semilunar (SL) valves.

An AV valve is found between each atrium and ventricle. When opened, it allows blood to flow into the ventricle. When closed, it prevents the backflow of blood into the atrium. The AV valves open and close with the help of the papillary muscles. These muscles are attached to the valve by the *chordae tendineae*, cordlike tendons. The AV valves are located as follows:

- *Bicuspid* or *mitral valve*: Found between the left atrium and ventricle and made up of two cusp or flaps (see Figure 40.2).
- *Tricuspid* valve: Found between the right atrium and ventricle and made up of three cusps.

The SL valves are found between the ventricles and the arteries leading out of the heart. The SL valves allow blood to flow out of the heart and prevent the backflow of blood into the ventricles. The valves are created by flaps from the pulmonary artery and aorta. The SL valves are located as follows:

- *Pulmonary valve*: Between the right ventricle and the pulmonary artery
- *Aortic valve*: Between the left ventricle and the aorta

CRITICAL THINKING APPLICATION 40.1

Rebecca is helping Lizzy review the blood flow through the body. She asks Lizzy to explain the blood flow through the pulmonary and systemic circulations, starting with the blood returning from the body. How should Lizzy answer her?

Heartbeat

A provider listens to the heart sounds with a stethoscope. The normal sound is a *lub dub*. The *lub* sound occurs when the AV valves close as the ventricles contract. This is a lower pitch and a longer sound, which is followed by a pause. The *dub* sound occurs when the SL valves close. With **incompetent valves**, the provider might hear additional abnormal noises.

A complete heartbeat or *cardiac cycle* can be divided into the diastole and systole phases. During the *diastole* phase, the heart is at rest, and the atria fill with blood. The *systole* phase occurs when the heart is contracting.

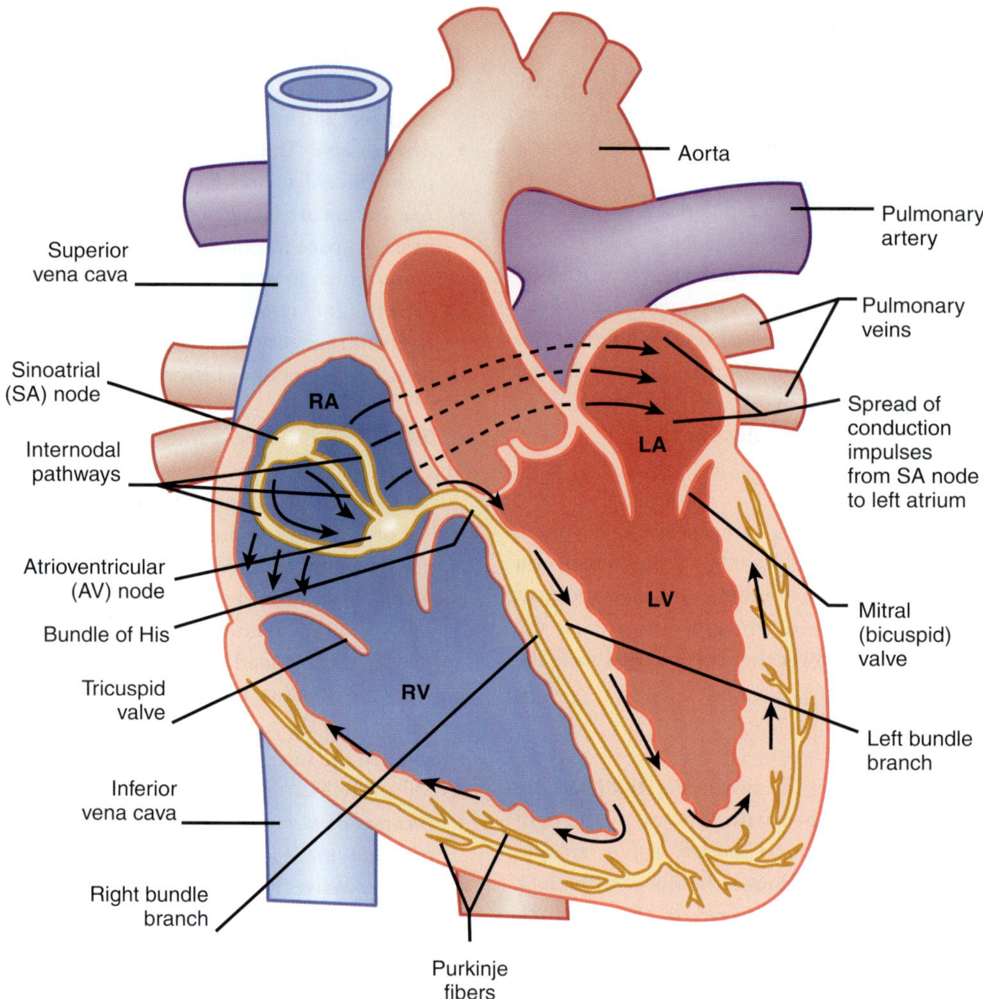

FIGURE 40.2 Structures of the heart (RA: right atrium; LA: left atrium; RV: right ventricle; LV: left ventricle.)

ANATOMY OF THE BLOOD FLOW

The body has several types of blood flow pathways, or circulations. The heart, being a double pump, sends blood in two different directions, resulting in two major circulatory pathways:

- *Pulmonary circulation*: **Deoxygenated** blood is pumped from the right side of the heart to the lungs, gas is exchanged, and oxygenated blood returns to the heart.
- *Systemic circulation*: Oxygenated blood is pumped from the left side of the heart and moves through the body. Oxygen, nutrients, and other substances are brought to the cells while the blood picks up waste products. The deoxygenated blood returns to the heart.

Because the pulmonary and the systemic circulation are closely tied, they will be discussed together. The *coronary circulation* (blood flow through the heart tissues) and *fetal circulation* (blood flow of a baby in utero) will also be examined.

Pulmonary and Systemic Circulations

Pulmonary circulation begins as the blood returns from the body. The superior vena cava and the inferior vena cava bring deoxygenated blood from the body to the right atrium. As the atria contract, the blood from the right atrium passes the tricuspid valve and empties into the right ventricle. When the ventricles contract, the blood in the right ventricle is pushed out past the pulmonary valve and enters the pulmonary artery trunk. The pulmonary artery trunk splits into the right and left pulmonary arteries. From there, the blood moves into the arterioles and then into the pulmonary capillaries in the lungs. The gas exchange occurs. Carbon dioxide leaves the blood and enters the lungs to be expelled. Oxygen enters the blood from the lungs. The oxygenated blood leaves the pulmonary capillaries and enters the pulmonary veins. The right and left pulmonary veins bring the blood back to the left atrium. This is the start of the systemic circulation.

When the atria are full of blood, they contract. The oxygenated blood in the left atrium moves past the bicuspid, or mitral, valve and empties into the left ventricle. When the ventricles contract, the blood in the left ventricle moves out of the heart, passing the aortic valve, and empties into the aorta. From here, the blood will move through the body before it returns to the heart. Blood from the head, neck, chest, and upper extremities empties into the superior vena cava before returning to the right atrium. Blood from the lower body empties into the inferior vena cava before returning to the right atrium.

CRITICAL THINKING APPLICATION **40.2**

Rebecca is helping Lizzy review the conduction system of the heart. To see what Lizzy can remember, Rebecca has her write down the five conduction system structures. What should Lizzy write down? What might be a creative way to remember these structures in order?

Coronary Circulation

The heart has its own blood vessels that support the tissues. The right and left coronary arteries are the first branches off the ascending aorta (Figure 40.3). The coronary arteries bring nutrients and oxygen to the heart tissue. The blood moves from the arteries to the capillaries in the myocardium. From there, the blood moves into the coronary veins. The coronary veins remove the waste products from the heart tissue. Blood from the coronary veins drains into the coronary sinus, which opens into the right atrium.

Coronary arteries have the important role of maintaining the myocardium. If a branch of the coronary artery becomes blocked, a person will experience a heart attack. The tissue supplied by the blocked artery will be deprived of oxygen and nutrients.

Hepatic Portal Circulation

In most cases, veins leaving an abdominal organ empty blood into the inferior vena cava as it heads to the heart. Veins from the spleen, gallbladder, pancreas, stomach, and intestines take an alternative route. Veins from these organs dump the blood into the hepatic portal vein, which takes the blood to the liver. In the liver, the blood moves through capillaries as it is filtered. Eventually, the blood drains into the hepatic veins before emptying into the inferior vena cava.

The liver has a special role in filtering the blood; it also metabolizes, or breaks down, substances. The hepatic portal system has many advantages:

- The **glucose** absorbed can be filtered and stored in the liver as glycogen. It will later be added back to the blood when the glucose levels are low.
- Toxic substances, such as alcohol and medications, can be partially filtered before moving to the rest of the body.

Fetal Circulation

Prior to birth, the baby is called a *fetus*. Fetal circulation differs from what we have discussed so far in this chapter. Before birth, the baby's lungs, gastrointestinal tract, and kidneys are not functioning as they will after birth. Toward the end of pregnancy, babies practice breathing as they breathe in the amniotic fluid. No gas exchange occurs. Babies also urinate, but the waste products in their blood are removed by their mothers' blood. Nutrients are passed through the blood from the mother.

During the early weeks of pregnancy, the placenta (reproductive organ) begins to grow. It attaches to the mother's uterus and connects to the growing baby via the umbilical cord. The umbilical cord contains two umbilical arteries and one umbilical vein. The arteries carry the fetal blood to the placenta. The umbilical vein carries oxygen and nutrient-rich blood to the baby. The waste, oxygen, and nutrient exchange occur in the placenta. There is a very thin wall separating the fetal blood from the mother's blood. There is no mixing of the two different blood supplies, although substances can pass between the separating wall. Oxygen and nutrients move from the mother's bloodstream to the fetal blood. Waste products (i.e., carbon dioxide) move from the fetal blood to the mother's blood.

Other structures that are unique to the growing baby in utero include the following:

- *Ductus venosus*: Shifts the majority of the blood from the umbilical vein and empties it into the inferior vena cava (Figure 40.4). This structure helps the blood bypass the immature liver. After birth, with the lack of blood flow from the umbilical vein, the ductus venosus **constricts**. Within 1 to 3 months after birth, it is permanently sealed.
- *Foramen ovale*: A small flaplike opening in the interatrial septum that allows blood to move from the right atrium to the left atrium (see Figure 40.4). This allows most of the blood to bypass the immature lungs. After birth, the flap opening is forced closed by the pressure of the blood pumping in the heart. During infancy, the flap should seal permanently.
- *Ductus arteriosus*: A short vessel that connects the pulmonary artery with the aorta. About 90% of the blood in the pulmonary artery is redirected to the aorta, bypassing the immature lungs. Usually, it closes at birth or shortly after.

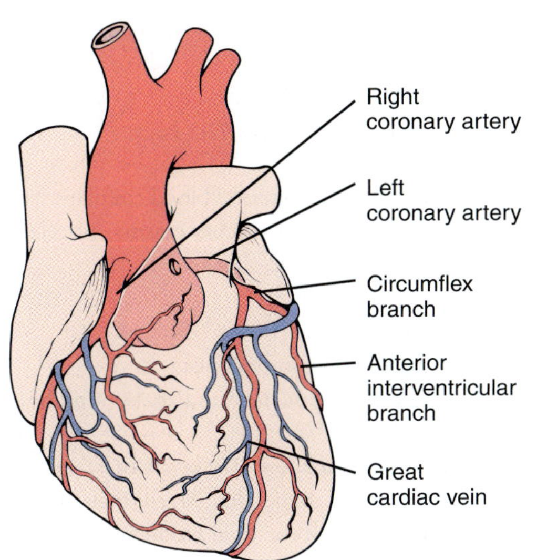

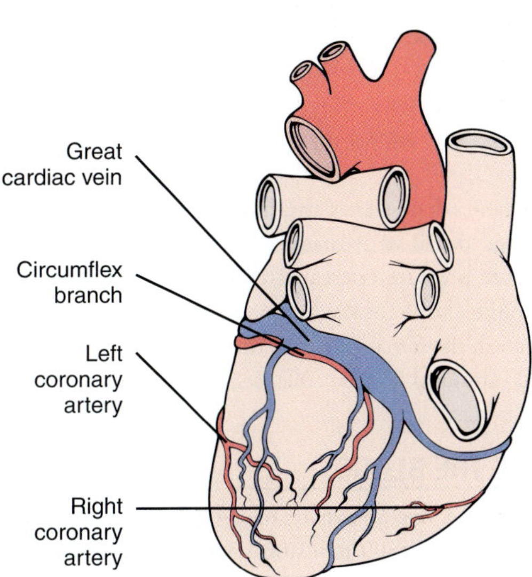

FIGURE 40.3 Coronary arteries. (From Frazier MS, et al: *Essentials of human diseases and conditions*, ed 5, St. Louis, 2013, Saunders.)

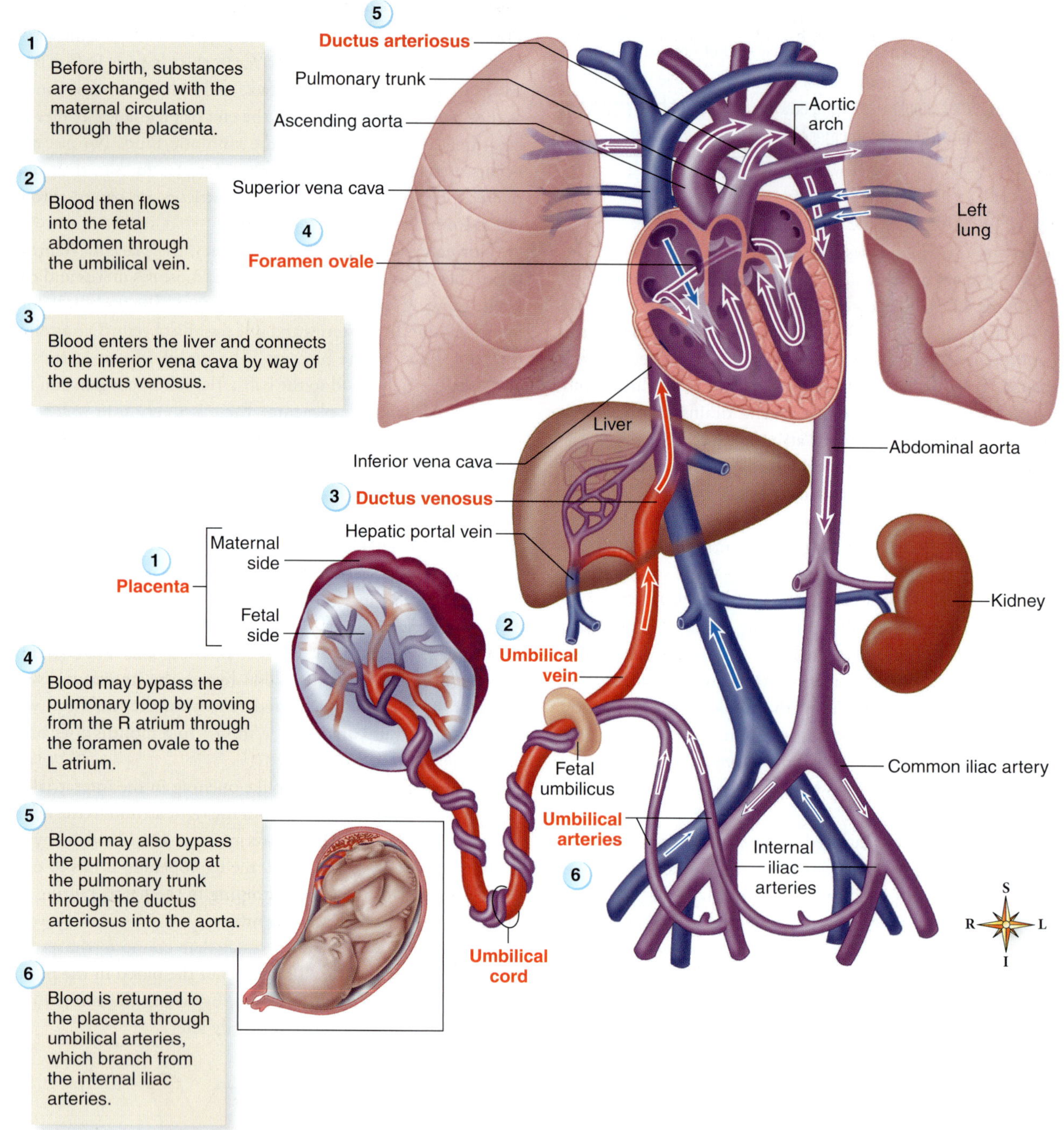

FIGURE 40.4 Fetal circulation. (From Patton KT, Thibodeau G: *The human body in health and disease*, ed 7, St. Louis, 2018, Mosby.)

At birth, when a baby takes the first breath and the umbilical cord is cut, these special structures are no longer needed. With the first breath, more pressure is created in the cardiovascular system. This helps with the closure of the foramen ovale. With the cutting of the umbilical cord, the remaining structures (ductus venosus, ductus arteriosus, and umbilical vessels) collapse.

ANATOMY OF THE BLOOD

A milliliter of blood has approximately 4.2 million to 6 million red blood cells (RBCs), 4500 to 11,000 white blood cells (WBCs), and 150,000 to 450,000 platelets. The average 150-pound (68-kg) person has approximately 5 liters of blood circulating throughout the body. The following sections discuss plasma, platelets, WBCs, and RBCs in more detail.

Blood Composition

Blood is made up of two components:

- *Liquid portion:* Called *plasma* and makes up about 55% of the total blood volume.
- *Formed elements:* Includes RBCs, WBCs, and platelets. The formed elements are suspended (freely float) in the plasma and make up about 45% of the total blood volume.

The following sections describe the components of the blood.

Plasma

Plasma is the liquid portion of **whole blood**. Plasma contains 90% water. Water is the **solvent** for all the dissolved substances that travel in the plasma. Plasma also contains the following components:

- *Plasma proteins*: Made in the liver; plasma proteins include the following:
  - *Albumin*: It is the most abundant protein in plasma, and it attracts water. It normally stays in the blood vessel; thus, it helps to maintain the blood volume.
  - *Globulins*: **Antibodies** are a type of globulin; they protect against infections.
  - *Clotting factors*: Include fibrinogen and prothrombin, which are important in the blood clotting or coagulation process.
  - *Complements*: **Enzymes** (proteins) that are normally inactive in the blood. When activated, they create protein rings that destroy pathogens.
- Inorganic substances and electrolytes (sodium, calcium, potassium, chloride, magnesium, bicarbonate).
- Organic substances (amino acids, glucose, fats, cholesterol, hormones).
- Waste products (urea, uric acid, ammonia, creatinine).

Organic and inorganic substances are needed for metabolism and cellular function, repair, and reproduction. Cellular metabolism waste products are dissolved in the plasma and are transported to the liver, kidneys, and lungs for excretion.

Plasma has a very narrow pH range (7.35 to 7.45), which is necessary to make sure that red blood cells can transport the optimal level of oxygen in the blood. The range also allows needed chemical reactions in the body to continue to work. Most chemical reactions in the body are pH dependent. Without a stable blood pH, homeostasis is unlikely to be maintained.

Thrombocytes

Thrombocytes, also called *platelets,* have an irregular round or oval shape. They are formed in the bone marrow from **stem cells**. They are just a small piece or fragment of a much larger cell called a *megakaryocyte,* which is in the bone marrow. Platelets aid in coagulation, the process of changing a liquid to a solid. When an injury to a blood vessel occurs, platelets rush to the area and *agglutinate*, or clump together. This stops or slows the bleeding, thus controlling the blood flow *(hemostasis).*

Leukocytes

Leukocytes, also called *white blood cells* (WBCs), protect the body from invading pathogens. There are two main types:

- *Granulocytes*: Have granules within the **cytoplasm**, and they also have a segmented or multilobed nucleus. There are three types of granulocytes: neutrophils, eosinophils, and basophils. Each has its own role in immunity (Table 40.2 and Figure 40.5).
- *Agranulocytes*: Lack granules in the cytoplasm, and they have one nucleus. Granulocytes originate in the bone marrow and mature after entering the lymphatic system. There are two types of agranulocytes: monocytes and lymphocytes (see Table 40.2 and Figure 40.5).

TABLE 40.2 Types of White Blood Cells

TYPE	DESCRIPTION	ROLE
Granulocytes		
Neutrophils	Also called segs, polys, or polymorphonucleocytes (PMNs); most abundant white blood cell (WBC)	Phagocytic (FAG uh sih tik) (protect by engulfing and destroying foreign substances); clean up the infection site and aid in the healing process
Eosinophils	Also called eos; make up about 1% of the WBCs	Increase in number when the body is defending against allergens and parasites
Basophils	Also called basos; make up 1% or less of the WBCs in the circulation	Respond to an allergic reaction by releasing histamine, which causes an inflammatory response; also release heparin (an anticoagulant)
Agranulocytes		
Monocytes	Also called *monos;* contain a single, large nucleus; largest phagocytic WBC; transform into macrophages when in lymphatic tissue	Very aggressive phagocytic cells that can destroy pathogens, malignant cells, and tumor cells in the body
Lymphocytes	Also called *lymphs;* two types: T lymphocytes (T cells) and B lymphocytes (B cells)	Involved in the immune response and destroy pathogens; B cells produce antibodies; T cells attack foreign substances and assist B cells

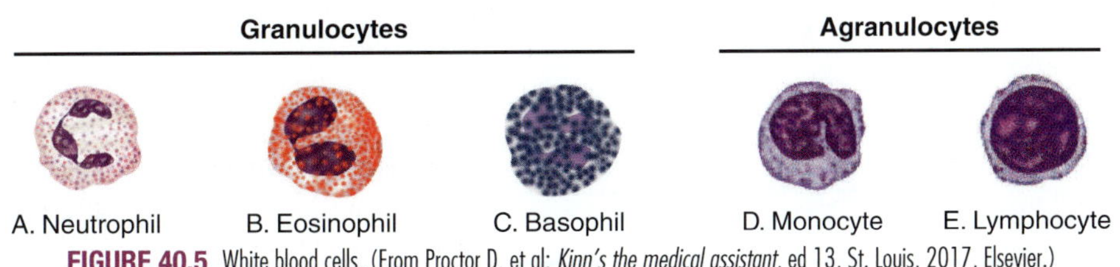

FIGURE 40.5 White blood cells. (From Proctor D, et al: *Kinn's the medical assistant,* ed 13, St. Louis, 2017, Elsevier.)

Erythrocytes

Erythrocytes, or red blood cells, have the important function of transporting oxygen (O_2) and carbon dioxide (CO_2) throughout the body. *Hemoglobin* (Hgb), a molecule on the RBC, is capable of binding, transporting, and releasing oxygen and carbon dioxide. Hemoglobin is made up of protein and iron.

RBC production is stimulated by *erythropoietin*, a hormone produced in the kidneys. **Hematopoiesis** of RBCs takes place in the red bone marrow. Stem cells produce immature RBCs that contain a nucleus. As an RBC matures, it loses its nucleus and is released into the bloodstream. RBCs are biconcave (curved inward on both sides), which allows for more surface area for the hemoglobin, thus allowing more O_2 and CO_2 to be carried (Figure 40.6). The shape also allows more flexibility as the RBC moves through the tiny capillaries.

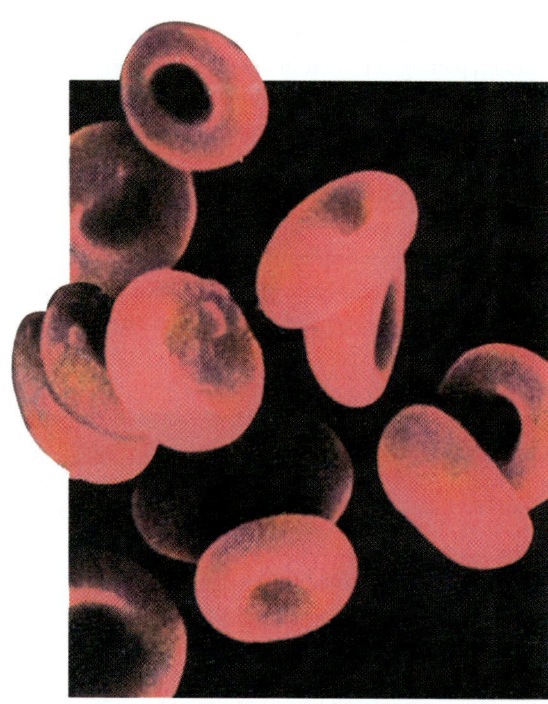

FIGURE 40.6 Red blood cells (RBCs). Color-enhanced scanning electron micrograph shows the detailed structure of normal RBCs. Note the biconcave shape of each RBC. (From Patton KT, Thibodeau GA: *The human body in health and disease*, ed 7, St. Louis, 2018, Elsevier.)

Red blood cells have a life span of approximately 120 days. When an RBC is no longer useful, it is broken down into iron and **bilirubin** in the spleen. The iron is stored mainly in the liver and is recycled into new RBCs. The bilirubin is further broken down into bile, which is excreted by the liver.

Blood Types

Two major classification systems are used with blood types, the ABO system and the Rh system. In the ABO system, each person has an A, a B, an ABO, or an O blood type. In the Rh system, a person is either Rh positive or Rh negative. For example, a person may have O-negative blood. In the ABO system, the person has type O blood and is Rh negative. These two systems are explained in more detail in the following sections.

ABO System

In the ABO system, each blood type is unique based on the specific **antigens** present or absent on the surface of the RBCs and specific antibodies circulating in the plasma (Table 40.3). Antigens are foreign substances to the body, and the immune system makes specific antibodies to fight off specific antigens. When a person receives a blood transfusion, the blood given must be compatible with the person's blood. If an antibody is present in the recipient's blood, the corresponding antigen cannot be in the donor's blood. For example, type O blood contains both A and B antibodies; thus blood with A or B antigens cannot be given. The only type of blood that is compatible with type O is type O. Another example is a person with type AB blood, which contains no antibodies. These people can receive all four blood types because they have no antibodies to attack the donor blood. Type AB blood is considered the universal recipient because it does not contain any antibodies. Type O is considered the universal donor because it does not contain any antigens, and everyone can receive type O blood.

Rh System

In the Rh system, there is a collection of 47 antigens that act together as a group and are referred to as the *Rh antigen* or *Rh factor.* When the Rh antigen is present, the person is said to be Rh positive. About 85% of the population in the United States is Rh positive, and 15% is Rh negative.

TABLE 40.3 Blood Types

TYPE	ANTIGENS PRESENT	ANTIBODIES PRESENT	CAN GIVE BLOOD TO	CAN RECEIVE BLOOD FROM
ABO System				
A	A antigen	B antibodies	A, AB	A, O
B	B antigen	A antibodies	B, AB	B, O
AB	A and B antigens	None	AB	AB, A, B, O
O	None	A and B antibodies	O, A, B, AB	O
Rh System				
Negative	Rh not present		Negative and positive	Negative
Positive	Rh present		Positive	Positive and negative

Rh antibodies are different from ABO antibodies. Rh antibodies are not preformed (present before antigen exposure), as are ABO antibodies. The first time a person is exposed to the Rh antigen, the immune system produces antibodies. This process is called *sensitization*. Nothing is noticeable during the first exposure, although subsequent exposures to the Rh antigen will cause lysis (destruction) of RBCs.

Blood typing is the process of determining a person's blood type using the ABO and Rh systems. If the person receives the wrong type of blood, a *transfusion reaction* can occur, which may be a serious, life-threatening situation. For instance, if a person with type A blood is transfused with type B blood, the anti-B antibodies in the recipient's blood will attack the B antigens in the donor's blood, causing *agglutination* (blood clumping) or *lysis* (blood cell rupture).

Erythroblastosis Fetalis

The Rh factor is an important consideration during pregnancy for Rh-negative mothers due to erythroblastosis fetalis (also called hemolytic disease of the newborn [HDN]). In this disorder, an Rh-negative mother who is carrying an Rh-positive fetus will develop antibodies to the Rh-positive blood if fetal blood exposure occurs. If another pregnancy occurs with an Rh-positive fetus, the mother's immune system produces antibodies that cross the placenta and destroy the fetal red blood cells.

To prevent this disorder, it is standard practice for the pregnant mother's blood to be tested *(typed)* early in pregnancy if the blood type is unknown. Mothers with Rh-negative blood receive an injection of RhoGAM (Rho[D] Immune Globulin [Human]) around weeks 26 to 28 of pregnancy. After the baby is born, the cord blood is tested. If the baby has Rh-positive blood, the mother receives another injection of RhoGAM within 72 hours of delivery.

MICRhoGam (a smaller dose of RhoGAM) should be given to Rh-negative women 72 hours after a threatened or actual termination of pregnancy (spontaneous [miscarriage] or induced) through week 12 of the pregnancy. For threatened or actual exposure to Rh-positive blood (e.g., through an invasive procedure, trauma, **ectopic pregnancy**, or pregnancy termination), Rh-negative women should receive RhoGAM within 72 hours. RhoGAM and MICRhoGAM are Rh_0 (D) human immune globulin, a blood product that prevents Rh immunization by binding to Rh-positive cells that sneak into the bloodstream, making them invisible to the mother's immune system.

PHYSIOLOGY OF THE CONDUCTION SYSTEM

To explore the physiology of the cardiovascular system, the action of the heart, blood vessels, and the blood components will be examined. The following sections discuss the conduction system, factors that affect blood pressure, and coagulation.

First it is necessary to learn the cardiac muscle characteristics and the three states they must undergo for each impulse to understand the conduction system. After this discussion, the conduction system and the blood volume will be examined.

Cardiac Muscle

There are two types of cardiac cells, electrical or conduction system cells and myocardial cells. The electrical cells are found in the conduction system. They have three unique characteristics:

- *Automaticity*: The cells create and discharge the electrical impulse.
- *Excitability*: The cells respond to the electrical impulse.
- *Conductivity*: The cells transmit electrical impulses to other cells.

The myocardial cells are found in the myocardium. They can shorten and lengthen their fibers for contraction (called *contractility*). The fibers made from the myocardial cells can contract for prolonged periods of time without fatigue and use less adenosine triphosphate (ATP) than other muscles. These features are beneficial for the heart.

Cardiac muscle fibers are electrically linked, forming one unit. A myocardial cell forms a strong, electrical connection to the next cells through special junctions called *intercalated discs*. The intercalated discs are responsible for the cell-to-cell communication that is required for coordinated muscle contraction. The intercalated discs help the muscle fibers form one unit that contracts all at once instead of a little at a time. The "one unit" approach is important because the atrial chambers need to contract together, and the ventricles need to contract at about the same time.

Conduction System Structures

As previously stated, the electrical cells make up the conduction system of the heart. These cells are found throughout the myocardium. They can respond to and transmit electronic impulses to neighboring cells. The conduction system is composed of five structures (see Figure 40.2):

- *Sinoatrial* (SA) *node*: Located in the posterior superior wall of the right atrium, the SA node is called the "pacemaker of the heart." This is because the electrical cells in the SA node generate the impulse that starts the heartbeat. When the SA node discharges the impulse, it travels in many directions through the heart muscle. The impulse also moves quickly across special bands of tissue called *internodal tracts*. The Bachmann bundle, a specialized internodal tract, takes the impulse to the left atrium. Other internodal tracts take the impulse quickly to the AV node. The impulse moving through the atrial chambers triggers the chambers to contract.
- *Atrioventricular* (AV) *node*: The AV node is located at the base of the interatrial septum. When the impulse reaches the AV node, it moves very slowly through it.
- *Bundle of His* (also called the *atrioventricular* [AV] *bundle*): The bundle of His is located in the upper interventricular septum. When the impulse leaves the AV node, it moves to the bundle of His.
- *Right and left bundle branches*: The bundle branches are located in the lower interventricular septum. After the impulse passes through the bundle of His, it enters the right and left bundle branches. The right bundle branch brings the impulse to the right ventricle. The left bundle branch brings the impulse to the left ventricle.
- *Purkinje fibers*: The bundle branches split into many Purkinje fibers. Purkinje fibers transmit the impulse quickly and efficiently to the ventricular myocardial cells. This causes the ventricular chambers to contract.

The cardiac muscle is different from other muscles in the body. The heart is controlled by the autonomic nervous system and the heart's own conduction system. When the heart rate needs to change to meet the demands of the body, the autonomic nervous system automatically kicks in.

CRITICAL THINKING APPLICATION 40.3

Rebecca is helping Lizzy review the conduction system of the heart. To see what Lizzy can remember, Rebecca has her write down the five conduction system structures. What should Lizzy write down? What might be a creative way to remember these structures in order?

States of Cardiac Cells

The cardiac cells cycle through three states or steps in the same sequence for each impulse:

1. *Polarized state*: Before the impulse hits the cells, they are in a polarized state. There is no electrical activity during the polarized state. Think of this as the "waiting" stage.
2. *Depolarized state*: When the impulse hits the cells, the cells' charges change. This is due to the movement of the ions (e.g., sodium, potassium, and calcium) across the cells' membrane. The change of the cells' charges allows the impulse to move through the cell, causing action potential (also called *depolarization*). Electrical activity can be recorded on an electrocardiogram (ECG) when the cells are in the depolarized state. (ECGs are discussed in Chapter 26.)
3. *Repolarized state*: After the impulse passes over the cells, the ions move back to their original location. This causes the cells' charge to change. This recovery phase is called the *repolarized state.* Electrical activity (less than the depolarized state) can also be recorded on an ECG during the repolarized state.

When you are discussing the three states and the chambers affected, the chamber (atrial, ventricular) comes before the state (e.g., atrial polarization, ventricular depolarization). This terminology will be used as we examine the blood flow and the conduction system together.

CRITICAL THINKING APPLICATION 40.4

Lizzy struggles with remembering what occurs with polarization, depolarization, and repolarization. Rebecca encourages her to keep the definitions simple, maybe using one to two words to summarize what is occurring. How might Lizzy define each of these words?

Conduction System and Blood Flow

The conduction system is the electrical system in the heart. As already mentioned, it is recorded on the ECG. Electrical impulses from the conduction system cause the chambers of the heart to contract. This contraction is a mechanical action, and, as a result, blood moves through the heart. The mechanical action can be seen with echocardiography (ECHO), described later in this chapter.

Table 40.4 summarizes an impulse's path through the conduction system and the resulting mechanical action with the blood flow movement. Notice that the atrial chamber state is always one step ahead of the ventricular chambers.

PHYSIOLOGY OF THE BLOOD

The components in the blood play an important role in the process of blood clotting or *coagulation*. Blood is also important because it carries nutrients and oxygen to the cells. Maintaining an adequate blood pressure helps with the delivery of nutrients and oxygen to the cells. Both the process of coagulation and an adequate blood

TABLE 40.4 Impulse Pathway through the Conduction System with the Triggered Mechanical Actions

IMPULSE MOVING THROUGH CONDUCTION SYSTEM	ATRIAL CARDIAC CELLS' STATE	VENTRICULAR CARDIAC CELLS' STATE	MECHANICAL ACTION TRIGGERED BY IMPULSE	
			RIGHT SIDE OF HEART	RIGHT SIDE OF HEART
SA node *(pacemaker)* generates the impulse, which travels to the AV node	Atrial depolarization	Ventricular polarization	Right atrium contracts; blood passes the tricuspid valves and empties into the right ventricle	Left atrium contracts; blood passes the bicuspid valves and empties into the left ventricle
Impulse moves slowly through AV node			Allows the atrial chambers to finish contracting	
Impulse leaves the AV node and moves to the bundle of His, to the right and left bundle branches, and to the Purkinje fibers	Atrial repolarization	Ventricular depolarization	Right ventricle contracts; blood passes the pulmonary valve before emptying into the pulmonary artery as it heads to the lungs	Left ventricle contracts; blood passes the aortic valve before emptying into the aorta as it goes to the body
(The impulse is now done.)	Atrial polarization	Ventricular repolarization (then moves into ventricular polarization)	Right atrium fills with deoxygenated blood from the body via the inferior vena cava and the superior vena cava	Left atrium fills with oxygenated blood from the lungs via the pulmonary vein

pressure are needed to sustain life. The following sections examine the process of coagulation and the factors that affect blood pressure.

Coagulation

The process required to form a blood clot is complicated, with many specific chemical reactions and clotting factors involved. What follows is a simplified version of this process.

First, a damaged vessel will constrict to slow the flow of blood through the vessel. In response to the injury, platelets become sticky and clump together *(aggregation).* Platelets then stick to the area of injury *(adhesion).* Because of platelet aggregation and adhesion, a platelet plug is formed over the injury, and platelets release clotting factors, which aid in the process of coagulation. The injured blood vessel tissue also activates clotting factors in the blood plasma. The interaction between the clotting factors works to form *fibrin*, a white, **filamentous**, tough protein strand that creates a netlike structure. The fibrin net traps red blood cells and more platelets to form a **thrombus**. This process is called *blood clotting* or *coagulation.* When the body stops the flow of blood through coagulation, the process is called *hemostasis.*

Factors Affecting the Blood Pressure

About 1 in 3 American adults has high blood pressure. This means that many of the patients seen in an ambulatory care center may be diagnosed with high blood pressure, or *hypertension.* More information on hypertension will be provided later in the chapter. By contrast, low blood pressure, or *hypotension*, can be life threatening in some cases.

The pressure of the blood is highest in the arteries and lowest in the veins. Thus, we measure arterial blood pressure. *Blood pressure* (BP) can be defined as the resulting force of blood against the walls of the arteries. Two measurements are taken during the cardiac cycle (a complete heartbeat):

- *Systole* or the *contractive phase*: Systolic pressure is measured when the heart is contracting and pumping out the blood.
- *Diastole* or the *relaxation phase*: Diastolic pressure is measured when the heart is resting between contractions.

You will learn more about the procedure to take blood pressure in Chapter 20. This section addresses the factors that can influence blood pressure.

Blood Volume

Blood volume, or the amount of circulating blood, has a direct influence on blood pressure. The greater the blood volume, the more force it exerts on the arterial walls. If the blood volume is low, less force or pressure will be put on the arterial walls. Think of a garden hose attached to a faucet. If you turn on the faucet to the maximum level, there will be a lot of water pressure in the hose. If you turn on the faucet to get a trickle, there is very little water pressure in the hose.

Let us briefly examine the factors that increase and decrease blood volume. The blood volume can be raised by the following actions:

- Blood, plasma, and fluid (intravenous [IV]) transfusions
- Increased sodium intake (because water follows sodium, more water will be drawn into the bloodstream due to the elevated sodium levels)

Blood volume can decrease due to *hemorrhaging* (bleeding), dehydration, and diuretic medications. Diuretics help pull water and sodium from the blood, thus lowering blood volume.

Strength of Ventricular Contractions

The left ventricle pumps blood to the body. The greater the force of the contraction, the more blood is pumped into the arteries. This increases the blood pressure. If the left ventricular contraction is weak, less blood is pumped out of the heart, and thus the blood pressure is lower. Digoxin is a medication that reduces the heart rate and strengthens the contractions of the heart.

With heart disease, tests are done to check how the left ventricle is functioning. The *stroke volume* is the amount of blood pushed out of the left ventricle compared to the total volume of blood that filled the ventricle. It is a measure of the ejection fraction of the cardiac output. As heart disease occurs, the stroke volume can decrease.

Resistance to Blood Flow

Any factor that increases the resistance to blood flow through the arteries will increase the blood pressure. Factors that increase resistance include the size of the *lumen* (inner opening) of the arteries, the elasticity of the arterial walls, and the **viscosity** of the blood.

The *peripheral resistance* of blood vessels refers to the size of the lumen and the amount of blood flowing through it. The smaller the vessel's lumen, the greater the resistance to blood flow, thus increasing blood pressure. Several dynamics lead to decreased lumen size, including the following:

- *Plaque* (waxy substance) builds up in the arteries and hardens over time. This buildup narrows the arteries and causes higher blood pressure.
- Smoking.
- Constriction of smooth muscles, causing vasoconstriction (VAE zoe kon strik shahn). Several medications—including benazepril, lisinopril, and losartan—relax smooth muscles, thus reducing blood pressure.

Another factor that increases blood flow resistance is the loss of vessel elasticity. The inner layer of an artery contains elastic-like fibers that allow the vessel to expand and contract. Arteries dilate as the blood is pumped out of the heart and narrows between heartbeats to help maintain blood pressure. Increasing age and plaque buildup reduce the elasticity of the vessels. To understand the effect of plaque on the vessels, think of dried glue on a balloon. The dried glue prevents that section of the balloon from expanding. The plaque is like the dried glue. It prevents the walls from expanding.

Lastly, the viscosity of blood influences the resistance to blood flow. As the viscosity of the blood increases, so does the resistance, and the blood pressure rises. The thickness of blood increases when more blood cells are present (e.g., **polycythemia** and blood transfusion).

In summary, blood pressure can be influenced by blood volume, the strength of ventricular contractions, and the resistance to blood flow. Resistance can be increased by the following:

- Narrowed lumen (e.g., due to plaque, smoking, and vasoconstriction)
- Loss of vessel elasticity due to aging and plaque
- Increased viscosity of the blood

CRITICAL THINKING APPLICATION 40.5

Because many of their patients have high blood pressure, Rebecca wants to make sure Lizzy understands the factors that affect blood pressure. She asks Lizzy to summarize factors that increase blood pressure. How might Lizzy respond?

LIFE SPAN CHANGES OF THE CARDIOVASCULAR SYSTEM

An unborn child receives oxygen and nutrients from the mother's blood through the placenta. As described earlier in this chapter, the ductus venosus, ductus arteriosus, foramen ovale, and umbilical vessels are special structures that help with fetal circulation. After birth, these structures are no longer necessary.

The heart rate decreases as a child grows and matures. The systemic vascular resistance increases with age. This means that the resistance for blood flow increases, and thus the blood pressure increases with age.

Changes in Pregnancy

During pregnancy, the mother's cardiovascular system undergoes changes:

- Cardiac output (the amount of blood pushed out of the heart in 1 minute) increases.
- Extracellular fluid volume increases; thus the blood volume is greater.
- Total peripheral resistance decreases, thus reducing the blood pressure.
- Blood flow to various organs increases.
- As the pregnancy progresses into the third trimester, the blood pressure increases.

Changes in Older Adults

As a person ages, the heart and blood vessels undergo change. The following heart changes occur:

- SA node loses some cells; thus, the heart rate can be slower.
- The left ventricle may increase in size, thus reducing the amount of blood it can hold.
- Normal ECG changes can occur with age.
- Valves can become thicker and stiffer, causing a heart murmur.
- Arterial walls become stiffer, thus increasing the blood pressure.

Baroreceptors in the carotid arteries and aorta detect changes in blood pressure and help maintain a fairly constant blood pressure with position changes. With age, the baroreceptors become less sensitive, making older people more at risk for orthostatic hypotension when changing positions.

Common Signs and Symptoms of Cardiovascular Diseases and Disorders

Many patients seen in the ambulatory care facility have cardiovascular diseases. Common signs and symptoms include the following:

- Angina pectoris (chest pain) and palpitations (fast, strong, or irregular heartbeats)
- Bradycardia (a pulse of fewer than 60 beats per minute [bpm]) and tachycardia (a pulse that is greater than 100 bpm)

Common Signs and Symptoms of Cardiovascular Diseases and Disorders—cont'd

- Bruit, an abnormal blowing or swishing sound heard over the artery when a Doppler ultrasound or stethoscope is used (Figure 40.7).
- Cardiomegaly (an enlargement of the heart) and edema (swelling)
- Cyanosis (a bluish discoloration of the skin, lips, and nail beds), pallor (paleness of the skin), and diaphoresis (profuse sweating)
- Dyspnea (difficulty breathing), orthopnea (dyspnea with lying flat, relieved when sitting up), and shortness of breath (SOB) (breathlessness)
- Venous distension (enlarged veins) and **syncope**

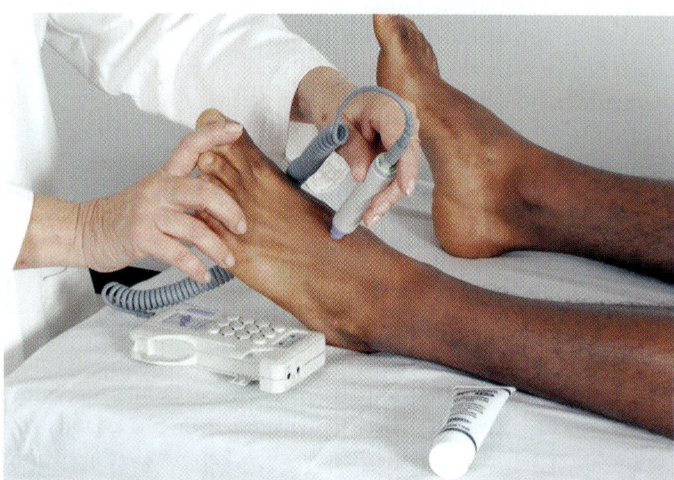

FIGURE 40.7 Using a Doppler to check the pulse. (From Jarvis C: *Physical examination and health assessment*, ed 7, St. Louis, 2016, Saunders.)

HEART DISEASES AND DISORDERS

Diseases and disorders of the heart affect the conduction system, the heart muscle, and the valves. The following sections describe common heart diseases and disorders.

Arrhythmias

An *arrhythmia* or dysrhythmia is an abnormal heart rate or rhythm. The rhythm may be irregular, or tachycardia or bradycardia may be occurring. The most common arrhythmia is *atrial fibrillation*, which means the rate is fast and the rhythm is irregular.

Arrhythmias are caused by an issue with the heart's conduction system, including an extra beat; the impulse is blocked, slowed, or takes a different pathway through the heart. Arrhythmias can be caused by diseases (e.g., heart failure), stress, substances (e.g., medications, caffeine), and electrolyte imbalances. Arrhythmias may be intermittent or constant. Signs and symptoms of arrhythmias include the following:

- Fast or slow heart rate
- Irregular, skipping, or uneven heartbeats
- Lightheadedness, dizziness, shortness of breath (SOB)
- Pallor, angina, sweating

The provider will listen to the heart with a stethoscope. An ECG is usually the first test done. Heart monitoring devices (e.g., the Holter monitor and an event monitor) provide ECG monitoring over days to weeks. Other tests ordered may include ECHO, coronary angiography, and an *electrophysiology study* (EPS), an in-depth study of the heart's electrical system. Treatment depends on the severity of the arrhythmia. Treatments may include *defibrillation* or *cardioversion*, which shocks the heart into a normal rhythm, or an implantable pacemaker to help establish a normal rate and rhythm. Antiarrhythmic medications, cardiac ablation, and an implantable **cardiac defibrillator** may also be used.

Cardiomyopathy

With cardiomyopathy, the heart muscle becomes abnormal. It may become thin and weakened, enlarged and thick, or rigid. As the disease worsens, the heart becomes less efficient at pumping blood and maintaining a normal electrical rhythm. Cardiomyopathy can lead to arrhythmias, heart failure, edema, and heart valve problems.

There are many types of cardiomyopathies; some develop due to other diseases, and others are inherited. This disease can affect people of all ages. Here are the major risk factors for cardiomyopathy:

- Diabetes mellitus, metabolic diseases, or severe obesity
- Diseases that cause heart damage (e.g., heart attack, coronary heart disease)
- A family history of cardiomyopathy
- Long-term alcoholism
- Long-term hypertension (high blood pressure)

Some people may never have symptoms, whereas others do not experience symptoms during the early stages of the disease. As the condition worsens, a person may experience SOB, especially after activity, edema in the legs, feet, ankles, abdomen, distension of neck veins, and fatigue.

The provider will obtain a history and perform a physical exam. Abnormal heart and lung sounds might be heard with a stethoscope. A heart murmur may be present. Crackling in the lungs may indicate fluid in the lungs. Swelling can also be seen, as mentioned in the previous section. A chest x-ray, an ECG, ECHO, and a stress test may be ordered. Further procedures may include cardiac catheterization, coronary angiography, or myocardial biopsy. Treatments depend on the severity of the condition. Treatments may include healthy lifestyle changes and medications, such as antiarrhythmics, anticoagulants, diuretics, and beta-blockers, which lower the heart rate. Surgery can also be done, including a septal myectomy (removal of the thickened septal muscle), a heart transplantation, and an implanted device.

Congenital Heart Defects

There are numerous congenital heart defects. Table 40.5 describes common defects. Depending on the type and severity of the defect, the newborn baby may require immediate surgery.

The cause of these congenital defects may be genetic, chromosomal, or unknown. The signs and symptoms of the defect will depend on its type and severity. For some, there are no symptoms, and the person may not realize the condition exists until adulthood. Other defects may cause the baby to have the following conditions:

- Cyanosis, increased respiration rate, or breathing difficulties
- Difficulty feeding, tiredness with feeding, or weight loss
- Abnormal heart murmur
- Sweating with feeding or crying

TABLE 40.5 Congenital Heart Defects

DEFECT	DESCRIPTION
Atrial septal defect (ASD)	A hole in the interatrial septum allows oxygen-rich blood from the left atrium to flow into the right atrium. May not have many symptoms. Hole may close on its own or with surgery.
Atrioventricular septal defect	Holes are between the right and left chambers, and the valves are malformed. Surgery is required to patch holes.
Coarctation of the aorta	Narrowing of the aorta, resulting in blood backflowing into the left ventricle, high blood pressure, and weakened pulses in the legs. Surgery or balloon angioplasty can correct the condition.
Dextro-transposition of the great arteries	The pulmonary artery and the aorta are switched. Oxygen-rich blood is pumped back to the lungs, and the deoxygenated blood is pumped back to the body. Requires emergency surgery.
Hypoplastic left heart syndrome	Structures on the left side of the heart are not correctly developed. Treated with medications and surgery to improve blood flow.
Patent foramen ovale (PFO)	Foramen ovale does not close during infancy but remains *patent* (open). May not have any symptoms and may not require treatment.
Patent ductus arteriosus (PDA)	Ductus arteriosus does not close soon after birth, causing too much blood to move into the pulmonary circulation. A heart murmur may be the only sign.
Pulmonary atresia	Pulmonary valve does not form, and blood cannot flow to the lungs. Requires immediate surgery after birth to improve blood flow to the lungs.
Tetralogy of Fallot (TOF)	Consists of four major conditions: ventricular septal defect, pulmonary stenosis, defective aortic valve, and ventricular hypertrophy. Requires immediate surgery.
Ventricular septal defect (VSD)	Septal wall is not fully developed between the ventricles, causing a hole. Blood tends to flow from the left ventricle into the right ventricle, stressing the pulmonary system.

Some of the defects may be identified during the pregnancy. Fetal echocardiography can be used on a baby in utero to detect cardiac abnormalities. After birth, ECHO, pulse oximetry, ECG, and chest x-rays may be performed to help diagnose the defect. Treatment for congenital heart defects depends on the type and severity of the defect. Some holes may close on their own, whereas others may require surgery to patch them. Some defects will be monitored, but no treatment will be required. Life-threatening defects will require emergency surgery after birth and follow-up throughout childhood.

Congestive Heart Failure

Congestive heart failure (CHF), also called *heart failure,* occurs when the heart does not efficiently pump blood. Blood backs up behind the failing pump (side of the heart). *Systolic heart failure* occurs when the heart muscle cannot pump the blood out of the heart. *Diastolic heart failure* occurs when the chamber muscle is stiff and does not completely fill up with blood. Heart failure can affect one or both sides of the heart. There are numerous types of heart failure:

- *Right-sided heart failure*: Fluid may back up into the body, causing swelling in the legs, feet, and abdomen.
- *Left-sided heart failure*: Fluid may back up into the lungs, causing shortness of breath and abnormal lung sounds.
- *Cor pulmonale*: Right-sided heart failure caused by high blood pressure in the right ventricle and pulmonary arteries.

Coronary artery disease (CAD) and high blood pressure are the most common causes of heart failure. Other causes include congenital problems, heart attack, faulty valves, arrhythmias, infections, and other diseases (e.g., thyroid problems). Symptoms can develop slowly or suddenly, depending on the cause. Symptoms can differ based on the side of the heart that is failing. The following are common signs and symptoms:

- Cough and shortness of breath with reclining or activity
- Fatigue, faintness, weakness, and loss of appetite
- Fast or irregular pulse and palpitations
- **Pitting edema** in the feet and legs
- Swollen liver and abdomen, weight gain

During the physical exam, the provider will listen for abnormal heart and lung sounds and check for edema (Figure 40.8). Echocardiography, imaging tests, and blood tests may be ordered. Treatment includes monitoring weight; limiting dietary cholesterol, salts, and fluids; and medications (e.g., diuretics, antihypertensives, and digoxin). Surgery, a pacemaker, an implantable defibrillator, or heart transplantation may also be needed.

Heart Valve Diseases

There are many types of valvular disease. Two types of heart valve disease can occur with each of the valves: either **stenosis** or **insufficiency** (also called *regurgitation* or *incompetence*). When you name the disease, the valve is followed by *stenosis* or *insufficiency* (e.g., tricuspid stenosis, tricuspid insufficiency). With stenosis, the heart may need to work harder to push blood through the smaller opening. With insufficiency, the valve does not close completely, and blood leaks backward across the valve into the prior chamber (Figure 40.9). The following sections discuss more common valvular diseases.

Aortic Insufficiency

With aortic insufficiency, the aortic valve does not close tightly. The blood backs up into the left ventricle. This is more common in males between the ages of 30 and 60.

Many conditions cause this disease, including high blood pressure, syphilis, congenital problems, and endocarditis. Signs and symptoms may not be present or may be slow to develop. They include a bounding pulse, angina, fainting, fatigue, palpitations, SOB, and swelling of the feet.

Besides the physical exam, a person may have an aortic angiography, ECHO, left heart catheterization, magnetic resonance imaging (MRI), and transthoracic echocardiography done to diagnose the condition. The treatment goal is to reduce blood pressure through medications. The patient may need surgery to replace the valve.

Mitral Valve Prolapse

Mitral valve prolapse occurs when one or both cusps of the mitral valve protrude back into the left atrium during ventricular systole.

This condition is congenital or genetic. The patient may experience palpitations, SOB, cough, fatigue, dizziness, anxiety, migraines, and chest discomfort.

The provider will do a physical exam, and additional tests will be ordered, including ECHO, Doppler ultrasound, chest x-ray, and an ECG. Treatment consists of medications (beta-blockers, diuretics, vasodilators) and surgery to repair or replace the valve.

Rheumatic Fever

Rheumatic fever is an inflammatory reaction that affects the heart valves (**valvulitis**) and causes swelling and scarring of the valves. Permanent damage to the valves leads to rheumatic heart disease.

Rheumatic fever occurs 2 to 4 weeks after a strep (group A *Streptococcus*) throat infection. Antibodies made by the body to attack the streptococcal infection start attacking the body tissues

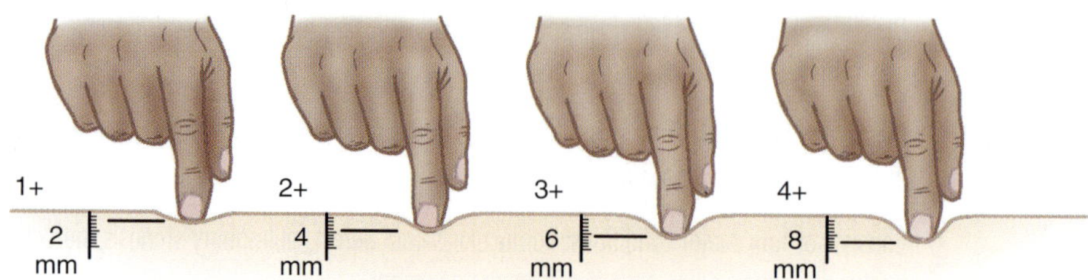

FIGURE 40.8 Providers measure pitting edema from 1+ to 4+. (From Ball J, et al: *Seidel's guide to physical examination*, St. Louis, 2019, Mosby.)

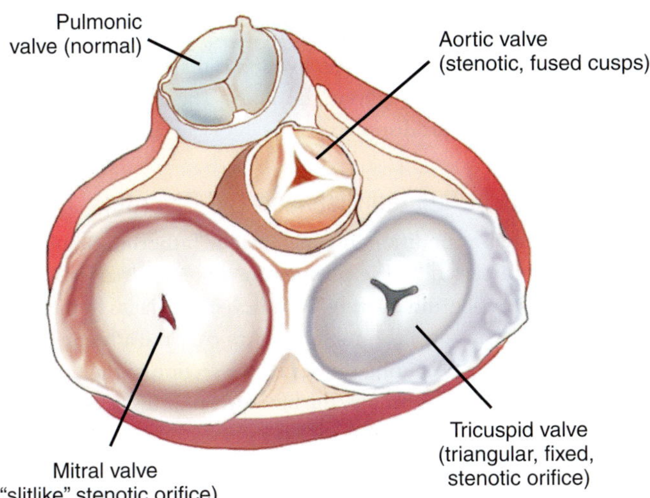

FIGURE 40.9 Valvular heart diseases. Disorders of the aortic, mitral, and tricuspid valves. (From Shiland B: *Medical terminology and anatomy for ICD-10 coding*, ed 2, St. Louis, 2016, Mosby.)

(joints and heart valves), causing inflammation, swelling, and scarring. The patient may have a fever, joint pain, stomach pain, weakness, SOB, *nodules* (small bumps) under the skin by the elbows and knees, and a rash on the chest, abdomen, or back.

After the physical exam, the provider may order blood tests, chest x-rays, ECHO, and an ECG. Treatment consists of antibiotics to address the infection and nonsteroidal anti-inflammatory drugs (NSAIDs) and corticosteroids to reduce the inflammation. Surgery may be needed to repair the valve.

Metabolic Syndrome

Metabolic syndrome is also called *metabolic syndrome X* and *insulin resistance syndrome.* Metabolic syndrome is a group of factors that increase a person's risk for heart disease, type 2 diabetes, and stroke.

Several causes act together. These include an inactive lifestyle, being overweight, obesity, and insulin resistance. With insulin resistance, the body cannot use insulin properly, which leads to elevated blood glucose levels. Other risk factors for metabolic syndrome include the following:

- Age: The risk increases with age.
- Ethnicity: Hispanic women have the greatest risk.
- Obesity: Carrying too much weight in the abdomen increases the risk.
- History of gestational diabetes, nonalcoholic fatty liver disease, polycystic ovary syndrome, or sleep apnea.
- Family history of type 2 diabetes.

The only signs include a large waist circumference and symptoms of diabetes if the blood glucose is elevated. These symptoms include increased thirst, frequent urination, fatigue, and blurred vision.

The provider will diagnose metabolic syndrome based on the physical exam findings and the blood test results. A patient must have at least three of these risk factors to be diagnosed with metabolic syndrome:

- A large waistline, which is defined as a waist measurement of 35 inches or more for females and 40 inches or more for males
- A triglyceride level of 150 mg/dL or higher
- A low high-density lipoprotein (HDL) cholesterol level of less than 50 mg/dL for females and less than 40 mg/dL for males
- High blood pressure (which is 130/85 mm/Hg or higher)
- A fasting blood glucose level of 100 mg/dL or higher

Treatment is focused on maintaining a heart-healthy lifestyle. This includes following a heart-healthy eating plan that limits the saturated and trans fats eaten. It also includes managing stress, getting regular physical activity, smoking cessation, and aiming for a healthy weight.

Myocardial Infarction

Myocardial **infarction** (MI), also called a *heart attack,* affects more than 1 million people in the United States each year, and about half of them die as a result. With an MI, the blood flow is limited or blocked, and the heart muscle cells die due to the lack of oxygen.

An MI can be caused by a blood clot or plaque buildup in the coronary arteries. The following risk factors can be changed:

- Smoking, drinking alcohol, lack of exercise, obesity, and stress
- High cholesterol, high blood pressure, and uncontrolled diabetes

These factors cannot be changed:

- Age: Risk increases with age.
- Sex: Males have a higher risk; after menopause, females have almost the same risk as males.
- Genetics: Family history increases risk.
- Race: African Americans, Mexican Americans, Native Americans, and Hawaiians have a greater risk.

The most common warning symptoms of MIs include these:

- Angina pectoris (chest pain): May also be described as mild or severe heaviness, squeezing, pressure, or heartburn; pain may be constant or intermittent.
- Upper body discomfort or pain in one or both arms, shoulders, neck, jaw, or upper part of the abdomen.
- Shortness of breath with activity or rest.
- Cold sweat, tiredness without a reason, nausea and vomiting, dizziness, lightheadedness, arrhythmias, or palpitations.
- Females may have sharp, burning chest pain or back pain; two-thirds have no symptoms.

Diagnostic tests for an MI include an ECG and blood tests (i.e., troponin, creatine kinase [CK], creatine kinase–MB [CK-MB], and serum myoglobin tests). *CK-MB* is an enzyme found in the heart muscle cell. Within hours of a heart attack, the CK-MB level increases in the blood. It peaks within 12 to 24 hours and returns to normal by 48 to 72 hours. The blood tests may be repeated over time to look for changes. Angiocardiography may be done to study the coronary blood flow and identify blockages. Immediate treatment involves the following:

- Chewing aspirin to prevent additional clots
- Nitroglycerin to dilate the coronary arteries and help increase the oxygen to the heart muscle
- Oxygen therapy

As soon as the diagnosis is determined, thrombolytic medications (also called "clot busters") are given. These medications help the body's natural process of dissolving blood clots. Percutaneous coronary intervention may be done to open the coronary artery. Medications, lifestyle changes, and cardiac rehabilitation may also be initiated.

CRITICAL THINKING APPLICATION **40.6**

Rebecca reviews the chest pain protocol with Lizzy. It states that patients with chest pain need to chew an aspirin. Nitroglycerin and oxygen must also be administered to the patient. Rebecca asks Lizzy why aspirin, nitroglycerin, and oxygen are important if a person is experiencing chest pain. How might Lizzy answer this question?

Additional Heart Diseases and Disorders

There are many cardiovascular diseases and disorders. The following list provides a brief description of some of them:

- *Cardiac tamponade*: Blood or fluid buildup in the pericardial sac, causing pressure on the heart.
- *Endocarditis*: Also called *infective endocarditis* (IE). The inner lining of the heart is inflamed. Bacterial endocarditis is most common and can damage the valves.
- *Pericarditis*: Inflammation of the pericardium.

BLOOD VESSELS DISEASES AND DISORDERS

Diseases and disorders of the blood vessels can affect the blood flow to various locations throughout the body. The following sections describe common heart disorders.

Atherosclerosis-Related Diseases and Disorders

Atherosclerosis is a condition in which plaque (**atheroma**) builds up and narrows the arteries. The plaque can prevent the arteries from properly constricting and dilating. At times, small cracks in the vessel wall can occur, causing a thrombus to form over the atheroma, partially or completely occluding the vessel. If a section of the thrombus breaks away and travels through the bloodstream, this is an **embolus** (Figure 40.10).

The cause of atherosclerosis is unknown. Studies have shown that it can develop in childhood and worsens with age. Risk factors for atherosclerosis include smoking, an unhealthy diet, lack of physical activity, high blood pressure, unhealthy cholesterol levels, and

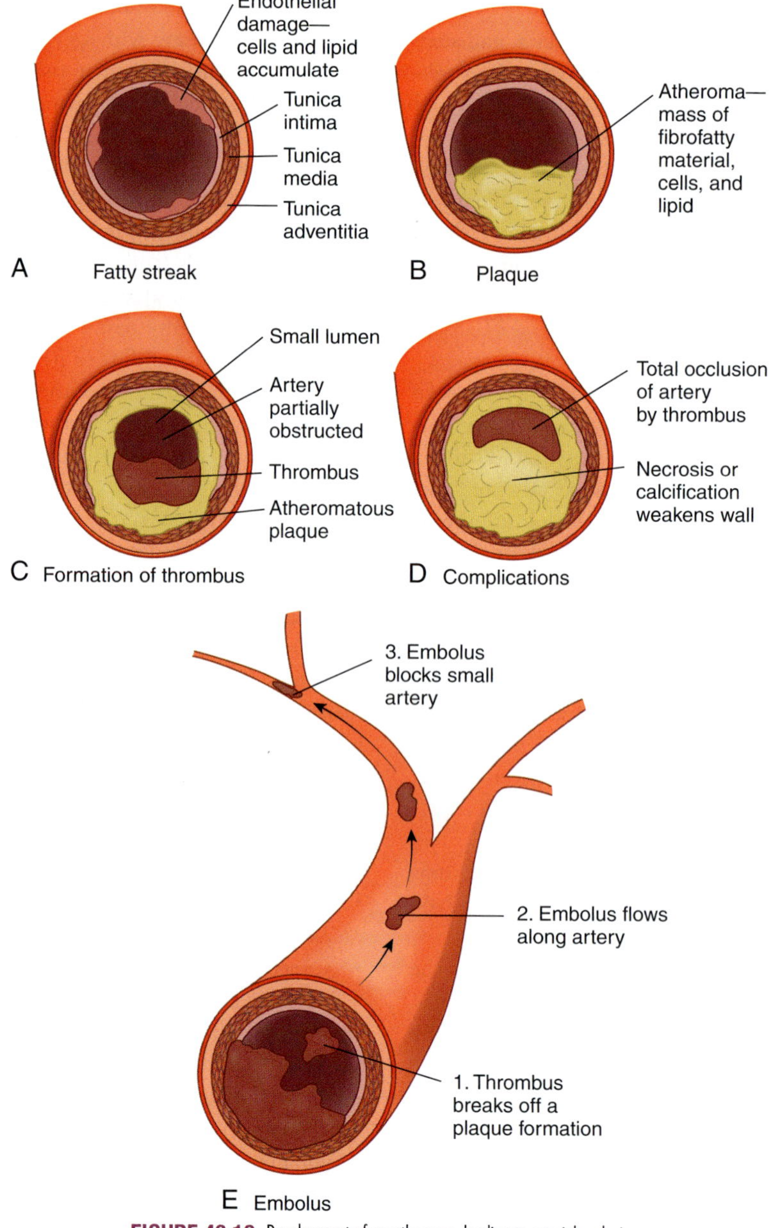

FIGURE 40.10 Development of an atheroma, leading to arterial occlusion.

TABLE 40.6 Atherosclerosis-Related Diseases

DISEASE	DESCRIPTION	SIGNS AND SYMPTOMS
Carotid artery disease	Plaque builds up in the carotid arteries and may lead to a stroke.	Sudden weakness or paralysis (inability to move), numbness, confusion, problems speaking or seeing, dizziness, and other symptoms of a stroke
Coronary heart disease (CHD) or coronary artery disease (CAD)	Plaque builds up in the coronary arteries. Can lead to angina (chest pain) or myocardial infarction (heart attack). Also known as ischemic heart disease.	Angina; pain in the shoulder, arm, neck, jaw or back; indigestion, shortness of breath, arrhythmias
Coronary microvascular disease (MVD)	Plaque builds up in the tiny coronary arteries, damaging the vessel walls.	Angina, shortness of breath, fatigue, lack of energy, sleep problems
Peripheral artery disease (PAD)	Plaque builds up in the large arteries of the legs, arms, and pelvis.	Numbness, pain, and life-threatening infections
Chronic kidney disease	Plaque builds up in the renal arteries and can cause kidney damage.	Tiredness, loss of appetite, nausea, swelling of hands or feet, numbness, changes in amount of urine

uncontrolled diabetes mellitus. The signs and symptoms depend on which arteries are affected by the plaque. In many cases, no symptoms are felt until the artery is severely narrowed or blocked. Several diseases can result from plaque buildup. Table 40.6 presents the descriptions, signs, and symptoms of atherosclerosis-related diseases.

Diagnostic procedures include blood tests to check the cholesterol, glucose, and protein levels. Additional tests include an ECG, echocardiography, chest x-ray, computed tomography (CT) scan, angiography, and a stress test. The goals of treatment are to lower the risk of blood clot formation, prevent diseases, and widen the affected arteries. Heart-healthy lifestyle changes will be encouraged. This involves exercise, a healthy diet, building stress-coping and management skills, maintaining a healthy weight, and smoking cessation. Medications that lower cholesterol levels may be used. Percutaneous coronary intervention, coronary artery bypass graft (CABG) surgery, or a carotid endarterectomy may also be performed (Figure 40.11).

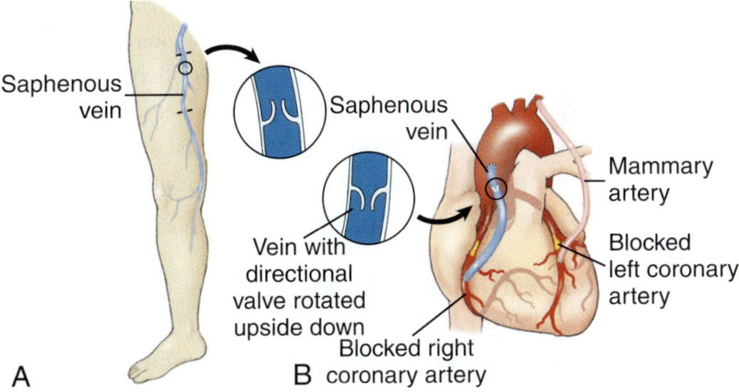

FIGURE 40.11 Coronary artery bypass graft (CABG) surgery. **(A)** A section of vein is harvested from the right leg and is anastomosed to a coronary artery to bypass an occlusion of the right coronary artery. **(B)** Bypass of the left coronary artery with a mammary artery. (From Shiland B: *Medical terminology and anatomy for ICD-10 coding*, ed 2, St. Louis, 2016, Mosby.)

CRITICAL THINKING APPLICATION 40.7

Lizzy is working with Ken Thomas, a patient. He asks her about plaque in the arteries and what can happen if a person has a lot of plaque. How might Lizzy answer Ken's questions?

Deep Vein Thrombosis

Deep vein thrombosis (DVT) or thrombophlebitis occurs when a thrombus forms in a vein deep in the body, usually in the legs. DVTs can occur at any age, but they most commonly occur in people over the age of 60. An embolus can occur from a DVT, which can lead to life-threatening conditions, including a pulmonary embolism (PE), cerebrovascular accident (*stroke*), or myocardial infarction (heart attack).

Blood clots can form when the vein's inner lining and valves are damaged by surgery, injuries, inflammation, or an immune response (Figure 40.12). Blood clots can also occur when the blood flow is slow or if the blood has an increase in viscosity. Estrogen, birth control pills, and inherited conditions can cause an increased risk for clotting. Here are some other risk factors for DVTs:

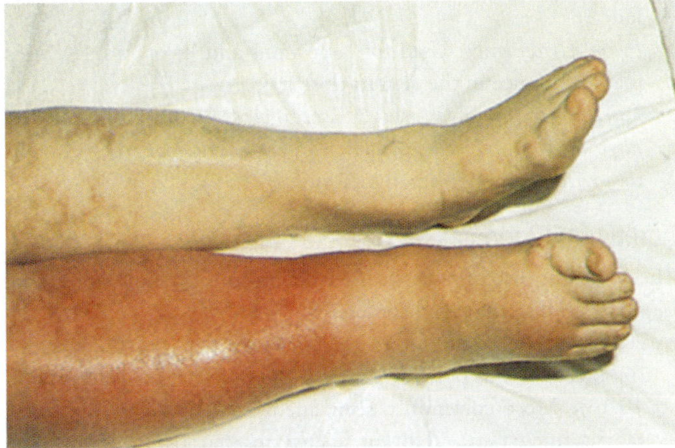

FIGURE 40.12 Deep vein thrombosis (DVT). (From Lewis SM: *Medical-surgical nursing: assessment and management of clinical problems*, ed 8, St. Louis, 2011, Mosby.)

- A family history of blood clots
- Medical conditions: Pregnancy or up to 6 months after delivery, pelvis and leg fractures, bed rest, polycythemia, surgery, indwelling catheter in a blood vessel, lupus, and cancer

- Certain medications (e.g., estrogen, birth control pills), smoking, and obesity
- Signs and symptoms that include leg pain, swelling, warmth, and redness

The provider will do a history and physical examination. An ultrasound may be ordered as well as blood tests (e.g., D-dimer blood test, antithrombin levels, and CBC). Treatment includes anticoagulant medications, compression stockings, and possibly surgery to remove the clot.

CRITICAL THINKING APPLICATION 40.8

Lizzy is preparing for a national exam. She is struggling to remember the difference between an embolus and a thrombus. What is a creative way to remember the differences between the two terms?

Varicose Veins

Varicose veins are swollen, twisted veins seen under the skin, usually in the legs or rectum (*hemorrhoids*). This is a common disorder.

The cause is the one-way valves in the veins, which keep blood flowing toward the heart. If the valves become weakened or damaged, the blood backs up or pools, leading to swollen or varicose veins. Risk factors include a family history of varicose veins, prolonged standing, heavy lifting, multiple pregnancies, and advancing age. Signs and symptoms include dark purple or blue twisty veins, swelling, and feelings of heaviness, fullness, aching, pain, fatigue, or cramping.

The provider will examine the legs and feet (or other areas involved) during the physical exam. An ultrasound may be ordered to check the functioning of the vein valves. Treatment includes wearing compression stockings, exercising, losing weight, avoiding standing for long periods of time, and elevating the legs. There are many other treatments for varicose veins:

- *Sclerotherapy*: Involves an injection of a substance that closes the vein, and within a few weeks, the varicose vein should fade.
- *Foam sclerotherapy*: Used for large veins and involves injecting a foam substance in the vein to close it.
- *Laser surgery*: Involves using a laser to close off small veins.
- *High ligation and vein stripping*: Involves tying off the vein and removing it through small incisions.

Additional Blood Vessel Diseases and Disorders

The following list provides a brief description of some additional blood vessel diseases and disorders:

- *Aneurysm*: A bulging of the arterial wall that can burst, causing bleeding and possible death of the blood vessel wall (Figure 40.13). Most commonly seen aneurysms occur in the aorta (aortic aneurysm). A brain aneurysm that ruptures causes a stroke.
- *Esophageal varices*: Enlarged veins in the esophagus that can rupture. Found in people with cirrhosis of the liver.
- *Raynaud disease*: Rare blood vessel disorder that affects the toes and fingers. With cold temperatures or stress, the blood vessels narrow, and blood cannot get to the surface of the skin. The toes and fingers affected turn white or blue (Figure 40.14). When the blood flow returns, the skin is red and painful.

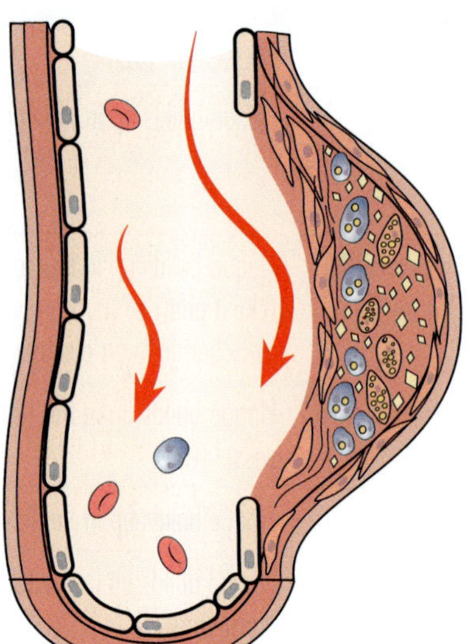

FIGURE 40.13 Aneurysm caused by weakening of the vessel wall. (From Damjanov I: *Pathology for the health-related professions*, ed 4, St. Louis, 2012, Saunders.)

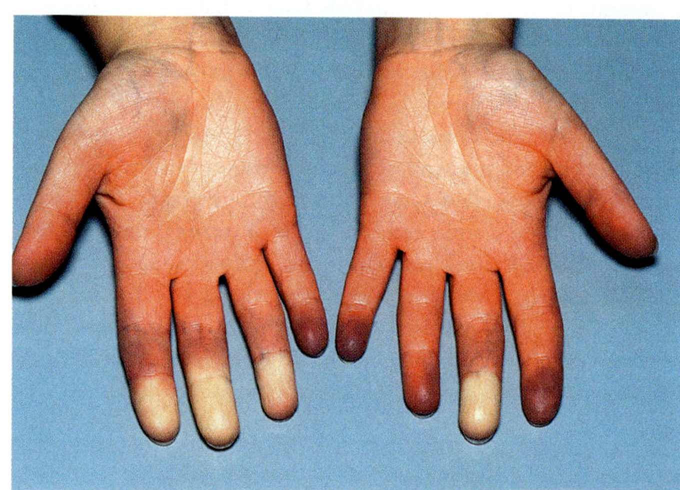

FIGURE 40.14 Raynaud disease. (From Hallett J, et al: *Comprehensive vascular and endovascular surgery*, ed 2, Philadelphia, 2009, Mosby.)

BLOOD PRESSURE–RELATED DISEASES AND DISORDERS

Hypertension is the most common blood pressure-related disease. According to the Centers for Disease Control and Prevention (CDC), about 45% of adults in the United States have hypertension. The following sections describe hypertension, hypotension, postural orthostatic tachycardia syndrome, and shock.

Hypertension

Hypertension (HTN) is high blood pressure. HTN occurs when the force of the blood pushing against the artery wall is elevated. There are three types of hypertension:

- *Primary hypertension* (or *essential hypertension*): The most common type with no identifiable cause; develops with age.
- *Secondary hypertension*: High blood pressure is caused by another disease, condition, or medication. If the disease is treated or the medication is removed, the high blood pressure resolves.

- *Malignant hypertension*: Very high blood pressure that causes organ damage.

Hypertension has many causes:

- *Genetics:* Hypertension tends to run in families.
- *Environmental factors*: High-sodium diet, alcohol, smoking, lack of exercise, obesity, and some medications can lead to hypertension.
- *Kidney fluid and salt balances*: The kidney regulates the electrolyte and water balance in the body. Kidney disease can lead to increased blood volume, which leads to hypertension.
- *Renin-angiotensin-aldosterone system*: A complex system that makes angiotensin, which constricts blood vessels. It also makes aldosterone, which affects kidney function and leads to increased blood volume. Both can cause hypertension.
- *Sympathetic nervous system*: Involved with blood pressure regulation.
- *Changes in blood vessels*: Loss of elasticity in the walls can lead to hypertension.

Hypertension has no symptoms. The only sign is a high blood pressure reading. However, it can cause serious problems, including stroke, heart attack, heart failure, and kidney failure.

Blood pressure is measured and recorded as two numbers. The top number is the systolic pressure, or the blood pressure during a heartbeat. The bottom number is the diastolic pressure, or the blood pressure when the heart rests. Blood pressure is measured in millimeters of mercury (mm Hg). Table 40.7 lists the stages of blood pressure. Treatment involves a low-salt or heart-healthy diet, maintaining a healthy weight, stopping smoking, exercising, limiting alcohol intake, and developing healthy strategies to cope with stress. Medications may also be used:

- Diuretics ("water pills"), which help the kidneys pull extra water and sodium from the blood, thus reducing blood volume
- Angiotensin II receptor blockers (ARBs), angiotensin-converting enzyme (ACE) inhibitors, calcium channel blockers (CCBs), and alpha-blockers, which relax blood vessels, thus reducing blood pressure

TABLE 40.7 Blood Pressure Stages for Adults

CATEGORY	SYSTOLIC	AND/OR	DIASTOLIC
Normal blood pressure	Less than 120 mm Hg		Less than 80 mm Hg
Elevated	120–129 mm Hg	*and*	Less than 80 mm Hg
Hypertension stage 1	130–140 mm Hg	*or*	80–89 mm Hg
Hypertension stage 2	At least 140 mm Hg	*or*	At least 90 mm Hg
Hypertensive crisis	More than 180 mm Hg	*and/or*	More than 120 mm Hg

mm Hg (millimeters of mercury).

Hypotension

Hypotension is lower than normal blood pressure. When the blood pressure is lower than normal, the heart, brain, and other organs are not getting enough blood. A drop of as little as 20 mm Hg can cause problems for some people.

Severe hypotension can be caused by a sudden loss of blood, severe infection, heart attack, or severe allergic reaction (**anaphylaxis**). Here are some additional causes of hypotension:

- **Orthostatic (postural) hypotension**, caused by a sudden change in body position, such as moving from sitting to standing
- Postprandial orthostatic hypotension, caused by eating
- *Neurally mediated hypotension* (NMH), which occurs when standing for a long time
- Medications, such as antianxiety drugs, antidepressants, and diuretics
- Drinking alcohol, heart failure, dehydration, and arrhythmias

Signs and symptoms of hypotension include blurry vision, confusion, dizziness, fainting, lightheadedness, nausea, vomiting, sleepiness, and weakness.

Besides a medical history, the provider will perform a physical exam. Laboratory tests, such as blood cultures, a complete blood count (CBC), and a urinalysis, might be done. An ECG and x-rays can also be done. Treatment depends on the cause of hypotension. With symptoms of hypotension, the patient should sit or lie down immediately and raise the feet above heart level. Medication dosages may be adjusted. Wearing compression stockings can prevent pooling of blood in the legs, keeping more blood in the upper body.

Postural Orthostatic Tachycardia Syndrome

Postural orthostatic tachycardia syndrome (POTS) is estimated to affect 1 million to 3 million Americans and can occur at any age, although it commonly affects females between 15 and 50 years of age. POTS is considered a dysautonomia, an abnormal condition of the autonomic nervous system (ANS). The ANS does not control the blood pressure or heart rate when a person is standing up.

Many times, the underlying cause of a person's POTS is unknown. Conditions that cause or are associated with POTS include autoimmune diseases, diabetes, infections (e.g., mononucleosis, Epstein-Barr virus, Lyme disease), multiple sclerosis, trauma, and vitamin deficiencies. The signs and symptoms can vary but may include *hypovolemia* (low blood volume), tachycardia, and orthostatic (postural) hypotension. Other symptoms include the following:

- Fatigue, exercise intolerance, nausea, headaches, and poor concentration
- Lightheadedness, blurred vision, syncope, heart palpitations, chest pain, and shortness of breath
- Cold or painful extremities (fingers and toes)
- Fainting with blood draws (phlebotomy) or deep breathing

For some people, the symptoms are mild and do not interfere with daily activity. Others experience significant symptoms that interfere with eating, moving, bathing, and working. About 25% of patients with POTS are disabled and cannot work.

Diagnostic testing for POTS includes the following:

- *Tilt table test*: A patient is strapped to a table; gradually, the table is tilted into the upright position, and the patient is monitored for the effects of the position changes.
- *Orthostatic vital signs*: Blood pressure and heart rate are obtained as the patient reclines, sits, and stands. In many cases, the blood pressure drops, and the heart rate increases.

Orthostatic (postural) hypotension occurs when there is a decrease in blood pressure within 3 minutes of standing up. The systolic blood pressure drops 20 or more mm Hg, and the diastolic blood pressure decreases 10 or more mm Hg. Treatment varies and may include medications to regulate the heart rate and blood pressure. Drinking plenty of fluids (2 to 3 L per day); eating a high-salt, low-carbohydrate diet; exercise; and compression stockings may also be encouraged as part of the treatment.

CRITICAL THINKING APPLICATION **40.9**

Rebecca and Lizzy are working with a patient who has been diagnosed with postural orthostatic tachycardia syndrome (POTS). Having never heard of POTS, Rebecca asks the patient to explain the disease. The patient explains that her blood volume is low. She needs to consume a lot of sodium and water to maintain her blood volume. The patient states that she faints with blood draws. Rebecca thanked the patient for her explanation. Why is it important for medical assistants to listen to their patients about their special needs?

Shock

Shock occurs when there is not enough blood and oxygen getting to the organs and tissues. It causes very low blood pressure.

Shock usually happens with a serious injury and can be life threatening. There are several types of shock:

- *Anaphylactic*: Severe allergic reaction; caused by exposure to an allergen (e.g., insect bites/stings, food allergy, drug allergy)
- *Cardiogenic*: Inability of the damaged heart to pump blood effectively; caused by a heart attack, arrhythmias, pulmonary embolism, or congestive heart failure
- *Hypovolemic*: Excessive loss of blood or body fluids from internal or external hemorrhage (bleeding); severe dehydration, burns, vomiting, or diarrhea
- *Neurogenic*: Peripheral vessels dilate due to a neurologic injury or disorder (e.g., spinal cord injury)
- *Septic*: Overwhelming infection; caused by bacteria, fungi, and rarely viruses

The following responses are signs and symptoms of shock:

- Weak, rapid pulse and rapid, shallow respirations
- Changes in the level of consciousness: confusion, lack of alertness, loss of consciousness
- Dizziness, lightheadedness, or faintness
- Sweaty, pale skin; cool hands and feet; bluish lips and fingernails
- Reduced or no urine output

Shock is diagnosed based on the history, exam, and vital signs of the patient. If time allows, additional testing may be done to identify the cause. The goals of medical treatment include increasing the cardiac output and blood pressure with medications, blood transfusions, and IV fluids. Additional treatments address the cause of the shock.

BLOOD DISEASES AND DISORDERS

These are some common signs and symptoms of blood diseases and disorders:

- Fatigue, weakness, pale skin, lightheadedness, and shortness of breath (SOB)
- Bruising and bleeding
- Fever and weight loss
- A deficiency in WBCs (*leukopenia*) or an elevated number of WBCs (*leukocytosis*)
- A deficiency of RBCs (anemia) or an elevated number of RBCs (*erythrocytosis*)
- A deficiency of platelets (*thrombocytopenia*) or an elevated number of platelets (*thrombocytosis*)

The following sections describe blood diseases and disorders.

Anemia

Anemia is a common blood disorder. It occurs when the blood does not have enough healthy red blood cells or enough hemoglobin, which carries oxygen to the rest of the body. Table 40.8 presents the types of anemia, along with their etiologies and treatments.

Signs and symptoms include weakness, fatigue, pale skin, arrhythmias, SOB, dizziness, lightheadedness, cold hands and feet, headache, and chest pain.

A physical exam and a complete blood count (CBC) will be done. Additional tests may be done to rule out or confirm the type of anemia.

Hemophilia

Hemophilia is a genetic bleeding disorder that can lead to spontaneous bleeding. About 20,000 males in the United States live with the disorder. There are two types of hemophilia:

- *Hemophilia A, or classic hemophilia:* Caused by a lack of or decrease in clotting factor VIII
- Hemophilia B, or Christmas disease: Caused by a lack of or decrease in clotting factor IX

Hemophilia is caused by a mutation in a gene that provides information to make clotting factor proteins needed for making a blood clot. Because the mutation is on the X chromosome, a male with the mutation will have the disease. A female must have two X chromosomes with the mutation to have the disease. She will be a carrier of hemophilia if she just has one X chromosome with the mutation. Signs and symptoms include bleeding within the joints, skin, mouth, nose, and gums. Blood can be in the urine or stool. Bleeding can occur after surgery or injury. Complications include chronic joint disease and pain, seizures, paralysis, and possibly death.

If hemophilia runs in the family, the provider will test the male newborn. Blood clotting tests are performed, and if the results are abnormal, clotting factor tests (factor assays) will be done. Treatment consists of infusing commercially prepared factor concentrates as prophylaxis (prevention) or when bleeding occurs.

Idiopathic Thrombocytopenic Purpura

Idiopathic thrombocytopenic **purpura** is also called *immune thrombocytopenia* and *immune thrombocytopenic purpura.* ITP is a rare autoimmune disease that results in the destruction of platelets.

The immune system produces antibodies that destroy platelets, thus causing ITP. In children, ITP sometimes occurs after a viral infection. In adults, ITP is a chronic disease that can occur after a viral infection, pregnancy, or infection with *Helicobacter pylori.* This disease can cause abnormally heavy menses, petechial rash (a rash with pinpoint red spots), easy bruising, nosebleeds, or bleeding (Figure 40.15).

TABLE 40.8 Types of Anemias

TYPE	DESCRIPTION	ETIOLOGY	TREATMENT
Aplastic anemia	Rare, life-threatening condition; the body does not produce enough red blood cells (RBCs)	Caused by infections, certain medications, exposure to toxic chemicals, and autoimmune disorders	Blood transfusions, stem cell transplantation, immunosuppressant medications, and bone marrow stimulants
Hemolytic anemia	Early destruction of RBCs occurs; bone marrow is not making enough RBCs to replace the destroyed RBCs	Autoimmune disorder, genetic RBC defect, infection, blood clots	Blood transfusions and treat the cause
Iron-deficiency anemia	Most common form; not enough iron to make RBCs	Heavy menstrual periods, intestinal disease (e.g., Crohn disease, cancer), use of aspirin, ibuprofen, or arthritis medication, ulcers; not enough dietary iron	Iron supplements or iron medications
Pernicious anemia	A type of vitamin B_{12}–deficiency anemia	Body destroys the cells that make intrinsic factor, which absorbs dietary vitamin B_{12} in the intestine	Monthly injections of vitamin B_{12}
Sickle cell anemia	Inherited disorder that causes the RBCs to form a sickle (crescent) shape, get stuck in the blood vessels, and break apart	Caused by a defective form of hemoglobin (hemoglobin S)	Manage and control the symptoms to prevent crises; folic acid supplements; blood transfusions, pain medications and fluids during crisis
Thalassemia	Inherited condition causing an abnormal form or inadequate amount of hemoglobin	Genetic condition	Blood transfusions and folate supplements
Vitamin B_{12}–deficiency anemia	A low RBC count due to a lack of vitamin B_{12}	Lack of dietary B_{12}, chronic alcoholism, Crohn disease, bariatric surgery, antacids	Depends on the cause; vitamin B_{12} supplements or monthly injections of vitamin B_{12}

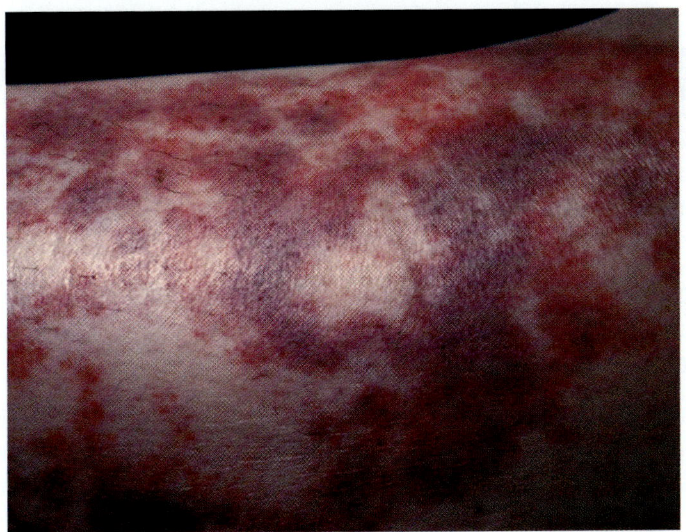

FIGURE 40.15 Purpura. (From Bolognia JL: *Dermatology*, ed 2, St. Louis, 2008, Mosby.)

After the physical exam, the provider will order a CBC to check the patient's platelet level and a platelet antibodies blood test. A biopsy or bone marrow aspiration may also be done. Treatment for adults consists of steroids and immunosuppressant medications, high-dose immune globulin infusions, drugs to stimulate the bone marrow, and a splenectomy.

Leukemia

Leukemia is cancer of the blood-forming tissues, such as the bone marrow and the lymphatic system. The bone marrow produces abnormal white blood cells. Leukemia is classified as either acute or chronic. The secondary classification of leukemia is the type of white blood cell affected by the disease. Table 40.9 describes different types of leukemia with the signs and symptoms.

The exact cause of leukemia is unknown, but scientists believe it is a combination of genetics and environmental factors. Risk factors for leukemia include prior cancer treatments, genetic disorders, exposure to certain chemicals, family history of leukemia, and a history of smoking. After the physical examination, a CBC will be ordered. A specific type of WBC will be elevated, depending on the type of leukemia. A bone marrow biopsy may also be done.

Treatment for acute leukemia is more aggressive and consists of chemotherapy, radiation, and in some cases, a splenectomy. With chronic leukemia, as the disease worsens, the patient may receive chemotherapy and radiation. Biological therapy can also be used for leukemia. It boosts the body's natural ability to fight cancer. In addition, targeted therapy may be used, which uses substances that fight cancer cells but do not harm normal cells.

Additional Blood Diseases and Disorders

The following are additional blood diseases and disorders:

- *Hemolytic disease of the fetus and newborn* (HDFN): Also called *erythroblastosis fetalis* and *hemolytic disease of the newborn* (HDN). A mismatch between the fetus and the mother involving the Rh factor can cause hemolytic disease in the newborn. The RBCs in the baby's blood break down at a faster rate.
- *Polycythemia vera*: A bone marrow disorder characterized by an increased number of red blood cells in the bloodstream. The number of WBCs and platelets may also be higher than normal.
- *Von Willebrand disease*: Most common inherited bleeding disorder in the United States. Affects both males and females. An inherited condition that results when the blood lacks functioning von Willebrand factor, a protein that helps blood clot.

THE MEDICAL ASSISTANT'S ROLE IN EXAMINATIONS, DIAGNOSTIC PROCEDURES, AND TREATMENTS

Patients with cardiovascular system concerns are seen in urgent care, primary care, and cardiology departments. Medical assistants working in these departments assist with examinations, diagnostic procedures, and treatments.

Assisting with the Examination

The cardiovascular examination begins with the medical assistant measuring the patient's height and weight, temperature, radial pulses, respirations, and blood pressure in both arms. Most cardiologists also want a complete list of the vitamins as well as the herbal, prescription, and over-the-counter (OTC) medications the patient is taking, including the strength and frequency of use for each.

A large part of the provider's examination focuses on subjective symptoms. The physical examination covers the chest, heart, and vascular systems. The patient's general appearance will be observed, as well as color of the skin, symmetry, temperature of the extremities, and breathing patterns. The veins in the neck may be examined for *distension* (enlargement). Using a stethoscope, the provider will listen to the lungs, because abnormal sounds may indicate *congestion* (fluid in the lungs), and the heart. A *murmur* (fluttering sound) is an abnormal heart sound. The provider may also use a Doppler to check the pulses. A *bruit* (blowing or swishing sound) can be heard over a

TABLE 40.9 Type of Leukemia

TYPE	DESCRIPTION	SIGNS AND SYMPTOMS
Acute lymphocytic leukemia (ALL)	Also called acute lymphoblastic leukemia; most common cause of cancer in children. Causes an increase in large, immature lymphocytes (lymphoblasts).	Weakness, fever, bleeding, shortness of breath, and weight loss; bone, stomach, or rib pain; painless lumps in the underarm, neck, and stomach.
Acute myeloid leukemia (AML)	Also called acute myelogenous leukemia. Most common type of acute leukemia in adults. Causes an elevated level of myeloblasts (immature cells of the bone marrow).	Fever, shortness of breath, bleeding, bruising, tiredness, weight loss.
Chronic lymphocytic leukemia (CLL)	Second most common type of leukemia in adults. Occurs during middle age. A slow-growing cancer that causes a gradual increase in B lymphocytes. Affects the lymph nodes, liver, and spleen. Eventually the bone marrow's function declines.	May not have symptoms. If present, may have painless swelling in the lymph nodes in the neck, stomach, groin, or underarm; fatigue, rib pain, fever, infection, and weight loss.
Chronic myeloid leukemia (CML)	Also called chronic granulocytic or chronic myelogenous leukemia. A slow-growing cancer that causes an increase in myeloblasts. An elevated level of myeloblasts can cause a decrease in RBCs and platelets.	May not have symptoms. If present, may have fatigue, fever, rib pain, night sweats, and weight loss.

carotid artery, aorta, or an organ and is caused by the blood flowing through a narrow artery.

Assisting with Diagnostic Procedures

The medical assistant can support the provider by doing some diagnostic tests in the exam room. Obtaining the blood pressure in both arms and performing orthostatic vital signs are common procedures (Procedure 40.1). The medical assistant can also perform **electrocardiography** and Holter monitor testing, which are discussed in Chapter 26. Besides these procedures, assisting with scheduling and preparing patients for procedures outside the department also fall into the medical assistant's scope of practice.

Tables 40.10 and 40.11 provide information on additional diagnostic procedures and tests. The medical assistant may need to screen the patient for specific allergies, medications, and so on prior to scheduling the procedure. For some procedures, a signed consent form is required. The patient should be notified of what will be experienced during the procedure and any follow-up care required after the test.

Angiography

Angiography is used to study blood vessels and detect occlusions, aneurysms, and structural defects. The procedure uses x-rays, computed tomography (CT), or magnetic resonance imaging (MRI) with contrast medium. The contrast medium makes the blood vessel visible on the x-ray images.

For regular angiography, the patient may be NPO (nothing by mouth) at midnight before the procedure. During the procedure, an intravenous (IV) line may be inserted and a sedative given to help relax the patient. The heart and blood pressure may be monitored during the procedure. After the area (e.g., groin) is shaved and cleansed, a small incision is made. A catheter is threaded into the blood vessel (e.g., femoral or carotid arteries) and advanced to the area that will be studied. Radiopaque contrast medium is injected to make the blood vessel appear on the x-ray. The patient may experience a burning or warming sensation in the location where the medium is given. A series of x-rays are taken. Some treatments can be done during the angiography. After the procedure, the patient is monitored as the medication wears off. The incision is monitored for bleeding. The patient needs to drink plenty of fluids to flush the dye from the body.

There are several types of angiographies:

- *Arteriography*: A type of angiography that involves the study of arteries.
- *Cerebral angiography*: Used to detect blood clots, aneurysms, and other vascular conditions in the brain.
- *Coronary angiography*: A series of x-rays are taken of the heart. The catheter can also monitor the blood pressure in the heart. Coronary angiography is part of a group of procedures known as cardiac catheterization, which will be discussed in a following section.
- *Pulmonary angiography*: This test is used to evaluate the pulmonary artery for blood circulation conditions (e.g., pulmonary embolism).

A computed tomography angiography (CTA) and magnetic resonance angiography (MRA) differ from a regular angiography. They are noninvasive and do not require recovery time, although

TABLE 40.10 Diagnostic Procedures for Cardiovascular Diseases and Disorders

PROCEDURE	DESCRIPTION
Cardiac computerized tomography (CT) scan	X-ray camera rotates around the body, taking projections creating a three-dimensional image of the heart. The patient is placed on a table inside of the doughnut-shaped machine.
Carotid ultrasound	Ultrasound of the carotid arteries on each side of the neck. Used to check for narrowed or blocked carotid arteries that can increase the risk of stroke.
Electrophysiology study	Used to test the conduction system of the heart when a patient has arrhythmias. Insulated electric catheters are threaded through a vein from the thigh to the heart for the study.
Magnetic resonance imaging (MRI)	Computerized imaging that uses radiofrequency pulses in a magnetic field to detect damaged areas and areas of blood flow.
Myocardial perfusion imaging	Use of radionuclide to diagnose coronary artery disease (CAD), valvular or congenital heart disease, and cardiomyopathy.
Nuclear ventriculography	A nuclear medicine test; a small amount of tracer (radioactive substance) is injected. X-ray video (fluoroscopy) shows the heart in motion and can measure the amount of blood pumped with each heartbeat (ejection fraction). Test is known by many names, including radionuclide angiogram (RNA), cardiac blood pooling scan, nuclear heart scan, multiple-gated acquisition (MUGA) scan, and radionuclide ventriculography.
Phlebography	X-ray imaging of a vein after the introduction of a contrast dye.
Positron emission tomography (PET)	Computerized nuclear medicine procedure that uses inhaled or injected radioactive substances to help identify how much a patient will benefit from revascularization procedures.
Swan-Ganz catheter	Long, thin cardiac catheter with a tiny balloon at the tip that is fed into the femoral artery near the groin and extended up to the left ventricle. Used to determine left ventricular function by measuring pulmonary capillary pressure.

TABLE 40.11 Medical Laboratory Tests for Cardiovascular Diseases and Disorders

TEST	DESCRIPTION
Cardiac enzymes test	Blood test that measures the level of cardiac enzymes, which characteristically released during a heart attack (myocardial infarction); determines the amount of lactate dehydrogenase (LDH) and creatine phosphokinase (CPK) in the blood.
Lipid profile	Blood test to measure the lipids (cholesterol and triglycerides) in the circulating blood. Some CLIA-waived tests available.
Prothrombin time	A prothrombin time (PT) measures the number of seconds it takes a clot to form after reagents are added to the blood sample. The PT is used to detect bleeding disorders or excessive clotting disorders. CLIA-waived tests are available.

CLIA, Clinical Laboratory Improvement Amendments.

no treatments can be done during the procedure. Caffeinated beverages may be restricted 12 hours before the test, and the patient may not eat for 4 hours before the test to prepare. The patient can drive before and after the test. A patient may receive a beta-blocker to slow the heartbeat or nitroglycerin to dilate the coronary arteries, making the images clearer. During the procedure, the contrast medium is given intravenously. Electrodes are placed on the patient's chest to monitor the heart during the procedure. After the test, the patient can resume normal activities, although it is important to increase the fluids consumed in order to flush the contrast medium from the body.

Cardiac Catheterization

Cardiac catheterization is a procedure used to diagnose and treat certain heart diseases. The patient preparation is similar to that for an angiography, although the patient may be restricted from eating and drinking for a longer period of time.

During the cardiac catheterization, a regular coronary angiography is done. The catheter is inserted into an artery in the groin and threaded to the heart (Figure 40.16). The contrast medium is injected, and narrowed or blocked arteries can be observed. The provider can also measure pressure, blood flow, and oxygen amounts in the chambers and large arteries. Blood samples and biopsies can be collected.

Based on what is found during the catheterization, the provider may also treat the condition. These treatments may include the following:

- Repair of congenital heart defects
- Angioplasty: A treatment to open narrowed blood vessels by expanding a small balloon at the site, which widens the vessel; a stent (small metal coil) may be inserted to help keep the vessel open (Figure 40.17)
- Replacement or repair of a heart valve

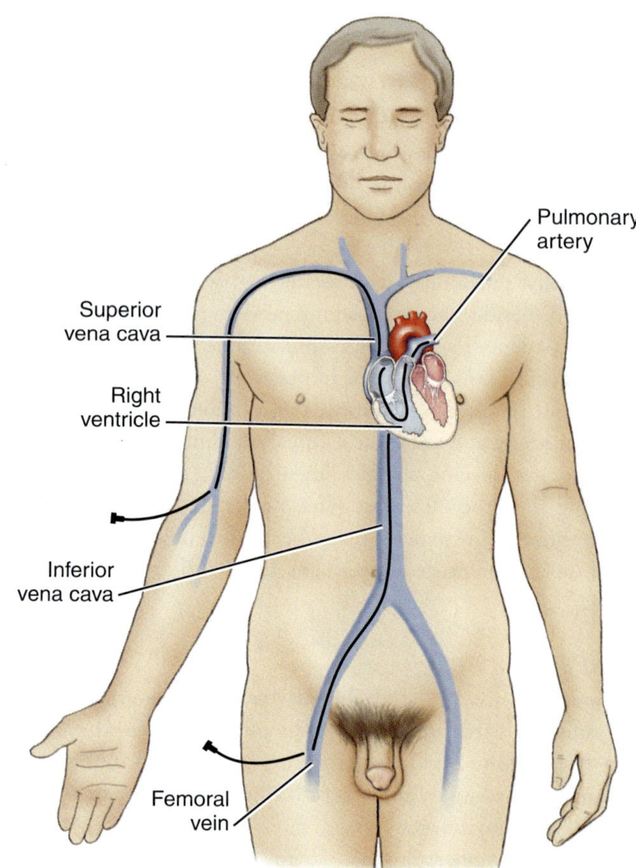

FIGURE 40.16 Cardiac catheterization. The catheter is inserted in the femoral or brachial vein and then is advanced through the right atrium and ventricle, into the pulmonary artery. (From Shiland B: *Medical terminology and anatomy for ICD-10 coding*, ed 2, St. Louis, 2016, Mosby.)

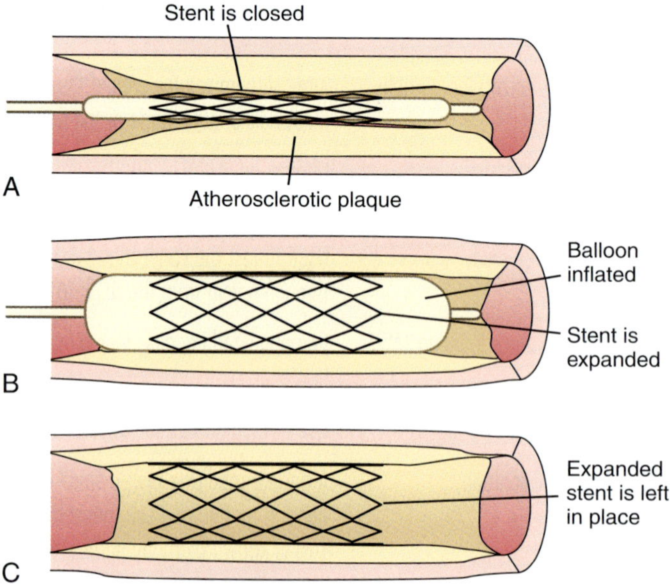

FIGURE 40.17 Angioplasty with stent placement. (From LaFleur Brooks M: *Exploring medical language*, ed 9, St. Louis, 2014, Mosby.)

- Balloon valvuloplasty: A treatment to open narrowed heart valves, using a catheter with a balloon
- Ablation: A treatment for arrhythmias that involves using a catheter with heat (radiofrequency energy or laser) or cold (nitrous oxide) to destroy abnormal tissue causing the arrhythmias

Doppler Ultrasound

The Doppler ultrasound exam provides information on the blood flow in the arms and legs. This test is used to help diagnose **arteriosclerosis**, arterial occlusion (from blood clots), peripheral artery disease, aneurysms, arterial stenosis, and venous insufficiency. There is no special preparation for this test. The patient needs to remove clothing on the extremity being tested.

During the test, the sonographer applies gel to the extremity and places a handheld transducer on the patient. The transducer directs ultrasound waves (high-frequency sound waves) over the vein or artery being checked, and the waves bounce off the circulating RBCs. This test helps the provider estimate the blood flow through the vein or artery. A *color Doppler* uses a computer to change sound waves into different colors. The colors show the speed and direction of the blood flow.

A simple handheld Doppler can often be used in the exam room to check the pulses in the extremities. An absent pulse means there is no blood flow through the artery, which is a medical emergency. With training, a medical assistant can use a handheld Doppler to check the pulses.

Echocardiography

An echocardiogram is a sonographic test that uses sound waves to create pictures of the heart structures. It shows the heart beating and the heart valves and other structures in motion.

Most people have a transthoracic echocardiogram (TTE). There is no special preparation for this test. The patient must remove any clothing and jewelry from the waist up and lie on the exam table in a supine position. A trained echocardiogram sonographer spreads warmed gel over the patient's chest and then moves a transducer slowly over the chest (Figure 40.18). The transducer releases high-frequency sound waves and picks up the waves. The waves are transmitted as electrical impulses that are converted by the echocardiography machine into moving pictures. During the process, the sonographer can take still pictures of the heart's structures.

A transesophageal echocardiogram (TEE) is done less often, and it requires the patient to not eat or drink for several hours before the test. The patient may be given a sedative for the procedure. The patient's throat is numbed before the provider guides a probe (a long flexible tube) with a small ultrasound transducer down the throat and to the stomach. The TEE can get clearer echocardiographic images of the heart than the TTE can.

Electrocardiography and Related Procedures

An *electrocardiography* (ECG, EKG) provides a recording of the electrical impulses of the heart as wave deflections. An *electrocardiograph* creates the record or recording, which is called the *electrocardiogram*. The patient is asked to remove jewelry and clothing above the waist to prepare for the test. Electrodes are applied to the skin, and lead wires from the electrocardiograph are attached to the electrodes.

ECGs are taken with other tests:

- *Exercise stress test* (EST) or *exercise electrocardiogram*: Tests the electrical activity of the heart during exercise on a treadmill. Patient coaching prior to the test includes having the patient dress for exercise. Food, drink, and nicotine are restricted 3 or more hours before the test, and no caffeine is allowed for 24 hours prior to the test. A consent form needs to be completed. Patients should let the provider know if any chest discomfort or pain, dizziness, palpitations, or shortness of breath occur during the test.
- *Nuclear stress test:* A nuclear imaging test that shows blood flow into the heart at rest and with activity. Many names for the test exist, which reflect the intravenous (IV) substance given (e.g., thallium or sestamibi stress test). Patient coaching prior to the procedure usually includes the following:
  - Caffeine is restricted 24 hours before the test.
  - The patient should dress for exercise if a treadmill will be used.
  - A camera takes pictures of the heart while the patient is at rest and when the heart rate is increased either with medication or activity.
- *Holter monitoring:* A portable electrocardiograph is worn to record the reaction of the heart to daily activities for a few days. Electrodes are applied to the chest. The patient receives information on how to complete the journal and use the monitor for the study.
- *Event recording:* A portable electrocardiograph is worn for several weeks. The patient presses a button on the recorder when symptoms occur.
- *Tilt table test:* The patient is placed on a tilt table and secured with straps. As the table is tilted in various positions, the patient's blood pressure and ECG are monitored. This test is used to diagnose orthostatic hypotension.

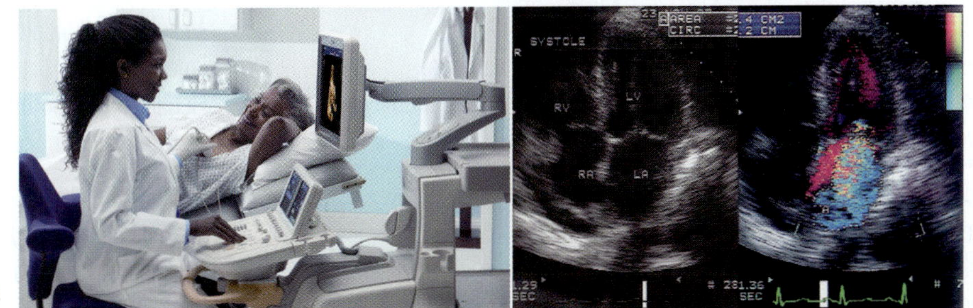

FIGURE 40.18 Person undergoing echocardiography (ECHO). (From Frank ED, Long BW, Smith BJ: *Merrill's atlas of radiographic positions and radiologic procedures,* ed 12, St. Louis, 2012, Mosby.)

Assisting with Treatments

Patients with cardiovascular diseases and disorders are prescribed a variety of medications. The following are some of the more common classifications of medications:

- *Antiarrhythmic:* Used to treat arrhythmias
- *Anticoagulant:* Used to prevent blood clots from forming
- *Antihypertensive:* Used to lower and control the blood pressure; several categories include the following:
  - *Beta-blocker*: Reduces the heart rate, the workload, and the output of the heart
  - *Angiotensin-converting enzyme* (ACE) *inhibitor*: Decreases angiotensin production, which causes blood vessels to dilate
  - *Angiotensin II receptor antagonist:* Blocks the effects of angiotensin, and blood vessels dilate
  - *Calcium channel blocker:* Prevents calcium from entering the heart and arteries' smooth muscles; decreases contraction force, dilates blood vessels, and reduces the heart rate
  - *Alpha-blocker*: Dilates arteries
- *Antiplatelet:* Used for post-treatment of stroke, heart attack, or angina
- *Cholesterol-lowering agent:* Reduces low-density lipoprotein (LDL) and triglycerides; increases high-density lipoprotein (HDL)
- *Diuretic:* Increases urinary output and lowers the blood pressure
- *Hematopoietic:* Treats anemia in patients undergoing chemotherapy
- *Hemostatic:* Controls acute or chronic blood-clotting disorder; promotes the formation of an absorbable, artificial clot

Refer to Table 40.12 for information on the medical classifications, including indications for use, desired effect, side effects, adverse reactions, and generic and trade names. Medical assistants should be familiar with medications that are prescribed to patients.

Pacemakers and Implantable Cardioverter-Defibrillators

A pacemaker uses low-energy electrical pulses to assist the heart when arrhythmias, tachycardia, or bradycardia occurs. There are two types of pacemakers:

- *Temporary pacemaker*: Used in an emergency until the permanent pacemaker can be placed. Also used for temporary conditions (e.g., heart attack and medication overdose).
- *Permanent pacemaker*: Surgically inserted into the chest or abdomen (Figure 40.19). Patients can use technology (e.g., smartphones) to transmit their pacemaker data to their providers.

An implantable cardioverter-defibrillator (ICD) is similar to a pacemaker in that it uses low-energy electrical pulses to treat arrhythmias. However, ICDs differ from pacemakers because they can also use high-energy pulses when a life-threatening arrhythmia occurs.

Patients with a pacemaker or ICD need to have the device checked on a routine basis. The batteries usually last 5 to 7 years, and a replacement requires a surgical procedure. When using a pacemaker or ICD, the person needs to stay away from magnets and strong electrical fields. This would include devices such as iPods, cell phones, microwaves, MRIs, power-generating equipment, and some metal detectors for screening. They should carry identification that indicates they have a pacemaker or an ICD.

CLOSING COMMENTS

Patient Coaching

According to the CDC, heart disease is the leading cause of death for adults. About 25% of all deaths are related to heart disease each year. Genetics, predisposition, and lifestyle factors—such as smoking, lack of exercise, and poor diet—play significant roles in the development of heart disease. Successful management of cardiovascular disease requires major lifestyle changes for most patients. The medical assistant can help by providing encouragement and support and using community resources to help the patient find assistance with these changes.

Sources for information include the American Heart Association (www.heart.org) and the US Department of Agriculture (USDA) (www.nutrition.gov and www.myplate.gov). Because many patients learn best through visual aids, providing them with pictures, brochures, and pamphlets is an effective means of helping them in this learning process. Education interventions are always documented so that the provider or medical assistant can clarify or expand on the information upon a return visit.

Legal and Ethical Issues

Diagnostic procedures can have a marked effect on the patient's treatment. When entrusted with performing testing procedures, the

TABLE 40.12 Medication Classifications

CLASSIFICATION	INFORMATION	GENERIC NAME (TRADE NAME)
Antiarrhythmic	Indications for use: Treats arrhythmias. Desired effects: Helps the heart work better, controls heart rate. Side effects and adverse reactions: Arrhythmias, weight gain, difficulty breathing, swelling of hands and feet.	• Amiodarone (Cordarone, Pacerone) • Procainamide • Flecainide (Tambocor) • Digoxin (Lanoxin, Digitek, Cardoxin)
Anticoagulant	Indication for use: Prevents blood clots from forming. Desired effects: Decreases blood clotting ability. Side effects and adverse reactions: Increased bleeding, blood irregularities, hypersensitivity.	• Beparin • Enoxaparin (Lovenox) • Dabigatran (Pradaxa) • Warfarin (Jantoven) • Rivaroxaban (Xarelto)

TABLE 40.12 Medication Classifications—*cont'd*

CLASSIFICATION	INFORMATION	GENERIC NAME (TRADE NAME)
Antihypertensive	Indications for use: Reduces and controls blood pressure. Desired effects: Lowers blood pressure Side effects and adverse reactions: Headache, vertigo, GI disturbances, rash, hypotension, nonproductive cough.	*Beta-Blockers* • Propranolol (Inderal XL, InnoPran XL) • Atenolol (Tenormin) *Angiotensin-Converting Enzyme (ACE) Inhibitors* • Quinapril (Accupril) • Benazepril (Lotensin) • Lisinopril • Metoprolol (Lopressor, Toprol XL) • Carvedilol (Coreg) *Angiotensin II Receptor Antagonists* • losartan (Cozaar) • Valsartan (Diovan, Prexxartan) *Calcium Channel Blockers* • Diltiazem (Cardizem, Cartia XT, Dilacor XR, Tiazac) • Amlodipine (Katerzia, Norvasc) *Alpha-Blockers* • Doxazosin (Cardura)
Antiplatelet	Indications for use: Post treatment of stroke, heart attack or angina. Desired effect: Inhibits the function of platelets (the formation of clots). Side effects and adverse reactions: GI distress, bleeding, weakness, or numbness	• Clopidogrel (Plavix)
Cholesterol lowering agent	Indications for use: Reduces low-density lipoprotein (LDL) and triglycerides; increases high-density lipoprotein (HDL). Desired effects: Prevents absorption of cholesterol in the intestine. Side effects and adverse reactions: GI discomfort, muscle pain and weakness, liver complications, hypersensitivity, cataracts, myopathy.	• Ezetimibe (Vytorin, Zetia) • Atorvastatin (Lipitor) • Rosuvastatin (Crestor, Ezallor) • Simvastatin (Flolipid, Zocor)
Diuretic	Indications for use: Increases urinary output; lower blood pressure. Desired effects: Inhibits reabsorption of sodium and chloride in the kidneys; promotes excretion of excess fluid in the body. Side effects and adverse reactions: Dehydration, muscle weakness, fatigue, electrolyte imbalance.	• Triamterene (Dyrenium) • Furosemide (Lasix) • Hydrochlorothiazide (Microzide, Oretic)
Hematopoietic	Indication for use: Treats low neutrophil levels and anemia. Desired effect: Promotes neutrophil and red blood cell production. Side effects and adverse reactions: Pain in the arms and legs, bone pain, injection site reaction, headache, weight loss, and insomnia.	*Colony-Stimulating Factor* • Pegfilgrastim (Neulasta) • Filgrastim (Neupogen) *Erythropoiesis-Stimulating Agents* • Epoetin alfa (Epogen, Procrit)
Hemostatic	Indications for use: Controls acute or chronic blood-clotting disorder; promotes formation of absorbable, artificial clot. Desired effects: Controls bleeding; acts as a blood coagulant (clots blood). Side effects and adverse reactions: Hypersensitivity reactions, transient flushing, dizziness; newborn hyperbilirubinemia.	• Phytonadione (Mephyton, Vitamin K_1)

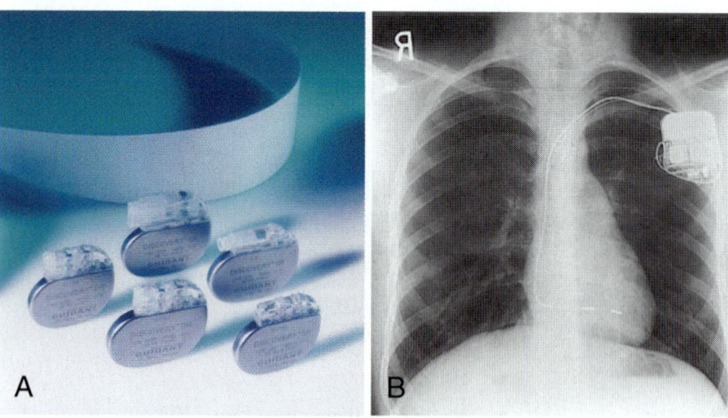

FIGURE 40.19 **(A)** Pacemakers. **(B)** Chest x-ray of a patient with a permanent implanted pacemaker. (From Frank ED, Long BW, Smith BJ: *Merrill's atlas of radiographic positions and radiologic procedures*, ed 12, St. Louis, 2012, Mosby.)

medical assistant assumes responsibility for the test's accuracy and for performing the test precisely. This is an important role because the results submitted could strongly influence the plan of treatment.

Patient-Centered Care

Two important aspects of patient-centered care are information and education. Many of the more common cardiovascular diseases require patients to be on medication for treatment. It is important that patients know the following:

- Name of the medication
- Reason for the medication
- Side effects/adverse reactions to report to the provider

When a patient is put on a new medication, providing information on the medication is important. The medical assistant should review the information with the patient. Also, giving the patient a handout to take home and a phone number to call if questions arise will promote patient-centered care.

Professional Behaviors

Critical thinking is a crucial part of professional behavior. The ability to question patients logically and comprehensively about possible cardiac signs and symptoms can greatly contribute to high-quality care. The provider relies on the medical assistant for initial information about the patient. Given the seriousness of cardiac conditions, medical assistants must use their knowledge about the topic to gather and analyze the patient's comments so that the provider is better prepared to make an accurate diagnosis and develop an effective treatment plan.

SUMMARY OF SCENARIO

During the weeks that followed, Lizzy became more independent in practicum. She was very excited to interview for a medical assistant position in a cardiology department in a nearby city. During her last day with Rebecca, they celebrated her completion of the practicum. Lizzy shared that she was offered the medical assistant position, which she accepted.

In the weeks that followed Lizzy's last day, Rebecca thought about all the information she had shared with Lizzy. She realized that she, too, had learned a lot from the practicum experience and found that she really enjoyed mentoring students. Rebecca plans to talk with her supervisor about future opportunities to mentor students in the department.

SUMMARY OF LEARNING OBJECTIVES

1. **Examine the anatomy of the cardiovascular system.**
   The cardiovascular system is a closed system that includes the following:
   - Blood vessels, consisting of arteries, arterioles, capillaries, venules, and veins that act as pipes to carry the blood around the body
   - A heart, which pumps the blood
   - Blood, which contains the nutrients for the cells and the waste products to be excreted

   The heart, which is the size of a fist, is a complex muscular organ that pumps blood around the body. It is located in the mediastinum of the thoracic cavity, slightly left of the midline. The *apex* (pointed tip) of the heart rests just above the diaphragm. The heart has two sets of chambers, the atria and ventricles. The septum divides the heart into a right and left section. The heart wall is composed of three layers: the endocardium, the myocardium, and the epicardium.
2. **Differentiate among the pulmonary, systemic, coronary, hepatic portal, and fetal circulations.**
   Pulmonary circulation begins as the blood returns from the body. The superior vena cava and the inferior vena cava bring deoxygenated blood from the body to the right atrium. The blood passes the tricuspid valve and empties into the right ventricle. When the ventricles contract, the blood in the right ventricle is pushed out past the pulmonary valve and enters the pulmonary artery trunk, which splits into the right and left pulmonary arteries. In the lungs, gas exchange occurs, and oxygenated blood returns to the lungs by the right and left pulmonary veins.

SUMMARY OF LEARNING OBJECTIVES—*continued*

Then the systemic circulation starts. The oxygenated blood in the left atrium moves past the bicuspid or mitral valve and empties into the left ventricle before passing the aortic valve and emptying into the aorta. From here, the blood will move through the body before it returns to the heart. Blood from the head, neck, and upper extremities empties into the superior vena cava before returning to the right atrium. Blood from the lower body empties into the inferior vena cava before returning to the right atrium.

The coronary veins remove waste products from the heart tissue, and the coronary arteries bring nutrients and oxygen to the heart tissue. The liver (hepatic circulation) has a special role in filtering the blood and metaboliizing or breaking down substances.

The umbilical cord contains two umbilical arteries and one umbilical vein. The arteries carry the fetal blood to the placenta. The umbilical vein carries oxygen and nutrient-rich blood to the baby. The waste, oxygen, and nutrient exchange occur in the placenta. Other structures that are unique to the growing baby include the following:

- *Ductus venosus*: Shifts the majority of the blood from the umbilical vein and empties it into the inferior vena cava, thus bypassing the immature liver
- *Foramen ovale*: A small flaplike opening in the interatrial septum that allows blood to move from the right atrium to the left atrium, thus bypassing the immature lungs
- *Ductus arteriosus*: A short vessel that connects the pulmonary artery with the aorta, and most of the blood is redirected from the pulmonary artery to the aorta, thus bypassing the immature lungs

3. **Examine the anatomy of the blood.**

Blood is made up of two components:

- *Liquid portion:* Plasma is the liquid portion of whole blood; it also contains plasma proteins (e.g., albumin, globulins, clotting factors, and complement), inorganic substances, electrolytes, organic substances, and waste products
- *Formed elements:* Includes red blood cells (RBCs), white blood cells (WBCs), and platelets

The two major classification systems for blood typing are the ABO and the Rh systems. With the ABO system, each person has the A, B, ABO, or O blood type. With the Rh system, a person is either Rh-positive or Rh-negative.

4. **Examine the physiology of the conduction system.**

The electrical cells in the SA node generate the impulse that starts the heartbeat. When the SA node discharges the impulse, it travels in many directions through the heart muscle. The Bachmann bundle, a specialized internodal tract, takes the impulse to the left atrium. Other internodal tracts take the impulse quickly to the atrioventricular (AV) node. In the AV node, the impulse moves very slowly and then moves to the bundle of His. After the impulse passes through the bundle of His, it enters the right and left bundle branches. The right bundle branch brings the impulse to the right ventricle. The left bundle branch brings the impulse to the left ventricle. The bundle branches split into many Purkinje fibers.

The cardiac cells cycle through three states or steps in the same sequence for each impulse:

- *Polarized state*: Before the impulse hits the cells, they are in a polarized or "waiting" state.
- *Depolarized state*: When the impulse hits the cells, the cells' charges change. The change of the cells' charges allows the impulse to move through the cell, causing *action potential*, also called depolarization.
- *Repolarized state*: After the impulse passes over the cell, the ions move back to their original location. This causes the cell's charge to change. This recovery phase is called the repolarized state.

5. **Examine the physiology of the blood, including coagulation and the factors that affect the blood pressure.**

The process required to form a blood clot is complicated. First, a damaged vessel will constrict to slow the flow of blood through the vessel. Aggregation of platelets will occur, and the platelets will adhere to the injured area, forming a platelet plug. Platelets release clotting factors, which aid in the process of coagulation. The injured blood vessel tissue also activates clotting factors in the blood plasma. The interaction between the clotting factors works to form fibrin. The fibrin net traps red blood cells and more platelets to form a thrombus.

The following factors affect the blood pressure:

- *Blood volume:* The amount of circulating blood has a direct influence on blood pressure. The greater the blood volume, the more force it makes on the arterial walls. If the blood volume is low, less force or pressure will be on the arterial walls.
- *Strength of ventricular contractions:* The greater the force of the contraction, the more blood is pumped into the arteries. This increases the blood pressure. If the left ventricular contraction is weak, less blood is pumped out of the heart, and thus the blood pressure is lower.
- *Resistance to blood flow:* Any factor that increases the resistance for blood to flow through the arteries will increase the blood pressure. Factors that increase resistance include the size of the lumen of the arteries, the elasticity of the arterial walls, and the viscosity of the blood.

6. **Analyze the life span changes to the cardiovascular system.**

As a child grows and matures, the heart rate decreases. The systemic vascular resistance increases with age. This means that the resistance for blood flow increases, and thus the blood pressure increases with age. As a person ages, the heart and blood vessels undergo changes. Heart changes that occur include a loss of some SA node cells and an increase in the left ventricle size. Normal ECG changes can occur with age. Valves can become thicker and stiffer, causing a heart murmur. Arterial walls become stiffer, thus increasing the blood pressure.

SUMMARY OF LEARNING OBJECTIVES—*continued*

7. **Examine heart diseases and disorders, including the signs, symptoms, etiology, diagnostic procedures, and treatments.**
Common signs and symptoms include angina, bradycardia, tachycardia, palpitation, cyanosis, pallor, dyspnea, orthopnea, shortness of breath, diaphoresis, edema, and syncope. Diseases and disorders of the heart include arrhythmias, cardiomyopathy, congenital heart defects, congestive heart failure, heart valve disorders (e.g., aortic insufficiency, mitral valve prolapse, and rheumatic fever), metabolic syndrome, and myocardial infarction. Additional diseases include cardiac tamponade, endocarditis, and pericarditis. Refer to this chapter for more information on these disorders.
8. **Examine blood vessel diseases and disorders, including the signs, symptoms, etiology, diagnostic procedures, and treatments.**
Diseases and disorders of the blood vessels include atherosclerosis-related diseases, deep vein thrombosis, and varicose veins. Additional diseases and disorders include aneurysms, esophageal varices, and Raynaud disease. Refer to this chapter for more information on these diseases.
9. **Examine blood pressure–related diseases and disorders, including the signs, symptoms, etiology, diagnostic procedures, and treatments.**
Blood pressure-related diseases and disorders include hypertension, hypotension, postural orthostatic tachycardia syndrome, and shock. There are several types of shock, including anaphylactic, cardiogenic, hypovolemic, neurogenic, and septic. Refer to this chapter for more information on these diseases.
10. **Examine blood diseases and disorders, including the signs, symptoms, etiology, diagnostic procedures, and treatments.**
Common signs and symptoms of blood diseases and disorders include fatigue, weakness, pale skin, lightheadedness, shortness of breath (SOB), bruising, bleeding, fever, weight loss, leukopenia, leukocytosis, anemia, erythrocytosis, thrombocytopenia, and thrombocytosis. Diseases of the blood include anemia (e.g., aplastic, hemolytic, iron deficiency, sickle cell, thalassemia, vitamin B_{12} deficiency, and pernicious), hemophilia, idiopathic thrombocytopenic purpura, and leukemia (e.g., acute lymphocytic, acute myeloid, chronic lymphocytic, and chronic myeloid). Additional blood disorders include hemolytic disease of the fetus and newborn, polycythemia vera, and Von Willebrand disease.
11. **Examine the medical assistant's role in assisting with examinations, diagnostic procedures, and treatments for cardiology diseases and disorders.**
The cardiovascular examination begins with the medical assistant measuring the patient's height and weight, temperature, radial pulses, respirations, and blood pressure in both arms. A large part of the provider's examination focuses on subjective symptoms.
Some of the diagnostic procedures include angiography, cardiac catheterization, Doppler ultrasound, echocardiogram, nuclear stress test, and nuclear ventriculography. An electrocardiography can be done as a resting ECG, an exercise stress test, or with a Holter monitor. Medical laboratory tests include cholesterol and prothrombin testing, cardiac enzymes test, and lipid profile.
Treatments include medication, pacemakers, and implantable cardioverter-defibrillators (ICDs). A pacemaker uses low-energy electrical pulses to assist the heart when arrhythmias, tachycardia, or bradycardia occurs. An implantable cardioverter-defibrillator (ICD) is similar to a pacemaker in that it uses low-energy electrical pulses to treat arrhythmias. However, ICDs differ from pacemakers because they can also use high-energy pulses when a life-threatening arrhythmia occurs.

PROCEDURE 40.1 Determine a Patient's Orthostatic Vital Signs

TASKS: Perform orthostatic vital signs and document them in the patient's health record.

EQUIPMENT and SUPPLIES

- Patient's health record
- Sphygmomanometer
- Stethoscope
- Watch with a second hand
- Alcohol wipes
- Exam table

PROCEDURAL STEPS

1. Wash hands or use hand sanitizer.
PURPOSE: To ensure infection control.
2. Assemble the equipment and supplies needed. Clean the earpieces and diaphragm of the stethoscope with alcohol wipes.
PURPOSE: For infection control and to follow Standard Precautions.
3. Greet the patient. Identify yourself. Verify the patient's identity with full name and date of birth. Explain the procedure to be performed in a manner that the patient understands. Answer any questions the patient may have about the procedure.
PURPOSE: Identification of the patient prevents errors, and explanations are a means of gaining implied consent and patient cooperation.
4. Help the patient lie comfortably in a supine position on the examination table. Pull out the table extender, if necessary, so that patients can rest their feet. Allow the patient to rest in this position for 5 minutes.
PURPOSE: Allowing the patient to rest before beginning will allow their blood pressure to come to baseline for this position.

PROCEDURE 40.1 Determine a Patient's Orthostatic Vital Signs—*continued*

5. Take the patient's pulse and blood pressure with the patient lying down. Do not remove the cuff from the arm.
   PURPOSE: Allowing the cuff to stay on the arm will allow the same arm to be used in additional measurements without putting it on and taking it off the arm.
6. Help the patient into a sitting position, and ask if the patient is experiencing any dizziness, weakness, or visual changes with the position change. Watch for any change in skin coloring or the patient's behavior.
   PURPOSE: This identifies any symptoms of hypotension the patient may be experiencing.
7. Once the patient has been sitting for 1 minute, repeat the pulse and blood pressure.
   PURPOSE: This will provide blood pressure readings in the new position.
   Note: If the patient has symptoms associated with the position change or the sitting blood pressure is less than 90 systolic and/or 60 diastolic, have the patient lay back down and immediately notify the provider.
8. Assist the patient to a standing position. Ask the patient about dizziness, weakness, or visual changes associated with the position change. Note any change in the patient's appearance or behavior.
9. Immediately repeat the blood pressure and pulse readings after the patient has stood up.
   PURPOSE: A quick change in positioning with an immediate read of BP and pulse will indicate if the patient is experiencing orthostatic hypotension.
10. Ask the patient to continue standing and repeat the pulse and blood pressure measurements after 3 minutes.
    PURPOSE: BP and pulse readings that return to normal after the patient has stood for a few minutes indicate a different problem than if the readings stay low (or high).
11. Clean the earpieces and the head of the stethoscope with an alcohol wipe, and return both the cuff and the stethoscope to storage.
12. Wash hands or use hand sanitizer.
    PURPOSE: To ensure infection control.
13. Clearly document each blood pressure and pulse reading, along with the position and any symptoms the patient experienced in the patient's health record.
    PURPOSE: Documenting the reading, along with the position and symptoms experienced, will allow the provider to make connections in positional BP/P and make diagnostic and treatment decisions.

Documentation Example

3/9/20XX 2:20 p.m. (Lying) BP 120/72 right arm, (adult cuff); P: 68 regular, 1+. (Sitting 1 min) BP 116/ 64; P: 84 regular, 1+. (Standing, initial VS) BP 110/58; P: 96 regular, 1+. (Standing 3 min) BP 112/66; P: 88 regular, 1+. Had dizziness initially after standing that resolved within 1 min. Pt resting on the exam table. Dr. Walden notified. ————————

———————————— Rebecca White, CMA (AAMA)

PULMONOLOGY 41

SCENARIO

Renee Thomas, CMA (AAMA), was hired 6 months ago. She assists the specialists who hold outreach clinics at Walden-Martin Family Medical (WMFM) Clinic. On Tuesdays, the pulmonologist from a local larger city comes to assist in the pulmonary outreach clinic. The pulmonologist brings his own equipment and one medical assistant, John.

Renee's job is to help the pulmonology medicine team because she knows the WMFM Clinic and the local community resources. Renee studied the anatomy and physiology of the respiratory system during her medical assistant training. She learned about common diseases but found that she has a lot more to learn. Besides obtaining patients' vital signs and medical histories, Renee performs a pulse oximetry. She has observed John performing a spirometry test, which she will learn to do in the future.

In her work with the pulmonologist and John, Renee sees patients with many interesting respiratory diseases. She continues to learn from her work with the specialist and the patients.

While studying this chapter, think about the following questions:

- What structures are in the respiratory system?
- What are the functions of the respiratory system?
- What are commonly diagnosed respiratory diseases and disorders? What are the etiologies, signs and symptoms, diagnostic processes, and treatments?
- What are the medical assistant's primary responsibilities when working with patients with respiratory diseases and disorders?

LEARNING OBJECTIVES

1. Differentiate among the structures of the upper respiratory tract.
2. Differentiate among the structures of the lower respiratory tract.
3. Examine the physiology of the respiratory system.
4. Analyze the life span changes to the respiratory system.
5. Differentiate between the signs and symptoms of respiratory system diseases and disorders.
6. Examine chronic respiratory diseases and disorders, including the signs, symptoms, etiology, diagnostic procedures, and treatments.
7. Examine respiratory system cancers, including the signs, symptoms, etiology, diagnostic procedures, and treatments.
8. Examine acute respiratory diseases and disorders, including the signs, symptoms, etiology, diagnostic procedures, and treatments.
9. Examine the medical assistant's role in examinations, diagnostic procedures, and treatments for respiratory conditions.

VOCABULARY

accessory muscles Muscles in the neck, abdomen, and back that assist in breathing.

analgesic (an ahl JEE zik) A drug that reduces or eliminates pain.

antipyretic (an tee pie RET ik) A drug that is used to reduce a fever.

aspirating The process of removing fluids or gases from the body using a suction device. Inhaling liquid (e.g., blood and vomitus) or a foreign object into the respiratory tract.

bronchodilator A drug that relaxes smooth muscle contractions in the bronchioles to improve lung ventilation.

clubbing Abnormal enlargement of the distal phalanges (fingers and toes) associated with chronic tissue hypoxia due to cyanotic heart disease or advanced chronic pulmonary disease.

corticosteroids (kor ti koe STER oids) A group of steroid hormones produced in the body or given as a medication. Some have metabolic functions, and others reduce tissue inflammation. Glucocorticoids and mineralocorticoids are two types.

decongestant A drug that is used for nasal congestion.

diaphragm (DIE uh fram) A broad, dome-shaped muscle used for breathing. It separates the thoracic and abdominopelvic cavities.

expectorate To cough up and spit out mucus from the lower respiratory tract.

expiration Exhaling; movement of waste gases from the alveoli into the atmosphere.

inspiration Inhaling; movement of oxygen from the atmosphere into the alveoli.

VOCABULARY—*continued*

intercostal muscles (in tur KOS tul) Muscles located between the ribs that help with quiet respiration.

mediastinum The space in the thoracic cavity that lies between the lungs, containing the heart, trachea, and esophagus.

paranasal sinuses (pair uh NAY zul SIE nus suhs) Hollow, air-filled cavities in the skull and facial bones. They lighten the weight of the skull and increase the tone, or resonance, of speech.

pharyngitis Inflammation or infection of the pharynx, usually causing the symptoms of a sore throat.

productive cough A cough that produces phlegm or mucus.

pulmonary hypertension High blood pressure that affects the pulmonary system (pulmonary arteries and the right side of the heart).

respiratory arrest Stoppage of breathing.

sputum Mucous secretion coughed up from the lungs and expectorated through the mouth.

surfactant (sur FACK tunt) A mixture of protein and fats that lines the alveoli and prevents the tissues from sticking together and collapsing during exhalation.

thoracentesis (thor ah sen TEE sis) Aspiration of a fluid from the pleural cavity.

INTRODUCTION

Pulmonology is the healthcare specialty that deals with respiratory diseases and disorders. A *pulmonologist* is a specialist involved in the diagnosis, treatment, and prevention of disorders of the respiratory system.

Pulmonary procedures and treatments are common in the ambulatory care area. Besides the pulmonary department, patients with respiratory concerns are typically seen in primary and urgent care departments. Medical assistants measure peak flow rates, perform spirometry, and assist with pulmonary treatments. Nebulizer treatments and oxygen therapy are the most frequent pulmonary treatments in ambulatory care.

The Respiratory Tract

The respiratory system is divided into the upper respiratory tract and the lower respiratory tract. The upper respiratory tract structures are considered passageways for the air, whereas the lower respiratory tract structures are involved in gas exchange.

ANATOMY OF THE UPPER RESPIRATORY TRACT

The upper respiratory tract is composed of structures from the nose to the larynx. These organs are located outside the chest cavity. The upper respiratory tract has several functions:

- Warming and cleaning the inspired air
- Serving as a passageway for air
- Providing the sense of smell

Nose and Paranasal Sinuses

Air can enter through the mouth or the two *nares* (nostrils) in the nose. The nasal septum separates the nares. The air then moves into the nasal cavity. The surface capillaries, mucous membrane, and *cilia* (small hairs) found in the nasal cavity clean, warm, and moisten the air. The cilia continually move in a wavelike motion to push mucus and debris out of the respiratory tract. Receptors for smell are in the nasal cavity. The nasal cavity is connected to four pairs of **paranasal sinuses**. The four pairs of paranasal sinuses are named for the bones they are found in: maxillary, frontal, sphenoid, and ethmoid.

Pharynx

Air continues to travel into the *pharynx* (throat) (Figure 41.1), which is divided into three sections:

- *Nasopharynx*: Located behind the nasal cavity. The *eustachian tube* connects the middle ear to the nasopharynx and equalizes the pressure in the ear with the air pressure outside the body.
- *Oropharynx*: Located behind the mouth and part of the respiratory and digestive systems.
- *Laryngopharynx*: Located between the epiglottis and the esophagus. The *epiglottis*, a flap of cartilage at the larynx opening, closes off the trachea when food is swallowed. As air passes out through the opening, the *larynx* (vocal cords) vibrates to produce speech. The vocal cords are paired bands of cartilaginous tissue.

CRITICAL THINKING APPLICATION **41.1**

Describe the structures that make up the upper respiratory tract.

ANATOMY OF THE LOWER RESPIRATORY TRACT

The lower respiratory tract consists of the trachea, bronchial tubes, and lungs (see Figure 41.1). These structures are lined with mucous membranes and cilia. The *trachea* (windpipe) lies in the space between the lungs, called the **mediastinum**. Air travels from the larynx through the trachea, and then the trachea branches into the right and left bronchi. The right bronchus is wider than the left bronchus.

Bronchioles and Alveoli

The bronchi divide into smaller branches, called *bronchioles*. These bronchioles end in microscopic ducts capped by air sacs, called *alveoli*. Each thin-walled alveolus is in contact with a blood capillary. This contact between the two structures allows the exchange of gases. It is at this point that oxygen (O_2) from the inspired air moves across the one-cell membrane into the blood cells. Carbon dioxide (CO_2) moves in the other direction, from the blood into the air to be expired. Each alveolus is coated with a substance called **surfactant**, which keeps it from collapsing. Without surfactant, the alveoli stick together during *exhalation* (breathing out) and deflate. *Inhalation* (breathing in) becomes more difficult, and less O_2 is able to move into the bloodstream. This condition is life threatening. Babies born before 37 to 39 weeks of gestation are at risk of not having enough surfactant. If time permits before delivery, steroids can be given to the mother to help mature the baby's lungs.

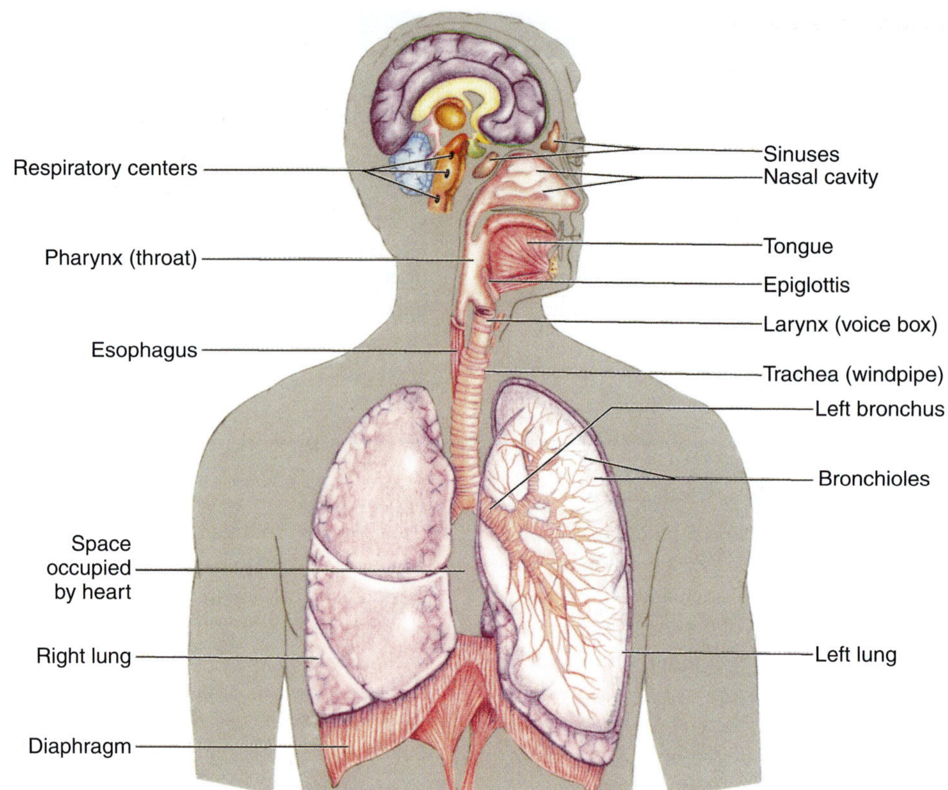

FIGURE 41.1 Anatomic structures of the respiratory system. (Modified from Solomon EP: *Introduction to human anatomy and physiology,* ed 3, St. Louis, 2009, Saunders.)

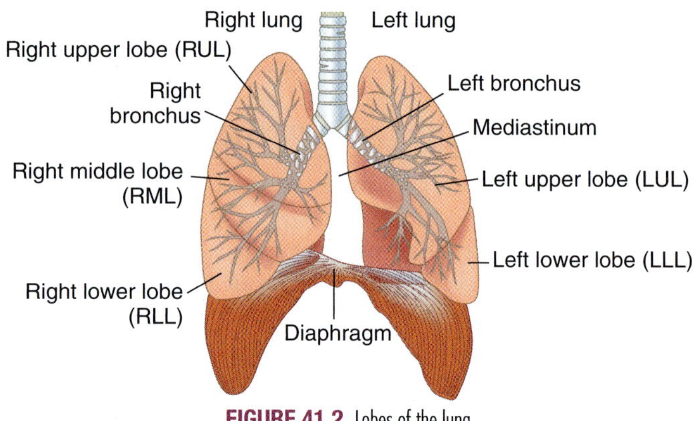

FIGURE 41.2 Lobes of the lung.

Lungs

The bronchial tree and alveoli are the major structures in the right and left lungs. The lungs are soft and spongy because of the air sacs that make up most of their mass. They hang on the right and left sides of the chest, separated by the pericardial sac, which contains the heart. Each lung is composed of sections called *lobes*. The right lung consists of three lobes, whereas the left has only two lobes (Figure 41.2).

Because each lobe has its own bronchus and blood supply, the removal of one lobe *(lobectomy)* results in little or no damage to the rest of the lung. The left lung is longer and narrower. It has a distinct indentation in its center, known as the *cardiac notch*. This is where the left ventricle of the heart is located and where an apical pulse is heard.

Pleura and Pleural Cavity

Pleura is a thin serous membrane found in the thoracic cavity. The pleura folds back on itself, creating a sac that surrounds the lung. The *visceral pleura* covers the lungs and adjoining structures. The *parietal pleura*, the outer portion of the pleura, lines the thoracic cavity and covers the **diaphragm** and mediastinum. Only the parietal pleura contains pain receptors, making it highly sensitive to pain. The right and left pleural sacs are entirely separate.

The *pleural cavity* is the space between the visceral and parietal pleurae. A small amount of pleural fluid is in the pleural cavity. When the lungs expand, moving the visceral pleura closer to the parietal pleura, friction is reduced between the tissues due to the pleural fluid.

Respiratory Muscles

The muscles responsible for normal, quiet respiration are the diaphragm and the **intercostal muscles.** On **inspiration,** the diaphragm is pulled down and flattened as it contracts, and the intercostal muscles expand, pulling air into the lungs. On **expiration,** the diaphragm relaxes and moves upward, pushing air out of the lungs.

PHYSIOLOGY OF THE RESPIRATORY SYSTEM

The two primary functions of the respiratory system are to exchange O_2 from the atmosphere for CO_2 waste and to maintain the acid-base balance in the body. Both functions involve *ventilation* (breathing), which is the movement of gases between the lungs and the environment. Ventilation includes the process of inspiration and expiration.

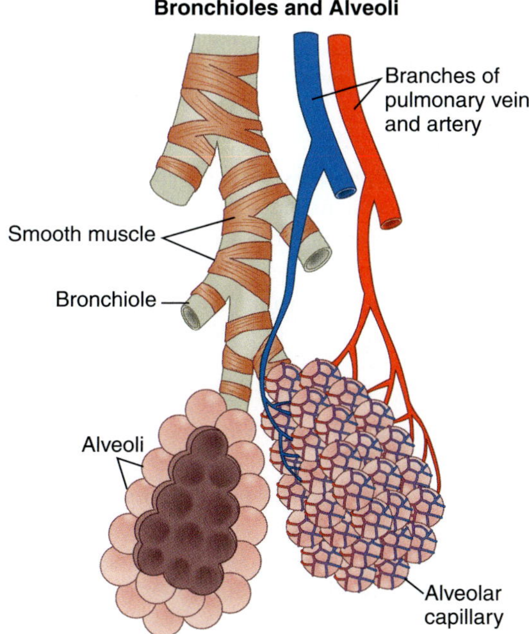

FIGURE 41.3 Alveoli with their capillary network.

Two types of respiration occur during the ventilation process:

- *External respiration* occurs when oxygenated air moves into the alveoli. Surrounding each alveolus is a pulmonary capillary network (Figure 41.3). The alveoli and the pulmonary capillaries are made of single-celled walls. This allows the O_2 to move easily across the alveoli and capillaries into the blood. CO_2 and other wastes are forced out of the capillaries and move into the alveoli.
- *Internal respiration* occurs when O_2 is exchanged for CO_2 between the cells in the body and the blood.

Inspiration

A healthy person breathes when the blood CO_2 level increases. A person with chronic obstructive pulmonary disease (COPD) has a constantly elevated blood CO_2 level. At some point, the body no longer uses the elevated blood CO_2 level as a trigger to breathe. A secondary system kicks in, and breathing is triggered by a decreased blood O_2 level.

When the breathing trigger is activated, it signals the respiratory center in the medulla oblongata, which is in the brainstem. The respiratory center causes a stimulus (i.e., signal) to be carried by the phrenic nerve to the diaphragm. When the diaphragm receives the signal, it flattens out and pulls downward. At the same moment, the intercostal muscles between the ribs contract, causing the ribs to move outward. The movement enlarges the chest cavity and causes the lungs to expand, increasing their volume. The greater the contraction, the deeper the inhalation and the greater the air volume.

CRITICAL THINKING APPLICATION 41.2

Renee sees many patients with chronic obstructive pulmonary disease (COPD) who use oxygen constantly. She realizes that the amount of oxygen is much lower than the amount providers order for patients without COPD. Confused, she asks John why patients with COPD use smaller amounts of supplemental oxygen. How would you answer this question?

Respiratory Distress Changes

When individuals are experiencing respiratory distress, they are unable to move enough air into the lungs. To help move additional air into their lungs, they use **accessory muscles**. To identify whether a person is using the accessory muscles, expose the chest and look for chest retractions with breathing. With intercostal retractions, the chest tissue between the ribs is indrawn or pulled in during breathing. Upper airway obstructions can cause the following retractions:

- *Suprasternal retractions*, sucking in of the skin just above the sternum
- *Supraclavicular retractions*, sucking in of the skin just above the clavicle

Lower airway obstructions can cause the following retractions:

- *Substernal retractions*, sucking in of the abdomen just below the sternum
- *Subcostal retractions*, sucking in of the abdomen just below the ribs

Using accessory muscles to breathe can tire a person. This can lead to **respiratory arrest**, a medical emergency. Typically, this occurs quicker in infants and young children.

CRITICAL THINKING APPLICATION 41.3

The pulmonologist asks Renee to review the signs of respiratory distress with the mother of an asthmatic patient. Discuss what Renee should review with the mother.

Expiration

The second half of ventilation is *expiration*. Once inspiration is complete, the diaphragm and intercostal muscles relax, which causes the diaphragm to move upward into the thoracic cavity and the ribs to move inward. This movement reduces the lung capacity and forces air out of the lungs. Typically, expiration requires very little energy. However, with some conditions (e.g., asthma and emphysema), the person has difficulty getting air out of the lungs. The accessory muscles are needed to help with complete exhalation.

Acid-Base Balance

The body attempts to keep the pH between 7.35 and 7.45. The respiratory system has an important role in acid-base balance. It regulates the amount of CO_2 in the blood. CO_2 in the blood can combine with water to form the buffer bicarbonate. If a person *hyperventilates* (breathes rapidly), the CO_2 and bicarbonate levels in the blood decrease. This causes the pH of the body to rise, resulting in *respiratory alkalosis*. This condition can be seen in patients with anxiety or an acute asthma attack. If hypoventilation occurs, the CO_2 in the blood increases (*hypercapnia*), and *respiratory acidosis* can occur. Respiratory alkalosis and respiratory acidosis are both life-threatening disorders if the underlying causes are not corrected.

LIFE SPAN CHANGES

Changes occur in the respiratory system over a person's lifetime. The following sections explain the changes that occur from infancy to adulthood.

Infant

An infant has a narrow airway with a shorter and softer trachea. If the neck is overextended, the airway can collapse. Infants tend to breathe through their noses, which means nasal congestion can make breathing difficult. Infants are abdominal breathers and have immature respiratory muscles, meaning fatigue with breathing difficulties can set in quickly. With a disproportionately larger tongue and epiglottis, infants and young children are at risk for airway obstruction.

Adult

At around age 20 to 25, the lungs reach maturity. By age 35, lung function starts to decline. People who smoke can increase the aging of their lungs. As a person ages, the following respiratory system changes occur:

- Chest wall and thoracic spine deformities cause increased work of breathing.
- The diaphragm grows weaker, leading to a decreased ability to inhale and exhale.
- Weakness in respiratory muscles causes the coughing reflex to be less effective.
- A decrease in tissue elasticity leads to an inability to keep the airway completely open.
- Alveoli lose their shape, which causes air to be trapped in the lungs. This leads to a decrease in gas exchange and lung capacity.

RESPIRATORY DISEASES

Besides cancer, most respiratory diseases can be divided into chronic or acute conditions. The disease sections of this chapter discuss these three categories of respiratory diseases. Prior to learning about the diseases, it is important for the medical assistant to understand the common signs and symptoms of respiratory diseases. Respiratory diseases can cause the following reactions:

- *Dyspnea*: Difficulty with breathing.
- *Shortness of breath* (SOB): Breathlessness
- *Hemoptysis*: **Expectorate** of blood or blood-streaked **sputum**
- *Hiccup*: Sound produced by the spasmodic involuntary contraction of the diaphragm that causes an uncontrolled breathing in of air followed by the rapid closure of the glottis
- *Epistaxis*: Nosebleed
- *Rhinorrhea*: Nasal discharge

Additional signs and symptoms relate to breathing, changes in the oxygen amount in the blood and tissues, and abnormal lung sounds.

Breathing Changes

Signs and symptoms of respiratory diseases that relate to abnormal breathing rate changes include the following:

- *Apnea*: Temporary absence of breathing
- *Bradypnea*: Abnormally slow breathing
- *Cheyne-Stokes respiration*: An increase in the depth and rate of breathing, followed by a decrease in breathing, and then a period of apnea
- *Hyperpnea*: An increase in the depth of breathing; the rate may also be increased.
- *Hyperventilation*: Abnormal increase in breathing
- *Orthopnea*: Difficulty breathing unless in an upright position (e.g., sitting or standing)
- *Tachypnea*: Rapid, shallow breathing

Oxygen Changes

Respiratory conditions can also change the amount of oxygen in the blood and tissues. These signs and symptoms include the following:

- *Cyanosis*: Lack of oxygen in the blood, causing a bluish color in the skin, nail beds, and lips
- *Hypoxemia*: Insufficient oxygen in the blood
- *Hypoxia*: Decrease in oxygen in the tissues

Abnormal Lung Sounds

Abnormal lung sounds are heard when using a stethoscope, which is placed over the lung field.

- *Pleural rub* or *pleuritic rub*: An auscultatory sound caused by the rubbing together of the visceral and costal pleurae.
- *Rales*: Inspiratory auscultatory sounds resembling crackles or popping sounds caused by fluid in the airway or alveoli. Can be described as moist, dry, fine, or coarse.
- *Rhonchi*: Auscultatory sounds resembling snoring. Occurs when airflow is partially blocked through the large airways.
- *Stridor*: High-pitched inspiratory sound due to a blockage in the upper airway; can be heard with or without a stethoscope.
- *Wheezing*: High-pitched sound produced by a narrowed airway; can be heard with or without a stethoscope.

CHRONIC RESPIRATORY DISEASES

A chronic disease, disorder, or syndrome that lasts longer than 6 months. Some chronic diseases last a lifetime. The following sections examine common chronic respiratory diseases.

Allergic Rhinitis

When a person is allergic to dust, animal dander, pollen, or foods, allergic rhinitis can occur. When the reaction is due to a pollen allergy, the person is said to have hay fever, seasonal allergies, or allergic rhinitis.

The cause of allergic rhinitis can be traced to an allergen that triggers an allergy in a person. When the allergen is breathed in, histamines in the body cause allergy symptoms to occur. Allergic rhinitis can cause the following:

- Itchy nose, mouth, eyes, and throat
- Problems smelling and runny nose
- Sneezing and watery eyes

Later symptoms may include nasal congestion, coughing, decreased sense of smell, and sore throat. Patients can also have dark circles and puffiness under the eyes. Fatigue and headaches are also common.

The provider will perform a physical exam and ask about the patient's allergy history. Allergy testing, a complete blood count (CBC), and other allergy-related tests (e.g., the IgE radioallergosorbent test [RAST] test) may be done. Treatment consists of avoiding the allergen or reducing exposure. A nasal wash may be recommended to remove mucus from the nose. Medications, such as antihistamines, **decongestants**, and **corticosteroids**, may also be ordered. Depending on the severity, the provider may also refer the

FIGURE 41.4 Inflammation and bronchospasm.

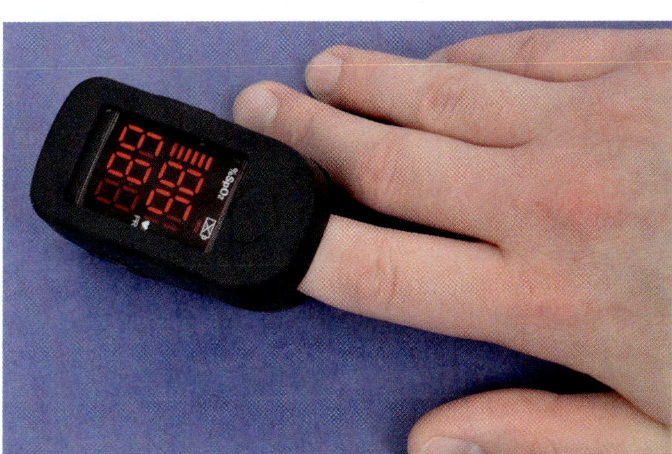

FIGURE 41.5 A pulse oximeter is used for oxygen saturation measurement.

patient to an allergy department for evaluation. Allergy shots *(immunotherapy)* are sometimes recommended.

Asthma

Asthma is a chronic disease that affects the airway. Bronchospasms and airway swelling narrows the passageway. Mucus in the lungs clogs the airway (Figure 41.4). Getting air into and out of the lungs becomes harder. The frequency of asthma episodes can vary. Severe asthma attacks are life threatening and require immediate emergency care.

Many different things can trigger an asthma episode:

- Allergens including foods (e.g., tree nuts), medications, and environmental substances, such as pollen, mold spores, pet dander, tobacco smoke, dust mites, cockroaches, wood smoke, and latex
- Environmental causes, such as chemical gases or fumes, dust, high humidity, and cold, dry air
- Strong emotional states
- Strenuous physical exercise

Asthma symptoms can vary in type and frequency. Typical symptoms include shortness of breath, chest tightness or pain, coughing or wheezing attacks, and early morning or nighttime coughing.

The provider may order peak flow monitoring, pulse oximetry (also called oxygen saturation measurement), and spirometry tests for diagnostic testing (Figure 41.5). Peak flow monitoring measures the amount of air exhaled. Peak flow monitoring can be used with at-home management of asthma. The provider can set up an asthma action plan to accompany the peak flow readings (Table 41.1).

TABLE 41.1 Asthma Action Plan

ZONE	SYMPTOMS	ACTION TO TAKE
Green Zone: Doing well	No asthma symptoms; peak flow is more than 80% of normal peak flow.	Take prescribed long-term control medications.
Yellow Zone: Asthma is getting worse	Asthma symptoms are present, or waking at night, or person cannot do usual activities, or peak flow is 50%–79% of normal peak flow.	Add quick-relief medication to the Green Zone medication. Continue to monitor. Contact provider if not improving.
Red Zone: Medical alert	Very short of breath, or quick-relief medications have not helped, or peak flow is less than 50% of best peak flow.	Take short-acting beta agonist medication and/or oral steroid. Contact the provider immediately.

Adapted from the National Institutes of Health. Asthma Action Plan, www.nhlbi.nih.gov/files/docs/public/lung/asthma_actplan.pdf.

Treatment for asthma is based on the severity of the disease. Asthma medications can be taken orally or inhaled. Inhaled medications are usually taken via a metered-dose inhaler with a spacer or a nebulizer. Long-term control medications are usually taken daily and may include inhaled corticosteroids, leukotriene modifiers, long-acting beta-agonists, and combination inhalers. Quick-relief medications are usually taken during the asthma episode because they provide rapid, short-term relief. Quick-relief medications include short-acting beta agonists supplied by metered-dose inhalers (MDIs), such as albuterol and levalbuterol. If the quick-relief medications do not reduce the episode, immediate emergency care is required.

Chronic Obstructive Pulmonary Disease

According to the Centers for Disease Control and Prevention (CDC), more than 16 million Americans have COPD and more

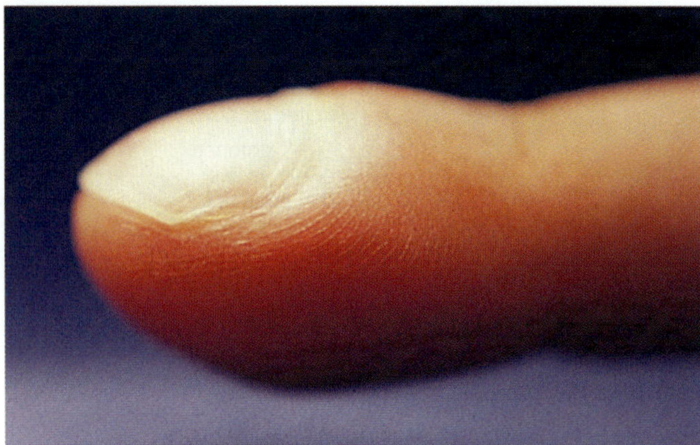

FIGURE 41.6 Finger clubbing. The nail is enlarged and curved. (From Ball J, et al: *Seidel's guide to physical examination,* ed 9, St. Louis, 2019, Mosby.)

than 150,000 Americans die of COPD each year. This condition is both treatable and preventable. COPD develops slowly, making it hard for the affected person to breathe. It includes two conditions:

- *Emphysema*: Thinning and eventual destruction of the alveoli. This usually accompanies chronic bronchitis.
- *Chronic bronchitis*: Inflammation of the bronchial tubes, excessive production of mucus, and diminished activity of the cilia.

The main cause of COPD is smoking tobacco. Other causes include secondhand smoke, air pollution, dust, and chemical fumes. COPD can also be caused by an alpha-1 antitrypsin (AAT) deficiency.

The symptoms of COPD often appear after damage has already been done to the lungs. With chronic bronchitis, a long-term, daily **productive cough** is seen. Additional symptoms of COPD include shortness of breath, chest tightness, breathlessness, wheezing, cyanosis of the lips and nail beds, and **clubbing** (Figure 41.6). The patient may experience a lack of energy and fatigue. Frequent respiratory infections are common.

Typical diagnostic tests include lung function tests (i.e., spirometry and pulse oximetry), chest x-ray, and chest computed tomography (CT) scan. An arterial blood gas test may be done to identify the severity of COPD. Because there is no cure for COPD, the goal of treatment is to slow the disease progression. Patients typically use **bronchodilators** and a bronchodilator-corticosteroid combination to reduce the inflammation. Patients may use low-level oxygen therapy. Adequate nutrition, vaccinations, and smoking cessation are also important in the treatment plan. With severe COPD, surgical options may be considered, such as lung volume reduction surgery (removal of damaged lung tissue) and lung transplantation.

Alpha-1 Antitrypsin Deficiency

Alpha-1 antitrypsin (AAT) deficiency is a rare inherited disorder that can increase a person's risk of developing lung and liver disease. The onset of lung disease occurs at a younger age than normal (around 30 to 41 years of age).

AAT is a protein in the blood and lungs. It protects the lungs from chronic obstructive pulmonary disease (COPD). Sometimes a person may not make enough of this protein, or the AAT that is made is abnormal. Genetic testing is available to determine a person's risk. There is no cure for AAT deficiency, although the lung disease can be managed.

Smoking and Smokeless Tobacco

Tobacco smoke contains more than 7000 chemicals. Of these, 250 are harmful, and at least 69 can cause cancer. It is estimated that 1 in 5 deaths are related to smoking. According to the Centers for Disease Control and Prevention (CDC), smokers are more likely to develop heart disease, lung cancer, and strokes. Smoking can cause the following effects:

- *Respiratory system*: Pneumonia, chronic obstructive pulmonary disease (COPD), tuberculosis, asthma, and cancer of the trachea, bronchus, and lung
- *Nervous system*: Stroke
- *Cardiovascular system*: Aortic aneurysm, early abdominal aortic atherosclerosis in young adults, coronary heart disease, atherosclerotic peripheral vascular disease, and acute myeloid leukemia
- *Sensory system*: Blindness, cataracts, and age-related macular degeneration
- *Digestive system*: Orofacial clefts (congenital defect from maternal smoking) and periodontitis; oropharynx, larynx, esophagus, stomach, liver, and colorectal cancers
- *Endocrine system*: Type 2 diabetes mellitus and pancreatic cancer
- *Musculoskeletal system*: Hip fractures and rheumatoid arthritis
- *Urinary system*: Cancer of the bladder, kidney, and ureters
- *Immune system*: Immune function issues
- *Reproductive system*: In females, reproductive effects (e.g., reduced fertility), ectopic pregnancy, and cervical cancer; in males, erectile dysfunction

Passive or *secondhand smoke*, which stays in the air and can be breathed in by others, causes lung cancer, strokes, low-birth-weight babies, and heart disease. Exposure to secondhand smoke increases a person's risk for lung cancer by 20%. Children exposed to secondhand smoke have an increased risk of sudden infant death syndrome (SIDS), ear infections, bronchitis, pneumonia, colds, and asthma. Secondhand smoke causes more than 53,000 deaths a year in the United States.

Thirdhand smoke is the residue or chemicals from the smoke that gets on skin, clothing, furniture, carpets, and so on. This can be harmful to little children and animals that spend time on the floor. Besides breathing in the residue, these chemicals can be ingested. They can transfer from the carpet, clothing, and so on to hands and then into the person's mouth.

The CDC reports that at least 28 cancer-causing chemicals have been found in smokeless tobacco (e.g., chew and dip). Smokeless tobacco can cause cancer of the mouth, pancreas, and esophagus.

E-cigarettes, which are used for vaping, are also considered tobacco products because they usually contain nicotine. E-cigarettes (also called *e-cigs, vape pens, mods,* or *e-hookahs*) are battery-operated devices that heat liquids to form an aerosol, which is then inhaled. The liquids typically contain nicotine, flavorings, and other additives. E-cigs can also be used for marijuana and other drugs. An e-cig may look like a cigarette, pipe, whiteout, marker, lipstick, pen, or USB (flash) drive. Compared to cigarettes, e-cigs are safer, but they still can be harmful. The aerosol can contain nicotine, heavy metals (e.g., lead), volatile organic compounds, and cancer-causing substances. One example of a health risk comes from diacetyl, which is found in many e-cigarette flavors. It has been known to cause bronchiolitis obliterans, commonly called "popcorn lung." Diacetyl was an ingredient in microwave popcorn and food flavorings until it was linked to hundreds of cases of bronchiolitis obliterans. Like COPD, this disease can cause wheezing, persistent cough, shortness of breath, and death. The alveoli become scarred, and the airway becomes narrowed.

According to the CDC, the advantages of giving up the use of tobacco products include the following:

- Blood pressure and heart rate begin to return to normal.
- Within a few hours, carbon monoxide levels in the blood decline.
- Within a few weeks, circulation improves and abnormal respiratory symptoms (e.g., cough, wheezing) decrease.
- One year after quitting, the cardiovascular risks decrease sharply.
- Two to 5 years after quitting, the risk for stroke returns to a nonsmoker's level.
- Five years after quitting, the risk of cancer of the esophagus, bladder, throat, and mouth is cut in half.
- Ten years after quitting, the lung cancer risk decreases by 50%.

Local resources and prescriptive medications are available to assist people who want to quit using these products. Websites (e.g., https://smokefree.gov) and quit lines are also available (e.g., National Cancer Institute Smoking Quitline: 1-877-44U-QUIT).

Cystic Fibrosis

Cystic fibrosis (CF) is a life-threatening, congenital disease. Mucus builds up in the lungs, pancreas, and other organs. The mucus blocks the airways and increases the risk of infections. In the pancreas, the mucus interrupts the release of digestive enzymes used to break down food.

More than 30,000 people in the United States have cystic fibrosis. The majority of people with CF are diagnosed by age 2. All states require newborn screening tests for cystic fibrosis. With improvements in treatments, people with CF can live, work, and play with a much greater quality of life than in the past.

CF is a genetic disease. Each parent gives one copy of a specific gene to the child. As a result, the child gets two copies of a specific gene. If one of the copies is defective, the person will be a carrier of that disease. If both copies are defective, the person will have the disease. CF can cause the following conditions:

- Higher than normal levels of salt in the sweat and electrolyte imbalances
- A persistent cough that produces a thick, sticky sputum
- Breathlessness, shortness of breath, wheezing, and frequent lung infections
- Poor growth and weight gain
- Intestinal blockage, severe constipation, and foul-smelling, greasy stools

One of the following tests can be done to diagnose CF:

- Two positive sweat tests (the tests must be performed on different days)
- Genetic testing, to detect two defective genes (for CF), and one positive sweat test

There is no cure for CF. Treatment centers on reducing the complications and symptoms. Treatment can include the following:

- Antibiotics for lung infections and anti-inflammatory medications can reduce the swelling in the lungs.
- Bronchodilators and mucus-thinning medication can help clear the lungs of mucus.
- Oral pancreatic enzymes are used to help with digestion.
- Chest physical therapy, vest therapy (vibrating vest), and O_2 therapy can be initiated.
- Surgical options for CF complications include lung transplantation and bowel surgery for obstructions.

Sleep Apnea

Sleep apnea occurs when a person stops breathing, or the breathing becomes very shallow. Breathing pauses may last a few seconds to minutes and can occur 30 or more times an hour. The cause of sleep apnea depends on the type:

- *Obstructive sleep apnea* (OSA): The most common type of sleep apnea; it causes breathing to pause during sleep. OSA results from a blockage or narrowing of the airway when the throat muscles relax. It can be caused by excessive weight, a thicker neck circumference, a narrowed airway, smoking, and nasal congestion. Males are twice as likely to have it, and age increases the risk.
- *Central sleep apnea*: The breathing repeatedly stops during sleep. The brain temporarily stops sending signals to the muscles that control breathing. This condition can be caused by brainstem injuries (including infections and stroke), congestive heart disease, and narcotic analgesics.
- *Complex sleep apnea syndrome*: Occurs when a person has both obstructive and central sleep apnea.

The most common signs and symptoms of these conditions include loud snoring, breathing cessation during sleep, dry mouth, sore throat, morning headache, difficulty staying asleep, excessive daytime sleepiness, irritability, and attention problems.

After an examination, the provider may refer the patient to a sleep specialist or order a sleep study. Treatments may include weight loss or stopping the use of alcohol or medications that may be causing the condition. Continuous positive airway pressure (CPAP) therapy is the most common treatment for OSA (Figure 41.7). It uses mild air pressure to keep the airway open.

RESPIRATORY SYSTEM CANCERS

Laryngeal and lung cancers are the most common cancers that impact the respiratory system. It is estimated that more than 12,000 people are diagnosed with laryngeal cancer yearly, and more than 3700 Americans die of it yearly. More than a half of million Americans

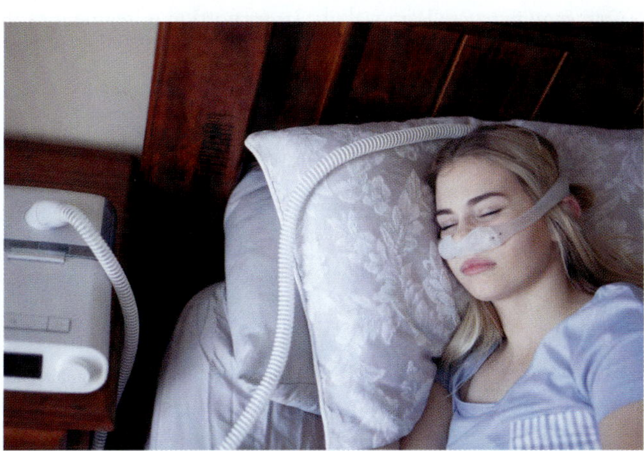

FIGURE 41.7 Adult using a CPAP machine.

have lung cancer. Lung cancer is one of the most common cancers in the United States.

Laryngeal Cancer

Laryngeal cancer is throat cancer that affects the vocal cords and larynx (voice box). In most cases, laryngeal cancer develops in adults older than 50, and males are more likely to get it than females. The causes of laryngeal cancer include tobacco and alcohol use. Laryngeal cancer can cause the following conditions:

- A constant sore throat and painful swallowing
- Ear pain and a lump in the neck or throat
- Hoarseness

After a physical exam, the provider may order a biopsy with laryngoscopy or endoscopy, a CT scan, magnetic resonance imaging (MRI), a positron emission tomography (PET) scan, a bone scan, and a barium swallow (or upper gastrointestinal series). Treatment consists of surgery, chemotherapy, and radiation therapy.

Lung Cancer

There are two main types of lung cancer: non–small cell and small cell. Non–small cell lung cancer is more prevalent. Lung cancer is the leading cause of cancer-related deaths in the United States.

The leading cause of lung cancer is cigarette smoking. The longer a person has smoked and the more a person has smoked, the more likely it is that the individual will contract lung cancer. High exposure levels of asbestos, radiation, and pollution can also increase a person's risk for lung cancer. Lung cancer can cause the following:

- A chronic, worsening cough with hemoptysis and constant chest pain
- Wheezing, breathlessness, shortness of breath, clubbing, and more frequent respiratory infections
- Fatigue, loss of appetite, weight loss, and swelling of the face and hands

Chest x-rays and CT scans, sputum cytology, bronchoscopy, and lung tissue biopsy are used to diagnose lung cancer. Treatment for lung cancer is based on the person's health, the stage of the disease, and the person's preferences. Treatments can include chemotherapy, radiation therapy, targeted drug therapy, and surgery. Here are some common surgical options for lung cancer:

- *Wedge resection*: Removal of a small portion of the lung tissue. It includes the tumor and the healthy tissue on the edge of the tumor.
- *Segmental resection*: Removal of a larger portion or segment of the lung.
- *Lobectomy*: Removal of a lobe of the lung.
- *Pneumonectomy*: Removal of the entire lung.

ACUTE RESPIRATORY DISEASES

An acute disease is a disease that has a severe, sudden onset. There are many acute respiratory diseases. The following sections examine common acute respiratory diseases.

Acute Bronchitis

Acute bronchitis is an inflammation of the lining of the bronchial tubes. The bronchial tubes become irritated and swollen, narrowing the airway. Excessive mucus is produced, leading to increased coughing.

Acute bronchitis is usually caused by a lower respiratory viral infection. Viral conditions, such as the common cold, influenza, and pertussis (whooping cough), can also cause acute bronchitis. In rare cases, a bacterial infection causes the disease. In addition, breathing in irritants or inhaling food or vomit can cause acute bronchitis. Acute bronchitis can cause a dry, hacking cough that can turn into a productive cough. The patient may also experience a low-grade fever, fatigue, and weakness.

After obtaining a medical history and performing an examination, the provider may order a chest x-ray. Pulse oximetry, which determines the oxygen saturation in the blood, may also be performed. In most cases, acute bronchitis is viral, so no antibiotics are prescribed. At-home treatments include using cough drops and a humidifier to soothe a dry throat. Patients are encouraged to drink plenty of fluids and get adequate rest. Over-the-counter (OTC) medications are used for fevers and body aches. Patients are encouraged to stop smoking and using e-cigarettes.

COVID-19

COVID-19 is also called coronavirus disease 2019 and SARS-CoV-2. This disease originated in China in 2019 and created a worldwide pandemic. Several vaccines have been approved and can prevent or decrease the severity of the illness should a person get COVID-19. Because this is a new disease, new information is being learned all the time.

COVID-19 is caused by the severe acute respiratory syndrome coronavirus 2 (SARS-CoV-2). Coronaviruses are a group of viruses that cause several illnesses, including the common cold and severe acute respiratory syndrome (SARS). The following factors put people at a higher risk of serious illness with COVID-19:

- Age over 65
- Lung disease, such as COPD, asthma, and cystic fibrosis
- Weakened immune system, from cancer treatments, transplants (e.g., bone marrow, solid organ), and chronic diseases
- Type 1 or type 2 diabetes mellitus, chronic kidney disease, liver disease, sickle cell disease, high blood pressure, heart disease, severe obesity, and nervous system conditions

The severity of the signs and symptoms can vary and can appear 2 to 14 days after exposure to the virus. COVID-19 can cause the following reactions:

- Fever, chills, muscle aches, and fatigue
- New loss of taste or smell, headache
- Rhinorrhea, sore throat, cough, shortness of breath, and chest pain
- Nausea, vomiting, and diarrhea
- Emergency warning signs: dyspnea, persistent chest pressure or pain, new confusion, inability to wake or stay awake, and cyanosis

A viral test is performed to diagnose a current infection. A nasal or throat specimen is obtained, and viral tests can be used to check for SARS-CoV-2, the virus that causes COVID-19. Nucleic acid amplification tests (NAATs) detect the virus's genetic material. NAATs are more accurate but take longer to process than the antigen test. Antigen tests detect viral proteins and are less sensitive; thus the test result may need to be confirmed with a NAAT. The antibody (serology) test is used to test for COVID-19 antibodies, indicating a past infection.

Treatments depend on the severity of the illness. Home care treatments include analgesics, cough medication, rest, and fluid intake.

Quarantining helps to minimize the spread of the disease. Severe cases can lead to hospitalization and oxygen therapy. Many clinical studies are underway, and additional treatments are being researched. COVID vaccines are available.

Most people return to normal health, but some people may have post-COVID conditions (or long COVID). They may experience many symptoms for weeks to months after the infection. Post-COVID signs and symptoms can include:

- Tiredness, fatigue, and fever
- Heart palpitations, difficulty breathing, cough, and chest pain
- Difficulty concentrating or thinking ("brain fog"), headache, sleep issues, lightheadedness, change in smell or taste, and depression
- Diarrhea and stomach pain
- Joint or muscle pain, rash, and changes in menstrual cycles

Croup

Croup is caused by inflammation of the trachea and larynx. It usually affects children ages 3 months to 5 years but can occur at any age. Croup is caused by bacteria and viruses, such as parainfluenza RSV, adenovirus, and influenza. Bacterial croup is more severe than viral croup. Usually, the person has a mild cold and low-grade fever for several days before the barking cough and hoarseness occur. As croup worsens, the child may have trouble breathing, such as inspiratory stridor, wheezing, and chest retractions.

The provider will complete a history and physical examination. Additional tests and chest x-rays may be completed. Treatment includes antipyretics, humidifier, bed rest, and increased fluid intake. Sitting up may help the person breathe easier. In severe cases, hospitalization with antibiotics and oxygen therapy may be necessary.

Epiglottis

Epiglottis, an upper respiratory system disease, is a life-threatening inflammation of the epiglottis. *Haemophilus influenzae* type b (*Hib*), *Streptococcus pneumoniae*, and viruses cause epiglottis. Signs and symptoms include a high fever, **pharyngitis**, stridor, cyanosis, drooling, difficulty breathing and swallowing, and hoarseness.

The provider will complete a history and physical examination. Blood and throat cultures, a complete blood count (CBC), and a neck x-ray may be ordered. Treatments for epiglottis include hospitalization, humidified oxygen, antibiotics, and corticosteroids.

Influenza

Influenza, also called the flu, is an acute contagious respiratory viral infection. Two main types of influenza include Types A and B. Influenza is spread mainly by droplets from coughing, sneezing, or talking. Signs and symptoms include a fever, cough, sore throat, nasal congestion, body aches, headache, and fatigue. Children may experience vomiting and diarrhea.

The provider will complete a history and physical examination. A nasopharyngeal swab is used to collect a specimen, and a rapid influenza diagnostic test (waived by the Clinical Laboratory Improvement Amendments [CLIA]) is done. Treatment involves bed rest, increased fluids, antiviral medications, and over-the-counter analgesics. A yearly vaccine is available for influenza.

Laryngitis

Laryngitis is inflammation of the voice box (larynx) and an upper respiratory system disease. The cause of laryngitis is overuse of the voice, irritation, or infection. Signs and symptoms include hoarseness, weakened (or loss of) voice, tickling sensation, sore or dry throat, and cough.

The provider will complete a history and physical examination. With chronic laryngitis, a laryngoscopy and biopsy may be done. Treatment consists of antibiotics and corticosteroids. The patient is encouraged to increase fluid intake, rest the voice, and breathe moist air,

Pertussis

Pertussis (also called whooping cough) is a contagious disease that is caused by *Bordetella pertussis*. Pertussis is spread by coughing or sneezing and develops within 5 to 10 days after exposure. Initially, the person may experience nasal drainage, a low-grade fever, and a mild, occasional cough. Later signs include a rapid coughing followed by a high-pitched "whoop" sound and vomiting. The person may be exhausted after the coughing fit. According to the CDC, infected people are most contagious up to about 2 weeks after the cough begins.

The provider will complete a history and physical examination. A nasopharyngeal specimen is obtained for a culture. A polymerase chain reaction (PCR) test can be done. Pertussis is treated with antibiotics. The person is encouraged to stay home, rest, and use a humidifier. Good hand washing helps to eliminate transmission. The DTaP and Tdap vaccines are used to help prevent pertussis.

Pneumonia

Pneumonia is an infection of the lungs. It may affect one or both lungs. The alveoli fill with fluid or pus. Young children, adults over 65 years of age, people who smoke, and those with chronic illnesses are at more risk for pneumonia. The severity of pneumonia can range from mild to life threatening. In the United States, about 1 million people have pneumonia yearly, and about 50,000 people die from the disease. Adults are at the most risk. Globally, it is the leading infectious disease killer of children under age 5.

Pneumonia can be caused by bacteria, viruses, and fungi (Table 41.2). If a person has viral pneumonia, there is also a risk of getting bacterial pneumonia. Various chemicals can also cause pneumonia. **Aspirating** fluid or a foreign material into the lungs can also cause pneumonia. Signs and symptoms of pneumonia vary based on the severity and type of pneumonia. Typically, pneumonia causes high fever, chills, productive cough, shortness of breath, and chest pain with coughing or breathing. A person may also experience decreased appetite and fatigue. Confusion may occur in older adults.

Providers will listen to a patient's lungs for abnormal sounds. Chest x-rays, a CBC, a sputum culture, and pulse oximetry are typical diagnostic procedures used to check for pneumonia. Treatment for pneumonia is based on the type of pneumonia a person has. Antibiotics are used for bacterial pneumonia, and antiviral medications are used for viral pneumonia. Patients are encouraged to drink plenty of fluids and get rest. OTC antipyretics and analgesics (e.g., ibuprofen and acetaminophen) may be recommended.

TABLE 41.2 Examples of Pathogens That Cause Pneumonia

TYPE OF PATHOGEN	PATHOGEN	DESCRIPTION
Bacteria	*Streptococcus pneumoniae*	Children under 2 years of age and adults 65 years or older are at most risk; pneumococcal vaccines are used for prevention.
	Haemophilus influenzae	Haemophilus influenza type b (Hib) vaccine is used as a prevention.
	Legionella pneumophila	Causes legionnaires disease and Pontiac fever.
	Mycoplasma pneumoniae	Called "walking pneumonia."
	Chlamydia pneumoniae	Most common in school-aged children.
	Chlamydia psittaci	Causes psittacosis; transmitted by infected pet birds and poultry.
Virus	Influenza virus	Prevention includes the yearly influenza vaccine.
	Respiratory syncytial virus (RSV)	Most common cause of pneumonia in children under 1 year of age.
Fungi	*Pneumocystis jirovecii*	More common in people with weakened immune systems.

CRITICAL THINKING APPLICATION **41.4**

Renee is rooming Carl Bowden. He is here today for a recheck appointment. He was diagnosed 10 days ago with pneumonia. As Renee gathers Carl's history, he tells her he has smoked two packs a day for the past 30 years. He also states that he has had pneumonia six times over the past 2 years. He asks Renee if smoking might have something to do with that. Thinking back to the respiratory structures and functions you have learned about in this chapter, how would you answer his question?

Pulmonary Embolism

Pulmonary embolism (PE) is a condition in which one of the pulmonary arteries is blocked. PE is a medical emergency and can be life threatening. Due to the blockage, blood flow may be interrupted to that section of the lung. This can lead to **pulmonary hypertension**. Oxygen can be limited to other body organs.

Often PE is a complication of deep vein thrombosis (DVT). Blood clots form in the veins, usually in the legs. Some of the clots break off and travel through the bloodstream. Eventually, the clot blocks a pulmonary artery. Risk factors for PE include the following:

- Current or past DVT
- Being bedridden, having surgery; breaking a bone
- Pregnancy
- Chronic illness (stroke, hypertension, chronic heart disease, obesity)
- Smoking
- Use of birth control pills or hormone therapy pills

Pulmonary embolism can cause problems breathing, unexplained shortness of breath, and rapid breathing. A patient may experience chest pain, coughing or coughing up blood, arrhythmias, lightheadedness, and fainting.

Besides a medical history and physical examination, the provider may order the following diagnostic procedures:

- Ultrasound: to detect DVT in the legs
- CT scan with contrast to detect PE or DVT
- Lung ventilation/perfusion scan (VQ scan)
- Pulmonary angiography
- Chest x-ray and chest MRI scan
- Echocardiography and electrocardiogram (ECG)

The goals of treatment include preventing more clots or larger clots from forming. Treatment includes the following:

- *Anticoagulants*: "Blood thinners" (e.g., warfarin [Coumadin] and heparin) to prevent clots from forming.
- *Thrombolytics*: Medications that break up the clot. These are used in emergencies. Thrombolytics can be delivered by a catheter to the site of the clot.
- *Compression stockings*: To help prevent blood from pooling and clotting in the legs.

Pulmonary Tuberculosis

Pulmonary tuberculosis (TB) is caused by bacteria that can affect the lungs. There are two TB-related conditions: latent TB infection and TB disease. Tuberculosis is caused by *Mycobacterium tuberculosis,* which is spread through the air. The following individuals are at risk for TB:

- Anyone who has lived in a country where TB is prevalent
- Anyone in frequent close contact with someone with TB disease
- Those working in healthcare, a homeless shelter, or a prison
- Those living in a nursing home, prison, or homeless shelter
- People who have latent TB infection and a weakened immune system because TB can become active under these conditions

There are differences regarding the spread and the signs/symptoms of the two TB-related conditions:

- With latent TB infection, a person cannot spread TB bacteria to others, and there are no signs or symptoms.
- With TB disease, a person can spread the disease by coughing, sneezing, singing, or talking. TB disease can cause a bad cough that lasts 3 or more weeks, pain in the chest, blood in the sputum, weakness, no appetite, weight loss, chills, fever, and night sweats.

Initially, the person is tested with either a Mantoux tuberculin skin test (TST) (also known as a purified protein derivative [PPD] test) or a TB blood test (e.g., QuantiFERON-TB Gold Plus [QFT-Plus], T-SPOT.TB). If the test is positive, then the person will have additional testing (e.g., chest x-ray and sputum smear/culture) to determine if it is latent TB infection or TB disease. With latent TB infection, the chest x-ray is normal, and the sputum smear/culture is negative. With TB disease, the chest x-ray is abnormal, and the sputum smear/culture is positive. Treatments include the following:

- For latent TB infections, isoniazid or rifapentine may be prescribed. The goal is to prevent TB disease; a weakened immune system can increase the risk of TB disease.

- For TB disease, isoniazid, rifampin, ethambutol, or pyrazinamide may be prescribed. With treatment, TB disease symptoms tend to diminish within 2 to 3 weeks, but medication treatment may last for 6 to 9 months.

CRITICAL THINKING APPLICATION **41.5**

Renee is confused about the two different types of tuberculosis (TB). She asks John to summarize the difference between latent TB infection and TB disease. How would you summarize the differences?

Respiratory Syncytial Virus

Respiratory syncytial virus (RSV) produces upper respiratory "cold" symptoms in healthy older children and adults. For young children and adults with medical problems, it can cause pneumonia and severe breathing problems.

RSV spreads by coughing or sneezing. The virus can survive for several hours on infected surfaces. Typical outbreaks of RSV occur in winter and early spring. RSV can cause nasal congestion, low-grade fevers, a runny nose, and a mild cough. Complications can include a barking cough from swelling near the vocal cords, high fevers, wheezing, apnea, cyanosis, and difficulty breathing.

During the physical exam, the provider listens to the lungs, checking for wheezing and other abnormal lung sounds. Additional diagnostic procedures include pulse oximetry, chest x-rays, and laboratory tests (e.g., a CLIA-waived RSV test, viral cultures of the respiratory secretions from the nose). Treatment consists of over-the-counter medication (e.g., acetaminophen [Tylenol]) for the fever and plenty of fluids to prevent dehydration. People with severe cases of RSV are hospitalized. Supplemental oxygen, albuterol breathing treatments, and inhaled epinephrine may be given.

Sinusitis

Sinusitis is the inflammation of the sinuses. It is an upper respiratory system disease and can be acute or chronic. The cause of sinusitis can include structural abnormalities, or a cold may cause mucus to pool and pathogens to grow.

Signs and symptoms of sinusitis include a fever, weakness, fatigue, nasal and sinus congestion, cough, bad breath, or loss of smell.

The provider will complete a history and physical examination. A sinus x-ray may be taken. Treatment includes antibiotics, decongestants, and over-the-counter **analgesics**. The patient may be encouraged to apply a warm pack to the sinus areas, administer saline nasal sprays, and use a vaporizer.

Strep Throat

Strep throat is a highly contagious bacterial infection of the throat. Untreated strep throat can cause kidney inflammation and rheumatic fever. Strep throat is common in children but can affect people of all ages.

Strep throat is caused by group A streptococcal bacteria, which spreads through droplets from coughing, sneezing, or sharing food or drink. Signs and symptoms of strep throat include a rash, nausea, vomiting, fever, headache, painful swallowing, sore throat, tiny red spots at the back of the throat, and white pus patches.

A history and physical will be done. A rapid antigen test (CLIA waived) and a throat culture can be done. Treatment consists of antibiotics, **antipyretics**, and over-the-counter analgesics. Patients are encouraged to rest, drink plenty of fluids, gargle with warm salt water, and use a humidifier. They should stay home until they have been on the antibiotics for 24 hours.

Additional Respiratory System Diseases and Disorders

There are many respiratory diseases. The following list provides a brief description of several of them:

- *Acute respiratory distress syndrome*: A life-threatening condition that prevents enough oxygen from getting into the blood. Fluid buildup in the lungs reduces the lungs' ability to expand and causes hypoxemia.
- *Anthracosis*: A loss of lung capacity caused by an accumulation of coal dust in the lungs; also called black lung disease.
- *Atelectasis*: A partial or complete collapse of the lung, which prevents normal oxygen absorption. Can be caused by lung disease, surgery, or a blockage.
- *Bronchiectasis*: An infection or other conditions that cause damage to the airway, leading to bronchial dilation and scarring.
- *Bronchiolitis*: A common viral infection in young children and infants. The bronchioles become inflamed, and mucus builds up in the airway, affecting breathing.
- *Bronchopulmonary dysplasia* (BPD): A chronic respiratory condition that affects premature infants or infants who are on a *ventilator* (breathing machine). Infants require high concentrations of oxygen and assisted ventilation. They may have lung damage and are at greater risk for repeated respiratory infections.
- *Deviated septum*: A shifting of the nasal septum from the midline.
- *Diphtheria*: A bacterial respiratory infection characterized by sore throat, fever, and headache.
- *Hemothorax*: A condition that results in a collection of blood in the space between the chest wall and the lung (the pleural cavity). Caused by chest trauma, blood clotting defect, thoracic surgery, lung cancer, and tuberculosis.
- *Histoplasmosis*: A fungal disease of the lungs caused by inhalation of *Histoplasma capsulatum*. H. capsulatum is found in soil and dust contaminated with bird or bat droppings.
- *Influenza A (H1N1) infection*: Results from transmission of the novel influenza A (H1N1) virus to humans, causing influenza symptoms, diarrhea, and vomiting. Also called swine flu.
- *Legionnaires' disease*: A serious, life-threatening type of pneumonia caused by breathing in mist or swallowing water containing *Legionella pneumophila* bacteria. Can come from water in hot tubs, showers, or air conditioning units. Also called legionellosis.
- *Nasal polyps*: Soft, saclike growths on the lining of the nose or sinuses. Can obstruct the airway and block drainage from the sinuses.
- *Nasopharyngeal carcinoma*: Malignant tumors in the pharynx, which can be related to diet or the Epstein-Barr virus. They cause a mass in the neck, nasal obstruction, epistaxis, and serous otitis media (middle ear infection).
- *Neonatal respiratory distress syndrome* (RDS): Often seen in premature babies born before 37 to 39 weeks of gestation. They lack enough surfactant in their lungs, which leads to respiratory

distress. Infants are given warm, moist oxygen and may be put on a ventilator.

- *Pleural effusion*: An abnormal, excessive buildup of fluid between the layers of tissue that line the lungs and chest cavity.
- *Pleurisy*: Infection of the pleura. Caused by bacteria, fungus, parasites, or viruses. Can also be caused by inhaling toxins. Causes stabbing pain with inspiration, cough, fever, chills, and dyspnea. A pleural friction rub is heard over the lung field. A chest x-ray, an ultrasound, and CT scan can be done. Treatment involves analgesics, anti-inflammatories, bed rest, and a **thoracentesis**.
- *Pneumothorax*: Air or gas in the pleural space causes the lung to collapse (atelectasis). Caused by a rupture of a small blister on the lung's surface or trauma. The person experiences a sudden, sharp pleuritic pain that increases with movement, breathing, or coughing. Shortness of breath, cyanosis, rapid pulse, and respiratory distress is also experienced. Breath sounds are decreased over the collapsed lung field. A chest x-ray, CT scan, pulse oximetry, and arterial blood gases may be done. Treatment depends on the cause of the collapse and may include bed rest and monitoring of vital signs, a chest tube, or surgical procedures to remove a portion of the pleura (pleurectomy).
- *Pulmonary abscess*: A localized collection of infectious material in the lungs.
- *Pulmonary edema*: An accumulation of fluid in the lung tissue caused by the inability of the heart to pump blood. It is often present in cases of congestive heart failure.
- *Pulmonary fibrosis*: Scarring of lung tissue, causing the tissues to get stiff and thick. Breathing can be difficult, and the person can have hypoxemia.
- *Pulmonary hypertension* (PH): The blood pressure is high in the pulmonary arteries, which affects the blood flow in the lungs. The blood vessels become hard and narrow, causing hypoxemia. PH may be related to genetics or other conditions, such as heart or lung disease.
- *Pyothorax*: Pus in the pleural cavity. Also called empyema.
- *Rhinomycosis*: A fungal infection of the nasal mucous membranes.
- *Sarcoidosis*: A condition that causes lesions to form in the lungs and chest lymph nodes. It can lead to chronic illness and organ damage. Its origin is unknown.
- *Severe acute respiratory syndrome* (SARS): A viral respiratory disorder caused by a coronavirus. It usually results in pneumonia.
- *Silicosis*: The loss of lung capacity caused by an accumulation of glass dust in the lungs.
- *Upper respiratory tract infection*: An inflammation or infection of the upper respiratory structures. Known as the common cold.

THE MEDICAL ASSISTANT'S ROLE IN EXAMINATIONS, DIAGNOSTIC PROCEDURES, AND TREATMENTS

Medical assistants in primary care, urgent care, and pulmonary departments work with patients with respiratory conditions. Medical assistants in occupational health are also involved with performing spirometry for preemployment physicals. The following sections describe the medical assistant's role in examinations, diagnostic procedures, and treatments.

Assisting with the Examination

Preparing a patient for a respiratory examination includes having the patient disrobe to the waist. The patient should put on a gown with the opening in the front or back, depending on the provider's preference. To assess the status of the respiratory system, the provider uses inspection, palpation, percussion, and auscultation on the anterior thorax, then repeats the process on the posterior and lateral thorax. The medical assistant is responsible for assisting the provider throughout the examination and providing privacy and support for the patient.

Assisting with Diagnostic Procedures

Table 41.3 lists common diagnostic procedures for respiratory diseases. Table 41.4 lists common medical laboratory tests for respiratory system diseases. Some diagnostic procedures are done in the clinic, whereas others are done in other departments (e.g., medical laboratory and radiology). The medical assistant may be responsible for coaching patients on diagnostic procedures done in other departments. As with other diagnostic procedures, the medical assistant should coach the patient regarding the following:

- Patient preparation (e.g., dietary restrictions and medications to hold)
- Location and time of the test
- What to expect during the procedure
- Any follow-up required after the procedure

The medical assistant performs the following diagnostic procedures.

CRITICAL THINKING APPLICATION **41.6**

Renee is working with a patient who needs to have an oxygen saturation measurement with a pulse oximeter. The patient asks Renee what this test shows. Thinking back to what you have learned already in this chapter, how would you answer the patient's question?

Peak Flow Rate Measurement

The peak flow meter measures the amount of air exhaled. A peak flow rate is measured using a manual or digital peak flow meter in an ambulatory care or home setting (see Figure 41.8A–B). It is used to diagnose acute conditions and manage chronic diseases, such as asthma. Procedure 41.1 describes the steps to take when measuring a peak flow rate. When a patient is performing a peak flow rate test, it is important that the medical assistant obtain three adequate readings.

For chronic disease management, providers encourage patients to use peak flow meters at home. The providers create asthma action plans for the patients to follow (see Table 41.1). Based on the patient's peak flow rate at home, the patient follows the directions on the plan.

CRITICAL THINKING APPLICATION **41.7**

Renee is working with an adult patient newly diagnosed with asthma. She has just explained how to use a peak flow meter at home, and the patient's "normal" peak flow volume was identified. As Renee explains the asthma action plan the pulmonologist has ordered, the patient begins to look confused. He asks, "Why can't I just call or come in if I don't feel good? Why do I need to bother with the asthma action plan?" What might be the benefits to the patient of using the asthma action plan? How might you respond to his question?

TABLE 41.3 Diagnostic Procedures for Respiratory System Diseases and Disorders

PROCEDURE	DESCRIPTION	PATIENT PREPARATION AND COACHING
Imaging Procedures		
Chest x-rays (CXRs)	Images taken from several directions, which provide a good outline of the heart and lungs. Abnormal air "pockets," fluid, and tumors can be seen on chest x-rays.	Metal must be removed (e.g., jewelry, glasses, cell phone). Patient should be screened for pregnancy and surgically implanted devices (e.g., heart valve and pacemaker).
Computed tomography (CT)	An imaging technique that can provide more information than chest x-rays.	Screen patient for pregnancy. All metal objects must be removed (e.g., glasses, dentures, jewelry). May have eating and drinking restrictions.
Lung positron emission tomography scan/ Computed tomography (PET/CT)	PET scans can be performed with CT scans. A tracer is given intravenously and after about an hour, a PET scan is taken.	Screen patient for pregnancy, claustrophobia, and an allergy to contrast dye or iodine. Patient may need to sign a consent form. May have eating and drinking restrictions.
Magnetic resonance imaging (MRI)	An imaging technique that can provide more information than chest x-rays.	Screen patient for pregnancy and implanted metal or electronic devices (e.g., pacemaker, valves, heart defibrillator, shrapnel, and cochlear implants). Darker inks used in tattoos may contain metal.
Pulmonary angiography	A procedure in which a catheter is inserted into the pulmonary blood vessels. Dye is injected, and x-ray pictures show the blood flow through the pulmonary vessels	Screen patient for pregnancy and an allergy to contrast dye or iodine. Patient may need to sign a consent form. May have eating and drinking restrictions.
Lung ventilation/ perfusion scan (VQ scan)	A procedure in which a radioisotope substance is inhaled and also injected; then a special x-ray scanner creates a picture of the blood flow and airflow in the lungs.	Screen patient for pregnancy. Usually needs a recent chest x-ray.
Pulmonary Function Tests		
Peak flow monitor	A handheld device that measures the exhaled air. It can also be used at home.	Need to loosen any restrictive clothing. Gum and loose dentures should be removed. Instruct patient on how to perform the test.
Pulse oximetry	A noninvasive test used to measure the oxygen saturation level in blood.	Remove nail polish or artificial nails to get an accurate reading.
Spirometry test	Measures the volume of inhaled and exhaled air, and the time required for each.	Patient will need instructions regarding taking or holding respiratory medications. Need to loosen any restrictive clothing. Gum and loose dentures should be removed. Instruct patient on how to perform the test.
Lung volume test	Determines lung volume after inhalation and exhalation. Also called plethysmography.	Patient may sit in a clear box and breathes in and out of a mouthpiece of the plethysmograph.
Lung diffusion capacity	Determines how effectively gas travels from the lungs to the bloodstream.	Patient breathes in a tracer gas (harmless gas), and the concentration of the gas is measured in the exhaled air.
Endoscopy		
Bronchoscopy	The insertion of an instrument (bronchoscope) through the mouth to visualize the trachea and bronchi.	Patient may need to stop anticoagulants and NSAIDs prior to procedure. Patient should not eat or drink (NPO) after midnight. Someone must drive the patient home after the test. Patient may need to sign a consent form.

Spirometry

Spirometry evaluates lung function as it is affected by respiratory, cardiac, and neuromuscular diseases. It can be ordered if the provider identifies abnormalities in the respiratory system. A spirometer can evaluate the amount of air you exhale and inhale. It looks at how quickly the air is exhaled and the rate at which air is breathed in. Several different tests can be done with spirometry (Table 41.5).

With spirometry testing, it is important that the medical assistant enter accurate patient data into the spirometer computer (Figure 41.9). Besides the patient's name, medical record number, and date

TABLE 41.4 Medical Laboratory Tests for Respiratory System Diseases and Disorders

PROCEDURE	DESCRIPTION	PATIENT PREPARATION AND COACHING
Arterial blood gas (ABG)	A test in which a blood specimen is collected from the artery in the wrist, and the pH of the blood, carbon dioxide (CO_2) and oxygen (O_2) content are measured.	Usually no restrictions for tests. Typically done in the hospital setting.
CLIA-waived tests	• Legionella urinary antigen test: for legionnaires' disease • Influenza A & B test: for influenza • Rapid strep A test: for strep throat • RSV test: for respiratory syncytial virus pneumonia	Usually no restrictions for tests.
Sputum cytology	A test in which sputum is collected and examined under a microscope for abnormal cells.	Provide patient with instructions on collecting sputum specimens.
Sputum culture	A test in which sputum is collected and analyzed in the lab for bacterial growth over a period of days.	

CLIA, Clinical Laboratory Improvement Amendments.

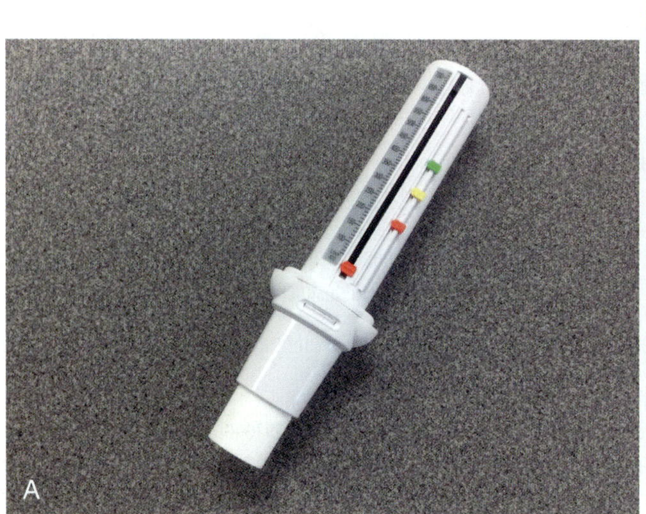

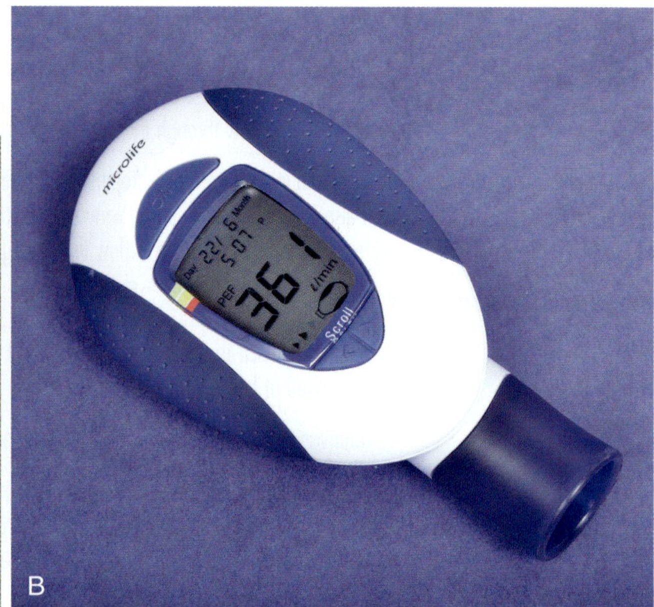

FIGURE 41.8 (A) Manual peak flow meter. **(B)** Digital peak flow meter.

of birth, the medical assistant may need to enter the person's sex, age, race, height, and weight. The patient's current height and weight need to be obtained prior to the spirometry. The computer pulls stored data and creates a "normal" person for those characteristics. After the patient has completed the test, the computer will print out the patient's results compared with the "normal" person's. This helps the provider identify areas of concern.

Procedure 41.2 describes the spirometry procedure. When performing the spirometry procedure, the following steps should be taken:

- Adults should exhale 6 seconds, and children should exhale 3 seconds for the forced vital capacity (FVC). For patients with obstructive breathing patterns, the FVC may take up to 15 seconds.
- Give patients at least 30 seconds between blows. Have patients indicate when they are ready for the next blow.
- Do a minimum of three blows and a maximum of eight blows (unless otherwise indicated by the facility's protocols).
- Make sure to follow the operators' manual for the machine you are using.
- Be encouraging yet respectful of patients when coaching them through the procedure.

CRITICAL THINKING APPLICATION 41.8

Renee's last patient of the day is Janine Butler, who is seeing the provider because of her asthma. After the provider sees Janine, he orders a spirometry test. Renee prepares the equipment and brings Janine into the testing room. However, Janine refuses to have her height and weight measured. Renee explains to Janine the importance of getting accurate height and weight measurements. Discuss how you would explain the importance of obtaining accurate height and weight measurements when doing a spirometry test.

TABLE 41.5 Spirometry Tests

TEST	DESCRIPTION	PATIENT COACHING
Tidal volume (TV)	Volume of air inhaled and exhaled during a normal respiration	Breathe in and out normally with lips pursed around the mouthpiece.
Forced vital capacity (FVC)	Amount of air that can be forcefully exhaled from a maximum inhalation	Inhale as deeply as possible, then quickly forcibly exhale as much as possible.
Forced expiratory volume in 1 second (FEV_1)	Volume of air exhaled in the first second of the FVC	
Expiratory reserve volume (ERV)	Maximal volume of air exhaled after normal exhalation	Breathe in and out normally, then exhale forcibly at the end of the TV.
Inspiratory reserve volume (IRV)	Maximal volume of air inhaled after normal inhalation	Breathe in normally, then forcibly inhale.
Vital capacity (VC)	Maximum amount of air that can be exhaled during a normal or slow exhalation after maximum inhalation	Inhale deeply and exhale completely.
Inspiratory capacity (IC)	Maximum amount of air that can be inhaled after a normal exhalation	Breathe in and out normally, then forcibly inhale at the end of the TV.
Functional residual capacity (FRC)	Amount of air remaining in the lungs at the end of a normal exhalation	None
Residual volume (RV)	Volume of air remaining in the lungs after a forced exhalation	None
Total lung capacity (TLC)	Maximum amount of air in the lungs with maximum inhalation	None
Maximum voluntary ventilation (MVV)	Maximum volume that is breathed in and out in 1 minute	Breathe in and out as deeply and as frequently as possible for 15 seconds.

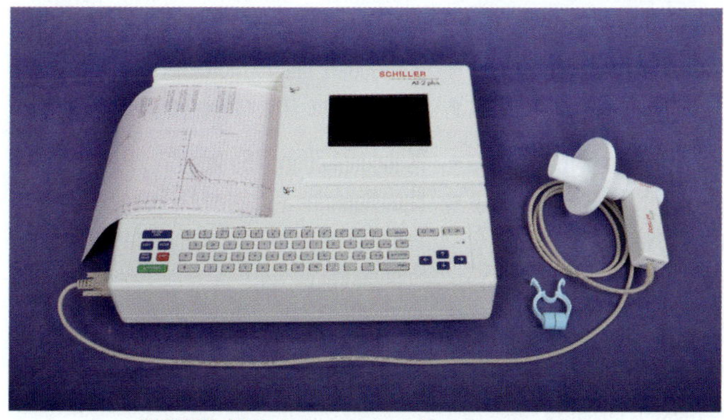

FIGURE 41.9 A spirometer is used for spirometry testing.

Assisting with Treatments

Patients with pulmonary conditions are prescribed a variety of medications. The following are some of the more common classifications:

- *Antihistamine:* Counteracts the effects of histamine
- *Antiviral:* Destroys or inhibits the growth and reproduction of viruses
- *Antitussive:* Inhibits the cough center
- *Bronchodilator:* Relaxes the smooth muscles of the bronchi
- *Corticosteroid (oral, nasal, and inhaled):* Reduces airway inflammation and bronchial resistance
- *Decongestant:* Relieves local congestion in the nasal and sinus tissues
- *Expectorant:* Thins the secretions in the bronchial tubes to make it easier to cough up the mucus
- *Leukotriene receptor antagonist:* Blocks the action of substances that cause asthma and allergic rhinitis

Refer to Table 41.6 for information on the medical classification, including the indication for use, desired effect, side effects, adverse reactions, and generic and trade names. Medical assistants should be familiar with medications that are prescribed to patients.

In the ambulatory care facility, common respiratory treatments include medication administration and oxygen therapy. Depending on the state's statutes and the facility's policies, the medical assistant may be able to administer nebulizer treatments and oxygen therapy when ordered by the provider. The medical assistant may also instruct patients on how to use metered-dose inhalers. The following sections cover metered-dose inhaler education, nebulizer treatments, and oxygen therapy.

Metered-Dose Inhalers

A metered-dose inhaler (MDI) provides aerosol medication that is breathed into the lungs. MDIs are typically ordered for conditions such as asthma and chronic obstructive pulmonary disease (COPD).

In many cases, the provider will order an MDI with a *spacer*. A spacer is a long tube that is attached to the mouthpiece of an MDI (Figure 41.10A). Spacers slow the delivery of medication from MDIs. Without a spacer, the MDI blasts the medication to the back of the throat and mouth. Inhaled corticosteroids can cause irritation and infections over time. When a spacer is used, the medication is blasted into the tube and, over several breaths, is pulled into the lungs. In an ambulatory care facility, the medical assistant may need to instruct the patient on the proper use of an MDI.

Using a Metered-Dose Inhaler. When teaching a patient to use an MDI, the medical assistant should instruct the patient to shake the

TABLE 41.6 Medication Classifications

CLASSIFICATION	INFORMATION	GENERIC NAME (TRADE NAME)
Antihistamine	Indications for use: Relieves allergies. Desired effects: Blocks the action of histamine, which causes allergic symptoms. Side effects and adverse reactions: CNS depression, muscle weakness, gastrointestinal distress, dry mouth.	• loratadine (Claritin, Alavert) • Diphenhydramine (Benadryl, Unisom) • Cetirizine (Zyrtec, Alleroff)
Antiviral	Indications for use: Treats viral infections, including oral and genital herpes, influenza, and HIV. Desired effects: Destroys or inhibits the growth and reproduction of viruses. Side effects and adverse reactions: Confusion, diarrhea, headache, kidney disease, urticaria, vomiting.	• Oseltamivir (Tamiflu) • Acyclovir (Zovirax)
Bronchodilator	Indications for use: Treats asthma, bronchospasm; promote bronchodilation. Desired effect: Relaxes the smooth muscle of the bronchi. Side effects and adverse reactions: CNS stimulation, tremors, tachycardia, increased blood glucose level, hypertension.	• Albuterol (Ventolin HFA, Proventil HFA, ProAir HFA) • Tiotropium (Spiriva HandiHaler)
Corticosteroid (oral)	Indications for use: Used to treat chronic inflammatory diseases (e.g., arthritis) and acute conditions (e.g., poison ivy, asthma). Desired effects: Reduces inflammation. Side effects and adverse reactions: Headache, mood changes, difficulty falling asleep or staying asleep, increased sweating, vision problems, depression, and weight gain.	• Prednisone (Prednisone Intensol, Sterapred) • Prednisolone (Flo-Pred, Orapred, Pediapred) • Methylprednisolone (Medrol)
Corticosteroid (nasal and inhaled)	Indications for use: Long-term relief of asthma symptoms; decrease frequency of asthma attacks; manage chronic obstructive pulmonary disease (COPD) and seasonal allergies. Desired effects: Reduces airway inflammation and bronchial resistance. Side effects and adverse reactions: Headache, pharyngitis, myalgia, hypersensitivity, oral candidiasis. Diskus products are contraindicated in patients with a milk allergy.	• Fluticasone and salmeterol (Advair Diskus) • Fluticasone (Flonase Allergy Relief Nasal Spray, Flovent Diskus, Flovent HFA) • Budesonide (Pulmicort Flexhaler, Pulmicort Respules, Rhinocort) • Budesonide and formoterol (Symbicort) • Mometasone (Asmanex, Nasonex)
Decongestant	Indications for use: Relieves nasal and sinus congestion caused by common cold, hay fever, or upper respiratory tract disorders. Desired effect: Relieves local congestion in the nasal and sinus tissues. Side effects and adverse reactions: Arrhythmias, hypertension, headache, nausea, dry mouth.	• Pseudoephedrine (Sudafed) • Phenylephrine (Sudafed PE Congestion, PediaCare Children's Decongestant, Suphedrin PE)
Expectorant	Indications for use: Relieves upper respiratory tract congestion. Desired effect: Thins the secretions in the bronchial tubes to make it easier to cough up the mucus. Side effects and adverse reactions: gastrointestinal distress.	• Guaifenesin
Leukotriene receptor antagonist	Indications for use: Treats asthma, exercise induced bronchospasms Desired effect: Blocks the action of substances that cause asthma and allergic rhinitis Side effects and adverse reactions: headache, dizziness, heartburn, stomach pain, tiredness, hypersensitivity, numbness in arms and legs, swelling of the sinuses	• Montelukast (Singulair)

MDI three or four times, then remove the cover from the mouthpiece. If using a spacer, the patient should do the following:

- Attach the spacer. Breathe out. Place the mouthpiece between the lips and close the lips around it.
- Press the top of the canister on the MDI.
- Breathe in very slowly, taking a full breath in. Some spacers will produce a whistle-like sound if the person is breathing in too fast.

Patients who are not using a spacer should do the following:

- Breathe out. Place the inhaler 1 to 2 inches (about 2 finger widths) in front of his or her opened mouth (Figure 41.10B).
- Press the top of the canister on the MDI.
- Breathe in very slowly, taking a full breath in.

After taking the medication, patients should hold their breath for 10 seconds (or count to 10) and then breathe out. When using an

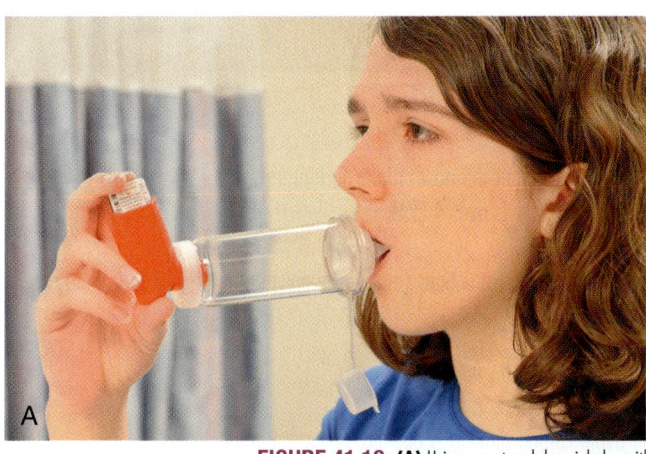
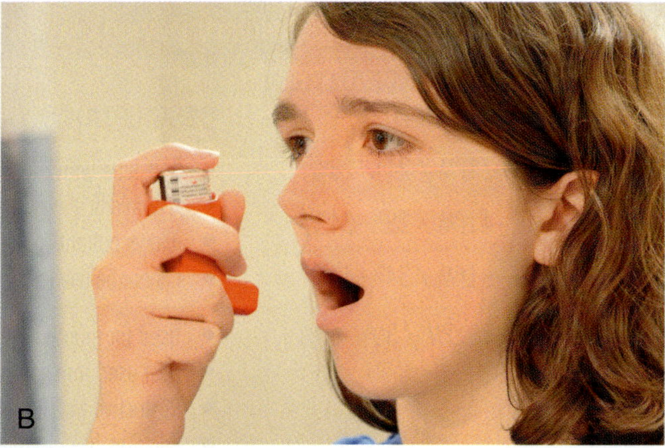

FIGURE 41.10 (A) Using a metered dose inhaler with spacer. **(B)** Using a metered dose inhaler without a spacer.

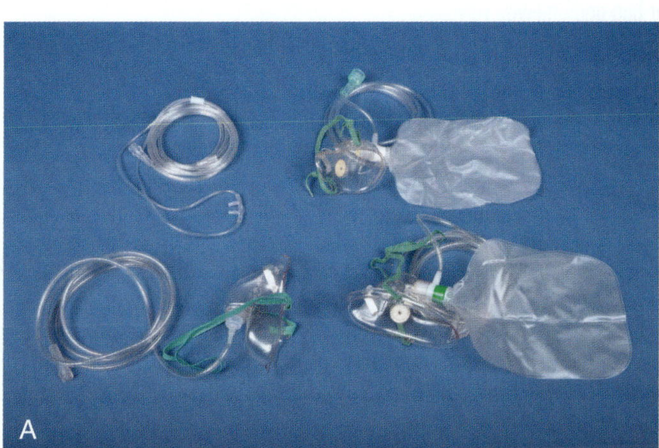
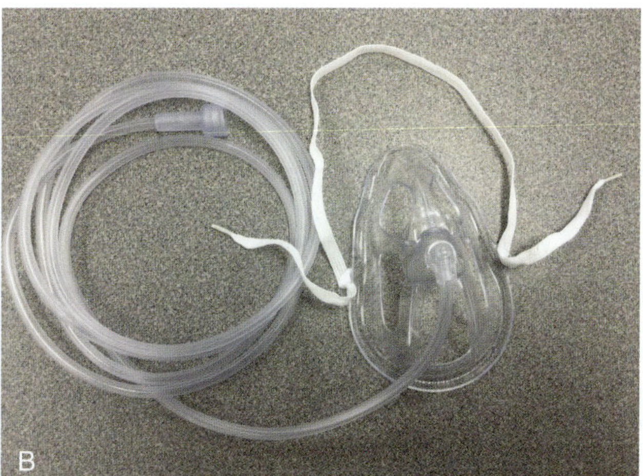

FIGURE 41.11 (A) *(Top left to right)* Nasal cannula and child non-rebreather mask. Non-rebreather masks have one-way valves (e.g., yellow circle on the mask). *(Bottom left to right)* Simple face mask and adult non-rebreather mask. **(B)** OxyMask is an open mask system that reduces the claustrophobic feeling. This mask can deliver 24% to 90% oxygen with flow rates from 1 to 15 L per minute.

inhaled, quick-relief medication (beta-agonists), the patient should wait 1 minute between puffs. These steps should be repeated until the dose is completed.

Nebulizer Treatment

Inhaled medication for asthma, COPD, and other lung diseases can be given using a nebulizer. A nebulizer treatment can be done in the ambulatory care setting and at home. A nebulizer is a small machine that turns liquid medication into a fine mist that can be inhaled. Typically, the medication used for nebulizers is much stronger than the same medication found in an MDI. When working with pediatric patients, a mask can be used instead of the mouthpiece. The mask should be an appropriate size so it covers their nose and mouth. Procedure 41.3 describes the steps for administering a nebulizer treatment.

Oxygen Therapy

When a patient comes to the ambulatory care facility with a cardiac or respiratory condition, the provider may order oxygen to be administered. Oxygen should be treated like a medication. The medical assistant must get the order from the provider for how much oxygen to administer and how to administer it. In the ambulatory care facility, oxygen may be available in the room by means of a wall-mounted flow meter or oxygen cylinders (portable tanks).

Room air is about 21% oxygen. Oxygen devices increase the concentration of oxygen for the patient to breathe in. Typically, a nasal cannula (NC) or a simple mask is used in the ambulatory care setting (Figure 41.11A). Other masks that deliver higher oxygen concentrations may also be available (Figure 41.11A–B).

Table 41.7 provides information on the more common oxygen delivery devices used in the ambulatory care setting. Procedure 41.4 presents the steps for administering oxygen.

CLOSING COMMENTS

Patient Coaching

Many patients who have chronic pulmonary conditions use MDIs as part of their treatments. It is important that patients learn how to clean their MDIs and spacers to prevent additional issues. A blocked or partially blocked MDI can prevent the patient from getting the proper dose of medication. To clean the MDI and spacer, do the following:

- Take the spacer apart. Clean the spacer with mild soap and allow it to air dry.

TABLE 41.7 Common Oxygen Delivery Devices

TYPE	FLOW RANGE/OXYGEN DELIVERED	DESCRIPTIONS
Nasal cannula	1–2 LPM / 24%–28% 2–4 LPM / 28%–34% 4–6 LPM / 34%–44%	• Soft tube with prongs that are placed in the nose; make sure prongs curve downward. • A humidification device is used if flow is over 4 LPM. • Allows patient to talk, drink, and eat. • Cannot be used with upper respiratory obstructions (e.g., nasal polyps); not helpful for mouth breathers.
Mask	5–10 LPM / 30%–60%	• Used for mouth breathers. • Best used for short-term situations (e.g., ambulatory care). • Restrictive for communication, coughing, and eating. • Requires 5–6 L/min to avoid carbon dioxide (CO2) accumulation in the mask.
Partial rebreathing mask	6–10 LPM / 41%–70%	• Oxygen feeds into a reservoir bag attached to a mask. • About one-third of expired air enters reservoir bag, and the rest exits the mask through exhalation ports.
Non-rebreathing face mask	10–15 LPM / Up to about 90%	• Mask with a reservoir bag and one-way valve. • One-way valve allows patient to inhale oxygen from the reservoir bag but prevents expired air from entering bag. • Before applying to patient, occlude valve and allow reservoir bag to fill with oxygen.

LPM, Liters per minute.

- Remove the medication canister and the mouthpiece cover from the MDI. Let warm water flow over the top and bottom of the MDI inhaler for about 30 seconds. Shake off and let air dry overnight. When assembling the device, spray twice in the air before taking a dose. Clean the MDI weekly to prevent medication from building up and blocking the sprayer.

Cleaning techniques can vary with medication products. Patients should be encouraged to check the product's website for directions.

Legal and Ethical Issues

Many times, with pulmonary disorders and treatments, patients may become dizzy. This can affect their balance or even cause them to faint. If a patient has a recent history of fainting or passing out, it is important for the medical assistant to keep the patient safe in the ambulatory care environment. Here are some ways to assist patients and prevent falls:

- Assist the patient as needed when stepping on and off the scale.
- Assist the patient on and off the exam table.
- Do not leave the patient on the exam table unattended.
- Ask if the patient would like a wheelchair.

Many lawsuits have been brought forward involving situations in which patients were injured from falls in the ambulatory care environment. Several cases have involved medical assistants not helping patients on and off equipment such as scales or having patients wait unattended on exam tables. Remember, safety is one of the most important concerns when caring for patients.

Patient-Centered Care

To provide patient-centered care, medical assistants need to do the following:

- Provide patients with clear instructions on the pulmonary procedure being done.
- Perform the procedure correctly so the patient's results are accurate.
- Be sensitive to patients' concerns and feelings regarding pulmonary diseases.
- Be respectful and empathetic when encouraging patients to breathe for spirometry tests. Remember, if the patient is short of breath or coughing due to an illness, blowing for a spirometry test can be difficult. Allow the patient to tell you when he or she is ready to do the next test.

Professional Behaviors

Part of being professional is one's appearance and grooming. When working with patients, it is essential that medical assistants have no odors on their bodies. Perfume, cologne, or scented lotions can trigger an allergic reaction in a patient. Patients with asthma can have flare-ups when they are around different scents, such as perfume, cologne, or scented lotions.

Medical assistants who smoke cigarettes need to be especially concerned with the odor. Research has shown that tobacco smoke contains more than 7000 chemicals, of which 250 are harmful. When the olfactory (sense of smell) system is exposed to these chemicals, reversible or permanent injuries can occur. The injury relates to the length of time the person has smoked and the tobacco toxicity. Ultimately, smoking tobacco can lead to a decrease in odor sensibility and recognition. This means people who smoke may not be able to smell the cigarette smoke on their clothing or body, yet it may be noticeable to others.

Many patients who have a chronic illness, such as cancer or chronic obstructive pulmonary disease (COPD), have quit smoking tobacco products. It is important that the healthcare professionals who care for these patients (and all other patients) do not smell of cigarette smoke.

SUMMARY OF SCENARIO

As Renee works with John, she realizes she has a lot more to learn. Pulmonary disease is common. Renee decides to research the diseases she encounters every week. She feels that to be professional, it is important to be up to date on the latest information. She likes to be confident in her skills and knowledge. This helps when patients have questions about diseases, procedures, or treatments.

Renee looks forward to her weekly pulmonary experiences. She is confident in rooming patients and performing oxygen saturation measurements. She is excited about learning how to do peak flow and spirometry tests in the coming weeks.

SUMMARY OF LEARNING OBJECTIVES

1. **Differentiate among the structures of the upper respiratory tract.**
   The upper respiratory tract is composed of the nose, pharynx, and larynx. These organs are located outside of the chest cavity. The main functions of the upper respiratory tract include warming and cleaning the inspired air, serving as a passageway for air, and providing the sense of smell.
2. **Differentiate among the structures of the lower respiratory tract.**
   The lower respiratory tract consists of the trachea, bronchial tubes, and lungs. The trachea (windpipe) lies in the space between the lungs, called the mediastinum. Air travels from the larynx through the trachea, and then the trachea branches into the right and left bronchi. The bronchi divide into smaller branches, called bronchioles. These bronchioles end in microscopic ducts capped by air sacs, called alveoli, which are involved with gas exchange.
3. **Examine the physiology of the respiratory system.**
   The two primary functions of the respiratory system are to exchange O_2 from the atmosphere for CO_2 waste and to maintain the acid-base balance in the body. Both functions involve ventilation (breathing), which is the movement of gases between the lungs and the environment. Ventilation includes the process of inspiration (air moving into the lungs) and expiration (air moving out of the lungs). Two types of respiration occur during the ventilation process: external and internal respiration.
4. **Examine the life span changes in the respiratory system.**
   An infant has a narrow airway with a shorter and softer trachea and tends to breathe through the nose. Infants are abdominal breathers and have immature respiratory muscles, meaning fatigue with breathing difficulties can set in quickly. As a person ages, the diaphragm grows weaker. The respiratory muscles become weaker, and there is a decrease in tissue elasticity. The alveoli lose their shape.
5. **Differentiate between the signs and symptoms of respiratory diseases and disorders.**
   Respiratory diseases can cause dyspnea, shortness of breath, hemoptysis, epistaxis, and rhinorrhea. Breathing changes include apnea, bradypnea, Cheyne-Stokes respirations, hyperpnea, hyperventilation, orthopnea, and tachypnea. Oxygen changes include cyanosis, hypoxemia, and hypoxia. Abnormal lung sounds include pleural rub, rales, rhonchi, stridor, and wheezing.
6. **Examine chronic respiratory diseases and disorders, including the signs, symptoms, etiology, diagnostic procedures, and treatments.**
   A chronic disease, disorder, or syndrome lasts longer than 6 months. Some chronic diseases last a lifetime. Chronic diseases discussed in this chapter include allergic rhinitis, asthma, chronic obstructive pulmonary disease, cystic fibrosis, and sleep apnea. Refer to each disease to learn about the signs, symptoms, etiology, diagnostic procedures, and treatments.

   This chapter discussed the hazards of using tobacco products. Cigarette smokers are more likely to develop heart disease, lung cancer, and strokes. Smoking impacts all body systems. Passive or secondhand smoke also causes health problems to others. Thirdhand smoke is the residue or chemicals from the smoke. This can be inhaled or ingested and can cause problems.
7. **Examine respiratory system cancers, including the signs, symptoms, etiology, diagnostic procedures, and treatments.**
   Respiratory system cancers discussed in this chapter include laryngeal cancer and lung cancer. Refer to each disease to learn about the signs, symptoms, etiology, diagnostic procedures, and treatments.
8. **Examine acute respiratory diseases and disorders, including the signs, symptoms, etiology, diagnostic procedures, and treatments.**
   An acute disease is one that has a severe, sudden onset. There are many acute respiratory diseases. Acute diseases discussed in this chapter include acute bronchitis, COVID-19, croup, epiglottis, influenza, laryngitis, pertussis, pneumonia, pulmonary embolism, pulmonary tuberculosis, respiratory syncytial virus, sinusitis, and strep throat. Refer to each disease to learn about the signs, symptoms, etiology, diagnostic procedures, and treatments.
9. **Examine the medical assistant's role in examinations, diagnostic procedures, and treatments for respiratory conditions.**
   Preparing a patient for a respiratory examination includes having the patient disrobe to the waist. The medical assistant is responsible for assisting the provider throughout the examination and providing privacy and support for the patient.

   The peak flow meter measures the amount of air exhaled. A peak flow rate is measured using a peak flow meter in an ambulatory care or home setting. It is used to diagnose acute conditions and manage chronic diseases, such as asthma. Procedure 41.1 describes the steps that must be taken to measure a peak flow rate.

   Spirometry is done to evaluate lung function as affected by respiratory, cardiac, and neuromuscular diseases. It can be ordered if the provider identifies abnormalities in the respiratory system. A spirometer can evaluate the amount of air inhaled and exhaled. Procedure 41.2 describes the spirometry procedure.

Continued

SUMMARY OF LEARNING OBJECTIVES—*continued*

A metered-dose inhaler (MDI) provides aerosol medication that is breathed into the lungs. MDIs are typically ordered for conditions such as asthma and chronic obstructive pulmonary disease (COPD).

A nebulizer treatment can be done in the ambulatory care setting and in the home. A nebulizer is a small machine that turns liquid medication into a fine spray that can be inhaled. Typically, the medication used for nebulizers is much stronger than the same medication found in an MDI. Procedure 41.3 describes the steps for administering a nebulizer treatment.

When a patient comes to the ambulatory care facility with a cardiac or respiratory condition, the provider may order oxygen to be administered. Oxygen should be treated like a medication. The medical assistant must get the order from the provider for how much to administer and how to administer it. Procedure 41.4 presents the steps for administering oxygen.

PROCEDURE 41.1 Measure a Peak Flow Rate

TASKS: Perform a peak flow measurement. Document the procedure in the patient's health record.

EQUIPMENT and SUPPLIES

- Peak flow meter
- Disposable mouthpiece
- Disinfection wipes
- Gloves
- Waste container
- Paper towel or denture cup (optional)
- Patient's health record

PROCEDURAL STEPS

1. Wash hands or use hand sanitizer.
   PURPOSE: Hand sanitization is an important step for infection control.
2. Assemble the equipment and supplies needed for the peak flow procedure. Place the mouthpiece on the peak flow meter. Move the indicator to the bottom of the calibration scale (if not using a digital meter).
   PURPOSE: Having the equipment ready reduces the patient's wait time. The indicator needs to be at the bottom of the scale before the test to get an accurate reading.
3. Greet the patient. Identify yourself. Verify the patient's identity with full name and date of birth. Make sure the patient's information matches the order and the record. Explain the procedure in a manner that the patient understands. Answer any questions the patient may have about the procedure.
   PURPOSE: It is important to identify the patient in two different ways to ensure that you have the correct patient. Explaining the procedure can make the patient feel more comfortable and reduces anxiety.
4. Ask the patient to loosen any restrictive clothing. Have the patient remove any gum and loose dentures. Make sure to provide a paper towel or denture cup if needed.
   PURPOSE: The patient needs to be able to take a large breath in before the test to get the most accurate results. Normally, dentures can be left in the mouth, but loose-fitting dentures may affect the results of the test and must be removed.
5. With patients in the seated position, ensure that their feet are flat on the floor and their legs are uncrossed. The patient should sit straight up and against the back of the chair.
   PURPOSE: It is important for the patient to be in a position in which the lungs can fully expand.
6. Describe how the patient should do the test. "Take the deepest breath possible. Seal your lips around the mouthpiece. Blow as hard and as fast as you can." Encourage patients to state when they are ready to start the test. Tell patients to seal their lips around the mouthpiece.
   PURPOSE: Clear directions will help the patient to understand what to do.
7. Coach the patient during the test. After the patient has blown through the meter, read the number next to the indicator. Write the number down. Reset the indicator to the bottom of the scale (if it is not a digital meter).
   PURPOSE: If the patient has breathing problems, it is important to allow the patient to indicate when he or she is ready.
8. Make any adjustments as needed. Repeat the test two additional times. Write down the last two numbers.
   PURPOSE: Three acceptable readings are needed for the peak flow procedure.
9. Put on gloves and remove the mouthpiece. Discard the mouthpiece in the waste container. Disinfect the peak flow meter. Remove your gloves and dispose of them in the waste container. Wash your hands or use hand sanitizer.
   PURPOSE: Wearing gloves and disinfecting the peak flow meter are important for infection control.
10. Notify the provider of the readings and document the readings in the patient's health record. Indicate the name of the provider who ordered the test, the procedure done, the results of the test, and how the patient tolerated the test.
    PURPOSE: Indicating who ordered the test and what was done is important for insurance reimbursement and legal reasons.

Documentation Example

08/07/20XX 1423 Per Dr. Angela Perez's order, a peak flow was performed. Pt stated she was "a little short of breath" on the third test. Peak flow readings: 200, 230, and 260 L/min. Dr. Perez was notified of results and patient's SOB complaint. ———————— Renee Thomas, CMA (AAMA)

PROCEDURE 41.2 Perform Spirometry Testing

TASKS: Perform a spirometry test. Document the procedure in the patient's health record.

EQUIPMENT and SUPPLIES

- Spirometry machine with paper (and users' guide if applicable)
- Disposable mouthpiece and tubing (if applicable)
- Nose clip
- Calibration equipment
- Disinfection wipes
- Gloves
- Waste container
- Paper towel or denture cup (optional)
- Patient's health record
- Scale (if no height and weight measurements were taken earlier that day)

PROCEDURAL STEPS

1. Wash hands or use hand sanitizer.
   PURPOSE: Hand sanitization is an important step for infection control.
2. Assemble the equipment and supplies needed for the spirometry procedure. Calibrate the machine according to the users' guide and the facility's procedures.
   PURPOSE: It is important to calibrate per the facility's procedures. Calibration ensures that the results are accurate and reliable.
3. Greet the patient. Identify yourself. Verify the patient's identity with full name and date of birth. Make sure the patient's information matches the order and the record. Explain the procedure in a manner that the patient understands. Answer any questions the patient may have about the procedure.
   PURPOSE: It is important to identify the patient in two different ways to ensure that you have the correct patient. Explaining the procedure can make the patient feel more comfortable and reduces anxiety.
4. Enter the patient's name, medical record number, age (or date of birth), race, sex, weight, and height into the machine. Enter any additional required information.
   PURPOSE: The information used for the spirometry calculations is current weight, height, age, race, and sex.
5. Ask the patient to loosen any restrictive clothing. Have the patient remove gum and loose dentures (if applicable). Make sure to provide a paper towel or denture cup if needed.
   PURPOSE: The patient needs to be able to take a large breath in before the test to get the most accurate results. Loose-fitting dentures can affect the results of the test.
6. With the patient in the seated position, ensure that the feet are flat on the floor and the legs are uncrossed. The patient should sit straight up and against the back of the chair.
   PURPOSE: The patient may get dizzy during the test, so standing can be problematic. The seated position provides the maximum lung expansion for the test.
7. Describe how the patient should do the test. "Take the deepest breath possible. Seal your lips around the mouthpiece. Blow as hard and as fast as you can. Blow until you empty the air from your lungs."
   PURPOSE: Clear directions will help the patient understand what to do.
8. Attach the mouthpiece to the machine. Explain the purpose of the nose clip to the patient. Apply the nose clip to the patient (Figure 1). Have patients state when they are ready to start. Start the test as directed by the users' guide.

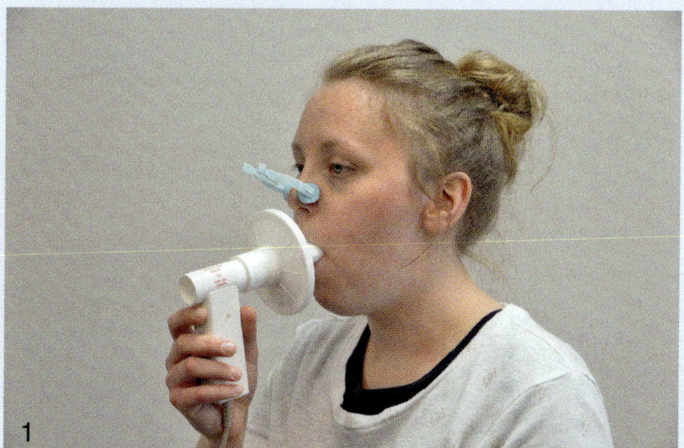
1

9. During the test, encourage the patient to empty the lungs. Repeat until three acceptable tests have been done. Allow patients to rest between tests if needed, and indicate when they are ready for the next test.
   PURPOSE: Usually, three test results are needed for comparison. If the patient is struggling and having difficulty breathing, ask the provider if three tests need to be done.
10. Put on gloves and remove the mouthpiece. Discard the mouthpiece in the waste container. Disinfect the spirometer as indicated in the users' guide. Remove your gloves and dispose of them in the waste container. Wash your hands or use hand sanitizer.
    PURPOSE: Wearing gloves and disinfecting the equipment are important for infection control.
11. Document that the test was performed. Indicate the name of the provider who ordered the test, the name of the test, how the patient tolerated the test, and what you did with the test results. Any patient instructions regarding follow-up can also be documented.
    PURPOSE: Indicating who ordered the test and what was done is important for insurance reimbursement and legal reasons.

Documentation Example

08/08/20XX 1423 Per Dr. James Martin's order, a spirometry test was performed. Pt stated she felt dizzy during the third attempt. The dizziness cleared within 5 minutes, and she stated she felt better. Pt was instructed to call the clinic tomorrow for the spirometry results. The spirometry results were given to Dr. Martin. ——————————— Renee Thomas, CMA (AAMA)

PROCEDURE 41.3 Administer a Nebulizer Treatment

TASKS: Administer a nebulizer treatment. Document the medication administration in the patient's health record.

ORDER: Levalbuterol 0.63 mg by nebulization

EQUIPMENT and SUPPLIES

- Nebulizer machine
- Disposable nebulizer patient kit (tubing, medication cup, mouthpiece or mask, flexible tube, and tee)
- Medication as ordered
- Provider's order
- Normal saline (as ordered or according to the facility's protocol)
- Disinfection wipes
- Gloves
- Waste container
- Patient's health record

PROCEDURAL STEPS

1. Wash hands or use hand sanitizer. Using the drug reference information and the order, review the information on the medication if needed. Clarify any questions you have with the provider.
   PURPOSE: Hand sanitization is an important step for infection control. It is important to be knowledgeable about the medication you are giving.
2. Select the right medication from the storage area. Check to see if the medication is concentrated and requires normal saline to dilute it. Check the medication label (and normal saline label, if used) against the order. Check for the right name, form, and route. Check the expiration date to make sure the drug has not expired. Verify that it is the right dose and time.
   PURPOSE: A provider's order is required for the nebulizer treatment. The medication needs to be verified three times before it is given. The nine rights of medication administration also need to be followed.
3. Assemble the equipment and supplies needed for the nebulizer treatment.
   PURPOSE: Having the equipment ready reduces the patient's wait time.
4. Perform the second medication check. Check the medication and normal saline label(s) against the order. Check for the right name, form, and route.
   PURPOSE: It is important to check the label(s) a second time before pouring the medication into the medication cup.
5. Add the medication and, if required, the normal saline to the medication cup (Figure 1). Secure the cover on the cup.
   PURPOSE: The medication cup holds the medication during the treatment.

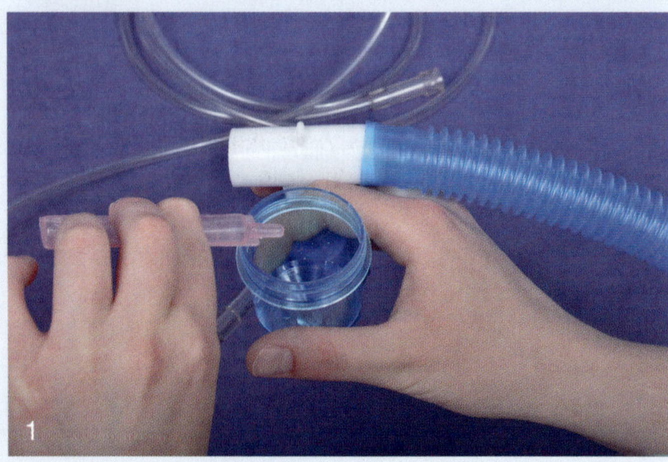

6. Perform the third medication check. Check the medication label and normal saline label (if used) against the order. Check for the right name, form, and route. Verify that the amount of medication in the cup is correct according to the order. Clean up the area.
   PURPOSE: It is important to check the label a third time before giving the medication.
7. Prior to entering the exam room, provide a courtesy knock on the door. Greet the patient. Identify yourself. Verify the patient's identity with full name and date of birth. Make sure the patient's information matches the order and the record.
   PURPOSE: It is important to identify the patient in two different ways to ensure that you have the correct patient. Explaining the procedure can make the patient feel more comfortable and reduces anxiety.
8. Provide the right education to the patient. Explain the medication ordered, the desired effect, and common side effects; also identify the provider who ordered it. Explain the procedure in a manner that the patient understands. Answer any questions the patient may have about the procedure. Ask if the patient has any allergies. If the patient refuses the medication, notify the provider.
   PURPOSE: The patient needs to be aware of what you are giving, the action and side effects, and who ordered it. It is also important to double-check the patient's allergies before administering the medication.
9. Attach the mouthpiece (or mask). Attach the tubing to the medication cup and the machine.
   PURPOSE: Use a mask if ordered by the provider.
10. Perform the right technique. The patient should be sitting upright on a chair. Instruct the patient to hold the mouthpiece between the teeth and seal the lips around the mouthpiece. Encourage the patient to take slow, deep breaths through the mouth. The patient should hold each breath 2 to 3 seconds before exhaling.
    PURPOSE: Sitting upright allows for total lung expansion. If patients breathe too deeply and too fast, they will become dizzy and may hyperventilate. Holding the breath in allows the medication to disperse through the lungs.
11. Turn on the nebulizer and give the medicine cup and mouthpiece to the patient to start the treatment. Instruct patients to put it into their mouths. If using a mask, position it securely and comfortably over the patient's nose and mouth.
    PURPOSE: It is important to make sure the mask is comfortable over the patient's face. If it is not comfortable, the patient may not tolerate the treatment.
12. Continue the treatment until the mist has stopped (approximately 10 minutes) (Figure 2). Turn off the nebulizer. Encourage the patient to take several deep breaths and cough.
    Note: After the treatment, it is common that patients will need to cough. Ensure that tissue is available if the patient needs it.

PROCEDURE 41.3 Administer a Nebulizer Treatment—*continued*

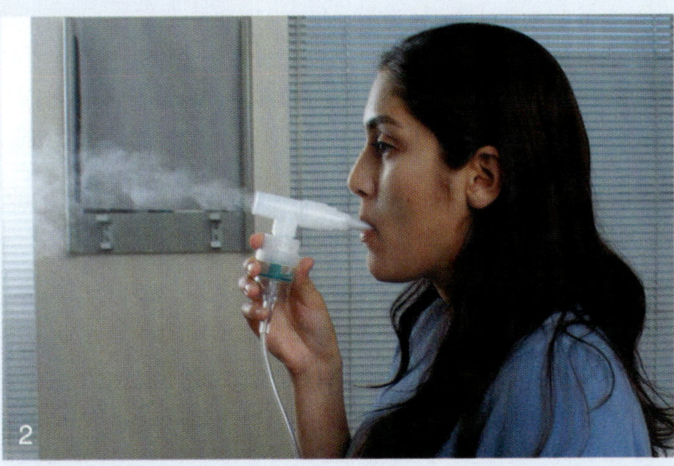

13. Put on gloves and dispose of the used supplies. Disinfect the nebulizer machine. Remove your gloves and dispose of them in the waste container. Wash your hands or use hand sanitizer.
    PURPOSE: To ensure infection control.
14. Document in the patient's health record. Include the name of the provider ordering the treatment, what was administered, how the patient tolerated the medication, and any follow-up assessments (e.g., vital signs).
    PURPOSE: Documentation is the last of the nine rights of medication administration.

Documentation Example

08/06/20XX 1120 P: 76 regular, 1+; R: 26 regular, shallow. Per Dr. Angela Perez's order, Levalbuterol 0.63 mg administered by nebulizer. Pt stated she felt a little shaky after the treatment and her lungs felt less tight. Pt is resting on the exam table. P: 86 regular, 1+; R: 20 regular, normal. Dr. Perez notified.
———————————— Renee Thomas, CMA (AAMA)

PROCEDURE 41.4 Administer Oxygen Using a Nasal Cannula or Mask

TASKS: Administer oxygen using a nasal cannula or mask. Document the oxygen administration in the patient's health record.

ORDER 1: Administer 2 LPM of oxygen using a nasal cannula.

ORDER 2: Administer 6 LPM of oxygen using a simple mask.

EQUIPMENT and SUPPLIES

- Oxygen cylinder with oxygen regulator or oxygen flow meter (wall unit)
- Adult nasal cannula or simple mask
- Provider's order
- Patient's health record
- Mannequin (optional)

PROCEDURAL STEPS

1. Wash hands or use hand sanitizer.
   PURPOSE: Hand sanitization is an important step for infection control.
2. Assemble the equipment and supplies needed for the provider's order. If an oxygen cylinder is used, identify the amount of oxygen left in the cylinder.
   PURPOSE: The order will include the amount to give and the device (e.g., cannula) to use for the administration. It is important to make sure the cylinder has enough oxygen for the patient.
3. Verify the order if you have any questions.
   PURPOSE: A provider's order is required for the oxygen administration.
4. Greet the patient. Identify yourself. Verify the patient's identity with full name and date of birth. Make sure the patient's information matches the order and the record. Explain the procedure in a manner that the patient understands. Answer any questions the patient may have about the procedure.
   PURPOSE: It is important to identify the patient in two different ways to ensure that you have the correct patient. Explaining the procedure can make the patient feel more comfortable and reduces anxiety.
5. Connect the nasal cannula or mask to the regulator or flow meter. Turn on the oxygen and adjust the flow rate to the correct amount per the provider's order. The ball should be centered on the number of liters ordered.
   PURPOSE: Oxygen needs to be flowing through the tubing before the cannula is applied to the patient.
6. Apply the mask or nasal cannula.
   a. Place the mask over the patient's nose, mouth, and chin. Place the elastic over the head. Adjust the elastic strap to tighten the mask on the face. Adjust the metal nasal bridge clamp, making sure it fits without obstructing the nose. Ensure that the mask fits tightly on the face.
   PURPOSE: A poorly fitting mask can cause oxygen to be directed into the eyes, causing additional problems.
   b. Insert the tips of the cannula into the nostrils. If the tips are curved, the curves face downward toward the bottom of the nose (Figure 1). Adjust the tubing around the back of the ears and then under the chin. Encourage the patient to breathe through the nose with the mouth closed.
   PURPOSE: The cannula needs to be inserted correctly into the nostrils. The cannula tips may be blocked by the top of the nostrils if they are inserted incorrectly. Breathing through the mouth when using a cannula is not as beneficial as breathing through the nose.

Continued

PROCEDURE 41.4 Administer Oxygen Using a Nasal Cannula or Mask—*continued*

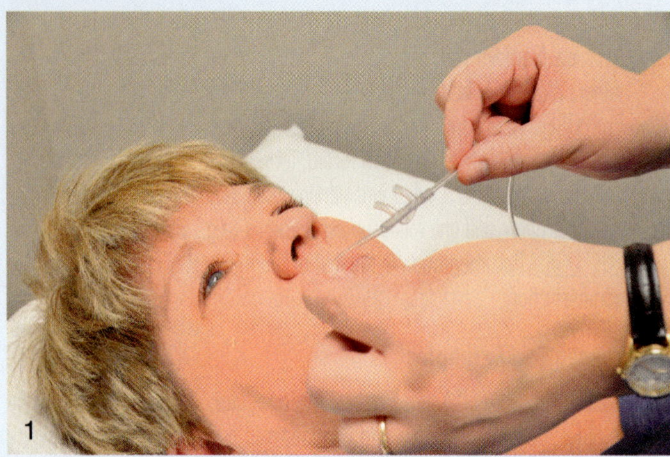

7. Make sure the patient is comfortable. Answer any questions the patient may have. Sanitize your hands.

   PURPOSE: Unanswered questions can cause anxiety. With breathing problems, it is important for the patient to be comfortable and calm.

8. Document the procedure. Include the name of the ordering provider, the number of liters of oxygen administered, the device used for administering the oxygen, and the patient's condition.

   PURPOSE: Indicating who ordered the oxygen and what was administered is important for insurance reimbursement and legal reasons.

Documentation Example

08/07/20XX 1541 R: 28 regular, shallow. Per Dr. Angela Perez's order, 2 L/min of oxygen administered via nasal cannula. Pt resting on exam table. ———————————— Renee Thomas, CMA (AAMA)

08/07/20XX 1555 R: 20 regular, normal. Pt stated she is "feeling better" with the oxygen and has less SOB. Dr. Angela Perez was notified. ———————————— Renee Thomas, CMA (AAMA)

UROLOGY AND MALE REPRODUCTION

42

SCENARIO

Hannah Yang, CMA (AAMA), was hired 4 months ago. She assists the specialists who hold outreach clinics at Walden-Martin Family Medical (WMFM) Clinic. She has been training with the urology staff that comes in to assist the outreach clinics four times a month.

Hannah's role is to help room patients and assist the urology staff. To prepare for working with the specialist, Hannah spent some time reviewing her medical assistant textbook. She had forgotten the process of urine formation. She had to brush up on how the urinary system affects the homeostasis of the body. Hannah knows that the urinary system is important and that if a person's kidneys are not functioning, the individual will need to go on dialysis. As part of her orientation to this specialty, she was able to spend 4 hours at the local dialysis clinic. There, the "regular" patients enjoyed telling her their experiences. Their experiences and the information from the dialysis technicians helped Hannah understand what patients go through with kidney disease.

By assisting the urologist, Dr. Ubert Riney, and his team, Hannah has learned a great deal. However, she knows she has more to learn about this specialty.

While studying this chapter, think about the following questions:

- What structures are in the urinary and male reproductive systems?
- What are the functions of the urinary and male reproductive systems?
- What are commonly diagnosed urinary and male reproductive systems diseases and disorders? What are the etiologies, signs and symptoms, diagnostic processes, and treatments?
- What are the medical assistant's primary responsibilities when working with patients who have urinary and male reproductive systems diseases and disorders?

LEARNING OBJECTIVES

1. Examine the anatomy of the urinary system.
2. Examine the physiology of the urinary system.
3. Analyze the life span changes to the urinary system.
4. Differentiate among the types of urinary system diseases and disorders, including the etiology, signs, symptoms, diagnostic procedures, and treatments.
5. Examine the anatomy of the male reproductive system.
6. Examine the physiology of the male reproductive system.
7. Analyze the life span changes of the male reproductive system.
8. Differentiate among the types of male reproductive diseases and disorders, including the etiology, signs, symptoms, diagnostic procedures, and treatments.
9. Examine the medical assistant's role in examinations and diagnostic procedures for urinary and male reproductive diseases and disorders.
10. Examine the medical assistant's role in treatments used for urinary and male reproductive diseases and disorders.

VOCABULARY

afferent (AF fur ent) Pertains to carrying toward a structure.

anticoagulant (an tee koe AG yoo lant) A substance (i.e., medication or chemical) that prevents the clotting of blood.

antihyperlipidemic (an tie hie per lip i DEE mik) A substance (i.e., medication) that lowers the lipid levels in the blood.

antihypertensive A drug that reduces high blood pressure.

arterioles (ar TEER ee ohlz) Small arteries.

arteriovenous graft (ahr teer ee oh VEE nuhs) A synthetic tube that connects an artery to a vein; also called an AV graft.

arteriovenous fistula An abnormal joining of an artery and a vein.

calculi (KAL kyuh lie) Stones formed in the kidneys, gallbladder, and other parts of the body.

catheter A hollow, flexible tube that can be inserted into a vessel, organ, or cavity of the body to withdraw or instill fluid, monitor information, and visualize a vessel or cavity.

corticosteroids A group of steroid hormones produced in the body or given as a medication; some have metabolic functions, and others reduce tissue inflammation. Glucocorticoids and mineralocorticoids are two types.

diuretic A substance (i.e., medication) that increases the amount of urine produced.

efferent (EF fur ent) Pertains to carrying away from a structure.

erythropoietin (eh rith roh POY eh tin) A hormone that is produced by the kidney cells and travels to the bone marrow to stimulate red blood cell formation.

VOCABULARY—*continued*

filtrate Fluid and substances that are filtered out of the blood in the Bowman capsule.

gamete (GAM eet) A mature sexual reproductive cell; spermatozoon or ovum.

gonad (GOH nads) Organs that produce sex cells in both males and females.

hyperlipidemia (hie per lip i DEE mee ah) An elevated level of lipids in the blood.

hypoalbuminemia (hie poh al byoo mi NEE mee ah) A decreased level of albumin (protein) in the blood.

in vitro fertilization An assisted reproductive technology procedure that involves removing mature eggs from the ovaries and fertilizing the eggs with sperm outside of the body. The fertilized eggs are then transferred to the uterus.

intermittent Occurring in intervals.

interstitial (in ter STISH uhl) Between the cells.

interstitial cells Testosterone-secreting cells of testes that are found in the spaces between the seminiferous tubules.

intravenous (IV) Through a vein; fluids and medications can be given through a vein.

metabolites (meh TAB uh lites) By-products of drug metabolism.

neuropathy (nu ROP a thee) A nervous system disorder of the peripheral nerves that causes discomfort, numbness, and weakness, especially in the extremities.

peritoneum (per i tuh NEE um) A serous membrane lining of the abdominal cavity, which folds inward to enclose the viscera (internal organs).

peritubular capillaries (per i TOO bu lar) Blood capillaries surrounding the proximal and distal convoluted tubules in the kidneys.

permeability A quality or characteristic of a material that allows another substance to pass through it.

puberty (PYOO bur tee) The stage of life in which males and females become functionally capable of sexual reproduction.

residual urine Urine that remains in the bladder after micturition or urination.

rugae (ROO gay) Folds in the wall of the organ; when the organ (e.g., stomach, bladder, uterus) fills or needs to expand, the rugae unfold.

septicemia (sep ti SEE mee ah) A systemic infection involving pathologic microbes in the blood as a result of an infection that has spread from elsewhere in the body.

spermatozoa (singular, spermatozoon) (spur mat ah ZOH ah) Mature male reproductive cells.

stoma (STOH mah) A temporary or permanent surgically created opening used for drainage (i.e., urine, stool).

stretch receptor A sensory nerve ending that responds to a stretch stimulus.

testis (plural, testes) (TES tis) The male gonad, also called a testicle (TES ti kul).

testosterone (tess TOS tuh rohn) Male sex hormone produced by the interstitial cells in the testes.

transitional epithelium A type of cell found in the lining of hollow organs. It has the ability to stretch with the contraction and distention of the organ.

urostomy (yoo ROS te mee) A surgically created opening on the abdominal wall used to drain urine.

vascular access A surgical procedure that creates a vein to remove and return blood during a hemodialysis procedure.

venule (VEN yuhl) A very small vein.

INTRODUCTION

Urology is the healthcare specialty that deals with most urinary diseases and disorders. A *urologist* is a specialist involved in the diagnosis, treatment, and prevention of disorders of the urinary system and the male reproductive system. *Nephrology* is the healthcare subspecialty that focuses on kidney function and disorders. A *nephrologist* diagnoses and treats kidney conditions.

Besides the urology department, patients with urinary and male reproductive concerns are typically seen in primary care, urgent care, and even specialty departments. Medical assistants should have a strong understanding of the common urinary signs, symptoms, diseases, diagnostic tests, and treatments. Sexually transmitted infections (STIs), which can impact both the urinary and male reproductive systems, are discussed in Chapter 33.

The anatomy, physiology, and pathology of the urinary system will be discussed before the male reproductive system is addressed.

ANATOMY OF THE URINARY SYSTEM

The urinary system is composed of two kidneys, two ureters, a urinary bladder, and a urethra (Figures 42.1 and 42.2). The kidneys filter the blood and eliminate waste through the passage of urine. The *ureters* move urine from the kidneys to the bladder. The urinary bladder stores the urine until it is excreted. The *urethra* is the tube that conducts the urine out of the bladder.

Kidneys

The kidneys are bean-shaped organs that are the size of a fist. The *hilum* (an indentation) is the location on the kidney where the ureter and renal vein leave the kidney and the renal artery enters. The kidneys are located posterior to the **peritoneum**, the muscles of the back, and between the T12 and L3 vertebrae. The left kidney is situated about 1 inch (2 cm) higher than the right because of the location of the liver.

The kidneys remove unwanted substances from the blood and form urine for excretion. Blood is delivered to the two kidneys by the renal arteries, which branch off the abdominal aorta (Figure 42.3). Blood flows from the renal arteries into **afferent arterioles** (smaller arteries) and through a network of capillaries called the *glomeruli.* Filtration of the blood occurs in the glomerulus. Blood from the glomerulus moves into the **efferent** arterioles and into the **peritubular** capillaries. As the blood leaves the kidneys, it moves from the

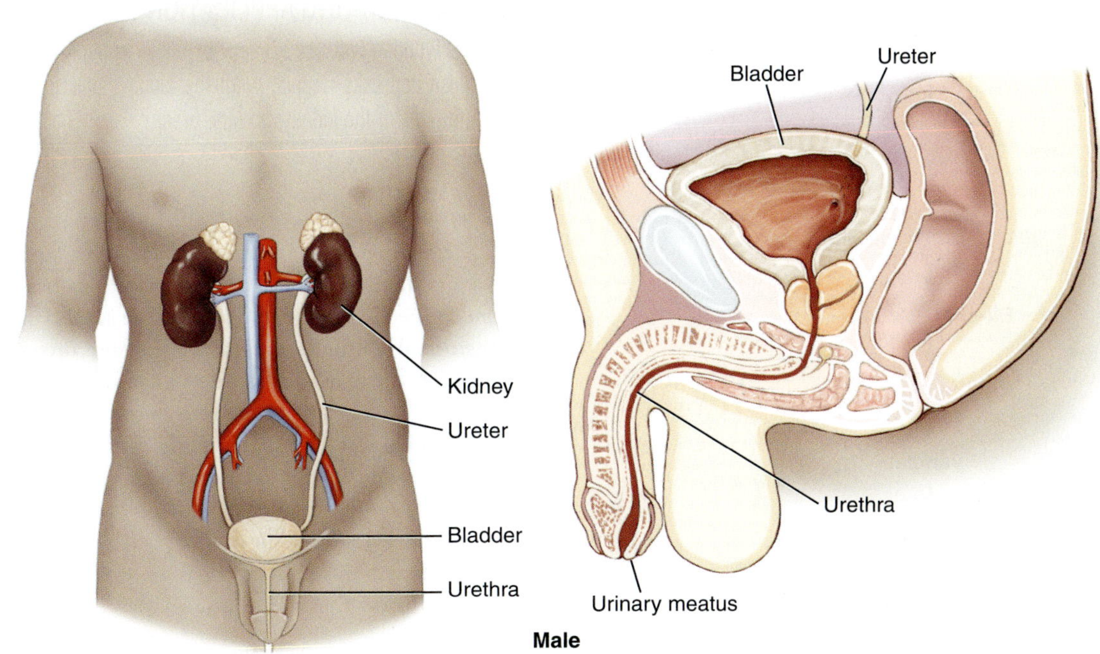

FIGURE 42.1 Male urinary system. (From Shiland B: *Medical terminology & anatomy for ICD-10 coding*, ed 2, St. Louis, 2016, Mosby.)

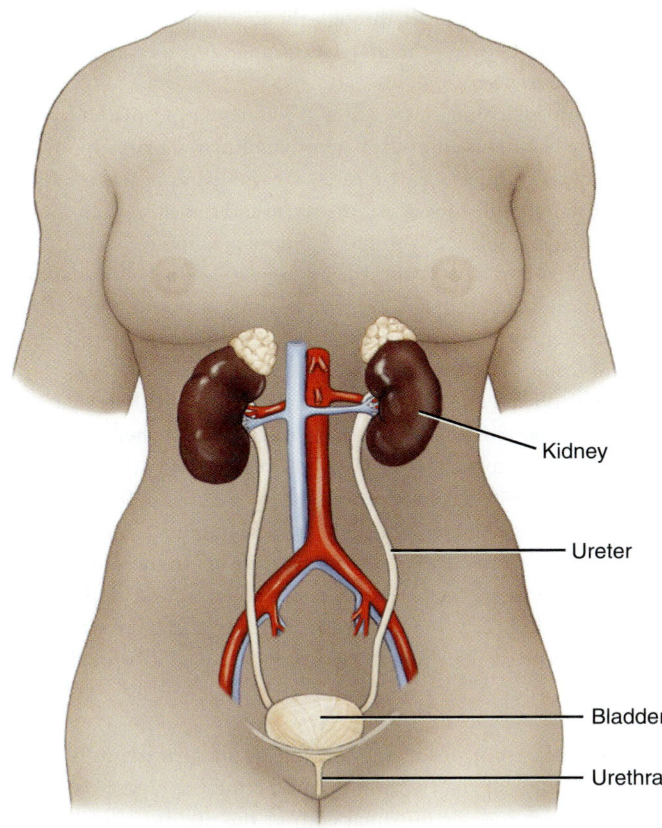

FIGURE 42.2 Female urinary system. (From Shiland B: *Medical terminology & anatomy for ICD-10 coding*, ed 2, St. Louis, 2016, Mosby.)

peritubular capillaries to **venules** and then empties into the renal veins. The renal veins take the blood out of the kidneys. Blood from the renal veins flows into the inferior vena cava as it heads to the heart to become oxygenated again (Figure 42.4).

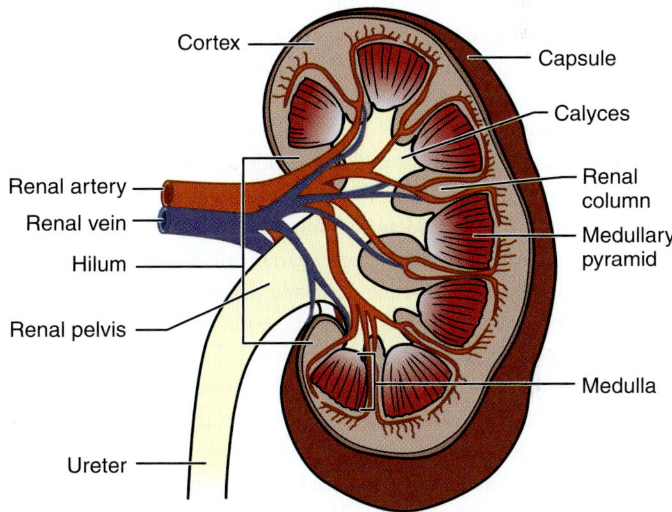

FIGURE 42.3 Cross section of a kidney.

The Kidney Structures

If a kidney were sliced open, you would see the following:

- *Capsule*: The fibrous outer covering of the kidney
- *Cortex*: The outer portion of the kidney
- *Renal column*: An extension of the cortex that dips down between the medullary pyramids
- *Medulla*: The inner portion that extends from the end of the cortex to the calyces
- *Medullary pyramid*: A cone-shaped structure located in the medulla and containing straight tubular structures and blood vessels
- *Minor and major calyces and the renal pelvis*: Extensions of the ureter inside the kidney

Nephrons

Each kidney contains tissue with millions of microscopic units called *nephrons*. Nephrons are the functional units of the kidneys. They are

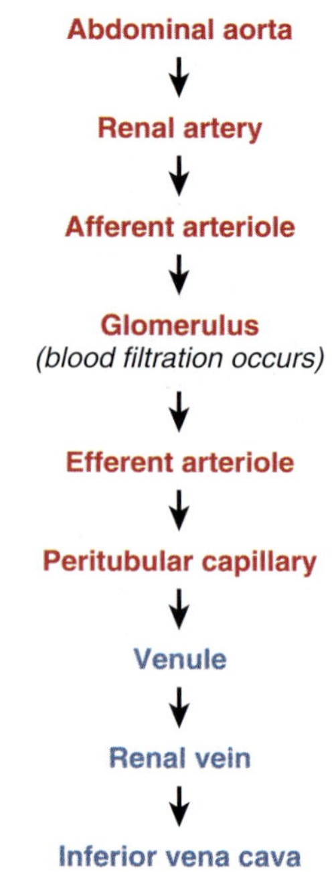

FIGURE 42.4 Blood flow to and from the kidney.

located in the cortex and extend into the medulla. Each nephron is a very long tube or *tubule*. One end of the nephron is the *renal corpuscle,* and the remaining section of the nephron is the *renal tubule*. The renal corpuscle consists of the following:

- *Bowman capsule*: A cup-shaped structure of the nephron that surrounds the glomerulus
- *Glomerulus*: A cluster of capillaries inside the Bowman capsule

The afferent arteriole brings blood into the glomerulus, and the efferent arteriole takes blood away from the glomerulus. The diameter of the afferent arteriole is much larger than the diameter of the efferent arteriole. The importance of the narrowed diameter will be discussed in the Physiology of the Urinary System section of this chapter.

The renal tubule is a long, thin, twisted tube that brings the **filtrate** (which will become urine) from the Bowman capsule to the renal pelvis. During the passage of filtrate from the Bowman capsule to the renal pelvis, water and electrolytes move between the urine and the blood to maintain homeostasis. The formation of urine will be discussed later in the chapter. The renal tubule is made up of the following:

- *Proximal (convoluted) tubule* (PCT): The first section of the renal tubule that is attached to the Bowman capsule.
- *Henle loop*: Follows the PCT and includes a straight descending section, a loop, and then a straight ascending section.
- *Distal (convoluted) tubule* (DCT): Follows the ascending section of the Henle loop.
- *Collecting duct* (CD): Multiple distal tubules join and form this straight collecting duct, which empties into the calyx.

To summarize, the nephron begins on one end with the Bowman capsule, which is filled with capillaries. The proximal tubule is the next section of the nephron. It is followed by the Henle loop, the distal tubule, and finally, the collecting duct. Many collecting ducts empty into one calyx. Many calyces merge into the renal pelvis, which is an extension of the ureter inside the kidney. The Bowman capsule, proximal tubules, and distal tubes are in the cortex. The Henle loop and the collecting ducts are in the medulla of the kidney.

CRITICAL THINKING APPLICATION 42.1

Hannah is working with Mrs. Green, a urology patient. Mrs. Green has kidney disease and asks Hannah what the kidneys do. How should Hannah explain the role of the kidneys to Mrs. Green?

Ureters

The bilateral ureters are thin, muscular tubes approximately 10 inches long. The tube's muscular layer creates peristaltic waves that help move the urine to the bladder. The ureters' walls are made of **transitional epithelium**, which allows the ureters to stretch to accommodate urine flow. Many nerve endings are also in the walls. A stone in the ureter can cause severe pain.

The point where the ureter enters the bladder is called the *ureterovesical junction*. The ureters enter the bladder at an angle. This creates a flap over the end of the ureter, which serves as a valve. Urine can empty into the bladder, but it cannot back up from the bladder and reenter the ureter. This mechanism also prevents bacteria from moving from the bladder up to the kidneys.

Bladder

The urinary bladder is a hollow organ in the pelvic cavity. It serves as a holding tank for urine. Urine enters the bladder through the ureters and leaves the bladder through the urethra. The triangular area in the bladder between the ureters' entrance and the urethral outlet is called the *trigone*.

Transitional epithelium creates the inner lining of the bladder. When the bladder is empty, it flattens, and the walls overlap in folds, also known as **rugae**. This creates a wrinkled appearance. As the bladder starts to fill with urine, the rugae and transitional epithelium allow for greater bladder volume. Think of a balloon that was blown up and then emptied of air. The balloon is smaller and wrinkly in appearance. When inflated, the wrinkles are gone, and it can accommodate a large volume of air. The same thing happens with the bladder and urine.

The bladder is also composed of smooth muscle fibers that make up the *detrusor muscle*. The detrusor muscle relaxes when the bladder fills. It contracts to push urine out of the bladder and into the urethra. Normally, the bladder holds about 1.5 to 2 cups (360 to 480 mL) of urine during the day and doubles that amount at night. As the bladder fills to about 150 mL, **stretch receptors** in the detrusor send a message to the central nervous system. As more urine enters the bladder, the urge to urinate increases. After urination or *micturition*, **residual urine** remains (usually less than 50 mL) in the bladder.

Urethra

The urethra is a mucous membrane–lined tube that drains urine out of the bladder. In males, the internal urethral sphincter is located at the bladder end (or proximal end) of the urethra. The sphincter is made of smooth involuntary muscles. The external sphincter is located in different places in males and females (Table 42.1). The external sphincter is made of skeletal muscles and is a voluntary muscle. A voluntary muscle provides you with the ability to control when you urinate. The distal end of the urethra is called the *urinary meatus*. The urinary meatus is the final structure before the urine leaves the body.

TABLE 42.1 Difference in the Urethra between the Genders

	FEMALE	MALE
Length	1–1.5 inches	8 inches
Function	Urination	Urination and ejaculation
Location of Internal Sphincter	None	At the proximal end (bladder end) of the urethra; may prevent semen from moving into the bladder
Location of External Sphincter	Extends up to the bladder, encircles the vagina and urethra	Under the prostate gland

CRITICAL THINKING APPLICATION 42.2

Hannah is working with Katrina, the urology medical assistant. Hannah asks Katrina what the major differences are between the male and female urinary systems. How would Katrina respond to Hannah's question?

PHYSIOLOGY OF THE URINARY SYSTEM

The urinary system has several important roles that help regulate homeostasis in the body:

- *Maintains fluid volume.* The urinary system increases fluid loss in urine when fluid volume is high. It decreases the fluid loss when the fluid volume is low (e.g., with dehydration).
- *Maintains the normal composition of body fluids.* The urinary system can increase or decrease the loss of certain electrolytes in the urine as it regulates the normal makeup of the body fluids. This helps to keep the pH of the blood within normal limits.
- *Maintains an adequate blood pressure. Renin,* an enzyme, is secreted in the urinary system and is involved in increasing the blood pressure.
- *Controls red blood cell production.* **Erythropoietin** is secreted by the urinary system, which triggers red blood cell production.
- *Activates vitamin D.* The kidneys are involved in the final step of vitamin D activation. Vitamin D is important in the absorption of calcium and phosphorus.

Many of these roles are performed during the formation of urine. The body rids itself of unneeded substances produced during the metabolic process. The process of urine formation includes three steps: filtration, reabsorption, and secretion. Each step will be described in more detail in the coming sections.

Filtration

Filtration is the first step in urine formation. It is a continual process that involves the renal corpuscle. If you recall, the renal corpuscle consists of a cup-shaped structure (Bowman capsule) that surrounds the network of capillaries (glomerulus).

The blood is brought to the kidneys by the renal arteries. The arteries branch into smaller vessels that transport the blood throughout the kidney. As the blood gets to the nephron, an afferent arteriole brings the blood into the glomerulus, and an efferent arteriole takes the blood away. Eventually, the blood moves into the renal vein and out of the kidney.

Let us focus on what occurs in the glomerulus. The diameter of the afferent arteriole is larger than the efferent arteriole's diameter. This means the blood moves into the glomerulus faster than it leaves. The pressure inside the glomerulus is high, with the quantity of blood moving into the glomerulus. This forces water and dissolved substances through the one-celled wall of the capillary and into the Bowman capsule. The substance in the Bowman capsule is known as filtrate. (Think of a garden hose that is wide at one part and narrow at the other. The pressure builds up behind the narrow section. Water can leak from any weakened areas in the wall of the hose. This is similar to what occurs in the glomerulus.)

Several dissolved substances can move through the capillary wall:

- Electrolytes (i.e., sodium, chloride, and potassium)
- Waste products (i.e., urea, **metabolites**)
- Other substances (i.e., amino acids and glucose)

White blood cells, red blood cells, and plasma proteins are too large to pass through the capillary wall. With normal kidney function, they remain in the capillary.

If the blood pressure falls (i.e., with hemorrhaging), the pressure in the glomerulus is not high enough to cause movement of the fluids, so little to no filtrate is created, and the person will have little to no urine output.

Reabsorption

Reabsorption means substances move from the filtrate back into the blood in the peritubular capillaries. As the filtrate moves out of the Bowman capsule and into the proximal tubule, the reabsorption process starts. Water (H_2O) and solutes (e.g., sodium [Na^+] ions and glucose) move back into the blood (Figure 42.5). See Table 42.2 for the list of solutes that move back into the blood.

In the Henle loop, the reabsorption process is a bit different. The Henle loop dips down into the medulla and then moves back up. The countercurrent flow occurs as the filtrate flows down and then moves back up. During this time, the chloride (Cl^-) and sodium ions move out of the filtrate and into the **interstitial** fluid and blood. This creates a salty interstitial fluid, which helps pull water from the distal tubule filtrate. Water, chloride, and sodium are reabsorbed into the blood as the filtrate passes through the distal tubule.

Action of Antidiuretic Hormone and Aldosterone

In the distal tubules, some sodium and chloride ions are reabsorbed from the filtrate. The walls of the distal tubules do not allow water to move out of the filtrate without special help. With the help of the *antidiuretic hormone* (ADH) (also called *vasopressin*), water moves out of the filtrate and into the bloodstream. ADH is a hormone stored in the posterior pituitary gland. ADH helps increase the water **permeability** of the walls of the distal tubule and collecting duct. Without ADH, a person would pass vast quantities of urine. An inadequate supply of ADH causes diabetes insipidus.

Besides ADH, another hormone called *aldosterone* works in the urinary system. Aldosterone is secreted by the adrenal cortex. This hormone increases the movement of sodium out of the filtrate in the distal tubule and collecting duct. See Table 42.2 for the complete list of substances reabsorbed in the distal tubule and collecting duct.

The kidneys retain (or reabsorb) what the body needs to maintain homeostasis. Substances in excessive concentrations and metabolism waste products remain in the filtrate. The filtrate becomes more concentrated as water is reabsorbed into the bloodstream. The kidneys create about 48 gallons (about 182 L) of filtrate a day. By the time reabsorption occurs, they produce only 1 to 2 quarts (about 0.9 to 1.9 L) of urine a day.

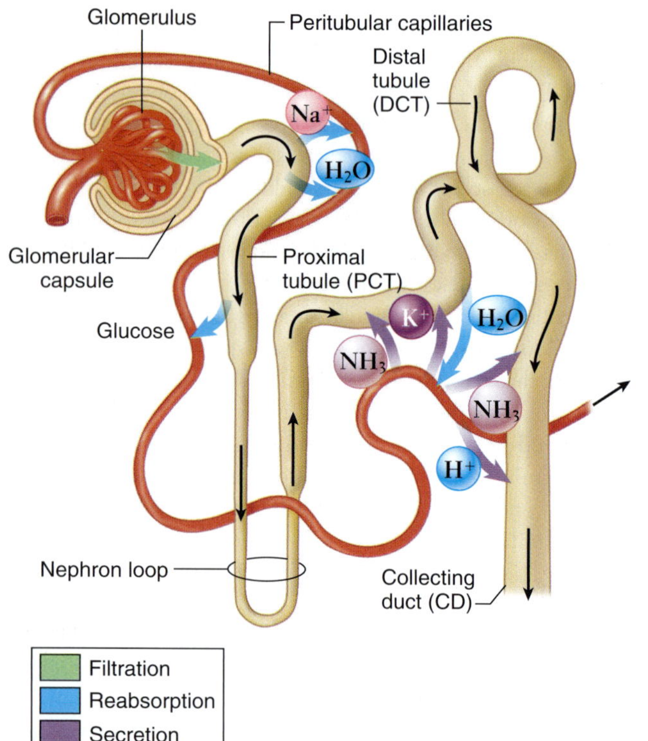

FIGURE 42.5 Formation of urine. Diagram shows examples of steps in urine formation in successive parts of a nephron: filtration, reabsorption, and secretion. (From Patton KT, Thibodeau G: *The human body in health and disease*, ed 7, St. Louis, 2019, Mosby.)

CRITICAL THINKING APPLICATION 42.3

Hannah is confused about diabetes insipidus. She always thought diabetes was related to insulin and blood glucose. She does not recall learning about diabetes insipidus in school. She asks Katrina, the urology medical assistant, to explain how diabetes insipidus affects the urinary system. How might Katrina respond to Hannah's question?

Secretion

Secretion means that substances move from the blood to the filtrate. This allows the body to maintain homeostasis and move unneeded substances back into the filtrate. Urea moves back to the filtrate in the Henle loop. As the filtrate moves through the distal tubule and collecting duct, more adjustments are made. Ammonia (NH_3), certain drugs, hydrogen (H^+), and potassium (K^+) move from the blood into the filtrate. The movement of potassium into the filtrate can be caused by aldosterone. After the filtrate or urine leaves the collecting ducts, no more adjustments are made. The urine then flows to the calyces and the ureter before going through the rest of the urinary system structures.

Renin and Blood Pressure

As mentioned before, the kidneys have an important role in maintaining blood pressure. The *juxtaglomerular cells* are smooth muscle cells in the afferent arterioles. These cells make and secrete the enzyme *renin.* When the arterial blood pressure decreases or there is a decrease in sodium, renin is released. Secreting renin is one of the first steps in the complex renin-angiotensin-aldosterone system (RAAS). Ultimately when renin is secreted, a series of events occur. The outcome increases the blood pressure in two different ways: by creating more blood plasma volume and by constricting blood vessels. Many **antihypertensive** medications impact the RAAS at various points in hopes of lowering blood pressure. Sometimes it takes

TABLE 42.2 Movement of Substances between the Blood and Filtrate in the Nephron

NEPHRON SECTIONS PROCESSES	RENAL CORPUSCLE *(BOWMAN CAPSULE AND GLOMERULUS)*	PROXIMAL TUBULE (PCT)	HENLE LOOP	DISTAL TUBULE (DCT)	COLLECTING DUCT (CD)
Filtration (moves from blood to create filtrate)	Water, electrolyte ions (sodium, chloride, potassium), urea, glucose, and amino acids				
Reabsorption (moves from filtrate to blood)	—	Water, glucose, amino acids, urea, and electrolyte ions (sodium, chloride, phosphate)	Water and electrolyte ions (chloride, sodium)	Electrolyte ions (chloride, sodium) and water (only in the presence of ADH)	Electrolyte ions (sodium), urea, water (only in the presence of ADH)
Secretion (moves from blood to filtrate)	—		Urea	Ammonium, potassium, hydrogen, some drugs	Ammonium, potassium, hydrogen, some drugs

ADH, Antidiuretic hormone.

more than one medication to lower a person's blood pressure to a safe level.

Erythropoietin

As the blood is moving through the kidneys, specialized kidney cells can detect low oxygen levels in the blood. When this occurs, a hormone called *erythropoietin* is released from the kidney cells. Erythropoietin travels to the bone marrow and stimulates the marrow to make more red blood cells.

Vitamin D

Vitamin D assists with calcium absorption and helps maintain calcium and phosphorus levels. These minerals are important for strong bones. We get vitamin D from exposure to sunlight, as well as from the consumption of supplements and food. The kidneys must convert vitamin D to an active form so the body can use it.

LIFE SPAN CHANGES OF THE URINARY SYSTEM

At about 10 to 12 weeks after conception, the kidneys start producing urine. While the baby is in utero, the mother's placenta performs most of the kidneys' function until the last few weeks before birth. When babies are born, they have the same number of nephrons as adults. The nephrons are immature and reach maturity by age 2. A baby's kidneys do not retain water like adult kidneys do. Thus, babies can lose water quickly, especially when they are hot or if they have diarrhea. During childhood, the bladder continues to grow. Bladder control is usually learned between ages 2 and 3.

During the adult years, males are more likely to develop kidney stones. This may be attributed to the amount of food they eat. They need to drink more water than females to clear the waste products from the body. Male kidneys also have an increased ability to concentrate urine, a risk factor for kidney stones. Females are at more risk for urinary tract infections (UTIs) than males. This is attributed to the anatomic differences. Most UTIs are caused by *Escherichia coli*, which is found near the vagina and rectum. The closeness of the urethra to these structures and the shortness of the urethra increase the risk of UTIs.

Changes with Pregnancy

During pregnancy, the filtration rate increases in females. The number of nephrons remains the same, but the filtration surface increases. This increase allows the kidneys to filter more blood, which is useful with the increased blood flow during pregnancy. In late pregnancy, the bladder may be twice as big. The anatomic and physiologic changes that occur during pregnancy put women at more risk for pyelonephritis at that time.

Changes in Older Adults

In older adults, the kidney tissue and number of nephrons are reduced by up to 20%. The renal arteries can harden. This causes the kidneys to filter blood slower. The kidneys become less able to regulate water balance. Older adults are at more risk of dehydration when the weather is hot or if they have diarrhea. The bladder wall becomes less stretchy with age. The bladder cannot hold as much urine as before. Bladder muscles weaken. The urethra may be obstructed by an enlarged prostate gland or a prolapse of the bladder or vagina. Older adults are at more risk for chronic kidney disease, UTIs, and incontinence.

URINARY SYSTEM DISEASES AND DISORDERS

Common urinary signs and symptoms include the following:

- *Dysuria*: Painful or difficult urination
- *Nocturia*: Urination at night
- *Polyuria*: Excessive excretion of urine may be accompanied by *polydipsia* (excessive thirst)
- *Frequency*: Urination at short periods without an increase in the daily volume of urine output
- *Urgency*: The sudden, almost uncontrollable need to urinate
- *Urinary incontinence*: Inability to hold urine
- *Urinary retention*: Inability to release urine

Typically, common signs of urinary system disorders found on medical imaging and laboratory tests include these:

- *Calculi*: Stones formed in the kidneys, gallbladder, and other parts of the body
- *Hydronephrosis*: A backup of urine that causes dilation of the ureters and calyces; can increase pressure on the nephron units
- *Azotemia*: An abnormal increase in nitrogenous waste products in the blood; also called uremia
- *Abnormal substances in the urine: Albuminuria* or *proteinuria* (albumin), *azoturia* (excessive nitrogen compounds), *bacteriuria* (bacteria), *glycosuria* (glycose [sugar]), *hematuria* (blood), and *pyuria* (pus)

The following sections describe cancers, genetic and congenital disorders, infectious and inflammatory disorders, and structural and functional disorders of the urinary system.

Urinary System Cancers

Bladder and kidney cancer are the most common types of urinary system cancers. The following sections discuss each of these types of cancers.

Bladder Cancer

Bladder cancer is the sixth most common cancer in the United States. Bladder cancer tends to recur, so follow-up testing is critical. Transitional cell carcinoma (also called urothelial carcinoma) is the most common type of bladder cancer in the United States.

Smoking, chemical exposure, family history of the disease, some chemotherapy medications, and chronic bladder infections can increase the risk of bladder cancer. People over 40 years of age, men, and Caucasians are also more at risk. Common signs and symptoms include hematuria, frequency, urgency, dysuria, pelvic pain, and low back pain.

The provider will do a physical exam. Urine testing, cystoscopy, and a biopsy may be done to diagnose bladder cancer. Additional imaging tests are done to check if the cancer has spread to other parts of the body. Treatments used for bladder cancer include surgery, radiation therapy, and chemotherapy. *Biological therapy* or *immunotherapy* can be useful, as it increases the body's ability to help fight the cancer.

Kidney Cancer

Kidney cancer or primary kidney cancer occurs when cancer starts in the kidney. There are three main types of primary kidney cancer:

TABLE 42.3 Common Types of Kidney Cancer

	RENAL CELL CARCINOMA	WILMS TUMOR	TRANSITIONAL CELL CANCER
Signs and Symptoms	Hematuria, lump in abdomen, side and back pain (below the ribs), loss of appetite, weight loss, anemia, **intermittent** fever	Hematuria, fever, and abdominal pain, mass, and swelling	Hematuria, back pain, extreme fatigue, weight loss, dysuria
Diagnostic Procedures	Physical exam, CBC, blood chemistry tests, UA, liver function tests, CT, MRI, US, biopsy	Physical exam, CBC, blood chemistry tests, UA, US, CT, MRI	Physical exam, CBC, blood chemistry tests, UA, ureteroscopy, IVP, CT, US, MRI, biopsy
Treatment	Surgery (nephrectomy), radiation, chemotherapy, biological therapy, targeted therapy	Surgery (nephrectomy), radiation, chemotherapy	Segmental resection of the ureter, nephroureterectomy, chemotherapy, radiation

CBC, Complete blood count; *CT,* computed tomography; *IVP,* intravenous pyelogram; *MRI,* magnetic resonance imaging; *UA,* urinalysis; *US,* ultrasonography.

- *Renal cell carcinoma* (RCC) (or *renal adenocarcinoma*): Most common type in adults; forms in the lining of the kidney tubules
- *Wilms tumor* (or *nephroblastoma*): Most common type in children younger than 5 years; occurs in the kidney tissue; improved treatments have increased the survival rate
- *Transitional cell cancer*: Occurs in adults; forms in the ureter and renal pelvis

It is unclear what causes the mutation of the kidney cell that leads to a tumor development. With kidney cancer, pain and hematuria can be key symptoms. See Table 42.3 for the symptoms of the three types of kidney cancer.

Diagnostic procedures for the three types of kidney cancer are similar (see Table 42.3). During the exam, the provider may identify a kidney mass. Urinalysis and blood work may be done to check for hematuria and the person's overall health. Once kidney cancer is diagnosed, imaging tests are done to check for cancer in other parts of the body. Treatment for kidney cancer can involve surgery. If no kidney function exists, then dialysis and a kidney transplant are done. If surgery is not an option, arterial embolization can be done. A **catheter** is inserted through an incision and passed into the main blood vessel of the kidney. A special gelatin sponge is inserted through the catheter into the blood vessel, creating a blockage and preventing blood flow, thus killing the tumor.

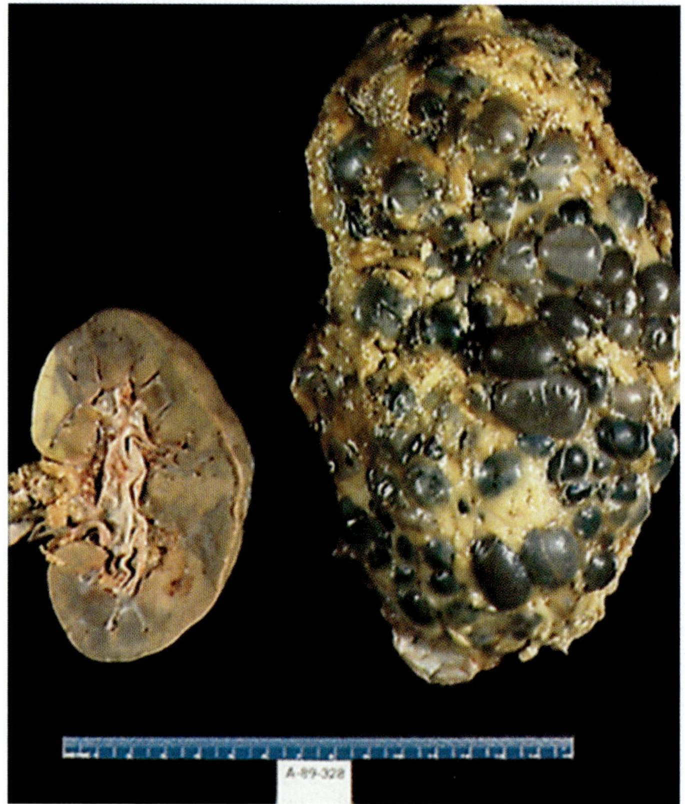

FIGURE 42.6 Comparison of a polycystic kidney *(right)* with a normal kidney *(left)*. (From Lewis SM: *Medical-surgical nursing: assessment and management of clinical problems,* ed 8, St. Louis, 2011, Mosby.)

Genetic and Congenital Urinary System Disorders

Genetic and congenital urinary system disorders cause kidney loss or malfunction later in life. Polycystic kidney disease is one of the more common genetic and congenital urinary system disorders.

Polycystic Kidney Disease

Polycystic kidney disease (PKD) is an inherited condition. Cysts form in the kidneys, causing the kidneys to become enlarged (Figure 42.6). A cyst-filled kidney can weigh up to 30 pounds. There are two types of PKD:

- *Autosomal dominant*: If the gene is inherited from one parent, the child will get the disease. Often the parent also has the disease. This is the most common form of PKD and inherited kidney disorder. It is typically identified between the ages of 30 and 50, although it can occur in childhood.
- *Autosomal recessive*: To get the disease, a person must get a copy of the defective gene from both parents.

People with PKD may also have cysts in their liver and pancreas. Aneurysms and diverticula of the colon may also be associated with PKD. Males can have cysts in their testes and tend to have more kidney failure. Women with PKD, *hypertension* (high blood pressure), and who have had three or more pregnancies are also more at risk for kidney failure. PKD can cause the following conditions:

- Pain in the flank, abdomen, and joints
- Nocturia and hematuria

- Drowsiness and nail abnormalities
- Pain or tenderness over the liver and an enlarged liver
- Heart murmur and hypertension

During the physical examination, the provider may order a computed tomography (CT), magnetic resonance imaging (MRI), and ultrasound (US) to check the cysts on the kidneys. PKD is a chronic condition that slowly gets worse. The treatment goals are to control symptoms and prevent complications. Treatment often includes antihypertensive medications, **diuretics**, and a low-salt diet. PKD can increase the risk of urinary tract infections due to blockages. UTIs should be treated quickly with antibiotics. Surgery to remove one or both kidneys may be required. The patient may also need dialysis or kidney transplantation. With the chronic nature of this condition, it is important for patients to get support. Sometimes, support groups can help the patient and family cope with the disease process.

Additional Genetic and Congenital Disorders

Besides PKD, there are several genetic and congenital disorders that affect the urinary system:

- *Hydronephrosis*: Distention of the renal pelvis and calyces due to urinary tract obstruction; caused by a congenital defect or renal calculi.
- *Prune belly syndrome* (PBS): Group of genetic birth defects usually occurring in boys; involves enlarged ureters and bladder, hydronephrosis (kidney swelling), poor development of the abdominal muscles, undescended testicles, and wrinkled skin over the abdomen.
- *Ureterocele*: End of ureter is malformed and bulges, creating a ureterocele, and may obstruct the ureter or bladder.
- *Ureteropelvic junction* (UPJ) *obstruction*: Blockage where the ureter joins the kidney, causing kidney swelling.
- *Vesicoureteral reflux* (VUR): Urine backs up into the ureter from the bladder due to a malformed or missing valve over the end of the ureter.

Infectious and Inflammatory Urinary System Diseases and Disorders

A urinary tract infection (UTI) is an infection in one or more of the urinary tract structures. There are several infections and inflammatory disorders that affect the urinary system. Examples of these disorders include the following:

- *Interstitial cystitis* (IC): Causes recurring bladder and pelvic region pain and discomfort, frequency, and urgency; also called *painful bladder syndrome* (PBS).
- *Interstitial nephritis*: Inflammation of the kidneys with an increase of interstitial tissue and thickening of blood vessel walls.
- *Membranous glomerulonephritis*: Inflammation occurs in the kidney due to glomerular changes, and large amounts of protein are excreted in the urine. The exact etiology is unknown.
- *Nephritis:* Inflammation of the kidney; can be chronic, acute, or nephrosis (also called nephrotic syndrome).
- *Urethritis*: Inflammation of the urethra due to bacteria, viruses, injury, or chemical sensitivity.

Acute cystitis, glomerulonephritis, and pyelonephritis are also conditions in this category and described in the following sections.

Acute Cystitis

Acute cystitis is an inflammation of the bladder. Due to the shorter urethra, women are more at risk than men of getting infections.

Typically, acute cystitis is caused by a bacterial infection, most commonly *Escherichia coli (E. coli)*. Other causes of inflammation can include medications, radiation therapy, spermicidal jellies, and long-term catheterization. Being pregnant, going through menopause, a catheter, urinary tract procedure, urinary retention, an obstruction, bowel incontinence, or diabetes can increase the risk of cystitis. Signs and symptoms include the following:

- Nocturia, dysuria, urgency, frequency, and urinary retention
- Cloudy, bloody, or strong/foul-smelling urine
- Low abdominal pressure or cramping, low-grade fever
- With older adults: confusion and mental changes

Usually, the provider will order a urinalysis, a urine culture, and a sensitivity (C&S) test (discussed in Chapter 47). The urinalysis provides information to help diagnose cystitis, and the C&S may take up to 3 days to identify the organism. If the urinalysis and culture come back negative for an infection, the provider may do additional tests (e.g., cystoscopy) to try to identify the cause of the symptoms. Treatment for bacterial cystitis consists of antibiotics.

Home care treatments may include drinking plenty of liquids; avoiding coffee, alcohol, and soft drinks; taking an analgesic, having a sitz bath, or using a heating pad to decrease the discomfort.

Glomerulonephritis

Several diseases affect kidney functioning because of their effects on the glomeruli. *Glomerulonephritis* is inflammation of the glomeruli. Damage to the glomeruli can cause protein and red blood cells to leak into the urine. Glomerulonephritis usually has an abrupt onset.

The cause is often unknown, and it can follow a streptococcal infection. Signs and symptoms include puffy eyes, fatigue, low-grade fever, headache, and pain in the kidney region. Hematuria, cola-colored urine, proteinuria, and oliguria can also be seen.

After the physical exam, the provider may order a urinalysis, blood urea nitrogen (BUN), creatinine, erythrocyte sedimentation rate (ESR), imaging tests (e.g., CT scan, x-ray, and ultrasound), and a renal biopsy. Treatment is based on the cause of the illness. Bed rest, antihypertensive medications, antibiotics, diuretics, and dietary restrictions (e.g., protein, salt, and potassium) may be ordered.

Pyelonephritis

Pyelonephritis is a urinary tract infection of one or both kidneys. Prompt treatment is required to prevent kidney damage and **septicemia**. The bacteria can spread to the bloodstream, causing an overwhelming infection that can be life threatening.

Pyelonephritis is caused by a bacterium or virus. The pathogen can move from the bladder to the kidneys, or carried by the bloodstream to the kidneys. An increased risk of pyelonephritis may be seen with structural defects, urinary reflux, obstruction, and bladder infection. The signs and symptoms consist of fever, chills, nausea, vomiting, dysuria, frequency, hematuria, foul-smelling urine, and low back, side (flank), or groin pain. Young children may only experience a fever, and some adults may have confusion and speech difficulties.

After the patient's history has been taken and the physical examination has concluded, the provider will usually order a urinalysis, urine culture, blood culture, and blood work. For the most accurate results, all cultures need to be obtained before the patient starts on antibiotics. Additional tests may include a US, a CT scan, a voiding cystourethrogram (VCUG), a digital rectal exam (DRE), and a dimercaptosuccinic acid (DMSA) scan. Initially, the provider will treat the infection with a broad-spectrum antibiotic. When the blood and urine culture results are known, the provider may have the patient take an antibiotic that is known to kill the pathogen. For severely ill patients, hospitalization, **intravenous** (IV) fluids and antibiotics, and close observation may be required. Repeat cultures may be taken after the antibiotics have been completed to ensure the infection is gone.

CRITICAL THINKING APPLICATION **42.4**

Hannah is working with Dr. Riney. He ordered an antibiotic for Mrs. Williams, who has a UTI. When the urine culture and sensitivity (C&S) report comes back to the department, he asks Hannah to call Mrs. Williams about a change in the antibiotic. Why might the provider change the antibiotic once the urine C&S report becomes available?

Structural and Functional Urinary System Diseases and Disorders

Several diseases cause structural or functional changes in the urinary system. Chronic kidney disease, end-stage renal disease, nephrotic syndrome, neurogenic bladder, renal calculi, and urinary incontinence are common disorders that cause structural or functional changes. Additional diseases include the following:

- *Acute tubular necrosis*: Rapid destruction of the tubular sections of the nephrons due to blood flow impairment or toxins.
- *Anterior prolapse*: Also called cystocele, prolapse, or dropped bladder. Anterior prolapse is a bulging or dropping of the bladder into the vagina caused by the weakening and stretching of supportive tissues and muscles (Figure 42.7).
- *Bladder outlet obstruction (BOO)*: Blockage at the opening of the bladder or in the urethra.
- *Minimal change disease*: Damage occurs to the glomeruli, though the cause is unknown.
- *Reflux nephropathy*: Urine backflows from the bladder, causing kidney damage. Can be due to a ureter defect, obstruction, or swelling.

The following sections describe the common diseases that cause structural or functional changes in the urinary system.

Chronic Kidney Disease

Chronic kidney disease is also called *chronic kidney failure.* With this condition, kidney function is gradually lost. During the early stage of chronic kidney disease, there may be few symptoms. As the kidney function diminishes, more symptoms occur.

Many diseases can lead to chronic kidney disease, including hypertension, diabetes mellitus, glomerulonephritis, interstitial nephritis, PKD, and vesicoureteral reflux. Signs and symptoms may be minimal at first. As the kidney function diminishes, the person may experience nausea, vomiting, loss of appetite, weakness, fatigue, muscle cramps, twitching, itching (*pruritus*), hypertension, decreased amounts of urine, sleep issues, and a reduction in mental sharpness.

After a history and examination, the provider may order urine and blood tests to assess the kidney function. Imaging tests may be done to assess the kidney size, shape, and structure. A kidney biopsy can also be done. For chronic kidney disease, there is no cure. Treatment is focused on slowing the progression of the disease and reducing complications. Underlying conditions, such as hypertension and diabetes, are also treated.

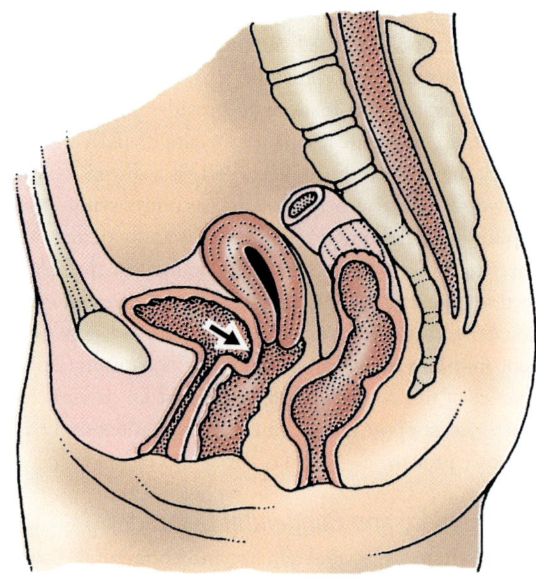

FIGURE 42.7 Anterior prolapse. The urinary bladder is displaced downward *(arrow)*, which causes bulging of the anterior vaginal wall. (From Ignatavicius DD, Workman ML: *Medical-surgical nursing: critical thinking for collaborative care*, ed 6, Philadelphia, 2011, Saunders.)

End-Stage Renal Disease

End-stage renal disease (ESRD), also called end-stage kidney disease and kidney failure, is advanced-stage chronic kidney disease. ESRD occurs when the kidneys are no longer filtering waste from the blood. Dangerous levels of electrolytes, waste products, and fluids build up in the bloodstream. More than 660,000 Americans have kidney failure. Over 44% of those patients are between the ages of 45 and 64.

The top two causes of ESRD are diabetes mellitus and hypertension. Additional causes include glomerulonephritis, polycystic kidney disease, prolonged obstructions, recurrent kidney infections, and vesicoureteral reflux. Using tobacco increases the risk of ESRD. Men, African Americans, and being 45 years or older can also increase the risk. The kidneys can slowly stop functioning over the course of 10 to 20 years before ESRD occurs. The signs and symptoms are the same as for chronic kidney disease.

Besides performing a physical exam, providers will order blood work and a bone density test. The blood work usually includes tests that evaluate the patient's complete blood count (CBC), electrolytes (e.g., potassium, sodium, calcium, and magnesium), albumin, and parathyroid hormone. The patient's blood pressure will be monitored closely.

ESRD is often treated with dialysis or kidney transplantation. Dialysis works like a kidney by filtering out the waste products, extra fluids, and electrolytes. There are two different types of dialysis:

- *Peritoneal dialysis*: A catheter is surgically placed in the abdomen. The patient can then infuse a special sterile solution through the catheter into the abdomen. The peritoneal membrane is used as a natural filter, and waste from the blood moves into the infused solution. After a few hours, the patient drains the fluid out of the abdomen via the catheter (Figure 42.8). New fluid is then infused into the abdomen.

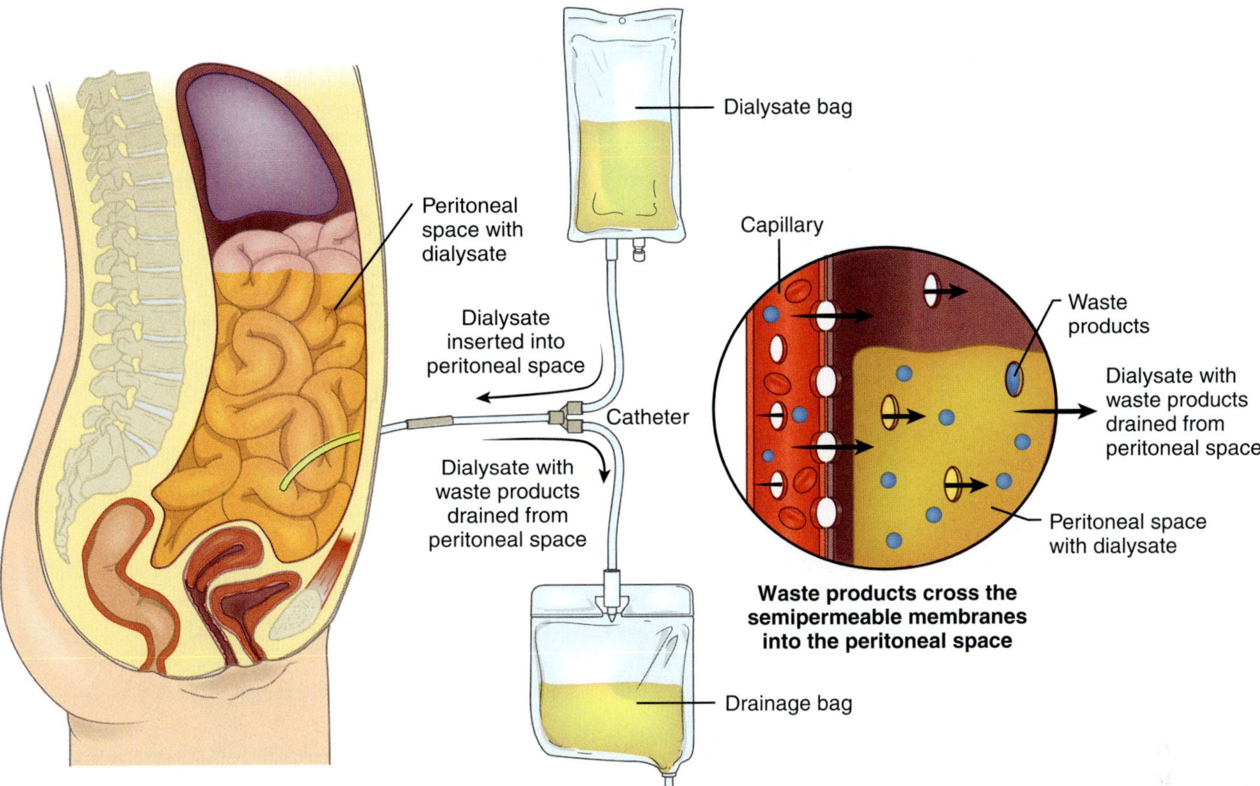

FIGURE 42.8 Peritoneal dialysis.

There may be four to six exchanges of fluid a day. This type of dialysis allows the person to work, travel, or sleep during the process.

- *Hemodialysis*: A **vascular access** (i.e., catheter, **arteriovenous** [ahr teer ee oh VEE nuhs] graft**, arteriovenous fistula**) is placed. The patient is hooked up to a dialysis machine using the vascular access. The person's blood flows through the special filter inside of the machine (Figure 42.9). The filter cleans the blood of waste products and extra fluids. Typically, patients need to have hemodialysis three times a week at the dialysis center.

Besides dialysis and kidney transplantation, other treatments are available:

- Dietary modifications, such as low protein, limiting fluids, and electrolyte supplements
- Antihypertensive medication and supplements (i.e., iron and vitamin D)

CRITICAL THINKING APPLICATION **42.5**

With Hannah's experience in the dialysis unit, she has learned that many people need to do hemodialysis three times a week for several hours each day. How might this affect a patient's lifestyle?

Nephrotic Syndrome

Nephrotic syndrome consists of a collection of symptoms that indicate kidney damage. The syndrome is caused by other disorders that eventually lead to kidney tissue destruction.

Nephrotic syndrome occurs more often in males than in females. It can affect children, usually 2 to 6 years of age, and adults. Minimal change disease is the most common cause of nephrotic syndrome in children. Membranous glomerulonephritis is the most common cause in adults. Nephrotic syndrome can also occur as the result of cancer, chronic disease (e.g., diabetes, systemic lupus erythematosus), infections, immune and genetic disorders, and with certain drugs. The most common sign is swelling of the face, extremities, and abdomen. Additional symptoms can include poor appetite, weight gain, seizures, skin sores, and foamy-appearing urine. Blood and urine tests show proteinuria, **hyperlipidemia**, and **hypoalbuminemia**.

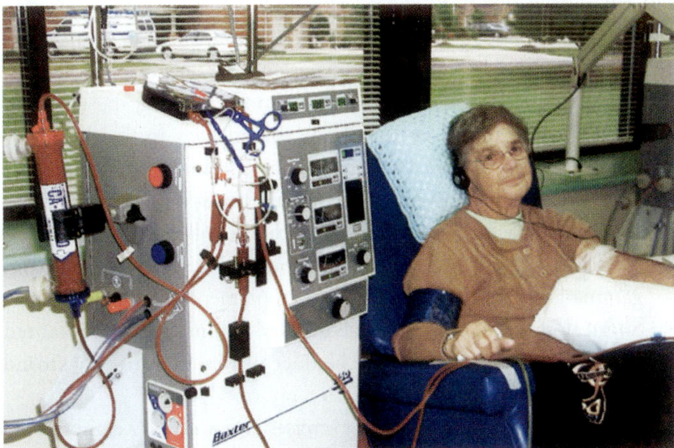

FIGURE 42.9 Hemodialysis machine. (From Ignatavicius DD, Workman ML: *Medical-surgical nursing: critical thinking for collaborative care*, ed 6, Philadelphia, 2011, Saunders.)

Providers will do a physical exam, laboratory testing (blood testing [albumin, blood chemistry tests, BUN, and creatinine] and urine testing [creatinine clearance and urinalysis]), and a kidney biopsy. Additional testing may be ordered to identify the specific cause of nephrotic syndrome. Infection with the human immunodeficiency virus (HIV), hepatitis, and syphilis are just a few of the diseases that could lead to nephrotic syndrome. The treatment goals are to reduce symptoms, delay kidney damage, and prevent additional complications. The following are common treatments:

- Antihypertensive medications to keep the blood pressure in the normal range
- Vitamin D supplements
- **Corticosteroids**, **anticoagulants**, **antihyperlipidemics**, and diuretics
- Dietary modifications, such as low-fat, low-cholesterol, low-salt, and low-protein diets

Neurogenic Bladder

The central nervous system, nerves that supply the bladder, and muscles work together for bladder control. Damage or disorders that impact the bladder nerves or the central nervous system can cause a neurogenic bladder. A person with a neurogenic bladder lacks bladder control, causing it to be *overactive* (the bladder muscles contract controllably) or *underactive* (the person does not have the urge to go even though the bladder is full).

The central nervous system disorders that can cause neurogenic bladder include birth defects, cerebral palsy, Alzheimer disease, brain or spinal cord tumors, multiple sclerosis (MS), Parkinson disease, stroke, and spinal cord injury. Damage and disorders of the bladder nerves can be caused by diabetes, syphilis, heavy alcohol use, **neuropathy**, nerve damage from pelvic surgery, herniated disk, or spinal canal stenosis. With an overactive bladder, urgency and frequency to urinate are common. With an underactive bladder, the bladder fills but the person does not have the urge to go, and *incontinence* (urine leakage) can occur. Problems with starting to urinate or completely emptying the bladder can also be experienced.

After a physical exam, additional procedures may be ordered, including a postvoid residual volume, blood tests to check kidney functioning (e.g., serum creatinine), renal ultrasonography, and cystoscopy. Treatment is aimed at managing the symptoms of neurogenic bladder. Possible treatments include the following:

- Medications: Antimuscarinic, anticholinergic, botulinum toxin, gamma-aminobutyric acid (GABA) supplements, and antiepileptics
- Surgical procedures: Artificial urinary sphincter, an implanted electronic device to stimulate bladder nerves, and urinary **stoma** (or **urostomy**)
- Additional procedures: Kegel exercises and a urinary catheter

Kegel Exercises

Kegel exercises are used to strengthen the pelvic floor muscles. Both males and females can do them. To use the right muscles, pretend you have to urinate but hold it. The muscles you tighten to stop urination help tighten the pelvic floor muscles. Muscles in the vagina (for females), rectum, and bladder should tighten. The muscles in the thighs, buttock, and abdomen should not be tightened. Kegel exercises should be done three times a day.

Take the following steps to perform Kegel exercises:

1. Empty your bladder.
2. Either sit or lie down while doing the exercises.
3. Tighten the pelvic floor muscles ("hold the urine"). Tighten as you count to 8.
4. Relax the muscles as you count to 10.
5. Repeat this sequence 10 times.

CRITICAL THINKING APPLICATION 42.6

Dr. Riney asks Hannah to coach Mrs. Smith on doing Kegel exercises. How might Hannah explain the process of doing Kegels to Mrs. Smith?

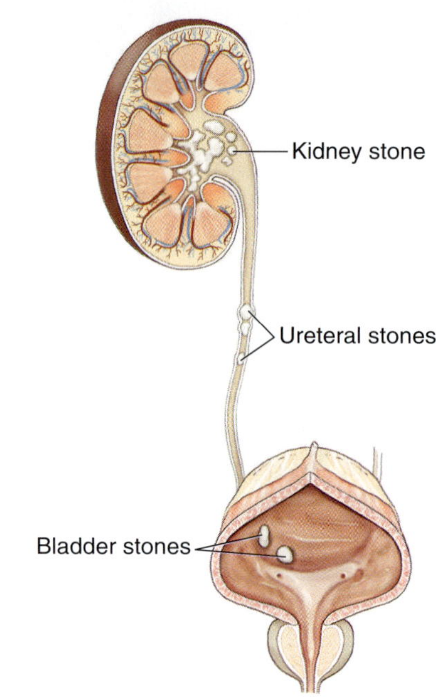

FIGURE 42.10 Locations of ureteral calculi. (From Shiland B: *Mastering healthcare terminology*, ed 5. St. Louis, 2016, Elsevier.)

Renal Calculi

Renal **calculi**, or kidney stones, are mineral pebbles that form in the kidney. Symptoms can occur if the calculi grow larger or move into the ureters or renal pelvis (Figure 42.10). If a stone blocks the flow of urine, infection can develop from the backflow of urine. This blockage also can result in hydronephrosis (Figure 42.11).

Renal calculi can occur when high levels of certain minerals, such as calcium, oxalate, and uric acid, collect in the kidney. Calculi can also form if fluid intake is low and the filtrate becomes highly concentrated. The tendency to develop kidney stones runs in families. With small stones, the person may not experience symptoms. With larger stones or stones that cause blockages, symptoms will be experienced. Signs and symptoms of kidney stones include dysuria, nausea, vomiting, fever, chills, and severe constant pain on either side of the lower back. The person may have cloudy, foul-smelling, or bloody urine.

After the physical exam is concluded, a urinalysis, blood tests, and imaging tests (e.g., CT scan and abdominal x-ray) are used to diagnose renal calculi. Treatment depends on the size, type, and location of the stones. Small stones may pass on their own. Analgesics may be encouraged for the pain and discomfort. Extra fluids are encouraged to flush the stone out. Typically, patients are asked to strain their urine. Kidney stone strainers should be supplied. If the patient finds a stone, it should be placed in a specimen container and brought to the lab to be analyzed (Figure 42.12). Additional procedures include the following:

- *Extracorporeal shock wave lithotripsy* (ESWL): Shock waves are used to break up the stones, so they pass without a problem (Figure 42.13).

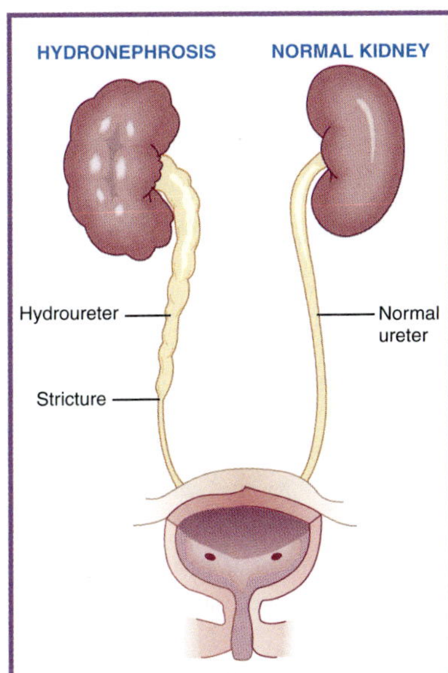

FIGURE 42.11 Hydronephrosis.

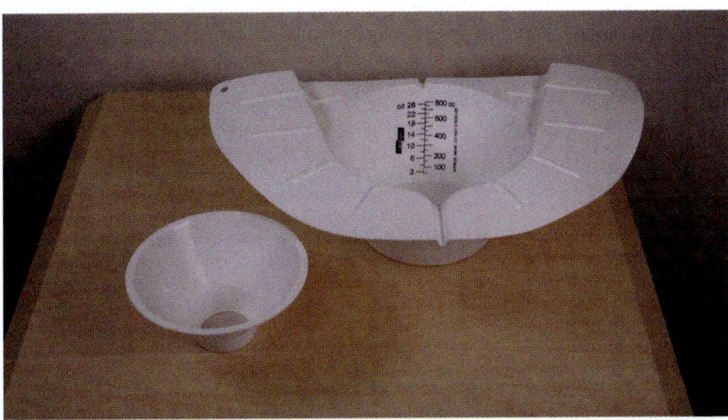

FIGURE 42.12 Urine strainer with a urine/stool collection container (also called a hat or a pan).

- *Ureteroscopy*: The ureteroscope is threaded up through the bladder and ureter. If the provider sees a stone, it can be removed during the procedure. Sometimes ESWL and ureteroscopy are both done. The stone is broken up before it is removed.
- *Nephrolithotomy:* A surgical incision is made, and the stones are removed by the tube. With *percutaneous nephrolithotripsy* (PNL), the stones are crushed and removed using suction.

CRITICAL THINKING APPLICATION **42.7**

Hannah receives a call from Zach Backstrom. He states that he has a kidney stone and wonders if he really needs to strain his urine and have it analyzed in the lab. What might be the benefit to Zach if he continues to strain his urine for the stones?

Urinary Incontinence

Urinary incontinence (UI) is the loss of bladder control, causing an accidental loss of urine. There are several types of urinary incontinence:

- *Stress incontinence*: Leakage of urine from stress on the bladder; caused by obesity, pregnancy, laughing, running, sneezing, coughing, or lifting heavy objects.
- *Urge incontinence*: Also called *overactive bladder;* strong sudden urge (urgency) before the accidental loss of urine.
- *Overflow incontinence*: Most often affects males; the person has difficulty emptying the bladder.
- *Functional incontinence*: Caused by a mental or physical disease; leakage occurs before the person can reach the toilet.
- *Mixed incontinence*: Typically affects females; leakage of urine due to overactive bladder and stress incontinence.
- *Total incontinence*: Severest type; constant urine leakage.
- *Enuresis*: Also known as "bed wetting." This condition is usually seen in children; the bladder fills during the night, and the child does not get up to urinate.

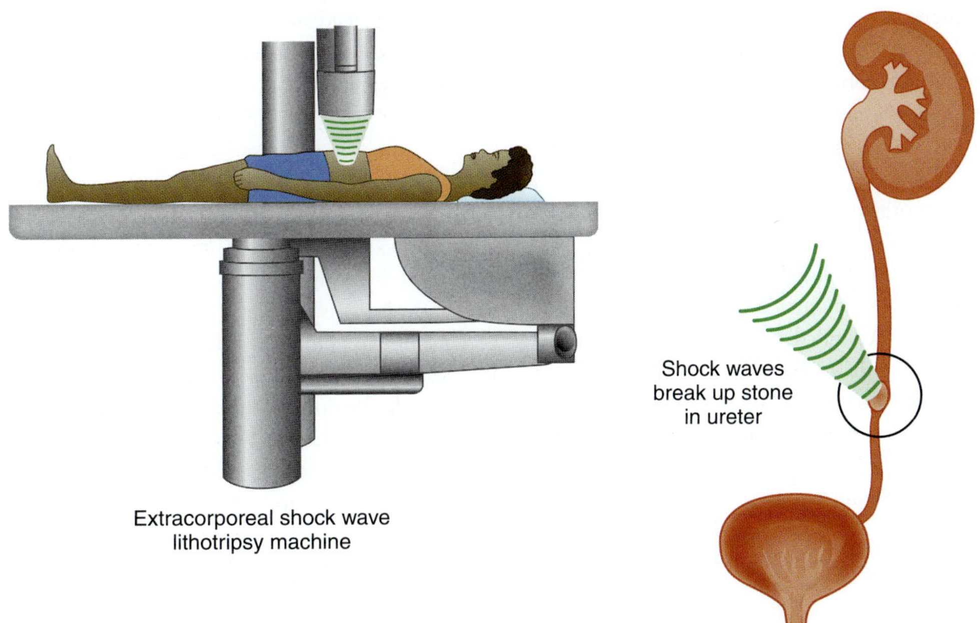

FIGURE 42.13 Extracorporeal shock wave lithotripsy. (From Linton AD: *Introduction to medical-surgical nursing,* ed 6, Philadelphia, 2016, Saunders.)

UI can occur for many reasons, including damage to the nerves that control the bladder, weak or overactive bladder muscles, diseases that limit mobility, urethral blockages (e.g., enlarged prostate), increase in urine volume, UTI, and constipation. Persistent incontinence can come from pregnancy, childbirth, menopause, pelvic surgery, aging, prostate diseases, obstructions, and neurologic disorders. Accidental leakage of urine, urgency, constant dribbling, and inability to empty the bladder are possible signs and symptoms.

Procedures used to diagnose incontinence include urinalysis, postvoid residual measurement, cystoscopy, cystogram, and pelvic ultrasound. The patient may keep a bladder diary, recording the amount of fluid consumed and urinated, the number of incontinence episodes, and frequency and urgency feelings. *Urodynamic testing* may also be done, which involves the bladder being filled via a catheter while the bladder pressure is measured. Treatments can vary based on the type of incontinence:

- *Behavior techniques:* Bladder training, double voiding, scheduled toilet trips, and management of fluid and diet.
- *Kegel exercises and electrical stimulation:* Used to strengthen pelvic floor muscles.
- *Medications:* Anticholinergics, mirabegron, alpha-blockers, Botox, and topical estrogen.
- *Surgical procedures:* Can also be performed to treat certain types of incontinence.
- *Medical devices*: A *urethral insert* is a disposable device inserted into the urethra before activities that trigger incontinence. A *pessary is a* stiff ring that is inserted into the vagina and holds up the bladder, related to a prolapsed bladder. A *nerve stimulator* is an implanted device that delivers electrical pulses to the nerves that control the bladder.

ANATOMY OF THE MALE REPRODUCTIVE SYSTEM

The male reproductive system is responsible for producing, transporting, and sustaining sperm cells. The sperm cells are called *sex cells* or **gametes**. A sperm cell contributes half of the genes of the new offspring. The gametes are produced in organs called **gonads**. Gonads are considered primary or *essential sex organs*. They are also responsible for producing hormones. The other organs in the reproductive system are secondary or *accessory organs*.

Testis

The primary reproductive organs in the male are the **testes**. Each **testis** is oval and measures about 1.6 inches (4 cm) long and 1 inch (2.5 cm) wide. The testes are surrounded by a white, fibrous capsule and are suspended together in a sac outside the body called the *scrotum*. Testes produce the gametes called **spermatozoa**. Spermatozoa are made up of three parts (Figure 42.14):

- *Head*: Contains the chromosomes in the nucleus; the acrosome covers the head of the sperm and contains enzymes to help penetrate the ovum.
- *Midpiece*: Contains mitochondria, which produce energy for movement.
- *Tail* or *flagellum*: Used for movement.

Spermatogenesis

The formation of sperm is called *spermatogenesis*. The spermatozoa are formed in a series of tightly coiled tiny tubes in each testis

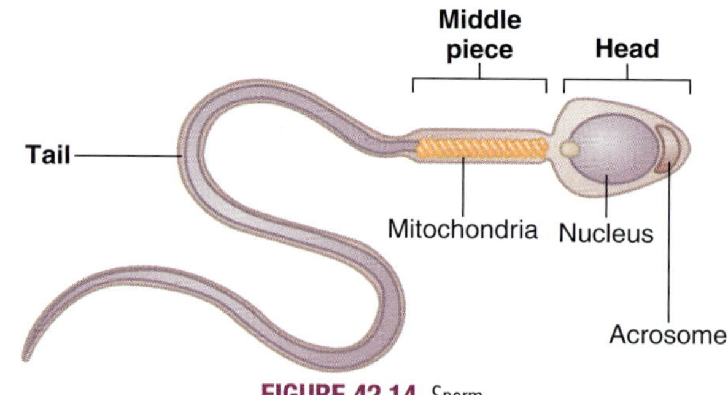

FIGURE 42.14 Sperm.

called the *seminiferous tubules*. From the seminiferous tubules, the formed spermatozoa travel to the *epididymis*, where they mature and are stored. The epididymis is a coiled tube almost 20 feet (6 meters) long and rests on top of and behind each testis.

From the epididymis, the spermatozoa move into the *vas deferens* or *ductus deferens* (Figure 42.15). Each vas deferens is a muscular tunnel about 18 inches (45 cm) long that connects to the base of the epididymis and passes along the side of the testis. The vas deferens travels into the pelvic cavity to just behind the bladder. Spermatozoa can stay in the vasa deferentia for several months in an inactive state.

The *prostate gland* is the size of a walnut and is found below the bladder in males. It surrounds part of the urethra. The prostate is considered a reproductive organ but it also affects the urinary system. When the prostate increases in size (as with benign prostatic hyperplasia [BPH]), it can obstruct the urethra, blocking the urine flow.

The prostate gland, seminal vesicles, and Cowper glands (or bulbourethral glands) provide fluid either to nourish or aid in motility and lubrication. The sperm and the fluid together make up a substance called *semen*. The ejaculatory duct begins where the seminal vesicles join the vas deferens, and this "tube" joins the urethra.

CRITICAL THINKING APPLICATION **42.8**

To review the anatomy of the male reproductive system, Hannah is writing down the process of spermatogenesis, including all the structures needed from the formation of the sperm until it leaves the body in semen. Can you do the same?

Urethra and Penis

The urethra is found within the penis and transports the semen to the outside of the body. The urethra also transports urine to the outside of the body.

The body is the shaft of the penis. The penis is composed of three columns of highly vascular erectile tissue. There are two columns of *corpora cavernosa* and one of *corpus spongiosum* that fill with blood through the dorsal veins during sexual arousal. During ejaculation, the sperm exit through the glans penis, the tip of the penis. At birth, the glans penis is surrounded by a fold of skin called the prepuce or foreskin, which can be removed by circumcision.

PHYSIOLOGY OF THE MALE REPRODUCTIVE SYSTEM

Several hormones are involved in the male reproductive system, including testosterone, follicle-stimulating, and luteinizing hormones.

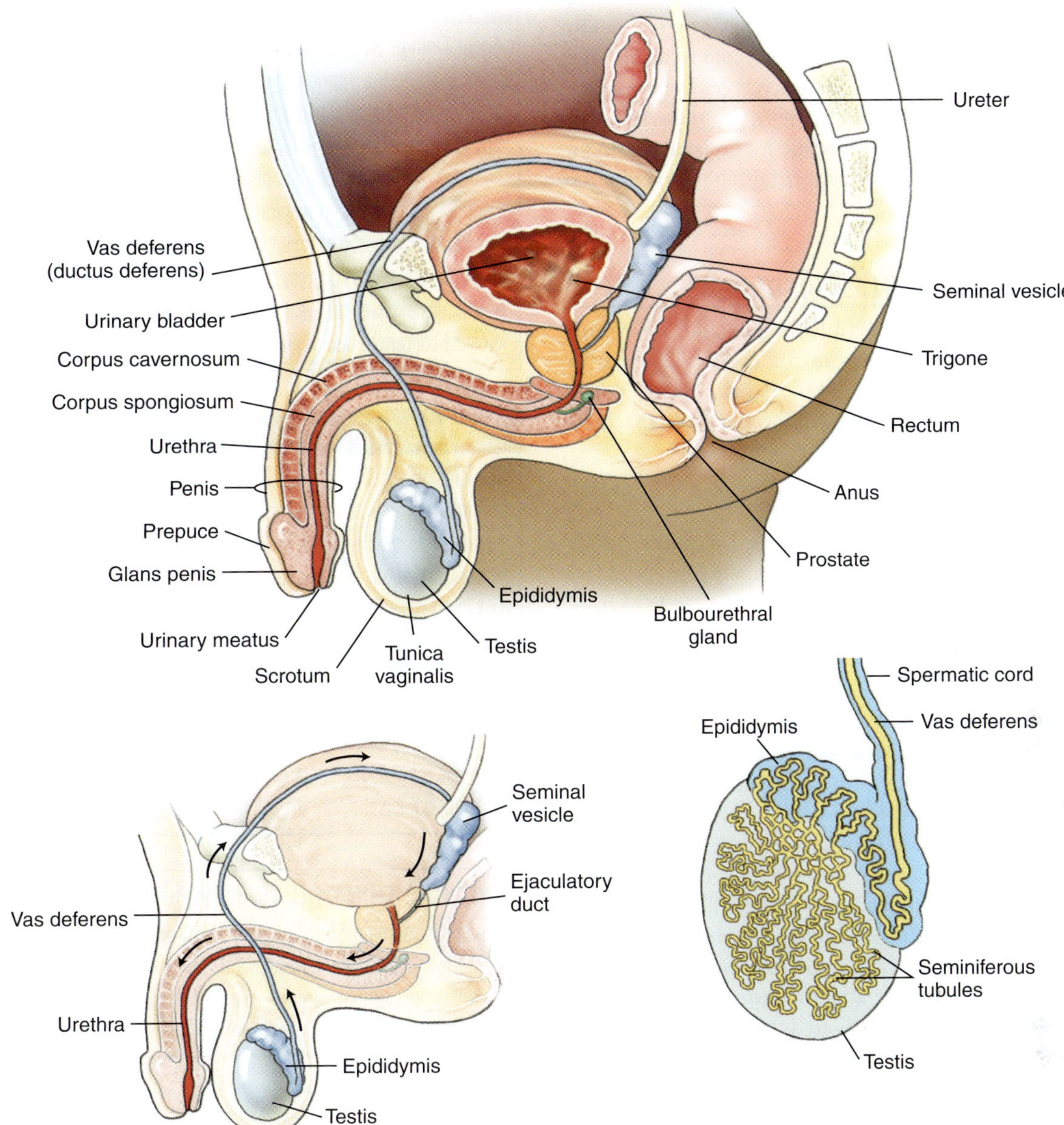

FIGURE 42.15 Male reproductive system with inset of sperm production. (From Shiland B: *Medical terminology & anatomy for ICD-10 coding*, ed 2, St. Louis, 2016, Mosby.)

Testosterone

At **puberty**, the **interstitial cells** in the testicles begin to produce **testosterone**. Testosterone is responsible for maintaining reproductive structures and for the development of sperm cells. Testosterone also helps with the development of secondary sex characteristics, which include a deep voice, broad shoulders, narrow hips, and additional body hair.

Follicle-Stimulating and Luteinizing Hormones

In addition to testosterone, *follicle-stimulating hormone* (FSH), secreted by the pituitary gland, promotes the formation of spermatozoa. The pituitary gland also produces *luteinizing hormone* (LH), which stimulates the interstitial cells to produce testosterone. Under the influence of these hormones, sperm cells develop and move into the epididymis to mature.

LIFE SPAN CHANGES OF THE MALE REPRODUCTIVE SYSTEM

The male reproductive system changes with age. The following sections discuss the changes to the male reproductive system over the life span.

Changes with Puberty

The testicle develops in the abdomen and starts its descent into the scrotum in utero around the seventh month. At puberty, usually between ages 9 to 15, the pituitary gland secretes luteinizing hormone, which stimulates the testicles to start producing testosterone. Testosterone is responsible for the development of sperm and the secondary sex characteristics. The male secondary sex characteristics include a deep voice, broad shoulders, narrow hips, and additional body hair.

Changes in Older Adults

As a male gets older, gradual aging changes begin. Changes occur in the testicular tissue, sperm production, and erectile function. The testicular tissue mass decreases. Testosterone levels gradually decrease and may cause issues with erections. The testes continue to create sperm but at a slower rate. Benign prostatic hyperplasia can occur, leading to issues with urine retention, ejaculation, and a slowed urine stream.

MALE REPRODUCTIVE SYSTEM DISORDERS

Common male reproductive disorder signs and symptoms include redness, swelling, or lumps in the organs. Changes in the urinary stream or issues during sexual intercourse (copulation) can also be seen. The following sections discuss male reproductive disorders.

Cancers of the Male Reproductive System

The most common cancers of the male reproductive system include prostate and testicular cancer. Penile cancer is a rare form of cancer and is highly curable in the early stages.

Prostate Cancer

Prostate cancer is one of the most common cancers among males, and the survival rate is very high. With prostate cancer, the gland can increase in size, obstruct the urethra, and cause additional urinary complications. About 1 in 8 men will be diagnosed with prostate cancer.

Cells in the prostate gland mutate, causing cancer. The risk for prostate cancer is increased in men over 60 years of age, African Americans, or those with a family history of the disease. Having a brother or father with the disease doubles the risk. The risk for the aggressive form of prostate cancer is increased in men who are tall, obese, lack exercise, have a family history of the disease, are African American, consume a high intake of calcium, and have been exposed to Agent Orange. Prostate cancer tends to be a silent disease in the early stages. It is not until the cancer grows large enough to obstruct the urethra that symptoms are noticeable. Advanced prostate cancer presents the following signs and symptoms:

- Problems with urination: slow, weak stream; frequency, nocturia
- Hematuria, blood in the semen
- Difficulty getting an erection
- Hip pain, back pain
- Loss of bladder or bowel control

The provider completes a DRE during the examination, and a PSA blood test is done. If the DRE is abnormal or the PSA blood test level has increased from the baseline, a needle biopsy of the prostate may be done. If cancer is detected, additional imaging tests will be ordered to determine the extent of the cancer. Treatment will be based on the type of prostate cancer. With nonaggressive cancers, the provider may suggest frequent checks to monitor the cancer growth. For aggressive prostate cancers, a prostatectomy and radiation may be done.

Agent Orange

Agent Orange was an herbicide used by the US military to remove dense foliage during the Vietnam War. It is presumed that any veteran who served in Vietnam was exposed to Agent Orange. The Veteran's Administration has attributed several diseases to Agent Orange. These diseases include diabetes mellitus, Hodgkin disease, multiple myeloma, hypothyroidism, Parkinson disease, and respiratory, bladder, and prostate cancers.

Veterans exposed to Agent Orange have a higher risk of developing prostate cancer, especially the aggressive form. Screening for prostate cancer is important in veterans exposed to Agent Orange. Male children of veterans with aggressive prostate cancer are also at greater risk of developing prostate cancer.

Prostate-Specific Antigen Blood Test

The prostate-specific antigen (PSA) blood test is used as a screening tool for prostate cancer. Both normal and cancerous prostate cells make the protein PSA. Often PSA levels increase in the blood when one has prostate cancer, prostatitis, or benign prostatic hyperplasia (BPH). Males are recommended to have a baseline PSA test at the age of 40. If the patient has an increased risk, the provider may decide to get a baseline PSA test earlier than age 40. The provider then checks the PSA level over time by comparing it to the baseline level. The higher the PSA level, the more likely it is the patient has prostate cancer. However, because the PSA level can be elevated with other disorders, one abnormal screening value is not enough to diagnose cancer. The reliability of the PSA blood test is debated, but it is the only screening tool available at this time.

CRITICAL THINKING APPLICATION **42.9**

Hannah is rooming Sam Fox, a 40-year-old father of three children. He is 6 feet tall. When Hannah obtains a family history on Sam, she learns that his father, a Vietnam veteran, was just diagnosed with aggressive prostate cancer. What risk factors does Sam have for prostate cancer?

Testicular Cancer

Testicular cancer is rare and highly treatable. It is the most common cancer in males between 15 and 35 years of age. It is more common in men with abnormal testicle development, an undescended testicle, and a family history of the cancer.

Many causes of testicular cancer are unknown. The patient usually discovers a lump or swelling in the testicle. There may also be complaints of a heavy sensation in the scrotum. The patient may also experience pain in a testicle, the scrotum, abdomen, or groin.

To determine if a lump is testicular cancer, a provider may order the following:

- Ultrasound and CT scan
- Biopsy of testicular tissue
- Blood tests to check the testicular cancer markers (alpha fetoprotein [AFP], beta-human chorionic gonadotropin [beta-hCG], and lactate dehydrogenase [LDH])

Treatment consists of surgery to remove the testicle (*radical inguinal orchiectomy*), radiation therapy, and chemotherapy.

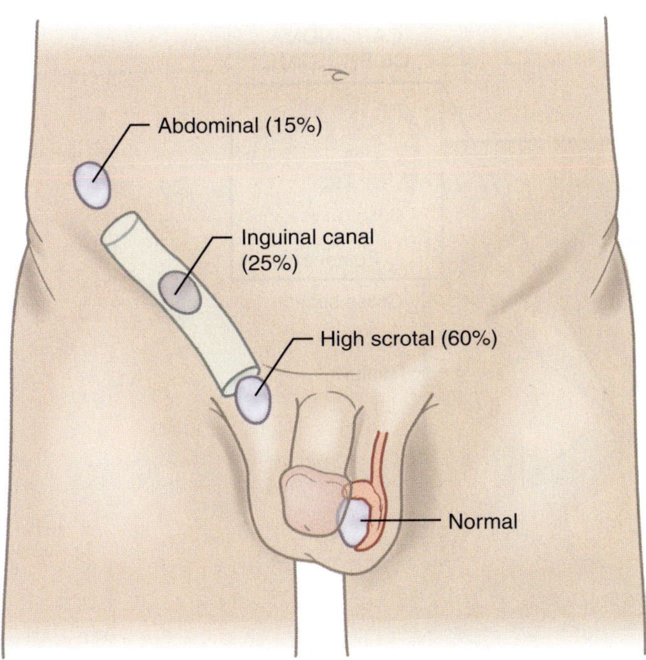

FIGURE 42.16 Cryptorchidism.

Congenital Male Reproductive System Diseases and Disorders

Several types of congenital conditions can affect the male reproductive system:

- *Anorchism*: The absence of one or both testes at birth
- *Chordee*: Downward curve of the penis due to a congenital condition such as hypospadias
- *Cryptorchidism*: Also called undescended testicle, or the testicle fails to descend into the scrotum (Figure 42.16); the testicle develops in the abdomen and starts its descent into the scrotum in utero around the seventh month; treatment for this condition consists of gonadotropic hormones and surgery (*orchiopexy*)
- *Epispadias*: Congenital malformation causing the urethra to open on top of the penis
- *Hypospadias*: Congenital malformation causing the urethra to open on the underside of the penis
- *Hydrocele*: Fluid-filled sac in the scrotum, common in newborn infants and may go away in a few months (Figure 42.17); often caused by an inguinal hernia
- *Phimosis*: Tightening of the penile foreskin that may result in the closure of the urethra opening, and the foreskin may not retract

Inflammatory Male Reproductive System Diseases and Disorders

Several types of inflammatory conditions can affect the male reproductive system:

- *Balanitis*: Inflammation of the head and foreskin of the penis
- *Epididymitis:* Inflammation of the epididymis; often caused by a bacterial infection that starts in the bladder, prostate, or urethra
- *Orchitis:* Inflammation of one or both testicles, usually caused by bacteria or viruses (e.g., mumps)
- *Prostatitis:* Inflammation of the prostate that can obstruct urinary flow

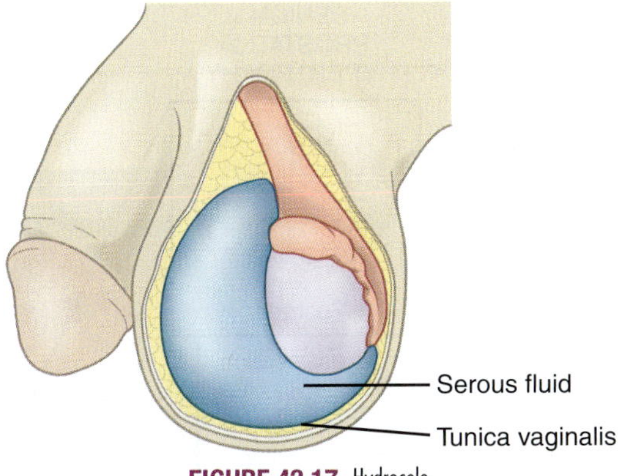

FIGURE 42.17 Hydrocele.

Structural and Functional Male Reproductive System Diseases and Disorders

Benign prostatic hyperplasia, erectile dysfunction, and male infertility are the most common structural and functional male reproductive disorders. The following sections describe these conditions along with additional disorders.

Benign Prostatic Hyperplasia

Benign prostatic hyperplasia (BPH) is a nonmalignant condition seen in about half of men over the age of 50 and more than 90% of men in their 70s and 80s.

As men age, the cells of the prostate gland surrounding the urethra can start to reproduce more rapidly, causing the organ to enlarge (*hyperplasia*). The enlarged prostate compresses the urethra, causing urgency, frequency, difficulty starting urination, urine retention, dribbling, hematuria, and repeated UTIs.

During the physical exam, the provider will do a digital rectal exam (DRE) by inserting a gloved finger in the rectum to palpate the prostate (Figure 42.18). Blood tests (e.g., prostate-specific antigen [PSA], tests of kidney function), urinalysis, transrectal biopsy, urodynamic tests, and cystoscopy may also be done. Treatments include the following:

- *Lifestyle changes*: Bladder training, avoiding caffeine and alcohol, and preventing constipation.
- *Medications*: Used independently or combined with other medications:
  - *Alpha-blockers*: Relax the smooth muscles of the prostate and the bladder neck to improve urine flow and reduce the blockage. Examples include terazosin, doxazosin (Cardura), tamsulosin (Flomax), alfuzosin (Uroxatral), and silodosin (Rapaflo).
  - *5-Alpha reductase inhibitors*: Prevent growth of or shrinks the prostate. Examples include finasteride (Proscar, Propecia) and dutasteride (Avodart).
- *Transurethral resection of the prostate (TURP) surgery*: A lighted scope is inserted into the urethra, and all but the outer part of the prostate is removed.
- *Laser therapy*: A high-energy laser is used to destroy the overgrown prostate tissue.

CRITICAL THINKING APPLICATION **42.10**

Hannah is working with Mr. Endl, who has BPH. He asks Hannah why the BPH impacts his urine flow. How should Hannah respond to Mr. Endl?

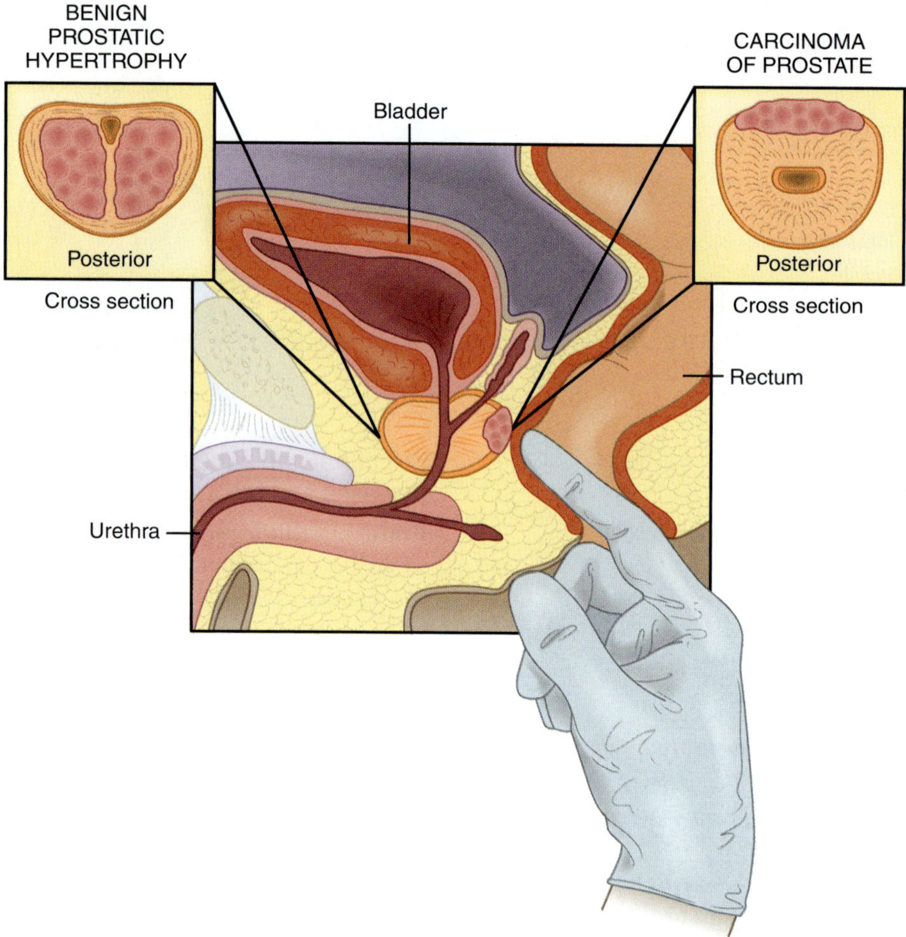

FIGURE 42.18 Digital rectal exam (DRE).

Erectile Dysfunction

Erectile dysfunction (ED), also called *impotence,* occurs when a male has trouble keeping or getting an erection. ED is an ongoing issue that impacts relationships, affects males' self-confidence, and can cause stress.

Common conditions that lead to ED include heart disease, hypertension, tobacco use, alcoholism, diabetes, metabolic syndrome, Parkinson disease, prior pelvic surgeries and treatments, obesity, depression, and stress. Male arousal involves hormones, emotions, muscles, blood vessels, nerves, and the brain; thus any change in these may lead to ED. The sign of ED is trouble keeping or getting an erection firm enough for intercourse.

After the physical exam, the provider may order tests to identify the cause of ED. Treatment consists of a healthy lifestyle and oral erectile dysfunction medications, including avanafil (Stendra), sildenafil (Viagra, Revatio), tadalafil (Adcirca, Cialis), and vardenafil (Levitra, Staxyn).

Male Infertility

Infertility is defined as not getting pregnant after 1 year or longer of unprotected sex. In about one-third of couples dealing with infertility issues, the cause is male infertility.

In about half of the male infertility cases, the cause is unknown. Known causes of infertility include infections, undescended testicles, inherited disorders, dilated veins around the testicle *(varicocele),* hormone imbalances, and blockages preventing sperm movement. Sperm production can be affected by heat, chemicals, and toxins (e.g., heavy metals, industrial chemicals). Stress, depression, and using drugs, alcohol, and nicotine can also cause infertility.

The main sign is not being able to conceive a child. Other signs and symptoms can include problems with sexual function, testicular swelling or pain, recurring respiratory infections, an inability to smell, low sperm counts, and decreased body and facial hair.

The provider will do a complete medical history and physical exam. Additional diagnostic testing includes a semen analysis, hormone testing, testicular biopsy, and scrotal and transrectal ultrasounds. Treatments depend on the cause of infertility. Treatments may include surgery, antibiotics to treat an infection, hormone treatments, and assisted reproductive technology (ART), such as **in vitro fertilization.**

Additional Structural and Functional Male Reproductive Disorders

Additional structural and functional male reproductive disorders include the following:

- *Peyronie disease*: Thick scar tissue develops in the penis, causing it to bend
- *Priapism*: Painful erection that does not go away
- *Gynecomastia:* Enlargement of breast tissue in males caused by an estrogen and testosterone imbalance
- *Spermatocele:* A cyst-like mass filled with fluid and dead sperm cells; located in the epididymis

- *Testicular torsion:* Twisting of the spermatic cord, causing the blood supply to be blocked off from the testicles; may occur after an injury to the area
- *Varicocele:* Enlargement of the veins in the scrotum; may cause low sperm production and quality, leading to infertility

ASSISTING WITH AN EXAMINATION AND DIAGNOSTIC PROCEDURES

As with other physical examinations, a careful history provides the physician with valuable information. The medical assistant should ask specific questions to gather important information on the patient's chief complaint for the visit. For instance, if a patient states, "I think I have a bladder infection," the medical assistant should focus on what signs and symptoms the patient is experiencing and not just document what the patient stated. For this type of situation, the medical assistant may ask the following questions:

- What is occurring now? When did it start?
- Have you had a history of bladder infections?
- Are you experiencing pain or discomfort? Where? When?
- Any urgency or the need to go "now"? Are you going more frequently?
- Is there blood in the urine?
- Any fevers? Chills?

Remember to start with more open-ended questions; in other words, use questions that encourage the patient to answer in more than just one or two words. To get specific details, the medical assistant can ask questions that are closed ended or those that require one- or two-word answers, such as yes or no.

Testicular Self-Exam

According to the American Cancer Society, males at any age can develop testicular cancer. About 50% of those diagnosed are between 20 and 34 years of age. It is estimated that 1 in 263 males will get testicular cancer. If the cancer is found early (before it has spread), there is a good chance of a cure.

The American Cancer Society recommends that providers perform a testicular exam as part of a routine physical exam. Some providers recommend that after puberty (around age 15), males should do a monthly testicular self-exam (TSE) after a shower (Procedure 42.1). The medical assistant may be involved in coaching a patient on how to do a TSE. Procedure 42.1 discusses how to coach a patient on the TSE. It is helpful for the patient to have a brochure and practice the technique on a TSE model during the coaching session.

Assisting with Diagnostic Procedures

The medical assistant helps with diagnostic procedures by scheduling and preparing patients for these procedures. If tests require restrictions of food or fluids, the medical assistant should address the following points with the patient after talking with the provider:

- Can the patient have water prior to the test?
- Which medications should the patient take prior to the test, or when can the patient resume the current medications?

Table 42.4 describes common diagnostic procedures used for urinary and male reproductive conditions. The medical assistant may need to screen the patient for specific allergies, medications, and pregnancy prior to scheduling the procedure. For some procedures, a signed consent form is required. The patient should be

TABLE 42.4 Common Diagnostic Procedures Used for Urinary System and Male Reproductive Diseases and Disorders

PROCEDURE	DESCRIPTION	PATIENT PREPARATION
Cystoscopy and ureteroscopy	Cystoscopy is used to examine the urethra and bladder, and procedures like removing small tumors may be done. A cystoscope is inserted into the urethra and advanced into the bladder. Ureteroscopy can be done at the same time. A smaller endoscope is used to examine the ureters.	The patient may need to take antibiotics prior to the procedure. For procedures requiring sedation or general anesthesia, there will be food and liquid restrictions prior to the procedure. The patient will not be able to drive. A consent form will be completed prior to the start of the procedure. To help with discomfort, local anesthetic medications may be used to numb the urethra.
Digital rectal examination (DRE)	Done during the physical examination. The provider inserts a gloved, lubricated finger into the rectum to feel for abnormalities in the prostate, bladder, ovaries, or uterus. For urinary tract issues, the DRE may be done to check if the prostate gland is swollen and obstructing the urinary tract structures.	Done during the physical examination. No advance preparation usually required. The patient may feel some discomfort during the test. Usually, taking some deep breaths will help.
Dimercaptosuccinic acid (DMSA) scan	A renal scan that uses the radioisotope, technetium-99m dimercaptosuccinic acid (DMSA), to evaluate the kidneys. The function, shape, position, size, and scarring can be observed. The radioisotope is injected, and a gamma camera is used to take pictures of the kidney.	If sedation is required, there will be food and fluid restrictions prior to the test. The medical assistant should screen the patient for allergies. An IV will be inserted, and the tracer will be injected. The patient may need to wait 2 to 4 hours before the test can occur. During the test, the person must remain still in a prone position.

Continued

TABLE 42.4 Common Diagnostic Procedures Used for Urinary System and Male Reproductive Diseases and Disorders—continued

PROCEDURE	DESCRIPTION	PATIENT PREPARATION
Intravenous pyelogram (IVP)	Intravenous (IV) Iodine contrast is given. Then x-ray images will be taken to see how the kidneys filter the contrast from the blood. The test can provide information on the functioning of the kidneys, bladder, and ureters.	The medical assistant will screen the patient for allergies (especially to iodine and shellfish), pregnancy, and a history of any reaction to x-ray dyes. Food and fluid restrictions prior to the test may be required. An IV will be placed, and the patient will need to be in a supine position on the exam table. The patient may be asked to urinate during the exam.
Postvoid residual (PVR) urine test	Measures the amount of urine in the bladder after urination. A straight catheter can be inserted to drain the remaining urine so the volume can be measured, but this procedure can increase the risk of urinary tract infections (UTIs). A portable ultrasound unit can also be used as a noninvasive test. The scan identifies the urine left, and the unit automatically calculates the volume of residual urine.	The patient will be asked to urinate prior to the test. The patient will experience some discomfort if a catheter is used for the test. With a catheter, the risk of a urinary tract infection increases. There is no discomfort if the test is done with a portable ultrasound unit.
Testicular exam	Done during the physical exam. The provider will check the penis, scrotum, and testicles for lumps, swelling, and other abnormalities.	No preparation is required.
Urodynamic testing	Using x-rays or ultrasound (US) scans, pictures or videos are taken as the bladder fills and empties. A catheter will be inserted in the bladder and contrast medium (for x-rays) or warm water (for the US scan) will be used to fill the bladder.	The patient will be asked to urinate prior to the test. During the test, the patient may have some discomfort as the catheter is inserted and the bladder is filled. After the test, the patient may experience some discomfort with urination and may need to take an antibiotic.
Voiding cystourethrogram (VCUG)	A minimally invasive test that involves fluoroscopy to visualize the urinary tract and bladder. Images are taken while the bladder is full and during urination. Contrast medium is used to help visualize the urinary structures on the x-ray image.	The patient may be asked to urinate prior to the test. Sedation may be used with children, and food and fluid restrictions prior to the test may be required. During the test, the patient may have some discomfort as the catheter is inserted and the bladder is filled. After the test, the patient may experience some discomfort with urination and may need to take an antibiotic.

notified of what they will experience during the procedure and any follow-up care required after the test. Table 42.5 lists common laboratory tests used for urinary and male reproductive conditions.

ASSISTING WITH TREATMENTS FOR URINARY AND MALE REPRODUCTIVE DISORDERS

Treatments for urinary and male reproductive disorders vary. The following sections examine treatments for both body systems.

Treatments for Urinary System Disorders

Common treatments used for urinary system disorders include the following:

- *Catheterization*: The insertion of a catheter to drain urine from the bladder. An indwelling catheter remains in, and a straight catheter is removed after the procedure.
- *Dialysis:* A technique in which filtration through a semipermeable membrane is used to remove metabolic wastes and extra fluid from the blood.
- *Extracorporeal shock wave lithotripsy (ESWL):* A nonsurgical approach that uses shock waves to break up stones in the ureters and kidneys.
- *Kidney transplantation:* Surgical transplantation of an entire kidney from a donor to a recipient.
- *Nephrectomy:* Surgical removal of a kidney. There are several types of surgical procedures:
    - *Partial nephrectomy*: Removal of cancer and surrounding tissue; kidney remains functional; used when the other kidney has been damaged or removed
    - *Simple nephrectomy*: Removal of the kidney
    - *Radical nephrectomy*: Removal of the kidney, adrenal gland, surrounding tissue, and local lymph nodes

TABLE 42.5 Medical Laboratory Tests for Urinary System and Male Reproductive Diseases and Disorders

TEST(S)	DESCRIPTION
Blood urea nitrogen (BUN)	Urea is a waste product in the blood that is filtered out by the kidneys. If the kidney function is abnormal, the blood level of urea will be increased.
Creatinine and creatinine clearance	Creatinine is a waste product from normal muscle breakdown. Creatinine is filtered out of the blood by the kidneys. The blood creatinine level indicates kidney function. The creatinine clearance rate shows how the kidneys filter creatinine from the blood.
Hormone testing	Blood tests to measure the levels of testosterone and other hormones.
Prostate-specific antigen (PSA)	Blood test used as a screening tool for prostate cancer.
Semen analysis	Measures the number of sperm present. Provides information on any abnormalities in *motility* (movement) and *morphology* (shape) of the sperm.
Urinalysis (UA)	A urine sample is collected in a special container. The urine is analyzed in the lab for abnormal levels of substances. Some of the substances that may be found in urine include blood, ketones, bilirubin, glucose, protein, and nitrites. The urinalysis is a CLIA-waived test. Specific CLIA-waived tests are also available, including glucose and ketones.
Urine culture	A urine sample is collected in a special container. The urine is analyzed in the lab for bacterial growth over a period of days (usually 1–3 days). Specific bacteria grown in the sample will be listed on the urine culture report.
Urine culture and sensitivity (C&S)	A urine culture is done as discussed above. The sensitivity results indicate if the pathogen is susceptible or resistant to specific antibiotics.

CLIA, Clinical Laboratory Improvement Amendments.

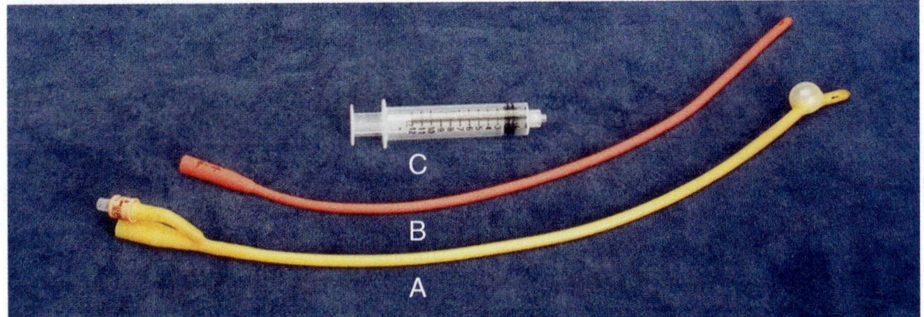

FIGURE 42.19 Urinary catheters. **(A)** Foley catheter with inflated balloon. **(B)** Straight catheter. **(C)** 12-mL Luer-Lok syringe used to inflate the balloon in the foley catheter. (From Proctor D, et al: *Kinn's the medical assistant*, ed 13, St. Louis, 2017, Elsevier.)

- *Nephrolithotomy:* A surgical incision of the kidney to remove a stone. The surgeon makes a small incision on the lower back to reach the kidney, and a nephroscope is inserted with other instruments to remove the stone. With *percutaneous nephrolithotripsy* (PNL), the stones are crushed and removed using suction.
- *Nephroureterectomy:* Surgical removal of the kidney and ureter.
- *Segmental resection of the ureter:* Surgical removal of the diseased section of the ureter; ureter is then reconnected.

Urinary Catheterization

A urinary catheter is a hollow, flexible tube that is inserted into the bladder through the urethra. It is used to collect urine. There are two primary types of urinary catheters (Figure 42.19A–B):

- An *indwelling Foley catheter* is used to help patients who are unable to ***void*** (urinate) on their own. It is placed with the tip in the bladder and left in place to allow urine to be removed from the body and drained in a collection bag. The tip of the catheter contains a balloon, which is filled using a syringe (Figure 42.19C). This holds the catheter in the bladder (Procedure 42.2). A coudé-tip catheter, which has a slightly curved tip, can be used if a person has an obstruction, such as enlarged prostate glands.
- A *straight catheter* is used to collect a sterile urine specimen. It is inserted into the bladder, a specimen is obtained, and then the catheter is removed (Procedure 42.3).

Some facilities and state statutes allow medical assistants to insert catheters. The medical assistant must use the correct-sized catheter to prevent tissue damage. Catheter sizes are measured in French gauge (Fr). Pediatric patients generally use 9-12 Fr, and adults may use 12-18 Fr catheters. The medical assistant should check with the provider if there is a question on the size of catheter to use. It is critical that the medical assistant insert the catheter using sterile technique to minimize the risk of a urinary tract infection (UTI).

Discontinuing Indwelling Catheters. Depending on the state statutes and the facility's policy, the medical assistant may discontinue indwelling catheters. Sometimes after an indwelling catheter is removed, the patient may have *urinary retention* (inability to void) or void small amounts, not emptying the bladder as normal. The patient may experience the following:

- Abdominal discomfort and pain
- If voiding, a weak stream, voiding small amounts
- Urinary incontinence

Patients should be instructed to monitor when and how much they void. Usually, a person should void 6 hours after the removal of an indwelling Foley catheter. Patients who suspect an issue should call the provider immediately.

Treatments for Male Reproductive Disorders

Common treatments used for male reproductive disorders include the following:

- *Circumcision:* Surgical removal of the foreskin (or *prepuce*) of the penis. (Commonly done on infants due to parental choice and unrelated to the treatment of disease. Studies have found male circumcision reduces the rate of certain sexually transmitted infections.)
- *Laser therapy:* A high-energy laser is used to destroy overgrown tissues, such as prostate tissue.
- *Prostatectomy:* Surgical removal of the prostate. With a *radical prostatectomy*, the prostate, nearby lymph nodes, and tissue, including the seminal vesicles, are removed.
- *Orchidectomy:* Surgical removal of the testicle.
- *Orchiopexy:* Surgical procedure for an undescended testicle (cryptorchidism). The testicle is brought down and implanted in the scrotum.
- *Transurethral resection of the prostate (TURP) surgery:* A lighted scope is inserted into the urethra, and all but the outer part of the prostate is removed.
- *Vasectomy:* A surgical procedure in which the vasa deferentia are cut, tied, and cauterized for the purpose of male sterilization.

Vasectomy

A vasectomy is a surgical procedure that is considered a permanent form of male birth control. The procedure involves cutting and sealing the vas deferens, which carry the sperm from the testicles. A vasectomy offers no protection from sexually transmitted infections.

The patient must stop taking any over-the-counter and prescription medications that may prevent blood clotting, such as aspirin, ibuprofen (Motrin, Advil), and anticoagulants (heparin, warfarin [Jantoven], enoxaparin [Lovenox]). The patient should shower the morning of the procedure, washing the genital area thoroughly. The provider may have the patient bring an athletic supporter or a pair of tight-fitting underwear to wear after the procedure to support the scrotum and minimize swelling at the site. The patient will not be able to drive after the procedure. A consent form needs to be signed after the provider discusses the procedure and alternatives with the patient.

Vasectomies are done in the ambulatory care facility, usually in urology or family medicine departments. They can also be done in ambulatory surgical centers under local anesthesia. The procedure may take about 30 minutes.

During the procedure, the provider will inject a local anesthetic into the skin of the scrotum. A small incision or a small puncture is made in the scrotum. The provider will locate the vas deferens and withdraw part of the tube through the incision or puncture. The vas deferens are cut and sealed either by tying it, cauterizing it with heat, or applying surgical clips (Figure 42.20). The provider returns the ends of the vas deferens into the scrotum and may close the hole with glue or stitches.

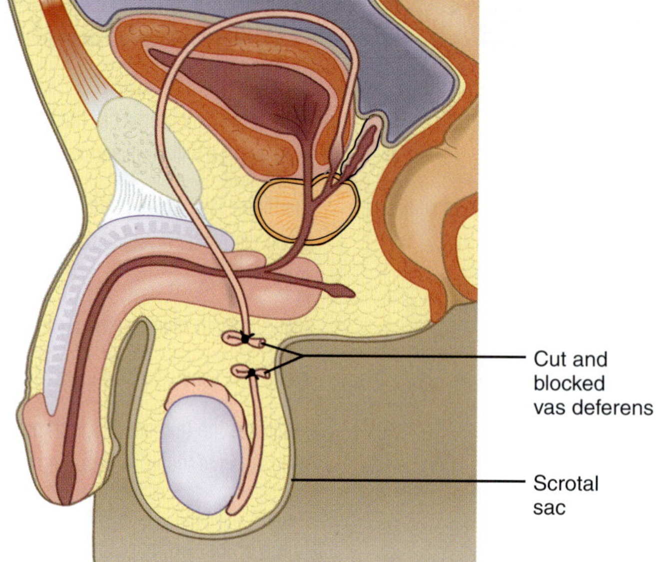

FIGURE 42.20 Vasectomy.

After the procedure, the patient will experience swelling, pain, and bruising in the area. Applying ice packs, limiting activity, and wearing tight-fitting underwear for 48 hours can minimize the pain and swelling. Sexual activity is limited for at least 1 week.

It is important for the patient to follow up with the provider. The provider will do a follow-up semen analysis 6 to 12 weeks after the surgery to ensure that no sperm exist in the semen. It is recommended that men use an alternative form of birth control during this period.

A vasectomy reversal can undo a vasectomy by reconnecting the vas deferens. Success rates range from 40% to 90%. The surgery is usually done in an ambulatory-care surgery center using general anesthesia.

Medications

Patients with urinary conditions are prescribed a variety of medications. The following are some of the more common classifications of medications for urinary conditions:

- *Antibiotic*: Destroys or inhibits the growth of bacteria. Used to treat bacterial infections.
- *Anticholinergic*: Stimulates the bladder to contract, which helps with urination. Used to treat overactive bladder and urge incontinence.
- *Antimuscarinic*: Relaxes the bladder muscle and decreases bladder contraction. Used to treat overactive bladder.
- *Diuretic*: Used to treat a variety of diseases such as hypertension; increases urinary output.
- *Electrolyte*: Used to treat certain diseases; may also be used in combination with other medications, such as diuretics.
- *Erectile dysfunction agent*: Used to facilitate an erection in patients with erectile dysfunction (impotence) and symptoms of benign prostatic hypertrophy (enlarged prostate).

Refer to Table 42.6 for information on the medical classification, including indication for use, desired effect, side effects, adverse reactions, and generic and trade names. Medical assistants should be familiar with medications that are prescribed to patients.

TABLE 42.6 Medication Classifications

CLASSIFICATION	INFORMATION	GENERIC NAME (TRADE NAME)
Antibiotic	Indications for use: Treats bacterial infections. Desired effects: Kills or inhibits bacteria growth. Side effects and adverse reactions: Hypersensitivity reaction, gastrointestinal distress.	*Penicillins* • Amoxicillin (Amoxil, Moxtag) • Amoxicillin and clavulanic acid (Augmentin) *Cephalosporins* • Cephalexin (Keflex) • Cefuroxime (Ceftin) *Macrolides* • Erythromycin (Ery-Tab, Erythocin) • Clarithromycin (Biaxin) • Azithromycin (Zithromax, Zithromax Z-Paks, Zmax) *Fluoroquinolones* • Ciprofloxacin (Cipro) • Levofloxacin *Sulfonamide* • Co-trimoxazole (Bactrim, Septra) • Trimethoprim (Primsol) *Tetracyclines* • Tetracycline (Achromycin V) • Doxycycline (Doryx, Oracea, Vibramycin) *Aminoglycosides* • Gentamicin • Tobramycin (Tobrex)
Anticholinergic	Indications for use: Dry secretions before surgery; prevents bronchospasm. Desired effects: Parasympathetic blocking agents; reduce spasms in smooth muscles. Side effects and adverse reactions: Blurred vision, confusion, reduced gastrointestinal and genitourinary motility, dilation of pupils, fever, flushing, headache, increased heart rate.	• Dicyclomine (Bentyl) • Propantheline (Pro-Banthine) • Glycopyrrolate (Cuvposa)
Antimuscarinic	Indications for use: Treats overactive bladder. Desired effects: Relaxes the bladder muscles. Side effects and adverse reactions: Blurred vision, dry mouth and eyes, gastrointestinal disturbances, headache, confusion, arrhythmias.	• Oxybutynin (Ditropan XL) • Solifenacin (VESIcare) • Fesoterodine (Toviaz) • Tolterodine (Detrol)
Diuretic	Indications for use: Increases urinary output; lower blood pressure. Desired effects: Inhibits reabsorption of sodium and chloride in the kidneys; promotes excretion of excess fluid in the body. Side effects and adverse reactions: Dehydration, muscle weakness, fatigue, electrolyte imbalance.	• Triamterene (Dyrenium) • Furosemide (Lasix) • Hydrochlorothiazide (Microzide, Oretic)
Electrolyte	Indications for use: Mineral supplement needed for certain diseases and medications. Desired effect: Maintains normal electrolyte level; proper functioning of the body systems. Side effects and adverse reactions: (depends on medication) confusion, listlessness, gray skin, black stools.	• Potassium (K-Tab, Klor-Con, K-Dur) • Ferrous sulfate (Feosol, Fer-in-Sol, Slow-Fe)
Erectile dysfunction agent	Indications for use: Facilitates an erection in patients with erectile dysfunction (impotence) and symptoms of benign prostatic hypertrophy (enlarged prostate). Desired effect: Facilitates an erection. Side effects and adverse reactions: Headache, flushing, nasal congestion, myalgia, prolonged erections, cerebrovascular accident (CVA), myocardial infarction (MI).	• Avanafil (Stendra) • Sildenafil (Viagra, Revatio) • Tadalafil (Cialis, Adcirca) • Vardenafil (Levitra, Staxyn)

CLOSING COMMENTS

Patient Coaching

Most men younger than 50 years of age have not seen a provider in years. Medical studies reveal that attitude, not biology, has a lot to do with the difference between men's and women's life spans. Men just do not go to the doctor as often as women do and tend to ignore symptoms of disease. The solution to maintaining good health is preventive care, and the first step is establishing a good rapport with a provider of choice. As a general rule, a man in good health should have three checkups in his 20s, three to four in his 30s, and a checkup every other year in his 40s. After the age of 50, a yearly checkup is recommended. In addition to testing for conditions such as cancer, heart disease, and diabetes, patient education can help male patients make responsible healthcare decisions.

The urinary system is a very private, personal part of the patient's body. Patients often feel embarrassed to ask questions about how to obtain the requested urine or semen sample. The medical assistant can provide this information in a sincere, confidential manner to relieve the patient's anxiety and worry. Diagrams, models, and handouts help the patient understand disease processes and treatments and encourage patient compliance.

Legal and Ethical Issues

When working in a urology office, the medical assistant must be very careful to ensure that patients have provided informed consent for ordered procedures. If the patient refuses a procedure, the assistant must have the patient sign the appropriate informed refusal forms, which are then included in the health record. All patient education should be done after the provider has completed the explanation and given the assistant instructions to do so. Never diagnose, prescribe, or offer comments about a patient's condition. Medical assistants who overstep their professional boundaries may place the provider and themselves in legal jeopardy. Remember that the patient who is legally informed and satisfied with the care received is less likely to take legal action.

Patient-Centered Care

Respecting a patient's preference is a key element of patient-centered care. When a medical assistant gathers a medical history on a patient regarding a male reproductive or a urology concern, the patient may hesitate to give information. These topics are sensitive, and the patient may only want to discuss concerns with the provider. Telling the patient, "If you would rather share the information with the provider, I will let them know," can show sensitivity. It is important for the medical assistant to respect the patient's wishes and help put the patient at ease.

Professional Behaviors

A urology practice manages many sensitive patient issues that require strict adherence to confidentiality guidelines. The Health Insurance Portability and Accountability Act of 1996 (HIPAA) protects the patient's confidential information, not just the paper or electronic records of that information. This means that verbal disclosure of a patient's information is limited to only the personnel who have the right to that information according to individual state laws.

SUMMARY OF SCENARIO

When Hannah started working with the urology team, she realized she knew very little about the urinary system. She had studied it during her medical assistant program but never appreciated what it might be like if her kidneys did not work. She was familiar with kidney cancer and UTIs but was amazed at all the other urinary diseases. As she learned more, she realized that hypertension (high blood pressure) could lead to kidney disease. She also figured out that kidney disease could lead to hypertension.

Looking back over the past weeks, Hannah realized that one of her favorite experiences was working with Mr. Rodgers. He had been on dialysis for the past 5 years and never had a vacation. He wanted to see his new grandson, who lived on the East Coast. Hannah found a dialysis unit in the city where he would be staying. She was able to get him scheduled for 2 weeks' worth of dialysis during his stay. She still can recall Mr. Rodgers' excitement when he realized he could do dialysis while on vacation. He started talking about other trips he was dreaming of taking.

Hannah is excited to continue her work with the urology team. She has learned so much in the short time she has worked with the patients.

SUMMARY OF LEARNING OBJECTIVES

1. **Examine the anatomy of the urinary system.**
   The urinary system is composed of two kidneys, two ureters, a urinary bladder, and a urethra. The kidneys are located posterior to the peritoneum, the muscles of the back, and between the T12 and L3 vertebrae. They filter the blood and eliminate waste through the passage of urine. The ureters move urine from the kidneys to the bladder. The urinary bladder, in the pelvic cavity, stores the urine until it is excreted. The urethra is the tube that conducts the urine out of the bladder.

2. **Examine the physiology of the urinary system.**
   The urinary system has several important roles that help regulate homeostasis in the body:
   - Maintains fluid volume
   - Maintains the normal composition of body fluids
   - Maintains an adequate blood pressure
   - Controls red blood cell production
   - Activates vitamin D

SUMMARY OF LEARNING OBJECTIVES—*continued*

Many of these roles are performed during the formation of urine. The body rids itself of unneeded substances produced during the metabolic process. The process of urine formation includes three steps:

- *Filtration*: During this phase in the glomerulus, substances from the blood such as electrolytes, waste products, and other substances move through the capillary wall into the filtrate.
- *Reabsorption*: This process starts as the filtrate moves out of the Bowman capsule and into the proximal tubule. Substances move from the filtrate back into the blood in the peritubular capillaries.
- *Secretion*: This process allows substances from the blood to move into the filtrate. This allows the body to maintain homeostasis and move unneeded substances back into the filtrate.

3. **Analyze the life span changes to the urinary system.**
When babies are born, they have the same number of nephrons as adults, though the nephrons are not mature until age 2. During childhood, the bladder continues to grow. Bladder control is usually learned between ages 2 and 3.

During pregnancy, the filtration rate increases in women. The number of nephrons remains the same, but the filtration surface increases. This increase allows the kidneys to filter more blood, which is useful with the increased blood flow during pregnancy. In late pregnancy, the bladder may be twice as big.

In older adults, the kidney tissue and number of nephrons are reduced by up to 20%. The renal arteries can harden, causing the kidneys to filter blood slower. The kidneys become less able to regulate water balance. Older adults are at more risk of dehydration when the weather is hot or if they have diarrhea. The bladder wall becomes less stretchy with age. The bladder cannot hold as much urine as before. Bladder muscles weaken. The urethra may be obstructed by an enlarged prostate gland or a prolapse of the bladder or vagina.

4. **Differentiate among the types of urinary system diseases and disorders, including the etiology, signs, symptoms, diagnostic procedures, and treatments.**
Common urinary signs and symptoms include the following: dysuria, nocturia, polyuria, frequency, urgency, urinary incontinence, and urinary retention. Typically, common signs of urinary system disorders found on medical imaging and laboratory tests include calculi, hydronephrosis, and azotemia. Abnormal substances in the urine include albuminuria or proteinuria (albumin), azoturia (excessive nitrogen compounds), bacteriuria (bacteria), glycosuria (glycose), hematuria (blood), and pyuria (pus).

Common urinary system disorders include bladder cancer, kidney cancer, polycystic kidney disease, acute cystitis, glomerulonephritis, pyelonephritis, chronic kidney failure, end-stage renal disease, nephrotic syndrome, neurogenic bladder, renal calculi, and urinary incontinence. Refer to the disease sections for more information regarding the signs, symptoms, etiology, diagnostic procedures, and treatments.

5. **Examine the anatomy of the male reproductive system.**
In the male reproductive system, the testes are surrounded by a white, fibrous capsule and are suspended together in a sac outside the body called the scrotum. The epididymis is a coiled tube that rests on top of and behind each testis. Each vas deferens connects to the base of the epididymis and passes along the side of the testis. The vas deferens travels into the pelvic cavity to just behind the bladder. The *prostate gland* is the size of a walnut and is found below the bladder in males. It surrounds part of the urethra.

The primary reproductive organs in the male are a pair of testes. Testes produce the gametes called spermatozoa. The prostate gland, seminal vesicles, and Cowper glands provide fluid either to nourish or aid in motility and lubrication. The sperm and the fluid together make up a substance called semen.

6. **Examine the physiology of the male reproductive system.**
At puberty, the interstitial cells in the testicles begin to produce testosterone. Testosterone is responsible for maintaining reproductive structures and for the development of sperm cells and secondary sex characteristics (e.g., deep voice, broad shoulders, narrow hips, and additional body hair).

In addition to testosterone, the follicle-stimulating hormone (FSH), secreted by the pituitary gland, promotes the formation of spermatozoa. The pituitary gland also produces luteinizing hormone (LH), which stimulates the interstitial cells to produce testosterone.

7. **Analyze the life span changes in the male reproductive system**
The testicle develops in the abdomen, start descending into the scrotum around the seventh month, and produce testosterone during puberty. As a male gets older, gradual aging changes begin. Changes occur in the testicular tissue, sperm production, and erectile function. The testicular tissue mass decreases. Testosterone levels gradually decrease and may cause issues with erections. The testes continue to create sperm but at a slower rate.

8. **Differentiate among the types of male reproductive diseases and disorders, including the etiology, signs, symptoms, diagnostic procedures, and treatments.**
Common male reproductive disorder signs and symptoms include redness, swelling, or lumps in the organs. Changes in the urinary stream or issues during sexual intercourse (copulation) can also be seen.

Common male reproductive system disorders include prostate cancer, testicular cancer, benign prostatic hyperplasia, erectile dysfunction, and male infertility. Refer to the disease sections for more information regarding signs, symptoms, etiology, diagnostic procedures, and treatments.

9. **Examine the medical assistant's role in examinations and diagnostic procedures for urinary and male reproductive diseases and disorders.**
As with physical examinations, a careful history provides the physician with valuable information, and the medical assistant should ask specific questions to gather important information on the patient's chief complaint for the visit.

The medical assistant can coach patients on doing the testicular self-exam. Procedure 42.1 outlines the steps followed to coach patients on the testicular self-exam. A TSE model and a brochure can be used to help with coaching. The patient should be given a TSE brochure to take home as a reference for the procedure.

Continued

SUMMARY OF LEARNING OBJECTIVES—*continued*

Diagnostic procedures for urology and male reproductive disorders include the following:

- *Cystoscopy*: Used to examine the urethra and bladder and for procedures like removing small tumors.
- *Ureteroscopy*: Can be done at the same time as cystoscopy. A smaller endoscope is used to examine the ureters.
- *Digital rectal examination (DRE):* The provider inserts a gloved, lubricated finger into the rectum to feel for abnormalities in the prostate, bladder, ovaries, or uterus.
- *DMSA scan:* A renal scan that uses the radioisotope, technetium-99m dimercaptosuccinic acid (DMSA), to evaluate the kidneys.
- *Intravenous pyelogram (IVP):* An intravenous iodine contrast is given, and then x-ray images are taken to see how the kidneys filter the contrast from the blood.
- *Postvoid residual (PVR) urine test:* Measures the amount of urine in the bladder after urination.
- *Urodynamic testing:* Using x-rays or US scans, pictures or videos are taken as the bladder fills and empties.
- *Voiding cystourethrogram (VCUG):* A minimally invasive test that involves fluoroscopy to visualize the urinary tract and bladder.

10. **Examine the medical assistant's role in treatments used for urinary and male reproductive diseases and disorders.**
    Treatments vary for the different diseases. Medications commonly prescribed in urology include antibiotics, antimuscarinics, diuretics, electrolytes, and erectile dysfunction agents. Vasectomies, a permanent form of male birth control, are also done in urology and family practice departments.

PROCEDURE 42.1 Coach a Patient on Testicular Self-Exam

TASKS: Coach a patient to do a testicular self-exam (TSE) while considering the patient's developmental life stage. Document your teaching in the patient's health record.

SCENARIO: You are working with Dr. David Kahn. For Truong Tran (DOB 05/30/19XX), he ordered testicular self-exam (TSE) coaching.

DIRECTIONS: Role-play this scenario with a peer, who will be the patient.

EQUIPMENT and SUPPLIES

- Testicular self-examination brochure (optional)
- Testicular model
- Provider's order
- Patient's health record

PROCEDURAL STEPS

1. Wash your hands or use hand sanitizer.
   PURPOSE: Hand sanitization is an important step for infection control.
2. Read the provider's order. Assemble the equipment.
   PURPOSE: It is important to know the provider's order before starting the procedure.
3. Greet the patient. Identify yourself. Verify the patient's identity with full name and date of birth. Explain the procedure to be performed in a manner that the patient understands. Answer any questions the patient may have about the procedure.
   PURPOSE: It is important to identify the patient in two different ways to ensure that you have the correct patient. Explaining the procedure can make the patient feel more comfortable and reduces anxiety.
4. Ask the patient what he knows about the self-exam. Clarify any inaccuracies. Build on the patient's prior knowledge of the topic during the session. Identify the patient's motivating factor for learning about the self-exam. Listen to the patient's concerns.
   PURPOSE: It is important to adapt the coaching to the patient's developmental stage. Because of the patient's age, identifying motivating factors is important.
5. Explain to the patient that the best time to do the self-exam is after a warm shower or bath.
   PURPOSE: The scrotal skin is more relaxed.
6. Demonstrate with the model while discussing the technique. Instruct the patient to examine each testicle gently with both hands. Roll the testicle between the thumb and fingers (Figure 1). Show the patient the epididymis, the soft curved structure behind and on top of the testicle (Figure 2). Then show the patient how to examine the vas deferens, which is the tube that runs up the epididymis (Figure 3).
   PURPOSE: This allows the person to do a better self-exam.

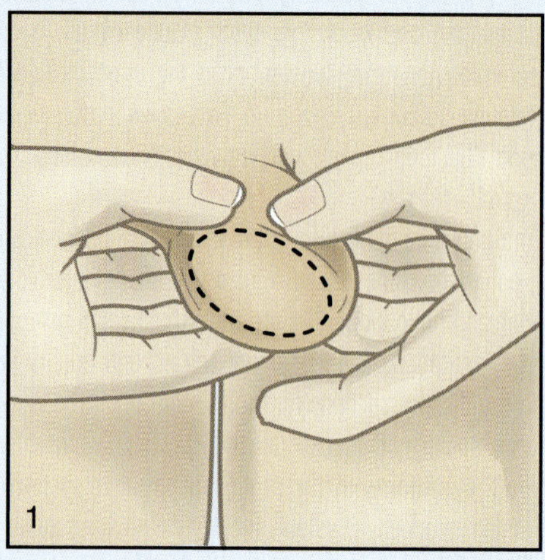

PROCEDURE 42.1 Coach a Patient on Testicular Self-Exam—*continued*

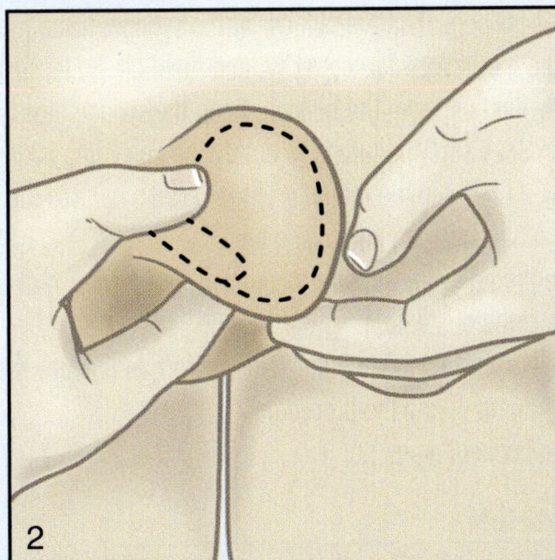

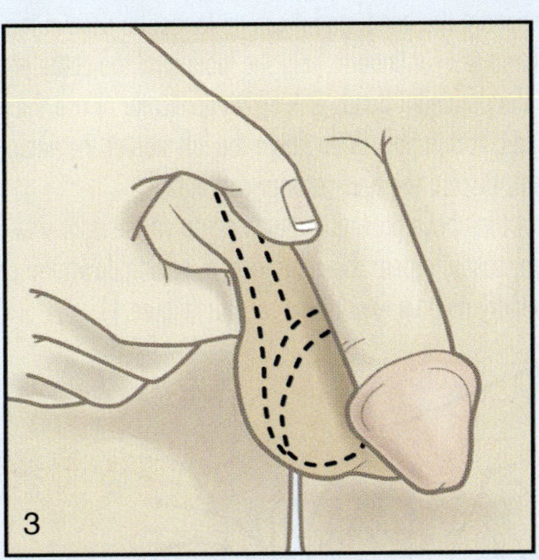

7. Instruct the patient to feel for any abnormalities and lumps. These could be painless or painful. Instruct the patient to look for changes in the size, texture, or shape.
   PURPOSE: Any changes should be reported to the provider for possible follow-up.
8. Have the patient demonstrate the technique on the model. Coach the patient on ways to improve the exam if needed.
   PURPOSE: It is important to have the patient demonstrate the teaching to check for accuracy of the technique and correct understanding.
9. Answer any questions the patient may have. Provide the patient with a brochure to take home (optional).
   PURPOSE: It is important to answer any questions the patient has and, if possible, provide him with a brochure to take home.
10. Document the patient education in the patient's health record. Include the provider's name, the order, what was taught, how the patient responded, how the patient did the demonstration, and any handouts provided.
    PURPOSE: It is important to document the patient education in the health record to show it was done.

Documentation Example

07/19/20XX 1505 Per Dr. Kahn's order, instructed pt on TSE. Instructed the patient on how to check for changes in the testes. Explained the technique and encouraged the patient to do monthly checks after a warm shower/bath. Pt provided an accurate return demonstration. His questions were answered. Gave pt the "TSE" brochure. ———————— Hannah Yang, CMA (AAMA)

PROCEDURE 42.2 Urinary Catheterization: Insert an Indwelling Foley Catheter

TASKS: Insert an indwelling catheter with a drainage bag using sterile technique. Remove an indwelling catheter. Document the procedures.

EQUIPMENT and SUPPLIES

- Patient's health record
- Gloves
- Waterproof pad (optional)
- Provider's order
- Straight catheterization tray kit containing the following items:
  - Waterproof pad
  - Fenestrated drape
  - Sterile gloves
  - Presaturated antiseptic applicators or antiseptic solution (povidone-iodine or chlorhexidine), sterile cotton balls, and sterile forceps
  - Water-soluble lubrication jelly packet or syringe
  - Indwelling urethral catheter connected to a urine drainage bag
  - Prefilled syringe with fluid
- Mayo stand
- Catheterization training model
- Waste container and biohazard waste container
- Disinfectant wipes for cleaning

PROVIDER'S ORDER

Insert Foley catheter.

PROCEDURAL STEPS

1. Wash your hands or use hand sanitizer. Read the provider's order. Assemble the necessary supplies.
   PURPOSE: A provider's order is required to insert a Foley catheter.
2. Greet the patient. Identify yourself. Verify the patient's identity with full name and date of birth. Explain the procedure to be performed in a manner that the patient understands. Answer any questions the patient may have about the procedure.

Continued

PROCEDURE 42.2 Urinary Catheterization: Insert an Indwelling Foley Catheter—*continued*

PURPOSE: It is important to answer the patient's questions before starting a procedure.

3. Place a waterproof pad on the lower part of the examination table. Provide a drape for the patient. Instruct the person to remove clothing from the waist down and sit on the examination table with the drape covering the patient's lap. Give the patient privacy.
   PURPOSE: To ensure cooperation during the procedure. Having the patient disrobe will allow access to the perineal area.
4. Before entering the room, give a courtesy knock. Ensure adequate lighting.
   PURPOSE: Adequate lighting is necessary to safely complete the procedure.
5. Position the patient. Place a drape to cover the patient and expose only the required anatomic areas.
   Female patient: On the back with the knees flexed and the thighs relaxed, so the hips rotate to expose the perineal area.
   Male patient: Supine with the legs extended and slightly apart.
   PURPOSE: This provides access to the urethra.
6. Put on gloves. Open the outer kit wrap.
   PURPOSE: Standard Precautions should be observed while cleaning the area and preparing the patient for the procedure.
7. Cleanse the perineal area with wipes from the kit or a washcloth, warm water, and soap or a perineal cleanser, according to facility policy.
   PURPOSE: Cleaning removes any secretions and reduces the risk of urinary tract infection (UTI).
8. Remove and dispose of gloves. Use hand sanitizer to perform hand hygiene.
9. Carefully open the catheterization kit, avoiding contaminating the sterile interior.
   PURPOSE: This will serve as your sterile field and keep supplies needed free of microbes.
10. Put on sterile gloves using sterile technique.
11. Using the waterproof pad from the kit, wrap the edges of the pad around your sterile gloved hands. Place it between the patient's legs, creating a sterile field.
    PURPOSE: Wrapping hands around the edges protects the sterile gloves from contamination.
12. Place the fenestrated drape on the patient, only exposing the perineum or penis.
    PURPOSE: This will provide a sterile surface around the patient, which works to minimize the risk of contamination of the supplies and the risk of UTI.
13. Working in the sterile field, prepare supplies. Open antiseptic applicators or open the antiseptic solution and pour it over the cotton balls. Open the lubricant packet or use the lubricant jelly syringe and place the water-soluble jelly on the tray. Remove the plastic upper tray from the bottom tray and place it nearby.
    PURPOSE: The upper plastic tray will remain as a sterile field.
14. In the lower tray, place the water-filled syringe to the inflation port on the catheter. If required by the facility's procedures, check the Foley catheter's balloon. Push the plunger of the syringe, filling the balloon. Make sure the balloon fills correctly, and there are no leaks or tears. Withdraw the fluid from the balloon. Keep the syringe attached to the catheter. Make sure the tubing to empty the Foley bag is closed.
    PURPOSE: Checking the integrity of the balloon reduces the risk of the catheter malfunctioning and falling out.
15. Lubricate the tip of the catheter about 1.5 to 2 inches. Make sure to keep the catheter sterile.
    PURPOSE: Lubricant will minimize discomfort and reduce the risk of urethral trauma during the procedure.
16. Clean the perineal area:

FEMALE PATIENT

- Separate the labia with the fingers of the nondominant hand; this will contaminate the hand, and it can no longer be used in the sterile field. This hand will continue to hold the labia until the catheter is inserted.
- With the dominant hand, pick up an applicator or use the forceps and pick up a cotton ball. Wipe down the left side of the vagina from top to bottom. Discard the applicator or cotton ball.
- Repeat the above procedure but wipe down the right side of the vagina. Lastly, repeat the same action, wiping down the center over the urinary meatus toward the rectum (Figure 1).

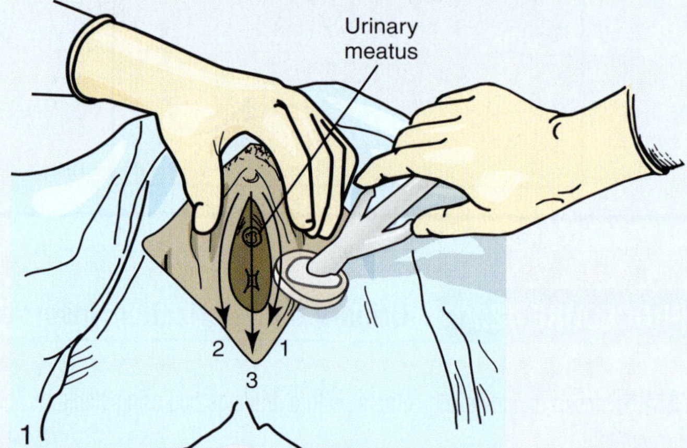

FIGURE 1 (From Laplant, N, Perry, AG, Potter, PA, and Ostendorf, WR: *Clinical nursing skills & techniques,* ed 10, St. Louis, 2022, Elsevier.)

MALE PATIENT

- Gently grasp the penis shaft and hold it at a right angle to the body with the nondominant hand. If the patient is uncircumcised, use this hand to gently retract the foreskin. (After the catheter is inserted, make sure to push the foreskin back to the original position.) This will contaminate the hand. This hand will continue to hold the penis until the catheter is inserted.
- With the dominant hand, pick up an applicator or use the forceps and pick up a cotton ball. Using the applicator or cotton ball, wipe the center of the urinary meatus and work outward in a circular manner (Figure 2). Discard the applicator or cotton ball. Repeat this cleaning technique two additional times, using a new applicator or cotton ball each time.

PROCEDURE 42.2 Urinary Catheterization: Insert an Indwelling Foley Catheter—*continued*

PURPOSE: This will reduce the number of microbes in the area of catheter insertion and minimize the transmission of microorganisms.

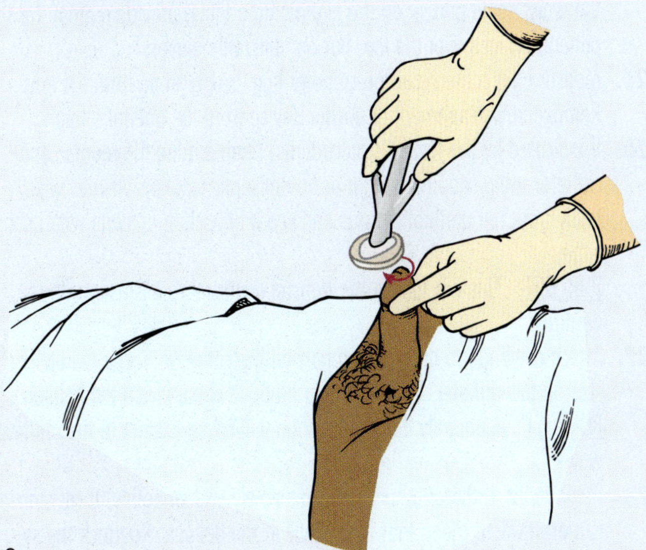

2

FIGURE 2 (From Laplant, N, Perry, AG, Potter, PA, and Ostendorf, WR: *Clinical nursing skills techniques*, ed 10, St. Louis, 2022, Elsevier.)

17. Pick up the catheter and the lower tray with the sterile dominant hand. Place the bottom tray between the patient's legs. Make sure hold the catheter approximately 2 to 3 inches from the tip.
PURPOSE: Holding the catheter closer to the tip will help control it during insertion. Holding it too close to the tip risks contaminating the sterile hand by touching the patient during insertion.

18. Insert the catheter. If you meet resistance while inserting the catheter, do not force it. Discontinue the procedure if continued resistance is met or the patient is having unusual discomfort or pain. Talk with the provider.

FEMALE

- Ask the patient to bear down gently to help expose the urethral meatus.
- Insert the catheter 2 to 3 inches into the meatus until urine starts to flow (Figure 3). Then advance the catheter an additional 1 to 2 inches to ensure it is in the bladder.
- Release the labia with the nondominant hand and hold the catheter in place as the dominant hand inflates the balloon. Disconnect the syringe and gently pull on the catheter until you feel resistance.

Note: If urine does not appear, the catheter may be in the patient's vagina. You may leave the catheter in place as a landmark and insert another sterile catheter into the urinary meatus. The catheter in the vagina is no longer sterile. Do not reuse that catheter. Do not allow the new catheter to come into contact with the previous catheter.

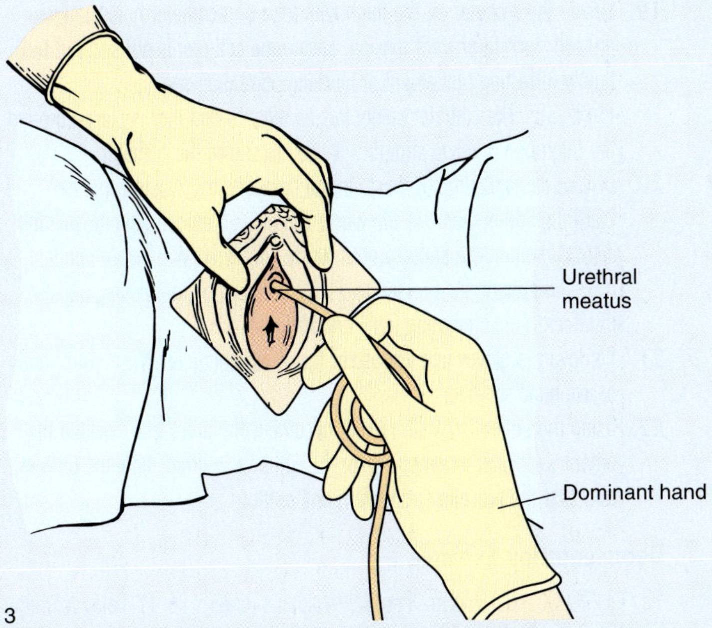

3

FIGURE 3 (From Stockert PA, Hall AM, Potter, PA, and Perry AG: *Essentials for nursing practice*, ed 9, St. Louis, 2019, Elsevier.)

MALE

- With the nondominant hand (which is holding the penis at a right angle to the body), pull up slightly on the shaft (Figure 4).
- Ask the patient to bear down gently and slowly insert the catheter through the urethral meatus. Advance the catheter 6 to 8 inches until urine flows. Then advance the catheter an additional 1 to 2 inches to ensure it is in the bladder.
- Hold the catheter in place with the nondominant hand while the dominant hand inflates the balloon. Disconnect the syringe and gently pull on the catheter until you feel resistance.

Note: If the catheter does not advance in the male patient, do not force it. The patient may have an enlarged prostate or urethral obstruction.

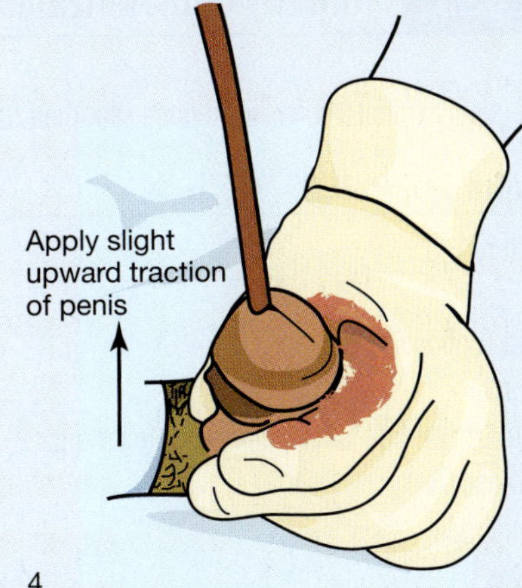

4

FIGURE 4 (From Stockert PA, Hall AM, Potter, PA, and Perry AG: *Essentials for nursing practice*, ed 9, St. Louis, 2019, Elsevier.)

Continued

PROCEDURE 42.2 Urinary Catheterization: Insert an Indwelling Foley Catheter—*continued*

19. Secure the catheter on the thigh with tape or a catheter holder. Allow enough slack to prevent tension. Ensure the catheter is not secured too tightly, affecting movement or blocking urine drainage.
    PURPOSE: The catheter holder has an elastic band that is placed around the thigh and a Velcro strip that is used to secure the catheter.
20. Discard all biohazardous waste in the biohazardous waste container. Discard all other waste in the waste container. Remove your gloves and discard them in the biohazardous waste container. Wash your hands. After the patient has dressed and left the room, put on gloves, and disinfect the examination table and Mayo stand.
21. Remove the gloves and dispose of them appropriately. Wash your hands or use hand sanitizer.
22. Using the patient's health record, document the procedure. Include the ordering provider's name, size of the catheter inserted, how the patient tolerated the procedure, and the urine output.

Documentation Example

12/11/20XX 10:10 a.m. Per Dr. Walden's order, 16 Fr Foley catheter inserted. Patient tolerated the procedure well with minimal discomfort. Within 5 minutes, 100 mL of clear, pale-yellow urine drained. Patient instructed on how to drain urine from bag and how to maintain Foley catheter system at home. ———————— Susie Rana, CMA (AAMA)

Scenario update: The patient returns for removal of the indwelling Foley catheter.

23. Wash your hands or use hand sanitizer. Read the provider's order. Assemble the necessary supplies. Place a waterproof pad on the lower part of the examination table.
    PURPOSE: A provider's order is required to remove a Foley catheter.
24. Greet the patient. Identify yourself. Verify the patient's identity with full name and date of birth. Explain the procedure to be performed in a manner that the patient understands. Answer any questions the patient may have about the procedure. Instruct the person to remove clothing from the waist down and sit on the examination table; provide a drape for the patient to place over the lap. Put on nonsterile gloves.
25. Measure the contents of the catheter bag. Empty urine from the bag. Remove any securement or anchor device from the patient's thigh.
26. If indicated by the facility's procedures, clean around the meatus and catheter using soap and water or an antiseptic solution. Always wipe away from the urethral meatus and use a new cloth or swab with each wipe.
    PURPOSE: This will reduce the transfer of microorganisms into the urethra.
27. Attach a syringe to the inflation port on the catheter. Verify the balloon size on the catheter. Withdraw that amount of fluid from the balloon.
    PURPOSE: A partially deflated balloon will cause trauma to the urethral wall.
28. Remove the catheter by pulling it out slowly and smoothly. If resistance is met, it might mean that fluid is still in the balloon. Reattach the syringe and pull back any remaining fluid. Continue to remove the catheter and wrap the used catheter in the waterproof pad.
    PURPOSE: This will prevent accidental spilling of urine from the catheter.
29. Discard waste in the appropriate waste containers. Wash or sanitize your hands. Using the patient's health record, document the procedure.

Documentation Example

12/28/20XX 10:10 a.m. Per Dr. Walden's order, indwelling Foley catheter removed. Patient tolerated the procedure well with minimal discomfort. Drained 250 mL of clear, pale yellow urine. ———————— Hannah Yang, CMA (AAMA)

PROCEDURE 42.3 Urinary Catheterization: Insert a Straight Catheter to Obtain a Urine Specimen

TASKS: Place a urinary catheter to collect a urine specimen using sterile technique and document the procedure.

EQUIPMENT and SUPPLIES

- Patient's health record
- Gloves
- Waterproof pad (optional)
- Provider's order
- Straight catheterization tray kit containing the following:
  - Waterproof pad
  - Fenestrated drape
  - Sterile gloves
  - Presaturated antiseptic applicators or antiseptic solution (povidone-iodine or chlorhexidine), sterile cotton balls, and sterile forceps
  - Water-soluble lubrication jelly packet
  - Specimen container with lid
  - Urethral catheter (properly sized)
  - Outer basin tray
- Specimen label
- Mayo stand
- Catheterization training model
- Waste container and biohazard waste container
- Disinfectant wipes for cleaning

PROVIDER'S ORDER

UA using a straight catheter for specimen collection.

PROCEDURE 42.3 Urinary Catheterization: Insert a Straight Catheter to Obtain a Urine Specimen—*continued*

PROCEDURAL STEPS

1. Wash your hands or use hand sanitizer. Read the provider's order. Assemble the necessary supplies.
   PURPOSE: A provider's order is required to gather a urine specimen by a straight catheterization.
2. Greet the patient. Identify yourself. Verify the patient's identity with full name and date of birth. Explain the procedure to be performed in a manner that the patient understands. Answer any questions the patient may have about the procedure.
   PURPOSE: It is important to answer the patient's questions before starting a procedure.
3. Place a waterproof pad on the lower part of the examination table (optional). Provide a drape for the patient. Instruct the person to remove clothing from the waist down and sit on the examination table with the drape over the patient's lap. Give the patient privacy.
   PURPOSE: To ensure cooperation during the procedure. Having the patient disrobe will allow access to the perineal area.
4. Before entering the room, give a courtesy knock. Ensure adequate lighting.
   PURPOSE: Adequate lighting is necessary to safely complete the procedure.
5. Position the patient. Place a drape to cover the patient and expose only required anatomic areas.
   Female patient: On the back with the knees flexed and the thighs relaxed, so the hips rotate to expose the perineal area.
   Male patient: Supine with the legs extended and slightly apart.
   PURPOSE: This provides access to the urethra.
6. Open the kit. Put on sterile gloves using sterile technique.
7. Using the waterproof pad from the kit, wrap the edges of the pad around your sterile gloved hands. Place the pad between the patient's legs, creating a sterile field.
   PURPOSE: Wrapping the hands around the edges of the pad protects the sterile gloves from contamination.
8. Working in the sterile field, prepare supplies. Open the antiseptic applicators or open the antiseptic solution and pour it over the cotton balls. Open the lubricant packet. Lubricate the tip of the catheter about 1.5 to 2 inches.
   PURPOSE: Lubricant will minimize discomfort and reduce the risk of urethral trauma during the procedure.
9. Clean the perineal area.

FEMALE PATIENT

- Separate the labia with the fingers of your nondominant hand. This will contaminate the hand, and it can no longer be used in the sterile field. This hand will continue to hold the labia until the catheter is inserted.
- With the dominant hand, pick up an applicator or use the forceps and pick up a cotton ball. Wipe down the center over the urinary meatus toward the rectum. Discard the applicator or cotton ball.
- Repeat the above but wipe down the right side of the vagina. Lastly, repeat the same action, but wipe down the center over the urinary meatus towards the rectum.

MALE PATIENT

- Gently grasp the penis shaft and hold it at a right angle to the body with the nondominant hand. If the patient is uncircumcised, use this hand to gently retract the foreskin. (After the catheter is inserted, make sure to push the foreskin back to the original position.) This will contaminate the hand. This hand will continue to hold the penis until the catheter is inserted.
- With the dominant hand, pick up an applicator or use the forceps and pick up a cotton ball. Using the applicator or cotton ball, wipe the center of the urinary meatus and work outward in a circular manner. Discard the applicator or cotton ball. Repeat this cleaning technique two additional times, using a new applicator or cotton ball each time.

PURPOSE: This will reduce the number of microbes in the area of catheter insertion and minimize the transmission of microorganisms.

10. Place the sterile collection cup in the sterile tray. Place the tray between the patient's legs. Place the end of the catheter in the sterile collection cup. Pick up the catheter with the sterile dominant hand approximately 2 to 3 inches from the tip.
    PURPOSE: The sterile cup will catch urine as it starts to flow. Holding the catheter closer to the tip will help control it during insertion. Holding the catheter too close to the tip risks contaminating the sterile hand by touching the patient during insertion.
11. Insert the catheter. If you meet resistance while inserting the catheter, do not force the catheter. Discontinue the procedure if continued resistance is met or the patient is having unusual discomfort or pain. Talk with the provider

FEMALE

- Ask the patient to bear down gently to help expose the urethral meatus.
- Insert the catheter 2 to 3 inches into the meatus until urine starts to flow.

Note: If urine does not appear, the catheter may be in the patient's vagina. You may leave the catheter in place as a landmark and insert another sterile catheter into the urinary meatus. The catheter in the vagina is no longer sterile. Do not reuse that catheter. Do not allow the new catheter to come into contact with the previous catheter.

MALE

- With the nondominant hand (which is holding the penis at a right angle to the body), pull up slightly on the shaft.
- Ask the patient to bear down gently and slowly insert the catheter through the urethral meatus. Advance the catheter 6 to 8 inches until urine flows.

Note: If the catheter does not advance in the male patient, do not force it. The patient may have an enlarged prostate or urethral obstruction.

12. Once the specimen is obtained, secure the cover on the container. Make sure not to touch the inside of the container or cover. Set the specimen container on the Mayo stand.

Continued

PROCEDURE 42.3 Urinary Catheterization: Insert a Straight Catheter to Obtain a Urine Specimen—*continued*

PURPOSE: The inner surface of the specimen container and cover are sterile and need to remain sterile.

13. Remove the catheter by pulling it out slowly and smoothly. Wrap the used catheter in the waterproof pad.
    PURPOSE: This will prevent accidental spilling of urine from the catheter.
14. Discard all biohazard waste in the biohazard waste container. Discard all other waste in the waste container. Remove your gloves and discard them in the biohazard waste container. Wash or sanitize your hands.
15. After the patient has dressed and left the room, put on gloves and disinfect the examination table and Mayo stand. Label the urine specimen.
16. Remove the gloves and dispose of them appropriately. Wash your hands or use hand sanitizer.
17. Using the patient's health record, document the procedure. Include the ordering provider's name, the size of the catheter inserted, how the patient tolerated the procedure, and the urine output.

Documentation Example

12/11/20XX 10:10 a.m. Per Dr. Walden's order, urine specimen obtained through use of 16 Fr straight catheter. Patient tolerated the procedure well with minimal discomfort. 50 mL of clear, pale-yellow urine obtained. Specimen sent to lab. ——————————— Hannah Yang, CMA (AAMA)

OBSTETRICS AND GYNECOLOGY 43

SCENARIO

Peggy St. John has been working in the obstetrics and gynecology (OB/GYN) department for about 5 years. She loves what she does and feels grateful that she can be there for her patients as they go through the pregnancy process. She also gets a lot of satisfaction from working with patients who come in with gynecologic issues. She especially likes the patient education that she can do with all her patients. Her supervisor recognizes that Peggy enjoys teaching and has asked her to mentor a medical assistant student, Jill Snow, who is just starting her practicum. Peggy is excited to share how she works with patients in the OB/GYN department.

While studying this chapter, think about the following questions:

- What is the basic anatomy and physiology of the female reproductive system?
- What does Jill need to learn about contraceptives to be able to answer patients' questions?
- Jill needs to become familiar with which gynecologic disorders?
- What are the primary malignancies of the female reproductive system?
- How should Peggy assist the provider with a Pap test?
- How can Peggy teach patients to perform breast self-examination?
- What are the stages of pregnancy and birth?
- How can Peggy help patients understand issues that can arise with menopause?
- What are the typical diagnostic procedures used in obstetrics and gynecology?

LEARNING OBJECTIVES

1. Examine the anatomy and physiology of the female reproductive system.
2. Analyze the life span changes that occur in the female reproductive system.
3. Examine the diseases and disorders of the female reproductive system.
4. Examine the cancers found in the female reproductive system.
5. Examine the medical assistant's role in assisting with examinations, diagnostic procedures, and treatments for the female reproductive system.
6. Examine the medical assistant's role in assisting with the obstetrical examination.

VOCABULARY

adhesions (ad HEE zhuns) Bands of scar tissue that can bind anatomic structures together.

amenorrhea (ey men uh REE uh) Lack of menstrual flow.

anencephaly (an en SEF uh lee) Congenital absence of part or all of the brain.

anovulation (an OV yuh ley shun) Failure of the ovaries to release an ovum at the time of ovulation.

Bartholin cyst (BAR thoh lin sist) A fluid-filled cyst in one of the vestibular glands located on either side of the vaginal orifice.

clitoris (KLIT uh ris) Sensitive, erectile tissue.

colposcopy (kol PAW skoh pee) Using a microscope with a light source, the vagina and cervix are visually examined to locate and evaluate abnormal cells. A biopsy of abnormal cells may be taken during this procedure.

cone biopsy An extensive cervical biopsy during which a cone-shaped wedge of tissue is removed from the cervix and examined under a microscope. Abnormal tissue, along with a small amount of normal tissue, is removed.

curettage (kyoo r I TAZH) A small, spoon-shaped instrument (curette) or a thin brush is used to scrape a tissue sample from the cervix.

cystic fibrosis (CF) A disorder that affects all the exocrine cells but affects the respiratory system the most. Mucus is abnormally thick and blocks the alveoli, causing dyspnea.

Down syndrome A genetic disorder in which abnormal cell division results in an extra chromosome 21.

dysmenorrhea (dis men uh REE uh) Painful menstrual flow, cramps.

dyspareunia (dis ph ROO nee ah) Painful or difficult intercourse.

ectopic pregnancy (eck TAH pick PREG nuhn se) Implantation of the embryo in any location other than the uterus.

gamete (GAM eet) A mature sexual reproductive cell; spermatozoa or ovum.

VOCABULARY—*continued*

gonads (GOH nadz) Organs that produce sex cells in both males and females.

hemophilia (hee moh FEE lee ah) A group of inherited blood disorders characterized by a deficiency of one of the factors necessary for the coagulation of blood.

hysterectomy Surgical removal of the uterus and cervix. The ovaries and fallopian tubes may also be removed.

labia majora (LAY bee ah muh JOR ah) The larger external folds of skin surrounding the opening of the vagina.

labia minora (LAY bee ah min NOR uh) The smaller inner folds of skin surrounding the opening of the vagina.

laparoscopy (lap ar AW scoh pee) A procedure used to visually examine the abdomen.

loop electrosurgical excision procedure (LEEP) After an anesthetic has been injected into the cervix, a high-frequency electrical current running through a wire is used to remove abnormal tissue from both the cervix and the endocervical canal.

lumpectomy (luhm PEK tuh mee) Removal of the breast tumor and a small amount of the surrounding tissue.

mastectomy (ma STEK tuh mee) Removal of the entire breast.

meningocele (meh NING goh seel) The protrusion of the meninges through an opening in the spinal column or skull.

menometrorrhagia (men oh meh troh RAH zsa) Excessive menstrual flow and uterine bleeding other than that caused by menstruation.

menorrhagia (men or RAH zsa) Abnormally heavy menstrual flow or prolonged menstrual periods.

necrosis (nuh KROH sis) Tissue death.

orifice (ORE ih fis) The vaginal opening.

osteoporosis (os tee oh phuh ROH sis) Abnormal thinning of the bone structure, causing bones to become brittle and weak.

ovulation (OV yuh ley shun) The release of the ovum from the ovarian follicle.

perineum (pair ih NEE um) The area between the opening of the vagina and the anus.

phenylketonuria (PKU) A deficiency in the enzyme phenylalanine hydroxylase, which is responsible for converting phenylalanine into tyrosine.

preeclampsia (pree eh KLAMP see ah) An abnormal condition of pregnancy of unknown cause, marked by hypertension, edema, and proteinuria.

purulent (PYOOR yoo lent) Pus like.

salpingo-oophorectomy (sal ping goh oh of or EK toh mee) Surgical removal of the fallopian tube and ovary.

sentinel node biopsy Removal of a limited number of lymph nodes to determine if the cancer has spread to the lymph nodes.

sickle cell anemia An inherited anemia characterized by crescent-shaped red blood cells (RBCs). It causes RBCs to block capillaries, reducing the oxygen supply to the cells.

spina bifida (SPY nah BIF id dah) A condition in which the spinal column has an abnormal opening that allows protrusion of the meninges or the spinal column.

symmetry (SIM i tree) Similarity in size, form, and arrangement of parts on opposite sides of the body.

viability Ability to live.

INTRODUCTION

The branch of medicine that deals with pregnancy, labor, and the postpartum period is known as *obstetrics*, and the branch of medicine that deals with diseases of the reproductive system in women is called *gynecology.* Frequently, a provider practices both specialties and is known as an *OB/GYN provider.* The assessment of the female reproductive system is an important part of healthcare. Patients are often hesitant and uncomfortable talking about sexual matters, so they wait until the symptoms are uncomfortable or the disease has advanced before they seek medical care. The medical assistant needs to be familiar with signs and symptoms of the diseases and conditions related to this specialty. In addition, the medical assistant must be aware of the patient's emotional state and must give support when needed.

In this chapter, we review the anatomy and physiology of the female reproductive system and diseases and disorders of the reproductive system. We will also discuss the medical assistant's role in gynecologic and obstetric procedures. A medical assistant has two roles in these situations:

- Assist the provider in any way needed
- Be there for the patient by helping her to be as comfortable as possible during her time in the healthcare facility

When we make patients feel comfortable, we help to establish a trusting relationship where patients will be able to share the information the provider needs in order to give them the best possible care.

ANATOMY AND PHYSIOLOGY OF THE FEMALE REPRODUCTIVE SYSTEM

The anatomy of the female reproductive system involves internal genitalia, external genitalia, and breasts. The gynecologic examination involves the assessment of each of those physical structures. The physiology of those structures can change depending on what is going on at the time. The anatomy and physiology of the female reproductive system are discussed in the following sections.

Anatomy of the Female Reproductive System

The anatomy of the female reproductive system can be divided into two parts. *Parenchymal* or *primary tissue* produces sex cells for reproduction. *Stromal* or *secondary tissue* includes all of the glands, nerves, ducts, and other tissues that serve a supportive function in producing, maintaining, and transmitting these sex cells.

In females, the **gonads** are the *ovaries.* They produce *ova,* the female **gametes**. From *menarche,* the first menstrual period, to *menopause,* the cessation of menstruation, mature ova are produced. The ovaries are small, almond-shaped, paired organs located on either side of the uterus in the female pelvic cavity. They are attached to the uterus by the ovarian ligaments. The ovaries lie close to the opening of the *fallopian tubes,* the ducts that convey the ova from the ovaries to the *uterus.* Fallopian tubes are also called *oviducts* or *uterine tubes.*

Once the mature ovum has been released, it is drawn into the *fimbriae*, the feathery ends of the fallopian tube. These tubes are about 1 cm in diameter and 10 to 12 cm long. The ovum travels down the fallopian tube to the uterus. The fallopian tubes and the ovaries make up what is called the *uterine adnexa*, or accessory organs, of the uterus.

Once the ovum has moved down the fallopian tube, it is secreted into the uterus or womb. The uterus is a pear-shaped organ that is designed to nurture a developing embryo/fetus. The uterus is composed of three layers:

- Outer layer, called the *perimetrium*
- Middle or muscle layer, called the *myometrium*
- Lining, called the *endometrium*

As a whole, it can be divided into several areas:

- *Corpus* or body, the large central area
- *Fundus*, the raised area at the top of the uterus between the outlets for the fallopian tubes
- *Cervix*, the narrowed lower area, often referred to as the neck of the uterus; the opening of the cervix is called the *cervical os*

CRITICAL THINKING APPLICATION 43.1

Many anatomic structures are involved in the ovulation process. Can you list them in order, starting with the structure that holds the ovum?

The *vagina* is a 10-cm (4-inch) muscular, tubelike structure that extends from the uterine cervix to the vulva (the external genitalia). It connects the internal reproductive structures with the external reproductive structures (Figure 43.1B). The vagina serves as the passageway for endometrium during menstruation, receives the penis during intercourse, and is the birth canal during the delivery of a baby.

The external female genitalia collectively are called the *vulva*; it consists of the **orifice**, *hymen*, **labia majora**, **labia minora**, **clitoris**, and **perineum**. The paired glands in the vulva that secrete a mucous lubricant for the vagina are the *Bartholin glands*. The *mons pubis* is a fatty cushion of tissue over the pubic bone (Figure 43.1A).

The *breasts*, or *mammary glands*, function to secrete milk. The breast tissue is composed of glandular, milk-producing, fatty, and fibrous tissue. The *nipple* of the breast is the *mammary papilla*, and the darker-colored skin surrounding the nipple is the *areola*.

Physiology of the Female Reproductive System

When a girl enters puberty, one of the many changes that occur is menarche. *Menstruation* is a normal body process that occurs in every female. It is the physiologic means by which the body rids itself of the thickened endometrial wall that develops during the average 28-day cycle. The menstrual cycle involves a series of events controlled by hormones from the pituitary gland and the ovaries. The cycle is divided into the follicular phase, the luteal phase, and the menstrual phase.

The follicular phase is also called the proliferative phase. In this phase, hormones are secreted to mature a Graafian follicle in an ovary that contains an ovum. The mature ovarian follicle secretes estrogen, which stimulates the growth of the endometrium. It takes approximately 9 days for the Graafian follicle to ripen and bulge out from the ovarian wall. The ovarian wall becomes thinner as the follicle enlarges until it bursts, releasing the ovum into the abdominal cavity. Expulsion of the ovum ends the follicular phase. The fallopian fimbriae begin their wavelike motion to fan the ovum into the fallopian tube. The rupture spot on the ovary, now called the *corpus luteum,* begins to secrete progesterone. **Ovulation** causes a rise in body temperature, and some women experience cramping and tenderness in the lower abdominal area at this time due to the rupture of the Graafian follicle.

The luteal phase is also called the secretory phase. Once ovulation is complete, the luteal phase begins. During this phase, progesterone secreted by the corpus luteum causes extensive growth of the endometrium as it prepares for a possible pregnancy. If conception occurs, the corpus luteum continues to secrete progesterone until the placenta is well established. The corpus luteum can secrete progesterone and human chorionic gonadotropin (hCG) to maintain the pregnancy. If conception does not occur, hCG is not secreted, and the corpus luteum atrophies. Without increased levels of progesterone and hCG, the endometrium breaks down, and menstruation begins.

In the menstrual phase, the uterus contracts to shed the lining of the uterus, made up of necrotic endometrial tissue, mucus, and blood from endometrial engorgement. A woman may experience cramping, pain, and irritability. This phase usually lasts approximately 5 days.

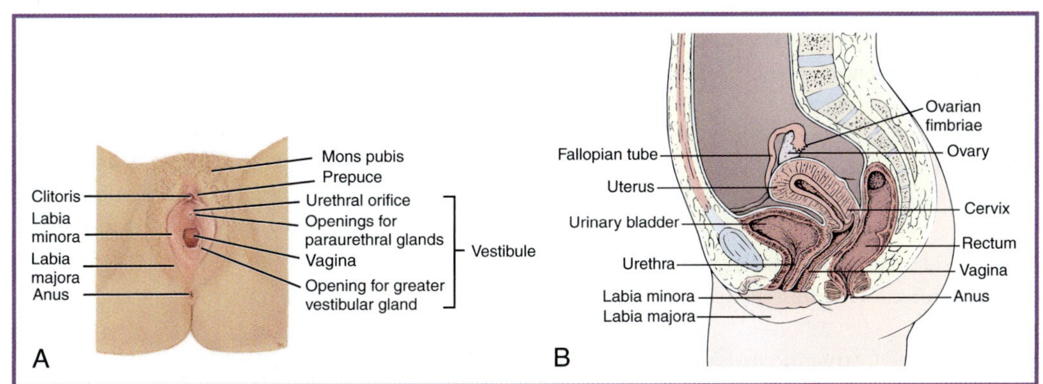

FIGURE 43.1 **(A)** Female external genitalia. **(B)** Normal female reproductive system. (A, from Applegate EJ: *The anatomy and physiology learning system*, ed 4, Philadelphia, 2011, Saunders; B, from Frazier MS, Drzymkowski JA: *Essentials of human diseases and conditions*, ed 5, St. Louis, 2013, Saunders.)

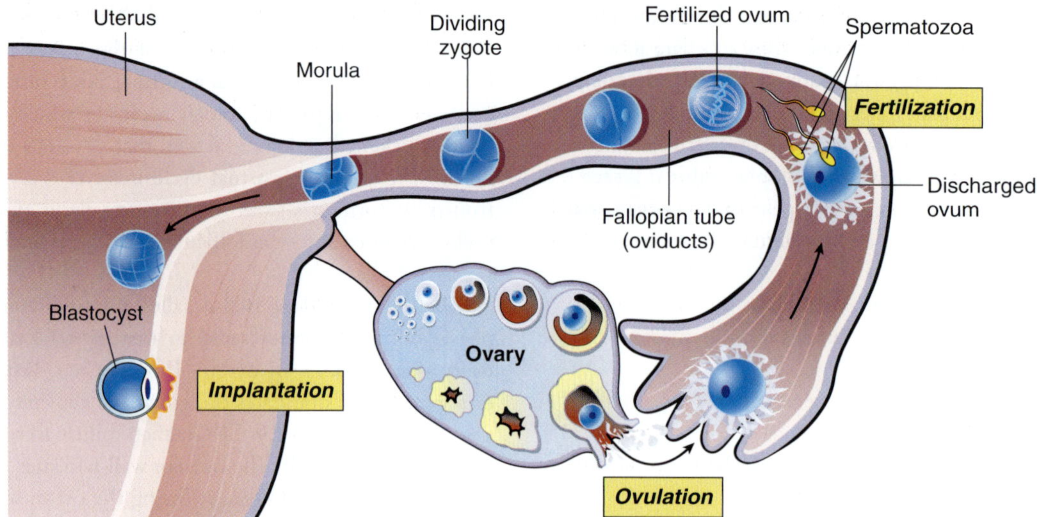

FIGURE 43.2 Ovulation, fertilization, and implantation. (From Salvo SG: *Massage therapy*, ed 3, St. Louis, 2007, Saunders.)

Pregnancy and Delivery

Pregnancy begins with the fertilization of an ovum by a sperm, often in the fallopian tube, as the ovum travels toward the uterus (Figure 43.2). Conception is usually the result of sexual intercourse. However, other methods of conception are possible if the couple has difficulty conceiving. These methods are discussed in the Disorders of the Female Reproductive System section.

CRITICAL THINKING APPLICATION **43.2**

After Peggy and Jill review the female reproductive anatomy, Jill asks Peggy to help her recall the phases of the menstrual cycle. Write down the different phases of the menstrual cycle and what occurs during each phase.

The fertilized egg, or *zygote*, divides as it moves through the fallopian tube to the uterus. In the first few days after fertilization, when the zygote has become a solid ball of cells from repeated divisions, it is called a *morula*. As it continues to develop, it moves from the fallopian tube into the uterus and implants into the uterine wall. At this point, it is called a *blastocyst*.

During implantation, the zygote functions as an endocrine gland by secreting hCG. The function of the hormone is to stop the corpus luteum from deteriorating. The corpus luteum allows the continued production of estrogen and progesterone to support the pregnancy and prevent menstruation. From the third to the eighth week of development, the organism is called an *embryo*. From the ninth through the thirty-eighth week of development (a normal length for *gestation*, or pregnancy), it is called a *fetus*.

At the same time that the embryo is developing, extraembryonic membranes are forming to sustain the pregnancy:

- The *amnion* and the *chorion* form the inner and outer sacs that contain the embryo.
- The fluid that forms inside the amnion is the *amniotic fluid*. It cushions the embryo, protects it against temperature changes, and allows it to move.
- The *placenta* is a highly vascular structure that acts as a physical communication between the mother and the embryo.
- The *umbilical cord* is the tissue that connects the embryo to the placenta (and hence to the mother). When the baby is delivered, the umbilical cord is cut, and the baby is then dependent on his or her own body for all physiologic processes. The remaining "scar" is the *umbilicus* or navel. The delivery of an infant is termed *parturition*.

LIFE SPAN CHANGES

As females age, several changes occur to the reproductive system. The following sections discuss some of those changes.

Changes in Children

Significant changes occur in the female reproductive system during puberty, typically between the ages of 10 and 14. These physical changes are driven by the levels of hormones that are produced by the pituitary gland; luteinizing hormone and follicle-stimulating hormone. Those hormones stimulate the production of the sex hormones. The increased level of estrogen stimulates the maturation of the breasts, ovaries, uterus, and vagina. In the United States, breast development usually occurs between the ages of 8 and 13. Two to three years later, menarche occurs. In addition, during puberty, body shape changes. There is an increase in body fat that accumulates in the hips and thighs.

Menstrual disorders are common problems during puberty. These include irregular menstruation, **dysmenorrhea,** and **amenorrhea**. It is not uncommon for periods to be irregular at the start of menstruation. Primary dysmenorrhea (not caused by another medical condition such as endometriosis) is usually treated with nonsteroidal anti-inflammatory drugs (NSAIDs) or oral contraceptives. Primary amenorrhea is when a girl, who is 16 years old, has never had a period. This can occur when there is an anatomic abnormality, which can be corrected with surgical intervention. If there are no anatomical abnormalities, amenorrhea treatments could include hormone treatments, oral contraceptives, changes in diet, and an evaluation for hormone-secreting tumors.

Changes in Adults

The changes in the female reproductive system as women age are also related to changing hormone levels. As women head into their 40s and 50s, signs of perimenopause occur and eventually, menopause takes place. Perimenopause and menopause are discussed in more depth later in this chapter. The changes in hormone levels can also cause physical changes in the reproductive tract. Vaginal walls become thinner, dryer, and less elastic. Sex can become painful because of these changes. There is a great risk for vaginal yeast infections.

Later in life, senior women are seen most often for neoplasms of the breast, uterus, cervix, and ovaries. In the United States, breast cancer alone will be diagnosed in one in eight women during their lifetime.

DISEASES AND DISORDERS OF THE FEMALE REPRODUCTIVE SYSTEM

The following sections discuss the common diseases and disorders of the female reproductive system, including the signs, symptoms, etiology, diagnostic procedures, and treatments.

Sexually Transmitted Infections

Many pathogens cause sexually transmitted infections (STIs), but what they have in common is all of them are most efficiently transmitted by *sexual contact.* Sexual contact refers to intercourse or any contact between the genitals of one person and the body of another person. No one is immune to these diseases. An individual can be infected with more than one STI at a time. No cure is available for viral STIs, such as human immunodeficiency virus (HIV) infection, herpes, and venereal warts. Bacterial infections are increasingly becoming resistant to antibiotic therapy. STIs are frequently asymptomatic in men, although they can cause serious health problems and are infectious regardless of whether symptoms are present. More information about STIs can be found in Chapter 33.

Endometriosis

With endometriosis, functional endometrial tissue is located outside of the uterus. It is commonly found attached to the ovaries, urinary bladder, fallopian tubes, uterosacral ligaments, intestines, and peritoneum. The endometrial tissue continues to act as it normally would during a menstrual cycle. It will thicken, break down, and bleed, just like the endometrium found in the uterus. This can cause inflammation at the implantation site that will recur with each cycle. Scar tissue and **adhesions** may form. Endometriosis can cause infertility and put women at higher risk for ovarian cancer.

The exact cause of endometriosis is not known, although there are some possible explanations: retrograde menstruation (the menstrual blood containing endometrial cells flows back through the fallopian tubes instead of leaving the uterus through the cervix), endometrial cells are transported through the blood vessels or lymphatic system to other parts of the body, and an immune system disorder in which the immune system does not recognize and destroy the endometrial tissue that is growing outside the uterus. Risk factors for endometriosis include never giving birth, menarche at a younger age, short menstrual cycles, low body mass index, alcohol consumption, family history of endometriosis, and uterine abnormalities. Common signs and symptoms of endometriosis include dysmenorrhea, **dyspareunia**, pain with bowel movements or urination, **menorrhagia**, **menometrorrhagia**, infertility, fatigue, diarrhea, constipation, bloating, and nausea.

To diagnose endometriosis, oftentimes, an ultrasound will be done. The ultrasound could be done through the abdomen or transvaginally. Another method of diagnosing endometriosis is **laparoscopy**. The surgeon will look inside the abdomen for signs of endometriosis. There are two methods for treating endometriosis: medications or surgery. Medications might include over-the-counter medications such as ibuprofen or naproxen sodium for pain; hormone therapy including contraceptives, gonadotropin-releasing hormone (GN-RH) agonists and antagonists, which block the production of ovarian-stimulating hormones, lowering estrogen levels and preventing menstruation; or progestin therapy, during which a progestin-only contraceptive such as an intrauterine device is used to stop menstrual periods and the growth of endometrial implants. Surgical options might include removal of the endometrial implants, which can be done laparoscopically or through an abdominal incision and will preserve the uterus and ovaries, or hysterectomy, which is removal of the uterus, cervix, and both ovaries.

Infections

The female genitalia provide an excellent environment for infections to occur. There is moisture, warmth, and plenty of nutrients that permit the infectious agents to flourish. The most common infections of the female reproductive system are discussed next.

Candidiasis

Commonly called a yeast infection. *Candida* organisms are part of the normal flora of the mouth, skin, intestinal tract, and vagina. Overgrowth of the organism can be caused by antibiotic use, high estrogen levels, oral contraceptive use, diabetes mellitus, pregnancy, and immunosuppressive disorders, including acquired immunodeficiency syndrome (AIDS).

This infection is caused by *Candida albicans* (fungus). Signs and symptoms include vulvovaginal itching; dry, bright red vaginal tissue; and an odorless, white, "cottage cheese" like vaginal discharge.

A diagnosis is made by means of a pelvic examination and a test of the vaginal secretions. Treatment includes antifungal medications, cream, ointments, tablets, and suppositories; some of these treatments may be available over the counter.

Cervicitis

Cervicitis is an inflammation of the cervix caused by an invading organism. This is caused by sexually transmitted infections, an allergic reaction, or a bacterial overgrowth. Signs and symptoms include thick, **purulent** discharge with odor, dysuria, dyspareunia, and vaginal bleeding after intercourse.

A diagnosis is made by means of a pelvic examination and test of the vaginal secretions. Treatment may not be needed unless the cervicitis is caused by an STI; then, both the patient and her partner must be treated for the STI.

Pelvic Inflammatory Disease

Pelvic inflammatory disease (PID) is an acute or chronic infection of the reproductive system that ascends from the vagina, cervix, uterus, fallopian tubes, and ovaries. These infections may cause the fallopian tubes to fill with pus, and chronic episodes can result in scarring of the fallopian tubes and the formation of adhesions.

PID is most often caused by gonorrhea or chlamydia (see Chapter 33), but many types of bacteria can cause PID. Initially, the patient may be asymptomatic. When signs and symptoms do occur, they could include fever, abdominal or pelvic pain, vaginal discharge, dysuria, and dyspareunia.

Diagnosis is made by means of a pelvic examination and test of the vaginal secretions. Treatment includes antibiotics for the patient and her partner and analgesics.

Menopause

Menopause is the permanent ending of menstruation as a result of the end of ovarian function. It usually occurs when a woman is between 45 and 55 years of age but can occur as early as the 30s and as late as the 60s. Menses may stop suddenly, the flow may decrease over time, or the time between menses may lengthen until menstruation completely stops. Menopause can be diagnosed only retrospectively. Only after 12 months of amenorrhea is a woman said to be in menopause, and the years after this are called *postmenopausal.*

Perimenopause begins when hormone-related changes start to appear, and it lasts until the final menses; this means it can be as long as 10 years before menopause occurs. During this time, women are still ovulating, but the uneven rise and fall of estrogen and progesterone may cause symptoms. Some women experience few or no symptoms, whereas others may have symptoms such as the following:

- Hot flashes
- Concentration problems
- Mood swings
- Irritability
- Migraines
- Vaginal dryness
- Urinary incontinence
- Dry skin
- Sleep disorders

Treatment focuses on relieving these signs and symptoms. The provider may prescribe very low-dose oral contraceptives to balance estrogen and progesterone levels or short-term hormone replacement therapy (HRT) to treat symptoms. The provider also may recommend that the patient consume soy products or take soy supplements for a plant source of estrogen. Vitamin E may help ease hot flashes, and vitamin B_6 helps create natural serotonin, a neurotransmitter that affects mood. Other methods that help with symptoms include the following:

- Avoiding caffeine and spicy foods (to reduce hot flashes)
- Using relaxation techniques (to aid with sleep disorders)
- Consuming a low-fat diet high in calcium and vitamin D
- Performing regular weight-bearing exercise (to help prevent **osteoporosis** and heart disease)

Medical treatment of menopause focuses on managing uncomfortable symptoms and preventing conditions associated with a drop in blood levels of estrogen, such as osteoporosis and coronary artery disease. Providers traditionally treated perimenopause and menopause with long-term HRT for most women; however, studies indicate that although HRT does protect the menopausal woman from osteoporosis, hip fracture, and colon cancer, at the same time, it increases the risk of heart attack, stroke, breast cancer, and blood clotting. It is now recommended that providers prescribe HRT to meet individual patients' needs over a short term (i.e., no longer than 5 years) rather than as a routine treatment for all menopausal women. Studies show that the risk for heart disease and other complications increases after 5 years of HRT. The medical assistant must be aware of the provider's recommendations regarding HRT.

Other medications that may be prescribed include antidepressants to prevent hot flashes. Gabapentin and clonidine also may be prescribed to reduce the frequency of hot flashes. Because the development of osteoporosis is a concern in perimenopausal and postmenopausal women, the provider may prescribe alendronate, risedronate, zoledronic acid, or ibandronate to reduce bone loss and the risk of fracture. Another drug that may be used to improve postmenopausal bone density is raloxifene; however, hot flashes are a common side effect of this medication. Vaginal dryness can be treated with estrogen administered locally by vaginal tablet, ring, or cream, or the patient can use K-Y Jelly or some other vaginal moisturizer as a lubricant.

CRITICAL THINKING APPLICATION **43.3**

Peggy and Jill room Janine Butler, a 53-year-old patient. Mrs. Butler is here to see Dr. Walden regarding her hormone replacement therapy, which she has been on for 3 years. Mrs. Butler is willing to have Jill in the room during her discussion with Dr. Walden so that Jill can observe and learn. Mrs. Butler recently read that her therapy may be dangerous. Dr. Walden agrees that if she is concerned, she can stop taking the medication; however, Dr. Walden recommends that Mrs. Butler try some alternative therapies. What suggestions might Dr. Walden make for the nonpharmaceutical treatment of perimenopausal symptoms?

Additional Female Reproductive System Diseases/ Disorders

There are additional female reproductive system diseases, and Table 43.1 provides information on many of them. Table 43.2 provides information on pregnancy-related conditions.

CRITICAL THINKING APPLICATION **43.4**

As Jill is working with more pregnant patients, she is becoming more familiar with the complications that can occur. She is still a bit confused between preeclampsia and eclampsia. How would you describe the differences?

CANCERS OF THE FEMALE REPRODUCTIVE SYSTEM

Cancer can be found in many different body systems, including the female reproductive system. The following sections discuss the most common cancers found in this system.

Breast Cancer

Breast cancer is the second leading cause of cancer deaths in women. According to the American Cancer Society, 1 in 8 women have a lifetime risk of developing breast cancer, and 1 in 39 risks of dying from the disease.

It is not known what causes breast cancer. Risk factors include being female, a family history of breast cancer, inherited genes, radiation exposure, obesity, menarche at a younger age, menopause at an

TABLE 43.1 Female Reproductive System Diseases

DISEASE	DESCRIPTION
Dysfunctional uterine bleeding (DUB)	Abnormal uterine bleeding not caused by a tumor, inflammation, or pregnancy.
Menopause	The cessation of menses.
Ovarian cyst	Benign, fluid-filled sac. Can be either a follicular cyst, which occurs when a follicle does not rupture at ovulation, or a cyst of the corpus luteum, which is caused when it does not continue its transformation.
Polycystic ovary syndrome	Bilateral presence of numerous cysts, caused by a hormonal abnormality leading to the secretion of androgens. Can cause acne, facial hair, and infertility.
Premenstrual dysphoric disorder (PMDD)	Mood disorder that includes depression, irritability, fatigue, changes in appetite or sleep, and difficulty in concentrating; occurs 1 to 2 weeks before the onset of the menstrual flow.
Premenstrual syndrome (PMS)	Poorly understood group of symptoms that occur in some women on a cyclical basis: breast pain, irritability, fluid retention, headache, and a lack of coordination are some of the symptoms.
Tumors fibroid/myoma	Fibroids are smooth muscle tumors of the uterus. They are usually nonpainful growths that may be removed surgically. Theses tumors may also be referred to as myomas.

TABLE 43.2 Pregnancy-Related Conditions

DISEASE	DESCRIPTION
Abruptio placentae	Premature separation of the placenta from the uterine wall; may result in a severe hemorrhage that can threaten both infant and maternal lives.
Eclampsia	Extremely serious form of hypertension secondary to pregnancy. Patients are at risk for coma, convulsions, and death.
Hemolytic disease of the newborn (HDN)	A mother with Rh– blood will develop antibodies to an Rh+ fetus during the first pregnancy. If another pregnancy occurs with an Rh+ fetus, the antibodies can destroy the fetal blood cells.
Hyperemesis gravidarum	Excessive vomiting that causes weakness, dehydration, and fluid and electrolyte imbalance.
Placenta previa	Placenta that is positioned in the uterus so that it covers the opening of the cervix.
Preeclampsia	Abnormal condition of pregnancy with unknown cause, marked by hypertension, edema, and proteinuria.
Zika virus	A mosquito-borne virus that typically causes a mild fever, rash, and joint pain. The virus can be passed to a fetus and is associated with certain birth defects such as microcephaly.

older age, having your first child at an older age, having never been pregnant, postmenopausal hormone therapy, and drinking alcohol. Signs and symptoms include a breast lump or thickening; change in the size, shape, or appearance of a breast; changes to the skin over the breast, such as dimpling, a newly inverted nipple, peeling, scaling, or flaking of the pigmented area of the skin surrounding the nipple (areola) or breast skin; and redness or pitting of the skin over the breast.

Diagnostic procedures start with a breast examination by the provider and may also include a mammogram, breast ultrasound, biopsy, or breast magnetic resonance imaging (MRI). Surgical treatment could consist of a **lumpectomy**, **mastectomy**, or **sentinel node biopsy**. Some women with cancer in one breast choose to have the other breast removed (contralateral prophylactic mastectomy). Treatment could also include radiation, chemotherapy, or hormone therapy.

Cervical Cancer

Almost all cervical carcinomas are caused by the human papillomavirus (HPV). The first stage of cervical cancer is asymptomatic, but early diagnosis of cervical cellular changes is possible with a Papanicolaou (Pap) test, and HPV can be detected with HPV testing.

The causes of cervical cancer are not known, but HPV is known to play a role. Risk factors include many sexual partners, early sexual activity, having other STIs, a weak immune system, and smoking. In the early stages of cervical cancer, the patient is asymptomatic. In the advanced stages, signs and symptoms include vaginal bleeding after intercourse, between periods, or after menopause; watery, bloody vaginal discharge that may be heavy and have a foul odor; and pelvic pain or pain during intercourse.

A Pap test is the most common screening test. From the same sample, an HPV test can be done. Diagnostic tests include a punch biopsy, endocervical **curettage**, **colposcopy**, and **loop electrosurgical excision procedure** (LEEP). The LEEP procedure can also be a treatment that removes all of the cancer cells. Other treatment options include **cone biopsy**, **hysterectomy**, radiation, and chemotherapy.

Ovarian Cancer

Ovarian cancer causes more deaths than any other cancer of the female reproductive system, but it accounts for only about 3% of all cancers in women. Most of the time, the cancer has already metastasized before the tumor is diagnosed.

It is not known what causes ovarian cancer. Risk factors include age, inherited gene mutation, estrogen hormone replacement therapy, menarche at a young age, menopause at an older age, having never been pregnant, fertility treatment, smoking, use of an intrauterine device, and polycystic ovary syndrome. In the early stages of ovarian cancer, the patient is asymptomatic. In the advanced stages, signs and symptoms can include abdominal bloating, quickly feeling full when eating, weight loss, discomfort in the pelvis area, changes in bowel habits, and a frequent need to urinate.

Diagnostic procedures include a pelvic examination, ultrasound, or computed tomography (CT) scan, cancer antigen 125 (CA-125) blood test (which looks for certain proteins in the blood), and a biopsy. Surgical treatments include hysterectomy, unilateral **salpingo-oophorectomy**, or bilateral salpingo-oophorectomy. Chemotherapy and targeted drug therapy may also be used in the treatment of ovarian cancer.

CRITICAL THINKING APPLICATION **43.5**

A patient is being seen in the OB/GYN department after having an abnormal Pap test, and Dr. Walden had recommended a LEEP procedure. Jill is wondering why a LEEP was recommended instead of a cone biopsy. Can you explain the difference between the two procedures?

THE MEDICAL ASSISTANT'S ROLE IN EXAMINATIONS, DIAGNOSTIC PROCEDURES, AND TREATMENTS

In this section, we discuss the medical assistant's role in gynecologic and obstetric procedures. A medical assistant has two roles in these situations:

- Assist the provider in any way needed
- Be there for the patient by helping her to be as comfortable as possible during her time in the healthcare facility

When we make the patient feel comfortable, we help establish a trusting relationship with her. This enables her to share the information the provider needs to give her the best possible care.

Assisting with the Gynecologic Examination

The need for an annual pelvic examination is being debated in the medical community. Currently, the American College of Obstetricians and Gynecologists (ACOG) recommends that pelvic and breast examinations be performed when indicated by medical history or symptoms. This examination is done to evaluate the reproductive organs and diagnose and treat any abnormalities of those organs.

A breast examination is considered part of the gynecologic examination. A clinical breast examination should be done every 1 to 3 years. The provider examines the breast, underarm area, and just below the clavicle.

Setting Up for a Gynecologic Examination

A medical assistant is responsible for setting up the examination room and making sure that all of the supplies are available for a gynecologic examination. The following is a list of supplies needed for a routine gynecologic examination:

- Patient's health record
- Laboratory requisition slips
- Patient gown and drape
- Lubricant
- Examination light
- Cervical spatula or cytobrush
- Microscope slides (direct smear method)
- Fixative (direct smear method)
- Plastic-fronded broom (liquid-based method)
- Liquid preparation container (liquid-based method)
- Vaginal speculum
- Sterile swabs
- Fecal occult blood test cards with developer
- Biohazard waste container

All items should be placed within easy reach for the provider and organized in a logical manner.

Preparation for the Gynecologic Examination

At the time the appointment was made, the patient should have been advised not to douche or have sexual intercourse for 24 hours before the examination. This allows the vaginal discharge to be properly evaluated and ensures accurate results of cytologic studies. Before the provider begins the pelvic examination, the medical assistant should obtain a complete gynecologic history. After documenting the patient's history and chief complaint, the medical assistant should prepare the room and the patient for the examination (Procedure 43.1).

The following should be included in the gynecologic history:

- Age at menarche
- Details about the regularity of the menstrual cycle, the amount and duration of menstrual flow, and a history of menstrual disturbances and their treatment
- Any current indicators of infection, including vaginal discharge, pelvic pain, and urinary difficulties
- Description of any breast abnormalities and the date of the patient's last mammogram
- Date of the last Pap test
- Sexual history; sexually transmitted infection (STI) history
- Number of times pregnant and the number of pregnancies carried to more than 20 weeks
- Date of last menstrual period (LMP)
- Lifestyle factors, including diet, exercise, smoking, and alcohol use

Assisting with an Examination

The pelvic and breast examination can be an embarrassing and emotionally difficult medical experience. In our society, reproduction is not openly talked about. Aside from the embarrassment, many women fear the provider's findings. By behaving in a professional manner, explaining what is going to happen, and showing a genuine interest in the patient's concerns, the medical assistant can help lay to rest most of the patient's anxieties and fears.

The medical assistant is responsible for supporting the patient and assisting the provider during the procedure. The procedure should be fully explained to the patient to prevent unnecessary embarrassment and discomfort. During the explanation, the medical assistant has the opportunity to provide patient education. This should be done using terms that are easy for the patient to understand. The medical assistant should remain in the examination room to provide reassurance to the patient and legal protection for the provider.

The patient should be instructed to empty her bladder, completely disrobe, and put on an examination gown. Some providers prefer that the patient put the gown on with the opening in the front, whereas others prefer the opening in the back. As the medical assistant, you should be aware of your provider's preference and instruct the patient accordingly.

Pap Test and Other Guidelines for Women

- Women ages 21 to 29 should have a Pap test alone every 3 years. HPV testing alone is not recommended
- Women ages 30 to 65 should have a Pap test and an HPV test (co-testing) every 5 years (preferred). It also is acceptable to have only a Pap test every 3 years or an HPV test every 5 years.
- If you have had a hysterectomy, you still may need screening. The decision is based on whether your cervix was removed, why the hysterectomy was needed, and whether you have a history of moderate or severe cervical cell changes or cervical cancer. Even if your cervix is removed at the time of hysterectomy, cervical cells can still be present at the top of the vagina. If you have a history of cervical cancer or cervical cell changes, you should continue to have a screening for 20 years after the time of your surgery.
- You can stop having cervical cancer screening after age 65 years if the following conditions apply:
  - You do not have a history of moderate or severe abnormal cervical cells or cervical cancer, and
  - You have had either three negative Pap test results in a row or two negative co-test results in a row within the past 10 years, with the most recent test performed within the past 5 years.

Cervical cancer screening. Patient Education FAQ085. Washington, DC: ACOG: 2017. Available at hwww.acog.org/Patients/FAQs/Cervical-Cancer-Screening.

Breast Examination. The first part of the gynecologic examination is the breast examination. The exam begins with the patient in the sitting position to allow for a visual check of the breasts. The gown should be adjusted so that the breast tissue can be easily exposed. After the visual inspection, the patient will be placed in the supine position. The medical assistant should be prepared to help the patient to lie down on the examination table. The footrest should be extended, and a small pillow may be placed under the patient's head for comfort. If needed, the gown and drape should be adjusted to protect the patient's modesty. Palpation will be used to determine if there is thickening or lumps in the breast and collar bone area. The provider will instruct the patient to place her arms above her head to allow assessment of the underarm area using palpation. When the examination is complete, the gown is readjusted to cover the breasts. The provider may choose to discuss breast self-examination with the patient at this time or may inform the patient that the medical assistant will explain the technique at the end of the examination.

According to the American Cancer Society, research has not shown a benefit for a patient or provider breast exam when women are also getting mammograms. It is recommended that women with an average risk of breast cancer start having yearly mammograms by age 45. It is optional to start earlier.

It is important for all women to know what is normal with their breasts. Any abnormality should be reported to their provider. Some providers still recommend monthly breast self-exams (BSEs) to be done after the menses. Procedure 43.2 describes how to perform a BSE. It is helpful for the medical assistant to provide the patient with a brochure showing the technique. It is also recommended to show the technique on a model (Figure 43.3). If possible, the patient should demonstrate the technique back to the medical assistant. This practice helps the medical assistant to determine if the patient understood the coaching.

Warning Signs of Breast Cancer

- Change in the skin (redness, warmth, darkening of the color, dimpling, puckering)
- Lump or hard area inside the breast or in the axilla area
- Change in the size or shape of the breast
- Change in the nipple (inverted or pulling in appearance, rash, sore, or drainage)
- Pain that does not go away

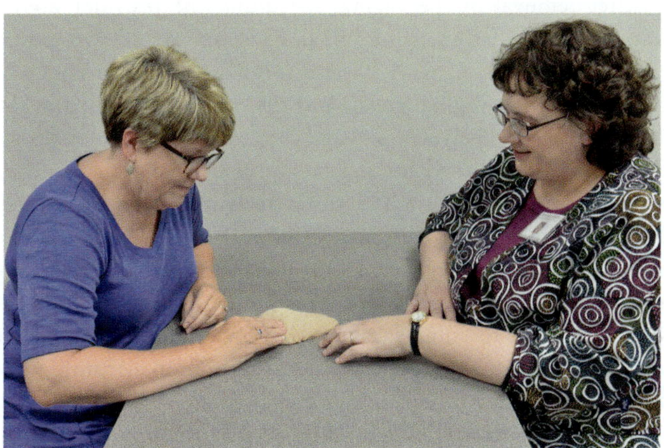

FIGURE 43.3 Coaching a patient regarding the breast self-exam.

Abdominal Examination. While the patient is in the supine position, the provider will palpate the abdomen. This is done to confirm normal **symmetry** of the pelvic organs and detect any masses. The provider also watches for any signs of discomfort or pain that could indicate a problem.

Pelvic Examination. For the pelvic examination, the patient is placed in the lithotomy position. This can be an awkward position for the patient to assume without assistance, and it may be embarrassing to the patient. If needed, the medical assistant should be available to help the patient into this position. Never place the patient in the lithotomy position until the provider is ready to begin the examination. When you assist the patient into the lithotomy position, always keep her totally covered.

You should stand at the patient's side so you can observe her yet still be able to move quickly (if needed by the provider). First, the provider inspects the external genitalia and palpates the perineal area. The patient may be asked to bear down to show any muscular weaknesses that may be the result of lacerations in the perineal body during childbirth. A third-degree laceration may have involved the rectal sphincter and may cause rectal incontinence.

Next, the vaginal speculum is inserted for examination of the cervix and the vaginal canal to obtain the Pap specimen. The speculum should be prewarmed with warm water. Have the patient take some deep breaths to help relax the abdominal muscles. The normal cervix points posteriorly and has smooth, pink, squamous epithelium. Abnormalities most frequently seen are ulcerations (erosions), **Bartholin cysts**, and cervical polyps. Because erosions cannot be palpated, inspection is the only method of detecting them. Healed lacerations from childbirth are common in a patient who has had multiple deliveries. Pregnancy increases the size of the cervix, and hormone deficiency causes it to atrophy. The vaginal wall is reddish pink and has a corrugated appearance from the overlapping tissue (rugae) lining. Vaginal infections change the appearance of the vaginal mucosa.

After inspecting the vaginal wall, the provider may collect a specimen for a Pap test. When the specimen has been obtained, the medical assistant may be responsible for labeling it and preparing it for transport to the cytology laboratory. Be sure to follow laboratory instructions during the preparation to avoid having to repeat the examination.

After removal of the vaginal speculum, the provider does a bimanual examination. For a bimanual examination, two gloved fingers are lubricated with a water-soluble jelly (lubricant) and inserted into the vaginal canal, and the other hand palpates the abdomen over the pelvic organs and the mons pubis (Figure 43.4). The uterus is examined for shape, size, and consistency, and its position is noted. A normal uterus is freely movable with limited discomfort. A laterally displaced uterus is usually the result of pelvic adhesions or displacement caused by a pelvic tumor. The fallopian tubes and ovaries are evaluated. Normal tubes and ovaries are difficult to palpate, which is why the provider may have to press firmly in the pelvic area, causing minor discomfort for the patient. A digital rectal exam may be done at this time. This involves the insertion of a gloved finger into the rectum. A small amount of stool is left on the glove and can be used for a fecal occult blood test.

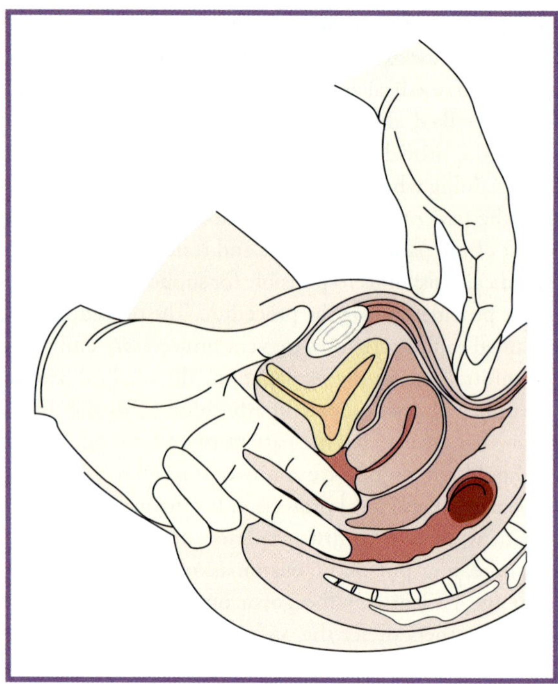

FIGURE 43.4 Bimanual examination.

Post-Examination Duties

When the examination is finished, help the patient into a sitting position and into the dressing room, if needed. Following the Standard Precautions established by the Occupational Safety and Health Administration (OSHA), remove the examination equipment and supplies while the patient is dressing so that when the provider returns to talk to the patient, the room is neat and clean. Once the patient has left, the room should be sanitized, disinfected, and restocked as necessary so it is ready for the next patient.

Contraception

At the time of a gynecologic examination, a provider may discuss contraception with the patient. A woman's choice of a contraceptive method is based on many factors. To make an informed choice, a patient should know the risks, benefits, side effects, costs, failure rates, and convenience of each available method. In addition, although condoms are only moderately successful at preventing pregnancy, they should be used consistently to prevent the transmission of STIs. The medical assistant may help provide patient education on contraceptive methods. Table 43.3 summarizes the characteristics of various contraceptive methods.

Barrier Methods. Barrier methods of contraception either kill sperm (through the use of a chemical spermicide) or prevent them from entering the cervical os. These methods, which are relatively inexpensive, include the condom, diaphragm, and cervical cap or sponge. Each method must be used every time the person has intercourse, which means the patient must be motivated to follow through on using it. Patient education on the use of a diaphragm includes the following instructions:

- Examine the diaphragm before each use by holding it up to a bright light to check for holes or cracks.
- Place 1 to 2 tablespoons of spermicidal jelly or cream into the diaphragm dome before insertion.

TABLE 43.3 Commonly Used Contraceptive Methods

	FAILURE RATE	CHARACTERISTICS	CONTRAINDICATIONS	SIDE EFFECTS
Male or female condom (barrier method)	2%–10%	No prescription or examination needed; easily available; inexpensive	Latex allergy in either partner	Possible allergic response to latex or spermicide
Diaphragm, cervical cap, cervical sponge (barrier method)	2%–19%	Must be fitted by clinician; requires instruction on how to insert and remove; spermicide must be used each time; diaphragm and sponge must be left in place for 6 hours after intercourse	Latex, rubber, or spermicide allergy; uterine prolapse; severe cystocele or rectocele	Increased risk for a urinary tract infection (diaphragm); increased risk of abnormal Pap test result (cap)
Intrauterine device (IUD)	2%–6%	Copper type releases copper, which slows sperm in the cervix; hormonal type releases progestin, which reduces sperm mobility and prevents thickening of the endometrial wall	Cervicitis, vaginitis, endometriosis, pelvic infection, history of STI or ectopic pregnancy	Copper type may temporarily increase vaginal bleeding and menstrual pain; hormonal intrauterine devices (IUDs) decrease menstrual flow and cramping
Birth control implants	1%	Flexible plastic implant inserted under skin of upper arm; releases progestin to prevent ovulation, thickens cervical secretions to block semen, thins endometrial wall; effective for up to 3 years	Certain antibiotics, HIV drugs, seizure medications may make it less effective; history of blood clots, liver disease, or breast cancer	Irregular bleeding in first 6–12 months; nausea, headache, sore breasts, scarring at implantation site
Depo-Provera (DMPA)	0.5%	Requires 150-mg intramuscular injection every 3 months	Intention of becoming pregnant within 1 year, breast cancer, liver disease	Return of fertility may be delayed 10–18 months; should not be used more than 2 years in a row because it can cause a temporary loss of bone density; headache, weight gain, possibly depression
Oral contraceptives (OCPs) Hormonal patch Vaginal ring	1%	Suppress ovulation; atrophy of the endometrium	Thrombolytic, liver, or coronary artery disease; breast, liver, reproductive tract cancer; smoker over age 35; diabetes; sickle cell disease	Nausea, breakthrough bleeding, breast tenderness, fluid retention; hypertension, elevated lipid levels, blood clots, strokes

- Leave the diaphragm in place for 6 hours after intercourse; do not douche until after you have removed it.
- Before repeated intercourse, add spermicide to the outside of the diaphragm with an applicator. Do not remove the diaphragm until 6 hours after the last intercourse.
- After removal, wash the diaphragm with soap and water, allow it to air dry and inspect it for breaks or holes before storing.
- Have the diaphragm refitted if the following occurs:
  - You gain or lose more than 10 to 15 pounds
  - You have a miscarriage, give birth, or undergo any type of pelvic surgery
  - You have difficulty voiding or moving your bowels with the diaphragm in place

The cervical cap is a thimble-sized, domed barrier device that fits over the end of the cervix. It also is used with spermicidal jelly (Figure 43.5).

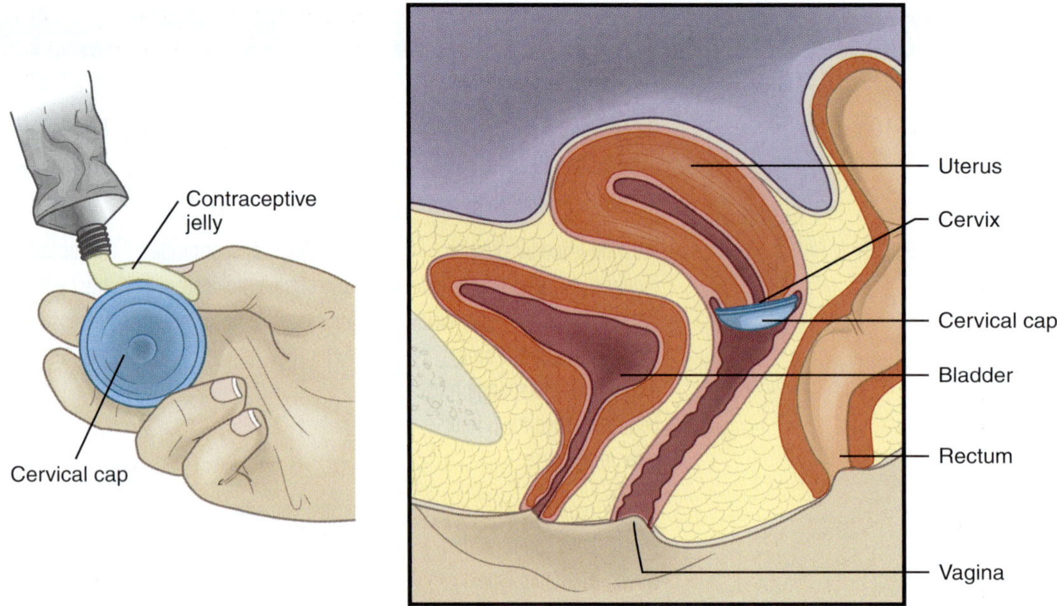

FIGURE 43.5 Cervical cap with spermicide.

If used properly, the cervical cap is 92% to 96% effective. An advantage of this barrier method is the cap can be inserted up to 12 hours before intercourse and can stay in place for up to 72 hours without a decrease in effectiveness or safety. The cervical sponge contains spermicide and can also be inserted hours before intercourse and is effective for 24 hours. If always used as directed, the sponge is 80% to 91% effective.

Hormonal Contraceptives. Hormonal contraceptives are a highly effective and reversible form of contraception. They work by preventing ovulation, changing the cervical mucosa, affecting sperm mobility, and preventing the thickening of the endometrial wall. Hormonal contraceptives include the following:

- Birth control pills or patch
- Vaginal ring
- Depo-Provera injections
- Hormonal implants

Besides being a highly effective method of birth control, oral contraceptives can be used to treat a wide range of gynecologic conditions, including menstrual irregularities, premenstrual syndrome (PMS) symptoms, and **anovulation**. They also can be used to prevent ovarian cysts and may be prescribed to increase bone density. However, to be effective, the pills must be taken daily, at the same time each day. Failure rates are associated with noncompliance and can range from less than 1% (in highly compliant women) to greater than 15% (in those who do not take the pills as prescribed). Oral contraceptive pills (OCPs) can have serious side effects. Patients should be informed of conditions that require immediate medical attention. These can be remembered with the mnemonic ACHES: *a*bdominal pain (new and severe), *c*hest pain (new and severe), *h*eadaches (new or more frequent), *e*ye problems (blurred vision or vision loss), and *s*evere leg pain. These symptoms may indicate the formation of a blood clot in the abdomen, chest, or leg. They may also be signs of a stroke. Blood clot formation and stroke are the most serious complications of OCPs.

A type of oral contraception, the extended cycle pill, limits the number of menstrual periods to four a year. Patients are more likely to have spotting and breakthrough bleeding with this hormone therapy than with the traditional 28-day birth control pill. The extended cycle pill is designed to be taken once a day for 84 days, and then an inactive dose is taken for a week, during which the woman would menstruate. A combination birth control pill that contains both estrogen and progestin may be prescribed for women suffering from premenstrual dysphoric disorder (PMDD); it is also useful for treating acne in female patients at least 14 years of age who have started menstruating.

As mentioned, hormonal contraception also can be delivered via a transdermal patch. The patch is a 1¾-inch square that slowly releases estrogen and progestin through the skin into the bloodstream. It is considered as effective as oral contraceptives in women who weigh less than 198 pounds; however, the patch is still a very effective method for women who weigh more than that. Current research shows that the risk of blood clots with the contraceptive patch is similar to the risks observed with oral contraceptives. However, cigarette smoking increases the risk of serious cardiovascular side effects, especially if the patient is over age 35. Patients should be told not to apply any creams or oils at the application site, change the patch weekly for 3 consecutive weeks, and go patch free the fourth week, allowing menstruation to occur. The patch can be applied to the buttocks, lower abdomen, and upper body but not to the breasts. The woman can bathe, shower, and swim while wearing the patch, but if it comes off, it should be replaced immediately.

The vaginal ring contraceptive device is made of flexible plastic and is inserted into the vagina. The ring slowly releases estrogen and progestin to prevent pregnancy and provide effective contraceptive action for 1 month after insertion. The device is 2 inches in diameter and can be inserted anywhere in the vagina; however, the deeper it is placed, the less likely it is to be felt after insertion. Side effects of the vaginal ring are similar to

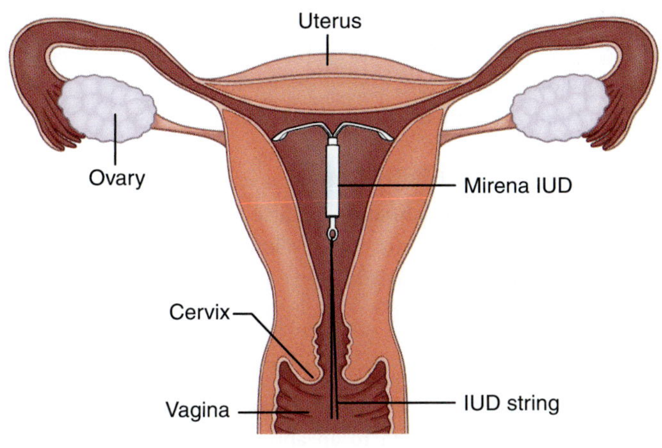

FIGURE 43.6 Intrauterine device.

those of other hormonal contraceptives, and it may increase the risk of heart attack, stroke, and blood clots. When the patient first starts using the ring, an additional method of birth control must be used for the first week. If the ring falls out, it should be rinsed with warm water and reinserted within 3 hours. If it is out for longer than 3 hours, contraception is not certain, and the patient should use another birth control method for 1 week.

Depo-Provera is an injectable contraceptive that contains high doses of progestin. Each dose prevents pregnancy for up to 3 months, but women must be compliant in returning to the healthcare facility for follow-up and repeat doses every 9 to 13 weeks. The first injection should be administered within the first 5 days of the menstrual period for birth control coverage. This is a highly effective method of contraception and is ideal for women who either do not comply with a birth control regimen or do not want to take a pill every day. However, using Depo-Provera for 2 years or longer may increase the risk of bone loss and the eventual development of osteoporosis. Almost all patients using the injections experience some menstrual irregularities, but these usually subside after two doses. Women using this form of hormonal contraception are not at risk for the side effects of estrogen exposure, such as the increased risk of blood clots and cardiovascular disease.

A birth control implant is a single, flexible rod, about the size of a match, that is inserted under the skin of the upper arm. The birth control implant releases a low, steady dose of progestin. This suppresses ovulation, thickens cervical mucus to block the passage of sperm, and thins the endometrial wall to prevent implantation. It prevents pregnancy for up to 3 years after insertion. Hormonal implants have risks and contraindications similar to those of other hormonal types of contraception.

Intrauterine Devices. The intrauterine device (IUD) (Figure 43.6) is a T-shaped plastic frame with threads attached that the provider inserts into the uterus to prevent pregnancy. Two general types of IUDs are available: the copper type and the hormonal type. Both products inhibit fertilization by blocking the sperm's journey to the fallopian tubes, and if fertilization does occur, they prevent the embryo from implanting into the uterine wall. In addition, the copper type of IUD releases copper, which acts to slow sperm in the cervix. The hormonal types of IUDs release progestin, which reduces sperm mobility and prevents the thickening of the endometrial wall during the menstrual cycle. Both types of IUDs are extremely effective at preventing pregnancy (over 99%); the copper type can remain in place for as long as 10 years, whereas the hormonal type must be replaced every 3 to 5 years. The copper IUD may temporarily increase vaginal bleeding and menstrual pain. The hormonal IUD results in both decreased menstrual flow and cramping. To remove an IUD, the provider gently withdraws it by pulling on the IUD string. In rare instances, it must be removed surgically.

Permanent Methods. Both male and female patients can undergo surgical procedures that are considered permanent contraceptive methods. Vasectomies in the male were addressed in Chapter 42. For the female, a bilateral tubal ligation can be performed in which a portion of both fallopian tubes is excised or ligated. The cost and rate of complications are higher for tubal ligations than for vasectomies. In addition, tubal ligations must be done on an outpatient basis with general anesthesia, so the woman has that additional risk. Both procedures can be reversed, but not always successfully.

CRITICAL THINKING APPLICATION 43.6

When directed by the provider, Peggy provides patient education regarding contraceptives. She has asked Jill to create a reference sheet that covers all birth control options, their characteristics and side effects, and any patient education details that might be appropriate. What should Jill include?

Assisting with Diagnostic Procedures

The medical assistant can play an important role when assisting with diagnostic procedures in obstetrics and gynecology. The following sections discuss that role.

Specimen Collection

During a pelvic examination, several types of specimens may be collected. If the pelvic exam is part of a wellness examination, a specimen for a Pap test may be collected. If the provider wants to evaluate endocrine function, a maturation index may be ordered. If the pelvic examination is for a possible vaginal infection, a specimen may be collected for culture or observation under a microscope.

Pap Test. The two methods of specimen collection for a Pap test are the direct smear method and the liquid-based method.

Direct Smear Method.

1. The specimen is collected with a cervical spatula.
2. The cells are placed (smeared) directly on a microscope slide.
3. A fixative must be applied immediately to the slide before it is sent to the laboratory.

Liquid-Based Method.

1. The specimen is collected with a plastic-fronded broom.
2. Cells are suspended in a bottle of preservative by rinsing the broom in the specimen vial.
3. The results of the Pap test are often reported using the Bethesda system.

PAP TEST RESULTS

The Bethesda system is often used to report the results of a Pap test. This system looks at the squamous cells and the glandular cells separately.

Squamous Cells

- Negative for intraepithelial lesion or malignancy: normal epithelial cells, no precancerous findings.
- Atypical squamous cells (ASC):
  - Atypical squamous cells of undetermined significance (ASC-US): Squamous cells do not appear completely normal but do not clearly suggest precancerous cells. Most often means there is an infection.
  - Atypical squamous cells cannot exclude a high-grade squamous intraepithelial lesion (ASC-H): Minor changes with unknown causes that are at risk of progressing to a high-grade lesion (HSIL).
- Low-grade squamous intraepithelial lesions (LSILs): Mild cell changes that may be classified as mild dysplasia. These abnormalities are often caused by human papillomavirus (HPV) infection.
- High-grade squamous intraepithelial lesions (HSILs): Severe abnormalities that have a higher likelihood of progressing to cancer if left untreated. May be classified as moderate or severe dysplasia. Includes carcinoma in situ (CIS), severe changes that appear similar to cervical cancer but have not spread beyond the surface of the cervix.
- Squamous cell carcinoma: Cervical cancer.

Glandular Cells

- Atypical glandular cells (ACG): Glandular cells do not appear normal, but it is not clear what is causing the changes.
- Endocervical adenocarcinoma in situ (AIS): Severely abnormal cells are found, but they have not spread beyond the glandular tissue of the cervix.
- Adenocarcinoma: Cancer of the endocervical canal and possibly endometrial, extrauterine, and other cancers.

Maturation Index. A *maturation index* is an endocrine evaluation that can assist in the diagnosis and treatment of infertility issues, amenorrhea, menopause, or postmenopausal bleeding. Cells are collected from the vaginal wall and treated much like a Pap test specimen. If the provider orders a maturation index, it must be indicated on the cytology request form.

Vaginal Infections. Earlier in this chapter, common vaginal infections were discussed. A pelvic exam needs to be done to determine what type of vaginal infection is occurring. For many vaginal infections, a sterile swab is used to collect a sample of the discharge. The secretion is then swabbed on the microscope slide, and the provider looks at it under a microscope. Common infections, the infectious agents, and the type of specimen and test used to identify each include the following:

- *Candidiasis (yeast infection):* The provider tests for the presence of *Candida albicans.* A small amount of discharge is placed on a slide, and a drop of a 10% solution of potassium hydroxide (KOH) is added. The KOH dissolves other cellular debris so that the provider can see the yeast buds.
- *Trichomoniasis:* A small amount of discharge is placed on a slide, and a drop of saline is added. The provider is looking for *Trichomonas vaginalis,* which appears as a pear-shaped organism with a flagellum (tail) that moves it around.
- *Chlamydia:* A sterile swab is used to collect a specimen from the endocervical canal. The swab is then placed in a tube containing a transport medium and sent to the lab for testing. The causative organism frequently is *Chlamydia trachomatis.*

Assisting with Treatments

As with diagnostic procedures, a medical assistant can have a role in assisting with treatments. The following sections discuss the medical assistant's role in assisting with treatments in obstetrics and gynecology.

Special Procedures

There are a number of gynecology-related special procedures that a patient may undergo related to an abnormal Pap test result. Let's look at the three most commonly performed procedures:

- Cryotherapy
- Colposcopy with or without a biopsy
- Loop electrosurgical excision procedure (LEEP)

Cryotherapy. Depending on the condition of the cervix, *cryotherapy*, or the application of freezing temperatures, may be used to treat chronic cervicitis and cervical erosion. Freezing causes cellular **necrosis**, and in approximately 1 month, the dead cells are replaced with healthy cells. The procedure involves placing a probe against the problem area on the cervix and applying liquid nitrogen to the area for approximately 3 to 4 minutes or until the site is frozen. The patient may experience some pain for about 30 minutes after the procedure and a slight watery discharge for up to a week. If any signs of infection, foul discharge, or pain develop, the patient should call the provider's office. Advise the patient not to engage in sexual intercourse for 1 month and to expect a heavier than usual menstrual flow for the first cycle after the procedure.

Colposcopy with or without a Biopsy. *Colposcopy* is the visual examination of the vagina and cervical surfaces with a colposcope (Figure 43.7). The *colposcope* is a microscope with a light source and a magnifying lens that can be used during a vaginal examination to do the following:

- Locate and evaluate abnormal cells
- Detect cancer of the cervix in the early stages
- Examine tissue from which an abnormal Pap test result has been obtained
- Monitor areas of the cervix where malignant lesions have been removed

The provider may wash the cervix with acetic acid to remove mucus and allow the provider to see abnormal areas more easily. In addition, the acetic acid will stain the abnormal areas white. An iodine solution (Schiller's or Lugol's solution) may also be used. This iodine solution will stain normal tissue brown, leaving abnormal tissue unchanged.

In combination with a colposcopy, a cervical biopsy may be performed. A major advantage of obtaining a biopsy during colposcopy is that the instrument permits visualization of the suspicious area so that the biopsy can be taken from the most atypical site. Multiple biopsies may be taken. The provider is looking for abnormalities on the cervix and will take a biopsy specimen when one is seen. You may be receiving the sample from the provider. It is very important to accurately label each specimen container with the location of the biopsy. The provider uses the face of a clock to determine the location of the biopsy. The specimen container label should indicate that

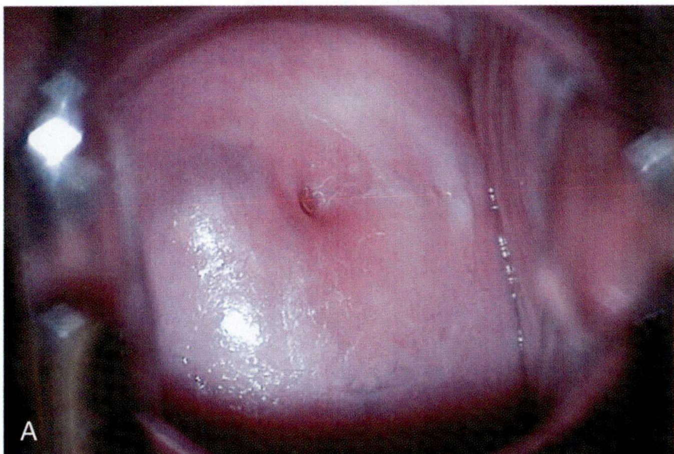

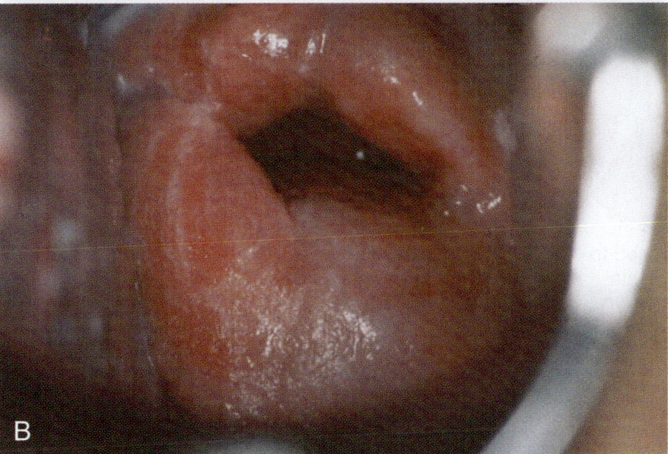

FIGURE 43.7 Colposcopic appearance of normal cervix (A) and abnormal cervix (B).

location (e.g., 2:00). Silver nitrate sticks or Monsel's paste may be used to stop the bleeding from the biopsies.

Colposcopy is a relatively safe, painless procedure performed in the provider's office. Discomfort may occur when the speculum is inserted into the vagina to improve visualization of the tissue. Discomfort and bleeding can occur when tissue is taken in a biopsy. The patient should be instructed to use a sanitary pad, as there may be bleeding from the procedure. The provider may recommend that the patient avoid using tampons, douching, or having intercourse for 7 to 10 days after the procedure.

Loop Electrosurgical Excision Procedure. Depending on the results of the cervical biopsy, the patient may need a more extensive procedure, *conization*, in which a cone-shaped wedge of cervical tissue is removed for treatment or further analysis. More often, a less-invasive LEEP is performed. For this technique, a local anesthetic is injected into the cervix, and a wire loop is inserted into the vagina. A high-frequency electrical current running through the wire is used to remove abnormal tissue from both the cervix and the endocervical canal. Like conization, LEEP can be used as a diagnostic tool to collect biopsy samples and as a treatment to remove abnormal tissue (Figure 43.8).

OBSTETRICS

Pregnancy can be the most exciting and terrifying experience for a patient, especially the first time around. As a medical assistant working in obstetrics, it is important to be able to reassure the patient while remaining professional. The next section discusses the examinations and procedures related to prenatal and postpartum care.

Assisting with the Prenatal Examination

During the prenatal examination, the medical assistant is responsible for setting up the prenatal and obtaining the necessary health history information during the initial prenatal visit. There will also be lab work to be completed and ordered. For subsequent visits, a less extensive history will be taken, as well as the routine tests described later.

Prenatal Record

At the first prenatal examination, an extensive health history will be taken. This history can help to identify any risk factors for the patient. Frequently, the first prenatal visit is the first comprehensive physical examination that the patient has had in a long time. The health history can point out pregnancy-related risk factors and overall health-related risk factors that can also be addressed. The following information should be collected when creating the prenatal record for a patient:

- Demographic information
- Menstrual history
- Obstetric history
- Medical and surgical history
- Family and social history

Menstrual History. The prenatal record should include the first day of the last menstrual period. This is used to determine the estimated date of delivery (EDD). It is also important to know the normal cycle length for the patient and if this last menstrual period was "normal." The medical assistant should also ask if the patient was using contraception when she became pregnant. If she was, the method being used should be documented.

Obstetric History. The provider will need to have a complete history of previous pregnancies. This will help to determine any risk factors for the current pregnancy. The following information should be included in the obstetric history (Figure 43.9):

- Dates of deliveries
- Types of deliveries (vaginal or cesarean); if cesarean, the type of incision should be noted
- Birth weight and gestational age of previous infants
- Complications of previous pregnancies

There are some specific terms related to an obstetric history that you should be familiar with. Table 43.4 lists those terms and their definitions.

A prenatal record includes documenting the gravida, para, and abortion information. As a medical assistant, you should be able to determine those numbers after obtaining the obstetric history from a patient. It is important to remember that gravida and para refer to the number of pregnancies, not the number of babies. A twin pregnancy is considered just one pregnancy. If this was the first pregnancy for the patient and the pregnancy went to term (38 to 40 weeks), she would be gravida: 1 and para: 1.

Gravida is the number of pregnancies, regardless of the number of weeks the patient was pregnant. If a patient has three children and had a spontaneous abortion at 8 weeks, her gravida number would 4.

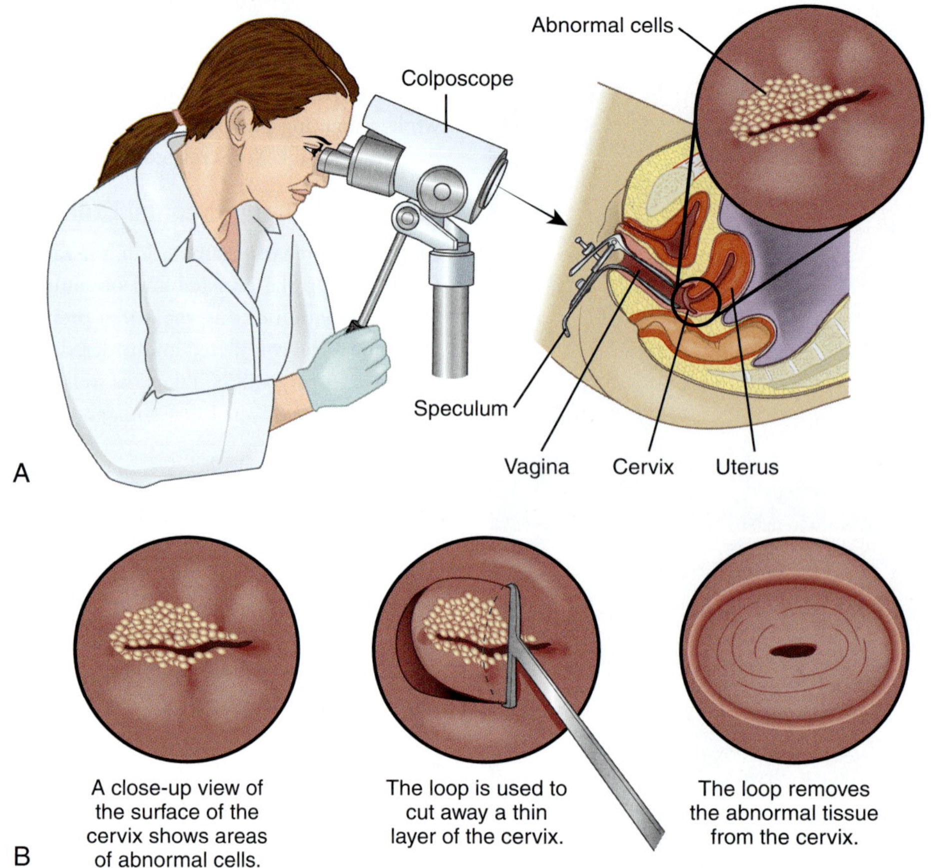

FIGURE 43.8 Colposcopic view of cervix **(A)** and LEEP biopsy of abnormal cells **(B)**.

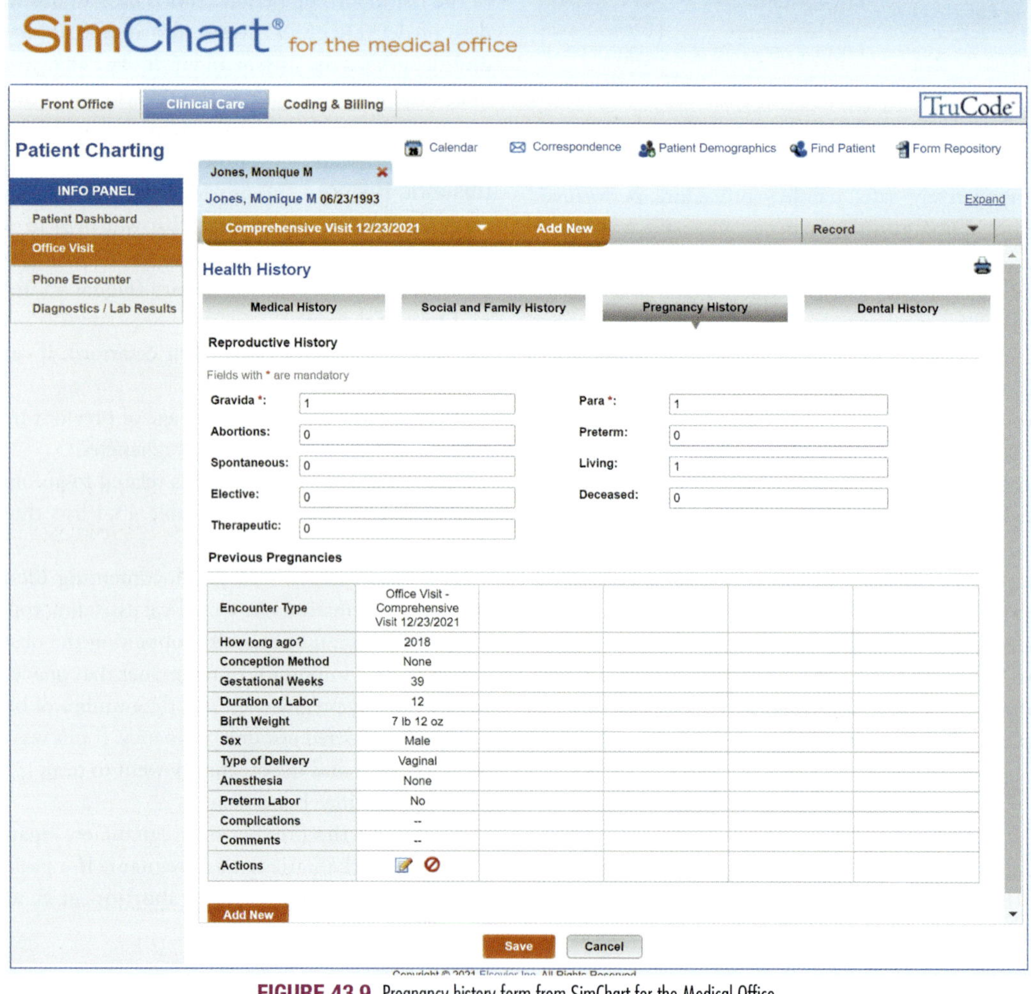

Reproductive History

Fields with * are mandatory

Gravida *:	1	Para *:	1
Abortions:	0	Preterm:	0
Spontaneous:	0	Living:	1
Elective:	0	Deceased:	0
Therapeutic:	0		

Previous Pregnancies

Encounter Type	Office Visit - Comprehensive Visit 12/23/2021				
How long ago?	2018				
Conception Method	None				
Gestational Weeks	39				
Duration of Labor	12				
Birth Weight	7 lb 12 oz				
Sex	Male				
Type of Delivery	Vaginal				
Anesthesia	None				
Preterm Labor	No				
Complications	--				
Comments	--				
Actions					

Add New

Save Cancel

FIGURE 43.9 Pregnancy history form from SimChart for the Medical Office.

TABLE 43.4 Obstetric History Terms

TERM	DEFINITION
Gravida	Number of pregnancies
Primigravida	A woman who is pregnant for the first time
Multigravida	A woman who has been pregnant two or more times
Nulligravida	A woman who has never been pregnant
Para	Number of pregnancies that have gone to the age of fetal viability (20 weeks' gestation)
Primipara	A woman who has carried one pregnancy to the age of fetal viability
Multipara	A woman who has carried two or more pregnancies to the age of fetal viability
Nullipara	A woman who has not carried a pregnancy to the age of fetal viability
Abortion	Termination of a pregnancy before the fetal age of viability Miscarriage, spontaneous, elective
Spontaneous abortion	Natural death of an embryo or fetus before the fetal age of viability; also called a miscarriage
Therapeutic or elective abortion	A procedure for the planned termination of a pregnancy
Stillbirth	Fetal death after 20 weeks' gestation; also called intrauterine fetal death (IUFD)

Para is the number of pregnancies that have gone to the age of **viability** (20 weeks). In the above scenario, the patient's para number would be 3, as the spontaneous abortion happened before 20 weeks.

The abortion information refers to the termination of a pregnancy before the age of viability (20 weeks). The abortion could be spontaneous, therapeutic, or elective. All would be included in this number. Some providers want this further defined as to which category of abortion. In our above scenario, the patient's abortion number would be 1.

CRITICAL THINKING APPLICATION 43.7

Jill is interviewing a new OB patient. The patient tells Jill that this is her fourth pregnancy, and she has two children. She had two early miscarriages. What would her gravida number be? What would her para number be? What would her abortion number be?

Medical and Surgical History. There are medical and surgical conditions that could affect a patient's current pregnancy. Common chronic conditions, such as diabetes, hypertension, asthma, and mitral valves prolapse, should be included in the prenatal record. The management of these conditions could change with pregnancy. Less common conditions, such as thyroid disorders, systemic lupus erythematosus, and bleeding disorders, can also affect the patient and the fetus. To help both, the provider needs to be aware of these conditions and the treatment being followed.

Certain infections can affect a pregnancy. A history of certain STIs can put the patient at risk for complications. Pelvic inflammatory disease (PID) can cause scarring of the fallopian tubes, which increases the risk of an **ectopic** pregnancy. Genital herpes and other infections can be transmitted to the newborn during delivery. If the provider is aware of those conditions, plans can be made to protect both the mother and the baby.

If the patient has had any type of abdominal surgical procedure, it could affect the pregnancy or delivery. If there is a history of a prior ectopic pregnancy, this would be a risk factor for another one. If there is a history of a uterine puncture or any uterine incision, the patient and provider will need to talk about a possible cesarean section.

Family and Social History. Many conditions have a genetic component. Obtaining an accurate family history can help determine if the patient or the infant is at risk. With this knowledge, the patient and the provider can be prepared. Additional testing may be included during the prenatal period for a patient with certain factors in the family history. Conditions that could be of concern include the following:

- Diabetes
- Hypertension
- Heart disease
- Kidney disease
- Seizures
- Depression
- Thyroid disease
- **Preclampsia**
- Autoimmune disorders (e.g. lupus, rheumatoid arthritis

A family history of genetic disorders should also be documented in the patient's family history. These disorders can include the following:

- **Down syndrome**
- Neural tube defects (**spina bifida**, **meningocele**, **anencephaly**)
- **Hemophilia**
- **Sickle cell anemia**
- **Cystic fibrosis (CF)**
- **Phenylketonuria (PKU)**

Other family history information that should be noted would include a history of twins in the family, food allergies, and a family history of recurrent miscarriages or stillbirths.

The social history includes tobacco, alcohol, and recreational drug use. This information can be used for patient education as it relates to pregnancy. Nutrition and exercise are an important part of pregnancy. Finding out if the pregnant patient follows a particular diet, such as vegan or vegetarian, will provide the opportunity for patient education regarding nutritional needs during pregnancy. Employment is also part of a social history. This can point out any occupational duties that could be affected by a pregnancy, such as working with certain chemicals or physical activities that should not be done when pregnant.

Collecting all of the components discussed previously is a great start to completing the patient's prenatal record, in addition to supplying the provider with the information needed to provide excellent care during the patient's pregnancy.

The prenatal record will continue to be updated throughout the pregnancy. Clinical data will be added at each prenatal visit. The medical assistant will also be checking with the patient to see if there have been any changes or additions to the initial demographic and historical information.

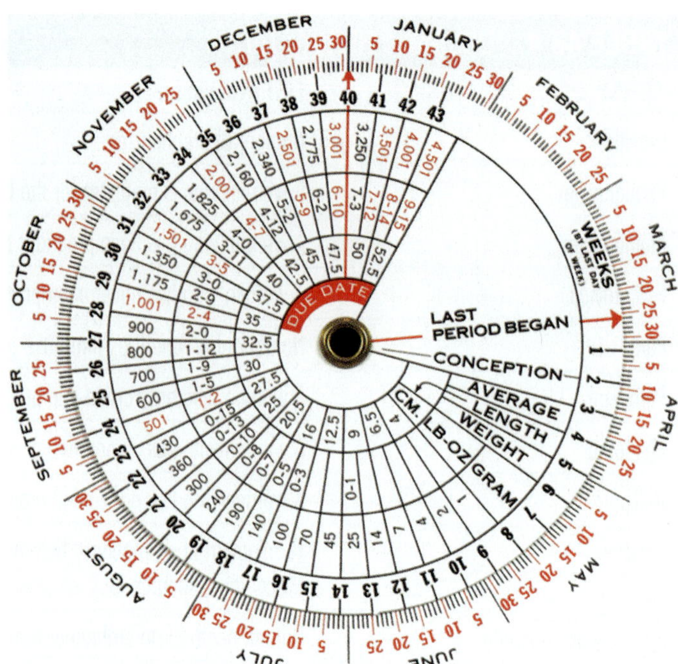

FIGURE 43.10 Gestational wheel. (From Jarvis C: *Physical examination and health assessment*, ed 6, St. Louis, 2012, Saunders.)

First Prenatal Examination

The physical examination during a first prenatal visit includes an overall assessment of the woman's health status. This would include vital signs, weight, and urinalysis. The medical assistant must prepare the patient. The patient should be asked if she needs to empty her bladder. If she does, she should collect a urine specimen for a routine urinalysis and a possible pregnancy test. The medical assistant should also prepare the exam room, ensuring that the supplies and equipment necessary to obtain pelvic measurements, perform serologic tests, and prepare for laboratory tests are available. The provider will assess the heart, lung, and thyroid. A physical examination will be done to rule out any other abnormalities. Next, the provider performs an obstetric examination that includes measurement of the height of the uterus and an internal or pelvic examination. A Pap test may be performed if one has not been done in the past year.

Pregnancy Test

There are two types of pregnancy tests. One is done with a urine sample, and the other is done with a blood sample. Both tests are looking for hCG levels. Blood tests are usually performed at the provider's office or laboratory. Urine tests can be performed at the provider's office, or the patient may do a home pregnancy test.

Whether the test is performed at home or in the office, the process is very much the same. A sample of the urine is placed on the test stick, and then the user waits for the results. Some test sticks will show a plus sign for a positive test and a minus sign for a negative test. Other tests will actually display the term *pregnant* for a positive test or *not pregnant* for a negative test.

The estimated date of delivery (EDD), or due date, will be determined at this visit. There are a number of ways to determine the due date. One method is using a gestational wheel (Figure 43.10). With this method, the arrow is lined up with the first date of the LMP, and the EDD is shown at the 40-week mark. The EDD may also be calculated by the electronic health record (EHR) or determined by ultrasound.

A series of blood tests are also performed during the initial prenatal visit. Prenatal blood and laboratory tests include the following:

- Hematocrit and hemoglobin levels to check for anemia.
- Blood type and Rh with antibody screening for possible Rh incompatibility (Figure 43.11).
- Rubella titer to determine whether the mother is immune to German measles; rubella infection during pregnancy can cause multiple birth defects, including deafness, vision disorders, and intellectual disability.
- Syphilis screening; if the result is positive, antibiotic treatment is initiated to protect the fetus from congenital syphilis.
- Hepatitis B screening because this virus can be passed to the fetus in utero.
- Human immunodeficiency virus (HIV) screening is suggested; if the result is positive, treatment of the mother greatly reduces the risk of transmission to the fetus.
- Gonorrhea and chlamydia cultures to prevent infection of the baby at birth.
- Urinalysis to detect protein, white blood cells, or glucose.

Any concerns that the patient has should be noted and reported to the provider. The medical assistant should be prepared to suggest community resources that can provide assistance to new parents, such as the following:

- Childbirth and parenting classes
- Infant cardiopulmonary resuscitation (CPR) courses
- Nutritional counseling, if needed
- Contact information for the Special Supplemental Nutrition Program for Women, Infants, and Children (WIC), which helps lower-income expectant mothers get nutritious food

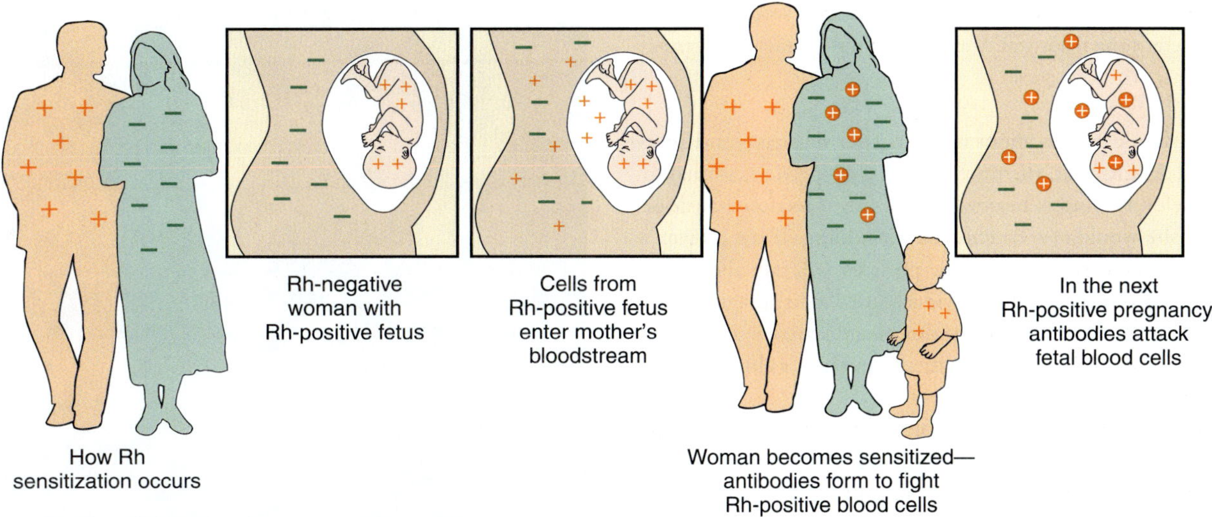

FIGURE 43.11 Hemolytic disease of the newborn. (From Hagen-Ansert SL: *Textbook of diagnostic sonography*, ed 7, St. Louis, 2012, Mosby)

Hemolytic Disease of the Newborn (HDN)

The blood is tested for the presence of D antigens to determine if someone's blood type is Rh positive or Rh negative. Rh-positive blood has D antigens; Rh-negative blood does not. If the blood type with Rh factor shows that the mother has Rh-negative blood, there is a concern that hemolytic disease of the newborn (HDN) could develop if the fetus is Rh positive. HDN is also known as *erythroblastosis fetalis.* If the mother is Rh negative and her fetus is Rh positive, the mother will form antibodies to the Rh-positive factor. Future Rh-positive pregnancies will be in jeopardy because the mother's anti-Rh antibodies will cross the placenta and destroy fetal blood cells (see Figure 43.11).

HDN can be prevented by giving the mother Rh immune globulin products. RhoGAM, or anti-D immune globulin, is given at 28 to 30 weeks of gestation to Rh-negative mothers, regardless of the father's Rh type. After delivery, the cord blood is tested, and a dose of RhoGAM is given within 72 hours of delivery, but only if the baby is Rh positive. RhoGAM is also given for miscarriages or abortions. The immune globulin prevents the infant's Rh-positive cells from stimulating the mother's immune system, thus preventing HDN.

Return Prenatal Visits

The return prenatal visits follow a regular schedule:

- Every 4 weeks through 28 weeks' gestation
- Every 2 weeks through 35 weeks' gestation
- Every 1 week until delivery

In follow-up prenatal visits, the medical assistant should collect a urine specimen for urinalysis, weigh the patient, measure her blood pressure, and answer questions about diet and health habits. The mother should gain approximately 10 to 12 pounds in the first half of pregnancy and another 15 to 17 pounds during the second half. Experts believe that a healthy weight gain is somewhere between 25 and 35 pounds.

Fetal Heart Tones. A Doppler monitor may be used to hear the baby's heart tones somewhere between 9- and 12-weeks' gestation. Once recorded, the fetal heart rate is assessed at each subsequent visit. It is important to remember that a fetal heart rate should be between 120 and 160 beats per minute. If you get a reading of between 60 and 100 beats per minute, you may be assessing the patient's heart rate and not the fetal heart rate.

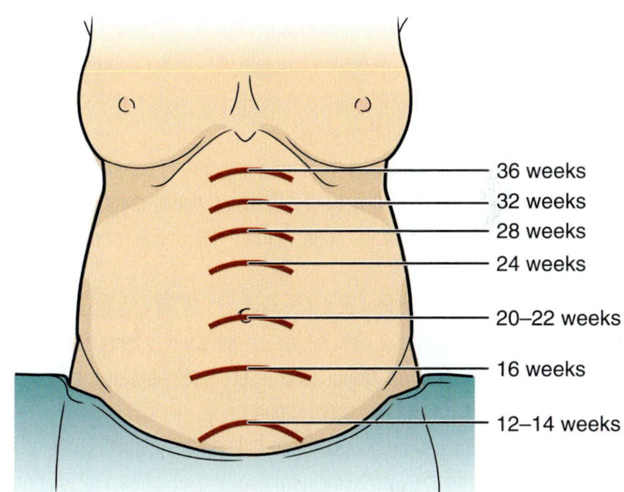

FIGURE 43.12 Fundal height measurement.

Fundal Height Measurement. Fundal height measurement is routinely done during the return prenatal visit. As the uterus grows during pregnancy, it will rise into the abdominal cavity. Between weeks 8 and 13, the fundus (the top of the uterus) can be palpated above the symphysis pubis. The fundal height measurement is taken with a flexible tape measure, measuring from the symphysis pubis to the fundus of the uterus. The height is measured in centimeters (cm) and most often matches the number of weeks the patient has been pregnant. For example, if the patient is 25 weeks pregnant, the provider would expect to see a fundal height measurement of 25 cm (Figure 43.12). This is only considered accurate for the first and second trimesters. If the fundal height measurement does not match the number of weeks pregnant, this could signal an issue with the pregnancy. Fundal height measurements that are either larger or smaller than expected could indicate the following:

- Slow fetal growth (intrauterine growth restriction)
- A significantly larger than average baby (*fetal macrosomia*)
- Too little amniotic fluid (*oligohydramnios*)
- Too much amniotic fluid (*polyhydramnios*)

If the provider suspects an issue, an ultrasound would likely be ordered to determine what was causing the unusual measurements.

Postpartum Visit

The patient should return about 6 weeks after delivery for a postpartum visit. At this visit, the provider will do a pelvic examination to make sure everything is healing. If a cesarean section was done, the incision site would also be checked for healing. If the patient is interested in using contraceptives, the provider will talk about contraceptive choices. If the patient previously used a diaphragm, the fit will need to be checked. There may also be a discussion about how breastfeeding is going. Any of the patient's questions about care for the baby should be answered at this visit.

The postpartum visit is also an opportunity to see how the patient is doing emotionally. The provider will ask questions about the patient's moods and check for signs of postpartum depression.

Postpartum Depression

- The incidence of postpartum depression (PPD) is not clear, but an estimated 10% to 20% of women struggle with major depression before, during, and after delivery of a baby. Fewer than half of these are diagnosed in routine office visits.
- Postpartum depression can be diagnosed a month to a year after childbirth. Women with a history of depression during pregnancy should be monitored for signs of postpartum depression for a minimum of 4 months.
- Risk factors include a history of depression, abuse, or mental illness; smoking or alcohol use; anxiety during pregnancy and fears over childcare; lack of financial resources and secure relationships; a fussy or colicky infant; and lack of social support.
- Symptoms of postpartum depression include anorexia and insomnia; irritability and anger; overwhelming fatigue; loss of interest in sex and lack of a feeling of joy in life; feelings of shame, guilt, or inadequacy; severe mood swings; difficulty bonding with the baby; withdrawal from family and friends; and thoughts of harming oneself or the baby.
- Postpartum depression must be detected as soon as possible so that treatment can begin; untreated postpartum depression may last for a year or longer. Treatment includes both counseling and antidepressant medication.

The 10-question Edinburgh Postnatal Depression Scale (EPDS) is a valuable and efficient way of identifying patients at risk for *perinatal* depression (between the 28th week of pregnancy and the 28th day after birth). Healthcare professionals working with the perinatal population should use the EPDS as a routine part of postnatal care because the EPDS is a valid and reliable means of detecting PPD. This screening tool is user-friendly, easy to administer, and easy to score. A score of 9 to 13 is considered the cutoff for PPD; the mother should be referred for further evaluation or treatment. Users may reproduce the scale without further permission, providing they respect the copyright by quoting the names of the authors and the title and the source of the paper in all reproduced copies. The EPDS can be accessed at the American Academy of Pediatrics website:

www.aap.org/en-us/advocacy-and-policy/aap-health-initiatives/practicing-safety/Documents/Postnatal%20Depression%20Scale.pdf.

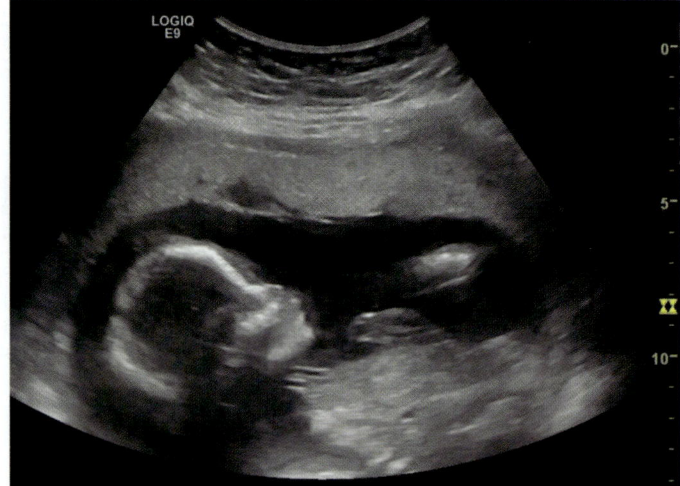

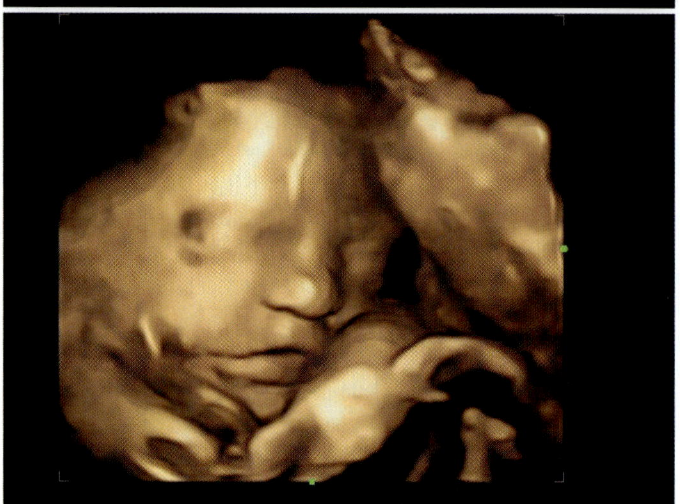

FIGURE 43.13 Ultrasound of a fetus. (Courtesy of Megan Pepper.)

Medical assistants should set up for this visit just as they would for a pelvic examination. You should also be aware of the patient's mood and body language. These can alert you to potential issues with postpartum depression. You should also have a list of provider-approved resources for the patient regarding postpartum depression or breastfeeding issues.

Assisting with Diagnostic Procedures

Throughout the pregnancy, there are special tests and procedures that may be done to assess the status of the pregnancy. In the next section, we will explore some of the more common tests and procedures.

Ultrasound

Ultrasound exams are typically done once during the first trimester and then again between weeks 18 and 20 to assess fetal development and thereby confirm the age of the fetus and proper growth (Figure 43.13). The sex of the baby can also be determined at that time. It is best if the patient has a full bladder for the ultrasound. The full bladder provides a great "window" for the sound waves to travel through, allowing for the best possible images. The patient should be instructed to drink two or three 8-ounce glasses of water 1 hour before the scheduled ultrasound.

Laboratory Testing

Between weeks 15 and 18 of pregnancy, the provider may suggest that the patient have a maternal blood screen in order to detect any risk of fetal and chromosomal disorders. This could be a triple screen test (also known as AFP Plus and multiple marker screening) or a quad screen test. Both tests screen for the following:

- Alpha-fetoprotein (AFP)
- Human chorionic gonadotropin (hCG)
- Estriol

The quad screen also tests for inhibin-A. These tests are used to evaluate if there is an increased chance of certain chromosomal conditions, such as Down syndrome. The alpha-fetoprotein evaluates the chances of neural tube defects, such as spina bifida.

If the patient is at risk for gestational diabetes, the provider will likely order a glucose challenge test. Risk factors for gestational diabetes include the following:

- A body mass index (BMI) before pregnancy of 30 or higher
- A mother, father, sibling, or child with diabetes

For a glucose challenge test, the patient must drink a glucose solution. One hour later, a blood test will be done to measure the glucose level. A blood glucose level of 130 to 140 milligrams per deciliter (mg/dL) is considered normal. If the result is higher than that, a glucose tolerance test may be ordered. The glucose tolerance test involves having the patient fast overnight before coming in for a blood glucose reading. The patient will then drink another glucose solution and have her blood glucose level checked every hour for the next 3 hours. If two out of the three readings are higher than normal, the patient would be diagnosed with gestational diabetes.

Group B streptococcus is a common bacterium found in the intestines. It is usually harmless in adults, but in newborns it can cause group B strep disease. This is a serious illness for newborns. A group B streptococcus culture of the lower vagina can be performed between weeks 32 and 36. If the result is positive, the mother is treated with intravenous (IV) antibiotics to prevent fetal exposure during vaginal birth.

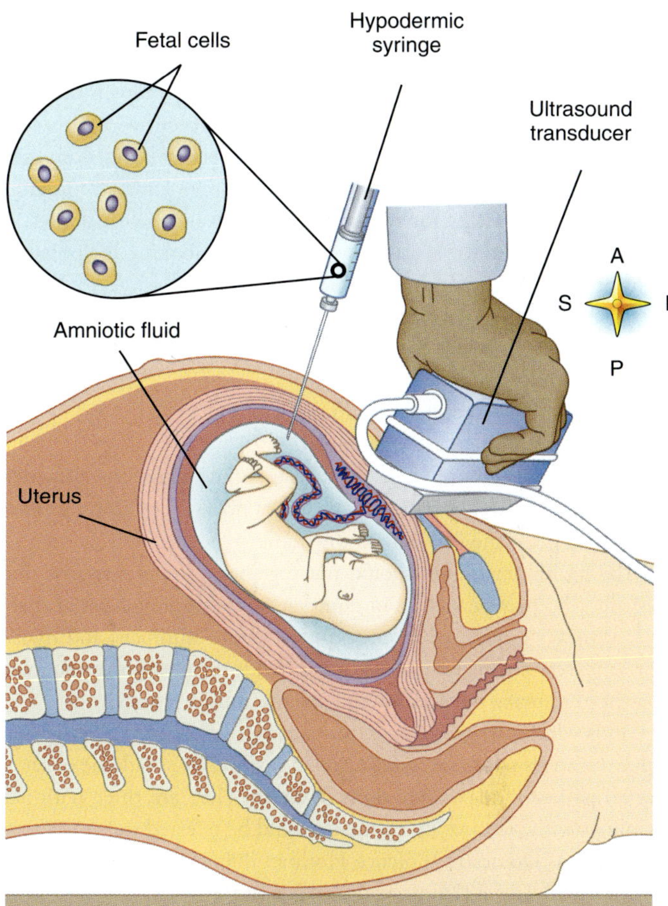

FIGURE 43.14 Amniocentesis. (From Shiland B: *Mastering healthcare terminology*, St. Louis, 2016, Elsevier.)

Amniocentesis

Amniocentesis involves needle aspiration of approximately 2 tablespoons of amniotic fluid after week 14 of pregnancy. The aim is to detect genetic and chromosomal abnormalities or inherited metabolic disorders (Figure 43.14). Potential complications include the following:

- Miscarriage
- Fetal injury
- Infection
- Premature labor
- Maternal hemorrhage

Results take up to 2 weeks.

Chorionic Villus Sampling

Chorionic villi are tiny placental projections, the cells of which have the same genetic material found in fetal cells. Chorionic villus sampling (CVS) involves the removal of a small piece of the chorionic villi, either transvaginally or through a small incision in the abdomen (Figure 43.15). Cellular screening at 8- to 12-week gestation provides early detection of genetic or chromosomal disorders. Potential complications include the following:

- Accidental abortion
- Infection, bleeding
- Fetal limb deformities

Results are available within several days.

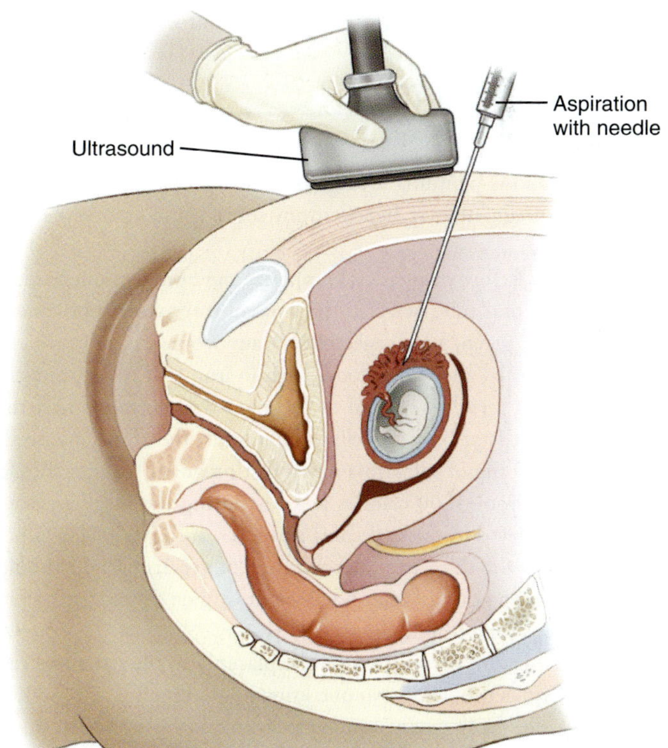

FIGURE 43.15 Chorionic villus sampling (CVS). (From Shiland B: *Medical terminology and anatomy for ICD-10 coding*, St. Louis, 2012, Mosby.)

Recognizing Domestic Abuse

There are federal laws in place that require many insurance plans to provide coverage for certain preventive health services without any cost-sharing for the patient. Included in the preventive health services are screening and counseling for interpersonal and domestic violence. Working in healthcare gives us an opportunity to provide support and resources for someone who is dealing with domestic violence. As a medical assistant, you should be looking for possible signs of abuse, such as the following:

- Unusual or frequent bruises or fractures
- Attempts to hide the bruises with makeup or clothing
- Low self-esteem
- Being extremely apologetic and meek
- References to the partner's temper

If you notice any of these signs, you should make the provider aware of them. Even a patient who shows no signs of abuse should be asked if he or she feels safe in the home.

The healthcare facility should put together a list of resources for patients who may be victims of domestic abuse. Having a list of shelters, advocacy groups, emergency contact phone numbers, and transportation services to give patients may provide them with the resources they need to make the decision to leave the abusive situation.

Abuse does not just happen in marriages or committed relationships; it can also occur in a dating relationship. We should be observing all patients for possible signs of abuse. Here are three national helplines with websites that patients could be referred to:

- National Domestic Violence Hotline: 800-799-SAFE (7233) or TTY 800-787-3224; www.thehotline.org
- National Dating Abuse Helpline: 866-331-9474 or TTY 866-331-8453; www.loveisrespect.org (live chat is available); text "loveis" to 77054
- Office on Women's Health: www.womenshealth.gov/relationships-and-safety/relationships-and-safety-resources

CLOSING COMMENTS

Patient Coaching

A woman who is planning a pregnancy or who has just found out that she is pregnant may benefit from some simple guidelines for healthy living:

- *Nutrition:* Before pregnancy, emphasize the need for folic acid to prevent neural tube defects. The woman can take a supplement or eat dark green, leafy vegetables. Many women have iron-deficiency anemia, and eating foods high in iron (red meat, spinach, or enriched cereal) is helpful. A pregnant woman must meet the calcium needs of both herself and her fetus; therefore, she needs about 1000 mg of calcium a day. Most pregnant women should consume about 1800 calories per day during the first trimester, 2200 per day during the second trimester, and 2400 calories per day during the third trimester. Women of average weight should gain 25 to 35 pounds, but underweight women should gain 35 to 45 pounds for a healthy infant.
- *Alcohol:* Alcohol passes through the placenta to the fetus and can cause serious problems. No one knows how much is safe, so it is a good idea for pregnant women to avoid alcohol completely.
- *Smoking:* Smoking can cause premature birth and low-birth-weight full-term infants. Smoking is linked to an increased risk of otitis media, heart problems, upper respiratory infection in infants, and also sudden infant death syndrome (SIDS). Pregnant women should not smoke and should not be exposed to secondhand smoke.
- *Medicine:* All chemicals pass through the placenta; therefore, a pregnant woman should never take any medicine (even over-the-counter drugs) without the knowledge and approval of her provider. If the medical assistant is managing telephone screening, having a list of provider-approved medications next to the phone helps answer patients' questions.
- *STI screening:* STI screening should be done before a woman becomes pregnant. Many STIs are asymptomatic in women but treatable. Infants are at risk for serious health problems if exposed to certain STIs in utero or during the birth process.

Legal and Ethical Issues

Many ethical and legal issues arise as a result of missed communication. Listen to what every patient reports and write down any information that will assist the provider in treating the patient. The issue may appear to be an insignificant problem, but to the patient, it may be a major concern. Let the provider be the judge of whether the problem is relevant. As the patient's advocate and the provider's assistant, the medical assistant plays an important role in establishing good communication as a vital link in patient care.

Confidentiality is crucial in dealing with obstetric and gynecologic disorders. Only healthcare professionals directly involved in the patient's care should know the purpose of the patient's visit, diagnosis, or treatment. Maintaining patient confidentiality is not just an ethical responsibility; it is a legal requirement.

Patient-Centered Care

When providing patient-centered care while working in obstetrics and gynecology, a medical assistant should do the following:

- Behave in a professional manner at all times because an OB/GYN visit can be an uncomfortable and embarrassing situation for the patient.
- During patient education sessions, make sure that the patient truly understands the content.
- Stay current with the new topics and technology related to obstetrics and gynecology.
- Treat all patients as you would want to be treated.

Professional Behaviors

When working in obstetrics and gynecology, it is important to remain nonjudgmental when dealing with different patient circumstances. Patients can present with situations that you have strong personal feelings about. It could be a young patient who is asking about birth control. It could be a patient who is being seen repeatedly for STIs. It could be a patient who is not following the prenatal care plan. In any of those situations, we must always do what is best for the patient and follow office policies and procedures. We cannot give our opinion on how we think the patient should behave. We have a responsibility to inform the provider of any patient issues that are presented.

SUMMARY OF SCENARIO

Jill Snow has enjoyed her time in the OB/GYN department and has learned a lot from Peggy. She was able to observe several procedures and saw how Peggy prepped the patient and the exam room for those procedures. Peggy has been an amazing mentor for Jill. She has taken the time to explain the reasons for how each procedure is done. Peggy's knowledge and expertise in OB/GYN, along with her willingness to teach others, have made Jill decide to pursue a position in this field after she graduates. Peggy's supervisor recognizes her talents in this area and has asked her to take over the practicum program for their department.

SUMMARY OF LEARNING OBJECTIVES

1. **Examine the anatomy and physiology of the female reproductive system.**
   There are two parts to the anatomy of the female reproductive system: parenchymal and stromal. Parenchymal or primary tissue produces sex cells for reproduction. The stromal or secondary tissues serve a supportive function for those sex cells.

   The ovaries, fallopian tubes, uterus, vagina, vulva, and breasts are the major organs of the female reproductive system.

   The menstrual cycle is divided into follicular, luteal, and menstrual phases. In the follicular phase, hormones are secreted to mature a Graafian follicle in the ovary. The mature follicle secretes estrogen that stimulates the growth of the endometrium. This phase ends when the ovum is released. In the luteal phase, progesterone is secreted to prepare the endometrium for a possible pregnancy. If pregnancy does not occur, the menstrual phase begins, and the uterus sheds the lining.

   Pregnancy begins with the fertilization of an ovum by a sperm. During implantation, the zygote functions as an endocrine gland by secreting hCG. At the same time that the embryo is developing, extraembryonic membranes are forming to sustain the pregnancy.
2. **Analyze the life span changes that occur in the female reproductive system.**
   Many changes happen to the female reproductive system during puberty. Hormonal changes stimulate the maturation of the breasts, ovaries, uterus, and vagina. Menarche occurs, and body shape changes. Irregular menstruations, dysmenorrhea, and amenorrhea are common menstrual disorders during this time.

   As women age, other changes occur that also relate to hormones. Many of these changes are related to perimenopause and menopause. Fertility decreases, and vaginal walls become thinner, dryer, and less elastic. Later in life, cancers of the breast, uterus, cervix, and ovaries can develop.
3. **Examine the diseases and disorders of the female reproductive system.**
   Sexually transmitted infections (STIs) are typically asymptomatic in men, although they can cause serious problems. Many pathogens cause STIs, but what they have in common is that they are most efficiently transmitted by sexual contact.

   With endometriosis, functional endometrial tissue is located outside the uterus. It is commonly attached to the ovaries, urinary bladder, fallopian tubes, uterosacral ligaments, intestines, or peritoneum. Common signs and symptoms of endometriosis include dysmenorrhea, dyspareunia, pain with bowel movements or urination, menorrhagia, menometrorrhagia, infertility, fatigue, diarrhea, constipation, bloating, and nausea.

   Common infections of the female reproductive system include candidiasis, cervicitis, and pelvic inflammatory disease (PID).

   Menopause is the permanent ending of menstruation caused by the cessation of ovarian function. Perimenopause begins when hormone-related changes start to appear and lasts until the final menses. Some women experience few or no symptoms, whereas others have hot flashes, concentration problems, mood swings, irritability, migraines, vaginal dryness, urinary incontinence, dry skin, and sleep disorders. The provider may prescribe low-dose oral contraceptives or HRT, weight-bearing exercise, soy products or vitamin supplements, dietary changes, and medication to manage hot flashes, mood swings, and vaginal dryness and prevent osteoporosis.
4. **Examine the cancers found in the female reproductive system.**
   Breast cancer is the second leading cause of cancer deaths in women. Risk factors include being female, a family history of breast cancer, genetics, radiation exposure, obesity, menarche at a younger age, menopause at an older age, having your first child at an older age, having never been pregnant, postmenopausal hormone therapy, and drinking alcohol. Diagnostic procedures start with a breast examination and mammogram. From there, additional imaging and a biopsy may be done. Treatment can include surgical options as well as radiation, chemotherapy, or hormone therapy.

   Cervical cancer is usually caused by HPV. Cervical cellular changes may be picked up with a Pap test, and HPV can be detected with specific HPV testing. Diagnostic procedures could include a biopsy, endocervical curettage, colposcopy, and LEEP. LEEP would also be considered a treatment option along with cone biopsy, hysterectomy, radiation, and chemotherapy.

   Ovarian cancer has often metastasized before the tumor is diagnosed. The causes of ovarian cancer are not known, but risk factors include age, inherited gene mutation, estrogen hormone replacement therapy, menarche at a young age, menopause at an older age, having never been pregnant, fertility treatment, smoking, use of an intrauterine device, and polycystic ovary syndrome. Diagnostic procedures include a pelvic examination ultrasound or CT scan, a CA-125 blood test (looks for certain proteins in the blood), and a biopsy.
5. **Examine the medical assistant's role in assisting with examinations, diagnostic procedures, and treatments for the female reproductive system.**
   The medical assistant prepares the patient for the examination, equips the room, makes sure supplies are available and properly prepared, positions and drapes the patient as needed, assists with the Pap smear or any

Continued

SUMMARY OF LEARNING OBJECTIVES—*continued*

other procedures, and provides support and understanding for the patient. (See Procedure 43.1.)

Barrier contraceptive methods include the use of condoms, a diaphragm, a cervical cap, or a cervical sponge; all of these are relatively inexpensive and reversible, but they must be used with each instance of intercourse. Two general types of intrauterine devices (IUDs) are available to inhibit fertilization and prevent the embryo from implanting in the uterine wall. Hormonal contraceptives include Depo-Provera injections, Implanon or Nexplanon implants, oral and patch contraceptives, and the vaginal ring, all of which are very effective but have side effects and contraindications. (See Table 43.3.)

A specimen for a Pap test can be collected in two ways. In the direct smear method, the cells are collected from the cervix with a cervical spatula and placed directly on a microscope slide; then, a fixative is applied. For the liquid-based method, a plastic-fronded broom is used to collect the cells from the cervix, and the broom is then rinsed in the specimen vial. The cells are prepared for viewing in the laboratory.

For a maturation index, cells are collected from the vaginal wall and are treated like a Pap test specimen.

For vaginal infections, a swab is used to collect a sample of the discharge. The sample is then placed on a microscope slide. If the provider suspects candidiasis, a drop of a 10% solution of potassium hydroxide (KOH) is added. If the provider is looking for trichomoniasis, a drop of saline is added. For chlamydia, the swab is sent to the lab for testing.

The patient should be helped into the sitting position and assistance offered for dressing. The examination room should be cleaned following Occupational Safety and Health Administration (OSHA) Standard Precautions.

Three of the most common gynecologic procedures performed in the medical office are as follows:

- *Cryotherapy:* Cryotherapy involves the application of freezing temperature to the cervix. This causes necrosis, and dead cells are replaced with healthy cells.
- *Colposcopy with or without a biopsy:* Colposcopy is the visual examination of the vagina and the cervical surfaces. A colposcope is used to locate and evaluate abnormal cells, detect cancer in the early stages, and monitor areas of the cervix where malignant lesions have been removed. If the provider identifies an area of concern, a biopsy will be obtained. Correct labeling of the biopsy specimen container is very important.
- *Loop electrosurgical excision procedure (LEEP):* In a LEEP procedure, a wire loop with an electrical current running through it is used to remove abnormal tissue from the cervix and the endocervical canal. This procedure can also be used to collect a biopsy sample.

6. Examine the medical assistant's role in assisting with the obstetrical examination.

At the first prenatal visit, a prenatal record will be created. It includes the following: demographic information, menstrual history, obstetric history, medical and surgical history, and family and social history.

The first prenatal examination includes an overall assessment of the woman's health status. A series of lab tests will be done, including a urinalysis and multiple blood tests. Return prenatal visits will follow a regular schedule and will include a check of vital signs, a test of hemoglobin, and a urinalysis.

The patient will return about 6 weeks after delivery for a postpartum visit. A pelvic examination will be done to assess healing; if the patient is interested in contraception, the options will be discussed.

An ultrasound is usually performed in the first trimester to assess fetal development, which is used to confirm the age of the fetus. The sex can also be determined between 18- and 20-weeks' gestation.

A number of laboratory tests can be ordered for an obstetric patient, including a triple screen test or a quad screen test. These tests are used to determine if there is an increased chance of certain chromosomal conditions, such as Down syndrome. The alpha-fetoprotein evaluates the chances of neural tube defects, such as spina bifida. If the patient is at risk for gestational diabetes, a glucose challenge test may be ordered. For this test, the patient must drink a glucose solution. One hour later, a blood test will be done to measure the glucose level. A blood glucose level of 130 to 140 milligrams per deciliter (mg/dL) is considered normal. If the result is higher than that, a glucose tolerance test may be ordered.

An amniocentesis may be done after week 14 of pregnancy to detect genetic and chromosomal abnormalities or inherited metabolic disorders. Chorionic villus sampling is another test that can be done to detect genetic or chromosomal disorders.

Signs of abuse include the following: unusual or frequent bruises or fractures, attempts to hide the bruises with makeup or clothing, low self-esteem, being extremely apologetic and meek, and references to the partner's temper. Medical assistants should be aware of the laws in their state regarding the reporting of domestic abuse.

PROCEDURE 43.1 Set Up for and Assist the Provider with a Gynecologic Examination

TASK: Prepare equipment for a gynecologic examination and assist the provider by placing the patient in the appropriate positions.

EQUIPMENT and SUPPLIES

- Disposable examination gloves
- Fecal occult blood test kit
- Water-soluble lubricant
- Vaginal speculum
- Slide and fixative or liquid preparation container
- Cervical spatula or plastic-fronded broom
- Laboratory requisition form
- Cotton-tipped applicator
- Patient gown
- Patient drape sheet
- Tray or Mayo stand

PROCEDURAL STEPS

1. Sanitize hands.
   PURPOSE: Hand sanitization is an important step for infection control.
2. Assemble equipment needed for the gynecologic examination. Place on a tray or Mayo stand in a logical order.
   PURPOSE: Having the equipment in a logical order allows you to assist the clinician in an efficient manner.
3. Change the table paper if needed.
   PURPOSE: Clean table paper prevents the transmission of microorganisms from one patient to another.
4. Greet the patient. Identify yourself. Verify the patient's identity with full name and date of birth. Explain the procedure to be performed in a manner that the patient understands. Answer any questions the patient may have.
   PURPOSE: It is important to identify the patient in two different ways to ensure that you have the correct patient. Explaining the procedure can make the patient feel more comfortable and reduces anxiety.
5. Ask if the patient needs to empty her bladder and collect a urine specimen if needed.
   PURPOSE: An empty bladder will make the pelvic examination more comfortable for the patient.
6. Instruct the patient to undress and put on the gown.
   PURPOSE: The patient will need to be completely undressed for the examination.
7. Assist the patient onto the examination table; she should remain in the sitting position. Place the drape across her lap.
   PURPOSE: The first position used for the gynecologic examination is the sitting position. While the patient is in this position, the provider will visually inspect the breasts.
8. Assist the patient into the supine position and provide a pillow to be placed under her head for comfort. Pull out the leg extension on the examination table.
   PURPOSE: For the rest of the breast examination and the abdominal examination, the patient will need to be in the supine position.
9. With the stirrups in place on the examination table, assist the patient into the lithotomy position. The leg extension should be pushed in.
   PURPOSE: The lithotomy position is used for the pelvic examination.
10. When the examination is complete, assist the patient into the sitting position. Instruct the patient that she can get dressed.
    PURPOSE: At the end of the examination, the patient can get dressed.
11. After the patient has dressed and left the exam room, clean the room and prepare specimens for transport to the laboratory.
    PURPOSE: By cleaning the examination room, you are preparing it for the next patient. It is the medical assistant's responsibility to properly prepare specimens for transport to the laboratory.

PROCEDURE 43.2 Coach a Patient on Breast Self-Examination

TASKS: Coach a patient to do a breast self-exam (BSE) while considering the patient's cultural beliefs and developmental life stage. Document this teaching in the patient's health record.

EQUIPMENT and SUPPLIES

- Breast self-examination brochure (optional)
- Breast model
- Provider's order
- Patient's health record

SCENARIO: You are working with Dr. David Kahn. He has ordered you to show Bihn, an 18-year-old Vietnamese patient, how to do a breast self-exam. She has a strong family history of breast cancer. The patient is fluent in speaking and understanding English.

PROCEDURAL STEPS

1. Wash hands or use hand sanitizer.
   PURPOSE: Hand sanitization is an important step for infection control.
2. Read the provider's order. Assemble the equipment.
   PURPOSE: It is important to know the provider's order before starting the procedure.
3. Greet the patient. Identify yourself. Verify the patient's identity with full name and date of birth. Explain the procedure to be performed in a manner that the patient understands. Answer any questions the patient may have.
   PURPOSE: It is important to identify the patient in two different ways to ensure that you have the correct patient. Explaining the procedure can make the patient feel more comfortable and reduces anxiety.
4. Provide privacy and independence during the session. Encourage the patient to ask questions and discuss her concerns.
   PURPOSE: It is important to adapt the coaching to the patient's developmental stage. Because this patient is 18, privacy and independence are important to her. Encouraging questions and discussions is also effective.
5. Ask the patient if she is familiar with breast self-examinations. Discuss her thoughts on illness and what she does for alternative therapies. Explain the importance of doing a self-exam.
   PURPOSE: In Vietnamese culture, illness is often explained by mystical beliefs. Asking the patient her thoughts might provide information that is helpful to the medical assistant during the coaching session.
6. Explain to the patient that she will need to undress and look at her breast in the mirror to identify any changes. She will need to check to see if they are the usual size, shape, and color and should look for any swelling, redness, rash, dimpling, puckering, or bulging of the skin. She will also need to see if the nipple position or appearance has changed. Also, explain that she should check to see if any fluid is coming from the nipple by placing her thumb and index finger on the tissue by the nipple and pulling outward toward the end of the nipple (Figure 1).
   PURPOSE: Changes in the appearance may indicate an issue.

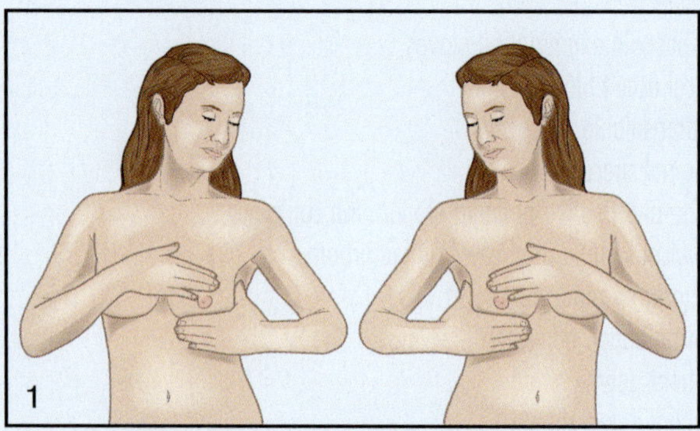

1

7. Instruct the patient that she needs to change positions and continue to check the appearance of the breast. She needs to place her hands on her hips and press down. This tightens the chest muscle under the breast. While in this position, she should turn from side to side to see the outer part of the breasts. Instruct her to clasp her hands behind her head or raise her arms and look at the outer part of the breast again (Figure 2).
   PURPOSE: Sometimes, changing the arm position may cause an abnormality to appear.

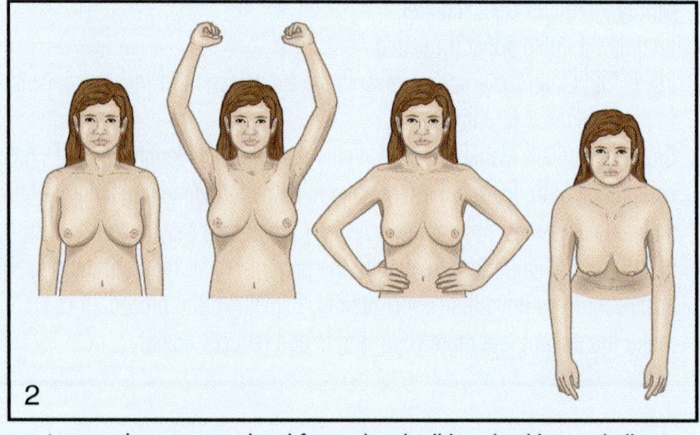

2

8. Instruct the patient to bend forward and roll her shoulders and elbows forward while tightening her chest muscles. While in this position, she can check for changes in the shape.
   PURPOSE: Sometimes, changing the arm position may cause an abnormality to appear.
9. Instruct the patient to palpate the breast using one of the two techniques. Use the model as you explain each technique.
   a. *Lying down technique*: Instruct the patient to check the breast while lying down. She should tuck a small pillow under the side being checked; then she can tuck one arm under the head and, with the other hand, check the opposite breast (e.g., the right hand checks the left breast). Instruct the patient to use the first two or three finger pads. With fingers together, she can use a circular motion and a firm, smooth touch to check the entire breast. Explain that she should start at the top of the breast and move around it in a circular pattern.

PROCEDURE 43.2 Coach a Patient on Breast Self-Examination—*continued*

When the top of the breast is reached again, she can move in 1 inch toward the nipple and complete another circle around the breast. Instruct her to work in a systematic method to cover the entire breast from the armpit to the cleavage. She can then place her fingers flat on the nipple and feel for any changes beneath the nipple. Explain that she will repeat this procedure on the other breast.

b. *Shower technique*: Instruct the patient to place her right hand on her right hip. With a soapy left hand, she can feel for changes in the right axilla area. Describe how she can use two or three finger pads to press on the breast. She will be moving in an up-and-down pattern over the breast tissue. Remind her to make sure to cover the area from the bra line to the collar bone. Explain that she will repeat this procedure on the opposite side.

PURPOSE: This position allows the patient to check the entire breast for changes, including under the arm and up to the collarbone.

10. Have the patient select a technique that she will use. Encourage the patient to demonstrate the technique on the breast model. Coach the patient on ways to improve the exam if needed.

PURPOSE: It is important to have the patient demonstrate the teaching to check for accuracy of technique and correct understanding.

11. Answer any questions the patient may have. Provide the patient with a brochure to take home (optional).

PURPOSE: It is important to answer any questions and, if possible, provide the patient with a brochure to take home.

12. Document the patient education in the patient health record. Include the provider's name, the order, what was taught to the patient, how the patient responded, how the patient did the demonstration, and any handouts provided.

PURPOSE: It is important to document the patient education in the health record to show it was done.

Documentation Example

07/19/20XX 1505 Per Dr. Kahn's order, instructed pt on the BSE. Instructed the patient on how to check for changes in the breast. Explained the lying and showering techniques. Pt opted for the showering technique. She demonstrated how to palpate the breast tissue correctly using a breast model. All her questions were answered. Provided her with the "BSE" brochure and encouraged her to perform it monthly. ———————————— Peggy St. John, CMA (AAMA)

PEDIATRICS

44

SCENARIO

Allison Kwong, who has 2 years of experience as a certified medical assistant (CMA) and has met the requirements of the American Association of Medical Assistants (AAMA), has accepted a new position with the pediatric department of the Walden-Martin Family Medical (WMFM) Clinic. Allison's primary responsibility will be to assist in the clinical area, but she also will have to rotate through the message screening center in the office. Office policy states that telephone screening employees should manage problems as much as possible. However, if patient callbacks are needed, they are to be referred to the provider on call that day by noon for morning calls and no later than 5 p.m. for afternoon calls. Although Allison has worked in the healthcare field for 2 years, she does not have much experience with pediatrics. She is glad that she has been assigned a mentor for the first few weeks.

While studying this chapter, think about the following questions:

- What are the expected growth and developmental patterns for children?
- When screening telephone calls from patients, which medical conditions should the screener call to the provider's attention right away and why?
- How does the schedule of immunizations presented by the Centers for Disease Control and Prevention (CDC) affect patient care?
- What is the importance of Vaccine Information Statements (VISs)?
- What information is needed when documenting immunizations?

LEARNING OBJECTIVES

1. Examine growth and developmental patterns of the pediatric patient.
2. Examine the common diseases and disorders found in the pediatric patient population, including the signs, symptoms, etiology, diagnostic procedures, and treatments
3. Examine the medical assistant's role in examinations and diagnostic procedures.
4. Explain the different types of pediatric visits.
5. Examine the common diagnostic procedures done during a pediatric visit.
6. Examine common treatments done with pediatric patients.
7. Contrast working with adolescent patients and younger pediatric patients.

VOCABULARY

attenuated (uh TEN yoo ayt ed) Weakened or changed.

autonomy (aw TON uh mee) The ability to function independently.

epiphyseal plate (eh pi FIZ ee uhl) A thin layer of cartilage located at the ends of a long bone where new bone forms.

excoriation (ik skawr ee AY shun) Inflammation and irritation of the skin.

fontanelle (fon tah NEL) A space covered by thick membranes between the sutures of an infant's skull; called the baby's "soft spots"; there are both anterior and posterior fontanelles.

hydrocephaly (hye droh SEF ul lee) Enlargement of the cranium caused by an abnormal accumulation of cerebrospinal fluid in the cerebral system.

lethargy (LETH er jee) The state of being drowsy and dull, listless and unenergetic.

microcephaly (mie kroh SEF ul lee) Abnormally small head associated with incomplete brain development.

nonorganic (nahn or GAN ik) Not having an organic or physiologic cause; a disorder that does not have a cause that can be found in the body.

serous (SEER uhs) A thin, watery, serum-like drainage.

suppurative (SUHP yuh ray tiv) Characterized by the formation or discharge of pus.

urticaria (ur ti KAYR ee ah) Hives.

INTRODUCTION

Pediatrics is the medical specialty that deals with the development and care of children and the treatment of childhood diseases. Pediatric patients range in age from newborn to puberty. Some practices continue to see the child until they graduate from high school. Subspecialties within pediatrics include surgery, cardiology, and psychiatry.

Approximately 50% of the patients in a pediatric office are there for well-baby or well-child visits. The roles of the provider and the medical office staff are to supervise and help maintain the health of these patients. The medical assistant can help by encouraging therapeutic communication among the patient, parents, caregivers, and medical staff. The trust that a child develops in these relationships and the consideration the family receives in the provider's office form the basis of good medical care.

Pediatric care actually starts before the child is born, with good prenatal care. The confidence and enthusiasm of the parents can have a significant impact on an infant's physical and emotional well-being.

NORMAL GROWTH AND DEVELOPMENT

The terms *growth* and *development* are often used together. They refer to the combination of changes a child goes through as they mature. *Growth* refers to measurable changes, such as height and weight. The first determinant of these physical characteristics is the genetics inherited from the parents; however, a child's growth can be influenced by many factors, including nutritional status, environmental factors, and the presence of disease. *Development* refers to the stages of physical, cognitive, and social growth. A provider looks at how the child is progressing in motor, mental, social, and language skills. A child's development is determined by a combination of prenatal, environmental, and caregiver factors. Each child has his or her own pattern of growth and development. Pediatric assessments are individualized for each child according to age, developmental level, health condition, family characteristics, and past experiences with healthcare professionals. National standards are used to help pinpoint irregularities in growth and development. The child's physical, intellectual, and social levels are compared with published national standards. This comparison indicates whether the child is at the appropriate stage of growth and development for his or her chronologic age.

Growth Patterns

Physical growth is one of the most visible changes in childhood. The average birth weight is 7 to 7 ½ pounds, and in 6 months, the baby's birth weight doubles. Growth then slows slightly over the next 6 months and even more over the next couple of years (Table 44.1). Between ages 2 and 3, most children slim down so that by the time the third birthday arrives, the potbellied toddler has become the characteristic preschooler.

By age 4, the child usually has doubled their birth length. During this time, the legs are the fastest-growing part; fatty connective tissue continues to increase slowly until approximately age 7. This same growth rate continues through the school-aged period (6 to 12 years), and as this period of development ends, the child usually is into a growth spurt that indicates impending puberty.

The growth spurt continues for approximately 2 years, and the child then reaches adolescence (ages 12 to 18 years). During this period, the adolescent gains almost half of his or her adult weight, and the skeleton and organs double in size. Weight increases in girls by 20 to 25 pounds and in boys by 15 to 20 pounds. Girls grow 5 to 6 inches, and boys grow 4 to 5 inches. As the growth spurt is completed, the teenager reaches sexual maturity. In girls, sexual maturity is signaled by the onset of the menstrual cycle; in boys, it is determined by the presence of sperm in the semen. The timing of sexual maturity in both genders varies greatly.

TABLE 44.1 Growth Patterns

6 months	Birth weight doubles
1 year	Birth weight triples, length increased by 50%
2 years	Gains 6 pounds in 1 year
3 years	Gains 3–5 pounds in 1 year and grows 2– 2 ½ inches
3–6 years	Gains 3–5 pounds per year, grows 1 ½ – 2 ½ inches per year

Skeletal growth is complete in girls between 15 and 16 years of age and boys between ages 17 and 18. Skeletal growth is considered complete when the **epiphyseal plates** (growth plates) of the long bones of the extremities have completely fused.

Growth charts are used to compare the child's individual growth pattern with national standards. The Centers for Disease Control and Prevention (CDC) has developed growth charts that track growth continuously through the age of 20. The growth charts are gender specific. Length, weight, and head circumference are tracked on the birth to 36 months growth chart. Stature and weight are tracked on the 2 to 20 years growth chart. There are also CDC growth charts used to track body mass index (BMI) in infants and young adults 2 to 20 years of age, giving providers another weapon in the fight against childhood obesity. BMI is a means of assessing the relationship between height and weight. BMI conversion charts are typically available or are calculated automatically in electronic health record (EHR) programs. The actual formula to calculate BMI is as follows:

$$\text{BMI} = \frac{\text{Weight (kg)}}{\text{Height(m)}^2}$$

For adults, the BMI itself is used as the screening tool. In pediatrics, the BMI needs to be plotted on the gender-specific growth chart, and the growth chart percentile is the screening tool. The CDC has developed four weight status categories.

Centers for Disease Control and Prevention (CDC) Weight Status Categories

WEIGHT STATUS CATEGORY	PERCENTILE RANGE
Underweight	Less than the 5th percentile
Normal or healthy weight	5th percentile to less than the 85th percentile
Overweight	85th percentile to less than the 95th percentile
Obese	Equal to or greater than the 95th percentile

Developmental Patterns

General patterns of child development occur rapidly during the first year of life as the infant progresses from reflex activities (e.g., grasping fingers and sucking) to learning to manipulate simple objects (e.g., pulling open drawers or throwing toys out of the crib). In addition to these motor skills, the child learns verbal patterns, progressing from cooing and crying for attention to speaking his or her first words.

By age 3, the child is showing increased **autonomy**. Now the child can walk, is toilet trained, sits at the table and eats with the family, makes simple sentences, understands the word *no*, and even imitates the parent by using gestures they have seen them use. The child's vocabulary consists of up to 900 words.

Therapeutic Approaches for Infants (Newborn to 12 Months)

- Crying is normal; use distraction, but do not overstimulate.
- It is important to keep the infant close to the caregiver; either have the parent hold the infant or keep the parent in the child's line of vision.
- Involve the parent as much as possible, depending on the task and the parent's level of comfort.
- Place a familiar object near the infant and keep frightening ones out of view.
- An infant's negative response to strangers usually develops at approximately 8 months; do not take the rejection personally.
- Do not restrain the infant any more than necessary but be ready to use restraint at times (e.g., when giving an injection) to keep the infant safe.
- Encourage the caregiver to cuddle and hug the child after the procedure is complete.
- Unpleasant procedures are associated with other objects, so do not use play areas for treatment, and do not use a favorite toy or object during the procedure; offer it afterward for comfort.

During the preschool stage, the child becomes increasingly independent and initiates activities. Preschoolers have mastered many gross motor skills and are perfecting their fine motor development. Verbal communication has increased to full, simple, and even complex sentences but remains quite literal. For example, if you tell a preschool child that you are going to fly to visit Aunt Sue, the child thinks you are going to flap your arms and fly. Nonverbal communication skills are also being mastered. The vocabulary now includes more than 2000 words. During this period, children need to develop social skills, such as sharing and taking part in peer-group activities.

Therapeutic Approaches for Toddlers and Preschoolers (2 to 6 Years)

- Toddlers and preschoolers often fear visits to the doctor; ignore temper tantrums and negative behavior.
- Praise the child as much as possible.
- Perform unpleasant procedures as quickly as possible; the fear of the procedure is worse than the actual discomfort.
- Allow the child to keep on as much clothing as possible for security and comfort.
- Use words familiar to the child, and do not use words the child could misinterpret. For example, "The test uses dye" (the child may think you mean "die"); "The doctor will put you to sleep so that it doesn't hurt" (the family dog may have been put to sleep).
- Explain a procedure as the child would sense it—what it will look like, how it will smell, how it will feel, and so on.
- Allow the child to handle equipment when possible.
- Do not use the child's favorite doll or stuffed animal to demonstrate; the child may believe the toy feels pain.
- Explain procedures to the parents away from the child when possible; the child may misinterpret the information.

CRITICAL THINKING APPLICATION **44.1**

Allison receives a call from the mother of a 6-month-old child. The woman is concerned that her child may not be reaching his developmental milestones. What type of information about the child's growth and development should Allison gather? If Allison is unable to answer the mother's questions, what should she do?

School-aged children have perfected fine motor skills and can paint, draw, and play an instrument. They enjoy team activities and are expanding their reading and writing skills. Their intellectual skills are developing, and social skills are going through refinement as a sense of self-achievement and self-worth is developed. During this time, the child learns and tests the rules for socializing outside the immediate family as an independent individual.

Therapeutic Approaches for School-Aged Children (7 to 11 Years)

- Allow choices when possible, such as which arm to use for an injection.
- A parent or caregiver should always be present during examinations.
- Remove only as much clothing as needed for the examination or procedure.
- Explain procedures in concrete terms; use pictures and diagrams when possible.
- Give the child time to ask questions.
- School-aged children often are curious, and can be cooperative if they know what is expected of them.
- Address the conversation to the child; involve the child in decision making as much as possible.
- Provide privacy.

Adolescence, or the transition stage, is the time when the individual attempts to establish an adult identity. The teenager proceeds by trial and error, experimenting with adult roles and behavior patterns. Traditional values learned in childhood may be questioned, and peer relationships take on new importance. During this time, teenagers must develop the emotional maturity and motivation to make reasonable decisions. They look to family members for encouragement and guidance in making decisions that will help them develop self-confidence and become patient, in addition to becoming less impulsive and self-centered.

Therapeutic Approaches for Adolescents (12 to 18 Years)

- Adolescents are self-conscious and strongly influenced by peers.
- Privacy is very important to them.
- Address how a procedure might affect the adolescent's appearance.
- Do not be judgmental; listen without condemning.
- Encourage the adolescent to verbalize his or her concerns and fears.
- The adolescent may regress to more childish behaviors when sick.
- Teenagers want to be treated as adults; they want to know what is being done and why.
- To promote an honest discussion about lifestyle issues, encourage the teenager to see the provider without the parent present.

CRITICAL THINKING APPLICATION **44.2**

Based on what you have learned about therapeutic approaches for the pediatric patient, what would be the best way to deal with the following patient situations?

1. A crying 3-month-old being seen for a well-child visit
2. A 10-month-old with otitis media
3. A 2-year-old who needs the dressing changed on an infected wound
4. A 5-year-old scheduled for vision and hearing screening
5. An 8-year-old who needs a throat culture to rule out a strep infection
6. A 12-year-old who needs a penicillin injection in the vastus lateralis site
7. A 15-year-old girl who complains of abdominal pain and is accompanied by her mother

Developmental Theory

Psychologists have been researching and developing theories about human behavior since the beginning of the 20th century. Erik Erikson, a developmental psychologist, expanded on Sigmund Freud's work. Erikson's theory recognizes the cultural and social influences on individual development. His theory is based on stages of development that the individual must pass through and master. Each stage focuses on a developmental crisis, starting in infancy and ending in old age. According to Erikson, children must master the following stages:

- *Trust versus mistrust:* Infants learn to rely on caregivers; mistrust occurs if needs are not met.
- *Autonomy versus shame and doubt:* Toddlers learn language skills and gain independence; they may feel shame and doubt if they cannot meet parental expectations or are overprotected.
- *Initiative versus guilt:* Preschoolers actively seek out new experiences; children become hesitant if restrictions or reprimands make them feel guilty or afraid to try more challenging skills.
- *Industry versus inferiority:* School-aged children enjoy finishing projects and receiving recognition; they develop feelings of inferiority if they are not accepted by peers or cannot please their parents.
- *Identity versus role confusion:* Adolescents face many physical and hormonal changes in this stage. Teenagers work at figuring out who they are and where they fit; they are seeking a direction for their lives. If they are unable to establish an identity and sense of direction, they become role confused.

When working in pediatrics, it can be helpful to understand Erikson's stages and how you can help someone master those stages.

PEDIATRIC DISEASES AND DISORDERS

The disease process in pediatric patients poses special problems because children are constantly changing both physically and functionally. As a child grows and develops, the immune system matures, and with the aid of routine prophylactic immunizations, the child acquires long-term protection against certain infectious diseases.

Colic

Colic usually is seen in the newborn period or early infancy. The problem is intermittent. The classic situation is an infant between 2 weeks and 4 months of age who has crying episodes that occur at least three times a week for longer than 3 hours a day and last 3 or more weeks. During an attack, the infant draws up the legs, clenches their fists, and cries inconsolably. The abdominal distress of colic usually occurs in the late afternoon and evening. Many theories have been suggested for why infants have colic, but none has been proven correct. If the baby is fed infant formula, providers recommend switching formulas to a non–cow's milk type because this may help relieve the infant's discomfort. Treatment involves trying to soothe the child as much as possible. Some recommended soothing strategies include using a pacifier, taking the infant for a car or stroller ride, giving the infant a warm bath, providing white noise, and rubbing the infant's stomach or back. Changing the way the baby is fed may also help. Bottle feeding in the upright position with frequent burping may help. If the infant is being breastfed, the mother may want to eliminate common food allergens such as dairy, eggs, nuts, and wheat. Potential irritating foods such as cabbage, onions and caffeine could also be eliminated. The provider will also try to determine the cause; however, the child frequently outgrows the condition before the causative agent can be identified. Drugs have not been found to be helpful. Parents need reassurance that they are not responsible for the child's discomfort and they may find counseling and assistance in developing coping techniques helpful.

Diarrhea

Diarrhea can be caused by a variety of microorganisms, including bacteria, viruses, and parasites. However, children sometimes can have diarrhea without having an infection. It could be caused by food allergies or certain medications, such as antibiotics. Diarrhea is diagnosed when the child has two or more watery or apparently abnormal stools within 24 hours. The child may not show other signs of illness or could have nausea, vomiting, stomach aches, headache, or fever. If the diarrhea continues for longer than 2 days, medical intervention is needed. Prolonged diarrhea can cause dehydration and an electrolyte imbalance because of excessive fluid loss. In addition, diarrhea can cause diaper rash and **excoriation**, which can be very painful.

CRITICAL THINKING APPLICATION **44.3**

Allison receives a call from the grandmother of a 3-year-old child who has had diarrhea since last night. What are some questions Allison should ask to determine the seriousness of the problem? Should the child be seen today, even though appointments are already overbooked?

Pediatric diarrhea needs to be followed closely. In the case of bloody stools, laboratory analysis should be ordered to determine the cause. If the patient is an infant or small child, a follow-up telephone call should be made after 12 hours and then daily until the diarrhea has stopped. Parents should know the indications of dehydration:

- Lack of tears when crying
- **Lethargy**
- Fewer wet diapers or decreased urination
- Dry mouth and lips
- Weight loss

The provider may recommend using oral rehydration therapy, such as Pedialyte or Enfalyte; small amounts (approximately 2 tablespoons) are offered at a time (i.e., every 15 minutes) to prevent vomiting. Soft drinks, juices, sports drinks, and tea should be avoided because they lack electrolytes and may lead to even more diarrhea. Parents should be informed that the child's diarrhea may not stop when the child is given oral rehydration therapy, but the fluids prevent the child from becoming dehydrated. It is important to continue to feed the child because lack of food can damage the villi in the small intestine. If breast-fed, the baby should continue to nurse because breast milk has been shown to protect the gastrointestinal lining.

The banana, rice, applesauce, and toast (BRAT) diet has been the traditional approach to treating children with diarrhea, but it is no longer recommended because there is no evidence that it is useful. In fact, the poor protein content of the BRAT diet may contribute to continued diarrhea and poor nutrition. Providers now recommend that children resume their prediarrhea diet as soon as possible so that they continue to eat something they prefer while the intestine heals. Probiotics found in certain yogurt products can also help to stabilize the child while the intestinal tract gets back to normal. The child should not be given over-the-counter (OTC) antidiarrheal medications, such as Pepto-Bismol, Kaopectate, Imodium, or Lomotil, because these can cause serious side effects, including decreased motility of the bowel, respiratory depression, and drowsiness. The provider may prescribe antibiotics if stool cultures test positive for pathogens. Children with severe dehydration require hospitalization and intravenous (IV) hydration to replace electrolytes and fluids.

Failure to Thrive

Failure to thrive refers to children whose current weight or rate of weight gain is much lower than that of other children of similar age and gender. It is a symptom more than a disease. An infant or a young child whose weight is consistently below the 3rd percentile on standardized growth charts, or who is 20% below the ideal body weight for length, may be diagnosed with failure to thrive. Physical, mental, and social skills also are delayed in these children. This could include failure to roll over, smile, coo, stand, or walk at age-appropriate developmental levels. Failure to thrive can be caused by a physiologic factor (e.g., malabsorption disease or cleft palate), or it may be related to a problem with the parent-child relationship. The provider needs an accurately recorded history of the child's birth weight and subsequent length, weight, and head circumference measurements. A comprehensive family history is important to rule out genetic growth abnormalities or a history of malabsorption problems, such as cystic fibrosis or celiac disease.

Children with failure to thrive need more calories than usual—approximately 150% of their normal calorie load—to catch up to their target weight. Both medical and social factors are evaluated in the treatment of children with this problem. Experts believe infants may suffer from this problem if they are being neglected; however, low weight gains are also possible with extremely attentive and cautious parents. The family must be considered as a whole to treat **nonorganic** causes effectively. Treatment may include the use of support groups and parental counseling.

Obesity

Just as with adult weight patterns, children are assessed according to their BMI. A child's level of body fat varies as the child grows; for example, children normally slim down as they reach school age, and very often, their weight increases as they mature from adolescence to adulthood. In addition, body fat levels vary between boys and girls as they reach puberty. Providers use growth charts that plot the child's BMI-for-age to determine whether the child's weight, in comparison with height, is within healthy limits. Obesity now affects more than 20% of all children and adolescents in the United States. Children who are overweight or obese as preschoolers are five times as likely as normal-weight children to be overweight or obese as adults. Studies have shown that a child who is obese between the ages of 10 and 13 has an 80% chance of becoming an obese adult.

The reasons for childhood obesity vary; they include a family history of obesity, inactivity, high-calorie diets, and stress. In rare cases, childhood obesity may be caused by metabolic or endocrine disorders. Overweight and obese children are at greater risk of developing serious health conditions, including asthma, diabetes mellitus type 2, sleep apnea, and hypercholesterolemia, which increases the risk of cardiovascular disease and hypertension. The psychosocial impact of obesity can be overwhelming for many children because isolation, loneliness, and lack of self-esteem are common. The provider can recommend a comprehensive diet and exercise program that emphasizes healthy living. The medical assistant can help by providing educational materials, encouragement for the child and parents, and referral to community education and support programs.

CRITICAL THINKING APPLICATION **44.4**

Juanita Johnston is a 12-year-old patient who was recently diagnosed as being obese. You are asked to help Juanita and her mother access online information about healthy nutrition options. What websites would be most appropriate for Juanita and her family? What other community resources can you recommend to support the family in making healthier nutrition decisions?

Otitis Media

Infection or inflammation of the middle ear usually is a side effect of a cold or other upper respiratory tract disorder, but it also can be caused by allergies. Otitis media usually occurs in children younger than 3 years of age. Signs include inflammation of the middle ear, with fluid building up behind the tympanic membrane. The child

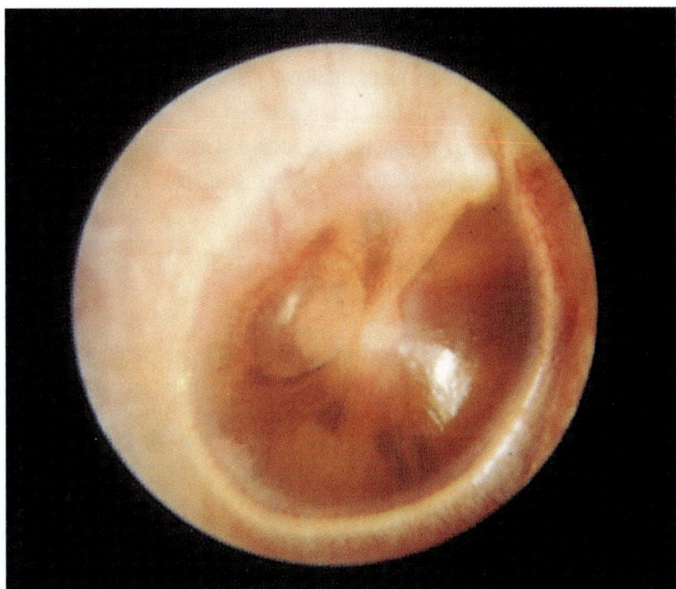

FIGURE 44.1 Serous otitis media. (From Swartz MH: *Textbook of physical diagnosis,* ed 5, Philadelphia, 2006, Saunders.)

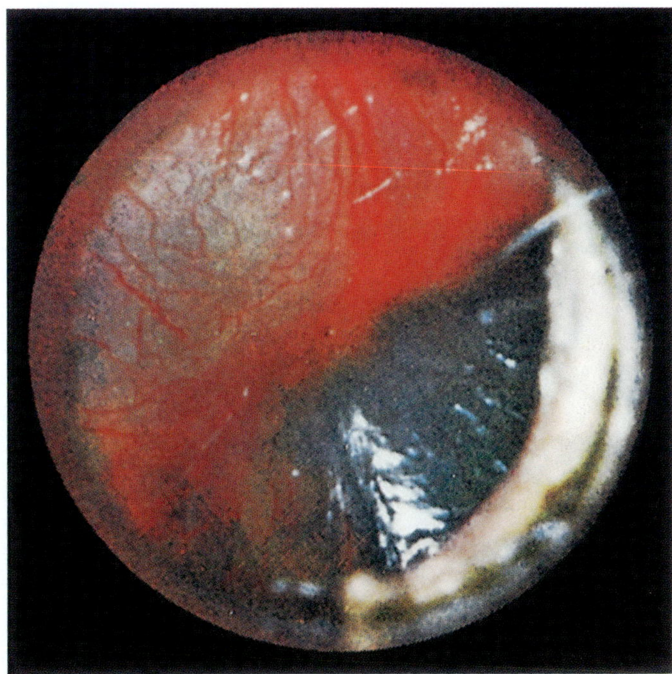

FIGURE 44.2 Suppurative otitis media. (Courtesy Dr. Richard A. Buckinham and Dr. George E. Shambaugh, Jr.)

may cry persistently, tug at the ear, have a fever, be irritable, and have diminished hearing in the affected ear. These symptoms sometimes may be accompanied by diarrhea, nausea, and vomiting.

Otitis media is classified as acute otitis media, otitis media with effusion (OME), or chronic otitis media with effusion. In all classifications, there is fluid trapped in the middle ear. This fluid is either **serous** (Figure 44.1) or **suppurative** (Figure 44.2). In Figure 44.2, pus is in the middle ear and shows up as white in the image. Acute otitis media has a sudden onset with swelling and redness of the tympanic membrane caused by fluid and mucus in the middle ear. Otitis media with effusion is when fluid and mucus continue to accumulate in the middle ear after the infection has subsided, causing a feeling of fullness and may affect hearing. With chronic otitis media with effusion, the fluid in the middle ear remains for an extended period of time or keeps returning without an infection.

Because otitis media may be caused by bacteria or a virus, determining the most appropriate treatment can be difficult. The American Academy of Pediatrics (AAP) and the American Academy of Family Physicians (AAFP) clinical practice guidelines for the diagnosis and management of otitis media in children age 6 months to 12 years state that antibiotics (typically amoxicillin or azithromycin [Zithromax]) should be prescribed for children 6 months or older who have severe signs and symptoms. Antibiotics can also be prescribed for patients younger than 24 months of age who are experiencing nonsevere bilateral infections. However, in children older than 6 months with nonsevere symptoms, observation and a follow-up within 48 to 72 hours before initiating antibiotics may be offered to assess patient improvement. If no improvement is noticed or symptoms have worsened, antibiotic therapy should be initiated. In all cases, if the child has not improved in 48 to 72 hours, the current antibiotic should be switched. Because antibiotics do not provide immediate relief from symptoms, children can be given oral acetaminophen or ibuprofen for pain relief.

If the fluid in the middle ear persists for longer than 3 months or if the child experiences hearing loss, the provider may recommend a *myringotomy;* in this operation, a small incision is made in the tympanic membrane, and a tube is inserted to drain the fluid and balance the pressure between the outer and middle ear. The tube typically stays in the eardrum for 6 to 12 months and falls out as the child grows.

Common Childhood Diseases

- Conjunctivitis—also called *pinkeye,* is a common infection in children and is highly contagious, especially in day care centers and schools. It can be caused by a bacterial or viral infection that produces white or yellowish pus, which may cause the eyelids to stick shut in the morning.
- Fifths disease—also called *erythema infectiosum, parvovirus infection,* or *slapped cheek disease,* is an infection caused by parvovirus B19. Outbreaks are most common in the winter and spring. Symptoms begin with a mild fever and general malaise. After a few days, the cheeks take on a flushed appearance, making the face look as if it has been slapped. A lacy rash also may be seen on the trunk, arms, and legs, but not all those infected develop the rash.
- Hand-foot-and-mouth disease—caused by the coxsackievirus, is transmitted by direct contact with nose and throat drainage, saliva, or the stool of an infected individual. The disease is seen most often in day care settings, where children can easily come in contact with infected bodily secretions. Symptoms include a combination of fever; sore throat; painful red blisters on the tongue, mouth, palms, and soles; headache; anorexia; and irritability (Figure 44.3).
- Reye syndrome—the cause of Reye syndrome is unknown, but the disorder has been linked to the use of aspirin during a viral illness. Reye syndrome is an acute and sometimes fatal illness characterized by fatty invasion of the inner organs, especially the liver, and swelling of the brain. It is most often seen in children from infancy through puberty (age 16). Prevention is the best treatment, which means children up to age 14 should never be given aspirin unless prescribed by a provider for a chronic condition such as juvenile rheumatoid arthritis.

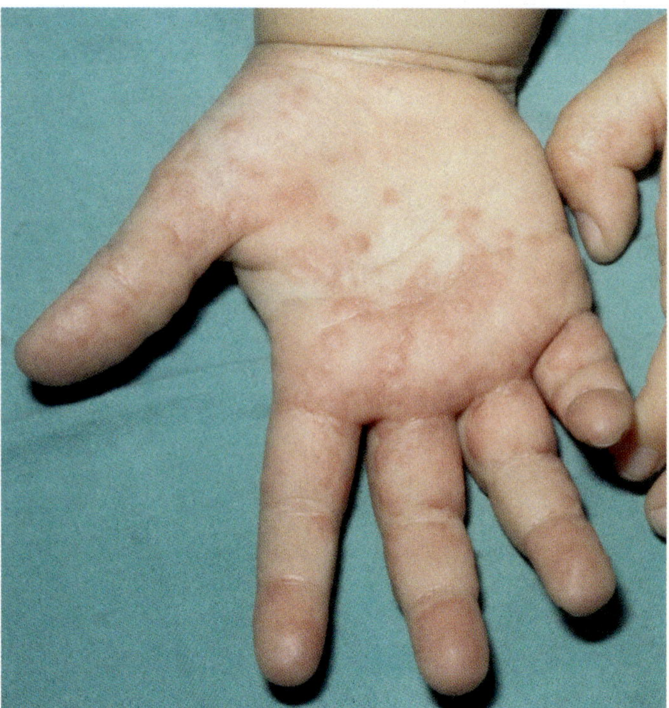

FIGURE 44.3 Vesicular palm lesions in hand-foot-and-mouth disease. (From Schachner LA, Hansen RC: *Pediatric dermatology*, ed 4, St. Louis, 2011, Mosby.)

Autism Spectrum Disorder

- Children diagnosed with autism spectrum disorder (ASD) show a wide range of neurologic and developmental behaviors. The most severe form is autism or classical ASD; a milder form may present as Asperger syndrome; sometimes, a child cannot be categorized into a specific diagnosis and is labeled as a pervasive developmental disorder (PDD).
- ASD occurs in all ethnic and socioeconomic groups and affects every age group.
- The Centers for Disease Control and Prevention (CDC) estimate the prevalence of ASD to be 1 in 44; it is almost four times more common among boys than among girls.
- Children with autism have impaired social interaction, do not respond to their names, avoid eye contact, and show limited interest in their surroundings. They rarely communicate with others and display repetitive movements or mannerisms, such as rocking or twirling. They may also have self-abusive behaviors, such as biting and head banging. Many children with autism have a very high pain tolerance but are extremely sensitive to noise, touch, or other sensory stimulation.
- The cause of this developmental disorder is unknown, but researchers believe it is due to a combination of genetic errors and environmental factors, perhaps a problem with fetal brain development. Although many parents are concerned about a connection with vaccines, extensive studies have failed to show a link between the two.
- The American Academy of Pediatrics (AAP) recommends a general developmental screening at every well-child visit and a developmental screening using a standardized tool at 9, 18, and 30 months or whenever a caregiver expresses concern. In addition, autism-specific screening is recommended for all children at the 18- and 24-month visits.
- Treatment involves coordinated educational and behavioral interventions to help the child develop social and language skills. Medications may be prescribed to treat depression, anxiety, and obsessive-compulsive behaviors.

From https://publications.aap.org/pediatrics/article/145/1/e20193447/36917/Identification-Evaluation-and-Management-of.

THE MEDICAL ASSISTANT'S ROLE IN THE PEDIATRIC EXAMINATION AND DIAGNOSTIC PROCEDURES

The medical assistant will play an active role in pediatric examination and diagnostic procedures. The following sections examine that role.

Examination

The medical assistant is responsible for the following:

- Assisting the provider with examinations
- Updating patient histories
- Performing ordered screening tests (e.g., vision, hearing, urinalysis, and hemoglobin checks)
- Measuring and weighing children as needed
- Administering immunizations
- Providing patient and caregiver support

When working in pediatrics, the medical assistant has an opportunity to develop a relationship with the pediatric patient that encourages cooperation and compliance with tests and treatment plans. Because the pediatric patient is seen on such a regular basis, the medical assistant can build trust with the patient and their caregivers. Using the therapeutic approaches to communication can help with building that relationship.

Diagnostic Procedures

Interacting with children requires special techniques, depending on the child's age. A calm, unhurried manner is essential to gaining cooperation. The tone of voice should be gentle but confident. Using a firm, direct approach about expected behavior is important to gain the cooperation of older children. Offer reasonable choices when possible, such as "Would you like your shot in your left leg or your right leg?" not "Are you ready for your shot now?" Offering sincere praise for the child during the examination or procedures helps ease anxiety and builds self-esteem. If the child is having an unusually difficult time, try to discover the reason. Children who have had a bad medical experience in the past may be afraid of what might happen. Each step should be explained in a language the child (and parent) can understand. Children younger than age 2 feel better when the parent holds them or remains very close (Figure 44.4). Preschool children enjoy playing, so making a game out of the situation is helpful (Figure 44.5). Whatever the child's age, the medical assistant should be sensitive to his or her individual needs and adapt the examination and procedures as much as possible to meet those needs.

The sequence of the provider's examination varies and frequently is based on the child's cooperation. The provider will probably leave procedures and tests that are likely to cause the most objections until

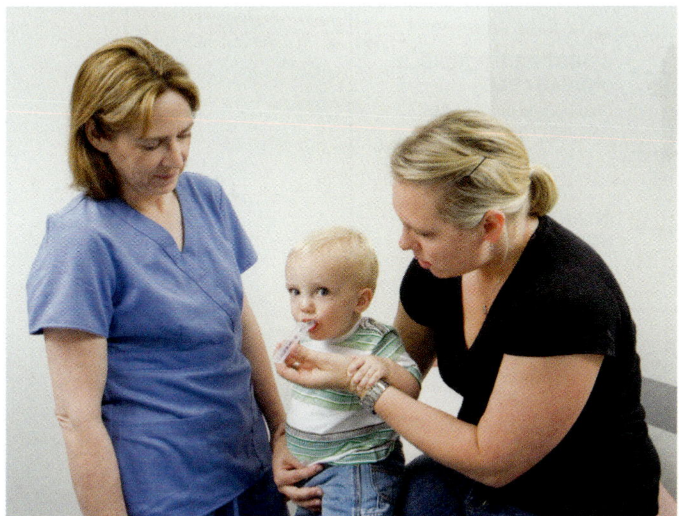

FIGURE 44.4 Sometimes a pediatric patient is more comfortable when held by a parent.

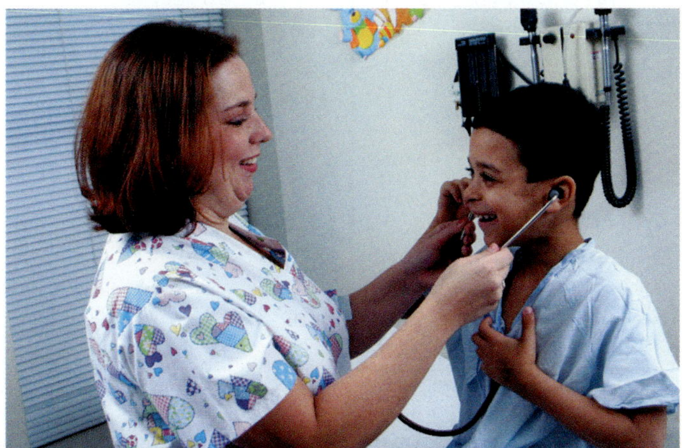

FIGURE 44.5 Making a game out of a procedure.

TABLE 44.2 Reference Ranges for Pediatric Vital Signs	
VITAL SIGN	REFERENCE RANGE
Temperature	
Oral	98.6°F (37°C)
Tympanic	99.6°F (37.6°C)
Axillary	97.6°F (36.4°C)
Pulse	
Newborn	100–180 beats per minute
3 mo–2 yr	80–150 beats per minute
2–10 yr	65–130 beats per minute
Respirations	
Newborn	• 30–50 breaths per minute
1–3 yr	• 25–30 breaths per minute
4–6 yr	• 23–25 breaths per minute
7+ yr	• 16–20 breaths per minute
Blood Pressure	
Newborn	• Systolic 90 mm Hg; diastolic 70 mm Hg
1–5 yr	• Systolic 100 mm Hg; diastolic 70 mm Hg
6–12 yr	• Systolic 120 mm Hg; diastolic 84 mm Hg
13+ yr	• Systolic, 100 mm Hg + age; diastolic, 30–40 mm Hg less

the end of the appointment. The provider is constantly evaluating the child's growth and development. A child's alertness and responses tell the provider a considerable amount. With infants and young children of preschool age, the parent is closely questioned about the child's eating, sleeping, and elimination habits. A school-aged child is usually a little more cooperative during an examination and can answer most questions without parental assistance. Adolescent patients should be given the option of not having parents present during an examination. This may permit teenagers to respond more honestly about lifestyle factors and also protect their privacy.

ASSISTING WITH THE EXAMINATION

The provider will have a designated set of procedures that the medical assistant completes before the provider sees the child. Vital signs are measured first (Table 44.2). Depending on the child's age and level of cooperation, the temperature may be obtained by the axillary, oral, rectal, tympanic, or temporal artery method. The rectal and temporal artery methods are considered most accurate in infants; however, the temporal artery method is easiest, quickest, and less invasive. It is important to remember that the younger the child, the more immature the ability to regulate body heat. Therefore, the temperature of an infant may fluctuate easily and rapidly. The child's pulse rate is affected similarly to that of an adult; it can increase due to activity, anxiety, illness, and environmental temperature. If the child is younger than age 2, the pulse is measured apically by placing the stethoscope on the left side of the chest medial to the nipple. Always count the beats for 1 full minute for accuracy.

An alternative method of obtaining the pulse of a very young child is to use the brachial artery in the upper arm. After age 2, the child's pulse may be taken at the radial pulse site. Anticipate a pulse rate higher than that of an adult; the younger the child, the faster the pulse. The respiratory rate is easily obtained in a child because the chest can be readily observed. Expect the rate to be increased according to the child's age (the younger the child, the faster the normal respiratory rate) and health. The ratio of 4 pulse beats to 1 respiration should remain constant in a healthy child.

It is recommended that blood pressure be checked for children aged 3 years or older. The cuff must be the appropriate width to obtain an accurate reading, and the bell of the stethoscope must be small enough to seal over the site. It is best to use a pediatric stethoscope with a pediatric bell when obtaining an infant's pressure. Blood pressure readings in a young child are lower than those in an adult (see Table 44.2).

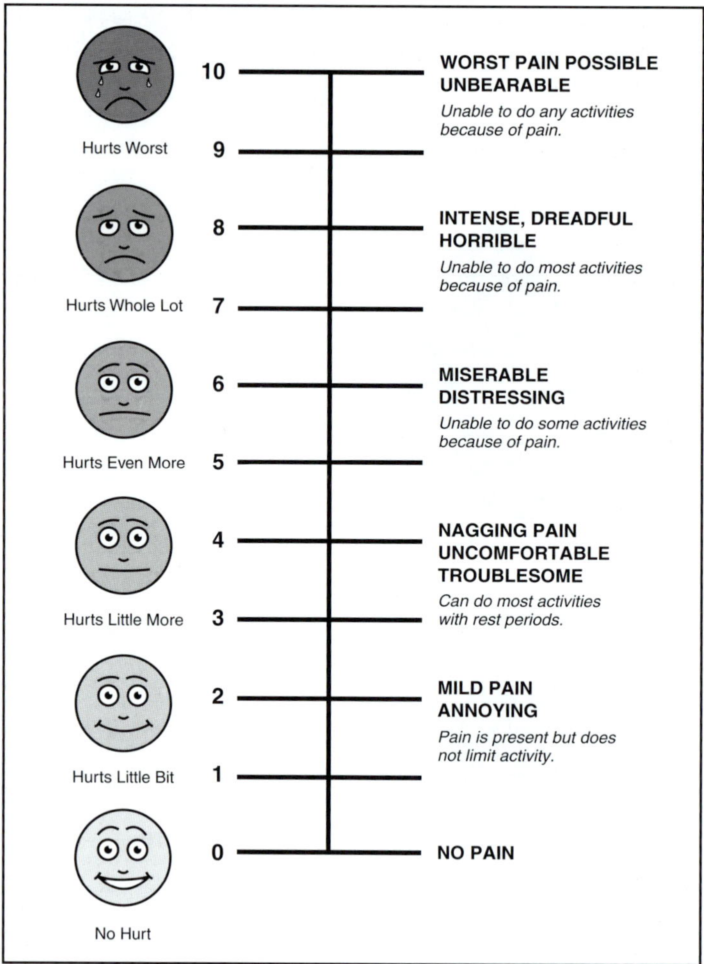

FIGURE 44.6 Wong-Baker FACES pain scale.

TABLE 44.3 Apgar Scoring System[a]

	ASSIGNED SCORE		
CLINICAL SIGN	**0**	**1**	**2**
Appearance: color	Blue and pale	Body pink and extremities blue	Pink all over
Pulse: heart rate	Absent	<100 beats per minute	>100 beats per minute
Grimace: reflex irritability	No response	Grimace	Coughing, sneezing, or vigorous cry
Activity: muscle tone	Limp	Some flexion of the arms and legs	Active movement
Respirations: breathing	Absent	Slow and irregular	Good and crying

[a]Readings are taken by the provider at 1 minute and 5 minutes after birth. At *1 minute:* If the score is 7 or lower, some nervous system problems are suspected. If the score is below 4, resuscitation usually is necessary. At *5 minutes:* If the score is at least 8, the child probably is reacting normally.

To prevent a small child or infant from rolling the head from side to side during the provider's examination, stand at the head of the table and support the child's head between your hands, taking care not to press on the ears or the anterior or posterior **fontanelles**. An infant need not be draped, but privacy is important to an older child. Sincere respect and friendly conversation at the child's level accomplish a great deal. Always be patient with children. Make sure they understand what is expected. Always involve the parents or caregivers as much as possible.

Accurately judging the level of pain a young patient is experiencing can be difficult. If the child is able to communicate, the Wong-Baker FACES Pain Scale could be used, which shows simple drawings of faces that express varying levels of pain on a 0-to-10 scale (Figure 44.6).

An infant's first physical assessment comes at the time of delivery when the provider assesses the newborn's ability to thrive outside the uterus. The Apgar score is a system for evaluating the infant's physical condition at 1 and 5 minutes after birth (Table 44.3). Developed by pediatrician Virginia Apgar, the scoring system evaluates the following: ***a***ppearance (color), ***p***ulse (heart rate), ***g***rimace (reflex; response to stimuli), ***a***ctivity (muscle tone), and ***r***espiration (breathing). These parameters are each rated 0, 1, or 2. The maximum total score is 10. Infants with low scores require immediate medical attention.

Well-Child Visits

The frequency of well-child visits varies with the provider and the community. The American Academy of Pediatrics recommends the following pattern:

- 2 to 5 days
- 1 month
- 2 months
- 4 months
- 6 months
- 9 months
- 12 months
- 15 months
- 18 months
- 2 years
- Annually

These visits focus on maintaining the child's health through basic system examinations, immunizations, and updating the child's medical history record.

The decision on whether the child is to be seen alone or with the parent depends on the provider and the child's age. Often the child looks to the parent for approval before answering or performing a skill; for this reason, the provider may want to assess the child alone. If this is the case, explain to the parent that the provider wants to evaluate the child's independent abilities and that as soon as testing is complete, the provider will explain the results of the tests.

The medical history is an essential guide to the pediatric examination. With an infant, the provider depends on the caregiver for the history, but as the child gets older, some history may be obtained from the child and clarified or amplified by the parent. When asking about things like lead paint, the child may not understand the question, and the parent may have to answer. Close observation also gives the provider considerable information.

Lead Paint Exposure

Children are especially vulnerable to lead levels in their environment. High blood lead levels can result in serious brain injury, including seizures, coma, and death. Lower levels can cause learning problems, stunted growth, and behavior disorders. The most common causes of lead exposure are lead-based paint in homes and on imported toys and chronic exposure to lead-contaminated dust and water. The Centers for Disease Control and Prevention (CDC) recommend a screening blood test for lead levels in all children between 1 and 2 years of age. For children who show elevated levels, follow-up should include home and school environmental testing to determine the cause of lead exposure.

Sick-Child Visits

Sick-child visits occur whenever needed, usually on short notice. For this reason, most pediatric offices keep open appointments in the schedule to accommodate calls for sick-child visits. The length and frequency of this type of visit depend entirely on the child and the illness. The medical assistant is frequently the first point of contact for a sick child and the child's caregiver.

TABLE 44.4 Important Questions for Telephone Screening of Pediatric Problems

COMPLAINT	SCREENING QUESTIONS
Pain	• What is the onset, frequency, and duration of the pain? • On a scale of 1 to 10, how severe is the pain? • Where is the exact location? • Was any accident involved (include details)? • Has the pain gotten worse over time? • Has the pain interfered with sleep? • Is there associated fever, vomiting, diarrhea, or rash?
Gastrointestinal	• What is the onset, duration, and frequency of the symptoms? Has the child been vomiting longer than 24 hours without improvement? • Is the child drinking and/or eating? • Is the child dehydrated (e.g., dry mouth, no urination in 8–10 hours, listless)? • If the child has diarrhea, have there been more than five or six watery stools in 12 hours? • Does the child have other symptoms (e.g., vomiting, fever of 101°F [38.3°C], rapid breathing)?
Respiratory	• What is the onset, duration, and frequency of the symptoms? • How would you describe the child's breathing? • Has the child been diagnosed with a breathing disorder? • Is a prescribed treatment being used? • Are any other signs or symptoms present (e.g., severe headache, stiff neck, fever, cough)? • If the child is coughing, what does it sound like? • Are there signs of a sore throat or earache?

Determining whether the child should be seen immediately or if the problem can wait for an opening in the schedule is crucial to pediatric care. Medical assistants should follow established office policies, but when in doubt about the seriousness of the problem, they should ask the office manager or provider for advice. Usually, providers prefer to see the child rather than delay seeing a patient with a potentially serious condition. Children younger than 2 years old should be seen right away, and the parent should report any of the following:

- Frequent cycles of crying, lethargy, or vomiting that have persisted longer than 24 hours
- Diarrhea (more than six stools in the past 12 hours)
- Fever of 101°F (38.3°C) or higher
- The child cannot verbalize associated pain or problems

Table 44.4 summarizes some important questions for telephone screening of an older child who can communicate symptoms. It is important to focus on the *onset* (when symptoms first started), *frequency* (whether symptoms are constant or cycle through recurrences), and *duration* (how long the episodes last) of the problem, in addition to attempted treatments and their effectiveness. As with any other patient, all telephone communication should be documented to record the reason for the call; the information gathered; the action taken, including whether the provider was consulted; any orders given; and whether and when an appointment was scheduled.

Measurements

Examination of the child during a routine well-child visit includes measuring the circumference of the infant's head to determine normal growth and development (Procedure 44.1). The size of the child's head reflects the growth of the brain. Brain growth is 50% complete by 1 year of age, 75% by age 3, and 90% by age 6. Routine head measurement is recommended in children until 36 months of age and in older children whose head size is not within norms. If the circumference of the head deviates greatly from normal measurements, **hydrocephaly** or **microcephaly** may be suspected. It is important to discover any congenital problems as early as possible so that appropriate treatment can be started.

Along with the head circumference, the medical assistant should record the child's length (or height) and weight (Procedure 44.2) on growth charts so that the provider can compare the child's measurement statistics with national standards. Growth charts consist of a series of percentile curves that illustrate the distribution of selected body measurements.

The CDC has gender-specific growth charts for the following:

- Birth to 36 months (Figure 44.7)
  - Length for age
  - Weight for age
  - Head circumference for age
  - Weight for length
- 2 to 20 years (Figure 44.8)
  - Stature for age
  - Weight for age
  - BMI for age

There are 20 CDC charts (10 for boys and 10 for girls). As mentioned previously, BMI is the recommended method of determining whether children or adults are overweight or obese. The BMI growth charts can be used beginning at 2 years of age when height can be measured accurately.

EHRs may automatically plot the measurements on the appropriate growth chart and calculate the percentile.

ASSISTING WITH DIAGNOSTIC PROCEDURES

The medical assistant that works with pediatric patients will also be involved in assisting with diagnostic procedures. The following sections examine the most common diagnostic procedures done in pediatrics.

Obtaining a Urine Sample

The easiest way to obtain a urine sample from a child who is toilet trained is to give the parent the container and instructions ahead of time. Then, when the child arrives at the office for the examination, the sample is available to be tested. If the sample is needed while the child is at the office, consult with the parent for the best method to use. If the child is not toilet trained, a pediatric urine collection device can be put on him or her to collect the sample (Figure 44.9). This device is placed as soon as the child is checked in to increase the chance of obtaining the needed sample before the child leaves. Once the device is in place, the child can be diapered to help hold it properly. Make sure the adhesive sticks tightly so that the specimen collects in the device when the child urinates.

In some cases, the child may need to be catheterized to obtain the specimen. Pediatric catheterization kits contain all the supplies needed for this procedure. When preparing the kit, always remember that this is a sterile procedure. The provider usually asks the parent to help with the infant while the medical assistant labels and prepares the specimen for the laboratory. In some practices, a registered nurse or a specially trained medical assistant may perform a catheterization procedure to collect a pediatric urine sample.

Vision Screening

The most common method of performing a distance vision screening with a pediatric patient is using a Snellen chart. You will likely see a variety of charts used. There is one with alphabetic characters, one with tumbling Es, and one with a picture of common objects instead of letters. Each row of characters shown on the chart gets smaller. As the child needs to be cooperative during this screening, it is important to make a game of it and make it fun. When working with the tumbling E chart, it can be helpful to have the E on an individual card and show it to the child before starting the evaluation. Ask the child to point in the direction that the "legs" of the E are pointing. You can rotate the card until you have covered all possible directions. Then when you move to the full chart, the child will have an understanding of what you want him or her to do.

Traditionally the Snellen chart has been mounted on the wall in a hallway that would allow for the 20-foot distance from the chart. There are now Snellen charts that can be displayed on a tablet computer and only require that the patient be 5 feet or less from the chart. For this screening test, patients cover one eye and read each line of the chart until they can no longer get the majority of the characters correct. Then the other eye is covered, and the process is repeated. Finally, patients can view the chart with both eyes and again read each line on the chart until they can no longer get the majority of the characters correct. Chapter 31 covers this process in more depth, and Procedure 31.1 explains the Snellen evaluation.

The Snellen chart will also have a green bar and red bar that can be used for a very basic color vision test. If a more expanded test is needed, a booklet of polychromatic plates made up of colored dots in a numeric pattern can be used. For pediatric patients who do not know their numbers, there are plates that have a trail the patient can trace (Figure 44.10). This booklet is referred to as the Ishihara color vision test. For the color vision screening, it is important to have a room with natural sunlight or lights that create that effect and will minimize distractions. More information about the Ishihara Color Vision test can be found in Chapter 31, and Procedure 31.2 explains how to assess color acuity using the Ishihara test.

If a problem with the patient's vision is found during either the acuity test or color vision test, the patient will likely be referred to an ophthalmologist.

Hearing Screening

Hearing screening is a common test for pediatric patients. It is usually accomplished by using an audiometer. The audiometer can assess hearing at various frequencies and intensities. The screening involves headphones placed over the child's ears. Before putting on the headphones, explain to children what to expect. They will hear sounds in

Birth to 36 months: Boys
Length-for-age and Weight-for-age percentiles

NAME ____________________

RECORD # ____________

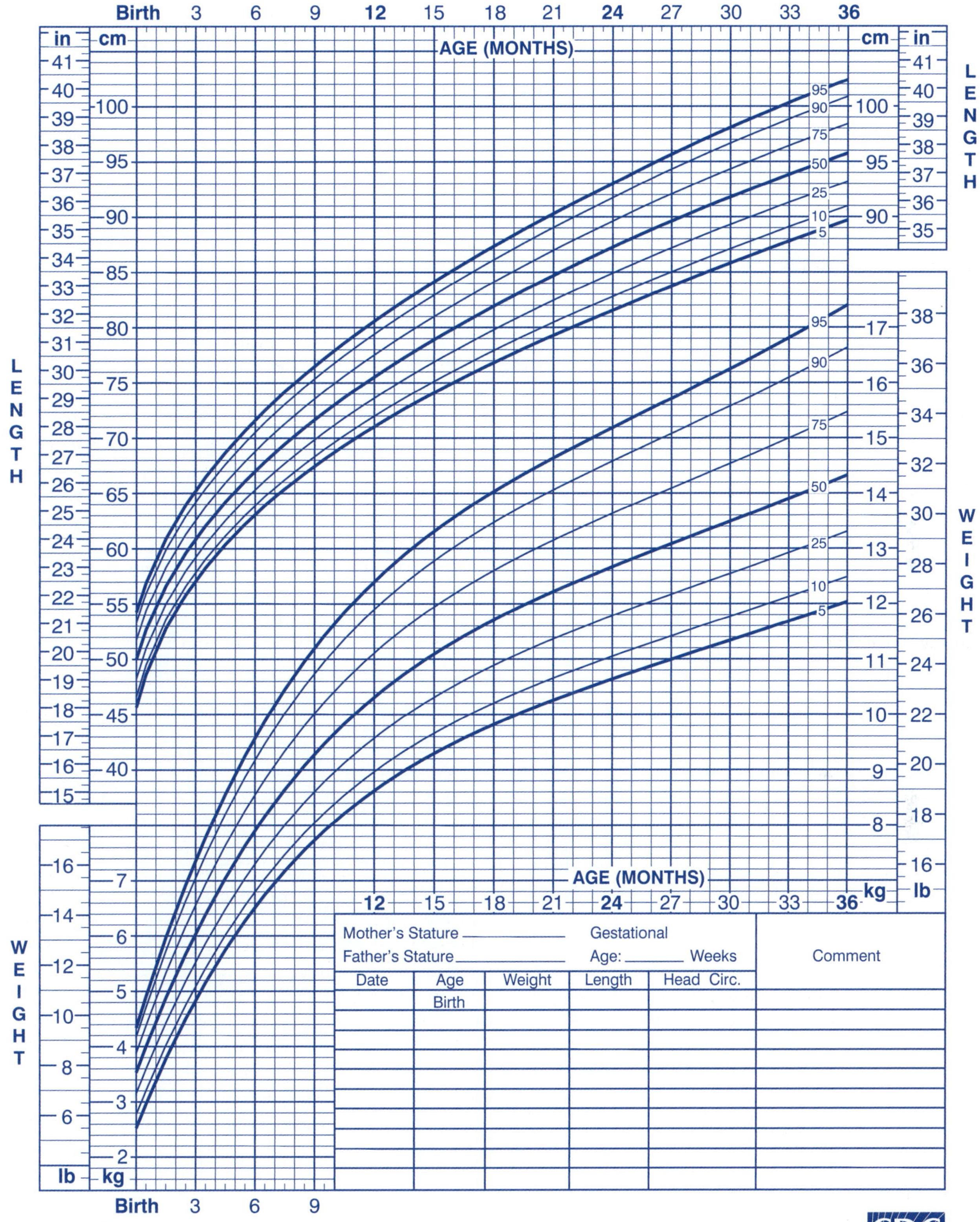

Birth 3 6 9 12 15 18 21 24 27 30 33 36

AGE (MONTHS)

LENGTH (in / cm) — WEIGHT (lb / kg)

Percentiles: 95, 90, 75, 50, 25, 10, 5

Mother's Stature ________			Gestational		Comment
Father's Stature ________			Age: ______ Weeks		
Date	Age	Weight	Length	Head Circ.	
	Birth				

Published May 30, 2000 (modified 4/20/01).
SOURCE: Developed by the National Center for Health Statistics in collaboration with
the National Center for Chronic Disease Prevention and Health Promotion (2000).
http://www.cdc.gov/growthcharts

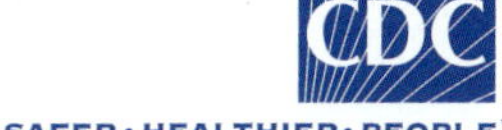

FIGURE 44.7 Growth chart: boys (birth to 36 months).

2 to 20 years: Girls
Stature-for-age and Weight-for-age percentiles

NAME ______________________

RECORD # ______________

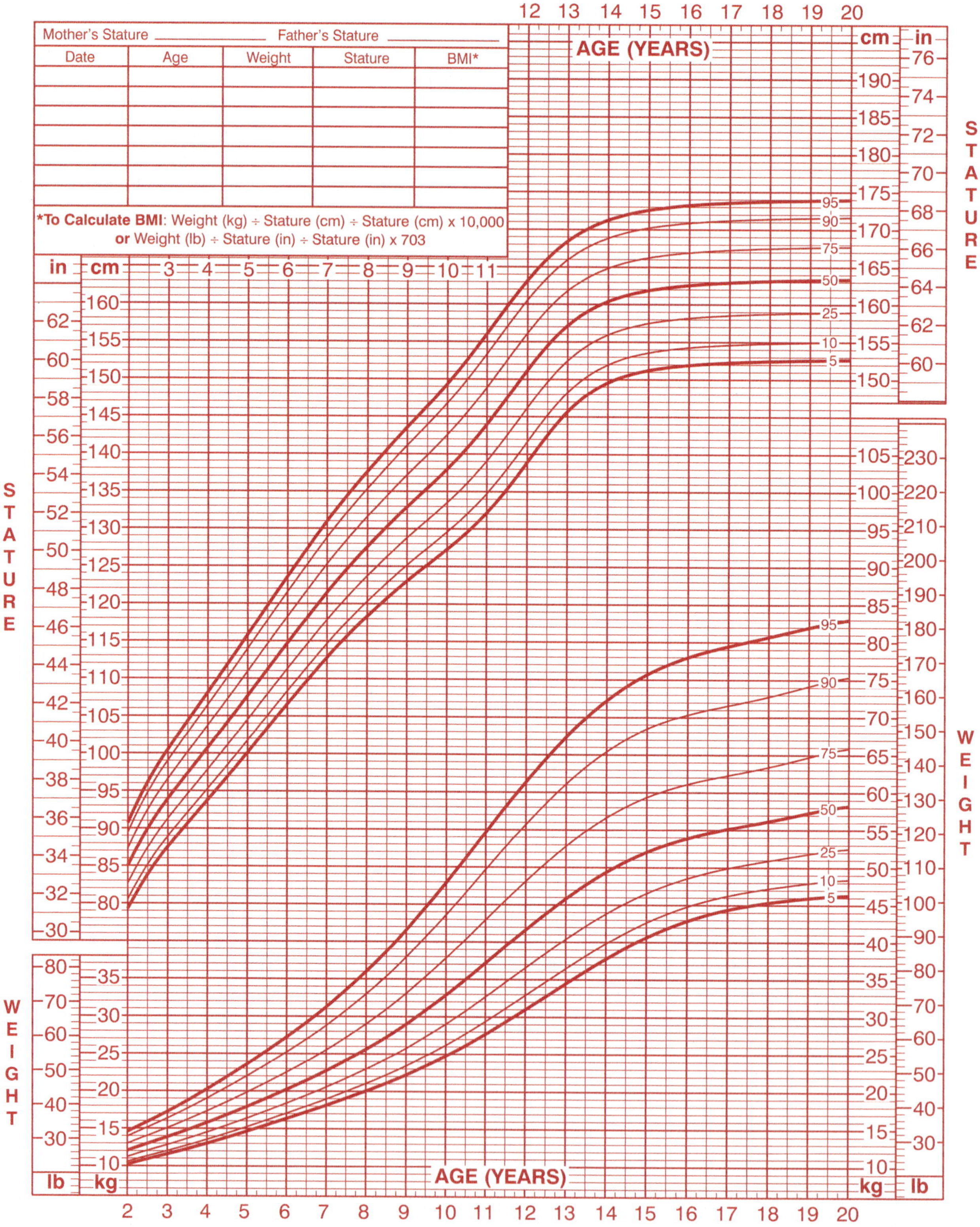

Mother's Stature ______________ Father's Stature ______________

Date	Age	Weight	Stature	BMI*

***To Calculate BMI**: Weight (kg) ÷ Stature (cm) ÷ Stature (cm) x 10,000
or Weight (lb) ÷ Stature (in) ÷ Stature (in) x 703

AGE (YEARS)
12 13 14 15 16 17 18 19 20
3 4 5 6 7 8 9 10 11

STATURE
in: 30 32 34 36 38 40 42 44 46 48 50 52 54 56 58 60 62 64 66 68 70 72 74 76
cm: 80 85 90 95 100 105 110 115 120 125 130 135 140 145 150 155 160 165 170 175 180 185 190

Percentiles: 95 90 75 50 25 10 5

WEIGHT
kg: 10 15 20 25 30 35 40 45 50 55 60 65 70 75 80 85 90 95 100 105
lb: 30 40 50 60 70 80 90 100 110 120 130 140 150 160 170 180 190 200 210 220 230

AGE (YEARS)
2 3 4 5 6 7 8 9 10 11 12 13 14 15 16 17 18 19 20

Published May 30, 2000 (modified 11/21/00).
SOURCE: Developed by the National Center for Health Statistics in collaboration with
the National Center for Chronic Disease Prevention and Health Promotion (2000).
http://www.cdc.gov/growthcharts

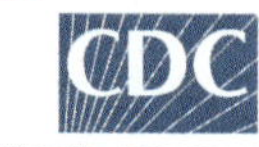

SAFER • HEALTHIER • PEOPLE™

FIGURE 44.8 Growth chart: girls (2 to 20 years).

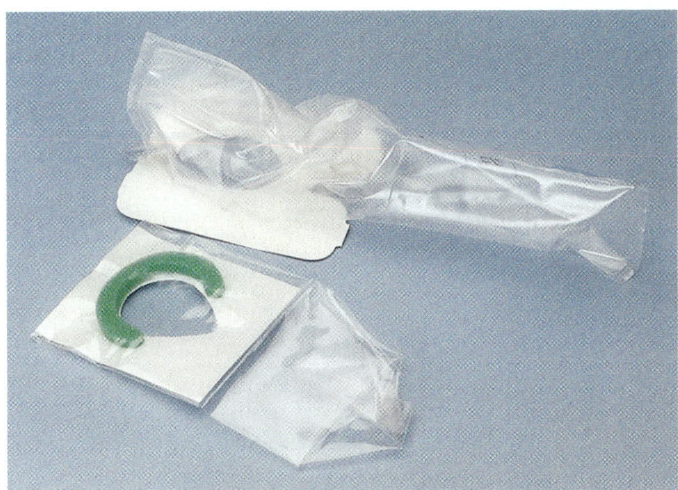

FIGURE 44.9 Urine collection devices.

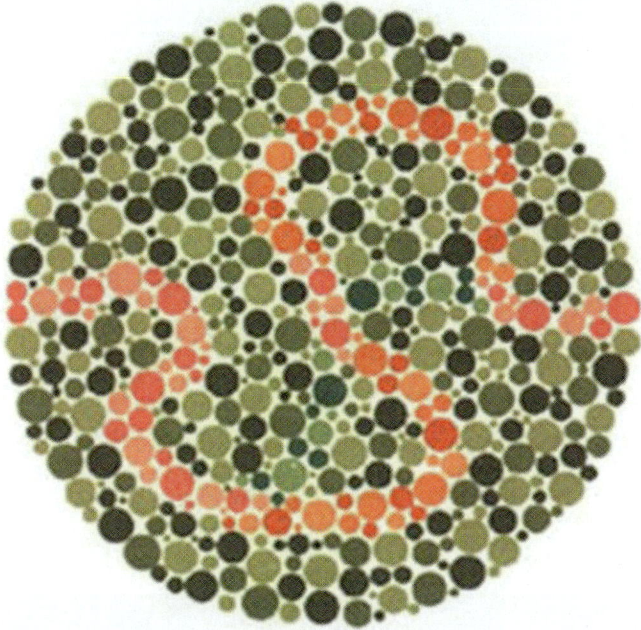

FIGURE 44.10 Ishihara Plate No. 37. (Image found at www.color-blindness.com/wp-content/images/Ishihara-Plate-37-38.jpg)

one ear or the other. When they hear the sound, they should raise that hand; if the sound is in the right ear, they should raise their right hand. Tell them that some of the sounds will be very quiet and some will be louder, so if they think they hear a sound, they should raise their hand. Chapter 31 and Procedure 31.5 provide more information about hearing screening and the steps for performing a hearing acuity test.

Audiometers may have the option to do the test manually or automatically. The medical assistant should be familiar with the provider's preference when performing the screening test. If a hearing deficit is indicated, the patient will likely be referred to an audiologist for further testing.

ASSISTING WITH TREATMENTS

The medical assistant may be involved in providing treatments for pediatric patients. The following sections examine two types of treatments.

Immunizations

Over the years, immunization has helped dramatically reduce potentially lethal childhood infections. Figure 44.11 shows the 2022 immunization schedule from the CDC for children 0 through 18 years of age. All of the immunization schedules can be found on the CDC's website at www.cdc.gov/vaccines/schedules/downloads/child/0-18yrs-child-combined-schedule.pdf.

The schedules are updated periodically as new vaccines become available, or research indicates a better method for giving the vaccine. The CDC recommends immunization against infectious diseases for all children, except those for whom a particular vaccination would pose a risk. However, each state develops its own immunization program and methods of enforcement. Parents/guardians do have the right to refuse immunizations.

The vaccines consist of a suspension of **attenuated** organisms or their toxins, which is administered to stimulate an active immune response in the body. This results in the production of antibodies against the specific pathogens. Booster doses are usually equivalent to a single dose of the initial immunization. For some immunizations (e.g., tetanus), boosters are prescribed at designated intervals to ensure the maintenance of immune levels.

Vaccine manufacturers have trade names for each product and have established protocols to ensure potency and stability. All vaccines are tested for safety and effectiveness. Every vaccine package has an insert that fully describes the following:

- The vaccine and its use
- The route of administration
- Adverse reactions
- Signs and symptoms the parent might observe after immunization that would indicate a potential problem

Unfavorable responses include high fever, swelling at the site of the injection, **urticaria**, breathing difficulties, severe headache, and convulsions. Any of these should be immediately reported to the provider. Vaccine storage should follow the manufacturer's guidelines (e.g., some vaccines must be refrigerated; others must not be exposed to sunlight).

Some vaccines are grown in birds' eggs or a medium made of animal organs, or they are weakened with chemicals. Therefore, a child who is allergic to eggs cannot receive some of the vaccines, such as influenza. The medical assistant must know the potential allergic problems, common symptoms, and adverse reactions to immunizations and must make sure the parent is informed. Table 44.5 details guidelines for childhood immunizations.

Before a child or adult receives a vaccine, the healthcare provider is required by the National Childhood Vaccine Injury Act (NCVIA) to provide a copy of a Vaccine Information Statement (VIS) to either the adult patient or the child's parent or legal guardian. A VIS provides information about the risks and benefits of each vaccine. If providing the parent or guardian with the VIS is the medical assistant's responsibility, the assistant should do the following (Procedure 44.3):

- Before administering the vaccine, give the parent the most current VIS available for that particular vaccine. Give the parent enough time to review the information, and then answer any questions or refer the parent's concerns to the provider before administering the vaccine. VIS forms are available online in a number of languages to meet the needs of a diverse patient population.

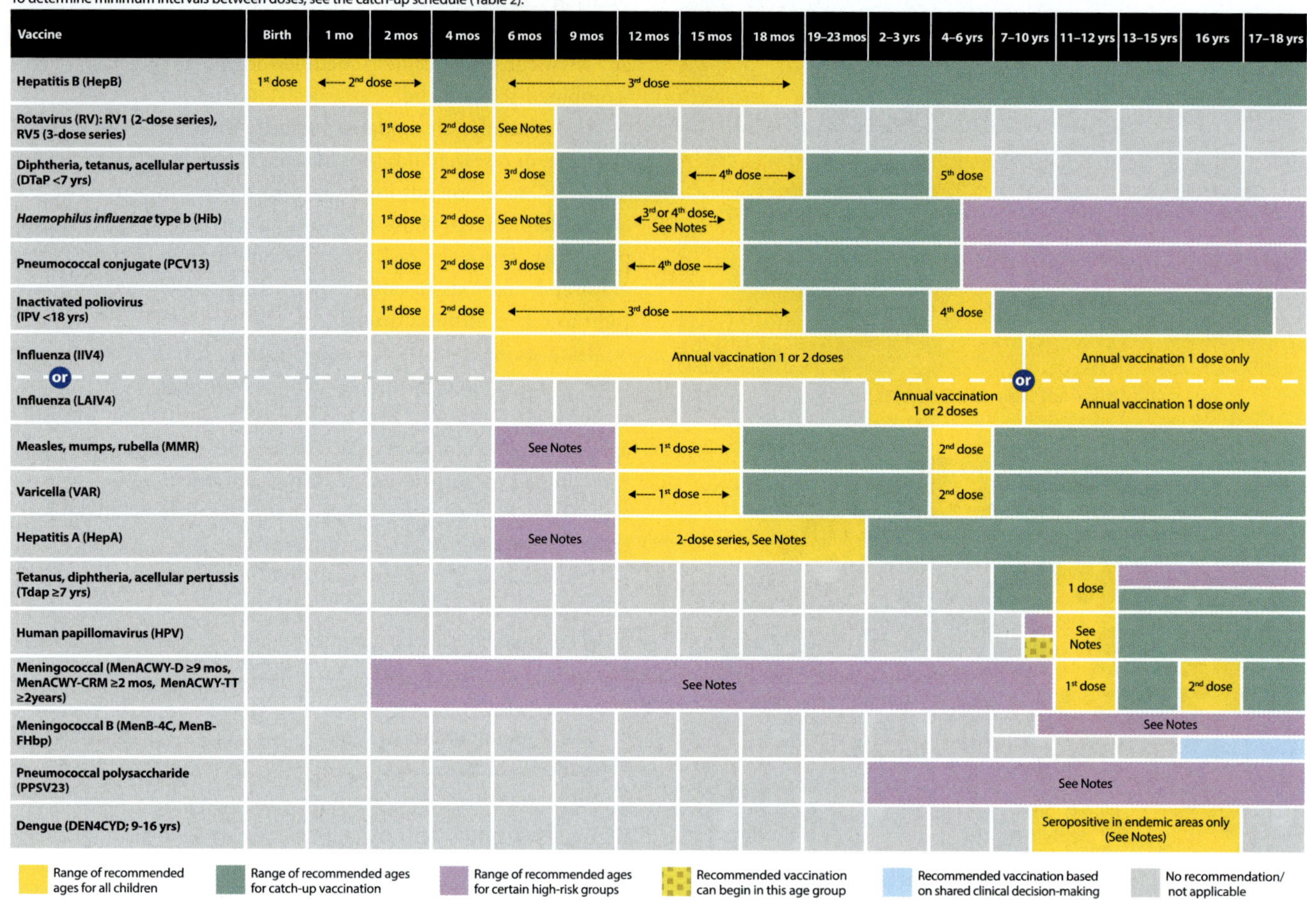
Table 1 Recommended Child and Adolescent Immunization Schedule for ages 18 years or younger, United States, 2022

These recommendations must be read with the notes that follow. For those who fall behind or start late, provide catch-up vaccination at the earliest opportunity as indicated by the green bars.
To determine minimum intervals between doses, see the catch-up schedule (Table 2).

Vaccine	Birth	1 mo	2 mos	4 mos	6 mos	9 mos	12 mos	15 mos	18 mos	19–23 mos	2–3 yrs	4–6 yrs	7–10 yrs	11–12 yrs	13–15 yrs	16 yrs	17–18 yrs
Hepatitis B (HepB)	1st dose	← 2nd dose →			← 3rd dose →												
Rotavirus (RV): RV1 (2-dose series), RV5 (3-dose series)			1st dose	2nd dose	See Notes												
Diphtheria, tetanus, acellular pertussis (DTaP <7 yrs)			1st dose	2nd dose	3rd dose			← 4th dose →				5th dose					
Haemophilus influenzae type b (Hib)			1st dose	2nd dose	See Notes		← 3rd or 4th dose, See Notes →										
Pneumococcal conjugate (PCV13)			1st dose	2nd dose	3rd dose		← 4th dose →										
Inactivated poliovirus (IPV <18 yrs)			1st dose	2nd dose	← 3rd dose →							4th dose					
Influenza (IIV4)					Annual vaccination 1 or 2 doses									Annual vaccination 1 dose only			
or																	
Influenza (LAIV4)											Annual vaccination 1 or 2 doses			Annual vaccination 1 dose only			
Measles, mumps, rubella (MMR)					See Notes		← 1st dose →					2nd dose					
Varicella (VAR)							← 1st dose →					2nd dose					
Hepatitis A (HepA)					See Notes		2-dose series, See Notes										
Tetanus, diphtheria, acellular pertussis (Tdap ≥7 yrs)														1 dose			
Human papillomavirus (HPV)														See Notes			
Meningococcal (MenACWY-D ≥9 mos, MenACWY-CRM ≥2 mos, MenACWY-TT ≥2years)			See Notes											1st dose		2nd dose	
Meningococcal B (MenB-4C, MenB-FHbp)															See Notes		
Pneumococcal polysaccharide (PPSV23)											See Notes						
Dengue (DEN4CYD; 9-16 yrs)														Seropositive in endemic areas only (See Notes)			

Range of recommended ages for all children; Range of recommended ages for catch-up vaccination; Range of recommended ages for certain high-risk groups; Recommended vaccination can begin in this age group; Recommended vaccination based on shared clinical decision-making; No recommendation/not applicable

FIGURE 44.11 Recommended immunization schedule for children ages birth to 18 years. (From the Centers for Disease Control and Prevention, https://www.cdc.gov/vaccines/schedules/downloads/child/0-18yrs-child-combined-schedule.pdf.)

TABLE 44.5 Guidelines for Childhood Immunizations

VACCINE	TRADE NAME	ROUTE OF ADMINISTRATION	CONTRAINDICATIONS[A]	SIDE EFFECTS
DTaP Diphtheria, tetanus, pertussis (whooping cough)	Daptacel, Infanrix	IM; Td (tetanus and diphtheria) boosters at 11–12 yr if at least 5 yr since last dose; subsequent booster every 10 yr	Moderate or severe acute illness; neurologic problem; complication after previous dose (e.g., fever, convulsions)	Mild fever, anorexia, irritability, drowsiness
HAV Hepatitis A (can use either Havrix or Vaqta)	Havrix, Vaqta	IM; all children 1 yr; 2 doses 6 mo apart	Hypersensitivity to product, acute infection or fever	Localized injection site reaction, fever, headache
HBV Hepatitis B	Engerix-B, Recombivax HB, HEPLISAV-B	IM; may give with all other vaccines but at a separate site; requires 3 injections	Moderate or severe acute illness; yeast allergy; severe cardiovascular disease	Fever, pain at injection site, headache, malaise, vomiting
Hib *Haemophilus influenzae* serotype B meningitis	COMVAX, PedvaxHIB, ActHIB, Hiberix	IM; may give with all other vaccines but at a separate site. Three doses of ActHIB, MenHibrix, or Pentacel at 2, 4, and 6 months or 2 doses of PedvaxHib or COMVAX at 2 and 4 months of age; booster dose at 12 through 15 months	Not routinely given to children older than 5; moderate or severe acute illness	Minimal

TABLE 44.5 Guidelines for Childhood Immunizations—*continued*

VACCINE	TRADE NAME	ROUTE OF ADMINISTRATION	CONTRAINDICATIONS[a]	SIDE EFFECTS
HPV Human papillomavirus	HPV2 (Cervarix) females only; HPV4 (Gardasil), HPV9 (Gardasil 9) males and females	IM; routine vaccination at age 11 or 12 years; second dose 1 to 2 months after first dose; third dose 16 weeks after second dose	Hypersensitivity to ingredients; pregnancy	Relatively few; mild headache and GI upset
Influenza Trivalent inactivated vaccine for 6 months; at 2 years, use live, attenuated vaccine	Afluria, Fluad, Flublok, Flucelvax, FluLaval, Fluarix, Fluvirin, Fluzone, FluMist (nasal spray)	IM; annually each fall	Allergy to eggs; recent fever	Uncommon; fever, local irritation at injection site, general malaise
IPV Inactive poliovirus for polio	Ipol	SC or IM; 4 doses; may give with all other vaccines but at a separate site	Moderate or severe acute illness; egg allergy	Uncommon
Meningococcal vaccine for meningitis (MCV4)	Menactra, Menomune, MenHibrix, Bexsero, or Trumenba	IM; single dose of Menactra or Menveo vaccine at age 11 through 12 years, with a booster dose at age 16 years; aged 16 through 23 years vaccinated with a 2-dose series of Bexsero or a 3-dose series of Trumenba vaccine to provide short-term protection	Moderate or severe acute illness; history of allergic reaction to MCV4	Uncommon
MMR Measles, mumps, rubella	M-M-R II	SC; may give with all other vaccines but at a separate site	Moderate or severe acute illness; immunocompromised patients (may be given if HIV positive); pregnancy or possible pregnancy in 3 mo; egg allergy	Fever
Pneumococcal (PCV) Pneumococcal pneumonia	Pneumovax 23, Prevnar 13	IM or SC; all children 2–23 mo; administer every 6 yr for high-risk patients	Moderate or severe acute illness; hypersensitivity	Drowsiness, local irritation at site, mild fever
Rotavirus (Rota) RotaTeq for prevention of rotavirus gastroenteritis	Rotarix	PO; 3 doses at 6–12 wk; subsequent doses at 4–10 wk intervals	Hypersensitivity	GI upset and blood disorders
Varicella (chickenpox)	Varivax	SC; may give with all other vaccines but at a separate site; 2-dose series at ages 12 through 15 mo and 4 through 6 yr	Confirmed history of chickenpox; pregnancy or possible pregnancy in 1 mo; moderate or severe acute illness; immunocompromised patients; egg allergy	No salicylates for 6 wk afterward to prevent risk of Reye syndrome
May give combination vaccine: measles, mumps, rubella, varicella (MMRV)	ProQuad	SC; may give with all other vaccines but at a separate site; all susceptible children 12 mo or older	Confirmed history of chickenpox; pregnancy or possible pregnancy in 1 mo; moderate or severe acute illness; immunocompromised patients; egg allergy	No salicylates for 6 wk afterward to prevent risk of Reye's syndrome

[a]Mild illness is not a contraindication.

GI, Gastrointestinal; *HIV,* human immunodeficiency virus; *IM,* intramuscular; *PO,* oral; *SC,* subcutaneous.

- Document in the child's health record the date the VIS was given and the publication date of the VIS (which appears on the bottom of the form).
- To make sure the office has the most current VIS forms, either call the state health department or refer to the CDC's website at www.cdc.gov/vaccines/hcp/vis/current-vis.html. Forms can be printed directly from the site.
- If an informed consent form is required in your state, it must be signed and attached to the child's health record or electronically signed in the child's EHR before immunizations are given. Documentation of immunization administration must include the date the vaccine was administered, the manufacturer of the vaccine, the manufacturer's lot number, the type of vaccine, the exact site of administration if an injection was given, any reported or observed side effects, the name and title of the person who administered the vaccine, and the address of the medical office where the vaccine was administered.
- An immunization record should be given to the parent. If it is in paper form (e.g., a booklet), it should be updated as needed to reflect the child's current immunization status. Most EHRs allow for the immunization record to be printed after each immunization. Medical assistants should not only document the required details in the patient's health record, but they should also complete the parent's immunization record each time the child receives another vaccination or booster (Procedure 44.4). These parent records help schools and day care centers determine the child's immunization status. Some states are developing computerized immunization record systems.
- It is very important that vaccine vials are handled and stored properly to maintain the compound's ability to fight disease. The CDC's recommendations for vaccine management practices can be found on its website at www.cdc.gov/vaccines/recs/storage.

CRITICAL THINKING APPLICATION 44.5

Allison will be administering pediatric immunizations during the well-baby visits scheduled for today. To prepare for this responsibility, she looked up the primary vaccinations, their routes of administration, contraindications, and possible side effects. The first child arrives for her 4-month checkup. She has received all of her previous immunizations on schedule. What immunizations should the child receive, and how should they be administered? The baby's father asks whether she will get sick from the vaccines. What should Allison tell him? What does Allison need to do to meet the requirements of the National Childhood Vaccine Injury Act?

Nebulizers

Nebulizers are used to administer medication in a form that can be inhaled. A small machine is used to turn liquid medication into a fine mist. This is a useful method for treating certain respiratory conditions such as asthma, croup, respiratory syncytial virus (RSV), or reactive airway disease. Often the first dose is administered during the office visit. This serves two purposes. The provider can see if the medication is helpful, and the caregiver can be instructed on how to use the nebulizer. This type of treatment can be done at home.

Safe Handling and Storage of Vaccines

The Centers for Disease Control and Prevention (CDC) has devised a list of important rules and steps to ensure safekeeping of a practice's vaccine supply. This list can be used as a checklist in the office.

1. One person should be in charge of handling and storing vaccines at the facility, with a backup person to ensure proper management.
2. A vaccine inventory log should be maintained that includes the following:
   (a) Vaccine name
   (b) Number of doses
   (c) Date vaccine was received
   (d) Condition of vaccine on arrival
   (e) Manufacturer
   (f) Lot number
   (g) Expiration date
3. Vaccines should be stored in separate, self-contained units that refrigerate or freeze only. A household-style combination unit can be used to store only refrigerated vaccines; frozen vaccines must be kept in a separate, stand-alone freezer.
4. The vaccine refrigerator and freezer should not be used for food or drinks.
5. Vaccines should be stored in the middle of the refrigerator or freezer, not in the door.
6. New supplies should be placed behind the vials with the closest expiration date; the vials with the nearest expiration date should be used first.
7. A sign should be posted on the refrigerator door identifying which vaccines should be stored in either the refrigerator or the freezer.
8. One thermometer should be kept in the refrigerator and one in the freezer; the refrigerator temperature should be maintained at 35° to 46°F (2° to 8°C) and the freezer temperature at −58° to 5°F (−50° to 15°C) or colder.
9. Containers of water should be kept in the refrigerator and ice packs in the freezer to help maintain cold temperatures.
10. A temperature log should be kept on the refrigerator door; the refrigerator and freezer temperatures should be recorded twice a day: first thing in the morning and at the end of the day.
11. A "Do Not Unplug" sign should be posted next to the refrigerator's electrical outlet.
12. If the refrigerator or freezer stops working, the following steps should be taken:
    - Immediately place the vaccines in another refrigerator or freezer and mark them so that they can be separated from vaccines that were not affected.
    - Record the temperature of the refrigerator or freezer and contact the vaccine manufacturer or state health department. Follow their instructions on the use, alteration of expiration dates, or disposal of the vaccines.
13. The facility should have a copy of the health department's general and emergency vaccine management policies.

The nebulizer treatment may be administered via a mask or a mouthpiece. Masks work better for younger patients because it is difficult for them to hold the mouthpiece in place. The medical assistant should provide written, detailed instructions to the caregiver and provide a phone number that the caregiver can call if they have questions. More information on nebulizer treatments can be found in Chapter 41 and Procedure 41.3.

THE ADOLESCENT PATIENT

One of the challenges of working in pediatrics is the wide age range of patients and the differing needs of those patients. Adolescent patients have different needs than younger patients. The following sections discuss how the medical assistant can meet the needs of the adolescent patient.

Examination

The adolescent patient may present the greatest challenge to health education and disease management. Adolescence begins with the onset of puberty, a time when the child's reproductive system matures. This is a period marked by rapid changes in the endocrine and musculoskeletal systems. The adolescent undergoes rapid growth spurts and the development of secondary sexual characteristics.

Health examinations for patients in this age group should include the following:

- Screening for height and weight
- Gathering details about diet and exercise routines
- Screening for sexually transmitted infections (STIs)
- Pap test (for sexually active female adolescents), especially to screen for infection with the human papillomavirus [HPV])
- Reviewing the vaccination history and administering boosters as indicated
- Assessing for high-risk behaviors, such as substance abuse, smoking, and sexual behavior

Developing a trusting relationship with the adolescent patient is key to being able to provide the best possible care. Many adolescents are embarrassed by the types of questions and conversations they have during their examination as well as the examination itself. By being professional and empathetic, you can ensure that your patient is getting the care and support they need.

Diseases and Disorders

Health problems most frequently seen in adolescent patients include eating disorders (anorexia nervosa and bulimia nervosa), obesity, and injury-related problems. Accidents are the leading cause of death and injury in adolescence, and suicide is the third leading cause of death. All healthcare personnel should be on the alert for indicators of suicide, including the following:

- Signs of depression, such as headaches, abdominal discomfort, anorexia, fatigue, aggressiveness, drug or alcohol abuse, and sexual promiscuity
- Verbal statements that hint at the adolescent's intention to commit suicide; talking about dying
- Actions such as giving away prized objects, withdrawing from social groups, suddenly changing normal behavior patterns, or writing a suicide note

This patient population can be challenging to work with, but it can also be rewarding as you help the adolescent patient handle the hurdles of becoming a healthy adult.

CLOSING COMMENTS

Patient Coaching

Unintentional injuries are the leading cause of death and disability in children in the United States. Injuries cause more childhood deaths than all diseases combined. The primary causes of childhood injuries are the following:

- Motor vehicle accidents
- Drowning
- Burns
- Falls
- Poisoning
- Aspiration with airway obstruction
- Firearm accidents

Childhood injuries are linked to the child's growth and development level and usually are preventable. Young children are totally dependent on caregivers to keep them safe, so constant supervision and a childproof environment are essential for this age group. Older children need to be aware of health hazards and should be encouraged to protect themselves from injury (e.g., they should use bike helmets, protective padding when skateboarding, seat belts, and so on). The highest incidence of accidental injuries is seen in children under age 9, but as children grow older, the percentage of deaths from injuries increases. In the United States, more than 9000 children die each year—about 25 deaths a day—from injuries. Healthcare workers play a major role in injury prevention. The medical assistant is responsible for making sure the ambulatory care office is safe, and parents are educated about potential hazards.

Legal and Ethical Issues

The Child Abuse Prevention and Treatment Act states that all threats to a child's physical or mental welfare must be reported. This means that every teacher, healthcare worker, and social worker, in fact, every citizen who suspects that a child is being neglected, abused, or exploited, must report this to the proper authority. The agency must record the report, and after three similar reports, the agency must investigate.

When suspected abuse, neglect, or exploitation is reported, the individual must provide his or her name. This is considered confidential information and is not given to the child's parent or guardian, nor is it given to the investigating officer. The individual making the report is also protected under the law from any liability for reporting suspicions of child abuse.

If the medical assistant suspects a child is a victim of abuse, neglect, or exploitation, she or he should consult with the provider immediately. In most states, the medical assistant and the provider can make separate reports to the authorities. However, state laws vary, so state and local reporting protocols should be outlined in the office procedures manual.

Signs of Child Abuse

Obvious Signs

- Previously filed reports of physical or sexual abuse of the child
- Documented abuse of other family members
- Different stories from the parents and the child on how an accident happened
- Stories of incidents and injuries that are suspicious
- Injuries blamed on other family members
- Repeated visits to the emergency department for injuries

Examination Findings

- Trauma to the nervous system
- Internal abdominal pain
- Discolorations/bruising on the buttocks, back, and abdomen
- Elbow, wrist, and shoulder dislocations

Changes in Child's Behavior

- Too eager to please the parent
- Overly passive and too compliant
- Aggressive and demanding
- Parenting the parent (role reversal)
- Delays in the normal growth and development patterns
- Erratic school attendance

Physical Indicators

- Poor hygiene
- Malnutrition
- Obvious dental neglect
- Neglected well-baby procedures (e.g., immunizations)

Patient-Centered Care

In a pediatric practice, the child usually is joined by one or both parents during visits to the provider. Parents need reinforcement, praise, and understanding in dealing with the health and welfare of their children. Provide parents with information to help them understand their children's behavior and improve their parenting skills. Understanding the normal behavioral characteristics of a particular developmental stage may increase the parents' confidence and reinforce expectations for the child.

The waiting room is an ideal place for parent education. Use the space and resources available to provide up-to-date information on child health issues and on local resources for support and assistance. If the provider has pamphlets available, discuss them with the parents. Answer questions when possible or alert the provider so that questions can be answered during the office visit. Every opportunity should be taken to teach parents about sound healthcare. Because so many ambulatory care visits involve infectious disorders, educating children and parents on the following infection control measures may reduce the spread of disease:

- Children should cover their mouth with a disposable tissue when they cough or cough into their bent arm rather than their hands.
- A tissue should be used only once and then immediately thrown away.
- Children should not be allowed to share toys they have put in their mouths.
- After a child has discarded a toy that was in their mouth, it should be placed in a bin for dirty toys that are out of the reach of others. Wash and disinfect these toys before allowing children to play with them again.
- Make sure all children and adults follow good handwashing practices. Have pump hand sanitizers available throughout the office.

Professional Behaviors

Working as a medical assistant in a busy pediatric practice can be very challenging. In essence, you are faced with two clients: a child who may be frightened and not feeling well and a caregiver who typically is stressed. When you are dealing with emotionally charged situations, it is easy to lose patience and act out yourself. Continuing to act professionally can help you manage these difficult situations. Consider the following suggestions:

- Routinely use active listening to get as much information as possible from the parents. Paying attention not only to the parents' words but also to their feelings helps the parents feel valued.
- Focus on age-appropriate methods for communicating with the child. Interacting with children on a level they can understand helps them feel more comfortable and hopefully promotes cooperative behavior.
- Use time management techniques to handle the work challenges you face each day. Staying organized keeps you from feeling overwhelmed.

SUMMARY OF SCENARIO

After working with the telephone screening staff, Allison has come to realize the importance of becoming familiar with childhood diseases and disorders and the management policy of her provider-employers. Many times Allison has had to refer to the office procedure manual to make sure she is asking the right questions and gathering all the information needed for the provider who will make the daily response calls. From working in the clinical area, Allison has also realized that a pediatric practice actually has two groups of patients: the child and the caregivers. She must be sensitive to the needs of both groups and develop communication skills that build trust with the child and his or her parents. Allison is working on developing a comprehensive education site in the office for interested parents and is creating a community resource guide for interested caregivers. She recognizes the need to stay up to date on the CDC's recommendations for childhood immunizations, and she routinely refers to the CDC's website to make sure the office has the most recently published VIS forms. Allison regularly attends her local American Association of Medical Assistants (AAMA) chapter meetings to maintain her certification and to continue to learn about the pediatric practice specialty.

SUMMARY OF LEARNING OBJECTIVES

1. **Examine growth and developmental patterns of the pediatric patient.**
By 6 months of age, a child's birth weight has doubled; at 1 year, it has tripled, and the child's length has increased by 50%. By age 2, the child has reached approximately 50% of adult height. This same growth rate continues throughout the school-age period, ages 6 to 12 years, which leads to a growth spurt that indicates impending puberty. In adolescence, ages 12 to 18 years, the adolescent gains almost half of his or her adult weight and the skeleton and organs double in size.
Using therapeutic approaches for infants, toddlers, school-age, and adolescent patients improve communication with a variety of patient age groups and promote quality patient care. Unnumbered boxes in the text discuss therapeutic approaches for pediatric patients.
Erik Erickson's developmental theory focuses on five stages that an individual must pass through and master: trust versus mistrust, autonomy versus shame and doubt, initiative versus guilt, industry versus inferiority, and identity versus role confusion.
2. **Examine the common diseases and disorders found in the pediatric patient population, including the signs, symptoms, etiology, diagnostic procedures, and treatments.**
Pediatric gastrointestinal disorders include infant colic; diarrhea, which can be caused by a variety of microorganisms and is medically treated when it continues for longer than 2 days; failure to thrive caused by a physiologic factor (e.g., malabsorption disease or cleft palate) or a nonorganic cause that is associated with the parent-child relationship; and obesity if the child's BMI is equal to or greater than the 95th percentile.
The common cold may lead to secondary bacterial infections, including strep throat or otitis media; croup is a viral disorder that affects the larynx; pertussis, commonly known as whooping cough, is caused by bacteria that attach to the cilia of the upper respiratory system and can cause violent, rapid coughing and apnea in infants; bronchiolitis is a viral infection of the bronchioles that causes acute onset of wheezing and dyspnea; respiratory syncytial virus (RSV) is a virus that infects the lungs and bronchioles; asthma causes bronchospasms and inflammation of the bronchioles; and influenza is an acute, highly contagious viral infection of the respiratory tract.
Pediatric infectious diseases include conjunctivitis, caused by a bacterial or viral infection; tonsillitis, typically caused by beta-hemolytic streptococci; fifth disease, also called *erythema infectiosum,* a mild infection caused by parvovirus B19; hand-foot-and-mouth disease, caused by the coxsackievirus, which leads to multiple symptoms, including painful blisters on the tongue, mouth, palms of the hands, and soles of the feet; and Reye syndrome, which is linked with the use of aspirin during a viral illness.
3. **Examine the medical assistant's role in examinations and diagnostic procedures.**
During the examination of the pediatric patient, the medical assistant is involved in assisting the provider, updating the patient history, performing screening tests, taking measurements and vital signs, and administering immunizations.
Many diagnostic procedures can be performed during the pediatric visit. It is important for the medical assistant to use appropriate techniques based on the child's age. Gaining the child's cooperation is key to having the visit go smoothly for the child, the caregiver, and the healthcare staff.
4. **Explain the different types of pediatric visits.**
The medical assistant assists the pediatrician with examinations; maintains patient histories; performs ordered screening tests, such as vision, hearing, urinalysis, and hemoglobin checks; administers immunizations; measures and weighs children as needed; documents accurately; and provides support to patients and caregivers.
Refer to Table 44.2 for reference ranges for pediatric vital signs
Apgar is used to evaluate a newborn's physical condition at 1 and 5 minutes after birth. The newborn is evaluated on appearance, pulse, grimace, activity, and respiration. Table 44.3 describes the scoring system.
Well-child visits are typically scheduled from age 2 weeks through 15 years to focus on maintaining the child's health with physical examinations, immunizations, and upgrading the child's medical health history record.
Sick-child visits occur whenever the child needs to be seen because of illness or injury. Table 44.4 summarizes important questions for telephone screening of pediatric problems.
5. **Examine the common diagnostic procedures done during a pediatric visit.**
The easiest way to obtain a urine sample from a child who is toilet trained is to give the parent the container and instructions ahead of time. In some cases, the child may need to be catheterized to obtain the specimen. Pediatric catheterization kits contain all the supplies needed for this procedure. When preparing the kit, always remember that this is a sterile procedure.
Vision screening is done using the Snellen distance visual acuity chart and the Ishihara color vision test. These tests should be done with natural light and few distractions for the pediatric patient. Explaining what the patient should do by using examples will ensure that accurate results are obtained.
Hearing screening is commonly done for the pediatric patient and uses an audiometer, which tests the patients hearing at different frequencies and intensities. As with vision screening, an explanation of the process will help get accurate results.

Continued

SUMMARY OF LEARNING OBJECTIVES—*Continued*

6. **Examine common treatments done with pediatric patients.**
The CDC's recommendations for childhood immunization are summarized in Table 44.5 and Figure 44.10.
Procedure 44.3 summarizes how to document immunizations in both the official vaccination record and the parent's immunization booklet. Documentation of immunization administration on the Vaccine Information Statement (VIS) form must include the date the vaccine was administered, the vaccine's manufacturer, the manufacturer's lot number, the type of vaccine, the route of administration and the exact site if an injection is given, any reported or observed side effects, the name and title of the person administering the vaccine, the address of the medical office where the vaccine was administered, and the date.
7. **Contrast working with adolescent patients and younger pediatric patients.**
Adolescents are going through extreme physical and emotional changes, and an extra measure of patience and understanding is required to establish therapeutic interactions. Ensuring their privacy, giving them the option of being seen without parents, and providing pertinent education materials are all important factors in patient-centered adolescent care.

PROCEDURE 44.1 Measure the Head Circumference of an Infant

TASKS: Obtain an accurate measurement of the circumference of an infant's head and plot the result on the patient's growth chart.

EQUIPMENT and SUPPLIES

- Patient's record
- Flexible disposable tape measure
- Age- and gender-specific growth chart
- Pen

PROCEDURAL STEPS

1. Wash hands or use hand sanitizer.
PURPOSE: Hand sanitization is necessary to ensure infection control.
2. Greet the patient and the parents or caregivers. Identify yourself. Verify the patient's identity with full name and date of birth. Explain the procedure to be performed in a manner that the patient (if old enough) or the parent or caregiver understands. Answer any questions. If the child is old enough, gain his or her cooperation through conversation.
PURPOSE: It is important to alleviate anxiety and gain the child's trust.
3. Place an infant in the supine position, or the infant may be held by the parent. An older infant may sit on the examination table.
4. Hold the tape measure with the zero mark against the infant's forehead, slightly above the eyebrows and the top of the ears. Ask the parent for assistance if necessary.
5. Bring the tape measure around the head, just above the ears, until it meets (Figure 1).

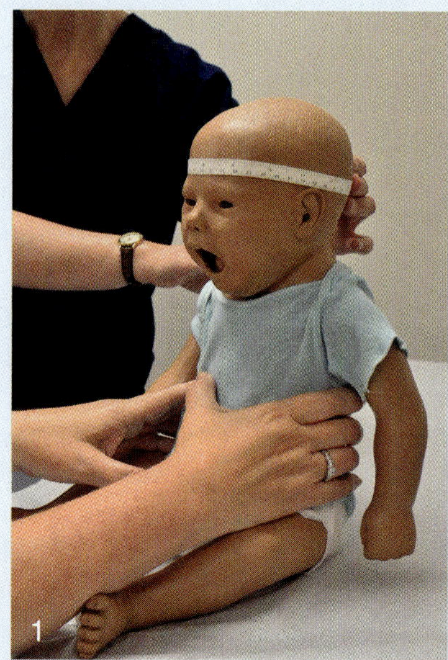
1

6. Read to the nearest 0.5 centimeter or quarter inch.
7. Record the measurement on the growth chart and the patient's health record.
PURPOSE: A procedure is not considered done until it is recorded.
8. Dispose of the tape measure.
9. Wash hands or use hand sanitizer.
PURPOSE: Hand sanitization is necessary to ensure infection control.

Documentation Example

10/21/20XX 10:20 am HC 39.5 cm ———————————— A. Kwong, CMA (AAMA)

PROCEDURE 44.2 Measure an Infant's Length and Weight

TASK: Measure an infant's length and weight accurately so that growth patterns can be monitored and recorded.

EQUIPMENT and SUPPLIES

- Patient's record
- Infant scale with paper cover
- Flexible measuring tape
- Examination table paper
- Pen
- Pediatric length board, if available
- Gender-specific infant growth chart
- Waste container

PROCEDURAL STEPS

MEASURING AN INFANT'S LENGTH

1. Wash hands or use hand sanitizer; assemble the necessary equipment.
   PURPOSE: Hand sanitization is necessary to ensure infection control.
2. Greet the patient and parents or caregivers. Identify yourself. Verify the patient's identity with full name and date of birth. Explain the procedure to be performed in a manner that the patient (if old enough) or the parent or caregiver understands. Answer any questions.
   PURPOSE: It is important to alleviate anxiety and gain the child's trust.
3. Undress the infant. The diaper may be left on.
4. Cover the examination table with smooth, flat paper. Ask the caregiver to place the infant on his or her back on the examination table. If using a pediatric table with a headboard, ask the caregiver to hold the infant's head gently against the headboard while you straighten the infant's leg and note the location of the heel on the measurement area. If there is no headboard, ask the caregiver to gently hold the infant's head still while you draw a line on the paper at the top of the baby's head and the heel after extending the leg (Figure 1).

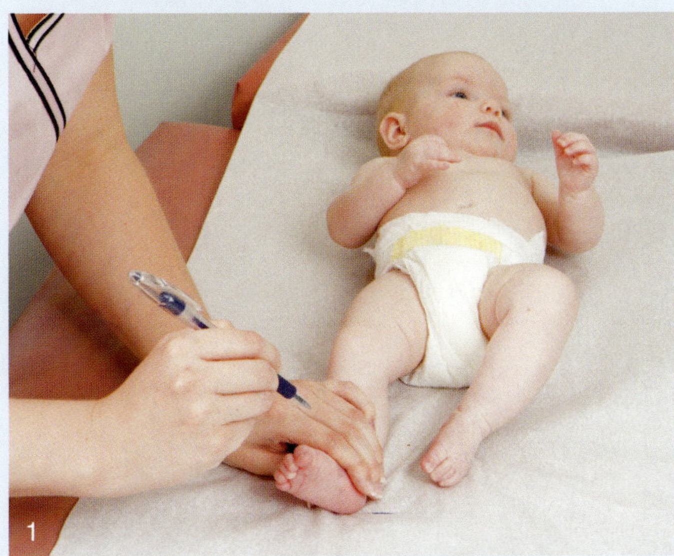

1

5. Measure the infant's length with the tape measure and record it.
6. Document the results in either inches or centimeters, depending on office policy, on the infant's growth chart, progress notes, and caregiver's record, if requested.

WEIGHING AN INFANT

1. Wash hands or use hand sanitizer, assemble the necessary equipment and explain the procedure to the infant's caregiver.
   PURPOSE: Hand sanitization is necessary to ensure infection control.
2. Greet the patient and parents or caregivers. Identify yourself. Verify the patient's identity with full name and date of birth. Explain the procedure to be performed in a manner that the patient understands. Answer any questions the parents or caregivers may have.
   PURPOSE: It is important to alleviate anxiety and gain the trust of the child and the parents or caregivers.
3. If the scale is not a digital model, prepare it by sliding weights to the left; line the scale with disposable paper to reduce the risk of pathogen transmission.
4. Completely undress the infant. If the diaper is clean and dry, it can remain on.
   PURPOSE: It is important to get the most accurate weight possible, and a wet diaper will add to the total weight.
5. Place the infant gently on the center of the scale, keeping your hand directly above the infant's trunk for safety (Figure 2).
   PURPOSE: This position will protect the infant from possible injury.

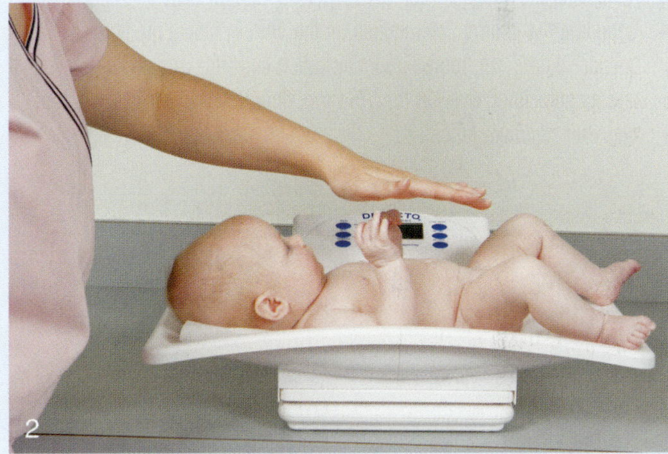

2

6. If the scale is not a digital model, slide the weights across until balance is achieved. Read the infant's weight while they are still.
7. If the scale is not a digital model, return the weights to the far left of the scale and remove the baby. Discard the paper lining the scale. If the scale becomes contaminated during the procedure, follow Occupational Safety and Health Administration (OSHA) guidelines for the use of gloves and disposal of contaminated waste. Disinfect the equipment according to the manufacturer's guidelines.
   PURPOSE: These steps will provide infection control.
8. Wash hands or use hand sanitizer.
9. Document the results in either pounds or kilograms, depending on office policy, the infant's growth chart, progress notes, and caregiver's record if requested.

Documentation Example

8/24/20XX 10:20 am Wt 17 lb 4 oz. Length 27 in. ———————————— A. Kwong, CMA (AAMA)

PROCEDURE 44.3 Document Immunizations

TASK: Document accurately the administration of a pediatric immunization.

EQUIPMENT and SUPPLIES

- Patient's record
- Vaccine administration record (VAR)
- Parent's immunization record (if used in the medical practice)
- Vaccine Information Statement (VIS) for hepatitis B (the current VIS forms can be accessed at www.cdc.gov/vaccines/hcp/vis/current-vis.html)

SCENARIO

Samantha Anderson, a 5-week-old infant, has just received her second dose of the hepatitis B (HBV) vaccine. Document the administration of the vaccine.

PROCEDURAL STEPS

1. Gather the necessary forms.
2. Make sure the provider obtained informed consent from the parent (if required by your state), that the hepatitis B VIS form was given, and that all the parent's questions were answered before the vaccine is dispensed and administered.
   PURPOSE: It is important to follow risk management practices.
3. Administer the vaccine intramuscularly (see Chapter 30).
4. Complete the information required on the VAR, including the name of the vaccine, date given, route of administration and site, vaccine lot number and manufacturer, date on the VIS form, date it was given to the parent, and your signature or initials.
   PURPOSE: This level of documentation is necessary to meet the legal requirements of the National Childhood Vaccine Injury Act.
5. On the parent's copy of the immunization record, record the date of administration, the name and address of the provider's practice, and the type of vaccine administered.
   PURPOSE: It is important to maintain an accurate and comprehensive parental record of childhood immunizations for school or day care purposes.
6. After administering the HBV vaccine, record the following details in the child's health record:
   - Date the vaccine was administered
   - Vaccine's manufacturer, batch and lot numbers, and expiration date
   - Type of vaccine administered and dose
   - Route of administration and exact site if an injection was given
   - Any reported or observed side effects
   - Publication date of the VIS form given to the parent (on the bottom of the form)
   - Parent education about possible side effects of the vaccine
   - Name and title of the person who administered the vaccine

Documentation Example

4/2/20XX 3:25 pm Mother given VIS form for Hep B. Had no questions. Administered second dose of Hep B IM to Ⓛ vastus lateralis per Dr. Walden's order. No problems noted after injection. ——————A. Kwong, CMA (AAMA)

PROCEDURE 44.3 Document Immunizations—*continued*

Vaccine administration record for children and teens

Patient name ______________________________

Birthdate ________________ Chart number ____________

PRACTICE NAME AND ADDRESS

Before administering any vaccines, give copies of all pertinent vaccine information statements (VISs) to the child's parent or legal representative and make sure he/she understands the risks and benefits of the vaccine(s). Always provide or update the patient's personal record card.

Vaccine	Type of vaccine[1]	Date vaccine given (mo/day/yr)	Funding source (F,S,P)[2]	Site[3]	Vaccine		Vaccine information statement (VIS)		Vaccinator[5] (signature or initials and title)
					Lot #	Mfr.	Date on VIS[4]	Date given[4]	
Hepatitis B[6] (e.g., HepB, Hib-HepB, DTaP-HepB-IPV) Give IM.[7]									
Diphtheria, Tetanus, Pertussis[6] (e.g., DTaP, DTaP/Hib, DTaP-HepB-IPV, DT, DTaP-IPV/Hib, DTaP-IPV, Tdap, Td) Give IM.[7]									
***Haemophilus influenzae* type b**[6] (e.g., Hib, Hib-HepB, DTaP-IPV/Hib, DTaP/Hib, Hib-MenCY) Give IM.[7]									
Polio[6] (e.g., IPV, DTaP-HepB-IPV, DTaP-IPV/Hib, DTaP-IPV) Give IPV Subcut or IM.[7] Give all others IM.[7]									
Pneumococcal (e.g., PCV7, PCV13, conjugate; PPSV23, polysaccharide) Give PCV IM.[7] Give PPSV Subcut or IM.[7]									
Rotavirus (RV1, RV5) Give orally (po).									

▶ **See page 2** to record measles-mumps-rubella, varicella, hepatitis A, meningococcal, HPV, influenza, and other vaccines (e.g., travel vaccines).

How to complete this record

1. Record the generic abbreviation (e.g., Tdap) or the trade name for each vaccine (see table at right).
2. Record the funding source of the vaccine given as either F (federal), S (state), or P (private).
3. Record the site where vaccine was administered as either RA (right arm), LA (left arm), RT (right thigh), LT (left thigh), or NAS (intranasal).
4. Record the publication date of each VIS as well as the date the VIS is given to the patient.
5. To meet the space constraints of this form and federal requirements for documentation, a healthcare setting may want to keep a reference list of vaccinators that includes their initials and titles.
6. For combination vaccines, fill in a row for each antigen in the combination.
7. IM is the abbreviation for intramuscular; Subcut is the abbreviation for subcutaneous.

Abbreviation	Trade name and manufacturer
DTaP	Daptacel (Sanofi Pasteur); Infanrix (GlaxoSmithKline [GSK]); Tripedia (Sanofi Pasteur)
DT (pediatric)	Generic (Sanofi Pasteur)
DTaP-HepB-IPV	Pediarix (GSK)
DTaP-IPV/Hib	Pentacel (Sanofi Pasteur)
DTaP-IPV	Kinrix (GSK); Quadracel (Sanofi Pasteur)
HepB	Engerix-B (GSK); Recombivax HB (Merck)
HepA-HepB	Twinrix (GSK); can be given to teens age 18 and older
Hib	ActHIB (Sanofi Pasteur); Hiberix (GSK); PedvaxHIB (Merck)
Hib-MenCY	MenHibrix (GSK)
IPV	Ipol (Sanofi Pasteur)
PCV13	Prevnar 13 (Pfizer)
PPSV23	Pneumovax 23 (Merck)
RV1	Rotarix (GSK)
RV5	RotaTeq (Merck)
Tdap	Adacel (Sanofi Pasteur); Boostrix (GSK)
Td	Decavac, Tenivac (Sanofi Pasteur); Generic (MA Biological Labs)

IMMUNIZATION ACTION COALITION Saint Paul, Minnesota • 651-647-9009 • www.immunize.org • www.vaccineinformation.org
www.immunize.org/catg.d/p2022.pdf • Item #P2022 (4/16)

PROCEDURE 44.4 Complete an Immunization Schedule for a Patient

TASKS: Complete an immunization schedule for a patient by reviewing a patient immunization record and determining what vaccines are needed. Document all vaccines that are given.

EQUIPMENT and SUPPLIES

- CDC Immunization Schedule (Figure 44.11)
- Vaccine Information Statement (VIS)
- Electronic health record or SimChart for the Medical Office (SCMO)

SCENARIO

In preparation for Daniel Miller's 2-year-old well-child visit tomorrow, you review his immunization record and see that he was up to date with his immunizations through 9 months of age, including the third dose of hepatitis B and inactivated poliovirus. His record doesn't show any immunizations since that time. A review of the statewide vaccination record system doesn't show any additional vaccines given elsewhere.

PROCEDURAL STEPS

1. Using the CDC Immunization Schedule, determine the vaccines needed to ensure that Daniel is current with all of his vaccinations.
   PURPOSE: The CDC Immunization Schedule will provide the information needed to determine what vaccines the child needs.

SCENARIO UPDATE

Daniel and his father have arrived for his well-care visit. The provider has discussed the needed vaccines with Daniel's father, and he has agreed that Daniel should get the missing vaccinations. He has given his consent. You provided Daniel's father with the required VIS, and he has no further questions or concerns. You administer the vaccines identified with the CDC Schedule review per the provider's orders and now need to document the vaccines.

1. Log in to the EHR or SCMO (using the Simulation Playground) and locate Daniel Miller's record (DOB 03/21/20XX). Create an office visit encounter for today's visit with Dr. Angela Perez.
   PURPOSE: An encounter is needed to document patient care.
2. Document that the patient has no allergies to drugs, food, or environmental items.
3. Using the Immunization screen, document the immunizations that were given today as ordered by Dr. Perez. All of the following information should be documented:
   - In the reaction field document, no reaction and the VIS edition date
   - Dose
   - Date (today's date)
   - Provider
   - Route/site (IM or subcut/vastus lateralis or anterolateral thigh)
   - Manufacturer (Elsevier)
   - Expiration date (one year from today's date)
   - Reaction
   - VIS edition (document in the Reaction field of SCMO)

   Note: When documenting combination vaccines, each vaccine must be documented separately.
4. Log out of EHR or SCMO.

45 GERIATRICS

SCENARIO

Bill Novelli, a certified medical assistant (CMA) who has met the requirements of the American Association of Medical Assistants (AAMA), works at Walden-Martin Family Medical (WMFM) Clinic. Although patients of all ages are seen in the practice, many patients are age 65 or older. Through his work with Dr. Angela Perez, Bill has learned to recognize the unique communication needs of aging individuals and the importance of using family and community resources to maintain optimum health in this special population.

While studying this chapter, think about the following questions:

- Do myths about aging and stereotypes about aging people negatively affect older individuals?
- What are the most common changes that occur in the aging body, and what recommendations can be made to promote health in this age group?
- What suggestions can be made to aging patients and their families to optimize older adults' health and protect them from injury and disease?
- How is Alzheimer disease diagnosed, and what are the stages of its development?
- Why is depression so common in aging individuals, and how is it diagnosed and treated?
- How can the medical assistant most effectively communicate with an older person?
- Why is the use of community resources such an important factor in the care of aging people?

LEARNING OBJECTIVES

1. Examine the changes in anatomy, physiology, and diseases of the cardiovascular and pulmonary systems.
2. Examine the changes in anatomy, physiology, and diseases of the endocrine and gastrointestinal systems.
3. Examine the changes in anatomy, physiology, and diseases of the integumentary and musculoskeletal systems.
4. Examine the changes in anatomy, physiology, and diseases of the nervous system and sensory organs.
5. Examine the changes in anatomy, physiology, and diseases of the urinary and reproductive systems.
6. Examine the role of the medical assistant in caring for aging patients.

VOCABULARY

collagen (KAHL ah jen) The most abundant structural protein found in skin and other connective tissues. It provides strength and cushioning to many parts of the body.

dermatome (DUR mah tome) Skin surface areas supplied by a single afferent spinal nerve.

elastin (ih LAS tin) A highly elastic protein in connective tissue that allows tissues to resume their shape after stretching or contracting; found abundantly in the dermis of the skin.

explicit (ek SPLIS it) Fully and clearly expressed or demonstrated; leaving nothing merely implied.

insidious (in SID ee uhs) Proceeding in a gradual, subtle way, but with harmful effects.

lacrimation (lak ri MAY shun) The secretion or discharge of tears.

Ménière disease (mayn YAIRZ) Chronic disease of the inner ear causing recurrent episodes of vertigo, progressive sensorineural hearing loss, and tinnitus.

mortality (mohr TAL i tee) The relative frequency of deaths in a specific population.

nocturia (nok TOOR ee uh) Frequent urination at night.

oophorectomy (oo for ECK tuh mee) Surgical removal of the ovaries.

orthostatic hypotension (or thuh STAT ik) A temporary fall in blood pressure when a person rapidly changes from a recumbent position to a standing position.

osteoporosis (os tee oh puh ROH sis) Abnormal thinning of the bone structure, causing bones to become brittle and weak.

ototoxic A medicine or substance capable of damaging cranial nerve VIII or the organs of hearing and balance.

peristalsis (per uh STAHL suhs) Rhythmic contraction of involuntary muscles lining the gastrointestinal tract.

postherpetic neuralgia (noo RAL juh) Nerve pain that occurs after a shingles outbreak that may become chronic.

pressure injuries Sores or ulcers that develop over a bony prominence as the result of ischemia from prolonged pressure; also called bed sores or pressure sores.

INTRODUCTION

According to the National Institutes of Health, the aging population in the United States (those age 65 or older) is expected to nearly double over the next 30 years. By 2050, it is projected that there will be 88 million people age 65 or older.

The average life expectancy of an individual who reaches age 65 is an additional 19.5 years (20.8 years for females and 18.2 years for males). A child born in 2021 can expect to live 78.99 years, about 30 years longer than a child born in 1900. Older women outnumber older men; 30 million women are over age 65, as are 24.1 million men. About 30% of older people who live outside of institutions live alone; half of women over age 75 live alone. More than half a million grandparents over the age of 65 are the primary caregivers for their grandchildren, who live with them. Most older people have at least one chronic medical condition, and many have multiple conditions. Hypertension, arthritis, heart disease, cancer, and diabetes are the health problems most commonly seen in the older adult population, and a significant number also suffer from strokes, asthma, emphysema, and chronic bronchitis. Many of these conditions require medications. If a patient has multiple conditions, they could be on multiple medications. Pillbox organizers are a great tool for patients to keep those medications straight (Figure 45.1). Some pharmacies will fill the pillbox organizers for patients. Medication bottles can be a challenge for older adults to open, especially when they have childproof caps on them. Patients can ask the pharmacy to use non-childproof caps (Figure 45.2).

What does all this mean to those who have chosen careers in healthcare? As the aging population expands, it will affect all aspects of society. One area, in particular, will be these individuals' increased use of health services. To provide quality care to aging patients, medical assistants must understand the aging process, including the physical and sensory changes that occur with aging (Procedure 45.1). This knowledge enables medical assistants to recognize the special needs of older adults and develop therapeutic management and communication skills that can help them effectively care for older patients. Ongoing research and education about the aging process have dispelled many of the old stereotypes.

Aging is a complex physiologic, psychological, and social process. Old age is not an illness but rather a normal life process that people experience in different ways. Lack of exercise, poor nutrition, substance abuse, continual stress, and air pollutants are all factors that cause a person to show the effects of aging decades earlier than someone who has practiced healthy living habits.

As people age, changes occur in their physical appearance and abilities, along with sensory changes in vision, hearing, taste, and smell. These changes do not occur at the same time in everyone; however, sensorimotor changes can have a profound effect on the individual's ability to interact with their environment.

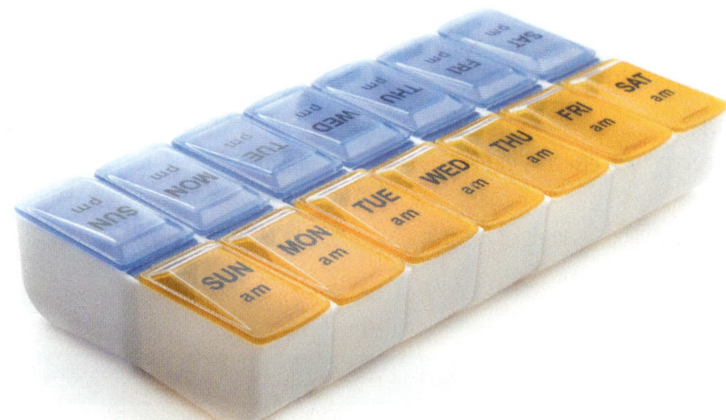

FIGURE 45.1 Pillbox organizer.

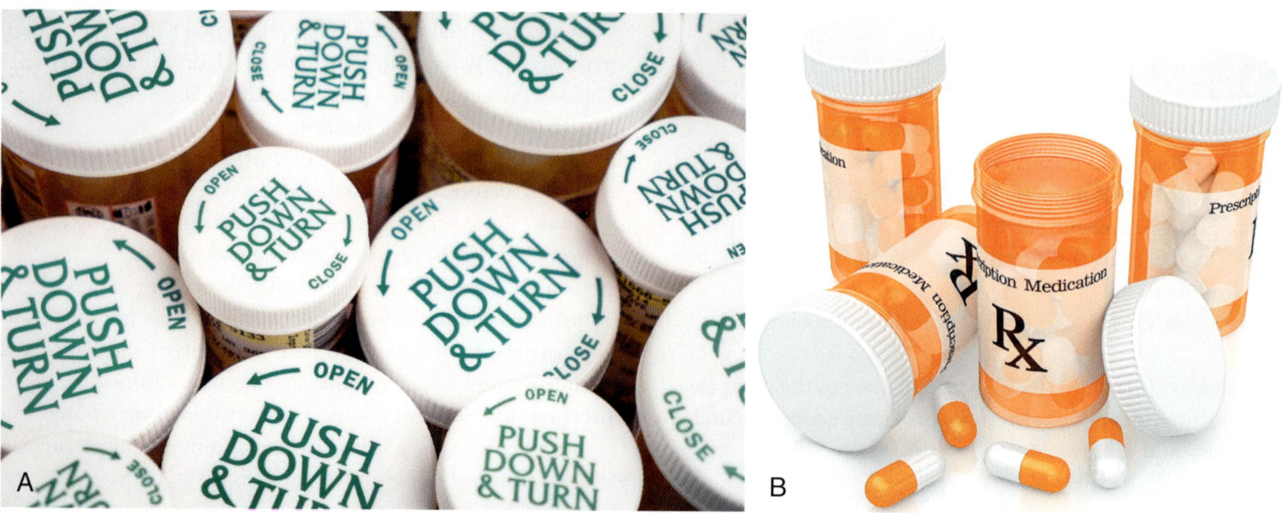

FIGURE 45.2 (A) Childproof medication bottles. **(B)** Non-childproof medication bottles.

Stereotypes and Myths about Aging

- *Most aging people will develop dementia.* Dementia is not part of the normal aging process. However, the older the person, the greater the risk of dementia. About 6% of those over age 65 and almost 50% of those over age 85 are diagnosed with significant memory and disorientation issues.
- *Disease is a normal and unavoidable part of the aging process.* Recent research verifies that individuals who have established healthy lifestyles as they age remain healthy well into their older years. Aging people are more likely to have health issues, but these are not inevitable for all persons over age 65.
- *Older workers are less productive than younger ones.* Individuals with a strong work ethic continue to perform in this way. It may take aging people longer to learn new material, but they continue to be capable of learning and applying new knowledge.
- *Most older people end up in long-term care facilities.* At any given time, approximately 5% of the aging population lives in long-term care facilities; 80% of aging individuals live independently, with or without a partner.
- *Most aging people have no interest in or capacity for sexual relations.* Sexual interest does not change significantly with age; a decrease in sexual activity is usually related to the loss of a partner.
- *Damage to health because of lifestyle factors is irreversible.* It is never too late to benefit from healthy lifestyle choices.

CRITICAL THINKING APPLICATION **45.1**

When Bill first started working with aging patients, he believed many of the stereotypes about people over age 65. Through his work with Dr. Perez, he has come to realize that many of these myths have no foundation in actual practice. Based on the myths mentioned in the text, what do you think about these beliefs on aging? Share your thoughts with your classmates.

CHANGES IN ANATOMY, PHYSIOLOGY, AND DISEASES OF THE CARDIOVASCULAR AND PULMONARY SYSTEMS

The aging process brings about changes in all of the body's systems. Table 45.1 summarizes the changes to the cardiovascular and pulmonary systems and what can be done to promote healthy aging. The following sections provide more detail about the changes to those systems.

Cardiovascular System

Cardiovascular disease is the most frequent cause of illness and disability in the aging population, and congestive heart failure (CHF) (see Chapter 40) is the most common reason for hospitalization. Age-related changes can occur in the cardiovascular system. Disease and lifestyle habits such as lack of exercise, poor diet, and stress can greatly contribute to these changes. Heart disease is ranked as the leading cause of death among men and women. Proper management of cardiovascular disease can help maintain the health of an aging population and reduce **mortality** rates.

The aging process causes structural changes in the heart. Myocardial cells enlarge, and deposits of fat and connective tissue increase. These combine to make the myocardial wall stiffer and increase the time needed for the relaxation phase of the cardiac cycle. As a result, cardiac output declines, making aging people more susceptible to CHF. The reduction in cardiac output leads to pooling of blood in the legs, cold extremities, and edema. In addition, the heart cannot respond as quickly or forcefully to an increased workload. Exercise, sudden movements, and changes in position can result in dizziness and loss of balance. Aging typically brings with it an increase in blood pressure, requiring the heart to work harder to pump blood into the systemic circulation. Hypertension increases the workload of the left ventricle, which may result in hypertrophy of the chamber and weakening of the myocardial wall. The valves of the heart tend to thicken and become more rigid, making it more difficult for blood to circulate through the cardiopulmonary vessels. With these cardiovascular problems, arrhythmias become more common.

Aging causes the walls of the veins to weaken and stretch. This damages the valves, especially in the veins of the legs, where the walls are subject to greater pressure as blood struggles to return to the heart against the force of gravity. As a result, edema and varicose veins of the lower extremities are common in older adults, increasing the risk of phlebitis and the formation of thrombi in the deep veins, or *deep vein thrombosis* (DVT).

Arteriosclerosis is considered part of the aging process. The vessel walls thicken and become less elastic because of the calcification and buildup of connective tissue. In addition, the artery's ability to dilate and contract diminishes. The heart must work harder to overcome the resistance caused by stiffened vessels to maintain an adequate

TABLE 45.1 System Changes Due to Aging of the Cardiovascular and Pulmonary Systems, and Measures to Promote Health

SYSTEM	AGE-RELATED CHANGES	HEALTH PROMOTION
Cardiovascular system	Arteriosclerosis and atherosclerotic plaque buildup reduces blood flow to major organs; 50% of the aging population have hypertension; CVD is the number one killer of women and men in their 60s.	Regular exercise; weight control; diet rich in fruits, vegetables, and whole grains; cholesterol, blood glucose monitoring
Pulmonary system	At age 55 the lungs become less elastic and the chest wall gradually stiffens, making oxygenation more difficult.	Quit smoking; regular aerobic exercise

blood supply throughout the body. Older adults have a higher incidence of **orthostatic hypotension**. The clinical criterion for alterations in blood pressure from sitting to standing is as follows:

- A drop of 20 mm Hg or more in the systolic pressure, or
- 10 mm Hg or more in the diastolic pressure, or
- Experiencing lightheadedness or dizziness

When a person with orthostatic hypotension stands, gravity causes blood to pool in the legs, resulting in a drop in the amount of blood returning to the heart for circulation. This decrease in circulating blood volume causes a sudden drop in blood pressure. The provider may have the medical assistant take orthostatic blood pressures as part of the routine intake protocol for aging patients. To perform this procedure, have the patient lie down for 5 minutes, apply a blood pressure cuff, and take the individual's blood pressure and pulse while the patient is lying down. Leave the cuff in place, have the patient stand, take the blood pressure and pulse after 1 minute of standing, and then again after 3 minutes. Record the blood pressure immediately, including the position for each of the readings.

Pulmonary System

Maximum lung function decreases with age. The rate of airflow through the bronchi slowly declines after age 30, and the maximum force one can achieve on inspiration and expiration declines. The lungs lose their elasticity because of changes in **elastin** and collagen. They become smaller and flabbier. The alveoli enlarge, their walls become thinner, and the number of capillaries is reduced. As a result, the area for gas exchange in the lungs is reduced. The chest wall may stiffen from osteoporosis of the ribs and vertebrae and calcification of the costal cartilage. The respiratory muscles become weaker, making it harder to move air into and out of the lungs. To compensate, older adults rely more on accessory muscles, such as the diaphragm. Weakening of the respiratory muscles and stiffening of the chest wall make it harder to cough deeply enough to clear mucus from the lungs. Pulmonary function tests reveal a decrease in vital capacity and an increase in residual volume. The incidence of sleep apnea and sleep disorders increases, causing a potential problem with nocturnal hypoxemia. All these factors combine to put the older adult at greater risk for pneumonia and aspiration and reactivation of tuberculosis.

The larynx also changes with aging, causing a change in the pitch and quality of the voice. The voice sounds quieter and slightly hoarse. The individual's voice may sound weaker, but it should not interfere with the ability to communicate effectively.

CHANGES IN ANATOMY, PHYSIOLOGY, AND DISEASES OF THE ENDOCRINE AND GASTROINTESTINAL SYSTEMS

Table 45.2 summarizes the changes to the endocrine and gastrointestinal systems and what can be done to promote healthy aging. The following sections provide more detail about the changes to those systems.

Endocrine System

Hormonal changes that occur with aging are related to a general decrease in hormone production combined with changes in tissue receptor binding. The most common endocrine system disorder seen in aging patients is *type 2 diabetes mellitus (DM).* As a person ages, insulin production by the beta cells in the pancreas decreases and insulin resistance at the tissue level increases. According to the National Institutes of Health, more than half of the 16 million Americans diagnosed with type 2 diabetes are over age 65. Older adult patients with diabetes are at increased risk of developing the following vascular diseases:

- Renal disorders
- Retinopathy
- Neuropathy
- Myocardial ischemia
- Angina
- Myocardial infarction
- Cerebrovascular accidents
- Peripheral vascular disease, such as lower extremity ulcers

Older patients do not always experience the classic symptoms of diabetes, which are polyuria, polydipsia, and polyphagia. They may show a variety of problems:

- Unexplained weight loss
- Slow wound healing
- Recurrent bacterial or fungal infections
- Changes in mental state
- Cataracts
- Macular disease
- Muscle weakness and pain
- Angina
- Foot ulcers
- Uremia

The range of symptoms is due to the **insidious** onset of diabetes in older people, who may have been gradually developing hyperglycemia for years before diagnosis.

TABLE 45.2 System Changes Due to Aging of the Endocrine and Gastrointestinal Systems, and Measures to Promote Health

SYSTEM	AGE-RELATED CHANGES	HEALTH PROMOTION
Endocrine system	After age 50, women have a sharp decline in estrogen; men have a more gradual decline in testosterone.	Possible hormone replacement therapy or natural soy supplements
Gastrointestinal system	Decline in gastric juices and enzymes by age 60; decreased peristalsis with increased constipation; some nutrients are not absorbed as well.	High-fiber diet and adequate fluid intake; regular exercise to prevent constipation

The treatment protocol for aging patients with diabetes is the same as for other age groups; however, special consideration must be given to the patient's ability to understand and comply with the therapeutic plan. In addition, the person may have other health problems that are being treated with medications. Therefore, an aging patient newly diagnosed with diabetes may face a complicated treatment plan that requires **explicit** instruction and continual follow-up in the ambulatory care setting.

The medical assistant must be aware of any sensory abnormalities, such as diminished vision or problems with fine motor skills that may interfere with the patient's ability to follow treatment guidelines. Coaching and treatment plans must be adapted to meet the individual needs of each patient. For example, if the patient has vision difficulties, an injector pen with audible clicks can be used to deliver a preset amount of insulin.

Factors That Can Affect Diabetes Management in Older People

- Modifying lifestyle risk factors may be more difficult because of poor nutrition, inability to exercise, and long-standing habits, such as smoking and a diet high in saturated fats and calories.
- Previously diagnosed health conditions, such as hypertension and heart disease, in addition to an age-related decline in kidney and liver function, increase the challenge of treating diabetes.
- Older people are more likely to be prescribed multiple medications, which increases the risk of adverse drug interactions.
- Older adult patients with diabetes are more prone to hypoglycemia and may not recognize and respond quickly to the signs of low blood glucose levels.
- Diabetic complications can develop quickly because of a long history of prediabetes before diagnosis.
- Older people may have decreased physical or mental abilities that make it difficult for them to understand and adhere to a complicated treatment regimen.
- Older patients may be unable to afford the medications and supplies needed to maintain health.

CRITICAL THINKING APPLICATION **45.2**

Quite a few of the older adult patients at WMFM Clinic have diabetes type 2. Based on what you have learned about the difficulty of managing diabetes in aging people, what factors do you need to consider when conducting patient education for an older adult with diabetes? Are there any community resources that might be useful for patients and their families?

Gastrointestinal System

Age-related changes in the gastrointestinal system begin in the mouth with dental problems:

- A decrease in the number of taste buds
- A decrease in the production of saliva
- A diminishing sense of smell

Older people generally find eating less pleasurable, have a reduced appetite, and are unable to chew and lubricate their food as well as younger people. This makes *dysphagia* (difficulty swallowing) a common age-related problem. Aging also brings a decrease in the production of hydrochloric acid, which affects the digestion of calcium and iron. Secretion of intrinsic factor, a protein needed to absorb vitamin B_{12}, also declines. This affects the function of the nervous system. It also affects the formation of red blood cells, resulting in excessive fatigue. It is not unusual for aging patients to be on regular vitamin B_{12} replacement therapy, either by oral dosage or injection.

Food passes more quickly through the small intestine, resulting in poorer absorption of vitamins and minerals. **Peristalsis** in the colon decreases, making aging patients more susceptible to constipation and diverticular disease. Poor eating habits, reduced fluid intake, and some medications (e.g., antidepressants, diuretics, antacids containing aluminum or calcium, and medications for Parkinson disease) also contribute to constipation. The liver decreases in size and weight after age 70. It is still able to perform vital functions, but more time is required to metabolize drugs and alcohol. All of these factors combine to increase the potential for adverse drug reactions in older adults.

Aging individuals have a higher incidence of several gastrointestinal system diseases, such as the following:

- Gastroesophageal reflux disease (GERD)
- Peptic ulcers
- Diverticulosis (related to lack of dietary fiber and constipation)
- Cholelithiasis
- Colorectal cancer

Dietary counseling and annual screenings should be part of the routine care of aging patients.

CHANGES IN ANATOMY, PHYSIOLOGY, AND DISEASES OF THE INTEGUMENTARY AND MUSCULOSKELETAL SYSTEMS

Table 45.3 summarizes the changes to the integumentary and musculoskeletal systems and what can be done to promote healthy aging. The following sections provide more detail about the changes to those systems.

Integumentary System

The skin is the body's first line of protection against infection, and it also is responsible for preventing the loss of body fluids and regulating body temperature. Changes in the appearance and function of the integumentary system are usually caused by a combination of ordinary age-related changes and environmental factors, especially the amount of sun exposure over time. Exposure to ultraviolet light from the sun frequently is the cause of the following skin conditions:

- Wrinkles
- Age spots
- Blotches
- Leathery, dry, loose skin

All of these conditions are associated with aging. Changes caused by the ultraviolet light from the sun or by the normal aging process can affect all three layers of the skin: the epidermis, dermis, and subcutaneous tissue.

The cells in the epidermis reproduce more slowly as people age, and this slower regeneration causes the skin to appear thinner. The skin becomes more prone to tearing and blistering. The risk of

TABLE 45.3 System Changes Due to Aging of the Integumentary and Musculoskeletal Systems, and Measures to Promote Health

SYSTEM	AGE-RELATED CHANGES	HEALTH PROMOTION
Integumentary system	Cells in the epidermis reproduce more slowly, dermis loses 20% of its mass, collagen cells decline, blood supply to the dermis decreases, atrophy of the subcutaneous layer.	Use a room humidifier, bathe less frequently using warm water instead of hot, use a mild soap, wear protective clothing in cold weather, moisturize dry skin
Musculoskeletal system	Muscle mass decreases; tendency to gain weight; gradual loss of bone density; deterioration of joint cartilage.	Strength training to increase muscle mass; stretching to remain limber; exercise; vitamin D and calcium supplements

infections increases, the healing process takes longer, and older people are more susceptible to bruising. Because the skin can be easily torn, it is important to be very careful when performing phlebotomy or covering a wound on an older patient. The use of tape should be avoided. Vitamin D synthesis, a major function of the epidermis, significantly declines in aged skin, and a decrease in the number of melanocytes increases photosensitivity.

The dermis loses 20% of its mass during the aging process, resulting in the paper-thin or transparent skin seen in older adults. The number of **collagen** cells in the dermis also declines with age, causing the skin to sag and wrinkle. Because both sweat and sebaceous glands decrease in number, aging people have difficulty tolerating higher temperatures because they perspire less. At the same time, the blood supply to the dermis decreases; this makes it difficult to regulate the body temperature and leads to an increased susceptibility to both hypothermia and heat stroke in aging individuals. Any situation in which an older adult would be exposed to extremes of cold or heat should be avoided. Make sure a blanket is available in the examining room if the air conditioning is on. Ask patients if they are too cold or too hot and take the necessary steps to make the patients feel more comfortable.

Atrophy of the subcutaneous layer increases the skin's susceptibility to trauma, so patients bruise much more easily. The skin is denied natural lubrication, and dry skin is one of the most common complaints among older people. In addition, fat deposits increase in the abdomen in men and in the abdomen and thighs in women as they age.

Here are some suggestions that might help older people to prevent and treat dry skin:

- Use a room humidifier to moisten the air
- Bathe less frequently and use warm rather than hot water
- Use a mild soap or cleansing cream (e.g., Aveeno, Basis, or Dove)
- Wear protective clothing in cold weather
- Moisturize dry skin

Pain receptors are distributed throughout the skin. Because of age-related changes in the receptors, older people have a higher pain threshold. They may not notice a cut or burn as quickly as a younger person would, so a more serious burn may occur before it is noticed. In addition, wound healing becomes a problem because of decreased blood flow to dermal tissues.

Other changes occur in the skin's appendages. Hair changes in color, growth, and distribution. Hair grays because of the decreased rate of melanin production and the replacement of pigmented hair with nonpigmented hair. Women lose hair on the trunk and have increased facial hair. Although *alopecia* (loss of hair) is caused by an inherited trait, aging also causes hair loss. Hair on the eyebrows and in the nose and ears becomes coarser and longer in men. The nails of older people take longer to grow and are more brittle. Nails, particularly toenails, thicken as a result of trauma or nutritional deficiencies. It is not unusual for nails to split, making them more susceptible to fungal infections.

Seborrheic keratoses, usually referred to as "age spots," are one of the most common benign skin disorders found in the aging population. They appear as waxy, scaly papules that vary from tan to dark brown (Figure 45.3) and typically are found in areas of sun exposure, such as the trunk, back, face, neck, extremities, and scalp. They are not dangerous but may be removed for cosmetic purposes.

Shingles is another condition that shows up on the skin. It is caused by the same virus that causes chickenpox. A person who has had chickenpox in the past is at risk of developing shingles.

Shingles Risk Reduction

The varicella-zoster virus causes both shingles and chickenpox. After an active chickenpox infection, the virus lies dormant in a nerve **dermatome**. As people age, their risk increases that the virus will reactivate, causing the formation of blisters and varying degrees of pain along the affected nerve pathway. It is estimated that 1 in 3 adults will develop shingles in their lifetime. There is currently one shingle vaccine approved in the United States.

Shingrix reduces the risk of shingles. Shingrix is a recombinant vaccine that also boosts immunity against the varicella-zoster virus. This vaccine is administered as an intramuscular injection. It is recommended that the two doses should be given 6 months apart. This vaccine is recommended for healthy adults 50 years and older. The two doses are 90% effective at preventing shingles and **postherpetic neuralgia**.

For individuals who develop shingles even though they were immunized, the duration of symptoms is shorter. The vaccine is recommended even if an individual has had shingles in the past to help prevent future occurrences of the disease.

A shingles vaccination can be quite expensive ($200 to $300). Therefore, it is important that the patient or the medical assistant first check with the individual's insurance carrier to see whether the injection is covered.

CRITICAL THINKING APPLICATION 45.3

Rose Deluca, a 71-year-old patient of Dr. Martin, is unhappy about the changes in her skin that have occurred in the past several years. Based on what Bill knows about the normal changes that occur in the skin as people age, how can he explain these changes to Mrs. Deluca, and what can he suggest to help with dryness and other typical aging changes?

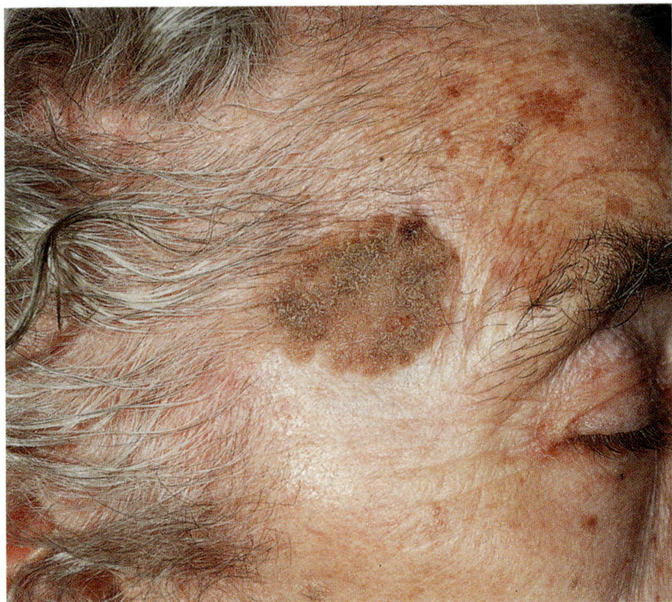

FIGURE 45.3 Seborrheic keratosis. (From Habif TP: *Clinical dermatology: a color guide to diagnosis and therapy*, ed 6, St. Louis, 2016, Mosby.)

Musculoskeletal System

As the body ages, changes in the muscles, bones, and joints affect the individual's appearance, strength, and mobility. The extent of change depends on the person's diet, exercise pattern, and heredity. Cartilage loss and degeneration, which produce osteoarthritis, commonly occur in the weight-bearing joints of older people. Joint range of motion is affected, and the intervertebral disc spaces are decreased, causing loss of height as a person ages. A breakdown in joint structures may lead to inflammation, pain, stiffness, and deformity.

Suggestions for Helping the Older Adult with Mobility, Dexterity, and Balance Problems

- Encourage the person to use assistive devices, such as adaptive silverware, a tub seat or shower chair, electric razor, and reaching devices.
- Assist the person with gripping devices as needed (wait for the patient to place their hand around a cup or help them with it before letting go).
- Provide older adults with enough time to complete tasks independently.
- For a post-stroke patient who is ambulatory but has one weak side, use a gait belt when transferring the patient from a chair to an examination table.
- The provider may recommend physical therapy for range-of-motion exercises.
- Encourage activity approved by the provider; lack of activity results in a decline in the ability to function.

Aging brings a decrease in the strength and speed of muscle contractions in the extremities but only a slight decline in overall muscle endurance. Muscular changes in the aging patient are directly related to the individual's activity level. Research shows that musculoskeletal disease is not an inevitable result of the aging process; however, 40% to 50% of women over age 50 have a serious problem with bone demineralization. Men also experience bone loss but at a later age, and a much slower rate than women.

Osteoporosis

Osteoporosis is the primary cause of hip fractures, which can lead to a loss of independence and complications that ultimately can end in death. The spinal vertebrae also can collapse, producing the stooped posture associated with "dowager's hump." Sometimes bones break because of the sheer weight of the body on them. Often people say they fell and broke a bone when in reality, the bone fractured, causing them to fall. Multiple factors contribute to the development of osteoporosis, but it is most common in postmenopausal women. Risk factors for osteoporosis include the following:

- Female gender (women have a five times greater risk than men)
- Thin; small-boned frame
- Family history of osteoporosis
- Estrogen deficiency before age 45, either from early menopause or **oophorectomy**
- Estrogen deficiency resulting from an abnormal absence of menses (eating disorders, excessive aerobic exercise, fibrocystic ovaries)
- Racial background (Caucasian and Asian women have the highest risk)
- Aging
- Extended use of anticonvulsant drugs, prednisone, and excessive thyroid hormone medications
- Sedentary lifestyle, smoking, excessive alcohol intake, and lack of calcium and vitamin D when growing up

Weight-bearing exercises and calcium and vitamin D supplements are recommended to prevent demineralization of the bones. A number of medications are used to prevent or treat osteoporosis:

- Alendronate (Fosamax) and risedronate (Actonel), which reduce the rate of demineralization
- Raloxifene (Evista) and ibandronate (Boniva), which slow bone thinning and cause some increase in bone thickness
- Denosumab (Prolia, Xgeva), an injectable medication that helps increase bone mass
- Teriparatide (Bonsity, Forteo), a daily injectable medication to increase bone density and decrease the risk for fractures.

Another option is an intravenous (IV) medication, zoledronic acid (Reclast), for the once-yearly treatment of postmenopausal women with osteoporosis. Reclast helps increase bone density in the spine and hip, thus reducing the risk of fractures.

Falls

The risk of injuries from falls increases with age; falls cause the greatest number of injuries in people over age 70. Aging individuals are at greater risk of falling because of sensorimotor changes in vision and mobility, osteoporosis, and cerebrovascular accidents (CVAs). Falls in older patients usually result in fractures because a large percentage of these individuals have osteoporosis. Serious fractures, such as those of the hip, require the patient to be immobile for extended periods, and this opens the door to a wide range of debilitating complications:

- **Pressure injuries**
- Pneumonia
- Placement in long-term care facilities
- Even death

Falls are largely preventable. The medical assistant can play an active role in helping family members and patients become aware of risk factors and safety measures. Here are some suggestions that can help patients prevent falls:

- Have regular vision tests.
- Understand the side effects of medications, especially those that cause vertigo.
- If you experience orthostatic hypotension, rise slowly and stand still for a moment with support before moving.
- Limit the use of alcohol.
- If needed, consistently use assistive devices, such as a cane or walker, for support.
- Wear low-heeled, rubber-soled shoes with good support.
- Avoid going outside in icy weather.
- Engage in regular weight-bearing exercise for muscle and bone strength.
- Keep hallways, stairs, and bathrooms well lit.
- Assess the home for possible danger areas, remove throw rugs, use handrails on steps and grab bars in bathrooms, and keep emergency numbers handy.

CRITICAL THINKING APPLICATION **45.4**

The family of Rita Schaeffer, a 73-year-old patient, is concerned about the risk of falls. Mrs. Schaeffer recently was diagnosed with osteoporosis, and she lives alone. What information should Bill give the family to help them prevent accidents in their mother's home? Also, Mrs. Schaeffer's 45-year-old daughter is concerned about developing osteoporosis. What steps should the daughter take to prevent the disease?

CHANGES IN ANATOMY, PHYSIOLOGY, AND DISEASES OF THE NERVOUS SYSTEM AND SENSORY ORGANS

Table 45.4 summarizes the changes to the nervous system and sensory organs and what can be done to promote healthy aging. The following sections provide more detail about the changes to those systems.

Nervous System

Cognitive ability (i.e., the ability of a person to think) is influenced by many factors, including a person's general state of health, educational background, and genetic code. The normal process of aging may contribute to a change in the thinking process. The brain begins to get smaller at approximately age 50 and continues to get smaller as we age because of a loss of fluid within the neurons and shrinkage of dendrites. Thinning of the dendrites makes transmitting messages from one neuron to the next more difficult. As a result of all these factors, the aging brain is smaller, weighs less, and has started to pull away from the sheath or cortical mantle. Older neurons process information more slowly, so retrieving old information and learning new information takes longer. Reaction time also slows, and aging individuals are distracted more easily; however, recent research shows that the loss of brain cells is minimal and that the older brain is still capable of generating new neurons. Researchers believe that continued, moderate physical and mental activity can maintain the cognitive abilities of aging individuals.

Dementia, the severe loss of intellectual ability, is not an inevitable part of aging but rather the result of an organic disorder. Most men and women remain mentally competent until the end of their lives. Sudden loss of memory, disorientation, and trouble performing the daily tasks of life indicate a problem that should be investigated. Many conditions can cause signs and symptoms of dementia:

- Depression
- Reactions to prescription and over-the-counter (OTC) drugs
- Alcoholism
- Malnutrition
- Thyroid, liver, heart, and vascular disorders
- Parkinson disease

Multiple factors can interfere with mental judgment and motor skills, giving the impression of decreased mental status.

TABLE 45.4 System Changes Due to Aging of the Nervous System and Sensory Organs, and Measures to Promote Health

SYSTEM	AGE-RELATED CHANGES	HEALTH PROMOTION
Central nervous system	Brain shrinks by 10% between ages 30 and 90; takes longer to learn new material; attention span and language remain the same; signs and symptoms may be caused by depression, vascular disease, and drug reactions.	Aerobic exercise to increase blood flow to CNS; maintaining mental activities (e.g., reading, interacting with others)
Sensory organs	Hearing is intact through the mid-50s but declines by 25% by age 80; oral problems are common; skin thins and loses elasticity; presbyopia after age 40; cataracts common after age 60.	Avoid exposure to loud noise, use hearing aids; good dental hygiene; prevention of sun damage to the skin; annual eye examinations; diet rich in dark green, leafy vegetables to prevent cataracts and macular degeneration

The best way to ensure mental functioning in later life is to remain mentally and physically stimulated. Exercise improves memory and thinking because of its positive effect on vascular health, increasing the amount of oxygen delivered to the aging brain. Other ways to maintain mental function are to keep socially active; practice stress-reduction activities; quit smoking; drink alcohol in moderation; use hearing aids and glasses, if needed, to stay in touch with the world; and receive treatment for depression, diabetes, hypertension, and high cholesterol levels. Risk factors for cognitive decline include the following:

- Hypertension, diabetes, and heart disease (these reduce blood flow to the brain)
- Environmental exposure to lead
- High stress levels
- Sedentary lifestyle and lack of social interaction
- Low education level
- Smoking and substance abuse

Alzheimer Disease

Alzheimer disease (AD) is a progressive deterioration of the brain caused by the destruction of central nervous system (CNS) neurons, leading to problems with memory, language, thinking, and behavior. Three major changes occur in the brain:

- Amyloid plaques form.
- Neurofibrillary tangles clump together, affecting neuron function (neurons eventually die).
- The connections between neurons that are responsible for memory and learning are lost, resulting in neuron destruction; as neurons die throughout the brain, the affected regions begin to atrophy, or shrink. By the final stage of AD, damage is widespread, and brain tissue has shrunk significantly.

Patients who show signs and symptoms of dementia are first evaluated for organic causes, such as systemic disease or depression. AD has no definitive diagnostic test because it can be confirmed only through examination of the brain at autopsy. If the patient shows a gradual onset of progressive difficulty with memory, functional abilities, and behavior, and has no evidence of other causes of these disturbances, the provider makes the diagnosis of AD. Imaging studies, including computed tomography (CT), magnetic resonance imaging (MRI), and positron emission tomography (PET), may help show the structural and functional changes in the brain associated with AD.

Researchers estimate that about 6 million Americans suffer from AD. The disease typically begins after age 60, and the risk of developing the disorder increases with age, although younger people as early as age 30 have been diagnosed with AD. Research shows that 1 in 9 Americans over age 65 have AD; almost 35% of people age 85 or older are diagnosed with the disease. Despite these statistics, AD is not considered a normal part of the aging process. AD is the sixth leading cause of death (across all ages) in the United States and the sixth leading cause of death for those age 65 to 85.

AD is a slowly progressive disease that begins with mild memory problems and ends with severe brain damage. The course the disease takes and how fast changes occur varies among individuals, but on average, patients live for 8 to 10 years after they have been diagnosed. Currently, no treatment can stop the progression of the disease. However, a great deal of research on the diagnosis and treatment of AD is under way.

The goal of treatment is to maintain normal activities as long as possible. In June of 2021, the US Food and Drug Administration (FDA) approved aducanumab to treat some cases of AD. This drug is aimed at treating the amyloid plaques in the brain by removing them. In addition, there are four medications for the treatment of AD symptoms (Table 45.5). These drugs help individuals carry out the activities of daily living by maintaining thinking, memory, or speaking skills. They can also help with some of the behavioral and

TABLE 45.5 Medications Approved for the Treatment of Alzheimer Disease Symptoms

DRUG	STAGE OF TREATMENT	COMMON ADVERSE EFFECTS
Cholinesterase Inhibitors		
Donepezil (Aricept)	All stages	• Appetite loss • Dizziness • Fatigue • Increased frequency of bowel movements and diarrhea • Insomnia • Muscle cramps • Nausea, vomiting • Weight loss
Galantamine (Razadyne)	Mild to moderate	
Rivastigmine (Exelon)—tablet, liquid, or topical patch	All stages	
Receptor Antagonist		
Memantine (Namenda)—prescribed alone or in combination with donepezil	Moderate to severe	• Confusion • Constipation • Diarrhea • Dizziness • Headache

personality changes associated with AD. However, they will not stop or reverse AD, and they appear to help individuals for only a few months to a few years. Cholinesterase inhibitors improve the production of neurotransmitters in the brain, which helps prevent memory loss from worsening for a limited time. These drugs do not help everyone (as many as 50% of patients show no improvement in mental function). Memantine (Namenda) was the first drug to be approved for the treatment of moderate to severe AD, although it also has limited effects. Individuals with AD frequently experience changes in behavior, so medications may be prescribed to help control sleeplessness, agitation, wandering, anxiety, and depression. Treating these problems helps make the patient more comfortable while easing the burden on caregivers.

Supportive care for family members is absolutely essential because they are faced with caring for a loved one who is suffering progressive memory loss. The medical assistant can be especially helpful in recommending educational workshops, support groups, and stress management skills for caregivers. Multiple resources are available, including online information and support groups, which family members may find helpful.

Sleep Disorders

Complaints of sleeping difficulties increase with age. The amount of time spent sleeping may be slightly longer than in a younger person, but the quality of sleep declines. Older people are often light sleepers and have periods of wakefulness in bed. Rapid eye movement (REM) sleep is the stage of sleep in which people experience dreaming. Non-REM sleep is the period of deepest sleep. The amount of time spent in the deepest stages of sleep decreases with age. Sleep that is disturbed or that leaves the person feeling tired is not part of the aging process and may indicate some underlying emotional or physical problem. Lack of sleep can result in restlessness, disorientation, "thick" speech, and mispronounced words. Often, these symptoms are mistaken for signs of dementia. Other factors that might influence sleep patterns are medications, caffeine, alcohol, depression, and environmental or physical changes.

Common sleep problems in older adults include dyssomnias, such as periodic limb movement disorder (PLMD), in which periodic jerking of the legs occurs during sleep, and sleep apnea. This is common among overweight individuals and can frequently occur during the night, interrupting sleep. Numerous medical conditions can interfere with sleep:

- Joint and bone pain
- Parkinson disease (because of difficulty changing positions)
- Congestive heart failure
- Chronic obstructive pulmonary disease (COPD)
- Diabetes mellitus, which increases **nocturia**
- Depression
- Certain medications (e.g., beta-blockers can cause nightmares, antidepressants increase PLMD, and barbiturates may result in nightmares or hallucinations)

It is important to be aware of the effect of sleep problems because often, these can be confused with dementia. Patients experiencing difficulty with sleeping should be encouraged to document their sleeping patterns, napping patterns, medications, diet, exercise routines, and any events that have resulted in a change of lifestyle. They should discuss this problem with their provider. A simple modification of behavioral patterns may resolve the problem. Taking fewer naps, completing exercise several hours before bedtime, changing eating times, reducing the amount of alcohol and caffeine ingested, drinking a glass of milk before bedtime, or changing medications or the time they are taken all are suggestions that might alter the factors responsible for sleep disturbances.

If behavioral approaches are not effective, medications may be considered for short-term use only because they have a high incidence of physical and psychological dependence. Older adults are especially susceptible to side effects from these drugs, such as next-day drowsiness and temporary memory loss. Sedatives or hypnotics that may be prescribed include zolpidem (Ambien), eszopiclone (Lunesta), zaleplon (Sonata), and ramelteon (Rozerem).

Sensory Organs

As we age, there are some expected changes to the sensory organs. These changes can impact the geriatric patient's quality of life. The next sections discuss those changes.

Vision

By the time a person reaches age 50, structural and functional changes in the eye become noticeable (Table 45.6). The eyebrows and eyelashes start to gray. The skin around the eyelids wrinkles, and the loss of orbital fat allows the eye to sink deeper into the orbit.

TABLE 45.6 Age-Related Changes to the Anatomic Structures of the Eye

STRUCTURE	AGE-RELATED CHANGE	EFFECTS
Lens	Thickens, becomes more opaque	Decreased refraction, causing blurred vision; decreased color acuity; cataracts
Anterior chamber	Decrease in size and volume	May develop increased intraocular pressure and glaucoma
Ciliary muscles	Affects pupil constriction and dilation	Limits light accommodation; night blindness
Cornea	Thickens, curve decreases	Problems with refraction
Retina	Decrease in number of rods and cones	Decreased clarity; requires increase in minimum amount of light needed to see clearly

The cornea increases in thickness and has reduced refractive power. A yellow-gray ring (arcus senilis) may develop on the periphery of the cornea. The iris loses pigmentation, and as a result, older people appear to have gray eyes.

The lens of the eye continues to grow. As new lens fibers grow, old lens fibers are compressed and pushed to the center, causing the lens to become denser. The lens becomes flatter, thicker, less elastic, and more opaque, progressively yellowing with age. By age 70, the lens has tripled in mass. Clouding of the lens causes light rays to scatter, creating glare.

The pupil is designed to adjust to control the amount of light entering the eye. The ciliary muscle that causes the pupil to dilate weakens during the aging process. As a result, a reduction in the size of the pupil occurs, limiting the amount of light available to reach the retina. Tear production normally decreases. Tear glands do not make enough tears, or the tears are of poor quality and do not keep the eyes wet enough. Eye irritation and excessive tearing are a result of decreased **lacrimation**.

By the early to mid-40s, *presbyopia* develops, which makes it difficult to focus in detail on objects close at hand. This requires the use of corrective lenses to accommodate age-related farsightedness. The ability to refocus quickly from far to near or near to far decreases. Also, the ability to follow a moving object is decreased. The yellowing of the lens causes it to act like a filter, making it difficult to distinguish certain color intensities. Blues, greens, and violets are hard to differentiate, whereas yellows, reds, and oranges are easier to identify. The loss in the ability to discriminate closely related colors can affect the older person's ability to judge distances or depth perception. This increases an aging person's susceptibility to falls and accidents. Stairs become a potential hazard because the edges of the steps cannot be seen clearly.

Older people need as much as six times more light to read; however, increasing the level of light does not completely compensate for visual decline because the older adult also experiences an increased sensitivity to glare. Glare is probably one of the most painful experiences for the aging eye. Exposed light bulbs, such as those used in chandeliers, and light from highly reflective surfaces, such as glass tables and floors, can produce excessive glare. The eye has a decreased ability to respond to abrupt changes from light to dark or dark to light. Going from a well-lit waiting room into a dim hallway or negotiating the way down dimly lit aisles in a movie theater could be treacherous for an older person.

Cataracts, Glaucoma, and Macular Degeneration. Eye diseases and disorders that frequently occur in older individuals are as follows:

- Cataracts
- Glaucoma
- Macular degeneration

Cataracts are cloudy or opaque areas in the lens that cause blurred vision, rings or halos around lights and objects, and a blue or yellow tint to the visual field (Figure 45.4). Surgical lens extraction and implantation with an artificial lens improves vision in 95% of cases. The procedure, which is performed in an outpatient facility, involves a small incision to remove the lens, laser therapy, or *phacoemulsification* (ultrasonic vibrations), which breaks up the lens and removes it without the need for an incision. After the procedure, patients must avoid bending or lifting heavy objects for 3 to 4 weeks; wearing an eye shield at night and glasses during the day helps protect the eye until it heals. Recovery takes about 2 weeks.

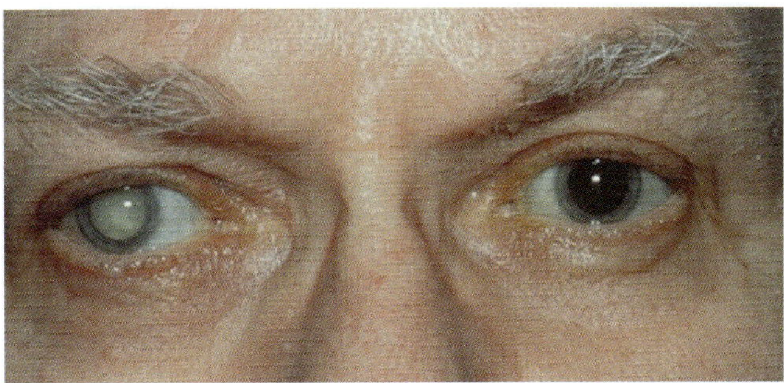

FIGURE 45.4 Cataracts. (From Mayo Foundation for Medical Education and Research. All Rights Reserved. Retrieved from www.mayoclinic.org/diseases-conditions/cataracts/symptoms-causes/syc-20353790#dialogId57162167.)

Glaucoma is a result of a blockage in the outflow of aqueous humor, which causes an increase in intraocular pressure and damage to the optic nerve. If not treated, glaucoma can cause progressive loss of peripheral vision and ultimately lead to blindness; however, it can be treated with medication.

The *macula* is the part of the eye responsible for sharp vision and color. Damage to or breakdown of the macula is called *macular degeneration,* which causes progressive loss of the central field of vision. Macular degeneration is the leading cause of blindness in aging people. (All three of these eye disorders are discussed in more detail in Chapter 31.)

Suggestions for Helping the Visually Impaired Older Adult

- Ask if the person wants assistance.
- When escorting an older person, regardless of whether the individual is visually impaired, allow the patient to place their hand above your elbow. It is easier for the person to follow your movements. This method also provides a source of support and security.
- Use high levels of evenly distributed glare-free light.
- Ask the pharmacist to use large lettering when labeling medicine bottles.
- Use paper with a nonglare finish and large print for forms and educational materials.
- Make distinct differences (e.g., size of containers or color coding with bright primary colors) for pills that are similar in size and color.
- Place all objects within the visual field and prevent clutter.

Hearing

Hearing loss can have a profound psychological effect on aging people, causing depression, social withdrawal, and feelings of isolation. Hearing loss occurs gradually over a long period and may go undetected by the older person and healthcare providers. Lack of attention when addressed, inappropriate responses, asking to have statements repeated, and speaking too loudly or too softly often are signs of hearing loss. Changes in hearing begin around age 30. By age 65, one out of three people has a hearing loss, and this increases to 65% of those over age 80. Age-related hearing loss usually is caused by a dysfunction or loss of cochlear cilia, resulting in an inability to hear high-frequency sounds and difficulty understanding speech.

GERIATRIC DEPRESSION SCALE (SHORT FORM)

Choose the best answer for how you have felt over the past week:

1. Are you basically satisfied with your life? YES / **NO**
2. Have you dropped many of your activities and interests? **YES** / NO
3. Do you feel that your life is empty? **YES** / NO
4. Do you often get bored? **YES** / NO
5. Are you in good spirits most of the time? YES / **NO**
6. Are you afraid that something bad is going to happen to you? **YES** / NO
7. Do you feel happy most of the time? YES / **NO**
8. Do you often feel helpless? **YES** / NO
9. Do you prefer to stay at home, rather than going out and doing new things? **YES** / NO
10. Do you feel you have more problems with memory than most? **YES** / NO
11. Do you think it is wonderful to be alive now? YES / **NO**
12. Do you feel pretty worthless the way you are now? **YES** / NO
13. Do you feel full of energy? YES / **NO**
14. Do you feel that your situation is hopeless? **YES** / NO
15. Do you think that most people are better off than you are? **YES** / NO

Answers in **bold** indicate depression. Although differing sensitivities and specificities have been obtained across studies, for clinical purposes, a score >5 points is suggestive of depression and should warrant a follow-up interview. Scores >10 almost always indicate depression.

FIGURE 45.5 Geriatric Depression Scale.

Hearing impairment is compounded by impacted cerumen, otitis media, otosclerosis, **Ménière disease**, long-term exposure to intense noise, and certain **ototoxic** drugs, such as aspirin.

Presbycusis is associated with normal aging and causes a decreased ability to hear high frequencies and discriminate sounds. Parts of a conversation may be missed because the sound of the word goes above the 2000-cycle frequency. Often words that sound similar are difficult to differentiate. Consonants such as *g, f, s, sh, t,* and *z* produce high-pitched sounds that are more difficult to hear and differentiate. Low-frequency pitched sounds, such as the vowels *a, e, i, o,* and *u,* may be more easily heard by people with presbycusis. Inability to hear different frequencies combined with low background noise from groups of people talking, noise from appliances, or busy public places compromises an older person's ability to hear clearly. Hearing aids, which can be used to amplify speech, may increase background noises, resulting in sensory overload.

Another hearing disorder common among older people is *tinnitus*, a ringing or buzzing in the ear. It can be caused by the following:

- Impacted cerumen
- Ear infection
- Use of antibiotics
- Reaction to a medication
- Nerve disorder

Tinnitus can cause difficulty understanding conversational speech and make sleeping difficult because of the continuous ringing sensation in the ears.

Hearing loss, with its resultant isolation, is directly related to the development of depression in older adults. Treatable depression often is overlooked in older adults because of coexisting physical illnesses that mask the symptoms of depression. The medical assistant may be able to contribute information about depression in older adult patients through conversations with the individual and family members. The provider may use or train the medical assistant to use the Geriatric Depression Scale Short Form, which includes questions for the patient about daily activities, interests, and feelings to help diagnose depression in the ambulatory setting (Figure 45.5).

Suggestions for Helping the Hearing-Impaired Older Adult

- Stand in the patient's direct line of vision and gently touch the person to get their attention.
- Use gestures, pictures, and large, bold print to communicate.
- Talk in short sentences into the ear with better hearing.
- Do not increase the volume of your speech; this also raises the frequency of the voice, which is the hearing most impaired in aging people. Use expanded speech; lower the tone of your voice and talk in distinct syllables.
- Avoid background noise. Give instructions in a quiet room with the door closed. If the patient has a hearing aid, make sure it is on.

Taste and Smell

During the aging process, the abilities to taste and smell decline subtly. Deterioration and atrophy of the taste buds are part of the aging process. The ability to taste salt and sweet flavors is reduced, whereas the ability to detect bitter and sour flavors remains relatively the same. As a result, food frequently tastes bland and unappetizing. Patients on salt-restricted diets and patients with diabetes must be cautioned about the use of excessive amounts of salt and sugar. A decrease in the sense of smell accompanies the decrease in taste. Not only does this affect the individual's enjoyment of food, it also puts them at risk of environmental dangers, such as gas leaks, smoke, and other dangerous odors that may go undetected. Checking for gas leaks around stoves and heaters and using smoke alarms reduce some of the danger. Also, dating food when it is put in the refrigerator is a good idea.

Nutritional Status. Because of the many environmental, social, economic, and physical changes of aging, older people are at greater risk for poor nutrition, which can adversely affect their health and energy levels. It is estimated that 25% of the aging population suffers from malnutrition. Nutrition screening should be part of routine primary care to identify nutritional deficiencies and correct them before a disease process develops or to assist in the treatment of chronic disease. Patients with chronic conditions, such as cardiovascular disease, hypertension, and diabetes, can benefit from nutrition assessments and interventions. Malnourished older patients get more infections, their injuries take longer to heal, surgery is riskier for them, and their hospital stays are longer and more expensive.

The most effective method of assessing a patient's nutritional status is conducting a comprehensive patient interview that considers all potential stumbling blocks to adequate nutrition. The medical assistant can help determine the nutritional status of older patients by considering the following factors when conducting patient interviews:

- *Oral health:* Does the patient wear dentures, and if so, do they fit properly? Does the patient have mouth pain? Can the patient swallow without difficulty?
- *Gastrointestinal complaints:* Does the patient have anorexia, nausea, vomiting, diarrhea, or constipation? Is the patient lactose intolerant (the incidence increases with age)?
- *Sensorimotor changes:* Does the patient have loss of vision or hearing or changes in taste and smell? Can the patient feed herself or himself? Does the patient need adaptive utensils?
- *Diet influences:* Can the patient afford, shop for, and prepare food? Are ethnic or religious influences a factor? Does the patient have any disease-related diet restrictions? What is the patient's alcohol consumption?
- *Social and mental influences:* Is the patient depressed, lonely, or isolated? Are support systems available?

CRITICAL THINKING APPLICATION 45.5

Multiple sensory changes occur as people age. Dr. Perez asks Bill to develop a handout for patients and family members to help them understand these normal, age-related sensorimotor changes and adaptations that can improve communication. What information should Bill include?

CHANGES IN ANATOMY, PHYSIOLOGY, AND DISEASES OF THE URINARY AND REPRODUCTIVE SYSTEMS

Table 45.7 summarizes the changes to the urinary and reproductive systems and what can be done to promote healthy aging. The following sections provide more detail about the changes to those systems.

Urinary System

As the body ages, structural changes in the kidneys cause the urinary system to become less efficient. Between the ages of 40 and 80, the kidney loses about 20% of its mass. The number of functional nephron units decreases. Blood flow to the kidneys is reduced because of a decrease in cardiovascular efficiency. Because of the reduced blood flow to the kidneys and the decreased number of nephrons, the kidneys become less efficient at filtering waste from the blood. This results in a more diluted, less concentrated urine. The kidneys require more water to excrete the same amount of waste. Medication takes longer to be removed from the body. Older adults are at increased risk for toxic levels of medication in the bloodstream because of this reduced filtration rate.

Fibrous connective tissue replaces the smooth muscle and elastic tissue in the bladder. This thickening of the bladder wall reduces the bladder's ability to expand. The bladder's capacity to store fluid comfortably is reduced from 400 to 250 mL. These structural changes lead to increased frequency of urination and urinary retention. Older adults are at increased risk of urinary tract infections because of residual urine. Sleep is interrupted by the need to void during the night. The sensation of bladder fullness is not recognized as quickly by the older brain. Reduced time between awareness of the need to void and involuntary urination can cause anxiety. Often, older adults reduce their fluid intake to prevent possible embarrassment. Unfortunately, this causes dehydration and an increased risk of urinary tract infections. Another change is the loss of muscle tone in the urethra. In addition, the pelvic floor muscles in an aging woman relax due to decreased estrogen levels or previous pregnancy and childbirth.

Despite these changes, the kidneys have great reserve capacity and are able to continue functioning normally. *Urinary incontinence*, the involuntary loss of urine, is a significant problem for aging patients but is not a normal part of the aging process. Changes in the urinary system make older people more vulnerable to incontinence, but factors such as infection, confusion, difficulty with mobility, and side effects of medications contribute to the development of the problem. Incontinence is both an emotional and a physical problem. To avoid the risk of an embarrassing accident, people with this problem may avoid social occasions or activities they enjoy. Often people are too embarrassed to admit they have this condition or believe it is just part of aging. Once the condition has been diagnosed by a urologist, pelvic floor muscle exercises, medication, or surgery may be recommended.

TABLE 45.7 System Changes Due to Aging of the Urinary and Reproductive Systems, and Measures to Promote Health

SYSTEM	AGE-RELATED CHANGES	HEALTH PROMOTION
Urinary system	Kidneys become less efficient; bladder muscles weaken; one-third of seniors experience incontinence; prostate enlargement is common.	Pelvic exercises, drugs, or surgery for incontinence; annual prostate-specific antigen (PSA) screening with digital rectal exam monitoring for men
Sexuality	*Men:* Impotence is not a symptom of normal aging; men over age 50 may have some altered function. *Women:* Menopause causes vaginal narrowing and dryness, resulting in painful intercourse.	*Men:* Maintenance of cardiovascular health with exercise, weight control, no smoking, diabetes management *Women:* Use of vaginal lubricants or estrogen cream

Reproductive System

Aging brings a decrease in circulating levels of the female hormones estrogen and progesterone, whereas androgen levels increase. The results of this decrease are changes in the genital tract. The vagina diminishes in width and length and becomes less elastic. The cervix, uterus, and ovaries decrease in size. Vaginal secretions decline; therefore, lubrication diminishes, resulting in vaginal dryness. Bacterial or yeast infections may occur because vaginal secretions are less acidic. Estrogen cream applied to vaginal tissue may be prescribed by the provider to help with dryness and thinning of the vaginal tissue. The patient should discuss the benefits and risks of estrogen replacement therapy with the provider to determine whether it should be used.

Even though sperm production may decline in men over age 50, men remain virile well into old age. However, they experience a change in hormonal levels of testosterone, and these changes can affect the prostate gland. The prostate enlarges over time and presses down on the urethra, causing difficulty with urination. Surgery may be required to remove excess portions of the gland. Unfortunately, the operation may cause impotence, which can be treated medically with erectile dysfunction medications.

Men experience some changes in sexual functioning as they age. It takes longer for the penis to become erect, longer for an orgasm to occur, and longer to recover. Direct stimulation may be required before an erection occurs, and when it does, it may be less firm than in younger years.

Some drugs and illnesses can interfere with sexual function. Drugs used to control high blood pressure, antihistamines, antidepressants, and some stomach acid blockers, in addition to the diseases diabetes, arthritis, and arteriosclerosis, can have an adverse effect on sexual function. People who have had heart surgery or a heart attack are often concerned about sexual activity. Patients need to feel comfortable and should not be embarrassed to discuss their concerns openly with their providers. It is important for healthcare practitioners to dismiss the myth that older patients have lost the desire for and interest in sexual intercourse.

THE MEDICAL ASSISTANT'S ROLE IN CARING FOR THE OLDER PATIENT

Older adult patients in the ambulatory care setting present a specific set of needs that require a certain amount of accommodation by the staff. For example, aging patients typically require more time to perform tasks and have questions answered. The office staff may want to hurry them so the day's schedule can be maintained. In the best interests of the patient, however, they should be treated with respect and given whatever time is needed to prepare for examinations, ask questions and receive answers, and have procedures explained. A system that is sensitive to the needs of older patients does the following:

- Schedules longer periods for appointments
- Has adequate lighting in the waiting room
- Provides forms in large print
- Has an examination room equipped with furniture, magazines, and treatment folders specifically designed for older adults
- Invites a professional in the management of older patients for in-service training

Communication

The primary issue in elder care is effective communication. How you communicate with people is often influenced by what you know or do not know about them. Older people are subject to many changes that affect how they are able to interact with their environment. It is important to recognize these changes and to investigate one's personal perception of older people to break down the barriers that prohibit effective communication.

As people age, they frequently experience a loss of control over their lives because of physical disabilities, economic constraints, and institutional living. Part of the medical assistant's job is to help aging people maintain their dignity and independence while in the ambulatory care setting. Remember, regardless of their education, socioeconomic status, or age, each patient deserves to be treated with compassion and respect. Ask the patient directly what is wrong rather than discussing the patient with family members. It is also important to listen carefully and be specific and sincere when responding. When a patient is talking, take time to allow them to complete the sentence; do not finish it for the person. Give the patient your full attention rather than continuing with other tasks while the person is speaking. Older people may take a little longer to process information, but they are capable of understanding. Do not hurry through explanations or questions; rather, take time to review a form or give instructions as needed.

Resources

When medical assistants work with the geriatric population, the subject of living arrangements will likely come up. At any given time, only 5% of the older adult population lives in long-term care facilities. According to information published by the National Institute on Aging, older people live close to their children and are in frequent contact with them. People prefer to age in place—that is, they want to live in their own home environment as long as possible. Individuals are admitted to nursing homes because they are no longer able to perform daily living activities, such as bathing, dressing, eating, walking, and maintaining bladder and bowel continence. They also have difficulty with grocery shopping, housekeeping, and money management. Chronic health conditions and accidents interfere with the older person's ability to perform these tasks.

Many resources are available to help seniors maintain their independence. Outreach programs, such as Meals on Wheels, deliver nutritious meals to the homes of older adults. Senior centers serve as a focal point for many activities and as a source of information. Transportation services provide rides to doctors' appointments, daycare centers, shopping centers, and community events. Home health agencies provide several types of services, including personal care, shopping, transportation, and meal preparation. Some home health agencies provide a range of activities, from patient education to IV therapy; medical social services; physical, speech, and occupational therapies; and nutrition and dietary counseling. Advanced technology allows people to receive services at home that formerly were provided only in a hospital or a physician's office.

Adult daycare centers provide socialization, recreation, meals, and, in some centers, physical therapy, occupational therapy, and transportation. These centers offer supervision for older adults who

Suggestions for Effective Communication with Aging Patients

- Address the patient as Mr., Mrs., or Ms. unless the patient has given you permission to use their first name.
- Introduce yourself and explain the purpose of a procedure before performing the procedure.
- Face the aging person and softly touch the individual to get their attention before beginning to speak.
- Use expanded speech, gestures, demonstrations, or written instructions in block print.
- If the message must be repeated, paraphrase or find other words to say the same thing.
- Observe the patient's nonverbal behavior for cues indicating whether the individual understands.
- Provide adequate lighting without glare.
- Allow patients time to process information and take care of themselves unless they ask for assistance.
- Conduct communication in a quiet room without distractions.
- Involve family members as needed for continuity of care.
- When leaving a telephone message, remember to speak slowly and clearly and repeat the message in the same manner. It is difficult to interpret a message, and even more difficult to write it down, if the message was delivered in a hurried manner.
- Use referrals and community resources for support, such as these:
  - Alzheimer's Association: www.alz.org (1-800-272-3900).
  - American Council of the Blind: http://acb.org (1-800-424-8666): Provides referrals to state and other organizations that provide services and equipment for the blind.
  - American Speech-Language-Hearing Association: www.asha.org (1-800-638-8255): Offers information on hearing aids, hearing loss, and communication problems in older people and provides a list of certified audiologists and speech pathologists.
  - Arthritis Foundation Information Line: www.arthritis.org (404-872-7100): Makes referrals to local chapters and provides information on various types of arthritis.
  - American Diabetes Association: www.diabetes.org (1-800-342-2383): Provides information and support for those with diabetes.
  - Eldercare Locator: www.eldercare.gov/Eldercare.NET/Public/Index.aspx (1-800-677-1116): Run by the National Association of Area Agencies on Aging; its helpline provides information on contacting local chapters that oversee services for older adults.
  - National Institute on Aging Information Center: www.nia.nih.gov (1-800-222- 2225): Provides information on aging health issues for patients, families, and healthcare professionals.
  - National Meals-on-Wheels Foundation: www.mowaa.org (1-888-998-6325).

may be taken care of by family members in the evening but need care during the day. They also serve as respite for a caregiver.

Assisted-living facilities can be retirement homes or board-and-care homes. These facilities are appropriate for older adults who need assistance with some activities of daily living, such as bathing, dressing, and walking. Skilled nursing facilities provide 24-hour medical care and supervision. In addition to medical care, residents receive care that may include physical, occupational, and speech therapies. The objective of treatment is to improve or maintain the person's abilities.

CLOSING COMMENTS

Patient Coaching

The medical assistant must keep in mind the sensorimotor changes that accompany aging and also must consider respectful patient communication when conducting patient education with older patients. Remember, the aging process does not affect a person's ability to learn; it just may take longer for the older patient to process the information, and the material may need to be repeated for understanding. Showing sensitivity to the needs of aging learners ensures successful patient education and improves compliance with prescribed treatment plans. The current aging population generally is respectful toward authority; therefore, if the medical assistant cannot gain the patient's cooperation, the provider may be able to provide authoritative reinforcement of the material. Here are some general guidelines for effective patient education with older adults:

- The patient may have short-term memory loss, so you may need to repeat the information using different words.
- The patient may be distracted more easily, so learning in a group may be difficult.
- The patient may take longer to process information, so teach at a pace that matches the patient's needs.
- Provide the patient with handouts that have large print and block letters for reviewing information at home.
- Involve family members as needed for continuity of care; supply provider-approved websites for reference.

Legal and Ethical Issues

One legal issue in the care of aging patients is the possibility of elder abuse, neglect, and exploitation. Mistreatment of aging people occurs at all social, racial, and economic levels. The abuse may be physical, mental, sexual, material, or financial; it may involve neglect or failure to provide adequate care, or it may involve self-neglect when aging people are unable or refuse to care for themselves. Abuse, neglect, and exploitation of elders by their caregivers may be difficult to identify. The aging victim could feel embarrassed, guilty, or afraid to report the abuse. Here are some indications that a patient may be the victim of elder abuse, neglect, or exploitation:

- Poor general appearance and poor hygiene
- Pattern of changing doctors and frequent emergency department visits
- Skin lesions, signs of dehydration, bruises (signs of new and old bruising together), abrasions, welts, burns, or pressure sores
- Recurrent injuries caused by accidents
- Signs of malnutrition and weight loss without related illness
- Any injury that does not fit the given history

If abuse, neglect, or exploitation is suspected, interviewing the caregiver and questioning the demands of care and self-reported perceptions of stress levels may help the provider detect the problem. Many states now have laws that require reporting of suspected elder abuse, neglect, or exploitation. Check your state laws to determine the requirements for healthcare workers.

Patient-Centered Care

When working with this patient population, it is important to include the patient and that individual's support system in the decision-making process. Although many geriatric patients are still making their own healthcare decisions, there are some who have others involved in the process. It might be a partner, family member, or a trusted friend. The medical assistant needs to be aware of HIPAA concerns about privacy and confidentiality. This means making sure that the patient has signed all of the appropriate forms regarding who can receive information about the patient's healthcare status. The disclosure authorization form will allow the healthcare facility to provide information to the designated representative. An advance directive will name the person who will make decisions for the patient when she or he is no longer able to.

Some patients just want another set of ears listening to what the provider says and any directions for care that may be given. The medical assistant will ask if the patient is comfortable with someone else being in the room, and when verbal consent is given, the visit can proceed. It can be comforting for patients to know they have someone they trust hearing the information. This person or persons may provide their opinion about the treatment but the patient will ultimately make the decision, unless the advance directive has been activated.

For certain situations, a meeting with the provider may need to be scheduled in a conference room setting to accommodate all that may need to attend. It is important to remember that we treat the whole patient, not just the patient's medical condition.

Professional Behaviors

Your future employers will expect you to use problem-solving techniques, including recognizing and defining a problem, analyzing the issue, and developing a plan of action. Older adult patients typically have multiple health problems that are frequently complicated by physical, psychological, and environmental factors. To provide quality care for these individuals, you must look at their health issues in a holistic way, taking into consideration all the factors that affect their eventual ability to follow treatment plans and improve their health status. Part of the process involves identifying resources that might help the aging person be better equipped to take care of himself or herself. Consistently using community and online resources may mean the difference between an aging person being able to stay in the home or having to go to a long-term care facility. The professional medical assistant can play a crucial role in providing assistance to aging clients.

SUMMARY OF SCENARIO

Bill has learned to understand the special needs of aging patients. He used to think that most older people were chronically sick and would ultimately end up in long-term care facilities. Now he understands that most aging people lead healthy, active lives and that the disorders that occur in later life are usually the result of lifestyle factors, such as diet and lack of exercise. Bill also has learned how to communicate effectively with older patients and conduct patient interviews to evaluate the patient's physical, mental, emotional, and nutritional health.

SUMMARY OF LEARNING OBJECTIVES

1. **Examine the changes in anatomy, physiology, and diseases of the cardiovascular and pulmonary systems.**
   Table 45.1 summarizes changes associated with aging that occur in the cardiovascular and pulmonary systems. Cardiovascular disease is often the cause of illness and disability in the geriatric patient population. The myocardial wall becomes stiffer due to structural changes, including enlarged myocardial cells, fat deposits, and an increase in connective tissue. Blood pressure typically increases, causing the heart to work harder. There is also damage to the blood vessels with the valves in the veins, causing edema and varicose veins of the legs. Arteriosclerosis impacts the arteries' ability to dilate and contract, causing the heart to work harder to pump the blood throughout the body.

   In the pulmonary system, the maximum lung function decreases as we age. The lungs lose their elasticity, resulting in less area for gas exchange to occur. Osteoporosis may cause the chest wall to stiffen, making it harder to move air in and out of the lungs. Weakening of the respiratory muscles makes it harder to cough deeply. There is also an increase in the incidence of sleep apnea. All those factors put the older adult at greater risk for pneumonia and aspiration.
2. **Examine the changes in anatomy, physiology, and diseases of the endocrine and gastrointestinal systems.**
   Table 45.2 summarizes changes associated with aging that occur in the endocrine and gastrointestinal systems. The most common endocrine system disorder seen in geriatric patients is diabetes mellitus (DM) type 2. Insulin production decreases and insulin resistance increases. DM type 2 increases the risk of developing vascular disease throughout the body.

   Within the gastrointestinal system, changes usually begin in the mouth. There is a decrease in taste buds and saliva, along with a diminished sense of smell. All of those factors can contribute to a lack of interest in eating, which can lead to nutritional issues. Also contributing to the nutritional status are the changes in the small intestine with poorer absorption of vitamins and minerals.

SUMMARY OF LEARNING OBJECTIVES—*continued*

3. **Examine the changes in anatomy, physiology, and diseases of the integumentary and musculoskeletal systems.**
   Table 45.3 summarizes changes associated with aging that occur in the integumentary and musculoskeletal systems. Many changes in the integumentary system are the result of exposure to ultraviolet light from the sun over time, such as wrinkles, age spots, and leathery skin. Skin regeneration becomes slower, causing skin to appear thinner and more prone to tearing or blistering. Atrophy of the subcutaneous layer decreases the natural lubrication and causes dry skin. Hair color, growth, and distribution change as we age. Nails take longer to grow and are more brittle.

   Shingles is a condition that can develop if the patient has had chicken pox, and it is commonly seen in the older patient population. There is a vaccine available, Shingrix, which can prevent shingles and postherpetic neuralgia.

   Within the musculoskeletal system, we see cartilage loss and degeneration producing osteoarthritis. There is also a decline in overall muscle endurance. Osteoporosis is a common concern, especially for small-boned, thin women. There are several medications that can be used to prevent or treat osteoporosis.
4. **Examine the changes in anatomy, physiology, and diseases of the nervous system and sensory organs.**
   Table 45.4 summarizes changes associated with aging that occur in the nervous system and sensory organs. Dementia is not an inevitable part of aging but is caused by an organic disorder. There are many conditions that have the same signs and symptoms as dementia and should be investigated as the cause of the new behavior.

   Alzheimer disease (AD) is a progressive disease the involves the destruction of the central nervous system neurons. The major changes that occur with AD are: amyloid plaque formation, neurofibrillary tangles clumping together, and the loss of the connection between neurons responsible for memory and learning. Recently a new drug was approved for the treatment of AD, and there are several drugs that are used to treat the symptoms.

   Aging can impact vision, hearing, taste, and smell. Cataracts are not uncommon in this age group and is easily corrected with surgery. Glaucoma can be treated with medication.

   Hearing loss can have a big impact on aging people. It can cause depression, social withdrawal, and feelings of isolation. Hearing aids may be helpful but can also amplify background noise, making it hard to hear clearly and creating sensory overload.

   As we age, we lose taste buds, and our ability to smell also decreases. This can impact the patient's interest in eating and can therefore affect the person's nutritional status. The decrease in the sense of smell can impact the safety of patients, as they may not smell smoke or natural gas leaks. They may not be able to smell when food has gone bad. Dating food that is put in the refrigerator can help.
5. **Examine the changes in anatomy, physiology, and diseases of the urinary and reproductive systems.**
   Table 45.7 summarizes changes associated with aging that occur in the urinary and reproductive systems. As we age, our kidneys become less efficient at filtering waste from the blood. Medication will remain in the body longer, creating an increased risk for toxic levels in the bloodstream. The bladder wall becomes thickened, reducing its ability to expand and its capacity, meaning that the patient will have to urinate more frequently at all times of the day and night. Due to urinary retention, an older adult is at increased risk for urinary tract infections.

   In the reproductive system of women, the vagina diminishes in width and length and becomes less elastic. Vaginal secretions decline, resulting in vaginal dryness. In men, there are changes in the prostate. It can enlarge and press on the urethra, causing difficulty with urination.
6. **Examine the role of the medical assistant in caring for aging patients.**
   The medical assistant's role in caring for the older patient is to develop effective communication skills that accommodate age-related sensorimotor changes, allow time for longer appointments, provide adequate lighting and forms in large print, and develop appropriate in-service training as requested by the provider. Examination rooms should have furniture and treatment folders specifically designed for older adult patients. Referrals and community resources should be used for patient and family support.

   Effective communication with aging patients includes addressing the patient with an appropriate title; introducing yourself and explaining the purpose of a procedure before touching the patient; establishing eye contact and getting the patient's attention before beginning to speak; using expanded speech, gestures, demonstrations, or written instructions in block print; repeating the message as needed for understanding; observing the patient's nonverbal behaviors for cues that indicate whether the patient understands; allowing time for the patient to process information; preventing distractions; involving family members as needed.

   Aging people prefer to remain in their home environment for as long as possible. Adult daycare centers can provide supervision for older adults who may be taken care of by family members in the evening but need care during the day. Assisted living facilities are appropriate for older adults who need assistance with some activities of daily living. Skilled nursing facilities provide 24-hour medical care and supervision.

PROCEDURE 45.1 Understand the Sensorimotor Changes of Aging

TASK: Role-play as an older adult to better understand the needs of aging people.

EQUIPMENT and SUPPLIES

- Yellow-tinted glasses, ski goggles, or laboratory goggles
- Pink, white, yellow "pills" (e.g., various colors of Tic Tac mints)
- Petroleum jelly (e.g., Vaseline)
- Cotton balls
- Eye patches
- Tape
- Utility gloves
- Tongue depressors
- Elastic bandages
- Medical forms in small print
- Pennies
- Button shirts
- Walker

PROCEDURAL STEPS

1. Role-play vision and hearing loss.
   - Put two cotton balls in each ear and an eye patch over one eye. Follow your partner's instructions.
   - *Partner:* Stand out of the line of vision (to prevent lip-reading). Without using gestures or changing your voice volume, tell your partner to cross the room and pick up a book.
2. Role-play yellowing of the lens of the eye.
   - Line up "pills" of different pastel colors.
   - *Partner:* Pick out the different colors while wearing the yellow-tinted glasses.
3. Role-play difficulty with focusing.
   - Put on goggles smeared with petroleum jelly and follow your partner's directions.
   - *Partner:* Stand at least 3 feet in front of your partner and motion for them to come to you (your partner is deaf, so talking will not help).
4. Role-play loss of peripheral vision.
   - Put on goggles with black paper taped to the sides.
   - *Partner:* Stand to the side, out of the field of vision, and motion for your partner to follow you.
5. Role-play aphasia and partial paralysis.
   - You are unable to use your right arm or leg. Place tape over your mouth. Let your partner know you need to go to the bathroom.
   - *Partner:* Stand at least 3 feet away with your back to your partner and wait for instructions.
6. Role-play problems with dexterity.
   - Put thick gloves on your hands and try to sign your name, button a shirt, tie your shoes, and pick up pennies.
7. Role-play problems with mobility.
   - Use the walker to cross the room.
   - *Partner:* After your partner starts to use the walker, hand them a book to carry.
8. Role-play changes in sensation.
   - Put on a rubber utility glove; turn on very warm water; test the difference in temperature between the gloved hand and the ungloved hand.
9. Summarize and share your impressions of the effects of age-related sensorimotor changes with the group.

INTRODUCTION TO THE CLINICAL LABORATORY 46

SCENARIO

Greg Stuart, CMA (AAMA), graduated from a medical assisting program 4 years ago and has been working at Walden-Martin Family Medical (WMFM) Clinic ever since. He enjoys working with patients and providers, but recently WMFM Clinic decided to expand its physician office laboratory (POL). A few weeks ago, Greg transferred into the phlebotomy/laboratory area, and he has really enjoyed it so far. He loves the patient contact he has during the phlebotomy procedures, and every day is just a little different. He really liked the laboratory portion of his medical assistant coursework in school and wanted a new challenge at work. It has been fun to brush up on his phlebotomy skills, and he has found that he has a real talent for putting people at ease.

He is working with another laboratory CMA, Julie Salter, as he trains in the laboratory. Julie has worked in the POL for about 8 years and is happy to expand the services that are provided at WMFM Clinic. Today she is going to reintroduce Greg to the laboratory.

While studying this chapter, think about the following questions:

- What is the role of the clinical laboratory in patient care?
- What is the medical assistant's role in coordinating laboratory tests and results?
- What are the three regulatory categories established by the Clinical Laboratory Improvement Amendments (CLIA)?
- Why is it important to have quality assurance practices in the laboratory?
- What is a laboratory flow sheet, and how is it used?
- What is a Safety Data Sheet (SDS), and why is it important?
- Why is it important to know safety techniques to minimize physical, chemical, and biological hazards in the clinical laboratory?
- Why is specimen collection, including the importance of sensitivity to patients' rights and feelings when collecting specimens, important in the laboratory?
- What metric units are used for measuring liquid volume, distance, and mass?
- What are the parts of a microscope?

LEARNING OBJECTIVES

1. Examine the organization of the clinical laboratory.
2. Examine the impact of the Clinical Laboratory Improvement Amendments on the clinical laboratory.
3. Examine quality assurance and quality control in the clinical laboratory setting.
4. Examine all aspects of laboratory safety.
5. Examine the process of completing laboratory requisitions, handling reports, specimen collection, processing, and storage in the clinical laboratory.
6. Examine how mathematics and measurements are used in the clinical laboratory.
7. Examine the common equipment found in the clinical laboratory.

VOCABULARY

aliquot A portion of a well-mixed sample removed for testing

analyte (AN e lit) The substance or chemical being analyzed or detected in a specimen.

anticoagulant (an tee koh AG yuh lunts) Category of medication or a chemical that prevents clotting of blood.

aseptically (ay SEP tick ah lee) Free from living pathogenic organisms.

aspirate (AS puh rayt) To withdraw fluid using suction; the material removed using suction—for example, a specimen that has been removed from the body using a needle and syringe.

calibration (kal uh BRAY shun) Determining the accuracy of an instrument by comparing its output with that of a known standard or another instrument known to be accurate.

caustic (KAW stik) Capable of burning, corroding, or damaging tissue by chemical action.

control materials Manufacturer-prepared samples that have a known quantity of a specific analyte. Used for quality control purposes. Testing results should fall within a manufacturer-defined range of results. Also called controls or quality controls.

corrosive (kuh ROH siv) Causing or tending to cause the gradual destruction of a substance by chemical action.

culture media A solid, liquid, or semisolid medium designed to support the growth of microorganisms, especially bacteria and fungi.

VOCABULARY—*continued*

cytology (sie TOL oh jee) The study of cells using microscopic methods.

exudates (EKS yoo dayts) Fluids with high concentrations of protein and cellular debris that have escaped from the blood vessels and have been deposited in tissues or on tissue surfaces.

forensic (fuh REN sik) Scientific tests or techniques used regarding the detection of crimes.

hemolyzed (HEE muh liezd) A blood sample in which the red blood cells have ruptured.

histology (hi STOL oh jee) The study of tissues.

inhalant (in HAY lunt) Any substance that can be breathed into the lungs.

International Normalized Ratio (INR) Also called prothrombin time (PT). Used to test the effectiveness of blood-thinning medication.

in vitro Latin term meaning "in glass" and commonly known as "in the laboratory."

pathologist (pah THOL uh jist) A physician specially trained in the nature and cause of disease.

pure culture The growth of only one microorganism in a culture or on a nutrient surface.

quality assurance Written policies and procedures that ensure monitoring of all processes involved before, during, and after a laboratory test is performed to produce reliable patient test results.

quality control A process to ensure the reliability of test results, often using manufactured samples with known values.

reagent (re AY jent) A substance for use in a chemical reaction.

referral laboratory A laboratory that performs testing for another laboratory. Testing varies from high-volume routine testing to low-volume unique or unusual testing. Also called reference, diagnostic, or commercial testing laboratories. Often privately owned.

sharps Medical term for devices with sharp points or edges that can puncture or cut skin. Examples include needles, scalpels, or broken glass.

specimen A biological sample such as blood, urine, body fluids, feces, or tissue collected for analysis and evaluation.

standard operating procedures (SOP) A set of step-by-step instructions to help employees carry out routine operations with efficiency, high quality, and uniformity of performance.

STAT The medical abbreviation for the Latin term *statum,* meaning immediately; at this moment.

sterile Free from all living organisms

toxicology (tok si KOL oh jee) The study and science that deal with the effects, antidotes, and detection of poisons or drugs.

INTRODUCTION

Laboratory medicine is the medical discipline that applies clinical laboratory science to the care and diagnosis of patients. Laboratory tests are used for four main purposes:

- To document the good health of a patient
- To screen patients for diseases and conditions such as diabetes, high cholesterol, or urinary tract infections (UTIs)
- To help the provider diagnose a medical disease, disorder, or condition
- To help the provider decide on the most appropriate treatment, to monitor the effects of medications and treatments, and to monitor a disease process

Healthcare providers order laboratory testing for patients. Patient **specimens** are collected at the laboratory, an ambulatory care facility, or home. A specimen is a sample of body fluid, waste product, or tissue collected for analysis. Once in the laboratory, the specimen is processed and directed to the proper laboratory department. Each department of the lab will analyze and evaluate the specimen based on specific tests ordered by the provider. Tests can be performed *manually* (by hand) or through a variety of specialized automated instruments. Once test results have been completed, they are reported to the provider.

Role of Medical Assistants

When the healthcare provider orders a laboratory test for a patient, the medical assistant can enter the provider's order into the laboratory ordering system. The medical assistant may also do the following:

- Provide the patient with specimen collection instructions.
- Collect and label patient specimens.
- Assist with preparing specimens to be transported to a laboratory for testing.
- Perform CLIA-waived testing.

The medical assistant must be knowledgeable about the patient preparations, testing procedures, and the normal range of results for common tests. The medical assistant must carefully follow all laboratory instructions. Excellent communication between the team members and the patient is very important. The medical assistant should make the patient feel at ease with these procedures and hopefully gain the patient's cooperation and trust.

ORGANIZATION OF THE CLINICAL LABORATORY

There are certain components found in all clinical laboratories. Personnel are needed to staff the laboratory; certain tests are performed in the laboratory, and there are different departments performing those tests. The following sections discuss each of those aspects of the clinical laboratory.

Personnel in the Clinical Laboratory

Medical laboratories are in hospitals, ambulatory care facilities, public health departments, health maintenance organizations, and **referral laboratories** (also called *reference laboratories*). The clinical laboratory is staffed with a variety of professionals, including the following:

- A director may be a **pathologist** or a clinical laboratory scientist with a doctorate degree. In ambulatory care facilities, the lab director may be the physician. This type of lab is referred to as a *physician's office laboratory* (POL).

TABLE 46.1 Certifying Agencies for Laboratory Personnel

AGENCY	TITLE	POSITION
American Society for Clinical Pathologists (ASCP)	MLS (ASCP)	Medical laboratory scientist
	MT (ASCP)	Medical technologist
	MLT (ASCP)	Medical laboratory technician—certificate
	MLT-AD (ASCP)	Medical laboratory technician—associate degree
American Medical Technologists (AMT)	CMLA (AMT)	Certified medical laboratory assistant
	MT (AMT)	Medical technologist
	MLT (AMT)	Medical laboratory technician
	RPT	Phlebotomy technician
	RMA	Registered medical assistant
American Association of Medical Assistants (AAMA)	CMA (AAMA)	Certified medical assistant
National Healthcareer Association (NHA)	CCMA	Certified clinical medical assistant
	CPT	Certified phlebotomy technician
	CMLA	Certified medical laboratory assistant

- Clinical laboratory scientists (CLSs) and clinical laboratory technicians (CLTs).
- Medical laboratory assistants (MLAs) and phlebotomists. MLAs and phlebotomists have received specialized training in the collection of blood samples and the preparation of laboratory specimens. The agencies granting certifications and titles are listed in Table 46.1.
- Medical assistants (CMAs, RMAs, CCMAs). Medical assistants are trained to properly collect patient specimens and perform specific testing procedures within the POL. They are also trained to properly collect specimens that are sent to outside reference laboratories for testing.

Clinical Laboratory Testing

Clinical laboratory testing is used in conjunction with a thorough health history and physical examination to obtain essential data for screening, diagnosis, or management of a patient's condition. The body is healthy when a state of equilibrium exists in the internal environment. This healthy state of equilibrium, called *homeostasis,* occurs when the physical and chemical characteristics of body substances are within a certain acceptable range, known as the *normal range* or *reference range*. A normal or reference range is a numeric range of test values for which the general population consistently shows similar results 95% of the time. A change in the internal environment of the body often results in abnormal test values, which are outside the population's reference range.

When a provider uses a laboratory test for diagnosis, the patient's results are compared with the reference range of values. Reference values are also useful for assessing the progress of a patient's course of treatment. Each medical institution will establish its own reference ranges. It is important for medical assistants to be familiar with the ranges for their institution.

Abnormal values for a test may be seen with more than one pathologic condition. For example, a decrease in a patient's hemoglobin level is seen in iron-deficiency anemia, but also in hyperthyroidism and cirrhosis of the liver. Therefore, providers cannot rely solely on one laboratory test to make a diagnosis. They must use a combination of results obtained from the history and physical exam and a number of diagnostic and laboratory tests.

Types of Clinical Laboratory Tests

Tests performed in a clinical laboratory range from simple screening tests of one **analyte** (e.g., measuring glucose to diagnose or monitor diabetes) to complex *profile testing*, where more than one analyte is tested from a single sample. The tests are all associated with an organ or disease (e.g., performing a lipid profile to determine the various fats in the blood).

A *screening test* examines a specimen for the presence of an analyte that may indicate a disease state. Screening tests are not necessarily diagnostic for one disease; rather, they indicate that a disease state may exist. Screening tests are routinely done on patients based on their age, history, or gender.

Types of Test Results

Clinical laboratory tests can be reported in three different ways:

- *Qualitative*: Test results are reported as positive or negative. A numeric value is not attached to the result. A CLIA-waived mononucleosis test is reported as either positive or negative.
- *Semi-quantitative*: Test results do not indicate a precise amount of a substance present but an estimate of how much is present. These test results are less precise than quantitative test results but they are more precise than qualitative test results. Semi-quantitative test results may be indicated as "trace amount" or "1+, 2+, or 3+". Urine dipsticks are examples of semi-qualitative tests.
- *Quantitative*: The test result is expressed as a number, usually with units of measure attached to numeric values. It is essential that quantitative test results be reported with the units of measure. A CLIA-waived blood glucose test is reported with a number followed by mg/dL (e.g., 120 mg/dL). The abbreviation mg/dL means milligrams per deciliter.

CRITICAL THINKING APPLICATION **46.1**

Julie and Greg have been going over general information on laboratory testing this morning. It is important to know some terms used in the laboratory. Julie asks Greg to define qualitative, semi-quantitative, and quantitative test results in his own words. How would you describe these three terms?

Departments of the Clinical Laboratory

Large laboratories are divided into various departments, which may include urinalysis, hematology, chemistry, microbiology, specimen collection and processing, blood bank (immunohematology), coagulation, immunology/serology, **histology**, **cytology**, **toxicology**, and special chemistry. A POL generally performs test procedures in urinalysis, hematology, chemistry, and microbiology.

Some larger laboratories use the *core laboratory* concept, which combines clinical hematology, immunochemistry, chemistry, toxicology, and coagulation into one automated process. The core concept provides for faster turnaround times.

Urinalysis

Urinalysis includes the physical, chemical, and microscopic examination of urine. As part of the physical examination, the color, clarity, and specific gravity are noted. The specimen's temperature may also be measured to verify that the sample is at body temperature and, therefore, recently collected. Urine is tested with a multiple test strip, also called a *dipstick*, which tests the following analytes in urine: glucose, protein, ketones, blood, bilirubin, urobilinogen, nitrites, and pH. We will go into the details of urinalysis in Chapter 47. Microscopically, the provider may examine urine for the presence of red blood cells (RBCs), white blood cells (WBCs), epithelial cells, mucus, casts, crystals, and microorganisms. Additional quantitative tests may be performed in the urinalysis department of a reference laboratory to confirm routine screening test results.

Hematology

Hematology is the study of blood cells and coagulation. Laboratory testing in the hematology department may be qualitative or quantitative. In a POL, screening tests for hemoglobin, hematocrit, and the **International Normalized Ratio** (**INR**, a coagulation test) are typically performed in the ambulatory setting. Reference laboratories will perform blood cell counts that determine the number of RBCs, WBCs, and platelets in a blood sample. Microscopic tests determine the characteristics of cells, such as size, shape, and maturity. In addition, the hematology department performs tests to determine the coagulating ability of blood.

Chemistry

The clinical chemistry department analyzes the chemicals found in blood, cerebrospinal fluid, urine, and joint fluid (synovial fluid). Specimen testing may be done manually or with complex chemistry instruments. In a POL, procedures may include single analyte tests (of blood glucose) or multitest profiles. Chemistry profiles include tests for a number of related analytes. Lipid profiles, for example, include assessments of total cholesterol, triglycerides, low-density lipoprotein (LDL), and high-density lipoprotein (HDL). POL chemistry analyzers are becoming more common in ambulatory care as technology becomes more compact and easier to use.

Microbiology

Microbiology involves the study of very small, infectious organisms such as bacteria, fungi, yeasts, parasites, and viruses. Specimens used in microbiology include blood, urine, sputum, cerebrospinal fluid (CSF), stool, wound material, and other biological sources. Specimens used for microbiology testing must be collected **aseptically** in **sterile** containers.

The goal of the microbiology department is to identify the microorganism causing the infection. The staff will also determine the most effective antimicrobial medications, which include antibiotics. This process is called identification and sensitivity (or susceptibility) testing.

Microbiology specimens may be grown on **culture media**. Once the organism is growing, and in **pure culture**, it can be identified. Organism identification tests have changed with technology and will continue to change in the future. A variety of methods and technologies are applied to identify the microorganism. Methods include biochemical, molecular, and antigen-antibody complex testing.

Sensitivity testing is performed on organisms to establish an appropriate antibiotic therapy for specific bacterium or fungi. Once again, a variety of techniques and technologies may be used to help determine which antibiotic would be most effective. In a POL, this may include the following:

- Rapid strep testing may be performed to screen for strep throat
- Microbiologic specimens may be aseptically collected and then sent to a reference laboratory
- Some microscope slides may be prepared for the provider to examine

Identification and sensitivity tests are usually performed in larger centralized ambulatory care, hospital, or reference laboratories.

CRITICAL THINKING APPLICATION **46.2**

Greg and Julie have reviewed the different areas that are common in a POL. WMFM is now doing testing in microbiology, a new area that has been added to the POL in the past 6 months. As they talk about microbiology, Julie asks, "Why do microbiology samples need to be collected aseptically in a sterile container?" How would you answer this question?

GOVERNMENT LEGISLATION AFFECTING CLINICAL LABORATORY TESTING

In 1988 Congress passed the *Clinical Laboratory Improvement Amendments* (CLIA). This law established quality standards for all clinical laboratory testing, and it is designed to ensure the accuracy, precision, reliability, and timeliness of patient test results, regardless of which laboratory performed the testing. A clinical laboratory is defined as any facility that performs laboratory testing on human specimens to provide information about the diagnosis, prevention, and treatment of disease or the impairment of health.

Clinical Laboratory Improvement Amendments

Under CLIA, all laboratories that perform even one type of test must meet certain federal requirements. They must register with the Centers for Medicare and Medicaid Services (CMS) as a laboratory. The registration application must be submitted to the CMS with information about the laboratory's operations. The type of certificate that is issued is based on the information provided in the application. (Note that most POLs are registered as CLIA-waived laboratories.)

The US Food and Drug Administration (FDA) is responsible for categorizing commercially marketed tests performed **in vitro** based on the CLIA guidelines. The FDA has assumed primary responsibility for determining the CLIA complexity of all laboratory tests. Every laboratory test product is assigned to one of three CLIA categories based on the product's potential risk to public health. The CLIA categories are as follows: waived tests, moderate-complexity tests, and high-complexity tests.

CLIA-Waived Tests and Laboratories

CLIA-waived tests are defined as laboratory tests and procedures that have been approved by the FDA for home use or that are simple laboratory tests and procedures to perform. Waived tests are designed to have straightforward directions and procedures, so they have a minimal risk of incorrect results. Waived tests include tests that do the following:

- Use methodologies that are simple and accurate so that the likelihood of incorrect user results is negligible
- Pose no unreasonable risk of harm to the patient if it is performed incorrectly

Table 46.2 shows some common CLIA-waived tests performed in ambulatory care facilities registered as CLIA-waived laboratories.

The FDA's CLIA-waived database of tests is available online. This database contains the commercially marketed laboratory test systems categorized by the FDA since January 31, 2000, and tests categorized by the Centers for Disease Control and Prevention (CDC) before that date. The database can be searched by test system name, specialty or subspecialty, analyte, document number, qualifier, effective date, and complexity. The application process for a CLIA waiver varies from state to state.

Moderate- and High-Complexity Tests and Laboratories

The CLIA program oversees the quality of nearly 200,000 laboratory procedures. Most laboratory tests are categorized by the FDA as moderate-complexity tests. Some moderate-complexity tests performed in POLs include the following:

- Hematology and chemistry: testing done on an automated analyzer
- Microbiology: Gram stain procedures
- Urinalysis: microscopic analysis of urine sediment

Moderate-complexity tests must be performed by qualified personnel as described by CLIA. High-complexity tests are generally not performed in a POL but rather in a hospital or reference laboratory.

Laboratories that perform moderate- to high-complexity testing must meet rigorous CLIA regulations and are subject to surprise inspections every 2 years. Each laboratory that performs these tests must do the following:

- Establish a system to maintain the identification of patients' specimens throughout the testing process and ensure accurate reporting of results.
- Establish and follow written **quality assurance** (QA), **quality control** (QC), and **standard operating procedures** (SOPs).
- Participate in *proficiency testing*, which is a form of external quality control. Three times a year, the laboratory must test samples provided by an approved proficiency-testing agency. The proficiency samples are tested in the same way as patient samples. Results are then reported to the proficiency-testing agency, and the accuracy of testing is verified. The College of American Pathologists (CAP) is an accrediting body for laboratories that offers proficiency testing.
- Employ personnel that meet CLIA regulations and specific qualifications for a moderate- to high-complexity laboratory. Requirements are most rigorous for high-complexity testing.

Medical assistants can perform all CLIA-waived tests and some specific moderate-complexity tests. Additional training will be required to perform moderate-complexity tests, depending on the certification of the POL where the medical assistant works. Although medical assistants cannot perform high-complexity tests, they can be involved in patient preparation, provider-directed patient education, specimen collection, and documenting results in the patient's health record.

CRITICAL THINKING APPLICATION 46.3

The laboratory at WMFM Clinic is a registered waived facility. List five commonly performed waived tests. What is the difference between waived testing and moderate- or high-complexity testing? List three differences and be ready to share them with your classmates.

QUALITY ASSURANCE AND QUALITY CONTROL

Quality assurance (QA) is a set of written policies and procedures that ensure monitoring of all the processes involved before, during, and after a laboratory test is performed in order to produce reliable patient test results. It is the promise of healthcare professionals to achieve the highest degree of excellence in the care given to every patient. QA includes a comprehensive set of policies developed to ensure excellent documentation and reliability of laboratory testing. These policies benefit the provider by reducing the liability for inaccurate reporting of test results. QA also focuses on establishing a series of operating procedures for the benefit of the patient and the medical assistant who does the laboratory testing. The QA system enables the laboratory to assess, verify, and document the quality of the laboratory processes. This documentation is a way of comparing *what is happening* with *what should be happening*.

As mandated by law, QA programs monitor all aspects of laboratory activity, from specimen collection to processing, testing, and reporting steps. Programs check supplies, reagents, machinery, and actual test performance. QA includes quality control, personnel orientation, laboratory documentation, knowledge of laboratory instrumentation, and enrollment in a proficiency testing program (if the lab performs moderate- or high-complexity tests).

The Three Stages of Quality Assurance in the Laboratory

The overall process required to ensure QA in the laboratory is divided into three stages. These three stages must be applied to each test or procedure that is performed in the laboratory. If any of these steps are missed or performed incorrectly, QA has been broken.

Preanalytic Stage

The preanalytic stage consists of the following actions:

1. The provider orders a test to screen, monitor, or diagnose a patient's condition.
2. A written or electronic requisition is filled out, showing the test requested, the specimen required, and where the specimen will be tested.
3. The specimen is collected, labeled, and processed.

TABLE 46.2 CLIA-Waived Tests and Their Purposes

SPECIMEN AND TEST	PURPOSE
Dipstick or tablet reagent urinalysis (manual or automated)	Urine screening to assess or diagnose diseases such as diabetes mellitus, kidney disease, and urinary tract infection
Urine pregnancy tests: visual color comparison tests	Diagnose pregnancy
Fecal occult blood	Colorectal screening to detect hidden blood in the stool
Erythrocyte sedimentation rate, nonautomated	Diagnoses inflammatory process; increases in arthritis, infection, leukemia, and most cancers
Spun microhematocrit	Measures red blood cells; screening for certain types of anemia
STAT-CRIT hematocrit	Screening for certain types of anemia
Hemoglobin	Measures hemoglobin level in whole blood
Blood glucose by glucose-monitoring devices cleared by the FDA specifically for home use	Monitor blood glucose levels
Hemoglobin A_{1c} by single analyte instruments with self-contained or component features to perform specimen-reagent interaction	Measure A_{1c} levels to assess and manage long-term care of patients with diabetes
Cholestech LDX	Measures total blood cholesterol, triglycerides, HDL, and glucose levels
Whole-Blood i-STAT Chem8+ Cartridge	Measures ionized calcium, carbon dioxide, chloride, creatinine, glucose, potassium, sodium, urea nitrogen, and hematocrit in whole blood
Whole-blood thyroid-stimulating hormone (TSH) assay	Qualitative determination of thyroid-stimulating hormone (TSH) in whole blood
Blood mononucleosis antibodies	Rapid whole-blood test to detect heterophile antibodies to help diagnose infectious mononucleosis
Helicobacter pylori antibodies	Rapid whole-blood test to detect *H. pylori* antibodies to determine the cause of peptic ulcer
Borrelia burgdorferi antibodies	Rapid whole-blood test to detect *B. burgdorferi* antibodies to diagnose Lyme disease
Trinity Biotech Uni-Gold Recombigen HIV Test	Detects HIV-1 in a blood specimen
Nasal influenza A and B	Quick qualitative diagnosis of influenza antigens in nasal secretions or swab
Streptococcus A throat swab	Rapid strep test
Urine or blood drug tests	Multiple tests for the presence of a variety of substance abuse agents
Urine fertility and menopause tests	Detect follicle-stimulating hormone in urine
Ovulation tests; visual color comparison tests for luteinizing hormone	Detect ovulation

CLIA, Clinical Laboratory Improvement Amendments; *FDA,* US Food and Drug Administration; *HDL,* high-density lipoprotein; *HIV-1,* human immunodeficiency virus type 1.
Information summarized from the Centers for Medicare and Medicaid Services, www.cms.gov/Regulations-and-Guidance/Legislation/CLIA/downloads/waivetbl.pdf.

4. The specimen is transported to the laboratory in the POL or properly prepared for offsite laboratory pickup.

Analytic Stage

The analytic stage includes the following actions:

1. Instruments are maintained and calibrated.
2. Controls are run and analyzed for each test method (part of ongoing quality control).
3. The specimen is tested, and the results are compared with reference ranges.
4. The test results are logged and documented in the patient's health record.

Postanalytic Stage

The postanalytic stage consists of the following actions:

1. Specimens are properly discarded.

2. Analyses of control results are compared over time.
3. Patient reports from outside laboratories are logged or documented.
4. The provider interprets and signs all lab reports.
5. The patient is notified of the results in the office or is contacted by laboratory personnel.
6. The final report and all communication with the patient are documented in the patient's health record.

Record Keeping. Accurate record keeping is one of the key responsibilities of a medical assistant. Various formats are available to record laboratory information. Most providers document patient information and testing results in electronic health records (EHRs). Some POLs still use paper records. In the case of paper records, the primary source of documentation is the *laboratory master logbook*. The logbook contains a written record for each procedure performed, the patient identification number, results obtained, the date performed, and personnel initials. The results are then sent to the provider for verification.

Testing Procedure. POLs are also required to have a procedure manual that describes how each test is performed and how the patient results are reported to the provider. Personnel are required to perform **calibration** or *optics checks* on laboratory instruments that use light detection or color change as part of the reaction process. An optics check is a specific type of calibration that assesses the optics of an electronic testing instrument or system.

In addition, they must run quality control or **control materials** each day before patient testing. Each manufacturer will include instructions for running control materials for its kit, procedure, or instrument. Quality control results must be documented and readily accessible. If errors or problems occur while completing quality control, the POL must perform and document remedial actions to correct errors or problems as they are identified. The requirement for when QC is to be done is a combination of management discretion and the manufacturer's recommendations. It may not be daily.

Preventive Maintenance. Preventive maintenance schedules must be followed and documented. *Preventive maintenance* is regularly scheduled care of equipment that will decrease the likelihood of failure. It is performed and documented at regular intervals while the equipment is in good working order. Preventive maintenance includes daily cleaning and adjustment, as well as replacement of parts when necessary. Each instrument should have a paper or electronic log or worksheet to record all changes, including daily maintenance details.

A preventive maintenance program for laboratory equipment includes the following duties:

- Follow the manufacturer's instructions for calibrating instruments.
- Read and understand the instructions for routine instrument care.
- Perform all preventive maintenance specified by the manufacturer's instructions.
- Keep spare parts available for immediate use.
- Record the name, address, and phone number of the contact person for maintenance or repair.
- Create a maintenance form, or use one provided by the manufacturer.

Ready? Set? Test! is an excellent online resource provided by the CDC for setting up and maintaining a CLIA-waived laboratory. Figure 46.1 shows the checklist summary of the steps needed to assure proper CLIA-waived testing in a POL.

Quality Control

A crucial step in the QA process is running quality control specimens (Procedure 46.1). The purpose of QC in the laboratory is to ensure the reliability of test results while detecting and eliminating errors. It is important to remember a few important terms:

- *Accuracy* is a measure of how close a test result is to the true value of the control material, as established by the manufacturer.
- *Precision* is the ability to consistently reproduce a test result.

When a series of control results show both accuracy and precision, the test is considered *reliable* and may be used for testing patients. QC monitoring is crucial because patient treatment is often based on or reinforced by the results of laboratory tests. Without QC monitoring, laboratory error is difficult to detect. Undetected laboratory errors may result in harm to the patient.

Quality Control Testing

Prepared QC test samples, called *controls*, are tested daily, along with patient samples. A normal control contains the normal level of the analyte, and an abnormal control contains a below or above normal level of the analyte being tested. Control test results must fall within a preestablished range of results before patient results can be reported. Controls are usually supplied with the manufacturer's prepackaged kits and should be analyzed at specified intervals as recommended by the manufacturer.

Internal controls are also provided in many CLIA-waived kit tests. Internal controls are part of the test cartridge, cassette, or card. These internal controls provide a mechanism for assuring that the test cartridge, cassette, or card is working properly and must meet the manufacturer's QC standards in order to report the results.

Quality Control Testing Examples. Examples of routine quality control testing in a POL include the following:

- Positive and negative controls supplied with pregnancy test kits are performed with each patient specimen or batch of patient specimens.
- Urinalysis dipstick controls (used for chemical examination of urine) should be checked daily before patient testing, and each time a new **reagent** container is opened.
- Controls for automated chemistry analyses should be performed before patient testing and at specified intervals during the day, depending on the number of tests run per day and the manufacturer's recommendations.

Recording Quality Control Testing

Every day that patient tests are performed, QC tests must also be performed and the results entered onto a paper or electronic graph or flow sheet. When new control materials are opened and used, the results and dates must be entered on a new flow sheet, along with the expiration dates of the controls. These records must be retained for several years; the exact number of years is determined by state law and CLIA mandates.

Using a Graph for Quality Control Results

Many laboratories will use a graph to display daily quality control results. A paper or electronic graph file can be updated with daily QC values. Graphing advantages include the following:

- A graph is a physical representation of the QC results that can display data irregularities in an easy-to-see format.
- It displays possible *trends* (data that continues to go upward or downward in value) and *shifts* (data results that show an abrupt change in value) over time.

See the labeled graph that follows.

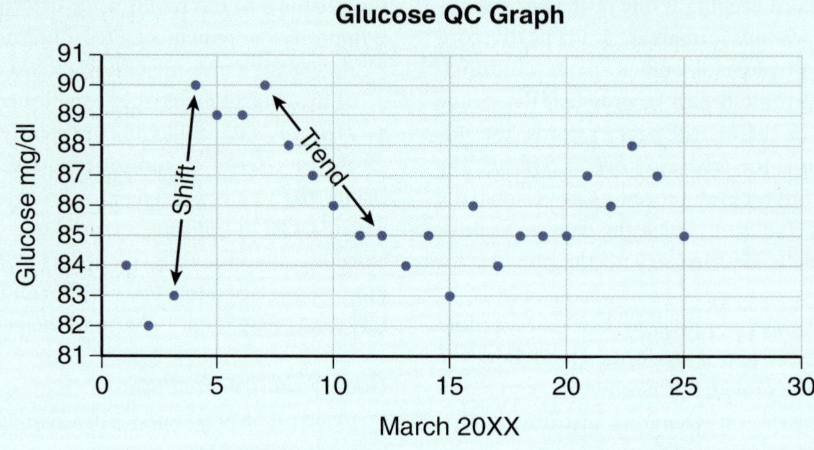

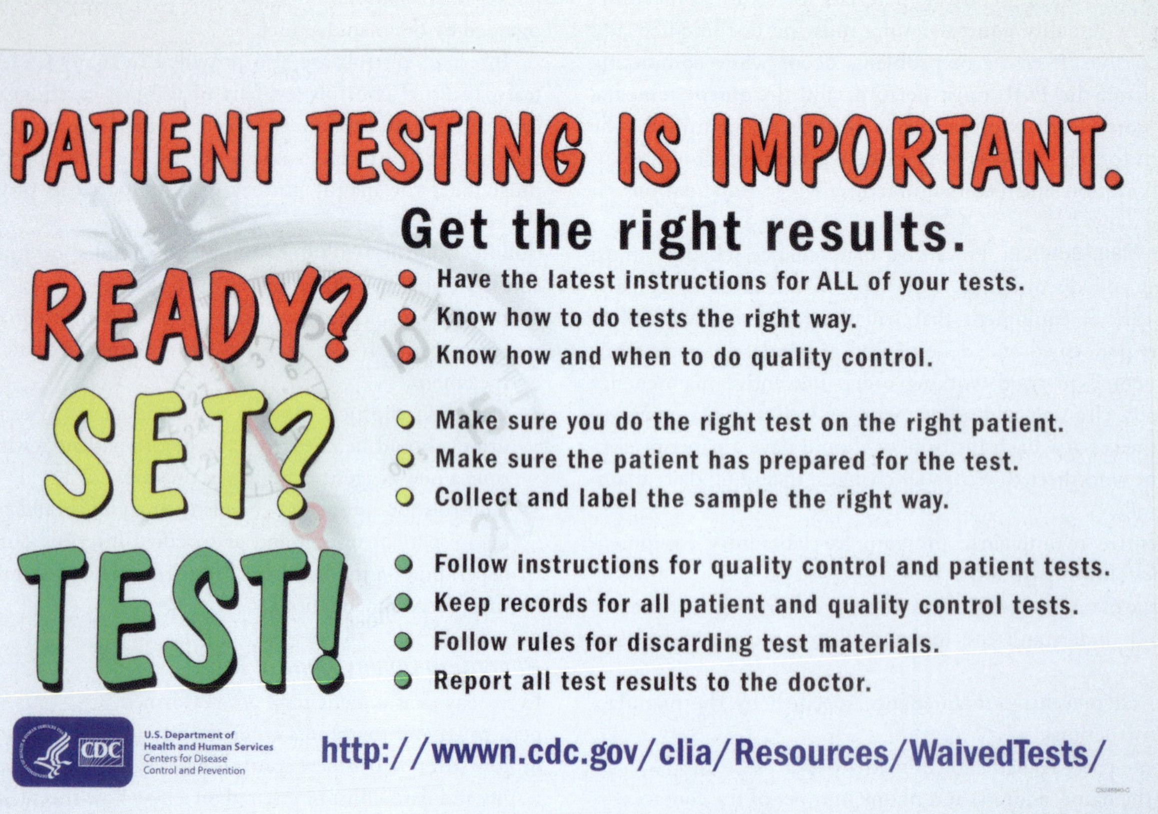

FIGURE 46.1 Summary checklist from Ready? Set? Test!

CRITICAL THINKING APPLICATION 46.4

As Greg and Julie are reviewing quality assurance and quality control, Greg asks Julie to clarify the differences between QA and QC. In your own words, define QA and QC. How are they different? Be ready to discuss your answer with your classmates.

LABORATORY SAFETY

The importance of safety in the laboratory cannot be overemphasized. Most laboratory accidents can be prevented using proper techniques and common sense. Following safe practices in the laboratory requires a personal commitment and concern for others. An unsafe act may also harm an innocent bystander without harming the person who performs the act.

Safety Standards and Governing Agencies

The US government created a system of safeguards and regulations under the Occupational Safety and Health Act of 1970. This system affects nearly every worker in the United States because the regulations apply to all businesses with one or more employees (the regulations are discussed in detail in Chapter 4). Two programs have been mandated by the Occupational Safety and Health Administration (OSHA) to ensure the safety of personnel working in clinical laboratories. One covers occupational exposure to chemical hazards; the other covers exposure to bloodborne pathogens.

The CDC also has established recommendations and resources in Standard Precautions and Transmission Precautions as they relate to specimen collection. (These recommendations are discussed in Chapter 19.)

Chemical Hazards

The clinical laboratory may have chemicals that are flammable, **caustic**, and potentially poisonous. Exposure to these dangerous chemicals can occur by breathing in fumes, direct absorption by contact with the skin, ingestion, direct contact with a mucous membrane, or entry through a cut, abrasion, or burn in the skin. OSHA is involved in regulating the standards directed at minimizing occupational exposure to hazardous chemicals in laboratories. OSHA's Hazard Communication Standard (HCS; known as the employee "right to know" rule) became law in 1991. It ensures that laboratory workers are made fully aware of the hazards associated with their workplace. The law requires the development of a comprehensive plan to put in place safe practices throughout the laboratory regarding chemicals. All workers must be provided with information and training.

Safety Data Sheet

A Safety Data Sheet (SDS) must also be on file for all chemicals used in the laboratory. OSHA requires the manufacturer of the chemicals to make these sheets available, usually as a package insert or online. Employers must ensure that SDSs are readily accessible to employees. SDSs supply information about chemical safety and hazard information in case of an accident, spill, or fire to the user or emergency personnel.

Since June 2015, OSHA has required all SDSs to use a uniform format that includes the following section numbers, headings, and information:

- Section 1. Identification
- Section 2. Hazard(s) identification
- Section 3. Composition/information on ingredients
- Section 4. First-aid measures
- Section 5. Fire-fighting measures
- Section 6. Accidental release measures
- Section 7. Handling and storage
- Section 8. Exposure controls/personal protection
- Section 9. Physical and chemical properties
- Section 10. Stability and reactivity
- Section 11. Toxicologic information
- Section 12. Ecologic information
- Section 13. Disposal considerations
- Section 14. Transport information
- Section 15. Regulatory information
- Section 16. Other information

Please note that Sections 12 through 15 are regulated by agencies other than OSHA and are required of the manufacturers, not the employees.

Proper Chemical Handling, Storage, and Disposal Procedures

In the POL, the most common hazardous chemicals are as follows:

- Sodium hypochlorite, commonly known as bleach, which is used for disinfecting laboratory work areas
- CaviWipes and glutaraldehyde, which are disinfectants
- Acetone and dyes, which are used for staining slides

It should be noted that all of these disinfectants and dyes are available in premixed sprays or wipes to reduce chemical exposure during dilution.

Common guidelines have been developed to reduce the risks associated with handling and storing chemicals in the clinical laboratory:

- Date the chemical containers when they are first opened and first received.
- Keep the laboratory doors closed at all times.
- Only use chemicals that you have been trained to use.
- Store large bottles of acids on low shelves. Store flammable substances away from sources of ignition.
- If a chemical produces toxic or flammable vapors, work under a fume hood that exhausts air to the outside

Chemical waste is regulated by state and federal laws. Chemicals must be disposed of in a safe manner and according to the laws. Chemicals should be disposed of following state and federal guidelines. General recommendations have been established for chemical waste disposal:

- Check the Safety Data Sheet for disposal considerations.
- Keep chemicals separated. Mixing chemicals can create toxic vapors and mixtures.
- Ensure the chemical waste is correctly identified and labeled.
- Contact a disposal company that handles chemical waste. The disposal company will transfer the chemical waste to the disposal site.

Chemical Labels. Chemical labels are workplace safeguards. Chemicals should be tightly sealed and properly marked with the original manufacturer's labels. A hazard identification system, developed by the National Fire Protection Association (NFPA), provides information at a glance on the potential health, flammability, and chemical reactivity hazards of materials. This identification system consists of four small, diamond-shaped, colored symbols grouped into a larger diamond shape (Figure 46.2):

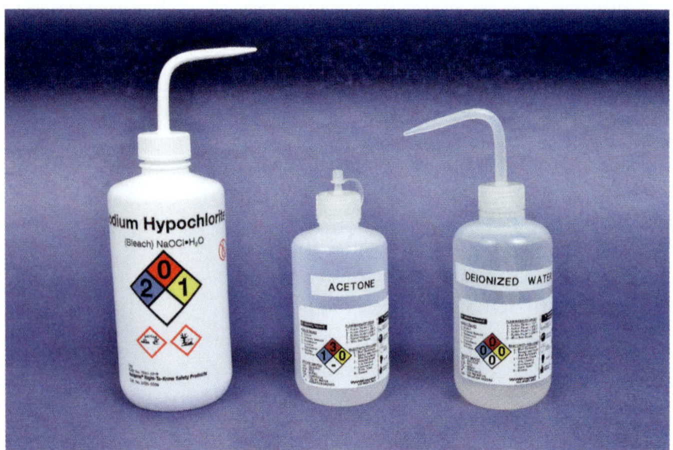

FIGURE 46.2 Laboratory bottles with chemical labels.

- The top diamond is red and indicates flammability (the potential to catch on fire).
- The diamond on the left is blue and indicates a health hazard such as a dangerous **inhalant** or **corrosive** acid.
- The bottom diamond is white and provides special hazard information, including recommended personal protective equipment (PPE) if biohazards are present and in other dangerous situations.
- The diamond on the right is yellow and indicates a reactivity or stability hazard. An example of reactivity is mixing an acid (e.g., bleach) with a base (e.g., ammonia), creating a dangerous gas.

The four-color system also indicates the severity of the hazard by using numbers imprinted in the diamonds from 0 to 4, with 0 representing no hazard and 4 representing an extremely hazardous substance (see Figure 46.2).

First Aid for Chemical Exposures

Prompt medical attention must be given to victims of chemical exposure. The SDS provides first-aid measures that untrained responders should give to individuals with a chemical exposure. Exposure routes include inhalation, skin and eye contact, and ingestion. Some SDSs provide recommendations for immediate medical care and special treatments needed.

General guidelines for chemical exposures include the following:

- With an accidental exposure of the skin, rinse the affected area under running water for at least 5 minutes. Remove any contaminated clothing.
- If chemicals are splashed in the eyes, flush the eyes with water from an eyewash station (Figure 46.3) for a minimum of 15 minutes. (See Procedure 46.2.)

CRITICAL THINKING APPLICATION **46.5**

Greg has a few hours to review WMFM Clinic's current laboratory safety policies and procedures on his own. There are a number of policies that apply to the laboratory only, but there are also many policies that apply to the entire facility. Why is it so important for employees to be aware of safety policies and procedures? Write down five reasons for being safety aware in the laboratory.

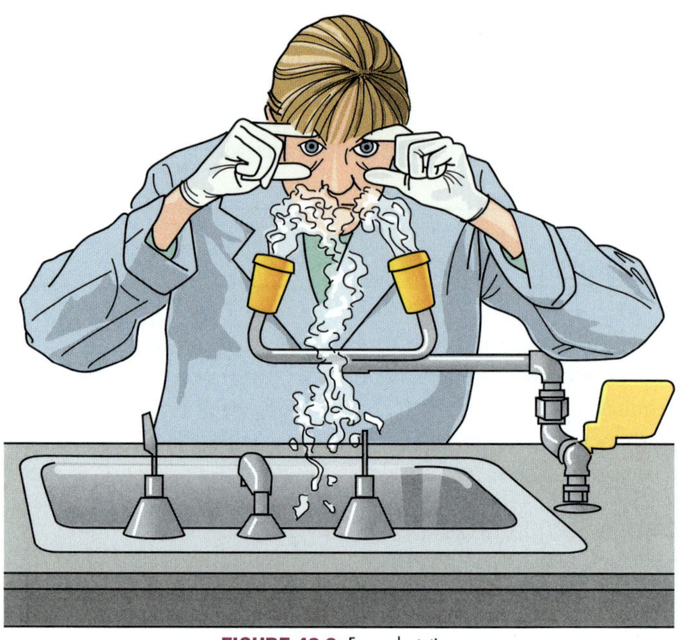
FIGURE 46.3 Eyewash station.

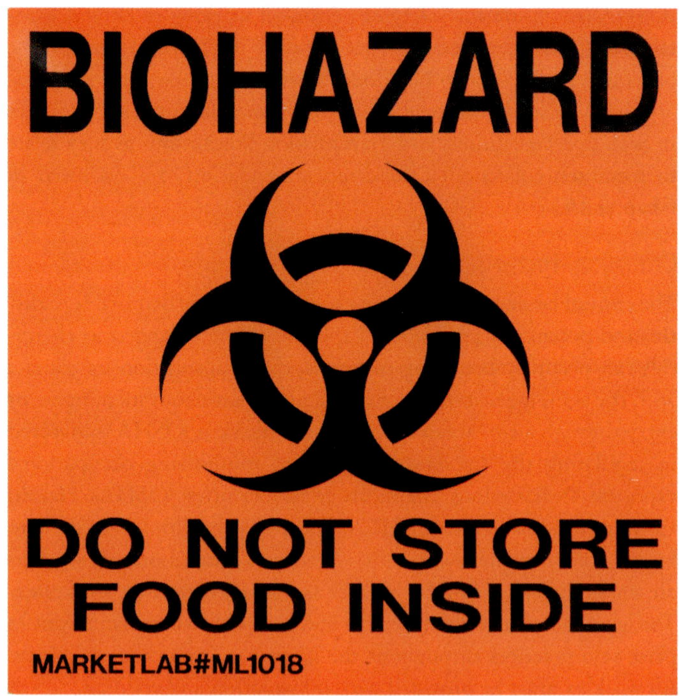

FIGURE 46.4 Biohazard symbol.

Biohazards and Infection Control

Biohazards, or biological hazards, are materials or situations that present the possible risk of infection (Figure 46.4). Infection with biohazard material can occur during specimen collection, handling, transportation, or testing. Specimens with the potential to be infectious include blood, body fluids, biological specimens, **exudates**, bacterial cultures, and smears. Infection can be introduced into the body in many ways; a few examples include the following:

- Breathing in a pathogen
- Accidental inoculation by a needlestick or **sharps** injury
- Aerosols created by uncapping specimen tubes
- Centrifuge accidents
- Entry of pathogens through a cut, abrasion, burn, or break in the skin

Standard Precautions

As described in Chapter 19, the CDC continuously monitors infection and disease in the United States. The CDC has also recommended preventive practices called Standard Precautions. These precautions apply to all patient care, regardless of the suspected or confirmed infection status of the patient. The precautions also apply to any setting where healthcare is delivered. The precautions are designed both to protect the healthcare provider and prevent the healthcare provider from spreading infections among patients.

Standard Precautions include the following five elements:

- Hand hygiene
- Use of PPE (e.g., gloves, gowns, masks, eye protection)
- Safe needle practices
- Safe handling of potentially contaminated equipment or surfaces in the patient environment
- Respiratory hygiene/cough etiquette

Hand Hygiene. According to the CDC, hand washing is the single most effective means of preventing infection. It is also the single most effective way of preventing the spread of infections. Proper hand sanitation protects you, your patient, and your co-workers because it removes or kills potentially pathogenic organisms from the skin surface. In the laboratory, it is essential to wash your hands with soap and water or use hand sanitizer in the following situations:

- When entering the laboratory or before leaving the laboratory
- Before putting on gloves and after removing gloves
- After contact with body fluid
- Before and after eating
- Before and after using the restroom

Bloodborne Pathogens Standard

In 1991 OSHA published the Bloodborne Pathogens Standard, which addressed ways to minimize or eliminate the risk of bloodborne pathogen exposures. The Bloodborne Pathogens Standard was created in response to the significant health risk associated with workplace exposure to blood and *other potentially infectious materials* (OPIMs) that may contain bloodborne pathogens. The Bloodborne Pathogens Standard covers all employees who could "reasonably anticipate contact with blood and other potentially infectious materials as the result of performing their job duties." Hepatitis B virus (HBV), hepatitis C virus (HCV), and human immunodeficiency virus (HIV) are constant hazards to clinical laboratory personnel.

Bloodborne pathogens are transmitted through exposure to blood and body fluids, which are the primary substances handled in the laboratory. Urine is the only fluid not specifically included in the standard. However, because blood and blood elements are frequently associated with urine, it must be included and considered a possible source of exposure.

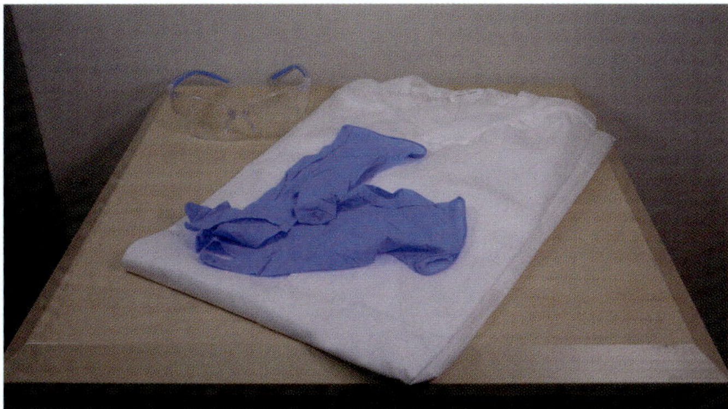

FIGURE 46.5 Personal protective equipment (PPE).

The Bloodborne Pathogens Standard requires that the laboratory employer have a written exposure control plan that proves steps have been taken so that the following information is available to protect employees:

- Written job categories of employees at risk of exposure to blood (laboratory workers are considered "high risk")
- HBV vaccination guidelines and records for each employee at risk
- Record of initial and annual bloodborne pathogens and safety training for each employee (including proper use of safety needles)
- Definition and listing of safe work practices: personal protective equipment (PPE) for all lab personnel (fluid-impermeable lab coats that do not leave the laboratory area, gloves, face protection [Figure 46.5]), and labeling of biohazard sharps and waste containers and their proper disposal.
- Sharps injury log of all work-related needlesticks and exposures to blood, with medical intervention after exposure incidents
- Written plan to maintain privacy of the individual exposed to blood
- Documentation of employee input on new safety devices

Proper Handling and Disposal Procedures for Blood and Other Potentially Infectious Materials

The following guidelines are required for handling blood and OPIMs:

- Use the appropriate PPE.
- Handle and process all specimens as if they contain infectious material.
- Wipe the outside of specimen containers with a germicide.
- Clean up spills using a disinfectant (see Chapter 19).
- Immediately dispose of any chipped or broken glassware into a sharps container using appropriate safety methods to prevent accidental punctures.

Dispose of all biohazardous waste according to state and federal guidelines. Disposal methods include treatment by heat, incineration, steam sterilization, chemical treatment, or other equivalent methods that will render the waste inactive before it is placed in a landfill. Disposal guidelines include the following:

- Infectious agents may be inactivated (such as using the autoclave) before disposal.
- Blood and potentially infectious materials mixed with chemicals are considered mixed waste. If possible, the infectious material should be inactivated, and the disposal should follow the chemical disposal procedure.

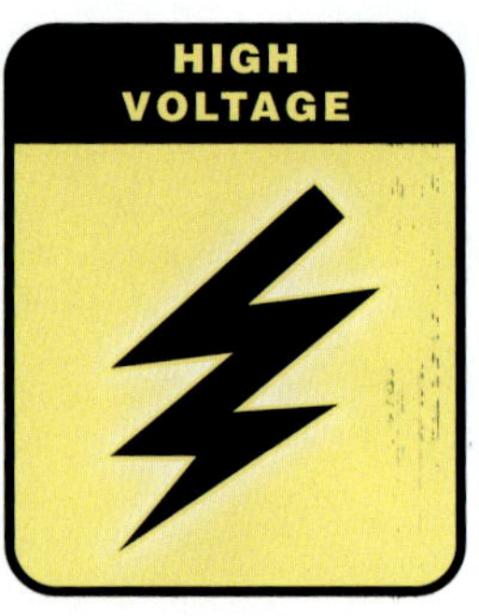

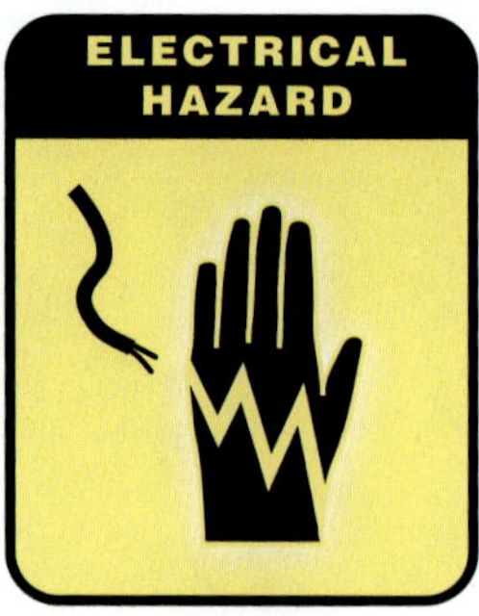

FIGURE 46.6 High voltage and electrical hazard labels.

- Biohazardous waste must be collected in impermeable, red polyethylene or polypropylene biohazard-labeled bags or containers and sealed.
- Used, disposable sharp items must be placed in a labeled, leakproof, puncture-resistant biohazard (sharps) container. When placing items into the sharps container, always place the sharp end in first. Never attempt to reach inside a sharps container. Sharps containers must be kept as close as possible to the work area. Sharps containers should be replaced when they are about 75% filled; never overfill them. Close the lid securely before removing and replacing the sharps container.
- Workers who handle biomedical waste should observe Standard Precautions.

First Aid Measures after an Exposure. If a blood or OPIM exposure occurs, a medical assistant must know the immediate steps to take. If you have an exposure to blood or OPIM, do the following:

- With a needlestick or an exposure to a cut or a body surface, wash the area with soap and warm, running water for 10 to 15 minutes as soon as possible after the exposure. Chlorine-based antiseptics and 10% iodine solution can also be used to clean the area.
- Flush splashes to the nose or mouth with water.
- Irrigate the eyes. Continuously flush them with water as soon as possible for a minimum of 15 minutes using an eyewash station.
- Report the incident to the supervisor and immediately seek medical treatment.

Physical Hazards

Physical hazards in the laboratory can be classified as electrical, fire, and mechanical hazards.

Electrical Hazards

Electric shock is a threat when any electrical equipment is in use. It is imperative to keep all electrical equipment in proper repair and always follow manufacturers' instructions.

To prevent electrical hazards, do the following:

- Use surge protectors.
- Inspect all cords and plugs frequently. Do not use damaged cords or plugs.
- Never use extension cords.
- Do not overload circuits.

Unplug the electrical device before servicing, and never operate electrical instruments with wet hands. If a sink is nearby, make sure electrical cords do not come in contact with the water supply. Workplace safeguards, such as signs and labels, should be placed on specific electrical hazards (Figure 46.6).

Fire Hazards

Open flames are rarely used in a laboratory anymore, but the potential for fire still exists. Fires may be ignited by smoking, heating elements, and sparks from electrical connections. Flammable materials should not be stored near any source of ignition. All laboratory personnel should be familiar with the locations of fire extinguishers and fire safety blankets. Fire extinguishers should be the carbon dioxide (CO_2), dry chemical, or halon type, known as the ABC type of extinguisher. ABC extinguishers can be used on all types of fires. Extinguishers should be inspected regularly by a licensed inspector and replaced or recharged if used. The medical assistant may be responsible for maintaining records on the care and maintenance of fire extinguishers (Procedure 46.3).

Fire safety blankets can be used to smother flames on burning clothing. However, a victim should not be wrapped in a fire blanket because it may intensify burns. Instead, the flames should be patted out or the victim directed to stop, drop, and roll on the blanket.

Emergency phone numbers should be posted on the wall near the telephone, and all personnel should know the locations of fire alarms, the fire escape routes, and procedures to follow if exits are blocked. Periodic fire drills should be conducted, and hallways and exits should be kept free of clutter.

Mechanical Hazards

Mechanical hazards arise from the use of laboratory equipment. Care should be exercised when using equipment with moving parts, such as a centrifuge. A laboratory centrifuge is a device that separates liquids from solids by rotating samples in a test tube at a high rate of speed. This forces heavier constituents of the sample to the bottom of the test tube and allows lighter constituents to remain at the top of the sample. Centrifuges present a hazard not only from moving parts but also from glassware that might break during centrifugation and from aerosols that might be created if tubes are not capped tightly.

Care should also be exercised when using equipment that relies on pressure, such as autoclaves. Autoclaves are used to sterilize metal instruments, microbiologic media, and some microbiologic waste. Autoclaves present a danger if opened prematurely before the pressure has come down to a safe level.

Although centrifuges and autoclaves often have built-in safeguards, such as locks that prevent entry until the environment is safe, improper care of the equipment can cause safety measures to fail.

SPECIMEN COLLECTION, PROCESSING, AND STORAGE

In the clinical laboratory setting, the medical assistant could be responsible for the specimen collection, processing, and storage. If any of those steps are done incorrectly, it can impact the results of the ordered tests. The following sections discuss those very important steps.

Laboratory Requisitions and Reports

When the provider orders laboratory testing, an electronic or paper requisition must be generated. Patient information on the requisitions must be complete, accurate, and legible. The patient is then directed to the POL, or the specimen is collected, prepared, and sent to an outside laboratory.

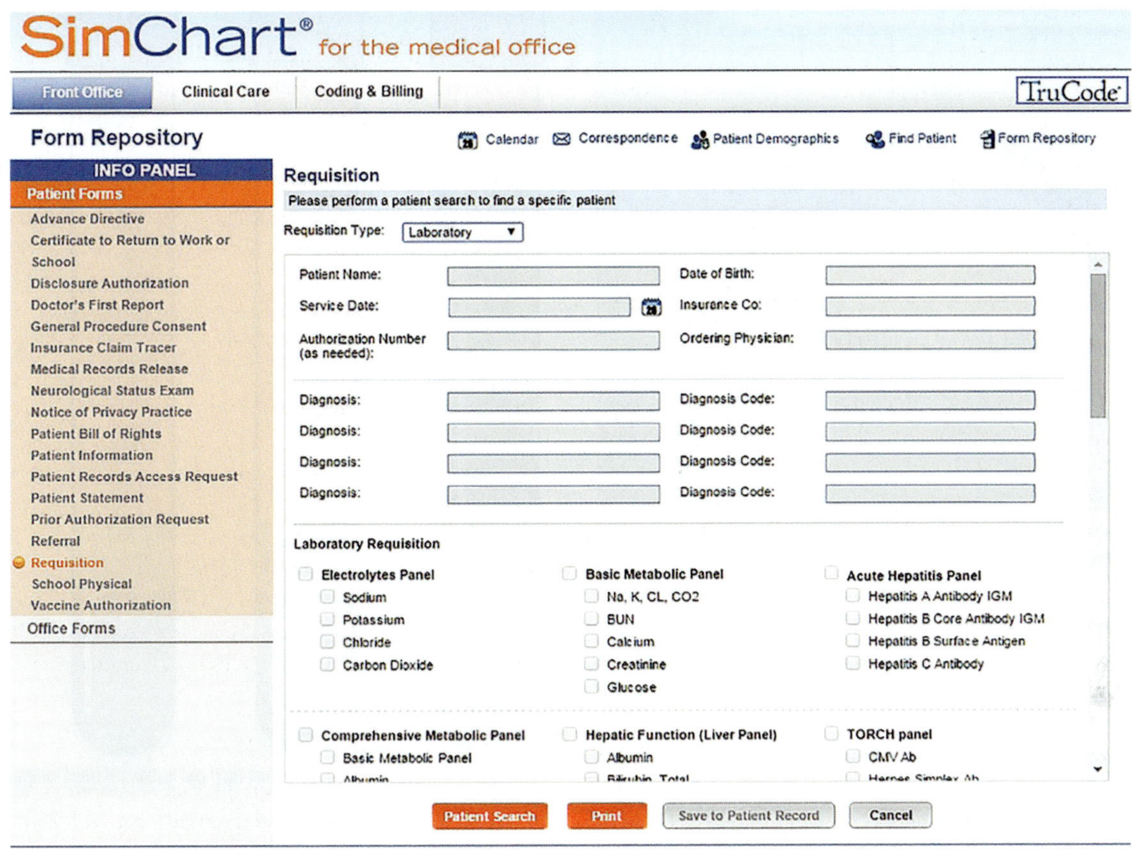

FIGURE 46.7 Electronic laboratory requisition form.

Figure 46.7 shows the electronic lab requisition form used in *SimChart for the Medical Office*. The following information typically is required on the requisition when specimens are sent to a reference laboratory:

- Provider's name, account number, address, and phone number
- Patient's full name, age, date of birth, gender, address, and insurance information
- Source of specimen
- Date and time of collection, and initials of the person collecting the specimen
- Specific test (or tests) requested
- Medications the patient is taking
- Whether the patient fasted or followed dietary restrictions if required, time of last intake
- Possible diagnosis
- Indication of whether the test is to be performed **STAT**

When the results of the tests are obtained, a laboratory report is sent to the office. The laboratory reports can be sent in two ways:

- Directly from the referral laboratory to the patient's EHR
- Electronically to the facility; then staff members upload the electronic document to the EHR or print it out for the paper medical record

A medical assistant is frequently responsible for making sure that all outside laboratory reports have been received and given to the provider for review. Testing results cannot be given to a patient until the provider has reviewed them. Any testing that is completed outside the POL at a reference lab must be tracked. This can be done by maintaining a master laboratory specimen log sheet or electronic file. This tracks patient specimens, tests ordered, designated lab results, and the provider's response.

Specimen Collection

The medical assistant is responsible for the collection of many different types of specimens. It is important to recognize that laboratory results are only as good as the specimen collected. The importance of proper specimen collection cannot be overemphasized. To ensure that test results are accurate indicators of the patient's state of health, it is critical that proper specimen collection procedures are understood and followed exactly. The most common specimens are blood, urine, and swab samples collected from wounds or mucous membranes. Specimens that may be collected less frequently include feces, gastric contents, CSF, tissue samples, semen, and **aspirates**.

Verifying the patient's identity before specimen collection is a critical step in the collection process. Patient identification should follow the written procedure for your institution. Using a minimum of two patient identifiers before specimen collection is standard. If the patient is not identified properly, the laboratory results that are generated will be useless.

Proper Choice of a Specimen Container

Another important step in specimen collection is the proper choice of a specimen container or collection tubes. For example, blood may be collected using a vacuum tube system. Blood collection tubes are available in a variety of sizes, depending on the collection needs. Blood collection tubes are also available with and without preservatives and **anticoagulants**. The tube stoppers are color coded. The

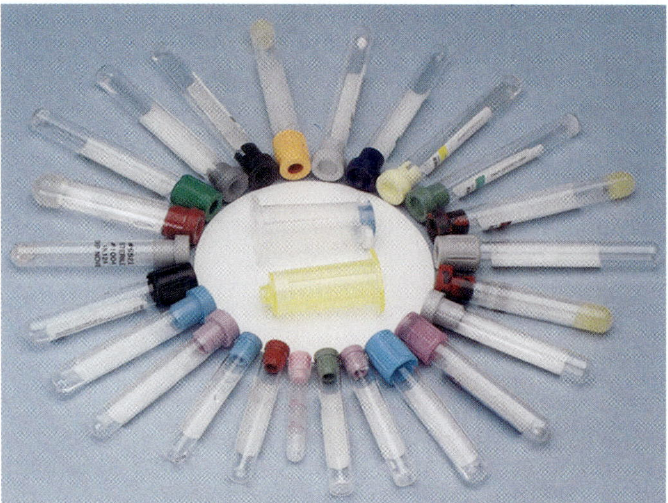

FIGURE 46.8 Vacutainer tubes with colored stoppers. (From Proctor D, et al: *Kinn's the medical assistant,* ed 13, St. Louis, 2017, Elsevier.)

color of the stopper indicates which additive is present, if any (Figure 46.8). Collection in an incorrect colored tube may result in an unacceptable specimen, and re-collection may be necessary.

If a specimen will be tested for the presence of microorganisms, a sterile container must be used. When a nonsterile container is used, it could cause contamination of the specimen. If patients are to collect the specimen at home, they should be provided with the appropriate container and complete instructions for collection. Patient education is an important role for the medical assistant. Each patient should receive clear instructions for proper home collection. Make sure your patients listen to the directions and ask them to repeat the instructions back to you so that you know they understand the information. Remember to be sensitive to individual patient factors (e.g., hearing, sight, primary language, cognitive capacity). These can affect the patient's understanding of the instructions, as well as his or her ability to follow through. Giving patients written directions to take home can also be helpful and reassuring.

Labeling. The specimen container or collection tube must be labeled properly at the time of collection. Unlabeled containers are not acceptable for laboratory testing and must be rejected. When labeling a sample container or collection tube, make sure you only use a black waterproof marker or pen, *never* pencil! All labels should include the following information, at a minimum:

- Patient's name: surname, first name, then middle initial
- Identification number
- Date (MM/DD/YYYY) and time of collection
- Specimen type
- Phlebotomist's or collector's initials

If affixing a computer-generated label, make sure to write the time and initial the specimen after the collection has been completed.

CRITICAL THINKING APPLICATION 46.6

As Greg has been working in phlebotomy, he has been reminded of the importance of patient identification. Write down three reasons why patient identification is critical to laboratory specimens. Be ready to share your reasons with the class.

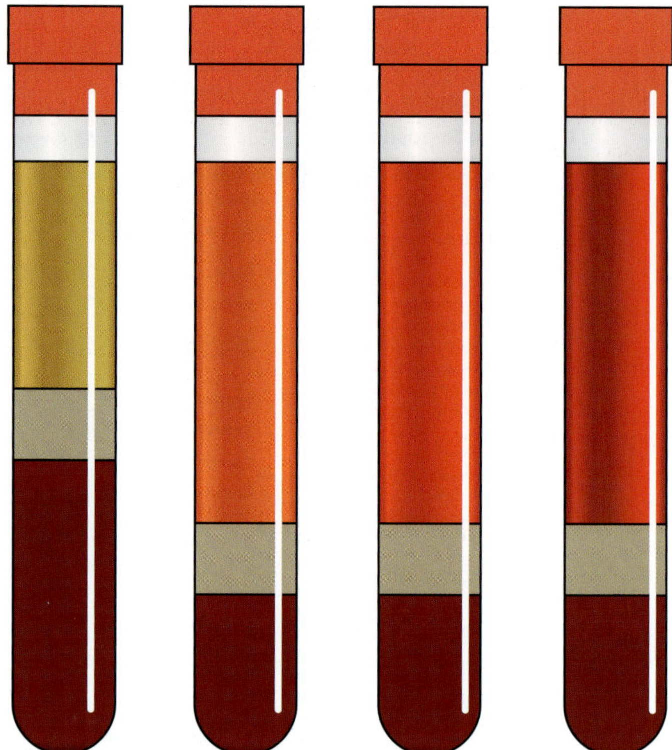

FIGURE 46.9 Normal *(left)* and hemolyzed blood samples.

Preventing Contamination

Medical assistants must take care to prevent the contamination of specimens and themselves. Expiration dates on swabs, tubes, transport media, and other collection containers should be checked before the items are used. Any expired materials should not be used and should be properly discarded. An improperly handled specimen may become contaminated or may contaminate the surrounding environment. Standard Precautions should be followed. Blood and body fluids from all patients should be considered infectious.

The specimen collected must be a true representative sample. A swab for a wound culture collected from the surface of the wound generally does not yield the same results as one taken from the depths of the wound. A **hemolyzed** blood specimen shows marked differences in many tests (Figure 46.9). If a large volume of specimen is collected (e.g., a 24-hour urine specimen), the total volume or weight must be carefully measured and recorded. The specimen must be well mixed before an **aliquot** is removed and submitted for testing.

Handling, Processing, and Storing Specimens

Specimens must be handled, processed, and stored according to test manufacturer's guidelines to prevent any changes that would affect test results. In Chapters 47 through 50, specimen handling, processing, and storage are discussed for each specific area of the laboratory. Each department in the lab has unique testing and specimen requirements. Some general guidelines to keep in mind include the following:

- The storage temperature of the specimen should follow manufacturer's testing requirements.
- Serum must be separated from red blood cells as soon as possible after the specimen has clotted to prevent changes caused by the metabolism of the blood cells.

- Specimens for chemistry and liver panels may need to be protected from light.
- Specimens may need to be frozen to prevent chemical constituents from changing. Follow manufacturer's guidelines for freezing a specimen.
- Manufacturers' package inserts or reference laboratory specimen requirements should be consulted to ensure that each specimen is handled and processed properly.

Using Reference Laboratories

The medical assistant should always check the laboratory's specimen requirements manual or reference laboratory website for any unfamiliar tests. A clear understanding of the specimen and collection requirements is very important. Any unanswered questions should be resolved by calling the reference laboratory before collecting the specimen.

Most offices have a laboratory courier service that picks up specimens periodically throughout the day. Specimens should be properly stored (some may require refrigeration) until the courier arrives. Instructions for properly obtaining, processing, and preparing a specimen for transport are usually supplied by the testing laboratory. If the instructions are not clear, or if you have a question about a particular test collection, the reference laboratory should be able to answer the question over the phone. Criteria for safe shipping of specimens include the following:

- Length of time acceptable for transport
- Recommended temperature range to maintain the specimen
- Appropriate material packaging if the specimen needs to be protected from light

If the specimen is to be mailed, it must be carefully packaged to prevent breakage, damage, or contamination during handling. Follow the instructions for transport supplied by the reference laboratory. Do not ship specimens without proper packaging and labeling as specified by the test laboratory.

Chain of Custody

When a specimen may be needed as evidence in a court case, certain procedures must be followed when collecting and handling the specimen. **Forensic** or legal specimens should be collected, handled, and stored in a manner consistent with established standards designated by law. Specimen processing must be documented precisely, ensuring no tampering with evidence has occurred. *Chain of custody* refers to the stepwise method used to collect, process, and test a specimen. The documentation must be signed by every person who had any contact with the specimen, from collection to the final reporting of results. Blood alcohol level testing and drug screening often require chain of custody handling. Everything needed for the collection of the specimen is provided in a kit: the gloves, the vacuum tube, and the needle used to collect the blood specimen. Documentation is included and must be signed by all personnel. Medical assistants and phlebotomists can be subpoenaed to testify in court about specimens they have collected. It is always in your best interest to follow chain of custody procedures exactly.

CRITICAL THINKING APPLICATION **46.7**

What is the difference between a patient specimen and a forensic specimen? In your own words, describe *chain of custody*.

TABLE 46.3 Greenwich Time and Military Time

GREENWICH TIME	MILITARY TIME
1:00 a.m.	0100 hours
3:00 a.m.	0300 hours
5:00 a.m.	0500 hours
7:00 a.m.	0700 hours
9:00 a.m.	0900 hours
11:00 a.m.	1100 hours
1:00 p.m.	1300 hours
3:00 p.m.	1500 hours
5:00 p.m.	1700 hours
7:00 p.m.	1900 hours
9:00 p.m.	2100 hours
11:00 p.m.	2300 hours
12:00 a.m. (midnight)	2400 hours

LABORATORY MATHEMATICS AND MEASUREMENT

All laboratory testing relies on the accurate use of values, units, and measurements. For example, values are used for reporting the time the sample was collected, the volume of the specimen, the amount of analyte found in a specimen, and dilutions used in sample preparation and for recording QC results.

Measuring Time

Time of day is a critical factor in patient care. Medications must be administered, diets must be followed, and specimens must be collected on a timed schedule. Many laboratories use the 24-hour clock when recording time; this method avoids the confusion that comes with the *Greenwich clock*, which uses a.m. (morning) and p.m. (afternoon) designations.

The 24-hour clock system, also known as *military time,* is expressed with four digits in terms of "hundred hours." Noon is referred to as 1200 (twelve hundred) hours; midnight is 0000 (zero hundred), or 2400 hours. The military clock is based on 24 60-minute hours, as is the Greenwich clock; therefore, 5:35 p.m. is expressed as 1735 (seventeen thirty-five) hours (Table 46.3).

CRITICAL THINKING APPLICATION **46.8**

If the time on the clock is 10 a.m., how would you write that in military time? If the time is 10 p.m., how would you write that in military time? If the time on a document is written as 1900 hours, how would you write it in Greenwich time? How would you write it if it had been documented as 0800 hours?

TABLE 46.4 Common Laboratory Temperature Settings

	FAHRENHEIT	CELSIUS
Refrigerator	35°–46°	2°–8°
Freezer	32°	0°
Room	59°–86°	15°–30°
Incubator	98.6°	37°
Body temperature	98.6°	37°
Autoclave	254°	121°

Measuring Temperature

Two scales are currently used for measuring temperature; each is divided into units called *degrees* (Table 46.4). The Fahrenheit scale is considered part of the *English system* of measurement and is the scale most commonly used in the United States. The *sys scale*, formerly called the centigrade scale, is used in countries that apply the *metric system*. On the Celsius (C) scale, water freezes at 0°C and boils at 100°C. On the Fahrenheit (F) scale, water freezes at 32°F and boils at 212°F. Almost all laboratories in the United States use the Celsius scale for temperature.

Converting Temperatures

To change from Fahrenheit to Celsius:

98.6°F = ____________°C	SOLUTION:
Step 1: Subtract 32 from F temp	98.6 – 32 = 66.6
Step 2: Divide number by 1.8	66.6 / 1.8 = 37°C

To change from Celsius to Fahrenheit:

100°C = ____________°F	SOLUTION:
Step 1: Multiply C temp by 1.8	100 × 1.8 = 180
Step 2: Add 32 to that number	180 + 32 = 212°F

Units of Measurement

The units of measurement we commonly use in the United States differ from those used in the laboratory. In everyday life, we use the English system of measurement (Table 46.5). In the laboratory, the metric system and the Système International (SI) are used. It is important for medical assistants to memorize and practice these systems so that they can communicate professionally.

The metric system is based on a decimal system, which consists of basic units and prefixes that indicate a system of division in multiples of 10. Prefixes are added to each symbol to reduce or enlarge them by units of 10. See Tables 46.6 and 46.7 for an overview of metric system measurements.

International organizations, such as the World Health Organization (WHO), officially recognize SI units. Many countries have adopted this system, but the United States has not completely converted to it. The SI is an adaptation of the metric system that uses several basic units, although some units are different for reporting results. For example, blood glucose is reported in millimoles per liter (mmol/L) using the SI system, but it is reported as milligrams per deciliter (mg/dL) using the metric system. Therefore, it is very important for the medical assistant to double-check the laboratory's standard and include the appropriate units of measurement when reporting test values.

TABLE 46.5 Comparing the English System of Measurement with the Metric System

	ENGLISH SYSTEM OF MEASUREMENT	METRIC SYSTEM
Weight	Ounces (oz) and pounds (lb)	Grams (g)
Length	Inches and feet	Meters (m)
Volume	Cups and quarts	Liters (L)

CRITICAL THINKING APPLICATION 46.9

If you had 3.2 grams of salt and you wanted to express it in milligrams, how would you write it? If the length of an item were 455 centimeters and you wanted to express it in meters, how would you write it?

Measuring Liquid Volume

Test tubes are used to test or hold liquid reagents, samples, or aliquots. Test tubes come in many sizes and are typically disposable. Test tubes may be sterile for use in microbiology. When liquids are measured into test tubes, the most common piece of glassware used is the *pipet*. A pipet is a hollow tube that can be made from glass or plastic. Pipets often have lines to indicate volume on the length of the tube. Some plastic pipets have a built-in bulb to help transfer fluids and are known as transfer pipets. This type of pipet usually does not have any measurement lines on the tube. Figure 46.10 shows a variety of transfer pipets that are used in the laboratory. Micropipets are used to deliver very small volumes of liquid (Figure 46.11). These pipetting devices must be fitted with an appropriate disposable tip. The device is equipped with a piston at the top, which must be depressed before the pipet is filled and when the pipet is drained. It is important to follow the manufacturer's instructions for use with all pipets and micropipets. Each type of pipet may be slightly different.

LABORATORY EQUIPMENT

The three most common pieces of equipment found in a clinical laboratory are a microscope, a centrifuge, and an incubator. It is important for medical assistants working in a clinical laboratory setting to have a basic understanding of these pieces of equipment. The following sections discuss them.

TABLE 46.6 Metric System: Prefixes of Measurements

PREFIXES	SIZE	OR ANOTHER WAY TO LOOK AT IT	
Kilo (k)	1000 base units	1 kilo = 1000 base units	Larger than the base unit
Hecto	100 base units	1 hecto = 100 base units	
Deka	10 base units	1 deka = 10 base units	
Base Units (Meter, Liter, or Gram)			
Deci	0.1 base unit	10 deci = 1 base unit	Smaller than the base unit
Centi (c)	0.01 base unit	100 centi = 1 base unit	
Milli (m)	0.001 base unit	1000 milli = 1 base unit	
Micro (mc)	0.000001 base unit	1,000,000 micro = 1 base unit	

TABLE 46.7 Common Units of Measure Seen in Healthcare

VOLUME	LENGTH	WEIGHT
Liter (L)	Meter (m)	Gram (g)
Milliliter (mL or ml)	Centimeter (cm)	Kilogram (kg)
Cubic centimeter (cc)	Millimeter (mm)	Milligram (mg)
cc = mL		Microgram (mcg)

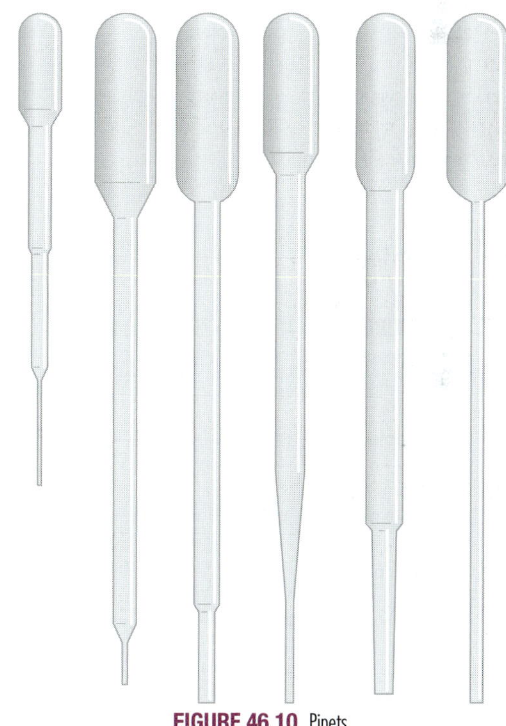

FIGURE 46.10 Pipets.

Microscope

Nearly every medical laboratory is equipped with a *microscope*. This indispensable instrument is used to view objects too small to be seen with the naked eye (Figure 46.12). The microscope is used to evaluate stained blood smears, urine sediment, vaginal secretions, and smears made from body fluids and microorganisms.

Microscopic procedures are not considered CLIA-waived tests because they require judgment and additional training. In addition, an error in reading microscopic tests may have a detrimental effect on the patient's care. Providers petitioned the CMS to create a new laboratory category that would allow them to perform a set of simple microscopic tests that could be performed in the ambulatory setting (Table 46.8). The CMS approved the list and created an additional CLIA category called *provider-performed microscopy procedures* (PPMP). Certified CLIA-PPMP laboratories must meet the same quality standards as laboratories that perform moderate-complexity tests, including passing three proficiency tests from an outside agency per year. The medical assistant is taught how to prepare the microscope slide and bring it into focus. The final analysis of a microscope slide must be made by one of the following personnel:

- Physician (medical doctor, doctor of osteopathy, or doctor of podiatric medicine)
- Midlevel practitioner (nurse midwife, nurse practitioner, or physician's assistant)
- Dentist (doctor of dental surgery or doctor of dental medicine) trained as a laboratory professional with CLIA moderate- or high-complexity training
- A CLS or CLT trained in moderate and highly complex testing

Microscopes have three components:

- The magnification system, which focuses the image
- The illumination system, which brings the image from the slide to the viewer
- The framework, which includes all components responsible for positioning the slide

The magnification system includes the ocular and objective lenses, plus the fine and coarse knobs used to adjust the clarity. Microscopes may be monocular or binocular. A monocular microscope has one eyepiece for viewing, and a binocular microscope has two. The eyepiece, or ocular, is located at the top of the microscope and contains a lens to magnify what is being viewed.

The usual ocular magnification is 10 times (10×). In addition to the ocular, compound microscopes have objective lenses that increase the magnification of the specimen. The objectives are attached to the revolving nosepiece. Most microscopes have four objectives, each with a different magnifying power:

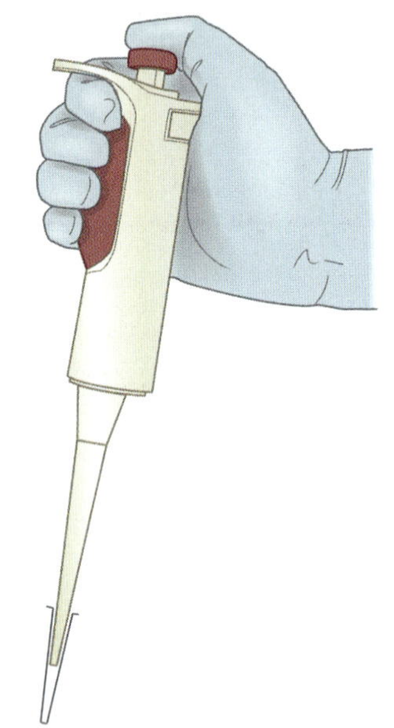

FIGURE 46.11 Micropipet with disposable tip.

- The shortest objective has the lowest power (4×) and is called the *scanning lens.* This lens is used to scan the field of interest and then focus on a particular object.
- Greater detail is observed with the next longest objective, which is low power (10×).
- The high or high dry objective usually has a magnification of 40× or 45×.
- The longest objective, oil immersion (100×), allows the finest focusing of the object and requires the use of a special oil that is placed directly on the slide. This special oil, called *immersion oil,* prevents refraction of the light and improves the resolution (clarity) of the magnified image. Oil immersion is used to view cells and extremely small materials (e.g., bacteria and platelets) and to examine stained specimens.

The total magnification of the specimen is determined by multiplying the magnification of the objective lens by 10 (the magnification of the ocular lens). Therefore, if you have the 10× objective in place when observing blood cells, you are magnifying the image 100 times. Just above the base are the focusing knobs. The coarse adjustment is used only with scanning and low-power lenses, and the fine adjustment is used with high-power and oil immersion lenses.

The arm of the microscope connects the objectives and the oculars to the base, which supports the microscope and contains its light source. The stage of the microscope holds the slide to be viewed. Under the stage is the light source, the condenser, and the iris diaphragm, which make up the illumination system. The condenser directs light up through the slide, and the iris diaphragm regulates the amount of light passing through the specimen.

Microscopes are very precise and expensive instruments that require careful handling. The amount of routine maintenance required depends on the amount of daily use. Dirt is the enemy

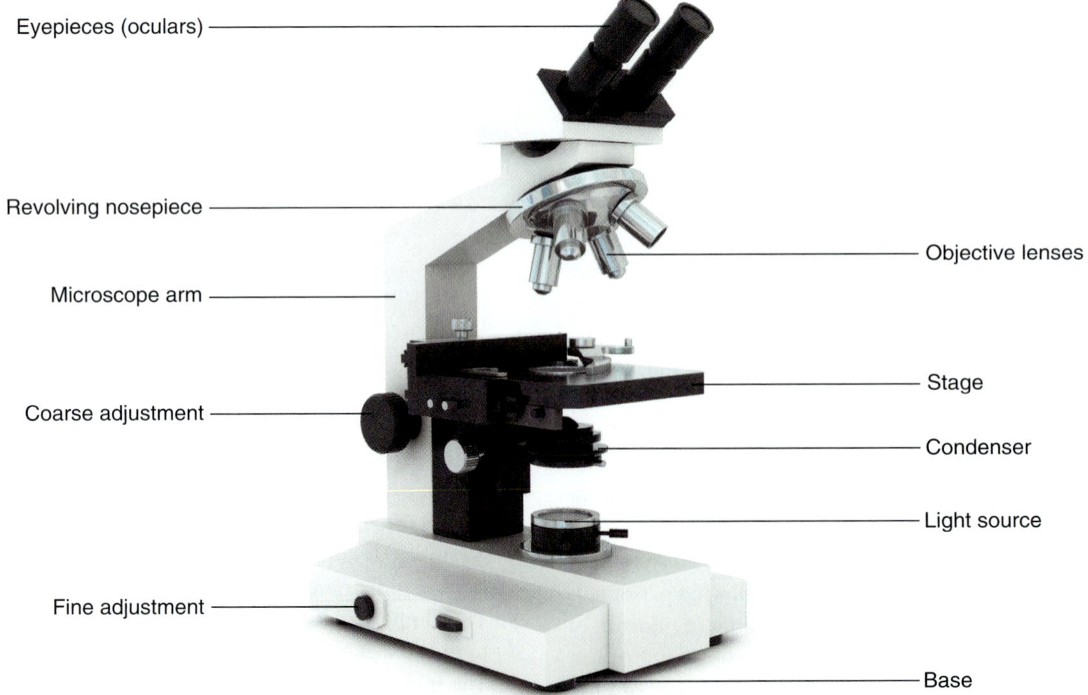

FIGURE 46.12 The parts of a microscope. (Courtesy urfinguss/iStock/thinkstock.)

TABLE 46.8 CLIA-Approved Procedures for Provider-Performed Microscopy (PPM)

TEST NAME	DESCRIPTION	EXAMPLE
Direct wet mount	Examination of specimens for the presence or absence of bacteria, fungi, parasites, and human cellular elements	Observing vaginal secretions for the presence of yeast to assist with diagnosis of vulvovaginal candidiasis
KOH preparation	Any preparation using potassium hydroxide	Observing skin scrapings for the presence of fungi
Fecal leukocyte examination	Simple stain of fecal specimen; assists in diagnosis of diarrheal disease	Leukocytes are found in stool in antibiotic-associated colitis, ulcerative colitis, shigellosis, and salmonellosis
Pinworm examination	Preparations are observed for the presence or absence of *Enterobius vermicularis* eggs	Performing a cellulose tape collection for pinworms
Postcoital direct, qualitative examinations	Vaginal or cervical mucus is examined 4–10 hours after intercourse for the presence of live, motile sperm	Assists in the diagnosis of infertility
Qualitative semen analysis	Semen is examined for the presence or absence of spermatozoa; motility of the sperm is noted	Assists in post vasectomy semen analysis and in the diagnosis of infertility
Urine sediment examination	Urine sediment is examined for the presence or absence of formed elements	Part of a routine urinalysis (see Chapter 47, Procedure 46.4, Prepare a Urine Specimen for Microscopic Examination)

CLIA, Clinical Laboratory Improvement Amendments; *KOH,* potassium hydroxide.

of the microscope, which must be kept very clean at all times. Oil, makeup, dust, and eye secretions can all obstruct vision through the lens and may transmit infective organisms. The microscope should always be stored in a plastic dust cover when not in use. Lenses should be cleaned before and after each use with lens paper and lens cleaner. Any other type of tissue scratches the lenses or leaves lint residue behind. Routine use of solvent cleaners, such as xylene, is not recommended because these cleaners may loosen a lens. The body of the microscope should be dusted with a soft cloth.

The microscope should be placed in a permanent location in the laboratory, on a sturdy table, in an area where it cannot be bumped. If a microscope must be moved, it should be carried securely, with one hand supporting the base and the other holding the arm. When the microscope is stored, it should be left covered with the low-power objective in the highest position. The stage should be centered.

Using a microscope involves focusing and illumination (Procedure 46.4). The image is focused by moving the objectives closer to the specimen using the fine and coarse knobs. Proper focusing begins with the objective at the lowest power. The coarse adjustment moves the objective quickly. This knob is used first to bring the specimen into approximate focus. The fine adjustment focus knob then brings the specimen into precise focus. The fine focus moves the objective more slowly to allow the viewer to zero in on the specimen with greater accuracy. Illumination is accomplished by raising or lowering the condenser and by opening and closing the diaphragm on the condenser.

If the microscope is a binocular model, the eyepieces may need to be adjusted to accommodate the distance between the pupils and the individual's point of greatest visual acuity. A gentle push inward or pull outward adjusts the distance between the eyepieces.

Centrifuge

A centrifuge is an instrument that is used to separate solids from liquids. A centrifuge works by rapidly spinning the specimen, which increases the gravitational force. The increased force pushes the heavier solids to the bottom of the specimen and lets lighter liquids remain at the top of the specimen. Centrifugation is used to separate blood cells from serum or plasma. It is also used to separate solid materials in urine specimens, such as cells and crystals.

Centrifuges (Figure 46.13) are designed for specific uses. They may be bench-top or floor models; some may be refrigerated. Some may have rotating parts or members known as *rotors* or heads that are interchangeable to accommodate different-sized sample tubes. Centrifuge configurations vary with the laboratory task that needs to be done. Here are the three common configurations used in the clinical laboratory:

- A centrifuge that has a fixed-angle *rotor,* where specimen cups are held in a rigid position at a fixed angle
- A centrifuge that has a horizontal head with buckets that swing out horizontally during centrifugation
- A centrifuge used for centrifuging capillary tubes for microhematocrit testing (see Chapter 48)

Directions for using a centrifuge usually are given in terms of revolutions per minute (rpm). Spinning generates centrifugal force, causing the heaviest particles in a liquid to migrate to the bottom of the tube. Centrifuges can be dangerous if not used correctly. The most important rule is to ensure that the centrifuge is balanced so that tubes of equal size and equal volume are directly across from one another in the rotor holders or buckets. Therefore, there must always be an even number of tubes in the

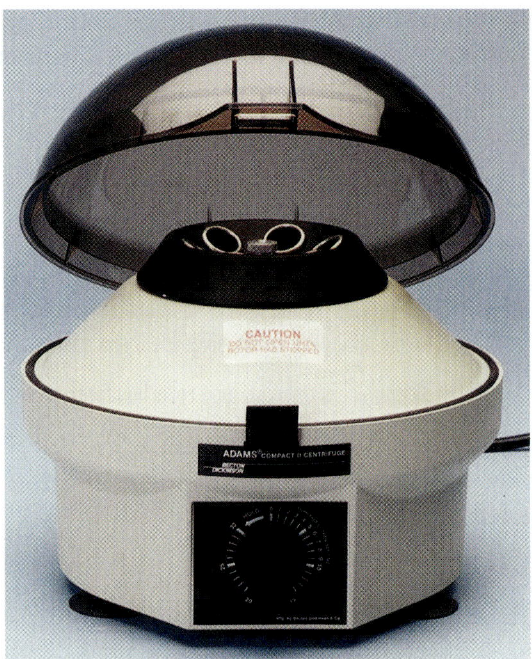

FIGURE 46.13 A centrifuge.

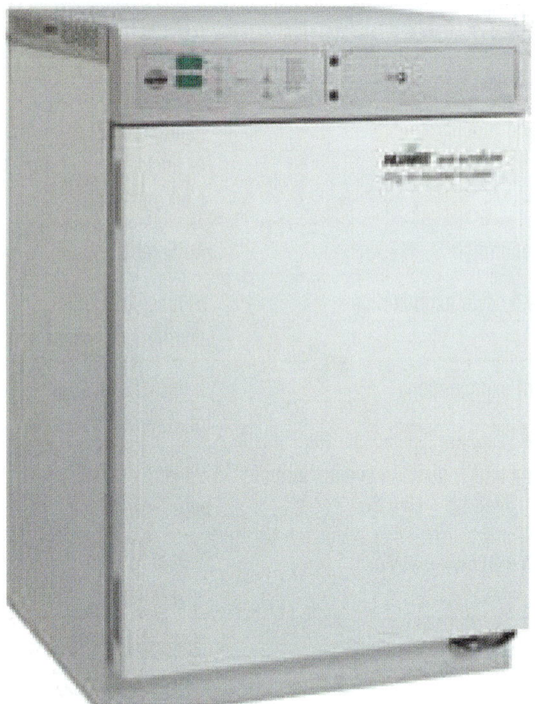

FIGURE 46.14 An incubator. (Courtesy NuAire, Plymouth, MN.)

centrifuge. An exception to this rule is if there is one empty space between each tube, then there can be an odd number of tubes. If a second specimen of the same volume in the same-sized tube is not available for balance, a tube of water may be used to balance the load. Tubes being centrifuged should be capped to prevent samples from creating aerosols during spinning. Rubber cups should be placed at the bottom of the carrier cups to prevent breakage of the glass tubes.

Centrifuges should never be opened while they are in operation, nor should you attempt to slow a centrifuge with your hands. Most centrifuges are equipped with a brake, which should be used only in an emergency, the most common of which is a broken glass tube. In this case, wait until the centrifuge comes to a complete stop and follow the manufacturer's instructions for disinfecting the unit; also, follow Standard Precautions to prevent injury and disease transmission.

Centrifuges should be regularly checked, cleaned, and lubricated to ensure proper operation. A certified technician must ensure the centrifuge's speed to comply with quality assurance guidelines set forth by the College of American Pathologists (CAP).

Incubator

Incubators are cabinets that maintain constant temperatures (Figure 46.14). Generally used in the microbiology laboratory, an incubator can be set to a specific temperature. Microbiology departments usually maintain a constant temperature of 35° to 37°C (95° to 98.6°F), although other temperatures may also be appropriate. Incubators usually have warning alarms that sound if the temperature exceeds or falls below a specified range. The temperature should be checked daily, and the cabinets should be cleaned regularly with a disinfectant approved by the manufacturer. These procedures should be documented every time they are completed.

See Figure 46.15 for an example of a laboratory maintenance log. All laboratory equipment that is temperature sensitive should have temperatures checked and recorded daily.

CLOSING COMMENTS

Patient Coaching

For many testing procedures, patients must be given a specific set of instructions to follow. The provider often communicates the instructions to the patient but may also ask the medical assistant to reinforce the information. For example, patients may be required to fast 8 to 12 hours before blood samples are collected.

Often, the medical assistant is responsible for communicating provider directions that need to be followed before laboratory testing. Make sure you have reviewed the provider's orders correctly before explaining the procedure to the patient. The patient should be given verbal and written instructions prior to testing. Also, include a phone number on the instruction sheet so the patient can call if he or she has questions after returning home.

Legal and Ethical Issues

If disease did not exist, there would be little need for clinical laboratories. The fact that the human body is susceptible to disease necessitates the existence of laboratory testing. All health and safety risks cannot be anticipated or eliminated, but the risks are greatly reduced when everyone who works in the laboratory is conscious of safety guidelines.

Use common sense, and document everything. If you are in doubt about the safety of a procedure, ask your supervisor. If you are

Medical clinic								
Daily maintenance control chart								
MONTH	YEAR							
DAY	Daily					Monthly		BY
	Refrig	Freezer	Room	Incubator	Bleach	Eyewash	Shower	
	2°–8°C	–0°–20°C	15°–30°C	34°–36°C	Counters	Checked	Checked	
1								
2								
3								
4								
5								

FIGURE 46.15 An example of a laboratory maintenance log.

aware of a potential safety problem, report it to the person in charge. Your welfare, the welfare of the patient, and your co-workers may depend on your commitment to safety.

Patient-Centered Care

Before the patient receives test results, the medical assistant must make sure the provider has reviewed and signed the results and has given permission for the patient to be told about them. Most providers personally inform patients of laboratory results, but some providers may delegate this duty to office staff. Regardless of who informs the patient of test results, the individual must make sure the specific guidelines for communication are followed as stipulated in the patient's Health Insurance Portability and Accountability Act (HIPAA) release form. Maintaining a patient's privacy and confidentiality are crucial factors that must be considered when dealing with test results.

Professional Behaviors

The next four chapters discuss the most common CLIA-waived tests performed in the POL. They cover patient education, preparation, specimen collection, and testing procedures, which are all aspects of professionalism you must develop as you work with others and document your results appropriately. Look over the professionalism evaluation form in your study guide to see what actions you should take to become a professional in the laboratory classroom. At the end of the laboratory chapters, your instructor may meet with you one-on-one to discuss your evaluation results, or you may do a self-evaluation of your performance.

SUMMARY OF SCENARIO

Greg has had a busy day in the laboratory. He has reviewed safety policies and procedures, reacquainted himself with waived laboratory testing, and had a refresher on units of measure. He is looking forward to another day of training in the lab tomorrow, when he will be running some urinalysis tests.

There is a lot to remember and learn, but with some extra effort, review with Julie, and hands-on testing practice, Greg will become more comfortable in his new department. He thinks the change will be a good move for him.

SUMMARY OF LEARNING OBJECTIVES

1. **Examine the organization of the clinical laboratory.**
Clinical laboratory personnel are responsible for analyzing blood and body fluids and sending the provider the test results, which become part of the essential data for diagnosing and managing a patient's condition. Medical assistants are responsible for collecting specimens, instructing patients, and performing tests that have been waived by the Clinical Laboratory Improvement Amendments (CLIA) and some moderately complex testing.
Most physician offices that perform laboratory testing do so in the areas of urinalysis, hematology, chemistry, and microbiology. Routine urinalysis, complete blood counts, glucose tests, and throat cultures are some of the tests that might be performed in a physician's office laboratory (POL).
2. **Examine the impact of the Clinical Laboratory Improvement Amendments on the clinical laboratory.**
A CLIA-waived test is one that has been approved by the Food and Drug Administration (FDA) for over-the-counter sales and may be performed in certified CLIA-waived laboratories (i.e., POLs). The test has been determined to pose no unreasonable risk of harm if performed incorrectly. More complex tests that require additional training or education may be performed only in CLIA-certified moderate- or high-complexity laboratories. *Note:* Providers may perform certain microscopic exams if they are certified to perform provider-performed microscopy (PPM) procedures.
CLIA established the standards of quality for laboratory testing. Medical assistants are allowed to perform and monitor all CLIA-waived tests. Table 46.2 summarizes the CLIA-waived tests that may be performed in a registered CLIA-waived laboratory and the common diseases or conditions in which they are used.
3. **Examine quality assurance and quality control in the clinical laboratory setting.**
Quality assurance (QA) involves all the procedures undertaken to ensure that each patient is provided excellent care. Quality control (QC), which determines whether a laboratory test is accurate, precise, and reliable, is one part of a QA program. Procedure 46.1 outlines the steps for analyzing the reliability of a test based on the results of running its control and documenting the results on a laboratory flow sheet.

Continued

SUMMARY OF LEARNING OBJECTIVES—*continued*

4. **Examine all aspects of laboratory safety.**
The importance of safety in the laboratory cannot be overemphasized. The US government created a system of safeguards and regulations under the Occupational Safety and Health Act of 1970. Two programs have been mandated by OSHA to ensure the safety of personnel working in clinical laboratories; one covers occupational exposure to chemical hazards and the other covers exposure to bloodborne pathogens.

All workers must be provided with information and training, and a Safety Data Sheet (SDS, formerly MSDS) must be on file for all chemicals used in the laboratory. OSHA requires the manufacturer of the chemical to make these sheets available, usually as a package insert or online.

The medical facility must do the following: provide an annual formal safety training program to review and update physical, biological, and chemical hazards that apply to the laboratory; maintain an up-to-date safety procedures manual; provide safety equipment (e.g., fire blankets, fire extinguishers, eyewash stations, and personal protective equipment) to all employees; make sure chemicals are clearly marked with the National Fire Protection Association (NFPA) diamond; make sure SDSs are bound in an accessible manual; reinforce the principles of Standard Precautions when any biological material is handled.

5. **Examine the process of completing laboratory requisitions, handling reports, specimen collection, processing, and storage in the clinical laboratory.**
The laboratory requisition must include all information needed to identify the patient, the ordering provider, the test ordered, insurance information, and the specific details regarding the collection of the specimen (e.g., time and source).

Identification of the patient is the first essential step. If the patient is to collect the specimen at home, he or she should be provided with the appropriate container and complete instructions for collection. Bear in mind the principles of patient education, and be sensitive to factors that can affect the patient's understanding of the instructions for specimen collection. Review the eight steps to follow when collecting specimens and informing patients of their results.

Chain of custody is a method used to ensure that a specimen provided by a patient who may be involved in a legal matter is handled in a fashion that does not compromise the test results. All individuals who handle or test the specimen must be identified in writing and must provide a signature.

6. **Examine how mathematics and measurements are used in the clinical laboratory.**
Many laboratories use the 24-hour clock when recording time, which avoids the confusion that comes with the Greenwich clock. Two scales are used for measuring temperature: Fahrenheit and Celsius. Almost all laboratories in the United States use the Celsius scale for temperature.

Liquid volume is measured in liters, distance is measured in meters, and mass is measured in grams. Prefixes commonly used in clinical laboratories include *deci-* (0.1), *centi-* (0.01), *milli-* (0.001), *micro-* (0.000001), and *kilo-* (1000).

7. **Examine the common equipment found in the clinical laboratory.**
The parts of the microscope can be divided into the illumination system (light source, condenser, and iris diaphragm lever), the frame (base, adjustment knobs, arm, stage, and stage control), and the magnification system (objective lenses on the revolving nosepiece and oculars). The illumination system controls the light that passes through the specimen to the eye, the frame provides the structure for the instrument and the components that allow for adjustment of the sample, and the magnification system provides the ground-glass lenses that magnify the specimen. Refer to Table 46.8 for a list of microscopy tests that may be performed in the ambulatory care setting.

To use a centrifuge safely, the proper tube must be used, and it must be protected from breakage. Centrifuge loads must be carefully balanced, and specimens must be capped to prevent aerosols. Under no circumstances should a centrifuge be opened while it is in operation.

Incubators are cabinets that maintain constant temperatures. They generally are used in a microbiology laboratory. The temperature should be checked daily.

PROCEDURE 46.1 Perform a Quality Control Measure on a Glucometer and Record the Results on a Flow Sheet

TASKS: Test and analyze the results of glucometer controls to see whether a glucometer is producing reliable test results, and record the results on the laboratory flow sheet.

EQUIPMENT and SUPPLIES

- Fluid-impermeable lab coat, gloves, and protective eyewear
- Glucometer
- Coded test strips designed for the glucometer used
- Control solution provided by the manufacturer
- Package insert showing directions on how to run the glucometer
- Biohazard waste container
- Waste container
- Glucose test-control flow sheet

The three color-coded bottles of controls (1, 2, and 3) in the figure will produce high, low, and normal test results. The test strip is to the right of the glucometer, and the container for the test strips is on the far right (Figure 1).

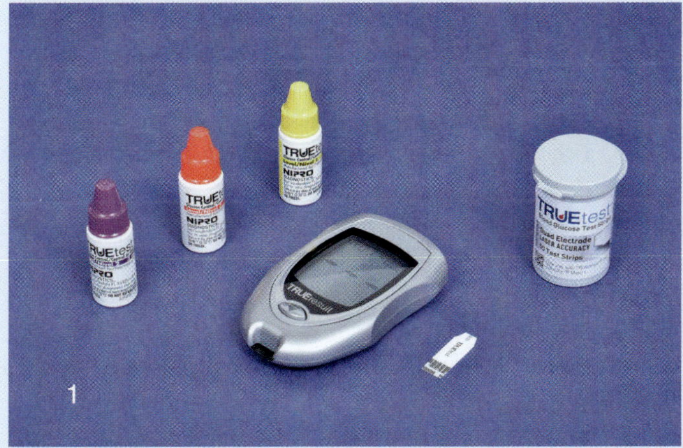

PROCEDURAL STEPS

1. Put on a lab coat. Wash your hands or use hand sanitizer. Put on gloves and eye protection. Comply with safety practices during the procedure.
   PURPOSE: Hand sanitization is an important step for infection control. PPE is necessary when working with any control or specimen material.
2. Take a coded strip out of the bottle and note the control level and range listed on the control bottle or the strip container. Close the coded strip bottle.
3. Review the directions on the glucometer package insert. Calibrate the meter by inserting the precoded test strip into the monitor or manually inserting the code number into the monitor (Figure 2).
   PURPOSE: Manufacturers must provide directions on how to calibrate light-sensitive meters every time a new container of test strips is used.
   Note: The newer test strips will code themselves when inserted into the meter.

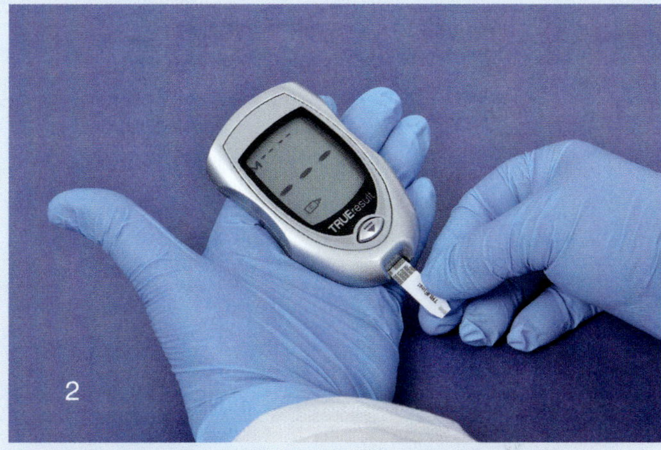

4. Check the expiration date on the liquid control bottle and mix well by inverting and rolling the bottle between the palms of your hands.
   PURPOSE: If the date on the control bottle shows that it has expired, the control cannot be run. It is crucial to have all the reagents in the bottle in suspension to produce reliable results.
5. Complete the top portion of the control log sheet with the test name, control lot number, expiration date, and the control's reference range based on whether it is a low-level, normal, or high-level control.
   PURPOSE: All of this information is checked each time a control is run to compare the results of the same control.
6. Insert the strip into the glucometer and apply a drop of the liquid control to the strip according to the directions.
   PURPOSE: The manufacturer must supply clear directions that ensure consistency every time a control or patient specimen is run.
7. Record the result on the glucose test-control flow sheet and note whether it falls within the manufacturer's reference range. If not, the test should be repeated with a new strip.
   PURPOSE: An occasional "out of range" result can occur. If the repeated test with a new strip is back in range, proceed with patient testing. If the second strip falls outside of the range, the patient may not be tested until the cause of the error is determined.
8. When you have finished running the controls, properly dispose of the strips as recommended by the manufacturer.
9. Remove your gloves and eyewear. Dispose of the gloves in the waste container. Wash your hands or use hand sanitizer.
   PURPOSE: This is necessary to ensure infection control.
10. Review the control results for the following:
    - *Accuracy:* Did all the results fall near the middle of the reference range?
    - *Precision:* Were the results consistently close to each other (without extreme highs and lows)?
    - Reliability: If both of the previous points are affirmed, the test is reliable, and the glucometer may be used to test patient samples.

Continued

PROCEDURE 46.1 Perform a Quality Control Measure on a Glucometer and Record the Results on a Flow Sheet—*continued*

GLUCOSE TEST CONTROL FLOW SHEET					
Control Lot #: ________			Expiration Date: ________		
Control Range: ________			Level: Low/Normal/High		
DATE	**STUDENT/MA INITIALS**	**RESULT**	**ACCEPT**	**REJECT**	**CORRECTIVE ACTION**

PROCEDURE 46.2 Use of the Eyewash Equipment: Perform an Emergency Eyewash

TASK: Minimize the risk of occupational exposure to pathogens if body fluids contact the eyes.

EQUIPMENT and SUPPLIES

- Plumbed or self-contained eyewash unit

PROCEDURAL STEPS

1. If a hazardous substance enters the eye, immediately go to the eyewash station and push the activation lever to discharge water into both eyes. If using an eyewash unit, follow the manufacturer's directions.
   PURPOSE: To ensure flushing of all materials from the eyes.
2. Quickly remove your gloves once irrigation has begun and is in an uninterrupted flow. Then hold the eyelids open with the thumb and index finger to ensure adequate rinsing of the entire eye and eyelid surface (Figure 1). If you have contacts in, gently remove them during the flushing process.
   PURPOSE: The normal reflex is to close the eyes tightly, which prevents removal of all of the contaminated material. Failure to remove contacts can result in improper irrigation of the eyes. It is important to *not* delay irrigating the eyes by first stopping to wash hands, donning gloves, and then taking them out. Go to the eyewash immediately, activate it, and then remove contacts once flushing has begun.
3. Flush the eyes and eyelids for a minimum of 15 minutes, rolling the eyes periodically to ensure complete removal of the foreign material.
   PURPOSE: To completely remove the potentially dangerous substance from the eyes.
4. After completion of the eyewash, wash your hands and complete the postexposure follow-up procedures.
   PURPOSE: The facility's policies may include provider completion of an exposure incident form and provider follow-up, depending on the type of exposure.

PROCEDURE 46.3 Evaluate the Laboratory Environment

TASKS: Evaluate the laboratory environment and identify unsafe working conditions. Identify compliance with safety practices, such as safety signs, symbols, and labels.

EQUIPMENT and SUPPLIES

- Laboratory environment evaluation form
- Pen

PROCEDURAL STEPS

1. Observe the use of workplace safeguards, such as safety signs, symbols, and labels, in the laboratory setting. Document what each sign, symbol, and label means. Document your findings on the work environment evaluation form.

PROCEDURE 46.3 Evaluate the Laboratory Environment—*continued*

PURPOSE: Workplace safeguards, such as safety signs, symbols, and labels, must be used in the laboratory setting.

2. Explain if the laboratory personnel are complying with the safety signs, symbols, and labels.
3. Observe the environment for safety risks. Document your findings.
   PURPOSE: Identifying and correcting safety risks is important in the workplace environment.
4. Based on your observations, summarize your findings. If risks are present, create a list of issues that need to be addressed. Describe what needs to be done for each risk.

PROCEDURE 46.4 Perform Routine Maintenance on a Microscope

TASKS: Focus the microscope properly using a prepared slide under low power, high power, and oil immersion. Then perform routine maintenance on the microscope before storing it.

EQUIPMENT and SUPPLIES

- Microscope
- Lens cleaner
- Lens tissue
- Slide containing specimen
- Immersion oil
- Waste container

PROCEDURAL STEPS

1. Wash your hands or use hand sanitizer.
   PURPOSE: Hand sanitization is necessary to ensure proper infection control practices.
2. Gather the needed materials.
   PURPOSE: Being prepared for the task will allow efficient use of your time.
3. Clean the lenses with lens tissue and lens cleaner.
   PURPOSE: Dust on lenses can obscure elements in the microscopic field.
4. Adjust the seating to a comfortable height.
   PURPOSE: Proper seat height will reduce back and neck strain.
5. Plug the microscope into an electrical outlet and turn on the light switch.
6. Place the slide specimen on the stage and secure it.
7. Turn the revolving nosepiece to engage the 4× or 10× lens.
   PURPOSE: Always begin microscopic observations at low power.
8. Carefully raise the stage while observing with the naked eye from the side.
   PURPOSE: Observing from the side prevents breaking of the slide if the coarse adjustment knob is advanced too far.
9. Focus the specimen using the coarse adjustment knob.
   PURPOSE: The coarse adjustment knob quickly brings the specimen into focus.
10. Adjust the amount of light by closing the iris diaphragm, bringing the condenser up or down, or adjusting the light from the source.
    PURPOSE: Too much light when the low-power objective is used can irritate the eyes.
11. Switch to the 40× lens. Use the fine adjustment knob to focus on the specimen in detail.
12. Turn the revolving nosepiece to the area between the high-power objective and oil immersion. Place a small drop of oil on the slide.
    PURPOSE: Immersion oil has nearly the same refractive index as glass and prevents refraction of the light, thus improving resolution.
13. Carefully rotate the oil immersion objective into place. The objective will be immersed in the oil. Adjust the focus with the fine adjustment knob.
    PURPOSE: The fine adjustment knob moves the objective slowly, preventing damage to the microscope and the slide.
14. Increase the light by opening the iris diaphragm and raising the condenser.
    PURPOSE: Lighting is crucial to microscopy; the higher the magnification, the more light that is needed.
15. Identify the specimen.
16. Return to low power, but do not drag the 40× lens through the oil. Remove the slide and dispose of it in a biohazard sharps container.
    PURPOSE: Getting oil on the 40x lens will cause blurriness the next time it is used. It will have to be cleaned again.
17. Lower the stage. Center the stage.
    PURPOSE: Returning the microscope to this position protects it during storage.
18. Switch off the light and unplug the microscope. Clean the lenses with lens tissue and remove oil with lens cleaner.
    PURPOSE: Dust and oil must be removed from the lenses after a procedure.
19. Wipe the microscope with a cloth. Cover the microscope.
    PURPOSE: Exposing the microscope to a minimum of dust will help maintain the equipment.
20. Place the trash in the waste container. Sanitize the work area. Wash your hands or use hand sanitizer.
    PURPOSE: Sanitization is necessary in order to follow proper infection control practices.

URINALYSIS

47

SCENARIO

Becca Rundle is a medical assistant student who is observing at the Walden-Martin Family Medical (WMFM) Clinic's physician office laboratory (POL) today. As part of an assignment, Becca needs to shadow an experienced medical assistant in an area that interests her. Becca is curious about the laboratory, so she will be spending a few hours with Julie Salter, CMA (AAMA). Julie is going to explain the tests that she will be performing in the urinalysis department. She has even saved a few interesting samples that came in earlier in the week.

While studying this chapter, think about the following questions:

- How would you describe urine collection procedures and common choices of collection containers?
- What would you say to instruct a patient in the proper collection of a 24-hour urine specimen and a clean-catch midstream urine specimen?
- How would you examine and report the physical and chemical aspects of urine?
- How would you test and record quality control and chemical urinalysis using methods that have been waived by the Clinical Laboratory Improvement Amendments (CLIA)?
- How would you prepare a urine specimen for microscopic evaluation?
- How would you explain the following CLIA-waived urine tests: urine pregnancy test, ovulation and menopause tests, and toxicology/drug tests?

LEARNING OBJECTIVES

1. Explain the formation and elimination of urine.
2. Explain the various methods used to collect urine specimens and the handling and transportation of specimens.
3. Examine the physical and chemical aspects of urine along with the limitations of reagent strip testing and quality control.
4. Explain the process of preparing urine for microscopic examination and what is seen in the microscopic examination of urine.
5. Explain additional CLIA-waived tests that can be performed on urine.

VOCABULARY

artificial insemination The injection of semen into the vagina or uterus using a catheter or syringe. Nonsexual.

catheter A hollow, flexible tube that can be inserted into a vessel, organ, or cavity of the body to withdraw or instill fluid, monitor information, and visualize a vessel or cavity.

creatinine clearance rates Result from a procedure used to evaluate the glomerular filtration rate of the kidneys.

crystals Solid substances with a regular shape due to the structure of molecules.

decanting Pouring a liquid gently so that it does not disturb the remaining sediment.

esterase Any enzyme that breaks down esters (a type of organic molecule) into alcohols and acids.

follicle-stimulating hormone (FSH) A glycoprotein hormone secreted by the anterior pituitary gland. It stimulates the growth of ova (eggs) in the ovary and induces the formation of sperm in the testis.

glomerulonephritis A kidney disease affecting the glomeruli of the nephron. Characterized by albumin in the urine, edema, and high blood pressure.

graduated cylinder A narrow, tube-shaped container marked with horizontal lines to represent units of measurement. Used to precisely measure the volume of liquids.

homeostasis The internal environment of the body that is compatible with life. A steady state that is created by all the body systems working together to provide a consistent and unvarying internal environment.

ion An electrically charged atom or the smallest component of an element. (A cation has a positive charge, and an anion has a negative charge.)

jaundice Yellow discoloration of the skin, whites of the eyes, and mucous membranes due to an increase of bilirubin in the blood.

luteinizing hormone (LH) A hormone produced by the anterior pituitary gland. LH stimulates ovulation and the development of the corpus luteum in females and the production of testosterone in males.

micturate Urinate.

meatus A body opening or passage, especially the external opening of a structure.

VOCABULARY—*continued*

myoglobin Type of hemoglobin found in the muscle.
nephrotoxic Damaging or destructive to the kidneys.
normal flora Microorganisms (mostly bacteria and yeast) that live on or in the body. Normal microscopic residents of the body.
phenylalanine An essential amino acid found in milk, eggs, and other foods.
protozoa Single-celled organisms that are the most primitive form of animal life. Most are microscopic. Examples are amoebas, ciliates, flagellates, and sporozoans.
quantitative Describes a test result that is expressed as a number, usually with units of measure attached to numeric values.
renal ischemia A blood flow deficiency to the kidney(s).
renal threshold The blood level of a substance above which the kidneys fail to reabsorb it, so the substance will appear in the urine.
sediment An insoluble material that settles to the bottom of a liquid specimen and the bottom of a centrifuged sample.
supernatant The clear liquid above the sediment in a centrifuged urine specimen.

INTRODUCTION

Urine is the second most common specimen analyzed in the laboratory. Only blood is tested more frequently. Urine is analyzed for several reasons:

- To detect diseases or disorders in which the kidneys are working normally but are excreting abnormal substances that are the result of an imbalance of **homeostasis** in the body. For example, an individual with diabetes mellitus may be excreting glucose.
- To detect diseases or disorders of the kidneys or urinary tract. Examples would be the presence of kidney stones or a urinary tract infection (UTI).
- To detect medications or drugs that are excreted by the kidneys.

URINE FORMATION AND ELIMINATION

Medical assistants must have a basic knowledge of kidney structure and urine formation to understand the results of a urinalysis (UA). For a helpful review of the urinary system, see Chapter 42.

Formation of Urine

The urinary tract consists of two kidneys, two ureters, one bladder, and one urethra. Blood passes through microscopic structures in the kidneys called *nephrons* (Figure 47.1). In the nephrons, blood is filtered to form a *filtrate*. The composition of the filtrate is adjusted as it passes through the renal tubules of the nephron. Selective reabsorption and secretion occur in the renal tubules until the filtrate reaches its final composition. The final filtrate is known as *urine*.

Elimination of Urine

Urine flows through a series of collection areas until it leaves the kidney through the ureter and is stored in the urinary bladder. Urine remains in the bladder until it is voided through the urethra. The average person voids about 1 to 2 liters of urine per day.

The largest component of urine is water. Normal waste products found in urine include urea, uric acid, creatinine, and electrolytes (sodium, chloride, potassium). Abnormal waste products that can be found in urine include protein, glucose, ketones, red blood cells (RBCs), white blood cells (WBCs), bacteria, nitrites, bilirubin, and urobilinogen. Protein and blood cells are too large to be filtrated by the glomerulus, so when these substances appear in the urine, it may indicate damage to one or more organs of the urinary system.

COLLECTING AND HANDLING OF A URINE SPECIMEN

The request for a urine specimen may create an uneasy moment for the patient. The request should be made in a private area, such as the exam room, if possible. The patient should be given clear instructions so that he or she understands what is expected. The medical assistant should clearly communicate and explain the details of the procedure.

Be observant and ask the patient to repeat the directions, so you know he or she understands the procedure. Answer any questions with patience and clear directions to avoid confusion. If a language barrier exists, be creative but respectful of the patient's needs. Use an interpreter if one is available. Posting a picture with directions in a variety of languages in the patient restroom could also help.

CRITICAL THINKING APPLICATION 47.1

Becca and Julie meet in the reception area and walk back to the POL. They talk about the need for proper personal protective equipment (PPE), and Julie gives Becca a lab coat and protective eyewear. She also shows Becca where the gloves are near the UA counter. Becca will not be performing tests today, but anyone in the lab should wear proper PPE even if they are observing.

There are a few specimens on the counter, and Julie asks Becca if she has practiced giving instructions for UA collection procedures in any of her classes. Becca replies that she has but thought it was a bit silly. Julie talks about how patients can be embarrassed about collecting specimens and may not want to ask too many questions. Julie asks Becca to write down three items that are important to include when explaining a UA collection procedure. Write down your own answer and be ready to share it with your class.

Containers

The POL should provide the appropriate urine container for the patient. Patients should not use containers from home. Disposable, nonsterile, plastic, or coated paper containers are the most frequently used and are available in many sizes with tight-fitting lids. Most routine UA tests, pregnancy tests, and tests for abnormal analytes are performed on urine collected in nonsterile containers. Special flexible polyethylene bags with adhesive are used to collect urine from infants and children who are not toilet trained (see Chapter 44). For specimens that must be collected over a stated time (24-hour urines), large, wide-mouth plastic containers with screw-cap tops are used (Procedure 47.1).

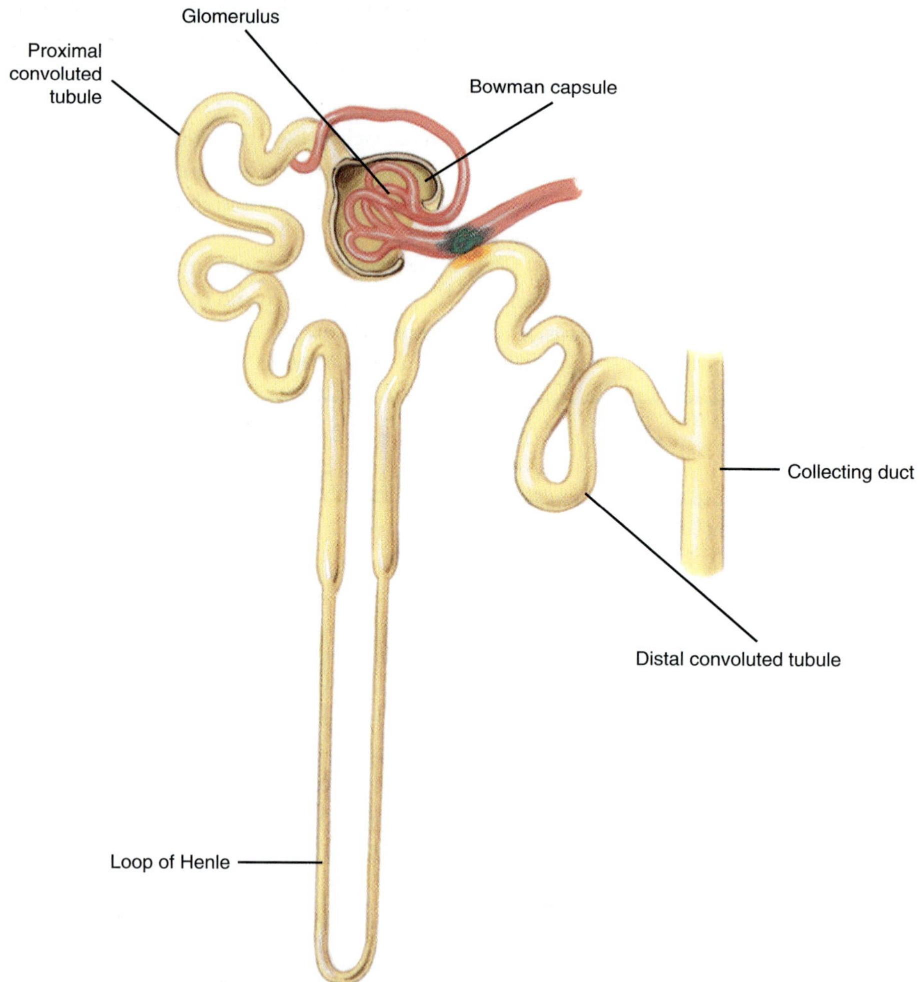

FIGURE 47.1 Nephron. Notice the blood vessels entering and exiting the glomerulus, where the small particles in the blood are filtered out of the blood into the surrounding capsule of the nephron. Then, follow the filtrate through the proximal convoluted tubule, the descending limb, the loop of Henle, and the ascending limb of the nephron. This is where water and substances from the filtrate are reabsorbed back into the blood vessels. Finally, in the distal convoluted tubule of the nephron, additional waste products are selectively secreted into the filtrate by the blood vessels. The collection duct continues to concentrate the filtrate to form urine ready for excretion. (From Applegate EJ: *The anatomy and physiology learning system*, ed 4, Philadelphia, 2011, Saunders.)

If the sample is being sent to the microbiology department of the laboratory for culture, it must be collected in a sterile container. Explain the collection procedure to the patient, and make sure the patient understands how to collect the specimen and handle the sterile specimen cup. Most sterile containers have a paper seal over the cap. If the seal is broken, the specimen cup may not be sterile and should be discarded (Figure 47.2).

Labeling

The label on all specimens must be printed in permanent marker or ink and include the patient's name, the date and time of collection, and the type of specimen. If available, computer-generated labels should be placed on the container so that the information is easy to read. Always put on gloves before handling filled specimen containers.

When a clinic sends specimens to multiple laboratories, it is important to have a system in place that meets the labeling and collection needs of all facilities. Each laboratory may require specific information and specific specimen containers. Double-check the laboratory name and specimen requirements before patient collection to avoid mistakes and possible specimen recollection issues. Patient insurance may direct laboratory usage or affiliation.

Methods of Specimen Collection

There are several types of urine specimens.

- *Random specimen*: Urine is collected in clean containers. Most tests use this type of specimen.
- *First-morning specimen*: A urine specimen is collected when the patient first wakes up in the morning. This type of specimen is more concentrated than a random sample. It is best used when testing for nitrite, protein, or pregnancy and microscopic examination. First-morning samples are also the preferred samples for possible UTI testing, but this is not a requirement.

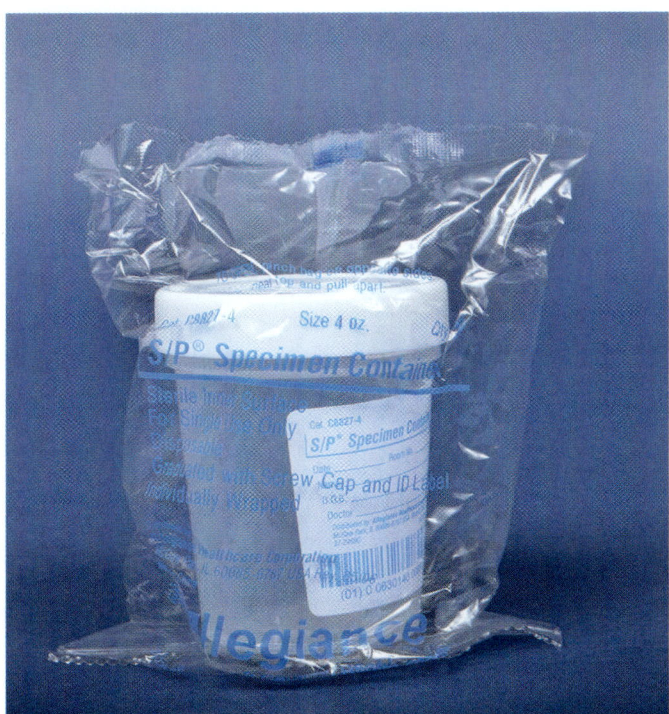

FIGURE 47.2 Sterile urine container.

- *Second-voided specimen:* The first void of the morning is discarded, and the second void of the day is collected for testing. The specimen is used to determine glucose levels in urine.
- *Two-hour postprandial urine specimens:* The specimen is collected 2 hours after a meal. This specimen is required for diabetes screening and home diabetes testing programs.
- *Catheterized specimen*: The provider, nurse, or specially trained medical assistant inserts a sterile **catheter** into the bladder to collect the specimen.

Besides these specimens, a 24-hour specimen collection and a clean-catch midstream specimen collection can also be required. The following sections describe these two collection methods.

24-Hour Specimen Collection

A *24-hour urine specimen* is collected over 24 hours to provide a **quantitative** chemical analysis, such as hormone levels and **creatinine clearance rates**. The patient must understand the proper way to collect a 24-hour urine specimen (see Procedure 47.1).

Patient instructions for an at-home 24-hour urine collection are as follows:

- Do not put anything but urine into the container.
- Do not pour out any liquid or powdered preservative from the container.
- If you accidentally spill some of the preservative on yourself, immediately wash with water and call the POL, provider's office, or testing laboratory.
- Always keep the collection container cool. Refrigerate the container or keep it in an ice-filled cooler or pail.
- Keep the cap on the container.

Clean-Catch Midstream Specimen Collection

A *clean-catch midstream specimen* (CCMS) is ordered when the provider suspects a urinary tract infection. When a UTI is possible, the provider will order a urine *culture and sensitivity* (C&S). For a C&S procedure, the specimen is cultured on microbiological media to detect bacterial or fungal growth. This is followed by screening the bacteria that grows for antibiotic sensitivity. A C&S is performed in the microbiology department of a referral laboratory.

The clean-catch technique is used to eliminate microorganisms from the urinary **meatus**. In the medical facility, collecting CCMS samples starts by instructing the patient to thoroughly cleanse around the meatus and then **micturate** a small amount into the toilet. This is done to flush out the distal portion of the urethra, where **normal flora** can accumulate. The patient then collects a CCMS specimen. Prior to collection, the medical assistant needs to give complete, understandable instructions to the patient on the method of collection (Procedure 47.2). Failure to do so may mean that the patient will have to return to the office to provide another specimen. For a urine C&S, the urine is collected either by catheterization or the clean-catch method into a sterile container.

CRITICAL THINKING APPLICATION 47.2

As Julie and Becca review the different types of UA specimens, Julie asks, "Why is it so important that a CCMS be collected midstream? Why not start collecting the sample as soon as the void starts?" What would your answer be to that question? Write down your answer and be ready to share it in class.

Handling and Transporting a Specimen

Proper handling of specimens is essential. The chemical and cellular components of urine change if the urine warms to room temperature (Table 47.1). Urine specimens should therefore be kept refrigerated and processed within 1 hour of collection. If the specimen must be transported to a referral laboratory, evacuated transport tubes are available (Figure 47.3). These tubes contain preservatives and look like blood collection tubes. The preservatives in the tube prevent the overgrowth of bacteria and will prevent chemical changes in the urine that may affect test results. Chemical reagent strip testing can be performed on preserved specimens within 72 hours. Tubes may be held at room temperature during this time.

A different preservative must be used for urine culture specimens. The preservative used for culture specimens helps maintain the number of bacteria present at the time of collection. This type of transport system should be used only for urine specimens that will be cultured. Results on the chemical reagent strip may be altered by the alternative preservatives. Culture and sensitivity testing should be performed within 72 hours. The C&S tubes can be held at room temperature.

A laboratory request form, paper or electronic, must be completed for all specimens being transported to another site for analysis. Typical forms include the following information:

- Patient's name and the date
- Type of urinalysis ordered
- Name of the provider requesting the examination
- Appropriate *Current Procedural Terminology* (CPT) code for the diagnosis
- A line on which the provider signs after they have reviewed the results

TABLE 47.1 Changes in Urine After 1 Hour at Room Temperature

CONSTITUENT	CHANGE
Clarity	Urine becomes cloudy as crystals precipitate and bacteria multiply
Color	May change if pH becomes alkaline
pH	Becomes alkaline as bacteria form ammonia from urea
Glucose	Decreases as it is metabolized by bacteria
Ketones	Decrease because of evaporation
Bilirubin and urobilinogen	Undergo degradation in light
Blood	May hemolyze; false-positive results are possible because of bacterial enzymes
Nitrite	Test result may change from negative to positive as bacteria multiply and reduce nitrates to nitrites
Casts	Lyse or dissolve in alkaline urine
Cells	Lyse or dissolve in alkaline urine
Bacteria	Multiply twofold approximately every 20 minutes
Yeasts	Multiply
Crystals	Precipitate as urine cools; may dissolve if pH changes

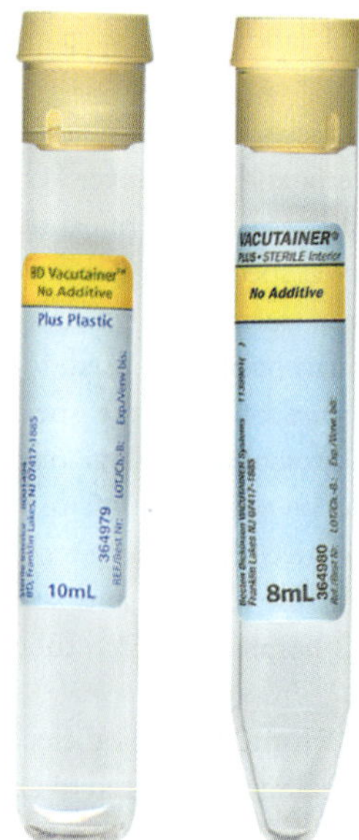

FIGURE 47.3 Urine transport tubes. (Courtesy Becton, Dickinson & Co., Franklin Lakes, NJ.)

- Always handle specimens by the container and not the lid to avoid accidental spills

Specimens are sent to the laboratory in a plastic biohazard bag that zips closed and has an outside pocket, where a paper laboratory request is placed if the order has not been placed in the electronic medical record, and the specimen is labeled with the appropriate order information. After the test has been performed, the lab physically sends a paper report or electronically sends the results to the provider.

TABLE 47.2 Components of Physical and Chemical Urinalysis

PHYSICAL PROPERTY	CHEMICAL COMPONENT
Color	Protein
Clarity	Glucose
Specific gravity	Ketones
Volume[a]	Bilirubin
Odor[a]	Blood
Foam[a]	Nitrite
	pH
	Urobilinogen
	Leukocyte enzyme

[a]Not always assessed.

ROUTINE URINALYSIS

The minimum volume needed for a routine UA usually is about 10 to 12 mL, but more is preferred. A complete UA is an assessment of the following:

- Physical properties of the urine
- Selected chemical measurements that are important for diagnosing diseases (Table 47.2).
- Microscopic contents of the urine and its **sediment**

Physical Examination of Urine: Appearance

The physical examination of urine involves observations regarding the appearance of the specimen (Procedure 47.3). This does not involve chemical analysis but rather observation of the characteristics of color, *turbidity* (cloudiness), volume, presence of foam or odor, and specific gravity.

Color

Normal urine is a shade of yellow that ranges from pale straw to yellow to amber (Figure 47.4). The color depends on the concentration of *urochrome*, a yellow pigment normally found in urine, and the amount of water in the specimen. A dilute specimen should be a pale straw color, and a more concentrated specimen should be a darker yellow or amber color. First morning specimens will likely be amber in color due to the concentration of the urochrome during the night. Variations in color may also be caused by diet, medication, and disease. Abnormal colors may be related to pathologic or nonpathologic factors (Table 47.3).

Turbidity

Both normal and abnormal urine specimens may range in appearance from clear to very cloudy (Figure 47.5). Turbidity may be caused by cells, bacteria, yeast, vaginal contaminants, or **crystals**. It is possible for a urine specimen to be clear when voided, but as crystals form and precipitate out of the liquid, it causes the urine to become cloudy as it cools.

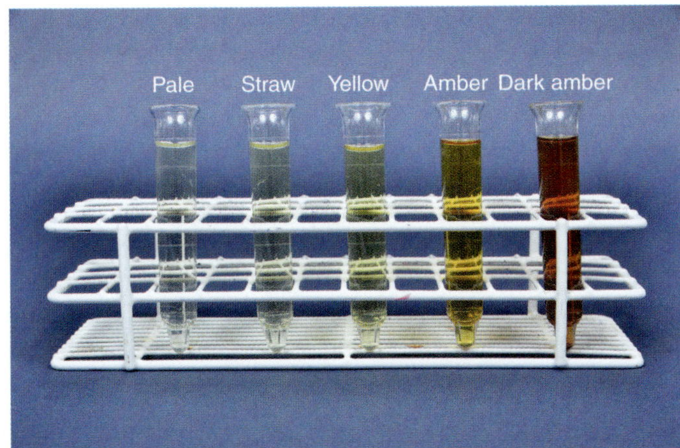

FIGURE 47.4 Color of urine specimens.

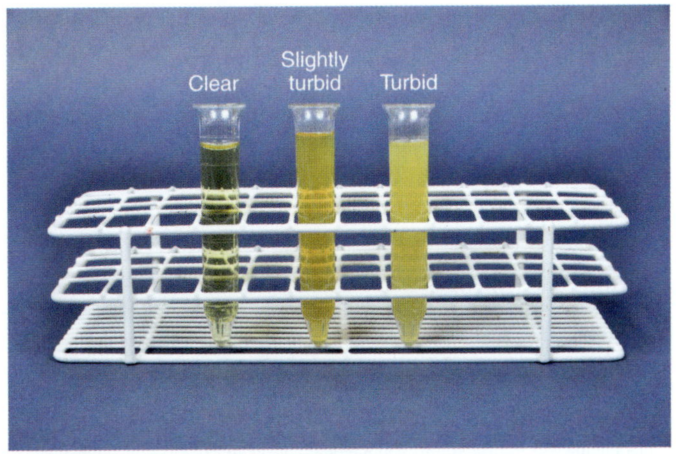

FIGURE 47.5 Turbidity of urine specimens.

TABLE 47.3 Possible Causes of Urine Colors

COLOR	PATHOLOGIC CAUSE	NONPATHOLOGIC CAUSE
Straw	Diabetes	Diuretics; high fluid intake (coffee, beer)
Amber	Dehydration	Concentrated first morning specimen; excessive sweating; low fluid intake
Bright yellow	—	Carotene, vitamins
Red	Blood, porphyrins	Menstruation, beets, drugs, dyes
Orange-yellow	Bile, hepatitis	Phenazopyridine (fen az oh PEER i deen) (Pyridium, Uristat), dyes, drugs
Greenish yellow	Bile, hepatitis	Senna (laxative), cascara (laxative), rhubarb
Reddish brown	Old blood, methemoglobin	—
Brownish black	Methemoglobin, melanin	Carbidopa-levodopa (kar bi DOH puh–lee vuh DOH puh) (Sinemet, Parcopa)
Salmon pink	—	Amorphous urates
White (milky)	Fats, pus	Amorphous phosphates
Blue-green	Biliverdin, infection with *Pseudomonas* organisms	Vitamin B, drugs, dyes, Amitriptyline, Indomethacin

Volume

The amount of urine is rarely measured in a random specimen. With a timed specimen such as a 24-hour collection, volume is measured by pouring the complete collection into a large, **graduated cylinder**. It is not accurate enough to use the markings on the side of the collection container. Once the volume has been measured and recorded, a portion of the well-mixed specimen, called an *aliquot,* is removed for testing. The remainder is discarded or stored, depending on the preference of the laboratory.

The normal volume of urine produced every 24 hours varies according to the age of the individual. Infants and children produce smaller volumes than adults. The normal adult volume of urine produced is approximately 800 to 2000 mL in 24 hours. Excessive production of urine is called *polyuria.* This is common in those who have diabetes mellitus, diabetes insipidus, and certain kidney disorders. *Oliguria* is an insufficient production of urine, which can be caused by dehydration, decreased fluid intake, shock, renal disease, or urinary tract infections. The absence of urine production, *anuria*, occurs when there is renal obstruction and renal failure.

CRITICAL THINKING APPLICATION 47.3

Write down, in your own words, definitions for these terms: *anuria, oliguria,* and *polyuria.* Be ready to share your definitions with the class.

Foam

Normally the presence of foam is not recorded, but careful observation of this property can detect a significant clue to an abnormality. Foam consists of small bubbles that persist for a long time after the specimen has been swirled to mix. Foam must not be confused with any bubbles that rapidly disappear. White foam can indicate the presence of increased protein (Figure 47.6). Greenish-yellow foam may indicate bilirubin in the urine. Care should be taken in handling such urine specimens because the greenish-yellow color may indicate that the patient has viral hepatitis, which is highly contagious. Always observe Standard Precautions and wear appropriate personal protective equipment (PPE) when handling specimens. If foam is observed and seems significant, add a note in the Comments field of a paper or electronic test report.

Odor

As with foam, odor is not normally recorded but can be an important clue to metabolic disorders. Normal urine is said to be *aromatic* or having a distinct smell. Changes in the odor of urine may be caused by disease, the presence of bacteria, or diet. A patient with diabetes may pass urine that has a fruity odor if he or she is excreting ketones in the urine. An ammonia or a *putrid* (foul or decaying) smell in the urine can be caused by an infection. An ammonia smell may also be noticed in urine that has been at room temperature for too long before it is tested. Foods such as asparagus and garlic also can produce an abnormal odor in the urine. Urine from a child with *phenylketonuria* (PKU) may smell "mousy." If the odor seems significant, add a note in the Comments field of a paper or electronic test report.

Phenylketonuria

Phenylketonuria (PKU) is a rare hereditary condition in which the amino acid **phenylalanine** is not properly metabolized or broken down in the body. PKU that is undiagnosed or untreated can lead to severe cognitive disabilities. An accumuation of phenylalanine in the blood and urine gives body fluids the odor of wet fur.

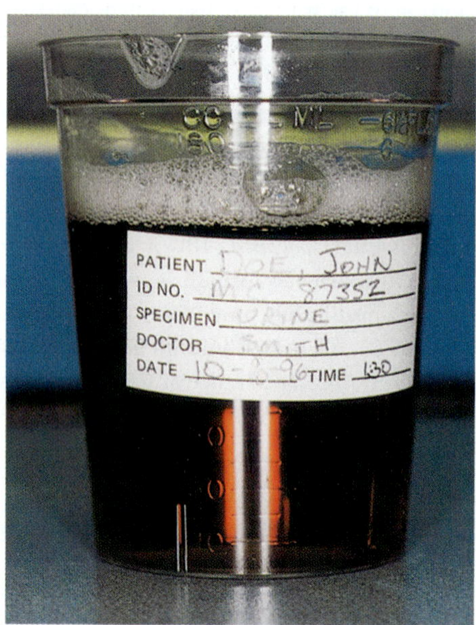

FIGURE 47.6 Urine with foam.

Specific Gravity

Specific gravity is defined as the weight of a substance compared with the weight of an equal volume of distilled water. In UA, specific gravity is the approximate measurement of the concentration of substances dissolved in the urine. The specific gravity of distilled water is 1.000. The normal specific gravity of urine ranges from 1.005 to 1.030, depending on the patient's fluid intake. Most samples fall between 1.010 and 1.025. The urine's specific gravity indicates whether the kidneys can concentrate the urine. A change in specific gravity is one of the first indications of kidney disease. Conditions such as **glomerulonephritis**, chronic renal insufficiency, or diabetes may lower the specific gravity. To measure specific gravity, laboratories may use a refractometer, but most use Clinical Laboratory Improvement Amendments (CLIA)-waived chemical reagent strips.

A *refractometer* measures the *refraction* (bending) of light through solids in a liquid. The result is called the *refractive index,* which, for our purposes, is the same as *specific gravity*. The refractometer requires only a drop of urine. One drop of well-mixed urine is placed under the hinged cover of the instrument. Then the value is read directly from a scale viewed through the eyepiece. Figure 47.7 shows the refractometer on the left and the visual results of the urine in the circle on the right. The scale on the left side of the circle shows a urine-specific gravity of 1.020. The refractometer must be calibrated daily with distilled water, which should read 1.000. Note that specific gravity carries no unit of measure after the number.

The analysis that uses a reagent strip, also called a urine *dipstick,* is a CLIA-waived test. A reagent strip test is the most common method used for measuring specific gravity in the POL. The pad on the strip contains a chemical that is sensitive to positively charged **ions**, such as sodium (Na^+) and potassium (K^+). The pad detects the urine's specific gravity. Various color changes indicate values between 1.000 and 1.030.

Chemical Examination of Urine

Tests can be performed on urine to detect the presence of certain chemicals, which can provide valuable information to the provider. In certain situations, these chemical test results can be critical to

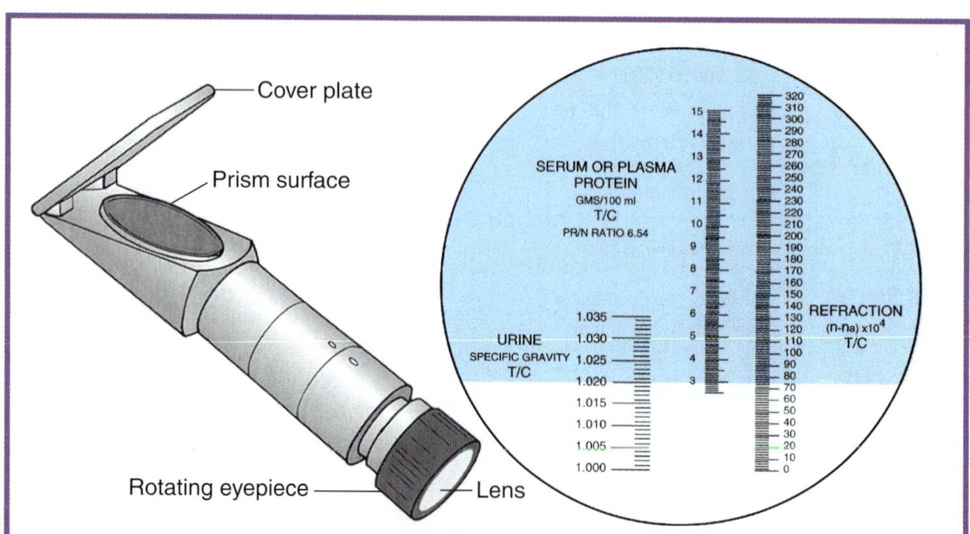

FIGURE 47.7 Refractometer. A drop of urine is placed on the prism surface of the refractometer *(left)*, and the cover plate is closed. When the examiner looks through the lens, two graphs are seen in the circular field of vision *(right)*. The urine specific gravity (SG) is read from the left scale, where the blue shadow meets the lighted bottom. The SG is 1.020.

a diagnosis. Also, some urine dipstick results will turn positive before a patient has specific symptoms of a disease or disorder. That is one reason a routine urinalysis can be a screening test for many conditions.

Reagent strip testing is the most widely used technique for detecting chemicals in the urine (Procedures 47.4 and 47.5). These strip tests are available in a variety of types (Figure 47.8). Dipsticks are plastic strips with paper pads attached. The paper pads contain chemical reagents. The reagents react chemically with analytes in the urine. The chemical reaction is read by looking for a color change on each individual pad. The presence or absence of these chemicals in the urine provides information on the status of carbohydrate metabolism, liver and kidney function, and the patient's acid-base balance.

Reagent strips are designed to be used once and then discarded in a biohazard waste container. The directions for each type of reagent strip test are included inside the package. Instructions must be followed exactly if accurate results are to be obtained. A color comparison chart is provided on the label of the container. In addition to reagent strips, a few tablet tests are available for chemically testing urine.

All strips and tablets must be kept in tightly closed containers in a cool, dry area and should be removed just before testing. To prevent contamination of the bottle, never touch a strip that has been exposed to urine against the color comparison chart on the bottle. If both a UA and C&S have been ordered for a specimen, separate the sample. The original sample in the sterile container will go to the microbiology department and be used for the C&S. Pour off an aliquot into a nonsterile urine tube for the UA. If you were to introduce a reagent strip into the sterile urine sample, it would contaminate the specimen and make it unfit for C&S testing.

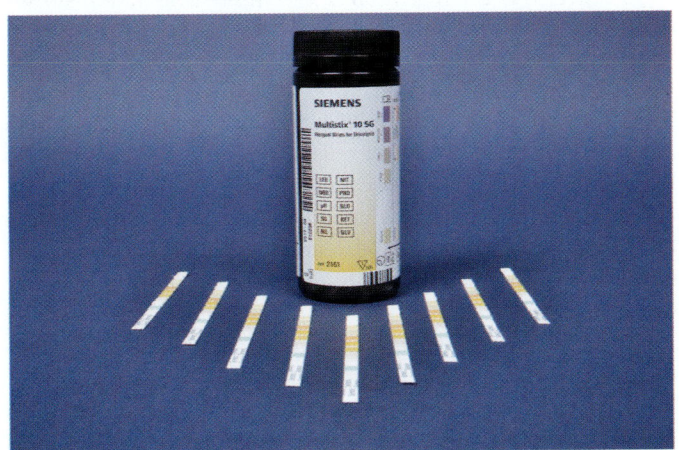

FIGURE 47.8 Urine reagent strip test.

pH

The pH is a measurement of the acidity or alkalinity of the urine. A urine specimen with a pH of 7 is neutral. A value below 7 indicates acidity and above 7 indicates alkalinity. Normal, freshly voided urine may have a pH range of 5.5 to 8 (Figure 47.9). The urinary pH varies with an individual's metabolic status, diet, drug therapy, and disease. In the case of bacteria in the urine, the urine pH is usually alkaline. Knowing the pH of the sample also helps when identifying crystals that may be found in the urine sediment.

Glucose

Glucose is filtered out of the blood in the glomerulus, and, under normal conditions, most glucose is reabsorbed in the tubules of the nephron. Detectable *glycosuria* (glucose in the urine) occurs when the filtered glucose in the renal tubules is so high it cannot be reabsorbed into the blood. A positive urine glucose may be the first indication that a patient is diabetic. The glucose pad on a reagent strip test is based on a specific enzyme reaction in which glucose, and no other sugar, causes a positive reaction. Because many types of bacteria use glucose for energy, specimens should be tested for glucose within an hour of collection or within 24 hours if refrigerated. This will reduce the amount of bacteria from overgrowing in the sample.

Glucose Reabsorption. The reabsorption of glucose depends on its **renal threshold**. The renal threshold for blood glucose is below 160 mg/dL. This means that all the glucose will be reabsorbed into the blood if the blood glucose level is below 160 mg/dL. If the blood glucose level is higher than 160 mg/dL, the blood will not reabsorb the glucose. The filtered glucose then remains in the urine, which will show up as a positive test result for glucose during urinalysis.

Ketones

Ketones are the end product of fat metabolism in the body. *Ketonuria* (ketones in the urine) is commonly seen in patients with diabetes mellitus that is not well controlled, in persons on a very-low-carbohydrate diet (in which case the presence of ketones would be an expected finding and not necessarily considered abnormal.), or after excessive vomiting. Because ketones evaporate at room temperature,

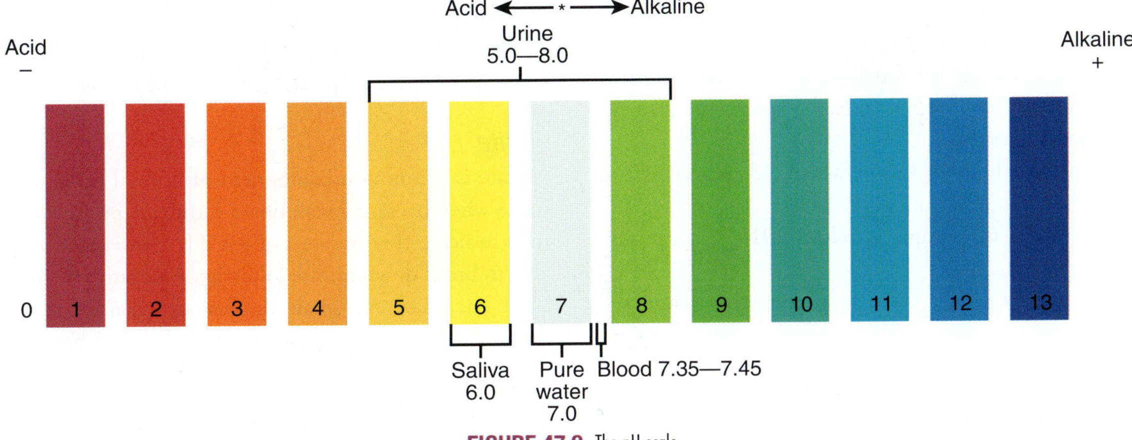

FIGURE 47.9 The pH scale.

urine should be tested immediately, or the specimen should be tightly covered and refrigerated. Examples of ketones include acetoacetate and acetone.

CRITICAL THINKING APPLICATION **47.4**

Julie performs routine urinalysis as Becca observes. One sample has a high glucose level and a low ketone level. Becca knows that both analytes are associated with diabetes. How would you explain a high urine glucose and low urine ketone result? Write down your answer. Could there be more than one explanation? Discuss this question with your class.

Protein

Protein in the urine in detectable amounts is called *proteinuria* and is one of the first signs of renal disease. We normally excrete a very small amount of protein every day that is undetectable.

Some causes of proteinuria may include the following:

- *Orthostatic proteinuria*: protein is excreted only when the patient is in an upright position.
- Pregnancy: a common finding in pregnancy that must be monitored along with excessive weight gain and increased blood pressure (there are three possible symptoms of preeclampsia; see Chapter 43).
- After heavy exercise

The reagent strip is highly sensitive to urinary albumin and is less sensitive to the other proteins.

Blood

The presence of blood in urine may indicate infection or trauma to the urinary tract. The blood test pad on the reagent strip reacts with three different blood constituents: *intact* (whole) red blood cells, hemoglobin from *lysed* (broken) red blood cells, and **myoglobin**.

Hematuria is the presence of intact red blood cells in urine. The color reaction on the reagent strip ranges from yellow to green to dark green when hematuria is present, revealing a speckled appearance. Hematuria can be caused by irritation of the kidneys, ureters, bladder, or urethra. It also is a common finding in *cystitis* (inflammation of the urinary bladder) and in individuals passing kidney stones. A random specimen may contain blood from vaginal contamination if the woman is menstruating.

Hemoglobinuria is the presence of *hemolyzed* (ruptured, broken) red blood cells in urine (Figure 47.10). True hemoglobinuria is not common. But urine specimens that contain blood may test positive for hemolyzed blood for a few reasons:

- The urine specimen has sat for too long at room temperature, causing the RBCs to lyse. Freshly collected specimens give the most accurate testing results.
- The pH of the urine is highly alkaline, which can cause RBCs to lyse.
- The specific gravity of the sample is below 1.010; this can also cause RBCs to lyse.
- Bacteria in the urine can also cause a false-positive hemolyzed blood test result.

Finding blood or hemolyzed blood on the urine dipstick should be confirmed by microscopic examination of the urine. If intact RBCs are seen microscopically, this should be noted on the UA report to the provider. (A medical assistant would not be doing the microscopic exam.) True hemoglobinuria is the result of intravascular red blood cell destruction and can be caused by blood transfusion reactions, malaria, drug reactions, snakebites, and severe burns.

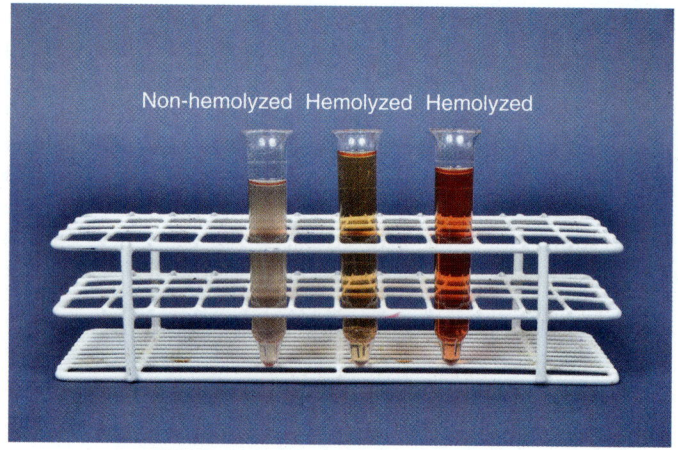

FIGURE 47.10 Hemolyzed and nonhemolyzed blood.

Myoglobinuria (myoglobin in the urine) occurs when muscle tissue is damaged or injured. This can occur with crushing injuries, myocardial infarctions, contact sports, or strenuous exercise. Patients with muscular dystrophy often have myoglobinuria. Hemoglobinuria cannot be distinguished from myoglobinuria by reagent strip testing. Both cause a uniform change in color from light green to dark green on the strip. Myoglobin testing is not normally part of the urine dipstick.

Bilirubin and Urobilinogen

Bilirubin is a product of the breakdown of hemoglobin. Hemoglobin is released from old red blood cells and is gradually converted to bilirubin in the liver. The liver continues to convert bilirubin to *urobilinogen*, which is sent to the intestines for excretion. Bilirubin is a bile pigment not normally found in urine. Its presence in urine is one of the first signs of liver disease or other diseases in which the liver may be involved.

Bilirubin in the urine (*bilirubinuria*) can occur even before **jaundice** or other symptoms of liver disease are evident. It is the result of liver cell damage or obstruction of the common bile duct by stones or tumors. Excessive bilirubin colors the urine yellow-brown to greenish orange. Because direct light causes bilirubin to break down, urine samples must be protected from light until testing is complete.

Urobilinogen normally is present in urine in small amounts. Elevated urobilinogen is seen with increased red blood cell destruction, liver disease, or total obstruction of the bile duct.

Nitrite

Nitrate is a common component of normal urine. *Nitrites* occur in urine when bacteria break down nitrate. A positive nitrite test result may indicate the presence of a UTI. However, not all bacteria are able to break down nitrate to nitrite. A negative nitrite test can occur when bacteria are in small numbers or when the urine has not been in the bladder long enough for the chemical breakdown to occur. *Escherichia coli* (*E. coli*), the bacteria that is the most common cause of UTIs, does break down nitrate to nitrite. A positive reaction is any pink color on the nitrite dipstick pad.

Leukocyte Esterase

Leukocytes (white blood cells) are present in the urine when a person has a UTI. The leukocyte **esterase** test pad on the reagent strip takes 2 minutes to release esterase from white blood cells. Wait a full 2 minutes before reading the leukocyte esterase result. The test does not react with small numbers of white blood cells found in normal urine. A false-positive result could be caused by WBC contaminants from the vagina, especially if the sample is allowed to sit at room temperature. Urine specimens should be tested as soon as possible after collection. If this is not possible, the specimen should be refrigerated.

CRITICAL THINKING APPLICATION **47.5**

One of yesterday's samples that Julie saved in the laboratory refrigerator is ready to test. The sample gives a bright pink positive result for nitrites and a moderate positive result for leukocytes on the reagent strip test. What condition would give this result on a dipstick UA? Could there be more than one answer?

Limitations of Reagent Strip Testing

The reagent strip is a reliable method of testing urine if used properly. The normal urine reference ranges for a reagent strip are presented in Table 47.4. Errors can arise from several sources:

- The test strip is soaked in the specimen, and chemicals in the pads may be overly diluted.
- The test strip is not held horizontally while read, and colors from one pad may bleed onto another.
- The test pads on the strip are not read at the proper time, or the chemical reaction may be read incorrectly.
- Certain chemicals, such as vitamin C, also called *ascorbic acid*, may affect the results of nitrite, glucose, bilirubin, and blood tests. Normal levels of vitamin C do not interfere with routine urinalysis, but large amounts can alter test results. Be sure to check the package insert for a list of all interfering substances.

Visual interpretation of the color on the reagent strip pads is likely to vary among individuals. Some laboratories use automated instruments to read the strips. Several companies manufacture instruments that detect the color change in the analysis of the reagent strip. Once the strip has been placed in the instrument, a microprocessor controls the movement of the strip into the instrument. Light of a specific wavelength is beamed onto each of the test areas on the strip. The color change on each pad is analyzed by the microprocessor and converted into a digital reading, and the results are printed out (Figure 47.11). The advantage of this method is that timing and color interpretation are consistent. The disadvantage is that the instrument is not able to identify and adjust for highly colored urine, leading to false results. The medical assistant should be aware of this and should manually test urine specimens that are darkly colored or send them to a reference lab for further testing.

Quality Assurance and Quality Control in Urinalysis

The US Food and Drug Administration (FDA) categorizes the chemical analysis of urine performed by an instrument or a reagent strip as a CLIA-waived test. The chemical analysis includes the reagent strip (dipstick) tests for bilirubin, glucose, hemoglobin or blood, ketones, leukocyte esterase, nitrite, pH, protein, specific gravity, and urobilinogen. A commercially available control strip should be used to determine the reliability of the reagent strips used in chemical analysis. One such control strip is the Chek-Stix. The plastic control strip has seven pads, each containing synthetic ingredients that mimic human urine when reconstituted in water. After reconstitution, a reagent test strip is immersed in the control solution, and the results are compared with a chart that accompanies the Chek-Stix. Both positive and negative Chek-Stix controls are available. The positive reconstituted control shows positive (abnormal) results when a test strip is inserted and read, whereas the negative reconstituted control shows normal urinalysis results along its test strip. It is important to observe and record the abnormal and normal results produced by the positive and negative controls. Also, make sure the test results are consistent with the Chek-Stix charts provided by the manufacturer before testing patient urine specimens.

The Chek-Stix is one type of commercial control, but other strips and prepared liquid controls are also available. Each POL should investigate the best commercial control for its needs and quality control program.

TABLE 47.4 Normal Urine Reference Ranges for Reagent Strips

PROPERTY	REFERENCE RANGE
Color	Pale yellow to amber
Clarity	Clear to slightly turbid
Specific gravity	1.001–1.035
pH	4.6–8
Protein (mg/dL)	NEG
Glucose (mg/dL)	NEG
Ketone (mg/dL)	NEG
Bilirubin (mg/dL)	NEG
Blood (mg/dL)	NEG
Nitrite (mg/dL)	NEG
Urobilinogen (Ehrlich units)	0.1–1
White blood cells	NEG

NEG, Negative.

MICROSCOPIC PREPARATION AND EXAMINATION OF URINE SEDIMENT

Microscopic examination of urine consists of categorizing and counting cells, casts, crystals, and miscellaneous constituents in the sediment of a urine sample. The sediment is obtained after a measured portion of urine is centrifuged. The sediment will be pushed to the bottom of the tube containing urine. The sediment will be prepared for a microscopic exam, and the remaining liquid urine will be poured off and disposed of properly.

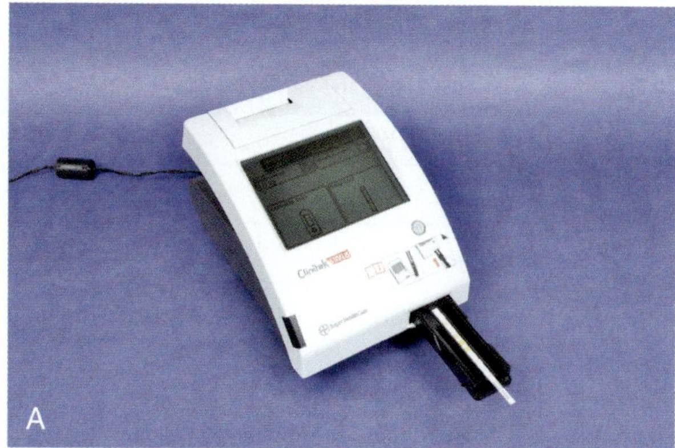

ID: Erika Seager
11-16-XX 5:37 PM
CLARITY: Clear
COLOR: YELLOW

MULTISTIX 10 SG

GLU	NEGATIVE
BIL	NEGATIVE
KET	NEGATIVE
SG	1.025
BLO	TRACE-LYSED
pH	5.5
PRO	NEGATIVE
URO	0.2 E.U./dl
NIT	NEGATIVE
LEU	NEGATIVE

B

FIGURE 47.11 **(A)** Clinitek 50 Urine Chemistry Analyzer. The reagent strip is placed on the tray before the test is begun. **(B)** Sample of the Clinitek results.

Many formed elements are found in the urine. Some are significant, and others are not. Most important, the microscopic examination should correlate with the physical and chemical analyses. For example, if the physical examination of the urine showed a reddish color and the chemical reagent strip tested positive for blood, then seeing red blood cells during the microscopic examination would be consistent with the physical and chemical results. Medical assistants should be familiar with the preparation of urine specimens for this test and with the possible test results (Procedure 47.6).

Microscopic Preparation of Urine

To perform the microscopic UA procedure, a laboratory must be certified to perform CLIA Provider-Performed Microscopy Procedures (PPMPs), a subcategory of CLIA moderate-complexity laboratories. Quality assurance is just as important in the microscopic examination as in the chemical analysis of urine. To ensure consistency and standardization, commercially available systems can be used, such as the KOVA System or the UriSystem. These systems may include specially designed, graduated centrifuge tubes with devices or pipets that allow easy **decanting** of **supernatant** and retention of an exact amount of sediment. They also use specially designed plastic slides with wells or coverslips that accept only a given volume of sediment. Control solutions containing preserved cells are also available from KOVA. This type of solution also provides quality control for cell identification. Whatever system is used, the Clinical and Laboratory Standards Institute (CLSI) recommends the following:

- The urine volume should be 12 mL.
- The specimen should be centrifuged for 5 minutes at a relative centrifugal force of 400 *g* (i.e., 400 times normal gravity).
- A standardized slide should be used to view the sediment.
- A consistent reporting format should be used.

When a urine sample is centrifuged, the clear upper portion of the specimen is called the supernatant. It is poured off, and a drop of the well-mixed sediment at the bottom of the centrifuged tube is examined under a microscope. The sediment may be stained to give greater contrast to the formed elements. The stain assists in the identification of formed elements by improving the detail of cellular structures.

Microscopic Examination of Urine

The examination of urine is not categorized as CLIA-waived; therefore it cannot be performed by a medical assistant without additional training, supervision, and rigid compliance with CLIA quality assurance protocols for the laboratory. Periodic proficiency testing must be successfully completed to maintain a PPMP laboratory certification. (See Chapter 46 for CLIA moderate complexity-approved.)

The three main categories of microscopic findings are casts, cells, and crystals.

Casts

Casts are created when protein accumulates and precipitates in the kidney tubules and is washed into the urine. The protein takes on the size and shape of the tubules, forming the casts. Casts are cylindric, with flat or rounded ends, and are classified according to the substances observed inside them. Certain types of casts are connected to specific renal diseases and disorders. Other casts are physiologic and are generally caused by strenuous exercise. Casts can dissolve in alkaline urine if the sample is not examined promptly. The microscopic exam should take place as soon as possible after specimen collection. The following paragraphs describe some of the casts that may be seen, but these are not all the possible casts. The presence of casts should be determined using a low-power objective such as the 10x.

Hyaline casts are pale, transparent, cylindric structures with rounded ends and parallel sides (Figure 47.12). They are formed when urine flow through individual nephrons is diminished. They can be found in the urine of individuals with kidney disease but also in the urine of people without such disease who have exercised heavily. Hyaline casts will be missed entirely if the light is not adjusted properly. Occasionally, hyaline casts have granular or cellular inclusions.

White blood cell casts are hyaline casts that contain leukocytes. White blood cells seen in casts usually have a multilobed nucleus. White blood cell casts are seen in pyelonephritis (Figure 47.13).

Red blood cell casts always indicate a pathologic condition and are highly diagnostic. These casts occur in glomerulonephritis. They are hyaline casts with embedded red blood cells. Their presence indicates damage to the glomerulus. They may appear brown due to the color of the red blood cells present (Figure 47.14).

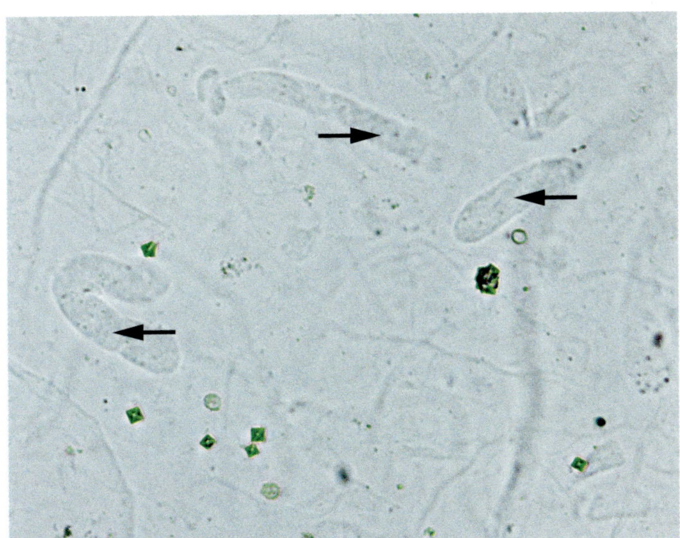

FIGURE 47.12 Hyaline cast. (From Brunzel NA: *Fundamentals of urine and body fluid analysis*, ed 3, Philadelphia, 2013, Saunders.)

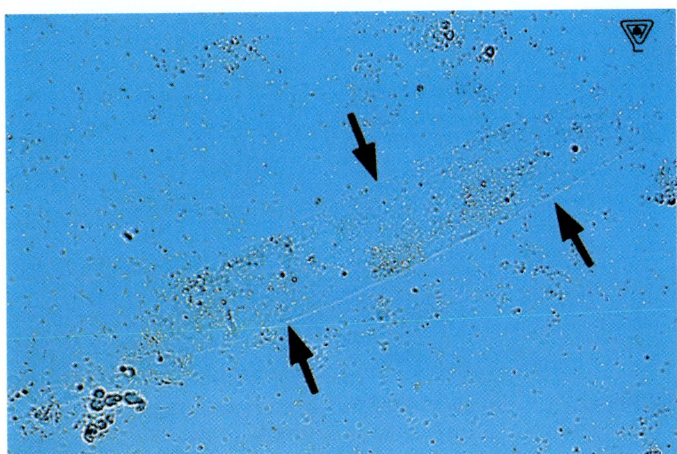

FIGURE 47.13 White blood cell cast. (From Stepp CA, Woods MA: *Laboratory procedures for medical office personnel*, Philadelphia, 1998, Saunders.)

Renal tubular epithelial cell casts contain embedded renal tubular epithelial cells. These casts are easily confused with white blood cell casts, particularly if the cells have started to degenerate. Renal tubular epithelial cell casts are found when excessive damage has occurred in the kidney. Causes include shock, **renal ischemia**, heavy-metal poisoning, certain allergic reactions, and **nephrotoxic** drugs (Figure 47.15).

Finely and coarsely granular casts may indicate renal disease. On close examination, granular casts show a hyaline cast with coarse or fine granular inclusions. The granules are thought to be caused by protein clusters or the breakdown of cellular inclusions (Figure 47.16).

Waxy casts are rarely seen. They appear as glassy, brittle, smooth, homogeneous structures. They usually are yellowish, have cracks or fissures, and have squared or broken ends. They are considered to be cellular casts that have broken down and are found in individuals with severe renal disease (Figure 47.17).

Occasionally more than one type of cell is found in a single cast. Mixed cellular casts have been reported, and it may be difficult to absolutely identify the cell types present. Cast identification is not a CLIA-waived procedure.

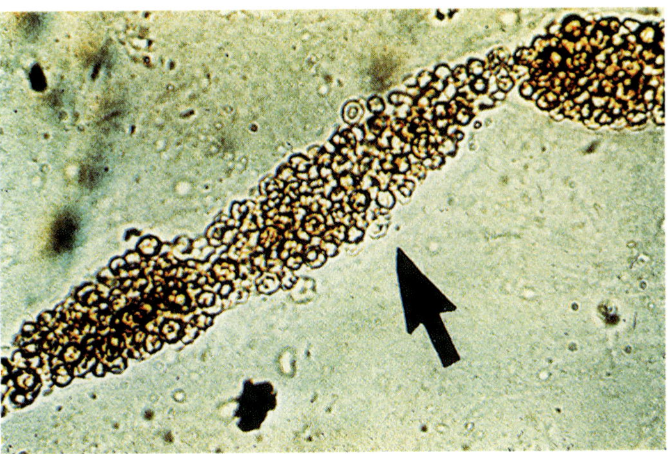

FIGURE 47.14 Red blood cell cast. (From Stepp CA, Woods MA: *Laboratory procedures for medical office personnel*, Philadelphia, 1998, Saunders.)

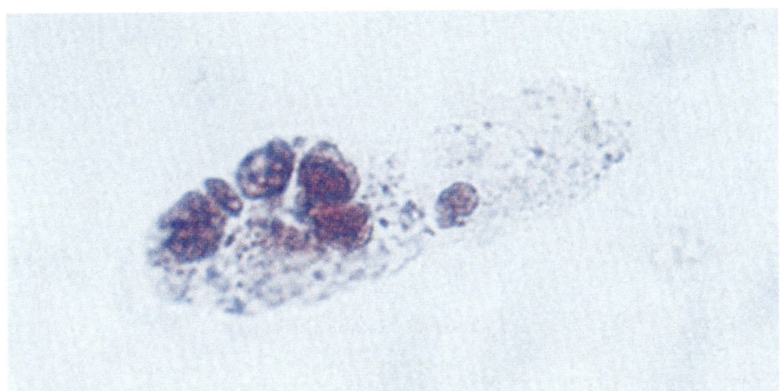

FIGURE 47.15 Renal tubular epithelial cell cast. (From Brunzel NA: *Fundamentals of urine and body fluid analysis*, ed 3, Philadelphia, 2013, Saunders.)

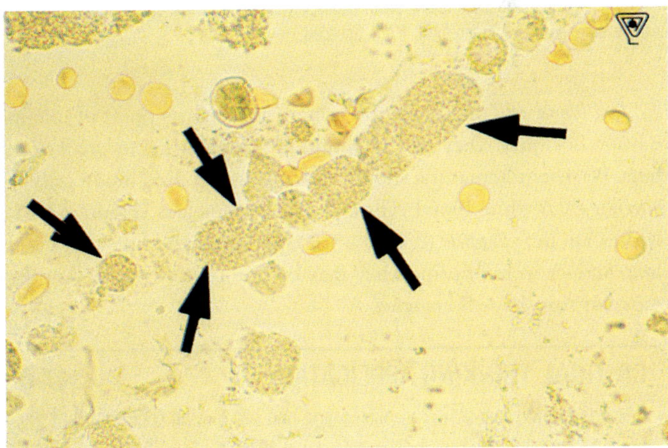

FIGURE 47.16 Granular cast. (From Stepp CA, Woods MA: *Laboratory procedures for medical office personnel*, Philadelphia, 1998, Saunders.)

Cells

Cells found in the urine include epithelial cells, which come from the lining of the genitourinary tract. Red blood cells and white blood cells, which come from the bloodstream, also may be seen. Cells are classified and counted under high-power magnification.

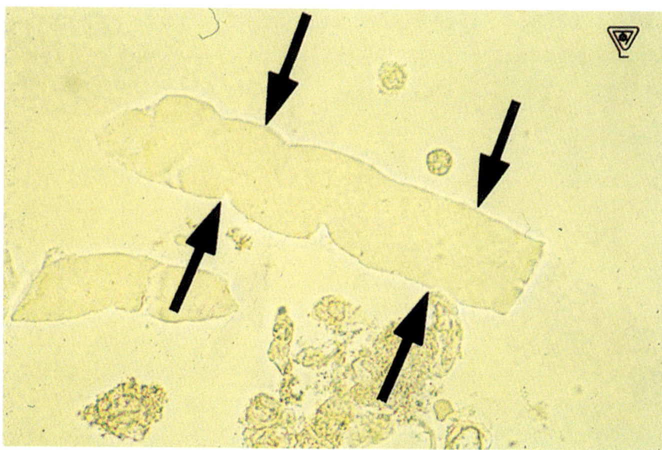

FIGURE 47.17 Waxy cast. (From Stepp CA, Woods MA: *Laboratory procedures for medical office personnel*, Philadelphia, 1998, Saunders.)

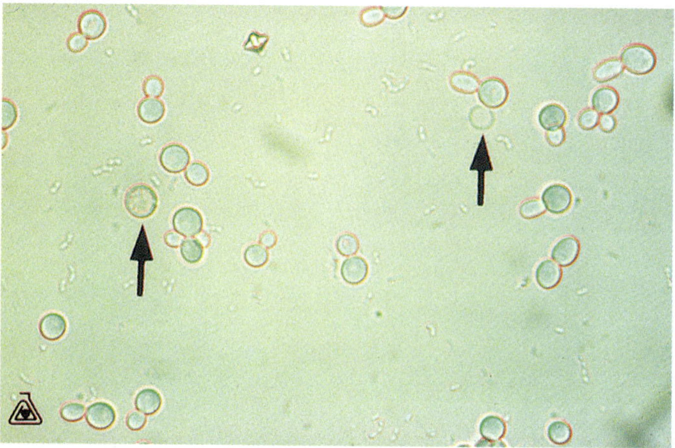

FIGURE 47.19 Yeast cells in urine. (From Stepp CA, Woods MA: *Laboratory procedures for medical office personnel*, Philadelphia, 1998, Saunders.)

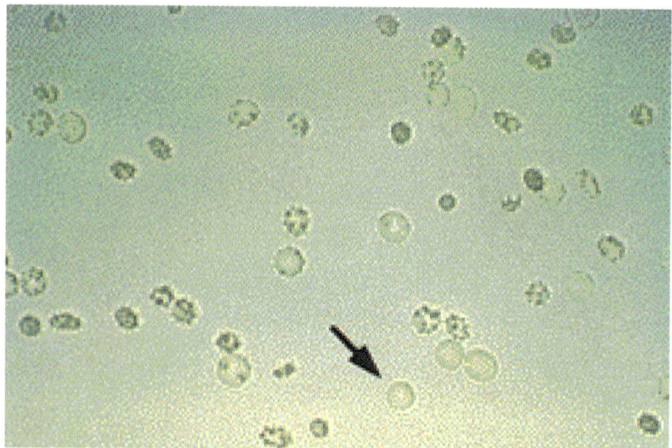

FIGURE 47.18 Red blood cells in urine. (From Stepp CA, Woods MA: *Laboratory procedures for medical office personnel*, Philadelphia, 1998, Saunders.)

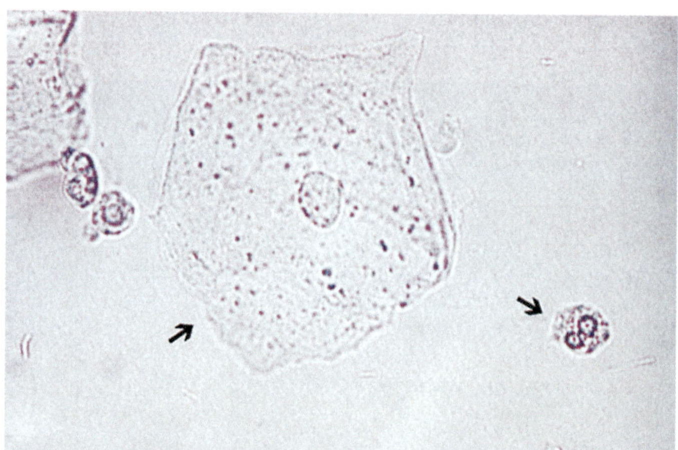

FIGURE 47.20 A large squamous epithelial cell *(left arrow)* and a white blood cell *(right arrow)* in urine. (From Ringsrud KM, Linne JJ: *Urinalysis and body fluids: a color text and atlas*, St. Louis, 1995, Mosby.)

Red blood cells may enter the urinary tract at any point of inflammation or injury. They may be found in normal urine in small numbers. Persistent hematuria should be investigated. Red blood cells are smaller than white blood cells and have no nucleus (Figure 47.18). If they are in *hypotonic* (dilute) urine, they swell and burst. In *hypertonic* (concentrated) urine, they may be bumpy or wrinkle. Another term for this shape is *crenated.*

CRITICAL THINKING APPLICATION **47.6**

Becca is excited to look in the microscope and see a urine sediment that has been prepared for the nurse practitioner at WMFM, Jean Burke. As Becca looks in the microscope's eyepiece, she sees quite a few red blood cells. What could cause red blood cells to be present in the urine? Discuss your thoughts with the class.

Yeast cells in the urine may indicate vaginal contamination or a urinary yeast infection (Figure 47.19). Yeast is common in the urine of patients with diabetes. Yeast cells are oval shaped and may show budding. Adding a drop of potassium hydroxide (KOH) will assist in distinguishing red blood cells from yeast, as it will cause all red blood cells to lyse but not yeast.

White blood cells may occasionally be found in normal urine, but increased numbers are associated with a UTI or vaginal contamination during specimen collection. White blood cells are larger than red blood cells and have a granular appearance. They may have a multilobed nucleus. Most white blood cells in the urine are neutrophils (Figure 47.20), but further testing will be needed to actually determine cell type.

Squamous epithelial cells line the lower portion of the genitourinary tract. When present in large numbers in female patients, they usually indicate vaginal contamination. Squamous epithelial cells are large, flat, and irregular. They have a single, small, round, centrally located nucleus and often occur in sheets or clumps (see Figure 47.20).

Transitional epithelial cells line most of the urinary tract. They are round or oval and may have a tail. Occasionally, two nuclei are seen. They may be seen in diseases of the urinary system (Figure 47.21).

Renal tubular epithelial cells are somewhat larger than white blood cells, are round or oval, and have a nucleus that is single, large, oval, and sometimes eccentric. A few may be found in normal urine

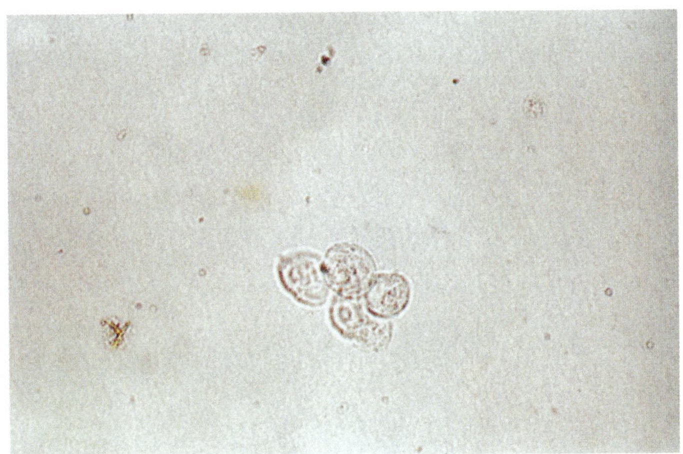

FIGURE 47.21 Small cluster of transitional epithelial cells in urine. (From Ringsrud KM, Linne JJ: *Urinalysis and body fluids: a color text and atlas,* St. Louis, 1995, Mosby.)

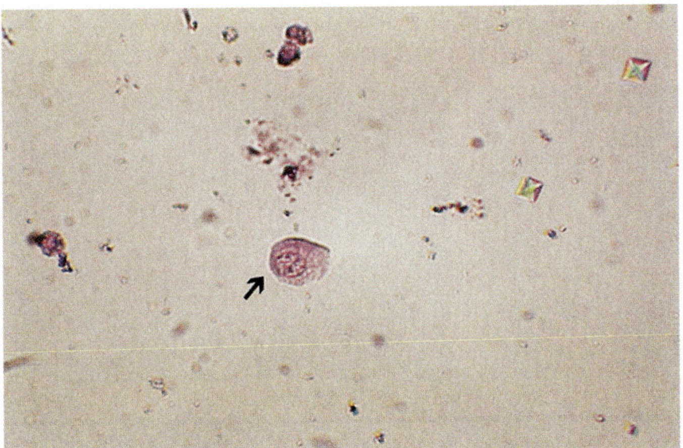

FIGURE 47.22 Renal tubular cell *(arrow)* in urine. (From Ringsrud KM, Linne JJ: *Urinalysis and body fluids: a color text and atlas,* St. Louis, 1995, Mosby.)

specimens, but their presence in increased numbers indicates tubular damage of the nephrons (Figure 47.22).

Crystals

Crystals are common in urine specimens, particularly if the specimen has been allowed to cool. Cooling causes solid crystals to precipitate out of the urine, which changes the urine's appearance from clear to cloudy. The presence of most crystals is not clinically significant unless the crystals are found in large numbers. With only rare exceptions, abnormal crystals are seen in acidic urine. Abnormal crystals may be present because of certain disease states or an inherited metabolic condition. They may also be *iatrogenic,* which means they are present because of medication or treatment. Identification of crystals begins with noting the pH of the urine specimen. A history of medications and recent diagnostic testing may be helpful too.

Crystals are reported as occasional, few, moderate, or many per high-power field (Table 47.5). At times, crystals can be *amorphous,* or lacking a defined shape. Frequently crystals are difficult to identify without additional chemical testing. Amorphous urates are found in acidic urine, whereas amorphous phosphates are found in alkaline samples.

Miscellaneous Findings

Oval fat bodies are formed when renal tubular epithelial cells or macrophages absorb fats. The fat droplets in the cells vary in size. They are characteristic of kidney distress (Figure 47.23).

A few *bacteria* may be found in normal urine specimens. High bacterial counts in a urine specimen without white blood cells may indicate that the specimen sat at room temperature and the bacteria multiplied. Urine specimens with a putrid odor, numerous white blood cells, and bacteria (Figure 47.24) are common in UTIs. Bacteria are seen under high-power magnification. They are often *motile* (moving).

Spermatozoa can be found in the urine specimens of both male and female patients. In a specimen from a female, their presence represents vaginal contamination. Sperm usually have pointed, oval heads and long, whiplike tails. They may be motile in fresh urine.

Trichomonas vaginalis is the most commonly encountered **protozoan** in urine (Figure 47.25). It is frequently a vaginal contaminant but may also be found in urine specimens from male patients. When urine is fresh and warm, trichomonas may be motile and move rapidly when viewed under the microscope. Trichomonas organisms are pear-shaped protozoa with four *flagella,* or whiplike tails. They are larger than round epithelial cells but smaller than squamous cells. Trichomonas organisms die when the specimen cools.

Mucous threads can be found in most urine specimens. They appear as pale, irregular, threadlike structures with tapered ends. Beginners often confuse hyaline casts with mucous threads. They are frequently seen in patients with inflammation and in specimens contaminated with vaginal secretions (Figure 47.26).

Artifacts and contaminants are often found in urine sediment. Training is required to tell them apart from significant structures. Fibers are common in the sediment and come from clothing, diapers, or digested plant material:

- Clothing fibers often are long and twisted and sometimes are colored. Diaper fibers can be confused with casts (Figure 47.27).
- Plant fibers appear in the urine because of fecal contamination (Figure 47.28).
- Hair is distinct not only because of the visible rough look to the strand but also because of the large size (Figure 47.29).
- Air bubbles are common if the coverslip was improperly placed over the sediment. Air bubbles are structureless, *refractile* (refracting light, causing a glow) and have a dark outline (Figure 47.30).

Understanding the Results of a Microscopic Examination

The medical assistant should understand how the microscopic findings of the sediment are reported. First, the sediment is examined under the low-power objective and low light to locate casts, generally found around the edges of the coverslip. From 10 to 15 low-power fields are scanned, and the number of casts is counted and reported.

TABLE 47.5 Normal and Abnormal Crystals Found in Urine

NORMAL CRYSTALS		
ACID URINE	**ALKALINE URINE**	**ABNORMAL CRYSTALS**
Calcium oxalate[a]	Ammonium biurate[b]	Sulfonamide
Uric acid[c]	Triple phosphate[a]	Cholesterol[a]

[a]From Stepp CA, Woods MA: *Laboratory procedures for medical office personnel,* Philadelphia, 1998, Saunders.
[b]From McPherson RA: *Henry's Clinical Diagnosis and Management by Laboratory Methods,* ed 24, St. Louis, 2022, Elsevier.
[c]From Brunzel NA: *Fundamentals of urine and body fluid analysis,* ed 3, Philadelphia, 2013, Saunders.

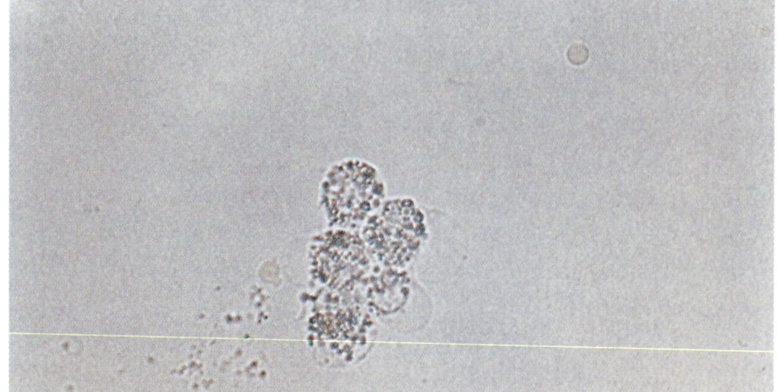

FIGURE 47.23 Small cluster of oval fat bodies in urine. (From Ringsrud KM, Linne JJ: *Urinalysis and body fluids: a color text and atlas,* St. Louis, 1995, Mosby.)

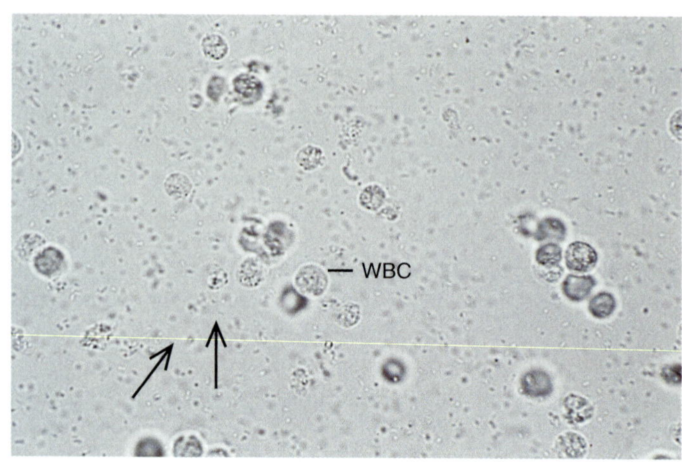

FIGURE 47.24 Many small bacteria *(arrows)* in urine. (From Ringsrud KM, Linne JJ: *Urinalysis and body fluids: a color text and atlas,* St. Louis, 1995, Mosby.)

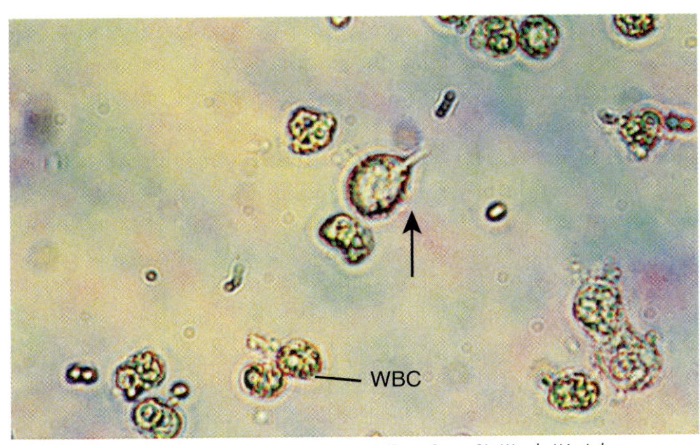

FIGURE 47.25 *Trichomonas* sp. *(arrow)* in urine. (From Stepp CA, Woods MA: *Laboratory procedures for medical office personnel,* Philadelphia, 1998, Saunders.)

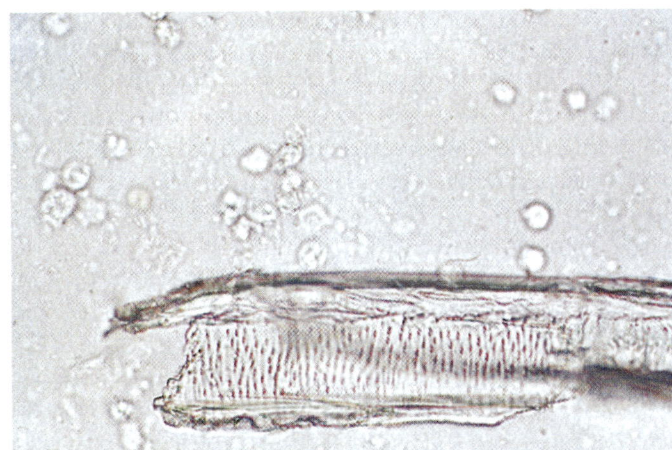

FIGURE 47.28 Plant fibers from fecal contamination; cells and bacteria are also present. (From Ringsrud KM, Linne JJ: *Urinalysis and body fluids: a color text and atlas,* St. Louis, 1995, Mosby.)

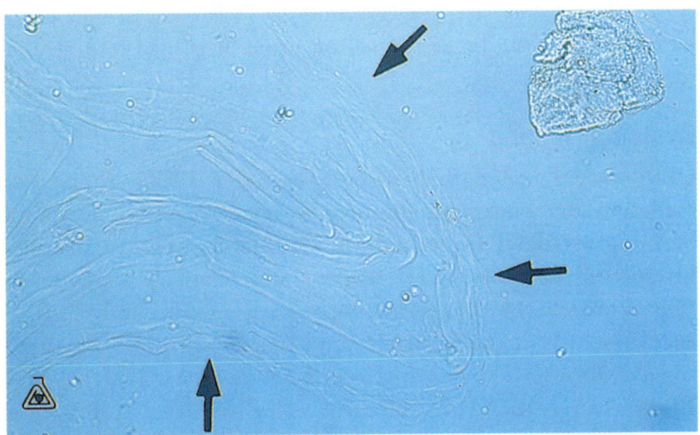

FIGURE 47.26 Mucous threads in urine. (From Stepp CA, Woods MA: *Laboratory procedures for medical office personnel,* Philadelphia, 1998, Saunders.)

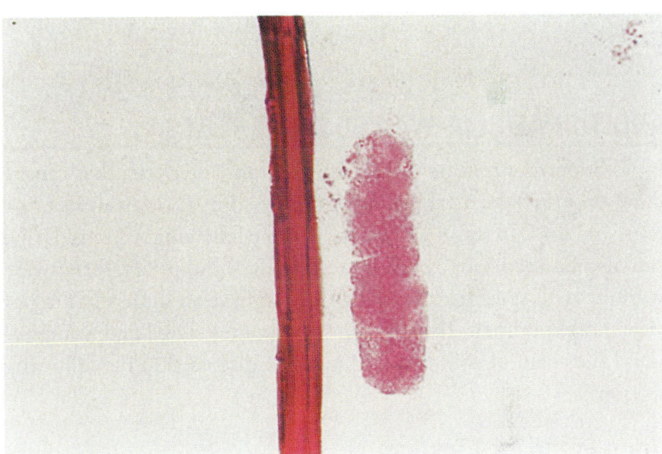

FIGURE 47.29 Fiber, probably hair *(left)* and waxy cast *(right)* in urine. (From Ringsrud KM, Linne JJ: *Urinalysis and body fluids: a color text and atlas,* St. Louis, 1995, Mosby.)

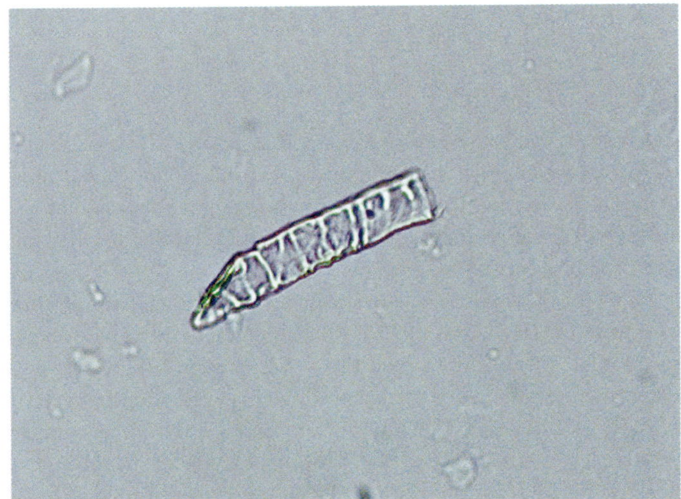

FIGURE 47.27 Diaper fibers in urine. (From Brunzel NA: *Fundamentals of urine and body fluid analysis,* ed 3, Philadelphia, 2013, Saunders.)

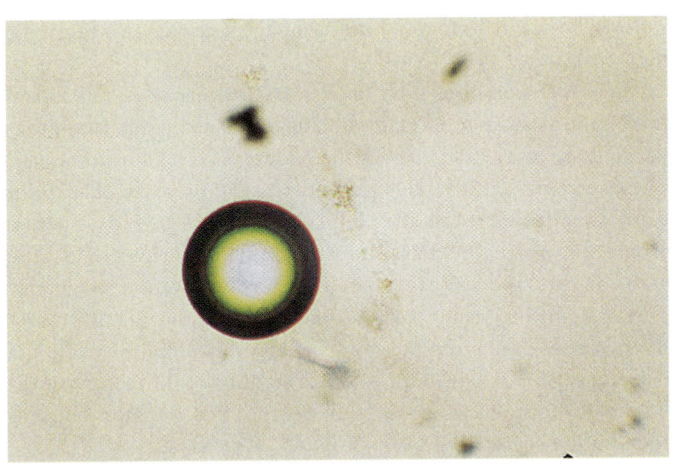

FIGURE 47.30 Large air bubble in urine. (From Ringsrud KM, Linne JJ: *Urinalysis and body fluids: a color text and atlas,* St. Louis, 1995, Mosby.)

Red and white blood cells, epithelial cells, yeasts, bacteria, and crystals are identified using the high-power objective and increased light. From 10 to 15 high-power fields should be scanned and the number counted, averaged, and reported. The method of counting varies considerably among laboratories. It is important that all workers in the same laboratory use the same counting and reporting systems.

The numbers of casts, RBCs, and WBCs are counted, totaled, and averaged. They are reported using numeric ranges based on the average seen (e.g., range of 0–1, 1–2, 2–5, 5–10, 10–20, and so forth; also, too numerous to count [TNTC]). Microscopic examination of epithelial cells is similar. Epithelial cells are counted, totaled, and averaged. Then they are reported as occasional, few, moderate, or many per high-power field (e.g., 1–3 occasional, 4–6 few, 7–12 moderate, >12 many). Miscellaneous elements seen in urine are counted, averaged, and estimated. Reports will be estimated as occasional (not seen in every field), few (covers less than one-fourth of the field), moderate (covers approximately one-half of the field), and many (covers the entire field).

ADDITIONAL CLIA-WAIVED URINE TESTS

In addition to a routine urinalysis, there are other tests that can be done on urine. Medical assistants can perform CLIA-waived urine tests, and some of those are discussed in the following sections. Urine can also be used for toxicology testing. It is important for anyone working with specimens for toxicology to have an understanding of how those specimens could potentially be adulterated and to understand the chain of command. This is also discussed in the following section.

Urine Pregnancy Testing

All pregnancy tests detect the presence of human chorionic gonadotropin (hCG), a hormone produced by the placenta and present in urine during pregnancy (see Procedure 47.7). After the fertilized egg has implanted in the uterus, the hCG levels in serum double every few days. This rapid rise occurs for approximately 7 weeks, and then the level begins to decline. Within 72 hours of delivery, the hormone disappears.

The most common type of test for pregnancy is the lateral flow immunoassay test. Many brands are available for laboratory use and are also available over the counter (OTC) for home use. These tests are sensitive enough to detect the presence of hCG in urine as early as 1 week after implantation, or 4 to 5 days before a missed menstrual period. The tests can be performed in as little as 5 minutes and are easy to interpret. CLIA-waived pregnancy tests or home pregnancy tests are read following the manufacturer's instructions. Evaluating the results is often as simple as reading a color change. For optimum results, the test should be performed on a first-morning urine specimen because it is the most concentrated urine of the day.

The test is based on reactions that occur between *antibodies* and *antigens*. Antibodies are proteins formed in response to a specific antigen (e.g., paired like a lock and key). Antigens are foreign substances that initiate the production of antibodies. When antibodies and antigens come in contact, the antibody binds to the antigen. This makes the antigen unable to cause disease. (See Chapter 33 for more information on antibodies and antigens.)

The pregnancy test cartridge contains a membrane with an absorbent pad. The urine sample is pipetted into the sample well of the test cartridge. The urine then moves along the absorbent pad, reaching the test area on the membrane. The following reactions can occur:

- All samples (positive or negative) cause the control zone (C) line to turn blue. The presence of this line indicates that the test has been carried out correctly. If the C control zone does not show a color reaction, the test is considered invalid (incorrect) and must be repeated using another test device.
- In a positive sample, the hCG antigen attaches to the antibodies in the test zone (T), forming a pink line.
- In a negative sample, there is no hCG antigen to attach to the antibodies in the test zone (T), and no line forms.

The Quick Vue test (see Procedure 47.7) is a lateral flow pregnancy test that can be performed on urine. It is used routinely in many POLs.

Ovulation Testing

CLIA-waived lateral flow urine tests are available to predict ovulation for women attempting to conceive either naturally or using **artificial insemination**. During the menstrual cycle, **luteinizing hormone (LH)** remains at a relatively stable level. Approximately 14 days before menstruation, the body experiences the "LH surge," a brief, rapid increase in LH. This surge triggers the release of an ovum (egg) from the ovary. Two to 3 days after the surge, the LH level returns to the base level. Conception is most likely to occur within 36 hours after the LH surge. The principle behind this test is similar to that of the pregnancy test. The absorbent membrane contains anti-LH antibodies. A positive test result indicates a urine LH level of 20 mIU/mL or higher. Testing usually is performed for 5 consecutive days in the middle of a woman's cycle. Once the surge is detected, ovulation can be expected within 2 to 3 days.

Menopause Testing

A woman is said to have reached *menopause* when she has not had a menstrual period for at least 12 months. The time before menopause, called *perimenopause,* can last for years, bringing with it uncomfortable symptoms such as irregular periods, hot flashes, vaginal dryness, and sleep problems.

Some of this may be due to an increase in **follicle-stimulating hormone (FSH)**. Levels of FSH increase temporarily each month to stimulate the ovaries to produce an ovum (egg). When a woman enters menopause, the ovaries stop producing eggs, and the levels of FSH rise. CLIA-waived lateral flow tests detect FSH in the urine. A positive test result indicates that a woman may be in menopause; a negative test result, along with symptoms of menopause, may indicate that a woman is in perimenopause.

The qualitative lateral flow test should never be used to direct a woman to stop using birth control methods if she does not want to conceive. Pregnancy is still possible during perimenopause.

TABLE 47.6 Commonly Abused Drugs and Body Retention Times

DRUG	RETENTION TIME
Alcohol	2–10 hours
Amphetamine	24–48 hours
Methamphetamine	3–5+ days
Barbiturates	
Phenobarbital	2–6 days
Secobarbital	24 hours
Cocaine, cocaine metabolites	12 hours–3 days
Opiates, heroin, morphine	3–4 days
Phencyclidine (PCP)	3–7+ days
Marijuana (tetrahydrocannabinol metabolites)	2 days up to 11 weeks (for daily users)
Oxycodone	3 days

CRITICAL THINKING APPLICATION 47.7

Becca thinks the immunoassays are so fun, watching the quality control samples flow through the kit and the results develop right in front of her. Take a few moments, and in your own words, describe how a lateral flow immunoassay works. What substances interact to create the reaction in the test kit?

Urine Toxicology

Toxicology is the study of poisonous substances and drugs and their effects on the body. The clinical laboratory performs tests on body fluids and tissues to monitor the use of therapeutic drugs, such as antibiotics, anticonvulsants, antidepressants, and barbiturates. They may also test for poisoning by herbicides, metals, animal toxins, and poisonous gases (e.g., carbon monoxide)

Laboratory testing for illegal drugs or alcohol is also done, most commonly due to employment, insurance, or legal requirement (Table 47.6). A urine specimen is the most reliable choice for most routine screening procedures. Urine drug tests detect drug *metabolites* and not the drugs themselves. A metabolite is a by-product of drug metabolism. Urine samples will remain positive even after the effects of the drugs are gone (see Procedure 47.8). For routine screening, a random specimen is usually collected.

Often, the following safeguards are used to ensure that a specimen is fresh and is truly from the patient:

- Water may be temporarily unavailable in the restroom.
- Bluing agents may be added to the toilets.
- A sealed container with a temperature-sensitive strip may be provided for collection.
- Someone of the same gender may accompany the patient into the restroom during the collection.

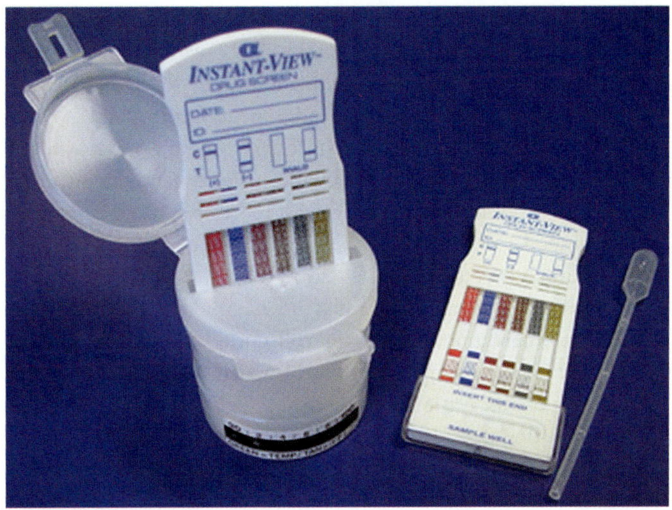

FIGURE 47.31 Instant View drug screening test. (Courtesy Alfa Scientific, Poway, CA.)

The *chain of custody* protocol is required for any legal specimen. This means that everyone handling the specimen must document their interaction with the sample. The drugs and their metabolites often remain in urine much longer than the physical impairment lasts. This is one reason urine screening is favored over blood screening.

As a medical assistant, you may be responsible for collecting specimens for toxicology tests and for performing certain laboratory tests. Rapid drug screening devices are about the size and shape of a credit card (Figure 47.31). The device is dipped into a urine sample, or urine is directly applied to the device. The results are read according to the manufacturer's instructions in just minutes. Negative results indicate that none of the targeted drugs were found in the urine sample at a detectable level. Inconclusive results indicate that the device reacted with something in the urine, and confirmatory testing is needed.

Urine multidrug screening tests are a type of lateral flow immunoassay that tests for urine metabolites of a variety of drugs. Common drugs tested include amphetamines, barbiturates, benzodiazepines, cocaine, morphine, methadone, phencyclidine (PCP), tricyclic antidepressants, marijuana, Ecstasy, methamphetamines, methadone, oxycodone, and opiates. This type of testing is also an immunoassay in which antibodies and antigens react to form a readable test result. By using antibodies specific to different drug classes, some test cartridges can simultaneously detect up to 10 different drugs from a single sample in 5 minutes.

Note: Unlike the lateral flow tests for pregnancy, ovulation, and menopause, the appearance of a line in the T band during a drug screening test indicates a negative result.

Adulteration Testing and Chain of Custody

Drug testing has legal consequences; therefore additional testing may be necessary to ensure that samples have not been adulterated. *Adulteration* is the intentional manipulation of a urine sample that allows someone to falsely pass a drug screening test. It may involve using urine from another person or an animal, diluting the sample with water, or adding other substances that would compromise the test procedure.

Sensitivity limits for drug screening are set by the US Substance Abuse and Mental Health Services Administration (SAMHSA), the National Institute on Drug Abuse (NIDA), and the US Department of Health and Human Services (DHHS). Positive results on urine drug samples should be confirmed with more specific confirmatory testing methods.

Chain of Custody Rules.

1. The individual being tested must provide photo identification.
2. Indirect observation of specimen collection is important to make sure the patient being tested has provided the sample. Indirect methods of observation include the following:
   - Measuring the specimen's temperature
   - Securing water faucets in the restroom so that urine cannot be diluted
   - Having the patient remove outer clothing and leave personal belongings in the examination room
   - Not allowing water to be run or the toilet to be flushed in the restroom during the collection

Note: If you suspect the sample has been adulterated, the patient may be asked to provide another specimen.

3. Within 4 minutes of receiving the specimen, check its temperature (the range should be 32° to 38°C [90° to 100°F]). The sample volume should be a minimum of 30 to 45 mL. Inspect the sample for any indications of adulteration (e.g., an unusual color, the presence of foreign materials).
4. Pour the specimen into a specimen bottle and seal the lid with the tamper-evident label/seal provided at the bottom of the chain of custody form. The donor should be present when this is done and should see you write the date and your initials on the label (Figure 47.32).
5. Ship the specimen to the testing laboratory as soon as possible. It must be sent the same day it was collected.
6. Individual testing method results may vary. Some tests have lower limits of detection, which can make some results positive at lower substance levels. Also, a person's diet, the volume of urine flow, and recent fluid intake can affect some results.
7. Because of the legal implications of drug testing, chain of custody must be strictly followed. Each step—from collecting the specimen to reporting the test results—must be strictly monitored and documented. Requirements include sealed specimen containers, supervised laboratory analysis throughout the process, and authorized signatures at each step.

CLOSING COMMENTS

Patient Coaching

Frequently, medical assistants are called on to explain specimen collection techniques to the patient. Patients want to do the procedure correctly but often lack knowledge of urinary terminology. They may be embarrassed or not know how to ask questions about cleaning the genital area. When explaining a urinary collection procedure, you should use pictures and words that the patient will understand. As you explain the procedure in terms the patient knows, he or she will feel comfortable telling you or asking you about pertinent details that may have a definite effect on treatment of the problem. Providing the patient with a clearly written instruction sheet also is helpful. The instruction sheet should be personalized with the patient's name, the time to begin collecting or testing (if applicable), what supplies should be used, and a phone number to call if questions arise.

Legal and Ethical Issues

Similar to all other procedures, the test is only as valid as the specimen and the procedure performed on that specimen. You, as the provider's agent, are responsible for that validity when you instruct the patient and perform the test.

A medical assistant responsible for office laboratory testing must clearly understand the basic concepts of laboratory medicine. Therefore, you must stay current with the rapid technologic advances in laboratory medicine and help establish a protocol of the tests best suited to your provider-employer.

You are responsible for properly collecting specimens and testing them accurately. In addition, you are responsible for strictly adhering to protocol when collecting and testing specimens, especially when legal ramifications are associated with the test results. Patient confidentiality is paramount when drug testing is performed, as is rigid conformation to all established rules and regulations.

Patient-Centered Care

Urine testing is frequently done in an ambulatory care setting. Knowing laboratory procedures helps medical assistants to ask informed and useful questions of their patients. Vitamin C can affect urine reagent strip testing, so asking a patient if he or she takes a vitamin C supplement is useful for obtaining correct testing results. If a person consumes large amounts of vitamin C, a special strip can be used to detect interfering levels of vitamin C. If an elevated level is found, the patient should be instructed to discontinue vitamin C intake for 24 hours, and then another urine specimen should be collected for testing.

Professional Behaviors

A laboratory professional performing urinalysis should have the following attributes:

- A discreet, respectful attitude when communicating with patients, co-workers, and supervisors.
- The ability to show sensitivity to patients' concerns and reassure patients of the accuracy of tests result (Procedure 47.9). When reassuring a patient, the medical assistant should listen to the patient's concerns and demonstrate therapeutic communication skills, respect, and empathy. Sometimes reassuring a patient involves educating the patient on the topic of concern. Increased understanding can help alleviate the patient's fears and calm the person.
- Good eyesight and manual dexterity.
- Accountability, honesty, and integrity when unsure of any procedure.
- Ability to multitask, manage his or her time, pay attention to details, and problem-solve if test results are unexpected.

FEDERAL DRUG TESTING CUSTODY AND CONTROL FORM

1A

SPECIMEN ID NO. 1234567 LAB ACCESSION NO.

OMB No. 0930-0158

STEP 1: COMPLETED BY COLLECTOR OR EMPLOYER REPRESENTATIVE

A. Employer Name, Address, I.D. No.

B. MRO Name, Address, Phone and Fax No.

C. Donor SSN or Employee I.D. No. ______

D. Reason for Test: ☐ Pre-employment ☐ Random ☐ Reasonable Suspicion/Cause ☐ Post Accident ☐ Return to Duty ☐ Follow-up ☐ Other (specify) ______

E. Drug Tests to be Performed: ☐ THC, COC, PCP, OPI, AMP ☐ THC & COC Only ☐ Other (specify) ______

F. Collection Site Address:

Collector Phone No. ______

Collector Fax No. ______

STEP 2: COMPLETED BY COLLECTOR

Read specimen temperature within 4 minutes. Is temperature between 90° and 100° F? ☐ Yes ☐ No, Enter Remark

Specimen Collection: ☐ Split ☐ Single ☐ None Provided (Enter Remark) ☐ Observed (Enter Remark)

REMARKS

STEP 3: Collector affixes bottle seal(s) to bottle(s). Collector dates seal(s). Donor initials seal(s). Donor completes STEP 5 on Copy 2 (MRO Copy)

STEP 4: CHAIN OF CUSTODY - INITIATED BY COLLECTOR AND COMPLETED BY LABORATORY

I certify that the specimen given to me by the donor identified in the certification section on Copy 2 of this form was collected, labeled, sealed and released to the Delivery Service noted in accordance with applicable Federal requirements.

X ______ Signature of Collector

______ AM PM Time of Collection

______ (PRINT) Collector's Name (First, MI, Last)

/ / Date (Mo./Day/Yr.)

SPECIMEN BOTTLE(S) RELEASED TO:

______ Name of Delivery Service Transferring Specimen to Lab

RECEIVED AT LAB:

X ______ Signature of Accessioner

______ (PRINT) Accessioner's Name (First, MI, Last)

/ / Date (Mo./Day/Yr.)

Primary Specimen Bottle Seal Intact

☐ Yes

☐ No, Enter Remark Below

SPECIMEN BOTTLE(S) RELEASED TO:

STEP 5a: PRIMARY SPECIMEN TEST RESULTS - COMPLETED BY PRIMARY LABORATORY

☐ NEGATIVE ☐ DILUTE ☐ REJECTED FOR TESTING

☐ POSITIVE for: ☐ MARIJUANA METABOLITE ☐ COCAINE METABOLITE ☐ PCP ☐ CODEINE ☐ MORPHINE ☐ 6-ACETYLMORPHINE ☐ AMPHETAMINE ☐ METHAMPHETAMINE

☐ ADULTERATED ☐ SUBSTITUTED ☐ INVALID RESULT

REMARKS ______

TEST LAB (if different from above) ______

I certify that the specimen identified on this form was examined upon receipt, handled using chain of custody procedures, analyzed, and reported in accordance with applicable Federal requirements.

X ______ Signature of Certifying Scientist

______ (PRINT) Certifying Scientist's Name (First, MI, Last)

/ / Date (Mo./Day/Yr.)

STEP 5b: SPLIT SPECIMEN TEST RESULTS - (IF TESTED) COMPLETED BY SECONDARY LABORATORY

______ Laboratory Name

______ Laboratory Address

☐ RECONFIRMED ☐ FAILED TO RECONFIRM - REASON ______

I certify that the split specimen identified on this form was examined upon receipt, handled using chain of custody procedures, analyzed, and reported in accordance with applicable Federal requirements.

X ______ Signature of Certifying Scientist

______ (PRINT) Certifying Scientist's Name (First, MI, Last)

/ / Date (Mo./Day/Yr.)

PEEL

1234567 A

SPECIMEN ID NO.

PLACE OVER CAP

1234567

SPECIMEN BOTTLE SEAL

/ / Date (Mo. Day Yr.)

Donor's Initials

PEEL

1234567 B (SPLIT)

SPECIMEN ID NO.

PLACE OVER CAP

1234567

SPECIMEN BOTTLE SEAL

/ / Date (Mo. Day Yr.)

Donor's Initials

PRESS HARD - YOU ARE MAKING MULTIPLE COPIES

0000-0000-0225

COPY 1 - LABORATORY

Drug Form Part 1
Face Inks: 000 BLK / 000 RED
Date: 05/09/00
Not To Use For Colormatch
Follow PMS Guide For Colors

FIGURE 47.32 First page of the Federal Drug Testing Custody and Control Form.

SUMMARY OF SCENARIO

Becca has had a fun and busy time in the laboratory at WMFM. She has enjoyed learning about the laboratory. She has had a chance to see some of the testing, PPE, quality assurance, and quality control processes that are part of a day in the lab. It was also nice to see the general workflow of the lab and the need for organization, attention to detail, and manual dexterity in laboratory testing.

With these observations fresh in her mind, Becca will finish her assignment later today. She is looking forward to graduating soon and working as a medical assistant. There are so many areas within ambulatory care to work as a medical assistant. Becca is excited for the future.

SUMMARY OF LEARNING OBJECTIVES

1. **Explain the formation and elimination of urine.**
   The urinary tract consists of two kidneys, two ureters, one bladder, and one urethra. The functional unit of the kidney is the nephron, and each nephron interacts with the blood by filtration, reabsorption, and secretion. Urine passes from the pelvis of the kidney down the ureter and into the bladder, where it remains until it is voided through the urethra.
2. **Explain the various methods used to collect urine specimens and the handling and transportation of specimens.**
   Some urine collections, such as the 2-hour postprandial specimen, must be timed around meals or fasts. Routine urinalysis (UA) requires no special preparation, whereas a clean-catch midstream specimen (CCMS) requires cleansing of the external genitalia. Only urine that will be cultured must be collected in a sterile container. Urine to be sent to a referral laboratory may require the addition of preservatives.

   Proper patient instruction is necessary for an acceptable CCMS. Both men and women are given instructions on cleaning the external genitalia to prevent contamination of the urine. Urine must be collected in a sterile container and refrigerated if it cannot be tested within 1 hour (see Procedure 47.2).

   If the specimen must be transported to a referral laboratory, evacuated transport tubes are often used. These tubes contain preservatives that prevent the overgrowth of bacteria and will prevent chemical changes in the urine that may affect test results. Chemical reagent strip testing can be performed on preserved specimens within 72 hours. Tubes may be held at room temperature during this time. A different preservative must be used for urine culture specimens. The preservative used for culture specimens helps maintain the number of bacteria present at the time of collection.
3. **Examine the physical and chemical aspects of urine along with the limitations of reagent strip testing and quality control.**
   The physical examination of urine involves determining the color, turbidity, and specific gravity. Odor and foam color also may be noted (see Procedure 47.3).
   - *Color:* Normal urine is a shade of yellow that ranges from pale straw to yellow to amber. The color depends on the concentration of the pigment urochrome and the amount of water in the specimen. Variations in color may also be caused by diet, medication, and disease.
   - *Turbidity:* Both normal and abnormal urine specimens may range in appearance from clear to very cloudy. Turbidity may be caused by cells, bacteria, yeast, vaginal contaminants, or crystals.

   The medical assistant should analyze and differentiate the normal and abnormal quality control results for the reagent strips before running the patient's chemical urinalysis (see Procedure 47.4).

   The chemical examination of urine involves determining the pH level and the levels of glucose, protein, ketones, blood, bilirubin, urobilinogen, and nitrite, in addition to specific gravity and leukocyte esterase, using a reagent strip. Most chemical urine testing requires reagent strips. It is essential that these supplies be stored in a dark, cool, moisture-free area.
   - *Reagent strip testing limitations can arise from several sources:*
     - The test strip is soaked in the specimen, and chemicals in the pads may be overly diluted.
     - The test strip is not held horizontally while read, and colors from one pad may bleed onto another.
     - The test pads on the strip are not read at the proper time, or the chemical reaction may be read incorrectly.
     - Certain chemicals may affect the results of nitrite, glucose, bilirubin, and blood tests.
     - Visual interpretation of color on the reagent strip pads is likely to vary among individuals.
   - *Quality assurance and quality control.*
     A commercially available control strip should be used to determine the reliability of chemical analysis. One such control strip is the Chek-Stix. After reconstitution, a reagent test strip is immersed in the control solution, and the results are compared with a chart that accompanies the Chek-Stix. Both positive and negative Chek-Stix controls are available (see Procedure 47.4). It is important to observe and record the abnormal and normal results produced by the positive and negative controls. Also, make sure the test results are consistent with the Chek-Stix charts provided by the manufacturer before testing patient urine specimens. There are many manufactured quality control (QC) liquids and strips that can be used for QC testing. The Chek-Stix is just one example.

SUMMARY OF LEARNING OBJECTIVES—*Continued*

4. **Explain the process of preparing urine for microscopic evaluation and what is seen in the microscopic examination of urine.**
   A complete UA involves physical, chemical, and microscopic assessment. The results of these three assessments must correlate with one another. Refer to Procedure 47.6.
5. **Examine additional CLIA-waived tests that can be performed on urine.**
   - *Urine pregnancy test:* Pregnancy tests detect hCG, a hormone produced by the placenta. Urine moves through the test (T) and control (C) areas of the test device by lateral absorption. Anti-hCG antibodies embedded in the test cartridge bind to hCG in the urine, causing a color change in the test area (see Procedure 47.7).
   - *Ovulation and menopause tests:* Fertility can be assessed using lateral flow tests that detect luteinizing hormone (LH), which increases in concentration in the urine shortly before ovulation. Menopause can be assessed using lateral flow tests that detect follicle-stimulating hormone (FSH), which increases as menopause approaches.
   - *Urine toxicology and drug testing:* Drug testing with lateral flow technology is similar to pregnancy testing, except it uses a competitive binding principle. Unlike with the pregnancy test, a line in the T region indicates a negative test result (see Procedure 47.8).

   Drinking excessive water before urinating, adding water to a urine specimen, and adding chemicals or products sold specifically to adulterate urine can render a drug test invalid. Adulteration test strips can detect most methods of adulteration.

PROCEDURE 47.1 Provide Instructions on How to Collect a 24-Hour Urine Specimen and Process the Sample

TASKS: Instruct a patient on how to collect a 24-hour urine specimen. Process a 24-hour specimen for a creatinine clearance test.

EQUIPMENT and SUPPLIES

- Patient's health record
- 2-4 L urine collection container
- Plastic cup or specimen collection pan for collecting urine (which is then poured into the collection container)
- Printed patient instructions
- Laboratory requisition
- Fluid-impermeable lab coat, protective eyewear, and gloves

PROCEDURAL STEPS

1. Greet the patient. Identify yourself. Verify the patient's identity with full name, ask the patient to spell the first and last name, and give his or her date of birth. Explain the procedure to be performed in a manner that the patient understands. Answer any questions the patient may have about the procedure.
   PURPOSE: It is important to identify the patient in two different ways to ensure that you have the correct patient. Explaining the procedure can make the patient feel more comfortable and reduces anxiety.
2. Label the container with the patient's name and the current date, identify the specimen as a 24-hour urine specimen, and include your initials. Check for preservative if needed.
   PURPOSE: Labeling the container prevents a possible mix-up of specimens.
3. Explain the following instructions to adult patients or the guardians of pediatric patients.

PATIENT INSTRUCTIONS: OBTAINING A 24-HOUR URINE SPECIMEN

a. Empty your bladder into the toilet in the morning without saving any of the specimen. Record the time you first emptied your bladder on the label.
b. For the next 24 hours, each time you empty your bladder, all the urine should be collected into the plastic cup or collection pan that is placed on the toilet (also called a nun's cap or toilet hat). Then pour all the collected urine directly into the large specimen container (see the following figure).
PURPOSE: Do not urinate directly into the large specimen container. It may contain a preservative that could be caustic. You do not want to splash any of the preservative while urinating.

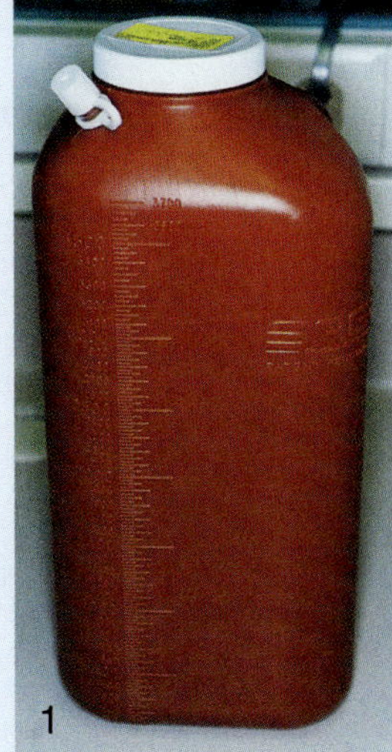

c. Put the lid back on the container after each urination and rinse out the plastic cup or collection pan; store the container in the refrigerator or at room temperature, as directed, throughout the 24 hours of the study.
PURPOSE: Refrigeration or the preservative inhibits microbial growth in the specimen.
d. If at any time you forget to collect your specimen or if some urine is accidentally spilled, you must begin the test over again with a new container and a newly recorded start time.
PURPOSE: The test will be inaccurate if you fail to collect all urine produced during the designated 24-hour period.

Continued

PROCEDURE 47.1 Provide Instructions on How to Collect a 24-Hour Urine Specimen and Process the Sample—*Continued*

e. Collect the final urine specimen at the same time you started the collection process on the previous day. This last collected specimen is placed in the large container. Collection ends with the voided morning specimen on the second day, which completes the 24-hour period.

f. As soon as possible after completing collection, return the specimen container to the provider's office or the designated laboratory.

4. Give the patient the specimen container and supplies with written instructions to confirm understanding.
PURPOSE: Ensuring correct supplies and instructions is essential to proper specimen collection.

5. Document details of the patient education session in the patient's record.
PURPOSE: Documentation confirms patient education was completed.

PROCESSING A 24-HOUR URINE SPECIMEN

6. Ask the patient whether he or she collected all voided urine throughout the 24-hour period or whether any problems occurred during the collection process.
PURPOSE: To confirm the accuracy of the specimen.

7. Complete the laboratory request form. Make sure that all the information is filled out on the container label.
PURPOSE: Proper labeling ensures specimen identification.

8. Wash hands or use hand sanitizer. Put on a fluid-impermeable lab coat, protective eyewear, and gloves before preparing the specimen for transport. Comply with safety practices.
PURPOSE: To ensure infection control.

9. Store the specimen in the refrigerator until it is picked up by the laboratory.
PURPOSE: Proper storage ensures the quality of the specimen.

10. Remove gloves and discard them appropriately. Remove protective eyewear and lab coat. Wash hands or use hand sanitizer.
PURPOSE: To ensure infection control.

11. Document that the specimen was sent to the laboratory, including the type of test ordered, the date and time, the type of specimen, and your initials.
PURPOSE: Properly documenting specimen collection and transport are essential parts of the process.

PROCEDURE 47.2 Provide Instructions on How to Collect a Clean-Catch Midstream Specimen and Process the Sample

TASKS: Instruct a patient on how to collect a clean-catch midstream specimen (CCMS). Process the specimen.

EQUIPMENT and SUPPLIES

- Patient's health record
- Patient written instructions
- Sterile container with a lid and label
- Antiseptic towelettes
- Laboratory requisition
- Biohazard specimen bag
- Fluid-impermeable lab coat, protective eyewear, and gloves

PROCEDURAL STEPS

1. Greet the patient. Identify yourself. Verify the patient's identity with full name, ask the patient to spell the first and last name and state his or her date of birth. Explain the procedure to be performed in a manner that the patient understands. Answer any questions the patient may have about the procedure.
PURPOSE: It is important to identify the patient in two different ways to ensure that you have the correct patient. Explaining the procedure can make the patient feel more comfortable and reduce anxiety.

2. Label the sterile sealed container (not the lid), and give the patient the towelette supplies (see the following figure) and patient instruction form, if needed.
PURPOSE: Labeling the container prevents a possible mix-up of specimens.

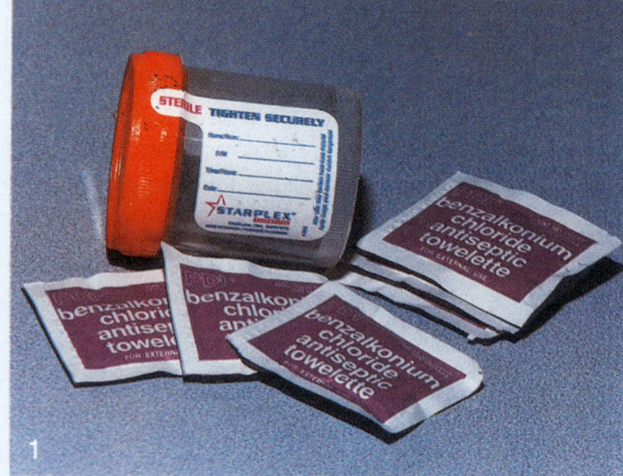

1

3. Using written directions, explain the following instructions to adult patients or the guardians of pediatric patients, making sure you show sensitivity to privacy issues.
PURPOSE: Instructions must be understood if they are to be followed correctly. By talking to the patient, you can determine whether the patient understands or has any questions.

PROCEDURE 47.2 Provide Instructions on How to Collect a Clean-Catch Midstream Specimen and Process the Sample—*Continued*

PATIENT INSTRUCTIONS: OBTAINING A CLEAN-CATCH MIDSTREAM SPECIMEN (FEMALE PATIENT)

a. Wash your hands and open the towelette packages for easy access.
PURPOSE: To wash away any contaminating bacteria from the hands
b. Remove the lid from the specimen container, being careful not to touch the inside of the lid or the inside of the container. Place the lid, facing up, on a paper towel.
PURPOSE: The lid and the container must be handled carefully to maintain the internal sterility of the container and prevent contamination of the urine sample.
c. Lower your underclothing and sit on the toilet.
d. Expose the urinary meatus by spreading apart the labia with one hand (see the following figure, part A).
PURPOSE: To allow for adequate cleansing.

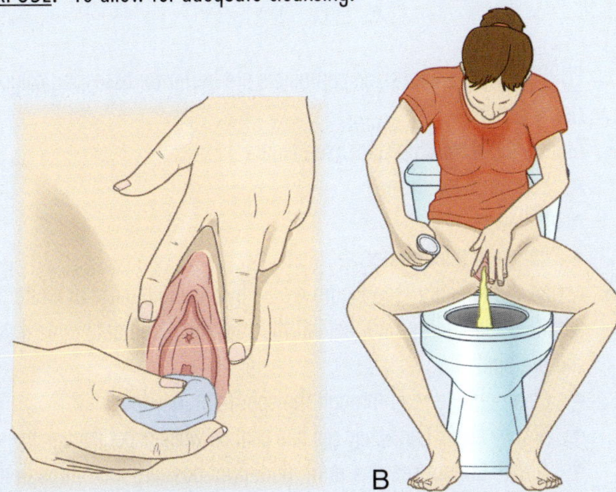

e. Cleanse each side of the urinary meatus with a front-to-back motion from the pubis toward the anus. Use a separate antiseptic wipe to cleanse each side of the meatus.
PURPOSE: Cleansing the area around the urinary meatus prevents contamination of the urine sample. Wiping in one stroke from front to back prevents the passage of microorganisms from the anal region to the area around the urinary meatus.
f. Cleanse directly across the meatus, front to back, using a third antiseptic wipe (see the preceding figure, part A).
g. Hold the labia apart throughout this procedure.
PURPOSE: To avoid specimen contamination.
h. Void a small amount of urine into the toilet (see the preceding figure, part B).
PURPOSE: Allowing the initial flow of urine to pass into the toilet flushes the opening of the urethra.
i. Move the specimen container into position and void the next portion of urine into it. Fill the container halfway. Remember, this is a sterile container. Do not put your fingers on the inside of the container.
PURPOSE: To avoid specimen contamination
j. Remove the cup and void the last amount of urine into the toilet. (This means that the first and last parts of the urinary flow have been excluded from the specimen. Only the middle portion of the flow is included.)
PURPOSE: To avoid specimen contamination.
k. Place the lid on the container, taking care not to touch the interior surface of the lid. Wipe in your usual manner, redress. Wash your hands and return the sterile specimen to the place designated by the medical facility.
PURPOSE: To avoid specimen contamination; to ensure infection control.

PATIENT INSTRUCTIONS: OBTAINING A CLEAN-CATCH MIDSTREAM SPECIMEN (MALE PATIENT)

a. Wash your hands and expose the penis.
b. Retract the foreskin of the penis (if not circumcised).
PURPOSE: To allow for adequate cleansing.
c. Cleanse the area around the glans penis (tip of the penis) and the urethral opening (meatus) by washing each side of the glans with a separate antiseptic wipe (see the following figure, part A).

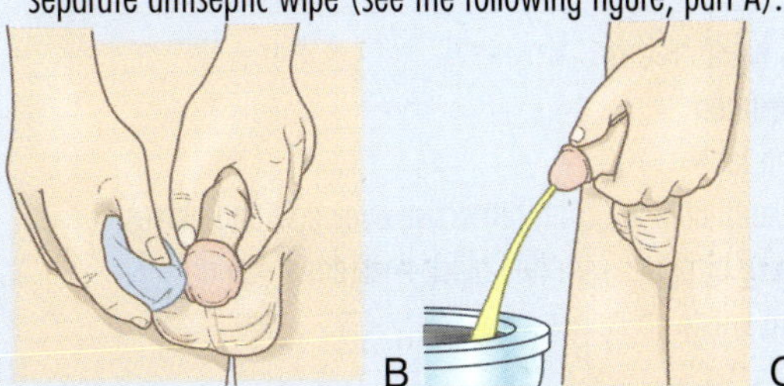

d. Cleanse directly across the urethral opening using a third antiseptic wipe.
PURPOSE: To cleanse the area of normal flora that may contaminate the specimen.
e. Void a small amount of urine into the toilet or urinal (see the preceding figure in step (c), part B).
f. Collect the next portion of the urine in the sterile container, filling the container halfway without touching the inside of the container with the hands or the penis (see the preceding figure in step [c], part C).
PURPOSE: To avoid specimen contamination
g. Void the last amount of urine into the toilet or urinal.
h. Place the lid on the container, taking care not to touch the interior surface of the lid. Wipe in your usual manner, redress. Wash your hands and return the sterile specimen to the place designated by the medical facility.
PURPOSE: To avoid specimen contamination. To ensure infection control.
i. Return the specimen to the designated area.

PROCESSING A CLEAN-CATCH URINE SPECIMEN

4. Document the date, time, and collection type.
PURPOSE: Essential information for specimen documentation.
5. Wash hands or use hand sanitizer. Put on the fluid-impermeable lab coat, protective eyewear, and gloves. Comply with safety practices.
PURPOSE: Hand sanitization is an important step for infection control. PPE is part of Standard Precautions.

Continued

PROCEDURE 47.2 Provide Instructions on How to Collect a Clean-Catch Midstream Specimen and Process the Sample—*Continued*

6. Process the specimen according to the provider's orders. Perform urinalysis in the office or prepare the specimen for transport to the laboratory. If it is to be sent to an outside laboratory, complete the following steps:
   a. Make sure the label is properly completed with the patient's information, the date, time, test ordered, and your initials.
   b. Place the specimen in a biohazard specimen bag.
   c. Complete a laboratory requisition and place it in the outside pocket of the specimen bag.
   d. Keep the specimen refrigerated until pickup.

   PURPOSE: Proper labeling, storage, and transport ensure the correct patient specimen and specimen quality.

7. Remove gloves, protective eyewear, and lab coat. Dispose of gloves appropriately. Wash hands or use hand sanitizer. Document that the specimen was sent.
   PURPOSE: To ensure infection control. A procedure is not completed until it is documented.

PROCEDURE 47.3 Assess Urine for Color and Turbidity: Physical Test

TASKS: Assess and record the color and clarity of a urine specimen.

EQUIPMENT and SUPPLIES

- Patient's health record
- Urine specimen
- Centrifuge tube
- Fluid-impermeable lab coat, protective eyewear, and gloves
- White piece of paper with thin black lines drawn on it
- Biohazard waste container

PROCEDURAL STEPS

1. Wash hands or use hand sanitizer. Put on the fluid-impermeable lab coat, protective eyewear, and gloves. Comply with safety practices.
   PURPOSE: Hand sanitization is an important step for infection control. Wearing PPE is part of Standard Precautions.

2. Mix the urine by gently swirling the specimen.
   PURPOSE: Suspended substances settle when urine stands. If urine is not mixed before its appearance is assessed, the finding will be incorrect.

3. Label a centrifuge tube if a complete urinalysis is to be done.
   PURPOSE: If a complete urinalysis is to be done, a portion of the specimen will be centrifuged for microscopic examination. The centrifuged specimen must be labeled to prevent specimen confusion.

4. Pour the specimen into a standard-sized centrifuge tube.
   PURPOSE: Standard-sized containers are better for assessing color and clarity results.

5. Assess and record the color (see Figure 47.4):
   - Pale straw or straw
   - Yellow
   - Amber or dark amber

6. Assess the turbidity (see Figure 47.5) by placing a piece of white paper with fine, dark black print behind the specimen, and determine if you can see the print:
   - *Clear:* Able to read through the specimen; no cloudiness
   - *Slightly turbid:* Can barely see fine print on white paper through the specimen
   - *Turbid:* Cannot see fine print, dark print possibly seen through the tube, or see no print at all through the tube

7. Clean the work area and dispose of procedure supplies in the biohazard waste container.
   PURPOSE: To ensure infection control.

8. Dispose of gloves. Remove your lab coat and protective eyewear. Wash hands or use hand sanitizer.
   PURPOSE: To ensure infection control.

9. Document the results in the patient's record.
   PURPOSE: A procedure is not considered complete until it is documented.

PROCEDURE 47.4 Perform Quality Control Measures to Determine the Reliability of Chemical Reagent Strips

TASKS: Reconstitute a control sample and test the reliability of the urinalysis chemical testing strip.

EQUIPMENT and SUPPLIES

- Chek-Stix control strips with reference ranges for urinalysis
- Distilled water
- Capped tube with milliliter markings
- Test tube rack
- Forceps
- Timer
- Urine chemical strips for urine testing
- Color chart for interpreting the chemical strip results
- Fluid-impermeable lab coat, protective eyewear, and gloves
- Biohazard waste container
- Control reference sheet and control flow sheet

PROCEDURE 47.4 Perform Quality Control Measures to Determine the Reliability of Chemical Reagent Strips—*Continued*

PROCEDURAL STEPS

1. Assemble the equipment and supplies. Record the lot number and the expiration date of the Chek-Stix on the control log sheet.
   PURPOSE: Chek-Stix cannot be used if the expiration date has passed. Recording the lot number and expiration date is an important part of quality assurance.
2. Wash hands or use hand sanitizer. Put on the fluid-impermeable lab coat, protective eyewear, and gloves. Comply with safety practices.
   PURPOSE: To ensure infection control. PPE is part of Standard Precautions.
3. Place a conical tube in a test tube rack, and remove the cap.
4. Pour 15 mL of distilled water into the tube.
5. Using forceps, remove one strip from the Chek-Stix bottle. Inspect the strips for mottling or discoloration.
   PURPOSE: The control strips have chemicals that you should not handle or contaminate with your hands. Any mottling or discoloration may mean that the strips have been exposed to moisture, light, or solvents. Improperly stored control strips should not be used.
6. Place the strip into the water and tightly cap the tube.
7. Invert the tube for 2 minutes.
   PURPOSE: Chemicals embedded in the pads must be thoroughly dissolved in the water.
8. Allow the tube to sit in the test tube rack for 30 minutes.
9. Invert the tube one time and remove the strip with forceps.
10. Discard the strip in the biohazard waste container. Once reconstituted, the control solution is stable for 8 hours at room temperature.
    PURPOSE: To ensure infection control.
11. Perform quality control of the chemical reagent strip by dipping it into the control solution (see Procedure 47.5).
    PURPOSE: Quality control is an essential step in assuring quality patient results.
12. Read and record the results.
    PURPOSE: Proper documentation is a necessity in all quality control procedures.
13. Compare the results with the control reference ranges provided on the Chek-Stix package insert.
    PURPOSE: Results should fall within a given range provided by the manufacturer. If they do not, the chemical reagent strips cannot be used to test patients' urine.
14. Discard the chemical reagent strip and the control solution in the biohazard waste container.
15. Clean up the work area and appropriately dispose of supplies and gloves in a biohazard waste container.
    PURPOSE: To ensure infection control; to maintain a proper work area.
16. Remove protective eyewear and lab coat. Wash hands or use hand sanitizer.
    PURPOSE: To ensure infection control.

PROCEDURE 47.5 Test Urine with Chemical Reagent Strips

TASK: Perform chemical testing on a urine sample.

EQUIPMENT and SUPPLIES

- Patient's health record
- Urine specimen
- Reagent strips
- Timer
- Fluid-impermeable lab coat, protective eyewear, and gloves
- Biohazard waste container

PROCEDURAL STEPS

1. Wash hands or use hand sanitizer. Put on the fluid-impermeable lab coat, protective eyewear, and gloves. Comply with safety practices.
   PURPOSE: To ensure infection control. PPE is part of Standard Precautions.
2. Check the time of collection, the container, and the mode of preservation.
   PURPOSE: Proper specimen identification and screening of specimens for appropriate collection containers and procedures prevent the testing of inappropriate specimens.
3. If the specimen has been refrigerated, allow it to warm to room temperature.
   PURPOSE: Certain tests are temperature dependent. Testing cold specimens may cause false-negative results.
4. Check the reagent strip container for the expiration date.
   PURPOSE: Do not use expired reagents.
5. Remove the reagent strip from the container. Hold it in your hand or place it on a clean, dry paper towel. Recap the container tightly.
   PURPOSE: Test strips are sensitive to moisture and light and must be stored in tightly-sealed containers. Contamination from chemical residues on countertops can affect results.
6. Compare nonreactive test pads with the negative color blocks on the color chart on the container. Discard strips that have discolored pads.
   PURPOSE: Discolored pads indicate that the product has not been properly stored and must not be used for testing.
7. Thoroughly mix the specimen by gently swirling the container.
   PURPOSE: If settling occurs, certain elements may not be detected.
8. Following the manufacturer's directions, note the time, dip the strip into the urine, and remove it.
   PURPOSE: Tests are time dependent. Some pads darken over time.
9. Quickly remove the excess urine from the strip by pulling the back of the strip across the lip of the specimen container and then blotting the edge of the strip on a clean, dry paper towel or the side of the specimen container.

Continued

PROCEDURE 47.5 Test Urine with Chemical Reagent Strips—*Continued*

PURPOSE: Excess urine on the strip or prolonged dipping time affects test results.

10. Hold the strip horizontally (see the following figure). At the required time, compare the strip with the appropriate color chart on the reagent container. *Do not touch the strip to the bottle.*
    Alternately, the strip can be placed on a clean, dry paper towel.

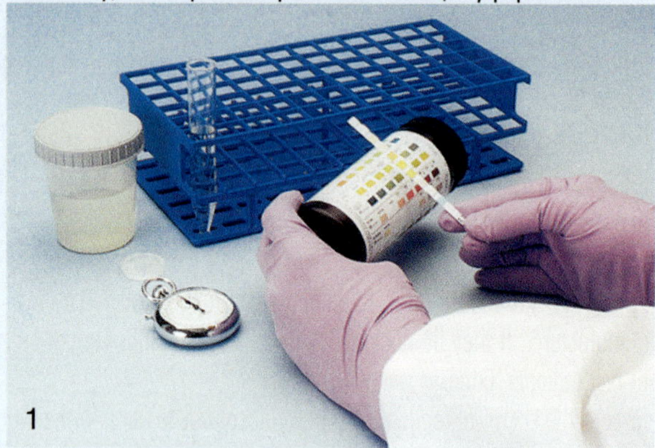

PURPOSE: Holding the strip horizontally prevents runover from one test pad to another and prevents interference from mixing chemicals in the test pads.

11. Read and record the first two results 30 seconds after dipping the strip (the indicated time to read the "Glucose" and "Bilirubin"). Compare the two reagent pads closest to your hand with the bottom two rows of the color chart (see the following figure). Continue reading and recording each row of possible results with its appropriate reagent pad at its designated time.
    PURPOSE: Timing is critical. Allowing the strip to touch the bottle contaminates the bottle.
12. Clean the work area. If a paper towel was used, dispose of it and the reagent strip in an appropriate biohazard waste container.
    PURPOSE: To ensure infection control.
13. Remove gloves and dispose of them appropriately. Remove protective eyewear and lab coat. Wash hands or use hand sanitizer.
    PURPOSE: To ensure infection control.
14. Document the results in the patient's health record.
    PURPOSE: A procedure is not complete until it has been documented.

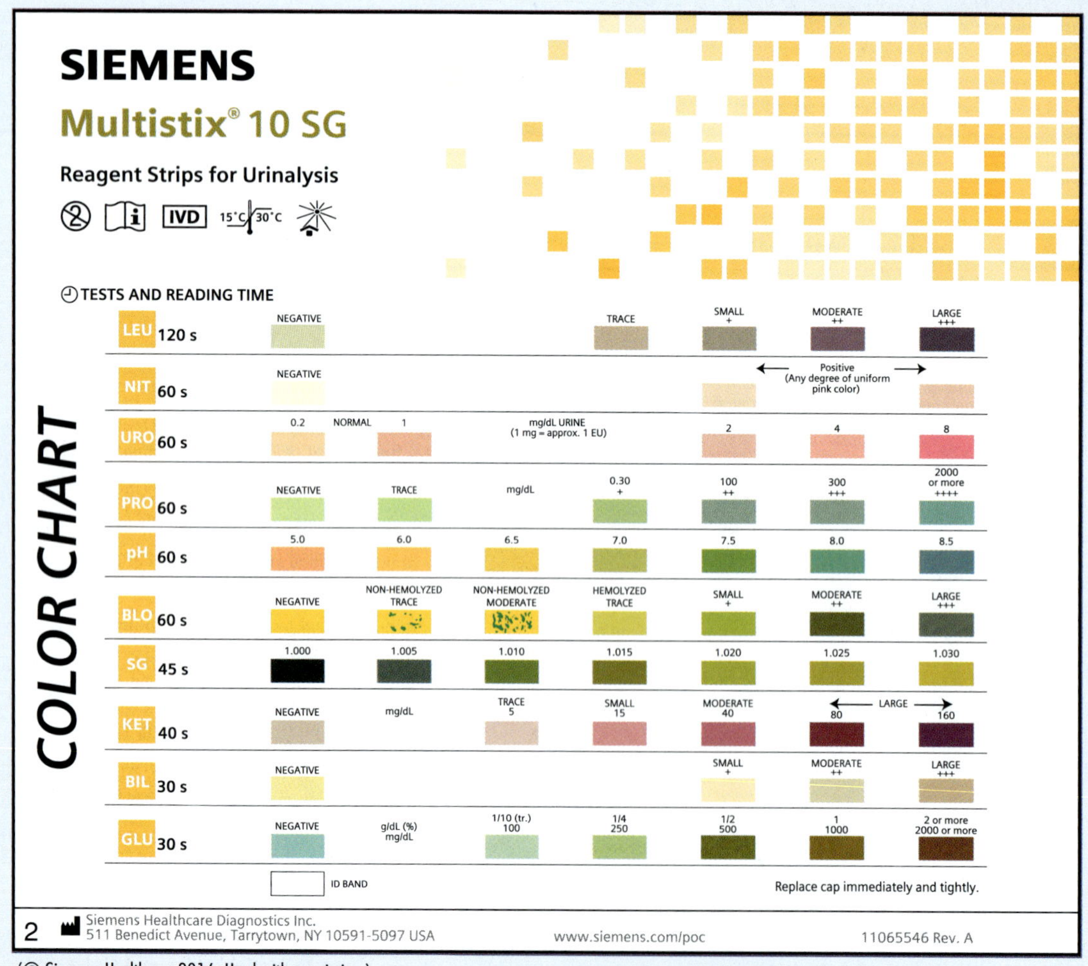

PROCEDURE 47.6 Prepare a Urine Specimen for Microscopic Examination

TASK: Prepare a urine specimen for the provider's microscopic examination to determine the presence of normal and abnormal elements.

EQUIPMENT and SUPPLIES

- Patient's health record
- Urine specimen
- Centrifuge tube
- Centrifuge
- Disposable pipet
- Sedi-Stain
- Microscope slide and coverslip
- Microscope
- Permanent marker
- Fluid-impermeable lab coat, protective eyewear, and gloves
- Biohazard waste container

PROCEDURAL STEPS

1. Wash hands or use hand sanitizer. Put on the fluid-impermeable lab coat, protective eyewear, and gloves. Comply with safety practices.
   PURPOSE: To ensure infection control. PPE is part of Standard Precautions.
2. Gently mix the urine specimen by swirling the covered specimen container.
   PURPOSE: If the urine is not well mixed, elements that have settled to the bottom of the specimen container will be missed.
3. Pour 12 mL of urine into a labeled centrifuge tube and cap the tube.
   PURPOSE: Label to ensure proper specimen identification.
4. Place the tube in the centrifuge (see the following figure).

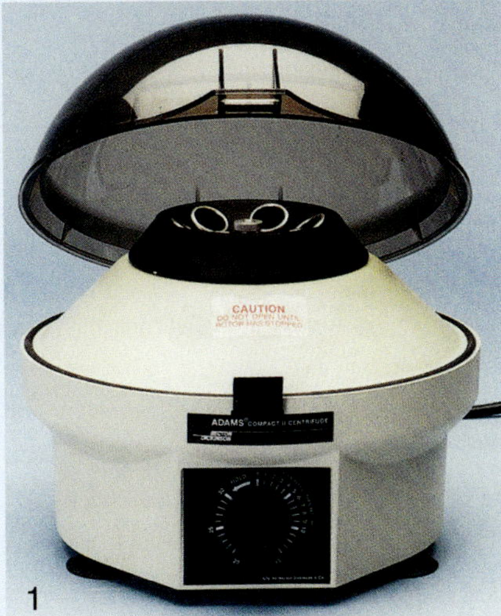

1

(From Stepp CA, Woods MA: *Laboratory procedures for medical office personnel*, Philadelphia, 1998, Saunders.)

5. Place another tube containing 12 mL of urine or water in the opposite cup.
   PURPOSE: For proper operation, centrifuges must be carefully balanced. If not properly balanced, damage to the instrument can occur.
6. Secure the lid and centrifuge for 5 minutes or the time specified for your instrument.
   PURPOSE: Timing varies according to the speed and the size of the centrifuge head.
7. Remove the tube from the centrifuge after the instrument has come to a full stop.
   PURPOSE: Wait for a full stop to safely operate the centrifuge.
8. Pour off the clear supernatant from the top of the specimen by inverting the centrifuge tube over the sink drain while allowing the running water from the faucet to flush the urine down the drain.
   PURPOSE: Decanting the supernatant creates a good sediment specimen.
9. Turn the tube upright when the supernatant has been decanted, allowing a small amount to return to the sediment on the bottom of the tube without losing sediment down the drain (see the following figure).
   PURPOSE: The sediment will be examined under the microscope.

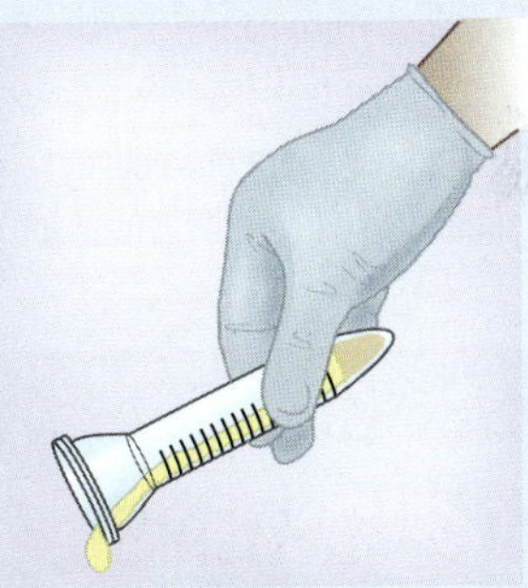

2

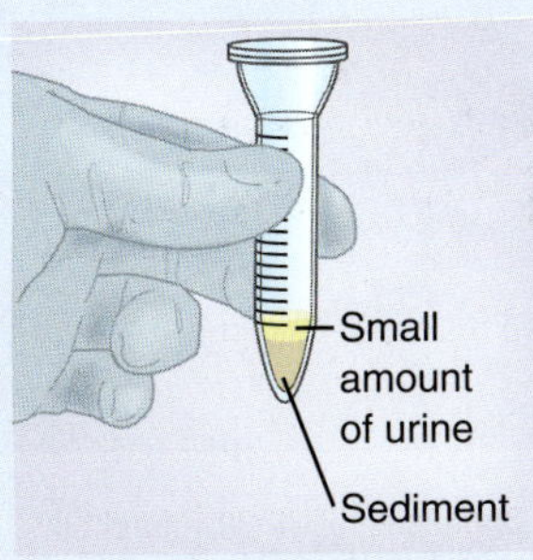

3

10. Thoroughly mix the sediment with a drop of Sedi-Stain by grasping the tube near the top and rapidly flicking it with the fingers of the other hand until all sediment is thoroughly resuspended.
    PURPOSE: Elements centrifuge at different rates. Failure to mix the entire sediment completely may result in evaluation errors. Sedi-Stain colors the sediment for easier viewing.
11. Transfer 1 drop of sediment to a clean, labeled slide using a clean, disposable transfer pipet. Transfer pipet should be disposed of in a sharps container.
    PURPOSE: A clean slide will not contaminate the specimen. Labeling ensures the correct patient specimen.
12. Place a clean coverslip over the drop and place the slide on the microscope stage. Remove eye protection.
    PURPOSE: The coverslip allows the specimen to be properly focused on the microscope.
13. Focus under low power and reduce the light.
    Note: Once the slide is focused under low power, the remaining steps of this procedure are performed by the trained healthcare provider or moderate/highly complex trained laboratory personnel.

PROCEDURE 47.7 Perform a CLIA-Waived Urinalysis: Perform a Pregnancy Test

TASK: Perform a pregnancy test on urine using the QuickVue pregnancy test method.

EQUIPMENT and SUPPLIES

- Patient's health record
- Urine specimen
- QuickVue test kit
- Fluid-impermeable lab coat, protective eyewear, and gloves
- Biohazard sharps container
- Biohazard waste container

PROCEDURAL STEPS

1. Wash hands or use hand sanitizer. Put on a fluid-impermeable lab coat, protective eyewear, and gloves. Comply with safety practices.
   PURPOSE: Hand sanitization is an important step for infection control. PPE is part of Standard Precautions.
2. Prepare the testing equipment (see the following figure). Check the expiration date of the kit before proceeding.
   PURPOSE: Expired kits should not be used for quality control or patient samples.

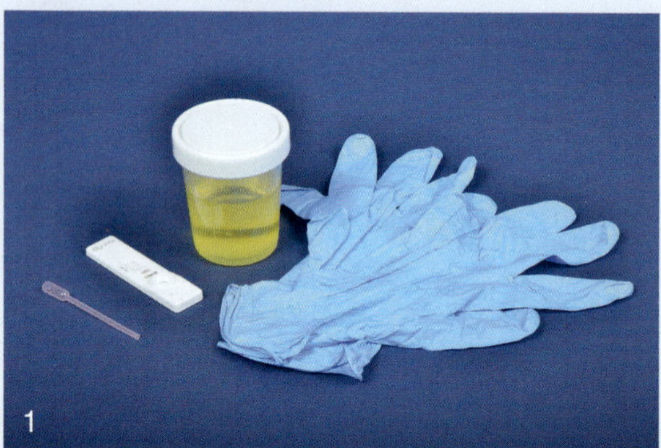

1

3. Obtain the proper patient specimen (preferably a first-morning specimen).
4. Remove the test cassette from the foil pouch.
5. Add 3 drops of urine using the transfer pipet (dropper) that accompanies the kit (see the following figure).
   PURPOSE: The specimen amount must be added as indicated by the manufacturer's written procedure to ensure accurate test results.

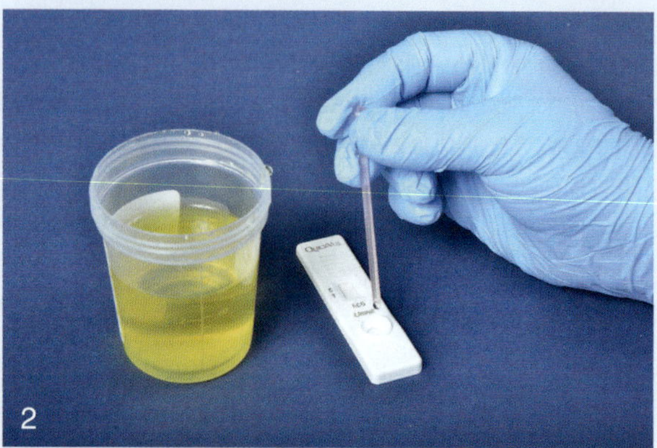

2

6. Dispose of the pipet in a biohazard sharps container.
   PURPOSE: To ensure infection control.
7. Wait 3 minutes and read the test results.
   PURPOSE: Timing must be accurate to ensure accurate test results.
8. Interpret the results (see the following figure):
   Negative: A blue control line is next to the letter C; no line is seen next to the letter T (see the cassette in the middle).
   Positive: A blue control line is next to the letter C; a pink line is next to the letter T (see the cassette on the right).
   Invalid: If a blue line does not appear in the C area, the test is invalid, and the specimen must be retested using another kit.

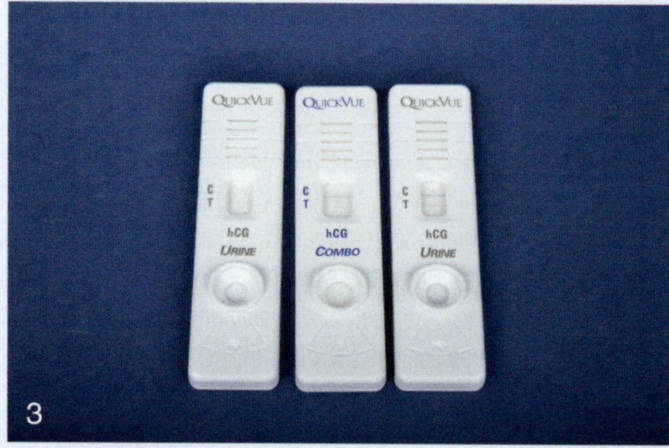

3

9. Discard the test cassette in the biohazard waste container, clean up the testing area, then remove and discard gloves in a biohazard waste container. Remove your lab coat and protective eyewear.
   PURPOSE: To ensure infection control.
10. Wash hands or use hand sanitizer.
    PURPOSE: To ensure infection control.
11. Document the results in the patient's health record as either positive or negative for pregnancy.
    PURPOSE: A procedure is not considered complete until it is documented.

Documentation Example

10/2/20XX 3:45 p.m.: Last menstrual period (LMP) 9/16/20XX. QuickVue pregnancy test: Positive. ————— Julie Salter, CMA (AAMA)

PROCEDURE 47.8 Obtain a Specimen and Perform a CLIA-Waived Urinalysis: Perform a Multidrug Screening Test on Urine

TASK: To screen a urine specimen for drugs or drug metabolites at their specified cutoff levels.

EQUIPMENT and SUPPLIES

- Patient's health record
- Multi-Drug Screen Urine Test in a sealed container
- Freshly voided urine sample
- Timer
- Fluid-impermeable lab coat, eye protection, and gloves
- Biohazard waste container

PROCEDURAL STEPS

1. Wash hands or use hand sanitizer. Put on the fluid-impermeable lab coat, eye protection, and gloves. Comply with safety practices.
   PURPOSE: To ensure infection control and use of Standard Precautions.
2. Assemble the equipment and specimen. Check the expiration date on the test kit.
   PURPOSE: An expired test strip may yield inaccurate results.
3. Determine the temperature of the urine (within 4 minutes of voiding). The temperature should be between 32° and 38°C (90° and 100°F).
   PURPOSE: If the urine temperature is below or above this range, the sample may have been adulterated. Once it has been determined that the sample is at the correct temperature, it may be stored at room temperature for 8 hours or in the refrigerator for up to 3 days before testing.
4. Bring the specimen and the testing device to room temperature.
   PURPOSE: Both the specimen and the device must be at room temperature to ensure accurate results.
5. Remove the device from the foil pouch and label it with the specimen identification.
   PURPOSE: To ensure correct specimen identification
6. Apply the specimen to the device by using one of two methods:
   a. *Dip method:* Remove the cap of the specimen and dip the device into the specimen for 10 seconds, making sure the surface of the urine is above the sample well and below the arrowheads in the window (see the following figure).
   PURPOSE: The pads must be saturated with urine.

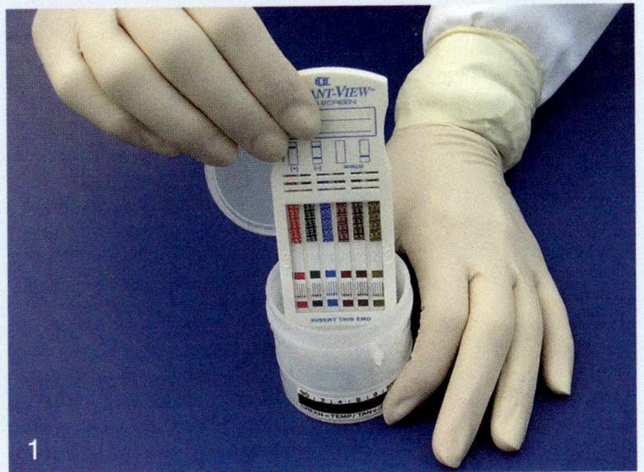

(Courtesy Alfa Scientific, Poway, CA.)

   b. *Alternate method:* Remove the pipet from the pouch and fill it to the line on the barrel with urine. Dispense the entire volume onto the sample well on the testing device (see the following figure).
   PURPOSE: If insufficient urine is available in the cup to use the dip method, this method applies urine directly to the device.

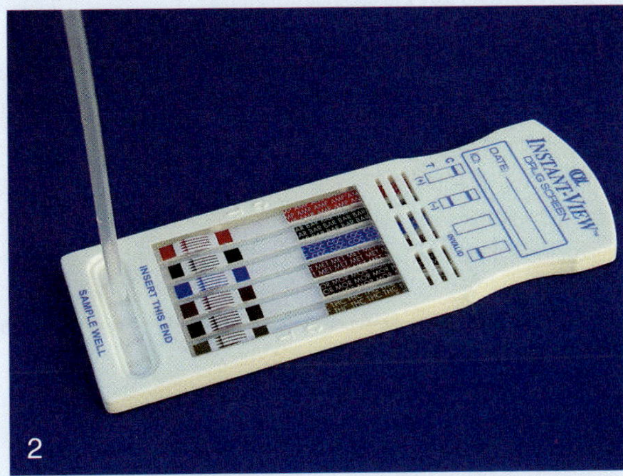

(Courtesy Alfa Scientific, Poway, CA.)

7. Recap the urine specimen.
   PURPOSE: To ensure no specimen spills.
8. Set the timer for the designated time. Do not read the results until after the maximum time as stated in the manufacturer's instructions.
   PURPOSE: Correct timing is essential for reliable, accurate test results.
9. Interpret the results (see the following figure):
   Positive: If the C line appears, but the T line does not, the result is positive for that drug.
   Negative: If both the C line and the T line appear, the level of the drug or its metabolites is below the cutoff level (i.e., negative for that drug).
   Invalid: If no C line develops within 5 minutes on any test strip, the assay is invalid. Repeat the assay with a new test device if invalid.

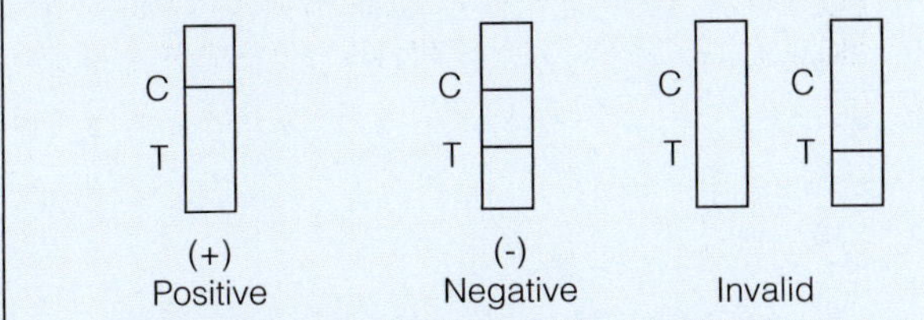

10. Discard the urine and the device in the biohazard container.
    PURPOSE: To ensure infection control.
11. Disinfect the area. Remove your gloves and dispose of them in a biohazard container. Remove your lab coat, and wash your hands or use hand sanitizer.
    PURPOSE: To ensure infection control.
12. Document the results in the patient's health record.
    PURPOSE: A procedure is not considered complete until it is documented.

PROCEDURE 47.9 Reassure a Patient of the Accuracy of the Test Results

TASK: Show empathy and communicate respectfully and professionally with a patient. Reassure the patient of the accuracy of the test result.

SCENARIO: Elyse is seeing Jean Burke, a nurse practitioner at WMFM Clinic today. Elyse has been feeling tired and slightly nauseous for the last few weeks. She and her husband use birth control, but her menstrual periods are very irregular. She did a home pregnancy test 2 weeks ago, and it was negative. But she is still feeling poorly. Jean Burke orders a urine pregnancy test. The lab runs a CLIA-waived urine pregnancy test, and it is positive. Elyse doesn't believe the result. You need to reassure her of the accuracy of the test result.

DIRECTIONS: Role-play the scenario with a peer. The peer is the patient, and you are the medical assistant.

PROCEDURAL STEPS

1. Encourage the patient to talk about her concerns and fears. Demonstrate active listening skills.
   PURPOSE: Understanding the patient's concerns is important when reassuring the patient.
2. Address the patient's concerns and notify the provider of any issues that are outside of the medical assistant's scope of practice. Reassure the patient by demonstrating respect and empathy while addressing the concerns.
   Scenario update: The patient indicates that she does not understand how the first test was negative and the second test was positive.
3. Describe the difference between the first and second tests. Use language that the patient can understand.
4. Answer any questions the patient has.

BLOOD COLLECTION

48

SCENARIO

Maggie Brandt, CMA (AAMA), has been a medical assistant with the Walden-Martin Family Medical (WMFM) Clinic for about 15 years. She has worked in many areas of the clinic, but for the past 8 years, she has been the primary phlebotomist each morning from 8 a.m. until noon. Maggie has the right combination of skills to be a wonderful phlebotomist:

- She is warm, friendly, and can easily talk to patients.
- She is detail oriented, a stickler for safety practices, and very organized.
- She has good small motor skills and a certain quality that makes her venipunctures so smooth that patients hardly feel the needle go through the skin.
- She can explain procedures well in understandable terms and is willing to listen to her patients and put them at ease.

It is Monday morning, and the phlebotomy area is usually busy with patients who have scheduled venipunctures in advance. Let's see what is happening in the phlebotomy area today.

While studying this chapter, think about the following questions:

- What equipment is needed to perform a venipuncture and a capillary puncture?
- What is different about each colored stopper venipuncture tube, and what is the correct order of the draw?
- What types of safety needles and collection devices are used in phlebotomy?
- What steps should be followed for the postexposure management of accidental needlesticks?
- How do you properly perform a venipuncture using evacuated tubes? How do you properly perform a venipuncture using a syringe or butterfly equipment?
- What are problem-solving strategies related to blood collection?
- How is pediatric phlebotomy unique? Consider patient behavior, parental involvement during phlebotomy, and general guidelines for pediatric blood collection.
- How do you properly perform a capillary puncture?

LEARNING OBJECTIVES

1. Examine the equipment needed to perform a venipuncture.
2. Examine needle safety when performing phlebotomy.
3. Examine the process for performing a routine venipuncture.
4. Examine the problems that can be associated with venipuncture.
5. Examine the process for performing phlebotomy on the pediatric patient.
6. Examine the process of performing a capillary puncture.
7. Explain the requirements for the handling of a specimen after collection.

VOCABULARY

anticoagulant (an tee koh AG yuh lant) A substance (i.e., medication or chemical) that prevents clotting of blood.

antiseptic (an tuh SEP tik) A substance that inhibits the growth of microorganisms on living tissue (e.g., alcohol and povidone-iodine solution [Betadine]); they are used to cleanse the skin, wounds, and so on.

aspirating (AS puh rayt ing) To draw off or remove by suction.

blood culture A microbiologic procedure ordered when a provider suspects a bacterial infection is causing a fever of unknown origin (FUO). A blood sample is collected into a nutrient media and held at body temperature. If bacteria are in the blood sample, the culture media should encourage the growth of the infecting bacteria in the laboratory.

clot activators Substances added to a venipuncture tube to enhance and speed up blood clotting.

evacuated Absence of air to create a vacuum in a tube, flask, or reaction vessel.

g-force A force acting on an object because of gravity. For example, a centrifuge spins and exerts g-force.

glycolysis (glie KOL uh sis) The chemical breakdown of carbohydrates (glucose) by enzymes, with the release of energy.

hematoma (hee mah TOH mah) An abnormal buildup of blood in an organ or tissue of the body caused by a leak or cut in a blood vessel.

hemoconcentration (hee muh kon sun TRAY shun) A condition in which the concentration of blood cells is increased in proportion to the plasma.

VOCABULARY—*continued*

hemolysis (hee MOL i sis) The breakdown of red blood cells with the release of hemoglobin.

interstitial (in ter STISH ul) Between the cells.

lymphostasis (lim foh STAY sis) Obstruction or interruption of normal lymph flow.

nosocomial (nos uh KOH mee ul) Also known as healthcare-acquired infections (HAI).

petechiae (peh TEE kee ah) A very small, round hemorrhage in the skin or mucous membrane.

plasma (PLAZ muh) The liquid portion of a whole blood sample that has not clotted due to an anticoagulant. The liquid portion of blood that contains clotting factors. The liquid portion of the blood found in the body.

postural orthostatic tachycardia syndrome (POTS) An autonomic nervous system condition that causes heart palpitations, lightheadedness, increased heart rate, low blood pressure, low blood volume, inability to concentrate, "brain fog," trouble sleeping, gastrointestinal symptoms, and dark red-blue discoloration of the legs.

reference laboratory A laboratory that performs testing for another laboratory. Testing varies from high-volume routine testing to low-volume unique or unusual testing. Also called a referral, diagnostic, or commercial testing laboratory.

serum (SEER um) The liquid portion of a clotted blood specimen. It no longer contains active clotting agents.

suction (SUHK shun) The production of a partial vacuum by the removal of air in order to force fluid into a vacant space.

syringe (suh RINJ) A device with a slender barrel and needle used to withdraw blood from a vein or artery.

vasovagal syncope A faint brought on by excessive activity of the vagus nerve, causing a sudden drop in the heart rate and blood pressure. Can be caused by stress, heat exposure, long periods of standing, or the sight of blood.

INTRODUCTION

Phlebotomy is performed primarily to do the following:

- Assist the provider in diagnosing disease
- Monitor a patient's condition, treatment, or medication levels
- Document the existing good health of a patient

According to the American Society of Clinical Pathologists (ASCP), nearly 80% of providers base at least part of their diagnostic decisions on the results of laboratory tests. The most common specimen used in the laboratory is blood. *Phlebotomy* is the process of acquiring blood from a patient. The most common method of obtaining a blood specimen is by *venipuncture*, which is when blood is taken directly from a surface vein. The vein is punctured with a needle, and the blood is collected directly into a stoppered vacuum tube or a **syringe** and then transferred into the vacuum tube. The procedure is safe when performed by a trained professional, but it must be performed with care. Practice is required to become skilled and confident in the technique of venipuncture.

When it comes to phlebotomy, safety is an important concern. Several bloodborne viral diseases can be spread by exposure to infected blood and body fluids. The viruses identified as possible bloodborne pathogen risks are hepatitis B virus (HBV), hepatitis C virus (HCV), and human immunodeficiency virus (HIV). These viruses are not the only diseases that can be spread by contaminated blood or body fluids, but they are considered a risk for healthcare workers and public safety personnel (such as firefighters, police, and other first responders). The high standards necessary for the safe practice of phlebotomy led to the creation of the Bloodborne Pathogens Standard (overseen by the Occupational Safety and Health Administration [OSHA]) and by different organizations that develop additional standards for training (see Chapter 19).

Training and Certification

Medical assistants are trained to perform phlebotomy as part of their education. They can choose to become certified phlebotomists by completing additional training, coursework, and passing a national certification examination. The following is a list of phlebotomy certifying agencies:

- American Society of Clinical Pathologists (ASCP)
- American Allied Health, Inc.
- American Certification Agency for Healthcare Professionals (ACA)
- American Medical Technologists (AMT)
- American Society of Phlebotomy Technicians (ASPT)
- National Center for Competency Testing (NCCT)
- National Healthcareer Association (NHA)
- National Phlebotomy Association (NPA)

Continuing education often is required to maintain a phlebotomy certification. It is important for medical assistants to become familiar with the guidelines of the states where they work because not all states require a certificate to perform phlebotomy.

VENIPUNCTURE EQUIPMENT

Proper collection of blood requires specialized equipment. Phlebotomists in hospitals generally carry the equipment in a portable tray (Figure 48.1). A physician's office laboratory (POL) often has a permanent location where the same supplies are stored, and venipuncture is performed. In such cases, you may use a phlebotomy chair with an adjustable locking armrest to protect patients if they should faint (Figure 48.2). However, if a patient has a history of *syncope* (fainting), it is best to perform phlebotomy while they are lying on an examination table or in a reclining phlebotomy chair.

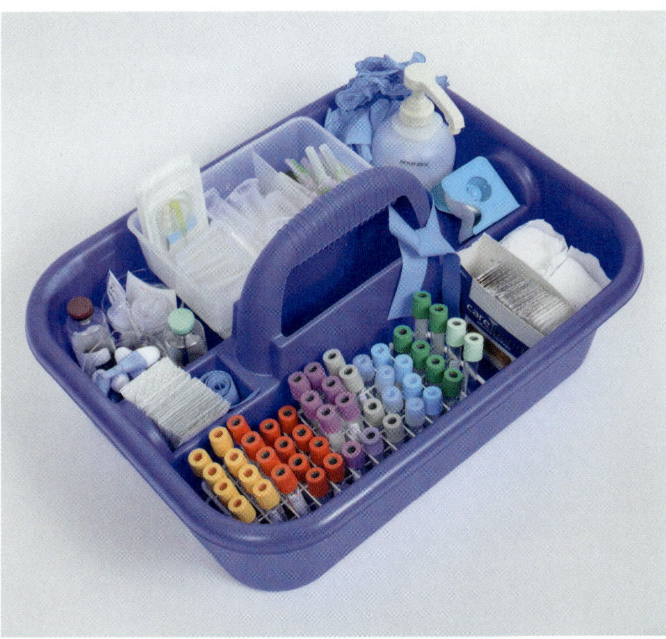

FIGURE 48.1 A stocked venipuncture tray.

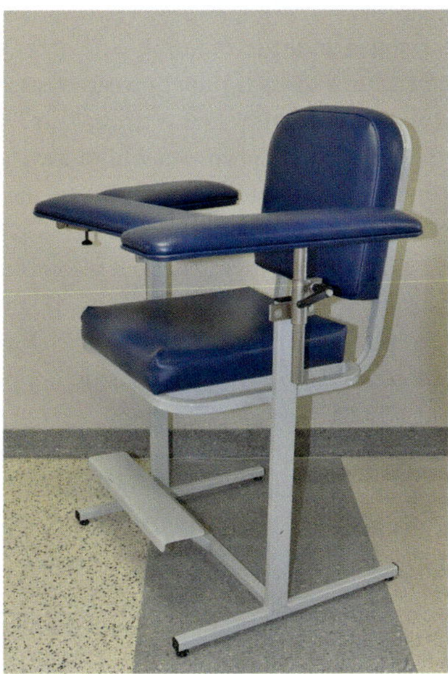

FIGURE 48.2 A phlebotomy chair.

Equipment Used in Routine Venipuncture

- Personal protective equipment (PPE): gloves, fluid-impermeable lab coat, protective eyewear, or face shield (if necessary)
- Permanent marker
- Alcohol wipes
- Gauze
- Hypoallergenic self-stick wrap, tape, or bandages
- Nonlatex tourniquets
- Double-pointed safety needles
- Winged infusion sets (butterfly needles)
- Disposable needle holders
- Evacuated, stoppered tubes
- Syringes and removable needles with safety devices
- Biohazard sharps container
- Biohazard waste container

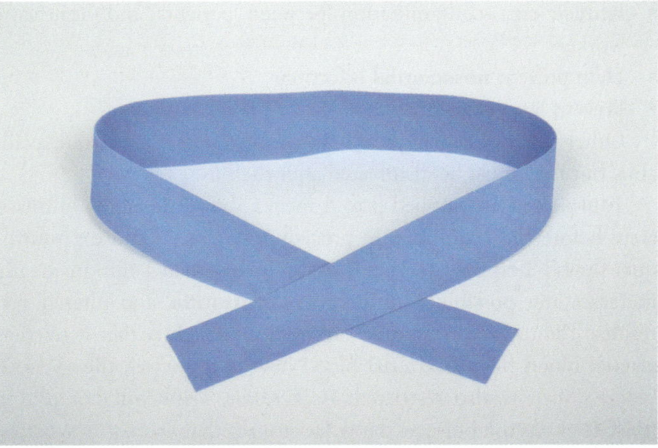

FIGURE 48.3 A latex-free tourniquet.

Personal Protective Equipment

Employers must provide employees with personal protective equipment (PPE), such as gloves, disposable fluid-impenetrable lab coats, protective eyewear, and face shields. All facilities must stock only latex-free supplies because of the potential for allergic responses in workers and patients. Some people with latex allergies can have life-threatening reactions to latex exposure.

OSHA requires healthcare workers to wear gloves during venipuncture. Because veins can be difficult to locate with gloved fingertips, the site may be palpated before gloves are put on, as long as the hands have been washed or sanitized. According to the standard procedure for venipuncture established by the Clinical and Laboratory Standards Institute (CLSI), gloves may be put on after vein palpation but before preparation of the site. Those who need the final assurance of one last palpation before the needle is inserted must remember that touching the prepared site, even with gloves, contaminates the area. To help yourself find the vein after the area has been cleansed, make note of any skin markers, such as creases, freckles, or scars. If the area is touched, *it must be cleansed again.* Keep in mind that the tourniquet should be tied for no longer than 1 minute at a time.

CRITICAL THINKING APPLICATION 48.1

Maggie is in a little early on a Monday morning. She knows that Monday is usually busy and wants to make sure all her supplies are adequately stocked. Maggie cleans her protective eyewear and has it ready at the phlebotomy station. Why is it important to wear protective eyewear whenever drawing blood? Can you think of a few reasons and share them with your class?

Tourniquets

Before blood can be drawn, a vein must be located. Most venipunctures are done in the *antecubital region* or inner bend in front of the elbow. Application of a *tourniquet* is very helpful for locating veins in the antecubital region and any other area that may be drawn for venipuncture. Tourniquets prevent the venous blood flow from the site, causing the veins to bulge or plump up. If the antecubital area is drawn, a tourniquet is tied around the upper arm so that it is tight but still comfortable and can be easily released with one hand. Single-use, nonlatex tourniquets are available (Figure 48.3) and currently are recommended to do the following:

- Reduce cross-contamination between patients and healthcare workers
- Help prevent **nosocomial** infections
- Prevent latex exposure

Other types of tourniquets with quick-release closures are available, but they must be disinfected after each use.

Tourniquets are applied 3 to 4 inches above the elbow immediately before the venipuncture procedure begins. Because a tourniquet slows blood flow, leaving it on for longer than 1 minute greatly increases the possibility of **hemoconcentration** and altered test results. The tourniquet should not be tied so tightly that it restricts arterial blood flow. If arterial blood flow is restricted, then venous blood return is also restricted. As a result, veins will not plump up. Checking the pulse at the wrist ensures that arterial flow is not restricted. Tourniquets are also used when blood is drawn from hand and foot veins and tied on the wrist or ankle, respectively.

Tourniquets can be uncomfortable for patients, especially those with heavy-set or hairy upper arms if they are not applied correctly. Make sure the tourniquet is flat against the skin, and, if necessary, tie it over the clothing if it is causing the patient discomfort. This may be especially important when blood is drawn from an older adult because of the thinness or fragility of the skin.

Antiseptics

A venipuncture site must be cleansed with an **antiseptic** to prevent infection. The most commonly used antiseptic is 70% isopropyl alcohol, also known as *rubbing alcohol.* Prepackaged alcohol wipes are the product used most often. An alcohol wipe is used to clean the puncture site, which is then allowed to air dry. Alcohol does not sterilize the skin but kills many existing bacteria that might contaminate the sample. The alcohol should remain on the skin for 30 to 60 seconds and allowed to air dry to be most effective. As the alcohol dries, it breaks open the bacterial cells and kills the bacteria. Alcohol wipes should not be used when collecting a blood alcohol sample. Sterile soap pads, benzalkonium chloride, or povidone-iodine (Betadine) can be used instead.

If a provider suspects a fever of unknown origin (FUO), a **blood culture** is frequently ordered. Additional preparation is needed at the venipuncture site to eliminate contaminating bacteria. First, 70% isopropyl alcohol wipes are used to clean the area, which is allowed to air dry. Then an iodine solution is used, such as povidone-iodine. Chlorhexidine gluconate or benzalkonium chloride can be used for patients who are allergic to iodine. The iodine prep is also allowed to air dry. Once the venipuncture site is properly prepared, the blood cultures must be drawn into a sterile tube or bottle specifically designed for the test (Figure 48.4).

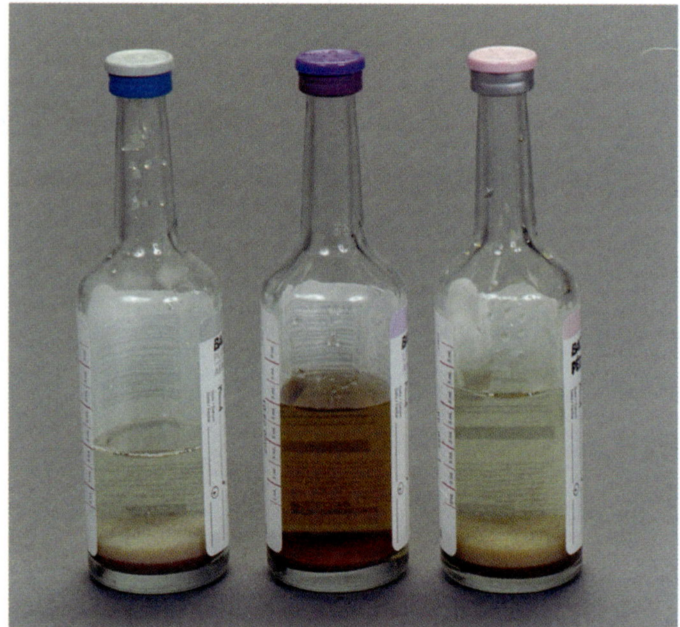

FIGURE 48.4 Blood culture bottles.

Evacuated Collection Tubes

The most common collection system is the **evacuated** tube system (these tubes are also called *vacuum tubes;* a particular brand of vacuum tubes is the Vacutainer). It consists of evacuated tubes of various sizes that have color-coded stoppers. The colored stoppers indicate the tube's contents (Table 48.1). Venipuncture tubes must be either shatter-resistant glass or plastic. More traditional rubber tube stoppers have been replaced by safer plastic *Hemogard* colored tops. Hemogard tops have the advantage of not splattering blood when removed from the tube (Figure 48.5). Table 48.1 lists the colored stoppers and the chemical additives, **anticoagulants**, **clot activators**, or thixotropic gel that are contained in each type of tube. The different stopper colors indicate the unique contents of that color-coded tube. The vacuum in each tube draws a measured amount of blood into the tube. Tube volumes range from 2 to 15 mL.

The size of the tube to be drawn depends on several factors. Each test performed in the laboratory requires a specific amount of blood. Blood volumes can often be combined, which reduces the number of tubes that must be drawn. For example, both a complete blood count and an erythrocyte sedimentation rate test (discussed in Chapter 49) are performed on a sample from a lavender-topped tube. The combined volume for both tests can be drawn with one lavender-topped tube, so you do not need to draw two tubes. When in doubt, refer to the appropriate laboratory manual for questions regarding specimen requirements and handling. Another option would be to call the laboratory. Keep in mind that blood is approximately half cells and half liquid. If a test requires 2 mL of serum, at least 4 mL of blood must be collected.

CRITICAL THINKING APPLICATION **48.2**

It is important to use a tourniquet to properly locate veins for phlebotomy. List three advantages of using a tourniquet to help locate veins. Be ready to share them with your class.

Tube Additives

Most vacuum tubes contain an additive. The plain, red-topped tube contains nothing. It is a plain tube with no additives, anticoagulants, or clot activator. A gold-topped tube contains silica to activate clotting and an inert thixotropic gel to separate serum and cells after the sample is centrifuged. Most other color-topped plastic tubes contain some form of anticoagulant, which prevents blood from clotting. The additive may be a powder, a liquid visible in the tube, or a liquid sprayed inside the tube by the manufacturer and allowed to dry. The choice of anticoagulant depends on the test to be completed.

Anticoagulant additives prevent blood from clotting, which allows the contents of the tube to be used in two ways. First, the sample can be used as whole blood; second, the sample can be centrifuged, and the liquid portion, called **plasma**, can be used for testing.

TABLE 48.1 Common Color-Coded Stoppers and Their Additives and Laboratory Uses

VACUUM TUBE COLOR[a]	COLOR	HEMOGARD COLOR[b]	ADDITIVE AND ITS FUNCTION[c]	LABORATORY USE
Blood culture bottles	No color for blood culture bottles (see Figure 48.4)	Yellow	Sodium polyanethole sulfonate (SPS); prevents blood from clotting and stabilizes bacterial growth. Yellow-topped tubes have specific uses. They cannot be used to collect all blood culture specimens.	Blood culture bottles—blood or body fluid cultures Yellow-topped tubes—mycobacteria, fungus, or acid-fast bacilli (AFB) blood cultures
Light blue		light blue	Sodium citrate; removes calcium to prevent blood from clotting.	Coagulation testing
Red		Red	None.	Serum tests; chemistry studies, blood bank, immunology
Red-gray (marbled)		Gold	No anticoagulant but contains silica particles to enhance clot formation; usually contain gel for serum separation.	Serum tests; chemistry studies, immunology
Green		Green	Heparin; inhibits thrombin formation to prevent clotting.	Chemistry tests
Green-gray (marbled)		Light green	Lithium heparin and gel; for plasma separation.	Plasma determinations in chemistry studies
Lavender		Lavender	Ethylenediaminetetraacetic acid (EDTA); removes calcium to prevent blood from clotting.	Hematology tests
Gray		Gray	Potassium oxalate and sodium fluoride; removes calcium to prevent blood from clotting; fluoride inhibits **glycolysis**.	Chemistry testing, especially glucose and alcohol levels

[a]Stopper colors are based on BD Vacutainer tubes.
[b]Hemogard closures provide a protective plastic cover over the rubber stopper as an additional safety feature.
[c]Additives, additive functions, and laboratory uses are the same for both pediatric and adult tubes.

An example of a test that uses whole blood would be a complete blood count (CBC). An example of a test that uses plasma would be a coagulation study.

Ethylenediaminetetraacetic acid (EDTA) is the anticoagulant found in the lavender-topped tube. It prevents platelet clumping and preserves the appearance of blood cells for microscopic examination.

Clot activators promote blood clotting in the tubes with either a marbled red-gray or a gold top. For example, silica particles in the gold tubes enhance clotting by providing a surface for platelet activation. Thrombin from the platelets quickly promotes clotting and is used in tubes drawn for chemistry testing or in the event a sample is needed from a patient taking a prescribed anticoagulant, such as heparin.

If blood clots and then is centrifuged, the liquid portion is referred to as **serum**. Without a clot activator, blood clots in 15 to 60 minutes, after which it must be centrifuged. The serum must be quickly separated from the cells because cells may continue to metabolize glucose or may release substances that interfere with testing.

Thixotropic gel can be found in some tubes, including *serum separator tubes* (SSTs). SST tubes are identified by the marbled red-gray rubber stopper or the gold Hemogard top. The *plasma separator tube* (PST) also contains thixotropic gel. The tubes have a marbled green-gray top, and the Hemogard tubes have a light green top. Thixotropic gel, a synthetic, chemically neutral gel, has a density that is between that of red cells and plasma or serum. The gel settles between the plasma/serum and cells during centrifugation. The gel forms a barrier that makes it easy to pour off the liquid portion of the sample without cells contaminating the specimen.

It is important to avoid a "short draw" (i.e., a tube that is not completely filled). Table 48.2 lists the consequences of underfilling tubes. Some tubes are designed to fill only partially, according to their preset vacuum. Having the proper ratio of blood to additive is crucial. Always check the tube for the expiration date. Outdated tubes may have a diminished vacuum, or the additive may have degraded and not be as effective.

CRITICAL THINKING APPLICATION 48.3

In your own words, define *plasma* and *serum*.

Order of the Draw. If more than one tube must be drawn during a venipuncture, a specified order must be followed. Carryover of additives from one tube to the next could cause sample alteration and incorrect results. CLSI has established a set of standards outlining the order to follow for a multitube draw. The same order applies to filling tubes when blood is collected in a syringe.

1. *Blood culture bottles:* These bottles are filled first because they are sterile and should not be contaminated by the other tubes. In addition to blood culture bottles, a yellow-topped tube can be drawn for blood cultures for mycobacteria, fungi, and acid-fast bacilli. These tubes are not drawn frequently in an ambulatory setting. If they are ordered, they would be drawn in the same place as blood culture bottles in the order of the draw.
2. *Light blue* top: These tubes, which contain sodium citrate, are next because other anticoagulants might contaminate the sample collected for coagulation studies. If no blood culture has been ordered, CLSI recommends that blood for the light blue–topped tube be drawn first if routine coagulation testing has been ordered. Examples of coagulation tests include prothrombin time with international normalized ratio (PT/INR) and activated partial thromboplastin time (APTT). See Chapter 49 for more details about coagulation testing. Some laboratories recommend that a red-topped "waste" tube with no additives be partially filled before the light blue–topped tube. This is done to remove any tissue thromboplastin that may be released during the venipuncture. Thromboplastin interferes with coagulation testing. CLSI also recommends that when a winged infusion (butterfly assembly) is used, blood should be drawn into the red-topped tube even if the order does not call for it. This is done to fill the tubing's dead air space with blood before drawing the light blue–topped sodium citrate tube. A light blue tube must have an exact blood-to-citrate dilution. It is not necessary to completely fill the waste tube because it will be discarded.
3. *Red* top or *gold* top: Red serum tubes without clot activator or gold serum tubes with clot activator are filled next. These tubes are drawn to test serum after the specimens have clotted and been centrifuged. SSTs with thixotropic gel are also drawn at this time. SST tubes have a marbled red-gray stopper or a gold Hemogard stopper.
4. *Green* top: These tubes are drawn next because the plasma in their anticoagulated specimen is used for testing when STAT results are needed (usually in chemistry). The dark green tops contain no thixotropic gel. The tubes with marbled green-gray tops and light green Hemogard tops both contain gel to help separate the plasma from the cells when centrifuged.
5. *Lavender* top: These tubes are drawn next. They contain an EDTA anticoagulant that preserves blood cell size and shape, otherwise known as morphology. EDTA tubes are drawn near the end of the draw because the additive interferes with chemistry and coagulation specimens.
6. *Gray* top: This tube is drawn last, and the blood is used to test glucose or blood alcohol levels. Its additives may elevate electrolyte levels and damage cells if passed into the other tubes.

It is important to gently mix the contents of the tubes after collection by inverting them (do not shake the tubes). Most tubes should be inverted eight times, but clot activator tubes should be inverted five times, and sodium citrate three to four times.

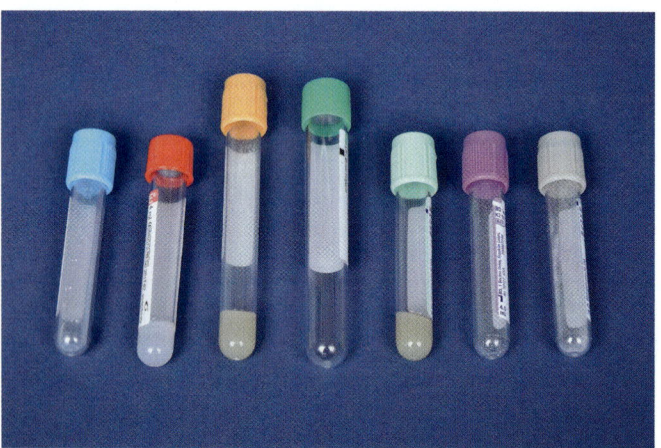

FIGURE 48.5 Hemogard tube stoppers.

TABLE 48.2 Effects of Underfilling Collection Tubes

STOPPER COLOR	EFFECTS OF UNDERFILLING
Yellow	Reduces possibility of bacterial recovery
Light blue	Coagulation test results falsely prolonged
Red	Insufficient sample
Marbled red-gray, and gold (SST tubes)	Poor barrier formation; insufficient sample
Green	False results because of excess heparin
Marbled green-gray, and light green (PST tubes)	False results because of excess heparin
Lavender	Falsely low blood cell counts and hematocrits; morphologic changes to red blood cells; staining changes
Gray	False results

CRITICAL THINKING APPLICATION 48.4

Sometimes making up a saying or sentence can help you remember the order of a process. Here are a few sayings that might help the medical assistant remember the order of the draw.

The order of the draw is as follows: **st**erile (blood culture bottles/tubes)–**l**ight blue–**r**ed/gold–**g**reen–**l**avender–**g**ray. Use the first letter for each tube color and make up a sentence that helps you remember the order of the draw.

Consider the following examples:

1. Stop light red. Green light go.
2. Stan's light red glasses look gray.
3. Stella's lecture reading gives little giggles.
4. Street lights reveal green little gardens.

Can you make up your own saying to remember the order of the draw? Share your saying with your classmates.

Needles and Supplies Used in Phlebotomy

A critical part of phlebotomy is knowing which needle and tube, or syringe, should be used in each situation. All needles used in phlebotomy are sterile and have a safety device that is activated immediately after withdrawal from the vein. The needle is then discarded in a biohazard sharps container. Each needle is housed in a protected cover, which should be inspected before use to ensure that sterility has not been compromised (i.e., the seal should be intact) and the needle has no manufacturing defects, such as burs, nicks, or bends.

Needles have two parts: the hub and the shaft. The hub of the needle is designed to attach the needle to the vacuum tube needle holder or a syringe. Shafts differ in length, ranging from ¾ inch to 1½ inches (Figure 48.6). The length of the shaft has no bearing on the venipuncture procedure. Some phlebotomists prefer a longer needle, and others prefer a shorter needle because it makes patients less uneasy. One end of the shaft is cut at an angle and forms the *bevel*, which creates a very sharp point. The bevel of the needle makes the entry into the skin much smoother (Figure 48.7)

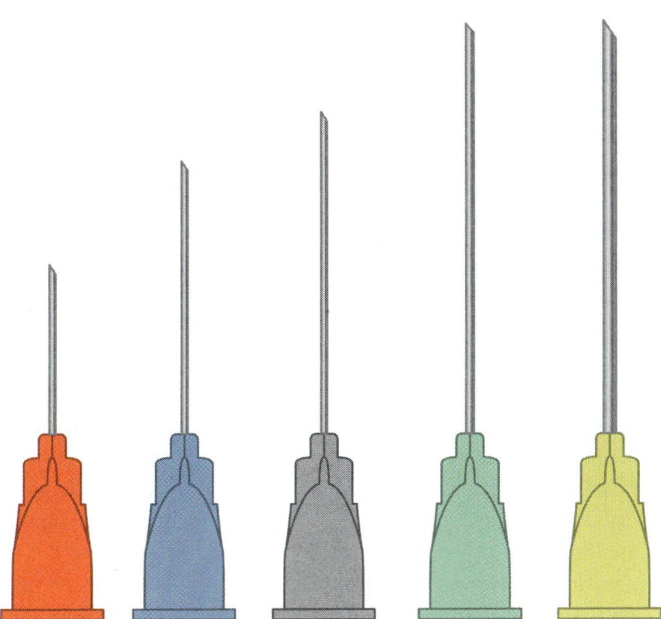

FIGURE 48.6 Venipuncture needles.

The bore, or hollow space, inside the needle is called the *lumen*. Lumen size is important and is referred to as the *gauge*. A numeric value designates the gauge of the needle. The higher the gauge number, the smaller the lumen. Be sure to match the needle gauge to the size of the tube. A large vacuum tube is more likely to hemolyze the blood if a high-gauge needle (i.e., small lumen) is used. For example, blood banks use a large, 16-gauge needle to collect pints of blood for transfusions. The lumen is wide, which reduces the chance of **hemolysis**. A small, 23-gauge needle is used to collect blood from small or fragile veins, such as those in older adults and very young patients. Routine adult venipuncture requires a 20- to 21-gauge needle.

Multisample Needles

Multisample needles are commonly used in routine adult venipuncture. They are used when several tubes need to be drawn during a single venipuncture. These needles are double pointed (see Figure 48.7). One point enters the patient's vein, and the other punctures the stopper of the collection tube. The point that enters the tube is sheathed with a retractable rubber sleeve that allows tubes to be changed without blood leaking into the needle holder or tube holder.

CRITICAL THINKING APPLICATION 48.5

Maggie has a few different gauge needles to use in phlebotomy. Why would she need different sized needles? If the process is the same for each patient, why would the needle size be important? Share your ideas with the class.

Needle Holders

Double-pointed needles must be firmly placed into a needle holder (Figure 48.8). Usually, needle holders are translucent cylinders, and they come in different sizes to accommodate different-sized tubes. The holders often have a ring that indicates how far the tube can be pushed onto the needle without losing the vacuum. To prevent accidental

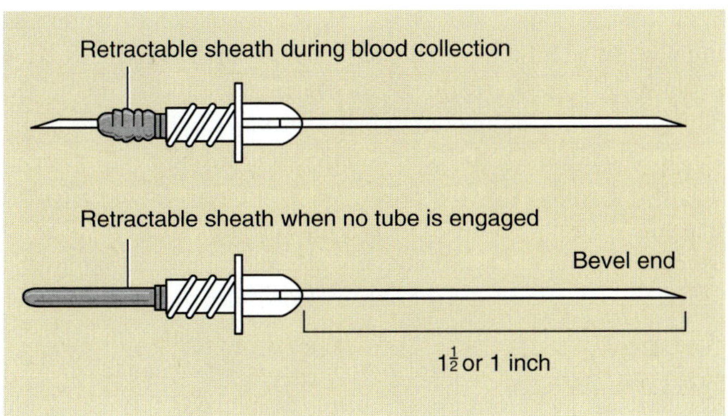

FIGURE 48.7 Bevel of a venipuncture needle.

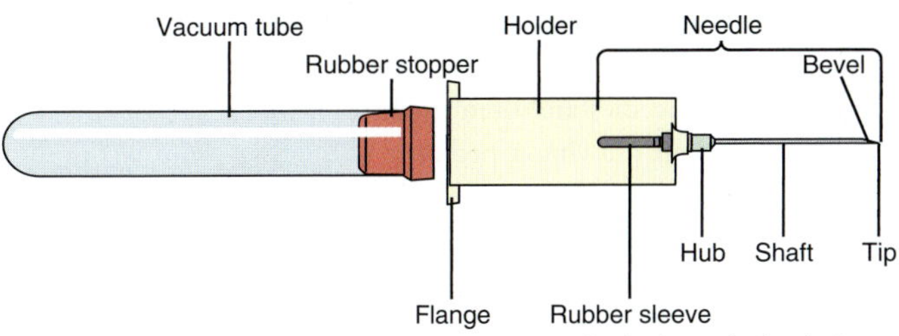

FIGURE 48.8 Venipuncture assembly. (From Hunt SA: *Saunders fundamentals of medical assisting*, revised reprint, St. Louis, 2007, Saunders.)

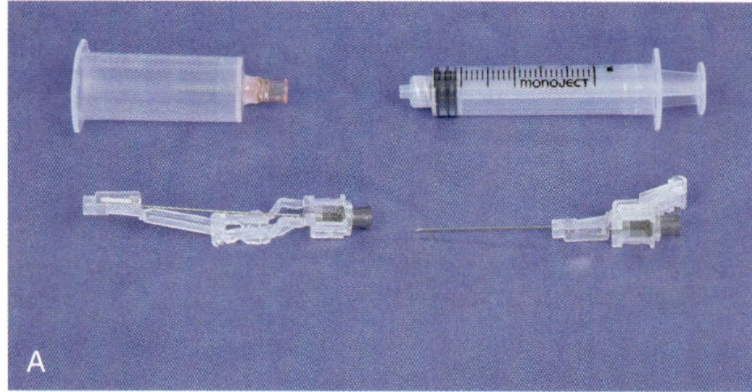

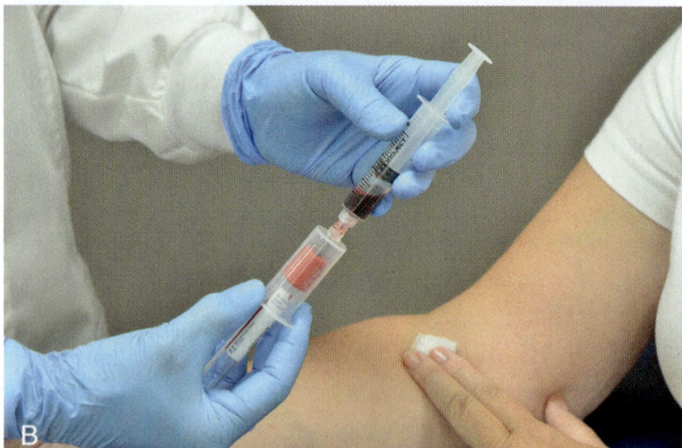

FIGURE 48.9 Syringe assembly. **(A)** Syringe, syringe safety needle, and safety transfer tube device. The needle on the lower left has the safety device activated, whereas the needle on the lower right does not. **(B)** Using a syringe safety transfer tube device.

needlesticks, OSHA requires that the needle holder, with its safety-activated needle still attached, must be discarded into a biohazard sharps container immediately after completing the venipuncture.

Syringes

Syringes are used when there is concern that the strong vacuum in a stoppered vacuum tube might collapse the vein. The syringe needle fits on the end of the syringe barrel. Syringe needles also come in different gauges. The amount of blood drawn into the syringe barrel depends on how much blood needs to be collected for testing. When blood is drawn into a syringe, it must be transferred immediately to the evacuated tube(s). Blood that sits in the syringe barrel could clot if not transferred quickly. The syringe needle safety device must be activated and discarded in the sharps container. A special transfer tube device is then used to transfer the blood to the vacuum tubes. This device connects to the top of the syringe; it contains an enclosed needle that punctures the vacuum tube's stopper and delivers the blood into the tube (Figure 48.9).

Winged Infusion Sets (Butterfly Assembly)

Butterfly assemblies (Figure 48.10) are designed for use on small veins. Butterfly needles are often used to draw veins in the back of the hand or when drawing a pediatric patient. The most common butterfly needle size is a 22 or 23 gauge with a needle length of ½ to ¾ inch. A butterfly needle has a plastic, flexible, butterfly-shaped grip attached to a short length of tubing. The hub end is fitted into a syringe or a needle holder tube adapter. Syringes are frequently paired with butterfly needles because the syringe can create a gentle vacuum that the phlebotomist can easily control. The syringe blood

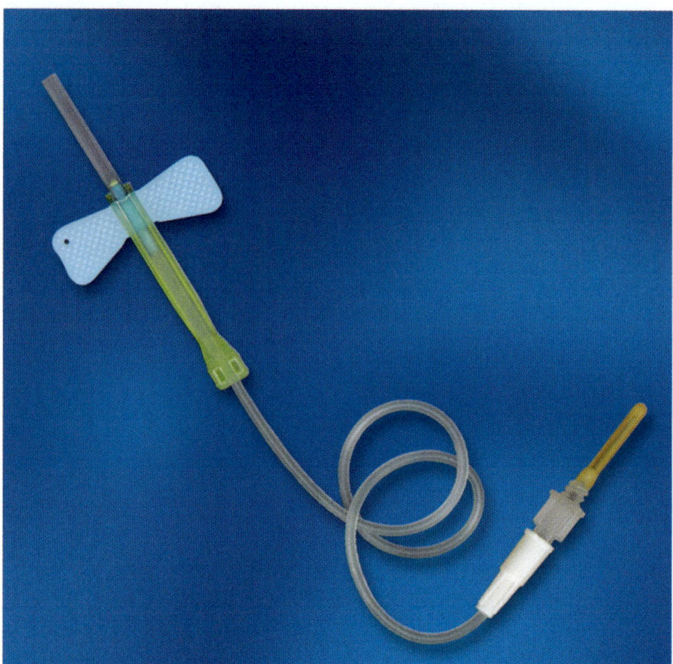

FIGURE 48.10 Butterfly assembly. (Courtesy Becton, Dickinson, Franklin Lakes, NJ.)

sample must be transferred to the evacuated tubes using the transfer device described previously.

> **CRITICAL THINKING APPLICATION — 48.6**
>
> Describe the difference between a syringe and a winged infusion assembly. List two situations when each type of equipment may be used.

NEEDLE SAFETY

Healthcare workers who use or may be exposed to needles are at increased risk of needlestick injury. Such injuries can lead to serious or fatal infections with blood-borne pathogens, such as HBV, HCV, and HIV. Needlestick injuries account for most accidental exposures to blood. Used needles should never be recapped. After use, needles should be covered with the appropriate engineered safety device that is part of the needle assembly and disposed of in a biohazard sharps container.

Using Safety Needles

According to OSHA, the best practice for preventing needlestick injuries after phlebotomy is to use safety needles that are activated with one hand immediately after use. The US Food and Drug Administration (FDA), which is responsible for approving medical devices marketed and sold in the United States, recommends devices that provide a barrier between the hands and the needle, after use, in which the phlebotomist's hands remain behind the needle at all times. Safety shields that can be activated before or immediately after removing of the needle from the vein and that remain in effect after disposal should also be an integral part of the device. Finally, these devices should be as simple as possible, requiring little or no training to use. Some examples of needle safety devices are as follows:

- *One-handed vacuum tube needle:* After the needle has been used and removed from the vein, the thumb holding the vacuum tube holder slides under the base of the pink safety device, causing it

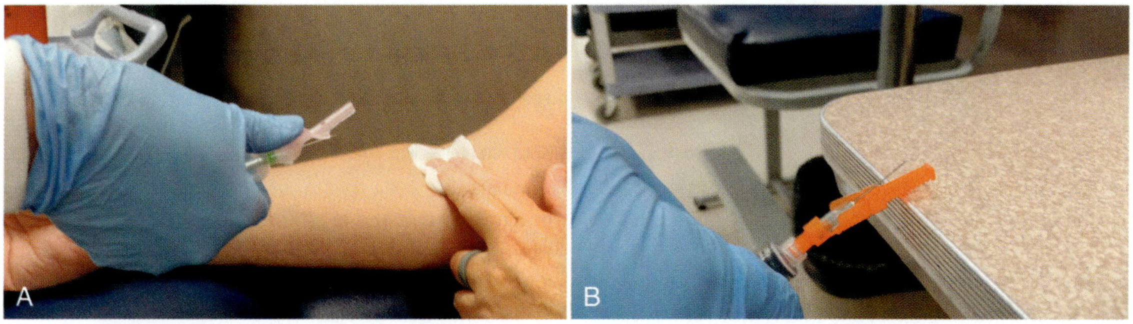

FIGURE 48.11 One-handed safety needles. **(A)** Activated by sliding the thumb up at the base of the guard, causing it to cover the needle. **(B)** Activated by pressing the orange guard against a solid surface, causing it to cover the needle.

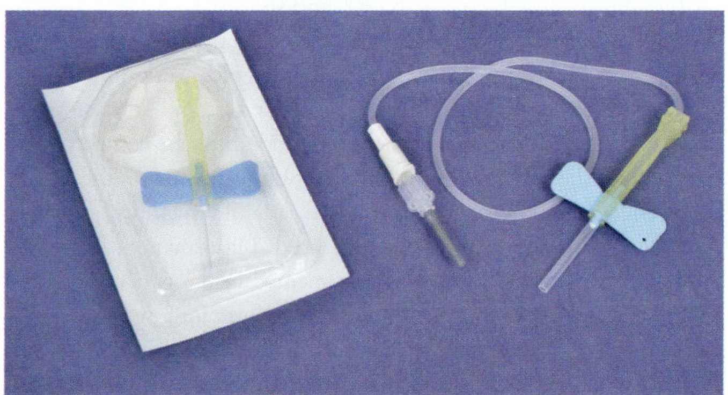

FIGURE 48.12 Safety-Lok butterfly needle.

to snap over the contaminated needle (Figure 48.11A). Or an orange needle shield on the holder is activated by pressing the device against a hard, flat surface (Figure 48.11B).

- *Syringe needle safety devices* (see Figure 48.9): These devices have a spring-activated shield attached to a disposable syringe needle. After the venipuncture, the phlebotomist activates the device with the thumb holding the syringe, and a spring locks a protective plastic tip into place, protecting the needle. The needle can then be removed and discarded. The syringe is attached to the safety transfer device to deliver the collected blood into the appropriate vacuum tubes (see Figure 48.9).
- *Butterfly needle safety lock* (Figure 48.12): After the venipuncture, the dominant hand holds the butterfly tail while the nondominant hand pulls back on the tubing, causing the needle to slide into the tubing and lock into place.
- *Push-button butterfly safety device* (Figure 48.13): With the needle still in the arm, the medical assistant grasps the tail of the butterfly with the dominant hand while the nondominant hand presses the button just below the wings, causing the needle to retract into the butterfly body as it leaves the vein.
- *Needle-blunting butterfly set* (Figure 48.14): A third wing is rotated after collection and before removal of the needle from the vein. As the third wing is rotated, it moves the blunt needle down the shaft before it is removed from the patient.

OSHA requires employers to establish and maintain a sharps injury log for recording injuries from contaminated sharps. This log should contain information about the device involved in the incident and the department or work area where the incident occurred, in addition to an explanation of the incident. Employee confidentiality must be maintained.

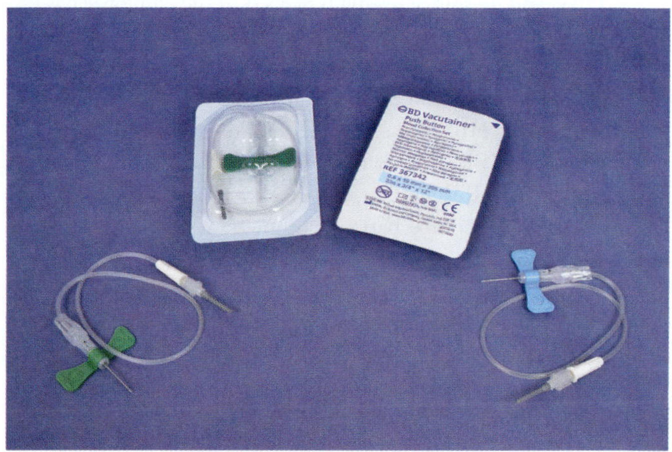

FIGURE 48.13 Push-button butterfly needle.

Protect against Needlestick Injuries

OSHA's Bloodborne Pathogens Standard emphasizes that phlebotomists should have direct input on the type of safety needles they will be using. The following steps should be taken to protect against needlestick injuries:

- Help your employer evaluate and select devices with safety features.
- Use devices with safety features provided by your employer.
- Never recap a contaminated needle except with a safety device.
- Plan for safe handling and disposal before beginning any procedure using needles.
- Dispose of used needles and needle holders promptly in appropriate biohazard sharps containers.
- Report all needlestick and other sharps-related injuries promptly to ensure that you receive appropriate follow-up care.
- Tell your employer about hazards from needles that you observe in your work environment.
- Participate in bloodborne pathogen training, and follow recommended infection prevention practices, including vaccination against hepatitis B virus (HBV).

Postexposure Needlestick Follow-Up

An accidental needlestick is a medical emergency. OSHA-recommended management procedures are discussed in Chapter 19. Effective management of an accidental sharps exposure includes the following measures:

- Immediately after injury, the wound is inspected and washed for 10 minutes with soap, 10% iodine solution, or chlorine-based antiseptic.

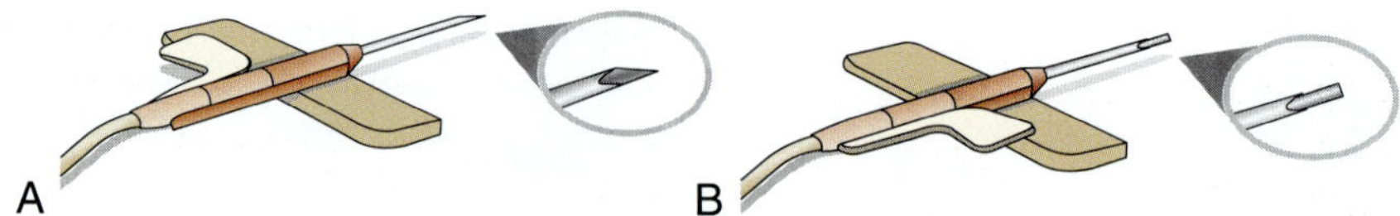

FIGURE 48.14 Needle-blunting butterfly needle.

- The injury is reported to the supervisor, and an incident report is completed.
- The employee is referred to a provider for confidential assessment and follow-up. Baseline testing for HBV, HCV, and HIV is recommended for both the employee and the source individual:
  - HBV: If the employee has been immunized for HBV and has a positive postimmunization titer, there is no risk of acquiring HBV, and no source testing is needed. If the employee has not been immunized or the postimmunization titer is negative, source testing for infection with HBV is recommended if the source is known and can be located. If the source patient tests positive for HBV, the employee should receive HBV immune globulin (HBIG), and a series of HBV immunizations should be initiated. If the source tests negative, no treatment is indicated. If the source patient cannot be tested, the employee should be treated as if the source patient were positive for HBV.
  - HCV: The source should also be tested for HCV. If the source is positive, the employee should be monitored for signs and symptoms of hepatitis for 6 months. No postexposure prophylaxis is recommended for HCV infection.
  - HIV: For HIV exposure, most employers recommend a 4-week regimen of antiretroviral drugs. To best protect the victim, antiretroviral therapy should be administered within hours of exposure. Early HIV drug therapy is now recommended for anyone who may be at risk of infection. Because these medications have side effects, the employee is the one who decides whether the medications are started. If the source is found to be negative, antiretroviral therapy can be discontinued.
- Interim testing may be performed if the healthcare worker experiences symptoms of acute HIV exposure or hepatitis. For HIV, antibody testing should be repeated at 6 weeks, 12 weeks, and 6 months if the source was HIV positive or the source's status remains unknown. Confidential follow-up care must include provisions for emotional support and counseling for the healthcare worker.

ROUTINE VENIPUNCTURE

Venipuncture involves a series of steps that are vital to collecting a good sample. In addition to learning good techniques, we also want to be able to make our patients as comfortable as possible. As you read through the information, you will start to become familiar with the venipuncture procedure and the details of the process.

The first step of the procedure is to select the proper method for venipuncture (evacuated tube, syringe, or butterfly assembly). Next, prepare your patient for the procedure. Then you are ready to collect the sample and process the specimen appropriately.

Patient Preparation

All blood collections begin with a requisition, a form from the patient's provider requesting a test. Requisitions may be computer-generated or handwritten, and at a minimum, they must include the following information:

- Patient's name
- Patient's date of birth
- Patient's identification number
- Name of the provider submitting the order
- Type of test requested
- Test status (timed, fasting, STAT, and so forth)

Begin the venipuncture procedure by greeting the patient and verifying his or her identity. According to CLSI, proper identification includes asking outpatients to (1) state and spell their first and last name and (2) state their birth date. All of the information must be compared and verified with the patient requisition. If communication with the patient is not effective due to any circumstances, a family member, guardian, or medical translator must provide the needed information. The name of the person assisting should be documented in the patient's medical record. Always follow your institution's procedures for assisted communication before completing the venipuncture procedure.

Briefly explain the venipuncture procedure to your patient, and make sure to ask him or her the following questions:

- Do you have any questions or concerns?
- Do you have an arm, vein, or site preference?
- Were you given any special instructions prior to the venipuncture (e.g., does the person need to be fasting)?
- Have you ever experienced any problems or complications with a routine venipuncture in the past?
- Do you take aspirin or blood thinners?

Answer questions and concerns, and take steps to prevent any past problems from recurring. If you cannot answer all the patient's questions, ask if the patient would like to talk to the provider for clarification. Obtain verbal consent to perform the venipuncture simply by asking whether you have permission to draw blood from the patient.

Your self-confidence in performing the procedure will help put your patient at ease. Act and speak professionally. Treat your patient with kindness and respect. Being pleasant and friendly is important. It makes your patients feel comfortable and shows that you take your role in their care seriously.

CRITICAL THINKING APPLICATION **48.7**

Why is patient identification so important in phlebotomy? List four reasons and be ready to share them with the class.

Preparing for the Venipuncture

Seat the patient in a phlebotomy area. Ask the patient to extend an arm and position his or her other hand under the elbow to help straighten the elbow, if necessary. Inspect both arms and ask whether the patient has an arm or site preference. Veins in the antecubital area are most commonly used for venipuncture (Figure 48.15). According to CLSI standards, the veins in the center of the antecubital area should be located as a first choice before alternative veins within the antecubital area are considered. The puncture site should be carefully selected after both arms have been

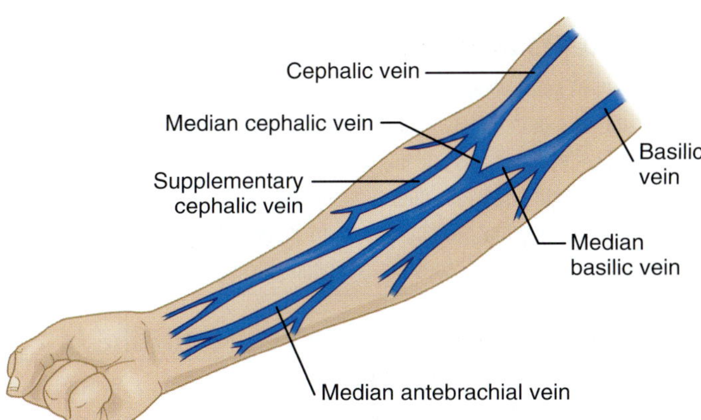

FIGURE 48.15 The veins of the forearm. (From Stepp CA, Woods MA: *Laboratory procedures for medical office personnel*, Philadelphia, 1998, Saunders.)

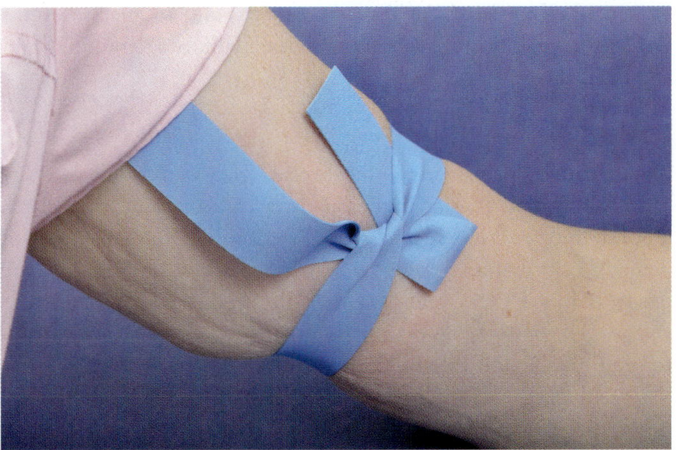

FIGURE 48.16 Placement of the tourniquet on the arm.

inspected. Alternative sites may be chosen if the area is scarred, bruised, burned, or swollen. You may use the veins on the back of the hand if the patient gives permission. Consult the provider for any other alternative site, and do not proceed without supervision.

When choosing the best available vein, palpate the area. Feel for a vein that has "bounce" when lightly palpated. Consider the three Ds of vein selection:

- **D**epth below the surface
- **D**iameter of the vein
- **D**irection through the antecubital region.

Correctly choosing a vein is one of the most important aspects of a venipuncture.

The medial veins generally run at a slight angle to the fold in the antecubital area. The cephalic veins are on the thumb side of the antecubital area. These are the veins of choice. The basilic vein, which lies on the inside of the antecubital area (the little finger side), is very close to the brachial artery and median nerves and should *not* be used! If the medial or cephalic veins are not accessible, consult the provider. Only the most experienced phlebotomists should ever attempt a basilic venipuncture. The chance of injury to the patient is too great.

The tourniquet should be placed about 3 to 4 inches above the patient's elbow. Make sure it is not twisted because that will cause discomfort to your patient (Figure 48.16). Grasp the tourniquet ends, one in each hand, close to the patient's skin. Pull the ends apart to gently stretch the tourniquet, then cross one end over the other while maintaining the tension. Tuck the top portion of the tourniquet underneath the bottom portion, creating a loop with the upper flap free. The free end will be tugged on to release the tourniquet later in the draw. The tourniquet should be tight without being uncomfortable or pinching the patient's skin. Both ends of the tourniquet should be pointing upward on the arm. This way, the end of the tourniquet does not contaminate the venipuncture site.

When the tourniquet is in place, ask the patient to place his or her other hand or fist under the elbow of the arm that will be drawn if this aids in palpating the vein. Ask the person to just relax the arm. Palpate for an acceptable vein using your gloved index finger. It is more efficient to put on gloves at the beginning of the procedure and continue. Also, if you learn to palpate veins with gloves on, you will train your finger to recognize the veins through the gloves from the beginning.

According to the CLSI, you can palpate veins without wearing gloves as long as the venipuncture site has not yet been cleaned. After locating the vein, clean the area with a 70% isopropyl alcohol wipe. While the site is drying, resanitize your hands, put on gloves, and continue with the rest of the procedure.

Performing the Venipuncture

When you have located a vein, remove the tourniquet. A tourniquet can remain in place for 1 minute. After its removal, wait 2 minutes before reapplying it. During this time, sanitize your hands and put on gloves (if they are not already on). Then cleanse the antecubital area with a 70% alcohol wipe. Clean the area by using a back-and-forth motion. CLSI guidelines recommend cleansing the site with friction and not in a circular motion. Do not touch this area after cleaning with alcohol. Assemble the equipment and place it within easy reach of the patient's arm.

Reapply the tourniquet. Do not have the patient clench or pump the fist. If the fist is relaxed, the venipuncture will feel less painful. Visually relocate the vein, and do not retouch the cleaned area. Anchor the vein by gently stretching the skin downward, about 2 to 3 inches below the collection site, with the thumb of the nondominant hand. Smoothly and quickly insert the needle into the vein at about a 15-degree angle, depending on the depth and position of the vein. The bevel should be facing up. Push the evacuated tube onto the double-pointed needle or pull back on the syringe plunger with your nondominant hand.

Angle of Needle Entry

Why is the angle of the needle so important? If the needle is inserted at an angle greater than 15 degrees, it penetrates the vein quickly and may pass through the back side of the vein and enter other structures. Formation of a hematoma is more likely then.

If the angle is less than 15 degrees, the needle may skim on the top of the vein and not create a clean puncture. If the vein is just skimmed or scratched, there is a greater chance of creating a hematoma on the front of the vein.

The depth and position of the vein may require angle adjustment, but a 15-degree angle is a good place to start. The angle of entry is very important to a successful venipuncture.

CRITICAL THINKING APPLICATION **48.8**

Maggie is drawing Ken Thomas this morning. The provider has ordered three different tests, so Maggie will need to draw three different-colored tubes. As Maggie puts on the tourniquet to locate a vein, Ken pumps his fist a few times to try to make the veins stand out. But Maggie asks him to just relax his hand. Why would relaxing his hand be better? List one or two reasons and be ready to share them with the class.

Completing the Venipuncture

Continue to draw the specimens, checking periodically on the patient's condition. As you remove each tube from the needle holder, gently invert it several times before placing it in a collection rack. Tubes with sodium citrate should be inverted three to four times. Tubes with clot activator should be inverted five times. Tubes with anticoagulant should be inverted eight times. If the tubes are not inverted immediately after collection, small clots can form in the specimen. When the last tube has started to fill, carefully release the tourniquet. Gently tug on the short portion of the tourniquet, and it should just fall open. Remove the final vacuum tube. Cover the venipuncture area with gauze, then smoothly and quickly remove the needle. Once the needle is out of the arm, apply pressure to the site. At the same time, activate the safety device to cover the needle. Dispose of the entire venipuncture assembly into a sharps container. Ask the patient to apply direct pressure to the gauze. *Do not* bend the arm.

While the patient applies pressure to the site, label the tubes with computer-generated labels or by writing the information in permanent marker. Make sure the label contains the following minimum information:

- Patient's last name, then first name
- Patient's date of birth
- Patient's ID number or medical insurance number
- Date and time of the draw and the phlebotomist's initials
- Provider's name; also indicate if the patient was fasting (optional)

Before putting on a bandage, perform a two-point check to make sure the site is not leaking. Observe the site for 5 to 10 seconds after releasing pressure and removing the gauze. If visible bleeding occurs or if the tissue around the puncture site rises, continue applying pressure until the bleeding has stopped. Special precautions must be taken for patients taking anticoagulants because the phlebotomy site will bleed longer than normal. Put on a pressure bandage by placing a folded gauze (not a cotton ball) over the site and applying a hypoallergenic self-stick wrap, stretchy gauze, or a bandage. Never leave the room or release an outpatient until all the tubes have been labeled. Make sure the patient is doing well, then escort them to the exit or reception area.

Procedures 48.1 and 48.2 outline the proper procedures for venipuncture using the evacuated tube method and the syringe method. Some patients may have small veins, and using a syringe or butterfly for venipuncture may work better than the standard evacuated assembly. Young children, chemotherapy patients, older adult patients, and people with veins that are difficult to draw may require syringe or butterfly equipment. Alternative equipment is always used to draw blood from hand veins (Procedure 48.3).

CRITICAL THINKING APPLICATION **48.9**

At the end of Ken's venipuncture, Maggie asks Ken to hold pressure on the draw site. She puts the computer-generated labels on the three tubes she drew and writes her initials and time of collection on the labels. Then Maggie checks Ken's arm and wraps gauze around the site.

Why is it important to label the tubes immediately after finishing the venipuncture? List two reasons this is a good practice for a phlebotomist.

PROBLEMS ASSOCIATED WITH VENIPUNCTURE

Issues associated with venipuncture include bruising, fainting, and potential tissue injury. Additionally, failure to obtain an adequate specimen can lead to the need to redraw a patient. Remaining calm helps you think clearly about the situation. Determining the cause of the problem will help you decide whether a second attempt is warranted. Knowing how and when to respond to adverse events during the venipuncture procedure is essential for patient safety and specimen integrity.

Hematoma

A **hematoma** is a large, painful, bruised area at the puncture site caused by blood leaking into the tissue, which causes the tissue around the puncture site to swell. The most common causes of hematoma formation during the draw are excessive probing with the needle to locate a vein, failure to insert the needle far enough into the vein, and passing the needle through the vein. A hematoma can also form after a draw if the tourniquet is not removed before removing the needle, if the vacuum tube is not removed from the hub of the needle before the needle is withdrawn, if adequate pressure is not applied at the puncture site, or if the elbow is bent while pressure is applied. If a hematoma forms, discontinue the procedure STAT, apply pressure to the area for a minimum of 3 minutes, and then apply an ice pack to the area. Notify the provider and observe the site to determine whether the bleeding has stopped. Depending on the facility's policy, an incident report may have to be completed and documented in the patient's record. A hematoma may also occur if the puncture reopens and bleeds into the tissue due to heavy lifting with the venipuncture arm. Instruct the patient to be careful with the arm for several hours after the procedure.

Nerve Damage and Other Complications

Nerve damage can be a consequence of venipuncture, but the risk is very small. Preventive measures include the following:

- Avoiding the basilic vein for phlebotomy
- Refraining from *blind probing* (moving the needle in the arm with the hope of finding a vein) if the vein is missed with the initial draw

Table 48.3 lists some workable solutions to complications. As a rule, it is wise to limit yourself to two venipuncture attempts for a patient. If a second attempt is unsuccessful, ask whether the patient would allow another phlebotomist to look at his or her arms. If another phlebotomist feels confident to attempt a venipuncture, that person will need to get permission from the patient first. If the patient does not give permission, it may be better to reschedule the venipuncture for another time. This strategy lets patients know that

TABLE 48.3 Managing Possible Blood Draw Complications

COMPLICATION	MANAGEMENT STRATEGIES
Burned area	Choose another site because these areas are prone to infection.
Convulsions	Stay calm. Remove the needle and quickly dispose of it in a sharps container. Then help guide the patient to the floor, protecting him or her from injury. Call for help.
Damaged or scarred veins or infected areas	Look for an alternative site; do not draw blood from scarred or infected areas.
Edema	Avoid the area; look for an alternative site.
Intravenous (IV) therapy or blood transfusion sites	Blood samples should not be drawn from an arm that is also the site for IV infusion or blood transfusion because of the dilution factor.
Mastectomy	Do not draw blood from the side of the mastectomy, because mastectomy surgery causes **lymphostasis**, which may produce false results.
Nausea	Place a cold cloth on the patient's forehead, give the patient a basin in case of vomiting, and instruct him or her to take deep breaths. Alert the provider.
No blood	Manipulate the needle slightly or remove the vacuum tube, and perform the blood draw again using a syringe or butterfly setup.
Petechiae	Loosen the tourniquet because this complication usually results from the tourniquet being in place longer than 2 minutes.

they have input into their care and some measure of control of the situation. At one time or another, everyone is unsuccessful in obtaining a blood sample, so do not have bad feelings about it. Make the best of the situation, learn from the experience, and treat the patient with kindness. We are all human, and our patients are usually quite understanding.

Fainting

Fainting, or syncope, can have serious consequences, so the phlebotomist must always be prepared to act quickly. Positioning the patient in a blood collection chair (by turning the armrest pad in front of the patient) prevents bodily injury if the person faints. Making eye contact and observing the patient before phlebotomy can help you estimate his or her level of comfort with the procedure. Constant light conversation with the patient during the venipuncture can help identify if the patient is distressed or anxious. As you finish the venipuncture, observe the patient's face, and assess the breathing rate if the patient seems anxious. Safety comes first. Make sure patients are not in a position in which they can be hurt.

According to CLSI, the procedure for a fainting patient or one who is nonresponsive is as follows:

- If the patient begins to faint, quickly remove the tourniquet and needle from the arm, immediately activate the needle safety device, apply pressure to the site, and dispose of the unit in a sharps container to prevent an accidental exposure.
- Notify staff members for assistance.
- Lay the patient flat or lower the head if the patient is sitting.
- Loosen tight clothing.
- Do not use ammonia inhalants/capsules because these are associated with adverse effects and are no longer recommended.
- Apply a cold compress or washcloth to the patient's forehead and back of the neck.
- Monitor the patient's pulse, blood pressure, and respiration rate.
- Stay with the patient until recovery is complete.
- Document the incident according to facility policies.
- When the patient regains consciousness, they must remain in the facility for at least 15 minutes and should not operate a vehicle for at least 30 minutes.

See Chapter 27 for more information on what to do if a patient faints.

Some patients have a history of fainting with venipunctures. Fainting can be related to several conditions, including **vasovagal syncope** and **postural orthostatic tachycardia syndrome (POTS)**. If a patient warns you that they might faint, anticipate that the patient will faint and take precautions before starting the procedure. Do not minimize what the patient states by telling the patient to "just relax." *Listen to your patient.*

CRITICAL THINKING APPLICATION 48.10

Two patients tell you they faint with venipunctures. Jane states that she frequently faints with venipunctures due to her anxiety. Chloe states she has POTS and faints with venipunctures. Describe similar actions you would take for both patients. Describe the differences in your actions between the patients.

Specimen Re-collection

Sometimes problems with a sample cannot be determined until the specimen is analyzed in the laboratory. Rejected specimens must be re-collected. The laboratory may reject a specimen for reasons that include the following:

- Unlabeled or mislabeled specimen
- Quantity not sufficient (QNS), which means there is an insufficient quantity of specimen for the test
- Defective tube
- Incorrect tube used for the test ordered (incorrect stopper color)
- Hemolysis (Table 48.4)
- Clotted blood in an anticoagulated specimen
- Improper handling

Hemolysis is the major cause of specimen rejection. It cannot be detected until the blood cells are separated from the plasma or serum. It is crucial to take steps to prevent red blood cell damage during collection. Hemolyzed serum or plasma appears rosy to bright red because of the release of hemoglobin from the cells. Some routine tests adversely affected by hemolysis are chemistry tests for electrolytes (e.g., potassium, sodium), bilirubin, total protein, and liver enzymes.

TABLE 48.4 Major Causes of Hemolysis during Collection

CAUSE	EXPLANATION	PREVENTION
Alcohol preparation	Transfer of alcohol into the specimen causes hemolysis.	Allow the venipuncture site to dry completely.
Incorrect needle size	A high-gauge needle causes the blood to go through a small lumen with great force, causing hemolysis. A very-low-gauge needle causes a large amount of blood to suddenly enter the tube with great force, causing frothing.	Choose the correct needle for the job, aiming for a 19- to 23-gauge needle.
Loose connections on the vacuum tube assembly	If the connection between the needle holder and the double-pointed needle or the syringe and the needle is loose, air can enter the sample and cause frothing.	Make sure all connections are tight before beginning the venipuncture.
Removing the needle from the vein with the tube intact	The remaining vacuum in the tube can cause air to be drawn forcefully into the tube, causing frothing.	Remove the final tube from the needle holder before withdrawing the needle from the patient's vein.
Underfilled tubes	Underfilling tubes leads to an improper blood/additive ratio.	Permit blood to flow into the tubes until no more movement can be seen.
Syringe collections	Pulling back too rapidly on the plunger draws blood too quickly through the needle. This causes hemolysis.	Loosen the plunger before use. Use the smallest syringe possible. Gently draw the plunger so no more than 1 mL of air space is present. When transferring blood into the vacuum tube, use a transfer device. *Never* push on the plunger when transferring blood.
Mixing tubes too vigorously	All tubes should be gently inverted. (See Table 48.3.)	Gently invert tubes immediately after the draw. Vigorous mixing can hemolyze cells.
Temperature and transport problems	Trauma and temperature extremes can damage cells. Freezing will cause hemolysis.	Tubes should be transported in the upright position with as little trauma as possible. Control the temperature.
Separation of plasma or serum from red blood cells	Removing the serum/plasma from cells lowers the risk of contaminating the specimen with red blood cells (RBCs).	Blood samples that are centrifuged should have cells and plasma/serum separated as soon as possible.
Prolonged tourniquet time	**Interstitial** fluid can leak into the veins and hemolyze RBCs.	Leave the tourniquet on for no longer than 1 minute.
Poor collection; blood flowing too slowly into the tube	The needle lumen may be blocked because it is too close to the inner wall of the vein.	Withdraw the needle slightly to center it within the vein.

PEDIATRIC PHLEBOTOMY

Obtaining blood from children and infants may be difficult and potentially hazardous. The procedure should be performed by personnel trained in pediatric phlebotomy. Successfully obtaining blood from children requires skill and an understanding of children and their development. Good communication skills are essential when dealing with children. The phlebotomist must gain the child's trust and often that of the parent or guardian. Parents frequently ask the phlebotomist to explain the tests being done and the reasons for testing. Be respectful when talking to parents. Defer to the provider if questions come up about specific information regarding possible diseases or conditions the child may have.

Role of the Parent or Guardian

A parent or guardian may be helpful during phlebotomy. Ask the parent or guardian about the child's previous phlebotomy experiences and how cooperative the child has been in the past. Respectfully determine whether the parent or guardian seems comfortable assisting in restraining an uncooperative child. Parental behavior greatly influences the child's behavior during the procedure. Children should never be restrained in a way that might cause physical injury or pain. If the parent or guardian is unable or unwilling to assist with the procedure, always refer to the office or laboratory policy on procedural holds for phlebotomy. Table 48.5 provides information on the typical fears and concerns of children during the procedure and suggested parental involvement.

Pediatric Concerns

Removing large amounts of blood, especially from premature infants, may result in anemia (Table 48.6). The amount of blood withdrawn must be recorded in the child's chart. Puncturing deep veins in children may result in serious complications, such as cardiac arrest, hemorrhage, venous thrombosis, damage to surrounding tissues, and infection.

In addition, the child could be harmed during restraint. To prevent these problems, blood should be collected only by dermal puncture from children younger than age 2 unless the procedure warrants venous collection (lead levels or blood culture). Venipuncture on

TABLE 48.5 Childhood Behavior and Parental Involvement during Phlebotomy

AGE	TYPICAL MENTAL STATE	SUGGESTED PARENTAL INVOLVEMENT
Newborns (0–12 months)	Trust that adults will respond to their needs	Parent should assist by cradling and comforting child.
Infants and toddlers (1–3 years)	Minimal fear of danger but fear of separation; limited language and understanding of procedure	Parent should assist by holding the child and providing emotional support.
Preschoolers (3–6 years)	Fearful of injury to body; still dependent on parent	Parent may be present to provide emotional support and to assist in obtaining child's cooperation.
School-aged children (7–12 years)	Less dependent on parent and more willing to cooperate; fear of loss of self-control (crying)	Child may not want parent present.
Teenagers (13–18 years)	Fully engaged in the process; embarrassed to show fear and may show hostility to cover emotions	Teen may not want parent present.

TABLE 48.6 General Guidelines for Pediatric Venipuncture

WEIGHT (LB)	SINGLE DRAW LIMIT
8–10	3.5 mL
11–15	5 mL
16–40	10 mL
41–60	20 mL
61–65	25 mL
66–80	30 mL

children younger than age 2 should be performed only on surface veins, including the dorsal hand vein, using a 23-gauge winged infusion set coupled to a syringe or a pediatric vacuum tube collection set.

Tips for Pediatric Phlebotomy

When required to perform pediatric phlebotomy, the medical assistant should remember to do the following:

- Wear a colorful, fluid-impermeable jacket lab coat, if possible.
- Be truthful about the discomfort the child will feel.
- Provide tokens and praise for bravery.
- Try to lessen the child's fears.

Topical anesthetics (e.g., ethyl chloride [EC] spray or EMLA cream) may be used to reduce pain at the puncture site. In most cases, a calm, professional phlebotomist who understands children and relates to them on their level can gain the trust needed. Work to perform a successful venipuncture or capillary puncture with minimal restraint and frustration.

CAPILLARY PUNCTURE

Capillaries are small blood vessels that connect small arterioles to small venules. A capillary puncture is an efficient means of collecting a blood specimen when only a small amount of blood is needed. Capillary punctures are also used when a patient's condition makes venipuncture difficult, such as in a patient undergoing chemotherapy. Also, capillary punctures are performed on infants (as a heel stick) and some young children. The test requisition may not specify a capillary collection, so be familiar with the advantages, limitations, and appropriate uses of this technique. Capillary puncture is warranted for the following patients:

- Older adult patients
- Pediatric patients (especially younger than age 2)
- Patients who require frequent glucose monitoring
- Patients with burns or scars in venipuncture sites
- Obese patients
- Patients receiving intravenous (IV) therapy or chemotherapy
- Patients who have had a mastectomy
- Patients at risk for venous thrombosis
- Patients who are severely dehydrated
- Patients who are undergoing tests that require a small volume of blood (i.e., some CLIA-waived tests)

Capillaries are connections between arteries and veins, so capillary blood is a mixture of the two. Small volumes of tissue fluid also are present in capillary blood, especially in the first drop. Analyte levels are usually the same in capillary and venous blood, with a few exceptions. Hemoglobin and glucose values are higher in capillary blood; potassium, calcium, and total protein are higher in venous blood.

Equipment

Capillary punctures are performed with specialized equipment. A look at the equipment is useful and can help you decide when a capillary puncture should be performed instead of a venipuncture.

Skin Puncture Devices

The device used to perform a dermal puncture is the *lancet*, which delivers a quick puncture to a preset depth (Figure 48.17). Puncture depths include the following:

- Finger stick: 3.0 mm depth, and the gauge of needle may vary by manufacturer
- Heel stick: 2.0 mm depth and the width should not exceed 2.5 mm; for premature infants, the heel stick depth is 0.65 to 0.85 mm, and a puncture width of 1.75 mm
- Bleeding time (BT) test: 1.0 mm depth and a length of 5 mm

OSHA has directed that lancets must have retractable blades. Safety lancets only puncture once and cannot be reused. Lancets are

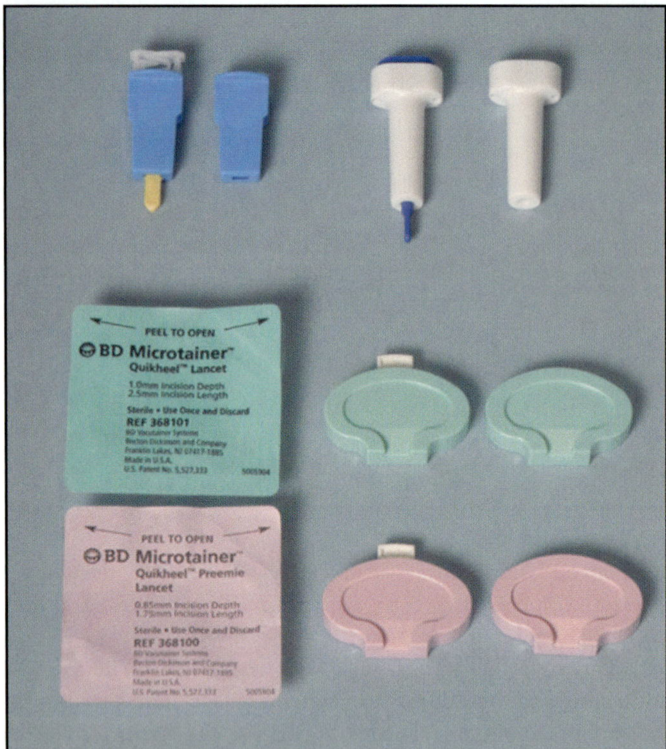

FIGURE 48.17 Dermal puncture devices. (Courtesy Becton, Dickinson, Franklin Lakes, NJ.)

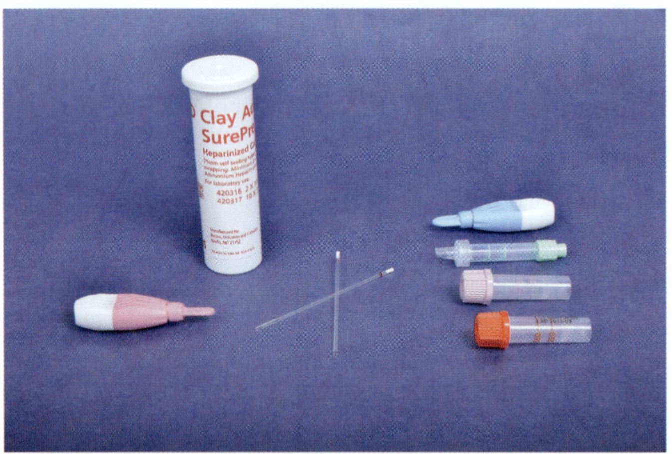

FIGURE 48.18 Capillary collection containers, Microtainers, and self-sealing microhematocrit tubes.

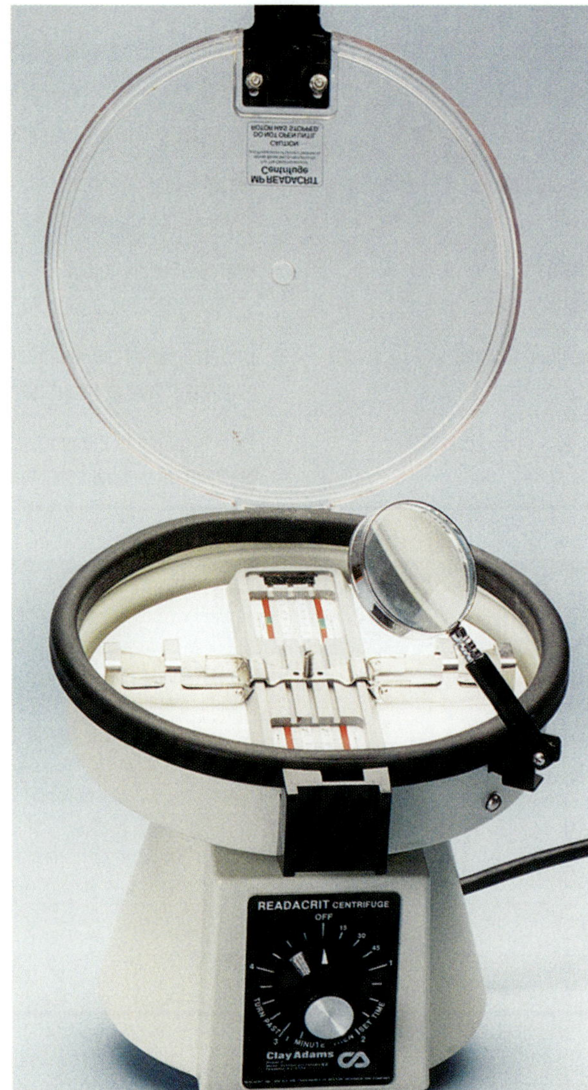

FIGURE 48.19 Microhematocrit centrifuge with indicators for capillary tube placement.

available as needle lancets and blade lancets. The choice of lancet should follow CLSI standards for puncture depth. Lancets should always be discarded in a sharps container immediately after use.

> **CRITICAL THINKING** APPLICATION **48.11**
>
> A capillary puncture is also called a fingerstick. What other term is used for this procedure?

Collection Containers

Different types of containers and collection devices are available, and the ones used depend on the test being performed. Microcollection tubes and Microtainers (Figure 48.18) are available with a variety of anticoagulants and additives. Their color-coded tops indicate the same additives as evacuated tubes. Blood drops are collected into the Microtainers through a funnel-like device.

Capillary tubes are another type of blood collection tube used to get a capillary sample. A capillary tube is a glass tube surrounded by a protective plastic coating for safety. The blood is pulled into the tube by *capillary action*; this means that the blood fills these small, narrow tubes without the help of **suction**. If the capillary tube is coated with the anticoagulant heparin, a red band will be seen at the top of the tube. A common, heparin-coated capillary tube is the microhematocrit tube. Microhematocrit tubes are used to determine the percentage of packed red blood cells in the blood (discussed in Chapter 49). Figure 48.19 shows a microhematocrit tube and centrifuge. Self-sealing capillary tubes are used in the microhematocrit test.

Manufacturers often provide collection devices for obtaining small amounts of blood for point-of-care testing (POCT), such as glucose, hemoglobin A1c, and cholesterol (see Chapter 49). Blood is pulled into the collecting device by capillary action after the puncture or applied to a reagent strip that has been inserted into the instrument to be analyzed.

Blood from a capillary puncture may also be deposited on paper cards. The Guthrie card (Figure 48.20) is used to test babies for certain metabolic disorders, such as phenylketonuria (PKU). Blood is deposited into circles on biologically inactive filter paper and is sent

A

DO NOT WRITE IN BLUE SHADED AREAS–DO NOT WRITE ON BARCODE

CC040H1088462C

ALL INFORMATION MUST BE PRINTED

Birthdate: MM/DD/YY Time (Use 24 hr time only)
Baby/s name: (last, first)
Hospital provider number: (mandatory)
Hospital name:
Mother's name: (last, first, Initial)
Mother's ID: Baby's ID:
Mother's address:
Mother's phone: ( ) -
Specimen date MM/DD/YY Time (Use 24 hr time only)
Physician's name:
Physician's address:
City: Ohio zip
Physician's phone: ( ) -
ODH COPY
Physician's provider number: (mandatory)
ODH COPY: SPECIAL:

TEST RESULTS
Screening test normal for PKU, HOM, GAL, Hypothyroidism
Screening test normal for PKU and HOM only
Screening test normal
PKU HOM GAL
Hypothyroidism
Screening test abnormal
See footnote ______ on back
Specimen rejected for reason:

Baby sex: Male Female
Birth weight: grams
Premature: Yes No
Antibiotics: Yes No
Transfusion: Yes No
Specimen: First Second
Submittor: Hospital
Physician
Health department
Other (name below)
HEA 2518

FILL ALL CIRCLES WITH BLOOD
BLOOD MUST SOAK COMPLETELY THROUGH
DO NOT APPLY BLOOD TO THIS SIDE

B

Correct

Incorrect

FIGURE 48.20 **(A)** Guthrie card used in neonatal screening. **(B)** Correctly and incorrectly filled cards. (From Warekois RS, Robinson R: *Phlebotomy: work text and procedures manual*, ed 4, St. Louis, 2016, Saunders.)

to a referral laboratory for analysis within 24 hours of sampling. Federal postal regulations for mailing biohazard material must be followed.

Site Selection

In adults and children (older than 1 year), capillary puncture sites include the ring or middle finger. Why do we collect capillary samples only from the middle and ring fingers? The thumb usually is too callused or thick-skinned, and the index finger has nerve endings that make the puncture more painful. The fifth finger (pinky finger) has too little tissue for a successful puncture.

Dermal puncture of an infant should be done on the heel of the foot (Figure 48.21). A capillary puncture is made on the palmar surface of the finger, near the tip, and slightly to the side of the finger. Punctures should be made across to the whorls of the finger. This

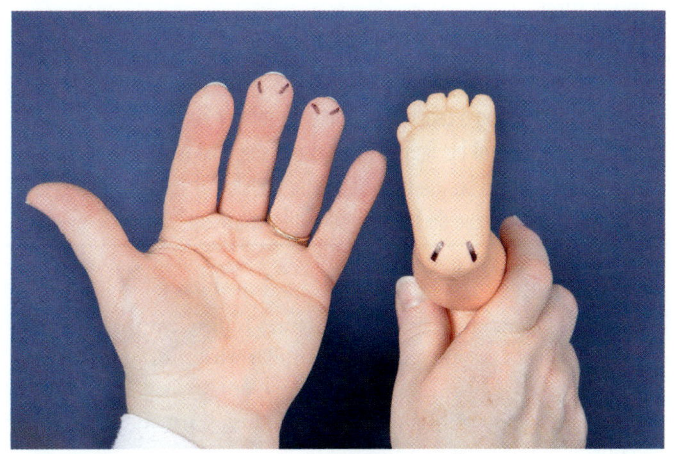

FIGURE 48.21 Dermal puncture site selection and lancet placement.

helps to create a nice drop of blood to collect. Avoid areas that are callused, scarred, burned, infected, cyanotic, or edematous.

For children younger than 2 years of age, a dermal puncture is performed on the medial or lateral areas of the *plantar surface* (bottom) of the heel or on the *palmar surface* of the ring or middle finger. Areas other than these are unsafe, and bone or nerve damage to an infant may occur. Blood flow from an infant's heel can be increased by applying a warm, moist towel (or other warming device) at a temperature no higher than 108°F (42°C) for 3 to 5 minutes. Never place bandages on the heel or anywhere on infants younger than age 2 because they may peel off and become a choking hazard.

Patient Preparation

Preparation for a capillary puncture is similar to that for a venipuncture. Put on a fluid-impermeable lab coat, wash your hands or use hand sanitizer, and wear gloves and protective eyewear.

You must work efficiently when performing a capillary puncture because blood flow stops quickly. Be sure to have the supplies organized and within easy reach. Because you are working with blood that is free flowing, make sure there are spare gloves, extra gauze, and disinfectant nearby. Be prepared if your gloves become contaminated with blood.

If the patient's hands are excessively soiled, ask the person to wash them before the procedure. If the patient's hands are cold, warm them in warm water and dry them thoroughly, or ask the person to rub or shake them vigorously. Cleanse the finger well with a 70% alcohol wipe.

Collecting the Specimen

The puncture must be on the palm-up surface of the distal fingertip of the middle or ring finger. The puncture should be made across the fingerprint, not parallel to it. Press the lancet firmly against the skin and quickly depress the plunger.

After the skin has been punctured, it is important to wipe away the first drop of blood with gauze. This drop contains tissue fluid that could interfere with test results. Fill the sampling containers according to the manufacturer's directions. Touch the container to the drop of blood as it is released from the puncture site, but do not touch the skin. If blood flow stops, wiping the site with gauze may restart the flow. After the containers have been filled, ask the patient to apply pressure to the gauze placed over the puncture site. Seal and mix the containers by gently inverting the tubes as recommended by the manufacturer.

CRITICAL THINKING APPLICATION **48.12**

Maggie is performing a capillary puncture on Johnny Parker, who is 7 years old. She is looking at his fingers to choose a site, and his hands are chilly. Which fingers would be the best choice for a child? If Johnny's hands are chilly, what can Maggie do to make sure they warm up?

Order of Draws

The order of draws for capillary punctures is different than phlebotomy. A medical assistant should be familiar with the order of draws:

1. *Capillary blood gas collection tubes*: Contain heparin additive. Used for capillary blood gas tests. (Must warm the site before collecting the specimen.)
2. *Blood smear*: Used for hematology blood counts.
3. *Lavender top*: Contains EDTA additive. Used for hematology blood counts.
4. *Green top*: Contains lithium heparin additive. Used for tests that require a heparinized plasma sample.
5. *Other tubes that contain anticoagulants.*
6. *Red or gold top*: Contain a clot activator additive. Used for tests that require a serum sample.
7. *Red top*: Contains no additive. Used for tests that require a serum sample without a clot activator.

Specimen Handling

Capillary collection containers are often too small for a label to be applied to the tube. The most efficient way to transport capillary tubes is to remove the stopper from a red-topped venipuncture tube, insert the capillary tubes, sealed-end down, replace the stopper, and label the red-topped tube. Microtainer tubes have plastic plugs that fit over the top. They may be placed in a labeled tube or a labeled zipper-lock bag for transport. Always decontaminate collection containers before delivering them to the laboratory if blood was deposited on the surface during collection. The procedure for routine capillary collection is outlined in Procedure 48.4.

HANDLING THE SPECIMEN AFTER COLLECTION

The laboratory testing results are only as good as the specimen sent for testing. Specimens handled improperly after collection may provide incorrect results. They may even compromise the patient's health. From the moment a specimen is collected, analytes in the blood begin to break down. By testing specimens as soon as possible, the laboratory tries to provide results that accurately represent the patient's condition at the time of blood collection. After collection, blood may need to be processed before the sample is tested. This may include separation of plasma or serum from the red blood cells. If the venipuncture tube contains no anticoagulant (i.e., tubes with a red, a marbled red-gray, or a gold stopper), blood starts the clotting process when it touches the tube. The "clot" tubes should sit upright in a rack for 30 to 60 minutes at room temperature while a solid clot forms. Tubes with a clot accelerator should form a dense clot within 30 minutes. The presence of anticoagulants in the patient's blood, such as warfarin (Coumadin) or heparin, may delay clotting. Once the clot has formed, every effort should be made to remove the clot from the serum within 2 hours.

Centrifugation

Removing the serum from a clot tube requires centrifugation. For thixotropic gel to form a barrier between the clot and the serum, certain requirements must be met. The tube must be centrifuged at a specified **g-force**, time, and temperature. A clinical centrifuge instruction manual should provide the appropriate settings for spinning blood specimens. The serum does not have to be removed from the tube after centrifugation because the gel has formed a barrier over the red blood cells. Once a tube with thixotropic gel has been centrifuged, it cannot be centrifuged again. The serum, however, can be decanted and centrifuged in another tube.

For tests that require plasma, the plasma should be removed from the cells as soon as possible. This can be done by centrifuging the tube and then **aspirating** the plasma off the cells. The plasma is then transferred to another tube using a disposable transfer pipet. You can also use a PST tube with a marbled green-gray top or a PST tube with a light green top. Both contain lithium heparin anticoagulant and a thixotropic gel, which form the necessary barrier when centrifuged.

Using Reference Laboratories

Certain blood tests, such as a CBC, require whole blood. It is wise to check the specimen requirements of the **reference laboratory** that will perform the test and follow the lab's instructions for transport and storage. The College of American Pathologists (CAP) recommends that whole blood for automated blood counts be refrigerated and tested within 72 hours.

Often specimens must be transported by courier to other facilities. The Hazardous Materials Shipping Regulations, established by the Department of Transportation, apply to the packaging and shipping of hazardous materials by ground transportation. POLs that ship human specimens must be trained to properly handle, pack, and ship biohazard materials. Reference laboratories will frequently have couriers who pick up specimens. The specimens and their requisitions are typically placed in individual biohazard bags and sorted according to which reference lab is affiliated with the patient's insurance.

Chain of Custody

Blood samples may be collected as evidence in legal proceedings. Blood may be drawn for drug and alcohol testing, DNA analysis, or paternity testing. These samples must be handled according to special procedures to prevent tampering, misidentification, or interference with the test results.

Chain of custody is a legal term that refers to the ability to guarantee the identity and integrity of the specimen from the time of collection to the time test results are reported. It is a process used to maintain and document the history of a specimen. Documents should include the name or initials of the individual collecting the specimen, the name of each person who tests or transports the specimen, the date the specimen was collected or transferred, the name of the employer or agency, the specimen number, the patient's or employee's name, and a brief description of the specimen.

Collection kits are available that contain everything needed for the venipuncture, including the tube, the needle, the chain of custody forms and seals, the antiseptic, and even the tourniquet. Familiarize yourself with these kits before using them. Phlebotomists may be required to testify at legal proceedings if they are involved in the collection or testing of a legal sample.

CLOSING COMMENTS

Patient Coaching

Phlebotomy can be a stressful event for some patients. Helping patients to remain calm and at ease is a high priority for the phlebotomist. Patients often express great concern when several tubes of blood must be drawn. It can seem like they are losing a lot of blood. You can put their fears to rest by explaining that the average adult has a little less than 5 L of blood (10 pints). Most adults can relate to donating a unit of blood, which is about 500 mL (1 pint). Because a large, red-topped tube contains 10 mL of blood, you would have to draw about 50 tubes to remove 500 mL of blood.

Provide as much explanation as needed to ease the patient's anxiety. Often the patient can help by identifying the site of the last successful blood venipuncture. When appropriate, follow the patient's suggestion in choosing the site for a venipuncture. When patients become active participants in the procedure, they remain more relaxed, talkative, and confident in your expertise as a phlebotomist.

Legal and Ethical Issues

Phlebotomy is an invasive procedure in which a sterile needle or lancet is inserted through the skin. Because the skin is penetrated, drawing blood becomes a surgical procedure and is subject to the laws and regulations of surgery. When a venipuncture is performed, the rules and regulations must be obeyed with no exceptions. Be sure to follow the written procedures in the laboratory. Become familiar with the regulations and standards established by CLSI and OSHA and by state and local agencies. Deviations from the standards leave the medical assistant open to malpractice. Document any situations in which the standard of care comes into question.

Patient-Centered Care

You may want to ask your patients how they would prefer to be addressed: By their first name? A nickname? Dr. Smith, Mr. Jones, Mrs. Blake, or Ms. Washington? Don't assume that patients want to be called by their first name. Also, do not call patients "sweetie," "honey," or "dear." Be respectful, professional, and patient focused.

Professional Behaviors

Your appearance and actions reflect your laboratory or facility. A patient's first impression of the facility often comes from the medical assistant. Clean fluid-impermeable laboratory coats and scrubs tell the patient the facility is clean; by sanitizing your hands in front of the patient and wearing gloves, you tell the patient you will treat him or her with care; and speaking knowledgeably provides the impression that the facility is staffed with professionals.

Medical assistants who perform venous and capillary blood collection must maintain a professional attitude yet remain sympathetic to the patient's fears and anxiety about the procedure (Procedure 48.5). Establishing an environment that encourages the person to relax can minimize the patient's pain and discomfort during the procedure. Always remember to verify your patient's identity and explain what you are going to do. Answer any questions the patient may have, and then make every effort to perform the procedure skillfully, quickly, and efficiently.

If your patient has a history of syncope when blood is drawn or if you suspect the patient may be very anxious during the procedure, have the person lie down. Assemble your equipment, and alert the provider before beginning the procedure. This type of professional care may help the patient get through the procedure without feeling anxious.

SUMMARY OF SCENARIO

Maggie has had a busy morning in the phlebotomy area. She likes it when it is busy. The morning seems to fly by. After the morning rush, Maggie restocks a few supplies and then is ready to sit down and take her lunch break. As she relaxes in the lunchroom for a few minutes, she thinks back on the morning with satisfaction. She helped a number of patients today. Norma Washington was in; she is in her fourth week of chemotherapy. She was nervous about today's venipuncture. Maggie calmed her fears and was able to do a capillary puncture instead of a venipuncture. That made Norma's day!

Every patient who came into the phlebotomy area this morning left with a smile. That does not happen every day, but Maggie was so happy that this Monday morning went well.

SUMMARY OF LEARNING OBJECTIVES

1. **Examine the equipment needed to perform a venipuncture.**
   Venipuncture requires a double-pointed safety needle, evacuated collection tubes, a needle holder or a syringe fitted with a safety needle, a tourniquet, an alcohol prep pad, gauze or cotton, a sterile bandage, nonlatex gloves, a fluid-impermeable lab coat, protective eyewear, and a biohazard sharps container.

   A tourniquet is used to hold back venous flow out of the site, which causes the veins to bulge. The tourniquet makes veins easier to locate and puncture. Tourniquets are applied snugly around the upper arm (or wrist for a hand draw) in a fashion that permits easy release.

   A venipuncture site must be cleansed with an antiseptic to prevent infection. The most commonly used antiseptic is 70% isopropyl alcohol or *rubbing alcohol.* Alcohol kills many of the existing bacteria that might contaminate the sample. The alcohol should remain on the skin for 30 to 60 seconds and allowed to air dry to be most effective.

   The various colors of vacuum tube stoppers indicate the contents of the tube. Certain additives are compatible with certain laboratory tests. The correct order of draw is (1) blood culture bottles or yellow, (2) light blue, (3) red top or gold top, (4) green, (5) lavender, and (6) gray. Vacuum tubes are collected in a specific order to prevent the carryover of tube additives.

   The venipuncture needle has a shaft with one end cut at an angle (bevel). The other end (the hub) attaches to the syringe or a needle holder. The inner bore or space in the needle is called the *lumen.* It is measured in gauge numbers (the higher the gauge number, the smaller the lumen). Double-pointed needles are used for the evacuated tube method in which the blood flows directly from the vein into the evacuated tube. Removable safety needles are used with disposable syringes. The collected blood in the syringe is then transferred to the appropriate evacuated tubes using a safety transfer device. Safety lancets are used for dermal puncture.
2. **Examine needle safety when performing phlebotomy.**
   The Food and Drug Administration (FDA) recommends devices that provide a barrier between the hands and the needle after use, so the phlebotomist's hands remain behind the needle at all times. Safety shields that can be activated before or immediately after removal of the needle from the vein and remain in effect after disposal should also be an integral part of the device.

   The Occupational Safety and Health Administration (OSHA) requires employers to have a postexposure plan in place for accidental sharps exposures. These plans generally include a means to cleanse the wound with an appropriate antiseptic cleanser; evaluation of the exposure to determine whether the employee is at risk for contracting HBV, HCV, or HIV, depending on the circumstance of the injury; gathering of information about the source of the blood involved; prophylactic care if necessary; confidential counseling for the injured; and follow-up on the exposure.
3. **Examine the process for performing a routine venipuncture.**
   Start the venipuncture by greeting the patient and verifying his or her identity. According to the Clinical and Laboratory Standards Institute (CLSI), proper identification includes asking outpatients to (1) state and spell their first and last name and (2) state their birth date. All the information must be compared and verified with the patient requisition. Briefly explain the venipuncture procedure to your patient, and make sure to ask him or her the necessary questions. Answer questions and concerns, and take steps to prevent any past problems from recurring. If you cannot answer all the patient's questions, ask if they would like to talk to the provider for clarification. Obtain verbal consent to perform the venipuncture simply by asking whether you have permission to draw blood from the patient.

   The medical assistant then sanitizes his or her hands, assembles the equipment and personal protective equipment (PPE), locates the vein, disinfects the area over the vein, allows the alcohol to dry, draws the blood into the correct vacuum tubes in the proper order of draw, removes and properly disposes of the needle, tends to the puncture site, labels the tubes, and delivers them to the laboratory. Standard Precautions are followed during the procedure.
4. **Examine the problems that can be associated with venipuncture.**
   The venipuncture procedure, even when performed correctly, can lead to adverse events. Recognizing these issues as they happen can keep patients safe. Syncope, hematomas, and nerve damage can result even when all steps of the procedure are completed appropriately. Reacting calmly and appropriately will ensure that the patient remains safe and the specimen maintains its integrity. Addressing these concerns will help to avoid the need for the patient to return for an additional blood draw.
5. **Examine the process for performing phlebotomy on the pediatric patient.**
   Obtaining blood from children and infants may be difficult and potentially hazardous. Refer to Table 48.5 for information on typical fears and concerns of children during the procedure and the suggested parental involvement. Refer to Table 48.6 for general guidelines for pediatric venipuncture.

SUMMARY OF LEARNING OBJECTIVES—*continued*

6. **Examine the process of performing a capillary puncture.**
When performing a capillary puncture, the medical assistant starts the procedure by sanitizing the hands. The equipment is gathered, and the patient is identified by asking for their first and last name and date of birth.
Have patients warm their hands by rubbing them together briskly or running warm water over them. Ask each patient which finger is preferred, and sanitize the chosen finger with a 70% isopropyl alcohol wipe. Allow the finger to dry before using a lancet to puncture the finger. The location for the puncture should be on the medial or lateral sides of the distal finger, avoiding the fat pad on the anterior aspect of the finger and avoiding the tip of the finger.
After the puncture, gently squeeze the finger and wipe away the first drop of blood. Squeeze the finger again and collect the subsequent blood that flows from the puncture site. The amount of blood to be collected will be determined by the tests that were ordered.
To finish the procedure, apply a gauze pad or cotton ball to the puncture site to stop the flow of blood. After a minute or two, remove the gauze or cotton and place a bandage over the puncture site. While the patient is applying pressure to the site, label the specimen with the patient's first and last name, birthdate, date, and time of draw, and the medical assistant's initials. Confirm that the patient tolerated the procedure well and inform the patient that the results will follow in a time frame dependent on the test that was ordered.
7. **Explain the requirements for the handling of the specimen after collection.**
From the moment the specimen is collected, analytes in the blood begin to decay, and it is a race against time to provide results that accurately represent a patient's condition at the time of the blood collection. There are various procedures based on the type of test performed.

PROCEDURE 48.1 Perform a Venipuncture: Collect a Venous Blood Sample Using the Vacuum Tube Method

TASKS: Collect a venous blood specimen using the vacuum tube technique. Document the results in the patient's health record.

EQUIPMENT and SUPPLIES

- Patient's health record
- Provider's order and/or lab requisition
- Vacuum tube needle, needle holder, and proper tubes for the requested tests
- 70% isopropyl alcohol wipes
- Gauze
- Tourniquet
- Hypoallergenic self-stick wrap, tape, or bandage
- Permanent marking pen or printed labels
- Fluid-impermeable lab coat, protective eyewear, and gloves
- Biohazard sharps container
- Biohazard waste container

PROCEDURAL STEPS

1. Check the provider's order and/or requisition form to determine the tests ordered. Gather the appropriate tubes and supplies. Put on a fluid-impermeable lab coat.
PURPOSE: Each test requires a specific tube color that is indicated on the requisition. Donning a lab coat is part of ongoing infection control.
2. Greet the patient. Identify yourself. Verify the patient's identity with their full name; ask the patient to spell the first and last names and give their date of birth. Explain the procedure to be performed in a manner that the patient understands. Answer any questions the patient may have on the procedure. Obtain permission for the venipuncture.
PURPOSE: Verifying the patient's identity ensures that you have the right patient. Explanations help gain the patient's cooperation and show awareness of a patient's concerns related to the procedure being performed.
3. Wash your hands or use hand sanitizer and wear gloves and protective eyewear.
PURPOSE: It is important to ensure infection control.
4. Ask the patient if they have a preference as to which arm is used for the venipuncture. Have the patient sit with his or her arm well supported in a slightly downward position.
PURPOSE: The veins of the antecubital area are more easily located when the elbow is straight. Asking about a patient's preference gives the patient a chance to participate in the procedure.
5. Apply the tourniquet around the patient's arm 3-4 inches above the elbow on the patient's preferred arm. The tourniquet should never be tied so tightly that it restricts blood flow in the artery (Figures 1 and 2). Tourniquets should remain in place no longer than 60 seconds.
PURPOSE: The tourniquet is used to make the veins more prominent.

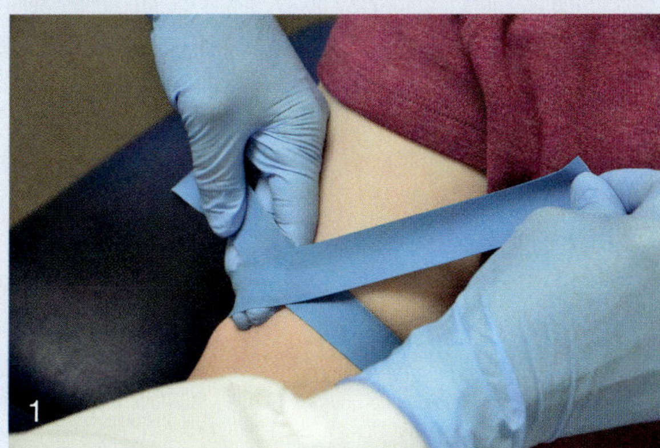

Continued

PROCEDURE 48.1 Perform a Venipuncture: Collect a Venous Blood Sample Using the Vacuum Tube Method—*continued*

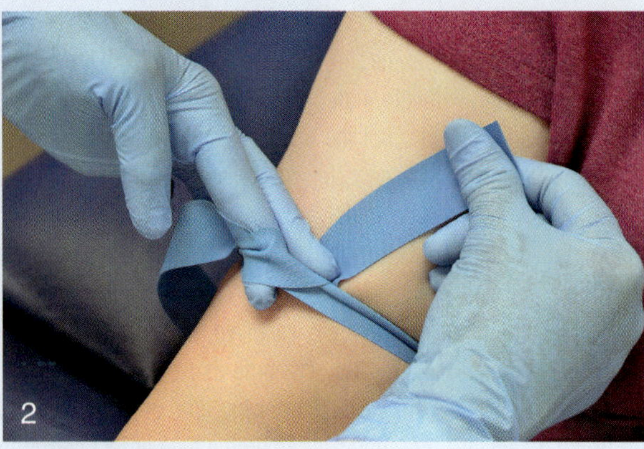
2

6. Select the venipuncture site by palpating the antecubital space. Use your index finger to trace the path of the vein and judge its depth. Look at both arms, and use your critical thinking skills to find the vein that will give you the greatest chance of success for the venipuncture.
   PURPOSE: The index finger is most sensitive for palpating the vein. Do not use the thumb because it has a pulse of its own. Spend time to properly locate the best vein available; your patient will thank you.
7. Remove the tourniquet and cleanse the site with a 70% alcohol wipe (Figure 3).
   PURPOSE: The tourniquet should be tied for only 60 seconds.

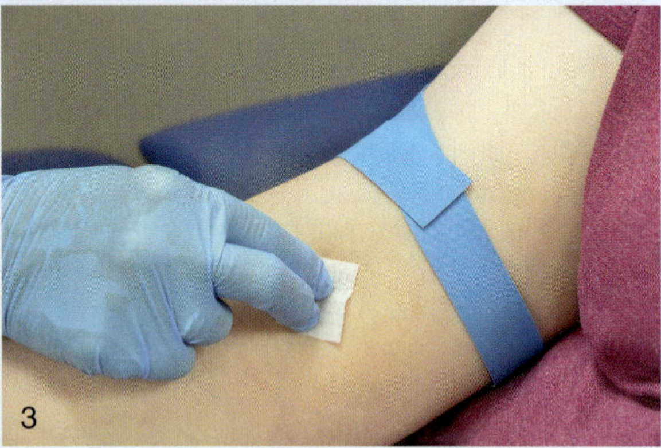
3

8. Assemble the equipment and supplies near your nondominant hand, next to the patient's arm for easy access during the procedure. Select an appropriate needle size and method of collection based on your inspection of the patient's veins. Attach the needle firmly to the vacuum tube holder. Keep the cover on the needle.
   PURPOSE: If the needle is loose, it may turn during the procedure, causing the bevel of the needle to turn away from its upward position.
9. Reapply the tourniquet when the alcohol is dry.
   PURPOSE: Puncturing an area still wet with alcohol stings and can cause hemolysis of the sample.
10. Hold the vacuum tube assembly in your dominant hand. Your thumb should be on top and your fingers underneath (Figure 4). Remove the needle sheath.
    PURPOSE: Positioning the hand in this manner provides the best visibility of the needle entering the vein and accessibility to insert and withdraw tubes with the nondominant hand. Pushing the tube into the double-pointed needle before it is in the arm causes air to rush into the tube, destroying the vacuum.

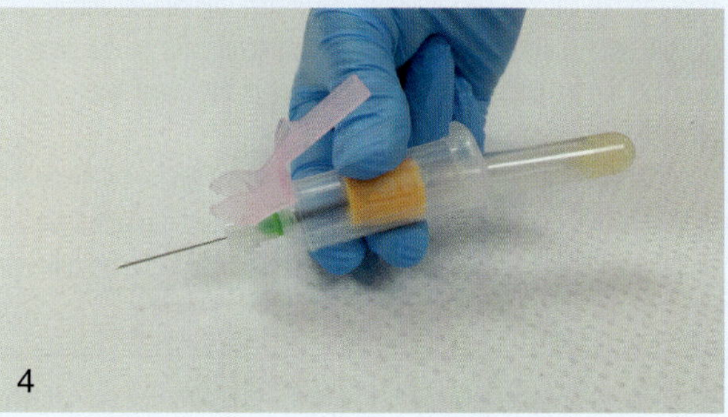
4

11. Grasp the patient's arm with the nondominant hand and anchor the vein with the thumb of your nondominant hand.
    PURPOSE: Failure to anchor the vein may cause it to move away from the needle as it enters the arm.
12. With the bevel up and the needle aligned parallel to the vein, insert the needle at a 15- to 20-degree angle through the skin and into the vein with a quick but smooth motion (Figure 5).
    PURPOSE: The sharpest point of the needle is inserted first. Inserting the needle quickly minimizes pain.

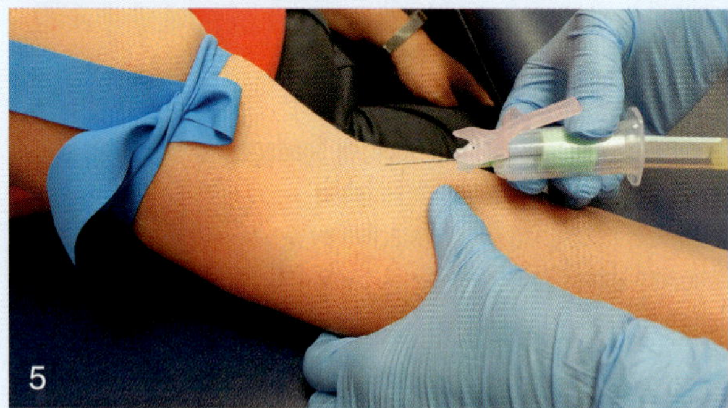
5

13. Hold the assembly in place with the dominant hand, steady through the venipuncture.
    PURPOSE: Holding the needle assembly steady will keep the needle from moving in the vein.
14. Place two fingers on the flanges of the needle holder and use the thumb to push the tube onto the double-pointed needle (Figure 6). Make sure you do not change the needle's position in the vein.
    PURPOSE: The thumb has the strength to push the needle swiftly through the stopper. Be careful and keep the position of the needle steady, so it is not pushed farther into the site when the tube is pushed.

PROCEDURE 48.1 **Perform a Venipuncture: Collect a Venous Blood Sample Using the Vacuum Tube Method—*continued***

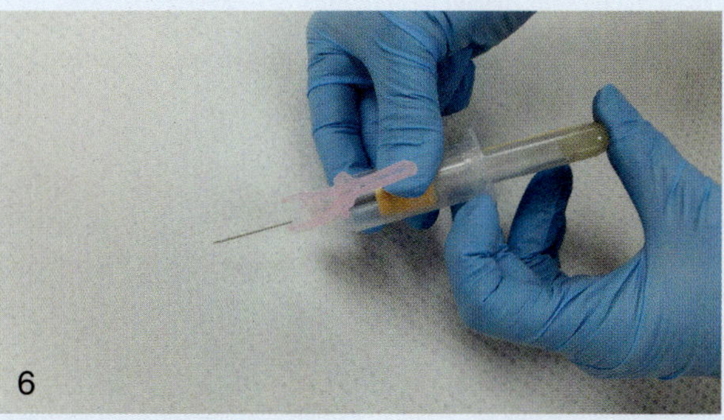

6

15. Allow the tube to fill to its maximum capacity. Remove the tube by placing the fingers at the end of the tube and pushing on the needle holder with the index finger (Figure 7). Do not move the needle when removing the tube. Immediately after removing the tube from the needle holder, gently invert the tube to mix the additives and the blood.
    PURPOSE: Tubes must be full to ensure the proper anticoagulant-to-blood ratio. Moving the needle may result in the needle advancing farther into the vein or slipping out of the vein. Gentle inversion prevents blood from clotting. Do not vigorously mix or shake the tubes because this may cause hemolysis.

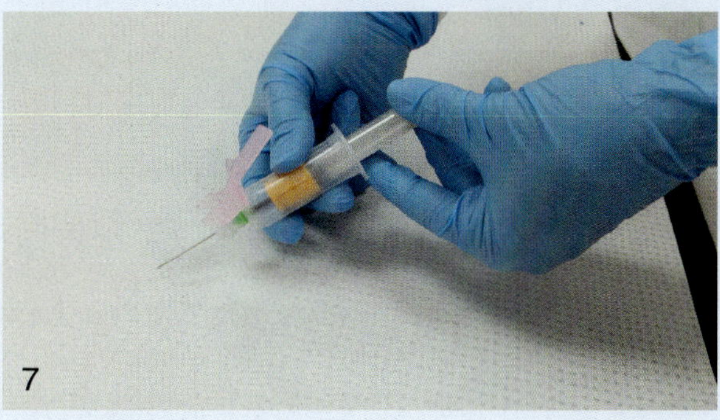

7

16. Insert the second tube into the needle holder, following the instructions in the previous steps. Continue filling tubes until the order on the requisition has been filled. Gently invert each tube after removing it from the needle holder.
17. As the last tube begins filling, release the tourniquet. The tourniquet must be released before the needle is removed from the arm (Figure 8).
    PURPOSE: The tourniquet should remain in place for no longer than 1 minute to prevent hemoconcentration.

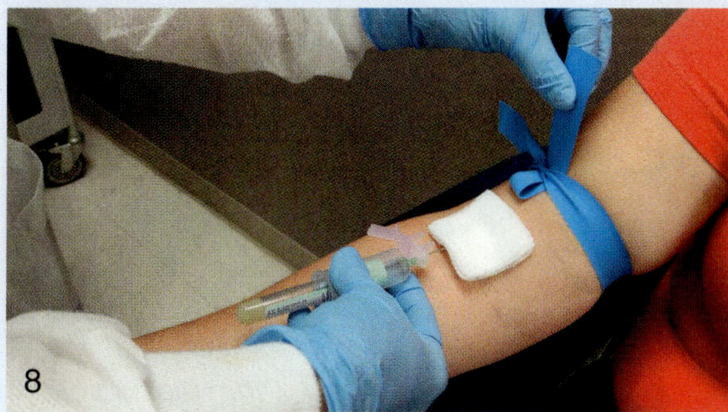

8

18. Remove the last tube from the holder. Place gauze over the puncture site and quickly remove the needle, engaging the safety device (Figure 9).
    PURPOSE: The gauze over the puncture site and activation of the safety needle ensure infection control.

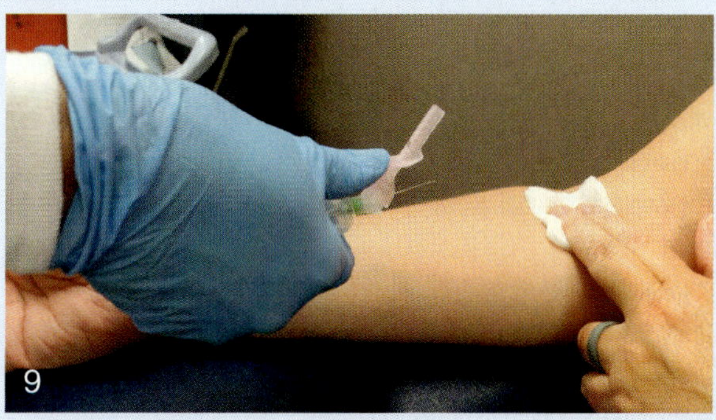

9

19. Dispose of the entire needle/holder assembly into the sharps container.
20. Apply pressure to the gauze or instruct the patient to do so. The patient may elevate the arm but should not bend the elbow.
    PURPOSE: Applying direct pressure and elevating the arm above the heart is the best method to stop bleeding.
21. While the patient is applying pressure to the site, label the tubes with the patient's name, date, time, and your initials, or affix the preprinted tube labels and print your initials and the time on the label.
    PURPOSE: Appropriate labeling will ensure proper specimen identification.
22. Check the venipuncture site. Make sure the bleeding has stopped. Apply a new folded gauze square to the puncture site. Secure the gauze to the site with a hypoallergenic self stick wrap, tape, or a bandage (Figure 10).

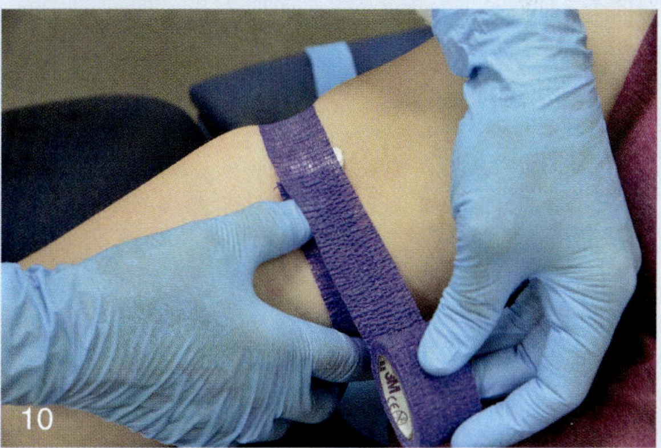

10

23. Disinfect the work area. Dispose of blood-contaminated materials in the biohazard waste container. Remove your protective eyewear and gloves.
24. Wash your hands or use hand sanitizer.
    PURPOSE: It is important to ensure infection control.
25. Complete the laboratory requisition form and route the specimen to the proper place. Record the procedure in the patient's health record.
    PURPOSE: A procedure is not considered done until it is recorded in the patient's record.

Documentation Example

10/05/20XX 1:45 p.m. Venous blood drawn from antecubital space of right arm. Lavender tube for CBC with differential, and red tube for Chemistry. Placed for pickup by Health Alliance Labs. ———— Maggie Brandt, CMA (AAMA)

PROCEDURE 48.2 Perform a Venipuncture: Collect a Venous Blood Sample Using the Syringe Method

TASKS: Collect a venous blood specimen using the syringe technique. Document the results in the patient's health record.

EQUIPMENT and SUPPLIES

- Patient's health record
- Provider's order and/or lab requisition
- Syringe with 21- or 22-gauge safety needle
- Vacuum tubes appropriate for tests ordered
- 70% isopropyl alcohol wipes
- Gauze
- Tourniquet
- Safety transfer device to transfer blood from the syringe to vacuum tubes
- Hypoallergenic self-stick wrap, tape, or bandage
- Permanent marking pen or printed labels
- Fluid-impermeable lab coat, protective eyewear, and gloves
- Biohazard sharps container
- Biohazard waste container

PROCEDURAL STEPS

1. Check the provider's order and/or requisition form to determine the tests ordered. Gather the appropriate tubes and supplies. Put on a fluid-impermeable lab coat.
   PURPOSE: Collect the specimen properly based on the tube requirements on the requisition. Donning a lab coat is part of ongoing infection control.
2. Greet the patient. Identify yourself. Verify the patient's identity with their full name; ask the patient to spell the first and last names and give their date of birth. Explain the procedure to be performed in a manner that the patient understands. Answer any questions the patient may have on the procedure. Obtain permission for the venipuncture.
   PURPOSE: It is important to identify the patient in two different ways to ensure that you have the correct patient. Explaining the procedure can make the patient feel more comfortable and reduces anxiety.
3. Wash your hands or use hand sanitizer. Put on gloves and protective eyewear.
   PURPOSE: It is important to ensure infection control.
4. Ask the patient if they have a preference as to which arm is used for the venipuncture. Have the patient sit with the arm well supported in a slightly downward position.
   PURPOSE: The veins of the antecubital area are more easily located when the elbow is straight. Asking about a patient's preference gives the patient a chance to participate in the procedure.
5. Apply the tourniquet around the patient's arm 3-4 inches above the elbow on the patient's preferred arm. The tourniquet should never be tied so tightly that it restricts blood flow in the artery (Figures 1 and 2). Tourniquets should remain in place no longer than 60 seconds.
   PURPOSE: The tourniquet is used to make the veins more prominent.

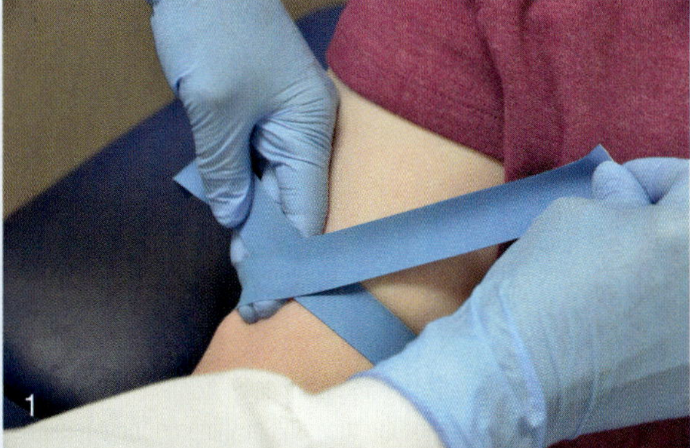

1

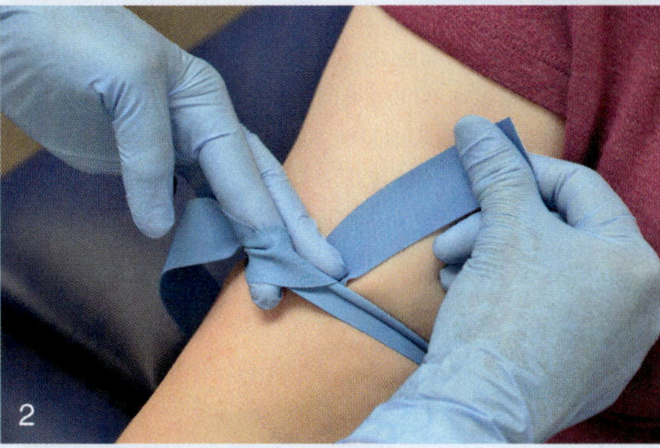

2

6. Select the venipuncture site by palpating the antecubital space. Use your index finger to trace the path of the vein and judge its depth. Look at both arms and use your critical thinking skills to find the vein that will give you the greatest chance of success for the venipuncture.
   PURPOSE: The index finger is most sensitive for palpating the vein. Do not use the thumb because it has a pulse of its own. Spend time to properly locate the best vein available; your patient will thank you.
7. Remove the tourniquet and cleanse the site with a 70% alcohol wipe (Figure 3).
   PURPOSE: The tourniquet should be tied for only 60 seconds.

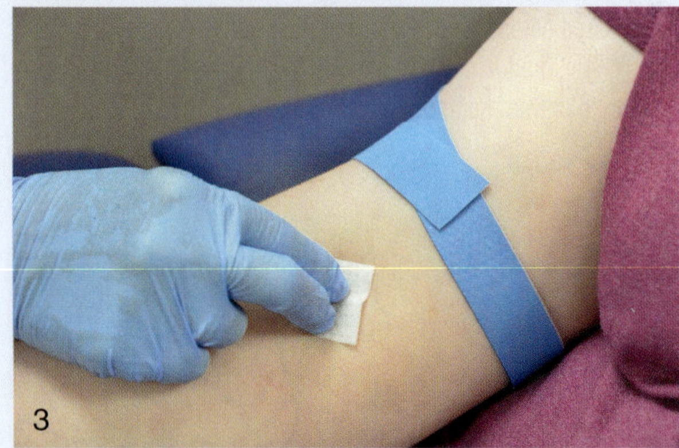

3

8. Assemble the equipment and supplies near your nondominant hand, next to the patient's arm, for easy access during the procedure. Use your critical thinking skills to choose the proper syringe barrel size and needle

PROCEDURE 48.2 Perform a Venipuncture: Collect a Venous Blood Sample Using the Syringe Method—*continued*

size. This depends on the amount of blood required for the ordered tests and your inspection of the patient's veins.
PURPOSE: Using the smallest syringe possible minimizes the chance of hemolysis. Engaging the plunger ensures that you will not have to use as much force to pull the blood into the barrel, thereby minimizing the chance of hemolysis.

9. Attach the needle firmly to the syringe. Pull and depress the plunger several times to loosen it in the barrel while keeping the cover on the needle (Figure 4). The plunger must be pushed in completely after you have loosened it in the barrel.

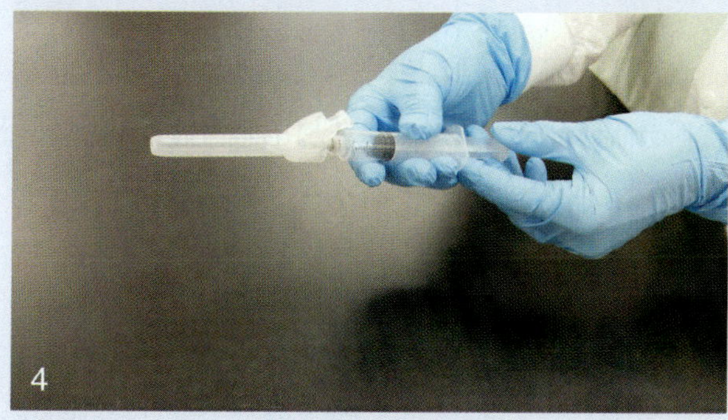

4

10. Reapply the tourniquet when the alcohol is dry.
PURPOSE: Puncturing an area still wet with alcohol stings and can cause hemolysis of the sample.
11. Hold the syringe in your dominant hand. Your thumb should be on top and your fingers underneath, the same as when using the vacuum tube method. Remove the needle sheath.
PURPOSE: Positioning the hand in this manner provides the best visibility of the needle entering the vein and accessibility to the syringe plunger.
12. Grasp the patient's arm with the nondominant hand and anchor the vein with the thumb of your nondominant hand.
PURPOSE: Failure to anchor the vein may cause it to move away from the needle when it is inserted, resulting in a missed vein.
13. With the bevel up and the needle aligned parallel to the vein, insert the needle at a 15- to 20-degree angle through the skin and into the vein with a quick but smooth motion (Figure 5). Observe for a flash of blood in the hub of the syringe.
PURPOSE: The sharpest point of the needle is inserted first. The angle ensures that the needle does not penetrate through the vein. The appearance (flash) of blood in the hub ensures that the needle is in the vein.

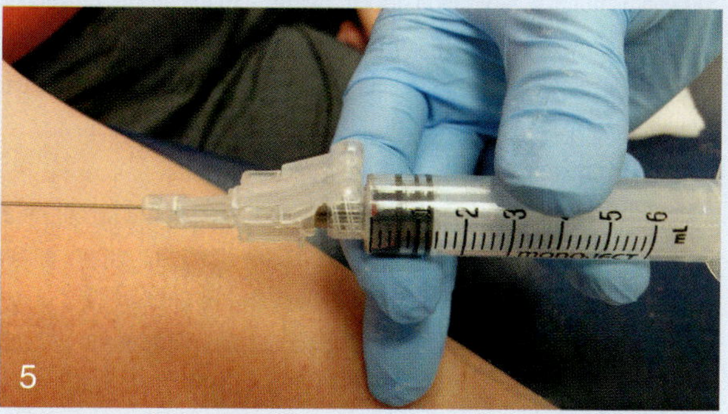

5

14. Slowly pull back the plunger of the syringe with the nondominant hand. Do not allow more than 1 mL of head space between the blood and the top of the plunger. Make sure you do not move the needle after entering the vein. Fill the barrel to the needed volume (Figure 6).
PURPOSE: Pulling back the plunger slowly allows for a consistent vacuum and less chance of vein collapse.

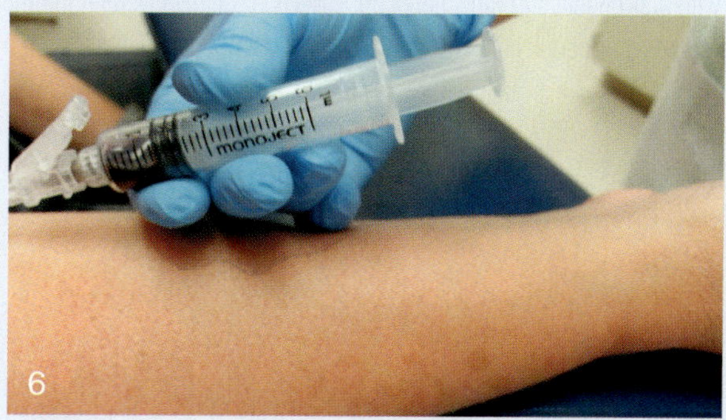

6

15. Release the tourniquet when the proper volume is reached. The tourniquet must be released before the needle is removed from the arm.
PURPOSE: Removal of the tourniquet releases pressure on the vein and helps prevent blood from getting into adjacent tissues, causing a hematoma.
16. Place sterile gauze over the puncture site at the time of needle withdrawal (Figure 7). Then immediately activate the needle safety device using the syringe hand and apply pressure to the site with the nondominant hand.
PURPOSE: The gauze over the puncture site and activation of the safety needle ensure infection control.

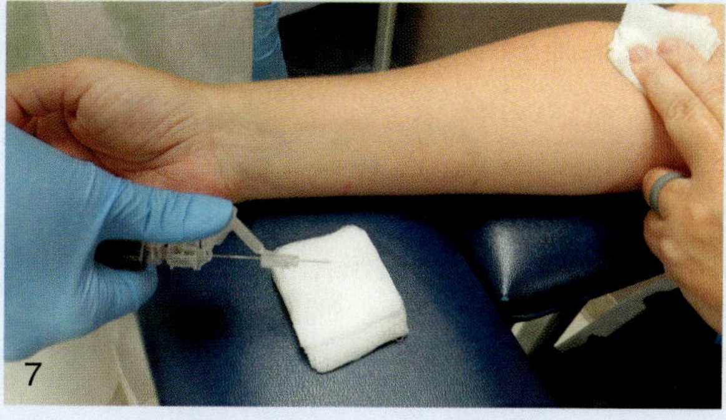

7

17. Instruct the patient to apply direct pressure on the puncture site with gauze. The patient may elevate the arm but should not bend the elbow.
PURPOSE: Applying direct pressure and elevating the arm above the heart is the best method to stop bleeding.
18. Remove the syringe safety needle and transfer the blood immediately to the required tube or tubes using a safety transfer device. Do not push on the syringe plunger during transfer.
19. Discard the entire unit in the sharps container when transfer is complete. Gently invert the tubes after the addition of blood.

Continued

PROCEDURE 48.2 Perform a Venipuncture: Collect a Venous Blood Sample Using the Syringe Method—*continued*

20. Label the tubes with the patient's name, date, time, and your initials, or affix the preprinted tube labels and print your initials and time on the label (Figure 8).
PURPOSE: The safety transfer device protects against accidental needlesticks and allows the correct amount of blood to be transferred into the tube by vacuum. Pushing the plunger hemolyzes the blood and may alter the amount of blood intended in each tube. Blood begins to clot shortly after collection, so it must be transferred into the vacuum tube and mixed with anticoagulant immediately after collection. Gently inverting the tubes ensures anticoagulation. Labeling ensures proper patient identification.

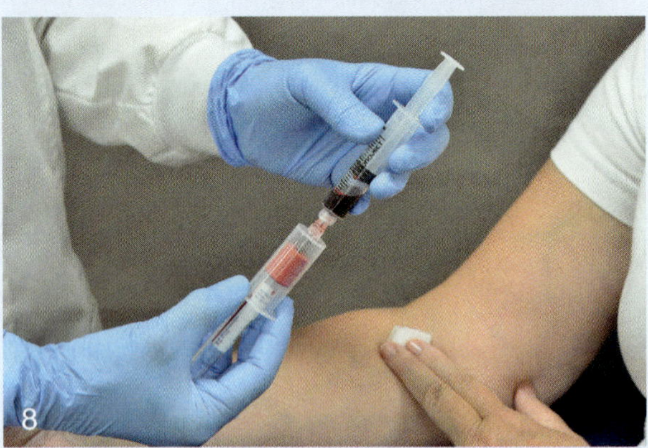

21. Check the venipuncture site. Make sure the bleeding has stopped. Apply a new folded gauze square to the puncture site. Secure the gauze to the site with a hypoallergenic self stick wrap, tape, or a bandage (Figure 9).

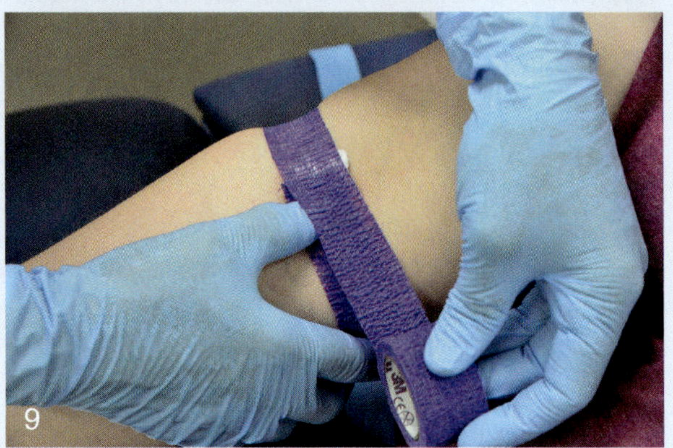

22. Disinfect the work area. Dispose of blood-contaminated materials in the biohazard waste container. Remove your eyewear and gloves.
23. Wash your hands or use hand sanitizer.
PURPOSE: It is important to ensure infection control.
24. Complete the laboratory requisition form and route the specimen to the proper place. Record the procedure in the patient's health record.
PURPOSE: A procedure is not considered complete until it is recorded in the patient's record.

PROCEDURE 48.3 Perform Venipuncture: Obtain a Venous Sample with a Safety Winged Butterfly Needle Assembly

TASKS: Obtain a venous sample accurately from a hand or arm vein using a butterfly needle and syringe. Document the results in the patient's health record.

EQUIPMENT and SUPPLIES

- Patient's health record
- Provider's order and/or lab requisition
- Safety winged (butterfly) needle set
- Syringe of appropriate volume for testing
- Vacuum tubes appropriate for tests ordered
- 70% isopropyl alcohol wipes
- Gauze
- Tourniquet
- Hypoallergenic self-stick wrap, tape, or bandage
- Permanent marking pen or printed labels
- Fluid-impermeable lab coat, protective eyewear, and gloves
- Biohazard waste container
- Biohazard sharps container

PROCEDURAL STEPS

1. Check the provider's order and/or requisition form to determine the tests ordered. Gather the appropriate tubes and supplies. Put on a fluid-impermeable lab coat.
PURPOSE: Collect the specimen properly based on the tube requirements on the requisition. Donning a lab coat is part of ongoing infection control.
2. Greet the patient. Identify yourself. Verify the patient's identity with their full name; ask the patient to spell the first and last names and give their date of birth. Explain the procedure to be performed in a manner that the patient understands. Answer any questions the patient may have on the procedure. Obtain permission for the venipuncture.
PURPOSE: It is important to identify the patient in two different ways to ensure that you have the correct patient. Explaining the procedure can make the patient feel more comfortable and reduces anxiety.
3. Wash your hands or use hand sanitizer. Put on gloves and protective eyewear.
PURPOSE: It is important to ensure infection control.
4. *If drawing from the antecubital region:* Ask if the patient has a preference as to which arm is used for the venipuncture. Have the patient sit with the arm well supported in a slightly downward position.
PURPOSE: The veins of the antecubital area are more easily located when the elbow is straight. Asking about a patient's preference gives the patient a chance to participate in the procedure.

PROCEDURE 48.3 Perform Venipuncture: Obtain a Venous Sample with a Safety Winged Butterfly Needle Assembly—*continued*

a. *If drawing from the back of the hand:* Have the patient place the venipuncture hand over the other, fisted hand with the fingers lower than the wrist.

PURPOSE: These positions help blood fill the veins in the hand; this makes it easier for you to identify the veins and choose the draw site.

5. *If drawing from the antecubital region*: Apply the tourniquet around the patient's arm 3-4 inches above the elbow on the patient's preferred arm. The tourniquet should never be tied so tightly that it restricts blood flow in the artery. Tourniquets should remain in place no longer than 60 seconds.

   PURPOSE: The tourniquet is used to make the veins more prominent.

   a. *If drawing from the back of the hand:* Apply the tourniquet above the wrist just proximal to the wrist bone (Figure 1). Do not apply the tourniquet so tightly that blood flow in the arteries is impeded.

   PURPOSE: The tourniquet is used to make the veins more prominent.

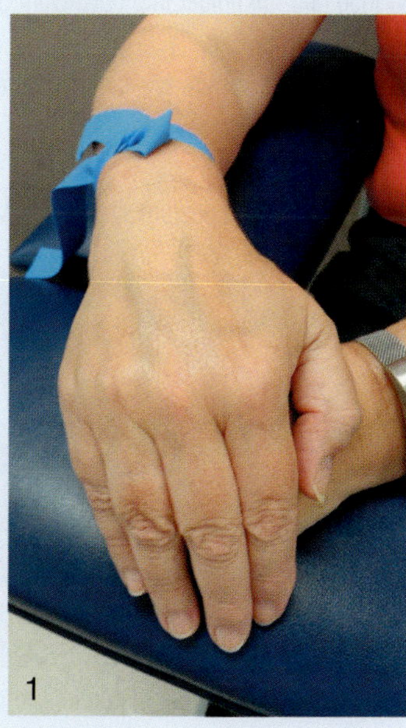

1

6. *If drawing from the antecubital region:* Select the venipuncture site by palpating the antecubital space. Use your index finger to trace the path of the vein and judge its depth. Look at both arms and use your critical thinking skills to find the vein that will give you the greatest chance of success for the venipuncture.

   PURPOSE: The index finger is most sensitive for palpating the vein. Do not use the thumb because it has a pulse of its own. Spend time to properly locate the best vein available; your patient will thank you.

   a. *If drawing from the back of the hand:* Select a vein on the back of the hand that is prominent, stable, and as straight as possible.

7. Remove the tourniquet and cleanse the site with a 70% alcohol wipe.

   PURPOSE: The tourniquet should be tied for only 60 seconds.

8. Assemble your equipment and supplies near your nondominant hand, next to the patient's arm for easy access during the procedure. Remove the butterfly device from the package and stretch the tubing slightly. Take care not to activate the needle-retracting safety device accidentally.

   PURPOSE: It is important to keep the butterfly tubing from recoiling.

9. Attach the butterfly device firmly to the syringe (Figure 2).

   a. If using a syringe, make sure to loosen the plunger a few times after the butterfly and syringe are attached.

   Note: The butterfly assembly can be attached to a needle holder *or* a syringe (see Figure 2). Make sure the connection is firmly in place.

   b. If using a needle assembly, lay the first tube in the vacuum tube holder and place the unit carefully where it will not roll away.

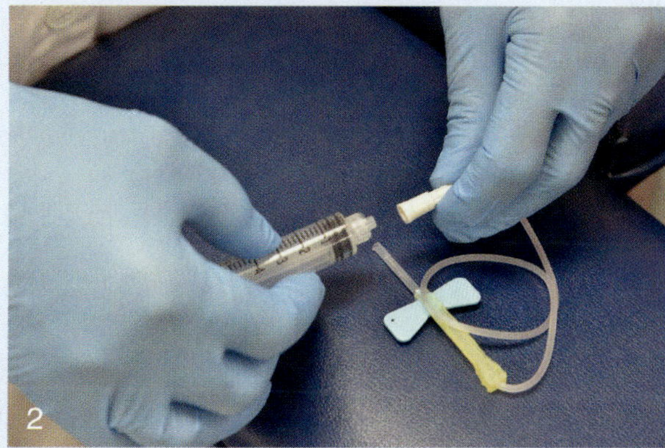

2

10. Reapply the tourniquet when the alcohol is dry.

    PURPOSE: Puncturing an area still wet with alcohol stings and can cause hemolysis of the sample.

11. Hold the butterfly wings pinched between your dominant hand thumb and index finger or hold the base of the needle (Figures 3 and 4). Remove the needle sheath.

    PURPOSE: Positioning the hand in this manner provides the best visibility of the needle entering the vein and accessibility to insert and withdraw tubes with the nondominant hand.

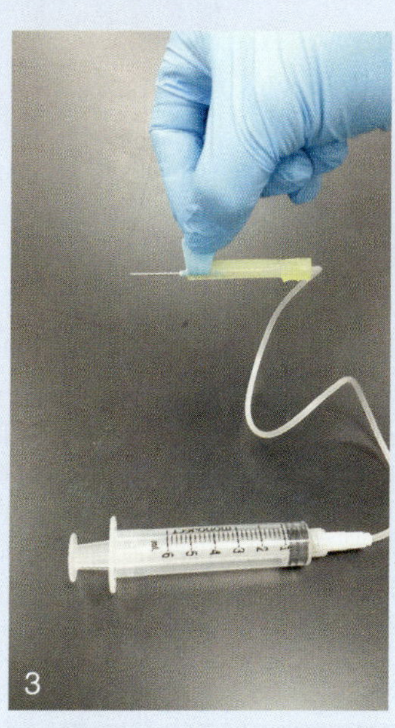

3

Continued

PROCEDURE 48.3 Perform Venipuncture: Obtain a Venous Sample with a Safety Winged Butterfly Needle Assembly—*continued*

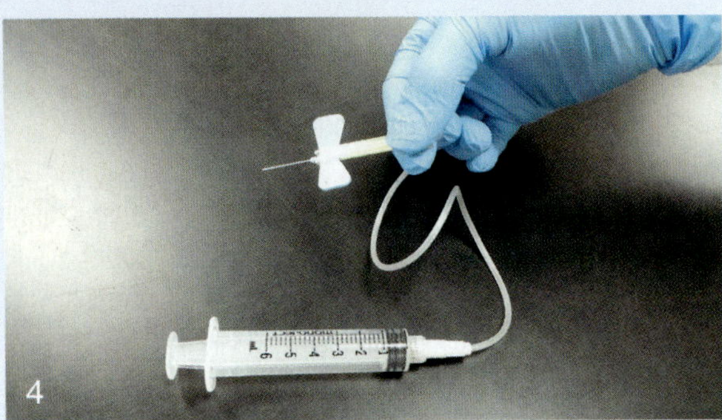
4

12. *If drawing from the antecubital region:* Grasp the patient's arm with the nondominant hand and anchor the vein by stretching the skin downward below the collection site with the thumb of the nondominant hand.
    PURPOSE: Failure to anchor the vein may cause it to move away from the needle when it is inserted, resulting in a missed vein.
    a. *If drawing from the back of the hand:* Using your thumb, pull the patient's skin taut over the knuckles.
    PURPOSE: Stretching the skin prevents the veins from rolling underneath.
13. With the bevel up and the needle aligned parallel to the vein, insert the needle at a 10- to15-degree angle through the skin and into the vein with a quick but smooth motion (Figure 5).
    Note: According to CLSI, after insertion of the needle, the wings should be held in place to keep the needle from moving until the butterfly needle is removed. Make sure the safety device is not activated.
    PURPOSE: The sharpest point of the needle is inserted first. The angle ensures that the needle does not penetrate through the vein.

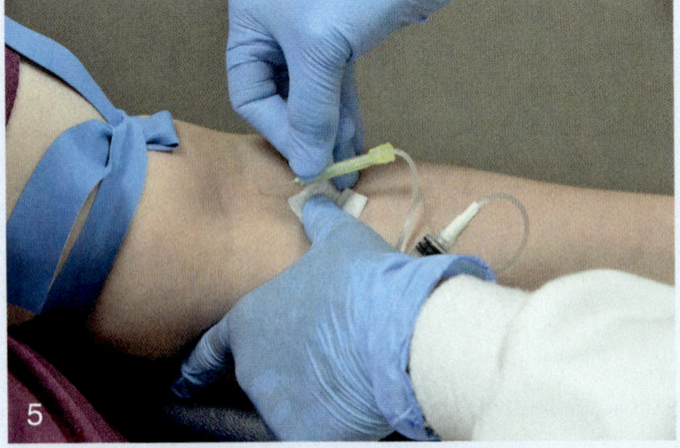
5

14. *If drawing with a needle holder assembly:* Push the blood collecting tube into the end of the holder with your nondominant hand.
    a. *If drawing with a syringe:* Make sure the vacuum you create is slow and steady and that no more than 1 mL of headspace exists between the blood and the plunger. Slowly pull back the plunger of the syringe with the nondominant hand. Fill the barrel of the syringe to the needed volume (Figure 6).PURPOSE: Drawing blood too forcefully into the syringe may collapse the vein or hemolyze the blood.

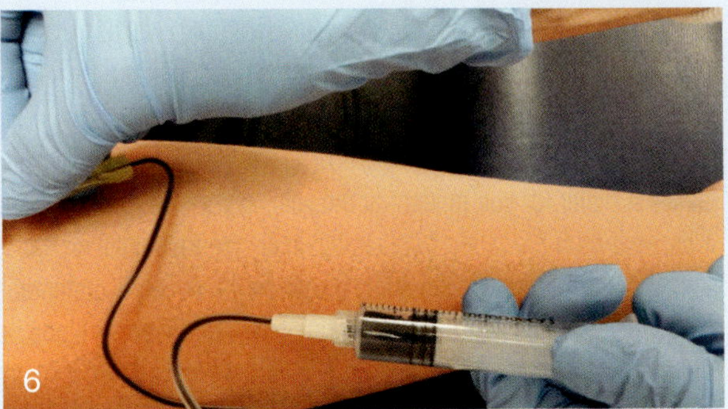
6

15. Release the tourniquet when the blood appears in the tubing or a flash of blood is seen in the hub of the syringe.
    PURPOSE: The tourniquet should remain in place no longer than 1 minute to prevent hemoconcentration.
16. Always keep the tube and the holder in a downward position so that the tube fills from the bottom up.
17. Place a gauze pad over the puncture site and gently remove the needle, engaging the safety device. Dispose of the entire unit in the sharps container (Figure 7).
    PURPOSE: The gauze over the puncture site and activation of the safety needle ensure infection control.

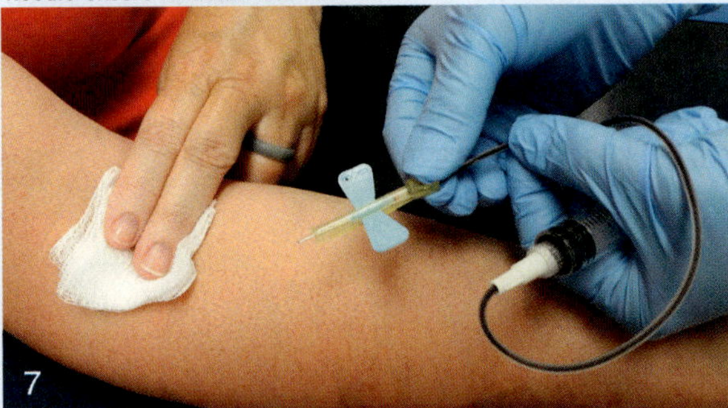
7

18. Apply pressure to the gauze or instruct the patient to do so. The patient may elevate the arm but should not bend the elbow.
19. *If drawing with a syringe:* Remove the syringe safety needle and transfer the blood immediately to the required tube or tubes using a safety transfer device. Do not push on the syringe plunger during transfer.
20. Discard the entire unit in the sharps container when transfer is complete. Gently invert the tubes after the addition of blood.
21. Label the tubes with the patient's full name, date, time, and your initials, or affix the preprinted tube labels and print your initials and time on the label.
22. Check the venipuncture site. Make sure the bleeding has stopped. Apply a new folded gauze square to the puncture site. Secure the gauze to the site with a hypoallergenic self stick wrap, tape, or a bandage.
23. Disinfect the work area. Dispose of blood-contaminated materials in the biohazard waste container. Remove your eyewear and gloves.
24. Wash your hands or use hand sanitizer.
25. Complete the laboratory requisition form and route the specimen to the proper place. Record the procedure in the patient's health record.

PROCEDURE 48.4 Perform a Capillary Puncture: Obtain a Blood Sample by Capillary Puncture

TASKS: Collect a blood specimen suitable for testing using the capillary puncture technique. Document the results in the patient's health record.

EQUIPMENT and SUPPLIES

- Patient's health record
- Provider's order and/or lab requisition
- Sterile, disposable safety lancet
- 70% isopropyl alcohol wipes
- Gauze
- Hypoallergenic self-stick wrap, tape, or bandage
- Fluid-impermeable lab coat, protective eyewear, and gloves
- Appropriate collection containers (e.g., capillary tubes, Microtainer tubes)
- Permanent marking pen or printed labels
- Biohazard sharps container
- Biohazard waste container

PROCEDURAL STEPS

1. Check the provider's order and/or requisition form to determine the tests ordered. Gather the appropriate tubes and supplies. Put on a fluid-impermeable lab coat.
   PURPOSE: Collect the specimen properly based on the tube requirements on the requisition. Donning a lab coat is part of ongoing infection control.
2. Greet the patient. Identify yourself. Verify the patient's identity with their full name; ask the patient to spell the first and last names and give their date of birth. Explain the procedure to be performed in a manner that the patient understands. Answer any questions the patient may have on the procedure. Obtain permission for the venipuncture.
   PURPOSE: It is important to identify the patient in two different ways to ensure that you have the correct patient. Explaining the procedure can make the patient feel more comfortable and reduces anxiety.
3. Wash your hands or use hand sanitizer. Put on gloves and protective eyewear.
   PURPOSE: It is important to ensure infection control.
4. Select a puncture site, depending on the patient's age and the sample to be obtained (e.g., palmar side of the middle or ring finger of the nondominant hand for an adult or child; medial or lateral curved surface of the plantar surface of the heel for an infant).
   PURPOSE: The nondominant hand may have fewer calluses. The palmar side of the finger is less sensitive, and the skin usually is not as thick. Use great caution when performing capillary punctures on infants (see Figure 48.21A–B).
5. Gently rub the finger or have your patient wiggle the fingers and open and close the hand.
   PURPOSE: Movement promotes circulation. If the finger is very cold, you may immerse it in warm water or moisten it with warm towels.
6. Once the finger is warm, clean the site with a 70% isopropyl alcohol pad and allow it to air dry (Figure 1).
   PURPOSE: Puncturing skin wet with alcohol will sting and can hemolyze the specimen.

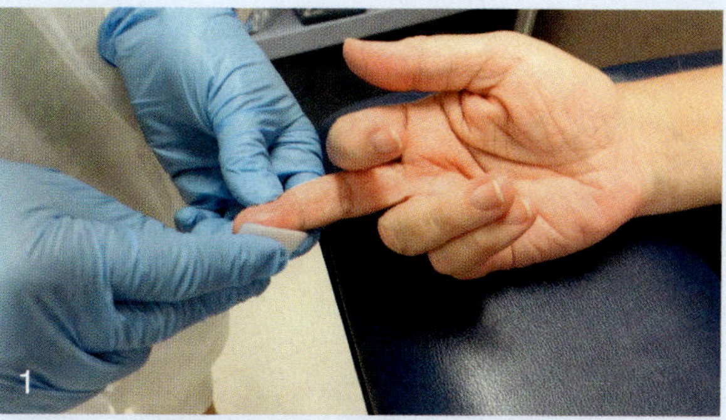
1

7. Hold onto the patient's finger above the puncture site with your nondominant hand. Select a site on the distal fingertip of the middle or ring finger. The puncture should be made across the fingerprint, not parallel to it.
   PURPOSE: Firmly holding the finger allows you to control the puncture and will not let the patient pull the hand away.
8. Hold the safety lancet firmly against the patient's finger and press down on the safety trigger that activates the needle or blade to penetrate the skin. The sharp will then automatically retract into the plastic housing of the lancet. (Figure 2).
   PURPOSE: Lancets are designed to puncture at specific depths that permit the free flow of blood.

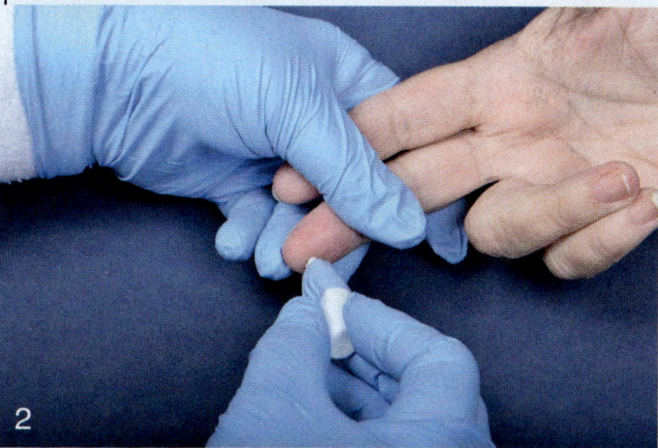
2

9. Dispose of the lancet in the sharps container. Wipe away the first drop of blood with gauze (Figure 3).
   PURPOSE: The first drop of blood contains tissue fluid, which may alter test results. If there is any residual alcohol on the finger, it will hemolyze the blood.

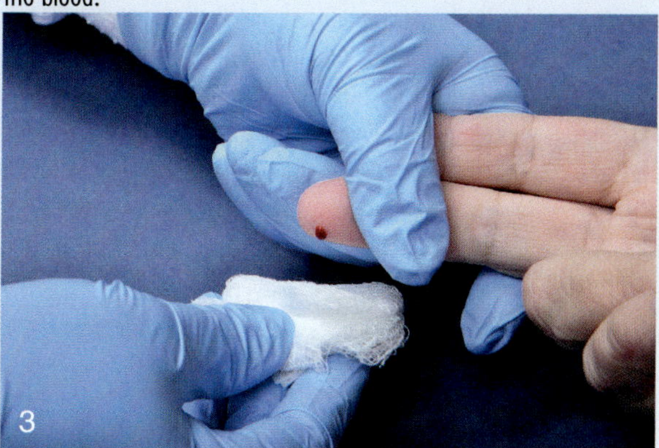
3

Continued

PROCEDURE 48.4 Perform a Capillary Puncture: Obtain a Blood Sample by Capillary Puncture—*continued*

10. Apply gentle, intermittent pressure to cause the blood to flow freely (Figure 4).
PURPOSE: Forceful squeezing liberates fluid that dilutes the blood and causes inaccurate results. *Do not* milk the finger.

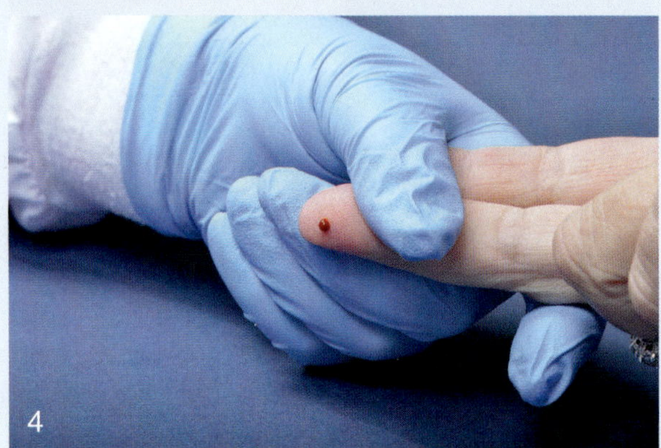

11. Collect the blood samples. Gently squeeze and release the finger two or three times to get a large drop of blood. Touch the capillary tube to the drop of blood. *Do not* scoop blood from the finger's surface. Fill the capillary tube to approximately three-fourths full or to the indicated line (Figure 5). Then tip the tube with the presealed end down. When the blood flows down and touches the sealant, hold it for 30 seconds to allow it to seal automatically.
PURPOSE: The specimen should be free of air bubbles and then sealed in preparation for centrifuging.

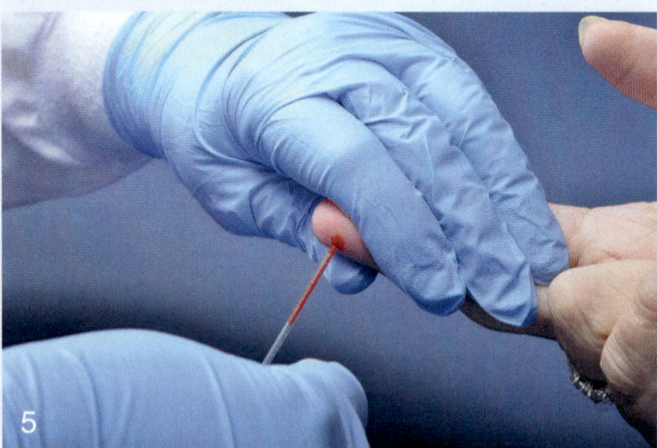

12. Wipe the patient's finger with gauze. Express another large drop of blood in the same way and fill a Microtainer (Figure 6). Do not touch the container to the finger. If more blood is needed, gently squeeze, and release the finger to get another drop. Cap the Microtainer tube when the collection is complete.
PURPOSE: Touching the container to the finger irritates the puncture site and may cause infection. Touching the container also smears the blood in the fingerprint and does not allow the blood to form a good hanging drop.

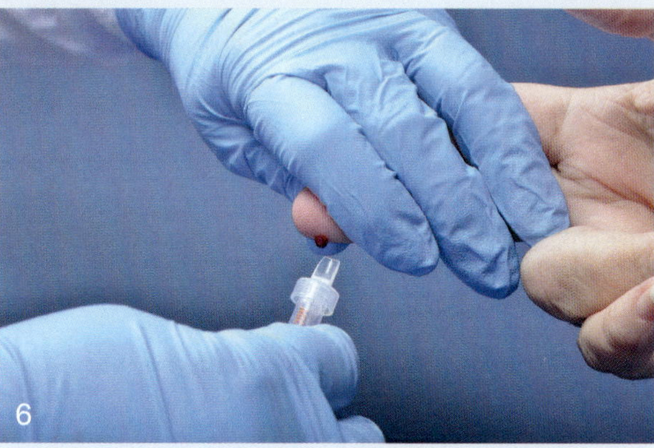

13. When the collection is complete, apply pressure to the site with gauze (Figure 7). The patient may be able to assist with this step.

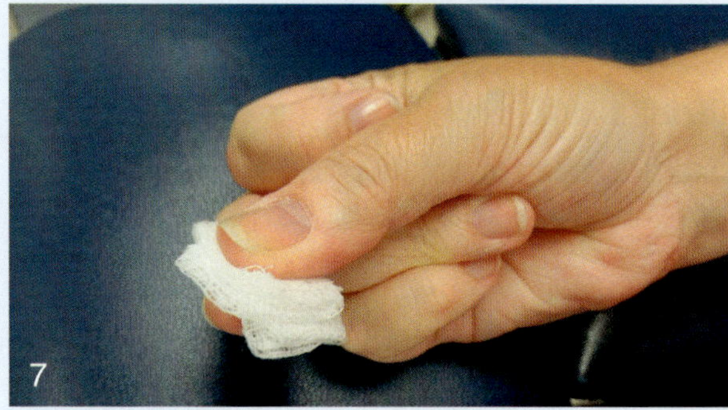

14. Select an appropriate means of labeling the containers. Sealed capillary tubes can be placed in a red-topped tube, which is then labeled. Microtainers can be placed in zipper-lock biohazard bags that are subsequently labeled. Follow your institution's procedures for labeling.
PURPOSE: Appropriate labeling will ensure proper patient identification.

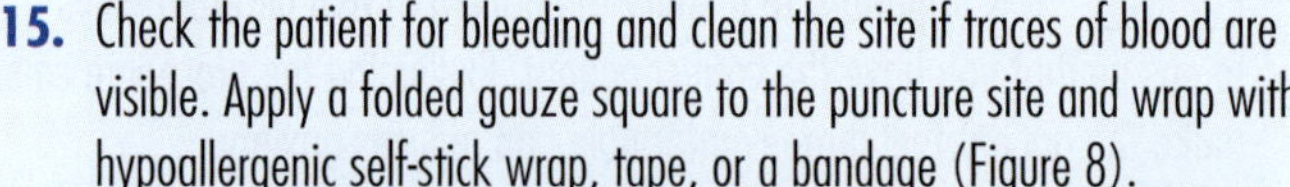

15. Check the patient for bleeding and clean the site if traces of blood are visible. Apply a folded gauze square to the puncture site and wrap with hypoallergenic self-stick wrap, tape, or a bandage (Figure 8).

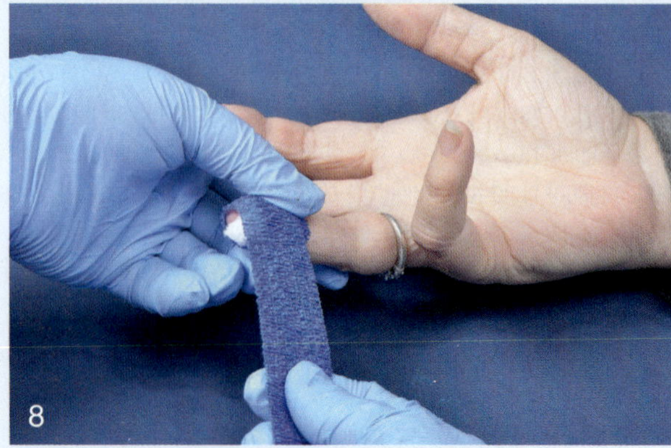

16. Disinfect the work area. Dispose of blood-contaminated materials in the biohazard waste container. Remove your protective eyewear.

17. Wash your hands or use hand sanitizer.
PURPOSE: It is important to ensure infection control.

18. Complete the laboratory requisition form and route the specimen to the proper location. Record the procedure in the patient's health record.
PURPOSE: A procedure is not considered done until it is recorded in the patient's record.

PROCEDURE 48.5 Demonstrate Empathy for a Patient's Concern Related to a Procedure

TASK: Demonstrate empathy for the patient's concern related to a venipuncture.

SCENARIO: You are a medical assistant working with Dr. Walden, who ordered bloodwork for Sam Brown. Your role includes performing venipuncture when bloodwork is ordered. You obtain the order, greet Sam, identify yourself, verify Sam's identity, and explain what you need to do. You notice that Sam appears to be uncomfortable and restless. Sam states she/he didn't really want the bloodwork done.

DIRECTIONS: Role-play this scenario with a peer. The peer will play Sam, and you are the medical assistant.

PROCEDURAL STEPS

1. Encourage patients to talk about their concerns. Demonstrate active listening skills.
   PURPOSE: Demonstrating active listening skills shows patients you are interested in their concerns.
2. Address the patient's concerns. Demonstrate respect and empathy while addressing the concerns.
3. Answer any questions the patient has.

ANALYSIS OF BLOOD

49

SCENARIO

Anita James, CMA (AAMA), has been working at the Walden-Martin Family Medical (WMFM) Clinic for 16 years. She loves her position as a medical assistant in a family medicine clinic. Every day is different. Each patient is unique. She has seen a number of children grow up over the years. Children who were toddlers when she started are now driving and thinking about college. The time has flown by.

Anita is working with Dr. Perez today, and they have a very busy schedule. A number of patients are in for follow-up visits, and a few new patients have appointments today, too.

While studying this chapter, think about the following questions:

- What is the purpose of the erythrocyte sedimentation rate (ESR) and coagulation testing?
- What tests are included in a complete blood count (CBC)? What are their reference ranges?
- When looking at hematology test results, can you differentiate between normal and abnormal test results?
- What is the medical assistant's role in blood transfusions?
- Why are the following test results important to a provider: blood glucose, hemoglobin A1c, cholesterol, liver enzymes, and thyroid hormones?
- What tests are part of a chemistry panel, and what are the reasons for performing each panel?

LEARNING OBJECTIVES

1. Analyze the role of blood and the components found in the blood.
2. Examine the hematology tests, including the erythrocyte sedimentation rate and coagulation testing, done in the physician office laboratory.
3. Examine the complete blood count, including the collection technique, components of the complete blood count, and the results.
4. Examine the hematology tests done in a reference laboratory.
5. Examine immunohematology.
6. Examine blood chemistry in the physician office laboratory.

VOCABULARY

albumin (al BYOO men) Most abundant plasma protein in human blood. It is important for regulating the water balance of blood.

anemia A deficiency of hemoglobin in the blood. Accompanied by a reduced number of red blood cells, pale skin, weakness, and shortness of breath, among other symptoms.

antibody Protein produced in the blood or tissues in response to a specific antigen that destroys or weakens the antigen. Part of the immune system.

antigen A substance that stimulates the production of an antibody when introduced into the body. Antigens include toxins, bacteria, viruses, and other foreign substances.

artifact A substance, structure, or event that does not naturally occur in a situation. Examples include interference, or electrical "garbage" on an ECG, or crystals, lint, or contamination of a staining technique.

atypical lymphs In many viral infections, stimulated or reactive lymphs are called atypical lymphs. They are commonly seen in infectious mononucleosis, or "mono."

autoimmune An immune response against a person's own tissues, cells, or cell parts.

buffy coat A white layer of WBCs and platelets that form between the plasma and the RBCs when anticoagulated blood is centrifuged.

centrifuge (SEN truh fyooj) A machine that rotates at high speed and separates substances of different densities by centrifugal force. For example, a tube of blood is separated into plasma/serum, white blood cells, platelets, and red blood cells.

cytoplasm (SYE toh plaz um) Jelly-like substance the surrounds the nucleus and fills the cells.

density Describes how compact or concentrated something is.

dilution Reducing the concentration of a mixture or solution by adding a known volume of liquid.

enzyme A special protein that speeds up a chemical reaction in the body.

hematologist (hee mah TOL uh jist) A person trained in the nature, function, and diseases of the blood and blood-forming organs. Can be a physician, trained laboratory personnel, or researcher.

VOCABULARY—*continued*

hemoglobin (HEE muh gloh bin) The oxygen-carrying pigment of red blood cells.

hormone A chemical substance produced in an endocrine gland and transported in the blood to a specific tissue, where it applies a specific effect.

immunoglobulins (im yuh noh GLOB yuh linz) A group of related proteins that function as antibodies. They are found in plasma and other body fluids.

intracellular pathogen A disease-causing organism that is within or inside a cell.

lateral flow immunoassay (im yuh noh AH say) A laboratory or clinical technique that uses the specific binding between an antigen and antibody to identify and quantify a substance in a sample. The sample in this technique moves in a sideways motion, usually on absorbent paper.

malignant A cell with uncontrolled growth that spreads rapidly, with the potential for serious harm.

metabolic Relating to or resulting from metabolism (the chemical process in which cells produce the substances and energy needed to sustain life).

microcuvette (MIE kroh koo vet) A small plastic or glass tube designed to hold samples for laboratory tests that detect light or color changes.

morphology The study of the form, shape, and structure of an organism or cell.

nucleus Control center of the cell; contains chromosomes that are made up of deoxyribonucleic acid (DNA), which carries genetic information.

pathologic Caused by or involving disease.

physiologic Consistent with the normal function of the body.

pipet (pie PET) A slender tube attached to or including a bulb, for transferring or measuring small amounts of a liquid, often used in a laboratory.

polycythemia (pohl ee sie THEE mee ah) A disorder characterized by an abnormal increase in the number of red blood cells in the blood.

reagent A substance used in a chemical reaction.

senescent cell (si NES ent) An old or aging cell that can no longer divide and reproduce.

INTRODUCTION

Blood tests are done routinely in the hematology, immunohematology (also referred to as the blood bank), chemistry, and immunology (also called *serology*) departments of the laboratory. The degree of blood testing performed by medical assistants depends on the level of service offered by the ambulatory care facility and the regulations established by the Clinical Laboratory Improvement Amendments (CLIA). As a medical assistant, you are qualified to perform CLIA-waived procedures described in the physician office laboratory (POL) sections of this chapter. More highly complex CLIA blood tests are performed at reference and hospital laboratories by medical laboratory personnel. This chapter explains more complex procedures to provide background information that is important for understanding the analysis of blood.

BLOOD

The average body holds 10 to 12 pints of blood. The heart circulates the blood through the circulatory system more than 1000 times every day. More than 70,000 miles of passageways, most of which are narrower than a human hair, carry blood throughout the body. The blood is contained in a closed system of vessels. The largest is the aorta, and the smallest are the capillaries. The capillaries are only one cell layer thick, and their thin, permeable walls allow certain substances to move back and forth between blood vessels and surrounding tissue. The circulating blood contains more than 25 trillion cells, and every second the body replaces 8 million old red blood cells (RBCs) with 8 million new RBCs.

Role of Blood in the Body

The circulating blood supplies the body's cells with nutrients and oxygen. The blood also distributes **enzymes**, **hormones**, and other chemicals needed for the regulation of body activities. In addition, the blood functions to maintain body temperature, keep body fluids in balance, and maintain pH. Maintaining a constant internal environment is called *homeostasis*.

Whole Blood

Whole blood is composed of visible formed elements suspended in *plasma* (a clear, yellow liquid). Plasma makes up approximately 55% of blood by volume. The remaining 45% consists of the following visible cellular elements: erythrocytes (RBCs), leukocytes (WBCs), and thrombocytes (platelets). The characteristics of blood and cellular components are reviewed in Chapter 40.

Plasma

Plasma is the highly complex liquid that transports the formed elements plus other substances, such as plasma proteins, throughout the body to every cell. Plasma proteins include **albumin**, the clotting proteins *prothrombin* and *fibrinogen*, and **immunoglobulins**. Plasma also transports nutrients (carbohydrates, fats, and amino acids), hormones, enzymes, mineral salts, gases, and waste products.

Plasma is composed of approximately 90% water, 9% protein, and 1% other chemical substances. The liquid portion of the blood in the body is plasma. In blood samples drawn for testing or other purposes, the body plasma must have an added anticoagulant to remain part of whole blood. The liquid that remains after blood has clotted is called *serum*.

HEMATOLOGY IN THE PHYSICIAN OFFICE LABORATORY

Hematology testing can occur in the POL or at a reference laboratory. For many POL hematology tests, an adequate blood sample can be obtained from a capillary puncture of the finger. If a larger sample is required, blood can be obtained via venipuncture.

Hematology tests done in the physician office laboratory can include the erythrocyte sedimentation rate, coagulation tests, and a complete blood count. These tests are described in the following sections.

Erythrocyte Sedimentation Rate

The *erythrocyte sedimentation rate* (ESR) is a laboratory test that measures the rate at which red blood cells gradually separate from plasma and settle to the bottom of a specially calibrated tube in 1 hour.

The ESR is not specific for any disease in particular but is used as a general indicator of inflammation. ESR and C-reactive protein (CRP) testing should correlate as indicators of inflammation. Normal values for males under age 64 are 0 to 15 mm/hr. Normal values for males over 64 and females are 0 to 20 mm/hr. A lower-than-normal ESR is not considered clinically significant. An increased ESR is significant to the provider because it indicates the presence of inflammation in the body. An increased ESR is seen in a number of conditions:

- Acute and chronic infections, such as tuberculosis and hepatitis
- **Autoimmune** conditions such as rheumatoid arthritis, lupus erythematosus, and rheumatic fever
- Multiple myeloma and other types of cancers

Several CLIA-waived methods of measuring the ESR are used, including the Sediplast procedure (Procedure 49.1). This closed system incorporates a pierceable stopper that ensures a leakproof seal when punctured by a **pipet**. An automatic self-zeroing cap and reservoir accurately bring the blood level to the zero mark and prevent overfilling. A prefilled vial of sodium citrate reagent is provided for **dilution** of blood before testing. A closed-tube Streck ESR method uses a Streck black-topped Vacutainer sample of blood that is directly placed in a Streck rack that provides results in 30 minutes (Figure 49.1).

Many factors can affect the ESR. The tube must be filled with blood and must not have air bubbles. The tube must be allowed to sit in a vertical position, undisturbed, for the full designated time—careful timing is important. Tilting a tube even slightly may increase the sedimentation rate. Jarring or vibrations from nearby machinery will falsely increase the ESR.

Coagulation Testing

Coagulation testing is used when a patient has a blooding disorder or when a patient is taking an anticoagulant, such as warfarin. Patient education is important to help patients regulate their coagulation test results when taking anticoagulants.

Prothrombin Time

Prothrombin time (PT or protime) is a blood test that measures the time it takes for the plasma of your blood to clot. PT test results are reported as the number of seconds blood takes to clot when mixed with the thromboplastin reagent. Prothrombin is a protein found in plasma that is converted to thrombin as part of the clotting process. Thrombin then causes fibrinogen to be converted to fibrin during the clotting process.

The normal range for a PT result is 11 to 13.5 seconds. A number lower than the normal range means the blood clots more quickly than normal, and a higher number means it takes longer for the blood to clot. Taking vitamin K supplements or estrogen-containing medications (e.g., oral contraceptives and hormone replacement medications) or eating foods high in vitamin K can cause the blood to clot too quickly. This means it decreases the clotting time or lowers the PT numeric value. Blood that clots too slowly can be caused from anticoagulant medication, liver disease, vitamin K deficiency, and clotting factor deficiencies.

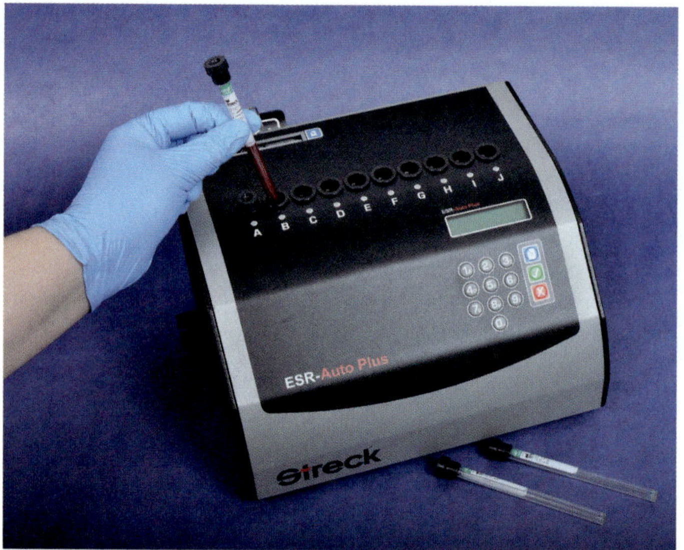

FIGURE 49.1 30-minute Streck ESR CLIA-waived test.

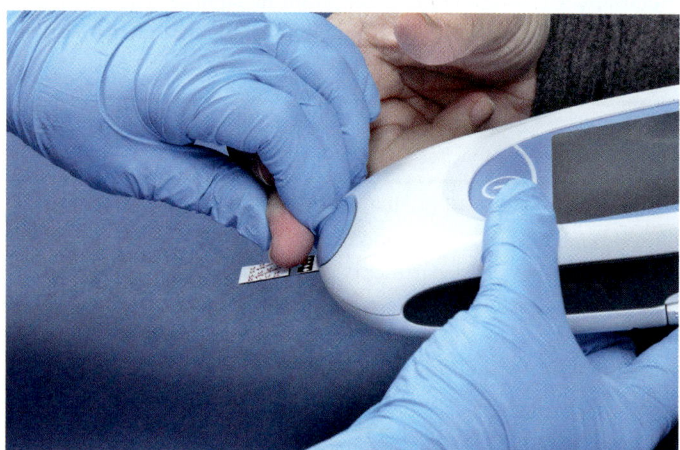

FIGURE 49.2 Applying a blood sample to the CoaguChek XS PT test monitor.

CLIA-waived tests for professional and home use are available for testing the PT. This test can be performed using a handheld, CLIA-waived instrument that uses whole blood from a fingerstick (Figure 49.2). The CLIA-waived CoaguChek XS PT measures the time it takes a blood sample to form a fibrin clot. A precise amount of capillary sample blood is dispensed into the channels of a testing strip. The blood is mixed with a thromboplastin reagent. The blood is pumped back and forth in the channel, and a series of light-emitting diodes (LEDs) detect the formation of a clot when blood movement in the channels stops (Procedure 49.2).

The PT is often used in combination with the partial thromboplastin time (PTT) to screen for hemophilia and other clotting disorders. The PT is also used to monitor patients taking anticoagulant drugs such as warfarin and similar anticoagulants. Warfarin is given to prevent clots in deep veins of the legs and to treat a pulmonary embolism.

International Normalized Ratio. The PT test results can vary by laboratory based on the thromboplastic reagent used. To standardize the reporting, the World Health Organization (WHO) created the international normalized ratio (INR). The INR is a conversion

Patient's name	______	DOB	______
Address	______	Health record #	______
Date warfarin started	______	Phone #	______
Dx for anticoagulation	______	ICD code	______
Outside lab phone #	______	INR goal	______

Date	Warfarin dose pre-test	PT	INR	Warfarin dose order	Next INR/PT	Signature

FIGURE 49.3 Warfarin flow sheet.

unit that considers the different sensitivities of reagents. It is widely accepted as the standard unit for reporting PT results rather than the actual clotting time.

The normal PT values are 11 to 13.5 seconds, or an INR of 0.8 to 1.1. Each increase in the INR of 0.1 means the blood is slightly thinner; thus it takes longer to clot. Patients who are taking warfarin to prevent the formation of blood clots or who have artificial heart valves should have an INR value of about 2.0 to 3.0. Their blood should take longer to clot than that of a normal healthy individual. An INR result higher than 3.0 puts a person at even higher risk of bleeding, and a result lower than 2.0 puts a person at risk for developing a blood clot.

It is important for the medical assistant to know how to accurately document INR follow-up and related warfarin dosages on a patient flow sheet. The provider will balance repeated INR levels with the warfarin dosage, so the INR is maintained at about 2.0 throughout the anticoagulant treatment (Figure 49.3).

Patient Education. Patient education is important when patients are being monitored with coagulation testing. Patients need to know the importance of the following:

- *Follow-up testing*: Patients who are taking the anticoagulant warfarin will need to follow up with the required lab work to monitor their PT/INR.
- *Vitamin K intake*: Vitamin K can increase blood clotting times. This means vitamin K works against the effects of warfarin. Helping patients identify foods high in vitamin K is crucial to maintaining a proper PT/INR value. Foods high in vitamin K include kale, mustard greens, Swiss chard, collards, spinach, brussels sprouts, broccoli, and beef liver. Most providers encourage patients to eat a consistent amount of vitamin K and not overindulge on foods high in vitamin K. A consistent level of vitamin K in the diet will help patients to maintain consistent PT/INR results.
- *Substances that can affect the PT/INR results*: Drinking large amounts of alcohol (three drinks per day) or taking aspirin, heparin, antihistamines, antibiotics, and vitamin C can change the results. If a patient is taking warfarin, many medications and over-the-counter products can interact with the medication. For example, garlic and Gingko biloba can increase the risk of bleeding, whereas St. John's wort and ginseng decrease the effects of warfarin. Patients should notify their providers of all prescribed and over-the-counter products they use.

PT/INR Home Monitoring. Some patients may need to monitor their PT/INR results at home. The PT/INR home monitors may be considered medically necessary durable medical equipment by the patient's insurance company if the person is on oral anticoagulation therapy for a variety of conditions. The medical assistant may be responsible for assisting the patient with the paperwork that must be completed to obtain the monitor and for coaching the patient on how to perform the test.

When coaching the patient on the process, it is useful to have the home machine available. The medical assistant should discuss how to get a successful blood sample by warming a cold finger, cleaning the site, and not squeezing the finger. The medical assistant should teach the patient the process (see Procedure 49.2). Then the patient should provide a return demonstration to ensure the patient knows the steps.

Typically, patients need to test every 1 to 4 weeks. They may need to report the results to the provider through their online patient portal or upload the monitor's history through the patient portal.

CRITICAL THINKING APPLICATION 49.1

Anita just roomed Janine Butler. She has an appointment today, and Dr. Perez would like to check her PT/INR results. Janine is on warfarin, but her INR is still a bit low. Anita checks her chart, and the INR completed in the lab is 1.7. Is this an acceptable result for someone who is on medication to prolong clotting time? Is it too high, too low, or normal?

HEMATOLOGY IN THE PHYSICIAN OFFICE LABORATORY: COMPLETE BLOOD COUNT

One of the most common hematology tests ordered is the CBC. The CBC is often used as a screening test to determine a patient's health status. It is used to screen for a variety of diseases and conditions, such as anemia, infection, and bleeding disorders. The CBC can be used to monitor the status of a condition. If a patient is undergoing chemotherapy, a CBC can also provide information on the impact of the treatment on the blood cells.

An automated hematology analyzer has been approved for CLIA-waived testing. This allowed CBCs to be done in the POL. If the results are abnormal or if the POL does not have the analyzer, the CBC is done in the reference (referral) laboratory. With abnormal results, a blood smear is examined using a microscope to identify additional information.

Collecting a Specimen for a Complete Blood Count

For a CBC, venous blood is collected in a lavender-topped tube containing ethylenediaminetetraacetic acid (EDTA), an anticoagulant that prevents whole blood from clotting. EDTA is the anticoagulant of choice for hematology testing because it also acts as a preservative for the blood cells. It is very important to prevent blood from being hemolyzed during collection for hematology testing.

Components of a Complete Blood Count

The CBC includes cell counts and provides information on the physical features of some of the cells. A standard CBC includes RBC, WBC, and platelet tests. The following sections discuss the components of the CBC.

CLIA-Waived Complete Blood Count

CLIA approved the Sysmex XW-100 for CLIA-waived CBC tests. This analyzer performs a three-part differential and includes the following:

- Total number of RBCs, WBCs, and platelets
- Hemoglobin and hematocrit
- Mean corpuscular volume (MCV)
- Total number and percentage of neutrophils, lymphocytes, and other WBCs

Red Blood Cell Tests

Part of the CBC incorporates RBC tests, including an RBC count, hematocrit, hemoglobin, and RBC indices (Table 49.1).

Red Blood Cell Count. The RBC count approximates the number of circulating RBCs in a person's blood. The function of an RBC is to transport oxygen to tissues and help carry some carbon dioxide away from the cells. RBCs have a life span of about 120 days.

The RBC count often is decreased in patients with anemia. Increased RBC counts are found in people with dehydration, polycythemia, severe burns, and those living at high altitudes. The normal RBC values range from approximately 4.4 million to 5.7 million/mm^3 in males and 3.9 million to 5.1 million/mm^3 in females.

Reticulocyte Count

Immature RBCs, also called *reticulocytes,* are RBCs that are still developing. They are made in the bone marrow and then sent to the bloodstream. Two days after forming, they develop into mature RBCs. A *reticulocyte count* (retic count) is done at a reference laboratory and can be part of the CBC. The reticulocyte count measures the number of reticulocytes in the blood. The normal value range for a reticulocyte count is 0.5% to 2.5%. An abnormally low or high count can indicate disorders of the bone marrow, liver, and kidneys. The retic count is also used to diagnose specific types of anemia.

Hematocrit. The *hematocrit* (Hct) is a measurement of the percentage of packed RBCs in a volume of blood. A spun microhematocrit test is based on the principle of separating the cellular elements from plasma using a **centrifuge** (Procedures 49.3 and 49.4).

Normal Hct values vary with sex and age (see Table 49.1). They range from a low of 36% in women to a high of 49% in men. Low microhematocrit values can indicate **anemia** or the presence of bleeding. High values may be caused by dehydration or **polycythemia**. Values can be influenced by **physiologic**, **pathologic**, and even geographic factors and by collection techniques. Normal Hct ranges are affected by a person's geographic location. For example, people living at high altitudes have a higher percentage of RBCs to compensate for the lower oxygen levels in the atmosphere.

Drops of blood are collected from a capillary puncture into two capillary tubes that are placed in a specially designed microhematocrit centrifuge (Figure 49.4). Capillary tubes can also be filled with EDTA-anticoagulated blood from a lavender-topped vacuum tube. As required by the Occupational Safety and Health Administration (OSHA), capillary tubes must be safe. They are made of either plastic or plastic-coated glass to avoid sharps injuries. The most common type of microhematocrit tube is self-sealing at one end. A less used type is open ended on both ends. If the tube is self-sealing, it must be tilted upright, causing the blood sample to flow down the tube and come into contact with the seal, and then held in place for 15 to 30 seconds. The open-ended tubes must be sealed with special clay before centrifugation.

After centrifugation, the packed RBCs are at the bottom of the tube against the sealant, the WBCs and platelets are in the center **buffy coat**, and plasma is on top (Figure 49.5). The microhematocrit is determined by comparing the volume of RBCs to the total volume of the whole blood sample. The percentage is read by placing the tubes on a special microhematocrit reader. Some microhematocrit centrifuges have a built-in reading scale that reads the calibrated capillary tubes. Microhematocrit tests should be performed in duplicate and the average of the two results reported.

The microhematocrit is a commonly performed test requested by providers either separately or as part of the CBC. Because it is a simple procedure that requires only a small amount of blood, it is an ideal screening test and often is part of a routine physical examination. Quality assurance includes care and maintenance of the microhematocrit instrument.

CRITICAL THINKING APPLICATION 49.2

One of Anita's patients today is Carl Bowden. Carl retired recently and has been enjoying his new, less hectic schedule. Carl is in good health, but he did mention at his physical today that he was feeling a little tired and lacked energy. Dr. Perez ordered a microhematocrit for Carl. The lab just sent the results to Carl's electronic health record.

Anita looks at the results and sees that his hematocrit is 38%. Is that value in the normal range for an adult male?

Hemoglobin. **Hemoglobin** (Hgb) determination is another way to measure the oxygen-carrying capacity of blood. The hemoglobin concentration can be part of the CBC or an individual test.

Normal hemoglobin values vary throughout a lifetime (see Table 49.1). The normal values for an adult male are 13.2 to 16.6 g/dL, and an adult female's range is 11.6 to 15 g/dL. Factors that affect the hemoglobin level include age, sex, diet, altitude, and existing disease states.

TABLE 49.1 Reference Ranges for Complete Blood Count (CBC) Values[a]

TEST	NEONATES (NEWBORN–1 MO)	CHILDREN (1 MO–23 MO)	CHILDREN (2–17 YR)	ADULTS (>17 YR)
Red blood cell (RBC) count	3.2–5.7 million/mm^3	2.9–5.1 million/mm^3	3.8–5.7 million/mm^3	Male: 4.4–5.7 million/mm^3 Female: 3.9–5.1 million/mm^3
Hematocrit (Hct)	31%–57%	27%–38%	31%–50%	Male: 39%–49% Female: 36%–45%
Hemoglobin (Hgb)	10–20 g/dL	8.9–12.7 g/dL	10.2–16.9 g/dL	Male: 13.2–16.6 g/dL Female: 11.6–15 g/dL
White blood cell (WBC) count	7,800–15,900/mm^3	6,000–15,000/mm^3	3,800–13,400/mm^3	3,400–9,600/mm^3
Platelet count	144,000–586,000/mm^3	206,000–597,000/mm^3	139,000–320,000/mm^3	150,000–450,000/mm^3
RBC Indices				
Mean corpuscular volume (MCV)	89–106 fL	70–96 fL	71–98 fL	80–100 fL
Mean corpuscular hemoglobin (MCH)	30–42 pg			26–34 pg
Mean corpuscular hemoglobin concentration (MCHC)	30–34 g/dL			32–36 g/dL
WBC Differential				
Neutrophils	25%–81%	15%–50%	20%–70%	55%–70%
Bands	—	—	—	0%–7%
Lymphocytes	21%–70%	41%–77%	25%–74%	20%–40%
Monocytes	0.2%–3.1%	0.2%–4%	0–0.8	2%–8%
Eosinophils	—	—	0%–3%	1%–4%
Basophils	—	—	1%–3%	0.5%–1%

[a]Lab reports, both electronic and paper, must supply their own reference ranges, along with each patient's results. This is because different methodologies may create different reference ranges and different units of measurement.
fL, Femtoliter; *MCH*, mean corpuscular hemoglobin; *MCHC*, mean corpuscular hemoglobin concentration; *MCV*, mean corpuscular volume; *pg*, picograms; *RBC*, red blood cell; *WBC*, white blood cell.

Hemoglobin and hematocrit tests are often performed together and are referred to as an *H&H.* A quick mental calculation should always be done before H&H results are reported: the hemoglobin value × 3 (± 3) should equal the hematocrit value. For example, if the hemoglobin is 15 g/dL, calculate the hematocrit as follows:

$$15 \times 3 = 45 \pm 3 = 42 - 48$$

The hematocrit should be between 42% and 48%.

CLIA-waived methods include use of the STAT-Site M Hgb, HemoPointH2, and HemoCue, all portable, battery-operated hemoglobin analyzers that fit in the palm of the hand (Figure 49.6 and Procedure 49.5). The HemoCue uses plastic **microcuvettes** that contain **reagents** that *lyse* (break apart) the RBCs in the sample, releasing the hemoglobin. The hemoglobin reacts with the reagents and forms a color. The color is detected and measured in the instrument, producing a digital readout. Capillary, venous, or arterial blood can be used in the disposable microcuvette. The cuvettes have a long shelf life.

Red Blood Cell Indices. A variety of calculations can be performed using the information obtained from the CBC. The red blood cell *indices* provide information about RBC disorders. The indices are used to classify anemias and to select additional tests that may help determine the cause of anemia. Red blood cell indices are also helpful to monitor the treatment of anemia. Because indices may change in response to treatment, they can be used as an indicator of how well the patient is responding to a treatment. The indices are mathematical calculations using the three red blood cell tests: Hct, Hgb, and the RBC count.

- *Mean corpuscular volume* (MCV): MCV = (Hct/RBC) × 10. The MCV is calculated to give the volume of the average RBC in a blood sample. The average size of the RBCs is the most important index for classifying anemias. (See Table 49.1.) Abnormal RBCs include these:
  - *Macrocytic:* Abnormally large RBCs and have a higher-than-normal MCV.

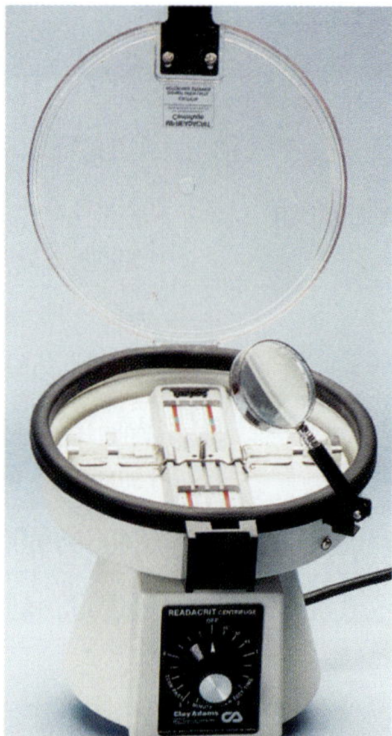

FIGURE 49.4 Microhematocrit centrifuge.

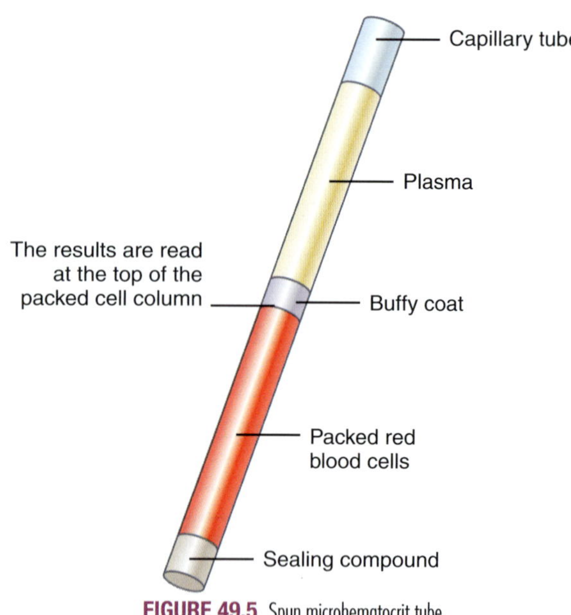

FIGURE 49.5 Spun microhematocrit tube.

- *Microcytic:* Small RBCs and have a lower-than-normal MCV. The normal reference range is 80 to 100 femtoliters (fL).
- *Mean corpuscular hemoglobin* (MCH): MCH = (Hgb/RBC) × 10. The MCH is calculated to give the average weight of hemoglobin in the RBC. The reference range is 26 to 34 picograms (pg).
- *Mean corpuscular hemoglobin concentration* (MCHC): MCHC = (Hgb × 100)/RBC. The MCHC indicates the average weight of hemoglobin compared with the cell size. A decreased MCHC shows *hypochromic* (pale, lacking color) RBCs in a stained blood smear. An increased MCHC is rare and should be flagged and brought to the attention of the provider.

White Blood Cell Tests

The white blood cell tests included in the CBC are the WBC count and a WBC differential. The following sections discuss these tests.

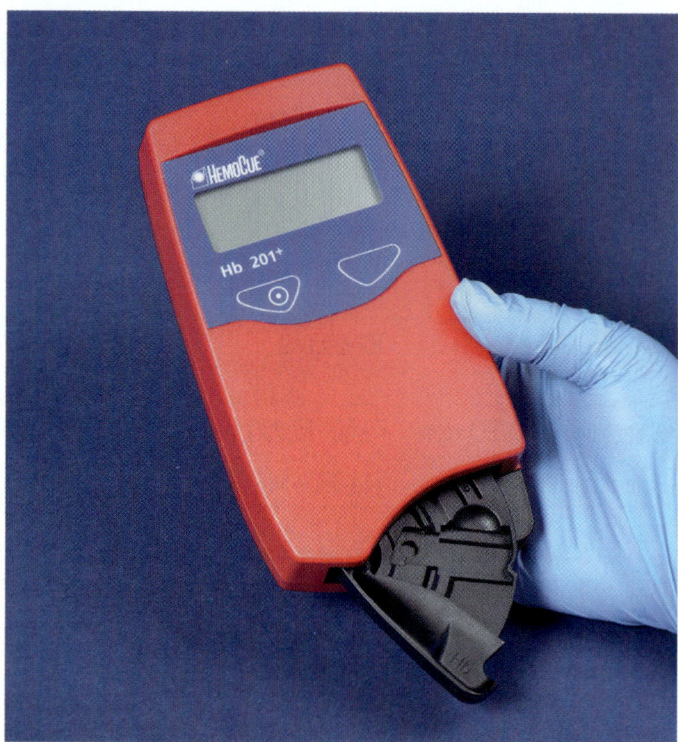

FIGURE 49.6 Handheld hemoglobin monitor.

White Blood Cell Count. The WBC count gives an estimate of the total number of leukocytes in circulating blood. The count is performed to help the provider determine whether an infection is present or to aid in the diagnosis of leukemia. It also may be used to follow the course of a disease and indicate if the patient is responding to treatment.

The normal WBC count varies with age. It is higher in newborns and decreases throughout a lifetime. The average adult range is 3400 to 9600 cells/mm^3. Many factors can affect the WBC count.

An increase in the number of normal WBCs is a condition called *leukocytosis*. Increased WBC counts may normally be seen with pregnancy, stress, anesthesia, exercise, and exposure to temperature extremes, and also after treatment with corticosteroids. Pathologic causes of leukocytosis include many bacterial infections, leukemia, appendicitis, and pneumonia.

A decrease in the WBC count is called *leukopenia*. This condition may be caused by a viral infection, by exposure to radiation and chemotherapy, or by certain chemicals and drugs.

White Blood Cell Differential. A CBC with differential (or diff) analyzes and counts the number of each type of WBC found in a sample of blood. In the POL, an automated instrument performs the differential. Automated cell counters have the ability to analyze the WBCs and gather information about cell size, internal structures, and **density**. (In the reference laboratory, the differential can be manually performed using a stained blood smear and a microscope.)

Table 49.2 describes the WBCs and a figure of the normal cell. There are five major types of WBCs:

- Granular WBCs
    - *Neutrophils (polymorphonuclear cells, PMNs, segs,* or *polys*): They are the most abundant WBC in the blood, with a normal adult range of 55% to 70% of the WBCs (see Table 49.1).

TABLE 49.2 Cells in a Differential

CELL NAME	DESCRIPTION	PHOTOGRAPH OF A NORMAL CELL
Red blood cell	Most numerous cell on diff. A small, red, biconcave disk with no nuclei.	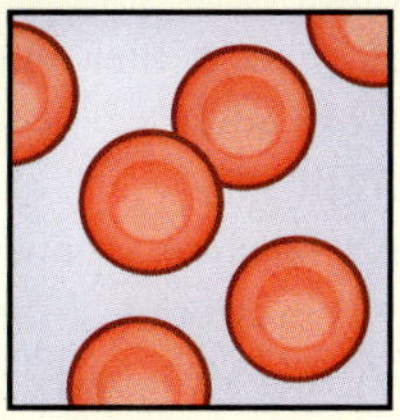
Platelet	Smallest cell on diff. May be round or oval. Has no nucleus. A fragment of cytoplasm from a large bone marrow cell called a *megakaryocyte*. Note the platelets, indicated by the arrows.	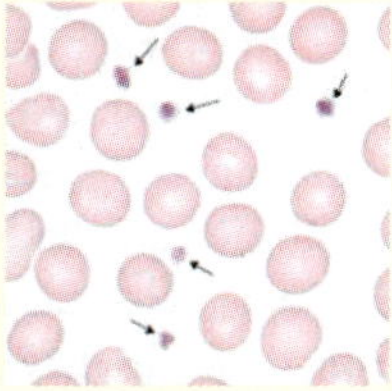
Neutrophil	Nucleus has many lobes. They travel to the site of an infection and release enzymes to fight off invading bacteria or viruses. Neutrophils engulf and destroy foreign substances, particularly bacteria. Increased numbers seen with bacterial infections.	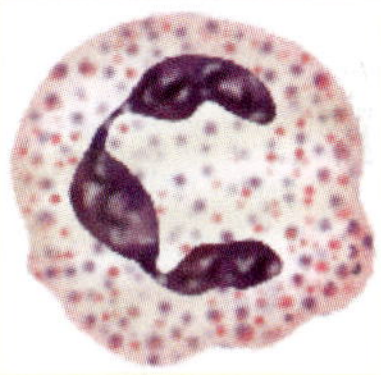
Bands	Horseshoe-shaped nucleus. An increase in bands is seen with severe bacterial infection, some types of leukemia, and inflammatory conditions.	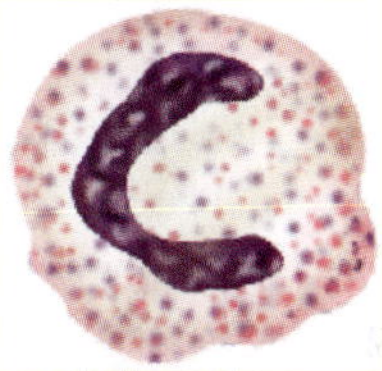
Eosinophil	Has large, red-orange granules. Increased numbers seen with allergies, asthma, cancer, and certain parasitic infections.	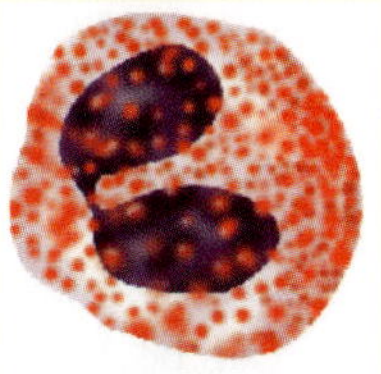
Basophil	Has large, dark blue/purple granules. Granules contain *histamine*, which is involved in the inflammatory response. Help in the destruction of allergens, by releasing enzymes to help control asthma attacks and allergic reactions. Have natural anticoagulant properties.	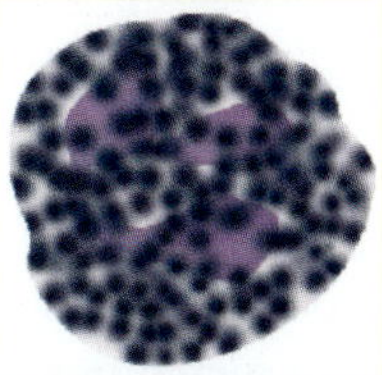
Monocyte	Largest WBC in the blood. Engulf, destroy, and remove destroy foreign substances, particularly **senescent** cells and **malignant** cells. They boost the body's immune system. Increased numbers seen with viral and some bacterial infections	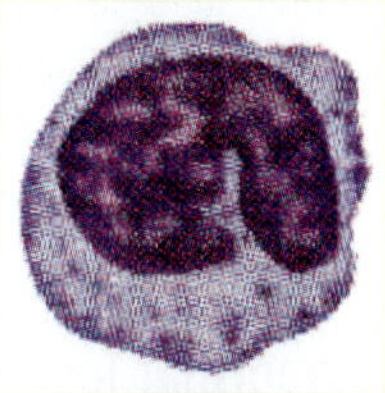
Lymphocyte	Smallest WBC, but most numerous in the blood. Large, dark blue/purple nucleus. Increased numbers seen with viral and some bacterial infections. Viral infections may show **atypical lymphs**.	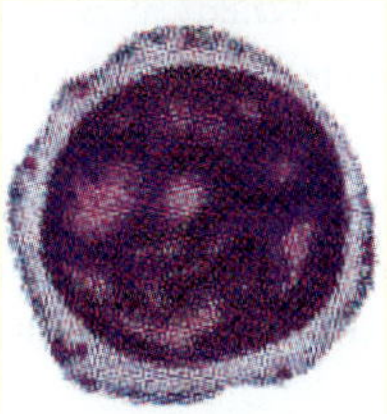

Bands are young neutrophils, and the normal range is 0% to 7% in an adult.
- *Eosinophils (eos):* They make up about 1% to 4% of the WBCs in an adult.
- *Basophils (basos):* They make up about 0.5% to 1% of the WBCs in an adult.

- Agranular WBCs
  - *Monocytes (monos):* Monocytes make up about 2% to 8% of the WBCs in an adult. Monocytes are found in the blood, but once they migrate into the tissues, they are called *macrophages.*
  - *Lymphocytes (lymphs):* Include two types: B cells and T cells. B cells destroy foreign substances (e.g., bacteria, toxins, or viruses) by producing **antibodies**. T cells target and destroy foreign substances, particularly **intracellular pathogens**. Thus, T cells destroy the body's own cells that have become infected with a disease-causing organism or cancer cells. B and T cells combined are the second most abundant WBC in the blood, making up about 20% to 40% of the WBCs.

Normal values for a WBC differential vary with age. A WBC differential test is used to diagnose a variety of conditions, including autoimmune diseases, inflammatory diseases, leukemia, infections, and anemia. It is a common screening test used as part of a general physical examination.

Platelet Count

Platelets are small and irregularly shaped and may vary considerably in size. They have a life span of about 10 days. Platelets are involved with blood clotting. Platelet tests done as part of a CBC include a platelet count, mean platelet volume, and platelet distribution width. These will be described in the following sections.

A platelet count measures how many platelets are in the blood sample. The normal platelet count for an adult is 150,000 to 450,000/mm^3. The number of platelets can indicate certain conditions, and it can also be used to monitor the effects of treatments, such as chemotherapy.

Thrombocytopenia is a lower-than-normal platelet count. Low platelet numbers can be related to not enough platelets being made in the bone marrow. It can also be related to the platelets being destroyed in the bloodstream, liver, or spleen. Drugs, medications, cancer treatments, and autoimmune disorders can cause thrombocytopenia.

Thrombocytosis is a higher-than-normal platelet count. Too many platelets can be the result of the following:
- Conditions: Including iron deficiency, infections, cancer, bone marrow disease
- Situations: After surgery, such as a splenectomy, and trauma
- Certain medications

Thrombocytosis can increase a person's risk for blood clots or other bleeding conditions.

Normal and Abnormal Test Results

It is important for medical assistants to understand the hematology laboratory reports (Figure 49.7). They should be able to distinguish between normal and abnormal results.

When laboratory test values are at a level that can be life threatening, they are considered *critical values*. Most ambulatory care facilities have policies and procedures regarding critical values. These values require the laboratory staff to take prompt action and notify the provider of the results. If critical values are called to the provider, the medical assistant may be involved in answering the call, documenting the values, and notifying the provider. When answering the call, usually at least two patient identifiers (e.g., name, date of birth [DOB], or health record number) must be obtained. The medical assistant must document the patient identifiers and the laboratory results and read the information back to the laboratory staff member to ensure the accuracy. The medical assistant must then notify the provider immediately of the results. Both the laboratory staff member and the medical assistant should document the actions they took regarding the critical results.

The medical assistant should never tell patients the laboratory results before the provider is notified of them. The provider will tell the medical assistant what to say to the patient.

CRITICAL THINKING APPLICATION **49.3**

Using the reference ranges in Table 49.1 and the lab report form in Figure 49.7, answer the following questions:
1. Grace Sifuentes, age 4, has a hematocrit of 38%. Is the result normal, high, or low?
2. Christian Washington, age 45, has a WBC count of 14,200/mm^3. Is the result normal, high, or low?
3. Brigitte Mulrooney, age 29, has a hematocrit of 32% and a hemoglobin of 10 g/dL. Is the result normal, high, or low?
4. Eleanor Jackson, age 81, has 23% bands in her white blood cell differential. Is the result normal, high, or low?
5. Using the lab report form (see Figure 49.7), describe information on the form. Also, what is the advantage of labeling results with "Low" and "High"?

HEMATOLOGY IN THE REFERENCE LABORATORY

The reference laboratory performs coagulation testing, blood smear preparation and microscopic examination, and platelet indices. As mentioned in a prior section, the reference laboratory may complete the automated CBC or perform a manual CBC if abnormalities are indicated. The following sections discuss tests done in the reference laboratory.

Partial Thromboplastin Time

A PTT test measures the time it takes for a blood clot to form. The PPT test is used to check the function of specific coagulation factors. If any factors are missing, it can take longer for the blood to clot. A PPT test is also used to monitor patients taking heparin, an anticoagulant. The reference range of the PTT is 60 to 70 seconds. If a patient is receiving anticoagulant therapy, the reference range is 1.5 to 2.5 times the normal reference range.

With the activated partial thromboplastin time (aPTT) test, an activator is added, which speeds up the clotting time. The reference range of the aPTT is 30 to 40 seconds.

Preparing and the Examination of Blood Smears

When blood must be microscopically examined, a blood smear needs to be created, and stain may be added. A blood smear enables the

WALDEN-MARTIN **FAMILY MEDICAL CLINIC** **1234 ANYSTREET I ANYTOWN, ANYSTATE 12345** **PHONE 123-123-1234 I FAX 123-123-5678**		**Date & time received**	**Accession number**
		10/30/20XX 1315	
		Date reported	10/30/20XX
		Patient name	Ken Thomas
		DOB	10/25/19XX
		Sex	Male
Physician	Dr. Martin	**Account #**	11594111

Test	Result		Reference range (adult)
Red blood cell count	3.8	LOW	4.4–5.7 million/mm^3 (M) 3.9–5.1 million/mm^3 (F)
Hematocrit	32	LOW	38%–51% (M) 36%–47% (F)
Hemoglobin	12.8	LOW	13.2–16.6 g/dL (M) 11.6–15 g/dL (F)
Mean corpuscular volume	39		80–100 fL
Mean corpuscular hemoglobin	31		26–34 pg
Mean corpuscular hemoglobin concentration	33.2		32–36 g/dL
Platelet count	475,000	HIGH	150,000–450,000/mm^3
White blood cell count	3,800		3,400–9,600/mm^3
Neutrophils	57		55%–70%
Bands	6		0%–7%
Lymphocytes	29		20%–40%
Monocytes	7		2%–8%
Eosinophils	1		1%–4%
Basophils	0.5		0.5%–1%
Protime			11–13.5 seconds
INR			0.8 to 1.1

FIGURE 49.7 Sample lab report with normal and abnormal patient results.

examiner to view the preserved cellular structures of blood. The **morphology** of WBCs, RBCs, and platelets can be studied. Their size, shape, and maturity can also be evaluated.

Preparing Blood Smears

A blood smear is prepared by placing a drop of blood from a fingerstick or an EDTA tube (using a DIFF-SAFE blood dispenser) onto a clean glass slide (Figure 49.8). The slide must be free of dust and grease. The best specimen for a blood smear is capillary blood that has no anticoagulant added. EDTA-anticoagulated blood can be used, provided the smear is made within 2 hours of specimen collection. Because timing is important, the medical assistant may be asked to prepare a smear during collection of the CBC specimen.

The wedge smear is used most frequently and is obtained by following these steps:

1. A small drop of blood is placed ½ inch from the frosted end (placed to the right) of a glass slide.
2. The end of a second glass spreader slide is placed in front (to the left) of the drop of blood at an angle of 30 to 35 degrees.

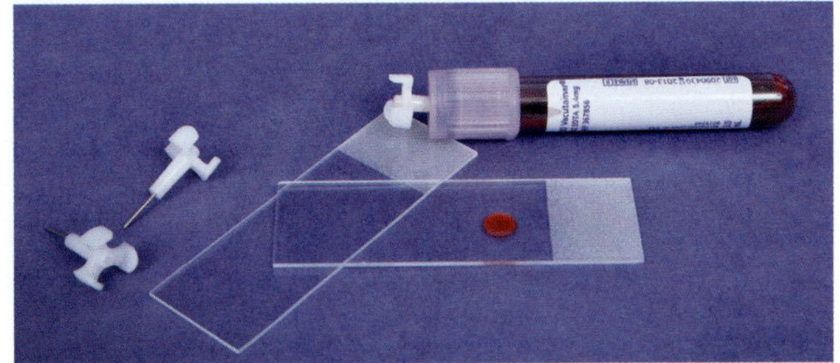

FIGURE 49.8 DIFF-SAFE device used to make a blood smear.

3. The spreader slide is brought back into the drop with a quick but smooth gliding motion until the blood spreads along the edge of the spreader slide.
4. The spreader slide is then pushed to the left with a quick, steady motion, spreading the blood across the slide (Figure 49.9).

A good wedge smear should cover one-half to three-quarters of the slide. It should show a gradual transition from a thick to a thin end with a feathered edge (Figure 49.10). It should have a smooth

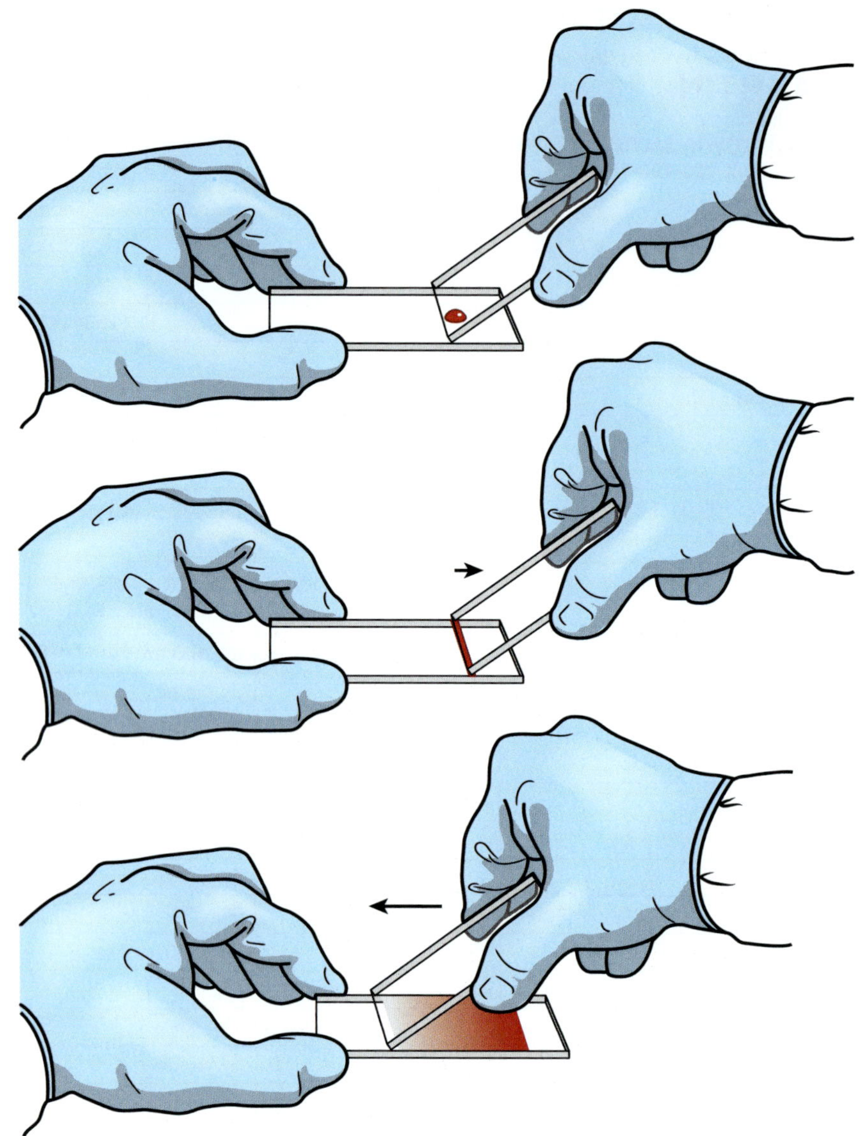

FIGURE 49.9 Making a differential wedge smear.

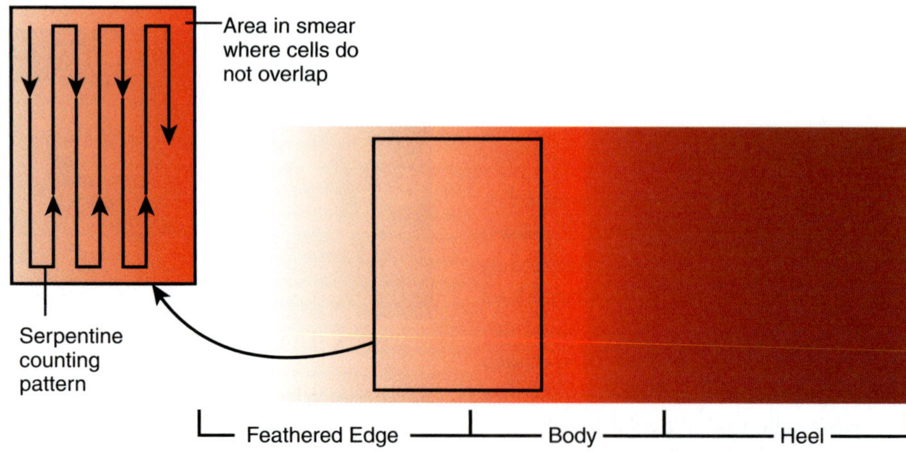

FIGURE 49.10 *Right,* Appearance of a properly prepared wedge smear. *Left,* Serpentine pattern used to count the cells.

appearance with no ridges, holes, lines, streaks, or clumps. On microscopic examination, the cells should be evenly distributed.

After the smear has been made, the patient's name is written on the frosted end of the slide with a pencil, and the smear is allowed to air-dry. The slide should be propped up to dry with the thick end down. Do not blow on the blood slide to dry it. The moisture in your breath can cause **artifacts** to form in the RBCs. Once dry, the slide is *fixed,* which preserves the cells and prevents changes in the cells. Many of the quick stains available on the market contain the fixative in the stain.

Staining Blood Smears. Stains commonly used to make blood smears are described as *polychromatic*. They contain dyes that stain cell components different colors. These stains are attracted to different parts of the cell, which makes the cells and their structures easier to see and tell apart. The most commonly used differential blood stain is Wright's stain.

Examination of a Blood Smear

As mentioned in Chapter 46, microscopic examination is outside of the medical assistant's scope of practice. It is important for the medical assistant to understand what occurs when blood smears are microscopically examined. Useful information can be gathered from a microscopic evaluation of blood cells in a stained smear.

Identification of Normal Blood Cells. The three features **hematologists** look for in blood cells are the cell size, the appearance of the **nucleus**, and the appearance of the **cytoplasm.** Table 49.2 presents a summary of the cells seen in a differential and a description of normal characteristics. To review additional information on blood cells, see Chapter 40.

Differential Examination. A specific area of a stained smear is examined under the microscope for a differential. The slide is examined near the feathered end of the smear, where cells are barely touching one another and are easiest to identify. Cells are examined with the oil immersion objective of the microscope. The differential involves counting and classifying 100 consecutive WBCs while moving in a winding pattern through the smear (see Figure 49.10). A count of the cells observed is kept on a differential cell counter or a computer.

Red Blood Cell Morphology. After the differential cell count has been determined, the RBCs are observed and evaluated. Normally, stained RBCs are the same size and shape and are well filled with hemoglobin. Any variations from the normal state are reported. (Figure 49.11 shows examples of abnormal cells.) The appearance of the RBCs should correlate with the RBC indices:

- *Size:* Normal-sized RBCs are said to be *normocytic.* If the cells are larger than normal, they are *macrocytic.* If the cells are smaller than normal, they are *microcytic.* The condition in which different sizes of RBCs are present is known as *anisocytosis.*
- *Shape:* Normal RBCs are round or slightly oval. Cells may be shaped like sickles, targets, crescents, or burs. *Poikilocytosis* is a significant variation in the shape of RBCs.
- *Content:* An RBC with a normal amount of hemoglobin is said to be *normochromic.* Pale-staining cells are *hypochromic* and have less hemoglobin than normal. Any inclusions within red blood cells should be reported.

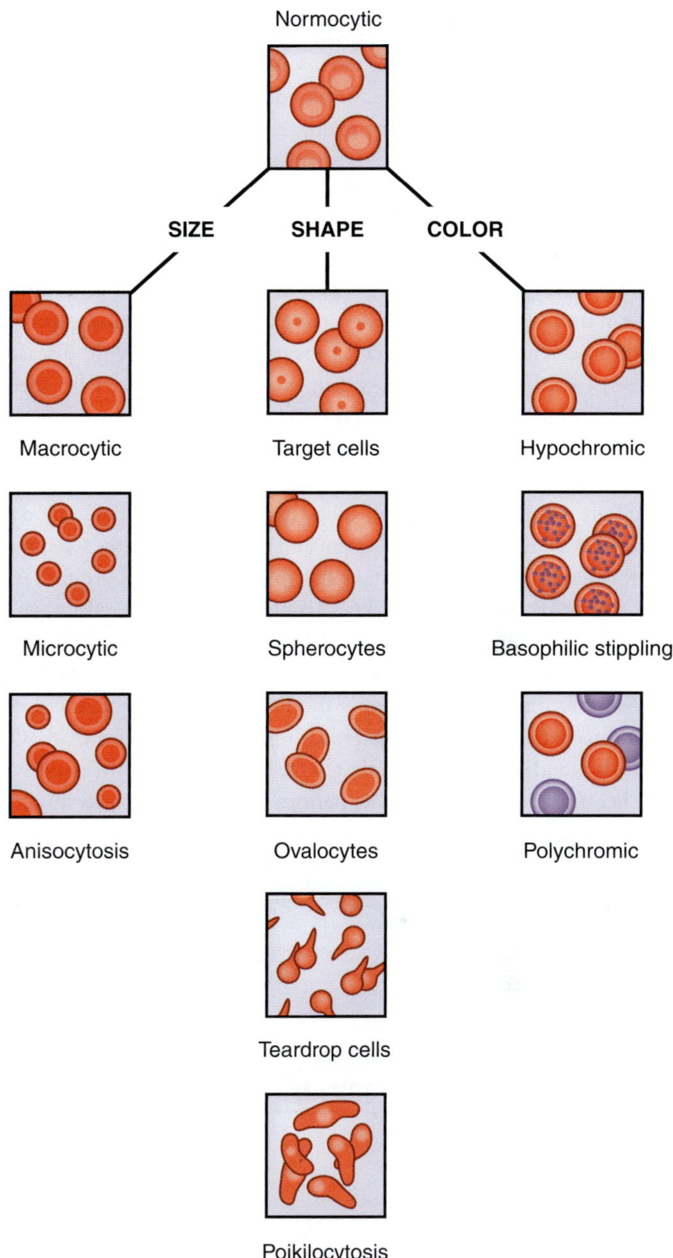

FIGURE 49.11 Abnormal red blood cells.

> **CRITICAL THINKING APPLICATION 49.4**
>
> Anita checks Reuven Ahmad's CBC and differential results as she prepares information for Dr. Perez. Reuven's RBC count is 5.1 million/mm^3. Is that a normal value for an adult male? In the notes from the differential, the laboratory technologist comments that Reuven's RBCs are normocytic and slightly hypochromic. Define *normocytic* and *hypochromic* in your own words. Be ready to share your definitions with the class.

Platelet Analysis. On a stained smear, the platelets are observed for any abnormalities. Excessive clumping of platelets may be an indication of a traumatic blood draw and a traumatic phlebotomy. It is also reported in a platelet analysis.

Platelet Indices

With automated hematology analyzers, platelet indices may be reported as part of the CBC. Platelet indices are helpful to providers when they are diagnosing thromboembolic diseases. There are several platelet indices:

- *Mean platelet volume (MPV):* Measures the average size of the platelets in the blood sample. The normal range for an adult is 7.2 to 11.8 fL.
- *Plateletcrit (Pct):* Measures the total mass of platelets as a percentage volume in the blood. The normal range is 0.22% to 0.24%.
- *Platelet distribution width (PDW):* Measures the variation in the platelet size. The normal range for an adult is 10% to 18%.

IMMUNOHEMATOLOGY

Formerly called the *blood bank,* the immunohematology department of the laboratory is responsible for blood typing and cross-matching blood units for transfusion. The major reason for performing immunohematology tests is to prevent problems caused by incompatible blood types during blood transfusions. Compatibility testing (also called *cross-matching*) is performed to prevent transfusion reactions in patients receiving blood from a donor. Identifying potential Rh incompatibility problems in expectant mothers is another procedure done in immunohematology. Rh incompatibility between an expectant mother and the unborn child may result in hemolytic disease of the newborn (HDN), also known as erythroblastosis fetalis. (See Chapter 43 for more details on HDN.)

Blood Typing

There are many blood antigen blood types. The two major blood **antigen** systems are the ABO system and the Rh system (see Chapter 40 for details). The ABO system has four major blood groups: A, B, O, and AB. Patients with type AB blood are considered universal recipients. Patients with type O blood are considered universal donors. Table 49.3 presents blood transfusion compatibility types.

Another major blood group is the Rh group. A person is either Rh positive (Rh+) or Rh negative (Rh–). Determinations of ABO and Rh blood groups are simple tests that can be performed easily. But because the consequences of performing the test incorrectly can be life threatening, blood typing is not a CLIA-waived test.

TABLE 49.3 Blood Compatibility

RBC ANTIGEN	PLASMA ANTIBODIES	COMPATIBLE WITH DONOR TYPES[A]
Type O (no antigens)	Anti-A and anti-B	O
Type A (type A antigen)	Anti-B	O and A
Type B (type B antigen)	Anti-A	O and B
Type AB (type AB antigen)	None	O, A, B, and AB

RBC, Red blood cell.

Blood Type Populations

This table gives you an idea of the blood type frequency in a few different populations in the United States.

TYPE	CAUCASIAN	AFRICAN-AMERICAN	ASIAN	LATINO-AMERICAN
O+	37%	47%	39%	53%
O–	8%	4%	1%	4%
A+	33%	24%	27%	29%
A–	7%	2%	0.5%	2%
B+	9%	18%	25%	9%
B–	2%	1%	0.4%	1%
AB+	3%	4%	7%	2%
AB–	1%	0.3%	0.1%	0.2%

Data from the American Red Cross. www.redcrossblood.org/learn-about-blood/blood-types.

CRITICAL THINKING APPLICATION 49.5

Griffin Jones is in for a physical today, but she would also like to have her blood type tested. She and her husband are thinking of starting a family soon and would like to know her ABO/Rh type. She thinks she is A–. If Griffin is A–, what antigen or antigens are on her RBCs?

Other Blood Types

In addition to the A and B antigens that characterize the ABO blood grouping, more than 600 antigens and more than 20 other blood antigen systems are known. Many are named after the person or family in which the blood antigen system was discovered. A medical assistant should be aware that other blood antigens exist. They may cause incompatibility issues in rare cases.

Legal and Ethical Issues Related to Blood Transfusion

The Blood Safety Act was passed in 1991 to ensure that all donor blood is tested for human immunodeficiency virus (HIV) and other blood-borne pathogens. The impact of this law can be seen in the ambulatory care environment. The law requires providers to explain to each elective surgery patient the chances that they may need a blood transfusion. The discussion must include positive and negative aspects of *autologous transfusion* (i.e., transfusion with a person's own blood). The pros and cons of transfusions from family, friends, or other donors should also be discussed. The conversation must be documented in the patient's health record. Before the surgery, the patient must sign a form giving consent to any needed blood transfusions. The medical assistant should be aware that certain populations (e.g., Jehovah's Witnesses) do not believe in blood transfusions.

If the patient decides to use autologous transfusions, this may require the patient to donate blood several weeks before the procedure. Usually, autologous transfusions are performed for stable patients undergoing major orthopedic, vascular, cardiac, or thoracic surgery. The medical assistant might need to help make arrangements for the blood donation. Another type of autologous transfusion can occur if the surgeon inserts an autologous drain in the surgical wound. The drain collects the blood from the surgical wound to prevent postoperative hematomas. The collected blood is then washed and reinfused into the patient.

BLOOD CHEMISTRY IN THE PHYSICIAN OFFICE LABORATORY

CLIA-waived chemistry tests using whole blood from capillary punctures have become popular in ambulatory practices. With the increase in diabetes and cardiovascular disease in the United States, patients with either (or both) of these **metabolic** diseases benefit from early diagnosis. Treatment is based on continued monitoring of glucose and hemoglobin A1c for diabetes and of cholesterol, lipid panels, and liver enzymes for cardiovascular diseases related to fatty deposits in the arteries.

Blood Glucose Testing

Glucose is used as a fuel by all body cells. Under normal circumstances, it is the only substance used to nourish brain cells.

Maintenance of blood glucose levels within a normal range is vital to homeostasis of the human body. Understanding the importance of glucose can help the medical assistant understand why glucose is the most frequently tested chemical analyte in the blood.

Elevated blood glucose levels are most often associated with diabetes mellitus. They also may indicate pancreatitis, endocrine disorders, or chronic renal failure. Diabetes mellitus is a disorder of carbohydrate metabolism that results in elevated blood and urine glucose levels. In diabetes mellitus, either the pancreas is unable to produce sufficient insulin to meet the body's needs, or insulin resistance develops at the cellular level (see Chapter 39).

For the initial screening of a patient for diabetes type 2, a fasting blood sample is usually taken in the morning, after a fast of 10 to 12 hours. The patient's fasting blood glucose (FBG) level should be less than 100 mg/dL. If it is higher than 105 mg/dL, the provider may request a blood *glucose tolerance test* (GTT). For this test, the fasting patient receives a sugary liquid to drink that contains 100 g of glucose. (The amount may be adjusted according to the patient's weight.) A blood glucose level of less than 140 mg/dL after 2 hours is normal. A reading of more than 200 mg/dL after 2 hours may indicate diabetes. A reading between 140 and 199 mg/dL indicates impaired glucose tolerance, or prediabetes.

Home Glucose Monitoring

Many CLIA-waived glucometers are available for professional and at-home use. The process the medical assistant uses in the ambulatory care facility for testing blood glucose is very similar to what the patient does at home (Procedure 49.6).

Home glucose monitoring is part of the treatment plan for diabetes mellitus (DM) management. Patients with type 1 DM or type 2 DM may need to test their blood glucose several times a day. Glucose levels may also be monitored by women with *gestational diabetes*, a condition seen during pregnancy in which the effect of insulin is partially blocked by hormones produced by the placenta (Figure 49.12).

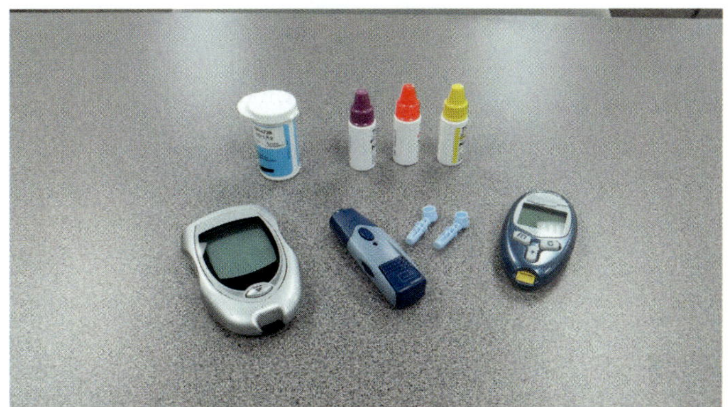

FIGURE 49.12 Glucometer and supplies.

The medical assistant may need to coach patients on how to test their blood glucose. If the patient's glucose monitor is available, it is helpful to demonstrate the procedure using the monitor the patient will use. The patient should also do a return demonstration so the medical assistant can ensure that the patient is performing the procedure accurately.

When coaching a patient on using the glucose monitor, the medical assistant should discuss the following topics:

- Equipment and supplies required, and how to dispose of sharps
- How to calibrate the monitor when using new container of test strips
- How to perform a capillary puncture, which includes finding and cleaning the site, lancets to use, disposal of lancets, and how to apply the blood to the test strip
- How to run the test, read the result, and how to document the results (if needed by the provider). Some monitors allow patients to upload their test results using the patient portal; thus the provider can see the results between visits.

Hemoglobin A1c Testing

Several methods can be used to measure the hemoglobin A1c level, including CLIA-waived handheld devices. Hemoglobin A1c is also described as *glycosylated hemoglobin* (sugar-coated hemoglobin). Glycosylated hemoglobin is the result of glucose irreversibly binding to the hemoglobin molecules in the RBCs. It is also referred to as the A1c.

RBCs have a life span of approximately 120 days. Measuring the amount of glucose that has been irreversibly bound to hemoglobin provides an assessment of the average blood glucose during the 60 to 90 days before the test. The A1c test is performed every 3 months in patients with diabetes to monitor the person's average blood glucose level during those months. An A1c value higher than normal indicates that the average blood glucose has been elevated during the past 2 to 3 months. A normal A1c level for a person without diabetes ranges from 4% to 5.6%. For patients with diabetes, the goal is to maintain the glycosylated hemoglobin level below 7%. In Table 49.4, glycosylated hemoglobin A1c levels are associated with blood glucose levels. With higher levels, the risk of developing complications from diabetes increases.

TABLE 49.4 Relationship between Glycosylated Hemoglobin Levels and Blood Glucose Levels

GLYCOSYLATED HEMOGLOBIN A1C (%)	BLOOD GLUCOSE (MG/DL)
14.0	355
13.0	326
12.0	298
11.0	269
10.0	240
9.0	212
8.0	183
7.0	154
6.0	125
5.0	97
4.0	68

Home A1c Monitoring

Home A1c monitoring does not replace home blood glucose monitoring. Home A1c monitoring is another tool for the management of DM. Patients can perform A1c testing at home using instruments approved by the US Food and Drug Administration (FDA), such as the A1CNow SelfCheck (Bayer) and the in2it (II) Self-Test A1c System (Bio-Rad). The medical assistant may need to coach the patient on home A1c monitoring. The same topics addressed in the Home Glucose Monitoring section would apply to home A1c monitoring.

Cholesterol Testing

Cholesterol is a fatlike substance (lipid) present in cell membranes. It is needed to form bile acids, steroid hormones, the coverings of our nerves, and some of our brain tissue. Cholesterol travels in the blood as distinct particles containing both lipids and proteins. These particles are called *lipoproteins.* The cholesterol level in the blood is determined partly by inheritance and partly by acquired factors, such as diet, calorie and nutrient balance, and level of physical activity.

Patients often are confused by cholesterol testing. *Cholesterol* is often a catchall term for both the cholesterol a person eats and the cholesterol that is produced in the body. A high blood level of low-density lipoprotein (LDL) cholesterol reflects an increased risk of heart disease. LDL cholesterol is often referred to as "bad" or "lousy" cholesterol. Lower levels of LDL cholesterol reflect a lower risk of heart disease. When too much LDL cholesterol circulates in the blood, it can slowly build up in the walls of arteries that feed the heart and brain. Together with other substances, it can form *plaque,* a thick and sticky deposit that can clog arteries. This condition is known as *atherosclerosis.* If a blood clot (thrombus) forms at the site of plaque, blood flow can be blocked in the coronary arteries of the heart muscle, causing a heart attack. If a clot blocks blood flow to part of the brain, a stroke may result. LDL results are often interpreted as follows:

LDL >100 mg/dL = Optimal
LDL 100–129 = Near or above optimal
LDL 130–159 = Borderline high
LDL 160–189 = High
LDL 190+ = Very high

About one-third to one-fourth of blood cholesterol is carried by high-density lipoprotein (HDL). HDL cholesterol is known as "good" or "healthy" cholesterol. High levels of HDL cholesterol seem to protect against heart attack. HDL can carry cholesterol away from the arteries and back to the liver. It is believed that cholesterol is removed from the lining of the arteries when high levels of HDL exist. Low levels of HDL cholesterol (i.e., lower than 40 mg/dL) may result in a greater risk of heart disease.

Adults older than 20 years of age should have a cholesterol test at least once every 5 years. Total cholesterol and the combination of LDL and HDL typically are screened and monitored. All three tests are considered screening tests, and elevated results require additional testing. In general, total cholesterol levels under 200 mg/dL are considered normal. Results over 240 mg/dL are considered elevated and may place a person in the high-risk category for coronary heart disease. An HDL cholesterol level of 40 mg/dL or higher is considered acceptable for men, and values of 50 or higher are acceptable for women. HDL levels below 40 mg/dL for men and below 50 mg/dL for women place a person at risk of coronary heart disease.

Although total cholesterol and HDL cholesterol levels are not significantly affected by food consumption, most providers prefer that patients fast from food and liquids, with the exception of water, for 12 hours before cholesterol levels are checked. If the total cholesterol is elevated, the provider is likely to order a *lipid profile,* which is a series of tests that measures the total cholesterol, HDL and LDL cholesterol levels, and triglyceride levels. *Triglycerides* are fat in the blood related to caloric intake. Therefore, the patient must be instructed to fast from all food and alcoholic beverages 12 hours before the triglyceride test or lipid profiles. Consistently high triglyceride levels may lead to heart disease, especially in people with low levels of "good" HDL cholesterol and high levels of "bad" LDL cholesterol and in people with diabetes type 2. Elevated levels of triglycerides are typically stored in belly fat and are associated with central obesity.

CLIA-waived cholesterol monitors can measure total cholesterol from a fingerstick specimen. The Cholestech LDX analyzer performs a lipid panel and provides a risk assessment using a capillary blood sample (Procedure 49.7). This system uses a cassette testing device capable of measuring glucose, total cholesterol (TC), HDL, LDL, very-low-density lipoprotein (VLDL), triglycerides, and the TC/HDL ratio. It uses a combination of testing methods to detect the color changes caused by each of the lipid panel analytes.

CRITICAL THINKING APPLICATION **49.6**

One of Anita's favorite patients is in today, Sophie McCoy. She is 86 years young, still lives in her own home, and works in her garden every chance she gets. Sophie had a cholesterol screen at a local senior citizens health fair recently, and her results were as follows:

Total cholesterol 202 mg/dL, LDL 104 mg/dL, HDL 42 mg/dL

Given Sophie's age and general good health, are the cholesterol results concerning? Are they normal, high, or low?

Thyroid Hormone Testing

The thyroid gland is located anterior to the trachea in the throat. It produces the hormones triiodothyronine (T_3) and thyroxine (T_4). These hormones are essential for life and regulate body metabolism, growth, and development. The thyroid gland is influenced by hormones produced by two other glands found in the brain, the pituitary gland and the hypothalamus. The pituitary gland produces thyroid-stimulating hormone (TSH), and the hypothalamus produces thyrotropin-releasing hormone (TRH). (Regulation of thyroid hormone production and thyroid disorders are discussed in Chapter 39.)

CLIA-waived rapid diagnostic tests are available to qualitatively measure TSH. These tests are available for point-of-care testing (POCT). Using whole blood from a fingerstick, CLIA-waived tests can screen patients for *hypothyroidism,* which is deficient activity of the thyroid gland. Hypothyroidism is indicated with elevated TSH levels. The tests use **lateral flow immunoassay** technology housed in a plastic cassette. One such commercially available test is the ThyroTest Whole Blood TSH Test.

Reference Laboratory Chemistry Panels and Single Analyte Testing and Monitoring

Automated blood chemistry analyzers are often used to perform blood chemistry testing in a reference laboratory. It is common for several analytes to be detected at once. A provider may order a chemistry panel, such as a renal or liver panel, to determine the levels of several related analytes (Figure 49.13). Analytes commonly detected in the chemistry department are listed in Table 49.5. In general, serum from a clotted specimen is needed to perform these tests. Typical panels are shown in Table 49.6. As noted previously, laboratory reports, both electronic and paper, must provide their own reference ranges, along with each patient's results. Different methodologies may generate different reference ranges and may use different units of measurement.

CLOSING COMMENTS

Patient Coaching

As with all other procedures, the laboratory test is only as valid as the specimen and the procedure performed on that specimen. You, as the provider's agent, are responsible for that validity when you instruct the patient and when you perform the test. Be clear in your instructions. Give written materials to reinforce your instructions. Ask if the patient has any questions, and take the time and effort to answer the questions in a way that is clear and understandable to the patient. If the patient has additional questions that you cannot answer, have the provider talk to the patient directly.

Legal and Ethical Issues

A medical assistant who is responsible for POL testing must clearly understand the basic concepts of laboratory medicine. Therefore, you must stay current with the rapid technologic advances in laboratory medicine and help establish a protocol for testing that best suits your provider-employer.

You are responsible for properly collecting specimens and testing them accurately. Patient confidentiality is paramount when testing is performed, as is strictly conforming to all established quality control procedures.

Patient-Centered Care

The CMA plays an important role in the laboratory and patient care. Often many different tests are needed to assess a patient's health. Many patients appreciate that they can have CLIA-waived tests done during a routine visit to their provider. With a simple fingerstick, a patient can have tests such as a hemoglobin and hematocrit, protime, A1c, blood glucose, cholesterol, and ALT/AST completed in the POL. Saving patients' time and the inconvenience of going to a different location are just a few benefits of having a CLIA-waived POL. Also, having test results available quickly and while patients are still in the clinic gives them the opportunity to ask questions and have them answered on the spot.

Professional Behaviors

An ever-increasing number of CLIA-waived hematology and chemistry blood tests are relatively simple to perform and require minimal training. This allows the provider to share the results with the patient quickly, which may lead to greater patient compliance with the prescribed treatment plan. Proper patient care demands attention to detail in all three areas of the testing process:

- *Preanalytic:* Proper care of the testing supplies and equipment, and proper patient identification and specimen collection
- *Analytic:* Running the tests according to the specific manufacturer's instructions; recording and analyzing the controls and the patient results
- *Postanalytic:* Proper disposal of biohazard supplies; routing of test results to the provider and patient

Medical assistants are involved in all three areas of testing. They are responsible for the organization and documentation of each performed test on the appropriate lab flow sheet and in the patient's health record.

Physician's Medical Center
77332 E. Capital Drive
Anytown, USA 11123

Ronald J. Haldor, M.D.
Kaye M. Jones, M.D.
Nicholas P. Stepp, M.D.

PATIENT – PLEASE NOTE

☐

If this box is checked, don't eat or drink anything, except water, for 14 hours before going to the lab.

PATIENT NAME ____________________ LAST FIRST M.I.

ADDRESS ____________________ DOB ____________

CITY ____________ STATE ______ ZIP ______ SEX: M F

TELEPHONE # ____________ SOCIAL SECURITY # ___ – ___ – ___

ORDERING PHYSICIAN ____________________ DATE ____________

BILLING: ☐ HMO ☐ MEDICARE ☐ MEDICAL ☐ OTHER # ____________

GUARANTOR (If other than patient) ____________________

☐ PHONE RESULTS TO ____________________

☐ SEND ADDITIONAL COPIES OF REPORT TO ____________________
(Please attach copy of eligibility card.)

Patient Diagnosis ____________________

☐ 906 ARTERIAL BLOOD GASES
ROOM AIR ____________
RESP. ASSIST ____________
☐ 105 BLOOD CELL PROFILE (Hgb + Hct)
☐ 862 BILIRUBIN (NEONATAL)
☐ 868 BILIRUBIN (TOTAL & DIRECT)
☐ 100 CBC (Complete Blood Count & Diff)
☐ 3000 ELECTROLYTES
☐ (NA, K, CO2, Cl)
☐ FANA
☐ GLUCOSE
☐ 915 GLUCOSE, PRE-NATAL DIABETIC SCR. (1 Hour Post-Glucola)
☐ GLUCOSE TOLERANCE TEST
\# OF HOURS ______ DOSE ______
☐ 3398 HEPATITIS PANEL (B-Surf Ag/Ab, B-Core Ab, A-Ab)
☐ 988 LIPID PROFILE (Chol, Trig, HDL, LDL, Cardiac Risk)
☐ 3380 LIVER PANEL (Alk Phos, Bili, TP, Alb, GGT, SGOT (AST) SGPT (ALT), & Consult)
☐ 3006 METABOLIC 7 (Na, K, CO2, Cl, Glu, Mg)

☐ 3035 PANEL 17 (Panel 13 + Na + K + Cl + CO2)
☐ 3020 METABOLIC 10 (Na, K, CO2, Cl, Glu, BUN, Creat)
☐ 3015 METABOLIC 11 (Met 10 & Phos)
☐ 3160 OBSTETRICAL PANEL 1 (CBC, UA, ABO/Rh, Antibody Screen, Rubella, RPR)
☐ 3172 OBSTETRICAL PANEL 3 (CBC, ABO/Rh, Antibody Screen, Rubella, RPR)
☐ 3445 OBSTETRICAL PANEL 7 (ABO/Rh, Antibody Screen, Rubella, RPR)
☐ 3447 OBSTETRICAL PANEL 7A (ABO/Rh, Antibody Screen, Rubella, RPR, Hepatitis B Surt Ag)
☐ 3025 PANEL 13 (Glu, BUN, Creat, Uric Acid, Ca, Tp, Alb, Bili, Chol, Alk, Phos, SGOT (AST), LDH, Phos)
☐ 3030 PANEL 15 (Panel 13 + Na + K)

☐ 3010 METABOLIC 8 (Na, K, CO2, Cl, Glu, BUN)
☐ 3040 PANEL 20 - SMAC (Panel 17 + SGPT (ALT) + GGT + Osmolality)
☐ 3043 S-1 Panel (Panel 20 + Triglyceride)
☐ 500 PROTHROMBIN TIME (PT)
☐ 505 Partial Thromboplastin Time (PPT)
☐ 7500 RPR
☐ 7515 RUBELLA
☐ 2030 THYROID SCREEN (T4, T3, Uptake, Adj T4)
☐ 704 URINALYSIS

BACTERIOLOGY

SPECIMEN SOURCE (REQUIRED)
COLLECTION DATE ____________
☐ ____ ROUTINE CULTURE
☐ 8919 AFB CULTURE
☐ 8921 FUNGAL CULTURE

ADDITIONAL LABORATORY TESTS: ____________________

2804 (4/2019)

LABORATORY OUTPATIENT REQUEST

OFFICE USE ONLY
Telephone Order per ____________
Order Received by ____________

FIGURE 49.13 Panel request form.

TABLE 49.5 Blood Chemistry Tests[a]

TEST	ABBREVIATION	NORMAL VALUES	DESCRIPTION	PURPOSE
Alanine aminotransferase (also called serum glutamic-pyruvic transaminase) *Some CLIA-waived available*	ALT (SGPT)	<45 units/L	Enzyme found predominantly in the liver but also in the kidney	To detect liver disease
Albumin *Some CLIA-waived available*		3.5–5 g/dL	Protein	To assess kidney function
Alkaline phosphatase *Some CLIA-waived available*	ALP	20–140 units/L	Enzyme found in several tissues	To detect liver and bone disease
Aspartate aminotransferase *Some CLIA-waived available*	AST (SGOT)	10–40 units/L	Enzyme found in several tissues	To detect tissue damage
Blood urea nitrogen *Some CLIA-waived available*	BUN	7–18 mg/dL *or* 2.5–6.4 mmol/L	Metabolic product of protein catabolism.	To detect renal disease
Calcium *Some CLIA-waived available*	Ca	8.4–10.2 mg/dL *or* 2.1–2.6 mmol/L	Electrolyte	To assess parathyroid function and calcium metabolism
Chloride *Some CLIA-waived available*	Cl	95–105 mmol/L	Electrolyte	To determine acid-base and water balance
Cholesterol *Some CLIA-waived available*	CH, Chol	*Total:* <200 mg/dL *LDL:* <130 mg/dL *HDL:* >40 mg/dL (males), >50 mg/dL (females)	Lipid	To screen for atherosclerosis related to heart disease
Creatine kinase *Some CLIA-waived available*	CK	39–308 units/L (males), 26–192 units/L (females)	Enzyme found in several tissues	CK-MB isoenzyme is used to assess source of muscle damage (CK-MB is used for myocardial infarct)
Creatinine *Some CLIA-waived available*	creat	0.74–1.35 mg/dL (males), 0.59–1.04 mg/dL (females)	Metabolic product of protein catabolism	To screen for renal function
Ferritin		40–400 ng/mL (males), 12–160 ng/mL (females)	Iron-carrying protein	To detect amount of iron stored in the body
Gamma glutamyl transferase *Some CLIA-waived available*	GGT	0–45 units/L	Enzyme found mainly in liver cells	To detect liver disease
Globulin	glob, Ig	Varies according to type	Protein	To detect abnormalities in protein synthesis and removal
Fasting blood glucose *Some CLIA-waived available*	FBS	70–99 mg/dL	Carbohydrate	To detect disorders of glucose metabolism (diabetes)
Glucose tolerance test	GTT	Varies with time	Carbohydrate	To detect disorders of glucose metabolism (diabetes)
Iron	Fe	50–160 mcg/dL	Mineral	To assist in diagnosis of anemia

Continued

TABLE 49.5 Blood Chemistry Tests[a]—*continued*

TEST	ABBREVIATION	NORMAL VALUES	DESCRIPTION	PURPOSE
Lactate dehydrogenase	LDH	140–280 units/L	Enzyme found in several tissues	To assist in confirmation of myocardial or pulmonary infarct
pH *Some CLIA-waived available*	pH	7.35–7.45	Measurement of the acid-base (acidity and alkalinity)	To assess acidity or alkalinity of blood
Phosphorus *Some CLIA-waived available*	P	3–4.5 mg/dL	Electrolyte	To assist in proper evaluation of calcium levels and to detect endocrine system disorders
Potassium *Some CLIA-waived available*	K	3.5–5.0 mmol/L	Electrolyte	To assist in diagnosis of acid-base and water balance
Sodium *Some CLIA-waived available*	Na	135–145 mmol/L	Electrolyte	To assist in diagnosis of acid-base and water balance
Total bilirubin *Some CLIA-waived available*	TB	0.1–1 mg/dL	Metabolic product of hemoglobin catabolism	To evaluate liver function and to aid in diagnosis of anemia
Total iron-binding capacity	TIBC	245–400 mcg/dL		A measure of the potential to transport iron
Total protein *Some CLIA-waived available*	TP	6–8 g/dL; 60–80 g/L		To assess the state of hydration; to screen for diseases that alter protein balance
Troponin I and T		<0.4	Cardiac-specific protein found only with heart muscle damage	To aid in diagnosis of myocardial infarction
Thyrotropin *Some CLIA-waived available*	TSH	0.3–4.2 milliunits/L	Hormone produced by the pituitary	To assess thyroid and pituitary gland function
Thyroxine	T_4	5–12 mcg/dL	Hormone produced by the thyroid gland	To assess thyroid function
Triglycerides *Some CLIA-waived available*	Trig	30–190 mg/dL	Lipid	To screen for atherosclerosis related to heart disease
Triiodothyronine, Total	T_3	80–200 ng/dL	Hormone produced by the thyroid gland	To assess thyroid function
Uric acid *Some CLIA-waived available*	UA	3.4–7 mg/dL (males), 2.4–6 mg/dL (females)	Metabolic product of protein catabolism	To evaluate renal failure, gout, and leukemia

[a]Lab reports, both electronic and paper, must supply their own reference ranges, along with each patient's results. This is because different methodologies may create different reference ranges and different units of measurement.
Ng/dL, nanogram/deciliter.

TABLE 49.6 Typical Chemistry Panels

PANEL	COMPONENT	PANEL	COMPONENT
Liver	Alkaline phosphatase (ALP) Gamma glutamyl transferase (GGT) Aspartate aminotransferase (AST) Alanine aminotransferase (ALT) Lactate dehydrogenase (LDH)	Cardiac	Creatine kinase (CK) Troponin I Troponin T
Anemia	Iron Total iron-binding capacity Ferritin Transferrin	Electrolyte	Sodium Potassium Chloride
Thyroid	Thyroid-stimulating hormone (TSH) Thyroxine (T_4) Triiodothyronine (T_3)	Renal	Creatinine Blood urea nitrogen (BUN) Uric acid Glucose

SUMMARY OF SCENARIO

It has been another busy day for Anita at WMFM Clinic. She had a chance to see a variety of patients with a variety of concerns. It was a normal day at work! Anita enjoys the variety. She also enjoys the work she does with the laboratory. Anita prepares specimens for transport to the reference lab. She checks on results once they are posted in patients' electronic medical records. She knows that Dr. Perez and all the providers at WMFM Clinic rely on lab results as part of patient diagnosis and treatment monitoring.

It has been another good day at work. Now Anita is going to go home and try to get a little gardening done!

SUMMARY OF LEARNING OBJECTIVES

1. **Analyze the role of blood and the components found in the blood.**
The circulating blood supplies the body's cells with nutrients and oxygen. The blood also maintains homeostasis. Whole blood is composed of visible formed elements suspended in plasma and cellular elements, including red blood cells (RBCs), white blood cells (WBCs), and platelets. Plasma transports the formed elements plus other substances, such as nutrients and plasma proteins, throughout the body to every cell.
2. **Examine the hematology tests, including the erythrocyte sedimentation rate and coagulation testing, done in the physician office laboratory.**
The erythrocyte sedimentation rate (ESR) test is a laboratory test that measures the rate at which red blood cells gradually separate from plasma and settle to the bottom of a specially calibrated tube in 1 hour. An ESR test is performed to assess inflammation and often is used to monitor rheumatoid arthritis. Refer to Procedure 49.1 for the steps in determining the ESR using a modified Westergren method.
Coagulation testing includes protime (PT) testing, which is a method of measuring how long it takes blood to clot. PT is used in combination with the partial thromboplastin time (PTT) to screen for hemophilia and other hereditary clotting disorders. It is important to educate patients who take warfarin about the need for follow-up laboratory monitoring of their protime/international normalized ratio (INR). Helping patients identify foods high in vitamin K is crucial to maintaining a balance between the warfarin dosage and the lab values. Refer to Procedure 49.2 for information on how you can reassure a patient of the accuracy of PT/INR test results.
3. **Examine the complete blood count, including the collection technique, components of the complete blood count, and the results.**
The most frequently ordered reference laboratory procedure for hematology is the complete blood count (CBC). This test requires a lavender-topped EDTA blood specimen. A CBC can be done in the physician office laboratory (POL) or the reference lab. The normal values for the CBC are found on Table 49.1. A CBC includes the following tests:
    - *Red blood cell tests*: Includes an RBC count, hematocrit, hemoglobin, and RBC indices. A reticulocyte count can be done at a reference laboratory as part of a CBC.
    - *White blood cell tests:* Includes a WBC count and a WBC differential.
    - *Platelet tests:* Includes a platelet count. Platelet indices, including mean platelet volume, plateletcrit, and platelet distribution width, can be done at a reference laboratory as part of a CBC.
4. **Examine the hematology tests done in a reference laboratory.**
Many hematology tests are done in the reference laboratory. When abnormal hematology results are obtained in the POL, further testing may be done in the reference laboratory. The partial thromboplastin

Continued

SUMMARY OF LEARNING OBJECTIVES—*Continued*

time test is a coagulation test done in the reference laboratory. The medical assistant may help with creating and staining a blood smear. Blood smears are used to microscopically examine the cells. They can be used for a manual WBC differential, RBC morphology, and platelet analysis.

With automated hematology analyzers, platelet indices may be reported as part of the CBC and used to diagnose thromboembolic disease. There are several platelet indices, including platelet volume (MPV), plateletcrit (Pct), and platelet distribution width (PDW).

5. **Examine immunohematology.**
Both the ABO blood type and the Rh type result from antigens on the surfaces of RBCs, and both groups are crucial when it comes to transfusion. There are four different ABO types (A, AB, B, and O). The body produces natural antibodies against the AB antigens that are not present in the blood cells. For example, if a person has type A antigens on the cells, there will be anti-B antibodies in the plasma. Type O blood has both anti-A antibodies and anti-B antibodies because they are both foreign to someone with type O blood. There are only two Rh types (positive and negative). Unlike the ABO group, an Rh-negative blood type does not have natural antibodies against Rh-positive cells. The Rh-negative individual must first be exposed to Rh-positive cells via transfusion or childbirth, which initiates the formation of anti-Rh antibodies that attack and destroy Rh-positive cells.

6. **Examine blood chemistry in the physician office laboratory.**
The blood glucose level is monitored routinely in patients with diabetes type 1 or type 2 and in women who have gestational diabetes during pregnancy (see Procedure 49.6). Hemoglobin A1c levels are measured to determine the average blood glucose level during the 2 to 3 months before the test; this test assists in the management of diabetes. Cholesterol testing generally refers to assessing levels of total cholesterol, HDL, and LDL (see Procedure 49.7). Cholesterol testing is done to help determine a patient's susceptibility to coronary artery disease. Liver enzyme testing (ALT and AST) is performed in the POL primarily to monitor the side effects of certain therapeutic drugs, such as those used to treat elevated cholesterol and diabetes. Thyroid testing is performed in the POL to detect elevated thyroid-stimulating hormone (TSH) levels and to assist in the diagnosis of hypothyroidism.

PROCEDURE 49.1 Perform CLIA-Waived Hematology Testing: Determine the Erythrocyte Sedimentation Rate Using a Modified Westergren Method

TASKS: Fill a Westergren tube properly and observe an erythrocyte sedimentation rate (ESR) obtained by using a modified Westergren method. Document the result on the lab flow sheet and in the patient's health record.

EQUIPMENT and SUPPLIES

- Patient's health record
- Provider's order or lab requisition
- Erythrocyte sedimentation rate (ESR) laboratory log
- Ethylenediaminetetraacetic acid (EDTA)–anticoagulated blood specimen
- Safety tube decapper (if tubes do not have Hemogard plastic tops)
- Disposable transfer pipet
- Sediplast ESR system (prefilled Sediplast vial)
- Sediplast rack
- Timer
- Fluid-impermeable lab coat, eye protection, and gloves
- Biohazard waste container
- Biohazard sharps container

PROCEDURAL STEPS

1. Wash hands or use hand sanitizer. Put on a fluid-impermeable lab coat, eye protection, and gloves. Comply with safety practices.
PURPOSE: To ensure infection control.
2. Assemble the materials needed.
3. Check the leveling bubble of the Sediplast rack.
PURPOSE: The rack must be horizontal on the table or bench to ensure that the tube is vertical.
4. Bring the blood sample to room temperature if it has been refrigerated, and mix the sample well by gently inverting the tube 6 to 8 times, making sure the tube has no bubbles.
PURPOSE: Cells settle when a specimen stands, and blood must always be well mixed before sampling. Test results will be altered if refrigerated blood is not brought to room temperature.
5. Remove the plastic Hemogard stopper on the blood sample by twisting and slowly pushing up on the stopper with your thumbs (or by using a tube decapper on rubber-stoppered blood tubes). Label with the patient's name and then remove the stopper on the prefilled Sediplast vial.
PURPOSE: Using the Hemogard cover or removing the rubber cap with a protective device blocks blood splashes and helps prevent aerosolization of the specimen.
6. Fill the Sediplast vial with blood to the indicated line using a disposable transfer pipet (see Figure 1). Replace the stopper on the prefilled vial and invert it several times to mix. Recap the blood collection tube with its stopper.
PURPOSE: This dilutes the blood in accordance with the Westergren procedure.

PROCEDURE 49.1 Perform CLIA-Waived Hematology Testing: Determine the Erythrocyte Sedimentation Rate Using a Modified Westergren Method—*Continued*

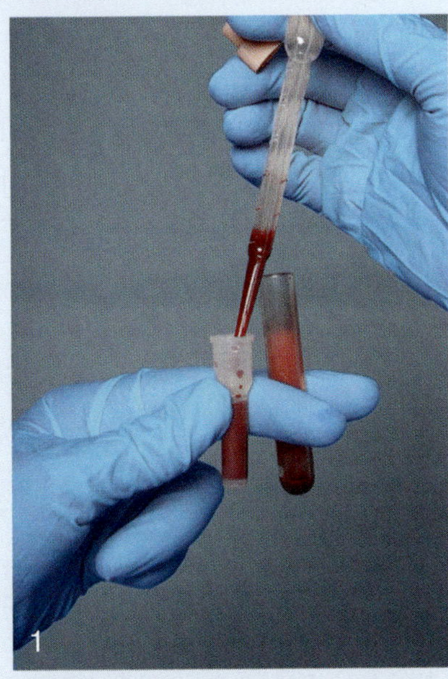
1

7. Insert a Sediplast pipet through the pierceable stopper on the prefilled vial and push down until the pipet touches the bottom of the vial. The pipet automatically draws the blood up and over the zero mark (see Figure 2).

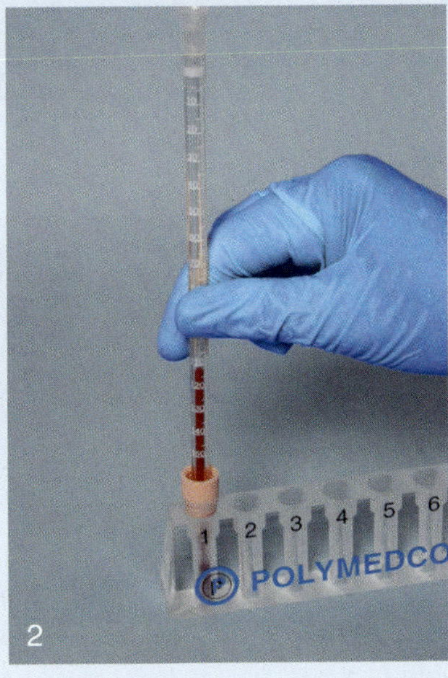

2

8. Insert the filled Sediplast pipet and its vial into the Sediplast rack, making sure the vial is vertical.
<u>PURPOSE:</u> A pipet that is not vertical produces incorrect results.

9. Note the start time on the ESR log sheet and allow the vial to stand undisturbed for 60 minutes.
<u>PURPOSE:</u> Jarring or moving the vial increases the sedimentation rate.

10. After 60 minutes, measure the distance the erythrocytes have fallen at the top of the tube. The scale reads in millimeters—each line is 1 mm.
<u>PURPOSE:</u> Precise timing is important with this test method.

11. Properly dispose of all biohazard materials. Dispose of the plastic Sediplast pipet and its vial into a biohazard sharps container. Disinfect the work area. Remove your gloves, protective eyewear, and lab coat. Wash hands or use hand sanitizer.
<u>PURPOSE:</u> To ensure infection control.

12. Record the findings in the lab's ESR log and the patient's health record. Remember that the Westergren ESR is reported in millimeters per hour (mm/hr). Using the normal range, determine if the test result is normal or abnormal.
<u>PURPOSE:</u> A procedure is not considered complete until it has been recorded.

ESR–SEDIPLAST PATIENT LOG

Hematocrit expected values: Adult male under age 64: 0–15 mm/hr			Adult male over age 64: 0–20 mm/hr Adult females: 0–20 mm/hr		
Date	Tech	Patient ID	Slot #	Results	Charted
10/07/20XX	AJ	@12345	2	15 mm/hr	✓

Documentation Example

10/09/20XX 9:30 a.m. ESR 15 mm/hour.
Anita James, CMA (AAMA)

PROCEDURE 49.2 Perform a CLIA-Waived Protime/INR Test

TASKS: Perform a capillary puncture and perform a coagulation test to determine PT/INR using the CoaguChek XS instrument with built-in quality control. Document the result on the lab flow sheet and in the patient's health record.

EQUIPMENT and SUPPLIES

- Patient's health record or flow chart (see Figure 49.3)
- Provider's order or lab requisition
- PT/INR lab log
- Gauze, alcohol wipes, bandage
- CoaguChek XS PT test monitor (see Figure 49.2)
- CoaguChek lancet
- CoaguChek test strip container and code chip
- Package insert or flow chart with directions
- Fluid-impermeable lab coat, protective eyewear, and gloves
- Biohazard waste container
- Biohazard sharps containers

PROCEDURAL STEPS

1. Wash hands or use hand sanitizer. Put on a fluid-impermeable lab coat, protective eyewear, and gloves. Comply with safety practices.
   PURPOSE: To ensure infection control.
2. Check the provider's order and collect the necessary equipment and supplies.
3. If you are using test strips from a new, unopened container, you must change the test strip code chip. The three-number code on the test strip container must match the three-number code on the code strip. To install the code strip, follow the instructions in the Code Chip section of the user's manual.
   PURPOSE: To ensure that the instrument is calibrated correctly, to produce accurate, precise, and reliable results.
4. Place the meter on a flat surface so that it will not vibrate or move during testing.
   PURPOSE: The test results are based on the back-and-forth movement of the blood sample that stops when the clot has formed. Vibrations or other movements will result in an error message, and the test will have to be repeated.
5. Greet the patient. Identify yourself. Verify the patient's identity with the patient's full name; ask patients to spell their first and last names and to state their date of birth.
   PURPOSE: It is important to identify the patient in two different ways to ensure that you have the correct patient.
6. Explain the procedure to be performed in a manner that the patient understands. Answer any questions the patient may have about the procedure. Obtain permission for the capillary puncture.
   PURPOSE: Explaining the procedure can make the patient feel more comfortable and reduces anxiety.
7. Examine the patient's fingers and choose the site to obtain the blood sample.
   PURPOSE: Proper site choice will help ensure a good sample.
8. Prepare the site:
   a. Warm the hand by placing it under the arm, using a hand warmer, or washing the hand in warm water.
   b. Have the patient hold his or her arm down to the side so that the hand is below the waist.
   c. Massage the palm of the hand toward the base of the finger and toward the tip until the fingertip has increased color.
   d. If necessary, immediately after lancing, gently squeeze the finger from its base to encourage blood flow.

PURPOSE: The hanging drop blood sample must be sufficient to travel down the three channels on the test strip. It must be free of contaminants, tissue fluids, and alcohol.

9. When you are ready to test, remove a test strip from the container and immediately close the container. Make sure it seals tightly. Do not open the container or touch the test strips with wet hands or wet gloves.
   PURPOSE: Exposure to moisture damages the test strips.
10. Insert the test strip as far as you can into the meter. This powers the meter ON (see Figure 1).

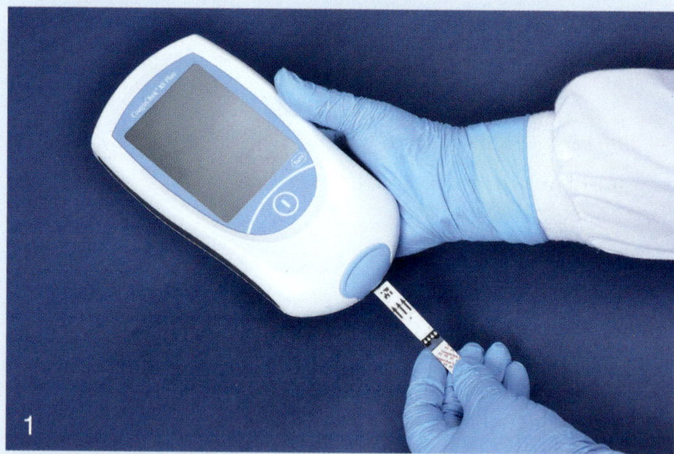
1

11. Disinfect the finger with an alcohol wipe and allow the finger to air-dry. Perform the fingerstick. If necessary, immediately after lancing, gently squeeze the finger to encourage blood flow. Do *not* wipe away the first drop of blood.
    PURPOSE: To ensure infection control
12. Hold the finger with a blood drop very close to the target (the clear area of the test strip). Apply one drop of blood to the top or side of the target area and wait until you hear the beep. *You must apply a hanging drop of blood to the test strip within 15 seconds of the fingerstick. Do not add more blood. Do not touch or remove the test strip while the test is in progress.* The flashing blood drop symbol changes to an hourglass symbol when the meter detects a sufficient sample (see Figure 49.2).

PROCEDURE 49.2 Perform a CLIA-Waived Protime/INR Test—*Continued*

13. Read the results.
    Note: The result appears in approximately 1 minute. It may be displayed in three ways: as the INR, as the protime (PT) in seconds, or as %Quick (a unit used mainly in Europe). Laboratory reports and manufacturers must supply their own reference ranges for PT results, along with each patient's results. This is because different methodologies may create different reference ranges and different units of measurement.
14. Dispose of the sharps into the biohazard sharps container. Dispose of regulated medical waste into the biohazard waste container. Disinfect the test area and remove your PPE.
15. Wash hands or use hand sanitizer.
16. Record the result in the lab's PT/INR log and in the patient's warfarin therapy flow sheet or patient's health record. Using the normal range, determine if the test result is normal or abnormal. For the paper log and paper patient health record, circle any results that do not fall into the desirable ranges. Identify critical values and take appropriate steps to notify the provider. Document the steps taken.
    PURPOSE: The provider needs to know the result while the patient is still in the office for proper follow-up with the patient.

Protime expected values for both normal and therapeutic whole blood:

	INR	PT SECONDS (ISI = 1.0)
Normal	0.8–1.1	11–13.5 sec
Low anticoagulation therapy	1.5–2	19.6–26.1 sec
Moderate anticoagulation therapy	2–3	26.1–39.2 sec
High anticoagulation therapy	3–4	39.2–52.2 sec

DATE	TECH	PATIENT ID	INR	PT SECONDS	CHARTED
10/07/20XX	AJ	@12345	1.5	19.6	✓

Documentation Example

10/07/20XX 9:30 a.m. INR = 1.5 and PT = 19.6 seconds. Patient is on low anticoagulation therapy.
Anita James, CMA (AAMA)

PROCEDURE 49.3 Perform Preventive Maintenance for the Microhematocrit Centrifuge

TASKS: Perform daily, monthly, semiannual, and annual maintenance on a microhematocrit centrifuge. Document the preventive maintenance in the laboratory logbook.

EQUIPMENT and SUPPLIES

- Microhematocrit centrifuge
- Maintenance logbook
- Utility gloves
- Fluid-impermeable lab coat, eye protection, and gloves
- Disinfectant
- Biohazard waste container

PROCEDURAL STEPS

1. Wash hands or use hand sanitizer. Put on a fluid-impermeable lab coat, eye protection, and gloves. In all maintenance procedures, gloves are worn under the utility gloves.
   Note: These are general recommendations. Always check the manufacturer's guidelines for specific instructions. Always unplug the power cord before cleaning or servicing the centrifuge.

DAILY MAINTENANCE

2. Clean the inside of the centrifuge and the gasket with a disinfectant recommended by the manufacturer. Plastic and nonmetal parts may be cleaned with a fresh solution of 5% sodium hypochlorite (bleach) mixed to a 1:10 dilution with water (1 part bleach plus 9 parts water).
   PURPOSE: To remove any dried blood or shattered glass. Do not use bleach on the gasket because it may harden the rubber.

MONTHLY MAINTENANCE

3. Check the reading device. Misuse and zeroing of reading devices can result in considerable error. Always use a second, simple reading device as a cross-check. Use a ruler or a flat plastic card specially made for this purpose. To use these cards, lay the spun hematocrit tube on the card and align the red blood cell with a line on the card to obtain the reading.
   PURPOSE: To ensure accuracy of quality control and patient results.
4. Check the rotor for cracks or corrosion and check the interior for signs of white powder.
   PURPOSE: Cracks, corrosion, or powder may indicate impending rotor failure; these findings require the immediate attention of a service technician.

SEMIANNUAL MAINTENANCE

5. Check the gasket for cuts and breaks.
   PURPOSE: Cut gaskets allow tubes to leak and must be replaced.
6. Check the timer with a stopwatch to verify timer accuracy.
   PURPOSE: To ensure timer accuracy.
7. Perform a maximum cell pack to verify the time required for complete packing by reading a sample after centrifugation and then recentrifuging for 1 minute. The results should be the same. If they are not, perform preventive maintenance or call the service technician.

Continued

PROCEDURE 49.3 Perform Preventive Maintenance for the Microhematocrit Centrifuge—*Continued*

PURPOSE: If the cells compact further during recentrifugation, the centrifuge is not rotating at the proper speed, and hematocrit results will be falsely elevated.

ANNUAL MAINTENANCE (OR MAINTENANCE PERFORMED AS NEEDED)

8. The centrifuge functions and maintenance verification should be performed by qualified personnel. This includes checking the centrifuge mechanism, rotors, timer, speed, and electrical leads.
   PURPOSE: To ensure proper centrifuge function.
9. Record all professional service calls in the laboratory logbook.
   PURPOSE: Proper documentation is essential for all laboratory maintenance.

MICROHEMATOCRIT CENTRIFUGE MAINTENANCE LOG

DATE	SERVICE	INITIALS
10/7/20XX	Performed routine daily, monthly, and annual preventive maintenance	AJ

PROCEDURE 49.4 Perform CLIA-Waived Hematology Testing: Perform a Microhematocrit Test

TASKS: Perform a microhematocrit test accurately. Document the result on the lab flow sheet and in the patient's health record.

EQUIPMENT and SUPPLIES

- Patient's health record
- Provider's order or lab requisition
- Microhematocrit lab log
- Fresh sample of blood collected in a tube containing ethylenediaminetetraacetic acid (EDTA) anticoagulant (or equipment for fingerstick specimen: lancet, alcohol wipe, gauze, bandage)
- Plastic-coated self-sealing capillary tubes or plain capillary tubes (blue-tipped)
- Sealing clay (if capillary tubes are not self-sealing)
- Gauze
- Microhematocrit centrifuge
- Fluid-impermeable lab coat, protective eyewear, and gloves
- Biohazard waste container
- Biohazard sharps containers

PROCEDURAL STEPS

1. Wash hands or use hand sanitizer. Put on fluid-impermeable lab coat, protective eyewear, and gloves. Comply with safety practices.
   PURPOSE: To ensure infection control.
2. Assemble the materials needed.
   a. *If the capillary tubes are self-sealing:* Fill two tubes by inserting the end opposite the sealed end into the well-mixed EDTA blood sample. *Note:* If the capillary tube and the EDTA tube are held almost parallel to the table, the capillary tubes fill easily by capillary action. When the self-sealing capillary tubes are two-thirds to three-fourths filled, tilt them upright, causing the blood sample to flow down the tube and meet the sealant. Continue to hold the tube vertical when the blood contacts the sealant for an additional 15 seconds.
   PURPOSE: Duplicates should always be done as a means of quality control.
   b. *Alternative:* Fill two plain (blue-tipped) capillary tubes two-thirds to three-fourths full of a well-mixed EDTA blood sample. Tip the blood tube slightly, touching the capillary tube into the blood using the side that is opposite the blue band. When enough blood has filled the capillary tube, tip the blue end of the tube down, causing the blood to flow toward the blue tip. Then readjust the tube horizontally while inserting the blue tip of the capillary tube into the clay sealant. Insert the tube as many times as needed to achieve a plug up to the blue band (Figure 1).

PURPOSE: Duplicates should always be done as a means of quality control. Tubes are not filled completely to provide space for the sealing clay.

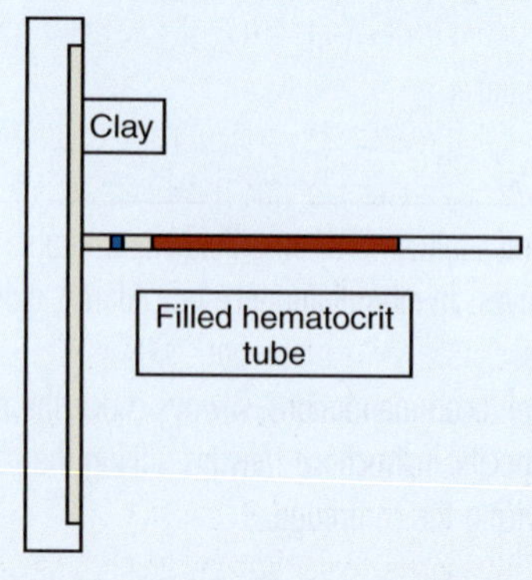

1

PROCEDURE 49.4 Perform CLIA-Waived Hematology Testing: Perform a Microhematocrit Test—*Continued*

3. Wipe the outside of the tubes with clean gauze without touching the wet open end of the tube.
   PURPOSE: Wiping the outside of the capillary tube removes any blood. Touching the blood inside the capillary tube with absorbent material removes more plasma than blood cells and can alter the hematocrit.
4. Place the tubes opposite each other in the centrifuge with the sealed ends securely against the gasket (see Figure 49.4).
   PURPOSE: The centrifuge must always be balanced to prevent damage. If the clay ends of the capillary tubes are not outermost against the gasket, the sample will spin out of the tubes, contaminating the centrifuge.
5. Note the numbers on the centrifuge slots and record the numbers on the log sheet, along with the patient's name
   PURPOSE: The sample must be identified throughout the entire procedure.
6. Secure the locking top, fasten the lid down, and lock it.
   PURPOSE: If the locking top is not firmly in place during the spinning cycle, the tubes will come out of their slots and break. The lid is always locked during centrifugation for safety purposes to prevent the ejection of aerosols or broken glass.
7. Set the timer to 3 to 5 minutes and adjust the speed to 11,000 to 12,000 rpm, or as indicated by the manufacturer's instructions.
   Note: Check the manufacturer's instructions for time and speed, as models vary.
8. Allow the centrifuge to come to a complete stop. Unlock the outer locking top and then remove the inner lid.
   PURPOSE: Opening the centrifuge before it has stopped could result in harm to the user.
9. Remove the tubes immediately and read the results. If this is not possible, store the tubes in an upright position.
   PURPOSE: Tubes left in the centrifuge will show altered results because RBC layer will spread out horizontally
10. Determine the microhematocrit values using one of the following methods:
    a. Centrifuge with built-in reader using calibrated capillary tubes.
       (1) Position the tubes as directed by the manufacturer's instructions.
       (2) Read both tubes.
       (3) The average of the two results is reported.
       (4) The two values should not vary by more than 2%.
    b. Centrifuge without a built-in reader.
       (1) Carefully remove the tubes from the centrifuge.
       (2) Place a tube on the microhematocrit reader.
       (3) Align the clay-RBC junction with the zero line on the reader. Align the plasma meniscus with the 100% line. The value is read at the junction of the red blood cell layer and the buffy coat. The buffy coat is not included in the reading (see Figure 2).
       (4) Read both tubes.
       (5) The average of the two results is reported.
       (6) The two values should not vary by more than 2%.

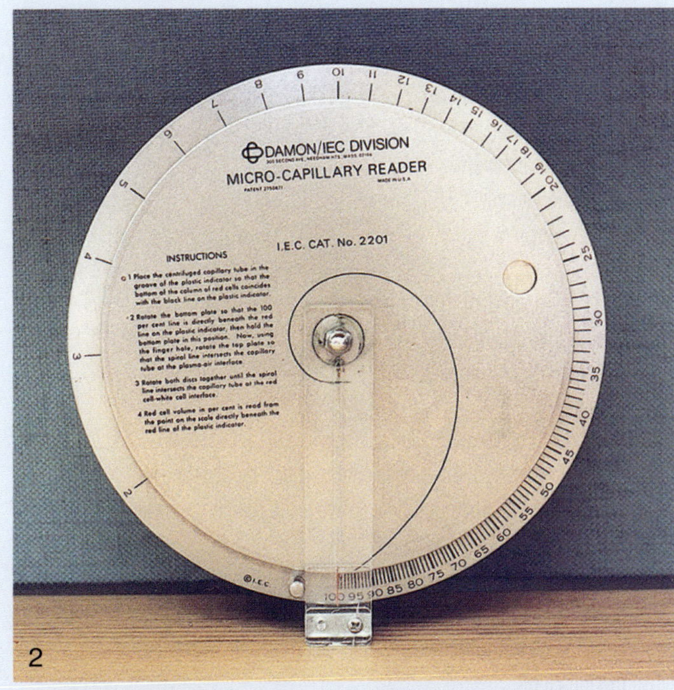

2

11. Dispose of the capillary tubes in a biohazard sharps container.
12. Disinfect the work area and properly dispose of all biohazard materials. Remove your gloves, eyewear, and lab coat.
13. Wash hands or use hand sanitizer.
    PURPOSE: To ensure infection control.
14. Record the results in the Hematocrit Patient Log and document the results in the patient's medical record. Using the normal range, identify if test results are normal or abnormal.
    PURPOSE: A procedure is not considered done until it is charted.

HEMATOCRIT PATIENT LOG

Hematocrit expected values:
Adult male: 39%–49%
Adult female: 36%–45%
Newborn–1 month: 31%–57%
Age:1 month–23 months: 27%–38%
Age 2–17 years: 31%–50%

DATE	TECH	PATIENT ID	SLOT #	RESULTS	CHARTED
10/07/20XX	AJ	@12345	1 & 4	44% and 44%	✓

Documentation Example

10/07/20XX 11:25 a.m. Hct 44%. ——————————————————— Anita James, CMA (AAMA)

PROCEDURE 49.5 Perform CLIA-Waived Hematology Testing: Perform a Hemoglobin Test

TASKS: Accurately determine the level of hemoglobin present in a blood sample using the HemoCue B-Hemoglobin System. Document the result on the lab flow sheet and in the patient's health record.

EQUIPMENT and SUPPLIES

- Patient's health record
- Provider's order or lab requisition
- Hemoglobin laboratory log
- HemoCue monitor
- HemoCue microcuvette
- Safety blood lancet
- Alcohol wipes
- Gauze
- Fluid-impermeable lab coat, protective eyewear, and gloves
- Biohazard waste container
- Biohazard sharps containers

PROCEDURAL STEPS

1. Perform an instrument quality control check by inserting the control cuvette into the instrument. Make sure the reading is within acceptable limits before proceeding.
   PURPOSE: Only instruments that record values within acceptable control limits can be used for patient testing. If the value is outside the control limits, refer to the troubleshooting guide for the instrument or contact the manufacturer.
2. Wash your hands or use hand sanitizer. Put on a fluid-impermeable lab coat, protective eyewear, and gloves. Comply with safety practices.
   PURPOSE: To ensure infection control.
3. Check the provider's order and collect the necessary equipment and supplies.
4. Greet the patient. Identify yourself. Verify the patient's identity with the patient's full name; ask patients to spell their first and last names and to state their date of birth.
   PURPOSE: It is important to identify the patient in two different ways to ensure that you have the correct patient.
5. Explain the procedure to be performed in a manner that the patient understands. Answer any questions the patient may have on the procedure. Obtain permission for the capillary puncture.
   PURPOSE: Explaining the procedure can make the patient feel more comfortable and reduces anxiety.
6. Examine the patient's fingers and choose the site to be used to obtain the blood sample.
   PURPOSE: The site must be free of trauma, calluses, and scarring.
7. Clean the site with an alcohol wipe or another recommended antiseptic preparation.
   PURPOSE: To ensure a properly cleaned puncture site; infection control.
8. Perform a capillary puncture and wipe away the first drop of blood.
   PURPOSE: This drop may contain tissue fluid or antiseptic that may hemolyze the blood.
9. Obtain a large drop of blood on the surface of the finger.
   PURPOSE: To ensure enough blood for an adequate sample.
10. Touch the microcuvette to the drop of blood. Do not touch the finger. The correct volume is drawn into the cuvette by capillary action. Wipe off any excess blood from the sides of the cuvette (Figures 1 and 2).
    PURPOSE: Blood on the cuvette may alter the readings or contaminate the instrument.

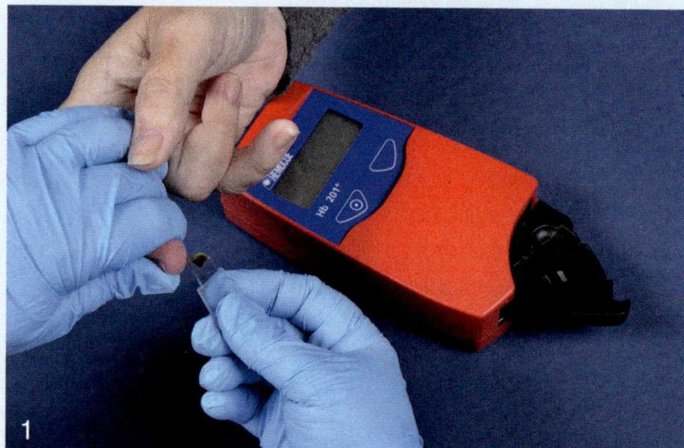
1

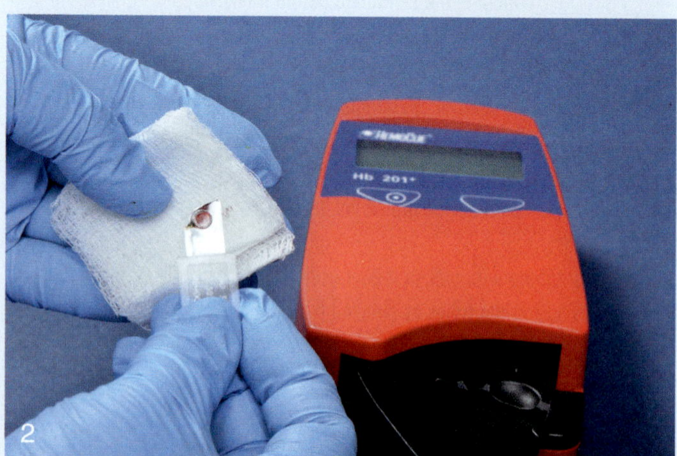

2

11. Place the cuvette in the cuvette holder of the HemoCue sample door and close the door of the instrument (Figure 3).
    PURPOSE: To begin the testing process.

PROCEDURE 49.5 Perform CLIA-Waived Hematology Testing: Perform a Hemoglobin Test—*Continued*

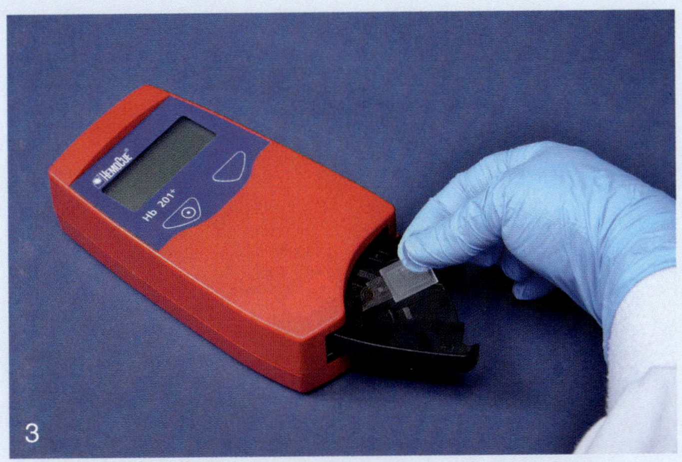

12. Read the result.
13. Dispose of biohazard waste in the biohazard waste container and the sharps in the biohazard sharps container. Turn off the instrument. Properly disinfect the work area.
14. Remove your gloves and dispose of them in the biohazard waste container. Remove the lab coat and protective eyewear.
15. Wash hands or use hand sanitizer.
    PURPOSE: To ensure infection control.
16. Record the result in the lab's hemoglobin log and the patient's health record. Using the normal range, determine if the test result is normal or abnormal.
    PURPOSE: A procedure is not completed until the result has been recorded.

Hemocue B Hemoglobin System Patient Log

Test:______________________ Kit Log #: ______________

Hemoglobin expected values: Newborn–1 month: 10–20 g/dL
Adult male: 13.2–16.6 g/dL Age:1 month–23 months: 8.9–12.7 g/dL
Adult female: 11.6–15 g/dL Age 2–17 years: 10.2–16.9 g/dL

DATE	TECH	PATIENT ID	RESULT	CHARTED
10/07/20XX	AJ	@12345	15.5 g/dL	✓

Documentation Example

10/09/20 9:30 a.m. Hgb 15.5 g/dL.———— Anita James, CMA (AAMA)

PROCEDURE 49.6 Perform a Blood Glucose Test

TASKS: Perform a blood test for blood glucose accurately. Document the result in the patient's health record.

EQUIPMENT and SUPPLIES

- Patient's health record
- Provider's order or lab requisition
- Glucometer glucose monitoring device
- Blood glucose test strip
- Lancet and autoloading finger-puncturing device
- Alcohol wipes
- Gauze
- Fluid-impermeable lab coat, protective eyewear, and gloves
- Biohazard waste container
- Biohazard sharps container

PROCEDURAL STEPS

1. Check the provider's order and collect the necessary equipment and supplies. Perform quality control measures according to the manufacturer's guidelines and office policy.
   Note: A variety of blood glucose monitors are available for testing blood glucose. Follow the specific instructions given by each individual manufacturer in the monitor/kit package insert.
2. Wash hands or use hand sanitizer. Put on a fluid-impermeable lab coat, protective eyewear, and gloves. Comply with safety practices.
   PURPOSE: To ensure infection control.
3. Greet the patient. Identify yourself. Verify the patient's identity with the patient's full name; ask patients to spell their first and last names and to state their date of birth.
   PURPOSE: It is important to identify the patient in two different ways to ensure that you have the correct patient.
4. Explain the procedure to be performed in a manner that the patient understands. Answer any questions the patient may have on the procedure. Obtain permission for the capillary puncture.
   PURPOSE: Explaining the procedure can make the patient feel more comfortable and reduces anxiety.

PROCEDURE 49.6 Assist the Provider with Patient Care: Perform a Blood Glucose Test—*Continued*

5. Ask the patient to wash his or her hands in warm, soapy water, then rinse them in warm water, and finally dry them completely.
   PURPOSE: To clean the area that will be punctured; also, warming the fingers may increase peripheral blood flow.
6. Check the patient's middle and ring fingers and select the site for puncture (both forearm and fingertip testing can be done).
   PURPOSE: To make sure the site of puncture is free of trauma.
7. Turn on the glucometer by pressing the ON button (Figure 1). Coding may or may not be necessary, depending on the monitor; follow the package insert directions for the specific glucose monitor you are using.

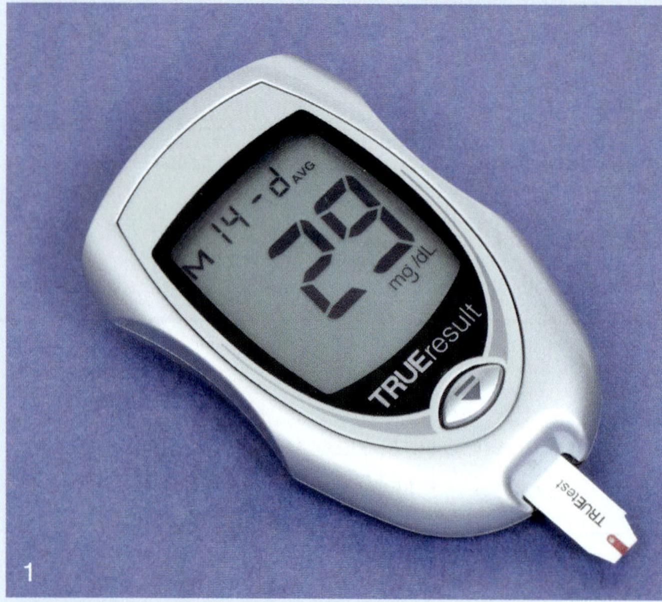

1

8. Check the expiration date on the test strip container. Take out a test strip and insert it into the glucometer.
   PURPOSE: Test strips should not be used if they have expired.
9. Cleanse the selected site on the patient's fingertip with an alcohol wipe and allow the finger to air-dry.
   PURPOSE: To ensure infection control.
10. Perform the capillary puncture and wipe away the first drop of blood.
    PURPOSE: Tissue fluid may be present in the first drop of blood.
11. Apply a small blood sample to the end of the test strip (Figure 2).

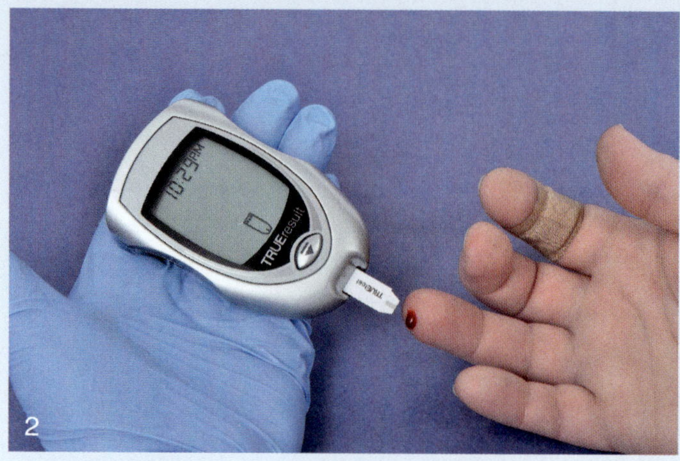

2

12. Give the patient gauze to hold securely over the puncture site; apply a hypoallergenic bandage or wrap if needed.
    PURPOSE: To aid in the stoppage of blood flow.
13. Read the test results before the glucometer turns off.
    Note: The glucometer automatically begins the measurement process, and results are obtained as soon as 4 seconds. The test result is shown in the display window in milligrams per deciliter (mg/dL) for most glucometers. Read the manufacturer's instructions to find out how the result is displayed. The glucometer will likely turn off automatically.
14. Discard all biohazard waste in biohazard waste containers and the sharps in the biohazard sharps container.
    PURPOSE: To ensure infection control.
15. Clean the glucometer according to the manufacturer's guidelines. Disinfect the work area.
16. Remove your gloves and dispose of them properly. Remove protective eyewear.
17. Wash hands or use hand sanitizer.
    PURPOSE: To ensure infection control.
18. Record the test results in the patient's health record.
    PURPOSE: A procedure is not complete until the patient's results have been recorded.

Documentation Example

08/16/20XX 1:00 p.m. Glucometer screening completed as ordered by Dr. Misha. NFBS 144. Pt took routine dose of 10 units Humalog insulin at noon. Pt had no questions. ———————————————— Anita James, CMA (AAMA)

PROCEDURE 49.7 Perform a CLIA-Waived Chemistry Test: Determine the Cholesterol Level or Lipid Profile Using a Cholestech Analyzer

TASKS: Perform a Cholestech test for total cholesterol level or a lipid panel and accurately report the results. Document the result on the lab flow sheet and in the patient's health record.

EQUIPMENT and SUPPLIES

- Patient's health record
- Provider's order or lab requisition
- Cholestech analyzer
- Package insert or flow chart with directions
- Optics check cassette
- Test cassettes (provided by Cholestech)
- Levels 1 and 2 liquid controls
- Capillary tubes and plungers for fingerstick sample (provided by Cholestech)
- Mini-Pet pipet and pipet tips for venipuncture sample (provided by Cholestech)
- Lancet, gauze, alcohol wipes, bandage for capillary blood, or lithium heparin (green-topped) tube for venous blood
- Safety tube decapper (if tubes do not have a Hemogard plastic top)
- Fluid-impermeable lab coat, protective eyewear, and gloves
- Biohazard waste container
- Biohazard sharps containers

PROCEDURAL STEPS

1. Check the provider's order and collect the necessary equipment and supplies. Allow refrigerated testing cassettes to come to room temperature (at least 10 minutes before opening).
   PURPOSE: The test is temperature and time sensitive when reading results.
2. Wash hands or use hand sanitizer. Put on a fluid-impermeable lab coat, protective eyewear, and gloves. Comply with safety practices. Assemble the materials needed.
   PURPOSE: To ensure infection control.
3. Perform quantitative quality control by performing a calibration check with the optics check cassette (Figure 1). Then test level 1 and level 2 liquid controls if using a new set of cassettes.
   PURPOSE: To ensure that the instrument is reading results accurately, precisely, and reliably.

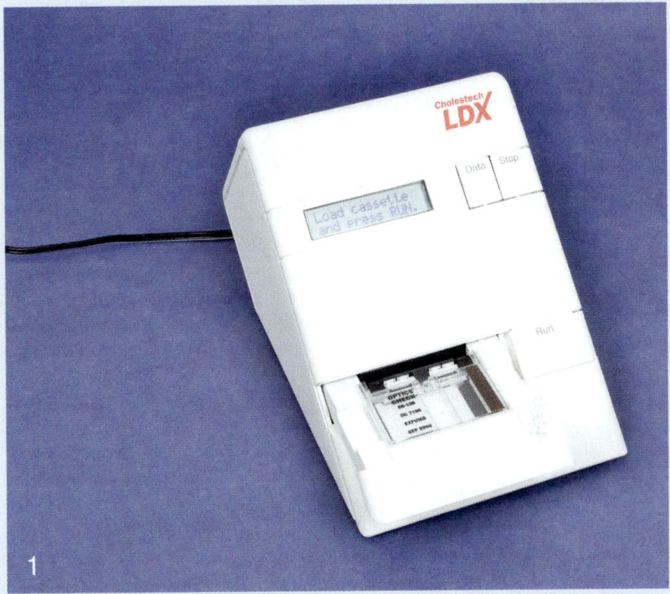

1

4. Greet the patient. Identify yourself. Verify the patient's identity with the patient's full name, ask the patient to spell the first and last name, and state the date of birth.
5. Explain the procedure to be performed in a manner that the patient understands. Answer any questions the patient may have on the procedure. Obtain permission for a capillary puncture.
6. Remove the cassette from its pouch and place it on flat surface without touching the black bar or magnetic strip.
   PURPOSE: The black bar is the testing area, and the magnetic strip must be read by the analyzer. Touching either may interfere with test results.
7. Press RUN on the analyzer, allowing it to do a self-test; this will be followed by OK on the screen, then the test drawer will open. The drawer will stay open for 4 minutes while the specimen is prepared.
   PURPOSE: Ensures the instrument's electronics are working properly before patient testing.
8. Perform a fingerstick and collect the capillary blood to the black line of the Cholestech capillary tube with its plunger inserted into the red end of the tube. *Or* collect the fresh venous whole blood with the Cholestech Mini-Pet pipet.

Continued

PROCEDURE 49.7 Perform a CLIA-Waived Chemistry Test: Determine the Cholesterol Level or Lipid Profile Using a Cholestech Analyzer—*Continued*

<u>PURPOSE:</u> Both collecting devices are provided by Cholestech to ensure that the exact volume of blood necessary is tested.

9. Place the whole blood sample into the well of the cassette.
   Note: The capillary specimen must be in the cassette within 5 minutes of collection (Figure 2).
   <u>PURPOSE:</u> Fingerstick blood will clot if not tested within 5 minutes.

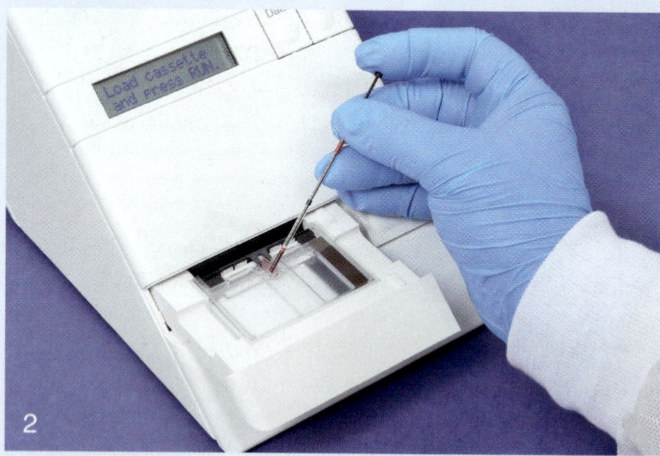

2

10. Immediately put the cassette into the drawer of the analyzer and press RUN. (*Note:* If the drawer has closed, press RUN again to open the drawer; load the specimen into the drawer and then press to close the drawer.) When the test is complete, the analyzer beeps. The screen displays and then prints out the results (Figure 3).
    <u>PURPOSE:</u> This is a test with a color reaction that continues to change over time.

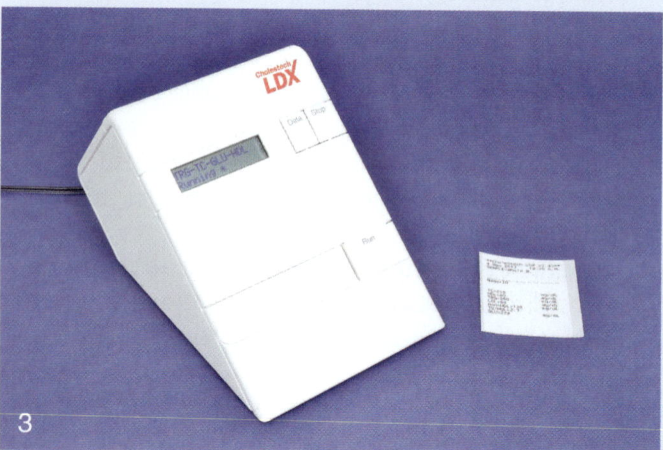

3

11. Dispose of all sharps in the biohazard sharps container (i.e., lancet and capillary pipet with plunger). Place all regulated medical waste into the biohazard waste container (i.e., gauze, alcohol wipes, and cassettes).
12. Disinfect test area, remove PPE, and dispose of gloves in biohazard waste container.
13. Wash hands or use hand sanitizer.
    <u>PURPOSE:</u> To ensure infection control.
14. Record the findings in the laboratory log and in the patient's health record. Using the normal range, determine if the test result is normal or abnormal. If using paper health records, circle the results that do not fall within the Desirable Ranges column of the following table. Identify critical values and take appropriate steps to notify the provider. Document the steps taken.
    <u>PURPOSE:</u> A procedure is not considered complete until it has been recorded.

CHOLESTECH LDX PATIENT/CONTROL LOG

Cassette Lot #: ____________ Expiration date: ____________
LDX Serial #: ____________

Date	Tech	PT ID	TC	HDL	LDL	TRG	TC/HDL	GLU	Charted
10/09/ 20XX	AJ	#12345	190	50	120	135	4.3	80	✓

Documentation Example

Attach a printed readout, or record results in the electronic chart.

TEST	RESULTS	DESIRABLE RANGES[a]
Total cholesterol (TC)	190	<200 mg/dL
HDL cholesterol	50	>40 mg/dL (males); >50 mg/dL (females)
LDL cholesterol	120	<130 mg/dL
Triglycerides	135	30–190 mg/dL
TC/HDL ratio	4.3	≤4.5
Other		
Glucose	80	Fasting: 70–99 mg/dL
		Nonfasting: <125 mg/dL

[a]Laboratory reports and manufacturers must supply their own reference ranges, along with each patient's results. This is because different methodologies may create different reference ranges and different units of measurement.

MICROBIOLOGY AND IMMUNOLOGY

50

SCENARIO

Laura Piper, CMA (AAMA), has worked at Walden-Martin Family Medical (WMFM) Clinic for 6 years. She has seen many infectious diseases diagnosed over that time. Bacterial and viral infections are common, but Laura also knows that not all microorganisms are bad. Some diseases have been controlled using vaccines. Other infections can be treated with antibiotics. Not all infectious diseases can be treated with antibiotics, and improper use of antibiotics can lead to bacteria that are resistant to those very useful drugs. Laura knows that it is important to identify pathogens quickly so that proper treatment can begin. The identification of pathogens can involve various types of tests, many of which can be performed in the physician office laboratory (POL) where she works.

While studying this chapter, think about the following questions:

- How are microorganisms classified?
- What are the various bacterial shapes, oxygen requirements, and physical structures?
- What are different types of pathogens?
- What are the common methods for the collection and transport of specimens?
- What are three common tests used for microbiology testing that have been waived by the Clinical Laboratory Improvement Amendments (CLIA)?
- What are three common CLIA-waived tests used for immunology testing?
- What is the importance of the Gram stain and acid-fast stains in microbiology?
- What are common stool-based tests?

LEARNING OBJECTIVES

1. Examine how microorganisms are identified.
2. Examine the characteristics of bacteria.
3. Differentiate among various pathogens.
4. Examine the procedures for specimen collection and transport in the physician office laboratory.
5. Examine CLIA-waived microbiology testing.
6. Examine CLIA-waived immunology testing.
7. Examine the reference laboratory process for the identification of pathogens.
8. Examine stool-based tests.

VOCABULARY

5% sheep's blood agar plate (BAP) A solid agar medium that contains nutrients and 5% washed sheep's blood. The blood is added as an extra nutrient source for bacteria.

acute phase The phase during which rapid multiplication of the pathogen takes place. Symptoms are very distinct. A strong response of the immune system takes place during this stage.

antibiotic A substance or medication that can destroy or inhibit the growth of bacteria.

antibody A protein substance produced in the blood or tissues in response to a specific antigen; antibodies destroy or weaken the antigen. Part of the immune system.

antigen A substance that stimulates the production of an antibody when introduced into the body. Antigens include toxins, bacteria, viruses, and other foreign substances.

antiseptic Substances that inhibit the growth of microorganisms on living tissue (e.g., alcohol and povidone-iodine [Betadine]); they are used to cleanse the skin, wounds, and so on.

arthropod Any animal that lacks a spine, such as insects, crustaceans, arachnids, and others.

asexual Describes reproduction that does not involve the fusion of male and female sex cells.

bacteria Microorganisms that are single celled, lack a nucleus, reproduce asexually, or can form spores. Some can cause disease. The most abundant life form on earth.

binary fission Asexual reproduction in single-celled organisms during which one cell divides into two daughter cells.

binomial A name consisting of a generic and a specific term.

VOCABULARY—*continued*

blood agar plate (BAP) A solid agar medium that contains nutrients and 5% washed sheep's blood. The blood is added as an extra nutrient source for bacteria.

bronchiolitis Occurs when the small airways of the lungs become inflamed because of a viral infection.

colony A discrete group of organisms, such as a group of bacteria, growing on a solid nutrient surface.

convalescent stage The phase during which the host recovers gradually and returns to baseline or normal health.

decolorizer A liquid that has the ability to wash out color.

diluent (DIL yoo uh nt) A liquid substance that dilutes or lessens the strength of a solution or mixture.

endospore An inactive form of certain bacteria that can withstand poor environmental conditions. When conditions improve, the bacteria become functional again.

eukaryote (yoo KAR ee oht) Any single-celled or multicellular organism that has genetic material contained in a distinct membrane-bound nucleus.

extract A certain substance that is taken out of a group or solution and is in a concentrated form.

extraction A process by which a specific substance is separated from a group or solution.

flagella A long, whiplike outgrowth from a cell that helps the cell move.

fomite Objects that are likely to carry infectious organisms.

fungi Single-celled organisms, including mushrooms, molds, mildew, smuts, rusts, and yeasts, and classified in the kingdom Fungi.

guaiac fecal occult blood test A test for fecal occult blood where glacial acetic acid and guaiac are mixed with the specimen.

healthcare-associated infections (HAIs) Infections that patients acquire while receiving treatment for other conditions within a healthcare setting (e.g., ambulatory care, long-term care, or rehabilitation facility).

hemoccult test A modified guaiac test using filter paper impregnated with guaiacum that turns blue if occult blood is present.

heterophile antibody An antibody that has an affinity for an antigen other than the specific antigen that stimulated its production.

infectious agents Living and nonliving pathogens—such as bacteria, viruses, fungi, protozoa, parasites, helminths, and prions—that can cause disease.

in vitro Latin term meaning "in glass" and commonly known as "in the laboratory."

macromolecules Molecules needed for metabolism: carbohydrates, lipids, proteins, amino acids, and nucleic acids.

microorganism Any living organism—such as bacterium, protozoan, fungi, parasite, or helminth—of microscopic size. Some definitions include viruses, which are not alive.

mold Growth of tiny fungi forming on a substance. Often looks downy or furry and is associated with dampness or decay.

molecule The simplest unit of a chemical compound that can exist, consisting of two or more atoms held together with chemical bonds.

mordant Having the ability to fix or set colors.

nasal wash Also called a nasal aspirate. A syringe is used to gently squirt a small amount of sterile saline into the nose, and the resulting fluid is collected into a cup (for a wash). Or after the saline is squirted into the nose, gentle suction is applied (for the aspirate).

nomenclature (NOH muh n kley cher) A system of names or terms, used in science and art to categorize items.

normal flora A microorganism (usually a bacterium or yeast) that lives on or in the body. A normal microscopic resident of the body.

occult Not visibly apparent or seen.

organelles Structures inside a cell that perform specific functions.

parasitic Pertaining to a parasite. (An organism that lives on or in another organism, known as the host. Benefits from the host; the host does not benefit from the parasite.)

pathogen A disease-causing organism or agent.

pneumonia Inflammation of the lungs with congestion of the air sacs (alveoli). Can be caused by a bacterium or virus.

prokaryote (proh KAR ee ote) Any organism that is made up of at least one cell and has genetic material that is not enclosed in a nucleus. Bacteria are prokaryotes, primitive organisms.

protozoa (pro tuh ZOH ah) Single-celled organisms that are the most primitive form of animal life. Most are microscopic. Examples are amoebas, ciliates, flagellates, and sporozoans.

pure culture The growth of only one microorganism in a culture or on a nutrient surface.

serologic Pertaining to the science involving the immune properties and actions of serum.

sputum Thick mucus often referred to as phlegm. It is coughed up from the lungs; not saliva that originates in the mouth.

stains Reagents or dyes used to prepare specimens for microscopic examination.

streaked for isolation To have produced isolated colonies of an organism on an agar plate. Using an inoculating loop, pick one colony and methodically spread it out onto solid nutrient media. The goal is to have colonies that are separate from other colonies.

subcultured Occurs when an organism (a bacterium) has been cultivated again on a new nutrient surface.

tissue culture The technique or process of keeping tissue alive and growing in a culture medium.

titer The lowest concentration of a serum solution containing a specific antibody where the antibody is still able to neutralize (or precipitate) an antigen.

transport medium A medium used to keep an organism alive during transport to the laboratory.

vector Arthropod (mosquito, tick, flea) that carries disease and transmits to another organism through a blood meal.

viable Able to live and grow.

wet mount A glass slide that holds a specimen suspended in a drop of liquid for microscopic examination.

yeast Any various single-celled fungi, which reproduce by budding and are able to ferment sugars.

INTRODUCTION

Infectious diseases caused by **microorganisms** and **infectious agents** have gotten a lot of publicity. We have heard news stories about COVID-19, influenza, Zika, and more. With news of foodborne illnesses, contaminated water supplies, tick-borne diseases, and communicable infections, it appears all microorganisms are harmful and can cause disease. **Healthcare-associated infections (HAIs)** are making it increasingly difficult to control methicillin-resistant *Staphylococcus aureus* (MRSA) and Clostridium difficile infections.

New strains of drug-resistant microorganisms are difficult to treat with existing **antibiotics**. Bioterrorism has become a real concern worldwide. Antimicrobial products line the pharmacy and supermarket shelves and are going to keep us "germ free." It is no wonder many people have the impression that all microorganisms are harmful. In reality, less than 1% of known microorganisms are pathogens.

Normal Flora

Most microorganisms are good. For example, *saprophytes* are beneficial microorganisms that are responsible for breaking down organic matter, such as plants and organic waste in farming, water purification, composting, and gardening. Without microorganisms, we could not survive. The **normal flora** in and on our bodies is needed for the following processes:

- Digesting food and making nutrients available to the body.
- Forming blood clots. Vitamin K is used in the clotting process and is made by **bacteria** in our intestines.
- Preventing pathogens from invading our skin, mucous membranes, and gastrointestinal and genitourinary tracts.

Normal flora takes up space, requires nutrients, and excretes waste. When pathogens try to populate the skin or areas of the body that have normal flora, they must compete with the existing organisms. This makes it harder for pathogens to cause disease. Normal flora discourages pathogen populations.

When the body's normal flora is weakened (e.g., by antibiotic overuse or hormonal changes), certain opportunistic organisms that are normally present in low numbers can overgrow. An example is Candida albicans, which is a **yeast** that is normally found in mucous membranes in the body. When a patient has been on broad-spectrum antibiotics for an infection, the antibiotics kill pathogens, along with some of the normal flora. For example, Candida albicans is not normally a problem in the vagina. If enough normal flora in the vagina is killed off, Candida albicans can increase in numbers, which causes a vaginal yeast infection.

Medical Assistant's Role

As a medical assistant, you need to understand basic microbiology and the role of microorganisms in both health and disease. The main objective of medical microbiology is to identify the organisms responsible for illness so that the provider can properly treat the patient. Your responsibilities will also include preventing HAIs by following infection control policies. Microbiology testing procedures may be performed in the physician office laboratory (POL) or in the microbiology department of a medical referral laboratory.

Immunology

Immunology is the study of the immune system, which is closely tied to microbiology. Invasive microorganisms stimulate an immune response, leading to the production of **antibodies** that come to our defense. Often a bacterial or viral infection is diagnosed by testing for a specific antibody that is produced to fight the infectious agent.

This chapter covers the following topics related to microbiology and immunology:

- Major categories of infectious agents
- Quality control issues regarding the collection and handling of microbiological specimens
- Common CLIA-waived microbiology and immunology testing

The chapter concludes with an overview of the more complex microbiology procedures and tests performed in hospitals and reference laboratories.

CLASSIFICATION OF MICROORGANISMS

Although the medical assistant is not responsible for identifying microorganisms, a working knowledge of the terminology used in the naming of microorganisms is essential.

Microorganisms

Microorganisms are too small to be seen without magnification. Bacteria, **fungi**, and **protozoa** are all microorganisms that can be seen with a microscope. **Parasitic** worm infections are also identified in the microbiology laboratory because their eggs are visible under the microscope. Viruses are the smallest microbe and are visible only with a highly magnified electron microscope.

Naming Microorganisms

Scientists use the **binomial** system of **nomenclature** developed by Swedish botanist Carl Linnaeus to name all living organisms: animals, plants, fungi, protozoa, and bacteria. This binomial system assigns two names, which are both either *italicized* or underlined when written:

- *Genus*: First name; begins with a capital letter. After the organism's full genus and species names are given once in a report, subsequent references can just use a single letter to represent the genus. For example, *Escherichia coli* is commonly referred to as *E. coli.*
- *Species*: Second name; begins with a lowercase letter.
- When microbiology laboratory results are reported, it is essential that both the genus and species names are recorded. Different species may cause different symptoms or require different antibiotic treatments. For example, *Streptococcus pyogenes* causes strep throat, whereas *Streptococcus viridans* is normal flora in the throat.

CHARACTERISTICS OF BACTERIA

As mentioned in a prior section, some bacteria can be helpful to the body, such as normal flora. Bacteria can also be harmful. Besides the helpful/harmful characteristic, bacteria have other characteristics. They are single-celled **prokaryote** organisms that reproduce **asexually**, by **binary fission**. This process of reproduction results in large numbers of bacteria being formed from a single cell. Because bacteria reproduce quickly, bacterial infections can swiftly overwhelm a person's immune system. Some bacteria reproduce in as little as 14 minutes, whereas other bacteria may take days. For example, a single *E. coli* cell reproduces about every 30 minutes to produce about 3.5 trillion offspring in 24 hours.

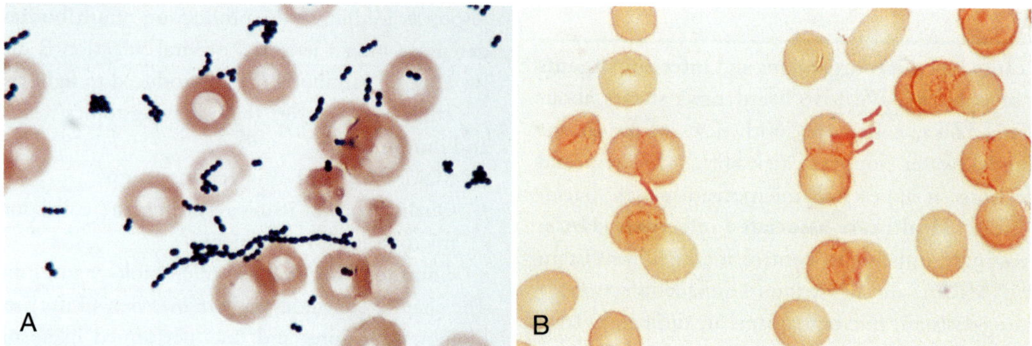

FIGURE 50.1 **(A)** Gram stain red blood cells (RBCs) and gram-positive cocci. **(B)** RBCs with gram-negative bacilli. (From De la Maza LM, Pezzlo MT, Baron EJ: *Color atlas of diagnostic microbiology,* St. Louis, 1997, Mosby.)

Bacteria often are classified according to their staining characteristics, shape, and the environmental conditions in which they thrive. Both shape and staining characteristics are direct results of their cell wall composition.

Bacterial Staining Properties

Three types of cell wall structures are found among pathogenic bacteria: gram-positive, gram-negative, and acid-fast structures. These labels are based on reactions to specialized **stains** used to see bacteria under a microscope. Bacterial cell walls are composed of *peptidoglycan* (PG), a **molecule** composed of carbohydrate and protein.

- *Gram-positive cells* contain a thick layer of PG, which looks deep blue/violet when stained with Gram stain (Figure 50.1A).
- *Gram-negative cells* contain a thin layer of PG, which looks pinkish red when stained with Gram stain (Figure 50.1B).
- *Acid-fast cells* contain a thin layer of PG surrounded by a thick layer of waxlike *lipids* (fats). Acid-fast bacteria do not stain well with a Gram stain, but they stain pink with the acid-fast stain (Figure 50.2).

Bacterial Shapes

Bacteria assume three different shapes:

- Round bacteria are called *cocci.*
- Rod-shaped bacteria are called *bacilli.*
- Spiral-shaped bacteria are called *spirilla.* Tightly coiled spirilla are called *spirochetes.*

Certain arrangements are also seen with different bacteria. For example, when bacteria are in a chain formation, the prefix *strepto-* is used; when bacteria are found in pairs, the prefix *diplo-* is used; and when they are found in grapelike clusters, the prefix *staphylo-* is used. Cocci in packets of 4 are called *tetrads,* and in packets of 8 or 16 they are called *sarcinae* (Figure 50.3).

Bacterial Oxygen Requirements

Bacteria are also classified according to oxygen requirements:

- *Aerobes*: Bacteria that require oxygen to live. An aerobic example is *Mycobacterium tuberculosis*, which thrives in white blood cells in the lungs
- *Anaerobes*: Bacteria that die in the presence of oxygen. An anaerobic example is *Bacteroides fragilis,* a gram-negative rod-shaped bacterium. *B. fragilis* is part of the normal flora in the colon.

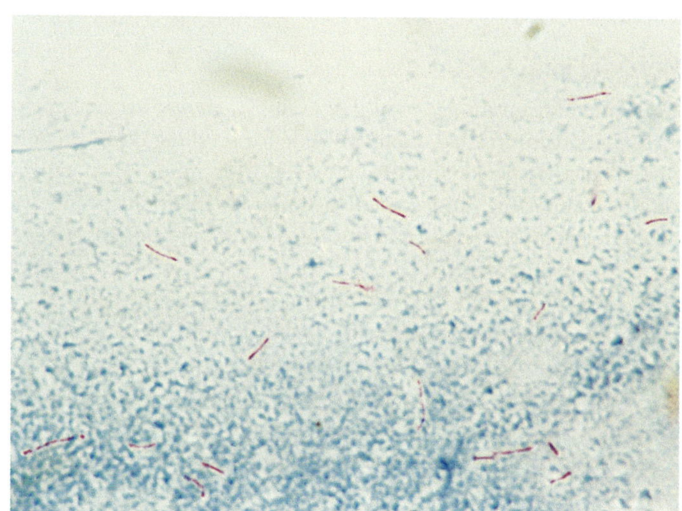

FIGURE 50.2 Acid-fast stain. (From De la Maza LM, Pezzlo MT, Baron EJ: *Color atlas of diagnostic microbiology,* St. Louis, 1997, Mosby.)

- *Facultative anaerobes*: Bacteria that are flexible regarding their oxygen needs; they can survive in the presence of oxygen but prefer to live without oxygen. *E. coli,* which is also found in the intestine, is an example of a facultative anaerobe.

Bacterial Physical Structures

Bacteria can be classified and identified according to additional physical structures. Some bacteria have long thin **flagella** that help them move. Some bacteria have a thick, jelly-like substance that surrounds the cell wall called a capsule, which can make the bacteria more pathogenic. Other bacteria form intracellular structures called an endospore. An **endospore** allows the bacteria to remain **viable** when environmental conditions are poor. *Clostridium tetani* produces spores; if spores enter a wound and grow, they cause the disease known as tetanus.

See Table 50.1 for a list of some important infectious diseases caused by pathogenic bacilli, cocci, and spirilla.

CRITICAL THINKING APPLICATION **50.1**

In your own words, write a brief description of the term *capsule.* What advantage does a bacterium have if a capsule surrounds it? Share your thoughts with the class.

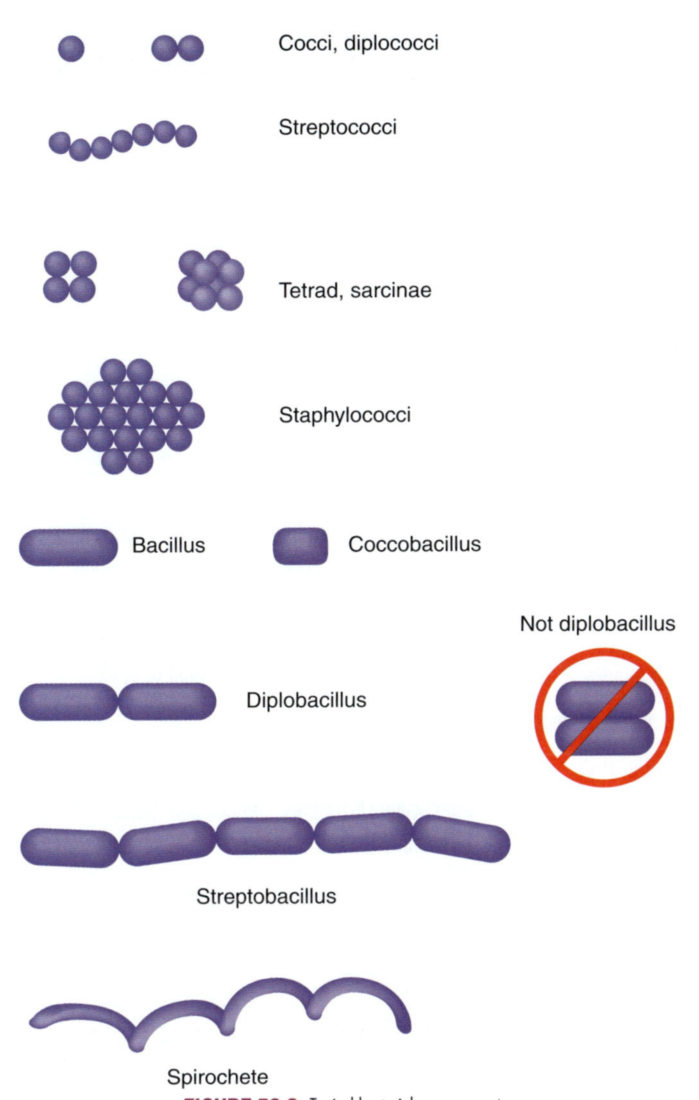

FIGURE 50.3 Typical bacterial arrangements.

PATHOGENS

Pathogens are disease-causing organisms. This section discusses several types of pathogens, including unusual pathogenic bacteria, fungi, protozoa, parasites, helminths, and viruses.

Unusual Pathogenic Bacteria

Typical pathogenic bacteria measure 1000 to 5000 nanometer (nm). Chlamydia, mycoplasma, and rickettsia are tiny, unusual bacteria that fall between the size ranges of typical pathogenic bacteria and viruses (Table 50.2).

- *Chlamydia*: Require host cells for growth.
- *Rickettsia*: Transmitted by blood-sucking insects and cannot multiply outside a living host cell.
- *Mycoplasmas*: Do not contain peptidoglycan in their cell wall. For example, *Mycoplasma pneumonia,* which causes "walking pneumonia," is a gram-negative bacterium that does not have a cell wall.

Pathogenic Fungi

Mycology is the study of fungi and the diseases they cause (see Table 50.2). Fungi are **eukaryotes** that are larger than bacteria and have a nucleus. Fungi include yeasts and **molds**. Fungi are present in the soil, air, and water, but only a few species cause disease. They are transmitted by the following:

- Direct contact with infected persons
- Prolonged exposure to a moist environment
- Inhalation of contaminated dust or soil

Some fungal infections affect the skin, hair, or nails. Tinea infections, such as ringworm and athlete's foot, are examples of these types of fungal infections. Some fungi can penetrate the tissues of the internal body structures and cause serious diseases of the mucous membranes, heart, and lungs.

A diagnosis of a fungal skin infection is usually based on culturing skin scrapings or microscopic observation of skin scrapings. Before

TABLE 50.1 Common Diseases Caused by Bacilli, Cocci, and Spirilla

CAUSED BY	DISEASE STATE	CAUSATIVE AGENT	TRANSMISSION
Bacilli	Botulism	*Clostridium botulinum*	Improperly cooked canned foods
	Clostridium difficile (C. diff)	*Clostridium difficile*	May be a healthcare-acquired infection (HAI), frequent antibiotic use increases likelihood; idiopathic
	Diphtheria	*Corynebacterium diphtheriae*	Inhalation
	Legionnaire's disease	*Legionella pneumophilia*	Grows readily in air-conditioning systems (standing water)
	Pertussis (whooping cough)	*Bordetella pertussis*	Respiratory secretions
	Salmonella infection	*Salmonella* species	Food-borne illness
	Tetanus (lockjaw)	*Clostridium tetani*	Open fractures, soil-contaminated wounds, open wounds, puncture wounds

continued

TABLE 50.1 Common Diseases Caused by Bacilli, Cocci, and Spirilla—continued

CAUSED BY	DISEASE STATE	CAUSATIVE AGENT	TRANSMISSION
	Tuberculosis	*Mycobacterium tuberculosis*	Airborne, inhalation
	Urinary tract infection (UTI)	Various, most common include the following: • Escherichia coli • Proteus species • Klebsiella species • Pseudomonas aeruginosa	Bacteria-contaminated urethra, catheterization
Cocci	Gonorrhea	*Neisseria gonorrhoeae*	Sexually transmitted
	Meningococcal meningitis	*Neisseria meningitidis*	Respiratory tract secretions
	Methicillin-resistant *Staphylococcus aureus* (MRSA) infection	Methicillin-resistant *Staphylococcus aureus*	Healthcare-acquired infection (HIA), direct contact, **fomites**, carriers, poor hand washing technique
	Pneumonia	*Streptococcus pneumoniae*	Direct contact, droplets
	Staphylococcal food poisoning	*Staphylococcus aureus*	Poor hygiene, improper refrigeration of foods
	Strep throat	*Streptococcus pyogenes*, also known as group A strep	Direct contact, droplets, fomites
	Wound infections, abscesses, boils	*Staphylococcus aureus*	Direct contact, fomites, carriers, poor hand washing technique
Spirilla	Food-borne illness (most commonly seen in the United States)	*Campylobacter jejuni*	Contaminated and undercooked food, contaminated water and milk
	Lyme disease	*Borrelia burgdorferi*	Tick bite
	Pyloric ulcers	*Helicobacter pylori*	Unknown, possibly food/water-borne
	Syphilis	*Treponema pallidum*	Sexually or congenitally

microscopic observation, the samples are treated with potassium hydroxide (KOH) to dissolve nonfungal material, making the fungal elements easier to observe. Fungal infections must be treated with antifungal medications.

CRITICAL THINKING APPLICATION 50.2

Fungi include two other types of organisms. Name these organisms. Share your answers with the class.

Pathogenic Protozoa

Protozoa are single-celled parasitic organisms that contain a nucleus. They range in size from microscopic to *macroscopic* (visible to the naked eye) (see Table 50.2). They are present in moist environments and in bodies of water, such as lakes and ponds. Protozoa are transmitted through contaminated feces, food, and drink. Some pathogenic protozoa inhabit the bloodstream; others inhabit the intestines and genital tract. Diagnosis usually is based on the patient's signs and symptoms and on microscopic examination of stool or blood.

Pathogenic Parasites

Parasitology includes the study of all parasitic organisms that live on or in the human body (see Table 50.2). In a parasitic relationship, the host is harmed, and the parasite thrives. Parasites are transmitted by ingestion, direct penetration of the skin, and injection by an **arthropod**, also referred to as a **vector**. A parasite cannot be identified accurately based on a single test or specimen. Parasites are frequently identified in feces, blood, urine, **sputum**, tissue fluid, or tissue biopsy samples.

Pathogenic Helminths

Helminths are parasites called worms. Helminths live on or in another living organism. They sustain themselves at the expense of the host organism. They can live in animals or humans. Worms are usually transmitted through the soil, by infected clothing or fingernails, after contact with infected persons, or through contaminated food/water. Helminths go through the same life cycle as other worms. The adult worm lays eggs (ova). The ova develop into larvae, which grow into adult worms, and the cycle begins again. Diagnosis usually is based on a microscopic examination of feces for ova (eggs) and parasites, and on patient signs and symptoms (Figure 50.4).

TABLE 50.2 Common Diseases Caused by Pathogens

CAUSED BY	DISEASE STATE	CAUSATIVE AGENT	TRANSMISSION
Rickettsia, mycoplasma, and chlamydia	Atypical or walking pneumonia	*Mycoplasma pneumoniae*	Respiratory secretions
	Inclusion conjunctivitis or pneumonia	*Chlamydia trachomatis*	During the birth process
	Nongonococcal urethritis or vaginitis	*Chlamydia trachomatis*	Sexually
	Rocky Mountain spotted fever	*Rickettsia rickettsii*	Tick bite
	Typhus (epidemic)	*Rickettsia prowazekii*	Body lice bite
	Typhus (endemic)	*Rickettsia typhi*	Flea bite
Fungi	Candidiasis, vulvovaginal, monilial (vaginal yeast)	*Candida* species (yeast)	After antibiotic therapy; using hormonal birth control; diabetes-type I, II; gestational; AIDS
	Cryptococcosis	*Cryptococcus neoformans*	Contact with poultry droppings
	Fungal infections; athlete's foot, jock itch, ringworm	*Tinea species and others*	Direct contact with an infected person or animal, damp surfaces
	Histoplasmosis	*Histoplasma capsulatum*	Inhaling dust contaminated with bird or bat droppings
	Pneumocystis pneumonia	*Pneumocystis jiroveci*	Contact with animals, most likely in immune-compromised patients, common in AIDS patients
	Thrush (in the mouth)	*Candida* species (yeast)	Possibly during birth process, after antibiotic therapy, diabetes, or weakened immune system
Protozoa and parasites	Amoebic dysentery	*Entamoeba histolytica*	Fecal contamination of food or water
	Giardiasis	*Giardia lamblia*	Contaminated water, opportunist in intestinal tract
	Lice	*Pediculus humanus* (head and body lice), *Phthirus pubis* (pubic lice)	Direct contact, contaminated clothing, bedding, furniture, personal items (combs, hats, etc.)
	Malaria	*Plasmodium* species	Bite of the *Anopheles* mosquito
	Pinworm	*Enterobius vermicularis*	Fecal-oral contamination
	Scabies	*Sarcoptes scabiei*	Direct contact, contaminated clothing, bedding
	Tapeworm: beef or pork	*Taenia* species	Eating undercooked beef or pork
	Tapeworm: fish	*Diphyllobothrium latum*	Eating undercooked fish
	Toxoplasmosis	*Toxoplasma gondii*	Fecal contamination from cat litter, congenitally
	Trichinosis	*Trichinella spiralis*	Eating undercooked pork or bear

Continued

TABLE 50.2 Common Diseases Caused by Pathogens—*continued*

CAUSED BY	DISEASE STATE	CAUSATIVE AGENT	TRANSMISSION
Viruses	Acquired immunodeficiency syndrome (AIDS)	Human immunodeficiency virus (HIV)	Sexual intercourse/contact, sharing needles, at-risk behavior
	Common cold	Rhinovirus most common among many possible	Direct contact, inhaling droplets, fomites
	Coronavirus disease (COVID-19)	Severe acute respiratory syndrome coronavirus 2 (SARS-CoV-2)	Airborne
	Ebola	Ebola virus species (five identified)	Direct contact with infected blood or body fluids (bloodborne)
	Human papillomavirus (HPV) infection	Human papillomavirus	Sexually, direct skin to skin and indirect contact
	Infectious mononucleosis	Epstein-Barr virus	Direct contact and airborne saliva/body fluids—kissing, same eating utensils
	Influenza	Myxovirus, influenza A and B	Droplet and fomites—cough, sneeze, or talk
	Measles	Paramyxovirus—measles virus	Direct contact, inhaling droplets
	Molluscum contagiosum warts	Molluscipoxvirus	Direct contact with an infected person—skin to skin
	Mumps	Paramyxovirus—mumps virus	Inhaling droplets, shared utensils with infected person
	Polio	Poliovirus	Direct contact, feces, via mouth (saliva), sneeze, cough
	Rubella (German measles)	Rubella virus	Direct contact, inhaling droplets from sneeze or cough, congenitally from mother

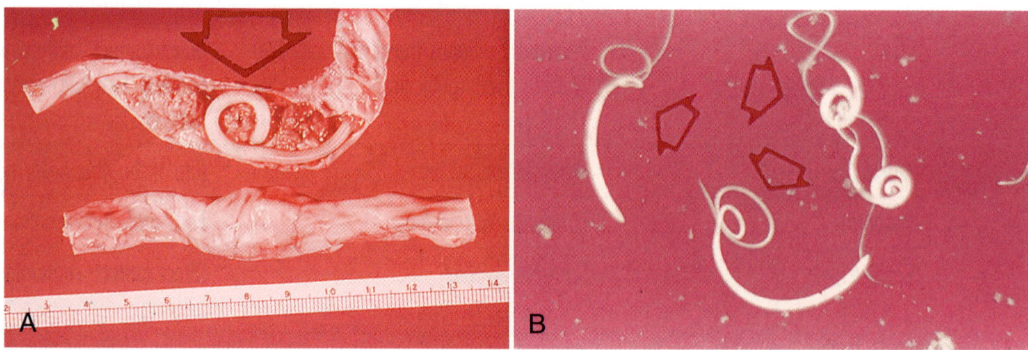

FIGURE 50.4 **(A)** Roundworms. **(B)** Whipworms. (From Stepp CA, Woods MA: *Laboratory procedures for medical office personnel*, Philadelphia, 1998, Saunders.)

Pathogenic Viruses

Many scientists do not consider viruses to be microorganisms because they are not alive. Viruses are not able to metabolize or reproduce unless they are inside of a host cell. Viruses have their own enzymes but must use the host cell **organelles** and **macromolecules** to reproduce and metabolize. Because of the absolute need for a host cell, a virus can be considered an obligate intracellular pathogen.

Viruses consist of a genetic core covered by a protein coat called a *capsid*. Some viruses have an additional spiked layer of protection over the capsid called an envelope. A viral genetic core is made up of either ribonucleic acid (RNA) or deoxyribonucleic acid (DNA). The RNA or DNA contains information about how and what the host cell needs to produce to form a new virus. The genetic material is like a recipe for a new viral particle.

A virus cannot be cultured on solid nutrient media, such as those used to culture bacteria and fungi. Viruses must be cultured in fertilized eggs or in a **tissue culture**, which is done by referral, research, or large hospital laboratories.

Usually, instead of culturing a specimen for a virus, the patient's blood sample is tested for a specific antibody related to the possible viral infection. For example, in the diagnosis of Lyme disease, patient serum is tested for the specific antibody produced in response to the Lyme **antigen**. This form of testing is referred to as serology or immunology testing (discussed later in the chapter). Table 50.2 lists common diseases caused by viruses.

CRITICAL THINKING APPLICATION 50.3

Looking at Table 50.2, pick four viral diseases that you are familiar with. Write down the disease, the virus that causes it, and two ways to prevent the infection. Be ready to share your answers with the class.

SPECIMEN COLLECTION AND TRANSPORT IN THE PHYSICIAN OFFICE LABORATORY

Specimen collection and handling are important considerations in patient care because the results are only as good as the quality of the sample. Ideally, specimens should be collected during the **acute phase** of an illness and before antibiotics are prescribed. Specimens for microbiology testing can include urine, stool, sputum, and blood. Sterile swabs can be used to collect samples from wounds and the upper respiratory tract.

Guidelines for Specimen Collection

Specimens must be collected carefully so that contaminating microorganisms are not introduced into the specimen. This means not only using sterile collection and transport devices, but also taking steps to prevent contamination. To prevent from contaminating the specimen, the person should do the following:

- Wash hands before collecting the sample.
- Cleanse the area involved with an **antiseptic**, if appropriate. For example, when obtaining a clean-catch midstream urine specimen, antiseptic wipes are used.
- Open sterile containers only when necessary and avoid touching the inside surfaces.
- Never touch a sterile swab or collection device to a nonsterile surface.

If patients are expected to collect a sample, it is crucial that they receive clear instructions on how to perform the procedure correctly and without contaminating the sample. The referral laboratory is responsible for providing a manual of written instructions to the POL. The POL is responsible for providing clear oral and written instructions to the patient. If the patient will be collecting the sample in private or at home, written instructions that are simple and straightforward should be supplied.

To protect from pathogen exposure, the medical assistant should wear the appropriate personal protective equipment (PPE) when collecting, handling, and processing specimens. The medical assistant should wear gloves, a fluid-impermeable lab coat, a surgical mask (for droplet or airborne pathogens), and protective eyewear or a face shield. Proper handwashing techniques are also important before and after the procedure.

The following sections discuss transporting specimens and how to collect different types of specimens.

Guidelines for Handling and Transporting Specimens

The transport of specimens to referral laboratories is also crucial. Different types of transport devices are available. Close attention must be given to their proper use. Microorganisms are living organisms, so they must be given conditions that ensure their survival. Care must also be taken so that any normal flora in the sample will not multiply and overgrow possible pathogens. The type and number of microorganisms in the sample should reflect the type and number of microorganisms at the site of collection and at the time of collection.

Specialized transport media are often included with specimen collection swabs or devices (Figure 50.5). Collection devices typically consist of a plastic tube that encases a sterile Dacron swab and a sealed vial of **transport medium**. After the specimen has been collected on the swab, it is placed in the plastic tube with the transport medium. It is essential to follow the manufacturer's directions to prevent the swab and specimen from drying out. Transport system swabs also have a label that must be filled out completely, indicating the patient's full name, the date and time of collection, the collector's initials, and the source of the specimen (e.g., deep wound sample from left leg abscess).

If possible, a specimen should be placed on culture media immediately after collection. If this is not possible, then the transport device must be sent to a referral laboratory or held in the POL until it can be cultured. For specimens that will be transported by a courier, make sure the specimen is safely packaged in a leak-proof container marked with warning labels (Figure 50.6). The proper time and temperature of storage are vital. Most pathogenic organisms prefer body temperatures, approximately 37°C (98.6°F). They will remain viable for up to 72 hours if held at room temperature or refrigerator temperature (4°C [39.2°F]). Some organisms die if exposed to cold temperatures. Always check the referral laboratory's procedure manual for directions regarding sample time and temperature of storage.

See Figure 50.7 for some commonly used microbiology collection devices. Devices used for both aerobic and anaerobic blood collection are shown in Figure 50.7A, and BACTEC blood culture bottles are pictured in Figure 50.7B. Two other commonly used transportation devices are the JEMBEC plate for transporting Neisseria gonorrhoeae (see Figure 50.7C) and a viral-chlamydial transport medium (see Figure 50.7D).

See Table 50.3 for a description of the specimens, containers, patient preparation processes, and storage of specimens commonly collected or handled by medical assistants.

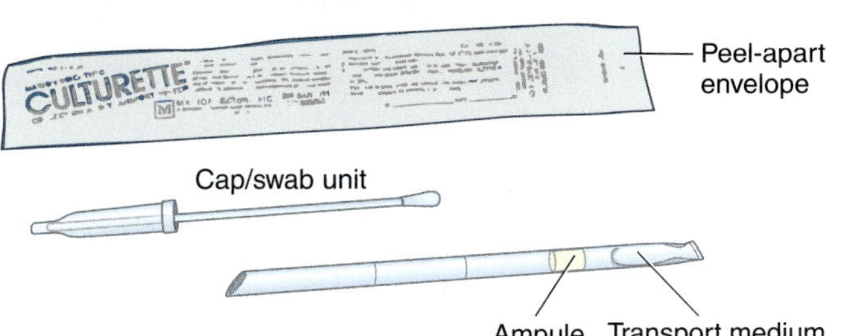

FIGURE 50.5 Collection and transport system for patient samples.

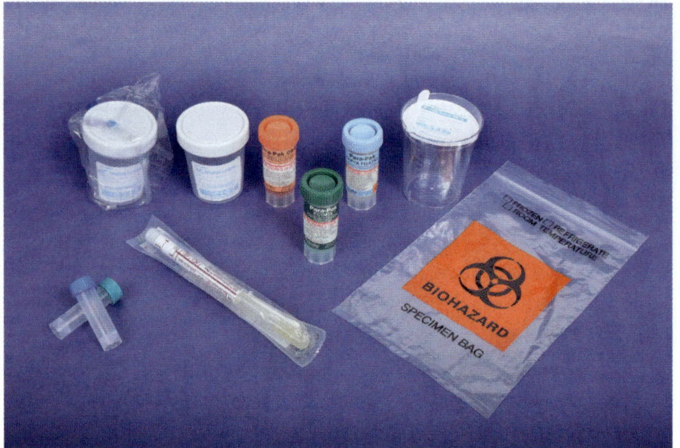

FIGURE 50.6 Microbiology specimen containers.

CRITICAL THINKING APPLICATION **50.4**

Each time Laura collects a wound swab that needs to be sent to the reference laboratory, she needs to put the swab in a transport medium. List three reasons why we use transport media when wound specimens cannot be tested immediately. Be ready to share your ideas with the class.

Stool Specimen Collection

Stool specimens are commonly examined for parasitic protozoa and helminths. The specimen is collected and placed into two vials, each with a preservative. From these preparations, a **wet mount** slide is made to observe moving organisms. A stained smear is made from a concentrated specimen. The smear is looked at under a microscope to observe protozoal cysts and helminth eggs. The medical assistant

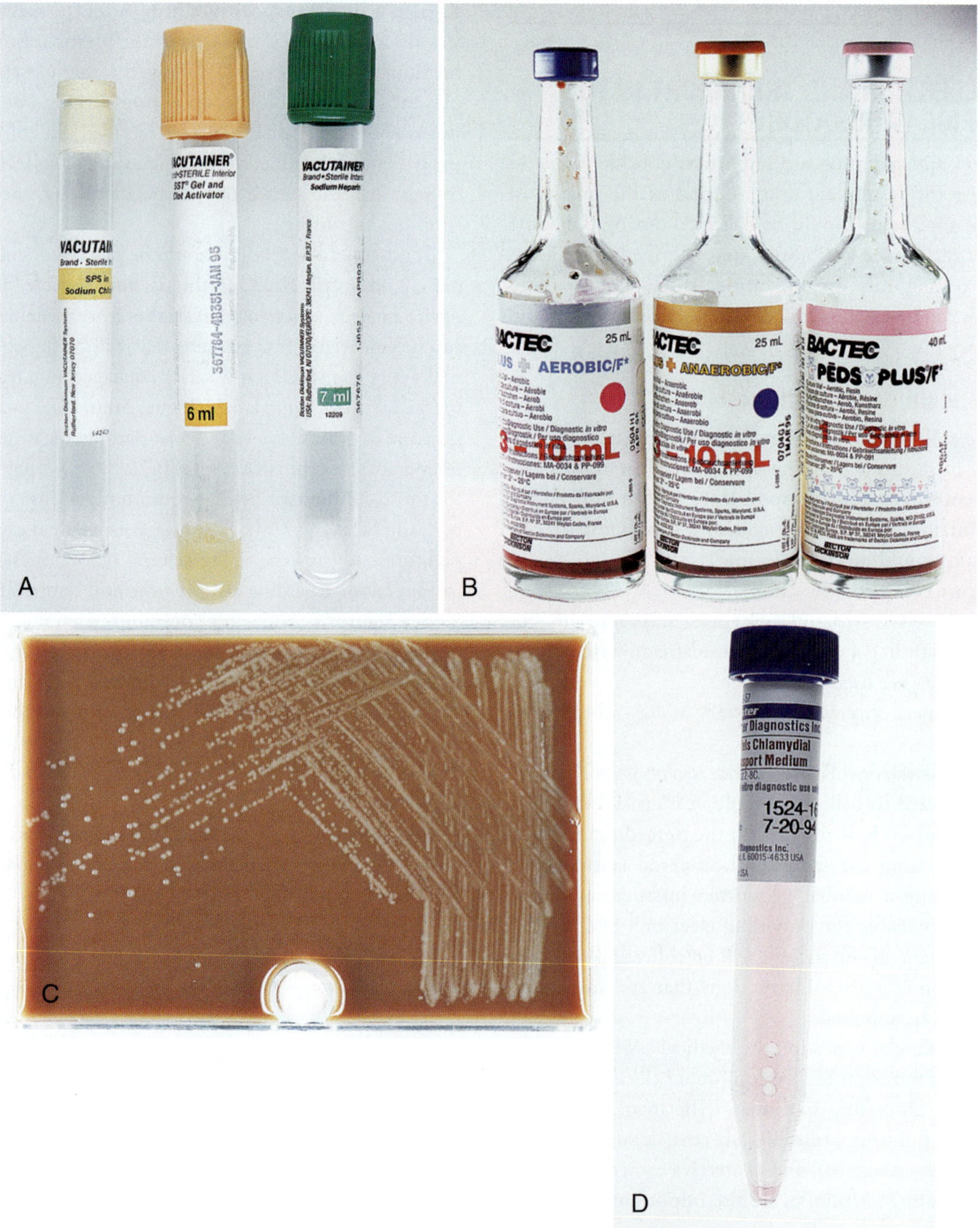

FIGURE 50.7 **(A)** Blood collection Vacutainer tubes, one for aerobic and one for anaerobic. **(B)** Bactec blood culture bottles. **(C)** Jembec plate. **(D)** Viral-chlamydial transport medium. (From De la Maza LM, Pezzlo MT, Baron EJ: *Color atlas of diagnostic microbiology*, St. Louis, 1997, Mosby.)

TABLE 50.3 Collection, Transport, and Processing of Specimens Commonly Collected in the Physician Office Laboratory[a]

SPECIMEN	CONTAINER	PATIENT PREPARATION	SPECIAL INSTRUCTIONS	STORAGE BEFORE PROCESSING
Throat	Transport swab (see Figure 50.5)	Have patient sitting with head tilted back	Swab pharynx and tonsils, not mouth, tongue, or teeth	Transport and plate within 24 hr; room-temperature storage
Superficial wound	Aerobic transport swab (see Figure 50.5)	Wipe area with sterile saline before collection	Rotate swab while gently swiping wound	Transport swab stored at room temperature
Eye	Aerobic transport swab (see Figure 50.5)	Pull lower lid down while gently collecting exudate along rim	Not applicable	Transport swab may be stored up to 24 hr at room temperature
Ova and parasite (O&P)	O&P transport containers (with formalin and PVA) (see Figure 50.6)	See Procedure 50.1 for collection of a stool specimen for ova and parasites	Wait 7–10 days if patient has been taking Pepto-Bismol, Kaopectate, or milk of magnesia	Store at room temperature and deliver to laboratory within 24 hr
Stool	Clean, leak-proof containers (see Figure 50.6)	Outpatients: At minimum, three specimens are collected every other day	Transport to laboratory within 24 hr if storing at 4°C (39.2°F)	Laboratory must plate within 72 hr if storing at 4°C (39.2°F)
Sputum	Sterile, screw-cap container (see Figure 50.6)	Patient should rinse or gargle with mouthwash before collection	Have patient collect from deep cough; do not collect saliva	Store at 4°C (39.2°F); laboratory must plate within 24 hr
Urine	Vacutainer collection system or sterile, screw-cap container (see Figure 50.6)	Instruct patient in clean-catch midstream collection	Hold at 4°C (39.2°F), and deliver to laboratory within 24 hr	Hold at 4°C (39.2° F), and plate within 24 hr
Skin scraping (fungal culture)	Clean, screw-top tube (see Figure 50.6)	Wipe skin with alcohol wipe	Scrape skin at leading edge of lesion	Can be held indefinitely at room temperature but best to process within 72 hr of collection
Blood	Blood culture tube with SPS medium (see Figure 50.7A) or Vacutainer blood culture medium (see Figure 50.7B)	Disinfect venipuncture site with alcohol wipe and Betadine	Draw blood during febrile episodes	Deliver to laboratory within 2 hr; incubate at 37°C (98.6°F) on receipt in the laboratory
Gonorrhea culture	Jembec transport system (see Figure 50.7C)	Wipe away exudate before obtaining culture specimen; obtain culture specimen with swab	Do not refrigerate	Transport to laboratory within 2 hr
Chlamydia culture	Specialized antibiotic *Chlamydia* transport medium (see Figure 50.7D)	Urogenital swabs preferred; necessary to obtain epithelial cells, not exudate	Transport immediately on ice to laboratory	Store up to 24 hr at 4°C (39.2°F); inoculate cultures within 15 min of collection if swab is not on ice
Body fluids (e.g., peritoneal, synovial, pleural)	Sterile, screw-cap container or anaerobic transporter	Disinfect aspiration site with alcohol wipe and Betadine	Needle aspirations are preferable to swab collections	Transport immediately to laboratory

Continued

TABLE 50.3 Collection, Transport, and Processing of Specimens Commonly Collected in the Physician Office Laboratory[a]—*continued*

SPECIMEN	CONTAINER	PATIENT PREPARATION	SPECIAL INSTRUCTIONS	STORAGE BEFORE PROCESSING
Rectal swab	Swab placed directly into enteric transport medium	Not applicable	Insert swab approximately 1 inch past anal sphincter	Store at 4°C (39.2°F), transport within 24 hr to laboratory, and plate within 72 hr
Deep wound or abscess	Anaerobic transport device	Wipe area with sterile saline or alcohol wipe before collection	Aspirate material, excise tissue, or insert swab deep into wound	Store at room temperature; transport to laboratory and plate within 4 hr

[a]Reference laboratories also have specific directions for collecting specimens based on their testing methods.
O&P, Ova and parasites; *PVA,* polyvinyl alcohol; *SPS,* Sodium polyanethole sulfonate.
Modified from Forbes BA, Sahm DF, Weissfeld AS: *Bailey and Scott's diagnostic microbiology,* ed 11, St. Louis, 2002, Mosby.

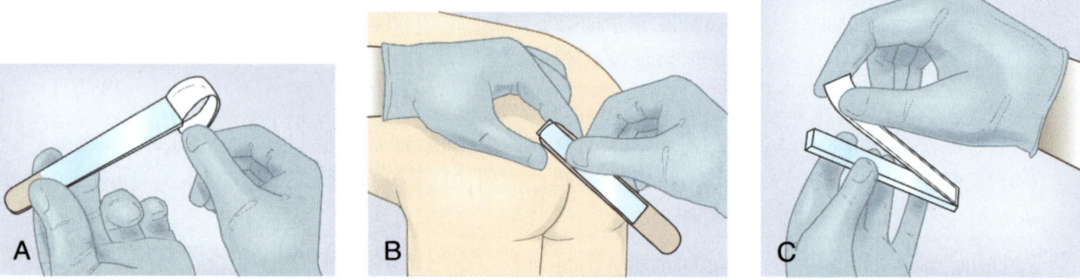

FIGURE 50.8 The three steps for collecting a pinworm specimen from a child. **(A)** Place cellulose tape over a tongue depressor with the sticky side out. **(B)** Press the tape firmly against the right and left anal folds. **(C)** Place the tape with adhesive side down onto the microscope slide.

should always consult the procedure manual provided by the referral laboratory when an ova and parasites stool examination (O&P) is ordered to make sure that proper specimen collection and transport takes place (Procedure 50.1).

Pinworm Collection

Enterobius vermicularis is commonly known as pinworm. The eggs hatch in the small intestine, and the females migrate out of the anus, usually at night, to deposit the eggs. The eggs adhere to the skin and hair surrounding the anus, sleeping garments, and other clothing. Pinworms cause itching in the anal area, which may cause the eggs to come in contact with the hands and fingernails of the host.

Pinworm infection is spread by the fecal-oral route. The infective pinworm eggs are transferred to the mouth directly by the hand or indirectly through contaminated clothing, food, liquids, and other articles. Since the pinworm eggs are so small, they can sometimes become airborne and are ingested while breathing.

In children, specimens are best collected late at night or early in the morning. Paraffin swabs impregnated with petroleum jelly or cellulose tape may be used to collect the eggs deposited by the adult worm during the night. The diagnosis is based on laboratory detection of the eggs in fecal smears. Some parents do not feel comfortable collecting the specimen. The medical assistant should instruct those parents to bring children to the office as soon as they wake up in the morning. Instruct the parents not to change the child's clothing or diaper before coming into the office. When the child arrives, have all the needed supplies ready to use, and perform the procedure immediately (Figure 50.8).

Nasal and Nasopharyngeal Specimen Collection

Nasal and nasopharyngeal specimens are obtained for several respiratory tests, including COVID-19. Depending on the state's medical assistant scope of practice, a medical assistant may be able to perform nasal and nasopharyngeal specimen collection (Procedure 50.2). The types of swabs used depend on the test and the collection site.

Three types of specimens can be collected:

- *Anterior nasal specimen:* The swab is inserted no more than 0.5 of an inch (1 cm) into the nostril (Figure 50.9).
- *Mid-turbinate nasal specimen*: With the patient's head tilted back at a 70-degree angle, the swab is inserted parallel to the nostril floor until resistance is met at the nasal turbinates. The swab is usually inserted no more than 1 inch (2 cm). This specimen is taken deeper into the nose than the anterior nasal specimen.
- Nasopha*ryngeal (NP) specimen:* When obtaining the specimen, the patient's head should be tilted back at a 70-degree angle. The minitip swab needs to be inserted through the nostril. Insert the swab so it is parallel to the palate, and continue to carefully insert it until resistance is encountered. The swab needs to be inserted the same distance as the nostril to the outer opening of the ear.

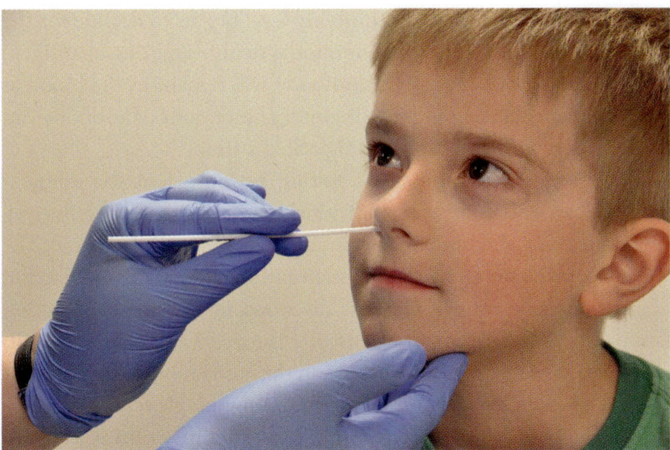

FIGURE 50.9 Obtaining an anterior nasal specimen.

The swab should be gently rolled and then left in place for several seconds to allow it to absorb secretions. A specimen is obtained from both nostrils unless the swab is saturated with secretions from the first nostril. If the patient has a nasal blockage or deviated septum, the unobstructed nostril should be used for the collection.

Sputum Specimen Collection

Sputum cultures may be ordered when patients have symptoms that may be related to infectious respiratory diseases. The following are examples of other sputum tests:

- Legionella testing for legionnaires' disease
- Acid-fast bacillus (AFB) testing for tuberculosis
- Gram stain for bacterial or fungal infections

The medical assistant may be responsible for coaching patients on how to collect sputum specimens. Many times, sputum specimens are collected in the morning. For some tests, three sputum samples may be collected over 3 days. When collecting a sputum specimen, patients should do the following:

1. Avoid food for 1 to 2 hours before collecting the sputum specimen.
2. Rinse your mouth well to remove food particles.
3. Open the container and avoid touching the inside of the container and cover.
4. Inhale two to three times, breathing out hard each time, then cough deeply.
5. Collect the sputum from the cough. Do not spit oral secretions into the cup.
6. Cover the container when enough sputum is collected.

The medical assistant should discuss how the specimen should be stored and brought to the healthcare facility for testing.

Throat Swab Specimen Collection

A throat swab specimen collection is a common procedure in the ambulatory care facility. This type of specimen is used to identify the cause of throat infections, such as strep throat. It is important that patients resist gagging and closing their mouths while the swabbing occurs. Procedure 50.3 describes the collection process. Patients should not use antiseptic mouthwash prior to the collection.

Wound Swab Specimen Collection

To perform a wound culture, the medical assistant will need the following items:

- A provider's order
- A culture swab with the patient's label, specimen bag for transport, and the laboratory requisition form
- Supplies to clean the wound (such as betadine)
- Dressing and bandages

The provider may have the medical assistant rinse the wound with normal saline to remove contaminated material (e.g., necrotic tissue and dried exudate). If the wound is dry, the swab should be moistened with sterile normal saline (NS). This helps with the collection process. If the wound is moist, no saline is needed.

To collect the specimen, the medical assistant should gently roll the swab stick from margin to margin using a zig-zag motion, using enough pressure to accumulate fluid on the swab. If pus is seen, it should be swabbed. The swab should only touch the wound. After the collection, the swab should be placed in a labeled tube. If the tube has formalin, squeeze the tube to release the formalin to preserve the specimen before sending it to the laboratory.

CLIA-WAIVED MICROBIOLOGY TESTING

Often, growing a pathogen on a nutrient media plate is difficult, and it takes time to grow and isolate the pathogen. A rapid direct immunology test demonstrates the presence of the antigen in a specimen that is placed in a test kit containing its specific antibody. If the pathogen is present, it produces a colored reaction, indicating a positive result.

POLs with appropriate CLIA-waived certification can perform many rapid identification tests for a variety of infectious diseases. Rapid tests are designed to give the provider positive test results quickly and efficiently so that treatment can be started. If the test result is negative, the provider may need to order additional referral laboratory tests:

The first step in performing these tests is to review the package insert provided by the manufacturer. This gives valuable information about the test:

- Principle on which the test is based
- Reagents and equipment needed
- Proper specimen collection techniques
- Patient preparation requirements
- Test procedures
- Any precautions or warnings pertaining to the procedure

The insert also provides information about quality control, interpretation of results, limitations of the procedure, and references.

Rapid Strep Testing

Rapid strep testing is commonly performed in the POL and can be completed while the patient waits. The patient's throat is swabbed. The test swab is placed in an **extraction** well, and the **extract** is tested for antigens found on the surface of *S. pyogenes* (also referred to as *Group A streptococcus* [GAS]). The test kit uses a lateral flow immunoassay. This means that the specimen "flows" into the test area. If the strep A pathogen is present, there will be an antigen-antibody reaction with the group A strep antibodies in the testing area. The reaction of the strep A antigen and the strep A antibodies cause a color change that can be seen (Procedure 50.4).

Negative test results should be confirmed with a throat culture performed in the microbiology laboratory (explained later in the chapter). The rapid strep tests are highly specific, so if the test results are positive, there is confidence that *S. pyogenes* is present in the sample. If the test results are negative, the organism may not have been present in high enough numbers to be detected. Then, a transport swab should be sent to the microbiology reference laboratory to be cultured.

CRITICAL THINKING APPLICATION **50.5**

Frankie Burns, a 10-year-old, has a raw, sore throat; fever of 101°F; and just feels awful. Laura is going to collect a throat swab from Frankie for a rapid strep test. What bacteria cause strep throat? What is the scientific name of the bacteria? Which of the two names is the genus, and which of the two names is the species?

Influenza A and B Testing

The *influenza* virus causes influenza, or "the flu." This is a highly contagious, acute viral infection of the respiratory tract. The infection is highly communicable through respiratory exposure, and outbreaks are typically seen in the fall and winter. Type A viruses usually are more common than type B viruses. Type A viruses typically are associated with epidemics, and type B viruses cause a milder infection. A rapid diagnosis of influenza can help with the decision to give antiviral medications. They should be given early in the infection cycle to be the most effective. CLIA-waived rapid lateral flow immunoassays detect both influenza A and influenza B antigens from **nasal washes** or nasopharyngeal swabs.

Respiratory Syncytial Virus Testing

Respiratory syncytial virus (RSV) is a major cause of upper and lower respiratory tract infections. It is the major cause of **bronchiolitis** and **pneumonia** in children and infants. Outbreaks typically occur yearly in the fall, winter, and spring and can be severe for very young children. The CLIA-waived rapid direct immunoassay for RSV uses a nasopharyngeal swab specimen or nasal washings to detect the virus. Because antiviral agents are available to treat RSV infection, rapid diagnosis can lead to the following:

- Shorter hospital stays
- Reduced need for antibiotic therapy to treat secondary bacterial infection
- Lower cost for hospital care

The tests are intended for children under age 5.

CLIA-WAIVED IMMUNOLOGIC TESTING

Immunology testing provides information about past or present infections with bacteria or viruses. It also detects certain types of cancers. Testing done in the immunology department is designed to demonstrate the reaction between an antigen and its specific antibody. Antibodies are formed when the body encounters a foreign agent.

In the acute stage of a disease, the antibody level starts to rise and increases fourfold over the next several weeks. Paired testing of sera from the acute stage of illness and 2 weeks later that demonstrate a fourfold increase indicate the presence of the disease. During the later **convalescent stage**, the antibody level begins to decline for the next 3 to 6 months. Once the immune system recognizes an antigen, then antibodies are made. The antibody will remain in the blood at a low but detectable level for a lifetime. The amount of antibody can be measured with **serologic** testing called a **titer**.

Most serologic/immunologic testing performed in the ambulatory care center is done using individual test kits (e.g., strep, influenza, mononucleosis, and human immunodeficiency virus [HIV] tests). The difference is the source of the specimen and what the test is looking for.

The direct immunologic tests discussed in the previous section (strep test and influenza test) used a throat swab and nasal swab specimen. The test kits were detecting the antigen or pathogen causing the disease directly. In the indirect immunologic tests, the specimen is the patient's blood or serum. The blood or serum is tested to see whether the patient has produced the specific antibody to the pathogen in question. CLIA-waived immunology tests that can be performed by a medical assistant to detect antibodies to a pathogen include infectious mononucleosis, *Helicobacter pylori*, Lyme disease, and HIV tests.

Infectious Mononucleosis Testing

Infectious mononucleosis, commonly called mono, is an acute infectious disease caused by the Epstein-Barr virus (EBV). EBV is one of the many herpes viruses. The virus is especially common in teenagers. It is found most frequently in people 10 to 25 years of age and is seen occasionally in adults over the age of 25. In the United States, about 95% of adults between 35 and 40 have already been infected.

In children, the infection may pass unrecognized or result in a mild illness lasting only a few days. It is marked by sore throat, fever, swollen tonsils, and enlarged lymph nodes in the neck. In young people, some of the most common complications include the abrupt onset of fatigue, headaches, very swollen tonsils, enlarged lymph glands, and loss of appetite often associated with nausea. There may be a short or prolonged period (days or weeks) after the initial illness when the fatigue continues. Occasionally, complications occur, including the development of a swollen spleen or liver, referred to as hepatosplenomegaly.

Testing for mononucleosis involves a complete blood count (CBC) and immunology tests, such a CLIA-waived mononucleosis test. The CBC should reveal an increased number of lymphocytes that appear atypical on the blood smear. Due to the abnormally high number of mononuclear leukocytes in the blood, the illness was called mononucleosis. Most patients exposed to EBV produce a nonspecific **heterophile antibody** response to the virus. These heterophile antibodies in the patient's blood react with the heterophile antigens supplied in the test kit, resulting in a positive color reaction in the testing area of the kit (Procedure 50.5).

CRITICAL THINKING APPLICATION **50.6**

Allyson Anderson is 15 years old. She came into the clinic today with signs and symptoms of infectious mononucleosis. Laura is going to do a fingerstick on Allyson and do a mono test. What are the typical signs and symptoms of mono in a teenager? What is the mono test checking for in Allyson's blood?

Helicobacter pylori Testing

H. pylori is a spiral-shaped bacterium that can infect the stomach's mucous layer or lining. *H. pylori* causes more than 90% of duodenal ulcers and more than 80% of stomach ulcers. Several methods can be used to diagnose *H. pylori* infection. Serologic tests that measure specific H. pylori antibodies can determine whether a person has been infected. CLIA-waived rapid immunoassay tests use whole blood applied to a well in a test cartridge. The blood migrates from the well through the testing area of the cartridge. The presence of a line in the test area of the cartridge indicates the presence of antibodies to the pathogen *H. pylori.*

Lyme Disease Testing

Lyme disease is the most common insect-borne infectious disease in North America, and it is a significant public health concern. The spirochete bacterium *Borrelia burgdorferi* is the most common causative agent in Lyme disease.

The disease is contracted from an infected tick that bites a person. The bacteria are in the saliva of the tick. These ticks typically are found on deer, mice, dogs, horses, and birds. Infection occurs when the bacteria enter the tick bite. A characteristic bull's-eye rash, known as erythema migrans (EM), develops at the bite site in 60% to 80% of patients. Lyme disease progresses in three stages. If the person is not treated, the disease progresses. The spirochete bacterium invades the skin, joints, central nervous system (CNS), heart, and other locations. Arthritic or CNS syndromes often accompany late-stage disease and may be the only clinical symptoms that indicate the infection.

Lyme disease can be detected early with a CLIA-waived test, such as the Wampole PreVue *B. burgdorferi* test. This immunoassay tests for antibodies in whole blood. A sample of blood is applied to a test cartridge, a **diluent** is added, and the results are read in 20 minutes. The microbiology reference laboratory should verify any positive results.

HIV Testing

HIV attacks and destroys the T-helper (CD4) lymphocytes. The T-helper lymphocytes play a critical role in protecting the body against infection. They work with the B lymphocytes to produce the specific antibodies that fight infections. As the HIV infection destroys more T-helper cells, the body becomes less able to fight off infections and more susceptible to opportunistic infections. If HIV is not treated with antiretroviral (ARV) medications, acquired immunodeficiency syndrome (AIDS) eventually develops. HIV infections become AIDS when life-threatening infections and cancers begin to appear.

In 2013 the Centers for Disease Control and Prevention (CDC) and the World Health Organization (WHO) both advised preventive measures to control the disease. This requires early detection and early treatment of individuals infected with HIV. The sooner the virus is detected via immunology testing, the sooner treatment with ARV medications may begin.

Two CLIA-waived HIV tests are readily available to detect the presence of HIV antibodies in blood and in oral specimens. Patients at risk of HIV infection are now strongly encouraged to take a blood test available in POLs or outpatient clinics. Note that HIV is a bloodborne pathogen. The medical assistant should always follow the Bloodborne Pathogens Standard established by the Occupational Safety and Health Administration (OSHA) when collecting and testing all patient blood and body fluids. Remember, all patients are treated the same when it comes to the Bloodborne Pathogens Standards and Standard Precautions.

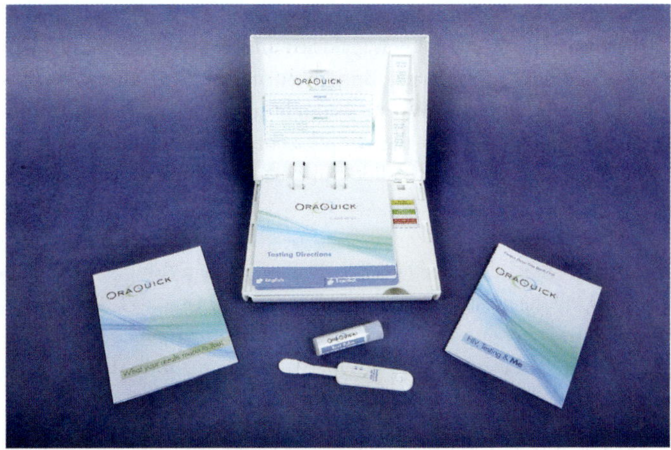

FIGURE 50.10 HIV home testing kit.

The patient may also choose to perform an oral self-test from a kit that is available at pharmacies (Figure 50.10). The test kit includes a testing device that is rubbed once over the upper and lower gums. It then is inserted into the test vial, which is placed in a plastic stand. The test results are read in 20 minutes. The test includes an internal control band that verifies a specimen was added and that the test was run correctly.

HIV Testing

For both HIV testing methods, it is important to provide the patient with information or counseling regarding HIV infection and its relationship to AIDS. Be aware that patients being tested may be fearful; therefore, proper knowledge presented in a therapeutic way can help them dispel the fear and take positive action toward preventive behavior and treatment. Positive HIV test results must be verified at a reference laboratory.

MICROBIOLOGY REFERENCE LABORATORY: IDENTIFICATION OF PATHOGENS

After receiving the specimens collected in the POL, the microbiology laboratory promptly inoculates the appropriate culture media first and then prepares a smear of the specimen on a slide to be stained (Figure 50.11). This ensures that the swab is not contaminated by the slide. If two swabs are received from the same source, one may be used for the culture and the other to make the smear. The equipment and supplies in a microbiology laboratory vary with the size of the facility. Most laboratories have a refrigerator, an autoclave, a safety cabinet, a microscope, and an incubator.

Staining

Pathogenic microorganisms generally are colorless, and a microscope is needed to see them. Special stains (e.g., Gram stain and acid-fast stain) are used to differentiate bacteria based on cell membrane differences. As discussed previously, Gram stain differentiates bacteria into two categories according to chemical makeup of the cell wall. The acid-fast stain differentiates bacteria into two categories based on the presence or absence of a waxy lipid in the cell wall.

Before staining can be done, the specimen must be applied to a labeled slide. The slide is then air-dried and fixed or adhered to the slide. Both heat (e.g., from a Bunsen burner or an incinerator) and methanol can be used to fix the sample to the slide. The heat and methanol cause protein in the sample to break down and stick to the slide. Note, overheating the slide can cause cell distortion.

Gram Stain

The Gram stain, developed by Dr. Hans Christian Gram in the late 1800s, is still the most commonly used stain in microbiology. This procedure involves applying a sequence of reagents: a primary stain, **mordant**, **decolorizer**, and *counterstain* (secondary stain) to the slide. The dyes are taken up differently according to the chemical composition of the bacterial cell walls. Bacteria react best in the Gram stain when they are less than 24 hours old. Gram-positive bacteria stain purple, and gram-negative bacteria stain pink or red (see Figure 50.1). It is useful for the medical assistant to understand the procedures and the microscopic results obtained. For example, when a Gram stain report is called in, the terms *GPCs* and *GNBs* mean "gram-positive cocci" (deeply blue-stained circular cells) and "gram-negative bacilli" (pink/red stained rod-shaped cells).

CRITICAL THINKING APPLICATION **50.7**

What are the four reagents used in the Gram stain? What color are gram-positive organisms? What color are gram-negative organisms? Share your answers with the class.

Acid-Fast Stain

The acid-fast stain is used in the identification protocol for Mycobacterium species. *M. tuberculosis* causes tuberculosis and can be isolated from sputum or tissue samples. *Mycobacterium avium complex (MAC)* is a common soil organism that enters through the respiratory tract and spreads throughout the body. MAC is one of the causes of death among patients with AIDS. An overview of the acid-fast stain is listed here:

- A red primary dye, carbolfuchsin, is applied first
- Then the decolorizer, acid-alcohol, is applied
- Followed by a counterstain, methylene blue

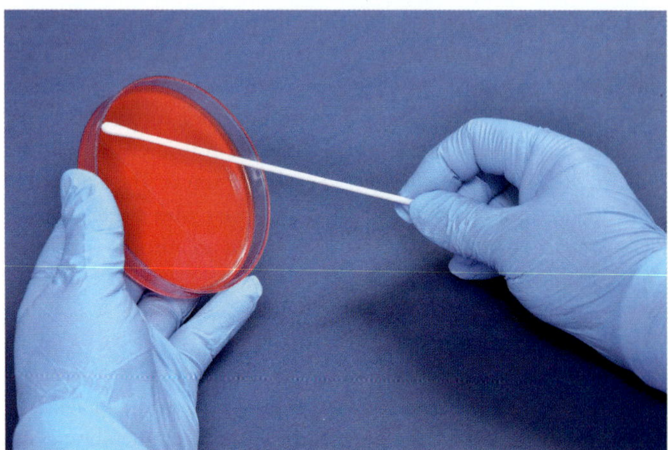

FIGURE 50.11 Inoculating a blood culture plate with a swab.

Acid-fast positive microbes stain fuchsia red. Acid-fast negative microbes stain baby blue. Bacilli that are acid-fast positive often are referred to as *acid-fast bacillus* (AFB) (see Figure 50.2).

Inoculating Equipment

Next, the specimen must be spread on specific culture media based on the source of the specimen. The inoculated culture media are placed in a body temperature incubator to grow overnight. Inoculating needles and loops (Figure 50.12) are used to transfer samples to culture media or microbes to slides for staining. Needles and loops may be disposable and presterilized. They may also be made of wire and can be heat sterilized before and after each transfer (Figure 50.13).

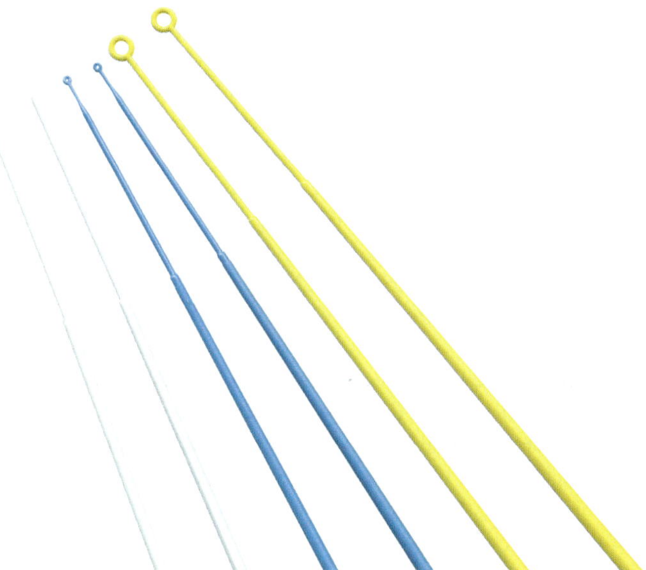

FIGURE 50.12 Inoculating needles *(left)*. Inoculating loops *(right)*. (Courtesy Simport Plastics, Beloeil, Quebec, Canada.)

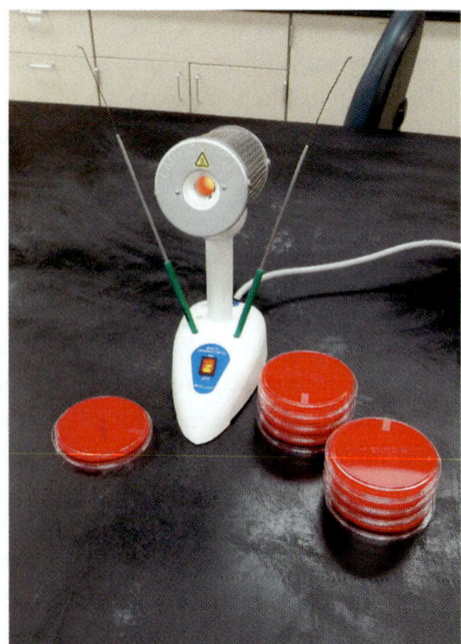

FIGURE 50.13 Incinerator for sterilizing wire loops and needles.

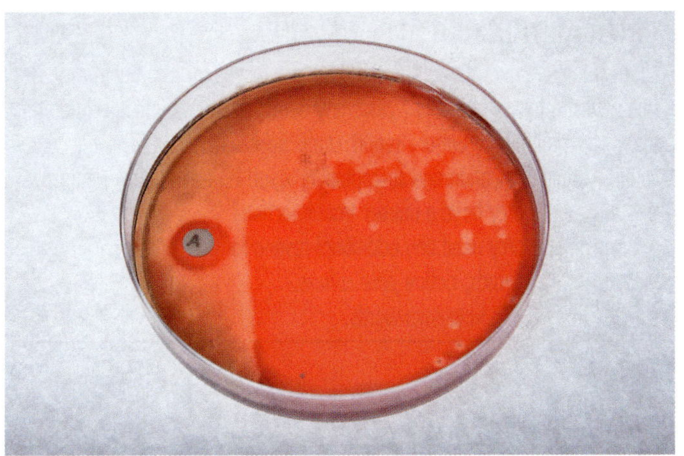

FIGURE 50.14 Positive strep test result on blood agar (*left side of plate*). *Group A streptococcus* (GAS) shows beta hemolysis (clearing) of the blood agar below the growing colonies. Notice there is no hemolysis or clearing of the blood around the white bacitracin disk. That is because bacitracin can destroy GAS.

An inoculating loop is shaped like a bubble wand, and a thin film of liquid adheres to the loop. The amount of fluid held by the loop can be calibrated. For example, a urine culture uses a loop that delivers a 1-mcL sample. The urine in the loop is spread across the culture medium and allowed to grow overnight. The next day, each bacterium becomes a visible **colony.** Colonies can then be counted and analyzed to determine the cause of a urinary tract infection.

Assessing a Culture

When the original (primary) culture has incubated at the appropriate temperature for 18 to 24 hours, it is examined for evidence of pathogens. Because normal flora is often present in samples in addition to pathogens, a trained eye is required to spot the organisms that might be causing an infection. Suspicious colonies are **subcultured** onto the appropriate medium to isolate them in **pure culture**. When the organism is in pure culture, staining and additional biochemical testing can be done to identify the organism. Throat and urine cultures may be performed in POLs that have been CLIA certified to perform moderately complex testing.

Throat Cultures

Streptococcus pyogenes, also known as *group A strep (GAS)* or *beta hemolytic streptococcus,* causes strep throat. If not diagnosed and treated promptly, this infection can cause severe complications, including scarlet fever, rheumatic fever, and glomerulonephritis. A throat swab is collected from the patient's throat. Then the swab is **streaked for isolation** on a **5% sheep'sblood agar plate (BAP)**. An antibiotic disk is placed on the first quadrant of the streaked plate (Figure 50.14) and incubated overnight at 37°C (98.6°F). The antibiotic disk contains bacitracin, which prevents the growth of *S. pyogenes*. Complete clearing of the agar around the colonies indicates *beta hemolysis*, which is caused by a toxin produced by *S. pyogenes*. The toxin breaks down the red blood cells in the agar, causing the agar to be a clear golden color around the colonies. The presence of beta hemolysis and a zone of no growth around the disk indicate that the patient has strep throat (see Figure 50.14). Additional testing may be needed to confirm the identity of the organism.

Streaking for Isolation

Streaking for isolation is also called a four-quadrant streak. It is a procedure that is performed with most microbiology specimens. By distributing bacteria across the agar plate and isolating bacterial colonies, laboratory personnel can see characteristics of the bacteria that are useful in the identification process.

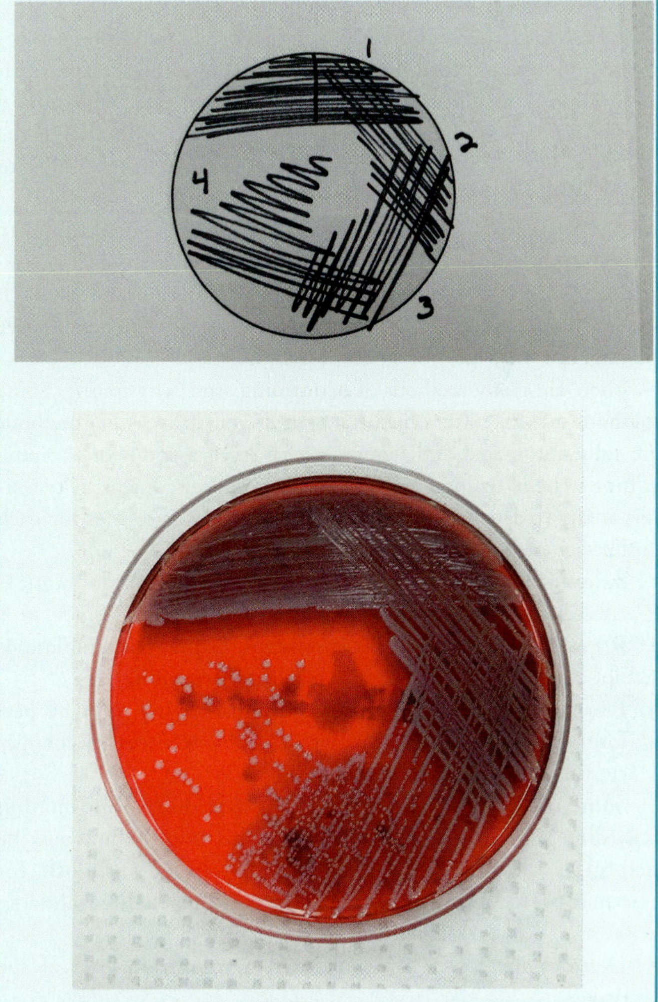

Urine Cultures

With urine cultures, the bacterial colonies that appear after incubation are counted. A calibrated inoculating loop is dipped into a well-mixed urine sample that was collected by the clean-catch midstream (CCMS) method or by catheterization. The urine from the loop is spread on solid culture media and incubated for 18 to 24 hours at 37°C (98.6°F). Each colony that grows on the plate represents 1000 colony-forming units (cfu) per milliliter. The final cfu results are interpreted as follows:

- Normal: <10,000 cfu/mL of urine; no urinary tract infection (UTI) is present
- Borderline: 10,000 to 100,000 cfu/mL of urine; a chronic or relapsing infection may be present, and the test should be repeated
- Positive: >100,000 cfu/mL of urine; a UTI is likely

The medical assistant needs to be aware of the terminology and values reported for urine cultures.

Microbiology Culture and Sensitivity Testing

Once a bacterial infection has been identified, additional steps are required for successful treatment. To determine the appropriate antibiotic to destroy the pathogen, the provider will order a culture and sensitivity (C&S) test. *Culture* refers to growing the organisms, and *sensitivity* refers to the organism's susceptibility to antibiotics.

The healthcare provider must decide which medication to order based on initial test results and the patient's physical examination. C&S test results provide vital information about which specific antibiotics work best against the particular infective pathogen.

There are many methods of performing sensitivity testing. Some methods involve culture media and antibiotic disks. Other methods are fully automated and require a very small amount of the pure culture to be tested. No matter what method is used, sensitivity testing is reported to the provider in one of three categories for each antibiotic tested:

- **S** means that the pathogen is susceptible, or that the antibiotic is effective in destroying that particular organism.
- **R** means that the pathogen is resistant, or that the antibiotic is not effective in destroying that particular organism.
- **I** means intermediate, or that additional testing must be performed to determine the dosage of antibiotic necessary for successful treatment.

Some testing methods may give additional information regarding the dosage tested **in vitro**. This information may be helpful as the providers choose the appropriate antibiotic for treatment. The appropriate antibiotic agent meets the following criteria:

- Destroys the infectious agent with a reasonable level of the drug
- Is the least toxic to the patient and has the least impact on normal flora of the body
- Has the desired pharmacologic characteristics (preparation, route of delivery, effectiveness)
- Is the most economical

CRITICAL THINKING APPLICATION **50.8**

Laura is looking over the reference laboratory results from the day. Mrs. Liz Darcy was in for an office visit yesterday and collected a urine specimen for C&S. Her preliminary culture report came back as 82,000 cfu/mL, pure culture. The identification and susceptibility report is due to follow tomorrow.

- Does Mrs. Darcy have a urinary tract infection?
- Does Mrs. Darcy need any additional testing for this condition?
- In your own words, define *pure culture.*
- Describe C&S in your own words.

STOOL-BASED TESTS

There are two main types of stool tests:

- *Fecal occult blood test (FOBT)*: Detects blood in the stool specimen
- *Stool DNA test*: Detects genetic material from polyps and cancerous tumors in the stool specimen

The following sections describe these tests.

Fecal Occult Blood Tests

The fecal **occult** blood test (FOBT) checks a sample of stool for occult blood. Blood in the stools can be caused by hemorrhoids, diverticulosis, ulcers, colitis, and polyps. There are two main types of FOBT: the **guaiac fecal occult blood test** (gFOBT) and the fecal immunochemical test (FIT).

Guaiac Fecal Occult Blood Test

The guaiac fecal occult blood test is a stool test that looks for the presence of occult blood. This is a common test in the ambulatory care environment. The medical assistant needs to coach the patient on both the preparations for the gFOBT and how to collect the stool specimens (Procedure 50.6). Usually, the patient is asked to collect samples from two or three stools on consecutive days. Each **hemoccult test** card has two locations (A and B) for samples. One card should be used on each day.

When the hemoccult test cards are returned to the lab, the company recommends that the test be developed no sooner than 3 days after the stool sample was applied. If immediate testing is required, wait 3 to 5 minutes for the sample to penetrate the test paper. Open the back of the slide and apply 2 drops of the hemoccult developer to the guaiac paper over each smear (Procedure 50.7). The medical assistant should read the results within 60 seconds. Any trace of blue on the specimen smear or near the edge is considered a positive test result for occult blood (Figure 50.15). The medical assistant must also apply 1 drop of the developer between the positive and negative Performance Monitors areas, for quality control. The results must be read within 10 seconds. The hemoccult card and the developer are functioning if a blue color appears in the positive Performance area and no blue appears in the negative Performance Monitors area.

Fecal Immunochemical Test

The fecal immunochemical test (FIT), also called the *immunochemical fecal occult blood test* (iFOBT), is a screening test for colon cancer. It only detects human hemoglobin from the large intestine (e.g., cecum, colon, or rectum). Hemoglobin from bleeding occurring

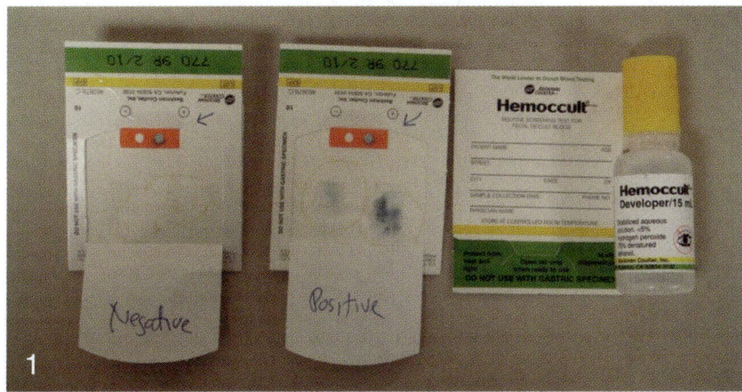

FIGURE 50.15 Negative and positive hemoccult results. (From Roberts J, Hedges J: *Clinical procedures in emergency medicine,* ed 5, Philadelphia, 2010, Saunders.)

from the mouth to the small intestine is generally degraded by the digestive and enzyme processes. Food and medications do not affect this test, so it tends to have fewer false-positive results than the gFOBT.

InSure ONE. InSure ONE is a FIT that detects human hemoglobin in samples of toilet bowel water collected around the feces. The toilet bowl water is collected after the person brushes the surface of the feces to release any blood into the water. The patient is given the test to take home, along with the following instructions:

1. Do not collect samples 3 days before, or during, or 3 days after the menstrual period; if the patient has bleeding hemorrhoids; or if there is visible blood in the urine.
2. Store the collection kit at room temperature away from heat and direct sunlight.
3. There are no preparations for the test.
4. Label the card as indicated.
5. Flush the toilet before starting. After having the bowel movement, put the used toilet paper in the wastebasket instead of the toilet.
6. Follow the kit instructions:
   a. Use the brush from the kit to brush the surface of the feces/stool for about 5 seconds.
   b. Then dip the brush into the toilet water before touching the brush to the space indicated on the test card.
   c. Wrap the brush in toilet paper and discard it in the wastebasket.
7. Seal the test card and return as directed to your provider or the laboratory.

Multitargeted Stool DNA Test

The multitargeted stool DNA test (MT-sDNA) detects abnormal DNA, along with the presence of occult hemoglobin in the stool. An example of a multitargeted stool DNA test (MT-sDNA) is the Cologuard, which tests stool for cancer and precancerous cells. Cologuard screens for DNA markers and the presence of occult hemoglobin in stool (Procedure 50.8). The patient is asked to obtain the sample at home and mail the test to the laboratory.

The patient is given the test to take at home, along with the following directions:

1. Do not obtain the sample if you have diarrhea or obvious blood in the urine or stool (e.g., bleeding hemorrhoids, bleeding wounds on the hands, or menstruation).
2. There is no preparation required for this test.

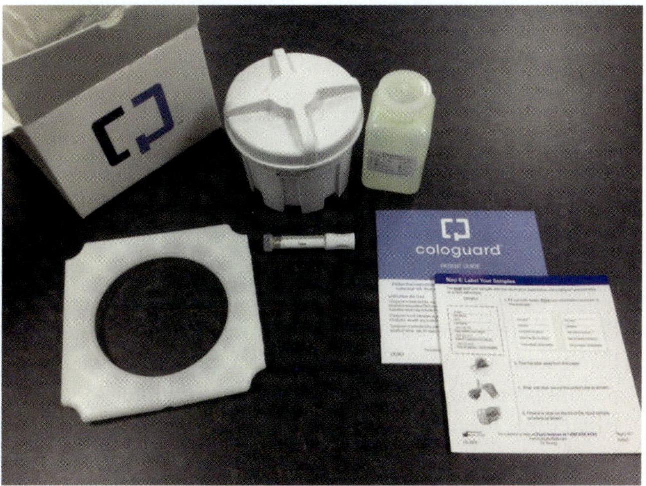

FIGURE 50.16 Cologuard Kit. Clockwise from upper left corner: shipping box, sample (specimen) container, bottle of preservative, patient direction booklet, shipping and specimen labels, tube, and bracket.

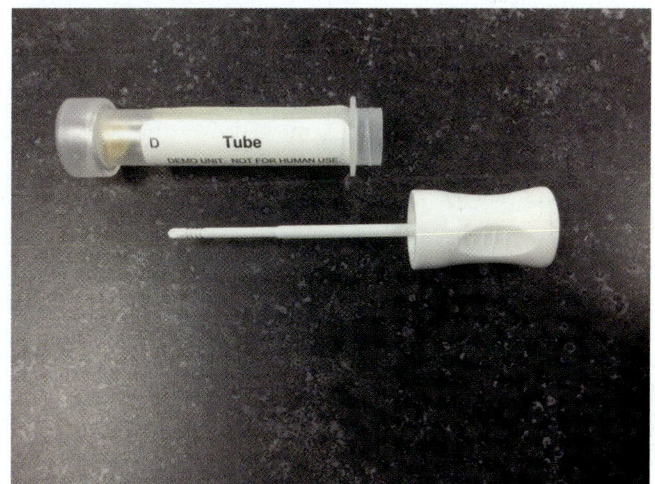

FIGURE 50.17 Probe and tube from the Cologuard kit.

3. Store the kit at room temperature, away from heat, direct sunlight, children, and pets.
4. The kit contains a bracket, sample container, tube with a probe, bottle of preservative, shipping label, and specimen labels (Figure 50.16).
5. The bracket is placed in the toilet. The lid is removed from the stool sample container, and the container is placed into the bracket.
6. When having the bowel movement, the person must avoid getting toilet paper and urine in the stool sample container.
7. Following the test directions, the person must scrape the stool sample with the probe to get a small sample (Figure 50.17). In addition, the preservative must be poured onto the stool in the stool sample container.
8. Both samples (sample probe tube and sample container) must be sealed tightly, labeled, packed in the special shipping box, and mailed to the lab within a day. The lab must get the sample within 3 days.

CLOSING COMMENTS

Patient Coaching

Microorganisms such as bacteria, viruses, fungi, and parasites are responsible for most human infectious diseases. Patient education plays an important role in helping the patient and family control the spread of infection. The teaching topics in the following list can help you educate a patient about infection control:

- An explanation of the patient's type of infection: bacterial, viral, fungal, or parasitic
- How infections spread
- Hand washing and sanitization, proper storage and cleaning of personal items, and disposal of contaminated supplies
- Risk factors for infection, such as poor nutritional habits or poor ventilation with airborne pathogens present
- The patient's role in specimen collection
- Patient preparation for laboratory tests, imaging tests, and other needed procedures

Explain to the patient that an infection can be transferred from person to person in many ways. Reinforce the importance of following directions for taking any medication. If patients do not follow the directions given to them by the provider or pharmacist, there is a real chance of the following:

- Developing complications
- Having a relapse of an infection
- Allowing an infection to spread to other areas or becoming systemic

Always listen to the patient. Be sure to answer all the patient's questions. Notify the provider of patient's concerns so that he or she can give further details or instructions before the patient leaves the facility.

Legal and Ethical Issues

Maintaining a laboratory in the office increases the physician's liability. By testing patients' specimens in the office, the physician assumes responsibility for the interpretation and accuracy of the results. As the person in the office who runs the tests and notes the results in the patient's record, you are responsible for maintaining optimum accuracy in testing results. A quality assurance (QA) program, including the running, interpreting, and recording of the internal controls supplied in each test kit, must be documented. Both microbiology and immunology tests allow the patient to benefit from the convenience of office testing. Strict confidentiality is essential. Never release information to anyone other than the patient or legal guardian.

Also note that certain infectious diseases must be reported to the CDC or local board of health. Each state legislature determines what diseases must be reported and how the data are to be reported. Additional data for nationally notifiable diseases is published weekly by the CDC in the *Morbidity and Mortality Weekly Report* (MMWR). For additional information on infectious disease reporting, please review the reporting procedure presented in Chapter 4.

Patient-Centered Care

Hand hygiene should be foremost in your mind with each patient encounter. Making sure that you wash hands or use hand sanitizer as you enter and leave an exam room should be part of your routine. Sanitizing hands before and after gloving is also a must. But also, remembering to sanitize hands when the patient is not in front of you is just as important. Anytime you handle specimens, containers, enter and leave a laboratory area, or put away laboratory supplies and equipment, you should also follow up with proper hand hygiene. The CDC states that the most effective means of stopping the transmission of disease is frequent and proper handwashing.

Professional Behaviors

Medicine is an ever-changing profession, and medical assistants need to remain current in all areas of their profession. The laboratory is no exception. Microbiology and immunology are areas of the laboratory where research, technical skills, and testing methods are changing rapidly. Making an effort to stay up to date with new ideas and concepts is critical to contributing to exceptional patient care.

SUMMARY OF SCENARIO

Laura has had another busy day at WMFM Clinic. Once again, she has seen infectious diseases in some of her patients today. Laura knows that most microorganisms are harmless, but knowing the signs and symptoms of common infectious diseases is important.

It is also important to diagnose and treat most infectious diseases. Laura knows that proper specimen collection is essential. She is also aware that rapid CLIA-waived tests can identify pathogens and help treat patients in a timely manner.

Microbiology and immunology tests have become useful in the physician office laboratory. Meeting the needs of patients and quickly addressing their concerns are benefits of CLIA-waived testing. Laura feels comfortable collecting specimens, testing patient samples, and reporting the results for the provider to review. As a certified medical assistant, she knows that the work she does throughout the day is helping every one of her patients.

SUMMARY OF LEARNING OBJECTIVES

1. **Examine how microorganisms are identified.**
   The naming of all living organisms uses a binomial system consisting of two names; the first "family" name is the *genus,* and the second is the *species.* Both names are either italicized or underlined when written. The genus begins with a capital letter, the species with a lowercase letter. Often the name reveals some characteristic about the organism.
2. **Examine the characteristics of bacteria.**
   Bacteria often are classified according to their staining characteristics, shape, and the environmental conditions in which they thrive. Their staining characteristics are gram positive (dark blue), gram negative (pink), and acid-fast (pink).
   Identification of bacteria begins with an observation of their morphology. Cocci are spherical organisms, bacilli are rod-shaped organisms, and

spirilla are spiral-shaped organisms. Staphylococci are cocci in clusters, streptococci and streptobacilli are organisms arranged in chains, and diplococci and diplobacilli are organisms arranged in pairs.

Organisms are classified by oxygen requirements as aerobic (needs oxygen to survive), anaerobic (lives without oxygen), or facultative (anaerobic but able to survive in the presence of oxygen). Table 50.1 can help explain the characteristics of common diseases caused by bacteria.

3. **Differentiate among various pathogens.**
Three are several types of pathogens, including unusual pathogenic bacteria, fungi, protozoa, parasites, helminths, and viruses. *Chlamydia* and *Rickettsia* organisms are tiny bacteria; however, unlike most bacteria, they require a host cell for replication. *Mycoplasmas* do not contain peptidoglycan in their cell wall.

Fungi are eukaryotes that are larger than bacteria, have a nucleus, and include yeasts and molds. Fungi are present in the soil, air, and water, but only a few species cause disease.

Protozoa are single-celled parasitic organisms that contain a nucleus and range in size. They are present in moist environments and in bodies of water. Parasites are transmitted by ingestion, direct penetration of the skin, and injection by an arthropod also referred to as a vector. Helminths are parasites called worms that live on or in animals or humans.

Viruses are not able to metabolize or reproduce unless they are inside of a host cell. Because of the absolute need for a host cell, a virus can be considered an obligate intracellular pathogen.

4. **Examine the procedures for specimen collection and transport in the physician office laboratory.**
Specimens must be collected carefully so that contaminating microorganisms are not introduced into the specimen. This means not only using sterile collection and transport devices, but also taking steps to prevent contamination. Specialized transport media are often included with specimen collection swabs or devices.

Stool specimens are commonly examined for parasitic protozoa and helminths. The specimen is collected and placed into two vials, each with a preservative (see Procedure 50.1). With pinworms, specimens are best collected late at night or early in the morning for children. Paraffin swabs impregnated with petroleum jelly or cellulose tape may be used to collect the eggs deposited by the adult worm during the night.

Nasal and nasopharyngeal specimens are obtained for several respiratory tests. Three types of specimens can be collected: anterior nasal specimen, mid-turbinate nasal specimen, and nasopharyngeal (NP) specimen (see Procedure 50.2). The swab should be gently rolled and then left in place for several seconds to allow it to absorb secretions. A specimen is obtained from both nostrils unless the swab is saturated with secretions from the first nostril.

Many times, sputum specimens are collected in the morning. For some tests, three sputum samples may be collected over 3 days. When collecting a sputum specimen, patients should avoid food for 1 to 2 hours and rinse their mouth. After coughing deeply, the sputum should be deposited into the cup.

A throat swab specimen collection is used to identify the cause of throat infections, such as strep throat. Procedure 50.3 describes the collection process. Patients should not use antiseptic mouthwash prior to the collection.

5. **Examine CLIA-waived microbiology testing.**
Often, growing a pathogen on a culture plate is difficult, and it takes time to grow and isolate the pathogen. A rapid "direct" immunology test demonstrates the presence of the pathogen's antigen in a specimen that is placed in a test kit containing its specific antibody. If the pathogen is present, it produces a colored reaction, indicating a positive result. The *rapid strep test* detects *S. pyogenes* and is used in the diagnosis of strep throat (see Procedure 50.4). The *influenza A and B rapid test* detects surface antigens of the viruses that cause influenza. The *RSV rapid test* detects antigens from the respiratory syncytial virus, which causes pneumonia and bronchiolitis in young children.

6. **Examine CLIA-waived immunology testing.**
"Indirect" immunology testing detects antibodies in whole blood, serum, or plasma that react to the specific antigen in the test kit, producing a colored reaction. A positive reaction indicates that the antibodies have been produced and attack the pathogen in question (e.g., heterophile antibodies seen in mononucleosis).

Mononucleosis testing detects the heterophile antibodies made in reaction to an infection of the Epstein-Barr virus (see Procedure 50.5). The *H. pylori test* detects antibodies to the bacterium that commonly causes stomach ulcers. Early detection of *Lyme disease* can be accomplished using a CLIA-waived test that detects the antibodies that attack the *B. burgdorferi* pathogen. Rapid HIV testing detects the HIV antibodies made in reaction to an HIV infection that could develop into AIDS.

7. **Examine the reference laboratory process for the identification of pathogens.**
After receiving the specimens collected in the POL, the microbiology laboratory promptly inoculates the appropriate culture media first and then prepares a smear of the specimen on a slide to be stained. Pathogenic microorganisms generally are colorless, and special stains are used to differentiate bacteria based on cell membrane differences. Gram-positive bacteria stain purple, and gram-negative bacteria stain pink or red. The acid-fast stain is used in the identification protocol for Mycobacterium species. Acid-fast positive microbes stain fuchsia red. Acid-fast negative microbes stain baby blue.

Next, the specimen must be spread on specific culture media based on the source of the specimen. The inoculated culture media are placed in a body temperature incubator to grow overnight. The next day, each bacterium becomes a visible colony. Colonies can then be counted and analyzed to determine the cause of an infection.

Once a bacterial infection has been identified, additional steps are required for successful treatment. To determine the appropriate antibiotic to destroy the pathogen, the provider will order a culture and sensitivity (C&S) test. *Culture* refers to growing the organisms, and sensitivity refers to the organism's susceptibility to antibiotics.

8. **Examine stool-based tests.**
There are two main types of stool tests:
Fecal occult blood test (FOBT): Detects blood in the stool specimen. There are two main types of FOBT:
   - *G*uaiac fecal occult blood test (gFOBT): A stool test that looks for the presence of occult blood.
   - Fecal immunochemical test (FIT): Also called the immunochemical fecal occult blood test (iFOBT). FIT is a screening test for colon cancer. It only detects human hemoglobin from the large intestine. InSure ONE is a FIT that detects human hemoglobin in samples of toilet bowel water collected around the feces.

Stool DNA test: Detects genetic material from polyps and cancerous tumors in the stool specimen. The multitargeted stool DNA test (MT-sDNA) detects abnormal DNA, along with the presence of occult hemoglobin in the stool. An example of a multitargeted stool DNA test (MT-sDNA) is the Cologuard, which tests stool for cancer and precancerous cells.

PROCEDURE 50.1 Coach a Patient on the Collection of Fecal Specimens to Be Tested for Ova and Parasites

TASK: Coach a patient in the proper collection of stool for an ova and parasite microscopic examination.

EQUIPMENT and SUPPLIES

- Patient's health record
- Provider's order or lab requisition
- Clean, dry container for stool collection
- Two parasitology collection vials*
- Plastic biohazard zipper-lock bag

PROCEDURAL STEPS

1. Greet the patient. Identify yourself. Verify the patient's identity with full name, then ask the patient to spell the first and last names and to state their date of birth.
2. Explain the procedure in a manner that the patient understands. Answer any general questions the patient may have about the collection procedures before you give detailed instructions.
3. Instruct the patient not to take any antacids, laxatives, or stool softeners before collecting the specimen. Instruct the patient that the liquid in the vials is extremely dangerous and to keep out of the reach of children.
   PURPOSE: Laxatives increase fecal transit time and may result in a false-negative test result.
4. Instruct the patient to urinate before collecting the specimen.
   PURPOSE: This eliminates the possibility of the stool becoming contaminated with urine.
5. The patient then collects the specimen.
   - *Adults:* Instruct the patient to defecate into the container. Stool cannot be retrieved from the toilet bowl.
   - *Children:* Loosely drape the toilet rim with plastic wrap and lower the seat. The child should have a bowel movement into the toilet, onto the wrap. Remove the stool using a disposable plastic spoon.

   PURPOSE: The stool cannot be contaminated by or diluted with water.
   - *Infants:* Fasten a "diaper" made of plastic wrap over the child, using tape. Remove the plastic wrap immediately after a bowel movement, and remove the stool using a plastic spoon. *Never leave the child unattended with the plastic wrap in place because of the risk of suffocation.*

   PURPOSE: Stool cannot be collected in a diaper.
6. Instruct the patient or parent/guardian to add stool to the collection containers.
   - If the stool is formed, use the scoop on the lid of the containers to add a large, jellybean–sized piece of stool to the liquid in the containers (Figure 1).
   - If the stool is liquid, pour it into the containers.
   - In both of the previous cases, keep adding the specimen until the liquid preservative in the vial reaches the indicated level on the containers.

   PURPOSE: Proper instructions will give patients confidence in what they need to do to ensure a proper specimen. (Image courtesy Meridian Bioscience.)

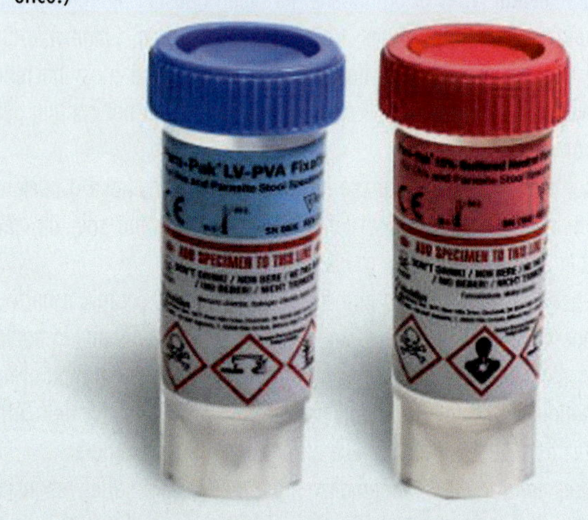

7. Instruct the patient or parent/guardian to tighten the caps completely and wipe the outside of the vials with rubbing alcohol or to wash carefully with soap and water.
   PURPOSE: These actions ensure infection control.
8. Instruct the patient or parent/guardian that the vials should be labeled, placed in a biohazard bag with a zippered closure, and transported to the laboratory immediately, if possible. The vials should not be refrigerated.
9. Instruct patients or parents/guardians to wash their hands after the specimen collection procedure.
   PURPOSE: It is important to ensure infection control.
10. Document the coaching in the patient's health record. Include the provider's name, what was taught, how the patient responded, and indicate the supplies and written directions sent home with the patient.
    PURPOSE: It is important to document the procedure in the health record to show it was done.

Documentation Example

08/14/20XX 1105 Per Dr. Kahn's order, instructed patient how to collect the ova and parasite specimen. Patient taught back the instructions accurately. Gave the patient the stool container, the O&P vials, and a biohazard bag. Patient will return the vials to the clinic later this week.
———————————— Laura Piper, CMA (AAMA)

* Please note that several types of preservatives are available. Check with the referral laboratory to make sure the patient is given the proper vials for collection. Preservatives include low-viscosity polyvinyl alcohol (LV-PVA), zinc sulfite polyvinyl alcohol (ZN-PVA), sodium acetate acetic acid formalin (SAF), and 10% neutral buffered formalin.

PROCEDURE 50.2 Collect a Nasal or Nasopharyngeal Specimen Using a Swab

TASKS: Collect an anterior nasal specimen, a mid-turbinate nasal specimen, or a nasopharyngeal specimen using a swab. Document the procedure in the patient's health record.

EQUIPMENT and SUPPLIES

- Patient's health record
- Provider's order or laboratory requisition
- Fluid-impermeable lab coat, mask, face shield, and gloves (or as indicated by healthcare facility)
- Collection kit or appropriate swab for test (e.g., sterile flocked or spun polyester tipped swab with a flexible shaft) and transport media tube
- Biohazard waste container

PROCEDURAL STEPS

1. Wash hands or use hand sanitizer. Put on the fluid-impermeable lab coat, mask, and face shield. Comply with safety practices.
   PURPOSE: To ensure infection control.
2. Review the order and gather the supplies needed.
3. Greet the patient. Identify yourself. Verify the patient's identity with full name, then ask the patient to spell the first and last names and to state their date of birth.
   PURPOSE: It is important to identify the patient in two different ways to ensure that you have the correct patient.
4. Explain the procedure in a manner that the patient understands. Answer any general questions the patient may have about the collection procedures before you give detailed instructions.
   PURPOSE: Explaining the procedure can make the patient feel more comfortable and reduces anxiety.
5. Obtain permission to perform the swab on the patient. Ask the patient if he or she has any nasal obstructions or a deviated septum. Have the patient blow his or her nose, if indicated.
   PURPOSE: If the patient has a nasal obstruction or a deviated septum, the opposite nostril should be used for the procedure.
6. Put on gloves.
7. Remove the sterile swab from the sterile wrap with your dominant hand.
8. Collect the specimen:
   a. For an anterior nasal swab:
      - Using the appropriate swab, insert the tip of the swab into the nostril, no more than 0.75 inch (1.9 cm).
      - Slowly rotate the swab, gently pressing against the nasal wall. Rotate four times for a total of 15 seconds. Remove the swab and insert it into the other nostril. Repeat the process.

   PURPOSE: Allows for the swab to absorb the secretions.

   b. For a mid-turbinate nasal specimen:
      - Have the patient tilt her or his head back 70 degrees.

   PURPOSE: Tilting the head helps the medical assistant position the swab in the correct location.
      - Using a tapered swab, rotate the swab while inserting it. Insert it less than 1 inch (2.5 cm) into the nostril along the nasal floor until resistance is met at the nasal turbinate (Figure 1). Rotate the swab for about 10 to 15 seconds. Hold in place for 5 seconds. Remove swab. Repeat process on the other nostril.

   c. For a nasopharyngeal specimen:
      - Have the patient tilt her or his head back 70 degrees.

   PURPOSE: Tilting the head helps the medical assistant position the swab in the correct location.
      - Using the unobstructed nostril, insert the swab parallel to the palate until resistance is encountered (Figure 2). A swab should be inserted about 3.1 to 3.9 inches (8 to 10 cm) in an adult and 2.4 to 2.8 inches (6 to 7 cm) in a child.

   PURPOSE: The swab needs to be inserted far enough back to be in the correct position.
      - Roll the swab gently, and then leave the swab in place for several sections. Rotate the swab as it is slowly removed. If the swab is not saturated with secretions, repeat the process using the other nostril if indicated by the testing procedure. The same swab can be used.

   PURPOSE: Leaving the swab in place allows it to absorb the nasopharyngeal secretions.
9. Place the swab in the transport medium. Snap or cut of the applicator stick if needed. Label the tube and send it to the laboratory.
   PURPOSE: A transport medium prevents the swab from drying. Labeling immediately after collection prevents specimens from getting mixed up.
10. Dispose of contaminated supplies in the biohazard waste container. Disinfect the work area.
    PURPOSE: To prevent the spread of infection.
11. Remove your gloves and discard them in the biohazard waste container. Remove face shield.
12. Wash hands or use hand sanitizer.
    PURPOSE: To ensure infection control.
13. Document the procedure in the patient's health record.
    PURPOSE: Procedures are not done until they are recorded.

Documentation Example

8/14/20XX 8:55 a.m. Nasopharyngeal specimen collected via swab. Sent to University Laboratories for strep testing. ____________ Laura Piper, CMA (AAMA)

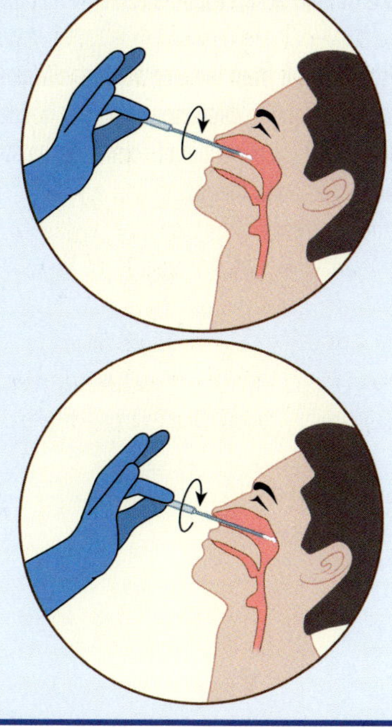

PROCEDURE 50.3 Collect a Specimen for a Throat Culture

TASKS: Collect a throat culture, using sterile technique, for immediate testing or for transportation to the laboratory. Document the procedure in the patient's health record.

EQUIPMENT and SUPPLIES

- Patient's health record
- Provider's order or laboratory requisition
- Fluid-impermeable lab coat, mask, face shield or protective eyewear, and gloves (or as indicated by healthcare facility)
- Sterile swab if transporting to a reference lab for culture, or sterile swab from the rapid strep test kit if testing patient in the POL
- Sterile tongue depressor
- Transport medium
- Biohazard waste container

PROCEDURAL STEPS

1. Wash hands or use hand sanitizer. Put on the fluid-impermeable lab coat and face shield. Put on a mask if required by the facility. Comply with safety practices.
   PURPOSE: To ensure infection control.
2. Review the order and gather the supplies needed.
3. Greet the patient. Identify yourself. Verify the patient's identity with full name, then ask the patient to spell the first and last names and to state their date of birth.
   PURPOSE: It is important to identify the patient in two different ways to ensure that you have the correct patient.
4. Explain the procedure in a manner that the patient understands. Answer any general questions the patient may have about the collection procedures before you give detailed instructions.
   PURPOSE: Explaining the procedure can make the patient feel more comfortable and reduces anxiety.
5. Obtain permission to perform the throat culture on the patient.
6. Put on gloves. Position the patient so that the light shines into the mouth.
   PURPOSE: To ensure infection control and to illuminate the area to be swabbed.
7. Remove the sterile swab from the sterile wrap with your dominant hand, and grasp the sterile tongue depressor with your nondominant hand.
   PURPOSE: These actions allow better control of the swabbing process.
8. Instruct the patient to open the mouth and say, "Ah." Depress the tongue with the depressor.
   PURPOSE: Saying "Ah" helps elevate the uvula and reduces the tendency to gag. The tongue is depressed so that you can see the back of the throat and prevent contamination of the sterile swab.
9. Swab the back of the throat between the tonsillar pillars in a figure-8 pattern, especially any reddened, patchy areas of the throat, white pus pockets, purulent areas, and the tonsils; take care not to touch any other areas in the mouth (Figure 1).
   PURPOSE: Pathogenic organisms are found in the back of the throat and on the tonsils.

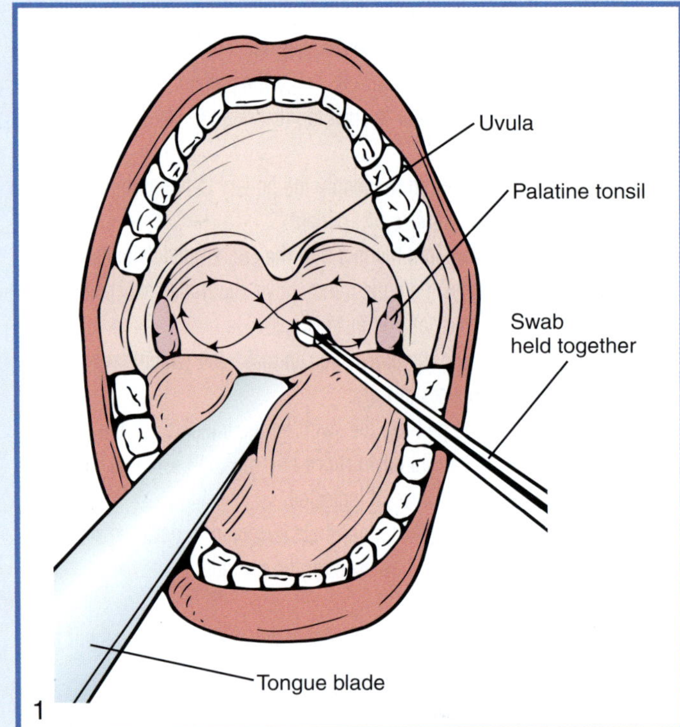

10. Place the swab in the transport medium, label it, and follow appropriate procedures to send it to the referral laboratory (Figure 2). If rapid strep testing is requested, it may be done in the POL or sent to a reference laboratory.
    PURPOSE: A transport medium prevents the swab from drying out. Labeling immediately after collection prevents specimen misidentification.

PROCEDURE 50.3 Collect a Specimen for a Throat Culture—*Continued*

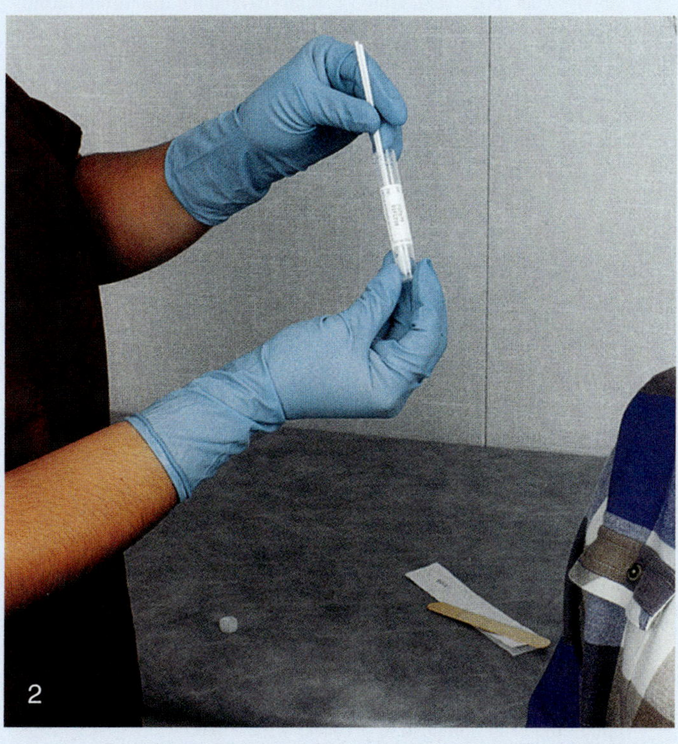
2

11. Dispose of contaminated supplies in the biohazard waste container. Disinfect the work area.
    PURPOSE: Disposing of contaminated supplies prevents the spread of infection.
12. Remove your gloves and discard them in the biohazard waste container. Remove the face shield.
13. Wash hands or use hand sanitizer.
    PURPOSE: Hand sanitization is an important step for infection control.
14. Document the procedure in the patient's health record.
    PURPOSE: Procedures are not complete until they are recorded.

Documentation Example

8/14/20 8:35 a.m. Throat specimen collected via swab from tonsillar area. Sent to University Laboratories for strep testing. ———————————————— Laura Piper, CMA (AAMA)

PROCEDURE 50.4 Perform a CLIA-Waived Microbiology Test: Perform a Rapid Strep Test

TASKS: Perform a rapid strep screening test to assist in the diagnosis of strep throat. Document the results in the patient's health record.

EQUIPMENT and SUPPLIES

- Patient's health record
- Provider's order or lab requisition
- QuickVue In-Line Strep A test kit contents (Figure 1):
  - Extraction solution bottles
  - Individually packaged test cassettes
  - Individually wrapped sterile rayon swabs provided in kit
  - Positive (+) control swab provided in kit
  - Visual flowchart outlining the steps of the test
- Rapid Strep Test Log Sheet
- Stopwatch or laboratory timer
- Fluid-impermeable lab coat, mask, face shield or protective eyewear, and gloves (or as indicated by healthcare facility)
- Biohazard waste container

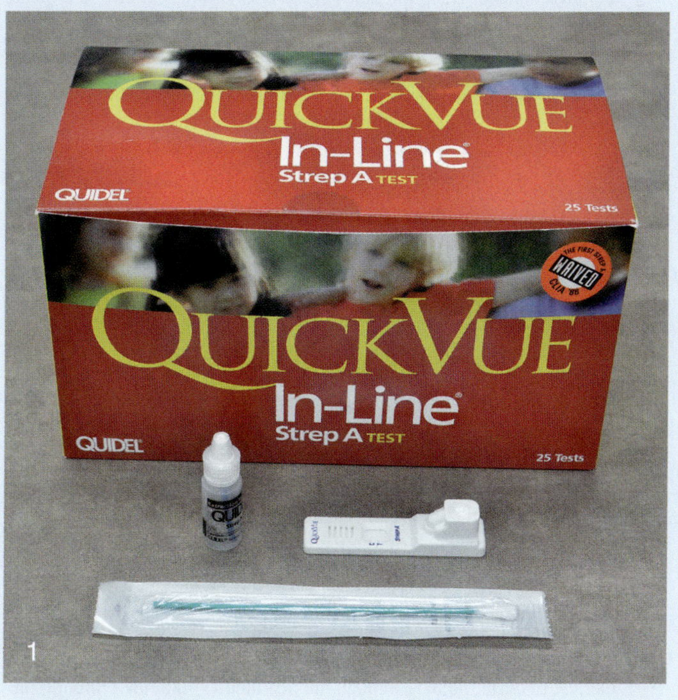

1

Continued

PROCEDURE 50.4 Perform a CLIA-Waived Microbiology Test: Perform a Rapid Strep Test—*Continued*

PROCEDURAL STEPS

1. Wash hands or use hand sanitizer. Put on the fluid-impermeable lab coat and face shield or protective eyewear. Put on a mask if required by the facility. Comply with safety practices.
   PURPOSE: To ensure infection control.
2. Collect all necessary supplies and equipment. Bring all reagents to room temperature. Check the expiration date on the test kit package.
   Note: Before running the first patient test from a new test kit, positive and negative controls must be run using the control swabs provided in the kit. Confirm that both controls reacted correctly and record the control results on the log sheet.
   PURPOSE: Both control swabs must be checked before patients are tested. If the controls show the appropriate results, the test kit is reliable.
3. Greet the patient. Identify yourself. Verify the patient's identity with full name, then ask the patient to spell the first and last names and to state their date of birth.
   PURPOSE: It is important to identify the patient in two different ways to ensure that you have the correct patient.
4. Explain the procedure in a manner that the patient understands. Answer any general questions the patient may have about the collection procedures before you give detailed instructions. Obtain permission to collect a throat culture.
   PURPOSE: Explaining the procedure can make the patient feel more comfortable and reduces anxiety.
5. Put on gloves. Collect a throat specimen using the rayon swab provided in the test kit.
   PURPOSE: The test kit provides a rayon swab to avoid the use of cotton swabs, which can kill bacteria, possibly causing a false-negative result.
6. Remove the test cassette from the foil pouch, and place it on a clean, dry, level surface. Using the notch at the back of the chamber as a guide, insert the patient's swab completely into the swab chamber (Figure 2).

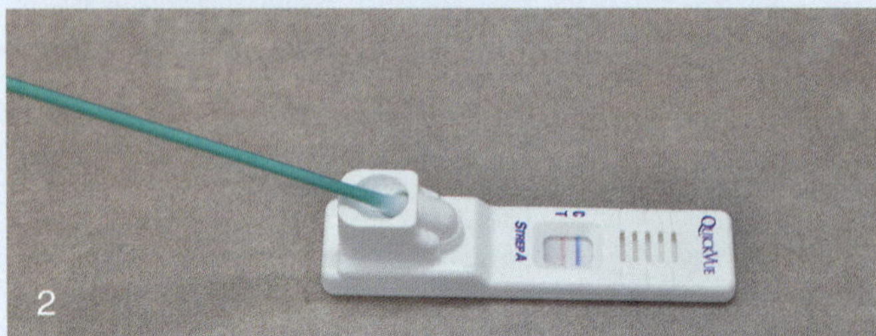

2

7. Place the extraction bottle between your thumb and forefinger, and squeeze once to break the glass ampule inside the extraction solution bottle. Vigorously shake the bottle five times to mix the solutions. The solution should turn green.
   PURPOSE: The color change is an indicator of extraction reagent integrity and that the extraction procedure was performed correctly.
8. Immediately remove the cap on the extraction solution bottle, hold the bottle vertically over the chamber, and quickly fill the chamber to the rim (approximately 8 drops).
   PURPOSE: The liquid extract reacts with the swab and then flows into the test cassette, passing through the test area (T) and then through the internal control area (C).
9. Remove your face shield. Wait 5 minutes to read the results and record them in the lab log.
   - *Positive result:* A pink line shows in the T area, indicating the presence of *Streptococcus pyogenes* antigen; a blue line appears in the C area, indicating that the fluid activated the internal control.
   - *Negative result:* No pink line appears in the T test area; a blue line appears in the C control area, indicating that the internal control worked.
   - *Invalid result:* The blue control line does not appear next to the letter C at 5 minutes. The test result cannot be reported.
10. Discard all the test materials in the appropriate biohazard waste container. Disinfect the work area.
    PURPOSE: Items that come in contact with samples are considered potentially infectious.
11. Remove your gloves. Wash hands or use hand sanitizer.
    PURPOSE: To ensure infection control.
12. Record the test results in the patient's health record.
    PURPOSE: A procedure is not considered complete until it has been properly documented.
13. If the test results are negative, a second throat swab should be obtained and sent to the reference laboratory for a throat culture. Often two swabs are used simultaneously when the sample is initially collected from the throat to prevent the need to re-collect a specimen.
    PURPOSE: Negative rapid strep test results should be confirmed with a throat culture.

QUALITATIVE CONTROL/PATIENT LOG SHEET

TEST: STREP A TEST
KIT NAME AND MANUFACTURER: QuickVue In-Line Strep A Test–Quidel
LOT # 12345 EXPIRATION DATE: 11/22/20XX
STORAGE REQUIREMENTS: Room Temp TEST FLOWCHART yes

DATE	SPECIMEN I.D. (CONTROL/ PATIENT)	RESULT (+ OR –)	INTERNAL CONTROL PASSED (Y OR N)	CHARTED IN PATIENT RECORD	TECH INITIALS
7/11/ 20XX	POSITIVE CONTROL	+	Y		LP
7/11/ 20XX	NEGATIVE CONTROL	–	Y		LP
7/11/ 20XX	PT ID: 5432	+	Y	✓	LP

Documentation in the Medical Record

10/9/20XX 9:30 a.m. Rapid Strep A Test performed with a positive result. ———————————— Laura Piper, CMA (AAMA)

PROCEDURE 50.5 Perform a CLIA-Waived Immunology Test: Perform the QuickVue+ Infectious Mononucleosis Test

TASKS: Perform a capillary puncture. Perform and interpret a rapid CLIA-waived test for infectious mononucleosis. Document the results in the patient's health record.

EQUIPMENT and SUPPLIES

- Patient's health record
- Provider's order or lab requisition
- CLIA-waived QuickVue+ test kit for infectious mononucleosis and blood collecting supplies (Figure 1):
  - Package with test kit supplies
  - Color-coded bottles of positive and negative controls and the developer
  - Test cassette in foil-wrapped protective pouch
  - Pipets supplied in kit with black line indicating amount of capillary blood to collect
- Alcohol prep pad, gauze, and bandage
- Lancet
- Laboratory timer, stopwatch, or wristwatch with sweep second hand
- Fluid-impermeable lab coat, eye protection, and gloves
- Biohazard waste container
- Qualitative Control/Patient Log Sheet

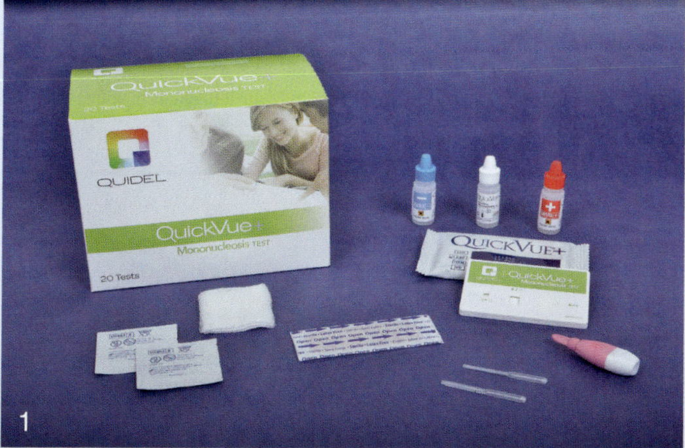

1

PROCEDURAL STEPS

1. Wash hands or use hand sanitizer. Put on the fluid-impermeable lab coat. Comply with safety practices.
   PURPOSE: To ensure infection control.
2. Remove the test kit from the refrigerator and allow the reagents to warm to room temperature. Check the expiration date of the kit.
   PURPOSE: Outdated or cold reagents do not react as expected.
3. Before running the first patient test from a new test kit, run the positive and negative liquid controls provided in the kit to see whether they react correctly. Record your control results on the log sheet.
   PURPOSE: Both control swabs must be checked before patients are tested. If the controls show the appropriate results, the test kit is reliable.
4. Greet the patient. Identify yourself. Verify the patient's identity with full name, then ask the patient to spell the first and last names and to state their date of birth.
5. Explain the procedure in a manner that the patient understands. Answer any general questions the patient may have about the collection procedures before you give detailed instructions. Obtain permission for the capillary puncture.
6. Put on gloves and protective eyewear.
   PURPOSE: To ensure infection control and safety.
7. Remove the test device from its protective pouch, and label it with the patient's identification.
   PURPOSE: Label the test kit to ensure proper identity of the test being run.
8. Disinfect the patient's finger with the alcohol wipe. Allow it to air-dry, and then perform a capillary puncture.
   PURPOSE: Disinfection will ensure infection control. If the alcohol is wet, the capillary puncture will sting and be uncomfortable for the patient.
9. Wipe away the first drop of blood, and then fill the disposable pipet provided in the kit to the calibration mark with capillary blood (Figure 2).
   PURPOSE: The plastic capillary tube measures the exact amount of sample, for accurate testing.

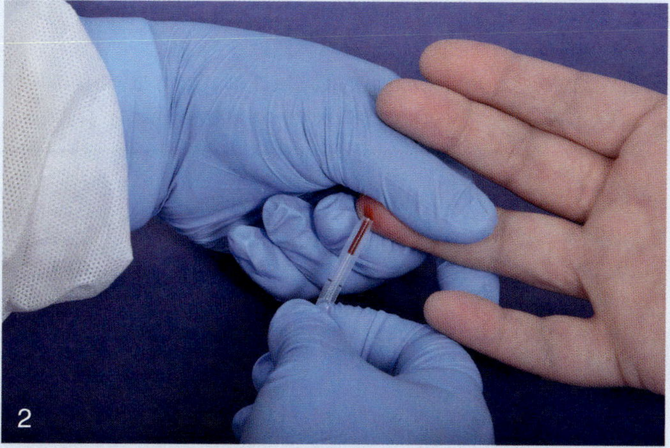
2

10. Dispense all the blood from the capillary tube into the "Add" well of the testing device. (Or, if you are using venous blood, transfer a large drop from the venous whole blood specimen using the longer capillary pipet provided in the kit.)
    PURPOSE: Proper specimen type and volume is required for accurate testing.
11. Hold the developer bottle vertically above the "Add" well and allow 5 drops to fall freely.
    PURPOSE: Holding a dropper vertically ensures delivery of the same-size drop. If the dropper touches other materials, it becomes contaminated, and the results will be inaccurate.
12. Read the results at 5 minutes. *Note:* The "Test Complete" box must be visibly colored by 10 minutes.
    - *Positive result:* A vertical line in any shade of blue forms a plus sign in the "Read Result" window, along with a blue "Test Complete" line. Even a faint blue plus sign should be reported as a positive.

Continued

PROCEDURE 50.5 Perform a CLIA-Waived Immunology Test: Perform the QuickVue+ Infectious Mononucleosis Test—*Continued*

- *Negative result:* No vertical blue line appears, leaving a minus sign in the "Read Result" window, along with a blue "Test Complete" line.
- *Invalid result:* After 10 minutes, no line is seen in the "Test Complete" window, or a blue color fills the "Read Result" window. If either of these is noted, the test must be repeated with a new testing device. If the problem continues, request technical support.

13. Dispose of biohazard waste in the biohazard waste container. Disinfect the work area.
PURPOSE: It is important to ensure infection control.
14. Remove your gloves and protective eyewear. Wash hands or use hand sanitizer.
15. Document control results in the appropriate laboratory log. Document patient results in the appropriate laboratory log and in the patient's health record.
PURPOSE: A procedure is not considered complete until it has been properly documented.

QUALITY CONTROL PROCEDURES

External positive and negative liquid controls are provided with each new kit. All new operators of the test should perform liquid positive and negative external controls once to confirm that their testing technique is correct. Also, external controls should be tested and charted when a new kit is used.

The *internal* control occurs in the "Test Complete" window built into each reaction unit. Chart the control results on the control log with the operator's initials.

QUALITATIVE CONTROL/PATIENT LOG SHEET

TEST: MONONUCLEOSIS RAPID TEST
KIT NAME & MANUFACTURER: QUICK VUE+ Infectious Mononucleosis Test -QUIDEL
LOT # 12345 EXPIRATION DATE: 11/22/20XX
STORAGE REQUIREMENTS: REFRIGERATOR TEST FLOWCHART yes

DATE	SPECIMEN I.D.(CONTROL/ PATIENT)	RESULT (+ OR –)	INTERNAL CONTROL PASSED (Y OR N)	CHARTED IN PATIENT RECORD	TECH INITIALS
7/11/ 20XX	POSITIVE CONTROL	+	Y		LP
7/11/ 20XX	NEGATIVE CONTROL	–	Y		LP
7/11/ 20XX	PT ID: 5432	–	Y	✓	LP

Documentation in the Medical Record

10/9/20XX 9:30 a.m. Mononucleosis rapid test performed with a negative result. Lavender-topped EDTA blood sample sent to lab for CBC and differential.
______________________ Laura Piper, CMA (AAMA)

PROCEDURE 50.6 Coach Patient on the Guaiac Fecal Occult Blood Test

TASKS: Coach a patient on the guaiac fecal occult blood test (gFOBT) while considering the patient's developmental life stage. Document the coaching in the patient's health record.

BACKGROUND: When coaching patients, it is important to consider their developmental life stage. When working with older adults, it is important to communicate with dignity and respect. Use simpler language. Speak clearly and allow time for the patient to respond. It is important to find out what patients know about the topic and respectfully correct any inaccuracies. Make sure to listen to their concerns and provide resources as needed.

SCENARIO: You work at WMFM Clinic. You are working with Dr. David Kahn, who asked you to coach Charles Johnson (date of birth [DOB] 03/03/19XX) on the gFOBT. He is to receive three hemoccult cards for stool smears.

DIRECTIONS: Role-play the scenario with a peer, who is the patient. Your instructor is the provider.

EQUIPMENT and SUPPLIES

- Hemoccult test kit (hemoccult cards, applicator sticks and, if available, flushable collection tissue)
- Patient instructions
- Patient's health record
- Pen

PROCEDURAL STEPS

1. Wash hands or use hand sanitizer.
PURPOSE: Hand sanitization is an important step for infection control.
2. Greet the patient. Identify yourself. Verify the patient's identity with full name and date of birth. Explain what you will be doing.

PROCEDURE 50.6 Coach Patient on the Guaiac Fecal Occult Blood Test—*Continued*

PURPOSE: It is important to identify the patient in two different ways to ensure that you have the correct patient. Explaining the procedure can make the patient feel more comfortable and reduces anxiety.

3. Use simple language when talking. Speak clearly. Communicate with dignity and respect. Allow time for the patient to respond. Listen to the patient's concerns.
   PURPOSE: When working with older patients, it is important to treat them with respect and dignity. Listening is important.
4. Ask the patient if he has ever taken a guaiac fecal occult blood test. If so, ask him what he remembers about it.
   PURPOSE: It is important to find out what the patient already knows about the topic.
5. Discuss the purpose of the test and the supplies needed (e.g., hemoccult cards, applicator kits, and, if available, flushable collection tissue). Show the supplies to the patient.
   PURPOSE: It is important that the patient knows what supplies will be used.
6. Discuss how the patient needs to prepare for the tests and refer to the written instructions.
   PURPOSE: Referring to the written directions that will be sent home with the patient helps eliminate confusion.
7. Discuss how the patient should collect and return the hemoccult cards. Use the written directions when coaching the patient. Write the patient's name, date of birth, and address on the hemoccult cards if required by the agency.
   PURPOSE: The cards need to be labeled with the patient's information. Having the medical assistant label the cards ensures that this step is completed.
8. Ask the patient to teach back the preparation and the collection procedures to you. Clarify any misconceptions or inaccuracies. Answer any questions the patient may have.
   PURPOSE: Using the "teach back" method to evaluate the patient's understanding will help identify any misunderstandings the patient may have.
9. Document the coaching in the patient's health record. Include the provider's name, what was taught, and how the patient responded, and indicate the supplies and written directions sent home with the patient.
   PURPOSE: It is important to document the procedure in the health record to show it was done.

Documentation Example

08/14/20XX 1105 Per Dr. Kahn's order, instructed patient on the gFOBT test including the preparation and collection. Patient taught back the instructions accurately. Gave the patient the hemoccult testing kit and the Hemoccult Patient Directions booklet. Patient will return the cards to the clinic later this week.
———————————— Laura Piper, CMA (AAMA)

PROCEDURE 50.7 Develop a Hemoccult Card and Perform Quality Control

TASKS: Develop a stool specimen using a hemoccult card, and perform a quality control test. Document the test results in the patient's health record.

SCENARIO: Charles Johnson (date of birth [DOB] 03/03/19XX) returns his hemoccult card(s). Dr. David Kahn is his provider. You need to develop (test) the sample.

EQUIPMENT and SUPPLIES

- Hemoccult card with stool smear applied
- Hemoccult developer
- Gloves
- Biohazard waste container
- Waste container
- Patient's health record
- Timer

PROCEDURAL STEPS

1. Wash hands or use hand sanitizer. Put on gloves.
   PURPOSE: Hand sanitization is an important step for infection control.
2. Identify when the specimen was applied and if testing can be done.
   PURPOSE: The company recommends a wait time of 3 days from when the sample was applied. This allows for the degradation of fruit and vegetable peroxidases from the sample. If immediate testing is required, wait 3 to 5 minutes to allow the sample to penetrate the test paper.
3. Open the back of the card and apply 2 drops of the hemoccult developer to the guaiac paper directly over each smear.
4. Within 60 seconds, read the result accurately.
   PURPOSE: Any trace of blue on or near the edge of the sample is considered positive for occult blood.
5. Perform quality control on the card by applying 1 drop of the hemoccult developer between the positive and negative Performance Monitors area.
   PURPOSE: This quality control test will indicate if the card and developer are functional.
6. Within 10 seconds, accurately read the results.
   PURPOSE: A blue color in the positive Performance Monitors area and no blue in the negative Performance Monitors area means the card and the developer are functional.
7. Discard the hemoccult card in the biohazard bag. Clean up the area. Remove gloves and discard in the waste container.
   PURPOSE: It is important to discard the hemoccult card in the biohazard bag for infection control.
8. Wash hands or use hand sanitizer.
9. Document the test result and the provider notified in the patient's health record.
   PURPOSE: It is important to document the procedure in the health record to show it was done.

Documentation Example

08/18/20XX 1105 Hemoccult card × 3 developed. All results were negative. Dr. Kahn notified. ———————————— Laura Piper, CMA (AAMA)

PROCEDURE 50.8 Coach Patient on Health Maintenance: Collecting a Stool Specimen for the Cologuard Test

TASKS: Coach a patient on collecting a stool specimen for a Cologuard test while considering the patient's developmental level. Document the coaching in the health record.

BACKGROUND: When coaching patients, it is important to consider their developmental life stage. When working with older adults, it is important to communicate with dignity and respect. Use simpler language. Speak clearly and allow time for the patient to respond. It is important to find out what they know about the topic and respectfully correct any inaccuracies. Make sure to listen to their concerns and provide resources as needed.

SCENARIO: You work at WMFM Clinic. You are working with Dr. David Kahn, who asked you to coach Charles Johnson (DOB 03/03/19XX) on the Cologuard test.

PATIENT EDUCATION:

- Purpose of the Cologuard test: to identify altered DNA and blood in the stool
- Do not collect a stool sample from patients who have diarrhea, bleeding hemorrhoids, rectal bleeding, menstrual period, or cuts or wounds on their hands.
- Make sure the sample can be returned within a day of collecting it. The laboratory must have the sample within 72 hours, so consider mailing delays such as holidays and weekends.
- Made sure patients are aware of the following instructions when collecting the sample:
  - Use the box, zippered plastic bag, and the tray to return the sample.
  - Remove the bracket from the box and unfold the sides. Place the bracket under the toilet seat near the back of the toilet. Lower the toilet seat.
  - Remove the sample container from the box. Remove the lid of the container and set the lid aside. Place the sample container in the hole in the center of the bracket.
  - Empty your bladder first. Avoid getting urine, toilet paper, or other material in the sample container.
  - Have a bowel movement. The stool sample should be no larger than the bottle of preservative, which is found in the box. Make sure the toilet paper is not placed in the container.
- After completing the bowel movement, patients should do the following:
  - Remove the sample (specimen) container from the bracket and place a counter or other stable surface.
  - Remove the bracket from the toilet and discard.
  - Remove the tube from the box and unscrew the cap. Pull the probe from the tube. Use the probe to scrap the surface of the stool in the container until the probe has stool on it. Make sure the grooves on the probe are filled with stool, but do not fill the tube with stool. Place the probe back into the tube and tighten the cap. Set the tube aside.
  - Remove the bottle of preservative out of the box and remove the cap. Pour all of the preservative into the sample container. The preservative bottle and cap can be discarded.
  - Place the lid on the sample container and tighten the lid.
  - Remove the Sample Label Card from the box and complete both labels. Write your first and last name, date of birth (MM/DD/YY), the date you collected the sample (MM/DD/YY) and the time you collected the sample. Circle AM or PM. Remove one of the labels from the paper and wrap the label around the tube. Remove the other label and place it on the sample container.
  - Place the tube and the sample container into the tray, which sits in the plastic bag in the box. Close the bag, removing the air. Close the box, peel the paper backing off the tape on the box lid, and secure the top of the box. Return the box within a day.

DIRECTIONS: Role-play the scenario with a peer, who is the patient. Your instructor is the provider.

EQUIPMENT and SUPPLIES

- Cologuard test kit (box with plastic bag, sample container, bottle of preservative, bracket, tube, sample labels, and directions)
- Patient instructions (optional)
- Patient's health record
- Pen

PROCEDURAL STEPS

1. Wash hands or use hand sanitizer.
   PURPOSE: Hand sanitization is an important step for infection control.
2. Greet the patient. Identify yourself. Verify the patient's identity with full name and date of birth. Explain what you will be doing.
3. Use simple language when talking. Speak clearly. Communicate with dignity and respect. Allow time for the patient to respond. Listen to the patient's concerns.
4. Ask the patient if he has ever collected a specimen for a Cologuard test. If so, ask him what he remembers about it.
5. Discuss the purpose of the test, the time to take the sample, and the supplies in the box.
6. Discuss how the patient should prepare to collect the sample.
7. Discuss the activities the patient needs to do after the collection, including the use of the probe, adding the preservative to the sample, and packing the box.
8. Ask the patient to teach back the preparation and the collection procedures to you. Clarify any misconceptions or inaccuracies. Answer any questions the patient may have.
9. Document the coaching in the patient's health record. Include the provider's name, what was taught, how the patient responded, and indicate the supplies and written directions sent home with the patient.

INTRAVENOUS THERAPY

51

SCENARIO

Gabe Garcia, CMA (AAMA), works at Walden-Martin Family Medical (WMFM) Clinic. Recently, state statutes were updated, and medical assistants now can insert and monitor intravenous (IV) fluid infusions. The statute stipulates that a medical assistant must pass a training course and the provider must be present at all times during the IV fluid therapy.

After talking with the providers, Gabe took a training course at the local college. He learned about the different types of IV fluids available, complications that can occur, and how to insert the IV catheter. During the training course, Gabe practiced giving IV fluid therapy. He learned how to prepare the equipment and supplies. Gabe practiced on an IV arm and then was able to insert an IV on his partner. By the end of the training course, Gabe was feeling more confident with IV fluid therapy. He is excited to assist the providers with IV fluid therapy at WMFM Clinic.

While studying this chapter, think about the following questions:

- What are the reasons for IV therapy in ambulatory care?
- What are the differences between isotonic, hypotonic, and hypertonic IV solutions, including potential complications with infusions?
- How are the infusion rate and flow rate calculated?
- How do you prime the infusion set, administer IV fluid, change an IV bag, and remove an IV catheter?
- What are issues related to IV infusions?

LEARNING OBJECTIVES

1. Differentiate among the three types of IV solutions, including the action of the fluid and risks associated with the fluids.
2. Differentiate between primary and secondary IV infusion sets.
3. Differentiate among the supplies and equipment used for IV therapy.
4. Calculate the total amount of fluid to be infused, the infusion rate, and the flow rate for IV solutions.
5. Demonstrate how to initiate an IV infusion, including priming the infusion set, preparing the site, and inserting the IV catheter.
6. Demonstrate how to monitor IVs and reduce the risk of complications.
7. Examine the complications of IV therapy, including the signs and symptoms, along with the actions that should be taken.

VOCABULARY

anesthetic (an ehs THET ik) An agent that causes partial or complete loss of sensation.

dextrose (DEK strose) A glucose solution administered intravenously.

extravasation (eks trav ah SAY shun) A discharge of fluid or blood from the blood vessel into the tissues.

flow rate The number of drops (gtt) in 1 minute required to infuse the ordered solution; also called the drip rate.

infusion rate The volume of fluid infused per hour; written as mL/hr.

interstitial fluid Liquid found between the cells of the body.

intravenous (in TRAH vee nus) Through a vein; fluids and medications can be given through a vein.

intravenous therapy Administration and monitoring of fluid and medication by intravenous infusion.

patency (PAT en see) Open condition of a body cavity or canal.

phlebitis (fle BYE tis) Inflammation of a vein.

solute A substance that is dissolved in a solvent (liquid) to form a solution.

solvent A liquid that is able to dissolve other substances.

vesicant (VES i kant) medicationA medication that can damage tissue and can produce blisters.

INTRODUCTION

The administration of **intravenous** (IV) fluids, medications, nutritional supplements, and blood components is common in the hospital setting. Over the years, more **intravenous therapy** has occurred in ambulatory healthcare facilities. Ambulatory care providers usually order IV therapy for the following reasons:

- *To provide fluids and electrolytes (also called hydration therapy):* One of the most common reasons for IV fluid (or solution) infusions is to treat dehydration. Dehydration can occur from reduced fluid intake, diarrhea, vomiting, and heat related illnesses.
- *To treat conditions:* IV medications can be used for many different conditions, including infections, cancer, osteoporosis, iron deficiency anemia, and autoimmune disorders (e.g., rheumatoid arthritis, psoriatic arthritis, and ulcerative colitis). IV medications reach the blood stream immediately, providing rapid action. Some medications only come as IV medications.
- *For diagnostic tests*: IV contrast media can be given for some diagnostic tests, including computerized axial tomography (CT) scans and intravenous pyelograms.

Providing IV therapy in ambulatory care facilities is an inexpensive option compared to hospitalizing patients.

State laws vary on the role of medical assistants regarding starting and monitoring IV fluid infusions and administering IV contrast media. It is important for medical assistants to know the state laws and the healthcare facility's policies before working with IVs. In this chapter, the techniques for preparing and administering IV fluids will be the primary focus. Administering IV medications, such as chemotherapy and antibiotics, is outside the medical assistant's scope of practice.

In previous chapters, you learned the basics of pharmacology and how to prepare and administer injections. To administer IV fluid therapy, you will need to apply the nine rights of medication administration you learned in Chapter 30.

INTRAVENOUS SOLUTIONS

IV solutions should be treated like medications. The medical assistant must follow the nine rights of medication administration. As part of these rights, the name of the IV solution must be checked three times before the IV therapy is started on the patient. The IV solution type, the amount of fluid in the bag, and the expiration date are all labeled on the bag and must be checked.

IV solutions come in plastic bags and are then connected to IV infusion sets. The IV solution bag has a hole at the top that is used to hang it from an IV pole or wall hook. Markings on the bag can help indicate the amount of fluid left. The medication port (also called the injection port) is located at the bottom of the bag and is used to inject medication into the IV fluid bag. (Injecting a medication into an IV solution bag is beyond the scope of a medical assistant.) The IV tubing port is located next to the medication port and is used to attach the IV infusion set. Once the IV bag is punctured by the infusion set, it is only good for 24 hours (unless otherwise stated by the healthcare facility).

When a patient requires IV fluid therapy in ambulatory care, the patient receives a crystalloid solution. **Solutes** such as electrolytes or **dextrose** are dissolved in a fluid, or **solvent**, creating a crystalloid solution. Crystalloid solutions can pass through semipermeable membranes, such as blood vessel walls and move into cells and tissues. Crystalloid solutions can be isotonic, hypotonic, or hypertonic.

Safety with IV Solutions

The IV solution should be discarded if the fluid has any of the following characteristics:

- Contains *precipitate* (solid particles) or looks cloudy
- Has expired
- Has become contaminated
- Is no longer needed or the patient's IV therapy has been completed

IV solutions, also called IV fluids, should be treated like medications. The medical assistant must follow the nine rights of medication administration. As part of these rights, the name of the IV solution must be checked three times before the IV therapy is started on the patient. The IV solution type, the amount of fluid in the bag, and the expiration date are all labeled on the bag and must be checked. Prior to starting the IV fluid infusion, the medical assistant should obtain the patient's vital signs. During the infusion, the patient's vital signs should be monitored due to potential side effects of the treatment.

CRITICAL THINKING APPLICATION 51.1

Describe the difference between a solute and a solvent.

Isotonic Solutions

Isotonic solutions and plasma have a similar dissolved particle concentration. When an isotonic solution is administered, it is distributed between the bloodstream, the **interstitial fluid**, and cells. Isotonic solutions are typically ordered when a patient is dehydrated. There are several types of isotonic IV solutions:

- 0.9% sodium chloride (also called 0.9% NaCl, normal saline, and NS)
- Lactated Ringer Solution (also called LR and Ringer Lactate)
- 5% dextrose in water (or D5W)
- Ringer Solution

Isotonic solutions can cause hypervolemia, or fluid volume overload. Signs and symptoms of hypervolemia include hypertension, pulmonary crackles, dyspnea, shortness of breath, and peripheral edema. If the patient experiences any of these, the medical assistant must immediately notify the provider.

Hypotonic Solutions

Hypotonic solutions have a lower concentration of dissolved particles than plasma. This causes the fluid to move out of the blood vessels and into the interstitial fluid and cells. Hypotonic solutions are typically ordered for patients with diabetic ketoacidosis. Types of hypotonic IV solutions include the following:

- 0.45% sodium chloride (also called 0.45% NS and 1/2 NS)
- 0.33% sodium chloride (or 0.33% NS)
- 2.5% dextrose in water (or D2.5W)

Because the hypotonic fluid moves out of the bloodstream, the patient has to be monitored for hypovolemia. Signs and symptoms of hypovolemia include hypotension, dizziness, and confusion. If the patient experiences any of these, the medical assistant must immediately notify the provider.

CRITICAL THINKING APPLICATION **51.2**

Describe why hypotonic solutions cause hypotension.

Hypertonic Solutions

Hypertonic solutions have a higher concentration of dissolved particles than plasma. This causes fluid from the cells to move into the bloodstream, increasing the blood volume and thus the blood pressure. Hypertonic solutions are typically ordered for patients with hypotension and *hyponatremia* (low sodium). Types of hypertonic IV solutions include the following:

- 3% sodium chloride (or 3% NS) and 5% sodium chloride (or 5% NS)
- Dextrose 5% in 0.45% sodium chloride (also called D5.45NS, D5 1/2 NS, Dextrose 5% in 0.45% NaCl)
- Dextrose 5% in 0.9% sodium chloride (also called D5NS, Dextrose 5% in 0.9% NaCl)
- Dextrose 5% in Lactated Ringer (or D5LR)
- 10% dextrose in water (or D10W)

Because the hypertonic solutions pull fluids into the bloodstream, the patient has to be monitored for hypervolemia. Signs and symptoms of hypervolemia include hypertension, pulmonary crackles, dyspnea, shortness of breath, and peripheral edema. If the patient experiences any of these, the medical assistant must immediately notify the provider.

CRITICAL THINKING APPLICATION **51.3**

Describe why hypertonic solutions cause hypertension.

IV INFUSION SETS

An IV infusion set is tubing with one end inserted into the IV solution bag, and the other end can be connected to the IV catheter. Depending on what is ordered for the IV therapy, both a primary and secondary infusion set may be used. The following sections describe the difference between primary and secondary infusion sets.

Primary Infusion Sets

A *primary infusion* set is also called an infusion set or a primary infusion administration set. The primary infusion set connects to the IV solution bag. The infusion set can be either a macro-drip or a micro-drip set. The difference between these two sets is the drop factor. The drop factor is the number of drops (gtt) per milliliter (mL) of fluid. The drop factor (gtt/mL) is listed on the infusion set packaging.

The *macro-drip infusion set* creates larger drops and comes in a variety of sizes, such as 10, 12, 15, or 20 gtt/mL. Macro-drip infusion sets are the most common set type to use for routine IV therapy in adults. These infusion sets are used when delivering a larger volume of fluid in an hour.

Micro-drip infusion sets create smaller drops and deliver 60 gtt/mL. These sets can deliver smaller amounts of fluid over a given time frame. Micro-drip infusion sets are used for pediatric patients and for an adult who needs a smaller volume of fluid (e.g., 40 mL/hr).

Parts of the Primary Infusion Set

The primary infusion set consists of the following parts:

- *Spike*: A sterile spike that is inserted into the IV bag using the IV tubing port.
- *Drip chamber*: Used to count the drip rate of the IV if an IV pump is not used. Counting the drips over 1 minute helps determine the **flow rate** of the IV fluid. The drip chamber needs to be one-third to one-half full of IV fluid at all times. If the drip chamber is too full, the drip rate cannot be counted. If the drip chamber is not full enough, air can get into the IV tubing and can be dangerous for the patient.
- *Roller clamp*: Used to control the rate at which the IV flows with a gravity infusion. If the roller clamp is moved down, the tubing is pinched, stopping the flow of fluid (Figure 51.1). As the roller clamp is moved toward the opposite side, the solution starts flowing. If the roller clamp is opened completely, the IV solution flows quickly into the patient, which can be dangerous if not ordered at that rate.
- *Slide clamp*: Used to completely stop the IV infusion. The slide clamp pinches off the tubing, stopping the solution flow. It can be helpful to use the slide clamp when the infusion must be stopped for a few minutes. It prevents having to readjust the flow rate with the roller clamp with gravity infusions.
- *Luer connector:* Also called Luer lock and Luer taper. Found at the end of the infusion tubing. The luer connects the infusion set to the IV catheter or extension tubing.

In addition to these parts, some primary infusion sets may also have:

- *Backcheck valve*: Prevents fluid or medications from traveling up the IV tubing and into the IV bag.
- *Injection ports*: Used to infuse IV medication. If the patient needs an IV medication, the medication can be infused either using a second IV solution bag or by IV push using a syringe. The injection port closest to the drip chamber is used to connect the secondary infusion set and bag. The injection port closer to the luer connector and patient is used for IV push medications. Administering IV medications is outside the scope of practice for medical assistants and is usually done by the registered nurse (RN) or provider.
- *Buretrol*: A cylinder holding device that limits the amount of IV solutions given; may be used in pediatrics.

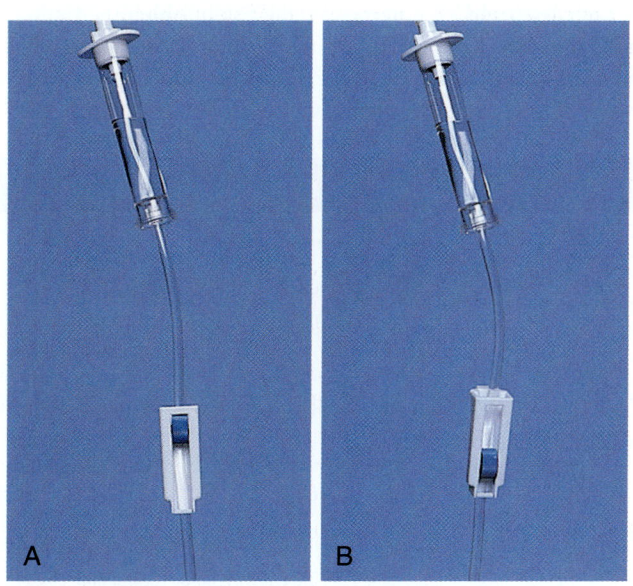

FIGURE 51.1 **(A)** Roller clamp in open position. **(B)** Roller clamp in closed or off position. (From Potter P, Perry A: *Basic nursing*, ed 7, St. Louis, 2011, Mosby.)

Secondary Infusion Sets

A secondary infusion set is used to give IV medications. The secondary infusion set has fewer features than the primary set, and the tubing is shorter. The secondary infusion set has a sterile spike, drip chamber, roller clamp, and a luer connector used to connect to the primary infusion set's injection port. When a secondary infusion set is used, the IV bag on the primary infusion set (or the primary IV bag) is hung lower. The secondary infusion bag is hung higher or piggybacked on the primary IV bag. The higher position creates greater gravitational pressure on the secondary IV bag, which will infuse first. After the secondary IV bag is empty, the primary IV bag infuses.

ADDITIONAL SUPPLIES AND EQUIPMENT FOR IV THERAPY

When initiating IV therapy, the medical assistant must gather the supplies needed. This section focuses on the supplies used to initiate and maintain IV therapy. Depending on the agency, supplies may vary.

IV Extension Tubing

An extension tubing can be used to connect the IV catheter with the primary infusion set. The extension tubing has a slide clamp, a male luer connector on one end, and a female luer connector on the other. The male luer connector connects with the primary infusion set, and the female connecter connects with the IV catheter. The length of the extension tubing can vary.

IV Catheters

Intravenous access can be done as either peripheral or central access. Commonly in ambulatory care, short peripheral IV catheters are inserted into a peripheral vein in the hand or arm. If allowed by the state laws and the agency's policy, this is the type of IV a medical assistant can insert. Table 51.1 describes the different types of IV access devices that may be seen in ambulatory care.

Usually, catheters 20 to 24-gauge are used for adult infusions in ambulatory care. For pediatric and older adult patients, 22 to 24-gauge catheters may be used. Catheters with a larger gauge than 20, such as 16 and 18, can increase the risk of **phlebitis**. Catheters with large diameter lumens allow the IV solution to flow at a faster rate than a catheters with smaller diameter lumens. The medical assistant must consider the patient and the type of treatment when selecting the IV catheter. With these factors in mind, the shortest catheter with the smallest diameter lumen should be used to decrease the risk of phlebitis.

The IV safety needle is beveled. The needle is covered with a catheter, a thin plastic tube. A clear flashback chamber behind the needle fills with blood when the needle enters the vein. Once the IV safety needle is inserted, the catheter is pushed into the vein, and the needle is withdrawn. The catheter is attached to extension tubing or the IV infusion set.

Safety Features

Two types of IV catheters seen in ambulatory care are straight and winged hub safety catheters. The wings vary in size and can be used to insert the needle and stabilize the catheter (Figure 51.2). Various features are available with IV catheters that improve the insertion success and the safety of the procedure.

The IV safety needles are passive or active. Passive IV safety needles are designed so the needle is automatically covered after use. Many IV needles are covered as the user pulls the needle from the catheter. The safety clamps onto the needle and protects against accidental needlesticks. Active IV safety needles require the healthcare professional to activate the safety device. Several active IV safety needles have buttons that retract the needle into the needle guard (Figure 51.3).

With the design of traditional IV catheters, blood backflows out of the catheter onto the patient's skin when the needle is removed. This causes a risk of contamination to the medical assistant. Newer IV safety catheters prevent blood from backflowing out of the catheter. Some catheters have a septum that closes as the needle is retracted, preventing blood from backflowing. The septum opens when the luer connector is joined to the catheter. Some winged hub catheters have preattached extension tubing that prevents blood from backflowing. With the wide variety of IV safety needle/catheter units on the market, the medical assistant needs to be trained on the types available in the facility before using them on patients.

CRITICAL THINKING APPLICATION **51.4**

Describe the safety features typically found in today's IV needle/catheter units. Why would these features be important for the medical assistant?

TABLE 51.1 Intravenous Access Devices

<table>
<tr><th>TYPES</th><th>PLACEMENT</th><th>LEFT IN PLACE FOR</th><th>USES</th></tr>
<tr><td>Peripheral IV line (PIV or IV)</td><td>Short catheter is placed in the hand or forearm.</td><td>3–4 days, depending on agency's policy; must be kept dry</td><td>Fluid and medication infusion; harsh medications can cause phlebitis and irritation</td></tr>
<tr><td>Peripherally inserted central line catheter (PICC)</td><td>Longer catheter is placed in the upper arm.</td><td rowspan="2">Weeks to months; must be kept dry and requires regular cleaning and maintenance to maintain patency</td><td rowspan="3">Usually requires a registered nurse to start the IV therapy, perform blood draws, and maintain the catheter</td></tr>
<tr><td>Central venous catheter (CVC)</td><td>Like the PICC but placed in the chest or neck.</td></tr>
<tr><td>Port</td><td>Catheter is surgically implanted under the skin in the chest; type of central line.</td><td>Years; requires limited maintenance. No limitation with showering or swimming</td></tr>
</table>

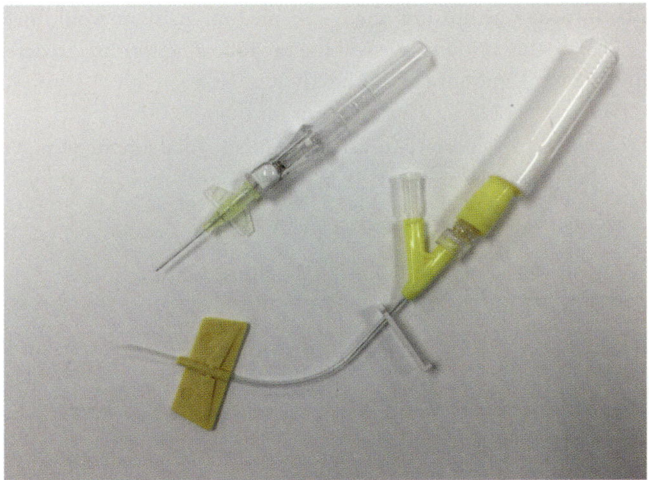

FIGURE 51.2 Examples of winged hub safety needles.

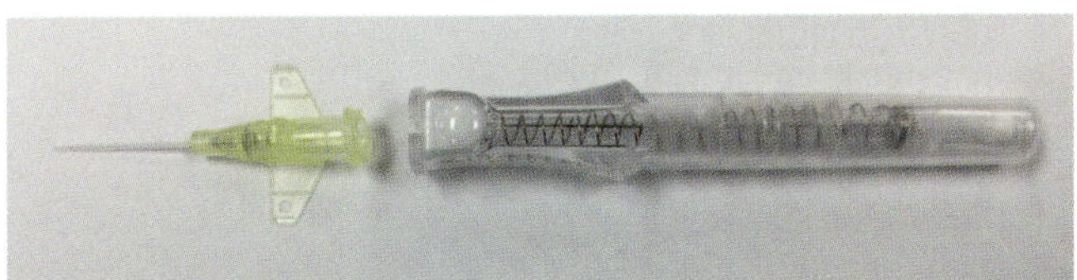

FIGURE 51.3 BD Insyte Autoguard IV catheter. When a button is pushed, the needle retracts into the needle guard.

IV Start Kits

Some ambulatory care facilities use IV start kits, which contain supplies needed to insert an IV. IV start kits may include (Figure 51.4) the following items:

- *A tourniquet*: To help engorge the vein during the insertion procedure.
- *Antiseptic swabs or applicators*: Chlorhexidine, Betadine, or alcohol is used to clean the insertion site prior to the catheter insertion.
- *Sterile gauze*: Used to apply pressure to the site if the insertion is unsuccessful. It can also be used to clean up any blood at the site when the needle is removed.
- *A transparent dressing*: Typically, a semipermeable membrane dressing. Used to cover the insertion site (Figure 51.5)
- *Tape*: Used to secure the catheter and tubing to the skin.

Topical Anesthetic

A topical **anesthetic** or vapocoolant may be ordered by the provider prior to the IV catheter insertion. This medication helps minimize the discomfort felt during the IV catheter insertion. Depending on the state law and the healthcare facility's policies and procedures, the medical assistant may be able to administer the medication. Prior to administration, always check the patient's allergies and be familiar with the medication, including the action, side effects, and administration techniques.

IV Pole and IV Infusion Pump

An IV pole or hook must be used to keep the IV bag higher than the patient to administer IV fluids. The IV tubing drip chamber should be about 3 feet above the level of the catheter insertion site. An infusion pump may also be used for IV infusions.

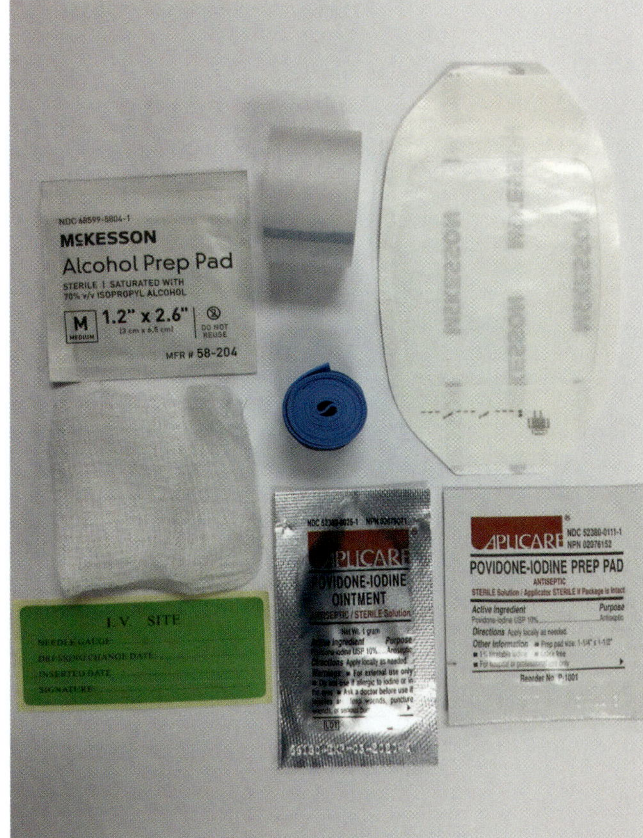

FIGURE 51.4 IV start kit.

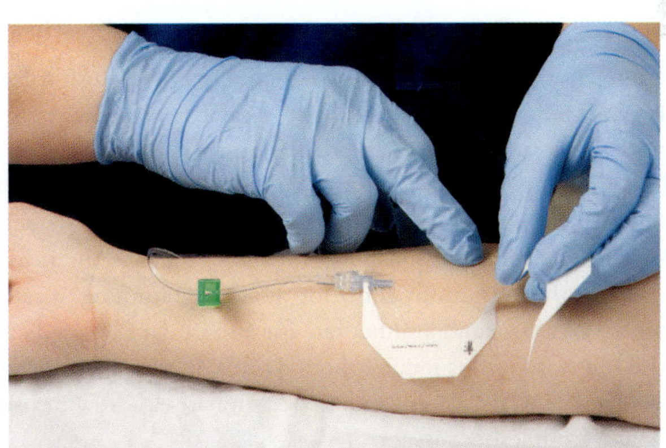

FIGURE 51.5 Applying a transparent dressing. (From Potter PA, Perry AG: *Fundamentals of nursing*, ed 9, St. Louis, 2017, Elsevier.)

Many ambulatory care facilities use IV infusion pumps to deliver the IV solution. The IV infusion pump regulates the IV solution infusion rate. Additional information on the IV infusion pump is discussed in the following section.

PUMP AND GRAVITY INFUSIONS

During the IV infusion, the goal is to deliver the solution at the rate ordered by the provider. The IV solution can be delivered by an infusion pump or by gravity. The medical assistant may need to perform calculations for the IV infusion.

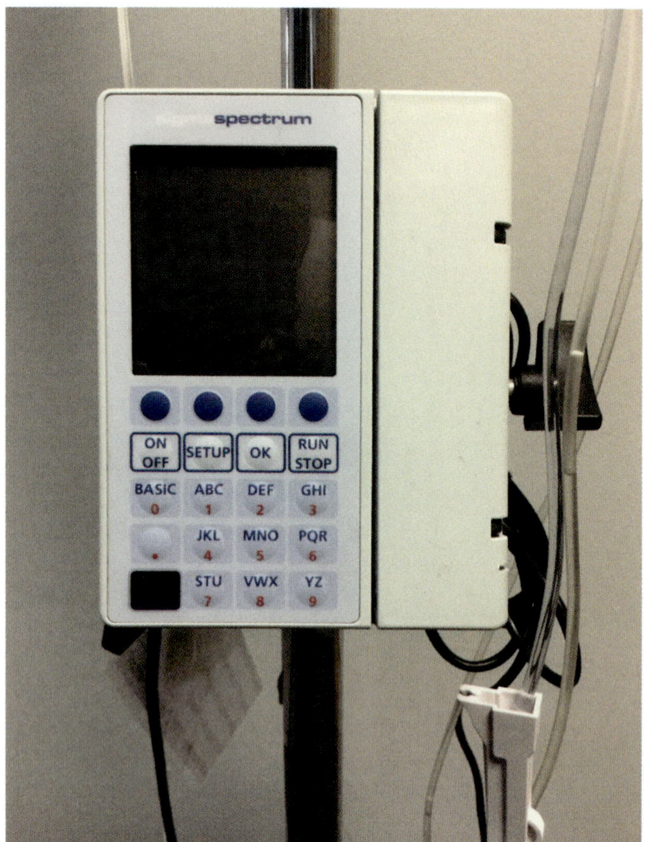

FIGURE 51.6 An example of an infusion pump. Many infusion pumps are available on the market.

Infusion Pump Delivery

Using an IV infusion pump is safer than a gravity infusion for IV fluids. Most infusion pumps have built-in safety features that prevent an accidental infusion of extra fluid. The pump regulates the amount of fluid the patient gets (Figure 51.6). The total amount of fluid infused and the rate of infusion are shown on the pump's screen. Locking mechanisms prevent unauthorized changes in the **infusion rate**. Most infusion pumps allow for dual programming, a rate for the primary IV bag, and another rate for a secondary IV medication bag. IV infusion pumps require specific infusion sets. If an IV pump is used, the medical assistant should be familiar with how to use the pump and troubleshoot issues.

Most IV infusion pumps require the healthcare professional to enter the following information:

- The total amount of fluid to be infused.
- The infusion rate

Both pieces of information may be in the provider's order. For example, the order may be written as "0.9% NS 1000 mL IV at 125 mL/hour." The total amount of fluid to be infused is 1000 mL. The infusion rate is 125 mL/hour. Sometimes the total amount of fluid to be infused or the infusion rate is not included in the order. In these cases, the medical assistant is required to calculate the information.

Calculate the Total Amount to Be Infused

A provider's order may be written as "0.9% NS IV 125 mL/hour for 6 hours." (Some providers may write "× 6 hours," which means "for 6 hours.") The infusion rate is 125 mL/hour, but the total amount to be infused was not indicated. The medical assistant would need to calculate this amount. We will use the following formula to determine the total amount to be infused:

Order: 0.9% NS IV 125 mL/hour for 6 hours

Formula: Infusion rate (mL/hr) × hours = Total amount (mL) to be infused

Solution: $\frac{125 \text{ mL}}{1 \text{ hr}} \times 6 \text{ hours} = 750 \text{ mL}$

The provider ordered 750 mL to be infused over 6 hours.

Practice Problems for Calculating the Total Amount to Be Infused

Find the total amount to be infused.

1. 0.9% NS IV 100 mL/hr for 8 hours.
2. 0.9% NS IV 75 mL/hr for 5 hours.
3. LR IV 50 mL/hr for 8 hours.
4. LR IV 125 mL/hr for 6 hours.
5. 0.9% NS IV 50 mL/hr for 2.5 hours.
6. 0.9% NS IV 100 mL/hr for 3 hours.
7. 0.9% NS IV 75 mL/hr for 3 hours.
8. LR IV 150 mL/hr for 3 hours.
9. LR IV 50 mL/hr for 4 hours.
10. 0.9% NS IV 50 mL/hr for 5 hours.

Calculate the Infusion Rate

Sometimes the medical assistant must calculate the infusion rate if the provider only indicates the volume of fluid to infuse over a set period of time. For example, a provider orders "0.9% NS IV 500 mL over 4 hours." The provider wants 500 mL to be given over a period of 4 hours. In this example, the medical assistant must calculate the infusion rate or number of mL to give over 1 hour. We will use the following formula to determine the infusion rate:

Order: 0.9% NS IV 500 mL over 4 hours

Formula: Total amount (mL) ÷ Hours = Infusion rate (mL/hour)

Solution: 500 mL ÷ 4 hours = 125 mL per hour

For this example, the patient receives 125 mL per hour for 4 hours.

In some cases, the medical assistant might receive an order for the IV solution to be infused in less than 1 hour. Infusions less than 1 hour are more common with IV medications than with IV fluids. A medical assistant performing IV fluid administration should be familiar with calculating infusion rates for infusions less than 1 hour. The following example demonstrates how to calculate the infusion rate:

Order: 0.9% NS IV 100 mL over 30 minutes

Formula: $\frac{\text{Total amount (mL)} \times 60 \text{ minutes}}{\text{Time (minutes)} \times 1 \text{ hour}} = \frac{\text{Infusion Rate}}{\text{(mL/ hour)}}$

Solution: $\frac{100 \text{ mL} \times 60 \text{ minutes}}{30 \text{ minutes} \times 1 \text{ hour}} = \frac{6000 \text{ mL}}{30 \text{ hour}} = \frac{200 \text{ mL}}{1 \text{ hour}}$

With this type of problem, you need to multiply the two *numerators* (the top numbers) and then multiply the two *denominators* (the bottom number). The minute labels cancel out, and your label is mL/hour.

Practice Problems for Calculating Infusion Rates

Find the infusion rate (mL/hr). Round to the nearest mL.

1. 0.9% NS IV 500 mL over 8 hours.
2. 0.9% NS IV 250 mL over 5 hours.
3. LR IV 1000 mL over 8 hours.
4. LR IV 500 mL over 6 hours.
5. 0.9% NS IV 250 mL over 2.5 hours.
6. 0.9% NS IV 100 mL over 30 minutes.
7. 0.9% NS IV 50 mL over 20 minutes.
8. LR IV 75 mL over 30 minutes.
9. LR IV 50 mL over 30 minutes.
10. 0.9% NS IV 50 mL over 40 minutes.

Gravity Infusions

When an IV is delivered by gravity, the medical assistant must use the roller clamp to regulate the IV flow. The roller clamp is used to adjust the rate of drops falling in the drip chamber. The speed of the drops relates to the amount of fluid delivered. The faster the drops fall in the drip chamber, the more fluid is being delivered. It is important that the IV solution be infused at the rate ordered, and the medical assistant should frequently check the IV flow rate. IV solution delivered too quickly or given too much fluid can harm the patient.

Calculate the Flow Rate

The *flow rate* (drip rate) is the number of drops (gtt) in 1 minute required to infuse the ordered solution. The flow rate is determined by the infusion rate and the infusion set drop factor. Once the flow rate is determined, the medical assistant must adjust the roller clamp, so the drops falling in the drip chamber for 1 minute match the flow rate. Usually, the drops are counted for 30 seconds and multiplied by 2.

To calculate the flow rate, the medical assistant must have the infusion set drop factor and the amount of fluid to infuse over x number of minutes. For example, let us take the following order and find the flow rate:

Order: 0.9% NS IV 50 mL over 30 min

Infusion set: Drop factor of 20 gtt/ml

Formula: $\frac{\text{Volume to infuse (mL)} \times \text{Drop factor (gtt)}}{\text{Time (min)} \times \text{(mL)}} = \frac{\text{Flow rate}}{\text{(gtt/min)}}$

Solution: $\frac{50\text{ mL} \times 20\text{ gtt}}{30\text{ min} \times 1\text{ mL}} = \frac{1000\text{ gtt}}{30\text{ min}} = \frac{33\text{ gtt}}{\text{min}}$ (flow rate)

With this type of problem, you need to multiply the two numerators and then multiply the two denominators. The mL labels cancel out, and your label is gtt/min. The medical assistant would need to regulate the roller clamp so that 33 drops fall in the drip chamber in 1 minute.

If the medical assistant does not have the number of minutes for the infusion, this can be calculated using the formula discussed earlier. For example, let us take the following order, find the number of minutes for the infusion, and then find the flow rate:

Order: 0.9% NS IV 150 mL over 2 hours

Infusion set: Drop factor of 15 gtt/ml.

- *Step 1:* Find the volume to infuse (mL) in 1 hour (the infusion rate)

Formula: Total amount (mL) ÷ hours = mL per hour

Solution: 150 mL ÷ 2 hours = 75 mL per hour

- *Step 2:* Switch 1 hour to 60 minutes (75 mL/60 min)
- *Step 3:* Find the flow rate.

Formula: $\frac{\text{Volume to infuse (mL)} \times \text{Drop factor (gtt)}}{\text{Time (min)} \times \text{(mL)}} = \frac{\text{Flow rate}}{\text{(gtt/min)}}$

Solution: $\frac{75\text{ mL} \times 15\text{ gtt}}{60\text{ min} \times 1\text{ mL}} = \frac{1125\text{ gtt}}{60\text{ min}} = 19\text{ gtt/min}$

With this type of problem, you need to multiply the two numerators and then multiply the two denominators. The mL labels cancel out, and your label is gtt/min. The answer is rounded to the nearest drop.

Practice Problems: Calculating the Flow Rate

Find the infusion rate and the flow rate. Round to the nearest gtt.

1. 0.9% NS IV 500 mL over 7 hours. Infusion set: drop factor of 10 gtt/ml.
2. 0.9% NS IV 250 mL over 5 hours. Infusion set: drop factor of 60 gtt/ml.
3. LR IV 1000 mL over 8 hours. Infusion set: drop factor of 10 gtt/ml.
4. LR IV 500 mL over 6 hours. Infusion set: drop factor of 20 gtt/ml.
5. 0.9% NS IV 250 mL over 2.5 hours. Infusion set: drop factor of 10 gtt/ml.

INITIATING IV INFUSIONS

When a medical assistant must initiate an IV infusion, preparation must be done before inserting the IV catheter. The medical assistant must prime the primary infusion set and prepare the site for the catheter insertion. After the catheter insertion, the medical assistant must document the procedure. The following sections discuss these procedures.

Priming the Primary Infusion Set

The preparation begins with an order from the provider. The order must include the following:

- Patient's name and date of birth (DOB)
- Type of IV solution
- Amount of fluid to infuse over a specific time period (e.g., 500 mL over 4 hours) or the rate of the infusion for a specific time period (e.g., 125 mL/hr × 4 hours)

As described earlier, IV orders may vary. The medical assistant must follow the nine rights of medication administration described in Chapter 30. The IV label must be compared to the order three times prior to the start of the infusion. The expiration date on the bag of fluid must also be checked.

The primary infusion set must be primed with the IV solution just before it is used. Priming means running IV fluid through the tubing to remove all of the air. This procedure prevents air from entering the patient's circulatory system, which can cause an air embolism. Deaths have been attributed to as little as 10 mL of air. Procedure 51.1 describes how to prime the infusion set.

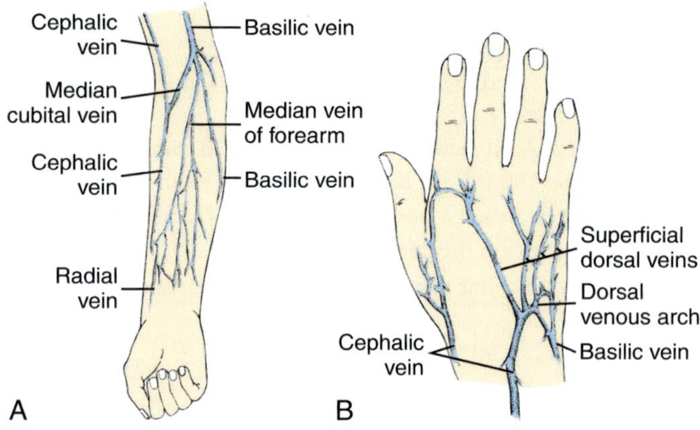

FIGURE 51.7 Common IV sites in adults. **(A)** Inner arm. **(B)** Dorsal surface of hand. (From Potter PA, Perry AG: *Fundamentals of nursing*, ed 9, St. Louis, 2017, Elsevier.)

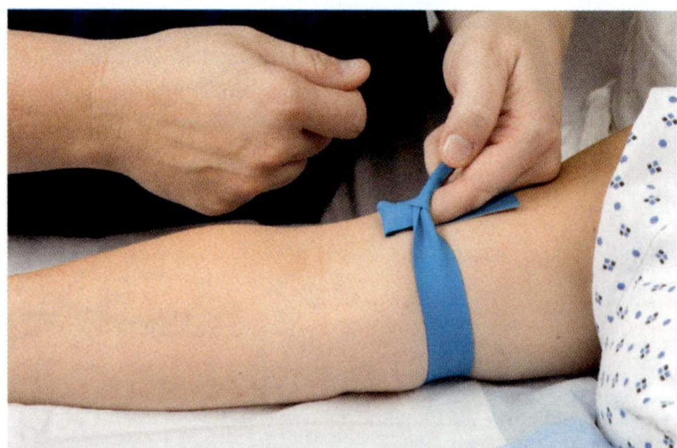

FIGURE 51.8 Tourniquet placed on arm for initial vein selection. (From Potter P, Perry A: *Basic nursing*, ed 7, St. Louis, 2011, Mosby.)

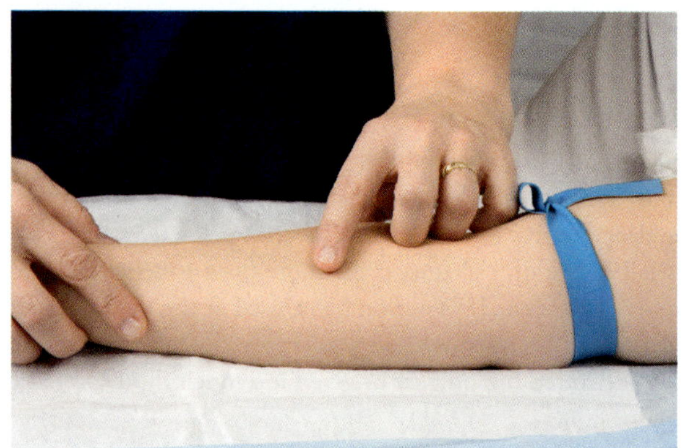

FIGURE 51.9 Palpate vein. (From Potter P, Perry A: *Basic nursing*, ed 7, St. Louis, 2011, Mosby.)

As the medical assistant prepares the IV supplies, it is important to use sterile technique. The sterile spike, which is used to spike the IV bag, must remain sterile. The luer connector, found on the opposite side of the infusion set, also must remain sterile.

Identifying a Vein

In ambulatory care, a peripheral IV is usually inserted in an upper extremity. When looking for a potential insertion site, the medical assistant should start distally and work up the hand and arm (Figure 51.7). If an IV attempt is unsuccessful, all future sites must be more proximal to that site. In other words, the medical assistant should start looking for a vein on the top of the hand and move up the arm. If a site on the arm is unsuccessful, the medical assistant cannot attempt a site more distal, such as on the hand. The IV catheter should not be inserted in the following locations:

- In an area that is painful, tender, infected, burned, or compromised (e.g., lymphedema)
- In an area with an open wound
- In an extremity that is paralyzed or affected by a stroke, contains a dialysis fistula, or on the same side of a mastectomy
- Distal to a previous IV site or infiltrated site
- In a fragile vein

The medical assistant should avoid inserting the catheter in areas of flexion. Inserting the catheter in the antecubital site, on the inside of the wrist (ventral surface), or in the cephalic vein at the wrist can increase the risk for nerve damage.

Typically, the IV catheter is inserted and removed during the same visit. If the patient needs the IV catheter to remain in for a longer period of time, the medical assistant must consider the following:

- If possible, use the nondominant hand/arm.
- Avoid inserting the catheter in the hand if the patient is using an assistive device, such as a walker or cane.
- Avoid inserting the catheter in a flexible area, such as near the wrist or elbow.

The medical assistant should look for a straight, nonbranched vein (Procedure 51.2). The tourniquet can be placed about 4 to 6 inches proximal to the site to help the vein engorge with blood (Figure 51.8). When using the tourniquet, the medical assistant must check the patient's radial pulse on the side with the tourniquet. If the radial pulse is diminished or absent, loosen the tourniquet. Here are some other strategies to help engorge the vein:

- Stroking the vessel
- Have the patient dangle their arm down on the side
- Applying a warm pack to the site for a few minutes
- Having the patient open and close the hand, making a fist

When the medical assistant palpates the vein, it should feel spongy (Figure 51.9). If the vessel is pulsing, it is likely to be an artery and should not be used. Some facilities use technology to help find a vein for catheter placement. Visible light devices transilluminate the vessel, and near infrared and ultrasound can also be used. Once the insertion site is determined, the tourniquet is removed.

Site Preparation

If the patient's skin is visibly soiled, it should be washed with soap and water and dried. If hair needs to be removed from the site, a disposable-head electric shaver can be used. Shaving is usually done for IVs that will remain in for a long period of time.

The skin can be cleaned using several different antiseptics. Always check the patient's allergies before starting the procedure. The most common antiseptics include chlorhexidine, povidone-iodine (Betadine), and alcohol. Chlorhexidine is the preferred antiseptic. When using chlorhexidine, place the applicator on the skin and do a friction scrub (Figure 51.10). Scrub back and forth and up and down for 30 seconds. Allow the product to dry on the skin for at least 30 seconds. If using Betadine or alcohol, place the applicator at the intended site of insertion and work outward in a circular pattern, making larger circles as the area is cleaned. Betadine must dry before

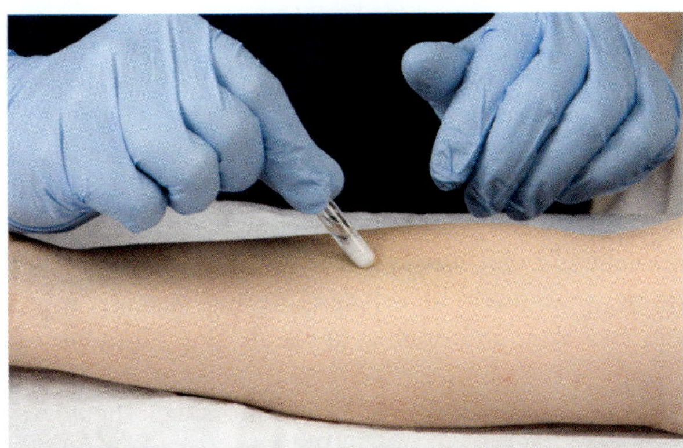

FIGURE 51.10 Cleanse site with chlorhexidine. (From Potter PA, Perry AG: *Fundamentals of nursing*, ed 9, St. Louis, 2017, Elsevier.)

starting the catheter insertion. The drying process kills the microorganisms. If the skin is touched with gloves or ungloved hands, the cleansing process needs to be repeated.

CRITICAL THINKING APPLICATION 51.5

A patient asks you why you need to clean the arm for so long before putting in the IV. How would you respond to this question?

Inserting the IV Catheter

Once the antiseptic is dried, the tourniquet is reapplied. Using the dominant hand, grasp the IV needle/catheter unit and place it parallel to the vein. Using the nondominant hand, hold the skin taut below the insertion site. The thumb should stabilize the vein in place during the insertion process.

With the bevel facing up, insert the needle/catheter unit directly on top of the vein using a 10- to 30-degree angle. Superficial veins require a lesser angle of insertion, whereas a deeper vein requires a greater angle. Once the needle enters the vein, a blood flashback is seen in the clear flashback chamber. The needle should be advanced a bit further. Then the catheter is pushed off the needle and advanced into the vein until the hub reaches the insertion site. A blood flashback may also be seen in the catheter as the catheter enters the vein. The needle is withdrawn, and the tubing is attached to the catheter. The catheter is taped to the arm, and a transparent or gauze dressing is applied. The infusion set is also secured to the arm with tape. After the IV catheter is inserted and the solution is infusing, the medical assistant should observe the site for a few minutes to ensure no complications occur.

If the patient experiences tingling or numbness during the insertion process or the infusion, the medical assistant should pause the infusion and notify the provider. This type of pain can indicate nerve damage.

If the medical assistant is unsuccessful with the insertion attempt, the entire cleansing process must be repeated in another location proximal to the attempted site. A new catheter must be used. The standard is two insertion attempts per person, with a total of four attempts.

CRITICAL THINKING APPLICATION 51.6

When inserting an IV, Gabe warns the patient, "You will feel a poke," just before he inserts the IV. Is this a good practice? Why or why not?

Documentation

After completing the catheter insertion and starting the IV infusion, the medical assistant must document the procedure. The documentation should include the following information:

- Date and time
- Ordering provider's name
- IV order, which includes the IV solution, amount, and rate per hour or over the number of hours
- Type and size of catheter inserted
- Location of insertion site
- Any issues with the insertion process, including the number of insertion attempts
- Type of IV fluid being infused and the infusion rate
- Name and credentials (e.g., registered medical assistant [RMA]) of the person who inserted the catheter
- Any other documentation required by the facility

MONITORING IV THERAPY

Once the IV is initiated, the medical assistant must monitor the IV infusion and the patient. The rest of the chapter addresses monitoring and maintaining IVs, identifying complications, and discontinuing IV therapy.

Monitoring the Infusion and the Patient

The patient should be checked at least every 30 to 60 minutes, depending on the situation and the facility's policy. The medical assistant should check on the patient and the site for complications. The medical assistant should obtain the vital signs, listen for changes in the patient's breathing, and ask how the patient is feeling. Concerns such as pain at or above the insertion site or difficulty breathing need to be reported to the provider. If a gravity infusion is used, the flow rate must be checked.

Even though a medical assistant sets the flow rate, frequent checking of the flow rate is critical to the safety of the IV infusion. If the IV catheter is inserted near an area of flexion, the flow rate can change if the patient bends the area. Sometimes patients change their positions, which can speed up or slow down the infusion rate. The hand and arm should be below the heart level. If raised above the heart, the flow rate can change. If the tubing becomes kinked, the infusion rate slows down. In some situations, the patient or family member may "adjust" the roller clamp, changing the flow rate. The patient should be instructed not to touch the roller clamp. Frequent checks can help prevent infusion issues.

Reducing the Risk of Complications

Many times, a patient receives a one-time treatment of IV solution. The catheter is inserted, the IV therapy is performed, and the catheter is removed. In some cases, the patient may need to return to the ambulatory care facility for additional infusions. In those cases, the medical assistant must know the guidelines for flushing the IV catheter and when to change the IV site, tubing, and IV solution bags. The following strategies are used to reduce the risk of complications.

- Use sterile technique when changing IV solution bags or priming IV tubing.
- IV tubing and the site are changed every 72 to 96 hours or per the healthcare facility's policies.

- The IV catheter is removed if the insertion site has any tenderness, redness, swelling, or drainage.
- If the IV catheter remains in for an extended period of time, the transparent semipermeable membrane dressing should be changed every 5 to 7 days. Gauze dressings should be changed every 2 days.
- IV solution bags are changed every 24 hours (Procedure 51.3).
- IV catheter and extension tubing not in use need to be flushed every 12 hours with 3 to 5 mL of sterile normal saline. This maintains the **patency** of the catheter. (Flushing IV catheters may be outside the medical assistant's scope of practice in some states.)

COMPLICATIONS OF IV THERAPY

Complications that can arise from IV therapy include infiltration, phlebitis, extravasation, hypersensitivity, local and systemic infections, pulmonary edema, and air embolism. With any suspicion of a complication, the medical assistant should notify the provider. If the medical assistant is helping the RN monitor the infusion, any suspicion of complications should be reported to the RN immediately.

Phlebitis

Phlebitis is inflammation of a vein. It is caused when the IV catheter rubs on the walls of the vein, with prolonged use of a site, or by trauma during the insertion process. Phlebitis can also be caused by the IV solution or medication, especially if it is acidic, alkaline, or hypertonic. Signs and symptoms of phlebitis include redness, tenderness or pain, heat, or swelling at the insertion site and tracking up the vein.

If phlebitis is suspected, the medical assistant must stop the infusion and remove the catheter. The extremity should be elevated above the heart level, and a warm compress can be applied. To help prevent phlebitis, the medical assistant should change the IV site according to the ambulatory care facility's policy. Frequent checks of the site during the IV infusion are important.

Infiltration

Infiltration occurs when the IV solution leaks or is administered into the surrounding tissues. It is caused when the IV catheter is placed improperly, slips out of the blood vessel, or punctures through the blood vessel. Usually, patient movement or a poorly secured catheter can lead to the catheter moving out of the vessel. Signs and symptoms of infiltration include the following:

- Swelling, discomfort, or pain at the site
- Coolness, blanching, and tightness of the skin at the site
- Slowed or stopped flow rate. This can trigger the alarm on IV infusion pumps.

If infiltration is suspected, the medical assistant needs to stop the infusion and remove the IV catheter. Elevating the extremity and applying a warm compress can help reduce the swelling. The medical assistant can prevent infiltration by avoiding joint areas when inserting an IV and properly securing the catheter. The site should be checked for infiltration when the IV infusion starts. Infiltration can occur anytime during the infusion; thus, the medical assistant must frequently check the site.

CRITICAL THINKING APPLICATION **51.7**

Describe the difference between the signs and symptoms of an infiltrated site and phlebitis.

Extravasation

Extravasation occurs when medication leaks into and damages the surrounding tissues. **Vesicant medications** (e.g., certain types of antineoplastic drugs) can cause extravasation. In most cases, administering vesicant medications is outside the medical assistant's scope of practice. However, the medical assistant may help the RN monitor infusions and thus should be aware of extravasation. Signs and symptoms of extravasation include blanching, burning, tenderness or pain, cool skin, and swelling at the IV site. Blistering may be seen.

If extravasation is suspected, the medical assistant should stop the IV flow and notify the provider or RN. The catheter should remain in if an antidote is to be administered. The arm should be elevated. Warm or cold compresses per the medication manufacturer should be applied. Larger veins should be used when a vesicant medication is given to prevent extravasation.

Hypersensitivity

Hypersensitivity is an immune response that causes the body to react with an exaggerated response to a foreign agent or antigen. The risk of hypersensitivity is higher when IV medications are given compared to IV solutions. Thus, medical assistants should be aware of hypersensitivity if they are helping to monitor medication infusions. A hypersensitivity reaction occurs when the patient is allergic to the medication being infused. The signs and symptoms of hypersensitivity include fever, bronchospasm, difficulty breathing, wheezing, rash, and urticaria.

If a hypersensitivity reaction is suspected, the medical assistant should stop the infusion and notify the provider or RN. The patient's vital signs should be monitored. Treatments ordered by the provider should be administered, such as epinephrine or diphenhydramine. A patient's allergy history should be obtained to prevent hypersensitivity. The patient should be monitored closely during the first 10 minutes of a medication infusion for signs of a hypersensitivity reaction. The medical assistant should remember that a hypersensitivity reaction can occur anytime during and after the infusion.

Local and Systemic Infections

A local infection at the IV insertion site may occur 2 to 3 days after the IV catheter is placed. The site may become tender and red; purulent drainage may be present. With a systemic infection (sepsis), the patient may experience a fever. Microorganisms may enter the blood through the insertion site or from contaminated IV tubing or solution.

If the IV catheter is in the extremity, it should be removed. The provider should be notified of the patient's symptoms. A blood culture and antibiotics may be ordered. Medical assistants should take the following steps to prevent a local or systemic infection:

- Wash their hands or use hand sanitizer before putting on gloves to start an IV.
- Use aseptic technique during IV insertion.
- Use sterile technique when priming the IV tubing and attaching the tubing to the catheter.
- Perform dressing, site, and tubing changes as indicated by the facility's policies.

Pulmonary Edema

Pulmonary edema (also called *circulatory overload* or *fluid overload*) is caused by fluid accumulation in the lungs. This condition can occur if IV fluids are given too quickly, or the patient receives too much fluid. The signs and symptoms of pulmonary edema are as follows:

- Shortness of breath and dyspnea
- Restlessness
- Productive cough and wheezing
- Labored and rapid breathing, rapid pulse, and a decreased blood pressure

If the patient experiences signs and symptoms of pulmonary edema, the medical assistant should notify the provider immediately. Typical treatments for pulmonary edema include having the person sit up, oxygen therapy, and monitoring vital signs. The provider may order additional treatments. To prevent pulmonary edema, the medical assistant must ensure the IV infusion is done at the ordered rate. Frequent checking on the patient may help identify early signs and symptoms of pulmonary edema.

Air Embolism

An air embolism occurs when air is introduced into the circulatory system and can block small arteries. Patients can usually tolerate small air bubbles, but 10 mL of air or more can lead to an air embolism and possible death. The signs and symptoms of an air embolism are as follows:

- Dyspnea, shortness of breath, wheezing, and coughing
- Shoulder, neck, or chest pain
- Light-headedness, agitation, confusion, and loss of consciousness
- Hypotension and tachycardia

If the patient experiences any of these signs or symptoms, the medical assistant should stop the entry of air, notify the provider immediately, and look for how air could have entered the system. Treatment includes oxygen therapy and monitoring of vital signs. To prevent an air embolism, the medical assistant must ensure all air is out of the tubing during the priming process and all connections are tight.

Discontinuing the IV

When the provider orders the IV to be discontinued, the medical assistant must stop the IV fluid infusion. Procedure 51.4 describes how to remove the catheter. The medical assistant must check the catheter tip to ensure it is intact. If a small part of the catheter breaks off, it can flow into the circulatory system, causing a catheter embolism. If the catheter is broken when removed, the provider should be notified immediately.

CLOSING COMMENTS

Patient Coaching

When initiating IV therapy, the medical assistant should coach the patient on what will happen and what the patient might feel during the procedure. The medical assistant should explain to the patient symptoms that would require the patient to immediately contact the medical assistant. Because the medical assistant will not stay continually at the patient's side during the infusion, there should be an easy way for the patient to notify the medical assistant of concerns. This should be explained to the patient before the medical assistant leaves the room.

Legal and Ethical Issues

When administering IV fluids, the medical assistant must be under the direct supervision of a provider. The provider needs to be present in the facility and readily available if needed, when the procedure is being done. The medical assistant must be aware of and follow the state's scope of practice for medical assistants, along with the facility's policies.

Patient-Centered Care

Providing patient-centered care includes providing education, emotional support, and assisting with the patient's physical comfort. When performing IV fluid therapy, the medical assistant needs to coach the patient on what to expect, the length of time for the infusion, and signs and symptoms of complications. This can help the patient understand what is occurring and reduce the anxiety the patient may be feeling. Because the infusion can take several hours, the medical assistant must do the following:

- Ensure the patient is comfortable.
- Provide something for the patient to do, such as watch television or read a magazine.
- Have blankets available if the patient becomes chilled, which is common during the therapy.
- Ensure the patient has something to drink if allowed by the provider.

Professional Behaviors

Inserting an IV catheter and managing IV fluid infusions are skills the medical assistant needs to practice to become confident and provide these services safely. Continuing education on IV fluid therapy is important if the medical assistant's duties include IV insertion and fluid infusion. A medical assistant should always be watchful of complications of IV therapy, regardless of the age of the patient. Skill refreshers and continuing education can help the medical assistant remain competent and confident with these skills.

SUMMARY OF SCENARIO

Gabe has had the opportunity to insert several IV catheters and perform IV fluid infusions. He is gaining more confidence with the insertion procedure. Gabe has worked with the providers to purchase an IV infusion pump and the required primary infusion sets. A representative from the company provided an in-service session on using the pump and troubleshooting issues. Gabe has found the pump easy to use and likes that it provides extra safety for IV infusions. Because the patients are in the facility for several hours for the infusions, Gabe has also worked with the providers to create a special room for IV infusions. The room includes a recliner, television, a few Mayo stands, and the infusion pump. Gabe is excited to continue to assist with IV therapy.

SUMMARY OF LEARNING OBJECTIVES

1. **Differentiate among the three types of IV solutions, including the action of the fluid and risks associated with the fluids.**
   Intravenous (IV) solution should be treated as a medication. The medical assistant must follow the nine rights of medication administration with IV therapy. The following are three types of IV fluids:
   - *Isotonic solutions:* Have a similar dissolved particle concentration as plasma. This means that isotonic solutions are distributed evenly among the bloodstream, the interstitial fluid, and cells.
   - *Hypotonic solutions:* Have a lower concentration of dissolved particles than plasma. This causes the fluid to move out of the blood vessels and into the interstitial fluid and cells.
   - *Hypertonic solutions:* Have a higher concentration of dissolved particles than plasma. This causes fluid from the cells to move into the bloodstream, increasing the blood volume and thus the blood pressure.
2. **Differentiate between primary and secondary IV infusion sets.**
   The primary infusion set can be either a macro-drip or a micro-drip set. The drop factor is the number of drops (gtt) per milliliter (mL) of fluid. The drop factor (gtt/mL) is listed on the infusion set packaging. The primary infusion set consists of a spike, drip chamber, roller clamp, slide clamp, and luer connector. A secondary infusion set is used to give IV medications.
3. **Differentiate among the supplies and equipment used for IV therapy.**
   An extension tubing can be used to connect the IV catheter with the primary infusion set. Straight and winged hub safety catheters are the types of catheters used. IV start kits contain the supplies needed to prepare the site and to secure the catheter once it is in place. An IV pole and an infusion pump are used for the infusion.
4. **Calculate the total amount of fluid to be infused, the infusion rate, and the flow rate for IV solutions.**
   When using an infusion pump, the medical assistant must know the total amount to be infused and the infusion rate. If one of these two pieces of information is missing from the provider's order, the following formulas can be used to calculate the information:
   - *Total amount to be infused formula:* Infusion rate (mL/hr) × hours = Total amount to be infused
   - *Infusion rate formula:* Total amount (mL) ÷ hours = mL per hour (infusion rate)

   For gravity infusions, the flow rate is required. To calculate the flow rate, the medical assistant must have the infusion set drop factor and the amount of fluid to infuse over × number of minutes. The formula for calculating the flow rate is as follows:

$$\frac{\text{Volume to infuse (mL)} \times \text{drop factor (gtt)}}{\text{Time (min)} \times \text{(mL)}} = \frac{\text{gtt}}{\text{min}} \text{ (flow rate)}$$

5. **Demonstrate how to initiate an IV infusion, including priming the infusion set, preparing the site, and inserting the IV catheter.**
   Procedure 51.1 describes how to prime the primary infusion set. When inserting an IV catheter in an adult, the medical assistant uses a site on an upper extremity. Procedure 51.2 details the steps involved in preparing the site and inserting a catheter.
6. **Demonstrate how to monitor IVs and reduce the risk of complications.**
   The patient should be checked at least every 30 to 60 minutes, depending on the situation and the facility's policy. The medical assistant should check on the patient and the site for complications. If a gravity infusion is used, the flow rate must be checked.
   The following strategies are used to reduce the risk of complications:
   - Use sterile technique when changing IV solution bags or priming IV tubing.
   - IV tubing and the site are changed every 72 to 96 hours or per the healthcare facility's policies. IV solution bags are changed every 24 hours (Procedure 51.3).
   - The IV catheter is removed if the insertion site has any tenderness, redness, swelling, or drainage.
   - IV catheter and extension tubing not in use need to be flushed every 12 hours with 3 to 5 mL of sterile normal saline. This maintains the patency of the catheter. (Flushing IV catheters may be outside of the medical assistant's scope of practice in some states.)
7. **Examine the complications of IV therapy, including the signs and symptoms, along with the actions that should be taken.**
   The medical assistant should monitor the patient for complications. Common complications that can arise from IV therapy include phlebitis, infiltration, extravasation, hypersensitivity, local and systemic infections, pulmonary edema, and air embolism. With any suspicion of a complication, the medical assistant should notify the provider.

PROCEDURE 51.1 Prime an IV Infusion Set

TASK: Prime an IV infusion set with IV solution.

SCENARIO: Dr. Martin ordered LR 500 mL over 5 hours for Celia Tapia (DOB 05/18/19XX). You need to administer the IV infusion.

EQUIPMENT and SUPPLIES

- Provider's order
- Patient's health record
- Primary IV infusion set
- IV fluid (LR 500 mL)
- Time label and marker or pen
- Waste container
- Sink or basin

PROCEDURAL STEPS

1. Wash your hands or use hand sanitizer. Review the order. Clarify any questions you have with the provider.
   PURPOSE: Hand sanitization is an important step for infection control. It is important to be knowledgeable about the medication you are giving.
2. Select the IV solution bag from the storage area. Check the IV solution label against the order. Check for the right name, form, and route. Check the expiration date to make sure the IV solution has not expired. Verify the right dose and the right time.
   PURPOSE: It is important to do the first check of the label when getting the IV solution bag from the cabinet.
3. Assemble the supplies required for the procedure. Remove the IV solution from the outer plastic packaging, if present.
   PURPOSE: Remember to split up the three medication checks with activities between each check.
4. Check the IV bag for leaks. Check the IV fluid for unusual color, precipitate, or cloudiness.
   PURPOSE: Do not use an IV bag with a leak or IV fluid that is cloudy or a different color than normal.
5. Remove the primary IV tubing from the packaging. Position the roller clamp about 1 inch below the drip chamber. Close the roller clamp. Keep the spike and luer connector sterile.
   PURPOSE: Closing the roller clamp prevents fluid from moving beyond the roller clamp.
6. Perform the second medication check. Check the IV solution label against the order. Check for the right name, form, and route.
   PURPOSE: It is important to check the label a second time before continuing with the procedure.
7. Remove the covers from the IV solution port and the IV tubing spike (Figure 1). Maintain the sterility of both during the removal process.

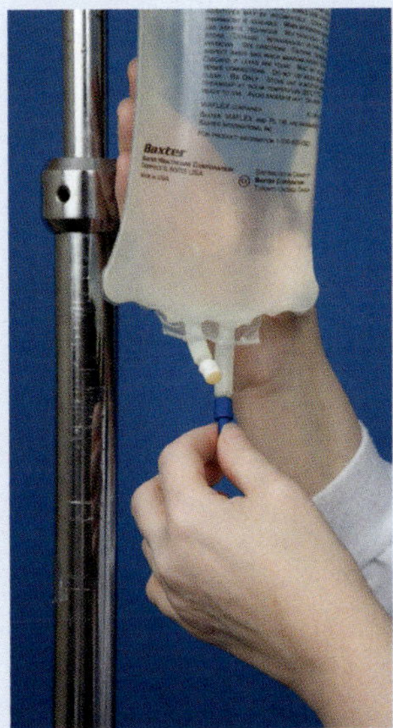

FIGURE 1 Remove protective covering from IV solution tubing port. (From Potter P, Perry A: *Basic nursing*, ed 7, St. Louis, 2011, Mosby.)

8. Insert the IV tubing spike into the IV solution port, using a twisting motion (Figure 2). Hang the IV solution bag on the IV pole or hook. Hold the luer connector end of the IV tubing.

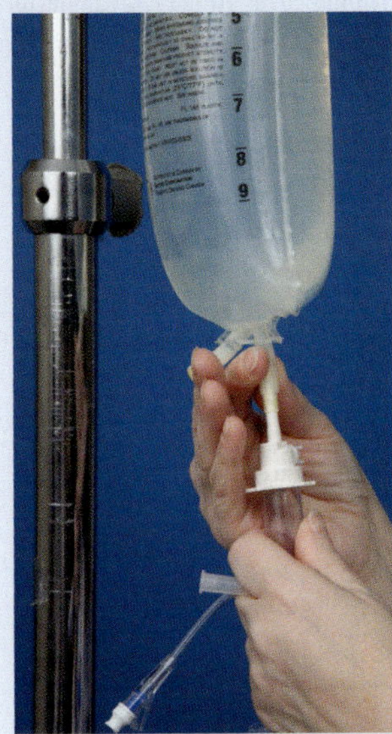

FIGURE 2 Insert tubing spike into IV container. (From Potter P, Perry A: *Basic nursing*, ed 7, St. Louis, 2011, Mosby.)

   PURPOSE: The IV solution bag must be higher than the patient for the fluid to infuse.

Continued

PROCEDURE 51.1 Prime an IV Infusion Set—*continued*

9. Gently squeeze the drip chamber so it fills about half full (Figure 3).
PURPOSE: If the drip chamber is too full, the medical assistant cannot count the drips. Filling the drip chamber with solution prevents air from getting into the tubing.

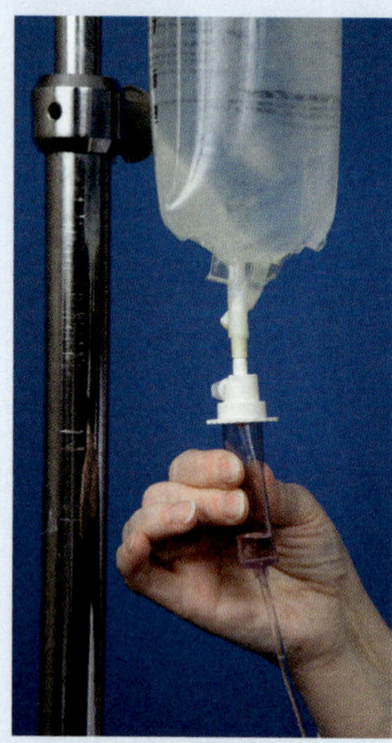

FIGURE 3 Squeeze drip chamber to fill with fluid. (From Potter P, Perry A: *Basic nursing*, ed 7, St. Louis, 2011, Mosby.)

10. Slowly open the roller clamp to prime the tubing. Invert the ports and any valves as the fluid passes. Tap the air out of the ports and valve (Figure 4). Remove the cover on the luer connector and keep the end sterile. Hold the luer connector end over a sink or basin and allow a small amount of fluid to drain out of the tubing.

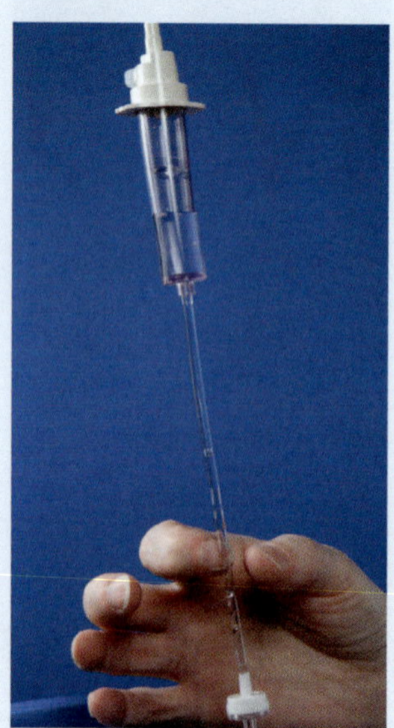

FIGURE 4 Remove air from the IV tubing. (From Potter P, Perry A: *Basic nursing*, ed 7, St. Louis, 2011, Mosby.)

PURPOSE: The air must be removed from the tubing to prevent an air embolism.

11. Close the roller clamp. Check the tubing for air. If air is found, reposition the tubing as needed to help move the air either to the drip chamber or out through the luer connector. Slowly open the roller clamp and allow a small amount of fluid to drain to remove the air. When the tubing is free of air, cover the luer connector end with the sterile cover.
PURPOSE: Air must be removed from the tubing to prevent an air embolism.

12. Place the tubing on the IV hook or pole. Perform the third medication check. Check the IV solution label against the order. Check for the right name, form, and route.
PURPOSE: Placing the tubing on the pole or hook helps to protect the tubing from touching the ground.

13. Following the healthcare facility's policy, complete the IV bag label with a pen or marker and place a label on the solution.
PURPOSE: The label provides important information needed when checking the infusion rate.

14. Clean up the work area. Packaging and other waste should be discarded in the waste container.
PURPOSE: It is professional to clean up after yourself. Never fill a biohazardous sharps container with uncontaminated waste (e.g., packaging).

PROCEDURE 51.2 Administer IV Fluids

TASKS: Insert an IV catheter, attach the primed IV tubing with the IV solution, and document in the patient's health record.

SCENARIO: Dr. Martin ordered LR 500 mL over 5 hours for Celia Tapia (DOB 05/18/19XX). You need to administer the IV infusion.

EQUIPMENT and SUPPLIES

- Provider's order
- Patient's health record
- Primed IV infusion set attached to the IV solution bag with an IV stand or hook
- Infusion pump (optional)
- Short extension tubing with syringe containing 1 to 3 mL of 0.9% sodium chloride (optional)
- IV safety catheter
- IV start kit
- Gloves
- Biohazardous sharps container
- Waste container

PROCEDURAL STEPS

1. Wash your hands or use hand sanitizer. Review the order. Clarify any questions you have with the provider.
   PURPOSE: Hand sanitization is an important step for infection control. It is important to be knowledgeable about the medication you are giving.
2. Calculate the infusion rate. Calculate the flow rate if needed.
   PURPOSE: The infusion rate is needed for the infusion pump. The infusion and flow rates are needed if doing a gravity infusion.
3. Gather the supplies and equipment needed, including the primed IV tubing with the IV solution and the IV pole or hook (see Procedure 51.1). If using a short extension tubing, remove any protective covers, prime with the 0.9% sodium chloride, and replace protective cover to maintain the sterility of the tubing.
   PURPOSE: Having all of the needed supplies and equipment is necessary before starting the procedure.
4. Prior to entering the exam room, knock on the door and wait a moment. Greet the patient. Identify yourself. Verify the patient's identity with full name and date of birth. Make sure the patient's information matches the order and the record. Explain what you are going to do.
   PURPOSE: It is important to identify the patient in two different ways to ensure that you have the correct patient. Explaining the procedure can make the patient feel more comfortable and reduces anxiety.
5. Provide the right education to the patient. Explain the medication ordered, the desired effect, and common side effects; also, identify the provider who ordered it. Answer any questions the parent/patient may have. Use language the parent/patient can understand. Ask if the patient has any allergies. If the parent/patient refuses the medication, notify the provider.
   PURPOSE: The patient needs to be aware of what you are giving, its action and side effects, and who ordered it. It is also important to double-check the patient's allergies before administering the medication.
6. Use hand sanitizer and put on gloves.
   PURPOSE: Hand sanitization is an important step for infection control.
7. Ask the patient which arm he or she prefers. Apply the tourniquet about 4 to 6 inches above the intended site. Do not apply the tourniquet too tight to avoid injuring the tissue. Check for a radial pulse. If the radial pulse is absent, loosen the tourniquet.
   PURPOSE: Some patients may have reasons for preferring certain arms. If a patient has lymphedema or had a recent mastectomy (under 3 years ago), the opposite arm should be used for the IV infusion if possible. A radial pulse should be present.
8. Palpate the vein with your index finger. Select a straight, well-dilated vein that is large enough for the IV catheter. Stroke the vessel or have the patient open and close the hand, making a fist.
   PURPOSE: A well-dilated vein is needed to insert the catheter.
9. Release the tourniquet.
   PURPOSE: The tourniquet needs to be released to prevent tissue damage.
   Note: If a topical anesthetic needs to be applied, it can be applied once the tourniquet is released.
10. Clean the intended site with the antiseptic swab or applicator as indicated by the facility's policies. If chlorhexidine is used, do a 30-second friction scrub back and forth and up and down at the site. Let the site dry. If using Betadine or alcohol, clean in a circular pattern working outwardly. Allow the Betadine to dry.
    PURPOSE: The site must be cleaned before the catheter is inserted. The drying process kills the microorganisms.
11. Using the dominant hand, firmly grip the catheter on each side of the hub. Use the non-dominant hand to hold the skin tautly. Apply distal traction and anchor the vein with the thumb.
    PURPOSE: Applying traction helps to stabilize the vein, and holding the skin tautly helps with a smooth insertion of the needle.
12. With the bevel up, position the needle unit parallel and directly above the vein. Inform the patient of the insertion.
13. Insert the needle in the skin using a 10- to 30-degree angle. Aim toward the vein and slowly advance it until blood flashback is seen in the clear flashback chamber (Figure 1A). Loosen the tourniquet.
    Note: If a drop of blood appears in the chamber, insert about 1 to 2 mm until the flash of blood is seen.

Continued

PROCEDURE 51.2 Administer IV Fluids—*Continued*

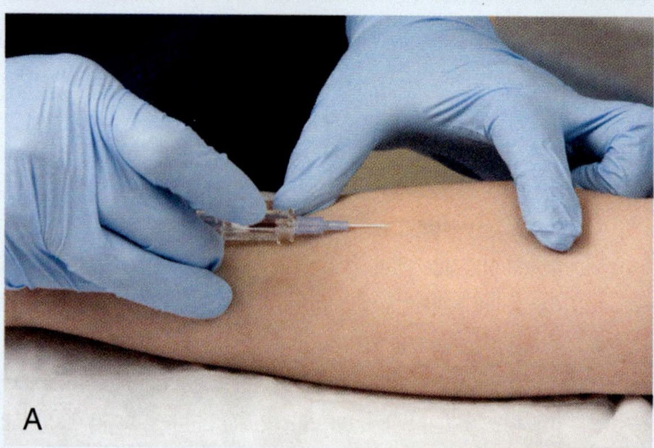

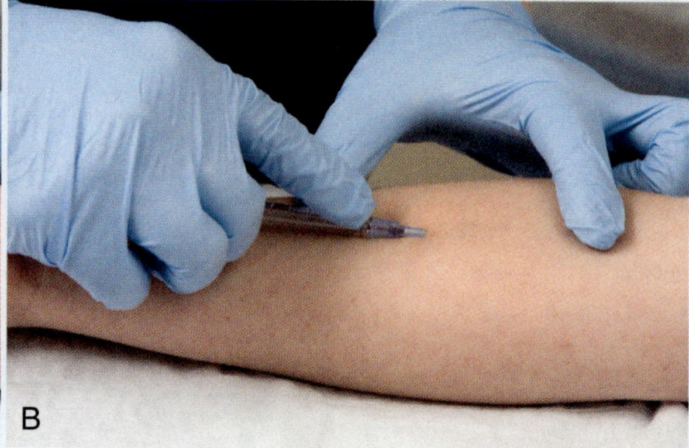

FIGURE 1 (From Potter PA, Perry AG: *Fundamentals of nursing*, ed 9, St. Louis, 2017, Elsevier.)

14. Lower the angle of the needle unit. Advance the cannula over the needle until the hub sits on the skin (Figure 1B).

15. Stabilize the catheter. With the dominant hand, withdraw the needle and activate the safety device if needed. Depending on the type of device used, apply pressure over the vein, above the catheter, if needed.
PURPOSE: The pressure occludes the vessel, preventing the blood from spilling out of the catheter as the tubing is connected.

16. Secure the luer connector on the tubing to the catheter hub without contaminating the hub. If the extension tubing is used, occlude the tubing with the slide clamp, remove the syringe, and connect the extension tubing to the primary infusion set.

17. Tape the catheter hub to the skin (Figure 2). Per the facility's policy, place the transparent dressing over the insertion site or place a 2 × 2-inch gauze dressing over the insertion site and the hub (Figure 3).

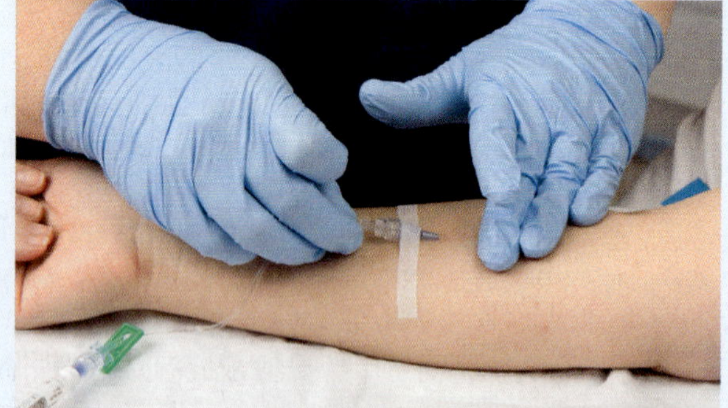

FIGURE 2 (From Potter PA, Perry AG: *Fundamentals of nursing*, ed 9, St. Louis, 2017, Elsevier.)

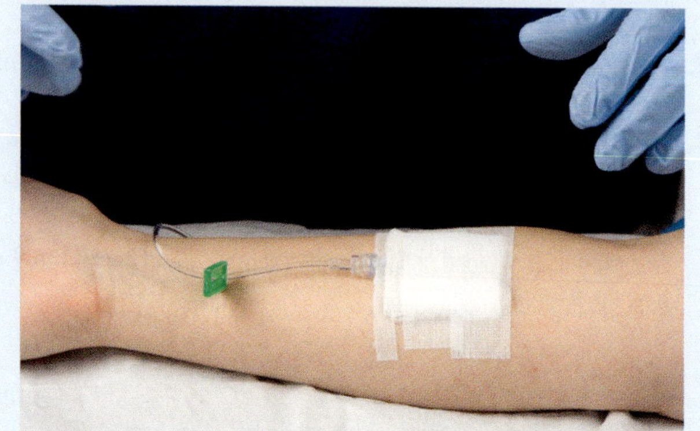

FIGURE 3 (From Potter PA, Perry AG: *Fundamentals of nursing*, ed 9, St. Louis, 2017, Elsevier.)

PURPOSE: Taping the hub prevents the catheter from being dislodged.

18. Create a loop with the IV tubing and secure the tubing to the skin with tape (Figure 4). If using extension tubing, connect it to the IV infusion set.
PURPOSE: Taping the tubing to the skin helps secure the IV and prevents the catheter from being dislodged.

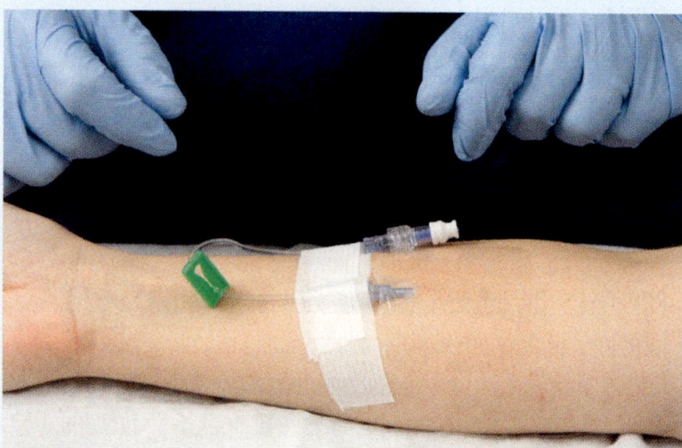

FIGURE 4 (From Potter PA, Perry AG: *Fundamentals of nursing*, ed 9, St. Louis, 2017, Elsevier.)

19. Set the infusion rate if using a pump and ensure the clamps are opened. If using gravity infusion, count the drops and adjust the roller clamp to get the correct flow rate.

20. Observe the site for swelling during the infusion of the fluid.
PURPOSE: If the site is infiltrated, the swelling will occur as the fluid infuses.

21. Discard the needle in the biohazard sharps container. Clean up the area. Discard the supplies per the facility's policy. Remove gloves and wash or sanitize hands.

22. Document the procedure, including the ordering provider's name, IV order, type and size of catheter inserted, number of attempts, IV solution, and the infusion rate.

Documentation Example

05/26/20XX 10:10 a.m. Per Dr. Martin's order, LR 500 mL over 5 hours started. Insyte Autoguard 20G 1-inch catheter inserted in right hand on first attempt. LR 100 mL/hr infusing per infusion pump. Patient tolerated the procedure without concerns. Patient resting in recliner. BP 112/72 right arm, sitting (adult cuff); P: 82 regular, 1+; R: 18, regular, normal.
———————————————— Gabe Garcia, CMA (AAMA)

PROCEDURE 51.3 Change an IV Bag

TASK: Change an IV bag.

SCENARIO: Dr. Martin ordered LR 500 mL over 5 hours for Celia Tapia (DOB 05/18/19XX). The first bag you hung was 250 mL, and now you need to switch bags to give the other 250 mL.

EQUIPMENT and SUPPLIES

- Provider's order
- IV bag

PROCEDURAL STEPS

1. Wash your hands or use hand sanitizer. Review the order. Clarify any questions you have with the provider.
   PURPOSE: Hand sanitization is an important step for infection control.
2. Select the IV solution bag from the storage area. Check the IV solution label against the order. Check for the right name, form, and route. Check the expiration date to make sure the IV solution has not expired. Verify the right dose and the right time.
   PURPOSE: It is important to do the first check of the label when getting the IV solution bag from the cabinet.
3. Remove the IV solution from the outer plastic packaging, if present. Check the IV bag for leaks. Check the IV fluid for unusual color, precipitate, or cloudiness.
   PURPOSE: Do not use an IV bag with a leak or IV fluid that is cloudy or a different color than normal.
4. Perform the second medication check. Check the IV solution label against the order. Check for the right name, form, and route.
   PURPOSE: It is important to do the second check of the label before continuing with the procedure.
5. Prior to entering the exam room, knock on the door and wait a moment. Greet the patient. Identify yourself. Verify the patient's identity with full name and date of birth. Make sure the patient's information matches the order and the record. Explain what you are going to do.
   PURPOSE: It is important to identify the patient in two different ways to ensure that you have the correct patient. Explaining the procedure can make the patient feel more comfortable and reduces anxiety.
6. Perform the third medication check. Hang the new IV solution bag on the IV pole.
7. Pause the IV infusion pump or close the roller clamp if giving the IV by gravity.
   PURPOSE: Pausing the pump or clamping the tubing prevents air from getting into the IV tubing.
8. Remove the protective plastic cover over the tubing port. Remove the old IV bag from the pole and turn the bag upside down. Using a twisting motion, remove the IV tubing spike from the IV bag (Figure 1A). Using a twisting motion, insert the spike into the new IV bag using the tubing port (Figure 1B). Keep the spike sterile during this procedure.

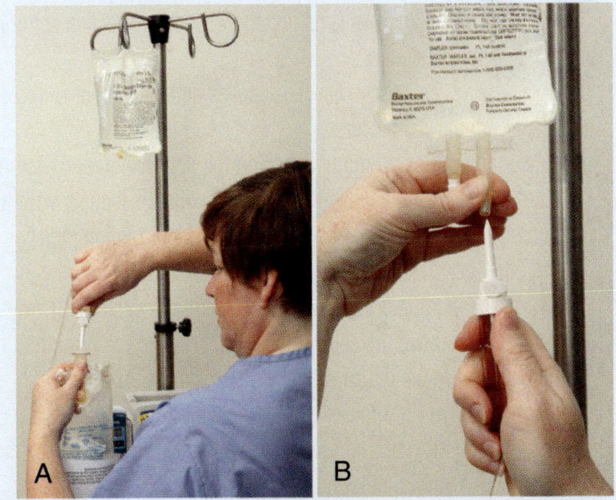

FIGURE 1 (From Potter PA, Perry AG: *Fundamentals of nursing*, ed 9, St. Louis, 2017, Elsevier.)

   PURPOSE: The spike must be kept sterile so that the fluid does not become contaminated.
9. If the drip chamber is less than one-third to one-half filled, squeeze the drip chamber to fill it to this level. Check for air in the tubing before restarting the infusion pump or opening and regulating the roller clamp.
10. Label the bag per the healthcare facility's policy. If the facility requires documentation when administering a new bag of fluid, document at this time.

PROCEDURE 51.4 Remove an IV Catheter

TASKS: Remove an IV catheter, and document the patient care.

SCENARIO: Dr. Martin ordered LR 500 mL over 5 hours for Celia Tapia (DOB 05/18/19XX). The fluid has been infused, and the IV needs to be discontinued or removed.

EQUIPMENT and SUPPLIES

- Provider's order
- Sterile gauze (e.g., 2 × 2s)
- Gloves
- Hypoallergenic self-stick wrap, tape, or bandage
- Patient's health record

PROCEDURAL STEPS

1. Wash your hands or use hand sanitizer. Review the order. Clarify any questions you have with the provider.
   PURPOSE: Hand sanitization is an important step for infection control.
2. Gather the supplies needed.
   PURPOSE: Having all of the needed supplies and equipment is necessary before starting the procedure.
3. Prior to entering the exam room, knock on the door and wait a moment. Greet the patient. Identify yourself. Verify the patient's identity with full name and date of birth. Make sure the patient's information matches the order and the record. Explain what you are going to do.
   PURPOSE: It is important to identify the patient in two different ways to ensure that you have the correct patient. Explaining the procedure can make the patient feel more comfortable and reduces anxiety.
4. Put on gloves. Open the supplies. If an IV is infusing, stop the flow.
5. Remove the tape that secured the tubing to the skin. Hold the IV catheter with one hand. With the other hand, start to remove the transparent dressing by loosening one side and stretching the dressing. Then loosen and stretch the dressing on the opposite side. Completely remove the transparent dressing.
   PURPOSE: Holding the catheter prevents additional tissue trauma when removing the dressing.
6. Hold the sterile gauze above the insertion site. Pull the IV catheter back and straight out.
7. Once the catheter is removed, place the sterile gauze over the site and hold pressure until the bleeding has stopped, which may be 2 to 3 minutes.
   Note: If a patient is taking an anticoagulant, it may take longer than 3 minutes to stop the bleeding.
8. Inspect the catheter tip for any breakage. Discard the catheter in the biohazardous sharps container.
   PURPOSE: If the tip of the catheter breaks off, it can cause a catheter embolism. The medical assistant must always inspect the catheter tip to ensure the end is intact before discarding the catheter into the biohazardous sharps container.
9. Once the bleeding has stopped, replace the gauze with a new piece of sterile gauze. Secure the gauze with a hypoallergenic self-stick wrap, tape, or bandage. Ensure the patient has adequate blood flow below the site.
10. Clean up the area. Discard the supplies per the facility's policy. Remove your gloves and wash or sanitize your hands.
11. Document the IV catheter removal. Include the ordering provider's name, the order, the amount of fluid infused, and the appearance of the catheter tip.

Documentation Example

05/26/20XX 3:20 p.m. Per Dr. Martin's order, the IV was discontinued. Catheter removed and tip intact. LR 500 mL infused. Patient stated she "feels better." ______________________ Gabe Garcia, CMA (AAMA)

RADIOLOGY BASICS

52

SCENARIO

Stephanie Hill has been a limited machine x-ray operator (LXMO) at Walden-Martin Family Medical (WMFM) Clinic for a month. She completed her training, passed the certification examination, and this is her first position as a LXMO. She is excited and nervous about her new position. Stephanie has learned how to conduct a patient assessment and perform x-ray examinations. Stephanie's first patient of the day is Martha Gordon. Mrs. Gordon is an older adult with knee pains who uses a wheelchair. Stephanie provides quality care when she is caring for her patients.

While studying this chapter, think about the following questions:

1. What is the scope of practice for limited x-ray machine operators?
2. What are the four essential requirements for the production of x-rays?
3. What are the prime factors for radiographic exposure?
4. What is the purpose of the inverse square law?
5. What is the importance of the exposure indicator?
6. How does pathology influence technical factors?
7. How do limited x-ray machine operators protect themselves from radiation exposure?

LEARNING OBJECTIVES

1. Examine the scope, education, and certification requirements of limited x-ray machine operators.
2. Differentiate between the primary x-ray beam and scatter radiation.
3. Examine radiographic equipment.
4. Examine basic radiation safety.
5. Examine basic physics for radiography.
6. Examine the components of x-ray production.
7. Examine the x-ray circuit.
8. Examine rectification.
9. Examine single-phase, three-phase, and high-frequency generators.
10. Explain the components of the x-ray control panel.
11. Examine the principles of exposure and image quality.
12. Examine digital imaging.

VOCABULARY

automatic exposure control (AEC) Terminates the exposure time when a certain quantity of radiation has been detected at the Image receptor.

bremsstrahlung radiation Radiation that is created when an electron enters the tungsten anode of the x-ray tube, misses the tungsten electrons, and gets very near the nucleus.

Bucky Contains a movable grid device that absorbs scatter radiation and also contains the image receptor.

central ray (CR) The center of the x-ray beam and perpendicular to the long axis of the x-ray tube.

characteristic radiation Radiation that is created when an electron enters the tungsten anode of the x-ray tube and knocks out a K-shell electron.

collimation (kol i MAY shun) The method of restricting and confiding the x-ray beam to a given area.

computed radiography A cassette-based digital imaging system where the image of the body part is obtained using storage phosphor plate.

digital radiography (DR) Cassetteless imaging system where the phosphor is bonded to a flat panel detector or the system converts x-ray energy directly to an electronic signal.

distortion The differences between the actual subject and its radiographic image.

energy The ability to do work.

exposure indicator (EI) A numeric value indicating the quantity of ionizing radiation received by a digital radiographic image receptor; also called an exposure index.

fog The unwanted image exposure caused by scatter radiation

generator Delivers the electrical power to the x-ray tube and permits the selection of x-ray energy, x-ray quantity, and exposure time.

image receptor (IR) The device that receives the energy of the x-ray beam and forms the image of the body part.

ionizing radiation Radiation that, when passing through the body, produces positively and negatively charged particles.

VOCABULARY—*continued*

kilovolts peak (kVp) The unit of measure used to assess the voltage; controls the penetrating power of the x-ray beam.
line focus principle The relationship between the actual focal spot on the anode surface and the effective focal spot size.
matter Anything that occupies space and has shape or form.
object-to-image receptor distance (OID) The distance between the subject and the image receptor.
primary radiation The radiation that leaves the tube.
radiation field The squared area of the x-ray beam that strikes the patient and x-ray table.
radiation protection The measures taken to safeguard patients, personnel, and the public from unnecessary exposure to ionizing radiation.
scatter radiation Radiation from the primary beam that is randomly scattered within or outside of the body.
source-to-image-receptor distance (SID) The distance between the tube target and the image receptor.
thermionic emission Electrons begin to "boil effect," when the filament is heated.
x-ray tube The source of x-rays; the x-rays are formed within the x-ray tube.

INTRODUCTION

On November 8, 1895, x-rays were discovered by Professor Wilhelm Conrad Roentgen at the University of Wurzburg in Germany. Roentgen had a particular interest in the conduction of high-voltage electricity through low-vacuum tubes. His discovery of the x-ray during an experiment was purely accidental. The first x-ray image by Roentgen was of his wife Bertha's hand using a 15-minute exposure. Physicians and inventors were the first to experiment with x-rays and create images of the human body (Figure 52.1). Shortly after that, these pioneers trained their assistants to take the "x-ray pictures," now called "images," and the radiography profession was born.

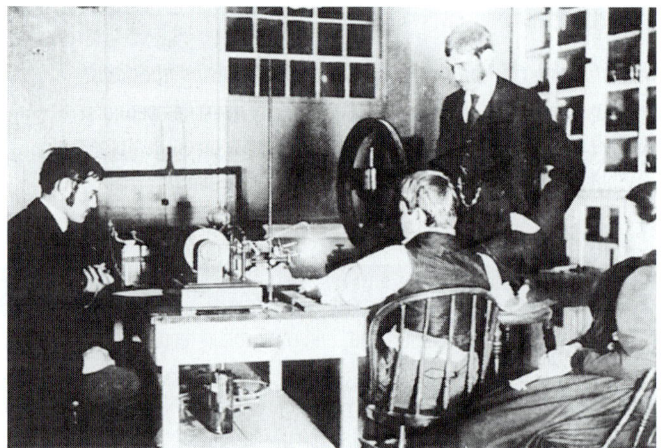

FIGURE 52.1 The first clinical radiograph in the United States was taken at Dartmouth College in 1896. (From Long BW, Frank ED, Ehrlich RA: *Radiography essentials for limited practice*, ed 6, St. Louis, 2021, Elsevier.)

LIMITED X-RAY MACHINE OPERATOR

A limited x-ray machine operator (LXMO) is an individual other than a radiologic technologist who performs diagnostic x-ray procedures on selected anatomy. Limited is used because the practice is limited when compared to a certified radiologic technologist. Limited x-ray practice does not involve the following:

- The use of contrast media for imaging blood vessels and abdominal organs
- The operation of complex radiographic equipment, such as computed tomography (CT), magnetic resonance imaging (MRI), mammography, and others.

Limited x-ray machine operators may perform radiographic exams at ambulatory care facilities, chiropractic offices, and hospitals. Limited scope x-ray machine operators prepare patients for exams, explain procedures, give clear instructions during the exam, and practice standards that ensure the highest level of **radiation protection** and safe operation of the x-ray machine. Limited x-ray machine operator members are certified limited practitioners or hold a restricted state license.

Education

Formal education is required to be eligible for certification as a limited x-ray machine operator. LXMO programs are typically certificate programs designed to prepare graduates for an entry-level position in ambulatory care. Programs emphasize developing clinical skills to train students for a career as a limited x-ray machine operator. Limited x-ray machine operators are restricted in terms of what parts of the body they can image. LXMOs are trained to perform imaging exams of the chest, upper and lower extremities, skull and sinuses, and spine and feet.

Curriculum

The American Society of Radiologic Technologists published the *Limited X-ray Machine Operator Curriculum* to support the education of limited operators of x-ray equipment. The curriculum allows states and faculty flexibility in developing limited curricula to meet the needs of individuals performing diagnostic x-ray procedures within a limited scope.

The LXMO curriculum is divided into specific content areas that represent the essential components of an LXMO program. The curriculum includes a minimum number of hours of didactic instruction and clinical instruction, along with the minimum number of required procedures (Table 52.1). Critical thinking must be fostered, developed, and assessed in the education process. The LXMO core curriculum is based on data relevant to today's healthcare environment and offers a foundation for lifelong learning and transition to general radiography studies. It is designed to meet the needs of individuals performing diagnostic x-ray procedures within a limited scope of practice.

Certification

Students must complete a program to be eligible for the certification examination written by the American Registry of Radiologic Technologists (ARRT) to earn their LXMO certification. LXMO

TABLE 52.1 Typical Curriculum for a Limited Machine X-ray Operator (LXMO) Program

ANATOMIC REGION	MINIMUM HOURS OF CLINICAL EXPERIENCE	MINIMUM PROCEDURES
Chest	160	100
Extremities • Upper extremity and pectoral girdle • Lower extremity	240 240	50 50
Skull/sinuses	240	50
Spine	240	50
Podiatric	160	50

certification means an individual has acquired the necessary training, has taken and passed the Limited Scope ARRT test, and received approval from the state. LXMOs are limited by the type of x-ray examinations they are permitted to perform. For example, limited scope x-ray machine operators who have taken and passed the Limited Scope ARRT extremity module may perform x-rays only on extremities.

The licensure of LXMOs varies from state to state. The majority of states have regulations for those who operate x-ray equipment. Currently, most states have laws requiring some licensure to practice radiography, and at least half of these include provisions for limited x-ray practice. State licensure is separate from ARRT credentialing. Depending on the state, limited x-ray may or may not be allowed. For example, Louisiana prohibits limited x-ray, whereas Missouri has no requirements for certification, and Wisconsin restricts limited x-ray to only the extremities, chest, and spine.

Legal requirements are subject to change, so you must inquire directly to your state's appropriate agency to determine the following:

- Whether limited x-ray is permitted
- Whether its practice is regulated
- How to obtain the necessary certification.

Each state that regulates limited x-ray has established standards for the scope of practice allowed. There are serious sanctions for practicing radiography outside the boundaries defined by state laws and regulations. Practicing without a valid license or permit or practicing outside the scope of one's credentials may result in fines, imprisonment, or both. In addition, a license or permit may be suspended or revoked. Employers may also be penalized in their employees practice radiography in violation of regulations. *All radiographers and limited operators must be aware of the legal standards that apply to them and ensure that their practice conforms to these standards.* The practice of radiography involves a variety of knowledge and skills. Although the scope of practice may be limited, there is no restriction on the knowledge and skill necessary for the practice. In other words, the limited operator is held to the same high standards as a registered radiologic technologist in performing procedures within the permitted scope of practice.

CRITICAL THINKING APPLICATION 52.1

Susan is a limited x-ray machine operator in Texas. However, she is originally from Wisconsin. Susan wants to move back to Wisconsin to help take care of her mother. Can Susan practice as a limited x-ray machine operator in Wisconsin? If Wisconsin certifies limited x-ray machine operators, will Susan need to take the ARRT certification examination for Wisconsin? Where can Susan locate this information?

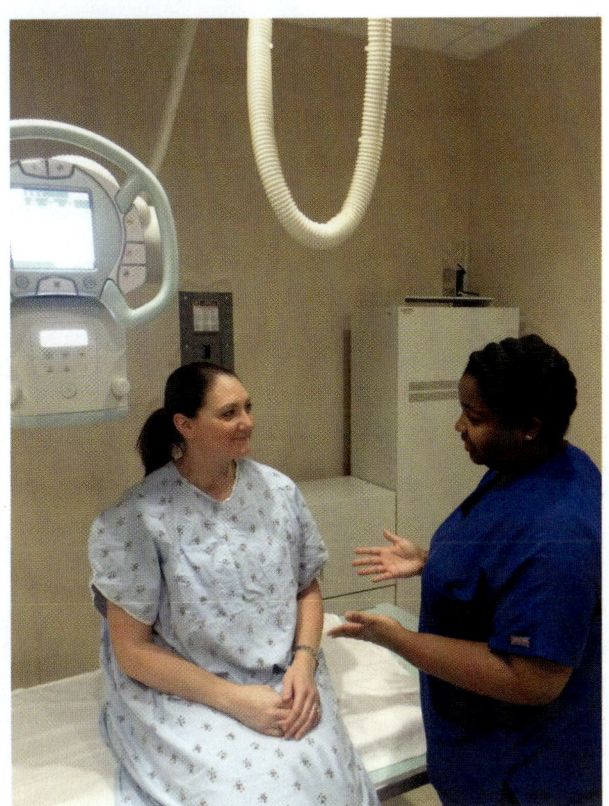

FIGURE 52.2 The limited operator explains the procedure to the patient. (From Sherer MAS, Visconti PJ, Ritenour ER, Haynes KW: *Radiation protection in medical radiography*, ed 8, St. Louis, 2018, Mosby.)

Typical Duties of a Limited X-ray Machine Operator

The limited operator encounters the patient after x-ray procedures are ordered by a provider. Usually, this occurs after the provider has examined the patient. Once the order is placed, the limited operator greets the patient and determines where the patient will need to undress. Many times the patient must change into a gown before radiography. Once the patients are appropriately dressed, they are taken into the x-ray room (Figure 52.2).

Then, the limited operator provides a brief explanation and answers any questions about the procedure. Often, the limited operator will have to discuss the examination with a radiographer to ensure that the appropriate x-ray projections will be made and the correct exposure techniques are used. The next step is to assist the patient in the general position required for the x-ray examination. For example, if a hand is to be x-rayed, the patient can be seated at the end of the table (Figure 52.3). For a spine examination, the patient may need to lie on the table (Figure 52.4). If a chest examination is ordered, the patient will stand at an upright **image receptor**

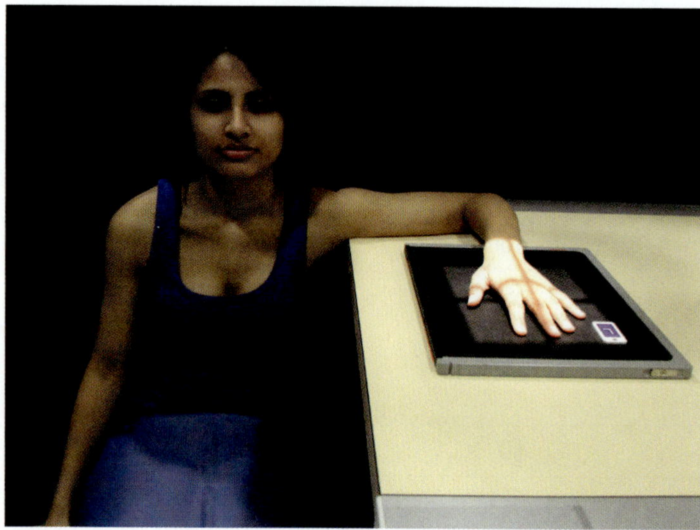

FIGURE 52.3 The patient is seated at the end of the x-ray examination table with hand on the image receptor placed on the table. (From Long BW, Rollins JH, Smith BJ: *Merrill's atlas of radiographic positioning and procedures*, ed 14, St. Louis, 2020, Mosby.)

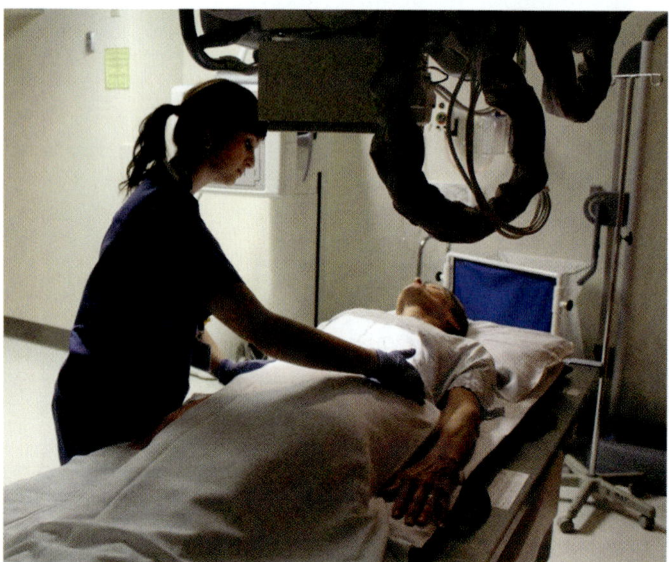

FIGURE 52.4 The patient is lying supine on the examination table.

(IR) (Figure 52.5). The limited operator then selects the IR and places it in position. Next, the patient is positioned precisely, and the **x-ray tube** is aligned with the body part and the IR at a specific distance. The operator sets the technical factors for the examination on the control panel. Final instructions are given to the patient, and the exposure is made. If more than one exposure is needed, the IR is changed, the patient is repositioned, and the steps are repeated until the examination is complete.

After ensuring that the patient is safe and comfortable, the operator processes the image. Once the image is viewed on the computer monitor and approved, it is sent for reading and then stored. Depending on the setting, the onsite or offsite radiologist will read the x-ray. In many ambulatory care settings, the treating provider reviews the x-ray and provides initial treatment, which is later evaluated when the final reading is completed.

The patient is returned to an examining room or dressing room. The operator then readies the x-ray room for the next examination and prepares the images for reading. The exact nature of a limited operator's duties will vary with the place of employment, the size of the staff, and the equipment available.

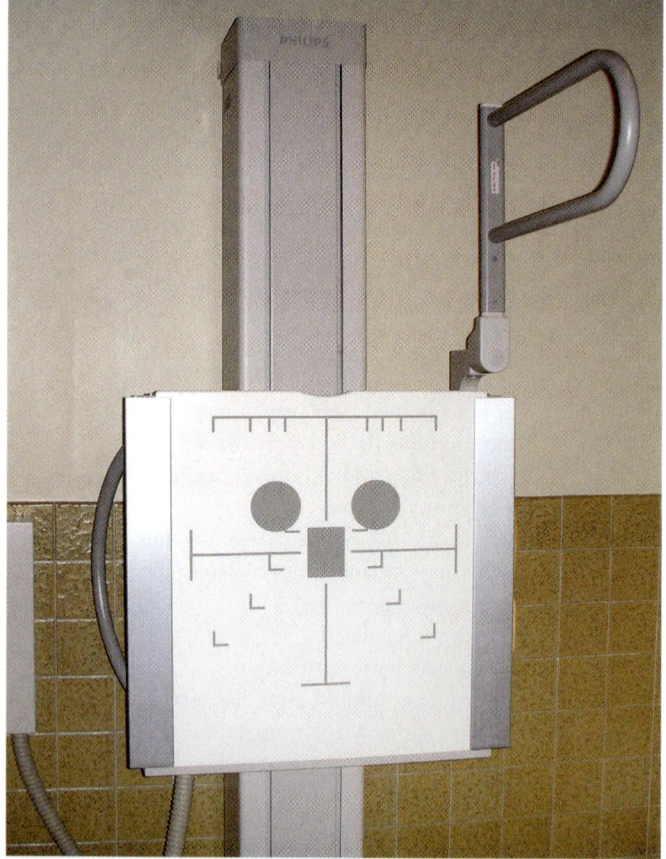

FIGURE 52.5 Upright vertical Bucky image receptor. (From Adler AM, Carlton RR: *Introduction to radiologic and imaging sciences and patient care*, ed 7, St. Louis, 2020, Saunders.)

PRIMARY X-RAY BEAM AND SCATTER RADIATION

Before we discuss the radiographic equipment, the following sections will discuss the primary x-ray beam and **scatter radiation**.

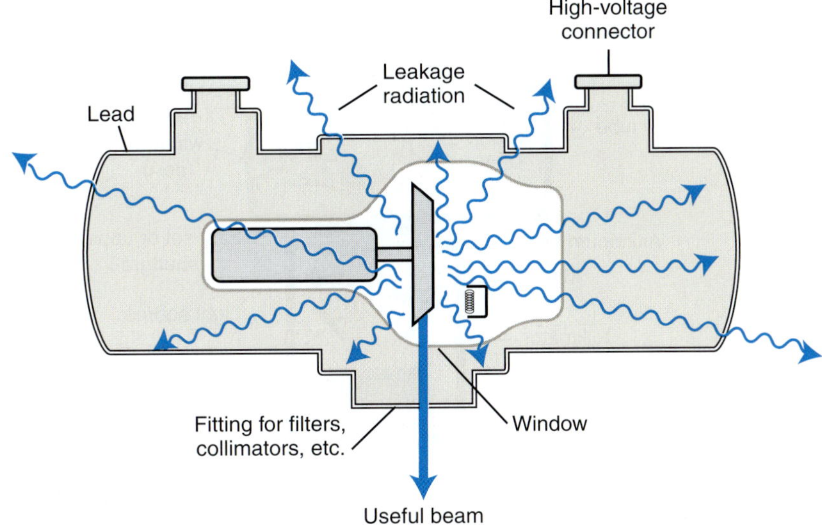

FIGURE 52.6 X-ray tube inside protective housing. (From Johnston J, Fauber TL: *Essentials of radiographic physics and imaging,* ed 3, St. Louis, 2020, Mosby.)

Primary X-ray Beam

The source of x-rays is the x-ray tube. X-rays are formed within a very small area inside the x-ray tube. Once the x-rays are created, they are directed to exit the tube and diverge as they travel toward the patient. A lead-lined tube housing surrounds the x-ray tube. X-rays that are created exit the housing through an opening called the *tube port* or window (Figure 52.6). The radiation that leaves the tube is known as **primary radiation**. The squared area of the x-ray beam that strikes the patient and x-ray table is the **radiation field**. The center of the x-ray beam and perpendicular to the long axis of the x-ray tube is the **central ray (CR)**. The CR is vital in positioning the patient because this point is used to align the x-ray tube to the body part to be imaged. Because the CR is essential, the limited operator knows exactly where to place the beam so that a light shines on the patient's body (Figure 52.7). The light field has crosshairs to identify the exact center of the x-ray beam, which is the central ray.

During a radiographic exposure, x-rays from the tube are directed through the patient to the IR (Figure 52.8). As x-rays pass through the patient, some of them are absorbed by the patient, and others are not. Some anatomy, such as bone, will absorb more radiation than other anatomy, such as muscle. Absorption is based on the density (mass) of the structure. This results in varying intensity in the x-ray beam as it exits the opposite side of the patient. The radiation, known as *remnant radiation*, then passes through to the IR. The IR now contains the *latent image*, which is the image until it is processed. The image remains stored in the IR until it is processed. Processing will convert the latent image into a *visible image*.

Tissue Densities on X-Rays

- *Bones*: Are dense and thus absorb more x-rays. Bones appear white on the image.
- *Fluid and soft tissue*: Blood and muscles absorb fewer x-rays than bones and appear darker on the image than bones.
- *Fat:* Appears darker than fluid and soft tissues.
- *Air:* Absorbs fewer x-rays and thus appears the darkest on images. Air is most visible in the lungs on chest x-rays.

Scatter Radiation

When the x-ray beam strikes the patient or the IR, part of its energy is absorbed in the patient or IR. Attenuation is the absorption of the x-ray beam. Attenuated x-rays can be absorbed within the body or scattered outside the body. The patient is the primary source of scatter radiation. Scatter radiation is radiation from the primary beam that is randomly scattered within or outside of the body. Scatter radiation has less energy than primary radiation, but it is not easily controlled. It travels from the absorbing matter in all directions, causing unwanted exposure to the IR or anyone in the room. This is why radiation safety is essential. Radiation safety will be discussed briefly later in this chapter. The unwanted image exposure caused by scatter radiation is called **fog**. See Table 52.2 for a summary of primary, remnant, and scatter radiation.

INTRODUCTION TO RADIOGRAPHIC EQUIPMENT

Radiographic equipment is used to create the x-ray beam and produce the image. Typical equipment in an x-ray room includes the IR system, x-ray tube, radiographic table, upright IR, control console, and the transformer cabinet.

Image Receptor System

For **computed radiography** systems, the IR consists of an image receptor that contains a phosphor imaging plate. The x-ray image is produced in digital format using computer technology. After the exposure is made, the IR is inserted into a *computed radiography reader*. A laser beam in the reader scans the phosphor on the plate, and the final image appears on a computer monitor. Then, the image can be manipulated and stored. The image will be sent to the radiologist for interpretation.

For **digital radiography (DR)** systems, a flat panel detector is used. *Flat-panel detectors* (FPDs) consist of a scintillation screen for a photoconductor, which converts the x-ray photons directly to electrical signals. The FPD is wired into the x-ray table or upright unit. Once the exposure is made, the image appears on the computer monitor in seconds. Then, the image can be manipulated, stored, and sent to the radiologist and possible treating provider for interpretation.

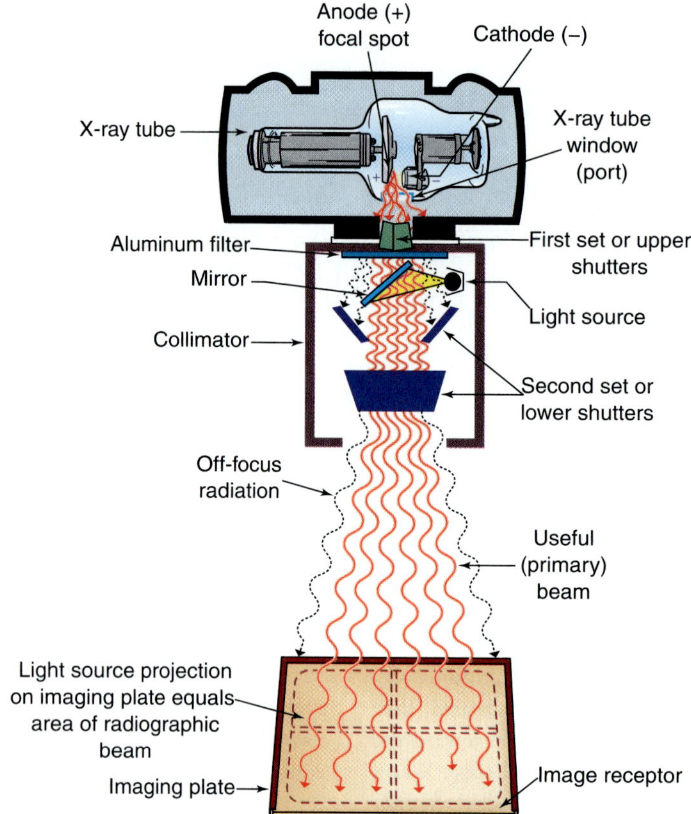

FIGURE 52.7 Diagram of typical collimator demonstrating a beam-defining system: Anode focal spot, x-ray tube window, upper lead shutters, aluminum filter, mirror, light source, and lower lead shutters. The metal shutters collimate the x-ray beam, so that is no larger than the image receptor. (From Sherer MAS, Visconti PJ, Ritenour ER, Haynes KW: *Radiation protection in medical radiography*, ed 8, St. Louis, 2018, Mosby.)

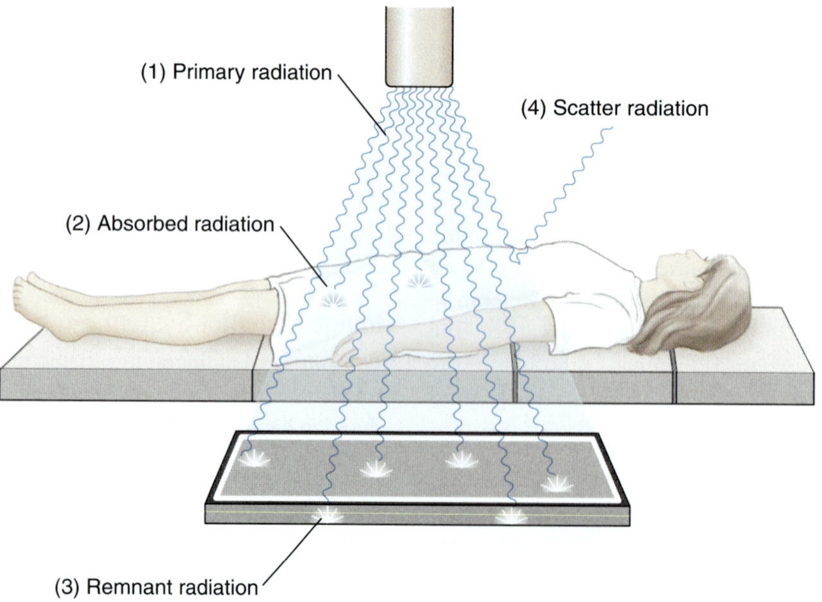

FIGURE 52.8 The path and attenuation of a beam of x-radiation. (1) The primary beam exits the x-ray tube. (2) The beam enters the patient, where the individual ex-ray photons' energies are altered (attenuated) by their passage through body tissues of varying characteristics. (3) The attenuated, or remnant, beam exits the patient, carrying energy representation of the body tissues traversed and striking the image receptor. (4) Some x-ray photons interact with matter and continue in a different direction, producing scatter radiation, which is nondiagnostic. (From Adler AM, Carlton RR: *Introduction to radiologic and imaging sciences and patient care*, ed 7, St. Louis, 2020, Saunders.)

TABLE 52.2 Summary of Primary, Remnant, and Scatter Radiation

TYPE OF RADIATION	DEFINITION	DESCRIPTION
Primary radiation	The x-ray beam that leaves the tube and travels into space	Its direction and location are predictable and controllable.
Remnant (exit) radiation	What remains of the primary beam after it has been attenuated by matter (the patient)	Tissue of different density, or atomic number, in the body absorbs x-rays differently and therefore emits x-rays differently. The remnant beam contains a varied pattern of x-ray energies that reflects the different absorption characteristics. The pattern of the remnant radiation creates the x-ray image.
Scatter radiation	Radiation from the primary beam that is randomly scattered within or outside of the body	Scatter radiation travels in all directions from the patient and is difficult to control. In general, it has less energy than the primary beam.

X-Ray Room

Figure 52.9 shows a typical x-ray room, including the x-ray equipment and a protective control booth. The x-ray machine consists of the x-ray tube, the tube support, the control console (located in the control booth), and the transformer cabinet. There is also a radiographic table and a wall-mounted IR for upright studies.

X-ray Machine

The x-ray machine consists of the transformer cabinet, x-ray tube, and collimator. Each of these is described in more depth in the following sections.

Transformer Cabinet. The transformer is an essential component of the x-ray machine. The function of the transformer is to produce the high voltage required for x-ray production and the low milliamperage (mA) needed in the x-ray tube. The transformer is located inside a cabinet in the x-ray room. The operator does not adjust or control the transformer.

X-Ray Tube. The x-ray tube is enclosed in a tube housing. The housing is lead-lined for radiation control. The housing protects the tube and the user. The housing may be mounted to the floor of the ceiling and is supported by a rail system. The rails allow for tube movement. Typical tube movement allows the following:

- *Longitudinal*: Along the long axis of the table
- *Transverse*: Across the table, at right angles to longitudinal
- *Vertical*: Up and down, increasing or decreasing the distance between the tube and table
- *Rotational*: Allows the entire x-ray tube to turn on its axis, changing the angle at which the tube arm is extended

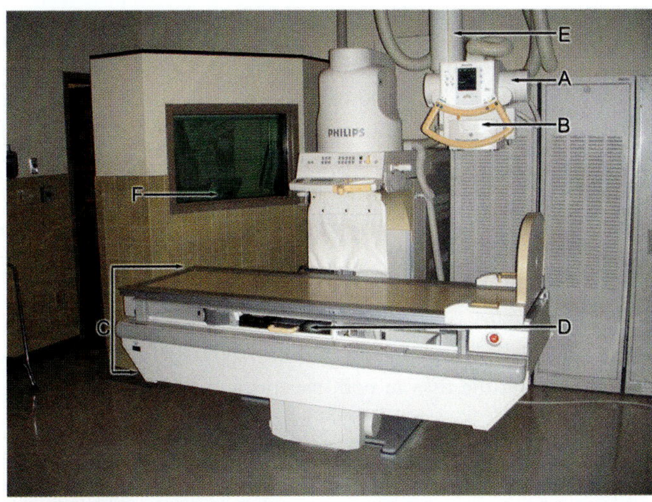

FIGURE 52.9 The generic components of diagnostic radiographic equipment include the x-ray tube **(A),** collimator **(B),** radiographic table **(C),** and image receptor tray (Bucky) **(D)**. The overhead tube crane support **(E)** is suspended from the ceiling, and the generator console is behind the leaded control booth **(F)**. (From Adler AM, Carlton RR: *Introduction to radiologic and imaging sciences and patient care*, ed 7, St. Louis, 2020, Saunders.)

- *Angular (tilt, roll)*: Permits angulation of the tube along the longitudinal axis of the table and allows the x-ray tube to be aimed at the wall rather than at the table

A system of locks holds the tube in place. To move the tube in any direction, a lock must be released. The *detent* is a special mechanism that allows the operator to position the tube at standard distances and when the x-ray tube and IR are correctly aligned.

Collimator. The *collimator* is a square-shaped device attached under the tube housing. It allows the operator to vary the size of the radiation field by adjusting the length and width of the primary beam. A centering light is used to align the CR to the **Bucky** tray.

Radiographic Table

The radiographic table is a support for the patient. The table typically has a floating tabletop and can be tilted and moved vertically. Mounted under the tabletop surface is a *grid* device used to absorb scatter radiation from the patient and prevent it from reaching the IR. For the CR, the IR is placed in the Bucky. For DR, the IR is housed below the grid.

Upright Image Receptor

The upright IR holds the IR in a vertical position for upright radiography. All rooms contain an upright IR because many x-rays are done with the patient standing or sitting upright. This unit is referred to as the *upright Bucky*.

Control Console

The control console is located in the *control booth*. This area is separated from the x-ray room by a lead barrier to protect the operator from scatter radiation exposure. There is usually a lead glass window so the operator can observe the patient from the control booth. The control console, or control panel, is the access point where the operator selects the exposure factors and initiates the exposure. A typical console has buttons for adjusting the milliamperage, exposure time, kilovoltage, Bucky, manual or **automatic exposure control (AEC)**, and anatomically programmed radiography control.

BASIC RADIATION SAFETY

Radiation exposure may pose a health hazard to operators if proper safety precautions are not followed. The potential risk is greater for the operator than the patient because the operator is often faced with the possibility of exposure. Scatter radiation is present throughout the x-ray room during exposure. The only time the potential for exposure exists is when the x-ray exposure is taken.

Risks Associated with Radiation

The general public does not sufficiently understand the health risks involved in radiation. Diagnostic radiography involves low doses of radiation, and the risks to both patients and limited operators are extremely small. It is essential to understand the risks associated with radiography and commit to radiation safety in all aspects of radiography work. When appropriately used, radiation from x-ray examinations also has benefits. The diagnostic information that the patient's physician receives from the x-ray examinations far outweighs the risks of exposure.

Ionizing radiation consists of particles, X-rays, or gamma rays with sufficient energy to cause ionization in the medium through which it passes. Radiation protection aims to reduce unnecessary radiation exposure to patients and operators. The biological effect of radiation exposure varies according to the type of radiation involved, its energy, and the types of cells that are exposed. Also, some cells are more sensitive to radiation than others. The *law of Bergonie and Tribondeau* states that cell sensitivity to radiation exposure depends on the following characteristics of cells:

1. *Age:* Immature (or younger) cells are more sensitive than mature cells. Younger tissue and organs are also more sensitive.
2. *Differentiation*: Undifferentiated (or simple) cells are more sensitive than differentiated (or specialized) cells.
3. *Metabolic rate*: Cells with a higher metabolic rate are more sensitive.
4. *Mitotic rate*: Rapidly dividing cells are more sensitive.

Highly radiosensitive tissues and organs are at a higher risk of injury from radiation. These include:

- Bone marrow and blood: Serious changes can occur with these cells.
- Intestines and lymphoid organs, such as the spleen, thymus gland, and lymph node.
- Gonads, such as the testes and ovaries. Permanent damage can occur that results in genetic mutations and sterility. Genetic mutations can be passed to offspring.

Organs and tissues that have a middle-range radiosensitivity include the epidermis, hair, eye lens, lungs, thyroid gland, liver, and kidneys. Tissues with lower radiosensitivity include muscles, bones, nerves, and blood vessels.

Protection for the Operator

The sources of radiation are the x-ray tube and the patient, as a source of scatter. There is the possibility of exposure to the operator from either the primary x-ray beam or from scatter radiation from the patient. The three principal methods used to protect limited operators from unnecessary radiation exposure are *time*, *distance*, and *shielding*. Time and distance apply principally to radiographers who are involved in fluoroscopy and mobile radiography. Shielding is employed to protect all radiographers.

The amount of exposure is directly proportional to the time spent in the radiation field, so the occupational dose is decreased when this time is minimized. The next method is distance. The operator should increase the distance from yourself and the source of radiation. This will decrease exposure proportionately to the square of the distance. Therefore, a small increase in distance will reduce operator dose significantly. The final, and most common method of protection is shielding. The walls of the x-ray room contain lead to reduce exposure to the operator. Other types of shielding include lead aprons, gloves, and thyroid shields. If the operator must be in the room during exposure, it is essential to wear a protective lead apron.

The limited operator must wear a device to monitor exposure to ionizing radiation. This device, a personnel dosimeter, is required whenever a radiation worker is likely to receive 10% or more of the annual occupational effective dose limit of 50 millisieverts (mSv).

CRITICAL THINKING APPLICATION **52.2**

Stephanie has an x-ray request for a chest x-ray examination. She brings the patient, Mrs. Jones, into the room. During her assessment of Mrs. Jones, Stephanie realizes that Mrs. Jones will not be able to stand unassisted for the chest x-ray. Therefore, Stephanie will be in the x-ray room during the exposure. How can Stephanie protect herself from radiation exposure?

Protection for the Patient

The guiding philosophy is the *ALARA principle*. The ALARA principle states that all radiation exposure should be limited to levels that are "as low as reasonably achievable." The limited operator can reduce radiation exposure to patients by reducing repeat exposures, using the smallest radiation field, using the highest kVP and the lowest possible mAs, and maintaining the **source-to-image-receptor distance (SID)** at a minimum of 40 inches.

BASIC PHYSICS FOR RADIOGRAPHY

Limited operators do not require an extensive background in physics, but some basic principles of physical science are essential to an understanding of x-rays and their use. This section covers the basic concepts of matter, energy, and electricity and relates these principles to radiography. Everything of a physical nature in the universe can be classified as either matter or energy. Both matter and energy can exist in several forms.

Matter

Matter is defined as anything that occupies space and has shape or form. The primary forms of matter are solids, liquids, and gases. All matter is composed of building blocks called *atoms*. The fundamental particles that constitute atoms are neutrons, protons, and electrons. The neutrons and protons form the nucleus of the atom, its center. The electrons circle the nucleus in orbits called shells.

The characteristic of an atom that determines its type is the number of protons in the nucleus. An element comprises only one kind of atom; all atoms of an element have the same atomic number. The atomic number of a material determines how it will absorb radiation and appear on an image.

When a neutral atom gains or loses an electron, the atom is said to be ionized. *Ionization* produces an atom with an electric charge. If an electron is added to a neutral atom, electrons will outnumber the protons, and the atom will have a negative charge. If an electron is removed, there will be more protons than electrons, so the atom will have a positive charge. Applying a small amount of energy to an outer orbital electron will remove the electron from the atom. Ionization is significant in radiology because x-rays cause ionization in the atoms of the human body.

Energy

Energy is the ability to do work. It occurs in several forms and can be changed from one form to another. *Electromagnetic energy* is the energy we deal with in radiology. The energy consists of light, x-rays, radio waves, microwaves, and other forms of energy. These energies have both electric and magnetic properties. Electromagnetic energy occurs in the form of a sine wave. The distance between the crest and the trough of the wave is the amplitude. The distance from one crest to another is the wavelength, and the frequency is the number of times per second that a crest passes a given point. X-rays with greater energy have shorter wavelengths but higher frequencies and are more penetrating. The smallest possible unit of electromagnetic energy is the *photon*, which can be thought of as a tiny bundle of energy. Photons come out of the x-ray tube as discrete bundles of energy.

Characteristics of X-Rays

X-rays and visible light are both forms of electromagnetic energy. They have some similar characteristics. Both travel in straight lines at the same velocity. X-rays and light can cause changes in living organisms (e.g., sunburn). X-rays are also different than visible light. X-rays are capable of producing more harmful effects than light because of their greater energy. X-rays can penetrate matter, dependent on the mass, atomic number, and thickness of the matter. X-rays come out of the x-ray tube and into space until they are absorbed or go into the human body.

Unique Characteristics of X-rays

X-rays exhibit the following characteristics:

- Have no mass
- Are highly penetrating and invisible
- Are electrically neutral
- Produce over a wide range of energies and wavelengths
- Travel in a straight line at the speed of light
- Can ionize matter
- Produce biological changes in tissue
- Produce secondary and scatter radiation

Electricity

X-ray energy is human made and is produced electrically. Electric current will flow in a vacuum, in particular liquids, and through certain metals called *conductors*. Copper wire is a common conductor. It is connected to form a circuit. Current will flow in the circuit when there is a difference in electric charge, known as a *potential difference*, between two points in the circuit.

Electric Circuits

Three electric factors are part of a circuit:

- *Resistance*: Hinders the flow of current.
- *Current*: The quantity of electrons flowing in a circuit. The *ampere (A)* is the unit of measure for current.
- *Potential difference*: The difference in electric potential between two points in an electric circuit. The *volt (V)* is the unit for potential difference. In radiology, we use *milliamperes (mA)* and **kilovolts peak (kVp)**.

An electric circuit is a continuous path for the flow of electric charges from the power source through one or more electrical devices and back to the source. The electricity provided by the utility company is in the form of an *alternating current* (AC). This means the current will flow in one direction and then alternate to another direction. Therefore, the current is constantly changing. As the voltage changes, the current flow increases, peaks, and decreases. AC can be converted so that it flows in one direction only. This process is called *rectification*. (Rectification will be discussed in more detail in a later section.) The x-ray tube cannot produce x-rays unless the current is rectified. Rectified AC is sometimes referred to as direct current (DC). The transformer of the x-ray machine will change AC to DC.

Electromagnetic Induction and Transformers

Magnetic fields and electric energy are interrelated. Magnetic fields can be used to produce electricity and, conversely, electric currents create magnetic fields. When a conductor is placed in a magnetic field, an electric current will flow in the conductor. This process is *electromagnetic induction*. When the direction of the movement changes, the direction of the current flow changes. Electromagnetic induction is the basis for the transformer, the device used to produce the high voltage required for x-ray production. A transformer consists of primary and secondary coils, usually surrounding an iron core. Current always flows from the primary to the secondary coils. When there are more turns, or "windings," in the secondary coil than in the primary coil, the voltage on the secondary side is greater, and the transformer is called a *step-up* transformer. On the other hand, if the secondary side has fewer turns, the secondary voltage and the transformer will be a *step-down* transformer.

A transformer can increase or decrease voltage, the change is based on the number of turns in the coil. This is known as the transformer ratio which is the ratio between turns on each side of the coil. The first number in the ratio is the number of windings on the secondary side. It is helpful to remember that both voltage and amperage flow in an electric circuit. Thus, amperage also flows through the transformer; however, kilovoltage and amperage are *inversely* proportional while flowing through the transformer. It is important to remember that as a step-up transformer increases the voltage from primary to secondary, amperage decreases. An x-ray machine uses both step-up and step-down transformers.

X-RAY PRODUCTION

This section discusses x-ray tube structure and function of how these factors affect the primary beam. The electric factors that control x-ray production are introduced. Roentgen accidentally discovered x-rays while experimenting with a Crookes cathode ray tube. In the late 19th century, these tubes were used in laboratory experiments. In 1913, a prototype for the modern x-ray tube was introduced by the General Electric Company.

X-Ray Tube

There are four essential requirements for the production of x-rays: (1) a vacuum, (2) a source of electrons, (3) a target, and (4) a high potential difference (voltage) between the electron source and the target.

The x-ray tube is contained within a glass structure made of Pyrex. The glass envelope contains the source of electrons and the target. The air is removed from the glass envelope to form a vacuum. The source of electrons is a filament at one end of the tube. The filament consists of a small coil of tungsten wire. An electric current flows through the filament to heat it. As the filament is heated, it begins to "boil off" electrons; this process is called **thermionic emission**. The electrons form an electron cloud called a space charge and are the source of free electrons for x-ray production.

At the opposite end of the tube is the anode (also referred to as the target), a slanted metal surface made of tungsten. The electrons are directed toward the target, which is where x-rays are generated. A high-voltage electric source provides acceleration of the electrons. A step-up transformer supplies the voltage required for x-ray production. The two ends of the x-ray tube are connected in the transformer circuit so that the filament end is positive during exposure. The positive end of the tube is the anode, and the negative end is the cathode. The high positive electric potential at the target attracts the negatively charged electrons of the space charge, which move rapidly across the tube, forming an electron stream. When these fast-moving electrons collide with the target, the kinetic energy of their motion is converted into heat (>99%), and only a small amount is converted into x-rays.

Bremsstrahlung and Characteristic Radiation

X-rays are produced at the target due to either a sudden deceleration (called **bremsstrahlung radiation**) or absorption of the electron stream (called **characteristic radiation**).

Bremsstrahlung Radiation

X-rays are produced when an incoming electron misses all the electrons in the tungsten atom, gets very close to the nucleus, and then suddenly slows down and abruptly changes direction. As a result, the electron loses energy and is converted into an x-ray photon. The new photon is a small bundle of electromagnetic energy. X-rays that are created by this interaction are *bremsstrahlung radiation*. *Bremsstrahlung* is a German word that means braking or slowing. Every x-ray exposure will contain photons produced from bremsstrahlung interactions in the anode.

Characteristic Radiation

Another type of radiation, characteristic radiation, is created when an incoming electron strikes the K-shell electron and ejects it out of orbit. The initial electron and the K-shell electron are eliminated. This creates a void in the K-shell which is filled with an electron from another orbit. The primary x-ray beam is made up of both bremsstrahlung and characteristic radiation. The wavelength and energy of the beam are known to be heterogeneous, which means that the beam is made up of many different wavelengths and energies. X-ray energy is measured in kiloelectron volts (keV).

Characteristics of the Cathode and Anode

The cathode, the negative side of the x-ray tube, contains two filaments, one large and one small (Figure 52.10). Only one filament is used at a time. Each filament is located in the cathode in the focusing cup. The focusing cup has a slightly negative charge and causes the electrons to be repelled in the direction of the target at the focal spot. Spatial resolution, the sharpness or detail seen in the image, is best with a small filament and small focal spot. For small-to-average sized patients, the small focal spot should be used on all body parts except the chest and abdomen. The chest and abdomen, because they are larger body parts require the use of the large focal spot.

Again, the majority of energy in the electron stream is converted to heat. This takes place at the anode, the positive side of the x-ray tube, which is made of tungsten. Tungsten is used because it has a high melting point and efficiently conducts heat away from the anode. The anode rotates during the exposure, so the heat is distributed all around the circumference of the disk. When the operator pushes the exposure button, there is a short delay before the exposure is made. This delay allows the rotor to accelerate and rotate, and the filament is heated. An audible sound is made during the exposure. When the sound ends, the exposure ends, and the operator releases the button. When the exposure is completed, the rotating anode slows down and stops. The anode is slanted or angled around the edges, forming a bevel. The slant, or angle, is typically between 7 and 17 degrees, with 12 degrees being the most common. The angle affects the tube's heat capacity, the sharpness of the image, and the maximum size of the x-ray beam.

Line Focus Principle

The term *actual focal spot* refers to the area on the target surface struck by the electron stream. A larger focal spot is best for heat capacity. The *effective focal spot* refers to the vertical projection of the actual focal spot onto the patient and IR. A smaller focal spot produces a smaller radiation field, which reduces the patient's radiation exposure.

The size of the effective focal spot influences the resolution of the image. This is known as the **line focus principle** (Figure 52.11). When vertical lines are drawn from each corner of the angled focal spot, these lines define an image of the focal spot as viewed from the IR. The effective focal spot is always smaller than the actual focal spot. A smaller effective focal spot will result in greater resolution in the image, and that a larger effective focal spot will have the opposite effect. The smaller the target angle, the greater the size difference between the actual and effective focal spots.

> **Line Focus Principle**
>
> - The size of the *effective* focal spot determines image resolution.
> - The target angle determines the relative size of the effective focal spot.
> - The steeper the target angle, the greater the difference between the actual and effective focal spot sizes.

Anode Heel Effect

Most x-rays are not produced on the surface of the target. Electrons from the beam may penetrate through multiple layers of atoms before interacting with any material. The interaction creates the x-ray and the x-ray will pass through, or exit, the target and travel toward the IR to create the image. Some of the x-rays will be absorbed by the target during this process. Because of the angle of the target, some x-rays will pass through more target material than others. The x-rays that are directed away from the cathode are more likely to be

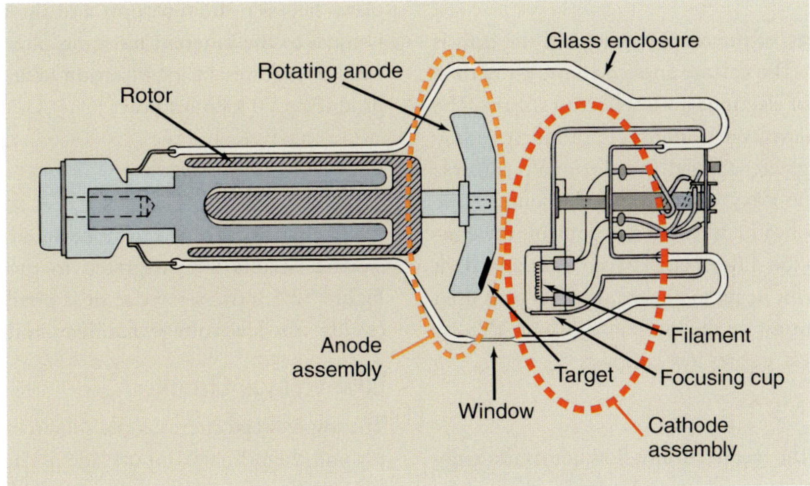

FIGURE 52.10 Principal parts of an x-ray tube. (From Bushong SC: *Radiologic science for technologists: physics, biology, and protection*, ed 12, St. Louis, 2021, Mosby.)

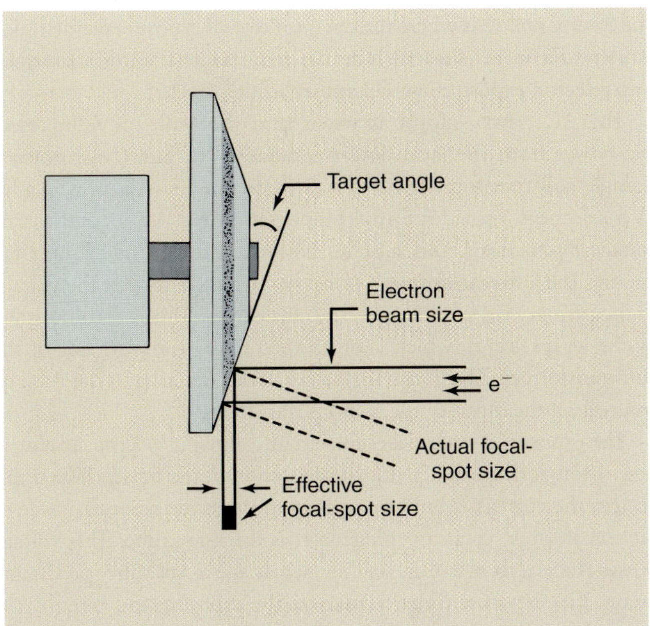

FIGURE 52.11 The line focus principle allows high anode heating with small effective focal spots As the target angle decreases, so does the effective focal spot size. (From Bushong SC: *Radiologic science for technologists: physics, biology, and protection*, ed 12, St. Louis, 2021, Mosby.)

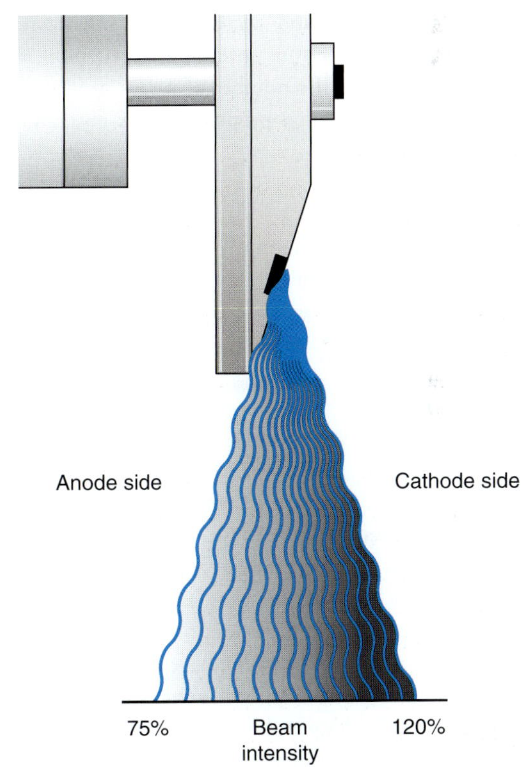

FIGURE 52.12 Anode heel effect. The anode heel effect is simply caused by photons produced on the anode side, which must penetrate the heel of the target before exiting the tube. This causes some photons to be weakened and some to be absorbed. The net effect is reduced intensity of the beam on the anode side. (From Johnston J, Fauber TL: *Essentials of radiographic physics and imaging*, ed 3, St. Louis, 2020, Mosby.)

absorbed. This results in an uneven distribution of radiation intensity in the x-ray beam, called the *anode heel effect* (Figure 52.12). If the anode heel effect is not used correctly, the thinner portions of the anatomy will appear too dark on the IR, and the thicker portions will be too light.

Anode Heel Effect

- Variation in radiation intensity across the length of the radiation field.
- Greater radiation intensity toward the cathode end of the field.
- Only significant with using the entire beam (14 × 17 IR at 40 inches or full spine at 72 inches).
- Place the thinner portion of the body part toward the anode end of the tube.

Electric Control of X-ray Production

Three terms describe electricity: amperes, volts, and watts (wattage). *Amperes* (also called *amps*) are simply the amount of electricity used by the item. Volts are the measure of the force of electricity. Amps multiplied by volts give you the total wattage (workload). In radiography, we are concerned with amperes and volts. However, to create an x-ray, the volts must be increased to kilovolts, and the amperes are decreased to milliamps.

Kilovoltage

Voltage is measured at the peak of the *electric* cycle, and the unit is stated as kilovolts peak (kVp). The voltage applied to the x-ray tube controls the speed and power of electrons in the electron stream. The electrons move faster when the voltage is increased, producing x-ray with shorter wavelengths and greater energy. Therefore, kVp controls the energy (wavelength) of the x-ray beam. The kVp controls the penetrating power of the x-ray beam. The kVp also controls the contrast in the image. *Contrast* is the difference between light and dark areas in an x-ray, which allows for detail to be seen. Low kVp, as used for extremities, creates low contrast on the image, while high kVp, as used for the chest and abdomen, creates low contrast.

Milliamperage

Milliamperage (mA) measures the rate of current flow across the x-ray tube, that is, the number of electrons flowing from the filament to target *each second*. The filament heat determines the number of available electrons. When filament heat is increased, more electrons are available each second to cross the tube. Therefore, increasing the mA increases the filament heat, and decreasing the mA decreases filament heat. When more electrons strike the target, more x-rays are produced, so mA controls the number of x-rays produced and the exposure rate. High mA settings produce more x-rays, and low mA settings produce fewer x-rays.

Exposure Time

Exposure time refers to the amount of time that x-rays are being produced. Most exposure times are measured in milliseconds (ms) because they are less than 1 second. The operator adjusts the time and a timer will end the exposure at the preset time.

Milliampere-Seconds

The total quantity of x-ray photons in an exposure cannot be determined by either mA or time alone. The quantity, or number, of x-rays created is determined by mA. However, mA does not dictate the length of the exposure. To establish the total quantity of radiation created during an exposure, the mA and the time are considered. Millliampere-seconds (mAs) is the unit used to indicate the quantity of exposure and mAs if the product of exposure time and mA:

mAs = Time (seconds) × mA

In the radiology department, most **generators** are designed so that the operator sets the kVp and the mAs. The operator can adjust the mA and time separately if needed.

X-Ray Beam Filtration

The x-ray beam contains photons of varying energies. This is known as heterogenous. Photons with a long wavelength are readily absorbed by the body and are less likely to penetrate through the body part and travel to the IR. The photons are absorbed by the patient and contribute to patient dose. To reduce radiation dose, the x-ray beam is filtered. Filtration removes the long-wavelength photons. Aluminum is placed between the x-ray tube and the patient and it will absorb unnecessary radiation and decrease patient dose. Filtration provided by the glass of the tube is called inherent filtration (built-in) and is approximately 0.5 mm Al equivalent. Filtration from the collimator is also considered inherent and equals about 1.0 mm Al. Additional filtration can be added by installing aluminum plates between the tube port and the collimator. The total filtration is equal to the inherent filtration plus the added filtration. The federal law requires a total filtration of at least 2.5 mm Al for machines producing 70 kVp or more.

X-RAY CIRCUIT

X-ray circuits help you to understand how three relatively complex electric circuits are integrated to produce x-rays. As indicated in Figure 52.13, the x-ray circuit is divided into three sections or subcircuits: the low-voltage, filament, and high-voltage.

Low-Voltage Circuit

The low-voltage circuit is the subcircuit between the AC power supply and the primary (input) side of the high-voltage (step-up) transformer. The current flows from the AC power supply to the step-up transformer. From the transformer, it returns to the power source, forming an enclosed loop. Except for the step-up transformer, all of the devices in the subcircuit are located within the control console. The *control console* is where the operator sets all exposure factors, such as kVp and mAs. They include the main switch, autotransformer, kVp selector, exposure switch, and exposure timer.

The AC power supply is wired into the wall, providing electric power from the local power company. The autotransformer is a single-coil transformer that serves three functions: it provides for kVp selection, provides form compensation for the incoming line voltage fluctuations, and supplies power to other parts of the x-ray circuit. The autotransformer's primary purpose is to vary the voltage to the primary side of the step-up transformer. This is accomplished by the kVp selector, which is on the secondary (output) side of the autotransformer. The autotransformer varies the kVp to the tube by controlling the input to the step-up transformer.

The exposure switch closes the circuit, allowing electric current to flow through the primary side of the step-up transformer. When this occurs, the current is induced to flow through the secondary side of the transformer, creating voltage across the x-ray tube. This voltage causes the electron stream to flow across the x-ray tube, producing x-rays. The exposure timer terminates the exposure and is set by the operator on the control console.

Filament Circuit

The *filament circuit* is another circuit within the main x-ray circuit as seen in Figure 52.13. This circuit is divided into two parts by the step-down transformer. The filament circuit supplies low current to heat the x-ray tube filament for thermionic emission. When the operator adjusts the mA on the control console, the filament circuit is activated.

The primary side of the circuit begins and ends with the contacts on the autotransformer. Current in this circuit flows from the autotransformer, the mA selector, the primary side of the step-down transformer, and back to the autotransformer. The secondary side begins and ends with the secondary side of the step-down transformer conducting current through the x-ray tube filament. The step-down transformer reduces the voltage on the secondary side, providing an appropriate current to heat the filament.

The mA selector controls amperage in the filament circuit. Because the current through this circuit controls filament heat, this

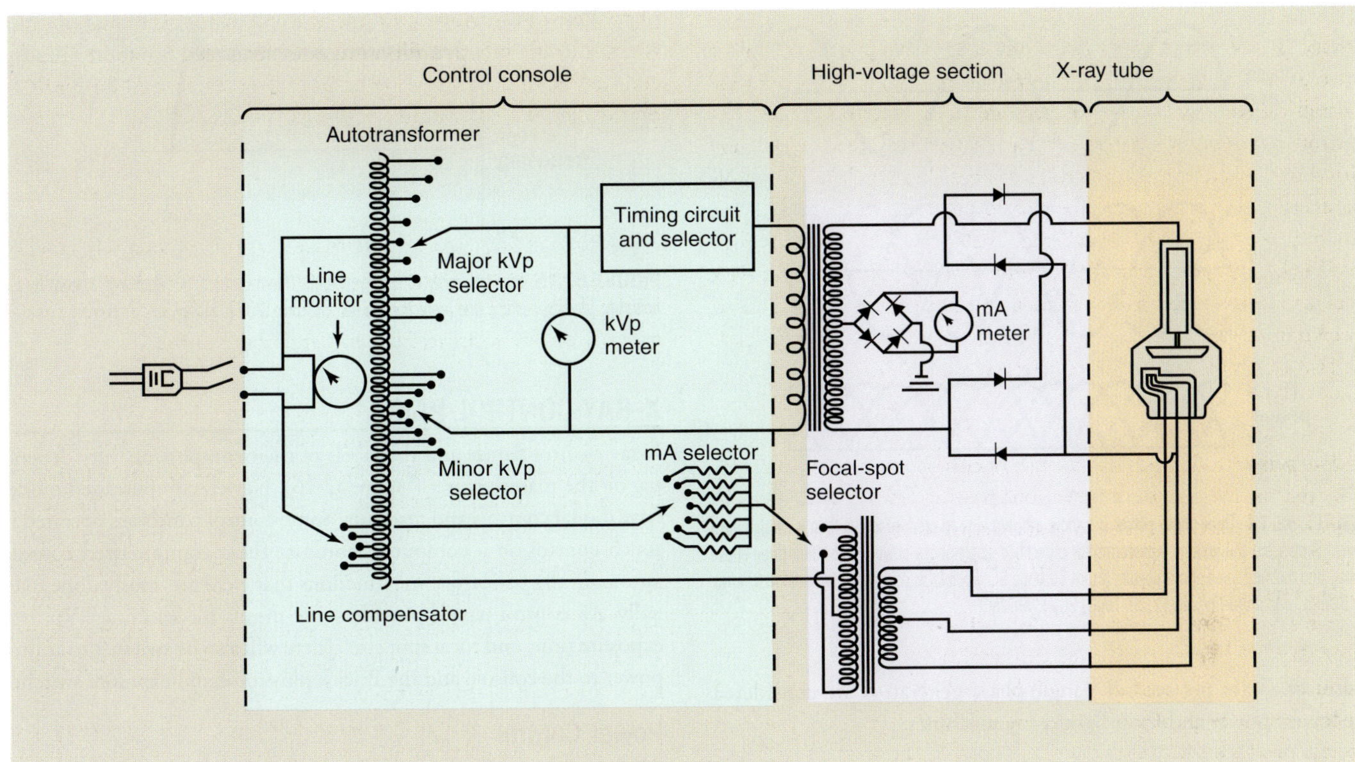

FIGURE 52.13 Schematic of a circuit of an x-ray imaging system. (From Bushong SC: *Radiologic science for technologists: physics, biology, and protection*, ed 12, St. Louis, 2021, Mosby.)

setting determines the number of available electrons at the x-ray tube filament. It determines the mA in the high-voltage section that includes the x-ray tube.

High-Voltage Circuit

The *high-voltage circuit* begins and ends with the secondary side of the step-up transformer. The rectifiers and the x-ray tube are located in the high-voltage section. During an exposure, the current is flowing. The high-voltage transformer is a step-up transformer because it increases the incoming voltage in proportion to the transformer ratio. The primary purpose of the high-voltage circuit is to supply the x-ray tube with voltage high enough to create x-rays. The autotransformer, step-down transformer, and high-voltage transformer are all located in a cabinet in the x-ray room.

RECTIFICATION

Rectification is changing AC into DC, so it flows in one direction only. This is done with the use of rectifiers. The rectification process prepares the current for x-ray production by ensuring that it flows in the right direction, in this case, from the filament to the target. There are three ways in which the current is rectified: self-rectification, half-wave rectification, and full-wave rectification. Self-rectification is no longer used.

Half-Wave Rectification

AC travels in copper wire as a sine wave. It moves in a pulsating manner from positive to negative. In half-wave rectification, the negative phase of the electric cycle is completely removed, and a gap remains. The x-rays are turned off during the eliminated (negative) phase. With only the positive phase remaining, the current is "direct" only or DC. The x-rays are pulsating on and off.

Full-Wave Rectification

During full-wave rectification, the current is redirected during the negative half of the electric cycle so that the current will flow in the same direction during the positive and negative halves of the cycle. So, full-wave rectification uses the entire electric cycle for x-ray production. The negative impulses are made positive rather than being eliminated. All modern general-purpose x-ray machines are full-wave rectified. The main advantage of full-wave rectification is that the exposure time can be cut in half because of the doubling in x-ray output compared with half-wave.

GENERATORS

The x-ray generator delivers the electrical power to energize the x-ray tube and permits the selection of x-ray energy, x-ray quantity, and exposure time. The generator's major internal components include transformers, diodes and rectifier circuits, filament circuits, timer switches, and kilovolt and milliampere meters. Single-phase, three-phase, and high-frequency generators produce different voltage waveforms (ripple) and x-ray beam spectra.

Single-Phase Generators

Single-phase generators, which are being phased out of operation due to their inefficiency, produce a pulsating current that alternates from negative to positive during the electric cycle, which results in a pulsating x-ray beam (Figure 52.14). In a single-phase current with full-wave rectification, 120 pulses of electricity per second create 120

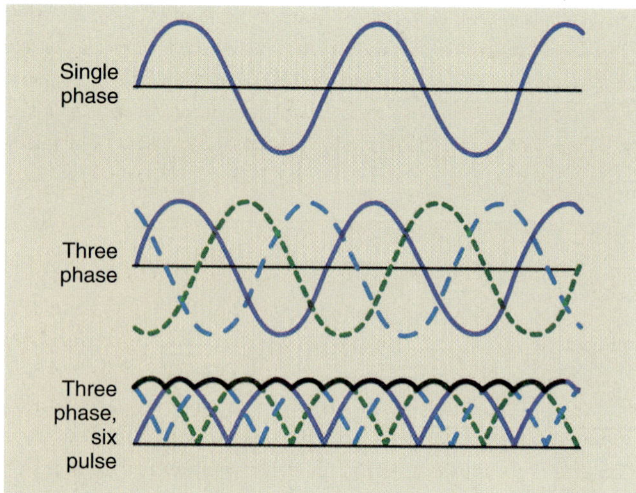

FIGURE 52.14 Three-phase power is a more efficient way to produce x-rays than is single-phase power. Shown are the voltage waveforms for unrectified single-phase power, unrectified three-phase power, and rectified three-phase power. (From Bushong SC: *Radiologic science for technologists: physics, biology, and protection*, ed 12, St. Louis, 2021, Mosby.)

pulses of x-rays per second. Single-phase generators are considered the lowest power and most basic x-ray machines.

Three-Phase Generators

Three-phase generators are powered by three separate sources of AC at the same time, which is a more constant and efficient voltage source. AC is generated over three overlapping cycles. When the current is rectified, its waveform appears as a "ripple" with no real low points. In a three-phase current with full-wave rectification, 360 pulses of electricity per second create 360 pulses of x-rays per second. An advantage of a three-phase current is that it is more efficient and produces approximately 40% more x-rays than a single-phase current. This greater output enables exposure times to be decreased by 40%.

High-Frequency Generators

High-frequency (HF) generators are the most common generators used today (Figure 52.15). They produce x-rays much more efficiently than single-phase or three-phase generators. The primary function in the complex HF circuitry is that the 60-Hz full-wave rectified circuit is converted to a significantly higher frequency of about 6000-Hz. The highest-powered HF units can convert the frequency to as high as 100,000 Hz. HF generators produce a near-constant voltage waveform, resulting in even less exposure time than three-phase. They produce the greatest number of x-rays for the same exposure technique. HF generators are also smaller than three-phase and single-phase generators.

CRITICAL THINKING APPLICATION **52.3**

At WMFM Clinic, the x-ray generator is a high-frequency generator. During Stephanie's clinical experience during training, she worked with a single-phase generator. She has learned the technical factors using the single-phase generator. What changes will Stephanie need to make to her technical factors now that she is using a high-frequency generator?

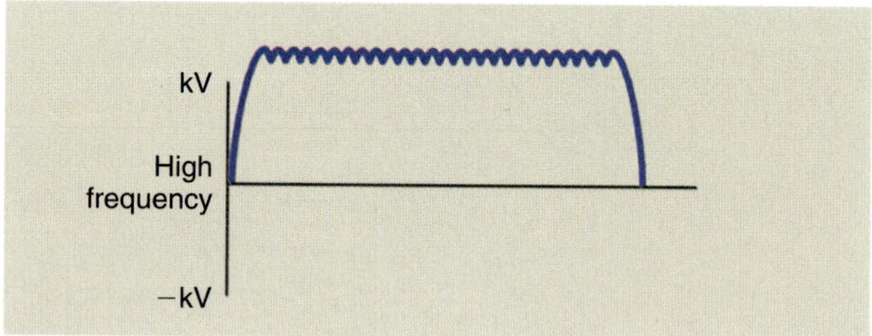

FIGURE 52.15 High-frequency voltage waveform. (From Bushong SC: *Radiologic science for technologists: physics, biology, and protection*, ed 12, St. Louis, 2021, Mosby.)

X-RAY CONTROL PANEL

X-ray control panels and the labels of their components vary depending on the manufacturer (Figure 52.16). Newer, computerized models have digital controls and readouts. Some control panels are operated by touch control on a computer monitor. These computerized consoles automatically perform some functions that were previously done manually. All control panels provide some means for selecting kVp, mA, exposure time, and focal spot size. There will also be switches to control power to the console and the Bucky, plus rotor and exposure switches.

Power Control

The on/off switch on the console corresponds to the main power switch in the schematic diagram (see Figure 52.13). This switch controls the power to the control panel and the entire x-ray generator.

Milliamperage Control and Exposure Time Control

Conventional panels have an mA selector, which provides options for choices of mA, known as mA stations. Each cathode filament in the x-ray tube is connected to specific mA stations. The filament and its associated focal spot are chosen automatically when the mA is selected. Usually, mA stations of 200 to 250 or less employ the small filament; the large filament supplies mA requirements of 250 or more. Digital readouts on the console will state the mAs setting and the exposure time.

All control consoles contain an exposure timer, whether it is set directly by the operator or not. The time set is the length of time the x-rays are turned on. Computerized controls may select the exposure time using an electronic timer. Electronic timers are more capable of ultrashort exposure times (1 ms or less).

Kilovoltage Control

Computerized controls have a digital read-out for the kVp setting and arrow buttons that can be pressed to increase or decrease the kVp.

Bucky Control

The *Bucky* is a moving grid used for radiography of larger body parts (Figure 52.17). The Bucky device incorporates a motor to oscillate the grid. The operator will select the wall Bucky, the table Bucky, or turn off the Bucky on the control panel. The grid will be turned off for tabletop exposures or removed for nongrid exposures.

Manual Exposure Time

Every x-ray exposure that is made will have three exposure factors set on the control panel: *kVp*, *mA*, and *exposure time*. These factors are typically selected manually by the operator.

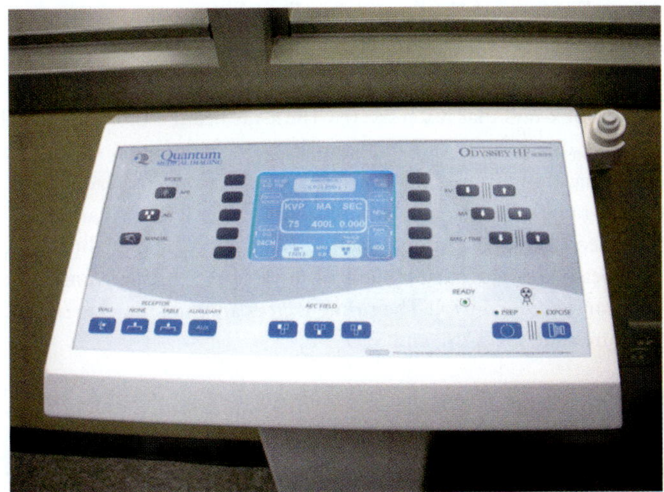

FIGURE 52.16 The control panel or control console. Exposure controls are convenient pushbuttons with a visual display of selected exposure factors. In this version, exposures may be made using prep and expose buttons. (From Adler AM, Carlton RR: *Introduction to radiologic and imaging sciences and patient care*, ed 7, St. Louis, 2020, Saunders.)

Automatic Exposure Control

Many x-ray machines provide AEC, which terminates the exposure when a certain quantity of radiation has been detected at the IR. The AEC system is a complex microprocessor circuit built into the generator and x-ray table and linked directly to the mA, kVp, and exposure time controls. When activating the AEC on the generator, the mA and kVp values are set, as usual; however, *the exposure time is automatically determined.*

A sensing device is located under the table and detects when a given amount of x-ray photons has been reached. When this happens, the sensor will terminate the exposure. The sensors under the table are referred to as detectors or sensors. The AEC system may contain three or five detectors, so the operator must choose which detectors to activate (Figure 52.18). Determining which sensors to activate depends on the anatomy being imaged. The kVp and mA are set manually. When using the AEC, patient positioning must be accurate. Otherwise, the sensor could cause overexposure or underexposure.

Anatomically Programmed Radiography Control

One of the most widely used electronic functions for exposure control is anatomically programmed radiography (APR). With this function, a microprocessor controls the exposure factors. The kVp, mA, time AEC detectors, body habitus, Bucky, and SID will be selected automatically by selecting the body part and the projection. For example, if there is an order for a pelvis, the operator selects "pelvis" and then selects "AP Projection," and the exposure is ready to be made. The operator does have the ability to override the automatic factor selection for specific patient situations. The AEC system can be used with the APR system. With proper and accurate positioning, APR systems can produce excellent images and fewer repeat examinations.

Exposure Controls

The control to make an exposure is located on the control console. Two separate switches are needed to make an exposure. The first is the rotor switch, which may be labeled "Rotor," "Prep," or "Ready." This switch has two functions. When activated, the rotating anode begins to spin, and heat is applied to the filament to create electrons via thermionic emission. When this switch is held in the "on" position for a few seconds, a signal will indicate that the tube is ready for exposure. When the x-ray tube is ready, the operator initiates the exposure by holding the rotor switch and pressing a second switch, the exposure switch. An **exposure indicator (EI)** on the control

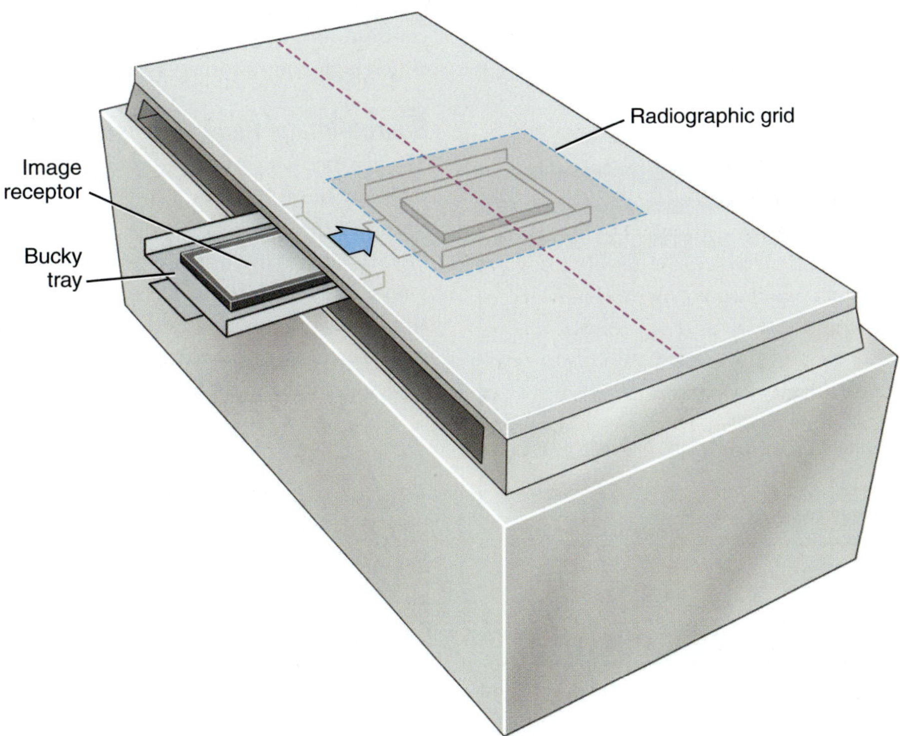

FIGURE 52.17 Bucky tray holding the IR. The Bucky tray is centered to the x-ray table under the grid. (From Adler AM, Carlton RR: *Introduction to radiologic and imaging sciences and patient care*, ed 7, St. Louis, 2020, Saunders.)

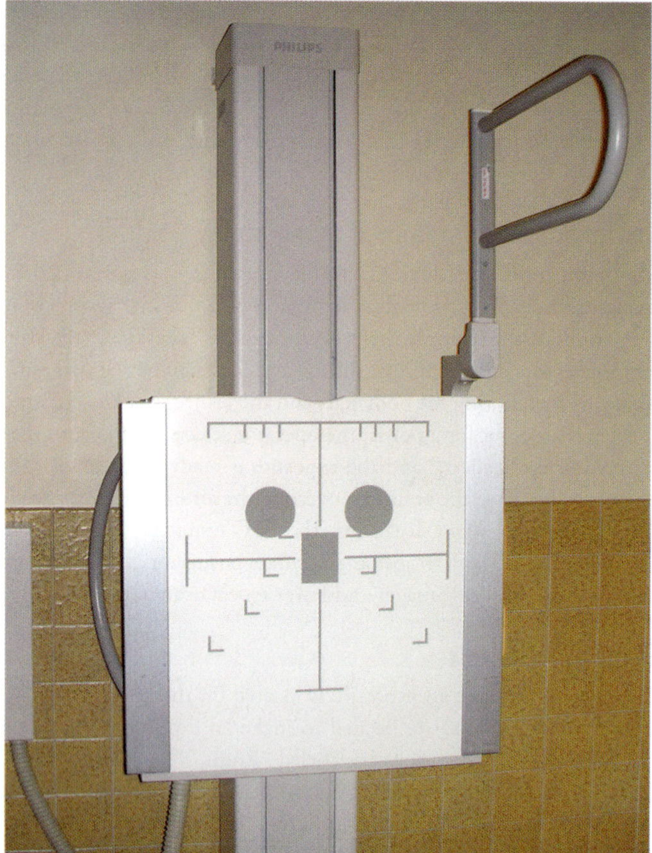

FIGURE 52.18 Automatic exposure control (AEC) system with upright Bucky unit. The locations of three AEC detector chambers are outlined on the face of the device. (From Fauber TL: *Radiographic imaging and exposure*, ed 3, St. Louis, 2009, Mosby.)

panel will indicate when the timer has terminated the exposure. Only then are the two buttons released. Most control panels have an exposure light, usually red, that is on during the exposure. When the light goes off, the exposure is complete, and an audible beep will be heard.

Setting the Control Panel on a Traditional Console

These are the steps for setting the controls and making exposure on a conventional console:

- Select mA.
- Select kVp.
- Set the Bucky.
- Activate and hold the rotor switch.
- Observe the exposure indicator to validate exposure and determine when it is complete.
- Release the rotor and exposure switches.

PRINCIPLES OF EXPOSURE AND IMAGE QUALITY

This section explains the prime factors of radiographic exposure and their radiographic effects. In addition, it introduces the primary factors of radiographic quality and the principal methods for controlling them.

Prime Factors of Radiographic Exposure

Exposure is a broad term used to describe the x-rays that the patient is exposed to, the amount of x-rays in the primary beam, and the amount of x-rays that reach the IR. The x-ray beam is often described in terms of quantity and quality. The principal factors that affect x-ray quantity are mAs, kVp, SID, and filtration. The factors that affect x-ray quality are kVp and filtration. Note that kVp and filtration affect both quantity and quality. The quantity and quality of the x-ray beam are controlled by four prime factors, which are under the operator's direct control. The prime factors are milliamperage (mA), exposure time (S), kVp, and SID.

Milliamperage, Exposure Time, and Milliampere-Seconds

As previously discussed, changes in mA affect the rate of exposure—that is, the number of photons produced per second during an exposure. An increase in mA increases the quantity of exposure, and a decrease in mA decreases the quantity of exposure. Exposure time controls the exposure to the IR and determines the length of the exposure. The number of mAs is the product of mA and exposure time (mA × time = mAs). Exposure is directly proportional to mAs; therefore, if mAs doubles, the quantity of exposure also doubles. The dose given to the patient is also directly proportional to the mAs.

Kilovoltage

The kVp controls both the quality and quantity of the x-ray beam. As the kVp increases, the energy of the photons in the beam increases, changing the quality. As the photon energy increases, the penetrating ability of the photons increases. kVp also affects the quantity of exposure to the IR. When the kVp is increased, the electrons from the filament reach the anode with more energy. More interactions then occur in the anode, and more x-rays are emitted.

The *contrast* of the image is directly affected by the kVp. A high kVp produces a low-contrast image, and a low kVp produces a high-contrast image. Low-contrast images have many shades of gray, which high-contrast images have fewer shades of gray.

Source-Image Receptor Distance

The distance between the tube target and the IR is the SID. Because the x-ray beam diverges, forming the shape of a cone, the photons spread farther apart as the distance from the target increases; thus, the SID affects the intensity of the x-ray beam and the quantity of x-rays. The *inverse square law* expresses the relationship between SID and intensity, which states that the intensity is *inversely proportional* to the square of the distance (Figure 52.19). The inverse square law is expressed mathematically as a formula:

$$\frac{I_2}{I_2} = \frac{(D_2)^2}{(D_1)^2}$$

In this formula, *I* represents radiation intensity, and *D* represents SID. For all SID calculations, the distance is always squared. As the distance increases, the intensity decreases and vice versa. For example, if the distance were doubled, the intensity would decrease to one-fourth of the original intensity. If the distance were reduced by 50%, the intensity would increase by four times. In Figure 52.20, suppose D_1 is 40 inches, and D_2 is 80 inches, or twice as great. If the original intensity at D_1 had a value of 100mR, the intensity at D_2 would be 25 mR. This value is determined by using the inverse square law formula as follows:

Insert values:

$$\frac{100}{X} = \frac{80^2}{40^2}$$

Square distances:

$$\frac{100}{X} = \frac{6400}{1600}$$

Cross multiply:

$$1600 \times 100 = 160,000$$

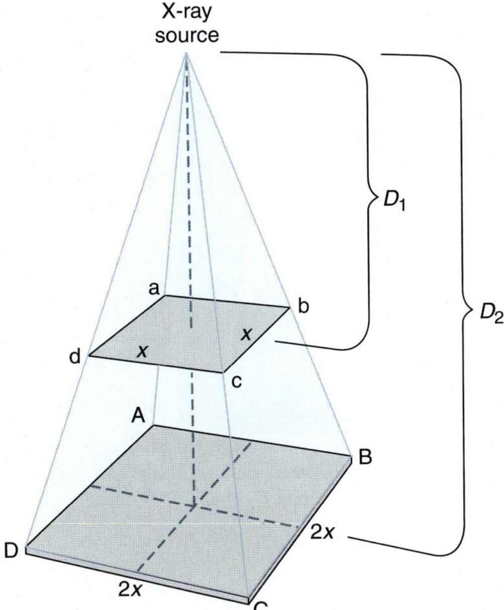

FIGURE 52.19 The Inverse Square Law. The radiation intensity at a given distance from a point source is inversely proportional to the square of the distance. (From Adler AM, Carlton RR: *Introduction to radiologic and imaging sciences and patient care*, ed 7, St. Louis, 2020, Saunders.)

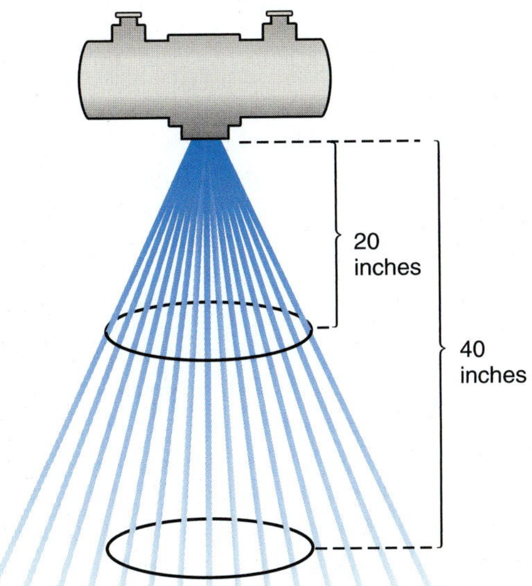

FIGURE 52.20 SID and Radiation Intensity. Source-to-image receptor distance affects both maximum field size and radiation intensity. At 40 inches, the field size is four times as large, and the x-ray intensity is four times less than at 20 inches. (From Johnston J, Fauber TL: *Essentials of radiographic physics and imaging*, ed 3, St. Louis, 2020, Mosby.)

Divide by x:

$$160,000/6400 = 25\text{mR}$$

It should be evident that the four prime factors are important technical elements in the production of an x-ray image. If the mA, exposure time, mAs, kVp, and SID are not set correctly, the body part will not have the correct contrast on the final image.

CRITICAL THINKING APPLICATION 52.4

Stephanie has a request for a chest x-ray on Mr. Hawkins. When she meets and assesses Mr. Hawkins, it is evident that Mr. Hawkins must remain seated in his wheelchair for his chest x-ray. A chest x-ray is typically performed at 72 inches, using 4 mAs. However, due to the patient's condition, the distance will be 60 inches. Using the inverse square law, how will Stephanie determine the mAs at 60 inches?

Prime Factors of Radiographic Exposure

Milliamperes (mA)

- Controls quantity of x-rays produced
- Quantity of exposure is directly proportional to mA

Exposure Time (Seconds)

- Controls quantity of x-ray produced
- Controls duration of the exposure
- Quantity of exposure is directly proportional to the exposure time

Kilovolts (kVp)

- Controls x-ray penetration
- Controls the quantity and quality of the x-ray beam
- Increased kVp results in an increased quantity of photons
- Increased kVp results in increased penetration of the body part

Source-to-Image Receptor Distance (SID)

- Affects the intensity of the x-ray beam
- Quantity of exposure is inversely proportional to the square of the distance
- Each dimension of the radiation field is proportional to the SID. Therefore, the field area is proportional to the square of the SID, and the radiation intensity is inversely proportional to the square of the SID.

Radiographic Geometric Factors

Two primary factors directly affect how the x-ray image looks: **distortion** and spatial resolution. An understanding of these factors is essential to the discussion and evaluation of x-ray images. Each factor is influenced and controlled differently. Knowledge of these concepts enables the radiographer to identify the nature of problems that relate to image quality and to solve these problems effectively.

Distortion

Distortion is a geometric property and refers to differences between the actual subject and its radiographic image. Because the subject is three-dimensional and the image is flat (two-dimensional), all

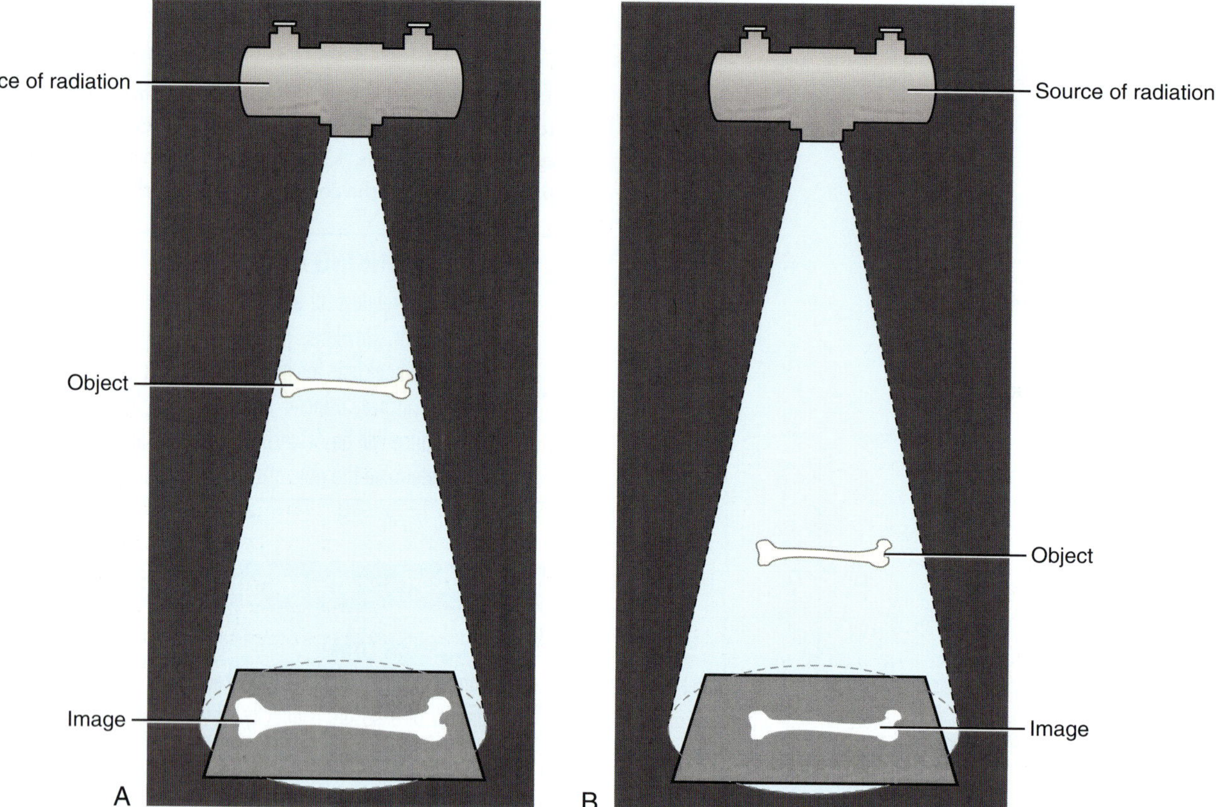

FIGURE 52.21 **OID and Size Distortion.** When the object is near the image receptor, the object and its image are nearly the same size. When the OID is increased, it causes more magnification than a short OID. The image in **(A)** is larger than **(B)** because the object is farther from the IR. (From Johnston J, Fauber TL: *Essentials of radiographic physics and imaging*, ed 3, St. Louis, 2020, Mosby.)

radiographic images have some distortion. Distortion is an unequal magnification of different portions of the same object. Radiographic distortion may be categorized by whether it primarily affects the size of the object or its shape. *Size distortion* is always in the form of magnification enlargement. *Shape distortion* is the result of unequal magnification of the actual shape of the structure.

Size Distortion

Size distortion occurs when the part is magnified. Magnification is a function of the relationship between the SID and the distance between the subject and the IR. This distance is the **object-to-image receptor distance (OID)**. As shown in Figure 52.21, there is little magnification distortion when the SID is great, and the OID is minimal. The object and its image are almost the same size.

As the OID is increased, the magnification increases, and distortion of the part occurs. Radiographic images can never be smaller than the actual size of the body. All images are magnified slightly because the body part is always above the IR. The goal is to keep the magnification as low as possible to prevent size distortion. Size distortion will occur when either the OID increases or the SID decreases from the standard positioning. Therefore, size distortion is controlled by positioning the body part as close as possible to the IR and using the longest practical SID.

Shape Distortion

Shape distortion, as mentioned previously, is the result of unequal magnification. The least amount of shape distortion occurs when the plane of the subject is parallel to the plane of the IR, and the CR is perpendicular to both. Angulation of the part in relation to the IR, or angulation of the x-ray beam, produces shape distortion. For these reasons, an effort should be made to position the patient so that the object of clinical interest is as parallel to the IR as possible and to minimize tube angulation.

Shape distortion displaces the projected image of an object from its actual position. It can be projected either shorter or longer; this is known as foreshortening and elongation. *Foreshortening* projects the part so it appears shorter than it actually is. This usually occurs when the body part is not correctly aligned. *Elongation* projects the object so it appears *longer* than it actually is. This distortion occurs when either the IR or the x-ray tube is not correctly aligned with the part. *Distortion is primarily controlled by the OID, SID, CR angle, part position, and IR position.*

Spatial Resolution

Spatial resolution refers to the sharpness of the image and is also referred to as resolution, sharpness, or detail. The edge sharpness of all portions of the image determines whether the image appears sharp or blurred. When the resolution is optimal, the edge sharpness of structures in the image is crisp. Poor resolution tends to appear fuzzy or unclear. Several key factors that affect spatial resolution are patient motion, OID, SID, and focal spot size.

To understand how spatial resolution is maintained or improved, the terms *umbra* and *penumbra* are used. Umbra is the actual anatomic area, body part, or structure shown in the radiographic image. The penumbra describes the unsharp edges of the umbra or body part. All body parts will have some unsharpness at the edges of the image.

TABLE 52.3 Effects of Image Geometry on Spatial Resolution

FACTOR	DIRECTION OF CHANGE	EFFECT ON RESOLUTION
Focal spot size	Decrease	Increase
Object-to-image receptor distance (OID)	Decrease	Increase
source-to-Image receptor distance (SID)	Increase	Increase

The goal is to reduce penumbra as much as possible. Penumbra is also referred to as blur or geometric unsharpness. When the OID decreases, the penumbra decreases, prompting greater spatial resolution. When the SID increases, the magnification and penumbra decrease, producing greater recorded detail; thus, there is also magnification of the penumbra whenever there is magnification of the image.

For this reason, magnification results in image unsharpness. These relationships are summarized in Table 52.3. Because only the OID and SID affect magnification, the shortest OID and the longest SID possible should be used.

Motion

Any movement during radiography will cause blurring of the image, reducing spatial resolution. This applies to patient motion, of course, and the movement of the IR or the x-ray tube. Patient motion may be categorized as either *voluntary* or *involuntary*. Voluntary motion usually is controllable, although some patients may be unable to control them. Involuntary motion involves movements over which the patient has no control, such as tremors, peristalsis, or heartbeats. The principal means of controlling involuntary motion is to use a shorter exposure time.

CRITICAL THINKING APPLICATION 52.5

Stephanie has an x-ray request for a hand x-ray on Mrs. Roberts. When she meets and assesses Mrs. Roberts, it is evident that Mrs. Roberts has Parkinson disease, which causes tremors. How can Stephanie adjust her technical factors based on the patient's condition?

Quantum Mottle

Quantum mottle is a term used to describe the situation in which a grainy or mottled (spotty) image is created. Quantum mottle occurs when either the mAs or the kVp is set too low. The result is a blotchy image with decreased spatial resolution. *Spatial resolution is primarily controlled by the OID, SID, focal spot, motion,* and *quantum mottle.*

CRITICAL THINKING APPLICATION 52.6

Stephanie has just completed imaging of Ms. Johnson's abdomen. Upon evaluation of the image, quantum mottle is visible, and it is evident that Stephanie will need to repeat the imaging process. What adjustments can Stephanie make to the technical factors to eliminate quantum mottle on the repeated image?

DIGITAL IMAGING

Digital imaging is the process of acquiring images of the body using x-rays, displaying them digitally, and viewing and storing them on a computer and in computer files. Today, more than 90% of radiology departments are using digital systems. It should be noted that *digital imaging* and *digital radiography* are terms that are used interchangeably.

Computed Radiography

Computed radiography is one of the two types of digital imaging systems. As previously mentioned, computed radiography uses an IR with an imaging plate that contains a photostimulable phosphor (PSP) that stores the latent image of the body part until it is processed. The phosphor absorbs the energy of the x-rays and the image of the body part. The computed radiography IR includes a barcode or label that allows the operator to match the image information with the patient-identifying barcode on the examination request. Five additional equipment components are required to process and view the image: a computed radiography reader, an operator workstation, a computer system with monitors for the radiologist to view the images, a printer (if images need to be printed), and a computer server to store the images.

After an IP is exposed, it is inserted into the computed radiography reader. Once the plate is inside the reader, the phosphor is scanned with a laser beam. This releases the stored energy in the form of visible light. Electronics convert the light into an electric signal to produce the digital image of the body part on a computer monitor. In computed radiography, the *sample frequency* is essential. As more signal is sampled, more information is obtained, and spatial resolution is improved. After the plate is scanned inside the reader, it is exposed to intense white light to erase it. The IP is sensitive to scatter; therefore, appropriate **collimation** and kVp must be used to achieve optimal images.

Digital Radiography

Digital radiography (DR) is the second type of digital imaging system. As previously mentioned, DR systems use a detector unit built into the table and the upright wall unit. Flat-panel detectors (FPDs) consist of either a scintillation screen or a photoconductor that converts the x-ray photons directly into electrical signals. The FPD is hard wired into the table and wall unit with DR, and a computed radiography reader is not required. DR systems can be divided into two categories: indirect conversion and direct conversion systems.

Indirect conversion DR is a two-step process in which the x-ray energy is converted into light and then converted into an electric signal. This method uses a scintillator to convert the x-ray energy into light. A scintillator is a device that glows when hit by high-energy x-ray photons and is often made of cesium iodide. A photodiode made of amorphous silicon then converts the light into an electric signal. The amorphous silicon collects electric charges as an array or matrix of pixel size elements (detector elements [DELs]). This sensing area has a fill factor. If the fill factor is 75%, the other 25% will be covered by electronics. Detectors with high fill factors present higher spatial resolution. This occurs with the use of an *analog-to-digital converter (ADC)*. The ADC takes the stored charge and converts it into digital values. From there, it is sent to the computer for processing and viewing.

The *charged coupled device* (CCD) is a type of indirect conversion detector. The CCD converts the light from the scintillator to the electric signal and uses optics and light. The FPD and CCD are built into the x-ray table and upright wall unit. Another type of indirect conversion detector is the *complementary metal oxide semiconductor* (CMOS). CMOS detectors convert light into electrons, similar to CCD technology. With CMOS, the electrons are stored in capacitors. The CMOS is silicon and is used with the ADC to convert the image into digital format.

Direct conversion is a one-step process. Detectors convert the x-ray energy directly to an electric signal through amorphous selenium detectors without the light conversion. DR images are available within seconds of making the exposure, whereas, with CR, the plate has to be manually inserted into the reader for processing before it can be viewed. *The ability to see x-ray images very fast is one of several advantages of computed and DR systems.* DR technology is now available in cassette form. Many manufacturers now build DR "plates" that have the FPD built into the cassette. Digital imaging starts when the x-rays exit the patient's body. With digital imaging, the x-ray image is produced, processed, viewed, and stored within a computer-based system, which provides many efficiencies for the radiology department.

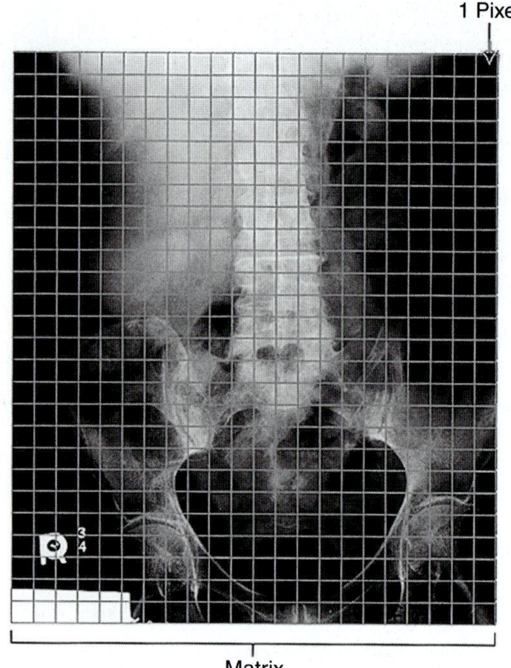

FIGURE 52.22 **Image Matrix.** The pixel's location within the image matrix corresponds to an area within the patient or volume of tissue. Note that the pixel size is not to scale and is used for illustration only. (From Fauber TL: *Radiographic imaging and exposure,* ed 3, St. Louis, 2009, Mosby.)

Digital Images

Matrix and *pixel* are digital terms used to describe the viewing monitor and the image (Figures 52.22 and 52.23). The *matrix* is thousands of tiny boxes or squares, known as picture elements or *pixels*. Each of these pixels presents a visual brightness level. A typical digital monitor may have a matrix of 2000 × 2500 pixels, which equals 5 million pixels to form the image.

Dead pixels are defects in the components, which may cause a loss of patient information. Pixels are complex components, and they are easily affected by dust, scratches, and interactions between materials. As the detector ages, the number of dead pixels increases. The software uses a method to fill in the dead pixels with information using the surrounding pixels.

Spatial resolution is a critical image quality factor. A basic definition of spatial resolution is the amount of detail or sharpness of an image as seen on the monitor. As previously mentioned, the larger the matrix and the smaller the pixels, the greater the spatial resolution.

Contrast resolution and dynamic range are two other image-quality factors that work together. *Contrast resolution* is the ability to distinguish anatomic structures of similar subject contrast, such as the liver and spleen. If contrast resolution is not adequate, it is challenging to see the difference between organs and other body structures, especially very small structures. *Dynamic range* is the response of the detector to different levels of radiation exposure. A digital image can be produced with a broader range of exposures. Because of this response, overexposures are underexposures may not need to be repeated. Contrast resolution and grayscale of the image are manipulated by adjusting the window level and width.

Signal-to-noise ratio (SNR) describes the ability of the digital system to convert the x-ray input electric signal into a useful radiographic image. *Signal* refers to the useful information image. *Noise* refers to the amount of information that is not useful. Noise can be caused by *quantum mottle* or inherent electric noise. Quantum mottle occurs when there are not enough photons in the detectors to provide a high-quality image, usually the result when mA or kVp is set to low (Figure 52.24). The goal of digital imaging is to reduce the amount of noise. The more signal that is present, the less noise, and the higher the quality of the image. Where there is a high SNR or low system noise, the greatest amount of information is captured. When the SNR is poor, contract resolution is directly affected.

In addition to the SNR, the *modulation transfer function* (MTF) plays a role in the system's efficiency. MTF is used to measure the capacity or accuracy of the digital detector to pass its spatial resolution characteristics to the final image. An MTF of 0 represents no signal and, therefore, no image, whereas an MTF of 1.0 would represent a perfect image.

Functions of the Processing System

When a digital image is processed, a histogram is created. The *histogram* is a graph of the minimum and maximum signals in the image (Figure 52.25). Each x-ray image has a histogram as part of its electronic file. The operator does not view the histogram directly; however, the histogram is adjusted when the contrast or brightness is adjusted. A *look-up table (LUT)* is used along with the histogram. The LUT is a file of stored images for each projection. These LUT files are referenced during processing. The LUT is used as a base image reference when adjustments are made to an image.

Postprocessing

An essential component of digital imaging is *postprocessing* because a repeat exposure may not be necessary. With postprocessing, any image can be further adjusted with computer software to enhance the image. Two standard postprocessing techniques are subtraction

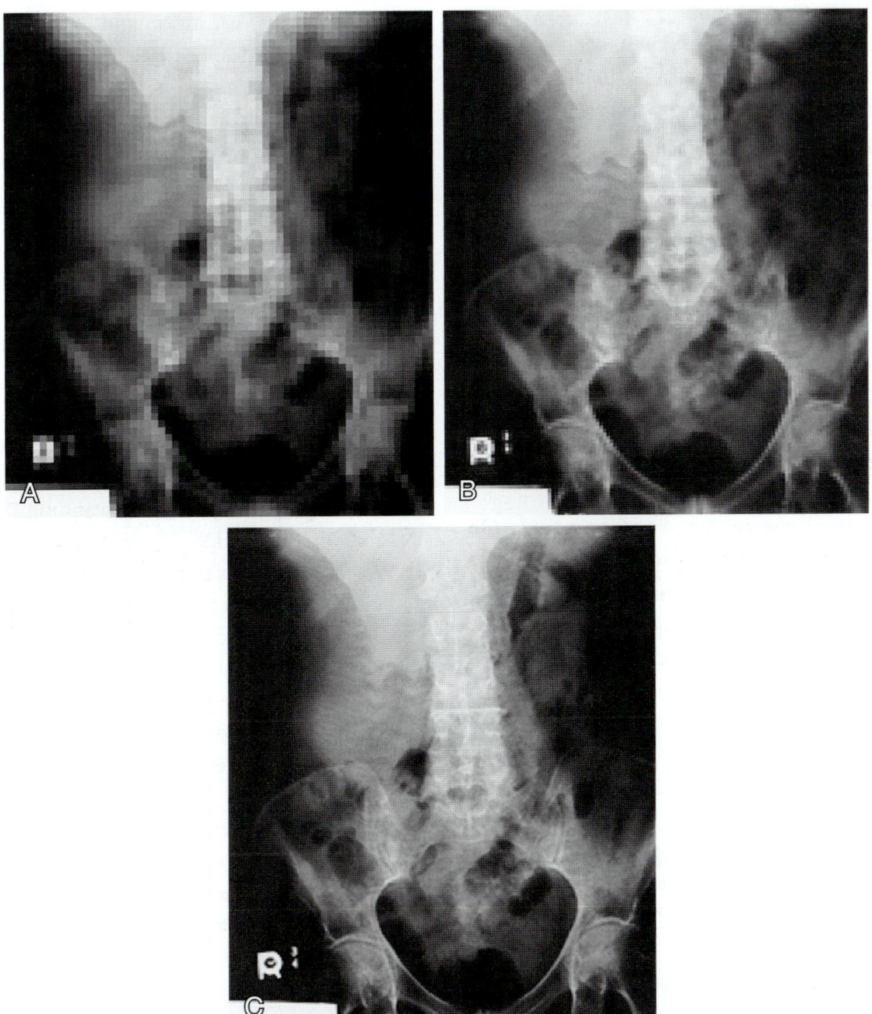

FIGURE 52.23 Matrix Size. The larger the matrix size, the greater the number of smaller individual pixels for a given field of view. Increasing the number of pixels improves the quality of the image. **(A)** The matrix size is 64 × 64. **(B)** The matrix size is 215 × 215. **(C)** The mtrix size is 2048 × 2048. (From Fauber TL: *Radiographic imaging and exposure,* ed 3, St. Louis, 2009, Mosby.)

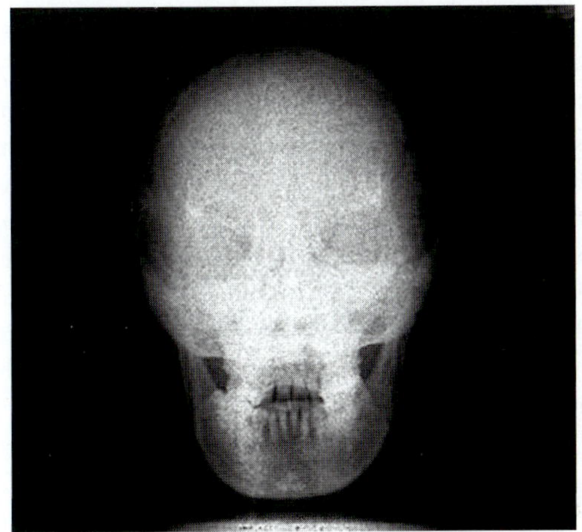

FIGURE 52.24 Grainy appearance because of insufficient light produced in the imaging plate. (From Carter C, Veale B: *Digital radiography and PACS*, ed 3, St. Louis, 2018, Mosby.)

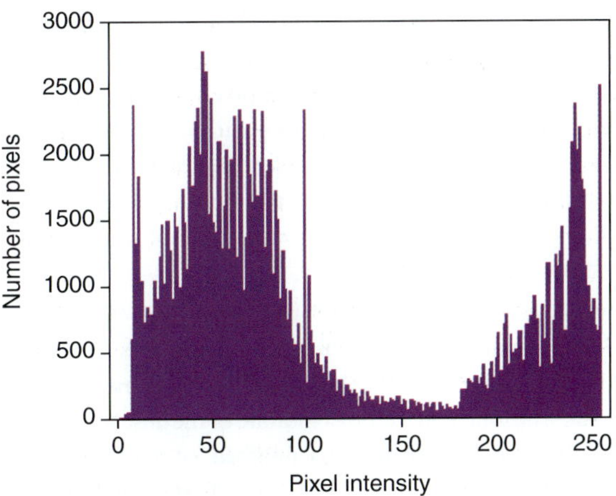

FIGURE 52.25 Simple Histogram Illustration. A graphical representation of the number of pixels with a particular intensity. (From Carter C, Veale B: *Digital radiography and PACS*, ed 3, St. Louis, 2018, Mosby.)

and contrast enhancement. The computer can remove anatomy with *subtraction* to visualize structures that may not otherwise be seen due to superimposition. With *contrast enhancement*, contrast can be changed from very high to very low. However, image manipulation should be kept to a minimum to avoid the loss of details.

Image Manipulation

The most common processing parameters are those for brightness and contrast. *Window level* controls the *brightness* in the image, and *window width* controls the contrast in the image. The operator can manipulate both of these controls by simply moving the mouse.

CRITICAL THINKING APPLICATION **52.7**

Stephanie has just completed an x-ray examination of Mr. Lambert's shoulder. Upon evaluation of the image, it is evident the proper exposure factors were used; however, the image does not appear bright on the monitor. How can Stephanie adjust the image without repeating the imaging process?

Electronic Cropping

When proper collimation is used, there is a clear area around the image. This clear or white area presents excess white light, which can interfere with viewing and interpretation. *Electronic cropping*, also known as masking, is used to blacken out the white collimation borders around the image. Many systems apply masking and cropping automatically, although it can be performed manually. Electronic cropping is not to be used to mask poor collimation.

Image Stitching

When anatomy is too large to fit on one IR, multiple images can be "stitched" together using a special computer technique called *image stitching*. This is often used for full-spine images for scoliosis. Two or three images are automatically stitched together to form one image.

Identification (ID) Markers and Image Annotation

ID markers, such as right (R) and left (L), should be placed directly on the IR or tabletop. Many times, information other than standard identification must be added to the image. *Image annotation* allows the operator to add helpful text to the image. *Annotation should never be used to place a right (R) or left (L) marker on the image.*

Edge Enhancement, Smoothing, and Rescaling

Edge enhancement is a computer processing technique in which images can be made sharper and have increased contrast; however, it does introduce some noise, resulting in the loss of small details. *Smoothing* is another processing technique used to average each pixel's frequency with surrounding tissue's pixel values. This is done to remove noise. When the x-ray exposure is greater or less than needed to produce an image, automatic rescaling occurs. This processing function is designed to display all the pixels for the area of interest. *Rescaling* means the images are created with uniform brightness and contrast, regardless of the amount of exposure. Rescaling is no substitute for appropriate technical factors.

Exposure Indicators (EI)

The amount of light given off by the phosphors in the IP results from the radiation exposure the plate has received. The light is converted into a signal to calculate the exposure indicator (EI), sometimes called an exposure index. The total signal is not a measure of the dose to the patient but indicates how much radiation was absorbed by the phosphors, which gives only an idea of what the patient received. The base EI for all manufacturers' systems designates the middle of the detector operating range. Unfortunately, the EI numbers are not standardized among the different digital systems manufacturers, and they can vary widely.

Digital Imaging and Communication in Medicine

Digital Imaging and Communication in Medicine (DICOM) is a universally accepted standard for exchanging medical radiographic images with the institution and in many areas where the images are viewed. DICOM specifies a standardized display function for the consistent display of grayscale images. Informatics in medical imaging are closely tied together. Each patient has an *electronic medical record*, sometimes referred to as the *electronic health record*. In radiology, a specific *radiology information system* is tied to these records for reports of the patient's x-ray examinations.

Artifacts

Computed and digital radiography systems produce unique artifact patterns in digital imaging. Generally, an *artifact* is considered an error on the image. Some of the most common artifacts are described here:

- *Quantum mottle* is caused by inadequate exposure techniques. Either low mAs or low kVp can cause this.
- *Moiré pattern* is an artifact that occurs when the grid lines are not aligned with the laser scanning frequency of the computed radiography reader.
- *Light spots* are usually caused by dust on the IP. Computed radiography phosphor plates should be cleaned carefully.
- *White line* artifacts appear along the length of travel on the image due to dust on the light guide.
- *Histogram analysis errors* may be caused by any of the following: improper collimation, importer technique, beam alignment error, scatter, and extreme subject density differences.
- *Phantom or ghost images* may appear as a result of incomplete IP erasure. This artifact requires troubleshooting of both the computed radiography plate and display systems. Extreme overexposure may require two erasure cycles to remove the image completely.
- *Scratches or tears* are permanent artifacts caused by damage to computed radiography plates. Replacement of computed radiography plates is costly but is the only solution to repair these artifacts.
- *Extraneous line patterns* are linear lines caused by noise in the image reader electronics. They can run lengthwise or crosswise.
- *Fogging* from background or scatter radiation can sometimes be seen on the computed radiography plates.

Picture Archival and Communication Systems

In a typical radiology department, thousands of x-ray images can be processed on a given day. With digital imaging, the images are contained within computer systems. The image management system used in radiology departments is the *picture archival and communication system (PACS)*, which consists of an extensive network of computers, servers, and archives. PACS will contain all the digital images produced in the department, including CT, MRI, ultrasound, and nuclear medicine images. This system allows multiple users inside and outside of the department to view images.

CLOSING COMMENTS

Patient Coaching

Communication is an interchange of ideas and information with others. Accurate communication is essential to quality patient care. The ability to give instructions depends on the speaker being clear and precise. The listener, on the other hand, is equally responsible for attentive and receptive behavior. The need to establish a rapport with patients is essential for a successful examination. Communication with a patient starts with an introduction and should continue until the completion of the examination.

Ethical and Legal Issues

Limited operators are taking the first steps toward making limited radiography a profession. Your work is closely associated with that of physicians, nurses, and other healthcare professionals. The public does not distinguish between limited operators (LXMOs) and professional radiologic technologists. All healthcare providers have a duty and obligation to perform competently and professionally. A high level of professionalism is expected of the limited operator. Strict adherence to professional standards is an expectation.

The *Standards of Ethics* for the radiologic technology profession is a two-part document that consists of a Code of Ethics and Rules of Ethics. Both are developed by the American Registry of Radiologic Technologists (ARRT). They are available on the ARRT website at www.arrt.org. The Code of Ethics is an aspirational document that establishes a high standard of professional conduct and assists the members of the profession in practicing ethical principles. The Rules of Ethics are mandatory standards of minimally acceptable professional conduct for all registered radiologic technologists.

Patient-Centered Care

As a limited operator, your work must be focused on the patients in your care, and your efforts must be devoted to providing high-quality service. Patient-centered care is the practice of caring for patients in ways that are meaningful and valuable to the individual patient. When in your care, you must treat a patient with courtesy and respect. Involve patients in decision making, recognizing they are individuals with unique values and preferences. Treat patients with dignity, respect, and sensitivity to each patient's cultural values and autonomy.

Professional Behaviors

Patients expect professionalism from healthcare workers and are most likely to respond with cooperation and confidence when these expectations are met. A professional attitude also promotes positive relationships with coworkers in the radiology department, as well as other departments in the healthcare facility. In radiography, as in any rapidly changing technical field, continuing education is necessary to learn about new practices and maintain competencies. As part of professional practice, limited operators are required to earn continuing education credits to maintain certification. There are many opportunities available for continuing education. Education may take the form of courses, workshops, seminars, or conferences. Failure to maintain competence and required certifications places both the employer and the employee at risk, resulting in a loss of employment and one's professional reputation. Knowing the credentials and keeping them current are essential professional responsibilities.

SUMMARY OF SCENARIO

Although Stephanie was initially apprehensive about Mrs. Gordon's x-ray examination, she was able to perform the examination with ease and made sure the patient was comfortable. Mrs. Gordon was not able to lie on the x-ray table. Stephanie was not deterred, and she was able to perform the x-ray examination while Mrs. Gordon remained in the wheelchair. Stephanie used a stool to prop Mrs. Gordon's knee on, and she was able to obtain the AP and lateral projections of Mrs. Gordon's knee. Stephanie learned she needs to rely on her skills to perform x-ray examinations.

SUMMARY OF LEARNING OBJECTIVES

1. **Examine the scope, education, and certification requirements of limited x-ray machine operators.**
   The limited x-ray machine operator (LXMO) is a role in the field of healthcare. Similar to radiographers, limited x-ray machine operators work closely with general physicians and work directly with radiologists, and their duties involve direct patient contact. Many are employed in ambulatory care clinics, and their work may vary considerably, depending on their place of employment. Many limited operators enjoy their work and later enter accredited programs to become radiologic technologists.
2. **Differentiate between the primary x-ray beam and scatter radiation.**
   The primary x-ray beam originates at a tiny point within the x-ray tube. It exits in one general direction through the tube port and diverges into space. Objects in its path attenuate the beam, forming scatter radiation. Scatter radiation is present throughout the x-ray room during exposure, creating a potential radiation hazard that requires proper precautions for safety.
3. **Examine radiographic equipment.**
   Radiographic equipment is used to create the x-ray beam and produce the image. Typical equipment in an x-ray room includes the IR system, x-ray tube, radiographic table, upright IR, control console, and the transformer cabinet.
4. **Examine basic radiation safety.**
   Radiation exposure may pose a health hazard to operators if proper safety precautions are not followed. The potential risk is greater for the operator than the patient because the operator is often faced with the possibility of exposure. Scatter radiation is present throughout the x-ray

Continued

SUMMARY OF LEARNING OBJECTIVES—cont'd

room during exposure. The only time the potential for exposure exists is when the x-ray exposure is taken.

5. **Examine basic physics for radiography.**
   Limited operators do not require an extensive background in physics, but some basic principles of physical science are essential to an understanding of x-rays and their use. LXMOs must understand the basic concepts of matter, energy, and electricity and muse be able to relate these principles to radiography. Everything of a physical nature in the universe can be classified as either matter or energy. Both matter and energy can exist in several forms.
6. **Examine the components of x-ray production.**
   There are four essential requirements for the production of x-rays: (1) a vacuum, (2) a source of electrons, (3) a target, and (4) a high potential difference (voltage) between the electron source and the target
7. **Examine the x-ray circuit.**
   An x-ray circuit diagram provides a means for studying the devices that make up the x-ray generators and understanding how they work together to meet the radiography requirements. The limited operator controls the functions of these devices utilizing a computer console. The control console provides the means for selecting the kVp and mAs and for making the x-ray exposure.
8. **Examine rectification.**
   Rectification is changing alternating current into direct current so that it flows in one direction only. The primary purpose of the rectifiers is to change the AC into direct current (DC). The rectification process prepares the current for x-ray production by ensuring that it flows in the right direction—pin this case, from the filament to the target.
9. **Examine single-phase, three-phase, and high-frequency generators.**
   The x-ray generator delivers the electrical power to energize the x-ray tube and permits the selection of x-ray energy, x-ray quantity, and exposure time. The generator's major internal components include transformers, diodes and rectifier circuits, filament circuits, timer switches, and kilovolt and milliampere meters. Single-phase, three-phase, and high-frequency generators produce different voltage waveforms (ripple) and x-ray beam spectra.
10. **Explain the components of the x-ray control panel.**
    All control panels provide some means for selecting kVp, mA, exposure time, and focal spot size. There will also be switches to control power to the console and the Bucky, plus rotor and exposure switches.
11. **Examine the principles of exposure and image quality.**
    The primary factors of exposure are mA, time, kVp, and source-to-image-receptor distance (SID). According to the inverse square law, the SID influences the quantity of exposure in a given area of the IR. Distortion refers to both magnification and changes in the shape of the image as compared with the object. Magnification, the enlargement of the image due to the relationship between the object-to-image receptor distance (OID) and SID, includes shape and size distortion.
12. **Examine digital imaging.**
    Computed and digital radiography systems are the most recent equipment used in radiography. The ability to manipulate images has improved the efficiency of imaging.

POSITIONING FOR RADIOLOGY 53

SCENARIO

Jonathan Nolan has been a limited machine x-ray operator (LXMO) for several years at Walden-Martin Family Medical (WMFM) Clinic. Jonathan performs x-rays on approximately 25 patients a day. His patients range in age from young children to older adults. Jonathan performs x-ray examinations of all extremities, the spine, and skull. When an x-ray is ordered by the orthopedic physician, Jonathan introduces himself to the patient and conducts a patient history. Jonathan's first patient of the day is Madeline Gallegos. Madeline is 18; she was in a motor vehicle collision and fractured her lower leg in several places. She has had surgery, and she has an open reduction internal fixator (ORIF) attached to her lower limb. She is in a wheelchair. Jonathan provides quality patient care when caring for his patients.

While studying this chapter, think about the following questions:

1. What is the correct terminology used in radiographic positioning?
2. What are the correct steps to prepare the room and the patient for a radiographic procedure?
3. What bones make up the upper limb and shoulder girdle?
4. What bones make up the lower limb and pelvis?
5. What bones make up the spine, bony thorax, chest, and abdomen?
6. What bones make up the skull, facial bones, and paranasal sinuses?
7. When evaluating the final image, what criteria should be considered?

LEARNING OBJECTIVES

1. Explain radiographic terminology, positions, and projections.
2. Explain how to prepare the room and the patient for performing the radiographic procedure.
3. Examine the process for performing upper limb and shoulder girdle images.
4. Examine the process for performing lower limb and pelvis images.
5. Examine the process for performing spinal images.
6. Examine the process for performing bony thorax, chest, and abdomen images.
7. Examine the process for performing skull, facial bones, and paranasal sinuses images.
8. Examine the process of image evaluation.

VOCABULARY

Bucky Contains a movable grid device that absorbs scatter radiation and also contains the image receptor.

central ray (CR) The center of the x-ray beam and perpendicular to the long axis of the x-ray tube.

collimation (kol i MAY shun) The method of restricting and confining the x-ray beam to a given area.

distortion The differences between the actual subject and its radiographic image.

exposure indicator (EI) A numeric value indicating the quantity of ionizing radiation received by a digital radiographic image receptor; also called an exposure index.

image receptor (IR) The device that receives the energy of the x-ray beam and forms the image of the body part.

landscape orientation The width is greater than its height.

object-to-image receptor distance (OID) The distance between the subject and the image receptor.

portrait orientation The height is greater than its width.

radiation protection The measures taken to safeguard patients, personnel, and the public from unnecessary exposure to ionizing radiation.

source-to-image-receptor distance (SID) The distance between the tube target and the image receptor.

INTRODUCTION

This chapter introduces the subjects of anatomy and radiographic positioning, including the terms to depict radiographic projections and body positions. Details of everyday tasks performed during radiographic procedures are also included. Details include selection, use, and alignment of the x-ray tube the image receptor (IR) and the body part, patient instructions and radiographic marker use and placement.

INTRODUCTION TO RADIOGRAPHIC POSITIONING

Radiographic positioning is placing the body or body part in the proper position to create the desired radiographic image. To properly perform a radiographic procedure, the limited operator must understand anatomic terms and terms for body positions, radiographic positions, and radiographic projections.

Terminology Review

Radiographic positioning instructions frequently include terms describing the relationship of body parts to each other and the location or orientation of body surfaces or structures in space. Terms that indicate these anatomic relationships are based on *anatomic position*. (Refer to Chapter 18 for more information on the anatomic position and medical terminology.) In addition to the terms covered in Chapter 18, limited operators must be familiar with the following terms to describe anatomic relationships, orientations, and relationships accurately:

- *Anterior:* Forward or front portion of the body or body part
- *Posterior:* Backward or back portion of the body or body part; opposite of anterior
- *Central:* Pertaining to the middle area or main part of an organ or body part
- *Caudal/caudad:* Away from the head
- *Cephalic/cephalad:* Pertaining to the head
- *Distal:* Away from the source or point or point of origin
- *Proximal:* Toward the source or point of origin
- *Peripheral:* Away from the central mass of an organ, toward its outer limits; the opposite of central
- *External:* To the outside, at or near the surface of the body or body part
- *Internal:* Deep, near the center of the body or a body part; opposite of external
- *Plantar:* Referring to the sole of the foot
- *Parietal:* Referring to the walls of a cavity
- *Visceral:* Pertaining to organs

Procedures for radiographic positioning are also described using body planes and body positions (see Chapter 18 for additional details).

Radiographic Positions

Radiographic positions describe the placement of the body part in relation to the radiographic table or IR.

For a *decubitus* position, the patient is recumbent with the central (CR) horizontal or parallel to the floor. This position is named according to the body surface on which the patient is lying: lateral decubitus (left or right), dorsal decubitus, or ventral decubitus.

A *lateral* position is accomplished by placing the body or body part with the sagittal plane parallel to the IR. It is named according to the side adjacent to the radiographic table or IR.

A *lordotic* position results in angulation of the coronal plane of the chest with the IR. This is achieved by having the upright patient lean back so that only the dorsal aspect of the shoulders is in direct contact with the IR.

An *oblique* position is achieved when the body or body part is placed so that the coronal plane is not parallel with the radiographic table or IR. The description is stated as a degree of rotation, either from a body plane or toward the affected side.

Radiographic Projections

A radiographic projection identifies the path of the CR from the radiographic tube through the patient to the IR. Most projections are named in anatomic terms based on the entrance and exit points of the CR in the body.

For *anteroposterior (AP) projections*, the CR enters the anterior surface and exits the posterior surface of the body or part.

For *posteroanterior (PA) projections*, the CR enters the posterior surface and exits the anterior surface of the body or part.

Lateral projections are those in which the sagittal plane of the body or body part is parallel to the IR. Lateral projections are always named for the side of the patient that is nearest the IR. Lateral projections of the extremities are further described with the lateral or medial entrance and exit of the CR: mediolateral or lateromedial.

Oblique projections are those in which the body is rotated so that the CR travels through the body on an oblique plane rather than following an anatomic plane. Oblique projections are named according to the entrance and exit points of the CR. For example, in an AP oblique position, the CR enters the anterior surface of the body and exits the posterior surface.

Axial projections are images taken with a longitudinal angulation of the CR of 10 degrees or more. The angle may either be cephalad (toward the head) or caudad (away from the head).

Tangential projections are produced by directing the CR to "skim" the profile of the subject. The tangential projection is typically utilized to demonstrate the patella and patellofemoral joint space.

RADIOGRAPHIC PROCEDURES

All radiographic procedures should be performed in a systematic, organized manner to ensure safe and effective performance. The approach to performing the procedure may vary based on the patient's condition, the anatomy of interest, the type of equipment, and departmental protocol. However, the following recommended actions will be effective for most common radiographic procedures.

Preparing the Room and the Patient

The following actions focus on preparing for the procedure:

- *Prepare the radiographic room*: The room should be clean and organized. Depending on the agency's policies, certain areas may need to be disinfected between patients.
- *Select the patient and projection from the computer worklist.*
- *Choose IR (CR cassette or digital radiography [DR] detector).*
- *Call the patient from the waiting area*: Make sure to identify the patient in a Health Insurance Portability and Accountability Act (HIPAA)–compliant manner. Ask the patient's first and last name along with the patient's birthdate. This information should match the information from the requisition.

- *Explain the procedure to the patient*: Use terminology and language that the patient can understand.
- *Assess the patient*: Obtain history to determine the correct procedure, ability to cooperate, and fall risk.
- *Prepare the patient*: Instruct the patient on what clothing and artifact items (e.g., jewelry) should be removed. Provide the patient with a gown. Prepare the patient as needed. Give the patient privacy to change or assist the patient as necessary to change into the gown.

Radiology Requisition

When an imaging study is required, the referring physician fills out a request form. The limited x-ray machine operator must become familiar with the information provided on the x-ray requisition. Every practice will have its specific version, but all requests must contain detailed information, such as the examination required, the patient's name, and patient location (Figure 53.1). Imaging procedures cannot be done without a physician's order. Performing a procedure without a request may lead to fines, disqualification of one's radiation license, dismissal, and possible litigation. This information will aid the LXMO in preparing for the examination. The requisition usually includes the following:

- Patient information: name, date of birth, a medical record number
- Clinical indication or details: signs and symptoms, previous imaging results
- Examination requested: specific body part to be imaged
- Mode of transport: ambulatory, wheelchair, or stretcher
- Additional information: background medical information (e.g., diabetic), allergies, communication impairments (e.g., hearing, vision)
- Ordering physician

CRITICAL THINKING APPLICATION 53.1

An x-ray requisition for an ankle x-ray just printed. What is the first step that Jonathan should complete to prepare for the imaging examination?

Preparing for Performing the Radiographic Procedure

The following actions focus on setting up the equipment, positioning the patient, performing the projections, and preparing the projections for the provider:

- *Set technical factors:* This would include kilovolts peak (kVp) and milliampere/seconds (mAs).
- Set the **source-to-image-receptor distance (SID)**.
- Align IR and CR.
- *Position of patient and position part.* Always make sure the patient is not at risk for falls or injuries.
- Collimate to the anatomy of interest.
- Place lead side marker (right or left).
- *Provide patient instructions*: For all projections, the patient must hold still to achieve a quality picture. Additional instructions include performing a deep breath or exhaling.
- *Orient IR,* either **portrait orientation** or **landscape orientation**.
- Expose IR.
- *Evaluate image*: Check the appearance, centering, positioning, and for the proper **exposure indicator (EI)** value.
- *Return the patient to the provider's department or release the patient*: Provide the patient with exit instructions, follow-up information, and post-procedure instructions, if applicable.

The procedural steps for a radiographic procedure include both technical and patient care aspects. These aspects should be discussed in detail for the operator to appreciate the need for each of these steps.

CRITICAL THINKING APPLICATION 53.2

Jonathan has an x-ray requisition for a hip x-ray. He has brought the patient into the x-ray room and positioned the patient on the table for the first projection. What is the first step that Jonathan should take when he steps up to the control console?

UPPER LIMB AND SHOULDER GIRDLE IMAGES

The bones of the upper limb are divided into the hand, forearm, upper arm, and shoulder girdle. This area also includes the wrist and elbow. Examinations of the upper limb from the fingertips to the elbow are usually done tabletop (the IR is placed on the radiographic table without a grid). Each image is created using a single IR. For example, the protocol for a hand examination is three projections. This will require three exposures and CR cassettes or the DR detector. To prepare for these exams, the patient must remove any clothing or jewelry from the area within the *radiation field*. Patients may need to remove clothing from the upper torso and don a gown to examine the shoulder region.

For the projections of the upper limb and shoulder girdle, use the following unless otherwise indicated:

- *IR:* Positioned by department protocol for proper anatomy orientation; CR plate 18 × 24 cm; portrait orientation.
- *Grid and SID:* No grid. SID 40 inches minimum.
- **Collimation***:* Adjust the light field to 2.5 cm on all sides of the anatomy. Place anatomic marker in the light field on the lateral side of the anatomy.
- *Patient instructions:* Do not move.

Positioning and Radiographic Examination of the Hand, Fingers, and Thumb

The hand and finger bones include the metacarpals and phalanges. The proximal phalanx is the first bone, next to the hand. The middle phalanx is the second section of the finger, and the distal phalanx makes up the tip of the finger. The thumb has a proximal phalanx and a distal phalanx (Figure 53.2).

Routine Examination of the Hand

The routine examination of the hand includes the PA, PA oblique-lateral rotation, and lateral projections.

- *Body and part position:* Seated at the end of the table with elbow flexed 90 degrees and arm resting on table.
  - *PA:* Hand open, fingers extended and moderately separated, palmar surface in contact with IR, fingers moderately separated (Figure 53.3A).

Doctor ordering ______________________________

Today's date ________________ ☐ Stat ☐ Routine ☐ ASAP

Date to be done ________________ Requested by ________________

Patient Label

RADIOGRAPHIC (X-RAY) PROCEDURES REQUISITION

Clinical indication ______________________________

Transportation ☐ Portable ☐ Stretcher ☐ Wheelchair ☐ Ambulatory

O_2 ☐ Yes / ☐ No | Diabetic ☐ Yes / ☐ No | Hearing deficit ☐ Yes / ☐ No

IV ☐ Yes / ☐ No | Seizure disorder ☐ Yes / ☐ No | Sight deficit ☐ Yes / ☐ No

Isolation ☐ Yes / ☐ No | Non-English speaking ☐ Yes / ☐ No

Write out the entire doctor's order

Comments ______________________________

☐ Abdomen ______________________________

☐ Bone age study ______________________________

☐ Bone x-ray order ______________________________

☐ Chest order ______________________________

☐ IVP ______________________________

☐ KUB / flat plate of abdomen ______________________________

☐ KUB order ______________________________

☐ Mammogram ______________________________

☐ Sinus series order ______________________________

☐ SNAT series ______________________________

☐ Spine order ______________________________

☐ BE ______________________________

☐ SBFT ______________________________

☐ UGI ______________________________

☐ Write in order ______________________________

FIGURE 53.1 Sample x-ray requisition. (From Seibel MMW, Gillingham EA: *LaFleur Brooks' health unit coordinating*, ed 7, St. Louis, 2014, Elsevier.)

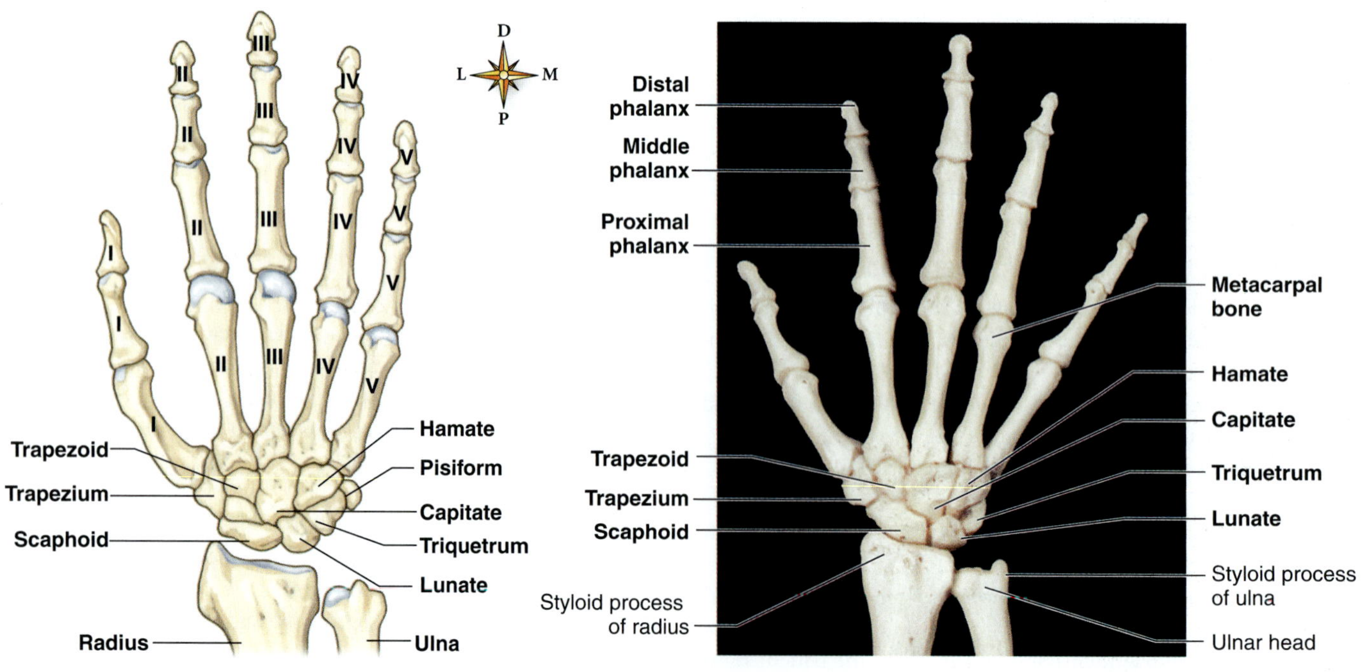

FIGURE 53.2 Right hand and wrist. Note that the phalanges of each respective finger are designated with a Roman numeral. (From Patton KT, Thibodeau GA: *The human body in health and disease*, ed 7, St. Louis, 2018, Elsevier.)

- *PA oblique:* From the PA, the hand is rotated laterally to please the anteromedial aspect in contact with the IR. Coronal plane of the hand forms a 45-degree angle with the IR. Stairstep sponge is used to support and maintain position of fingers so that interphalangeal (IP) joints are clearly visualized separated (Figure 53.3B).
- *Lateral:* Medial aspect of hand is in contact with IR with coronal plane of hand perpendicular to IR. Thumb is positioned as for PA projection and supported on a sponge. Wrist will be slightly pronated. Fingers may be spread to prevent superimposition separated (Figure 53.3C).

- **Central ray (CR)**: PA and PA oblique—perpendicular to the third metacarpophalangeal (MCP) joint; lateral—perpendicular to the second MCP joint.
- *Structures seen:* Anatomy of entire hand (including fingertips), carpus, distal radius and ulna.
  - *PA:* No overlap of metacarpals or digits.
  - *PA oblique:* No or minimal overlap of metacarpal shafts, with some overlap of metacarpal heads and bases. IP joint spaces open.
  - *Lateral:* Superimposition of the second through fifth metacarpals. Superimposition of the second through fifth phalanges (extension), or phalanges individual demonstrated (fanned). Thumb is seen in PA projection.

Routine Examination of the Fingers

Although the fingers are included in the examination of the hand, separate finger studies are often performed when the area of clinical interest is a specific finger. The routine for fingers may include a PA projection of the entire hand plus oblique and lateral projections of the affected finger, or the examination may be limited to the PA, oblique, and lateral projections of the affected finger only. Each projection of the finger should include the entire digit and the distal portion of the corresponding metacarpal. Position the finger as close to the IR as possible, and parallel to the IR. A stairstep sponge is a desirable aid for oblique and lateral positioning because it supports the finger parallel to the IR, decreasing **distortion** and improving visualization of the IP joints.

The routine examination of the fingers includes the PA, PA oblique-lateral rotation, and lateral projections.

- *Body and part position:* Seated at the end of the table with elbow flexed 90 degrees and arm resting on table.
  - *PA:* Hand open, fingers extended and moderately separated, palmar surface in contact with IR
  - *PA oblique:* From the PA, the hand is rotated laterally to please the anteromedial aspect in contact with the IR. Coronal plane of the hand forms a 45-degree angle with the IR. Stairstep sponge is used to support and maintain position of fingers so that IP joints are clearly visualized.
  - *Lateral:* Medial or lateral surface of hand is in contact with IR, depending on the finger of interest. Other fingers are flexed or extended as necessary to leave affected finger free of superimposition. Affected finger is supported parallel to IR.
- *CR:* Perpendicular to proximal IP joint.
- *Structures seen:* Entire digit and distal portion of metacarpal with IP and MCP joint spaces open and clearly visualized.

Routine Examination of the Thumb

Examination of the thumb is different than examinations of the other fingers because the thumb attaches to the hand at an angle. Images of the thumb must include the entire first metacarpal rather than only a portion of it. As with the finger, the thumb examination may include a PA projection of the entire hand. When this is the case, the PA hand position results in an oblique position of the thumb. The routine examination of the thumb includes the AP, PA oblique, and lateral projections.

- Body and part position:
  - *AP:* Seated at the end of the table, leaning forward, arm abducted 90 degrees, with forearm rotated internally into an exaggerated degree of pronation. Doral surface of thumb in contact with IR. Coronal plane of thumb in parallel to IR. Plane of palm of hand is perpendicular to IR.
  - *PA oblique and lateral:* Seated at the end of the table with the elbow flexed 90 degrees, arm fully supported, and palm resting on the IR. With the PA oblique, the palmar surface of the hand is in contact with IR as for PA projection of hand. Coronal plane of thumb will be 45 degrees to plane of IR. With the lateral project, begin with hand positioned for PA oblique thumb, patient flexes MCP joints 2 through 5 with the fingers extended, "tenting" hand until thumb is in lateral position.
- *CR:* Perpendicular to MCP joint.
- *Structures seen:* Entire thumb and first metacarpal with all joint spaces open and clearly visualized.

Positioning and Radiographic Examination of the Wrist

The wrist is made up of eight carpal bones, which include the scaphoid, lunate, triquetrum, trapezoid, trapezium, capitate, hamate, and pisiform (see Figure 53.2). The bones of the forearm, radius, and ulna articulate with the bones of the wrist.

Routine Examination of the Wrist

The wrist contains many small bones and joints. Although the routine projections are usually sufficient, there are supplemental projections designed to demonstrate specific bones and joints of this region.

The routine examination of the wrist includes the PA, PA oblique-lateral rotation, and lateral projections.

- *Body and part position:* Seated at the end of the table with elbow flexed 90 degrees and forearm resting on table.
  - *PA:* Anterior surface of wrist is on the IR. Fingers are flexed to form a loose fist, placing wrist in firmer contact with IR and opening intercarpal joints (Figure 53.4A).
  - *PA oblique:* Anteromedial surface of wrist is in contact with IR so that the coronal plane of wrist forms a 45-degree angle with IR. Position may be supported by wedge sponge, stairstep sponge, or patient's thumb separated (Figure 53.4B).
  - *Lateral:* Medial surface of wrist is in contact with IR. Coronal plane of wrist is perpendicular to IR.
- *CR:* Perpendicular to midcarpal area.
- *Structures seen:* Distal portion of radius and ulna, carpal bones, and proximal halves of metacarpals.

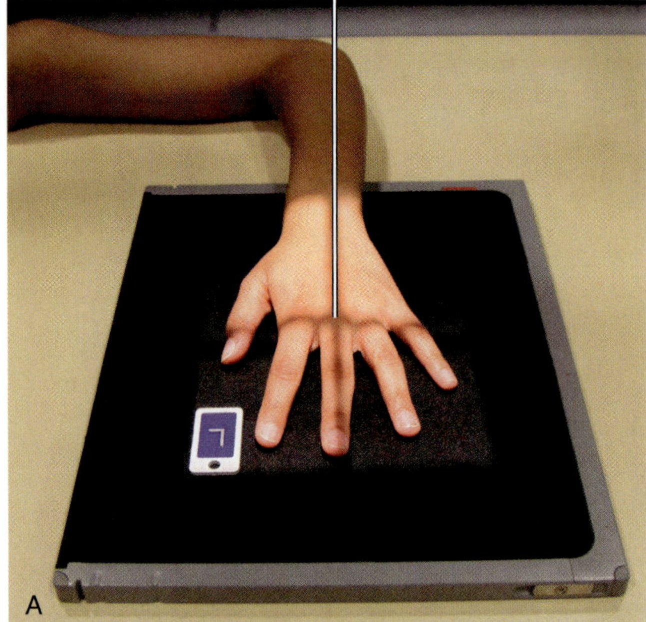

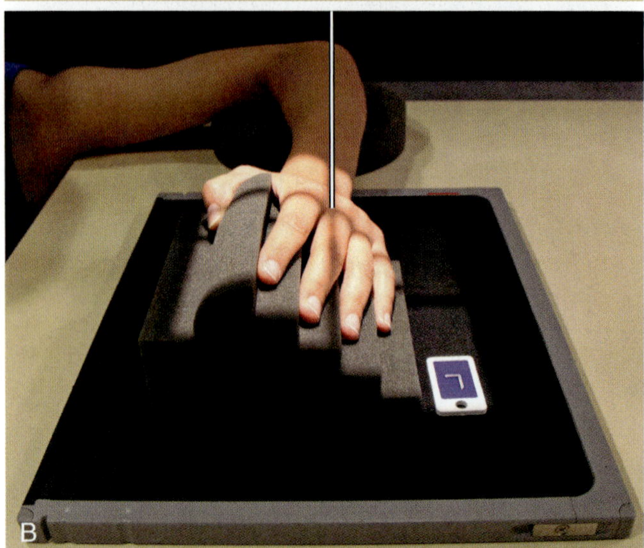

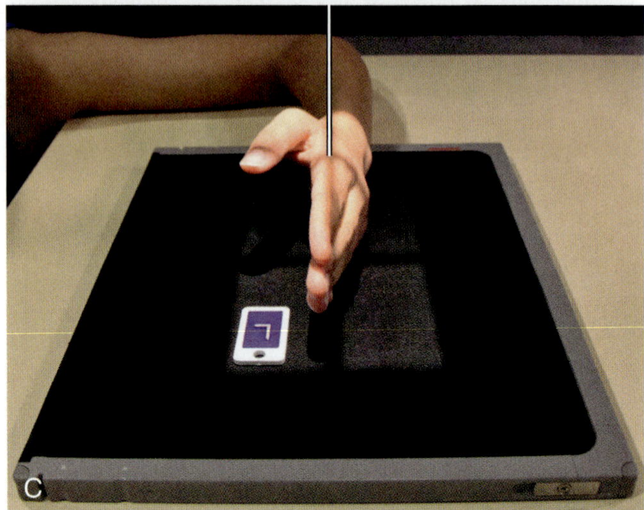

FIGURE 53.3 Hand. **(A)** Position for PA projection. **(B)** Position for PA oblique projection-lateral rotation, using stairstep sponge. **(C)** Position for lateral projection. (From Long BW, Frank ED, Ehrlich RA: *Radiography essentials for limited practice*, ed 6, St. Louis, 2021, Elsevier.)

Supplemental Projections of the Wrist

These supplemental projections may be added individually to the routine examination according to the area of clinical interest and the instructions of the physician.

AP Oblique Projection—Medial Rotation. The AP oblique projection with medial rotation is the opposite of the routine oblique. It is useful for the demonstration of the medial aspect of the carpus, particularly the lunate and the pisiform.

- *Body and part position:* Same as for other wrist projections. Posteromedial surface of the wrist is in contact with IR so that the coronal plane forms a 45-degree angle with IR.
- *CR:* Perpendicular to midcarpal area.
- *Structures seen:* Distal portion of radius and ulna, carpal bones, and proximal halves of metacarpals.

PA Projection—Ulnar Deviation. The PA projection with ulnar deviation is performed when a scaphoid fractured is suspected. It reduces foreshortening of the scaphoid.

- *Part position:* Same as PA wrist with fingers extended. Hand is then deviated outward, in the direction of ulna, to the extent that patient can tolerate.
- *CR:* Perpendicular, centered to scaphoid (a point slightly proximal and medial to first metacarpal base).
- *Structures seen:* Scaphoid seen with minimal foreshortening. Distal portion of radius and ulna, carpal bones, and proximal metacarpals deviated toward ulna are also demonstrated.

CRITICAL THINKING APPLICATION 53.3

An x-ray requisition for a wrist x-ray was just printed. When Jonathan approaches the patient and begins his assessment, he discovers the patient has a suspected scaphoid fracture. Which supplemental projection should be performed in addition to the routine projections for a wrist?

PA Axial Projection (Stecher Method). The Stecher method projection is also performed for a suspected schaphoid fracture. It reduces foreshortening of the scaphoid. It is preferred when ulna deviation is too painful for the patient.

- *Part position:* Arm is extended and parallel to long axis of table for correct alignment with angled x-ray beam. One end of the IR is elevated so the plane of the IR is 20 degrees with respect to tabletop. Wrist is positioned with anterior aspect of IR as for PA wrist, with the fingers oriented to the elevated end of the IR.
- *CR:* Perpendicular to table directed to enter the scaphoid (a point slightly proximal and medial to first metacarpal base).
- *Structures seen:* Scaphoid seen with minimal foreshortening. Distal portion of radius and ulna, carpal bones, and proximal metacarpals deviated toward ulna are also demonstrated.

Tangential Projection (Gaynor-Heart Method). The Gaynor-Heart method is used to demonstrate the carpal canal, usually in patients with symptoms of carpal tunnel syndrome or suspected fracture.

- *Part position:* Arm is extended and parallel to long axis of table for correct alignment with angled x-ray beam. Wrist is extended to place the palm of hand perpendicular to IR, if possible.
- *CR:* Directed to the palm at a point approximately 2.5 cm distal to the base of the third metacarpal and at an angle of 25 degrees

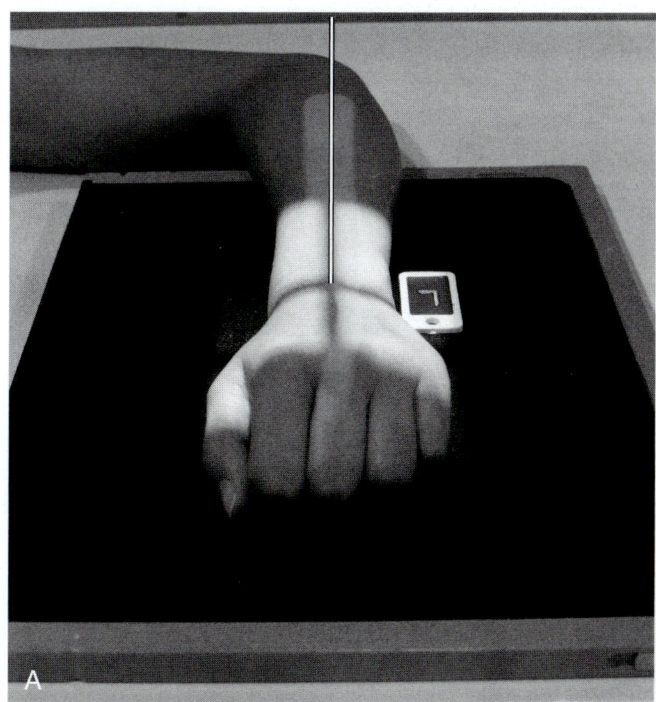

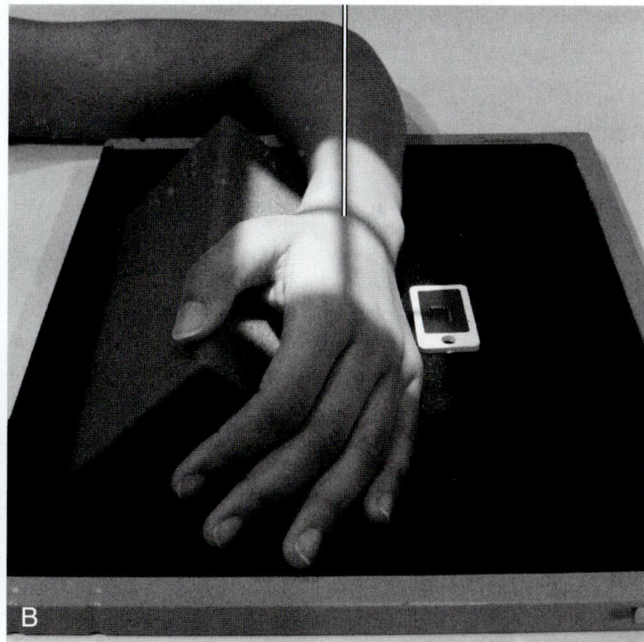

FIGURE 53.4 Wrist. **(A)** Position for PA projection. **(B)** Position for PA oblique projection—lateral rotation. (From Long BW, Frank ED, Ehrlich RA: *Radiography essentials for limited practice*, ed 6, St. Louis, 2021, Elsevier.)

to 30 degrees in direction of elbow. Greater angle may be required when the wrist cannot be extended.

- *Structures seen:* Carpal canal—anterior arch of carpal bones, including portions of the scaphoid, trapezium, pisiform, and hook of hamate.

Positioning and Radiographic Examination of the Forearm

Examination of the forearm is ordered when the area of interest is in the shaft of the radius or ulna (Figure 53.5). The examination should include the entirety of the radius and ulna and their articular surfaces. Visualization of both joints is preferable. If this is not possible, additional images that include the other joint will be needed.

The routine examination of the forearm includes the AP and lateral projections.

- *IR:* CR plate 24× 30 cm diagonal or 35 × 43 cm, portrait orientation.
- *Body and part position:* Seated at the end of the table with axilla (armpit) at table level; this may be achieved by lowering the seat or by instructing the patient lean toward the table.
  - *AP:* Arm is fully extended with hand supinated and posterior surface resting upon the IR. The wrist and the elbow are supinated with coronal plane of arm parallel to IR. This is accomplished by adjusting the coronal plane of the humeral epicondyles parallel to the plan of the IR (Figure 53.6A). A small sandbag in the palm of the hand can help maintain the position.
  - *Lateral:* Elbow is flexed 90 degrees with medial surface in contact with IR. Wrist is in lateral position.
- *CR:* Perpendicular to midpoint of the forearm.
- *Structures seen:* Entire forearm, including elbow and wrist joints in their entirety.

Positioning and Radiographic Examination of the Elbow

The routine examination of the elbow is the same as the forearm. Because it is often impossible for patients with an injured elbow to fully extend the elbow joint, alternatives are presented for the AP projection with the elbow partially flexed. Supplemental projections may be added for further visualization of specific aspects of the joint.

Routine Examination of the Elbow

The routine examination of the elbow includes the AP and lateral projections.

- *Body and part position:* Seated at the end of the table with axilla at level of table, as for AP forearm.
  - *AP:* Arm is fully extended with hand supinated and posterior surface in contact with IR. Coronal plane of humeral epicondyle parallel to IR. If patient is unable to fully extend arm, substitute alternate positions for AP projection with flexed elbow.
  - *Lateral:* Elbow is flexed 90 degrees with medial surface in contact with IR. Coronal plane of humeral epicondyles perpendicular to IR. Wrist is in lateral position to degree patient can achieve (Figure 53.6B).
- *CR:* Perpendicular to elbow joint. For AP projection, CR is midway between humeral epicondyles. For lateral projection, CR is at lateral epicondyle.
- *Structures seen:* Elbow joint with portions of distal humerus and proximal forearm.

Alternative Positions for AP Projections

If the patient is unable to fully extend the elbow joint for an AP projection, both of the following AP projections with flexed elbow are necessary to substitute for the routine AP projection.

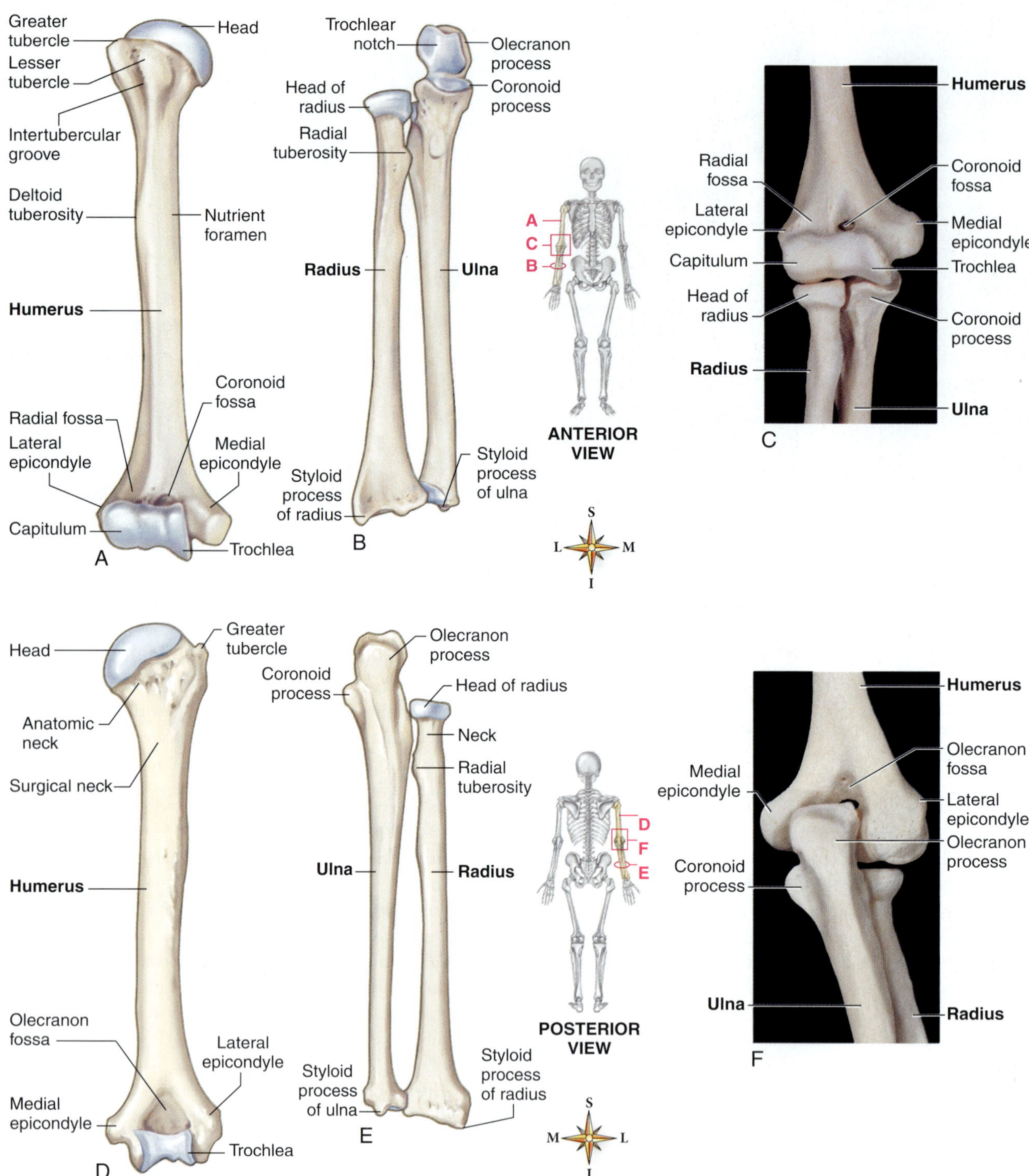

FIGURE 53.5 Right arm and forearm. Anterior view: A, Humerus; B, Radius and Ulna; and C, Elbow. Posterior view: D, Humerus; E, Radius and Ulna; and F, Elbow. (From Patton KT, Thibodeau GA: *The human body in health and disease,* ed 7, St. Louis, 2018, Elsevier.)

AP Elbow, Proximal Forearm

- *Body and part position:* Standing and leaning over the table, if possible. Posterior aspect of forearm rests on IR and elbow is extended as much as possible. Rotate the forearm so the so coronal plane of humeral epicondyles is parallel to IR.
- *CR:* Perpendicular to center of elbow. If the elbow is flexed 90 degrees or more, it is necessary to angle CR 5 to 15 degrees in proximal direction to avoid superimposing distal humerus over proximal forearm.
- *Structures seen:* Proximal forearm portion of elbow joint. Distal humerus will be distorted.

AP Elbow, Distal Humerus

- *Body position:* With axilla at table level as for routine AP projection, elbow is extended as much as possible, and forearm is

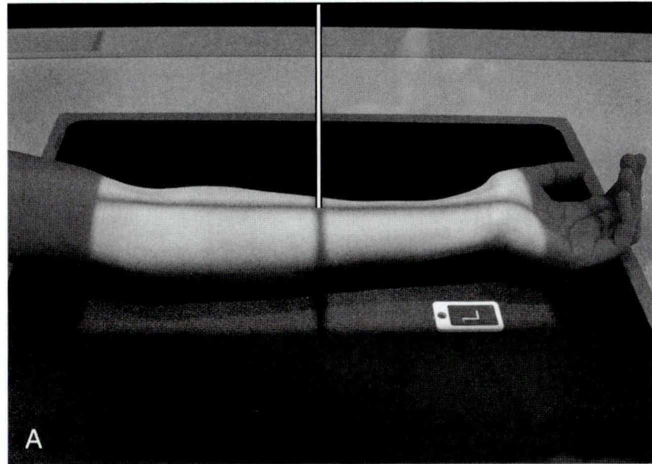

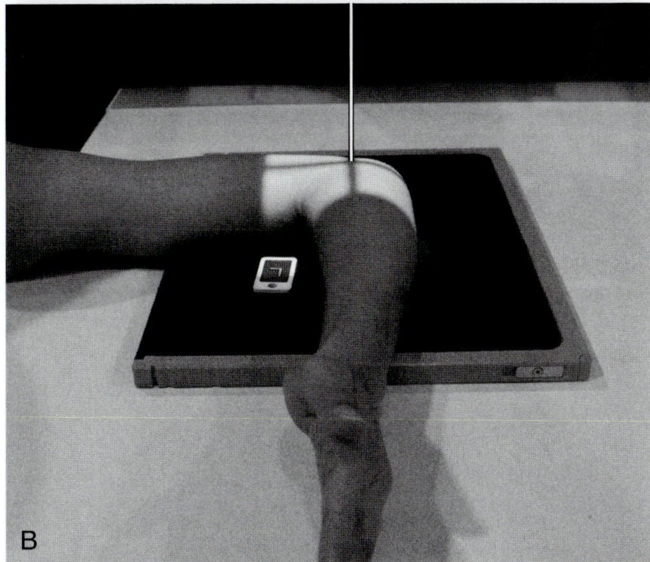

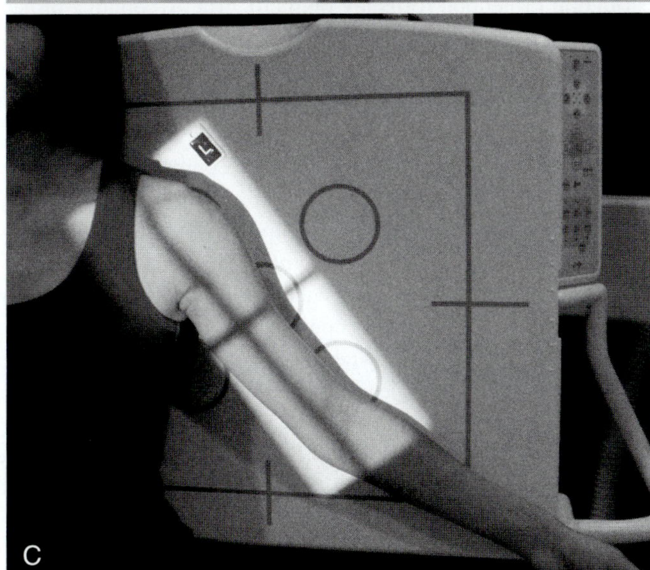

FIGURE 53.6 **(A)** Forearm. Position for AP projection. **(B)** Elbow. Position for lateral projection. **(C)** Humerus. Position for AP projection. (From Long BW, Frank ED, Ehrlich RA: *Radiography essentials for limited practice*, ed 6, St. Louis, 2021, Elsevier.)

supported. Arm is rotated to place coronal plane of humeral epicondyles parallel to IR.

- *CR:* Directed to center of joint. If the elbow is flexed 90 degrees or more, it is necessary to angle CR 5 to 15 degrees in distal direction to avoid superimposing proximal forearm over distal humerus.
- *Structures seen:* Distal humerus portion of elbow joint. Proximal forearm will be distorted.

CRITICAL THINKING APPLICATION 53.4

An x-ray requisition for an elbow x-ray was just printed. When Jonathan approaches the patient and begins his assessment, he discovers the patient has a cast on his elbow, so he cannot extend his elbow. Which supplemental projections should be performed in addition to the routine projections for an AP elbow?

Supplemental Projections of the Elbow

If the patient is unable to perform the typical projections for the elbow, due to trauma or pathology, supplemental projections may be performed. Supplemental projections utilize modified positioning to obtain the needed projections.

AP Oblique-Lateral Rotation. Performed when injury to the lateral portion of the elbow (radial head or capitulum) is suspected.

- *Body and part position:* From AP position, leaning laterally and rotating shoulder externally so that posterior lateral aspect of elbow is in contact with IR. Coronal plane of elbow forms angle of 45 degrees with IR.
- *CR:* Directed to enter elbow joint.
- *Structures seen:* Radial head and capitulum without superimposition of ulna.

AP Oblique-Medial Rotation. Performed when injury to the medial portion of the elbow (coronoid process or trochlea) is suspected.

- *Body and part position:* Same as for AP projection. Hand pronated, which allows coronal plane of elbow to assume a 45-degree angle with IR.
- *CR:* Directed to enter elbow joint.
- *Structures seen:* Coronoid process and trochlea without superimposition.

Positioning and Radiographic Examination of the Humerus

Depending on the patient's condition, the patient may be upright or supine for imaging of the humerus. Both methods are presented here. The thickness of the shoulder joint usually dictates that this study be done using a **Bucky** or grid. For relatively small patients, however, a grid is not necessarily required.

The routine examination of the humerus, with the patient upright, includes AP and lateral projections.

- *IR:* CR plate 35 × 43 cm, portrait orientation.
- *Grid:* Yes.
- *Body and part position:* For upright patient, patient is seated or standing with back to upright Bucky. The body position, whether

oblique or facing away from the IR, is not critical as long as the epicondyles are oriented appropriately for the projection. The procedure for imaging the humerus in the recumbent position is similar to that used for upright studies. The recumbent examination is done with the humerus nearer the trunk of the body, and the lateral projection is done without flexing the elbow. The upper margin of the IR should be about 3.8 cm above the head of the humerus.

- *AP:* Arm slightly abducted with palm of hand supinated. Coronal plane of humeral epicondyles parallel to IR (Figure 53.6C).
- *Lateral:* Elbow flexed approximately 45 degrees and palm of hand against hip and elbow is lateral with coronal plane of humeral epicondyles perpendicular to IR.

- *CR:* Perpendicular to midhumerus.
- Patient Instructions: Stop breathing.
- *Structures seen:* Entire humerus, shoulder joint, and elbow joint.

CRITICAL THINKING APPLICATION **53.5**

An x-ray requisition for a humerus x-ray was just printed. When Jonathan approaches the patient and begins his assessment, he discovers the patient will not be able to stand for the x-ray projections. What modifications must Jonathan make to the positioning protocol to obtain the images for the humerus on the table?

Positioning and Radiographic Examination of the Shoulder

Again, the patient's condition will determine if the shoulder girdle is imaged with the patient upright or recumbent. The shoulder examination requires that the patient be able to rotate the humerus. It is desirable to examine the entire shoulder girdle, so the routine study should include the scapula, clavicle, and proximal humerus. The IR is placed in landscape orientation.

Routine Examination of the Shoulder

The routine examination of the shoulder includes the AP projections with both internal and external humerus rotation.

- *IR:* CR plate 24 × 30 cm, landscape orientation.
- *Grid:* Yes.
- *Body and part position:* Standing or seated with back to upright Bucky or supine on table; coronal plane of body parallel to IR.
  - *External rotation:* Arm slightly abducted with palm of hand supinated. Arm adjusted to place coronal plane of humeral epicondyles parallel to IR. Figure 53.7A shows the patient in the upright position, and Figure 53.7B shows the patient in the recumbent position.
  - *Internal rotation:* Humerus and arm rotated internally until back of hand is against thigh. Arm adjusted to place coronal plane of humeral epicondyles perpendicular to IR.
- *CR:* Perpendicular to a point 2.5 cm inferior to coracoid process.
- *Patient instructions:* Stop breathing.
- *Structures seen:* Entire clavicle and scapula and proximal third of humerus. External rotation demonstrates greater tubercule in profile; internal rotation demonstrates lesser tubercule in profile.

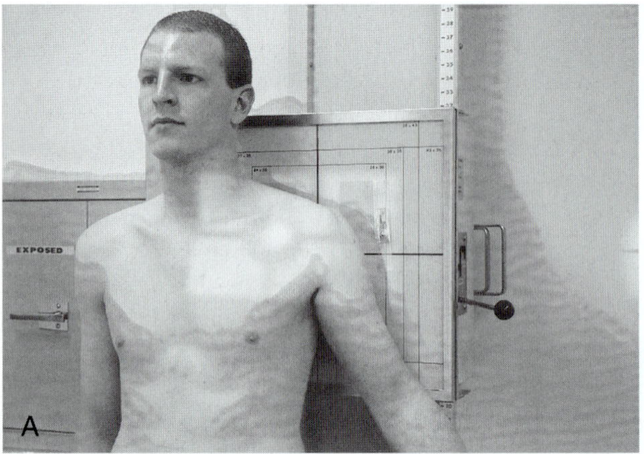

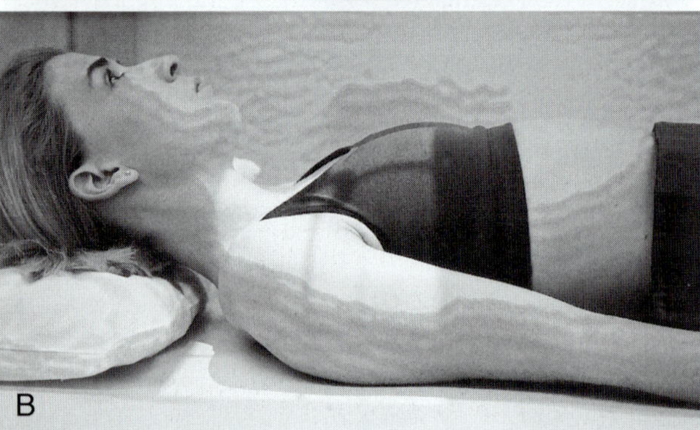

FIGURE 53.7 Shoulder. Position for AP projection—external (arm) rotation. **(A)** Patient upright. **(B)** Patient recumbent. (From Long BW, Frank ED, Ehrlich RA: *Radiography essentials for limited practice*, ed 6, St. Louis, 2021, Elsevier.)

Additional Shoulder Projection

At times, additional projections are needed to focus on an area of interest that may not be well visualized in the typical projections.

AP Oblique Projection (Grashey Method). The AP oblique projection demonstrates the glenoid fossa in profile, allowing evaluation of the glenohumeral joint.

- *IR, grid, and patient instructions:* Same as routine examination of the shoulder.
- *Body and part position:* Patient upright or recumbent. Coronal plane of body aligned 35 to 45 degrees with respect to IR. Posterolateral aspect of shoulder in contact with upright Bucky; scapular body parallel to IR; arm in internal, external, or neutral rotation.
- *CR:* Perpendicular through glenohumeral joint, a point 5 cm medial and 5 cm inferior to superolateral border of shoulder.
- *Structures seen:* Glenohumeral joint with open joint space and glenoid process in profile; coracoid process will usually obscure superior aspect of joint space.

Alternate Examination for Acute Shoulder Injury. The routine examination for acute injury to the shoulder may include AP and transthoracic lateral or PA oblique (scapular Y) projections.

- *IR and grid:* Same as routine examination of the shoulder.
- *Body and part position:* Standing or seated at upright Bucky.
  - *AP:* With back against the upright Bucky and the coronal plane of the body is parallel to IR.
  - *Transthoracic lateral:* Coronal plane of body is perpendicular to IR with affected side against Bucky. Unaffected arm is raised above head.

- *PA oblique (scapular Y):* Anterolateral aspect of shoulder against Bucky. Coronal plane of body 45 to 60 degrees to IR. Body rotation adjusted to place scapular body perpendicular to IR.

- *CR:* Perpendicular to center of IR, with top of IR 2.5 to 3.5 cm above top of shoulder.
- *Patient instructions:* For the AP and PA oblique, the patient must stop breathing during the exposure. For the transthoracic lateral projection, use the "breathing technique." (Exposure is made during slow, deep breathing. This technique effectively blurs superimposing rib and lung structures, improving visualization of humerus.)
- *Structures seen:* Proximal half of humerus and portions of scapula and clavicle. Demonstrates fractures of upper humerus and aids in evaluation of glenohumeral dislocation.

Routine Examination of the Clavicle

The routine projections for the clavicle are the PA and PA axial projections. The clavicle should be as close to the IR as possible. However, if the clavicle is injured, a supine position is more comfortable, performing AP and AP axial projections instead of PA and PA axial.

The routine examination of the clavicle includes the upright PA and PA axial projections or recumbent AP and AP axial projections.

- *IR:* CR plate 24 × 30 cm, landscape orientation.
- *Grid:* Yes.
- *Body and part position:*
  - *Upright:* Standing or seated facing Bucky with coronal plane parallel to IR. Head turned away from side of interest. Arm at side.
  - *Recumbent:* Supine.
- *CR:*
  - *PA or AP:* Perpendicular to midclavicle.
  - *PA axial:* 15 to 30 degrees caudad to midclavicle (Figure 53.8A).
  - *AP axial:* 15 to 30 degrees cephalad to midclavicle.
- *Patient instructions:* Stop breathing when image is taken.
- *Structures seen:* Entire clavicle and its articulations.

Routine Examination of the Scapula

The routine examination of the scapula includes AP and lateral projections.

- *IR:* CR plate 24 × 30 cm, portrait orientation.
- *Grid:* Yes.
- *Body and part position:* Standing or seated at upright Bucky, or recumbent on table.
  - *AP:* Arm abducted so that humerus is perpendicular to long axis of body. Elbow is flexed 90 degrees. When patient is upright, patient may support position by grasping a pole (Figure 53.8B).
  - *Upright lateral:* Anterior oblique body position with affected side nearest IR. Adjust rotation of body (45 to 60 degrees) so that the body of scapula is perpendicular to IR. Patient's forearm is positioned behind back with elbow flexed 90 degrees. Alternatively, arm may be positioned over head or across chest, depending on structures of interest and patient's ability to cooperate.

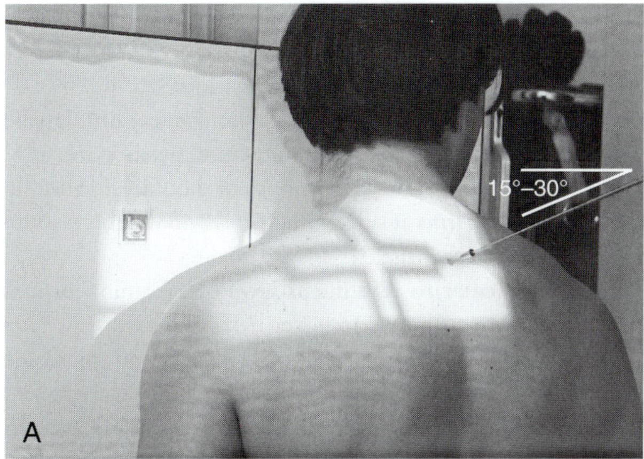

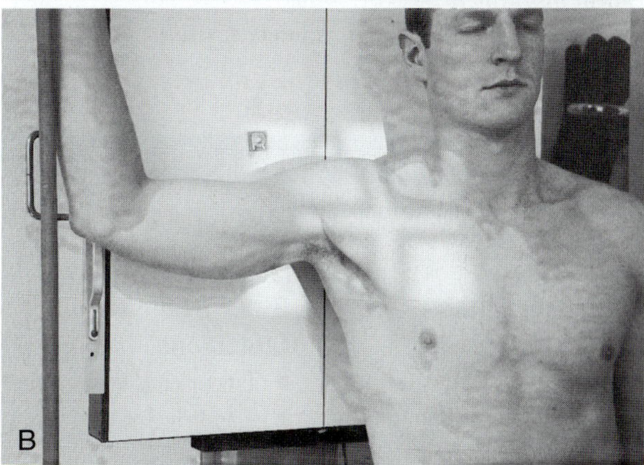

FIGURE 53.8 **(A)** Clavicle. Position for PA axial projection, patient upright. **(B)** Scapula. Position for AP projection, patient upright. (From Long BW, Frank ED, Ehrlich RA: *Radiography essentials for limited practice*, ed 6, St. Louis, 2021, Elsevier.)

  - *Recumbent lateral:* Posterior oblique body position with unaffected side in contact with table. Rotation of body adjusted (45 to 60 degrees) so that blade (body) of scapula is perpendicular to IR. Patient's arm may be positioned across chest.
- *CR:* Perpendicular to midscapula. For the AP, this point is ~5 cm inferior to coracoid process. For the lateral, this point is the middle of the medial border of the scapular body.
- *Patient instructions:* Stop breathing during the exposure.
- *Structures seen:* Entire scapula and its articulations with clavicle and humerus. AP projection demonstrates portions of scapula not obscured by ribs and clavicle. Lateral projections demonstrate body of scapula free of superimposition by ribs, acromion, and coracoid process. Position of arm will determine portion of scapula obscured by proximal humerus.

Routine Examination of the Acromioclavicular Joints

The routine examination of the AC joints includes the bilateral AP projections, performed with and without weights. The purpose is to determine ligament integrity by demonstrating a change in relative positions of the acromion and clavicle when under stress.

- *IR:* CR plate 35 × 43 cm, landscape orientation or two 24 × 30 cm, portrait landscape, one for each shoulder.

- *Grid and SID:* Grid may not be required but may be used. SID 40 inches minimum (or more as needed for wide shoulders).
- *Body and part position:* Standing with back to IR.
  - *First exposure (no weights):* Back of shoulders against lower half of IR(s). Arms relaxed at sides in neutral position.
  - *Second exposure (with weights):* Back of shoulders against upper half of IR(s). Arms at sides with 5- to 10-lb weights (sandbags) attached to each wrist.
- *CR:* Perpendicular to midline at level of acromion processes. Exposure field collimated to cover half of the IR.
- *Collimation:* Adjust the light field to 15 × 43 cm on collimator for large, single IR. Adjust light field to 15 × 20 cm for two smaller IRs. Place side marker in the light field on the lateral side of the anatomy.
- *Patient instructions:* Stop breathing.
- *Structures seen:* Both AC joints for comparison to evaluate ligament integrity.

Pathology

The most significant pathology affecting the upper limb is trauma. Fractures and other injuries to this portion of anatomy may vary greatly.

Common Fractures

- Boxer's fracture of the fifth metacarpal
- Scaphoid fracture
- Colles fracture of distal radius
- Monteggia fracture of ulna with dislocation of radial head
- Radial head fracture
- Surgical neck of humerus

Other Trauma Conditions

- Dislocation of the shoulder
- Foreign bodies

Nontraumatic Conditions

- Bursitis
- Tendonitis
- Arthritis
- Osteoarthritis
- Osteomyelitis

LOWER LIMB AND PELVIS IMAGES

The bones of the lower limb are divided into the foot, lower leg (tibia and fibula), upper leg (femur), and pelvis. This area also includes the ankle, knee, and hip.

The examinations of the hip and pelvis are typically performed in the table Bucky. Examinations of the lower limb from the toes up to the femur are usually done tabletop (nongrid), with the patient sitting or lying on the radiographic table. The shoe and sock should be removed from the affected leg. Pants should be removed from the radiation field.

For all lateral positions, the coronal plane of the pelvis is perpendicular to the table, the knee is flexed ~ 45 degrees, and the ankle is dorsiflexed so that the foot forms an angle of 90 degrees with the lower leg. The unaffected leg is supported to prevent rotation of the pelvis. However, when the patient is unable to attain this position, the unaffected leg can be placed behind the affected leg as long as the lateral position is maintained.

For the projections of the lower limb and pelvis, use the following unless otherwise indicated:

- *IR:* Positioned by department protocol for proper anatomy orientation; CR plate 18 × 24 cm; portrait orientation.

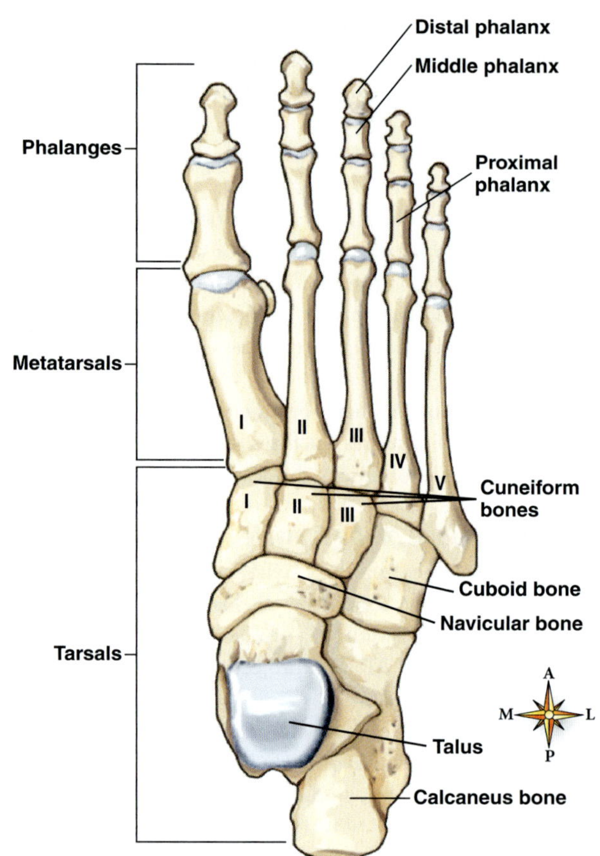

FIGURE 53.9 Right foot. (From Patton KT, Thibodeau GA: *The human body in health and disease*, ed 7, St. Louis, 2018, Elsevier.)

- *Grid and SID:* No grid. SID 40 inches minimum.
- *Collimation:* Adjust the light field to 2.5 cm on all sides of the anatomy. Place side marker in the light field on the lateral side of the anatomy.
- *Patient instructions:* Do not move.

Positioning and Radiographic Examinations of the Toes and Foot

The toes have three phalanges and the great toe has two. The 10 metatarsals form part of the foot near the toes. The 14 tarsal bones form the heel and the posterior part of the foot. The calcaneus is the largest tarsal bone (Figure 53.9).

Routine Examination of the Toes

Although the toes are included in the examination of the foot, separate studies of the toes may be performed when the area of clinical interest is a specific toe. Each projection of the toe should include the entire digit and the distal portion of the corresponding metatarsal. Toes 2 to 5 tend to curl downward. When the toes are angled in relation to the IR, visualization of the joint spaces is compromised. When this is the case, an AP axial projection is recommended. For lateral projections of the toes, the foot may be positioned with either its medial or lateral surface in contact with the IR, depending on which toe is involved. Keep the toe as close to the IR as possible, and maintain the toe in a position parallel to the IR.

The routine examination of the toe includes the AP or AP axial, AP oblique (medial rotation), and lateral projections.

- *Body and part position:* Seated or recumbent on table with knee flexed.
  - *AP axial:* Plantar surface supported on 15-degree wedge sponge.
  - *AP:* Plantar surface is in contact with IR.
  - *AP oblique:* Medial plantar surface of toe and forefoot is in contact with IR. Plantar surface of foot and toes forms a 30 to 45 degrees with IR.
  - *Lateral:* The lateral or medial aspect surface of foot may rest on the IR, depending on which brings toe of interest nearest to IR. Other toes are flexed or extended as needed to isolate the affected toe free of superimposition. Affected toe is supported parallel to IR. Toes may be held in position with tape. Variations may be required depending on which toe is involved, the configuration of the toe, and movements tolerable for the patient.
- *CR:*
  - *AP axial:* Angled 15 degrees posteriorly (toward heel) to metatarsophalangeal (MTP) joints.
  - *AP, AP oblique, and lateral:* Perpendicular to MTP joints.
- *Structures seen:* Entire digit and distal half of metatarsal with IP and MTP joint spaces open and clearly visualized.

Routine Examination of the Sesamoids

The sesamoid bones of the foot are located on the plantar aspect of the first MTP joint. These small bones are occasionally injured and are usually demonstrated on foot images. However, special positioning is required to demonstrate them without superimposition of other bones of the foot.

The routine examination of the sesamoids includes the tangential projection.

- *Body and part position:* Standing, facing away from x-ray tube, or prone. Plantar surface of foot resting on IR in a position of dorsiflexion and adjusted to place the ball of the foot perpendicular to the IR. If the patient can't stand, the tangential projection can be performed with the patient seated, the foot pointing up, and the plantar surface at an angle of ~ 70 degrees with the plane of the IR.
- *CR:* Perpendicular and tangential to the first MTP joint.
- *Structures seen:* Sesamoids and first metatarsal head in profile.

Routine Examination of the Foot

The top of the foot is its *dorsal aspect,* and the bottom is the *plantar surface*. The AP axial projection would more correctly be a dorsoplantar (DP) axial projection and is most commonly used in podiatric medicine. The CR is angled posteriorly (toward the heel) for this projection to reduce the foreshortening of the metatarsals and to better demonstrate the intertarsal articulations.

The routine examination of the foot includes the AP axial, AP oblique (medial), and lateral projections.

- *Body and part position:* Seated or recumbent on table with knee flexed. In podiatric practice, the AP (DP) and AP (DP) oblique are performed with the patient standing. For all projections, foot is centered with regard to IR so that toes, heel, and both malleoli are within field.
  - *AP axial:* Plantar surface of foot rests upon IR (Figure 53.10A).
  - *AP oblique:* Leg is rotated medially so that medial plantar aspect of foot is in contact with IR. Plantar surface of foot forms 30-degree angle with IR (Figure 53.10B).
  - *Lateral:* Lateral aspect of foot is in contact with IR and foot is in true lateral position with plantar aspect of forefoot perpendicular to IR. Ankle is dorsiflexed so that long axis of foot is perpendicular to tibia (Figure 53.10C).

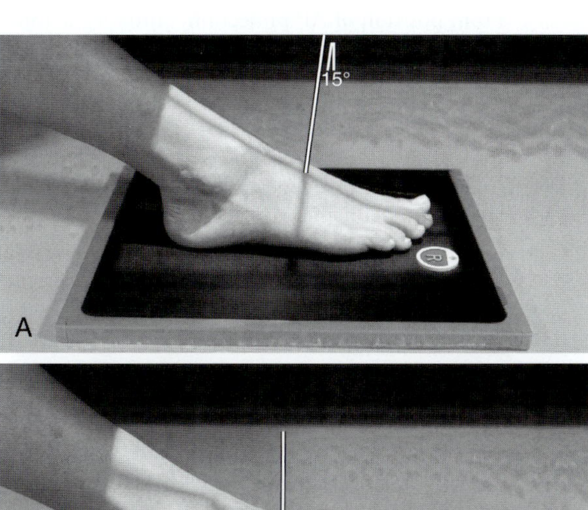

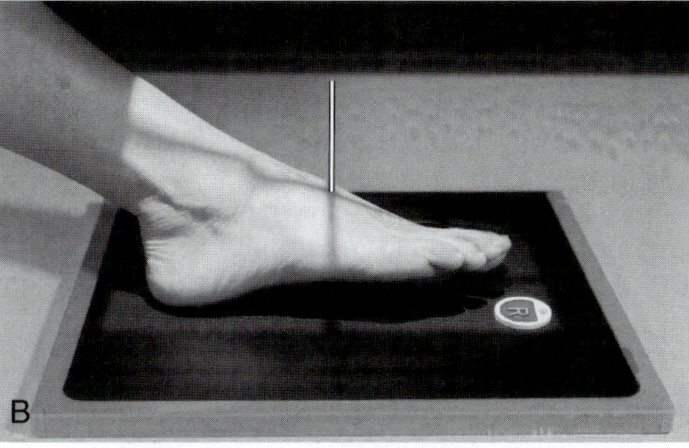

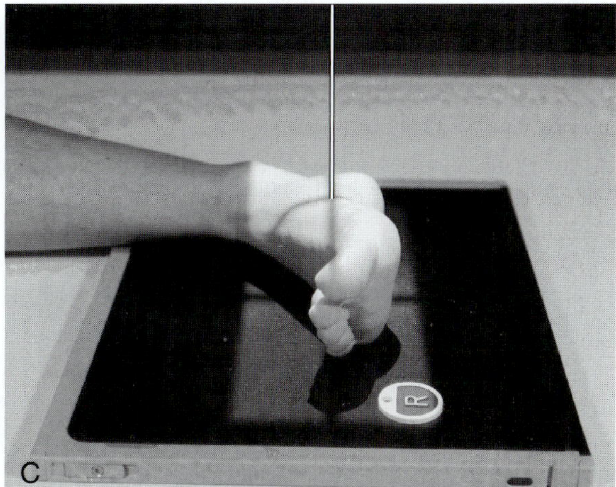

FIGURE 53.10 Foot. **(A)** Position for AP axial projection. **(B)** Position for AP oblique projection—medial rotation. **(C)** Position for lateral projection. (From Long BW, Frank ED, Ehrlich RA: *Radiography essentials for limited practice*, ed 6, St. Louis, 2021, Elsevier.)

- *CR:*
  - *AP axial:* Angled 10 degrees posteriorly (toward heel) and entering base of third metatarsal.
  - *AP oblique and lateral:* Perpendicular to base of third metatarsal.
- *Structures seen:* Entire foot, including toes, metatarsals, and tarsal bones. The calcaneus is obscured by superimposition of lower leg on the AP axial projection. AP oblique projection with medial rotation should demonstrate the metatarsals and some tarsals (cuboid, navicular, lateral cuneiform) with minimal superimposition. Lateral projection demonstrates superimposition of metatarsals, more proximal than distal. It should include the ankle joint.

CRITICAL THINKING APPLICATION **53.6**

An x-ray requisition for a foot x-ray was just printed. When Jonathan approaches the patient and begins his assessment, he determines this procedure will be a typical foot procedure. What are the steps for performing an x-ray of the foot? Which projections are included as part of the routine series?

Routine Examination of the Calcaneus

The routine examination of the calcaneus includes the axial (plantodorsal) and lateral projections.

- Body and part position:
  - *Axial (plantodorsal):* Seated or recumbent on table with leg extended. Posterior surface of ankle and heel rests on the IR. Adjust foot so the malleoli are centered to the center of the IR. Sagittal plane of foot is perpendicular to IR. Foot is dorsiflexed as much as possible and held in position by patient using a strap or other accessory (Figure 53.11).
  - *Lateral:* Seated or recumbent on table with knee flexed. Lateral surface of heel rests on IR. Part is positioned as for lateral projection of foot but with calcaneus centered to IR.
- *CR:*
  - *Axial (plantodorsal):* Angled 40 degrees cephalad to center of IR, entering base of third metatarsal.

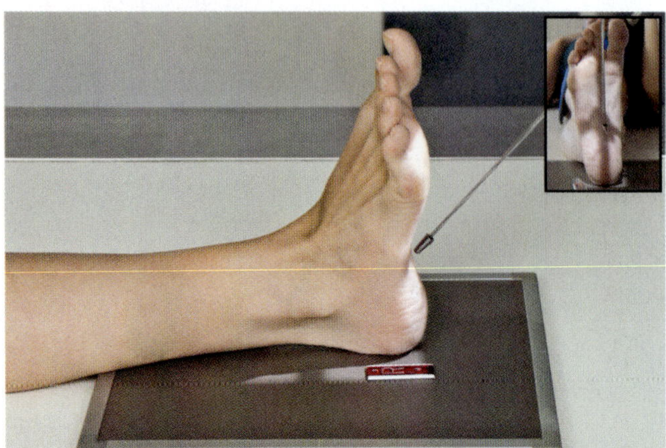

FIGURE 53.11 Calcaneus. Position for axial (plantodorsal) projection. (From Lampignano J, Ehrlich RA: *Bontrager's textbook of radiographic positioning and related anatomy*, ed 10, St. Louis, 2021, Mosby.)

  - *Lateral:* Perpendicular to center of IR, entering about 2.5 cm to medial malleolus.
- *Structures seen:* Entire calcaneus and its articulation with talus. Lateral projection also shows calcaneal articulations with cuboid and navicular anteriorly.

Positioning and Radiographic Examinations of the Ankle and the Lower Leg

The tibia is one of the two lower leg bones. The medial malleolus is the rounded projection at the lower end of the tibia. The fibula is the second lower leg bone. The lateral malleolus is the rounded projection at the lower end of the fibula (Figure 53.12).

Routine Examination of the Ankle

There are two medial oblique projections, one that best demonstrates the ankle mortise joint and one that demonstrates the tibiofibular joint. The projections that constitute a routine examination must be determined by the physician who will interpret the images.

The routine examination of the ankle includes the AP, AP oblique (medial rotation), AP oblique (medial rotation—mortise joint), and lateral projections.

- *IR:* CR plate 24 × 30 cm, portrait orientation.
- *Body and part position:*
  - *AP:* Seated or recumbent on the table with the affected leg extended. Posterior surface of heel and lower leg rests on IR. Midpoint between malleoli is centered to IR. Foot is dorsiflexed so that plantar surface of foot forms a 90-degree angle with coronal plane of lower leg. Sagittal planes of leg and foot are perpendicular to IR. Foot may be held in position by strap or other accessory (Figure 53.13).
  - *AP oblique (medial rotation):* (Same body position as AP.) From position of AP projection, entire leg is rotated medially 45 degrees. Sagittal planes of foot and leg must remain aligned to each other.
  - *AP oblique (medial rotation—mortise joint):* (Same body position as AP.) From position of AP projection, entire leg is rotated medially 15 to 20 degrees. Sagittal plane of foot and leg must remain aligned with each other.
  - *Lateral:* Recumbent on affected side with knee flexed 35 to 40 degrees. Lateral surface (medial surface, if upright) of ankle is in contact with IR. Sagittal plane of foot and leg must remain aligned with each other.
- *CR:*
  - *AP and AP obliques:* Perpendicular to point midway between malleoli.
  - *Lateral:* Perpendicular to medial malleolus.
- *Structures seen:* Superior portion of talus and distal portions of tibia and fibula. AP oblique projection with 45 degrees medial rotation demonstrates tibiofibular joint without superimposition. AP oblique projection with 15 to 20 degrees medial rotation demonstrates mortise joint spaces without superimposition. Lateral projection demonstrates tibiotalar and subtalar joints and includes base of the fifth metatarsal.

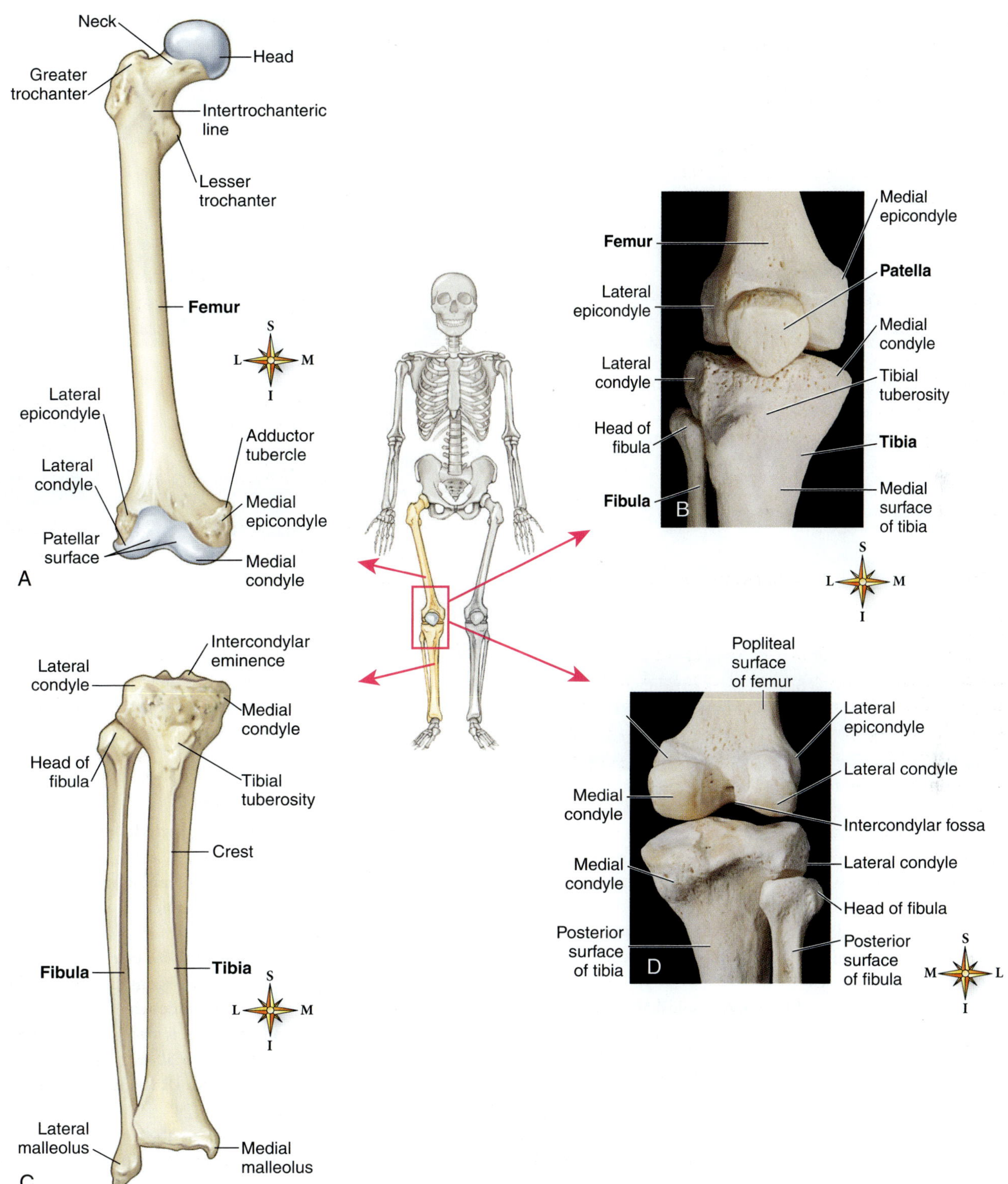

FIGURE 53.12 Right thigh, knee joint, and leg. **(A, B,** and **C)** Anterior views. **(D)** Posterior view. (From Patton KT, Thibodeau GA: *The human body in health and disease,* ed 7, St. Louis, 2018, Elsevier.)

Routine Examination of the Lower Leg

The routine examination of the lower leg includes the AP and lateral projections.

- *IR:* CR plate 35 × 43 cm, portrait or diagonal orientation.
- *Body and part position:*
  - *AP:* Seated or recumbent on the table. Leg is fully extended with posterior surface of lower leg resting on IR. Margin of IR is placed 1 to 2 inches beyond joint of primary interest. Foot is dorsiflexed so that plantar surface of foot forms a 90-degree angle with coronal plane of lower leg. Sagittal planes of leg and foot are perpendicular to IR. Foot may be held in position by patient using a strap or other accessory (Figure 53.14).
  - *Lateral:* Recumbent on affected side with unaffected leg anterior or posterior to affected leg. Knee may be flexed, if

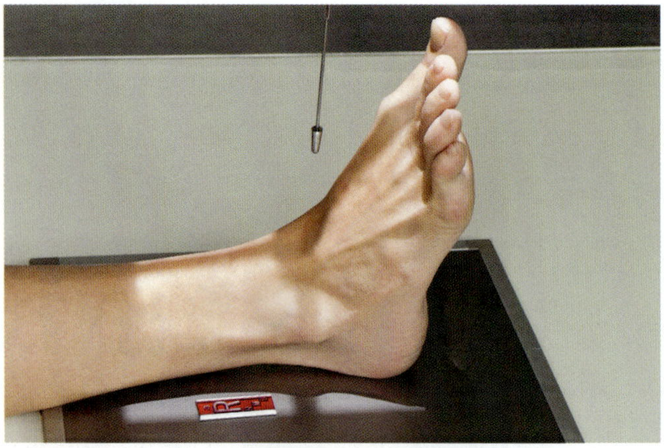

FIGURE 53.13 Ankle. Position for AP projection. (From Lampignano J, Ehrlich RA: *Bontrager's textbook of radiographic positioning and related anatomy*, ed 10, St. Louis, 2021, Mosby.)

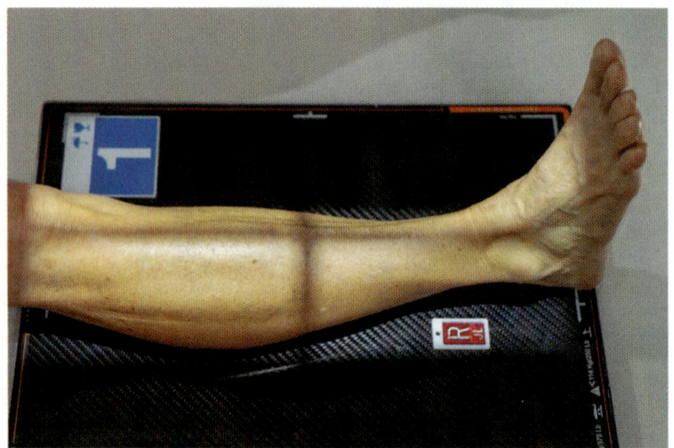

FIGURE 53.14 Lower leg. Position for AP projection. (From Lampignano J, Ehrlich RA: *Bontrager's textbook of radiographic positioning and related anatomy*, ed 10, St. Louis, 2021, Mosby.)

necessary, to ensure a true lateral position. Lateral surface of lower leg rests on IR. Leg is rotated to place sagittal plane of leg parallel to IR and coronal plane through patella perpendicular to IR. Margin of IR is placed 1 to 2 inches beyond joint of primary interest.

- *CR:* Perpendicular to center of IR entering midshaft of tibia.
- *Structures seen:* Entire lower leg and at least one joint.

Positioning and Radiographic Examinations of the Knee

The routine examination of the knee consists of AP and lateral projections. However, an axial projection of the intercondylar fossa ("tunnel" or "notch") and a tangential projection of the patella are frequently requested for the evaluation of chronic knee complaints.

When the area of clinical interest is the patella, the routine examination includes PA and lateral projections. A tangential projection of the patella may be added for chronic conditions but should not be included when there is suspicion of patellar fracture. *Do not flex the knee more than 10 degrees when there is suspicion of fracture of the patella.* In this instance, the lateral projection is taken with the knee extended.

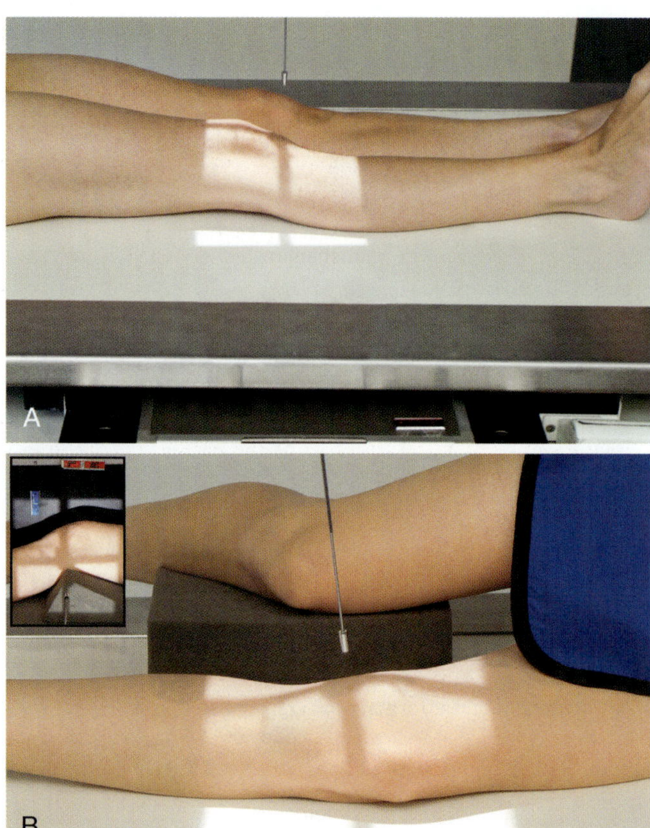

FIGURE 53.15 Knee. **(A)** Position for AP projection. **(B)** Position for lateral projection. (From Lampignano J, Ehrlich RA: *Bontrager's textbook of radiographic positioning and related anatomy*, ed 10, St. Louis, 2021, Mosby.)

Routine Examination of the Knee

The routine examination of the knee includes the AP and lateral projections.

- *IR:* CR plate 24 × 30 cm, portrait orientation.
- *Grid:* With or without grid is acceptable.
- *Body and part position:*
  - *AP:* Seated or supine on table with leg extended so the sagittal plane of leg perpendicular to IR (Figure 53.15A).
  - *Lateral:* Recumbent on affected side with femur aligned with center of table. Unaffected leg is anterior or posterior to affected leg. Knee is flexed 20 to 30 degrees. Sagittal plan of femur and lower leg is parallel to IR (Figure 53.15B).
- *CR:*
  - *AP:* Entering 0.5 inch distal to apex of patella. The angle of the CR is dependent on the measurement between the anterior superior iliac spine (ASIS) and the tabletop, as follows:
    - < 19 cm (thin patient) 3–5 degrees *caudad*
    - 19–24 cm 0 degrees (perpendicular)
    - > 24 cm (large pelvis) 3–5 degrees *cephalad*
  - *Lateral:* Angled 5–7 degrees cephalad entering 1 inch distal to medial epicondyle of femur.
- *Structures seen:* Knee joint with portions of distal femur and proximal lower leg. Lateral projection includes a profile of tibial tuberosity. Distal femur with condyles superimposed and joint

space free of superimposition. Entire patella and retropatellar joint space should also be clearly visualized.

Alternative Projection of the Knee

When the patella is the clinical interest, the PA projection can be performed.

- *IR and grid:* Same as for routine knee projections.
- *Body and body position:* Patient is prone. Affected leg extended and sagittal plane of leg perpendicular to IR; foot on affected side is plantar flexed and rests on its dorsal aspect.
- *CR:* Directed 5 to 7 degrees caudad to exit 0.5 inch (1.3 cm) inferior to the patellar apex.
- *Structures seen:* Knee joint with portions of distal femur and proximal lower leg. Greater visibility of the patella than on the AP projection.

Supplemental Projections of the Knee

If the patient is unable to perform the routine projections of the knee due to trauma or pathology, supplemental projections may be performed.

Two methods are presented for demonstration of the intercondylar fossa ("tunnel"). The Holmblad method, in which there is less distortion caused by tube angulation, is often preferred. The Camp-Coventry method may be desirable if the patient is unable to assume the correct position for the Holmblad method.

The tangential or "sunrise" projection is also an option. For all three of these supplemental projections, the IR and grid are the same as routine knee projections.

PA Axial Projection—Holmblad Method.

- *Body and part position:* Patient is on hands and knees on radiographic table with affected knees flexed so that the angle between the femur and table is 70 degrees. Contralateral knee is flexed to provide support. Pelvis must remain level, and sagittal plane of affected leg must remain perpendicular to the IR.
- *CR:* Perpendicular to center of IR through center of knee joint.
- *Structures seen:* Knee joint with portions of distal femur and proximal lower leg. Open intercondylar fossa.

PA Axial Projection—Camp-Coventry Method.

- *Body and part position:* Prone with affected knee flexed to form angle of 40 to 50 degrees between tibia and table.
- *CR:* Angled 40 degrees caudad through knee joint to center of IR if leg is 40 degrees, and 50 degrees if leg is 50 degrees.
- *Structures seen:* Knee joint with portions of distal femur and proximal lower leg. Open intercondylar fossa.

Tangential ("Sunrise") Projection of the Patella: Settegast Method.

- *Body and part position:* Prone with affected knee flexed as much as possible or until the patella is perpendicular to IR. Sagittal plane of femur is perpendicular to IR. Position may be supported by a strap around the ankle that is extended over the patient's shoulder and held by the patient. Alternatively, patient may be seated on the radiographic table.
- *CR:* Angled 15 to 20 degrees cephalad and centered to inferior margin of patella. Angulation is adjusted so that CR passes between patella and distal femur.
- *Structures seen:* Patella in profile and open patellofemoral joint.

CRITICAL THINKING APPLICATION **53.7**

An x-ray requisition for a knee x-ray was just printed. The x-ray requisition states, "Knee with Sunrise." What is a sunrise projection? What is the purpose of the sunrise projection? As an LXMO, will Jonathan be able to perform the sunrise projection?

Positioning and Radiographic Examinations of the Femur

For most adults, the entire femur is too long to be included on a 35 × 43 cm IR, so a choice must be made regarding which joint to include. Images of the distal femur include the knee, whereas those of the proximal femur include the hip joint. When the entire femur is imaged, AP and lateral images of both the proximal and distal femur are included.

Routine Examination of the Distal Femur

The routine examination of the distal femur includes the AP and lateral projections.

- *IR:* CR plate 35 × 43 cm, portrait orientation.
- *Grid:* Yes.
- *Body and part position:*
  - *AP:* Supine with affected femur aligned with center of table. Leg is extended with sagittal plane perpendicular to IR. Ensure plane through epicondyles is parallel with IR. Inferior margin of IR is placed 1 to 2 inches below knee joint (Figure 53.16).
  - *Lateral:* Recumbent on affected side with femur aligned with center of table. Knee and hip of unaffected limb are flexed, and leg is supported anterior to the body. Knee of affected leg is flexed 30 to 45 degrees. Sagittal plane of femur is parallel to IR. Inferior margin of IR is placed 1 to 2 inches below knee joint.
- *CR:* Perpendicular to midpoint of IR.
- *Structures seen:* Knee joint and distal three-fourths of femur.

Routine Examination of the Proximal Femur

The routine examination of the proximal femur includes the AP and lateral projections.

- *IR and grid:* Same as routine examination of distal femur.
- *Body and part position:*
  - *AP:* Supine with affected femur aligned with center of table. Leg is extended with sagittal plane perpendicular to IR. Rotate the limb internally 10 to15 degrees to place the femoral neck in profile. Superior margin of IR is placed at level of ASIS.
  - *Lateral:* Recumbent in oblique position on affected side with support under affected hip. Affected femur aligned to center of table. Knee and hip of unaffected limb are flexed, and leg is supported posterior to the body. Rotate pelvis posteriorly 10 to 15 degrees from lateral position to prevent superimposition. Sagittal plane of femur is parallel to IR as much as possible. Superior margin of IR is placed at level of ASIS.
- *CR:* Perpendicular to midpoint of IR.
- *Structures seen:* Hip joint and proximal three-fourths of femur.

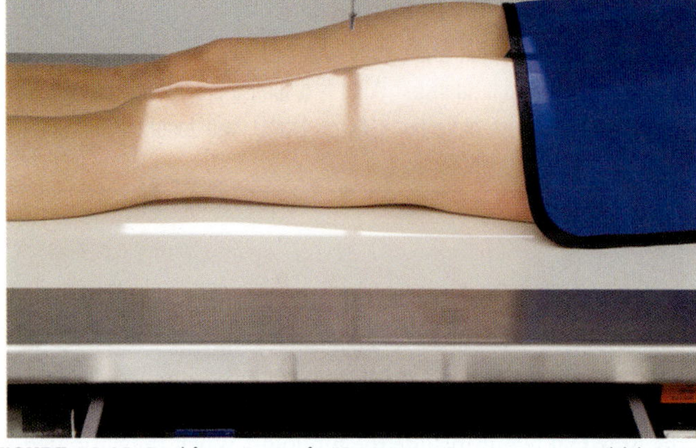

FIGURE 53.16 Distal femur. Position for AP projection. (From Lampignano J, Ehrlich RA: *Bontrager's textbook of radiographic positioning and related anatomy*, ed 10, St. Louis, 2021, Mosby.)

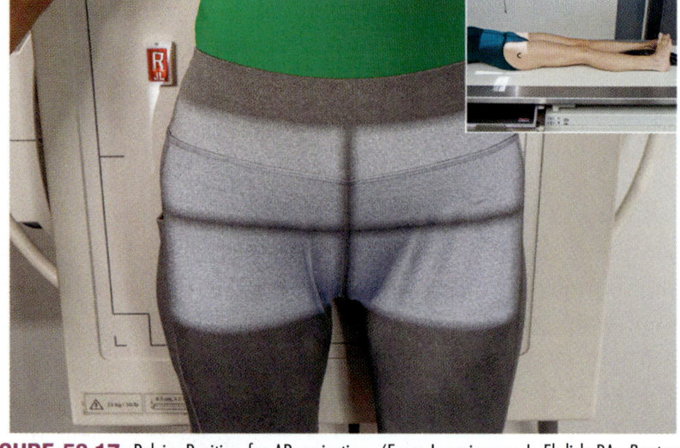

FIGURE 53.17 Pelvis. Position for AP projection. (From Lampignano J, Ehrlich RA: *Bontrager's textbook of radiographic positioning and related anatomy*, ed 10, St. Louis, 2021, Mosby.)

Positioning and Radiographic Examinations of the Pelvis

The routine examination of the pelvis includes the AP projection.

- *IR:* Positioned by department protocol for proper anatomy orientation; CR plate 35 × 43 cm, landscape orientation
- *Grid:* Yes.
- *Body and part position:* Supine on table. Coronal plane of body is parallel to IR. If there is no suspicion of recent fracture, femurs are rotated medially 15 to 20 degrees to place femoral necks parallel to IR. The heels will be 8 to 10 inches apart (Figure 53.17).
- *IR placement:* Center IR midway between ASIS and pubic symphysis.
- *CR:* Perpendicular to midpoint of IR.
- *Structures seen:* Entire pelvis and proximal portion of femurs.

Positioning and Radiographic Examinations of the Hip

If a hip fracture is suspected, begin the examination with an AP projection of the entire pelvis. *Do not move the affected leg, regardless of its position,* until a physician has checked the pelvis image. If a lateral projection is needed in cases of a recent hip fracture, an axiolateral projection is made without moving the affected leg. Routine hip examinations are commonly performed as follow-up studies after treatment for hip fracture or evaluation of chronic hip complaints.

Figure 53.18 illustrates the method to locate the hip joint, the long axis of the femoral neck, and the centering point for hip images. The midpoint of an imaginary line between the ASIS and the pubic symphysis determines the superior margin of the acetabulum which must be included in examinations of the proximal femur and in all hip studies. When a perpendicular line is drawn inferior to the center of this line, forming a T, this second line will indicate the long axis of the femoral neck. The center of the femoral neck is approximately 2.5 inches inferior to the junction and is the centering point for radiographic examinations of the hip.

Routine Examination of the Hip

The routine examination of the hip includes the AP and lateral projections.

- *IR:* CR plate 24 × 30 cm, portrait orientation.
- *Grid:* Yes.

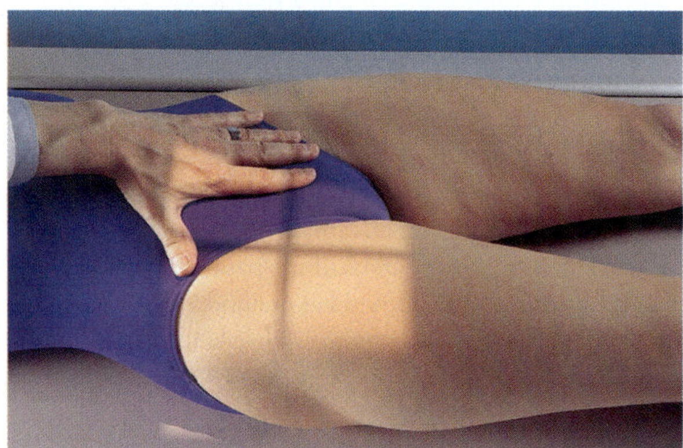

FIGURE 53.18 Suggested method of locating the right hip. The left thumb is on the ASIS, and the second finger is on the superior margin of the pubic symphysis. The central ray is positioned 1.5 inches distal to center of the line drawn between the ASIS and pubic symphysis. (From Long BW, Rollins JH, Smith BJ: *Merrill's atlas of radiographic positioning and procedures*, ed 14, St. Louis, 2020, Mosby.)

- *Body and part position:* Supine on table.
  - *AP:* Femur is medially rotated 15 degrees as for pelvis (Figure 53.19).
  - *Lateral ("frog-leg" position):* Hip is flexed as much as possible, and femur abducted 45 degrees. If patient cannot abduct femur sufficiently from supine position, pelvis may be rotated toward affected side.
- *CR:* Perpendicular to midfemoral neck.
- *Structures seen:* Proximal fourth of femur, acetabulum, and portion of pelvis surrounding acetabulum.

Alternative Lateral Projection of the Hip

When there is a known or suspected hip fracture, the lateral projection is modified for the axiolateral projection (Danelius-Miller method), also called the *cross-table lateral* or *surgical lateral projection,* is substituted for the frog-leg lateral projection. This image is taken without moving or rotating the affected leg.

- *IR and grid:* Same as routine examination of the hip.
- *Body and part position:* Supine on table. The hip and knee of the unaffected limb are flexed 90 degrees and supported above table. A grid cassette is used. The IR is oriented vertically and landscape, angled parallel to the long axis of the

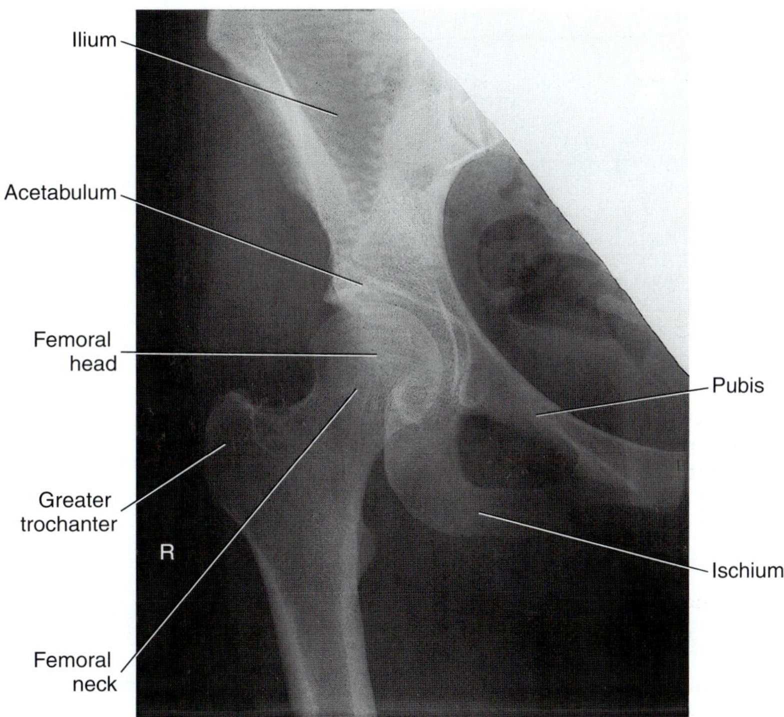

FIGURE 53.19 Hip. AP projection. (From Long BW, Frank ED, Ehrlich RA: *Radiography essentials for limited practice,* ed 6, St. Louis, 2021, Elsevier.)

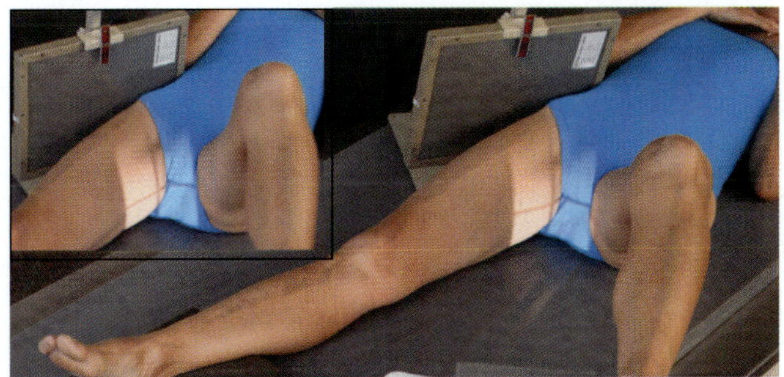

FIGURE 53.20 Hip. Position for axiolateral inferosuperior projection (Danelius-Miller method.). (From Lampignano J, Ehrlich RA: *Bontrager's textbook of radiographic positioning and related anatomy,* ed 10, St. Louis, 2021, Mosby.)

femoral neck, and the medial margin of the IR is placed solidly into the soft tissue just proximal to the iliac crest (Figure 53.20).

- *CR:* Horizontal and perpendicular to the center of the IR, entering through the patient's groin.
- *Structures seen:* Proximal fourth of femur, acetabulum, and portion of pelvis surrounding acetabulum.

CRITICAL THINKING APPLICATION **53.8**

An x-ray requisition for a hip x-ray was just printed. When Jonathan approaches the patient and begins his assessment, he discovers the patient has recently had hip surgery. Due to the surgery, the patient is unable to perform the positioning for the lateral hip projection. Which alternative projection should be performed instead of the routine projection for a lateral hip?

Pathology

Probably, the most significant pathology affecting the lower limb is trauma. Fractures and other conditions affecting this portion of anatomy may vary greatly.

Common Fractures

- Stress fractures in the feet and long bones
- Injury to meniscus cartilage or ligaments connecting the tibia to the femur
- Femoral and hip fractures

Nontraumatic Conditions

- Arthritis, including osteoarthritis, rheumatoid, and gouty
- Osteomyelitis
- Neoplastic and metastatic bone disease

SPINE

The bones of the spine are divided into the cervical spine, thoracic spine, and lumbar spine. This area also includes the sacrum, coccyx, and sacroiliac joints. The examinations of the cervical spine are most commonly performed at the wall Bucky with the patient upright, whereas those for the thoracic spine and lumbar spine are typically performed in the table Bucky with the patient recumbent.

Landmarks are used in positioning of the spine. Figure 53.21A demonstrates the landmarks of the cranium and face that are helpful for imaging the cervical spine. Figure 53.21B demonstrates the topographic anatomy that corresponds to specific vertebral levels of the spine. The limited operator must correctly identify the location of any vertebra when a tightly collimated image is necessary.

For the projections of the spine, use the following unless otherwise indicated:

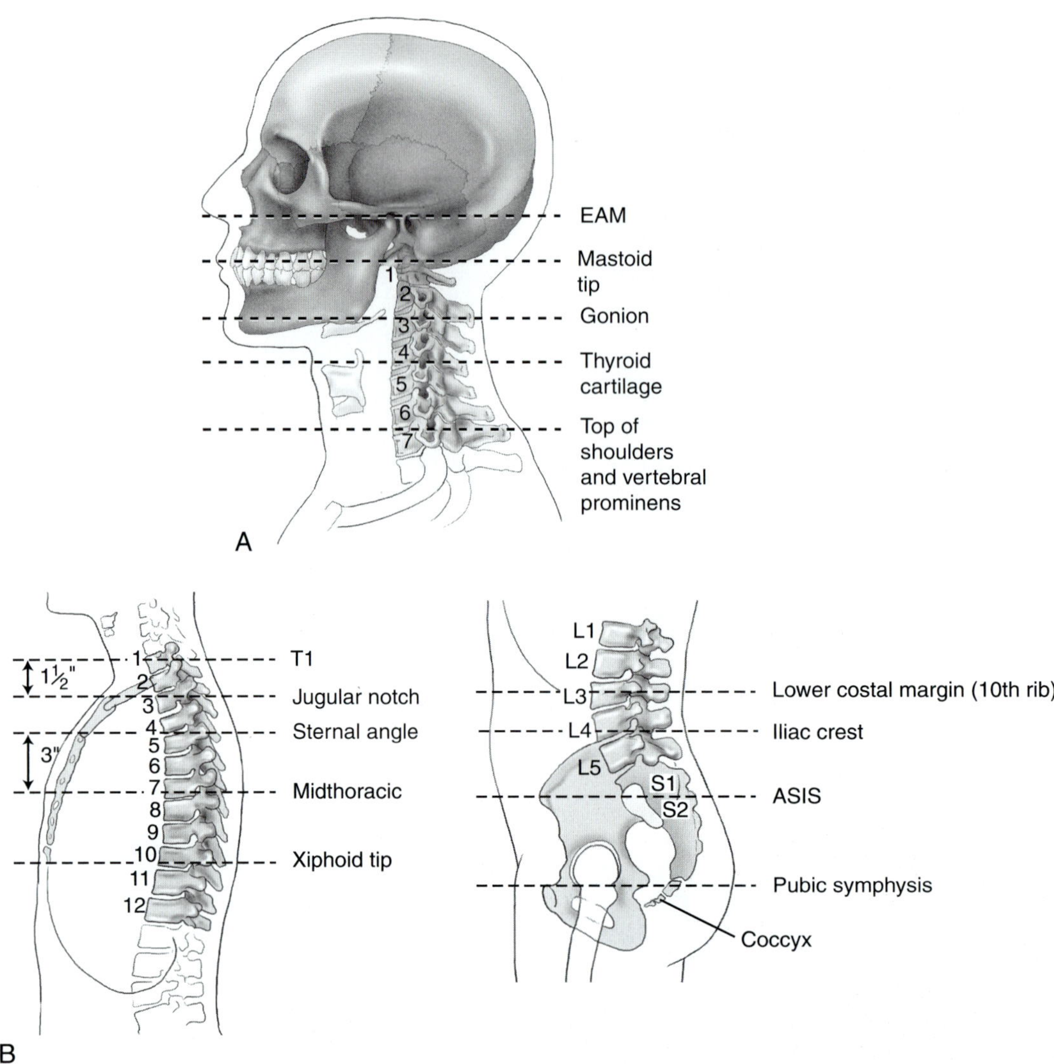

FIGURE 53.21 Palpable landmarks. **(A)** For cervical spine positioning. **(B)** For spine positioning. (From Long BW, Frank ED, Ehrlich RA: *Radiography essentials for limited practice*, ed 6, St. Louis, 2021, Elsevier.)

- *IR:* Positioned by department protocol for proper anatomy orientation; CR plate 18 × 24 cm; portrait orientation.
- *Grid and SID:* Grid is used. SID 40 inches minimum
- *Collimation:* Adjust the light field to 2.5 cm on all sides of the anatomy. Place anatomical marker in the light field on the lateral side of the anatomy.
- *Patient instructions:* Do not move.

Positioning and Radiographic Examination of the Cervical Spine

Two images are needed to illustrate the entire cervical spine in the AP projection. The AP axial projection of the lower cervical spine demonstrates C3 through C7, but the lower jaw and teeth are superimposed over the atlas and axis. To demonstrate the upper cervical vertebrae, a second AP projection is taken through the open mouth. This projection is sometimes referred to as the AP *open-mouth* or the *odontoid* projection.

For the lateral projection, the inferior margin of the IR must be below the level of the upper surface of the shoulder to demonstrate all of C7. This results in a large **object-to-image distance (OID)**. To minimize magnification and improve detail, a 72-inch SID is used with a small focal spot.

Prior to cervical spine imaging, the patient must remove eyeglasses, earrings, hairpins, necklaces, and any clothing with fasteners that may be within the radiation field. Dentures and hearing aids should also be removed.

Routine Examination of the Cervical Spine

The routine examination of the cervical spine includes the AP axial (lower cervical), AP (upper cervical), and lateral projections.

AP Axial Projection of the Lower Cervical Spine

- *Body and part position:* Seated, standing, or supine. Midsagittal plane of both body and head are aligned perpendicular to center of IR, with patient facing the x-ray tube. The head is adjusted so that a line between mental point and base of skull forms an angle of 15 degrees with the horizontal plane. If desired position cannot be attained in this way, a radiolucent wedge sponge is placed under/behind head for stability (Figure 53.22).
- *CR:* Centered to IR at an angle of 15 degrees cephalad through thyroid cartilage.

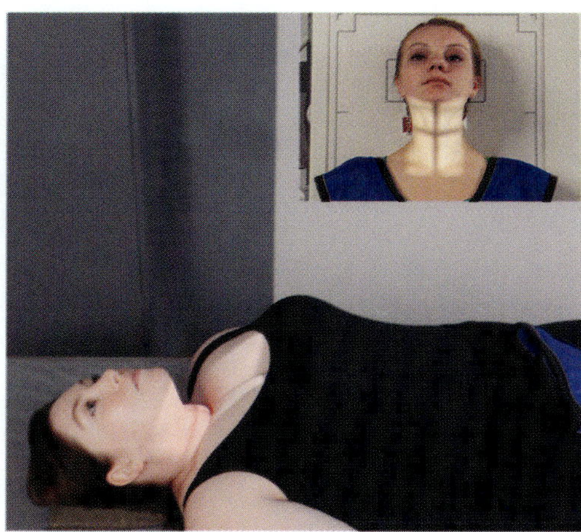

FIGURE 53.22 Cervical spine. Position for AP Axial projection. (From Lampignano J, Ehrlich RA: *Bontrager's textbook of radiographic positioning and related anatomy*, ed 10, St. Louis, 2021, Mosby.)

- *Patient instructions:* Do not breathe during the exposure.
- *Structures seen:* Vertebrae C3-T2, including bodies, articular pillars, and intervertebral disk spaces.

AP Projection Open Mouth Technique (Upper Cervical Spine).

- *Body and part position:* Seated, standing, or supine. Patient faces the x-ray tube with midsagittal plane of both body and head are aligned perpendicular to center of IR. Head is adjusted so that a line between mental lower surface of upper teeth (occlusal plane) and base of skull is parallel to horizontal plane.
- *CR:* Perpendicular to center of IR, through midpoint of open mouth.
- *Patient Instructions:* Open mouth as wide as possible. Do not breathe during the exposure.
- *Structures seen:* Lateral masses and transverse processes of atlas, dens, and upper half of body of axis, seen between upper and lower teeth.

Lateral Projection (Grandy Method).

- *SID:* 60 to 72 inches is recommended due to the increased OID
- *Body and part position:* Seated or standing. Midsagittal planes of body and head are parallel to IR with infraorbital line parallel to floor. Shoulders must be relaxed and depressed. IR is positioned so that the upper margin is about 1 inch above the external auditory meatus (EAM).
- *CR:* Perpendicular to center of IR through body of C4.
- *Patient instructions:* Do not breathe during the exposure.
- *Structures seen:* All seven cervical vertebrae and soft tissues of anterior neck, including spinal alignment, bodies, disk spaces, spinous processes, and zygapophyseal joints.

Supplemental Projections of the Cervical Spine

If the patient is unable to perform the routine projections for the cervical spine due to trauma, supplemental projections may be performed. Supplemental projections utilize modified positioning to obtain the needed projections.

Lateral Projection in Flexion and Extension. Lateral projections with cervical spine in flexion and extension are performed to evaluate intersegmental stability.

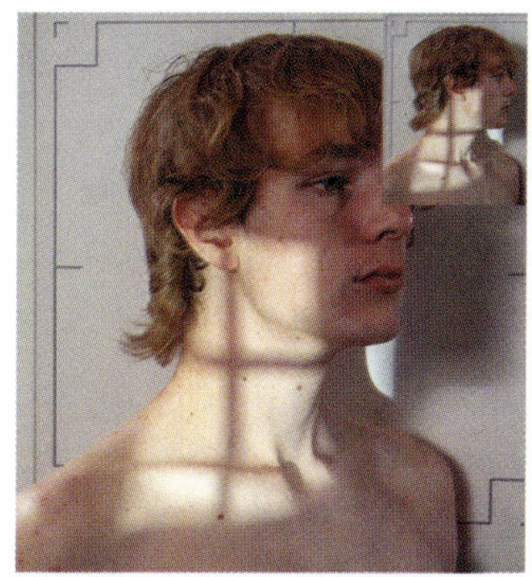

FIGURE 53.23 Cervical spine. Position for AP oblique projection. (From Lampignano J, Ehrlich RA: *Bontrager's textbook of radiographic positioning and related anatomy*, ed 10, St. Louis, 2021, Mosby.)

- *IR:* CR plate 24 × 30 cm, portrait orientation.
- *SID:* 60 to 72 inches is recommended due to the increased OID.
- *Body and part position:*
  - *Position for flexion:* Patient is positioned as for routine lateral projection. Patient is then instructed to tuck chin close to neck and then to flex neck, attempting to look at a spot midsternum.
  - *Position for extension:* Patient is positioned as for routine lateral projection. Patient is then instructed to extend neck, looking at a spot on ceiling directly above head.
- *CR:* Perpendicular to center of IR through body of C4.
- *Structures seen:* All seven cervical vertebrae and soft tissues of anterior neck, including spinal alignment, bodies, disk spaces, spinous processes, and zygapophyseal joints. Head tilted face down in flexion and tilted face up in extension.

Oblique Projections. Bilateral oblique projections are taken. Patient may be positioned PA (right and left anterior oblique) or AP (right and left posterior oblique). They may be done recumbent, with a 40-inch SID, or upright, with either a 40-inch or 72-inch SID.

- *SID:* SID 60 to 72 inches is recommended due to the increased OID.
- *Body and part position:* Seated, standing, or recumbent. Coronal plane of the body forms an angle of 45 degrees with plane of IR. Sagittal plane of skull is perpendicular to coronal plane of body. Have patient elevate and, if necessary, protrude the chin so that the mandible does not overlap the spine (Figure 53.23).
- *CR:*
  - *AP obliques:* Angled 15 degrees cephalad to center of IR through body of C4.
  - *PA obliques:* Angled 15 degrees caudad to center of IR through body of C4.
- *Structures seen:* AP obliques demonstrate intervertebral foramina on side farthest from IR. PA obliques demonstrate intervertebral foramina on side nearest IR.

Lateral Projection of Cervicothoracic Region. The lateral projection of the cervicothoracic region is commonly called the swimmer's lateral projection. It is used when routine lateral projections of either the cervical or the thoracic spine fail to demonstrate this area adequately. The shoulder positions create a small window between the shoulders, and the cervicothoracic spine is projected into this relatively open area.

- *IR:* CR plate 24 × 30 cm, portrait orientation.
- *Body and part position:* Seated, standing, or recumbent. Sagittal planes of body and head are parallel to IR. Arm nearest IR is raised above the head, and shoulder is rounded anteriorly. Opposite shoulder is depressed and slightly posterior.
- *CR:* Perpendicular to IR at C7-T1 interspace. CR enters at level of C7 spinous process.
- *Structures seen:* Vertebrae C6-T3 (C5-T5 with larger IR) in lateral projection without significant rotation. Bodies, disk spaces, spinous processes, and zygapophyseal joints are demonstrated between shoulders.

Positioning and Radiographic Examination of the Thoracic Spine

There is significant variation in tissue density between the extreme ends of the thoracic spine. Near the neck, there is much less tissue to penetrate than at the level of T12 in the upper abdominal region. Therefore, the anode heel effect should be utilized. For recumbent studies, the patient should be instructed to lie on the table with the head toward the anode end of the x-ray tube.

In the lateral projection, the density variation is reversed. The proximal thoracic spine is more difficult to penetrate due to the bone and muscle mass of the shoulders. The inferior portion is easily penetrated because its mass is largely air-containing lung. The first three thoracic vertebrae are rarely seen well on the lateral projection. When the upper thoracic vertebrae are the area of clinical interest, it is customary to include the swimmer's lateral projection of the cervicothoracic region.

For this examination, the patient should undress down to the waist and don a gown that opens in the back. This will facilitate visualization and palpation of the spine. Jewelry should be removed.

The routine examination of the thoracic spine includes the AP and lateral projections.

AP Projection

- *IR:* CR plate 35 × 43 cm, portrait orientation.
- *Body and part position:* Seated, standing, or supine. Midsagittal plane of body is perpendicular to IR and centered on it, with patient facing the x-ray. Superior border is aligned 1.5 to 2 inches above the shoulders. When patient is supine, it is helpful to bolster the knees. When patient is standing, feet should be shoulder width apart and patient's back should be firmly against IR holder.
- *CR:* Perpendicular to center IR at T7. This point is midline at the approximate midpoint of sternum.
- *Patient instructions:* Suspend breathing on expiration.
- *Structures seen:* All 12 thoracic vertebrae, particularly the bodies, disk spaces, and transverse processes. C7 and at least a portion of L1 are usually also seen.

Lateral Projection

- *IR:* CR plate 35 × 43 cm, portrait orientation.
- *Body and part position:* Seated, standing, or supine. Sagittal plane of body is parallel to IR. Center the posterior half of the thorax to the midline of the IR. Arms should be elevated overhead or anterior to the body with shoulders rounded anteriorly. The superior border of the IR is aligned 1.5 to 2 inches above the shoulders. The entire length of thoracic spine should be parallel to IR. When patient is recumbent, it is helpful to support the knees with a sponge under the waist (Figure 53.24).
- *CR:* Perpendicular to center IR at T7. CR enters at inferior angle of scapula through middle of posterior half of thorax.
- *Patient instructions:* Perform shallow breathing during exposure.
- *Structures seen:* T3 through T12 with blurring of ribs and lung markings when breathing technique is used.

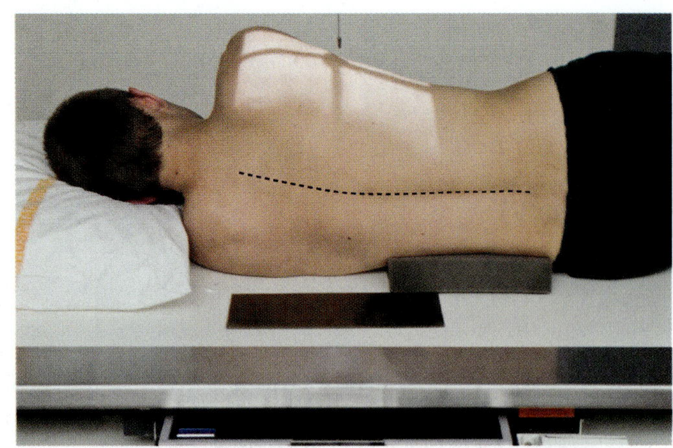

FIGURE 53.24 Thoracic spine. Position for lateral projection. (From Lampignano J, Ehrlich RA: *Bontrager's textbook of radiographic positioning and related anatomy*, ed 10, St. Louis, 2021, Mosby.)

Positioning and Radiographic Examination of the Lumbar Spine

Patients should remove outer clothing from the torso for lumbar spine imaging and don a gown opening in the back. Female patients must remove under garments.

Routine Examination of the Lumbar Spine

The routine examination of the lumbar spine includes AP or PA and lateral projections.

AP and PA Projection.

- *IR:* CR plate 35 × 43 cm, portrait orientation.
- *Body and part position:* Standing or supine.
  - *AP:* Patient faces the x-ray with midsagittal plane of body perpendicular to IR and centered on it. When patient is supine, knees are flexed and may be supported with a bolster. When patient is standing, feet should be shoulder-width apart and patient's back should be firmly against IR holder.
  - *PA:* Patient stands facing IR or lies prone, with midsagittal plane perpendicular to IR and centered to it.
- *CR:* Perpendicular to center IR at L4 and midline at the level of iliac crest.
- *Patient instructions:* Suspend breathing on expiration.
- *Structures seen:* All five lumbar vertebrae, intervertebral disk spaces, proximal portion of the sacrum, and sacroiliac SI joints. This projection demonstrates the bodies, disk spaces, and transverse processes. The pedicles are seen on end.

Lateral Projection.

- *IR, CR, and patient instructions:* Same as the AP projection.
- *Body and part position:* Standing or supine.
  - *Supine:* Spine is parallel to center of Bucky with arms anterior to body. Radiolucent sponges may be used to elevate waist to align the spine. Knees are flexed. A pad between knees helps keep pelvis lateral and maintains lateral position of the spine (Figure 53.25).
  - *Upright:* Feet are shoulder-width apart, and torso is stabilized against upright IR. Arms are crossed over chest with hands supported on shoulders.
- *Structures seen:* All five lumbar vertebrae and superior half of sacrum, including intervertebral foramina, spinous processes and profile of the bodies, and intervertebral disk spaces.

Supplemental Projections of the Lumbar Spine

If the patient is unable to perform the routine projections of the lumbar spine due to trauma, supplemental projections may be performed. Supplemental projections utilize modified positioning to obtain the needed projections.

AP Oblique Projection. Bilateral oblique projections are taken. AP obliques (right posterior oblique [RPO] and left posterior oblique [LPO] positions), rather than PA obliques, are most common because they demonstrate the pars interarticularis and the zygopophyseal joints of the side nearest the IR, providing better detail.

- *IR:* CR plate 35 × 43 cm, portrait orientation.
- *Body and part position:* Standing or supine. Sagittal plane is aligned 45 degrees to IR.
  - *Supine:* From supine position, patient is rotated 45 degrees toward the side being imaged. Position may be supported by a large 45-degree radiolucent sponge. The entire spine is rotated the same amount so there is no torsion (twist) of the spine (Figure 53.26A).
  - *Upright*: From AP position, patient is rotated 45 degrees toward the side being imaged. Feet are shoulder-width apart, and torso is stabilized against upright IR.
- *CR:* Perpendicular to center IR at L3. CR enters a point 2 inches medial to ASIS farthest from IR and 1.5 inches superior to iliac crest.
- *Patient instructions:* Suspend breathing on expiration.
- *Structures seen:* All five lumbar vertebrae and upper portion of the sacrum, including zygapophyseal joints and pars interarticularis on side nearest the IR.

Lateral Projection of L5-S1 Lumbosacral Junction. If there is poor visualization of the lumbosacral junction in the routine lateral projection, a collimated image of the area is recommended. This projection is important because this junction is a common site of chronic low back pain. Although this projection may be taken with the patient upright, the recumbent position produces superior results.

- *Body and part position:* Same as routine lateral lumbar projection, with care taken that spine is parallel to IR (Figure 53.26B).
- *CR:* Perpendicular to center IR through lumbosacral junction. This centering point is 2 inches posterior to ASIS and 1.5 inches inferior to iliac crest on coronal line midway between ASIS and posterior prominence of sacrum. When spine cannot be aligned, angle 5 degrees for males and 8 degrees for females.
- *Patient instructions:* Suspend breathing on expiration.
- *Structures seen:* The lower one or two lumbar vertebrae, the upper sacrum, and an open lumbosacral junction.

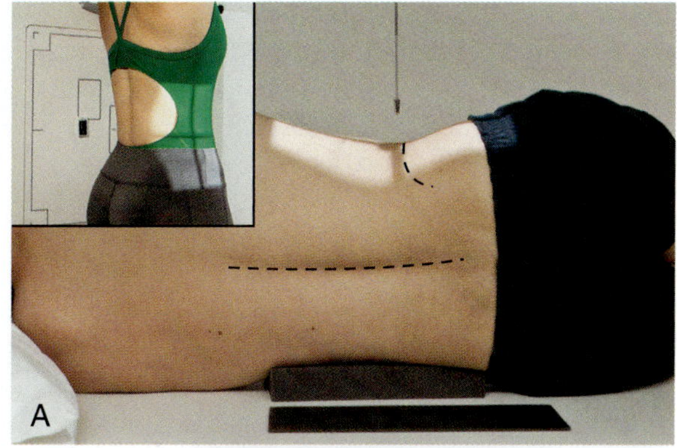

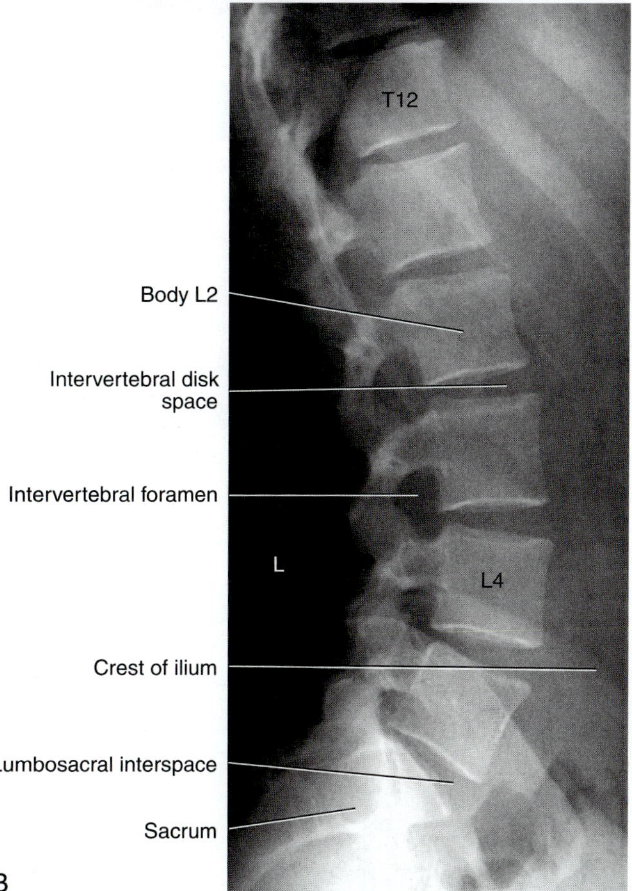

FIGURE 53.25 Lumbar spine. **(A)** Position for lateral projection. **(B)** Lateral projection. (A, from Lampignano J, Ehrlich RA: *Bontrager's textbook of radiographic positioning and related anatomy*, ed 10, St. Louis, 2021, Mosby. B, from Long BW, Frank ED, Ehrlich RA: *radiography essentials for limited practice*, ed 6, St. Louis, 2021, Elsevier.)

Positioning and Radiographic Examination of the Lumbar Spine and Sacroiliac Joints

The examinations of the lumbar spine and sacroiliac (SI) joints are most commonly performed in the table Bucky.

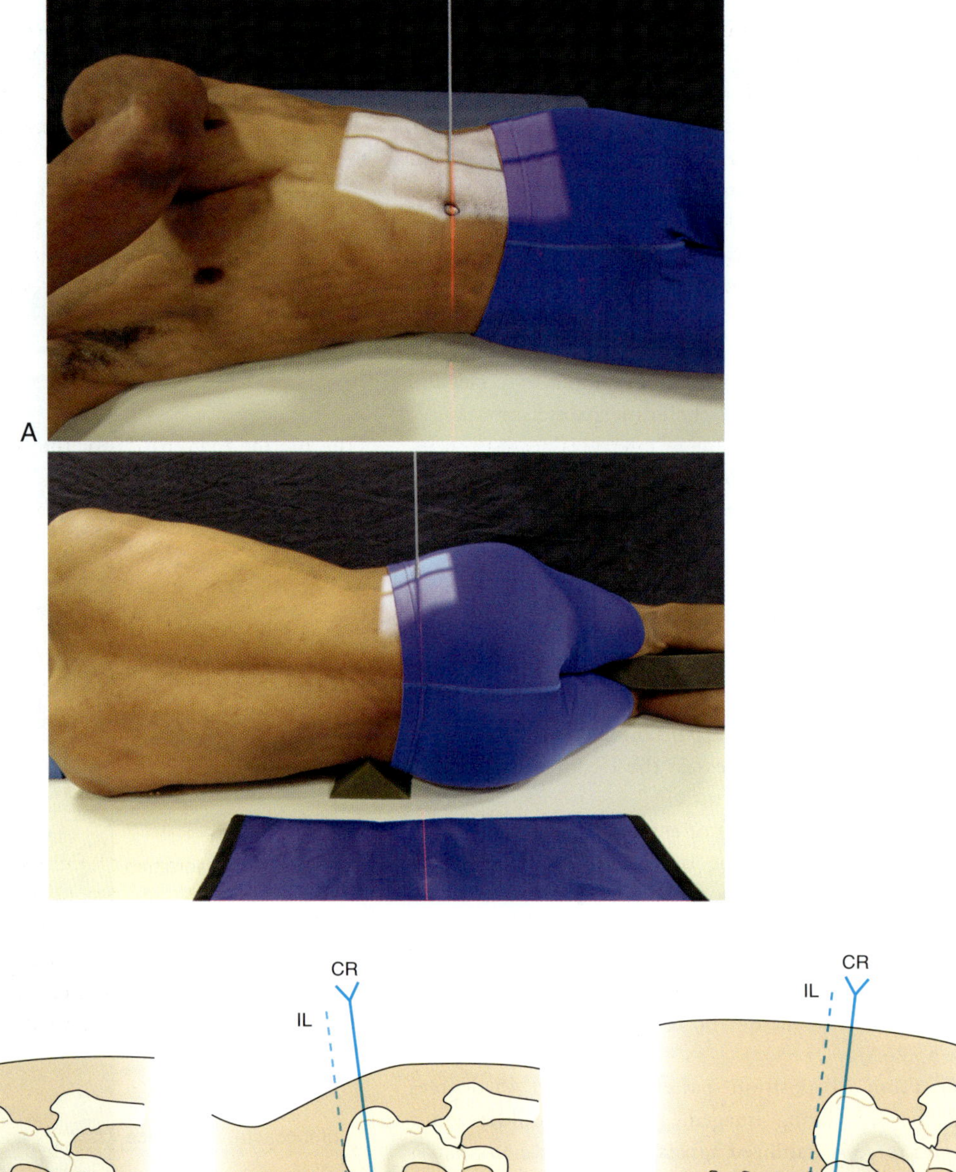

FIGURE 53.26 Lumbar spine. **(A)** Position for AP oblique (RPO) projection. **(B)** Position for lateral projection of L5-S1 lumbosacral junction. (A, from Long BW, Rollins JH, Smith BJ: *Merrill's atlas of radiographic positioning and procedures*, ed 14, St. Louis, 2020, Mosby. B, in Long BW, Rollins JH, Smith BJ: *Merrill's atlas of radiographic positioning and procedures*, ed 14, St. Louis, 2020, Mosby; modified from Francis C: Method improves consistency in L5–S1 joint space films, *Radiol Technol* 63:302, 1992.)

AP Axial Projection of Lumbosacral Junction and Sacroiliac Joints

Because of the sacral base angle, the lumbosacral junction is not well seen on the routine AP projection of the lumbar spine. The AP axial projection directs the CR parallel to the sacral base. This projection is also useful for demonstration of the SI joints.

- *Body position:* Supine, same as routine recumbent lumbar spine, with knees flexed and supported.
- *CR:* Angled 30 degrees cephalad for males and 35 degrees for females. CR is directed to center of IR through lumbosacral junction. CR enters in midline, 1 inch inferior to the ASIS.
- *Structures seen:* Open lumbosacral junction, sacral alae, and SI joints.

Sacroiliac Joints

The routine examination of the SI joints includes the AP oblique projections. The AP axial projection of the lumbosacral junction and the SI joints may also be included.

- *Body and part position:* Recumbent.
    - *AP obliques (RPO, LPO positions):* From supine position, body is rotated so that the coronal plane is aligned at an angle of 25 to 30 degrees to IR. The side of interest is elevated, farthest from IR. Position may be supported by a radiolucent sponge under hip and lumbar area of elevated side. The entire spine is rotated the same amount so that there is no torsion of the spine.
    - *PA obliques (RPO, LPO positions):* From prone position, body is rotated so that the coronal plane is aligned at an angle of 25 to 30 degrees to IR. The side of interest is nearest the IR. Position may be supported by a radiolucent sponge under hip on opposite side. The entire spine is rotated the same amount so that there is no torsion of the spine.
- *CR:*
    - *AP obliques:* Perpendicular to center of IR through point 1 inch medial to ASIS farthest from IR.
    - *PA obliques:* Perpendicular to center of IR through point 1 inch medial to ASIS nearest the IR.
- *Patient instructions:* Suspend breathing on expiration.
- *Structures seen:*
    - *AP obliques:* SI joint farthest from IR.
    - *PA obliques:* SI joint nearest IR.

Positioning and Radiographic Examination of the Sacrum

The routine examination of the sacrum includes the AP axial and lateral projections. Patient should be instructed to stop breathing during the exposure.

AP Axial Projection

- *IR:* CR plate 24 × 30 cm, portrait orientation.
- *Body and part position:* Supine or recumbent. Midsagittal plane is perpendicular to IR and centered to it. Knees are flexed and supported with a bolster, if needed (Figure 53.27).
- *CR:* Angled 15 degrees cephalad to enter body at midline, 1 inch inferior to the ASIS.
- *Structures seen:* Entire sacrum and SI joints.

Lateral Projection

- *IR:* Same as the AP axial projection.
- *Body and part position:* Recumbent. Sagittal plane is parallel to IR. Spine is aligned parallel to center of Bucky with arms anterior to body. Radiolucent sponges may be used to elevate waist or hips to align the spine. Knees are flexed. A pad between knees helps maintain lateral positions of pelvis and spine.
- *CR:* Perpendicular to center of IR through center of sacrum. CR enters a point 3.5 inches posterior to ASIS.
- *Structures seen:* Entire sacrum and lumbosacral junction. Coccyx is sometimes seen.

Positioning and Radiographic Examination of the Coccyx

The routine examination of the coccyx includes the AP axial and lateral projections.

AP Axial Projection

- *Body and part position:* Recumbent. Coronal plane is parallel to IR with patient facing the x-ray tube. Midsagittal pane is centered to midline of Bucky. Knees are flexed and supported with a bolster, if needed.
- *CR:* Angled 10 degrees caudad to enter body at midline, 1 inch inferior to the ASIS.
- *Structures seen:* Entire coccyx and distal portion of sacrum.

Lateral Projection

- *Body and part position:* Recumbent. Sagittal plane is parallel to IR. Knees are flexed and may be supported by a sponge.
- *CR:* Perpendicular to center of IR through center of coccyx. CR enters a point 2 inches inferior to ASIS.
- *Patient instruction:* Stop breathing during the exposure.
- *Structures seen:* Entire coccyx and distal portion of sacrum.

Positioning and Radiographic Examination of the Full Spine

It is sometimes desirable to demonstrate the entire spine in one image. This is useful for the evaluation of scoliosis. Some chiropractic physicians also use it for the evaluation of the entire spine with the patient weight bearing. The routine examination of the full spine includes the PA only, however, lateral projections may be performed for abnormal spinal curvatures.

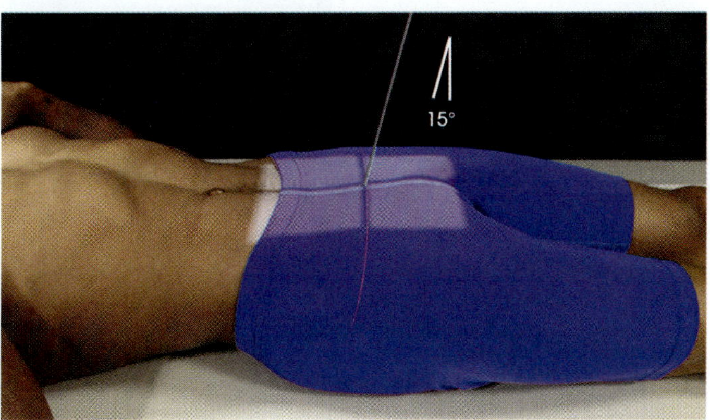

FIGURE 53.27 Sacrum. Position for AP axial projection. (From Long BW, Rollins JH, Smith BJ: *Merrill's atlas of radiographic positioning and procedures*, ed 14, St. Louis, 2020, Mosby.)

PA Projection

- *IR:* CR plate 14 × 36 cm, portrait orientation.
- *SID:* SID 60 inches minimum
- *Body position:* Standing. Height of grid and IR is adjusted to include area from top of patient's ears to level of greater trochanters. Head is positioned as for AP axial projection of upper cervical spine, with neck extended slightly to allow for angulation of diverging x-ray beam at upper extreme of exposure field.
- *CR:* Perpendicular to center of IR, entering at midline approximately at level of xiphoid process.
- *Patient instructions:* Stop breathing during the exposure.
- *Structures seen:* Portion of mandible, entire spine, portion of pelvis.

Lateral Projection

- *IR, SID, CR, and patient instructions:* Same as with full spine.
- *Body position:* Same as for upright lateral projection of thoracic spine. Shoulders are rounded anteriorly, and arms are extended anterior to body and supported
- *Structures seen:* Portion of mandible and skull, entire spine, portion of pelvis.

Pathology

Radiographic examination of the spine is critical for evaluating pathology.

Congenital Abnormalities

The spine is a common site for congenital abnormalities and deformities. A transitional vertebra occurs when a vertebra of one region takes on features of the adjacent region. Sacralization of L5 occurs when one or both spinous processes of L5 become fused to the sacrum. When the first sacral segment fails to fuse with the remainder of the sacrum, this is known as lumbarization.

Another congenital deformity of the spine is spina bifida, which results when the posterior portions of the neural arches fail to close during the embryo's development.

Spinal Fractures

Spinal fractures typically are the result of trauma. Fractures of vertebral bodies are often compression fractures with anterior wedging. Pathologic fractures are fractures that occur with little or no trauma, the bones are weakened by disease processes. Pathologic compression fractures of the thoracic spine caused by osteoporosis are often seen in older women.

Spondylosis, Spondylitis, Spondylolysis, Spondylolisthesis, and Spondyloschisis

All of these refer to different conditions, but the words look and sound very much alike. They all have the same root, *spondylo-*, which simply means "vertebra."

- *Spondylosis:* Fixation or fusion of vertebrae.
- *Spondylitis:* Often applies specifically to tuberculosis disease of the vertebrae, which is also called *Potts disease.* Spondylitis is also seen with rheumatoid arthritis.
- *Spondylolysis:* The breakdown of the structure of the bone, which occurs with osteoporosis, with some metastatic lesions, and other conditions that cause atrophy and bony destruction.
- *Spondylolisthesis:* Anterior displacement of one vertebra on another. It occurs most often at the lumbosacral joint and is usually caused by a defect or a fracture of the pars interarticularis or the pedicle.
- *Spondyloschisis:* A congenital fissure (split or cleft) in the neural arch (e.g., spina bifida occulta).

Disk Pathology

The pulpy center of intervertebral disks is normally a gel-like, semiliquid material. With the pressure of spinal movement, Its mass shifts to change the shape of the disk. With advancing age and repeated minor trauma to the spine, the disks tend to degenerate. The nucleus may dry out and become atrophied, which causes narrowing of the disk space. Without adequate cushioning, the joint becomes inflamed, and the surrounding bony structures show signs of degeneration. This condition is known as *degenerative disk disease (DDD)* and is usually associated with osteoarthritis.

Disk herniation or herniated nucleus pulposus (HNP) is the condition often called "slipped disk." The annulus fibrosus ruptures, and the nucleus is forced into the area posterior to the disk space.

BONY THORAX, CHEST, AND ABDOMEN

Radiographic imaging of the chest is the most common radiographic procedure (Procedure 53.1). Imaging of the chest and abdomen are performed to visualize structures and organs of the chest and abdomen.

The radiographic examinations of the thorax and abdomen typically require a 35 × 43 cm IR. Although the thorax and abdomen may have a similar thickness, imaging requires the application of different technical factors: high kVp for the large variations in the chest, moderate kVp to demonstrate the minor differences in tissue densities in the abdomen, and low kVp for the thin bones of the thoracic cage.

For the projections of the bony thorax, chest, and abdomen, use the following unless otherwise indicated:

- *IR:* Positioned by department protocol for proper anatomy orientation; CR plate 35 × 43 cm; portrait orientation.
- *Grid and SID:* Grid is used. SID 40 inches minimum.
- *Collimation:* Adjust the light field to 2.5 cm on all sides of the anatomy. Place anatomical marker in the light field on the lateral side of the anatomy.
- *Patient instructions:* Stop breathing on second deep inspiration.

Body Habitus

Accurate imaging of the chest and abdomen requires an awareness of body habitus—the general shape of the patient's body. Organs vary significantly in size, shape, and location according to body types. The four basic types of body habitus are as follows(Figure 53.28):

- *Sthenic:* Considered the be average; about 50% of the population has this body type.
- *Hyposthenic:* Thought of as slender; about 35% of the population has this type.
- *Asthenic:* Considered very slender; about 10% of the population has this body type.
- *Hypersthenic:* Considered massive and stocky; about 5% of the population has this body type.

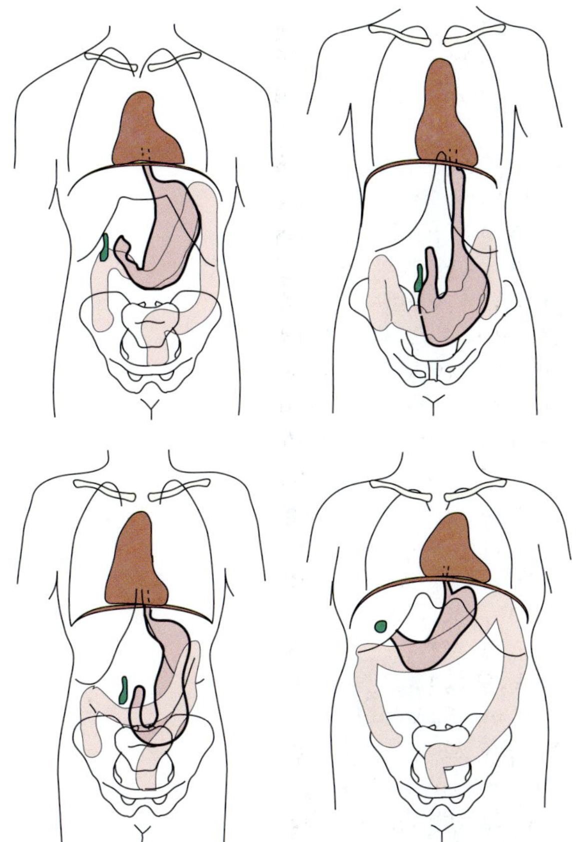

FIGURE 53.28 Four types of body habitus. (From Long BW, Rollins JH, Smith BJ: *Merrill's atlas of radiographic positioning and procedures*, ed 14, St. Louis, 2020, Mosby.)

Positioning and Radiographic Examinations of the Chest

Chest radiography is done at 72 inches SID to minimize magnification of the heart. Exposures of the chest are made on inspiration to expand the lung fields. It is good practice to have patients take two deep inspirations, holding their breath in on the second inspiration. The greater the inspiration, the greater the depression of the diaphragm. Evidence of full inspiration is seen on a chest image when 10 ribs can be counted superior to the diaphragm. In preparation for chest examinations, the patient is instructed to remove all clothing and jewelry from the waist up and to don a gown that opens in the back.

Routine Examination of the Chest

The routine examination of the chest includes the PA and left lateral projections. When a patient is unable to stand for the PA projection, the AP projection can be substituted.

- *SID:* 72 inches if possible.
- *Body and part position:* Standing, facing IR holder.
  - *PA:* Anterior surface of the chest is against upright Bucky with coronal plane parallel to IR. The backs of hands are placed on hips, and shoulders are rotated anteriorly. This arm position rotates the scapulae out of the lung fields. IR is aligned 1.5 to 2 inches above the spinous process of C7 (Figure 53.29).
  - *AP:* Patient supine or seated (typically in a wheelchair) with arms at side. IR is aligned so that upper margins are 1.5 to 2 inches above level of shoulders.
  - *Lateral:* Both arms are raised overhead, with the patient grasping opposite elbows. Left side of body is in contact with IR, and midcoronal plane is perpendicular to center of IR. IR is unchanged from PA projection (Figure 53.30).
- *CR:*
  - *PA:* Perpendicular to center of IR, entering at midline approximately at level of T7, which corresponds to the level of the inferior angle of the scapulae.
  - *AP:* Perpendicular to center of IR. Center point should be on the midsagittal plane at a level 3 inches below the jugular notch.
  - *Lateral:* Perpendicular to center of IR. Center point should be on the midcoronal plane at the level of T7.
- *Patient instruction:* Stop breathing on second deep inspiration.
- *Structures seen:* Heart, lungs, and mediastinum. No rotation of the sternoclavicular joints on the PA projection. Superimposition of the posterior ribs, indicating no rotation, on the lateral projection.

Supplemental Projections of the Chest

If the patient cannot perform the typical projections for the chest, supplemental projections may be performed due to trauma or pathology. Supplemental projections utilize modified positioning to obtain the needed projections.

AP or PA Projection (Lateral Decubitus Position)

- *SID and patient instructions:* Same as the routine examination of the chest.
- *Body and part position:* Recumbent, lying on side of interest. Midsagittal plane of chest horizontal. Chest elevated 2 to 3 inches on a radiolucent pad. Anterior or posterior surface of chest against a vertical grid device.
- *CR:* Horizontal and perpendicular to center of IR. Center point should midsagittal and at the level of T7.
- *Structures seen:* Heart, lungs, and mediastinum. Sternoclavicular joints equidistant from spine, which indicates no rotation. Any free fluid will be demonstrated along the independent chest wall.

Chest (Lung Apices)

The lungs' apical zone (apices) is one of the four chest radiographic zones and an important location for missed diagnoses when reporting a PA chest. The other three areas are behind the heart, below the diaphragm, and the bones and soft tissues.

AP Axial Projection (Lordotic Position).

- *SID and patient instructions:* Same as the routine examination of the chest.
- *Body and part position:* Standing. Patient stands facing the x-ray tube, 8 to 12 inches in front of upright Bucky; patient then arches back and places shoulders against Bucky. Sagittal plane is perpendicular to IR. Backs of hands are placed on hips, and shoulders are rotated anteriorly, which rotates the scapulae out of the lung fields. IR is aligned so that upper margin is 3 inches above border of shoulder.
- *CR:* Perpendicular to center of IR. Center point should be midsagittal and at the level of the sternum.
- *Structures seen:* Apices of both lungs, free of superimposition by the clavicles.

Positioning and Radiographic Examination of the Ribs

Rib studies may be done with the patient recumbent or upright. Upright positions are usually most comfortable for patients with rib injuries.

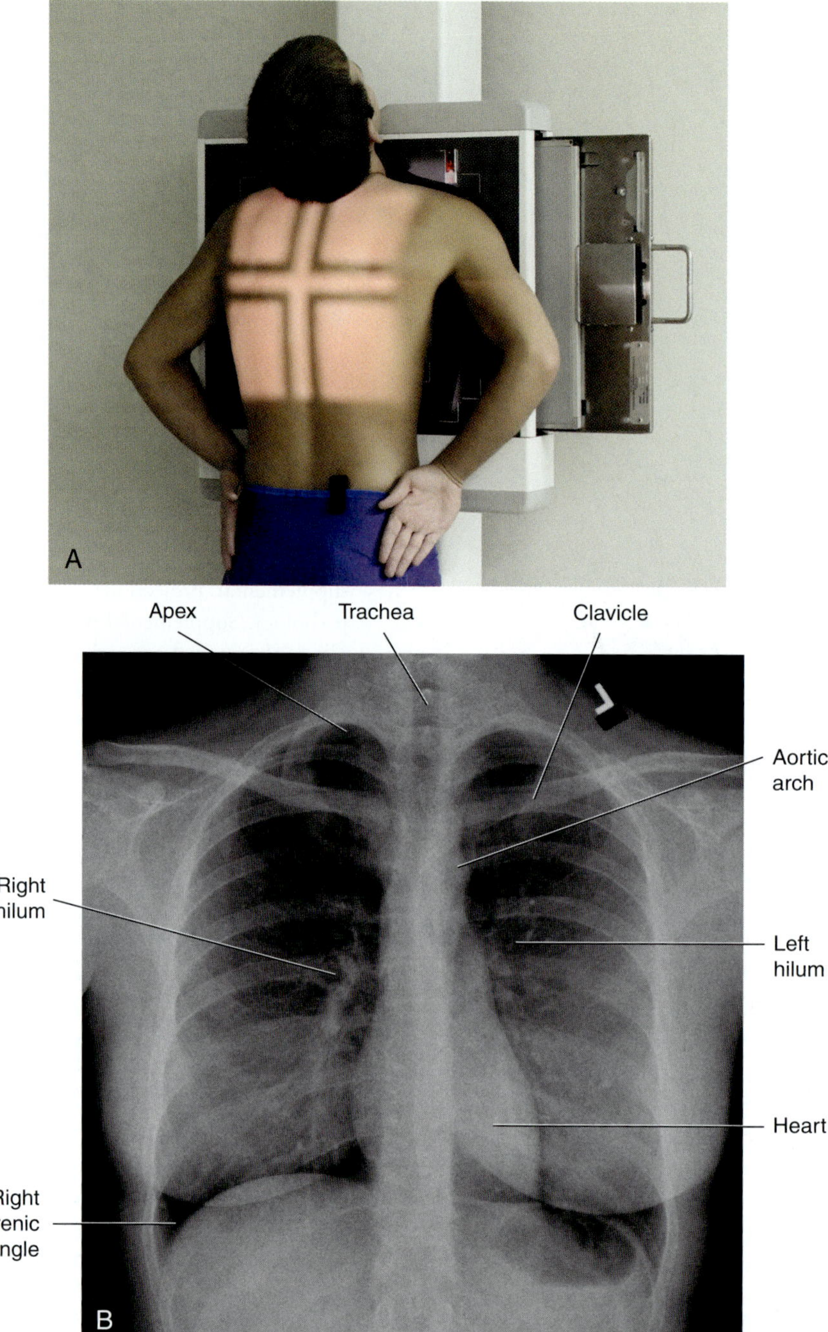

FIGURE 53.29 Chest. **(A)** Position for PA projection. **(B)** PA projection. (A, from Long BW, Rollins JH, Smith BJ: *Merrill's atlas of radiographic positioning and procedures*, ed 14, St. Louis, 2020, Mosby. B, from Long BW, Frank ED, Ehrlich RA: *Radiography essentials for limited practice*, ed 6, St. Louis, 2021, Elsevier.)

Ribs are named both by anatomic location and in relation to the diaphragm. The upper ribs are cephalad to the diaphragm, and the lower ribs are below the diaphragm. The anterior aspects of the ribs are *anterior ribs,* and the posterior aspects are *posterior ribs.* The lateral aspects are *axillary ribs* because they are located within or near the axillary region.

A rib examination usually consists of AP or PA and oblique projections. The ribs nearest the IR are the area of interest. It is customary to perform AP projections when the area of clinical interest is primarily posterior and to perform PA projections for greater detail of the anterior ribs. AP or PA projections demonstrate the anterior and posterior portions of the ribs in the coronal plane. Oblique projections are used to demonstrate the axillary portions of the ribs. Lateral projections are not useful because they result in the superimposition of the right and left ribs. For posterior ribs, RPO is used for right ribs, and the left posterior oblique (LPO) is used for left ribs. The RAO is used for the left ribs, and the LAO is used for the right ribs.

Upper Posterior Ribs: AP and AP Oblique Projections

- *Body and part position:* Standing or recumbent.
  - *AP:* Supine on table or upright with posterior surface of chest against upright Bucky. Coronal plane is parallel to IR. Upper margin of IR is 1.5 to 2 inches above level of spinous process of C7.

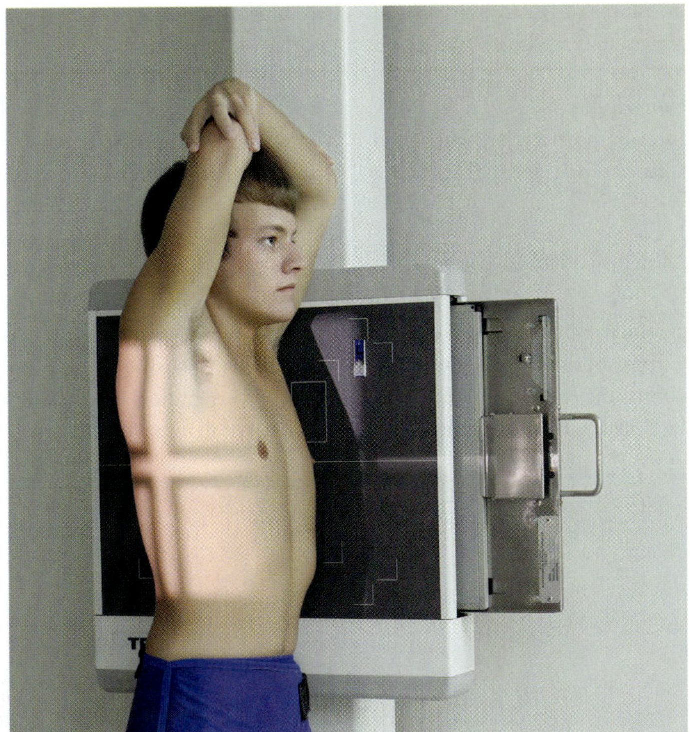

FIGURE 53.30 Chest. Position for lateral projection. (From Long BW, Rollins JH, Smith BJ: *Merrill's atlas of radiographic positioning and procedures*, ed 14, St. Louis, 2020, Mosby.)

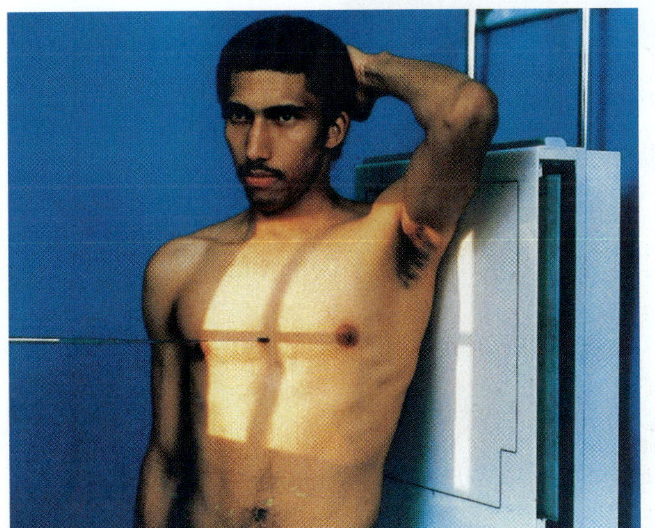

FIGURE 53.31 Ribs. Position for AP oblique projection. (From Long BW, Rollins JH, Smith BJ: *Merrill's atlas of radiographic positioning and procedures*, ed 14, St. Louis, 2020, Mosby.)

- *AP oblique:* RPO position for right ribs or LPO position for left ribs. Coronal plane forms a 45-degree angle with IR plane. Upper margin of IR is 1.5 to 2 inches above level of spinous process of C7 (Figure 53.31).
- *CR:*
  - *AP:* Perpendicular to center of IR. Center point should be in midclavicular line at approximate level of axillary fold.
  - *AP oblique:* Perpendicular to center of IR. CR enters at a point midline of anterior surface at approximate level of axillary fold.
- Patient instruction: Stop breathing.
- Structures seen: Ribs 1 to 10. Posterior portions are best seen on AP projection; axillary portions are best seen on oblique projection.

Upper Anterior Ribs: PA and PA Oblique Projections

- *Body and part position:* Standing or recumbent.
  - *PA:* Supine on table or upright with anterior surface of chest against upright Bucky. Coronal plane is parallel to IR. Upper margin of IR is 1.5 to 2 inches above level of spinous process of C7.
  - *PA oblique:* RAO position for right ribs or LAO position for right ribs. Coronal plane forms a 45-degree angle with IR plane. Upper margin of IR is 1.5 to 2 inches above level of spinous process of C7.
- *CR:*
  - *PA:* Perpendicular to center of IR. Center point should be in midclavicular line at approximate level of axillary fold.
  - *PA oblique:* Perpendicular to center of IR. CR enters at a point midline of posterior surface midway between spine and midaxillary line of affected side at approximate level of axillary fold.
- *Patient instruction:* Stop breathing on inspiration.
- *Structures seen:* Ribs 1 to 10. Anterior portions are best seen on PA projection; axillary portions are best seen on oblique projection.

Lower Posterior Ribs: AP and AP Oblique Projections

- Body and part position: Standing or recumbent.
  - *AP:* Supine on table or upright with posterior surface of chest against upright Bucky. Coronal plane is parallel to IR. Lower margin of IR is at level of iliac crest.
  - *AP oblique:* RPO position for right ribs or LPO position for left ribs. Coronal plane forms a 45-degree angle with IR plane. Lower margin of IR is at level of iliac crest.
- *CR:*

  AP: Perpendicular to center of IR. Center point should be in midclavicular line at approximate level of tip of xiphoid process.

- *AP oblique:* Perpendicular to center of IR. CR enters at a point midline of anterior surface at approximate level of tip of xiphoid process.
- *Patient instruction:* Stop breathing on expiration.
- *Structures seen:* Ribs 8 to 12. Posterior portions are best seen on AP projection; axillary portions are best seen on oblique projection.

Positioning and Radiographic Examinations of the Abdomen

Radiographic examinations of the abdomen may consist of one or more projections, depending on the purpose of the examination. The primary projection is the AP projection in the supine position, also called a "kidneys, ureters, and bladder" (or KUB) projection. Also, decubitus projections may be performed to evaluate the abdominal aorta.

Routine Examination of the Abdomen

The routine examination of the abdomen includes the AP projection in the supine position. Supplemental images are produced in the upright and left lateral decubitus positions.

- *Body and part position:* The patient is supine. Sagittal plane is perpendicular to IR, and the knees may be flexed moderately and supported by a bolster. The IR is centered at the level of iliac crests. The inferior margin of IR should be at the level of the greater trochanter to ensure inclusion of pelvic floor (Figure 53.32).
- *CR:* Perpendicular to center of IR through a point in midline at level of iliac crest.

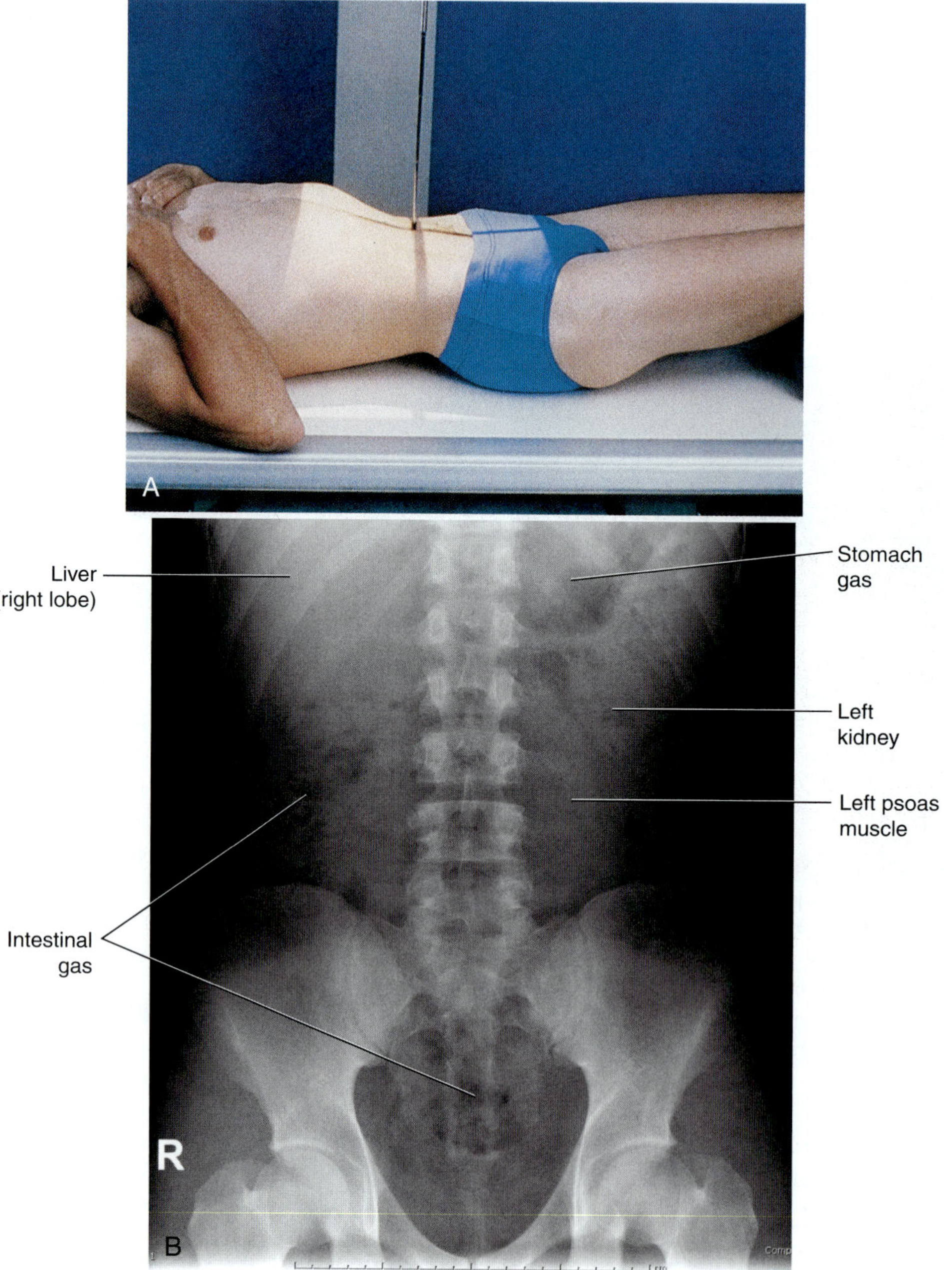

FIGURE 53.32 Abdomen. **(A)** Position for AP projection. **(B)** AP projection, patient recumbent. (A, from Long BW, Rollins JH, Smith BJ: *Merrill's atlas of radiographic positioning and procedures*, ed 14, St. Louis, 2020, Mosby. B, from Long BW, Frank ED, Ehrlich RA: *Radiography essentials for limited practice*, ed 6, St. Louis, 2021, Elsevier.)

- *Collimation:* Adjust the light field to 2.5 cm on all sides of the anatomy. Place anatomical marker in the light field on the lateral side of the anatomy.
- *Patient instruction:* Stop breathing on expiration.
- *Structures seen:* Abdominal contents between diaphragm and pelvic floor. When exposure is correct, psoas muscles, liver margin, and kidney shadows should be visible.

Supplemental Projections

If the patient cannot perform the routine projections for the abdomen, supplemental projections may be performed due to trauma or pathology. Supplemental projections utilize modified positioning to obtain the needed projections. For these projections, the patient must stop breathing on inspiration during the exposure.

AP Projection (Upright Position).

- *Body and part position:* Standing, facing the x-ray tube. Midsagittal plane is perpendicular and centered to IR.
- *CR:* Perpendicular to center of IR through a point in midline approximately 2 inches superior to level of iliac crest.
- *Structures seen:* Abdominal contents between diaphragm and pelvic floor included. Diaphragms must be seen at top of IR. Air-fluid levels will be visible in intestines, if present. Free intraperitoneal air, if present, may be seen beneath diaphragm.

AP Projection (Left Lateral Decubitus Position).

- *Body and part position:* Recumbent on left side on radiographic table or stretcher. Midsagittal plane of abdomen is horizontal and is centered vertically oriented to IR and perpendicular to it.
- *CR:* Horizontal and perpendicular to center of IR through a point in midline approximately 2 inches superior to level of iliac crest.
- *Structures seen:* Abdominal contents between diaphragm and pelvic floor. Diaphragm must be seen. Air-fluid levels will be visible in intestines, if present. Free intraperitoneal air, if present, may be seen near top of IR, along right abdominal wall adjacent to liver.

Pathology

Radiographic examination of the abdomen is critical for evaluating pathology. Abdominal x-rays can be utilized to determine the cause of abdominal pain, such as kidney stones, intestinal blockage, masses, or blockages.

- *Bony thorax*: The most common reason for imaging the bony thorax is trauma. Nontraumatic pathology includes malignant bone disease, multiple myeloma, metastatic bone lesions, and osteochondroma.
- *Air-fluid levels*: When fluid is present in a space usually occupied by air, it is a meaningful diagnostic sign of pathology. The interface between air and fluid is clearly visible radiographically. The possibility of abnormal air-fluid levels exists in the chest, abdomen, and paranasal sinuses. A horizontal x-ray beam is necessary to demonstrate air-fluid levels.
- *Chest:* Many acute and chronic conditions may affect the organs of the chest and can be evaluated radiographically. Trauma of the chest may result in lung collapse or atelectasis. Other pathology includes pneumothorax, pneumonia, pneumoconiosis, lung cancer, emphysema, tuberculosis, congenital malformations, and pleural effusion.
- *Abdomen:* Many abdominal structures, mainly the internal contours of abdominal organs, cannot be seen radiographically without contrast media. Contrast media is a liquid suspension of barium sulfate, and it can be ingested or injected. Conditions that may be diagnosed by abdomen imaging include enlargement of the liver and kidneys, displacement of the kidneys, abnormal gas patterns in the bowel, free intraperitoneal air, and calcifications such as kidney stones, gallstones, and calcification in arteries.

SKULL, FACIAL BONES, AND PARANASAL SINUSES

Images of the skull, facial bones, and paranasal sinuses are typically performed with the patient erect at the upright Bucky. Imaging of the skull may be performed to diagnose fractures of the bones of the skull, congenital disabilities, infection, foreign bodies, pituitary tumors, and certain metabolic and endocrine disorders that cause bone defects of the skull.

Figure 53.33 illustrates the landmarks used for radiographic positioning of the skull, facial bones, and paranasal sinuses. Positioning

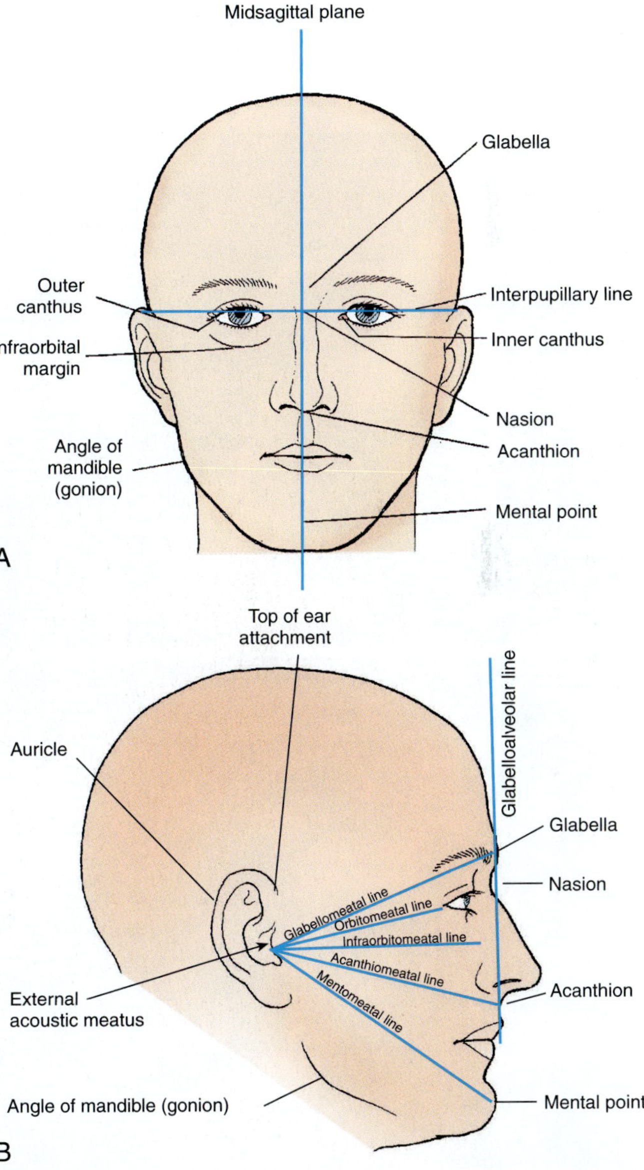

FIGURE 53.33 Common landmarks for positioning of the cranium and facial bones. **(A)** Anterior aspect. **(B)** Lateral aspect. (From Long BW, Rollins JH, Smith BJ: *Merrill's atlas of radiographic positioning and procedures*, ed 14, St. Louis, 2020, Mosby.)

lines that are used are the orbitomeatal line (OML), the infraorbitomeatal line (IOML), and the mentomeatal line (MML). Accurate positioning of the skull requires precise attention to all three body planes, coronal, sagittal, and transverse. The coronal and sagittal planes are adjusted by body position and rotation of the head. The transverse plane alignment depends on the flexion or extension of the neck.

For the projections of the skull, facial bones, and paranasal sinuses, use the following unless otherwise indicated:

- *IR:* Positioned by department protocol for proper anatomy orientation; CR plate 24 × 30 cm; portrait orientation.
- *Grid and SID:* Grid is used. SID 40 inches minimum.
- *Collimation:* Adjust the light field to 2.5 cm on all sides of the anatomy. Place side marker in the light field on the lateral side of the anatomy.
- *Patient instructions:* Stop breathing during the exposure.

Positioning and Radiographic Examinations of the Cranium

The cranial bones include the frontal bone, two parietal bones, two temporal bones, an occipital bone, a sphenoid bone, and an ethmoid bone.

The projections for skull imaging depend on the physician's preferences and the ability of the patient to assume the required body positions. Although the side nearest the IR is best demonstrated on the lateral projection, some physicians prefer a series that includes right and left lateral projections.

Routine Examination of the Cranium

The routine examination of the cranium includes the PA or PA axial (Caldwell method), AP axial (Towne method), and lateral projections.

PA and PA Axial Projection (Caldwell Method).

- *Body and part position:* Prone or seated facing upright Bucky. Sagittal plane of skull is perpendicular to center of IR, with forehead and nose resting on table or against upright Bucky. Neck flexion adjusted to place OML perpendicular to IR (Figure 53.34A).
- *CR:*
  - *PA:* Perpendicular to center of IR through nasion.
  - *PA axial (Caldwell method):* Angled 15 degrees caudad to center of IR through nasion.
- *Structures seen:* Frontal bone and outer contours of cranium. When perpendicular CR is used, petrous pyramids are projected

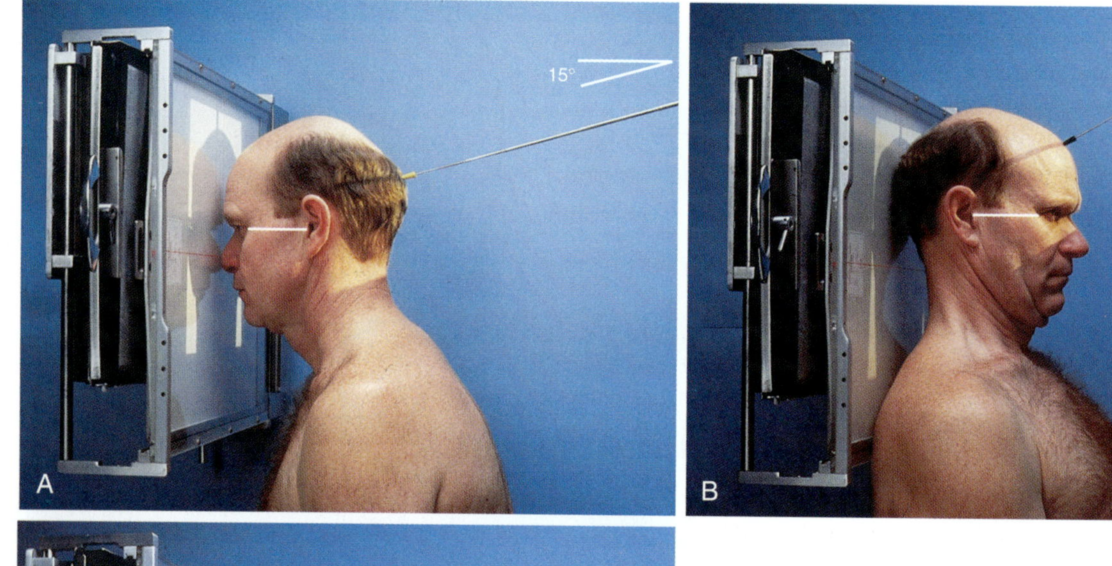

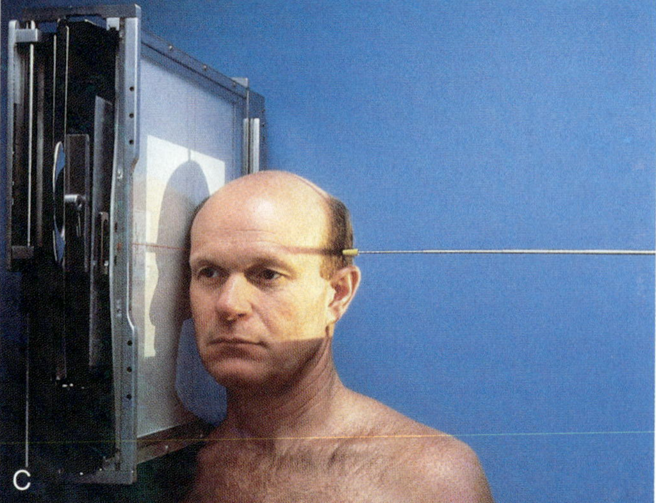

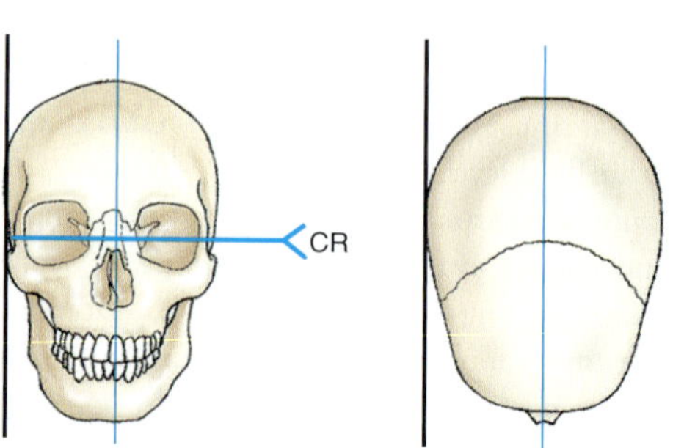

Figure 53.34 Cranium. **(A)** Position for PA axial (Caldwell method) projection. **(B)** Position for AP axial projection (Towne method). **(C)** Position for lateral projection. (From Long BW, Rollins JH, Smith BJ: *Merrill's atlas of radiographic positioning and procedures*, ed 14, St. Louis, 2020, Mosby.)

within orbits. When a 15-degree caudad angle with the Caldwell method is used, petrous pyramids are projected through the lower third of the orbit, and orbital margins are more clearly demonstrated.

AP Axial Projection (Towne Method).

- *Body and part position:* Supine or seated. Sagittal plane of skull is perpendicular to center of IR, with back of head resting on table or against upright Bucky. Neck flexion adjusted to place OML perpendicular to IR (Figure 53.34B).
- *CR:* Angled 30 degrees caudad to center of IR through foramen magnum at the level of the external acoustic meatus. CR enters skull in midsagittal plane, approximately 2.5 inches superior to glabella.
- *Structures seen:* Occipital bone and posterior parietal bones, foramen magnum, and petrous portions of temporal bones.

Lateral Projection.

- *Body and part position:* Recumbent or seated in an anterior oblique body position with side of interest nearest IR. Sagittal plane of skull is parallel to center of IR, and interpupillary line is perpendicular to it. Neck flexion adjusted to place IOML parallel to long axis of the IR (Figure 53.34C).
- *CR:* Perpendicular to center of IR through a point approximately 2 inches superior to EAM.
- *Structures seen:* Lateral image of entire cranium. Sella turcica is seen in profile. There should be no rotation or tilt of the cranium. The side nearest the IR is most clearly seen.

Alternative Projections of the Cranium

If the patient cannot perform the routine projections for the cranium (skull), supplemental projections may be performed due to trauma or pathology. Supplemental projections utilize modified positioning to obtain the needed projections.

AP and AP Axial ("Reverse" Caldwell Method) Projections. If the patient is unable to obtain the prone position, an AP projection may be substituted for the PA or PA axial (Caldwell method) projection.

- *Body and part position:* Supine or seated. Sagittal plane of skull is perpendicular to center of IR, with back of head resting on table or against upright Bucky. Neck flexion adjusted to place OML perpendicular to IR.
- *CR:*
  - *AP:* Perpendicular to center of IR through the nasion.
  - *AP axial ("reverse" Caldwell method):* Angled 15 degrees cephalad to enter through nasion.
- *Structures seen:* Frontal bone and outer contours of the cranium. When a perpendicular CR is used, petrous pyramids are projected within the orbits. With "reverse" Caldwell method, using a 15-degree cephalad angle, petrous pyramids are projected through the lower third of the orbit, and orbital margins are more clearly demonstrated. The orbits and other anterior structures are magnified in comparison with PA projections.

PA Axial (Haas Method) Projection. The PA axial (Haas method) projection may be used instead of the AP axial projection (Towne method). The Haas method is useful when obesity of exaggerated kyphosis of the thoracic spine makes it difficult for the patient to assume the supine position with the OML perpendicular to the IR. Both the patient position and the tube angle are reversed.

- *Body and part position:* Prone or seated facing IR. Sagittal plane of skull is perpendicular to center of IR, with forehead and nose resting on table or against upright Bucky. Neck flexion adjusted to place OML perpendicular to IR (Figure 53.35).
- *CR:* Angled 25 degrees cephalad to center of IR through a point 1.5 inches below external occipital protuberance. CR exits skull midsagittal plane at approximately 1.5 inches superior to nasion.
- *Structures seen:* Occipital bone, posterior parietal bones, foramen magnum, and petrous portions of the temporal bones.

Positioning and Radiographic Examinations of the Facial Bones

The routine examination of the facial bones includes the PA axial (Caldwell method), parietoacanthial (Waters method), and lateral projections.

PA Axial Projection (Caldwell Method)

The PA axial projection (Caldwell method) is performed in the same manner as the PA axial projection of the cranium (Caldwell method) described earlier.

- *Structures seen:* Orbits, zygomatic bones, maxilla, nasal septum, and a portion of the mandible. The petrous ridges are projected into the lower third of the orbits.

Parietoacanthial Projection (Waters Method)

- *IR:* CR plate 18 × 24 cm, portrait orientation.
- *Body and part position:* Standing, seated, or recumbent. The neck is extended with the chin resting on the table or upright Bucky, neck flexion adjusted so that the MML is perpendicular to the IR, and the OML forms a 37-degree angle to the IR. The sagittal plane is perpendicular to the IR.
- *CR:* Perpendicular to center of IR to exit at the acanthion.
- *Structures seen:* Maxilla, orbits, zygomatic arches, and nasal septum.

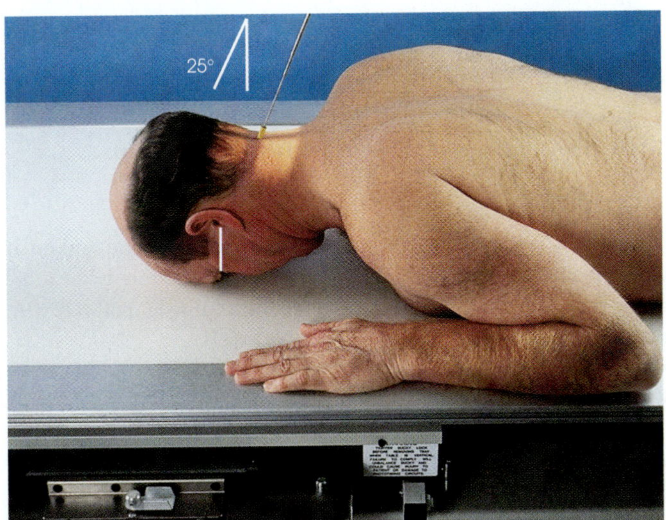

FIGURE 53.35 Cranium. Position for PA axial projection (Haas method). (From Long BW, Rollins JH, Smith BJ: *Merrill's Atlas of radiographic positioning and procedures*, ed 14, St. Louis, 2020, Mosby.)

Lateral Projection

The lateral projection is performed in the same manner as for the lateral projection of the cranium, with the following exceptions:

- *IR:* CR plate 18 × 24 cm, portrait orientation.
- *CR:* Perpendicular to center of IR through a point approximately halfway between the outer canthus and the EAM.
- *Structures seen:* Lateral image of all facial bones, with superimposition of paired bones.

Lateral Projection of Nasal Bones. The nasal bones are very thin, so exposure factors simulate those used for a finger.

- *IR:* CR plate 18 × 24 cm, portrait orientation.
- *Body and part position:* Same as for cranium and facial bones.
- *CR:* Perpendicular to IR to midpoint of nasal bone.
- *Structures seen:* Lateral image of the nasal bone closest to the IR, the anterior nasal spine, and associated soft tissue. Both lateral projections are usually taken.

Positioning and Radiographic Examinations of the Mandible

The routine examination of the mandible includes the PA, lateral, and axiolateral projections. It also may consist of AP axial projections for mandibular condyles and temporomandibular joints.

- *IR:* CR plate 18 × 24 cm, portrait orientation.
- *Body and part position:* Prone or seated facing IR. Sagittal plane of skull is perpendicular to center of IR with forehead and nose resting on table or against upright Bucky. Neck flexion is adjusted to place OML perpendicular to IR.
- *CR:* Perpendicular to center of IR to exit through acanthion.
- *Structures seen:* Entire mandible. Rami are symmetric.

Axiolateral Projection

The axiolateral projection is a projection in the mandible series. This projection can also be achieved by placing the head in a true lateral position and angling the CR 25 degrees caudal.

- *IR:* CR plate 18 × 24 cm, landscape orientation.
- *Body and part position:* Seated, facing IR with coronal plane of body somewhat oblique, as for lateral projection. Neck is extended somewhat and flexed laterally so that sagittal plane of skull forms a 15-degree angle to IR.
- *CR:* Angled 10 degrees cephalad through the mandible.
- *Structures seen:* Mandibular ramus and portion of body nearest IR. Mandibular condyle should be well demonstrated.

AP Axial Projection

An AP axial projection may be used to demonstrate the mandibular condyles and temporomandibular joints. The procedure is the same as for the AP axial projection of the cranium (Towne method) with the following exceptions:

- *IR:* CR plate 18 × 24 cm, portrait orientation.
- *CR:* Directed 35 degrees caudad through midsagittal plane, entering at a point approximately 3 inches above the nasion.
- *Structures seen:* Mandibular condyles and mandibular fossae of the temporal bones.

Positioning and Radiographic Examinations of the Paranasal Sinuses

The routine examination of the paranasal sinuses includes the PA axial (Caldwell method), parietoacanthial (Waters method), and lateral projections. All projections must be performed with the patient upright to demonstrate air-fluid levels if they are present. The PA axial projection (Caldwell method) is the same as this projection of the facial bones in the upright position, with the following exceptions:

- *Part position:* Extend the patient's neck, with the tip of the nose touching the IR and the nasion centered to the IR. Position the patient's head so the OML forms a 15-degree caudal angle with the horizontal CR. A radiolucent sponge may be placed between the forehead and grid to provide support.
- *CR:* Directed horizontal to exit the nasion.
- *Structures seen:* Frontal and ethmoid sinuses. The parietoacanthial projection (Waters method) demonstrates the maxillary and ethmoid sinuses. The lateral projection demonstrates all of the paranasal sinuses, with right and left chambers superimposed on each other.

Pathology

- *Trauma:* A blow to the head that causes brief unconsciousness or disorientation is called a cerebral concussion. Cranial fractures may or may not represent serious injuries. The most common facial fracture is that of the nasal bones. The weakest areas of the orbit are the medial and inferior walls, and a blow to the eye can cause sufficient pressure to fracture these fragile bones. A fracture of the orbital floor is called a blowout fracture.
- *Nontraumatic conditions:* Allergies or upper respiratory tract infections may cause inflammation of the paranasal sinuses, which are common infection sites. Air-fluid levels of the sinuses can be seen radiographically.

IMAGE EVALUATION

Critical image review contributes to your patient's care and to the physician who will interpret (read) the images. Each image should be evaluated to determine whether or not it has sufficient diagnostic quality to meet the minimum requirements of the examination. If not, the image must be repeated. When a projection must be repeated, your review provides information to ensure that the new image is satisfactory. Radiography is a science and an art, and your ability to consistently create high-quality images will develop with time and practice.

Viewing Images

Viewing images includes viewing conditions and image orientation. Image evaluation is an essential aspect of evaluative, effective radiography. It is the process of assessing the radiographic image to ensure it meets a high level of diagnostic standard. The limited x-ray machine operator must review an image and determine if the image is acceptable or not.

Viewing Conditions

You will be viewing images on a computer monitor. It is best to view images in a dimly lit room. Too much light causes the pupils to contract, admitting less light to the eyes and causing images to appear dark. A black frame, known as a mask, usually surrounds each image, enhancing your ability to perceive its detail accurately. Bright lights may cause glare on the monitor screen.

Image Orientation

Images are generally viewed right side up, with the most superior aspect of the anatomy at the top. Regardless of the patient's position, when the IR is exposed, it is customary to view both AP and PA projections as if the patient were facing the viewer in *anatomic position*. This is where the patient is standing erect, with the face directed forward and the toes pointing anteriorly. The patient's right side is the viewer's left side.

Systematic Image Review

With practice, you will learn to evaluate an image rapidly. However, it is essential not to rush this process, or important details may be overlooked. An accurate assessment of image quality requires a systematic approach. Here are some key items that you should look for in your images:

- Is the image labeled with the correct patient and body part?
- Is there evidence of collimation on at least three margins of the image?
- Marking: Is the correct right or left marker clearly visible and in the proper location?
- Is the anatomy of interest included in the image?
- Is the imaged marked with the correct anatomical marker?
- Were the exposure factors appropriate? Is the exposure indicator within the appropriate range?
- Does the image contain any artifacts?
- Is a repeat image needed? If so, what changes are necessary for the repeat to be successful?

Anatomy and Positioning Errors

During image evaluation, the limited x-ray machine operator must be able to identify anatomy and positioning errors.

Exclusion of Anatomy

There are times when some important anatomic details may be excluded because of inaccurate centering, collimation, or variations in patient anatomy. During positioning, make sure that the outer margins of the structures to be included are within the light field. The image should include the surrounding soft tissue and the bony structures. A small amount of light (about 1 inch) is typically extended beyond the skin shadow to allow for slight variation between the location of the light field and the actual radiation field.

Incorrect Positioning

Routine positions have been established for all body parts to ensure a complete evaluation of the anatomy. Misdiagnosis can occur when structures are not well demonstrated or when incorrect positioning prevents comparison with the typical image appearance. Some patients cannot assume routine positions for imaging. Therefore, the operator will need to modify their approach. When a modified position is used, the limited operator should strive to obtain at least two projections that are at ninety degrees of each other. All limb examinations must include at least one joint, which should appear on all images. Images taken in nonstandard positions should be shown to the physician before concluding that the examination is complete.

Exposure Factors

Image quality factors such as image brightness, radiographic contrast, spatial resolution, and distortion must be evaluated in the image.

Image Brightness Problems

With CR and DR systems, it can be difficult to determine incorrect exposure factors due to the wide exposure latitude of the electronic systems. The EI (Exposure Indicator) should be noted to ensure it is in range. The ranges are specific to each manufacturer, so, unfortunately, there is no current standard. The limited operator must become familiar with the proper exposure indicator numbers for the system in use and must check this number for each image during image evaluation.

Lack of Spatial Resolution (Detail)

When evaluating the image's resolution, note whether the margins and small details of the image are sharp and clear. Spatial resolution is affected by SID, object-image distance (OID), focal spot size, and motion. Because SID and focal spot size are usually established in advance to provide the required resolution, blurring or unsharpness is most likely caused by patient motion during the exposure.

CLOSING COMMENTS

Patient Coaching

During a radiographic imaging procedure, the limited machine x-ray operator takes the lead in the examination. The LXMO must explain the examination to the patient and provide instructions regarding positioning. Effective communication is critical to achieve quality patient care. Positive interactions ensure a cooperative patient and successful examination.

Legal and Ethical Issues

A limited x-ray machine operator performs radiographic procedures within the limited scope of practice, producing images at the request of and for interpretation by a licensed physician. Limited x-ray machine operators are individuals other than radiographers who perform diagnostic images on selected anatomic sites. They must demonstrate an understanding of anatomy, pathology, and medical terminology. Limited x-ray machine operators must possess, use, and maintain a high degree of accuracy in positioning and exposure techniques. They must possess, apply, and maintain knowledge of **radiation protection** and safety.

Radiologic technology is an evolving profession. Radiographers are expected to adhere to the field's particular ethical and legal standards. Any persons who do not comply with this code may lose their license and the privileges of the profession. Limited x-ray machine operators must practice within the established scope of practice and practice standards. A profession's practice standards serve as a guide for appropriate practice. The practice standards define the practice and establish general criteria to determine compliance. Practice standards are authoritative statements established by the profession for evaluating the quality of practice, service, and education provided by individuals within the profession.

PATIENT-CENTERED CARE

Medical imaging professionals are the primary liaison between patients, licensed practitioners, and other support team members. These professionals must remain sensitive to patients' needs through good communication, patient assessment, patient monitoring, and patient care skills. As members of the healthcare team, medical imaging professionals participate in quality improvement processes and continually assess their professional performance.

Professional Behaviors

Professionalism is defined by sets of attitudes and behaviors specific to professions. Professionalism has been described as the behavior, purposes, or traits that exemplify or differentiate a profession or a professional person and is a calling, demanding specialized knowledge and rigorous academic preparation. The practice standards published by the American Society of Radiologic Technologists (ASRT) and the standards of ethics published by the American Registry of Radiologic Technologists (ARRT) serve as guides for the professional behavior of radiographers.

SUMMARY OF SCENARIO

When Jonathan reviews the x-ray requisition for Madeline Gallegos, he becomes apprehensive regarding the ORIF. He has x-rayed patients with an ORIF in the past, and he knows they have limited mobility. However, he is confident he will be able to perform the x-ray examination. While obtaining the patient's history, Jonathan asked Madeline if she could stand and transfer to the radiographic examination table. Madeline assured Jonathan she would be able to do so. Once Madeline and Jonathan entered the x-ray room, Madeline was able to transfer to the table, and Jonathan could perform the imaging examination. Even though the ORIF appears cumbersome, Jonathan can use his skills to perform the x-ray examination of the lower limb successfully.

SUMMARY OF LEARNING OBJECTIVES

1. **Explain radiographic terminology, positions, and projections.**
   In preparation for the study of radiographic positioning, the limited operator must understand radiographic terminology for body positions, radiographic positions, and radiographic projections.
2. **Explain how to prepare the room and the patient for performing the radiographic procedure.**
   All radiographic procedures consist of steps designed to provide an organizational plan to ensure safe and effective performance. The order and details of these steps will vary depending on the anatomy of interest, the patient's condition, the type of equipment, and departmental protocol.
3. **Examine the process for performing upper limb and shoulder girdle images.**
   Examinations of the upper limb are usually done tabletop. Each upper limb image is created using a single image receptor (IR). To prepare for these exams, patients may need to remove clothing from the upper torso and don a gown for examination of the shoulder region.
4. **Examine the process for performing lower limb and pelvis images.**
   The bones of the lower limb are divided into the foot, lower leg (tibia and fibula), upper leg (femur), and pelvis. This area also includes the ankle, knee, and hip. The examinations from the toes to the femur are commonly performed tabletop, whereas the hip and pelvis are typically examined on the table Bucky.
5. **Examine the process for performing spinal images.**
   The bones of the spine are divided into the cervical spine, thoracic spine, and lumbar spine. This area also includes the sacrum, coccyx, and sacroiliac joints. The cervical spine examinations are most commonly performed at the wall Bucky, whereas the thoracic spine and lumbar spine are typically examined on the table Bucky.
6. **Examine the process for performing bony thorax, chest, and abdomen images.**
   Radiographic imaging of the chest is the most common radiographic procedure. Imaging of the chest and abdomen is performed to visualize structures and organs of the chest and abdomen.
7. **Examine the process for performing skull, facial bones, and paranasal sinuses images.**
   Images of the skull, facial bones, and paranasal sinuses are typically performed with the patient erect at the upright Bucky. Imaging of the skull may be performed to diagnose fractures of the bones of the skull, congenital disabilities, infection, foreign bodies, pituitary tumors, and certain metabolic and endocrine disorders that cause bone defects of the skull.
8. **Examine the process of image evaluation.**
   Critical image review contributes to your patient's care and to the physician who will interpret (read) the images. Image evaluation is the process by which you determine whether each projection is correctly identified and marked and whether it has sufficient diagnostic quality to meet the minimum requirements of the order or if the process must be repeated.

PROCEDURE 53.1 Perform a Two-View Chest X-ray Examination

TASK: Perform the two-view chest x-ray examination.

SCENARIO: You are working with Jean Burke, NP. She just finished seeing Ken Thomas (date of birth [DOB] 10/25/19XX) and orders a two-view chest x-ray examination.

DIRECTIONS: Role-play the scenario with a peer. You are the limited x-ray machine operator, and the peer is the patient.

EQUIPMENT and SUPPLIES

- Patient's x-ray requisition
- Image receptor

PROCEDURAL STEPS

1. Read the provider's order. Assemble supplies needed for the provider's order. Ensure that the patient can read and understand the directions. Verify the order if you have any questions.
   PURPOSE: It is important to clarify any questions you have prior to the procedure.
2. Greet the patient. Identify yourself. Verify the patient's identity with the full name and date of birth. Explain the order from the provider. Obtain a patient history. Answer any questions the patient may have.
   PURPOSE: It is important to identify the patient in two different ways to ensure that you have the correct patient.
3. Accurately instruct the patient on the procedure. Use words that the patient can understand. Refrain from jargon and medical terminology. Use professional verbal and nonverbal communication
   PURPOSE: Explaining the order can make the patient feel more comfortable and reduces anxiety.

Scenario update: After explaining the procedure, Mr. Thomas states he is not sure he will be able to extend his arm for the examination.

4. Using therapeutic communication techniques (e.g., reflection, restatement, and summarizing), show the patient you are aware of her concerns.
   PURPOSE: Therapeutic communication reduces patient anxiety and helps the healthcare professional provide the best patient care.
5. Based on the patient's concerns, provide positioning alternatives that would meet the requirements for the examination.
6. Evaluate the patient's understanding of the teaching by asking the patient to summarize the positioning plan. Answer any questions the patient may have
7. Position the patient for the first projection for the examination.
8. Step up to the control console, set the technical factors for the exposure, and take the exposure.
9. Position the patient for the second projection for the examination.
10. Step up to the control console, set the technical factors for the exposure, and take the exposure.
11. Evaluate the images and make adjustments as needed. Send the images to the picture archival and communication system (PACS).
12. Dismiss the patient and provide follow-up instructions (if needed).

SKILLS AND STRATEGIES

54

SCENARIO

Michelle, Krysia, and Zacarias (or "Zac" to his friends) met during their first semester of college. They have developed a great friendship over the past few months. They will be graduating from the medical assistant program in less than 6 weeks. Michelle just graduated from high school a year ago. Krysia entered the military just after her high school graduation. She spent 10 years in the Marines. Zac has been out of high school for several years and worked in a factory. He started as a line worker and gradually advanced to supervisory positions. Due to downsizing, his position was eliminated. He went back to school. These friends are looking forward to graduation and getting jobs as medical assistants.

As these three friends discuss finding a job, Michelle is hesitant about the job search experience. Her only work experience is 2 years as a waitress at a local restaurant. She has never created a résumé or a cover letter. She had only an informal interview with the restaurant owner before she was given the job. Krysia is concerned about her military career. The positions she held were not related to healthcare. She managed inventory and supervised others. She was also deployed to many hot spots around the world. Zac has a lot of experience in the factory setting, but he feels that that world is so different from healthcare. As they talk with each other, it is clear that each person has a unique situation, and they all must take a closer look at their past experiences as they prepare for their job search adventure.

While studying this chapter, think about the following questions:

- What personality traits are important to employers?
- What are the best job search methods?
- How do you develop a résumé and cover letter?
- How do you complete a job application?
- How do you prepare for an interview?

LEARNING OBJECTIVES

1. Examine personality traits in employees that are important to employers.
2. Examine how to assess your strengths and skills that are applicable to a job.
3. Examine the process of identifying career objectives and personal needs.
4. Examine strategies for finding job openings.
5. Create a professional résumé.
6. Create a professional cover letter.
7. Examine the use of online profiles and job applications.
8. Create a customized career portfolio.
9. Explain strategies for preparing for an interview.
10. Differentiate among the types of interviews, including strategies to use.
11. Examine how to be professional during and after the interview.
12. Examine strategies to improve your opportunities for more interviews and job offers.
13. Examine the typical requirements when starting a new position, including performance appraisals.

VOCABULARY

clarification Allows the listener to get additional information by explaining a specific statement or topic.

collaboration (kuh lab uh RAY shun) The act of working with another or multiple individuals.

counteroffer Return offer made by one who has rejected an offer or a job.

dignity The inherent worth or state of being worthy of respect.

interpersonal skills The ability to communicate and interact with others; sometimes referred to as "soft skills."

job boards Websites where employers post jobs; job seekers can use them to identify open positions.

mock Simulated; intended for imitation or practice.

paraphrasing Rewording a statement to check the meaning and interpretation; also shows you are listening to and understanding the speaker.

proofread To read and mark corrections.

reflecting Putting words to the patient's emotional reaction, which acknowledges the person's feelings.

reverse chronologic order The most recent item is listed first, and the oldest item is last.

skill set A person's abilities, skills, or expertise in an area.

summarizing Allowing the listener to recap and review what was said.

INTRODUCTION

As you move toward graduation, you may be experiencing many emotions. You might be excited about finishing your medical assistant program. You might be scared of future changes. The thought of finding a job might be overwhelming. These are common feelings of all graduates. The important step before graduation is to prepare for the next phase: getting a job.

Preparing for the job-seeking phase is very important. This chapter will help you to do the following:

- Understand the characteristics that employers want
- Identify your strengths, experiences, and skills
- Develop your career objectives

When you have done these things, you are ready to market yourself to potential employers. You will market yourself through your résumé and interview experiences. Remember that an early job search, even before graduation, can be the key to landing a job soon after graduation.

UNDERSTANDING PERSONALITY TRAITS IMPORTANT TO EMPLOYERS

It is important to understand what employers are looking for in employees. Employers spend money and time training new employees. It is critical that they initially find the right employees. Many employers will agree that they can help refine technical skill proficiencies. It is more difficult to help grow or change personality traits. We will examine the five personality traits that are most important to employers. These include collaboration, interpersonal skills, professionalism, compassion, and a genuine interest in the job.

Collaboration and Interpersonal Skills

Collaboration and **interpersonal skills** are crucial to the efficiency of the healthcare environment. Employers look for people who can blend well with the current staff. New employees need to be flexible, dependable, supportive of peers, and remain calm under pressure. Employers want employees who will provide excellent customer service by having outstanding interpersonal skills, including the following:

- *Effective verbal communication*: Involves using clear, thoughtful, and easily understood language.
- *Professional nonverbal communication*: Relays more information to patients and peers than any words you could use. Eye contact, posture, voice, and gestures provide insights into a person's attitude. Being focused, calm, polite, and interested in the other person are traits of effective nonverbal communication.
- *Good listening skills*: Critical when working with peers and patients. For effective communication to occur, listening must occur. Appropriate questions can draw others into the conversation and show others you are listening and care. Communication techniques such as **reflecting**, **paraphrasing**, **summarizing**, and asking for **clarification** are also excellent ways of demonstrating active listening skills.
- *Good manners*: Are essential, along with a basic understanding of the diversity of your patient population.

Professionalism

A person's professionalism is being evaluated from the cover letter to the interview and beyond. Employers are looking for employees who project a professional image in all situations. Professionalism includes a person's appearance (i.e., dress and grooming habits) and behaviors. The behaviors include a person's flexibility, punctuality, honesty, attention to detail, time management skills, ability to follow directions, and ability to prioritize.

Compassion

Compassion is another trait employers look for. *Compassion* means to have a deep awareness of another's suffering and the desire to lessen it. **Dignity** and respect are part of providing compassionate care to others. Many people go into healthcare to help others. They may like the technical skills involved with patient care. Providing dignity and respect during patient care is just as important. Compassion and respect help healthcare employees connect to patients and their families. Patients welcome acts of kindness and thoughtfulness that lessen stress.

Dignity and Respect Example

Imagine being a patient in your 70s. You have a walker. You spent 4 months in a wheelchair recovering from a stroke. You are proud to be walking today, even if you are slow. You know that walking is important, so you do not get stiff and cannot walk.

The medical assistant calls you in for your visit. You slowly walk to her, and she takes you down the hall. She is far ahead of you as you slowly make your way. It appears the room is at the end of the long hall. You hear the medical assistant calling for a peer to get a wheelchair. She looks back at you and states, "We have a wheelchair for you to speed things up." How do you feel? Do you feel that she values you? Is she showing you respect?

If you reverse the roles, how could you, as a medical assistant, show that you respect and value the patient?

Genuine Interest

Employers also look for people genuinely interested in the job. This trait can be seen during the interview. Does the person ask thoughtful questions regarding the position and the facility? Genuine interest in the job extends beyond the hiring phase into day-to-day operations. Being interested in one's job is critical. Looking for ways to improve procedures and provide better patient care is an important behavior to demonstrate to the employer. This genuine interest is reflected in your attitude and performance in the workplace. It helps ease your transition into a new job and promotes your success.

ASSESSING YOUR STRENGTHS AND SKILLS

As you prepare to market yourself to potential employers, you need to examine your strengths and skills in three different areas. What personality traits do you possess? What technical skills are your strengths? What transferable job skills do you possess?

Personality Traits

Besides the five personality traits previously discussed, the job posting may list extra traits, including additional personality traits. Which of these skills and strengths do you possess? Many people will tell potential employers what they think employers want to hear. They claim to be "a team player," to "communicate well," to be "dependable," and so on. Listing these phrases on your résumé or during the interview is not enough to convince the potential employer that you truly have those characteristics. Employers like supporting evidence.

Early in the preparation phase, make a list of the qualities that you believe you possess. For each quality, provide one or two pieces of evidence to support your claims. Your evidence may be a past job review or the evaluation from your student clinical experience (e.g., practicum, internship, apprenticeship, or externship focusing on administrative or clinical duties). The review or evaluation may indicate your strengths and characteristics. These are excellent documents to include in your portfolio, which will be discussed later in the chapter. Using stories of situations in which you portrayed those characteristics is another way to illustrate your qualities. It is important to share these during the interview if pertinent to the questions asked.

CRITICAL THINKING APPLICATION **54.1**

Think of the three friends in the scenario. Michelle just graduated from high school and has 2 years of waitressing experience. Krysia spent 10 years in the military, where she managed inventory, supervised others, and was deployed to many hot spots around the world. Zac has been working in a factory, advancing to supervisory positions. Now think about the personality traits that employers want. What personality traits might each friend possess? Explain your answer.

- Create your own list of the personality traits that employers want and you possess.

Technical Skills

Employers are also interested in your technical skills. Technical skills for medical assistants can be related to clinical procedures, such as phlebotomy, injections, electrocardiograms (ECGs), and obtaining vital signs. Technical skills can also be related to administrative procedures, including software proficiency, keyboard speed, reception duties, and coding procedures.

You may be able to provide supporting documentation of your technical skills through the use of the student clinical experience skill checklists or a portfolio. Technical skills might also include skills you developed outside the medical assistant program, but that still relate to your chosen career. For instance, if you worked as a pharmacy technician at a local hospital, several of the technical skills you acquired may relate to a clinic position.

Transferable Job Skills

Transferable job skills are the last area to examine. A person develops these skills in one job or experience. The skills can be "transferred" to another job. This means the person will use these skills in other occupations. Many of these skills may sound familiar. They are also characteristics employers are looking for. Potentially transferable skills include these:

- Customer service
- Compassion and empathy
- Strong communication and listening skills
- Computer skills
- Leadership skills
- Organizational skills
- Teamwork skills
- Time management and prioritizing skills
- Creativity
- Grace under pressure
- Problem-solving skills

Identifying transferable job skills can be difficult for many people. Job descriptions for past experiences can be useful. To start, make a list of your past jobs, military experience, and volunteer opportunities. Make a list of potentially transferable skills you developed and used for each experience. Here are some examples of transferable skills for different jobs and situations:

- *Wait staff jobs:* Strong communication and listening skills, prioritizing, and customer service skills
- *Factory jobs:* Communication skills, teamwork, and problem-solving
- *Military experience:* Strong communication skills, grace under pressure, and prioritizing
- *Stay-at-home parent:* Organization, prioritizing, budgeting, time management, and problem solving

You can use this list of transferable job skills as you create your résumé and prepare for your interview.

CRITICAL THINKING APPLICATION **54.2**

What might be some transferable skills that the three friends, Michelle, Krysia, and Zac, possess? Explain your answer.

- Using the list you have already started, add the personality traits, technical skills, and transferable job skills that you possess. Also, indicate why you believe you have these skills (e.g., identify the job or experience that helped you develop the skill).

IDENTIFYING CAREER OBJECTIVES AND PERSONAL NEEDS

One of the steps in seeking a job for a graduate involves identifying career objectives and personal needs. Knowing what you want to do in the future and what you need currently are two important considerations when looking for employment.

Developing Career Objectives

Each medical assistant has a reason for entering the healthcare field. This basic desire should influence decisions concerning the person's career choices. Because medical assisting is such a versatile profession, a medical assistant has numerous options after graduation.

Medical assistant students should take some time to think about what they want from their careers. While the medical assistant is attending school and subsequently completing the student clinical experience, ideas may surface about the area of healthcare or a specific facility in which she or he most wants to work.

When developing career objectives, the medical assistant should start by asking several questions:

- What areas and skills did I enjoy in the student clinical experience?
- Where do I want to be in 5 years?
- Where do I want to be in 10 years?
- What additional skills do I need to get to where I want to go?

Write down the questions and answers and go into specific detail. Set realistic goals and develop a plan for how and when they will be reached. Remember, career objectives are reached over time. It is important to know where you want to be, so you can start down the right path to reach your goals. Keep your list of goals available and visible so you can revisit it frequently.

CRITICAL THINKING APPLICATION 54.3

For the following four questions, write down your answers and explain them. These answers will help you as you start the job search process.

- What areas and skills did I enjoy in the student clinical experience?
- Where do I want to be in 5 years?
- Where do I want to be in 10 years?
- What additional skills do I need to get to where I want to go?

Identifying Personal Needs

The next step in the process is to identify personal needs. What do you need in a job? Do you need a specific wage to meet your living expenses? What benefits do you need? What hours do you need to work? Some people need to consider day care and school hours for their children. How far are you willing to travel for a job? Do you have a reliable mode of transportation? Evaluating your personal needs will help you find a job that matches your requirements.

CRITICAL THINKING APPLICATION 54.4

What are your personal needs? Make a list that identifies the needs you must consider when seeking a new position.

FINDING JOB OPENINGS

Finding employment and staying employed in healthcare are typically not difficult tasks. Usually, healthcare employment needs remain high, even in a poor economy. However, graduation from a medical assisting program does not guarantee employment. Completion of the program gives the medical assistant the job skills needed to work. A good attitude and positive outlook are essential for success in the job search. The medical assistant should always be open to new and better opportunities.

Depending on the location, some job seekers assume that potential employers will not interact with students until they have passed a credentialing examination. Here are some common credentialing examinations for medical assistants:

- Certified medical assistant (CMA) through the American Association of Medical Assistants (AAMA)
- Registered medical assistant (RMA) through the American Medical Technologists (AMT)
- Certified clinical medical assistant (CCMA) through the National Healthcareer Association (NHA)
- National certified medical assistant (NCMA) through the National Center for Competency Testing (NCCT)
- Clinical Medical Assistant Certification (CMAC) through the American Medical Certification Association (AMCA)

Searching for a job before graduation is a smart idea. Some employers do not require credentialing examinations. Others may hire a medical assistant before the exam is taken. They may have an agreement that the medical assistant will obtain the credential within a specified period of time. Many employers are interested in hiring new graduates. They consider new graduates to be teachable. This means that employers can train and mold graduates into the employees they require. Employers recognize that new graduates have more current knowledge and skills.

Two Best Job Search Methods

There are many ways to find employment. Networking and checking **job boards** are the best and most effective methods.

Networking

Networking is the exchange of information with others in your field. For medical assistant graduates or students searching for a job, networking involves meeting individuals in healthcare. It also involves sharing information on available opportunities. Through the medical assistant program, a student forms a network of friends and acquaintances (Figure 54.1). Staying in contact with these people allows for networking opportunities. Email, LinkedIn, Facebook, Twitter, and other social networking advances make staying in touch easy.

Another networking technique is to join a medical assistant organization. The members who often attend regular meetings know about job leads in the area. Creating connections with currently employed medical assistants can be helpful in the job search process.

The student clinical experience gives medical assistant students opportunities to network. During the experience, you will be working with many healthcare professionals. It is crucial that you look at the clinical experience as a continuous job interview. It is important to be professional, follow the guidelines, and strive to do your very best. It is not uncommon that when staff members find a student who portrays the characteristics of a professional medical assistant, they are willing to help the student find a job.

During the student clinical experience, medical assistant students can do the following:

- Inquire about potential job openings through their mentor, supervisor, or the facility's human resource department.
- Ask their mentors if they would be willing to provide a reference or a letter of recommendation.
- Show their gratitude by formally thanking their mentors for the opportunity. In most cases, the clinical agencies provide assistance to help train the medical assistant student. It is important to send a thank-you note to the mentor, the supervisor, and the department.
- Provide the supervisor with a résumé and cover letter.

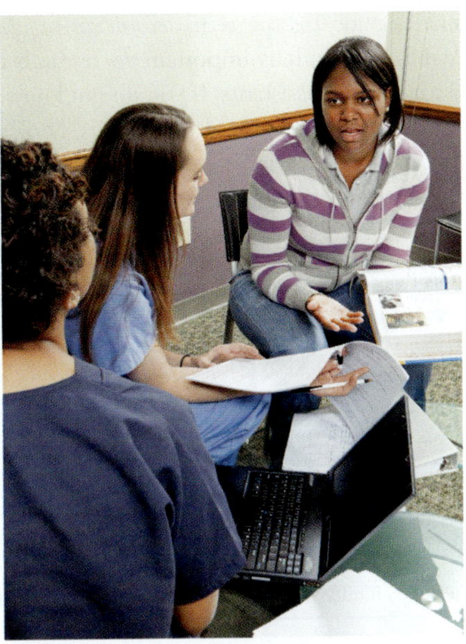

FIGURE 54.1 Stay in touch with classmates. They are excellent networking contacts and may be able to provide job leads.

CRITICAL THINKING APPLICATION **54.5**

Michelle, Krysia, and Zac know that networking is a great way to find employment. They make a list of people with whom they can share their résumé or whom they can inform that they are now ready to seek employment as a medical assistant.

- Who among your relatives would be good prospects for networking?
- Who among your professional contacts would be good prospects for networking?

Job Boards

Job boards are websites where employers post job openings. There are two types of job boards:

- *Facility job boards*: Larger healthcare facilities post job openings on their own websites. The employment website can use different tools that make the process easier for the job seeker and the employer. Some sites allow the job seeker to register for a specific type of job. The software will generate emails to job seekers when new jobs are posted. Some websites allow job seekers to complete online profiles or applications and upload a résumé and cover letter. These tools are useful to both the job seeker and the facility.
- *Public job boards*: These job boards include jobs from a variety of employers. The job boards can be local, state, or national. Local job boards may be found through your school or your community's media (i.e., newspaper, television, radio) agencies. These websites target the local audience. They are usually cheaper for employers. Smaller healthcare organizations tend to advertise using these boards. The Department of Workforce Development in each state addresses unemployment. It provides a job board for job seekers. National job boards provide job seekers the ability to search for openings across the country. Examples include the following:
  - www.monster.com
  - www.indeed.com
  - www.alliedhealthjobcafe.com
  - www.glassdoor.com/index.htm
  - www.usajobs.gov (federal government jobs)
- Many positions for medical assistants use alternative job titles. Some agencies may use the term *technician* or *coordinator* for medical assistant jobs. It is important to research the local job titles used for medical assistants. If you do not know the local job title, try looking at the allied health positions. Look at a job posting. What are the educational requirements? Are the duties skills you have? Make a list of job titles related to medical assisting, and search by those as you identify potential openings.

CRITICAL THINKING APPLICATION **54.6**

Michelle, Krysia, and Zac make a list of possible job boards to review frequently for medical assistant postings. They know that sometimes the postings are available for only a short time, so they develop a schedule to review the sites.

- Make a list of five job boards you would like to check for potential jobs.
- What other titles are used for medical assistants in your area?

Additional Job Search Methods

Besides networking and checking job boards, the medical assistant can find job postings through other, more traditional methods. The school's placement office resources, newspaper ads (online and print), and employment agencies also can have medical assistant job postings.

School Career Placement Offices

Students usually have lifetime access to their school placement offices. Students and graduates should take advantage of the opportunities offered. Many schools offer résumé building aids, job search classes, and interviewing assistance. School placement offices may also work with local employers to advertise their openings online to graduates. The school has a vested interest in helping you find employment. The placement office should be the first resource for the student's job search.

Newspaper Ads

Smaller healthcare facilities usually use newspaper ads to find potential employees. Many newspaper companies post their ads online. This allows more job seekers to view those positions.

Employment Agencies

Employment agencies hire staff to fill in at healthcare facilities. The facility pays the employment agency to staff different positions. Some employment agencies hire and pay the medical assistant. The medical assistants work in a healthcare facility as employment agency employees. After a period of time, if the medical assistant proves to be a good employee, the healthcare facility then hires that person. This allows the employment agency to do the hiring, firing, and managing of employees until the employees prove themselves to the healthcare facility.

Being Organized in Your Job Search

As you submit your résumé and cover letter for various positions, it is important that you stay organized and track the jobs you applied for. You should also keep the original electronic files of your customized documents.

Create a handwritten or electronic log of the jobs you apply for. Include the job title, number, and facility name. When you submit your résumé and cover letter, update the log with the date of those activities. As you are notified about an interview, add the interview information (e.g., date, time, location, interview team members) to your log. Continually update the status of each job in the log.

It is important for you to save the customized documents for each job position. If you are called for an interview, it is important to bring copies of your customized résumé and cover letter. The easiest method is to create a job-seeking folder on your computer. For each job you apply for, create a subfolder in the job-seeking folder. Save your customized résumé and cover letter in the subfolder. Save any other documents related to that job in that subfolder, including the job posting. If you are called for an interview, print the customized résumé and cover letter for your interview portfolio and the interviewer(s). You may also want to print the job posting as a reference during the interview.

One of the most important things to remember when job searching is that it takes time, stamina, and persistence to find a job. Do not expect to get a job with the first résumé and cover letter you send or with the first interview you have. By keeping good records, you will not apply for the same job twice or overlook job opportunities because you thought you had applied for them already.

DEVELOPING A RÉSUMÉ

The purpose of a résumé is to market yourself. You want an employer interested in you. You want your résumé to be included in those selected for an interview. A résumé summarizes your qualifications, education, and experience. Medical assistants must determine what to include in the résumé. The résumé should be developed before the cover letter is written. Strengths for the posted job must be identified and emphasized on all documents. These documents include the résumé, cover letter, and application.

Résumé Formats

There are three commonly used résumé formats: chronologic, combination, and targeted résumés. The résumé format used will depend on the medical assistant's situation.

A *chronologic résumé* is the most popular format used. It is useful when people are seeking employment in the same field as the one in which they have their education or previous experience. The chronologic résumé focuses on the person's employment history. Job duties for each position are bulleted out (Figure 54.2). See Procedure 54.1 for the steps in creating a chronologic résumé.

The *combination résumé* is sometimes called a *hybrid résumé*. A combination résumé lists a person's abilities and skill sets, along with

Michelle Marison

1234 Cedar Way, Mytown, OH 45458
Home phone: 715.555.1899
Cell phone: 715.555.1355
mmarison@elsevier.net

Education

Community College, Mytown, OH
Medical Assistant Diploma, 20XX
- GPA 3.6

Healthcare Experience

Family Practice Associates, Mytown, OH
Medical Assistant Practicum, April 20XX to May 20XX (220 hours)
- Performed injections, electrocardiogram, wound care, phlebotomy, throat swabs, and waived tests.
- Obtained vital signs and measurements on children and adults.
- Utilized an electronic health record to document patients' histories, test results, and treatments.
- Answered calls, checked-in patients, and updated patients' demographic and insurance information.

Mytown Hospital, Mytown, OH
Volunteer, January 20XX to May 20XX
- Provided hospital information to visitors.
- Maintained confidentiality of patients.
- Assisted with deliveries of mail and flowers to patients.
- Assisted nursing staff as needed.

Work Experience

Mytown Family Diner, Mytown, OH
Waitress, June 20XX to present
- Provide efficient, accurate, and timely service to customers.
- Prioritize duties to meet customer needs.
- Provide exceptional customer service.

Special Skills

Fluent in Spanish
Keyboarding speed: 73 wpm
Proficient in word processing and spreadsheet software

Credentials

Certified Medical Assistant, American Association of Medical Assistants (expires May 20XX)
BLS for Healthcare Providers, American Heart Association (expires March 20XX)

FIGURE 54.2 Chronologic résumé.

listing the employment history. A combination résumé may be ideal for the following job seekers:

- People who are switching careers
- New medical assistants, so they can indicate the skills they practiced during their student clinical experience, such as vital signs, injections, and obtaining patient information
- Applicants who have a gap in their work history

Those who are using a combination résumé should emphasize the transferable skills that relate to the new position. The focus is on the person's skills and ability rather than the employment history (Figure 54.3).

The third type of résumé is the *targeted résumé.* This type of résumé is customized to a unique job posting (Figure 54.4). A targeted résumé does the following:

- Details key skills required for the position
- Indicates how the applicant has demonstrated those skills
- Takes longer to create but can be the most effective format

CRITICAL THINKING APPLICATION **54.7**

The three friends have very different backgrounds. Michelle has waitressing experience, Krysia was in the military, and Zac worked in a factory. What type of résumé might each use? Explain your answers.

- What type of résumé would work best for you with your experience and background?

Zacarias Garcia

523 River Way, Mytown, OH 45459

Cell phone: 715.555.5472
ZacGarcia@elsevier.net

Education

Community College, Mytown, OH

Medical Assistant Diploma, 20XX

- Medical Assistant Practicum at Mytown Orthopedic and Massage Center, Mytown, OH
  - Obtained and charted history and vital signs in the electronic health record.
  - Assisted providers with tests and treatments.

Credentials

Certified Medical Assistant, American Association of Medical Assistants, expires May 20XX.

BLS for Healthcare Providers, American Heart Association, expires March 20XX.

Skills and Achievement

Strong communication skills

- Supervised 60 employees in a factory setting for over 3 years.
- Initiated procedures to improve communication between employees and management.
- Promoted in the union to assist with negotiations with upper management.
- Fluent in Spanish.

Excellent problem-solving skills

- Problem-solved factory issues that delayed shipments to customers.
- Initiated solutions to expedite shipments and increased the profit margin of the company.

Excel in Teamwork

- Assisted team on assembly line, helping fill in when others were absent.
- Promoted to Team Lead within 6 months of hire.
- Received "Outstanding Employee" award in 20XX, 20XX, and 20XX.

Work Experience

Mytown Doors, Mytown, OH

Supervisor (March 20XX – January 20XX)

Team Lead – Door Assembly (January 20XX – March 20XX)

Door Assembler (August 20XX – January 20XX)

FIGURE 54.3 Combination résumé.

Krysia Debski
111 Mall Drive • Mytown, OH 45457
Cell phone: 715.555.6956 • Email: KDebski@elsevier.net

Education
Community College, Mytown, OH
A.S. in Medical Assisting, 20XX
- Medical Assistant Practicum at Mytown Associates, Mytown, OH
  - o Obtained and charted patients' histories and vital signs in the electronic health record.
  - o Assisted providers with tests and treatments in a busy internal medicine practice.
  - o Performed injections, throat swabs, and phlebotomy.

Skills
ORGANIZATION SKILLS
- Organized supplies to expedite restocking procedures and decrease financial loss.
- Exceptional organizational and filing skills utilized to maintain purchase and delivery records from over 300 suppliers.
- Assisted with the install and training of inventory tracking software for warehouse.

TEAMWORK
- Refined teamwork skills with over ten years in the U.S. Marines.
- Taught teambuilding courses.
- Promoted teamwork among staff by incorporating incentives.

COMMUNICATION SKILLS
- Assertive when working with suppliers to meet deadlines.
- Utilized excellent listening skills to identify the needs of various teams that impact the warehouse.
- Composed frequent emails and letters for supervisors.
- Fluent in Spanish and Polish.

Credentials
Certified Medical Assistant, American Association of Medical Assistants, (expires May 20XX)

BLS for Healthcare Providers, American Heart Association (expires March 20XX)

Work Experience
United States Marines
Supply Administration and Operations Specialist (May 20XX – September 20XX)
Warehouse Clerk (August 20XX – May 20XX)

FIGURE 54.4 Targeted résumé customized for a medical assistant posting. The medical assistant should possess strong organizational skills, experience with teamwork, and exceptional communication skills. The posting indicated it required a person with a certified medical assistant (CMA) credential and a current basic life support (BLS) certification.

Résumé Content

There are similarities and differences in the information presented among the résumé formats. The following discussion describes the content found in the different sections of a résumé. See Procedure 54.1 for the steps in creating a chronologic résumé.

Header

The person's contact information is found in the header of the document. This includes the person's name, mailing address, professional email address, phone number, and personal websites (e.g., LinkedIn). This information or a variation of the information should appear on each sheet if the résumé is more than one page long.

Professional email addresses may include your first and last name or first initial and last name. Email addresses that include expressions such as "one_hot_chick" or "party_dude" are not professional and are not used on résumés. An old email format may indicate that you are not knowledgeable about the current technology. If you do not have a professional email address or have an old email address, free email sites are available (e.g., gmail.com). Like professional emails, personal websites should be professional and contain a professional image of you.

Before you give your phone number to potential employers, make sure your voice mail message is appropriate and sounds professional. State your name clearly in the message so that callers know they have reached the right person.

Education

The education section includes information on the schooling that the person received after high school. The information should appear in **reverse chronologic order**. Information should include the following:

- *If a diploma was obtained*: List the school's name, city, and state, the degree, and the year it was obtained.
- *If no degree was obtained*: Summarize the coursework completed. List the school's name, city, state, and the years of the coursework.
- *Student clinical experience information*: Include the location, dates, and duties performed during the experience. This is optional. Some will include this information in the Healthcare Experience section, discussed later in the chapter.
- *Academic recognition*: Include such things as academic awards and scholarships.

The location of the education section can differ based on the person's situation. For new graduates, the education section should appear toward the top of the résumé. If the degree is not related to the position or the degree is older, the education section would come toward the end of the résumé. Moving education to the end allows the person's achievements and work history to be emphasized.

Work Experience

This section can be titled several different ways. If a person strictly includes job information, then "Work Experience" or "Job Experience" can be used. Using the word *job* or *work* implies the person got paid for the position. If a person wants to include volunteer positions with job positions, then the section should be titled "Related Experience" or "Other Experience." *Related* means it relates to the position the person is applying for. If the section contains unrelated experience, then use "Other Experience." It is recommended that those who were in the military add a special section to discuss the military experience.

If you have prior healthcare experience, you may want to separate your volunteer and job experiences into two sections. First, use "Healthcare Experiences." Include any healthcare jobs and volunteer positions you have had. Some students may opt to include their student clinical experience in this section. Second, use a topic header, such as "Other Experience" or "Additional Experience." Include all of your non-healthcare jobs and volunteer positions. Do not repeat information you included in prior sections.

The information in this section should be presented in reverse chronologic order. All three résumés discussed require the following elements for each position:

- Name of the facility
- City and state of the facility
- Title of position or positions held at that facility
- Dates in that position (include start date [month and date] and end date [month and date]; for a current position, include the start date and use "to present")

For those in the workforce for 10 years or longer, employers want to see 10 years of employment information. For those working at the same facility for longer than 10 years, it is important to list changes and advancements in the position over the duration of employment. Any gaps in the employment history should be explained to the potential employer during the interview or discussed in the cover letter.

For the chronologic résumé, the most relevant job duties need to be listed. For instance, if you worked as a housekeeper in a motel, making beds is not related to medical assisting. Providing customer service would be relevant.

The statements regarding the duties should be bulleted and begin with an active verb. For present positions, use active verbs in the present tense (e.g., administer, provide). For past positions, use active verbs in the past tense (e.g., administered, provided).

The position of the work experience section is dependent on the résumé format. Chronologic résumés typically have work experience near the top, whereas combination and targeted résumés list it toward the end of the résumé.

Action Verbs in the Past Tense

Administered	Composed	Listened	Provided
Advocated	Computed	Logged	Purchased
Aided	Contacted	Mailed	Reconciled
Answered	Coordinated	Maintained	Restocked
Arranged	Copied	Monitored	Reviewed
Assigned	Developed	Operated	Scanned
Assisted	Distributed	Ordered	Scheduled
Balanced	Documented	Organized	Sorted
Calculated	Established	Performed	Supported
Cared	Filed	Posted	Taught
Coded	Guided	Prepared	Trained
Collected	Helped	Processed	Wrote
Compiled	Instructed		

Summary and Skills

A "Summary" section appears at the top of the targeted résumé. This section summarizes why the applicant is the best candidate for the job. It is helpful to use key words from the job posting when describing the skills one possesses. This helps the reader to make the connection between the job requirements and why this particular person is the best candidate for the job.

A "Skills" or "Skills and Achievements" section is found in combination résumés. It showcases specific transferable skills that relate to the new position. These transferable skills may have been obtained in the military, by a stay-at-home parent, or by a person switching careers. This section can also include the skills learned during the student clinical experience.

A "Special Skills" section is found in a chronologic résumé. Information that may appear in this section includes the following:

- Fluency in another language (e.g., fluent in Spanish)
- Keyboarding speed (e.g., keyboarding speed: 85 wpm)
- Computer skills and experiences (e.g., used electronic health records during the student clinical experience)

Certifications

Many employers may require specific certifications or credentials for a job. It is important to include those that relate to the position. When listing the information, include these items:

- Title of the certification or license
- Awarding agency
- Expiration date

An example for all résumé formats would be "BLS for Healthcare Providers, American Heart Association, expires 10/2027" to show that you are trained in basic life support.

Appearance of the Résumé

As you create your résumé, keep in mind the eye appeal or interest the résumé will create for the reader. Boldface only important information. A job title should be bold, whereas the facility should not be bold. Simple bullets help organize information and provide a neat appearance to the résumé. Changing the font size in certain areas can emphasize more important elements and help keep content on one page.

Spacing is crucial to the appearance of a résumé. Too much white space can give the reader a negative impression of the résumé. Too little spacing creates a busy, text-heavy résumé that is difficult to read. Make sure to use the same spacing between the sections. Use less spacing, but be consistent between subsections (e.g., different employment positions).

It is important to have résumé paper available. Even if you submit your résumé online, you should bring copies of your résumé on résumé paper to the interview. Use a light, solid-colored résumé paper (e.g., cream, light gray). The light colors will duplicate better than a pattern or dark-colored paper.

Before submitting your résumé, have another person review it. Obtain the person's initial impression of the résumé's appearance. Is there too much white space? Does the résumé look too wordy? Does it look too plain? Does it look too busy? Then have the person read the content in the résumé and provide you with feedback. Use the feedback to revise your résumé.

Here are some tips for creating a résumé:

- Do not add clipart or other pictures.
- Do not include personal information (e.g., married, children, and religious affiliation).
- Do not lie or exaggerate the truth.
- Do not add unrelated content, such as hobbies and interests.
- Do not include "References available upon request" or a similar statement because it is understood references will be requested and required.
- Do not use personal pronouns, such as "I."
- Do not repeat content.
- Do not include any pay/salary information.
- Always keep the résumé to one page unless you have been in the workforce for multiple years. Then use an additional page, but your content must fill both pages.
- Be concise and clear.
- Use key terms found in the job posting or job description in your résumé.
- Put important details first.
- Perform a grammar and spelling check on your résumé.
- Limit abbreviations to only the abbreviations used in the job posting (e.g., BLS for basic life support or CPR for cardiopulmonary resuscitation).

CRITICAL THINKING APPLICATION 54.8

Zac, Michelle, and Krysia drafted their résumés. They read each other's résumés and provided feedback. Who else could they give their résumés to for proofreading and feedback?

Think of your circle of family and friends. List three people who might be great candidates to provide feedback on your résumé.

DEVELOPING A COVER LETTER

A cover letter should always accompany the résumé (Figure 54.5). The cover letter is a critical tool that gains the reader's attention. The goal is to have the cover letter create enough interest that the reader wants to look at the résumé. The cover letter gives the reader more information on the applicant's personality than the factual résumé. Cover letters allow applicants to express themselves.

Strategies When Writing a Cover Letter

To create a professional cover letter, it is important to follow these strategies:

- *Match the appearance of the cover letter and résumé.*
  - Headers on both documents should be identical.
  - Font type and margins should be identical.
  - If using paper, use the same paper for both documents.
- *Address the inside address and the salutation (greeting) to a specific person.*
  - Address the letter to the person who is hiring the new employee. This shows that you took the time to find out the details.
  - Use the person's name and job title in the inside address.
  - Use a formal salutation (e.g., Dear Mr. Jones:).
  - Call the healthcare facility or use online resources, such as LinkedIn, to find out the information.
- *Start the body of your cover letter with a bang.*
  - In the first paragraph: Show enthusiasm as you summarize why you believe you are the best candidate for the job. Also include the job title and the number for easy reference for the reader.
  - For example: "Because I have a strong customer service background and a degree in medical assisting, I am confident that I can fulfill your expectations for the family practice medical assistant position (#123)."
- *Sell yourself to the reader.*
  - In the second paragraph, provide a snapshot of your experiences.
  - Weave in the key requirement words from the job posting. Address the requirements first, followed by the lesser requirements or "would like" qualities. Some experts recommend using bold font for these key words.
  - You can bullet your qualifications and abilities, but limit the bullets to four or five points.
  - Be concise yet clear. Do not repeat the résumé. You want the reader to move on to the résumé for the details.

Michelle Marison

1234 Cedar Way, Mytown, OH 45458
Home phone: 715.555.1899
Cell phone: 715.555.1355
mmarison@elsevier.net

May 15, 20XX

Ms. Alex Brown
Medical Assistant Supervisor
Mytown Medical Clinic
555 Clover Drive
Mytown OH 45457

Dear Ms. Brown:

I was excited to see the posting on the Mytown Telegram job board for the medical assistant position (#1243) and would like to be considered for that position. I am graduating from Community College on May 30, 20XX, and will be taking my AAMA CMA exam on June 2, 20XX.

With two years of customer service experience and five months as a hospital volunteer, I have learned the importance of prioritizing, teamwork, and communication. During my medical assistant practicum, I have utilized these skills along with my attention to detail and my medical assistant knowledge as I assist providers with procedures and treatments. The knowledge and skills I am learning in practicum, combined with the skills I have developed as a waitress and volunteer, will help me provide the best care to my future patients.

I have heard excellent things about Mytown Medical Clinic and would love to be a part of the staff of such a caring agency. I am available for interviews whenever it is convenient for you. I can be reached by either phone or email.

Thank you so much for considering me for this position.

Sincerely,

Michelle Marison

Enclosure: 1

FIGURE 54.5 Basic cover letter.

- Reaffirm that you are an excellent match for the job.
  - In the final paragraph: Use such phrases as "I believe I have the qualities you require" or "I am confident I will meet your expectations."
  - If you include an action you will take (e.g., "I will call the week of…"), do not be overly aggressive in your tone.
  - Finish the paragraph by expressing your interest in and enthusiasm for an interview (e.g., "I am very excited about this opportunity and would enjoy meeting with you to explore how my qualifications could meet your needs.").
- Be professional.
  - Express your thanks for the reader's consideration.

Proofreading the Cover Letter

After writing the cover letter, review it for inaccuracies. Use the spell-check tool in your word processing software to help identify errors. Also, **proofread** your letter. Make sure your spelling, punctuation, grammar, and sentence structure are correct. Avoid these common cover letter weaknesses:

- Starting a majority of sentences with "I."
- Introducing yourself in the first sentence (for instance, "Hi, I am Sally Green.")
- Spelling, grammar, punctuation, and sentence structure errors.
- Missing parts of the letter (e.g., date, inside address).
- Not including the position title and posting number.
- Too busy (overuse of font styles), too wordy, or too much white space.
- Inappropriate spacing that leads to the body of the letter being too high or too low on the page. Remember, the body should be centered vertically on the page.
- Creating a generic letter that does not contain the key-requirement words from the job posting. (Many larger employers use software to screen letters and résumés for key words. Those with key words are reviewed more closely. Those lacking the key words are discarded.)

Create an error-free cover letter. It must have a professional tone and appearance. Also, have a few people proofread your letter. Use their advice as you make your changes. Refer to Chapter 7 if you need assistance with composing a business letter. Procedure 54.2 will guide you in writing a professional cover letter.

COMPLETING ONLINE PROFILES AND JOB APPLICATIONS

Many healthcare agencies use the internet during the employment process. The online human resource software may require applicants to create a profile before applying for open positions. The online profile collects the information that previously was collected by paper applications.

Online Profiles

Online profiles have many advantages over paper applications for both the employer and the applicant. An applicant completes the profile once and updates the information as needed. Typically, the agencies keep the profiles active for years. Employers can take several actions:

- Track the activities of applicants.
- Easily read a person's information.
- Advertise new postings to potential applicants whose profiles meet certain requirements.

If a healthcare facility does not use online profiles, the applicant will need to complete a job application (Figure 54.6). Some organizations require the application to be submitted with the cover letter and résumé. Others have applicants complete the application when they arrive for the interview. If you need to complete an application before an interview, come prepared with your information. Arrive at least 20 minutes before the interview so you can complete the application. See Procedure 54.3 for the steps in completing a job application.

Information Required for Online Profiles and Applications

Regardless of whether you need to complete a profile or an application, you will need to provide the same information. Even if you have the information on your résumé, you still need to add it to the application or profile. Having the reference information in a word-processed document will save you time. If you are providing the information online, the copy-and-paste feature will speed

APPLICATION FOR EMPLOYMENT

Date:____________________

Name: (First, Middle Initial, Last)____________________

Social Security No.:____________________ Phone: ____________________

Address:____________________

EDUCATION

	Name, City, State	Graduation Date	Degree Obtained
High School:			
College:			
Other:			

LICENSURE/CERTIFICATION/REGISTRATION

Type of Certification, License or Registration	Agency/State	Registration Name

List any special skills or qualifications that you possess and feel are relevant to healthcare and the position for which you are applying.____________________

EMPLOYMENT HISTORY

May we contact and communicate with your present employer? ☐ Yes ☐ No

Employer:	Phone:
Address:	Supervisor:
Employed	Hourly Pay:
Position title and responsibilities:	
Reason for leaving:	

FIGURE 54.6 Application for employment.

up completion time. You should include certain information in the word-processed document:

- *Education*: Institution's name and address; dates and titles of coursework or diploma
- *Past and present jobs*: Facility name and address; supervisors' names, titles, and contact information; job title, duties, start and end salary, start and end dates; and reason for leaving
- *Certifications and credentials*: Certifying agency's name and address; certification/credential; expiration date (the employer may require a copy of your certification and BLS card)
- *References*: Name, title, facility, address, phone number, and email address

References

An interested employer and many online profiles will require your references. This means you need to ask specific people if they would be a reference for you. If they agree, then obtain their contact information. It is not professional to use people's names without asking them.

Your reference list should include three or four names of people who know you as a person and a professional. Select references based on someone who can speak to the following areas:

- Your skills and interactions with patients (e.g., clinical mentors)
- Your performance in the medical assistant program (e.g., instructors)
- Your work ethic, motivation, and professionalism (e.g., past and current co-workers or supervisors)

Answering Questions

When filling out the application or profile, answer the questions carefully. When addressing your current and past employment, keep these points in mind:

- When giving your availability date, make sure you know how long you have to give notice at your current position. Most employers have a 2-week notice policy. If you are hired, your new employer will understand that you need to give a 2-week notice.
- When giving the reason you left prior positions, make sure to write the reason using a positive tone. For instance, "Obtained a position that would advance my skill set" or "Resigned to focus on my education" sounds more professional than "I hated the job."

If you have a unique situation (e.g., sick parent, new baby), ask the advice of your school's placement counselor if you are unsure what to say in these sections. Most employers require an explanation for time not employed.

As you complete the online profile or paper application, you will be required to read important legal statements and add your signature (or electronic signature). This is a legal document. It should be filled out accurately and completely.

CAREER PORTFOLIOS

Many job seekers claim to have the skill sets required by the potential employer. Very few actually show the employer evidence of those qualifications. A career portfolio is a fantastic tool to show that you have the skills required for the job.

Customizing a Career Portfolio

The portfolio should be developed along with the cover letter and résumé. Creating a different portfolio for each type of job applied for is a great strategy. A receptionist portfolio would look different from a phlebotomy portfolio. There will be similarities in the information for all portfolios, but different evidence of skills will be in each. The medical assistant should be prepared to leave the portfolio with the interviewer, so no originals should be included.

Just before an interview, the medical assistant should customize the portfolio for that employer (Procedure 54.4). A copy of the cover letter and résumé sent to the employer should be in the portfolio. A list of references should also be included. All three of these documents should be printed on the same type of résumé paper. The medical assistant should do additional customization of the portfolio. The examples of work or the summary of projects should reflect the skills required and key words in the job posting.

Creating a Career Portfolio

The documents placed in the career portfolio binder should be positive and helpful to you in your mission of getting a job. Using a three-ring binder with plastic sheet protectors and divider tabs, put together a career portfolio that includes the following:

- Table of contents at the beginning with identified tabbed sections
- Cover letter and résumé (a copy of what was sent to that facility)
- References
- Certifications (e.g., copy of BLS card, copy of credentials [e.g., CMA or RMA card])
- Education-related documents
  - Copies of letters of recommendation
  - Copies of transcripts, awards, and honors (optional)
  - A list of the courses successfully completed with a short description of each course (optional, but consider doing this if you are moving to another location where your institution may not be known)
  - Copies of student clinical experience evaluation forms and skill document forms
  - Documentation of scholarships awarded
  - Copies/details of school-related activities (e.g., officer in student medical assistant group, athlete, volunteer activities)
- Prior employment documents
  - Copies of past employment evaluations
  - Copies of letters of recommendations
- Documentation showing that the student was able to balance work and education (this can help exhibit a strong work ethic, organizational skills, and prioritizing skills)
- Examples of work or summaries of projects that can provide evidence of abilities and skills
- Criminal background documentation, blood titers, vaccination history, and current tuberculosis (TB) skin or blood tests results (optional)

Be creative as you prepare your portfolio, keeping the appearance professional and neat.

PREPARING FOR THE INTERVIEW

When preparing for an interview, the job seeker needs to do the following:

- Research the facility.
- Practice answering potential questions.
- Select interview attire.
- Prepare for the day of the interview.

We will discuss each of these in depth. The better prepared the job candidate is, the more comfortable that person will be during the interview.

Research the Healthcare Facility

The job seeker should learn everything possible about the employer. The organization's website is an excellent source of information. A job seeker should research the following topics:

- Mission and value statements
- Size of the organization
- Size of the department with the open position
- Names and types of providers in the department

It is important to ask questions during the interview. Possible questions can relate to your research on the facility:

- "I see that there are two providers in this department. Would I be working with both of them?"
- "There are three locations for your clinic on your website; how will I interact with the other locations?"
- "Given the size of your organization, is there an opportunity to interact with the other departments?"

Questions that relate to your research show the interviewer you are truly interested in the position. They also show that you prepared for the interview.

Practice Answers to Questions

Organizations need to follow federal and state hiring laws. The agencies cannot discriminate. During the interview phase, most organizations use a preset list of questions. All candidates are asked the same questions. You will not know the exact questions that will be asked. It is important to practice answering some standard interview questions (Figure 54.7). This practice will help you prepare for the interview and also appear more confident during the actual interview.

1. Tell me about yourself.	16. What do you know about this facility and our competitors?
2. Why do you want to work for this company?	17. What has been your most rewarding experience at work?
3. Why should I hire you?	18. What was your single most important accomplishment for the company in your last job?
4. How do you work under pressure?	19. What was the toughest problem you have ever solved, and how did you do it?
5. How do you handle criticism?	20. How do you see yourself fitting in with our company?
6. What do you think your co-workers think about you?	21. What skills did you learn in your last job that can be used here?
7. Describe your last supervisor.	22. What immediate contribution could you make if you came to work for us today?
8. What would you like to change about yourself?	23. Do you prefer working with others or by yourself?
9. What is your best asset?	24. Can you take instructions or criticism without being upset?
10. What adjectives would you use to describe yourself?	25. What job in this company would you choose if you could?
11. How would you describe the perfect job?	26. What have you done that shows initiative and a willingness to work?
12. Why did you leave your last job?	27. What will previous supervisors say about you?
13. Why did you choose this type of profession?	28. Why would you be successful in this job?
14. What are your strongest and weakest personal qualities?	29. Can you explain the gap in your employment history?
15. What personal characteristics are necessary for success in your chosen field?	30. Are you a member of any professional organizations?

FIGURE 54.7 Top 30 interview questions.

When practicing your answers to standard interview questions, start by writing down your answer. Review your response. Does it answer the question? What perception might you be giving to the interviewers by your answer? Is it the perception you want to be giving? How might you strengthen your answer? Is it really short, or does it ramble on? Be clear and concise. Expand on the topic, but do not get too wordy. Provide examples to support what you say. When you have refined your answers, practice your answers before the interview.

Decide on Your Interview Attire

Prior to the interview, it is important to select an interview outfit. Be conservative and professional with wardrobe choices.

- Females: Business suit; skirt or dress pants and blouse. Skirt or dress should be of modest length (i.e., at the knee or longer). Blouse should not be sheer or show cleavage.
- Males: Business suit; dress pants and shirt. Conservative tie.

Be sure clothing is clean, wrinkle free, and well fitting and that shoes are clean and shined. For a medical assistant, scrubs may be acceptable for an interview. (It is appropriate to ask the person arranging the interview if scrubs can be worn.) Take care in washing and ironing your scrubs, and use a lint roller on them before wearing them on an interview.

Pay particular attention to other aspects of appearance. Make sure your hair is clean and styled attractively, your teeth are clean, and your breath is fresh. Nails should be clean and well-groomed. Nails should not be excessively long or painted in highly visible colors. Do not wear perfumes or colognes. Do not wear excessive jewelry or makeup. Do not chew gum during the interview. Do not smoke in your interview attire. Remember the appearance guidelines that applied to the student clinical experience. Some employers will react negatively to tattoos, piercings, extravagant hairstyles, unnatural hair colors, or other excessive wardrobe choices. Always dress appropriately and conservatively for an interview. Once hired, the new employee may be allowed to wear more diverse styles that comply with the employee handbook or procedures manual.

Prepare for the Interview Day

Do a test run before the day of the interview to identify the travel time if the interview is in person. Always arrive 15 minutes early for the interview. Never take anyone along on a job interview, especially children. Expect to be a little nervous. An interview can be a stressful situation. If necessary, practice stress-relieving strategies (e.g., deep breathing) that you can use before the interview. The better prepared a person is, the more successful the interview will be.

You should also prepare what you need to bring for the interview:

- An interview portfolio
- A copy of your cover letter and résumé for each interviewer
- A notepad and pen to take notes
- A list of references on résumé paper
- A list of questions for the interviewer

If you will be completing an application, bring the information discussed in the prior section regarding completing online profiles and applications.

TYPES OF INTERVIEWS

Face-to-face interviews have been the normal method for interviewing job candidates until recently. Over the last few years, phone interviews have gained in popularity. These are common for prescreening candidates for face-to-face or virtual interviews. Virtual interviews have also become popular.

Face-to-Face Interview

When you meet the interviewers, greet each person and shake hands. A firm handshake is recommended. Ensure each person has a copy of your résumé and cover letter before the interview begins.

During the actual interview, maintain good eye contact. Many supervisors refuse to hire people who seem uncomfortable looking them directly in the eyes. Never take control of the interview. Allow the supervisor or panel members to ask questions at their own pace. Do not fidget in the chair or display any nervous habits (e.g., tapping your pen) (Procedure 54.5).

Phone Interview

Phone interviews are usually conducted by the supervisor or the human resource representative. A phone interview may be the selected option in order to do the following:

- Screen applicants and narrow the candidate pool
- Provide additional information (e.g., benefits, job description) and verify that the applicant wants an interview
- Replace a face-to-face interview, especially if the candidate is from out of town

Phone interviews are becoming more prevalent. It is important to treat a phone interview like a face-to-face interview. Here are some tips for a phone interview:

- Prepare for the interview just as you would for a face-to-face interview.
- Take the call in a quiet environment. Make sure no dogs or children are close enough to be overheard. Be alone in the room.
- Pay attention to the caller. Do not use other electronic devices or use the bathroom during the call.
- Have a copy of your résumé and cover letter.
- Have your list of questions.
- Have a glass of water available should you need it.
- Make sure to thank the interviewer at the end of the call.

Virtual Interview

Virtual or video interviews use technology such as Microsoft Teams and Zoom. As with a phone interview, a virtual interview works well when the candidate is from out of town or if face-to-face interviews are not being held. There is a certain amount of technology needed for a virtual interview. Your school's placement office may be able to help you with that. The organization may have contacts for you to arrange your end of the interview. The benefit of a virtual interview over a phone interview is that the interviewer can actually see the interviewee. This allows the interviewer to assess the body language and the verbal message being presented.

Here are some tips for a virtual interview:

- Prepare like you would for a face-to-face interview. Research the company, and create a list of questions to ask.
- Dress like you would for a face-to-face interview.

- Practice with the technology. Be familiar with the software that will be used for the interview.
- Identify an appropriate location for the interview. During the interview, the microphone and camera will be on. Choose a quiet area without pets and other people. Choose a neutral background, such as a blank wall. If this is not available, select the least distracting environment. Limit the distractions behind you that will be visible to the interviewer. Cluttered counters with dirty dishes, inappropriate pictures, dirty laundry, and so on do not create the professional image you are striving for.
- Make sure the camera is positioned appropriately. The interviewer should be able to see your head and shoulders. Make sure you are not sitting too close or too far from the camera. The camera should be positioned so you can appear to be making eye contact with the interviewer. Make sure there is no glare. Adjust the light source if needed.
- Have the same materials ready that you would have for a phone interview so that you can access them if needed.
- Refrain from nervous habits that the interviewer can observe.

PROFESSIONALISM DURING AND AFTER THE INTERVIEW

Employers want to hire medical assistants who demonstrate professionalism. The interviewee's actions during and after the interview provide the interviewers with information about the person's professionalism.

During the Interview

Interviewers can consist of one or two people or a panel of employees. The job seeker may interview with a human resource employee, the office manager, the provider, or potential peers. The job seeker may have a number of interviews before the actual decision is made.

During the interview, it is important to be professional. Your professionalism may be tested if the interviewer asks illegal questions. We will discuss how to answer interview questions. We will also discuss professionalism during the different types of interviews.

Answering Interview Questions

It is important to give the interviewers a good impression of you. As discussed in a prior section, it is important to practice answering questions before the interview. This will help you to prepare and feel more confident during the interview.

Many times, the interview will start with a statement such as "Tell me about yourself." The temptation is to focus on your personal life. For example, you may be tempted to say, "I'm a recent graduate, and I am married and have two children." Your response should not reflect information about personal issues. Reply instead with "I am a recent graduate and completed a 6-week clinical experience in a family practice." Focus all responses on your career, strengths and attributes, and what skills you have to bring to the healthcare setting. Be able to prove the skills you claim. You can provide examples either by relating professional situations you have handled well or using your interview portfolio. Before the interview ends, the medical assistant should ask when a decision will be made and if it would be acceptable to call to follow up (see Procedure 54.5).

Tips for All Interviews

- For simple, straightforward questions, do not pause before you answer. Any pause would hint at insincerity.
- For complex questions, pause for a few seconds as you think about your answer. Write down some key words to help you focus and answer the question.
- Refrain from saying "um."
- Do not volunteer any negative information.
- Be honest, and do not exaggerate experiences or lengths of employment.
- Never speak negatively about former employers.
- Write down the names of the interviewers to help you as you follow up after the interview.
- Avoid a "know-it-all" attitude, which indicates overconfidence and a reluctance to take direction.
- Express a genuine interest in the employer and the organization's projects rather than in what the employer can do for you as the employee.
- Ask intelligent questions at the end of the interview if given the opportunity. Your first question should never be, "How much will I be paid?" Money, although important, cannot appear to be your primary concern.

Illegal Interview Questions

The interviewer should not ask any illegal questions. Table 54.1 lists such topics and potentially illegal questions. Employers may either intentionally or accidentally ask illegal questions. The way that the medical assistant answers the questions can influence the employer's hiring decision. Here are some points to consider:

- *If the medical assistant is openly offended:* Employers may negatively conclude that the applicant will be offended by abrasive comments from patients.
- *If the illegal question is answered:* Discrimination may occur in the hiring process. The employer may use the information to weed out the medical assistant as a candidate.

The best approach is to politely address the question. Either answer the question or redirect the interviewer back to the job requirements. For example, suppose an interviewer asks if the candidate plans to put her or his children in day care. This may be a way of determining the age of the dependent children. It could also provide information on the likelihood of absenteeism because of the children's illnesses. The medical assistant could answer, "I will be able to meet the work schedule and the responsibilities that this job requires."

Some questions that might normally be considered illegal, such as "What organizations are you a member of?" might be job related. The employer may be interested in knowing if the medical assistant is a member of various professional organizations, such as the AAMA or the AMT.

CRITICAL THINKING APPLICATION 54.9

Krysia is enjoying a good interview when the interviewer, a male supervisor, asks her if she is married. When Krysia replies that she is not, he asks if she has a steady boyfriend.

- What might the supervisor's motive be with this line of questioning?
- How should Krysia respond?
- Are these questions inappropriate, or do they serve a purpose?

TABLE 54.1 Illegal versus Legal Interview Questions

TOPIC	EXAMPLES OF ILLEGAL QUESTIONS	EXAMPLES OF LEGAL QUESTIONS
Birthplace, ancestry, or national origin	When did you move to the United States?	Are you eligible to work in this state?
Marital status, children, or pregnancy	Who will look after your child when she or he is born?	Are you able to work an 8 a.m. to 5 p.m. schedule?
Physical disability, health or medical history	What medications are you on?	Can you perform the essential job functions of a medical assistant with or without reasonable accommodation?
Religion or religious days observed	Where do you attend church services?	Can you work on weekends?
Age, race, ethnicity, gender, or color	How old are you?	Are you 18 or older? (or whatever the minimum age is for the facility)
Criminal record	Have you ever been arrested?	Have you ever been convicted of a crime?

Follow-up after the Interview

Follow-up is critical after an interview. Always send a thank-you note, letter, or email to the person who conducted the interview (Procedure 54.6). It can be challenging to figure out what to send to the interviewer.

- *Send an email if* the decision is going to be made quickly. Send an email later the day of the interview.
- *Send a written thank-you note or a letter if* the facility is more conservative and formal. Also, it can be sent if the decision is going to be made in a week or two. Send the thank-you note within 24 hours of the interview.

Many employers see the thank-you as an expression of gratitude and professionalism. Even if you do not see yourself in that position, it is still important to send a thank you. This may be their last perception of you, and it may help you in the future at that facility.

Typically, at the end of the interview, there will be a discussion of how quickly the decision will be made. Many agencies using online hiring software will indicate the status of the job on the posting. Candidates not selected for the position usually receive an email or letter.

After the initial interviews are completed with all the candidates, several things can occur. With some employers, the list of interviewed candidates will be narrowed. The top two or three may be asked to come back for a second interview with additional team members (e.g., providers, medical assistants). With other employers, the top candidate is selected, and references are checked. These processes take time, and the deadline may be extended if vacations or out-of-office times occur.

If the interviewer indicates a decision will be made in 2 weeks, wait to hear from the facility. Allow a few days after the deadline before you follow up. At that time, you can call and ask about the status of the job. Remember, following up prior to the deadline may not be in your best interest. The employer may perceive that you do not follow directions if you make extra phone calls. If you receive a job offer from another facility but are waiting for a decision on your favorite position, it is appropriate to contact the interviewer. Explain that you were offered another position and wondered about the status of this position. Many employers will let you know if you are in the running for the position.

Never place all your hope in one job. Make sure to continue to search and interview until an offer is made and accepted. In addition, always be on the lookout for the next job opportunity.

Negotiation

The negotiation stage of job acceptance can be as stressful as the actual interviews. The medical assistant must be professional during this process.

When a job offer is made, there should also be a discussion of the other benefits. If the salary offered is a bit lower than expected, but the employee's share of the health insurance premium is less than expected, the salary offer becomes more attractive. Medical assistants should know the lowest salary/benefit combination they can afford. They should ask for a little more than that figure.

Bracket salary requests are often helpful in expressing this amount. Instead of asking for $13 per hour, ask for a salary in the "mid to high twenties." Let the employer mention a figure or a range of salary first. Usually, the person who mentions a salary range first has the disadvantage. For example, if the medical assistant requests $15 per hour, but the facility was willing to pay $18 per hour, the medical assistant probably will get $15.

Many organizations have a starting pay level for new medical assistants. If you hope to get a higher pay level, you may need to do the following:

- Obtain a national medical assistant credential (e.g., CMA [AAMA] or RMA)
- Show an advanced skill level acquired from previous work experience in healthcare. Having a well-designed interview portfolio will allow you to show the interviewer all that you have accomplished.

Never say no to a job offer on the spot. Request at least 24 hours to consider the offer. Before accepting or rejecting a job offer, consider whether the position carries any authority, the benefits, the hours, the distance from home, and the potential for advancement. People accept jobs for reasons other than the salary; remember the value of experience.

CRITICAL THINKING APPLICATION 54.10

Michelle has been on several interviews and likes the prospect of working for three different physicians. If each office makes an offer, how can Michelle decide which to accept? What will help Michelle make this decision?

IMPROVING YOUR OPPORTUNITIES

When looking for a new position, sometimes job postings may appear to be sparse. By using different strategies, you may find additional job postings and ultimately have more interviews and job offers. We will examine ways to improve your opportunities for finding a job.

Finding Job Postings

Some students and graduates may not find job postings. This can be stressful, but it is important not to give up. Those who are not having success with the job search may want to reevaluate their search methods. Consider these questions:

- *Am I looking for a selective opportunity?* For instance, are you looking for a dermatology medical assistant position in a specific facility? Those positions may be limited. Try to broaden your search to other possible opportunities.
- *Am I looking for the correct job title?* Remember, employers may use a wide range of titles for a medical assistant.
- *Am I looking at all agencies that could potentially hire a person with my skill sets?* Depending on your area, medical assistants can be employed in many agencies besides medical clinics, including nursing homes, hospitals, schools, assisted-living facilities, and insurance companies.
- *Can I increase the geographic search area for employment opportunities? Can I relocate to an area with greater employment opportunities?*
- *Where can I network to increase my awareness of job openings?*
- *What job boards are local employers using?*

Increasing Interview Opportunities

People who apply for jobs but never get calls for interviews must reevaluate the information given to employers. Consider these questions:

- *Is your cover letter, résumé, online profile, or application negatively affecting the job search?* It may be important to get another opinion on the content and presentation. Often the school career placement officer will provide improvement tips.
- *Do you have spelling and grammar errors in your information?* Some employers may perceive those details are not important to you, so they may not be interested in hiring you for the position.
- *Do your cover letter and résumé need to be reformatted or revised?* Applicants need their letter and résumé to stand out from the crowd. People get very creative in how they make this occur.
- *Are your cover letter and résumé customized to the job posting?* Do your documents reflect the key words in the posting? Or do your documents look generic? Generic-looking documents lead employers to perceive that the person is not into details and was not interested enough to spend the time to customize the documents.
- *Are you following the directions in the job posting?* For instance, an employer may want a handwritten cover letter to be included. Sometimes the employer provides a mailing address and states that no calls or visits will be allowed. If applicants do not follow the directions, they may not be considered for the job.
- *Are you providing a professional image with your email address and social media sites, such as Facebook?* Graduates struggling to find positions may want to review their social media sites. Consider tighter security settings to limit outside viewers. You may want to remove any questionable content and pictures.

Increasing Job Offers

If you are getting interviews but no job offers, reevaluate your interview strategies. Again, the school's career placement office may have interview assistance. **Mock** interviews can help you refine your interview skills and behavior.

The following is a ranked list of reasons interviewers do not hire job candidates, as expressed by surveyed career consultants and reported on the website http://careers.workoplis.com:

- Based on social media postings
- Bad attitude, not interested, or appeared not to care
- Not researching a potential employer/company
- Smelled bad: heavy cologne or perfume use, reeked of cigarette smoke
- Sloppy documents: misused and misspelled words, inappropriate grammar and punctuation, and failed to proofread the résumé and cover letter
- Appeared desperate for the job
- Failed to have references that provided work and professional information
- Unrealistic salary expectations

It is always important to prepare for the interview, show enthusiasm for the position, and ask the right questions. Other factors may have negatively affected the decision as well:

- Inappropriate interview attire and grooming: The outfit was too tight, the neckline was too low, pants were dragging on the ground, or the shoes were too casual (e.g., flip-flops). The perfume or cologne was too strong. The hairstyle or color was too extreme.
- Did not fit in the environment: Each facility has a corporate environment. The interviewer looks to see which candidate would fit best. A candidate who is too shy, too talkative, or too loud might not be the best fit. Or a person may have worn too many piercings, or too many tattoos were visible.
- Used poor grammar: Some employers correlate good grammar with intelligence. Employers look for candidates who sound intelligent and who will positively represent their facility.

If you have heard or feel that your résumé indicates that you lack the skills needed for the specific positions you want to obtain, you may want to improve your **skill sets**. This can occur through education and experience. Some people improve their job history and skill sets by obtaining temporary employment through temp agencies. Temporary jobs can provide experience and also help you refine your skills. Another way to better your skill sets through experience is volunteering at a healthcare facility or free clinic. Depending on the volunteer position, it may help enhance your skill sets and provide you with potential job leads. Volunteer activities should be added to the résumé because these valuable experiences can often be used in a healthcare setting. It does not matter that the position was not a paid job, experience counts, whether paid or not.

STARTING AND KEEPING YOUR JOB

When you get a job offer and accept it, you will have mandatory activities to complete. The human resources department will have required paperwork for you to fill out. You will have to become oriented to the facility and your role. It is important for a medical assistant to demonstrate professionalism in the role and when they are leaving to move on to another position.

Human Resource Requirements

When you obtain a job, you will be required to complete a number of documents (Table 54.2). You will be asked to bring in proof of identity and employment authorization (e.g., US passport, Social Security card, and driver's license). These documents are required for the employer's portion of the Form I-9. Form I-9 must be completed within the set time period to meet governmental regulations. Make sure to complete all the required forms in a timely manner. Meet the deadlines given to you by the human resource representative.

Starting Strong

When you get your first job, it can be an exciting and scary time. You may feel excited about the new opportunities yet scared of the new responsibilities. With any job, it takes time to learn the position. Most healthcare agencies have *probationary periods* for new employees. This time frame can vary. The purpose of the probationary period is to see if the new employee is the right fit for the job. If the employee is not able to do the job or is not the right person for the position, the employer can terminate the employee during the probationary period.

It is important for the medical assistant to do well during the probationary period. The first weeks to months of the job are usually devoted to orientation. The new employee learns the processes and becomes efficient and confident in the role. To be successful, it is important for the medical assistant to adopt the following practices:

- Arrive 10 to 15 minutes prior to the start of the day. Limit absences, especially during the probationary period.
- Be groomed appropriately according to the facility's dress code.
- Be honest, trustworthy, and respectful in all interactions with peers, patients, and providers.
- Be willing to try new things and ask questions.
- Take feedback professionally and with a positive attitude.
- Be motivated to do a good job and be willing to keep learning.
- Be a team player and be willing to help others.
- Provide safe care to patients, always working within the medical assistant's scope of practice.
- Be open to new ideas, concepts, and procedures.
- Attempt to resolve simple differences with peers before involving the supervisor.
- Work with the supervisor to improve oneself and the department.
- Finish all assigned tasks in a timely manner and look for additional duties if time is available.

Performance Appraisals

For the medical assistant to continue with the facility, it is important to be a reliable employee. It is also important to improve one's weaknesses. The medical assistant will get regular feedback from supervisors through performance appraisals. The performance appraisals inform employees of their strengths and weaknesses on the job. These appraisals are done after the probationary period and annually thereafter. Types of performance appraisals include the following:

- *180-degree style*: Supervisors evaluate their employees based on their observations of job performance over a given time period.
- *360-degree style*: Supervisors gather input from your co-workers and others whom you interact with on a regular basis.

Do not expect to receive a perfect appraisal. Employees are seldom perfect in all aspects of their jobs. If the supervisor gives perfect scores to an employee, there is no room for growth or improvement. The areas for growth are usually discussed during a meeting with the supervisor. You may be asked where you want to grow or improve and your goals for the coming year. It is important to consider these topics prior to the meeting with the supervisor.

TABLE 54.2 Forms to Complete When Hired

FORM	DESCRIPTION
Form I-9: Employment Eligibility Verification Form	Form I-9 is used to verify a person's identity and employment authorization. All US employers must ensure the form is completed by both the new hire and the employer. The form requires the new hire to provide the employer with documents that prove identity and employment authorization proof.
Form W-4: Employee's Withholding Certificate	New hires must provide their tax status (e.g., single) and how many withholding allowances they are claiming. This information is used when the employer withholds money from their paycheck for income taxes.
Insurance benefit form	Most agencies have health and life insurance benefits that the new hire can participate in. Completion of paperwork is required as part of the enrollment activities.
Background check form	Many healthcare providers will pay for background checks on new hires. Some hiring may be contingent based on a clean background check. Some types of background checks include those that look at one's criminal record, presence on a sex offender registry or database, and caregiver history.
Emergency contact form	The new employee gives the employer information on whom to contact in case of an emergency.
Handbook acknowledgement form	Some agencies have handbooks for each employee. They may require that the employee sign a form to acknowledge receiving the handbook.
Direct deposit form	Most healthcare agencies will pay the employees using the direct deposit method. Funds are transferred into the employee's bank account instead of the employee receiving a paper paycheck.
Agreement forms	The newly hired employee must sign agreement forms related to the Health Insurance Portability and Accountability Act (HIPAA) and computer security.

Professional development is also important in maintaining one's job. Medical assistants must keep updated and current in the healthcare industry. It is important to meet the continuing education units (CEUs) needed to maintain your certification or registration. Information on the requirements can be found on the credentialing agency's website.

Leaving a Job

Always offer at least 2 weeks' notice when resigning from a job since you would want a 2-week notice from your employer if your job were terminated. Prepare a written notice of resignation and take it to the supervisor in person. Do not just leave it on a desk or place it in the interoffice mail.

Resigning from a job just as an attempt to get a salary increase is a dangerous practice. Once the employer doubts the employee's loyalty, the future is not usually bright for the employee at that facility. Only resign after a final decision has been made. If the medical assistant is resigning to take another position, the current employer may be expected to make a **counteroffer.** However, be wary about accepting counteroffers. What led you to look for a new job in the first place? Has the situation been resolved? Ask yourself these questions before agreeing to stay with your current employer. Often employees who accept a counteroffer and stay at their original job find that few changes are made, and the employee ends up leaving the position in the long run.

CLOSING COMMENTS

As you finish your medical assistant program, embrace the challenge of finding a job. Spend time preparing for the search. Design a professional résumé and cover letter that positively sets you apart from the other graduates. Network and check job boards for job openings. Apply for any jobs that interest you. Keep organized in your search, so you do not overlook opportunities. Work with employment resources at your school to increase your confidence in interviewing. Your preparation and hard work will help you find your first medical assistant job!

Legal and Ethical Issues

Always be completely honest when completing a job application and offering information on a résumé. Most facilities stipulate that if an individual is not truthful on these documents, employment can be terminated when the deception is discovered. Employers are more interested in honesty and a forthright explanation than in minor problems that affect job performance.

Professional Behaviors

In many ambulatory care facilities, the supervisor will have medical assistants in the department participate in the interview team. The interview team members ask each interviewee the same set of questions. At the end of the interviews, the interview team members provide feedback to the supervisor about the interviewees. The information discussed is confidential. The interview team members should not discuss the interview process with others.

If a medical assistant has had some brush with the law that requires disclosure on the job application, the best policy is to be honest and deal with the ramifications of telling the truth. Most businesses can verify whether a potential employee has any type of criminal record. A solid explanation of the facts, admission of a past mistake, and excellent current references often prompt an employer to have faith and make a positive decision about offering employment.

SUMMARY OF SCENARIO

Before graduation, Michelle was offered a job at Walden-Martin Family Medical (WMFM) Clinic. She took her instructor's advice and sent a thank-you note to those who interviewed her. When she was offered the job, the supervisor mentioned how thoughtful the note was. During the call, the supervisor summarized the benefits and the starting salary. She mentioned to Michelle that all medical assistants start at the same wage, but after they pass the CMA (AAMA) certification examination, they get a raise. Michelle took 2 days to consider the position and decided to accept the job offer. The wage was lower than she was hoping for, but the benefits were much better.

Krysia has interviewed for several medical assistant positions over the past few weeks. She found that employers respected her service to her country and valued the skills she learned in military service. She just received her third job offer within the past few days and has decided to accept the position at the local Veterans Affairs (VA) clinic. It is a full-time position with great benefits. The higher wage will help offset the extra mileage she will be driving to work. She is excited to be working with other veterans.

Zac has struggled to identify what type of clinic he wants to work for. With his strong leadership skills, he hopes to find a position where he can advance to a supervisory position. Zac has interviewed for job positions at small and large clinics. He is finding that he is more interested in working with surgeons than with family practitioners. He also likes the complexity involved with surgical patients. Zac is hoping to receive a job offer shortly after graduation. He has decided that if his dream job is not offered to him, he will pursue a position in family medicine or internal medicine. This will give him a solid foundation for his new career, and then someday, he can move into orthopedics or surgery.

SUMMARY OF LEARNING OBJECTIVES

1. **Examine personality traits in employees that are important to employers.**
Because of the cost of training new employees, employers must find the best person to hire. Many employers struggle with assisting new employees in evolving or changing personality traits. Thus, employers seek people who already have collaboration and interpersonal skills, professionalism, compassion, and a genuine interest in the job. Collaboration and interpersonal skills allow the new employee to blend well with the current staff. Being flexible, dependable, supportive of peers, remaining calm under pressure, listening, and having good manners are just some of the characteristics of a person with great collaboration and interpersonal skills. Being professional includes proper dress and grooming habits, punctuality, honesty, attention to detail, and the ability to follow directions, prioritize, and manage time efficiently. Providing compassionate and respectful care and supporting the patient's dignity are crucial to good patient care. Lastly, being genuinely interested in the position positively affects the person's attitude and performance in the job.
2. **Examine how to assess your strengths and skills that are applicable to a job.**
Medical assistants must identify the personality traits, technical skills, and transferable job skills they possess. Using a portfolio will help interviewees to showcase the qualities that they have. Technical skills consist of the administrative and clinical skills the person has developed during the medical assistant program. Transferable job skills are skills that were used in an unrelated position but did relate or transfer to the new position.
3. **Examine the process of identifying career objectives and personal needs.**
Medical assistants should take some time to think about what they want from their career and develop a career objective. Your personal needs (e.g., wage, benefits, hours, locations) help you determine what job might be right for you so that you can focus your job search.
4. **Examine strategies for finding job openings.**
The two best methods to identify jobs are networking and using job boards. When networking, the medical assistant exchanges information with other professionals and family members in hopes of obtaining possible job leads. Job boards are online sites that list positions posted by employers. They can be specific to the healthcare facilities, or they can be managed by local media organizations. National job boards can be very helpful for those who want to relocate to another part of the country. Traditional job search sources include school career placement offices, newspaper ads, and employment agencies.
5. **Create a professional résumé.**
The three commonly used résumé formats are chronologic, combination, and targeted résumés. Procedures 54.1 describe the steps involved in preparing a résumé. A résumé contains information on the person's education, work experience, skills, and certifications. As you create your résumé, keep in mind the eye appeal or interest the résumé will create in the reader.
6. **Create a professional cover letter.**
A cover letter should always accompany a résumé, and as much attention to detail is necessary. Procedures 54.2 describe the steps involved with preparing a cover letter. Follow these strategies when creating a cover letter:
   - Match the appearance of the cover letter and résumé.
   - Address the inside address and the salutation (greeting) to a specific person.
   - Start the body of your cover letter with a bang.
   - Sell yourself to the reader.
   - Reaffirm that you are an excellent match for the job.
   - Be professional.
7. **Examine the use of online profiles and job applications.**
Many healthcare agencies use the internet during the employment process, and an online profile can have many advantages over paper applications. However, not every employer uses online profiles, and students also may have to fill out job applications. Procedure 54.3 describes the steps involved in completing a job application.
8. **Create a customized career portfolio.**
Just before an interview, the medical assistant should customize the portfolio for that employer (see Procedure 54.4). Using a three-ring binder with plastic sheet protectors and divider tabs, put together a career portfolio that includes the following:
   - Table of contents at the beginning with identified tabbed sections
   - Cover letter and résumé
   - References
   - Certifications
   - Education-related documents
   - Prior employment documents
   - Documentation showing that the student can balance work and education
   - Examples of work or summaries of projects that can provide evidence of abilities and skills
   - Criminal background documentation, blood titers, vaccination history, and current tuberculosis (TB) skin or blood tests results (optional)
9. **Explain strategies for preparing for an interview.**
When preparing for an interview, the job seeker needs to do the following:
   - *Research the facility*: Identify the mission and value statement, size of the organization and department, and the providers in the department.
   - *Practice answering potential questions.* This practice will help you prepare for the interview and appear more confident during the actual interview.
   - *Select interview attire.* Be conservative and professional with wardrobe choices.
   - *Prepare for the day of the interview.* Do a test run and prepare what you will bring to the interview.
10. **Differentiate among the types of interviews, including strategies to use.**
With face-to-face interviews, greet each person and shake hands. Ensure that each person has a copy of your résumé and cover letter before the interview begins. Phone interviews are usually done by the supervisor or the human resource representative. Virtual or video interviews use technology such as Microsoft Teams or Zoom. As with a phone interview, a virtual interview works well when the candidate is from out of town or if face-to-face interviews are not being held. The interviewee should prepare for phone and virtual interviews just like one would for

SUMMARY OF LEARNING OBJECTIVES—*continued*

a face-to-face interview. The interview should occur in a quiet environment, and the interviewee should pay attention to the interviewer.

11. **Examine how to be professional during and after the interview.**
Focus all answers on your career, strengths, and attributes, and what skills you have to bring to the healthcare setting. You can provide examples for your claims by either relating professional situations you have handled well or using your interview portfolio. The interviewer should not ask any illegal questions. Table 54.1 lists such topics and potentially illegal questions. The way that the medical assistant answers the questions can influence the employer's hiring decision.
Writing a thank-you note for an interview is a way to make you stand out from the other people who have interviewed for the same position. It shows that you are a courteous and conscientious person and also gives you another opportunity to show why you are the right person for the job. Refer to Procedure 54.6.
12. **Examine strategies to improve your opportunities for more interviews and job offers.**
When looking for additional job offers, it is important to identify if one is being too selective and using the correct job title. Expanding the geographic search area may net additional job possibilities. People who apply for jobs but never get calls for interviews must reevaluate the information given to employers. People getting interviews but no job offers must reevaluate their interview strategies.
13. **Examine the typical requirements when starting a new position, including performance appraisals.**
When you obtain a job, you will be required to complete a number of documents, including Form I-9, Form W-4, an insurance benefits form, a background check form, an emergency contact form, a handbook acknowledgment form, a direct deposit form, and an agreement form. You will be asked to bring in proof of identity and employment authorization (e.g., US passport, Social Security card, and driver's license). These documents are required for the employer's portion of Form I-9.
Most healthcare agencies have probationary periods for new employees. The medical assistant will get regular feedback from supervisors through performance appraisals. The performance appraisals inform employees of their strengths and weaknesses on the job. These appraisals are done after the probationary period and annually thereafter.

PROCEDURE 54.1 Prepare a Chronologic Résumé

TASK: Write an effective résumé to use as a tool for obtaining employment.

EQUIPMENT and SUPPLIES

- Computer with word processing software and a printer
- Current job posting
- Résumé paper
- Paper and pen

PROCEDURAL STEPS

1. Apply critical thinking skills as you create a list of the personality traits (wanted by employers), technical skills, and transferrable job skills that you possess. Also, write down your career goal(s).
PURPOSE: To determine the strongest aspects of your abilities so you can emphasize them on your résumé.
2. Using the current job posting, identify the required and recommended qualifications and credentials needed for the position.
PURPOSE: Identifying what the employer requires and would like will help you tailor your résumé to address these qualifications and credentials.
3. Using a computer with word processing software, create a professional-looking header for your document. Include your name, address, telephone number(s), and email address. Select an appropriate font style for your name and a smaller font size for your contact information.
PURPOSE: To make sure potential employers have a means of contacting you. Using a font style that is bold and a larger size for your name will help your name stand out. Make sure your contact information is presented in a smaller, nonbold style so it will not detract from your name.
4. Create a section header for "Education." For the learning institution(s) you attended, list the school's name, city and state, degree obtained or coursework successfully completed, and the year. Include any additional educational information, such as awards and the student clinical experience information.
PURPOSE: It is important to provide the school's name, city, and state, along with the degree. Some employers may need to verify the information.
5. Create a section header for "Healthcare Experience" and/or "Work Experience." Provide details about your work experience, including the facility's name, city and state, title of your position, start and end date (month and year), and job duties. The job duties must start with an active verb using the appropriate tense (e.g., a past job would have past tense verbs, and a current job would include present tense verbs).
PURPOSE: The potential employer will need to know your employment history and all the details.
6. Create a section header for "Special Skills," and list your special language skills, computer proficiencies, and other unique skills you possess that relate to the position.
PURPOSE: This section can be thought of as a marketing area where you emphasize the unique skills you possess.
7. Create a section header for "Certifications and Credentials," and list the active credentials and certifications you have. Include the title of the certification, awarding agency, and the expiration date.
Note: You may want to consider adding the date you are taking a credentialing examination. Employers like to know the status of your credentialing examination.

Continued

PROCEDURE 54.1 Prepare a Chronologic Résumé —*continued*

PURPOSE: Employers need to know if you have your medical assistant credential (e.g., CMA, RMA). They also might like to know if you have an active cardiopulmonary resuscitation (CPR) card.

8. All information on the résumé needs to appear in reverse chronologic order (i.e., newest information is listed first). Work experiences should include both the start and end month and year.
   PURPOSE: Employers need to know how long you worked at a specific place. If the position was seasonal or temporary, it is important to note that.
9. The résumé needs to look professional and interesting. Use font styles (e.g., bold, underline, italic) to emphasize important words and phrases. Use professional-looking bullets to list job duties and other information. Use the key words from the posting throughout the résumé.
   PURPOSE: The more professional and interesting a résumé appears, the better the chance that the potential employer will review it.
10. Proofread the résumé. Correct any spelling, grammar, punctuation, or sentence structure errors you find. If time allows, have another person review your résumé and use the feedback to revise it.
    PURPOSE: Résumés submitted with errors often are discarded without consideration.
11. Print the résumé on résumé paper, and proofread it one final time. Any errors should be corrected, and the document should be reprinted or emailed to the instructor.

PROCEDURE 54.2 Create a Cover Letter

TASK: Write an effective cover letter that will accompany the résumé.

EQUIPMENT and SUPPLIES

- Computer with word processing software and a printer
- Current job posting
- Résumé paper
- Pen

PROCEDURAL STEPS

1. Using the job posting, read through the job description. With a pen, circle the position requirements and the key phrases.
   PURPOSE: Your letter should contain the key phrases and position requirements that are found in the job posting.
2. Using a computer with word processing software, create a professional-looking header in the document's header that matches your résumé header. Include your name, address, telephone number(s), and email address.
   PURPOSE: To ensure potential employers have a means of contacting you. You can enhance the professional appearance of your documents by having the same header on each document.
3. Type the date in the correct location using the correct format. Have one blank line between the dateline and the last line of the letterhead.
   PURPOSE: All letters require a date for legal purposes. The correct format would be month, date, and year (e.g., May 14, 2025).
4. Type the inside address using the correct spelling, punctuation, and location for the information. Leave one to nine blank lines between the date and the inside address, depending on the location of the body of the letter.
   PURPOSE: The body of the letter needs to be centered vertically from top to bottom of the document. More blank lines can be added to move the body to the correct location.
5. Starting on the second line below the inside address, type the salutation using the correct format. Use a colon after the person's name.
   PURPOSE: A proper greeting helps set the tone of the letter.
6. Type the message in the body of the letter using the proper location and format. There should be a blank line after the salutation and between each paragraph. The message should be clear, concise, and professional. Use proper grammar, punctuation, capitalization, and sentence structure.
   PURPOSE: Proper grammar usage helps convey the message more accurately and professionally.
7. The first paragraph should contain the title and number of the job posting. The middle paragraph(s) should summarize your strengths and include key phrases from the posting. The final paragraph should discuss your availability for an interview. The body should end with an expression of gratitude to the reader.
   PURPOSE: It is important to thank the reader for considering you for the position.
8. Type a proper closing, leaving one blank line between the last line of the body and the closing. Use the correct format and location.
   PURPOSE: The closing helps end the message with a proper tone.
9. Type the signature block using the correct format and location. There should be four blank lines between the closing and the signature block.
   PURPOSE: The four blank lines will provide you with space to sign your name.
10. Spell-check and proofread the document. Check for proper tone, grammar, punctuation, capitalization, and sentence structure. Check for proper spacing between the parts of the letter.
    PURPOSE: The spell-check tool will identify only certain errors; proofreading will help identify incorrect word usage, improper tone, and errors in formatting. The tone of the letter should be professional but not aggressive.
11. Make any final corrections. Print the document on résumé paper and sign the letter or email the document to your instructor or employer.
    PURPOSE: It is professional to use résumé paper when submitting a résumé and cover letter to an employer.

PROCEDURE 54.3 Complete a Job Application

TASK: Complete an accurate, detailed job application legibly to secure a job offer.

EQUIPMENT and SUPPLIES

- Pen
- Application form
- Information regarding your past education, job experiences, and the skill sets you have developed (e.g., computer skills, keyboarding speed)
- Contact information for former supervisors and references
- Current résumé

PROCEDURAL STEPS

1. Read the entire job application before completing any part of the document.
   PURPOSE: Reading through the entire application helps prevent errors when filling out the document.
2. Refer to your information on past jobs, education experiences, and skill sets you have developed as you complete the application. Answers to the questions need to be accurate and honest.
   PURPOSE: The application is a legal document, and the answers must be correct and true.
3. Use proper grammar, sentence structure, punctuation, spelling, and capitalization. Handwriting should be legible to the reader.
   PURPOSE: Errors on the application or illegible sections may affect whether you are hired.
4. Do not leave any space blank. Answer each question on the document. If the question does not apply, write "not applicable."
   PURPOSE: Leaving a space blank on the application may suggest that the candidate did not want to answer a certain question or accidentally overlooked it. By writing "not applicable" on such questions, the candidate demonstrates competence and attention to detail.
5. Do not write "See résumé" anywhere on the document.
   PURPOSE: Many supervisors view this practice as laziness. Always fill out the job application completely, and do not leave blank spaces.
6. Include information on the application that exhibits dependability, punctuality, teamwork, attention to detail, a positive work ethic and initiative, the ability to adapt to change, a responsible attitude, and the use of technology.
   PURPOSE: These phrases send an important message to employers. It is important to use the words they are looking for.
7. Sign and date the document.
   PURPOSE: Because this is a legal document, read the fine print before signing the document and dating it.
8. Proofread the document, and make sure none of the information conflicts with the résumé.PURPOSE: Proofreading helps the candidate catch any errors before submitting the application.

PROCEDURE 54.4 Create a Career Portfolio

TASK: Create a custom portfolio that provides potential employers with evidence of your skills and knowledge as a medical assistant.

EQUIPMENT and SUPPLIES

- Three-ring binder or folder
- Plastic sleeves for the three-ring binder
- Dividers with tabs for the three-ring binder
- Current résumé and cover letter
- Documents providing evidence of your skills and knowledge (e.g., transcripts, job evaluations, student clinical experience evaluation forms and skill checklist, projects completed in school, letters of recommendation, and copies of certifications [e.g., CPR card])

PROCEDURAL STEPS

1. Group documents in a logical manner, putting similar documents together. Identify the arrangement for the portfolio. An arrangement could include a cover letter and résumé, education section (e.g., transcript, evaluation form and skills checklist, awards), prior job-related documents (e.g., evaluations), reference letters, and work products (e.g., projects you created in your medical assistant program).
   PURPOSE: Organizing the documents in a logical manner will help the reader identify the important documents. The arrangement will also show the reader your ability to organize content.
2. Insert one document per plastic pocket. Place all documents in plastic pockets.
   PURPOSE: The plastic pockets will keep the documents clean and neat.
3. Neatly write the topic area on the tab of the dividers. Insert the tabbed dividers in the binder or folder.
   PURPOSE: This will help the reader find the content easier.
4. Place all documents in the binder or folder behind the correct divider. Place your cover letter and résumé in the front of all the other documents.
   PURPOSE: The reader can review the letter and résumé as needed before looking at the other documents in the portfolio.
5. Create a table of contents to identify the tabbed areas.
   PURPOSE: Organizing the documents in a logical manner will help the reader identify the important documents. The arrangement will also show the reader your ability to organize content.
6. After the portfolio is assembled, review the entire portfolio to ensure it looks professional, and the documents provide positive support for your skill set and knowledge.
   PURPOSE: Minimize the negative documents in your portfolio. They will not help you obtain a job as much as the positive, supporting documents.

PROCEDURE 54.5 Practice Interview Skills during a Mock Interview

TASKS: Project a professional appearance during a job interview and be able to express the reasons the medical assistant is the best candidate for the position.

EQUIPMENT and SUPPLIES

- Current job posting
- Résumé
- Cover letter
- Interview portfolio (optional)
- Application (optional)
- Interviewer
- Mock interview questions

PROCEDURAL STEPS

1. Wear interview-appropriate attire and be groomed professionally.
   PURPOSE: Your appearance will influence the first impression made on this potential employer. Most medical facilities prefer conservative dress.
2. Portray a professional image by shaking hands firmly prior to the start of the interview. Ensure that each interviewer has a copy of your résumé and cover letter. Refrain from nervous behaviors (e.g., saying "um," tapping a pen or your foot) during the interview.
   PURPOSE: Many employers feel a firm handshake is important. Each interviewer may need a copy of your documents to reference during the interview.
3. Answer introductory questions by providing only professional information. This may include information about your education, experience, and career goals.
   PURPOSE: Many people are tempted to answer with personal information (e.g., if they are married or have children). Personal information should not be discussed during the interview.
4. Answer interview questions with open, honest, and positive responses. Completely answer questions, provide information or examples, and do not answer in single sentences or with limited responses.
   PURPOSE: The goal of the interview is for the employer to get to know you. Limited responses negatively affect this goal.
5. Use key words from the job posting when answering the interview questions.
   PURPOSE: This helps prove the interviewee has exactly what the organization is looking for.
6. Ask the interviewer two to three appropriate questions about the facility or the position.
   PURPOSE: This demonstrates an interest in the organization and the position.
7. Express interest in the job and politely complete the interview by shaking hands and thanking the interviewer for the opportunity for the interview.
   PURPOSE: The employer wants to know that you are interested in the job. It is professional to thank the interviewer for the interview opportunity.

PROCEDURE 54.6 Create a Thank-You Note for an Interview

TASK: Create a meaningful, thank-you note to be sent after the interview process.

EQUIPMENT and SUPPLIES

- Computer with word processing software and a printer
- Job description
- Contact name from the interview

PROCEDURAL STEPS

1. Using word processing software, compose a professional letter using the business letter format. Include all of the required elements in the letter. Use correct spacing between the elements.
   PURPOSE: Creating a professional business letter shows the employer that you pay attention to detail.
2. Emphasize the particulars of the interview in the body of the letter.
   PURPOSE: Providing highlights of the interview will assure the employer that you took the time to write an individual thank-you letter.
3. Include positive information you wish you had covered in the interview.
   PURPOSE: This allows you to present any missed skills or details in a professional manner.
4. Create a message that is concise and to the point.
   PURPOSE: Keep the letter short and concise. Employers look for employees who can summarize a message and communicate that message.
5. Proofread the letter, and make any revisions as needed. Sign and send the thank-you note.
   PURPOSE: It is important to make sure your note is written correctly. You want to leave a positive perception with the employer.

GLOSSARY

5% Sheep's Blood Agar Plate (BAP) A solid agar medium that contains nutrients and 5% washed sheep's blood. The blood is added as an extra nutrient source for bacteria.

Abscess A localized collection of pus, which may be under the skin or deep in the body, that cause tissue destruction.

Abstract Collecting important information from the health record.

Abuse An action that purposely harms another person.

Accessory Muscles Muscles in the neck, abdomen, and back that assist in breathing.

Accommodation An adjustment of the eye that allows a person to see various sizes of objects at different distances.

Accounts Payable Money owed by a company to other companies for services and goods; pertains to paying the facility's bills.

Acetylcholinesterase (ah SEET l KOE leh nes teeh RASE) An enzyme that destroys acetylcholine and counteracts its action.

Acronym An abbreviation formed from the first letter of each word of a phrase and pronounced as a word.

Acute Phase The phase during which rapid multiplication of the pathogen takes place. Symptoms are very distinct. A strong response of the immune system takes place during this stage.

Acute Stage The phase during which rapid multiplication of the pathogen takes place. Symptoms are very distinct. A strong response of the immune system takes place during this stage.

Addiction A disease that occurs when a person cannot stop or limit the use of a drug, even after negative consequences have been experienced.

Adenosine Triphosphate (ATP) A high-energy molecule, found in every cell, that supplies large amounts of energy for various biochemical processes.

Adherence The act of sticking to something.

Adhesions (ad HEE zhuns) Bands of scar tissue that can bind anatomic structures together.

Adjudicate (uh JOO di kayt) To settle or determine judicially.

Advance Directives Written instructions about healthcare decisions in case a person is unable to make them.

Aerobic Occurring in the presence of oxygen

Afferent (AF er uhnt) Pertaining to carrying toward a structure.

Age of Majority The age at which the law recognizes a person to be an adult; it varies by state.

Albumin (al BYOO men) Most abundant plasma protein in human blood. It is important for regulating the water balance of blood.

Aliquot A portion of a well-mixed sample removed for testing.

Allopathic (al uh PATH ik) A system of medical practice that treats disease by the use of remedies, such as medications and surgery, to produce effects different from those caused by the disease under treatment; medical doctors (MDs) and osteopaths (DOs) practice allopathic medicine; also called conventional medicine.

Alphabetic Filing Any system that arranges names or topics according to the sequence of the letters in the alphabet.

Alphanumeric Describes systems made up of combinations of letters and numbers.

Amblyopia (am blee OH pee ah) Dull or dim vision, with no apparent organic defect.

Ambu Bag A self-refilling bag-valve-mask unit used for artificial respiration that is effective for ventilating and oxygenating intubated patients. Acronym for artificial manual breathing unit.

Amenorrhea (ey men uh REE uh) Lack of menstrual flow.

Amino Acids (ah MEE noe) Found in protein-containing foods and released during the digestion process in the intestines; carried by the blood to cells, where they are used to make proteins. Used for growth, maintenance, and repair of cells; they also transport nutrients.

Amnesia (am NEE zhah) Memory loss.

Amygdala (ah MIG dah lah) A small mass of gray matter found in each temporal lobe of the cerebrum and involved with memories, emotions, and activating the fight-or-flight response; part of the limbic system.

Amyloid Plaques Masses or clumps of proteins that form between neurons and disrupt cellular function.

Anaerobic Occurring without the presence of oxygen.

Analgesic (an ahl JEE zik) A drug that prevents or alleviates heart pain.

Analyte (AN e lit) The substance or chemical being analyzed or detected in a specimen.

Anaphylaxis (an ah fah LAK sis) A rapidly progressing, life-threatening allergic reaction; characterized by hives, swelling of the mouth and airway, difficulty breathing, wheezing, and loss of consciousness.

Anaplastic (an uh PLAS tic) A rapidly dividing cancer cell that has little to no similarity to normal cells.

Anastomosis (ah nas tih MOH sis) The surgical connection of separate or severed tubular hollow organs to form a continuous channel.

Anemia A deficiency of hemoglobin in the blood. Accompanied by a reduced number of red blood cells, pale skin, weakness, and shortness of breath among other symptoms.

Anencephaly (an en SEF uh lee) The congenital absence of part or all of the brain.

Anesthetic (an ehs THET ik) An agent that causes partial or complete loss of sensation.

Aneurysm (AN yeh rizm) An abnormal blood-filled sac formed by a localized dilation of the wall of a vein, artery, or heart.

Anhedonia (an hee DOE nee ah) The inability to feel or experience pleasure during a pleasurable activity.

Anisometropia (an EYE soh mi TROE pee ah) A condition in which the refraction (focus) is different in both eyes.

Anovulation Failure of the ovaries to release an ovum at the time of ovulation.

Answering Service A commercial service that answers telephone calls for its clients.

Antiarrhythmic (an tee ah RITH mik) A drug that prevents or alleviates heart arrhythmias.

Antibiotic (an ti bie OT ik) A drug that destroys or inhibits the growth of bacteria.

Antibody (AN tih bod ee) A protein substance, produced in the blood or tissues in response to a specific antigen, that destroys or weakens the antigen. Part of the immune system.

Anticoagulant (an tee koe AG yuh lant) A substance (i.e., medication or chemical) that prevents the clotting of blood.

Anticonvulsant (an tee kahn VUL sahnt) A drug used to prevent or treat seizures.

Antigen (an TIE jen) A substance that stimulates the production of an antibody when introduced into the body. Antigens include toxins, bacteria, viruses, and other foreign substances.

Antihistamine (an tee HIS tah meen) A drug that counteracts the effects of histamine.

Antihyperlipidemic (an tie hie per lip i DEE mik) A substance (i.e., medication) that lowers the lipid levels in the blood.

Antihypertensive A drug that reduces high blood pressure.

Anti-inflammatory (an tee in FLAM ah tor ee) A medication that prevents or reduces inflammation.

Antimalarial (an tee mah LAR ee ahl) A drug used to treat or prevent malaria.

Antipyretic (an tee pie RET ik) A drug used to reduce a fever.

Antiseptic (an ti SEP tik) A substance that inhibits the growth of microorganisms on living tissue (e.g., alcohol and povidone-iodine solution [Betadine]).

Antioxidant (an tee OK si dahnt) A synthetic or natural substance found in food and supplements; may prevent or delay some types of cell damage.

Antiseptics (an ti SEP tiks) Substances that inhibit the growth of microorganisms on living tissue (e.g., alcohol and povidone-iodine solution [Betadine]); they are used to cleanse the skin, wounds, and so on.

Anthropometric (an thruh po ME trik) Pertaining to the measurement of the size and proportions of the human body.

Aphasia (ah FAY zhah) The partial or complete loss of the ability to articulate ideas or understand written or spoken language.

Apnea (AP nee ah) Abnormal, periodic cessation of breathing.

Aponeurosis A tough, fibrous connective tissue that attaches muscles to muscles.

Approximated (uh PROK si may ted) Near, close together.

Arbitration (ahr bi TRAE shuhn) The process in which conflicting parties in a dispute submit their differences to a court-appointed person (arbitrator), who submits a legally binding decision.

Arrhythmia (ah RITH mee ah) An abnormal heart rate or rhythm.

Arterioles (ar TEER ee ohlz) Small arteries.

Arteriosclerosis (ar teer ee oh sklah ROH sis) Thickening, decreased elasticity, and calcification of arterial walls.

Arteriovenous (ahr teer ee oh VEE nuhs) Graft A synthetic tube that connects an artery to a vein; also called AV graft.

Arteriovenous Fistula An abnormal joining of an artery and vein.

Arthropod Any animal that lacks a spine, such as insects, crustaceans, arachnids, and others.

Artifact A substance, structure, or event that does not naturally occur in a situation. Examples include interference, or electrical "garbage," on an ECG, or crystals, lint, or contamination of a staining technique.

Artificial Insemination The injection of semen into the vagina or uterus using a catheter or syringe. Nonsexual.

Aseptically (ay SEP tick ah lee) Free from living pathogenic organisms.

Asexual Describes reproduction that does not involve the fusion of male and female sex cells.

Aspirate (AS puh rayt) To withdraw fluid using suction; the material removed using suction. One example is a specimen that has been removed from the body using a needle and syringe.

Aspiration The process of removing fluids or gases from the body using a suction device. Inhalation of a liquid (e.g., blood and vomitus) or a foreign object into the respiratory tract.

Assets All property available for the payment of debts.

Astigmatism (ah STIG mah tiz um) Inability of the cornea to focus, causing blurred vision.

Ataxia Loss of the ability to coordinate muscular movement.

Atheroma (ath uh ROH mah) A waxy lesion, made up of cholesterol, fat, calcium, cells, and other substances, that builds up on the inner wall of an artery.

Attenuated (uh TEN yoo ayt ed) Weakened or changed.

Atypical Lymphs In many viral infections, stimulated or reactive lymphs are called *atypical lymphs.* They are commonly seen in infectious mononucleosis, or "mono."

Audible (AW di buhl) Capable of being heard.

Audiologist (aw dee OL uh jist) An allied healthcare professional who specializes in the evaluation of hearing function, detection of hearing impairment, and determination of the anatomic site of impairment.

Audit A process completed before a claims submission in which claims are examined for accuracy and completeness.

Auditory Cortex The region of the cerebral cortex that receives auditory data.

Auscultate (AW skuhl tayt) To listen with a stethoscope.

Auscultated (AW skuhl tay ted) Listening to the sounds within the body with a stethoscope.

Authorized Agent A person who has written documentation that he or she can accept a shipment for another individual.

Autoimmune A disease in which the body produces antibodies that attack its own tissues and cells, leading to the deterioration of structure or function.

Automatic Call Routing A system that distributes incoming calls to a specific group or person based on customer need; for example, the customer presses 1 for appointments, 2 for billing questions, and so on.

Automatic Exposure Control (AEC) Terminates the exposure time when a certain quantity of radiation has been detected at the image receptor.

Autonomy (aw TON uh mee) The ability to function independently.

Axon (AK son) A long extension of a nerve fiber that conducts the impulse away from the nerve cell body; white matter.

Backordered An order placed for an item that is temporarily out of stock and will be sent later.

Bacteria Microorganisms that are single celled, lack a nucleus, reproduce asexually, or can form spores. Some can cause disease. The most abundant life form on earth.

Bartholin (BAR thoh lin) Cyst A fluid-filled cyst in one of the vestibular glands located on either side of the vaginal orifice.

Basal Bottom layer.

Belligerent (buh LIG er ent) Hostile and aggressive.

Beneficiary A designated person who receives funds from an insurance policy.

Benign A noncancerous condition; not malignant, harmless.

Biconvex (bie KON veks) Having two outward curving surfaces, on a lens.

Bilaterally (bie LAT er uhl ee) Pertaining to, involving, or affecting two or both sides.

Bilingual (bie LING gwuhl) Ability to communicate effectively in two languages.

Bilirubin (bil i ROO bin) A reddish-yellow pigment that results from the breakdown of red blood cells in the liver.

Billable Service Assistance (i.e., service) that is delivered by a healthcare provider and can be billed to the insurance company or patient.

Binary Fission Asexual reproduction in single-celled organisms during which one cell divides into two daughter cells.

Binocular (buh NOK yuh ler) Involving, relating, or seeing with both eyes.

Binomial A name consisting of a generic and a specific term.

Bioethicists (BYE oh eth I sists) People who study the ethical effect of biomedical advances (e.g., drugs and genetic engineering).

Biomarkers Detectable cellular indicators used as a marker for a substance or disease process.

Biopsy (BIE op see) Process of viewing living tissue that has been removed for the purpose of diagnosis or treatment.

Bipolar Having two poles or electrical charges.

Blood Agar Plate (BAP) A solid agar medium that contains nutrients and 5% washed sheep's blood. The blood is added as an extra nutrient source for bacteria.

Blood Culture A microbiologic procedure ordered when a provider suspects a bacterial infection is causing a fever of unknown origin (FUO). A blood sample is collected into a nutrient media and held at body temperature. If bacteria are in the blood sample, the culture media should encourage the growth of the infecting bacteria in the laboratory.

Bonded A term describing employees for whom an employer has obtained a fidelity bond from an insurance company, which will cover losses from any dishonest acts (e.g., embezzlement, theft) committed by those employees.

Bookkeeping The process of recording financial transactions.

Boot The process of starting or restarting a computer when the operating system is loaded.

Bounding Describes a pulse that feels full because of the increased power of cardiac contraction or as a result of increased blood volume.

Bradycardia (brad ee KAHR dee uh) A slow heartbeat; a pulse below 60 beats per minute.

Bradypnea (brad IP nee ah) Abnormally slow breathing.

Breach Disclosure of protected health information without a reason or permission, which compromises the security or privacy of the information.

Bremsstrahlung Radiation Radiation that is created when an electron enters the tungsten anode of the x-ray tube, misses the tungsten electrons, and gets very near the nucleus.

Bronchiolitis Occurs when the small airways of the lungs become inflamed because of a viral infection.

Bronchodilator A drug that relaxes smooth muscle contractions in the bronchioles to improve lung ventilation.

Bruit (broot) An abnormal sound or murmur heard on auscultation of an organ, vessel (e.g., carotid artery), or gland.

Bucky Contains a movable grid device that absorbs scatter radiation and also contains the image receptor.

Business Associate A person or business that provides a service to a covered entity that involves access to protected health information. Examples include legal, billing, and management services; accreditation agencies; consulting firms; and claims processing organizations.

Buying Cycle Refers to how often an item is purchased and depends on how frequently the item is used and the storage space available for it.

Calcium A naturally occurring element that is necessary for many body functions, including strong bones and teeth, proper blood clotting, nerve conduction, and muscle contractions.

Calculi (KAL kyuh lie) Stones formed in the kidneys, gallbladder, and other parts of the body.

Calibrated (KAL uh bray ted) Determined by or checked against a standard (as in readings).

Calibration (kal uh BRAY shun) Determining the accuracy of an instrument by comparing its output with that of a known standard or another instrument known to be accurate.

Caliper A pocket-sized tool used for measuring the height and width of the ECG waves and intervals.

Call Forwarding A telephone feature that allows calls made to one number to be forwarded to another specified number.

Caller ID A feature that identifies and displays the telephone numbers of incoming calls made to a particular line.

Callus Hard bony tissue that forms at the ends of fractured bones during the healing process.

Candidiasis (kan di DIE i sis) An infection caused by a yeast, *Candida albicans,* that typically affects the vaginal mucosa and skin.

Cannula (KAN yuh la) A rigid tube that surrounds a blunt trocar or a sharp, pointed trocar, which is inserted into the body; when the trocar is withdrawn, fluid may escape from the body through the cannula, depending on the insertion site.

Capitation (ka pi TAY shun) A payment arrangement for healthcare providers. The provider is paid a set amount for each enrolled person assigned to him or her, per period of time, whether or not that person has received services.

Caption A heading, title, or subtitle under which records are filed.

Cardiac Defibrillator An external or implantable device that provides an electric shock to the heart to restore a normal sinus rhythm.

Cardiopulmonary Resuscitation (ri sus i TAY shun) (CPR) The application of manual chest compressions and ventilations (also called *rescue breathing*) to patients who are not breathing or do not have a pulse; also known as *basic life support (BLS).*

Cartilage (KAR tih lij) Flexible connective tissue that covers the ends of many bones at the joint.

Cash on Hand The amount of money the healthcare facility has in the bank that can be withdrawn as cash.

Cataplexy (KAT ah PLEK see) A sudden loss of muscle strength and tone associated with an emotional stimulus.

Cataract (KAT ur ackt) Progressive loss of transparency of the lens of the eye.

Catheter A hollow, flexible tube that can be inserted into a vessel, organ, or cavity of the body to withdraw or instill fluid, monitor information, and visualize a vessel or cavity.

Caustic (KAW stik) Capable of burning, corroding, or destroying living tissue.

Central Ray (CR) The center of the x-ray beam and perpendicular to the long axis of the x-ray tube.

Centrifuge (SEN truh fyooj) A machine that rotates at high speed and separates substances of different densities by centrifugal force. For example, a tube of blood is separated into plasma/serum, white blood cells, platelets, and red blood cells.

Certified Registered Nurse Anesthetist (CRNA) A nursing healthcare professional who is certified to administer anesthesia.

Cerumen (si ROO muhn) A waxy secretion in the ear canal; commonly called ear wax.

Cessation (se SAY shuhn) Bringing to an end.

Characteristic Radiation Radiation that is created when an electron enters the tungsten anode of the x-ray tube and knocks out a K-shell electron.

Cheyne-Stokes Respiration Deep, rapid breathing followed by a period of apnea.

Chief Complaint A statement in the patient's own words that describes the reason for the visit.

Cholecystitis Inflammation of the gallbladder.

Choroid Plexus (KOR oid PLEK sus) A network of capillaries found in the lateral ventricles and the third and fourth ventricles that secrete cerebrospinal fluid.

Chromosomes (KROE mah somes) Rod-shaped structures found in the cell's nucleus; they contain genetic information.

Chronic Developing slowly and lasting for a long time, generally 3 or more months.

Chronologic (kron ih LOJ ic) Arranged in the order of time.

Cicatrix (SIK uh triks) Early scar tissue that appears pale, contracted, and firm.

Claim An itemized statement of services and costs from a healthcare facility submitted to the health (insurance) plan for payment.

Claims Clearinghouse An organization that accepts the claim data from the provider, reformats the data to meet the specifications outlined by the insurance plan, and submits the claim.

Claim Scrubbers Software that finds common billing errors before the claim is sent to the insurance company.

Clarification (klar i fi KAY shuhn) Allows the listener to get additional information.

Clitoris (KLIT uh ris) Sensitive, erectile tissue.

Clot Activators Substances added to a venipuncture tube to enhance and speed up blood clotting.

Clubbing Abnormal enlargement of the distal phalanges (fingers and toes) associated with cyanotic heart disease or advanced chronic pulmonary disease.

CMS-1500 Health Insurance Claim Form (CMS-1500) The standard insurance claim form used for all government and most commercial insurance companies.

Coaching Providing information in a supportive environment that allows people to grow, change, or improve their situation.

Code A term used in healthcare settings to indicate an emergency situation and to summon the trained team to the scene.

Coding System A system designed to use characters (i.e., numbers and letters) to represent something, such as a medical procedure or a disease.

Cohesive (koh HEE siv) Sticking together tightly; exhibiting or producing cohesion.

Collaboration (kuh lab uh RAY shun) The act of working with another or multiple individuals.

Collagen (KAH lah jen) The most abundant structural protein found in skin and other connective tissues. It provides strength and cushioning to many parts of the body.

Collimation (kol i MAY shun) The method of restricting and confiding the x-ray beam to a given area.

Colonoscopy (kohl uh NOS kuh pee) A procedure in which a fiberoptic scope is used to examine the large intestine.

Colony A discrete group of organisms, such as a group of bacteria, growing on a solid nutrient surface.

Colostomy (koh LOS tuh mee) A surgical procedure in which the large intestine is brought though the abdominal wall, creating either a temporary or a permanent opening (stoma) to allow stool to pass out of the body.

Colposcopy (kol PAW skoh pee) Using a microscope with a light source, the vagina and cervix are visually examined to locate and evaluate abnormal cells. A biopsy of abnormal cells may be taken during this procedure.

Coma A state of deep, often prolonged unconsciousness, usually the result of a head injury, neurologic disease, intoxication, or metabolic abnormalities.

Common Law Unwritten laws that come from judicial decisions based on societal traditions and customs.

Communicable (kuh MYOO ni kuh buhl) Diseases Diseases spread from person to person by either direct contact or indirect contact (e.g., via insects).

Compact Bone Consists of tightly packed osteons; denser and heavier compared to spongy bone.

Compartment Syndrome A serious condition that involves increased pressure, usually in the muscles; it leads to compromised blood flow and muscle and nerve damage.

Compassion Having a deep awareness of the suffering of another and the wish to ease it.

Complementary and Alternative Medicine (CAM) A group of diverse medical and healthcare systems, practices, and products that are not generally considered part of conventional medicine. Complementary medicine is used in combination with conventional medicine (allopathic or osteopathic); alternative medicine is used instead of conventional medicine.

Compliance (kuhm PLIE uhns) Meeting the standards and regulations of the practice's established policies and procedures. Can also mean cooperation.

Compliant (kum PLIE unt) Obeying, obliging, or yielding.

Computed Radiography A cassette-based digital imaging system where the image of the body part is obtained using storage phosphor plate.

Computer Network A system that links personal computers and peripheral devices to share information and resources.

Concise (kuhn SICE) Using as few words as possible to express a message.

Concussion A type of traumatic brain injury resulting from a hit to the head or body that causes the brain to move rapidly back and forth.

Cone Biopsy An extensive cervical biopsy during which a cone-shaped wedge of tissue is removed from the cervix and examined under a microscope. Abnormal tissue, along with a small amount of normal tissue, is removed.

Conference Call A telephone call in which a caller can speak with several people at the same time.

Congruence (kun GROO uhns) Agreement; the state that occurs when the verbal expression of the message matches the sender's nonverbal body language.

Conscientious (kon shee EN shuhs) Meticulous, careful.

Consensus (kun SEN sus) General agreement.

Constrict To contract or shrink.

Contamination (kun tam i NAY shun) The process by which something becomes harmful or unusable through contact with something unclean.

Continuity of Care The smooth continuation of care from one provider to another. This allows the patient to receive the most benefit with no interruption or duplication of care.

Contraindicate (kon truh IN di kayt) To specify that an agent or procedure should not be used.

Controlled Substances A behavior-altering or addictive drug or chemical substance whose possession and use are prohibited by or regulated under the federal Controlled Substances Act.

Control Materials Manufacturer-prepared samples that have a known quantity of a specific analyte. Used for quality control purposes. Testing results should fall within a manufacturer-defined range of results. Also called controls or quality controls.

Convalescent Stage The phase during which the host recovers gradually and returns to baseline or normal health.

Copayment (Copay) A set dollar amount that the patient must pay for each office visit. There can be one copayment amount for a primary care provider, and a different copayment amount (usually higher) to see a specialist or to be seen in the emergency department.

Coping Mechanisms Behavioral and psychological strategies used to deal with or minimize stressful events.

Correlate (CORE uh layt) To establish an orderly relationship or connection.

Corrosive (kuh ROH siv) Causing or tending to cause the gradual destruction of a substance by chemical action.

Corticosteroids (kor ti koe STER oids) A group of steroid hormones produced in the body or given as a medication. Some have metabolic functions, and others reduce tissue inflammation. Glucocorticoids and mineralocorticoids are two types.

Counterfeit (KOWN ter fit) An imitation intended to be passed off fraudulently or deceptively as genuine; forgery.

Counteroffer A return offer made by one who has rejected an offer or a job.

Covered Entity (KUV er ed EN ti tee) A healthcare facility, healthcare provider, pharmacy, health (insurance) plan, or claims clearinghouse that transmits protected health information electronically.

CPT Assistant An online version of the *Current Procedural Terminology* (CPT) coding journal, supported by the American Medical Association (AMA), that addresses subjects such as appealing insurance denials, validating coding to auditors, training staff members, and answering day-to-day coding questions.

Crash Cart Emergency and equipment (e.g., oxygen, intravenous [IV] and airway supplies) stored in a cart and ready for an emergency.

Creatinine Clearance Rates Results from a procedure used to evaluate the glomerular filtration rate of the kidneys.

Credential (kri DEN shul) Evidence of authority, status, rights, entitlement to privileges.

Crepitation (krep i TAY shun) A dry, crackling sound or sensation.

Critical Thinking The constant practice of considering all aspects of a situation when deciding what to believe or what to do.

Cryosurgery The technique of exposing tissue to extreme cold to produce a well-defined area of cell destruction.

Crystals Solid substances with a regular shape that is due to the structure of molecules.

Culture Media A solid, liquid, or semisolid medium designed to support the growth of microorganisms, especially bacteria and fungus.

Curettage (kyoo reh TAHZH) The act of scraping a body cavity with a surgical instrument, such as a curette.

Cryopreservation (KRIE oh pri zur vae shun) To preserve by freezing at low temperatures.

Cystic Fibrosis (CF) A disorder that affects all the exocrine cells, but affects the respiratory system the most. Mucus is abnormally thick and blocks the alveoli, causing dyspnea.

Cytology (sie TOL oh jee) The study of cells using microscopic methods.

Cytoplasm The cell substance that fills the area between the nucleus and the cell membrane. It contains the organelles of the cell.

Damages A monetary settlement the defendant pays the plaintiff in a civil case for loss or injury. Also, one of the 4 Ds of negligence, meaning the patient suffers a legally recognized injury.

Debridement The surgical removal of dead, damaged, or infected tissue to improve the function of healthy tissue.

Debris (duh BREE) The remains of anything broken down or destroyed; ruins, rubble.

Decanting Pouring a liquid gently so that it does not disturb the remaining sediment.

Declaratory Judgment A court judgment that defines the legal rights of the parties involved.

Decolorizer A liquid that has the ability to wash out color.

Decongestant A drug that is used for nasal congestion.

Decryption (dee KRIP shun) The computer process of changing encrypted text to readable or plain text after a user enters a secret key or password.

Decubitus Ulcers (deh KYOO bi tus) Sores or ulcers that develop over a bony prominence as the result of ischemia from prolonged pressure; also called *bed sores* or *pressure sores.*

De-escalating Reducing the level or intensity; bringing down a person's anger or elevated emotions.

Defecation (def i KAY shun) The act of voiding waste from the bowels through the anus; the act of having a bowel movement.

Defendant (dih FEN dant) An individual or a business against whom a lawsuit is filed.

Defense (di FENS) A strategy used by the defendant to avoid liability in a lawsuit.

Defense Mechanisms Unconscious mental processes that protect people from anxiety, loss, conflict, or shame.

Degenerative (dih JEN er uh tiv) An illness resulting from the deterioration of tissues and organs.

Delegate To appoint a person as a representative.

Delusion (de LOO zhun) An unshakable belief in something untrue; may be accompanied by hallucinations or paranoia.

Demeanor (dih MEE ner) Behavior toward others; outward manner.

Dementia (di MEN shah) A mental disorder in which the individual experiences a progressive loss of memory, personality alterations, confusion, loss of touch with reality, and stupor (seeming unawareness of, and disconnection with, one's surroundings).

Demographics Statistical data of a population. In healthcare this includes the patient's name, address, date of birth, employment, and other details.

Density Describes how compact or concentrated something is.

Deoxygenated Oxygen deficient; oxygen was removed.

Deposition (dep ah ZISH uhn) A sworn testimony made before a court-appointed officer; it is used in the discovery process and may be used in the trial.

Dependent Adults People between the ages of 18 and 64 who have a mental or physical impairment that prevents them from doing normal activities or from protecting themselves.

Depersonalization Alternative perception of the self; a person's own reality is lost. People feel they are not in control of their own actions or speech.

Depreciate To diminish in value (e.g., the value of an item) over a period of time; a concept used for tax purposes.

Derealization The loss of sensation of the reality of one's surroundings.

Dermatome (DUR mah tome) Skin surface areas supplied by a single afferent spinal nerve.

Detrimental (de truh MEN tl) Harmful.

Dextrocardia (dek stro KAHR dee ah) The condition in which the heart is located on the right side of the chest, and the apex is pointing to the right.

Dextrose (DEK strose) A glucose solution administered intravenously.

Diabetic Retinopathy (die ah BET ik reh tin OP ah thee) Damages the blood vessels in the retina, leading to loss of vision and eventual blindness.

Diagnosis (die ag NOH sis) Determining the cause of a condition, illness, disease, injury, or congenital defect.

Diagnostic Statement Information about a patient's diagnosis or diagnoses that has been taken from the medical documentation.

Diaphragm A broad, dome-shaped muscle used for breathing that separates the thoracic and abdominopelvic cavities.

Dictation (dik TEY shuhn) To say something aloud for another person to write down.

Differentiate (dif uh REN shee ayt) To distinguish one thing from another. To make a distinction between items.

Differentiated (dif uh REN shee ayt ed) Describes how malignant tissue or cells looks like the normal tissue or cells it came from; poorly differentiated means it does not look like the normal tissue or cells, and well differentiated means it looks like the normal tissue or cells.

Diffuse To spread, scatter, disperse, or move.

Digital Radiography (DR) Cassetteless imaging system where the phosphor is bonded to a flat panel detector or the system converts x-ray energy directly to an electronic signal.

Dignity (DIG ni tee) The inherent worth or state of being worthy of respect.

Dilation (die LAY shuhn) The opening or widening of the circumference of a body orifice with a dilating instrument.

Diluent (dye LU ent) A liquid substance that dilutes or lessens the strength of a solution or mixture; it is added to vials of powdered medications to create a solution of the drug for injection.

Dilution Reducing the concentration of a mixture or solution by adding a known volume of liquid.

Direct Filing System A filing system in which materials can be located without consulting another source of reference.

Discipline A branch of knowledge, learning, or instruction; for instance, medicine, nursing, social work, and physical therapy.

Discrepancy A lack of similarity between what is stated and what is found; for instance, the computer inventory count is different from the physical count.

Discretionary Income Money in a bank account that is not assigned to pay for any office expenses.

Disinfect The process of cleaning in order to destroy or prevent the growth of disease-causing microorganisms.

Disinfectant (dis in FEK tant) Any chemical agent used on nonliving objects to destroy or inhibit the growth of harmful organisms; not effective against bacterial spores.

Disparaging (di SPAR a jing) Slighting; having a negative or degrading tone.

Disruption An unexpected event that throws a plan into disorder; an interruption that prevents a system or process from continuing as usual or as expected.

Dissect To cut or separate tissue with a cutting instrument or scissors.

Distortion The differences between the actual subject and its radiographic image.

Diuretic A substance (i.e., medication) that increases the amount of urine produced.

Diurnal (die UR nl) Variation Fluctuations that occur during each day.

Diversity The differences and similarities in identity, perspective, and points of view among people.

Docking Station Also known as a *universal port replicator*; this hardware device allows laptops to connect with other devices, making it into a desktop computer.

Dongle A small hardware device that connects to a computer device and allows access to wireless devices, such as headsets, mice, and keyboards.

Dosage May also be referred to as dose; the quantity of medication to be administered at one time.

Down Syndrome A genetic disorder in which abnormal cell division results in an extra chromosome 21.

Downtime The interval of time during which something, such as hardware or software, is not functioning.

Drive A computer device that reads data from and may write data to a storage medium.

Dynamic (die NAM ik) Equilibrium Relating to balance when moving at an angle or rotating.

Dysmenorrhea (dis men uh REE uh) Painful menstrual flow, cramps.

Dyspareunia (dis ph ROO nee ah) Painful or difficult intercourse.

Dysphagia Difficulty swallowing.

Dyspnea (DISP nee ah) Difficult or painful breathing.

Ecchymosis (ek i MOH sis) Discoloration of the skin caused by the escape of blood into the tissues from ruptured blood vessels; typically caused by bruising.

Echocardiography (ECHO) (eck oh KAR dee ah gruh fee) The use of ultrasonic waves directed through the heart to study the structure and motion of the heart. The visual record produced is called an *echocardiogram.*

Ectopic (eck TAH pick) Pregnancy Implantation of the embryo in any location other than the uterus.

Efferent (EF er uhnt) Pertaining to carrying away from a structure.

Egress (EE gress) Leaving a place; exit route.

Elastin (ee LAS tin) A highly elastic protein in connective tissue that allows tissues to resume their shape after stretching or contracting. It is found abundantly in the dermis of the skin.

Electrocardiogram (ECG, EKG) (ee leck troh KAR dee ah gram) A record or recording of electrical impulses of the heart as produced by an electrocardiograph.

Electrocardiography The recording of electrical impulses of the heart as wave deflections on an instrument called an *electrocardiograph*. The record, or recording, is called an *electrocardiogram*.

Electrodes Adhesive patches that conduct electricity from the body to the ECG machine wires.

Electrolyte (ee LEK troe lite) A chemical substance that separates into ions in solution (water) and is capable of conducting an electric current. Electrolytes found in body fluids include sodium, potassium, calcium, magnesium, chloride, bicarbonate, and phosphate.

Electronic Health Record (EHR) An electronic record that conforms to nationally recognized standards and contains health-related information about a specific patient. It can be created, managed, and consulted by authorized clinicians and staff from more than one healthcare organization.

Electronic Medical Record (EMR) An electronic record of health-related information about an individual that can be created, gathered, managed, and accessed by authorized clinicians and staff members within a single healthcare organization. An EMR is an electronic version of a paper record.

Electronic Transaction The electronic exchange of information between two agencies to accomplish financial or administrative healthcare activities.

Eligibility (el i ji BILL i tee) Meeting the stipulated requirements to participate in the healthcare plan.

Emancipated Minor (i MANS i pa ted MIE nohr) A minor who has been granted emancipation by the court; the minor can assume the rights and responsibilities of adulthood.

Embezzlement (em BEZ ul ment) The misuse of funds for personal gain.

Embolus (EM boh lus) An air bubble, blood clot, or foreign body that travels through the bloodstream and blocks a blood vessel.

Embryo (EM bree oh) A developing organism from the moment of conception through the eighth week of development.

Emergency An unexpected, life-threatening situation that requires immediate action.

Empathy (EM pah thee) The ability to understand another's perspective, experiences, or motivations.

Emphysema (em fuh ZEE mah) Thinning and eventual destruction of the alveoli; usually accompanies chronic bronchitis.

Emulsifies (ee MUL sih fyez) When a substance suspends tiny droplets of one liquid in a second liquid. By creating an emulsion, you can mix two liquids that usually do not mix well, such as oil and water.

EMV Chip Technology Global technology that includes imbedded microchips that store and protect cardholder data; also called *chip and PIN* and *chip and signature*.

Encoder Software that will apply diagnostic or procedure codes to medical conditions or procedures.

Encounter Form A document used to capture the services/ procedures and diagnoses for a patient visit. The fees for the services/procedures are usually included on the encounter form.

Endocrine A glandular secretion that is released into the blood or lymph directly (does not go through a duct).

Endoscope A scope with a camera attached to a long, thin tube that can be inserted into the body.

Endoscopy (en DOS kuh pee) Nonsurgical procedure that uses an endoscope to view inside of the body.

Endospore An inactive form of certain bacteria that can withstand poor environmental conditions. When conditions improve, the bacteria become functional again.

Endotracheal (en doe TRAY kee al) (ET) Tube. A catheter that is inserted into the trachea through the mouth; provides a patent airway.

Enema Fluid introduced into the rectum for a therapeutic or diagnostic purpose.

Energy The ability to do work.

Enriched Nutrients are added back into a food after they were lost during food processing.

Enunciation (ih nuhn see EY shuhn) The use of articulate, clear sounds when speaking.

Enzymes (EN zimes) Special proteins that speed up chemical reactions in the body.

Epidemiology (ep i dee mee OL uh jee) The branch of medicine dealing with the incidence, distribution, and control of disease in a population. It also involves the prevalence of disease in large populations, in addition to detection of the source and cause of epidemics of infectious disease.

Epiglottis (ep i GLOT is) Lidlike structure over the glottis that prevents food and liquids from entering the trachea when swallowing occurs.

Epiphyseal Plate (eh pi FIZ ee uhl) A thin layer of cartilage located at the ends of a long bone where new bone forms.

Epithelial Cells (ep i THEE lee al) Form cellular sheets that cover surfaces, both inside and outside the body. Epithelial cells are closely packed, take on different shapes, and strongly stick to each other.

Eponym (EP uh nim) In medical terms, a medical diagnosis or procedure named for the person who discovered it.

E-Prescribing The use of electronic software to communicate with pharmacies and send prescribing information. It takes the place of writing a prescription by hand and giving it to a patient; most new or refill prescriptions can be submitted electronically, cutting down on fraud and errors.

Equilibrium (ee kwi LIB ree uhm) A state of rest or balance due to the equal action of opposing forces.

Ergonomics (ur guh NOM iks) An applied science concerned with designing and arranging things needed to do your job in an efficient and safe way.

Erythropoietin (eh rith roh POY eh tin) A hormone that is produced by the kidney cells and travels to the bone marrow to stimulate red blood cell formation.

Essential Hypertension Elevated blood pressure of unknown cause that develops for no apparent reason; sometimes called primary hypertension.

Established Patient A patient who has been treated by the healthcare provider within the past 3 years.

Esterase Any enzyme that breaks down esters (a type of organic molecule) into alcohols and acids.

Ethernet (EE thuhr net) A communication system for connecting several computers so information can be shared.

Ethics (ETH iks) Rules of conduct that differentiate between acceptable and unacceptable behavior.

Ethics Committee A group composed of members from a variety of disciplines that analyze ethical issues.

Etiology (ee tee OL uh jee) The study of the causes or origin of diseases.

Eukaryote (yoo KAR ee oht) Any single-celled or multicellular organism that has genetic material contained in a distinct membrane-bound nucleus.

Euphoria (yoo FOR ee ah) An exaggerated sense of physical and mental well-being.

Evacuated Absence of air to create a vacuum in a tube, flask, or reaction vessel.

Evert (ih VURT) To turn the eyelid inside out; the provider typically does this to inspect the area for foreign bodies.

Evidence-Based Practice Healthcare practice that incorporates the most current and valid research results, thus providing the best patient care.

Evoked Potential Test A nerve response test that uses electrodes, which are placed on the scalp to measure brain reaction to a stimulus.

Exclusivity (ik skloo SIV i tee) The sole right to market an approved medication granted by the Food and Drug Administration (FDA); may occur with the patent.

Excoriated (ik SKOHR ee ay ted) To strip off or remove the skin from an area.

Excoriation (ik skawr ee AY shun) Inflammation and irritation of the skin.

Executor An individual assigned to make financial decisions about the estate of a deceased patient.

Exocrine A glandular secretion released through a duct.

Expectorate To cough up and spit out mucus from the lower respiratory tract.

Expediency (ik SPEE dee uhn see) A means of achieving a particular end, as in a situation requiring urgency or caution.

Expert Witnesses People who are educated and knowledgeable in the area of concern; they testify in court and provide an expert opinion on the topic of concern.

Expiration Exhaling; movement of waste gases from the alveoli into the atmosphere.

Explanation of Benefits (EOB) A document sent by the insurance company to the provider and the patient explaining the allowed charge amount, the amount reimbursed for services, and the patient's financial responsibilities.

Expletive (EK sple tiv) An oath or a swear word.

Explicit (ek SPLIS it) Fully and clearly expressed or demonstrated; leaving nothing merely implied.

Exploitation (eks ploi TAY shuhn) The act of using another person for one's own advantage.

Exposure Indicator (EI) A numeric value indicating the quantity of ionizing radiation received by a digital radiographic image receptor; also called an exposure index.

Extension The process of stretching out; increasing the angle of a joint.

Extract A certain substance that is taken out of a group or solution and is in a concentrated form.

Extraction A process by which a specific substance is separated from a group or solution.

Extravasation (eks trav ah SAY shun) A discharge of fluid or blood from the blood vessel into the tissues.

Exudates (EKS yoo dayts) Fluids with high concentrations of protein and cellular debris that have escaped from the blood vessels and have been deposited in tissues or on tissue surfaces.

Fact Witnesses People who observed the situation and testify in court about the facts of the case.

Familial (fah MIL ee uhl) Occurring in or affecting members of a family more than would be expected by chance.

Fasciculations (fah SIK yeh LAE shuhns) Involuntary muscle tremors and fine movements.

Fatigue (fuh TEEG) Extreme tiredness.

Fatty Acids Result when fats are broken down; used by the body for energy and tissue development.

Febrile (FEB ruhl) Pertaining to an elevated body temperature.

Federal Reserve Bank The central bank of the United States. The Federal Reserve system consists of a seven-member board of governors with headquarters in Washington, DC, and 12 Federal Reserve banks in major cities throughout the country.

Fee Schedule A list of fixed fees for services.

Filamentous (fil ah MEN tuhs) Composed of or containing filaments or strands of a substance.

File A collection of data or program records stored as a unit with a specific name.

Filtrate Fluid and substances that are filtered out of the blood in the Bowman capsule.

Fire Doors Doors made of fire-resistant materials; close manually or automatically during a fire to prevent it from spreading.

Fissure A crack, cleft, or narrow opening.

Flagella A long, whiplike outgrowth from a cell that helps the cell move.

Flexion The process of decreasing the angle of a joint.

Flow Rate The number of drops (gtt) in 1 minute required to infuse the ordered solution; also called the drip rate.

Fluctuate (FLUHK choo ayt) To shift back and forth.

Fog The unwanted image exposure caused by scatter radiation.

Follicle-Stimulating Hormone (FSH) A glycoprotein hormone secreted by the anterior pituitary gland. It stimulates the growth of ova (eggs) in the ovary and induces the formation of sperm in the testis.

Follow-Up (Recheck) Appointment An appointment type used when a patient needs to see the provider after a condition should have been resolved or to monitor an ongoing condition, such as hypertension. Also known as a recheck appointment.

Fomite Objects that are likely to carry infectious organisms.

Fontanel (fon tah NEL) A soft membranous gap between the incompletely formed cranial bones of an infant; also called a *soft spot.*

Foramen Magnum (for AY men MAG num) A large opening in the base of the skull. It forms a passageway for the spinal cord.

Forensic (fuh REN sik) Scientific tests or techniques used regarding the detection of crime.

Form Physical characteristics of a medication (e.g., tablet and suspension).

Fornix (FORE niks) A recess in the upper part of the vagina caused by protrusion of the cervix into the vaginal wall.

Fortified The addition of one or more substances to a food to increase its nutrient density.

Fungi Single-celled organisms, including mushrooms, molds, mildew, smuts, rusts, and yeasts, and classified in the kingdom Fungi.

Gait The manner or style of walking.

Gamete (GAM eet) A mature sexual reproductive cell; spermatozoon or ovum.

Gatekeeper The primary care provider, who is in charge of a patient's treatment. Additional treatment, such as referrals to a specialist, must be approved by the gatekeeper.

Generator Delivers the electrical power to the x-ray tube and permits the selection of x-ray energy, x-ray quantity, and exposure time.

Germicides (JUR muh sides) Agents that destroy pathogenic organisms.

Germline Cells Sperm and egg cells.

G-Force A force acting on an object because of gravity. For example, a centrifuge spins and exerts g-force.

Girth The measurement around something; when referring to mail, it is the measurement around the middle of the package that is being shipped.

Glasgow Coma Scale A scale used to measure the level of consciousness and severity of a head injury; the ability to open the eyes, verbal response, and motor response are evaluated, and the score is determined based on the findings.

Glaucoma (glou KOE mah) An increase in the fluid pressure in the eye; can lead to blindness if not treated.

Global Services For purposes of *Current Procedural Terminology* (CPT) coding, medical services and procedures performed for the patient, before, during, and after a surgical procedure, that are included with the assigned CPT code.

Glomerulonephritis (gloh mer yuh loh neh FRIE tis) Kidney disease affecting the capillaries of the nephron (glomeruli); characterized by albuminuria, edema, and hypertension.

Glucagon (GLOO kah gon) A hormone produced by the alpha cells in the pancreas; works in the liver to release glycogen and thereby prevent dangerously low blood glucose levels.

Glucose Results when carbohydrates are broken down; main sugar found in the blood and used as the main source of energy in the body.

Glycolysis (glie KOL uh sis) The chemical breakdown of carbohydrates (glucose) by enzymes, with the release of energy.

Gonad (GOH nads) Organs that produce sex cells in both males and females.

Goniometer (go nee OHM eh ter) A calibrated device designed to measure the arc, angle, or range of motion of a joint.

Gonioscopy (goh nee AH skuh pee) Used to diagnose glaucoma and to inspect ocular movement.

Graduated Cylinder A narrow, tube-shaped container marked with horizontal lines to represent units of measurement. Used to precisely measure the volume of liquids.

Gray Matter Nerve tissue that lacks the insulation that causes a white appearance to other nerves; thus, gray matter looks gray.

Gross The amount earned before any tax deductions or adjustments.

Guaiac Fecal Occult Blood Test A test for fecal occult blood where glacial acetic acid and guaiac are mixed with the specimen.

Guarantor The person legally responsible for the entire bill. This is usually the patient, but in the case of a minor it would be a parent or legal guardian.

Gyri (JIE rie) Folds or convolutions on the surface of the cerebral hemisphere, which increase the gray matter surface area. Gyrus (JIE rus) is the singular form.

Hackers Unauthorized users who attempt to break into computer networks.

Hallucination (hah LOO si nae shun) A sensory experience (e.g., a smell, sound, sight, touch, or taste) involving something that is not present.

Harassment (hah RAS ment) Continued, unwanted, and annoying actions done to another person.

Hardware Physical equipment of the computer system required for communication and data processing functions.

Headset A set of headphones with a microphone attached, used especially in telephone communication.

Healthcare-Associated Infections (HAIs) Infections that patients acquire while receiving treatment for other conditions within a healthcare setting (e.g., ambulatory care, long-term care, or rehabilitation facility).

Health Insurance Exchange An online marketplace where people can compare and buy individual health insurance plans. State health insurance exchanges were established as part of the Affordable Care Act.

Hematologist (hee mah TOL uh jist) A person trained in the nature, function, and diseases of the blood and blood-forming organs. Can be a physician, trained laboratory personnel, or researcher.

Hematoma (hee mah TOH mah) An abnormal buildup of blood in an organ or tissue of the body, caused by a leak or cut in a blood vessel.

Hematopoiesis (hee mah toh poh EE sis) The formation of the blood cells and platelets.

Hemoccult Test A modified guaiac test using filter paper impregnated with guaiacum that turns blue if occult blood is present.

Hemoconcentration (hee muh kon sun TRAY shun) A condition in which the concentration of blood cells is increased in proportion to the plasma.

Hemoglobin (HEE muh gloh bin) The oxygen-carrying pigment of red blood cells.

Hemolysis (hee MOL i sis) The breakdown of red blood cells with the release of hemoglobin.

Hemolytic Uremic Syndrome A kidney disorder that can occur after a digestive infection with *Escherichia coli,* shigella, or salmonella; red blood cells are destroyed and block the kidneys' filtering system, causing acute kidney failure.

Hemolyzed (HEE muh liezd) A blood sample in which the red blood cells have ruptured.

Hemophilia (hee moh FEE lee ah) A group of inherited blood disorders characterized by a deficiency of one of the factors necessary for the coagulation of blood.

Hemostasis (hee muh STAY sis) The stoppage of bleeding.

Hereditary (huh RED i ter ee) Passed from parents to offspring through the genes.

Hertz (hurts) The unit of measurement used in hearing examinations; a wave frequency equal to one cycle per second.

Heterophile Antibody An antibody that has an affinity for an antigen other than the specific antigen that stimulated its production.

Hierarchy (HIE er ar kee) Things arranged in order and rank.

Hippocampus (hip oh KAM pus) A ridge in the floor of the lateral ventricle; composed of gray matter. Involved with the limbic system and with creating and filing new memories.

Histologic Pertaining to the study of body tissues.

Histology (hi STOL oh jee) The study of tissues.

History of Present Illness (HPI) Describes the signs and symptoms from the time of onset.

Holistic (hoh LIS tik) Considering the patient as a whole; includes the physical, emotional, social, economic, and spiritual needs of the person.

Homeostasis (hoh mee uh STAY sis) The internal environment of the body that is compatible with life. A steady state that is created by all the body systems working together to provide a consistent and unvarying internal environment.

Hormone A chemical substance produced in an endocrine gland and transported in the blood to a specific tissue, where it applies a specific effect.

Hospice (HOS pis) A concept of care that involves health professionals and volunteers who provide medical, psychological, and spiritual support to terminally ill patients and their loved ones.

Human Resources File (HR file) Contains all documents related to an individual's employment.

Hydrocephalus (hi droe SEF ah luhs) An abnormal accumulation of cerebrospinal fluid that causes enlargement of the skull and compression of the brain.

Hydrocephaly (hye droh SEF ul lee) Enlargement of the cranium caused by an abnormal accumulation of cerebrospinal fluid in the cerebral system.

Hyperlipidemia (hie per lip i DEE mee ah) An elevated level of lipids in the blood.

Hyperopia (hye pur OH pee ah) Farsightedness.

Hyperplasia (hahy per PLEY zhee uh) Enlargement due to an abnormal multiplication of cells.

Hyperventilation (hie pur ven ti LAY shun) Abnormally increased breathing.

Hypoalbuminemia (hie poh al byoo mi NEE mee ah) A decreased level of albumin (protein) in the blood.

Hypotension Blood pressure that is below normal (systolic pressure below 90 mm Hg and diastolic pressure below 50 mm Hg).

Hysterectomy Surgical removal of the uterus and cervix. The ovaries and fallopian tubes may also be removed.

Idiopathic (id ee uh PATH ik) Of unknown cause.

Image Receptor (IR) The device that receives the energy of the x-ray beam and forms the image of the body part.

Immunoglobulins (im yuh noh GLOB yuh linz) A group of related proteins that function as antibodies. They are found in plasma and other body fluids.

Immunosuppressant A drug used to suppress the immune system.

Impending A term used in the diagnosis of a condition that can be imminently threatening. For example, a patient showing signs of prediabetes may in the near future develop diabetes; therefore, in this case, diabetes is an impending condition.

Impervious (im PUR vee uhs) Not permitting penetration.

Inanimate Not animate; lifeless.

Incarcerated Confined or trapped.

Incentive Things that incite or spur to action; rewards or reasons for performing a task.

Incidence (IN si duhns) How often something happens or occurs.

Incompetence (in KOM pi tahns) The state of being incompetent or lacking the ability to manage personal affairs due to mental deficiency; an appointed guardian or conservator manages the person's affairs.

Incompetent Valves Valves that do not close completely and allow blood to leak backward into the prior chamber; also called "leaky valves."

Inconspicuous (in kuhn SPIK yoo uhs) Not noticeable or prominent.

Incurred To come into or acquire.

Indicator (IN di kay ter) An important point or group of statistical values that, when evaluated, indicates the quality of care provided in a healthcare facility.

Indigent (IN di jent) Poor, needy, impoverished.

Infarction (in FARK shuhn) Tissue death.

Infection Invasion of body tissues by microorganisms, which then multiply and damage tissues.

Infectious Agents Living and nonliving pathogens—such as bacteria, viruses, fungi, protozoa, parasites, helminths, and prions—that can cause disease.

Inflammation (in fluh MAY shuhn) A pathology characterized by redness, swelling, pain, tenderness, heat, and disturbed function of an area of the body. Especially a reaction of tissues to injury.

Infusion Rate The volume of fluid infused per hour; written as mL/hr.

Ingested Taken, as food, into the body.

Inhalant (in HAY lunt) Any substance that can be breathed into the lungs.

Inhalation (in huh LAY shuhn) The act of breathing in.

Initiative (i NISH eh tive) The ability to determine what needs to be done and to take action on your own.

Injunction (in JUNGK shuhn) A court order by which an individual or institution is required to perform or refrain from performing a certain act.

Insidious (in SID ee uhs) Proceeding in a gradual, subtle way, but with harmful effects.

Inspiration Inhaling; movement of O_2 from the atmosphere into the alveoli.

Insufficiency Also called *regurgitation* or *incompetence;* the valve does not close completely, and blood leaks backward across the valve into the prior chamber.

Insulin (IN suh lin) A hormone produced by the beta cells in the pancreas; moves glucose into the cells so it can be used for energy.

Intact (in TAKT) Complete or whole. Not altered; unbroken.

Intangible (in TAN juh buhl) Something of value that cannot be touched physically.

Integral (IN ti gruhl) Essential; being an indispensable part of a whole.

Integrity (in TEG ri tee) Adhering to ethical standards or right conduct standards.

Intercellular Located between cells.

Intercom A two-way communication system with a microphone and loudspeaker at each station; often a feature of business telephones.

Intercostal (in tur KOS tul) Muscles Muscles located between the ribs that help with quiet respiration.

Interest Money the bank pays the account holder, on the amount in his or her account, for using the money in the account.

Interface An interconnection between systems.

Interferon (in ter FEER on) A protein formed when a cell is exposed to a virus; the protein blocks viral action on the cell and protects against viral invasion.

Intermittent Occurring in intervals.

Intermittent Pulse A pulse in which beats occasionally are skipped.

International Normalized Ratio (Inr) Also called prothrombin time (PT). Used to test the effectiveness of a blood-thinning medication.

Interoperability (in ter op er uh BIL i tee) The ability to work with other systems.

Interpersonal Skills The ability to communicate and interact with others; sometimes referred to as "soft skills."

Interrogatory (IN tah rog ah TOOR ee) Written or oral questions that must be answered under oath.

Interstitial (in ter STISH uhl) Between the cells.

Interstitial Cells Testosterone-secreting cells of testes that are found in the spaces between the seminiferous tubules.

Interstitial Fluid Liquid found between the cells of the body.

Interval Space of time between events.

Intracellular Pathogen A disease-causing organism that is within or inside a cell.

Intranet (IN trah net) A private computer network that can only be accessed by authorized people (e.g., employees of the facility that owns the network).

Intraosseous (in tra OS ee us) Within bone; route for delivery of fluids and medications through a needle inserted into the marrow of certain bones (e.g., humerus, tibia, and femur).

Intravenous (in TRAH vee nus) Through a vein; fluids and medications can be given through a vein.

Intravenous Therapy Administration and monitoring of fluid and medication by intravenous infusion.

Intrinsic Factor Secreted by the parietal cells of the stomach; necessary for the absorption of vitamin B12 to prevent pernicious anemia.

Inventory A detailed list of equipment and supplies owned and stored; the process of counting the supplies in stock.

In Vitro Latin term meaning "in glass" and commonly known as "in the laboratory."

In Vitro Fertilization An assisted reproductive technology procedure that involves removing mature eggs from the ovaries and fertilizing the eggs with sperm outside of the body. The fertilized eggs are then transferred to the uterus.

Invoices Billing statements that list the amount owed for goods or services purchased.

Ion (AHY ons) An electrically charged atom, or the smallest component of an element.

Ionizing Radiation Radiation that, when passing through the body, produces positively and negatively charged particles.

Jargon (JAHR guhn) The vocabulary of a particular profession, as opposed to common, everyday terms.

Jaundice A yellow discoloration of the skin and mucous membranes caused by deposits of bile.

Job Boards Websites where employers post jobs; job seekers can use them to identify open positions.

Judicious (joo DISH uhs) Using good judgment; being discreet, sensible.

Kilovolts Peak (kVp) The unit of measure used to determine the voltage; controls the penetrating power of the x-ray beam.

Kwashiorkor (kwah shee ORE kore) A severe protein deficiency syndrome that leads to edema, pigmentation changes of the skin and hair, impaired growth and development, abdominal distension, and liver changes. Typically seen in infants and children.

Labia Majora (LAY bee ah muh JOR ah) The larger external folds of skin surrounding the opening of the vagina.

Labia Minora (LAY bee ah min NOR uh) The smaller inner folds of skin surrounding the opening of the vagina.

Lacrimation (lak ri MAY shun) The secretion or discharge of tears.

Landscape Orientation The width is greater than its height.

Laparoscopy (lap ar AW scoh pee) A procedure used to visually examine the abdomen.

Larynx (LAR inks) The voice box.

Lateral Flow Immunoassay (im yuh noh AH say) A laboratory or clinical technique that uses the specific binding between an antigen and antibody to identify and quantify a substance in a sample. The sample in this technique moves in a sideways motion, usually on absorbent paper.

Learning Style The way an individual perceives and processes information to learn new material.

Lethargy (LETH er jee) The state of being drowsy and dull, listless and unenergetic.

Leukoderma Lack of skin pigmentation, especially in patches.

Liability (LIE ah bil i tee) The state of being liable or responsible for something.

Liable Legally responsible or obligated.

Libido Sexual drive or instinct.

Licensure (LIE sen shur) A mandatory process established by state law that ensures a person has met the legal standards for practicing an occupation in that state.

Ligaments (LIH gah ments) Supportive connective tissue that connects bones at a joint.

Limbic System Consists of several structures, including the amygdala, hippocampus, and hypothalamus; plays an important role in behavior, memories, and emotions.

Line Focus Principle The relationship between the actual focal spot on the anode surface and the effective focal spot size.

Litigious (LI ti jehs) Prone to lawsuits.

Local Affecting the area where applied.

Locum tenens (LOE kuhm TEE nenz) Latin for "to substitute for"; the term refers to physicians or advanced practice professionals who temporarily contract to provide healthcare services when a facility has a vacancy, vacation, or a leave of absence.

Loop Electrosurgical Excision Procedure (LEEP) After an anesthetic has been injected into the cervix, a high-frequency electrical current running through a wire is used to remove abnormal tissue from both the cervix and the endocervical canal.

Lumen The cavity, channel, or open space within a tube or tubular organ.

Lumpectomy (luhm PEK tuh mee) Removal of the breast tumor and a small amount of the surrounding tissue.

Luteinizing Hormone (LH) A hormone produced by the anterior pituitary gland. LH stimulates ovulation and the development of the corpus luteum in females and the production of testosterone in males.

Lymph (limf) A clear, yellowish fluid containing white blood cells in a liquid similar to plasma. The fluid comes from the tissues of the body and is moved through the lymphatic vessels and the bloodstream.

Lymphedema (lim fuh DEE mah) A condition in which extra lymph fluid builds up in tissues and causes swelling. It may occur in an arm or leg if lymph vessels are blocked, damaged, or removed by surgery.

Lymphocyte (LIM fuh site) A type of white blood cell that has a large, round nucleus that is surrounded by a thin layer of agranular cytoplasm.

Lymphostasis (lim foh STAY sis) Obstruction or interruption of normal lymph flow.

Macromolecules Molecules needed for metabolism: carbohydrates, lipids, proteins, amino acids, and nucleic acids.

Macrophages (MACK roh fay jehs) Large white blood cells that live in the tissues. They engulf foreign particles, microorganisms, and cell debris.

Malaise (ma LAYZ) A condition of general bodily weakness or discomfort, often marking the onset of a disease.

Malignant A descriptive term for things or conditions that threaten life or well-being. Malignant is the opposite of benign.

Malpractice (mal PRAK tis) A type of negligence in which a licensed professional fails to provide the standard of care, causing harm to a person.

Malware (MAL wair) Malicious software designed to damage or disrupt a system (e.g., a virus).

Mania (MAY nee ah) Abnormally elated mental state; the person may have feelings of euphoria, lack of inhibitions, sleeplessness, talkativeness, risk-taking behaviors, and irritability.

Manipulation Movement or exercise of a body part by means of an externally applied force.

Mastectomy (ma STEK tuh mee) Removal of the entire breast.

Matrix (MEY triks) The environment in which something is created or takes shape. A base on which to build.

Matter Anything that occupies space and has shape or form.

Mature Minor A person under the age of adulthood who demonstrates the maturity to make a personal healthcare decision and can give informed consent for treatment.

Meatus A body opening or passage, especially the external opening of a structure.

Media (ME de ah) Types of communication (e.g., social media sites); with computers, the term refers to data storage devices.

Mediastinum (mee dee AH sti nuhm) The space in the thoracic cavity that lies between the lungs, containing the heart, trachea, and esophagus.

Mediation (MEE dee ae shuhn) The process of facilitating conflicting parties to make an agreement, settlement, or compromise.

Medically Necessary Accepted healthcare services that are appropriate for the evaluation and treatment of a disease, condition, illness, or injury and are consistent with the applicable standard of care.

Medical Necessity Services or supplies (*Current Procedural Terminology* [CPT] and *Healthcare Common Procedure Coding System* [HCPCS] codes) used to treat the patient's diagnosis (*International Classification of Diseases* [ICD] codes) that meet the accepted standard of medical practice.

Medulla Oblongata (muh DUHL uh ob lawng GAH tah) The lowest part of the brain, continuous with the top of the spinal cord.

Melanocytes (meh LAN oh sites) Cells of the stratum germinativum that produce a brownish pigment called *melanin.* Melanin gives us our skin color.

Ménière Disease (mayn YAIRZ) Chronic disease of the inner ear causing recurrent episodes of vertigo, progressive sensorineural hearing loss, and tinnitus.

Meninges (meh NIN jeez) A protective covering around the brain and spinal cord.

Meningocele (meh NING goh seel) The protrusion of the meninges through an opening in the spinal column or skull.

Menometrorrhagia (men oh meh troh RAH zsa) Excessive menstrual flow and uterine bleeding other than that caused by menstruation.

Menorrhagia (men or RAH zsa) Abnormally heavy menstrual flow or prolonged menstrual periods.

Mentor A steady employee whom a new staff member can approach with questions and concerns.

Metabolic Relating to or resulting from metabolism (the chemical process in which cells produce the substances and energy needed to sustain life).

Metabolism (me TAB oh lizm) The chemical process that occurs within a living organism to maintain life; the process the body uses to obtain or make energy from the food eaten.

Metabolites (muh TAB uh lites) By-products of drug metabolism

Metastasize (MEH tas tuh sizes) To spread from one part of the body (the primary tumor) to another part of the body, forming a secondary tumor.

Microbiome (mIE kroh BIE ohm) The total collection of microorganisms, and their genetic material, present on or in the human body or a specific site in the human body.

Microcephaly (mie kroh SEF ul lee) Abnormally small head associated with incomplete brain development.

Microcuvette (MIE kroh koo vet) A small plastic or glass tube designed to hold samples for laboratory tests that detect light or color changes.

Microorganisms Any living organisms of microscopic size. Examples include bacteria, protozoa, fungi, parasites, and helminths. Some definitions include viruses, which are not alive.

Micturate Urinate Minim (MIN im) An apothecary unit of measurement for liquid; approximately equal to one drop.

Minor One who has not reached adulthood; usually age 18 or 21, depending on the jurisdiction.

Miotic (my OT ik) Any substance or medication that causes constriction of the pupil.

Mnemonic (ni MON ik) A learning device (e.g., an image, a rhyme, or a figure of speech) that a person uses to help him or her remember information.

Mock Simulated; intended for imitation or practice.

Modalities (moe DAL i tees) Therapeutic treatments for a disorder.

Modem (MOE duhm) Peripheral computer hardware that connects to the router to provide internet access to the network or computer.

Mold A growth of tiny fungi forming on a substance. Often looks downy or furry and is associated with dampness or decay.

Molecule The simplest unit of a chemical compound that can exist, consisting of two or more atoms held together with chemical bonds.

Monocyte (MON uh site) Agranulocyte that engulfs foreign particles, microorganisms, and cell debris.

Monotone (MON uh tohn) A succession of syllables, words, or sentences spoken in an unvaried key or pitch.

Morale (muh RAL) An emotional or mental condition with respect to cheerfulness or confidence.

Morals (MORE ahls) Internal principles that distinguish between right and wrong.

Morbidity (more BID i tee) The rate of a disease in a population.

Mordant Having the ability to fix or set colors.

Mortality The relative frequency of deaths in a specific population.

Mucous Membrane A mucus-producing membrane that lines tracts and structures of the body (e.g., gastrointestinal tract, respiratory tract); also called mucosa.

Multiple-Line Telephone System A business telephone system that allows for more than one telephone line.

Murmur An abnormal sound heard during auscultation of the heart that may or may not have a pathologic origin; it is associated with valve disease or a congenital heart defect.

Myelin Sheath (MIE uh lin sheeth) A protective insulation that covers the axons and helps with the transmission of nerve impulses.

Myocardium (mie oh KAR dee um) The middle layer, and thickest layer, of the heart; composed of cardiac muscles.

Myoglobin Type of hemoglobin found in the muscle.

Myopia (mye OH pee ah) Nearsightedness.

Myxedema (mick suh DEE mah) Advanced hypothyroidism in adulthood.

Nasal Wash Also called a nasal aspirate. A syringe is used to gently squirt a small amount of sterile saline into the nose, and the resulting fluid is collected into a cup (for a wash). Or after the saline is squirted into the nose, gentle suction is applied (for the aspirate).

Nasopharyngeal (nae zoe fah RIN jee ahl) Airway (NPA) A soft flexible tube that is inserted into the nose and provides a patent airway; also known as a *nasal trumpet.*

National Provider Identifier (NPI) An identifier assigned by the Centers for Medicare and Medicaid Services (CMS) that classifies the healthcare provider by license and medical specialties.

Necrosis (nuh KROH sis) Tissue death.

Negative Feedback Loop A process in which a change from the normal ranges causes a response that opposes or decreases the change, thus helping to maintain homeostasis.

Neglect Failure to provide proper attention or care to another person.

Negligence (NEG li jens) Failure to act as a reasonably prudent person would under similar circumstances; such conduct falls below the standards of behavior established by law for the protection of others against unreasonable risk of harm.

Negotiable (ni GOH shee uh buhl) Instrument A document guaranteeing payment of a specific amount of money to the payer named on the document.

Nephrotoxic Damaging or destructive to the kidneys.

Net The amount someone is paid after taxes and other deductions have been subtracted.

Neuralgia (noo RAL jah) Sharp, spasm-like pain in a nerve or along the course of one or more nerves.

Neurofibrillary Tangles Abnormal structures composed of twisted protein fibers within nerve cells.

Neuropathy (nu ROP a thee) A nervous system disorder of the peripheral nerves that causes discomfort, numbness, and weakness, especially in the extremities.

Neurotransmitters Chemicals that help a nerve cell communicate with another nerve cell or muscle.

Nocturia (nok TOOR ee uh) Frequent urination at night.

Nodules (NOD jools) Small lumps, lesions, or swellings that are felt when the skin is palpated.

Nomenclature (NOH muh n kley cher) A system of names or terms, used in science and art to categorize items.

Noninvasive Procedures Procedures that do not penetrate human tissue.

Nonorganic (nahn or GAN ik) Not having an organic or physiologic cause; a disorder that does not have a cause that can be found in the body.

Nonverbal Communication A type of communication that occurs through body language and expressive behaviors rather than with verbal or written words.

Normal Flora Microorganisms (mostly bacteria and yeast) that live on or in the body. Normal microscopic residents of the body.

No-Show To fail to keep an appointment without giving advance notice.

Nosocomial (nos uh KOH mee uhl) Infections Infections acquired in a healthcare setting.

Notice of Privacy Practices (NPP) A written document describing the healthcare facility's privacy practices. The patient must be provided with the NPP and sign an acknowledgment of receipt.

Nucleus A specialized organelle of a cell that is encased in a membrane and directs growth, metabolism, and reproduction of the cell.

Numeric Filing The filing of records, correspondence, or cards by number.

Objective Information Data obtained through physical examination, laboratory and diagnostic testing, and by measurable information.

Object-to-Image Receptor Distance (OID) The distance between the subject and the image receptor.

Obliteration (ub lit uh REY shun) To remove or destroy all traces of; do away with; destroy completely.

Obturator (OB tuh rayt oar) A metal rod with a smooth, rounded tip that is placed in hollow instruments to reduce injury to body tissues during insertion.

Occlude To close, shut, or stop up.

Occult Hidden or unseen.

Oncologist (on KOL uh jest) A specially trained doctor who diagnoses and treats cancer.

Online Insurance Web Portal An online service provided by various insurance companies that allows providers to look up a patient's insurance benefits, eligibility, claims status, and explanation of benefits.

Oocyte (OO eh site) An immature ovum (egg).

Oophorectomy (oo for ECK tuh mee) Surgical removal of the ovaries.

Opaque (oh PAYK) Not transparent, cloudy or murky.

Operating System Software; it acts as the computer's software administrator by managing, integrating, and controlling application software and hardware. Windows is an example.

Organelle Structures inside of the cell that have specific functions to maintain the cell.

Orientation Awareness of one's environment, with reference to people, place, and time.

Orifice (ORE ih fis) The vaginal opening.

Orthopnea (or THOP nee ah) A condition of difficult breathing unless in an upright position.

Orthostatic (Postural) Hypotension A temporary fall in blood pressure when a person rapidly changes from a recumbent position to a standing position.

Osteoporosis (os tee oh phuh ROH sis) Abnormal thinning of the bone structure, causing bones to become brittle and weak.

Otitis Externa Inflammation or infection of the external auditory canal; commonly called swimmer's ear.

Otosclerosis (oh tuh skleh ROH sis) The ossicles of the middle ear (malleolus, incus, and stapes) become fused and act as a single unit instead of individual bones.

Ototoxic (oh tuh TOK sik) A medicine or substance capable of damaging cranial nerve VIII or the organs of hearing and balance.

Out Guides Sturdy cardboard or plastic file-sized cards used to replace a folder temporarily removed from the filing space.

Output Device Computer hardware that displays the processed data from the computer (e.g., monitors and printers).

Overlearn To learn or memorize beyond the point of proficiency or immediate recall.

Ovulation (OV yuh ley shun) The release of the ovum from the ovarian follicle.

Packing Slip A document that accompanies purchased merchandise and shows what is in the box or package.

Palpation (pal PAY shuhn) The use of touch during the physical examination to assess the size, consistency, and location of certain body parts.

Pandemic A disease that is prevalent throughout an entire country, continent, or the whole world.

Paralysis A loss of muscle function or sensation causing the inability to move or use a body part.

Parameters (puh RAM it ers) Rules that control how something should be done; guidelines or boundaries.

Paranasal Sinuses (pair uh NAY zul SIE nus suhs) Hollow, air-filled cavities in the skull and facial bones. They lighten the weight of the skull and increase the tone, or resonance, of speech.

Paranoia An unfounded or excessive suspicion of the motives of others.

Paraphrasing Rewording a statement to check the meaning and interpretation; also shows you are listening to and understanding the speaker.

Parasitic Pertaining to a parasite (an organism that lives on or in another organism, known as the host; benefits from the host; the host does not benefit from the parasite).

Parenteral (pa REN ter uhl) Taken into the body by any route other than the digestive tract (e.g., subcutaneous, intravenous, or intramuscular administration).

Participating Provider A physician or other healthcare provider who enters into a contract with a specific insurance company or program and by doing so agrees to abide by certain rules and regulations set forth by that particular third-party payer.

Patency (PAT en see) Open condition of a body cavity or canal.

Patent (PAT ent) Open. Also, a grant from the government that gives a creator (or manufacturer) of an invention the sole right to produce, use, and sell the product for a set period of time.

Pathogen A disease-causing organism.

Pathogenic Capable of producing disease.

Pathologic Caused by or involving disease.

Pathologist (pa THOL uh jest) A physician specially trained in the nature and cause of disease.

Pathology The study of disease.

Patient Abandonment A form of medical malpractice, also called negligent termination; the provider ends the provider-patient relationship without reasonable or adequate notification.

Patient Account A running balance of all financial transactions for a specific patient.

Patient Navigator A person who identifies patients' needs and barriers, then assists by coordinating care and identifying community and healthcare resources to meet the needs. May also be called a *care coordinator*.

Patient Portal A secure online website that gives patients 24-hour access to personal health information using a username and password.

Pegboard System A manual bookkeeping system that uses a day sheet to record all financial transactions for the date of service and maintains patient account balances by using physical ledger cards.

Perceiving (per SEEV ing) How an individual looks at information and sees it as real.

Performance Measurement The regular collection of data to assess whether the correct processes are being performed and desired results are being achieved.

Perineal (pair ih NEE uhl) Pertaining to the area between the vaginal opening and the rectum (perineum).

Perineum (pair ih NEE um) The area between the opening of the vagina and the anus.

Peripheral (puh RIF er uhl) Refers to an area outside of or away from an organ or structure.

Peripheral Neuropathy (puh RIF er uhl noo ROP uh thee) A problem with the function of the nerves outside the spinal cord; symptoms include weakness, burning pain, and loss of reflexes; a frequent complication of diabetes mellitus.

Peristalsis (per uh STAHL suhs) Rhythmic contraction of involuntary muscles lining the gastrointestinal tract; wavelike movement from alternate circulate contraction and relaxation of a tubular structure (e.g., intestine), which propels the content forward.

Peritoneum (per i tuh NEE um) A serous membrane lining of the abdominal cavity, which folds inward to enclose the viscera (internal organs).

Peritubular (per i TOO bu lar) Capillaries Blood capillaries surrounding the proximal and distal convoluted tubules in the kidneys.

Permeable (PUR mee ah buhl) A substance or structure that can be passed through, especially by liquids or gases.

Permeability (pur mee ah BIL i tee) A quality or characteristic of a material that allows another substance to pass through it.

Personal Ethics An individual's code of conduct.

Petechiae (peh TEEK kee ah) Very small, round hemorrhage in the skin or mucous membrane.

Peyer Patches (PAYH urh PACH ehz) Small masses of lymphatic tissue found mostly in the ileum of the small intestine. They are an important part of the immune system, because they monitor intestinal bacteria populations and prevent the growth of pathogenic bacteria in the intestines.

Pharyngitis Inflammation or infection of the pharynx, usually causing the symptoms of a sore throat.

Phenylalanine An essential amino acid found in milk, eggs, and other foods.

Phenylketonuria (PKU) A deficiency in the enzyme phenylalanine hydroxylase, which is responsible for converting phenylalanine into tyrosine.

Phishing A generic cyberattack toward many individuals or organizations with the intent to steal confidential data or install malware on the user's device.

Photophobia (foh toh FOH bee ah) Extreme sensitivity to light.

Phlebitis (fle BYE tis) Inflammation of a vein.

Physiologic Consistent with the normal function of the body.

Physiology (fi zee ALL uh jee) The study of body functions.

Pineal Gland A small organ in the brain that secretes melatonin, a hormone that regulates the sleep/awake cycle.

Pipet (pie PET) A slender tube attached to or including a bulb, for transferring or measuring small amounts of a liquid, often used in a laboratory.

Pitch The depth of a tone or sound; a distinctive quality of sound.

Pitting Edema Excessive fluid in the intercellular spaces in the tissue; when external pressure (e.g., socks, finger pressure) is relieved, a depression is seen in the tissue.

Place Value The numeric value that a digit has based on its position in a number.

Plaintiff (PLAIN tif) An individual or a party who brings a lawsuit to court.

Plasma (PLAZ muh) The liquid portion of a whole blood sample that has not clotted due to an anticoagulant. Liquid portion of blood that contains clotting factors. Liquid portion of the blood found in the body.

Plasma Membrane Outer covering surrounding the cell that allows certain substances to enter the cell and blocks other substances. Can also be called the cell membrane.

Plaque Sticky substance made of mucus, food particles, and bacteria that builds up on the exposed part of the tooth.

Plume Vapor, smoke, and particle debris produced by laser procedures.

Pneumonia Inflammation of the lungs with congestion of the air sacs (alveoli). Can be caused by a bacterium or virus.

Pocket Face Mask A device used to deliver a rescue breath.

Point-of-Care Something designed to be used at or near where the patient is seen; point-of-care tools and apps are resources for the provider to use when working directly with the patient.

Poised (poizd) Having a composed and self-assured manner; feeling confident, being patient, and maintaining good posture (standing and sitting up straight).

Policy A written agreement between two parties in which one party (the insurance company) agrees to pay another party (the patient) if certain specified circumstances occur.

Polycythemia (pol ee sie THEE mee ah) A condition caused by an abnormally large number of red blood cells (RBCs) in the blood.

Polyp A growth or mass protruding from a mucous membrane (e.g., nose, bladder, intestine).

Pores Tiny openings in the surface of the skin that allow gases, liquids, or microscopic particles to pass.

Portrait Orientation The most common layout for a printed page; the height of the paper is greater than its width.

Positive Feedback Loop A process in which a change causes a response that enhances that change.

Postherpetic Neuralgia (noo RAL juh) Nerve pain that occurs after a shingles outbreak and may become chronic.

Postural Orthostatic Tachycardia Syndrome (POTS) An autonomic nervous system condition that causes heart palpitations, lightheadedness, increased heart rate, low blood pressure, low blood volume, inability to concentrate, "brain fog," trouble sleeping, gastrointestinal symptoms, and dark red-blue discoloration of the legs.

Practice Management Software A type of software that allows the user to enter demographic information, schedule appointments, maintain lists of insurance payers, perform billing tasks, and generate reports.

Preauthorization A process required by some insurance carriers in which the provider obtains permission to perform certain procedures or services or refers a patient to a specialist.

Precedence (PRES i dehns) The top priority.

Precedent (PRES i dent) A prior court decision that serves as a model for similar legal cases in the future.

Precertification The process of determining if a procedure or service is covered by the insurance plan and what the reimbursement is for that procedure or service.

Precipitate (pri SIP i tayt) Solid particles that settle out of a liquid.

Preeclampsia (pree ih KLAMP see ah) A form of toxemia during pregnancy, characterized by high blood pressure, fluid retention, and protein in the urine. May progress to eclampsia.

Preexisting Condition A health problem that was present before new health insurance coverage started.

Premium The amount paid or to be paid by the policyholder for coverage under the contract, usually in periodic installments.

Presbyopia (pres bee oh pee- uh) Farsightedness due to ciliary weakness and loss of elasticity in the lens.

Primary Radiation The radiation that leaves the tube.

Privileged Communication Communication that cannot be disclosed without the authorization of the person involved; includes provider-patient and lawyer-client communications.

Process A prominence or projection on a bone.

Processing (prah CES ing) How an individual internalizes new information and makes it his or her own.

Product The number obtained by multiplying two or more numbers together.

Productive Cough A cough that produces phlegm or mucus.

Proficiency (pruh FISH uhn see) Skilled as a result of training or practice.

Prognosis (prog NOH sis) The likely outcome of a disease, including the chance of recovery.

Progress Notes Documentation in the medical record to track the patient's condition and progress.

Prokaryote (proh KAR ee ote) Any organism that is made up of at least one cell and has genetic material that is not enclosed in a nucleus. Bacteria are prokaryotes, primitive organisms.

Proofread To read and mark corrections.

Protected Health Information (PHI) Individually identifiable health information stored or transmitted by covered entities or business associates. Includes verbal, paper, or electronic information.

Protozoa (pro tuh ZOH ah) Single-celled organisms that are the most primitive form of animal life. Most are microscopic. Examples are amoebas, ciliates, flagellates, and sporozoans.

Provider An individual or company that provides medical care and services to a patient or the public.

Provider Network An approved list of physicians, hospitals, and other providers.

Provider Web Portal A secure online website that gives contracted providers a single point of access to insurance companies. This allows the provider to determine patient eligibility and deductible status, submit preauthorizations/precertifications, and check the status of claims.

Pruritus (proo RIE tuss) Itching.

Psoriasis (suh RIE i sis) A usually chronic, recurrent skin disease marked by bright red patches covered with silvery scales.

Psychiatrists Medical doctors who have been specially trained to diagnose and treat patients with mental, emotional, and behavioral conditions.

Psychotherapy (sie KOE ther ah pee) The treatment of behavioral health disorders through the use of psychological techniques, which encourage communication of conflicts and insights into the person's problems. The goals of this treatment include symptom relief, changes in behavior leading to improved social and vocational function, and personality growth.

Psychotherapy Notes Patient-provider details from private, group, or family therapy, including what the patient stated and the provider's analysis of the statements and situation.

Puberty (PYOO bur tee) The stage of life in which males and females become functionally capable of sexual reproduction.

Pulmonary Hypertension High blood pressure that affects the pulmonary system (pulmonary arteries and the right side of the heart).

Pulse Deficit A condition in which the radial pulse is less than the apical pulse; it may indicate a peripheral vascular abnormality.

Pulse Pressure The difference between the systolic and diastolic blood pressures (30 to 50 mm Hg is considered normal).

Purchase Order (PO) Number A unique number assigned by the ordering facility that allows the facility to track or reference the order.

Pure Culture The growth of only one microorganism in a culture or on a nutrient surface.

Purpura A condition characterized by hemorrhages in the tissues, causing the appearance of purplish spots.

Purulent (PYOOR yoo lent) Pus like.

Pyemia (pie EE mee uh) The presence of pus-forming organisms in the blood.

Pyrexia (pie REK see ah) A febrile condition or fever.

Qualified Medicare Beneficiaries (QMBs) Low-income Medicare patients who qualify for Medicaid for their secondary insurance.

Quality Assurance Written policies and procedures that ensure monitoring of all of the processes involved before, during, and after a laboratory test is performed to produce reliable patient test results.

Quality Control A process to ensure the reliability of test results, often using manufactured samples with known values.

Quantitative Describes a test result that is expressed as a number, usually with units of measure attached to numeric values.

Radiation Field The squared area of the x-ray beam that strikes the patient and x-ray table.

Radiation Protection The measures taken to safeguard patients, personnel, and the public from unnecessary exposure to ionizing radiation.

Rales (rayls) An abnormal lung sound heard on auscultation, characterized by discontinuous bubbling noises.

Rapport (ra PORE) A relationship of harmony and accord between the patient and the healthcare professional.

Reagent (re AY jent) A substance for use in a chemical reaction.

Rebound Pain Pain felt when the pressure on the abdomen is released.

Receptors Structures or sites on or in a cell that bind with substances such as hormones, antigens, or drugs.

Recommended Dietary Allowance (RDA) The average daily food intake needed to meet the nutrient requirements of most healthy people.

Reconciliation (rek uh n sill ee AY shun) To bring into agreement.

Reconciling Comparing a document with another document to ensure that they are consistent.

Reconstituted (ree KON sti toot ed) A dried substance (powder) that has been restored to a fluid form so that it can be injected.

Recovery Position A position on the person's side that helps to keep the airway open and clear.

Red Bone Marrow Soft, gelatinous tissue that consists of blood stem cells that can become white or red blood cells or platelets. Found at the center of most bones.

Reference Laboratory A laboratory that performs testing for another laboratory. Testing varies from high-volume routine testing to low-volume unique or unusual testing. Also called a referral, diagnostic, or commercial testing laboratory.

Referral An order from a primary care provider for the patient to see a specialist or to get certain medical services.

Referral Laboratory A laboratory that performs testing for another laboratory. Testing varies from high-volume routine testing to low-volume unique or unusual testing. Also called a reference, diagnostic, or commercial testing laboratory. Often privately owned.

Referred Pain Pain that is felt at a site in the body at a distance from the cause (e.g., the injury or diseased part).

Reflecting Putting words to the patient's emotional reaction, which acknowledges the person's feelings.

Reflection (ree FLEK shun) The process of thinking about new information so as to create new ways of learning.

Reflexes Movements or processes caused by a reflex response; a reflex is an automatic response that does not require thought.

Registered Dietitian (die eh TISH an) A credentialed healthcare professional who is trained in nutrition and is able to apply the information to the dietary needs of healthy and ill patients.

Regular Diet The food and drink a person typically consumes when there are no dietary limitations.

Reimbursement (ree im BURS ment) To make repayment for an expense or a loss incurred.

Relapse The recurrence of the symptoms of a disease after apparent recovery.

Release of Information A form completed by the patient that authorizes the medical office to release medical records to the insurance company for health insurance reimbursement.

Reliable (ree LIE ah bul) Dependable, able to be trusted.

Remission The partial or complete disappearance of the clinical and subjective characteristics of a chronic or malignant disease.

Renal Ischemia A blood flow deficiency to the kidney(s).

Renal Threshold The blood level of a substance, above which the kidneys fail to reabsorb it, so the substance will appear in the urine.

Replication The production of exact copies of a complex molecule, such as DNA.

Rescue Breathing A life-saving maneuver to resuscitate a person who has stopped breathing. The rescuer forces air into the victim's lungs at intervals by exhaling into the victim's mouth, nose, or stoma from a laryngectomy.

Resection Surgical removal of all or part of an organ.

Resident A physician who has graduated from medical school and is finishing specialized clinical training.

Residual Urine Urine that remains in the bladder after micturition or urination.

Res Ipsa Loquitur **(RASE ipsah low kwah tuhr)** A Latin term meaning "the thing speaks for itself." A legal concept under which the plaintiff's burden to prove malpractice is minimal because the jury can clearly understand the details of the injury (for example, a surgical instrument was left in the body during surgery).

Res Judicata **(RASE JOO di kah tah)** Latin for "a thing decided." Once a case has been decided by the court, it cannot be litigated again.

Respect To show consideration or appreciation for another person.

Respiration A metabolic process by which cells break down substances (e.g., carbohydrates, amino acids, and fats) to produce adenosine triphosphate (ATP).

Respiratory Arrest Stoppage of breathing.

Respondeat Superior **(re SPON dee at soo PIR ee ahr)** Latin for "let the master answer"; a legal doctrine by which the employer/provider is legally responsible for the wrongful actions or lack of actions of employees if done within the scope of employment.

Restock The process of replacing the supplies that were used.

Retaliation (ree tal ee A shuhn) Getting back at others for something they did to you.

Retention A term referring to actions taken by management to keep good employees.

Retention Schedule A method or plan for retaining or keeping health records and for their movement from active to inactive to closed.

Retractions (re TRAK shuns) The sucking in of tissues between the intercostal spaces and neck due to respiratory distress; classic sign of severe asthma.

Retribution (reh trih BYOU shuhn) Punishment inflicted on someone as vengeance for a wrong or criminal act; the act of taking revenge.

Revenue (REV eh noo) Money collected for providing a product or service.

Reverse Chronologic Order The most recent item is on top, and the oldest item is last.

Review of Systems (ROS) A list of questions related to each organ system, designed to uncover potential disease processes.

Rhonchi (RON kie) An abnormal rumbling sound heard on auscultation, caused by airways blocked by secretions or muscle contractions.

Route The means by which a drug enters the body.

Rugae (ROO gah) Folds in the wall of an organ; when an organ (e.g., stomach, bladder, uterus) fills or needs to expand, the rugae unfold.

Salary A fixed compensation periodically paid to a person for regular work.

Salpingo-Oophorectomy (sal ping goh oh of or EK toh mee) Surgical removal of the fallopian tube and ovary.

Sanitize The process of cleaning equipment and instruments with detergent and water in order to remove debris and reduce the number of microorganisms.

Scatter Radiation Radiation from the primary beam that is randomly scattered within or outside of the body.

Sclera (SKLER uh) The white part of the eye that forms the orbit.

Scope of Practice Range of responsibilities and practice guidelines that determine the boundaries within which a healthcare worker practices.

Scored Tablet A tablet with a groove on the surface, used for splitting it in half.

Screening A system for examining and separating into different groups; in the healthcare facility, it means determining the severity of illness that patients experience and prioritizing appointments based on that severity.

Seborrhea (seb uh REE ah) An excessive discharge of sebum from the sebaceous glands, forming greasy scales or crusty areas on the body.

Secondary Storage Devices Media (e.g., jump drive, flash drive, hard drive) capable of permanently storing data until it is replaced or deleted by the user.

Sediment An insoluble material that settles to the bottom of a liquid specimen and to the bottom of a centrifuged sample.

Senescent (si NES ent) Cell An old or aging cell that can no longer divide and reproduce.

Sensorineural (sen suh ree NOOR uhl) Involving the sensory nerves, especially as they affect hearing.

Sentence A penalty imposed by a court of law or other authority when a person is found guilty of a crime or other offense.

Sentinel Node Biopsy Removal of a limited number of lymph nodes to determine if the cancer has spread to the lymph nodes.

Septicemia (sep ti SEE mee ah) A systemic infection involving pathologic microbes in the blood as a result of an infection that has spread from elsewhere in the body.

Sequela (si KWEL uh) (singular), sequelae (plural) An abnormal condition resulting from a previous disease.

Serologic Pertaining to the science involving the immune properties and actions of serum.

Serous (SEER uhs) A thin, watery serum-like drainage.

Serum (SEER um) The liquid portion of a clotted blood specimen. It no longer contains active clotting agents.

Server Computer hardware and software that perform data analysis, storage, and archiving; accepts and responds to requests from devices (clients) made over a network. Also called a database server or data server.

Shaken Baby Syndrome Condition resulting from internal head injuries that occur when a baby or young child is violently shaken.

Sharps Medical term for devices with sharp points or edges that can puncture or cut skin. Examples include needles, scalpels, or broken glass.

Sickle Cell Anemia An inherited anemia characterized by crescent-shaped red blood cells (RBCs). It causes RBCs to block capillaries, reducing the oxygen supply to the cells.

Side Effects Unpleasant effects of a drug in addition to the desired or therapeutic effect.

Signs Objective findings determined by a clinician, such as a fever, hypertension, or rash.

Sinus Arrhythmia An irregular heartbeat that originates in the sinoatrial node (pacemaker).

Skill Set A person's abilities, skills, or expertise in an area.

Small Claims Court A special court established to handle small claims or debts without the services of lawyers.

Software A set of electronic instructions to operate and perform different computer tasks.

Solute A substance that is dissolved in a solvent (liquid) to form a solution.

Solvent (SOL vent) Able to pay all debts. Also, a liquid that can dissolve other substances.

Somatic cells (soe MAT ik) Nonreproductive cells; they do not include sperm and egg cells.

Source-to-Image-Receptor Distance (SID) The distance between the tube target and the image receptor.

Speakerphone A telephone with a loudspeaker and a microphone; it can be used without having to pick up and hold the handset.

Spear Phishing A customized cyberattack toward an individual or organization with the intent to steal confidential data or install malware on the user's device.

Special Report Additional medical documentation required to confirm the need for the use of unlisted, unusual, or newly adopted medical procedures code.

Specificity (spes uh FIS i tee) The quality or state of being specific.

Specimen A biological sample such as blood, urine, body fluids, feces, or tissue collected for analysis and evaluation.

Speed Dialing A telephone function in which a selected stored number can be dialed by pressing only one key.

Spermatozoa (spur mat ah ZOH ah) (singular, spermatozoon) Mature male reproductive cells.

Sphincter (SFINGK ter) A circular muscle that either constricts and closes the opening or relaxes and allows substances to pass through the opening.

Spina Bifida (SPY nah BIF id dah) A condition in which the spinal column has an abnormal opening that allows protrusion of the meninges or the spinal column.

Spongy Bone Lighter and less dense than compact bone; also called cancellous bone. Usually found at the ends of bones and contains red bone marrow.

Spoof To assume or mimic the identity of another user to gain access to a computer system.

Spore A thick-walled, dormant form of bacteria that is very resistant to disinfection measures.

Sputum Thick mucus often referred to as phlegm. It is coughed up from the lungs; not saliva that originates in the mouth.

Stains Reagents or dyes used to prepare specimens for microscopic examination.

Standard of Care The level and type of care an ordinary, prudent healthcare professional with the same training and experience in a similar practice would have provided under a similar situation.

Standard Operating Procedures Also known as SOP, a set of step-by-step instructions to help employees carry out routine operations with efficiency, high quality, and uniformity of performance.

Standard Precautions A set of infection control practices used to prevent the transmission of diseases that can be acquired by contact with blood, body fluids, nonintact skin, and mucous membranes.

Stat The medical abbreviation for the Latin term *statum*, meaning immediately; at this moment.

Static (STAT ik) Equilibrium Relating to balance when moving in a straight line.

Stem Cells Undifferentiated cells that can become specialized cells in the body.

Stenosis (sten OH sis) Occurs when the heart valve flaps are stiff or fused together, thus narrowing the valve.

Sterile (STER il) Free of all microorganisms, pathogenic and nonpathogenic.

Sterilize The process of removing all microorganisms.

Stertorous (STUR ter uhs) Heavy, as related to snoring.

Stoma (STOH mah) A temporary or permanent surgically created opening used for drainage (i.e., urine, stool).

Strangulation Constriction of a tubular structure, such as an intestine or vessel, leading to a lack of blood supply to the tissues.

Strata Naturally or artificially formed layers of material, usually multiple layers.

Streaked for Isolation To have produced isolated colonies of an organism on an agar plate. Using an inoculating loop, pick one colony and methodically spread it out onto solid nutrient media. The goal is to have colonies that are separate from other colonies.

Stretch Receptor A sensory nerve ending that responds to a stretch stimulus.

Stylus (STI luhs) A pen-shaped device with a variety of tips that is used on touchscreens to write, draw, or input commands.

Subcultured Occurs when an organism (a bacterium) has been cultivated again on a new nutrient surface.

Subjective Information Data or information obtained from the patient, including the patient's feelings, perceptions, and concerns; this information is obtained through interviews or written questions.

Subpoena (suh PEE nuh) A court order requiring a person to appear in court at a specific time to testify in a legal case.

***Subpoena Duces Tecum* (suh PEE nuh DOO seez TEE kuhm)** A legal document commanding a person to bring a piece of evidence (e.g., the plaintiff's health record) to court.

Subsequent (SUHB si kwuhnt) Occurring later or after.

Suction (SUHK shun) The production of a partial vacuum by the removal of air in order to force fluid into a vacant space.

Sulci (SUL sie) Grooves or depressions on the surface of the brain between the gyri.

Sulcus (SUL kus) The singular form of *sulci.*

Summarizing Allowing the listener to recap and review what was said.

Supernatant The clear liquid above the sediment in a centrifuged urine specimen.

Suppurative (SUHP yuh ruh tiv) Characterized by the formation or discharge of pus.

Surfactant (sur FACK tunt) A mixture of protein and fats that lines the alveoli and prevents the tissues from sticking together and collapsing during exhalation.

Surrogate (SUR ah git) A person who acts on behalf of another person or takes the place of another person. Examples include a surrogate mother or a healthcare agent.

Symmetry (SIM ih tree) Similarity in size, form, and arrangement of parts on opposite sides of the body.

Symptoms Subjective complaints reported by the patient, such as pain or nausea.

Synapse (SIN aps) A point of communication between two cells.

Syncope Loss of consciousness and postural tone caused by diminished blood flow to the brain.

Synthesis (SIN theh sis) Formation of a chemical compound from simpler compounds or elements.

Syringe (suh RINJ) A device with a slender barrel and needle used to withdraw blood from a vein or artery.

Systemic Affecting the entire body.

Tachycardia (tak i KAHR dee ah) A rapid but regular heart rate; one that exceeds 100 beats per minute.

Tachypnea (tack ip NEE ah) Rapid, shallow breathing.

Tactful The quality of having a sense of what to do or say to maintain good relations with others or to prevent offense.

Target Cell A cell selectively affected by a specific agent, such as a drug, hormone, or virus.

Target Tissue The destination, or intended tissue, in the nervous impulse (e.g., a muscle).

Telehealth Refers to remote clinical services and nonclinical services, such as provider training, meetings, and continuing education.

Telemedicine (TEL i med i sin) The use of telecommunication technology to provide healthcare services to patients at a distance; it is usually used in rural communities.

Template (TEM plit) A document or file that has a preset format; this is used as a starting point for composing something and eliminates the need to recreate it each time it is used.

Tendons (TEN duns) Connective tissue that attaches muscles to bone.

Termination Letters Documents sent to patients explaining that the provider is ending the physician-patient relationship and the patient needs to see other providers.

Testis (TES tis) (plural, testes) The male gonad, also called a *testicle* (TES ti kul).

Testosterone (tess TOS tuh rohn) Male sex hormone produced by the interstitial cells in the testes.

Thalamus (THAL uh muhs) The middle part of the brain through which sensory impulses pass to reach the cerebral cortex.

Therapeutic Range The blood concentrations of a medication that are high enough to produce the drug's therapeutic effect.

Thermionic Emission Electrons begin to "boil effect," when the filament is heated.

Third-Party Administrator (TPA) An organization that processes claims and provides administrative services for another organization. Often used by self-funded plans.

Thoracentesis (thor ah sen TEE sis) Aspiration of a fluid from the pleural cavity.

Thready Describes a pulse that is thin and feeble.

Thrombus (THRAHM bus) A blood clot that blocks the flow of blood.

Tickler File A chronologic file used as a reminder that something must be dealt with on a certain date.

Tinea (TIN ee uh) Any fungal skin disease that results in scaling, itching, and inflammation; examples include ringworm and athlete's foot.

Tinnitus (TIN it uhs) A noise sensation of ringing heard in one or both ears.

Tissue Culture The technique or process of keeping tissue alive and growing in a culture medium.

Titer The lowest concentration of a serum solution containing a specific antibody where the antibody is still able to neutralize (or precipitate) an antigen.

Tonometer (toh NOM i ter) An instrument used to measure intraocular pressure.

Tort A civil wrongdoing that causes harm to a person or property; excludes breach of contract.

Tortfeasor (TORTE fee zahr) The individual or entity who committed the tort, either intentionally or as a result of negligence.

Toxicity The harmful and deadly effect of a medication that can develop due to the buildup of medication or by-products in the body.

Toxicology (tok si KOL oh jee) The study and science that deal with the effects, antidotes, and detection of poisons or drugs.

Toxins (TOK sins) Substances created by microorganisms, plants, or animals that are poisonous to humans.

Tract A system of tissues (e.g., neuronal axons) or organs (e.g., intestines) that function together.

Transcription (tran SKRIP shuhn) A typed or written copy of dictated material.

Transient (TRAN zee uhnt) Not lasting, enduring, or permanent; transitory.

Transillumination (trans ih LOO muh nay shun) Inspection of a cavity or organ by passing light through its walls.

Transitional Epithelium A type of cell found in the lining of hollow organs. It has the ability to stretch with the contraction and distention of the organ.

Transmission The passage or spread of disease.

Transport Medium A medium used to keep an organism alive during transport to the laboratory.

Trauma (TRAW muh) A physical injury or wound caused by external force or violence.

Triage (tree AHZH) The process of sorting patients to determine medical need and the priority of care.

Triaging Flow Map A written flow map to make triage decisions; based on answers to questions, the person moves through the map until a triage decision is made.

Tripod Position The standing position when using crutches; crutch tips are 4 to 6 inches to the side and front of each foot.

Trustee The coordinator of financial resources assigned by the court during a bankruptcy case.

Turgor (TUR ger) Referring to normal skin tension; the resistance of the skin to being grasped between the fingers and released. Turgor decreases with dehydration and increases with edema.

Unipolar Having one pole or electrical charge.

Unit Dose Packaging A packaging method for drugs; holds a specified quantity of medication in a single-use container (e.g., syringe, blister pack).

Unsecured Debt Debt that is not guaranteed by something of value; credit card debt is the most common type of unsecured debt.

Urgent An acute situation that requires immediate attention but is not life threatening.

Urostomy (yoo ROS te mee) A surgically created opening on the abdominal wall used to drain urine.

Urticaria (ur ti KAYR ee ah) Hives.

Utilization Management A decision-making process used by managed care organizations to manage healthcare costs. It involves case-by-case assessments of the appropriateness of care.

Valvulitis The inflammatory condition of a valve that results in valve stenosis and obstructed blood flow; caused most commonly by rheumatic fever, bacterial endocarditis, or syphilis.

Vascular (VAS kyuh ler) Having (blood) vessels that conduct or circulate liquids (blood).

Vascular Access A surgical procedure that creates a vein to remove and return blood during the hemodialysis procedure.

Vasoconstriction (vay zoh kuhn STRIK shuhn) Contraction of the muscles causing the narrowing of the inside tube of the vessel.

Vasovagal Syncope A faint brought on by excessive activity of the vagus nerve, causing a sudden drop in the heart rate and blood pressure. Can be caused by stress, heat exposure, long periods of standing, or the sight of blood.

Vector An arthropod (mosquito, tick, flea) that carries disease and transmits to another organism through a blood meal; an animal or insect (e.g., tick, rodent, mosquito) that transmits a pathogen.

Vendors Companies that sell supplies, equipment, or services to other companies or individuals.

Venule (VEN yuhl) A very small vein.

Verification of Eligibility The process of confirming health insurance coverage for the patient.

Vertebrae (VUR teh bray) A series of small, irregularly shaped bones that form the spine. Each vertebra has several projections, joint surfaces, areas for muscle attachment, and a hole where the spinal cord passes.

Vertigo (VUR tih goh) Dizziness; an abnormal sensation of movement when there is none.

Vesicant (VES i kant) Medication A medication that can damage tissue and can produce blisters.

Vested Granted or endowed with a particular authority, right, or property; to have a special interest in.

Viability (vie a BIL ih tee) The ability to live.

Viable Able to live and grow.

Vigilance (VIJ uh lahns) Keen watchfulness to detect danger.

Viscosity (vis KOS i tee) Resistance to flow; the thicker the liquid, the higher the viscosity.

Voice Mail An electronic system that allows messages from telephone callers to be recorded and stored.

Waiting Period The length of time a patient waits for disability insurance to pay after the date of injury.

Water Deprivation Test A test to measure the amount and concentration of urine produced when water is withheld from a patient for a period of time.

Wet Mount A glass slide that holds a specimen suspended in a drop of liquid for microscopic examination.

Wheal A raised mark on the skin.

Wheezing (WHEE zing) A whistling sound made during breathing.

Whistleblower A person (usually an employee) who reports a violation of the law within an organization. The person reports the information to the public or to a person in authority.

Whole Blood Plasma and the formed elements of blood in a free-flowing liquid form.

Workplace Emergencies Unforeseen situations that threaten the employees and visitors; can disrupt services provided.

X-ray Tube The source of x-rays; the x-rays are formed within the x-ray tube.

Yeast Any various single-celled fungi, which reproduce by budding and are able to ferment sugars.

Zollinger-Ellison Syndrome A rare condition that causes tumors to form in the pancreas or duodenum. Tumors secrete large amounts of gastrin, which causes an increase in acid production.

Zone A region or geographic area used for shipping.

ABBREVIATIONS

%TBSA percent of total burn surface area
°C Celsius
°F Fahrenheit
$\bar{s}$ without
3D three-dimensional

A

A&Ox3 alert and oriented to person, place, and time
A/P accounts payable
A/R accounts receivable
A1c glycated hemoglobin
$\overline{aa}$ of each (used in prescriptions)
AAA abdominal aortic aneurysm
AAFP American Academy of Family Physicians
AAMA American Association of Medical Assistants
AAMT American Association for Medical Transcriptions
AAP American Academy of Pediatrics
AAT alpha-1 antitrypsin
ABG arterial blood gas
ABHES Accrediting Bureau of Health Education Schools
ac before meals
ACA The Affordable Care Act
ACE inhibitor angiotensin converting enzyme inhibitor
Ach acetylcholine
ACL anterior cruciate ligament
ACTH adrenocorticotropic hormone
AD Alzheimer disease
ad lib as desired
ADA American Diabetes Association; Americans with Disabilities Act
ADAAA Americans with Disabilities Act Amendment Act
ADF scanner automatic document feeder
ADH antidiuretic hormone
ADHD attention deficit hyperactivity disorder
ADLs activities of daily living
ADR alternative dispute resolution
AED automated external defibrillator
AFB acid-fast bacilli
AFP alpha-fetoprotein
$AgNO_3$ silver nitrate
AHA American Heart Association
AHRQ Agency for Healthcare Research and Quality
AIDS acquired immunodeficiency syndrome
AK astigmatic keratotomy
ALL acute lymphocytic leukemia
ALP alkaline phosphatase
ALS amyotrophic lateral sclerosis
ALT alanine aminotransferase
AM, a.m. morning
AMA American Medical Association
AML acute myelogenous leukemia; acute myeloid leukemia
AMT American Medical Technologists
ANA antinuclear antibody test
ANLL acute non-lymphocytic leukemia
ANS autonomic nervous system
Anti-CCP anti-cyclin citrullinated peptide
AP anteroposterior
APAP acetaminophen
APRN advanced practice registered nurse
aq water
ARB angiotensin II receptor blocker
ART assistive reproductive technology
ARV antiretroviral
ASA Anesthesia Society of America; aspirin
ASCP American Society of Clinical Pathologists
ASD atrial septal defect; autism spectrum disorder
AST aspartate aminotransferase
ATP adenosine triphosphate
AUD alcohol use disorder
AV atrioventricular
aV augmented voltage

B

BAP blood agar plate
BBB blood-brain barrier
BBPS bloodborne pathogen standard
BCG bacille Calmette-Guérin
BD Blu-Ray disc
beta-hCG beta human chorionic gonadotropin
bid twice a day
BLS basic life support
BMI body mass index
BMR basal metabolic rate
BOO bladder outlet obstruction
BP blood pressure
BPD bronchopulmonary dysplasia
BPH benign prostatic hyperplasia
BSE breast self-examination
BTL bottle
BUN blood urea nitrogen
BX box

C

$\bar{c}$ with
C Celsius
c centi
C&S culture and sensitivity
Ca calcium
CAAHEP Commission on Accreditation of Allied Health Education Programs
CABG coronary artery bypass graft
CAD coronary artery disease
CAM complementary and alternative medicine

cap capsule
CAP College of American Pathologists
CAPTA Child Abuse Prevention and Treatment Act
CARD check, assign, reverse, define
CAT computerized axial tomography
CBC complete blood count
CBT cognitive behavioral therapist
CC chief complaint
cc cubic centimeter
CCB calcium channel blocker
CCK cholecystokinin
CCMA certified clinical medical assistant
CCMS clean-catch midstream urine
CD collecting duct; compact disc; conduct disorder
CDC Centers for Disease Control and Prevention
CEJA Council of Ethical and Judicial Affairs
CEU continuing education unit
CF cystic fibrosis
cfu colony-forming units
CHAMPVA Civilian Health and Medical Program of the Department of Veterans Affairs
CHD coronary heart disease
CHF congestive heart failure
CHIP Children's Health Insurance Program
Chol cholesterol
CIS clinically isolated syndrome
CK creatine kinase
CKD chronic kidney disease
CK-MB creatine kinase-MB
Cl chloride
CLIA Clinical Laboratory Improvement Amendments
CLL chronic lymphocytic leukemia
CLS clinical laboratory scientist
CLSI Clinical and Laboratory Standards Institute
CLT clinical laboratory technician/technologist
cm centimeter
CMA certified medical assistant
CML chronic myeloid leukemia
CMLA certified medical laboratory assistant
CMP comprehensive metabolic profile
CMPs civil monetary penalties
CMS Centers for Medicare and Medicaid Services
CNM certified nurse midwife
CNS central nervous system; clinical nurse specialist
CO_2 carbon dioxide
COPD chronic obstructive pulmonary disease
CoW certificate of waiver
COW computer on wheels
CPAP continuous positive airway pressure
CPK creatinine phosphokinase
CPOE computerized provider/physician order entry
CPR cardiopulmonary resuscitation
CPT certified phlebotomy technician; current procedural terminology
CPU central processing unit
Creat creatinine
CRNA certified registered nurse anesthetist
CRP C-reactive protein
CS case
CSF cerebrospinal fluid
CSMT color, sensation, motion, and temperature
CT computed tomography
CTA computerized tomography angiography
CVA cerebrovascular accident
CVS chorionic villus sampling; cyclic vomiting syndrome
CWP coal workers' pneumoconiosis
CXR chest x-ray

D

d day
DAP test draw-a-person test
DASH Dietary Approaches to Stop Hypertension
DBS deep brain stimulation
DBT dialectical behavioral therapy
DC doctor of chiropractic
DCT distal (convoluted) tubule
DDL digital data loggers
DEA Drug Enforcement Agency
DHE dihydroergotamine
(D)HHS Department of Health and Human Services
DI diabetes insipidus
DJD degenerative joint disease
DKA diabetic ketoacidosis
DM diabetes mellitus
DMARDs disease-modifying antirheumatic drugs
DNA deoxyribonucleic acid
DNR do not resuscitate
DO doctor of osteopathy
DOB date of birth
DRE digital rectal exam
DSL modem digital subscriber line modem
DSM Diagnostic and Statistical Manual of Mental Disorders
DTP diphtheria-tetanus-pertussis
DUB dysfunctional uterine bleeding
DV daily value
DVD digital versatile/video disc
DVT deep vein thrombosis

E

E/M evaluation and management
EA each
EAP employee assistance program
EBV Epstein-Barr virus
ECG electrocardiogram
ECHO echocardiography
ED emergency department; erectile dysfunction
EDTA ethylenediaminetetraacetic acid
EEG electroencephalography
EFT electronic funds transfers
EGD esophagogastroduodenoscopy
EHR electronic health record
EIA enzyme immunoassay
EIN employer identification number
EKG electrocardiogram

ELISA enzyme-linked immunosorbent assay
EM erythema migrans (sometimes called erythema chronicum migrans)
EMDR eye movement desensitization and reprocessing
EMG electromyography; emergency
EMR electronic medical record
EMS emergency medical services
EMTs emergency medical technicians
ENT ear, nose, throat
EOB explanation of benefits
EOM extraocular movement
EP established patient
EPA Environmental Protection Agency
EPDS Edinburgh Postnatal Depression Scale
ePHI electronic protected health information
EPO exclusive provider organization
EPS electrophysiology study
EPSDT early and periodic screening, diagnosis, and treatment
ER endoplasmic reticulum
ERCP endoscopic retrograde cholangiopancreatography
ERV expiratory reserve volume
ESR erythrocyte sedimentation rate
ESRD end-stage renal disease
ESU electrosurgical unit
ESWL extracorporeal shock wave lithotripsy
ET endotracheal

F

F Fahrenheit
FAERS FDA adverse event reporting system
FBG fasting blood glucose
FBS fasting blood sugar
FDA Food and Drug Administration
Fe iron
FECA Federal Employees Compensation Act
FEV_1 forced expiratory volume in 1 second
FH family history
FIT fecal immunochemical test
fl oz fluid ounce
FOB fecal occult blood
FOBT fecal occult blood test
FRC functional residual capacity
FSH follicle-stimulating hormone
FTC Federal Trade Commission
FUO fever of unknown origin
FVC forced vital capacity

G

g gram
G gauge
GAD generalized anxiety disorder
GAS general adaptation syndrome; group A streptococcus
GB gigabyte
GER gastroesophageal reflux
GERD gastroesophageal reflux disease
gFOBT guaiac fecal occult blood test
GGT gamma glutamyl transferase
GH growth hormone
GHRL ghrelin
GI gastrointestinal; glycemic index
GINA Genetic Information Nondiscrimination Act
GMOs genetically modified organisms
GNB gram-negative bacilli
GN-RH gonadotropin-releasing hormone
GPC gram-positive cocci
GPOs group purchasing organizations
gr grain
GTT glucose tolerance test
gtt(s) drop(s)

H

H&H hemoglobin and hematocrit
H&P history and physical
h, hr hour
H^+ hydrogen
HAV hepatitis A virus
HbA1C or A1C glycosylated hemoglobin
HBV hepatitis B virus
hCG human chorionic gonadotropin
HCPCS Healthcare Common Procedure Coding System
HCS hazard communication standard
HCT hematocrit
HCV hepatitis C virus
HD hoarding disorder; Huntington disease
HDD hard disk drive
HDL high-density lipoprotein
HDN hemolytic disease of the newborn
HDV hepatitis D virus
HEV hepatitis E virus
Hgb hemoglobin
HHR hybrid health record
HHS Department of Health and Human Services
HIDA scan hepatobiliary iminodiacetic acid scan
HIE health information exchange
HIPAA Health Insurance Portability and Accountability Act
HITECH Health Information Technology for Economic and Clinical Health Act
HIV human immunodeficiency virus
HMIS hazardous materials information system
HMO health maintenance organization
HPI health plan identifier; history of present illness
HPV human papilloma virus
HRT hormone replacement therapy
HSV herpes simplex virus
HSV-1 herpes simplex virus-1
HZV herpes zoster vaccine

I

I&D incision and drainage
IAPS International Academy of Phlebotomy Sciences
IBD inflammatory bowel disease
IBS irritable bowel syndrome
IC inspiratory capacity; interstitial cystitis
ICD implantable cardioverter defibrillator; *International Classification of Diseases*

ICD-10-CM *International Classification of Diseases, 10th revision, Clinical Modification*
ICP intracranial pressure
ICS intercostal space
ID identification; intradermal
IDS integrated delivery system
IE infective endocarditis
IFA immunofluorescence assay
iFOBT immunochemical fecal occult blood test
Ig Immunoglobulin
IM intramuscular
INR international normalized ratio
IOL intraocular lens
IPA independent practice associations
IPAA ileal pouch-anal anastomosis
IPT interpersonal psychotherapy
IQ intelligent quotient
IRV inspiratory reserve volume
ISCLT International Society of Clinical Laboratory Technology
ISP internet service provider
IT information technology
ITP idiopathic thrombocytopenic purpura
IUD intrauterine device
IUFD intrauterine fetal death
IUI intrauterine insemination
IV intravenous
IVIg intravenous immunoglobulin
IVP intravenous pyelogram

J

JA juvenile arthritis
JIA juvenile idiopathic arthritis

K

k kilo
K potassium
KB kilobyte
kg kilogram
KOH potassium hydroxide
KS Kaposi sarcoma

L

L liter
LA left arm
LAGB laparoscopic adjustable gastric band
LAN local area network
LASIK laser-assisted in-situ keratomileusis
lb pound
LCD monitor liquid crystal display monitor
LCL lateral collateral ligament
LCSW licensed clinical social worker
LDH lactate dehydrogenase
LDL low-density lipoprotein
LED light-emitting diodes
LEEP loop electrosurgical excision procedure
LES lower esophageal sphincter
LH luteinizing hormone
LICSW license independent clinical social worker
LL left leg
LLQ left lower quadrant
LP lumbar puncture
LPN licensed practical nurse
LSW licensed social worker
LUQ left upper quadrant

M

m meter; milli
MA medical assistant
MAC Mycobacterium avium complex
MB megabyte
mc micro
mcg microgram
MCH mean cell hemoglobin
MCHC mean cell ratio of hemoglobin and hematocrit
MCL medial collateral ligament
MCO managed care organization
MCV mean cell volume
MD doctor of medicine; muscular dystrophy
MDI metered-dose inhaler
med medicine
mg milligram
MGUS monoclonal gammopathy of undetermined significance
mHealth mobile health
MI myocardial infarction
min minute
mL milliliter
MLA medical laboratory assistant
MLT medical laboratory technician
mm millimeter
MMPI Minnesota Multiphasic Personality Inventory
MMR measles-mumps-rubella
MOM milk of magnesia
Mono infectious mononucleosis
MPM medical practice management
MRA magnetic resonance angiography
MRI magnetic resonance imaging
MS multiple sclerosis; musculoskeletal system
MSAFP maternal serum alpha-fetoprotein (test)
MT medical technologist
MT-sDNA multi-targeted stool DNA (test)
MUGA multiple-gated acquisition
MVD coronary microvascular disease
MVV maximum voluntary ventilation
MY myopia

N

Na sodium
NAFLD nonalcoholic fatty liver disease
NAS nasal
NCA National Certification Agency for Medical Laboratory Personnel
NCCI National Corrective Coding Initiative
NCCT National Center for Competency Testing
NCMA National Certified Medical Assistant

NCQA National Committee for Quality Assurance
NCV nerve conduction velocity
NCVIA National Childhood Vaccine Injury Act
NDC National Drug Code
NH_3 ammonia
NHA National Healthcareer Association
NHI National Institutes of Health
NIDA National Institute on Drug Abuse
NIH National Institutes of Health
NK natural killer
NKA no known allergies
NKDA no known drug allergies
nm nanometer
NMJ neuromuscular junction
noc, noct night
NOTA National Organ Transplant Act
NP new patient; nurse practitioner
NPA National Phlebotomy Association
NPI national provider identifier
NPO nothing by mouth
NPP notice of privacy practices
NS normal saline
NSAID nonsteroidal anti-inflammatory drug
NTM nontuberculous mycobacteria
NUCC National Uniform Claim Committee

O

O&P ova and parasite
O_2 oxygen
OA osteoarthritis
OAE otoacoustic emission
OB/GYN obstetrics and gynecology
OCD obsessive-compulsive disorder
OCP oral contraceptive pills
OCR Office for Civil Rights; optical character recognition
ODD oppositional defiant disorder
OGTT oral glucose tolerance test
OMT osteopathic manipulative therapy
ONC The Office of the National Coordinator for Health Information Technology
OPIM other potentially infectious materials
OPTN Organ Procurement and Transplant Network
ORIF open reduction and internal fixation
OSA obstructive sleep apnea
OSH Act Occupational Safety and Health Act
OSHA Occupational Safety and Health Administration
OT oxytocin
OTC over-the-counter (drugs)
OUI operating under the influence
OWI operating while intoxicated
oz ounce

P

$\bar{p}$ after
P phosphorus
PA physician assistant; posteroanterior
PA-C physician assistant-certified
PACs premature atrial contractions
PAD peripheral artery disease
PAP Papanicolaou
PAR participating provider
PBGs physician buying groups
PBS painful bladder syndrome; prune belly syndrome
pc after meals
PC personal computer
PCL posterior cruciate ligament
PCMH patient-centered medical home
PCP primary care provider
PCT proximal (convoluted) tubule
PCV13 13-valent pneumococcal conjugate vaccine
PD Parkinson disease
PDA patent ductus arteriosus
PDD pervasive developmental disorder
PDR Physician Desk Reference; proliferative diabetic retinopathy
PDT photodynamic therapy
PE pulmonary embolism
PEP post-exposure prophylaxis
PET positron emission tomography
PFO patent foramen ovale
PG peptidoglycan
PH past history; pulmonary hypertension
PHI protected health information
PHQ-2 Patient Health Questionnaire-2
PHQ-9 Patient Health Questionnaire-9
PHR personal health record
PID pelvic inflammatory disease
PIN personal identification number
PKD polycystic kidney disease
PKG package
PKU phenylketonuria
PLMD periodic limb movement disorder
PM, p.m. afternoon
PMDD premenstrual dysphoric disorder
PMH past medical history
PMN polymorphonucleocyte
PMS practice management software; premenstrual syndrome
PNL percutaneous nephronlithotripsy
PNS peripheral nervous system
po, PO by mouth; oral (route)
PO purchase order
POCT point-of-care testing
POL physician office laboratory
POLST Physician Orders for Life-Sustaining Treatment
POR problem-oriented record
POS place of service; point-of-sale
POTS postural orthostatic tachycardia syndrome
PPD postpartum depression; prepaid; purified protein derivative (tuberculin skin test)
PPE personal protective equipment
PPI proton pump inhibitor
PPM(P) provider-performed microscopy (procedures)
PPMS primary progressive multiple sclerosis
PPO preferred provider organizations
PPP 2-hour postprandial urine specimen

PPSA Physician Payments Sunshine Act
PPSV23 or PPSV 23-valent pneumococcal polysaccharide vaccine
PRL prolactin
prn as needed
PSA prostate-specific antigen
PSDA Patient Self-Determination Act
PSI pounds per square inch
PST plasma separator tubes
Pt, pt patient
pt pint
PT prothrombin time; protime
PTH parathyroid hormone
PTSD post-traumatic stress disorder
PTT partial thromboplastin time
PTT activated partial thromboplastin time
PUVA psoralen plus ultraviolet A
PVCs premature ventricular contractions
PYMT payment

Q

q2h every 2 hours
q3h every 3 hours
q4h every 4 hours
q6h every 6 hours
q8h every 8 hours
QA quality assurance
qam every morning
QC quality control
QFT QuantiFERON-TB
QFT-GIT QuantiFERON-TB Gold In-Tube
qh every hour
qid four times a day
QMBs qualified Medicare beneficiaries
qs quantity sufficient
qt quart
QTY quantity

R

RA remittance advice; rheumatoid arthritis; right arm
RAAS renin-angiotensin aldosterone system
RAIU radioactive iodine uptake
RAM random access memory
RBC red blood cell
RBRVS resource-based relative value system
RCC renal cell carcinoma
RDS respiratory distress syndrome
REM rapid eye movement
RF rheumatoid factor
RICE rest, ice, compression, and elevation
RL right leg
RLQ right lower quadrant
RLS restless leg syndrome
RLS/WED restless legs syndrome/Willis-Ekborn disease
RMA registered medical assistant
RMT registered medical technician
RN registered nurse
RNA ribonucleic acid
ROM range of motion; read-only memory
ROS review of systems
RPM remote patient monitoring; revolutions per minute
RRMS relapsing-remitting multiple sclerosis
RSV respiratory syncytial virus
RUQ right upper quadrant
RV residual volume
RVG relative value guide
RW read/write
Rx take

S

SA sinoatrial
SA node sinoatrial node
SAFER Safety Assurance Factors for EHR Resilience
SAMHSA Substance Abuse and Mental Health Services Administration
SBS shaken baby syndrome
SDS safety data sheet
SH social history
SI Système International
SIBO small intestinal bacterial overgrowth
SIDS sudden infant death syndrome
Sig give the following directions
SL semilunar; sublingual
SLADH syndrome of inappropriate antidiuretic hormone
SLE systemic lupus erythematosus
SNRI serotonin and norepinephrine reuptake inhibitor
SOB shortness of breath
sol, soln solution
SOP standard operating procedure
SOR source-oriented record
SPECT single-photon emission computerized tomography
SPMS secondary progressive multiple sclerosis
SpO_2 pulse oximetry
SR systems review
SS symptom severity (score)
SSD solid-state disk or drive
SSN Social Security number
SSRI selective serotonin reuptake inhibitors
SST serum separator tubes
STAT immediately
STI sexually transmitted infection
subcut subcutaneous

T

T_3 triiodothyronine
T_4 thyroxine
tab(s) tablet(s)
TAT thematic apperception test
TB terabyte; total bilirubin; tuberculosis
TBI traumatic brain injury
Tbs, tbsp tablespoon
TC total cholesterol
Td tetanus and diphtheria
Tdap tetanus-diphtheria-pertussis (vaccine)
TEE transesophageal echocardiogram

TENS transcutaneous electrical nerve stimulation
TFT thyroid function test
TIA transient ischemic attack
TIBC total iron-binding capacity
tid three times a day
TILA Truth in Lending Act
TIM topical immunomodulators
tinct tincture
TLC total lung capacity
TM tympanic membrane
TNF tumor-necrosis factor
TNM tumor, number of lymph nodes, metastasized
TOF tetralogy of Fallot
TP total protein
TPA third-party administrator
TPR temperature, pulse, respirations
TRH thyrotropin-releasing hormone
Trig triglyceride
TSE testicular self-exam; testicular self-examination
TSH thyroid-stimulating hormone
tsp teaspoon
T-Spot T-SPOT *TB* (test)
TST tuberculin skin test
TTE transthoracic echocardiogram
TTM transtelephonic monitor
TURP transurethral resection of the prostate
TV tidal volume

U

UA uric acid; urinalysis
UAGA Uniform Anatomical Gift Act
UCD or UCHD usual childhood diseases
UCR usual, customary, and reasonable
UDDA Uniform Determination of Death Act
UES upper esophageal sphincter
UGI upper gastrointestinal
ung ointment
UNHS universal newborn hearing screening test
UPJ ureteropelvic junction
US ultrasound
USAN US adopted name (council)
USB universal serial bus
USDA US Department of Agriculture
USMLE US Medical Licensing Examination
USP-NP US Pharmacopeia and the National Formulary
USPS US Postal Service
UTI urinary tract infection
UV ultraviolet

V

VA visual acuity
VAERS vaccine adverse event reporting system
VC vital capacity
V-fib ventricular fibrillation
VICP Vaccine Injury Compensation Program
VIS vaccine information statement
VLDL very low-density lipids
VO verbal order
VQ scan lung ventilation/perfusion scan
VS vital signs
VSD ventricular septal defect
V-tach ventricular tachycardia
VUR vesicoureteral reflux

W

WAIS Wechsler Adult Intelligent Scale
WAN wide area network
WBC white blood cell
WHO World Health Organization
WOW workstation on wheels
WPI widespread pain index (score)

X

x (×) times

INDEX

Page numbers followed by "*f*" indicate figures, "*t*" indicate tables, and "*b*" indicate boxes.

C

D

F

H

I

T

U

V

W

X

Y

Z